Dear colleague,

I am delighted to be able to provide you as a medical student member of the BMA with this copy of *Clinical Evidence* free as a major benefit of membership. I am sure you will find it invaluable during your studies and that you will continue to refer to subsequent issues after you qualify.

Clinical Evidence is a comprehensive international source of evidence on the effects of clinical interventions in virtually all therapeutic areas from cardiovascular disorders, through infectious diseases to sexual health, women's health and wounds. It is continuously updated and you can always gain access to the very latest information online.

Should any of your colleagues, who are not members, like a free copy of *Clinical Evidence*, then please encourage them to join the BMA by calling our membership department on 020 7383 6598 to request a membership application form. Once we have received their completed application form we will be happy to send them a copy too. Alternatively, they can request an application form by email at **membership@bma.org.uk** or apply for membership on the BMA website **www.bma.org.uk**

I hope that you will find this issue of *Clinical Evidence* useful along with all the other benefits on offer to medical student members of the BMA.

I would like to wish you every success with your studies and your future career in medicine.

Jeremy Strachan

BMA Secretary

10 ISSUE

DECEMBER 2003

clinical evidence

The international source of the best available evidence for effective health care

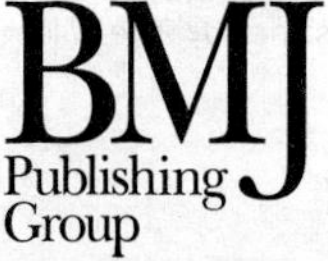

Editorial Office
BMJ Publishing Group, BMA House, Tavistock Square, London, WC1H 9JR, United Kingdom.
Tel: +44 (0)20 7387 4499 • Fax: +44 (0)20 7383 6242 • www.bmjpg.com

Subscription prices for *Clinical Evidence*
Clinical Evidence and *Clinical Evidence Concise* (with companion CD-ROM) are both published six monthly (June/December) by the BMJ Publishing Group. The annual subscription rates (for December, Issue 10 and June, Issue 11) are:

Concise edition
Personal: £90 • €145 • US$145 • Can$200
Institutional: £190 • €305 • US$305 • Can$420
Student/nurse: £40 • €65 • US$65 • Can$90

Full edition
Personal: £100 • €160 • US$160 • Can$220
Institutional: £210 • €335 • US$335 • Can$460
Student/nurse: £45 • €70 • US$70 • Can$100

All individual subscriptions (personal, student, nurse) include online access at no additional cost. Institutional subscriptions are for print editions only. Institutions may purchase online site licences separately. For information on site licences and individual electronic subscriptions please visit the subscription pages of our website www.clinicalevidence.com or email us at CEsubscriptions@bmjgroup.com (UK and ROW) or clinevid@pmds.com (Americas). You may also telephone us or fax us on the following numbers:

UK and ROW Tel: +44 (0)20 7383 6270 • Fax: +44 (0)20 7383 6402
Americas Tel: +1 800 373 2897/240 646 7000 • Fax: +1 240 646 7005

Bulk subscriptions for societies and organisations
The Publishers offer discounts for any society or organisation buying bulk quantities for their members/specific groups. Please contact Miranda Lonsdale, Sales Manager (UK) at mlonsdale@bmjgroup.com or Maureen Rooney, Sales Manager (USA) at mrooney@bmjgroup.com.

Contributors
If you are interested in becoming a contributor to *Clinical Evidence* please contact us at clinicalevidence@bmjgroup.com.

Rights
For information on translation rights, please contact Daniel Raymond-Barker at draymond-barker@bmjgroup.com.

British Library Cataloguing in Publication Data. A catalogue record for this book is available from the British Library. ISSN 1462-3846 ISBN 0-7279-1801-X

Permission to reproduce
Please contact Alan Thomas at athomas@bmjgroup.com when requesting permission to reprint all or part of any contribution in *Clinical Evidence*.

Categories presented in *Clinical Evidence* indicate a judgement about the strength of the evidence available and the relative importance of benefits and harms. The categories do not indicate whether a particular treatment is generally appropriate or whether it is suitable for individuals.

Printed by William Clowes Ltd, Beccles, Suffolk, UK
Designed by Pete Wilder, The Designers Collective Limited, London, UK

Team and Advisors

Executive Editor Fiona Godlee **Deputy Editor** David Tovey **Clinical Editors** Mike Bedford, Luis Gabriel Cuervo Amore, Anjana Patel, Bazian Ltd **Quality Assurance Editor** James Woodcock **Content Editor** Karen Pettersen **Assistant Content Editor** Polly Brown **North American Editor** David Goldmann **Publishing Manager** Josephine Woodcock **Production Editor** Alan Thomas **Editorial/Production Assistants** Claire Folkes, Rachael Kriefman **Technical Editors** Andy Baker, Jemma Carter, Maysoon Delahunty, Anne Lawson, Adrienne Penfield, Andrea Porter **Indexer** Angela Cottingham **Digital Production** Cassara Burgess, Karen Caillé, Kourosh Mojar, BMJ Electronic Production **Print Production** Catherine Harding-Wiltshire **Information Specialist Manager** Andrea Lane **Information Specialists** Mick Arber, Olwen Beaven, Sarah Greenley, Jane McHugh, Tamara Rader **Information Specialist Administrator** Varsha Mistry **Business Manager** Rachel Armitage **Technical Manager** Jonathan Peterson **Department Administrator** Hannah Lawrence **Marketing and Sales Manager** Diane Harris **Marketing and Sales Team** Jaspal Chaggar, Miranda Lonsdale, Daniel Raymond-Barker

SECTION ADVISORS

Cardiovascular disorders Nick Hicks, UK **Child health** Mary Rudolf, UK and Virginia Moyer, USA **Digestive system disorders** David Cave, USA, John McDonald, Canada, and David Metz, USA **Ear, nose, and throat disorders** George Browning, UK **Endocrine disorders** Shereen Ezzat, Canada and Victor Montori, Canada **Eye disorders** Andrew Dick, UK **HIV and AIDS** Nandi Siegfried, South Africa **Infectious diseases** Paul Garner, UK **Kidney disorders** Fred Coe, USA and Michael Conlin, USA **Men's health** Peter Schlegal, USA and Robyn Webber, UK **Mental health** John Geddes, UK **Musculoskeletal disorders** Troels Mork Hansen, Denmark and John Stothard, UK **Neurological disorders** Tony Marson, UK **Oral health** Aubrey Sheiham, UK **Perioperative care** Andrew Smith, UK and Valerie Palda, USA **Poisoning** Robin Ferner, UK and Allister Vale, UK **Pregnancy and childbirth** Metin Gulmezoglu, Switzerland **Sexual health** George Schmid, USA **Skin disorders** Hywel Williams, UK and Jane McGregor, UK **Sleep disorders** Michael Hensley, Australia **Women's health** Mike Dixon, UK **Wounds** Nicky Cullum, UK

EDITORIAL BOARD

Acknowledgements

The BMJ Publishing Group thanks the following people and organisations for their advice and support: The Cochrane Collaboration, and especially Iain Chalmers, Mike Clarke, Phil Alderson, Peter Langhorne, and Carol Lefebvre; the National Health Service (NHS) Centre for Reviews and Dissemination, and especially Jos Kleijnen and Julie Glanville; the NHS, and especially Tom Mann, Sir John Patteson, Ron Stamp, Veronica Fraser, Muir Gray, Nick Rosen, and Ben Toth; the British National Formulary, and especially Dinesh Mehta, Eric Connor, and John Martin; Martindale: The Complete Drug Reference, and especially Sean Sweetman; the Health Information Research Unit at McMaster University, and especially Brian Haynes and Ann McKibbon; the United Health Foundation (UHF), and especially Dr Reed Tuckson and Yvette Krantz; Bazian Ltd, and especially Anna Donald and Vivek Muthu; Dr Paul Dieppe, Dr Tonya Fancher, and Professor Richard Kravitz who are working with Clinical Evidence to explore ways of presenting evidence on the usefulness of diagnostic test; previous staff who have contributed to this issue; the clinicians, epidemiologists, and members of patient support groups who have acted as peer reviewers.

The BMJ Publishing Group values the ongoing support it has received from the global medical community for *Clinical Evidence*. In addition to others, we wish to acknowledge the efforts of the UHF and the NHS who have provided educational funding to support the wide dissemination of this valuable resource to many physicians and health professionals in the USA (UHF) and UK (NHS). We are grateful to the clinicians and patients who spare time to take part in focus groups, which are crucial to the development of *Clinical Evidence*. Finally, we would like to acknowledge the readers who have taken the time to send us their comments and suggestions.

Contents

*These topics appear on the website but not in this paper edition.

Welcome to Issue 10

Welcome to Issue 10 of *Clinical Evidence*, the international source of the best available evidence on the effects of common clinical interventions. *Clinical Evidence* summarises the current state of knowledge and uncertainty about the prevention and treatment of clinical conditions, based on thorough searches and appraisal of the literature. It is neither a textbook of medicine nor a set of guidelines. It describes the best available evidence from systematic reviews and RCTs, and if there is no good evidence it says so.

HOW MUCH DO WE KNOW?

Clinical Evidence aims to help people make informed decisions about which treatments to use. It can also show where more research is needed. For clinicians and patients we wish to highlight treatments that work and for which the benefits outweigh the harms, especially those treatments that may currently be underused. We also wish to highlight treatments that do not work or for which the harms outweigh the benefits. For the research community our intention is to highlight gaps in the evidence — where there are currently no good RCTs or no RCTs that look groups of people or at important patient outcomes.

So what can *Clinical Evidence* tell us about the state of our current knowledge? What proportion of commonly used treatments are supported by good evidence, what proportion should not be used or used only with caution, and how big are the gaps in our knowledge? A quick scan of the 1851 treatments covered in Issue 10 shows that 270 (15%) are rated as beneficial, 392 (21%) likely to be beneficial, 139 (7%) as trade off between benefits and harms, 96 (5%) unlikely to be beneficial, 88 (4%) likely to be ineffective or harmful, and 866 (47%), the largest proportion) as unknown effectiveness (see figure 1). Dividing treatments into categories is never easy. It always involves a degree of subjective judgement and is sometimes controversial. We do it because users tell us it is helpful, but judged by its own rules the categorisation is certainly of unknown effectiveness and may well have trade offs between benefits and harms. However, the figures above suggest that the research community has a large task ahead and that most decisions about treatments still rest on the individual judgements of clinicians and patients.

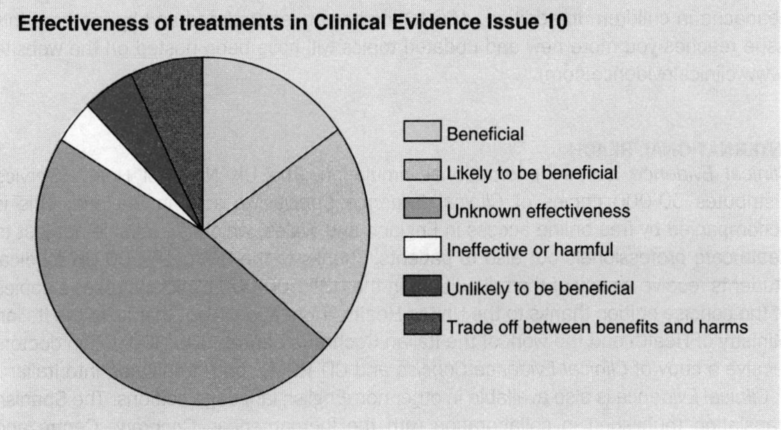

Figure 1

UPDATING AND EXPANSION

Clinical Evidence undergoes a continual process of updating, expansion, and improvement to include new evidence, cover new questions, and respond to user feedback. Each topic is completely updated with a full literature search every 8 months and published on the website as soon as peer review and editing allow, the aim being to minimise the interval between search and publication. The most recent search date for topics included in this issue is June 2003. Figure 2 shows a distribution of the search dates for each topic.

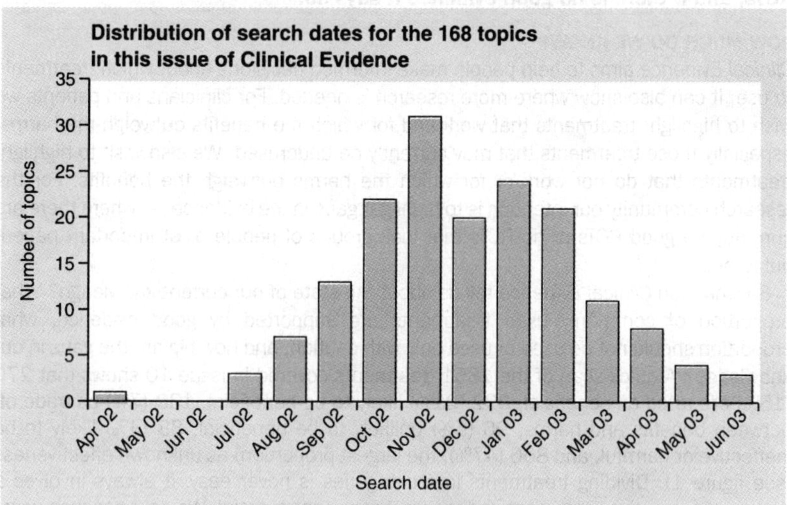

Figure 2

The content of *Clinical Evidence* Issue 10 is a snapshot of all content that was ready for publication in August 2003. Eleven new topics have been added since Issue 9: acute sinusitis, acute bronchitis, otitis externa, acute gout, bipolar disorder, deliberate self harm, domestic violence, hepatitis B, halitosis, sickle cell disease, and migraine headache in children. In addition, 106 topics have been updated and by the time this issue reaches you more new and updated topics will have been posted on the website (www.clinicalevidence.com).

INTERNATIONAL REACH

Clinical Evidence has an international circulation. The UK National Health Service distributes 50 000 copies of *Clinical Evidence Concise* to staff in England. This is accompanied by free online access in England and Wales, which is available not just to healthcare professionals but also to patients. Thanks to the BMA, 14 000 UK medical students receive a copy of the full edition. In the USA 500 000 clinicians receive copies of the concise edition thanks to the United Health Foundation. Also, thanks to the Italian Ministry of Health and the work of the Italian Cochrane Centre, 300 000 Italian doctors receive a copy of *Clinical Evidence Conciso* and CD-ROM,[1] both translated into Italian.

Clinical Evidence is also available in other non-English language editions. The Spanish translation (published in collaboration with the Iberoamerican Cochrane Centre and Legis) now comes in all formats: full, concise, CD-ROM, and online.[2] The full text is available in Japanese[3] and Russian[4] (seven broad speciality editions). The concise edition is available in German[5] and French[6] (both with CD-ROM in English).

Finally, *Clinical Evidence* online continues to be available free to people in developing countries as part of an initiative spearheaded by the World Health Organization and the BMJ Publishing Group. Details of those countries that qualify are available from the *Clinical Evidence* website (www.clinicalevidence.com).

FEEDBACK

If you have any comments on any of the material in *Clinical Evidence*, think that important evidence has been missed, or have suggestions for new topics or questions please let us know. You can contact us at CEfeedback@bmjgroup.com. Many thanks to all of you who have already sent in your comments.

REFERENCES

1. *Clinical Evidence Conciso: La fonte delle migliori prove de efficacia per la pratica clinica*. Milan, Italy: Centro Cochrane Italiano/Editore Italiano/Editore Zadig, 2003.
2. *Evidencia Clinica*. Barcelona, Spain/Bogotá, Colombia: Asociación Colaboración Cochrane Iberoamerican/Legis, 2003.
3. *Clinical Evidence (Japanese edition)*. Tokyo, Japan: Nikkei Medical, 2002.
4. *Dokazatel'naya meditsina*. Moscow, Russia: Media Sphera Publishing Group, 2003.
5. *Kompendium evidenzbasierte Medizin*. Bern, Switzerland Verlag Hans Huber, 2003.
6. *Décider pour traiter abrégé*. Meudon, France: RanD, 2002.

About Clinical Evidence

The inspiration for *Clinical Evidence* came in a phone call in 1995. Tom Mann and his colleagues at the NHS Executive asked the BMJ Publishing Group to explore the possibility of developing an evidence "formulary" along the lines of the *British National Formulary*. They recognised that clinicians were under increasing pressure to keep up to date and to base their practice more firmly on evidence, but that few had the necessary time or skills to do this. Their idea was to provide a pocketbook containing concise and regularly updated summaries of the best available evidence on clinical interventions. However, they didn't think that the NHS could develop such a formulary itself. "It would be marvellous", said Tom Mann, "if somebody would just do it." A small team at the BMJ set to work to produce a pilot version of what was then called the *Clinical Effectiveness Directory*.

Since that pilot, a great deal has changed. In collaboration with the American College of Physicians–American Society of Internal Medicine, we convened an international advisory board, held focus groups of clinicians, talked to patient support groups, and adopted countless good ideas from early drafts by our contributors. Throughout we kept in mind an equation set out by Slawson et al.[1] This states that the usefulness of any source of information is equal to its relevance, multiplied by its validity, divided by the work required to extract the information. In order to be as useful as possible, we aimed for high relevance, high validity, and low work in terms of the reader's time and effort. We also kept in mind principles of transparency and explicitness. Readers needed to understand where our information came from and how it was assembled.

A UNIQUE RESOURCE

Clinical Evidence is one of growing number of sources of evidence-based information for clinicians. But it has several features that make it unique.

- Its contents are driven by questions rather than by the availability of research evidence. Rather than start with the evidence and summarise what is there, we identify important clinical questions, and then search for and summarise the best available evidence to answer them.
- It identifies but does not try to fill important gaps in the evidence. In a phrase used by Jerry Osheroff, who has led much of the research on clinicians' information needs,[2] *Clinical Evidence* presents the dark as well as the light side of the moon. We feel that it is helpful for clinicians to know when their uncertainty stems from gaps in the evidence rather than gaps in their own knowledge.
- It is continuously updated, with full literature searches in each topic every eight months. Print copies containing the latest version of each topic are published every six months and the website is refreshed, with new and updated content, every month.
- It specifically aims not to make recommendations. The experience of the clinical practice guideline movement has shown that it is nearly impossible to make recommendations that are appropriate in every situation. Differences in individual patients' baseline risks and preferences, and in the local availability of interventions, will always mean that the evidence must be individually interpreted rather than applied across the board. *Clinical Evidence* provides the raw material for developing locally applicable clinical practice guidelines, and for clinicians and patients to make up their own minds on the best course of action. We supply the evidence, you make the decisions.

COMPLEMENTARY BUT DIFFERENT

We are often asked how *Clinical Evidence* differs from two other high quality sources of evidence-based information: The *Cochrane Library*; and the evidence-based journals *ACP Journal Club, Evidence-Based Medicine, Evidence-Based Mental Health,* and *Evidence-Based Nursing*.

Clinical Evidence is complementary to but different from the work of the Cochrane Collaboration (www.cochrane.org), which produces and publishes high quality systematic reviews of controlled trials. *Clinical Evidence* has been called the friendly front end of the *Cochrane Library*, because it takes this and other high quality information and pulls it together in one place in a concise format. Many of our advisors and contributors are active members of the Cochrane Collaboration, and we are exploring closer ties between *Clinical Evidence* and the Collaboration in the way the evidence is searched for, summarised, and accessed by users.

Clinical Evidence is also complementary to but different from the evidence-based journals, which select and abstract the best and most clinically relevant articles as they appear in the world's medical literature. Together these journals form a growing archive of high quality abstracts of individual articles. *Clinical Evidence* takes a different approach. It begins not with the journals but with clinical questions. It is able to answer some. For others it simply reports that no good evidence was found.

A WORK IN PROGRESS

Clinical Evidence continues to evolve. We knew when we started that we were undertaking an enormous task, and the more we work on it, the more we realise its enormity. Although we have made every effort to ensure that the searches are thorough and that the appraisals of studies are objective (see Searching and appraising the literature), we will inevitably have missed some important studies. In order not to make unjustified claims about the accuracy of the information, we use phrases such as "we found no systematic review" rather than "there is no systematic review". In order to be as explicit as possible about the methods used for each contribution, we have asked each set of contributors to provide a brief methods section, describing the searches that were performed and how individual studies were selected.

Clinical Evidence is now a family of products, appearing in different formats and languages for different audiences. Our expectation is that *Clinical Evidence* will evolve further over the next few years, in response to the needs of clinicians and patients.

REFERENCES

1. Slawson DC, Shaughnessy AF, Bennett JH. Becoming a medical information master: feeling good about not knowing everything. *J Fam Pract* 1994;38:505–513.
2. Ely JW, Osheroff JA, Ebell MJ, et al. Analysis of questions asked by family doctors regarding patient care. *BMJ* 1999;319:358–361.

A guide to the text

SUMMARY PAGE

The summary page for each topic presents the questions addressed, key messages, and a list of the interventions covered (in alphabetical order), categorised according to whether we have found evidence that they are effective or not. We have developed categories of effectiveness based on those used in the Cochrane Collaboration's *A guide to effective care in pregnancy and childbirth*.[1] The categories we now use are explained in the table below:

TABLE Categorisation of treatment effects in *Clinical Evidence*

Beneficial	Interventions for which effectiveness has been demonstrated by clear evidence from RCTs, and for which expectation of harms is small compared with the benefits.
Likely to be beneficial	Interventions for which effectiveness is less well established than for those listed under "beneficial".
Trade off between benefits and harms	Interventions for which clinicians and patients should weigh up the beneficial and harmful effects according to individual circumstances and priorities.
Unknown effectiveness	Interventions for which there are currently insufficient data or data of inadequate quality.
Unlikely to be beneficial	Interventions for which lack of effectiveness is less well established than for those listed under "likely to be ineffective or harmful".
Likely to be ineffective or harmful	Interventions for which ineffectiveness or harmfulness has been demonstrated by clear evidence.

Fitting interventions into these categories is not always straightforward. For one thing, the categories represent a mix of several hierarchies: the size of benefit (or harm), the strength of evidence (RCT or observational data), and the degree of certainty around the finding (represented by the confidence interval). Another problem is that much of the evidence that is most relevant to clinical decisions relates to comparisons between different interventions rather than to comparison with placebo or no intervention. Where necessary, we have indicated the comparisons. A third problem is that interventions may have been tested, or found to be effective, in only one group of people, such as those at high risk of an outcome. Again, we have indicated this where possible. But perhaps most difficult of all has been trying to maintain consistency across different topics. We continue to work on refining the criteria for putting interventions under each category. Interventions that cannot be tested in an RCT for ethical or practical reasons are sometimes included in the categorisation table and are identified with an asterisk.

NEGATIVE FINDINGS

A surprisingly hard aspect to get right is the reporting of negative findings. Saying that there is no good evidence that a treatment works is not, of course, the same as saying that the treatment doesn't work. In trying to get this right, we may have erred too much on the side of caution; when in doubt, instead of saying, for example, that "the review found no difference", we say that "the review found no evidence of a difference". We recognise that to get this right, we need a better handle on the power of individual systematic reviews and trials to demonstrate statistically significant differences between groups, and better information on what constitutes clinically important differences in the major outcomes for each intervention.

In the meantime, we hope that the text makes a clear distinction between lack of benefit and lack of evidence of benefit.

OUTCOMES

Clinical Evidence focuses on outcomes that matter to patients, meaning those that patients themselves are aware of, such as symptom severity, quality of life, survival, disability, walking distance, and live birth rate. We are less interested in proxy outcomes such as blood lipid concentrations, blood pressure, or ovulation rates. Each topic includes a list of the main patient oriented outcomes, and where possible describes how these are measured. We have for the moment decided not to address the vexed question of what constitutes a clinically important change in an outcome, but we would welcome suggestions on how to do this.

EFFECTS, NOT EFFECTIVENESS

A key aim of *Clinical Evidence* is to emphasise the important trade offs between advantages and disadvantages of different treatment options. We therefore talk about the effects of interventions, both positive and negative, rather than the effectiveness, and for each question or intervention option we present data on benefits and harms under separate headings.

HARMS

Information about harms is often more difficult to synthesize than information about benefits.[2] Most controlled trials are designed to investigate benefits. Many either fail to document harms or present the information in a form that is difficult to analyse or interpret. When drugs are licensed they may have been used clinically in only a few thousand people; the absence of documented harms is not strong evidence that harms will not be discovered in the years after licensing.

Clinical Evidence recognises that the evidence about harms is often weaker than that about benefits. In an attempt to correct for this bias, *Clinical Evidence* has lowered the threshold for evidence to be included in the harms section. Much of the evidence for harms comes from observational studies ranging from prospective controlled cohort studies to case reports, and these are included when the harm is serious or when there is good corroborating evidence that the harm can be attributed to the treatment.

DRUG NAMES

Clinical Evidence has an international audience. Difficulties can arise when different names for the same drug are used in different parts of the world. We state the recommended or proposed International Name where possible and give only the generic or non-proprietary names of drugs rather than the brand names. Where an international name for a drug is not available we use the most common name (e.g. aspirin). A regularly updated table of equivalent drug names, put together by *Martindale: The Complete Drug Reference*,[1] is available on the *Clinical Evidence* website (www.clinicalevidence.com).

INFORMATION ON COST

We have decided not to include information on the cost or cost effectiveness of interventions. This is not because we believe cost to be unimportant, but because the question of what constitutes good evidence on cost is much disputed and because costs vary greatly both within and between countries. However, we believe that it will become increasingly untenable for clinicians to act without paying attention to the cost of treatments. Future companion publications of *Clinical Evidence* may provide relevant information on costs.

NUMERICAL DATA

Whenever possible, data are presented in the same form as in the original studies. However, sometimes we have changed the units or type of information in an attempt to present the results in a systematic and easily interpretable form.

AN INTERNATIONAL APPROACH

Clinical Evidence takes an international approach to the evidence. This means including drugs that are not licensed in some countries. It also means keeping in mind the practicalities of treating people in poorer countries, by covering some interventions even if they have been superseded (for example, single drug treatment for HIV infection as opposed to three drug treatment).

COMPETING INTERESTS

In line with the *BMJ*'s policy,[2] our aim is not to try to eliminate conflicts of interest but to make them explicit so that readers can judge for themselves what influence, if any, these may have had on the contributors' interpretation of the evidence. We therefore ask all contributors (and peer reviewers) to let us know about any potential competing interests, and we append any that are declared to the end of the contribution. Where the contributor gives no competing interests, we record "none declared".

CHANGES SINCE THE LAST UPDATE

Substantive changes since the last update are listed at the end of each topic. These are defined as:

- Presentation of additional evidence that either confirms or alters the conclusions
- Re-evaluation of the evidence
- Correction of an important error

WEB ONLY TOPICS AND WEB ARCHIVE

Some topics appear only on the website and not in the paper edition. These include topics whose search date is more than 13 months before an editorial deadline for the paper edition (February for the June edition and August for the December edition each year). The "web only" topics are listed on the contents page. We also have a web archive for topics that we are no longer updating.

REFERENCE LINKS TO FULL TEXT

Clinical Evidence references link to the full text on PubMed or the Cochrane Library, as appropriate.

EMAIL ALERTING SERVICE

If you wish to be notified by email about new topics, updates, or corrections, you can register for our alerting service on our website.

HOW TO USE THE INFORMATION IN CLINICAL EVIDENCE

The type of information contained in *Clinical Evidence* is necessary but not sufficient for the provision of effective, high quality health care. It is intended as an aid to clinical decision making, to be used in conjunction with other important sources of information. These other sources include estimates of people's baseline risk of a condition or outcome based on history, physical examination and clinical investigations; individual preferences; economic arguments; availability of treatments; and local expertise.
Some guidance on how to apply research evidence in practice is available on our website (www.clinicalevidence.com) and in appendix 3.

REFERENCES

1. Enkin M, Keirse M, Renfrew M, et al. *A guide to effective care in pregnancy and childbirth*. Oxford: Oxford University Press, 1998.
2. Derry S, Loke YK, Aronson JK. Incomplete evidence: the inadequacy of databases in tracing published adverse drug reactions in clinical trials. *BMC Medical Research Methodology* 2001;1:7. http://www.biomedcentral.com/1471-2288/1/7 (last accessed 13 October 2003). Sweetman SC (Ed). *Martindale: The Complete Drug Reference*. 33rd ed. London: Pharmaceutical Press, 2002. http://www.pharmpress.com (last accessed 13 October 2003) or contact martindale@rpsgb.org.uk.
3. Smith R. Beyond conflict of interest. *BMJ* 1998;317:219–292.

How Clinical Evidence is put together

The summaries in *Clinical Evidence* result from a rigorous process aimed at ensuring that they are both reliable and relevant to clinical practice.

SELECTING TOPICS
Clinical Evidence aims to cover common or important clinical conditions seen in primary and hospital care. To decide which conditions to cover we review national data on consultation rates, morbidity and mortality, we take account of national priorities for health care such as those outlined in the UK National Service Frameworks and in the US Institute of Medicine reports, and we take advice from generalist clinicians and patient groups. Our website (www.clinicalevidence.com) provides a list of conditions that we are planning to cover in future issues. Further suggestions are welcome.

SELECTING THE QUESTIONS
The questions in *Clinical Evidence* concern the benefits and harms of preventative and therapeutic interventions, with emphasis on outcomes that matter to patients. Questions are selected for their relevance to clinical practice by section advisors and contributors, in collaboration with primary care clinicians and patient groups. Each new issue of *Clinical Evidence* includes new questions as well as updates of existing questions. Readers can suggest new clinical questions using the feedback slips to be found at the back of the book and on the *Clinical Evidence* website (www.clinicalevidence.com), or by writing directly to *Clinical Evidence*.

SEARCHING AND APPRAISING THE LITERATURE
For each question, the literature is searched using the Cochrane Library, Medline, Embase and, occasionally, other electronic databases, looking first for good systematic reviews of RCTs; then for good RCTs published since the search date of the review. Where we find no good recent systematic reviews, we search for individual RCTs back to 1966. The date of the search is recorded in the methods section for each topic. Of the studies that are identified in the search, we select and summarise only a small proportion. The selection is done by critically appraising the abstracts of the studies identified in the search, a task performed independently by information scientists using validated criteria similar to those of Sackett et al[1] and Jadad.[2 3] Where the search identifies more than one or two good reviews or trials, we select those we judge to be the most robust or relevant. Where we identify few or no good reviews or trials, we include other studies but highlight their limitations. Contributors, chosen for their clinical expertise in the field and their skills in epidemiology, are asked to review our selection of studies and to justify any additions or exclusions they wish to make.

Our search strategy and critical appraisal criteria are available on our website (www.clinicalevidence.com).

SUMMARISING THE EVIDENCE, PEER REVIEW, AND EDITING
The contributors summarise the evidence relating to each question. Each topic is then peer reviewed by the section advisors, by at least two external expert clinicians, and by an editorial committee, including external expert clinicians and epidemiologists. The revised text is then extensively edited by editors with clinical and epidemiological training, and data are checked against the original study reports. Bazian Ltd has authored several topics, as acknowledged in each, and has provided additional content and support.

FEEDBACK AND ERROR CORRECTIONS

Despite the extensive peer review and quality checks, we expect that the text will contain some errors and inconsistencies. Please let us know if you find any, either by using the comment card at the back of the book or by emailing us at CEfeedback@bmjgroup.com.

REFERENCES

1. Sackett DL, Haynes RB, Guyatt GH, et al. *Clinical Epidemiology: A basic science for clinical medicine*. 2nd ed. Boston: Little Brown, 1991.
2. Jadad A. Assessing the quality of RCTs: Why, what, how and by whom? In: Jadad A, ed. *Randomised Controlled Trials*. London: BMJ Books, 1998:45–60.
3. Jadad AR, Moore RA, Carroll D, et al. Assessing the quality of reports of randomized clinical trials: is blinding necessary? *Control Clin Trials* 1996;17:1–12.

Glossary

Absolute risk (AR) The probability that an individual will experience the specified outcome during a specified period. It lies in the range 0 to 1, or is expressed as a percentage. In contrast to common usage, the word "risk" may refer to adverse events (such as myocardial infarction) or desirable events (such as cure).

Absolute risk increase (ARI) The absolute difference in risk between the experimental and control groups in a trial. It is used when the risk in the experimental group exceeds the risk in the control group, and is calculated by subtracting the AR in the control group from the AR in the experimental group. This figure does not give any idea of the proportional increase between the two groups: for this, relative risk (RR) is needed (see below).

Absolute risk reduction (ARR) The absolute difference in risk between the experimental and control groups in a trial. It is used when the risk in the control group exceeds the risk in the experimental group, and is calculated by subtracting the AR in the experimental group from the AR in the control group. This figure does not give any idea of the proportional reduction between the two groups: for this, relative risk (RR) is needed (see below).

Allocation concealment A method used to prevent selection bias by concealing the allocation sequence from those assigning participants to intervention groups. Allocation concealment prevents researchers from (unconsciously or otherwise) influencing which intervention group each participant is assigned to.

Applicability The application of the results from clinical trials to individual people. A randomised trial only provides direct evidence of causality within that specific trial. It takes an additional logical step to apply this result to a specific individual. Individual characteristics will affect the outcome for this person.

Baseline risk The risk of the event occurring without the active treatment. Estimated by the baseline risk in the control group.

Best evidence Systematic reviews of RCTs are the best method for revealing the effects of a therapeutic intervention.

Bias Systematic deviation of study results from the true results, because of the way(s) in which the study is conducted.

Blinding/blinded A trial is fully blinded if all the people involved are unaware of the treatment group to which trial participants are allocated until after the interpretation of results. This includes trial participants and everyone involved in administering treatment or recording trial results.

Block randomisation Randomisation by a pattern to produce the required number of people in each group.

Case control study A study design that examines a group of people who have experienced an event (usually an adverse event) and a group of people who have not experienced the same event, and looks at how exposure to suspect (usually noxious) agents differed between the two groups. This type of study design is most useful for trying to ascertain the cause of rare events, such as rare cancers.

Case series Analysis of series of people with the disease (there is no comparison group in case series).

Cluster randomisation A cluster randomised study is one in which a group of participants are randomised to the same intervention together. Examples of cluster randomisation include allocating together people in the same village, hospital, or school. If the results are then analysed by individuals rather than the group as a whole bias can occur.

Cohort study A non-experimental study design that follows a group of people (a cohort), and then looks at how events differ among people within the group. A study that examines a cohort, which differs in respect to exposure to some suspected risk factor (e.g. smoking), is useful for trying to ascertain whether exposure is likely to cause specified events (e.g. lung cancer). Prospective cohort studies (which track participants forward in time) are more reliable than retrospective cohort studies.

Completer analysis Analysis of data from only those participants who remained at the end of the study. Compare with intention to treat analysis, which uses data from all participants who enrolled (see below).

Confidence interval (CI) The 95% confidence interval (or 95% confidence limits) would include 95% of results from studies of the same size and design in the same population. This is close but not identical to saying that the true size of the effect (never exactly known) has a 95% chance of falling within the confidence interval. If the 95% confidence interval for a relative risk (RR) or an odds ratio (OR) crosses 1, then this is taken as no evidence of an effect. The practical advantages of a confidence interval (rather than a P value) is that they present the range of likely effects.

Controlled clinical trial (CCT) A trial in which participants are assigned to two or more different treatment groups. In Clinical Evidence, we use the term to refer to controlled trials in which treatment is assigned by a method other than random allocation. When the method of allocation is by random selection, the study is referred to as a randomised controlled trial (RCT; see below). Non-randomised controlled trials are more likely to suffer from bias than RCTs.

Controls In a controlled trial, controls refer to the participants in the comparison group, who may be allocated to placebo, no treatment, or a standard treatment.

Correlation coefficient A measure of association that indicates the degree to which two variables change together in a linear relationship. It is represented by r, and varies between –1 and +1. When r is +1, there is a perfect positive relationship (when one variable increases, so does the other, and the proportionate difference remains constant). When r is –1 there is a perfect negative relationship (when one variable increases the other decreases, or vice versa, and the proportionate difference remains constant). This, however, does not rule out a relationship—it just excludes a linear relationship.

Crossover randomised trial A trial in which participants receive one treatment and have outcomes measured, and then receive an alternative treatment and have outcomes measured again. The order of treatments is randomly assigned. Sometimes a period of no treatment is used before the trial starts and in between the treatments (washout periods) to minimise interference between the treatments (carry over effects). Interpretation of the results from crossover randomised controlled trials (RCTs) can be complex.

Cross sectional study A study design that involves surveying a population about an exposure, or condition, or both, at one point in time. It can be used for assessing prevalence of a condition in the population.

Disability Adjusted Life Year (DALY) A method for measuring disease burden, which aims to quantify in a single figure both the quantity and quality of life lost or gained by a disease, risk factor, or treatment. The DALYs lost or gained are a function of the expected number of years spent in a particular state of health, multiplied by a coefficient determined by the disability experienced in that state (ranging from 0 [optimal health] to 1 [deaths]). Later years are discounted at a rate of 3 per year, and childhood and old age are weighted to count for less.

Effect size (standardised mean differences) In the medical literature, effect size is used to refer to a variety of measures of treatment effect. In *Clinical Evidence* it refers to a standardised mean difference: a statistic for combining continuous variables (such as pain scores or height), from different scales, by dividing the difference between two means by an estimate of the within group standard deviation.

Event The occurrence of a dichotomous outcome that is being sought in the study (such as myocardial infarction, death, or a four-point improvement in pain score).

Experimental study A study in which the investigator studies the effect of intentionally altering one or more factors under controlled conditions.

Factorial design A factorial design attempts to evaluate more than one intervention compared with control in a single trial, by means of multiple randomisations.

False negative A person with the target condition (defined by the gold standard) who has a negative test result.

False positive A person without the target condition (defined by the gold standard) who has a positive test result.

Fixed effects The "fixed effects" model of meta-analysis assumes, often unreasonably, that the variability between the studies is exclusively because of a random sampling variation around a fixed effect (see random effects below).

Hazard ratio (HR) Broadly equivalent to relative risk (RR); useful when the risk is not constant with respect to time. It uses information collected at different times. The term is typically used in the context of survival over time. If the HR is 0.5 then the relative risk of dying in one group is half the risk of dying in the other group.

Heterogeneity In the context of meta-analysis, heterogeneity means dissimilarity between studies. It can be because of the use of different statistical methods (statistical heterogeneity), or evaluation of people with different characteristics, treatments or outcomes (clinical heterogeneity). Heterogeneity may render pooling of data in meta-analysis unreliable or inappropriate.

Homogeneity Similarity (see heterogeneity above).

Incidence The number of new cases of a condition occurring in a population over a specified period of time.

Intention to treat (ITT) analysis Analysis of data for all participants based on the group to which they were randomised and not based on the actual treatment they received.

Likelihood ratio The ratio of the probability that an individual with the target condition has a specified test result to the probability that an individual without the target condition has the same specified test result.

Meta-analysis A statistical technique that summarises the results of several studies in a single weighted estimate, in which more weight is given to results of studies with more events and sometimes to studies of higher quality.

Morbidity Rate of illness but not death.

Mortality Rate of death.

Negative likelihood ratio (NLR) The ratio of the probability that an individual with the target condition has a negative test result to the probability that an individual without the target condition has a negative test result. This is the same as the ratio (1-sensitivity/specificity).

Negative predictive value (NPV) The chance of not having a disease given a negative test result (not to be confused with specificity, which is the other way round; see below).

Non-systematic review A review or meta-analysis that either did not perform a comprehensive search of the literature and contains only a selection of studies on a clinical question, or did not state its methods for searching and appraising the studies it contains.

Not significant/non-significant (NS) In *Clinical Evidence*, not significant means that the observed difference, or a larger difference, could have arisen by chance with a probability of more than 1/20 (i.e. 5%), assuming that there is no underlying difference. This is not the same as saying there is no effect, just that this experiment does not provide convincing evidence of an effect. This could be because the trial was not powered to detect an effect that does exist, because there was no effect, or because of the play of chance. If there is a potentially clinically important difference that is not statistically significant then do not say there was a non-significant trend. Alternative phrases to describe this type of uncertainty include, "Fewer people died after taking treatment x but the difference was not significant" or "The difference was not significant but the confidence intervals covered the possibility of a large beneficial effect" or even, "The difference did not quite reach significance."

Number needed to harm (NNH) One measure of treatment harm. It is the average number of people from a defined population you would need to treat with a specific intervention for a given period of time to cause one additional adverse outcome. NNH can be calculated as 1/ARI. In *Clinical Evidence*, these are usually rounded downwards.

Number needed to treat (NNT) One measure of treatment effectiveness. It is the average number of people who need to be treated with a specific intervention for a given period of time to prevent one additional adverse outcome or achieve one additional beneficial outcome. NNT can be calculated as 1/ARR (see appendix 2). In *Clinical Evidence*, NNTs are usually rounded upwards.

NNT for a meta-analysis Absolute measures are useful at describing the effort required to obtain a benefit, but are limited because they are influenced by both the treatment and also by the baseline risk of the individual. If a meta-analysis includes individuals with a range of baseline risks, then no single NNT will be applicable to the people in that meta-analysis, but a single relative measure (odds ratio or relative risk) may be applicable if there is no heterogeneity. In *Clinical Evidence*, an NNT is provided for meta-analysis, based on a combination of the summary odds ratio (OR) and the mean baseline risk observed in average of the control groups.

Odds The odds of an event happening is defined as the probability that an event will occur, expressed as a proportion of the probability that the event will not occur.

Odds ratio (OR) One measure of treatment effectiveness. It is the odds of an event happening in the experimental group expressed as a proportion of the odds of an event happening in the control group. The closer the OR is to one, the smaller the difference in effect between the experimental intervention and the control intervention. If the OR is greater (or less) than one, then the effects of the treatment are more (or less) than those of the control treatment. Note that the effects being measured may be adverse (e.g. death or disability) or desirable (e.g. survival). When events are rare the OR is analagous to the relative risk (RR), but as event rates increase the OR and RR diverge.

Odds reduction The complement of odds ratio (1-OR), similar to the relative risk reduction (RRR) when events are rare.

Open label trial A trial in which both participant and assessor are aware of the intervention allocated.

Placebo A substance given in the control group of a clinical trial, which is ideally identical in appearance and taste or feel to the experimental treatment and believed to lack any disease specific effects. In the context of non-pharmacological interventions, placebo is usually referred to as sham treatment (see sham treatment below).

Positive likelihood ratio (LR+) The ratio of the probability that an individual with the target condition has a positive test result to the probability that an individual without the target condition has a positive test result. This is the same as the ratio (sensitivity/1-specificity).

Positive predictive value (PPV) The chance of having a disease given a positive test result (not to be confused with sensitivity, which is the other way round; see below).

Power A study has adequate power if it can reliably detect a clinically important difference (i.e. between two treatments) if one actually exists. The power of a study is increased when it includes more events or when its measurement of outcomes is more precise.

Pragmatic study An RCT designed to provide results that are directly applicable to normal practice (compared with explanatory trials that are intended to clarify efficacy under ideal conditions). Pragmatic RCTs recruit a population that is representative of those who are normally treated, allow normal compliance with instructions (by avoiding incentives and by using oral instructions with advice to follow manufacturers instructions), and analyse results by "intention to treat" rather than by "on treatment" methods.

Prevalence The proportion of people with a finding or disease in a given population at a given time.

Publication bias Occurs when the likelihood of a study being published varies with the results it finds. Usually, this occurs when studies that find a significant effect are more likely to be published than studies that do not find a significant effect, so making it appear from surveys of the published literature that treatments are more effective than is truly the case.

P value The probability that an observed or greater difference occurred by chance, if it is assumed that there is in fact no real difference between the effects of the interventions. If this probability is less than 1/20 (which is when the P value is less than 0.05), then the result is conventionally regarded as being "statistically significant".

Quality Adjusted Life Year (QALY) A method for comparing health outcomes, which assigns to each year of life a weight from 1 (perfect health) to 0 (state judged equivalent to death) dependent on the individual's health related quality of life during that year. A total score of years multiplied by weight can then be compared across different interventions. There is disagreement about the best methods for measuring health-related quality of life.

Quasi randomised A trial using a method of allocating participants to different forms of care that is not truly random; for example, allocation by date of birth, day of the week, medical record number, month of the year, or the order in which participants are included in the study (e.g. alternation).

Random effects The "random effects" model assumes a different underlying effect for each study and takes this into consideration as an additional source of variation, which leads to somewhat wider confidence intervals than the fixed effects model. Effects are assumed to be randomly distributed, and the central point of this distribution is the focus of the combined effect estimate (see fixed effects above).

Randomised controlled trial (RCT) A trial in which participants are randomly assigned to two or more groups: at least one (the experimental group) receiving an intervention that is being tested and another (the comparison or control group) receiving an alternative treatment or placebo. This design allows assessment of the relative effects of interventions.

Regression analysis Given data on a dependent variable and one or more independent variables, regression analysis involves finding the "best" mathematical model to describe or predict the dependent variable as a function of the independent variable(s). There are several regression models that suit different needs. Common forms are linear, logistic, and proportional hazards.

Relative risk (RR) The number of times more likely (RR > 1) or less likely (RR < 1) an event is to happen in one group compared with another. It is the ratio of the absolute risk (AR) for each group. It is analogous to the odds ratio (OR) when events are rare.

Relative risk increase (RRI) The proportional increase in risk between experimental and control participants in a trial.

Relative risk reduction (RRR) The proportional reduction in risk between experimental and control participants in a trial. It is the complement of the relative risk (1-RR).

Sensitivity The chance of having a positive test result given that you have a disease (not to be confused with positive predictive value [PPV], which is the other way around; see above).

Sensitivity analysis Analysis to test if results from meta-analysis are sensitive to restrictions on the data included. Common examples are large trials only, higher quality trials only, and more recent trials only. If results are consistent this provides stronger evidence of an effect and of generalisability.

Sham treatment An intervention given in the control group of a clinical trial, which is ideally identical in appearance and feel to the experimental treatment and believed to lack any disease specific effects (e.g. detuned ultrasound or random biofeedback).

Significant By convention, taken to mean statistically significant at the 5% level (see statistically significant below). This is the same as a 95% confidence interval not including the value corresponding to no effect.

Specificity The chance of having a negative test result given that you do not have a disease (not to be confused with negative predictive value [NPV], which is the other way around; see above).

Standardised mean difference (SMD) A measure of effect size used when outcomes are continuous (such as height, weight, or symptom scores) rather than dichotomous (such as death or myocardial infarction). The mean differences in outcome between the groups being studied are standardised to account for differences in scoring methods (such as pain scores). The measure is a ratio; therefore, it has no units.

Statistically significant Means that the findings of a study are unlikely to have arisen because of chance. Significance at the commonly cited 5% level ($P < 0.05$) means that the observed difference or greater difference would occur by chance in only 1/20 similar cases. Where the word "significant" or "significance" is used without qualification in the text, it is being used in this statistical sense.

Subgroup analysis Analysis of a part of the trial/meta-analysis population in which it is thought the effect may differ from the mean effect.

Systematic review A review in which specified and appropriate methods have been used to identify, appraise, and summarise studies addressing a defined question. It can, but need not, involve meta-analysis (see meta-analysis). In *Clinical*

Evidence, the term systematic review refers to a systematic review of RCTs unless specified otherwise.

True positive A person with the target condition (defined by a gold standard) who also has a positive test result.

Validity The soundness or rigour of a study. A study is internally valid if the way it is designed and carried out means that the results are unbiased and it gives you an accurate estimate of the effect that is being measured. A study is externally valid if its results are applicable to people encountered in regular clinical practice.

Weighted mean difference (WMD) A measure of effect size used when outcomes are continuous (such as symptom scores or height) rather than dichotomous (such as death or myocardial infarction). The mean differences in outcome between the groups being studied are weighted to account for different sample sizes and differing precision between studies. The WMD is an absolute figure and so takes the units of the original outcome measure.

Non-Hodgkin's lymphoma

Search date October 2002

Graham Mead, James Woodcock, and Charles Young

QUESTIONS

INTERVENTIONS

To be covered in future updates

Different chemotherapy for advanced stage aggressive non-Hodgkin's lymphoma

Granulocyte colony stimulating factor as supportive therapy

High dose chemotherapy with stem cell support

Maintenance treatment for aggressive non-Hodgkin's lymphoma in remission

Treatments for follicular non-Hodgkin's lymphoma

Treatments for relapsed aggressive non-Hodgkin's lymphoma

See glossary, p 15

Key Messages

Early stage disease

- **ACVBP versus m-BACOD** One RCT, mostly in people with early stage disease, found no significant difference in 5 year survival between ACVBP and m-BACOD.
- **Chemotherapy versus radiotherapy** We found no systematic review or RCTs of chemotherapy compared with radiotherapy.
- **CVP versus BACOP** One RCT found no significant difference in 5 year survivial between CVP and BACOP. Subgroup analysis in people with aggressive disease found no significant difference in complete remission between CVP and BACOP.

- **Short schedule CHOP plus radiotherapy versus longer schedule CHOP alone** One RCT found that short schedule CHOP plus radiotherapy significantly improved 5 year survival with the addition of radiotherapy compared with longer schedule CHOP alone. It included many older people. Longer schedule CHOP increased the risk of congestive heart failure and possibly the risk of myelosuppression.

Advanced stage disease

- **CHOP versus BCOP** One RCT compared CHOP with BCOP. Subgroup analysis of people with advanced stage disease found significantly higher complete response with CHOP. Subgroup analysis in people under 60 years of age found similar results but the difference was not significant. However, 20% of people were excluded for poorly defined reasons.
- **CHOP versus CHOP-B** One RCT in a population of mixed ages found no significant difference in 5 year mortality between CHOP and CHOP-B.
- **CHOP versus CHOP-M** One poorly reported RCT in a population of mixed ages and disease stages found similar mortality at 36 months with CHOP and CHOP-M.
- **CHOP versus CHOP plus interferon** We found no systematic review or RCTs of CHOP versus CHOP plus interferon.
- **CHOP versus CHOP plus monoclonal antibodies** We found one systematic review, which found no RCTs of CHOP versus CHOP plus monoclonal antibodies.
- **CHOP versus CHOP/VIA** One RCT, including people with stage II disease, found no significant difference in 3 year survival between CHOP and CHOP/VIA.
- **CHOP versus CIOP** One RCT of people with Kiel classification intermediate grade lymphoma, including some people with stage II disease and some people over 65 years of age, found similar overall survival at 42 months with CHOP and CIOP.
- **CHOP versus HOP** One poorly reported RCT, including people with all grades of non-Hodgkin's lymphoma, found significantly higher complete response with CHOP with HOP. However, 20% of people were excluded for a variety of reasons.
- **CHOP versus MACOP-B** One RCT, including some people aged over 65 years, found no significant difference in 3 year survival between four chemotherapy regimens: CHOP, MACOP-B, m-BACOD, and ProMACE-CytaBOM. It found limited evidence of greater toxicity with MACOP-B and m-BACOD compared with CHOP and ProMACE-CytaBOM. A second RCT, including some people with early stage disease and some older people, found no significant difference in complete response. Subgroup analysis in younger people found significantly improved 5 year survival with MACOP-B. A third RCT, including people with stage II disease, found no significant difference in complete response. Subgroup analysis from one centre found better quality of life and physical function with CHOP compared with MACOP-B. These two RCTs found a different range of adverse events with CHOP compared with MACOP-B.
- **CHOP versus m-BACOD** We found one RCT comparing four different chemotherapy regimens (see CHOP *v* MACOP-B above). A second RCT comparing CHOP with m-BACOD, including older adults and with a high withdrawal rate, found no significant difference in mortality at 4 or 5.3 years.
- **CHOP versus MEV** One RCT, including some older people and people who relapsed after treatment for early stage disease, found weak evidence of a survival benefit with CHOP compared with MEV. Subgroup analysis in people with advanced disease found that more people achieved complete response with CHOP.

- **CHOP versus PACEBOM** One RCT of people with intermediate grade lymphoma, including some people with stage II disease, found no difference in 5 or 8 year mortality in the total population. Subgroup analysis found mortality was lower with PACEBOM than CHOP in people with stage IV disease at 8 years' follow up, but the difference was not significant.
- **CHOP versus ProMACE-CytaBOM** We found one RCT comparing four different chemotherapy regimens (see CHOP v MACOP-B above). A second RCT, including some people with stage II disease and some people over 65 years of age, found longer median survival with CHOP compared with ProMACE-CytaBOM, but significance was not assessed.

DEFINITION Non-Hodgkin's lymphoma (NHL) consists of a complex group of cancers arising mainly from B lymphocytes and occasionally from T lymphocytes (15% of cases). NHL usually develops in lymph nodes but can arise in other tissues almost anywhere in the body. NHL is divided according to histology and stage (spread). **Histology:** Historically histology was divided into aggressive (see glossary, p 15) and low grade disease. This chapter focuses on the most common aggressive lymphoma — diffuse large B cell lymphoma in the WHO (see table 1, p 18)[1] and REAL classification systems (see glossary, p 16). Interpretation of older studies is complicated by changes in classification systems and diagnostic techniques. We have included studies using older systems if they are primarily in people with the following types of aggressive lymphoma: Working Formulation classification — primarily intermediate grades (grades E–H [see table 2, p 18]);[2] Kiel classification — centroblastic, immunoblastic, and anaplastic (see table 3, p 19);[3] Rappaport classification — diffuse histiocytic, diffuse lymphocytic poorly differentiated, and diffuse mixed (lymphocytic and histiocytic [see table 4, p 19]).[4] There is no direct correspondence between the terms used in the different classification systems and attempts to generalise results must be treated with caution.[1–4] **Stage:** Historically, NHL has been staged according to disease spread using the Ann Arbor (see glossary, p 15) system (see table 5, p 20).[5] Ann Arbor stages I and II correspond to early disease, whereas stages III and IV are advanced disease (see glossary, p 15). However, people with bulky disease will usually be treated as having advanced disease even if the stage is only I or II. There is also substantial variation in prognosis within each stage. More recent studies assess stage using a prognostic indicator. We excluded RCTs that were primarily in children (< 16 years old), older people (> 65 years old), people with HIV infection, and people who had received prior treatment other than local radiotherapy. We also excluded RCTs of maintenance treatment and RCTs with fewer than 50 people in each arm. In RCTs of mixed populations we have reported subgroup analysis in the population of interest, if available.

INCIDENCE/ PREVALENCE NHL occurs more commonly in males than females, and is increasing in incidence in the Western world at about 4% a year. It is the seventh most common cancer in the UK consisting of 8680 new cases in 1998 (3% of cancers) and causing 4500 deaths in 2000.[6]

AETIOLOGY/ RISK FACTORS Unknown for most people. Surveys have implicated pesticides and hair dyes. Incidence is higher in people who are immunosuppressed.

PROGNOSIS Relates to histological type, stage, age, performance status, and lactate dehydrogenase levels. High grade lymphomas, particularly diffuse large B cell lymphoma and Burkitt's lymphoma, have a high cure rate, with both initial and salvage (high dose) chemotherapy.[7] CHOP (see glossary, p 15) is the standard treatment for aggressive NHL (but not Burkitt's lymphoma) and placebo controlled trials would be considered unethical.

AIMS OF INTERVENTION To achieve cure if possible, to palliate by achieving remission and prolonging survival, to minimise adverse effects of treatment, to maximise quality of life.

OUTCOMES Mortality at 5 or 10 years, median survival, duration of remission, quality of life, treatment mortality, other adverse effects of treatment. Only one RCT reported any quality of life results. The main secondary outcome is complete response, variously defined in different studies but usually measured at 1 or 2 months.

METHODS *Clinical Evidence* search and appraisal October 2002.

QUESTION **What are the effects of treatments for early stage aggressive non-Hodgkin's lymphoma in younger adults?**

OPTION **CHEMOTHERAPY (VERSUS CHEMOTHERAPY)**

One RCT found no significant difference in 5 year survival between CVP and BACOP. Subgroup analysis in people with aggressive disease found no significant difference in complete response between CVP and BACOP. One RCT, mostly in people with early stage disease, found no significant difference in 5 year survival between ACVBP and m-BACOD.

Benefits: We found one systematic review (search date 1998, no RCTs)[8] and two additional RCTs.[9,10] The first RCT compared CVP versus BACOP (see glossary, p 15).[9] It included 177 people with Rappaport system diffuse histiocytic, diffuse lymphocytic, diffuse mixed, lymphoblastic, and Burkitt's lymphoma, with stage I and II disease (including people with involvement of extranodal sites). About 80% were younger than 60 years. It found no significant difference in 5 year survival (73% with CVP *v* 85% with BACOP; P = 0.07). The RCT did not provide absolute data for the subgroup of people with aggressive (see glossary, p 15) lymphoma (see comment below) for mortality, survival, or disease free survival. *Clinical Evidence* subgroup analysis in people with aggressive lymphoma (including Burkitt's) found no significant difference in complete response rates at the end of the treatment (59/63 [94%] with CVP *v* 63/65 [97%] with BACOP; RR 1.00, 95% CI 0.89 to 1.04).[9] The second RCT compared ACVBP versus m-BACOD (see glossary, p 15).[10] It included 673 people aged 16–69 years with Working Formulation E, F, G, and H lymphomas and Kiel classification anaplastic large cell. About two thirds of people had stages I and II disease. It excluded people with high tumour burden (≥ 10 cm) or two or more extranodal sites. People who responded to ACVBP either partially (50–75% regression of tumour size) or completely received consolidation treatment of two courses each of methotrexate, etoposide, asparaginase, and cytarabine. The RCT did not provide absolute data for the subgroup of people with stages I and II disease. Overall, the RCT found no significant difference in 5 year survival (75% with ACVBP *v* 73% with m-BACOD; $P = 0.44$) or 5 year failure free survival (65% with ACVBP *v* 61% with m-BACOD; $P = 0.016$).

Harms: The RCT comparing CVP versus BACOP did not report comparative harms.[9] The RCT comparing ACVBP versus m-BACOD found no significant difference in the risk of treatment related deaths (12/332 [4%] with ACVBP *v* 16/341 [5%] with m-BACOD; RR 0.80, 95% CI 0.37 to 1.60), but found that ACVBP significantly increased the risk of severe or life threatening reactions ($P < 0.0001$), whereas m-BACOD significantly increased pulmonary toxicity (> 1% with ACVBP *v* 19% with m-BACOD; $P < 0.001$).[10] Other adverse effects included cardiac, hepatic, and neurological toxicity and the development of second cancers.

Comment: Subgroup analysis provides a weaker method of assessing the effects of an intervention than overall analysis and should be treated with caution. The RCT of CVP versus BACOP enrolled people according to the Rappaport system but provided subgroup analysis according to the Working Formulation.

OPTION CHEMOTHERAPY VERSUS RADIOTHERAPY

We found no systematic review or RCTs of chemotherapy versus radiotherapy.

Benefits: We found no systematic review or RCTs.

Harms: We found no systematic review or RCTs.

Comment: None.

OPTION CHEMOTHERAPY PLUS RADIOTHERAPY VERSUS CHEMOTHERAPY ALONE

One RCT comparing longer schedule CHOP with short schedule CHOP plus radiotherapy alone found significantly improved 5 year survival with combined treatment. It included many older people. Longer schedule CHOP increased the risk of congestive heart failure and possibly the risk of myelosuppression.

Benefits: We found one systematic review (search date 1998, no RCTs).[8] We found one RCT of chemotherapy versus chemotherapy plus radiotherapy.[11] It compared eight cycles of CHOP (see glossary, p 15) versus three cycles of CHOP plus radiotherapy (total dose 4000–5500 cGy). It included 401 people with Working Formulation intermediate or high grade lymphomas D, E, F, G, H, I, and J, with stages I and II disease. Just over half were younger than 60 years. It did not report subgroup analysis by age or grade. It found that radiotherapy significantly improved progression free survival (estimated 77% with CHOP plus radiotherapy *v* 64% with CHOP; HR 1.5, 95% CI 1.0 to 2.2) and overall 5 year survival (estimated survival 82% with CHOP plus radiotherapy *v* 72% with CHOP; estimated HR 1.7, 95% CI 1.1 to 2.7; median follow up 4.4 years).

Non-Hodgkin's lymphoma

Harms: The RCT found that two people died as a result of treatment.[11] One person treated with CHOP alone died of sepsis associated with neutropenia and one person treated with CHOP plus radiotherapy died of liver failure, consistent with radiation induced hepatitis. Life threatening toxic events were more common in people treated with CHOP alone but the difference was not significant (80/201 [40%] with CHOP *v* 61/200 [31%] with CHOP plus radiotherapy; P = 0.06). The most common life threatening adverse event was myelosuppression, which caused grade 4 neutropenia (absolute neutrophil count < 500 mm) in 71/201 (35%) with CHOP alone compared with 54/200 (27%) with CHOP plus radiotherapy (P = 0.09). The RCT also found symptoms or signs of congestive heart failure or more than a 20% decrease from baseline in the left ventricular ejection fraction in significantly more people with CHOP alone (7 with CHOP alone *v* 0 with CHOP plus radiotherapy, P = 0.02). It did not describe other life threatening events.

Comment: Subgroup analysis provides a weaker method of assessing the effects of an intervention than overall analysis and should be treated with caution. The systematic review reported only some results of interest and has been used solely as a source of references.[8]

QUESTION **What are the effects of treatments for advanced stage aggressive non-Hodgkin's lymphoma in younger adults?**

OPTION **CHOP VERSUS MACOP-B**

One RCT, including some people aged over 65 years, found no significant difference in 3 year survival between four chemotherapy regimens: CHOP, MACOP-B, m-BACOD, and ProMACE-CytaBOM. It found limited evidence of greater toxicity with MACOP-B and m-BACOD versus CHOP and ProMACE-CytaBOM. A second RCT, including some people with early stage disease and some older people, found no significant difference in complete response. Subgroup analysis in younger people found significantly improved 5 year survival with MACOP-B. A third RCT, including people with stage II disease, found no significant difference in complete response. Subgroup analysis from one centre found better quality of life and physical function with CHOP compared with MACOP-B. The RCTs found a different range of adverse events with CHOP versus MACOP-B.

Benefits: We found three systematic reviews (search dates 1998,[8] 2000,[12] and not stated;[13] see comment below). We found three RCTs comparing CHOP and MACOP-B (see glossary, p 15).[14–18] The first RCT compared four treatment groups (CHOP [225 people] *v* m-BACOD [223 people] *v* ProMACE-CytaBOM [233 people] *v* MACOP-B [218 people]).[14,15] It included people with Working Formulation intermediate or high grade lymphomas D, E, F, G, H, and J (about 15% of people had grade group D or E lymphoma). Participants had bulky stage II, stage III, and IV disease and were aged 15–81 years, with about 75% aged under 65 years. The RCT did not report results at 5 years or more by age or grade. It found no significant difference in estimated 3 year survival (43% with CHOP *v* 43% with m-BACOD *v* 44% with ProMACE-CytaBOM *v* 40% with MACOP-B; overall P = 0.90) or 3 year disease free survival (43%

with CHOP *v* 43% with m-BACOD *v* 44% with PMCB *v* 40% with MACOP-B; overall P = 0.40; absolute numbers not reported). The RCT reported no significant difference in complete response (44% with CHOP *v* 48% with m-BACOD, *v* 56% with PMCB, *v* 51% with MACOP-B) although P values or CIs were not reported.[14,15] The second RCT compared MACOP-B versus CHOP.[16,17] It included 304 people with Working Formulation intermediate grade or high grade D, E, F, G, or H lymphoma; 15/236 (6.4%) had Working Formulation grade D lymphoma. Participants had bulky stage I–IV disease and were aged 16–72 years. About two thirds had stages III or IV disease, and about two thirds were aged under 60 years. Overall, it found no significant difference in complete response (64/125 [51%] with MACOP-B *v* 65/111 [59%] with CHOP; RR 0.87, 95% CI 0.69 to 1.10). Subgroup results by stage or grade were not reported at 5 years. Subgroup analysis in people aged 60 years or less (159 people) found MACOP-B significantly improved 5 year survival (58% with MACOP-B *v* 43% with CHOP; P = 0.03).[16,17] The third RCT compared CHOP versus MACOP-B.[18] It included 405 people with the Kiel classification aggressive (see glossary, p 15) lymphomas — centroblastic, immunoblastic, anaplastic large cell, and peripheral T cell. Participants were aged 18–67 years. Just over half of people had stage III or IV disease (51.6%). More people treated with CHOP had stage I disease (27/193 [14%] with CHOP *v* 6/181 [3%] with MACOP-B). Overall, it found no significant difference in complete response (72/193 [37%] with CHOP *v* 74/181 [41%] with MACOP-B; RR 0.91, 95% CI 0.71 to 1.18). It did not report subgroup analysis for people by stage. One centre investigated quality of life (92/106 [87%] people participated). It found significantly lower quality of life with MACOP-B at 12 weeks (P = 0.04; European Organisation for Research into Treatment of Cancer 30, modified Q of L score) and worse physical function (P = 0.01). However, at 56 weeks the difference was no longer significant (quantified results not reported). Subgroup analyses in people aged 60 years or less were presented graphically. It found no significant difference in estimated 5 year survival (59% with CHOP *v* 60% with MACOP-B; absolute numbers not presented), or estimated 5 year failure free survival (44% with CHOP *v* 47% with MACOP-B; absolute numbers not presented).[18]

Harms: The first RCT[14,15] found fatal toxicity in 1% of people treated with CHOP, 3% with ProMACE-CytaBOM, 5% with m-BACOD, and 6% with MACOP-B. It found life threatening toxicity in 31% with CHOP, 54% with m-BACOD, 29% with ProMACE-CytaBOM, and 43% with MACOP-B. Combining these two outcomes found significantly lower toxicity for CHOP and Pro-MACE-CytaBOM than m-BACOD and MACOP-B (P = 0.001). The second RCT found CHOP compared with MACOP-B significantly reduced grade 3 or 4 haematologic toxicity (P = 0.04), stomatitis (9% *v* 45%; P ≤ 0.0001), cutaneous toxicity (0% with CHOP *v* 11% with MACOP-B; P = 0.0001), and gastrointestinal ulceration (4% with CHOP *v* 12% with MACOP-B; P = 0.03), although CHOP significantly increased alopecia (71% with CHOP *v* 48% with MACOP-B; P = 0.0006).[16,17] It found no significant difference in nausea and vomiting, infection, constipation, diarrhoea, peripheral neuropathy, cardiovascular events, or myopathy. The RCT reported that people aged over 60 years tolerated MACOP-B poorly (46% of older people completed treatment *v* 83% of younger people; P = 0.0001), with significantly more taken off treatment because of toxicity (37% of older people *v* 10% of younger people; P = 0.01). The third RCT found no significant difference in treatment related mortality (1.9% with CHOP *v* 1.7% with MACOP-B).[18] It reported on other adverse events for the people enrolled in the quality of life study. It found less appetite loss with MACOP-B but more fatigue. Beyond 12 weeks (at which time treatment with CHOP was still ongoing but MACOP-B had finished), it found more constipation and diarrhoea, nausea and vomiting, dizziness, hair loss, headache, fatigue, dryness of mouth, and heart burn with CHOP. At 56 weeks, it found more neuropathic symptoms and mucositis with MACOP-B. Absolute numbers and significance were not reported and some results were presented graphically.

Comment: Subgroup analysis provides a weaker method of assessing the effects of an intervention than overall analysis and should be treated with caution. The systematic reviews reported only some results of interest and have been used solely as a source of references.[8,12,13] In the first RCT of the initial 1138 people, 239 were excluded after randomisation when histology was reassessed to low grade lymphoma.[14,15] The second RCT excluded 65 people on histological or other grounds.[16,17] In the third RCT, 31 people were excluded for non-lymphoid tumours, non-eligible lymphoma categories, insufficient biopsy, or central nervous system involvement.[18]

OPTION CHOP VERSUS PACEBOM

One RCT of people with intermediate grade lymphoma, including some people with stage II disease, found no difference in 5 or 8 year mortality. Subgroup analysis found mortality was lower with PACEBOM than CHOP in people with stage IV disease at 8 years' follow up, but the difference was not significant.

Benefits: We found three systematic reviews (search dates 1998,[8] 2000,[12] and not stated;[13] see comment below). We found one RCT comparing CHOP versus PACEBOM (see glossary, p 16).[19,20] It included 459 people aged 16–69 years with Working Formulation F and G grade lymphoma. About two thirds had stage III or IV disease. It found no significant difference in complete response (57% with CHOP *v* 64% with PACEBOM; P = 0.14; absolute numbers not reported; see comment below). It found no significant difference in overall estimated relapse free survival at 5 years (59% with CHOP *v* 67% with PACEBOM; P > 0.05; absolute numbers not reported; results presented graphically), or at 8 years (60% with CHOP *v* 65% with PACEBOM, P = 0.65), or overall estimated survival at 5 years (50% with CHOP *v* 60% with PACEBOM; P = 0.18; results presented graphically) or at 8 years (41% with CHOP *v* 51% with PACEBOM; P = 0.11). Subgroup analysis found lower actuarial mortality with PACEBOM than with CHOP for people with stage IV disease at 8 years' follow up but the difference was not significant (42% with PACEBOM *v* 25% with CHOP; P = 0.06; absolute and relative risks not reported). Other subgroup analysis by stage was not reported.

Harms: The RCT reported three treatment related deaths with CHOP and four treatment related deaths with PACEBOM. It found PACEBOM significantly increased severe haematological toxicity (WHO 3 or 4 haematological toxicity 34% with CHOP *v* 50% with PACEBOM; P = 0.02).[19,20]

Comment: Subgroup analysis provides a weaker method of assessing the effects of an intervention than overall analysis and should be treated with caution. The systematic reviews reported only some results of interest and have been used solely as a source of references.[8,12,13] Criteria for complete response were stricter than for most RCTs (required normal results at 3 months after the completion of treatment).[19,20]

OPTION CHOP VERSUS PROMACE-CYTABOM

One RCT, including some people aged over 65 years, found no significant difference in 3 year survival between four chemotherapy regimens: CHOP, MACOP-B, m-BACOD, and ProMACE-CytaBOM. It found limited evidence of greater toxicity with MACOP-B and m-BACOD versus CHOP and ProMACE-CytaBOM. One RCT, including some people with stage II disease and some people aged over 65 years, found longer median survival with CHOP versus ProMACE-CytaBOM, but significance was not assessed.

Benefits: We found three systematic reviews (search dates 1998,[8] 2000,[12] and not stated;[13] see comment below) and two RCTs.[14,15,21] The first RCT compared CHOP versus m-BACOD versus ProMACE-cytaBOM versus MACOP-B (see glossary, p 15) (see benefits of CHOP v MACOP-B, p 6).[14,15] The second RCT compared CHOP versus ProMACE-cytaBOM.[21] It included people with Working Formulation intermediate or high grades E, F, G, and H lymphoma and a few people with group D lymphoma (11/148 [7%]). About three quarters had stage III or IV disease. Just under half of participants were younger than 60 years (70/148 [47%]). It found no significant difference in complete response (42/73 [57.5%] with CHOP *v* 38/61 [62.3%] with ProMACE-CytaBOM, see comment below). It found longer median survival with CHOP versus ProMACE-CytaBOM (45 months with CHOP *v* 27 months with ProMACE-CytaBOM; P value not reported). The RCT did not report sufficient data on disease free survival. The RCT did not report results by stage, age, or grade.

Harms: The first RCT compared CHOP versus m-BACOD versus ProMACE-CytaBOM versus MACOP-B (see benefits of CHOP v MACOP-B, p 7).[14,15] The second RCT found no significant difference in toxicity between CHOP and ProMACE-CytaBOM.[21] More people died from treatment toxicity with ProMACE-CytaBOM compared with CHOP but the difference was not significant (6/72 [8%] with CHOP *v* 1/76 [1%] with ProMACE-CytaBOM; P = 0.126).

Comment: Subgroup analysis provides a weaker method of assessing the effects of an intervention than overall analysis and should be treated with caution. The systematic reviews reported only some results of interest and have been used solely as a source of references.[8,12,13] In the RCT comparing CHOP versus ProMACE-cytaBOM, 28 people were excluded after randomisation for unclear reasons and 14 people who died before evaluation or refused treatment were excluded from the analysis.[21]

OPTION CHOP VERSUS M-BACOD

One RCT, including some people aged over 65 years, found no significant difference in 3 year survival between four chemotherapy regimens: CHOP, MACOP-B, m-BACOD, and ProMACE-CytaBOM. It found limited evidence of greater toxicity with MACOP-B and m-BACOD versus CHOP and ProMACE-CytaBOM. A second RCT comparing CHOP with m-BACOD, including older adults and with a high withdrawal rate, found no significant difference in mortality at 4 or 5.3 years. It reported similar results in younger people.

Benefits: We found three systematic reviews (search dates 1998,[8] 2000,[12] and not stated;[13] see comment below) and two RCTs.[14,15,22] The first RCT compared CHOP versus m-BACOD versus ProMACE-CytaBOM versus MACOP-B (see glossary, p 15) (see benefits of CHOP v MACOP-B, p 6).[14,15] The second RCT compared CHOP versus m-BACOD.[22] It included 392 people with Working Formulation (see table 2, p 18) groups F–H lymphoma and stages III and IV disease. Just over half of participants were over 60 years old (167/325 [51%] aged ≥ 60 years). It found no significant difference in mortality at median follow up of 4 years (91/174 [52.3%] with CHOP *v* 71/151 [47.0%] with m-BACOD; RR 1.1, 95% CI 0.9 to 1.4) or at 5.3 years (results presented graphically; 286 people available for analysis). It found no significant difference in complete response rates (88/174 [51%] with CHOP *v* 85/151 [56%] with m-BACOD; P = 0.32). It found no significant difference in the duration of complete response at median follow up of 4 years (numbers not reported). In the subgroups of people aged 50–60 years and aged 50 years or less, results for complete response were reported as similar (aged < 50 years, 47% with CHOP *v* 40% with m-BACOD; aged 50–59 years, 58% with CHOP *v* 61% with m-BACOD; absolute numbers and significance not reported).

Harms: The first RCT compared CHOP versus m-BACOD versus ProMACE-cytaBOM versus MACOP-B (see benefits of CHOP v MACOP-B, p 6).[17,18] The second RCT[22] found significantly more toxic reactions with m-BACOD versus CHOP. This included grades 2–4 of the following conditions: anaemia, leukopenia, infection, pulmonary toxicity, and thrombocytopenia. Most notably for grades 2–4 pulmonary toxicity (3% with CHOP *v* 23% with m-BACOD; P < 0.001), infection grades 3 and 4 (13% with CHOP *v* 35% with m-BACOD; P < 0.001), grades 3 and 4 thrombocytopenia (2% with CHOP *v* 13% with m-BACOD; P = 0.003), and stomatitis grades 3 and 4 (2% with CHOP *v* 37% with m-BACOD; P < 0.001). It found no significant difference in treatment related deaths (8 with CHOP *v* 9 with m-BACOD; percentages not clear).

Comment: Subgroup analysis provides a weaker method of assessing the effects of an intervention than overall analysis and should be treated with caution.[8,12,13] The systematic reviews reported only some results of interest and have been used solely as a source of references. The second RCT excluded 67 people from analysis after randomisation, primarily for incorrect pathological assessment.[22]

OPTION CHOP VERSUS HOP

One poorly reported RCT, including people with all grades of non-Hodgkin's lymphoma, found significantly higher complete response with CHOP versus HOP. However, 20% of participants were excluded from analysis.

Benefits: We found three systematic reviews (search dates 1998,[8] 2000,[12] and not stated;[13] see comment below). We found one old RCT that compared CHOP versus HOP (see glossary, p 15).[23] It included 506 people with stage III or IV lymphoma. It included people with all kinds of non-Hodgkin's lymphoma, according to the Rappaport system. About two thirds had no prior treatment; a quarter had previous radiation treatment and 8% had previous chemotherapy. Ages were not reported. People who achieved complete response were rerandomised to different consolidation regimens. The RCT found no significant difference in expected survival at 1 year (81% with CHOP *v* 76% with HOP; see comment below). It found CHOP significantly increased complete response (144/204 [70%] with CHOP *v* 132/216 [61%] with HOP; RR 1.15, 95% CI 1.01 to 1.35). The RCT did not report longer term results.

Harms: The RCT reported that the most common adverse event was myelosuppression but there was no significant difference between groups (numbers not reported).[23] It found more cardiac arrhythmia with HOP (12 with HOP *v* 8 with CHOP; percentages not calculable). Drug related congestive heart failure occurred in two people in both groups but improved following discontinuation of doxorubicin.

Comment: Subgroup analysis provides a weaker method of assessing the effects of an intervention than overall analysis and should be treated with caution. The systematic reviews reported only some results of interest and have been used solely as a source of references.[8,12,13] The RCT excluded nearly 20% of participants after randomisation for a variety of reasons, including early death and loss to follow up.[23]

OPTION CHOP VERSUS BCOP

One RCT compared CHOP with BCOP. Subgroup analysis of people with advanced stage disease found significantly higher complete response with CHOP. Subgroup analysis in people younger than 60 years found similar results but the difference was not significant. However, 20% of participants were excluded for poorly defined reasons.

Benefits: We found three systematic reviews (search dates 1998,[8] 2000,[12] and not stated;[13] see comment below). We found one RCT that compared CHOP versus BCOP (see glossary, p 15).[24] It included 368 people with Rappaport nodular histiocytic, diffuse lymphocytic poorly differentiated, diffuse mixed, diffuse histiocytic, diffuse lymphoblastic, and diffuse undifferentiated non-Hodgkin's lymphoma. Some people had prior minimal local radiotherapy. Most people had stage III or IV disease (251/283 [89%]). More than half of participants were aged 60 years or older (57%). The RCT allowed crossover in people not responding. It found no significant difference in overall survival (follow up length apparently ≥5 years; P = 0.09). The median duration of complete response was not reached. It found significantly more people achieved complete response with CHOP (67/153 [44%] with CHOP *v* 44/142 [31%] with BCOP; RR 1.41, 95% CI 1.04 to 1.92; see comment below). Subgroup analysis in people with stages III or IV disease found significantly more people achieved complete response with CHOP (recalculation by *Clinical Evidence* 54/132 [41%] with CHOP *v* 32/119 [27%] with BCOP; RR 1.52, 95% CI 1.06 to 2.18). Subgroup analysis in people younger than 60 years old (recalculation by *Clinical Evidence*) found a higher proportion of people had complete response with CHOP but the difference was not significant (33/73 [45%] with CHOP *v* 19/64 [30%] with BCOP; RR 1.52, 95% CI 0.97 to 2.40).

Harms: The RCT found similar rates of adverse events considered life threatening for both groups (including granulocytes 5% with CHOP *v* 9% with BCOP; platelets 3% with CHOP *v* 2% with BCOP).[24]

Comment: Subgroup analysis provides a weaker method of assessing the effects of an intervention than overall analysis and should be treated with caution. The systematic reviews reported only some results of interest and have been used solely as a source of references.[8,12,13] The RCT excluded 72 people (20%) after randomisation (23 people for being ineligible, 21 for major protocol variations, 28 for not receiving adequate treatment; details of these criteria were not explained).[24]

OPTION CHOP VERSUS MEV

One RCT, including some older people and people who relapsed after treatment for early stage disease, found weak evidence of a survival benefit with CHOP versus MEV. Subgroup analysis in people with advanced disease found that more people achieved complete response with CHOP.

Benefits: We found three systematic reviews (search dates 1998,[8] 2000,[12] and not stated;[13] see comment below). We found one RCT of CHOP versus MEV (see glossary, p 16).[25] It included 153 adults with Rappaport system diffuse histiocytic, nodular histiocytic, or diffuse mixed lymphoma. The median age of participants was 65 years for CHOP and 63 years for MEV. Inclusion criteria were stages III or IV or systemic relapse after local radiotherapy for stage I or II disease. People with progressive disease and who relapsed were taken off protocol but included in intention to treat results. Overall results found that at follow up (duration not stated) significantly more people were still alive and in first complete remission with CHOP (23/67 [34%] with CHOP *v* 7/74 [9%] with MEV; P < 0.001). However, it found no significant difference in actuarial survival at 36 months (results presented graphically). Subgroup analysis in people with stage III or IV disease found significantly higher complete response with CHOP versus MEV (38/57 [66%] with CHOP *v* 16/65 [25%] with MEV; $P < 0.001$; see comment below). Results by grade were not reported.

Harms: The RCT of CHOP versus MEV did not report on adverse events.[25]

Comment: Subgroup analysis provides a weaker method of assessing the effects of an intervention than overall analysis and should be treated with caution. The systematic reviews reported only some results of interest and have been used solely as a source of references.[8,12,13] Eight people were excluded after randomisation as the diagnosis was changed.[25]

OPTION CHOP VERSUS CIOP

One RCT, including some people with stage II disease and some people over 65 years, found similar overall survival at 42 months with CHOP versus CIOP.

Benefits: We found three systematic reviews (search dates 1998,[8] 2000,[12] and not stated;[13] see comment below). We found one RCT that compared CHOP versus CIOP (see glossary, p 15).[26] It included 103 people with stage II–IV (84% stage III or IV) Kiel classification intermediate grade non-Hodgkin's lymphoma (see comment below). Participants were aged 26–69 years. It found no significant difference in complete response (33/52 [63%] with CHOP *v* 30/51 [59%] with CIOP, RR 1.1, 95% CI 0.8 to 1.5). It found similar overall survival at 42 months (85% with CHOP *v* 90% with CIOP; absolute numbers and significance not reported). The RCT did not report results by stage or grade.

Harms: The RCT found significantly more grade 3 or 4 alopecia with CHOP versus CIOP (58% with CHOP *v* 20% with CIOP).[26] It found no significant difference in other grade 3 or 4 toxicities, including neutropenia (17% with CHOP *v* 15.5% with CIOP), nausea and vomiting (8% with CHOP *v* 8% with CIOP), oral mucositis (8% with CHOP *v* 4% with CIOP), peripheral neurotoxicity (6% with CHOP *v* 6% with CIOP), and hepatic toxicity (2% with CHOP *v* 2% with CIOP). There were no treatment related deaths.

Comment: Subgroup analysis provides a weaker method of assessing the effects of an intervention than overall analysis and should be treated with caution. The systematic reviews reported only some results of interest and have been used solely as a source of references.[8,12,13] It is unclear exactly which histologies correspond to intermediate grade Kiel classification.[26]

OPTION CHOP VERSUS CHOP VARIATIONS

One poorly reported RCT in a population of mixed ages and disease stages found similar mortality at 36 months with CHOP and CHOP-M. One RCT in a population of mixed ages found no significant difference in 5 year mortality between CHOP and CHOP-B. One RCT, including people with stage II disease, found no significant difference in 3 year survival between CHOP and CHOP/VIA.

Benefits: We found one systematic review (search date 1998; see comment below)[8] and three RCTs.[27–29] **CHOP versus CHOP-M:** We found one RCT reported as an abstract only.[27] It included 221 people aged 17–75 years with high grade non-Hodgkin's lymphoma (classification system unclear). Most people had stage III or IV disease (165/212 [78%]). Previous treatment status was not stated. It found similar complete response (59% with CHOP *v* 61% with CHOP-M (see glossary, p 15); absolute numbers and significance not reported). Complete response was not defined. Estimated survival at 36 months was also similar (30% with CHOP *v* 31% with CHOP-M; significance not reported). It did not report subgroup analysis. **CHOP versus CHOP-B:** We found one RCT.[28] It included 274 people with stage III and IV non-Hodgkin's lymphoma. It included people with Working Formulation group D, E, F, G, and H lymphomas. About 10% had prior radiotherapy. Under half were aged younger than 60 years. The RCT rerandomised responders to high or normal dose methotrexate. Overall results were not reported fully. The RCT found no significant difference in estimated survival at 5 years (37% with CHOP *v* 39% with CHOP-B (see glossary, p 15); P = 0.73) in people with diffuse large cell lymphoma (177 people, group G and H). It also found no significant difference in failure free survival at 5 years for people with group E and F lymphoma (17% with CHOP *v* 15% with CHOP-B; P = 0.34). **CHOP versus CHOP/VIA:** We found one RCT.[29] It included 132 people with Working Formulation E, F, G, or H lymphoma, with mean age 55 years. It included people with disease stages II (34%), III, or IV. Radiotherapy was given to people with a tumour mass of 10 cm or more. It found no significant difference in complete remission (64% with CHOP *v* 63% with CHOP/VIA (see glossary, p 15); P = NS, absolute numbers not reported; 114 people evaluated). It reported no difference in response between treatment groups for the different stages (numbers not reported). Actuarial survival at 36 months from diagnosis was 53.5% with CHOP *v* 48% with CHOP/VIA. The difference was reported as non-significant, but absolute numbers were not reported.

Harms: **CHOP versus CHOP-M:** The RCT did not report on harms.[27] **CHOP versus CHOP-B:** The RCT found no significant difference in treatment related deaths (4/92 [4%] with CHOP *v* 4/85 [5%] with CHOP-B); it did not report comparative results for other adverse events.[28] **CHOP versus CHOP/VIA:** In the RCT, one person with CHOP and two with CHOP/VIA died during initial treatment phase. It found rates of WHO grade 3 or 4 toxicities varied by drug (anaemia 6% with CHOP *v* 9% with CHOP/VIA; neutropenia 15.5% with CHOP *v* 22% with CHOP/VIA; thrombocytopenia 4% with CHOP *v* 11.5% with CHOP/VIA; nausea and vomiting 8% with CHOP *v* 9% with CHOP/VIA; gastrointestinal 0% with CHOP *v* 2% with CHOP/VIA; neurological 10% with CHOP *v* 4.5% with CHOP/VIA).[29]

Comment: Subgroup analysis provides a weaker method of assessing the effects of an intervention than overall analysis and should be treated with caution. The systematic reviews reported only some results of interest and have been used solely as a source of references.[8,12,13] RCTs of high dose CHOP plus granulocyte colony stimulating factor versus standard dose CHOP and those with bone marrow transplantation will be included in future *Clinical Evidence* updates. The RCT of CHOP compared with CHOP-M excluded nine people from analysis on histology grounds. The RCT of CHOP versus CHOP/VIA excluded 11 people on histology, two for lack of data, and one for prior treatment.[29]

OPTION CHOP VERSUS CHOP PLUS INTERFERON

We found no systematic review or RCTs.

Benefits: We found no systematic review or RCTs

Harms: We found no systematic review or RCTs.

Comment: None.

OPTION CHOP VERSUS CHOP PLUS MONOCLONAL ANTIBODIES

We found one systematic review, which found no RCTs.

Benefits: We found one systematic review (search date 1999, no RCTs).[30]

Harms: We found no RCTs.

Comment: None.

GLOSSARY

ACVBP Doxorubicin, cyclophosphamide, vindesine, bleomycin, prednisone.

Aggressive disease Diffuse large B cell lymphoma has been classified variously as diffuse histiocytic lymphoma and occasionally as diffuse mixed lymphocytic–histiocytic lymphoma (Rappaport), centroblastic lymphoma, and large cell anaplastic (B cell) lymphoma (Kiel) and diffuse large cell lymphoma, diffuse large cell lymphoma immunoblastic, and occasionally diffuse mixed small and large cell lymphoma (Working Formulation).[1,3,6]

Ann Arbor See table 5, p 20.

BACOP Bleomycin, doxorubicin, cyclophosphamide, vincristine, prednisone.

BCOP 1,3-bis(2-chloroethyl)-1-nitrosourea carmustine (now accepted more), cyclophosphamide, vincristine, prednisone.

CHOP Cyclophosphamide, doxorubicin, vincristine, prednisone.

CHOP-B Cyclophosphamide, doxorubicin, vincristine, prednisone plus low dose bleomycin.

CHOP-M Cyclophosphamide, doxorubicin, vincristine, prednisone, methotrexate.

CHOP/VIA Alternate administration of CHOP (cyclophosphamide, doxorubicin, vincristine, prednisone) with VIA (etoposide, ifosfamide, cytarabine).

CIOP Idarubicin, cyclophosphamide, vincristine, prednisone.

CVP Cyclophosphamide, vincristine, prednisone.

Early and advanced disease Staging is historically done by the Ann Arbor system (see table 5, p 20). We have treated people with stage I or stage II non-bulky disease as having early disease, whereas stage III or IV, or bulky are included as advanced disease. It is recognised that there will be substantial variation even within these groups and that in more recent trials participants stage will be assessed by use of the International Prognostic Index (IPI score).

HOP Doxorubicin, vincristine, prednisone.

MACOP-B Methotrexate, leucovorin rescue, doxorubicin, cyclophosphamide, vincristine, prednisone, bleomycin.

m-BACOD Low dose methotrexate, leucovorin rescue, doxorubicin, cyclophosphamide, vincristine, prednisone, bleomycin.

MEV Cyclophosphamide, vincristine, methotrexate.
PACEBOM Prednisolone, doxorubicin, cyclophosphamide, etoposide, bleomycin, vincristine, methotrexate.
ProMACE-CytaBOM Prednisone, methotrexate, doxorubicin, cyclophosphamide, etoposide, cytarabine, bleomycin, vincristine, methotrexate, with leucovorin rescue.
REAL A precursor to the present WHO classification system.
WHO The World Health Organization classify lymphomas on the basis of standard stains (e.g. H and E, and reticulin) supplemented by immunophenotyping using an increasing battery of monoclonal antibodies. Where possible fresh tissue is also obtained for cytogenetic analysis. The classification then consists of an amalgamation of the above data with clinical information, ideally in a multidisciplinary team setting (see table 1, p 18).[1]

REFERENCES

1. Harris N, Jaffe E, Diebold J, et al. The World Health Organization Classification of Neoplastic Diseases of the Hematopoietic and Lymphoid Tissues. *Ann Oncol* 1999;10:1419–1432.
2. The Non-Hodgkin's Lymphoma Pathologic Classification Project. National Cancer Institute Sponsored Study of Classification of Non-Hodgkin's Lymphomas. *Cancer* 1982;49:2112–2135.
3. Stansfeld AG, Diebold J, Noel H, et al. Updated Kiel classification for lymphomas. *Lancet* 1988;8580:292–293. [Erratum appears in *Lancet* 1988;8581:372].
4. Rappaport H. Tumors of the hematopoietic system. In: *Atlas of Tumor Pathology*, section 3, fascicle 8. Washington, DC: Armed Forces Institute of Pathology, 1966.
5. Carbone PP, Kaplan HS, Musshoff K, et al. Report of the committee on Hodgkin's Disease Staging Classifcation. *Cancer Res* 1971;31:1860–1861.
6. http://www.cancerresearchuk.org/aboutcancer/statistics/?version=3 (last accessed 20 Feb 2003).
7. International Non-Hodgkin's Lymphoma Prognostic Factor Project. A predictive model for aggressive Non-Hodgkin's Lymphoma. *New Engl J Med* 1993;329:987–994.
8. Kimby E, Brandt L, Nygren P, et al. A systematic overview of chemotherapy effects in aggressive non-Hodgkin's lymphoma. [Review] *Acta Oncol* 2001;40:198–212. Search date 1998; primary sources Medline, Cancerlit, review of reference lists of relevant articles, expert identification of adequate reports from the "grey" literature (mostly symposium meetings), the PDQ database, current issues of comprehensive oncology textbooks, personal knowledge of experts involved.
9. Bajetta E, Valagussa P, Bonadonna G, et al. Combined modality treatment for stage I–II non-Hodgkin's lymphomas: CVP versus BACOP chemotherapy. *Int J Radiat Oncol Biol Physics* 1988;15:3–12.
10. Tilly H, Mounier N, Lederlin P, et al. Randomized comparison of ACVBP and m-BACOD in the treatment of patients with low-risk aggressive lymphoma: the LNH87–1 study. Groupe d'Etudes des Lymphomes de l'Adulte. *J Clin Oncol* 2000;18:1309–1315.
11. Miller TP, Dahlberg S, Cassady JR, et al. Chemotherapy alone compared with chemotherapy plus radiotherapy for localized intermediate- and high-grade non-Hodgkin's lymphoma. *N Engl J Med* 1998;339:21–26.
12. Messori A, Vaiani M, Trippoli S, et al. Survival in patients with intermediate or high grade non-Hodgkin's lymphoma: meta-analysis of randomized studies comparing third generation regimens with CHOP. *Br J Cancer* 2001;84:303–307. Search date 2000; primary sources PubMed, Iowa Drug Information System (IDIS) compact-disc, consultation of reviews, textbooks and experts in the field of study, and a review of all references listed in the trials found.
13. Meyer RM, Hryniuk WM, Goodyear MD. The role of dose intensity in determining outcome in intermediate-grade non-Hodgkin's lymphoma. *J Clin Oncol* 1991;9:339–347. Search date not stated; primary sources Medline, references from review articles, a review of abstracts from the American Society of Clinical Oncology and the American Association of Cancer Research 1983–1989, and the American Society of Hematology 1983–1988.
14. Fisher RI, Gaynor ER, Dahlberg S, et al. A Phase III comparison of CHOP vs. m-BACOD vs. ProMACE-CytaBOM vs. MACOP-B in patients with intermediate- or high-grade non-Hodgkin's lymphoma: results of SWOG-8516 (Intergroup 0067), the National High-Priority Lymphoma Study. *Ann Oncol* 1994;5(S2):91–95.
15. Fisher RI, Gaynor ER, Dahlberg S, et al. Comparison of a standard regimen (CHOP) with three intensive chemotherapy regimens for advanced non-Hodgkin's lymphoma. *New Engl J Med* 1993;328:1002–1006.
16. Cooper IA, Wolf MM, Robertson TI, et al. Randomized comparison of MACOP-B with CHOP in patients with intermediate-grade non-Hodgkin's lymphoma. The Australian and New Zealand Lymphoma Group. *J Clin Oncol* 1994;12:769–778.
17. Wolf M, Matthews JP, Stone J, et al. Long-term survival advantage of MACOP-B over CHOP in intermediate-grade non-Hodgkin's lymphoma. The Australian and New Zealand Lymphoma Group. *Ann Oncol* 1997;8(S1):71–75.
18. Jerkeman M, Anderson H, Cavallin-Stahl E, et al. CHOP versus MACOP-B in aggressive lymphoma — a Nordic Lymphoma Group randomised trial. *Ann Oncol* 1999;10:1079–1086.
19. Linch DC, Smith P, Hancock BW, et al. A randomized British National Lymphoma Investigation trial of CHOP vs. a weekly multi-agent regimen (PACEBOM) in patients with histologically aggressive non-Hodgkin's lymphoma. *Ann Oncol* 2000;11 Suppl 1:87–90.
20. Linch DC, Vaughan HB, Hancock BW, et al. A randomised comparison of a third-generation regimen (PACEBOM) with a standard regimen (CHOP) in patients with histologically aggressive

non-Hodgkin's lymphoma: a British National Lymphoma Investigation report. *Br J Cancer* 1996;74:318–322.

21. Montserrat E, Garcia-Conde J, Vinolas N, et al. CHOP vs. ProMACE-CytaBOM in the treatment of aggressive non-Hodgkin's lymphomas: long-term results of a multicenter randomized trial.(PETHEMA: Spanish Cooperative Group for the Study of Hematological Malignancies Treatment, Spanish Society of Hematology). *Eur J Haematol* 1996;57:377–383.
22. Gordon LI, Harrington D, Andersen J, et al. Comparison of a second-generation combination chemotherapeutic regimen (m-BACOD) with a standard regimen (CHOP) for advanced diffuse non-Hodgkin's lymphoma. *New Engl J Med* 1992;327:1342–1349.
23. McKelvey EM, Gottlieb JA, Wilson HE, et al. Hydroxyldaunomycin (Adriamycin) combination chemotherapy in malignant lymphoma. *Cancer* 1976;38:1484–1493.
24. Gams RA, Rainey M, Dandy M, et al. Phase III study of BCOP *v* CHOP in unfavorable categories of malignant lymphoma: a Southeastern Cancer Study Group trial. *J Clin Oncol* 1985;3:1188–1195.
25. Hagberg H, Bjorkholm M, Glimelius B, et al. CHOP vs MEV for the treatment of non-Hodgkin's lymphoma of unfavourable histopathology: a randomized clinical trial. *Eur J Cancer Clin Oncol* 1985;21:175–179.
26. Zinzani PL, Martelli M, Storti S, et al. Phase III comparative trial using CHOP vs CIOP in the treatment of advanced intermediate-grade non-Hodgkin's lymphoma. *Leuk Lymph* 1995;19:329–335.
27. Hagberg H, Lindemalm C, Cavallin-Stahl E. CHOP vs CHOP-M in the treatment of high grade malignant lymphomas in adults: a Swedish national randomized study. *Proc Am Soc Clin Oncol* 1988;7:243–243.
28. Gottlieb AJ, Anderson JR, Ginsberg SJ, et al. A randomized comparison of methotrexate dose and the addition of bleomycin to CHOP therapy for diffuse large cell lymphoma and other non-Hodgkin's lymphomas. Cancer and Leukemia Group B study 7851. *Cancer* 1990;66:1888–1896.
29. Lopez-Guillermo A, Garcia-Conde J, Alvarez-Carmona A, et al. Comparison of CHOP and CHOP/VIA chemotherapy regimens for the treatment of aggressive non-Hodgkin's lymphomas: a randomised, multicentre study in 132 patients. *Med Clin* 1998;16:601–604.
30. Imrie K, Esmail R, Buckstein R, et al. Use of rituximab in the treatment of lymphoma: an evidence summary. *Curr Oncol* 1999;6:228–235. Search date 1999; primary sources Medline, Cancerlit, Healthstar, Cinahl, Pubmed, the Cochrane Library, search of abstracts (American Society of Clinical Oncology 1997–1999, American Society of Hematology 1998, and the 1999 Lugano conference proceedings), the Physician Data Query database, the European Organization for Research and Treatment of Cancer database, and review of selected article reference lists.

Graham Mead
Department of Medical Oncology
Southampton General Hospital
UK

James Woodcock
London
UK

Charles Young
London
UK

Competing interests: CY and GM none declared. JDW is an editor on the journal *Clinical Evidence*.

Non-Hodgkin's lymphoma

TABLE 1 **WHO Classification 2001 (see text, p 3).[1]**

Precursor B-cell neoplasm
Precursor B-lymphoblastic leukemia/lymphoma (precursor B-cell acute lymphoblastic leukemia)

Mature (peripheral) B-cell neoplasms
B-cell chronic lymphocytic leukemia/small cell lymphocytic lymphoma
Lymphoplasmacytic lymphoma
Splenic marginal zone B-cell lymphoma (± villous lymphocytes)
Hairy cell leukemia
Plasma cell myeloma/plasmacytoma
Extranodal marginal zone B-cell lymphoma of MALT type
Nodal marginal zone B-cell lymphoma (± monocytoid B cells)
Follicular lymphoma
Mantle cell lymphoma
Diffuse large B-cell lymphoma
- Mediastinal large B-cell lymphoma
- Primary effusion lymphoma
Burkitt's lymphoma/Burkitt's cell leukemia

MALT, mucosa-associated lymphoid tissue; WHO, World Health Organization.
Reproduced with permission of the copyright holder. Harris N, Jaffe E, Diebold J, et al. The World Health Organization Classification of Neoplastic Diseases of the Hematopoietic and Lymphoid Tissues.*Ann Oncol* 1999; 10:1419–1432.

TABLE 2 **International Working Formulation Classification (see text, p 3).[2]**

Grade	Working formulation	Classification
Low grade		
A	Small lymphocytic, consistent with chronic lymphocytic leukaemia	SL
B	Follicular, predominantly small cleaved cell	FSC
C	Follicular, mixed small cleaved and large cell	FM
Intermediate grade		
D	Follicular, predominately large cell	FL
E	Diffuse, small cleaved cell	DSC
F	Diffuse mixed, small and large cell	DM
G	Diffuse, large cell cleaved or non cleaved cell	DL
High grade		
H	Immunoblastic, large cell	BL
I	Lymphoblastic, convoluted or non-convoluted cell	LL
J	Small non-cleaved cell, Burkitt's or non-Burkitt's	SNC

TABLE 3 Updated Kiel classification (see text, p 3).[3]

B Cell lymphoma	T cell lymphoma
Low grade	
Lymphocytic, chronic lymphocytic, and prolymphocytic leukaemia; hairy cell leukaemia	Lymphocytic, chronic lymphocytic, and prolymphocytic leukaemia
Lymphoplasmacytic/cytoid	Small, cerebriform cell mycosis fungoides, Sezary's syndrome
Plasmacytic	Lymphoepithedloid (Lennert's syndrome)
Centroblastic/centrocytic, follicular, and diffuse	Angioimmunioblastic T zone
High grade	
Centrocytic	Pleomorphic, small cell
Immunoblastic	Immunoblastic
Large cell anaplastic	Large cell anaplastic
Burkitt's lymphoma	
Lymphoblastic	Lymphoblastic

TABLE 4 Rappaport classification (see text, p 3).[4]

Desciption	Classification
Diffuse lymphocytic, well differentiated	DLWD
Nodular lymphocytic poorly differentiated	NLPD
Nodular mixed, lympocytic and histiocytic	NM
Nodular histiocytic	NH
Diffuse lymphocytic poorly differentiated	DLDP
Diffuse mixed, lymphocytic and histiocytic	DM
Diffuse histiocytic	DH
Diffuse lymphoblastic	DL
Diffuse undifferentiated, Burkitt's or non-Burkitt's	DU

Non-Hodgkin's lymphoma

TABLE 5 Ann Arbor classification (see text, p 3).[5]

Stage	Description
I	Involvement of a single lymph node region or of a single extralymphatic organ or site.
II	Involvement of two or more lymph node regions on the same side of diaphragm or localised involvement of extralymphatic organ or site of one or more lymph node regions on the same side of the diaphragm.
III	Involvement of lymph node regions on both sides of the diaphragm, which may also be accompanied by localised involvement extralymphatic organ or site or by involvement of the spleen of both.
IV	Diffuse or disseminated involvement of one or more extralymphatic organs of tissues with or without associated lymph node involvement.

Reproduced with permission of American Association of Cancer Research (Cancer Research, 31: 1860–1861, 1971) in paper format only.

Sickle cell disease

Search date January 2003

Martin M Meremikwu

QUESTIONS

INTERVENTIONS

To be covered in future updates

Bone marrow transplantation
Cetiedil
Chronic blood tranfusions
Chronic ulcers
Hormonal contraceptives
Contraception, pregnancy, and child birth
Neonatal screening
Piracetam
Phytomedicine and alternative medicine
Pre-/intra-operative management
Priapism
Psychological therapies
Rehydration for prevention
Urea infusion
Zinc sulphate

Covered elsewhere in *Clinical Evidence*

Non-steroidal anti-inflammatory drugs, p 1393
Malaria: prevention in travellers, p 911

See glossary, p 34

Key Messages

Prevention

- **Penicillin prophylaxis in children under 5 years of age** One systematic review found that penicillin prophylaxis in children younger than 5 years reduced the risk of invasive pneumococcal infections and related deaths.

Clin Evid 2003;10:21–36.

Sickle cell disease

- **Hydroxyurea** Two RCTs found that hydroxyurea reduced the risk of acute chest syndrome and the need for blood transfusion in people with sickle cell disease. A non-significant reduction was also found for stroke, hepatic sequestration, and death related to sickle cell disease. Hydroxyurea has been associated with neutropenia, hair loss, skin rash, and gastrointestinal disturbances. We found no evidence on the long term effects of hydroxyurea.
- **Avoidance of cold environment; limiting physical exercise** We found no RCTs or observational studies of sufficient quality about the effects of these interventions in preventing sickle cell crisis and other life threatening complications.
- **Malaria chemoprophylaxis** We found no RCTs of malaria chemoprophylaxis in people with sickle cell disease.
- **Pneumococcal vaccine** One RCT found insufficient evidence to determine whether polysaccharide pneumococcal vaccine is effective. We found no RCTs of conjugate pneumococcal vaccine in sickle cell disease. Three RCTs found that pneumococcal vaccines caused local reaction and fever but no severe adverse events.

Treatment

- **Controlled release oral morphine given after an intravenous bolus dose of morphine** One RCT found that controlled release oral morphine was as effective as intravenous morphine after an intravenous loading dose of morphine at onset of treatment.
- **Corticosteroid as adjunct to narcotic analgesics** One RCT found that intravenous methylprednisolone improved pain relief as an adjunct to intravenous morphine, but was associated with a high rate of recurrence of crisis.
- **Patient controlled analgesia** Two small RCTs found no significant difference between patient controlled analgesia using either meperidine or morphine and intermittent parenteral treatment. The incidence of adverse effects was also equal in both regimens.
- **Acupuncture** We found no systematic reviews or RCTs on the effects of acupuncture in sickle cell disease.
- **Codeine** We found no systematic reviews or RCTs on the effects of codeine in sickle cell disease.
- **Diflunisal** One RCT found no significant difference between oral diflunisal and placebo as an adjunct to meperidine in sickle cell crisis.
- **Ketorolac** Four RCTs found insufficient and conflicting evidence on the pain relieving effect of ketorolac in sickle cell crisis.
- **Oxygen** Two RCTs found insufficient evidence on the effects of oxygen therapy as an adjunct to analgesics. The RCTs excluded patients with acute chest syndrome.
- **Rehydration** We found no systematic reviews or RCTs on the effects of rehydration in sickle cell crisis.
- **Aspirin; ibuprofen; paracetamol** We found no RCTs on the effects of these analgesics in sickle cell crisis.

DEFINITION **Sickle cell disease** refers to a group of disorders caused by inheritance of a pair of abnormal haemoglobin genes, including the sickle cell gene. It is characterised by chronic haemolytic anaemia and episodic clinical events called "crises".[1] Vaso-occlusive painful crisis is the most common and occurs when abnormal red cells clog small vessels causing tissue ischaemia. The others are hyper haemolytic crisis (excessive haemolysis), acute chest syndrome, sequestration crisis, and aplastic crisis (see glossary, p 34). Infections such as pneumonia, septicaemia, meningitis, and osteomyelitis are common in people with sickle cell disease. A common variant of sickle cell disease, also characterised by haemolytic anaemia, occurs in people with one sickle and one thalassaemia gene. **Sickle cell trait** occurs in people with one sickle gene and one normal gene. People with sickle cell trait do not have any clinical manifestation of illness. This topic covers people with sickle cell disease with or without thalassaemia.

INCIDENCE/ PREVALENCE Sickle cell disease is most common among people living in or originating from sub-Saharan Africa.[2] The disorder also affects people of Mediterranean, Caribbean, Middle Eastern, and Asian origin. Sickle cell trait affects about 10–30% of Africa's tropical populations.[3] Sickle cell disease affects an estimated 1–2% (120 000) of newborns in Africa. About 60 000 people in the USA[4] and 10 000 in the UK suffer from the disease.[5] The sickle cell gene is most common in areas where malaria is endemic: sickle cell trait effects about 10–30% of people in tropical Africa.[3] Sickle cell disease effects an estimated 1–2% (120 000) of newborns in Africa[3] and 250 000 newborns worldwide. About 60 000 people in the USA[4] and 10 000 in the UK[5] suffer from the disease.

AETIOLOGY/ RISK FACTORS Factors that precipitate or modulate the occurrence of sickle cell crisis are not fully understood, but infections, hypoxia, dehydration, acidosis, stress (such as major surgery or childbirth), and cold are believed to play some role. In tropical Africa, malaria is the most common cause of anaemic and vaso-occlusive crisis.[3] High levels of fetal haemoglobin is known to ameliorate the severity and incidence of sickle cell crisis and other complications of the disease.

PROGNOSIS People affected by sickle cell disease are predisposed to bacterial infections, especially to those caused by encapsulated organisms such as *Pneumococcus*, *Haemophilus influenzae*, *Meningococcus*, and *Salmonella* species. Severe bacterial infections such as pneumonia, meningitis, and septicaemia are common causes of morbidity and mortality, especially among young children.[6] About 10% of children with sickle cell anaemia may develop a stroke, and more than half of these may suffer recurrent strokes.[7] Abnormal features of cerebral blood vessels shown by transcranial Doppler scan predict a high risk of stroke in children with sickle cell disease.[8] Frequent episodes of crisis, infections, and organ damage reduce the quality of life of people with sickle cell disease. High rate of painful crisis is an index of clinical severity that correlates with early death. Life expectancy remains low, especially in communities with poor access to health services. In some parts of Africa, about 50% of children with sickle cell disease die before their first birthday.[3] The average life expectancy for men and women with sickle cell disease in the USA is about 42 and 48 years, respectively.[9] Frequent blood transfusions could increase the risk of immune reactions and infections, such as HIV and hepatitis B or C viruses, and Chagas' disease.

AIMS OF INTERVENTION To reduce the incidence and severity of sickle cell crisis and other acute complications; to prevent organ damage; to improve quality of life and increase life expectancy; to achieve effective pain relief during painful crises, with minimal adverse events.

OUTCOMES Mortality; quality of life; adverse effects of treatment (e.g. gastrointestinal bleeding due to non-steroidal anti-inflammatory drugs, addiction to narcotic analgesics, immune reactions and infections due to blood transfusions such as HIV, viral hepatitis, and Chagas' disease); incidence of life threatening complications (e.g. stroke, acute chest syndrome, and sequestration crisis — see glossary, p 34); and incidence of painful crisis. Secondary outcomes include duration of painful crisis, days out of school or work, blood transfusion for severe anaemia, and infectious complications (invasive pneumococcal infection or acute osteomyelitis). Fetal and total haemoglobin levels are considered proxy outcomes and are not addressed in this chapter.

METHODS *Clinical Evidence* search and appraisal January 2003; this included a search for observational studies on limiting physical exercise and avoidance of cold environment.

QUESTION **What are the effects of interventions to prevent sickle cell crisis and other acute complications of sickle cell disease?** New

OPTION **ANTIBIOTIC PROPHYLAXIS**

One systematic review found that penicillin prophylaxis in children younger than 5 years reduced the risk of invasive pneumococcal infections and related deaths.

Benefits: We found one systematic review (search date 2001, 3 RCTs, 857 children with sickle cell anaemia).[10] One of the RCTs (242 children in Jamaica, aged 6–36 months) had a factorial design (see main glossary) comparing monthly intramuscular penicillin injection (dose not specified) versus no injection. Half of the children receiving penicillin and half of those not receiving penicillin also received either polysaccharide pneumococcal vaccine or *H influenzae* vaccine, while half in each group received no vaccine. No details were given about the method of allocation for the vaccine. The second RCT (215 children in the USA, aged 3–36 months) compared oral penicillin (125 mg twice daily) versus placebo. All children received polysaccharide pneumococcal vaccine (see glossary, p 35) at the ages of 1 and 2 years. Meta-analysis of both RCTs showed that penicillin prophylaxis reduced the risk of pneumococcal infections regardless of vaccination status (9/248 [3.6%] with penicillin prophylaxis *v* 19/209 [9.1%] without penicillin prophylaxis; RR 0.39, 95% CI 0.17 to 0.88). There was no significant difference in risk of death between those given penicillin and those not given penicillin (0/105 [0.0%] with penicillin *v* 4/110 [3.6%] without penicillin; RR 0.12, 95% CI 0.01 to 2.14).[11] The wide confidence interval indicates low precision; small size of sample may be responsible. Penicillin prophylaxis was discontinued earlier than planned because of a significant reduction in the risk of pneumococcal infection in the penicillin group compared with placebo (RR 0.16, 95% CI 0.04 to 0.70), which made it unethical to continue recruitment. The third RCT (400 children in the USA) identified in the systematic review was meant to assess of the effect of stopping penicillin prophylaxis after the age of 5 years. It found that stopping penicillin prophylaxis was not associated with an increase in the risk of pneumococcal infections (RR 0.99, 95% CI 0.14 to 7.08) or in the risk of dying (RR 0.99, 95% CI 0.14 to 6.96).[12]

Harms: The systematic review found no severe adverse effects. One RCT recorded minor adverse effects, including localised reactions to vaccine (2 cases) and nausea/vomiting (3 cases); the difference between the penicillin prophylaxis group (4/210) and placebo group (1/199) was not statistically significant (RR 3.84, 95% CI 0.43 to 34.70).

Comment: Antibiotic prophylaxis and pneumococcal vaccines are recommended to reduce morbidity and mortality from pneumococcal infections in vulnerable groups, including children with sickle cell disease.[13] The effectiveness of antibiotic prophylaxis could be diminished by high incidence of *S pneumoniae* resistance. Allergy to penicillin is a contraindication. Erythromycin is usually the recommended alternative to penicillin but its value in sickle cell disease has not been evaluated in an RCT.

OPTION MALARIA CHEMOPROPHYLAXIS

We found no RCTs of malaria chemoprophylaxis in people with sickle cell disease.

Benefits: We found no systematic reviews or RCTs of malaria chemoprophylaxis in people with sickle cell disease.

Harms: We found no systematic review or RCTs. Adverse effects of drugs commonly used for malaria prophylaxis (chloroquine, proguanil, doxycycline, mefloquine and atovoquone–proguanil) are described elsewhere (see malaria: prevention in travellers, p 911).

Comment: Because falciparum malaria is known to precipitate sickle cell crisis, and increase the risk of death in children with sickle cell anaemia, regular chemoprophylaxis with antimalarial drugs is advocated.[3] See malaria: prevention in travellers, p 911.

OPTION PNEUMOCOCCAL VACCINES

We found no systematic review or RCTs evaluating the clinical effects of pneumococcal vaccines in sickle cell disease. Three RCTs found that pneumococcal vaccines caused local reaction and fever but no severe adverse events.

Benefits: We found no systematic review. **Polysaccharide pneumococcal vaccine:** We found one RCT (123 Zambian residents with sickle cell anaemia aged > 2 years; 106 aged 2–15 years). It compared polyvalent polysaccharide pneumococcal vaccine (see glossary, p 35) versus placebo for a period of 2 years, but reported no data on clinical effects.[14] **Pneumococcal conjugate vaccine:** We found no systematic reviews or RCTs evaluating the clinical effects of pneumococcal conjugate vaccine (see glossary, p 34) in people with sickle cell disease.

Harms: **Polyvalent polysaccharide vaccine:** The RCT of pneumococcal polysaccharide vaccine found a non-significant increase in adverse effects (sore arm, induration at the site of injection, and fever) with the vaccine (3/61 [5%] with vaccine *v* 0/62 [0%] with no vaccine; ARI +4.9%, 95% CI –3.7% to +11.6%).[14] One RCT of pneumococcal polysaccharide vaccine assessed the incidence of reactions following booster immunisation in 32 children with sickle cell disease aged < 5 years who had been immunised with the same vaccine 2 or more years before the booster.[15] Post-vaccination reactions (muscle pain, fever, headache, or rash) were found in 16 (50%) children after booster vaccine and in 7 (21.9%) after placebo (RR 2.29, 95% CI 1.09 to 4.79) **Pneumococcal conjugate vaccine:** One RCT (22 children, 11 allocated to each intervention) comparing a combined schedule of 7 valent pneumococcal conjugate vaccine followed by 23 valent polysaccharide pneumococcal vaccine versus 23 valent vaccine alone found post-vaccination fever in 27.3% and 18.1% of the groups, respectively; the relative risk is not significantly different (RR 1.50, 95% CI 0.31 to 7.30).[16]

Comment: Antibiotic prophylaxis and pneumococcal vaccines are recommended to reduce morbidity and mortality from pneumococcal infections in vulnerable groups, including children with sickle cell disease.[13] An increase in penicillin resistant strains of *Streptococcus pneumoniae* has highlighted the potential for pneumococcal vaccination as an alternative. Polyvalent polysaccharide pneumococcal vaccine offers no protective immunity to children younger than 2 years, who have the highest rates of invasive pneumococcal infections.[13] Newly developed pneumococcal conjugate vaccines show protective efficacy in children younger than 2 years and are recommended for routine use in young infants,[17] but this has not been demonstrated in infants with sickle cell disease.

OPTION HYDROXYUREA

Two RCTs found that hydroxyurea reduced the risk of acute chest syndrome and the need for blood transfusion in people with sickle cell disease. A non-significant reduction was also found for stroke, hepatic sequestration, and death related to sickle cell disease. Hydroxyurea has been associated with neutropenia, hair loss, skin rash, and gastrointestinal disturbances. We found no evidence on the long term effects of hydroxyurea.

Benefits: We found one systematic review (search date 2001, 2 RCTs).[18] Both of the included RCTs compared hydroxyurea versus placebo (25 children, crossover design;[19] 299 adults, parallel group design[20]). **Painful crisis:** Both RCTs found a significant reduction in the incidence of painful crisis. The parallel RCT found that hydroxyurea reduced the number of painful crises compared with placebo after a mean follow up of 21 months (mean number of episodes during follow up 5.1 with hydroxyurea v 7.9 with placebo; WMD −2.8, 95% CI −4.74 to −0.86).[20] The crossover study reported a reduced duration of hospital stay with hydroxyurea compared with placebo by the sixth month of follow up (mean duration of hospital stay 5.3 days with hydroxyurea v 15.2 days with placebo); available data were insufficient to test for statistical significance.[19] **Death and life threatening complications:** The parallel RCT found that hydroxyurea significantly reduced the risk of acute chest syndrome (see glossary, p 34) (RR 0.44, 95% CI 0.28 to 0.68) and the need for blood transfusion (RR 0.67, 95% CI 0.52 to 0.87).[20] No significant reductions were found for stroke (RR 0.64, 95% CI 0.11 to 3.80), hepatic sequestration (RR 0.32, 95% CI 0.03 to 3.06), and death related to sickle cell disease (RR 0.48, 95% CI 0.09 to 2.60), although the trend favoured hydroxyurea. The study was too small to rule out clinically relevant effects. **Quality of life:** The parallel RCT reported data on quality of life collected at 6 monthly intervals using the Health Status Survey, Profile of Mood States, and the Ladder of Life.[20] Lower scores reflect lower quality of life in all scales. Scores on all the quality of life scales assessed at baseline and by the 12th month were higher with hydroxyurea compared with placebo, but the weighted mean differences were not statistically significant (general health perception: WMD +0.6, 95% CI −0.18 to +1.38; social function: WMD +0.2, 95% CI −0.36 to +0.76; pain recall: WMD +0.4, 95% CI −0.18 to +0.98; and Ladder of Life: WMD +0.4, 95% CI −0.15 to +0.95).

Harms: Neutrophil count was significantly lower with hydroxyurea compared with placebo at the end of the parallel RCT (WMD −1.9, 95% CI −2.57 to −1.29).[20] Neutropenia (neutrophil count 2500 x 109/L) was reported in 79% of the people in the hydroxyurea group compared with 37% of the people allocated to placebo, but no case of infection was related to neutropenia among participants. Some participants suffered hair loss, skin rash, and gastrointestinal disturbances, but these did not differ significantly between groups. The long term safety of hydroxyurea in sickle cell disease remains uncertain.

Comment: Data extracted from the crossover RCT were obtained during the sixth month before crossover.[19] Hydroxyurea in adults was given at 15 mg/kg daily, and the dose increased at 12 weekly intervals by 2.5 mg/kg daily until mild bone marrow suppression was detected (not stated how). Dose in children was 20 mg/kg daily and increased to a maximum of 25 mg/kg daily.

OPTION LIMITING PHYSICAL EXERCISE

We found no RCTs or observational studies of sufficient quality about the effects of limiting exercise to prevent sickle cell crisis and other life threatening complications of sickle cell disease.

Benefits: We found no systematic reviews, RCTs, or observational studies that met our inclusion criteria.

Harms: We found no RCTs or observational studies that met our inclusion criteria.

Comment: Moderate exercise is generally accepted to be beneficial, especially in reducing risk of cardiovascular disease. Moderate exercise is therefore unlikely to cause harm in people with sickle cell disease. Strenuous exercise is suspected to lead to factors that may precipitate sickle cell crisis, such as low tissue oxygen saturation, dehydration, and stress.

OPTION AVOIDANCE OF COLD ENVIRONMENT

We found no RCTs or observational studies of sufficient quality about the effects of avoiding exposure to cold environment to prevent crisis and other life threatening complications of sickle cell disease.

Benefits: We found no systematic reviews, RCTs, or observational studies that met our inclusion criteria.

Harms: We found no RCTs or observational studies that met our inclusion criteria.

Comment: A 10 year retrospective study found a close correlation between cold weather and admissions for sickle cell painful crisis.[21] One observational study in 60 men with sickle cell disease and 30 adults with normal haemoglobin genotype found that vasoconstriction induced by skin cooling was significantly more likely to occur in people with sickle cell disease than in those with normal haemoglobin genotype (83% *v* 60%; P = 0.03).[22] Among people with sickle cell disease, the frequency of painful crises was significantly greater in those prone to cooling induced vasoconstriction than those less prone (0.36 crises per year *v* 0.12 crises per year; P = 0.04).[22]

QUESTION What are the effects of interventions to treat pain in sickle cell crisis? New

OPTION PARACETAMOL

We found no RCTs of paracetamol (acetaminophen) in sickle cell crisis.

Benefits: We found no systematic review or RCTs.

Harms: We found no evidence on the adverse effects of paracetamol relating to its use in treating pain in sickle cell crisis.

Comment: Paracetamol is widely used by clinicians to relieve mild pain and fever. Standard clinical dosage of paracetamol is well tolerated and unlikely to cause harm, but overdose is known to cause liver toxicity. See paracetamol (acetaminophen) poisoning, p 1664.

OPTION ASPIRIN

We found no RCTs of aspirin in sickle cell crisis.

Benefits: We found no systematic reviews or RCTs.

Harms: We found no evidence on the adverse effects of aspirin in relation to its use in treating pain in sickle cell crisis.

Comment: Aspirin is widely used by clinicians to relieve mild pain and fever, although there is concern about using it in children because it has been associated with Reye's syndrome. The adverse effects of aspirin in different populations are discussed in other *Clinical Evidence* topics (see primary prevention, p 154; stroke prevention, p 246; and non-steroidal anti-inflammatory drugs, p 1393). Studies on long term aspirin prophylaxis address a different question to that addressed here on treating acute pain in sickle cell crisis.

OPTION IBUPROFEN

We found no RCTs of ibuprofen for treating pain in sickle cell crisis.

Benefits: We found no systematic reviews or RCTs.

Harms: Ibuprofen is widely used by clinicians to relieve mild pain and fever. The adverse affects of ibuprofen in other populations are discussed in other *Clinical Evidence* topics (see acute otitis media, p 301; carpal tunnel syndrome, p 1271; and migraine headache, p 1538).

Comment: Adverse events associated with non-steroidal anti-inflammatory drugs have been reviewed elsewhere in *Clinical Evidence* (see non-steroidal anti-inflammatory drugs, p 1393; low back pain and sciatica [acute, p 1343 and chronic, p 1359]; osteoarthritis, p 1402; tennis elbow, p 1493; and dysmenorrhoea, p 2058).

OPTION DIFLUNISAL

One RCT found that diflunisal had no narcotic sparing effect and did not enhance the pain relieving effect of intramuscular meperidine.

Benefits: We found no systematic review. We found one RCT (32 adults, 46 episodes of crisis, randomisation based on the episodes), which compared oral diflunisal (1000 mg loading dose followed by 500 mg 12 hourly for 5 days) versus placebo in people having a sickle cell painful crisis.[23] Intravenous meperidine (1.0–1.5 mg/kg) and hydroxyzine (0.5 1.0 mg/kg) were given every 3–4 hours as necessary for pain relief in all people. A categorical pain scale ranging from 0–5 was used to assess response to treatment. No significant difference was found in the mean total amount of meperidine administered (1400 mg with diflunisal *v* 1000 mg with placebo; WMD +400.0, 95% CI –28.6 to +828.6). Average pain intensity difference scores did not differ significantly between diflunisal and placebo groups.

Harms: We found no systematic reviews or RCTs assessing harms of diflunisal in people with sickle cell disease. Adverse events associated with non-steroidal anti-inflammatory drugs have been reviewed elsewhere in *Clinical Evidence* (see non-steroidal anti-inflammatory drugs, p 1393; low back pain and sciatica [acute, p 1343 and chronic, p 1359]; osteoarthritis, p 1402; tennis elbow, p 1493; and dysmenorrhoea, p 2058).

Comment: None.

OPTION KETOROLAC

Four RCTs found insufficient evidence on the effects of parenteral ketorolac in relieving pain in sickle cell crisis.

Benefits: We found no systematic review. We found four small RCTs of ketorolac compared with placebo. **Versus meperidine:** One crossover RCT (20 adolescents aged 11–19 years) compared parenteral ketorolac (1.0 mg/kg) versus parenteral meperidine (1.5 mg/kg) in sickle cell vaso-occlusive crisis in the first phase (150 minutes) before crossover.[24] Pain was measured in a visual analogue scale (VAS) ranging from 0–80 mm where 0 mm denotes "no pain" and 80 mm denotes "the worst pain I've ever had". Measurements were taken at 30 minutes and 150 minutes. It found that ketorolac significantly reduced pain compared with meperidine at 30 minutes (mean VAS 39 mm with ketorolac *v* 54 mm with meperidine; $P < 0.01$) and at 150 minutes (mean VAS 33 mm with ketorolac *v* 56 mm with meperidine; $P < 0.01$). No significant reduction was found in the number of pain free people at 150 minutes with ketorolac compared with meperidine (4/10 [40%] with ketorolac *v* 2/10 [20%] with meperidine; RR 2.0, 95% CI 0.47 to 8.56), but the study was too small to rule out clinically important differences. Data obtained after crossover were not included because it is deemed unsuitable to confirm the effect of either drug. **Ketorolac plus meperidine versus placebo plus meperidine:** One RCT (18 adults with sickle cell crisis) found no significant difference in the pain relieving effects of a single dose of intramuscular ketorolac (60 mg) compared with placebo given as a supplement to repeated doses of intravenous meperidine.[25] Another RCT (21 people with sickle cell crisis, aged > 14 years) found intravenous infusion of ketorolac (150 mg first day, 120 mg subsequent days for total of 5 days) to be more effective than placebo as a supplement to intermittent intramuscular meperidine (100 mg every 3 hours if pain level is moderate or severe).[26] The intravenous ketorolac group required a significantly lower amount of meperidine to control pain compared with placebo (WMD –937.8 mg of meperidine, 95% CI –1803.2 mg to –72.4 mg). **Ketorolac plus morphine sulphate versus placebo plus morphine sulphate:** One RCT (29 people, 41 episodes of sickle cell crisis, age 5–17 years; basis for randomisation episodes of crisis) compared intravenous ketorolac (0.9 mg/kg) versus placebo as supplements to simultaneous treatment with parenteral morphine sulphate (0.1 mg/kg).[27] Morphine was repeated every 2 hours based on pain intensity rated on the VAS. No significant differences were found in the need for morphine (0.28 mg/kg with ketorolac *v* 0.32 mg/kg with placebo; WMD –0.04 mg/kg, 95% CI –0.09 mg/kg to +0.01 mg/kg). No significant differences were found in the proportion of people requiring admission for further management of severe pain (9/22 [41%] with ketorolac *v* 10/19 [53%] with placebo; RR 0.78, 95% CI 0.40 to 1.50).

Harms: No severe adverse events were reported apart from one case of epistaxis in a person that received ketorolac.[26] Other adverse events (mostly gastrointestinal disturbances) did not differ remarkably between treatment groups.

Comment: None.

OPTION CODEINE

We found no RCTs of codeine for treating pain in sickle cell crisis.

Benefits: We found no systematic reviews or RCTs.

Harms: Codeine is widely used by clinicians to relieve moderate pain. Prolonged use of narcotic analgesics may lead to addiction. Codeine is known to be less addictive than other narcotic analgesics like morphine and meperidine.

Comment: None.

OPTION MORPHINE

One RCT found that controlled release oral morphine is as good as intravenous morphine in relieving pain in sickle cell crisis following a loading of parenteral morphine at onset of treatment.

Benefits: We found no systematic review. We found one double blind placebo controlled RCT (56 children aged 5–17 years) of controlled release morphine given orally (1.9 mg/kg every 12 hours) plus intravenous placebo (saline) compared with intravenous morphine (0.04 mg/kg) plus placebo tablets for sickle cell vaso-occlusive crisis.[28] No significant differences were found in the Children's Hospital of Eastern Ontario Pain Scale (see glossary, p 34) (WMD +0.10 units, 95% CI –0.09 units to +0.70 units) and clinical scales (Oucher, faces or clinical pain scales: –0.20 units, 95% CI –0.54 units to +0.14 units) throughout the observation period (at 0900, 1300, 1700, and 2100 every day). No significant differences were found for the mean frequency of rescue analgesia (WMD –0.12 doses/day, 95% CI –0.30 doses/day to +0.06 doses/day) and the mean duration of pain (WMD +1.2 days, 95% CI –0.01 days to +2.41 days) between the oral and intravenous morphine groups.

Harms: Frequency of spontaneously reported adverse events did not differ significantly between the groups (62 for oral *v* 52 for intravenous; 16 *v* 19 for severe intensity events). Common adverse events were fever, pruritus, nausea, vomiting, and constipation; these did not differ significantly between study groups.

Comment: None.

OPTION PATIENT CONTROLLED ANALGESIA

Two small RCTs found no ignificant difference between patient controlled analgesia using either meperidine or morphine and intermittent parenteral treatment. The incidence of adverse effects was also equal in both regimens.

Benefits: We found no systematic review. **Meperidine:** One RCT (20 adults, age range 17–39 years) compared patient controlled analgesia meperidine (infusion of 25–30 mg/hour plus oral hydroxyzine 50 mg every 6 hours) versus intermittent analgesia (intramuscular meperidine 75–100 mg plus intramuscular hydroxyzine 50–75 mg given as necessary every 3–4 hours).[29] No significant differences in pain were observed over 3 days in mean scores on categorical and analogue pain scales (categorical scores on day 2: WMD +4.0 mm, 95% CI –1.09 mm to +9.09 mm; analogue scores: WMD +68.0 mm, 95% CI –25.35 mm to +161.35 mm); no significant differences were found in the amount of meperidine used each day after 3 days (WMD +451 mg, 95% CI –70 mg to +972 mg). The units being measured in the pain scales were not defined. **Morphine:** One RCT compared patient controlled analgesia (PCA) versus intermittent intravenous injections of morphine in two phases of high and low dose regimen, respectively, in adult patients with sickle cell crisis pain.[30] In the first phase (20 people), the intermittent therapy group received either 4 mg intravenous bolus of morphine sulphate every 30–60 minutes as needed to achieve a linear analogue pain intensity score < 50 mm. The PCA group received 2 mg bolus of intravenous morphine sulphate followed by 1 mg intravenous controlled by the patient with 6 minute lock out. The dose of morphine was increased to 6 mg for the intermittent therapy group, and 1.5 mg for the PCA group if pain control by the end of the first 30 minutes was inadequate (pain score > 50 mm). The second phase (25 people) was similar but used higher doses of morphine for the PCA (2.7 mg with 10 minutes' lock out) and the intermittent intravenous group (8 mg every 30–60 minutes). There was marked reduction in pain scores on the linear analogue scale, with no significant difference between treatment groups in both the first phase (WMD –0.10 mm, 95% CI –27.03 mm to +26.83 mm) and the second phase (WMD +9.0 mm, 95% CI –18.25 mm to +36.25 mm). The total amount of morphine administered did not differ significantly between the intermittent intravenous and PCA group in the first phase (WMD –6.70 mg, 95% CI –23.35 mg to +9.95 mg) and the second phase of the study (WMD +6.40 mg, 95% CI –8.71 mg to +12.51 mg).

Harms: Nausea, vomiting, and pruritus were common events observed with both high and low dose morphine, with 44% and 31% requiring antiemetic therapy (prochlorperazine) in the intermittent intravenous and PCA groups, respectively. The frequency of side effects did not differ significantly between treatment groups. Incidence of adverse effects was 53% and 47%, respectively, but no details were given about the types of adverse effects or their severity. Respiratory depression or clinically significant hypotension was not observed during the study. Respiratory depression is a well known adverse effect of narcotic drugs. The meperidine study reported no significant adverse event. Some severe advents like seizures and respiratory depression have been commonly associated with meperidine. There are concerns of possible addiction to narcotic analgesics, but some studies show a relatively low rate of addiction (0–11%) in sickle cell disease.[31]

Comment: None.

OPTION ACUPUNCTURE

We found no RCTs of acupuncture for treating pain in sickle cell crisis.

Benefits: We found no systematic reviews or RCTs.

Harms: Acupuncture is widely used to relieve pain. Adverse effects of acupuncture in different populations are discussed in other *Clinical Evidence* topics (see low back pain and sciatica acute, p 1343 and chronic, p 1359 and nausea and vomiting in early pregnancy, p 1671).

Comment: None.

OPTION OXYGEN

Two RCTs found insufficient evidence on the effects of oxygen therapy in sickle cell crisis.

Benefits: We found no systematic review. One RCT (25 children aged 3–18 years) compared 50% oxygen versus air as an adjunct to continuous intravenous morphine infusion.[32] There was no significant difference between 50% oxygen and air in the duration of severe pains (0.94 days with 50% oxygen *v* 0.95 days with air; WMD –0.19, 95% CI –0.91 to +0.89), amount of narcotic analgesic administered, or further hospitalisation for pain. No significant differences were found in the proportion of people with progression of crisis indicated by appearance of new pain sites (5/14 [36%] with 50% oxygen *v* 4/11 [36%] with air; RR 1.47, 95% CI 0.42 to 5.14).

Harms: None reported.

Comment: The RCT was reported twice.[32,33] Low tissue oxygen saturation is a dominant factor in the mechanism that results in sickling. Given that increased sickling is a key component of the pathophysiology of acute painful complications of sickle cell disease, namely vaso-occlusive crisis and acute chest syndrome (see glossary, p 34), oxygen therapy is expected to ameliorate these conditions. Oxygen therapy is recommended routinely for treatment of sickle cell acute chest syndrome. Patients with acute chest syndrome were excluded from the RCT appraised in this topic section.[32] That study was small and inadequately powered. The result should be interpreted with caution.

OPTION REHYDRATION

We found no systematic reviews or RCTs on the effects of rehydration in sickle cell crisis.

Benefits: We found no systematic review or RCTs.

Harms: We found insufficient evidence.

Comment: None.

OPTION CORTICOSTEROIDS

One RCT found that high dose intravenous methylprednisolone, given as an adjunct to intravenous morphine in sickle cell crisis, reduced the duration of inpatient analgesic therapy compared with placebo, but was associated with more episodes of recurrent pain shortly after discontinuation of treatment.

Benefits: We found no systematic review. We found one RCT of high dose intravenous methylprednisolone compared with placebo, given as an adjunct to narcotic analgesia (intravenous morphine followed by oral codeine plus paracetamol) in 56 acute episodes of severe sickle cell painful crisis in 34 people aged 2–19 years. Pain episodes were the basis for randomisation.[34] A significant reduction in duration of inpatient analgesia was found with methylprednisolone compared with placebo (41.3 hours with methylprednisolone *v* 71.3 hours with placebo; P = 0.01).

Harms: No significant increase was found in readmissions associated with recurrent pain with methylprednisolone compared with placebo (4/26 [15%] with prednisolone *v* 1/30 [3%] with placebo; RR 4.62, 95% CI 0.55 to 38.74). However, the study may have lacked power to rule out clinically important differences. No complication related to corticosteroid use was observed in the study participants. Some of the known adverse effects of steroid therapy are increased risk of infections, weight gain, hypertension, poor glucose metabolism, cataracts, and poor growth in children.

Comment: There is evidence from one RCT that dexamethasone, another type of corticosteroid, reduced the number of doses and duration of analgesia in acute sickle cell chest syndrome.[35]

GLOSSARY

Acute chest syndrome Acute chest syndrome is a life-threatening complication of sickle cell disease characterised by fever, cough, chest pain, difficult breathing, worsening anaemia, and new pulmonary infiltrates on radiography. It is difficult to differentiate acute chest syndrome clinically from pneumonia and pulmonary infarctions.

Aplastic crisis Sudden cessation of the bone marrow from making new blood cells.

CHEOPS scale (Children's Hospital of Eastern Ontario Pain scale) A behavioural scale used to evaluate postoperative pain. It was initially validated in children aged 1–5 years, and subsequently validated in children from other populations and ages.[36] CHEOPS scale is used to monitor the effectiveness of interventions for reducing the pain and discomfort. Scores obtained from adding points from six different parameters range from 4–13.

Fetal haemoglobin (Hb F) This is the predominant type of normal haemoglobin (i.e. the oxygen carrying molecule in the human red blood cell) in the unborn child. Following birth, another type of normal haemoglobin (HbA) replaces HbF and remains predominant throughout life. HbF binds oxygen stronger than HbA and maintains higher tissue oxygen tension than HbA.

Haemoglobin S (Hb S) This is an inherited type of abnormal haemoglobin that has a tendency to form crystals when oxygen saturation is low. Under such conditions, red blood cells become deformed (many shaped like "sickle"), more rigid, and easily breakable. This is the main disorder responsible for the clinical syndrome experienced by people with sickle cell anaemia. People affected by sickle cell anaemia who also have high level of fetal haemoglobin (see glossary, p 34) tend to have fewer episodes of crisis because fetal hemoglobin maintains a higher level of tissue oxygen saturation.

Pneumococcal conjugate vaccines These are polysaccharide pneumococcal vaccines linked with proteins such as those of the outer membrane meningococcus, tetanus, or diphtheria toxoids. The conjugate pneumococcal vaccines have been shown to be immunogenic in children younger than 2 years, and is recommended for routine use in infants beginning from the age of 2 months.[16,37]

Polyvalent polysaccharide pneumococcal vaccine (PPV) This type of vaccine contains the purified capsular polysaccharides of several *S pneumoniae* serotypes. Many of the polysaccharides contained in the vaccines do not induce protective immunity in children younger than 2 years. This type of pneumococcal vaccine is recommended for children aged 2 years and older affected by conditions that predispose them to increased risk of invasive pneumococcal infection.[37]

Sequestration crisis Sudden pooling of blood in spleen and liver, with the result that the patient becomes very anaemic and hypotensive, with the affected organ becoming remarkably enlarged and painful.

REFERENCES

1. Akinyanju OO. A profile of sickle cell disease in Nigeria. *Ann N Y Acad Sci* 1989;565:126–136.
2. Serjeant GR. *Sickle cell disease*, 2nd revised ed. Oxford: Oxford University Press, 1992.
3. Ohene-Frempong K, Nkrumah FK. Sickle cell disease in Africa. In: Embury SH, Hebbel RP, Mohandas N, Steinberg MH, eds. *Sickle cell disease: basic principles and clinical practice*. 1994; New York: Raven Press Ltd.
4. Hickman M, Modell B, Greengross P, et al. Mapping the prevalence of sickle cell and beta thalassaemia in England: estimating and validating ethnic-specific rates. *Br J Haematol* 1999;104:860–867.
5. Davies SC, Oni L. The management of patients with sickle cell disease. *BMJ* 1997;315:656–660.
6. Overtuff GD, Powars D, Baraff LJ. Bacterial meningitis and septicemia in sickle cell disease. *Am J Dis Child* 1977;131:784–787.
7. Cohen AR, Norris CF, Smith-Whitley K. Transfusion therapy for sickle cell disease. In: Capon SM, Chambers LA, eds. *New directions in pediatric hematology*. Bethesda MD: American Association of Blood Banks, 1996:39–85.
8. Adams RJ, Nichols FT, Figueroa R, McKie V, Lott T. Transcranial Doppler correlation with cerebral angiography in sickle cell disease. *Stroke* 1992;23:1073–1077.
9. Platt OS, Brambilla DJ, Rosse WF, et al. Mortality in sickle cell disease: life expectancy and risk factors for early death. *N Engl J Med* 1994;330:1639–1643.
10. Riddington C, Owusu-Ofori S. Prophylactic antibiotics for preventing pneumococcal infection in children with sickle cell disease. In: The Cochrane Library, Issue 4, 2002. Oxford: Update Software. Search date 2001; primary sources Cochrane Cystic Fibrosis and Genetic Disorders Group specialised trials register on haemoglobinopathies and hand searches of bibliographic references of all retrived literature.
11. Gaston MH, Verter JI, Woods G, et al. Prophylaxis with oral penicillin in children with sickle cell anemia: a randomized trial. *N Engl J Med* 1986;314:1593–1599.
12. Falletta JM, Woods GM, Verter JI, et al. Discontinuing penicillin prophylaxis in children with sickle cell anemia. *J Pediatr* 1995;127:685–690.
13. Overturf GD. Pneumococcal vaccination in children. *Semin Pediatr Infect Dis* 2002;13:155–164.
14. Chintu C, Gupta K, Osborne C, et al. Clinical trial of the protective role of polyvalent pneumococcal vaccine in sickle cell anaemia patients in Zambia. *Med J Zambia* 1983;17:73–76.
15. Rigau-Perez JG, Overtuff GD, Chan LS, et al. Reactions to booster pneumococcal vaccination in patients with sickle cell disease. *Pediatr Infect Dis* 1983;2:199–202.
16. Vernacchio L, Neufeld EJ, MacDonald K, et al. Combined schedule of 7-valent pneumococcal conjugate vaccine followed by 23-valent pneumococcal vaccine in children and young adults with sickle cell disease. *J Pediatr* 1998;133:275–278.
17. Pai VB, Heyman CA, Erramouspe J, et al. Conjugated heptavalent pneumococcal vaccine. *Ann Pharmacother* 2002;36:1403–1413.
18. Davies S, Olujohungbe A. hydroxyurea for sickle cell disease. In: The Cochrane Library, Issue 4, 2002. Oxford: Update Software. Search date 2001; primary sources Cochrane Cystic Fibrosis and Genetic Disorders Group specialised trials register on haemoglobinopathies and hand searches of bibliographic references of all retrieved studies and reviews and personal contact with the pharmaceutical manufacturer.
19. Ferster A, Vermylen C, Cornu G, et al. Hydroxyurea for treatment of severe sickle cell anemia: a pediatric clinical trial. *Blood* 1996;88:1960–1964.
20. Charache S, Terrin M, Moore RD, et al. Effect of hydroxyurea on the frequency of painful crisis in sickle cell anemia. *N Engl J Med* 1995;332:1317–1322.
21. Redwood AM, Williams EM, Desal P, et al. Climate and painful crisis of sickle-cell disease in Jamaica. *BMJ* 1976;1:66–68.
22. Mohan J, Marshall JM, Reid HL, et al. Peripheral vascular response to mild indirect cooling in patients with homozygous sickle cell (SS) disease and the frequency of painful crisis. *Clin Sci* 1998;94:111–120.
23. Perlin E, Finke H, Castro O, et al. Treatment of sickle cell pain crisis: a clinical trial of diflunisal (Dolobid). *Clin Trials J* 1988;25:254–264.
24. Grisham JE, Vichinsky EP. Kekorolac versus meperidine in vaso-occlusive crisis: a study of safety and efficacy. *Int J Pediatr Hematol Oncol* 1996;3:239–247.
25. Wright SW, Norris RL, Mitchell TR. Ketorolac for sickle cell vaso-occlusive crisis pain in the emergency department: lack of a narcotic-sparing effect. *Ann Emerg Med* 1992;21:925–928.
26. Perlin E, Finke H, Castro O, et al. Enhancement of pain control with ketorolac tromethamine in patients with sickle cell vaso-occlusive crisis. *Am J Hematol* 1994;46:43–47.
27. Hardwick WE, Givens TG, Monroe KW, et al. Effect of ketorolac in pediatric sickle cell vaso-occlusive pain crisis. *Pediatr Emerg Care* 1999;15:179–182.
28. Jacobson SJ, Kopecky EA, Joshi P, Babul N. Randomised trial of oral morphine for painful episodes of sickle-cell disease in children. *Lancet* 1997;350:1358–1361.

29. Perlin E, Finke H, Castro O, et al. Infusional/patient-controlled analgesia in sickle-cell vaso-occlusive crises. *Pain Clinic* 1993;6:113–119.
30. Gonzalez ER, Bahal N, Hansen LA, et al. Intermittent injection vs patient-controlled analgesia for sickle cell crises pain: comparison in patients in the emergency department. *Arch Intern Med* 1991;151:1373–1378.
31. Shapiro BS, Ballas SK. The acute painful episode. In: Embury SH, Hebbel RP, Mohandas N, Steinberg MH, eds. *Sickle cell disease: principles and clinical practice*. New York: Raven Press Ltd.
32. Robieux IC, Kellner JD, Coppes MJ, et al. Analgesia in children with sickle cell crisis: comparison of intermittent opioids vs. continuous intravenous infusion of morphine and placebo-controlled study of oxygen inhalation. *Pediatr Hematol Oncol* 1992;9:317–326.
33. Zipursky A, Robieux IC, Brown EJ, et al. Oxygen therapy in sickle cell disease. *Am J Pediatr Hematol Oncol* 1992;14:222–228.
34. Griffin TC, McIntire D, Buchanan GR. High-dose intravenous methylprednisolone therapy for pain in children and adolescents with sickle cell disease. *N Engl J Med* 1994;330:733–737.
35. Bernini JC, Rogers ZR, Sandler ES, et al. Beneficial effect of intravenous dexamethasone in children with mild to moderately severe acute chest syndrome complicating sickle cell disease. *Blood* 1998;92:3082–3089.
36. Suraseranivongse S, Santawat U, Kraiprasit K, et al. Cross-validation of a composite pain scale for preschool children within 24 hours of surgery. *Br J Anaesth* 2001;87:400–5 [link: http://bja.oupjournals.org/cgi/content/full/87/3/400]
37. American Academy of Pediatrics. Technical report: Prevention of pneumococcal infections, including the use of pneumococcal conjugate and polysaccharide vaccines and antibiotics prophylaxis. *Pediatrics* 2000;106;(Pt 1/3):367–376.

Martin Meremikwu
Dr
Department of Paediatrics
College of Medical Sciences
University of Calabar
Calabar
Nigeria

Competing interests: None declared.

Acute myocardial infarction

Search date February 2003

Nicolas Danchin, Edoardo De Benedetti, and Philip Urban

QUESTIONS

INTERVENTIONS

See glossary, p 54

Key Messages

Improving outcomes in acute myocardial infarction

- **Angiotensin converting enzyme inhibitors** One systematic review in people treated within 14 days of acute myocardial infarction has found that angiotensin converting enzyme inhibitors reduce mortality after 6 weeks compared with placebo. However, a non-systematic review found that angiotensin converting enzyme inhibitors increase persistent hypotension and renal dysfunction at 6 weeks compared with placebo.

Acute myocardial infarction

- **Aspirin** One systematic review in people with acute myocardial infarction has found that aspirin reduces mortality, reinfarction, and stroke at 1 month compared with placebo.
- **β Blockers** We found evidence from systematic reviews and one subsequent RCT that β blockers reduced mortality compared with no β blockers. One RCT in people receiving thrombolytic treatment found that immediate treatment with metoprolol reduced rates of reinfarction and chest pain at 6 days compared with delayed treatment, but had no significant effect on mortality at 6 days or at 1 year.
- **Primary percutaneous transluminal coronary angioplasty versus thrombolysis (performed in specialist centres)** One systematic review has found that primary percutaneous transluminal coronary angioplasty reduces a combined outcome of death, non-fatal reinfarction, and stroke compared with thrombolysis.
- **Thrombolysis** Two non-systematic reviews in people with acute myocardial infarction and ST segment elevation or bundle branch block on their initial electrocardiogram found that prompt thrombolytic treatment (within 6 hours and perhaps up to 12 hours and longer after the onset of symptoms) reduces mortality compared with placebo. RCTs comparing different types of thrombolytic agents versus each other found no significant difference in mortality. One non-systematic review found that thrombolytic treatment increased the risk of stroke or major bleeding compared with control. The review also found that intracranial haemorrhage is more common in people of advanced age and low body weight, those with hypertension on admission, and those given tissue plasminogen activator rather than another thrombolytic agent. One non-systematic review found conflicting results for intracerebral haemorrhage with bolus treatment compared with infusion of thrombolytic agents.
- **Nitrates (in the absence of thrombolysis)** One systematic review of the trials conducted in the prethrombolytic era found that nitrates reduced mortality in people with acute myocardial infarction compared with placebo.
- **Nitrates (in addition to thrombolysis)** Two RCTs in people with acute myocardial infarction (after thrombolysis was introduced) found no significant difference in mortality between nitrates and placebo.
- **Glycoprotein IIb/IIIa inhibitors** Two large RCTs have found that combined treatment with half dose thrombolysis plus abciximab does not reduce mortality at 1 month compared with full dose thrombolysis in people with acute myocardial infarction, but may prevent non-fatal cardiovascular events. However, the RCTs found that combined treatment with abciximab increased bleeding complications, particularly extracranial haemorrhage. Three RCTs found conflicting evidence about the benefits of adding abciximab to primary coronary angioplasty or stenting in people with acute myocardial infarction, although all found that adding abciximab increased bleeding risk.
- **Calcium channel blockers** We found evidence that neither dihydropyridines nor verapamil reduce mortality compared with placebo. One RCT found limited evidence that, in people with left ventricular dysfunction, nifedipine given in the first few days after myocardial infarction may increase mortality compared with placebo.

Treating cardiogenic shock after acute myocardial infarction

- **Early invasive cardiac revascularisation** One large RCT has found that early invasive cardiac revascularisation reduces mortality after 6 and 12 months compared with medical treatment alone in people with cardiogenic shock within 48 hours of acute myocardial infarction. A second smaller RCT found similar results, although the difference was not significant.
- **Intra-aortic balloon counterpulsation** We found limited evidence from an abstract of an RCT of no significant difference in mortality at 6 months between intra-aortic balloon counterpulsation plus thrombolysis with thrombolysis alone in people with cardiogenic shock.
- **Thrombolysis** Subgroup analysis of one RCT found no significant difference in mortality after 21 days between thrombolysis and no thrombolysis in people with cardiogenic shock.
- **Early cardiac surgery; positive inotropes and vasodilators; pulmonary artery catheterisation; ventricular assistance devices and cardiac transplantation** We found no evidence from RCTs about the effects of these interventions.

DEFINITION **Acute myocardial infarction (AMI):** The sudden occlusion of a coronary artery leading to myocardial cell death. **Cardiogenic shock:** Defined clinically as a poor cardiac output plus evidence of tissue hypoxia that is not improved by correcting reduced intravascular volume.[1] When a pulmonary artery catheter is used, cardiogenic shock may be defined as a cardiac index (see glossary, p 54) below 2.2 L/minute/m^2 despite an elevated pulmonary capillary wedge pressure (≥ 15 mm Hg).[1–3]

INCIDENCE/ PREVALENCE **AMI:** Acute myocardial infarction is one of the most common causes of mortality worldwide. In 1990, ischaemic heart disease was the world's leading cause of death, accounting for about 6.3 million deaths. The age standardised incidence varies among and within countries.[4] Each year, about 900 000 people in the USA experience AMI, about 225 000 of whom die. About half of these people die within 1 hour of symptoms and before reaching a hospital emergency room.[5] Event rates increase with age for both sexes and are higher in men than in women and in poorer than richer people at all ages. The incidence of death from AMI has fallen in many Western countries over the past 20 years. **Cardiogenic shock:** Cardiogenic shock occurs in about 7% of people admitted to hospital with AMI.[6] Of these, about half have established cardiogenic shock at the time of admission to hospital, and most of the others develop it during the first 24–48 hours after their admission.[7]

AETIOLOGY/ RISK FACTORS **AMI:** See aetiology/risk factors under primary prevention, p 154. The immediate mechanism of AMI is rupture or erosion of an atheromatous plaque causing thrombosis and occlusion of coronary arteries and myocardial cell death. Factors that may convert a stable plaque into an unstable plaque (the "active plaque") have yet to be fully elucidated. Shear stresses, inflammation, and autoimmunity have been proposed. The changing rates of coronary heart disease in different populations are only partly explained by changes in the standard risk factors for ischaemic heart disease (particularly a fall in blood pressure and smoking). **Cardiogenic shock:** Cardiogenic shock after AMI usually follows a reduction in functional ventricular myocardium, and is caused by left ventricular infarction (79% of people with cardiogenic shock) more often than by right ventricular infarction (3% of people with cardiogenic shock).[8] Cardiogenic shock after AMI may also be caused by cardiac structural defects, such as mitral valve regurgitation due to papillary muscle dysfunction (7% of people with cardiogenic shock), ventricular septal rupture (4% of people with cardiogenic shock), or cardiac tamponade after free cardiac wall rupture (1% of people with cardiogenic shock). Major risk factors for cardiogenic shock after AMI are previous myocardial infarction, diabetes mellitus, advanced age, hypotension, tachycardia or bradycardia, congestive heart failure with Killip class II–III (see glossary, p 54), and low left ventricular ejection fraction (ejection fraction < 35%).[7,8]

PROGNOSIS **AMI:** May lead to a host of mechanical and cardiac electrical complications, including death, ventricular dysfunction, congestive heart failure, fatal and non-fatal arrhythmias, valvular dysfunction, myocardial rupture, and cardiogenic shock. **Cardiogenic shock:** Mortality rates for people in hospital with cardiogenic shock after AMI vary between 50–80%.[2,3,6,7] Most deaths occur within 48 hours of the onset of shock (see figure 1, p 61). People surviving until discharge from hospital have a reasonable long term prognosis (88% survival at 1 year).[10]

AIMS OF INTERVENTION To relieve pain; to restore blood supply to heart muscle; to reduce incidence of complications (such as congestive heart failure, myocardial rupture, valvular dysfunction, and fatal and non-fatal arrhythmia); to prevent recurrent ischaemia and infarction; to decrease mortality, and with minimal adverse effects of treatments.

OUTCOMES **Efficacy outcomes:** Rates of major cardiovascular events, including death, recurrent acute myocardial infarction, refractory ischaemia, and stroke. **Safety outcomes:** Rates of major bleeding and intracranial haemorrhage.

METHODS *Clinical Evidence* search and appraisal February 2003.

QUESTION Which treatments improve outcomes in acute myocardial infarction?

Nicolas Danchin

OPTION ASPIRIN

One systematic review in people with acute myocardial infarction has found that aspirin reduces mortality, reinfarction, and stroke at 1 month compared with placebo.

Benefits: **Versus placebo:** We found one systematic review (search date 1990, 9 RCTs, 18 773 people) that compared antiplatelet agents begun soon after the onset of acute myocardial infarction (AMI) and for at least 1 month afterwards with placebo.[11] Almost all (> 95%) of the people in these studies were randomised to either aspirin or placebo. The absolute and relative benefits found in the systematic review are shown in figure 2, p 62. The largest of the RCTs identified by the review (17 187 people with suspected AMI) compared aspirin 162.6 mg versus placebo chewed and swallowed on the day of AMI and continued daily for 1 month.[12] There was a 2.4% absolute reduction in vascular death at 35 days. The survival benefit was maintained for up to 4 years.[13] In the systematic review, the most widely tested aspirin regimens were 75–325 mg daily.[11] Doses throughout this range seemed similarly effective, with no evidence that "higher" doses were more effective (500–1500 mg/day aspirin *v* placebo; odds reduction for all vascular events 21%, 95% CI 14% to 27%) than "medium" doses (160–325 mg/day aspirin *v* placebo; odds reduction for all vascular events 28%, 95% CI 22% to 33%), or "lower" doses (75–160 mg/day aspirin *v* placebo; odds reduction 26%, 95% CI 5% to 42%). The review found insufficient evidence for efficacy of doses below 75 mg daily. One RCT identified by the review found that a loading dose of 160–325 mg daily achieved a prompt antiplatelet effect.[14]

Harms: The largest RCT identified by the review found no significant difference between aspirin and placebo in rates of cerebral haemorrhage or bleeds requiring transfusion (0.4% on aspirin and placebo).[12] It also found a small absolute excess of "minor" bleeding (ARI 0.6%, CI not reported; $P < 0.01$).

Comment: None.

OPTION THROMBOLYSIS

Two non-systematic reviews in people with acute myocardial infarction and ST segment elevation or bundle branch block on their initial electrocardiogram found that prompt thrombolytic treatment (within 6 hours and perhaps up to 12 hours and longer after the onset of symptoms) reduces mortality compared with placebo. RCTs comparing different types of thrombolytic agents with each other found no significant difference in mortality. One non-systematic review found that thrombolytic treatment increased the risk of stroke or major bleeding compared with control. The review also found that intracranial haemorrhage is more common in people of advanced age and low body weight, those with hypertension on admission, and those given tissue plasminogen activator rather than another thrombolytic agent. One non-systematic review found conflicting results for intracerebral haemorrhage with bolus treatment compared with infusion of thrombolytic agents.

Benefits: **Versus placebo:** We found one non-systematic review (9 RCTs, 58 600 people with suspected acute myocardial infarction [AMI]) comparing thrombolysis versus placebo.[15] Baseline electrocardiograms showed ST segment elevation in 68% of people and ST segment depression, T wave abnormalities, or no abnormality in the rest. The review found that thrombolysis reduced short term mortality compared with placebo (9.6% with thrombolysis *v* 11.5% with placebo; RR 0.82, 95% CI 0.77 to 0.87). The greatest benefit was found in the large subgroup of people presenting with ST elevation (RR 0.79, CI not reported) or bundle branch block (RR 0.75, CI not reported). Reduced death rates were seen in people with all types of infarction, but the benefit was several times greater in those with anterior infarction (ARR 3.7%) compared with those with inferior infarction (ARR 0.8%) or infarctions in other zones (ARR 2.7%). One of the RCTs included in the overview found that thrombolysis significantly reduced mortality after 12 years compared with placebo (36/107 [34%] died with thrombolysis *v* 55/112 [49%] with placebo; ARR 15.0%, 95% CI 2.4% to 29.0%; RR 0.69, 95% CI 0.49 to 0.95; NNT 7, 95% CI 4 to 41).[16] **Timing of treatment:** The non-systematic review found that the earlier thrombolytic treatment was given after the onset of symptoms, the greater the absolute benefit of treatment (see figure 3, p 63).[15,17] For each hour of delay in thrombolytic treatment, the absolute risk reduction for death decreased by 0.16% (ARR for death if given within 6 hours of symptoms 3%; ARR for death if given 7–12 hours after onset of symptoms 2%).[15,17] Too few people in the review received treatment more than 12 hours after the onset of symptoms to determine whether the benefits of thrombolytic treatment given after 12 hours would outweigh the risks (see comment below). **Streptokinase versus tissue plasminogen activator (tPA):** We found one non-systematic review (3 RCTs;[18–20] see table 1, p 58)[17] comparing streptokinase versus tPA. The first RCT, in people with ST segment elevation and symptoms of AMI for less than 6 hours, was unblinded.[18] People were first randomised to intravenous tPA 100 mg over 3 hours or streptokinase 1.5 MU over 1 hour and then further randomised to subcutaneous heparin 12 500 U twice daily beginning 12 hours later, or no heparin. It found no significant difference in mortality between thrombolysis plus heparin and thrombolysis plus no heparin (AR of death in hospital 8.5% with thrombolysis plus heparin *v* 8.9% with thrombolysis plus no heparin; RR 0.95, 95% CI 0.86 to 1.04). There was no significant difference in mortality between tPA 100 mg and streptokinase (8.9% with tPA 100 mg *v* 8.5% with streptokinase; RR 1.05, 95% CI 0.95 to 1.16). In the second RCT, people with suspected AMI presenting within 24 hours of symptoms were first randomised to receive either streptokinase 1.5 MU over 1 hour, tPA 0.6 MU/kg every 4 hours, or anisoylated plasminogen streptokinase activator complex 30 U every 3 minutes, and then further randomised to subcutaneous heparin 12 500 U starting at 7 hours and continued for 7 days, or no heparin.[19] All people received aspirin on admission. The RCT found no significant difference between thrombolytic agents in mortality (streptokinase 10.6%, anisoylated plasminogen streptokinase activator complex 10.5%, tPA 10.3%) and no significant difference in mortality after 35 days between thrombolysis plus heparin and thrombolysis plus no heparin (AR of death 10.3% with thrombolysis plus heparin *v* 10.6% with thrombolysis plus no heparin). The third RCT was unblinded and included people with ST segment elevation presenting within 6 hours of symptom onset.[20] People were randomised to one of four regimens: streptokinase 1.5 MU over 1 hour plus subcutaneous heparin 12 500 U twice daily starting 4 hours after thrombolytic treatment; streptokinase 1.5 MU over 1 hour plus intravenous heparin 5000 U bolus followed by 1000 U every hour; accelerated tPA 15 mg bolus then 0.75 mg/kg over 30 minutes followed by 0.50 mg/kg over 60 minutes, plus intravenous heparin 5000 U bolus then 1000 U every hour; or tPA 1.0 mg/kg over 60 minutes, 10% given as a bolus, plus streptokinase 1.0 MU over 60 minutes.[20] Meta-analysis of the three trials, weighted by sample size, found no significant difference between treatments in the combined outcome of any stroke or death (AR 9.4% for streptokinase only regimens *v* 9.2% for tPA based regimens, including the combined tPA and streptokinase arm in the third trial; ARR for tPA *v* streptokinase +0.2%, 95% CI –0.2% to +0.5%).[17] **Tissue plasminogen activator versus other thrombolytics:** We found two RCTs that compared tPA versus other thrombolytic agents in people with AMI also receiving treatment with aspirin and heparin.[21,22] The first RCT (15 059 people from 20 different countries with AMI evolving for < 6 hours, with ST segment elevation or with the appearance of a new left bundle branch block on their electrocardiogram) compared tPA (accelerated iv administration according to the GUSTO regimen) versus reteplase (recombinant plasminogen activator; two 10 MU iv boluses, 30 minutes apart).[21] It found no significant difference in mortality after 30 days (OR 1.03, 95% CI 0.91 to 1.18). The second RCT (16 949 people; see comment below) compared tPA (accelerated iv administration) versus tenecteplase (a genetically engineered variant of tPA; 30–50 mg iv according to body weight as a single bolus).[22] It found no significant difference between treatments in total mortality after 30 days (6% with tenecteplase *v* 6% with tPA; RR 1.0, 95% CI 0.91 to 1.10).

Harms: **Stroke/intracerebral haemorrhage:** The overview found that thrombolytic treatment significantly increased the risk of stroke compared with control (ARI 0.4%, 95% CI 0.2% to 0.5%; NNH 250, 95% CI 200 to 500).[15] In the third RCT comparing streptokinase versus tPA, the overall incidence of stroke was 0.7%, of which 31% were severely disabling and 50% were intracerebral haemorrhages.[20] The RCT also found that tPA significantly increased the risk of haemorrhagic stroke compared with streptokinase plus subcutaneous heparin or streptokinase plus intravenous heparin (AR for combined streptokinase 0.54%; P = 0.03 for tPA compared with combined streptokinase arms). The RCT comparing reteplase with tPA found that the incidence of stroke was similar with both treatments, and the odds ratio for the incidence of death or disabling stroke was 1.0.[21] The RCT comparing tenecteplase with tPA found no significant difference between treatments in the rate of stroke or death (7% with tenecteplase *v* 7% with tPA; RR 1.01, 95% CI 0.91 to 1.13).[22] We found one non-systematic review that compared bolus thrombolytic treatment versus infusion treatment.[23] Meta-analysis of nine small phase II trials (3956 people) found no significant difference between bolus and standard infusion thrombolysis for intracerebral haemorrhage (bolus *v* infusion: OR 0.53, 95% CI 0.27 to 1.01). However, meta-analysis of six larger phase III trials (62 673 people) found that bolus treatment significantly increased the risk of intracerebral haemorrhage (OR 1.25, 95% CI 1.06 to 1.49). **Predictive factors for stroke/intracranial haemorrhage:** Multivariate analysis of data from a large database of people who experienced intracerebral haemorrhage after thrombolytic treatment identified four independent predictors of increased risk of intracerebral haemorrhage: age 65 years or older (OR 2.2, 95% CI 1.4 to 3.5); weight less than 70 kg (OR 2.1, 95% CI 1.3 to 3.2); hypertension on admission (OR 2.0, 95% CI 1.2 to 3.2); and use of tPA rather than another thrombolytic agent (OR 1.6, 95% CI 1.0 to 2.5).[21] Absolute risk of intracranial haemorrhage was 0.26% on streptokinase in the absence of risk factors and 0.96%, 1.32%, and 2.17% in people with one, two, or three risk factors.[24] Analysis of 592 strokes in 41 021 people from the trials found seven factors to be predictors of intracerebral haemorrhage: advanced age, lower weight, history of cerebrovascular disease, history of hypertension, higher systolic or diastolic pressure on presentation, and use of tPA rather than streptokinase.[25,26] **Major bleeding:** The overview also found that thrombolytic treatment significantly increased the risk of major bleeding compared with placebo (ARI 0.7%, 95% CI 0.6% to 0.9%; NNH 143, 95% CI 111 to 166).[15] Bleeding was most common in people undergoing procedures (coronary artery bypass grafting or percutaneous transluminal coronary angioplasty). Spontaneous bleeds were observed most often in the gastrointestinal tract.[20]

Comment: Extrapolation of the data from the overview (see figure 3, p 63) suggests that, at least for people suspected of having an AMI and with ST segment elevation on their electrocardiogram, there may be some net benefit of treatment between 12–18 hours after symptom onset (ARR for death 1%).[15] The evidence from the RCT comparing reteplase versus tPA is consistent with a similar efficacy for both treatments, although formal equivalence cannot be established because the trial was designed as a superiority trial.[21] The evidence suggests that it is far more important to give prompt thrombolytic treatment than to debate which thrombolytic agent should be used. A strategy of rapid thrombolysis in a broad population is likely to lead to the greatest impact on mortality. When the results of RCTs are taken together, tPA based regimens do not seem to confer a significant advantage over streptokinase in the combined outcome of any stroke and death (unrelated to stroke). The legitimacy of combining the results of the three trials can be questioned, as the selection criteria and protocols differed in important aspects (see review for arguments to justify combining the results of these trials despite their apparent differences).[17]

OPTION GLYCOPROTEIN IIB/IIIA INHIBITORS

Two large RCTs have found that combined treatment with half dose thrombolysis plus abciximab does not reduce mortality at 1 month in people with acute myocardial infarction compared with full dose thrombolysis, but may prevent more non-fatal cardiovascular events. However, the RCTs found that combined treatment with abciximab increased bleeding complications, particularly extracranial haemorrhage. Three RCTs found conflicting evidence about the benefits of adding abciximab to primary coronary angioplasty or stenting in people with acute myocardial infarction, although all found that adding abciximab increased bleeding risk.

Benefits: We found two RCTs.[27,28] The first RCT (16 588 treated within 6 hours of ST segment elevation myocardial infarction; unblinded design) compared half dose reteplase plus abciximab (0.25 mg/kg bolus plus 0.125 μg/kg/minute for 12 hours) versus standard dose reteplase (total dose 20 U).[27] It found no significant difference in all cause mortality or stroke at 30 days between combined treatment with abciximab and full dose reteplase (mortality: AR 5.9% for reteplase alone *v* 5.6% for combined treatment; OR 0.95, 95% CI 0.83 to 1.08; any stroke: AR 0.9% for reteplase *v* 1.0% for combined treatment; OR 1.10, 95% CI 0.80 to 1.51). It found that combined treatment reduced the composite end point of mortality or non-fatal reinfarction at 30 days (AR 8.8% for thrombolysis alone *v* 7.4% for combined treatment; OR 0.83, 95% CI 0.74 to 0.93). At one year, there was no significant difference in mortality between combination treatment and standard dose reteplase (692/8260 [8.4%] with standard reteplase *v* 698/8328 [8.4%] with combined therapy; HR 1.0, 95% CI 0.90 to 1.11).[29] The second RCT (6095 people treated within 6 hours of ST segment elevation myocardial infarction; unblinded design) compared three treatments: full dose tenecteplase (30–50 mg according to body weight) plus unfractionated heparin (60 U/kg bolus plus 12 U/kg/hour); full dose tenecteplase plus enoxaparin (30 mg immediately then 1 mg/kg every 12 hours); or half dose tenecteplase plus full dose abciximab (0.25 mg/kg bolus plus 0.125 μg/kg/minute for 12 hours).[28] It found no significant difference among groups in mortality at 30 days (AR 6.0% with unfractionated heparin *v* 5.4% with enoxaparin *v* 6.6% with abciximab; P = 0.25). It found that abciximab increased composite risk of death, non-fatal cardiovascular events, or haemorrhage at 30 days compared with enoxaparin but reduced risk compared with unfractionated heparin (AR 13.8% with enoxaparin, 14.2% with abciximab, 17.0% with unfractionated heparin). **Primary percutaneous transluminal coronary angioplasty with or without glycoprotein IIb/IIIa inhibitors:** We found three RCTs.[30–32] The first RCT (483 people with ST segment elevation myocardial infarction in the past 12 hours referred for primary angioplasty) compared abciximab (bolus + 12 hour infusion) versus placebo, given before the procedure. It found no significant difference between abciximab and placebo in the composite end point of death, reinfarction, or need for revascularisation of the target vessel at 6 months (AR 28% in both groups; OR 1.01, 95% CI 0.68 to 1.50; P = 0.90).[30] The second RCT (300 people with acute myocardial infarction in the past 12 hours referred for primary coronary angioplasty) found that abciximab significantly reduced the composite end point of death, reinfarction, or urgent revascularisation of the target vessel at 30 days compared with placebo (AR 6.0% with abciximab *v* 14.6% with placebo; RR 0.41, 95% CI 0.18 to 0.93).[31] The third RCT (2082 people with acute myocardial infarction) compared percutaneous transluminal coronary angioplasty with or without stenting and with or without abciximab given during the procedure (2 x 2 unblinded factorial design).[32] At 6 months, it found that adding abciximab to angioplasty or stenting significantly reduced the risk of the composite end point of death, reinfarction, disabling stroke, or ischaemia-driven revascularisation of the target vessel compared with either procedure alone (AR 20.0% after angioplasty alone *v* 16.5% after angioplasty plus abciximab; CI and P values not reported; AR 11.5% after stenting alone *v* 10.2% after stenting plus abciximab; CI and P values not reported).

Harms: **Glycoprotein IIb/IIIa inhibitors plus thrombolysis versus thrombolysis alone:** The first RCT found that abciximab plus half dose thrombolysis increased severe or moderate extracranial bleeding at 30 days compared with full dose thrombolysis (AR 4.6% with combined treatment *v* 2.3% with full dose thrombolysis; OR 2.03, 95% CI 1.70 to 2.42).[27] However, it found no significant difference in rates of intracranial haemorrhage (AR 1.0% with combined treatment *v* 0.9% with thrombolysis alone; OR 1.10, 95% CI 0.80 to 1.81). The second RCT found that rates of any stroke and of intracranial haemorrhage were similar for thrombolysis plus abciximab, enoxaparin, or unfractionated heparin (AR for any stroke about 1.5%, AR for intracranial haemorrhage about 0.9%).[28] **Primary percutaneous transluminal coronary angioplasty with or without glycoprotein IIb/IIIa inhibitors:** The largest RCT found that abciximab given during percutaneous angioplasty or stenting increased transfusion requirements compared with no abciximab (5.4% *v* 3.4%; P = 0.02; RR and CI not reported).[32] The remaining two RCTs found that giving abciximab before percutaneous angioplasty increased minor bleeding[31] and major bleeding[29] compared with no abciximab (minor bleeding: AR 12% *v* 3%; RR 3.7, 95% CI 1.3 to 10.1;[31] major bleeding: AR 16.6% *v* 9.5%; P = 0.02; CI not reported[30]).

Comment: None.

OPTION β BLOCKERS

We found evidence from systematic reviews and one subsequent RCT that β blockers reduced mortality compared with no β blockers. One RCT in people receiving thrombolytic treatment found that immediate treatment with metoprolol reduced rates of reinfarction and chest pain at 6 days compared with delayed treatment, but had no significant effect on mortality at 6 days or at 1 year.

Benefits: **Versus no β blocker:** We found two systematic reviews (search dates 1997[33] and not stated[34]) of β blockers in people with acute myocardial infarction (AMI) and one subsequent RCT.[35] The first review (27 RCTs) found that, within 1 week of treatment, β blockers significantly reduced the risk of death and major vascular events (for the combined outcome of death, non-fatal cardiac arrest, or non-fatal reinfarction: 1110 events *v* 1298 events; RR 0.84, CI not reported; P < 0.001).[34] The more recent review (82 RCTs, 54 234 people) separately analysed 51 short term RCTs (people within 6 weeks after the onset of pain) and 31 long term RCTs (people treated for up to 48 months after AMI).[33] In most of the RCTs, the participants did not receive thrombolysis. In the short term studies, seven RCTs reported no deaths and many reported only a few. The short term RCTs reporting at least one death found no significant difference in mortality between β blockers and no β blockers (ARR 0.4%; OR 0.96, 95% CI 0.85 to 1.08). In the longer term RCTs, β blockers significantly reduced mortality over 6 months to 4 years compared with no β blockers (OR 0.77, 95% CI 0.69 to 0.85). See β blockers under secondary prevention of ischaemic cardiac events, p 188. No significant difference in effectiveness was found between different types of β blocker (based on cardioselectivity or intrinsic sympathomimetic activity). Most evidence was obtained with propranolol, timolol, and metoprolol. The subsequent RCT (1959 people within 3–21 days of AMI and with left ventricular dysfunction, of whom 46% had received thrombolysis or percutaneous transluminal coronary angioplasty at the acute stage of their infarction, of whom 97% received angiotensin converting enzyme inhibitors) compared carvedilol (6.25 mg increased to a maximum of 25 mg over 4–6 weeks) versus placebo.[35] It found that carvedilol significantly reduced mortality (12% with carvedilol v 15% with placebo; HR 0.77, 95% CI 0.60 to 0.98) and non-fatal AMI (HR 0.59, 95% CI 0.39 to 0.90), but found no difference between treatments in the combined end point of total mortality and hospital admission for any cardiovascular event (HR 0.92, 95% CI 0.80 to 1.07) after a median of 1.3 years. **Early versus delayed treatment:** We found one RCT (1434 people with AMI who had received tissue plasminogen activator thrombolysis), which compared early versus delayed metoprolol treatment.[36] Early treatment began on day 1 (iv then oral) and delayed treatment on day 6 (oral). It found that early treatment significantly reduced rates of reinfarction (AR 2.7% with early treatment v 5.1% with delayed treatment; CI not reported; P = 0.02) and recurrent chest pain (AR 18.8% with early treatment v 24.1% with delayed treatment; P < 0.02) after 6 days. There were no significant differences observed in mortality or left ventricular ejection fraction between the two groups at 6 days or 1 year.

Harms: People with asthma or severe congestive cardiac failure were excluded from most trials. One RCT found that people given immediate versus delayed β blockers after tissue plasminogen activator experienced increased frequency of heart failure during the initial admission to hospital, although the result was not statistically significant (15.3% with immediate v 12.2% with delayed; P = 0.10).[36] The presence of first degree heart block and bundle branch block was associated with more adverse events.

Comment: Until recently, trials involving the use of β blockers in AMI were conducted mostly in people considered to be at low risk of heart failure (because of the supposed deleterious effect of β blockers on left ventricular function), and many of these trials took place in the prethrombolytic era. β Blockers may reduce rates of cardiac rupture and ventricular fibrillation. This may explain why people older than 65 years and those with large infarcts benefited most, as they have higher rates of these complications. The trial comparing early versus delayed β blockade after thrombolysis was too small to rule out an effect on mortality of β blockers when added to thrombolysis.[36]

OPTION ANGIOTENSIN CONVERTING ENZYME INHIBITORS

One systematic review in people treated within 14 days of acute myocardial infarction has found that angiotensin converting enzyme inhibitors reduce mortality after 6 weeks compared with placebo. However, a non-systematic review found that angiotensin converting enzyme inhibitors increase persistent hypotension and renal dysfunction at 6 weeks compared with placebo.

Benefits: We found one systematic review (search date 1997, 15 RCTs with at least ≥6 weeks' follow up, 15 104 people) that compared angiotensin converting enzyme (ACE) inhibitors started within 14 days of myocardial infarction versus placebo.[37] It found that ACE inhibitors decreased overall mortality and sudden cardiac death compared with placebo after 2 to 42 months (overall mortality: 1105/7658 [14.4%] with ACE inhibitors *v* 1251/7446 [16.8%] with placebo; OR 0.83, 95% CI 0.71 to 0.97). Sudden cardiac death was also decreased (OR 0.80, 95% CI 0.70 to 0.92).[37]

Harms: One non-systematic review of RCTs (search date not stated, 4 RCTs, 98 496 people within 36 hours of acute myocardial infarction [AMI]) found that ACE inhibitors significantly increased persistent hypotension and renal dysfunction at 6 weeks compared with placebo (hypotension: AR 17.6% with ACE inhibitor *v* 9.3% with control; CI for difference not reported; P < 0.01; renal dysfunction: AR 1.3% *v* 0.6%; P < 0.01).[38] The relative and absolute risks of these adverse effects were uniformly distributed across both the high and lower cardiovascular risk groups. The systematic review did not report on harms.[37]

Comment: ACE inhibitors in people with AMI work best when treatment is started within 24 hours. The evidence does not answer the question of which people with an AMI should be offered ACE inhibitors, nor for how long after AMI it remains beneficial to start treatment. We found one systematic review (search date not stated; based on individual data from about 100 000 people in RCTs of ACE inhibitors) that found that people receiving both aspirin and ACE inhibitors had the same relative risk reduction as those receiving ACE inhibitors alone (i.e. there was no evidence of a clinically relevant interaction between ACE inhibitors and aspirin).[39] Of the 12 RCTs in the systematic review that reported on left ventricular function among participants, all reported a mean left ventricular ejection fraction of 54% or less. Six of these RCTs reported a mean left ventricular ejection fraction of 40% or less. However, there is debate over whether the benefits of ACE inhibitors also benefit people with normal left ventricular function after AMI.

OPTION NITRATES

One systematic review in people with acute myocardial infarction in the prethrombolytic era found that nitrates reduce mortality compared with placebo. Two RCTs in people with acute myocardial infarction (after thrombolysis was introduced) found no significant difference in mortality between nitrates and placebo.

Benefits: **Without thrombolysis:** We found one systematic review (search date not stated, 10 RCTs, 2000 people with acute myocardial infarction [AMI] who did not receive thrombolysis) that compared intravenous glyceryl trinitrate or sodium nitroprusside versus placebo.[40] The review found that nitrates significantly reduced mortality (RR 0.65, 95% CI 0.45 to 0.84). **With aspirin/thrombolysis:** We found two RCTs that compared nitrates (given acutely) versus placebo in people with AMI, of whom 90% received aspirin and about 70% received thrombolytic treatment.[41,42] The first RCT (58 050 people with AMI) compared oral controlled release isosorbide mononitrate 30–60 mg daily versus placebo.[41] It found no significant difference in mortality between isosorbide mononitrate and placebo (ARR nitrates *v* placebo 0.20%; OR 0.97, 95% CI 0.91 to 1.03). The other RCT (17 817 people with AMI) compared intravenous glyceryl trinitrate for 24 hours, followed by transdermal glyceryl trinitrate, versus placebo. It found no significant difference in mortality between nitrates and placebo (ARR nitrates *v* placebo 0.4%; OR 0.94, 95% CI 0.84 to 1.05). Neither RCT found significant differences in mortality in subgroups of people with different risks of dying.

Harms: The systematic review and the large RCTs found no significant harm associated with routine use of nitrates.[40–42]

Comment: Results for the two large RCTs were limited because a large proportion of people took nitrates outside the study, there was a high rate of concurrent use of other hypotensive agents, people were relatively low risk, and nitrates were not titrated to blood pressure and heart rate.[41,42] The RCTs found that nitrates were a useful adjunctive treatment to help control symptoms in people with AMI.

OPTION CALCIUM CHANNEL BLOCKERS

We found evidence that neither dihydropyridines nor verapamil reduce mortality compared with placebo. One RCT found limited evidence that, in people with left ventricular dysfunction, nifedipine given in the first few days after myocardial infarction may increase mortality compared with placebo.

Benefits: **Dihydropyridine calcium channel blockers:** We found two RCTs that compared short acting nifedipine versus placebo within the first few days of acute myocardial infarction (AMI).[43,44] The first RCT (4491 people) was terminated prematurely because of concerns about safety.[43] It found that nifedipine increased mortality by 33% compared with placebo, although the increase did not reach statistical significance. The second RCT (1006 people) found no significant difference in mortality between nifedipine and placebo (18.7% with nifedipine *v* 15.6% with placebo; OR 1.60, 95% CI 0.86 to 3.00).[44] We found no RCTs about sustained release nifedipine, amlodipine, or felodipine in this setting. **Verapamil:** We found one systematic review (search date 1997, 7 RCTs, 6527 people with AMI).[45] It found no significant difference in mortality between verapamil and placebo (RR 0.86, 95% CI 0.71 to 1.04).

Harms: Two systematic reviews (search dates not stated; included both randomised and observational trials) in people with AMI investigating the use of calcium channel blockers found non-significant increases in mortality of about 4% and 6%.[46,47] One RCT (2466 people with AMI) compared diltiazem (60 mg orally 4 times daily starting 3–15 days after AMI) versus placebo.[48] It found no significant difference in total mortality or reinfarction between diltiazem and placebo. Subgroup analysis in people with congestive heart failure found that diltiazem significantly increased death and reinfarction (RRI 1.41, 95% CI 1.01 to 1.96).

Comment: None.

OPTION PRIMARY PERCUTANEOUS TRANSLUMINAL CORONARY ANGIOPLASTY VERSUS THROMBOLYSIS

One systematic review has found that primary percutaneous transluminal coronary angioplasty reduces a combined outcome of death, non-fatal reinfarction, and stroke compared with thrombolysis.

Benefits: We found one systematic review (search date not stated, published 2003, 23 RCTs, 7739 people with or without cardiogenic shock) that compared primary percutaneous transluminal coronary angioplasty (PTCA) versus thrombolysis (streptokinase and fibrin specific agents) in people with acute ST segment myocardial infarction.[49] It found that PTCA significantly reduced the combined end point of death, non-fatal reinfarction, and stroke at 4–6 weeks compared with thrombolysis (253/3089 [8%] with PTCA *v* 442/3085 [14%] with thrombolysis; OR 0.53, 95% CI 0.45 to 0.63; no significant heterogeneity was detected; P = 0.35). It also found that PTCA significantly reduced the combined outcome at 6–18 months (approximately 11% *v* 20%, results presented graphically; P < 0.0001). Results were similar for PTCA compared with streptokinase and for PTCA compared with fibrin specific agents (PTCA *v* streptokinase, 8 RCTs, 1837 people: OR 0.40, 95% CI 0.28 to 0.58; PTCA *v* fibrin specific agents, 15 RCTs, 5902 people: OR 0.57, 95% CI 0.48 to 0.63). The review also found that emergent hospital transfer for primary PTCA (average delay 39 minutes) significantly reduced the combined outcome compared with on-site thrombolysis (5 RCTs, 2909 people: 8% with PTCA *v* 15% with thrombolysis, results presented graphically; P < 0.0001).

Harms: **Stroke:** The review found that PTCA reduced the risk of all types of stroke compared with thrombolysis (all stroke: 1.0% with PTCA *v* 2.0% with thrombolysis; P < 0.001; haemorrhagic stroke: 0.05% with PTCA *v* 1.1 % with thrombolysis; P = 0.03).[49] **Major bleeding:** The review also found that PTCA increased major bleeding at 4–6 weeks compared with thrombolysis (7% with PTCA *v* 5% with thrombolysis; OR 1.30, 95% CI 1.02 to 1.56).[49]

Comment: Although collectively the trials found an overall short term and long term reduction in deaths with PTCA compared with thrombolysis, there were several pitfalls common to individual RCTs, most of which may have inflated the benefit of PTCA.[50] RCTs comparing PTCA versus thrombolysis could not be easily blinded, and ascertainment of end points that required some judgement, such as reinfarction or stroke, may have been influenced by the investigators' knowledge of the treatment allocation (the vast majority of the earlier trials did not have blinded adjudication events committees). In addition, the RCTs conducted before the GUSTO RCT (published 1997[51]) should be viewed as hypothesis generating, in that the composite outcome (death, reinfarction, and stroke) was not prospectively defined, and attention was only placed on these end points after there seemed to be some benefit on *post hoc* analysis. The lower mortality and reinfarction rates reported with primary PTCA are promising but not conclusive, and the real benefits may well be smaller. Only in a minority of centres (such as those who participated in the randomised trials) that perform a high volume of

PTCA, and in the hands of experienced interventionists, may primary PTCA be clearly superior to thrombolytic treatment. Elsewhere, primary PTCA may be of greatest benefit in people with contraindications to thrombolysis, in people in cardiogenic shock, or in people in whom the mortality reduction with thrombolysis is modest and the risk of intracranial haemorrhage is increased, for example elderly people.[52] The value of PTCA over thrombolysis in people presenting to hospital more than 12 hours after onset of chest pain remains to be tested. In one large RCT, the collective rate of haemorrhagic stroke in people given thrombolysis was 1.1%, substantially higher than that observed in trials comparing thrombolysis versus placebo.[51] This may have been because the trials summarised above were in older people and used tissue plasminogen activator. However, the lower rates of haemorrhagic stroke with primary PTCA were consistent across almost all trials, and this may be the major advantage of PTCA over thrombolysis.

QUESTION Which treatments improve outcomes for cardiogenic shock after acute myocardial infarction?

Edoardo De Benedetti and Philip Urban

OPTION EARLY INVASIVE CARDIAC REVASCULARISATION

One large RCT has found that early invasive cardiac revascularisation reduces mortality after 6 and 12 months compared with medical treatment alone in people with cardiogenic shock within 48 hours of acute myocardial infarction. A second smaller RCT found similar results, although the difference was not significant.

Benefits: We found no systematic review. We found two RCTs in people with cardiogenic shock within 48 hours of acute myocardial infarction comparing early invasive cardiac revascularisation (see glossary, p 54) versus initial medical treatment alone (see comment below).[2,3,53] The first RCT (302 people) found that early invasive cardiac revascularisation significantly reduced mortality after 6 and 12 months (see table 2, p 60).[2,53] The second RCT (55 people) found that early invasive cardiac revascularisation reduced mortality after 30 days and at 12 months, although the difference was not significant (see table 2, p 60).[3] **Percutaneous transluminal coronary angioplasty versus coronary artery bypass graft:** We found no RCTs in people with cardiogenic shock after acute myocardial infarction comparing percutaneous transluminal coronary angioplasty versus coronary artery bypass grafting.

Harms: The first RCT (56 people aged ≥ 75 years) found that there was a non-significant increase in 30 day mortality with early invasive cardiac revascularisation compared with initial medical treatment alone (18/24 [75%] with early invasive cardiac revascularisation *v* 17/32 [53%] with medical treatment alone; RR 1.41, 95% CI 0.95 to 2.11).[2,53] The first RCT also found that acute renal failure (defined as a serum creatinine level > 265 μmol/L) was significantly more common in the medical treatment alone group than the early cardiac revascularisation group (36/150 [24%] *v* 20/152 [13%];

RR 1.82, 95% CI 1.1 to 3.0; NNH 9, 95% CI 5 to 48). Other harms reported by the RCT included major haemorrhage, sepsis, and peripheral vascular occlusion, although comparative data between groups for these harms were not provided. The second RCT did not report harms.[3]

Comment: In the first RCT, medical treatment included intra-aortic balloon counterpulsation (see glossary, p 54) and thrombolytic treatment.[2,53] In the second RCT, medical treatment was not defined.[3] The second RCT was stopped prematurely because of difficulties with recruitment. Both RCTs were conducted in centres with expertise in early invasive cardiac revascularisation. Their results may not necessarily be reproducible in other settings.[2,3,53]

OPTION THROMBOLYSIS

Subgroup analysis of one RCT found no significant difference in mortality after 21 days between thrombolysis and no thrombolysis in people with cardiogenic shock.

Benefits: We found no systematic review. We found one RCT (11 806 people with acute myocardial infarction) that compared streptokinase versus no thrombolysis and performed a subgroup analysis on people with cardiogenic shock (see comment below).[54] The subgroup analysis found no significant difference in inpatient mortality after 21 days (280 people; 102/146 [70%] with thrombolysis *v* 94/134 [70%] with no thrombolysis; RR 1.0, 95% CI 0.85 to 1.16).

Harms: The RCT did not specifically report harms in the subgroup of people with cardiogenic shock.[54] Overall, adverse reactions attributed to streptokinase were found in 705/5860 (12%) people either during or after streptokinase infusion. These adverse reactions included minor and major bleeding (3.7%), allergic reactions (2.4%), hypotension (3.0%), anaphylactic shock (0.1%), shivering/fever (1.0%), ventricular arrhythmias (1.2%), and stroke (0.2%). See harms of thrombolysis in acute myocardial infarction, p 43.

Comment: The RCT was not blinded.[54] Data presented are from a retrospective subgroup analysis. Randomisation was not stratified by the presence of cardiogenic shock.

OPTION POSITIVE INOTROPES (DOBUTAMINE, DOPAMINE, ADRENALINE [EPINEPHRINE], NORADRENALINE [NOREPINEPHRINE], AMRINONE) AND VASODILATORS (ANGIOTENSIN CONVERTING ENZYME INHIBITORS, NITRATES)

We found no RCTs comparing inotropes with placebo or comparing vasodilators with placebo.

Benefits: **Positive inotropes:** We found no systematic review or RCTs. We found three non-systematic reviews that did not include RCTs evaluating positive inotropes in people with cardiogenic shock after acute myocardial infarction.[1,55,56] **Vasodilators:** We found no systematic review or RCTs.

Harms: Positive inotropes may worsen cardiac ischaemia and induce ventricular arrhythmias.[1,55,56] We found no studies of harms specifically in people with cardiogenic shock after acute myocardial infarction (see harms of positive inotropic drugs and vasodilators under heart failure, p 118).

Comment: There is consensus that positive inotropes are beneficial in cardiogenic shock after acute myocardial infarction. We found no evidence to confirm or reject this view. The risk of worsening hypotension has led to concern about treating acute cardiogenic shock with any vasodilator.[56]

OPTION PULMONARY ARTERY CATHETERISATION

We found no RCTs comparing pulmonary artery catheterisation versus no catheterisation.

Benefits: We found no systematic review and no RCTs.

Harms: Observational studies have found an association between pulmonary artery catheterisation and increased morbidity and mortality, but it is unclear whether this arises from an adverse effect of the catheterisation or because people with a poor prognosis were selected for catheterisation.[57] Harms such as major arrhythmias, injury to the lung, thromboembolism (see thromboembolism, p 273), and sepsis occur in 0.1–0.5% of people undergoing pulmonary artery catheterisation.[57]

Comment: Pulmonary artery catheterisation helps to diagnose cardiogenic shock, guide correction of hypovolaemia, optimise filling pressures for both the left and right sides of the heart, and adjust doses of inotropic drugs.[1] There is consensus that pulmonary artery catheterisation benefits people with cardiogenic shock after acute myocardial infarction,[58,59] although we found no evidence to confirm or reject this view.

OPTION INTRA-AORTIC BALLOON COUNTERPULSATION

We found limited evidence from an abstract of an RCT of no significant difference in mortality at 6 months between intra-aortic balloon counterpulsation plus thrombolysis and thrombolysis alone in people with cardiogenic shock.

Benefits: We found no systematic review. We found one abstract of an RCT (57 people) that compared intra-aortic balloon counterpulsation (see glossary, p 54) plus thrombolysis versus thrombolysis alone in people with cardiogenic shock after acute myocardial infarction (AMI; see comment below).[60] The RCT found no significant difference in mortality after 6 months (22/57 [39%] with thrombolysis plus balloon counterpulsation *v* 25/57 [43%] with thrombolysis alone; RR 0.90, 95% CI 0.57 to 1.37; P = 0.3).

Harms: Harms were not reported in the abstract of the RCT.[60]

Comment: The abstract did not describe detailed methods for the trial, making interpretation of results difficult.[56] We also found two additional small RCTs (30 people[61] and 20 people[62]) that compared intra-aortic balloon counterpulsation versus standard treatment in people after AMI. Neither RCT specifically recruited or identified data from people with cardiogenic shock after AMI. Neither RCT found a reduction in mortality with intra-aortic balloon counterpulsation. There is consensus that inra-aortic balloon counterpulsation is beneficial in people with cardiogenic shock after AMI. We found no evidence to confirm or reject this view.

OPTION VENTRICULAR ASSISTANCE DEVICES AND CARDIAC TRANSPLANTATION

We found no RCTs evaluating either ventricular assistance devices or cardiac transplantation.

Benefits: We found no systematic review and no RCTs.

Harms: We found no evidence of harms specifically associated with ventricular assistance devices (see glossary, p 55) or cardiac transplantation in people with cardiogenic shock after acute myocardial infarction.

Comment: Reviews of observational studies[1,56,63] and retrospective reports[64,65] have suggested that ventricular assistance devices may improve outcomes in selected people when used alone or as a bridge to cardiac transplantation. The availability of ventricular assistance devices and cardiac transplantation is limited to a few specialised centres. Results may not be applicable to other settings.

OPTION EARLY CARDIAC SURGERY

We found no RCTs evaluating early surgical intervention for ventricular septal rupture, free wall rupture, or mitral valve regurgitation complicated by cardiogenic shock after acute myocardial infarction.

Benefits: We found no systematic review and no RCTs.

Harms: We found no evidence about the harms of surgery in people with cardiogenic shock caused by cardiac structural defects after acute myocardial infarction.

Comment: Non-systematic reviews of observational studies have suggested that death is inevitable after free wall rupture without early surgical intervention and that surgery for both mitral valve regurgitation and ventricular septal rupture is more effective when carried out within 24–48 hours.[1,56]

GLOSSARY

Cardiac index A measure of cardiac output derived from the formula: cardiac output/unit time divided by body surface area (L/minute/m^2).

Intra-aortic balloon counterpulsation A technique in which a balloon is placed in the aorta and inflated during diastole and deflated just before systole.

Invasive cardiac revascularisation A term used to describe either percutaneous transluminal coronary angioplasty or coronary artery bypass grafting.

Killip class A categorisation of the severity of heart failure based on easily obtained clinical signs. The main clinical features are Class I: no heart failure; Class II:

crackles audible half way up the chest; Class III: crackles heard in all the lung fields; Class IV: cardiogenic shock.

Ventricular assistance device A mechanical device placed in parallel to a failing cardiac ventricle that pumps blood in an attempt to maintain cardiac output. Because of the risk of mechanical failure, thrombosis, and haemolysis, ventricular assistance devices are normally used for short term support while preparing for a heart transplant.

Substantive changes

Glycoprotein IIb/IIIa inhibitors One RCT added;[29] conclusions unchanged.

Percutaneous transluminal coronary angioplasty versus thrombolysis One systematic review added;[49] conclusions unchanged.

REFERENCES

1. Califf RM, Bengtson JR. Cardiogenic shock. *N Engl J Med* 1994;330:1724–1730.
2. Hochman JS, Sleeper LA, Webb JG, et al, for the SHOCK investigators. Early revascularization in acute myocardial infarction complicated by cardiogenic shock. *N Engl J Med* 1999;341:625–634.
3. Urban P, Stauffer JC, Khatchatrian N, et al. A randomized evaluation of early revascularization to treat shock complicating acute myocardial infarction. The (Swiss) Multicenter Trial of Angioplasty SHOCK — (S)MASH. *Eur Heart J* 1999;20:1030–1038.
4. Murray C, Lopez A. Mortality by cause for eight regions of the world: global burden of disease study. *Lancet* 1997;349:1269–1276.
5. National Heart, Lung, and Blood Institute. *Morbidity and mortality: chartbook on cardiovascular, lung, and blood diseases.* Bethesda, Maryland: US Department of Health and Human Services, Public Health Service, National Institutes of Health; May 1992.
6. Goldberg RJ, Samad NA, Yarzebski J, et al. Temporal trends in cardiogenic shock complicating acute myocardial infarction. *N Engl J Med* 1999;340:1162–1168.
7. Hasdai D, Califf RM, Thompson TD, et al. Predictors of cardiogenic shock after thrombolytic therapy for acute myocardial infarction. *J Am Coll Cardiol* 2000;35:136–143.
8. Hochman JS, Buller CE, Sleeper LA, et al. Cardiogenic shock complicating acute myocardial infarction — etiology, management and outcome: a report from the SHOCK trial registry. *J Am Coll Cardiol* 2000;36(3 suppl A):1063–1070.
9. Urban P, Bernstein M, Costanza M, et al. An internet-based registry of acute myocardial infarction in Switzerland. *Kardiovasculaäre Medizin* 2000;3:430–441.
10. Berger PB, Tuttle RH, Holmes DR, et al. One year survival among patients with acute myocardial infarction complicated by cardiogenic shock, and its relation to early revascularisation: results of the GUSTO-1 trial. *Circulation* 1999;99:873–878.
11. Antiplatelet Trialists' Collaboration. Collaborative overview of randomised trials of antiplatelet therapy I: prevention of death, myocardial infarction, and stroke by prolonged antiplatelet therapy in various categories of people. *BMJ* 1994;308:81–106. Search date 1990; primary sources Medline and Current Contents.
12. Second International Study of Infarct Survival (ISIS-2) Collaborative Group. Randomized trial of intravenous streptokinase, oral aspirin, both or neither among 17 187 cases of suspected acute myocardial infarction. *Lancet* 1988;ii:349–360.
13. Baigent BM, Collins R. ISIS-2: four year mortality of 17 187 patients after fibrinolytic and antiplatelet therapy in suspected acute myocardial infarction study [abstract]. *Circulation* 1993;88(suppl I):I-291–I-292.
14. Patrignani P, Filabozzi P, Patrono C. Selective cumulative inhibition of platelet thromboxane production by low-dose aspirin in healthy subjects. *J Clin Invest* 1982;69:1366–1372.
15. Fibrinolytic Therapy Trialists' (FTT) Collaborative Group. Indications for fibrinolytic therapy in suspected acute myocardial infarction: collaborative overview of early mortality and major morbidity results of all randomized trials of more than 1000 patients. *Lancet* 1994;343:311–322.
16. French JK, Hyde TA, Patel H, et al. Survival 12 years after randomization to streptokinase: the influence of thrombolysis in myocardial infarction flow at three to four weeks. *J Am Coll Cardiol* 1999;34:62–69.
17. Collins R, Peto R, Baigent BM, et al. Aspirin, heparin and fibrinolytic therapy in suspected acute myocardial infarction. *N Engl J Med* 1997;336:847–860.
18. Gruppo Italiano per lo studio della streptochinasi nell'infarto miocardico (GISSI). GISSI-2: a factorial randomised trial of alteplase versus streptokinase and heparin versus no heparin among 12–490 patients with acute myocardial infarction. *Lancet* 1990;336:65–71.
19. Third International Study of Infarct Survival (ISIS-3) Collaborative Group. ISIS-3: a randomised comparison of streptokinase vs tissue plasminogen activator vs anistreplase and of aspirin plus heparin vs aspirin alone among 41–299 cases of suspected acute myocardial infarction. *Lancet* 1992;339:753–770.
20. The GUSTO Investigators. An international randomized trial comparing four thrombolytic strategies for acute myocardial infarction. *N Engl J Med* 1993;329:673–682.
21. The Global Use of Strategies to Open Occluded Coronary Arteries (GUSTO III) investigators. A comparison of reteplase with alteplase for acute myocardial infarction. *N Engl J Med* 1997;337:1118–1123.
22. Assessment of the Safety and Efficacy of a New Thrombolytic (ASSENT-2) investigators. Single bolus tenecteplase compared to front-loaded alteplase in acute myocardial infarction: the ASSENT-2 double-blind randomised trial. *Lancet* 1999;354:716–722.
23. Eikelboom JW, Mehta SR, Pogue J, et al. Safety outcomes in meta-analyses of Phase 2 vs Phase 3 randomized trials: intracranial hemorrhage in trials of bolus fibrinolytic therapy. *JAMA* 2001;285:444–450.

24. Simoons MI, Maggioni AP, Knatterud G, et al. Individual risk assessment for intracranial hemorrhage during thrombolytic therapy. *Lancet* 1993;342:523–528.
25. Gore JM, Granger CB, Simoons MI, et al. Stroke after thrombolysis: mortality and functional outcomes in the GUSTO-1 trial. *Circulation* 1995;92:2811–2818.
26. Berkowitz SD, Granger CB, Pieper KS, et al. Incidence and predictors of bleeding after contemporary thrombolytic therapy for myocardial infarction. *Circulation* 1997;95:2508–2516.
27. The GUSTO V investigators. Reperfusion therapy for acute myocardial infarction with fibrinolytic therapy or combination reduced fibrinolytic therapy and platelet glycoprotein IIb/IIIa inhibition: the GUSTO V randomised trial. *Lancet* 2001;357:1905–1914.
28. The Assessment of the Safety and Efficacy of a New Thrombolytic regimen (ASSENT) 3 investigators. Efficacy and safety of tenecteplase in combination with enoxaparin, abciximab, or unfractionated heparin: the ASSENT-3 randomised trial in acute myocardial infarction. *Lancet* 2001;358:605–613.
29. Lincoff AM, Califf RM, Van de Werf F, et al. Mortality at 1 year with the combination platelet glycoprotein IIb/IIIa inhibition and reduced-dose fibrinolytic therapy vs conventional fibrinolytic therapy for acute myocardial infarction: GUSTO V randomized trial. *JAMA* 2002;288:2130–2135.
30. Brener SJ, Barr LA, Burchenal JEB, et al. Randomized, placebo-controlled trial of platelet glycoprotein IIb/IIIa blockade with primary angioplasty for acute myocardial infarction. *Circulation* 1998;98:734–741.
31. Montalescot G, Barragan P, Wittenberg O, et al. for the ADMIRAL investigators. Platelet glycoprotein IIb/IIIa inhibition with coronary stenting for acute myocardial infarction. *N Engl J Med* 2001;344:1895–1903.
32. Stone GW, Grines CL, Cox DA, et al. Comparison of angioplasty with stenting, with or without abciximab, in acute myocardial infarction. *N Engl J Med* 2002;346:957–966.
33. Freemantle N, Cleland J, Young P, et al. Beta blockade after myocardial infarction: systematic review and meta regression analysis. *BMJ* 1999;318:1730–1737. Search date 1997; primary sources Medline, Embase, Biosis, Healthstar, Sigle, IHTA, Derwent drug file, dissertation abstracts, Pascal, international pharmaceutical abstracts, science citation index, and hand searches of reference lists.
34. Yusuf S, Peto R, Lewis S, et al. Beta-blockade during and after myocardial infarction: an overview of the randomized trials. *Prog Cardiovasc Dis* 1985;27:355–371. Search date not stated; primary sources computer-aided search of the literature, manual search of reference lists, and enquiries to colleagues about relevant papers.
35. The CAPRICORN investigators. Effect of carvedilol on outcome after myocardial infarction in patients with left-ventricular dysfunction: the CAPRICORN randomized trial. *Lancet* 2001;357:1385–1390.
36. Roberts R, Rogers WJ, Mueller HS, et al. Immediate versus deferred beta-blockade following thrombolytic therapy in patients with acute myocardial infarction: results of the thrombolysis in myocardial infarction (TIMI) II-B study. *Circulation* 1991;83:422–437.
37. Domanski MJ, Exner DV, Borkowf CB, et al. Effect of angiotensin converting enzyme inhibition on sudden cardiac death in patients following acute myocardial infarction. A meta-analysis of randomized clinical trials. *J Am Coll Cardiol* 1999;33:598–604. Search date 1997; primary sources Medline and hand searches of reference lists.
38. ACE Inhibitor Myocardial Infarction Collaborative Group. Indications for ACE inhibitors in the early treatment of acute myocardial infarction: systematic overview of individual data from 100 000 patients in randomised trials. *Circulation* 1998;97:2202–2212. Search date not stated; primary source collaboration group of principal investigators of all randomised trials who collated individual patient data.
39. Latini R, Tognoni G, Maggioni AP, et al. Clinical effects of early angiotensin-converting enzyme inhibitor treatment for acute myocardial infarction are similar in the presence and absence of aspirin. Systematic overview of individual data from 96 712 randomized patients. *J Am Coll Cardiol* 2000;35:1801–1807. Search date not stated; primary source individual patient data on all trials involving more than 1000 patients.
40. Yusuf S, Collins R, MacMahon S, et al. Effect of intravenous nitrates on mortality in acute myocardial infarction: an overview of the randomised trials. *Lancet* 1988;1:1088–1092. Search date not stated; primary sources literature, colleagues, investigators, and pharmaceutical companies.
41. Fourth International Study of Infarct Survival (ISIS-4) Collaborative Group. ISIS-4: a randomised factorial trial assessing early oral captopril, oral mononitrate, and intravenous magnesium sulphate in 58 050 patients with suspected acute myocardial infarction. *Lancet* 1995;345:669–685.
42. Gruppo Italiano per lo studio della streptochinasi nell'infarto miocardico (GISSI). GISSI-3: effects of lisinopril and transdermal glyceryl trinitrate singly and together on 6-week mortality and ventricular function after acute myocardial infarction. *Lancet* 1994;343:1115–1122.
43. Wilcox RG, Hampton JR, Banks DC, et al. Early nifedipine in acute myocardial infarction: the TRENT study. *BMJ* 1986;293:1204–1208.
44. Goldbourt U, Behar S, Reicher-Reiss H, et al. Early administration of nifedipine in suspected acute myocardial infarction: the Secondary Prevention Reinfarction Israel Nifedipine Trial 2 Study. *Arch Intern Med* 1993;153:345–353.
45. Pepine CJ, Faich G, Makuch R. Verapamil use in patients with cardiovascular disease: an overview of randomized trials. *Clin Cardiol* 1998;21:633–641. Search date 1997; primary sources Medline, Science Citation Index, Current Contents, and hand searches of reference lists.
46. Yusuf S, Furberg CD. Effects of calcium channel blockers on survival after myocardial infarction. *Cardiovasc Drugs Ther* 1987;1:343–344. Search dates not stated and primary sources not stated.
47. Teo KK, Yusuf S, Furberg CD. Effects of prophylactic antiarrhythmic drug therapy in acute myocardial infarction: an overview of results from randomized controlled trials. *JAMA* 1993;270:1589–1595. Search date not stated; primary sources Medline and correspondence with investigators and pharmaceutical companies.
48. The Multicenter Diltiazem Post Infarction Trial Research Group. The effect of diltiazem on mortality and reinfarction after myocardial infarction. *N Engl J Med* 1988;319:385–392.
49. Keeley EC, Boura JA, Grines CL. Primary angioplasty versus intravenous thrombolytic therapy for acute myocardial infarction: a quantitative review of 23 randomised trials. *Lancet* 2003;361:13–20.

50. Yusuf S, Pogue J. Primary angioplasty compared to thrombolytic therapy for acute myocardial infarction [editorial]. *JAMA* 1997;278:2110–2111.
51. The GUSTO IIb Angioplasty Substudy Investigators. A clinical trial comparing primary coronary angioplasty with tissue plasminogen activator for acute myocardial infarction. *N Engl J Med* 1997;336:1621–1628.
52. Van de Werf F, Topol EJ, Lee KL, et al. Variations in patient management and outcomes for acute myocardial infarction in the United States and other countries: results from the GUSTO trial. *JAMA* 1995;273:1586–1591.
53. Hochman JS, Sleeper LA, White HD, et al. One year survival following early revascularization for cardiogenic shock. *JAMA* 2001;285:190–192.
54. GISSI-1. Effectiveness of intravenous thrombolytic treatment in acute myocardial infarction. *Lancet* 1986;1:397–401.
55. Herbert P, Tinker J. Inotropic drugs in acute circulatory failure. *Intensive Care Med* 1980;6:101–111.
56. Hollenberg SM, Kavinsky CJ, Parrillo JE. Cardiogenic shock. *Ann Int Med* 1999;131:47–59. Search date 1998; primary sources Medline and hand searches of bibliographies of relevant papers.
57. Bernard GR, Sopko G, Cerra F, et al. Pulmonary artery catheterization and clinical outcomes. *JAMA* 2000;283:2568–2572.
58. Hollenberg SM, Hoyt J. Pulmonary artery catheters in cardiovascular disease. *New Horiz* 1977;5:207–213. Search date 1996; primary sources not stated.
59. Participants. Pulmonary artery catheter consensus conference: consensus statement. *Crit Care Med* 1997;25:910–925.
60. Ohman EM, Nanas J, Stomel R, et al. Thrombolysis and counterpulsation to improve cardiogenic shock survival (TACTICS): results of a prospective randomized trial [abstract]. *Circulation* 2000;102(suppl II):II-600.
61. O'Rourke MF, Norris RM, Campbell TJ, et al. Randomized controlled trial of intraaortic balloon counterpulsation in early myocardial infarction with acute heart failure. *Am J Cardiol* 1981;47:815–820.
62. Flaherty JT, Becker LC, Weiss JL, et al. Results of a randomized prospective trial of intraaortic balloon counterpulsation and intravenous nitroglycerin in patients with acute myocardial infarction. *J Am Coll Cardiol* 1985;6:434–446.
63. Frazier OH. Future directions of cardiac assistance. *Semin Thorac Cardiovasc Surg* 2000;12:251–258.
64. Pagani FD, Lynch W, Swaniker F, et al. Extracorporeal life support to left ventricular assist device bridge to cardiac transplantation. *Circulation* 1999;100(suppl 19):II-206–210.
65. Mavroidis D, Sun BC, Pae WE. Bridge to transplantation: the Penn State experience. *Ann Thorac Surg* 1999;68:684–687.

Nicolas Danchin
Professor of Medicine Université Paris VI
H pital Européen Georges Pompidou, Paris, France

Philip Urban
Director, Interventional Cardiology
H pital de la Tour, Meyrin-Geneva, Switzerland

Edoardo De Benedetti
Cardiologist
C.H.U.V., Lausanne, Switzerland

Competing interests: PU has received funds for research and public speaking from a variety of pharmaceutical and device companies, both related and unrelated to products discussed here. EDB and ND none declared.

The following previous contributors of this topic would also like to be acknowledged: Shamir Mehta and Salim Yusuf.

TABLE 1 Direct randomised comparisons of the standard streptokinase regimen with various tissue plasminogen activator based fibrinolytic regimens in people with suspected acute myocardial infarction in the GISSI-2, ISIS-3, and GUSTO-1 trials (see text, p 41).[18–20]

Trial and treatment	Number of people randomised	Any stroke Absolute number (%)	Any death Absolute number (%)	Death not related to stroke* Absolute number (%)	Stroke or death Absolute number (%)
GISSI-2†[18]					
Streptokinase	10 396	98 (0.9)	958 (9.2)	916 (8.8)	1014 (9.8)
tPA	10 372	136 (1.3)	993 (9.6)	931 (9.0)	1067 (10.3)
Effect/1000 people treated with tPA instead of streptokinase		3.7 ± 1.5 more	3.6 ± 4.0 more	1.7 ± 4.0 more	5.3 ± 4.2 more
ISIS-3‡[19]					
Streptokinase	13 780	141 (1.0)	1455 (10.6)	1389 (10.1)	1530 (11.1)
tPA	13 746	188 (1.4)	1418 (10.3)	1325 (9.6)	1513 (11.0)
Effect/1000 people treated with tPA instead of streptokinase		3.5 ± 1.3 more	2.4 ± 3.7 fewer	4.4 ± 3.6 fewer	1.0 ± 3.8 fewer
GUSTO-1§[20]					
Streptokinase (sc heparin)	9841	117 (1.2)	712 (7.3)	666 (6.8)	783 (8.0)
Streptokinase (iv heparin)	10 410	144 (1.4)	763 (7.4)	709 (6.8)	853 (8.2)
tPA alone	10 396	161 (1.6)	653 (6.3)	585 (5.6)	746 (7.2)
tPA plus streptokinase	10 374	170 (1.6)	723 (7.0)	647 (6.2)	817 (7.9)
Effect/1000 people treated with tPA-based regimens instead of streptinokinase		3.0 ± 1.2 more	6.6 ± 2.5 fewer	8.6 ± 2.4 fewer	5.5 ± 2.6 fewer

TABLE 1 **continued**

chi²/2 heterogeneity of effects between 3 trials	0.7	5.6	7.0	5.4
P value	0.3	0.06	0.03	0.07
Weighted average of all 3 trials¶				
Effect/1000 people treated with tPA-based regimens instead of streptokinase	3.3 ± 0.8 more	2.9 ± 1.9 fewer	4.9 ± 1.8 fewer	1.6 ± 1.9 fewer
P value	< 0.001	> 0.1	0.01	0.4

Values are numbers (%). This table should not be used to make direct non-randomised comparisons between the absolute event rates in different trials, because the patient populations may have differed substantially in age and other characteristics. Deaths recorded throughout the first 35 days are included for GISSI-2 and ISIS-3 and throughout the first 30 days for GUSTO-1. Numbers randomised and numbers with follow up are from the ISIS-3 report[19] and GUSTO-1[20] (supplemented with revised GUSTO-1 data from the National Auxiliary Publications Service), and numbers with events and the percentages (based on participants with follow up) are from the ISIS-3 report[19] and Van de Werf, et al.[59] Plus-minus values are ± standard deviation. In all three trials, streptokinase was given in intravenous infusions of 1.5 MU over a period of 1 hour.

AMI, acute myocardial infarction; iv, intravenous; tPA, tissue plasminogen activator; sc, subcutaneous.

*Death not related to stroke was defined as death without recorded stroke.

†In the GISSI-2 trial, the tPA regimen involved an initial bolus of 10 mg, followed by 50 mg in the first hour and 20 mg in each of the second and third hours.

‡In the ISIS-3 trial, the tPA regimen involved 40 000 clot-lysis U/kg of body weight as an initial bolus, followed by 360 000 U/kg in the first hour and 67 000 U/kg in each of the next 3 hours.

§In the GUSTO-1 trial, the tPA alone regimen involved an initial bolus of 15 mg, followed by 0.75 mg/kg (up to 50 mg) in the first 30 minutes and 0.5 mg/kg (up to 35 mg) in the next hour; in the GUSTO-1 trial the other tPA based regimen involved 0.1 mg/kg of tPA (up to 9 mg) as an initial bolus and 0.9 mg/kg (up to 81 mg) in the remainder of the first hour, plus 1 MU of streptokinase in the first hour.

¶The weights are proportional to the sample sizes of the trials, so this average gives most weight to the GUSTO-1 trial and least to the GISSI-2 trials.[17]

Reproduced with permission from Collins R, Peto R, Baigent BM, et al. Aspirin, heparin and fibrinolytic therapy in suspected AMI. *N Engl J Med* 1997;336:847–860.

TABLE 2 Comparison of early invasive cardiac revascularisation versus initial medical treatment on mortality at 30 days, 6 months, and 12 months (see text, p 51).[2,3,53]

Time after AMI	Mortality in early invasive cardiac revascularisation group Number dead/total number (%)	Mortality in medical treatment alone group Number dead/total number (%)	ARR (95% CI)	RR (95% CI)	NNT (95% CI)
SHOCK study[2,60]					
30 days	71/152 (47)	84/150 (56)	9.3% (–2 to +20.2)	0.83 (0.67 to 1.04)	NA
6 months	76/152 (50)	94/150 (63)	12.7% (1.5 to 23.4)	0.80 (0.65 to 0.98)	8 (5 to 68)
12 months	81/152 (53)	99/150 (66)	12.7% (1.6 to 23.3)	0.80 (0.67 to 0.97)	8 (5 to 61)
SMASH study[3]					
30 days	22/32 (69)	18/23 (78)	9.5% (–14.6 to +30.6)	0.88 (0.64 to 1.2)	NA
12 months	23/32 (74)	19/23 (83)	10.7% (–12.7 to +30.9)	0.87 (0.65 to 1.16)	NA

AMI, acute myocardial infarction; NA, not applicable.

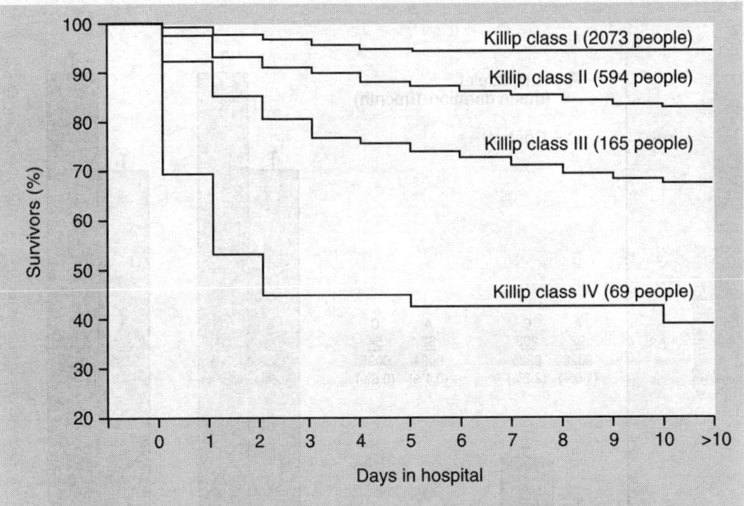

FIGURE 1 **The AMIS registry Kaplan–Meier survival curves as a function of Killip class (see glossary, p 54) at hospital admission for 3138 people (2901 evaluable) admitted in 50 Swiss hospitals between 1977 and 1998. Published with permission: Urban P, Bernstein MS, Costanza MC, et al, for the AMIS investigators. An internet-based registry of acute myocardial infarction in Switzerland. *Kardiovac Med* 2000;3:430–440 (see text, p 40).[9]**

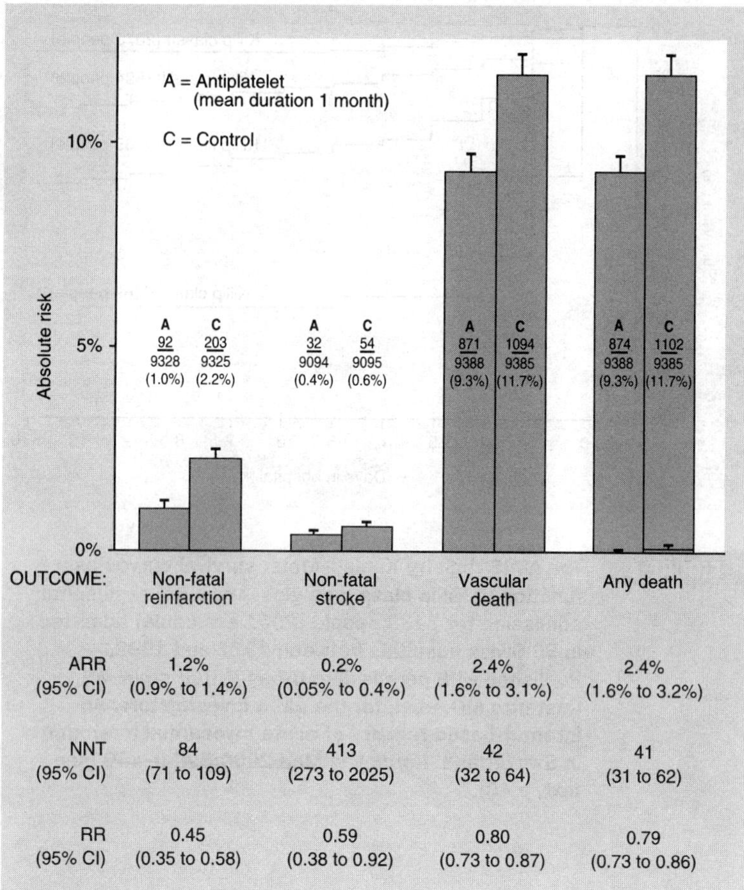

OUTCOME:	Non-fatal reinfarction	Non-fatal stroke	Vascular death	Any death
ARR (95% CI)	1.2% (0.9% to 1.4%)	0.2% (0.05% to 0.4%)	2.4% (1.6% to 3.1%)	2.4% (1.6% to 3.2%)
NNT (95% CI)	84 (71 to 109)	413 (273 to 2025)	42 (32 to 64)	41 (31 to 62)
RR (95% CI)	0.45 (0.35 to 0.58)	0.59 (0.38 to 0.92)	0.80 (0.73 to 0.87)	0.79 (0.73 to 0.86)

FIGURE 2 **Absolute effects of antiplatelet treatment on outcomes in people with a prior suspected or definite acute myocardial infarction (AMI).[11] The columns show the absolute risks over 1 month for each category; the error bars are the upper 95% CI. In the "any death" column, non-vascular deaths are represented by lower horizontal lines. The table displays for each outcome the absolute risk reduction (ARR), the number of people needing treatment for 1 month to avoid one additional event (NNT), and the risk reduction (RR), with their 95% CI values (see text, p 40). Published with permission.[11]**

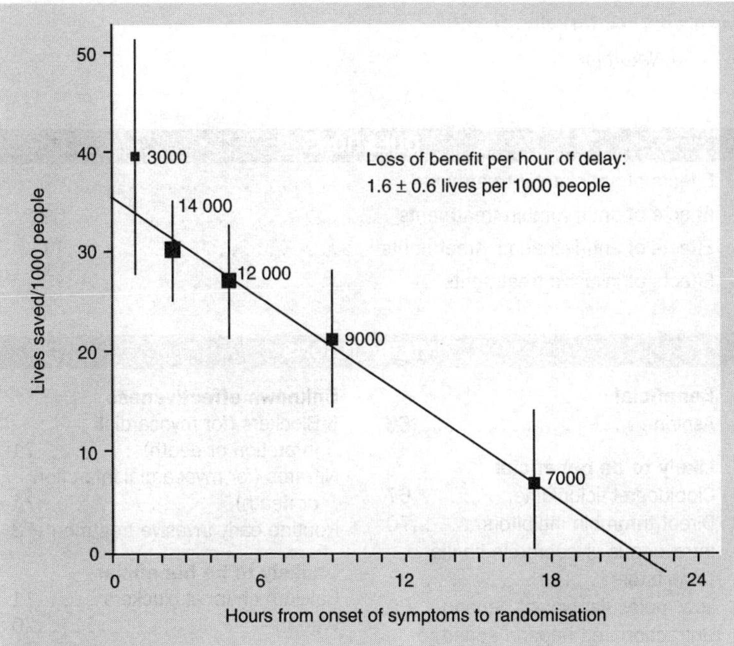

FIGURE 3 **Absolute number of lives saved at 1 month/1000 people receiving thrombolytic treatment plotted against the time from the onset of symptoms to randomisation among 45 000 people with ST segment elevation or bundle branch block.[15] Numbers along the curve are the number of people treated at different times (see text, p 41). Published with permission: Collins R, Peto R, Baigent BM, et al. Aspirin, heparin and fibrinolytic therapy in suspected AMI. *N Engl J Med* 1997;336:847–860. Copyright © 1997 Massachusetts Medical Society. All rights reserved.[17]**

Angina (unstable)

Search date November 2002

Madhu Natarajan

QUESTIONS

INTERVENTIONS

See glossary, p 74

Key Messages

- **Aspirin** One systematic review has found that aspirin reduces the risk of death, myocardial infarction, and stroke compared with placebo in people with unstable angina. The evidence suggests no added cardiovascular benefit, and possible added harm, from doses of aspirin over 325 mg daily.
- **Clopidogrel/ticlopidine** Two RCTs have found that clopidogrel or ticlopidine reduce mortality and myocardial infarction compared with placebo or conventional treatment alone. One RCT found that clopidogrel increased major bleeding, but not haemorrhagic strokes compared with placebo after 6–9 months. Ticlopidine may cause reversible neutropenia. These drugs may be an alternative in people who are intolerant of or allergic to aspirin.
- **Direct thrombin inhibitors** One systematic review has found that treatment with direct thrombin inhibitors for 7 days reduces death and myocardial infarction compared with heparin after 30 days.
- **Intravenous glycoprotein IIb/IIIa inhibitors** One systematic review found that intravenous glycoprotein IIb/IIIa inhibitors reduced the risk of death or myocardial infarction compared with placebo but increased the risk of major bleeding complications.

Clin Evid 2003;10:64–75.

- **Low molecular weight heparins** One systematic review in people taking aspirin has found that adding low molecular weight heparin reduces the risk of death or myocardial infarction compared with placebo or no treatment and does not significantly increase bleeding complications in the first 7 days after unstable angina. However, it found that longer term treatment with low molecular weight heparin did not significantly reduce death or myocardial infarction compared with placebo. One systematic review found no significant difference between low molecular weight heparin and unfractionated heparin in death or myocardial infarction. Long term low molecular weight heparin increased major bleeding compared with placebo, but not compared with unfractionated heparin.
- **Unfractionated heparin added to aspirin** One systematic review has found that adding unfractionated heparin to aspirin for 7 days in people with unstable angina reduced death or myocardial infarction at 1 week. However, a second review found no significant effect after 12 weeks.
- **β Blockers; nitrates** We found insufficient evidence of effects of these interventions on myocardial infarction or death rates. However, RCTs found that those interventions may reduce frequency and severity of chest pain.
- **Routine early invasive treatment** We found five RCTs that reported on different composite outcomes. Two of these found that early invasive treatment reduced death and other cardiac events compared with conservative treatment at 6 months. However, the remaining three RCTs found no significant difference in death or other cardiac events between early invasive treatment and conservative treatment at 12 months or more.
- **Calcium channel blockers** One systematic review found no significant difference between calcium channel blockers and either placebo or standard treatment on mortality or myocardial infarction. Observational studies suggest that short acting dihydropyridine calcium channel blockers may increase mortality.
- **Warfarin** One RCT found that adding warfarin to aspirin reduced cardiac events and death after 12 weeks. However, four RCTs found no significant effect after 5 months or more and one RCT found that warfarin was associated with an increase in major bleeding.
- **Oral glycoprotein IIb/IIIa inhibitors** One systematic review found that the oral glycoprotein IIb/IIIa inhibitor sibrafiban did not reduce the combined outcome of death, myocardial infarction, and recurrent ischaemia compared with aspirin. However, it found that oral glycoprotein IIb/IIIa inhibitors with or without aspirin increased bleeding compared with aspirin alone.

DEFINITION Unstable angina is distinguished from stable angina, acute myocardial infarction, and non-cardiac pain by the pattern of symptoms (characteristic pain present at rest or on lower levels of activity), the severity of symptoms (recently increasing intensity, frequency, or duration), and the absence of persistent ST segment elevation on a resting electrocardiogram. Unstable angina includes a variety of different clinical patterns: angina at rest of up to 1 week of duration; angina increasing in severity to moderate or severe pain; non-Q wave myocardial infarction; and post-myocardial infarction angina continuing for longer than 24 hours.

INCIDENCE/ PREVALENCE In industrialised countries, the annual incidence of unstable angina is about 6/10 000 people in the general population.

AETIOLOGY/ RISK FACTORS Risk factors are the same as for other manifestations of ischaemic heart disease: older age, previous atheromatous cardiovascular disease, diabetes mellitus, smoking cigarettes, hypertension, hypercholesterolaemia, male sex, and a family history of ischaemic heart disease. Unstable angina can also occur in association with other disorders of the circulation, including heart valve disease, arrhythmia, and cardiomyopathy.

PROGNOSIS In people taking aspirin, the incidence of serious adverse outcomes (such as death, acute myocardial infarction, or refractory angina requiring emergency revascularisation) is 5–10% within the first 7 days and about 15% at 30 days. Between 5% and 14% of people with unstable angina die in the year after diagnosis, with about half of these deaths occurring within 4 weeks of diagnosis. No single factor identifies people at higher risk of an adverse event. Risk factors include severity of presentation (e.g. duration of pain, speed of progression, evidence of heart failure), medical history (e.g. previous unstable angina, acute myocardial infarction, left ventricular dysfunction), other clinical parameters (e.g. age, diabetes), electrocardiogram changes (e.g. severity of ST segment depression, deep T wave inversion, transient ST segment elevation), biochemical parameters (e.g. troponin concentration), and change in clinical status (e.g. recurrent chest pain, silent ischaemia, haemodynamic instability).

AIMS OF INTERVENTION To relieve pain and ischaemia; to prevent death and myocardial infarction; to identify people at high risk who require revascularisation; to facilitate early hospital discharge in people at low and medium risk; to modify risk factors; to prevent death, myocardial infarction, and recurrent ischaemia after discharge from hospital, with minimum adverse effects.

OUTCOMES Rate of death or myocardial infarction (often measured at 2, 7, and 30 days, and 6 months after randomisation); and adverse effects of treatment. Some RCTs include rates of refractory ischaemia or readmission for unstable angina.

METHODS *Clinical Evidence* search and appraisal November 2002.

QUESTION What are the effects of antiplatelet treatments?

OPTION ASPIRIN

One systematic review has found that aspirin reduces the risk of death, myocardial infarction, and stroke compared with placebo in people with unstable angina. The evidence suggests no added cardiovascular benefit, and possible added harm, from doses of aspirin over 325 mg daily.

Benefits: One systematic review (search date 1990, 145 RCTs, 100 000 people) compared antiplatelet treatment versus placebo.[1] Seven of these trials included a total of 4000 people with unstable angina. The review found that antiplatelet treatment (mostly medium dose aspirin, 75–325 mg/day) reduced the combined outcome of vascular death, myocardial infarction, or stroke at 6 months compared with placebo (AR 14% with placebo *v* 9% with antiplatelet treatment; RR 0.65, 95% CI 0.51 to 0.79; NNT 20, 95% CI 15 to 34). Individual trials within the systematic review found consistent benefit from daily aspirin in terms of reduced deaths and myocardial infarction.

Harms: The review found that people taking doses of aspirin of 75–1200 mg daily had no significant adverse events, including gastrointestinal intolerance or bleeding.[1] However, the sum of the evidence suggests no added cardiovascular benefit, and greater incidence of gastrointestinal effects, for aspirin doses greater than 325 mg daily. Some people are allergic to aspirin.

Comment: The systematic review covered a wide range of people with different morbidities and levels of risk. Its results probably generalise to routine practice.[1] People with unstable angina who are allergic or who do not respond to aspirin will need alternative antiplatelet treatment.

OPTION CLOPIDOGREL/TICLOPIDINE

Two RCTs have found that clopidogrel or ticlopidine reduce mortality and myocardial infarction compared with placebo or conventional treatment alone. One RCT found that clopidogrel increased major bleeding, but not haemorrhagic strokes, compared with placebo after 6–9 months. Ticlopidine may cause reversible neutropenia. These drugs may be an alternative in people who are intolerant of or allergic to aspirin.

Benefits: We found no systematic review. We found two RCTs comparing clopidogrel or ticlopidine versus placebo or conventional treatment.[2,3] The first RCT (12 562 people) compared clopidogrel (300 mg orally within 24 hours of onset of symptoms followed by 75 mg/day) versus placebo.[2] It found that clopidogrel significantly reduced the combined outcome of death, myocardial infarction, and stroke after 9 months compared with placebo (AR 9% with clopidogrel *v* 11% with placebo; OR 0.8, 95% CI 0.7 to 0.9). The second RCT (652 people) found that ticlopidine plus conventional treatment significantly reduced the combined outcome of vascular deaths and myocardial infarction after 6 months compared with conventional treatment alone (RR 0.5, 95% CI 0.2 to 0.9; NNT 16, 95% CI 9 to 62).[3]

Harms: In the first RCT, clopidogrel increased major bleeding complications compared with placebo, but not haemorrhagic strokes (major bleeding 3.7% with clopidogrel *v* 2.7% with placebo, OR 1.4, 95% CI 1.1 to 1.7; haemorrhagic stroke 0.1% with clopidogrel *v* 0.1% with placebo; P value and OR not provided).[2]

Comment: Reversible neutropenia has been reported in 1–2% of people taking ticlopidine. Clopidogrel and ticlopidine are also associated with other adverse effects, including diarrhoea and rash.

OPTION INTRAVENOUS GLYCOPROTEIN IIB/IIIA PLATELET RECEPTOR INHIBITORS

One systematic review found that intravenous glycoprotein IIb/IIIa inhibitors reduced death or myocardial infarction compared with placebo, but increased major bleeding complications.

Benefits: We found one systematic review (search date 2001, 8 RCTs, 30 006 people) comparing intravenous glycoprotein IIb/IIIa inhibitors (abciximab, eptifibatide, lamifiban, and tirofiban) with placebo.[4] It found that intravenous glycoprotein IIb/IIIa inhibitors significantly reduced the combined outcome of death and myocardial infarction at 30 days and 6 months compared with placebo (at 30 days: 8 RCTs, AR 10.8% with inhibitors *v* 11.8% with placebo; OR 0.91, 95% CI 0.85 to 0.98; at 6 months: 4 RCTs, AR 13.3% with inhibitors *v* 14.6% with placebo; OR 0.88, 95% CI 0.81 to 0.95).[4]

Harms: The systematic review found that intravenous glycoprotein IIb/IIIa inhibitors (abciximab, eptifibatide, lamifiban, and tirofiban) increased major bleeding complications at 30 days compared with placebo (AR 4.2% with inhibitors *v* 3.2% with placebo; OR 1.38, 95% CI 1.04 to 1.85).[4]

Comment: One small trial found limited evidence that in people receiving standard treatment, a "dose ceiling" may exist, beyond which dose escalation of added glycoprotein IIb/IIIa inhibitor increases bleeding complications with no increase in efficacy.[5]

OPTION ORAL GLYCOPROTEIN IIB/IIIA PLATELET RECEPTOR INHIBITORS

One systematic review found that the oral glycoprotein IIb/IIIa inhibitor sibrafiban did not significantly reduce the combined outcome of death, myocardial infarction, and recurrent ischaemia compared with aspirin. However, it found that oral glycoprotein IIb/IIIa inhibitors with or without aspirin increased bleeding compared with aspirin alone.

Benefits: We found one systematic review (search date not stated, 4 RCTs, 26 462 people) comparing oral glycoprotein IIb/IIIa inhibitors with or without aspirin (sibrafiban with and without aspirin, orbofiban plus aspirin, and lefradafiban plus aspirin) versus aspirin alone.[5] Three of the RCTs were reported as abstracts only. The systematic review found that oral glycoprotein IIb/IIIa inhibitors did not reduce the combined outcome of death, myocardial infarction, and severe ischaemia compared with aspirin after 90 days (results from fully reported RCT: AR 10.1% with sibrafiban *v* 9.8% with aspirin; difference not statistically significant; OR and P value not reported).

Harms: The fully reported RCT in the systematic review found that sibrafiban increased major bleeding compared with aspirin (AR 27% with low dose sibrafiban *v* 19% with aspirin; OR and P value not provided). One RCT in the systematic review comparing sibrafiban plus aspirin versus placebo plus aspirin was stopped early because of the findings of the fully reported RCT. A further RCT in the systematic review comparing orbofiban plus aspirin versus placebo plus aspirin was stopped early because orbofiban plus aspirin increased mortality compared with placebo plus aspirin at 30 days (quantitative data not reported). One RCT in the systematic review comparing different doses of lefradafiban plus aspirin with placebo plus aspirin stopped recruiting to the high dose lefradafiban plus aspirin group because of increased bleeding (AR 11% with high dose lefradafiban *v* 3% with low and medium dose lefradafiban *v* 1% with placebo; P value not reported).

Comment: None.

QUESTION What are the effects of antithrombin treatments?

OPTION UNFRACTIONATED HEPARIN

One systematic review has found that adding unfractionated heparin to aspirin for 7 days in people with unstable angina reduced death or myocardial infarction at 1 week. However, a second review found no significant effect after 12 weeks.

Benefits: **Added to aspirin:** We found two systematic reviews (search dates 1995[6] and not stated[7]). Both included the same six RCTs in 1353 people with unstable angina who were treated with either unfractionated heparin plus aspirin or aspirin alone for 2–7 days. The more recent review found that unfractionated heparin plus aspirin reduced the risk of death or myocardial infarction after 7 days compared with aspirin alone (AR 8% with unfractionated heparin plus aspirin *v* 10% with aspirin alone; OR 0.67, 95% CI 0.45 to 0.99).[7] The older systematic review found that heparin plus aspirin did not reduce death or myocardial infarction after 12 weeks compared with aspirin alone (AR 12% with unfractionated heparin plus aspirin *v* 14% with aspirin; RR 0.82, 95% CI 0.56 to 1.20).[6] **Versus low molecular weight heparin:** See benefits of low molecular weight heparin, p 69.

Harms: The older systematic review found that heparin plus aspirin did not significantly increase major bleeding compared with aspirin alone (AR 1.5% with unfractionated heparin plus aspirin *v* 0.4% with aspirin; RR 1.89, 95% CI 0.66 to 5.38).[6]

Comment: None.

OPTION LOW MOLECULAR WEIGHT HEPARINS

One systematic review in people taking aspirin has found that adding low molecular weight heparin reduces death or myocardial infarction compared with adding placebo or no treatment and does not significantly increase bleeding complications in the first 7 days after unstable angina. However, it found that longer term treatment with low molecular weight heparin did not significantly reduce death or myocardial infarction compared with placebo. One systematic review found no significant difference between low molecular weight heparin and unfractionated heparin in death or myocardial infarction. Long term low molecular weight heparin increased major bleeding compared with placebo, but not compared with unfractionated heparin.

Benefits: **Versus placebo or no heparin treatment:** We found one systematic review (search date not stated, 7 RCTs) comparing low molecular weight heparin (LMWH) versus placebo or no heparin treatment.[7] The systematic review found two RCTs (1639 people already taking aspirin) comparing LMWH versus no heparin or placebo for up to 7 days. It found that LMWH reduced death or myocardial infarction compared with no heparin or placebo during treatment (OR 0.34, 95% CI 0.20 to 0.58). The systematic review found five RCTs (12 099 people) comparing longer term LMWH (≤ 90 days) versus placebo. It found that LMWH did not reduce death or myocardial infarction after 90 days compared with placebo (OR 0.98, 95% CI 0.81 to 1.17). **Versus unfractionated heparin:** We found one systematic review (search date not stated, 5 RCTs, 12 171 people) comparing an equal duration (maximum 8 days) of LMWH versus unfractionated heparin.[7] It found that LMWH did not significantly reduce the combined outcome of death or myocardial infarction compared with unfractionated heparin (OR 0.88, 95% CI 0.69 to 1.12).

Harms: The systematic review found no significant difference between LMWH and unfractionated heparin in the frequency of major bleeds (OR 1.00, 95% CI 0.64 to 1.57)[7] (see harms of unfractionated heparin, p 69). Long term LMWH significantly increased the risk of major bleeding compared with placebo (OR 2.26, 95% CI 1.63 to 3.14): equivalent to an excess of 12 bleeds for every 1000 people treated.[7]

Comment: LMWH may be more attractive than unfractionated heparin for routine short term use because coagulation monitoring is not required and it can be self administered after discharge. A Cochrane systematic review comparing LMWH and unfractionated heparin for acute coronary syndromes has been published since the *Clinical Evidence* search date for this update, and will be included in the next update.[8]

OPTION DIRECT THROMBIN INHIBITORS

One systematic review has found that treatment with direct thrombin inhibitors for 7 days reduces death and myocardial infarction compared with heparin after 30 days.

Benefits: We found one systematic review (search date not stated, 11 RCTs, 35 070 people) comparing 7 days' treatment with direct thrombin inhibitors (hirudin, argatroban, bivalirudin, efegatran, inogatran) versus heparin.[9] It found that direct thrombin inhibitors reduced death or myocardial infarction compared with heparin after 30 days (AR 7.4% with direct thrombin inhibitors *v* 8.2% with heparin; RR 0.91, 95% CI 0.84 to 0.99).

Harms: The systematic review found that direct thrombin inhibitors reduced major bleeding during treatment compared with heparin (major bleeding; AR 1.9% with direct thrombin inhibitors *v* 2.3% with heparin; OR 0.75, 95% CI 0.65 to 0.87), and found no significant difference between the risk of stroke at 30 days (stroke; AR 0.6% with direct thrombin inhibitors *v* 0.6% with heparin; OR 1.01, 95% CI 0.78 to 1.31).[9]

Comment: None.

OPTION WARFARIN

One RCT found that adding warfarin to aspirin reduced cardiac events and death after 12 weeks. However, four RCTs found no significant effect after 5 months or more. One RCT found that warfarin was associated with an increase in major bleeding.

Benefits: We found no systematic review. We found five RCTs comparing warfarin versus no warfarin in addition to usual treatment.[10–13] Two of the RCTs were reported in the same journal article.[11] The first RCT (214 people) compared warfarin plus aspirin versus aspirin alone.[10] It found that warfarin (target international normalised ratio [see glossary, p 74] 2.0–2.5) plus aspirin reduced the combined outcome of recurrent angina, myocardial infarction, or death after 12 weeks, but the difference was not significant (AR 13% with warfarin plus aspirin *v* 25% with aspirin alone; P = 0.06). The second RCT (309 people) compared warfarin (fixed dose 3 mg/day) plus aspirin versus aspirin alone.[11] It found no significant difference between warfarin plus aspirin and aspirin alone in the combined outcome of refractory angina, myocardial infarction, and death after 6 months (AR 7% with warfarin plus aspirin *v* 4% with aspirin alone; RR 1.66, 95% CI 0.62 to 4.44).[11] The third RCT (197 people) compared warfarin (target international normalised ratio 2.0–2.5) plus aspirin versus aspirin alone.[11] It found no significant difference with adding warfarin to aspirin in the combined outcome of refractory angina, myocardial infarction, and death after 6 months (AR 5% with warfarin plus aspirin *v* 12% with aspirin alone; RR 0.42, 95% CI 0.15 to 1.15). The fourth RCT (3712 people) compared adding warfarin (target international normalised ratio 2.0–2.5) to standard treatment versus no warfarin.[12] It found no significant difference with adding warfarin in the combined outcome of death, myocardial infarction, and stroke after 5 months (8% with warfarin *v* 8% with no warfarin; RR 0.90, 95% CI 0.72 to 1.14).[12] The fifth RCT (135 people with prior coronary artery bypass grafts) compared warfarin plus aspirin, warfarin plus placebo, and aspirin plus placebo.[13] It found no significant difference between treatments in the combined outcome of death, myocardial infarction, and hospital admission for unstable angina after 1 year (AR 11% with warfarin plus aspirin *v* 14% with warfarin plus placebo *v* 12% with aspirin plus placebo; P = 0.76).[13]

Harms: In the fourth RCT, warfarin increased major bleeding compared with standard treatment alone (AR 2.7% with warfarin *v* 1.3% with no warfarin; RR 1.99, 95% CI 1.23 to 3.22; NNH 71; CI not provided).[12]

Comment: None.

QUESTION What are the effects of anti-ischaemic treatments?

OPTION NITRATES, β BLOCKERS, AND CALCIUM CHANNEL BLOCKERS

We found insufficient evidence on the effects of nitrates and β blockers on mortality or myocardial infarction, although RCTs suggested that these interventions may reduce frequency and severity of chest pain. One systematic review found no significant difference between calcium channel blockers and either placebo or standard treatment on mortality or myocardial infarction. Observational studies suggest that short acting dihydropyridine calcium channel blockers may increase mortality.

Benefits: We found no systematic review. **Nitrates:** We found one RCT (162 people) comparing intravenous glyceryl trinitrate versus placebo for 48 hours.[14] It found that glyceryl trinitrate significantly reduced the proportion of people with more than two episodes of chest pain and one new episode lasting more than 20 minutes (18% with glyceryl trinitrate *v* 36% with placebo; RR 0.50, 95% CI 0.25 to 0.90) and the proportion of people needing more than two additional sublingual glyceryl trinitrate tablets (16% with glyceryl trinitrate *v* 31% with placebo; RR 0.52, 95% CI 0.26 to 0.97). We found one RCT (200 people within 6 months of percutaneous transluminal coronary angioplasty) comparing intravenous glyceryl trinitrate alone, heparin alone, glyceryl trinitrate plus heparin, and placebo.[15] It found that recurrent angina occurred significantly less frequently in people treated with glyceryl trinitrate alone and glyceryl trinitrate plus heparin compared with placebo, but there was no benefit from heparin alone or additional benefit from combination treatment ($P < 0.003$ for glyceryl trinitrate alone and for glyceryl trinitrate plus heparin *v* placebo; CI not reported). **β Blockers:** We found two RCTs.[16,17] The first RCT (338 people with rest angina not receiving a β blocker) compared nifedipine, metoprolol, both, or neither versus placebo.[16] It found that metoprolol significantly reduced the composite outcome of recurrent angina and myocardial infarction within 48 hours compared with nifedipine (28% with metoprolol *v* 47% with nifedipine; RR 0.66, 95% CI 0.43 to 0.98). The second RCT (81 people with unstable angina on "optimal doses" of nitrates and nifedipine) compared propranolol (≥ 160 mg/day) versus placebo.[17] It found no significant difference in death, myocardial infarction, and requirement for coronary artery bypass grafting or percutaneous coronary interventions at 30 days (38% with propranolol *v* 46% with placebo; RR 0.83, 95% CI 0.44 to 1.30). People taking propranolol had a lower cumulative probability of experiencing recurrent rest angina over the first 4 days of the trial. The mean number of clinical episodes of angina, duration of angina, glyceryl trinitrate requirement, and ischaemic ST changes by continuous electrocardiogram monitoring was also lower. **Calcium channel blockers:** We found one systematic review (search date not stated, 6 RCTs, 1109 people)[18] comparing calcium channel blockers versus control treatment (3 RCTs used propranolol as a control and 3 used placebo). The duration of the RCTs ranged from 48 hours (4 RCTs) to 4 months (2 RCTs). The review found no significant difference between calcium channel blockers and control in rates of myocardial infarction or death.

Harms: Hypotension is a potential adverse effect of nitrates. Both older and more recent large RCTs in people with other ischaemic conditions showed that nitrates were safe and well tolerated when used judiciously in clinically appropriate doses. Potential adverse effects of β blockers include bradycardia, exacerbation of reactive airways disease, and hypoglycaemia in people with diabetes. Observational studies have reported increased mortality with short acting calcium channel blockers (such as nifedipine) in people with coronary heart disease.[19,20]

Comment: We found no good evidence that anti-ischaemic drugs (nitrates, β blockers, calcium channel blockers) prevent death or myocardial infarction. Consensus suggests that until further data are available, intravenous nitrates remain the preferred treatment together with heparin and aspirin in unstable angina.

QUESTION What are the effects of invasive treatments?

OPTION EARLY ROUTINE CARDIAC CATHETERISATION AND REVASCULARISATION

We found five RCTs that reported on different composite outcomes. Two of these found that early invasive treatment reduced death and other cardiac events compared with conservative treatment at 6 months. However, the remaining three RCTs found no significant difference in death or other cardiac events between early invasive treatment and conservative treatment at 12 or more months.

Benefits: We found no systematic review. We found five RCTs (6 articles) comparing early routine angiography and revascularisation if appropriate versus medical treatment alone.[21–26] The first RCT (2457 people) compared invasive treatment within the first 7 days and non-invasive treatment plus planned coronary angiography.[21] Invasive treatment significantly reduced the combined outcome of death and myocardial infarction compared with non-invasive treatment after 6 months (AR 9% with invasive treatment *v* 12% with non-invasive treatment; RR 0.78, 95% CI 0.62 to 0.98; NNT 38; CI not provided). The second RCT (2220 people) compared cardiac catheterisation at 4–48 hours and revascularisation (if appropriate) after a cardiovascular event versus standard treatment.[22] It found that cardiac catheterisation reduced the combined outcome of death, myocardial infarction, and readmission for unstable angina after 6 months (AR 16% with catheterisation *v* 19% with standard treatment; OR 0.78, 95% CI 0.62 to 0.97; NNT 34; CI not reported). The third RCT (1473 people) compared early cardiac catheterisation at 18–48 hours versus standard treatment.[23,24] Early cardiac catheterisation did not significantly reduce death or myocardial infarction but did reduce hospital admissions after 1 year (death or myocardial infarction: 11% with cardiac catheterisation *v* 12% with standard treatment, P = 0.42; hospital admissions: 26% with cardiac catheterisation *v* 33% with standard treatment; P < 0.005; NNT 14; CI not reported). The fourth RCT (920 people) compared invasive with conservative treatment.[25] Invasive treatment did not significantly reduce the combined outcome of death or myocardial infarction compared with conservative treatment after 12–44 months (RR 0.87, 95% CI 0.68 to 1.10). The fifth RCT (1810 people) found that early intervention significantly reduced the composite outcome of death, non-fatal myocardial infarction, or refractory angina compared with conservative treatment at 4 months (4 months: 86/895 [9.6%] with early intervention *v* 133/915 [14.5%] with conservative treatment, RR 0.66, 95% CI 0.51 to 0.85).[26] The difference was mainly due to reduced refractory angina with early intervention. The RCT found no significant difference in a combined outcome of death and myocardial infarction between early intervention and conservative treatment at 1 year (68/895 [7.6%] with early intervention *v* 76/915 [8.3%] with conservative treatment, RR 0.91, 95% CI 0.67 to 1.25).[26]

Harms: The first RCT found that early invasive treatment increased major bleeding, but not stroke, compared with non-invasive treatment (major bleeds: AR 1.6% with invasive treatment *v* 0.7% with non-invasive treatment; NNH 111; CI not reported).[21] The second RCT found that cardiac catheterisation increased bleeding compared with standard treatment (6% with cardiac catheterisation *v* 3% with standard treatment; $P < 0.01$: NNH 34; CI not reported).[22] The third RCT found that early cardiac catheterisation did not increase complication rates (death, myocardial infarction, emergency coronary artery bypass grafting, abrupt vessel closure, haemorrhage, serious hypotension) compared with conservative treatment (AR 14% with cardiac catheterisation *v* 13% with conservative treatment; $P = 0.38$; NNH 100; CI not reported).[23,24]

Comment: All trials have reported only short term and medium term follow up, so we cannot exclude a long term difference in effect between early invasive and early non-invasive strategies. There may be subgroups of people who benefit particularly from either invasive or conservative treatment. Advances in catheterisation and revascularisation technology and periprocedural management may reduce the early risks of invasive treatment in the future.

GLOSSARY

International normalised ratio (INR) A value derived from a standardised laboratory test that measures the effect of an anticoagulant. The laboratory materials used in the test are calibrated against internationally accepted standard reference preparations, so that variability between laboratories and different reagents is minimised. Normal blood has an international normalised ratio of 1.0. Therapeutic anticoagulation often aims to achieve an international normalised ratio value of 2.0–3.5.

Substantive changes

Early revascularisation One RCT added;[26] conclusions unchanged.

REFERENCES

1. Antiplatelet Trialists' Collaboration. Collaborative overview of randomised trials of antiplatelet therapy. I: Prevention of death, myocardial infarction, and stroke by prolonged antiplatelet therapy in various categories of patients. *BMJ* 1994;308:81–106. Search date 1990; primary sources Medline and Current Contents.
2. Yusuf S, Zhao F, Mehta S, et al. The Clopidogrel in Unstable angina to prevent Recurrent Events (CURE) trial. *N Engl J Med* 2001;345:494–502.
3. Balsano F, Rizzon P, Violi F, et al, and the Studio della Ticlopidina nell'Angina Instabile Group. Antiplatelet treatment with ticlopidine in unstable angina: a controlled multicentre clinical trial. *Circulation* 1990;82:17–26.
4. Bosch X, Marrugat J. Platelet glycoprotein IIb/IIIa blockers for percutaneous coronary revascularization, and unstable angina and non-ST-segment elevation myocardial infarction (Cochrane Review). In: The Cochrane Library, Issue 2, 2002. Oxford: Update Software. Search date 2001; primary sources Cochrane Library, Medline, Embase, reference lists of articles, medical internet sites, and hand searches of abstracts from cardiology congresses.
5. McDonagh MS, Bachmann LM, Golder S, et al. A rapid and systematic review of the clinical effectiveness and cost-effectiveness of glycoprotein IIb/IIIa antagonists in the medical management of unstable angina. *Health Technol Assess* 2000;4:1–95. Search date not stated; primary sources Cochrane Library, Embase, Medline, National Research Register, and various Internet and online resources.
6. Oler A, Whooley MA, Oler J, et al. Adding heparin to aspirin reduces the incidence of myocardial infarction and death in patients with unstable angina: a meta-analysis. *JAMA* 1996;276:811–815. Search date 1995; primary sources Medline, hand searches of reference lists, and consultation with experts.

7. Eikelboom JW, Anand SS, Malmberg K, et al. Unfractionated heparin and low molecular weight heparin in acute coronary syndrome without ST elevation: a meta-analysis. *Lancet* 2000;355:1936–1942. Search date not stated; primary sources Medline and Embase, reference lists of published papers, and experts canvassed for unpublished trials, and personal data.
8. Magee KD, Sevcik W, Moher D, et al. Low molecular weight heparins versus unfractionated heparin for acute coronary syndromes (Cochrane Review). In: The Cochrane Library, Issue 1, 2003. Oxford: Update Software. Search date 2000; primary sources Cochrane Controlled Trials Register, Medline, Embase, Cinahl, reference lists of articles, and pharmaceutical companies.
9. The Direct Thrombin Inhibitor Trialists' Collaborative Group. Direct thrombin inhibitors in acute coronary syndromes: principal results of a meta-analysis based on individual patients' data. *Lancet* 2002;359:294–302. Search date not stated; primary sources Medline, Embase, Cochrane Library, and conference abstracts and proceedings.
10. Cohen M, Adams PC, Parry G, et al. Combination antithrombotic therapy in unstable rest angina and non-Q-wave infarction in nonprior aspirin users. Primary end points analysis from the ATACS trial. Antithrombotic Therapy in Acute Coronary Syndromes Research Group. *Circulation* 1994;89:81–88.
11. Anand SS, Yusuf S, Pogue J, et al. Long-term oral anticoagulant therapy in patients with unstable angina or suspected non-Q-wave myocardial infarction: organization to assess strategies for ischaemic syndromes (OASIS) pilot study results. *Circulation* 1998;98:1064–1070.
12. OASIS Investigators. Effects of long-term, moderate-intensity oral anticoagulation in addition to aspirin in unstable angina. *J Am Coll Cardiol* 2001;37:475–484.
13. Hunyh T, Theroux P, Bogaty P, et al. Aspirin, warfarin, or the combination for secondary prevention of coronary events in patients with acute coronary syndromes and prior coronary artery bypass surgery. *Circulation* 2001;103:3069–3074.
14. Karlberg KE, Saldeen T, Wallin R, et al. Intravenous nitroglycerine reduces ischaemia in unstable angina pectoris: a double-blind placebo-controlled study. *J Intern Med* 1998;243:25–31.
15. Douchet S, Malekianpour M, Theroux P, et al. Randomized trial comparing intravenous nitroglycerin and heparin for treatment of unstable angina secondary or restenosis after coronary artery angioplasty. *Circulation* 2000;101:955–961.
16. HINT Research Group. Early treatment of unstable angina in the coronary care unit: a randomized, double blind, placebo controlled comparison of recurrent ischaemia in patients treated with nifedipine or metoprolol or both. *Br Heart J* 1986;56:400–413.
17. Gottlieb SO, Weisfeldt ML, Ouyang P, et al. Effect of the addition of propranolol to therapy with nifedipine for unstable angina pectoris: a randomized, double-blind, placebo-controlled trial. *Circulation* 1986;73:331–337.
18. Held PH, Yusuf S, Furberg CD. Calcium channel blockers in acute myocardial infarction and unstable angina: an overview. *BMJ* 1989;299:1187–1192. Search date not stated; primary sources not specified in detail.
19. Furberg CD, Psaty BM, Meyer JV. Nifedipine: dose-related increase in mortality in patients with coronary heart disease. *Circulation* 1995;92:1326–1331. Search date and primary sources not stated.
20. WHO-ISH Study. Ad hoc subcommittee of the liaison committee of the World Health Organization and the International Society of Hypertension: effects of calcium antagonists on the risks of coronary heart disease, cancer and bleeding. *J Hypertens* 1997:15:105–115.
21. FRISC II Investigators. Invasive compared with non-invasive treatment in unstable coronary-artery disease: FRISC II prospective randomised multicentre study. Fragmin and Fast Revascularisation during Instability in Coronary artery disease Investigators. *Lancet* 1999;354:694–695.
22. Cannon CP, Weintraub WS, Demopoulos LA, et al. Treat angina with Aggrastat and determine Cost of Therapy with an Invasive or Conservative Strategy (TACTICS). *New Engl J Med* 2001;344:1879–1887.
23. The TIMI IIIB Investigators. Effects of tissue plasminogen activator and a comparison of early invasive and conservative strategies in unstable angina and non-Q-wave myocardial infarction. Results of the TIMI IIIB trial. *Circulation* 1994;89:1545–1556.
24. Anderson V, Cannon CP, Stone PH, et al, for the TIMI IIIB Investigators. One-year results of the thrombolysis in myocardial infarction (TIMI) IIIB clinical trial: a randomized comparison of tissue-type plasminogen activator versus placebo and early invasive versus early conservative strategies in unstable angina and non-Q wave myocardial infarction. *J Am Coll Cardiol* 1995;26:1643–1650.
25. Boden WE, O'Rourke RA, Crawford MH, et al, for the VANQWISH Trial Investigators. Outcomes in patients with acute non-Q-wave myocardial infarction randomly assigned to an invasive as compared with a conservative management strategy. *N Engl J Med* 1998;338:1785–1792.
26. Fox KAA, Poole-Wilson PA, Henderson RA, et al. Interventional versus conservative treatment for patients with unstable angina or non-ST-elevation myocardial infarction; the British Heart Foundation RITA 3 randomised trial. *Lancet* 2002;360:743–751.

Madhu Natarajan
Division of Cardiology
McMaster University
Hamilton
Canada

Competing interests: None declared.

Atrial fibrillation (acute)

Search date February 2003

Gregory Y H Lip and Bethan Freestone

QUESTIONS

INTERVENTIONS

See glossary, p 91

Key Messages

Prevention of embolism

- **Antithrombotic treatment before cardioversion** We found no RCTs of aspirin, heparin, or warfarin as thromboprophylaxis before attempted cardioversion in acute atrial fibrillation.

Conversion to sinus rhythm

- **Flecainide** One RCT found that compared with placebo, intravenous flecainide increased the proportion of people who reverted to sinus rhythm within 1 hour and in whom the sinus rhythm was maintained after 6 hours. Flecainide has been associated with serious adverse events such as severe hypotension and torsades de point. Two RCTs found that compared with intravenous amiodarone, oral flecainide increased the proportion of people who reverted to sinus rhythm within 8 hours. We found insufficient evidence to draw any conclusions about comparisons between intravenous flecainide and intravenous amiodarone and flecainide versus quinidine. Two RCTs found no significant difference between flecainide and propafenone. Flecainide and propafenone are not used in people with known or suspected ischaemic heart disease due to possible proarrhythmic effects.

- **Propafenone** One systematic review and subsequent RCTs have found that compared with placebo, propafenone increased the proportion of people converting to sinus rhythm within 1–4 hours. One RCT found no significant difference between intravenous propafenone and amiodarone in the proportion of people converting to sinus rhythm within 1 hour in people with onset of atrial fibrillation of less than 48 hours. Another RCT found that compared with amiodarone, a higher proportion of people converted to sinus rhythm with oral propafenone within 2.5 hours but the difference did not remain significant at 24 hours in people with onset of atrial fibrillation of less than 2 weeks. Two RCTs found no significant difference between flecainide and propafenone. Propafenone and flecainide are not used in people with known or suspected ischaemic heart disease due to possible proarrhythmic effects.
- **Amiodarone** We found insufficient evidence from three RCTs about the effects of amiodarone as a single agent compared with placebo for conversion to sinus rhythm in people with acute atrial fibrillation. Four small RCTs found no significant difference between amiodarone versus digoxin in rate of conversion to sinus rhythm at 24–48 hours, although the studies may have lacked power to exclude clinically important differences. We found insufficient evidence from one small RCT to compare amiodarone versus verapamil. We found no RCTs comparing amiodarone with either DC cardioversion or diltiazem.
- **DC cardioversion** We found no RCTs of DC cardioversion in acute atrial fibrillation. It may be unethical to conduct RCTs in people with acute atrial fibrillation and haemodynamic compromise.
- **Quinidine** We found no RCTs comparing quinidine versus placebo. One small RCT in people with onset of atrial fibrillation of less than 48 hours found that compared with sotalol, quinidine plus digoxin increased the proportion of people converting to sinus rhythm within 12 hours.
- **Sotalol** We found no systematic review or RCTs comparing sotalol versus placebo. One small RCT in people with onset of atrial fibrillation of less than 48 hours found that compared with sotalol, quinidine plus digoxin increased the proportion of people converting to sinus rhythm within 12 hours.
- **Digoxin** Three RCTs found no significant difference between digoxin and placebo in conversion to sinus rhythm in people with atrial fibrillation of up to 7 days' duration. Four small RCTs found no significant difference between amiodarone versus digoxin for conversion to sinus rhythm in people with acute atrial fibrillation, although the trials might have lacked power to exclude clinically important differences.

Heart rate control

- **Digoxin** We found no RCTs only in people with acute atrial fibrillation. Two RCTs found that digoxin versus placebo reduced ventricular rate within 2 hours in people with atrial fibrillation of up to 7 days' duration.
- **Diltiazem** One RCT in people with atrial fibrillation or atrial flutter found that intravenous diltiazem (a calcium channel blocker) reduced heart rate over 15 minutes compared with placebo. Another RCT in people with acute atrial fibrillation or atrial flutter found that intravenous diltiazem reduced heart rate within 5 minutes compared with intravenous diltiazem.

Atrial fibrillation (acute)

- **Timolol** One small RCT in people with atrial fibrillation of unspecified duration found that intravenous timolol (a β blocker) reduced ventricular rate within 20 minutes compared with placebo.
- **Verapamil** Two RCTs found that intravenous verapamil (a calcium channel blocker) reduced heart rate at 10 or 30 minutes compared with placebo in people with atrial fibrillation or atrial flutter. One RCT found no significant difference in rate control or measures of systolic function with intravenous verapamil versus intravenous diltiazem in people with atrial fibrillation or atrial flutter, but verapamil caused hypotension in some people.
- **Amiodarone** We found no RCTs examining effects of amiodarone alone on heart rate in people with acute atrial fibrillation.
- **Sotalol** We found no systematic review or RCTs comparing sotalol with placebo.

DEFINITION Acute atrial fibrillation is rapid, irregular, and chaotic atrial activity of less that 48 hours' duration. It includes both the first symptomatic onset of persistent atrial fibrillation and episodes of paroxysmal atrial fibrillation (see glossary, p 92). It is sometimes difficult to distinguish episodes of new onset atrial fibrillation from long standing atrial fibrillation that was previously undiagnosed. Atrial fibrillation within 72 hours of onset is sometimes called recent onset atrial fibrillation. By contrast, chronic atrial fibrillation is a more sustained form of atrial fibrillation, which in turn can be described as paroxysmal, persistent, or permanent atrial fibrillation (see glossary, p 92). Intermittent atrial fibrillation, with spontaneous recurrences/termination and with sinus rhythm between recurrences is known as paroxysmal atrial fibrillation. More sustained atrial fibrillation, which is considered amenable to cardioversion, is called persistent atrial fibrillation. If cardioversion is considered inappropriate, then the atrial fibrillation is known as "permanent". In this review we have excluded episodes of atrial fibrillation that arise during or soon after cardiac surgery, and we have excluded management of chronic atrial fibrillation.

INCIDENCE/ PREVALENCE We found limited evidence of the incidence or prevalence of acute atrial fibrillation. Extrapolation from the Framingham study[1] suggests an incidence in men of 3/1000 person years at age 55 years, rising to 38/1000 person years at 94 years. In women, the incidence was 2/1000 person years at age 55 years and 32.5/1000 person years at 94 years. The prevalence of atrial fibrillation ranged from 0.5% for people aged 50–59 years to 9% in people aged 80–89 years. Among acute emergency medical admissions in the UK, 3–6% have atrial fibrillation and about 40% were newly diagnosed.[2,3] Among acute hospital admissions in New Zealand, 10% (95% CI 9% to 12%) had documented atrial fibrillation.[4]

AETIOLOGY/ RISK FACTORS Paroxysms of atrial fibrillation are more common in athletes.[5] Age increases the risk of developing acute atrial fibrillation. Men are more likely to develop atrial fibrillation than women (38 years' follow up from the Framingham Study, RR after adjustment for age and known predisposing conditions 1.5).[6] Atrial fibrillation can occur in association with underlying disease (both cardiac and non-cardiac) or can arise in the absence of any other condition. Epidemiological surveys have found that risk factors for the development of acute atrial fibrillation include ischaemic heart disease, hypertension, heart failure, valve disease, diabetes, alcohol abuse, thyroid disorders, and disorders of the lung and pleura.[1] In a UK survey of acute hospital admissions with atrial fibrillation, a history of ischaemic heart disease was present in 33%, heart failure in 24%, hypertension in 26%, and rheumatic heart disease in 7%.[3] In some populations, the acute effects of alcohol explain a large proportion of the incidence of acute atrial fibrillation.

PROGNOSIS We found no evidence about the proportion of people with acute atrial fibrillation who develop more chronic forms of atrial fibrillation (e.g. paroxysmal, persistent, or permanent atrial fibrillation). Observational studies and placebo arms of RCTs have found that more than 50% of people with acute atrial fibrillation revert spontaneously within 24–48 hours, especially if atrial fibrillation is associated with an identifiable precipitant such as alcohol or myocardial infarction. We found little evidence about the effects on mortality and morbidity of acute atrial fibrillation where no underlying cause is found. Acute atrial fibrillation during myocardial infarction is an independent predictor of both short term and long term mortality.[7] Onset of atrial fibrillation reduces cardiac output by 10–20% irrespective of the underlying ventricular rate[8,9] and can contribute to heart failure. People with acute atrial fibrillation who present with heart failure have worse prognosis. Acute atrial fibrillation is associated with a risk of imminent stroke.[10–13] One case series used transoesophageal echocardiography in people who had developed acute atrial fibrillation within the preceding 48 hours; it found that 15% had atrial thrombi.[14] An ischaemic stroke associated with atrial fibrillation is more likely to be fatal, have a recurrence, and leave a serious functional deficit among survivors, than a stroke not associated with atrial fibrillation.[15]

AIMS OF INTERVENTION To reduce symptoms, morbidity, and mortality, with minimum adverse effects.

OUTCOMES Major outcomes include measures of symptoms, recurrent stroke or transient ischaemic attack, thromboembolism, mortality, and major bleeding. Proxy measures include heart rhythm, ventricular rate, and timing to restoration of sinus rhythm. Frequent spontaneous reversion to sinus rhythm makes it difficult to interpret short term studies of rhythm; treatments may accelerate restoration of sinus rhythm without increasing the proportion of people who eventually convert. The clinical importance of changes in mean heart rate is also unclear.

METHODS *Clinical Evidence* search and appraisal February 2003. Current Contents, textbooks, review articles, and recent abstracts were reviewed. Many studies were not solely in people with acute atrial fibrillation. The text indicates where results have been extrapolated from studies of paroxysmal, persistent, or permanent atrial fibrillation. Atrial fibrillation that follows coronary surgery has been excluded. We found no RCTs that reported on quality of life, functional capacity, or mortality.

QUESTION **What are the effects of interventions to prevent embolism?**

OPTION **ANTITHROMBOTIC TREATMENT BEFORE CARDIOVERSION**

We found no RCTs on use of aspirin, heparin, or warfarin as thromboprophylaxis before cardioversion in acute atrial fibrillation.

Benefits: We found no RCTs on use of aspirin, heparin, or warfarin as thromboprophylaxis before cardioversion in acute atrial fibrillation.

Harms: We found no RCTs.

Comment: For acute atrial fibrillation, there is consensus to give heparin to people undergoing cardioversion within 48 hours of arrhythmia onset but we found insufficient evidence. The decision for anticoagulation both short term and after cardioversion is usually based on individual intrinsic risk of thromboembolism.[16] Warfarin is not used as an anticoagulant in acute atrial fibrillation because of its slow onset of action. One transoesophageal echocardiography study in people with a recent embolic event found left atrial thrombus in 15% of people with acute atrial fibrillation of less than 3 days' duration.[14] This would suggest that people with atrial fibrillation of less than 3 days' duration may benefit from formal anticoagulation or require evaluation by transoesophageal echocardiography before safe cardioversion. One ongoing trial is assessing the feasibility and effects of such a strategy by comparing low molecular weight and unfractionated heparin in people with atrial fibrillation of more than 2 days' duration undergoing transoesophageal echocardiographically guided early electrical or chemical cardioversion.[17]

QUESTION **What are the effects of interventions for conversion to sinus rhythm and to control heart rate?**

OPTION **DC CARDIOVERSION**

We found no RCTs of DC cardioversion in acute atrial fibrillation. It may be unethical to conduct RCTs of DC cardioversion in people with acute atrial fibrillation and haemodynamic compromise.

Benefits: We found no RCTs of DC cardioversion in acute atrial fibrillation.

Harms: We found no RCTs of DC cardioversion in acute atrial fibrillation. Adverse events from synchronised DC cardioversion include those associated with a general anaesthetic, generation of a more serious arrhythmia, superficial burns, and thromboembolism. Cardioversion may be unsuccessful. The atrial fibrillation might recur.

Comment: It might be unethical to conduct RCTs of DC cardioversion in people with acute atrial fibrillation and haemodynamic compromise. The only evidence for DC cardioversion in acute atrial fibrillation is extrapolated from its use in chronic atrial fibrillation (see glossary, p 91). DC cardioversion has been used for the treatment of atrial fibrillation since the 1960s.[18] There is a consensus[16] that immediate DC cardioversion for acute atrial fibrillation should be attempted only if there are signs of haemodynamic compromise. Otherwise full anticoagulation is recommended (warfarin for 3 weeks before and 4 weeks after cardioversion) to reduce the risk of thromboembolism in people with acute atrial fibrillation of more than 48 hours' duration.[16] We found insufficient evidence on whether cardioversion or rate control is superior for acute atrial fibrillation.

OPTION AMIODARONE

Two small RCTs found no significant difference in rates of conversion to sinus rhythm at 8 hours between amiodarone as a single agent and placebo. However, one small RCT found higher cardioversion rates for amiodarone compared with placebo. Four small RCTs have found no significant difference in rate of conversion to sinus rhythm at 24–48 hours for amiodarone compared with digoxin, although the studies may have lacked power to exclude clinically important differences. One small RCT found that compared with verapamil, amiodarone increased cardioversion rate at 3 hours. We found no RCTs comparing amiodarone with either DC cardioversion or diltiazem.

Benefits: **Versus placebo:** We found two systematic reviews (search dates 2001, 2 RCTs comparing amiodarone as a single agent with placebo, 104 people with acute onset atrial fibrillation)[19,20] and one subsequent RCT.[21] Both RCTs included in the reviews found no significant difference in rates of conversion from atrial fibrillation to sinus rhythm between intravenous amiodarone and placebo at 8 hours (first RCT: 40 people; cardioversion rate 37% with amiodarone 5 mg/kg bolus plus 1800 mg/day *v* 48% with placebo; second RCT: 64 people; cardioversion rate 59% with amiodarone 7 mg/kg bolus *v* 56% with placebo).[22,23] The subsequent RCT (72 people) found higher cardioversion rates with oral amiodarone compared with placebo at 8 hours (50% cardioverted with amiodarone 30 mg/kg/day *v* 20% with placebo; $P < 0.0001$).[21] **Versus digoxin:** We found two systematic reviews (search date 2001, 3 RCTs, 148 people with acute onset atrial fibrillation;[19] search date 2001, 3 RCTs, 114 people, no statistical pooling of results[20]). Together, the reviews identified four small RCTs (34, 45, 50, and 30 people). None found any statistically significant difference in rates of conversion to sinus between amiodarone and digoxin at 24–48 hours. **Versus diltiazem:** We found no systematic review or RCTs in people with acute atrial fibrillation. **Versus verapamil:** We found two systematic reviews (both search dates 2001, 1 RCT, 24 people).[19,20] The included RCT found that amiodarone increased conversion to sinus rhythm compared with verapamil at 3 hours (AR for cardioversion 77% with amiodarone *v* 0% with iv verapamil; $P < 0.05$).[24] **Versus DC cardioversion:** We found no systematic review or RCTs.

Harms: One systematic review found that the most common adverse effects of intravenous amiodarone were phlebitis, hypotension, and bradycardia.[20] Pooled adverse event rates were higher with amiodarone than placebo (AR for any adverse effect 17% with amiodarone *v* 11% with placebo). Other reported adverse effects of amiodarone in the acute setting include heart failure and arrhythmia.

Comment: The RCTs were small. Those that found no significant difference between treatments might have lacked power to detect clinically important effects.

OPTION DIGOXIN

We found no RCTs only in people with acute atrial fibrillation. Three RCTs found no significant difference between digoxin and placebo in conversion to sinus rhythm in people with atrial fibrillation of up to 7 days' duration. Two RCTs found that compared with placebo, digoxin reduced ventricular rate after 30 minutes and after 2 hours in people with atrial fibrillation. Four RCTs found no significant difference between amiodarone and digoxin in conversion to sinus rhythm at 24–48 hours, although these trials may have lacked power to detect clinically important differences.

Benefits: We found no systematic review but found three RCTs.[25–27] **Versus placebo:** One RCT (239 people within 7 days of onset of atrial fibrillation, mean age 66 years, mean ventricular rate 122 beats/minute) found that intravenous digoxin (mean 0.88 mg) versus placebo did not increase the restoration of sinus rhythm by 16 hours (51% with digoxin *v* 46% with placebo).[25] It found a rapid and clinically important reduction in ventricular rate at 2 hours (to 105 beats/minute with digoxin *v* 117 beats/minute with placebo; $P = 0.0001$). The second RCT (40 people within 7 days of the onset of atrial fibrillation, mean age 64 years, 23 men) compared high dose intravenous digoxin 1.25 mg versus placebo. Restoration to sinus rhythm was not significantly different (9/19 [47%] with digoxin *v* 8/20 [40%] with placebo; $P = 0.6$). The ventricular rate after 30 minutes was significantly lower with digoxin versus placebo ($P < 0.02$).[26] The third RCT (36 people within 7 days of the onset of atrial fibrillation) compared oral digoxin (doses of 0.6, 0.4, 0.2, and 0.2 mg at 0, 4, 8, and 14 hours, or until conversion to sinus rhythm, whichever occurred first) versus placebo. Conversion to sinus rhythm by 18 hours was not significantly different (50% with digoxin *v* 44% with placebo; ARR +6%, 95% CI −11% to +22%).[27] **Versus amiodarone:** See benefits of amiodarone, p 81.

Harms: In one RCT, some people developed asymptomatic bradycardia and one person with previously undiagnosed hypertrophic cardiomyopathy suffered circulatory distress.[25] In the second RCT, two people developed bradyarrhythmias.[26] No adverse effects were stated in the third RCT.[27] Digoxin at toxic doses could result in visual, gastrointestinal, and neurological symptoms, heart block, and arrhythmias.

Comment: The peak action of digoxin is delayed for up to 6–12 hours. We found one systematic review (search date 1998)[28] and RCTs of digoxin versus placebo in people with chronic atrial fibrillation (see glossary, p 91), which found that control of the ventricular rate control during exercise was poor unless a β blocker or rate limiting calcium channel blocker (verapamil or diltiazem) was used in combination.[29,30] The evidence suggests that digoxin is no better than placebo for restoring sinus rhythm in people with recent onset atrial fibrillation.

OPTION DILTIAZEM

One RCT found that compared with placebo, intravenous diltiazem reduced heart rate in people with atrial fibrillation or atrial flutter. One RCT found that compared with digoxin, intravenous diltiazem reduced heart rate within 5 minutes in people with acute atrial fibrillation and atrial flutter.

Benefits: We found no systematic review but found three RCTs.[31–33] **Versus placebo:** One RCT (113 people; 89 with atrial fibrillation and 24 with atrial flutter [see glossary, p 91]; ventricular rate > 120 beats/minute; systolic blood pressure ≥ 90 mm Hg without severe heart failure; 108 people with at least 1 underlying condition that may explain atrial arrhythmia; mean age 64 years) compared intravenous diltiazem (a calcium channel blocker) versus placebo.[31] After randomisation, a dose of intravenous diltiazem (or equivalent placebo) 0.25 mg/kg every 2 minutes was given; if the first dose had no effect after 15 minutes, then the code was broken and diltiazem 0.35 mg/kg every 2 minutes was given regardless of randomisation. The RCT found that intravenous diltiazem versus placebo significantly decreased heart rate during a 15 minute observation period (ventricular rate below 100 beats/minute 42/56 [75%] with diltiazem *v* 4/57 [7%] with placebo; $P < 0.001$; average decrease in heart rate, 22% with diltiazem *v* 3% with placebo; median time from start of drug infusion to maximal decrease in heart rate 4.3 minutes; mean rate decreased from 139 beats/minute to 114 beats/minute with diltiazem).[31] The RCT found no difference in response rate to diltiazem in people with atrial fibrillation versus those with atrial flutter. **Versus digoxin:** One RCT (30 consecutive people, 10 men, mean age 72 years, 26 with acute atrial fibrillation, 4 with atrial flutter, unspecified duration) compared intravenous diltiazem versus intravenous digoxin versus both given on admission to the Accident and Emergency Department.[32] Heart rate control was defined as a ventricular rate of less than 100 beats/minute. Intravenous digoxin (25 mg given as a bolus at 0 and 30 minutes) and intravenous diltiazem (initially 0.25 mg/kg over the first 2 minutes, followed by 0.35 mg/kg at 15 minutes and then a titratable infusion at a rate of 10–20 mg/hour) were given to maintain heart rate control. The dosing regimens were the same whether the drugs were given alone or in combination. The RCT found that diltiazem versus digoxin significantly decreased ventricular heart rate within 5 minutes ($P = 0.0006$; mean rates 111 beats/minute with diltiazem *v* 144 beats/minute with digoxin). The decrease in heart rate achieved with digoxin did not reach statistical significance until 180 minutes ($P = 0.01$; mean rates 90 beats/minute with diltiazem *v* 117 beats/minute with digoxin). No additional benefit was found with the combination of digoxin and diltiazem. **Versus verapamil:** See benefits of verapamil, p 91.

Harms: In one RCT, in the diltiazem treated group, seven people developed asymptomatic hypotension (systolic blood pressure < 90 mm Hg), three developed flushing, three developed itching, and one developed nausea and vomiting; these were not significantly different from placebo.[31] The second RCT was not large enough to adequately assess adverse effects, and none were apparent.[32] Rate limiting calcium channel blockers may exacerbate heart failure and hypotension.

Comment: The evidence suggests that calcium channel blockers such as verapamil and diltiazem reduce ventricular rate in acute or recent onset atrial fibrillation, but they are probably no better than placebo for restoring sinus rhythm. We found no studies of the effect of rate limiting calcium channel blockers on exercise tolerance in people with acute or recent onset atrial fibrillation, but studies in people with chronic atrial fibrillation (see glossary, p 91) have found improved exercise tolerance.

OPTION FLECAINIDE New

One RCT found that compared with placebo, intravenous flecainide increased the proportion of people who reverted to sinus rhythm within 1 hour and in whom sinus rhythm was maintained after 6 hours. Flecainide has been associated with serious adverse events such as severe hypotension and torsades de point. Two RCTs found that compared with intravenous amiodarone, oral flecainide increased the proportion of people who reverted to sinus rhythm within 8 hours. We found insufficient evidence to draw any conclusions about comparisons between intravenous flecainide and intravenous amiodarone and flecainide versus quinidine. Two RCTs found no significant difference between flecainide and propafenone. Flecainide and propafenone are not used in people with known or suspected ischaemic heart disease due to possible proarrhythmic effects.

Benefits: **Versus placebo:** We found one RCT.[34] The RCT found that compared with placebo, intravenous flecainide significantly increased the proportion of people who reverted to sinus rhythm within 1 hour and in whom the sinus rhythm was maintained after 6 hours (1 RCT, 102 people with recent onset atrial fibrillation [< 72 hours]; reversion to sinus rhythm within 1 hour of starting treatment: 29/51 [57%] with flecainide *v* 7/51 [14%] with placebo; OR 8.3, 95% CI 2.9 to 24.8; maintenance of sinus rhythm after 6 hours: 34/51 [67%] *v* 18/51 [35%]; OR 3.67, 95% CI 1.50 to 9.10). Participants were randomised to receive either flecainide 2 mg/kg over 30 minutes (maximum dose 150 mg) or a placebo and were monitored in intensive care or coronary care units. Intravenous digoxin 500 μg over 30 minutes was given to all people who had not previously received digoxin.[34] **Versus amiodarone or propafenone:** We found five RCTs.[35–39] The first RCT found no significant difference between oral flecainide and intravenous amiodarone in the proportion of people converting to sinus rhythm at 1 and 3 hours but found a higher rate of conversion to sinus rhythm with oral flecainide at 8 hours (1 RCT, 5 arm study, 417 people, onset of atrial fibrillation ≤ 7 days; conversion to sinus rhythm at 1 hour: 9/69 [13%] with oral flecainide *v* 3/51 [6%] with iv amiodarone; RR 2.2, 95% CI 0.6 to 7.8; at 3 hours: 39/69 [57%] with oral flecainide *v* 13/51 [25%] with iv amiodarone; RR 2.20, 95% CI 0.96 to 1.51; at 8 hours: 52/69 [75%] with oral flecainide *v* 29/51 [57%] with iv amiodarone; RR 1.30, 95% CI 1.01 to 1.74).[35] The other groups in the RCT were placebo, intravenous propafenone, and oral propafenone. The RCT found no significant difference between oral flecainide and oral propafenone in the proportion of people converting to sinus rhythm at 1, 3, or 12 hours (1 RCT, 5 arm study, 417 people, onset of atrial fibrillation ≤ 7 days; conversion to sinus rhythm at 1 hour: 9/69 [13%] with oral flecainide *v* 10/119 [8%] with oral propafenone; RR 1.55, 95% CI 0.66 to 3.63; at 3 hours: 39/69 [57%] with oral flecainide *v* 54/119 [45%] with oral propafenone; RR 1.25, 95% CI 0.94 to 1.66; at 8 hours: 52/69 [75%] with oral flecainide *v* 91/119 [76%] with oral propafenone; RR 0.99, 95% CI 0.83 to 1.17).[35] The second RCT found that compared with intravenous amiodarone, oral flecainide significantly increased the proportion of people converting to sinus rhythm at 8 hours (1 RCT, 3 arm study, 62 people aged > 75 years, onset of atrial fibrillation ≤ 7 days; conversion to sinus rhythm at 8 hours: 20/22 [91%] with flecainide *v* 7/19 [37%] with amiodarone; RR 2.47, 95% CI 1.35 to 4.51).[36] The RCT also found that significantly higher proportion of people converted to sinus rhythm with flecainide compared with placebo (P < 0.01).[36] The third RCT found that compared with intravenous amiodarone, intravenous flecainide significantly increased the proportion of people converting to sinus rhythm at 1, 8, and 12 hours (1 RCT, 3 arm study, 150 people, onset of atrial fibrillation ≤ 48 hours; conversion to sinus rhythm at 1 hour: 29/50 [58%] with flecainide *v* 7/50 [14%] with amiodarone; RR 4.14, 95% CI 2.00 to 8.57; at 8 hours: 41/50 [82%] with flecainide *v* 21/50 [42%] with amiodarone; RR 1.95, 95% CI 1.38 to 2.77; at 12 hours: 45/50 [90%] with flecainide *v* 32/50 [64%] with amiodarone; RR 1.41, 95% CI 1.12 to 1.77).[39] The RCT found no significant difference between intravenous flecainide and intravenous propafenone in the proportion of people converting to sinus rhythm at 1 and 8 hours. It found a significantly higher conversion rate at 12 hours with flecainide compared with propafenone (1 RCT, 3 arm study, 150 people, onset of atrial fibrillation ≤ 48 hours; conversion to sinus rhythm at 1 hour: 29/50 [58%] with flecainide *v* 30/50 [60%] with propafenone; RR 0.97, 95% CI 0.70 to 1.34; at 8 hours: 41/50 [82%] with flecainide *v* 34/50 [68%] with propafenone; RR 1.21, 95% CI 0.96 to 1.51; at 12 hours: 45/50 [90%] with flecainide *v* 36/50 [72%] with propafenone; RR 1.25, 95% CI 1.03 to 1.52).[39] The fourth RCT found no significant difference between intravenous flecainide and intravenous amiodarone in the proportion of people who converted to sinus rhythm within 2 hours (1 RCT, 3 arm study, 98 people, onset of atrial fibrillation ≤ 72 hours; conversion to sinus rhythm within 2 hours: 20/34 [59%] with flecainide *v* 11/32 [34%] with amiodarone; RR 1.71, 95% CI 0.98 to 2.98). The RCT also found that significantly higher proportion of people converted to sinus rhythm with flecainide compared with placebo (conversion to sinus rhythm within 2 hours: 20/34 [59%] with flecainide *v* 7/32 [22%] with placebo; RR 2.69, 95% CI 1.32 to 5.48).[37] The fifth RCT found significantly faster conversion to sinus rhythm with intravenous flecainide within 1 hour after treatment (1 RCT, 3 arm study, 352 people; restoration to sinus rhythm at 1 hour, 72.5% with flecainide *v* 54.3% with propafenone, P = 0.05; absolute numbers not provided).[38] **Versus quinidine:** One small RCT found insufficient evidence to draw any conclusions about effectiveness of flecainide versus quinidine for conversion to sinus rhythm (60 people aged 16–92 years, of whom 36 people had atrial fibrillation < 10 days; conversion to sinus rhythm [time period not provided]: 18/21 [86%] with flecainide *v* 12/15 [80%] with quinidine; RR 1.07, 95% CI 0.79 to 1.46).[40]

Harms: One RCT found that a higher proportion of people developed severe hypotension (a decrease in systolic arterial pressure by ≥ 33%) with flecainide compared with placebo (11/51 [22%] with flecainide *v* 3/51 [6%] with placebo; OR 4.40, 95% CI 1.03 to 18.60). One person in the flecainide group with no history of ventricular arrhythmia and a normal QT interval developed torsades de pointes.[34]

Comment: Following the increased mortality observed in post-myocardial infarction patients randomised to flecainide or ecainide in the Cardiac Arrhythmia Suppression Trial, flecainide is not used for the treatment of atrial fibrillation in patients with known ischaemic heart disease because of the risk of proarrhythmia.[41]

OPTION PROPAFENONE *New*

One systematic review and subsequent RCTs have found that compared with placebo, propafenone increased the proportion of people converting to sinus rhythm within 1–4 hours. One RCT in people with onset of atrial fibrillation of less than 48 hours found no significant difference between intravenous propafenone and amiodarone in conversion to sinus rhythm within 1 hour. Another RCT in people with onset of atrial fibrillation of less than 2 weeks found that compared with amiodarone, a higher proportion of people converted to sinus rhythm with oral propafenone within 2.5 hours but the difference did not remain significant at 24 hours. Propafenone and flecainide are not used in people with known or suspected ischaemic heart disease due to possible proarrhythmic effects.

Benefits: **Versus placebo:** We found one systematic review (search date 1997, 27 controlled clinical trials including some non-randomised trials, 1843 people),[42] one additional RCT,[43] and five subsequent RCTs.[44–47] The systematic review found that compared with placebo, people treated with propafenone were more likely to convert to sinus rhythm at 4 and 8 hours after initial treatment but the difference between the groups did not remain significant after 24 hours (1 SR, conversion to sinus rhythm at 4 hours: ARR 31.5%, 95% CI 24.5% to 38.5%; at 8 hours: ARR 32.9%, 95% CI 24.3% to 41.5%; P < 0.01 for both time points; conversion to sinus rhythm at 24 hours: ARR +11.0% 95% CI –0.6% to +22.4%; absolute numbers not provided).[42] In the trials included in the systematic review, propafenone was given either intravenously (2 mg/kg as initial bolus followed by infusion) or orally (450–600 mg).[42] The systematic review included people with either acute or chronic fibrillation (see glossary, p 91) but did not stratify the data. The number of RCTs is not clearly stated. The additional RCT found that compared with placebo, intravenous propafenone significantly increased the proportion of people converting to sinus rhythm within 3 hours (1 RCT, 75 people aged 18–75 years, onset of atrial fibrillation < 72 hours; conversion to sinus rhythm within 3 hours: 24/41 [58.5%] with propafenone *v* 10/34 [29.4%] with placebo; OR 3.2, 95% CI 1.3 to 7.9).[43] The first subsequent RCT found that compared with placebo, propafenone significantly increased the proportion of people in sinus rhythm at 3 and 6 hours after treatment (1 multicentre RCT, 240 people [mean age 59 years] with atrial fibrillation duration < 7 days; conversion to sinus rhythm at 3 hours: 54/119 [45%] with propafenone *v* 22/121 [18%] with placebo; ARR 27%, 95% CI 17% to 39%; RR 2.5, 95% CI 1.6 to 3.8; conversion to sinus rhythm at 8 hours: 91/119 [76%] with propafenone *v* 45/121 [37%] with placebo; ARR 39%, 95% CI 29% to 52%; RR 2.1, 95% CI 1.6 to 2.6).[44] After stratification by age (≤ 60 years or > 60 years of age) the RCT found that conversion to sinus rhythm with propafenone versus placebo was more likely in people less than 60 years old compared with older people (conversion to sinus rhythm in people ≤ 60 years of age, at 3 hours, OR 3.78, 95% CI 1.80 to 7.92; at 8 hours, OR 4.74, 95% CI 2.12 to 10.54; conversion to sinus rhythm in people > 60 years of age, at 3 hours, OR 5.03, 95% CI 2.08 to 12.12; at 8 hours, OR 6.75 95% CI 3.38 to 73.86).[48] The second subsequent RCT found that compared with placebo, a significantly higher proportion of people converted to sinus rhythm within 2 hours with propafenone and the significant difference was maintained up to 6 hours but not at 12 or 24 hours (1 RCT, 55 people [mean age 59 years] atrial fibrillation duration < 7 days; conversion to sinus rhythm at 2 hours: 12/29 [41%] with propafenone *v* 2/26 [8%] with placebo; P = 0.005; conversion to sinus rhythm at 6 hours, 65% with propafenone *v* 31% with placebo, P = 0.015; at 12 hours, 69% with propafenone *v* 31% with placebo, P = 0.06; at 24 hours, 79% with propafenone *v* 73% with placebo, P = 0.75).[45] The third subsequent RCT found that compared with placebo, intravenous propafenone significantly increased the proportion of people converting to sinus rhythm within 2 hours (156 people aged 18–80 years, onset of atrial fibrillation < 72 hours; conversion to sinus rhythm within 3 hours: 57/81 [70.3%] with propafenone *v* 13/75 [17.3%] with placebo; ARR 53%, 95% CI 42% to 68%; RR 4.06, 95% CI 2.43 to 6.79).[46] The fourth subsequent RCT found that compared with placebo, intravenous or oral propafenone significantly increased the proportion of people converting to sinus rhythm within 1 and 4 hours but not at 8 hours after initial treatment (1 RCT, 123 people, onset of atrial fibrillation < 72 hours; conversion to sinus rhythm within 1 hour: 25/81[31%] with propafenone *v* 7/42 with placebo [17%]; RR 1.85, 95% CI 0.87 to 3.92; within 4 hours: 49/81 [61%] with propafenone *v* 14/42 [33%] with placebo; RR 1.82, 95% CI 1.14 to 2.88; within 8 hours: 53/81 [65%] *v* 20/42 [48%]; RR 1.37, 95% CI 0.96 to 1.96).[47] The RCT also found that compared with oral propafenone, the time to conversion to sinus rhythm was significantly shorter with intravenous propafenone (conversion to sinus rhythm 1 hour: 19/40 [48%] with iv propafenone *v* 6/41 [15%] with oral propafenone; RR 3.25, 95% CI 1.45 to 7.28; within 4 hours: 20/40 [50%] with iv propafenone *v* 29/41 [71%] with oral propafenone; RR 0.71, 95% CI 0.49 to 1.02).[47] The fifth subsequent RCT found that significantly higher proportion of people converted to sinus rhythm with propafenone versus placebo but found no significant difference between digoxin and placebo (1 RCT, 3 arm study, conversion to sinus rhythm with 1 hour: 20/41 [49%] with propafenone *v* 6/42 [14%] with placebo; RR 3.42, 95% CI 1.53 to 7.63; 13/40 [33%] with digoxin *v* 6/42 [14%] with placebo; RR 2.28, 95% CI 0.96 to 5.40). After 1 hour, people who had not converted to sinus rhythm were switched over to the alternative drug.[49] **Versus amiodarone:** We found two RCTs.[50,51] The first RCT found no significant difference between intravenous propafenone and amiodarone in proportion of people converting to sinus rhythm within 1 hour (1 RCT, 3 arm study, 143 people, onset of atrial fibrillation < 48 hours; conversion to sinus rhythm within 1 hour: 36/46 [78.2%] with propafenone *v* 40/48 [83.3%] with amiodarone; RR 0.94, 95% CI 0.77 to 1.15).[50] The RCT also found that compared with placebo, a significantly higher proportion of people converted to sinus rhythm with propafenone and amiodarone (conversion to sinus rhythm within 1 hour: 36/46 [78.2%] with propafenone *v* 27/49 [55.1%] with placebo; RR 1.42, 95% CI 1.06 to 1.91; 40/48 [83.3%] with amiodarone *v* 27/49 [55.0%] with placebo; RR 1.51, 95% CI 1.14 to 2.01). Intravenous propafenone was given as 2 mg/kg in 15 minutes then 10 mg/kg in 24 hours. Amiodarone was given as 300 mg in 1 hour then 20 mg/kg over 24 hours plus 1800 mg daily in three oral doses.[50] The second RCT found a faster rate of conversion to sinus rhythm with oral propafenone compared with amiodarone but found no significant difference in the proportion of people converting to sinus rhythm at 24 and 48 hours (1 RCT, 86 people, onset of atrial fibrillation < orally 2 weeks; median time to sinus rhythm 2.4 hours with propafenone *v* 6.9 hours with amiodarone, P = 0.05; conversion to sinus rhythm at 24 hours, 56% with propafenone *v* 47% with amiodarone, NS, results presented graphically).[51]

Harms: **Versus placebo:** One systematic review did not comment on adverse events.[42] One RCT that included people with structural heart disease and hypertension found no significant difference between propafenone and placebo in terms of adverse events (sustained atrial flutter [see glossary, p 91] or tachycardia lasting > 1 minute: 8/119 [7%] with propafenone *v* 7/121 [6%] with placebo, P > 0.2; pauses of > 2 seconds: 1/119 [1%] with propafenone *v* 3/121 [2%] with placebo, P > 0.2). No cases of ventricular proarrhythmia were reported.[44] Five other RCTs comparing propafenone versus placebo reported no serious adverse events.[43,45–47,49] **Versus amiodarone:** One RCT found no serious adverse events.[51] **Other comparisons:** We found one RCT (246 people with onset of atrial fibrillation AF < 48 hours) evaluating the safety of oral loading dose of propafenone (600 mg for > 60 kg body weight, then 300 mg if persistent) compared with digoxin plus propafenone, digoxin plus quinidine, or placebo.[52] The RCT found no serious adverse events. The RCT found transient atrial flutter (13/66 [20%] with propafenone *v* 12/70 [17%] with digoxin plus propafenone *v* 9/70 [13%] with digoxin plus quinidine *v* 3/40 [8%] with placebo), asymptomatic salvos of up to 4 ventricular beats (4/70 [6%] with digoxin plus propafenone *v* 1/70 [1%] with digoxin plus quinidine), transient left bundle branch block (3/66 [5%] with propafenone *v* 2/70 [3%] with digoxin plus propafenone *v* 2/70 [3%]

digoxin plus quinidine), transient Wenkebach 2 : 1 heart block (2/66 [3%] with propafenone *v* 2/70 [3%] with digoxin plus quinidine), and transient mild hypotension (5/66 [8%] propafenone *v* 1/70 [1%] digoxin plus quinidine). The RCT found no significant difference between groups for non-cardiac adverse events such as nausea, headache, gastrointestinal disturbance, dizziness, and paraesthesia.[52]

Comment: Extrapolation of the results of the CAST trial,[41] mean that other class Ic antiarrhythmic agents including propafenone tend not to be used in patients with ischaemic heart disease due to concerns over a possible increase in proarrhythmic effects in this group of people. Also, the increased frequency of cardiac adverse events with long-term propafenone noted in people with structural heart disease,[53] means that trials in acute atrial fibrillation have for the main part, excluded people with significant heart disease.

OPTION QUINIDINE *New*

We found no RCTs comparing quinidine versus placebo. One small RCT in people with onset of atrial fibrillation of less than 48 hours found that quinidine plus digoxin increased the proportion of people converting to sinus rhythm within 12 hours compared with sotalol.

Benefits: **Versus placebo:** We found no RCTs comparing quinidine versus placebo. **Quinidine plus digoxin versus sotalol:** One small RCT found that compared with sotalol, quinidine plus digoxin significantly increased the proportion of people converting to sinus rhythm within 12 hours (1 RCT, 61 people aged 18–75 years [mean age about 54 years] with recent onset atrial fibrillation of < 48 hours; conversion to sinus rhythm within 12 hours: 24/28 [85.7%] with quinidine plus digoxin *v* 17/33 [51.5%] with sotalol; ARR 34%, 95% CI 16% to 58%; RR 1.66, 95% CI 1.16 to 2.39; NNT 3, 95% CI 2 to 6).[54] Quinidine was given as quinidine 200 mg orally up to three times with 2 hour intervals and up to 0.75 mg of digoxin was given intravenously if the initial heart rate was greater than 100 beats/minute. Sotalol 80 mg was given orally and the dose was repeated at 2, 6, and 10 hours after the initial dose if sinus rhythm was not achieved.[54] **Versus flecainide:** See benefits of flecainide, p 84.

Harms: One RCT reported broad complex tachycardia in 7/28 (27%) people with quinidine plus digoxin compared with 4/33 (13%) people with sotalol. Electrocardiogram R-R interval prolongation was also reported in both groups, (total 3 people, longest R–R 3.8 seconds with digoxin plus quinidine *v* 6.4 seconds with sotalol).[54]

Comment: None.

OPTION SOTALOL *New*

We found no systematic review or RCTs comparing sotalol versus placebo. One small RCT in people with onset of atrial fibrillation of less than 48 hours found that compared with sotalol, quinidine plus digoxin increased the proportion of people converting to sinus rhythm within 12 hours.

Benefits: We found no systematic review or RCTs comparing sotalol versus placebo in people with acute atrial fibrillation for conversion to sinus rhythm or heart rate control. **Versus quinidine plus digoxin:** See benefits of quinidine, p 89.

Harms: We found no RCTs comparing sotalol versus placebo.

Comment: We found one systematic review (search date 1996) that identified one open label RCT in people with acute atrial fibrillation.[55] The RCT compared oral sotalol 80 mg versus quinidine but digoxin was also given to people with a heart rate of less than 100 beats/minute in the quinidine group. The RCT found insufficient evidence to draw any conclusions.[55] We also found another systematic review comparing β blockers with placebo in people with either acute or chronic atrial fibrillation (see glossary, p 91).[28] See comment of timolol, p 90.

OPTION TIMOLOL

One small RCT found that, timolol (a β blocker) reduced ventricular rate within 20 minutes compared with placebo.

Benefits: We found no systematic review. **Versus placebo:** We found one RCT (61 people with atrial fibrillation of unspecified duration, ventricular rate > 120 beats/minute) that compared intravenous timolol 1 mg (a β blocker) versus intravenous placebo given immediately and repeated twice at 20 minute intervals if sinus rhythm was not achieved.[56] It found that 20 minutes after the last injection, intravenous timolol versus placebo significantly increased the proportion of people who had a ventricular rate below 100 beats/minute (41% with timolol *v* 3% with placebo; $P < 0.01$).

Harms: In the RCT, the most common adverse effects were bradycardia (2%) and hypotension (9%).[56] β Blockers may exacerbate heart failure and hypotension in acute atrial fibrillation. β Blockers plus rate limiting calcium channel blockers (diltiazem, verapamil) may increase the risk of asystole and sinus arrest.[57–59] β Blockers can precipitate bronchospasm.[60]

Comment: In addition to the evidence from people with acute atrial fibrillation, we found one systematic review of β blockers versus placebo in people with either acute or chronic atrial fibrillation (see glossary, p 91).[28] It found that in 7/12 (58%) comparisons at rest and in all during exercise, β blockers reduced ventricular rate compared with placebo.

OPTION VERAPAMIL

Two RCTs found that intravenous verapamil (a calcium channel blocker) reduced heart rate at 10 or 30 minutes compared with placebo in people with atrial fibrillation or atrial flutter. One RCT found no significant difference between intravenous verapamil and intravenous diltiazem (both calcium channel blockers) in rate control or measures of systolic function in people with atrial fibrillation or atrial flutter, but verapamil caused hypotension in some people.

Benefits: We found no systematic review in people with acute atrial fibrillation. **Versus placebo:** We found two RCTs.[61,62] The first RCT (21 men with atrial fibrillation and a rapid ventricular rate, age 37–70 years) was a crossover comparison of intravenous verapamil versus placebo (saline).[61] It found that intravenous verapamil versus placebo reduced ventricular rate within 10 minutes (reduction > 15% of the initial rate: 17/20 [85%] with verapamil *v* 2/14 [14%] with saline). The second RCT (double blind, crossover study of 20 people with atrial fibrillation or atrial flutter [see glossary, p 91] for 2 hours to 2 years) compared intravenous low dose verapamil 0.075 mg/kg versus placebo.[62] A positive response was defined as conversion to sinus rhythm or a decrease of the ventricular response to less than 100 beats a minute, or by more than 20% of the initial rate. If a positive response did not occur within 10 minutes, then a second bolus injection was given (placebo for people who initially received verapamil, and verapamil for people who initially received placebo). It found no significant difference between low dose verapamil versus placebo. With the first bolus injection, verapamil versus placebo significantly reduced ventricular rate (mean heart rate 118 beats/minute with verapamil *v* 138 beats/minute with placebo), and more people converted to sinus rhythm within 30 minutes but the difference was not significant (3/20 [15%] with verapamil *v* 0/15 [0%] with placebo; P = 0.12). **Versus diltiazem:** We found one small double blind, crossover RCT (17 men, 5 with acute atrial fibrillation, 10 with atrial flutter, and 2 with combination of atrial fibrillation and atrial flutter; ventricular rate ≥ 120 beats/minute, systolic blood pressure > 100 mm Hg) compared intravenous verapamil versus intravenous diltiazem.[33] It found no significant differences in rate control or measures of systolic function. **Versus amiodarone:** See amiodarone, p 81.

Harms: One RCT reported that intravenous verapamil caused a transient drop in systolic and diastolic blood pressure greater than with placebo (saline), which did not require treatment, but it did not state the number of people affected.[61] The second RCT reported development of 1 : 1 flutter in one person with previous Wolff Parkinson White syndrome (see glossary, p 92) and 2 : 1 flutter.[62] In the third RCT, comparing verapamil versus diltiazem, 3/17 (18%) of people receiving verapamil as the first drug developed symptomatic hypotension and were withdrawn from the study before crossover.[33] Two people recovered, but the episode in the third person was considered to be life threatening. In people with Wolff Parkinson White syndrome, verapamil may increase the ventricular rate and can cause ventricular arrhythmias.[63] Rate limiting calcium channel blockers may exacerbate heart failure and hypotension.

Comment: See comment of diltiazem, p 84.

GLOSSARY

Atrial flutter A similar arrhythmia to atrial fibrillation but the atrial electrical activity is less chaotic and has a characteristic saw tooth appearance on an electrocardiogram.

Chronic atrial fibrillation Refers to more sustained or recurrent forms of atrial fibrillation, which can be subdivided into paroxysmal, persistent, or permanent atrial fibrillation.

Atrial fibrillation (acute)

Paroxysmal atrial fibrillation If the atrial fibrillation recurs intermittently with sinus rhythm, with spontaneous recurrences or termination, it is designated as "paroxysmal", and the objective of management is suppression of paroxysms and maintenance of sinus rhythm.

Permanent atrial fibrillation If cardioversion is inappropriate, and has not been indicated or attempted, atrial fibrillation is designated as "permanent", where the objective of management is rate control and antithrombotic treatment.

Persistent atrial fibrillation When atrial fibrillation is more sustained, atrial fibrillation is designated "persistent", necessitating termination with pharmacological treatment or electrical cardioversion.

Torsades de point A form of ventricular tachycardia with atypical QRS complexes ECG pattern.

Wolff Parkinson White syndrome Occurs when an additional electrical pathway exists between the atria and ventricles as a result of anomalous embryonic development. The extra pathway may cause rapid arrhythmias. Worldwide it affects about 0.2% of the general population. In people with Wolff Parkinson White syndrome, β blockers, calcium channel blockers, and digoxin can increase the ventricular rate and cause ventricular arrhythmias.

REFERENCES

1. Benjamin EJ, Wolf PA, Kannel WA. The epidemiology of atrial fibrillation. In: Falk RH, Podrid P, eds. *Atrial fibrillation: mechanisms and management.* 2nd ed. Philadelphia: Lippincott-Raven Publishers, 1997:1–22.
2. Lip GYH, Tean KN, Dunn FG. Treatment of atrial fibrillation in a district general hospital. *Br Heart J* 1994;71:92–95.
3. Zarifis J, Beevers DG, Lip GYH. Acute admissions with atrial fibrillation in a British multiracial hospital population. *Br J Clin Pract* 1997;51:91–96.
4. Stewart FM, Singh Y, Persson S, et al. Atrial fibrillation: prevalence and management in an acute general medical unit. *Aust N Z J Med* 1999;29:51–58.
5. Furlanello F, Bertoldi A, Dallago M, et al. Atrial fibrillation in elite athletes. *J Cardiovasc Electrophysiol* 1998;9(8 suppl):63–68.
6. Kannel WB, Wolf PA, Benjamin EJ, et al. Prevalence, incidence, prognosis, and predisposing conditions for atrial fibrillation: population-based estimates. *Am J Cardiol* 1998;82:2N–9N.
7. Pedersen OD, Bagger H, Kober L, et al. The occurrence and prognostic significance of atrial fibrillation/flutter following acute myocardial infarction. TRACE Study group. TRAndolapril Cardiac Evaluation. *Eur Heart J* 1999;20:748–754.
8. Clark DM, Plumb VJ, Epstein AE, et al. Hemodynamic effects of an irregular sequence of ventricular cycle lengths during atrial fibrillation. *J Am Coll Cardiol* 1997;30:1039–1045.
9. Schumacher B, Luderitz B. Rate issues in atrial fibrillation: consequences of tachycardia and therapy for rate control. *Am J Cardiol* 1998;82:29N–36N.
10. Peterson P, Godfredson J. Embolic complications in paroxysmal atrial fibrillation. *Stroke* 1986;17:622–626.
11. Sherman DG, Goldman L, Whiting RB, et al. Thromboembolism in patients with atrial fibrillation. *Arch Neurol* 1984;41:708–710.
12. Wolf PA, Kannel WB, McGee DL, et al. Duration of atrial fibrillation and imminence of stroke: the Framingham study. *Stroke* 1983;14:664–667.
13. Corbalan R, Arriagada D, Braun S, et al. Risk factors for systemic embolism in patients with paroxysmal atrial fibrillation. *Am Heart J* 1992;124:149–153.
14. Stoddard ME, Dawkins PR, Prince CR, et al. Left atrial appendage thrombus is not uncommon in patients with acute atrial fibrillation and a recent embolic event: a transesophageal echocardiographic study. *J Am Coll Cardiol* 1995;25:452–459.
15. Lin HJ, Wolf PA, Kelly-Hayes M, et al. Stroke severity in atrial fibrillation. The Framingham Study. *Stroke* 1996;27:1760–1764.
16. Fuster V, Ryden LE, Asinger RW, et al. ACC/AHA/ESC guidelines for the management of patients with atrial fibrillation: executive summary. *Circulation* 2001;104:2118–2150.
17. Murray RD, Shah A, Jasper SE, et al. Transoesophageal echocardiography guided enoxaparin antithrombotic strategy for cardioversion of atrial fibrillation: the ACUTE II pilot study. *Am Heart J* 2000;139:1–7.
18. Lown B, Amarasingham R, Neuman J. Landmark article Nov 3, 1962: new method for terminating cardiac arrhythmias. Use of synchronised capacitator discharge. *JAMA* 1986:256;621–627.
19. Slavik RS, Tisdale JE, Borzak S. Pharmacological conversion of atrial fibrillation: a systematic review of available evidence. *Prog Cardiovasc Dis* 2001;44:121–152. Search date 2001; primary sources Medline, Embase, Current Contents, reference lists, recent review articles, personal files, experts in the field, and manual searching.
20. Hilleman DE, Spinler SA. Conversion of recent onset atrial fibrillation with intravenous amiodarone: a meta-analysis of randomised control trials. *Pharmacotherapy* 2002;22:66–74. Search date 2001; primary sources Medline, pertinent reviews, and references.
21. Peuhkurinen K, Niemela M, Ylitalo A, et al. Effectiveness of amiodarone as a single oral dose for recent onset atrial fibrillation. *Am J Cardiol* 2000;85:462–465.
22. Capucci A, Lenzi T, Boriani G, et al. Effectiveness of loading oral flecainide for converting recent onset atrial fibrillation to sinus rhythm in patients without organic heart disease or with only systemic hypertension. *Am J Cardiol* 1992;70:69–72.

23. Donovan KD, Power BM, Hockings BE, et al. Intravenous flecainide versus amiodarone for recent onset atrial fibrillation. *Am J Cardiol* 1995;75:693–697.
24. Noc M, Stager D, Horrat M. Intravenous amiodarone versus verapamil for acute cardioversion of paroxysmal atrial fibrillation to sinus rhythm. *Am J Cardiol* 1990;65:679–680.
25. Digitalis in Acute AF (DAAF) Trial Group. Intravenous digoxin in acute atrial fibrillation. Results of a randomized, placebo-controlled multicentre trial in 239 patients. *Eur Heart J* 1997;18:649–654.
26. Jordaens L, Trouerbach J, Calle P, et al. Conversion of atrial fibrillation to sinus rhythm and rate control by digoxin in comparison to placebo. *Eur Heart J* 1997;18:643–648.
27. Falk RH, Knowlton AA, Bernard SA, et al. Digoxin for converting recent-onset atrial fibrillation to sinus rhythm. *Ann Intern Med* 1987;106:503–506.
28. McNamara RL, Bass EB, Miller MR, et al. Management of new onset atrial fibrillation. Evidence Report/Technology Assessment No. 12 (prepared by the John Hopkins University Evidence-based Practice Center in Baltimore, MD, under contract no. 290–97-0006). AHRQ publication number 01-E026. Rockville, MD: Agency for Healthcare Research and Quality. January 2001. Search date 1998; primary sources The Cochrane Library, Medline, Pubmed's "related links" feature, reviews of Cochrane hand search results, hand searches of reference lists, and scanning of tables of contents from relevant journals.
29. Farshi R, Kistner D, Sarma JS, et al. Ventricular rate control in chronic atrial fibrillation during daily activity and programmed exercise: a crossover open-label study of five drug regimens. *J Am Coll Cardiol* 1999;33:304–310.
30. Klein HO, Pauzner H, Di Segni E, et al. The beneficial effects of verapamil in chronic atrial fibrillation. *Arch Intern Med* 1979;139:747–749.
31. Salerno DM, Dias VC, Kleiger RE, et al. Efficacy and safety of intravenous diltiazem for treatment of atrial fibrillation and atrial flutter: the Diltiazem-Atrial Fibrillation/Flutter Study Group. *Am J Cardiol* 1989;63:1046–1051.
32. Schreck DM, Rivera AR, Tricarico VJ. Emergency management of atrial fibrillation and flutter: intravenous diltiazem versus intravenous digoxin *Ann Emerg Med* 1997;29:135–140.
33. Phillips BG, Gandhi AJ, Sanoski CA, et al. Comparison of intravenous diltiazem and verapamil for the acute treatment of atrial fibrillation and atrial flutter. *Pharmacotherapy* 1997;17:1238–1245.
34. Donovan KD, Dobb GJ, Coombs LJ, et al. Efficacy of flecainide for the reversion of acute onset atrial fibrillation. *Am J Cardiol* 1992;70:50A–55A.
35. Boriani G, Biffa M, Cappuci A, et al. Conversion of recent-onset atrial fibrillation to sinus rhythm: effects of different drug protocols. *Pacing Clin Electrophysiol* 1998;21:2470–2474.
36. Capucci A, Lenzi T, Boriani G, et al. Effectiveness of loading oral flecainide for converting recent-onset atrial fibrillation to sinus rhythm in patients without organic heart disease or with only systemic hypertension. *Am J Cardiol* 1992;70:69–72.
37. Donovan KD, Power BM, Hockings BE, et al. Intravenous flecainide versus amiodarone for recent-onset atrial fibrillation. *Am J Cardiol* 1995;75:693–697.
38. Romano S, Fattore L, Toscano G, et al. Effectiveness and side effects of the treatment with propafenone and flecainide for recent-onset atrial fibrillation. *Ital Heart J* 2001;2(suppl):41–45. [Italian]
39. Martinez-Marcos FJ, Garcia-Garmendia JL, Ortega-Carpio A, et al. Comparison of intravenous flecainide, propafenone, and amiodarone for conversion of acute atrial fibrillation to sinus rhythm. *Am J Cardiol* 2000;86:950–953.
40. Borgeat A, Goy JJ, Maendley R, et al. Flecainide versus quinidine for the conversion of atrial fibrillation to sinus rhythm. *Am J Cardiol* 1986;58:496–498.
41. Akiyama T, Pawitan Y, Greenberg H, et al. Increased risk of death and cardiac arrest from encainide and flecainide in patients after non-Q-wave acute myocardial infarction in the Cardiac Arrhythmia Suppression Trial. CAST Investigators. *Am J Cardiol* 1991;68:1551–1555.
42. Reimold SC, Maisel WH, Antman EM, et al. Propafenone for the treatment of supraventricular tachycardia and atrial fibrillation: a meta-analysis. *Am J Cardiol* 1998;82:66N–71N. Search date 1997; primary sources Medline and Paperchase.
43. Fresco P, Proclemer A, Pavan A, et al. Intravenous propafenone in paroxysmal atrial fibrillation: a randomized, placebo-controlled, double-blind multicenter clinical trial. Paroxysmal Atrial Fibrillation Italian Trial (PAFIT)-2 Investigators. *Clin Cardiol* 1996;19:409–412.
44. Boriani G, Biffi M, Capucci A, et al. Oral propafenone to convert recent-onset atrial fibrillation in patients with and without underlying heart disease. A randomized, controlled trial. *Ann Intern Med* 1997;126:621–625.
45. Azpitarte J, Alverez M, Baun O, et al. Value of a single oral loading dose of propafenone in converting recent-onset atrial fibrillation. Results of a randomized, double-blind controlled study. *Eur Heart J* 1997;18:1649–1654.
46. Ganau G, Lenzi T. Intravenous propafenone for converting recent onset atrial fibrillation in emergency departments: a randomized placebo-controlled multicentre trial. FAPS Investigators Study Group. *J Emerg Med* 1998;16:383–387.
47. Botto GL, Bonini W, Broffoni T, et al. Randomized, crossover comparison of oral loading versus intravenous infusion of propafenone in recent-onset atrial fibrillation. *Pacing Clin Electrophysiol* 1998;21:2480–2484.
48. Boriani G, Biffi M, Capucci A, et al. Oral loading with propafenone: a placebo-controlled study in elderly and nonelderly patients with recent onset atrial fibrillation. *Pacing Clin Electrophysiol* 1998;21:2465–2469.
49. Bianconi L, Mennuni M. Comparison between propafenone and digoxin administered intravenously to patients with acute atrial fibrillation. PAFIT-3 Investigators. The Propafenone in Atrial Fibrillation Italian Trial. *Am J Cardiol* 1998;82:584–588.
50. Kochiadakis GE, Igoumenidis NE, Simantirakis EN, et al. Intravenous propafenone versus intravenous amiodarone in the management of atrial fibrillation of recent onset: a placebo-controlled study. *Pacing Clin Electrophysiol* 1998;21:2475–2479.
51. Blanc JJ, Voinov C, Maarek M. Comparison of oral loading dose of propafenone and amiodarone for converting recent-onset atrial fibrillation. PARSIFAL Study Group. *Am J Cardiol* 1999;84:1029–1032.
52. Capucci A, Villani GQ, Aschieri D, et al. Safety of oral propafenone in the conversion of recent onset atrial fibrillation to sinus rhythm: a prospective parallel placebo-controlled multicentre study. *Int J Cardiol* 1999;68:187–196.

53. Podrid PJ, Anderson JL, for the Propafenone Multicenter Study Group. Safety and tolerability of long term propafenone therapy for supraventricular tachyarrhythmias. *Am J Cardiol* 1996;78:430–434.
54. Halinen MO, Huttunen M, Paakinen S, et al. Comparison of sotalol with digoxin–quinidine for conversion of acute atrial fibrillation to sinus rhythm (the Sotalol-Digoxin-Quinidine Trial). *Am J Cardiol* 1995;76:495–498.
55. Ferreira E, Sunderji R, Gin K. Is oral sotalol effective in converting atrial fibrillation to sinus rhythm. *Pharmacotherapy* 1997;17:1233–1237. Search date 1996; primary sources Medline and hand searches of reference lists.
56. Sweany AE, Moncloa F, Vickers FF, et al. Antiarrhythmic effects of intravenous timolol in supraventricular arrhythmias. *Clin Pharmacol Ther* 1985;37:124–127.
57. Lee TH, Salomon DR, Rayment CM, et al. Hypotension and sinus arrest with exercise-induced hyperkalemia and combined verapamil/propranolol therapy. *Am J Med* 1986;80:1203–1204.
58. Misra M, Thakur R, Bhandari K. Sinus arrest caused by atenolol–verapamil combination. *Clin Cardiol* 1987;10:365–367.
59. Yeh SJ, Yamamoto T, Lin FC, et al. Repetitive sinoatrial exit block as the major mechanism of drug-provoked long sinus or atrial pause. *J Am Coll Cardiol* 1991;18:587–595.
60. Doshan HD, Rosenthal RR, Brown R, et al. Celiprolol, atenolol and propranolol: a comparison of pulmonary effects in asthmatic patients. *J Cardiovasc Pharmacol* 1986;8(suppl 4):105–108.
61. Aronow WS, Ferlinz J. Verapamil versus placebo in atrial fibrillation and atrial flutter. *Clin Invest Med* 1980;3:35–39.
62. Waxman HL, Myerburg RJ, Appel R, et al. Verapamil for control of ventricular rate in paroxysmal supraventricular tachycardia and atrial fibrillation or flutter: a double-blind randomized cross-over study. *Ann Intern Med* 1981;94:1–6.
63. Strasberg B, Sagie A, Rechavia E, et al. Deleterious effects of intravenous verapamil in Wolff-Parkinson-White patients and atrial fibrillation. *Cardiovasc Drugs Ther* 1989;2:801–806.

Bethan Freestone
Research Fellow

Gregory Y H Lip
Professor of Cardiovascular Medicine

Haemostasis Thrombosis
and Vascular Biology Unit
University Department of Medicine
City Hospital
Birmingham
UK

Competing interests: GYHL has been reimbursed by various pharmaceutical companies for attending several conferences, and running educational programmes and research projects. BF none declared.

Changing behaviour

Search date January 2003

Margaret Thorogood, Melvyn Hillsdon, and Carolyn Summerbell

QUESTIONS

INTERVENTIONS

Categorisation relates to producing the intended behavioural change

See glossary, p 114

Key Messages

- **Advice from physicians and trained counsellors to quit smoking** Systematic reviews have found that simple, one off advice from a physician during a routine consultation is associated with 2% of smokers quitting smoking without relapse for 1 year. Advice from trained counsellors who are neither doctors nor nurses also increases quit rates compared with minimal intervention.
- **Advice on cholesterol lowering diet** Systematic reviews have found that advice on cholesterol lowering diet (i.e. advice to lower total fat intake or increase the ratio of polyunsaturated : saturated fatty acid) leads to a small reduction in blood cholesterol concentrations in the long term (≥ 6 months).
- **Advice on diet and exercise supported by behavioural therapy for the encouragement of weight loss** Systematic reviews and subsequent RCTs have found that a combination of advice on diet and exercise supported by behavioural therapy is probably more effective than either diet or exercise advice alone in the treatment of obesity, and might lead to sustained weight loss.
- **Advice on reducing sodium intake to reduce blood pressure** One systematic review has found that, compared with usual care to reduce sodium intake, intensive interventions, unsuited to primary care or population prevention programmes, provide only small reductions in blood pressure. Effects on deaths and cardiovascular events are unclear.
- **Bupropion as part of a smoking cessation programme** One systematic review of antidepressants used as part of a smoking cessation programme has found that bupropion increases quit rates at 1 year.
- **Counselling people at high risk of disease to quit smoking** Systematic reviews and one subsequent RCT have found that antismoking advice improves smoking cessation in people at high risk of smoking related disease.
- **Counselling pregnant women to quit smoking** Two systematic reviews have found that antismoking interventions in pregnant women increase abstinence rates during pregnancy. Interventions without nicotine replacement were as effective as nicotine replacement in healthy non-pregnant women.
- **Exercise advice to women over 80 years** One RCT found that exercise advice delivered in the home by physiotherapists increased physical activity and reduced the risk of falling in women over 80 years.
- **Nicotine replacement in smokers who smoke at least 10 cigarettes daily** One systematic review and one subsequent RCT have found that nicotine replacement is an effective additional component of cessation strategies in smokers who smoke at least 10 cigarettes daily. We found no evidence that any method of delivery of nicotine is more effective than others. We found limited evidence from three RCTs with follow up of 2–6 years that the additional benefit of nicotine replacement treatment on quit rates reduced with time.
- **Advice from nurses to quit smoking** One systematic review has found that advice to quit smoking increased quitting at 1 year compared with no advice.
- **Counselling sedentary people to increase physical activity** We found weak evidence from systematic reviews and subsequent RCTs that counselling sedentary people increases physical activity compared with no intervention. Limited evidence from RCTs suggests that consultation with an exercise specialist rather than a physician may increase physical activity at 1 year. We found limited evidence that interventions delivered by new media can lead to short term changes in physical activity.

- **Self help materials for people who want to stop smoking** One systematic review found that self help materials slightly improve smoking cessation compared with no intervention. It found that individually tailored materials were more effective than standard or stage based materials and that telephone counselling increased the effectiveness of postal self help materials.
- **Physical exercise to aid smoking cessation** One systematic review found limited evidence that exercise may increase smoking cessation.
- **Training health professionals to give advice on smoking cessation (increases frequency of antismoking interventions, but may not improve effectiveness)** One systematic review has found that training professionals increases the frequency of antismoking interventions being offered. It found no good evidence that antismoking interventions are more effective if the health professionals delivering the interventions received training. One RCT found that a structured intervention delivered by trained community pharmacists increased smoking cessation rates compared with usual care delivered by untrained community pharmacists.
- **Acupuncture for smoking cessation** One systematic review has found no significant difference between acupuncture and control in smoking cessation rates at 1 year.
- **Anxiolytics for smoking cessation** One systematic review found no significant difference in quit rates with anxiolytics compared with control.

DEFINITION Cigarette smoking, diet, and level of physical activity are important in the aetiology of many chronic diseases. Individual change in behaviour has the potential to decrease the burden of chronic disease, particularly cardiovascular disease. This topic focuses on the evidence that specific interventions lead to changed behaviour.

INCIDENCE/ PREVALENCE In the developed world, the decline in smoking has slowed and the prevalence of regular smoking is increasing in young people. A sedentary lifestyle is becoming increasingly common and the prevalence of obesity is increasing rapidly.

AIMS OF INTERVENTION To encourage individuals to reduce or abandon unhealthy behaviours and to take up healthy behaviours; to support the maintenance of these changes in the long term.

OUTCOMES Ideal outcomes are clinical, and relate to the underlying conditions (longevity, quality of life, and rate of stroke or myocardial infarction). However, the focus of this topic and the outcomes reported by most studies are proxy outcomes, such as the proportion of people changing behaviour (e.g. stopping smoking) in a specified period.

METHODS *Clinical Evidence* search and appraisal January 2003.

QUESTION **Which interventions reduce cigarette smoking?**

OPTION **ADVICE TO QUIT SMOKING**

Systematic reviews have found that simple, one off advice from a physician during a routine consultation is associated with at least 2% of smokers quitting smoking and not relapsing for 1 year. Additional encouragement or support may increase the effectiveness of the advice (by a further 3%). Individual advice from a psychologist achieves a similar quit rate (3%), and advice from trained nurse counsellors, or from trained

counsellors who are neither doctors nor nurses, increases quit rates compared with minimal intervention or no advice. We found limited evidence from one systematic review that telephone counselling may improve quit rates compared with interventions with no personal contact. One systematic review found that self help materials slightly improve smoking cessation compared with no intervention. It found that individually tailored materials were more effective than standard or stage based materials and that telephone counselling increased the effectiveness of postal self help materials.

Benefits: We found five systematic reviews[1–4,6] and one subsequent RCT.[5] **Physicians:** The first review (search date 2000, 34 RCTs, 28 000 smokers) considered advice given by physicians, most often in the primary care setting, but also in hospitals and other clinics.[1] It found that brief advice improved quit rates compared with no advice (16 trials, 12 with follow up for at least 1 year; 451/7705 [5.9%] with brief advice *v* 241/5870 [4.1%] with no advice; meta-analysis OR 1.69, 95% CI 1.45 to 1.98). Intensive advice slightly improved quit rates compared with minimal advice among smokers not at high risk of disease (10 trials, 7 with follow up for at least 1 year; OR with intensive *v* minimal advice 1.23, 95% CI 1.02 to 1.49). One subsequent RCT tested a brief (10 minute) intervention given by general practitioners who had received 2 hours of training.[5] The intervention increased the abstinence rate at 12 months (7.3% with control *v* 13.4% with intervention; $P < 0.05$). **Counsellors:** The second systematic review (search date 2002, 15 RCTs) examined individual counselling of at least 10 minutes by professionals trained in smoking cessation (social work, psychology, psychiatry, health education, and nursing).[2] Follow up was at 6–12 months. The review found that counselling increased the rate of quitting (rate of quitting 340/2590 [13%] with counselling *v* 232/2592 [9%] with control; OR of quitting 1.64, 95% CI 1.33 to 2.01).[2] The authors did not find a greater effect of intensive counselling compared with brief counselling (3 RCTs; OR 0.98, 95% CI 0.61 to 1.56). **Nurses:** The third review (search date 2001, 22 RCTs, 5 with follow up for < 1 year) considered the effectiveness of smoking interventions delivered by a nurse. It found that advice from a nurse increased the rate of quitting by the end of follow up (meta-analysis of 18 studies: 646/4836 [13.4%] quit with advice *v* 405/3356 [12.1%] with control; OR 1.50, 95% CI 1.29 to 1.73).[3] **Telephone advice:** The fourth systematic review (search date 2000, 23 RCTs) considered counselling delivered by telephone.[4] Ten of the included trials (9 with follow up for at least 12 months) compared proactive telephone counselling versus minimum intervention (involving no person to person contact). Pooled analysis was not possible because of statistical heterogeneity among trials. However, three trials found that telephone counselling was significantly more effective than minimum intervention; four trials found a non-significant benefit, and none of the trials found significant harms of telephone counselling. **Self help materials:** We found one systematic review (search date 2002, 51 RCTs) that examined effects of providing materials giving advice and information to smokers attempting to give up on their own.[6] The review found that self help materials without face to face contact slightly improved smoking cessation compared with no intervention (11 RCTs, including 8 RCTs with at least 12 months' follow up; OR 1.24, 95% CI 1.07 to 1.49). Individually tailored materials were more effective than standard or stage based materials (10 RCTs; OR for cessation 1.36, 95% CI 1.13 to 1.64).

Harms: We found no evidence of harm.

Comment: The effects of advice may seem small, but a year on year reduction of 2% in the number of smokers would represent a significant public health gain (see smoking cessation under primary prevention, p 154). In the systematic review of advice provided by nurses,[3] there was significant heterogeneity of the study results and many studies may not have been adequately randomised (7/18 studies [39%] did not specify the randomisation method and 3/18 [17%] used an inadequate form of randomisation).

OPTION NICOTINE REPLACEMENT

One systematic review and one subsequent RCT have found that nicotine replacement is an effective additional component of cessation strategies in smokers who smoke at least 10 cigarettes daily. We found no evidence of any particular method of nicotine delivery having superior efficacy. We found limited evidence from three RCTs (follow up 2–6 years) that the benefit of nicotine replacement treatment on quit rates decreased with time.

Benefits: **Abstinence at 12 months:** We found one systematic review (search date 2002)[7] that identified 51 trials of nicotine chewing gum, 34 trials of nicotine transdermal patches, four of nicotine intranasal spray, four of inhaled nicotine, and three of sublingual tablets. All forms of nicotine replacement were more effective than placebo. When the abstinence rates for all trials were pooled according to the longest duration of follow up available, nicotine replacement increased the odds of abstinence compared with placebo (3335/19 783 [16.8%] with nicotine replacement *v* 1835/17 977 [10.2%] with placebo; OR 1.74, 95% CI 1.64 to 1.86). The review found no significant difference in abstinence with different forms of nicotine replacement in indirect comparisons (OR 1.66 for nicotine chewing gum *v* 2.27 for nicotine nasal spray) or direct comparisons (1 RCT, inhaler *v* patch; OR 0.57, 95% CI 0.19 to 1.65). In trials that directly compared 4 mg with 2 mg nicotine chewing gum, the higher dose improved abstinence in highly dependent smokers (OR 2.18, 95% CI 1.49 to 3.17). High dose patches slightly increased abstinence compared with standard dose patches (6 RCTs; OR 1.21, 95% CI 1.03 to 1.42). The review found no significant difference in effectiveness for 16 hour compared with 24 hour patches, and no difference in effect in trials where the dose was tapered compared with those where the patches were withdrawn abruptly. Use of the patch for 12 weeks was as effective as longer use and there was suggestive evidence that repeated use of nicotine replacement treatment in people who have relapsed after an initial course may produce further quitters, though the absolute effect was small. One included RCT (3585 people) found that abstinence at 1 week was a strong predictor of 12 month abstinence (25% of those abstinent at 1 week were abstinent at 12 months *v* 2.7% of those not abstinent at 1 week).[8] One meta-analysis of relapse rates in nicotine replacement trials found that nicotine replacement increased abstinence at 12 months, but that continued nicotine replacement did not significantly affect relapse rates between 6 weeks and 12 months.[9] **Longer term abstinence:** We found three RCTs[10–12] that found nicotine replacement does not affect long term abstinence. In one RCT that compared nicotine spray with placebo, 47 people abstinent at 1 year were followed for up to a further 2 years and 5 months, after which there was still a significant, although smaller, difference in abstinence (in the longer term 15.4% abstinent with nicotine spray *v* 9.3% with placebo; NNT [for 1 extra person to abstain] 7 at 1 year *v* 11 at 3.5 years).[10] The second RCT compared 5 months of nicotine patches plus nicotine spray versus the same patches plus a placebo spray. It found no significant difference between treatments after 6 years (16.2% abstinent with nicotine spray *v* 8.5% with placebo spray; P = 0.08).[11] The third RCT compared patches delivering different nicotine doses versus placebo patches. The trial followed everyone that quit at 6 weeks for a further 4–5 years and found no significant difference in relapse between the groups. Overall, 73% of people who quit at 6 weeks relapsed.[12]

Harms: Nicotine chewing gum has been associated with hiccups, gastrointestinal disturbances, jaw pain, and orodental problems. Nicotine transdermal patches have been associated with skin sensitivity and irritation. Nicotine inhalers and nasal spray have been associated with local irritation at the site of administration. Nicotine sublingual tablets have been reported to cause hiccups, burning, smarting sensations in the mouth, sore throat, coughing, dry lips, and mouth ulcers.[13]

Comment: Nicotine replacement may not represent an "easy cure" for nicotine addiction, but it does improve the cessation rate. The evidence suggests that the most of smokers attempting cessation fail at any one attempt or relapse over the next 5 years. Multiple attempts may be needed.

OPTION ACUPUNCTURE

One systematic review has found no significant difference between acupuncture and control in smoking cessation rates at 1 year.

Benefits: We found one systematic review (search date 2002, 22 RCTs, 4158 adults, 330 young people aged 12–18 years)[14] comparing acupuncture with sham acupuncture, other treatment, or no treatment. Seven RCTs (2701 people) reported abstinence after at least 12 months. The review found no significant difference in smoking cessation with acupuncture compared with control at 12 months (OR 1.08, 95% CI 0.77 to 1.52).

Harms: None were documented.

Comment: None.

OPTION PHYSICAL EXERCISE

One systematic review found limited evidence that physical exercise may increase smoking cessation.

Benefits: We found one systematic review (search date 1999, 8 RCTs)[15] of exercise versus control interventions. Four small RCTs in the review reported point prevalence of non-smoking at 12 months and found no significant benefit from exercise, but these studies were insufficiently powered to exclude a clinically important effect. One RCT (281 women) found that three exercise sessions a week for 12 weeks plus a cognitive behavioural programme (see glossary, p 114) improved continuous abstinence from smoking at 12 months compared with the behavioural programme alone (16/134 [12%] with exercise *v* 8/147 [5%] with control; ARR +6.5%, 95% CI –19% to 0%; RR 2.2, 95% CI 0.98 to 4.5).[16]

Harms: None were documented.

Comment: None.

OPTION ANTIDEPRESSANT AND ANXIOLYTIC TREATMENT

Systematic reviews have found that quit rates are increased by bupropion, but not by moclobemide or anxiolytics.

Benefits: **Antidepressants:** We found one systematic review of antidepressants (search date 2001, 18 RCTs).[17] Eight of the RCTs (2649 people) reported 12 month cessation rates. It found that bupropion increased quit rates compared with placebo at 6–12 months (calculated by combining results of 4 RCTs with 12 month follow up and 3 RCTs with 6 month follow up; OR of quitting with bupropion *v* placebo 2.54, 95% CI 1.90 to 3.41). The review found no evidence of statistical heterogeneity between the two follow up times.[17] One RCT included in the review compared combined bupropion plus a nicotine patch versus patch alone. It found that combined treatment improved cessation compared with patch alone (OR 2.65, 95% CI 1.58 to 4.45), but was not more effective than bupropion alone. Another included RCT compared different doses of bupropion (100–300 mg/day) and found that cessation rate was linearly related to dose. Three other included RCTs (2 with 6 months' and 1 with 12 months' follow up) found that nortriptyline improved long term (6–12 month) abstinence rates compared with placebo (OR 2.77, 95% CI 1.73 to 4.44). One RCT of moclobemide found no significant difference in abstinence at 12 months. **Anxiolytics:** We found one systematic review of anxiolytics (search date 2000, 6 RCTs).[18] Four of the RCTs (626 people) reporting 12 month cessation rates found no significant increase in abstinence between anxiolytics and control treatment.[18]

Harms: Headache, insomnia, and dry mouth were reported in people using bupropion.[18] Nortriptyline can cause sedation and urinary retention, and can be dangerous in overdose. One large RCT found that discontinuation rates caused by adverse events were 3.8% with placebo, 6.6% for nicotine replacement treatment, 11.9% for bupropion, and 11.4% for bupropion plus nicotine replacement treatment.[19] Anxiolytics may cause dependence and withdrawal problems, tolerance, paradoxical effects, and impair driving ability. Allergic reactions to bupropion have been reported in about 1/1000 people.

Comment: None.

QUESTION **Are smoking cessation interventions more effective in people at high risk of smoking related disease?**

OPTION **IN PREGNANT WOMEN**

Two systematic reviews have found that antismoking interventions in pregnant women increase abstinence rates during pregnancy. Interventions without nicotine replacement were as effective as nicotine replacement in healthy non-pregnant women.

Benefits: We found two systematic reviews[20,21] and three additional RCTs.[22–24] The most recent review (search date 1998, 44 RCTs) assessed smoking cessation interventions in pregnancy. It found that smoking cessation programmes improved abstinence (OR of continued smoking in late pregnancy with antismoking programmes *v* no programmes 0.53, 95% CI 0.47 to 0.60).[21] The findings were similar if the analysis was restricted to trials in which abstinence was confirmed by means other than self reporting. The review calculated that of 100 smokers attending a first antenatal visit, 10 stopped spontaneously and a further six or seven stopped as the result of a smoking cessation programme. Five included trials examined the effects of interventions to prevent relapse in 800 women who had quit smoking. Collectively, these trials found no evidence that the interventions reduced relapse rate.[21] One earlier systematic review (search date not stated, 10 RCTs, 4815 pregnant women)[20] of antismoking interventions included one trial of physician advice, one trial of advice by a health educator, one trial of group sessions, and seven trials of behavioural therapy based on self help manuals. Cessation rates among trials ranged from 1.9–16.7% in the control groups and from 7.1–36.1% in the intervention groups. The review found that antismoking interventions significantly increased the rate of quitting (ARI with intervention *v* no intervention 7.6%, 95% CI 4.3% to 10.8%).[20] One additional RCT found that nicotine patches did not significantly alter quit rates in pregnant women compared with placebo.[22] The second additional RCT (1120 pregnant women) compared a brief (10–15 minute) smoking intervention delivered by trained midwives at booking interviews versus usual care.[23] It found no significant difference in smoking behaviour between women receiving intervention compared with usual care (abstinence in final 12 weeks of pregnancy until birth 17% in each group; abstinence for 6 months after birth 7% with intervention *v* 8% with control). The intervention was difficult to implement (see comment below). The third RCT compared motivational interviewing (see glossary, p 114) with usual care in 269 women in their 28th week of pregnancy who had smoked in the past month.[24] It found no significant differences in cessation rate between intervention and control group at 34th week or at 6 months post partum.

Harms: None documented.

Comment: The recent review found that some women quit smoking before their first antenatal visit, and most of these will remain abstinent.[21] Recruitment to the RCT comparing midwife delivered intervention versus usual care was slow. Midwives reported that the intervention was difficult to implement because of a lack of time to deliver the intervention at the booking appointment.[23]

OPTION IN PEOPLE AT HIGH RISK OF DISEASE

Systematic reviews and one subsequent RCT have found that antismoking advice improves smoking cessation in people at high risk of smoking related disease.

Benefits: We found no trials in which the same intervention was used in high and low risk people. We found one systematic review (search date not stated, 4 RCTs, 13 208 healthy men at high risk of heart disease),[20] one systematic review among people admitted to hospital (search date 2002, 17 RCTs),[25] and one subsequent RCT.[26] The first review found that antismoking advice improved smoking cessation rates compared with control interventions among healthy men at high risk of heart disease (ARI of smoking cessation 21%, 95% CI 10% to 31%; NNT 5, 95% CI 4 to 10).[20] One early trial (223 men) that was included in the review used non-random allocation after myocardial infarction. The intervention group was given intensive advice by the therapeutic team while in the coronary care unit. The trial found that the self reported cessation rate at 1 year or more was higher in the intervention group than the control group (63% quit in the intervention group *v* 28% in the control group; ARI of quitting 36%, 95% CI 23% to 48%).[27] The second review included seven trials (6 of them with at least 12 months' duration) of high intensity behavioural interventions (defined as contact in hospital plus active follow up for at least 1 month) among smokers admitted to hospital. The review found that active intervention increased quit rates compared with usual care (OR 1.82, 95% CI 1.49 to 2.22).[25] The subsequent RCT compared postal advice on smoking cessation versus no intervention in men aged 30–45 years with either a history of asbestos exposure, or forced expiratory volume in 1 second in the lowest quartile for their age. Postal advice increased the self reported sustained cessation rate at 1 year compared with no intervention (5.6% with postal advice *v* 3.5% with no intervention; $P < 0.05$).[26]

Harms: None were documented.

Comment: There was heterogeneity in the four trials included in the review among healthy men at high risk of heart disease, partly because of a less intense intervention in one trial and the recording of a change from cigarettes to other forms of tobacco as success in another.[20] One of the included trials was weakened by use of self reported smoking cessation as an outcome and non-random allocation to the intervention.[27]

QUESTION **Does training of professionals increase the effectiveness of smoking cessation interventions?**

One systematic review has found that training professionals increases the frequency of antismoking interventions being offered, but found no good evidence that antismoking interventions are more effective if the health professionals delivering the interventions received training. One RCT found that a structured intervention delivered by trained community pharmacists increased smoking cessation rates compared with usual care delivered by untrained community pharmacists.

Benefits: We found one systematic review[28] and one subsequent RCT.[29] The review (search date 2000, 9 RCTs) included eight RCTs of training medical practitioners and one RCT of training dental practitioners to give antismoking advice.[28] All the trials took place in the USA. The training was provided on a group basis, and variously included lectures, videotapes, role plays, and discussion. The importance of setting quit dates and offering follow up was emphasised in most of the training programmes. The review found no good evidence that training professionals leads to higher quit rates in people receiving antismoking interventions from those professionals, although training increased the frequency with which such interventions were offered. Three of the trials used prompts and reminders to practitioners to deploy smoking cessation techniques, and found that prompts increased the frequency of health professional interventions.[28] The later RCT compared a structured smoking cessation intervention delivered by community pharmacists, who had received 3 hours of training versus no specific training or antismoking intervention.[29] Intervention delivered by trained pharmacists improved abstinence compared with usual care (AR of abstinence at 12 months 14.3% with intervention *v* 2.7% with usual care; RR 5.3; NNT 9; CIs not reported; $P < 0.001$).

Harms: None were documented.

Comment: The results of the systematic review should be interpreted with caution because there were variations in the way the analysis allowed for the unit of randomisation.

QUESTION **Which interventions increase physical activity in sedentary people?**

OPTION **COUNSELLING**

We found weak evidence from systematic reviews and subsequent RCTs that counselling sedentary people increases physical activity compared with no intervention. Limited evidence from RCTs suggests that consultation with an exercise specialist rather than a physician may increase physical activity at 1 year. We found limited evidence that interventions delivered by new media can lead to short term changes in physical activity.

Benefits: We found three systematic reviews that focused on different types of interventions[30–32] and seven subsequent RCTs.[33–39] The first review (search date 1996, 11 RCTs based in the USA, 1699 people) assessed the effect of single factor physical activity promotion on exercise behaviour.[30] Seven trials evaluated advice to undertake exercise from home (mainly walking, but including jogging and swimming), and six evaluated advice to undertake facility based exercise (including jogging and walking on sports tracks, endurance exercise, games, swimming, and exercise to music classes). An increase in activity in the intervention groups was seen in trials in which home based moderate exercise was encouraged and regular brief follow up of participants was provided. In most of the trials, participants were self selected volunteers, so the effects of the interventions may have been exaggerated. The second systematic review (search date not stated, 3 RCTs, 420 people) compared "lifestyle" physical activity interventions with either standard exercise treatment or a control group.[31] Lifestyle interventions were defined as those concerned with the daily accumulation of moderate or vigorous exercise as part of everyday life. The first RCT in the review (60 adults, 65–85 years old) found significantly more self reported physical activity in the lifestyle group than a standard exercise group. The second RCT in the review (235 people, 35–60 years old) found no significant difference in physical activity between the groups. The third RCT in the review (125 women, 23–54 years old) of encouraging walking found no significant difference in walking levels at 30 months' follow up between people receiving an 8 week behavioural intervention and those receiving a 5 minute telephone call and written information about the benefits of exercise, although both groups increased walking. The third review (search date 2002, 7 RCTs and 1 quasi-randomised trial, 9054 people) examined the efficacy of exercise counselling from a primary care clinician compared with a control or comparison group.[32] Counselling was delivered using advice only, the promotion of self efficacy, posted educational materials, referral to community resources, and written exercise prescriptions. The review found equivocal results and at least one methodological limitation in most studies. There was limited evidence that the interventions in these studies led to short term (< 3 months) improvements in physical activity. There were insufficient studies to consider the relationship between the components of the interventions and the reported efficacy. Only two RCTs were rated as good quality. One good quality RCT (874 people) compared 3 minutes of physician advice plus educational materials, all the above plus behavioural counselling plus interactive mail, and all the above plus telephone counselling plus classes.[40] It found no significant difference in self reported activity between interventions at 24 months. The other good quality RCT (355 sedentary people) compared a brief 5 minute message, a prescription for exercise, and a follow up visit with usual care. It found no significant difference in the proportion of people meeting the Healthy People 2010 goal after 8 months (28% with advice or prescription *v* 23% with usual care; difference +5%, 95% CI –6% to +14%).[41] All but one of the subsequent trials[39] involved primary care delivered interventions, although they were not restricted to clinician led interventions.[33–38] Two of the three trials in which advice was delivered by an exercise specialist rather than a physician found significant improvement in self reported physical activity at long term (> 6 months) follow up compared with controls.[35,36] A third RCT (1658 people in a primary care setting), which compared a client centred, negotiating style to direct advice and a no intervention control group, did not find any significant difference in changes in physical activity.[38] Short term improvement was found in two further trials, but not maintained at 9 months or 1 year.[33,34] One RCT (298 people) compared physical activity counselling with nutrition counselling, both delivered with automated telephone conversations using digitised human speech.[39] The system used information about current behaviour and some known determinants to counsel people on either physical activity or nutrition. The percentage of individuals meeting current physical activity recommendations at 3 months follow up was significantly greater in the physical activity group compared with the nutrition group at 3 months, but there was no significant difference at 6 months (3 months 26% with activity counselling *v* 19.6% with dietary counselling; P = 0.04). One RCT (229 women) of encouraging women to increase walking found significantly increased walking in the intervention group at 10 years' follow up (86% of women available for follow up, median estimated calorie expenditure from self reported amount of walking 1344 kcal/week with encouragement *v* 924 kcal/week with no encouragement; P = 0.01).[42] A further RCT (260 people in a primary care setting) compared the additional offer of community walks (led by lay people) with fitness tests and advice alone.[37] It found no significant difference in physical activity at 12 months' follow up (ARR for achieving at least 120 minutes of moderate intensity activity a week +6%, 95% CI –5% to +16.4%).

Harms: Insufficient detail is available from these studies to judge the potential harm of exercise counselling. In the RCT comparing behavioural counselling with brief advice, 60% of participants experienced a musculoskeletal event during the 2 years of the study.[40] About half of these required a visit to the physician. About 5% of all participants were admitted to hospital for a suspected cardiovascular event. The trial lacked a non-intervention control group. We found no evidence that counselling people to increase activity levels increased adverse events compared with no counselling.

Comment: Self reporting of effects by people in a trial, especially where blinding to interventions is not possible (as is the case with advice or encouragement), is a potential source of bias. Few studies conduct intention to treat analyses, which may lead to an exaggeration of the true effect of interventions. Methodological problems in RCTs included in the third review included only moderate follow up rates, highly motivated providers, differences in physical activity levels at baseline between intervention groups, uncertain or low provided adherence, inclusion of some counselling advice in usual care control groups, and inadequate power to detect a clinically important difference.[32]

QUESTION **What are effects of exercise advice in high risk people?**

OPTION **IN WOMEN AGED OVER 80 YEARS**

One RCT found that exercise advice increased physical activity in women aged over 80 years and decreased the risk of falling.

Benefits: We found no systematic review. One RCT (233 women > 80 years old, conducted in New Zealand) compared four visits from a physiotherapist who advised a course of 30 minutes of home based exercises three times a week that was appropriate for the individual versus a similar number of social visits.[43] After 1 year, women who had received physiotherapist visits were significantly more active than women in the control group, and 42% were still completing the recommended exercise programme at least three times a week. The mean annual rate of falls in the intervention group was 0.87 compared with 1.34 in the control group, a difference of 0.47 falls a year (95% CI 0.04 to 0.90).

Harms: No additional harms in the intervention group were reported.

Comment: None.

QUESTION **What are the effects on blood cholesterol of dietary advice to reduce fat, increase polyunsaturated fats, and decrease saturated fats?**

OPTION **COUNSELLING**

Systematic reviews have found that advice on eating a cholesterol lowering diet (i.e. advice to reduce fat intake or increase the polyunsaturated : saturated fatty acid ratio in the diet) leads to a small reduction in blood cholesterol concentrations in the long term (≥ 6 months). We found no evidence to support the effectiveness of such advice in primary care.

Benefits: **Effects on blood cholesterol:** We found three systematic reviews[13,44,45] and two subsequent RCTs[46,47] that reported biochemical rather than clinical end points. None of the reviews included evidence after 1996. One review (search date 1993) identified five trials of cholesterol lowering dietary advice (principally advice from nutritionists or specially trained counsellors) with follow up for 9–18 months.[44] It found a reduction in blood cholesterol concentration in the intervention group of 0.22 mmol/L (95% CI 0.05 mmol/L to 0.39 mmol/L) compared with the control group. There was significant heterogeneity ($P < 0.02$), with two outlying studies — one showing no effect and one showing a larger effect. This review excluded trials in people at high risk of heart disease. Another systematic review (search date 1994) identified 13 trials of more than 6 months' duration and included people at high risk of heart disease.[13] It found that dietary advice reduced blood cholesterol (mean reduction in blood cholesterol concentration with advice 4.5%, 95% CI 3.9% to 5.1%; given a mean baseline cholesterol of 6.3 mmol/L, mean AR about 0.3 mmol/L). The third systematic review (search date 1996, 1 trial,[48] 76 people) found no significant difference between brief versus intensive advice from a general practitioner and dietician on blood cholesterol at 1 year.[45] The first subsequent RCT (186 men and women at high risk of coronary heart disease) compared advice on healthy eating versus no intervention. At 1 year it found no significant differences between groups in total and low density lipoprotein cholesterol concentrations for either sex, even though the reported percentage of energy from fat consumed by both women and men in the advice group decreased significantly compared with that reported by the women and men in the control group.[46] These results may reflect bias caused by self reporting of dietary intake. The second RCT, in 531 men with hypercholesterolaemia (with and without other hyperlipidaemias) and fat intake of about 35%, compared dietary advice aimed at reducing fat intake to 30% versus 26% versus 22%. All interventions were similarly effective for reducing fat intake (total fat intake after intervention about 26% in all groups).[47] **Effects on clinical outcomes:** We found two systematic reviews that reported on morbidity and mortality.[13,49] The first review (search date 1994) compared 13 separate and single dietary interventions.[13] It found no significant effect of dietary interventions on total mortality or coronary heart disease mortality but found a reduction in non-fatal myocardial infarction (total mortality: OR 0.93, 95% CI 0.84 to 1.03; coronary heart disease mortality: OR 0.93, 95% CI 0.82 to 1.06; non-fatal myocardial infarction: OR 0.77, 95% CI 0.67 to 0.90). The second review (search date 1999, 27 studies including 40 intervention arms, 30 901 person years) found dietary advice to reduce or modify dietary fat had no significant effect on total mortality or cardiovascular disease mortality compared with no dietary advice but significantly reduced cardiovascular disease events (total mortality: HR 0.98, 95% CI 0.86 to 1.12; cardiovascular disease mortality: HR 0.98, 95% CI 0.77 to 1.07; cardiovascular disease events: HR 0.84, 95% CI 0.72 to 0.99).[49] RCTs in which people were followed for more than 2 years showed significant reductions in the rate of cardiovascular disease events. The relative protection from cardiovascular disease events was similar in both high and low risk groups, but was significant only in high risk groups.

Harms: We found no evidence about harms.

Comment: The finding of a 0.2–0.3 mmol/L reduction in blood cholesterol in the two systematic reviews accords with the findings of a meta-analysis of the plasma lipid response to changes in dietary fat and cholesterol.[50] The analysis included data from 244 published studies (trial duration 1 day to 6 years), and concluded that adherence to dietary recommendations (30% energy from fat, < 10% saturated fat, and < 300 mg cholesterol/day) compared with average US dietary intake would reduce blood cholesterol by about 5%.

QUESTION Does dietary advice to reduce sodium intake lead to a sustained fall in blood pressure?

One systematic review has found that, compared with usual care, intensive interventions to reduce sodium intake, unsuited to primary care or population prevention programmes, provide only small reductions in blood pressure, and effects on deaths and cardiovascular events are unclear.

Benefits: We found one systematic review (search date 2000).[51] The review (5 RCTs in 2326 normotensive people and 3 RCTs in 801 people being treated for hypertension with follow up of ≥6 months) compared the effects of advice to restrict dietary sodium (involving intensive group or individual nutrition counselling programmes) versus usual or control diet. It found that systolic blood pressure was significantly reduced at 13–60 months (reduction 1.1 mm Hg, 95% CI 0.4 mm Hg to 1.8 mm Hg). It found no significant difference in diastolic blood pressure (reduction +0.6 mm Hg, 95% CI +1.5 mm Hg to –0.3 mm Hg). Mortality and cardiovascular deaths were inconsistently reported, and effects were unclear.[51]

Harms: None reported.

Comment: None.

QUESTION What are the effects of lifestyle interventions to achieve sustained weight loss?

Systematic reviews and subsequent RCTs have found that combined advice on diet and exercise, supported by behavioural therapy, is probably more effective in achieving weight loss than either diet or exercise advice alone. A low energy diet is the most effective lifestyle intervention for weight loss. Combined personal and computerised tailoring of weight loss programmes may improve maintenance of weight loss. RCTs have found no significant differences in weight loss between interventions to promote physical activity. Weight regain is likely, but weight loss of 2–6 kg may be sustained over at least 2 years.

Benefits: We found three systematic reviews[52–54] and 19 additional RCTs.[55–73] One systematic review (search date 1995) identified one relevant RCT that found that the combination of diet and exercise in conjunction with behavioural therapy produced significantly greater weight loss than diet alone at 1 year (mean weight loss: 7.9 kg with diet and exercise *v* 3.8 kg with diet alone; significance result not reported).[52] The second systematic review of the detection, prevention, and treatment of obesity (search date 1999) included eight RCTs comparing dietary prescriptions versus exercise, counselling, or behavioural therapy for the treatment of obesity, and three RCTs comparing dietary counselling alone versus no intervention. In both comparisons, initial weight loss was followed by gradual weight regain once treatment had stopped (mean difference in weight change at least 2 years after baseline, 2–6 kg with dietary prescription and 2–4 kg with dietary counselling).[53] The third systematic review (search date 1997) of RCTs and observational studies similarly found that a combination of diet and exercise, supported by behavioural therapy, was more effective than any one or two of these individual interventions.[54] The first additional RCT compared advice on an energy restricted diet to advice on a fat restricted diet.[60] Weight loss was greater on an energy restricted diet than on the fat restricted diet at 6 months (–11.2 kg with energy restricted diet *v* –6.1 kg with fat restricted diet; $P < 0.001$) and at 18 months (–7.5 kg with energy restricted diet *v* –1.8 kg with fat restricted diet; $P < 0.001$). The next seven additional RCTs focused on physical activity.[56–58,62–64,67] The heterogeneity of interventions makes pooling of data inappropriate, but no major differences were found between the various behavioural therapies and exercise regimes. The ninth additional RCT found behavioural choice therapy increased weight loss at 12 months compared with standard behavioural therapy (see glossary, p 114) (–10.1 kg with behavioural choice therapy *v* –4.3 kg with standard behavioural therapy; $P < 0.01$).[59] The 10th additional RCT (166 people) compared standard behavioural therapy plus support from friends with standard behavioural therapy without support. It found no additional weight loss at 16 months with social support from friends (–4.7 kg with behavioural therapy plus support *v* –3.0 kg with behavioural therapy without support, $P > 0.05$).[61] The 11th additional RCT (results from 89 overweight women with impaired glucose tolerance analysed) published only in abstract form compared three interventions: behaviour modification plus nutritional information at quarterly visits; dietary advice only at quarterly visits; and one dietary advice session only.[65] It found that weight reduction after 2 years was greater with the behaviour modification programme but levels of statistical significance were not reported (percentage weight change from baseline: –5.5% with behaviour modification *v* –3.2% with dietary advice quarterly *v* –1.2% with one diet session only). The 12th additional RCT (76 women, 58 analysed) found no statistically significant difference between a 10 week standard cognitive behavioural programme (see glossary, p 114) compared with a modified cognitive behavioural programme after 1 year follow up (weight change from baseline: –2.1 kg with modified programme *v* –3.8 kg with standard programme; P value not reported).[66] The 13th additional RCT[68] has found that adding meal replacements to a dietician led group intervention improved weight loss at 1 year (9.1% weight loss with replacements *v* 4.1% without) although the 14th additional RCT[69] found that adding body image treatment did not significantly improve weight loss compared with dietician led treatment alone. The 15th and 16th RCTs examined effects of advice to lose weight among people who were overweight and hypertensive.[55,70] The 15th RCT (1191 people) found that weight loss advice reduced weight and hypertension more than no weight loss advice at 3 years (weight change at 3 years: –0.2 kg with advice *v* +1.8 kg with control; RR for hypertension with advice *v* control 0.81, 95% CI 0.70 to 0.95).[70] Subgroup analysis of the 16th RCT (585 overweight elderly people with hypertension) found that weight loss advice reduced body weight more than no weight loss advice, but the statistical significance of the difference was not reported (weight change at 30 months –4.7 kg with weight loss programme *v* –0.9 kg with no weight loss programme).[55] The 17th RCT (588 overweight people) compared three different cognitive behavioural approaches for tailoring lifestyle modification goals:

workbook alone (no tailoring of goals); adding computerised tailoring using computer kiosks with touch screen monitors to help participants tailor goals; and adding both computers and staff consultation to tailor goals.[71] After 12 months, it found that all groups achieved a statistically significant mean weight loss from baseline. It found that combined personal and computerised tailoring improved weight loss compared with workbook alone (mean weight change –1 kg with workbook *v* –2.1 kg with computerised tailoring *v* –3.3 kg with combined personal and computerised tailoring; P = 0.02 for workbook *v* combined group). The 18th additional RCT (78 obese female chronic dieters, 52 analysed) compared the effects of a 24 week "non-diet" wellness programme intervention with a traditional "weight loss" programme. It found that the weight loss programme increased weight loss compared with the non-diet programme at 1 year (diet 101.1 kg at baseline to 95.2 kg at 1 year *v* non-diet 99.6 kg at baseline to 99.9 kg at 1 year; P < 0.001).[72] The 19th additional RCT (101 obese men and women) compared the effects of a moderate fat (based on the Mediterranean diet), low energy diet compared with a low fat, low energy diet.[73] It found that the moderate fat diet increased weight loss compared with the low fat diet after 18 months (difference in weight change 7.0 kg, 95% CI 5.3 kg to 8.7 kg). There was a mean decrease in body weight of 4.1 kg in the moderate fat group compared with an increase in body weight of 2.9 kg in the low fat group.

Harms: The systematic reviews and RCTs provided no evidence about harms resulting from diet or exercise for weight loss.

Comment: In one RCT (78 obese women), the withdrawal rate for a diet programme was 41% compared with 8% in a non-diet control.[72]

QUESTION **What are the effects of lifestyle interventions to maintain weight loss?**

One systematic review and additional RCTs have found that most types of maintenance strategy result in smaller weight gains or greater weight losses compared with no contact. Strategies that involve personal contact with a therapist, family support, walking training programmes, or multiple interventions, or are weight focused, seem most effective.

Benefits: We found one systematic review[52] and nine additional RCTs.[74–82] The systematic review (search date 1995, 21 studies) compared different types and combinations of interventions. It found that increased contact with a therapist in the long term produced smaller weight gain or greater weight loss, and that additional self help peer groups, self management techniques, or involvement of the family or spouse may increase weight loss. The largest weight loss was seen in programmes using multiple strategies. Two additional small RCTs (102 people[74] and 100 people in two trials[78]) assessed simple strategies without face to face contact with a therapist. Frequent telephone contacts, optional food provision, continued self monitoring, urge control, or relapse prevention did not reduce the rate of weight regain. One small RCT (117 people) found that telephone contacts plus house visits did reduce the rate of weight regain compared with no intervention (3.65 kg with telephone contacts plus house visits *v* 6.42 kg with no intervention;

P = 0.048).[75] One further small RCT (80 obese women) found no difference in weight change at 1 year between participants offered relapse prevention training or problem solving compared with no further contact.[80] One RCT (82 women) compared two walking programmes (4.2 or 8.4 MJ/week) plus diet counselling versus diet counselling alone after a 12 week intensive weight reduction programme.[79] Both walking programmes reduced weight regain at 1 year (reduction in weight gain compared with dietary counselling alone 2.7 kg, 95% CI 0.2 kg to 5.2 kg with low intensity programme and 2.6 kg, 95% CI 0 kg to 5.1 kg with high intensity programme). At 2 years, weight regain was not significantly different between high intensity programme and control, but was reduced in the low intensity group (reduction in weight gain 3.5 kg, 95% CI 0.2 kg to 6.8 kg with low intensity programme and +0.2 kg, 95% CI –3.1 kg to +3.6 kg with high intensity programme). One additional small RCT (67 people) found that people on a weight focused programme maintained weight loss better than those on an exercise focused programme (0.8 kg with weight focused programme *v* 4.4 kg with exercise focused programme; $P < 0.01$).[76] One 5 year RCT (489 menopausal women) compared behavioural intervention in two phases aimed at lifestyle changes in diet and physical activity with lifestyle assessment. People in the intervention group were encouraged to lose weight during the first 6 months (phase I), and thereafter maintain this weight loss for a further 12 months (phase II). The intervention resulted in weight loss compared with control during the first 6 months (–8.9 lb [–4.0 kg] *v* –0.8 lb [–0.4 kg]; $P < 0.05$), most of which was sustained over phase II (–6.7 lb [–3.0 kg] *v* –0.6 lb [–0.3 kg]; $P < 0.05$).[77] One RCT (90 obese men) compared the effects of walking, resistance training of moderate dose 6 at months, and no increase in exercise control after a 2 month weight loss programme with a very low energy diet.[82] It found no significant difference in long term weight maintenance between walking and resistance training programmes and control at 23 months (adjusted mean difference in weight compared with control: +0.8 kg with walking, 95% CI –4.0 kg to +5.6 kg *v* –0.5 kg with resistance, 95% CI –5.0 kg to +4.0 kg; P between interventions = 0.8). There was poor adherence to prescribed exercise (82% with walking *v* 66% with resistance).[82] One RCT (122 overweight men and women, 101 analysed) compared the effects of a weight maintenance programme conducted in person (frequent support or minimal support) or over the Internet for 1 year, after a 6 month weight loss programme.[81] It found significantly less weight loss with Internet support compared with in person support (weight loss: –5.7 kg with Internet support *v* –10.4 kg with minimal in person support *v* –10.4 kg with frequent in person support, $P < 0.05$).[81]

Harms: We found no direct evidence that interventions designed to maintain weight loss are harmful.

Comment: Weight regain is common. The resource implication of providing long term maintenance of any weight loss may be a barrier to the routine implementation of maintenance programmes. One RCT (122 obese people) comparing in person and Internet support for weight maintenance, found attrition rates of 18% after 6 months and 24% after 18 months.[81]

QUESTION **What are the effects of lifestyle advice to prevent weight gain?**

One small RCT found that low intensity education increased weight loss. A second RCT found no significant effect on weight gain from a postal newsletter with or without a linked financial incentive. One RCT found that lifestyle advice prevented weight gain in perimenopausal women compared with assessment alone.

Benefits: We found three systematic reviews (search dates 1995,[52] 1999,[53] and not stated[83]) that included the same two RCTs[84,85] and two subsequent RCTs.[86,87] The first RCT (219 people) compared low intensity education with a financial incentive to maintain weight versus an untreated control group. It found significantly greater average weight loss in the intervention group than in the control group (–0.95 kg with intervention *v* –0.14 kg with control; P = 0.03).[84] The second RCT (228 men and 998 women) compared a monthly newsletter versus the newsletter plus a lottery incentive versus no contact. There was no significant difference in weight gain after 3 years between the groups (1.6 kg with newsletter *v* 1.5 kg with newsletter plus lottery incentive *v* 1.8 kg with no contact).[85] The first subsequent RCT (535 perimenopausal women) found that lifestyle advice reduced weight gain over 2 years compared with assessment alone (weight gain 0.5 kg with advice *v* 11.5 kg with assessment alone).[86] The second small subsequent RCT (40 female students, 33 analysed) compared the effects of a one semester nutrition course (4 months) with no such course.[87] It found no significant change from mean baseline weight in either group 1 year after the end of intervention (66.7 kg at baseline to 67.7 kg at 1 year with course *v* 65.7 kg at baseline to 68.9 kg at 1 year with no course).

Harms: None reported.

Comment: None.

QUESTION **What are the effects of training professionals in promoting reduction of body weight?**

One systematic review of poor quality RCTs found little evidence on the sustained effect of interventions to improve health professionals' management of obesity. One subsequent small RCT found limited evidence that training for primary care doctors in nutrition counselling plus a support programme reduced body weight of the people in their care over 1 year.

Benefits: We found one systematic review (search date 2000, 18 RCTs, 8 with follow up > 1 year)[88] and one subsequent RCT.[89] The studies in the review were heterogeneous and poor quality. The subsequent RCT (45 people) compared nutrition counselling training plus a support programme for primary care doctors versus usual care.[89] The nutrition supported intervention compared with usual care increased weight loss at 1 year (additional weight loss 2.3 kg; P < 0.001).

Harms: None reported.

Comment: The doctors were randomly allocated to treatment but the analysis of results was based on the people in the care of those doctors. No allowance was made for cluster bias. This increases the likelihood that the additional weight loss could have occurred by chance.

GLOSSARY

Behavioural choice therapy A cognitive behavioural intervention based on a decision making model of women's food choice. This relates situation specific eating behaviour to outcomes and goals using decision theory. The outcomes and goals governing food choice extend beyond food related factors to include self esteem and social acceptance.
Cognitive behavioural programme Traditional cognitive behavioural topics (e.g. self monitoring, stimulus control, coping with cravings and high risk situations, stress management, and relaxation techniques) along with topics of particular importance to women (e.g. healthy eating, weight management, mood management, and managing work and family).
Motivational interviewing A goal directed counselling style that helps participants to understand and resolve areas of ambivalence that impede behavioural change.
Standard behavioural therapy A behavioural weight management programme that incorporates moderate calorie restriction to promote weight loss.

Substantive changes

Counselling One systematic review and two RCTs added;[32] conclusions unchanged.
Diet and blood pressure One systematic review added;[51] conclusions unchanged.
Achieving weight loss Two RCTs added;[72,73] conclusions unchanged.
Maintaining weight loss Two RCTs added;[81,82] conclusions unchanged.
Prevention of weight gain One RCT added;[87] conclusions unchanged.

REFERENCES

1. Silagy C, Stead LF. Physician advice for smoking cessation. In: The Cochrane Library, Issue 2, 2002. Oxford: Update Software. Search date 2000; primary sources Cochrane Tobacco Addiction Group Trials Register and the Cochrane Controlled Trials Register.
2. Lancaster T, Stead LF. Individual behavioural counselling for smoking cessation. In: The Cochrane Library, Issue 1, 2003. Oxford: Update Software. Search date 2002; primary sources Cochrane Tobacco Addiction Group Trials Register.
3. Rice VH, Stead LF. Nursing interventions for smoking cessation. In: The Cochrane Library, Issue 2, 2002. Oxford: Update Software. Search date 2001; primary sources Cochrane Tobacco Addiction Group Trials Register and Cinahl.
4. Stead LF, Lancaster T. Telephone counselling for smoking cessation. In: The Cochrane Library Issue 2, 2002. Oxford: Update Software. Search date 2000; primary source Cochrane Tobacco Addiction Group Trials Register.
5. Pieterse ME, Seydel ER, de Vries H, et al. Effectiveness of a minimal contact smoking cessation program for Dutch general practitioners: a randomized controlled trial. *Prev Med* 2001;32:182–190.
6. Lancaster T, Stead LF. Self-help interventions for smoking cessation (Cochrane review). In: The Cochrane Library Issue 1, 2003. Oxford: Update Software. Search date 2002; primary sources previous reviews and meta-analyses, the Tobacco Addiction Review Group register of controlled trials identified from Medline Express (Silverplatter) to March 2002 and the Science Citation Index to 7 March 2002.
7. Silagy C, Mant D, Fowler G, et al. Nicotine replacement therapy for smoking cessation. In: The Cochrane Library, Issue 1, 2003. Oxford: Update Software. Search date 2002; primary source Cochrane Tobacco Addiction Group Trials Register.
8. Tonneson P, Paoletti P, Gustavsson G, et al. Higher dose nicotine patches increase one year smoking cessation rates: results from the European CEASE trial. *Eur Respir J* 1999;13:238–246.
9. Stapleton J. Cigarette smoking prevalence, cessation and relapse. *Stat Methods Med Res* 1998;7:187–203.
10. Stapleton JA, Sutherland G, Russell MA. How much does relapse after one year erode effectiveness of smoking cessation treatments? Long term follow up of a randomised trial of nicotine nasal spray. *BMJ* 1998;316:830–831.
11. Blondal T, Gudmundsson J, Olafsdottir I, et al. Nicotine nasal spray with nicotine patch for smoking cessation: randomised trial with six years follow up. *BMJ* 1999;318:285–289.
12. Daughton DM, Fortmann SP, Glover ED, et al. The smoking cessation efficacy of varying doses of nicotine patch delivery systems 4 to 5 years post-quit day. *Prev Med* 1999;28:113–118.
13. Ebrahim S, Davey Smith G. Health promotion in older people for the prevention of coronary heart disease and stroke. *Health promotion effectiveness reviews series*, No 1. London: Health Education Authority, 1996. Search date 1994;

primary sources Medline, hand searches of reference lists, and citation search on Bids for Eastern European trials.

14. White AR, Rampes H, Ernst E. Acupuncture for smoking cessation (Cochrane review) In: The Cochrane Library Issue 2, 2002. Oxford: Update Software. Search date 2002; primary sources Cochrane Tobacco Addiction Group Register, Medline, Psychlit, Dissertation Abstracts, Health Planning and Administration, Social SciSearch, Smoking and Health, Embase, Biological Abstracts, and Drug.
15. Ussher MH, Taylor AH, West R, et al. Does exercise aid smoking cessation? *Addiction* 2000;95:199–208. Search date 1999; primary sources Medline, Psychlit, Dissertation Abstracts, Sports Discus, hand searches of reference lists, and personal contact with research colleagues.
16. Marcus BH, Albrecht AE, King TK, et al. The efficacy of exercise as an aid for smoking cessation in women. *Arch Intern Med* 1999;159:1229–1234.
17. Hughes JR, Stead LF, Lancaster T. Antidepressants for smoking cessation. In: The Cochrane Library, Issue 2, 2002. Oxford: Update Software. Search date 2001; primary source Cochrane Tobacco Addiction Group Trials Register.
18. Hughes JR, Stead LF, Lancaster T. Anxiolytics for smoking cessation. In: The Cochrane Library, Issue 2, 2002. Oxford: Update Software. Search date 2000; primary source Cochrane Tobacco Addiction Group Trials Register.
19. Jorenby DE, Leischow SJ, Nides MA, et al. A controlled trial of sustained-release bupropion, a nicotine patch, or both for smoking cessation. *N Engl J Med* 1999;340:685–691.
20. Law M, Tang JL. An analysis of the effectiveness of interventions intended to help people stop smoking. *Arch Intern Med* 1995;155:1933–1941. Search date not stated; primary sources Medline and Index Medicus.
21. Lumley J, Oliver S, Waters E. Interventions for promoting smoking cessation during pregnancy. In: The Cochrane Library, Issue 2, 2002. Oxford: Update Software. Search date 1998; primary source Cochrane Tobacco Addiction Group Trials Register.
22. Wisborg K, Henriksen TB, Jespersen LB, et al. Nicotine patches for pregnant smokers: a randomized controlled study. *Obstet Gynecol* 2000;96:967–971.
23. Hajek P, West R, Lee A, et al. Randomized trial of a midwife-delivered brief smoking cessation intervention in pregnancy. *Addiction* 2001;96:485–494.
24. Stotts A, DiClememte CC, Dolan-Mullen P. One-to-one. A motivational intervention for resistant pregnant smokers *Addict Behav* 2002;27:275–292.
25. Rigotti NA, Munafro MR, Murphy MFG, et al. Interventions for smoking cessation in hospitalised patients. In: The Cochrane Library, Issue 1, 2003. Oxford: Update Software. Search date 2002; primary sources Cochrane Controlled Trials Register, Centre for Disease Control Smoking and Health database, Cinahl, and experts.
26. Humerfelt S, Eide GE, Kvale G, et al. Effectiveness of postal smoking cessation advice: a randomized controlled trial in young men with reduced FEV_1 and asbestos exposure. *Eur Respir J* 1998;11:284–290.
27. Burt A, Thornley P, Illingworth D, et al. Stopping smoking after myocardial infarction. *Lancet* 1974;1:304–306.
28. Lancaster T, Silagy C, Fowler G. Training health professionals in smoking cessation. In: The Cochrane Library, Issue 2, 2002. Oxford: Update Software. Search date 2000; primary source Cochrane Tobacco Addiction Group Trials Register.
29. Maguire TA, McElnay JC, Drummond A. A randomized controlled trial of a smoking cessation intervention based in community pharmacies. *Addiction* 2001;96:325–331.
30. Hillsdon M, Thorogood M. A systematic review of physical activity promotion strategies. *Br J Sports Med* 1996;30:84–89. Search date 1996; primary sources Medline, Excerpta Medica, Sport SciSearch, and hand searches of reference lists.
31. Dunn AL, Anderson RE, Jakicic JM. Lifestyle physical activity interventions. History, short- and long-term effects and recommendations. *Am J Prev Med* 1998;15:398–412. Search date not stated; primary sources Medline, Current Contents, Biological Abstracts, The Johns Hopkins Medical Institutions Catalog, Sport Discus, and Grateful Med.
32. Eden KB, Orleans CT, Mulrow CD, et al. Does counseling by clinicians improve physical activity? A summary of the evidence for the U.S. Preventive Services Task Force. *Ann Intern Med* 2002;137:208–215. Search date: 2002; primary sources: the Cochrane Database of Systematic Reviews, Cochrane Controlled Trials Register, Medline, HealthStar, contact with experts, and hand searches of reference lists.
33. Harland J, White M, Drinkwater C, et al. The Newcastle exercise project: a randomised controlled trial of methods to promote physical activity in primary care. *BMJ* 1999;319:828–832.
34. Taylor, A, Doust, J, Webborn, N. Randomised controlled trial to examine the effects of a GP exercise referral programme in Hailsham, East Sussex, on modifiable coronary heart disease risk factors. *J Epidemiol Community Health* 1998;52:595–601.
35. Stevens W, Hillsdon M, Thorogood M, et al. Cost-effectiveness of a primary care based physical activity intervention in 45–74 year old men and women; a randomised controlled trial. *Br J Sports Med* 1998;32:236–241.
36. Halbert JA, Silagy CA, Finucane PM, et al. Physical activity and cardiovascular risk factors: effect of advice from an exercise specialist in Australian general practice. *Med J Aust* 2000;173:84–87.
37. Lamb SE, Bartlett HP, Ashley A, et al. Can lay-led walking programmes increase physical activity in middle aged adults? A randomised controlled trial. *J Epidemiol Community Health* 2002;56:246–252.
38. Hillsdon M, Thorogood M, White I, et al. Advising people to take more exercise is ineffective: a randomized controlled trial of physical activity promotion in primary care. *Int J Epidemiol* 2002;31:808–815.
39. Pinto BM, Friedman R, Marcus BH, et al. Effects of a computer-based, telephone-counseling system on physical activity. *Am J Prev Med* 2002;23:113–120.
40. The Writing Group for the Activity Counseling Trial Research Group. Effects of physical activity counseling in primary care: the Activity Counseling Trial: a randomised controlled trial. *JAMA* 2001;286:677–687.
41. Norris SL, Grothaus LC, Buchner DM, et al. Effectiveness of physician-based assessment and counseling for exercise in a staff model HMO. *Prev Med* 2000;30:513–523.
42. Pereira MA, Kriska AN, Day RD, et al. A randomized walking trial in postmenopausal women. *Arch Intern Med* 1998;158:1695–1701.
43. Campbell AJ, Robertson MC, Gardner MM, et al. Randomised controlled trial of a general practice

programme of home based exercise to prevent falls in elderly women. *BMJ* 1997;315:1065–1069.
44. Brunner E, White I, Thorogood M, et al. Can dietary interventions change diet and cardiovascular risk factors? A meta-analysis of randomised controlled trials. *Am J Public Health* 1997;87:1415–1422. Search date 1993; primary sources computer and manual searches of databases and journals.
45. Tang JL, Armitage JM, Lancaster T, et al. Systematic review of dietary intervention trials to lower blood total cholesterol in free living subjects. *BMJ* 1998;316:1213–1220. Search date 1996; primary sources Medline, Human Nutrition, Embase, Allied and Alternative Health, and hand searches of *Am J Clin Nutr* and reference lists.
46. Stefanick ML, Mackey S, Sheehan M, et al. Effects of diet and exercise in men and postmenopausal women with low levels of HDL cholesterol and high levels of LDL cholesterol. *N Engl J Med* 1998;339:12–20.
47. Knopp RH, Retzlaff B, Walden C, et al. One year effects of increasingly fat-restricted, carbohydrate-enriched diets in lipoprotein levels in free living subjects. *Proc Soc Exp Biol Med* 2000;225:191–199.
48. Tomson Y, Johannesson M, Aberg H. The costs and effects of two different lipid intervention programmes in primary health care. *J Intern Med* 1995;237:13–17.
49. Hooper L, Summerbell CD, Higgins JPT, et al. Reduced or modified dietary fat for preventing cardiovascular disease. In: The Cochrane Library, Issue 2, 2002. Oxford: Update Software. Search date 1999; primary sources Cochrane Library, Medline, Embase, CAB Abstracts, CVRCT registry, related Cochrane Groups' Trial Registers, trials known to experts in the field, and biographies.
50. Howell WH, McNamara DJ, Tosca MA, et al. Plasma lipid and lipoprotein responses to dietary fat and cholesterol: a meta-analysis. *Am J Clin Nutr* 1997;65:1747–1764. Search date 1994; primary sources Medline, and hand searches of selected review publications and bibliographies.
51. Hooper L, Bartlett C, Davey Smith G, et al. Systematic review of long term effects of advice to reduce dietary salt in adults. *BMJ* 2002;325:628. Search date 2000; primary sources The Cochrane Library, Medline, Embase, CAB abstracts, CVRTC registry, Sigle to May 1998 plus Medline, Embase and the Cochrane Library to July 2000, and bibliographies.
52. Glenny A-M, O'Meara S, Melville A, et al. The treatment and prevention of obesity: a systematic review of the literature. *Int J Obesity* 887:21;715–737. Published in full as NHS CRD report 1997, No 10. A systematic review of interventions in the treatment and prevention of obesity. http://www.york.ac.uk/inst/crd/obesity.htm (last accessed 24 June 2003). Search date 1995; primary sources Medline, Embase, DHSS data, Current Research in UK, Science Citation Index, Social Science Citation Index, Conference Proceedings index, Sigle, Dissertation Abstracts, Sport, Drug Info, AMED (Allied and alternative medicine), ASSI (abstracts and indexes), CAB, NTIS (national technical information dB), Directory of Published Proceedings (Interdoc), Purchasing Innovations database, Health promotion database, S.S.R.U., DARE (CRD, database of systematic reviews, NEED, CRD, database of health economic reviews), and all databases searched from starting date to the end of 1995.
53. Douketis JD, Feightner JW, Attia J, et al. Periodic health examination, 1999 update. Detection, prevention and treatment of obesity. Canadian Task Force on Preventive Health Care. *Can Med Assoc J* 1999;160:513–525. Search date 1999; primary sources Medline, Current Contents, and hand searches of reference lists.
54. The National Heart, Lung, and Blood Institute. Clinical guidelines on the identification, evaluation, and treatment of overweight and obesity in adults. Bethesda, Maryland: National Institutes of Health, 1998; http://www.nhlbi.nih.gov/guidelines/obesity/ob_home.htm (last accessed 24 June 2003). Search date 1997; primary sources Medline, and hand searches of reference lists.
55. Whelton PK, Appel LJ, Espeland MA, et al. Sodium reduction and weight loss in the treatment of hypertension in older persons. A randomized controlled Trial of Nonpharmacologic Interventions in the Elderly (TONE). *JAMA* 1998;279:839–846.
56. Wing RR, Polley BA, Venditti E, et al. Lifestyle intervention in overweight individuals with a family history of diabetes. *Diabetes Care* 1998;21:350–359.
57. Anderson RE, Wadden TA, Barlett SJ, et al. Effects of lifestyle activity v structured aerobic exercise in obese women. *JAMA* 1999;281:335–340.
58. Jakicic JM, Winters C, Lang W, et al. Effects of intermittent exercise and use of home exercise equipment on adherence, weight loss, and fitness in overweight women. *JAMA* 1999;282:1554–1560.
59. Sbrocco T, Nedegaard RC, Stone JM, et al. Behavioural choice treatment promotes continuing weight loss. *J Consult Clin Psychol* 1999;67:260–266.
60. Harvey-Berino J. Calorie restriction is more effective for obesity treatment than dietary fat restriction. *Ann Behav Med* 1999;21:35–39.
61. Wing RR, Jeffery RW. Benefits of recruiting participants with friends and increasing social support for weight loss and maintenance. *J Consult Clin Psychol* 1999;67:132–138.
62. Jeffery RW, Wing RR, Thorson C, et al. Use of personal trainers and financial incentives to increase exercise in a behavioural weight loss program. *J Consult Clin Psychol* 1998;66:777–783.
63. Craighead LW, Blum MD. Supervised exercise in behavioural treatment for moderate obesity. *Behav Ther* 1989;20:49–59.
64. Donnelly JE, Jacobsen DJ, Heelan KS, et al. The effects of 18 months of intermittent vs. continuous exercise on aerobic capacity, body weight and composition, and metabolic fitness in previously sedentary, moderately obese females. *Int J Obesity* 2000;24:566–572.
65. Kunz K, Kreimel K, Gurdet C, et al. Comparison of behaviour modification and conventional dietary advice in a long-term weight reduction programme for obese women [abstract]. *Diabetologia* 1982;23:181.
66. Rapoport L, Clark M, Wardle J. Evaluation of a modified cognitive-behavioural programme for weight management. *Int J Obesity* 2000;24:1726–1737.
67. Wing R, Epstein LH, Paternostro-Bayles M, et al. Exercise in a behavioural weight control program for obese patients with type 2 (non insulin dependent) diabetes. *Diabetologica* 1988;31:902–909.
68. Ashley LM, St Jeor ST, Schrage JP, et al. Weight control in the physicians office. *Arch Intern Med* 2001;161:1599–1604.
69. Ramirez EM, Rosen JC. A comparison of weight control and weight control plus body image therapy for obese men and women. *J Consult Clin Psychol* 2001;69:444–446.

70. Stevens VJ, Obarzanek E, Cook NR, et al. for the Trials of Hypertension Prevention Research Group. Long term weight loss and changes in blood pressure: Results of the Trials of Hypertension Prevention, Phase II. *Ann Intern Med* 2001;134:1–11.
71. Wylie-Rosett J, Swencionis C, Ginsberg M, et al. Computerized weight loss intervention optimises staff time: the clinical and cost results of a controlled clinical trial conducted in a managed care setting. *J Am Dietetic Assoc* 2001;101:1155–1162.
72. Bacon L, Keim NL, Van Loan MD, et al. Evaluating a 'non-diet' wellness intervention for improvements of metabolic fitness, psychological well-being and eating and activity behaviours. *Int J Obes Relat Metab Disord* 2002;26:854–865.
73. McManus K, Antinoro L, Sacks F. A randomized controlled trial of a moderate-fat, low-energy diet compared with a low-fat, low-energy diet for weight loss in overweight adults. *Int J Obes Relat Metab Disord* 2001;25:1503–1511.
74. Bonato DP, Boland FJ. A comparison of specific strategies for long-term maintenance following a behavioural treatment program for obese women. *Int J Eat Disord* 1986;5:949–958.
75. Hillebrand TH, Wirth A. Evaluation of an outpatient care program for obese patients after an inpatient treatment. *Pravention und Rehabilitation* 1996;8:83–87.
76. Leermakers EA, Perri MG, Shigaki CL, et al. Effects of exercise-focused versus weight-focused maintenance programs on the management of obesity. *Addict Behav* 1999;24:219–227.
77. Simkin-Silverman LR, Wing RR, Boraz MA, et al. Maintenance of cardiovascular risk factor changes among middle-aged women in a lifestyle intervention trial. *Women's Health* 1998;4:255–271.
78. Wing RR, Jeffery RW, Hellerstedt WL, et al. Effect of frequent phone contacts and optional food provision on maintenance of weight loss. *Ann Behav Med* 1996;18:172–176.
79. Fogelholm M, Kukkonen-Harjula K, Nenonen A, et al. Effects of walking training on weight maintenance after a very-low-energy diet in premenopausal obese women: a randomized controlled trial. *Arch Intern Med* 2000;160:2177–2184.
80. Perri MG, Nezu AM, McKelvey WF, et al. Relapse prevention training and problem-solving therapy in the long-term management of obesity. *J Consult Clin Psychol* 2001;69:722–726.
81. Harvey-Berino J, Pintauro S, Buzzell P, et al. Does using the Internet facilitate the maintenance of weight loss? *Int J Obes Relat Metab Disord* 2002;26:1254–1260.
82. Borg P, Kukkonen-Harjula K, Fogelholm M, et al. Effects of walking or resistance training on weight loss maintenance in obese, middle-aged men: a randomized trial. *Int J Obes Relat Metab Disord* 2002;26:676–683.
83. Hardeman W, Griffin S, Johnston M, et al. Interventions to prevent weight gain: a systematic review of psychological models and behaviour change methods. *Int J Obesity* 2000;4:131–143. Search date not stated; primary sources Medline, Embase, Psychlit, The Cochrane Library, Current Contents, ERIC, HealthStar, Social Science Citation Index, and hand searches of reference lists.
84. Forster JL, Jeffery RW, Schmid TL, et al. Preventing weight gain in adults: a pound of prevention. *Health Psychol* 1988;7:515–525.
85. Jeffery RW, French SA. Preventing weight gain in adults: the pound of prevention study. *Am J Public Health* 1999;89:747–751.
86. Kuller LH, Simkin-Silverman LR, Wing RR, et al. Women's health lifestyle project: a randomized clinical trial. *Circulation* 2001;103:32–37.
87. Matvienko O, Lewis DS, Schafer E. A college science nutrition course as an intervention to prevent weight gain in female college freshmen. *J Nutr Educ* 2001;33:95–101.
88. Harvey EL, Glenny A, Kirk SFL, et al. Improving health professionals' management and the organisation of care for overweight and obese people. In: The Cochrane Library, Issue 2, 2002. Oxford: Update Software. Search date 2000; primary sources Specialised Registers of the Cochrane Effective Practice and Organisation of Care Group; the Cochrane Depression, Anxiety and Neurosis Group; the Cochrane Diabetes Group; the Cochrane Controlled Trials Register; Medline; Embase; Cinahl; Psychlit; Sigle; Sociofile; Dissertation Abstracts; Resource Database in Continuing Medical Education; and Conference Papers Index.
89. Ockene IS, Hebert JR, Ockene JK, et al. Effect of physician-delivered nutrition counseling training and an office-support program on saturated fat intake, weight, and serum lipid measurements in a hyperlipidemic population: Worcester area trial for counseling in hyperlipidemia (WATCH). *Arch Intern Med* 1999;159:725–731.

Margaret Thorogood
Professor of Epidemiology
Warwick Medical School University of Warwick, Coventry, UK

Melvyn Hillsdon
Lecturer in Health Promotion
London School of Hygiene and Tropical Medicine University of London, London, UK

Carolyn Summerbell
Reader in Human Nutrition
School of Health University of Teesside, Middlesbrough, UK

Competing interests: None declared.

Heart failure

Search date October 2002

Robert Samuel

QUESTIONS

INTERVENTIONS

See glossary, p 138

Key Messages

Non-drug treatments

- **Exercise** One systematic review has found that exercise training improved physiological measures compared with control. One included RCT assessed clinical outcomes and found that exercise versus control improved quality of life and reduced cardiac events, mortality, and hospital admission for heart failure at 12 months. One subsequent RCT found no significant difference for 3 months of supervised aerobic and resistance training followed by 9 months of home based training versus usual care in 6 minute walk distance or quality of life at 12 months.
- **Multidisciplinary interventions** One systematic review has found that multidisciplinary programmes significantly reduce admissions to hospital but did not significantly reduce mortality. The review found that telephone contact plus improved coordination of primary care had no significant effect on admission

rate. Two included RCTs found that that home based support versus usual care significantly reduced cardiovascular events at 3–6 years. Subsequent RCTs found that education and nurse led support reduced death and hospital readmission and improved quality of life at 12 weeks to 1 year.

Drug and invasive treatments

- **Amiodarone** Systematic reviews have found weak evidence suggesting that amiodarone versus placebo may reduce mortality. However, we were not able to draw firm conclusions about effects of amiodarone in people with heart failure.
- **Angiotensin converting enzyme inhibitors** Systematic reviews and RCTs have found that angiotensin converting enzyme inhibitors versus placebo significantly reduce ischaemic events, mortality and hospital admission for heart failure. Relative benefits are similar in different groups of people, but absolute benefits are greater in people with severe heart failure. RCTs in people with asymptomatic left ventricular systolic dysfunction have found that angiotensin converting enzyme inhibitors versus placebo significantly delay the onset of symptomatic heart failure and reduce cardiovascular events over 40 months.
- **Angiotensin II receptor blockers** One systematic review has found that angiotensin receptor blockers versus placebo reduced all cause mortality and hospital admission in people with New York Heart Association class II–IV heart failure, although the difference was not significant. It found no significant difference in all cause mortality or hospital admission with angiotensin receptor blockers versus angiotensin converting enzyme inhibitors. It found that angiotensin receptor blockers plus angiotensin converting enzyme inhibitors versus angiotensin converting enzyme inhibitors alone reduced admission for heart failure but did not significantly reduce all cause mortality.
- **Anticoagulation** A preliminary report from one RCT found no significant difference for warfarin versus no antithrombotic treatment or for warfarin versus aspirin for the combined outcome of death, myocardial infarction, and stroke after 27 months. However, the study may have lacked power to detect a clinically important difference.
- **Antiplatelet agents** A preliminary report from one RCT found no significant difference for aspirin versus no antithrombotic treatment or for aspirin versus warfarin for the combined outcome of death, myocardial infarction, and stroke after 27 months. However, the study may have lacked power to detect a clinically important difference.
- **β Blockers** Systematic reviews have found strong evidence that adding a β blocker to an angiotensin converting enzyme inhibitor significantly decreases mortality and hospital admission. Limited evidence from a subgroup analysis of one RCT found no significant effect on mortality in black people.
- **Calcium channel blockers** One systematic review has found no significant difference in mortality with second generation dihydropyridine calcium channel blockers versus placebo. RCTs comparing other calcium channel blockers versus placebo found no evidence of benefit.
- **Digoxin (improves morbidity in people already receiving diuretics and angiotensin converting enzyme inhibitors)** One large RCT in people already receiving diuretics and angiotensin converting enzyme inhibitors found that digoxin versus placebo significantly reduced the number of people admitted to hospital for worsening heart failure at 37 months, but did not significantly reduce mortality.

- **Implantable cardiac defibrillators (in people with heart failure and near fatal arrhythmia)** One RCT has found good evidence that an implantable cardiac defibrillator reduces mortality in people with heart failure who have experienced a near fatal ventricular arrhythmia.
- **Non-amiodarone antiarrhythmic drugs** Evidence extrapolated from one systematic review in people treated after a myocardial infarction suggests that other antiarrhythmic drugs (apart from β blockers) may increase mortality.
- **Positive inotropes (ibopamine, milrinone, and vesnarinone)** RCTs found that positive inotropic drugs (other than digoxin) versus placebo significantly increased mortality over 6–11 months.
- **Prophylactic use of implantable cardiac defibrillators in people at high risk of arrhythmia** Two RCTs have found that implantable cardiac defibrillators versus medical treatment reduce mortality in people with heart failure and at high risk of arrhythmia, whereas one RCT found no significant difference in mortality.
- **Spironolactone in severe heart failure** One RCT in people with severe heart failure taking diuretics, angiotensin converting enzyme inhibitors, and digoxin has found that adding spironolactone versus placebo significantly reduces mortality after 2 years.
- **Treatments for diastolic heart failure** We found no RCTs in people with diastolic heart failure.

DEFINITION Heart failure occurs when abnormality of cardiac function causes failure of the heart to pump blood at a rate sufficient for metabolic requirements under normal filling pressure. It is characterised clinically by breathlessness, effort intolerance, fluid retention, and poor survival. It can be caused by systolic or diastolic dysfunction and is associated with neurohormonal changes.[1] Left ventricular systolic dysfunction (LVSD) is defined as a left ventricular ejection fraction below 0.40. It may be symptomatic or asymptomatic. Defining and diagnosing diastolic heart failure can be difficult. Recently proposed criteria include: (1) clinical evidence of heart failure; (2) normal or mildly abnormal left ventricular systolic function; and (3) evidence of abnormal left ventricular relaxation, filling, diastolic distensibility, or diastolic stiffness.[2] However, assessment of some of these criteria is not standardised.

INCIDENCE/ PREVALENCE Both the incidence and prevalence of heart failure increase with age. Studies of heart failure in the USA and Europe found that under 65 years of age the incidence is 1/1000 men a year and 0.4/1000 women a year. Over 65 years, incidence is 11/1000 men a year and 5/1000 women a year. Under 65 years the prevalence of heart failure is 1/1000 men and 1/1000 women; over 65 years the prevalence is 40/1000 men and 30/1000 women.[3] The prevalence of asymptomatic LVSD is 3% in the general population.[4–6] The mean age of people with asymptomatic LVSD is lower than that for symptomatic individuals. Both heart failure and asymptomatic LVSD are more common in men.[4–6] The prevalence of diastolic heart failure in the community is unknown. The prevalence of heart failure with preserved systolic function in people in hospital with clinical heart failure varies from 13–74%.[7,8] Less than 15% of people with heart failure under 65 years have normal systolic function, whereas the prevalence is about 40% in people over 65 years.[7]

AETIOLOGY/ RISK FACTORS Coronary artery disease is the most common cause of heart failure.[3] Other common causes include hypertension and idiopathic dilated congestive cardiomyopathy. After adjustment for hypertension, the presence of left ventricular hypertrophy remains a risk factor for the development of heart failure. Other risk factors include cigarette smoking, hyperlipidaemia, and diabetes mellitus.[4] The common causes of left ventricular diastolic dysfunction are coronary artery disease and systemic hypertension. Other causes are hypertrophic cardiomyopathy, restrictive or infiltrative cardiomyopathies, and valvular heart disease.[8]

PROGNOSIS The prognosis of heart failure is poor, with 5 year mortality ranging from 26–75%.[3] Up to 16% of people are readmitted with heart failure within 6 months of first admission. In the USA, heart failure is the leading cause of hospital admission among people over 65 years of age.[3] In people with heart failure, a new myocardial infarction increases the risk of death (RR 7.8, 95% CI 6.9 to 8.8). About a third of all deaths in people with heart failure are preceded by a major ischaemic event.[9] Sudden death, mainly caused by ventricular arrhythmia, is responsible for 25–50% of all deaths, and is the most common cause of death in people with heart failure.[10] The presence of asymptomatic LVSD increases an individual's risk of having a cardiovascular event. One large prevention trial found that for a 5% reduction in ejection fraction, the risk ratio for mortality was 1.20 (95% CI 1.13 to 1.29). For hospital admission for heart failure, the risk ratio was 1.28 (95% CI 1.18 to 1.38) and the risk ratio for heart failure was 1.20 (95% CI 1.13 to 1.26).[4] The annual mortality for people with diastolic heart failure varies in observational studies (1.3–17.5%).[7] Reasons for this variation include age, the presence of coronary artery disease, and variation in the partition value used to define abnormal ventricular systolic function. The annual mortality for left ventricular diastolic dysfunction is lower than that found in people with systolic dysfunction.[11]

AIMS OF INTERVENTION To relieve symptoms; to improve quality of life; to reduce morbidity and mortality, with minimum adverse effects.

OUTCOMES Functional capacity (assessed by the New York Heart Association (see glossary, p 138) functional classification or more objectively by using standardised exercise testing or the 6 min walk test);[12] quality of life (assessed with questionnaires);[13] mortality; adverse effects of treatment. Proxy measures of clinical outcome (e.g. left ventricular ejection fraction and hospital readmission rates) are used only when clinical outcomes are unavailable.

METHODS *Clinical Evidence* search and appraisal October 2002. Generally, RCTs with less than 500 people have been excluded because of the number of large RCTs available. If for any comparison very large RCTs exist then much smaller RCTs have been excluded, even if they have more than 500 people.

QUESTION What are the effects of non-drug treatments?

OPTION MULTIDISCIPLINARY INTERVENTIONS

One systematic review has found that multidisciplinary programmes significantly reduce admissions to hospital but did not significantly reduce mortality. The review found that telephone contact plus improved coordination of primary care had no significant effect on admission rate. Two included RCTs found that that home based support versus usual care significantly reduced cardiovascular events at 3–6 years. Subsequent RCTs found that education and nurse led support reduced death and hospital readmission and improved quality of life at 12 weeks to 1 year.

Benefits: We found one systematic review (search date 1999, 11 RCTs, 2067 people with heart failure)[14] and three subsequent RCTs.[15–17] Multidisciplinary programmes in the review included non-drug treatments such as nutrition advice, counselling, patient education, and exercise training. The review found that multidisciplinary interventions significantly reduced hospital admission (406/1001 [40.6%] with multidisciplinary programme *v* 474/1011 [46.9%] with conventional care; RR 0.87, 95% CI 0.79 to 0.96; 11 RCTs), but did not significantly reduce mortality (104/534 [19.5%] with multidisciplinary programme *v* 121/572 [21.2%] with conventional care; RR 0.94, 95% CI 0.75 to 1.19; 7 RCTs). However, the hospital admission results were heterogeneous by intervention. Specialised follow up by a multidisciplinary team substantially reduced admissions to hospital (RR 0.77, 95% CI 0.68 to 0.86; 1366 people with heart failure; 9 RCTs), but there was no benefit from telephone contact plus improved coordination of primary care services (RR 1.15, 95% CI 0.96 to 1.37; 646 people with heart failure; 2 RCTs). One subsequent report of two RCTs included in the review (297 people living at home with at least 1 hospital admission for heart failure) found that home based support versus usual care significantly increased event free survival at 3–6 years (median event free survival: 7 months with support *v* 3 months with usual care, $P < 0.01$).[17] However, it found no significant difference in mortality for support versus usual care at 5 years (83/149 [56%] with support *v* 96/148 [65%] with usual care; $P = 0.06$). We found three subsequent RCTs.[15–17] The first RCT (88 people recently discharged after admission for heart failure) found that, compared with usual care, nurse led education and support significantly reduced the number of people who either died or had at least one readmission at 1 year (25/44 [57%] with support *v* 36/44 [82%] with usual care; RR 0.69, 95% CI 0.52 to 0.92).[15] The second subsequent RCT (200 people admitted with chronic heart failure) found no significant difference for protocol driven support and management by nurses versus usual care in mortality at 6 months (7/102 [7%] with support *v* 13/98 [13%] with usual care; $P = 0.14$).[16] It found that support improved quality of life compared with usual care at 6 months (Minnesota Living with Heart Failure Questionnaire: final score 35.7 with support *v* 45.3 with usual care; $P = 0.01$). The third subsequent RCT (98 people) found that nurse led education plus specialist dietician advice significantly reduced readmission rate for heart failure compared with usual care at 12 weeks (readmission for heart failure: 1/51 [2%] with support *v* 11/47 [23%] with usual care; $P < 0.01$; OR 0.07, 95% CI 0.01 to 0.53).[18]

Harms: The review and subsequent RCTs did not report on harms (see comment below).

Comment: Studies in the review were small, involved highly selected patient populations, lasted less than 6 months, and were usually performed in academic centres, so results may not generalise to longer term outcomes based in smaller community centres. The review suggested that disease management programmes may fragment care such that peoples' other conditions are overlooked.[14] However, it did not provide evidence to support this.

OPTION EXERCISE

One systematic review has found that exercise training improved physiological measures compared with control. However, we found that clinical effects are uncertain. One included RCT assessed clinical outcomes and found that exercise versus control improved quality of life and reduced cardiac events, mortality, and hospital readmission for heart failure at 12 months. One subsequent RCT found no significant difference for 3 months of supervised aerobic and resistance training followed by 9 months of home based training versus usual care in 6 minute walk distance or quality of life at 12 months.

Benefits: We found one systematic review (search date 2000, 14 parallel group RCTs, 582 people)[19] and one subsequent RCT.[20] The included RCTs predominantly excluded people with other illnesses and most used a cycle ergometer or combined exercise programme. Only one identified RCT lasted longer than 6 months. The review did not include a meta-analysis. Overall, the review reported that 12 of the 14 RCTs found a positive effect for exercise training versus control on physiological measures.[19] One RCT (99 people with heart failure, 88 men) evaluated clinical outcomes.[21] It compared 12 months of exercise training versus no exercise training and found that exercise improved quality of life, reduced fatal or non-fatal cardiac events, and reduced mortality and hospital readmission for heart failure at 12 months (quality of life assessed using Minnesota Living with Heart Failure Questionnaire, $P < 0.001$ in favour of exercise; fatal or non-fatal cardiac events 17/50 [34%] with exercise *v* 37/49 [76%] without exercise; ARR 42%, 95% CI 20% to 58%; RR 0.45, 95% CI 0.23 to 0.73; NNT 2, 95% CI 2 to 5; mortality 9/50 [18%] with exercise *v* 20/49 [41%] without exercise; RR 0.44, 95% CI 0.20 to 0.87; NNT 4, 95% CI 3 to 19; hospital readmission for heart failure 5/50 [10%] with exercise *v* 14/49 [29%] without exercise; ARR 19%, 95% CI 3% to 25%; RR 0.35, 95% CI 0.12 to 0.88; NNT 5, 95% CI 4 to 30).[21] The subsequent RCT (181 people with New York Heart Association [see glossary, p 138] class I–III) found no significant difference between aerobic and resistance training (3 months supervised followed by 9 months home based) versus usual care in 6 minute walk distance or quality of life at 12 months (not by intent to treat; increase in walk distance from baseline in 139 people: 17 m with exercise *v* 20 m with usual care, P = 0.81; change in Minnesota Living with Heart Failure Questionnaire score for 124 people: –3.4 points with exercise *v* –3.3 points with usual care, P = 0.98).[20] It also found no significant difference for total mortality or admission to hospital for heart failure (results presented graphically; mortality about 30% for both groups, P = 0.95; death or admission to hospital about 40% for both groups, P = 0.73).[20]

Harms: The review and RCTs reported no important adverse effects associated with prescribed exercise training.[19–21]

Comment: The studies were small, involved highly selected patient populations, and were performed in well resourced academic centres. The results may not generalise to smaller community centres. The specific form of exercise training varied among studies and the relative merits of each strategy are unknown. The studies generally lasted less than 1 year and long term effects are unknown. Larger studies over a longer period are needed.

QUESTION **What are the effects of drug treatments in heart failure?**

OPTION **ANGIOTENSIN CONVERTING ENZYME INHIBITORS**

Two systematic reviews and recent RCTs have found that angiotensin converting enzyme inhibitors reduce mortality, hospital admission for heart failure, and ischaemic events in people with heart failure. Relative benefits are similar in different groups of people, but absolute benefits are greater in people with severe heart failure.

Benefits: We found two systematic reviews (search dates 1994[22] and not stated[23]) of angiotensin converting enzyme (ACE) inhibitors versus placebo in heart failure. The first systematic review (search date 1994, 32 RCTs, duration 3–42 months, 7105 people, New York Heart Association [see glossary, p 138] class III or IV) found that ACE inhibitors versus placebo reduced mortality (611/3870 [16%] with ACE inhibitors *v* 709/3235 [22%] with placebo; ARR 6%, 95% CI 4% to 8%; OR 0.77, 95% CI 0.67 to 0.88; NNT 16).[22] Relative reductions in mortality were similar in different subgroups (stratified by age, sex, cause of heart failure, and New York Heart Association class). The second systematic review (search date not stated, 5 RCTs, 12 763 people with left ventricular dysfunction or heart failure of mean duration 35 months) analysed long term results from large RCTs that compared ACE inhibitors versus placebo.[23] Three RCTs examined effects of ACE inhibitors in people for 1 year after myocardial infarction. In these three postinfarction trials (5966 people), ACE inhibitor versus placebo significantly reduced mortality (702/2995 [23.4%] with ACE inhibitor *v* 866/2971 [29.1%] with placebo; OR 0.74, 95% CI 0.66 to 0.83), readmission for heart failure (355/2995 [11.9%] with ACE inhibitor *v* 460/2971 [15.5%] with placebo; OR 0.73, 95% CI 0.63 to 0.85), and reinfarction (324/2995 [10.8%] with ACE inhibitor *v* 391/2971 [13.2%] with placebo; OR 0.80, 95% CI 0.69 to 0.94). For all five trials, ACE inhibitors versus placebo reduced mortality (1467/6391 [23.0%] with ACE inhibitor *v* 1710/6372 [26.8%] with placebo; OR 0.80, 95% CI 0.74 to 0.87), reinfarction (571/6391 [8.9%] with ACE inhibitor *v* 703/6372 [11.0%] with placebo; OR 0.79, 95% CI 0.70 to 0.89), and readmission for heart failure (876/6391 [13.7%] with ACE inhibitor *v* 1202/6372 [18.9%] with placebo; OR 0.67, 95% CI 0.61 to 0.74). The relative benefits began soon after the start of treatment, persisted in the long term, and were independent of age, sex, and baseline use of diuretics, aspirin, and β blockers. Although there was a trend towards greater relative reduction in mortality or readmission for heart failure in people with lower ejection fraction, benefit was apparent over the range examined. **Other ischaemic events:** RCTs that studied high risk groups found that ACE inhibitors significantly reduced some ischaemic event rates. One RCT in people with left ventricular dysfunction found that ACE inhibitors reduced myocardial infarction (combined fatal or non-fatal myocardial infarction: 9.9% with ACE inhibitor *v* 12.3% with placebo; RR 0.77, 95% CI 0.61 to 0.98), hospital admission for angina (15% with ACE inhibitor *v* 19% with placebo; RR 0.73, 95% CI 0.60 to 0.88), and the combined end point of cardiac death, non-fatal myocardial infarction, or hospital admission for angina (43% with ACE inhibitor *v* 51% with placebo; RR 0.77, 95% CI 0.68 to 0.86).[9] Effects on hospital readmissions were observed shortly after starting ACE inhibitor treatment, although effects on ischaemic events were not apparent for at least 6 months and peaked at 36 months. **Dose:** We found one large RCT (3164 people with New York Heart Association class II–IV heart failure) that compared low dose lisinopril (2.5 or 5.0 mg/day) versus high dose lisinopril (32.5 or 35.0 mg/day).[24] It found no significant difference in mortality (717/1596 [44.9%] with low dose *v* 666/1568 [42.5%] with high dose; ARR 2.4%; CI not provided; HR 0.92, 95% CI 0.80 to 1.03; P = 0.128), but found that high dose lisinopril reduced the combined outcome of death or hospital admission for any reason (1338/1596 [83.8%] events with low dose *v* 1250/1568 [79.7%] events with high dose; ARR 4.1%; CI not provided; HR 0.88, 95% CI 0.82 to 0.96), and reduced admissions for heart failure (1576/1596 [98.7%] admissions with low dose *v* 1199/1568 [76.5%] admissions with high dose; ARR 22.2%; CI not provided; P = 0.002). **Comparison of different angiotensin converting enzyme inhibitors:** The first systematic review found similar benefits with different ACE inhibitors.[22]

Harms: We found no systematic review. The main adverse effects in large trials were cough, hypotension, hyperkalaemia, and renal dysfunction. Compared with placebo, ACE inhibitors increased cough (37% with ACE inhibitor *v* 31% with placebo; ARI 7%, 95% CI 3% to 11%; RR 1.23, 95% CI 1.11 to 1.35; NNH 14), dizziness or fainting (57% with ACE inhibitor *v* 50% with placebo; ARI 7%, 95% CI 3% to 11%; RR 1.14, 95% CI 1.06 to 1.21; NNH 14), increased creatinine concentrations above 177 μmol/L (10.7% with ACE inhibitor *v* 7.7% with placebo; ARI 3.0%, 95% CI 0.6% to 6.0%; RR 1.38, 95% CI 1.09 to 1.67; NNH 34), and increased potassium concentrations above 5.5 mmol/L (AR 6.4% with ACE inhibitor *v* 2.5% with placebo; ARI 4%, 95% CI 2% to 7%; RR 2.56, 95% CI 1.92 to 3.20; NNH 26).[25] Risk of angio-oedema was similar with ACE inhibitors and placebo (3.8% with enalapril *v* 4.1% with placebo; ARI +0.3%, 95% CI –1.4% to +1.5%).[25] The trial comparing low and high doses of lisinopril found that most adverse effects were more common with high dose (no P value provided; dizziness: 12% with low dose *v* 19% with high dose; hypotension: 7% with low dose *v* 11% with high dose; worsening renal function: 7% with low dose *v* 10% with high dose; significant change in serum potassium concentration: 7% with low dose *v* 7% with high dose), although there was no difference in withdrawal rates between groups (18% discontinued with low dose *v* 17% with high dose). The trial found that cough was less commonly experienced with high dose compared with low dose lisinopril (cough: 13% with low dose *v* 11% with high dose).

Comment: The relative benefits of ACE inhibitors were similar in different subgroups of people with heart failure. Most RCTs evaluated left ventricular function by assessing left ventricular ejection fraction, but some studies defined heart failure clinically, without measurement of left ventricular function in people at high risk of developing heart failure (soon after myocardial infarction). It is unclear whether there are additional benefits from adding ACE inhibitor to antiplatelet treatment in people with heart failure (see antiplatelet agents, p 135).

OPTION ANGIOTENSIN II RECEPTOR BLOCKERS

One systematic review has found that angiotensin receptor blockers versus placebo reduced all cause mortality and hospital admission in people with New York Heart Association class II–IV heart failure, although the difference was not significant. This may be explained by the small numbers of deaths and admissions reported. It found no significant difference in all cause mortality or hospital admission with angiotensin receptor blockers versus angiotensin converting enzyme inhibitors. It found that angiotensin receptor blockers plus angiotensin converting enzyme inhibitors versus angiotensin converting enzyme inhibitors alone reduced admission for heart failure but did not significantly reduce all cause mortality.

Benefits: **Versus placebo:** We found one systematic review (search date 2001, 11 RCTs, 2259 people with New York Heart Association [see glossary, p 138] class II–IV, follow up 4 wks to 2 years).[26] It found that angiotensin receptor blockers versus placebo reduced all cause mortality and admission for heart failure, although the differences were not significant (all cause mortality: 7 RCTs; AR 2% with angiotensin receptor blockers *v* 3% with placebo; OR 0.68, 95% CI 0.38 to 1.22; admission for heart failure: 1 RCT; 8% with angiotensin receptor blockers *v* 12% with placebo; OR 0.67, 95% CI 0.29 to 1.51). The numbers of deaths and admissions were small, which may explain why the difference did not reach significance. **Versus angiotensin converting enzyme inhibitors:** The systematic review identified six RCTs (4682 people with New York Heart Association class II–IV, follow up 4 wks to 1.5 years) comparing angiotensin receptor blockers versus angiotensin converting enzyme (ACE) inhibitors.[26] It found no significant difference between treatments for all cause mortality or rate of admission for heart failure (all cause mortality: 6 RCTs; OR 1.09, 95% CI 0.92 to

1.29; admission for heart failure: 3 RCTs; OR 0.95, 95% CI 0.8 to 1.13). **Plus angiotensin converting enzyme inhibitors versus ACE inhibitors alone:** The systematic review identified six RCTs (5712 people with New York Heart Association class II–IV heart failure) comparing angiotensin receptor blockers plus ACE inhibitors versus ACE inhibitors alone.[26] It found that combined treatment significantly reduced hospital admission for heart failure (3 RCTs; OR 0.74, 95% CI 0.64 to 0.86). However, it found no significant difference between treatments for all cause mortality (6 RCTs; OR 1.04, 95% CI 0.91 to 1.20).

Harms: The systematic review did not report on harms.[26]

Comment: In people who are truly intolerant of ACE inhibitors the evidence supports the use of angiotensin II receptor blockers, with the expectation of at least symptomatic improvement of the heart failure.

OPTION POSITIVE INOTROPIC AGENTS

One well designed RCT found that digoxin decreased the rate of hospital admissions for worsening heart failure in people already receiving diuretics and angiotensin converting enzyme inhibitors, although it found no evidence of an effect on mortality. RCTs found evidence that positive inotropic drugs other than digoxin increased mortality in people with heart failure; evidence on morbidity was less clear.

Benefits: **Digoxin:** We found one systematic review (search date 1992, 13 RCTs, duration 3–24 wks, 1138 people with heart failure and sinus rhythm)[27] and one subsequent large RCT.[28] The systematic review found that six of the 13 RCTs enrolled people without assessment of ventricular function and may have included some people with mild or no heart failure. Other limitations of the older trials included crossover designs and small sample sizes. In people who were in sinus rhythm with heart failure, the systematic review found fewer people with clinical worsening of heart failure (52/628 [8.3%] with digoxin *v* 131/631 [20.8%] with placebo; ARR 12.5%, 95% CI 9.5% to 14.7%; RR 0.40, 95% CI 0.29 to 0.54) but did not find a definite effect on mortality (16/628 [2.5%] with digoxin *v* 15/631 [2.4%] with placebo; ARR –0.2%, 95% CI –2.6% to +1.1%; RR 1.07, 95% CI 0.53 to 2.23). The subsequent large RCT (6800 people, 88% male, mean age 64 years, New York Heart Association [see glossary, p 138] class I–III, 94% already taking angiotensin converting enzyme inhibitors, 82% taking diuretics) compared blinded additional treatment with either digoxin or placebo for a mean of 37 months.[28] Digoxin did not reduce all cause mortality compared with placebo (1181/3397 [34.8%] with digoxin *v* 1194/3403 [35.1%] with placebo; ARR +0.3%, 95% CI –2.0% to +2.6%; RR 0.99, 95% CI 0.93 to 1.06). Digoxin reduced admission rates for heart failure over 37 months (910/3397 [27%] with digoxin *v* 1180/3403 [35%] with placebo; ARR 8%, 95% CI 6% to 10%; RR 0.77, 95% CI 0.72 to 0.83; NNT 13, 95% CI 10 to 17) and reduced combined outcome of death or hospital admission caused by worsening heart failure (1041/3397 [31%] with digoxin *v* 1291/3403 [38%] for placebo; ARR 7.3%, 95% CI 5.1% to 9.4%; RR 0.81, 95% CI 0.75

to 0.87; NNT 14). **Other inotropic agents:** One non-systematic review (6 RCTs, 8006 people) of RCTs found that non-digitalis inotropes increased mortality compared with placebo.[10] The largest RCT in the review (3833 people with heart failure) found increased mortality with vesnarinone (60 mg/day) versus placebo over 9 months (292/1275 [23%] with vesnarinone *v* 242/1280 [19%] with placebo; ARI 4%, 95% CI 1% to 8%; RR 1.21, 95% CI 1.04 to 1.40; NNH 25).[10,29] Another large RCT (1088 people with heart failure) found milrinone versus placebo increased mortality over 6 months (168/561 [30%] with milrinone *v* 127/527 [24%] with placebo; ARI 6.0%, 95% CI 0.5% to 12.0%; RR 1.24, 95% CI 1.02 to 1.49; NNH 17).[30] A third large RCT (1906 people with heart failure) compared ibopamine versus placebo over 11 months.[31] It found that ibopamine increased mortality (232/953 [25%] with ibopamine *v* 193/953 [20%] with placebo; RR 1.26, 95% CI 1.04 to 1.53). The review found that some studies reported improved functional capacity and quality of life, but this was not consistent across all studies.

Harms: We found no systematic review. **Digoxin:** The RCT (6800 people) found that more people had suspected digoxin toxicity in the digoxin group versus placebo (11.9% with digoxin *v* 7.9% with placebo; ARI 4.0%, 95% CI 2.4% to 5.8%; RR 1.50, 95% CI 1.30 to 1.73; NNH 25).[28] The RCT found no evidence that digoxin increased the risk of ventricular fibrillation or tachycardia compared with placebo (37/3397 [1.1%] with digoxin *v* 27/3403 [0.8%] with placebo; ARI +0.3%, 95% CI –0.1% to +1.0%; RR 1.37, 95% CI 0.84 to 2.24). Digoxin compared with placebo increased rates of supraventricular arrhythmia (2.5% with digoxin *v* 1.2% with placebo; ARI 1.3%, 95% CI 0.5% to 2.4%; RR 2.08, 95% CI 1.44 to 2.99; NNH 77) and second or third degree atrioventricular block (1.2% with digoxin *v* 0.4% with placebo; ARI 0.8%, 95% CI 0.2% to 1.8%; RR 2.93, 95% CI 1.61 to 5.34; NNH 126). **Other inotropic agents:** Most RCTs found that inotropic agents other than digoxin increased risk of death (see benefits above).

Comment: None.

OPTION β BLOCKERS

We found strong evidence from systematic reviews that adding β blockers to standard treatment with angiotensin converting enzyme inhibitors in people with moderate or severe heart failure reduces the rate of hospital admission or death. Subgroup analysis in black people found no significant effect on mortality.

Benefits: We found two systematic reviews (search dates 2000[32] and not stated[33]) and two subsequent RCTs[34,35] of the effects of β blockers in heart failure. **In people with any severity of heart failure:** The first systematic review (search date 2000, 22 RCTs, 10 315 people with heart failure) found that β blockers versus placebo significantly reduced the risk of death and hospital admission (death 444/5273 [8.4%] with β blockers *v* 624/4862 [12.8%] with placebo; OR 0.65, 95% CI 0.53 to 0.80; hospital admissions: 540/5244 [10.3%] with β blockers *v* 754/4832 [15.6%] with placebo; OR 0.64, 95%

CI 0.53 to 0.79).[32] This is equivalent to three fewer deaths and four fewer hospital admissions per 100 people treated for 1 year. The results were consistent for selective and non-selective β blockers. Sensitivity analysis and funnel plots found that publication bias was unlikely. **In people with severe heart failure:** We found one systematic review[31] and two subsequent RCTs.[32,33] The systematic review (search date not stated, 4 RCTs, 635 people with class IV heart failure) found that β blockers versus placebo significantly reduced the risk of death (56/313 [17.9%] with β blockers *v* 81/322 [25.1%] with placebo; RR 0.71, 95% CI 0.52 to 0.96). The two subsequent RCTs compared β blockers versus placebo in people with New York Heart Association (see glossary, p 138) class III or IV heart failure.[34,35] The first RCT (2289 people with class IV heart failure, who were euvolaemic [defined as the absence of rales and ascites and the presence of no more than minimal peripheral oedema] and who had an ejection fraction of < 25%, but were not receiving intensive care, iv vasodilators, or positive inotropic drugs) compared carvedilol versus placebo over 10.4 months. It was stopped early because of a significant beneficial effect on survival that exceeded the pre-specified interim monitoring boundaries.[34] It found that β blockers significantly reduced mortality (130/1156 [11.2%] with β blockers *v* 190/1133 [16.8%] with placebo; RR 0.65, 95% CI 0.52 to 0.81) and the combined outcome of death or hospital admission (425/1156 [36.8%] with β blockers *v* 507/1133 [44.7%] with placebo; RR 0.76, 95% CI 0.67 to 0.87). The second RCT compared bucindolol versus placebo in people with severe heart failure (2708 people class III or IV heart failure and ejection fraction ≤ 35%; about 70% of the people were white and 24% were black).[35] The RCT was stopped early because of accumulated evidence from other studies. It found that death was more common with placebo, but the difference did not reach significance (411/1354 [30.4%] with bucindolol *v* 449/1354 [33.1%] with placebo; HR 0.90, 95% CI 0.78 to 1.02). The RCT found a significant interaction of treatment effect with race (black *v* non-black). There was no evidence of benefit in black people (HR 1.17, 95% CI 0.89 to 1.53), although there was a significant effect for non-black people (HR 0.82, 95% CI 0.70 to 0.96).[35]

Harms: One subsequent RCT found that fewer people with carvedilol versus placebo required permanent discontinuation of treatment because of adverse events other than death (P = 0.02).[34] Cumulative withdrawals at 1 year were 14.8% with carvedilol versus 18.5% with placebo. For the subgroup of people with recent or recurrent cardiac decompensation or severely depressed cardiac function the difference in withdrawal rates was greater (17.5% with carvedilol *v* 24.2% with placebo). The subsequent RCT comparing bucindolol versus placebo found that 23% in the bucindolol group and 25% of people in the placebo group permanently discontinued the medication.[35]

Comment: Fears that β blockers may cause excessive problems with worsening heart failure, bradyarrhythmia, or hypotension have not been confirmed. Good evidence was found for β blockers in people with moderate symptoms (New York Heart Association class II or III) receiving standard treatment, including angiotensin converting enzyme inhibitors. The value of β blockers is uncertain in heart failure with preserved ejection fraction and in asymptomatic left ventricular systolic dysfunction. One recent RCT (1959 people) has found that carvedilol reduced all cause mortality compared with placebo (AR for death: 12% with carvedilol *v* 15% with placebo; HR 0.77, 95% CI 0.60 to 0.98) in people with acute myocardial infarction and left ventricular ejection fraction 40% or less.[36] The RCTs of β blockers have consistently found a mortality benefit, but it is not clear whether or not this is a class effect. One recent small RCT (150 people) of metoprolol versus carvedilol found some differences in surrogate outcomes, but both drugs produced similar improvements in symptoms, submaximal exercise tolerance, and quality of life.[37] The results for non-black people were consistent between bucindolol and carvedilol. The lack of observed benefit for black people in one RCT[35] raises the possibility that there may be race specific responses to pharmacological treatment for cardiovascular disease.

OPTION CALCIUM CHANNEL BLOCKERS

One systematic review of second generation dihydropyridine calcium channel blockers found no evidence of benefit. RCTs of other calcium channel blockers found no evidence of benefit.

Benefits: **After myocardial infarction:** See calcium channel blockers under acute myocardial infarction, p 037. **Other heart failure:** We found one systematic review (search date not stated, 18 RCTS, 3128 people with moderate to advanced heart failure for > 2 months) of second generation dihydropyridine calcium channel blockers,[38] one non-systematic review of all calcium channel blockers (3 RCTs, 1790 people with heart failure),[10] and one subsequent RCT.[39] Meta-analysis found no significant difference in mortality (2 RCTs, 1603 people; OR 0.94, 95% CI 0.79 to 1.12; significant heterogeneity was found; $P = 0.48$).[38] The largest RCT in the non-systematic review (1153 people, [New York Heart Association (see glossary, p 138) class III or IV], left ventricular ejection fraction < 0.30, using diuretics, digoxin, and angiotensin converting enzyme inhibitors) found that amlodipine versus placebo had no significant effect on the primary combined end point of all cause mortality and hospital admission for cardiovascular events over 14 months (222/571 [39%] with amlodipine *v* 246/582 [42%] with placebo; ARR +3.4%, 95% CI –2.3% to +8.8%; RR 0.92, 95% CI 0.79 to 1.06).[10,40] Subgroup analysis of people with primary cardiomyopathy found a reduction in mortality (45/209 [22%] with amlodipine *v* 74/212 [35%] with placebo; ARR 13%, 95% CI 5% to 20%; RR 0.62, 95% CI 0.43 to 0.85; NNT 7). There was no significant difference in the group with heart failure caused by coronary artery disease. The second RCT (186 people, idiopathic dilated cardiomyopathy, New York Heart Assocation class I–III) compared diltiazem versus placebo.[10] It found no evidence of a difference in survival with diltiazem versus placebo in those who did not have a heart transplant, although people on diltiazem had improved cardiac function, exercise capacity, and subjective quality of life. The third RCT (451 people with mild heart failure, New York Heart Assocation class II or III) compared felodipine versus placebo.[10] It found no significant effect. The subsequent RCT (2590 people with New York Heart Assocation class II–IV heart failure, mean follow up of 1.5 with mibefradil and 1.6 years with placebo) found no significant difference in death rates between mibefradil and placebo (350/1295 [27.0%] with mibefradil *v* 319/1295 [24.6%] with placebo; RR 1.10, 95% CI 0.96 to 1.25).[39]

Harms: Calcium channel blockers have been found to exacerbate symptoms of heart failure or increase mortality in people with pulmonary congestion after myocardial infarction or ejection fraction less than 0.40 (see calcium channel blockers under acute myocardial infarction, p 37).[10] One RCT found mibefradil versus placebo increased risk of death in people taking digoxin, class I or II antiarrhythmics, amiodarone, or drugs associated with torsade de pointes.[39] The review found that second generation dihydropyridine calcium channel blockers did not cause significant adverse effects.[38]

Comment: Many of the RCTs were underpowered and had wide confidence intervals. One RCT of amlodipine in people with primary dilated cardiomyopathy is in progress.

OPTION ALDOSTERONE RECEPTOR ANTAGONISTS

One large RCT of people with severe heart failure (on usual treatment, including angiotensin converting enzyme inhibitors) has found that adding an aldosterone receptor antagonist (spironolactone) reduces death rates compared with placebo after 2 years.

Benefits: We found no systematic review. We found one RCT of spironolactone (25 mg/day) versus placebo (1663 people with heart failure, New York Heart Association [see glossary, p 138] class III or IV, left ventricular ejection fraction < 0.35, all taking angiotensin converting enzyme inhibitors and loop diuretics, and most taking digoxin).[41] The trial was stopped early because spironolactone significantly reduced all cause mortality with spironolactone compared with placebo after 2 years (mortality: 284/822 [35%] with spironolactone *v* 386/841 [46%] with placebo; ARR 11%, 95% CI 7% to 16%; RR 0.75, 95% CI 0.66 to 0.85; NNT 9, 95% CI 6 to 15).[41]

Harms: The RCT found no evidence that adding spironolactone to an angiotensin converting enzyme inhibitor increases risk of clinically important hyperkalaemia. Gynaecomastia or breast pain were reported in 10% of men given spironolactone and 1% of men given placebo.[41]

Comment: The RCT was large and well designed. As only people with New York Heart Association functional class III or IV were included, these results cannot necessarily be generalised to people with milder heart failure.

OPTION ANTIARRHYTHMIC DRUG TREATMENT

Systematic reviews found weak evidence that amiodarone reduced total mortality in people with heart failure. Extrapolation from one systematic review in people treated after a myocardial infarction suggests that other antiarrhythmic agents may increase mortality in people with heart failure.

Benefits: **Amiodarone:** We found two systematic reviews of the effects of amiodarone versus placebo in heart failure.[42,43] The most recent review (search date 1997, 10 RCTs, 4766 people) included people with a wide range of conditions (symptomatic and asymptomatic heart failure, ventricular arrhythmia, recent myocardial infarction, and recent cardiac arrest).[42] Eight of these RCTs reported the number of deaths. The review found that treatment with amiodarone over 3–24 months reduced the risk of death from any cause compared with placebo or conventional treatment (436/2262 [19%] with amiodarone *v* 507/2263 [22%] with control; ARR 3.0%, 95% CI 0.8% to 5.3%; RR 0.86, 95% CI 0.76 to 0.96; NNT 32). This review did not perform any subgroup analyses in people with heart failure. The earlier systematic review (search date not stated) found eight RCTs (5101 people after myocardial infarction) of prophylactic amiodarone versus placebo or usual care and five RCTs (1452 people) in people with heart failure.[43] Mean follow up was 16 months. Analysis of results from all 13 RCTs found a lower total mortality with amiodarone than control (annual mortality: 10.9% with amiodarone *v* 12.3% with control). The effect was significant with some methods of calculation (fixed effects model: OR 0.87, 95% CI 0.78 to 0.99) but not with others (random effects model: OR 0.85, 95% CI 0.71 to 1.02). The effect of amiodarone was significantly greater in RCTs that compared amiodarone versus usual care than in placebo controlled RCTs. Amiodarone significantly reduced arrhythmic death or sudden death compared with placebo (OR 0.71, 95% CI 0.59 to 0.85). Subgroup analysis found that amiodarone significantly reduced mortality in the five heart failure RCTs (annual mortality: 19.9% with amiodarone *v* 24.3% with placebo; OR 0.83, 95% CI 0.70 to 0.99). **Other antiarrhythmics:** Apart from β blockers, other antiarrhythmic drugs increase mortality in people at high risk (see class I antiarrhythmic agents under secondary prevention of ischaemic cardiac events, p 188).

Harms: **Amiodarone:** Amiodarone did not significantly increase non-arrhythmic death rate (OR 1.02, 95% CI 0.87 to 1.19).[43] In placebo controlled RCTs, after 2 years, 41% of people in the amiodarone group and 27% in the placebo group had permanently discontinued study medication.[43] In 10 RCTs of amiodarone versus placebo, amiodarone increased the odds of reporting adverse drug reactions compared with placebo (OR 2.22, 95% CI 1.83 to 2.68). Nausea was the most common adverse effect. Hypothyroidism was the most common serious adverse effect (7.0% with amiodarone *v* 1.1% with placebo). Hyperthyroidism (1.4% with amiodarone *v* 0.5% with placebo), peripheral neuropathy (0.5% with amiodarone *v* 0.2% with placebo), lung infiltrates (1.6% with amiodarone *v* 0.5% with placebo), bradycardia (2.4% with amiodarone *v* 0.8% with placebo), and liver dysfunction (1.0% with amiodarone *v* 0.4% with placebo) were all more common in the amiodarone group.[43] **Other antiarrhythmics:** These agents (particularly class I antiarrhythmics) may increase mortality (see class I antiarrhythmic agents under secondary prevention of ischaemic cardiac events, p 188).

Comment: **Amiodarone:** RCTs of amiodarone versus usual treatment found larger effects than placebo controlled trials.[43] These findings suggest bias; unblinded follow up may be associated with reduced usual care or improved adherence with amiodarone. Further studies are required to assess the effects of amiodarone treatment on mortality and morbidity in people with heart failure.

OPTION IMPLANTABLE CARDIAC DEFIBRILLATORS

One RCT has found good evidence that implantable cardiac defibrillator reduces mortality in people with heart failure who have experienced a near fatal ventricular arrhythmia. Two RCTs have found that implantable cardiac defibrillators reduce mortality compared with medical treatment in people with heart failure and at high risk of arrhythmia, whereas one RCT found no significant difference in mortality.

Benefits: We found no systematic review. We found four RCTs examining the effects of implantable cardiac defibrillators (ICDs) in people with left ventricular dysfunction.[44–47] The first RCT (1016 people resuscitated after ventricular arrhythmia and either syncope or other serious cardiac symptom and left ventricular ejection fraction ≤ 0.40) compared an ICD versus an antiarrhythmic drug (mainly amiodarone).[44] ICDs improved survival at 1, 2, and 3 years (1 year survival: 89.3% with ICD *v* 82.3% with antiarrhythmic; 2 year survival: 81.6% with ICD *v* 73.7% with antiarrhythmic; 3 year survival: 75.4% with ICD *v* 64.1% with antiarrhythmic). The second RCT included 196 people with New York Heart Association (see glossary, p 138) class I–III heart failure and previous myocardial infarction, a left ventricular ejection fraction 0.35 or less, a documented episode of asymptomatic unsustained ventricular tachycardia, and inducible non-suppressible ventricular tachyarrhythmia on electrophysiological study.[45] Ninety five people received an ICD and 101 received conventional medical treatment. The trial found that ICDs reduced mortality over a mean of 27 months (deaths: 15/95 [16%] with ICD [11 from cardiac cause] *v* 39/101 [39%] with conventional treatment [27 from cardiac cause]; HR 0.46, 95% CI 0.26 to 0.82). The third RCT included 1055 people aged less than 80 years who were scheduled for coronary artery bypass surgery, had a left ventricular ejection fraction less than 0.36, and had electrocardiographic abnormalities. It found that ICD (446 people) at the time of bypass surgery versus no ICD (454 people) produced no significant difference in mortality over a mean of 32 months (deaths: 101/446 [23%] with ICD [71 from cardiac causes] *v* 95/454 [21%] with control [72 from cardiac causes]; HR 1.07, 95% CI 0.81 to 1.42).[46] The fourth RCT (1232 people with prior myocardial infarction and left ventricular ejection fraction < 0.30) compared an ICD (742 people) versus conventional medical treatment (490 people).[47] It found that ICD reduced all cause mortality after 20 months' mean follow up (AR 14.2% with ICD *v* 19.8% with conventional treatment; HR 0.69, 95% CI 0.51 to 0.93).

Harms: The RCTs found that the main adverse effects of ICDs were infection (about 5%), pneumothorax (about 2%), bleeding requiring further operation (about 1%), serious haematomas (about 3%), cardiac perforation (about 0.2%), problems with defibrillator lead (about 7%), and malfunction of defibrillator generator (about 3%).[44–47]

Comment: The RCTs were in people with reduced left ventricular function and included people with and without previous cardiac arrest or inducible arrhythmia. It is uncertain whether asymptomatic ventricular arrhythmia is in itself a predictor of sudden death in people with moderate or severe heart failure.[48] Several RCTs of prophylactic ICD treatment in people with heart failure and in survivors of acute myocardial infarction are ongoing.[49]

OPTION ANTICOAGULATION

A preliminary report from one RCT found no significant difference for warfarin versus no antithrombotic treatment or for warfarin versus aspirin for the combined outcome of death, myocardial infarction, and stroke after mean follow up of 27 months. However, the study may have lacked power to detect clinically important effects.

Benefits: **Versus placebo:** We found one systematic review (search date 2000, 1 RCT, 279 people, 70% with New York Heart Association [see glossary, p 138] class III).[50] The RCT identified by the review was a pilot study comparing warfarin (international normalised ratio 2.5), aspirin (300 mg/day), and no antithrombotic treatment.[51] The RCT found no significant difference for warfarin versus no antithrombotic treatment for the combined outcome of death, myocardial infarction, and stroke after mean follow up of 27 months (combined outcome: 26% with warfarin *v* 27% with no antithrombotic treatment; P value not reported).[51] **Versus antiplatelets:** See antiplatelets, p 135.

Harms: The RCT found four haemorrhagic events with warfarin versus none with no antithrombotic treatment (total number of people in each group not reported).[51]

Comment: The systematic review (search date 2000)[50] found three additional non-randomised trials. Meta-analysis of these trials and the RCT[51] found that anticoagulant versus control significantly reduced death from all causes, cardiovascular event rates (death from all causes in 1087 people: OR 0.64, 95% CI 0.45 to 0.90; cardiovascular event rates in 1130 people: OR 0.26, 95% CI 0.16 to 0.43).[50] Meta-analysis of two non-randomised trials (645 people) found no significant difference in bleeding complications for warfarin versus no warfarin (OR 1.52, 95% CI 0.56 to 4.10).[50] The non-randomised controlled studies were performed in the early 1950s in hospitalised people with a high prevalence of rheumatic heart disease and atrial fibrillation and the methods used may be considered unreliable today. One retrospective analysis assessed the effect of anticoagulants used at the discretion of individual investigators in RCTs on the incidence of stroke, peripheral arterial embolism, and pulmonary embolism.[52] The first cohort was from one RCT (642 men with chronic heart failure) comparing hydralazine plus isosorbide dinitrate versus prazosin versus placebo. The second cohort was from another RCT (804 men with chronic heart failure) comparing enalapril versus hydralazine plus isosorbide dinitrate. All people were given digoxin and diuretics. The retrospective analysis found that without treatment the incidence of all thromboembolic events was low (2.7/100 patient years in the first RCT; 2.1/100 patient years in the second RCT) and that anticoagulation did not reduce the incidence of thromboembolic events (2.9/100 patient years in the first RCT; 4.8/100 patient years in the second RCT). In this group of people, atrial fibrillation was not found to be associated with a higher risk of thromboembolic events. The second retrospective analysis was from two large RCTs (2569 people with symptomatic and asymptomatic left ventricular dysfunction) that compared enalapril versus placebo.[53] The analysis found that people treated with warfarin at baseline had significantly lower risk of death during follow up (HR adjusted for baseline differences 0.76, 95% CI 0.65 to 0.89). Warfarin use was associated with a reduction in the combined outcome of death plus hospital admission for heart failure (adjusted HR 0.82, 95% CI 0.72 to 0.93). The benefit with warfarin use was not significantly influenced by the presence of symptoms, randomisation to enalapril or placebo, sex, presence of atrial fibrillation, age, ejection fraction, New York Heart Association classification, or cause of heart failure. Warfarin reduced cardiac mortality, specifically deaths that were sudden, or associated with either heart failure or myocardial infarction. Neither of the retrospective studies was designed to determine the incidence of thromboembolic events in heart failure or the effects of treatment. Neither study included information about the intensity of anticoagulation or warfarin use. We found several additional cohort studies that showed a reduction in thromboembolic events with anticoagulation, but they all reported results for too few people to provide useful results. An RCT is needed to compare anticoagulation versus no anticoagulation in people with heart failure.

OPTION ANTIPLATELET AGENTS

A preliminary report from one RCT found no significant difference for aspirin versus no antithrombotic treatment or for aspirin versus warfarin for the combined outcome of death, myocardial infarction, and stroke after mean follow up of 27 months.

Benefits: We found one systematic review (search date 2000, 1 RCT, 279 people, 70% with New York Heart Association (see glossary, p 138) class III).[50] The RCT identified by the review was a pilot study comparing aspirin (300 mg/day) versus warfarin (international normalised ratio 2.5) versus no antithrombotic treatment.[51] **Versus placebo:** The RCT found no significant difference for aspirin versus no antithrombotic treatment for the combined outcome of death, myocardial infarction, and stroke after mean follow up of 27 months (combined outcome: 32% with aspirin *v* 27% with no antithrombotic treatment; P value not reported).[51] It found that aspirin significantly increased all cause hospital admission compared with placebo ($P < 0.05$; no data reported). **Versus warfarin:** The RCT found no significant difference for aspirin versus warfarin for the combined outcome of death, myocardial infarction, and stroke after mean follow up of 27 months (combined outcome: 32% with aspirin *v* 24% with warfarin; P value not reported).[51] It found that all cause hospital admissions were significantly higher for aspirin versus warfarin ($P = 0.05$; no data reported).

Harms: Preliminary information on one RCT reported five haemorrhagic events with aspirin versus four with warfarin (total number of people in each group not reported).[51] The total number of serious adverse reactions were similar in all groups (198 with aspirin, 173 with warfarin, and 178 with no antithrombotic treatment).[54]

Comment: **In people not taking angiotensin converting enzyme inhibitors:** We found no systematic review and no RCTs. We found one retrospective cohort analysis within one RCT in 642 men with heart failure.[52] The RCT compared hydralazine plus isosorbide dinitrate versus prazosin versus placebo in men receiving digoxin and diuretics. Aspirin, dipyridamole, or both were used at the discretion of the investigators. The number of thromboembolic events was low in both groups (1 stroke, 0 peripheral, and 0 pulmonary emboli in 184 people years of treatment with antiplatelet drugs *v* 21 strokes, 4 peripheral, and 4 pulmonary emboli in 1068 people years of treatment without antiplatelet drugs; 0.5 events/100 people years with antiplatelet agents *v* 2.0 events/100 patient years without antiplatelet agents; P = 0.07). **In people taking angiotensin converting enzyme inhibitors:** We found no RCTs. We found two large retrospective cohort studies.[52,55] The first retrospective analysis assessed the effect of antiplatelet agents used at the discretion of individual investigators on the incidence of stroke, peripheral arterial embolism, and pulmonary embolism within one RCT.[52] The RCT (804 men with chronic heart failure) compared enalapril versus hydralazine plus isosorbide dinitrate. It found that the incidence of all thromboembolic events was low without antiplatelet treatment and found no significant difference between groups (1.6 events/100 patient years with antiplatelet treatment *v* 2.1 events/100 people years with no antiplatelet treatment; P = 0.48). The second cohort analysis was from two large RCTs that compared enalapril versus placebo (2569 people with symptomatic and asymptomatic left ventricular dysfunction). It found that people treated with antiplatelet agents at baseline had a significantly lower risk of death (HR adjusted for baseline differences 0.82, 95% CI 0.73 to 0.92).[55] Subgroup analysis suggested that antiplatelet agents might have an effect in people randomised to placebo (mortality HR for antiplatelet treatment at baseline *v* no antiplatelet treatment at baseline 0.68, 95% CI 0.58 to 0.80), but not in people randomised to enalapril (mortality HR for antiplatelet treatment *v* no antiplatelet treatment 1.00, 95% CI 0.85 to 1.17). Both retrospective studies have important limitations common to studies with a retrospective cohort design. One study did not report on the proportions of people taking aspirin and other antiplatelet agents.[52] The other study noted that more than 95% of people took aspirin, but the dosage and consistency of antiplatelet use was not recorded.[55] One retrospective non-systematic review (4 RCTs, 96 712 people) provided additional evidence about the effect of aspirin on the benefits of early angiotensin converting enzyme inhibitors in heart failure.[56] It found a similar reduction in 30 day mortality with angiotensin converting enzyme inhibitor versus control for those people not taking aspirin compared with those taking aspirin (aspirin: OR 0.94, 95% CI 0.89 to 0.99; no aspirin: OR 0.90, 95% CI 0.81 to 1.01). However, the analysis may not be valid because the people who did not receive aspirin were older and had a worse baseline prognosis than those taking aspirin. The effects of antiplatelet treatment in combination with angiotensin converting enzyme inhibitors in people with heart failure requires further research.

QUESTION **What are the effects of angiotensin converting enzyme inhibitors in people at high risk of heart failure?**

RCTs have found good evidence that angiotensin converting enzyme inhibitors can delay development of symptomatic heart failure and reduce the frequency of cardiovascular events in people with asymptomatic left ventricular systolic dysfunction, and in people with other cardiovascular risk factors for heart failure.

Benefits: **In people with asymptomatic left ventricular systolic dysfunction:** We found no systematic review but found two RCTs. One large RCT (4228 people) examined an angiotensin converting enzyme (ACE) inhibitor (enalapril) versus placebo over 40 months in people with asymptomatic left ventricular systolic dysfunction (ejection fraction < 0.35).[57] It found no significant difference for enalapril versus placebo in total mortality and cardiovascular mortality (all cause mortality: 313/2111 [14.8%] with ACE inhibitor *v* 334/2117 [15.8%] with placebo; ARR +0.9%, 95% CI –1.3% to +2.9%; RR 0.94, 95% CI 0.81 to 1.08; cardiovascular mortality: 265/2111 [12.6%] with ACE inhibitor *v* 298/2117 [14.1%] with placebo; ARR +1.5%, 95% CI –0.6% to +3.3%; RR 0.89, 95% CI 0.76 to 1.04). During the study more people assigned to the placebo received digoxin, diuretics, or ACE inhibitors that were not part of the study protocol, which may have contributed to the lack of significant difference in mortality between the two groups. Compared with placebo, enalapril reduced symptomatic heart failure, hospital admission for heart failure, and fatal or non-fatal myocardial infarction (symptomatic heart failure: 438/2111 [21%] with ACE inhibitor *v* 640/2117 [30%] with placebo; ARR 9.5%, 95% CI 7.0% to 12.0%; RR 0.69, 95% CI 0.61 to 0.77; NNT 11; admission for heart failure: 306/2111 [15%] with ACE inhibitor *v* 454/2117 [21%] with placebo; ARR 7%, 95% CI 5% to 9%; RR 0.68, 95% CI 0.59 to 0.77; NNT 14; fatal or non-fatal myocardial infarction: 7.6% with ACE inhibitor *v* 9.6% with placebo; ARR 2%, 95% CI 0.4% to 3.4%; RR 0.79, 95% CI 0.65 to 0.96).[9,57] A second RCT in asymptomatic people after myocardial infarction with documented left ventricular systolic dysfunction found that an ACE inhibitor (captopril) reduced mortality and reduced the risk of ischaemic events compared with placebo.[58] **In people with other risk factors:** We found one large RCT comparing ramipril (10 mg/day) versus placebo, for a mean of 5 years, in 9297 high risk people (people with vascular disease or diabetes plus one other cardiovascular risk factor) who were not known to have left ventricular systolic dysfunction or heart failure.[59] It found that ramipril reduced the risk of heart failure (9.0% with ramipril *v* 11.5% with placebo; RR 0.77, 95% CI 0.67 to 0.87; $P < 0.001$). Ramipril also reduced the combined risk of myocardial infarction or stroke or cardiovascular death, the risk of these outcomes separately, and all cause mortality (see ACE inhibitors under secondary prevention of ischaemic cardiac events, p 188). During the trial, 496 people had an echocardiography; 2.6% of these people were found to have ejection fraction less than 0.4. Retrospective review of charts found that left ventricular function had been documented in 5193 people; 8.1% had a reduced ejection fraction.

Harms: We found no systematic review. The first RCT over 40 months found that a high proportion of people in both groups reported adverse effects (76% with enalapril *v* 72% with placebo).[57] Dizziness or fainting (46% with enalapril *v* 33% with placebo) and cough (34% with enalapril *v* 27% with placebo) were reported more often in the enalapril group (P value not reported). The incidence of angio-oedema was the same in both groups (1.4%). Study medication was permanently discontinued by 8% of the people in the enalapril group versus 5% in the placebo group (P value not reported).

Comment: Asymptomatic left ventricular systolic dysfunction is prognostically important, but we found no prospective studies that have evaluated screening to detect its presence.

QUESTION **What are the effects of treatments for diastolic heart failure?**

We found no RCTs in people with diastolic heart failure.

Benefits: We found no systematic review or RCTs in people with diastolic heart failure.

Harms: We found no evidence on the harms of treatments for diastolic heart failure.

Comment: The causes of diastolic dysfunction vary among people with diastolic heart failure. Current treatment is empirical, based on the results of small clinical studies and consists of treating the underlying cause and coexistent conditions with interventions optimised for individuals.[6,60,61] RCTs with clinically relevant outcome measures are needed to determine the benefits and harms of treatment in diastolic heart failure.

GLOSSARY

New York Heart Association classification Classification of severity by symptoms. Class I: no limitation of physical activity; ordinary physical activity does not cause undue fatigue or dyspnoea. Class II: slight limitation of physical activity; comfortable at rest, but ordinary physical activity results in fatigue or dyspnoea. Class III: limitation of physical activity; comfortable at rest, but less than ordinary activity causes fatigue or dyspnoea. Class IV: unable to carry out any physical activity without symptoms; symptoms are present even at rest; if any physical activity is undertaken, symptoms are increased.

REFERENCES

1. Poole-Wilson PA. History, definition, and classification of heart failure. In: Poole-Wilson PA, Colucci WS, Massie BM, et al, eds. *Heart failure. Scientific principles and clinical practice.* London: Churchill Livingston, 1997:269–277.
2. Working Group Report. How to diagnose diastolic heart failure: European Study Group on Diastolic Heart Failure. *Eur Heart J* 1998;19:990–1003.
3. Cowie MR, Mosterd A, Wood DA, et al. The epidemiology of heart failure. *Eur Heart J* 1997;18:208–225.
4. McKelvie RS, Benedict CR, Yusuf S. Prevention of congestive heart failure and management of asymptomatic left ventricular dysfunction. *BMJ* 1999;318:1400–1402.
5. Bröckel U, Hense HW, Museholl M. Prevalence of left ventricular dysfunction in the general population [abstract]. *J Am Coll Cardiol* 1996;27(suppl A):25.
6. Mosterd A, deBruijne MC, Hoes A. Usefulness of echocardiography in detecting left ventricular dysfunction in population-based studies (the Rotterdam study). *Am J Cardiol* 1997;79;103–104.
7. Vasan RS, Benjamin EJ, Levy D. Congestive heart failure with normal left ventricular systolic function. *Arch Intern Med* 1996;156:146–157.
8. Davie AP, Francis CM, Caruana L, et al. The prevalence of left ventricular diastolic filling abnormalities in patients with suspected heart failure. *Eur Heart J* 1997;18:981–984.

9. Yusuf S, Pepine CJ, Garces C, et al. Effect of enalapril on myocardial infarction and unstable angina in patients with low ejection fractions. *Lancet* 1992;340:1173–1178.
10. Gheorghiade M, Benatar D, Konstam MA, et al. Pharmacotherapy for systolic dysfunction: a review of randomized clinical trials. *Am J Cardiol* 1997;80(8B):14H–27H.
11. Gaasch WH. Diagnosis and treatment of heart failure based on LV systolic or diastolic dysfunction. *JAMA* 1994;271:1276–1280.
12. Bittner V, Weiner DH, Yusuf S, et al, for the SOLVD Investigators. Prediction of mortality and morbidity with a 6-minute walk test in patients with left ventricular dysfunction. *JAMA* 1993;270:1702–1707.
13. Rogers WJ, Johnstone DE, Yusuf S, et al, for the SOLVD Investigators. Quality of life among 5025 patients with left ventricular dysfunction randomized between placebo and enalapril. The studies of left ventricular dysfunction. *J Am Coll Cardiol* 1994;23:393–400.
14. McAlister FA, Lawson FME, Teo KK, et al. A systematic review of randomized trials of disease management programs in heart failure. *Am J Med* 2001;110:378–384. Search date 1999; primary sources Medline, Embase, Cinahl, Sigle, Cochrane Controlled Trials Register, the Cochrane Effective Practice and Organization of Care Study Register, hand searches of bibliographies of identified studies, and personal contact with content experts.
15. Krumholz HM, Amatruda J, Smith GL, et al. Randomized trial of an education and support intervention to prevent readmission of patients with heart failure. *J Am Coll Cardiol* 2002;39:83–89.
16. Kasper EK, Gerstenblith G, Hefter G, et al. A randomized trial of the efficacy of multidisciplinary care in heart failure outpatients at high risk of hospital readmission. *J Am Coll Cardiol* 2002;39:471–480.
17. Stewart S, Horowitz JD. Home-based intervention in congestive heart failure: long-term implications on readmission and survival. *Circulation* 2002;105:2861–2866.
18. McDonald K, Ledwidge M, Cahill J, et al. Heart failure management: multidisciplinary care has intrinsic benefit above the optimization of medical care. *J Card Fail* 2002;8:142–148.
19. Lloyd-Williams F, Mair FS, Leitner M. Exercise training and heart failure: a systematic review of current evidence. *Br J Gen Pract* 2002;52:47–55. Search date 2000; primary sources Medline, Science Citation Index, Social Sciences Citation Index, Bids, Bandolier, Cochrane Database of Systematic Reviews, NHS National Research Register, Current Research in Britain, and latest editions of 10 relevant journals.
20. McKelvie RS, Teo KK, Roberts R, et al. Effects of exercise training in patients with heart failure: the Exercise Rehabilitation Trial (EXERT). *Am Heart J* 2002;144:23–30.
21. Belardinelli R, Georgiou D, Cianci G, et al. Randomized, controlled trial of long-term moderate exercise training in chronic heart failure. Effects on functional capacity, quality of life, and clinical outcomes. *Circulation* 1999;99:1173–1182.
22. Garg R, Yusuf S, for the Collaborative Group on ACE Inhibitor Trials. Overview of randomized trials of angiotensin-converting enzyme inhibitors on mortality and morbidity in patients with heart failure. *JAMA* 1995;273:1450–1456. Search date 1994; primary sources Medline and correspondence with investigators and pharmaceutical companies.
23. Flather M, Yusuf S, Kober L, et al, for the ACE-Inhibitor Myocardial Infarction Collaborative Group. Long-term ACE-inhibitor therapy in patients with heart failure or left-ventricular dysfunction: a systematic overview of data from individual patients. *Lancet* 2000;355:1575–1581. Search date not stated; primary sources Medline, Ovid, hand searches of reference lists, and personal contact with researchers, colleagues, and principal investigators of the trials identified.
24. Packer M, Poole-Wilson PA, Armstrong PW, et al, on behalf of the ATLAS Study Group. Comparative effects of low and high doses of the angiotensin-converting enzyme inhibitor, lisinopril, on morbidity and mortality in chronic heart failure. *Circulation* 1999;100:2312–2318.
25. SOLVD Investigators. Effect of enalapril on survival in patients with reduced left ventricular ejection fractions and congestive heart failure. *N Engl J Med* 1991;325:293–302.
26. Jong P, Demers C, McKelvie RS, et al. Angiotensin receptor blockers in heart failure: meta-analysis of randomized controlled trials. *J Am Coll Cardiol* 2002;39:463–470. Search date 2001; primary sources Medline, Embase, Biological Abstracts, International Pharmaceutical Abstracts, Cochrane Controlled Trials Database, McMaster Cardiovascular Randomized Clinical Trial Registry, and Science Citation Index.
27. Kraus F, Rudolph C, Rudolph W. Wirksamkeit von Digitalis bei Patienten mit chronischer Herzinsuffizienz und Sinusrhythmus. *Herz* 1993;18:95–117. Search date 1992; primary source Medline.
28. Digitalis Investigation Group. The effect of digoxin on mortality and morbidity in patients with heart failure. *N Engl J Med* 1997;336:525–533.
29. Cohn J, Goldstein S, Greenberg B, et al. A dose-dependent increase in mortality with vesnarinone among patients with severe heart failure. *N Engl J Med* 1998;339:1810–1816.
30. Packer M, Carver JR, Rodeheffer RJ, et al, for the PROMISE Study Research Group. Effect of oral milrinone on mortality in severe chronic heart failure. *N Engl J Med* 1991;325:1468–1475.
31. Hampton JR, van Veldhuisen DJ, Kleber FX, et al. Randomised study of effect of ibopamine on survival in patients with advanced severe heart failure. *Lancet* 1997;349:971–977.
32. Brophy JM, Joseph L, Rouleau JL. β-blockers in congestive heart failure: a Bayesian meta-analysis. *Ann Intern Med* 2001;134:550–560. Search date 2000; primary sources Medline, Cochrane Library, Web of Science, and hand searches of reference lists from relevant articles.
33. Whorlow SL, Krum H. Meta-analysis of effect of β-blocker therapy on mortality in patients with New York Heart Association class IV chronic congestive heart failure. *Am J Cardiol* 2000;86:886–889. Search date not stated; primary sources Medline and hand searches of reference lists from relevant reviews.
34. Packer M, Coats A, Fowler MB. Effect of carvedilol on survival in severe chronic heart failure. *Engl J Med* 2001;344:1651–1658.
35. The Beta-Blocker Evaluation of Survival Trial Investigators. A trial of the β-blocker bucindolol in patients with advanced chronic heart failure. *N Engl J Med* 2001;344:1659–1667.
36. The CAPRICORN Investigators. Effect of carvedilol on outcome after myocardial infarction in patients with left ventricular dysfunction: the CAPRICORN randomized trial. *Lancet* 2001;357:1385–1390.
37. Metra M, Giubbini R, Nodari S, et al. Differential effects of β-blockers in patients with heart failure: a prospective, randomized, double-blind

comparison of the long-term effects of metoprolol versus carvedilol. *Circulation* 2000;102:546–551.
38. Cleophas T, van Marum R. Meta-analysis of efficacy and safety of second-generation dihydropyridine calcium channel blockers in heart failure. *Am J Card* 2001;87:487–490. Search date not stated; primary source Medline.
39. Levine TB, Bernink P, Caspi A, et al. Effect of mibefradil, a T-type calcium channel blocker, on morbidity and mortality in moderate to severe congestive heart failure. The MACH-1 study. *Circulation* 2000;101:758–764.
40. Packer M, O'Connor CM, Ghali JK, et al, for the Prospective Randomized Amlodipine Survival Evaluation Study Group. Effect of amlodipine on morbidity and mortality in severe chronic heart failure. *N Engl J Med* 1996;335:1107–1114.
41. Pitt B, Zannad F, Remme WJ, et al, for the Randomized Aldactone Evaluation Study Investigators. The effects of spironolactone on morbidity and mortality in patients with severe heart failure. *N Engl J Med* 1999;341:709–717.
42. Piepoli M, Villani GQ, Ponikowski P, et al. Overview and meta-analysis of randomised trials of amiodarone in chronic heart failure. *Int J Cardiol* 1998;66:1–10. Search date 1997; primary source unspecified computerised literature database.
43. Amiodarone Trials Meta-analysis Investigators. Effect of prophylactic amiodarone on mortality after acute myocardial infarction and in congestive heart failure: meta-analysis of individual data from 6500 patients in randomised trials. *Lancet* 1997;350:1417–1424. Search date not stated; primary sources literature reviews, computerised literature reviews, and discussion with colleagues.
44. The Antiarrhythmic versus Implantable Defibrillators (AVID) Investigators. A comparison of antiarrhythmic-drug therapy with implantable defibrillators I patients resuscitated from near-fatal ventricular arrhythmias. *N Engl J Med* 1997;337:1576–1583.
45. Moss AJ, Hall WJ, Cannom DS, et al. Improved survival with an implanted defibrillator in patients with coronary disease at high risk for ventricular arrhythmia. *N Engl J Med* 1996;335:1933–1940.
46. Bigger JT for The Coronary Artery Bypass Graft (CABG) Patch Trial Investigators. Prophylactic use of implanted cardiac defibrillators in patients at high risk for ventricular arrhythmias after coronary-artery bypass graft surgery. *N Engl J Med* 1997;337:1569–1575.
47. Moss AJ, Zoreba W, Hall J, et al, for the Multicenter Automatic Defibrillator Implantation Trial II Investigators. Prophylactic implantation of a defibrillator in patients with myocardial infarction and reduced ejection fraction. *N Engl J Med* 2002;346:877–883.
48. Teerlink JR, Jalaluddin M, Anderson S, et al. Ambulatory ventricular arrhythmias in patients with heart failure do not specifically predict an increased risk of sudden death. *Circulation* 2000;101:40–46.
49. Connolly SJ. Prophylactic antiarrhythmic therapy for the prevention of sudden death in high-risk patients: drugs and devices. *Eur Heart J* 1999;(suppl C):31–35.
50. Lip GYH, Gibbs CR. Anticoagulation for heart failure in sinus rhythm (Cochrane Review). In: The Cochrane Library, Issue 4, 2001. Oxford: Update Software. Search date 2000; primary sources Cochrane Controlled Trials Register, Medline, Embase, NHS Database of Abstracts of Reviews of Effectiveness, abstracts from national and international cardiology meetings, authors of identified studies, and reference lists.
51. Jones CG, Cleland JGF. Meeting report: the LIDO, HOPE, MOXCON, and WASH studies. *Eur J Heart Fail* 1999;1:425–431.
52. Dunkman WB, Johnson GR, Carson PE, et al, for the V-HeFT Cooperative Studies Group. Incidence of thromboembolic events in congestive heart failure. *Circulation* 1993;87:94–101.
53. Al-Khadra AS, Salem DN, Rand WM, et al. Warfarin anticoagulation and survival: a cohort analysis from the studies of left ventricular dysfunction. *J Am Coll Cardiol* 1998;31:749–753.
54. Lip GYH, Gibbs CR. Antiplatelet agents versus control or anticoagulation for heart failure in sinus rhythm (Cochrane Review). In: The Cochrane Library, Issue 4, 2001. Oxford: Update Software. Search date not stated; primary sources Medline, Embase, Dare, abstracts from national and international meetings, and contact with relevant authors.
55. Al-Khadra AS, Salem DN, Rand WM, et al. Antiplatelet agents and survival: a cohort analysis from the Studies of Left Ventricular Dysfunction (SOLVD) Trial. *J Am Coll Cardiol* 1998;31:419–425.
56. Latini R, Tognoni G, Maggioni AP, et al, on behalf of the Angiotensin-converting Enzyme Inhibitor Myocardial Infarction Collaborative Group. Clinical effects of early angiotensin-converting enzyme inhibitor treatment for acute myocardial infarction are similar in the presence and absence of aspirin. Systematic overview of individual data from 96 712 randomized patients. *J Am Coll Cardiol* 2000;35:1801–1807.
57. SOLVD Investigators. Effect of enalapril on mortality and the development of heart failure in asymptomatic patients with reduced left ventricular ejection fractions. *N Engl J Med* 1992;327:685–691.
58. Rutherford JD, Pfeffer MA, Moyé LA, et al. Effects of captopril on ischaemic events after myocardial infarction. *Circulation* 1994;90:1731–1738.
59. The Heart Outcome Prevention Evaluation Study Investigators. Effects of an angiotensin-converting-enzyme inhibitor, ramipril, on cardiovascular events in high-risk patients. *N Engl J Med* 2000;342:145–153.
60. The Task Force of the Working Group on Heart Failure of the European Society of Cardiology. The treatment of heart failure. *Eur Heart J* 1997;18:736–753.
61. Tendera M. Ageing and heart failure: the place of ACE inhibitors in heart failure with preserved systolic function. *Eur Heart J* 2000;2(suppl I):I8–I14.

Robert McKelvie
Associate Professor of Medicine
McMaster University, Hamilton, ON, Canada

Competing interests: RM has been paid by AstraZeneca and Bristol-Myers Squibb to serve on steering committees and has been paid by AstraZeneca and Merck Frosst to give presentations.

Peripheral arterial disease

Search date August 2002

Bazian Ltd

QUESTIONS

INTERVENTIONS

To be covered in future updates
Anticoagulation
Beraprost
β Blockers
Buflomedil
Defibrotide
Ginkgo biloba
Improved glycaemic control in people with diabetes
Indobufen
Levocarnitine
Lipid lowering therapy
Naftidrofuryl
Thrombolysis for acute limb ischaemia
Vitamin E

See glossary, p 150

Key Messages

- **Antiplatelet treatment** Systematic reviews have found that antiplatelet agents versus control treatments significantly reduce the rate of major cardiovascular events over about 2 years. Systematic reviews have found that antiplatelet agents versus placebo or no treatments significantly reduce the risk of arterial occlusion and reduce the risk of revascularisation procedures. The balance of benefits and harms is in favour of treatment for most people with symptomatic peripheral arterial disease, because as a group they are at much greater risk of cardiovascular events.
- **Bypass surgery (v percutaneous transluminal angioplasty)** One systematic review found that surgery versus percutaneous transluminal angioplasty significantly improved primary blood vessel patency after 12–24 months, but found no significant difference after 4 years. The review found no significant difference in mortality after 12–24 months. Although the consensus view is that bypass surgery is the most effective treatment for people with debilitating symptomatic peripheral arterial disease, we found inadequate evidence from RCTs reporting long term clinical outcomes to confirm this view.

- **Bypass surgery (*v* thrombolysis in people with acute limb ischaemia)** One systematic review found that surgery versus thrombolysis significantly reduced the risk of ongoing ischaemic pain, but found no significant difference in mortality after 1 year.
- **Cilostazol** RCTs in people with intermittent claudication have found that cilostazol versus placebo significantly improves initial claudication distance and absolute claudication distance measured on a treadmill and significantly reduces the proportion of people with symptoms that do not improve. One RCT with a high withdrawal rate found that pentoxifylline versus cilostazol reduced initial and absolute claudication distance. Adverse effects are common and include headache, diarrhoea, and palpitations.
- **Exercise** Systematic reviews and one subsequent RCT in people with chronic stable claudication have found that regular exercise at least three times weekly versus no exercise significantly improves total walking distance and maximal exercise time after 3–12 months.
- **Pentoxifylline** One systematic review and one subsequent RCT have found insufficient evidence to compare pentoxifylline versus placebo. One RCT found that pentoxifylline reduced absolute claudication distance compared with cilostazol.
- **Percutaneous transluminal angioplasty (transient benefit only)** Two small RCTs in people with mild to moderate intermittent claudication found limited evidence that angioplasty versus no angioplasty significantly improved walking distance after 6 months but found no significant difference after 2 or 6 years. Four RCTs in people with femoral to popliteal artery stenoses have found no significant difference with angioplasty alone versus angioplasty plus stent placement in patency rates, occlusion rates, or clinical improvement.
- **Smoking cessation (based on consensus of opinion)** We found no RCTs of smoking cessation in people with peripheral vascular disease. The consensus view is that smoking cessation improves symptoms in people with intermittent claudication. One systematic review has found observational evidence that continued cigarette smoking by people with intermittent claudication is associated with progression of symptoms, poor prognosis after bypass surgery, amputation, and need for reconstructive surgery.

DEFINITION Peripheral arterial disease arises when there is significant narrowing of arteries distal to the arch of the aorta. Narrowing can arise from atheroma, arteritis, local thrombus formation, or embolisation from the heart or more central arteries. This topic includes treatment options for people with symptoms of reduced blood flow to the leg that are likely to arise from atheroma. These symptoms range from calf pain on exercise (intermittent claudication — see glossary, p 151), to rest pain, skin ulceration, or ischaemic necrosis (gangrene) in people with critical ischaemia.

INCIDENCE/ PREVALENCE Peripheral arterial disease is more common in people aged over 50 years than in younger people, and is more common in men than women. The prevalence of peripheral arterial disease of the legs (assessed by non-invasive tests) is about 3% in people under the age of 60 years, but rises to over 20% in people over 75 years.[1] The overall annual incidence of intermittent claudication is 1.5–2.6/1000 men a year and 1.2–3.6/1000 women a year.[2]

AETIOLOGY/ RISK FACTORS Factors associated with the development of peripheral arterial disease include age, gender, cigarette smoking, diabetes mellitus, hypertension, hyperlipidaemia, obesity, and physical inactivity. The strongest association is with smoking (RR 2.0–4.0) and diabetes (RR 2.0–3.0).[3] Acute limb ischaemia (see glossary, p 150) may result from thrombosis arising within a peripheral artery or from embolic occlusion.

PROGNOSIS The symptoms of intermittent claudication can resolve spontaneously, remain stable over many years, or progress rapidly to critical limb ischaemia (see glossary, p 150). About 15% of people with intermittent claudication eventually develop critical leg ischaemia, which endangers the viability of the limb. The incidence of critical limb ischaemia in Denmark and Italy in 1990 was 0.25–0.45/1000 people a year.[4,5] Coronary heart disease is the major cause of death in people with peripheral arterial disease of the legs. Over 5 years, about 20% of people with intermittent claudication have a non-fatal cardiovascular event (myocardial infarction or stroke).[6] The mortality rate of people with peripheral arterial disease is two to three times higher than that of age and sex matched controls. Overall mortality after the diagnosis of peripheral arterial disease is about 30% after 5 years and 70% after 15 years.[6]

AIMS OF INTERVENTION To reduce symptoms (intermittent claudication), local complications (arterial leg ulcers, critical leg ischaemia), and general complications (myocardial infarction and stroke).

OUTCOMES **Local outcomes:** Proportion of people with adverse outcomes including shorter claudication distance, amputation, or adverse effects of treatment, the mean improvement in claudication distance measured on a treadmill or by some other specified means. **General outcomes:** Rates of myocardial infarction, stroke, and other major cardiovascular events.

METHODS *Clinical Evidence* search and appraisal August 2002.

QUESTION **What are the effects of treatments for people with chronic peripheral arterial disease?**

OPTION **ANTIPLATELET AGENTS**

Systematic reviews have found strong evidence that antiplatelet agents versus control treatments significantly reduce the rate of major cardiovascular events over an average of about 2 years. Systematic reviews have found that antiplatelet agents versus placebo or no treatments significantly reduce the risk of arterial occlusion and the risk of revascularisation procedures. The balance of benefits and harms is in favour of treatment for most people with symptomatic peripheral arterial disease, because as a group they are at much greater risk of cardiovascular events.

Benefits: **Peripheral arterial disease complications:** We found two systematic reviews,[7,8] one of which has subsequently been updated.[9] The first systematic review (search date 1997, 42 RCTs; 9506 people with intermittent claudication [see glossary, p 151], bypass surgery of the leg, or peripheral artery angioplasty) found that antiplatelet treatment compared with no additional treatment significantly reduced the risk of arterial occlusion over 19 months

(RRR 30%; P < 0.00001).[9] The second systematic review (search date 1998, 54 RCTs) found that aspirin versus placebo reduced the number of arterial occlusions and that ticlopidine reduced the risk of revascularisation procedures.[8] **Cardiovascular events:** We found two systematic reviews.[9,10] The first review (search date 1997, 42 RCTs; 9506 people) found that antiplatelet treatment versus control treatment significantly reduced the combined outcome of vascular death, myocardial infarction, or stroke over an average of 2 years (280/4844 [6.0%] with antiplatelet treatment *v* 347/4662 [7%] with control; RR 0.78, 95% CI 0.67 to 0.90; NNT 61, 95% CI 38 to 153).[9] The second systematic review (search date 1999, 39 RCTs) found that antiplatelet treatment versus control significantly reduced the absolute event rate for the combined end point of myocardial infarction, stroke, or vascular death (6.5% with antiplatelet treatment *v* 8.1% with control; OR 0.78, 95% CI 0.63 to 0.96).[10]

Harms: The first review (prior to updating, search date 1990; 35 RCTs; 8098 people with peripheral arterial disease) found no significant difference with antiplatelet treatment versus control treatment in the risk of non-fatal major bleeds (14/2545 [0.55%] *v* 9/2243 [0.40%]; RR 1.37, 95% CI 0.60 to 3.16).[7] The second review (search date 1999, 36 RCTs, 8449 people with peripheral disease) found no significant difference with antiplatelet treatment versus placebo in major bleeding (47/4349 [1%] with antiplatelet treatment *v* 33/4100 [< 1%] with placebo; OR 1.40, 95% CI 0.90 to 2.20), and found no significant difference with aspirin versus other antiplatelet agents in major bleeding (68/3467 [2%] with aspirin *v* 59/3561 [2%] with other antiplatelet agents; RR 1.18, 95% CI 0.84 to 1.67).[10] The number of events was too low to exclude a clinically important increase in major bleeding.[7,10] Across a wide range of people, antiplatelet agents have been found to significantly increase the risk of major haemorrhage (see harms of antiplatelet agents under primary prevention, p 154).

Comment: We found no evidence about the effects of combined clopidogrel and aspirin versus a single antiplatelet agent in people with peripheral arterial disease. Peripheral arterial disease increases the risk of cardiovascular events, so for most people the risk of bleeding is outweighed by the benefits of regular antiplatelet use.

OPTION EXERCISE

Systematic reviews and one subsequent RCT in people with chronic stable claudication have found that regular exercise at least three times weekly versus no exercise significantly improves total walking distance and maximal exercise time after 3–12 months.

Benefits: **Walking exercise versus no exercise:** We found two systematic reviews of exercise versus no exercise in people with chronic stable intermittent claudication (see glossary, p 151) (search dates 1996,[11] and not stated;[12] see comment below). The first review found that exercise programmes (at least 30 min walking as far as claudication permits, at least 3 times weekly, for 3–6 months in people also being treated with surgery, aspirin, or dipyridamole) versus no exercise significantly increased both the initial claudication distance (4 RCTs; 94 people; mean difference 139 m, 95% CI 31 m to 247 m) and the absolute claudication distance (see glossary, p 150) (5 RCTs; 115 people; mean difference 179 m, 95% CI 60 m to 298 m) after 3–12 months.[11] Control treatments were placebo tablets (2 RCTs) or "instructed to continue with normal lifestyle". The second review (10 RCTs, including all those in the first review) found that exercise versus no exercise increased maximal exercise time (3 RCTs; 53 people: WMD 6.5 min, 95% CI 4.4 to 8.7 min).[12] We found one subsequent RCT (52 people), which compared a 24 week programme of initially supervised, regular polestriding (walking exercise using modified ski poles) versus no exercise programme.[13] All participants received standard medical treatment. At 24 weeks, it found that regular exercise significantly increased exercise tolerance compared with no exercise on a controlled work treadmill test (tolerance to exercise, walking at 1.8 miles/h with a 12% gradient: mean increase in exercise duration about 28 min with exercise programme *v* 11 min without exercise programme, $P < 0.0001$).[13] **Different types of exercise:** All the RCTs included in the systematic reviews involved walking exercise. We found one RCT (67 people with moderate to severe intermittent claudication), which compared arm versus leg exercise of similar intensity.[14] A third group of 15 people was given no exercise, but this group was not created by random allocation. The RCT found no significant difference with arm versus leg exercises in improvement in initial claudication distance (improvement in initial claudication distance 122% with arm exercise *v* 93% with leg exercise) and absolute claudication distance (47% with arm exercise *v* 50% with leg exercise) although both groups improved after 6 weeks.

Harms: The reviews and subsequent RCT did not report on harms of the exercise programmes.[11,13,15]

Comment: The RCTs in the systematic reviews had low withdrawal rates and it is unclear whether those assessing the outcomes were blind to the group allocation. Concealment of the allocation to participants was not possible.[11,12] Most (5/6) exercise programmes in the second review occurred under supervision.[12] We found one further systematic review (search date 1993, 21 observational studies or RCTs of exercise, 564 people with peripheral arterial disease).[15] It calculated effects based on the differences in claudication distance after and before exercise treatment, but it made no allowance for any spontaneous improvement that might have occurred in the participants. It reported large increases with exercise in the initial claudication distance (126–351 m) and in the absolute claudication distance (325–723 m), but these estimates were based on observational data. An ongoing Australian RCT is examining the effect of exercise treatment in 1400 men.[12] The benefit from arm exercise remains unconfirmed, but suggests that improved walking may be caused by generally improved cardiovascular function rather than local changes of the peripheral circulation.

OPTION SMOKING CESSATION

RCTs of advice to stop smoking are unlikely to be conducted. The consensus view is that smoking cessation improves symptoms in people with intermittent claudication. One systematic review has found observational evidence that continued cigarette smoking by people with intermittent claudication is associated with progression of symptoms, poor prognosis after bypass surgery, amputation, and need for reconstructive surgery.

Benefits: We found no RCTs.

Harms: We found no RCTs.

Comment: RCTs of advice to stop smoking are unlikely to be conducted, although the consensus view is that smoking cessation improves symptoms in people with intermittent claudication (see glossary, p 151). We found one systematic review (search date 1996; 4 observational studies; 866 people) of advice to quit cigarette smoking versus no advice.[11] One large observational study in the systematic review found no significant increase in absolute claudication distance (see glossary, p 150) after cessation of smoking.[11] Two other studies found conflicting results about the risk of deteriorating from moderate to severe claudication in people who successfully quit smoking compared with current smokers. The fourth study provided no numerical results. Overall, the review found no good evidence to confirm or refute the consensus view that advice to stop smoking improves symptoms in people with intermittent claudication.

OPTION CILOSTAZOL

Five RCTs in people with intermittent claudication have found that cilostazol versus placebo improves initial claudication distance and absolute claudication distance measured on a treadmill and reduces the proportion of people with symptoms that do not improve. One RCT with a high withdrawal rate found that cilostazol increased the proportion of people reporting improvement in claudication distance and improved initial and absolute claudication distance compared with cilostazol. Adverse effects are common and include headache, diarrhoea, and palpitations.

Benefits: We found no systematic review. **Versus placebo:** We found five RCTs comparing cilostazol (200 mg daily) versus placebo (see comment below) (see table 1, p 153).[16–20] Overall, the RCTs found that cilostazol versus placebo reduced the proportion of people who rated their claudication unchanged, worsened, or who were unsure of any change at the end of each trial. They found that cilostazol versus placebo significantly improved the initial claudication distance (by 38–80 m) and the absolute claudication distance (see glossary, p 150) (by 28–84 m). One of the RCTs also evaluated a lower dose of cilostazol (100 mg daily).[20] It found no significant difference between this dose of cilostazol versus placebo for mean maximum walking distance (167 metres with cilostazol 100 mg daily v 141 m with placebo; P = 0.18). **Versus pentoxifylline:** See benefits of pentoxifylline, p 147.

Harms: One recent RCT reported that cilostazol versus placebo significantly increased risk of withdrawal from the trial because of adverse effects or concerns about safety (39/227 [17%] with cilostazol *v* 24/239 [10%] with placebo; RR 1.71, 95% CI 1.06 to 2.75; NNH 14, 95% CI 8 to 111).[16] Adverse effects of cilostazol included headache (28% *v* 12% with placebo), diarrhoea (19% *v* 8%), abnormal stools (15% *v* 5%), palpitations (17% *v* 2%), and dizziness.[16–20] Cilostazol is a phosphodiesterase inhibitor; RCTs have found that other phosphodiesterase inhibitors (milrinone, vesnarinone) are associated with increased mortality in people with heart failure. However, results aggregated from other studies have not found an excess of cardiovascular events with cilostazol.[21]

Comment: Although the overall results of cilostazol versus placebo indicate a significant effect of cilostazol on increasing walking distance, the RCTs have some weakness of their methods, which may limit the applicability of the results.[16–19] Firstly, none of the RCTs evaluated cilostazol beyond 24 weeks. In addition, the RCTs all had high withdrawal rates after randomisation (up to 29%).[17] All the RCTs found that withdrawals were more common with cilostazol than placebo.[16–19] To allow for these problems, the authors performed an intention to treat analysis using "last available observation carried forward". However, the analysis did not include people with no observations to carry forward, and the effects of the difference in withdrawals between the groups was not explored adequately. If people with worsening claudication were more likely to withdraw, then the observed differences might have been artefactual. We found one further trial written in Chinese, which compared cilostazol versus dipyridamole in 32 people with peripheral vascular disease and type 2 diabetes.[22] This study is awaiting translation and appraisal for inclusion in *Clinical Evidence*. Although cilostazol appears promising, the balance of its benefits and harms remains unclear.

OPTION PENTOXIFYLLINE

One systematic review and one subsequent RCT have found insufficient evidence to compare pentoxifylline versus placebo. One RCT found that pentoxifylline reduced absolute claudication distance compared with cilostazol.

Benefits: We found one systematic review (search date 1999)[23] and one subsequent RCT.[16] The review found two RCTs (192 people) that met its reliability criteria for inclusion, but did not pool results. Both RCTs found no significant difference between pentoxifylline versus placebo for change in pain free walking distance or maximum walking distance (follow up time not stated; improvement in mean pain free walking distance for pentoxifylline *v* placebo 15 m, 95% CI –5 to +35 m and –30 m, 95% CI –138 to +78 m; improvement in mean maximum walking distance +21 m, 95% CI –10 to +52 m and +69 m, 95% CI –44 to 182 m).[23] The subsequent RCT (438 people; see comment below) similarly found no significant difference with pentoxifylline versus placebo in the proportion of people who had no change or deterioration in the claudication distance (72/212 [34%] with pentoxifylline *v* 68/226 [30%] with placebo;

RR 1.13, 95% CI 0.86 to 1.48).[16] **Versus cilostazol:** The subsequent RCT (see comment below) found that pentoxifylline versus cilostazol significantly increased the proprotion of people who had no change or deterioration in the claudication distance (72/212 [34%] with pentoxifylline *v* 47/205 [23%] with cilostazol; RR 1.48, 95% CI 1.08 to 2.03; ARR 11%, 95% CI 2.4% to 20%; NNT 9, 95% CI 5 to 42), the initial claudication distance (202 m with pentoxifylline *v* 218 m with cilostazol; mean difference –16 m; P = 0.0001), and the absolute claudication distance (see glossary, p 150) (308 m with pentoxifylline *v* 350 m with cilostazol; mean difference –42 m; P = 0.0005) after 24 weeks.[16]

Harms: The subsequent RCT found that pentoxifylline versus placebo significantly increased the risk of withdrawal from the RCT because of adverse effects or concerns about safety (44/232 [19%] with pentoxifylline *v* 24/239 [10%] with placebo; RR 1.89, 95% CI 1.19 to 3.00; NNH 12, 95% CI 7 to 39).[16] Side effects of pentoxifylline included sore throat (14% *v* 7%), dyspepsia, nausea, diarrhoea (8% *v* 5% with placebo; P = 0.31), and vomiting.[16] No life threatening adverse effects of pentoxifylline have been reported, although RCTs have been too small to date to assess this reliably.

Comment: Results from the subsequent RCT[16] have been published in many articles without stating clearly whether any contain additional results.[17–19] The subsequent RCT had a high withdrawal rate after randomisation, which could be a source of bias (60/232 [26%] with pentoxifylline *v* 61/237 [26%] with cilostazol).

OPTION PERCUTANEOUS TRANSLUMINAL ANGIOPLASTY

Two small RCTs in people with mild to moderate intermittent claudication found limited evidence that percutaneous angioplasty versus no angioplasty significantly improved walking distance after 6 months but found no significant difference after 2 or 6 years. Four RCTs in people with femoral to popliteal artery stenoses have found no significant difference with angioplasty alone versus angioplasty plus stent placement in patency rates, occlusion rates, or clinical improvement. The RCTs may lack power to rule out an important clinical effect.

Benefits: **Percutaneous transluminal angioplasty (PTA) versus no PTA:** We found one systematic review (search date not stated; 2 RCTs; 78 men and 20 women with mild to moderate intermittent claudication [see glossary, p 151]) of PTA of the aortoiliac or femoral-popliteal arteries versus no angioplasty.[24] The first RCT identified by the review found that PTA versus no PTA significantly increased the median claudication distance after 6 months (667 m *v* 172 m; P < 0.05), but found no significant difference in median claudication distance or quality of life after 2 years.[25] The second RCT found that PTA versus an exercise programme significantly increased the absolute claudication distance (see glossary, p 150) at 6 months (130 m *v* 50 m; WMD 80 m), but found no significant difference in absolute claudication distance after 6 years (180 m *v* 130 m; WMD 50 m; P > 0.05).[26,27] **PTA versus PTA plus stents:** We found no systematic review, but found five RCTs.[28–32] One RCT (279 people with intermittent claudication and iliac artery stenosis) compared

PTA plus routine stent placement versus PTA plus selective stent placement.[28] It found no significant difference in short or long term patency rates. The other four RCTs included people with femoral to popliteal artery stenoses and compared PTA plus stent placement versus PTA alone.[29–32] The first of these four RCTs (51 people) found no significant differences in patency assessed by colour flow duplex ultrasound (62% with PTA plus stent *v* 74% with PTA alone; P = 0.22) or in the occlusion rate (5/24 [21%] with PTA plus stent *v* 7% [2/27] with PTA alone; P = 0.16).[29] The second RCT (53 people) found no significant difference in primary patency after 34 months' follow up (62% with PTA plus stent placement *v* 68.4% with PTA). The third RCT (32 people) found no significant difference in "clinical improvement" after 1 year (60% with PTA plus stent placement *v* 71% with PTA; P = 0.17).[32] The fourth RCT (141 people, 154 limbs) found no significant difference in primary patency as determined by angiography after 1 year (63% of limbs with PTA plus stent placement *v* 63% with PTA).[30] **PTA versus surgery:** See surgery option, p 149.

Harms: Prospective cohort studies have found that PTA complications include puncture site major bleeding (3.4%), pseudoaneurysms (0.5%), limb loss (0.2%), renal failure secondary to intravenous contrast (0.2%), cardiac complications such as myocardial infarction (0.2%), and death (0.2%).[33,34]

Comment: This limited evidence suggests transient benefit from angioplasty versus no angioplasty. The longer term effects of angioplasty or stent placement on symptoms, bypass surgery, and amputation remain unclear and the available RCTs are to small to rule out clinically important effects of stent placement. The long term patency of femoral–popliteal angioplasties is poor, and there is no evidence that the addition of stents confers any additional benefit.[30–32]

OPTION BYPASS SURGERY

One systematic review found that surgery versus percutaneous transluminal angioplasty in people with chronic progressive peripheral arterial disease significantly improved primary patency after 12–24 months, but found no significant difference after 4 years. The review found no significant difference in mortality after 12–24 months. One systematic review found that surgery versus thrombolysis significantly reduced the number of amputations and the number of people reporting ongoing ischaemic pain, but found no significant difference in mortality after 1 year. Although the consensus view is that bypass surgery is the most effective treatment for people with debilitating symptomatic peripheral arterial disease, we found inadequate evidence from RCTs reporting long term clinical outcomes to confirm this view.

Benefits: **Surgery versus exercise:** We found no RCTs (see comment below). **Surgery versus percutaneous transluminal angioplasty (PTA):** We found one systematic review (search date 2001, 2 RCTs, 365 people with chronic progressive peripheral arterial disease), which found no significant difference with surgery versus PTA in mortality after 12–24 months (OR 1.08,

95% CI 0.61 to 1.89).[35] The review found that surgery versus PTA significantly improved patency after 12–24 months (OR 0.62, 95% CI 0.39 to 0.99), but found no significant difference in primary patency after 4 years (P = 0.14). The review found no significant difference in mortality or amputation rates. **Surgery versus thrombolysis:** We found one systematic review (search date 2001, 1 RCT in people with acute limb ischaemia (see glossary, p 150)), which compared surgery versus thrombolysis using tissue plasminogen activator or urokinase.[35] The review found no significant difference in mortality after 1 year (OR 1.59, 95% CI 0.70 to 3.59). The review found that surgery versus thrombolysis significantly reduced the number of amputations (OR 0.19, 95% CI 0.06 to 0.59) and significantly reduced the number of people reporting ongoing ischaemic pain (OR 0.30, 95% CI 0.17 to 0.50) after 1 year. **Surgery versus PTA plus stent placement:** We found no RCTs of surgery versus PTA plus stent placement that reported long term outcomes.

Harms: Surgery versus PTA increased early procedural complications. Among people having aortoiliac surgery, perioperative mortality (within 30 days of the procedure) was 3.3%, and complications having a major health impact occurred in 8.3%.[36] Among people having infrainguinal bypass surgery, perioperative mortality was about 2% and serious complications occurred in 8%.[37] Among people having PTA with or without stent placement, perioperative mortality was about 1% and serious complications occurred in about 5%.[38]

Comment: The RCTs are small, have different follow up periods, and assessed different outcomes. Indirect comparisons from observational studies of proxy outcomes (primary patency rates) suggest that for aortoiliac stenosis or occlusion, greater patency rates 5 years after intervention are achieved with surgery (6250 [89%] people) compared with PTA (1300 [34–85%] people) or compared with combined PTA and stent placement (816 [54–74%] people).[32–34] Too few people with infrainguinal lesions were included in the RCTs to provide good evidence about surgical management. Indirect comparisons of proxy outcomes in people with infrainguinal lesions suggest worse results after PTA (after 5 years patency 38%, range 34–42%) compared with surgery (patency 80%).[39] Although the consensus view is that bypass surgery is the most effective treatment for people with debilitating symptomatic peripheral arterial disease, we found inadequate evidence from RCTs reporting long term clinical outcomes to confirm this view.

GLOSSARY

Absolute claudication distance Also known as the total walking distance; the maximum distance a person can walk before stopping.

Acute limb ischaemia An ischaemic process that threatens the viability of the limb, and is associated with pain, neurological deficit, inadequate skin capillary circulation, and/or inaudible arterial flow signals by Doppler examination. This acute process often leads to hospitalisation.

Critical limb ischaemia results in a breakdown of the skin (ulceration or gangrene) or pain in the foot at rest. Critical limb ischaemia corresponds to the Fontaine classification III and IV (see below).

Fontaine's classification I: asymptomatic; II: intermittent claudication (see below); II-a: pain free, claudication walking more than 200 metres; II-b: pain free, claudication walking less than 200 metres; III: rest/nocturnal pain; IV: necrosis/gangrene.

Initial claudication distance The distance a person can walk before the onset of claudication symptoms.

Intermittent claudication Pain, stiffness, or weakness in the leg that develops on walking, intensifies with continued walking until further walking is impossible, and is relieved by rest.

REFERENCES

1. Fowkes FGR, Housely E, Cawood EH, et al. Edinburgh Artery Study: prevalence of asymptomatic and symptomatic peripheral arterial disease in the general population. *Int J Epidemiol* 1991;20:384–392.
2. Kannel WB, McGee DL. Update on some epidemiological features of intermittent claudication. *J Am Geriatr Soc* 1985;33:13–18.
3. Maurabito JM, D'Agostino RB, Sibersschatz, et al. Intermittent claudication: a risk profile from the Framingham Heart Study. *Circulation* 1997;96:44–49.
4. Catalano M. Epidemiology of critical limb ischemia: north Italian data. *Eur J Med* 1993;2:11–14.
5. Ebskov L, Schroeder T, Holstein P. Epidemiology of leg amputation: the influence of vascular surgery. *Br J Surg* 1994:81:1600–1603.
6. Leng GC, Lee AJ, Fowkes FG, et al. Incidence, natural history and cardiovascular events in symptomatic and asymptomatic peripheral arterial disease in the general population. *Int J Epidemiol* 1996;25:1172–1181.
7. Antiplatelet Trialists' Collaborative overview of randomized trials of antiplatelet therapy. Collaborative meta-analysis of randomised controlled trials of antiplatelet therapy for prevention of death, myocardial infarction, and stroke in high risk patients. *BMJ* 2002;324:71–8. Search date 1997; primary sources Medline, Embase, Derwent, Scisearch, and Bioisis; in addition trials registers of Cochrane Stroke and Peripheral Vascular Diseases Group, hand searches of journals, abstracts and conference proceedings, and contact with experts.
8. Girolami B, Bernardi E, Prins MH, et al. Antithrombotic drugs in the primary medical management of intermittent claudication: a meta-analysis. *Thromb Haemost* 1999;81:715–722. Search date 1998; primary sources Medline and hand searches.
9. Antithrombotic, Trialists' Collaboration Collaborative meta-analysis of randomised trials of antiplatelet therapy for prevention of death, myocardial infarction, and stroke in high risk patients. *BMJ* 2002; 324:71–86. Search date 1997; primary sources Medline, Embase, Derwent, Scisearch, Biosis, the Cochrane Stroke and Peripheral Vascular Disease Group Registers, handsearching of journals, abstracts, and proceedings of meetings, reference lists of trials and review articles, and personal contact with colleagues, including representatives of pharmaceutical companies.
10. Robless P, Mikhailidis D, Stansby G. Systematic review of antiplatelet therapy for the prevention of myocaridial infarction, stroke, or vascular death in patients with peripheral vascular disease. *Br J Surg* 2001;88:787–800. Search date January 1999; primary sources Medline, Embase, Antiplatelet Trialists Collaboration register of trials, Cochrane Controlled Trials Register, proceedings from vascular surgical society meetings (Vascular Surgical Society of Great Britain and Ireland, European Vascular Surgical Society, North American Society of Vascular Surgery), contact with pharmaceutical companies that market antiplatelet agents for details of any trials (Bristol Myers Squibb, Sanofi Winthrop).
11. Girolami B, Bernardi E, Prins M, et al. Treatment of intermittent claudication with physical training, smoking cessation, pentoxifylline, or nafronyl: a meta-analysis. *Arch Intern Med* 1999;159:337–345. Search date 1996; primary sources Medline and hand searches of reference lists.
12. Leng GC, Fowler B, Ernst E. Exercise for intermittent claudication In: The Cochrane Library, Issue 3, 2000. Oxford: Update Software. Search date not stated; primary sources Cochrane Peripheral Vascular Diseases Group trials register, Embase, reference lists of relevant articles, and personal contact with principal investigators of trials.
13. Langbein WE, Collins EG, Orebaugh C, et al. Increasing exercise tolerance of persons limited by claudication pain using polestriding. *J Vasc Surg* 2002;35:887–893.
14. Walker RD, Nawaz S, Wilkinson CH, et al. Influence of upper- and lower-limb exercise training on cardiovascular function and walking distances in patients with intermittent claudication. *J Vasc Surg* 2000;31:662–669.
15. Gardner A, Poehlman E. Exercise rehabilitation programs for the treatment of claudication pain. *JAMA* 1995;274:975–980. Search date 1993; primary sources Medline and hand searches of bibliographies of reviews, textbooks, and studies located through the computer search.
16. Dawson DL, Cutler BS, Hiatt WR, et al. A comparison of cilostazol and pentoxifylline for treating intermittent claudication. *Am J Med* 2000;109:523–530.
17. Money SR, Herd A, Isaacsohn JL, et al. Effect of cilostazol on walking distances in patients with intermittent claudication cause by peripheral vascular disease. *J Vasc Surg* 1998;27:267–275.
18. Beebe HG, Dawson D, Cutler B, et al. A new pharmacological treatment for intermittent claudication. *Arch Intern Med* 1999;159:2041–2050.
19. Dawson D, Cutler B, Meeisner M, et al. Cilostazol has beneficial effects in treatment of intermittent claudication. *Circulation* 1998;98:678–686.
20. Strandness DE, Dalman RL, Panian S, et al. Effect of cilostazol in patients with intermittent claudication: A randomized, double-blind, placebo controlled study. *Vasc Endovasc Surg* 2002;36:83–91.
21. Hiatt WR. Medical treatment of peripheral arterial disease and claudication. *N Engl J Med* 2001;344:1608–1621.

22. Yuan G-H, Gao Y, Feng Q, et al. Clinical evaluation of cilostazol in treatment of peripheral vascular disease with type 2 diabetes. *Chin J Clin Pharmacol* 1999;15:425–430.
23. De Backer TL, Vander Stichele RH, Warie HH, et al. Oral vasoactive medication in intermittent claudication: utile or futile? *Eur J Clin Pharmacol* 2000;56:199–206. Search date 1999; primary sources Medline, International Pharmaceutical Abstracts, the Cochrane Library, direct contact with marketing companies and key authors, snowballing and Science Citation Index search.
24. Fowkes FG, Gillespie IN. Angioplasty (versus non surgical management) for intermittent claudication. In: The Cochrane Library, Issue 3, 2002. Oxford: Update Software. Search date not stated; primary sources Cochrane Peripheral Vascular Diseases Group Trials Register, Embase, reference lists of relevant articles and conference proceedings, and personal contact with principal investigators of trials.
25. Whyman MR, Fowkes FGR, Kerracher EMG, et al. Randomized controlled trial of percutaneous transluminal angioplasty for intermittent claudication. *Eur J Vasc Endovasc Surg* 1996;12:167–172.
26. Creasy TS, McMillan PJ, Fletcher EWL, et al. Is percutaneous transluminal angioplasty better than exercise for claudication? Preliminary results of a prospective randomized trial. *Eur J Vasc Surg* 1990;4:135–140.
27. Perkins JMT, Collin J, Creasy TS, et al. Exercise training versus angioplasty for stable claudication. Long and medium term results of a prospective, randomized trial. *Eur J Vasc Endovasc Surg* 1996;11:409–413.
28. Teteroo E, van der Graef Y, Bosch J, et al. Randomized comparison of primary stent placement versus primary angioplasty followed by selective stent placement in patients with iliac artery occlusive disease. *Lancet* 1998;351:1153–1159.
29. Vroegindeweij D, Vos L, Tielbeek A, et al. Balloon angioplasty combined with primary stenting versus balloon angioplasty alone in femoropopliteal obstructions: a comparative randomized study. *Cardiovasc Intervent Radiol* 1997;20:420–425.
30. Cejna M, Thurnher S, Illiasch H, et al. PTA versus palmaz stent placement in femeropopliteal artery obstructions: a multicenter prospective randomised study. *J Vasc Interv Radiol* 2001;12:23–31.
31. Grimm J, Muller-Hulsbeck S, Jahnke T, et al. Randomized study to compare PTA alone versus PTA with Palmaz stent placement for femoropopliteal lesions. *J Vasc Interv Radiol* 200;12:935–42.
32. Zdanowski Z, Albrechtsson U, Lundin A, et al. Percutaneous transluminal angioplasty with or without stenting for femoropopliteal occlusions? A randomized controlled study. *Int Angiol* 1999;18:251–5.
33. Becker GJ, Katzen BT, Dake MD. Noncoronary angioplasty. *Radiology* 1989;170:921–940.
34. Matsi PJ, Manninen HI. Complications of lower-limb percutaneous transluminal angioplasty: a prospective analysis of 410 procedures on 295 consecutive patients. *Cardiovasc Intervent Radiol* 1998;21:361–366.
35. Leng GC, Davis M, Baker D. Bypass surgery for chronic lower limb ischemia. Cochrane Library Issue 2, 2002. Oxford: Update Software. Search date 2001; primary sources Cochrane Peripheral Vascular Diseases Group Trials Register, Medline, Embase, reference lists of various articles and contact with trial investigators.
36. De Vries SO, Hunink MG. Results of aortic bifurcation grafts for aortoiliac occlusive disease: a meta-analysis. *J Vasc Surg* 1997;26:558–569. Search date 1996; primary sources Medline and hand searches of review articles, original studies, and a vascular surgery textbook.
37. Johnston KW, Rae M, Hogg-Johnston SA, et al. Five-year results of a prospective study of percutaneous transluminal angioplasty. *Ann Surg* 1987;206:403–413.
38. Bosch J, Hunink M. Meta-analysis of the results of percutaneous transluminal angioplasty and stent placement for aortoiliac occlusive disease. *Radiology* 1997;204:87–96. Search date not stated; primary sources Medline and hand searches of reference lists.
39. Johnson KW. Femoral and popliteal arteries: reanalysis of results of balloon angioplasty. *Radiology* 1992;183:767–771.

Bazian Ltd
London
UK

Competing interests: None declared.

TABLE 1 Cilostazol 200 mg daily versus placebo (see text pp 146, 147).

Ref	Duration (weeks)	Number of people: Randomised	Protocol violation	Withdrawn	People self rated as worsened, unchanged, or unsure	Absolute claudication distance (m)	Initial claudication distance (m)
16	24	466	35	64	47/205 (23%) *v* 68/226 (30%); RR 0.76 (95% CI 0.55 to 1.05)	350 *v* 300 (P < 0.001)	218 *v* 180 (P = 0.02)
17	16	298	59	27	53/119 (45%) *v* 78/120 (65%); RR 0.68 (95% CI 0.54 to 0.87)	333 *v* 281	NA
18	24	516	23	75	80/171 (47%) *v* 106/169 (63%); RR 0.75 (95% CI 0.61 to 0.91)	259 *v* 175 (P < 0.001)	138 *v* 96 (P < 0.001)
19	12	81	4	15	27/54 (50%) *v* 22/27 (81%); RR 0.61 (95% CI 0.45 to 0.85)	113 *v* 85 (P = 0.007)	232 *v* 152 (P = 0.002)
20	24	394*	17	59	N/A	196 *v* 141 (P=0.0003)	N/A

*133 people allocated to 200 mg cilostazol daily; 132 allocated to cilostazol 100 mg daily; 129 allocated to placebo. Results presented only for comparison between high dose cilostazol v placebo;
m, metres; NA, not available; Ref, reference.

Primary prevention

Search date November 2002

Charles Foster, Michael Murphy, Julian J Nicholas, Michael Pignone, and Bazian Ltd

QUESTIONS

INTERVENTIONS

Covered elsewhere in *Clinical Evidence*

See prevention of cardiovascular events in diabetes, p 690

Clin Evid 2003;10:154–187.

Key Messages

Exercise

- **Physical activity** One RCT and many observational studies have found that moderate to high physical activity reduces coronary heart disease and stroke. They also found that sudden death soon after strenuous exercise was rare, more common in sedentary people, and did not outweigh the benefits.

Diet

- **Eating more fruit and vegetables** Observational studies found limited evidence that eating fruit and vegetables reduces ischaemic heart disease and stroke. The size and nature of effects are uncertain.
- **Antioxidants (other than β carotene and vitamin E)** We found insufficient evidence on the effects of vitamin C, copper, zinc, manganese, or flavonoids.
- **β Carotene** Systematic reviews of RCTs found no evidence of benefit from β carotene supplements, and RCTs suggest that they may be harmful.
- **Vitamin E** Systematic reviews of RCTs found no evidence of benefit from vitamin E supplements, and RCTs suggest that they may be harmful.

Smoking

- **Smoking cessation** We found no direct evidence from RCTs that advice to stop smoking reduces cardiovascular risk compared with no advice. However, we found robust evidence from observational studies that smoking is an important risk factor for overall mortality, coronary heart disease, and stroke, and that smoking cessation should therefore be encouraged. The evidence is strongest for stroke.

Antithrombotic drugs

- **Anticoagulant treatment (warfarin)** One RCT found that the benefits and harms of oral anticoagulation (to a target international normalised ratio of 1.5) among people without symptoms of cardiovascular disease were finely balanced, and that net effects were uncertain.
- **Aspirin in low risk people** We found insufficient evidence to identify which asymptomatic individuals would benefit overall and which would be harmed by regular treatment with aspirin. Benefits are likely to outweigh risks in people at higher risk.

Interventions aimed at lowering blood pressure

- **Antihypertensive drug treatments in people with hypertension** Systematic reviews have found that initial treatment with diuretics, angiotensin converting enzyme inhibitors, or β blockers reduce morbidity and mortality compared with placebo, with minimal adverse effects. RCTs found no significant differences in morbidity or mortality among these agents. We found limited evidence from two systematic reviews that diuretics, β blockers, and angiotensin converting enzyme inhibitors reduced coronary heart disease and heart failure more than calcium channel antagonists. However, calcium channel antagonists reduced risk of stroke more than the other agents. One RCT found that a thiazide diuretic reduced cardiovascular events, particularly congestive heart failure, compared with an α blocker. One RCT found that losartan (an angiotensin receptor blocker) reduced cardiovascular events compared with atenolol in people with hypertension and left ventricular hypertrophy.

- **Diuretics in high risk people** Systematic reviews have found that diuretics decrease the risk of fatal and non-fatal stroke, cardiac events, and total mortality compared with placebo. The biggest benefit is seen in people with the highest baseline risk. Systematic reviews have found no significant difference in mortality or morbidity between diuretics and β blockers.
- **Dietary salt restriction** We found no RCTs of the effects of salt restriction on morbidity or mortality. One systematic review has found that a low salt diet may lead to modest reductions in blood pressure compared with a usual diet, with more benefit in people older than 45 years than in younger people.
- **Fish oil supplementation** We found no RCTs examining the effects of fish oil supplementation on morbidity or mortality in people with primary hypertension. One systematic review has found that fish oil supplementation in large doses of 3 g daily modestly lowers blood pressure.
- **Low fat, high fruit and vegetable diet** We found no systematic review and no RCTs examining the effects of low fat, high fruit and vegetable diet on morbidity or mortality of people with raised blood pressure. One RCT found that a low fat, high fruit and vegetable diet modestly reduced blood pressure compared with control diet.
- **Physical activity** We found no RCTs in people with primary hypertension examining the effects of exercise on morbidity or mortality. One systematic review has found that aerobic exercise reduces blood pressure compared with no exercise.
- **Potassium supplementation** We found no RCTs examining the effects of potassium supplementation on morbidity or mortality in people with primary hypertension. One systematic review has found that a daily potassium supplementation of about 60 mmol (2 g, which is about the amount contained in 5 bananas) reduces blood pressure by small amounts.
- **Smoking cessation** Observational studies have found that smoking is a risk factor for cardiovascular disease. We found no direct evidence in people with hypertension that stopping smoking decreases blood pressure.
- **Weight loss** We found no RCTs examining the effects of weight loss on morbidity and mortality. One systematic review and additional RCTs have found that modest weight reduction in obese people with hypertension leads to a modest reduction in blood pressure.
- **Calcium supplementation** We found insufficient evidence about the effects of calcium supplementation on blood pressure, morbidity, or mortality specifically in people with hypertension. One systematic review in people with and without hypertension found that calcium supplementation may reduce systolic blood pressure by a small amount.
- **Magnesium supplementation** We found no RCTs examining the effects of magnesium supplementation on morbidity or mortality in people with hypertension. We found limited and conflicting evidence on the effect of magnesium supplementation on blood pressure in people with hypertension and normal magnesium concentrations.
- **Reduced alcohol consumption** We found no RCTs examining the effects of reducing alcohol consumption on morbidity or mortality. One systematic review in moderate drinkers (25–50 drinks/week) found inconclusive evidence regarding effects of alcohol reduction on blood pressure.

Interventions aimed at lowering cholesterol

- **Cholesterol reduction in high risk people** Systematic reviews have found that reducing cholesterol concentration in asymptomatic people lowers the rate of cardiovascular events. RCTs have found that the magnitude of the benefit is related to an individual's baseline risk of cardiovascular events, and to the degree of cholesterol lowering, rather than to the individual's cholesterol concentration.
- **Low fat diet** Systematic reviews and RCTs have found that combined use of cholesterol lowering diet and lipid lowering drugs reduces cholesterol concentration more than lifestyle interventions alone.

DEFINITION Primary prevention in this context is the long term management of people at increased risk but with no evidence of cardiovascular disease. Clinically overt ischaemic vascular disease includes acute myocardial infarction, angina, stroke, and peripheral vascular disease. Many adults have no symptoms or obvious signs of vascular disease, even though they have atheroma and are at increased risk of ischaemic vascular events because of one or more risk factors (see aetiology below). In this topic, we have taken primary prevention to apply to people who have not had clinically overt cardiovascular disease, or people at low risk of ischaemic cardiovascular events. Prevention of cerebrovascular events is discussed in detail elsewhere in *Clinical Evidence* (see stroke prevention topic, p 246).

INCIDENCE/ PREVALENCE According to the World Health Report 1999, ischaemic heart disease was the leading single cause for death in the world, the leading single cause for death in high income countries, and second to lower respiratory tract infections in low and middle income countries. In 1998 it was still the leading cause for death, with nearly 7.4 million estimated deaths a year in member states of the World Health Organization. This condition had the eighth highest burden of disease in the low and middle income countries (30.7 million disability adjusted life years).[1]

AETIOLOGY/ RISK FACTORS Identified major risk factors for ischaemic vascular disease include increasing age, male sex, raised low density lipoprotein cholesterol, reduced high density lipoprotein cholesterol, raised blood pressure, smoking, diabetes, family history of cardiovascular disease, obesity, and sedentary lifestyle. For many of these risk factors, observational studies show a continuous gradient of increasing risk of cardiovascular disease with increasing levels of the risk factor, with no obvious threshold level. Although by definition event rates are higher in high risk people, most ischaemic vascular events that occur in the population are in people with intermediate levels of absolute risk because there are many more of them than there are people at high risk; see Appendix 1.[2]

PROGNOSIS A study carried out in Scotland found that about half of people who suffer an acute myocardial infarction die within 28 days, and two thirds of acute myocardial infarctions occur before the person reaches hospital.[3] The benefits of intervention in unselected people with no evidence of cardiovascular disease (primary prevention) are small because in such people the baseline risk is small. However, absolute risk of ischaemic vascular events varies widely, even among people with similar levels of blood pressure or cholesterol. Estimates of absolute risk can be based on simple risk equations or tables; see Appendix 1.[4,5]

AIMS OF INTERVENTION To reduce morbidity and mortality from cardiovascular disease, with minimum adverse effects.

OUTCOMES Incidence of fatal and non-fatal cardiovascular events (including coronary, cerebrovascular, renal, and eye disease, and heart failure). Surrogate outcomes include changes in levels of individual risk factors, such as blood pressure.

METHODS *Clinical Evidence* search and appraisal November 2002.

QUESTION **Does physical activity reduce the risk of vascular events in asymptomatic people?**

Charles Foster and Michael Murphy

We found one RCT and strong observational evidence that moderate to high levels of physical activity reduce the risk of non-fatal and fatal coronary heart disease and stroke. People who are physically active (those who undertake moderate levels of activity daily or almost daily, e.g. walking) typically experience 30–50% reductions in relative risk of coronary heart disease compared with people who are sedentary after adjustment for other risk factors. The absolute risk of sudden death after strenuous activity is small (although greatest in people who are habitually sedentary) and does not outweigh observed benefits.

Benefits: **Effects of physical activity on coronary heart disease:** One systematic review (search date 2001)[6] identified one RCT (196 women aged 50–65 years with no previous heart disease). The RCT found that an exercise programme consisting of regular walking significantly reduced coronary heart disease (CHD) compared with no exercise programme at 10 years (RR for participants reporting that their physician had diagnosed heart disease 0.18, 95% CI 0.04 to 0.80). The systematic review also identified 11 further observational studies, although it was not clear that they were only in people with no previous heart disease (see comment below). This systematic review[6] and three further systematic reviews (search dates 1995[7] and not stated[8,9]) evaluated observational studies and found increased risk of CHD in sedentary compared with active people. Since 1992, 17 large, well conducted prospective, non-randomised studies, with follow up periods ranging from 18 months to 29 years, have specifically examined the association between physical activity and risk of non-fatal or fatal CHD.[10–26] The studies found that risk declined with increasing levels of physical activity (for examples of activity levels see table 1, p 184) (AR for CHD death in people with sedentary lives [rare or no physical activity] 70/10 000 person-years *v* 40/10 000 person-years in people with the highest level of activity [> 3500 kcal/week]; absolute benefit of high levels of physical activity 30 lives saved/10 000 person-years). One subsequent observational study of women found that at least 1 hour of walking a week predicted lower risk compared with no walking a week (OR 0.49, 95% CI 0.28 to 0.86).[27] **Effects of physical fitness on coronary heart disease:** We found no RCTs. One systematic review (search date not stated)[28] identified seven large, well designed, prospective, non-randomised studies of the effects of physical fitness on CHD. All used reproducible measures of physical fitness. Five studies adjusted for other CHD risk factors. These found an increased risk of death from CHD in people with low levels of physical fitness compared with those with high levels (RR of death lowest quartile *v* highest quartile ranged from 1.2–4.0). Most studies reported only baseline measures of physical fitness and thus not could assess effects of changes in fitness. One large follow up study found lower risk among people who increased their fitness level (RR for cardiovascular disease death compared with those whose level of fitness did not change 0.48, 95% CI 0.31 to 0.74).[29] One study showed that high fitness levels seem to slow down the development of atherosclerosis compared with lower levels of fitness.[30] A new meta-analysis examining fitness and activity as separate risk factors for CHD concluded that being unfit warrants consideration as a risk factor.[31] **Effects of physical activity on stroke:** We found no RCTs and no systematic review of observational studies. We found 12 observational studies (published between 1990 and 1999), based on people with a total of 3680 strokes among North American, Japanese, and European populations.[32–45] Most of these found that moderate activity was associated with reduced risk of stroke compared with inactivity (RR of stroke, moderate activity *v* inactivity about 0.5). One cohort study from Japan found that "heavy" physical activity reduced the risk of stroke compared with "moderate" activity (RR of stroke, "heavy" *v* "moderate" activity about 0.3; $P < 0.05$).[43] In most studies, the benefits were greater in older people and in men. Most studies were conducted in white men in late middle age, which potentially limits their applicability to other groups of people. The results usually persisted after adjustment for other known risk factors for stroke (blood pressure, blood lipids, body mass index, and smoking) and after exclusion of people with pre-existing diseases that might limit physical activity and increase risk of stroke. The more recent studies found maximum reduction in the risk of stroke with moderate as opposed to high levels of physical exercise levels. See stroke prevention topic, p 246.

Harms: The identified studies provided no direct evidence of harm from exercise. Injury is likely to be the most common adverse event, but we found too few population data to measure its risk. We found two studies in people who had experienced non-fatal myocardial infarction, conducted in the USA and Germany. Each involved more than 1000 events and found that 4–7% of these events occurred within 1 hour of strenuous physical activity.[46–48] Strenuous activity was estimated to have raised the relative risk of acute myocardial infarction between two- and sixfold in the hour after activity, with risks returning to baseline after that. However, the absolute risk remained low, variously estimated at six deaths per 100 000 middle aged men a year[49] or 0.3–2.7 events per 10 000 person-hours of exercise.[50] Both studies found that the relative risk of acute myocardial infarction after strenuous activity was much higher in people who were habitually sedentary (RR 107, 95% CI 67 to 171) compared with the relative risk in those who engaged in heavy physical exertion on five or more occasions a week (RR 2.4, 95% CI 1.5 to 3.7).[47]

Comment: The most recent systematic review (search date 2001) also identified nine prospective cohort studies and two case-control studies in about 20 000 older adults, mostly men.[6] It reported that increased physical activity or cardiovascular fitness significantly reduced CHD in five out of 11 studies, and non-significantly reduced CHD in three further studies.[6] Findings from observational studies identified by all the reviews should be interpreted with caution. The studies varied in definitions of levels of activity and fitness. The level of activity or fitness experienced by each person was not experimentally assigned by an investigator (as in an RCT) but resulted from self selection. Active (or fit) people are likely to differ from inactive (or unfit) people in other ways that also influence their risk of cardiovascular disease. Confounding of this type can be partially controlled by adjustment for other known risk factors (such as age, smoking status, and body mass index), but it is likely that some residual confounding will remain, which could overestimate the effect of exercise. The studies have found that the absolute risk of sudden death during or immediately after physical activity is small and does not outweigh the observed benefits.

QUESTION What intensity and frequency of physical activity improves fitness?

Charles Foster and Michael Murphy

Small RCTs found that at least moderate intensity exercise (equivalent to brisk walking) is necessary to improve fitness. We found insufficient evidence on the effects of short bouts of exercise several times daily compared with longer daily bouts.

Benefits: **Intensity:** We found no systematic review. Numerous small RCTs of varying quality have been conducted in different subpopulations. In general, these found that over a period of 6–12 months low intensity activity programmes produced no measurable changes in maximum oxygen consumption (Vo_2max), whereas moderate intensity activity programmes (equivalent to brisk walking) typically produced improvements of 20% in oxygen consumption in sedentary people. Table 1, p 184 gives the intensity of effort required for a range of physical activities. Two recent RCTs compared structured aerobic exercise (such as step and aerobics classes) with lifestyle activity programmes (such as regular walking and using stairs instead of lifts) among obese women[51] and sedentary men and women.[52] Both studies reported similar, significant changes in measures of cardiovascular fitness and blood pressure with each intervention, and these changes were sustained for at least 2 years after intervention. One prospective follow up study of women previously involved in a randomised trial of physical activity found that women who start a programme of regular walking maintain higher levels of physical activity 10 years after the intervention.[53]

Frequency: We found no systematic review. One RCT (36 men) compared 8 weeks of a single daily session of 30 minutes of exercise versus three daily sessions of 10 minutes each.[54] It found no significant difference in fitness between groups after the end of the programme.

Harms: None reported.

Comment: None.

QUESTION **What are the effects of dietary interventions on the risk of myocardial infarction and stroke in asymptomatic people?**

Bazian Ltd

OPTION **EATING MORE FRUIT AND VEGETABLES**

Cohort studies have found that eating more fruit and vegetables reduces the risk of myocardial infarction and stroke. The size and nature of any protective effect is uncertain.

Benefits: **Ischaemic heart disease:** We found no RCTs. We found three systematic reviews of observational studies.[55–58] With addition of recently published studies[59–67] to those reported in the first review (search date 1995),[55] a protective association was observed for ischaemic heart disease in 14/25 (56%) cohort studies. In the second review (search date not stated),[56] the authors calculated a summary measure of the protective association of 15% between those above the 90th centile and those below the 10th centile for fruit and vegetable consumption. In the third review (search date 1998),[57,58] the authors estimated that increased intake of fruit and vegetables of about 150 g daily was associated with a reduced risk of coronary heart disease of 20–40%. The validity of these estimates has been questioned. One large, high quality cohort study found that eating more vegetables was associated with decreased coronary mortality (≥ 117 g vegetables/day *v* < 61 g vegetables/day: RR 0.66, 95% CI 0.46 to 0.96); for fruit, the association was more modest and not significant (≥ 159 g fruit/day *v* < 75 g fruit/day: RR 0.77, 95% CI 0.54 to 1.12).[68] **Stroke:** We found no RCTs but we found two systematic reviews examining the evidence from observational studies for stroke.[55,57,58] With addition of recently published studies[59–66,68] to those reported in the first review (search date 1995),[55] a protective association was observed in 10/16 (63%) cohort studies for stroke. In the second review (search date not stated),[57,58] the authors estimated that increased intake of fruit and vegetables of about 150 g daily was associated with a reduced risk of stroke of 0–25%. The basis for this estimate is not clear. One large, high quality cohort study in US health professionals found that increased fruit and vegetable intake was associated with a decreased risk of ischaemic stroke (RR per daily serving of fruit and vegetables 0.94, 95% CI 0.90 to 0.99; RR in the fifth of the population eating the most fruit and vegetables *v* the fifth eating the least 0.69, 95% CI 0.52 to 0.92).[69]

Harms: None were identified.

Comment: Lack of RCT evidence and deficiencies in the data available from observational studies mean that the size and nature of any real protective effect is uncertain.[70,71] The observed associations could be the result of confounding as people who eat more fruit and vegetables often come from higher socioeconomic groups and have other healthy lifestyles.[72]

OPTION ANTIOXIDANTS

Systematic reviews of RCTs found no evidence of benefit from β carotene or vitamin E supplements, and RCTs suggest that they may be harmful. We found insufficient evidence about effects of other antioxidants.

Benefits: **β Carotene:** We found two systematic reviews of prospective studies and RCTs (search date not stated, published in 1997[73] and search date 2001[74]). The most recent systematic review (6 RCTs, 86 056 people) found no significant difference between β carotene and control for cardiovascular disease (OR 1.02, 95% CI 0.96 to 1.08).[74] However, β carotene was combined with other antioxidants in some treatment groups, and it was not clear whether the systematic review accounted for effects of multiple interventions compared with control. It was also not clear whether all control groups received placebo only. **Vitamin C (ascorbic acid):** We found three systematic reviews (search dates not stated,[73] 1996,[75] and 2001[74]). The most recent systematic review (2 RCTs; 16 700 people, most people from 1 large RCT) found no significant difference between vitamin C and control for cardiovascular disease risk (OR 0.98, 95% CI 0.75 to 1.26).[74] However, vitamin C was combined with molybdenum in the larger trial, which may have contributed to the observed effect. It was also not clear from the review whether all control groups received placebo only. **Vitamin E:** We found two systematic reviews and additional prospective studies.[72,74] The most recent systematic review (4 RCTs, 48 346 people) compared vitamin E versus control.[74] It found no significant difference between vitamin E and control for cardiovascular disease (OR 0.96, 95% CI 0.88 to 1.04). However, vitamin E was combined with other antioxidants in some treatment groups, which may have contributed to the observed effect. It was also not clear whether all control groups received placebo only. **Antioxidant minerals:** We found little epidemiological evidence about the cardioprotective effect of copper, zinc, or manganese on the heart.[76] Cohort studies reported an increased risk of ischaemic heart disease in people with low blood selenium concentrations.[77] Most of these were carried out in Finland, a country with low intakes of antioxidants.[78] **Flavonoids:** We found no systematic review. We found five cohort studies,[78–82] three of which reported a reduced risk of ischaemic heart disease with increased flavonoid intake.[78–80] One of four observational studies reported a reduced risk of stroke with increased flavonoid intake.[58,79,83,84]

Harms: One of the RCTs identified in the most recent systematic review found that vitamin E may increase death from subarachnoid haemorrhage compared with control (RR for subarachnoid haemorrhage

1.50, 95% CI 0.97 to 2.32; RR death 2.81, 95% CI 1.37 to 5.79).[74,85] Pooled analysis of four of the β carotene RCTs found that β carotene may increase cardiovascular mortality (RR for cardiovascular death 1.12, 95% CI 1.04 to 1.22).[86] Effects may be dependent on the isomer or dose.[87,88]

Comment: RCTs of antioxidants such as β carotene and vitamin E have not found any evidence of benefit. Routine use of antioxidant supplements is not justified by the currently available evidence. Most of the RCTs identified in the most recent systematic review were designed to investigate whether antioxidants protect against cancer, and not specifically to investigate their effect on cardiovascular disease. Some of the trials were limited to smokers and there may be an interaction between antioxidants and smoking. Further RCTs of antioxidant supplementation are under way.[89]

QUESTION By how much does smoking cessation, or avoiding starting smoking, reduce risk?

Julian J Nicholas

We found no direct evidence from RCTs that advice to stop smoking reduces cardiovascular risk compared with no advice. However, we found robust evidence from observational studies that smoking is an important risk factor for overall mortality, coronary heart disease, and stroke, and that smoking cessation should therefore be encouraged. The evidence is strongest for stroke.

Benefits: We found one RCT of advice encouraging smoking cessation in 1445 men aged 40–59 years that found that more men given advice to stop smoking gave up cigarettes (mean absolute reduction in men continuing to smoke after advice *v* control 53%).[90] The RCT found no evidence that men given advice to stop smoking had a significantly lower mortality from coronary heart disease (CHD; RR 0.82, 95% CI 0.57 to 1.18). However, it is not clear how many people advised to stop smoking actually quit. The wide confidence intervals mean that there could have been anything from a 43% decrease to an 18% increase in rates of CHD death in men given advice to quit, regardless of whether they actually gave up smoking. We found strong observational evidence that smoking is an important risk factor for cardiovascular disease. Several large cohort studies examining the effects of smoking have been reviewed extensively by the US Surgeon General[91] and the UK Royal College of Physicians.[92] The reviews concluded that cigarette smoking was causally related to disease and that smoking cessation substantially reduced the risk of cancer, respiratory disease, CHD, and stroke. **Death from all causes:** The longest prospective cohort study, in 34 439 male British doctors whose smoking habits were periodically assessed over 40 years (1951–1991), found a strong association between smoking and increased mortality.[93] It found that smokers were about three times more likely to die in middle age (45–64 years) and twice as likely to die in older age (65–84 years) compared with lifelong non-smokers (CI not reported). The prospective nurses' health study followed 117 001 middle aged female nurses for 12 years.[94] It found that the total mortality in current smokers was nearly twice that in lifelong non-smokers (RR of death

1.87, 95% CI 1.65 to 2.13). **Coronary heart disease:** One review (published in 1990) identified 10 cohort studies, involving 20 million person-years of observation.[91] All studies found a higher incidence of CHD among smokers (pooled RR of death from CHD compared with non-smokers 1.7, CI not reported). People smoking more than 20 cigarettes daily were more likely to have a coronary event (RR 2.5, CI not provided).[92] Middle aged smokers were more likely to experience a first non-fatal acute myocardial infarction compared with people who had never smoked (RR in men 2.9, 95% CI 2.4 to 3.4; RR in women 3.6, 95% CI 3.0 to 4.4).[95,96] **Stroke:** One systematic review (search date 1998) found 32 studies (17 cohort studies with concurrent or historical controls, 14 case control studies, and one hypertension intervention RCT).[97] It found good evidence that smoking was associated with an increased risk of stroke (RR of stroke in cigarette smokers *v* non-smokers 1.5, 95% CI 1.4 to 1.6). Smoking was associated with an increased risk of cerebral infarction (RR 1.92, 95% CI 1.71 to 2.16) and subarachnoid haemorrhage (RR 2.93, 95% CI 2.48 to 3.46), and a reduced risk of intracerebral haemorrhage (RR 0.74, 95% CI 0.56 to 0.98). The relative risk of stroke in smokers compared with non-smokers was highest in those aged under 55 years (RR 2.90, 95% CI 2.40 to 3.59) and lowest in those aged over 74 years (RR 1.11, 95% CI 0.96 to 1.28).

Harms: We found no evidence that stopping smoking increases mortality in any subgroup of smokers.

Comment: We found no evidence of publication or other overt bias that may explain the observed association between smoking and stroke. There was a dose related effect between the number of cigarettes smoked and the relative risk for stroke, consistent with a causal relation. The absolute risk reduction from stopping smoking will be highest for those with the highest absolute risk of vascular events. Effects on quit rates of different methods of encouraging people to stop smoking are discussed elsewhere in *Clinical Evidence* (see changing behaviour topic, p 95).

QUESTION How quickly do risks diminish when smokers stop smoking?

Julian J Nicholas

Observational studies have found that the risk of death and cardiovascular events falls when people stop smoking. The risk can take many years to approach that of non-smokers, particularly in those with a history of heavy smoking.

Benefits: **Death from all causes:** In people who stopped smoking, observational studies found that death rates fell gradually to lie between those of lifelong smokers and people who had never smoked. Estimates for the time required for former smokers to bring their risk of death in line with people who had never smoked varied among studies but may be longer than 15 years.[98] Actuarial projections from one study among British doctors predicted that life expectancy would improve even among people who stopped smoking in later life (≥ 65 years).[93] **Coronary heart disease:** Observational studies found that, in both male and female ex-smokers, the risk of coronary events rapidly declined to a level comparable with that of people who had never smoked after 2–3 years and was independent of the number of cigarettes smoked before quitting.[91] **Stroke:** The US Surgeon General's review of observational studies found that the risk of stroke decreased in ex-smokers compared with smokers (RR of stroke, smokers *v* ex-smokers 1.2, CI not reported) but remained raised for 5–10 years after cessation compared with those who had never smoked (RR of stroke, ex-smokers *v* never smokers 1.5, CI not reported).[91] One recent study in 7735 middle aged British men found that 5 years after smoking cessation the risk of stroke in previously light smokers (< 20 cigarettes/day) was identical to that of lifelong non-smokers, but the risk in previously heavy smokers (> 20 cigarettes/day) was still raised compared with lifelong non-smokers (RR of stroke, previously heavy smokers *v* never smokers 2.2, 95% CI 1.1 to 4.3).[99] One observational study in 117 001 middle aged female nurses also found a fall in risk on stopping smoking and found no difference between previously light and previously heavy smokers (RR in all former smokers 2–4 years after stopping smoking 1.17, 95% CI 0.49 to 2.23).[94]

Harms: We found no evidence that stopping smoking increases mortality in any subgroup of smokers.

Comment: For a review of the evidence on methods of changing smoking behaviour, see secondary prevention of ischaemic cardiac events, p 188.

QUESTION What are the effects of lifestyle changes in asymptomatic people with primary hypertension?

Michael Pignone

OPTION PHYSICAL ACTIVITY

One systematic review has found that aerobic exercise reduces blood pressure.

Benefits: We found no RCTs in people with primary hypertension examining the effects of exercise on morbidity, mortality, or quality of life. One systematic review (search date 2001, 54 RCTs, 2419 sedentary adults aged > 18 years) examined the effects on blood pressure of at least 2 weeks of regular exercise compared with no exercise.[100] Compared with non-exercising control groups, groups randomised to aerobic exercise reduced their systolic blood pressure by 3.8 mm Hg (95% CI 2.7 mm Hg to 5.0 mm Hg) and diastolic blood pressure by 2.6 mm Hg (95% CI 1.8 mm Hg to 3.4 mm Hg). Reductions in blood pressure were seen in hypertensive and non-hypertensive people, and in overweight and normal weight people. RCTs with interventions lasting longer than 6 months in adults aged 45 years or over with hypertension found non-significant mean reductions in blood pressure, with wide confidence intervals (systolic reduction 0.8 mm Hg, 95% CI 5.9 mm Hg reduction to 4.2 mm Hg increase).[101]

Harms: Musculoskeletal injuries can occur, but their frequency was not documented.

Comment: Many adults find aerobic exercise programmes difficult to sustain. The clinical significance of the observed reductions in blood pressure is uncertain. The type and amount of exercise most likely to result in benefits are unclear, with some recent studies showing some benefits with simple increases in lifestyle activity. One cohort study (173 men with hypertension) found that "regular heavy activity several times weekly" compared with no or limited spare time physical activity reduced all cause and cardiovascular mortality (all cause mortality RR 0.43, 95% CI 0.22 to 0.82; cardiovascular mortality RR 0.33, 95% CI 0.11 to 0.94).[102]

OPTION LOW FAT, HIGH FRUIT AND VEGETABLE DIET

We found no systematic review and no RCTs examining the effects of low fat, high fruit and vegetable diet on morbidity or mortality in people with primary hypertension. One RCT found that a low fat, high fruit and vegetable diet modestly reduced blood pressure.

Benefits: We found no systematic review and no RCTs examining the effects of low fat, high fruit and vegetable diet on morbidity or mortality in people with primary hypertension. For evidence in asymptomatic people in general see question on effects of dietary interventions, p 161. One RCT (459 adults with systolic blood pressures of < 160 mm Hg and diastolic blood pressures of 80–90 mm Hg) compared effects on blood pressure of three diets (control diet low in both magnesium and potassium *v* fruit and vegetable diet high in both potassium and magnesium *v* combination of the fruit and vegetable diet with a low fat diet high in both calcium and protein).[103] After 8 weeks the fruit and vegetable diet reduced systolic and diastolic blood pressure compared with the control diet (mean change in systolic blood pressure –2.8 mm Hg, 97.5% CI –4.7 mm Hg to –0.9 mm Hg; mean change in diastolic blood pressure –1.1 mm Hg, 97.5% CI –2.4 mm Hg to +0.3 mm Hg). The combination diet also reduced systolic and diastolic blood pressure compared with the control diet (mean change in systolic blood pressure –5.5 mm Hg, 97.5% CI –7.4 mm Hg to –3.7 mm Hg; mean change in diastolic blood pressure –3.0 mm Hg, 97.5% CI –4.3 to –1.6 mm Hg).[103]

Harms: We found no direct evidence that a low fat, high fruit and vegetable diet is harmful.

Comment: The RCT was of short duration and people were supplied with food during the intervention period.[103] Other studies have found that long term maintenance of particular diets is difficult for many people, although low fat, high fruit and vegetable diets may have multiple benefits (see changing behaviour, p 95).

OPTION REDUCED ALCOHOL CONSUMPTION

One systematic review found inconclusive evidence regarding effects of alcohol reduction on blood pressure among people with primary hypertension and moderate to high alcohol intake.

Benefits: We found no RCTs examining the effects of reducing alcohol consumption on morbidity or mortality in people with primary hypertension. Over 60 population studies have reported associations between alcohol consumption and blood pressure. The relation was found to be generally linear, although several studies reported a threshold effect at about two to three standard drinks daily.[104] Any adverse effects of up to two drinks daily on blood pressure was found to be either small or non-existent. One systematic review (search date 1999, 7 RCTs, 751 people with hypertension; mainly men) found that data were inconclusive on the benefits of reducing alcohol among moderate to heavy drinkers (25–50 drinks/week).[105]

Harms: We found no direct evidence that reducing alcohol intake to as few as two drinks daily was harmful.

Comment: Most data were from observational studies. RCTs were small and lacked reliable information about adherence. Substantial reductions in alcohol use in both control and intervention groups were observed, with limited ability to detect differences between groups.

OPTION SALT RESTRICTION

One systematic review has found that salt restriction may lead to modest reductions in blood pressure, with more benefit in people older than 45 years than in younger people.

Benefits: We found no RCT examining the effects of salt restriction on morbidity or mortality in people with primary hypertension. We found one systematic review (search date 1997, 58 RCTs, 2161 people with hypertension, age 23–73 years)[106] and two subsequent RCTs,[107,108] which examined the effects of salt restriction on blood pressure. Interventions were low salt diets with or without weight reduction. People in the control groups took their usual diet. Changes in salt intake varied among RCTs in the systematic review; a mean reduction in sodium intake of 118 mmol (6.7 g) daily for 28 days led to reductions of 3.9 mm Hg (95% CI 3.0 mm Hg to 4.8 mm Hg) in systolic blood pressure and 1.9 mm Hg (95% CI 1.3 mm Hg to 2.5 mm Hg) in diastolic blood pressure.[106] One RCT (875 people with hypertension, age 60–80 years, duration 30 months) found that a mean decrease in salt intake of about 40 mmol (2.4 g) daily reduced systolic blood pressure by 2.6 mm Hg (95% CI 0.4 mm Hg to 4.8 mm Hg) and diastolic blood pressure by 1.1 mm Hg (95% CI 0.3 mm Hg rise in diastolic to 2.5 mm Hg fall).[107] Another RCT (412 people with systolic/diastolic blood pressure > 120/80 mm Hg, mean age 48 years, duration 30 days) that tested three different target levels of sodium intake (150, 100, and 50 mmol/day [8.6, 5.7, and 2.9 g/day]) found significantly lower systolic blood pressure levels with lower sodium intakes.[108] An earlier systematic review (search date 1994) identified 28 RCTs in 1131 people with hypertension. It found that lesser reductions of 60 mmol (3.4 g) daily led to smaller reductions in systolic/diastolic blood pressure of 2.2/0.5 mm Hg and found greater effects in RCTs in which mean age was over 45 years (6.3/2.2 mm Hg).[109]

Harms: We found no direct evidence that low salt diets may increase morbidity or mortality.

Comment: Small RCTs tended to report larger reductions in systolic and diastolic blood pressure than larger RCTs. This may be explained by publication bias or less rigorous methodology in small RCTs.[109]

OPTION SMOKING CESSATION

We found no direct evidence that stopping smoking decreases blood pressure in people with hypertension. However, we found robust epidemiological data that smoking is an important risk factor for cardiovascular disease.

Benefits: We found no direct evidence that stopping smoking reduces blood pressure in people with hypertension, although we found good evidence that smoking is an important risk factor for cardiovascular disease (see question on how much does smoking cessation, or avoiding starting smoking, reduce risk, p 163).

Harms: We found insufficient evidence in this context.

Comment: None.

OPTION WEIGHT LOSS

One systematic review and additional RCTs have found that modest weight reductions of 3–9% of body weight are achievable in motivated middle aged and older adults, and lead to modest reductions in blood pressure in obese people with hypertension. Many adults find it difficult to maintain weight loss.

Benefits: We found no RCTs examining the effects of weight loss on morbidity and mortality in people with primary hypertension. We found one systematic review (search date 1998, 18 RCTs, 2611 middle aged people, mean age 50 years, mean weight 85 kg, mean systolic/diastolic blood pressure 152/98 mm Hg, 55% men)[110] and two subsequent RCTs[111,112] that examined the effects of weight loss on blood pressure. In the systematic review, caloric intakes ranged from 450–1500 kcal daily. Most diets led to weight reductions of 3–9% of body weight. Combined data from the six RCTs that did not vary antihypertensive regimens during the intervention period found that reducing weight reduced systolic and diastolic blood pressures (mean reduction in systolic pressure, weight loss *v* no weight loss 3.0 mm Hg, 95% CI 0.7 mm Hg to 6.8 mm Hg; mean reduction in diastolic blood pressure, weight loss *v* no weight loss 2.9 mm Hg, 95% CI 0.1 mm Hg to 5.7 mm Hg). RCTs that allowed adjustment of antihypertensive regimens found that lower doses and fewer antihypertensive drugs were needed in the weight reduction groups compared with control groups. The two subsequent RCTs found that sustained weight reduction of 2–4 kg significantly reduced systolic blood pressure at 1–3 years by about 1 mm Hg.[111,112]

Harms: We found no direct evidence that intentional gradual weight loss of less than 10% of body weight is harmful in obese adults with hypertension.

Comment: None.

OPTION POTASSIUM SUPPLEMENTATION

One systematic review has found that a daily potassium supplementation of about 60 mmol (2 g, which is about the amount contained in 5 bananas) is feasible for many adults and reduces blood pressure by small amounts.

Benefits: We found no RCTs examining the effects of potassium supplementation on morbidity or mortality in people with primary hypertension. One systematic review (search date 1995, 21 RCTs, 1560 adults with hypertension, age 19–79 years) compared the effects on blood pressure of potassium supplements (60–100 mmol/day [2–3 g/day] potassium chloride) versus placebo or no supplement.[113] It found that, compared with the control interventions, potassium supplements reduced systolic and diastolic blood pressures (mean decrease in systolic blood pressure with potassium supplements 4.4 mm Hg, 95% CI 2.2 mm Hg to 6.6 mm Hg; mean decrease in diastolic blood pressure 2.5 mm Hg, 95% CI 0.1 mm Hg to 4.9 mm Hg).

Harms: We found no direct evidence of harm in people without kidney failure and in people not taking drugs that increase serum potassium concentration. Gastrointestinal adverse effects such as belching, flatulence, diarrhoea, or abdominal discomfort occurred in 2–10% of people.[113]

Comment: None.

OPTION FISH OIL SUPPLEMENTATION

One systematic review has found that fish oil supplementation in large doses of 3 g daily modestly lowers blood pressure.

Benefits: We found no RCTs examining the effects of fish oil supplementation on morbidity or mortality in people with hypertension. One systematic review (search date not stated, 7 brief RCTs, 339 people with hypertension, mainly middle aged white men, mean age 50 years) compared effects on blood pressure of fish oil (usually 3 g/day as capsules) versus no supplements or "placebo".[114] The contents of placebo capsules varied among RCTs. Some used oil mixtures containing omega-3 polyunsaturated fatty acids, some did not. The review found that fish oil supplements reduced blood pressure compared with control interventions (mean decrease in systolic blood pressure in treatment *v* control 4.5 mm Hg, 95% CI 1.2 mm Hg to 7.8 mm Hg, and mean decrease in diastolic blood pressure in treatment *v* control 2.5 mm Hg, 95% CI 0.6 mm Hg to 4.4 mm Hg).

Harms: Belching, bad breath, fishy taste, and abdominal pain occurred in about a third of people taking high doses of fish oil.[114]

Comment: The RCTs were of short duration and used high doses of fish oil. Such high intake may be difficult to maintain. We found no evidence of beneficial effect on blood pressure at lower intakes.

OPTION **CALCIUM SUPPLEMENTATION**

We found insufficient evidence on the effects of calcium supplementation specifically in people with hypertension. One systematic review in people both with and without hypertension found that calcium supplementation may reduce systolic blood pressure by small amounts.

Benefits: We found no RCTs examining the effects of calcium supplementation on morbidity or mortality in people with primary hypertension. One systematic review (search date 1994, 42 RCTs, 4560 middle aged people with and without hypertension) compared the effects on blood pressure of calcium supplementation 500–2000 mg daily versus placebo or no supplements.[115] It found that calcium supplements reduced blood pressure by a small amount (mean systolic blood pressure reduction, supplement *v* control 1.4 mm Hg, 95% CI 0.7 mm Hg to 2.2 mm Hg; mean diastolic reduction 0.8 mm Hg, 95% CI 0.2 mm Hg to 1.4 mm Hg).

Harms: Adverse gastrointestinal effects, such as abdominal pain, were generally mild and varied among particular preparations.

Comment: Data relating specifically to people with hypertension are limited by few studies with small sample sizes and short durations.

OPTION **MAGNESIUM SUPPLEMENTATION**

We found no RCTs examining the effects of magnesium supplementation on morbidity or mortality in people with hypertension. We found limited and conflicting evidence on the effect of magnesium supplementation on blood pressure in people with hypertension and normal magnesium concentrations.

Benefits: We found no RCTs examining the effects of magnesium supplementation on morbidity or mortality. A few small, short term RCTs found mixed results on effects on blood pressure reduction in people with hypertension and normal magnesium levels.

Harms: We found insufficient evidence.

Comment: None.

QUESTION **What are the effects of drug treatment in primary hypertension?**

Michael Pignone

OPTION **ANTIHYPERTENSIVE DRUGS VERSUS PLACEBO**

Many systematic reviews have found that antihypertensive drug treatment decreases the risk of fatal and non-fatal stroke, cardiac events, and total mortality in people with primary hypertension. The greatest benefit is seen in people with highest baseline risk of cardiovascular disease.

Benefits: We found many systematic reviews. One review (search date 1997, 17 RCTs with morbidity and mortality outcomes, duration > 1 year, 37 000 people) found that antihypertensive drugs produced variable reductions of systolic/diastolic blood pressure that averaged about 12–16/5–10 mm Hg compared with placebo.[116] It found evidence of benefit in total death rate, cardiovascular death rate, stroke, major coronary events, and congestive cardiac failure, but the absolute results depended on age and the severity of the hypertension (see target diastolic blood pressure below). The biggest benefit was seen in those with the highest baseline risk. The RCTs mainly compared placebo versus diuretics (usually thiazides with the addition of amiloride or triamterene) and versus β blockers (usually atenolol or metoprolol) in a stepped care approach. One systematic review (search date 1999, 8 RCTs, 15 693 people) found that, in people aged over 60 years with systolic hypertension, treatment of systolic pressures greater than 160 mm Hg decreased total mortality and fatal and non-fatal cardiovascular events.[117] Absolute benefits were greater in men than women, in people aged over 70 years, and in those with prior cardiovascular events or wider pulse pressure. The relative hazard rates associated with a 10 mm Hg higher initial systolic blood pressure were 1.26 (P = 0.0001) for total mortality, 1.22 (P = 0.02) for stroke, but only 1.07 (P = 0.37) for coronary events. Active treatment reduced total mortality (RR 0.87, 95% CI 0.78 to 0.98; P = 0.02).[117] **Target diastolic blood pressure:** We found one RCT (18 790 people, mean age 62 years, diastolic blood pressures 100–115 mm Hg), which aimed to evaluate the effects on cardiovascular risk of target diastolic blood pressures of 90, 85, and 80 mm Hg.[118] However, mean achieved diastolic blood pressures were 85, 83, and 81 mm Hg, which limited power to detect differences among groups. There were no significant differences in major cardiovascular events among the three groups.

Harms: **Mortality and major morbidity:** One systematic review (search date 1997)[116] comparing diuretics and β blockers versus placebo found no increase in non-cardiovascular mortality in treated people. **Quality of life and tolerability:** One systematic review (search date 1990)[119] and several recent RCTs found that quality of life was not adversely affected and may be improved in those who remain on treatment.[120]

Comment: RCTs included people who were healthier than the general population, with lower rates of cardiovascular risk factors, cardiovascular disease, and comorbidity. People with higher cardiovascular risk can expect greater short term absolute risk reduction than seen in the RCTs, whereas people with major competing risks such as terminal cancer or end stage Alzheimer's disease can expect smaller risk reduction. In the systematic review,[116] five of the RCTs were in middle aged people with mild to moderate hypertension. Seven of the RCTs were in people older than 60 years. On average, every 1000 person-years of treatment in older adults prevented five strokes (95% CI 2 to 8), three coronary events (95% CI 1 to 4), and four cardiovascular deaths (95% CI 1 to 8). Drug treatment in middle aged people prevented one stroke (95% CI 0 to 2) for every 1000 person-years of treatment and did not significantly affect coronary events or mortality. One meta-analysis (7 RCTs, 40 233 people with hypertension) found an increased risk of total and cardiovascular mortality with diastolic blood pressure levels below 85 mm Hg that was not related to antihypertensive treatment.[121]

OPTION COMPARING ANTIHYPERTENSIVE DRUG TREATMENTS

Systematic reviews have found that initial treatment with diuretics, angiotensin converting enzyme inhibitors, or β blockers reduce morbidity and mortality, with minimal adverse effects. RCTs found no significant differences in morbidity or mortality among these agents. We found limited evidence from two systematic reviews that diuretics, β blockers, and angiotensin converting enzyme inhibitors reduced coronary heart disease and heart failure more than calcium channel antagonists. However, calcium channel antagonists reduced risk of stroke more than the other agents. One RCT found that a thiazide diuretic reduced cardiovascular events, particularly congestive heart failure, compared with an α blocker. One RCT found that losartan (an angiotensin receptor blocker) reduced cardiovascular events compared with atenolol in people with hypertension and left ventricular hypertrophy.

Benefits: **β Blockers versus diuretics:** One systematic review (search date 1995, > 48 000 people) identified RCTs comparing effects of high and low dose diuretics versus β blockers.[122] A second systematic review (search date 1998) was limited to 10 RCTs in 16 164 elderly people.[123] These reviews did not summarise direct comparisons of diuretics versus β blockers but compared results of RCTs that used diuretics as preferred treatment versus results of RCTs that used β blockers as preferred treatment. The reviews found no significant difference between diuretics and β blockers for lowering blood pressure. They found that diuretics reduced coronary events, but found no evidence that β blockers reduced coronary events. **Comparison of β blockers, diuretics, angiotensin converting enzyme inhibitors, and calcium channel antagonists:** One systematic review (search date 2000, 8 RCTs) compared different antihypertensive regimens, and found no significant differences in outcome among people initially treated with β blockers, diuretics, or angiotensin converting enzyme (ACE) inhibitors.[124] However, it found that β blockers or diuretics decreased coronary events compared with calcium channel antagonists and increased stroke rate, although there was no significant difference for all cause mortality (OR for mortality, β blockers or diuretics *v* calcium channel antagonists 1.01, 95% CI 0.92 to 1.11). ACE inhibitors did not significantly alter all cause mortality or stroke rate compared with calcium channel antagonists (OR for ACE inhibitors *v* calcium channel antagonist 1.03, 95% CI 0.91 to 1.18 for all cause mortality; 1.02, 95% CI 0.85 to 1.21 for stroke). However, ACE inhibitors decreased coronary events (OR for ACE inhibitors *v* calcium channel antagonist 0.81, 95% CI 0.68 to 0.97 for coronary events).[124] A second review of similar trials (search date 2001, 9 RCTs, 62 605 hypertensive people) found that diuretics, β blockers, ACE inhibitors, and calcium channel antagonists were all associated with similar reductions in cardiovascular risk.[125] However, calcium channel antagonists reduced risk of stroke and increased risk of myocardial infarction compared with other agents (RR for stroke

0.87, 95% CI 0.76 to 0.99; RR for myocardial infarction 1.19, 95% CI 1.04 to 1.37).[125] **Comparison of α blockers and diuretics:** One double blind RCT (24 335 high risk people with hypertension), which was included in the systematic review,[125] found no significant differences in coronary heart disease outcomes between doxazosin, an α blocker, and chlorthalidone (chlortalidone). However, doxazosin increased the total number of cardiovascular events after 4 years compared with chlorthalidone (25% with doxazosin *v* 22% with chlorthalidone; HR 1.25, 95% CI 1.17 to 1.33) and, in particular, increased congestive heart failure (8% with doxazosin *v* 4% with chlorthalidone; HR 2.04, 95% CI 1.79 to 2.32).[126] **Comparison of angiotensin receptor blockers and β blockers:** We found one RCT (9193 people aged 55–80 years with primary hypertension and left ventricular hypertrophy, but with no history of coronary events), which compared losartan versus atenolol.[127] It found that losartan reduced cardiovascular events compared with atenolol after 4 years (composite of death, myocardial infarction, or stroke: 11% with losartan *v* 13% with atenolol; RR 0.87, 95% CI 0.77 to 0.98). **Drug treatment in people with diabetes:** See prevention of cardiovascular events in diabetes, p 690.

Harms: **Quality of life and tolerability:** In the three long term, double blind comparisons of low dose diuretics, β blockers, ACE inhibitors, and calcium channel antagonists, tolerability and overall quality of life indicators tended to be more favourable for diuretics and β blockers than for newer drugs.[128–130] One systematic review (search date 1998) of RCTs comparing thiazides versus β blockers found that thiazides were associated with fewer withdrawals because of adverse effects (RR 0.69, 95% CI 0.63 to 0.76).[131] Adverse effects are agent specific. The recent unblinded RCT comparing diuretics, β blockers, calcium channel antagonists, and ACE inhibitors found that after 5 years' follow up, 26% of people receiving felodipine or isradipine (calcium channel antagonists) reported ankle oedema, 30% receiving enalapril or lisinopril (ACE inhibitors) reported cough, and 9% receiving diuretics, β blockers, or both reported cold hands and feet.[118] **Major harm controversies:** Case control, cohort, and randomised studies suggest that short and intermediate acting dihydropyridine calcium channel antagonists, such as nifedipine and isradipine, may increase cardiovascular morbidity and mortality.[132]

Comment: None.

QUESTION What are the effects of lowering cholesterol concentration in asymptomatic people?

Michael Pignone

Systematic reviews have found that in people with an annual risk of coronary heart disease events of 0.6–1.5% a year, cholesterol reduction reduces non-fatal myocardial infarction (see cholesterol reduction under secondary prevention of ischaemic cardiac events for additional information, p 188). RCTs have found that absolute benefit is related to an individual's baseline risk of cardiovascular events and to the degree of

cholesterol lowering rather than to the individual's cholesterol concentration. The effect of lipid lowering therapies in people with low short to medium term risk of coronary heart disease events (< 0.6%/year) has not been well studied to date.

Benefits: **Cholesterol lowering drug treatment:** We found two systematic reviews which compared any type of cholesterol lowering drug treatment versus placebo or no treatment in people without a diagnosis of coronary heart disease (CHD).[133,134] Both systematic reviews found similar results. The most recent systematic review (search date 1999) found four RCTs (2 with statins, 1 with fibrates, and 1 with cholestyramine, 21 087 people).[133] It found that cholesterol reduction treatment significantly reduced CHD events and CHD mortality compared with placebo, but found no significant effect on overall mortality (OR for treatment *v* placebo; 0.70, 95% CI 0.62 to 0.79 for CHD events; 0.71, 95% CI 0.56 to 0.91 for CHD mortality; 0.94, 95% CI 0.81 to 1.09 for overall mortality). **Statins:** We found five systematic reviews (search dates 1995,[135] 1997,[136] 1998,[137] 1999,[133] and not stated[134]) and two subsequent RCTs[138,139] that considered the effect of 3-hydroxy-3-methylglutaryl coenzyme A reductase inhibitors (statins) on clinical outcomes in people given long term (≥6 months) treatment compared with placebo. All the systematic reviews included the same two RCTs of statins in primary prevention (13 200 people).[140,141] All the systematic reviews found similar results. After 4–6 years of treatment for primary prevention, statins did not reduce significantly all cause mortality or CHD mortality compared with placebo (all cause mortality: OR 0.87, 95% CI 0.71 to 1.06). However, they did reduce major coronary events and cardiovascular mortality (CHD mortality OR 0.73, 95% CI 0.51 to 1.05; major coronary events OR 0.66, 95% CI 0.57 to 0.76; cardiovascular mortality OR 0.68, 95% CI 0.50 to 0.93).[137] The absolute risk reduction for CHD events, CHD mortality, and total mortality varied with the baseline risk (see figure 1, p 187). The first subsequent RCT (15 454 men and 5082 women) included 7150 people with no diagnosis of CHD but at high risk (1820 had cerebrovascular disease, 2701 had peripheral arterial disease, and 3982 had diabetes).[138] In people with no diagnosis of CHD, simvastatin reduced the risk of a major vascular event (major coronary event, stroke, or revascularisation) after 5 years compared with placebo (risk of major vascular event: event rate ratio 0.75, 95% CI 0.67 to 0.84). The second subsequent RCT (246 men with hyperlipidaemia) compared three treatments: diet alone, diet with pravastatin, and diet and probucol. It found that pravastatin reduced cardiovascular events compared with diet alone after 2 years (AR for any cardiovascular event 4.8% with pravastatin *v* 13.6% with diet alone, P value and CI not reported).[139] **Low fat diet:** See changing behaviour topic, p 95.

Harms: Specific harms of statins are discussed under secondary prevention of ischaemic cardiac events topic, p 188.

Comment: The CHD event rate in the placebo group of the two large primary prevention RCTs using statins was 0.6%[140] and 1.5%[141] a year. If the 17% relative reduction in total mortality observed in the higher risk west of Scotland RCT is real, then about 110 high risk people without known CHD would need to be treated for 5 years to save one life. One regression analysis of all the major statin trials found that mortality benefits of statins outweigh risks in people with a 10 year CHD risk of more than 13%.[145] **Cholesterol lowering treatment in older people:** We found no RCTs specifically evaluating the effect of cholesterol lowering treatment in asymptomatic people aged over 75 years. One large RCT comparing statin with placebo included more than 5000 people over the age of 70 years.[138] It found major vascular events were reduced to a similar extent in people above and below the age of 70 years. **Cholesterol lowering treatment in women:** Subgroup analyses of two RCTs have found conflicting results. One RCT (5608 men, 997 women) compared statins with placebo for primary prevention in women.[140] It found that lovastatin reduced the risk of CHD events in women but this was not statistically significant (RR 0.54, 95% CI 0.22, 1.35). In the second RCT, the reduction in major event rate was similar in men and women (quantitative results not reported).[138] Other treatments are discussed under changing behaviour, p 95, or were performed in people with known CHD (see secondary prevention of ischaemic cardiac events, p 188). We found one systematic review (search date 1996, 59 RCTs, 173 160 people receiving drug treatments, dietary intervention, or ileal bypass), which did not differentiate primary and secondary prevention and included RCTs of any cholesterol lowering intervention, irrespective of duration, as long as mortality data were reported.[146] Overall, baseline risk was similar in people allocated to all interventions. Among non-surgical treatments, the review found that only statins reduced CHD mortality (RR *v* control 0.69, 95% CI 0.59 to 0.80 for statins; 0.44, 95% CI 0.18 to 1.07 for n-3 fatty acids; 0.98, 95% CI 0.78 to 1.24 for fibrates; 0.71, 95% CI 0.51 to 0.99 for resins; 1.04, 95% CI 0.93 to 1.17 for hormones; 0.95, 95% CI 0.83 to 1.10 for niacin; 0.91, 95% CI 0.82 to 1.01 for diet), and that only statins and n-3 fatty acids reduced all cause mortality (RR *v* control 0.79, 95% CI 0.71 to 0.89 for statins; 0.68, 95% CI 0.53 to 0.88 for n-3 fatty acids; 1.06, 95% CI 0.78 to 1.46 for fibrates; 0.85, 95% CI 0.66 to 1.08 for resins; 1.09, 95% CI 1.00 to 1.20 for hormones; 0.96, 95% CI 0.86 to 1.08 for niacin; 0.97, 95% CI 0.81 to 1.15 for diet).[146] The effect of lipid-lowering therapies in people with low short to medium term risk of CHD events (< 0.6%/year) has not been well studied to date.

QUESTION **What is the role of antithrombotic treatment in asymptomatic people?**

Michael Pignone

OPTION **ASPIRIN**

We found the role of antiplatelet treatment in individuals without symptoms of cardiovascular disease to be uncertain. We found insufficient evidence from RCTs to identify which individuals would benefit overall and which would be harmed by regular treatment with aspirin, although those at high and intermediate rather than low risk, would be more likely to gain benefit.

Primary prevention

Benefits: We found five systematic reviews,[147–151] which included five large RCTs comparing regular aspirin versus control among individuals with no prior history of vascular disease, with or without vascular risk factors.[118,152–155] The earliest two trials recruited a total of about 30 000 healthy, mainly middle aged, male doctors (5139 in the UK, randomised between aspirin 500 mg/day and control, and 22 071 in the USA, randomised between aspirin 325 mg every other day and placebo).[153,154] Three later RCTs included asymptomatic people with identifiable risk factors for vascular events. All three had a factorial design. The first compared aspirin 75 mg daily versus placebo and low intensity warfarin versus placebo in 5000 middle aged men with coronary heart disease risk score in the top 20–25% of the population distribution.[156] The second compared aspirin 75 mg daily versus placebo in three groups with different intensities of blood pressure reduction in a total of about 19 000 people with hypertension, most of whom had no history of vascular disease.[118] The third compared aspirin 100 mg daily versus placebo and vitamin E versus placebo in about 4500 people aged more than 50 years, with at least one major cardiovascular risk factor (hypertension, hypercholesterolaemia, diabetes, obesity, family history of premature myocardial infarction, or age ≥ 65 years).[77] The average control group risk of a serious vascular event (myocardial infarction, stroke, or death from a vascular cause) in each of these trials was low (about 1% a year). Data from these five RCTs were pooled in our own meta-analysis, which currently includes about 55 000 low risk people. Results are summarised in table 2, p 185 and table 3, p 186. We found that, overall, aspirin slightly reduced the risk of a serious vascular event (OR 0.86, 95% CI 0.80 to 0.90; ARR 1/1000 people/year), reduced the relative risk of myocardial infarction by about a third (OR 0.71, 95% CI 0.60 to 0.80), but had an uncertain effect on stroke (OR 1.05, 95% CI 0.90 to 1.20). The systematic reviews found similar results.[147–151] One of these systematic reviews[147] also included an RCT in about 3000 people with diabetes[155] who were at substantially higher average risk of vascular events (about 4% a year) than the low risk individuals in the primary prevention RCTs included in our meta-analysis.

Harms: Serious, potentially life threatening bleeding is the most important adverse effect of aspirin. **Intracranial haemorrhage:** These are uncommon, but they are often fatal or cause substantial disability in survivors. We found one relevant systematic review (search date 1997)[158] in which people were randomised to aspirin or control treatment for at least 1 month. It found that aspirin produced a small increased risk of intracranial haemorrhage in about 1/1000 (0.1%) people treated for 3 years.[158] Our meta-analysis of the primary prevention RCTs found a somewhat smaller absolute overall excess of about 0.1/1000 (0.01%) people treated with aspirin a year (see table 3, p 186). **Extracranial haemorrhage:** Major extracranial bleeds occur mainly in the gastrointestinal tract and may require hospital admission or blood transfusion, but do not generally result in permanent disability and are rarely fatal. We found one relevant systematic review of aspirin versus control with a scheduled treatment duration of at least 1 year. It found the relative excess risk of gastrointestinal bleeding with aspirin to be about 70% (OR 1.7, 95% CI 1.5 to 1.9).[159] A recent overview of 15 observational studies, including over 10 000 cases of upper gastrointestinal bleeding or perforation requiring admission to hospital, found the relative risk with aspirin to be 2.5 (95% CI 2.4 to 2.7). If only those studies that had a prospective (and so methodologically more rigorous) design were considered, the relative risk fell to 1.9 (95% CI 1.7 to 2.1), similar to that found in the RCTs.[160] Meta-analysis of primary prevention RCTs found a similar relative excess risk of major extracranial (mainly gastrointestinal) haemorrhage and an absolute excess of about 0.7 major extracranial haemorrhages per 1000 people treated with aspirin a year (see table 3, p 186).

Comment: Currently available information suggests that some asymptomatic individuals would gain net benefit whereas others would experience net harm with regular aspirin treatment. People at intermediate risk of vascular disease (≥ 1%/year risk of coronary heart disease events) may benefit overall, but we found insufficient evidence to be certain.[149,150] One large overview of randomised trials of antiplatelet treatment among people at high risk of vascular events (> 3%/year), including people with diabetes, found clear evidence of net benefit (see stroke prevention, p 246, secondary prevention of ischaemic cardiac events, p 188, and prevention of cardiovascular events in diabetes, p 690).[161]

OPTION ANTICOAGULANT TREATMENT

We found evidence from one RCT that the benefits and risks of low intensity oral anticoagulation among individuals without evidence of cardiovascular disease are finely balanced, and the net effects are uncertain.

Benefits: We found no systematic review. We found one RCT assessing anticoagulation (with a low target international normalised ratio of 1.5) among people without evidence of cardiovascular disease.[156] It found that the proportional effects of warfarin were similar among people allocated aspirin or placebo, and overall warfarin non-significantly reduced the odds of a vascular event over about 6.5 years compared with placebo (253 events in 2762 people allocated to warfarin, AR 9.2% *v* 288 events in 2737 people allocated to placebo, AR 10.5%; mean ARR warfarin *v* placebo about 2 events/1000 individuals/year; reduction in odds of vascular event warfarin *v* placebo +14%, 95% CI –2% to +28%). Compared with placebo, warfarin produced a relative reduction in the rate of all ischaemic heart disease (RRR 21%, 95% CI 4% to 35%), but had no significant effect on the rate of stroke (increase in RR +15%, 95% CI –22% to +68%) or other causes of vascular death.[156]

Harms: Warfarin was associated with a non-significant excess of about 0.4 intracranial bleeds per 1000 individuals a year (14/2762 [0.5%] with warfarin *v* 7/2737 [0.3%] with placebo) and a non-significant excess of extracranial bleeds of about 0.5/1000 individuals a year (21/2545 [0.8%] with warfarin *v* 12/2540 [0.5%] with placebo; RR 1.75, 95% CI 0.86 to 3.50).[156]

Comment: As for aspirin, the benefits and risks of low intensity oral anticoagulation among people without evidence of cardiovascular disease are finely balanced. The proportion of individuals randomised to date is only about 10% of the number included in primary prevention RCTs of aspirin (see aspirin, p 175), and so the reliable identification of those who may benefit from such treatment will require further large scale, randomised evidence.

Substantive changes

Reduced alcohol consumption Recategorised from Likely to be beneficial to Unknown effectiveness after reassessing the evidence.

Physical activity in asymptomatic adults One systematic review added;[6] conclusions unchanged.

Antioxidants One systematic review added;[74] vitamin E recategorised from Unknown effectiveness to Likely to be ineffective or harmful.

Comparing antihypertensive drug treatments One RCT added;[127] conclusions unchanged.

Antithrombotics One systematic review added;[151] conclusions unchanged.

REFERENCES

1. World Health Organization. The world health report 1999: making a difference. The World Health Organization. Geneva. 2000. http://www.who.int/whr2001/2001/archives/1999/en/index.htm (last accessed 7 August 2003).
2. Heller RF, Chinn S, Pedoe HD, et al. How well can we predict coronary heart disease? Findings of the United Kingdom heart disease prevention project. *BMJ* 1984;288:1409–1411.
3. Tunstall-Pedoe H, Morrison C, Woodward M, et al. Sex differences in myocardial infarction and coronary deaths in the Scottish MONICA population of Glasgow 1985 to 1991: presentation, diagnosis, treatment, and 28-day case fatality of 3991 events in men and 1551 events in women. *Circulation* 1996;93:1981–1992.
4. Anderson KV, Odell PM, Wilson PWF, et al. Cardiovascular disease risk profiles. *Am Heart J* 1991;121:293–298.
5. National Health Committee. Guidelines for the management of mildly raised blood pressure in New Zealand. Wellington Ministry of Health, 1993. http://www.nzgg.org.nz/library/gl_complete/bloodpressure/table1.cfm (last accessed 7 August 2003).
6. Batty GD. Physical activity and coronary heart disease in older adults. A systematic review of epidemiological studies. *Eur J Public Health* 2002;12:171–176. Search date 2001; primary sources Pubmed and reference sections of identified papers.
7. Powell KE, Thompson PD, Caspersen CJ, et al. Physical activity and the incidence of coronary heart disease. *Ann Rev Public Health* 1987;8:253–287. Search date 1995; primary sources computerised searches of personal files, *J Chronic Dis* 1983–1985, and *Am J Epidemiol* 1984–1985.
8. Berlin JA, Colditz GA. A meta-analysis of physical activity in the prevention of coronary heart disease. *Am J Epidemiol* 1990;132:612–628. Search date not stated; primary sources review articles and Medline.
9. Eaton CB. Relation of physical activity and cardiovascular fitness to coronary heart disease. Part I: a meta-analysis of the independent relation of physical activity and coronary heart disease. *J Am Board Fam Pract* 1992;5:31–42. Search date not stated; primary source Medline.
10. Fraser GE, Strahan TM, Sabate J, et al. Effects of traditional coronary risk factors on rates of incident coronary events in a low-risk population: the Adventist health study. *Circulation* 1992;86:406–413.
11. Lindsted KD, Tonstad S, Kuzma JW. Self-report of physical activity and patterns of mortality in Seventh-Day Adventist men. *J Clin Epidemiol* 1991;44:355–364.
12. Folsom AR, Arnett DK, Hutchinson RG, et al. Physical activity and incidence of coronary heart disease in middle-aged women and men. *Med Sci Sports Exerc* 1997;29:901–909.
13. Jensen G, Nyboe J, Appleyard M, et al. Risk factors for acute myocardial infarction in Copenhagen, II: smoking, alcohol intake, physical activity, obesity, oral contraception, diabetes, lipids, and blood pressure. *Eur Heart J* 1991;12:298–308.
14. Simonsick EM, Lafferty ME, Phillips CL, et al. Risk due to inactivity in physically capable older adults. *Am J Public Health* 1993;83:1443–1450.
15. Haapanen N, Miilunpalo S, Vuori I, et al. Association of leisure time physical activity with the risk of coronary heart disease, hypertension and diabetes in middle-aged men and women. *Int J Epidemiol* 1997;26:739–747.
16. Sherman SE, D'Agostino RB, Cobb JL, et al. Does exercise reduce mortality rates in the elderly? Experience from the Framingham Heart Study. *Am Heart J* 1994;128:965–672.
17. Rodriguez BL, Curb JD, Burchfiel CM, et al. Physical activity and 23-year incidence of coronary heart disease morbidity and mortality among middle-aged men: the Honolulu heart program. *Circulation* 1994;89:2540–2544.
18. Eaton CB, Medalie JH, Flocke SA, et al. Self-reported physical activity predicts long-term coronary heart disease and all-cause mortalities: 21-year follow-up of the Israeli ischemic heart disease study. *Arch Fam Med* 1995;4:323–329.
19. Stender M, Hense HW, Doring A, et al. Physical activity at work and cardiovascular disease risk: results from the MONICA Augsburg study. *Int J Epidemiol* 1993;22:644–650.

20. Leon AS, Myers MJ, Connett J. Leisure time physical activity and the 16-year risks of mortality from coronary heart disease and all-causes in the Multiple Risk Factor Intervention Trial (MRFIT). *Int J Sports Med* 1997;18(suppl 3):208–315.
21. Rosolova H, Simon J, Sefrna F. Impact of cardiovascular risk factors on morbidity and mortality in Czech middle-aged men: Pilsen longitudinal study. *Cardiology* 1994;85:61–68.
22. Luoto R, Prattala R, Uutela A, et al. Impact of unhealthy behaviors on cardiovascular mortality in Finland, 1978–1993. *Prev Med* 1998;27:93–100.
23. Woo J, Ho SC, Yuen YK, et al. Cardiovascular risk factors and 18-month mortality and morbidity in an elderly Chinese population aged 70 years and over. *Gerontology* 1998;44:51–55.
24. Gartside PS, Wang P, Glueck CJ. Prospective assessment of coronary heart disease risk factors: the NHANES I Epidemiologic Follow-up Study (NHEFS) 16-year follow-up. *J Am Coll Nutr* 1998;17:263–269.
25. Dorn JP, Cerny FJ, Epstein LH, et al. Work and leisure time physical activity and mortality in men and women from a general population sample. *Ann Epidemiol* 1999;9:366–373.
26. Hakim AA, Curb JD, Petrovitch H, et al. Effects of walking on coronary heart disease in elderly men: the Honolulu heart program. *Circulation* 1999;100:9–13.
27. Pate RR, Pratt M, Blair SN, et al. Physical activity and public health. A recommendation from the Centers for Disease Control and Prevention and the American College of Sports Medicine. *JAMA* 1995;273:402–407.
28. Lee IM, Rexrode KM, Cook NR, et al. Physical activity and coronary heart disease in women: is "no pain, no gain" passe? *JAMA* 2001;285:1447–1454.
29. Eaton CB. Relation of physical activity and cardiovascular fitness to coronary heart disease, Part II: cardiovascular fitness and the safety and efficacy of physical activity prescription. *J Am Board Fam Pract* 1992;5:157–165. Search date not stated; primary sources Medline and hand searches.
30. Blair SN, Kohl HW 3rd, Barlow CE, et al. Changes in physical fitness and all-cause mortality: a prospective study of healthy and unhealthy men. *JAMA* 1995;273:1093–1098.
31. Lakka TA, Laukkanen JA, Rauramaa R, et al. Cardiorespiratory fitness and the progression of carotid atherosclerosis in middle-aged men. *Ann Intern Med* 2001;134:12–20.
32. Williams PT. Physical fitness and activity as separate heart disease risk factors: a meta-analysis. *Med Sci Sports Exerc* 2001;33:754–761.
33. Sacco RL, Gan R, Boden-Albala B, et al. Leisure-time physical activity and ischemic stroke risk: the Northern Manhattan stroke study. *Stroke* 1998;29:380–387.
34. Shinton R. Lifelong exposures and the potential for stroke prevention: the contribution of cigarette smoking, exercise, and body fat. *J Epidemiol Community Health* 1997;51:138–143.
35. Gillum RF, Mussolino ME, Ingram DD. Physical activity and stroke incidence in women and men. The NHANES I epidemiologic follow-up study. *Am J Epidemiol* 1996;143:860–869.
36. Kiely DK, Wolf PA, Cupples LA, et al. Physical activity and stroke risk: the Framingham study [correction appears in *Am J Epidemiol* 1995;141:178]. *Am J Epidemiol* 1994;140:608–620.
37. Abbott RD, Rodriguez BL, Burchfiel CM, et al. Physical activity in older middle-aged men and reduced risk of stroke: the Honolulu heart program. *Am J Epidemiol* 1994;139:881–893.
38. Haheim LL, Holme I, Hjermann I, et al. Risk factors of stroke incidence and mortality: a 12-year follow-up of the Oslo study. *Stroke* 1993;24:1484–1489.
39. Wannamethee G, Shaper AG. Physical activity and stroke in British middle aged men. *BMJ* 1992;304:597–601.
40. Menotti A, Keys A, Blackburn H, et al. Twenty-year stroke mortality and prediction in twelve cohorts of the seven countries study. *Int J Epidemiol* 1990;19:309–315.
41. Lindenstrom E, Boysen G, Nyboe J. Risk factors for stroke in Copenhagen, Denmark. II. Lifestyle factors. *Neuroepidemiology* 1993;12:43–50.
42. Lindenstrom E, Boysen G, Nyboe J. Lifestyle factors and risk of cerebrovascular disease in women: the Copenhagen City heart study. *Stroke* 1993;24:1468–1472.
43. Folsom AR, Prineas RJ, Kaye SA, et al. Incidence of hypertension and stroke in relation to body fat distribution and other risk factors in older women. *Stroke* 1990;21:701–706.
44. Nakayama T, Date C, Yokoyama T, et al. A 15.5-year follow-up study of stroke in a Japanese provincial city: the Shibata study. *Stroke* 1997;28:45–52.
45. Lee IM, Hennekens CH, Berger K, et al. Exercise and risk of stroke in male physicians. *Stroke* 1999;30:1–6.
46. Evenson KR, Rosamond WD, Cai J, et al. Physical activity and ischemic stroke risk: the atherosclerosis in communities study. *Stroke* 1999;30:1333–1339.
47. Mittleman MA, Maclure M, Tofler GH, et al. Triggering of acute myocardial infarction by heavy physical exertion. Protection against triggering by regular exertion: determinants of myocardial infarction onset study investigators. *N Engl J Med* 1993;329:1677–1683.
48. Willich SN, Lewis M, Lowel H, et al. Physical exertion as a trigger of acute myocardial infarction: triggers and mechanisms of myocardial infarction study group. *N Engl J Med* 1993;329:1684–1690.
49. Thompson PD. The cardiovascular complications of vigorous physical activity. *Arch Intern Med* 1996;156:2297–2302.
50. Oberman A. Exercise and the primary prevention of cardiovascular disease. *Am J Cardiol* 1985;55:10–20.
51. Andersen RE, Wadden TA, Bartlett SJ, et al. Effects of lifestyle activity vs structured aerobic exercise in obese women: a randomized trial. *JAMA* 1999;281:335–340.
52. Dunn AL, Marcus BH, Kampert JB, et al. Comparison of lifestyle and structured interventions to increase physical activity and cardiorespiratory fitness: a randomized trial. *JAMA* 1999;281:327–434.
53. Pereira MA, Kriska AM, Day RD, et al. A randomized walking trial in postmenopausal women: effects on physical activity and health 10 years later. *Arch Intern Med* 1998;158:1695–1701.
54. DeBusk RF, Stenestrand U, Sheehan M, et al. Training effects of long versus short bouts of exercise in healthy subjects. *Am J Cardiol* 1990;65:1010–1013.
55. Ness AR, Powles JW. Fruit and vegetables and cardiovascular disease: a review. *Int J Epidemiol* 1997;26:1–13. Search date 1995; primary sources Medline, Embase, and hand searches of personal bibliographies, books, reviews, and citations in located reports.

56. Law MR, Morris JK. By how much does fruit and vegetable consumption reduce the risk of ischaemic heart disease? *Eur J Clin Nutr* 1998;52:549–556. Search date not stated; primary sources Medline, Science Citation Index, and hand searches of review articles.
57. Klerk M, Jansen MCJF, van't Veer P, et al. Fruits and vegetables in chronic disease prevention. Wageningen: Grafisch Bedrijf Ponsen and Looijen, 1998. Search date 1998; primary sources Medline, Current Contents, and Toxline.
58. Knekt P, Isotupa S, Rissanen H, et al. Quercetin intake and the incidence of cerebrovascular disease. *Eur J Clin Nutr* 2000;54:415–417.
59. Key TJA, Thorogood M, Appleby PN, et al. Dietary habits and mortality in 11 000 vegetarians and health conscious people: results of a 17 year follow up. *BMJ* 1996;313:775–779.
60. Pietinen P, Rimm EB, Korhonen P, et al. Intake of dietary fibre and risk of coronary heart disease in a cohort of Finnish men. *Circulation* 1996;94:2720–2727.
61. Mann JI, Appleby PN, Key TJA, et al. Dietary determinants of ischaemic heart disease in health conscious individuals. *Heart* 1997;78:450–455.
62. Geleijnse M. Consumptie van groente en fruit en het risico op myocardinfarct 1997. Basisrapportage. Rotterdam: Erasmus Universiteit (cited in appendix XIII of review by Klerk).
63. Todd S, Woodward M, Tunstall-Pedoe H, et al. Dietary antioxidant vitamins and fiber in the etiology of cardiovascular disease and all-cause mortality: results from the Scottish heart health study. *Am J Epidemiol* 1999;150:1073–1080.
64. Bazzano L, Ogden LG, Vupputuri S, et al. Fruit and vegetable intake reduces cardiovascular mortality: results from the NHANES I Epidemiologic Follow-up Study (NHEFS). Abstract presented at the 40th Annual conference on Cardiovascular Epidemiology and Prevention, San Diego California 1–4 March 2000.
65. Liu S, Lee I-M, Ajani U, et al. Intake of vegetables rich in carotenoids and risk of coronary heart disease in men: the Physicians' Health Study. *Int J Epidemiol* 2001;30:130–135.
66. Lui S, Manson JE, Lee I-M, et al. Fruit and vegetable intake and risk of cardiovascular disease: the Women's Health Study. *Am J Clin Nutr* 2000;72:922–928.
67. Cox BD, Whichelow MJ, Prevost AT. Seasonal consumption of salad vegetables and fresh fruit in relation to the development of cardiovascular disease and cancer. *Public Health Nutr* 2000;3:19–29.
68. van't Veer P, Jansen MCJF, Klerk M, et al. Fruits and vegetables in the prevention of cancer and cardiovascular disease. *Public Health Nutr* 2000;3:103–107.
69. Joshipura KJ, Ascherio A, Manson JE, et al. Fruit and vegetable intake in relation to risk of ischemic stroke. *JAMA* 1999;282:1233–1239.
70. Ness AR, Powles JW. Does eating fruit and vegetables protect against heart attack and stroke? *Chem Indus* 1996;792–794.
71. Ness AR, Powles JW. Dietary habits and mortality in vegetarians and health conscious people: several uncertainties exist. *BMJ* 1997;314:148.
72. Serdula MK, Byers T, Mokhad AH, et al. The association between fruit and vegetable intake and chronic disease risk factors. *Epidemiology* 1996;7:161–165.
73. Lonn EM, Yusuf S. Is there a role for antioxidant vitamins in the prevention of cardiovascular disease? An update on epidemiological and clinical trials data. *Can J Cardiol* 1997;13:957–965. Search date not stated; primary sources Medline, Science Citation Index, and hand searches.
74. Asplund K. Antioxidant vitamins in the prevention of cardiovascular disease: a systematic review. *J Intern Med* 2002;251:372–392. Search date 2001; primary sources Medline, Science Citation Index, and reference lists of published articles.
75. Ness AR, Powles JW, Khaw KT. Vitamin C and cardiovascular disease — a systematic review. *J Cardiovasc Risk* 1997;3:513–521. Search date 1996; primary sources Medline, Embase, and hand searches of personal bibliographies, books, reviews, and citations in located reports.
76. Houtman JP. Trace elements and cardiovascular disease. *J Cardiovasc Risk* 1996;3:18–25.
77. Nève J. Selenium as a risk factor for cardiovascular disease. *J Cardiovasc Risk* 1996;3:42–47.
78. Hertog MGL, Feskens EJM, Holliman PCH, et al. Dietary antioxidant flavonoids and risk of coronary heart disease: the Zutphen elderly study. *Lancet* 1993;342:1007–1011.
79. Yochum L, Kushi LH, Meyer K, et al. Dietary flavonoid intake and risk of cardiovascular disease in postmenopausal women. *Am J Epidemiol* 1999;149:943–949.
80. Knekt P, Jarvinen R, Reunanen A, et al. Flavonoid intake and coronary mortality in Finland: a cohort study. *BMJ* 1996;312:478–481.
81. Rimm EB, Katan MB, Ascherio A, et al. Relation between intake of flavonoids and risk for coronary heart disease in male health professionals. *Ann Intern Med* 1996;125:384–389.
82. Hertog MGL, Sweetnam PM, Fehily AM. Antioxidant flavonols and ischemic heart disease in a Welsh population of men: the Caerphilly study. *Am J Clin Nutr* 1997;65:1489–1494.
83. Hirvonen T, Virtamo J, Korhonen P, et al. Intake of flavonoids, carotenoids, vitamin C and E, and risk of stroke in male smokers. *Stroke* 2000;31:2301–2306.
84. Keli SO, Hertog MGL, Feskens EJM, et al. Dietary flavonoids, antioxidant vitamins, and incidence of stroke. *Arch Intern Med* 1996;156:637–642.
85. Leppälä JM, Virtamo J, Fogelholm R, et al. Controlled trial of α-tocopherol and β-carotene supplements on stroke incidence and mortality in male smokers *Arterioscler Thromb Vasc Biol* 2000;20:230–235.
86. Egger M, Schneider M, Davey Smith G. Spurious precision? Meta-analysis of observational studies. *BMJ* 1998;316:140–144.
87. Doering WV. Antioxidant vitamins, cancer, and cardiovascular disease. *N Engl J Med* 1996;335:1065.
88. Pietrzik K. Antioxidant vitamins, cancer, and cardiovascular disease. *N Engl J Med* 1996;335:1065–1066.
89. Hennekens CH, Gaziano JM, Manson JE, et al. Antioxidant vitamin cardiovascular disease hypothesis is still promising, but still unproven: the need for randomised trials. *Am J Clin Nutr* 1995;62(suppl):1377–1380.
90. Rose G, Hamilton PJ, Colwell L, et al. A randomised controlled trial of anti-smoking advice: 10-year results. *J Epidemiol Community Health* 1982;36:102–108.
91. US Department of Health and Human Services. The health benefits of smoking cessation: a report of the Surgeon General. Rockville, Maryland: US Department of Health and Human Services, Public Health Service, Centers for Disease Control, 1990. DHHS Publication (CDC) 90–8416.
92. Royal College of Physicians. *Smoking and health now*. London: Pitman Medical and Scientific Publishing, 1971.

93. Doll R, Peto R, Wheatley K, et al. Mortality in relation to smoking: 40 years' observations on male British doctors. *BMJ* 1994;309:901–911.
94. Kawachi I, Colditz GA, Stampfer MJ, et al. Smoking cessation in relation to total mortality rates in women: a prospective cohort study. *Ann Intern Med* 1993;119:992–1000.
95. Rosenberg L, Kaufman DW, Helmrich SP, et al. The risk of myocardial infarction after quitting smoking in men under 55 years of age. *N Engl J Med* 1985;313:1511–1514.
96. Rosenberg L, Palmer JR, Shapiro S. Decline in the risk of myocardial infarction among women who stop smoking. *N Engl J Med* 1990;322:213–217.
97. Shinton R, Beevers G. Meta-analysis of relation between cigarette smoking and stroke. *BMJ* 1989;298:789–794. Search date 1988; primary source index references from three studies on cigarette smoking and stroke on medicine.
98. Rogot E, Murray JL. Smoking and causes of death among US veterans: 16 years of observation. *Public Health Rep* 1980;95:213–222.
99. Wannamethee SG, Shaper AG, Ebrahim S. History of parental death from stroke or heart trouble and the risk of stroke in middle-aged men. *Stroke* 1996;27:1492–1498.
100. Whelton SP, Chin A, Xin X, et al. Effect of aerobic exercise on blood pressure: a meta-analysis of randomized, controlled trials. *Ann Intern Med* 2002;136:493–503.
101. Ebrahim S, Davey Smith G. Lowering blood pressure: a systematic review of sustained non-pharmacological interventions. *J Public Health Med* 1998;20:441–448. Search date 1995; primary source Medline.
102. Engstom G, Hedblad B, Janzon L. Hypertensive men who exercise regularly have lower rate of cardiovascular mortality. *J Hypertens* 1999;17:737–742.
103. Appel LJ, Moore TJ, Obarzanek E, et al. A clinical trial of the effects of dietary patterns on blood pressure. *N Engl J Med* 1997;336:1117–1124.
104. Beilin LJ, Puddey IB, Burke V. Alcohol and hypertension: kill or cure? *J Hum Hypertens* 1996;10(suppl 2):1–5.
105. Xin X, HE J, Frontini MG, et al. Effects of alcohol reduction on blood pressure: a meta-analysis of randomized controlled trials. *Hypertension* 2001;38:1112–1117. Search date 1999; primary sources Medline and reference lists of retrieved articles.
106. Graudal NA, Galloe AM, Garred P. Effects of sodium restriction on blood pressure, renin, aldosterone, catecholamines, cholesterols, and triglyceride. *JAMA* 1998;279:1383–1391. Search date 1997; primary source Medline.
107. Whelton PK, Appel LJ, Espelland MA, et al. Sodium reduction and weight loss in the treatment of hypertension in older persons: a randomized controlled trial of non pharmacologic interventions in the elderly (TONE). *JAMA* 1998;279:839–846.
108. Sacks FM, Svetkey LP, Vollmer WM, et al. Effects on blood pressure of reduced dietary sodium and the Dietary Approaches to Stop Hypertension (DASH) diet. *N Engl J Med* 2001;344:3–10
109. Midgley JP, Matthew AG, Greenwood CMT, et al. Effect of reduced dietary sodium on blood pressure. *JAMA* 1996;275:1590–1597. Search date 1994; primary sources Medline and Current Contents.
110. Mulrow CD, Chiquette E, Angel L, et al. Dieting to reduce body weight for controlling hypertension in adults. In: The Cochrane Library, Issue 1, 2003. Oxford: Update Software. Search date 1998; primary source Cochrane Library, Medline, and contact with experts in the field.
111. Metz JA, Stern JS, Kris-Etherton P, et al. A randomized trial of improved weight loss with a prepared meal plan in overweight and obese patients. *Arch Intern Med* 2000;160:2150–2158.
112. Stevens VJ, Obarzanek E, Cook NR, et al. Long-term weight loss and changes in blood pressure: results of the Trials of Hypertension Prevention, Phase II. *Ann Intern Med* 2001;134:1–11.
113. Whelton PK, He J, Cutler JA, et al. Effects of oral potassium on blood pressure: meta-analysis of randomized controlled clinical trials. *JAMA* 1997;277:1624–1632. Search date 1995; primary source Medline.
114. Morris MC, Sacks F, Rosner B. Does fish oil lower blood pressure? A meta-analysis of controlled clinical trials. *Circulation* 1993;88:523–533. Search date not stated; primary source Index Medicus.
115. Griffith LE, Guyatt GH, Cook RJ, et al. The influence of dietary and nondietary calcium supplementation on blood pressure. *Am J Hypertens* 1999;12:84–92. Search date 1994; primary sources Medline and Embase.
116. Gueyffier F, Froment A, Gouton M. New meta-analysis of treatment trials of hypertension: improving the estimate of therapeutic benefit. *J Hum Hypertens* 1996;10:1–8. Search date 1997; primary source Medline.
117. Staessen JA, Gasowski J, Wang JG, et al. Risks of untreated and treated isolated systolic hypertension in the elderly: meta-analysis of outcome trials. *Lancet* 2000;355:865–872. Search date 1999; primary sources other systematic reviews and reports from collaborative trialists.
118. Hansson L, Zanchetti AZ, Carruthers SG, et al. Effects of intensive blood pressure lowering and low-dose aspirin in patients with hypertension: principal results of the Hypertension Optimal Treatment (HOT) trial. *Lancet* 1998;351:1755–1762.
119. Beto JA, Bansal VK. Quality of life in treatment of hypertension: a meta-analysis of clinical trials. *Am J Hypertens* 1992;5:125–133. Search date 1990; primary sources Medline and ERIC.
120. Croog SH, Levine S, Testa MA. The effects of antihypertensive therapy on quality of life. *N Engl J Med* 1986;314:1657–1664.
121. Boutitie F, Gueyffier F, Pocock S, et al. J-Shaped relationship between blood pressure and mortality in hypertensive patients: new insights from a meta-analysis of individual-patient data. *Ann Intern Med* 2002;136:438–448.
122. Psaty BM, Smith NS, Siscovick DS, et al. Health outcomes associated with antihypertensive therapies used as first line agents: a systematic review and meta-analysis. *JAMA* 1997;277:739–745. Search date 1995; primary source Medline.
123. Messerli FH, Grossman E, Goldbourt U. Are beta blockers efficacious as first-line therapy for hypertension in the elderly? A systematic review. *JAMA* 1998;279:1903–1907. Search date 1998; primary source Medline.
124. Blood Pressure Lowering Treatment Trialists' Collaboration. Effects of ACE inhibitors, calcium antagonists, and other blood-pressure-lowering drugs: results of prospectively designed overviews of trials. *Lancet* 2000;356:1955–1964. Search date 2000; primary sources WHO-International Society of Hypertension registry of randomised trials; trials were sought that had not published or presented their results before July 1995.

125. Staessen JA, Wang JG, Thijs L. Cardiovascular protection and blood pressure reduction: a meta-analysis. *Lancet* 2001;358:1305–1315. Search date 2001; primary sources Medline and hand searches of reference lists of overviews.
126. The ALLHAT Officers and Coordinators for the ALLHAT Collaborative Research Group. Major cardiovascular events in hypertensive patients randomized to doxazosin vs chlorthalidone: the Antihypertensive and Lipid-Lowering treatment to prevent Heart Attack Trial (ALLHAT). *JAMA* 2000;283:1967–1975.
127. Dahlof B, Devereux RB, Kjeldsen SE, et al. Cardiovascular morbidity and mortality in the Losartan Intervention For Endpoint reduction in hypertension study (LIFE): a randomised trial against atenolol. *Lancet* 2002;359:995–1003.
128. Neaton JD, Grimm RH, Prineas RJ, et al. Treatment of mild hypertension study: final results. *JAMA* 1993;270:713–724.
129. Materson BJ, Reda DJ, Cushman WC, et al. Single drug therapy for hypertension in men. *N Engl J Med* 1993;328:914–921.
130. Philipp T, Anlauf M, Distler A, et al. Randomised, double blind, multicentre comparison of hydrochlorothiazide, atenolol, nitrendipine, and enalapril in antihypertensive treatment: results of the HANE study. *BMJ* 1997;315:154–159.
131. Wright JM, Lee CH, Chambers CK. Systematic review of antihypertensive therapies: does the evidence assist in choosing a first line drug? *Can Med Assoc J* 1999;161:25–32. Search date 1998; primary sources Medline and Cochrane Library.
132. Cutler JA. Calcium channel blockers for hypertension — uncertainty continues. *N Engl J Med* 1998;338:679–680.
133. Pignone M, Phillips C, Mulrow C. Use of lipid lowering drugs for primary prevention of coronary heart disease: meta-analysis of randomised trials. *BMJ* 2000;321:983–986. Search date 1999; primary sources Medline, Cochrane Library, and hand searches of bibliographies of systematic reviews and clinical practice guidelines.
134. Cucherat M, Lievre M, Gueyffier F. Clinical benefits of cholesterol lowering treatments. Meta-analysis of randomized therapeutic trials. *Presse Med* 2000 May 13;29:965–976. Search date and primary sources not stated.
135. Katerndahl DA, Lawler WR. Variability in meta-analytic results concerning the value of cholesterol reduction in coronary heart disease: a meta-meta-analysis. *Am J Epidemiol* 1999;149:429–441. Search date 1995; primary sources Medline and meta-analysis bibliographies.
136. Ebrahim S, Davey Smith G, McCabe CCC, et al. What role for statins? A review and economic model. *Health Technol Assess* 1999;3(10):i–iv, 1–91. Search date 1997; primary sources Medline, Cochrane Controlled Trials Register, and personal contact with investigators working in the field of cholesterol lowering.
137. LaRosa JC, He J, Vupputuri S. Effect of statins on risk of coronary disease: a meta-analysis of randomized controlled trials. *JAMA* 1999;282:2340–2346. Search date 1998; primary sources Medline, bibliographies, and authors' reference files.
138. Heart Protection Study Collaborative Group MRC/BHF Heart Protection Study of cholesterol lowering with simvastatin in 20536 high-risk individuals: a randomised placebo-controlled trial. *Lancet* 2002;360:7–22.
139. Sawayama Y, Shimuzu C, Maeda N, et al. Effects of probucol and pravastatin on common carotid atherosclerosis in patients with asymptomatic hypercholesterolemia. Fukuoka Atherosclerosis Trial (FAST). *J Am Coll Cardiol* 2002;39:610–616.
140. Downs JR, Clearfield M, Weis S, et al. Primary prevention of acute coronary events with lovastatin in men and women with average cholesterol levels: results of the AFCAPS/TexCAPS. *JAMA* 1998;279:1615–1622.
141. Shepherd J, Cobbe SM, Ford I, et al. Prevention of coronary heart disease with pravastatin in men with hypercholesterolemia. *N Engl J Med* 1995;333:1301–1307.
142. Scandinavian Simvastatin Survival Study Group. Randomized trial of cholesterol lowering in 4444 patients with coronary heart disease: the Scandinavian simvastatin survival study (4S). *Lancet* 1995;344:1383–1389.
143. Long-term Intervention with Pravastatin in Ischemic Disease (LIPID) Study Program. Prevention of cardiovascular events and death with pravastatin in patients with coronary heart disease and a broad range of initial cholesterol levels. *N Engl J Med* 1998;339:1349–1357.
144. Sacks FM, Pfeffer MA, Moye LA, et al. Effect of pravastatin on coronary events after myocardial infarction in patients with average cholesterol levels. *N Engl J Med* 1996;335:1001–1009.
145. Jackson PR, Wallis EJ, Haq IU, et al. Statins for primary prevention: at what coronary risk is safety assured? *Br J Clin Pharmacol* 2001;52:439–446.
146. Bucher HC, Griffith LE, Guyatt G. Systematic review on the risk and benefit of different cholesterol-lowering interventions. *Arterioscler Thromb Vasc Biol* 1999:19;187–195. Search date 1996; primary sources Medline, Embase, and hand searches of bibliographies.
147. Hart RG, Halperin JL, McBride R, et al. Aspirin for the primary prevention of stroke and other major vascular events. Meta-analysis and hypotheses. *Arch Neurol* 2000;57:326–332. Search date 1998; primary sources unspecified computerised medical databases, Cochrane Collaboration Registry, and hand searches of references of Antiplatelet Trialists' Collaboration publications.
148. Hebert PR, Hennekens CH. An overview of the 4 randomized trials of aspirin therapy in the primary prevention of vascular disease. *Arch Int Med* 2000;160:3123–3127. Search date and primary sources not stated.
149. Sanmuganathan PS, Ghahramani P, Jackson PR, et al. Aspirin for primary prevention of coronary heart disease: safety and absolute benefit related to coronary risk derived from a meta-analysis of randomised trials. *Heart* 2001;85:265–271. Search date not stated; primary sources Medline and previous meta-analyses and review articles.
150. Hayden M, Pignone M, Phillips C, et al. Aspirin for the primary prevention of cardiovascular events: a summary of the evidence for the US preventive services task force. *Ann Intern Med* 2002;136:161–172. Search date 2001; primary source Medline.
151. Boltri JM, Akerson MR, Vogel RL. Aspirin prophylaxis in patients at low risk for cardiovascular disease: a systematic review of all-cause mortality. *J Fam Pract* 2002; 51:700–704. Search date not stated; primary sources Medline, the Cochrane Library, the Internet and reference lists of identified trials and reviews.
152. Collaborative group of the Primary Prevention Project (PPP). Low-dose aspirin and vitamin E in people at cardiovascular risk: a randomised trial in general practice. *Lancet* 2001;357:89–95.

153. Peto R, Gray R, Collins R, et al. Randomised trial of prophylactic daily aspirin in British male doctors. *BMJ* 1988;296:313–316.
154. Steering Committee of the Physicians' Health Study Research Group. Final report on the aspirin component of the ongoing physicians' health study. *N Engl J Med* 1989;321:129–135.
155. ETDRS Investigators. Aspirin effects on mortality and morbidity in patients with diabetes mellitus. Early Treatment Diabetic Retinopathy Study report 14. *JAMA* 1992;268:1292–1300.
156. Medical Research Council's General Practice Research Framework. Thrombosis prevention trial: randomised trial of low-intensity anticoagulation with warfarin and low dose aspirin in the primary prevention of ischaemic heart disease in men at increased risk. *Lancet* 1998;351:233–241.
157. Antiplatelet Trialists' Collaboration. Collaborative overview of randomised trials of antiplatelet therapy — I: prevention of death, myocardial infarction, and stroke by prolonged antiplatelet therapy in various categories of patients. *BMJ* 1994;308:81–106. Search date 1990; primary sources Medline, Current Contents, hand searches of reference list of trials and review articles, journal abstracts and meeting proceedings, trial register of the International Committee on Thrombosis and Haemostasis, and personal contacts with colleagues and antiplatelet manufactures.
158. He J, Whelton PK, Vu B, et al. Aspirin and risk of hemorrhagic stroke: a meta-analysis of randomized controlled trials. *JAMA* 1998;280:1930–1935. Search date 1997; primary sources Medline, the authors' reference files, and reference lists from original communications and review articles.
159. Derry S, Loke YK. Risk of gastrointestinal haemorrhage with long term use of aspirin: meta-analysis. *BMJ* 2000;321:1183–1187. Search date not stated; primary sources Medline, Embase, and reference lists from previous review papers and retrieved trials.
160. Garc a Rodr guez LA, Hernández-D az S, De Abajo FJ. Association between aspirin and upper gastrointestinal complications: a systematic review of epidemiologic studies. *Br J Clin Pharmacol Zool* 2001;52:563–571.
161. Antithrombotic Trialists' Collaboration. Collaborative meta-analysis of randomised trials of antiplatelet therapy for prevention of death, myocardial infarction, and stroke in high risk patients. *BMJ* 2002;324:71–86.

Michael Murphy
Director, ICRF General Practice Research Group

Charles Foster
British Heart Foundation Scientist

University of Oxford
Oxford
UK

Julian J Nicholas
Resident Physician
Staub Clinic and Hospital
Honolulu
USA

Michael Pignone
Assistant Professor of Medicine
Division of General Internal Medicine
University of North Carolina
Chapel Hill
USA

Bazian Ltd
London
UK

Competing interests: CF, MM, and JN none declared. MP has received research support, consulting fees, and licensing fees from Bayer Inc. and Pfizer Inc.

The following previous contributors of this topic would like to be acknowledged: David Whiteman, Tom Kottke, Rod Jackson, Jeffery Probstfield, Colin Baigent, Cathie Sudlow, Cindy Mulrow, and Andy Ness.

TABLE 1 **Examples of common physical activities by intensity of effort required in multiples of the resting rate of oxygen consumption during physical activity (see text, p 158). Published in *JAMA* 1995;273:402–407.[27]**

Activity type	Light activity (< 3.0 METs)	Moderate activity (3.0–6.0 METs)	Vigorous activity (> 6.0 METs)
Walking	Slowly (1–2 mph)	Briskly (3–4 mph)	Briskly uphill or with a load
Swimming	Treading slowly	Moderate effort	Fast treading or swimming
Cycling	NA	For pleasure or transport (≤ 10 mph)	Fast or racing (> 10 mph)
Golf	Power cart	Pulling cart or carrying clubs	NA
Boating	Power boat	Canoeing leisurely	Canoeing rapidly (> 4 mph)
Home care	Carpet sweeping	General cleaning	Moving furniture
Mowing lawn	Riding mower	Power mower	Hand mower
Home repair	Carpentry	Painting	NA

METs, work metabolic rate/resting metabolic rate; 1 MET represents the rate of oxygen consumption of a seated adult at rest; mph, miles per hour; NA, not applicable.

TABLE 2 **Effects of aspirin on vascular events (myocardial infarction, stroke, or vascular death) in RCTs among individuals without evidence of cardiovascular disease (see text, p 175).**

Trials (duration)	Annual risk of vascular event (control)	Vascular events: Antiplatelet, control, and odds ratio* (CI†)	Events avoided per 1000 person-years	Myocardial infarction: Antiplatelet, control, and odds ratio* (CI†)	Stroke: Antiplatelet, control, and odds ratio* (CI†)
UK doctors[153] (70 months)	1.5%	288/3429, 280/3420‡, 1.03 (0.6 to 2.3)	–0.4	169/3429, 176/3420‡, 0.96 (0.7 to 1.4)	91/3429, 78/3420‡, 1.16 (0.7 to 1.9)
US physicians[154] (60 months)	0.7%	321/11 037, 387/11 034, 0.82 (0.7 to 1.0)	1.2	139/11 037, 239/11 034, 0.58 (0.5 to 0.8)	119/11 037, 98/11 034, 1.22 (0.9 to 1.7)
TPT[156] (76 months)	1.8%	239/2545, 270/2540, 0.87 (0.7 to 1.1)	2.0	154/2545, 190/2540, 0.80 (0.7 to 1.1)	47/2545, 48/2540, 0.98 (0.6 to 1.7)
HOT[118] (46 months)	1.0%	315/9399, 368/9391, 0.85 (0.7 to 1.0)	1.5	82/9399, 127/9391, 0.65 (0.5 to 0.9)	146/9399, 148/9391, 0.99 (0.7 to 1.3)
PPP[152] (44 months)	0.8%	45/2226, 64/2269, 0.71 (0.4 to 1.2)	2.2	19/2226, 28/2269, 0.69 (0.3 to 1.5)	16/2226, 24/2269, 0.68 (0.3 to 1.6)
All trials (56 months)	1.0%	1208/28 636 (4.2%), 1369/28 654 (4.8%), 0.86§ (0.8 to 0.9)	1.2	563/28 636 (2.0%), 760/28 654 (2.4%), 0.71§ (0.6 to 0.8)	419/28 636 (1.5%), 396/28 654 (1.4%), 1.05§ (0.9 to 1.2)

Data from individual trial publications and from the APT overview (1994).[157] The effects of aspirin were similar in the absence or presence of warfarin, so the data presented are not stratified by warfarin allocation. * Odds ratios calculated using the "observed minus expected" method;[157] † 99% CI for individual trials 95% CI for "All trials"; ‡ Number of patients in control group was 1710 (randomisation ratio 2 : 1); numerator and denominator multiplied by 2 to calculate totals for absolute differences between antiplatelet and control group event rates; actual numbers of events used to calculate odds ratios and confidence intervals; § Heterogeneity of odds ratios between five trials not significant ($P > 0.05$).

TABLE 3 **Effects of aspirin on intracranial and major extracranial haemorrhages in RCTs among individuals without evidence of cardiovascular disease (see text, p 175).**

Trials	Antiplatelet	Control	Summary odds ratio* (95% CI)	Excess bleeds per 1000 patients treated per year
Intracranial bleeds				
UK doctors[149]	13/3429	12/3420†		
US physicians[150]	23/11 037	12/11 034		
TPT[155]	12/2545	6/2540		
HOT[121]	14/9399	15/9391		
PPP[81]	2/2226	3/2269		
All trials	**64/28 636 (0.22%)**	**48/28654 (0.17%)**	**1.4 (0.9 to 2.0)**	**0.1 (P = 0.1)**
Major extracranial bleeds				
UK Doctors[149]	21/3429	20/3420†		
US Physicians[150]	48/1037	28/11 034		
TPT[155]	20/2545	13/2540		
HOT[121]	122/9399	63/9391		
All trials	**211/26 410 (0.8%)**	**134/28 095 (0.5%)**	**1.7 (1.4 to 2.1)**	**0.7 (P < 0.00001)**

Data from individual trial publications. *Odds ratios calculated using the "observed minus expected" method.[157]
†Number of patients in control group was 1710 (randomisation ratio 2 : 1); numerator and denominator multiplied by 2 to calculate totals for absolute differences between antiplatelet and control group event rates; actual numbers of events used to calculate odds ratios and confidence intervals.

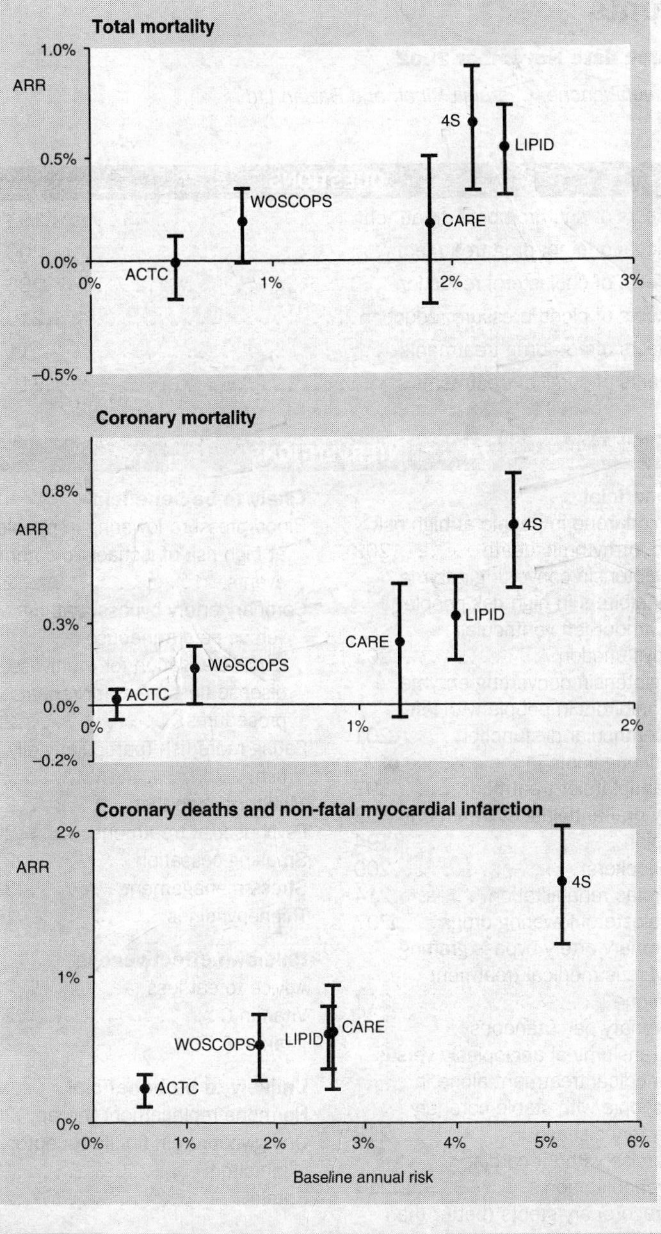

FIGURE 1 **Effects of cholesterol lowering: relation between the ARR (for annual total mortality, coronary heart disease mortality, coronary deaths, and non-fatal myocardial infarction) and the baseline risk of those events in the placebo group for five large statin trials (ACTC = AFCAPS/TexCAPS,[140] 4S,[142] LIPID,[143] CARE,[144] WOSCOPS[141]) (see text, p 173).**

Secondary prevention of ischaemic cardiac events

Search date November 2002

Michael Pignone, Charanjit Rihal, and Bazian Ltd

QUESTIONS

INTERVENTIONS

Likely to be ineffective or harmful	To be covered in future updates
Adding anticoagulants to antiplatelet treatment. 198	Alcohol intake
β Carotene 212	Implantable cardioverter defibrillators
Calcium channel blockers 204	
Class I antiarrhythmic agents . .203	See glossary, p 222

Key Messages

Antithrombotic treatment

- **Anticoagulants in the absence of antiplatelet treatment** One systematic review and subsequent RCTs have found that high or moderate intensity oral anticoagulants given alone reduce the risk of serious vascular events compared with placebo or no anticoagulants in people with coronary artery disease, but are associated with substantial risk of haemorrhage.
- **Any oral antiplatelet treatment** One systematic review has found that prolonged antiplatelet treatment compared with placebo or no antiplatelet treatment reduces the risk of serious vascular events in people at high risk of ischaemic cardiac events.
- **Aspirin** One systematic review has found that, for prolonged use, aspirin 75–150 mg daily is as effective as higher doses, but found insufficient evidence that doses below 75 mg daily are as effective.
- **Thienopyridines** One systematic review has found that clopidogrel is at least as safe and effective as aspirin in people at high risk of cardiovascular events.
- **Oral glycoprotein IIb/IIIa receptor inhibitors** Systematic reviews in people with acute coronary syndromes or undergoing percutaneous coronary interventions have found that oral glycoprotein IIb/IIIa receptor inhibitors (with or without aspirin) increase risk of mortality and bleeding compared with aspirin alone.
- **Adding anticoagulants to antiplatelet treatment** One systematic review and subsequent RCTs found no consistent evidence that addition of oral anticoagulation at low (international normalised ratio < 1.5) or moderate (international normalised ratio 1.5–3.0) intensity to aspirin reduced risk of death or recurrent cardiac events, but found an increased risk of major haemorrhage compared with aspirin alone.

Other drug treatments

- **Amiodarone in people at high risk of arrhythmic death** Two systematic reviews have found that amiodarone reduces the risk of sudden cardiac death and overall mortality at 1 year compared with placebo in people at high risk of arrhythmic death after myocardial infarction.
- **Angiotensin converting enzyme inhibitors in high risk people without left ventricular dysfunction** One large RCT in high risk people without left ventricular dysfunction found that ramipril reduced the combined outcome of cardiovascular death, stroke, and myocardial infarction compared with placebo after about 5 years.
- **Angiotensin converting enzyme inhibitors in people with left ventricular dysfunction** One systematic review has found that, in people who have had a myocardial infarction and have left ventricular dysfunction, angiotensin converting enzyme inhibitors reduce mortality, admission to hospital for congestive heart failure, and recurrent non-fatal myocardial infarction compared with placebo after 2 years' treatment.

- **β Blockers** Systematic reviews in people after myocardial infarction have found that long term β blockers reduce all cause mortality, coronary mortality, recurrent non-fatal myocardial infarction, and sudden death. One RCT found that about 25% of people suffer adverse effects.
- **Hormone replacement therapy** Large RCTs found no significant difference between hormone replacement therapy and placebo in major cardiovascular events in postmenopausal women with established coronary artery disease. Observational studies and one large RCT found that hormone replacement therapy increased risk of breast cancer, venous thromboembolism, and gall bladder disease compared with placebo.
- **Sotalol** One RCT found limited evidence that sotalol increased mortality within 1 year compared with placebo.
- **Calcium channel blockers** One systematic review found non-significantly higher mortality with dihydropyridines compared with placebo. One systematic review found no benefit from calcium channel blockers in people after myocardial infarction or with chronic coronary heart disease. Diltiazem and verapamil may reduce rates of reinfarction and refractory angina in people after myocardial infarction who do not have heart failure.
- **Class I antiarrhythmic agents** One systematic review has found that class I antiarrhythmic agents given after myocardial infarction increase the risk of cardiovascular mortality and sudden death compared with placebo.

Cholesterol reduction

- **Cholesterol lowering drugs** Systematic reviews and large subsequent RCTs have found that lowering cholesterol in people at high risk of ischaemic coronary events substantially reduces overall mortality, cardiovascular mortality, and non-fatal cardiovascular events. We found good evidence from systematic reviews and subsequent RCTs that statins were the only non-surgical treatment for cholesterol reduction that reduced mortality. One systematic review has found that the absolute benefits increase as baseline risk increases, but are not additionally influenced by the person's absolute blood cholesterol concentration.

Blood pressure reduction

- **Blood pressure lowering in people at high risk of ischaemic coronary events** We found no direct evidence of the effects of blood pressure lowering in people with established coronary heart disease. Observational studies, and extrapolation of primary prevention trials of blood pressure reduction, support the lowering of blood pressure in those at high risk of ischaemic coronary events. The evidence for benefit is strongest for β blockers, although not specifically in people with hypertension. The optimum target blood pressure in people with hypertension is not clear. Effects of angiotensin converting enzyme inhibitors, calcium channel blockers, and β blockers are discussed separately.

Non-drug treatments

- **Cardiac rehabilitation** One systematic review has found that cardiac rehabilitation including exercise reduces the risk of major cardiac events. One subsequent RCT found no significant difference in quality of life between standard rehabilitation and early return to normal activities, although the study may have lacked power to detect a clinically important difference between groups.
- **Exercise without cardiac rehabilitation** One systematic review has found that exercise alone reduces mortality compared with usual care.

- **Eating more fish (particularly oily fish)** One RCT has found that advising people with coronary heart disease to eat more fish (particularly oily fish) reduced mortality at 2 years. A second RCT found that fish oil capsules reduced mortality at 3.5 years.
- **Mediterranean diet** One RCT has found that advising people with coronary artery disease to eat more bread, fruit, vegetables, and fish, and less meat, and to replace butter and cream with rapeseed margarine reduces mortality at 27 months.
- **Psychosocial treatment** RCTs found limited evidence that psychosocial treatments reduced cardiac events or cardiac death compared with no psychosocial treatment in people with coronary heart disease. Two RCTs found that psychological treatments improved quality of life compared with no psychological treatment.
- **Smoking cessation** We found no RCTs of the effects of smoking cessation on cardiovascular events in people with coronary heart disease. Moderate quality evidence from epidemiological studies indicates that people with coronary heart disease who stop smoking rapidly reduce their risk of recurrent coronary events or death. Treatment with nicotine patches seems safe in people with coronary heart disease.
- **Stress management** One systematic review of mainly poor quality RCTs found that stress management may decrease rates of myocardial infarction or cardiac death in people with coronary heart disease.
- **Advice to eat less fat** RCTs found no strong evidence that low fat diets reduced mortality at 2 years.
- **Vitamin C** We found insufficient evidence about effects of vitamin C alone.
- **Vitamin E** We found no consistent evidence from four RCTs about effects of vitamin E versus placebo or other antioxidants in people with high cardiovascular risk.
- **β carotene** Four large RCTs of β carotene supplementation in primary prevention found no cardiovascular benefits, and two of the RCTs raised concerns about increased mortality.

Surgical treatments

- **Coronary artery bypass grafting versus medical treatment alone** One systematic review found that coronary artery bypass grafting reduced the risk of death from coronary artery disease at 5 and 10 years compared with medical treatment alone. Greater benefit occurred in people with poor left ventricular function. One subsequent RCT in people with asymptomatic disease found that revascularisation with coronary artery bypass grafting or coronary percutaneous transluminal angioplasty reduced mortality at 2 years compared with medical treatment alone.
- **Coronary percutaneous transluminal angioplasty versus medical treatment alone in people with stable coronary artery disease** One systematic review found that coronary percutaneous transluminal angioplasty improved angina compared with medical treatment alone, but was associated with a higher rate of coronary artery bypass grafting. The review found higher mortality and rates of myocardial infarction with percutaneous transluminal angioplasty than with medical treatment but the difference was not significant. RCTs have found that percutaneous transluminal angioplasty is associated with increased risk of emergency coronary artery bypass grafting and myocardial infarction during and soon after the procedure. One RCT found that percutaneous transluminal angioplasty reduced cardiac events and improved angina severity compared with medical treatment alone in people over the age of 75 years.

- **Intracoronary stents (better than coronary percutaneous transluminal angioplasty alone)** One systematic review found that intracoronary stents reduce the need for repeat vascularisation compared with coronary percutaneous transluminal angioplasty alone. It found no significant difference in mortality or myocardial infarction, but crossover rates from angioplasty to stent were high. RCTs found that intracoronary stents improved outcomes after 4–9 months compared with percutaneous transluminal angioplasty in people with previous coronary artery bypass grafting, chronic total occlusions, and for treatment of restenosis after initial percutaneous transluminal angioplasty.
- **Coronary artery bypass grafting versus percutaneous revascularisation for multivessel disease (less need for repeat procedures)** One systematic review has found no significant difference between coronary artery bypass grafting and percutaneous transluminal angioplasty in death, myocardial infarction, or quality of life. Percutaneous transluminal angioplasty is less invasive but increased the number of repeat procedures.

DEFINITION Secondary prevention in this context is the long term management of people with a prior acute myocardial infarction, and of people at high risk of ischaemic cardiac events for other reasons, such as a history of angina or coronary surgical procedures.

INCIDENCE/ PREVALENCE Coronary artery disease is the leading cause of mortality in developed countries and is becoming a major cause of morbidity and mortality in developing countries. There are pronounced international, regional, and temporal differences in death rates. In the USA, the prevalence of overt coronary artery disease approaches 4%.[1]

AETIOLOGY/ RISK FACTORS Most ischaemic cardiac events are associated with atheromatous plaques that can cause acute obstruction of coronary vessels. Atheroma is more likely in elderly people, in those with established coronary artery disease, and in those with risk factors (such as smoking, hypertension, high cholesterol, and diabetes mellitus).

PROGNOSIS Of people admitted to hospital with acute myocardial infarction, 7–15% die in hospital and another 7–15% die during the following year. People who survive the acute stage of myocardial infarction fall into three prognostic groups, based on their baseline risk (see table 1, p 228);[2–4] high (20% of all survivors), moderate (55%), and low (25%) risk. Long term prognosis depends on the degree of left ventricular dysfunction, the presence of residual ischaemia, and the extent of any electrical instability. Further risk stratification procedures include assessment of left ventricular function (by echocardiography or nuclear ventriculography) and of myocardial ischaemia (by non-invasive stress testing).[4–8] Those with low left ventricular ejection fraction, ischaemia, or poor functional status can be assessed further by cardiac catheterisation.[9]

AIMS OF INTERVENTION To improve long term survival and quality of life; to prevent (recurrent) myocardial infarction, unstable angina, left ventricular dysfunction, heart failure, and sudden cardiac death; and to restore and maintain normal activities.

OUTCOMES Mortality (total, cardiovascular, coronary, sudden death, non-cardiovascular); morbidity (myocardial infarction, severe angina, stroke); quality of life.

METHODS *Clinical Evidence* search and appraisal November 2002.

QUESTION What are the effects of antithrombotic treatment?

Bazian Ltd

OPTION ANY ORAL ANTIPLATELET TREATMENT

One systematic review has found that prolonged antiplatelet treatment reduces the risk of serious vascular events in people at high risk of ischaemic cardiac events.

Benefits: **Oral antiplatelet treatment versus no antiplatelet treatment:** We found one systematic review (search date 1997, 195 RCTs, > 140 000 high risk people) comparing an antiplatelet regimen (mostly aspirin) versus no antiplatelet treatment (including placebo).[10] It found that antiplatelet treatment reduced the odds of a serious vascular event (myocardial infarction, stroke, or vascular death) by 25% among all types of high risk people (OR 0.75, 95% CI 0.72 to 0.78), excluding those with acute ischaemic stroke (among whom the proportional benefits were smaller).[10] The proportional effects of antiplatelet treatment were similar regardless of whether the people were included on the basis of a prior or acute myocardial infarction, prior stroke or transient ischaemic attack, stable or unstable angina, peripheral arterial disease, atrial fibrillation, or other high risk condition. Most of these people were at high risk of ischaemic cardiac events, and some (including those with a history of myocardial infarction, those with stable angina, and those who had undergone coronary revascularisation procedures) were at particularly high risk. Among the 20 000 people with a prior myocardial infarction it was estimated that antiplatelet treatment prevented 18 non-fatal recurrent myocardial infarctions, five non-fatal strokes, and 14 vascular deaths per 1000 people treated for about 2 years. The review also found that antiplatelet treatment reduced the risk of all cause mortality (see figure 1, p 229).

Harms: **Oral antiplatelet treatment:** The most important adverse effect of antiplatelet treatment is haemorrhage, particularly intracranial haemorrhage because it is frequently fatal or disabling. The systematic review (search date 1997) found a proportional increase in the risk of intracranial haemorrhage of about a quarter (OR 1.22, 95% CI 1.03 to 1.44). However, the absolute excess risk was no more than one or two events per 1000 people a year.[10] Antiplatelet treatment was associated with about a 60% increased odds of extracranial haemorrhage (mainly from the gastrointestinal tract) (OR 1.6, 95% CI 1.4 to 1.8) corresponding to an absolute excess risk of about 1–2/1000 people treated a year with a prior myocardial infarction. Most of the extracranial haemorrhages were non-fatal.[10]

Comment: Among people at high risk of cardiac events, the large absolute reductions in serious vascular events associated with antiplatelet treatment far outweigh any absolute risks.

OPTION ASPIRIN

One systematic review has found that for prolonged use, aspirin 75–150 mg daily is as effective as higher doses, but found insufficient evidence that doses below 75 mg daily are as effective. It found no clear evidence that any alternative antiplatelet regimen reduced recurrent vascular events compared with aspirin in the long term, but found that clopidogrel is at least as effective and as safe as aspirin.

Benefits: **Versus no aspirin:** We found one systematic review (search date 1997, 195 RCTs, > 140 000 high risk people) comparing an antiplatelet regimen versus no antiplatelet treatment (including placebo).[10] Aspirin was by far the most widely studied antiplatelet drug in the systematic review. Among almost 60 000 people (excluding those with acute ischaemic stroke) aspirin reduced the odds of a serious vascular event by about a quarter compared with control (OR 0.77, 95% CI 0.73 to 0.81).[10] **Different daily doses:** Direct comparisons (3197 high risk people) between daily doses of 500–1500 mg versus 75–325 mg found no significant difference in effect (OR higher versus lower dose 0.97, 95% CI 0.79 to 1.19).[10] A subsequent RCT (2849 high risk people) compared four doses of aspirin, two lower doses of 81 or 325 mg daily, and two higher doses of 650 or 1300 mg daily. It found that the combined rate of myocardial infarction, stroke, or death was slightly lower in the lower dose than in the higher dose groups at 3 months (AR 6.2% with lower doses *v* 8.4% with higher doses; P = 0.03).[11] Direct comparisons (3570 people in the review) between daily doses of 75 mg or more and less than 75 mg daily found no significant difference, but the confidence intervals included a potentially clinically important difference (OR higher *v* lower doses 1.08, 95% CI 0.90 to 1.31).[10] Indirect comparisons of trials in the review comparing different daily aspirin doses versus control among people at high risk (excluding those with acute ischaemic stroke) found similar reductions in serious vascular events for the higher daily doses 500–1500 mg daily (OR 0.81, 95% CI 0.75 to 0.87), 160–325 mg daily (OR 0.74, 95% CI 0.69 to 0.80), 75–150 mg daily (OR 0.68, 95% CI 0.59 to 0.79), but somewhat smaller effect with less than 75 mg daily (OR 0.87, 95% CI 0.74 to 1.03) (see figure 2, p 230).[10] **Versus or with thienopyridines:** See benefits of thienopyridines, p 195. **Versus or with anticoagulants:** See benefits of oral anticoagulants in absence of antiplatelet treatment, p 197 and benefits of oral anticoagulants in addition to antiplatelet treatment, p 198.

Harms: **Intracranial haemorrhage:** A systematic review of aspirin versus control for at least 1 month found that aspirin produced a small increased risk of intracranial haemorrhage of about 1/1000 (0.1%) people treated for 3 years.[12] There was no clear variation in risk with the dose of aspirin used. In RCTs directly comparing different daily doses there was no significant difference in the risk of intracranial haemorrhage, but the number of events was small and the confidence intervals wide.[11,13,14] Two observational studies (1 case control and 1 cohort study) found a dose dependent association between aspirin and intracranial haemorrhage, but the methods of these studies prevent firm conclusions being drawn.[15,16] **Extracranial haemorrhage:** The systematic review (search date 1997) found that aspirin slightly increased the risk of major extracranial haemorrhage, similar to the risk for antiplatelet treatment in general (see harms of antiplatelet treatment, p 193). It found that the risk of major extracranial haemorrhage was similar with different daily doses (numerical results not presented).[10] **Gastrointestinal haemorrhage:** A systematic review (search date 1999) of aspirin versus control found an increased risk of gastrointestinal haemorrhage with aspirin (OR 1.68, 95% CI 1.51 to 1.88), with no definite variation in risk between doses or different formulations.[17] RCTs directly comparing different doses of aspirin found a trend towards more gastrointestinal haemorrhages with high (500–1500 mg/day) versus medium (75–325 mg/day) doses (OR 1.7, 95% CI 0.9 to 2.1). There was no difference between medium (283 mg/day) and low (30 mg/day) doses (OR 1.2, 95% CI 0.7 to 2.0).[11,13,14] A recent overview of 15 observational studies including over 10 000 cases of upper gastrointestinal haemorrhage or perforation requiring admission to hospital, found a more than doubled increased risk with aspirin (RR 2.5, 95% CI 2.4 to 2.7).[18] Restricting the analysis to prospective studies gave a lower risk (RR 1.9, 95% CI 1.7 to 2.1), similar to that found in the RCTs.[17,18] **Upper gastrointestinal symptoms:** RCTs directly comparing different doses of aspirin found that high dose (500–1500 mg/day) significantly increased the odds of upper gastrointestinal symptoms compared with medium dose (75–325 mg/day; OR 1.3, 95% CI 1.1 to 1.5),[11,13] and that medium dose (283 mg/day) aspirin was associated with non-significantly higher odds of upper gastrointestinal upset compared with low dose (30 mg/day; OR 1.1, 95% CI 0.9 to 1.4).[14]

Comment: Among people at high risk of cardiac events, the large absolute reductions in serious vascular events associated with aspirin far outweigh any absolute risks.

OPTION THIENOPYRIDINES (CLOPIDOGREL OR TICLOPIDINE)

One RCT has found that clopidogrel is at least as effective at preventing vascular events and is at least as safe as aspirin in people with a history of cardiovascular disease.

Benefits: **Versus aspirin:** One RCT (19 185 people with a history of myocardial infarction, stroke, or peripheral arterial disease) compared clopidogrel 75 mg daily versus aspirin 325 mg daily.[19] It found that clopidogrel reduced the odds of a serious vascular event by 10% (OR 0.90, 95% CI 0.82 to 0.99). One systematic review found similar, but non-significant results for ticlopidine (a thienopyridine similar to clopidogrel) versus aspirin (search date 1997, 4 RCTs, 3791 high risk people; RR 0.88, 95% CI 0.75 to 1.03).[10] We found one subsequent RCT comparing ticlopidine versus aspirin.[20] It found a non-significant lower risk of a vascular event (OR 0.69, 95% 0.31 to 1.48). A separate systematic review comparing ticlopidine or clopidogrel versus aspirin (search date 1999, 4 RCTs, 22 656 people at high risk of vascular disease, most of whom were included in the trial comparing clopidogrel with aspirin[20]) found that ticlopidine or clopidogrel reduced the odds of a vascular event compared with aspirin (OR 0.91, 95% CI 0.84 to 0.98).[21] However, there was substantial uncertainty about the absolute size of any additional benefit (average 11 events prevented/1000 people treated for 2 years, 95% CI 2 events prevented/1000 people treated to 19 events prevented/1000 people treated). **Thienopyridines plus aspirin versus aspirin alone:** We found no completed long term trials of the effects of adding clopidogrel to aspirin among people at high risk of occlusive arterial disease but without an acute cardiovascular event. We found one RCT in people with acute coronary syndromes (see comment below).

Harms: One systematic review of randomised trials of the thienopyridine derivatives versus aspirin found that the thienopyridines produced significantly less gastrointestinal haemorrhage and upper gastrointestinal upset than aspirin.[21] However, the odds of skin rash and diarrhoea were doubled with ticlopidine and increased by about a third with clopidogrel. Ticlopidine (but not clopidogrel) increased the odds of neutropenia. Observational studies have also found that ticlopidine is associated with thrombocytopenia and thrombotic thrombocytopenic purpura.[22,23] However, we found no clear evidence of an excess of haematological adverse effects with clopidogrel.[24,25] Three RCTs (about 2700 people undergoing coronary artery stenting) of clopidogrel plus aspirin versus ticlopidine plus aspirin suggested better safety and tolerability with clopidogrel versus ticlopidine.[26–28]

Comment: One RCT (about 12 500 people within 24 hours of onset of an acute coronary syndrome without ST segment elevation) compared clopidogrel plus aspirin versus placebo plus aspirin.[29] After 3–12 months' treatment, it found that adding clopidogrel to aspirin significantly reduced the risk of a major vascular event (RR 0.88, 95% CI 0.72 to 0.90).[29] See antiplatelets under angina (unstable), p 64. The trial found that combined treatment increased risk of major haemorrhages (mainly gastrointestinal) and bleeding at sites of arterial punctures (RR 1.38, 95% CI 1.13 to 1.67), but did not increase intracranial, life-threatening, or fatal haemorrhages compared with aspirin alone.[29] An RCT of the effects of adding clopidogrel to aspirin in people with acute myocardial infarction is underway.[30]

OPTION ORAL GLYCOPROTEIN IIB/IIIA RECEPTOR INHIBITORS

Systematic reviews in people with acute coronary syndromes or undergoing percutaneous coronary interventions have found that oral glycoprotein IIb/IIIa receptor inhibitors (with or without aspirin) increase mortality and bleeding compared with aspirin alone.

Benefits: We found two systematic reviews in people with acute coronary syndrome or undergoing percutaneous coronary intervention (search dates 2000[31] and 2001[32]). Both reviews identified the same four RCTs (33 326 people). They both found that oral glycoprotein IIb/IIIa receptor inhibitors (with or without aspirin) significantly increased mortality. They did not significantly affect the risk of myocardial infarction compared with aspirin alone after 3–10 months (results taken from first review[31]; mortality: pooled OR 1.37, 95% CI 1.13 to 1.66; myocardial infarction: pooled OR 1.04, 95% CI 0.93 to 1.16).

Harms: The first review found that oral glycoprotein IIb/IIIa receptor inhibitors with or without aspirin increased all cause mortality and major bleeding compared with aspirin.[31] One subsequent RCT (9200 people with a recent myocardial infarction, unstable angina, ischaemic stroke/transient ischaemic attack, or peripheral arterial disease) assessing the effects of adding an oral glycoprotein IIb/IIIa receptor inhibitor to aspirin was stopped early because of safety concerns.[33]

Comment: None.

OPTION ORAL ANTICOAGULANTS IN THE ABSENCE OF ANTIPLATELET TREATMENT

One systematic review and subsequent RCTs have found that high or moderate intensity oral anticoagulants given alone reduce the risk of serious vascular events in people with coronary artery disease, but are associated with substantial risks of haemorrhage compared with placebo or no anticoagulants. Oral anticoagulants require regular monitoring for intensity of anticoagulant effect.

Benefits: We found one systematic review (search date 1999) of the effects of oral anticoagulation in people with coronary artery disease.[34] It identified 16 RCTs of high intensity anticoagulation (international normalised ratio [INR — see glossary, p 223] > 2.8) versus control (either no anticoagulation or placebo) in 10 056 people, and four RCTs of moderate intensity anticoagulation (INR 2–3) versus control in 1365 people. Antiplatelet treatment was not routinely given in any of these 20 trials. The review found that high intensity anticoagulation reduced the odds of the combined outcome of mortality, myocardial infarction, or stroke compared with control (OR 0.57, 95% CI 0.51 to 0.63; about 98 events avoided/1000 people treated). Compared with control, moderate intensity anticoagulation was associated with a smaller non-significant reduction.[34] In direct comparisons of high or moderate intensity oral anticoagulation with aspirin, the effects on mortality, myocardial infarction, or stroke were similar (OR 1.04, 95% CI 0.80 to 1.34).[34] One subsequent RCT (3630 people with previous acute myocardial infarction) compared three treatments: warfarin alone (to target INR 2.8–4.2); aspirin 160 mg daily; and warfarin (to target INR 2.0–2.5) plus aspirin 75 mg daily.[35] After 4 years, it found that warfarin alone significantly reduced cardiovascular events (death, myocardial infarction, or cerebral infarction) compared with aspirin alone (cardiovascular event rate 203/1216 [16.7%] with warfarin *v* 241/1206 [20%] with aspirin alone; RR 0.81, 95% CI 0.69 to 0.83). However, warfarin was associated with increased bleeding compared with aspirin (see harms below). A second subsequent

RCT (999 people after acute coronary syndrome) similarly compared three treatments: aspirin 80 mg daily; oral anticoagulants (to target INR 3.0–4.0); and aspirin 80 mg daily plus oral anticoagulants (to target INR 2.0–2.5).[36] It found that oral anticoagulants reduced cardiovascular events compared with aspirin, although the result was of borderline significance (17/325 [5%] with anticoagulants *v* 31/336 [9%] with aspirin; HR 0.55, 95% CI 0.30 to 1.00).

Harms: Compared with control, high intensity anticoagulation increased the odds of major (mainly extracranial) haemorrhage about six-fold (OR 6.0, 95% CI 4.4 to 8.2; absolute increase 39 events/1000 people treated), and moderate intensity anticoagulation increased the odds of major haemorrhage about eight-fold (OR 7.7, 95% CI 3.3 to 17.6).[34] Compared with aspirin, high or moderate intensity oral anticoagulation increased the odds of major haemorrhage more than two-fold (OR 2.4, 95% CI 1.6 to 3.6).[34] The first subsequent RCT found that warfarin significantly increased major nonfatal bleeding compared with aspirin (0.68% a year with warfarin *v* 0.17% a year with aspirin; RR 4.00, 95% CI 1.67 to 10.00).[35] The second subsequent RCT found no significant difference in major bleeding between aspirin and combination treatment, although the study may have lacked power to detect a clinically important difference (1% with combination *v* 1% with aspirin; HR 1.03, 95% CI 0.21 to 5.08).[36]

Comment: Oral anticoagulants provide substantial protection against vascular events in the absence of antiplatelet treatment, but the risks of serious haemorrhage are higher than for antiplatelet treatment and regular monitoring is required. Aspirin provides similar protection, but is safer and easier to use (see harms under antiplatelet treatment, p 193).

OPTION ORAL ANTICOAGULANTS IN ADDITION TO ANTIPLATELET TREATMENT

One systematic review found no evidence that the addition of low intensity oral anticoagulation (target international normalised ratio < 1.5) to aspirin reduced mortality, myocardial infarction, and stroke. We found no consistent evidence from RCTs that moderate intensity oral anticoagulation (target international normalised ratio 1.5–3.0) plus aspirin reduced recurrent cardiovascular events or mortality compared with aspirin alone, although we found consistent evidence that it increased the risk of major haemorrhage.

Benefits: We found one systematic review (search date 1999, 6 RCTs, 8915 people with coronary artery disease) of adding an oral anticoagulant regimen to aspirin.[34] Three of these RCTs assessed the addition of a low intensity (target international normalised ratio [INR — see glossary, p 223] < 1.5) regimen to aspirin in a total of 8435 people, and found no significant reduction in the odds of mortality, myocardial infarction, or stroke (OR 0.91, 95% CI 0.79 to 1.06).[34] Trials assessing the addition of a moderate intensity (INR 2–3) oral anticoagulant regimen to aspirin were too small (480 people) to produce reliable estimates of efficacy and safety.[34] We found four subsequent RCTs.[35–38] The first subsequent RCT (3712 people with unstable angina) compared 5 months' oral anticoagulant treatment (target INR 2.0–2.5) plus standard treatment (usually including aspirin) versus standard treatment alone.[37] When this trial was included in a meta-analysis with the previous trials assessing the addition of moderate intensity oral anticoagulation to aspirin, oral anticoagulation was associated with a non-significant reduction in mortality, myocardial infarction, or stroke (OR 0.83, 95% CI 0.66 to 1.03).[34] The second subsequent RCT (5059 people with myocardial infarction in the previous 14 days; unblinded) compared warfarin (target INR 1.5–2.5) plus aspirin 81 mg daily versus aspirin 162 mg daily alone.[38] It found no significant differences between treatments in mortality, recurrent myocardial infarction, or stroke after a median of 2.7 years (mortality 17.6% with warfarin plus aspirin *v* 17.3% with aspirin alone, P = 0.8; AR for recurrent myocardial infarction 13.3% with warfarin plus aspirin *v* 13.1% with aspirin alone, P = 0.8; AR for stroke 3.1% with warfarin plus aspirin *v* 3.5% with aspirin alone, P = 0.5). The third subsequent RCT (3630 people with previous acute myocardial infarction) compared three treatments: warfarin alone (target INR 2.8–4.2); aspirin 160 mg daily; and warfarin (target INR 2.0–2.5) plus aspirin 75 mg daily.[35] After 4 years, it found that warfarin plus aspirin significantly reduced cardiovascular events (death, myocardial infarction, or cerebral infarction) compared with aspirin alone (cardiovascular event rate 181/1208 [15%] with warfarin plus aspirin *v* 241/1206 [20%] with aspirin alone; RR 0.71, 95% CI 0.60 to 0.83). However, warfarin plus aspirin was associated with increased bleeding compared with aspirin alone (see harms below).[35] The fourth subsequent RCT (999 people after acute coronary syndrome) similarly compared three treatments: aspirin 80 mg daily; oral anticoagulants (to target INR 3.0–4.0); and aspirin 80 mg daily plus oral anticoagulants (to target INR 2.0–2.5).[36] It found that combination treatment significantly reduced cardiovascular events compared with aspirin alone (16/332 [5%] with combination *v* 31/336 [9%] with aspirin; HR 0.50, 95% CI 0.27 to 0.92).[36]

Harms: The systematic review found a non-significant excess of major haemorrhage with the addition of low intensity oral anticoagulation to aspirin (OR 1.29, 95% CI 0.96 to 1.75).[34] An updated meta-analysis assessing the addition of moderate intensity oral anticoagulation to aspirin included the RCTs from the systematic review[34] and one subsequent trial[37] (total of 4192 people with coronary artery disease). It found a clear excess of major haemorrhage in people allocated oral anticoagulation (OR 1.95, 95% CI 1.27 to 2.98).[37] The second subsequent RCT (5059 people) examining the addition of moderate intensity anticoagulation to aspirin also found that combined treatment increased risk of major haemorrhage (RR 1.78, 95% CI 1.27 to 2.72).[38] The third subsequent RCT found similar results at 4 years (non-fatal major bleeding: 0.57% a year with warfarin plus aspirin *v* 0.17% a year with aspirin; RR, CI, and significance not stated).[35] The fourth subsequent RCT found no significant difference in major bleeding between aspirin and combination treatment, although the study may have lacked power to detect a clinically important difference (2% with combination *v* 1% with aspirin alone; HR 2.35, 95% CI 0.61 to 9.10).[36]

Comment: The issue of whether adding a moderately intense oral anticoagulant regimen to aspirin provides additional net benefit to people at high risk of ischaemic cardiac events is being assessed in several ongoing RCTs. One RCT (135 people with unstable angina or non-ST segment myocardial infarction, with prior coronary artery bypass grafting) compared three treatments: aspirin 80 mg daily alone plus placebo; warfarin (target INR 2.0–2.5) plus placebo; and aspirin plus warfarin.[39] It found no significant difference among treatments for rates of primary end point (death or myocardial infarction or unstable angina requiring admission to hospital at 1 year; AR 14.6% with warfarin alone v 11.5% with aspirin alone v 11.3% with combination, P = 0.76).[39] However, it found no significant difference for major haemorrhage among people taking warfarin compared with those who were not. Event rates were low and the study may have lacked power to detect a clinically important difference for adverse effects.[39]

QUESTION What are the effects of other drug treatments?

Bazian Ltd

OPTION β BLOCKERS

Systematic reviews have found strong evidence that β blockers reduce the risk of all cause mortality, coronary mortality, recurrent non-fatal myocardial infarction, and sudden death in people after myocardial infarction. Most benefit was seen in those at highest risk of mortality after a myocardial infarction (> 50 years old; previous myocardial infarction, angina pectoris, hypertension, or treatment with digitalis; transient mechanical or electrical failure; higher heart rate at study entry). About 25% of people suffered adverse effects.

Benefits: **Survival and reinfarction:** One systematic review (search date 1993, 26 RCTs, > 24 000 people) compared oral β blockers versus placebo within days or weeks of an acute myocardial infarction (late intervention trials) and continued for between 6 weeks and 3 years.[40] Most RCTs followed people for 1 year. The review found improved survival in people given β blockers (RR 0.77, 95% CI 0.70 to 0.86).[40] One prior systematic review (search date not stated, 24 RCTs) found that long term use of β blockers versus placebo after myocardial infarction reduced total mortality (RR about 0.80), sudden death (RR about 0.70), and non-fatal reinfarction (RR about 0.75).[41] **Anginal symptoms:** We found no good RCTs assessing the antianginal effects of β blockers in people after myocardial infarction. One trial found atenolol more effective than placebo in people with chronic stable effort angina or silent ischaemia.[42] **Different types of β blockers:** The earlier review found no differences between β blockers with and without cardioselectivity or membrane stabilising properties, but it raised concerns about the lack of efficacy of β blockers with intrinsic sympathomimetic activity in long term management after myocardial infarction.[41] One RCT (607 people after myocardial infarction) found that acebutolol, a β blocker with moderate partial agonist activity, decreased 1 year mortality compared with placebo (AR of death: 11% with placebo v 6% with acebutolol; RR 0.52, 95% CI 0.29 to 0.91).[43] **Effects in**

different subgroups: One systematic review (search date 1983, 9 RCTs) compared β blockers versus placebo started more than 24 hours after onset of symptoms of acute myocardial infarction and continued for 9–24 months.[44] Pooled analysis of individual data (13 679 people) found that the benefits of β blockers versus placebo on mortality seemed comparable in men and women. The highest absolute benefit from β blockers was found in subgroups with the highest baseline risks (i.e. those with the highest mortality on placebo), those over 50 years of age; those with a history of previous myocardial infarction, angina pectoris, hypertension, or treatment with digitalis; those with transient signs or symptoms of mechanical or electrical failure in the early phases of myocardial infarction; and those with a higher heart rate at study entry. Low risk subgroups had smaller mean absolute benefit.

Harms: Adverse effects include shortness of breath, bronchospasm, bradycardia, hypotension, heart block, cold hands and feet, diarrhoea, fatigue, reduced sexual activity, depression, nightmares, faintness, insomnia, syncope, and hallucinations. Rates varied among studies. One RCT reported an absolute risk increase for any adverse effect of 24% with propranolol compared with placebo (no CI available). Serious adverse effects were uncommon and only a small proportion of people withdrew from the study as a result.[45] We found one systematic review (search date 2001; 15 RCTs; > 35 000 people) that examined harms of β blockers compared with placebo in people with previous myocardial infarction, heart failure, or hypertension.[46] It found no significant difference between β blockers and placebo in depressive symptoms or sexual dysfunction (depressive symptoms: RR 1.12, 95% CI 0.89 to 1.41; sexual dysfunction 1.10, 95% CI 0.96 to 1.25). However, it found a small but significant increase in fatigue with β blockers compared with placebo (RR 1.15, 95% CI 1.05 to 1.25)

Comment: Continued benefit has been reported from β blockers up to 6 years after myocardial infarction (ARR for mortality: 5.9%, P = 0.003; RR 0.82, CI not available). However, the study was not blinded after 33 months.

OPTION ANGIOTENSIN CONVERTING ENZYME INHIBITORS

One systematic review has found that in people who have had a myocardial infarction and have left ventricular dysfunction, angiotensin converting enzyme inhibitors reduce mortality, admission to hospital for congestive heart failure, and recurrent non-fatal myocardial infarction compared with placebo. One large RCT in people without left ventricular dysfunction found that ramipril versus placebo reduced cardiovascular death, stroke, and myocardial infarction.

Benefits: **In people with left ventricular dysfunction:** One systematic review (search date not stated, 3 RCTs, 5966 people)[47] compared angiotensin converting enzyme (ACE) inhibitors (captopril, ramipril, or trandolapril) versus placebo started 3–16 days after acute myocardial infarction and continued for 15–42 months. It analysed individual data from 5966 people with a recent myocardial infarction and with clinical manifestations of congestive heart failure or moderate left ventricular dysfunction (left ventricular ejection fraction ≥ 35–40%). ACE inhibitors versus placebo significantly reduced mortality (702/2995 [23.4%] with ACE inhibitors *v* 866/2971 [29.1%] with control; OR 0.74, 95% CI 0.66 to 0.83; NNT 17 people treated for about 2 years to prevent 1 death, CI not provided), admission to hospital for congestive heart failure (355/2995 [11.9%] with ACE inhibitors *v* 460/2971 [15.5%] with control; OR 0.73, 95% CI 0.63 to 0.85; NNT 28, CI not available), and recurrent non-fatal myocardial infarction (324/2995 [10.8%] with ACE inhibitors *v* 391/2971 [13.1%] with control; OR 0.80, 95% CI 0.69 to 0.94; NNT 43, CI not provided). **In people without impaired ventricular function or evidence of congestive heart failure:** We found no systematic review but found one large RCT (9297 people at high risk of cardiovascular events).[48] It found that ramipril 10 mg daily versus placebo reduced the composite primary outcome of cardiovascular death, myocardial infarction, or stroke over an average of 4.7 years (RR for composite outcome 0.78, 95% CI 0.70 to 0.86; NNT 27, 95% CI 20 to 45; RR for cardiovascular death 0.74, 95% CI 0.64 to 0.87; NNT 50, CI not available; RR for myocardial infarction 0.80, 95% CI 0.70 to 0.90; NNT 42, CI not available; RR for stroke 0.68, 95% CI 0.56 to 0.84; NNT 67, CI not available; RR for death from all causes 0.84, 95% CI 0.75 to 0.95; NNT 56, CI not available). The RCT found that ramipril reduced the need for revascularisation procedures and reduced heart failure related outcomes (need for revascularisation: RR 0.85, CI not available; heart failure related outcomes: RR 0.77, CI not available). Ramipril versus placebo produced benefit in all subgroups examined, including women and men; people aged over and under 65 years; those with and without a history of coronary artery disease, hypertension, diabetes, peripheral vascular disease, cerebrovascular disease, and those with and without microalbuminuria at study entry.[48] **In people with diabetes:** See antihypertensive treatment under prevention of cardiovascular events in diabetes, p 690.[49]

Harms: The major adverse effects reported in these trials were cough (ARI 5–10% with ACE inhibitors *v* placebo), dizziness, hypotension (ARI with 5–10% with ACE inhibitors *v* placebo), renal failure (ARI < 3% with ACE inhibitors *v* placebo), hyperkalaemia (ARI < 3% with ACE inhibitors *v* placebo), angina, syncope, diarrhoea (ARI 2% with ACE inhibitors *v* placebo), and, for captopril, alteration in taste (2% of captopril users).[47]

Comment: There are several other ongoing large RCTs assessing ACE inhibitors in people without clinical manifestations of heart failure and with no or with mild impairment in left ventricular systolic function. These include one trial of trandolapril in 8000 people with coronary artery disease, and one trial of perindopril in 10 500 people with stable coronary artery disease.[50]

OPTION CLASS I ANTIARRHYTHMIC AGENTS (QUINIDINE, PROCAINAMIDE, DISOPYRAMIDE, ENCAINIDE, FLECAINIDE, AND MORACIZINE)

One systematic review has found that class I antiarrhythmic agents after myocardial infarction increase the risk of cardiovascular mortality and sudden death.

Benefits: One systematic review has found that class I antiarrhythmics are harmful in people who have had an acute coronary event (see harms below).

Harms: One systematic review (search date 1993, 51 RCTs, 23 229 people) compared class I antiarrhythmic drugs versus placebo given acutely and later in the management of myocardial infarction.[40] The review found that the antiarrhythmic agents increased mortality (AR of death 5.6% with class I antiarrhythmic *v* 5.0% with placebo; OR 1.14, 95% CI 1.01 to 1.28). One RCT (1498 people with myocardial infarction and asymptomatic or mildly symptomatic ventricular arrhythmia) found that encainide or flecainide versus placebo increased the risk of death or cardiac arrest after 10 months (RR 2.38, 95% CI 1.59 to 3.57; NNH 17).[51]

Comment: The evidence implies that class I antiarrhythmic drugs should not be used in people after myocardial infarction or with significant coronary artery disease.

OPTION CLASS III ANTIARRHYTHMIC AGENTS (AMIODARONE, SOTALOL)

Systematic reviews have found that amiodarone reduces the risk of sudden death and marginally reduces mortality in people at high risk of arrhythmic death after myocardial infarction compared with placebo. One RCT found limited evidence that sotalol increased mortality within 1 year compared with placebo.

Benefits: **Amiodarone:** We found two systematic reviews.[52,53] The first systematic review (search date not stated, individual data from 6553 high risk people in 13 RCTs) compared amiodarone versus control treatments.[52] People were selected with a recent myocardial infarction and a high risk of death from cardiac arrhythmia (based on low left ventricular ejection fraction, frequent ventricular premature depolarisation, or non-sustained ventricular tachycardia, but no history of sustained symptomatic ventricular tachycardia or ventricular fibrillation); 78% of people from eight RCTs had a recent myocardial infarction, and 22% of people from five RCTs had congestive heart failure.[52] Most trials were placebo controlled with a mean follow up of about 1.5 years. The people with congestive heart failure were symptomatic but stable and had not had a recent myocardial infarction, although in most cases the heart failure was ischaemic in origin. All RCTs used a loading dose of amiodarone (400 mg/day for 28 days or 800 mg/day for 14 days) followed by a maintenance dose (200–400 mg/day). Amiodarone significantly reduced total mortality compared with placebo (AR for total mortality: 10.9% a year with amiodarone *v* 12.3% a year with placebo; RR 0.87, 95% CI 0.78 to 0.99) and rates of sudden cardiac death

(RR 0.71, 95% CI 0.59 to 0.85). Amiodarone had similar effects in the studies after myocardial infarction and congestive heart failure.[52] The second systematic review (search date 1997, 5864 people with myocardial infarction, congestive heart failure, left ventricular dysfunction, or cardiac arrest) found similar results.[53] **Sotalol:** We found one RCT (3121 people with myocardial infarction and left ventricular dysfunction), which found increased mortality with the class III antiarrhythmic agent sotalol versus placebo (AR for death: 5.0% with sotalol *v* 3.1% with placebo; RR 1.65, 95% CI 1.15 to 2.36). The trial was terminated prematurely after less than 1 year.[54]

Harms: Adverse events leading to discontinuation of amiodarone were hypothyroidism (expressed as events per 100 person-years: 7.0 with amiodarone *v* 1.1 with placebo; OR 7.3), hyperthyroidism (1.4 with amiodarone *v* 0.5 with placebo; OR 2.5), peripheral neuropathy (0.5 with amiodarone *v* 0.2 with placebo; OR 2.8), lung infiltrates (1.6 with amiodarone *v* 0.5 with placebo; OR 3.1), bradycardia (2.4 with amiodarone *v* 0.8 with placebo; OR 2.6), and liver dysfunction (1.0 with amiodarone *v* 0.4 with placebo; OR 2.7).[52]

Comment: The conclusions of the review are probably specific to amiodarone.[52,53] The two largest RCTs of amiodarone after myocardial infarction found a favourable interaction between β blockers and amiodarone, with additional reduction in cardiac mortality.[55,56]

OPTION CALCIUM CHANNEL BLOCKERS

One systematic review found no benefit from calcium channel blockers in people after myocardial infarction or with chronic coronary heart disease. Diltiazem and verapamil may reduce rates of reinfarction and refractory angina in people after myocardial infarction who do not have heart failure. The review found non-significantly higher mortality with dihydropyridines compared with placebo.

Benefits: One systematic review (search date 1993, 24 RCTs) compared calcium channel blockers (including dihydropyridines, diltiazem, and verapamil) versus placebo given early or late during the course of acute myocardial infarction or unstable angina and continued in the intermediate or long term.[40] Two of the RCTs used angiographic regression of coronary stenosis as an outcome in people with stable coronary heart disease treated with calcium channel blockers. The review found no significant difference in the absolute risk of death compared with placebo (AR 9.7% with calcium channel blockers *v* 9.3% with placebo; ARI with calcium channel blockers *v* placebo +0.4%, 95% CI –0.4% to +1.2%; OR 1.04, 95% CI 0.95 to 1.14). **Diltiazem and verapamil:** The review found no significant effect compared with placebo (OR 0.95, 95% CI 0.82 to 1.09).[40] Three RCTs comparing diltiazem or verapamil versus placebo found decreased rates of recurrent infarction and refractory angina with active treatment but only for those people without signs or symptoms of heart failure. For those with clinical manifestations of heart failure, the trends were towards harm.[57–59] **Dihydropyridines:** The review found non-significantly higher mortality with dihydropyridines

Benefits: **All cholesterol treatments:** We found one systematic review (search date 1996, 59 RCTs, 173 160 people), which did not differentiate primary and secondary prevention, and included RCTs of any cholesterol lowering intervention, irrespective of duration, as long as mortality data were reported.[69] It included drug treatments (statins, n-3 fatty acids, fibrates, resins, hormones, or niacin), dietary intervention alone, or surgery (ileal bypass) alone. Overall, baseline risk was similar among all intervention groups. Among non-surgical treatments, the review found that only statins reduced coronary heart disease mortality, and that only statins and n-3 fatty acids significantly reduced all cause mortality (RR of coronary heart disease mortality: statins *v* control 0.69, 95% CI 0.59 to 0.80; n-3 fatty acids *v* control 0.44, 95% CI 0.18 to 1.07; fibrates *v* control 0.98, 95% CI 0.78 to 1.24; resins *v* control 0.71, 95% CI 0.51 to 0.99; hormones *v* control 1.04, 95% CI 0.93 to 1.17; niacin *v* control 0.95, 95% CI 0.83 to 1.10; diet *v* control 0.91, 95% CI 0.82 to 1.01. RR of all cause mortality: statins *v* control 0.79, 95% CI 0.71 to 0.89; n-3 fatty acids *v* control 0.68, 95% CI 0.53 to 0.88; fibrates *v* control 1.06, 95% CI 0.78 to 1.46; resins *v* control 0.85, 95% CI 0.66 to 1.08; hormone *v* control 1.09, 95% CI 1.00 to 1.20; niacin *v* control 0.96, 95% CI 0.86 to 1.08; diet *v* control 0.97, 95% CI 0.81 to 1.15).[69] **Statins:** We found one systematic review (search date 1998, 5 RCTs, 30 817 people) that compared long term (≥ 4 years) treatment with statins versus placebo.[70] Combining the three secondary prevention trials, the review found that statins reduced coronary heart disease mortality, cardiovascular mortality, and all cause mortality compared with placebo over a mean of 5.4 years (coronary heart disease mortality: OR 0.71, 95% CI 0.63 to 0.80; cardiovascular mortality: OR 0.73, 95% CI 0.66 to 0.82; all cause mortality: OR 0.77, 95% CI 0.70 to 0.85). One subsequent RCT (20 536 adults with total cholesterol > 3.5 mmol/L [an inclusion threshold lower than previous statin trials], including > 5000 women and > 5000 people over 70 years of age) compared simvastatin 40 mg versus placebo. The study included both primary and secondary prevention populations.[71] After a mean of 5.5 years follow up, simvastatin reduced total mortality and major vascular events compared with placebo (all cause mortality: 12.9% with simvastatin *v* 14.7% with placebo, RR 0.87, 95% CI 0.81 to 0.94; major vascular events 19.8% with simvastatin *v* 25.2% with placebo, RR 0.76, 95% CI 0.72 to 0.81). We found one subsequent RCT (1600 people with established coronary heart disease).[72] It found that atorvastatin (10–80 mg/day, titrated to achieve low density lipoprotein cholesterol < 2.6 mM [100 mg/dL]) significantly reduced recurrent coronary events or death, and all cause mortality compared with management not involving statins at 3 years (coronary events or death: 12.0% with atorvastatin *v* 24.5% without statins; RR 0.49, 95% CI 0.27 to 0.73; all cause mortality: 2.9% with atorvastatin *v* 5.0% without statins; RR 0.57, 95% CI 0.39 to 0.78).[72] **Effects of statins in different groups of people:** Combining results from primary and secondary prevention trials, the review found that, compared with placebo, statins reduced coronary events by a similar proportion in men (OR 0.69, 95% CI 0.65 to 0.74; ARR 3.7%, 95% CI 2.9% to 4.4%), in women (OR 0.71, 95%

CI 0.64 to 0.76; ARR 3.3%, 95% CI 1.3% to 5.2%), in people under 65 years (OR 0.69, 95% CI 0.64 to 0.76; ARR 3.2%, 95% CI 2.4% to 4.0%), and in people over 65 years (OR 0.68, 95% CI 0.61 to 0.77; ARR 4.4%, 95% CI 3.0% to 5.8%). The reduction of coronary heart disease events in women involved more non-fatal and fewer fatal events than in men. One large RCT found no significant difference in mortality with statins versus placebo for the subgroup of women, but the confidence interval was wide (28/407 [6.9%] with simvastatin *v* 25/420 [6.0%] with placebo; RR 1.16, 95% CI 0.68 to 1.99).[73] One recent RCT that was not included in the review found that relative risk reductions were similar for people with initial total cholesterol levels of under 5.0 mmol/L compared with people with levels over 5.0 mmol/L and for women and the elderly compared with younger men.[71] One RCT compared early initiation of atorvastatin (80 mg/day started 1–4 days after admission) versus placebo in people with unstable angina or non-Q wave myocardial infarction.[74] After 3 months, it found no significant difference between treatments for coronary event rates, although atorvastatin reduced readmission rate for recurrent ischaemia compared with placebo (AR for readmission for ischaemia: 6.2% with atorvastatin *v* 8.4% with placebo; RR 0.74, 95% CI 0.57 to 0.95). One further RCT compared fluvastatin 80 mg daily versus placebo in 1677 people with total cholesterol 135–270 mg/dL (3.5–7.0 mM) and cardiac ischaemia after percutaneous coronary intervention.[75] It found that fluvastatin significantly reduced major cardiac events (cardiac death, non-fatal myocardial infarction, or reintervention) compared with placebo after 3–4 years (21.4% with fluvastatin *v* 26.7% with placebo; RR 0.78, 95% CI 0.64 to 0.95). **Intensity of statin treatment:** We found one RCT (1351 people with a history of saphenous vein coronary artery bypass grafting) that compared aggressive reduction of cholesterol with lovastatin and, if necessary, cholestyramine (colestyramine) (aiming for target low density lipoprotein cholesterol 1.6–2.2 mmol/L [60–85 mg/dL]) with more moderate reduction (target low density lipoprotein cholesterol 3.4–3.7 mmol/L [130–140 mg/dL]) with the same drugs.[76] The trial found that aggressive treatment reduced the risk of needing repeat revascularisation at 4 years (6.5% with aggressive treatment *v* 9.2% with moderate treatment, P = 0.03). After an additional 3 years, aggressive treatment reduced the risk of revascularisation and cardiovascular death compared with moderate treatment (AR of revascularisation 19% with aggressive treatment *v* 27% with moderate treatment, P = 0.0006; AR for cardiovascular death, 7.4% with aggressive treatment *v* 11.3% with moderate treatment, P = 0.03).[76] **Fibrates:** We found one systematic review (search date not stated, 4 RCTs)[77] and two additional RCTs.[78,79] The systematic review compared fibrates versus placebo in people with known coronary heart disease. The review identified one RCT (2531 men with coronary heart disease and a level of high density lipoprotein cholesterol > 1 mmol/L) that found gemfibrozil versus placebo reduced the composite outcome of non-fatal myocardial infarction plus death from coronary heart disease after a median of 5.1 years (AR 219/1264 [17%] for gemfibrozil *v* 275/1267 [22%] for placebo; ARR 4.4%, 95% CI 1.4% to 7.0%; RR 0.80, 95% CI 0.68 to 0.94; NNT 23, 95% CI 14 to 73). The review identified three trials comparing clofibrate versus placebo, which found no consistent difference between groups. The two additional RCTs[78,79] both compared bezafibrate versus placebo. The larger RCT (3090 people selected with previous myocardial infarction or stable angina, high density lipoprotein cholesterol < 45 mg/dL, and low density lipoprotein cholesterol < 180 mg/dL) found that bezafibrate versus placebo did not significantly reduce all cause mortality or the composite end point of myocardial infarction plus sudden death (AR for myocardial infarction or sudden death: 13.6% with bezafibrate *v* 15.0% with placebo; cumulative RR 0.91; P = 0.26).[78] The smaller RCT (92 young male survivors of myocardial infarction) found that bezafibrate versus placebo significantly reduced the combined outcome of death, reinfarction, plus revascularisation (3/47 [6%] with bezafibrate *v* 11/45 [24%]; RR 0.26, 95% CI 0.08 to 0.88).[79]

Cholesterol lowering versus angioplasty: We found no systematic review. One RCT found that aggressive lipid lowering treatment was as effective as percutaneous transluminal angioplasty for reducing ischaemic events, although anginal symptoms were reduced more by percutaneous transluminal angioplasty (see percutaneous transluminal angioplasty *v* medical treatment, p 218).

Harms: Total non-cardiovascular events, total and tissue specific cancers, and accident and violent deaths have been reported in statin trials. However, the systematic review of long term statin trials found no significant difference between statins and placebo in terms of non-cardiovascular mortality, cancer incidence, asymptomatic elevation of creatine kinase (> 10 times upper reference limit), or elevation of transaminases (> 3 times upper reference limit) during a mean of 5.4 years of treatment (OR of event, statin *v* placebo for non-cardiovascular mortality 0.93, 95% CI 0.81 to 1.07; for cancer 0.99, 95% CI 0.90 to 1.08; for creatine kinase increase 1.25, 95% CI 0.83 to 1.89; for transaminase increase 1.13, 95% CI 0.95 to 1.33).[73] We found one meta-analysis of three large RCTs (19 592 people) examining safety of pravastatin compared with placebo in primary or secondary prevention.[80] It found no clinically important difference between pravastatin and placebo for any adverse effects after a mean follow up of 5 years (primary cancer: 9.6% with pravastatin *v* 9.3% with placebo, P = 0.48; musculoskeletal adverse effects: < 0.1% in both groups, P = 0.02; gastrointestinal adverse effects: 1.4% *v* 1.5%, P = 0.48; hepatobiliary adverse effects: ≤ 0.1% in both groups, P = 0.45; dermatological adverse effects: 3.6% with pravastatin *v* 3.4% with placebo, P = 0.31; renal adverse effects: 2.7% with pravastatin *v* 2.5% with placebo, P = 0.42).[80] We found no evidence of additional harm associated with cholesterol lowering in elderly people, or in people after acute myocardial infarction.

Comment: Multivariate analysis in one systematic review (search date 1996) indicates that in a wide range of clinical contexts the relative risk reduction depends on the percent reduction in total or low density lipoprotein cholesterol and is not otherwise dependent on the method by which cholesterol is lowered. The absolute benefit over several years of lowering cholesterol will therefore be greatest in people with the highest baseline risk of an ischaemic cardiac event. Even if the relative risk reduction attenuates at older age, the absolute risk reduction for ischaemic cardiac events may be higher in elderly people than in younger people. The Women's Health Initiative (48 000 people, completion 2007, diet, up to age 79 years),[81] and the Antihypertensive and Lipid Lowering Treatment to Prevent Heart Disease Trial (10 000 people, completion 2002, pravastatin, no upper age limit) are ongoing.[82] We found no large direct comparisons of cholesterol modifying drugs; it remains unclear whether any one drug has advantages over others in subgroups of high risk people with particular lipid abnormalities. Because the main aim of treatment is to reduce absolute risk (rather than to reduce the cholesterol to any particular concentration), treatments aimed at lowering cholesterol need assessing for effectiveness in comparison and in combination with other possible risk factor interventions in each individual. People in the large statin trials in both treatment and placebo groups were given dietary advice aimed at lowering cholesterol.

QUESTION What are the effects of blood pressure reduction?

Bazian Ltd

We found no direct evidence of the effects of blood pressure lowering in people with established coronary heart disease. Observational studies, and extrapolation of primary prevention trials of blood pressure reduction, support the lowering of blood pressure in those at high risk of ischaemic coronary events. The evidence for benefit is strongest for β blockers, although not specifically in people with hypertension. The optimum target blood pressure in people with hypertension is not clear.

Benefits: We found no systematic review and no RCTs designed specifically to examine blood pressure reduction in those with established coronary heart disease. Prospective epidemiological studies have established that blood pressure continues to be a risk factor for cardiovascular events in people who have already experienced myocardial infarction. Prospective follow up of 5362 men who reported prior myocardial infarction during screening for one large RCT found no detectable association between systolic blood pressure and coronary heart disease mortality, and increased coronary heart disease mortality for those with lowest diastolic blood pressure in the first 2 years.[83] After 15 years there were highly significant linear associations between both systolic and diastolic blood pressure and increased risk of coronary heart disease mortality (stronger relation for systolic blood pressure), with apparent benefit for men with blood pressure maintained at levels lower than the arbitrarily defined "normal" levels. Experimental evidence of benefit from lowering of blood pressure in those with coronary heart disease requires extrapolation from primary prevention trials, because trials of antihypertensive treatment in elderly people[84–86] are likely to have included those with preclinical coronary heart disease. Mortality benefit has been established for β blockers after myocardial infarction (see β blockers, p 200), for verapamil and diltiazem after myocardial infarction in those without heart failure (see calcium channel blockers, p 204), and for angiotensin converting enzyme inhibitors after myocardial infarction, especially in those with heart failure (see angiotensin converting enzyme inhibitors, p 201).

Harms: Some observational studies have found increased mortality among those with low diastolic blood pressure.[87] Trials in elderly people of blood pressure lowering for hypertension or while treating heart failure[88] found no evidence of a J-shaped relation between blood pressure and death.

Comment: Without specific studies comparing different antihypertensive treatments, the available evidence is strongest for a beneficial effect of β blockers when treating survivors of a myocardial infarction who have hypertension. We found no specific evidence about the target level of blood pressure.

QUESTION What are the effects of non-drug treatments?

Bazian Ltd

OPTION DIET

One RCT found that advising people with coronary heart disease to eat more fruit and vegetables, bread, pasta, potatoes, olive oil, and rapeseed margarine (i.e. a Mediterranean diet) may result in a substantial survival benefit. We found no strong evidence from RCTs for a beneficial effect of low fat or high fibre diets on major non-fatal coronary heart disease events or coronary heart disease mortality. One RCT has found that advising people with coronary heart disease to eat more fish (particularly oily fish) significantly reduces mortality at 2 years. A second RCT found that fish oil capsules reduced mortality at 3.5 years.

Benefits: **Low fat diets:** One systematic review (search date not stated) found no evidence that allocation to a low fat diet reduced mortality from coronary heart disease in people after myocardial infarction (RR 0.94, 95% CI 0.84 to 1.06).[89] One large RCT included in the review (2033 middle aged men with a recent myocardial infarction) compared three dietary options: fat advice (to eat less fat), fibre advice (to eat more cereal fibre), and fish advice (to eat at least 2 portions of oily fish a week).[90] Advice to reduce fat was complicated and, though fat intake reduced only slightly in the fat advice group, fruit and vegetable intake increased by about 40 g daily.[91] However, there was no significant reduction in mortality (unadjusted RR at 2 years for death from any cause 0.97, 95% CI 0.75 to 1.27). **High fibre diets:** In the RCT, people advised to eat more fibre doubled their intake, but survival was non-significantly worse (unadjusted RR at 2 years for death from any cause 1.23, 95% CI 0.95 to 1.60).[90] **High fish diets:** In the RCT, those advised to eat more fish ate three times as much fish, although about 14% could not tolerate the fish and were given fish oil capsules. Those given fish advice were significantly less likely to die within 2 years (94/1015 [9.3%] with fish advice *v* 130/1018 [12.8%] with no fish advice; NNT 29, 95% CI 17 to 129; RR 0.71, 95% CI 0.54 to 0.93).[90] In a second trial, 11 324 people who had survived a recent myocardial infarction were randomised to receive 1 g daily of n-3 polyunsaturated fatty acids (fish oil) or no fish oil. Those given fish oil were less likely to die within 3.5 years (RR 0.86, 95% CI 0.76 to 0.97).[92] **Mediterranean diet:** One RCT (605 middle aged people with a recent myocardial infarction) compared advice to eat a Mediterranean diet (more bread, fruit and vegetables, fish, and less meat, and to replace butter and cream with rapeseed margarine) versus usual dietary advice.[93] There were several dietary differences between the groups. Fruit intake, for example, was about 50 g daily higher in the intervention group than the control group. After 27 months, the trial was stopped prematurely because of significantly better outcomes in the intervention group (mortality: 8/302 [2.6%] with intervention *v* 20/303 [6.6%] with usual dietary advice, adjusted RR of death 0.24, 97% CI 0.15 to 0.91 [97% CI to allow for early stopping]; NNT 25, 95% CI 14 to 299 over 27 months).[93]

Harms: No major adverse effects have been reported.

Comment: Diets low in saturated fat and cholesterol can lead to 10–15% reductions in cholesterol concentrations in highly controlled settings, such as in metabolic wards.[94] In people in the community the effects are smaller: 3–5% reductions in cholesterol concentrations in general population studies and 9% reductions in people after myocardial infarction.[89,95–97] Several RCTs of intensive dietary intervention in conjunction with multifactorial risk reduction treatment found decreased progression of anatomic extent of coronary heart disease on angiography.[98] A trial of advice to eat more fruit and vegetables in men with angina is underway (Burr M, personal communication 2001). **Effect on cardiovascular risk factors:** Other studies have investigated the effects of dietary interventions on cardiovascular risk factors rather than the effect on cardiovascular morbidity and mortality. One systematic review (search date 1992) suggested that garlic may reduce cholesterol by about 10%.[99] Some trials in this review had problems with their methods. More recent reports (published in 1998) found no effects of garlic powder or garlic oil on cholesterol concentrations.[100,101] One systematic review (search date 1991) reported modest reductions in cholesterol levels of 2–5% from oats and psyllium enriched cereals (high fibre diets), although we found no evidence that high fibre diets reduce mortality in people with coronary heart disease.[102] One systematic review (search date 1991) of soy protein also reported modest reductions in cholesterol concentrations.[102]

OPTION ANTIOXIDANT VITAMINS (VITAMIN E, β CAROTENE, VITAMIN C)

We found no consistent evidence from four RCTs about effects of vitamin E versus placebo or other antioxidants in people with high cardiovascular risk. We found insufficient evidence about effects of vitamin C alone. Four large RCTs of β carotene supplementation in primary prevention found no cardiovascular benefits, and two of the RCTs raised concerns about increased mortality.

Benefits: **Vitamin E:** We found four large RCTs of vitamin E in people with coronary artery disease.[92,103–105] The first RCT (2002 people with angiographically proved ischaemic heart disease)[103] used a high dose of vitamin E (400 or 800 IU) and follow up was brief (median 510 days). The RCT found that vitamin E reduced non-fatal coronary events (RR 0.23, 95% CI 0.11 to 0.47), but also found a non-significant increase in coronary death (RR 1.18, 95% CI 0.62 to

2.27) and all cause mortality. The second RCT (29 133 male Finnish smokers) compared β carotene supplements versus vitamin E supplements versus both versus placebo.[104] The dose of vitamin E (50 mg/day) was smaller than that used in the first trial. In the subgroup analysis of data from the 1862 men with prior myocardial infarction, the trial found that vitamin E reduced non-fatal myocardial infarction (RR 0.62, 95% CI 0.41 to 0.96) but non-significantly increased coronary death (RR 1.33, 95% CI 0.86 to 2.05).[104] The third RCT (11 324 people ≤3 months after myocardial infarction)[102] used a factorial design to compare vitamin E 300 mg daily versus no vitamin E (as well as fish oil *v* no fish oil). After 3.5 years there was a small and non-significant reduction in the risk of cardiovascular death and deaths from all causes in those who received vitamin E compared with those who did not (all cause mortality: RR 0.92, 95% CI 0.82 to 1.04). There was no significant change in the rate of non-fatal coronary events in those who received vitamin E (RR 1.04, 95% CI 0.88 to 1.22).[102] The fourth RCT (9541 people at high cardiovascular risk, 80% with prior clinical coronary artery disease, remainder with other atherosclerotic disease or diabetes with ≥1 additional cardiovascular risk factor) compared natural source vitamin E (D-α tocopherol acetate, 400 IU/day) versus placebo and followed people for an average of 4.7 years.[105] It found no significant differences in any cardiovascular outcomes between vitamin E and placebo (AR for major fatal or non-fatal cardiovascular event 16.2% with vitamin E *v* 15.5% with placebo, P > 0.05; AR for cardiovascular death 7.2% with vitamin E *v* 6.9% with placebo, P > 0.05; AR for non-fatal myocardial infarction 11.2% with vitamin E *v* 11.0% with placebo, P > 0.05; AR for stroke 4.4% with vitamin E *v* 3.8% with placebo, P > 0.05; AR for death from any cause 11.2% with vitamin E *v* 11.2% with placebo, P > 0.05). One additional smaller RCT (196 people on haemodialysis, aged 40–75 years) compared high dose vitamin E (800 IU/day) versus placebo.[106] After a median of 519 days, it found that vitamin E reduced the rate of combined cardiovascular end points but found no significant effect for all cause mortality (cardiovascular end points: vitamin E *v* placebo RR 0.54, 95% CI 0.23 to 0.89; mortality: vitamin E *v* placebo RR 1.09, 95% CI 0.70 to 1.70).[106] **Vitamin C:** We found no RCTs examining effects of vitamin C alone in people with coronary heart disease. **β Carotene:** See harms below.

Harms: Two of the trials of vitamin E found non-significant increases in the risk of coronary death (see benefits above).[103,107] **β Carotene:** One systematic review (search date 1996) identified four large RCTs of β carotene supplementation. All were primary prevention studies, and so have not been included in the benefits section above. None found evidence of cardiovascular benefits, although two of the trials suggested that β carotene may increase mortality compared with placebo (cardiovascular death: β carotene *v* placebo RR 1.12, 95% CI 1.04 to 1.22) and cancer rates.[107]

Comment: One systematic review (search date 1996) of epidemiological studies found consistent associations between increased dietary intake, supplemental intake of vitamin E, or both, and lower cardiovascular risk and less consistent associations for β carotene and vitamin C.[107] Most observational studies of antioxidants have excluded people with pre-existing disease.[108,109] The results of the trial in people on haemodialysis raises the possibility that high dose vitamin E supplementation may be beneficial in those at high absolute risk of coronary events.[106] Further trials in such groups are required to confirm or refute this finding. The Heart Protection Study (results not fully published at time of search, 20 536 people aged 40–80 years with prior cardiovascular events or at high risk for vascular disease) compared a combination of antioxidant vitamins (daily doses: vitamin C 250 mg, vitamin E 600 mg, and β carotene 20 mg) versus placebo. After 5.5 years, the antioxidant treatment had no significant effect on total mortality and major cardiovascular events.[110]

OPTION CARDIAC REHABILITATION INCLUDING EXERCISE

One systematic review has found that cardiac rehabilitation including exercise reduces the risk of major cardiac events in people after myocardial infarction. It found that exercise alone reduced the risk of a major cardiac event, and probably reduced mortality. One subsequent RCT found no significant difference in quality of life between standard rehabilitation and early return to normal activities, although the study may have lacked power to detect clinically important differences between groups.

Benefits: We found one systematic review (search date 1998).[111] **Cardiac rehabilitation:** The review identified 42 RCTs of cardiac rehabilitation including exercise versus usual care (7683 people, who have had myocardial infarction, coronary artery bypass grafting [CABG], or percutaneous transluminal coronary angioplasty, or who have angina pectoris or coronary artery disease defined by angiography). It found that cardiac rehabilitation including exercise reduced the composite end point of mortality, non-fatal myocardial infarction, CABG, and percutaneous transluminal angioplasty (636/3863 [16.5%] with cardiac rehabilitation *v* 734/3820 [19.2%] with usual care; RR 0.85, 95% CI 0.77 to 0.93). It found limited evidence of a reduction in mortality but significance was sensitive to the quality of the trials.[111] We found one subsequent RCT.[112] The RCT (142 people with acute myocardial infarction in the previous week) compared 6 weeks of standard rehabilitation versus early return to normal activities.[112] It found no significant difference between groups in quality of life (measured on the cardiovascular extension of the Health Measurement Questionnaire; results presented graphically). However, the trial may have lacked power to exclude clinically important differences between groups.[111] **Exercise alone:** The review identified 12 RCTs of exercise alone versus usual care (2582 people, who have had myocardial infarction, CABG, or percutaneous transluminal angioplasty, or who have angina pectoris or coronary artery disease defined by angiography). It found that exercise significantly reduced mortality (93/1297 [7.2%] with exercise *v* 122/1285 [9.5%] with usual care; RR 0.76, 95% CI 0.59 to 0.98). It was associated with a reduction in the composite end point of mortality, non-fatal myocardial infarction, CABG, and percutaneous transluminal angioplasty, but the difference was not significant (183/1297 [14.1%] with exercise *v* 216/1285 [16.8%] with usual care; RR 0.85, 95% CI 0.71 to 1.01).[111]

Harms: Rates of adverse cardiovascular outcomes (syncope, arrhythmia, myocardial infarction, or sudden death) were low (2–3/100 000 person-hours) in supervised rehabilitation programmes, and rates of fatal cardiac events during or immediately after exercise training, were reported in two older surveys as ranging from 1/116 400 to 1/784 000 person-hours.[113]

Comment: The review included some RCTs performed before the widespread use of thrombolytic agents and β blockers after myocardial infarction.[113] Most people were white men, without comorbidity, and under 70 years of age. Other interventions aimed at risk factor modification were often provided in the intervention groups (including nutritional education, counselling in behavioural modification, and, in some trials, lipid lowering medications). We found no strong evidence that exercise training and cardiac rehabilitation programmes increased the proportion of people returning to work after myocardial infarction.

OPTION SMOKING CESSATION

We found no RCTs of the effects of smoking cessation on cardiovascular events in people with coronary heart disease. Moderate quality evidence from epidemiological studies indicates that people with coronary heart disease who stop smoking rapidly reduce their risk of recurrent coronary events or death. Treatment with nicotine patches seems safe in people with coronary heart disease.

Benefits: We found no RCTs assessing the effects of smoking cessation on coronary morbidity and mortality. Many observational studies have found that people with coronary heart disease who stop smoking rapidly reduce their risk of cardiac death and myocardial infarction (recurrent coronary events or premature death compared with continuing smokers: RR about 0.50).[114] See smoking cessation under primary prevention for more details, p 154. The studies found that about 50% of the benefits occur in the first year of stopping smoking, followed by a more gradual decrease in risk, reaching the risk of never smokers after several years of abstinence.[114] Among people with peripheral arterial disease and stroke, smoking cessation has been shown in observational studies to be associated with improved exercise tolerance, decreased risk of amputation, improved survival, and reduced risk of recurrent stroke.

Harms: Two recent RCTs found no evidence that nicotine replacement using transdermal patches in people with stable coronary heart disease increased cardiovascular events.[115,116]

Comment: One RCT compared the impact of firm and detailed advice to stop smoking (125 survivors of acute myocardial infarction) versus conventional advice (85 people).[117] Allocation to the intervention or control group was determined by day of admission. At over 1 year after admission, 62% of the intervention group and 28% of the control group were non-smokers. Morbidity and mortality were not reported. (See psychological and stress management, p 216).

OPTION PSYCHOLOGICAL AND STRESS MANAGEMENT

RCTs found limited evidence that psychosocial treatments decreased cardiac events or cardiac death compared with no psychosocial treatment in people with coronary heart disease. Two RCTs found that psychological treatments improved quality of life compared with no psychological treatment.

Benefits: One systematic review (search date not stated, 23 RCTs, 3180 people with coronary artery disease) compared a diverse range of psychosocial treatments (2024 people) versus usual treatment (1156 people).[118] Mortality results were available in only 12 RCTs. Psychosocial interventions versus control interventions significantly reduced mortality (OR survival 1.70, 95% CI 1.09 to 2.64) and non-fatal events in the first 2 years after myocardial infarction (OR for no event 1.84, 95% CI 1.12 to 2.99).[118] We found three subsequent RCTs.[119–121] The first RCT (142 people with newly diagnosed angina managed in primary care) compared a self management plan versus a single nurse-led educational session.[119] The self management plan consisted of a work book and relaxation programme, which was introduced and explained to participants by a primary care nurse. The RCT found that the self management plan significantly improved depression and anxiety scores compared with the educational session at 6 months (measured by Hospital Anxiety and Depression Scale (see glossary, p 222); change in anxiety score from baseline –1.03 with angina plan *v* 0 with educational session, $P = 0.05$; change in depression score –0.48 with angina plan *v* 0.41 with educational session, $P = 0.01$).[119] The second RCT (114 people after acute myocardial infarction) compared usual care versus an individualised cognitive behavioural programme based on national guidelines, which involved discussion of worries, establishing goals, repeated consultation to discuss progress, and a range of written materials and a relaxation tape.[120] The trial found that the individualised cognitive behavioural programme significantly improved health related quality of life compared with usual care (proportion of people with improved Dartmouth COOP score, measured on a scale from 1 [best quality of life] to 5 [worst quality of life]: 59% with intervention *v* 33% with usual care; OR 0.34, 95% CI 0.16 to 0.73; NNT 4, 95% CI 3 to 12).[120] The third RCT (65 people with recent acute myocardial infarction) compared standard care versus a brief in-hospital intervention to alter illness perception, consisting of three 30–40 minute interviews with a psychologist.[121] In these interviews, participants' worries were discussed; participants' causal models of coronary heart disease were discussed and challenged; implications for lifestyle were discussed, and a staged self management plan established and reviewed. At 3 months, the in-hospital intervention significantly reduced angina compared with standard care (self report of angina: 14.3% with intervention *v* 39.3% with standard care, $P < 0.05$).[121] However, it was not clear whether this difference was due to altered perception of symptoms or because of different rates of genuine ischaemia.[121]

Harms: No specific harms were reported.

Comment: These results should be interpreted with caution because of limits of the methods of the individual RCTs and the diversity of interventions (relaxation, stress management, counselling). The RCTs were generally small, with short follow up, and used non-uniform outcome measures. Methods of concealment allocation were not assessed. The authors of the review acknowledged the strong possibility of publication bias but made no attempt to measure it. The results were inconsistent across trials.[122] Several observational studies have found that depression and social isolation (lack of social and emotional support) are independent predictors of mortality and non-fatal coronary heart disease events in people after myocardial infarction.[123]

QUESTION What are the effects of surgical treatments?

Charanjit Rihal

OPTION CORONARY ARTERY BYPASS GRAFTING VERSUS MEDICAL TREATMENT ALONE

One systematic review found that coronary artery bypass grafts reduced the risk of death from coronary artery disease at 5 and 10 years compared with medical treatment alone. Greater benefit occurred in people with poor left ventricular function. One subsequent RCT in people with asymptomatic disease found that revascularisation with coronary artery bypass grafting or coronary percutaneous transluminal angioplasty reduced mortality compared with medical treatment alone at 2 years.

Benefits: We found one systematic review comparing coronary artery bypass grafting (CABG) with medical treatment alone[124] and one subsequent RCT in asymptomatic people of revascularisation with CABG or coronary percutaneous transluminal angioplasty versus medical treatment alone.[125] In the systematic review (search date not stated, 7 RCTs, individual results from 2649 people with coronary heart disease) most people were middle aged men with multivessel disease but good left ventricular function who were enrolled from 1972–1984 (97% were male; 82% 41–60 years old; 80% with ejection fraction > 50%; 60% with prior myocardial infarction; and 83% with 2 or 3 vessel disease).[124] People assigned to CABG also received medical treatment, and 40% initially assigned to medical treatment underwent CABG in the following 10 years. The systematic review found that CABG versus medical treatment reduced deaths at 5 and 10 years (death at 5 years: RR 0.61 95% CI 0.48 to 0.77; death at 10 years: RR 0.83, 95% CI 0.70 to 0.98).[124] Most trials did not collect data on recurrent angina or quality of life. **Effects in people with reduced versus normal left ventricular function:** The systematic review found that the relative benefits were similar in people with normal versus reduced left ventricular function (death: OR 0.61, 95% CI 0.46 to 0.81 if left ventricular function was normal; OR 0.59. 95% CI 0.39 to 0.91 if left ventricular function was reduced).[124] The absolute benefit of CABG was greater in people with a reduced left ventricular function because the baseline risk of death was higher. **Effects in people with different numbers of diseased vessels:** The systematic review found lower mortality with CABG versus medical treatment in people with single vessel, two vessel, three vessel, and left main stem disease, but for single vessel and two vessel disease the difference was not statistically significant, possibly because the number of deaths was small (RR with single vessel disease 0.54, 95% CI 0.22 to 1.33; with two vessel disease 0.84, 95% CI 0.54 to 1.32; with three vessel disease 0.58, 95% CI 0.42 to 0.80; with left main stem disease 0.32, 95% CI 0.15 to 0.70).[124] **Effects in asymptomatic people:** We found one RCT (558 people) of revascularisation with CABG or percutaneous transluminal angioplasty versus symptom guided treatment versus electrocardiogram and symptom guided treatment in people with asymptomatic ischaemia identified by exercise test or ambulatory electrocardiogram.[125] It found that revascularisation versus medical treatment alone reduced death or myocardial infarction at 2 years (death or myocardial infarction: AR 4.7% with revascularisation *v* 8.8% with symptom guided treatment *v* 12.1% with symptom plus electrocardiogram guided treatment; $P < 0.04$).

Harms: In the systematic review, of the 1240 people who underwent CABG, 40 (3.2%) died and 88 (7.1%) had documented non-fatal myocardial infarction within 30 days of the procedure. At 1 year, the estimated incidence of death or myocardial infarction was significantly higher with CABG versus medical treatment (11.6% with CABG *v* 8% with medical treatment; RR 1.45, 95% CI 1.18 to 2.03).[124] The diagnosis of myocardial infarction after CABG is difficult, and true incidence may be higher.

Comment: The results of the systematic review may not be easily generalised to current practice. People were 65 years or younger, but more than 50% of CABG procedures are now performed on people over 65 years of age. Almost all people were male. High risk people, such as those with severe angina and left main coronary artery stenosis, were under-represented. Internal thoracic artery grafts were used in fewer than 5% of people. Lipid lowering agents (particularly statins) and aspirin were used infrequently (aspirin used in 3% of people at enrolment). Only about 50% of people were taking β blockers. The systematic review may underestimate the real benefits of CABG in comparison with medical treatment alone because medical and surgical treatment for coronary artery disease were not mutually exclusive; by 5 years, 25% of people receiving medical treatment had undergone CABG surgery and by 10 years, 41% had undergone CABG surgery. The underestimate of effect would be greatest among people at high risk. People with previous CABG have not been studied in RCTs, although they now represent a growing proportion of those undergoing CABG.

OPTION CORONARY PERCUTANEOUS TRANSLUMINAL ANGIOPLASTY VERSUS MEDICAL TREATMENT ALONE

One systematic review found that coronary percutaneous transluminal angioplasty improved angina compared with medical treatment alone, but was associated with a higher rate of coronary artery bypass grafting. The review found higher mortality and rates of myocardial infarction with percutaneous transluminal angioplasty than with medical treatment but the difference was not significant. RCTs have found that percutaneous

transluminal angioplasty was associated with increased risk of emergency coronary artery bypass grafting and myocardial infarction during and soon after the procedure. One RCT found that percutaneous transluminal angioplasty reduced cardiac events and improved angina severity compared with medical treatment alone in people over the age of 75 years.

Benefits: We found one systematic review (search date 1998, 6 RCTs, 1904 people with stable coronary artery disease) comparing coronary percutaneous transluminal angioplasty (PTA) versus medical treatment alone.[126] Follow up varied from 6–57 months. It found that PTA versus medical treatment alone reduced angina, but increased subsequent coronary artery bypass grafting (CABG) (angina: RR 0.70, 95% CI 0.50 to 0.98; CABG: RR 1.59, 95% CI 1.09 to 2.32). It found higher mortality and myocardial infarction with PTA versus medical treatment alone but the difference was not significant (death: RR 1.32, 95% CI 0.65 to 2.70; myocardial infarction: RR 1.42, 95% CI 0.90 to 2.25). The review found significant heterogeneity between trials. The largest RCT identified by the review (1018 people) found that PTA versus medical treatment improved physical functioning, vitality, and general health at 1 year (proportion of people rating their health "much improved": 33% of people treated with PTA *v* 22% with medical treatment alone; P = 0.008), but found no significant difference at 3 years.[127] The improvements were related to breathlessness, angina, and treadmill tolerance. High transfer (27%) from the medical to PTA group may partly explain the lack of difference between groups at 3 years. **Effects in elderly people:** One RCT (305 people aged > 75 years with chronic refractory angina) compared PTA versus medical treatment alone.[128] It found that PTA reduced all adverse cardiac events and decreased anginal severity compared with medical treatment, but had no significant effect on deaths or non-fatal myocardial infarctions after 6 months (adverse cardiac events: AR 19% with PTA *v* 49% with medical treatment alone, P < 0.0001; change in angina class: –2.0 with PTA *v* –1.6 with medical treatment alone, P < 0.0001; deaths: AR 8.5% with PTA *v* 4.1% with medical treatment alone, P = 0.15; non-fatal infarctions: AR 7.8% with PTA *v* 11.5% with medical treatment alone, P = 0.46). **Effects in people with different angina severity:** One of the RCTs in the systematic review found that antianginal benefit from PTA was limited to people with moderate to severe (grade 2 or worse) angina (20% lower incidence of angina and 1 minute longer treadmill exercise times compared with medical treatment).[129] People with mild symptoms at enrolment derived no significant improvement in symptoms. **Effects in asymptomatic people:** We found one RCT (558 people) of revascularisation with CABG or PTA versus symptom-guided treatment versus electrocardiogram- and symptom-guided treatment in people with asymptomatic ischaemia identified by exercise test or ambulatory electrocardiogram[125] (see benefits of coronary artery bypass grafting *v* medical treatment alone, p 217).

Harms: Procedural death and myocardial infarction, as well as repeat procedures for restenosis, are the main hazards of PTA. Four RCTs included in the review reported complications of PTA. In the first RCT, two (1.9%) emergency CABG operations and five (4.8%) myocardial infarctions occurred at the time of the procedure. By 6 months, the PTA group had higher rates of CABG surgery (7% with PTA *v* 0% with medical treatment alone) and non-protocol PTA (15.2% with PTA *v* 10.3% with medical treatment alone).[129,130] In the second RCT, the higher mortality or rate of myocardial infarction with PTA was attributable to one death and seven procedure related myocardial infarctions.[128] The third RCT found a procedure related CABG rate and myocardial infarction rate of 2.8% each, and the fourth found rates of 2.0% for CABG and 3.0% for myocardial infarction.[125]

Comment: We found good evidence that PTA treats the symptoms of angina, but we found no evidence that it reduces the overall incidence of death or myocardial infarction in people with stable angina. This could be because of the risk of complications during and soon after the procedure, and because most PTAs are performed for single vessel disease.

OPTION CORONARY PERCUTANEOUS TRANSLUMINAL ANGIOPLASTY VERSUS CORONARY ARTERY BYPASS GRAFTING

One systematic review has found no significant difference in mortality, risk of myocardial infarction, or quality of life between percutaneous transluminal angioplasty and coronary artery bypass grafting. Percutaneous transluminal angioplasty is less invasive but increased the number of repeat procedures. The relevant RCTs were too small to exclude a 20–30% relative difference in mortality.

Benefits: We found one systematic review (search date not stated, 8 RCTs, 3371 people),[131] one subsequent RCT,[132] one subsequent non-systematic review (including the subsequent RCT),[133] which compared percutaneous transluminal angioplasty (PTA) versus coronary artery bypass grafting (CABG). **Angina:** The systematic review found that the prevalence of moderate to severe angina (grade 2 or worse) was significantly higher after PTA than after CABG at 1 year (RR 1.6, 95% CI 1.3 to 1.9).[131] After 3 years this difference had decreased (RR 1.2, 95% CI 1.0 to 1.5). **Mortality:** The systematic review found that PTA did not reduce deaths compared with CABG after 1 year (RR 1.08, 95% CI 0.79 to 1.50),[131] the subsequent RCT (392 people) found no significant difference in deaths between CABG versus PTA after 8 years, although the trial was too small to exclude a clinically important difference (AR for survival 83% with CABG *v* 79% with PTA; P = 0.40).[133] The subsequent non-systematic review found that mortality was not significantly different between PTA versus CABG (OR 1.09, 95% CI 0.88 to 1.35).[132] **Repeat procedures:** The systematic review found that PTA increased subsequent procedures compared with CABG (subsequent CABG: RR 1.59, 95% CI 1.09 to 2.32; subsequent PTA: RR 1.29, 95% CI 0.71 to 3.36).[131] **Quality of life:** Two of the RCTs included in the systematic review found no difference in quality of life between people who had PTA and people who had CABG over 3–5 years.[134,135]

Harms: See harms under percutaneous transluminal angioplasty versus medical treatment, p 219. CABG is more invasive than PTA, but PTA is associated with a greater need for repeat procedures.

Comment: Although no major differences in death or myocardial infarction were observed in the systematic review[131] these trials enrolled people at relatively low risk of cardiac events, so it is premature to conclude that PTA and CABG are equivalent for people with multi-vessel disease. Fewer than 20% of people had left ventricular dysfunction, almost 70% had one or two vessel disease, and observed mortality was only 2.6% for the first year and 1.1% for the second year. People enrolled in the largest trial more closely approximated to moderate risk people, but this was caused primarily by the higher proportion of people with diabetes mellitus.[136] Even in that trial nearly 60% of people had two vessel coronary artery disease. The total number of people enrolled in the nine trials so far is not adequate to show anything less than a 20–30% difference in mortality between PTA and CABG. Subgroup analysis of one RCT (1829 people) found that in people with diabetes (353 people) CABG reduced deaths compared with PTA after 7 years[136] (see coronary artery bypass grafting versus percutaneous transluminal angioplasty in prevention of cardiovascular events in diabetes, p 690). This difference was not found in people without diabetes or any other subgroup (deaths in people without diabetes: AR 13.6% with CABG *v* 13.2% with PTA; P = 0.72).[136]

OPTION — INTRACORONARY STENTS VERSUS CORONARY PERCUTANEOUS TRANSLUMINAL ANGIOPLASTY ALONE

One systematic review has found that intracoronary stents alone reduce the need for repeat vascularisation compared with coronary percutaneous transluminal angioplasty. It found no significant difference in mortality or myocardial infarction, but crossover rates from angioplasty to stent were high. RCTs found that intracoronary stents improved outcomes after 4–9 months compared with percutaneous transluminal angioplasty in people with previous coronary artery bypass grafting, chronic total occlusions, and for treatment of restenosis after initial percutaneous transluminal angioplasty.

Benefits: We found one systematic review (search date 1999, 11 RCTs with 4–11 months' follow up, 4815 people) of stents versus percutaneous transluminal angioplasty (PTA) alone.[137] It found a significant reduction in cardiac event rates after 4–11 months with stents compared with PTA alone (composite of death, myocardial infarction, or repeat vascularisation; 17.9% with stent *v* 24.1% with PTA; OR 0.68, 95% CI 0.59 to 0.78). Stents reduced repeat vascularisation compared with PTA alone (12.4% with stent *v* 20.6% with PTA alone; OR 0.54, 95% CI 0.45 to 0.65), whereas there was no significant difference in deaths (0.9% with stent *v* 1.3% with PTA alone; OR 0.68, 95% CI 0.40 to 1.14) or myocardial infarctions (4.4% with stent *v* 3.6% with PTA alone; OR 1.23, 95% CI 0.88 to 1.72). Seven RCTs with follow up over 1 year found a significant reduction in cardiac events with stents compared with PTA alone (19.5% with stent *v* 28.1% with PTA alone; OR 0.62, 95% CI 0.52 to 0.74). **In saphenous vein graft lesions in people with prior coronary artery bypass grafting:** We found one RCT (220 people) comparing stents with PTA alone for stenosed saphenous vein grafts.[138] There was no significant difference in rates of restenosis (37% with stent *v* 46% with PTA alone; P = 0.24) after 6 months, but stents compared with PTA alone reduced death, myocardial infarction, coronary artery bypass grafting, or repeat PTA (27% with stent *v* 42% with PTA alone; P = 0.03). **In people with total**

occlusions: We found three RCTs comparing stents with PTA alone in people with chronic totally occluded coronary arteries.[139–141] The first RCT (119 people) found that stent compared with PTA alone reduced angina, angiographic restenosis, and repeat procedures (angina free at 6 months: 57% with stent *v* 24% with PTA alone, P < 0.001; > 50% stenosis on follow up angiography: 32% with stent *v* 74% with PTA alone, P < 0.001; repeat procedures: 22% with stent *v* 42% with PTA alone, P = 0.03).[139] The second RCT (110 people) found that stents compared with PTA alone reduced restenosis and repeat procedures after 9 months (restenosis: 32% with stent *v* 68% with PTA alone, P < 0.001; repeat procedures: 5% with stent *v* 22% with PTA alone, P = 0.04).[140] The third RCT (110 people) found that stents versus PTA alone reduced restenosis and repeat PTA after 4 months (restenosis: 26% with stent *v* 62% with PTA alone, P = 0.01; repeat PTA: 24% with stent *v* 55% with PTA alone, P = 0.05). No deaths or coronary artery bypass grafting operations occurred in either group. The incidence of myocardial infarction was low in both groups (0% with stent *v* 2% with PTA alone, P > 0.05).[141] **For treatment of restenosis after initial percutaneous transluminal angioplasty:** We found one RCT (383 people) of coronary stent versus PTA alone for treatment of restenosis.[142] It found that stents versus PTA alone reduced restenosis and repeat procedures, and increased survival free of myocardial infarction and repeat revascularisation after 6 months (restenosis: 18% with stent *v* 32% with PTA alone, P = 0.03; repeat procedures: 10% with stent *v* 27% with PTA alone, P = 0.001; survival free of myocardial infarction or repeat revascularisation: 84% with stent *v* 72% with PTA alone, P = 0.04).[142]

Harms: Initially, aggressive combination antithrombotic and anticoagulant regimens were used after stenting because of a high incidence of stent thrombosis and myocardial infarction. These regimens led to a high incidence of arterial access site haemorrhage.[133] More recently, improved stent techniques and use of aspirin and ticlopidine have reduced both stent thrombosis and arterial access site haemorrhage.[138,142] Currently, the risk of stent thrombosis is less than 1%.[143–145] Haemorrhage (particularly femoral artery haemorrhage) was more frequent after stenting than PTA alone,[146] but occurred in less than 3% after stenting when antiplatelet drugs were used without long term anticoagulants.

Comment: It is unclear whether stenting influences the relative benefits and harms of percutaneous procedures compared with coronary artery bypass grafting. Coronary stents are associated with fewer repeat revascularisation procedures and less angiographic restenosis than PTA. Rates of death and myocardial infarction are low in the RCTs and are not significantly different between stents and PTA. However, any potential differences may be masked by the crossover to stents after poor results (such as dissection) immediately after PTA.

GLOSSARY

Hospital anxiety and depression scale (HADS) A self report questionnaire designed to assess anxiety and depression in hospital inpatients. It has subscales for anxiety and depression, each comprising seven questions, which are scored from 0–3.

International normalised ratio (INR) A value derived from a standardised laboratory test that measures the effect of an anticoagulant. The laboratory materials used in the test are calibrated against internationally accepted standard reference preparations, so that variability between laboratories and different reagents is minimised. Normal blood has an INR of 1. Therapeutic anticoagulation often aims to achieve an INR value of 2.0–3.5.

Substantive changes

Oral glycoprotein IIb/IIIa receptor inhibitors One systematic review added;[32] conclusions unchanged.
Oral anticoagulants in addition to antiplatelet treatment Two RCTs added;[35,36] conclusions unchanged.
Oral anticoagulants in the absence of antiplatelet treatment Two RCTs added;[35,36] conclusions unchanged.
β blockers One systematic review of harms added;[46] conclusions unchanged.
Hormone replacement therapy Extended follow up of existing RCT reported[61,65] and one RCT added;[62] conclusions unchanged.
Cholesterol reduction Two RCTs and one safety meta-analysis added;[72,75,80] conclusions unchanged.
Cardiac rehabilitation One subsequent RCT added;[112] conclusions unchanged.
Psychological and stress management Three RCTs added;[119–121] conclusions unchanged.

REFERENCES

1. Greaves EJ, Gillum BS. 1994 Summary: national hospital discharge survey. Advance data from Vital and Health Statistics, no. 278. Hyattsville, Maryland, USA: National Center for Health Statistics, 1996.
2. Shaw LJ, Peterson ED, Kesler K, et al. A meta-analysis of predischarge risk stratification after acute myocardial infarction with stress electrocardiographic, myocardial perfusion, and ventricular function imaging. *Am J Cardiol* 1996;78:1327–1337. Search date 1995; primary sources Medline and hand searches of bibliographies of review articles.
3. Kudenchuk PJ, Maynard C, Martin JS, et al. Comparison, presentation, treatment and outcome of acute myocardial infarction in men versus women (the Myocardial Infarction Triage and Intervention Registry). *Am J Cardiol* 1996;78:9–14.
4. The Task Force on the Management of Acute Myocardial Infarction of the European Society of Cardiology. Acute myocardial infarction: pre-hospital and in-hospital management. *Eur Heart J* 1996;17:43–63.
5. Peterson ED, Shaw LJ, Califf RM. Clinical guideline: part II. Risk stratification after myocardial infarction. *Ann Intern Med* 1997;126:561–582.
6. The Multicenter Postinfarction Research Group. Risk stratification and survival after myocardial infarction. *N Engl J Med* 1983;309;331–336.
7. American College of Cardiology/American Heart Association Task Force on Practice Guidelines (Committee on Exercise Testing). ACC/AHA guidelines for exercise testing. *J Am Coll Cardiol* 1997;30:260–315.
8. Fallen E, Cairns J, Dafoe W, et al. Management of the postmyocardial infarction patient: a consensus report — revision of the 1991 CCS guidelines. *Can J Cardiol* 1995;11:477–486.
9. Madsen JK, Grande P, Saunamaki, et al. Danish multicenter randomized study of invasive versus conservative treatment in patients with inducible ischemia after thrombolysis in acute myocardial infarction (DANAMI). DANish trial in Acute Myocardial Infarction. *Circulation* 1997;96:748–755.
10. Antithrombotic Trialists' Collaboration. Collaborative meta-analysis of randomised trials of antiplatelet therapy for prevention of death, myocardial infarction and stroke in high risk patients. *BMJ* 2002;324:71–86. Search date 1997; primary sources Medline, Embase, Derwent, Scisearch, and Biosis, in additional trials registers of Cochrane Stroke and Peripheral Vascular Diseases Group, hand searches of journals, abstracts, and conference proceedings, and contact with experts.
11. Taylor DW, Barnett HJM, Haynes RB, et al. Low-dose and high-dose acetylsalicylic acid for patients undergoing carotid endarterectomy: a randomised controlled trial. *Lancet* 1999;353:2179–2184.
12. He J, Whelton PK, Vu B, et al. Aspirin and risk of hemorrhagic stroke. A meta-analysis of randomised controlled trials. *JAMA* 1998;280:1930–1935.
13. Farrell B, Godwin J, Richards S, et al. The United Kingdom transient ischaemic attack (UK-TIA) aspirin trial: final results. *J Neurol Neurosurg Psychiatry* 1991;54:1044–1054.
14. Dutch TIA Trial Study Group. A comparison of two doses of aspirin (30 mg vs 283 mg a day) in patients after a transient ischemic attack or minor ischemic stroke. *N Engl J Med* 1991;325:1261–1266.
15. Thrift AG, McNeil JJ, Forbes A, et al. Risk factors for cerebral hemorrhage in the era of well-controlled hypertension. Melbourne Risk Factor Study (MERFS) Group. *Stroke* 1996;27:2020–2025.
16. Iso H, Hennekens CH, Stampfer MJ, et al. Prospective study of aspirin use and risk of stroke in women. *Stroke* 1999;30:1764–1771.
17. Derry S, Loke YK. Risk of gastrointestinal haemorrhage with long term use of aspirin:

meta-analysis. *BMJ* 2000;321:1183–1187. Search date 1999; primary sources Medline, Embase, and reference lists of existing systematic reviews.
18. Garc a Rodr guez LA, Hernández–D az S, de Abajo FJ. Association between aspirin and upper gastrointestinal complications. Systematic review of epidemiologic studies. *Br J Clin Pharmacol* 2001;52:563–571.
19. CAPRIE Steering Committee. A randomised, blinded, trial of clopidogrel versus aspirin in patients at risk of ischaemic events. *Lancet* 1996;348:1329–1339.
20. Scrutinio D, Cimminiello C, Marubini E, et al. Ticlopidine versus aspirin after myocardial infarction (STAMI) trial. *J Am Coll Cardiol* 2001;37:1259–1265.
21. Hankey GJ, Sudlow CLM, Dunbabin DW. Thienopyridine derivatives (ticlopidine, clopidogrel) versus aspirin for preventing stroke and other serious vascular events in high vascular risk patients. In: The Cochrane Library, Issue 4, 2002. Oxford: Update Software. Search date 1999; primary sources Medline, Embase, Cochrane Stroke Group Register, Antithrombotics Trialists' database, authors of trials, and drug manufacturers.
22. Moloney BA. An analysis of the side effects of ticlopidine. In: Hass WK, Easton JD, eds. *Ticlopidine, platelets and vascular disease*. New York: Springer, 1993:117–139.
23. Bennett CL, Davidson CJ, Raisch DW, et al. Thrombotic thrombocytopenic purpura associated with ticlopidine in the setting of coronary artery stents and stroke prevention. *Arch Int Med* 1999;159:2524–2528.
24. Bennett CL, Connors JM, Carwile JM, et al. Thrombotic thrombocytopenic purpura associated with clopidogrel. *N Engl J Med* 2000;342:1773–1777.
25. Hankey GJ. Clopidogrel and thrombotic thrombocytopenic purpura. *Lancet* 2000;356:269–270.
26. Müller C, Büttner HJ, Petersen J, et al. A randomized comparison of clopidogrel and aspirin versus ticlopidine and aspirin after the placement of coronary-artery stents. *Circulation* 2000;101:590–593.
27. Bertrand ME, Rupprecht H-J, Urban P, et al, for the CLASSICS Investigators. Double-blind study of the safety of clopidogrel with and without a loading dose in combination with aspirin compared with ticlopidine in combination with aspirin after coronary stenting. The Clopidogrel Aspirin Stent International Cooperative Study (CLASSICS). *Circulation* 2000;102:624–629.
28. Taniuchi M, Kurz HI, Lasala JM. Randomized comparison of ticlopidine and clopidogrel after intracoronary stent implantation in a broad patient population. *Circulation* 2001;104:539–543.
29. The Clopidogrel in Unstable Angina to Prevent Recurrent Events (CURE) Trial Investigators. Effects of clopidogrel in addition to aspirin in patients with acute coronary syndromes without ST-segment elevation. *N Engl J Med* 2001;345:494–502.
30. Second Chinese Cardiac Study (CCS-2) Collaborative Group. Rationale, design and organisation of the Second Chinese Cardiac Study (CCS-2): a randomised trial of clopidogrel plus aspirin, and of metoprolol, among patients with suspected acute myocardial infarction. *J Cardiovasc Risk* 2000;7:435–441.
31. Chew DP, Bhatt DL, Sapp S, et al. Increased mortality with oral platelet glycoprotein IIb/IIIa antagonists. *Circulation* 2001;103:201–206. Search date 2000; primary source Medline.
32. Newby LK, Califf RM, White HD, et al. The failure of orally administered glycoprotein IIb/IIIa inhibitors to prevent recurrent cardiac events. *Am J Med* 2002;112:647–658. Search date 2001.
33. SoRelle R. SmithKline Beecham halts tests of lotrafiban, an oral glycoprotein IIb/IIIa inhibitor. *Circulation* 2001;103:E9001–E9002.
34. Anand SS, Yusuf S. Oral anticoagulant therapy in patients with coronary artery disease: a meta-analysis. *JAMA* 1999;282:2058–2067. Search date 1999; primary sources Medline, Embase, Current Contents, hand searches of reference lists, and contact with experts and pharmaceutical companies.
35. Hurlen M, Abdelnoor M, Smith P et al. Warfarin, aspirin, or both after myocardial infarction. *N Engl J Med* 2002;347:969–974.
36. van Es RF, Jonker JJ, Verheugt FW, et al, for the Antithrombotics in the Secondary Prevention of Events in Coronary Thrombosis-2 (ASPECT-2) Research Group. Aspirin and coumadin after acute coronary syndromes (the ASPECT-2 study): a randomised controlled trial. *Lancet* 2002;360:109–113.
37. The Organization to Assess Strategies for Ischemic Syndromes (OASIS) Investigators. Effects of long-term, moderate intensity oral anticoagulation in addition to aspirin in unstable angina. *J Am Coll Cardiol* 2001;37:475–484.
38. Fiore LD, Ezekowitz MD, Brophy MT, et al, for the Combination Hemotherapy and Mortality Prevention (CHAMP) Study Group. Department of Veterans Affairs Cooperative Studies Program clinical trial comparing combined warfarin and aspirin with aspirin alone in survivors of acute myocardial infarction. Primary results of the CHAMP study. *Circulation* 2002;105:557–563.
39. Huynh T, Theroux P, Bogaty P, et al. Aspirin, warfarin, or the combination for secondary prevention of coronary events in patients with acute coronary syndromes and prior coronary artery bypass surgery. *Circulation* 2001;103:3069–3074.
40. Teo KK, Yusuf S, Furberg CD. Effects of prophylactic antiarrhythmic drug therapy in acute myocardial infarction. *JAMA* 1993;270:1589–1595. Search date 1993; primary sources Medline, hand searches of reference lists, and details of unpublished trials sought from pharmaceutical industry/other investigators.
41. Yusuf S, Peto R, Lewis J, et al. Beta blockade during and after myocardial infarction: an overview of the randomized trials. *Prog Cardiovasc Dis* 1985;27:335–371. Search date and primary sources not stated.
42. Pepine CJ, Cohn PF, Deedwania PC, et al. Effects of treatment on outcome in mildly symptomatic patients with ischemia during daily life: the atenolol silent ischemia study (ASIST). *Circulation* 1994;90:762–768.
43. Boissel J-P, Leizerovicz A, Picolet H, et al. Secondary prevention after high-risk acute myocardial infarction with low-dose acebutolol. *Am J Cardiol* 1990;66:251–260.
44. The Beta-Blocker Pooling Project Research Group. The Beta-Blocker Pooling Project (BBPP): subgroup findings from randomized trials in post infarction patients. *Eur Heart J* 1988;9:8–16. Search date 1983; primary sources not stated.
45. Beta-blocker Heart Attack Trial Research Group. A randomized trial of propranolol in patients with acute myocardial infarction: I. mortality results. *JAMA* 1982;247:1707–1714.
46. Ko DT, Hebert PR, Coffey CS et al. Beta-blocker therapy and symptoms of depression, fatigue, and sexual dysfunction. *JAMA* 2002;288:351–357.

47. Flather MD, Yusuf S, Kober L, et al. Long-term ACE-inhibitor therapy in patients with heart failure or left-ventricular dysfunction: a systematic overview of data from individual patients. ACE-Inhibitor Myocardial Infarction Collaborative Group. *Lancet* 2000 6;355:1575–81. Search date not stated; primary sources Medline, hand searches of reference lists, and contact with experts.
48. The Heart Outcomes Prevention Evaluation (HOPE) Investigators. Effects of an angiotensin-converting enzyme inhibitor, ramipril, on cardiovascular events in high-risk patients. *N Engl J Med* 2000;342;145–153.
49. Heart Outcomes Prevention Evaluation (HOPE) Investigators. Effects of ramipril on cardiovascular and microvascular outcomes on people with diabetes mellitus: results of the hope study and MICRO-HOPE substudy. *Lancet* 2000;355:253–259.
50. Yusuf S, Lonn E. Anti-ischaemic effects of ACE inhibitors: review of current clinical evidence and ongoing clinical trials. *Eur Heart J* 1998;19:J36–J44.
51. Echt DS, Liebson PR, Mitchell LB, et al. Mortality and morbidity in patients receiving encainide, flecainide, or placebo. The Cardiac Arrhythmia Suppression Trial. *N Engl J Med* 1991;324:781–788.
52. Amiodarone Trials Meta-Analysis Investigators. Effect of prophylactic amiodarone on mortality after acute myocardial infarction and in congestive heart failure: meta-analysis of individual data from 6500 patients in randomised trials. *Lancet* 1997;350:1417–1424. Search date and primary sources not stated.
53. Sim I, McDonald KM, Lavori PW, et al. Quantitative overview of randomized trials of amiodarone to prevent sudden cardiac death. *Circulation* 1997;96:2823–2829. Search date 1997; primary sources Medline and Biosis.
54. Waldo AL, Camm AJ, de Ruyter H, et al, for the SWORD Investigators. Effect of d-sotalol on mortality in patients with left ventricular dysfunction after recent and remote myocardial infarction. *Lancet* 1996;348:7–12.
55. Cairns JA, Connolly SJ, Roberts R, et al, for the Canadian Amiodarone Myocardial Infarction Arrhythmia Trial Investigators. Randomized trial of outcome after myocardial infarction in patients with frequent or repetitive ventricular premature depolarisations: CAMIAT. *Lancet* 1997;349:675–682.
56. Julian DG, Camm AJ, Janse MJ, et al, for the European Myocardial Infarct Amiodarone Trial Investigators. Randomised trial of effect of amiodarone on mortality in patients with left-ventricular dysfunction after recent myocardial infarction: EMIAT. *Lancet* 1997;349:667–674.
57. Gibson R, Boden WE, Theroux P, et al. Diltiazem and reinfarction in patients with non-Q-wave myocardial infarction. Results of a double-blind, randomized, multicenter trial. *N Engl J Med* 1986;315:423–429.
58. The Multicenter Diltiazem Postinfarction Trial Research Group. The effect of diltiazem on mortality and reinfarction after myocardial infarction. *N Engl J Med* 1988;319:385–392.
59. The Danish Study Group on Verapamil in Myocardial Infarction. Effect of verapamil on mortality and major events after acute myocardial infarction: the Danish verapamil infarction trial II (DAVIT II). *Am J Cardiol* 1990;66:779–785.
60. Hulley S, Grady D, Bush T, et al. Randomized trial of estrogen plus progestin for secondary prevention of coronary heart disease in postmenopausal women. *JAMA* 1998;280:605–613.
61. Grady D, Herrington D, Bittner V, et al. Cardiovascular disease outcomes during 6.8 years of hormone therapy: Heart and Estrogen/progestin Replacement Study follow up (HERS II). *JAMA* 2002;288:49–57.
62. Clarke SC, Kelleher J, Lloyd-Jones H, et al. A study of hormone replacement therapy in postmenopausal women with ischaemic heart disease: the Papworth HRT atherosclerosis study. *Br J Obstet Gynaecol* 2002;109:1056–1062.
63. Coronary Drug Research Project Research Group. The coronary drug project: initial findings leading to modifications of its research protocol. *JAMA* 1970;214:1303–1313.
64. Daly E, Vessey MP, Hawkins MM, et al. Risk of venous thromboembolism in users of hormone replacement therapy. *Lancet* 1996;348:977–980.
65. Hulley S, Furberg C, Barret-Connor E, et al. Noncardiovascular disease outcomes during 6.8 years of hormone therapy: Heart and estrogen/progestin replacement study follow up (HERS II). *JAMA* 2002;288:58–66.
66. Newton KM, LaCroix AZ, McKnight B, et al. Estrogen replacement therapy and prognosis after first myocardial infarction. *Am J Epidemiol* 1997;145:269–277.
67. Sullivan JM, El-Zeky F, Vander Zwaag R, et al. Effect on survival of estrogen replacement therapy after coronary artery bypass grafting. *Am J Cardiol* 1997;79:847–850.
68. The Writing Group for the PEPI Trial. Effects of estrogen or estrogen/progestin regimens on heart disease risk factors in postmenopausal women. *JAMA* 1995;273:199–208.
69. Bucher HC, Griffith LE, Guyatt G. Systematic review on the risk and benefit of different cholesterol-lowering interventions. *Arterioscler Thromb Vasc Biol* 1999;19:187–195. Search date 1996; primary sources Medline, Embase, and bibliographic searches.
70. Miettinen TA, Pyorala K, Olsson AG, et al. Cholesterol-lowering therapy in women and elderly patients with myocardial infarction or angina pectoris: findings from the Scandinavian Simvastatin Survival Study (4S). *Circulation* 1997;96:4211–4218.
71. Heart Protection Study Collaborative Group. MRC/BHF Heart Protection Study of cholesterol lowering with simvastatin in 20 536 high-risk individuals: a randomised placebo-controlled trial. *Lancet* 2002;360:7M–22M.
72. Athyros VG, Papageorgriou AA, Mercouris BR, et al. Treatment with atorvastatin to the National. Cholesterol Educational Program goal versus 'usual' care in secondary coronary heart disease prevention. The GREek Atorvastatin and coronary-heart-disease evaluation (GREACE) study. *Curr Med Res Opin* 2002;18:220–228.
73. LaRosa JC, He J, Vupputuri S. Effect of statins on risk of coronary disease: a meta-analysis of randomized controlled trials. *JAMA* 1999;282:2340–2346. Search date 1998; primary sources Medline, bibliographies, and authors' reference files.
74. Schwartz GG, Olsson AG, Ezekowitz MD, et al. Effects of atorvastatin on early recurrent ischemic events in acute coronary syndromes: the MIRACL study: a randomized controlled trial. *JAMA* 2001;285:1711–1718.
75. Serruys PW, de Feyter P, Macaya C, et al. Fluvastatin for prevention of cardiac events following successful first percutaneous coronary intervention: a randomized controlled trial. *JAMA* 2002;287:3215–3222.

76. Knatterud GL, Rosenberg Y, Campeau L, et al. Long-term effects on clinical outcomes of aggressive lowering of low-density lipoprotein cholesterol levels and low-dose anticoagulation in the post coronary artery bypass graft trial. Post CABG Investigators. *Circulation* 2000;102:157–165.
77. Montagne O, Vedel I, Durand-Zaleski I. Assessment of the impact of fibrates and diet on survival and their cost-effectiveness: evidence from randomized, controlled trials in coronary heart disease and health economic evaluations. *Clin Ther* 1999;21:2027–2035. Search date not stated; primary sources Medline and hand searches of reference lists and systematic reviews.
78. Schlesinger Z, Vered Z, Friedenson A, et al. Secondary prevention by raising HDL cholesterol and reducing triglycerides in patients with coronary artery disease: the Bezafibrate Infarction Prevention (BIP) study. *Circulation* 2000;102:21–27.
79. Ericsson CG, Hamsten A, Nilsson J, et al. Angiographic assessment of effects of bezafibrate on progression of coronary artery disease in young male postinfarction patients. *Lancet* 1996;347:849–853.
80. Pfeffer MA, Keech A, Scks FM, et al. Safety and tolerability of pravastatin in long term clinical trials: Prospective Pravastatin Pooling (PPP) project. *Circulation* 2002;105:2341–2346.
81. The Women's Health Initiative Study Group. Design of the women's health initiative clinical trial and observational study. *Control Clin Trials* 1998;19:61–109.
82. Davis BR, Cutler JA Gordon DJ, et al, for the ALLHAT Research Group. Rationale and design for the antihypertensive and lipid lowering treatment to prevent heart attack trial (ALLHAT). *Am J Hypertens* 1996;9:342–360.
83. Flack JM, Neaton J, Grimm R, et al. Blood pressure and mortality among men with prior myocardial infarction. *Circulation* 1995;92;2437–2445.
84. Dahlof B, Lindholm LH, Hansson L, et al. Morbidity and mortality in the Swedish trial in old patients with hypertension (STOP-hypertension). *Lancet* 1991;338:1281–1285.
85. Medical Research Council Working Party. MRC trial on treatment of hypertension in older adults: principal results. *BMJ* 1992;304:405–412.
86. Systolic Hypertension in Elderly Patients (SHEP) Cooperative Research Group. Prevention of stroke by antihypertensive treatment in older persons with isolated systolic hypertension. *JAMA* 1991;265:3255–3264.
87. D'Agostini RB, Belanger AJ, Kannel WB, et al. Relationship of low diastolic blood pressure to coronary heart disease death in presence of myocardial infarction: the Framingham study. *BMJ* 1991;303:385–389.
88. Pfeffer MA, Braunwald E, Moye LA, et al. Effect of captopril on mortality and morbidity in patients with left ventricular dysfunction after myocardial infarction: results of the survival and ventricular enlargement trial. *N Engl J Med* 1992;327:669–677.
89. NHS Centre for Reviews and Dissemination, University of York. Cholesterol and coronary heart disease: screening and treatment. *Eff Health Care* 1998;4:1. Search date and primary sources not stated.
90. Burr ML, Fehily AM, Gilbert JF, et al. Effects of changes in fat, fish, and fibre intakes on death and myocardial reinfarction: Diet And Reinfarction Trial (DART). *Lancet* 1989;2:757–761.
91. Fehily AM, Vaughan-Williams E, Shiels K, et al. The effect of dietary advice on nutrient intakes: evidence from the Diet And Reinfarction Trial (DART). *J Hum Nutr Diet* 1989;2:225–235.
92. GISSI-Prevenzione Investigators. Dietary supplementation with n-3 polyunsaturated fatty acids and vitamin E after myocardial infarction: results of the GISSI-Prevenzione. *Lancet* 1999;354:447–455.
93. De Lorgeril M, Renaud S, Mamelle N, et al. Mediterranean alpha-linolenic acid-rich diet in secondary prevention of coronary heart disease. *Lancet* 1994;343:1454–1459.
94. Clarke R, Frost C, Collins R, et al. Dietary lipids and blood cholesterol: quantitative meta-analysis of metabolic ward studies. *BMJ* 1997;314:112–117. Search date 1995; primary sources Medline and hand searches of reference lists and nutrition journals.
95. Tang JL, Armitage JM, Lancaster T, et al. Systematic review of dietary intervention trials to lower blood total cholesterol in free-living subjects. *BMJ* 1998;316:1213–1220. Search date 1997; primary sources Medline, Human Nutrition, Embase, and Allied and Alternative Medicine, and hand searches the *Am J Clin Nutr* and references of review articles.
96. Brunner E, White I, Thorogood M, et al. Can dietary interventions change diet and cardiovascular risk factors? A meta-analysis of randomized controlled trials. *Am J Public Health* 1997;87:1415–1422. Search date 1993; primary sources Medline and hand searches of selected journals.
97. Ebrahim S, Davey SG. *Health promotion in older people for the prevention of coronary heart disease and stroke*. London: Health Education Authority, 1996.
98. Waters D. Lessons from coronary atherosclerosis "regression" trials. *Cardiol Clin* 1996;14:31–50.
99. Silagy C, Neil A. Garlic as a lipid lowering agent: a meta-analysis. *J R Coll Physicians Lond* 1994;28:39–45. Search date 1992; primary sources Medline, Alternative Medicine database, contact with authors of published studies, manufacturers, and hand searches of references.
100. Isaacsohn JL, Moser M, Stein EA, et al. Garlic powder and plasma lipids and lipoproteins. *Arch Intern Med* 1998;158:1189–1194.
101. Berthold HK, Sudhop T, von Bergmann K. Effect of a garlic oil preparation on serum lipoproteins and cholesterol metabolism. *JAMA* 1998;279:1900–1902.
102. Ripsin CM, Keenan JM, Jacobs DR Jr, et al. Oat products and lipid lowering: a meta-analysis. *JAMA* 1992;267:3317–3325. Search date 1991; primary sources Medline and unpublished trials solicited from all known investigators of lipid–oats association.
103. Stephens NG, Parsons A, Schofield PM, et al. Randomised controlled trial of vitamin E in patients with coronary disease: Cambridge Heart Antioxidant Study (CHAOS). *Lancet* 1996;347:781–786.
104. Rapola JM, Virtamo J, Ripatti S, et al. Randomised trial of alpha-tocopherol and beta-carotene supplements on incidence of major coronary events in men with previous myocardial infarction. *Lancet* 1997;349:1715–1720.
105. The Heart Outcomes Prevention Evaluation Study Investigators. Vitamin E supplementation and cardiovascular events in high-risk patients. *N Engl J Med* 2000;342:154–160.
106. Boaz M, Smetana S, Weinstein T, et al. Secondary prevention with antioxidants of cardiovascular disease in endstage renal disease (SPACE): randomised placebo-controlled trial. *Lancet* 2000;356:1213–1218.

107. Lonn EM, Yusuf S. Is there a role for antioxidant vitamins in the prevention of cardiovascular diseases? An update on epidemiological and clinical trials data. *Can J Cardiol* 1997;13:957–965. Search date 1996; primary sources Medline and one reference from 1997.
108. Jha P, Flather M, Lonn E, et al. The antioxidant vitamins and cardiovascular disease: a critical review of epidemiologic and clinical trial data. *Ann Intern Med* 1995;123:860–872.
109. Ness AR, Powles JW, Khaw KT. Vitamin C and cardiovascular disease: a systematic review. *J Cardiovasc Risk* 1997;3:513–521. Search date not stated; primary sources Medline, contact with experts, and hand searches of references.
110. Collins R, Peto R, Armitage J. The MRC/BHF heart protection study: preliminary results. *Int J Clin Pract* 2002;56:53–56).
111. Jolliffe JA, Rees K, Taylor RS, et al. Exercise-based rehabilitation for coronary heart disease. In: The Cochrane Library, Issue 4, 2002. Oxford: Update Software. Search date 1998; primary sources Cardiovascular RCT register at McMaster University, Cochrane Controlled Trials Register, Medline, Embase, Cinahl, Amed, Bids, ISI, and Sportsdiscus, hand searches of reference lists and conference proceedings, and contact with experts.
112. Hall JP, Wiseman VL, King MT, et al. Economic evaluation of a randomised trial of early return to normal activities versus cardiac rehabilitation after acute myocardial infarction. *Heart Lung Circ* 2002;11:10–18.
113. Wenger NK, Froelicher NS, Smith LK, et al. *Cardiac rehabilitation and secondary prevention*. Rockville, Maryland: Agency for Health Care Policy and Research and National Heart, Lung and Blood Institute, 1995. Search date and primary source not stated.
114. US Department of Health and Human Services. *The health benefits of smoking cessation: a report of the surgeon general*. Bethesda, Maryland: US DHSS, 1990.
115. Working Group for the Study of Transdermal Nicotine in Patients with Coronary Artery Disease. Nicotine replacement therapy for patients with coronary artery disease. *Arch Intern Med* 1994;154:989–995.
116. Joseph AM, Norman SM, Ferry LH, et al. The safety of transdermal nicotine as an aid to smoking cessation in patients with cardiac disease. *N Engl J Med* 1996;335:1792–1798.
117. Burt A, Thornley P, Illingworth D, et al. Stopping smoking after myocardial infarction. *Lancet* 1974;1:304–306.
118. Linden W, Stossel C, Maurice J. Psychosocial interventions in patients with coronary artery disease: a meta-analysis. *Arch Intern Med* 1996;156:745–752. Search date and primary sources not stated.
119. Lewin RJ, Furze G, Robinson J, et al. A randomised controlled trial of a self-management plan for patients with newly diagnosed angina. *Br J Gen Pract* 2002;52:194–201.
120. Mayou RA, Thompson DR, Clements A et al. Guideline based early rehabilitation after myocardial infraction – a pragmatic randomised controlled trial. *J Psychosom Res* 2002;52:89–95.
121. Petrie KJ, Cameron LD, Ellis CJ et al. Changing illness perceptions after myocardial infarction: an early intervention randomized controlled trial. *Psychosom Med* 2002;64;580–586.
122. US Department of Health and Human Services. Cardiac rehabilitation. AHCPR Publication No 96–0672, 1995;121–128.
123. Hemingway H, Marmot M. Psychosocial factors in the primary and secondary prevention of coronary heart disease: a systematic review. In: Yusuf S, Cairns JA, Camm AJ, et al, eds. *Evidence based cardiology*. London: BMJ Books, 1998. Search date 1996; primary sources Medline, and manual searches of bibliographies of retrieved articles and review articles.
124. Yusuf S, Zucker D, Peduzzi P, et al. Effect of coronary artery bypass graft surgery on survival: overview of 10-year results from randomized trials by the Coronary Artery Bypass Graft Surgery Trialists Collaboration. *Lancet* 1994;344:563–570. Search date and primary sources not stated.
125. Davies RF, Goldberg AD, Forman S, et al. Asymptomatic Cardiac Ischemia Pilot (ACIP) study two-year follow-up: outcomes of patients randomized to initial strategies of medical therapy versus revascularization. *Circulation* 1997;95:2037–2043.
126. Bucher HC, Hengstler P, Schindler C, et al. Percutaneous transluminal coronary angioplasty versus medical treatment for non-acute coronary heart disease: meta-analysis of randomised controlled trials. *BMJ* 2000;321:73–77. Search date 1998; primary sources Medline, Embase, Cochrane Library, Biological Abstracts, Health Periodicals Database, Pascal, and hand searches of references.
127. Pocock SJ, Henderson RA, Clayton T, et al. Quality of life after coronary angioplasty or continued medical treatment for angina: three-year follow-up in the RITA-2 trial. Randomized Intervention Treatment of Angina. *J Am Coll Cardiol* 2000;35:907–914.
128. TIME investigators. Trial of invasive versus medical therapy in elderly patients with chronic symptomatic coronary-artery disease (TIME): a randomised trial. *Lancet* 2001;358:951–957.
129. RITA-2 Trial Participants. Coronary angioplasty versus medical therapy for angina: the second randomized intervention treatment of angina (RITA-2) trial. *Lancet* 1997;350:461–468.
130. Parisi AF, Folland ED, Hartigan P. A comparison of angioplasty with medical therapy in the treatment of single-vessel coronary artery disease. *N Engl J Med* 1992;326:10–16.
131. Pocock SJ, Henderson RA, Rickards AF, et al. Meta-analysis of randomized trials comparing coronary angioplasty with bypass surgery. *Lancet* 1995;346:1184–1189. Search date and primary sources not stated.
132. Rihal CS, Gersh BJ, Yusuf S. Chronic coronary artery disease: coronary artery bypass surgery vs percutaneous transluminal coronary angioplasty vs medical therapy. In: Yusuf S, Cairns JA, Camm JA, et al, eds. *Evidence based cardiology*. London: BMJ Books, 1998.
133. King SB, Kosinski AS, Guyton RA, et al. Eight-year mortality in the Emory Angioplasty versus Surgery Trial (EAST). *J Am Coll Cardiol* 2000;35:1116–1121.
134. Hlatky MA, Rogers WJ, Johnstone I, et al. Medical care costs and quality of life after randomization to coronary angioplasty or coronary bypass surgery. *N Engl J Med* 1997;336:92–99.
135. Währborg P. Quality of life after coronary angioplasty or bypass surgery. *Eur Heart J* 1999;20:653–658.
136. Bypass Angioplasty Revascularization Investigation (BARI) Investigators. Comparison of coronary bypass surgery with angioplasty in patients with multivessel disease. *N Engl J Med* 1996;335:217–225.

137. National Institute of Clinical Excellence http://www.nice.org.uk/pdf/HTAReport-Stents.pdf (last accessed 8 June 2003). Search date 1999; primary sources Medline, Embase, Bids, Cochrane Library, and York HTA.
138. Savage MP, Douglas JS Jr, Fischman DL, et al. Stent placement compared with balloon angioplasty for obstructed coronary bypass grafts. *N Engl J Med* 1997;337:740–747.
139. Sirnes P, Golf S, Yngvar M, et al. Stenting In Chronic Coronary Occlusion (SICCO): a randomized controlled trial of adding stent implantation after successful angioplasty. *J Am Coll Cardiol* 1996;28:1444–1451.
140. Rubartelli P, Niccoli L, Verna E, et al. Stent implantation versus balloon angioplasty in chronic coronary occlusions: results from the GISSOC trial. Gruppo Italiano di Studio sullo Stent nelle Occlusioni Coronariche. *J Am Coll Cardiol* 1998;32:90–96.
141. Sievert H, Rohde S, Utech A, et al. Stent or Angioplasty after Recanalization of Chronic Coronary Occlusions? (The SARECCO trial). *Am J Cardiol* 1999;84:386–390.
142. Erbel R, Haude M, Hopp HW, et al. Coronary artery stenting compared with balloon angioplasty for restenosis after initial balloon angioplasty. *N Engl J Med* 1998;23:1672–1688.
143. Versaci F, Gaspardone A, Tomai F, et al. A comparison of coronary-artery stenting with angioplasty for isolated stenosis of the proximal left anterior descending coronary artery. *N Engl J Med* 1997;336:817–822.
144. Schomig A, Neumann FJ, Kastrati A, et al. A randomized comparison of antiplatelet and anticoagulation therapy after the placement of intracoronary stents. *N Engl J Med* 1996;334:1084–1089.
145. Leon MB, Baim DS, Gordon P, et al. Clinical and angiographic results from the Stent Anticoagulation Regimen Study (STARS). *Circulation* 1996;94(suppl S):4002.
146. Witkowski A, Ruzyllo W, Gil R, et al. A randomized comparison of elective high-pressure stenting with balloon angioplasty: six-month angiographic and two-year clinical follow-up. *Am Heart J* 2000;140:264–271.

Michael Pignone
Division of General Internal Medicine
University of North Carolina
Chapel Hill
USA

Charanjit Rihal
Consultant Cardiologist
Mayo Clinic and Mayo Foundation
Rochester
USA

Bazian Ltd
London
UK

Competing interests: CR and Bazian Ltd none declared. MP has received honoraria, consulting fees and licensing income from Bayer, Inc. He has received research support from Bayer, Inc. and Pfizen, Inc.

The following previous contributors of this topic would also like to be acknowledged: Colin Baigent, Jeffrey Probstfield, Cathie Sudlow, Andy Ness, and Eva Lonn.

TABLE 1 **Prognostic groups for people who survive the acute stage of myocardial infarction (see text, p 192).**

Baseline risk	1 year mortality	Clinical markers[2–4]
High	10–50%	Older age; history or previous myocardial infarction; reduced exercise tolerance (New York Heart Association functional classes II–IV) before admission; clinical signs of heart failure in the first 2 days (Killip classes IIb, III, and IV) or persistent heart failure on days 3–5 after infarction; early increased heart rate; persistent or early appearance of angina at rest or with minimal exertion; and multiple or complex ventricular arrhythmias during monitoring in hospital.
Moderate	10%	ND
Low	2–5%	Younger age (< 55 years), no previous myocardial infarction, an event free course during the first 5 days after myocardial infarction.[2]

ND, no data.

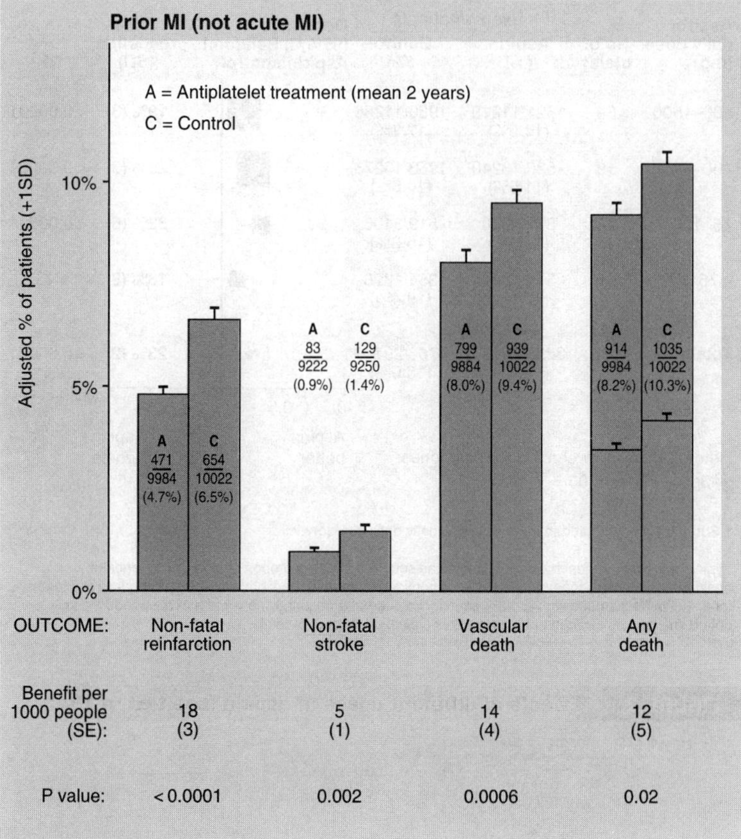

FIGURE 1 **The absolute effects of antiplatelet treatment on various outcomes in people with prior myocardial infarction: results of a systematic review.[10] The columns show the absolute risks over 2 years for each outcome. The error bars represent standard deviations. In the "any death" column, non-vascular deaths are represented by lower horizontal lines (see text, p 193).**

Aspirin daily dose (mg)	No of trials†	Events/patients Aspirin (%)	Events/patients Control (%)	Odds ratio (95% CI Random) Aspirin:control	Odds reduction (SD)	2P
500–1500	34	1621/11215 (14.5%)	1930/11236 (17.2%)		19% (3)	< 0.00001
160–325	19	1526/13240 (11.5%)	1963/13273 (14.8%)		25% (3)	< 0.00001
75–150	12	370/3370 (11.0%)	519/3406 (15.2%)		32% (6)	< 0.00001
< 75	3	316/1827 (17.3%)	354/1828 (19.4%)		13% (8)	NS
Total	65	3833/29652 (12.9%)	4766/29743 (16.0%)		23% (2)	< 0.00001

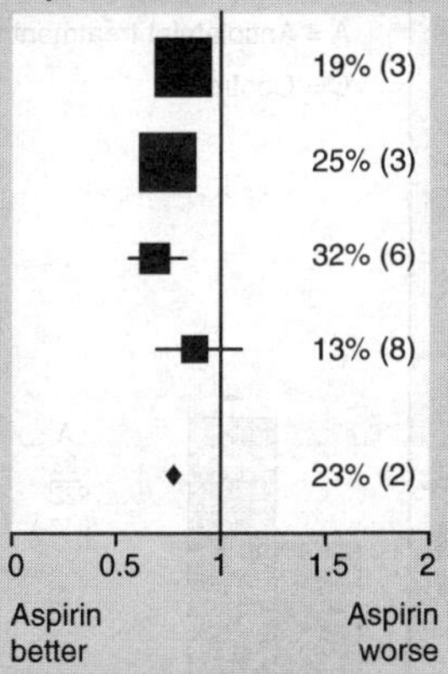

0 0.5 1 1.5 2

Aspirin better — Aspirin worse

Heterogeneity between 4 dose categories: χ^2 3df = 7.7: P = 0.06

† Some trials contributed to more than one daily dose category.

Typical odds ratio for each category shown as square (with area proportional to the variance of observed - expected) together with its 99% confidence interval (horizontal line). Typical odds ratio for the total shown as diamond with its 95% confidence interval (horizontal line = width of diamond). Vertical dotted line passes through point estimate of typical odds ratio for total.

FIGURE 2 **Effects of different doses of aspirin (see text, p 194).**

Stroke management

Search date September 2002

Elizabeth Warburton

QUESTIONS

INTERVENTIONS

See glossary, p 242

Key Messages

Acute ischaemic stroke

- **Acute reduction in blood pressure** One systematic review in people with acute stroke found insufficient evidence about the effects of lowering blood pressure versus placebo on clinical outcome, but RCTs have suggested that people treated with antihypertensive agents may have a worse clinical outcome and increased mortality.
- **Aspirin** One systematic review in people with ischaemic stroke confirmed by computerised tomography scan has found that aspirin versus placebo within 48 hours of stroke onset significantly reduces death or dependency at 6 months and significantly increases the number of people making a complete recovery. One prospective combined analysis of two large RCTs found indirect evidence that aspirin should not be delayed if a computerised tomography scan is not available within 48 hours and ischaemic stroke is suspected. Subgroup analysis of results from the two large RCTs found no significant difference in further stroke or death with aspirin versus placebo in people who were subsequently found to have haemorrhagic rather than ischaemic stroke.

Stroke management

- **Immediate systemic anticoagulation** One systematic review comparing systemic anticoagulants (unfractionated heparin, low molecular weight heparin, heparinoids, oral anticoagulants, or specific thrombin inhibitors) versus usual care without systemic anticoagulants found no significant difference in death or dependence after 3–6 months. One systematic review has found that immediate systemic anticoagulation significantly reduces the risk of deep venous thrombosis and symptomatic pulmonary embolus, but increases the risk of intracranial haemorrhage or extracranial haemorrhage. One RCT in people with acute ischaemic stroke and atrial fibrillation found no significant difference with low molecular weight heparin versus aspirin in recurrent ischaemic stroke within 14 days. One RCT in people within 48 hours of stroke onset found no significant difference with high or low dose tinzaparin versus aspirin in people achieving functional independence at 6 months.
- **Neuroprotective agents (calcium channel antagonists, γ-aminobutyric acid agonists, lubeluzole, glycine antagonists, tirilazad, N-methyl-D-aspartate antagonists)** RCTs found no evidence that, compared with placebo, calcium channel antagonists, tirilazad, lubeluzole, γ-aminobutyric acid agonists, glycine antagonists, or N-methyl-D-aspartate antagonists significantly improve clinical outcomes. One systematic review found that lubeluzole versus placebo was associated with a significant increase in the risk of having Q-T prolongation to more than 450 ms on electrocardiography.
- **Specialised care** One systematic review has found that specialist stroke rehabilitation units versus conventional (less specialised) care significantly reduces death or dependency after a median follow up of 1 year.
- **Thrombolysis** One systematic review in people with ischaemic stroke (without cerebral haemorrhage) which was excluded by computerised tomography scan) has found that thrombolysis versus placebo significantly reduces the risk of the composite outcome of death or dependency after 1–6 months, but significantly increases the risk of death from intracranial haemorrhage measured in the first 7–10 days.

Intracerebral haematomas

- **Evacuation** We found that the balance between benefits and harms has not been clearly established for the evacuation of supratentorial haematomas. We found no evidence from RCTs on the role of evacuation or ventricular shunting in people with infratentorial haematoma whose consciousness level is declining.

DEFINITION Stroke is characterised by rapidly developing clinical symptoms and signs of focal, and at times global, loss of cerebral function lasting more than 24 hours or leading to death, with no apparent cause other than that of vascular origin.[1] Ischaemic stroke is stroke caused by vascular insufficiency (such as cerebrovascular thromboembolism) rather than haemorrhage.

INCIDENCE/ PREVALENCE Stroke is the third most common cause of death in most developed countries.[2] It is a worldwide problem; about 4.5 million people die from stroke a year. Stroke can occur at any age, but half of all strokes occur in people over 70 years old.[3]

AETIOLOGY/ RISK FACTORS About 80% of all acute strokes are caused by cerebral infarction, usually resulting from thrombotic or embolic occlusion of a cerebral artery.[4] The remainder are caused either by intracerebral or subarachnoid haemorrhage.

PROGNOSIS About 10% of all people with acute ischaemic strokes will die within 30 days of stroke onset.[5] Of those who survive the acute event, about 50% will experience some level of disability after 6 months.[6]

AIMS OF INTERVENTION To minimise impairment, disability, secondary complications, and adverse effects from treatment.

OUTCOMES Risk of death or dependency (generally assessed as the proportion of people dead or requiring physical assistance for transfers, mobility, dressing, feeding, or toileting 3–6 months after stroke onset);[6] quality of life.

METHODS *Clinical Evidence* search and appraisal September 2002.

QUESTION **What are the effects of specialised care in people with stroke?**

One systematic review has found that specialist stroke rehabilitation units versus conventional (less specialised) care significantly reduces death or dependency after a median follow up of 1 year. Prospective observational data suggest these findings may be reproducible in routine clinical settings.

Benefits: We found one systematic review (search date 2001, 23 RCTs, 4911 people with stroke) comparing specialised stroke rehabilitation versus conventional care.[7] In most trials, the specialised stroke rehabilitation unit consisted of a designated area or ward, although some trials used a mobile "stroke team". People in these trials were usually transferred to stroke unit care within the first or second week after stroke onset. It found people cared for in a stroke rehabilitation unit versus alternative (less organised) care had significantly lower rates of death or dependency after a median follow up of 1 year (AR 60.5% without stroke unit *v* 55.8% with stroke unit; ARR 4.7%, 95% CI 1.6% to 7.8%; NNT 21, 95% CI 13 to 63; OR 0.78, 95% CI 0.68 to 0.89; [see figure 1, p 245]).[7] The duration of stay was calculated differently for many of the trials, so heterogeneity among results limits generalisability. However, overall, duration of stay in the stroke unit was about 6 days (95% CI 2 to 10 days) shorter than duration of stay in a non-stroke unit setting. Two RCTs included in the review extended follow up to 5 years post stroke. The review found that organised stroke unit care versus alternative service significantly reduced death or dependency at 5 years' follow up (2 RCTs; 223/286 [78%] with organised stroke unit care *v* 214/249 [86%] with alternative care; RR 0.91, 95% CI 0.84 to 0.99).[7] One RCT (220 people) included in the review found that care in a combined acute and rehabilitation unit compared with care in general wards increased the proportion of people able to live at home 10 years after their stroke (ARI 11%, 95% CI 1.9% to 20%; NNT 9, 95% CI 5 to 52).[11] We found one additional RCT, which randomised 76 people 2–10 days after their stroke to either an integrated care pathway (see glossary, p 242) or to conventional multidisciplinary care on a stroke rehabilitation unit in the UK.[12] All received similar occupational and physical therapy. Conventional treatment versus the integrated care pathway produced more improvement in the Barthel Index from 4–12 weeks (CI not provided; $P < 0.01$), and higher scores on the Euroquol (Quality of Life Scale) after 6 months ($P < 0.05$). It found no significant difference between the two treatments in mortality, duration of hospital stay, or the proportion of people requiring long term institutional care.

Harms: No detrimental effects attributable to stroke units were reported.[7]

Comment: Although the proportional reduction in death or dependency seems larger with thrombolysis (see thrombolysis option, p 234), stroke unit care is applicable to most people with stroke whereas thrombolysis is applicable only to a small proportion. The systematic review did not provide evidence about which aspects of the multidisciplinary approach led to improved outcome,[7] although one limited retrospective analysis of one of the RCTs found that several factors, including early mobilisation, increased use of oxygen, intravenous saline solutions, and antipyretics, might have been responsible.[13] Most RCTs excluded the most mild and severe strokes. After publication of the systematic review,[7] prospective observational data have been collected in one large series of over 14 000 people in 80 Swedish hospitals.[14] In this series, people admitted to stroke units had reduced dependence at 3 months (RRR 6%, 95% CI 1% to 11%). Although biases are inherent in such observational data, the findings suggest that the results of the meta-analysis may be reproducible in routine clinical settings.

QUESTION What are the effects of medical treatment in acute ischaemic stroke?

OPTION THROMBOLYSIS

One systematic review in people with ischaemic stroke (without cerebral haemorrhage, which was excluded by computerised tomography scan) has found that thrombolysis versus placebo significantly reduces the risk of the composite outcome of death or dependency after 1–6 months, but significantly increases the risk of death from intracranial haemorrhage measured in the first 7–10 days and risk of death after 1–6 months. The excess in deaths was offset by fewer people being alive but dependent 6 months after stroke onset and the net effect was a reduction in people who were dead or dependent.

Benefits: We found one systematic review (search date 1999, 17 RCTs, 5216 highly selected people) comparing thrombolysis versus placebo given soon after the onset of stroke.[8] All trials used computerised tomography or magnetic resonance imaging before randomisation to exclude intracranial haemorrhage or other non-stroke disorders. Results for three different thrombolytic agents (streptokinase, urokinase, and recombinant tissue plasminogen activator) were included, but direct comparison of different thrombolytic drugs was not possible. Two trials used intra-arterial administration and the rest used the intravenous route. Thrombolysis significantly reduced the risk of death or dependency at the end of the studies (1–6 months: ARR 4.2%, 95% CI 1.2% to 7.2%; RRR 7%, 95% CI 3% to 12%; NNT 24, 95% CI 14 to 83) (see figure 1, p 245 and figure 2, p 245).[8] In the subset of trials that assessed intravenous recombinant tissue plasminogen activator, the findings were similar (ARR 5.7%, 95% CI 2.0% to 9.4%; RRR 10%, 95% CI 4% to 16%; NNT 18, 95% CI 11 to 50). One meta-analysis (4 RCTs, individual results of 1292 people with acute ischaemic stroke treated with streptokinase or placebo) found that streptokinase versus placebo had no clear effect on the proportion of people dead or dependent at 3 months, and included the possibility of both substantial benefit or substantial harm (RRR +1%, 95% CI –6% to +8%).[15] People allocated to streptokinase were more likely to be dead after 3 months (RRI 46%, 95% CI 24% to 73%). The combination of aspirin plus streptokinase significantly increased mortality at 3 months (P = 0.005), but this did not affect the combined risk of death or severe disability (CI not provided; P = 0.28).

Harms: **Fatal intracranial haemorrhage:** In the systematic review, thrombolysis increased fatal intracranial haemorrhage compared with placebo measured in the first 7–10 days (ARI 4.4%, 95% CI 3.4% to 5.4%; RRI 396%, 95% CI 220% to 668%; NNH 23, 95% CI 19 to 29).[8] In the subset of trials that assessed intravenous recombinant tissue plasminogen activator, the findings were similar (ARI 2.9%, 95% CI 1.7% to 4.1%; RRI 259%, 95% CI 102% to 536%; NNH 34, 95% CI 24 to 59). **Death:** In the systematic review, thrombolysis compared with placebo increased the risk of death by the end of the follow up (1–6 months: ARI 3.3%, 95% CI 1.2% to 5.4%; RRI 23%, 95% CI 10% to 38%; NNH 30, 95% CI 19 to 83).[8] This excess of deaths was offset by fewer people being alive but dependent 6 months after stroke onset. The net effect was a reduction in the number of people who were dead or dependent.

Comment: There was no significant heterogeneity of treatment effect overall, but heterogeneity of results was noted for the outcomes of death, and death or dependency at final follow up among the eight trials of intravenous recombinant tissue plasminogen activator.[8] Explanations may include the combined use of antithrombotic agents (aspirin or heparin within the first 24 h of thrombolysis), stroke severity, the presence of early ischaemic changes on computerised tomography scan, and the time from stroke onset to randomisation. Most trials reported outcomes at 3 months; only one trial reported 1 year outcome data.[16] We found little evidence about which people are most and least likely to benefit from thrombolysis. A subgroup analysis suggested that thrombolysis may be more beneficial if given within 3 hours of symptom onset, but the duration of the "therapeutic time window" could not be determined reliably. A recent preliminary pooling of three RCTs (1734 people) suggested that recombinant tissue plasminogen activator versus placebo given between 3 and 6 hours may reduce death or dependency in some people.[17] However, there is currently no consensus about giving thrombolysis after 3 hours. Newer magnetic resonance imaging techniques, such as diffusion/perfusion weighted imaging, may be helpful in patient selection, but studies using these techniques have so far been small.[18] A number of trials of different thrombolytic regimens are under way.[19] In addition, preliminary information from a meta-analysis of individual patient data from the recombinant tissue plasminogen activator trials by the ECASS, NINDS, and ATLANTIS investigators was recently reported at the 27th International Stroke Conference; when published, data will be presented in future *Clinical Evidence* updates (B Thomas, personal communication, 2002).

OPTION ASPIRIN

One systematic review in people with ischaemic stroke confirmed by computerised tomography scan has found that aspirin versus placebo within 48 hours of stroke onset significantly reduces death or dependency at 6 months and significantly increases the number of people making a complete recovery. One prospective combined analysis of two large RCTs found indirect evidence that aspirin should not be delayed if a computerised tomography scan is not available within 48 hours and ischaemic stroke is suspected. Subgroup analysis of results from the two large RCTs found no significant difference in further stroke or death with aspirin versus placebo in people who were subsequently found to have haemorrhagic rather than ischaemic stroke.

Benefits: **Early use of aspirin:** We found one systematic review (search date 1999, 8 RCTs, 41 325 people with definite or presumed ischaemic stroke), which compared antiplatelet treatment started within 14 days of the stroke versus placebo.[20] Of the data in the systematic review, 98% came from two large RCTs of aspirin (160–300 mg daily) started within 48 hours of stroke onset.[9,10] Most people had an ischaemic stroke confirmed by computerised tomography scan before randomisation, but people who were conscious could be randomised before computerised tomography scan if the stroke was very likely to be ischaemic on clinical grounds. Treatment duration varied from 10–28 days. Aspirin started within the first 48 hours of acute ischaemic stroke reduced death or dependency at 6 months' follow up (RRR 3%, 95% CI 1% to 5%; NNT 77, 95% CI 43 to 333) (see figure 1, p 245) and increased the number of people making a complete recovery (NNT 91, 95% CI 50 to 500). A prospective combined analysis[21] of the two large RCTs[9,10] found a significant reduction in the outcome of further stroke or death with aspirin versus placebo (ARR 0.9%, 95% CI 0.75% to 1.85%; NNT 111, 95% CI 54 to 133). The effect was similar across subgroups (older *v* younger; male *v* female; impaired consciousness or not; atrial fibrillation or not; blood pressure; stroke subtype; timing of computerised tomography scanning). For the 773 people subsequently found to have had a haemorrhagic stroke rather than an ischaemic stroke, the subgroup analysis found no difference in the outcome of further stroke or death between those who were randomised to aspirin versus placebo (16% *v* 18%; ARR +2.0%, 95% CI −4.0% to +6.6%).[21] **Long term treatment:** See aspirin under stroke prevention, p 246.

Harms: Aspirin caused an excess of about two intracranial and four extracranial haemorrhages per 1000 people treated, but these small risks were more than offset by the reductions in death and disability from other causes both in the short term[20] and in the long term.[22] Common adverse effects of aspirin (such as dyspepsia and constipation) were dose related.[23]

Comment: We found no clear evidence that any one dose of aspirin is more effective than any other in the treatment of acute ischaemic stroke. One recent meta-regression analysis of the dose–response effect of aspirin on stroke found a uniform effect of aspirin in a range of doses from 50–1500 mg daily.[24] People unable to swallow safely after a stroke may be given aspirin as a suppository.

OPTION IMMEDIATE SYSTEMIC ANTICOAGULATION

One systematic review comparing systemic anticoagulants (unfractionated heparin, low molecular weight heparin, heparinoids, oral anticoagulants, or specific thrombin inhibitors) versus usual care without systemic anticoagulants has found no significant difference in death or dependence after 3–6 months. One systematic review has found that immediate systemic anticoagulation significantly reduces the risk of deep venous thrombosis and symptomatic pulmonary embolus, but increases the risk of intracranial haemorrhage or extracranial haemorrhage. One RCT in people with acute ischaemic stroke and atrial fibrillation found no significant difference with low molecular weight heparin versus aspirin in recurrent ischaemic stroke within 14 days. One RCT comparing four different doses of a low molecular weight heparin within 12 hours of stroke onset found no significant differences in neurological outcomes after 3 months. One RCT in people within 48 hours of stroke onset found no significant difference with high or low dose tinzaparin versus aspirin in people achieving functional independence at 6 months.

Benefits: **Death or dependency:** We found one systematic review (search date 1999, 21 RCTs, 23 427 people)[25] and three subsequent RCTs.[26–28] The systematic review compared unfractionated heparin, low molecular weight heparin, heparinoids, oral anticoagulants, or specific thrombin inhibitors versus usual care without systemic anticoagulants.[25] Over 80% of the data came from one trial, which randomised people with any severity of stroke to either subcutaneous heparin or placebo, usually after exclusion of haemorrhage by computerised tomography scan.[10] The systematic review found no significant difference in the proportion of people dead or dependent in the treatment and control groups at the end of follow up (3–6 months after the stroke: ARR +0.4%, 95% CI –0.9% to +1.7%; RRR 0%, 95% CI –2% to +3%).[25] There was no clear short or long term benefit of anticoagulants in any prespecified subgroups (stroke of presumed cardioembolic origin *v* others; different anticoagulants). The first subsequent RCT (449 people with acute stroke and atrial fibrillation) found no significant difference between dalteparin (a low molecular weight heparin) versus aspirin for the primary outcome of recurrent ischaemic stroke during the first 14 days (ARI +1.0%, 95% CI –3.6% to +6.2%) or for secondary outcomes, including functional outcome at 3 months.[26] The second RCT randomised 404 people to one of four different doses of certoparin (a low molecular weight heparin) within 12 hours of stroke onset.[27] There was no difference in neurological outcome between the four groups 3 months after treatment. The third RCT (1486 people) compared aspirin versus two different doses of tinzaparin (a low molecular weight heparin) within 48 hours of stroke onset.[28] It found no significant difference among the three groups for achieving functional independence at 6 months (AR for independence 41.5% with tinzaparin 175 anti-Xa IU/kg daily *v* 42.4% with tinzaparin 100 anti-Xa IU/kg daily *v* 42.5% with aspirin 300 mg/daily). **Deep venous thrombosis and pulmonary embolism:** We found three systematic reviews.[25,29,30] The first systematic review (search date 1999) included 10 small heterogeneous RCTs (22 000 people), which assessed anticoagulants in 916 people at high risk of deep venous thrombosis after their stroke.[25] Anticoagulation compared with control reduced the risk of deep vein thrombosis (ARR 29%, 95% CI 24% to 35%; RRR 64%, 95% CI 54% to 71%; NNT 3, 95% CI 2 to 4) and reduced symptomatic pulmonary embolism (ARR 0.3%, 95% CI 0.1% to 0.6%; RRR 38%, 95% CI 16% to 54%; NNT 333, 95% CI 167 to 1000). No RCT performed investigations in all people to rule out silent events. The frequency of reported pulmonary emboli was low and varied among RCTs, so there may have been under ascertainment. Two other systematic reviews (search dates 1999[30] and 2001,[29] same 5 RCTs in each review, 705 people with acute ischaemic stroke) found that low molecular weight heparins or heparinoids versus unfractionated heparin significantly reduced deep venous thrombosis (AR 13% with low molecular weight heparins or heparinoids *v* 22% with unfractionated heparin; ARR 9%, 95% CI 4.5% to 16%). The number of events was too small to estimate the effects of low molecular weight heparins or heparinoids versus unfractionated heparin on death, intracranial haemorrhage, or functional outcome in survivors.

Harms: One systematic review found that anticoagulation slightly increased symptomatic intracranial haemorrhages within 14 days of starting treatment compared with control (ARI 0.93%, 95% CI 0.68% to 1.18%; RRI 163%, 95% CI 95% to 255%; NNH 108, 95% CI 85 to 147).[25] The large trial of subcutaneous heparin found that this effect was dose dependent (symptomatic intracranial haemorrhage by using medium dose compared with low dose heparin for 14 days; RRI 143%, 95% CI 82% to 204%; NNH 97, 95% CI 68 to 169).[10] The review also found a dose dependent increase in major extracranial haemorrhages after 14 days of treatment with anticoagulants (ARI 0.91%, 95% CI 0.67% to 1.15%; RRI 231%, 95% CI 136% to 365%; NNH 109, 95% CI 87 to 149).[25] The subsequent RCT of dalteparin versus aspirin for people with acute stroke and atrial fibrillation found no difference in adverse events, including symptomatic or asymptomatic intracerebral haemorrhage, progression of symptoms, or early or late death.[26] As in the systematic review,[25] the RCT comparing different doses of certoparin found that intracranial haemorrhage occurred more often in those receiving a higher dose of anticoagulant.[27] However, the overall number of people experiencing haemorrhagic complications in the RCT may have been artificially lowered because the study protocol was changed during the trial period so as to exclude people with early ischaemic changes on computerised tomography scan. The RCT comparing different doses of tinzaparin found that high dose tinzaparin versus aspirin significantly increased symptomatic intracranial haemorrhage (AR 1.5% with high dose tinzaparin *v* 0.2% with aspirin; OR 7.2, 95% CI 1.1 to 163).[28]

Comment: Alternative treatments to prevent deep venous thrombosis and pulmonary embolism after acute ischaemic stroke include aspirin and compression stockings. The evidence relating to these will be reviewed in future *Clinical Evidence* updates.

OPTION BLOOD PRESSURE REDUCTION

One systematic review in people with acute stroke found insufficient evidence about the effects of lowering blood pressure versus placebo on clinical outcome, but RCTs have suggested that people treated with antihypertensive agents may have a worse clinical outcome and increased mortality.

Benefits: We found one systematic review (search date 2000, 5 RCTs, 281 people with acute stroke) comparing blood pressure lowering treatment with placebo.[31] Several different antihypertensive agents were used. The trials collected insufficient clinical data to allow an analysis of the relation between changes in blood pressure and clinical outcome.

Harms: Two placebo controlled RCTs have suggested that people treated with antihypertensive agents may have a worse clinical outcome and increased mortality.[32,33] The first RCT (295 people with acute ischaemic stroke) compared nimodipine (a calcium channel antagonist) versus placebo.[32] The RCT was stopped prematurely because of an excess of unfavourable neurological outcomes in the nimodipine treated group. Exploratory analyses confirmed that this negative correlation was related to reductions in mean arterial blood pressure (CI not provided; $P = 0.02$) and diastolic blood pressure ($P = 0.0005$). The second RCT (302 people with acute ischaemic stroke) assessed β blockers (atenolol or propranolol).[33] There was a non-significant increase in death for people taking β blockers, and no difference in the proportion of people achieving a good outcome. One systematic review (search date 1994, 9 RCTs, 3719 people with acute stroke) compared nimodipine versus placebo; no net benefit was found.[34] A second review (24 RCTs, 6894 people) found a non-significant increase in the risk of death with calcium channel antagonists versus placebo (RRI 8%, 95% CI 1% reduction to 18% increase).[35] Although treatment with calcium channel antagonists in these trials was intended for neuroprotection, blood pressure was lower in the treatment group in several trials.

Comment: Population based studies suggest a direct and continuous association between blood pressure and the risk of recurrent stroke.[36] However, acute blood pressure lowering in acute ischaemic stroke may lead to increased cerebral ischaemia. The systematic review[31] identified several ongoing RCTs. We identified one additional ongoing RCT not included in the review.[37]

OPTION NEUROPROTECTIVE AGENTS

RCTs found no evidence that compared with placebo, calcium channel antagonists, lubeluzole, γ-aminobutyric acid agonists, tirilazad, glycine antagonists, or N-methyl-D-aspartate antagonists significantly improved clinical outcomes. One systematic review found that lubeluzole versus placebo was associated with a significant increase in the risk of having Q-T prolongation to more than 450 ms on electrocardiography.

Benefits: We found no systematic reviews assessing the general effectiveness of neuroprotective agents in acute ischaemic stroke. **Calcium channel antagonists:** We found two systematic reviews comparing calcium channel antagonists with placebo.[38,39] The first review (search date 1999, 28 RCTs, 7521 people with acute ischaemic stroke) found that calcium channel antagonists did not significantly reduce the risk of poor outcome (including death) at the end of the follow up period compared with placebo (ARI of poor outcome +4.9%, 95% CI –2.5% to +7.3%; RRI +4%, 95% CI –2% to +9%).[38] The second review (search date 1999)[39] includes one additional RCT (454 people)[40] that was stopped prematurely because of publication of the first review.[38] Inclusion of its data does not change the results of the first review. **γ-Aminobutyric acid agonists:** We found one systematic review (search date not stated, 3 RCTs, 1002 people with acute ischaemic stroke), which found no significant difference between piracetam (a γ-aminobutyric acid agonist) and control groups for the number of people dead or dependent at the end of follow up (ARI +0.2%, 95% CI –6.0% to +6.4%; RRI 0%, 95% CI –11% to +9%).[41] We found one RCT (1360 people with acute stroke), which identified no significant effect of clomethiazole (chlormethiazole; a γ-aminobutyric acid agonist) versus placebo on functional independence (ARR +1.5%, 95% CI –4.0% to +6.6%; RRR +3.0%, 95% CI –7% to +13%).[42] **Lubeluzole:** We found one systematic review (search date 2001, 5 RCTs, 3510 people) that compared lubeluzole (5, 10, or 20 mg daily for 5 days) versus placebo.[43] It found no significant difference with any dose of lubeluzole versus placebo in death or dependency at the end of follow up (after 4–12 wks' follow up, AR 54.6% with lubeluzole *v* 53.4% with placebo; ARI +1.2%, 95% CI –2.5% to +6.2%). **Glycine antagonists:** We found two RCTs.[44,45] One RCT (1804 conscious people with limb weakness assessed within 6 h of stroke onset) found no significant difference between gavestinel (a glycine antagonist) versus placebo in survival and outcome at 3 months as measured using the Barthel Index (ARR +1.0%, 95% CI –3.5% to +6.0%).[44] The second RCT (1367 people with predefined level of limb weakness and functional independence before stroke) also found no significant difference in survival and outcome at 3 months, measured using the Barthel Index (ARI +1.9%, 95% CI –3.8% to +6.4%).[45] **N-methyl-D-aspartate antagonists:** Two recent RCTs assessing the N-methyl-D-aspartate antagonist (see glossary, p 242) selfotel found no significant difference in the proportion of people with a Barthel Index over 60, but data were limited as the trials were terminated because of adverse outcomes after only 31% of the total planned patient enrolment.[46] Similarly, an RCT comparing the N-methyl-D-aspartate antagonist aptiganel versus placebo was terminated early because of lack of efficacy and a potential imbalance in mortality.[47] The RCT found a larger proportion of people with favourable outcomes in the placebo group and a non-significant trend favouring placebo in mortality rates.[47] **Tirilazad:** We found one systematic review (search date 2001, 6 RCTs, 1757 people) comparing tirilazad (a steroid derivative) versus placebo in people with acute ischaemic stroke.[48]

Tirilazadincreased death and disability at 3 months' follow up when measured using the expanded Barthel Index (ARI +3.9%, 95% CI −0.8% to +8.6%).[48]

Harms: In the systematic review of calcium channel antagonists, indirect and limited comparisons of intravenous versus oral administration found no significant difference in adverse events (ARI of adverse events, iv *v* oral, +2.3%, 95% CI −0.9% to +3.7%; RRI +17%, 95% CI −3% to +41%).[38] In the systematic review of piracetam, there was a non-significant increase in death with piracetam versus placebo, which was no longer apparent after correction for imbalance in stroke severity.[41] The systematic review of lubeluzole found that, at any dose, lubeluzole was associated with a significant increase in the risk of having a heart conduction disorder (Q-T prolongation to more than 450 ms on electrocardiography) at the end of follow up (AR with lubeluzole 11.9% *v* 9.74% with control; ARI 2.2%, 95% CI 0.1% to 4.2%; NNH 45, 95% CI 23 to 1000).[43] Lubeluzole did not significantly increase heart rhythm disorders (atrial fibrillation, ventricular tachycardia or fibrillation, torsade de pointes) at the end of the scheduled follow up (OR 1.28, 95% CI 0.97 to 1.69). The trials of selfotel were terminated after enrolling 567 people because of greater early mortality in the selfotel groups.[46] The systematic review of tirilazad found an increased risk of injection site phlebitis compared with placebo (ARI 12.2%, 95% CI 8.7% to 15.7%).[48]

Comment: The effects of the cell membrane precursor citicholine have been assessed in small trials, and a systematic review is in progress.[49] Systematic reviews are being developed for antioxidants and for excitatory amino acid modulators.[50] Several RCTs are ongoing, including one of intravenous magnesium sulphate[51] and another of diazepam (a γ-aminobutyric acid agonist).[52]

QUESTION What are the effects of surgical treatment for intracerebral haematomas?

OPTION EVACUATION

We found that the balance between benefits and harms has not been clearly established for the evacuation of supratentorial haematomas. We found no evidence from RCTs on the role of evacuation or ventricular shunting in people with infratentorial haematoma whose consciousness level is declining.

Benefits: **For supratentorial haematomas:** We found three systematic reviews.[53–55] The first review (search date 1998)[53] and second review (search date 1997)[54] both assessed the same four RCTs comparing surgery (craniotomy in 3 trials and endoscopy in 1 trial) versus best medical treatment in 354 people with primary supratentorial intracerebral haemorrhage. The second review also assessed information from case series.[54] Overall, neither review found significant short or long term differences between surgical and medical treatment for death or disability (ARI +3.3%, 95% CI −5.9% to +12.5%; RRI +5%, 95% CI −7% to +19%). The third review (search date 1999)[55] includes several analyses. The first analysis includes results from seven RCTs (530 people), including two RCTs not included in either of the first two systematic reviews. The overall results are similar to those of the first two systematic reviews, with no significant difference in death or disability for surgically treated people (ARI +3.5%, 95% CI –4.4% to +11.4%). A further analysis of results from only recent, post-computerised tomography, well constructed, balanced trials (5 trials, 224 people in total) did not find a significant difference between the two groups (ARR +9.3%, 95% CI –2.6% to +21.2%). **For infratentorial haematomas:** We found no evidence from systematic reviews or RCTs on the role of surgical evacuation or ventricular shunting.[56]

Harms: The two earlier reviews undertook subgroup analyses separating results for craniotomy and endoscopy. They found that for the 254 people randomised to craniotomy rather than best medical treatment, there was increased death and disability (ARI 12%, 95% CI 1.8% to 22%; RRI 17%, 95% CI 2% to 34%; NNH 8, 95% CI 5 to 56).[53,54] For the 100 people randomised to endoscopy rather than best medical practice, there was no significant effect on death and disability (RRR 24%, 95% CI –2% to +44%). The third systematic review did not evaluate these adverse outcomes.[55]

Comment: Current practice is based on the consensus that people with infratentorial (cerebellar) haematomas whose consciousness level is declining probably benefit from evacuation of the haematoma. We identified one ongoing multicentre trial comparing a policy of "early surgical evacuation" of haematoma versus "initial conservative treatment" in people with spontaneous intracerebral haemorrhage.[57]

GLOSSARY

Integrated care pathway A model of care that includes definition of therapeutic goals and specification of a timed plan designed to promote multidisciplinary care, improve discharge planning, and reduce the duration of hospital stay.

N-methyl-D-aspartate antagonist Glutamate can bind to N-methyl-D-aspartate receptors on cell surfaces. One hypothesis proposed that glutamate released during a stroke can cause further harm to neurones by stimulating the N-methyl-D-aspartate receptors. N-Methyl-D-aspartate antagonists block these receptors.

REFERENCES

1. Hatano S. Experience from a multicentre stroke register: a preliminary report. *Bull World Health Organ* 1976;54:541–553.
2. Bonita R. Epidemiology of stroke. *Lancet* 1992;339:342–344.
3. Bamford J, Sandercock P, Dennis M, et al. A prospective study of acute cerebrovascular disease in the community: the Oxfordshire community stroke project, 1981–1986. 1. Methodology, demography and incident cases of first ever stroke. *J Neurol Neurosurg Psychiatry* 1988;51:1373–1380.
4. Bamford J, Dennis M, Sandercock P, et al. A prospective study of acute cerebrovascular disease in the community: the Oxfordshire community stroke project, 1981–1986. 2. Incidence, case fatality rates and overall outcome at one year of cerebral infarction, primary intracerebral and subarachnoid haemorrhage. *J Neurol Neurosurg Psychiatry* 1990;53:16–22.
5. Bamford J, Dennis M, Sandercock P, et al. The frequency, causes and timing of death within 30 days of a first stroke: the Oxfordshire community stroke project. *J Neurol Neurosurg Psychiatry* 1990;53:824–829.
6. Wade DT. Functional abilities after stroke: measurement, natural history and prognosis. *J Neurol Neurosurg Psychiatry* 1987;50:177–182.
7. Stroke Unit Trialists' Collaboration. Organised inpatient (stroke unit) care for stroke. In: The Cochrane Library, Issue 3, 2002. Oxford: Update Software. Search date 2001; primary sources Cochrane Stroke Group Specialised Trials Register and hand searches of reference lists of relevant articles and personal contact with colleagues.
8. Wardlaw JM, del Zoppo G, Yamaguchi T. Thrombolysis for acute ischaemic stroke. In: The Cochrane Library, Issue 3, 2002. Oxford: Update Software. Search date 1999; primary sources Cochrane Stroke Group Specialised Register of Controlled Trials, Embase, hand searches of relevant journals and references listed in relevant papers, and personal contact with pharmaceutical companies and principal investigators of trials.

9. CAST (Chinese Acute Stroke Trial) Collaborative Group. Randomised placebo-controlled trial of early aspirin use in 20 000 patients with acute ischaemic stroke. *Lancet* 1997;349:1641–1649.
10. International Stroke Trial Collaborative Group. The international stroke trial (IST): a randomised trial of aspirin, heparin, both or neither among 19 435 patients with acute ischaemic stroke. *Lancet* 1997;349:1569–1581.
11. Indredavik B, Bakke RPT, Slordahl SA, et al. Stroke unit treatment. 10-year follow-up. *Stroke* 1999;30:1524–1527.
12. Sulch D, Perez I, Melbourn A, et al. Randomized controlled trial of integrated (managed) care pathway for stroke rehabilitation. *Stroke* 2000;31:1929–1934.
13. Indredavik B, Bakke RPT, Slordahl SA, et al. Treatment in a combined acute and rehabilitation stroke unit. Which aspects are most important. *Stroke* 1999;30:917–923.
14. Stegmayr B, Asplund K, Hulter-Asberg K, et al. Stroke units in their natural habitat: can results of randomized trials be reproduced in routine clinical practice? For the risk-stroke collaboration. *Stroke* 1999;30:709–714.
15. Cornu C, Boutitie F, Candelise L, et al. Streptokinase in acute ischemic stroke: an individual patient data meta-analysis: the thrombolysis in acute stroke pooling project. *Stroke* 2000;31:1555–1560.
16. Kwiatkowski T, Libman R, Frankel M, et al. Effects of tissue plasminogen activator for acute ischemic stroke at one year. National Institute of Neurological Disorders and stroke recombinant tissue plasminogen activator stroke study group. *N Engl J Med* 1999;340:1781–1787.
17. Ringleb PA, Schellinger PD, Schranz C, et al. Thrombolytic therapy within 3 to 6 hours after onset of ischemic stroke. Useful or harmful? *Stroke* 2002;33:1437–1441.
18. Parsons MW, Barber PA, Chalk J, et al. Diffusion — and perfusion — weighted MRI response to thrombolysis in stroke. *Ann Neurol* 2002;51:28–37.
19. Internet Stroke Center. http://www.strokecenter.org/trials (last accessed 24 February 2003).
20. Gubitz G, Sandercock P, Counsell C. Antiplatelet therapy for acute ischaemic stroke. In: The Cochrane Library, Issue 3, 2002. Oxford: Update Software. Search date 1999; primary sources Cochrane Stroke Group Specialised Register of Controlled Trials, the Register of the Antiplatelet Trialists' Collaboration, MedStrategy, and personal contact with pharmaceutical companies.
21. Chen Z, Sandercock P, Pan H, et al. Indications for early aspirin use in acute ischemic stroke: a combined analysis of 40 000 randomized patients from the Chinese Acute Stroke Trial and the International Stroke Trial. *Stroke* 2000;31:1240–1249.
22. Antithrombotic Trialists' Collaboration. Collaborative meta-analysis of randomised trials of antiplatelet therapy for prevention of death, myocardial infarction, and stroke in high risk patients. *BMJ* 2002;324:71–86. Search date 1997; primary sources Medline, Embase, Derwent, Scisearch, Biosis, Cochrane Stroke Group Controlled Trials Register, Cochrane Peripheral Vascular Disease Group Controlled Trials Register, hand searches of journals, abstracts and proceedings of meetings, reference lists from relevant articles, and personal contact with colleagues and pharmaceutical companies.
23. Slattery J, Warlow CP, Shorrock CJ, et al. Risks of gastrointestinal bleeding during secondary prevention of vascular events with aspirin — analysis of gastrointestinal bleeding during the UK-TIA trial. *Gut* 1995;37:509–511.
24. Johnson ES, Lanes SF, Wentworth CE, et al. A metaregression analysis of the dose–response effect of aspirin on stroke. *Arch Intern Med* 1999;159:1248–1253.
25. Gubitz G, Counsell C, Sandercock P, et al. Anticoagulants for acute ischaemic stroke. In: The Cochrane Library, Issue 3, 2002. Oxford: Update Software. Search date 1999; primary sources Cochrane Stroke Group Specialised Register of Controlled Trials, trials register held by the Antithrombotic Therapy Trialist's Collaboration, MedStrategy, and personal contact with pharmaceutical companies.
26. Berge E, Abdelnoor M, Nakstad P, et al. Low-molecular-weight heparin versus aspirin in people with acute ischaemic stroke and atrial fibrillation: a double-blind randomised study. HAEST Study Group. Heparin in Acute Embolic Stroke Trial. *Lancet* 2000;355:1205–1210.
27. Diener H, Ringelstein E, von Kummer R, et al. Treatment of acute ischemic stroke with the low-molecular-weight heparin certoparin: results of the TOPAS Trial. *Stroke* 2001;32:22–29.
28. Bath P, Lindenstrome E, Bioysen G, et al. Tinzaparin in acute ischaemic stroke (TAIST): a randomised aspirin-controlled trial. *Lancet* 2001;358:702–710.
29. Counsell C, Sandercock P. Low-molecular-weight heparins or heparinoids versus standard unfractionated heparin for acute ischaemic stroke. In: The Cochrane Library, Issue 3, 2002. Oxford: Update Software. Search date 2001; primary sources Cochrane Stroke Group Specialised Trials Register, MedStrategy, and personal contact with pharmaceutical companies.
30. Bath P, Iddenden R, Bath F. Low-molecular-weight heparins and heparinoids in acute ischemic stroke: a meta-analysis of randomized controlled trials. *Stroke* 2000;31:1770–1778. Search date 1999; primary sources Cochrane Stroke Group Database of Trials in Acute Stroke, Cochrane Library, and hand searches of reference lists of identified publications.
31. Blood pressure in Acute Stroke Collaboration (BASC). Interventions for deliberately altering blood pressure in acute stroke. In: The Cochrane Library, Issue 3, 2002. Oxford: Update Software. Search date 2000; primary sources Cochrane Stroke Group Specialised Register of Controlled Trials, Cochrane Library (CDSR, CCTR), Medline, Embase, Bids, ISI-Science Citation Index, hand searches of reference lists of existing reviews and the ongoing trials section of the journal *Stroke*, and personal contact with research workers in the field and pharmaceutical companies.
32. Wahlgren NG, MacMahon DG, DeKeyser J, et al. Intravenous nimodipine west European stroke trial (INWEST) of nimodipine in the treatment of acute ischaemic stroke. *Cerebrovasc Dis* 1994;4:204–210.
33. Barer DH, Cruickshank JM, Ebrahim SB, et al. Low dose beta blockade in acute stroke (BEST trial): an evaluation. *BMJ* 1988;296:737–741.
34. Mohr JP, Orgogozo JM, Harrison MJG, et al. Meta-analysis of oral nimodipine trials in acute ischaemic stroke. *Cerebrovasc Dis* 1994;4:197–203. Search date 1994; primary source Bayer database.
35. Horn J, Orgogozo JM, Limburg M. Review on calcium antagonists in ischaemic stroke; mortality data. *Cerebrovasc Dis* 1998;8(suppl 4):27.Search date not stated; primary sources Medline, and hand searches of Congress reports and references

lists and personal contact with the Cochrane Collaboration Stroke Review Group and the Ottawa Stroke Registry.
36. Rodgers A, MacMahon S, Gamble G. Blood pressure and risk of stroke patients with cerebrovascular disease. *BMJ* 1996;313:147.
37. Schrader J, Rothemeyer M, Luders S, et al. Hypertension and stroke – rationale behind the ACCESS trial. *Basic Res Cardiol* 1998;93(suppl 2):69–78.
38. Horn J, Limburg M. Calcium antagonists for acute ischemic stroke. In: The Cochrane Library, Issue 3, 2002. Oxford: Update Software. Search date 1999; primary sources Cochrane Stroke Group Specialised Register of Controlled Trials and personal contact with trialists.
39. Horn J, Limburg M. Calcium antagonists for ischemic stroke: a systematic review. *Stroke* 2001;32:570–576. Search date 1999; primary sources Cochrane Collaboration Stroke Group Specialized Register of Controlled Trials, and personal contact with principal investigators and company representatives.
40. Horn J, de Haan R, Vermeulen M, et al. Very Early Nimodipine Use in Stroke (VENUS). A randomized, double-blind, placebo-controlled trail. *Stroke* 2001;32:461–465.
41. Ricci S, Celani MG, Cantisani AT, et al. Piracetam for acute ischaemic stroke (Cochrane Review). In: The Cochrane Library, Issue 3, 2002. Oxford: Update Software. Search date not stated; primary sources Cochrane Stroke Review Group trials register, Medline, Embase, BIDIS ISI, hand searches of relevant journals, and personal contact with the manufacturer.
42. Wahlgren NG, Ranasinha KW, Rosolacci T, et al. Clomethiazole acute stroke study (CLASS): results of a randomised, controlled trial of clomethiazole versus placebo in 1360 acute stroke patients. *Stroke* 1999;30:21–28.
43. Gandolfo C, Sandercock P, Conti M. Lubeluzole for acute ischaemic stroke. In: The Cochrane Library, Issue 3, 2002. Oxford: Update Software. Search date 2001; primary sources Cochrane Stroke Group Specialised Register of Controlled Trials, Cochrane Controlled Trials Register (CENTRAL/CCTR), Medline, Embase, Pascal BioMed, Current Contents, hand searches of all references in relevant papers, and personal contact with Janssen Research Foundation.
44. Lees K, Asplund K, Carolei A, et al. Glycine antogonist (gavestinel) in neuroprotection (GAIN International) in people with acute stroke: a randomised controlled trial. *Lancet* 2000;355:1949–1954.
45. Sacco R, DeRosa J, Haley E Jr, et al. for the GAIN Americas Investigators. Glycine Antagonist in Neuroprotection for Patients with Acute Stroke. GAIN Americas: a randomized controlled trial. *JAMA* 2001;285:1719–1728.
46. Davis S, Lees K, Albers G, et al, for the ASSIST Investigators. Selfotel in acute ischemic stroke. Possible neurotoxic effects of an NMDA antagonist. *Stroke* 2000;31:347–354.
47. Albers GW, Goldstein LB, Hall D, et al. Aptiganel hydrochloride in acute ischemic stroke. A randomised controlled trial. *JAMA* 2001;286:2673–2682.
48. The Tirilazad International Steering Committee. Tirilazad for acute ischaemic stroke. In: The Cochrane Library, Issue 3, 2002. Oxford: Update Software. Search date 2001; primary sources Cochrane Stroke Group Specialised Trials Register, Cochrane Controlled Trials Register (CENTRAL/CCTR), the Cochrane Library, hand searches of a publication on the quality of acute stroke RCTs, and personal contact with Pharmacia & Upjohn.
49. Saver JL, Wilterdink J. Choline precursors for acute and subacute ischemic and hemorrhagic stroke (Protocol for a Cochrane Review). In: The Cochrane Library, Issue 3, 2002. Oxford: Update Software.
50. Cochrane Stroke Review Group. Department of Clinical Neurosciences, Western General Hospital, Crewe Road, Edinburgh, UK EH4 2XU. http://www.dcn.ed.ac.uk/csrg (last accessed 24 February 2003).
51. Muir KW, Lees KR. IMAGES. Intravenous magnesium efficacy in stroke trial [abstract]. *Cerebrovasc Dis* 1996;6:75P383.
52. Lodder J, van Raak L, Kessels F, et al. Early GABA-ergic activation study in stroke (EGASIS). *Cerebrovasc Dis* 2000;10(suppl 2):80.
53. Prasad K , Shrivastava A. Surgery for primary supratentorial intracerebral haemorrhage. In: The Cochrane Library, Issue 3, 2002. Oxford: Update Software. Search date 1998; primary sources Cochrane Stroke Group Trials Register and hand searches of reference lists of articles identified, three relevant monographs and issues of *Curr Opin Neurol Neurosurg* and *Neurosurg Clin N Am*.
54. Hankey G, Hon C. Surgery for primary intracerebral hemorrhage: is it safe and effective? A systematic review of case series and randomised trials. *Stroke* 1997;28:2126–2132. Search date 1997; primary sources Medline, and hand searches of reference lists of identified articles, published epidemiological studies, and reviews.
55. Fernandes HM, Gregson B, Siddique S, et al. Surgery in intracerebral hemorrhage: the uncertainty continues. *Stroke* 2000;31:2511–2516. Search date 1999; primary sources Ovid databases (unspecified), Medline, and hand searches of the reference lists of identified articles and relevant cited references.
56. Warlow CP, Dennis MS, van Gijn J, et al, eds. Treatment of primary intracerebral haemorrhage. In: *Stroke: a practical guide to management*. Oxford: Blackwell Science, 1996:430–437.
57. Mendelow A. International Surgical Trial in Intracerebral Haemorrhage (ISTICH). *Stroke* 2000;31:2539.

Elizabeth Warburton
Consultant in Stroke Medicine
Neuroscience's
Addenbrookes Hospital
Cambridge
UK

Competing interests: EAW has received funding for a stroke nurse from Servier and has also been reimbursed for attending a stroke conference.

The following previous contributors of this topic would also like to be acknowledged: Gord Gubitz, and Peter Sandercock.

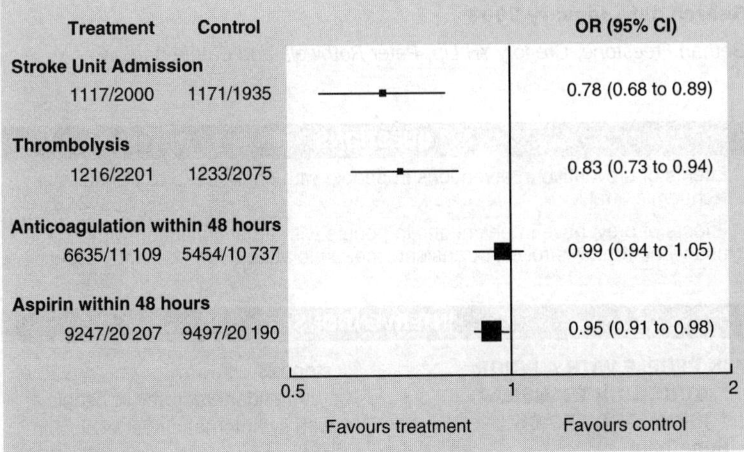

FIGURE 1 Proportional effects on "death or dependency" at the end of scheduled follow up: results of systematic reviews.[7–10] Data refer only to benefits and not to harms (see text, p 236).

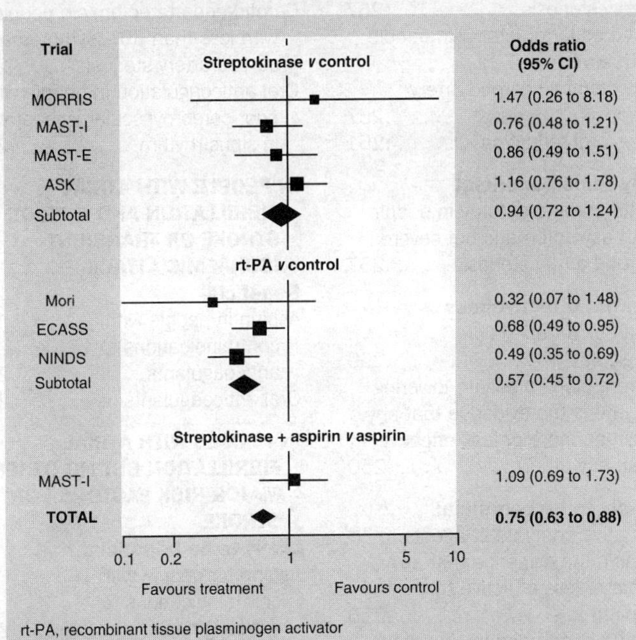

FIGURE 2 Effect of thrombolysis on death and dependency at end of trial: results of review (see text, p 234). Figure reproduced with permission. Wardlaw JM, Warlow CP, Counsell C. Systematic review of evidence on thrombolytic therapy for acute ischaemic stroke. *Lancet* 1997;350:607–614. © by The Lancet Ltd, 1997.

Stroke prevention

Search date January 2003

Bethan Freestone, Gregory YH Lip, Peter Rothwell, and Cathie Sudlow

QUESTIONS

INTERVENTIONS

See glossary, p 266

Key Messages

In people with a prior stroke or transient ischaemic attack

- **Antiplatelet treatment** One systematic review has found that antiplatelet treatment reduces the risk of serious vascular events in people with prior stroke or transient ischaemic attack compared with placebo or no antiplatelet treatment.
- **Blood pressure reduction** One systematic review and one subsequent RCT found that antihypertensive treatment reduced stroke among people with a prior stroke or transient ischaemic attack, whether or not they were hypertensive.
- **Carotid endarterectomy in people with moderately severe (50–69%) symptomatic carotid artery stenosis** Evidence from a pooled analysis of individual patient data from three RCTs found that carotid endarterectomy reduced stroke and death compared with no endarterectomy in symptomatic people with 50–69% carotid stenosis.
- **Carotid endarterectomy in people with severe (> 70%) symptomatic carotid artery stenosis** Evidence from three RCTs has found that carotid endarterectomy reduces stroke and death compared with no endarterectomy in symptomatic people with more than 70% carotid stenosis, although no benefit was found in people with near-occlusion. Benefit in symptomatic people with more than 70% stenosis is greater than in people with lower grade stenosis.
- **Cholesterol reduction** One large RCT has found that, compared with placebo, simvastatin reduced major vascular events, including stroke, in people with prior stroke or transient ischaemic attack. RCTs found no evidence that non-statin treatments reduced stroke compared with placebo or no treatment.
- **Carotid endarterectomy in people with asymptomatic but severe carotid artery stenosis** Two systematic reviews found that carotid endarterectomy reduced perioperative stroke, death, and subsequent ipsilateral stroke in people with asymptomatic but severe stenosis. However, because the risk of stroke without surgery in asymptomatic people is relatively low, the benefit from surgery is small.
- **Carotid or vertebral angioplasty** We found insufficient evidence about the effects of carotid or vertebral percutaneous transluminal angioplasty or stenting compared with medical treatment or carotid endarterectomy in people with a recent carotid or vertebral territory transient ischaemic attack or non-disabling ischaemic stroke who have severe stenosis of the ipsilateral carotid or vertebral artery.
- **Different blood pressure lowering regimens (no evidence that any regimen more or less effective than any other)** Systematic reviews found no clear evidence of a difference in effectiveness between different antihypertensive drugs. One systematic review found that more intensive treatment reduced stroke and major cardiovascular events, but not mortality, compared with less intensive treatment.
- **Alternative antiplatelet agents to aspirin (no evidence that any more or less effective than aspirin)** Systematic reviews have found no good evidence that any antiplatelet treatment is superior to aspirin for long term secondary prevention of serious vascular events.
- **Carotid endarterectomy in people with moderate (30–49%) symptomatic carotid artery stenosis** Evidence from a pooled analysis of individual patient data from three RCTs suggests that carotid endarterectomy is of no benefit in symptomatic people with 30–49% stenosis.

- **Carotid endarterectomy in people with symptomatic near-occlusion of the carotid artery** We found limited evidence from three RCTs that carotid endarterectomy increases the risk of stroke or death due to surgery in symptomatic people with near occlusion of the ipsilateral carotid artery.
- **High dose versus low dose aspirin (no additional benefit but may increase harms)** One systematic review and one subsequent RCT have found that low dose aspirin (75–150 mg/day) is as effective as higher doses for preventing serious vascular events. It found insufficient evidence that doses lower than 75 mg daily are as effective. Systematic reviews found no evidence of an association between aspirin dose and risk of intracranial, major extracranial, or gastrointestinal haemorrhage. RCTs found that high dose aspirin (500–1500 mg/day) increased the risk of upper gastrointestinal upset compared with medium dose aspirin (75–325 mg/day).
- **Carotid endarterectomy in people with less than 30% symptomatic carotid artery stenosis** Evidence from a pooled analysis of individual patient data from three RCTs suggests that carotid endarterectomy increases the risk of stroke or death due to surgery in symptomatic people with less than 30% carotid stenosis.
- **Oral anticoagulation in people with prior cerebrovascular ischaemia and sinus rhythm** Systematic reviews found no significant difference between anticoagulation and placebo or antiplatelet treatment for preventing recurrent stroke after presumed ischaemic stroke in people in normal sinus rhythm. Anticoagulants increased the risk of fatal intracranial and extracranial haemorrhage compared with placebo. High intensity anticoagulation increased the risk of major bleeding compared with antiplatelet treatment.

In people with atrial fibrillation and a prior stroke or transient ischaemic attack

- **Aspirin in people with contraindications to anticoagulants** Systematic reviews have found that aspirin reduces the risk of stroke compared with placebo, but found that aspirin is less effective than anticoagulants. These findings support the use of aspirin in people with atrial fibrillation and contraindications to anticoagulants.
- **Oral anticoagulation** Systematic reviews have found that adjusted dose warfarin reduces the risk of stroke compared with placebo. Systematic reviews have also found that warfarin reduces the risk of stroke in people with previous stroke or transient ischaemic attack compared with aspirin.

In people with atrial fibrillation but no other major risk factors for stroke

- **Aspirin in people with contraindications to anticoagulants** One systematic review has found that aspirin reduces the risk of stroke compared with placebo, but another review found no significant difference. These findings support the use of aspirin in people with atrial fibrillation and contraindications to anticoagulants.
- **Oral anticoagulation** One systematic review has found that warfarin reduces fatal and non-fatal ischaemic stroke compared with placebo, provided there is a low risk of bleeding and careful monitoring. The people in the review had a mean age of 69 years. One overview in people less than 65 years old has found no significant difference in the annual stroke rate between warfarin and placebo.

DEFINITION Prevention in this context is the long term management of people with a prior stroke or transient ischaemic attack, and of people at high risk of stroke (see glossary, p 266) for other reasons such as atrial fibrillation. **Stroke:** See definition under stroke management, p 231. **Transient ischaemic attack:** This is similar to a mild ischaemic stroke except that symptoms last for less than 24 hours.[1]

INCIDENCE/ PREVALENCE See incidence/prevalence under stroke management, p 231.

AETIOLOGY/ RISK FACTORS See aetiology under stroke management, p 231. Risk factors for stroke include prior stroke or transient ischaemic attack, increasing age, hypertension, diabetes, cigarette smoking, and emboli associated with atrial fibrillation, artificial heart valves, or myocardial infarction. The relation with cholesterol is less clear. One overview of prospective studies among healthy middle aged people found no association between total cholesterol and overall stroke risk.[2] However, one review of prospective observational studies in eastern Asian people found that cholesterol was positively associated with ischaemic stroke but negatively associated with haemorrhagic stroke.[3]

PROGNOSIS People with a history of stroke or transient ischaemic attack are at high risk of all vascular events, such as myocardial infarction, but are at particular risk of subsequent stroke (about 10% in the first year and about 5% each year thereafter); see figure 1, p 272, and figure 1 in secondary prevention of ischaemic cardiac events, p 188.[4,5] People with intermittent atrial fibrillation treated with aspirin should be considered at similar risk of stroke, compared with people with sustained atrial fibrillation treated with aspirin (rate of ischaemic stroke/year: 3.2% with intermittent *v* 3.3% with sustained).[6]

AIMS OF INTERVENTION To prevent death or disabling stroke, as well as other serious non-fatal outcomes, especially myocardial infarction, with minimal adverse effects from treatment.

OUTCOMES Stroke, myocardial infarction; mortality, and dependency.

METHODS *Clinical Evidence* search and appraisal January 2003. Options authored by Cathie Sudlow were searched May 2002 (including hand searches of vascular, neurology, and general medical journals). The six journals that contained the largest number of relevant papers were hand searched (search dates 1994–2000).

QUESTION **What are the effects of interventions in people with prior stroke or transient ischaemic attack?**

OPTION **BLOOD PRESSURE REDUCTION VERSUS NO BLOOD PRESSURE REDUCTION**

Cathie Sudlow

One systematic review and one subsequent RCT found that antihypertensive treatment reduced stroke in people with a prior stroke or transient ischaemic attack, whether or not they were hypertensive.

Benefits: We found one systematic review[7] and one subsequent RCT[8] comparing antihypertensive treatment versus placebo, no treatment, or usual care in people with a prior stroke or transient ischaemic attack. The systematic review (search date not stated, 9 RCTs, 6753 people with a prior stroke or transient ischaemic attack) found that antihypertensive treatment significantly reduced stroke and major cardiovascular events compared with placebo, no treatment, or usual care over 2–7 years (stroke: RR 0.72, 95% CI 0.61 to 0.85; major cardiovascular events: RR 0.79, 95% CI 0.68 to 0.91).[7] Over 80% of people in the review were included in a single large RCT, the results of which have only been published in preliminary form.[9] The subsequent RCT (6105 people with a prior stroke or transient ischaemic attack with and without hypertension) compared the angiotensin converting enzyme inhibitor perindopril plus indapamide (added at the discretion of the physician) versus placebo.[8] It found that active treatment reduced stroke compared with placebo but found no significant difference in mortality after about 4 years (stroke: AR 10% with treatment *v* 14% with placebo; RR 0.72, 95% CI 0.62 to 0.83; deaths: AR 10% with treatment *v* 10% with placebo; RR 0.96, 95% CI 0.82 to 1.12). Relative risks were similar in people with and in those without hypertension.

Harms: In people with a history of stroke, reports of an apparently J-shaped relationship between blood pressure and subsequent stroke have led to concerns that blood pressure reduction may increase the risk of recurrent stroke, perhaps because of reduced cerebral perfusion, particularly among people with extracranial carotid or vertebral artery stenosis.[10] However, observational studies found no evidence of a threshold of diastolic blood pressure below which there was no reduction in stroke.[10,11]

Comment: The systematic review found that the effects of blood pressure lowering were similar in people with and without a history of stroke or transient ischaemic attack.[7]

OPTION DIFFERENT BLOOD PRESSURE LOWERING REGIMENS

Cathie Sudlow

Systematic reviews found no clear evidence of a difference in effectiveness between different antihypertensive drugs. One systematic review found that more intensive treatment reduced stroke and major cardiovascular events, but not mortality, compared with less intensive treatment.

Benefits: We found no RCTs comparing different antihypertensive regimens specifically among people with a prior stroke or transient ischaemic attack. We found three systematic reviews[12–14] and one subsequent RCT[15] that compared the effects of different antihypertensive treatments on stroke and other vascular outcomes in people with hypertension. One systematic review (search date 1997, 5 RCTs, about 18 000 people) found no significant difference between diuretics and β blockers in death, stroke, or coronary artery disease.[12] The second systematic review (search date not stated, 15 RCTs) compared more intensive versus less intensive treatment (3 RCTs, about 20 000 people), angiotensin converting enzyme inhibitors versus diuretics or β blockers (3 RCTs, about 16 000 people), calcium channel blockers versus diuretics or β blockers (5 RCTs, about 23 000 people), and angiotensin converting enzyme inhibitors versus calcium channel blockers (2 RCTs, about 5000 people).[13] It found that more intensive treatment (target diastolic blood pressure 75–85 mm Hg) significantly reduced stroke and major cardiovascular events but not death compared with less intensive treatment (target diastolic blood pressure 85–105 mm Hg) (stroke: RR 0.80, 95% CI 0.65 to 0.98; major cardiovascular events: RR 0.85, 95% CI 0.76 to 0.96; death: RR 0.97, 95% CI 0.85 to 1.11). It found no significant difference between angiotensin converting enzyme inhibitors and diuretics or β blockers in stroke, other vascular outcomes, or death (stroke: RR 1.05, 95% CI 0.92 to 1.19; death: RR 1.03, 95% CI 0.93 to 1.14). Calcium channel blockers reduced stroke compared with diuretics or β blockers, but they slightly increased coronary heart disease and had no significant effect on death or other vascular outcomes (stroke: RR 0.87, 95% CI 0.77 to 0.98; coronary heart disease: RR 0.81, 95% CI 0.68 to 0.97; death: RR 1.01, 95% CI 0.92 to 1.11). Angiotensin converting enzyme inhibitors reduced coronary heart disease compared with calcium channel blockers, but they had no significant effect on stroke or death (coronary heart disease: RR 0.81, 95% CI 0.68 to 0.97; stroke: RR 1.02, 95% CI 0.85 to 1.21; death: RR 1.03, 95% CI 0.91 to 1.18). However, the RCTs included in this comparison were statistically heterogeneous, and so the results of the analysis should be treated with caution. The third systematic review (search date not stated) found similar results to those of the second review.[14] It suggested that results for different antihypertensive drugs could be explained by the blood pressure differences between randomised groups. The subsequent RCT (9193 people with hypertension, 728 of whom had a history of cerebrovascular disease) compared an angiotensin II receptor blocker (losartan) versus a β blocker (atenolol).[15] It found that losartan significantly reduced the combined outcome of cardiovascular death, myocardial infarction, and stroke after 5 years compared with atenolol (AR 14% with atenolol *v* 12% with losartan; HR 0.85, 95% CI 0.76 to 0.96). Blood pressure reduction was similar in both treatment groups (systolic/diastolic: about 30/17 mm Hg).

Harms: See harms under blood pressure reduction, p 250.

Comment: It has been suggested that both angiotensin converting enzyme inhibitors and angiotensin II receptor blockers produce reductions in vascular outcomes beyond what might be expected from their effects on blood pressure.[15,16]

OPTION CHOLESTEROL REDUCTION

Cathie Sudlow

One large RCT has found that, compared with placebo, simvastatin reduced major vascular events, including stroke, in people with prior stroke or transient ischaemic attack. RCTs have found no evidence that non-statin treatments reduced stroke compared with placebo or no treatment.

Benefits: **Statins:** We found several systematic reviews (about 38 000 people with and without a history of coronary heart disease) that assessed the effects of reducing cholesterol with a statin on coronary heart disease and that reported on stroke as an outcome. The RCTs included did not specifically aim to include people with a prior stroke or transient ischaemic attack (TIA). One systematic review (search date 1995, 14 RCTs)[17] and one additional RCT[18] included all of the relevant results, which are summarised in table 1, p 271. The review found that reducing mean total cholesterol with a statin by 21% over an average of 4 years reduced the relative odds of stroke by 24% (see table 1, p 271). We found one subsequent RCT (20 536 people with coronary heart disease, other occlusive vascular disease, or diabetes, 3280 of whom had a history of cerebrovascular disease and over 4000 of whom had a pretreatment cholesterol of < 5.0 mmol/L) that compared simvastatin 40 mg daily versus placebo (see table 1, p 271).[19] It found that simvastatin reduced mean total cholesterol by 24%, and reduced stroke, major vascular events (major coronary events, strokes, and coronary or non-coronary revascularisations), and deaths over 5 years compared with placebo (stroke: AR 4% with simvastatin *v* 6% with placebo; RR 0.75, 95% CI 0.66 to 0.85; major vascular events: AR 20% with simvastatin *v* 25% with placebo; RR 0.76, 95% CI 0.72 to 0.81; deaths: AR 13% with simvastatin *v* 15% with placebo; RR 0.87, 95% CI 0.81 to 0.94). The relative risk of major vascular events was similar and separately significant in people with and without a history of coronary artery disease, among those with a history of ischaemic stroke or TIA, peripheral vascular disease, and diabetes, and among those with different pretreatment concentrations of cholesterol and triglycerides. **Non-statin treatments:** We found one overview,[20] one subsequent RCT,[21] and one additional RCT[22] that assessed the outcome of stroke. The overview (11 RCTs) compared reducing cholesterol with a non-statin treatment (fibrate, resin, or diet) versus placebo or no treatment.[20] It found no significant difference between a non-statin treatment and placebo in the risk of stroke (OR 0.99, 95% CI 0.82 to 1.21). Results for people with previous stroke or TIA were not reported separately. The subsequent RCT (2531 men with coronary heart disease) found no significant difference between gemfibrozil and placebo in the risk of stroke (AR 5% with gemfibrozil *v* 6% with placebo; RRR +25%, 95% CI –6% to +47%).[21] Results for people with previous stroke or TIA were not reported separately. The additional RCT (532 men who had a previous stroke or TIA) found no significant difference between clofibrate and placebo in death after 3.5 years (AR 13% with clofibrate *v* 19% with placebo; P value not reported).[22]

Harms: Although it has been suggested that statins may increase haemorrhagic stroke,[3,17] the subsequent RCT found that simvastatin did not increase haemorrhagic stroke.[19]

Comment: An RCT comparing atorvastatin versus placebo in 4200 people with minor stroke or TIA is in progress.[23] A planned overview of individual participant data from all RCTs of cholesterol reduction aims to summarise the effects of reducing cholesterol in different groups of people, including those with a prior stroke or TIA.[24]

OPTION ANTIPLATELET TREATMENT VERSUS NO ANTIPLATELET TREATMENT

Cathie Sudlow

One systematic review has found that prolonged antiplatelet treatment reduces the risk of serious vascular events in people with prior stroke or transient ischaemic attack compared with placebo or no antiplatelet treatment.

Benefits: We found one systematic review (search date 1997, 195 RCTs, about 135 640 people at high risk of vascular disease: previous stroke or transient ischaemic attack [TIA], acute stroke, ischaemic heart disease, heart failure, cardiac valve disease, atrial fibrillation, peripheral arterial disease, diabetes, and haemodialysis) comparing antiplatelet treatment (mostly aspirin) versus placebo or no antiplatelet treatment.[25] It found that in people with prior stroke or TIA (21 RCTs, 18 270 people) antiplatelet treatment reduced serious vascular events (stroke, myocardial infarction, or vascular death) compared with placebo or no antiplatelet treatment after 3 years (AR 18% with antiplatelet *v* 21% with placebo or no antiplatelet treatment; OR 0.78, 95% CI 0.73 to 0.85). Antiplatelet treatment also reduced the separate outcomes of stroke, myocardial infarction, vascular death, and death (see figure 1, p 272). For every 1000 people with a prior stroke or TIA treated for about 3 years, antiplatelet treatment prevented 25 non-fatal strokes, six non-fatal myocardial infarctions, and 15 deaths.[25]

Harms: The systematic review found that antiplatelet treatment in people with prior stroke or TIA increased major extracranial haemorrhage (haemorrhages requiring hospital admission or blood transfusion) and intracranial haemorrhage compared with no antiplatelet treatment (intracranial haemorrhage: AR 0.64% with antiplatelet *v* 0.56% with no antiplatelet; OR 1.2, CI not reported; major extracranial haemorrhage: AR 0.97% with antiplatelet *v* 0.47% with no antiplatelet; OR 2.0, CI not reported).[25] We found one systematic review (search date 1999, 24 RCTs) that assessed the effects of aspirin on gastrointestinal bleeding.[26] It found that aspirin increased gastrointestinal bleeding compared with placebo or no aspirin (OR 1.68, 95% CI 1.51 to 1.88). Another systematic review (search date 1997, 16 RCTs, 55 462 people) found that aspirin increased intracranial haemorrhage by about one event per 1000 people treated for 3 years.[27]

Comment: In people at high risk of vascular disease, including those with a prior ischaemic stroke or TIA, the large absolute reductions in serious vascular events produced by antiplatelet treatment far outweighed any absolute hazards.

OPTION HIGH DOSE VERSUS LOW DOSE ASPIRIN

Cathie Sudlow

One systematic review and one subsequent RCT have found that low dose aspirin (75–150 mg/day) is as effective as higher doses for preventing serious vascular events. It found insufficient evidence that doses lower than 75 mg daily are as effective. Systematic reviews found no evidence

of an association between aspirin dose and risk of intracranial, major extracranial, or gastrointestinal haemorrhage. RCTs found that high dose aspirin (500–1500 mg/day) increased the risk of upper gastrointestinal upset compared with medium dose aspririn (75–325 mg/day).

Benefits: We found one systematic review (search date 1997; 7225 people at high risk of vascular disease in RCTs comparing different doses of aspirin; about 60 000 people at high risk of vascular disease, excluding those with acute stroke, in RCTs comparing different doses of aspirin versus placebo or no aspirin) that compared the effects of higher versus lower dose aspirin on stroke.[25] The results in people with prior stroke or transient ischaemic attack were not presented separately. The systematic review found no significant difference between aspirin 500–1500 mg daily and 75–325 mg daily in serious vascular events (stroke, myocardial infarction, or vascular death; OR 0.97, 95% CI 0.79 to 1.19). It also found that doses of 75 mg or more did not reduce serious vascular events compared with doses lower than 75 mg (OR 1.08, 95% CI 0.90 to 1.31). However, the comparison lacked power to exclude a clinically important difference. The systematic review also found that different aspirin doses compared with placebo or no antiplatelet treatment reduced serious vascular events by similar amounts for the higher daily doses (500–1500 mg/day *v* placebo or no antiplatelet treatment: OR 0.81, 95% CI 0.75 to 0.87; 160–325 mg/day *v* placebo or no antiplatelet treatment: OR 0.74, 95% CI 0.69 to 0.80; 75–150 mg/day *v* placebo or no antiplatelet treatment: OR 0.68, 95% CI 0.59 to 0.79) but by a smaller amount for lower doses (< 75 mg/day *v* placebo or no antiplatelet treatment: OR 0.87, 95% CI 0.74 to 1.03). See figure 2 in secondary prevention of ischaemic cardiac events, p 188. People with acute stroke were excluded from these analyses.

Harms: **Extracranial haemorrhage:** The systematic review found that the proportional increase in risk of major extracranial haemorrhage was similar with all daily aspirin doses. In direct comparisons, 75–325 mg aspirin did not increase major extracranial haemorrhage compared with doses lower than 75 mg (AR 2.5% with 75–325 mg/day *v* 1.8% with < 75 mg/day; $P > 0.05$).[25] We found one systematic review (search date 1999, 24 RCTs) of the effects of aspirin on gastrointestinal bleeding.[26] Indirect comparisons in a meta-regression analysis found no association between dose of aspirin and risk of gastrointestinal bleeds. RCTs directly comparing different daily doses of aspirin have found a trend toward more gastrointestinal haemorrhage and a significant increase in upper gastrointestinal symptoms with high (500–1500 mg) than with medium (75–325 mg) doses (upper gastrointestinal symptoms: OR 1.3, 95% CI 1.1 to 1.5), but no significant difference in these outcomes between 283 mg and 30 mg daily.[28–30] We found one systematic review of observational studies (search date 2001, 5 studies) of the effects of different doses of aspirin on the risk of upper gastrointestinal complications (bleeding, perforation, or upper gastrointestinal event leading to hospital admission or visit to specialist).[31] It found greater risks of upper gastrointestinal complications with doses of aspirin greater than 300 mg daily. **Intracranial haemorrhage:** We found one systematic review (search date 1997, 16 RCTs, 55 462 people) of the effects of aspirin on intracranial haemorrhage.[27] It found no clear variation in risk with the dose of aspirin used. Three RCTs directly compared different daily doses of aspirin and found no significant differences in the risk of intracranial haemorrhage, but they lacked power to detect clinically important differences.[28–30]

Comment: None.

OPTION ALTERNATIVE ANTIPLATELET AGENTS TO ASPIRIN

Cathie Sudlow

Systematic reviews have found no good evidence that any antiplatelet regimen is superior to aspirin for long term secondary prevention of serious vascular events.

Benefits: **Thienopyridines (clopidogrel and ticlopidine) versus aspirin:** We found two systematic reviews (search dates 1997[25] and 1999[32]) that compared thienopyridines versus aspirin. The first systematic review (4 RCTs, 3791 people at high risk of vascular disease) found no significant difference between ticlopidine and aspirin in serious vascular events (stroke, myocardial infarction, or vascular death: AR 21% with ticlopidine *v* 23% with aspirin; OR presented graphically; P value not reported).[25] It also found that the risk of serious vascular events was similar with clopidogrel and aspirin (1 RCT, 19 185 people: AR 10% with clopidogrel *v* 11% with aspirin; OR 0.90, 95% CI 0.82 to 0.99). The second systematic review (4 RCTs) found that ticlopidine or clopidogrel marginally reduced vascular events after about 2 years compared with aspirin (OR 0.91, 95% CI 0.84 to 0.98; ARR 1.1%, 95% CI 0.2% to 1.9%).[32] **Dipyridamole plus aspirin:** We found one systematic review (search date 1997, 25 relevant RCTs, 10 404 people) comparing dipyridamole plus aspirin versus aspirin alone.[25] It found no significant difference in serious vascular events (stroke, myocardial infarction, or vascular death) between dipyridamole plus aspirin and aspirin alone (AR 11.8% with combination treatment *v* 12.4% with aspirin alone; OR 0.94, 95% CI 0.83 to 1.06).

Harms: **Thienopyridines (clopidogrel and ticlopidine):** The second systematic review comparing thienopyridines versus aspirin found that the thienopyridines reduced gastrointestinal haemorrhage and upper gastrointestinal symptoms compared with aspirin (gastrointestinal haemorrhage: OR 0.71, 95% CI 0.59 to 0.86; indigestion, nausea, or vomiting: OR 0.84, 95% CI 0.78 to 0.90).[32] However, thienopyridines increased the incidence of skin rash and diarrhoea compared with aspirin (skin rash: clopidogrel *v* aspirin OR 1.3, 95% CI 1.2 to 1.5; ticlopidine *v* aspirin OR 2.2, 95% CI 1.7 to 2.9; diarrhoea: clopidogrel *v* aspirin OR 1.3, 95% CI 1.2 to 1.6; ticlopidine *v* aspirin OR 2.3, 95% CI 1.9 to 2.8). Ticlopidine (but not clopidogrel) increased neutropenia compared with aspirin (OR 2.7, 95% CI 1.5 to 4.8). Observational studies have found ticlopidine to be associated with thrombocytopenia and thrombotic thrombocytopenic purpura.[33,34] **Dipyridamole:** One RCT found that combination treatment with dipyridamole plus aspirin was discontinued more frequently for adverse effects than was aspirin alone.[35]

Comment: One large RCT has assessed effects of adding clopidogrel to aspirin among people with unstable angina (see benefits of antiplatelet treatments in angina [unstable], p 64).[36] A further large RCT is currently assessing the effects of alternative antiplatelet regimens among people with acute myocardial infarction.[37] One ongoing RCT is comparing effects of oral anticoagulation, aspirin plus dipyridamole, and aspirin alone among 4500 people with a prior transient ischaemic attack or minor ischaemic stroke.[38]

OPTION LONG TERM ORAL ANTICOAGULATION IN PEOPLE WITH RECENT CEREBRAL ISCHAEMIA AND IN SINUS RHYTHM

Systematic reviews have found no significant difference between anticoagulation and placebo or antiplatelet treatment for preventing recurrent stroke after presumed ischaemic stroke in people in normal sinus rhythm. Anticoagulants increased the risk of fatal intracranial and extracranial haemorrhage compared with placebo. High intensity anticoagulation increased the risk of major bleeding compared with antiplatelet treatment.

Benefits: **Versus placebo:** We found one systematic review (search date not stated, 9 small RCTs, 1214 people in sinus rhythm with previous non-embolic presumed ischaemic stroke or transient ischaemic attack, mean duration 1.8 years).[39] It found no clear benefit of oral anticoagulants (warfarin, dicoumarol, or phenindione) on death or dependency compared with placebo, or on mortality or recurrent stroke (death or dependency: ARR +4%, 95% CI –6% to +14%; RRR +5%, 95% CI –9% to +18%). **Versus antiplatelet treatment:** We found one systematic review (search date 2001, 4 RCTs, 1870 people) comparing long term (> 6 months) treatment with oral anticoagulants (warfarin, phenprocoumarin, or acenocoumarol [nicoumalone]) versus antiplatelet treatment in people with a history of transient ischaemic attack or minor stroke of presumed arterial (non-cardiac) origin in the past 6 months.[40] It found no significant difference between high intensity (international normalised ratio [INR — see glossary, p 266] 3.0–4.5) or low intensity (INR 2.1–3.5) anticoagulation compared with antiplatelet treatment for preventing recurrent stroke (low intensity anticoagulation *v* antiplatelet treatment: ARR +0.2%, 95% CI –4.0% to +4.3%; RR 0.96, 95% CI 0.38 to 2.42; high intensity anticoagulation *v* antiplatelet treatment: ARR –0.1%, 95% CI –1.7% to +1.5%; RR 1.02, 95% CI 0.49 to 2.13).

Harms: **Versus placebo:** The first review found that anticoagulants increased the risk of fatal intracranial haemorrhage (ARI 2.0%, 95% CI 0.4% to 3.6%; RR 2.51, 95% CI 1.12 to 5.60; NNH 49 people treated with anticoagulants over 1.8 years for 1 additional non-fatal extracranial haemorrhage, 95% CI 27 to 240).[39] The risk of fatal and non-fatal extracranial haemorrhage was also increased by anticoagulants compared with placebo (ARI 5.1%, 95% CI 3.0% to 7.2%; RR 5.86, 95% CI 2.39 to 14.3; NNH 20, 95% CI 14 to 33). **Versus antiplatelet treatment:** The review comparing anticoagulants versus antiplatelet treatment found no significant difference in risk of major intracranial or extracranial bleeding between low intensity anticoagulation (INR 2.1–3.6) and antiplatelet treatment (RR 1.19, 95% CI 0.59 to 2.41).[40] However, high intensity anticoagulation (INR 3.0–4.5) significantly increased the risk of major intracranial or extracranial bleeding (RR 1.08, 95% CI 1.03 to 1.20).

Comment: **Versus placebo:** The trials in the systematic review all had major problems with their methods, including poor monitoring of anticoagulation.[39] All were completed before introducing routine computerised tomography scanning, which means that people with primary haemorrhagic strokes could have been included. The systematic review could not therefore provide a reliable and precise overall estimate of the balance of risk and benefit regarding death or dependency. Most people in the trial comparing warfarin and aspirin did have a computerised tomography scan, but an adverse outcome was still seen with anticoagulants. Two further RCTs are in progress: one is comparing a lower intensity of adjusted dose warfarin (to maintain an INR of 1.4–2.8) versus aspirin 325 mg four times daily within 30 days after stroke and treated for at least 2 years;[41] whereas the other is comparing warfarin (to maintain an INR of 2.0–3.0) versus aspirin (any dose between 30–325 mg/day) versus aspirin plus dipyridamole (400 mg/day).[42]

OPTION CAROTID ENDARTERECTOMY FOR PEOPLE WITH RECENT CAROTID TERRITORY ISCHAEMIA

Peter Rothwell

Evidence from a pooled analysis of individual patient data from three RCTs in people with symptomatic carotid artery stenosis suggests that carotid endarterectomy increases the risk of stroke or death due to surgery in people with less than 30% stenosis, is of no benefit in people with 30–49% stenosis, and is of increasing benefit in people with higher grade stenosis. The RCTs found that carotid endarterectomy is of greatest benefit in people with less than 70% stenosis, although it may be ineffective in people with near-occlusion. Two systematic reviews found that carotid endarterectomy reduced perioperative stroke, death, and subsequent ipsilateral stroke in people with asymptomatic but severe stenosis. However, benefit from surgery is small because the absolute risk of stroke in asymptomatic people is low. One systematic review found no evidence that eversion carotid endarterectomy is more beneficial than conventional carotid endarterectomy.

Benefits: **People with symptomatic stenosis:** We found one pooled analysis[43] of individual patient data from the three large RCTs (4 publications) that examined the effects of endarectomy in people with symptomatic carotid stenosis.[44–47] The RCTs used different methods to measure the degree of carotid stenosis, studied different populations, and used different definitions of outcome events. However, the pooled analysis adjusted for these differences. The pooled analysis (3 RCTs, 6092 people, 35 000 person years of follow up) found that surgery increased the 5 year risk of any stroke or surgical death in people with less than 30% stenosis, had no significant effect in patients with 30–49% stenosis, was of some benefit in patients with 50–69% stenosis, and was highly beneficial in patients with 70% or more stenosis without near-occlusion

(< 30% stenosis, 1746 people: RR 1.17, 95% CI 0.90 to 1.43; 30–49% stenosis, 1429 people: RR 0.90, 95% CI 0.75 to 1.04; 50–69% stenosis, 1549 people: RR 0.72, 95% CI 0.58 to 0.86; ≥ 70% stenosis without near-occlusion, 1095 people: RR 0.52, 95% CI 0.40 to 0.64).[43] However, there was no evidence of benefit in people with the most severe disease (near-occlusion of ipsilateral carotid artery, 262 people: RR compared with control 0.98, 95% CI 0.61 to 1.59). **People with asymptomatic stenosis:** We found two systematic reviews (search dates 1998) assessing carotid endarterectomy for asymptomatic carotid stenosis (no carotid territory transient ischaemic attack or minor stroke within the past few months).[48,49] One review included results from five RCTs (2440 people).[48] The other review included results from 2203 people from four of these five RCTs, after excluding the fifth RCT because of weak methods.[49] Both reviews found similar results. Carotid endarterectomy reduced the risk of perioperative stroke, death, or subsequent ipsilateral stroke (for the review of 4 RCTs:[49] AR 4.9% over 3 years in the surgical group *v* 6.8% in the medical group; ARR 1.9%, 95% CI 0.1% to 3.9%; NNT 52, 95% CI 26 to 1000; for the review of 5 RCTs:[48] 4.7% over 3 years in the surgical group *v* 7.4% in the medical group; ARR 2.7%, 95% CI 0.8% to 4.6%; NNT 37, 95% CI 22 to 125). Although the risk of perioperative stroke or death from carotid surgery for people with asymptomatic stenosis appears to be lower than in people with symptomatic stenosis, the risk of stroke or death without surgery in asymptomatic people is low and so the absolute benefit from surgery is small, and for most people the balance of risk and benefit from surgery remains unclear.[48,49] **Eversion carotid endarterectomy versus conventional carotid endarterectomy:** We found one systematic review (search date 1999, 5 RCTs, 2645 people, 2590 carotid arteries) that compared eversion carotid endarterectomy versus conventional carotid endarterectomy (see glossary, p 266) performed either with primary closure or patch angioplasty.[50] Overall, the review found no significant differences in the rate of perioperative stroke, stroke or death, local complication rate, and rate of neurological events (for stroke or death: AR 1.7% with eversion *v* 2.6% with conventional; ARR +0.9%, 95% CI –0.3% to +2.1%; for stroke: AR 1.4% with eversion *v* 1.7% with conventional, ARR +0.3%, 95% CI –0.7% to +1.3%).

Harms: **People with symptomatic stenosis:** The pooled analysis (3248 people randomised to surgery a median of 6 days after randomisation) reported 229 strokes or deaths within 30 days of surgery (7.1%, 95% CI 6.3 to 8.1).[43] Operative risk was not related to the degree of stenosis. The risk of death within 30 days of endarterectomy was 1.1% (36/3248; 95% CI 0.8% to 1.5%), and among 209 people who had an operative stroke 20 people (9.6%) died (95% CI 5.9% to 14.4%). One earlier systematic review (search date 1996, 36 studies) identified several risk factors for operative stroke and death from carotid endarterectomy, including female sex, occlusion of the contralateral internal carotid artery, stenosis of the ipsilateral external carotid artery, and systolic blood pressure greater than 180 mm Hg.[51] Endarterectomy is also associated with other postoperative complications, including wound infection (3%), wound haematoma (5%), and lower cranial nerve injury (5–7%). **People with asymptomatic stenosis:** Given the low prevalence of severe carotid stenosis in the general population, there is concern that screening and surgical intervention in asymptomatic people may result in more strokes than it prevents.[52]

Comment: **People with symptomatic stenosis**: The RCTs included in the pooled analysis found different results.[44–47] This may be partly due to differences in the methods of measurement of the degree of carotid stenosis on the pre-randomisation catheter angiograms; the method used in one RCT[44] produced higher values than the method used in the other trials.[45,46,53] There were also other differences, such as in the definitions of outcome events. Meta-analyses of the overall trial results have been reported but these took no account of the differences between the trials.[54,55] The subsequent meta-analysis reported here analysed individual participant data and was designed to determine the effectiveness and durability of endarterectomy according to degree of carotid stenosis.[43] The degree of carotid stenosis is the single most important factor influencing effects of endarterectomy.[44] A preliminary report based on subgroup analyses of the three RCTs[44–47] suggested that benefits of carotid endarterectomy were greatest within 2 weeks of an ischaemic event and that benefits reduced if surgery was delayed (interaction; P=0.009).[56] There was also evidence of reduced benefit in women (interaction; P=0.003) and trend towards increasing benefit with age (P=0.03). These observations were consistent across the individual trials. **People with asymptomatic stenosis:** A large scale trial is ongoing and is due to report initial results in 2003.[57]

OPTION CAROTID AND VERTEBRAL PERCUTANEOUS TRANSLUMINAL ANGIOPLASTY

Peter Rothwell

We found insufficient evidence about effects of carotid or vertebral percutaneous transluminal angioplasty or stenting compared with medical treatment or carotid endarterectomy in people with a recent carotid or vertebral territory transient ischaemic attack or non-disabling ischaemic stroke who have severe stenosis of the ipsilateral carotid or vertebral artery.

Benefits: **Carotid percutaneous transluminal angioplasty versus medical treatment:** We found one RCT.[58] The RCT (504 people with a recent carotid territory transient ischaemic attack or non-disabling ischaemic stroke with stenosis of the ipsilateral carotid artery) compared "best medical treatment" plus carotid percutaneous transluminal angioplasty (PTA) versus "best medical treatment" plus carotid endarterectomy.[58] It found no significant difference between endovascular treatment and surgery for disabling stroke or death within 30 days of first treatment (AR for disabling stroke or death 6.4% with PTA *v* 5.9% with surgery; AR for stroke lasting more than 7 days or death 10.0% with PTA *v* 9.9% with surgery). The trial found no significant difference between treatments for ipsilateral stroke rate up to 3 years after randomisation (adjusted HR 1.04, 95% CI 0.63 to 1.70; P = 0.9). **Carotid angioplasty plus stenting versus endarterectomy:** We found two RCTs in symptomatic people.[59,60] The first RCT (219 people with carotid stenosis of

60–90%) found that carotid stenting significantly increased the combined outcome of ipsilateral stroke, procedure related death, or vasular death at 1 year compared with carotid endarterectomy (12.1% with stent *v* 3.6% with endarterectomy, P = 0.022).[59] The second RCT (104 people with > 70% carotid stenosis) found no significant difference between carotid angioplasty plus stenting and carotid endarterectomy for death or cerebral ischaemia (1 transient ischaemic attack with angioplasty *v* 1 death for endarterectomy; P not reported).[60] **Vertebral artery angioplasty:** The RCT also compared vertebral angioplasty versus "best medical treatment" in 16 people, but did not provide enough data for reliable estimates of efficacy to be made.[58]

Harms: The RCT comparing carotid angioplasty versus medical treatment found that cranial neuropathy was more common with surgery (22 people [8.7%] undergoing surgery *v* 0 people after endovascular treatment; P < 0.0001).[58] Major groin or neck haematoma occurred less often after endovascular treatment than after surgery (3 people with endovascular treatment [1.2%] *v* 17 people with surgery [6.7%]; P < 0.0015).[58] Harms data are not yet available from the other trial, which is still to be published in full.[59]

Comment: The RCTs comparing endovascular treatment versus surgery had low power, and results lacked precision.[58] Several ongoing RCTs are comparing carotid endarterectomy versus primary stenting in people with recently symptomatic severe carotid stenosis. **Carotid percutaneous transluminal angioplasty:** The two RCTs comparing angioplasty (with or without stenting) and endarterectomy suggest that angioplasty with or without stenting is associated with a higher procedural risk than endarterectomy, and a higher rate of restenosis during follow up.[59,60] However, improvements in cerebral protection devices may reduce the procedural risks,[61] and several other RCTs comparing angioplasty plus stenting with cerebral protection versus endarterectomy are currently ongoing. The use of angioplasty is likely to increase in future, but trial results will help to decide whether increased use will be confined to people in whom endarterectomy is technically difficult.

QUESTION What are the effects of anticoagulant and antiplatelet treatment in people with atrial fibrillation?

Gregory YH Lip and Bethan Freestone

Systematic reviews have found that people with atrial fibrillation at high risk of stroke and with no contraindications are likely to benefit from anticoagulation. However, one recent systematic review has questioned the quality of existing RCTs and reviews, and suggested that more trials are needed to establish the effects of anticoagulation. Antiplatelet agents are less effective than warfarin, but they are associated with a lower bleeding risk and are a reasonable alternative if warfarin is contraindicated. The best time to begin anticoagulation after an ischaemic stroke is unclear.

Benefits: **Adjusted dose warfarin versus placebo in people with atrial fibrillation and high risk of stroke:** We found two systematic reviews examining the effect of warfarin in different groups of people with atrial fibrillation at high risk of stroke (see glossary, p 266).[62,63] The first systematic review (search date 1999, 16 RCTs, 9874 people) included six RCTs (2900 people) of adjusted dose warfarin versus placebo (5 RCTs) or versus control (1 RCT) in high risk people (45% had hypertension, 20% had experienced a previous stroke or transient ischaemic attack [TIA]).[62] These six RCTs included five trials in people without prior cerebral ischaemia (primary prevention trials) and one RCT in people with prior cerebral ischaemia (secondary prevention trial).[64] Target international normalised ratio (INR), varied among RCTs (2.0–2.6 in primary prevention RCTs and 2.9 in the secondary prevention RCT). The results of this systematic review were similar to the others. The meta-analysis found that adjusted dose warfarin reduced the risk of stroke (5 primary prevention RCTs: ARR 4.0%, 95% CI 2.3% to 5.7%; NNT 25, 95% CI 18 to 43; 1 secondary prevention RCT: ARR 14.5%, 95% CI 7.7% to 21.3%; NNT 7, 95% CI 5 to 13; combined primary and secondary prevention RCTs: ARR 5.5%, 95% CI 3.7% to 7.3%; NNT 18, 95% CI 14 to 27). The second systematic review (search date 1999, 14 RCTs) identified the same trials of warfarin compared with placebo and found similar results.[63] **Adjusted dose warfarin versus minidose warfarin in people with atrial fibrillation and high risk of stroke:** We found no systematic review or RCTs of low dose warfarin regimens in people with atrial fibrillation and a recent TIA or acute stroke. We found one RCT that compared low, fixed dose warfarin plus aspirin versus standard adjusted dose warfarin;[65] three RCTs that compared adjusted dose warfarin versus low dose warfarin plus aspirin;[66–68] and one RCT that compared conventional intensity warfarin versus low intensity warfarin.[69] The first RCT (1044 people with atrial fibrillation at high risk of stroke) found that adjusted dose warfarin (target international normalised ratio [INR — see glossary, p 266] 1.2–1.5) significantly reduced the combined rate of ischaemic stroke or systemic embolism, and reduced disabling or fatal stroke compared with low, fixed dose warfarin (target INR 1.2–1.5) plus aspirin (325 mg/day) (stroke or embolism: ARR 6.0%, 95% CI 3.4% to 8.6%; NNT 17, 95% CI 12 to 29; disabling or fatal stroke: ARR 3.9%, 95% CI 1.6% to 6.1%; NNT 26, 95% CI 16 to 63).[65] The three RCTs comparing adjusted dose warfarin versus low dose warfarin plus aspirin[66–68] were stopped prematurely when the results of the earlier trial[65] were published. Analyses of the optimal anticoagulation intensity for stroke prevention in atrial fibrillation found that stroke risk was substantially increased at INR levels below 2.[64,70] The fourth RCT (115 people with ischaemic stroke in the previous 1–6 months) found no significant difference between conventional (target INR 2.2–3.5) and low intensity (target INR 1.5–2.1) warfarin in ischaemic stroke rate after mean follow up of around 1 year (AR 1/55 [1.1%] with conventional intensity *v* 2/60 [1.7%] with low intensity warfarin).[69] The RCT was terminated prematurely because of significantly more bleeding complications with conventional intensity warfarin (see harms and comment, below). **Adjusted dose warfarin versus aspirin in people with atrial fibrillation and high risk of stroke:** We found one systematic review comparing warfarin versus different antiplatelet regimens in people at high risk of stroke[62] and one subsequent individual patient meta-analysis.[71] The systematic review (search date 1999, 16 RCTs, 9874 people) included five RCTs (4 primary prevention and 1 secondary prevention RCTs; 2837 people) of adjusted dose warfarin versus aspirin in high risk people (45% had hypertension, 20% had experienced a previous stroke or TIA).[62] Target INR varied among RCTs (2.0–4.5 in primary prevention RCTs; 2.5–4.0 in the secondary prevention RCT). Adjusted dose warfarin reduced the overall risk of stroke compared with aspirin (ARR 2.9%, 95% CI 0.9% to 4.8%; NNT 34, 95% CI 21 to 111). The effect varied widely among the five RCTs, none of which were blinded. The recent individual patient meta-analysis (5 RCTs of primary and secondary prevention, 2633 people at high risk of ischaemic stroke) compared full dose oral anticoagulation (largely coumarin derivatives) versus aspirin (75–325 mg).[71] It found that anticoagulation significantly decreased strokes compared with aspirin in people at high risk of ischaemic stroke (ARR 3.3% per year). **Adjusted dose warfarin versus other antiplatelet treatment in people with atrial fibrillation and high risk of stroke:** One systematic review (search date 1999) compared adjusted dose warfarin versus other antiplatelet agents such as indobufen.[62] One RCT included in the review (916 people within 15 days of stroke onset) compared warfarin (target INR 2.0–3.5) versus indobufen.[72] It found no significant difference in the rate of recurrent stroke between the two groups (5% for indobufen *v* 4% for warfarin; ARR +1.0%, 95% CI –1.7% to +3.7%). **Oral anticoagulant versus oral anticoagulant plus aspirin in people with atrial fibrillation and high risk of stroke:** We found one RCT (157 people at high risk) that compared oral fluindione (active dose 5–25 mg) versus fluindione plus aspirin (100 mg).[73] It found no significant difference between fluindione alone and fluindione plus aspirin for a combined outcome of stroke, myocardial infarction, systemic arterial embolism, vascular death, or haemorrhagic complications after mean follow up of 8 months (2/81 [2.5%] with fluindione *v* 5/76 [6.6%] with fluindione plus aspirin; P = 0.21). The study was insufficiently powered to detect clinically important differences between treatments. **Aspirin versus placebo in people with atrial fibrillation and high risk of stroke:** We found one systematic review (search date 1999, 4 RCTs, 2769 people with atrial fibrillation and prior stroke or TIA).[63] It found no significant difference between aspirin and placebo for stroke or death (stroke: OR 0.68, 95% CI 0.29 to 1.57; death: OR 0.87, 95% CI 0.68 to 1.12). **In people with atrial fibrillation at moderate risk of stroke:** See glossary, p 266. We found no RCT that considered this group specifically. **Anticoagulants in people with atrial fibrillation at low risk of stroke:** See glossary, p 266. We found one systematic review[74] and one overview[75] comparing warfarin versus placebo in people with atrial fibrillation and a variety of stroke risks. Both reviews included the same five RCTs. The overview (2461 people) found that, for people younger than 65 years with atrial fibrillation (but no history of hypertension, stroke, TIA, or diabetes), the annual stroke rate was the same with warfarin or placebo (subgroup analysis among 17% of people on warfarin and 15% on placebo; stroke rate 1% per year in each group).[75] The systematic review (search date 1999, 2313 people, mean age 69 years, 20% aged > 75 years; 45% had hypertension, 15% diabetes, and 15% a prior history of myocardial infarction) found that warfarin (INR 2.0–2.6) reduced fatal and non-fatal ischaemic stroke, reduced all ischaemic strokes or intracranial haemorrhage, and reduced the combined outcome of disabling or fatal ischaemic stroke or intracranial haemorrhage compared with placebo after mean follow up of 1.7 years (fatal and non-fatal ischaemic stroke: ARR 4.0%, 95% CI 2.4% to 5.6%; NNT 25, 95% CI 18 to 42; all ischaemic strokes or intracranial haemorrhage: ARR 4.5%, 95% CI 2.8% to 6.2%; NNT 22, 95% CI 16 to 36; combined outcome: ARR 1.8%, 95% CI 0.5% to 3.1%; NNT 56, 95% CI 32 to 200).[74] **Antiplatelet treatment in people with atrial fibrillation and low risk of stroke:** We found two systematic reviews in people with atrial fibrillation at low risk of stroke.[62,76] The first review (search date 1999, 2 RCTs, 1680 people with either paroxysmal or sustained non-valvular atrial fibrillation confirmed by electrocardiogram but without previous stroke or TIA, 30% aged > 75 years) compared aspirin versus placebo.[76] In primary prevention, aspirin did not significantly reduce ischaemic stroke, all stroke, all disabling or fatal stroke, or the composite end point of stroke, myocardial infarction, or vascular death after mean follow up of 1.3 years (ischaemic stroke: OR 0.71, 95% CI 0.46 to 1.10; ARR +1.6%, 95% CI –0.5% to +3.7%; all stroke: OR 0.70, 95% CI 0.45 to 1.08; ARR +1.8%, 95% CI –0.5% to +3.9%; all disabling or fatal stroke: OR 0.88, 95% CI 0.48 to 1.58; ARR +0.4%, 95% CI –1.2% to +2.0%; composite end point: OR 0.76, 95% CI 0.54 to 1.05; ARR +2.3%, 95% CI –0.4% to +5.0%). The second systematic review (search date 1999) included three RCTs of primary prevention.[62] The average rate of stroke among people taking placebo was 5.2%. Meta-analysis of the three RCTs found that antiplatelet treatment reduced the risk of stroke compared with placebo after mean follow up from 1.2–2.3 years (ARR 2.2%, 95% CI 0.3% to 4.1%; NNT 45, 95% CI 24 to 333).

Harms: The major risk associated with anticoagulants and antiplatelet agents was haemorrhage. In the overview assessing elderly people with variable risk factors for stroke, the absolute risk of major bleeding was 1% for placebo, 1% for aspirin, and 1.3% for warfarin.[75] Another systematic review found the absolute risk of intracranial haemorrhage increased from 0.1% a year with control to 0.3% a year with warfarin, but the difference was not significant.[62] The absolute risks were three times higher in people who had bled previously. Both bleeding and haemorrhagic stroke were more common in people aged over 75 years. The risk of death after a major bleed was 13–33%, and risk of subsequent morbidity in those who survived a major bleed was 15%. The risk of bleeding was associated with an INR greater than 3, fluctuating INRs, and uncontrolled hypertension. In a systematic review (search date not stated, 2 RCTs) major extracranial bleeding was more frequent with anticoagulation treatment than with placebo (ARI 4.9%, 95% CI 1.6% to 8.2%; RR 6.2, 95% CI 1.4 to 27.1; NNH 20, 95% CI 12 to 63).[77] The studies were too small to define the rate of intracranial haemorrhage (none occurred). In a systematic review (search date not stated) comparing anticoagulants versus antiplatelet treatment, major extracranial bleeding was more frequent with anticoagulation (ARI 4.9%, 95% CI 1.6% to 8.2%; RR 6.4, 95% CI 1.5 to 28.1; NNH 20, 95% CI 12 to 63).[78] The studies were too small to define the rate of intracranial haemorrhage (in 1 RCT, none of the people on anticoagulant and 1 person on aspirin had an intracranial bleed). In the systematic review of oral anticoagulants versus placebo in low risk people, the number of intracranial haemorrhages was small, with a non-significant increase in the treatment group (5 in the treatment group and 2 in the control group).[74] Likewise, in the systematic review assessing antiplatelet treatment in low risk people with atrial fibrillation, too few haemorrhages occurred to characterise the effects of aspirin.[76] One more recent systematic review found no evidence that warfarin significantly increased the risk of major haemorrhage compared with placebo among people with no prior TIA or stroke (5 RCTs, 2415 people: ARI for major haemorrhage warfarin *v* placebo +0.8%, 95% CI −1.3% to +2.9%).[63] However, if people with prior stroke or TIA were included then warfarin significantly increased major haemorrhage (6 RCTs: ARI warfarin *v* placebo 1.3%, 95% CI 0.4% to 2.2%; NNH 77, 95% CI 45 to 250). The systematic review found no evidence of a difference in major haemorrhage between warfarin and aspirin; warfarin and any antiplatelet agent; warfarin and low dose warfarin plus aspirin; and low molecular weight heparin and placebo. However, the review may have lacked power to detect a clinically important difference.[63] One small RCT (157 people) found that full dose anticoagulation (target INR 2–2.6) plus aspirin significantly increased haemorrhagic complications compared with aspirin alone (13/76 [17%] with fluindione plus aspirin *v* 2/81[2.5%] with fluindione alone; P = 0.0021).[73] **Adjusted dose warfarin versus minidose warfarin in people with atrial fibrillation and high risk of stroke:** One RCT (115 people) found that conventional intensity warfarin significantly increased major haemorrhagic complications compared with low intensity warfarin after about 1 year (6/55 [10.9%] with conventional v 0/60 [0%] with low intensity; P = 0.01).[69]

Comment: The three risk strata used above have been identified based on evidence derived from one overview of five RCTs[75] and one subsequent RCT.[65] Most reviews have stratified effects of treatment in terms of these risk categories. However, one recent systematic review (search date 1999), which did not stratify for perceived risk, has suggested that RCTs may be too heterogeneous to determine effects of long term oral anticoagulation compared with placebo among people with non-rheumatic atrial fibrillation (see comment below).[79] The review (search date 1999, 5 RCTs, 3298 people) has found results that conflict with those of previous reviews.[79] The review questions the methods and highlights the heterogeneity of RCTs of oral anticoagulation in people with non-rheumatic atrial fibrillation. People in the RCTs were highly selected (< 10%, range 3–40% of eligible people were randomised); many were excluded after assessments for the absence of contraindications and physicians' refusal to enter them into the study. Many of the studies were not double blinded, and in some studies there was poor agreement between raters for "soft" neurological end points. The frequent monitoring of warfarin treatment under trial conditions and motivation of people/investigators was probably more than that seen in usual clinical practice. The review has suggested that considerable uncertainty remains about benefits of long term anticoagulation in people with non-rheumatic atrial fibrillation. The review has different inclusion and exclusion criteria than previously published reviews, having excluded data from two RCTs and including a trial not included in previous reviews.[65] Unlike previous reviews, the recent systematic review did not stratify people for perceived stroke risk and identified no significant difference between anticoagulant and placebo with either a fixed effects model or a random effects model, which was employed to account for heterogeneity of underlying trials (fixed effects: OR 0.74, 95% CI 0.39 to 1.40 for stroke deaths; OR 0.86, 95% CI 0.16 to 1.17 for vascular deaths; random effects: OR 0.79, 95% CI 0.61 to 1.02 for combined fatal and non-fatal events).[79] The publication of this review has led to debate and uncertainty about clinical effectiveness of long term anticoagulation in people with non-rheumatic atrial fibrillation. Decisions to treat should be informed by considering trade offs between benefits and harms, and each person's treatment preferences.[80–85] We found net benefit of anticoagulation for people in atrial fibrillation who have had a TIA or stroke, or who are over 75 years of age and at a high risk of stroke. We found less clear cut evidence for those aged 65–75 years at high risk, and for those with moderate risk (i.e. > 65 years and not in a high risk group or < 65 years with clinical risk factors) or for those at low risk (< 65 years with no other risk factors). The benefits of warfarin in the RCTs may not translate into effectiveness in clinical practice.[79,86,87] In the RCTs, most strokes in people randomised to warfarin occurred while they were not in fact taking warfarin, or were significantly underanticoagulated at the time of the event. A recent systematic review (search date not stated, 410 people) identified three trials comparing the outcomes of people treated with anticoagulants in the community versus the pooled results of the RCTs.[88] The authors confirmed that people who undergo anticoagulation for atrial fibrillation in actual clinical practice are generally older and have more comorbid conditions than people enrolled in RCTs. However, both groups had similar rates of stroke and major bleeding. This risk of minor bleeding was higher in the community group, and it was suggested that these people may require more intensive monitoring in routine practice. **Adjusted dose warfarin versus minidose warfarin in people with atrial fibrillation and high risk of stroke:** The RCT comparing conventional versus low intensity warfarin found no significant difference between treatments.[69] This may be due to insufficient power; premature termination of the trial because of significantly more bleeding complications in the conventional intensity anticoagulation group; the low rate of ischaemic stroke observed in both groups in this population, possibly contributed to by different ethnicity from original anticoagulation trial cohorts; or the similar anticoagulation range reached in the two groups (1.9 with low intensity *v* 2.2 with conventional).[69] **Timing of anticoagulation:** The best time to start anticoagulation after an ischaemic stroke is unclear, but aspirin reduces the risk of recurrent stroke in such people with or without atrial fibrillation, suggesting that it is reasonable to use aspirin until it is considered safe to start oral anticoagulants.[89]

Stroke prevention

GLOSSARY

Conventional carotid endarterectomy This is more commonly employed and involves a longitudinal arteriotomy of the carotid artery.

Eversion carotid endarterectomy This involves a transverse arteriotomy and reimplantation of the carotid artery.

International normalised ratio (INR) A value derived from a standardised laboratory test that measures the effect of an anticoagulant such s warfarin. The laboratory materials used in the test are calibrated against internationally accepted standard reference preparations, so that variability between laboratories and different reagents is minimised. Normal blood has an INR of 1. Therapeutic anticoagulation often aims to achieve an INR value of 2.0–3.5.

People at high risk of stroke People of any age with a previous transient ischaemic attack or stroke or a history of rheumatic vascular disease, coronary artery disease, congestive heart failure, and impaired left ventricular function or echocardiography; and people aged 75 years and over with hypertension, diabetes, or both.

People at moderate risk of stroke People aged over 65 years who are not in the high risk group; and people aged under 65 years with clinical risk factors, including diabetes, hypertension, peripheral arterial disease, and ischaemic heart disease.

People at low risk of stroke All other people aged less than 65 years with no history of stroke, transient ischaemic attack, embolism, hypertension, diabetes, or other clinical risk factors.

Substantive changes

Carotid endarterectomy for people with recent carotid territory ischaemia One meta-analysis added;[43] conclusions refined for different subgroups according to degree of stenosis.

Carotid and vertebral percutaneous transluminal angioplasty Two RCTs added;[59,60] conclusions unchanged.

Prevention in atrial fibrillation Two RCTs[69,73] and one meta-analysis added;[71] conclusions unchanged.

REFERENCES

1. Hankey GJ, Warlow CP. *Transient ischaemic attacks of the brain and eye*. London: WB Saunders, 1994.
2. Prospective Studies Collaboration. Cholesterol, diastolic blood pressure, and stroke: 13 000 strokes in 450 000 people in 45 prospective cohorts. *Lancet* 1995;346:1647–1653.
3. Eastern Stroke and Coronary Heart Disease Collaborative Research Group. Blood pressure, cholesterol, and stroke in eastern Asia. *Lancet* 1998;352:1801–1807.
4. Warlow CP, Dennis MS, Van Gijn J, et al. Predicting recurrent stroke and other serious vascular events. In: *Stroke. A practical guide to management.* Oxford: Blackwell Science, 1996:545–552.
5. Antiplatelet Trialists' Collaboration. Collaborative overview of randomised trials of antiplatelet therapy — I: prevention of death, myocardial infarction, and stroke by prolonged antiplatelet therapy in various categories of patients. *BMJ* 1994;308:81–106. Search date 1990; primary sources Medline, Current Contents, hand searches of journals, reference lists, and conference proceedings, and contact with authors of trials and manufacturers.
6. Hart RG, Pearce LA, Rothbart RM, et al. Stroke with intermittent atrial fibrillation: incidence and predictors during aspirin therapy. Stroke Prevention in Atrial fibrillation Investigators. *J Am Coll Cardiol* 2000;35:183–187.
7. The INDANA Project Collaborators. Effect of antihypertensive treatment in patients having already suffered from stroke. *Stroke* 1997;28:2557–2562. Search date not stated; primary sources electronic medical databases; survey of specialised and general medical journals and congress proceedings and consultanting experts.
8. PROGRESS Collaborative Group. Randomised trial of a perindopril-based blood-pressure-lowering regimen among 6105 individuals with previous stroke or transient ischaemic attack. *Lancet* 2001;358;1033–1041.
9. PATS Collaborating Group. Post-stroke antihypertensive treatment study: a preliminary result. *Chinese Med J* 1995;108:710–717.
10. Rodgers A, MacMahon S, Gamble G, et al, for the United Kingdom Transient Ischaemic Attack Collaborative Group. Blood pressure and risk of stroke in patients with cerebrovascular disease. *BMJ* 1996;313:147.
11. Neal B, Clark T, MacMahon S, et al, on behalf of the Antithrombotic Trialists' Collaboration. Blood pressure and the risk of recurrent vascular disease. *Am J Hypertension* 1998;11:25A–26A.
12. Wright JM, Lee C-H, Chambers GK. Systematic review of antihypertensive therapies: does the evidence assist in choosing a first-line drug? *Can Med Assoc J* 1999;161:25–32. Search date 1997; primary sources Medline, Cochrane Library

(Issue 2, 1998), and references from previous meta-analyses published between 1980 and 1997.
13. Blood Pressure Lowering Treatment Trialists' Collaboration. Effects of ACE inhibitors, calcium antagonists, and other blood-pressure-lowering drugs: results of prospectively designed overviews of randomised trials. *Lancet* 2000;356:1955–1964. Search date not stated; primary sources result from a collaboration of trialists providing a limited data set for inclusion in the overview analyses.
14. Staessen JA, Wang J-G, Thijs L. Cardiovascular protection and blood pressure reduction: a meta-analysis. *Lancet* 2001;358:1305–1315. Search date not stated; primary sources Medline and hand searches of reference lists of previous overviews.
15. Dahlöf B, Devereux RB, Kjeldsen SE, et al, for the LIFE study group. Cardiovascular morbidity and mortality in the Losartan Intervention for Endpoint reduction in hypertension study (LIFE): a randomised trial against atenolol. *Lancet* 2002;359:995–1003.
16. Sleight P, Yusuf S, Pogue J, et al, for the Heart Outcomes Prevention Evaluation (HOPE) study investigators. Blood-pressure reduction and cardiovascular risk in HOPE study. *Lancet* 2001;358:2130–2131.
17. Hebert PR, Gaziano JM, Chan KS, et al. Cholesterol lowering with statin drugs, risk of stroke, and total mortality: an overview of randomized trials. *JAMA* 1997;278:313–321. Search date 1995; primary sources electronic databases, reference lists, authors of trials and funding agencies. Cholesterol and Current Events (CARE) data added in 1996.
18. The Long-term Intervention with Pravastatin in Ischaemic Disease (LIPID) study group. Prevention of cardiovascular events and death with pravastatin in patients with coronary heart disease and a broad range of initial cholesterol levels. *N Engl J Med* 1998;339:1349–1357.
19. Heart Protection Study Collaborative Group. MRC/BHF Heart Protection Study of cholesterol lowering with simvastatin in 20 536 high-risk individuals: a randomised placebo-controlled trial. *Lancet* 2002;360:7–22.
20. Hebert PR, Gaziano M, Hennekens CH. An overview of trials of cholesterol lowering and risk of stroke. *Arch Intern Med* 1995;155:50–55.
21. Rubins HB, Robins SJ, Collins D, et al. Gemfibrozil for the secondary prevention of coronary heart disease in men with low levels of high-density lipoprotein cholesterol. *N Engl J Med* 1999;341:410–418.
22. Anonymous. The treatment of cerebrovascular disease with clofibrate. Final report of the Veterans' Administration Cooperative Study of Atherosclerosis, neurology section. *Stroke* 1973;4:684–693.
23. Welch KMA. Stroke Prevention by Aggressive Reduction in Cholesterol Levels (SPARCL). *Stroke* 2000;31:2541.
24. Cholesterol Treatment Trialists' Collaboration. Protocol for a prospective collaborative overview of all current and planned randomized trials of cholesterol treatment regimens. *Am J Cardiol* 1995;75:1130–1134.
25. Antithrombotic Trialists' Collaboration. Collaborative meta-analysis of randomised trials of antiplatelet therapy for prevention of death, myocardial infarction, and stroke in high risk patients. *BMJ* 2002;324:71–86. Corrections: *BMJ* 2002;324:141. Search date 1997; primary sources Medline, Embase, Derwent, SciSearch, Biosis, searching the trials registers of the Cochrane Stroke and Peripheral Vascular Disease Groups trials registers, and hand searches of selected journals, proceedings of meetings, reference lists of trials and review articles, and personal contact with colleagues and representatives of pharmaceutical companies.
26. Derry S, Loke YK. Risk of gastrointestinal haemorrhage with long term use of aspirin: meta-analysis. *BMJ* 2000;321:1183–1187. Search date 1999; primary sources Medline, Embase, and hand searches of reference lists from previous review papers and retrieved trials.
27. He J, Whelton PK, Vu B, et al. Aspirin and risk of hemorrhagic stroke. A meta-analysis of randomised controlled trials. *JAMA* 1998;280:1930–1935. Search date 1997; primary sources Medline and hand searches of reference lists of relevant articles.
28. The Dutch TIA Study Group. A comparison of two doses of aspirin (30 mg vs 283 mg a day) in patients after a transient ischaemic attack or minor ischaemic stroke. *N Engl J Med* 1991;325:1261–1266.
29. Farrell B, Godwin J, Richards S, et al. The United Kingdom transient ischaemic attack (UK-TIA) aspirin trial: final results. *J Neurol Neurosurg Psychiatry* 1991;54:1044–1054.
30. Taylor DW, Barnett HJM, Haynes RB, et al, for the ASA and Carotid Endarterectomy (ACE) Trial Collaborators. Low-dose and high-dose acetylsalicylic acid for patients undergoing carotid endarterectomy: a randomised controlled trial. *Lancet* 1999;353:2179–2184.
31. Garc a Rodr guez LA, Hernández-D az S, de Abajo FJ. Association between aspirin and upper gastrointestinal complications. Systematic review of epidemioligic studies. *Br J Clin Pharmacol* 2001;52;563–571. Search date 2001; primary sources Medline and hand searches of reference lists of reviews.
32. Hankey GJ, Sudlow CLM, Dunbabin DW. Thienopyridine derivatives (ticlopidine, clopidogrel) versus aspirin for preventing stroke and other serious vascular events in high vascular risk patients. In: The Cochrane Library, Issue 3, 2001. Oxford: Update Software. Search date 1999; primary sources Cochrane Stroke Group Trials Register, Antithrombotic Trialists' Collaboration database, and personal contact with the Sanofi pharmaceutical company.
33. Moloney BA. An analysis of the side effects of ticlopidine. In: Hass WK, Easton JD, eds. *Ticlopidine, platelets and vascular disease.* New York: Springer, 1993:117–139.
34. Bennett CL, Davidson CJ, Raisch DW, et al. Thrombotic thrombocytopenic purpura associated with ticlopidine in the setting of coronary artery stents and stroke prevention. *Arch Int Med* 1999;159:2524–2528.
35. Diener HC, Cunha L, Forbes C, et al. European secondary prevention study 2: dipyridamole and acetylsalicylic acid in the secondary prevention of stroke. *J Neurol Sci* 1996;143:1–13.
36. The Clopidogrel in Unstable Angina to Prevent Recurrent Events (CURE) Trial Investigators. Effects of clopidogrel in addition to aspirin in patients with acute coronary syndromes without ST-segment elevation. *N Engl J Med* 2001;345:494–502.
37. Second Chinese Cardiac Study (CCS-2) Collaborative Group. Rationale, design and organisation of the Second Chinese Cardiac Study (CCS-2): a randomised trial of clopidogrel plus aspirin, and of metoprolol, among patients with suspected acute myocardial infarction. *J Cardiovasc Risk* 2000;7:435–441.
38. De Schryver ELLM, on behalf of the European/Australian Stroke Prevention in

Reversible Ischaemia Trial (ESPRIT) Group. Design of ESPRIT: an international randomized trial for secondary prevention after non-disabling cerebral ischaemia of arterial origin. *Cerebrovasc Dis* 2000;10:147–150.

39. Liu M, Counsell C, Sandercock P. Anticoagulants for preventing recurrence following ischaemic stroke or transient ischaemic attack. In: The Cochrane Library, Issue 3, 2001. Oxford: Update Software. Search date not stated; primary sources Cochrane Stroke Group Trials Register, and contact with companies marketing anticoagulant agents.
40. Algra A, De Schryver ELLM, van Gijn J, et al. Oral anticoagulants versus antiplatelet therapy for preventing further vascular events after transient ischaemic attack or minor stroke of presumed arterial origin (Cochrane Review). In: The Cochrane Library, Issue 2, 2002. Oxford: Update Software. Search date 2001; primary sources Cochrane Stroke Group Trials Register and personal contact with authors of published trials.
41. Mohr J, for the WARSS Group. Design considerations for the warfarin-antiplatelet recurrent stroke study. *Cerebrovasc Dis* 1995;5:156–157.
42. De Schryvfer E, for the ESPRIT Study Group. ESPRIT: mild anticoagulation, acetylsalicylic acid plus dipyridamole or acetylsalicylic acid alone after cerebral ischaemia of arterial origin [abstract]. *Cerebrovasc Dis* 1998;8(suppl 4):83.
43. Rothwell PM, Gutnikov SA, Eliasziw M, et al, for the Carotid Endarterectomy Trialists' Collaboration. Analysis of pooled data from the randomised controlled trials of endarterectomy for symptomatic carotid stenosis. *Lancet* 2003;361:107–116.
44. European Carotid Surgery Trialists' Collaborative Group. Randomised trial of endarterectomy for recently symptomatic carotid stenosis: final results of the MRC European carotid surgery trial. *Lancet* 1998;351:1379–1387.
45. North American Symptomatic Carotid Endarterectomy Trial Collaborators. Beneficial effect of carotid endarterectomy in symptomatic patients with high-grade carotid stenosis. *N Engl J Med* 1991;325:445–453.
46. Barnett HJ, Taylor DW, Eliasziw M, et al. Benefit of carotid endarterectomy in patients with symptomatic moderate or severe stenosis. North American symptomatic carotid endarterectomy trial collaborators. *N Engl J Med* 1998;339:1415–1425.
47. Mayberg MR, Wilson E, Yatsu F, et al, for the Veterans Affairs Cooperative Studies Program 309 Trialist Group. Carotid endarterectomy and prevention of cerebral ischaemia in symptomatic carotid stenosis. *JAMA* 1991;266:3289–3294.
48. Benavente O, Moher D, Pham B. Carotid endarterectomy for asymptomatic carotid stenosis: a meta-analysis. *BMJ* 1998;317:1477–1480. Search date 1998; primary sources Medline, Cochrane Controlled Trials Register, Ottawa Stroke Trials Register, Current Contents, and hand searches.
49. Chambers BR, You RX, Donnan GA. Carotid endarterectomy for asymptomatic carotid stenosis. In: The Cochrane Library, Issue 3, 2001. Oxford: Update Software. Search date 1998; primary sources Cochrane Stroke Group Trials Register, Medline, Current Contents, hand searches of reference lists, and contact with researchers in the field.
50. Cao PG, De Rango P, Zannetti S, et al. Eversion versus conventional carotid endarterectomy for preventing stroke. In: The Cochrane Library, Issue 4, 2001. Oxford: Update Software. Search date 1999; primary sources Medline, Cochrane Stroke Group Trials Register, hand searches of surgical journals and conference proceedings, and contact with experts.
51. Rothwell P, Slattery J, Warlow C. Clinical and angiographic predictors of stroke and death from carotid endarterectomy: systematic review. *BMJ* 1997;315:1571–1577. Search date 1996; primary sources Medline, Cochrane Collaboration Stroke database, and hand searches of reference lists.
52. Whitty C, Sudlow C, Warlow C. Investigating individual subjects and screening populations for asymptomatic carotid stenosis can be harmful. *J Neurol Neurosurg Psychiatry* 1998;64:619–623.
53. Rothwell PM, Gibson RJ, Slattery J, et al. Equivalence of measurements of carotid stenosis: a comparison of three methods on 1001 angiograms. *Stroke* 1994;25:2435–2439.
54. Cina C, Clase C, Haynes R. Carotid endarterectomy for symptomatic stenosis. In: The Cochrane Library, Issue 3, 2001. Oxford: Update Software. Search date 1999; primary sources Cochrane Stroke Group Specialised Register of Trials, Medline, Embase, Healthstar, Serline, Cochrane Controlled Trials Register, DARE, and Best Evidence.
55. Goldstein LB, Hasselblad V, Matchar DB, et al. Comparison and meta-analysis of randomised trials of endarterectomy for symptomatic carotid artery stenosis. *Neurology* 1995;45:1965–1970.
56. Rothwell PM, Gutnikov SA, Mayberg MR, et al. A pooled analysis of individual patient data from trials of endarterectomy for symptomatic carotid stenosis: efficacy of surgery in important subgroups. *Stroke* 2001;32:328.
57. Halliday A, Thomas D, Manssfield A. The asymptomatic carotid surgery trial (ACST). Rationale and design. *Eur J Vascular Surg* 1994;8:703–710.
58. CAVATAS Investigators. Endovascular versus surgical treatment in patents with carotid stenosis in the Carotid and Vertebral Artery Transluminal Angioplasty Study (CAVATAS): a randomised trial. *Lancet* 2001;357;1729–1737.
59. Alberts M.J, for the Publications Committee of the WALLSTENT. Results of a multicentre prospective randomised trial of carotid artery stenting vs. carotid endarterectomy. *Stroke* 2001;32:325.
60. Brooks WH, McClure RR, Jones MR, et al. Carotid angioplasty and stenting versus carotid endarterectomy: randomized trial in a community hospital. *J Am Coll Cardiol* 2001;38:1589–1595.
61. Reimers B, Corvaja N, Moshiri S, et al. Cerebral protection with filter devices during carotid artery stenting. *Circulation* 2001;104:12–15.
62. Hart R, Benavente O, McBride R, et al. Antithrombotic therapy to prevent stroke in patients with atrial fibrillation: a meta-analysis. Ann Intern Med 1999;131:492–501. Search date 1999; primary sources Medline, Cochrane Database, and Antithrombotic Trialists' Collaboration database.
63. Segal JB, McNamara RL, Miller MR, et al. Anticoagulants or antiplatelet therapy for non-rheumatic atrial fibrillation and flutter. In: The Cochrane Library, Issue 2, 2002. Oxford: Update Software. Search date 1999; primary sources Medline, Embase, Cochrane Heart Group Trials Register, hand searches of selected journals and conference proceedings, and contact with experts.
64. The European Atrial Fibrillation Trial Study Group. Optimal oral anticoagulant therapy in patients with non-rheumatic atrial fibrillation and recent cerebral ischemia. *N Engl J Med* 1995;333:5–10.
65. Stroke Prevention in Atrial Fibrillation Investigators. Adjusted-dose warfarin versus low-intensity,

fixed-dose warfarin plus aspirin for high-risk patients with atrial fibrillation: stroke prevention in atrial fibrillation III randomised clinical trial. *Lancet* 1996;348:633–638.
66. Pengo V, Zasso Z, Barbero F, et al. Effectiveness of fixed minidose warfarin in the prevention of thromboembolism and vascular death in nonrheumatic atrial fibrillation. *Am J Cardiol* 1998;82:433–437.
67. Gullov A, Koefoed B, Petersen P, et al. Fixed minidose warfarin and aspirin alone and in combination vs adjusted-dose warfarin for stroke prevention in atrial fibrillation. Second Copenhagen Atrial Fibrillation, Aspirin, and Anticoagulation Study. *Arch Intern Med* 1998;158:1513–1521.
68. Hellemons B, Langenberg M, Lodder J, et al. Primary prevention of arterial thrombo-embolism in non-rheumatic atrial fibrillation in primary care: randomised controlled trial comparing two intensities of coumarin with aspirin. *BMJ* 1999;319:958–964.
69. Yamaguchi T. Optimal intensity of warfarin therapy for secondary prevention of stroke in patients with non-valvular atrial fibrillation: a multicenter, prospective randomised trial. Japanese Nonvalvular Atrial Fibrillation-Embolism Secondary Prevention Cooperative Study Group. *Stroke* 2000;31:817–821.
70. Hylek EM, Skates SJ, Sheehan MA, et al. An analysis of the lowest effective intensity of prophylactic anticoagulation for patients with non-rheumatic atrial fibrillation. *N Engl J Med* 1996;335:540–546.
71. Van Walraven C, Hart RG, Singer DE, et al. Oral anticoagulants vs aspirin in nonvalvular atrial fibrillation. An individual patient meta-analysis. *JAMA* 2002;288:2441–2448.
72. Morocutti C, Amabile G, Fattapposta F, et al, for the SIFA Investigators. Indobufen versus warfarin in the secondary prevention of major vascular events in non-rheumatic atrial fibrillation. *Stroke* 1997;28:1015–1021.
73. Lechat P, Lardoux H, Mallet A, et al. Anticoagulant (fluindione)–aspirin combination in patients with high risk atrial fibrillation. A randomised trial (Fluindione, fibrillation Auriculaire, Aspirin et Contraste Spontane; FFAACS). *Cerebrovasc Dis* 2001;12:245–252.
74. Benavente O, Hart R, Koudstaal P, et al. Oral anticoagulants for preventing stroke in patients with non-valvular atrial fibrillation and no previous history of stroke or transient ischemic attacks. In: The Cochrane Library, Issue 2, 2002. Oxford: Update Software. Search date 1999; primary sources Cochrane Stroke Group Specialised Register of Trials, Medline, Antithrombotic Trialists' Collaboration database, and hand searches of reference lists of relevant articles.
75. Atrial Fibrillation Investigators. Risk factors for stroke and efficacy of antithrombotic therapy in atrial fibrillation. *Arch Intern Med* 1994;154:1449–1457.
76. Benavente O, Hart R, Koudstaal P, et al. Antiplatelet therapy for preventing stroke in patients with non-valvular atrial fibrillation and no previous history of stroke or transient ischemic attacks. In: The Cochrane Library, Issue 2, 2002. Oxford: Update Software. Search date 1999; primary sources Medline, Cochrane Specialised Register of Trials, and hand searches of reference lists of relevant articles.
77. Koudstaal P. Anticoagulants for preventing stroke in patients with non-rheumatic atrial fibrillation and a history of stroke or transient ischemic attacks. In: The Cochrane Library, Issue 2, 2002. Oxford: Update Software. Search date not stated; primary source Cochrane Stroke Group Trials Register and contact with trialists.
78. Koudstaal P. Anticoagulants versus antiplatelet therapy for preventing stroke in patients with non-rheumatic atrial fibrillation and a history of stroke or transient ischemic attacks. In: The Cochrane Library, Issue 2, 2002. Oxford: Update Software. Search date not stated; primary sources Cochrane Stroke Group Trials Register and contact with trialists.
79. Taylor F, Cohen H, Ebrahim S. Systematic review of long term anticoagulation or antiplatelet treatment in patients with non-rheumatic atrial fibrillation. *BMJ* 2001;322:321–326. Search date 1999; primary sources Cochrane Central database, Embase, Medline, Cinahl, Sigle, hand searches of reference lists, and personal contact with experts.
80. Lip G. Thromboprophylaxis for atrial fibrillation. *Lancet* 1999;353:4–6.
81. Ezekowitz M, Levine J. Preventing stroke in patients with atrial fibrillation. *JAMA* 1999;281:1830–1835.
82. Hart R, Sherman D, Easton D, et al. Prevention of stroke in patients with non-valvular atrial fibrillation. *Neurology* 1998;51:674–681.
83. Feinberg W. Anticoagulation for prevention of stroke. *Neurology* 1998;51(suppl 3):20–22.
84. Albers G. Choice of antithrombotic therapy for stroke prevention in atrial fibrillation. Warfarin, aspirin, or both? *Arch Intern Med* 1998;158:1487–1491.
85. Nademanee K, Kosar E. Long-term antithrombotic treatment for atrial fibrillation. *Am J Cardiol* 1998;82:37N–42N.
86. Green CJ, Hadorn DC, Bassett K, et al. Anticoagulation in chronic non-valvular atrial fibrillation: a critical appraisal and meta-analysis. *Can J Cardiol* 1997;13:811–815.
87. Blakely J. Anticoagulation in chronic non-valvular atrial fibrillation: appraisal of two meta-analyses. *Can J Cardiol* 1998;14:945–948.
88. Evans A, Kalra L. Are the results of randomized controlled trials on anticoagulation in patients with atrial fibrillation generalizable to clinical practice? *Arch Intern Med* 2001;161:1443–1447. Search date not stated; primary sources Medline, Cochrane Library, and hand searches of reference lists of relevant retrieved articles.
89. Chen ZM, Sandercock P, Pan HC, et al. Indications for early aspirin use in acute ischemic stroke: a combined analysis of 40 000 randomized patients from the Chinese acute stroke trial and the international stroke trial. On behalf of the CAST and IST collaborative groups. *Stroke* 2000;31:1240–1249.

Bethan Freestone
Research Fellow
City Hospital
Birmingham
UK

Gregory YH Lip
Consultant Cardiologist and Professor of Cardiovascular Medicine, Director of Haemostasis Thrombosis and Vascular Biology Unit
City Hospital
Birmingham
UK

Peter Rothwell
Reader in Clinical Neurology
Department of Clinical Neurology
Oxford
UK

Cathie Sudlow
Wellcome Clinician Scientist
Department of Clinical Neurosciences
University of Edinburgh
Edinburgh
UK

Competing interests: CS on one occasion received a fee from Sanofi-Synthelabo for giving a talk at a GP meeting. GYHL, PR, and BF none declared.

The following previous contributors of this topic would also like to be acknowledged: Colin Baigent, Gord Gubitz, and Peter Sandercock.

TABLE 1 Effects of cholesterol reduction with a statin on risk of stroke: results of systematic review[18] and RCTs.[19,20]

	Number of		Mean pretreatment cholesterol	Average follow up duration	Mean reduction in cholesterol*	Summary OR (95% CI) for active treatment v control	
	People	Strokes	(mmol/L)*	(years)*	(%)	Fatal or non-fatal stroke	Fatal stroke
1997 overview (14 RCTs)[18] + LIPID trial[19]	38 000	827	6.3	4	21	0.76† (0.66 to 0.87)	0.99† (0.67 to 1.45)
Heart Protection Study[20]	20 000	1029	5.9	5	24	0.75 (0.66 to 0.85)	0.81 (0.62 to 1.1)
All trials	58 000	1856	6.2	4.4	23	0.75 (0.67 to 0.83)	0.86 (0.69 to 1.1)

*Weighted by trial size; †the findings of other published overviews were consistent with the results shown here.

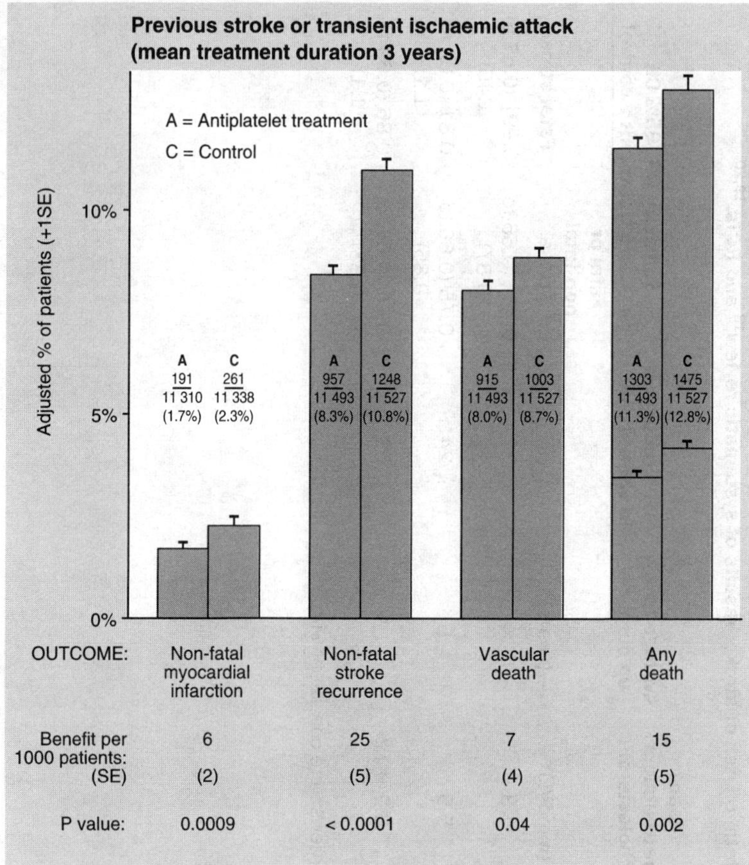

FIGURE 1 **Absolute effects of antiplatelet treatment on various outcomes in 21 trials in people with a prior (presumed ischaemic) stroke or transient ischaemic attack. The columns show the absolute risks over 3 years for each outcome. The error bars represent standard deviations. In the "any death" column, non-vascular deaths are represented by lower horizontal lines (see text, p 253). Adapted with permission.[4]**

Thromboembolism

Search date November 2002

David Fitzmaurice, FD Richard Hobbs, and Richard McManus

QUESTIONS

INTERVENTIONS

To be covered in future updates

Aspirin
Inferior vena cava filters
Oral antithrombotic agents (such as glycoprotein IIb/IIIa antagonists)
Thromboembolism in pregnancy

See glossary, p 286

Key Messages

Proximal deep vein thrombosis

- **Unfractionated and low molecular weight heparin** Systematic reviews have found that low molecular weight heparin reduces the incidence of recurrent thromboembolic disease and decreases the risk of major haemorrhage compared with unfractionated heparin. One systematic review found no significant difference between long term low molecular weight heparin and oral anticoagulation in recurrent thromboembolism, major haemorrhage, or mortality. One systematic review of RCTs found no significant difference in recurrence of thromboembolism between heparin treatment at home and in hospital.
- **Warfarin** We found no RCTs comparing warfarin versus placebo. One RCT found that fewer people had recurrence of proximal deep vein thrombosis within 6 months with combined acenocoumarol (nicoumalone) plus intravenous unfractionated heparin than with acenocoumarol alone; as a result, the trial was stopped. Systematic reviews have found that longer duration of anticoagulation reduces recurrence of deep vein thrombosis compared with

shorter duration of anticoagulation. One non-systematic review found limited evidence that longer compared with shorter duration of warfarin was associated with an increased risk of major haemorrhage, but another non-systematic review found no significant difference in major haemorrhage. The absolute risk of recurrent venous thromboembolism decreases with time, but the relative risk reduction with treatment remains constant. Harms of treatment, including major haemorrhage, continue during prolonged treatment. Individuals have different risk profiles and it is likely that the optimal duration of anticoagulation will vary.

- **Compression stockings** We found no RCTs of standard compression stockings for treating people with proximal deep vein thrombosis. One RCT found that made to measure knee length graduated compression stockings reduced post-thrombotic syndrome over 5–8 years compared with no stockings.

Isolated calf vein thrombosis

- **Warfarin plus heparin** One unblinded RCT found no significant difference in recurrent thromboembolism or rates of major haemorrhage between 6 and 12 weeks of anticoagulation. One RCT found that warfarin plus intravenous unfractionated heparin (international normalised ratio 2.5–4.2) reduced the rate of proximal extension compared with heparin alone.

Pulmonary embolism

- **Oral anticoagulants** We found no direct evidence about the optimum intensity and duration of anticoagulation in people with pulmonary embolism. The best available evidence requires extrapolation of results from studies of people with proximal deep vein thrombosis (see above).
- **Unfractionated and low molecular weight heparin** One small RCT in people with pulmonary embolism found that heparin plus warfarin reduced mortality compared with no anticoagulation at 1 year. One RCT in people with symptomatic pulmonary embolism who did not receive thrombolysis or embolectomy found no significant difference between low molecular weight heparin and unfractionated heparin in mortality or new episodes of thromboembolism. Another RCT in people with proximal deep vein thrombosis without clinical signs or symptoms of pulmonary embolism but with high probability lung scan findings found that fixed dose low molecular weight heparin reduced the proportion of people with new episodes of venous thromboembolism compared with intravenous heparin.
- **Thrombolysis** RCTs identified by one systematic review found no significant difference in mortality between thrombolysis plus heparin and heparin alone, and found that thrombolysis may increase the incidence of intracranial haemorrhage. One small RCT identified by the review found limited evidence that adding thrombolysis to heparin may reduce mortality in people with shock due to massive pulmonary embolism.

Computerised decision support

- **Computerised decision support in oral anticoagulation** We found no RCTs comparing computerised decision support versus usual management of oral anticoagulation that used clinically important outcomes (major haemorrhage or death).
- One systematic review and three subsequent RCTs have found that, compared with usual care, computerised decision support in oral anticoagulation increases time spent in the target international normalised ratio range. Another subsequent RCT found no significant difference between computerised decision support and standard manual support in the time spent in the target

international normalised ratio range. A subsequent RCT of initiation of warfarin found that computerised decision support reduced the mean time taken to reach therapeutic levels of anticoagulation compared with usual care. Most RCTs were small and brief.

DEFINITION **Venous thromboembolism** is any thromboembolic event occurring within the venous system, including deep vein thrombosis and pulmonary embolism. **Deep vein thrombosis** is a radiologically confirmed partial or total thrombotic occlusion of the deep venous system of the legs sufficient to produce symptoms of pain or swelling. **Proximal deep vein thrombosis** affects the veins above the knee (popliteal, superficial femoral, common femoral, and iliac veins). **Isolated calf vein thrombosis** is confined to the deep veins of the calf and does not affect the veins above the knee. **Pulmonary embolism** is radiologically confirmed partial or total thromboembolic occlusion of pulmonary arteries, sufficient to cause symptoms of breathlessness, chest pain, or both. **Post-thrombotic syndrome** is oedema, ulceration, and impaired viability of the subcutaneous tissues of the leg occurring after deep vein thrombosis. **Recurrence** refers to symptomatic deterioration owing to a further (radiologically confirmed) thrombosis, after a previously confirmed thromboembolic event, where there had been an initial partial or total symptomatic improvement. **Extension** refers to a radiologically confirmed new, constant, symptomatic intraluminal filling defect extending from an existing thrombosis.

INCIDENCE/ PREVALENCE We found no reliable study of the incidence/prevalence of deep vein thrombosis or pulmonary embolism in the UK. A prospective Scandinavian study found an annual incidence of 1.6–1.8/1000 people in the general population.[1,2] One postmortem study estimated that 600 000 people develop pulmonary embolism each year in the USA, of whom 60 000 die as a result.[3]

AETIOLOGY/ RISK FACTORS Risk factors for deep vein thrombosis include immobility, surgery (particularly orthopaedic), malignancy, smoking, pregnancy, older age, and inherited or acquired prothrombotic clotting disorders.[4] The oral contraceptive pill is associated with increased risk of death due to venous thromboembolism (ARI with any combined oral contraception: 1–3/million women a year).[5] The principal cause of pulmonary embolism is a deep vein thrombosis.[4]

PROGNOSIS The annual recurrence rate of symptomatic calf vein thrombosis in people without recent surgery is over 25%.[6,7] Proximal extension develops in 40–50% of people with symptomatic calf vein thrombosis.[8] Proximal deep vein thrombosis may cause fatal or non-fatal pulmonary embolism, recurrent venous thrombosis, and the post-thrombotic syndrome. One case series (462 people) published in 1946 found 5.8% mortality from pulmonary emboli in people in a maternity hospital with untreated deep vein thrombosis.[9] One non-systematic review of observational studies found that, in people after recent surgery who have an asymptomatic deep calf vein thrombosis, the rate of fatal pulmonary embolism was 13–15%.[10] The incidence of other complications without treatment is not known. The risk of recurrent venous thrombosis and complications is increased by thrombotic risk factors.[11]

AIMS OF INTERVENTION	To reduce acute symptoms of deep vein thrombosis and to prevent morbidity and mortality associated with thrombus extension, post-thrombotic syndrome, and pulmonary embolisation; to reduce recurrence; to minimise any adverse effects of treatment.
OUTCOMES	Rates of symptomatic recurrence, post-thrombotic syndrome, symptomatic pulmonary embolism, and death. Proxy outcomes include radiological evidence of clot extension or pulmonary embolism.
METHODS	*Clinical Evidence* search and appraisal November 2002. Observational studies were used for estimating incidence, prevalence, and adverse event rates. RCTs were included only if participants were included and outcomes defined on the basis of objective tests, and if the trial provided dose ranges (with adjusted dosing schedules for oral anticoagulation and unfractionated heparin) and independent, blinded outcome assessment.

QUESTION **What are the effects of treatments for proximal deep vein thrombosis?**

OPTION **WARFARIN**

We found no RCTs comparing warfarin versus placebo. One RCT found that fewer people had recurrence of proximal deep vein thrombosis within 6 months with acenocoumarol (nicoumalone) plus intravenous unfractionated heparin as initial treatment than with acenocoumarol alone; as a result, the trial was stopped. Systematic reviews have found fewer deep vein thrombosis recurrences with longer versus shorter duration of anticoagulation. One non-systematic review found limited evidence that prolonged compared with shorter anticoagulation significantly increased major haemorrhage, but another non-systematic review found no significant difference in major haemorrhage.

Benefits: **Versus placebo:** We found no systematic review and no RCTs. **Acenocoumarol (nicoumalone) plus intravenous unfractionated heparin versus acenocoumarol alone for initial treatment:** We found no systematic review. One RCT (120 people with proximal deep vein thrombosis) found that fewer people had recurrence at interim analysis at 6 months with combined intravenous unfractionated heparin plus acenocoumarol than with acenocoumarol alone; as a result, the trial was stopped. The difference in recurrence did not quite reach significance (4/60 [7%] with combined treatment *v* 12/60 [20%] with warfarin alone; P = 0.058).[12] **Longer versus shorter duration of anticoagulation:** We found two systematic reviews[13,14] and two subsequent open label RCTs.[15,16] The first systematic review (search date 2000, 4 RCTs, 1500 people) included two RCTs of people with a first episode of venous thromboembolism, one RCT in people with a second episode of venous thromboembolism, and one RCT in people with acute proximal deep vein thrombosis.[13] The periods of treatment compared were different in all four RCTs: 4 weeks versus 3 months, 6 weeks versus 6 months, 3 months versus 27 months, and 6 months versus 4 years. In all RCTs, warfarin doses were adjusted to achieve an international normalised ratio (see glossary, p 286) of 2.0–3.0. The review found that prolonged compared with shorter warfarin treatment significantly reduced thromboembolic complications (AR 7/758 [0.9%] in the long arm v 91/742 [12.3%] in the short arm; RR 0.08, 95% CI 0.04 to 0.16; NNT 9, 95% CI 8 to 12). However, it found no significant reduction in mortality between prolonged and shorter treatment (AR 37/758 [4.9%] in the long arm v 50/742 [6.7%] in the short arm; RR 0.72, 95% CI 0.48 to 1.08).[13] The second systematic review (search date not stated, 7 RCTs, 2304 people) included three of the same RCTs as the first systematic review plus four RCTs that had been excluded from the first systematic review on methodological grounds (either because of problems with blinding of outcomes or lack of an objective test to confirm thromboembolism).[14] There was wide variation in the duration of short term (3–12 weeks) and longer term (12 weeks to 2 years) RCTs. This review also found that longer compared with shorter duration of warfarin reduced the risk of recurrent thromboembolism (74/1156 [6.4%] events per person with longer duration v 127/1148 [11.1%] with shorter duration; RR 0.60, 95% CI 0.45 to 0.79; NNT 22, 95% CI 15 to 43). The first subsequent RCT (736 people, including 539 with proximal deep vein thrombosis, pulmonary embolism, or both; open label) comparing fluindione for 3 months versus 6 months found no significant difference in the risk of recurrent thromboembolism, although the confidence interval was wide (AR 21/270 [7.8%] with 3 months v 23/269 [8.6%] with 6 months; ARR +0.8%, 95% CI –3.9% to +5.4%; RR 0.93, 95% CI 0.53 to 1.65).[15] The second subsequent RCT (267 people with a first episode of symptomatic proximal deep vein thrombosis; open label) compared warfarin or acenocoumarol treatment for 3 months versus 12 months.[16] It found no significant difference in recurrence of venous thromboembolism over a mean of 3 years between longer and shorter treatment (21/134 [15.7%] with 12 months v 21/133 [15.8%] with 3 months; RR 0.99, 95% CI 0.57 to 1.73). However, it found that mean time to recurrence was shorter with 3 months' than with 12 months' treatment (11.2 months with 3 months v 16 months with 12 months; no further data reported).[16] **Intensity of anticoagulation:** We found one RCT (96 people with a first episode of idiopathic venous thromboembolism) comparing international normalised ratio targets of 2.0–3.0 versus 3.0–4.5 over 12 weeks' treatment with warfarin after an initial course of intravenous heparin.[17] It found similar recurrence rates at 10 months for both international normalised ratio target ranges (1/47 [2.1%] with lower range v 1/49 [2.0%] with higher range; $P > 0.05$), but found significantly fewer haemorrhagic events with the lower target range (2/47 [4.3%] with lower range v 11/49 [22.4%] with higher range; ARR 18%, 95% CI 5% to 32%; RR 0.19, 95% CI 0.04 to 0.81; NNT 6, 95% CI 4 to 23).[17] **Abrupt versus gradual discontinuation of anticoagulation:** One RCT (41 people with deep vein thrombosis who had received iv heparin for 3–5 days followed by warfarin for 3–6 months) compared abrupt withdrawal of warfarin versus an additional month of warfarin at a fixed low doseof 1.25 mg daily.[18] It found similar recurrence with abrupt compared with gradual discontinuation (3 people with abrupt withdrawal v 1 person with gradual withdrawal; CI not reported).[18]

Harms: **Warfarin:** Two non-systematic reviews of RCTs and cohort studies found annual bleeding rates of 0–5% (fatal bleeding) and 2–8% (major bleeds).[19,20] Rates depended on how bleeding was defined and the intensity of anticoagulation. **Acenocoumarol plus intravenous unfractionated heparin versus acenocoumarol alone for initial treatment:** In the RCT comparing acenocoumarol plus heparin versus acenocoumarol alone, one person in the combined treatment group committed suicide at 6 months.[12] There were two cancer related deaths, confirmed by postmortem examination, in the group treated with warfarin alone: one in week 11 and the other in week 12. **Longer versus shorter duration of anticoagulation:** No individual RCT in either review comparing length of anticoagulation found a significant increase in bleeding complications during prolonged compared with shorter treatment for venous thromboembolism.[13,14] Both reviews included studies with different periods of treatment and the populations studied had different types of venous thromboembolism (see benefits above). The first review found that prolonged compared with shorter anticoagulation significantly increased the risk of major haemorrhage (see glossary, p 287) (19/758 [2.5%] with prolonged anticoagulation *v* 4/742 [0.5%] with shorter anticoagulation; OR 3.75, 95% CI 1.63 to 8.62).[13] The second review found a greater risk of major haemorrhage with prolonged compared with shorter anticoagulation, but the difference was not significant (10/917 [1.1%] with prolonged anticoagulation *v* 6/906 [0.7%] with shorter anticoagulation; RR 1.43, 95% CI 0.51 to 4.01).[14]

Comment: **Studies assessing harm:** These varied in regard to diagnostic criteria, definitions of adverse events, and intensity of anticoagulation, making interpretation difficult.[13,14] **Duration of anticoagulation:** The absolute risk of recurrent venous thromboembolism decreases with time, whereas the relative risk reduction with treatment remains constant. Observed recurrence of venous thromboembolism is therefore dependent on length of follow up. Harms of treatment, including major haemorrhage, continue during prolonged treatment. Individuals have different risk profiles and it is likely that the optimal duration of anticoagulation will vary.

OPTION UNFRACTIONATED AND LOW MOLECULAR WEIGHT HEPARIN

Systematic reviews have found that low molecular weight heparin reduces the incidence of recurrent thromboembolic disease and decreases the risk of major haemorrhage compared with unfractionated heparin. One systematic review found no significant difference between long term low molecular weight heparin and oral anticoagulation in recurrent thromboembolism, major haemorrhage, or mortality. One systematic review of weak RCTs found no significant difference in recurrence of thromboembolism between heparin treatment at home and in hospital.

Benefits: **Low molecular weight heparin versus unfractionated heparin in people with proximal deep vein thrombosis:** We found one systematic review[21] and one subsequent RCT[22] in people with symptomatic proximal deep vein thrombosis, and one systematic review[23] in people with symptomatic venous thromboembolism that included two RCTs in people with proximal deep vein thrombosis. The first review (search date 1994, 10 RCTs, 1424 people) found that low molecular weight heparin (LMWH) (see glossary, p 286) significantly reduced symptomatic thromboembolic complications compared with unfractionated heparin (5 RCTs: 17/540 [3%] with LMWH *v* 36/546 [7%] with unfractionated heparin; RR 0.47, 95% CI 0.27 to 0.82) and mortality (21/540 [4%] with LMWH *v* 39/546 [7%] with unfractionated heparin; RR 0.53, 95% CI 0.31 to 0.90).[21] The second review[23] (search date not stated, 16 unblinded and blinded RCTs, 6042 people with symptomatic venous thromboembolism) included two RCTs[24,25] in people with proximal deep vein thrombosis published after the search date of the first review. Results for people with proximal deep vein thrombosis alone were not analysed separately.[23] The first RCT included in the review (961 people, unblinded) compared LMWH twice daily for 1 week versus LMWH once daily for 4 weeks versus intravenous unfractionated heparin.[24] It found that both LMWH regimens significantly increased thrombus regression at 21 days compared with unfractionated heparin (167/312 [53.5%] with once daily LMWH *v* 129/321 [40.2%] with unfractionated heparin; RR 1.29, 97.5% CI 1.08 to 1.53; 175/328 [53.4%] with twice daily LMWH *v* 129/321 [40.2%] with unfractionated heparin; RR 1.28, 97.5% CI 1.08 to 1.52). It found that twice daily LMWH significantly reduced recurrent thromboembolism at 90 days compared with unfractionated heparin (7/388 [1.8%] with twice daily LMWH *v* 24/375 [6.4%] with unfractionated heparin; RR 0.28, 97.5% CI 0.11 to 0.74), but found no significant difference between once daily LMWH and unfractionated heparin (13/374 [3.5%] with once daily LMWH *v* 24/375 [6.4%] with unfractionated heparin; RR 0.55, 97.5% CI 0.24 to 1.16). The second RCT included in the review (538 people, unblinded) compared fixed dose LMWH versus adjusted dose unfractionated heparin for 12 days.[25] It found no significant difference in thrombus regression at 7–15 days between LMWH and unfractionated heparin (RR 0.93, 95% CI 0.82 to 1.05). It found that LMWH significantly reduced recurrent venous thromboembolism compared with unfractionated heparin (ARs not provided; OR 0.66, 95% CI 0.51 to 0.86).[25] The subsequent RCT (294 people with acute proximal deep vein thrombosis, unblinded) compared intravenous unfractionated heparin in hospital versus LMWH twice daily given mainly at home (outpatients) or alternatively in hospital versus subcutaneous heparin calcium given at home.[22] It found no significant difference in recurrent deep vein thrombosis (6/98 [6%] with unfractionated heparin *v* 6/97 [6%] with LMWH *v* 7/99 [7%] with subcutaneous heparin calcium).[22] See systematic anticoagulation under stroke management, p 231. **Once daily versus twice daily LMWH:** We found one systematic review (search date 1999, 5 RCTs, 1522 people with symptomatic proximal deep vein thrombosis) comparing once versus twice daily LMWH for 5–10 days.[26] It found no significant difference in the proportion of people with symptomatic or asymptomatic venous thromboembolism at 10 days or 3 months between once and twice daily LMWH (symptomatic venous thromboembolism at 10 days: 5 RCTs, OR 0.82, 95% CI 0.26 to 2.49; at 3 months: 3 RCTs, OR 0.85, 95% CI 0.48 to 1.49). **Long term low molecular weight**

heparin versus oral anticoagulation: We found one systematic review (search date 2001, 7 RCTs, 1137 people with proximal deep vein thrombosis treated initially with LMWH or unfractionated heparin for 5–10 days) comparing long term oral anticoagulation versus long term LMWH.[27] It found no significant difference between LMWH and oral anticoagulation in recurrent symptomatic thromboembolism (27/568 [4.8%] *v* 38/569 [6.7%]; OR 0.70, 95% CI 0.42 to 1.16) or mortality (21/568 [3.7%] *v* 14/569 [2.5%]; OR 1.51, 95% CI 0.77 to 2.97).[27] **Home versus hospital treatment with short term heparin:** We found one systematic review (search date 2000, 3 RCTs, 1104 people).[28] Two of the RCTs in the systematic review compared LMWH at home versus unfractionated heparin in hospital, and the other RCT compared LMWH both at home and in hospital. The RCTs had methodological problems, including high exclusion rates and partial hospital treatment in the home treatment arms. The systematic review found no significant difference between treatments in recurrence of thromboembolism, minor bleeding, major haemorrhage (see glossary, p 287), or mortality.[28]

Harms: **Haemorrhage and mortality with low molecular weight heparin versus unfractionated heparin:** We found two systematic reviews.[21,23] The first review found that unfractionated heparin was associated with significantly higher rates of clinically important bleeding compared with LMWH (21/759 [3%] with unfractionated heparin *v* 6/753 [0.8%] with LMWH; RR 3.47, 95% CI 1.41 to 8.55).[21] One RCT (538 people with proximal deep vein thrombosis) included in the second review[23] found that LMWH significantly reduced the composite end point of death, recurrent venous thromboembolism, or major bleeding at 6 months compared with unfractionated heparin (18/265 [7%] with LMWH *v* 35/273 [13%] with unfractionated heparin; RR 0.53, 95% CI 0.31 to 0.90).[25] **Thrombocytopenia with low molecular weight heparin versus unfractionated heparin:** We found one systematic review[29] and one subsequent RCT.[30] The review (3306 people treated for at least 5 days) found no significant difference between LMWH and unfractionated heparin in the risk of thrombocytopenia (RR 0.85, 95% CI 0.45 to 1.62).[29] The subsequent RCT (1137 people with symptomatic venous thromboembolism, unblinded) assessed the risk of thrombocytopenia with three treatments: LMWH for 5–7 days; LMWH for 26–30 days; or unadjusted dose unfractionated heparin for 5–7 days.[30] It found that short term LMWH was associated with less thrombocytopenia compared with long term LMWH or unfractionated heparin (0/388 [0%] with short term LMWH *v* 2/374 [0.53%] with long term LMWH *v* 2/375 [0.53%] with unfractionated heparin). The RCT did not assess the significance of the difference between groups. **Long term low molecular weight heparin versus anticoagulation:** One systematic review found that long term anticoagulation significantly reduced major haemorrhage compared with long term LMWH (7 RCTs; 5/568 [0.9%] *v* 14/569 [2.5%]; OR 0.38, 95% CI 0.15 to 0.94) but, when only high quality RCTs were included, it found no significant difference in major haemorrhage between long term LMWH and anticoagulation (3 RCTs; 4/236 [1.7%] with long term LMWH *v* 5/241 [2.1%] with anticoagulation; OR 0.80, 95% CI 0.21 to 3.00).[27]

Comment: **Studies assessing harm:** These varied in their diagnostic criteria and definitions of adverse events, making interpretation difficult.

OPTION COMPRESSION STOCKINGS New

We found no RCTs of standard compression stockings for treating people with proximal deep vein thrombosis. One RCT found that made to measure knee length graduated compression stockings significantly reduced post-thrombotic syndrome over 5–8 years compared with no stockings.

Benefits: We found no systematic review but found one RCT (194 people with a first episode of venogram proven proximal deep vein thrombosis) comparing made to measure knee length graduated compression stockings (see comment below) versus no stockings for 2 years.[31] Median follow up was 76 months (range 60–96 months). It found that, compared with no stockings, compression stockings significantly reduced mild to moderate post-thrombotic syndrome (19/94 [20%] with compression stockings *v* 46/94 [47%] with no stockings; $P < 0.001$) and severe post-thrombotic syndrome (11/100 [11%] with stockings *v* 23/100 [23%] with no stockings; $P < 0.001$).[31]

Harms: The RCT gave no information on harms.[31]

Comment: The compression stockings evaluated in the RCT were made to measure rather than the standard sized stockings generally used in clinical practice.[31]

QUESTION What are the effects of treatment for isolated calf vein thrombosis?

OPTION WARFARIN

We found no RCTs comparing warfarin versus placebo. One RCT found that warfarin plus intravenous unfractionated heparin reduced rates of proximal extension compared with heparin alone. One unblinded RCT found no significant difference in recurrent thromboembolism or rates of major haemorrhage between 6 and 12 weeks of warfarin.

Benefits: **Versus placebo:** We found no systematic review and no RCTs. **Plus heparin versus warfarin alone:** We found no systematic review. We found one RCT that compared intravenous unfractionated heparin (international normalised ratio [see glossary, p 286] 2.5–4.2) for at least 5 days with or without 3 months of warfarin. It found that heparin plus warfarin significantly reduced proximal extension of clot at 1 year compared with heparin alone (1/23 [4%] people with heparin plus warfarin *v* 9/28 [32%] people with heparin alone; ARR 28%, 95% CI 9% to 47%).[6] **Duration of anticoagulation:** We found one unblinded RCT (736 people, including 197 with isolated calf vein thrombosis) comparing 6 weeks versus 12 weeks of warfarin, which found no significant difference in recurrence of venous thromboembolism (AR 2/105 [1.9%] with 6 weeks *v* 3/92 [3.3%] with 12 weeks; RR 0.58, 95% CI 0.10 to 3.36).[15]

Harms: See harms of anticoagulation under treatments for proximal deep vein thrombosis, p 278. **Duration of anticoagulation:** One RCT (197 people) found no significant difference in rate of haemorrhage between 6 weeks and 12 weeks of warfarin (AR 13/105 [12.4%] with 6 weeks *v* 19/92 [20.6%] with 12 weeks; RR 0.59, 95% CI 0.31 to 1.26).[15]

Comment: Many reported cases of isolated calf vein thrombosis are asymptomatic but detected radiologically for research purposes. We found limited evidence about the clinical importance of asymptomatic calf vein thrombosis. Similarly, studies into the incidence of pulmonary embolism associated with isolated calf vein thrombosis detected asymptomatic embolism by ventilation–perfusion scanning, and the clinical relevance of these findings is unclear.

QUESTION What are the effects of treatments for pulmonary embolism?

OPTION ANTICOAGULATION

We found no direct evidence in people with pulmonary embolism about the optimum intensity and duration of anticoagulation. Evidence for intensity and duration of treatment has been extrapolated from RCTs in people with proximal deep vein thrombosis and any venous thromboembolism. One small RCT found that heparin plus warfarin significantly reduced mortality in people with pulmonary embolism compared with no anticoagulation. One RCT in people with symptomatic pulmonary embolism who did not receive thrombolysis or embolectomy found no significant difference between low molecular weight heparin and unfractionated heparin in mortality or new episodes of thromboembolism. Another RCT in people with proximal deep vein thrombosis without clinical signs or symptoms of pulmonary embolism but with high probability lung scan findings found that low molecular weight heparin reduced the proportion of people with new episodes of venous thromboembolism compared with intravenous heparin.

Benefits: We found no RCTs comparing heparin versus placebo, warfarin versus placebo, or heparin plus warfarin versus heparin alone or versus warfarin alone. **Heparin plus warfarin versus no anticoagulation:** We found no systematic review. We found one RCT (published 1960; 35 people with pulmonary embolism) comparing heparin plus warfarin versus no anticoagulation.[32] It found that anticoagulation significantly reduced mortality at 1 year compared with no anticoagulation (0/16 [0%] deaths with anticoagulation *v* 5/19 [26%] deaths with no anticoagulation; NNT 4, 95% CI 2 to 16).[32] **Duration and intensity of anticoagulation:** We found no direct evidence in people with pulmonary embolism. Evidence for intensity and duration of treatment has been extrapolated from RCTs in people with proximal deep vein thrombosis and any venous thromboembolism. These trials found that bleeding rates were increased by higher international normalised ratio (see glossary, p 286) target ranges (international normalised ratio 3.0–4.5), but recurrence rates were not significantly different compared with a lower range (international normalised ratio 2.0–3.0), and that longer courses of anticoagulation reduced recurrence compared with shorter courses (see benefits of anticoagulation under treatments for proximal deep vein thrombosis, p 276). **Low molecular weight heparin versus unfractionated heparin:** We found no systematic review but found two RCTs.[33,34] The first RCT (612 people with symptomatic pulmonary embolism who did not receive thrombolysis or embolectomy) found no significant difference in mortality between low molecular weight heparin (LMWH — tinzaparin) and intravenous heparin (AR 12/304 [3.9%] with tinzaparin *v* 14/308 [4.5%] with heparin; P = 0.7) or recurrent thromboembolism (5/304 [1.6%] with tinzaparin *v* 6/308 [1.9%] with heparin; P = 0.8).[33] The second RCT (200 people with proximal deep vein thrombosis without clinical signs or symptoms of pulmonary embolism but with high probability lung scan findings) found that fixed dose LMWH (see glossary, p 286) given once daily significantly reduced the proportion of people with new episodes of venous thromboembolism compared with dose adjusted intravenous heparin (AR 0/97 [0%] with LMWH *v* 7/103 [6.8%] with iv heparin; P = 0.01).[34]

Harms: The first RCT comparing LMWH versus unfractionated heparin found no significant difference in the rate of major haemorrhage (see glossary, p 287) (3/304 [1.0%] with LMWH *v* 5/308 [1.6%] with unfractionated heparin; P = 0.5).[33] The second RCT also found no significant difference in the risk of major haemorrhage (1/97 [1%] with LMWH *v* 2/103 [2%] with iv heparin; P = 0.6).[34] See harms of anticoagulation under treatments for proximal deep vein thrombosis, p 278. However, in both RCTs, the incidence of major haemorrhage was low and the number of people is likely to have been too small to detect a clinically important difference.[33,34]

Comment: None.

OPTION THROMBOLYSIS

RCTs identified by a systematic review found no significant difference in mortality between thrombolysis plus heparin and heparin alone, and found that thrombolysis may increase the incidence of intracranial haemorrhage. One small RCT identified by the review found limited evidence that adding thrombolysis to heparin may reduce mortality in people with shock owing to massive pulmonary embolism.

Benefits: We found one systematic review,[35] one subsequent RCT,[36] and one large, non-randomised trial (see comment below).[37] **Plus heparin versus heparin alone:** One systematic review (search date 1998) identified nine RCTs comparing various thrombolytic agents versus heparin.[35] The review did not perform a meta-analysis. The largest RCT (160 people with angiographically documented pulmonary embolism) identified by the review compared a 12 hour infusion of urokinase followed by heparin versus heparin alone. It found no significant difference between treatments in mortality (6/82 [7%] with combined treatment *v* 7/78 [9%] with heparin alone; RR 1.23, 95% CI 0.43 to 3.49) or recurrent pulmonary embolism at 12 months (12/82 [15%] with combined treatment *v* 15/78 [19%] with heparin alone; RR 1.31, 95% CI 0.66 to 2.63).[35] Seven short term RCTs identified by the review compared urokinase, streptokinase, or recombinant tissue-type plasminogen activator followed by heparin versus heparin alone, where heparin was adjusted to maintain a therapeutic partial thromboplastin time. They found no significant difference in mortality or recurrent embolism at 24 hours to 30 days. One small RCT identified by the review (8 people with shock related to pulmonary embolism) comparing bolus streptokinase versus heparin found limited evidence that streptokinase may reduce mortality (0/4 [0%] with streptokinase *v* 4/4 [100%] with heparin).[35] However, these results should be interpreted with caution as people receiving heparin alone had a much longer delay between onset of symptoms and initiation of treatment than people receiving streptokinase. One subsequent RCT (256 people) comparing alteplase plus heparin versus placebo plus heparin for 2 days found no significant difference in in-hospital mortality over a mean 16.7 days (4/118 [3.4%] with alteplase plus heparin *v* 3/118 [2.2%] with heparin alone; P = 0.71).[36] However, it also found that people given heparin alone compared with heparin plus alteplase were significantly more likely to receive rescue thrombolysis (P = 0.004). This makes the results difficult to interpret.[36] **Versus each other:** The systematic review identified six RCTs (491 people) comparing different thrombolytic agents versus each other.[35] It found no significant difference in mortality or recurrent pulmonary embolism with different thrombolytics.

Harms: One systematic review (search date not stated)[38] assessing haemorrhagic complications of anticoagulation identified the same 16 RCTs as the review above.[35] It found a similar range of major bleeding event rates with thrombolysis compared with thrombolytics plus heparin or heparin alone (0–48% with thrombolytics *v* 0–45% with thrombolytics plus heparin *v* 0–27% with heparin alone).[38] It also found similar rates of major bleeding events with different thrombolytics (9–14%). It found that intravenous thrombolytics increased the proportion of people who had an intracranial haemorrhage compared with heparin (896 people; 1.2% with thrombolytics [half of which were fatal] *v* 0% with heparin alone).[38]

Comment: **Versus heparin:** One additional, non-randomised trial (719 people), which excluded people with shock, found limited evidence that thrombolytics reduced overall mortality (8/169 [5%] with thrombolytics *v* 61/550 [11%] with heparin; RR 0.43, 95% CI 0.21 to 0.87) and recurrent pulmonary embolism over 30 days compared with heparin (13/169 [8%] with thrombolytics *v* 103/550 [19%] with heparin; RR 0.25, 95% CI 0.13 to 0.51).[37] However, these results should be interpreted with caution as people receiving heparin were older and more likely to have underlying cardiac or pulmonary disease than those receiving thrombolytics.

QUESTION What are the effects of computerised decision support on oral anticoagulation management?

We found no RCTs comparing computerised decision support versus usual management of oral anticoagulation that used clinically important outcomes (major haemorrhage or death). One systematic review and three subsequent RCTs have found that, compared with usual care, computerised decision support in oral anticoagulation significantly

increases time spent in the target international normalised ratio range. Another subsequent RCT found no significant difference between computerised decision support and standard manual support in the time spent in the target international normalised ratio range. A subsequent RCT of initiation of warfarin found that computerised decision support significantly reduced the mean time taken to reach therapeutic levels of anticoagulation compared with usual care. Most RCTs were small and brief.

Benefits: **Clinical outcomes:** We found no systematic review and no RCTs. **Laboratory outcomes:** We found one systematic review[39] and five subsequent RCTs.[40–44] The review (search date 1997, 9 RCTs, 1336 people) included eight RCTs using warfarin and one using heparin.[39] The computer systems advised the doses for initiation of anticoagulation (2 RCTs) and for maintenance of anticoagulation (6 RCTs). Follow up was short (15 days to 12 months). Indications for treatment included cardiac diseases and venous thrombosis. The outcome reported by 7/9 RCTs (693 people) in the systematic review was the proportion of days within the target range of anticoagulation. The review found that computerised decision support (see glossary, p 286) increased the time that the international normalised ratio (see glossary, p 286) was in the target range compared with usual care (OR 1.29, 95% CI 1.12 to 1.49). Reanalysis excluding one trial that introduced significant heterogeneity found similar results (OR for remaining RCTs 1.25, 95% CI 1.08 to 1.45). The first subsequent RCT (285 people) compared a computerised decision support dosing system versus physician adjusted dosing in five hospitals.[40] People who were taking warfarin for at least 6 days were selected and followed for at least 3 months (results from 254 people [89%] were analysed). People managed by computerised decision support spent significantly more time with their international normalised ratio in the target range than people managed conventionally (63% with computerised decision support *v* 53% with conventional management; $P < 0.05$).[40] The second subsequent RCT (244 people) compared a package of care that included computerised decision support versus traditional hospital outpatient management.[41] The intervention was based in primary care: a practice nurse clinic that included near patient international normalised ratio testing and computerised decision support. It found significantly more time spent in the target range after 12 months with packaged care versus traditional outpatient management (69% with packaged care *v* 57% with traditional care; $P < 0.001$), but found no significant difference in the proportion of tests in range (61% with packaged care *v* 51% with traditional care; reported as non-significant, no further data provided) or in the point prevalence of tests in range (71% with packaged care *v* 62% with traditional care; reported as non-significant, no further data provided).[41] The third subsequent RCT (101 people receiving oral anticoagulation after heart valve replacement) compared a computerised decision support system versus standard manual monitoring of international normalised ratio over 315 days.[42] It found no significant difference in the proportion of international normalised ratios in the target range or time spent in the target range (no further data and no mean follow up time provided). It found that people had significantly fewer dose changes with computerised than with standard manual monitoring (31% with computerised *v* 47% with manual; P = 0.02). The fourth subsequent RCT (335 people receiving initiation, 916 people receiving maintenance anticoagulation treatment for a variety of indications) compared a computerised decision support system for both dosing and appointment scheduling versus standard manual monitoring by "expert physicians".[43] It found that significantly more people managed by computerised decision support compared with standard monitoring achieved a stable international normalised ratio in the first month (39% with computerised decision support *v* 27% with standard monitoring; P < 0.01) and spent more time with their international normalised ratio in the target range over 3 months (71% with computerised decision support *v* 68% with standard monitoring; P < 0.001). The fifth subsequent RCT (122 people on warfarin after hip replacement) compared usual care versus computerised decision support.[44] Only initiation of warfarin was studied. It found that computerised decision support significantly reduced the mean time taken to reach therapeutic levels of anticoagulation compared with usual care (2.8 days with computerised decision support *v* 4.7 days with usual care; P = 0.002).[44]

Harms: One systematic review (search date 1997, 9 RCTs, 1336 people) found major haemorrhages (see glossary, p 287) in 14/700 (2%) people with computerised decision support compared with 25/636 (4%) in the standard monitoring group.[39] Most of the events occurred in one study, making meta-analysis inappropriate. One RCT found no significant difference in overall mortality or serious adverse events with computerised decision support versus usual care.[40]

Comment: We found limited evidence (from small trials with short follow up of proxy outcomes) on the use of computerised decision support in oral anticoagulation management. Computerised decision support for oral anticoagulation seems to be at least as effective as human performance in terms of time spent in the target international normalised ratio range. It is not clear if this will translate to improved clinical outcomes. Larger and longer trials that measure clinical outcomes (particularly harms) are needed.

GLOSSARY

Computerised decision support system A computer program that provides advice on the significance and implications of clinical findings or laboratory results.

International normalised ratio (INR) A value derived from a standardised laboratory test that measures the effect of an anticoagulant. The laboratory materials used in the test are calibrated against internationally accepted standard reference preparations, so that variability between laboratories and different reagents is minimised. Normal blood has an international normalised ratio of 1. Therapeutic anticoagulation often aims to achieve an international normalised ratio value of 2.0–3.5.

Low molecular weight heparin (LMWH) is made from heparin using chemical or enzymatic methods. The various formulations of LMWH differ in mean molecular weight, composition, and anticoagulant activity. As a group, LMWHs have distinct properties and it is not yet clear if one LMWH will behave exactly like another. Some LMWHs given subcutaneously do not require monitoring.

Major haemorrhage Exact definitions vary between studies but usually a major haemorrhage is one involving intracranial, retroperitoneal, joint, or muscle bleeding leading directly to death or requiring admission to hospital to stop the bleeding or provide a blood transfusion. All other haemorrhages are classified as minor.

Substantive changes

Unfractionated and low molecular weight heparin Two RCTs added;[25,30] conclusions unchanged.

REFERENCES

1. Nordstrom M, Linblad B, Bergqvist D, et al. A prospective study of the incidence of deep-vein thrombosis within a defined urban population. *Arch Intern Med* 1992;326:155–160.
2. Hansson PO, Werlin L, Tibblin G, et al. Deep vein thrombosis and pulmonary embolism in the general population. *Arch Intern Med* 1997;157:1665–1670.
3. Rubinstein I, Murray D, Hoffstein V. Fatal pulmonary emboli in hospitalised patients: an autopsy study. *Arch Intern Med* 1988;148:1425–1426.
4. Hirsh J, Hoak J. Management of deep vein thrombosis and pulmonary embolism. *Circulation* 1996;93:2212–2245.
5. Farley TMM, Meirik O, Chang CL, et al. Effects of different progestogens in low oestrogen oral contraceptives on venous thromboembolic disease. *Lancet* 1995;346:1582–1588.
6. Lagerstedt C, Olsson C, Fagher B, et al. Need for long term anticoagulant treatment in symptomatic calf vein thrombosis. *Lancet* 1985;334:515–518.
7. Lohr J, Kerr T, Lutter K, et al. Lower extremity calf thrombosis: to treat or not to treat? *J Vasc Surg* 1991;14:618–623.
8. Kakkar VV, Howe CT, Flanc C, et al. Natural history of postoperative deep vein thrombosis. *Lancet* 1969;ii:230–232.
9. Zilliacus H. On the specific treatment of thrombosis and pulmonary embolism with anticoagulants, with a particular reference to the post thrombotic sequelae. *Acta Med Scand* 1946;s171:1–221.
10. Giannoukas AD, Labropoulos N, Burke P, et al. Calf deep vein thrombosis: a review of the literature. *Eur J Vasc Endovasc Surg* 1995;10:398–404.
11. Lensing AWA, Prandoni P, Prins MH, et al. Deep-vein thrombosis. *Lancet* 1999;353:479–485.
12. Brandjes DPM, Heijboer H, Buller HR, et al. Acenocoumarol and heparin compared with acenocoumarol alone in the initial treatment of proximal-vein thrombosis. *N Engl J Med* 1992;327:1485–1489.
13. Hutten BA, Prins MH. Duration of treatment with vitamin K antagonists in symptomatic venous thromboembolism. In: The Cochrane Library, Issue 1, 2002. Oxford: Update Software. Search date 2000; primary sources Medline, Embase, hand searches of relevant journals, and personal contacts.
14. Pinede L, Duhaut P, Cucherat M, et al. Comparison of long versus short duration of anticoagulant therapy after a first episode of venous thromboembolism: a meta-analysis of randomized, controlled trials. *J Intern Med* 2000;247:553–562. Search date not stated; primary sources Medline, Embase, Cochrane Controlled Trials Register, and hand searches of reference lists.
15. Pinede L, Ninet J, Duhaut P, et al. Comparison of 3 and 6 months of oral anticoagulant therapy after a first episode of proximal deep vein thrombosis or pulmonary embolism and comparison of 6 and 12 weeks of therapy after isolated calf deep vein thrombosis. *Circulation* 2001;103:2453–2460.
16. Agnelli G, Prandoni P, Santamaria MG, et al. Three months versus one year of oral anticoagulant therapy for idiopathic deep venous thrombosis. Warfarin Optimal Duration Italian Trial Investigators. *N Engl J Med* 2001;345:165–169.
17. Hull R, Hirsh J, Jay RM, et al. Different intensities of oral anticoagulant therapy in the treatment of proximal vein thrombosis. *N Engl J Med* 1982;307:1676–1681.
18. Ascani A, Iorio A, Agnelli G. Withdrawal of warfarin after deep vein thrombosis: effects of a low fixed dose on rebound thrombin generation. *Blood Coagul Fibrinolysis* 1999;10:291–295.
19. Landefeld CS, Beyth RJ. Anticoagulant related bleeding: clinical epidemiology, prediction, and prevention. *Am J Med* 1993;95:315–328.
20. Levine MN, Hirsh J, Landefeld CS, et al. Haemorrhagic complications of anticoagulant treatment. *Chest* 1992;102(suppl):352–363.
21. Lensing AWA, Prins MH, Davidson BL, et al. Treatment of deep venous thrombosis with low-molecular weight heparins. *Arch Intern Med* 1995;155:601–607. Search date 1994; primary sources Medline, and manual and hand searches of references.
22. Belcaro G, Nicolaides AN, Cesarone MR, et al. Comparison of low-molecular-weight heparin, administered primarily at home, with unfractionated heparin, administered in hospital, and subcutaneous heparin, administered at home for deep-vein thrombosis. *Angiology* 1999;50:781–787.
23. Van der Heijden JF, Prins MH, Buller HR. For the initial treatment of venous thromboembolism: are all low-molecular-weight heparin compounds the same? *Thromb Res* 2000;10:V121–V130. Search date not stated; primary sources Medline, Embase, and Current Contents.
24. Breddin HK, Hach-Wunderle V, Nakov R, et al. Effects of a low-molecular-weight heparin on thrombus regression and recurrent thromboembolism in patients with deep-vein thrombosis. *N Engl J Med* 2001;344:626–631.
25. Harenberg J, Schmidt JA, Koppenhagen K, et al. Fixed-dose, body weight-independent subcutaneous LMW heparin versus adjusted dose unfractionated intravenous heparin in the initial treatment of proximal venous thrombosis. EASTERN Investigators. *Thromb Haemost* 2000;83:652–656.
26. Couturaud F, Julian JA, Kearon C. Low molecular weight heparin administered once versus twice daily in patients with venous thromboembolism: a meta-analysis. *Thromb Haemost* 2001;86:980–984. Search date 1999; primary sources Medline, The Cochrane Library, hand searches of reference lists, and personal files of local experts.
27. Van Der Heijden JF, Hutten BA, Buller HR, et al. Vitamin K antagonists or low-molecular-weight

heparin for the long term treatment of symptomatic venous thromboembolism. In: The Cochrane Library, Issue 1, 2002. Oxford: Update Software. Search date 2001; primary sources Medline, Embase, Current Contents, hand searches of relevant journals, and personal contacts.
28. Schraibman IG, Milne AA, Royle EM. Home versus in-patient treatment for deep vein thrombosis. In: The Cochrane Library, Issue 1, 2002. Oxford: Update Software. Search date 2000; primary sources Medline, Embase, Cochrane Controlled Trials Register, and hand searches of relevant journals.
29. Dolovich LR, Ginsberg JS, Douketis JD, et al. A meta-analysis comparing low-molecular-weight heparins with unfractionated heparin in the treatment of venous thromboembolism. *Arch Intern Med* 2000;160:181–188. Search date 1996; primary sources Medline, HEALTH, The Cochrane Library, and hand searches of references.
30. Lindhoff-Last E, Nakov R, Misselwitz F, et al. Incidence and clinical relevance of heparin-induced antibodies in patients with deep vein thrombosis treated with unfractionated or low-molecular-weight heparin. *Br J Haematol* 2002;118:1137–1142.
31. Brandjes DPM, Büller HR, Heijboer H, et al. Randomised trial of effect of compression stockings in patients with symptomatic proximal-vein thrombosis. *Lancet* 1997;349:759–762.
32. Barrit DW, Jordan SC. Anticoagulant drugs in the treatment of pulmonary embolism: a controlled trial. *Lancet* 1960;i:1309–1312.
33. Simonneau G, Sors H, Charbonnier B, et al. A comparison of low-molecular weight heparin with unfractionated heparin for acute pulmonary embolism. *N Engl J Med* 1997;337:663–669.
34. Hull RD, Raskob GE, Brant RF, et al. Low-molecular-weight heparin vs heparin in the treatment of patients with pulmonary embolism. American–Canadian Thrombosis Study Group. *Arch Intern Med* 2000;160:229–236.
35. Arcasoy SM, Kreit JW. Thrombolytic therapy for pulmonary embolism. A comprehensive review of current evidence. *Chest* 1999;115:1695–1707. Search date 1998; primary sources Medline and hand searches of reference lists of retrieved articles.
36. Konstantinides S, Geibel A, Heusel G, et al. Heparin plus alteplase compared with heparin alone in patients with submassive pulmonary embolism. *N Engl J Med* 2002;347:1143–1150.
37. Konstantinides S, Geibel A, Olschewski M, et al. Association between thrombolytic treatment and the prognosis of haemodynamically stable patients with major pulmonary embolism: results of a multicentre registry. *Circulation* 1997;96:882–888.
38. Levine MN, Goldhaber SZ, Gore JM, et al. Haemorrhagic complications of thrombolytic therapy in the treatment of myocardial infarction and venous thromboembolism. *Chest* 1995;108:291S–301S. Search date not stated; primary sources not stated.
39. Chatellier G, Colombet I, Degoulet P. An overview of the effect of computer-assisted management of anticoagulant therapy on the quality of anticoagulation. *Int J Med Inf* 1998;49:311–320. Search date 1997; primary source Medline.
40. Poller L, Shiach CR, MacCallum PK, et al. Multicentre randomised study of computerised anticoagulant dosage. European Concerted Action on Anticoagulation. *Lancet* 1998;352:1505–1509.
41. Fitzmaurice DA, Hobbs FDR, Murray ET, et al. Oral anticoagulation management in primary care with the use of computerized decision support and near-patient testing. Randomized Controlled Trial. *Arch Intern Med* 2000;160:2343–2348.
42. Ageno W, Turpie AG. A randomized comparison of a computer-based dosing program with a manual system to monitor oral anticoagulant therapy. *Thromb Res* 1998;91:237–240.
43. Manotti C, Moia M, Palareti G, et al. Effect of computer-aided management on the quality of treatment in anticoagulated patients: a prospective, randomized, multicenter trial of APROAT (Automated PRogram for Oral Anticoagulant Treatment). *Haematologica* 2001;86:1060–1070.
44. Motykie GD, Mokhtee D, Zebala LP, et al. The use of a Bayseian Forecasting Model in the management of warfarin therapy after total hip arthroplasty. *J Arthroplasty* 1999;14:988–993.

David Fitzmaurice
Senior Lecturer

FD Richard Hobbs
Professor

Richard McManus
Clinical Research Fellow

Department of Primary Care and General Practice
The Medical School University of Birmingham
Birmingham
UK

Competing interests: RM none declared. FDRH is a member of the European Society of Cardiology (ESC) Working Party on Heart Failure, Treasurer of the British Society for Heart Failure, and Chair of the British Primary Care Cardiovascular Society (PCCS). He has received travel sponsorship and honoraria from several multinational biotechnology and pharmaceutical companies with cardiovascular products for plenary talks and attendance at major cardiology scientific congresses and conferences. DF has been reimbursed by LEO Laboratories for speaking at and attending symposia.

Varicose veins

Search date November 2002

Bazian Ltd

QUESTIONS

INTERVENTIONS

See glossary, p 294

Key Messages

- **Compression stockings** One crossover RCT found no significant difference in symptoms between compression stockings for 4 weeks versus no treatment in people with varicose veins. However, the study may have lacked power to exclude clinically important effects.
- **Injection sclerotherapy** One systematic review has found no RCTs comparing injection sclerotherapy versus no treatment or compression stockings in people with varicose veins. One RCT has found no significant difference between injection sclerotherapy with polidocanol versus sodium tetradecyl sulphate for improving appearance of varicose veins not due to saphenofemoral or saphenopopliteal incompetence at 16 weeks.
- **Surgery (*v* injection sclerotherapy)** We found no RCTs comparing surgery versus no treatment or compression stockings. One RCT found that surgery significantly improved cure of varicose veins compared with injection sclerotherapy at 5 years in people with varicose veins from saphenofemoral, saphenopopliteal, and perforator incompetence. The RCT did not report separately on effects of surgery for each site of venous incompetence.

Varicose veins

DEFINITION Although we found no consistent definition of varicose veins,[1] the term is commonly taken to mean veins that are distended and tortuous. Any vein may become varicose, but the term "varicose veins" conventionally applies to varices of the superficial leg veins. The condition is caused by poorly functioning valves within the lumen of the veins. Blood flows from the deep to the superficial venous systems through these incompetent valves, causing persistent superficial venous hypertension, which leads to varicosity of the superficial veins. Common sites of valvular incompetence include the saphenofemoral and saphenopopliteal junctions and perforating veins connecting the deep and superficial venous systems along the length of the leg. Sites of venous incompetence are determined by clinical examination or, more reliably, by Doppler ultrasound. Symptoms of varicose veins include distress about cosmetic appearance, pain, itch, limb heaviness, and cramps. This review focuses on uncomplicated, symptomatic varicose veins. We have excluded treatments for chronic venous ulceration and other complications. We have also excluded studies that solely examine treatments for small, dilated veins in the skin of the leg, known as thread veins, spider veins, or superficial telangiectasia.

INCIDENCE/ PREVALENCE One large US cohort study found the annual incidence of varicose veins to be 2.6% in women and 1.9% in men.[2] Incidence was constant over the age of 40 years. The prevalence of varicose veins in Western populations is about 25–30% among women and 10–20% in men.[3]

AETIOLOGY/ RISK FACTORS One large case control study found that women with two or more pregnancies were at increased risk of varicose veins compared with women with fewer than two pregnancies (RR about 1.2–1.3 after adjustment for age, height, and weight).[2] It found that obesity was also a risk factor, although only among women (RR about 1.3). One narrative systematic review found insufficient evidence about effects of other suggested risk factors, including genetic predisposition; prolonged sitting or standing; tight undergarments; low fibre diet; constipation; deep vein thrombosis; and smoking.[3]

PROGNOSIS We found no reliable data about prognosis, nor about the frequency of complications, which include chronic inflammation of affected veins (phlebitis), venous ulceration, and rupture of varices.

AIMS OF INTERVENTION Treating varicose veins aims to reduce symptoms; improve appearance; and prevent recurrence and complications, with minimal adverse effects.

OUTCOMES Symptoms, including pain, ache, itch, heaviness, cramps, and cosmetic distress or cosmetic appearance (self or physician rated); quality of life; recurrence rates; complications of treatment, including haematoma formation; pigmentation; ulceration; superficial thrombophlebitis; and deep venous and pulmonary thromboembolism. Retreatment rates were only considered if other outcomes were unavailable and are described only in comments.

METHODS *Clinical Evidence* search and appraisal November 2002.

QUESTION What are effects of treatments in adults with varicose veins?

OPTION COMPRESSION STOCKINGS

One crossover RCT found no significant difference in symptoms between compression stockings for 4 weeks versus no treatment in people with varicose veins. However, the study may have lacked power to exclude clinically important effects.

Benefits: **Versus no treatment:** We found one crossover RCT (72 people aged < 65 years with ≥ 2 of the following symptoms: pain, heaviness, itch, night cramps, swelling, or cosmetic distress).[4] People with a history of deep vein thrombosis were excluded. The study did not specify the sites of venous incompetence. It compared four treatments: a pharmacological agent (O-[beta-hydroxyethyl]-rutosides, 1 g/day orally); placebo alone; stockings plus placebo; and stockings plus the drug. Stockings were fitted to apply a pressure of 30–40 mm Hg to each ankle. Each treatment was given for 4 weeks before crossover to another treatment. The trial found no significant difference between stockings plus placebo versus placebo alone for any symptom scores after each treatment (analysis not by intention to treat; 6 people excluded from analysis; symptom scores measured on 100 point visual analogue scale [high score = more severe]; pain: mean score 35 with stockings *v* 38 with placebo, $P = 0.06$; heaviness: 34 *v* 36, $P = 0.39$; itch: 32 *v* 31, $P = 0.56$; swelling: 28 *v* 35, $P = 0.13$; night cramps: 22 *v* 25, $P = 0.24$; cosmetic distress: 43 *v* 41, $P = 0.43$). The RCT may have lacked power to exclude clinically important effects. **Versus injection sclerotherapy:** See benefits of injection sclerotherapy, p 291. **Versus surgery:** See benefits of surgery, p 292.

Harms: The RCT did not report on harms of compression stockings.

Comment: **Versus no treatment:** The RCT did not report whether investigators were blinded to treatment allocation and did not report on the validity and reliability of symptom scales.[4] Reliability of results may be reduced because previous treatments may continue to have effects even after crossover. The study did not report the duration of any washout period, which may have reduced such an effect between treatment periods.

OPTION INJECTION SCLEROTHERAPY

One systematic review has found no RCTs comparing injection sclerotherapy versus no treatment or compression stockings in people with varicose veins. One RCT has found no significant difference between injecting polidocanol versus sodium tetradecyl sulphate for improving appearance of varicose veins that are not due to saphenofemoral or saphenopopliteal incompetence at 16 weeks.

Benefits: **Versus no treatment:** One systematic review (search date 2001) found no RCTs.[1] **Versus compression stockings:** One systematic review (search date 2001) found no RCTs.[1] **Different types of**

sclerosant: One systematic review (search date 2001) found no RCTs reporting clinical outcomes in people with varicose veins (see comment below).[1] We found one subsequent RCT (129 people with a total of 169 varicose veins; 58 veins < 1 mm diameter; 55 veins 1–3 mm diameter; 54 veins 3–6 mm diameter).[5] People with saphenofemoral or saphenopopliteal incompetence were excluded. Each vein, rather than each person, was randomly allocated to injection sclerotherapy with polidocanol versus sodium tetradecyl sulphate. The strength of solution depended on size of vein being treated (veins < 1 mm diameter: polidocanol 0.5% or sodium tetradecyl sulphate 0.5%; veins 1–3 mm diameter: polidocanol 1% or sodium tetradecyl sulphate 0.5%; veins 3–6 mm diameter: polidocanol 3% or sodium tetradecyl sulphate 1.5%). The study found no significant difference between polidocanol or sodium tetradecyl sulphate for change in photographic appearance of veins 16 weeks after treatment (mean score on a scale of 1 to 5 [1 = worse than pretreatment photograph; 5 = complete disappearance] 4.5 with both treatments; P = 0.12). **Versus surgery:** See benefits of surgery, p 292.

Harms: **Different types of sclerosant:** The systematic review found no RCTs examining the effect of sclerosant in veins other than thread veins.[1] The subsequent RCT only reported local reactions.[5] It found that both treatments were associated with similar rates of ecchymosis (70% of veins treated with sodium tetradecyl sulphate *v* 58% with polidocanol), hyperpigmentation (64% *v* 53%), and thrombosis (46% *v* 42%; significance not stated for any comparison). Polidocanol reduced local urticaria and skin necrosis compared with sodium tetradecyl sulphate (skin necrosis 7% with sodium tetradecyl sulphate *v* 0% with polidocanol; urticaria 36% *v* 23%, P value not stated). **Versus surgery:** See harms of surgery, p 292.

Comment: **Different types of sclerosant:** In the subsequent RCT, assessors were blinded to treatment allocation.[4] **Versus surgery:** See comment under surgery, p 292.

OPTION SURGERY VERSUS NON-SURGICAL TREATMENT

We found no RCTs comparing surgery versus no treatment or compression stockings. One RCT found that surgery significantly improved cure of varicose veins compared with injection sclerotherapy at 5 years in people with varicose veins from saphenofemoral, saphenopopliteal, and perforator incompetence. The RCT did not report separately on effects of surgery for each site of venous incompetence.

Benefits: **Versus no treatment:** We found no RCTs. **Versus compression stockings:** We found no RCTs. **Versus injection sclerotherapy:** We found two RCTs comparing surgical versus non-surgical treatments for varicose veins.[5–7] The first RCT (164 people with symptomatic primary varicose veins, aged 21–65 years) compared surgery versus injection sclerotherapy (hydroxypolyaethoxydodecan 30 mg/mL; 0.5–0.75 mL injected into each varicosity, repeated after 1–2 wks if required).[6] People were allocated to treatments without regard for site of venous incompetence (53 legs with saphenofemoral or saphenopopliteal incompetence alone; 97 legs with saphenofemoral or saphenopopliteal incompetence combined with perforator incompetence; 17 with perforator incompetence only). Among people allocated to surgery, the surgical technique depended on the site of venous incompetence (see comment below). The trial found that surgery improved physician rated cure rate compared with injection sclerotherapy at 5 years ("cure" defined as no varicose veins; 55% with surgery *v* 3% with sclerotherapy; see comment below). The second RCT (249 people with varicose veins but no prior treatment, aged 15–64 years) compared surgery versus injection sclerotherapy.[7] The study did not specify the proportions of people with saphenofemoral, saphenopopliteal, or perforator incompetence. The extent and type of surgery depended on the site of venous incompetence (see comment below). The trial did not report on symptoms, quality of life, or recurrence (see comment below).

Harms: **Versus injection sclerotherapy:** The first RCT reported postoperative wound infection in 6% and symptoms of sural or saphenous nerve injury in 10% of surgically treated patients (rates not reported in sclerotherapy group).[6] Five people (proportion not stated) in the sclerotherapy group had migratory thrombophlebitis and 28% developed haematoma (rates not reported in surgical group). Duration of sick leave was greater with surgery versus sclerotherapy (mean duration 20 days with surgery *v* 1 day with sclerotherapy; significance not stated). One person in the surgical arm had a symptomatic pulmonary embolism that resolved without complications. No thromboembolic events occurred in the sclerotherapy group. The second RCT reported that one person in the surgically treated group had severe bronchospasm under anaesthetic.[7] The 5 year follow up study reported that during surgery one person had a myocardial infarction and one person had a pulmonary embolus.[8]

Comment: The effects of surgery versus injection sclerotherapy or other treatments may vary according to the sites of venous incompetence. However, none of the identified RCTs reported relative effects with regard to sites of venous incompetence. In the surgical groups of both RCTs, varicose veins from saphenofemoral or saphenopopliteal incompetence were treated by ligation and stripping (see glossary, p 294). Incompetent perforator veins were treated by avulsion (see glossary, p 294). **Versus injection sclerotherapy:** The first RCT did not report whether the investigators were blinded to treatment allocation.[6] It was not clear whether analysis was by intention to treat. The follow up rate at 5 years was about 77%. The second RCT found that surgery reduced retreatment rates compared with sclerotherapy at 3 years (14% with surgery *v* 22% with sclerotherapy; significance not stated).[7] Five year follow up of the same RCT also found that surgery reduced retreatment rates (24.2% with surgery *v* 40% with sclerotherapy; significance not stated; no blinding of assessors).[8] We found one published protocol for an ongoing systematic review on surgery for varicose veins.[9] Results will be reported in *Clinical Evidence* following publication of the completed review.

GLOSSARY

Avulsion is typically used to treat multiple varicosities, typically caused by perforator incompetence. Small incisions are made in the skin overlying each varicosity and the affected vein excised.

Ligation involves tying off a vein close to the site of incompetence to prevent blood flowing from the deep to the superficial system.

Stripping A wire is passed along the lumen of the saphenous vein and is then used to strip the entire vein out of the leg. This disconnects any superficial veins from the deep venous system.

REFERENCES

1. Tisi PV, Beverley CA. Injection sclerotherapy for varicose veins (Cochrane Review). In: The Cochrane Library, Issue 4, 2002. Oxford: Update Software. Search date 2001; primary sources Embase, Medline, hand searches of references and relevant journals, and contact with manufacturers.
2. Brand FN, Dannenberg AL, Abbott RD, et al. The epidemiology of varicose veins: the Framingham study. *Am J Prev Med* 1988;4:99–101.
3. Kurz X, Kahn SR, Abenhaim L, et al. Chronic venous disorders of the leg: epidemiology, outcomes, diagnosis and management. Summary of an evidence-based report of the VEINES* task force. *Int Angiol* 1998;18:83–102.
4. Anderson JH, Geraghty JG, Wilson YT, et al. Paroven and graduated compression hosiery for superficial venous insufficiency. *Phlebology* 1990;5:271–276.
5. Goldman MP. Treatment of varicose and telangiectatic leg veins: double blind prospective comparative trial between aethoxyskerol and sotradecol. *Dermatol Surg* 2002;28:52–55.
6. Einarsson E, Eklof B, Neglen P. Sclerotherapy or surgery as treatment for varicose veins: a prospective randomized study. *Phlebology* 1993;8:22–26.
7. Chant ADB, Jones HO, Weddell JM. Varicose veins: a comparison of surgery and injection/compression sclerotherapy. *Lancet* 1972;2:1188–1191.
8. Beresford SAA, Chant ADB, Jones HO, et al. Varicose veins: a comparison of surgery and injection/compression sclerotherapy. *Lancet* 1978;29:921–924.
9. Michaels JA, Kendall RJ. Surgery for varicose veins (protocol for a Cochrane review). In: The Cochrane Library, Issue 3, 2001. Oxford. Update Software.

Bazian Ltd
London
UK

Competing interests: None declared.

Absence seizures in children

Search date January 2003

Ewa Posner

QUESTIONS

INTERVENTIONS

*We found no RCT evidence for valproate or ethosuximide versus placebo but there is consensus belief that valproate and ethosuximide are beneficial in typical absence seizures.

See glossary, p 300

Key Messages

- **Ethosuximide** We found no systematic review or RCTs comparing ethosuximide versus placebo. There is consensus that ethosuximide is beneficial. Ethosuximide is associated with rare but serious adverse effects, including aplastic anaemia, skin reactions, and renal and hepatic impairment. We found no RCTs comparing ethosuximide versus other anticonvulsants (except valproate) in children with typical absence seizures.
- **Lamotrigine** One RCT found that, compared with placebo, lamotrigine increased the proportion of children who remained seizure free. However, lamotrigine is associated with serious skin reactions. We found no RCTs comparing lamotrigine versus other anticonvulsants.
- **Valproate** We found no RCTs comparing valproate versus placebo. There is consensus that valproate is beneficial. Valproate is associated with rare but serious adverse effects, including behavioural and cognitive abnormalities, liver necrosis, and pancreatitis. Three small RCTs found no significant difference between valproate and ethosuximide. We found no RCTs comparing valproate versus other anticonvulsants (except ethosuximide) in children with typical absence seizures.
- **Gabapentin** One brief RCT found no significant difference between gabapentin versus placebo in the frequency of typical absence seizures.

Absence seizures in children

DEFINITION Absence seizures are sudden episodes of unconsciousness lasting a few seconds. Depending on electroencephalogram findings, they are divided into typical and atypical seizures. Typical absence seizures are associated with an electroencephalogram showing regular symmetrical generalised spike and wave complexes with a frequency of 3 Hz. Absence seizures may be the only type of seizures experienced by a child and this then constitutes an epileptic syndrome (see glossary, p 300) called childhood absence epilepsy. In many children, typical absence seizures coexist with other types of seizures. Atypical absence seizures do not show the characteristic electroencephalogram pattern of typical absence seizures; are usually one of many types of seizures in a child with a background of learning disability and severe epilepsy; and tend to be less defined in time.[1] This differentiation into typical versus atypical seizures is important as the natural history and response to treatment varies in the two groups. Interventions for atypical absence seizures are not included in this topic.

INCIDENCE/ PREVALENCE About 10% of seizures in children with epilepsy are typical absence seizures.[1] Annual incidence has been estimated at 0.7–4.6/100 000 people in the general population and 6–8/100 000 in children aged 0–15 years. Prevalence is 5–50/100 000 people in the general population.[2] Age of onset ranges from 3–13 years with a peak at 6–7 years.

AETIOLOGY/ RISK FACTORS The cause is presumed to be genetic.

PROGNOSIS In childhood absence epilepsy, in which typical absence seizures are the only type of seizures suffered by the child, seizures cease spontaneously after a few years. In other epileptic syndromes (in which absence seizures may coexist with other types of seizures) prognosis is varied, depending on the syndrome. Absence seizures have significant impact on quality of life. The episode of unconsciousness may occur at any time. Absence seizures usually occur without warning. Affected children need to take precaution to prevent injury during absences. Often school staff are the first to notice the recurrent episodes of absence seizures and treatment is needed because of the impact on learning.

AIMS OF INTERVENTION Cessation or decrease in the frequency of seizures, with minimum adverse effects of treatment.

OUTCOMES Seizure frequency measured as normalisation of the electroencephalogram; adverse effects of treatment with anticonvulsants. We found no studies assessing quality of life.

METHODS *Clinical Evidence* search and appraisal January 2003.

QUESTION **What are the effects of treatments for typical absence seizures in children?**

OPTION **VALPROATE**

We found no RCTs comparing valproate versus placebo. There is consensus that valproate is beneficial. Valproate is associated with rare but serious adverse effects, including behavioural and cognitive

abnormalities, liver necrosis, and pancreatitits. Three small RCTs found no significant difference between valproate and ethosuximide. We found no RCTs comparing valproate versus other anticonvulsants (except ethosuximide) in children with typical absence seizures.

Benefits: We found no systematic review. **Versus placebo:** We found no RCTs comparing valproate (sodium valproate or valproic acid) versus placebo. **Versus ethosuximide:** We found three RCTs.[3–5] The first RCT (45 children and adolescents aged 4–18 years with absence seizures, including children with other seizure types, children refractory to anticonvulsant treatment, and children who had not previously received any anticonvulsant treatment [naïve children]) compared valproic acid versus ethosuximide followed by a crossover after 6 weeks.[4] Response to treatment was defined as no generalised spike-wave discharges on 12 hour telemetered electroencephalogram. The RCT found no significant difference in response with valproic acid versus ethosuximide at 6 weeks (naïve: 6/7 [85.7%] with valproic acid *v* 4/9 [44.4%] with ethosuximide; RR 1.93, 95% CI 0.88 to 4.25; refractory: 3/15 [20%] with valproic acid *v* 4/14 [28.6%] with ethosuximide; RR 0.70, 95% CI 0.19 to 2.59).[4] The second RCT (28 naïve children and adolescents aged 4–15 years with typical absence seizures) compared sodium valproate versus ethosuximide for up to 4 years. Response was measured by 6 hour telemetry at two intervals of 6 months and parent and teacher reports of seizure frequency. The RCT found no significant difference with sodium valproate versus ethosuximide in overall improvement (> 50% decrease in the seizure frequency over 6 months, 12/14 [85.7%] with sodium valproate *v* 11/13 [84.6%] with ethosuximide; RR 1.01, 95% CI 0.74 to 1.39).[3] The third RCT (20 children aged 5–8 years) compared sodium valproate versus ethosuximide for up to 2 years in children with recent (< 6 months) onset of absence seizures.[5] Seizure frequency was assessed using parent-completed record cards and electroencephalogram recordings. The RCT found no significant difference in complete remission of seizures with sodium valproate versus ethosuximide (7/10 [70%] with sodium valproate *v* 8/10 [80%] with ethosuximide; RR 0.88, 95% CI 0.53 to 1.46).[5] **Versus other anticonvulsants:** We found no RCTs.

Harms: **Versus placebo:** We found no RCTs comparing valproate versus placebo. Common adverse effects associated with valproic acid include dyspepsia, weight gain, tremor, transient hair loss, and haematological abnormalities. Rare adverse effects include behavioural and cognitive abnormalities, potentially fatal liver necrosis, and pancreatitis.[1] **Versus ethosuximide:** One RCT reported adverse events in children who had not previously received any anticonvulsant treatment. The adverse events with valproic acid and ethosuximide included nausea, vomiting, poor appetite, drowsiness, dizziness, headache, and leukopenia. Transient thrombocytopenia occurred in two children with valproic acid. No child withdrew from the trial because of these events.[4] Another RCT reported acute pancreatitis (1 child) and weight gain not responding to dietary restriction (1 child) with sodium valproate, and drowsiness (1 child receiving a high dose of ethosuximide).[3] A third RCT reported infrequent adverse events with both sodium valproate (transient nausea and vomiting, decreased number of platelets without thrombocytopenia) and ethosuximide (tiredness).[5]

Comment: The RCTs comparing sodium valproate versus ethosuximide suggest a beneficial effect with sodium valproate and ethosuximide.[3–5] We found one study (crossover, 35 children with typical absence seizures) comparing sodium valproate versus ethosuximide or placebo for 4 weeks.[6] This is an old study reported in Japanese. A summary of the results in English reported together with another RCT[3] suggests that it found no significant difference between sodium valproate versus ethosuximide.[6]

OPTION ETHOSUXIMIDE

We found no systematic review or RCTs comparing ethosuximide versus placebo. There is consensus that ethosuximide is beneficial. Ethosuximide is associated with rare but serious adverse effects, including aplastic anaemia, skin reactions, and renal and hepatic impairment. We found no RCTs comparing ethosuximide versus other anticonvulsants (except valproate) in children with typical absence seizures.

Benefits: We found no systematic review. **Versus placebo:** We found no systematic review or RCTs comparing ethosuximide versus placebo. **Versus valproate:** See benefits of valproate, p 297. **Versus other anticonvulsants:** We found no RCTs.

Harms: **Versus placebo:** We found no RCTs comparing ethosuximide versus placebo. Common adverse effects associated with ethosuximide include gastrointestinal disturbances, anorexia, weight loss, drowsiness, photophobia, headache, and behaviour and psychotic disturbances. Rare adverse effects include aplastic anaemia, serious skin reactions, and renal and hepatic impairment.[1] **Versus valproate:** See harms of valproate, p 297.

Comment: None.

OPTION LAMOTRIGINE

One RCT found that, compared with placebo, lamotrigine increased the proportion of children who remained seizure free. However, lamotrigine is associated with serious skin reactions. We found no RCTs comparing lamotrigine versus other anticonvulsants.

Benefits: We found no systematic review. **Versus placebo:** We found one RCT (45 children and adolescents aged 3–15 years with newly diagnosed typical absence seizures) comparing lamotrigine versus placebo for 4 weeks.[7] Response was measured with 24 hour ambulatory electroencephalogram and a hyperventilation test during the electroencephalogram. The RCT found that lamotrigine versus placebo significantly increased the number of children who remained seizure free for 4 weeks (64% with lamotrigine *v* 21% with placebo; $P = 0.03$).[7] **Versus other anticonvulsants:** We found no RCTs.

Harms: The RCT reported abdominal pain, headache, nausea, anorexia, dizziness, and hyperkinesia with lamotrigine.[7] Skin rash was reported in 10/29 (35%) children, but only in one did the investigator consider it to be causally related to lamotrigine.[7] The children from this RCT were recruited into another study that looked at long term tolerability of lamotrigine.[8] It found that the most common adverse events were dizziness (23/252 [9.1%]), somnolence (20/252 [7.9%]), nausea (16/252 [6.3%]), vomiting (13/252 [5.2%]), and headache (13/252 [5.2%]). The study was an open label continuation phase of several short term clinical trials. It enrolled 252 children (43 [17%] with absence seizures, type unspecified) but 125 of them discontinued, mostly because of inadequate response or administrative reasons. The average duration of lamotrigine exposure was 96.7 weeks. A total of 17% had absence seizures. We found two open label add on studies reporting on adverse events with lamotrigine.[9,10] One add on study (117 children aged 0–17 years with various drug resistant epilepsies) reported adverse events in 25/117 (21%) children during treatment with lamotrigine, including skin rash (mainly in children also receiving sodium valproate), ataxia, drowsiness, headache, and vomiting. Skin rash was reported as the main adverse event, occurring in 12 children (10 children were receiving valproic acid) 1–18 days after initiation of lamotrigine. No correlation was found with lamotrigine blood levels.[10] Another add on study (285 children aged < 13 years with refractory epilepsies and ≥ 2 seizure types) found that rash was the most common adverse event leading to discontinuation of lamotrigine (withdrawal of 21/285 [7.4%] from the study).[9] A higher rate of withdrawal was reported from the group receiving concomitant sodium valproate (occurrence of rash according to concomitant medication, sodium valproate 22.8%, carbamazepine 11.7%, and phenytoin 10.8%). Other adverse events leading to withdrawal of two or more children treated with lamotrigine were increased seizure frequency (1.8%), somnolence (1.1%), agitation (0.7%), ataxia (0.7%), fever (0.7%), and vomiting (0.75%).[9] Serious skin rash leading to admission to hospital has been found in 1% of children.[1]

Comment: The RCT randomised a group of children who responded to treatment with lamotrigine in an open label trial (potentially introducing selection bias).[7]

OPTION GABAPENTIN

One brief RCT found no significant difference between gabapentin versus placebo in frequency of typical absence seizures.

Benefits: We found no systematic review. **Versus placebo:** We found one RCT (33 children aged 4–16 years with absence seizures) comparing gabapentin (15–20 mg/kg daily) versus placebo.[11] The study consisted of a 2 week double blind treatment phase followed by a 6 week open label phase. Response was assessed as the change from baseline in seizure frequency (measured with quantified electroencephalogram) after 2 weeks. The RCT found no significant difference between gabapentin versus placebo in frequency of typical absence seizures after 2 weeks.[11] **Versus other anticonvulsants:** We found no RCTs.

Absence seizures in children

Harms: The RCT found that somnolence and dizziness were the most frequent adverse events.[11] All reported adverse events were mild to moderate and no children withdrew from the study because of adverse events of treatment. This is consistent with the adverse effect profile of gabapentin reported by one other study.[12]

Comment: The RCT was of short duration and used relatively small doses of gabapentin.[11] The target dosage range was 15–20 mg/kg daily, although the current maintenance dose used in children with other epilepsies is 30 mg/kg daily.

GLOSSARY

Epileptic syndrome The term used in the classification of childhood seizure disorders. It relates to a recognisable clinical and electroencephalogram pattern.

Substantive changes

Lamotrigine One study added;[8] conclusions unchanged.

REFERENCES

1. Panayiotopoulos CP. Treatment of typical absence seizures and related epileptic syndromes. *Paediatr Drugs* 2001;3:379–403.
2. Duncan JS, Panayiotopoulos CP. Typical absences and related epileptic syndromes. London: Churchill Communications Europe, 1995.
3. Callaghan N, O'Hare J, O'Driscoll D, et al. Comparative study of ethosuximide and sodium valproate in the treatment of typical absence seizures (petit mal). *Dev Med Child Neurol* 1982;24:830–836.
4. Sato S, White BG, Penry JK, et al. Valproic acid versus ethosuximide in the treatment of absence seizures. *Neurology* 1982;32:157–163.
5. Martinovic Z. Comparison of ethosuximide with sodium valproate as monotherapies of absence seizures. In: Parsonage M, et al. *Advances in epileptology: 14th Epilepsy International Symposium.* New York: Raven Press, 1983:301–305.
6. Suzuki M, Maruyama H, Ishibashi Y, et al. The clinical efficacy of sodium dipropylacetate and ethosuximide for infantile epilepsy by double-blind method: especially focusing on pure minor seizure. *Igakunoayum* 1972;82:470–488.
7. Frank LM, Enlow T, Holmes GL, et al. Lamictal (lamotrigine) monotherapy for typical absence seizures in children. *Epilepsia* 1999;40:973–979.
8. Duchowny M, Gilman J, Messenheimer J, et al. Long-term tolerability and efficacy of lamotrigine in pediatric patients with epilepsy. *J Child Neurol* 2002;17:278–285.
9. Besag FM, Wallace SJ, Dulac O, et al. Lamotrigine for the treatment of epilepsy in childhood. *J Pediatr* 1995;127:991–997.
10. Schlumberger E, Chavez F, Palacios L, et al. Lamotrigine in treatment of 120 children with epilepsy. *Epilepsia* 1994;35:359–367.
11. Trudeau V, Myers S, LaMoreaux L, et al. Gabapentin in naïve childhood absence epilepsy: results from two double-blind, placebo-controlled, multicenter studies. *J Child Neurol* 1996;11:470–475.
12. Anhut H, Ashman P, Feuerstein TJ, et al. Gabapentin (Neurontin) as add-on therapy in patients with partial seizures: a double-blind, placebo-controlled study. *Epilepsia* 1994;35:795–801.

Ewa Posner
Specialist Registrar in Paediatrics
Royal Victoria Infirmary
Newcastle upon Tyne
UK

Competing interests: None declared.

Acute otitis media

Search date October 2002

Paddy O'Neill and Tony Roberts

QUESTIONS

INTERVENTIONS

Key Messages

Treatment

- **Antibiotics versus placebo** We found four systematic reviews comparing antibiotics versus placebo in acute otitis media but using different inclusion criteria and outcome measures. One review in children aged 4 months to 18 years found a significant reduction in symptoms with a range of antibiotics (cephalosporins, erythromycin, penicillins, trimethoprim–sulfamethoxazole [co-trimoxazole]) versus placebo after 7–14 days of treatment. Another review in children aged less than 2 years found no significant difference in clinical improvement with antibiotics (penicillins, sulphonamides, co-trimoxazole) versus placebo alone or versus placebo with myringotomy. A third review in children aged 4 weeks to 18 years found that antibiotics (ampicillin, amoxicillin) versus placebo or observational treatment significantly reduced clinical failure rate within 2–7 days. The final review in children aged 6 months to 15 years found that early use of antibiotics (erythromycin, penicillins) versus placebo significantly reduced the proportion of children still in pain 2–7 days after presentation and reduced the risk of developing contralateral acute otitis media. This review also found that antibiotics increased the risk of vomiting, diarrhoea, or rashes.

- **Choice of antibiotic regimen** One systematic review in children aged 4 months to 18 years found no significant difference between a range of antibiotics in rate of treatment success at 7–14 days or of middle ear effusion at 30 days. Another systematic review in children aged 4 weeks to 18 years found no significant difference between antibiotics in clinical failure rates within 7–14 days. The second review also found that adverse effects, primarily gastrointestinal, were more common with cefixime versus amoxicillin or ampicillin, and were more common with amoxicillin/clavulanate (original formulation) versus azithromycin.
- **Ibuprofen** One RCT in children aged 1–6 years receiving antibiotic treatment found that ibuprofen versus placebo significantly reduced earache as assessed by parental observation after 2 days.
- **Immediate versus delayed antibiotic treatment** One RCT in children aged 6 months to 10 years found that immediate versus delayed antibiotic treatment significantly reduced the number of days of earache, ear discharge, and amount of daily paracetamol used after the first 24 hours of illness but found no difference in daily pain scores. It also found a significant increase in diarrhoea with immediate versus delayed antibiotic treatment.
- **Myringotomy** One RCT in infants aged 3 months to 1 year found no significant difference in resolution of clinical symptoms with myringotomy only versus antibiotic only or myringotomy plus antibiotic but found higher rates of persistent infection with myringotomy only. A second RCT in children aged 2–12 years found no significant difference in reduction of pain at 24 hours or 7 days with myringotomy versus no treatment. A third RCT in children aged 7 months to 12 years found significantly higher rates of initial treatment failure (resolution of symptoms within 12 hours) for severe episodes of acute otitis media treated by myringotomy and placebo versus antibiotic.
- **Paracetamol** One RCT in children aged 1–6 years receiving antibiotic treatment found that paracetamol versus placebo significantly reduced earache as assessed by parental observation after 2 days.
- **Short versus longer courses of antibiotics** One systematic review and two subsequent RCTs have found that 10 day versus 5 day courses of antibiotics significantly reduce treatment failure, relapse, and reinfection at 8–19 days, but found no significant difference at 20–30 days.

Prevention of recurrence

- **Long term antibiotic prophylaxis** One systematic review in children and adults has found that long term antibiotic prophylaxis versus placebo significantly reduces recurrence of acute otitis media after 1 month. However, one subsequent RCT in children aged 3 months to 6 years found no significant difference between antibiotic prophylaxis and placebo in preventing recurrence. We found insufficient evidence on which antibiotic to use, for how long, and how many previous episodes of acute otitis media justify starting preventive treatment.
- **Tympanostomy (ventilation tubes)** One small RCT found that tympanostomy tube insertion versus myringotomy alone or no surgery significantly reduced the mean number of acute otitis media episodes during the first 6 month period after treatment but not during the subsequent 18 months. It also found a trend for more recurrent infections and worse hearing, after tube extrusion, in those treated with tympanostomy.

- **Xylitol chewing gum or syrup** One RCT found that xylitol syrup or chewing gum versus control significantly reduced the incidence of acute otitis media over 3 months. It found no significant difference with xylitol lozenges versus control gum. More children taking xylitol versus control withdrew because of abdominal pain or other unspecified reasons.

DEFINITION Otitis media is an inflammation in the middle ear. Subcategories include acute otitis media (AOM), recurrent AOM, and chronic suppurative otitis media. AOM is the presence of middle ear effusion in conjunction with rapid onset of one or more signs or symptoms of inflammation of the middle ear. Uncomplicated AOM is limited to the middle ear cleft.[1] AOM presents with systemic and local signs, and has a rapid onset. The persistence of an effusion beyond 3 months without signs of infection defines otitis media with effusion (also known as "glue ear"). Chronic suppurative otitis media is characterised by continuing inflammation in the middle ear causing discharge (otorrhoea) through a perforated tympanic membrane.

INCIDENCE/ PREVALENCE AOM is common and has a high morbidity and low mortality in otherwise healthy children. In the UK, about 30% of children under 3 years of age visit their general practitioner with AOM each year and 97% receive antimicrobial treatment.[2] By 3 months of age, 10% of children have had an episode of AOM. It is the most common reason for outpatient antimicrobial treatment in the USA.[3]

AETIOLOGY/ RISK FACTORS The most common bacterial causes for AOM in the USA and UK are *Streptococcus pneumoniae*, *Haemophilus influenzae*, and *Moraxella catarrhalis*.[2] Similar pathogens are found in Colombia.[4] The incidence of penicillin resistant *S pneumoniae* has risen, but rates differ between countries. The most important risk factors for AOM are young age and attendance at daycare centres, such as nursery schools. Other risk factors include being white; male sex; a history of enlarged adenoids, tonsillitis, or asthma; multiple previous episodes; bottle feeding; a history of ear infections in parents or siblings; and use of a soother or pacifier. The evidence for an effect of environmental tobacco smoke is controversial.[2]

PROGNOSIS In about 80% of children the condition resolves in about 3 days without antibiotic treatment. Serious complications are rare in otherwise healthy children but include hearing loss, mastoiditis (see glossary, p 312), meningitis, and recurrent attacks.[2] The World Health Organization estimates that each year 51 000 children under the age of 5 years die from complications of otitis media in developing countries.[5]

AIMS OF INTERVENTION To reduce the severity and duration of pain and other symptoms, to prevent complications, and to minimise adverse effects of treatment.

OUTCOMES Pain control (in infants this can be assessed by surrogate measures such as parental observation of distress/crying and analgesic use); incidence of complications such as deafness (usually divided into short and long term hearing loss), recurrent attacks of AOM, mastoiditis, and meningitis; resolution of otoscopic appearances; incidence of adverse effects of treatment.

METHODS *Clinical Evidence* search and appraisal October 2002.

QUESTION **What are the effects of treatments?**

OPTION **ANALGESICS**

One RCT in children receiving antibiotic treatment found that ibuprofen or paracetamol versus placebo significantly reduced earache as assessed by parental observation after 2 days.

Benefits: We found no systematic review but found one RCT (219 children aged 1–6 years with otoscopically diagnosed acute otitis media and receiving antibiotic treatment with cefaclor for 7 days) comparing the effect of three times daily treatment with ibuprofen or paracetamol versus placebo for 48 hours on earache (otalgia) and related outcomes.[6] It found that ibuprofen versus placebo significantly reduced earache after 2 days as assessed by parental observation (AR 5/71 [7%] with ibuprofen *v* 19/75 [25%] with placebo; RR 0.28, 95% CI 0.11 to 0.71; NNT 5, 95% CI 3 to 15) and with paracetamol versus placebo (AR 7/73 [10%] *v* 19/75 [25%] with placebo; RR 0.38, 95% CI 0.17 to 0.85; NNT 6, 95% CI 3 to 28). It found no difference between paracetamol and ibuprofen for reducing earache, and no difference between ibuprofen or paracetamol and placebo for other outcomes (appearance of the tympanic membrane; rectal temperature; and parental assessment of appetite, sleep, and playing activity).

Harms: The RCT found that 11 children experienced mild nausea, vomiting, and abdominal pain (5 [7%] taking ibuprofen, 3 [4%] taking paracetamol, and 3 [4%] taking placebo). None were withdrawn from treatment.[6]

Comment: The evidence from this RCT is limited because the assessment of the child's pain relief was based on parental observation using a scale of 0 or 1.[6] The paracetamol versus placebo result has been recalculated by *Clinical Evidence* from data in the original publication, and corrects the stated conclusions of the RCT.

OPTION **ANTIBIOTICS**

We found four systematic reviews comparing antibiotics versus placebo in acute otitis media, which used different inclusion criteria and outcome measures. Three reviews found that a range of antibiotics versus placebo significantly reduced symptoms, clinical failure rate, and pain in children aged 4 weeks to 18 years. One of these three reviews also found that antibiotics increased the risk of vomiting, diarrhoea, or rashes. Another review found no significant difference in clinical improvement with antibiotics versus placebo alone or versus placebo with myringotomy in children under 2 years of age.

Benefits: We found four systematic reviews.[1,7–9] **Versus placebo or no treatment:** One systematic review (search date 1992, 33 RCTs, 5400 children aged 4 months to 18 years) identified four RCTs (535 children receiving analgesics or other symptomatic relief).[7] Acute otitis media (AOM) was defined as bulging or opacification of the tympanic membrane with or without erythema, accompanied by at least one of the following signs: fever, otalgia, irritability, otorrhoea, lethargy, anorexia, vomiting, diarrhoea, and mobility of the tympanic membrane absent or markedly decreased. It found a significant reduction in symptoms with a range of antibiotics (cephalosporins, erythromycin, penicillins, trimethoprim–sulfamethoxazole [co-trimoxazole]) versus placebo after 7–14 days of treatment (4 RCTs; ARR 13.7%, 95% CI 8.2% to 19.2%; NNT 7, 95% CI 5 to 12).[7] The second systematic review (search date 1997, 741 children aged < 2 years) identified four RCTs comparing antibiotics (penicillins, sulphonamide, amoxicillin/clavulanic acid [co-amoxiclav]) versus placebo alone or versus placebo with myringotomy (see glossary, p 312).[8] Three RCTs used diagnosis of AOM based on otoscopic appearance of the tympanic membrane and clinical signs of acute infection and one RCT used otoscopy alone. The systematic review found no significant difference between antibiotics versus placebo in symptomatic clinical improvement within 7 days (OR 1.31, 95% CI 0.83 to 2.08). Otoscopic appearance, middle ear effusion, and bacteriology were not considered as end points.[8] A third systematic review (search date 1999, 5 RCTs, 1518 children aged 4 wks to 18 years) compared the effects of antibiotics (ampicillin, amoxicillin [amoxycillin]) versus placebo or observational treatment on clinical failure rate.[1] AOM was defined as the presence of middle ear effusion in conjunction with rapid onset of one or more signs or symptoms of inflammation of the middle ear, and was categorised as uncomplicated AOM when limited to the middle ear cleft. Clinical failure was defined as the presence of pain, fever, middle ear effusion, clinical signs of otitis media, or suppurative complications such as mastoiditis (see glossary, p 312). The review found that antibiotics (ampicillin, amoxicillin) versus placebo or observational treatment significantly reduced clinical failure rate within 2–7 days (reduction of 12.3%, 95% CI 21.8% to 2.8%; NNT 8, 95% CI 5 to 36).[1] A fourth systematic review (search date 2000, 9 RCTs, 2288 children aged 6 months to 15 years) compared early use of antibiotics (erythromycin, penicillins, sulphonamides) versus placebo.[9] AOM was defined as acute earache with at least one abnormal eardrum, otoscopic middle ear effusion, and general signs and symptoms. Pain was assessed using parental report/score card/diary or clinician assessment at 4 days. The review found that antibiotics versus placebo significantly reduced the proportion of children still in pain 2–7 days after presentation (175/1160 [15.1%] with antibiotics *v* 234/1128 [20.7%] with placebo; ARR 5.6%, 95% CI 2.5% to 8.7%; RR 0.72, 95% CI 0.62 to 0.85; NNT 17, 95% CI 11 to 40). In addition, fewer children experienced contralateral AOM (35/329 [10.6%] with antibiotics *v* 56/337 [16.6%] with placebo; ARR 5.9%, 95% CI 1.0% to 10.8%; RR 0.65, 95% CI 0.45 to 0.94). The review found no difference in the rate of subsequent recurrence of AOM (187/864 [21.6%] with antibiotics *v* 175/804 [21.8%] with placebo; RR 0.99, 95% CI 0.83 to 1.19), abnormal tympanometry at 1 month (85/234 [36.3%] with antibiotics *v* 91/238 [38.2%] with placebo; RR 0.94, 95% CI 0.74 to 1.19), or abnormal tympanometry at 3 months (38/182 [20.9%] with antibiotics *v* 49/188 [26.1%] with placebo; RR 0.80, 95% CI 0.55 to 1.16). Four RCTs (717 children) reported pain outcomes (parental report of pain or symptom diary) 24 hours after presentation. All four found no difference in pain outcomes with antibiotics versus placebo (RR 1.02, 95% CI 0.85 to 1.22). Most RCTs did not state the time interval between onset of symptoms and starting treatment; the two RCTs that did, stated 1–24 hours and about 30 hours. Only 1/2202 children developed mastoiditis (in a penicillin treated group).[9]

Harms: Two systematic reviews gave no information on adverse events.[7,8] The third systematic review found that adverse effects, primarily gastrointestinal, were more common in children on cefixime than in those on amoxicillin or ampicillin (5 RCTs, rate difference 8.4%, 95% CI 3.8% to 13.1%; NNH 12, 95% CI 8 to 27) and were more common in children on amoxicillin/clavulanate (original formulation) than in those on azithromycin (3 RCTs, rate difference −18.0, 95% CI −28.0 to −8.0; NNH 6, 95% CI 4 to 13).[1] The fourth systematic review found that antibiotics increased the risk of vomiting, diarrhoea, or rashes (AR 57/345 [17%] with antibiotics *v* 38/353 [11%] with control; RR 1.55, 95% CI 1.11 to 2.16; NNH 17, 95% CI 9 to 152).[9]

Comment: One systematic review[7] excluded two placebo controlled trials that were included in another review[9] because they included myringotomy as part of the treatment. This may have biased the results in favour of antibiotic treatment and may explain the higher absolute risk reduction quoted in the first review.[7] Another systematic review commented on the difficulty of performing meta-analyses because of the varying criteria between studies for defining AOM and outcome measures.[1] The variation between the systematic reviews that provide numbers needed to treat for the effect of antibiotics versus placebo is because of differences in entry criteria and outcome measures. We found inadequate evidence for the effectiveness of antibiotics in countries where the incidence of complicating mastoiditis is high.

OPTION CHOICE OF ANTIBIOTIC REGIMEN

One systematic review in children aged 4 months to 18 years found no significant difference between a range of antibiotics in rate of treatment success at 7–14 days or of middle ear effusion at 30 days. Another systematic review in children aged 4 weeks to 18 years found no significant difference between antibiotics in clinical failure rates within 7–14 days. The second review also found that adverse effects, primarily gastrointestinal, were more common in children on cefixime than in those on amoxicillin or ampicillin, and were more common in children on amoxicillin/clavulanate (original formulation) than in those on azithromycin.

Benefits: We found two systematic reviews.[1,7] One systematic review (search date 1992, 33 RCTs, 5400 children aged 4 months to 18 years) compared a range of antibiotics (cephalosporins, erythromycin, penicillins, co-trimoxazole).[7] Acute otitis media was defined as bulging or opacification of the tympanic membrane with or without erythema, accompanied by at least one sign (fever, otalgia, irritability, otorrhoea, lethargy, anorexia, vomiting, diarrhoea, mobility of the tympanic membrane absent or markedly decreased). Treatment success was defined as the absence of all presenting signs and symptoms of acute otitis media at the evaluation point closest to 7–17 days after start of treatment. The systematic review found no significant differences between different antibiotics in rate of treatment success at 7–14 days or of middle ear effusion at 30 days.[7] A second systematic review (search date 1999) found no significant difference between penicillin versus ampicillin or amoxicillin (amoxycillin) in clinical failure rates within 7–14 days (3 RCTs, 491 children aged 4 wks to 18 years; clinical failure rate difference +4.5%, 95% CI –1.8% to +10.7%).[1] The same review found no significant difference in clinical failure rates within 3–7 days with cefaclor versus ampicillin or amoxicillin (4 RCTs, 56 children aged 4 wks to 18 years; clinical failure rate difference –5.4%, 95% CI –15.2% to +4.4%). Clinical failure was defined as the presence of pain, fever, middle ear effusion, clinical signs of otitis media, or suppurative complications such as mastoiditis (see glossary, p 312).[1]

Harms: See harms of antibiotics, p 306.

Comment: None.

OPTION IMMEDIATE VERSUS DELAYED ANTIBIOTIC TREATMENT

One RCT in children aged 6 months to 10 years found that immediate versus delayed antibiotic treatment significantly reduced the number of days of earache, ear discharge, and amount of daily paracetamol used after the first 24 hours of illness, but found no significant difference in daily pain scores. It also found a significant increase in diarrhoea with immediate versus delayed antibiotic treatment.

Benefits: We found one RCT (315 children aged 6 months to 10 years) comparing immediate versus delayed antibiotic (amoxicillin [amoxycillin] or erythromycin) use.[10] Acute otitis media was defined as acute otalgia and otoscopic evidence of acute inflammation of the ear drum, such as dullness or cloudiness with erythema, bulging, or perforation. Immediate antibiotic treatment was defined as a prescription given to parents at the initial consultation. Delayed antibiotic treatment was defined as parents asked to wait 72 hours after seeing the doctor before using the prescription and only if the child still had substantial otalgia or fever, or was not starting to get better. Earache was assessed from daily diary of symptoms and perceived severity of pain scores (1 = no pain to 10 = extreme pain). The RCT found that, after the first 24 hours of illness, immediate versus delayed antibiotic use reduced the duration of earache (mean difference –1.10 days, 95% CI –0.54 to –1.48 days), duration of ear discharge (mean difference –0.66 days, 95% CI –0.19 to –1.13 days), number of disturbed nights (mean difference –0.72 days, 95% CI –0.30 to –1.13 days), number of days crying (mean difference –0.69 days, 95% CI –0.31 to –1.08 days), and the number of teaspoons of paracetamol used (mean difference –0.52 teaspoons daily, 95% CI –0.26 to –0.79 teaspoons daily). The RCT found no significant difference in mean daily pain score (mean difference –0.16, 95% CI –0.42 to +0.11), number of daily episodes of distress (mean difference –0.12, 95% CI –0.34 to +0.11), or days absence from school (mean difference –0.18 days, 95% CI –0.76 to +0.41 days).

Harms: The RCT found that immediate treatment increased diarrhoea (AR 25/135 [19%] with immediate *v* 14/150 [9%] with delayed; RR 1.9, 95% CI 1.08 to 3.66; NNH 11, 95% CI 5 to 125), but had no significant effect on rash (AR 6/133 [5%] with immediate *v* 8/149 [5%] with delayed; RR 0.84, 95% CI 0.30 to 2.36).[10]

Comment: None.

OPTION SHORT VERSUS LONGER COURSES OF ANTIBIOTICS

One systematic review has found that 10 day versus 5 day courses of antibiotics reduce treatment failure, relapse, or reinfection in the short term (at 8–19 days), but found no significant difference in the long term (at 20–30 days). Two subsequent RCTs found similar results.

Benefits: We found one systematic review[11] and two subsequent RCTs.[12,13] The systematic review (search date 1998, 30 RCTs in children aged 4 wks to 18 years with acute otitis media) found that treatment failure, relapse, or reinfection at an early evaluation (8–19 days) was more likely to occur with shorter courses of antibiotics (5 days) than with longer courses (8–10 days; summary OR *v* longer courses 1.52, 95% CI 1.17 to 1.98).[11] However, by 20–30 days there were no differences between treatment groups (summary OR 1.22, 95% CI 0.98 to 1.54).[11] The first subsequent RCT (385 younger children with newly diagnosed acute otitis media, mean age 13.3 months, range 4.0–30.0 months) compared amoxicillin (amoxycillin)/clavulanate in three divided doses for 10 days versus 5 days followed by 5 days of placebo.[12] Clinical success or failure was assessed at 12–14 days and again at 28–42 days after starting treatment. Intention to treat analysis found that the 10 day versus the 5 day regimen increased clinical success on days 12–14 (AR 158/186 [85%] for 10 days *v* 141/192 [73%] for 5 days; RR 1.16, 95% CI 1.04 to 1.28; NNT 8, 95% CI 5 to 30). However, by days 28–42 there was no significant difference in clinical success between the two groups (AR 108/185 [58%] for 10 days *v* 102/190 [54%] for 5 days; RR 1.09, 95% CI 0.91 to 1.30). The second subsequent RCT compared cefpodoxime/proxetil twice daily at 8 mg/kg daily for 10 days versus for 5 days followed by 5 days of placebo. It found that success rates were higher with the 10 day versus the 5 day treatment group after 12–14 days (AR 199/222 [90%] for 10 day treatment *v* 180/226 [80%] for 5 day treatment; RR 1.13, 95% CI 1.04 to 1.22; NNT 10, 95% CI 6 to 30), but no significant difference was found after 28–42 days (AR 149/222 [67%] for 10 day treatment *v* 141/226 [62%] for 5 day treatment; RR 1.08, 95% CI 0.94 to 1.23).[13]

Harms: The systematic review[11] and the two subsequent RCTs[12,13] found no difference with short versus long courses of antibiotics in diarrhoea and/or vomiting and rash.

Comment: None.

OPTION MYRINGOTOMY

One RCT in infants aged 3 months to 1 year found no significant difference in resolution of clinical symptoms with myringotomy only versus antibiotic only or myringotomy plus antibiotic, but found higher

rates of persistent infection with myringotomy only. A second RCT in children aged 2–12 years found no significant difference in reduction of pain at 24 hours or 7 days with myringotomy versus no treatment. A third RCT in children aged 7 months to 12 years found significantly higher rates of initial treatment failure (resolution of symptoms within 12 h) for severe episodes of acute otitis media treated by myringotomy and placebo versus antibiotic.

Benefits: We found no systematic review but found three RCTs.[14–16] The first RCT (105 infants aged 3 months to 1 year with acute otitis media [AOM]) compared antibiotic only (co-amoxiclav), myringotomy (see glossary, p 312) plus placebo (35 infants), or myringotomy plus antibiotic (co-amoxiclav). AOM was defined as the presence of middle ear effusion and bulging (with or without redness of the tympanic membrane) associated with recent irritability or fever. It found that after 3–6 days of treatment, irritability and fever had resolved in more than three quarters of the children, with no significant differences between groups receiving antibiotic (co-amoxiclav) only, or myringotomy plus placebo, or both.[15] The second RCT (171 children aged 2–12 years with AOM) compared no treatment (40 children), myringotomy only (36 children), amoxicillin (250 mg 3 times daily for 7 days) only (47 children), or amoxicillin plus myringotomy (48 children). AOM was diagnosed by the general practitioner on the basis of history and clinical picture. Diffuse redness and/or bluging of the eardrum was taken as decisive. The RCT found no significant difference with myringotomy alone versus no treatment in pain at 24 hours (26/36 [72%] *v* 29/40 [72%]) or pain at 7 days (31/35 [89%] *v* 34/38 [90%]).[14] The third RCT (536 infants and children stratified 7–23 months, 2–5 years and 6–12 years with AOM or recurrent AOM) compared children receiving antibiotics (amoxycillin 40 mg/kg per day in 3 divided doses for 14 days), or myringotomy, or in children aged over 2 years, myringotomy and placebo.[16] AOM was diagnosed on the basis of fever, otalgia, or irritability with redness and/or bulging of the eardrum. An episode of AOM was classified as severe or non-severe according to the child's temperature and an otalgia score. The RCT found significantly higher rates of initial treatment failure (no resolution of symptoms within 12 h) for severe episodes of AOM treated by myringotomy or placebo versus antibiotic (8/34 [23.5%] *v* 1/32 [3.1%]). It found no significant difference in the percentage of children who developed ultimate treatment failure defined as more than 180 days of ear effusion, more than four episodes of severe AOM, protocol defined need for fourth myringotomy, or a fifth myringotomy within 12 months, or a suppurative complication (16/88 [18.2%] *v* 13/80 [16.3%] for non severe episodes, and 1/13 [7.7%] *v* 3/12 [25%] for severe episodes).

Harms: In the first RCT, children in the myringotomy alone or placebo group were more likely than those receiving myringotomy plus antibiotics to have persistent ear infection (28/35 [80%] *v* 11/35 [31%]; NNH 2, 95% CI 1 to 3). At 9–11 days those in the myringotomy/placebo group compared with those receiving antibiotics had higher rates of persistent ear infection (21/30 [70%] *v* 2/30 [7%]; NNH 3,

95% CI 2 to 12) and lower rates of otoscopic recovery (7/32 [23%] *v* 18/32 [60%]; NNH 3, 95% CI 2 to 5).[15] The second RCT reported no difference in harm between the two groups.[14] The third RCT did not comment on adverse effects beyond treatment failures in the three arms of the study.[16]

Comment: Two RCTs provided results in the form of children or ears as the unit measured. As randomisation was based on children, the figures reported here exclude those based on ears.[14,15]

QUESTION **What are the effects of interventions to prevent recurrence?**

OPTION **LONG TERM ANTIBIOTIC TREATMENT**

One systematic review in children and adults has found that long term antibiotic prophylaxis versus placebo reduces recurrence of acute otitis media. However, one subsequent RCT in children aged 3 months to 6 years found no significant difference between antibiotic prophylaxis and placebo. We found insufficient evidence on which antibiotic to use, for how long, and how many episodes of acute otitis media justify starting preventive treatment.

Benefits: **Versus placebo:** We found one systematic review[17] and one subsequent RCT.[18] The systematic review (search date 1993) identified 33 RCTs comparing antibiotics versus placebo to prevent recurrent acute otitis media (AOM) and otitis media with effusion.[17] Nine of the trials (945 people) looked at recurrent AOM only. It was not clear from the review which of the studies referred only to children; four either included the word "children" in the title or appeared in paediatric journals. Most studies defined recurrent AOM as at least three episodes of AOM in 6 months. The most commonly used antibiotics were amoxicillin (amoxycillin), co-trimoxazole, and sulfamethoxazole (sulphamethoxazole) given for 3 months to 2 years. All nine studies showed a lower rate of recurrence with antibiotic treatment, although in seven of the studies the difference was not significant. Overall, the review found that antibiotics significantly reduced recurrence of AOM (AR of recurrence per person per month 8% with antibiotics *v* 19% with placebo; ARR 11%, 95% CI 3% to 19%; NNT per month to prevent 1 acute episode 9, 95% CI 5 to 33). The subsequent RCT (194 children aged 3 months to 6 years with 3 documented episodes of AOM within the preceding 6 months) compared amoxicillin (20 mg/kg/day) versus placebo.[18] The children were followed up monthly if asymptomatic or within 3–5 days if they had symptoms of upper respiratory tract infection for up to 90 days. The RCT found no significant difference between antibiotics versus placebo in preventing recurrent AOM (RR of remaining AOM free, diagnosed by otoscopy and tympanometry 1.00, 95% CI 0.66 to 1.52 using completer analysis, 36 children lost to follow up). Calculations including those children lost to follow up yielded similar results whether the outcomes were assumed in favour of placebo or in favour of antibiotics. **Choice and duration of antibiotic:** The systematic review found no significant difference in rate of recurrence between antibiotics.[17]

Harms: The studies gave no information on harms.

Comment: None.

OPTION XYLITOL CHEWING GUM OR SYRUP

One RCT found that xylitol syrup or chewing gum versus control reduced the incidence of acute otitis media. It found no significant difference with xylitol lozenges versus control gum. More children taking xylitol versus control withdrew because of abdominal pain or other unspecified reasons.

Benefits: We found no systematic review but found one RCT (857 children, 54% boys) comparing xylitol (either as chewing gum, syrup, or lozenges) versus control (syrup or chewing gum) for 3 months.[19] The RCT randomised children into two groups according to their ability to chew gum. Children who could chew gum received xylitol gum (8.4 g/day, 179 children), xylitol lozenges (10 g/day, 176 children), or control gum (xylitol 0.5 g/day, 178 children). Children who could not chew gum received xylitol syrup (10 g/day, 159 children) or control syrup (0.5 g day, 165 children). Each time the child showed any signs of acute respiratory infection, acute otitis media (AOM) was excluded using tympanometry and otoscopy. In the first group, xylitol gum versus control gum significantly reduced the proportion of children with at least one episode of AOM (AR 29/179 [16%] *v* 49/178 [28%]; RR 0.59, 95% CI 0.39 to 0.89; NNT 8, 95% CI 5 to 36) but no significant difference was found with xylitol lozenges versus control gum (AR 39/176 [22%] *v* 49/178 [28%]; RR 0.81, 95% CI 0.56 to 1.16). In the second group, xylitol syrup versus control syrup significantly reduced the proportion of children with at least one episode of AOM (AR 46/159 [29%] *v* 68/165 [41%]; RR 0.70, 95% CI 0.52 to 0.95; NNT 8, 95% CI 4 to 53).

Harms: The RCT found that more children taking xylitol lozenges or syrup versus control treatment withdrew from the trial (xylitol lozenges *v* control gum, 26/176 [15%] *v* 8/178 [5%], $P < 0.001$; xylitol syrup *v* control syrup, 30/159 [19%] *v* 17/165 [10%]; CI not provided; $P < 0.03$).[19] Most withdrawals were because of either an unwillingness to take the intervention, having left the area, or because of abdominal discomfort. We found no evidence on the long term effects of xylitol.

Comment: The children in this study received xylitol or the control intervention five times daily — a regimen that might be difficult to maintain long term.[19] The incidence of AOM in those who withdrew from the trial was not described; therefore, the reported effect of xylitol may be underestimated or overestimated.

OPTION TYMPANOSTOMY (VENTILATION) TUBES

One small RCT found that tympanostomy tube insertion versus myringotomy alone or no surgery significantly reduced the mean number of acute otitis media episodes during the first 6 month period after treatment but not during the subsequent 18 months. It also found a trend for more recurrent infections and worse hearing, after tube extrusion, in those treated with tympanostomy.

Benefits: We found no systematic review but found one RCT.[20] The RCT (44 children aged 9 months to 7 years with bilateral recurrent acute otitis media of equal severity in each ear despite over 3 months of antibiotic prophylaxis) compared tympanostomy (see glossary, p 312) with ventilation tube insertion into a randomly selected ear, with the contralateral ear receiving either no surgery, or myringotomy (see glossary, p 312) alone. Recurrent acute otitis media was defined as the recurrent presence (more than 4 episodes) of otalgia with red and bulging tympanic membranes. The RCT found that tympanostomy tube insertion versus myringotomy alone or no surgery significantly reduced the mean number of AOM episodes during the first 6 month period after treatment (–1.2, 95% CI –2.2 to –0.9), but not during the subsequent 18 months.

Harms: The RCT reported a non-significant trend ($P = 0.30$) for more recurrent infections and worse hearing in ears that had received tympanostomy tubes, which became apparent after tube extrusion.[20] Anatomical abnormalities (tympanosclerosis, atrophy, or retraction and chronic perforation, though not thought to be clinically significant) were more common in the ears receiving tympanostomy tubes. There was more tympanosclerosis in ears that received ventilating tubes than those that received myringotomy alone (35/61 [57.4%] *v* 5/26 [19.2%]; $P = 0.004$) or no surgery (35/61 [57.4%] *v* 2/27 [7.4%]; $P \le 0.0001$). At the 2 year evaluation the hearing was poorer in ears with anatomical abnormalities.

Comment: This RCT included some children with otitis media with effusion, though the results concerning benefits presented here refer only to those children in the study with recurrent acute otitis media. It was not possible from the data available to differentiate out the evidence on harms into children with recurrent acute otitis media versus otitis media with effusion. Medical treatment and antibiotic prophylaxis were allowed "whenever indicated". It was not possible from the data presented to tell whether the different groups differed in the amount of medical treatment and prophylactic antibiotics.

GLOSSARY

Mastoiditis The presence of infection in mastoid cavity.
Myringotomy The surgical creation of a perforation in tympanic membrane.
Tympanostomy The surgical creation of a perforation in tympanic membrane for the purpose of inserting a ventilation tube.

REFERENCES

1. Marcy M, Takata G, Shekelle P, et al. *Management of Acute Otitis Media. Evidence Report/Technology Assessment No.15*. (Prepared by the Southern California Evidence Based Practice Centre under contract No. 290–97-0001.) AHRQ Publication No. 01-E010. Rockville, MD: Agency for Healthcare Research and Quality, May 2001. Search date 1999; primary sources Medline, Cochrane library, Health STAR, International Pharmaceutical Abstracts, CINAL, BIOSS, EMBASE.
2. Froom J, Culpepper L, Jacobs M, et al. Antimicrobials for acute otitis media? A review from the International Primary Care Network. *BMJ* 1997;315:98–102.
3. Del Mar C, Glasziou P, Hayem M. Are antibiotics indicated as initial treatment for children with acute otitis media? A meta-analysis. *BMJ* 1997;314:1526–1529. Search date 1994; primary sources Medline and Current Contents.
4. Berman S. Otitis media in developing countries. *Pediatrics* 1995;96:126–131.
5. World Health Organization. *World Development Report 1993: Investing in Health*. Oxford: Oxford University Press, 1993:215–222.
6. Bertin L, Pons G, d'Athis P, et al. A randomized double blind multicentre controlled trial of ibuprofen versus acetaminophen and placebo for symptoms of acute otitis media in children. *Fundam Clin Pharmacol* 1996;10:387–392.
7. Rosenfeld RM, Vertrees JE, Carr J, et al. Clinical efficacy of antimicrobial drugs for acute otitis media: meta-analysis of 5400 children from

thirty-three randomised trials. *J Pediatr* 1994;124:355–367. Search date 1992; primary sources Medline and Current Contents.
8. Damoiseaux RA, van Balen FAM, Hoes AW, et al. Antibiotic treatment of acute otitis media in children under two years of age: evidence based? *Br J Gen Pract* 1998;48:1861–1864. Search date 1997; primary sources Medline, Embase, and hand searched references.
9. Glasziou PP, Del Mar CB, Sanders SL. Antibiotics for acute otitis media in children (Cochrane Review). In: The Cochrane Library, Issue 1, 2002. Oxford: Update Software. Search date 2000; primary sources Medline, Current Contents, and reference lists.
10. Little P, Gould C, Williamson I, et al. Pragmatic randomised controlled trial of two prescribing strategies for childhood acute otitis media. *BMJ* 2001;322:336–342.
11. Kozyrskyj AL, Hildes-Ripstein GE, Longstaffe SEA, et al. Short course antibiotics for acute otitis media. In: The Cochrane Library, Issue 1, 2002. Oxford: Update Software. Search date 1998; primary sources Medline, Embase, Science Citation Index, Current Contents, hand searches of reference lists, and personal contacts.
12. Cohen R, Levy C, Boucherat M, et al. A multicenter randomized, double blind trial of 5 versus 10 days of antibiotic therapy for acute otitis media in young children. *J Pediatr* 1998;133:634–639.
13. Cohen R, Levy C, Boucherat M, et al. Five vs. ten days of antibiotic therapy for acute otitis media in young children. *Pediatr Infect Dis J* 2000;19:458–463.
14. van Buchem FL, Dunk JH, van't Hof MA. Therapy of acute otitis media: myringotomy, antibiotics, or neither? A double blind study in children. *Lancet* 1981;2:883–887.
15. Engelhard D , Cohen D, Strauss N, et al. Randomised study of myringotomy, amoxycillin/clavulanate, or both for acute otitis media in infants. *Lancet* 1989;2:141–143.
16. Kaleida PH, Casselbrant ML, Rockette HE, et al. Amoxicillin or myringotomy or both for acute otitis media: results of a randomised clinical trial. *Pediatrics* 1991;87:466–474.
17. Williams RL, Chalmers TC, Stange KC, et al. Use of antibiotics in preventing recurrent acute otitis media and in treating otitis media with effusion: a meta-analytic attempt to resolve the brouhaha. *JAMA* 1993;270:1344–1351. (Published erratum appears in *JAMA* 1994;27:430.) Search date 1993; primary sources Medline and Current Contents.
18. Roark R, Berman S. Continuous twice daily or once daily amoxycillin prophylaxis compared with placebo for children with recurrent acute otitis media. *Pediatr Infect Dis J* 1997;16:376–378.
19. Uhari M, Kontiokari T, Niemela MA. Novel use of xylitol sugar in preventing acute otitis media. *Pediatrics* 1998;102:879–884.
20. Le TC, Freeman DW, Fireman BH. Evaluation of ventilating tubes and myringotomy in the treatment of recurrent or persistent otitis media. *Pediatr Infect Dis J* 1991;10:2–11.

Paddy O'Neill
General Practitioner
Norton Medical Centre
Stockton on Tees
UK

Tony Roberts
Clinical Effectiveness Advisor and
Honorary Research Fellow
South Tees Hospitals Trust
North Tees Primary Care Trust
and The University of Durham
UK

Competing interests: None declared.

Asthma and other wheezing disorders of childhood

Search date October 2002

Duncan Keeley and Michael McKean

QUESTIONS

INTERVENTIONS

Unknown effectiveness
Inhaled ipratropium bromide . .338
Inhaled short acting β_2 agonist 339
Lower dose inhaled corticosteroids 339

Unlikely to be beneficial
Addition of inhaled corticosteroid to short acting β_2 agonist 339

To be covered in future updates
Allergen avoidance
Education and self management

Continuous oral theophylline and inhaled sodium cromoglicate for prophylaxis in wheezing infants

Covered elsewhere in *Clinical Evidence*
Bronchiolitis (see bronchiolitis, p 345)

*No RCT, but observational evidence and strong consensus belief that oxygen is beneficial.

See glossary, p 341

Key Messages

Treating acute asthma in children

- **Oxygen** An RCT of oxygen versus no oxygen treatment in acute severe asthma would be considered unethical. One prospective cohort study and clinical experience support the need for oxygen in acute asthma.
- **High dose inhaled corticosteroids** We found one systematic review that identified four RCTs comparing high dose inhaled versus oral corticosteroids in children. Three RCTs found no significant difference in hospital admission with nebulised budesonide or dexamethasone versus oral prednisolone in children with mild to moderate asthma. One RCT in children with moderate to severe asthma found that oral prednisolone versus inhaled fluticasone significantly reduced hospital admission and improved lung function at 4 hours. A subsequent RCT in children aged 4–16 years found that nebulised fluticasone versus oral prednisolone significantly improved lung function over 7 days. Another RCT in children aged 5–16 years admitted to hospital with severe asthma found no significant difference with nebulised budesonide versus oral prednisolone in lung function at 24 hours or 24 days after admission.
- **Inhaled ipratropium bromide added to β_2 agonists (after initial stabilisation)** One RCT in children admitted to hospital with initially stabilised severe asthma found no significant difference in clinical asthma scores during the first 36 hours with nebulised ipratropium bromide versus placebo added to salbutamol and corticosteroid (hydrocortisone or prednisone).
- **Inhaled ipratropium bromide added to β_2 agonists (in emergency room)** One systematic review has found that in children aged 18 months to 17 years multiple doses of inhaled ipratropium bromide plus an inhaled β_2 agonist (fenoterol or salbutamol) versus the β_2 agonist alone reduce hospital admissions and improve lung function in children with severe asthma exacerbations. In children with mild to moderate asthma exacerbations, a single dose of inhaled ipratropium bromide plus a β_2 agonist (fenoterol, salbutamol, or terbutaline) versus a β_2 agonist alone significantly improves lung function for up to 2 hours, but does not significantly reduce hospital admissions.

- **Intravenous theophylline** One systematic review found that in children aged 1–19 years admitted to hospital with severe asthma, intravenous theophylline versus placebo significantly improved lung function and symptom scores 6–8 hours after treatment but found no significant difference in number of bronchodilator treatments required or length of hospital stay. A subsequent RCT in children aged 1–17 years admitted to intensive care unit with severe asthma found that intravenous theophylline versus control significantly decreased the time to reach clinical asthma score of 3 or less but found no significant difference in length of stay in intensive care unit.
- **Metered dose inhaler plus spacer devices for delivery of β_2 agonists (as effective as nebulisers)** One systematic review in children with acute but not life threatening asthma who were old enough to use a spacer has found no significant difference in hospital admission rates with a metered dose inhaler plus a spacer versus nebulisation for delivering β_2 agonists (fenoterol, salbutamol, or terbutaline) or β agonist (orciprenaline). Children using metered dose inhaler with spacer may have shorter stays in emergency departments, less hypoxia, and lower pulse rates compared with children receiving β_2 agonist by nebulisation.
- **Oral corticosteroids** One systematic review has found that oral corticosteroids (prednisone or prednisolone) versus placebo within 45 minutes of an acute asthma attack significantly reduce hospital admission.

Single agent prophylaxis in childhood asthma

- **Inhaled corticosteroids** One systematic review has found that inhaled corticosteroids (betamethasone, beclometasone, budesonide, flunisolide, or fluticasone) versus placebo improve symptoms and lung function in children with asthma. Two systematic reviews of studies with long term follow up and a subsequent long term RCT have found no evidence of growth retardation in children with asthma treated with inhaled corticosteroids. Some shorter term studies found reduced growth velocity.
- One RCT in children aged 6–16 years found no significant difference in improvement of asthma symptoms with inhaled beclometasone versus theophylline, but found less use of bronchodilators and oral corticosteroids with inhaled beclometasone.
- Small RCTs have found inhaled corticosteroids to be more effective than sodium cromoglicate in improving symptoms and lung function.
- RCTs in children aged 5–16 years have found that inhaled corticosteroids (beclometasone, budesonide, or fluticasone) versus inhaled long acting β_2 agonists (salmeterol) or inhaled nedocromil improve symptoms and lung function in children with asthma.
- **Inhaled nedocromil** Two RCTs in children aged 6–17 years found that inhaled nedocromil versus placebo significantly reduces asthma symptom scores, asthma severity, bronchodilator use, and lung function. One large RCT in children aged 5–12 years with mild to moderate asthma found no significant difference with nedocromil versus budesonide versus placebo in lung function, hospital admission rate, or the symptom score on diary cards, but found that budesonide was superior to nedocromil, and that nedocromil was superior to placebo in several measures of asthma symptoms and morbidity.
- **Inhaled salmeterol** Two RCTs in children aged 4–14 years found that inhaled salmeterol versus placebo significantly improved lung function but found conflicting evidence about a reduced salbutamol use. One RCT comparing inhaled salmeterol versus beclometasone found that salmeterol was associated with a significant deterioration in bronchial reactivity.

- **Inhaled sodium cromoglicate** One systematic review found insufficient evidence for prophylactic treatment with sodium cromoglicate in children aged less than 1 year to 18 years. Several small comparative RCTs have found sodium cromoglicate to be less effective than inhaled corticosteroids in improving symptoms and lung function.
- **Oral montelukast** One RCT in children aged 6–14 years found that oral montelukast versus placebo significantly increased (from baseline) the mean morning forced expiratory volume in 1 second and significantly reduced the total daily β_2 agonist use but found no significant difference in daytime asthma symptom score or in nocturnal awakenings with asthma. Another RCT in children aged 2–5 years found that oral montelukast versus placebo significantly improved average daytime symptom scores and reduced the need for rescue oral steroid courses but found no significant difference in average overnight asthma symptom scores. We found no RCTs directly comparing oral montelukast versus inhaled corticosteroids.
- **Oral theophylline** One small RCT in children aged 6–15 years found that oral theophylline versus placebo significantly increased mean morning peak expiratory flow rate and significantly reduced the mean number of acute night time attacks and doses of bronchodilator used. Another RCT in children aged 6–16 years found no significant difference in improvement of asthma symptoms with oral theophylline versus inhaled beclometasone, but found greater use of bronchodilators and oral corticosteroids with theophylline over 1 year. Theophylline has serious adverse effects (cardiac arrhythmia, convulsions) if therapeutic blood concentrations are exceeded.

Additional treatments in childhood asthma inadequately controlled by standard dose inhaled corticosteroids

- **Increased dose of inhaled corticosteroid** One RCT in children aged 6–16 years taking inhaled beclometasone comparing the addition of a second dose of inhaled corticosteroid (beclometasone) versus placebo found no significant difference in lung function, symptom scores, exacerbation rates, or bronchial reactivity but found significant reduction of growth velocity at 1 year.
- **Long acting β_2 agonists** One RCT in children aged 6–16 years found that addition of a long acting β_2 agonist (salmeterol) increased peak expiratory flow rates in the first few months of treatment but found no increase after 1 year. A second short term RCT in children aged 4–16 years also found increased morning peak expiratory flow rates and more symptom free days at 3 months with addition of a long acting β_2 agonist (salmeterol).
- **Oral leukotriene receptor antagonists** One crossover RCT in children aged 6–14 years with persistent asthma who had been taking inhaled budesonide for at least 6 weeks found that the addition of oral montelukast versus placebo significantly improved lung function and decreased the proportion of days with asthma exacerbations over 4 weeks. These differences were statistically significant but modest in clinical terms.
- **Oral theophylline** One small RCT found that addition of theophylline versus placebo to previous treatment significantly increased the proportion of symptom free days and significantly reduced the use of additional β agonist (orciprenaline) and additional corticosteroid (beclometasone or prednisolone) over 4 weeks.

Treating acute wheeze in infants

- **Addition of ipratropium bromide to long acting β_2 agonist** One RCT identified by a systematic review in infants aged 3–24 months found that addition of ipratropium bromide to fenoterol versus fenoterol alone significantly reduced the proportion of infants receiving further treatment 45 minutes after initial treatment.
- **High dose inhaled corticosteroids** One systematic review found that high dose inhaled corticosteroids versus placebo reduced the requirement for oral corticosteroids but the difference was not statistically significant. The review also found a clear preference for the inhaled corticosteroids by the children's parents over placebo. The clinical importance of these results is unclear.
- **Inhaled ipratropium bromide** We found no RCTs comparing inhaled ipratropium bromide versus placebo for treating acute wheeze.
- **Oral corticosteroids** One small RCT found no significant difference in daily symptom scores with oral prednisolone versus placebo.
- **Short acting β_2 agonists** One RCT in infants aged 3 months to 2 years found that nebulised salbutamol versus placebo significantly improved respiratory rate but found no significant difference in hospital admission. Another RCT that included infants aged less than 18 months to 36 months found no significant difference in change from baseline in clinical symptom scores with nebulised salbutamol versus placebo.
- **Short acting β_2 agonists delivered by metered dose inhaler/spacer versus nebuliser** Two RCTs in children aged up to 5 years found no significant difference in hospital admission with delivery of salbutamol through a metered dose inhaler plus spacer versus nebulised salbutamol. Another RCT in infants aged 1–24 months found no significant difference in improvement of symptoms with delivery of terbutaline through a metered dose inhaler plus spacer versus nebulised terbutaline. Nebulised β_2 agonists may cause tachycardia, tremor, and hypokalaemia.

Prophylaxis in wheezing infants

- **Addition of inhaled corticosteroid to short acting β_2 agonist** One RCT found no significant improvement in symptoms with addition of inhaled beclometasone versus placebo to inhaled salbutamol
- **Higher dose inhaled corticosteroids** One RCT in infants aged 6–30 months found that higher prophylactic doses of inhaled corticosteroids (budesonide) versus placebo significantly reduced symptoms and the proportion of children with acute wheezing episodes during a 12 week period but found no significant reduction in the proportion of wheezing episodes per infant. Another RCT in infants aged 11–36 months found that higher prophylactic doses of inhaled corticosteroid (budesonide) significantly reduced the proportion of days requiring oral prednisolone and symptoms of wheezing and sleep disturbance but found no significant improvement for cough. Higher doses of inhaled corticosteroids have the potential for adverse effects.
- **Inhaled ipratropium bromide** One small RCT identified by a systematic review found no significant difference in relief of symptoms with nebulised ipratropium bromide versus placebo. The study may have lacked power to exclude a clinically important difference between treatments.
- **Inhaled short acting β_2 agonist** Two RCTs identified by a systematic review in infants aged up to 2 years found no significant improvement in symptoms with inhaled salbutamol versus placebo.

- **Lower dose inhaled corticosteroids** Three RCTs found no clear evidence of effectiveness with lower prophylactic doses of inhaled corticosteroids (budesonide) in children aged 1 week to 6 years with recurrent wheeze.
- **Oral short acting β_2 agonist** One RCT identified by a systematic review in infants aged 3–14 months found that oral salbutamol versus placebo significantly reduced treatment failures.

DEFINITION **Childhood asthma** is characterised by chronic or recurrent cough and wheeze. The diagnosis is confirmed by demonstrating reversible airway obstruction in children old enough to perform peak flow measurements or spirometry. Diagnosing asthma in children requires exclusion of other causes of recurrent respiratory symptoms. **Wheezing in infants** is characterised by a high pitched purring or whistling sound produced predominantly during breathing out and is commonly associated with an acute viral infection such as bronchiolitis (see bronchiolitis, p 345) or asthma. These are not easy to distinguish clinically.

INCIDENCE/ PREVALENCE **Childhood asthma:** Surveys have found increasing prevalence in children diagnosed with asthma. The increase is more than can be explained by an increased readiness to diagnose asthma. One questionnaire study from Aberdeen, Scotland, surveyed 2510 children aged 8–13 years in 1964 and 3403 children in 1989. Over the 25 years, diagnosis of asthma rose from 4% to 10%.[1] The increase in prevalence of childhood asthma from the 1960s to 1980s was accompanied by an increase in hospital admissions over the same period. In England and Wales this was a sixfold increase.[2] **Wheezing in infants** is common and seems to be increasing though the magnitude of any increase is not clear. One Scottish cross-sectional study (2510 children aged 8–13 years in 1964 and 3403 children in 1989) found that prevalence of wheeze rose from 10% in 1964 to 20% in 1989 and episodes of shortness of breath rose from 5% to 10% over the same period.[1] Difficulties in defining clear groups (phenotypes) and the transient nature of the symptoms, which often resolve spontaneously, have confounded many studies.

AETIOLOGY/ RISK FACTORS **Childhood asthma:** Asthma is more common in children with a personal or family history of atopy; severity and frequency of wheezing episodes and presence of variable airway obstruction or bronchial hyperresponsiveness. Precipitating factors for symptoms and acute episodes include infection, house dust mites, allergens from pet animals, exposure to tobacco smoke, and anxiety. **Wheezing in infants:** Most wheezing episodes in infancy are precipitated by viral respiratory infections.

PROGNOSIS **Childhood asthma:** A British longitudinal study of children born in 1970 found that 29% of 5 year olds wheezing in the past year were still wheezing at the age of 10 years.[3] Another study followed a group of children in Melbourne, Australia from age 7 years (in 1964) into adulthood. The study found a large proportion (73%) of 14 year olds with infrequent symptoms had little or no symptoms by the age of 28 years, whereas two thirds of those 14 year olds with frequent wheezing still had recurrent attacks at the age of 28 years.[4] **Wheezing in infants:** The results of one cohort study (826 infants followed from birth to 6 years) suggests that there may be at least three different prognostic categories for wheezing in infants.[5] The study found one group (14% of total, with risk factors for atopic asthma such as elevated immunoglobulin E levels and maternal history of asthma) were "persistent wheezers" who initially suffered wheeze during viral infections, but the wheezing persisted into school age.[5] A second group (20% of total, with reduced lung function as infants but no early markers of atopy) were "transient wheezers" who also suffered wheeze during viral infections but stopped wheezing after the first 3 years of life. A third group (15% of total) were "late onset wheezers" who did not wheeze when aged under 3 years but had developed wheeze by school age.[5] Another retrospective cohort study found that 14% of children with one attack and 23% of children with four or more attacks in the first year of life had experienced at least one wheezing illness in their past year at age 10 years.[3] Administering inhaled treatments to young children can be difficult. Inconsistencies in results could reflect the effects of the differences in the drugs used, delivery devices used, dosages used, and the differences in the pattern of wheezing illnesses and treatment responses among young children.

AIMS OF INTERVENTION To reduce or abolish cough and wheeze; to attain best possible lung function; to reduce the risk of severe attacks; to minimise sleep disturbance and absence from school; to minimise adverse effects of treatment; and to allow normal growth.

OUTCOMES **Asthma in children:** Wheeze, cough, nights disturbed by asthma, days lost from school or normal activities, diary card symptom scores, lung function tests (peak expiratory flow rates and forced expiratory volume in 1 second), airway hyperresponsiveness (measured using methacholine challenge tests), service usage measures (emergency consultations, casualty attendances, hospital admissions). In acute episodes — blood oxygen saturation, admission rate from casualty, duration of admission, need for intensive care unit admission or intubation, mortality. **Wheezing in infants:** There are no suitable objective outcome parameters by which a response can be adequately measured as assessment of lung function is impractical in the clinical setting. Clinical symptoms and signs are usually subjective, vary between observers, and can be affected by short term changes. Parental preference is considered to be a relevant outcome.

METHODS *Clinical Evidence* search and appraisal October 2002. We have excluded studies with heterogeneous groups of infants (those with bronchiolitis as well as those with episodic of viral wheeze [see glossary, p 341] and those with chronic, persistent wheeze).

QUESTION **What are the effects of treatments for acute asthma in children?**

Duncan Keeley

OPTION **OXYGEN**

One prospective cohort study and clinical experience support the need for oxygen in acute asthma.

Benefits: We found no systematic review or RCTs. One double blind, prospective cohort study (280 children) found that decreased oxygen saturation upon entry to an emergency department was correlated with increased treatment with intravenous aminophylline (see glossary, p 341) and corticosteroids, and increased rates of hospital admission or subsequent readmission (arterial oxygen saturation $\leq$91% *v* arterial oxygen saturation $\geq$96%: OR 35, 95% CI 11 to 150; for arterial oxygen saturation 92–95% *v* $\geq$96%: OR 4.2, 95% CI 2.2 to 8.8).[6]

Harms: We found no evidence about harms.

Comment: An RCT of oxygen versus no oxygen treatment in acute severe asthma would be considered unethical. The cohort study does not address directly whether oxygen should be given therapeutically but it does suggest, along with clinical experience, that oxygen should continue to be given promptly to children with acute asthma.[6]

OPTION INHALED IPRATROPIUM BROMIDE ADDED TO β_2 AGONISTS

One systematic review has found that in children aged 18 months to 17 years multiple doses of inhaled ipratropium bromide plus an inhaled β_2 agonist (fenoterol or salbutamol) versus the β_2 agonist alone reduce hospital admissions and improve lung function in children with severe asthma exacerbations. In children with mild to moderate asthma exacerbations, a single dose of inhaled ipratropium bromide plus a β_2 agonist (fenoterol, salbutamol, or terbutaline) versus a β_2 agonist alone significantly improves lung function for up to 2 hours, but does not significantly reduce hospital admissions. A subsequent RCT in children aged 1–18 years with initially stabilised severe asthma found no significant difference in clinical asthma scores during the first 36 hours with nebulised ipratropium bromide versus placebo added to salbutamol and corticosteroid (hydrocortisone or prednisone).

Benefits: We found one systematic review[7] and one subsequent RCT.[8] **Single dose:** The systematic review (search date 2000, 13 RCTs, children aged 18 months to 17 years with acute asthma)[7] found that in children with mild to moderate exacerbations, adding a single dose of inhaled ipratropium bromide to inhaled β_2 agonists (fenoterol, salbutamol [see glossary, p 341] or terbutaline) versus the β_2 agonist alone significantly improved forced expiratory volume in 1 second (FEV_1) at 1 hour (3 RCTs: standardised mean difference 0.57, 95% CI 0.21 to 0.93) and at 2 hours (3 RCTs: standardised mean difference 0.53, 95% CI 0.17 to 0.90), but found no significant reduction in hospital admission (3 RCTs: RR 0.93, 95% CI 0.65 to 1.32).[7] **Multiple doses:** The systematic review found that in children with mild, moderate, or severe exacerbations, adding multiple doses of inhaled ipratropium bromide to an inhaled β_2 agonist (fenoterol or salbutamol) improved FEV_1 (4 RCTs: WMD 9.7% of predicted FEV_1, 95% CI 5.7% to 13.7%, 1 h after last ipratropium bromide inhalation) and reduced hospital admissions (6 RCTs: RR 0.75, 95% CI 0.62 to 0.89; NNT 13, 95% CI 8 to 32). Subgroup analysis found significant reduction in children with only severe exacerbations (baseline FEV_1 < 50% of predicted or change of 7 to 9 in baseline clinical score after last combined inhalation;

RR 0.71, 95% CI 0.58 to 0.89; NNT 7, 95% CI 5 to 20).[7] The subsequent RCT (80 children and adolescents aged 1–18 years admitted to hospital with moderate to severe asthma, FEV_1 25–85% predicted or clinical asthma score [see glossary, p 341] of 3–9, initially stabilised in emergency department) compared addition of nebulised ipratropium bromide versus placebo (sodium chloride) to nebulised salbutamol and intravenous hydrocortisone or oral prednisone.[8] The RCT found no significant difference during the first 36 hours in clinical asthma scores, oxygen saturation, or number of nebulisations needed with ipratropium bromide versus placebo.

Harms: The systematic review found no significant increase in risk of nausea (3 RCTs: RR 0.59, 95% CI 0.30 to 1.14), vomiting (3 RCTs: RR 1.03, 95% CI 0.37 to 2.87), or tremor (4 RCTs: RR 1.01, 95% CI 0.63 to 1.63) in children treated with multiple doses of ipratropium bromide.[7] The subsequent RCT found a significant increase in heart rate with ipratropium bromide versus placebo ($P = 0.01$).[8]

Comment: None.

OPTION METERED DOSE INHALER PLUS SPACER DEVICES VERSUS NEBULISERS FOR DELIVERING β_2 AGONISTS

One systematic review, in children with acute but not life threatening asthma who were old enough to use a spacer, has found no significant difference in hospital admission rates with a metered dose inhaler plus a spacer versus nebulisation for delivery of β_2 agonists (fenoterol, salbutamol, or terbutaline) or β agonist (orciprenaline). Children using a metered dose inhaler with a spacer may have shorter stays in emergency departments, less hypoxia, and lower pulse rates compared with children receiving β_2 agonist by nebulisation.

Benefits: We found one systematic review (search date 2001, 13 RCTs, 880 children with acute asthma but excluding life threatening asthma) comparing spacer/holding chamber attached to a metered dose inhaler versus single or multiple treatment with nebuliser for delivery of β_2 agonists (fenoterol, salbutamol (see glossary, p 341) or terbutaline) or β agonist (orciprenaline [see glossary, p 341]).[9] The review found no significant difference between spacer and multiple treatments with nebulisers in hospital admission rates (OR 0.65, 95% CI 0.40 to 1.06). It found a significant increase in pulse rate with nebulisers (WMD 7.8% from baseline, 95% CI 5.3% to 10.2%). One RCT (152 children $\geq$ 2 years) found that the time spent in the emergency department was shorter in children using metered dose inhaler plus spacer (WMD –37 min, 95% CI –50 min to –24 min).[10] Two small RCTs included in the review comparing delivery of β_2 agonists (salbutamol or terbutaline) through a spacer versus single treatment with nebuliser found less deterioration in blood gases with the spacer.[9]

Harms: The systematic review found no significant deterioration in any of the outcome measures with delivery of β_2 agonists using metered dose inhaler plus a spacer versus nebulisation.[9]

Comment: These findings suggest that, in children old enough to use a spacer, metered dose inhaler with spacer could be substituted for nebulisation in the treatment of acute asthma in emergency departments and hospital wards.

OPTION ORAL CORTICOSTEROIDS

One systematic review has found that early oral corticosteroids (prednisone or prednisolone) versus placebo reduce hospital admission in children with acute asthma exacerbations.

Benefits: We found one systematic review (search date 1999, 3 RCTs comparing corticosteroid *v* placebo within 45 min of arrival at the emergency department).[11] It found that oral corticosteroid (1–2 mg/kg prednisone or prednisolone) versus placebo significantly reduced hospital admission rates in children with acute asthma exacerbations (OR 0.24, 95% CI 0.11 to 0.53).[11]

Harms: The systematic review included RCTs in adults and did not report separately on adverse reactions in children given oral corticosteroids; overall it found no significant difference with oral corticosteroids versus placebo.[11] We found few reports of adverse effects with short courses of systemic corticosteroids. Several case reports have associated systemic corticosteroid treatment with severe varicella infection. One case control study (167 cases, 134 controls) in otherwise immunocompetent children with complicated and uncomplicated varicella infection did not find significant risk attributable to corticosteroid exposure (OR 1.6, 95% CI 0.2 to 17.0), but it was too small to exclude a clinically important risk.[12]

Comment: None.

OPTION HIGH DOSE INHALED CORTICOSTEROIDS

We found one systematic review that identified four RCTs comparing high dose inhaled versus oral corticosteroids in children. Three RCTs found no significant difference in hospital admission with nebulised budesonide or dexamethasone versus oral prednisolone in children with mild to moderate asthma. One RCT in children with moderate to severe asthma found that oral prednisolone versus inhaled fluticasone significantly reduced hospital admission and improved lung function at 4 hours. A subsequent RCT in children aged 4–16 years found that nebulised fluticasone versus oral prednisolone significantly improved lung function over 7 days. Another RCT in children aged 5–16 years admitted to hospital with severe asthma found no significant difference with nebulised budesonide versus oral prednisolone in lung function at 24 hours or 24 days after admission.

Benefits: **Versus oral corticosteroids:** We found one systematic review (search date 2000, 4 RCTs),[13] one subsequent RCT,[14] and one additional RCT.[15] The systematic review compared effects of initial treatment with high dose inhaled corticosteroids versus oral corticosteroids in hospital emergency departments on admission rates.[13] The results from the four RCTs were not pooled because of marked heterogeneity between studies. One RCT (100 children with moderate to severe asthma, aged 5–16 years, mean initial flow expiratory volume in 1 second 45%) compared fluticasone (2 mg through metered dose inhaler with spacer) versus prednisone (2 mg/kg orally).[16] It found that prednisone reduced hospital admission (31% with fluticasone *v* 10% with prednisone; P = 0.01) and increased mean flow expiratory volume in 1 second at 4 hours (9% with fluticasone *v* 19% with prednisone; P ≤ 0.001).[16] The second RCT (111 children with mild to moderate asthma, aged 1–17 years) compared dexamethasone (1.5 mg/kg through nebuliser) versus prednisone (2 mg orally).[17] It found no significant difference between nebulised dexamethasone versus oral prednisone in hospital admission (12/56 [21%] with dexamethasone *v* 17/55 [31%] with prednisone; ARR 9.5%, 95% CI –8.0% to 21.0%; RR 0.69, 95% CI 0.36 to 1.27), but found fewer relapses with nebulised dexamethasone within 48 hours after discharge (0/44 [0%] *v* 6/38 [16%]; ARR –16.0%, 95% CI –27.0% to –4.5%); however, all children in the RCT received a 5 day course of prednisone (2 mg/kg/day) on discharge.[17] Two other RCTs (104 children with mild to moderate asthma) compared budesonide (800 μg through nebuliser at 1, 30, and 60 min; 1600 μg through turbohaler) versus prednisolone (2 mg/kg orally).[18,19] Overall, no significant differences were found between the groups in admission rates (OR for inhaled corticosteroids *v* oral corticosteroids 0.49, 95% CI 0.22 to 1.07).[18,19] The subsequent RCT (321 children aged 4–16 years, peak expiratory flow rate 40–75% predicted) compared nebulised fluticasone (1 mg twice daily for 7 days) versus oral prednisolone (2 mg/kg for 4 days then 1 mg/kg for 3 days). It found that nebulised fluticasone versus oral prednisolone significantly improved mean morning peak expiratory flow rate over 7 days (difference 9.5 L/min, 95% CI 2.0 L/min to 17.0 L/min). No significant differences were found in symptom scores, withdrawals, or adverse events.[14] The additional RCT (46 children, aged 5–16 years, admitted to hospital with severe exacerbations of asthma) compared nebulised budesonide (2 mg/h) with oral prednisolone (2 mg/kg) at admission and after 24 hours.[15] It found no significant difference between groups in flow expiratory volume in 1 second at 24 hours or at 3 and 24 days after admission. All children in this trial were treated with budesonide (800 μg/day) after discharge from hospital.

Harms: The systematic review found no significant adverse effects with inhaled corticosteroids.[13] The subsequent RCT found no significant difference in the profile of adverse events with inhaled fluticasone versus oral prednisolone except a slightly higher frequency of oral candidiasis with fluticasone (8% with fluticasone *v* 3% with prednisolone).[14]

Comment: These RCTs suggest that high dose inhaled corticosteroids may be substituted for oral corticosteroids in the initial phase of treatment of moderately severe acute asthma. This may be useful for children who vomit oral corticosteroids or for children with frequent exacerbations where there is concern about the cumulative dose of oral steroids. One RCT was funded by the manufacturers of fluticasone.[14]

OPTION INTRAVENOUS THEOPHYLLINE

One systematic review found that in children aged 1–19 years admitted to hospital with severe asthma, intravenous theophylline versus placebo significantly improved lung function and symptom scores 6–8 hours after treatment but found no significant difference in number of bronchodilator treatments required or length of hospital stay. A subsequent RCT in children aged 1–17 years admitted to intensive care unit with severe asthma, found that intravenous theophylline versus control significantly decreased the time to reach clinical asthma score of 3 or less but found no significant difference in length of stay in intensive care unit.

Benefits: We found one systematic review[20] and one subsequent RCT.[21] The systematic review (search date 2001, 7 RCTs, 380 children and adolescents aged 1–19 years admitted to hospital with severe asthma, flow expiratory volume in 1 second 35–45% predicted) compared the effects of intravenous theophylline versus placebo on lung function (measured as change from baseline in flow expiratory volume in 1 second).[20] The review found that at 6–8 hours, intravenous theophylline versus placebo significantly improved lung function (2 RCTs; WMD 8.4%, 95% CI 0.8% to 15.9%) and clinical symptom scores (WMD −0.71, 95% CI −0.82 to −0.60) but found no significant difference in number of nebulised bronchodilator treatments required (2RCTs; WMD +0.15; 95% CI −0.52 to +0.83) or length of hospital stay (3 RCTs; WMD +4.29; 95% CI −4.16 to +12.74). The subsequent RCT (47 children aged 1–17 years admitted to intensive care unit with severe asthma receiving salbutamol (see glossary, p 341), ipratropium, and methylprednisolone) compared intravenous theophylline versus controls on time to reach clinical asthma score of 3 or less.[21] The RCT found that intravenous theophylline versus control significantly decreased the time to reach clinical asthma score of 3 or less (18.6 h with theophylline *v* 31 h with control; $P < 0.05$) but found no significant difference in length of stay in intensive care unit.

Harms: The systematic review found that theophylline versus placebo significantly increased the risk of vomiting (5 RCTs; RR 3.69, 95% CI 2.15 to 6.33) but found no significant differences for headache, tremor, seizures, and arrhythmia. There were no deaths reported in the included studies.[20] The subsequent RCT found significantly higher incidence of emesis with theophylline and tremor with control (both $P < 0.05$).[21] Theophylline can cause serious adverse effects (cardiac arrhythmia or convulsion) if therapeutic blood concentrations are exceeded.

Comment: None.

QUESTION What are the effects of single agent prophylaxis in childhood asthma?

Duncan Keeley

OPTION INHALED CORTICOSTEROIDS

One systematic review has found that prophylactic inhaled corticosteroids (betamethasone, beclometasone, budesonide, flunisolide, or fluticasone) versus placebo improve symptoms and lung function in

children with asthma. Two systematic reviews of studies with long term follow up and a subsequent long term RCT have found no evidence of growth retardation in children with asthma treated with inhaled corticosteroids. Some shorter term studies found reduced growth velocity. One RCT in children aged 6–16 years found no significant difference in improvement of asthma symptoms with inhaled beclometasone versus theophylline, but found less use of bronchodilators and oral corticosteroids with inhaled beclometasone. Several RCTs have found inhaled corticosteroids to be more effective than sodium cromoglicate in improving symptoms and lung function. RCTs in children aged 5–16 years have found that inhaled corticosteroids (beclometasone, budesonide, or fluticasone) versus inhaled long acting β_2 agonists (salmeterol) or inhaled nedocromil improve symptoms and lung function in children with asthma.

Benefits: **Versus placebo:** We found one systematic review (search date 1996, 24 RCTs, 1087 children, 10/24 RCTs in preschool children, duration 4–88 wks) comparing effects of regular inhaled corticosteroids (betamethasone, beclometasone, budesonide, flunisolide, or fluticasone) versus placebo on asthma symptoms (see comment below), concomitant drug use, and peak expiratory flow rate (PEFR).[22] It found that corticosteroids significantly improved symptom score (overall weighted relative improvement in symptom score 50%, 95% CI 49% to 51%), reduced β_2 agonist use (RR 0.37, 95% CI 0.36 to 0.38), reduced oral corticosteroid use (RR 0.68, 95% CI 0.66 to 0.70), and improved peak flow rate (weighted mean improvement in PEFR 11% predicted, 95% CI 9.5% to 12.5%). **Versus theophylline:** We found no systematic review. We found one RCT (195 children aged 6–16 years, followed for 12 months) comparing inhaled beclometasone (360 μg/day) versus oral theophylline.[23] It found no significant difference with inhaled beclometasone versus oral theophylline in the mean asthma symptom score (0 = no symptoms, 6 = incapacitating symptoms: mean score 0.5–0.8 for beclometasone *v* 0.6–0.9 for theophylline) with less use of bronchodilators and oral corticosteroids with inhaled beclometasone.[23] **Versus sodium cromoglicate:** We found no systematic review. We found four RCTs comparing inhaled corticosteroids (betamethasone, budesonide, fluticasone) versus inhaled sodium cromoglicate.[24–27] One RCT (20 children aged 6–14 years) found that betamethasone versus sodium cromoglicate significantly improved symptoms and lung function (mean PEFRs, $P < 0.001$).[24] The second RCT (crossover, 75 children aged 5–15 years) found that budesonide or fluticasone versus sodium cromoglicate significantly reduced bronchodilator use ($P < 0.05$) and lung function (forced expiratory volume in 1 second [FEV_1], $P < 0.01$).[25] The third RCT (unblinded, 335 children aged 2–6 years) found that budesonide versus sodium cromoglicate significantly reduced rate of asthma exacerbations over 52 weeks ($P \leq 0.001$). Asthma exacerbations were defined as use of systemic corticosteroids or additional maintenance treatment, emergency department or urgent care visit, or admission to hospital.[26] The fourth RCT (unblinded, multicentre, 225 children aged 4–12 years) found that fluticasone versus sodium cromoglicate significantly improved mean percentage PEFR (at 6–8 wks, $P = 0.0001$) and symptoms (at 6–8 wks, $P < 0.05$) but found no significant difference for relief medication use or FEV_1.[27] **Versus nedocromil:** We found one RCT (1041 children aged 5–12 years, with mild to moderate asthma, mean prestudy FEV_1 94% predicted, all using salbutamol [see glossary, p 341] for asthma symptoms) that compared inhaled budesonide (200 µg twice daily) and inhaled nedocromil (8 mg twice daily) versus placebo for 4–6 years.[28] It found no significant difference with budesonide versus nedocromil versus placebo in lung function, hospital admission rate, or the symptom score on diary cards but found that budesonide was superior to nedocromil, and that nedocromil was superior to placebo in several measures of asthma symptoms and morbidity (see table 1, p 344). The mean change in post-bronchodilator FEV_1 over the study period was not significantly different among the three groups. **Versus inhaled long acting β_2 agonists:** We found no systematic review but found two RCTs of beclometasone (200 µg twice daily) versus salmeterol (50 µg twice daily) for 1 year.[29,30] The first RCT (67 children aged 6–16 years) found that beclometasone was more effective than salmeterol in improving FEV_1 (mean change of FEV_1 −4.5% of predicted with salmeterol, 95% CI −9.0% to +0.1% *v* 10% with beclometasone, 95% CI not provided; mean difference beclometasone *v* salmeterol 14.2%, 95% CI 8.3% to 20.0%), reducing use of rescue salbutamol (0.44 uses/day with salmeterol *v* 0.07 uses/day with beclometasone; $P \leq 0.001$).[29] Both treatments improved symptom scores (before trial 3% of children asymptomatic with salmeterol *v* 6% with beclometasone; at 1 year 36% with salmeterol *v* 55% with beclometasone) and PEFR (improvement in morning PEFR 49 L/min with salmeterol *v* 61 L/min with beclometasone), but there was no significant difference between treatments at 1 year. There were two exacerbations in the beclometasone group compared with 17 in the salmeterol group.[29] The second RCT (241 children aged 6–14 years) compared beclometasone (81 children) versus salmeterol (80 children) versus placebo (80 children).[30] It found that beclometasone reduced airway hyperresponsiveness more than salmeterol (methacholine PC20 36 hours after study medication 12 months into the study, 2.1 mg/mL with beclometasone *v* 0.9 mg/mL with salmeterol; $P = 0.009$). Beclometasone versus placebo reduced rescue bronchodilator use (92% with beclometasone *v* 83% with placebo days and nights without need for salbutamol; $P \leq 0.001$) and treatment withdrawals because of exacerbations (5 with beclometasone *v* 15 with placebo; $P = 0.03$). Salmeterol versus placebo did not significantly reduce the use of a rescue bronchodilator (88% with salmeterol *v* 83% with placebo days and nights without need for salbutamol; $P = 0.09$) or treatment withdrawals because of exacerbations (15 with salmeterol *v* 15 with placebo; $P = 0.55$). Both salmeterol and beclometasone improved FEV_1 compared with placebo, but the difference between beclometasone and salmeterol was not significant (10% with beclometasone *v* 10% with salmeterol *v* 5% with placebo). **Versus oral montelukast:** We found no RCTs comparing directly inhaled corticosteroids versus oral montelukast in children. A systematic review of mainly adult studies comparing inhaled corticosteroids with leukotriene receptor antagonists found similar exacerbation rates, but greater improvement in lung function and symptoms with inhaled steroids.[31] (See benefits section of leukotriene antagonists in adults with mild to moderate, persistent asthma option in asthma in adults topic, p 1757.)

Harms: **Versus placebo:** One systematic review (search date 1996) found no significant difference with inhaled corticosteroids (betamethasone, budesonide, flunisolide, or fluticasone) versus placebo in adrenal function (12 RCTs) and found clinical cases of oral candidiasis (4 RCTs).[22] Case reports[32] and a national survey of paediatricians and endocrinologists[33] have indicated the possibility of adrenal suppression leading to adrenal crisis associated with hypoglycaemia in children on high dose inhaled corticosteroids. Most cases involved fluticasone, in daily doses of 500–2000 μg. Observational studies have found little or no biochemical evidence of change in bone metabolism with inhaled corticosteroids.[34,35] Two cross-sectional studies using a slit lamp to screen for lenticular changes in children taking long term inhaled corticosteroids (beclometasone, budesonide) found no posterior subcapsular cataracts.[36,37] The systematic review identified eight RCTs reporting growth velocity and found no significant difference with inhaled corticosteroids versus placebo.[22] One systematic review (search date 1993, 21 studies) reported height for age in 810 children with asthma treated with oral or inhaled corticosteroids. It found no evidence of growth impairment with inhaled beclometasone (12 studies, 331 children).[38] A second systematic review (search date 1999, 3 RCTs) identified one RCT (94 children, aged 7–9 years) comparing effect of inhaled beclometasone (400 μg/day) versus placebo on growth as a primary outcome measure in children with recurrent viral induced wheeze.[39] It found a significant decrease in growth with beclometasone versus placebo (mean growth at end of 7 month treatment period, 2.7 cm with beclometasone *v* 3.7 cm with placebo; 95% CI −1.4 to −0.6; P < 0.0001) and found no significant catch up growth during a follow up 4 month washout period.[40] **Versus theophylline or sodium cromoglicate:** One RCT compared inhaled beclometasone (360 μg/day) versus oral theophylline for 1 year.[23] It found a significantly higher rate of growth (more notable in boys) with the theophylline group (mean rate of growth in prepubescent boys 4.3 cm/year with beclometasone *v* 6.2 cm/year with theophylline). This effect was not sufficient to be noticed by the children or by their parents, and no child was withdrawn from the study on this account.[23] One controlled, prospective study compared 216 children treated with budesonide (400–600 μg/day) with 62 children treated with theophylline or sodium cromoglicate over 3–5 years' follow up.[41] No significant changes in growth velocity were found at doses up to 400 μg/day (5.5 cm/year with budesonide *v* 5.6 cm/year with controls). The adult height of 142 of these budesonide treated children (mean treatment period 9.2 years, mean dosage 412 μg/day) was compared with 18 controls never treated with inhaled corticosteroids and 51 healthy siblings. There were no significant differences. Children in all groups attained their target adult height (mean difference between measured and target adult height: +0.3 cm, 95% CI −0.6 cm to +1.2 cm for budesonide treated children;

−0.2 cm, 95% CI −2.4 cm to +2.1 cm for control children with asthma; +0.9 cm, 95% CI −0.4 cm to +2.2 cm for healthy siblings).[42] Two RCTs found no clinically relevant differences between inhaled corticosteroids (betamethasone, budesonide) and sodium cromoglicate.[24,26] One RCT found that budesonide versus fluticasone or sodium cromoglicate significantly reduced growth (decrease in height standard deviation score > 2 standard deviation compared with mean height standard deviation score change during preceding year, $P < 0.05$).[25] Another RCT found that a higher proportion of children taking sodium cromoglicate withdrew because of adverse events (breathlessness and wheeze, burning sensation in chest, sore throat, sickness) compared with fluticasone.[27] **Versus nedocromil:** A large RCT (1041 children with mild to moderate asthma) compared budesonide (400 μg/day) versus nedocromil versus placebo with 4–6 years' follow up.[28] The mean increase in height in the budesonide group was 1.1 cm less than in the placebo group (22.7 cm with budesonide *v* 23.8 cm with placebo; $P = 0.005$); the difference occurred mainly within the first year of treatment.[28] **Versus inhaled long acting β_2 agonists:** Two RCTs comparing beclometasone with salmeterol found slowing in linear growth with beclometasone (growth over year of treatment 5.4 cm[29] and 6.1 cm[30] in the salmeterol groups; 4.0 cm[29] and 4.7 cm[30] in the beclometasone groups; $P = 0.004$;[29] $P = 0.007$[30]). One RCT comparing inhaled beclometasone versus salmeterol found that symptom improvement in the salmeterol group was accompanied by significant deterioration in bronchial reactivity indicating a failure to control underlying bronchial inflammation.[29]

Comment: Treatment with inhaled corticosteroids should be reviewed regularly and the dose gradually reduced to the lowest that is compatible with good symptom control.

OPTION INHALED SODIUM CROMOGLICATE

One systematic review found insufficient evidence for prophylactic treatment with inhaled sodium cromoglicate in children aged 1–18 years. Several small comparative RCTs have found sodium cromoglicate to be less effective than inhaled corticosteroids in improving symptoms and lung function.

Benefits: **Versus placebo:** We found one systematic review (search date 1999, 24 RCTs, about 1000 children aged 0–18 years with moderate to severe asthma) comparing inhaled sodium cromoglicate versus placebo.[43] The RCTs differed in design, severity of asthma, number of children included, age of children, duration of intervention, and follow up period. The review found heterogeneity between RCTs but did not separately analyse RCTs in terms of asthma severity, age of children, or the outcome measured. The review found that sodium cromoglicate versus placebo significantly improved symptom scores for cough (point estimate not provided; 95% CI 0.11 to 0.26) and wheeze (point estimate not provided; 95% CI 0.13 to 0.27) but also found significant publication bias by the absence of small, negative trials (P = 0.01 for cough and wheeze). The review concluded that there is insufficient evidence for prophylactic treatment with sodium cromoglicate in children with asthma. **Versus inhaled corticosteroids:** See benefits of inhaled corticosteroids, p 326.

Harms: **Versus placebo:** Fifteen RCTs included in the systematic review reported adverse effects described as minor and of low incidence, including cough, bitter taste, wheezing, sneezing, throat irritation, and perioral eczema.[43] **Versus inhaled corticosteroids:** See harms of inhaled corticosteroids, p 328.

Comment: The conclusions of the systematic review[43] have been criticised in correspondence and the assertion made that analysis of trials using sodium cromoglicate by spinhaler in children over 5 years of age was consistent with a beneficial effect of sodium cromoglicate compared with placebo.[44]

OPTION INHALED NEDOCROMIL

Two RCTs in children aged 6–17 years found that inhaled nedocromil versus placebo significantly reduces asthma symptom scores, asthma severity, bronchodilator use, and lung function. One large RCT in children aged 5–12 years with mild to moderate asthma found no significant difference with nedocromil versus budesonide versus placebo in lung function, hospital admission rate, or the symptom score on diary cards, but found that budesonide was superior to nedocromil, and that nedocromil was superior to placebo in several measures of asthma symptoms and morbidity.

Benefits: We found no systematic review. **Versus placebo:** We found two RCTs.[45,46] The first RCT (209 children and adolescents aged 6–7 years allowed to continue using usual medication) compared inhaled nedocromil (4 mg 4 times daily) versus placebo for 12 weeks. Symptoms were recorded by the children in daily diary cards, including scoring day and night time asthma and cough severity, use of all medication, and morning and evening peak expiratory flow rate. The RCT found that inhaled nedocromil versus placebo significantly reduced total symptom scores, clinician assessed asthma severity, β_2 agonist use, and lung function (forced expiratory volume in 1 second).[45] The second RCT (parallel group study, 79 children aged 6–12 years recovering acute asthma and allowed to use inhaled bronchodilators) compared inhaled nedocromil (2 mg 3 times daily) versus placebo for 12 weeks.[46] Symptoms were recorded by the children in daily diary cards, including day and night time asthma severity, morning and evening peak expiratory flow rate, and usage of bronchodilators. The RCT found that after 6 weeks, inhaled nedocromil versus placebo significantly improved (from baseline) the morning peak expiratory flow rate (difference, 20 L/min; P = 0.036), evening peak expiratory flow rate (difference, 22 L/min; P = 0.033), night time asthma score (difference on a 5 point scale, 0.48, P = 0.001), and daytime asthma score (difference on a 5 point scale, 0.38, P = 0.03). The RCT found no significant difference before 6 weeks of treatment. **Versus inhaled corticosteroids:** See benefits of inhaled corticosteroids, p 326.

Harms: **Versus placebo:** Sore throat and headache were reported marginally more often with nedocromil than placebo in the first RCT.[45] The second RCT found no significant difference between nedocromil and placebo in adverse event rates except for more frequent respiratory adverse events with placebo.[46] **Versus inhaled corticosteroids:** See harms of inhaled corticosteroids, p 328.

Comment: None.

OPTION INHALED LONG ACTING β_2 AGONISTS

Two RCTs in children aged 4–14 years found that inhaled salmeterol versus placebo significantly improved lung function but found conflicting evidence about a reduced salbutamol use. One RCT comparing inhaled salmeterol versus beclometasone found that salmeterol was associated with a significant deterioration in bronchial reactivity.

Benefits: We found no systematic review. **Versus placebo:** We found two RCTs.[30,47] The first RCT (241 children aged 6–14 years with clinically stable asthma and < 1 month of prior glucocorticoid use) compared inhaled salmeterol (80 children) versus beclometasone (81 children) versus placebo (80 children) for 1 year.[30] The RCT found that salmeterol versus placebo significantly improved lung function (mean change in force expiratory volume in 1 second as percentage predicted 10% with salmeterol *v* 5% with placebo; P < 0.001) but found no significant difference in the use of a rescue salbutamol (see glossary, p 341) (P = 0.09) or withdrawals because of exacerbations (P = 0.55).[30] The second RCT (parallel group study, 207 children aged 4–11 years with asthma diagnosed according to American Thoracic Society guidelines, forced expiratory volume in 1 second [without medication] 50–80% predicted) compared inhaled salmeterol (50 µg twice daily) versus placebo for 12 weeks.[47] The RCT found that salmeterol versus placebo significantly improved lung function (change in mean morning peak expiratory flow 25 L/min with salmeterol *v* 13.2 L/min with placebo; P < 0.001; change in mean evening peak expiratory flow 20 L/min with salmeterol *v* 10.1 L/min with placebo; P = 0.01) and reduced salbutamol use (–0.8 with salmeterol *v* –0.3 with placebo; P = 0.004). It found no significant difference in the number of nights without awakenings between salmeterol versus placebo.[47] **Versus inhaled corticosteroids:** See benefits of inhaled corticosteroids, p 326.

Harms: **Versus placebo:** One RCT found no evidence of adverse effects from salmeterol over 1 year.[30] The second RCT found no significant difference between salmeterol and placebo for adverse effects.[47] **Versus inhaled corticosteroids:** See harms of inhaled corticosteroids, p 328. Long acting β_2 agonists occasionally cause tremor or tachycardia.

Comment: Monotherapy with long acting β_2 agonists is not advised because of the possibility of significant deterioration in bronchial reactivity indicating a failure to control underlying bronchial inflammation (see harms of inhaled corticosteroids, p 328).

Asthma and other wheezing disorders of childhood

OPTION ORAL THEOPHYLLINE

One small RCT in children aged 6–15 years found that oral theophylline versus placebo significantly increased mean morning peak expiratory flow rate and significantly reduced the mean number of acute night time attacks and doses of bronchodilator used. Another RCT in children aged 6–16 years found no significant difference in improvement of asthma symptoms with oral theophylline versus inhaled beclometasone, but found greater use of bronchodilators and oral corticosteroids with theophylline over 1 year. Theophylline has serious adverse effects (cardiac arrhythmia, convulsions) if therapeutic blood concentrations are exceeded.

Benefits: We found no systematic review. **Versus placebo:** We found one RCT (crossover study, 24 children aged 6–15 years experiencing at least 2 night awakenings/wk) comparing once daily oral sustained release theophylline (mean theophylline level of 11.2 mg/L) versus placebo for 6 weeks.[48] The RCT found that theophylline versus placebo significantly increased mean morning peak expiratory flow (244 L/min with theophylline *v* 207 L/min with placebo, $P < 0.001$) and significantly reduced the mean number of acute night time attacks (3.2 with theophylline *v* 10.7 with placebo, $P < 0.001$) and the mean number of doses of bronchodilator used (6.5 with theophylline *v* 23.7 with placebo, $P < 0.001$). **Versus inhaled corticosteroids:** See benefits of inhaled corticosteroids, p 326.

Harms: **Versus placebo:** One RCT found significantly higher rates of gastric symptoms including dyspepsia, nausea, and vomiting with oral sustained release theophylline versus placebo (30% with theophylline *v* 6% with placebo, $P < 0.001$).[48] One systematic review (search date not stated, 12 studies, 340 children) of the behavioural and cognitive effects of theophylline found no evidence of significant adverse effects.[49] Theophylline has serious adverse effects (cardiac arrhythmia, convulsions) if therapeutic blood concentrations are exceeded.[50] **Versus inhaled corticosteroids:** See harms of inhaled corticosteroids, p 328.

Comment: None.

OPTION ORAL LEUKOTRIENE RECEPTOR ANTAGONISTS

One RCT in children aged 6–14 years found that oral montelukast versus placebo significantly increased (from baseline) the mean morning forced expiratory volume in 1 second and significantly reduced the total daily β_2 agonist use but found no significant difference in daytime asthma symptom score or in nocturnal awakenings with asthma. Another RCT in children aged 2–5 years found that oral montelukast versus placebo significantly improved average daytime symptom scores and reduced the need for rescue oral steroid courses but found no significant difference in average overnight asthma symptom scores. We found no RCTs directly comparing oral montelukast versus inhaled corticosteroids.

Benefits: We found no systematic review. **Versus placebo:** We found two RCTs.[51,52] The first RCT (parallel group study, 336 children aged 6–16 years with mean forced expiratory volume in 1 second 72%

predicted, concomitant inhaled steroid treatment in 33% of placebo group and 39% of montelukast group) compared oral montelukast (5 mg/day) versus placebo for 8 weeks.[51] The RCT found that montelukast versus placebo significantly increased (from baseline) the mean morning flow expiratory volume in 1 second (8.2% with montelukast *v* 3.6% with placebo, $P < 0.001$) and significantly reduced the total daily β_2 agonist use (reduced by 13% with montelukast and increased by 9.5% with placebo, $P = 0.01$).[51] The RCT found no significant difference between montelukast versus placebo in daytime asthma symptom score or in nocturnal awakenings with asthma.[51] The second RCT (parallel group study, 689 children aged 2–5 years, concomitant inhaled steroid treatment in 29% of placebo group, 27% of montelukast group, 2 : 1 ratio montelukast : placebo group) compared oral montelukast (4 mg/day) versus placebo for 12 weeks.[52] The RCT found that montelukast versus placebo significantly improved average daytime symptom scores (improved by 0.37 with montelukast *v* 0.26 with placebo on a 6 point scale, $P = 0.003$) and reduced the need for rescue oral steroid courses (needed in 19% with montelukast *v* 28% with placebo, $P = 0.008$). The RCT found no significant difference between montelukast versus placebo in average overnight asthma symptom scores.[52] **Versus inhaled corticosteroids:** We found no RCTs comparing oral montelukast versus inhaled corticosteroids directly.

Harms: **Versus placebo:** Two RCTs found no significant difference in incidence of adverse effects with montelukast versus placebo.[51,52]

Comment: None.

QUESTION What are the effects of additional treatments in childhood asthma inadequately controlled by standard dose inhaled corticosteroids?

Duncan Keeley

OPTION INCREASED DOSE OF INHALED CORTICOSTEROID

One RCT in children aged 6–16 years taking inhaled beclometasone comparing the addition of a second dose of inhaled corticosteroid (beclometasone) versus placebo found no significant differences in lung function, symptom scores, exacerbation rates, or bronchial reactivity, and found significant reduction of growth velocity at 1 year.

Benefits: We found no systematic review but found one RCT (177 children, age 6–16 years, 1 year of follow up, mean pre-bronchodilator flow expiratory volume in 1 second 86% predicted) comparing beclometasone (200 μg twice daily), salmeterol (50 μg twice daily), and placebo in children already taking beclometasone (200 μg twice daily).[53] No significant differences were found at 1 year in lung function (mean change in flow expiratory volume in 1 second 5.8% of predicted, 95% CI 2.9% to 8.7% with double dose beclometasone *v* 4.3%, 95% CI 2.1% to 6.5% with placebo), symptom scores, exacerbation rates, bronchial reactivity, or changes in airway responsiveness (1.30 units of methacholine, 95% CI 0.73 to 1.87 with salmeterol *v* 0.80, 95% CI 0.33 to 1.27 with placebo). No benefit of either adding salmeterol or a second dose of beclometasone was found in this group of children whose compliance with pre-existing medication was good.

Harms: Growth was significantly slower in children receiving higher dose inhaled corticosteroids (3.6 cm, 95% CI 3.0 cm to 4.2 cm with double dose beclometasone *v* 5.1 cm, 95% CI 4.5 cm to 5.7 cm with salmeterol *v* 4.5 cm, 95% CI 3.8 cm to 5.2 cm with placebo).

Comment: Higher dose inhaled corticosteroids are frequently used despite lack of evidence of benefit. In some children, higher prescribed doses may compensate for poor compliance or incorrect inhaler technique.

OPTION ADDITION OF REGULAR LONG ACTING β_2 AGONIST

One RCT in children aged 6–16 years found that addition of inhaled salmeterol increased peak expiratory flow rates in the first few months of treatment but found no increase after 1 year. A second short term RCT in children aged 4–16 years also found increased morning peak expiratory flow rates and more symptom free days at 3 months with addition of inhaled salmeterol.

Benefits: We found no systematic review but found two RCTs.[53,54] One RCT (177 children) found that at 1 year the addition of inhaled salmeterol did not improve lung function, airway responsiveness, symptom scores, exacerbation rates, or bronchial reactivity.[53] Salmeterol versus placebo increased mean morning peak expiratory flow rates slightly after 3 months (difference: +12 L/min). There were no significant differences in symptom scores at any time. The second RCT (210 children aged 4–16 years, 12 weeks' follow up, mean morning peak flow expiratory rate 79% predicted) compared salmeterol (50 µg twice daily) versus placebo in children inadequately controlled on inhaled corticosteroids (average dose 750 µg/day).[54] At 12 weeks, mean morning peak expiratory flow rate (relative to the predicted peak flow expiratory rate) was 4% higher in the salmeterol group. Mean evening peak expiratory flow rate was not significantly different. The median proportion of symptom free days improved more with salmeterol than with placebo (60% with salmeterol *v* 30% with placebo for the third month of treatment).

Harms: The RCTs found no significant adverse effects associated with salmeterol.[53,54]

Comment: The second RCT was organised and funded by the manufacturer of salmeterol. Studies of adults with poor control on low dose inhaled corticosteroids have found greater benefit with additional long acting β_2 agonists than with higher doses of inhaled steroid (see salmeterol v high dose inhaled corticosteroids in asthma in adults topic, p 1757).

OPTION ADDITION OF ORAL THEOPHYLLINE

One small brief RCT found that addition of theophylline versus placebo to previous treatment significantly increased the number of symptom free days and significantly reduced the use of additional β agonist and additional corticosteroid medication. We found insufficient evidence to weigh these short term benefits and possible long term harms.

Benefits: We found no systematic review but found one RCT (double blind crossover trial, 33 children, age 6–19 years, recruited from a hospital asthma clinic, 22 children used inhaled beclometasone [mean 533 μg/day], 11 used oral prednisolone [mean 30 mg alternate days]).[42] It found that the addition for 4 weeks of oral theophylline (serum concentration 10–20 μg/mL) versus placebo increased the mean number of symptom free days (63% with theophylline *v* 42% with placebo; $P \leq 0.01$). Inhaled β agonist (orciprenaline — see glossary, p 341) was needed twice as often with placebo (0.5 doses/day with theophylline *v* 1.0 with placebo; $P \leq 0.01$). Additional daily prednisolone was needed by fewer children while on theophylline than while on placebo (3/32 [9%] with theophylline *v* 10/32 [31%] with placebo; P = 0.02).

Harms: In the RCT, short term adverse effects included mild transient headache and nausea in six children after the crossover from placebo to the theophylline dose that they had previously tolerated.[55]

Comment: One child was excluded from the analysis because of poor compliance. The RCT was too brief to assess long term harms.

OPTION ADDITION OF ORAL LEUKOTRIENE RECEPTOR ANTAGONISTS

One crossover RCT in children aged 6–14 years with persistent asthma who had been taking inhaled budesonide for at least 6 weeks found that the addition of oral montelukast versus placebo significantly improved lung function and decreased the proportion of days with asthma exacerbations over 4 weeks. These differences were statistically significant but modest in clinical terms.

Benefits: We found no systematic review but found one crossover RCT (279 children aged 6–14 years previously treated with inhaled corticosteroid for at least 6 wks, with mean forced expiratory volume in 1 second 78% predicted after 1 month run-in with budesonide 200 μg) comparing adding oral montelukast versus placebo to inhaled budesonide over 4 weeks.[56] It found variable changes in forced expiratory volume in 1 second with montelukast versus placebo (primary efficacy analysis of 251 children, relative change of forced expiratory volume in 1 second, relative to baseline: 4.6% with montelukast *v* 3.3% with placebo, 95% CI –0.1% to +2.7%; per-protocol analysis of 205 children, 6.0% with montelukast *v* 4.1% with placebo, 95% CI 0.5% to 3.4%). It found fewer asthma exacerbation days (decrease from baseline peak flow of > 20%, or increase from baseline of β_2 agonist use of > 70%) with montelukast versus placebo (12.2% with montelukast *v* 15.9% with placebo; P = < 0.001). No significant differences were found in quality of life measurements, global evaluations, or asthma attacks requiring unscheduled medical intervention or treatment with oral corticosteroid.

Harms: The RCT found no significant difference with montelukast versus placebo in asthma exacerbation, upper respiratory tract infection, headache, cough, pharyngitis, and fever.[56]

Comment: The RCT in children was brief (4 wks treatment).[56] We found one large RCT of montelukast added to beclometasone in adults with inadequately controlled asthma that found benefit over a 16 week period.[57] Both RCTs were funded by the manufacturers of montelukast.

QUESTION What are the effects of treatments for acute wheezing in infants?

Michael McKean

OPTION SHORT ACTING β_2 AGONISTS

One RCT in infants aged 3 months to 2 years found that nebulised salbutamol versus placebo significantly improved respiratory rate and clinical symptom score but found no significant difference in hospital admission. Another RCT in children aged less than 18 months to 36 months found no significant difference in change from baseline in clinical symptom scores with nebulised salbutamol versus placebo. Two RCTs in children aged up to 5 years found no significant difference in hospital admission with delivery of salbutamol through a metered dose inhaler plus spacer versus nebulised salbutamol. Another RCT in infants aged 1–24 months found no significant difference in improvement of symptoms with delivery of terbutaline through a metered dose inhaler plus spacer versus nebulised terbutaline. Nebulised β_2 agonists may cause tachycardia, tremor, and hypokalaemia.

Benefits: **Nebulised salbutamol versus placebo:** We found one systematic review (search date not stated)[58] that identified two RCTs in children with an acute exacerbation of wheeze in hospital emergency room settings.[59,60] One RCT (28 infants aged 3 months to 2 years) compared nebulised salbutamol (see glossary, p 341) (0.3 mg/kg in 2 doses over 1 h) versus placebo on respiratory rate and symptom score (assessment of heart rate, respiratory rate, wheeze, and accessory muscle score).[59] The RCT found that nebulised salbutamol versus placebo significantly improved respiratory rate (WMD –5.10 breaths/min, 95% CI –9.45 breaths/min to –0.75 breaths/min) and total clinical symptom score for heart rate, respiratory rate, wheezing, and accessory muscle use (clinical symptom score on scale 0 [none] to 3 [severe], WMD –2.50, 95% CI –3.88 to –1.12) but found no significant difference in hospital admission (OR 1.95, 95% CI 0.27 to 13.98).[59] The second RCT (28 infants aged < 18 months and 13 infants aged 18–36 months with acute wheeze) found no significant difference in change from baseline in clinical symptom scores with nebulised salbutamol (2 doses of 0.15 mg/kg) versus placebo groups. Some improvement was observed in children aged more than 18 months, but this was not statistically significant.[60] **Delivery through metered dose inhaler versus nebuliser:** We found three RCTs comparing delivery of short acting β_2 agonists through metered dose inhaler versus nebuliser.[61–63] The first RCT (64 children aged 1–5 years with acute recurrent wheezing) found no significant difference in hospital admission with delivery of salbutamol (50 μg/kg) through a metered dose inhaler plus spacer versus nebulised salbutamol (150 μg/kg).[61] The second RCT (42 infants, mean age < 2 years with acute wheezing) found no significant difference in hospital admission with delivery of salbutamol (400 μg) through a metered dose inhaler plus spacer versus nebulised salbutamol (2.5 mg).[62] The third RCT (34 infants aged 1–24 months) found no significant difference in the rate of improvement from baseline of a clinical score (assessing respiratory rate, wheezing, retractions, degree of cyanosis, colour, and pulse oximetry data) with delivery of terbutaline (500 μg) through a metered dose inhaler plus spacer versus nebulised terbutaline (4 mg).[63]

Harms: **Nebulised salbutamol versus placebo:** The systematic review did not comment on any adverse effects of nebulised salbutamol in infants with acute wheezing.[58] Nebulised β_2 agonists may cause tachycardia, tremor, and hypokalaemia.[62] **Delivery through metered dose inhaler versus nebuliser:** Three RCTs found no clinically significant adverse events.[61–63]

Comment: None.

OPTION INHALED IPRATROPIUM BROMIDE

We found no RCTs comparing inhaled ipratropium bromide versus placebo. One RCT identified by a systematic review in infants aged 3–24 months found that addition of ipratropium bromide to fenoterol versus fenoterol alone significantly reduced the proportion of infants receiving further treatment 45 minutes after initial treatment.

Benefits: **Versus placebo:** We found no RCTs. **Addition to long acting β_2 agonist:** We found one systematic review (search date not stated), which identified one RCT in infants aged under 2 years with wheeze.[64] The RCT (61 infants aged 3–24 months with acute wheeze) found that addition of ipratropium bromide (50 μg) to fenoterol (0.1 mg/kg) versus fenoterol (0.1 mg/kg) alone significantly reduced the proportion of infants receiving further treatment 45 minutes after initial treatment (OR 0.22, 95% CI 0.08 to 0.61).

Harms: The systematic review found no evidence of harm specific to the use of ipratropium bromide.[64]

Comment: The results of the review do not support the widespread, indiscriminate use of anticholinergic agents in the treatment of children under the age of 2 years with airways obstruction and wheeze. It is possible that infants did obtain symptomatic relief but that this was not always identified by the outcomes chosen.

OPTION ORAL CORTICOSTEROIDS

One small RCT found no significant difference in daily symptom scores with oral prednisolone versus placebo.

Benefits: We found one RCT (38 acutely wheezing infants aged 3–17 months with wheezing episode lasting ≥ 48 h, including 30 infants who had previously been admitted to hospital with wheeze)[65] comparing oral prednisolone (2 mg/kg/day) versus placebo given for 5 days during an acute wheezing episode. It found no significant difference in daily symptom scores (cough, wheeze, breathlessness) for the 56 acute wheezing episodes studied.[65]

Harms: The RCT found no adverse effects.[65]

Comment: None.

OPTION HIGH DOSE INHALED CORTICOSTEROIDS

One systematic review found that high dose inhaled corticosteroids versus placebo reduced the requirement for oral corticosteroids but the difference was not statistically significant. The review also found a clear preference for the inhaled corticosteroids by the children's parents over placebo. The clinical importance of these results is unclear.

Benefits: We found one systematic review (search date not stated, 2 RCTs in infants with acute viral wheeze (see glossary, p 341)).[66] The primary outcome for the review was wheeze episodes requiring oral corticosteroids. The review found that episodic high dose inhaled corticosteroids (budesonide, beclometasone) versus placebo reduced the need for oral corticosteroids but the difference was not statistically significant (2 crossover RCTs, 67 infants; RR 0.53, 95% CI 0.27 to 1.04). The review also found a clear preference for the inhaled corticosteroids by the children's parents over placebo (2 crossover RCTs, 67 infants; RR 0.64, 95% CI, 0.48 to 0.87).[66]

Harms: The systematic review did not report any adverse events. See harms of inhaled corticosteroids, p 328.[66]

Comment: Most of the RCTs included in the systematic review were carried out before the 1990s when it was commonly thought that wheeze was synonymous with asthma and different patterns of wheeze in young children were seldom recognised. Although there is some evidence to support the use of high dose inhaled corticosteroids in acute episodes of viral wheeze, the practicalities of delivering treatment may limit applicability.

QUESTION What are the effects of prophylactic treatments for wheezing in infants?

Michael McKean

OPTION INHALED IPRATROPIUM BROMIDE

One small RCT identified by a systematic review found no significant difference in relief of symptoms with nebulised ipratropium bromide versus placebo. The study may have lacked power to exclude a clinically important difference between treatments.

Benefits: We found one systematic review (search date not stated),[64] which found one RCT of high quality although the power of the RCT was low.[67] The RCT (crossover, 23 infants aged 4–23 months) compared nebulised ipratropium bromide versus placebo or sodium cromoglicate. The RCT found no significant difference in relief of symptoms as defined by diary cards for ipratropium bromide versus placebo (OR 0.60, 95% CI 0.19 to 1.88).[67]

Harms: The RCT reported no significant adverse effects with ipratropium bromide.[67]

Comment: The study may have lacked power to exclude a clinically important difference between treatments. We found insufficient data to support the use of ipratropium bromide as a prophylactic agent for wheezing in infants.

OPTION SHORT ACTING β_2 AGONISTS

Two RCTs identified by a systematic review in infants aged up to 2 years found no significant improvement in symptoms with inhaled salbutamol versus placebo. Another RCT identified by the same systematic review in infants aged 3–14 months found that oral salbutamol versus placebo significantly reduced treatment failures.

Benefits: We found one systematic review (search date not stated), which identified three RCTs in infants aged under 2 years with recurrent wheeze but no apparent history of acute viral bronchiolitis.[58] **Inhaled short acting β_2 agonists:** One RCT (crossover, 80 infants aged < 1 year with persistent or recurrent wheeze and a personal or family history of atopy) compared inhaled salbutamol (see glossary, p 341) (200 μg/day) versus placebo for 4 weeks. It found no significant difference between salbutamol versus placebo in symptoms (recorded in a diary) or lung function.[68] Another RCT (29 infants aged 2–18 months with a history of recurrent wheeze) compared inhaled salbutamol (600 μg) plus inhaled beclometasone (300 μg) versus inhaled salbutamol (600 μg) alone or placebo for 6 weeks.[69] It found no significant improvement in symptoms (cough, wheezing, sleep problems, expectorations) with salbutamol versus placebo.[69] **Oral short acting β_2 agonists:** One RCT (59 infants aged 3–14 months with at least 1 previous wheezy episode) compared oral salbutamol plus placebo, placebo plus prednisolone, and placebo plus placebo for 14 days.[70] It found that oral salbutamol versus placebo significantly reduced treatment failures (RR 2.51, 95% CI 1.09 to 5.79) and found no significant difference between salbutamol alone and the combination of salbutamol plus prednisolone.[70]

Harms: **Inhaled short acting β_2 agonists:** The RCTs did not report any adverse events.[68,69] **Oral short acting β_2 agonists:** The RCTs did not report any adverse events.[70]

Comment: None.

OPTION INHALED CORTICOSTEROIDS

Three RCTs found no clear evidence of effectiveness with lower prophylactic doses of inhaled corticosteroids (budesonide) in children aged 1 week to 6 years with recurrent wheeze. One RCT in infants aged

6–30 months found that higher prophylactic doses of inhaled corticosteroids (budesonide) versus placebo significantly reduced symptoms and the proportion of children with acute wheezing episodes during a 12 week period but found no significant reduction in the proportion of wheezing episodes per infant. Another RCT in infants aged 11–36 months found that higher prophylactic doses in inhaled corticosteroid (budesonide) significantly reduced the proportion of days requiring oral prednisolone and symptoms of wheezing and sleep disturbance but found no significant improvement for cough. Higher doses of inhaled corticosteroids have the potential for adverse effects. One RCT found no significant improvement in symptoms with addition of inhaled beclometasone versus placebo to inhaled salbutamol.

Benefits: We found one systematic review (search date not stated)[66] and four additional RCTs.[71–74] **Lower dose versus placebo:** The systematic review identified one RCT.[75] The RCT (57 children aged 8 months to 6 years) found no significant difference after 4 months in acute episodes of wheeze with inhaled budesonide (400 μg/day by metered dose inhaler) versus placebo.[75] The RCT did not analyse infants separately. The first additional RCT (29 infants aged 4–17 months with recurrent wheeze) found that inhaled budesonide (150 μg through a metered dose inhaler) versus placebo significantly improved some symptoms (breathlessness, daytime wheeze, daytime cough) but not others (night time wheeze and cough), and found no significant difference in the need for bronchodilators.[73] The second additional RCT (60 infants aged 1–42 wks ready for discharge after an episode of acute viral bronchiolitis requiring hospital admission) compared inhaled budesonide (200 μg/day through a metered dose inhaler) versus placebo for 12 months.[74] Symptoms of coughing and wheezing were recorded in a diary kept by parents. The RCT found no significant difference after 6 months in symptoms of coughing and wheezing with inhaled budesonide versus placebo.[74] **Higher dose versus placebo:** One additional RCT (40 infants aged 6–30 months with severe asthma) compared nebulised budesonide (1 mg twice daily) versus placebo for 12 weeks.[71] The RCT found that nebulised budesonide versus placebo significantly reduced the proportion of children with acute wheezing episodes (40% with budesonide *v* 83% with placebo; $P < 0.01$), incidence of daytime wheezing (2.2% with budesonide *v* 11.6% with placebo; $P < 0.05$), and incidence of night time wheezing (0.6% with budesonide *v* 6.5% with placebo; $P < 0.01$) but did not significantly reduce the number of acute wheezing episodes per child (0% with budesonide *v* 1% with placebo; $P = 0.13$). The second additional RCT (77 infants aged 11–36 months with moderate to severe recurrent wheezing) compared inhaled budesonide (400 μg twice daily) versus placebo for 12 weeks.[72] The RCT found that budesonide versus placebo significantly improved symptom scores from baseline for wheezing and sleep disturbance ($P < 0.05$ for both symptoms) but found no significant difference for cough or for restriction in physical activity because of coughing or wheezing. It also found that inhaled budesonide versus placebo significantly reduced the proportion of days requiring oral prednisolone.[72] **Addition of inhaled corticosteroid to short acting β_2 agonist:** We found one RCT (31 infants aged 13–18 months with recurrent wheeze) comparing addition of inhaled beclometasone (200 μg twice daily) to inhaled salbutamol (see glossary, p 341) (taken when needed) versus addition of inhaled placebo to inhaled salbutamol (as needed).[75] It found no significant difference between adding beclometasone versus placebo in clinical score, number of salbutamol doses, sleep disturbance, or number of symptom free days.[76]

Harms: The RCTs did not report any adverse events.[71–76] Higher doses of inhaled corticosteroids have the potential for adverse effects (see harms of inhaled corticosteroids, p 328).

Comment: None.

GLOSSARY

Aminophylline A stable combination of theophylline and ethylenediamine; the ethylenediamine is added to increase the solubility of theophylline in water.

Clinical asthma score is used to assess asthma severity. It involves five clinical variables (respiratory rate, wheezing, inspiratory–expiratory ratio, indrawing, dyspnoea), which are scored 0, 1, or 2. The scores for each variable are added together with a possible total score of 10.[77]

Orciprenaline is known as metaproterenol in USA; it is a non-selective β agonist.

Salbutamol is known as albuterol in USA; it is a short acting selective β_2 agonist.

Viral wheeze is defined as wheeze in association with nasal congestion and discharge but minimal or no intercurrent lower respiratory tract symptoms.

REFERENCES

1. Russell G, Ninan TK. Respiratory symptoms and atopy in Aberdeen school children: evidence from two surveys 25 years apart. *BMJ* 1992;304:873–875.
2. Kabesh M, Von Mutius E. Epidemiology and public health. In: Silverman M ed. *Childhood asthma and other wheezing disorders*. 2nd ed. London: Arnold, 2002.
3. Park ES, Golding J, Carswell F, et al. Pre-school wheezing and prognosis at 10. *Arch Dis Child* 1986;61:642–646.
4. Kelly WJW, Hudson I, Phelan PD, et al. Childhood asthma in adult life: a further study at 28 years of age. *BMJ* 1987; 294:1059–1062.
5. Martinez FD, Wright AL, Taussig L, et al. Asthma and wheezing in the first six years of life. *N Engl J Med* 1995;333:133–138.
6. Geelhoed GC, Landau LI, Le Souef PN. Evaluation of SaO2 as a predictor of outcome in 280 children presenting with acute asthma. *Ann Emerg Med* 1994;23:1236–1241.
7. Plotnick LH, Ducharme FM. Combined inhaled anticholinergics and β_2 agonists in the initial management of acute paediatric asthma. In: The Cochrane Library, Issue 3, 2002. Oxford: Update Software. Search date 2000; primary sources Medline, Embase, Cinahl, hand searches of bibliographies of references, and contact with pharmaceutical companies for details of unpublished trials and personal contacts.
8. Goggin N, Macarthur C, Parkin PC. Randomized trial of the addition of ipratropium bromide to albuterol and corticosteroid therapy in children hospitalized because of an acute asthma exacerbation. *Arch Pediatr Adolesc Med* 2001;155:1329–1334.
9. Cates CJ. Holding chambers versus nebulisers for β-agonist treatment of acute asthma. In: The Cochrane Library, Issue 3, 2002. Oxford: Update Software. Search date 2001; primary sources Medline and Cochrane Airways Review Group Register.
10. Chou KJ, Cunningham SJ, Crain EF. Metered-dose inhalers with spacers vs nebulizers for pediatric asthma. *Arch Pediatr Adolesc Med* 1995;149:201–205.
11. Rowe BH, Spooner C, Ducharme FM, et al. Early emergency department treatment of acute asthma with systemic corticosteroids (Cochrane Review) In: The Cochrane Library, Issue 3, 2002. Oxford: Update Software. Last amended November 2000. Search date 1999; primary sources Cochrane Airways Review Group Register, Embase, Medline, Cinahl, and hand searches.
12. Patel H, Macarthur C, Johnson D. Recent corticosteroids use and the risk of complicated varicella in otherwise immunocompetent children. *Arch Pediatr Adolesc Med* 1996;150:409–414.
13. Edmonds ML, Camargo CA Jr, Pollack CV Jr, et al. Early use of inhaled corticosteroids in the emergency department treatment of acute asthma. In: The Cochrane Library, Issue 3, 2002. Oxford: Update Software. Search date 2000; primary sources Cochrane Airways Group Register, and hand searches of bibliographies.
14. Manjra AI, Price J, Lenney W, et al. Efficacy of nebulised fluticasone propionate compared with oral prednisolone in children with an acute exacerbation of asthma. *Respir Med* 2000;94:1206–1214.
15. Matthews EE, Curtis PD, McLain B, et al. Nebulized budesonide versus oral steroid in severe exacerbations of childhood asthma. *Acta Paediatr* 1999;88:841–843.
16. Schuh S, Resiman J, Alshehri M, et al. A comparison of inhaled fluticasone and oral prednisone for children with severe acute asthma. *N Engl J Med* 2000;343:689–694.
17. Scarfone RJ, Loiselle JM, Wiley JF II, et al. Nebulized dexamethasone versus oral prednisone in the emergency treatment of asthmatic children. *Ann Emerg Med* 1995;26:480–486.
18. Volowitz B, Bentur L, Finkelstein Y, et al. Effectiveness and safety of inhaled corticosteroids in controlling acute asthma attacks in children

who were treated in the emergency department: a controlled comparative study with oral prednisolone. *J Allergy Clin Immunol* 1998;102:1605–1609.
19. Devidayal S, Singhi S, Kumar L, et al. Efficacy of nebulized budesonide compared to oral prednisolone in acute bronchial asthma. *Acta Paediatr* 1999;88:835–840.
20. Mitra A, Bassler D, Ducharme FM. Intravenous aminophylline for acute severe asthma in children over 2 years using inhaled bronchodilators (Cochrane Review). In: The Cochrane Library, Issue 1, 2002. Oxford: Update Software. Search date 2001; primary sources Cochrane Airways Group Register and reference lists of relevant articles.
21. Ream RS, Loftis LL, Albers GM, et al. Efficacy of IV theophylline in children with severe status asthmaticus. *Chest* 2001;119:1480–1488.
22. Calpin C, Macarthur C, Stephens D, et al. Effectiveness of prophylactic inhaled steroids in childhood asthma: a systematic review of the literature. *J Allergy Clin Immunol* 1997;100:452–457. Search date 1996; primary source Medline.
23. Tinkelman DG, Reed C, Nelson H, et al. Aerosol beclomethasone diproprionate compared with theophylline as primary treatment of chronic, mild to moderately severe asthma in children. *Pediatrics* 1993;92:64–77.
24. Ng SH, Dash CH, Savage SJ. Betamethasone valerate compared with sodium cromoglycate in asthmatic children. *Postgrad Med J* 1977;53:315–320.
25. Kannisto S, Voutilainen R, Remes K, et al. Efficacy and safety of inhaled steroid and cromone treatment in school-age children: a randomized pragmatic pilot study. *Pediatr Allergy Immunol* 2002;13:24–30.
26. Leflein JG, Szefler SJ, Murphy KR, et al. Nebulized budesonide inhalation suspension compared with cromolyn sodium nebulizer solution for asthma in young children: results of a randomized outcomes trial. *Pediatrics* 2002;109:866–872.
27. Price JF, Weller PH. Comparison of fluticasone propionate and sodium cromoglycate for the treatment of childhood asthma (an open parallel group study). *Respir Med* 1995;89:363–368.
28. The Childhood Asthma Management Program Research Group. Long-term effects of budesonide or nedocromil in children with asthma. *N Engl J Med* 2000;343:1054–1063.
29. Verberne A, Frost C, Roorda R, et al. One year treatment with salmeterol compared with beclomethasone in children with asthma. *Am J Respir Crit Care Med* 1997;156:688–695.
30. Simons FER and the Canadian Beclomethasone Diproprionate–Salmeterol Xinafoate Study Group. A comparison of beclomethasone, salmeterol and placebo in children with asthma. *N Engl J Med* 1997;337:1659–1665.
31. Ducharme FM, Hicks GC. Anti-leukotriene agents compared to inhaled corticosteroids in the management of recurrent and/or acute asthma. In: The Cochrane Library, Issue 3, 2002. Search date 1999; primary sources Medline, Embase, Cinahl, hand searches of reference lists, and personal contact with colleagues and internal headquarters of leukotriene producers.
32. Drake AJ, Howells RJ, Shield JPH, et al. Symptomatic adrenal insufficiency presenting with hypoglycaemia in children with asthma receiving high dose inhaled fluticasone proprionate. *BMJ* 2002;324:1081–1083.
33. Todd GR, Acerini CL, Ross-Russell R, et al. Survey of adrenal crisis associated with inhaled corticosteroids in the United Kingdom. *Arch Dis Child* 2002;87:457–461.
34. Wolthers OD, Riis BJ, Pedersen S. Bone turnover in asthmatic children treated with oral prednisolone or inhaled budesonide. *Pediatr Pulmonol* 1993;16:341–346.
35. Reilly SM, Hambleton G, Adams JE, et al. Bone density in asthmatic children treated with inhaled corticosteroids. *Arch Dis Child* 2001;84:183–184.
36. Simons FE, Persaud MP, Gillespie CA, et al. Absence of posterior subcapsular cataracts in young patients treated with inhaled corticosteroids. *Lancet* 1993;342:776–778.
37. Abuektish F, Kirkpatrick JN, Russell G. Posterior subcapsular cataract and inhaled steroid therapy. *Thorax* 1995;50:674–676.
38. Allen DB, Mullen M, Mullen B. A meta-analysis of the effect of oral and inhaled steroids on growth. *J Allergy Clin Immunol* 1994;93:967–976. Search date 1993; primary sources literature searches of leading medical journals 1956–1993.
39. Sharek PJ, Bergman DA. Beclomethasone for asthma in children: effects on linear growth. In: The Cochrane Library, Issue 3, 2002. Oxford: Update Software. Search date 1999; primary source Cochrane Airways Group Asthma Trials Register.
40. Doull 1995, Freezer NJ, Holgate ST. Growth of prepubertal children with mild asthma treated with inhaled beclometasone dipropionate. *Am J Resp Crit Care Med* 1995;151:1715–1719.
41. Agertoft L, Pedersen S. Effects of long-term treatment with an inhaled corticosteroid on growth and pulmonary function in asthmatic children. *Respir Med* 1994;88:373–381.
42. Agertoft L, Pedersen S. Effect of long-term treatment with inhaled budesonide on adult height in children with asthma. *N Engl J Med* 2000;343:1064–1069.
43. Tasche M, Uijen J, Bernsen R, et al. Inhaled disodium cromoglycate (DSCG) as maintenance therapy in children with asthma: a systematic review. *Thorax* 2000;55:913–920. Search date 1999; primary sources Medline, Embase, Cochrane Controlled Trials Register, database of manufacturers of disoduim cromoglicate, and hand searched referecnes.
44. Edwards A, Holgate S, Howell J, et al. Sodium cromoglycate in childhood asthma [Letter]. *Thorax* 2001;56:331.
45. Armenio L, Baldini C, Bardare M, et al. Double blind placebo controlled study of nedocromil sodium in asthma. *Arch Dis Child* 1993;68:193–197.
46. Edwards AM, Lyons J, Weinberg E, et al. Early use of inhaled nedocromil sodium in children following an acute episode of asthma. *Thorax* 1999;54:308–315.
47. Weinstein S, Pearlman D, Bronsky E, et al. Efficacy of salmeterol xinafoate powder in children with chronic persistent asthma. *Ann Allergy Asthma Immunol* 1998;81:51–58.
48. Pedersen S. Treatment of nocturnal asthma in children with a single dose of sustained release theophylline taken after supper. *Clin Allergy* 1985;15:79–85.
49. Stein MA, Krasowski M, Leventhal BL, et al. Behavioural and cognitive effects of theophylline and caffeine. *Arch Pediatr Adolesc Med* 1996;50:284–288. Search date not stated; primary sources Medline, Psychlit, Dissertation Abstracts, and hand searched references.
50. Tsiu SJ, Self TH, Burns R. Theophylline toxicity: update. *Ann Allergy* 1990;64:241–257.
51. Knorr B, Matz J, Bernstein JA, et al. Montelukast for chronic asthma in 6–14 year old children. *JAMA* 1998;279:1181–1186.
52. Knorr B. Franchi LM, Bisgaard H, et al. Montelukast, a leukotriene receptor antagonist for

the treatment of persistent asthma in children aged 2–5 years. *Pediatrics* 2001;108:E48.
53. Verberne A, Frost C, Duiverman E, et al. Addition of salmeterol versus doubling the dose of beclomethasone in children with asthma. *Am J Respir Crit Care Med* 1998;158:213–219.
54. Russell G, Williams DAJ, Weller P, et al. Salmeterol xinafoate in children on high dose inhaled steroids. *Ann Allergy Asthma Immunol* 1995;75:423–428.
55. Nassif EG, Weinberger M, Thompson R, et al. The value of maintenance theophylline in steroid dependent asthma. *N Engl J Med* 1981;304:71–75.
56. Simons FER, Villa JR, Lee BW, et al. Montelukast added to budesonide in children with persistent asthma: a randomized double blind crossover study. *J Pediatr* 2001;138:694–698.
57. Laviolette M, Malmstrom K, Lu S, et al. Montelukast added to inhaled beclomethasone in treatment of asthma. *Am J Respir Crit Care Med* 1999;160:1862–1868.
58. Chavasse R, Seddon P, Bara A, et al. Short acting beta agonists for recurrent wheeze in children under 2 years of age. In: The Cochrane Library, 2002. Oxford: Update Software. Search date not stated; primary sources Medline and Pubmed.
59. Bentur L, Canny GJ, Shields MD, et al. Controlled trial of nebulised albuterol in children younger than 2 years of age with acute asthma. *Pediatrics* 1992;89:133–137.
60. Prahl P, Petersen NT, Hornsleth A. Beta2-agonists for the treatment of wheezy bronchitis. *Ann Allergy* 1986;57:439–441.
61. Ploin D, Chapuis FR, Stamm D, et al. High-dose albuterol by metered dose inhaler plus a spacer device versus nebulization in preschool children with recurrent wheezing: a double-blind randomized equivalence trial. *Pediatrics* 2000;106:311–317.
62. Mandelberg A, Tsehori S, Houri S, et al. Is nebulized aerosol treatment necessary in the pediatric emergency department? *Chest* 2000;117:1309–1313.
63. Closa RM, Ceballos JM, Gomez-Papi A, et al. Efficacy of bronchodilators administered by nebulizers versus spacer devices in infants with acute wheezing. *Pediatr Pulmonol* 1998;26:344–348.
64. Everard ML, Bara A, Kurian M, et al. Anticholinergic drugs for wheeze in children under the age of two years. In: The Cochrane Library, Issue 3, 2002. Oxford: Update Software. Search date not stated; primary sources Cochrane Airways Group Register and hand searches of respiratory care and paediatric journals.
65. Webb M, Henry R, Milner AD. Oral corticosteroids for wheezing attacks under 18 months. *Arch Dis Child* 1986;61:15–19.
66. McKean M, Ducharme F. Inhaled steroids for episodic viral wheeze of childhood. Cochrane Database Syst Rev 2000:3. Search date not stated; primary sources Cochrane Airways Group Register and reference lists of articles.
67. Henry RL, Hiller EJ, Milner AD, et al. Nebulised ipratropium bromide and sodium cromoglycate in the first two years of life. *Arch Dis Child* 1984;59:54–57.
68. Chavasse RJ, Bastian-Lee Y, Richter H, et al. Inhaled salbutamol for wheezy infants: a randomised controlled trial. *Arch Dis Child* 2000;82:370–375.
69. Kraemer R, Graf Bigler U, Casaulter Aebischer C, et al. Clinical and physiological improvement after inhalation of low- dose beclomethasone dipropionate and salbutamol in wheezy infants. *Respiration* 1997;64:342–349.
70. Fox GF, Marsh MJ, Milner AD. Treatment of recurrent acute wheezing episodes in infancy with oral salbutamol and prednisolone. *Eur J Pediatr* 1996;155:512–516.
71. de Blic J, Delacourt C, Le Bourgeois M, et al. Efficacy of nebulized budesonide in treatment of severe infantile asthma: a double-blind study. *J Allergy Clin Immunol* 1996;98:14–20.
72. Bisgaard H, Munck SL, Nielsen JP, et al. Inhaled budesonide for treatment of recurrent wheezing in early childhood. *Lancet* 1990;336:649–651.
73. Noble V, Ruggins NR, Everard ML, et al. Inhaled budesonide for chronic wheezing under 18 months of age. *Arch Dis Child* 1992;67:285–288.
74. Fox GF, Everard ML, Marsh MJ, et al. Randomised controlled trial of budesonide for the prevention of post-bronchiolitis wheezing. *Arch Dis Child* 1999;80:343–347.
75. Wilson N, Sloper K, Silverman M. Effect of continuous treatment with topical corticosteroid on episodic viral wheeze in preschool children. *Arch Dis Child* 1995;72:317–320.
76. Barrueto L, Mallol J, Figueroa L. Beclomethasone dipropionate and salbutamol by metered dose inhaler in infants and small children with recurrent wheezing. *Pediatr Pulmonol* 2002;34:52–57.
77. Parkin PC, Macarthur C, Saunders NR, et al. Development of clinical asthma score for use in hospitalized children between 1 and 5 years of age. *J Clin Epidemiol* 1996;49:821–825.

Duncan Keeley
General Practitioner
Thame
UK

Michael McKean
Consultant in Respiratory Paediatrics
Newcastle-upon-Tyne
UK

Competing interests: DK has received occasional consultancy fees or assistance with organisation of, or travel to, meetings from companies including Allen and Hanburys, Astra, MSD, Zeneca, 3M, and Boots. MM none declared.

TABLE 1 **Comparison of inhaled budesonide, nedocromil, and placebo over 4–6 years on several measures of asthma symptoms and morbidity (see text, p 325).[28]**

Intervention	Budesonide (311 children)	Nedocromil (312 children)	Placebo (418 children)
Prednisone courses per 100 person years	70	102	122
Urgent care visits due to asthma per 100 person years	12	16	22
Hospital admissions due to asthma per 100 person years	2.5	4.3	4.4
Beclometasone or other asthma medications added	6.6%	17.1%	18.7%

Bronchiolitis

Search date February 2003

Juan Manuel Lozano

QUESTIONS

INTERVENTIONS

To be covered in future updates
Oxygen
Surfactant, in the context of bronchopulmonary dysplasia

See glossary, p 355

Key Messages

Prevention

- **Respiratory syncytial virus immunoglobulins or palivizumab (monoclonal antibody) in children at high risk** One systematic review has found that, in children born prematurely, in children with bronchopulmonary dysplasia, and in children with a combination of risk factors, prophylactic respiratory syncytial virus immunoglobulin or palivizumab (monoclonal antibody) reduces admission rates to hospital and intensive care units compared with placebo or no prophylaxis.
- **Nursing interventions (cohort segregation, handwashing, gowns, masks, gloves, and goggles) in children admitted to hospital** We found no RCTs about the effects of these interventions to prevent spread of bronchiolitis to other children.

Treatment

- **Bronchodilators (inhaled salbutamol, inhaled adrenaline [epinephrine])** Systematic reviews have found that, inhaled bronchodilators achieve short term improvement in overall clinical scores compared with placebo in children treated in hospital, emergency departments, and outpatient clinics. They have found no evidence that bronchodilators reduce admission rates or produce a clinically important improvement in oxygen saturation. Subsequent RCTs found no evidence that nebulised adrenaline, changed short term outcomes during the first 4 days of illness in infants or the duration of hospital stay compared with 0.9% sodiumk chloride. One small RCT found that nebulised adrenaline reduced the rate of hospital admission compared with salbutamol. However, we were unable to draw reliable conclusions from this small study.

- **Corticosteroids** One systematic review and 10 additional RCTs found limited and conflicting evidence on the effects of corticosteroids compared with placebo.
- **Routine broad spectrum antibiotics** We found no evidence in children with bronchiolitis alone. One unblinded RCT in children with bronchiolitis and uncomplicated pneumonia (crackles on auscultation or consolidation on a chest radiograph) found no significant difference in clinical scores with routine use of antibiotics (ampicillin, penicillin, or erythromycin) compared with placebo. However, the RCT may have lacked power to exclude a clinically important effect.
- **Ribavirin** One systematic review found insufficient evidence that ribavirin reduced mortality, risk of respiratory deterioration, or duration of hospital stay in children admitted to hospital with respiratory syncytial virus bronchiolitis. It found some evidence that ribavirin reduced the duration of mechanical ventilation. Two subsequent RCTs found no evidence that ribavirin reduced duration of hospital stay, admission rate because of lower respiratory tract symptoms during the first year after the acute episode, or the frequency of recurrent wheezing illness over 1 year of follow up.
- **Respiratory syncytial virus immunoglobulins, pooled immunoglobulins, or palivizumab (monoclonal antibody)** RCTs found insufficient evidence on the effects of immunoglobulin treatment.

DEFINITION Bronchiolitis is a virally induced acute bronchiolar inflammation that is associated with signs and symptoms of airway obstruction. Diagnosis is based on clinical findings. Clinical manifestations include fever, rhinitis (inflammation of the nasal mucosa), tachypnoea, expiratory wheezing, cough, rales, use of accessory muscles, apnoea (absence of breathing), dyspnoea (difficulty in breathing), alar flaring (flaring of the nostrils), and retractions (indrawing of the intercostal soft tissues on inspiration). Disease severity (see glossary, p 355) of bronchiolitis may be classified clinically as mild, moderate, or severe.

INCIDENCE/ PREVALENCE Bronchiolitis is the most common lower respiratory tract infection in infants, occurring in a seasonal pattern with highest incidence in the winter in temperate climates,[1] and in the rainy season in warmer countries. Each year in the USA, about 21% of infants have lower respiratory tract disease and 6–10/1000 infants are admitted to hospital for bronchiolitis (1–2% of children < 12 months of age).[2] The peak rate of admission occurs in infants aged 2–6 months.[3]

AETIOLOGY/ RISK FACTORS Respiratory syncytial virus is responsible for bronchiolitis in 70% of cases. This figure reaches 80–100% in the winter months. However, in early spring, parainfluenza virus type 3 is often responsible.[1]

PROGNOSIS **Morbidity and mortality:** Disease severity is related to the size of the infant, and to the proximity and frequency of contact with infective infants. Children at increased risk of morbidity and mortality are those with congenital heart disease, chronic lung disease, history of premature birth, hypoxia, and age less than 6 weeks.[4]

Other factors associated with a prolonged or complicated hospital stay include a history of apnoea or respiratory arrest, pulmonary consolidation seen on a chest radiograph, and (in North America) people of Native American or Inuit race.[5] The risk of death within 2 weeks is high for children with congenital heart disease (3.4%) or chronic lung disease (3.5%) as compared with other groups combined (0.1%).[4] Rates of admission to intensive care units (range 31–36%) and need for mechanical ventilation (range 11–19%) are similar among all high risk groups.[4] The percentage of these children needing oxygen supplementation is also high (range 63–80%).[4] In contrast, rates of intensive care unit admission (15%) and ventilation (8%) in such children are markedly lower.[6] **Long term prognosis:** Information on long term prognosis varies among studies. One small prospective study of two matched cohorts (25 children with bronchiolitis; 25 children without) found no evidence that bronchiolitis requiring outpatient treatment is associated with an increased risk of asthma in the long term.[7] Possible confounding factors include variation in illness severity, smoke exposure, and being in overcrowded environments.[8] We found one prospective study in 50 randomly selected infants admitted with bronchiolitis, followed up by questionnaires for 5 years and a visit in the fifth year. It found a doubling of asthma incidence compared with the general population, although there was large (30%) loss to follow up and no matched control group.[9]

AIMS OF INTERVENTION To decrease morbidity and mortality, shorten hospital stay, and prevent transmission of infection, with minimum adverse effects.

OUTCOMES Death rate; rates of hospital admission; rate of intubation or admission to intensive care units; clinical score (clinical score is a subjective, unvalidated measure that is based on judgements made by the clinician); rates of clinical and serological infection. Oxygen saturation is a proxy outcome, but the clinical significance and sensitivity of this outcome are unclear.

METHODS *Clinical Evidence* search and appraisal February 2003.

QUESTION What are the effects of prophylactic measures in high risk children?

OPTION IMMUNOGLOBULINS

One systematic review has found that, in children born prematurely or children with bronchopulmonary dysplasia, prophylactic respiratory syncytial virus immunoglobulin or palivizumab (monoclonal antibody) given monthly reduces hospital admission and admission to intensive care compared with placebo or no prophylaxis. Treatment duration varied between 4 and 6 months across studies.

Benefits: We found one systematic review (search date 1999, 4 RCTs, 2598 children) comparing monthly respiratory syncytial virus immunoglobulin (RSV Ig) or palivizumab (monoclonal antibody) with placebo or no prophylaxis.[10] Three of the RCTs used intravenous RSV Ig and one used intramuscular palivizumab. Two of the RCTs using RSV Ig were unblinded and both of them used no prophylaxis as the control intervention. The review found that RSV Ig or palivizumab compared with placebo reduced admission to hospital. (95/1535 [6%] for RSV Ig or palivizumab *v* 138/1063 [13%] with placebo; OR 0.48, 95% CI 0.37 to 0.64) and intensive care unit (27/1535 [2%] for RSV Ig or palivizumab *v* 43/1063 [4%] with placebo; OR 0.47, 95% CI 0.29 to 0.77), but did not reduce the incidence of mechanical ventilation (16/1535 [1%] for RSV Ig or palivizumab *v* 14/1063 [1%] with placebo; OR 0.99, 95% CI 0.48 to 2.07). Follow up duration varied across studies in the systematic review from 150 days up to 17 months.[10]

Harms: See harms of immunoglobulins, p 355.

Comment: Premature infants included in the RCTs were children under 6 months old, with gestational age at birth of less than either 32 or 35 weeks. Children with bronchopulmonary dysplasia were under 2 years old and still undergoing treatment for this anomaly. Planned subgroup analysis in the review found that prophylaxis reduced hospital admission in children whose only risk factor was prematurity (OR 0.27, 95% CI 0.15 to 0.49) and in children with bronchopulmonary dysplasia alone (OR 0.54, 95% CI 0.37 to 0.80), but not in children with cardiac comorbidity alone (OR 0.64, 95% CI 0.37 to 1.10).[10] A cost-effectiveness analysis suggests that the clinical effect of palivizumab when used in all children who meet the licensed indication for it is small, and its benefits are likely to be clinically and economically relevant in children at the highest risk.[11]

QUESTION What are the effects of measures to prevent transmission in hospital?

OPTION NURSING INTERVENTIONS (COHORT SEGREGATION, HANDWASHING, GOWNS, MASKS, GLOVES, AND GOGGLES)

We found no direct evidence from RCTs that cohort segregation, handwashing, use of gowns, masks, gloves, or goggles reduced nosocomial transmission of respiratory syncytial virus to other children.

Benefits: We found no systematic review and no good quality RCTs examining effects of cohort segregation (see glossary, p 355), handwashing, gowns, masks, gloves, or goggles, used either singly or in combination, on nosocomial transmission of bronchiolitis in children.

Harms: **Cohort segregation:** Potential risks associated with cohort segregation include misdiagnosing respiratory syncytial virus infection and putting non-infected people at risk by subsequent placement into the wrong cohort. **Handwashing:** Dermatitis is a potential adverse effect of repeated handwashing with some products, affecting care providers. **Other interventions:** No harms reported.

Comment: Handwashing is a well established technique for reducing cross-infection in other contexts, and so RCTs may not be ethically feasible. **Single nursing interventions:** We found four observational studies comparing nosocomial infection rates in separate series of children before and after introduction of cohort segregation, handwashing, gowns and masks, and goggles.[12–15] No study adjusted results for variations in baseline incidence. Three studies found a lower incidence of transmission after introduction of cohort segregation alone, handwashing alone, and eye–nose goggles alone.[12–14] The fourth study found no significant difference in transmission after introducing gowns and masks.[15] **Combinations of nursing interventions:** We found one RCT (58 medical personnel caring for children admitted with bronchiolitis), which found no significant difference in nosocomial infection rate in staff when they used gowns and masks in addition to handwashing (5/28 [18%] of those using gowns, masks, and handwashing *v* 4/30 [13%] in the control group; RR 1.3, 95% CI 0.4 to 3.6).[16] The RCT did not report transmission rates in the children. One non-randomised prospective trial (233 children at risk of severe nosocomial infection) compared transmission rates in wards using different nursing policies.[17] It found that a combination of cohort segregation, gowns, and gloves reduced nosocomial transmission rates compared with all other policies (cohort segregation alone, gown and gloves alone, no special precautions) taken together. However, the control interventions did not remain constant throughout the trial, the results were based on an interim analysis, and the definition of "at risk" children was not stated clearly.

QUESTION **What are the effects of treatment for children with bronchiolitis?**

OPTION **BRONCHODILATORS (INHALED SALBUTAMOL, INHALED ADRENALINE [EPINEPHRINE])**

Good quality systematic reviews have found that, inhaled bronchodilators overall clinical scores in the short term compared with placebo in children treated in hospital, emergency departments, and outpatient clinics. They have found no evidence that bronchodilators reduce admission rates or produce a clinically important improvement in oxygen saturation. Subsequent RCTs found no evidence that nebulised adrenaline, changed short term outcomes during the first 4 days of illness in infants or the duration of hospital stay compared with 0.9% sodium chloride. One small RCT found that nebulised adrenaline reduced the rate of hospital admission when compared with salbutamol.

Benefits: **Compared with placebo:** We found two systematic reviews[18,19] and two subsequent RCTs.[20,21] The first review (search date 1998, 8 RCTs, 485 children) evaluated children in outpatient clinics or the emergency department and after admission to hospital.[18] The second review (search date 1995, 5 RCTs, 251 children) considered children treated in outpatient clinics.[19] Four RCTs were common to both reviews. The first review found that, in the short term, bronchodilators improved clinical scores in children with mild and moderately severe bronchiolitis (lack of improvement in clinical score, bronchodilator *v* placebo; RR 0.76, 95% CI 0.60 to 0.95).[18] Both reviews found evidence that bronchodilators improved oxygen saturation by a clinically unimportant amount (mean difference in oxygen saturation +1.2%, 95% CI +0.8% to +1.6%[19]). Both reviews found no evidence that bronchodilators compared with placebo reduced admission rates in children treated in outpatient clinics or emergency departments (RR 0.85, 95% CI 0.47 to

1.53;[18] 23/97 [24%] children treated with bronchodilator admitted v 21/90 [23%] with placebo; RR 1.0, 95% CI 0.6 to 1.7[19]). The first subsequent RCT (38 infants without previous wheezing episodes) compared a single dose (3 mg in 3 mL) of nebulised levo-adrenaline (epinephrine) compared with 0.9% sodium chloride placebo during the first 4 days of their respiratory illness.[20] There were no significant differences in respiratory and heart rates, oxygen saturation, and the RDAI (see glossary, p 355) measured during the following 60 minutes. Results were reported graphically. The second RCT (149 hospitalised infants without previous history of wheezing and with a clinical diagnosis of acute viral bronchiolitis) compared nebulisations of racemic adrenaline (0.03 mL/kg/dose of a 2.25% solution), salbutamol (0.03 mL/kg/dose of a 5 mg/mL solution), and placebo (0.03 mL/kg/dose of 0.9% sodium chloride) given every 1–6 hours, at the discretion of the attending medical team. There were no significant differences in the length of hospital stay (placebo v adrenaline: mean difference +3.5 hours, 95% CI –18.6 hours to +25.6 hours; placebo v salbutamol: mean difference +1.9 hours, 95% CI –18.3 hours to +22.1 hours) or in the mean time to normal oxygenation, adequate fluid intake, RDAI of 4 or less, or infrequent nebulisations.[21] **Compared with other treatments:** We found four RCTs comparing nebulised adrenaline with salbutamol (see table 1, p 358).[21–24] The first RCT (24 sedated, hospitalised infants without previous wheeze) found a significant improvement in clinical scores after administration of racemic adrenaline, as compared with baseline score (mean difference 1.80, 95% CI 0.79 to 2.80), which was not present after salbutamol inhalation (mean difference +0.40, 95% CI –0.61 to +1.40).[22] However, the clinical importance of this finding is not clear, and a comparison between groups was not provided. The second RCT (42 infants aged 6 weeks to 1 year seen in the emergency department) compared inhaled adrenaline with salbutamol.[23] It found a significant improvement in oxygen saturation after 60 minutes of treatment in favour of adrenaline (mean difference 2%, CI not provided; P = 0.02). The clinical importance of this finding is unclear, given that this was one of many statistical comparisons and because the change is below the 3% difference in oxygen saturation that the authors had previously established as clinically important. It also found a significant reduction in admissions (7/20 [35%] with adrenaline v 17/21 [81%] with salbutamol; RR 0.43, 95% CI 0.23 to 0.81; NNT 3, 95% CI 2 to 7). The third RCT (100 infants aged 1–24 months, randomised in the emergency department to 4 treatments: nebulised racemic adrenaline followed by 0.9% sodium chloride placebo; nebulised salbutamol followed by 0.9% sodium chloride placebo; 0.9% sodium chloride placebo followed by racemic adrenaline; 0.9% sodium chloride placebo followed by salbutamol) found no significant differences in RDAI scores between the four groups during the study.[24] The fourth RCT that compared racemic adrenaline, salbutamol, and placebo did not find differences between adrenaline and salbutamol in any of the study outcomes (see above).[21]

Harms: One systematic review reported tachycardia, increased blood pressure, decreased oxygen saturation, flushing, hyperactivity, prolonged cough, and tremor after use of bronchodilators.[18] The review did not report the frequency of adverse events. The second review did not report harms.[19] One RCT reported a higher incidence of pallor in children treated with adrenaline than in those receiving salbutamol (at 30 minutes: 10/20 [50%] with adrenaline *v* 3/21 [14%] with salbutamol; RR 3.50, 95% CI 1.12 to 10.90; NNH 3, 95% CI 2 to 8).[23] Three RCTs made no mention of harms.[20,22,24] One RCT reported asymptomatic transient (< 1 hour) tachycardia, mild hypertension, and slight tremor which were equally frequent in all treatment groups (figures not provided).[21]

Comment: None of the RCTs considered respiratory failure as an outcome. One systematic review found significant heterogeneity among RCTs in the effects of bronchodilators on oxygen saturation.[18] Discrepancies in primary studies included differences in study populations such as inclusion of sedated children, short duration of follow up, and validity of clinical scores. Bronchodilators may improve the clinical appearance of a child through a general stimulatory effect rather than by improving respiratory function.[25]

OPTION CORTICOSTEROIDS

One systematic review and 10 additional RCTs found limited and conflicting evidence on the effects of corticosteroids compared with placebo.

Benefits: We found one systematic review (search date 1999, 6 RCTs, 347 children in hospital)[26] and 10 additional RCTs (969 children) of corticosteroids compared with placebo in children with bronchiolitis.[27–36] Three of the additional RCTs had been mentioned in the systematic review but excluded because of data inconsistency,[31] treatment outside hospital,[32] or failure to report the outcome markers sought by the systematic review.[33] The systematic review found no significant difference in the mean duration of stay (5 RCTs, 229 children: WMD –0.43 days, 95% CI –1.05 days to +0.18 days), in the RCTs with clearly identified randomisation methods (4 RCTs, 253 children: WMD –0.35 days, 95% CI –0.84 days to +0.14 days), and after exclusion of RCTs that included children with previous wheezing (4 RCTs, 264 children: WMD –0.29 days, 95% CI –0.71 days to +0.13 days).[26] Interpretation of the effect of corticosteroids compared with placebo on clinical symptoms found by the systematic review is difficult (see comment below). The RCTs in the systematic review reported different clinical scales at varying times after starting treatment. The scales usually included measurements of oxygen saturation, wheezing, accessory muscle use, and respiratory rate. Results reported 72 hours after starting treatment were too heterogeneous for analysis. Only three RCTs (197 children) provided results for 24 hours after starting treatment. The systematic review pooled the standardised effect size for clinical scores from these three RCTs and found that corticosteroids produced a significant improvement, compared with placebo.[26] Although statistically significant, the clinical importance of such an improvement is not clear because different scales are combined across studies. Seven of the nine additional RCTs that compared the clinical score found no significant benefit from corticosteroids (see table 2, p 359).[27–30,32–34] One RCT found a significant transient improvement in a "bronchiolitis score" with oral prednisolone for 2 days.[34] This change, limited to the clinical score, is of doubtful clinical importance. One subsequent RCT (70 children aged between 8 weeks and 23 months old without previous wheezing episodes) compared oral dexamethasone 1 mg/kg with placebo in the emergency department, along with nebulised salbutamol. After a 4 hour observation period, children were discharged to their homes and continued to receive either daily oral dexamethasone 0.6 mg/kg/dose or placebo for 5 days, as well as inhaled salbutamol. Compared with placebo, a significant reduction in the RACS (see glossary, p 355) measured after 4 hours was found in the dexamethasone group (means difference –1.8, 95% CI –0.175 to –3.425), but no significant difference was found at day 7 (difference in means +0.4, 95% CI –2.1 to +2.8). Admission rates measured at the emergency ward were significantly reduced with dexamethasone (7/36 [19%] with dexamethasone *v* 15/34 [44%] with placebo; RR 0.44, 95% CI 0.21 to 0.95).[35] Another subsequent RCT (41 children aged < 24 months with respiratory syncytial virus-positive infection who required mechanical ventilation) compared intravenous dexamethasone 0.5 mg/kg/dose or an equal volume of placebo every 12 hours for 4 days. No significant difference was found in median number of ventilator days (median 5.50 days [interquartile range 4.0 days] with dexamethasone *v* 6.0 days [interquartile range 4.5 days] with placebo; P = 0.86), duration of intensive care unit stay (median 7.0 days [interquartile range 7.0 days] with dexamethasone *v* 8.0 days [interquartile range 4.0 days] with placebo; P = 0.76), or duration of hospital stay (median 11.0 days [interquartile range 6.0 days] with dexamethasone *v* 10.0 days [interquartile range 5.5 days] with placebo; P = 0.40). However, this study, aimed at detecting differences in virus quantities in tracheal aspirates, had a power of 80% to exclude differences of 50% or more in ventilator days, or 40% or more in hospital days with a power of 80%. Therefore it is not possible to rule out smaller but still clinically important differences in these outcomes.[36] Three small long term follow up RCTs (3 years,[37] 3–5 years,[38] and 2 years[39]) used telephone questionnaires to examine the effect of corticosteroids during the acute episode on subsequent wheezing. Two of the three RCTs did not observe any benefit from corticosteroids. The third was an unblinded RCT in which 117 hospitalised infants (mean age 2.6 months, requiring hospital treatment because of respiratory syncytial virus bronchiolitis) were allocated to be in a control group (41 infants), and received inhaled budesonide for 7 days (40 infants) or inhaled budesonide for 2 months (36 infants).[39] However, this RCT had several problems that compromised its validity (see comment below).

Harms: The acute adverse effects of oral corticosteroids are well documented, and include hyperglycaemia and immunosuppression.[40] The RCTs did not give information on these.[27–36] See harms of corticosteroids in asthma and other wheezing disorders of childhood, p 314.

Comment: The evidence presented in the systematic review[26] is difficult to interpret because some of the RCTs did not exclude children with a history of wheezing who may have asthma, a condition likely to respond to corticosteroids. The clinical scales used in the RCTs included oxygen saturation, but the clinical relevance of changes in this parameter are unclear. Even if the results are accepted at face value, the clinical significance of an effect size is unclear. Furthermore, eight RCTs with more than double the number of people were not included in the meta-analysis. All of these RCTs, except one, did not find a benefit of corticosteroids, and the single RCT that did, only observed a transient improvement in clinical score at one time point. Another systematic review is underway (Lozano JM, personal communication, 2003). We found inadequate evidence to evaluate the effects of systemic compared with inhaled corticosteroids. The unblinded RCT comparing two different regimens of inhaled budesonide in hospitalised children had several problems that further compromised its validity.[39] Diagnosis of asthma was based only on a telephone survey; the children were not assessed to establish whether they had received additional interventions or exposures that could explain the results.

OPTION ROUTINE BROAD SPECTRUM ANTIBIOTICS

We found no evidence in children with bronchiolitis alone. One unblinded RCT in children with bronchiolitis and uncomplicated pneumonia (crackles on auscultation or consolidation on a chest radiograph) found no significant difference in clinical scores with routine use of antibiotics (ampicillin, penicillin, or erythromycin) compared with placebo. However, the RCT may have lacked power to exclude a clinically important effect.

Benefits: We found no systematic review. We found one unblinded RCT (138 children admitted to hospital with clinically apparent pneumonia, 45% of whom were diagnosed with respiratory syncytial virus infection) comparing the routine use of antibiotics (ampicillin, penicillin, or erythromycin) to no antibiotics (no placebo, see comment below).[41] It found no significant difference between treatment groups in the proportion of children infected with respiratory syncytial virus. It found no evidence that antibiotics reduced duration of hospital stay or respiratory rate, or improved clinical symptoms, clinical signs, or radiographic assessment scores for pulmonary disease.

Harms: The RCT did not report harms,[41] although potential risks include superinfection with resistant bacteria and drug reactions.[42]

Comment: The RCT was unblinded and used block randomisation (children were randomised in groups of 20).[41] This reduces confidence in the results. The RCT may have been too small to exclude a clinically important effect. Two children initially treated without antibiotics were switched to antibiotics because of complicating purulent infections. Analysis was by intention to treat.

OPTION RIBAVIRIN

One systematic review found no good evidence that ribavirin reduced mortality, risk of respiratory deterioration, or duration of hospital stay in children admitted to hospital with respiratory syncytial virus bronchiolitis. It found some evidence that ribavirin reduced the duration of mechanical ventilation. Two subsequent RCTs found no evidence that ribavirin

reduced duration of hospital stay or admission rate because of lower respiratory tract symptoms during the first year after the acute episode or the frequency of recurrent wheezing illness over 1 year of follow up.

Benefits: We found one systematic review (search date 1999, 10 small RCTs)[43] and two subsequent RCTs.[44,45] The review found that, in children and infants hospitalised with respiratory syncytial virus bronchiolitis, ribavirin (tribavirin) compared with placebo did not significantly reduce mortality (5/86 [6%] with ribavirin *v* 7/72 [10%] with placebo; RR 0.61, 95% CI 0.21 to 1.75), respiratory deterioration (4/56 [7%] with ribavirin *v* 11/60 [18%] with placebo; RR 0.42, 95% CI 0.15 to 1.17), or duration of hospital stay (–1.9 days with ribavirin *v* placebo, 95% CI –0.9 to +4.6 days), but duration of ventilation was reduced significantly (–1.2 days, 95% CI –0.2 days to –3.4 days).[43] The high mortality in both groups may have been because of severe disease at baseline. The first subsequent RCT (40 hospitalised infants who received ribavirin or placebo within 12 hours of admission) found no significant differences in outcomes measured during the acute episode, such as the duration of oxygen supplementation need (ribavirin 2.72 days *v* placebo 1.92 days; mean difference +0.80 days, 95% CI –0.73 days to +2.32 days) or hospital stay (ribavirin 4.94 days *v* placebo 3.36 days; mean difference +1.58 days, 95% CI –0.18 days to +3.35 days).[44] That RCT also followed the infants for 1 year after the initial episode. It found no significant differences in admission rates associated with recurrent lower respiratory illness (2/16 [13%] with ribavirin *v* 3/19 [16%] with placebo; RR 0.79, 95% CI 0.15 to 4.17) or use of bronchodilators (5/16 [31%] with ribavirin *v* 8/19 [42%] with placebo; RR 0.74, 95% CI 0.30 to 1.82). However, the sample size may have been too small to rule out a clinically important difference.[44] A second RCT (45 previously healthy infants < 180 days old and hospitalised because of severe respiratory syncytial virus confirmed bronchiolitis) compared nebulised ribavirin (60 mg/mL over 3 2-hour periods for a total of 6 g/100 mL every 24 hours for 3 days) with no ribavirin in an open manner. There were no significant differences in the frequency of recurrent wheezing illness over 1 year of follow up (15/24 [63%] with ribavirin *v* 17/21 [81%] with placebo; RR 0.78, 95% CI 0.53 to 1.12).[45]

Harms: We found no results from prospective studies. The review and the two RCTs did not report harms.[43–45] We found case reports of headaches and contact lens dysfunction in carers.[46] Ribavirin has been reported to be associated with acute bronchospasm in treated children. The standard aerosol is sticky, and clogging of ventilatory equipment has been reported.[47]

Comment: We found one small prospective study comparing pulmonary function tests in 54 children previously randomised to inpatient treatment with ribavirin or placebo.[48] It found no evidence of long term differences in outcome, although the study was not sufficiently powerful to rule out a clinically important difference.

OPTION IMMUNOGLOBULINS

Small, low powered RCTs found insufficient evidence about the effects of immunoglobulins compared with albumin solution or with 0.9% sodium chloride in children admitted to hospital with bronchiolitis.

Benefits: We found no systematic review but found five RCTs (4 using albumin solution as control, 1 using 0.9% sodium chloride, 335 children in total).[49–53] Two RCTs used pooled immunoglobulins, two RCTs used respiratory syncytial virus immunoglobulin (RSV Ig), and one RCT used palivizumab (synthetic monoclonal antibody). Neither RCT using RSV Ig found evidence that RSV Ig shortened duration of hospital stay compared with albumin (in high risk children [see glossary, p 355]: mean duration of hospital stay 8.41 days with RSV Ig *v* 8.89 days with albumin, P = NS; in non-high risk children: mean stay 4.58 days with RSV Ig *v* 5.52 days with albumin, P = NS; CIs not reported).[49,50] The third RCT (35 children) found no evidence that palivizumab reduced duration of hospital stay (mean 14.5 days, 95% CI 12.4 days to 16.6 days with RSV Ig *v* 11.5 days, 95% CI 10.0 days to 13.0 days with placebo; P = 0.25), duration of ventilation (mean 8.8 days, 95% CI 6.5 days to 11.1 days with palivizumab *v* 6.2 days, 95% CI 4.7 days to 7.7 days with placebo; P = 0.45), or duration of treatment with supplemental oxygen (mean 12.3 days, 95% CI 10.0 days to 14.6 days with palivizumab *v* 9.5 days, 95% CI 7.9 days to 11.1 days with placebo; P = 0.47).[51] Neither of the remaining RCTs found any evidence that pooled immunoglobulins improved outcome in children with bronchiolitis.[52,53]

Harms: The RCTs found that RSV Ig was associated with elevation in liver enzymes and anoxic spells (no frequencies provided).[49] One unblinded RCT (249 children) of prophylactic RSV Ig found that adverse effects occurred in about 3% of treated children.[10] That RCT and a subsequent analysis of the data found that effects included increased respiratory rate, mild fluid overload during the first infusion, urticarial reaction at the infusion site, mild decreases in oxygen saturation, and fever (no frequencies provided).[10,54]

Comment: Four RCTs used albumin as control. The effects of albumin in bronchiolitis are not known.

GLOSSARY

Cohort segregation Children infected with different viral strains are segregated from each other and treated separately, with the aim of preventing cross infection.

Disease severity Mild: not requiring admission to hospital. Moderate: requiring admission to hospital but not intubation. Severe: requiring intubation or artificial ventilation.

High risk children Premature infants with or without bronchopulmonary dysplasia, or infants and children with congenital heart disease.

RACS Respiratory Assessment Change Score.

RDAI Respiratory Distress Assessment Instrument.

Bronchiolitis

Substantive changes

Bronchodilators One RCT added;[21] conclusions unchanged.

Corticosteroids One RCT added;[36] conclusions unchanged.

Ribavirin One RCT added;[45] conclusions unchanged.

REFERENCES

1. Phelan P, Olinsky A, Robertson C. *Respiratory illness in children.* 4th ed. London: Blackwell Scientific Publications, 1994.
2. Gruber W. Bronchiolitis. In: Long S, Pickering L, Prober C, eds. *Principles and practice of pediatric infectious diseases.* 1st ed. New York: Churchill Livingstone, 1997:1821.
3. Glezen WP, Taber LH, Frank AL, et al. Risk of primary infection and reinfection with respiratory syncytial virus. *Am J Dis Child* 1986;140:543–546.
4. Navas L, Wang E, de Carvalho V, et al. Improved outcome of respiratory syncytial virus infections in a high-risk hospitalized population of Canadian children. *J Pediatr* 1992;121:348–354.
5. Wang EEL, Law BJ, Stephens D, et al. Pediatric Investigators Collaborative Network on Infections in Canada (PICNIC) study of morbidity and risk factors with RSV disease. *J Pediatr* 1995;126:212–219.
6. Wang EEL, Law BJ, Boucher F, et al. Pediatric Investigators Collaborative Network on Infections in Canada (PICNIC) study of admission and management variation in patients hospitalized with respiratory syncytial viral lower respiratory infection. *J Pediatr* 1996;129:390–395.
7. McConnochie KM, Mark JD, McBride JT, et al. Normal pulmonary function measurements and airway reactivity in childhood after mild bronchiolitis. *J Pediatr* 1985;107:54–58.
8. McConnochie KM, Roghmann KJ. Parental smoking, presence of older siblings and family history of asthma increase risk of bronchiolitis. *Am J Dis Child* 1986;140:806–812.
9. Sly PD, Hibbert ME. Childhood asthma following hospitalization with acute viral bronchiolitis in infancy. *Pediatr Pulmonol* 1989;7:153–158.
10. Wang EEL, Tang NK. Immunoglobulin for preventing respiratory syncytial virus infection. In: The Cochrane Library, Issue 3, 2001. Oxford: Update Software. Search date 1999; primary sources Cochrane Acute Respiratory Infections Trials Register, Medline, abstracts from the Pediatric Academy Meetings and the Intersciences Conference on Antimicrobial Agents and Chemotherapy from 1994–1997.
11. Simpson S, Burls A. *A systematic review of the effectiveness and cost-effectiveness of palivizumab (Synagis®) in the prevention of respiratory syncytial virus (RSV) infection in infants at high risk of infection*. Birmingham: West Midlands Health Technology Assessment Group, University of Birmingham, 2001.
12. Krasinski K, LaCouture R, Holzman R, et al. Screening for respiratory syncytial virus and assignment to a cohort at admission to reduce nosocomial transmission. *J Pediatr* 1990;116:894–898.
13. Isaacs D, Dickson H, O'Callaghan C, et al. Handwashing and cohorting in prevention of hospital acquired infections with respiratory syncytial virus. *Arch Dis Child* 1991;66:227–231.
14. Gala CL, Hall CB, Schnabel KC, et al. The use of eye-nose goggles to control nosocomial respiratory syncytial virus infection. *JAMA* 1986;256:2706–2708.
15. Hall CB, Douglas RG. Nosocomial respiratory syncytial virus infections: should gowns and masks be used? *Am J Dis Child* 1981;135:512–515.
16. Murphy D, Todd JK, Chao RK, et al. The use of gowns and masks to control respiratory illness in pediatric hospital personnel. *J Pediatr* 1981;99:746–750.
17. Madge P, Paton JY, McColl JH, et al. Prospective controlled study of four infection-control procedures to prevent nosocomial infection with respiratory syncytial virus. *Lancet* 1992;340:1079–1083.
18. Kellner JD, Ohlsson A, Gadomski AM, et al. Bronchodilators for bronchiolitis. In: The Cochrane Library, Issue 3, 2001. Oxford: Update Software. Search date 1998; primary sources Medline, Embase, Reference Update, reference lists of articles, and files of the authors.
19. Flores G, Horwitz RI. Efficacy of beta 2-agonists in bronchiolitis: a reappraisal and meta-analysis. *Pediatrics* 1997;100:233–239. Search date 1995; primary sources Medline and hand searches of references and selected journals.
20. Abul-Ainine A, Luyt D. Short term effects of adrenaline in bronchiolitis: a randomised controlled trial. *Arch Dis Child* 2002;86:276–279.
21. Patel H, Platt RW, Pekeles GS, et al. A randomized, controlled trial of the effectiveness of nebulized therapy with epinephrine compared with albuterol and saline in infants hospitalized for acute viral bronchiolitis. *J Pediatr* 2002;141:818–824.
22. Sanchez I, De Koster J, Powell RE, et al. Effect of racemic epinephrine and salbutamol on clinical score and pulmonary mechanics in infants with bronchiolitis. *J Pediatr* 1993;122:145–151.
23. Menon K, Sutcliffe T, Klassen TP. A randomized trial comparing the efficacy of epinephrine with salbutamol in the treatment of acute bronchiolitis. *J Pediatr* 1995;126:1004–1007.
24. Reijonen T, Korppi M, Pitkakangas S, et al. The clinical efficacy of nebulized racemic epinephrine and albuterol in acute bronchiolitis. *Arch Pediatr Adolesc Med* 1995;149:686–692.
25. Gadomski AM, Lichenstein R, Horton L, et al. Efficacy of albuterol in the management of bronchiolitis. *Pediatrics* 1994;93:907–912.
26. Garrison MM, Christakis DA, Harvey E, et al. Systemic corticosteroids in infant bronchiolitis: a meta-analysis. *Pediatrics* 2000;105:e44. Search date 1999; primary sources Medline, Embase, and Cochrane Clinical Trials Registry.
27. Richter H, Seddon P. Early nebulized budesonide in the treatment of bronchiolitis and the prevention of postbronchiolitic wheezing. *J Pediatr* 1998;132:849–853.
28. Bulow SM, Nir M, Levin E. Prednisolone treatment for respiratory syncytial virus infection: a randomized controlled trial of 147 infants. *Pediatrics* 1999;104:77.
29. Tal A, Bavilski C, Yohai D, et al. Dexamethasone and salbutamol in the treatment of acute wheezing in infants. *Pediatrics* 1983;71:13–18.
30. Cade A, Brownlee KG, Conway SP. Randomised placebo-controlled trial of nebulised corticosteroids in acute respiratory syncytial viral bronchiolitis. *Arch Dis Child* 2000;82:126–130.
31. Connolly JH, Field CM, Glasgow JF, et al. A double blind trial of prednisolone in epidemic bronchiolitis due to respiratory syncytial virus. *Acta Paediatr Scand* 1969;58:116–120.

32. Berger I, Argaman Z, Schwartz SB. Efficacy of corticosteroids in acute bronchiolitis: short-term and long-term follow-up. *Pediatr Pulmonol* 1998;26:162–166.
33. Leer JA, Green JL, Heimlich EM, et al. Corticosteroid treatment in bronchiolitis. A controlled collaborative study in 297 infants and children. *Am J Dis Child* 1969;117:495–503.
34. Goebel J, Estrada B, Quinonez J, et al. Prednisolone plus albuterol versus albuterol alone in mild to moderate bronchiolitis. *Clin Pediatr* 2000;39:213–220.
35. Schuh S, Coates AL, Binnie R, et al. Efficacy of oral dexamethasone in outpatients with acute bronchiolitis. *J Pediatr* 2002;140:27–32.
36. Buckingham SC, Jafri HS, Bush AJ, et al. A randomized, double-blind, placebo-controlled trial of dexamethasone in severe respiratory syncytial virus (RSV) infection: effects on RSV quantity and clinical outcome. *J Infect Dis* 2002;185:1222–1228.
37. Reijonen TM, Kotaniemi-Syrjanen A, Korhonen K, et al. Predictors of asthma three years after hospital admission for wheezing in infancy. *Pediatrics* 2000;106:1406–1412.
38. Van Woensel JBM, Kimpen JLL, Sprikkelman AB, et al. Long-term effects of prednisolone in the acute phase of bronchiolitis caused by respiratory syncytial virus. *Pediatr Pulmonol* 2000;30:92–96.
39. Kajosaari M, Syvanen P, Forars M, et al. Inhaled corticosteroids during and after respiratory syncytial virus-bronchiolitis may decrease subsequent asthma. *Pediatr Allergy Immunol* 2000;11:198–202.
40. Schimmer BP, Parker KL. Adrenocorticotropic hormone; adrenocortical steroids and their synthetic analogs; inhibitors of the synthesis and actions of adrenocortical hormones. In: Hardman JG, Limbird LE, eds *Goodman & Gilman's The pharmacological basis of therapeutics*. 10th ed. New York: McGraw-Hill, 2001:1649–1677.
41. Fris B, Andersen P, Brenoe E, et al. Antibiotic treatment of pneumonia and bronchiolitis: a prospective randomised study. *Arch Dis Child* 1984;59:1038–1045.
42. Chambers HF. Antimicrobial agents. General considerations. In: Hardman JG, Limbird LE, eds *Goodman & Gilman's The pharmacological basis of therapeutics*. 10th ed. New York: McGraw-Hill, 2001:1143–1170.
43. Randolph AG, Wang EEL. Ribavirin for respiratory syncytial virus lower respiratory tract infection. In: The Cochrane Library, Issue 3, 2001. Oxford: Update Software. Search date 1999; primary sources Medline, hand searches of references, and contact of noted experts.
44. Everard ML, Swarbrick A, Rigby AS, et al. The effect of ribavirin to treat previously healthy infants admitted with acute bronchiolitis on acute and chronic respiratory morbidity. *Respir Med* 2001;95:275–280.
45. Edell D, Khoshoo V, Ross G, et al. Early ribavirin treatment of bronchiolitis: effect on long-term respiratory morbidity. *Chest* 2002;122:935–939.
46. Edelson PJ. Reactions to ribavirin. *Pediatr Infect Dis J* 1991;10:82.
47. Johnson EM. Developmental toxicity and safety evaluations of ribavirin. *Pediatr Infect Dis J* 1997;9(suppl):85–87.
48. Long CE, Voter KZ, Barker WH, et al. Long term follow-up of children hospitalized with respiratory syncytial virus lower respiratory tract infection and randomly treated with ribavirin or placebo. *Pediatr Infect Dis J* 1997;16:1023–1028.
49. Rodriguez WJ, Gruber WC, Welliver RC, et al. Respiratory syncytial virus (RSV) immune globulin intravenous therapy for RSV lower respiratory tract infection in infants and young children at high risk for severe RSV infections. *Pediatrics* 1997;99:454–461.
50. Rodriguez WJ, Gruber WC, Groothuis JR, et al. Respiratory syncytial virus immune globulin treatment of RSV lower respiratory tract infection in previously healthy children. *Pediatrics* 1997;100:937–942.
51. Malley R, DeVincenzo J, Ramilo O, et al. Reduction of respiratory syncytial virus (RSV) in tracheal aspirates in intubated infants by use of humanized monoclonal antibody to RSV F protein. *J Infect Dis* 1998;178:1555–1561.
52. Hemming VG, Rodriguez W, Kim HW, et al. Intravenous immunoglobulin treatment of respiratory syncytial virus infections in infants and young children. *Antimicrob Agents Chemother* 1987;31:1882–1886.
53. Rimensberger PC, Burek-Kozlowska A, Morell A, et al. Aerosolized immunoglobulin treatment of respiratory syncytial virus infection in infants. *Pediatr Infect Dis J* 1996;15:209–216.
54. Groothuis JR, Levin MJ, Rodriguez W, et al. Use of intravenous gamma globulin to passively immunize high-risk children against respiratory syncytial virus: safety and pharmacokinetics. *Antimicrob Agents Chemother* 1991;35:1469–1473.

Juan Manuel Lozano
Titular Professor
Department of Paediatrics and
Clinical Epidemiology Unit
School of Medicine
Universidad Javeriana
Bogotá DC
Colombia

Competing interests: None declared.

The following previous contributors of this topic would also like to be acknowledged: Nancy Tang and Elaine Wang.

TABLE 1 Studies of adrenaline (epinephrine) compared with salbutamol in bronchiolitis: results of RCTs (see text, p 349).

Ref	Allocation/blinding	Intervention	Number of children	Outcome	Results
21	Random/blinded	Nebulised racemic adrenaline or salbutamol	101 inpatients	Length of hospital stay, time to normal oxygenation adequate fluid intake, RDAI < 4, or infrequent nebulisations	No differences
22	Random/blinded, crossover design	Nebulised racemic adrenaline or salbutamol	24 inpatients	Clinical score at 20–30 minutes	Improvement with adrenaline
23	Random/blinded	Nebulised adrenaline or salbutamol	42 emergency room patients	Pulse oximetry; RDAI scores at 30, 60, and 90 minutes; admission rate	Transient effect at 60 minutes; fewer admissions
24	Random/blinded, factorial design	Nebulised racemic adrenaline, salbutamol or saline placebo	100 emergency room patients	RDAI and RACS scores at 15 and 30 minutes	Unclear differences

Min, minutes; RACS, Respiratory Assessment Change Score; RDAI, Respiratory Distress Assessment Instrument; Ref, reference.

TABLE 2 Studies of corticosteroids compared with placebo in bronchiolitis: results of RCTs (see text, p 351).

Ref	Allocation/blinding	Intervention	Number of children	Outcome	Results
27	Random/blinded	Nebulised budesonide	40	Clinical score and condition at 6 months	No benefit
28	Random/blinded	Prednisolone/ methylprednisolone	147	Hospital stay; supportive measures in hospital; condition at 1 month and 1 year after discharge	No benefit
29	Random/blinded, factorial design	Dexamethasone/placebo salbutamol/placebo	32	Clinical score and hospital stay	No benefit
30	Random/blinded	Budesonide	161	Hospital stay; time taken to be symptom free; readmission rates; GP consultation	No benefit
31	Random/blinded	Prednisolone	95	Duration of illness after hospitalisation	No benefit
32	Random/blinded	All had salbutamol; prednisone	38	Clinical score; oxygen saturation; condition at 7 days and 2 years later	No benefit
33	Random/blinded	Betamethasone	297	Nine respiratory tract signs; fever and complications after admission	No benefit
34	Random/blinded	All children received salbutamol (oral or inhaled) prednisolone	48	Bronchiolitis score at day 2	Transient effect only on day 2
35	Random/blinded	Oral dexamethasone	70	Clinical score and admission rate	Improvement in clinical score and admission rate
36	Random/blinded	iv dexamethason e/placebo	41	Number ventilator, ICU, or hospital days	No benefit

GP, general practitioner; ICU, intensive care unit; Ref, reference.

Cardiorespiratory arrest in children

Search date October 2002

Kate Ackerman and David Creery

QUESTIONS

INTERVENTIONS

*Although we found no direct evidence to support their use, widespread consensus holds that, on the basis of indirect evidence and extrapolation from adult data, these interventions should be universally applied to children who have arrested. Placebo controlled trials would be considered unethical.

See glossary, p 366

Key Messages

- **Bag–mask ventilation** We found no RCTs. One controlled clinical trial in children requiring airway management in the community found no significant difference between endotracheal intubation and bag–mask ventilation in survival or neurological outcome.
- **Bystander cardiopulmonary resuscitation** It is widely accepted that cardiopulmonary resuscitation should be undertaken in children who have arrested. Placebo controlled trials would be considered unethical. One systematic review of observational studies found that children who received bystander cardiopulmonary resuscitation versus no bystander cardiopulmonary resuscitation were more likely to survive to hospital discharge.
- **Intubation** See bag–mask ventilation.
- **Airway management and ventilation; direct current cardiac shock (for ventricular fibrillation or pulseless ventricular tachycardia); standard dose intravenous adrenaline (epinephrine)** Although we found no direct evidence to support their use, widespread consensus based on indirect evidence and extrapolation from adult data holds that these interventions should be universally applied to children who have arrested. Placebo controlled trials would be considered unethical.

Clin Evid 2003;10:360–368.

- **High dose intravenous adrenaline (epinephrine); intravenous sodium bicarbonate; intravenous calcium; training parents to perform cardiopulmonary resuscitation** We found no RCTs or prospective cohort studies on the effects of these interventions in children who have arrested in the community.

DEFINITION Non-submersion out of hospital cardiorespiratory arrest in children is a state of pulselessness and apnoea occurring outside of a medical facility and not caused by submersion in water.[1]

INCIDENCE/ PREVALENCE We found 12 studies (3 prospective, 9 retrospective) reporting the incidence of non-submersion out of hospital cardiorespiratory arrest in children (see table 1, p 368).[2–13] Eleven studies reported the incidence in both adults and children, and eight reported the incidence in children.[2–9,11–13] Incidence of arrests in the general population ranged from 2.2–5.7/100 000 people a year (mean 3.1, 95% CI 2.1 to 4.1). Incidence of arrests in children ranged from 6.9–18.0/100 000 children a year (mean 10.6, 95% CI 7.1 to 14.1).[8] One prospective study (300 children) found that about 50% of out of hospital cardiorespiratory arrests occurred in children under 12 months, and about two thirds occurred in children under 18 months.[11]

AETIOLOGY/ RISK FACTORS We found 26 studies reporting the causes of non-submersion pulseless arrests (see glossary, p 366) in a total of 1574 children. The commonest causes of arrest were undetermined causes as in sudden infant death syndrome (see glossary, p 366) (39%), trauma (18%), chronic disease (7%), and pneumonia (4%) (see table 2, p 368).[1,3–12,14–28]

PROGNOSIS We found no systematic review that investigated non-submersion arrests alone. We found 27 studies (5 prospective, 22 retrospective; total of 1754 children) that reported out of hospital arrest.[1–12,14–28] The overall survival rate following out of hospital arrest was 5% (87 children). Nineteen of these studies (1140 children) found that of the 48 surviving children, 12 (25%) had no or mild neurological disability and 36 (75%) had moderate or severe neurological disability. We found one systematic review (search date 1997), which reported outcomes after cardiopulmonary resuscitation for both in hospital and out of hospital arrests in children of any cause, including submersion.[29] Studies were excluded if they did not report survival. The review found evidence from prospective and retrospective observational studies that out of hospital arrest of any cause in children carries a poorer prognosis than arrest within hospital (132/1568 children [8%] survived to hospital discharge after out of hospital arrest *v* 129/544 children [24%] after in hospital arrests). About half of the survivors were involved in studies that reported neurological outcome. Of these, survival with "good neurological outcome" (i.e. normal or mild neurological deficit) was higher in children who arrested in hospital compared with those who arrested elsewhere (60/77 surviving children [78%] in hospital *v* 28/68 [41%] elsewhere).[29]

AIMS OF INTERVENTION To improve survival and minimise neurological sequelae in children suffering non-submersion out of hospital cardiorespiratory arrest.

OUTCOMES Out of hospital death rate; rate of death in hospital without return of spontaneous circulation; return of spontaneous circulation with subsequent death in hospital; and return of spontaneous circulation with successful hospital discharge with mild, moderate, severe, or no neurological sequelae; adverse effects of treatment.

METHODS *Clinical Evidence* search and appraisal October 2002. In addition, the authors searched citation lists of retrieved articles and relevant review articles. Studies reporting out of hospital arrest in adults that listed "adolescent" as a MeSH heading were also reviewed. Both authors reviewed the retrieved studies independently and differences were resolved by discussion. Studies were excluded if data relating to submersion could not be differentiated from non-submersion data (except where we found no data relating exclusively to non-submersion arrest; in such cases we have included studies that did not differentiate these types of arrest and indicated their limitation in this regard). Some features of cardiorespiratory arrest in adults appear to be different from arrest in children, so studies were excluded if data for adults could not be differentiated from data for children.

QUESTION What are the effects of treatments for non-submersion out of hospital cardiorespiratory arrest?

OPTION AIRWAY MANAGEMENT AND VENTILATION

It is widely accepted, based on indirect evidence and extrapolation from adult data, that good airway management and rapid ventilation should be undertaken in a child who has arrested, and it would be considered unethical to test its role in a placebo controlled trial. We found no RCTs or prospective observational studies of airway management and ventilation.

Benefits: We found no systematic review, RCTs, or prospective observational studies of airway management and ventilation.

Harms: We found no prospective evidence.

Comment: It would be considered unethical to test the role of airway management and ventilation in a placebo controlled trial. Widespread consensus based on indirect evidence and extrapolation from adult data suggests that airway management and ventilation should be undertaken.

OPTION INTUBATION VERSUS BAG–MASK VENTILATION

We found no RCTs. One controlled trial found no significant difference in survival or neurological outcome with endotracheal intubation versus bag–mask ventilation in children with non-submersion cardiorespiratory arrest requiring airway management in the community.

Benefits: We found no systematic review or RCTs. We found one controlled trial (830 children requiring airway management in the community, including 98 children who had arrested after submersion) comparing (using alternate day allocation) bag–mask ventilation versus endotracheal intubation (given by paramedic staff trained in these techniques).[30] Treatments were not randomised; each was allocated on alternate days. Analysis was by intention to treat (see comment below). The trial found no significant difference in rates of survival or good neurological outcome (normal, mild deficit, or no change from baseline function) between the two treatment groups in children with non-submersion cardiorespiratory arrest (105/349 [30%] survived after bag–mask ventilation *v* 90/373 [24%] after intubation; OR 1.36, 95% CI 0.97 to 1.89; good neurological outcome achieved in 80/349 [23%] of children after bag–mask ventilation *v* 70/373 [19%] after intubation; OR 1.27, 95% CI 0.89 to 1.83; ORs for non-submersion cardiorespiratory arrest calculated by author).

Harms: The trial found that time spent at the scene of the arrest was longer when intubation was intended, and this was the only significant determinant of a longer total time from dispatch of paramedic team to arrival at hospital (mean time at scene: 9 min with bag–mask *v* 11 min with intubation; $P < 0.001$; mean total time: 20 min with bag–mask *v* 23 min with intubation; $P < 0.001$).[30] However, it found no significant difference with bag–mask ventilation versus intubation in complications (complications in 727 children for whom data were available: gastric distension 31% with bag–mask *v* 7% with intubation; $P = 0.20$; vomiting 14% *v* 14%; $P = 0.82$; aspiration 14% *v* 15%; $P = 0.84$; oral or airway trauma 1% with bag–mask *v* 2% with intubation; $P = 0.24$). A total of 186 children across both treatment groups were thought by paramedical staff to be successfully intubated. Of these, oesophageal intubation occurred in three children (2%); the tube became dislodged in 27 children (14%; unrecognised in 12 children, recognised in 15); right main bronchus intubation occurred in 33 children (18%); and an incorrect size of tube was used in 44 children (24%). Death occurred in all but one of the children with oesophageal intubation or unrecognised dislodging of the tube.[30]

Comment: **Population characteristics:** The baseline characteristics of children did not differ significantly between groups in age, sex, ethnicity, or cause of arrest. The trial did not report the frequency of pulseless arrest versus respiratory arrest (see glossary, p 366). **Intention to treat:** Intubation and bag–mask ventilation were not mutually exclusive in the trial.[30] The trial protocol allowed bag–mask ventilation before intubation and after unsuccessful intubation. Of 420 children allocated to intubation, 115 received bag–mask ventilation before intubation, 128 received bag–mask ventilation after attempted intubation, four were lost to follow up, and the remainder received intubation that was believed to be successful. Of 410 children allocated to bag–mask ventilation, 10 children were intubated successfully (although in violation of study protocol), nine received bag–mask ventilation after attempted intubation, six were lost to follow up, and the remainder received bag–mask ventilation in accordance with study protocol.[30]

OPTION INTRAVENOUS ADRENALINE (EPINEPHRINE)

Intravenous adrenaline (epinephrine) at "standard dose" (0.01 mg/kg) is a widely accepted treatment for establishing return of spontaneous circulation and it would be considered unethical to test its role in a

placebo controlled trial. We found no RCTs or prospective observational studies in children who have arrested in the community comparing adrenaline versus placebo or comparing standard or single doses versus high or multiple doses of adrenaline.

Benefits: We found no systematic review, RCTs, or prospective observational studies on the effects of intravenous adrenaline.

Harms: We found no prospective evidence.

Comment: **Versus placebo:** Standard dose adrenaline (epinephrine) is a widely accepted treatment for arrests in children. Placebo controlled trials would be considered unethical. **High versus low dose:** Two small retrospective studies (128 people) found no evidence of a difference in survival to hospital discharge between low or single dose and high or multiple dose adrenaline, although the studies were too small to rule out an effect.[8,12]

OPTION INTRAVENOUS SODIUM BICARBONATE

We found no RCTs or prospective cohort studies on the effects of intravenous bicarbonate in out of hospital cardiorespiratory arrest in children.

Benefits: We found no systematic review, RCTs, or prospective observational studies on the effects of intravenous sodium bicarbonate.

Harms: We found no prospective evidence.

Comment: Sodium bicarbonate is widely believed to be effective in arrest associated with hyperkalaemic ventricular tachycardia or fibrillation, but we found no prospective evidence supporting this.

OPTION INTRAVENOUS CALCIUM

We found no RCTs or prospective observational studies on the effects of intravenous calcium in out of hospital cardiorespiratory arrest in children.

Benefits: We found no systematic review, RCTs, or prospective observational studies.

Harms: We found no prospective evidence.

Comment: Calcium is widely believed to be effective in arrest associated with hyperkalaemic ventricular tachycardia or fibrillation, but we found no prospective evidence supporting this.

OPTION BYSTANDER CARDIOPULMONARY RESUSCITATION

It is widely accepted that cardiopulmonary resuscitation and ventilation should be undertaken in children who have arrested. Placebo controlled trials would be considered unethical. We found no RCTs on the effects of training parents to perform cardiopulmonary resuscitation. One systematic review of observational studies has found that children whose arrest was witnessed and who received bystander cardiopulmonary resuscitation were more likely to survive to hospital discharge.

Benefits: We found no RCTs. We found one systematic review (search date 1997, 1420 children who had arrested outside hospital) of prospective and retrospective studies.[29] This concluded that survival was improved in children who were witnessed to arrest and received cardiopulmonary resuscitation from a bystander. Of 150 witnessed arrests outside hospital, 28/150 (19%) survived to hospital discharge. Of those children who received bystander cardiopulmonary resuscitation, 20/76 (26%) survived to discharge.[29] The review did not report survival rates in children whose arrests were not witnessed, but the overall survival rate for out of hospital cardiac arrest was 8%. **Training parents to perform cardiopulmonary resuscitation:** We found no systematic review, RCTs, or prospective observational studies examining the effects of training parents to perform cardiopulmonary resuscitation in children who have arrested outside hospital.

Harms: Potential harms include those resulting from unnecessary chest compression after respiratory arrest with intact circulation.

Comment: The review of observational studies found that children who received bystander cardiopulmonary resuscitation had a hospital discharge rate of 20/76 (26%) versus 8/74 (11%) in children whose arrest was witnessed but had not received cardiopulmonary resuscitation.[29] Cardiopulmonary resuscitation was not randomly allocated and children resuscitated may be systematically different from those who did not receive resuscitation. The apparent survival rates for witnessed arrests and arrests with bystander initiated cardiopulmonary resuscitation may be artificially high because of inappropriate evaluation of true arrest. However, assuming confounding variables were evenly distributed between groups, then the best estimate of the benefit of cardiopulmonary resuscitation is a 15% absolute increase in the probability that children will be discharged alive from hospital.

OPTION DIRECT CURRENT CARDIAC SHOCK

It is widely accepted that children who arrest outside hospital and are found to have ventricular fibrillation or pulseless ventricular tachycardia should receive direct current cardiac shock treatment. Placebo controlled trials would be considered unethical. We found no RCTs or prospective observational studies on the effects of direct current cardiac shock in children who have arrested in the community, regardless of the heart rhythm.

Benefits: We found no systematic review, RCTs, or prospective observational studies.

Harms: We found no prospective evidence.

Comment: **In children with ventricular fibrillation:** One retrospective study (29 children with ventricular fibrillation who had arrested out of hospital from a variety of causes, including submersion) found that of 27 children who were defibrillated, 11 survived (5 with no sequelae, 6 with severe disability). The five children with good outcome all received defibrillation within 10 minutes of arrest (time to defibrillation not given for those who died). Data on the two children who were not defibrillated were not presented.[31] **In children with asystole:** One retrospective study in 90 children with asystole (see glossary, p 366) (including those who had arrested after submersion) found that 49 (54%) had received direct current cardiac shock treatment. None of the children survived to hospital discharge, regardless of whether or not direct current cardiac shock was given.[32] We found one systematic review of observational studies that recorded electrocardiogram rhythm (search date 1997, 1420 children who had arrested outside hospital).[29] Bradyasystole or pulseless electrical activity (see glossary, p 366) were found in 73%, whereas ventricular fibrillation or pulseless ventricular tachycardia (see glossary, p 366) were found in 10%.[29] The review found that survival after ventricular fibrillation or ventricular tachycardia arrest was higher than after asystolic arrest in children. Survival to discharge reported in the systematic review was 39/802 (5%) for children with initial rhythm asystole (see glossary, p 366) and 30% (29/97) with initial rhythm ventricular fibrillation (see glossary, p 366) or ventricular tachycardia.[29]

GLOSSARY

Asystole The absence of cardiac electrical activity.

Bradyasystole Bradycardia clinically indistinguishable from asystole.

Initial rhythm asystole The absence of cardiac electrical activity at initial determination.

Initial rhythm ventricular fibrillation Electrical rhythm is ventricular fibrillation at initial determination.

Pulseless arrest Absence of palpable pulse.

Pulseless electrical activity The presence of cardiac electrical activity in absence of a palpable pulse.

Pulseless ventricular tachycardia Electrical rhythm of ventricular tachycardia in absence of a palpable pulse.

Respiratory arrest Absence of respiratory activity.

Sudden infant death syndrome The sudden unexpected death of a child, usually between the ages of 1 month and 1 year, for which a thorough postmortem examination does not define an adequate cause of death. Near miss sudden infant death syndrome refers to survival of a child after an unexpected arrest of unknown cause.

REFERENCES

1. Schindler MB, Bohn D, Cox PN, et al. Outcome of out of hospital cardiac or respiratory arrest in children. *N Engl J Med* 1996;335:1473–1479.
2. Broides A, Sofer S, Press J. Outcome of out of hospital cardiopulmonary arrest in children admitted to the emergency room. *Isr Med Assoc J* 2000;2:672–674.
3. Eisenberg M, Bergner L, Hallstrom A. Epidemiology of cardiac arrest and resuscitation in children. *Ann Emerg Med* 1983;12:672–674.
4. Applebaum D, Slater PE. Should the Mobile Intensive Care Unit respond to pediatric emergencies? *Clin Pediatr (Phila)* 1986;25:620–623.
5. Tsai A, Kallsen G. Epidemiology of pediatric prehospital care. *Ann Emerg Med* 1987;16:284–292.
6. Thompson JE, Bonner B, Lower GM. Pediatric cardiopulmonary arrests in rural populations. *Pediatrics* 1990;86:302–306.
7. Safranek DJ, Eisenberg MS, Larsen MP. The epidemiology of cardiac arrest in young adults. *Ann Emerg Med* 1992;21:1102–1106.
8. Dieckmann RA, Vardis R. High-dose epinephrine in pediatric out of hospital cardiopulmonary arrest. *Pediatrics* 1995;95:901–913.
9. Kuisma M, Suominen P, Korpela R. Paediatric out of hospital cardiac arrests — epidemiology and outcome. *Resuscitation* 1995;30:141–150.
10. Ronco R, King W, Donley DK, et al. Outcome and cost at a children's hospital following resuscitation for out of hospital cardiopulmonary arrest. *Arch Pediatr Adolesc Med* 1995;149:210–214.
11. Sirbaugh PE, Pepe PE, Shook JE, et al. A prospective, population-based study of the demographics, epidemiology, management, and outcome of out of hospital pediatric cardiopulmonary arrest. *Ann Emerg Med* 1999;33:174–184.
12. Friesen RM, Duncan P, Tweed WA, et al. Appraisal of pediatric cardiopulmonary resuscitation. *Can Med Assoc J* 1982;126:1055–1058.

13. Hu SC. Out of hospital cardiac arrest in an Oriental metropolitan city. *Am J Emerg Med* 1994;12:491–494.
14. Barzilay Z, Somekh E, Sagy M, et al. Pediatric cardiopulmonary resuscitation outcome. *J Med* 1988;19:229–241.
15. Bhende MS, Thompson AE. Evaluation of an end-tidal CO_2 detector during pediatric cardiopulmonary resuscitation. *Pediatrics* 1995;95:395–399.
16. Brunette DD, Fischer R. Intravascular access in pediatric cardiac arrest. *Am J Emerg Med* 1988;6:577–579.
17. Clinton JE, McGill J, Irwin G, et al. Cardiac arrest under age 40: etiology and prognosis. *Ann Emerg Med* 1984;13:1011–1015.
18. Hazinski MF, Chahine AA, Holcomb GW, et al. Outcome of cardiovascular collapse in pediatric blunt trauma. *Ann Emerg Med* 1994;23:1229–1235.
19. Losek JD, Hennes H, Glaeser P, et al. Prehospital care of the pulseless, nonbreathing pediatric patient. *Am J Emerg Med* 1987;5:370–374.
20. Ludwig S, Kettrick RG, Parker M. Pediatric cardiopulmonary resuscitation. A review of 130 cases. *Clin Pediatr (Phila)* 1984;23:71–75.
21. Nichols DG, Kettrick RG, Swedlow DB, et al. Factors influencing outcome of cardiopulmonary resuscitation in children. *Pediatr Emerg Care* 1986;2:1–5.
22. O'Rourke PP. Outcome of children who are apneic and pulseless in the emergency room. *Crit Care Med* 1986;14:466–468.
23. Rosenberg NM. Pediatric cardiopulmonary arrest in the emergency department. *Am J Emerg Med* 1984;2:497–499.
24. Sheikh A, Brogan T. Outcome and cost of open- and closed-chest cardiopulmonary resuscitation in pediatric cardiac arrests. *Pediatrics* 1994;93:392–398.
25. Suominen P, Rasanen J, Kivioja A. Efficacy of cardiopulmonary resuscitation in pulseless paediatric trauma patients. *Resuscitation* 1998;36:9–13.
26. Suominen P, Korpela R, Kuisma M, et al. Paediatric cardiac arrest and resuscitation provided by physician-staffed emergency care units. *Acta Anaesthesiol Scand* 1997;41:260–265.
27. Torphy DE, Minter MG, Thompson BM. Cardiorespiratory arrest and resuscitation of children. *Am J Dis Child* 1984;138:1099–1102.
28. Walsh R. Outcome of pre-hospital CPR in the pediatric trauma patient [abstract]. *Crit Care Med* 1994;22:A162.
29. Young KD, Seidel JS. Pediatric cardiopulmonary resuscitation: a collective review. *Ann Emerg Med* 1999;33:195–205. Search date 1997; primary sources Medline and bibliographic search.
30. Gausche M, Lewis RJ, Stratton SJ, et al. Effect of out of hospital pediatric endotracheal intubation on survival and neurological outcome. *JAMA* 2000;283:783–790.
31. Mogayzel C, Quan L, Graves JR, et al. Out of hospital ventricular fibrillation in children and adolescents: causes and outcomes. *Ann Emerg Med* 1995;25:484–491.
32. Losek JD, Hennes H, Glaeser PW, et al. Prehospital countershock treatment of pediatric asystole. *Am J Emerg Med* 1989;7:571–575.

Kate Ackerman
The Children's Hospital
Boston
USA

David Creery
Children's Hospital of Eastern Ontario
Ottawa
Canada

Competing interests: None declared.

Cardiorespiratory arrest in children

TABLE 1 **Incidence of non-submersion out of hospital cardiorespiratory arrest in children* (see text, p 361).**

Ref	Location	Year	Incidence / 100 000 people in total population	Incidence / 100 000 children
12	Manitoba, Canada	1982	2.9	ND
3	King County, USA	1983	2.4	9.9
4	Jerusalem, Israel	1986	2.5	6.9
5	Fresno, USA	1987	5.7	ND
6	Midwestern USA	1990	4.7	ND
7	King County, USA	1992	2.4	10.1
13	Taipei, Taiwan	1994	1.3	ND
8	San Francisco, USA	1995	2.2	16.1
9	Helsinki, Finland	1995	1.4	9.1
10	Birmingham, USA	1995	ND	6.9
11	Houston, USA	1999	4.9	18.0
2	Southern Israel	2000	3.5	7.8

*Incidence represents arrests per 100 000 population per year. ND, no data.

TABLE 2 **Causes of non-submersion out of hospital cardiorespiratory arrest in children* (see text, p 361).**

Cause	Number of arrests (%)	Number of survivors (%)
Undetermined	691 (43.9)	1 (0.1)
Trauma	311 (19.8)	10 (3.2)
Chronic disease	126 (8.0)	9 (7.1)
Pneumonia	75 (4.8)	6 (8.0)
Non-accidental injury	23 (1.5)	2 (8.7)
Aspiration	20 (1.3)	0 (0)
Overdose	19 (1.2)	3 (15.8)
Other	309 (19.6)	28 (9.1)
Total	**1574 (100)**	**59 (3.7)**

*Figures represent the numbers of arrests/survivors in children with each diagnosis.

Constipation in children

Search date April 2003

Gregory Rubin

QUESTIONS

INTERVENTIONS

*Not widely licensed for use in children. Clinical use in adults was recently restricted because of heart rhythm abnormalities. See comments on cisapride under gastro-oesophageal reflux in children, p 397.

Key Messages

- **Medical treatment plus toilet training or biofeedback (compared with medical treatment alone)** One small, short term RCT in children with encopresis found that adding toilet training or biofeedback to medical treatment (enemas and osmotic or stimulant laxatives) reduced soiling compared with medical treatment alone.
- **Cisapride** Two RCTs in people aged 2–18 years found that cisapride improved stool frequency and symptoms of constipation after 8–12 weeks of treatment in an outpatient setting compared with placebo. We found no evidence from primary care settings. Use of cisapride has been restricted in some countries because of adverse cardiac effects.
- **Biofeedback training** One systematic review found no significant difference between biofeedback plus conventional treatment and conventional treatment alone in persisting defecation problems at 12 months.
- **Increased dietary fibre** We found no RCTs in children on the effects of increasing dietary fibre.
- **Osmotic laxatives** We found no RCTs that compared osmotic laxatives with placebo in children. Two small RCTs found no significant difference in stool frequency or consistency between lactulose and lactitol after 2–4 weeks in children aged 8 months to 16 years. One of these RCTs found that lactulose increased abdominal pain and flatulence compared with lactitol. One small, short term RCT in children with encopresis found that adding toilet training or biofeedback to stimulant or osmotic laxatives reduced soiling compared with medical treatment alone.
- **Stimulant laxatives** One systematic review found no reliable RCTs comparing stimulant laxatives versus placebo or other treatments in children. One small, short term RCT found that adding toilet training or biofeedback to stimulant or osmotic laxatives reduced soiling compared with medical treatment alone.

Constipation in children

DEFINITION Constipation is characterised by infrequent bowel evacuations; hard, small faeces; or difficult or painful defecation. The frequency of bowel evacuation varies from person to person.[1] Encopresis is defined as involuntary bowel movements in inappropriate places at least once a month for 3 months or more, in children aged 4 years and older.[2]

INCIDENCE/ PREVALENCE Constipation with or without encopresis is common in children. It accounts for 3% of consultations to paediatric outpatient clinics and 25% of paediatric gastroenterology consultations in the USA.[3] Encopresis has been reported in 2% of children at school entry. The peak incidence is at 2–4 years of age.

AETIOLOGY/ RISK FACTORS No cause is discovered in 90–95% of children with constipation. Low fibre intake and a family history of constipation may be associated factors.[4] Psychosocial factors are often suspected, although most children with constipation are developmentally normal.[3] Chronic constipation can lead to progressive faecal retention, distension of the rectum, and loss of sensory and motor function. Organic causes for constipation are uncommon, but include Hirschsprung's disease (1/5000 births; male to female ratio of 4 : 1; constipation invariably present from birth), cystic fibrosis, anorectal physiological abnormalities, anal fissures, constipating drugs, dehydrating metabolic conditions, and other forms of malabsorption.[3]

PROGNOSIS Childhood constipation can be difficult to treat and often requires prolonged support, explanation, and medical treatment. In one long term follow up study of children presenting under the age of 5 years, 50% recovered within 1 year and 65–70% recovered within 2 years; the remainder required laxatives for daily bowel movements or continued to soil for years.[3] It is not known what proportion continue to have problems into adult life, although adults presenting with megarectum or megacolon often have a history of bowel problems from childhood.

AIMS OF INTERVENTION To remove faecal impaction and to restore a bowel habit in which stools are soft and passed without discomfort.

OUTCOMES Number of defecations per week; number of episodes of soiling per month; gut transit time as measured by timing the passage of radio-opaque pellets, which may be ingested within a gelatin capsule; use of laxatives.

METHODS *Clinical Evidence* search and appraisal April 2003. Keywords: constipation, diet therapy, diagnosis, therapy, psychology, stimulant laxatives, dietary fibre, and lactulose. The search was limited to infants and children. Trials were selected for inclusion if they focused on the management of constipation or encopresis, or both; if they were relevant to primary health care; and if they included children without an organic cause for constipation.

QUESTION **What are the effects of treatments?**

OPTION **INCREASED DIETARY FIBRE**

We found no RCTs on the effects of increasing dietary fibre in children.

Benefits: We found no systematic review or RCTs.

Harms: We found no good evidence.

Comment: None.

OPTION CISAPRIDE

Two RCTs in people aged 2–18 years found that cisapride improved stool frequency and symptoms of constipation after 8–12 weeks of treatment in an outpatient setting compared with placebo. We found no evidence from primary care settings. Use of cisapride has been restricted in some countries because of adverse cardiac effects.

Benefits: We found no systematic review but found two RCTs.[5,6] One RCT (69 people aged 4–18 years, attending hospital with constipation defined as pain, difficulty in defecation, or ≤ 3–4 bowel movements/week for at least 3 months in the absence of a history of bowel disease) compared cisapride 0.3 mg/kg daily (as a syrup) versus placebo following clearance of accumulated stool.[5] It found that after 8 weeks cisapride significantly increased stool frequency and decreased gut transit time (mean stool frequency/week 6.75 with cisapride *v* 1.31 with placebo). The second RCT (40 children aged 2–16 years with a history of chronic constipation referred for evaluation to a paediatric hospital gastroenterology clinic) found significant benefit for cisapride compared with placebo at 12 weeks, measured by a composite of improved stool frequency, absence of faecal soiling, and no use of other laxatives (improvement in composite index 14/20 [70%] with cisapride *v* 7/20 [35%] with placebo; RR 2.00, CI 1.03 to 3.88; NNT 3, 95% CI 1 to 24).[6]

Harms: The RCTs did not report harms (see comment below).[5,6]

Comment: Use of cisapride has been restricted in some countries because of its association with heart rhythm abnormalities in adults. See comments on cisapride under gastro-oesophageal reflux in children, p 397. An RCT comparing cisapride plus magnesium oxide versus magnesium oxide alone is being translated.[7]

OPTION OSMOTIC LAXATIVES

We found no RCTs that compared osmotic laxatives with placebo in children. Two small RCTs found no significant difference in stool frequency or consistency between lactulose and lactitol after 2–4 weeks in children aged 8 months to 16 years. One of these RCTs found that lactulose increased abdominal pain and flatulence compared with lactitol. One small, short term RCT in children with encopresis found that adding toilet training or biofeedback to stimulant or osmotic laxatives reduced soiling compared with medical treatment alone.

Benefits: **Versus placebo:** We found no systematic review and no placebo controlled RCTs of osmotic laxatives in children. We found two small RCTs comparing effects of lactitol versus lactulose on stool frequency and consistency.[8,9] The first RCT (51 children, aged 8 months to 16 years visiting a physician for chronic idiopathic constipation) found no significant difference in stool frequency or consistency of stools between lactitol and lactulose at 4 weeks (stool frequency per week increased from 2.5 to 5.6 with lactitol *v* 2.0 to 4.8 for lactulose; stool consistency normal or soft in 15/23 [65%] children with lactitol *v* 16/19 [84%] with lactulose).[8] The second RCT (39 children, aged 11 months to 13 years) compared lactitol 150–350 mg/kg daily versus lactulose 150 mg/kg daily over 2 weeks.[9] It found no significant difference in stool frequency between lactulose and lactitol (stool frequency in both groups was 1–1.5/day). A third RCT (220 non-breastfed, constipated infants aged 0–6 months) compared 2% and 4% lactulose mixed with an artificial milk preparation.[10] At 14 days over 90% of parents in both groups reported easy passage of normal or thin consistency stools. However, the RCT did not compare outcomes between treatment groups. **With toilet training or biofeedback:** One RCT (87 children with encopresis) compared medical treatment (enemas and osmotic or stimulant laxatives) plus toilet training versus medical treatment plus biofeedback versus medical treatment alone.[11] Children receiving toilet training used significantly fewer laxatives and required fewer treatment sessions than did those in the other two groups. Toilet training and biofeedback produced similar reductions in rates of soiling, which were greater than those achieved by medical treatment alone ($P < 0.04$).

Harms: The first RCT found that significantly fewer children taking lactitol had abdominal pain or flatulence compared with lactulose (abdominal pain: 22% with lactitol *v* 58% with lactulose; $P < 0.005$; flatulence: 30% with lactitol *v* 63% with lactulose; $P < 0.01$).[8]

Comment: The benefits shown in the third RCT are comparisons of outcomes before and after treatment, and were not necessarily because of the treatments.[10] Toilet training consisted of reinforcement and scheduling to promote response to the urge to defaecate, and instruction and modelling to promote appropriate straining.[11]

OPTION STIMULANT LAXATIVES

One systematic review found no reliable RCTs comparing stimulant laxatives versus placebo or other treatments in children. One small, short term RCT found that adding toilet training or biofeedback to stimulant or osmotic laxatives reduced soiling compared with medical treatment alone.

Benefits: We found one systematic review (search date 2001), which found no RCTs of adequate methodological rigour comparing stimulant laxatives with either placebo or alternative treatment in children.[12] We found no placebo controlled RCTs of the effects of stimulant laxatives in children. **With toilet training or biofeedback:** See osmotic laxatives, p 371.

Harms: None identified.

Comment: The studies identified by the review were all comparative, used multiple interventions, and had small sample sizes.[12] One quasi-randomised study (using last hospital number digit to allocate patients) compared senna versus mineral oil concentrate in 37 children (aged 3–12 years) with chronic constipation.[13] The study found that senna versus mineral oil was less effective in reducing involuntary faecal soiling after 6 months (8/18 [44%] with senna *v* 1/19 [5%] with mineral oil; RR 8.44, 95% CI 1.52 to 16.70). No significant differences were found in the number of children with relapses of constipation symptoms during the treatment period (12/19 [63%] with senna *v* 16/18 [89%] with mineral oil; RR 0.71, 95% CI 0.48 to 1.04).

OPTION BIOFEEDBACK TRAINING

One systematic review found no significant difference between biofeedback plus conventional treatment and conventional treatment alone in persisting defecation problems at 12 months.

Benefits: We found one systematic review (search date 2001, 8 RCTs).[14] The review found no significant difference in rates of persisting problems between conventional treatment plus biofeedback and conventional treatment alone at 12 months (OR 1.34, 95% CI 0.92 to 1.94). There was heterogeneity of borderline significance (P = 0.087). One included RCT (41 children) found a different trend from the other seven RCTs for reasons that were not apparent.[15] After exclusion of this RCT, results were no longer heterogeneous. Meta-analysis excluding this RCT found that biofeedback plus conventional treatment increased rates of persisting problems compared with conventional treatment alone (OR 1.59, 95% CI 1.07 to 2.35; heterogeneity P = 0.53). **With medical treatment:** See osmotic laxatives, p 371.

Harms: The review did not report any information on adverse effects.[14]

Comment: In the systematic review, sample sizes were generally small, and interventions and outcomes varied among trials.[14]

Substantive changes

Biofeedback training One systematic review added;[14] conclusions changed from Likely to be beneficial to Unknown effectiveness.

REFERENCES

1. Nelson R, Wagget J, Lennard-Jones JE, et al. Constipation and megacolon in children and adults. In: Misiewicz JJ, Pounder RE, Venables CW, eds. *Diseases of the gut and pancreas*. 2nd ed. Oxford: Blackwell Science, 1994; 843–864.
2. American Psychiatric Association. *Diagnostic and statistical manual of mental disorders*. 4th ed. Washington, DC: American Psychiatric Association, 1994.
3. Loening-Baucke V. Chronic constipation in children. *Gastroenterology* 1993;105:1557–1563.
4. Roma E, Adamidis D, Nikolara R, et al. Diet and chronic constipation in children: the role of fiber. *J Pediatr Gastroenterol Nutr* 1999;28:169–174.
5. Halibi IM. Cisapride in the management of chronic pediatric constipation. *J Pediatr Gastroenterol Nutr* 1999;28:199–202.
6. Nurko MD, Garcia-Aranda JA, Worona LB, et al. Cisapride for the treatment of constipation in children: a double blind study. *J Pediatr* 2000;136:35–40.
7. Ni YH, Lin CC, Chang SH, et al. Use of cisapride with magnesium oxide in chronic pediatric constipation. *Acta Paediatr Taiwan* 2001;42:345–349.
8. Pitzalis G, Mariani P, Chiarini-Testa MR, et al. Lactitol in chronic idiopathic constipation of childhood. *Pediatr Med Chir* 1995;17:223–226.
9. Martino AM, Pesce F, Rosati U. The effects of lactitol in the treatment of intestinal stasis in childhood. *Minerva Pediatr* 1992;44:319–323.
10. Hejlp M, Kamper J, Ebbesen F, et al. Infantile constipation and allomin-lactulose. Treatment of infantile constipation in infants fed with breast milk substitutes: a controlled trial of 2% and 4% allomin-lactulose. *Ugeskr Laeger* 1990;152:1819–1822.
11. Cox DJ, Sutphen J, Borowitz S, et al. Contribution of behaviour therapy and biofeedback to laxative therapy in the treatment of pediatric encopresis. *Ann Behav Med* 1998;20:70–76.
12. Price KJ, Elliott TM. What is the role of stimulant laxatives in the management of childhood constipation and soiling? In: The Cochrane Library, Issue 1, 2003. Oxford: Update Software. Search date 2001; primary sources Cochrane database of randomised controlled clinical trials, hand searching of paediatric journals, and contact with experts in the field.
13. Sondheimer JM, Gervaise EP. Lubricant versus laxative in the treatment of chronic functional

constipation of children: a comparative study. *J Pediatr Gastroenterol Nutr* 1982;1:223–226.

14. Brazzelli M, Griffiths P. Behavioural and cognitive interventions with or without other treatments for defaecation disorders in children (Cochrane Review). In: The Cochrane Library, Issue 1, 2003. Oxford: Update Software. Search date 2001; primary sources Cochrane Incontinence Group Trials Register, Cochrane Controlled Trials Register, hand searching of journals, and the Enuresis Resource and Information Centre Register.
15. Loening-Baucke V. Modulation of abnormal defecation dynamics by biofeedback treatment in chronically constipated children with encopresis. *J Pediatr* 1990;116:214–222.

Gregory Rubin
Professor of Primary Care
University of Sunderland
Sunderland
UK

Competing interests: None declared.

Depression in children and adolescents

Search date September 2002

Philip Hazell

QUESTIONS

INTERVENTIONS

See glossary, p 383

Key Messages

- **Cognitive therapy (depressed adolescents with depressed parent)** One RCT in depressed adolescents with depressed parents found no significant difference in recovery from depression with cognitive behavioural therapy plus usual care versus usual care alone over 2 years.
- **Cognitive therapy (in mild to moderate depression)** One systematic review in children and adolescents with mild to moderate depression has found that cognitive behavioural therapy significantly improves symptoms compared with non-specific support.
- **Electroconvulsive therapy** We found no RCTs on electroconvulsive therapy in children and adolescents with depression.
- **Interpersonal therapy in adolescents (in mild to moderate depression)** Two RCTs found that interpersonal therapy versus clinical monitoring or waiting list control significantly increased recovery rate over 12 weeks in adolescents with mild to moderate depression.
- **Intravenous clomipramine (adolescents)** One RCT found that, in non-suicidal adolescents, intravenous clomipramine versus placebo significantly reduced depression scores at 6 days. However, the trial was too small and brief for us to draw reliable conculsions.

- **Lithium** One RCT found no significant difference with lithium versus placebo in global assessment or depression scores after 6 weeks in children with depression and a family history of bipolar affective disorder. Lithium was associated with adverse effects.
- **Long term effects of treatments** We found no systematic review or RCTs examining long term outcomes of interventions for depression in children and adolescents.
- **Monoamine oxidase inhibitors** One RCT found insufficient evidence to compare moclobemide versus placebo in children aged 9–15 years with major depression. We found no RCTs of non-reversible monoamine oxidase inhibitors in children or adolescents.
- **Oral tricyclic antidepressants** One systematic review found no significant difference with oral tricyclic antidepressants (amitriptyline, desipramine, imipramine, nortriptyline) versus placebo in depression scores in adolescents and children with depression. Subgroup analyses found that oral tricyclic antidepressants versus placebo significantly reduced symptoms in adolescents but not in children. However, the review also found that oral tricyclic antidepressants were associated with adverse effects.
- **Selective serotonin reuptake inhibitors** One RCT found no significant difference, one RCT found equivocal results (statistically significant differences on some depression measures but not others), and one RCT found a significant improvement in depressive symptoms with fluoxetine versus placebo after 8–9 weeks. One RCT found that, in adolescents with major depression, paroxetine versus placebo significantly improved remission after 8 weeks. We found no RCTs on other selective serotonin reuptake inhibitors. Selective serotonin reuptake inhibitors are frequently associated with dizziness, lightheadedness, drowsiness, poor concentration, nausea, headache, and fatigue if treatment is reduced or stopped.
- **St John's Wort** We found no RCTs on St John's Wort (*Hypericum perforatum*) in children or adolescents with depression.
- **Venlafaxine** One RCT found no significant difference with venlafaxine versus placebo in improvement of depressive symptoms in children and adolescents with major depression after 6 weeks.
- **Family therapy; group treatments other than cognitive behavioural therapy** We found insufficient evidence in children and adolescents about the effects of these interventions.

DEFINITION Compared with adult depression, depression in children (6–12 years) and adolescents (13–18 years) may have a more insidious onset, may be characterised more by irritability than sadness, and occurs more often in association with other conditions such as anxiety, conduct disorder, hyperkinesis, and learning problems.[1]

INCIDENCE/ PREVALENCE Estimates of prevalence of depression among children and adolescents in the community range from 2–6%.[2,3] Prevalence tends to increase with age, with a sharp rise at around the onset of puberty. Pre-adolescent boys and girls are affected equally by the condition, but depression is seen more frequently among adolescent girls than boys.[4]

AETIOLOGY/ RISK FACTORS The aetiology is uncertain, but may include genetic vulnerability,[5] childhood events, and current psychosocial adversity.[4]

PROGNOSIS In children and adolescents, the recurrence rate following a first depressive episodes in childhood or adolescence is 70% by 5 years, which is similar to the recurrence rate in adults. It is not clear whether this is related to the severity of depression.[4] Young people experiencing a moderate to severe depressive episode may be more likely than adults to have a manic episode within the next few years.[4,6] Trials of treatments for child and adolescent depression have found high rates of spontaneous remission (as much as two thirds of people in some inpatient studies).

AIMS OF INTERVENTION To improve mood, social and occupational functioning, and quality of life; to reduce morbidity and mortality; to prevent recurrence of depressive disorder; and to minimise adverse effects of treatment.

OUTCOMES In children and adolescents there are developmentally specific pseudo-continuous measures such as the Children's Depression Rating Scale and the Children's Depression Inventory, although some studies of adolescents use scales developed for use in adults such as the Hamilton Rating Scale for Depression. Parent report pseudo-continuous measures such as the Children's Depression Inventory for Parents are also used. Categorical outcomes are sometimes expressed as people no longer meeting specified criteria for depression on a structured psychiatric interview such as the Kiddie-SADS, which combines data from children and their parents. Global improvement in symptoms as judged by an investigator is sometimes reported using the Clinical Global Impressions scale or the Clinical Global Assessment scale. Severity of depression is defined in some studies using cut-off scores on pseudo-continuous measures such as the Children's Depression Rating scale and the Children's Depression Inventory, but this is often not stated.

METHODS *Clinical Evidence* search and appraisal September 2002, plus additional references identified by contributor.

QUESTION What are the effects of treatments?

OPTION TRICYCLIC ANTIDEPRESSANTS

One systematic review found no significant difference with oral tricyclic antidepressants (amitriptyline, desipramine, imipramine, nortriptyline) versus placebo in depression scores in children and adolescents with depression. Subgroup analyses found that oral tricyclic antidepressants versus placebo significantly reduced symptoms in adolescents but not in children. The review also found that oral tricyclic antidepressants were associated with adverse effects. One small RCT found that, in non-suicidal adolescents, intravenous clomipramine versus placebo significantly reduced depression scores at 6 days.

Benefits: **Oral tricyclic antidepressants:** We found one systematic review (search date 2000, 13 RCTs, 506 children and adolescents aged 6–18 years, severity of depression not stated) comparing oral tricyclic antidepressants (amitriptyline, desipramine, imipramine, and nortriptyline) versus placebo.[7] It found no significant difference in overall improvement (depression checklist scores) with tricyclic antidepressants versus placebo (OR 0.84, 95% CI 0.56 to 1.25). Subgroup analyses found a significant reduction in symptoms with tricyclic antidepressants versus placebo in adolescents (7 RCTs: effect size SMD –0.47, 95% CI –0.92 to –0.02) but no significant difference in children (3 RCTs: effect size SMD –0.15, 95% CI –0.64 to +0.34). **Pulsed intravenous clomipramine:** See glossary, p 384. We found one RCT (16 non-suicidal adolescent outpatients, aged 14–18 years, with major depression [21-item Hamilton Rating Scale for Depression score ≥18]) comparing intravenous clomipramine (200 mg) versus placebo.[8] The RCT found that intravenous clomipramine versus placebo significantly decreased depression scores at 6 days (decrease in Hamilton Rating Scale for Depression score from baseline of ≥50%: 7/8 people with iv clomipramine *v* 3/8 with placebo).[8]

Harms: **Oral tricyclic antidepressants:** The systematic review found that tricyclic antidepressants were more commonly associated with vertigo (OR 8.47, 95% CI 1.40 to 51.0), orthostatic hypotension (OR 4.77, 95% CI 1.11 to 20.5), tremor (OR 6.29, 95% CI 1.78 to 22.17), and dry mouth (OR 5.19, 95% CI 1.15 to 23.5) than was placebo.[7] The review found no significant differences for other adverse effects (tiredness: OR 1.52, 95% CI 0.63 to 3.67; sleep problems: OR 1.87, 95% CI 0.84 to 4.14; headache: OR 1.15, 95% CI 0.68 to 1.95; palpitations: OR 1.20, 95% CI 0.17 to 8.68; perspiration: OR 2.01, 95% CI 0.39 to 10.44; constipation: OR 1.94, 95% CI 0.72 to 5.24; or problems with micturition: OR 0.30, 95% CI 0.01 to 7.89). **Pulsed intravenous clomipramine:** The RCT did not report any adverse effects.[8]

Comment: We found single case reports and case series of toxicity and mortality from tricyclic antidepressants in overdose and therapeutic doses. Further research is needed to determine long term effects of intravenous clomipramine.

OPTION MONOAMINE OXIDASE INHIBITORS

One RCT found insufficient evidence to compare moclobemide versus placebo in children aged 9–15 years with major depression, some of whom had a comorbid disorder. We found no RCTs on non-reversible monoamine oxidase inhibitors in children or adolescents.

Benefits: We found no systematic review. **Reversible monoamine oxidase inhibitors:** We found one RCT (20 Turkish children aged 9–15 years with major depression, including 13 children with a comorbid disorder) comparing moclobemide versus placebo for 5 weeks.[9] The RCT found significant improvement with moclobemide versus placebo in one clinician rated scale (Clinical Global Impressions-investigator assessment of severity of depression, adverse effects, and global recovery) after 5 weeks but not on parent rated (Children's Depression Inventory for Parents) and self reported measures (Children's Depression Inventory).[9] **Non-reversible monoamine oxidase inhibitors:** We found no RCTs.

Harms: The RCT found no significant difference with moclobemide versus placebo in adverse effects assessed using Clinical Global Impression of adverse effects scale and self assessed adverse effects forms.[9] We found no information on the safety of moclobemide usage in children younger than 9 years.

Comment: The small sample size limits the conclusions that may be drawn from this RCT.[9]

OPTION SELECTIVE SEROTONIN REUPTAKE INHIBITORS

One RCT found no significant difference, one RCT found equivocal difference (statistically significant results on some depression measures but not others), and one RCT found a significant improvement in depressive symptoms with fluoxetine versus placebo after 8–9 weeks. One RCT found that, in adolescents with major depression, paroxetine versus placebo significantly improved remission after 8 weeks. We found no RCTs on other selective serotonin reuptake inhibitors. Selective serotonin reuptake inhibitors are frequently associated with dizziness, lightheadedness, drowsiness, poor concentration, nausea, headache, and fatigue if treatment is reduced or stopped.

Benefits: **Fluoxetine:** We found one systematic review[10] (search date 1998, 2 RCTs[11,12]) and one subsequent RCT.[13] The systematic review did not pool results.[10] The first RCT identified by the review (40 adolescents, aged 13–18 years, of whom 30 completed the trial, severity of depression not stated) found no significant difference after 8 weeks with fluoxetine (20–60 mg) versus placebo in mean number of depression symptoms or psychosocial functioning (Clinical Global Impressions scale).[11] The second RCT identified by the review (96 children and adolescents aged 7–17 years with major depression) found that fluoxetine (20 mg) versus placebo significantly improved depressive symptoms after 8 weeks in terms of Clinical Global Impressions scale (27/48 [56%] improved with fluoxetine *v* 16/48 [33%] with placebo; RR of failure to recover 0.66, 95% CI 0.45 to 0.96) and self reported Children's Depression Rating Scale (34% improved *v* 18%; $P < 0.01$), but that it did not improve other measures.[12] The subsequent RCT (219 children and adolescents aged 8–17 years with major depression) found that fluoxetine versus placebo did not significantly increase rate response defined a priori as on the Children's Depression Rating Scale (≥ 30% decrease in score, 71/109 [65%] with fluoxetine *v* 54/101 [54%] with placebo; $P = 0.093$).[13] The RCT found a significant difference in mean change for Children's Depression Rating Scale (mean change 7.1, 95% CI 3.3 to 10.9) and Clinical Global Impressions Severity scale with fluoxetine versus placebo (mean change 0.6, 95% CI 0.3 to 1.0). **Paroxetine:** We found one RCT (180 adolescents, aged 12–18 years, of whom 133 completed the trial, severity of depression score of at least 12 on the Hamilton Rating Scale for Depression and < 60 on the Children's Global Assessment scale) that compared paroxetine (20–40 mg) versus placebo versus imipramine for 8 weeks with respect to end point response (Hamilton Rating Scale for Depression score ≤ 8 or a 50% reduction from baseline score) and change from baseline score (Hamilton Rating Scale for Depression).[14] The RCT did not include a direct statistical comparison of paroxetine versus imipramine. The RCT found that paroxetine versus placebo significantly improved remission (Hamilton Rating Scale for Depression: AR for failure to recover 37% with paroxetine *v* 54% with placebo; ARI 17%, no CI available; RR 0.68, 95% CI 0.49 to 0.95; $P = 0.02$). Among adolescents who completed treatment, paroxetine versus placebo significantly improved remission (Clinical Global Impressions scale among 133 people completing the study: AR for remission 66% with paroxetine *v* 48% with placebo; ARR 18%; P = 0.02). **Other selective serotonin reuptake inhibitors:** We found no RCTs.

Harms: **Fluoxetine:** One RCT found significantly more weight loss with fluoxetine versus placebo (data not provided).[11] The other RCT did not report on adverse effects.[12] The third RCT found that headache was reported significantly more often with fluoxetine versus placebo (P = 0.017). **Paroxetine:** The RCT reported more serious adverse events with paroxetine (12%) versus placebo (2%).[14] The most frequent adverse effects were somnolence (17% with paroxetine *v* 3% with placebo) and tremor (11% with paroxetine *v* 2% with placebo) but no statistical analyses were reported. A discontinuation syndrome following abrupt cessation or reduction in the dose of selective serotonin reuptake inhibitors has been described in a series of six cases.[15] The most frequent symptoms included dizziness, lightheadedness, drowsiness, poor concentration, nausea, headache, and fatigue.[15]

Comment: There is insufficient information provided in one of the RCTs[11] to make an informed comparison with the other RCT.[12]

OPTION VENLAFAXINE

One RCT found no significant difference with venlafaxine versus placebo in improvement of depressive symptoms in children and adolescents with major depression after 6 weeks.

Benefits: We found one systematic review (search date 1998,[10] 1 RCT[16]). The RCT (33 children and adolescents aged 8–17 years with major depression and on psychotherapy) compared venlafaxine (37.5–75.0 mg/day in divided doses) versus placebo for 6 weeks.[16] It found no significant difference with venlafaxine versus placebo in improvement of depressive symptoms (Children's Depression Inventory, Hamilton Rating Scale for Depression, Children's Depression Rating Scale).

Harms: The RCT reported nausea in a subgroup of participants aged ≥ 13 years.[16]

Comment: The RCT lacked power to rule out a clinically important difference.

OPTION LITHIUM

One RCT found no significant difference with lithium versus placebo in global assessment or depression scores after 6 weeks in children with depression and family history of bipolar affective disorder. Lithium was associated with adverse effects.

Benefits: We found no systematic review. We found one RCT (30 children, aged 6–12 years, with depression and family history of bipolar affective disorder) comparing lithium versus placebo for 6 weeks.[17] The RCT found no significant difference with lithium versus placebo in global assessment or depression scores (9 depression items of the Kiddie-SADS interview).

Harms: Of the 17 children randomised to lithium treatment, four were withdrawn because of adverse effects (3 had confusion, 1 had nausea and vomiting).[17]

Comment: The RCT lacked power to rule out a clinically important difference.

OPTION ST JOHN'S WORT (*HYPERICUM PERFORATUM*)

We found no RCTs on St John's Wort (*H perforatum*) in children or adolescents with depression.

Benefits: We found no RCTs on St John's Wort (*H perforatum*) in children or adolescents with depression.

Harms: We found no RCTs.

Comment: None.

OPTION ELECTROCONVULSIVE THERAPY

We found no RCTs on electroconvulsive therapy in children and adolescents with depression.

Benefits: We found no RCTs on electroconvulsive therapy in children and adolescents with depression.

Harms: We found no specific evidence on harms in children or adolescents. Known adverse effects in adults include memory impairment.

Comment: None.

OPTION SPECIFIC PSYCHOLOGICAL TREATMENTS

One systematic review has found that cognitive behavioural therapy increases resolution of symptoms compared with non-specific supportive therapies for children and adolescents with mild to moderate depression. One RCT in depressed adolescents with depressed parents found no significant difference in recovery from depression with cognitive behavioural therapy plus usual care versus usual care alone over 2 years. We found limited evidence from two small RCTs that interpersonal therapy versus clinical monitoring alone or placement on a waiting list increases recovery in adolescents with mild to moderate depression. We found insufficient evidence that family therapy or group treatments other than cognitive behavioural therapy are effective treatments for depression in children and adolescents.

Benefits: **Cognitive behavioural therapy:** See glossary, p 383. We found one systematic review (search date 1997, 6 RCTs, 376 people) of cognitive behavioural therapy versus other treatments ranging from waiting list control to supportive psychotherapy,[18] and one subsequent RCT.[19] The systematic review found that cognitive behavioural therapy increased the rate of resolution of symptoms of depression (OR 3.2, 95% CI 1.9 to 5.2; NNT 4, 95% CI 3 to 5).[18] This finding is consistent with three non-systematic meta-analytic studies.[20–22] The subsequent RCT (88 adolescents aged 13–18 years with major depression or dysthymia) compared cognitive behavioural therapy (16 sessions) plus usual care versus usual care alone in depressed adolescents with depressed parents over 2 years.[19] The RCT found no significant difference between cognitive behavioural therapy plus usual care versus usual care alone in recovery rate (≥ 8 weeks with few or no depressive symptoms, 13/41 [31.7%] with cognitive behavioural therapy plus usual care *v* 14/47 [29.8%] with usual care alone). A factor that could have contributed to the absence of a treatment effect was the higher level of impairment in the participants compared with other RCTs. **Interpersonal therapy:** See glossary, p 383. We found two RCTs comparing 12 weekly sessions of interpersonal therapy versus clinical monitoring or waiting list control in adolescents with depression.[23,24] The first RCT (48 adolescents aged 12–18 years with major depressive disorder) found that interpersonal therapy versus clinical monitoring significantly increased recovery rate (Hamilton Rating Scale for Depression < 6 or Beck Depressive Inventory < 9: 18/24 [75%] with interpersonal therapy *v* 11/24 [46%] with clinical monitoring alone; RR 1.64, 95% CI 1.00 to 2.68; ARR 0.29, 95% CI 0.03 to 0.56).[23] The second RCT (46 adolescents with major depression) comparing interpersonal therapy versus being on a waiting list found no significant difference in proportion of adolescents not manifesting severe depression (defined by a cut-off score on the Children's Depression Inventory: 17/19 [89%] with interpersonal therapy *v* 12/18 [67%] with waiting list; RR 1.33, 95% CI 0.94 to 1.93; ARR +0.22, 95% CI –0.03 to +0.49).[24] However, if the Children's Depression Inventory score was considered as a continuous measure, then the mean Children's Depression Inventory score was significantly lower after interpersonal therapy versus waiting list (P < 0.01). **Systemic behavioural family therapy:** See glossary, p 384. We found one RCT (78 adolescents with major depressive disorder) comparing family therapy versus non-specific supportive therapy.[25] The RCT found no significant difference in remission rates (combination of no longer meeting DSM-III-R criteria for major depression as determined by the Kiddie-SADS interview and Beck Depression Inventory score < 9: 29% with family therapy *v* 34% with non-specific supportive therapy). **Group administered cognitive behavioural therapy:** We found one RCT (123 adolescents aged 14–18 years with major depression or dysthymia) comparing group administered cognitive behavioural therapy versus waiting list.[26] It found that cognitive behavioural therapy significantly increased the remission rate (Longitudinal Interval Follow-up Evaluation interview for DSM-III-R diagnoses: 46/69 [67%] with group cognitive behavioural therapy *v* 13/27 [48%] on a waiting list; P < 0.05). **Group therapeutic support versus group social skills training:** We found one RCT (66 adolescents aged 13–17 years, of whom 47 completed the protocol; 58 with major depression, 8 with dysthymia) comparing group therapeutic support versus group social skills training.[27] In 26 adolescents (pre-treatment scores in the clinical range for the Kiddie-SADS, Child Depression Inventory, and a self esteem instrument), the RCT found no significant difference in remission rates (score of < 4 on Kiddie-SADS dysphoria and anhedonia symptoms: 8/16 [50%] with group therapeutic support *v* 4/10 [40%] with group social skills training).

Harms: The RCTs did not report any adverse events.[19–27] We found no report of harms specifically for children and adolescents. In adults, there have been case reports suggesting that "imaginal flooding" (a form of cognitive behavioural therapy) worsens symptoms, leading for calls for caution in the use of this treatment.

Comment: Large RCTs are needed in more representative groups of people in a range of clinical settings, including primary care. In the first RCT of interpersonal therapy, sessions were augmented by telephone contact.[23]

QUESTION Which treatments are most effective at improving long term outcome?

We found no systematic review or RCTs looking at long term outcomes of interventions for depression in children and adolescents.

Benefits: We found no systematic review and no RCTs. We found no RCTs comparing structured psychotherapy with pharmacotherapy in children and adolescents. We found no RCTs comparing combined pharmacotherapy and psychotherapy with either treatment alone. We found no RCTs comparing different psychotherapies.

Harms: We found no RCTs.

Comment: We found one prospective cohort study, in which adolescents with depression had been randomised to cognitive behavioural therapy, systemic behavioural family therapy, or non-directive supportive therapy (see glossary, p 384).[28] After the initial trial phase of 16 weeks, they were allowed booster treatments and also had access to open treatment in any modality for the 2 years of follow up. They were assessed at 3 monthly intervals for the first 12 months and then again at 24 months. The study found no significant difference between the groups. Of 106 adolescents, 38% experienced sustained recovery, 21% experienced persistent depression, and 41% had a relapsing course.[28]

GLOSSARY

Cognitive behavioural therapy A brief structured treatment (20 sessions over 12–16 wks) aimed at changing the dysfunctional beliefs and negative automatic thoughts that characterise depressive disorders.[29] Cognitive behavioural therapy requires a high level of training for the therapist, and has been adapted for children and adolescents suffering from depression. A course of treatment is characterised by 8–12 weekly sessions, in which the therapist and the child collaborate to solve current difficulties. The treatment is structured and often directed by a manual. Treatment generally includes cognitive elements, such as the challenging of negative thoughts, and behavioural elements, such as structuring time to engage in pleasurable activity.

Interpersonal therapy A standardised form of brief psychotherapy (usually 12–16 weekly sessions) intended primarily for outpatients with unipolar non-psychotic depressive disorders. It focuses on improving the individual's interpersonal functioning and identifying the problems associated with the onset of the depressive episode.[30] In children and adolescents, interpersonal therapy has been adapted for adolescents to address common adolescent developmental issues, for example separation from parents, exploration of authority in relationship to parents, development of dyadic interpersonal relationships, initial experience with the death of a relative or friend, and peer pressure.

Non-directive supportive therapy Helping people to express feelings, and clarify thoughts and difficulties; therapists suggest alternative understandings and do not give direct advice but try to encourage people to solve their own problems.

Pulsed intravenous clomipramine An intravenous loading procedure for clomipramine.

Systemic behavioural family therapy A combination of two treatment approaches that have been used effectively for dysfunctional families. In the first phase of treatment, the therapist clarifies the concerns that brought the family into treatment, and provides a series of reframing statements designed to optimise engagement in therapy and identification of dysfunctional behaviour patterns (systemic therapy). In the second phase, the family members focus on communication and problem solving skills and the alteration of family interactional patterns (family behaviour therapy).

REFERENCES

1. Birmaher B, Ryan ND, Williamson DE, et al. Childhood and adolescent depression: a review of the past 10 years, Part I. *J Am Acad Child Adolesc Psychiatry* 1996;35:1427–1439.
2. Costello EJ, Angold A, Burns BJ, et al. The Great Smoky Mountains Study of Youth. Goals, design, methods, and the prevalence of DSM-III-R disorders. *Arch Gen Psychiatry* 1996;53:1129–1136.
3. Costello EJ. Developments in child psychiatric epidemiology. *J Am Acad Child Adolesc Psychiatry* 1989;28:836–841.
4. Lewinsohn PM, Rohde P, Seely JR. Major depressive disorder in older adolescents: prevalence, risk factors, and clinical implications. *Clin Psychol Rev* 1998;18:765–794.
5. Rice F, Harold G, Thapar A. The genetic aetiology of childhood depression: a review. *J Child Psychol Psychiatry* 2002;43:65
6. Geller B, Fox LW, Fletcher M. Effect of tricyclic antidepressants on switching to mania and on the onset of bipolarity in depressed 6- to 12-year-olds. *J Am Acad Child Adolesc Psychiatry* 1993;32:43–50.
7. Hazell P, O'Connell D, Heathcote D, et al. Tricyclic drugs for depression in children and adolescents. In: The Cochrane Library, Issue 3, 2002. Oxford: Update Software. Search date 2002; primary sources Medline, Excerpta Medica, and Cochrane trials database.
8. Sallee FR, Vrindavanam NS, Deas-Nesmith D, et al. Pulse intravenous clomipramine for depressed adolescents: double-blind, controlled trial. *Am J Psychiatry* 1997;154:668–673.
9. Avci A, Diler RS, Kibar M, et al. Comparison of moclobemide and placebo in young adolescents with major depressive disorder. *Ann Med Sci* 1999;8:31–40.
10. Williams JW, Mulrow CD, Chiquette E, et al. A systematic review of newer pharmacotherapies for depression in adults: evidence report summary. *Ann Intern Med* 2000;132:743–756. Search date 1998; primary sources Medline, Embase, Psychlit, Lilacs, Psyindex, Sigle, Cinahl, Biological Abstracts, Cochrane Controlled Trials, hand searches, and personal contacts.
11. Simeon JG, Dinicola VF, Ferguson HB, et al. Adolescent depression: a placebo-controlled fluoxetine treatment study and follow-up. *Prog Neuropsychopharmacol Biol Psychiatry* 1990;14:791–795.
12. Emslie GJ, Rush AJ, Weinberg WA, et al. A double-blind, randomized, placebo-controlled trial of fluoxetine in children and adolescents with depression. *Arch Gen Psychiatry* 1997;54:1031–1037.
13. Emslie GJ, Heiligenstein JH, Wagner KD, et al. Fluoxetine for acute treatment of depression in children and adolescents: a placebo-controlled, randomized clinical trial. *J Am Acad Child Adolesc Psychiatry* 2002;41:1205–1215.
14. Keller MB, Ryan ND, Strober M, et al. Efficacy of paroxetine in the treatment of adolescent major depression: a randomized, controlled trial. *J Am Acad Child Adolesc Psychiatry* 2001;40:762–772.
15. Diler RS, Avci A. Selective serotonin reuptake inhibitor discontinuation syndrome in children: six case reports. *Curr Ther Res Clin Exp* 2002;63:188–197.
16. Mandoki MW, Tapia MR, Tapia MA, et al. Venlafaxine in the treatment of children and adolescents with major depression. *Psychopharmacol Bull* 1997;33:149–154.
17. Geller B, Cooper TB, Zimerman B, et al. Lithium for prepubertal depressed children with family history predictors of future bipolarity: a double-blind, placebo-controlled study. *J Affect Disord* 1998;51:165–175.
18. Harrington R, Whittaker J, Shoebridge P, et al. Systematic review of efficacy of cognitive behavioural therapies in childhood and adolescent depressive disorder. *BMJ* 1998;316:1559–1563. Search date 1997; primary sources Medline, Psychlit, Cochrane, and hand searches of reference lists, book chapters, conference proceedings, and relevant journals in the field.
19. Clarke GN, Hornbrook M, Lynch F, et al. Group cognitive-behavioral treatment for depressed adolescent offspring of depressed patients in a Health Maintenance Organization. *J Am Acad Child Adolesc Psychiatry* 2002;41:305–313.
20. Lewinsohn PM, Clarke GN. Psychosocial treatments for adolescent depression. *Clin Psychol Rev* 1999;19:329–342.
21. Reinecke MA, Ryan NE, DuBois DL. Cognitive-behavioral therapy of depression and depressive symptoms during adolescence: a review and meta-analysis. *J Am Acad Child Adolesc Psychiatry* 1998;37:26–34.
22. Mendez Carrillo FX, Moreno PJ, Sanchez-Meca J, et al. Effectiveness of psychological treatment for

child and adolescent depression: a qualitative review of two decades of research. *Psicol Conductual* 2000;8:487–510.
23. Mufson L, Weissman MM, Moreau D, et al. Efficacy of interpersonal psychotherapy for depressed adolescents. *Arch Gen Psychiatry* 1999;56:573–579.
24. Rossello J, Bernal G. The efficacy of cognitive-behavioral and interpersonal treatments for depression in Puerto Rican adolescents. *J Consult Clin Psychol* 1999;67:734–745.
25. Brent DA, Holder D, Kolko D, et al. A clinical psychotherapy trial for adolescent depression comparing cognitive, family, and supportive therapy. *Arch Gen Psychiatry* 1997;54:877–885.
26. Clarke GN, Rohde P, Lewinsohn PM, et al. Cognitive-behavioral treatment of adolescent depression: efficacy of acute group treatment and booster sessions. *J Am Acad Child Adolesc Psychiatry* 1999;38:272–279.
27. Fine S, Forth A, Gilbert M, et al. Group therapy for adolescent depressive disorder: a comparison of social skills and therapeutic support. *J Am Acad Child Adolesc Psychiatry* 1991;30:79–85.
28. Birmaher B, Brent DA, Kolko D, et al. Clinical outcome after short-term psychotherapy for adolescents with major depressive disorder. *Arch Gen Psychiatry* 2000;57:29–36.
29. Haaga DAF, Beck AT. Cognitive therapy. In: Paykel ES, ed. *Handbook of affective disorders*. Edinburgh: Churchill Livingstone, 1992;511–523.
30. Klerman GL, Weissman H. Interpersonal psychotherapy. In: Paykel ES, ed. *Handbook of affective disorders*. Edinburgh: Churchill Livingstone, 1992;501–510.

Philip Hazell
Conjoint Professor of Child and Adolescent Psychiatry/Director Child and Youth Mental Health Service
University of Newcastle
New South Wales
Australia

Competing interests: The author has been paid a fee by Pfizer, the manufacturer of sertraline, for speaking to general practitioners about the evidence for the treatment of depression in young people. The author's service has been in receipt of funding from Eli Lilly to participate in a relapse prevention trial of atomoxetine for attention deficit hyperactivity disorder.

Gastroenteritis in children

Search date February 2003

Jacqueline Dalby-Payne and Elizabeth Elliott

QUESTIONS

INTERVENTIONS

See glossary, p 390

Key Messages

- **Oral rehydration solutions (as effective as iv fluids)** One systematic review and two additional RCTs in children with mild to moderate dehydration in developed countries found no significant difference between oral rehydration solutions versus intravenous fluids in duration of diarrhoea, time spent in hospital, or weight gain at discharge. One small RCT in children with mild to moderate dehydration managed in the emergency department found that oral rehydration reduced length of stay in the department but did not significantly reduce admission to hospital compared with intravenous fluids. One RCT in children with severe dehydration in a developing country found that oral rehydration solutions reduced the duration of diarrhoea and increased weight gain at discharge, and was associated with fewer adverse effects compared with intravenous fluids.
- **Lactose-free feeds (for duration of diarrhoea)** We found evidence from one systematic review and subsequent RCTs that lactose-free feeds versus feeds containing lactose reduce the duration of diarrhoea in children with mild to severe dehydration.
- **Loperamide (reduces duration of diarrhoea, but adverse effects unclear)** Two RCTs found that, in children with mild to moderate dehydration, loperamide versus placebo significantly reduces the duration of diarrhoea. Another RCT found no significant difference with loperamide versus placebo in the duration of diarrhoea. We found insufficient evidence about adverse effects.
- **Clear fluids (other than oral rehydration solutions)** We found no systematic review or RCTs on "clear fluids" (water, carbonated drinks, and translucent fruit juices) versus oral rehydration solutions for treatment of mild to moderate dehydration caused by acute gastroenteritis.

DEFINITION Acute gastroenteritis is characterised by rapid onset of diarrhoea with or without vomiting, nausea, fever, and abdominal pain.[1] In children, the symptoms and signs can be non-specific.[2] Diarrhoea is defined as the frequent passage of unformed liquid stools.[3]

INCIDENCE/ PREVALENCE Worldwide, about 3 billion–5 billion cases of acute gastroenteritis occur in children under 5 years of age each year.[4] In the UK, acute gastroenteritis accounts for 204/1000 general practitioner consultations each year in children under 5 years of age.[5] Gastroenteritis leads to hospital admission in 7/1000 children under 5 years of age a year in the UK[5] and 13/1000 in the USA.[6] In Australia, gastroenteritis accounts for 6% of all hospital admissions in children under 15 years of age.[7]

AETIOLOGY/ RISK FACTORS In developed countries, acute gastroenteritis is predominantly caused by viruses (87%), of which rotavirus is most common;[8–11] bacteria cause most of the remaining cases, predominantly Campylobacter, Salmonella, Shigella, and *Escherichia coli*. In developing countries, bacterial pathogens are more frequent, although rotavirus is also a major cause of gastroenteritis.

PROGNOSIS Acute gastroenteritis is usually self limiting but if untreated can result in morbidity and mortality secondary to water and electrolyte losses. Acute diarrhoea causes 4 million deaths a year in children under 5 years of age in Asia (excluding China), Africa, and Latin America, and over 80% of deaths occur in children under 2 years of age.[12] Although death is uncommon in developed countries, dehydration secondary to gastroenteritis is a significant cause of morbidity and need for hospital admission.[6,7,13]

AIMS OF INTERVENTION To reduce the duration of diarrhoea and quantity of stool output, and duration of hospital stay; to prevent and treat dehydration; to promote weight gain after rehydration; to prevent persistent diarrhoea associated with lactose intolerance (see glossary, p 390).

OUTCOMES Total stool volume; duration of diarrhoea (time until permanent cessation); failure rate of oral rehydration treatment (as defined by individual RCTs); weight gain after rehydration; length of hospital stay; mortality.

METHODS *Clinical Evidence* search and appraisal February 2003.

QUESTION What are the effects of treatments for acute gastroenteritis?

OPTION CLEAR FLUIDS

We found no systematic review or RCTs on "clear fluids" (water, carbonated drinks, and translucent fruit juices) versus oral rehydration solutions for treatment of mild to moderate dehydration caused by acute gastroenteritis.

Benefits: We found no systematic review or RCTs of "clear fluids" versus oral rehydration solutions (see comment below).

Harms: We found no RCTs.

Comment: In this review, oral rehydration solutions are defined as glucose plus electrolyte or food (e.g. rice) based electrolyte solutions. Fruit juices and carbonated drinks are low in sodium and potassium, and usually have a high sugar content, which can exacerbate diarrhoea.

OPTION ORAL VERSUS INTRAVENOUS FLUIDS

One systematic review and two additional RCTs in children with mild to moderate dehydration in developed countries found no significant difference between oral rehydration solutions versus intravenous fluids in duration of diarrhoea, time spent in hospital, or weight gain at discharge. One RCT in children with mild to moderate dehydration managed in the emergency department found that oral rehydration reduced length of stay in the department but did not significantly reduce length of hospital stay compared with intravenous fluids. One RCT in children with severe dehydration in a developing country found that oral rehydration solutions reduced the duration of diarrhoea and increased weight gain at discharge, and was associated with fewer adverse effects compared with intravenous fluids.

Benefits: **Mild to moderate dehydration:** We found one systematic review[14] (search date 1993, 6 RCTs,[15–20] 371 children in developed countries with acute gastroenteritis, most with mild to moderate dehydration and in hospital), two additional RCTs[21,22] and one subsequent RCT[23] comparing oral rehydration solutions versus intravenous fluids (see table 1, p 393). The review and the additional RCTs found no significant difference with oral versus intravenous fluids in the duration of diarrhoea, time spent in hospital, or weight gain at discharge. If children responded poorly to oral fluids, they were given intravenous fluids, which was used as a measure of failure of oral fluids. However, the failure rate of intravenous treatment was not recorded. The subsequent RCT (34 children managed in the emergency department) did not report on duration of diarrhoea, length of hospital stay, or weight gain.[23] However, it found that oral rehydration significantly reduced length of stay in the emergency department compared with intravenous fluids, but found no significant difference for hospitalisation rate (mean length of stay in emergency department: 225 minutes with oral rehydration *v* 358 minutes with iv rehydration, $P < 0.01$; hospitalisation rate: 11% with oral rehydration *v* 25% with iv rehydration, $P = 0.2$).
Severe dehydration: We found one RCT (470 children in Iran with acute gastroenteritis with severe dehydration) comparing oral rehydration solutions versus intravenous fluids (see table 1, p 393).[24] It found that oral versus intravenous treatment significantly reduced the duration of diarrhoea (4.8 days with oral rehydration *v* 5.5 days with iv rehydration; difference 0.7 days; $P < 0.01$), and increased weight gain at discharge (percentage increase in admission weight 9% with oral rehydration *v* 7% with iv rehydration; $P < 0.001$). Failure of oral treatment (defined as the need to move to intravenous treatment) occurred in 1/236 children (0.4%; CI not reported). It found no significant difference in mortality between oral and intravenous fluids (2/236 [1%] with oral rehydration *v* 5/234 [2%] with iv rehydration; RR 0.40, 95% CI 0.08 to 2.02). Causes of death were not reported.

Harms: **Mild to moderate dehydration:** The systematic review reported no adverse effects.[14] One additional RCT (100 children in Afghanistan) reported fever and rigors in 9/50 children (18%) receiving intravenous fluids versus none receiving oral fluids.[21] **Severe dehydration:** The RCT in children in Iran found that significantly more children receiving intravenous treatment vomited during the first 6 hours of rehydration (47/236 [20%] with oral rehydration *v* 70/234 [30%] with iv rehydration; RR 0.64, 95% CI 0.46 to 0.89).[24] There was no significant difference in the risk of peri-orbital oedema (RR 0.99, 95% CI 0.25 to 3.92) or abdominal distension (RR 8.90, 95% CI 0.48 to 164.00). Phlebitis at the injection site requiring antibiotics occurred in 5/234 (2%) children. In the same RCT, subgroup analysis of 58 children with hypernatraemia found that fewer children taking oral versus intravenous fluids developed seizures during rehydration, although the difference did not quite reach significance (2/34 [6%] with oral rehydration *v* 6/24 [25%] with iv rehydration; RR 0.23, 95% CI 0.05 to 1.07).

Comment: The quality of the RCTs was difficult to assess because of poor reporting. Two RCTs reported the method of allocation concealment[17,23] and two reported the method of randomisation.[21,23] Blinding of outcomes was impossible owing to the nature of the intervention. Intention to treat analysis was used in all but one RCT.[17] The RCT in children managed in the emergency department was small and may have lacked power to detect clinically important effects.

OPTION LOPERAMIDE

Two RCTs found that, in children with mild to moderate dehydration, loperamide reduced the duration of diarrhoea compared with placebo. Another RCT found no significant difference between loperamide and placebo in the duration of diarrhoea. We found insufficient evidence to assess the risk of adverse effects.

Benefits: We found no systematic review. We found five RCTs in children with acute diarrhoea (701 children, most with mild to moderate dehydration) (see table 2, p 395).[25–29] Of the three RCTs that assessed the duration of diarrhoea, two[25,27] found that loperamide significantly reduced duration of diarrhoea compared with placebo (largest RCT, 315 children; risk of having diarrhoea at 24 hours, 36/100 [36%] with loperamide *v* 112/203 [55%] with placebo; RR 0.83, 95% CI 0.73 to 0.94).[25] Another RCT found no significant difference.[26] The results of other outcomes are included in table 2, p 395.

Harms: Four RCTs reported no adverse effects from loperamide.[25–27,29] One RCT found significantly more mild abdominal distension, excessive sleep, and lethargy in children taking loperamide versus placebo (3/16 [19%] with loperamide 0.8 mg/kg *v* 1/18 [6%] with 0.4 mg/kg *v* 0/18 [0%] with placebo; RR loperamide *v* placebo 4.90, 95% CI 0.28 to 86.00). Adverse effects caused one child to withdraw from the trial.[28] We found one evidence based guideline that identified case studies reporting lethargy, intestinal ileus, respiratory depression, and coma, especially in infants.[2]

Comment: We found insufficient evidence to estimate accurately the risk of adverse effects of loperamide in children.

OPTION LACTOSE-FREE FEEDS

We found evidence from one systematic review and subsequent RCTs that lactose-free feeds reduce the duration of diarrhoea compared with lactose-containing feeds in children with mild to severe dehydration.

Benefits: We found one systematic review (search date not stated, 13 RCTs, 873 children with mild to severe dehydration)[30] and four subsequent RCTs[31–34] comparing feeds containing lactose versus lactose-free feed. The review was limited by flaws in its methods (see comment below). It found that feeds containing lactose versus lactose-free feeds significantly increased "treatment failure" (89/399 [22%] with lactose *v* 56/474 [12%] with lactose-free; RR 2.1, 95% CI 1.6 to 2.7). The definition of treatment failure varied among trials and included increasing severity or persistence of diarrhoea or recurrence of dehydration. It found that lactose-free feeds versus feeds containing lactose significantly reduced the duration of diarrhoea (9 RCTs; 826 children with mild or no dehydration receiving oral rehydration treatment; 92 hours with lactose *v* 88 hours with lactose-free; SMD 0.2 hours after initiation of the study; P = 0.001). When the three RCTs that included children given additional solid food were excluded, it found that lactose-free versus feeds containing lactose significantly reduced the duration of diarrhoea (6 RCTs; 604 children; 95 hours with lactose *v* 82 hours with lactose-free; SMD 0.3 hours; P < 0.001). Children receiving lactose-free versus feeds containing lactose had significantly reduced stool frequency (4 RCTs; 387 children; 4.0 stool movements/day with lactose *v* 3.5 stool movements/day with lactose-free; SMD 0.3 stool movements/day; P < 0.004). Total stool volume was greater in children who received feeds containing lactose (4 RCTs; 209 children; SMD 0.4 g; P = 0.002). Differences in weight gain during treatment could not be assessed because of the use of solid food in two studies and considerable heterogeneity among studies. We found four subsequent RCTs (see table 3, p 396).[31–34] Two found that lactose-free versus feeds containing lactose significantly reduced the duration of diarrhoea,[31,34] and the other two found no significant difference.[32,33] The results of other outcomes are summarised in table 3, p 396.

Harms: The one RCT assessing adverse effects reported none in the treatment or control groups.[33]

Comment: Although the systematic review stated criteria for inclusion and exclusion of RCTs, only published studies were included and the method of determining RCT quality was not stated.[30] There was considerable heterogeneity among studies. Lactose-free feeds were superior to feeds containing lactose for the duration of diarrhoea. Differences for other outcomes, although statistically significant, were not clinically important.

GLOSSARY

Lactose intolerance Malabsorption of lactose can occur for a short period after acute gastroenteritis because of mucosal damage and temporary lactase deficiency.

Substantive changes

Oral versus intravenous fluids One RCT added;[23] conclusions unchanged.

REFERENCES

1. Armon K, Elliott EJ. Acute gastroenteritis. In: Moyer VA, Elliott EJ, Davis RL, eds. *Evidence based pediatrics and child health*. London: BMJ Books, 2000;273–286.
2. American Academy of Pediatrics (APP). Practice parameter: the management of acute gastroenteritis in young children. American Academy of Pediatrics, Provisional Committee on Quality Improvement, Subcommittee on Acute Gastroenteritis. *Pediatrics* 1996;97:424–435.
3. Critchley M. *Butterworths medical dictionary second edition*. London: Butterworths, 1986.
4. OPCS. *Mid-1993 population estimates for England and Wales*. London: HMSO, 1994.
5. OPCS. *Morbidity statistics from general practice. Fourth national study, 1991–1992*. London: HMSO, 1993.
6. Glass RI, Lew JF, Gangarosa RE, et al. Estimates of morbidity and mortality rates for diarrheal diseases in American children. *J Pediatr* 1991;118:S27–S33.
7. Elliott EJ, Backhouse JA, Leach JW. Pre-admission management of acute gastroenteritis. *J Paediatr Child Health* 1996;32:18–21.
8. Conway SP, Phillips RR, Panday S. Admission to hospital with gastroenteritis. *Arch Dis Child* 1990;65:579–584.
9. Finkelstein JA, Schwartz JS, Torrey S, et al. Common clinical features as predictors of bacterial diarrhea in infants. *Am J Emerg Med* 1989;7:469–473.
10. DeWitt TG, Humphrey KF, McCarthy P. Clinical predictors of acute bacterial diarrhea in young children. *Pediatrics* 1985;76:551–556.
11. Ferson MJ. Hospitalisations for rotavirus gastroenteritis among children under five years of age in New South Wales. *Med J Aust* 1996;164:273–276.
12. Anonymous. *A manual for the treatment of diarrhoea. Programme for the control of diarrhoeal diseases*. Geneva: WHO, 1990.
13. Conway SP, Phillips RR, Panday S. Admission to hospital with gastroenteritis. *Arch Dis Child* 1990;65:579–584.
14. Gavin N, Merrick N, Davidson B. Efficacy of glucose-based oral rehydration therapy. *Pediatrics* 1996;98:45–51. Search date 1993; primary sources Medline and experts and organisations involved in diarrhoea treatment contacted.
15. Santosham M, Daum RS, Dillman L, et al. Oral rehydration therapy of infantile diarrhea: a controlled study of well-nourished children hospitalized in the United States and Panama. *N Engl J Med* 1982;306:1070–1076.
16. Listernick R, Zieserl E, Davis AT. Outpatient oral rehydration in the United States. *Am J Dis Child* 1986;140:211–215.
17. Mackenzie A, Barnes G. Randomised controlled trial comparing oral and intravenous rehydration therapy in children with diarrhoea. *BMJ* 1991;303:393–396.
18. Tamer AM, Friedman LB, Maxwell SR, et al. Oral rehydration of infants in a large urban US medical center. *J Pediatr* 1985;107:14–19.
19. Vesikari T, Isolauri E, Baer M. A comparative trial of rapid oral and intravenous rehydration in acute diarrhoea. *Acta Paediatr Scand* 1987;76:300–305.
20. Issenman RM, Leung AK. Oral and intravenous rehydration of children. *Can Fam Physician* 1993;39:2129–2136.
21. Singh M, Mahmoodi A, Arya LS, et al. Controlled trial of oral versus intravenous rehydration in the management of acute gastroenteritis. *Indian J Med Res* 1982;75:691–693.
22. Oritiz A. Rehidratacion oral: Experiencia en el manejo de pacientes con gastroenteritis aguda en la sala de emergencia hospital pediatrico. *Bol Asoc Med P R* 1990;82:227–233.
23. Atherly-John YC, Cunningham SJ, Crain EF. A randomized trial of oral vs intravenous rehydration in a pediatric emergency department. *Arch Pediatr Adolesc Med* 2002;156:1240–1243.
24. Sharifi J, Ghavami F, Nowrouzi Z, et al. Oral versus intravenous rehydration therapy in severe gastroenteritis. *Arch Dis Child* 1985;60:856–860.
25. Diarrhoeal Diseases Study Group (UK). Loperamide in acute diarrhoea in childhood: results of a double blind, placebo controlled multicentre clinical trial. *BMJ Clin Res Ed* 1984;289:1263–1267.
26. Owens JR, Broadhead R, Hendrickse RG, et al. Loperamide in the treatment of acute gastroenteritis in early childhood. Report of a two centre, double-blind, controlled clinical trial. *Ann Trop Paediatr* 1981;1:135–141.
27. Kassem AS, Madkour AA, Massoud BZ, et al. Loperamide in acute childhood diarrhoea: a double blind controlled trial. *J Diarrhoeal Dis Res* 1983;1:10–16.
28. Karrar ZA, Abdulla MA, Moody JB, et al. Loperamide in acute diarrhoea in childhood: results of a double blind, placebo controlled clinical trial. *Ann Trop Paediatr* 1987;7:122–127.
29. Bowie MD, Hill ID, Mann MD. Loperamide for treatment of acute diarrhoea in infants and young children. A double-blind placebo-controlled trial. *S Afr Med J* 1995;85:885–887.
30. Brown KH, Peerson JM, Fontaine O. Use of nonhuman milks in the dietary management of young children with acute diarrhea: a meta-analysis of clinical trials. *Pediatrics* 1994;93:17–27. Search date not stated; primary sources Medline, hand searches of reference lists, and contact with researchers.
31. Allen UD, McLeod K, Wang EE. Cow's milk versus soy-based formula in mild and moderate diarrhea: a randomized, controlled trial. *Acta Paediatr* 1994;83:183–187.
32. Clemente YF, Tapia CC, Comino AL, et al. Lactose-free formula versus adapted formula in acute infantile diarrhea. *An Esp Pediatr* 1993;39:309–312.
33. Lozano JM, Cespedes JA. Lactose vs. lactose free regimen in children with acute diarrhoea: a randomized controlled trial. *Arch Latinoam Nutr* 1994;44:6–11.
34. Fayad IM, Hashem M, Husseine A, et al. Comparison of soy-based formulas with lactose and with sucrose in the treatment of acute diarrhoea in infants. *Arch Pediatr Adolesc Med* 1999;153:675–680.

Jacqueline Dalby-Payne
Lecturer
Discipline of Paediatrics and Child Health
University of Sydney
Consultant Paediatrician
The Children's Hospital at Westmead
Sydney
Australia

Elizabeth Elliott
Associate Professor
Discipline of Paediatrics and Child Health
University of Sydney
Consultant Paediatrician
The Children's Hospital at Westmead
Sydney
Australia

Competing interests: None declared.

TABLE 1 **Oral versus intravenous fluids in mild to moderate[15–23] and severe dehydration[24] (see text, p 388).**

Intervention (saline concentration in %, unless otherwise stated)	Participants (age)	Duration of diarrhoea (days)	Stay in hospital (days)	Weight gain	Stool output (mL/kg body weight)	Failure of oral treatment (defined as the need to revert to iv treatment)*
Oral versus iv fluids in mild to moderate dehydration						
ORS (90, 50) *v* iv[15]	52 children from US and 94 children in Panama with acute diarrhoea (3–24 months)	NS	NR	NS	US: ORS (90) *v* iv (NS); ORS (50) *v* iv (193 *v* 112; P < 0.02). Panama: ORS (90) *v* iv (90 *v* 168; P < 0.001); ORS (50) *v* iv (NS)	1/98 (1%)
ORS (60) *v* iv[16]	29 children with acute diarrhoea (3–24 months)	NR	NR	NS	NR	2/15 (13%)
ORS (50) *v* iv[17]	111 children with acute diarrhoea (3–36 months)	NR	NS	NR	NR	2/52 (4%)
ORS (75, 50) *v* iv[18]	100 children with acute diarrhoea (3–33 months)	NR	NS	NS	NR	3/50 (6%)
ORS (60) *v* iv[19]	37 children with acute diarrhoea (< 5 years)	ORS < iv (1.0 ± 0.5 *v* 2.6 ± 1.6; P < 0.001)	ORS < iv (2.7 ± 1.0 *v* 3.9 ± 1.7; P < 0.001)	ORS > iv + 314 g *v* –16 g; P < 0.05)	NS	2/20(10%)
ORS (45, 74) *v* iv[20]	42 children with acute diarrhoea (6–31 months)	NR	NR	NS	NR	4/22 (18%)
ORS (3.5 g/L) *v* iv[21]	100 children with acute diarrhoea (mean age 11 years)	NS	NR	NS	NR	NR

TABLE 1 continued

Intervention (saline concentration in %, unless otherwise stated)	Participants (age)	Duration of diarrhoea (days)	Stay in hospital (days)	Weight gain	Stool output (mL/kg body weight)	Failure of oral treatment (defined as the need to revert to iv treatment)*
ORS (75) *v* iv[22]	31 children with acute diarrhoea (mean age 4–5 years)	NS	NR	NS	NR	NR
ORS (NR) *v* iv[23]	34 children with acute diarrhoea (3 months to 17 years)	NR	NR	NR	NR	3/18 (17%)
Oral versus iv fluids in severe dehydration						
ORS (80, 40) *v* iv[24]	470 children with acute diarrhoea (1–18 months)	ORS < iv (4.8 *v* 5.5; $P < 0.01$)	NR	ORS > iv (8.9% *v* 7.3%; $P < 0.001$)	NR	1/236 (0.4%)

*Although this outcome measures treatment failure of oral treatment it is not a comparative outcome as the number of children responding poorly to was not recorded. iv, intravenous; NR, not reported; NS, non-significant; ORS, oral rehydration solution

TABLE 2 Loperamide in mild to moderate dehydration: results of placebo controlled RCTs (see text, p 389).[25–29]

Intervention (loperamide dose mg/kg/day)	Participants (age)	Duration of diarrhoea	Stay in hospital	Weight gain	Stool output
Loperamide (0.4, 0.8) *v* placebo[25]	315 children with acute diarrhoea and mild to moderate dehydration (3 months to 3 years)	L < placebo; risk of having diarrhoea at 24 hours; RR 0.83, 95% CI 0.73 to 0.94.	NS	L > placebo; children with increased weight at 3 days: loperamide 0.8 mg *v* 0.4 mg *v* placebo: 58% *v* 51% *v* 36%	NR
Loperamide (0.2) *v* placebo[26]	50 children with acute diarrhoea (1–4 years)	NS	NS	NS	NR
Loperamide (0.2) *v* placebo[27]	100 children with acute diarrhoea and mild to moderate dehydration (< 2 years)	L < placebo; 59.1 hours *v* 81.1 hours; $P < 0.05$	NR	NS	NS
Loperamide (0.4, 0.8) *v* placebo[28]	53 children with acute diarrhoea (3 months to 3 years)	NR	NR	L > placebo; children with increased weight at 3 days: loperamide 0.8 mg *v* 0.4 mg *v* placebo: 88% *v* 50% *v* 39%; RR 0.53, 95% CI 0.29 to 0.97	NR
Loperamide (0.8) *v* placebo[29]	185 children with acute gastroenteritis and mild to moderate dehydration (3–18 months).	NR	NS	NR	NR

L, loperamide; NR, not reported; NS, non-significant.

TABLE 3 **Feeds containing lactose versus lactose-free feeds in children with mild to severe dehydration: results of subsequent RCTs (see text, p 390).[31–34]**

Intervention	Participants (age)	Duration of diarrhoea	Weight gain	Total stool output (mL/kg body weight)	Treatment failure
Cow's milk *v* soy-based formula[31]	76 children with acute diarrhoea and mild to moderate dehydration (2–12 months)	L > LF; 6.6 *v* 4.5 days; $P < 0.01$	NS	NR	NS
Lactose *v* lactose-free formula[32]	60 children with acute diarrhoea (< 1 year)	NS	NS	NR	NR
Lactose *v* lactose-free formula[33]	52 children with acute diarrhoea and mild to moderate dehydration (1–24 months)	NS	NS	NR	NS
Soy-based formula with lactose *v* soy-based formula with sucrose[34]	200 boys with acute diarrhoea (3–18 months)	L > LF; 39 hours *v* 23 hours; $P < 0.001$	NS	L > LF; mean 164 (95% CI 131 to 208) *v* 69 (95% CI 55 to 87); $P < 0.001$	NS

NR, not recorded; NS, non-significant; L, lactose-containing; LF, lactose-free.

Gastro-oesophageal reflux in children

Search date January 2003

Yadlapalli Kumar and Rajini Sarvananthan

QUESTIONS

INTERVENTIONS

*Not widely licensed for use in children. Clinical use in adults has been restricted because of heart rhythm abnormalities.

Key Messages

- **Sodium alginate** Two RCTs in infants and in children under 2 years old found that sodium alginate reduced the frequency of regurgitation at 8–14 days compared with placebo.
- **Domperidone** We found insufficient evidence from one small RCT about effects of domperidone in children with gastro-oesophageal reflux.
- **Feed thickeners** One systematic review of feed thickeners in newborn infants found no RCTs. One small RCT in older infants aged 1–16 weeks found no significant difference between carob flour and placebo thickening after 1 week, although the study may have lacked power to detect a clinically important difference.
- **H_2 antagonists** We found insufficient evidence from two small RCTs about effects of H_2 antagonists in children with gastro-oesophagael reflux. Neither RCT reported clinically meaningful results.
- **Metoclopramide** We found insufficient evidence from three small RCTs about the clinical effects of metoclopramide compared with placebo or other treatments.
- **Positioning (left lateral or prone)** We found insufficient evidence about clinical effects. Small crossover RCTs in children aged under 6 months found limited evidence that prone or left lateral positioning improved oesophageal pH variables compared with supine positioning. Both prone and left lateral positions may be associated with a higher risk of sudden infant death syndrome compared with supine positioning.
- **Proton pump inhibitors** We found no RCTs about proton pump inhibitors for gastro-oesophageal reflux in children.
- **Surgery** We found no RCTs about surgery for gastro-oesophageal reflux in children.

- **Cisapride** One systematic review found no significant difference between cisapride and placebo in the proportion of children with improved symptoms at the end of treatment. Cisapride has been withdrawn or restricted in several countries because of an association with heart rhythm abnormalities.

DEFINITION Gastro-oesophageal reflux disease is the passive transfer of gastric contents into the oesophagus due to transient or chronic relaxation of the lower oesophageal sphincter.[1] A survey of 69 children (median age 16 months) with gastro-oesophageal reflux disease attending a tertiary referral centre found that presenting symptoms were recurrent vomiting (72%), epigastric and abdominal pain (36%), feeding difficulties (29%), failure to thrive (28%), and irritability (19%).[2] However, results may not be generalisable to younger children or children presenting in primary care, who make up the majority of cases. Over 90% of children with gastro-oesophageal reflux disease have vomiting before 6 weeks of age.[1]

INCIDENCE/ PREVALENCE Gastro-oesophageal regurgitation is considered a problem if it is frequent, persistent, and is associated with other symptoms such as increased crying, discomfort with regurgitation, and frequent back arching.[1,3] A cross-sectional survey of parents of 948 infants attending 19 primary care paediatric practices found that regurgitation of at least one episode a day was reported in 51% of infants aged 0–3 months. "Problematic" regurgitation occurred in significantly fewer infants (14% *v* 51%; $P < 0.001$).[3] Peak regurgitation reported as "problematic" was reported in 23% of infants aged 6 months.[3]

AETIOLOGY/ RISK FACTORS Risk factors for gastro-oesophageal reflux disease include immaturity of the lower oesophageal sphincter, chronic relaxation of the sphincter, increased abdominal pressure, gastric distension, hiatus hernia, and oesophageal dysmotility.[1] Premature infants and children with severe neurodevelopmental problems or congenital oesophageal anomalies are particularly at risk.[1]

PROGNOSIS Regurgitation is considered benign, and most cases resolve spontaneously by 12–18 months of age.[4] In a cross-sectional survey of 948 parents, the peak age for reporting four or more episodes of regurgitation was at 5 months of age (23%), which decreased to 7% at 7 months ($P < 0.001$). One cohort study found that those infants with frequent spilling (see glossary, p 404) in the first 2 years of life (90 days or more in the first 2 years) were more likely to have symptoms of gastro-oesophageal reflux at 9 years of age than those with no spilling (RR 2.3, 95% CI 1.3 to 4.0).[5] The prevalence of "problematic" regurgitation also reduced from 23% in infants aged 6 months to 3.25% in infants aged 10–12 months.[3] Rare complications of gastro-oesophageal reflux disease include oesophagitis with haematemesis and anaemia, respiratory problems (such as cough, apnoea, and recurrent wheeze), and failure to thrive.[1] A small comparative study (40 children) suggested that, when compared with healthy children, infants with gastro-oesophageal reflux disease had slower development of feeding skills and had problems affecting behaviour, swallowing, food intake, and mother–child interaction.[6]

AIMS OF INTERVENTION To relieve symptoms, maintain normal growth, prevent complications such as oesophagitis, and minimise adverse effects of treatment.

OUTCOMES Clinical condition (in terms of improvement in symptoms of vomiting and regurgitation); growth; parental distress; and incidence of complications (e.g. oesophagitis). Reflux Index, a measure of the percentage of time with a low oesophageal pH (frequently < pH 4), is a surrogate outcome that is often used in RCTs. Clinical interpretation of the resulting data is problematic. We have only reported Reflux Index findings where clinical outcomes are unavailable.

METHODS *Clinical Evidence* search and appraisal January 2003. The authors also searched Cinahl for studies on incidence and prevalence. Studies did not often discuss whether breastfeeding was also undertaken or withdrawn in treatment groups. Presence or absence of concomitant breastfeeding may have confounded study results.

QUESTION What are the effects of treatment for symptomatic gastro-oesophageal reflux?

OPTION DIFFERENT SLEEP POSITIONS

Three crossover RCTs in children aged under 6 months found limited evidence that prone or left lateral positioning improved oesophageal pH variables compared with supine positioning. Both prone and left lateral positions may be associated with a higher risk of sudden infant death syndrome compared with supine positioning.

Benefits: We found no systematic review or RCTs on the effect of posture on clinical symptoms, but found three small crossover RCTs on the effect of posture on oesophageal pH variables such as Reflux Index.[7–9] The first RCT (crossover, 24 infants, age < 5 months) assessed four sleep positions (supine, prone, left lateral, right lateral) over 48 hours; for the first 24 hours the infant was held horizontally, and for the remaining 24 hours the infant's head was elevated.[7] It found that the prone and left lateral positions significantly reduced the Reflux Index over 48 hours compared with the supine and right lateral positions ($P < 0.001$); it found no significant difference in the Reflux Index with horizontal positioning compared with head elevation. The second RCT (crossover, 15 infants, age < 6 months) alternated placing infants for 2 hours in a prone position (head elevated in a harness) and placing infants for 2 hours in a supine position (in an infant seat where the head and trunk were elevated to 60°) after a feed of apple juice.[8] It found that prone positioning significantly reduced the Reflux Index over 72 normal hours compared with supine positioning ($P < 0.001$). The third RCT (crossover, 18 infants, < 37 weeks gestation but > 7 days old) compared prone versus left lateral versus right lateral positions over 24 hours. It found that prone and left lateral positions significantly reduced Reflux Index compared with right lateral position ($P < 0.001$), the number of reflux episodes ($P < 0.001$), and duration of longest reflux episode ($P < 0.001$).[9]

Harms: The RCTs gave no information on adverse effects (see comment below).[7–9]

Comment: All three RCTs measured the surrogate outcome of Reflux Index, and it is difficult to interpret the clinical importance of the observed changes.[7–9] The results of these RCTs should be interpreted with caution because oesophageal pH variable may change over time, and the results were not assessed prior to crossover. Both prone and left lateral positioning have been associated with an increased risk of sudden infant death syndrome (see sudden infant death syndrome for prone positioning, p 457). One large, prospective cohort study found that the left lateral sleeping position compared with the supine position increased the risk of sudden infant death syndrome (at 2 months, adjusted OR 6.6, 95% CI 1.7 to 25.2).[10]

OPTION FEED THICKENERS

One systematic review of feed thickeners found no RCTs in newborn infants. One small RCT in older infants aged 1–16 weeks found no significant difference between carob flour and placebo thickening after 1 week, although the study may have lacked power to detect a clinically important difference.

Benefits: We found one systematic review (search date 2001), which examined the use of feed thickeners for newborn infants (defined as full-term infants < 28 days of age and preterm infants up to 44 weeks postmenstrual corrected age).[11] It identified no RCTs that reported results separately for neonates. We found one small RCT in older infants.[12] **Versus placebo:** The RCT (20 infants aged 1–16 weeks with regurgitation > 5 times daily, receiving formula feeds, parental reassurance and prone positioning) compared carob flour thickened feeds with placebo thickening (Saint John's bread, which is free of fibre and polysaccharides).[12] It found no significant difference in regurgitation rates between carob flour and placebo thickening after 1 week of treatment (mean regurgitation score 2.2 with carob flour *v* 3.3 with placebo; P = 0.14).

Harms: One RCT (24 children, age 0–6 months with gastro-oesophageal reflux disease) assessing the effects of feed thickeners on cough found that feeds thickened with dry rice cereal significantly increased coughing after feeding compared with isocaloric unthickened feeds (mean cough salvos/hour 3.1 with thickened feeds *v* 2.0 with unthickened feeds; P = 0.034).[13]

Comment: The clinical significance of changes in regurgitation scores in the first RCT is unclear.[12] One small crossover RCT (24 infants, age 5–11 months) found that carob flour significantly reduced a symptom score and the frequency of vomiting recorded by parents compared with traditional formula thickened with rice after 2 weeks (symptom score: mean relative reduction 70% with carob flour *v* 49% with traditional formula plus rice, P < 0.01; frequency of vomiting as recorded by parents, P < 0.05).[14] The results of this crossover RCT should be treated with caution because symptoms may change over time and the results were not assessed before crossover.[14]

OPTION SODIUM ALGINATE

Two RCTs in infants and in children under 2 years found that sodium alginate reduced the frequency of regurgitation at 8–14 days compared with placebo. A third RCT of children under 17 years of age comparing sodium alginate with metoclopramide and placebo found no significant difference among treatments.

Benefits: We found no systematic review but we found three RCTs.[15–17] The first RCT (90 infants aged 0–12 months attending 25 general practices) found that aluminium-free alginate reduced the number of episodes of vomiting after 14 days and increased the number of symptom free days compared with placebo (median number of episodes in previous 24 hours: 3.0 with alginate *v* 5.0 with placebo, P = 0.009; at least 10% symptom free days: 31% with alginate *v* 11% with placebo, P = 0.027).[15] The second RCT (20 children, mean age 28 months) found that sodium alginate reduced the total number of reflux episodes per 24 hours, as detected with pH monitoring, compared with baseline (episodes: alginate 131.6 at baseline to 65.0 after treatment; placebo 87 at baseline to 91 post-treatment; between treatment comparisons were not reported).[16] The third RCT (30 children aged 4 months to 17 years) found no significant difference in the frequency of regurgitation episodes over 24 hours with sodium alginate, metoclopramide, or placebo given before a meal (episode defined as pH < 4) or in Reflux Index over 24 hours (reported as non-significant; no further data provided).[17]

Harms: One RCT found no significant difference between aluminium-free alginate and placebo in diarrhoea, teething syndrome, emesis, pyrexia of unknown origin, constipation, colic or acute nasopharyngitis.[15] One other RCT found no adverse effects.[16]

Comment: The high sodium content of sodium alginate may be inappropriate in preterm babies.[18]

OPTION CISAPRIDE

One systematic review found no significant difference between cisapride and placebo in the proportion of children with improved symptoms at the end of treatment. Cisapride has been withdrawn or restricted in several countries because of an association with heart rhythm abnormalities.

Benefits: We found one systematic review (search date 2000, 8 RCTs).[19] It found no significant difference between cisapride and placebo in the proportion of children whose symptoms had improved at the end of treatment (7 RCTs, 236 children; 51/123 [41%] with cisapride *v* 64/113 [57%] with placebo; RR 0.72, 95% CI 0.54 to 0.96).

Harms: The review found a non-significant increase in adverse effects with cisapride compared with placebo (4 RCTs, 190 children; 56/95 [59%] with cisapride *v* 45/95 [47%] with placebo; RR 1.19, 95% CI 0.96 to 1.47), but it did not describe specific adverse effects.[19] See comment below.

Gastro-oesophageal reflux in children

Comment: The systematic review reported that results may be biased.[19] It found evidence of publication bias in favour of cisapride. Trials were statistically heterogeneous for symptom improvement, perhaps due to inconsistent definitions of degrees of improvement among studies. The clinical validity and reliability of outcome measures such as Reflux Index and severity scores were poorly described. Cisapride has been withdrawn or its use restricted in several countries because of an increased frequency of heart rhythm abnormalities that are associated with sudden death.[20] One case control study (201 children, age 1–12 months) found that cisapride significantly prolonged the QTc interval on electrocardiogram in a subgroup of infants younger than 3 months, but in older infants the difference was not significant.[21] A second case control study (252 infants) found similar results.[22] A third case control study (120 children) found prolonged QT interval in some normal children with or without cisapride.[23] Gastrointestinal adverse effects (borborygmi, cramps, and diarrhoea) occurred in 2% of infants.[21] Rash, pruritus, urticaria, bronchospasm, extrapyramidal effects, headache, dose-related increases in urinary frequency, hyperprolactinaemia, and reversible liver function abnormalities were extremely rare. Most macrolide antibiotics and cimetidine elevate plasma cisapride levels and may increase the clinical risk.[21]

OPTION DOMPERIDONE

We found insufficient evidence from one small RCT about effects of domperidone in children with gastro-oesophageal reflux.

Benefits: We found no systematic review. One small RCT (17 children, age 5 months to 11 years) found no significant difference in symptoms (vomiting, spitting, irritability, heartburn, coughing, choking), as assessed by daily parent record or Reflux Index, after 4 weeks of treatment between domperidone and placebo.[24] The RCT might have been too small to exclude a clinically important difference.

Harms: The RCT found that four children taking domperidone had mild self limiting diarrhoea compared with two children taking placebo.[24]

Comment: None.

OPTION H_2 ANTAGONISTS

We found insufficient evidence from two small RCTs about effects of H_2 antagonists on children with gastro-oesopgaheal reflux.

Benefits: We found no systematic review but found two small RCTs.[25,26] The first RCT (double blind, 37 children aged 1 month to 14 years with gastro-oesophageal reflux disease complicated by oesophagitis, 32 analysed) found that cimetidine 30–40 mg/kg daily significantly increased the proportion of children who improved compared with placebo at 12 weeks (67.4% improved in clinical score from baseline with cimetidine *v* 29.6% with placebo; $P < 0.01$).[25] The clinical score was developed for the study and the clinical importance of this result is unclear. The second small RCT (27 children, aged 3–14 years with gastro-oesophageal reflux disease) compared different doses of cimetidine but reported only physiological outcomes (gastric pH, gastric acid suppression).[26] We found no RCTs of ranitidine in children.

Harms: The RCTs found no adverse effects.[25,26]

Comment: Cimetidine has been reported to cause bradycardia in a small subgroup of people and may increase cisapride plasma levels.[21] Uncontrolled studies of ranitidine have reported bronchospasm, acute dystonic reactions, sinus node dysfunction, bradycardia, and vasovagal reactions.[21] Both RCTs were small and provide insufficient evidence about clinical effects.

OPTION METOCLOPRAMIDE

We found insufficient evidence from three small RCTs about the clinical effects of metoclopramide compared with placebo or other treatments.

Benefits: We found no systematic review but found three RCTs.[17,27,28] The first RCT (crossover; 30 infants aged 1–9 months receiving formula feed) found that metoclopramide 1 mg/kg four times daily significantly reduced the Reflux Index over 2 weeks compared with placebo ($P < 0.001$), but it found no significant difference in average daily symptoms (see comment below).[27] A second RCT (44 infants aged under 1 year) found no significant difference in the Reflux Index at 14 days between metoclopramide 0.2 mg three times daily and placebo before a meal.[28] A third RCT (30 infants aged 4 months to 17 years) compared three treatments: metoclopramide sodium alginate, and placebo (see benefits of sodium alginate, p 401).[17]

Harms: The RCTs gave no information on adverse effects.[17,27,28]

Comment: The results of the crossover RCT should be treated with caution as it did not assess the effects of metoclopramide versus placebo before crossover.[27] In the second RCT 5/44 (11%) of infants withdrew from the study, three because of lack of efficacy and two for unknown reasons; the results given are not intention to treat.[28] One observational study (42 infants), which assessed the effect of metoclopramide 0.2 mg or 0.3 mg on pH parameters, found that metoclopramide was associated with dystonia in one infant and increased irritability in three infants.[29]

OPTION PROTON PUMP INHIBITORS

We found no RCTs about proton pump inhibitors for gastro-oesophageal reflux in children.

Benefits: We found no systematic review or RCTs on proton pump inhibitors for gastro-oesophageal reflux in children. One small case series did not report clinical outcomes.[30]

Harms: We found no systematic review or RCTs.

Comment: Proton pump inhibitors have been reported to cause hepatitis, and omeprazole chronically elevates serum gastrin.[30]

Gastro-oesophageal reflux in children

OPTION SURGERY

We found no RCTs about surgery for gastro-oesophageal reflux in children.

Benefits: We found no systematic review or RCT comparing surgery versus medical interventions, or one surgical procedure versus another.

Harms: A retrospective review (106 children) of modified Nissen's fundoplication found a failure rate of 8% and, when neurologically impaired children were included, a long term mortality of 8%.[31] If only neurologically normal children were considered, then the mortality was 2% in the immediate postoperative period and 3% on long term follow up (3 deaths in 62 children; all deaths were in children with congenital abnormalities).

Comment: We found a cohort study of 22 children who had undergone anterior gastric fundoplication.[32] Twenty children (91%) remained asymptomatic at 2 years. Complications of surgical treatment include dumping, retching, intestinal obstruction, "gas bloat", and recurrence of gastro-oesophageal reflux disease.[18]

GLOSSARY

Spilling When liquid or substance in small particles falls or spills out of the mouth.

Substantive changes

Feed thickeners One systematic review added;[11] conclusion unchanged.

Sodium alginate One RCT added;[15] intervention recategorised from Unknown effectiveness to Likely to be beneficial.

REFERENCES

1. Herbst JJ. *Textbook of Gastroenterology and Nutrition in Infancy*. 2nd ed. New York: Raven Press, 1989:803–813.
2. Lee WS, Beattie RM, Meadows N, et al. Gastro-oesophageal reflux: Clinical profiles and outcome. *J Paediatr Child Health* 1999;35:568–571.
3. Nelson SP, Chen EH, Syniar GM, et al. Prevalence of symptoms of gastroesophageal reflux during infancy. *Arch Pediatr Adolesc Med* 1997;151:569–572.
4. Vandenplas Y, Belli D, Benhamou P, et al. A critical appraisal of current management practices for infant regurgitation — recommendations of a working party. *Eur J Pediatr* 1997;156:343–357.
5. Martin JA, Pratt N, Kennedy D, et al. Natural history and familial relationships of infant spilling to 9 years of age. *Paediatrics* 2002;109:1061–1067.
6. Mathisen B, Worrall L, Masel J, et al. Feeding problems in infants with gastro-oesophageal reflux disease: a controlled study. *J Paediatr Child Health* 1999;35:163–169.
7. Tobin JM, McCloud P, Cameron DJS. Posture and gastro-oesophageal reflux: a case for left lateral positioning. *Arch Dis Child* 1997;76:254–258.
8. Orenstein SR, Whitington PF. Positioning for prevention of infant gastroesophageal reflux. *J Pediatr* 1983;103:534–537.
9. Ewer AK, James ME, Tobin JM. Prone and left lateral positioning reduce gastro-oesophageal reflux in preterm infants. *Arch Dis Child Fetal Neonatal Ed* 1999;81:F201–205.
10. Dwyer T, Ponsonby AB, Newman NM, et al. Prospective cohort study of prone sleeping position and sudden infant death syndrome. *Lancet* 1991;337:1244–1247.
11. Huang RC, Forbes DA, Davies MW. Feed thickener for newborn infants with gastro-oesophageal reflux. In: The Cochrane Library, Issue 3, 2002. Oxford: Update software. Search date 2001; primary sources Medline, Cochrane Controlled Trials Register, Cochrane Library, Cinahl, conference and symposia proceedings published in *Paediatric Research* 1990–1994, and conference proceedings for the European Society for Paediatric Gastroenterology and Nutrition and the North American Society for Paediatric Gastroenterology and Nutrition.
12. Vandenplas Y, Hachimi-Idrissi S, Casteels A, et al. A clinical trial with an "anti-regurgitation" formula. *Eur J Pediatr* 1994;153:419–423.
13. Orenstein SR, Shalaby TM, Putnam PE. Thickening feedings as a cause of increased coughing when used as therapy for gastroesophageal reflux in infants. *J Pediatr* 1992;121:913–915.
14. Borrelli O, Salvia G, Campanozzi A, et al. Use of a new thickened formula for treatment of symptomatic gastroesophageal reflux in infants. *Ital J Gastroenterol Hepatol* 1997;29:237–242.
15. Miller S. Comparison of the efficacy and safety of a new aluminium-free paediatric alginate preparation and placebo in infants with recurrent gastro-oesophageal reflux. *Curr Med Res Opin* 1999;15:160–168.
16. Buts JP, Barudi C, Otte JB. Double-blind controlled study on the efficacy of sodium alginate (Gaviscon) in reducing gastroesophageal reflux

assessed by 24 hour continuous pH monitoring in infants and children. *Eur J Pediatr* 1987;146:156–158.
17. Forbes D, Hodgson M, Hill, R. The effects of gaviscon and metoclopramide in gastroesophageal reflux in children. *J Pediatr Gastroenterol Nutr* 1986;5:556–559.
18. Davies AEM, Sandhu BK. Diagnosis and treatment of gastro-oesophageal reflux. *Arch Dis Child* 1995;73:82–86.
19. Augood C, MacLennan S, Gilbert R, et al. Cisapride treatment for gastro-oesophageal reflux. In: The Cochrane Library, Issue 2, 2002. Oxford: Update Software. Search date 2000; primary sources Cochrane Central Trials Register, Cochrane Specialised Trials register of the Cochrane Upper Gastrointestinal and Pancreatic Diseases Group, Medline, Embase, Science Citation Index, and hand searched reference lists.
20. WHO Pharmaceuticals Newsletter, No.3, 2000. http://www.who.int/medicines/library/pnewslet/pn32000.html (last accessed 20 June 2003).
21. Vandenplas Y, Belli DC, Benatar A, et al. The role of cisapride in the treatment of pediatric gastroesophageal reflux. *J Pediatr Gastroenterol Nutr* 1999;28:518–528.
22. Benatar A, Feenstra A, Decraene T, et al. Effects of cisapride on corrected QT interval, heart rate, and rhythm in infants undergoing polysomnography. *Pediatrics* 2000;106:E85.
23. Ramirez-Mayans J, Garrido-Garcia LM, Huerta-Tecanhuey A, et al. Cisapride and QTc interval in children. *Pediatrics* 2000;106:1028–1030.
24. Bines JE, Quinlan JE, Treves S, et al. Efficacy of domperidone in infants and children with gastroesophageal reflux. *J Pediatr Gastroenterol Nutr* 1992;14:400–405.
25. Cucchiara S, Gobio-Casali L, Balli F, et al. Cimetidine treatment of reflux esophagitis in children: An Italian multicentre study. *J Pediatr Gastroenterol Nutr* 1989;8:150–156.
26. Lambert J, Mobassaleh M, Grand RJ. Efficacy of cimetidine for gastric acid suppression in pediatric patients. *J Pediatr* 1992;120:474–478.
27. Tolia V, Calhoun J, Kuhns L, et al. Randomized, double-blind trial of metoclopramide and placebo for gastroesophageal reflux. *J Pediatr* 1989;115:141–145.
28. Bellisant E, Duhamel JF, Guillot M, et al. The triangular test to assess the efficacy of metoclopramide in gastroesophageal reflux. *Clin Pharm Ther* 1997;61:377–384.
29. Hyams JS, Leichtner AM, Zamett LO, et al. Effect of metoclopramide on prolonged intraoesophageal pH testing in infants with gastroesophageal reflux. *J Pediatr Gastroenterol Nutr* 1986;5:716–720.
30. Gunasekaran TS, Hassall EG. Efficacy and safety of omeprazole for severe gastroesophageal reflux in children. *J Pediatr* 1993;123:148–154.
31. Spillane AJ, Currie B, Shi E. Fundoplication in children: Experience with 106 cases. *Aust NZ J Surg* 1996;66:753–756.
32. Bliss D, Hirschl R, Oldham K, et al. Efficacy of anterior gastric fundoplication in the treatment of gastroesophageal reflux in infants and children. *J Paediatr Surg* 1994;29:1071–1075.

Yadlapalli Kumar
Consultant Paediatrician
Royal Cornwall Hospital
Treliske Truro Cornwall
UK

Rajini Sarvananthan
Specialist Registrar in Paediatrics
Bradford Royal Infirmary
Bradford
UK

Competing interests: None declared.

Infantile colic

Search date January 2003

Teresa Kilgour and Sally Wade

QUESTIONS

INTERVENTIONS

See glossary, p 415

Key Messages

- **Whey hydrolysate milk** One RCT found limited evidence that replacing cows' milk formula with whey hydrolysate formula reduced crying recorded in a parental diary.
- **Dicycloverine** Two systematic reviews of RCTs of variable quality found limited evidence that dicycloverine reduced crying in infants with colic compared with placebo. RCTs found that dicycloverine increased drowsiness, constipation, and loose stools compared with placebo, but the difference did not reach significance. Case reports of harms in infants have included breathing difficulties, seizures, syncope, asphyxia, muscular hypotonia, and coma.
- **Car ride simulation device** One RCT comparing a car ride simulation device plus non-specific reassurance, counselling mothers about specific management techniques plus non-specific reassurance, and non-specific reassurance alone, found no significant difference among groups in maternal anxiety or hours of infant crying over 2 weeks.
- **Casein hydrolysate milk** Two RCTs found insufficient evidence about the effects of replacing cows' milk formula with casein hydrolysate hypoallergenic formula.
- **Cranial osteopathy** We found no RCTs about the effects of cranial osteopathy in infants with colic.

- **Focused counselling** One RCT comparing counselling mothers about specific management techniques (responding to crying with gentle soothing motion, avoiding over stimulation, using a pacifier, and prophylactic carrying) plus non-specific reassurance, a car ride simulation device plus non-specific reassurance, and non-specific reassurance alone, found no significant difference among groups in maternal anxiety or hours of infant crying over 2 weeks. Another small RCT found that focused counselling decreased duration and extent of crying compared with substitution of soya or cows' milk with casein hydrolysate formula.
- **Herbal tea** One small RCT found that herbal tea (containing extracts of camomile, vervain, liquorice, fennel, and balm mint in a sucrose solution) improved symptoms of colic rated by parents at 7 days compared with sucrose solution alone. However, we were unable to draw reliable conclusions from this small study.
- **Infant massage** One RCT found no significant difference between massage and a crib vibrator in colic related crying or parental rating of symptoms of infantile colic, but it may have lacked power to detect a clinically important difference.
- **Low lactose (lactase treated) milk** Four small crossover RCTs found insufficient evidence on the effects of low lactose (lactase treated) milk in infants with colic.
- **Reduction of stimulation of the infant** One RCT found limited evidence that advice to reduce stimulation (by not patting, lifting, or jiggling the baby, or by reducing auditory stimulation) reduced crying after 7 days in infants under 12 weeks of age compared with an empathetic interview. However, we were unable to draw reliable conclusions from this small study.
- **Soya based infant feeds** One small RCT found that soya based infant feeds reduced the duration of crying in infants with colic compared with standard cows' milk formula. However, we were unable to draw reliable conclusions from this small study.
- **Spinal manipulation** Two RCTs found insufficient evidence about the effects of spinal manipulation.
- **Sucrose solution** One small crossover RCT found limited evidence that sucrose solution improved symptoms of colic as rated by parents after 12 days compared with placebo. However, we were unable to draw reliable conclusions from this small study.
- **Increased carrying** One RCT found no significant difference in daily crying time between carrying the infant, even when not crying, for at least an additional 3 hours a day and a general advice group (to carry, check baby's nappy, feed, offer pacifier, place baby near mother, or use background stimulation such as music). The "advice to carry" group carried their babies for 4.5 hours daily compared with 2.6 hours daily in the general advice group.
- **Simethicone (activated dimeticone)** One RCT found no significant difference between simethicone (activated dimeticone) and placebo in colic rated by carers. Another RCT found no significant difference between simethicone and placebo in improvement as rated by parental interview, 24 hour diary, or behavioural observation. Another poor quality RCT found that simethicone reduced the number of crying attacks on days 4–7 of treatment compared with placebo.

DEFINITION Infantile colic is defined as excessive crying in an otherwise healthy baby. The crying typically starts in the first few weeks of life and ends by 4–5 months. Excessive crying is defined as crying that lasts at least 3 hours a day, for 3 days a week, for at least 3 weeks.[1] Due to the natural course of infantile colic it can be difficult to interpret trials which do not include a placebo or no treatment group for comparison.

INCIDENCE/ PREVALENCE Infantile colic causes 1/6 (17%) families to consult a health professional. One systematic review of 15 community based studies found a wide variation in prevalence, which depended on study design and method of recording.[2] Two prospective studies identified by the review yielded prevalence rates of 5% and 19%.[2] One RCT (89 breast and formula fed infants) found that, at 2 weeks of age, the prevalence of crying more than 3 hours a day was 43% among formula fed infants and 16% among breastfed infants. The prevalence at 6 weeks was 12% (formula fed) and 31% (breast fed).[3]

AETIOLOGY/ RISK FACTORS The cause of infantile colic is unclear and, despite its name, might not have an abdominal cause. It may reflect part of the normal distribution of infantile crying. Other possible explanations are painful intestinal contractions, lactose intolerance, gas, or parental misinterpretation of normal crying.[1]

PROGNOSIS Infantile colic improves with time. One study found that 29% of infants aged 1–3 months cried for more than 3 hours a day, but by 4–6 months of age the prevalence had fallen to 7–11%.[4]

AIMS OF INTERVENTION To reduce infant crying and distress, and the anxiety of the family, with minimal adverse effects of treatment.

OUTCOMES Duration of crying or colic, as measured on dichotomous, ordinal, or continuous scales; parents' perceptions of severity (recorded in a diary).

METHODS *Clinical Evidence* search and appraisal January 2003. The contributors also searched Cinahl up to 1999 for publications using reduction in crying or colic as the main outcome. Trials were excluded for the following reasons: infants studied had normal crying patterns, infants were older than 6 months, interventions lasted less than 3 days, trials had no control groups, or had low scores on the Jadad Scale (see glossary, p 416).[5]

QUESTION What are the effects of treatments for infantile colic?

OPTION DICYCLOVERINE

Two systematic reviews of RCTs of variable quality found limited evidence that dicycloverine reduced crying in infants with colic compared with placebo. RCTs found that dicycloverine increased drowsiness, constipation, and loose stools compared with placebo, but the difference did not reach significance. Case reports of harms in infants have included breathing difficulties, seizures, syncope, asphyxia, muscular hypotonia, and coma.

Benefits: We found two systematic reviews.[1,6] The first systematic review (search date 1996)[1] identified five RCTs (134 infants) comparing the effect of dicycloverine (dicyclomine) (see glossary, p 415) versus placebo on crying or the presence of colic. It found that dicycloverine (most frequently 5 mg 4 times daily) significantly reduced crying compared with placebo (5 RCTs; effect size 0.46, 95% CI 0.33 to 0.60).[1] The clinical importance of this result is unclear (see comment below).[6] The second systematic review (search date 1999)[6] identified three RCTs included in the first systematic review,[1] but did not pool results. One RCT[7] identified by the review found that, compared with placebo (cherry syrup), dicycloverine significantly reduced colic (elimination of colic: 63% with dicycloverine *v* 25% with placebo; RR 0.50, 95% CI 0.28 to 0.88; NNT 3, CI not provided).[6] The other two RCTs identified by the review used definitions of colic that included symptoms but not duration and frequency, and reported results in terms of clinical scores.[6] The review reported that both RCTs found significantly better mean clinical scores with dicycloverine than with placebo (P values not stated).

Harms: Two of five RCTs[8,9] in the systematic reviews[1,6] assessed harms of dicycloverine compared with placebo. The first RCT (crossover design, 30 infants) found more drowsiness with dicycloverine compared with placebo (4/30 [13%] with dicycloverine *v* 1/30 [3%] with placebo; ARI +10%, 95% CI –4% to +24%).[8] The second RCT (crossover design, 25 infants) found more loose stools or constipation in infants taking dicycloverine compared with placebo (3/25 [12%] with dicycloverine *v* 1/25 [4%] with placebo; ARI +8%, 95% CI –7% to +23%).[9] Case reports of harms in infants have included breathing difficulties, seizures, syncope, asphyxia, muscular hypotonia, and coma.[10]

Comment: The first review is limited because it pooled different outcome measures from RCTs and included crossover studies.[1] The crossover design is unlikely to provide valid evidence because infantile colic has a naturally variable course, and the effects of dicycloverine may continue even after a washout period.[11] Only one RCT identified by the reviews stated measures to make the control syrup taste the same as the drug syrup.[8]

OPTION SIMETHICONE (ACTIVATED DIMETICONE)

One RCT found no significant difference between simethicone (activated dimeticone) and placebo in colic rated by carers. Another RCT found no significant difference between simethicone and placebo in improvement as rated by parental interview, 24 hour diary, or behavioural observation. Another, poor quality RCT found that simethicone reduced the number of crying attacks on days 4–7 of treatment compared with placebo.

Benefits: We found two systematic reviews (search dates 1996,[1] 1999,[6] same 3 RCTs in each review, 136 infants) comparing the effect of simethicone (see glossary, p 416) versus placebo on the duration of crying or the presence of colic. The first RCT identified by the reviews (double blind, crossover, 83 infants aged 2–8 weeks) compared 0.3 mL of simethicone versus placebo before feeds.[12] It found no significant difference in colic when rated by carers (28% improved with simethicone *v* 37% with placebo *v* 20% with both; effect size for simethicone versus placebo –0.10, 95% CI –0.27 to +0.08).[1,12] The second RCT identified by the reviews (double blind, crossover trial, 27 infants aged 2–8 weeks) found no significant difference between simethicone and placebo in improvement as rated by parental interview, 24 hour diary, or behavioural observation (effect size +0.06, 95% CI −0.17 to +0.28).[1,13] The third poor quality RCT identified by the reviews (26 infants aged 1–12 weeks) reported no details on how cases of colic were defined.[14] It found that simethicone significantly reduced the number of crying attacks on days 4–7 of treatment compared with placebo (effect size 0.54, 95% CI 0.21 to 0.87).[1,14]

Harms: None of the RCTs reported adverse effects with either simethicone or placebo.[12–14]

Comment: The crossover design of two of the RCTs limits their validity and clinical utility because infantile colic has a naturally variable course, and the effects of simethicone may continue even after a washout period.[12,13]

OPTION REPLACEMENT OF COWS' MILK WITH SOYA BASED INFANT FEEDS

One small RCT found that soya based infant feeds reduced the duration of crying in infants with colic compared with standard cows' milk formula.

Benefits: We found two systematic reviews (search dates 1996[1] and 1999,[6] 2 RCTs). One RCT (19 infants) found that soya based infant feeds (see glossary, p 416) significantly reduced the duration of crying compared with standard cows' milk formula (4.3–12.7 hours with soya based infant feeds *v* 17.3–20.1 hours with cows' milk; mean difference −10.3 hours, 95% CI −16.2 hours to −4.3 hours).[15] The other RCT provided insufficient evidence as it considered infants admitted to hospital for colic and used weak methods (Jadad [see glossary, p 416] score 1).[16]

Harms: None reported in the RCTs.[15,16]

Comment: In the first RCT, mothers were not told which milk the babies received, but differences between the milks may have been detected from smell and texture.[15] We were unable to draw reliable conclusions from the second small RCT.

OPTION REPLACEMENT OF COWS' MILK WITH CASEIN HYDROLYSATE MILK

Two RCTs found insufficient evidence about the effects of replacing cows' milk formula with casein hydrolysate hypoallergenic formula.

Benefits: We found two systematic reviews (search dates 1996[1] and 1999[6]), which identified the same two RCTs.[17,18] The first RCT (double blind, crossover, 17 infants) included in the reviews studied the effect of each of three changes of infant diet over 4 days.[17] Bottle fed infants received casein hydrolysate milk (see glossary, p 415) and cows' milk alternately. By the third change, it found no notable difference in the incidence of colic between groups. A total of 8/17 (47%) infants left the study before completion. The second RCT (122 infants) included in the reviews compared bottle fed infants (38 infants) given casein hydrolysate milk (active diet) versus cows' milk formula and breast fed infants (77 infants) with mothers on a hypoallergenic diet (see glossary, p 415) (active diet) versus controls on an unmodified diet.[18] Fifty four infants received the active diet, but the RCT did not specify which of these were bottle fed and which were breast fed. The RCT pooled the results of breast and bottle fed babies and found that the active diet versus control diet reduced infant distress as measured by parents on a validated chart. The number of bottle fed infants was too small to establish or exclude important effects in infants bottle fed casein hydrolysate milk versus cows' milk.

Harms: None reported in the RCTs.[17,18]

Comment: None.

OPTION REPLACEMENT OF COWS' MILK FORMULA BY WHEY HYDROLYSATE FORMULA

One RCT found limited evidence that replacing cows' milk formula with whey hydrolysate formula reduced crying recorded in a parental diary.

Benefits: We found two systematic reviews (search dates 1996[1] and 1999[6]) and one subsequent RCT.[19] The systematic reviews found no RCTs of adequate quality. The subsequent, double blind RCT (43 infants) found that whey hydrolysate formula (see glossary, p 416) (23 infants) compared with standard cows' milk formula reduced the time that babies cried each day, measured by a validated parental diary (crying reduced by 63 minutes/day, 95% CI 1 minute/day to 127 minutes/day).[19]

Harms: None identified in the subsequent RCT.[19]

Comment: In the subsequent RCT, parents may not have been blind to the intervention. When asked, six indicated that they were aware of allocation, but two of these falsely identified the formula. When these infants' results were removed from the analysis, the crying time with whey hydrolysate formula was significantly reduced compared with standard cows' milk formula (crying reduced by 58 minutes/day; $P = 0.03$).[19]

OPTION LOW LACTOSE (LACTASE TREATED) MILK

Four small crossover RCTs found insufficient evidence on the effects of low lactose (lactase treated) milk in infants with colic.

Benefits: We found two systematic reviews (search dates 1996[1] and 1999,[6] 2 RCTs) and two additional RCTs.[20,21] The first RCT included in the reviews (double blind, crossover, 10 weaned infants) compared four interventions: bottle feeding using pooled breast milk; low lactose (lactase treated) breast milk; cows' milk; and low lactose (lactase treated) cows' milk.[22] It found no evidence that low lactose milk reduced the timing, severity, or duration of colic recorded by parents (days with colic: lactose containing milks *v* lactase treated milks, $P > 0.05$; duration and severity of colic: lactose containing milks *v* lactase treated milk, $P > 0.05$).[22] The second RCT (12 breast fed infants) included in the reviews compared low lactose versus placebo drops given within 5 minutes of feeding.[6] It found no significant difference in time spent feeding, sleeping, or crying. The first additional RCT (crossover, 13 infants) compared low lactose milk versus placebo treated milk.[20] It found a significant reduction in crying time with low lactose milk (1.1 hours/day, 95% CI 0.2 hours/day to 2.1 hours/day); however, caution should be applied interpreting the results because of the small number of infants in the trial and the crossover design (see comments below). The second additional RCT (crossover, 53 infants) found that low lactose formula/breast milk reduced cry time after crossover at 25 days compared with untreated formula/breast milk, but the difference was not significant (median 11.0 hours with lactase *v* 14.1 hours with no lactase; median difference in crying time 23%; P = 0.09).[21]

Harms: None reported in the RCTs.[1,6,20,21]

Comment: It is difficult to make firm conclusions from these RCTs.[1,6,20,21] The babies were not selected on the basis of confirmed lactose intolerance. The crossover design of three of the RCTs limits their validity and clinical utility because infantile colic has a naturally variable course.[20–22]

OPTION SUCROSE SOLUTION

One small crossover RCT found limited evidence that sucrose solution increased parent rated improvement in symptoms of infantile colic after 12 days compared with placebo.

Benefits: We found one systematic review (search date 1999,[6] 1 RCT[23]). The small crossover RCT (19 infants) included in the review compared 2 mL of 12% sucrose solution versus placebo given to babies when they continued to cry despite comforting.[23] Parents, blind to the intervention, scored the effect of the treatment on a scale of 1–5. Treatments were crossed over after 3–4 days and again after 6–8 days. The RCT found that sucrose significantly increased parent rated improvement after 12 days compared with placebo (12/19 [63%] with sucrose *v* 1/19 [5%] with placebo; ARI 58%, 95% CI 10% to 89%; NNT 2, 95% CI 1 to 10; RR 12, 95% CI 3 to 19).[23]

Harms: None reported in the RCT.[23]

Comment: We were unable to draw reliable conclusions from this small study.

OPTION HERBAL TEA

One small RCT found that herbal tea (containing extracts of chamomile, vervain, licorice, fennel, and balm mint in a sucrose solution) improved symptoms of colic rated by parents at 7 days compared with sucrose solution alone.

Benefits: We found two systematic reviews (search dates 1996[1] and 1999,[6] 1 RCT[24]). The RCT included in the reviews compared herbal tea (containing extracts of chamomile, vervain, licorice, fennel, and balm mint in a sucrose solution) (33 infants) versus sucrose solution alone (35 infants) given by parents up to three times daily in response to episodes of colic.[24] Coding was only known to the pharmacist and the taste and smell of the tea and placebo were similar. Parents rated the response using a symptom diary. The RCT found that, at 7 days, herbal tea eliminated colic significantly more frequently than sucrose solution (number of infants colic free: 19/33 [58%] with herbal tea *v* 9/35 [26%] with sucrose; ARI 32%, 95% CI 7% to 53%; RR 2.2, 95% CI 1.3 to 3.1; NNT 3, 95% CI 2 to 14).

Harms: None reported in the RCT.[24]

Comment: The RCT did not state the exact proportion of the herbs used in the preparation.[24] We were unable to draw reliable conclusions from this small study.

OPTION BEHAVIOURAL MODIFICATION

One RCT comparing counselling mothers about specific management techniques (responding to crying with gentle soothing motion, avoiding over stimulation, using a pacifier, and prophylactic carrying) plus non-specific reassurance, a car ride simulation device plus non-specific reassurance, and non-specific reassurance alone, found no significant difference among groups in maternal anxiety or hours of infant crying over 2 weeks. Another small RCT found that focused counselling decreased duration and extent of crying compared with substitution of soya or cows' milk with casein hydrolysate formula. One RCT found limited evidence that advice to reduce stimulation (by not patting, lifting, or jiggling the baby, or by reducing auditory stimulation) reduced crying after 7 days in infants under 12 weeks compared with an empathetic interview. One RCT found no significant difference in daily crying time between carrying the infant, even when not crying, for at least an additional 3 hours a day and a general advice group (to carry, check baby's nappy, feed, offer pacifier, place baby near mother, or use background stimulation such as music).

Benefits: We found two systematic reviews (search dates 1996[1] and 1999,[6] 4 RCTs). **Focused counselling plus non-specific reassurance or car ride simulation device plus non-specific reassurance or non-specific reassurance alone:** One RCT (38 infants) assessed maternal anxiety and the hours of crying each day by questionnaire.[25] The RCT compared three interventions: counselling mothers about specific management techniques (responding to crying with gentle soothing motion, avoiding over stimulation, using a pacifier, and prophylactic carrying) plus non-specific reassurance (see glossary, p 416) and support; car ride simulation device plus non-specific reassurance and support; and non-specific reassurance and support alone. It found no significant difference among groups in maternal anxiety or hours of infant crying over 2 weeks (mean hours of crying: results presented graphically, P value not provided; mean maternal anxiety score: results presented graphically, P value not provided).[25] **Focused counselling versus elimination of cows' milk protein:** One RCT (20 infants) found that counselling parents to respond to their baby's cries by feeding, holding, offering a pacifier, stimulating, or putting the baby down to sleep, decreased duration and extent of crying significantly more than substitution of soya or cows' milk with casein hydrolysate formula (mean decrease in crying, recorded by parent diary, 2.1 hours/day with counselling *v* 1.2 hours/day with dietary change;

P = 0.05).[26] **Increased carrying versus general advice:** One RCT (66 infants) randomised mothers of babies with colic to carry their infant, even when not crying, for at least an additional 3 hours a day or to a general advice group (to carry, check baby's nappy, feed, offer pacifier, place baby near mother, or use background stimulation such as music).[27] The "advice to carry" group carried their babies for 4.5 hours daily compared with 2.6 hours daily in the general advice group. The RCT found no significant difference in daily crying time (mean difference 3 minutes less, 95% CI 37 minutes less to 32 minutes more).[27] **Reducing stimulation versus non-specific interview:** One RCT (42 infants, median age 10 weeks) allocated mothers of infants to advice to reduce stimulation (mothers were advised to reduce stimulation by not patting, lifting, or jiggling the baby, or reducing auditory stimulation) or to an empathetic interview.[28] For infants under 12 weeks, advice to reduce stimulation significantly improved a change rating scale for more infants compared with no advice (after 7 days: 14/15 [93%] improved with advice *v* 6/12 [50%] with control; ARI 43%, 95% CI 8% to 49%; RR 1.9, 95% CI 1.2 to 2.0; NNT 2, 95% CI 2 to 13).[28] Improvement in the change rating scale was defined as a score of +2 or better on a scale from –5 to +5 that indicated a perceived change in crying since the start of the trial. It is unclear whether this scale has been validated (see comment below).

Harms: None reported in the RCTs identified by the reviews.[1,6]

Comment: Behavioural modification involves interventions to change the way in which parents respond to their babies crying from colic. Mothers given advice to reduce stimulation were also given permission to leave their infants if they felt they could no longer tolerate the crying. It is unclear whether the improved change score represents a true change in the hours that the baby cried, or altered maternal perception.

OPTION CRANIAL OSTEOPATHY

We found no RCTs on the effects of cranial osteopathy in infants with colic.

Benefits: We found no systematic review and no RCTs on the effects of cranial osteopathy (see glossary, p 415) in infants with colic.

Harms: We found no RCTs.

Comment: None.

OPTION INFANT MASSAGE

One RCT found no significant difference between massage and a crib vibrator for colic related crying or parental rating of symptoms of infantile colic, but it may have lacked power to detect a clinically important difference.

Benefits: We found no systematic review. **Versus usual care:** We found no RCTs. **Versus other care:** We found one RCT (58 infants, 47% with colic; see comment below) comparing massage versus a crib vibrator over a 4 week period.[29] Infant massage (performed 3 times daily) included gentle stroking of the skin over different parts of the head, body, and limbs, using olive oil and while maintaining eye contact. The crib vibrator was used for 25 minute periods at least three times daily (see comment below). Colic symptom ratings were obtained from parental diaries of crying. The RCT found no significant difference between massage and a crib vibrator for colic related crying or parental rating of symptoms (AR for less colicky crying: 64% with massage *v* 52% with crib vibrator; P = 0.24).[29]

Harms: None reported in the RCT.[29]

Comment: Only 47% of infants in the RCT had colic, so the results may not apply to infants with colic.[29] The RCT stated that "use of a crib vibrator was chosen for control intervention or placebo treatment because it had been ineffective in a previous study".[29] It is unclear whether reduced crying in this RCT reflects the natural course of infantile colic or the specific effect of interventions.[29] The RCT may have lacked power to detect clinically important effects.

OPTION SPINAL MANIPULATION

Two RCTs found insufficient evidence about the effects of spinal manipulation.

Benefits: We found no systematic review. We found two RCTs that considered the effects of spinal manipulation (see glossary, p 416).[30,31] **Versus simethicone (activated dimeticone [dimethicone]):** One RCT (41 infants) compared 2 weeks of spinal manipulation versus 2 weeks of daily treatment with simethicone (see glossary, p 416); parents recorded length of crying in a colic diary. It found that spinal manipulation significantly reduced crying compared with simethicone (mean reduction in crying for days 4–7: 2.4 hours with spinal manipulation *v* 1.0 hours with simethicone; P = 0.04).[30] Parents were not blinded to treatment. **Versus holding:** One RCT (86 infants) compared spinal palpation by a chiropractor versus holding of the infant by a nurse (3 times over 8 days).[31] The parents, who were blind to the intervention, rated symptom severity on a five point scale and recorded crying in a diary. The RCT found no significant difference between spinal palpation and holding for crying reduction (by day 8, mean reduction 3.1 hours for both groups; P = 0.98).

Harms: None reported in the RCTs.[30,31]

Comment: It is unclear whether reduced crying reflected effects of interventions or spontaneous improvement.

GLOSSARY

Casein hydrolysate milk Contains casein protein; it is used in the same way as soya based infant feeds.

Cranial osteopathy Involves gentle manipulation of the tissues of the head by an osteopath.

Dicycloverine (dicyclomine) This has direct antispasmodic action on the gastrointestinal tract and anticholinergic effects, which are similar to atropine.

Hypoallergenic diet In bottle fed infants, a hypoallergenic diet uses a casein hydrolysate formula. In breast fed infants, a hypoallergenic diet involves a maternal diet, free of artificial colourings, preservatives, and additives, and low in common allergens (e.g. milk, egg, wheat, and nuts).

Jadad Scale This measures factors that impact on trial quality. Poor description of the factors, rated by low figures, are associated with greater estimates of effect. The scale includes three items: was the study described as randomised? (0–2); was the study described as double blind? (0–2); was there a description of withdrawals and drop outs? (0–1).[5]

Reassurance Informing the parent that infantile colic is a self limiting condition resolving by 3–4 months of age, and is not caused by disease or any fault in parental care.

Simethicone (activated dimeticone [dimethicone]) It has defoaming properties, which can aid dispersion of gas in the gastrointestinal tract.

Soya based infant feeds Contain proteins from soya beans; the feeds are used as lactose free vegetable milks for those with lactose or cows' milk protein intolerance.

Spinal manipulation Chiropractic manual treatment of the infant's vertebral column.

Whey hydrolysate milk Contains whey protein; it is used in the same way as soya based infant feeds.

REFERENCES

1. Lucassen, PLBJ, Assendelft WJJ, Gubbels JW, et al. Effectiveness of treatments for infantile colic: a systematic review. *BMJ* 1998;316:1563–1569. Search date 1996: primary sources Cochrane Controlled Trials Register, Embase, Medline, and hand searches of reference lists.
2. Lucassen PLBJ, Assendelft WJJ, Van Eijk JTHM, et al. Systematic review of the occurrence of infantile colic in the community. *Arch Dis Child* 2001;84:398–403. Search date 1998; primary sources Embase and Medline.
3. Lucas A, St James-Roberts I. Crying, fussing and colic behaviour in breast and bottle-fed infants. *Early Hum Dev* 1998;53:9–19.
4. St James-Roberts I, Halil A. Infant crying patterns in the first year: normal community and clinical findings. *J Child Psychol Psychiatry* 1991;32:951–968.
5. Jadad AR, Moore RA, Carroll D, et al. Assessing the quality of reports of randomized clinical trials: is blinding necessary? *Control Clin Trials* 1996;17:1–12.
6. Garrison MM, Christakis DA. A systematic review of treatments for infant colic. *Pediatrics* 2000;106:184–190. Search date 1999; primary sources Medline, Cochrane Clinical Trials Registry, hand searches of reference lists, and authors.
7. Weissbluth M, Christoffel KK, Davis AT. Treatment of infantile colic with dicyclomine hydrochloride. *J Pediatr* 1984:104:951–955.
8. Hwang CP, Danielsson B. Dicyclomine hydrochloride in infantile colic. *BMJ* 1985;291:1014.
9. Gruinseit F. Evaluation of the efficacy of dicyclomine hydrochloride ("Merbentyl") syrup in the treatment of infantile colic. *Curr Med Res Opin* 1977;5:258–261.
10. Williams J, Watkin Jones R. Dicyclomine: worrying symptoms associated with its use in some small babies. *BMJ* 1984;288:901.
11. Fleiss JL. The crossover study. In: Fleiss JL, ed. *The design and analysis of clinical experiments.* New York: Wiley and Sons, 1986.
12. Metcalf TJ, Irons TG, Sher LD, et al. Simethicone in the treatment of infantile colic: a randomized, placebo-controlled, multicenter trial. *Pediatrics* 1994;94:29–34.
13. Danielsson B, Hwang CP. Treatment of infantile colic with surface active substance (simethicone). *Acta Paediatr Scand* 1985;74:446–450.
14. Sethi KS, Sethi JK. Simethicone in the management of infant colic. *Practitioner* 1988;232:508.
15. Campbell JPM. Dietary treatment of infantile colic: a double-blind study. *J R Coll Gen Pract* 1989;39:11–14.
16. Lothe L, Lindbert T, Jakobsson I. Cow's milk formula as a cause of infantile colic: a double-blind study. *Pediatrics* 1982;70:7–10.
17. Forsythe BWC. Colic and the effect of changing formulas: a double blind, multiple-crossover study. *J Pediatr* 1989;115:521–526.
18. Hill DJ, Hudson IL, Sheffield LJ, et al. A low allergen diet is a significant intervention in infantile colic: results of a community based study. *J Allergy Clin Immunol* 1995;96:886–892.
19. Lucassen PLBJ, Assendelft WJJ, Gubbels LW, et al. Infantile colic: crying time reduction with a whey hydrolysate; a double blind, randomized placebo-controlled trial. *Pediatrics* 2000;106:1349–1354.
20. Kearney PJ, Malone AJ, Hayes T, et al. A trial of lactase in the management of infant colic. *J Hum Nutr Diet* 1998;11:281–285.
21. Kanabar D, Randhawa M, Clayton P. Improvement of symptoms of infant colic following reduction of lactose load with lactase. *J Hum Nutr Diet* 2001,14;359–363.
22. Stahlberg MR, Savilahti E. Infantile colic and feeding. *Arch Dis Child* 1986;61:1232–1233.
23. Markestad T. Use of sucrose as a treatment for infant colic. *Arch Dis Child* 1997;77:356–357.
24. Weizman Z, Alkrinawi S, Goldfarb D, et al. Herbal teas for infantile colic. *J Pediatr* 1993;123:670–671.
25. Parkin PC, Schwartz CJ, Manuel BA. Randomised controlled trial of three interventions in the management of persistent crying of infancy. *Pediatrics* 1993;92;197–201.

26. Taubman B. Parental counselling compared with elimination of cow's milk or soy milk protein for the treatment of infant colic syndrome: a randomized trial. *Pediatrics* 1988;81:756–761.
27. Barr RG, McMullen SJ, Spiess H, et al. Carrying as a colic "therapy": a randomized controlled trial. *Pediatrics* 1991;87:623–630.
28. McKenzie S. Troublesome crying in infants: effect of advice to reduce stimulation. *Arch Dis Child* 1991;66:1461–1420.
29. Huhtala V, Lehtonen L, Heinonen R, et al. Infant massage compared with crib vibrator in the treatment of colicky infants. *Pediatrics* 2000;105:e84.
30. Wiberg JMM, Nordsteen J, Nilsson N. The short term effect of spinal manipulation in the treatment of infant colic: a randomized controlled clinical trial with a blinded observer. *J Manip Physiol Therap* 1999;22:517–522.
31. Olafsdottir E, Forshei S, Fluge G, et al. Randomised controlled trial of infant colic treated with chiropractic spinal manipulation. *Arch Dis Child* 2001;84:138–141.

Teresa Kilgour
Staff Grade Community Paediatrician
City Hospitals Sunderland
Sunderland
UK

Sally Wade
Staff Grade Community Paediatrician
Archer Street Clinic
Darlington
UK

Competing interests: None declared.

Measles

Search date December 2002

Bazian Ltd

QUESTIONS

INTERVENTIONS

Beneficial

See glossary, p 426

Key Messages

Live combined measles, mumps, and rubella vaccine; live monovalent measles vaccine

- Large cohort studies, large time series, and population surveillance data from different countries have all found that combined measles, mumps, and rubella (MMR) and live monovalent measles vaccination programmes reduce the risk of measles infection to near zero, especially in populations in which vaccine coverage is high.
- We found no RCTs comparing the effects of MMR versus no vaccination or placebo on measles infection rates. Such trials are likely to be considered unethical because of the large body of whole-population evidence finding benefit from vaccination.
- Unlike live monovalent measles vaccine, MMR additionally protects against mumps and rubella, which themselves cause serious complications (mumps causes orchitis, pancreatitis, infertility, meningoencephalitis, deafness, and congenital fetal abnormalities; rubella causes deafness, blindness, heart defects, liver, spleen and brain damage, and stillbirth).
- One systematic review, one RCT, one large population based survey, and one population based study found no evidence that MMR was associated with acute developmental regression. Large time series studies have consistently found no evidence that MMR or live monovalent measles vaccine was associated with autism.
- One large, long term population surveillance study and one population based case control study found no evidence that either MMR or monovalent measles vaccine was associated with inflammatory bowel disease. One large cohort study and two population based case control studies found no association between monovalent measles vaccine and inflammatory bowel disease.
- One systematic review and one additional RCT found that MMR and monovalent measles vaccine were associated with a small and similar risk of self limiting fever within 3 weeks of vaccination compared with 100% risk of acute fever in people with measles.

DEFINITION Measles is an infectious disease caused by a ribonucleic acid paramyxovirus. The illness is characterised by an incubation period of 10–12 days; a prodromal period of 2–4 days with upper respiratory tract symptoms; Koplik's spots on mucosal membranes and high fever; followed by continuing fever, and a widespread maculopapular rash that persists for 5–6 days.[1]

INCIDENCE/ PREVALENCE Measles incidence varies according to vaccination coverage. Worldwide, there are an estimated 30 million cases of measles each year,[2] but an incidence of only 0–10/100 000 people in countries with widespread vaccination programmes such as the USA, UK, Mexico, India, China, Brazil, and Australia.[3] In the USA, before licensing of effective vaccines, more than 90% of people were infected by the age of 15 years. After licensing in 1963, incidence fell by about 98%.[1] Mean annual incidence in Finland was 366/100 000 in 1970,[4] but declined to about zero by the late 1990s.[5] Similarly, annual incidence declined to about zero in Chile, the English speaking Caribbean, and Cuba during the 1990s when vaccination programmes were introduced.[6,7]

AETIOLOGY/ RISK FACTORS Measles is highly contagious. The virus is spread through airborne droplets that persist for up to 2 hours in closed areas. As with other infectious diseases, risk factors include overcrowding, low herd immunity (see glossary, p 426), and immunosuppression. People with immunosuppression, children younger than 5 years of age, and adults older than 20 years of age have a higher risk of severe complications and death, although these also occur in healthy people (see prognosis below).[1] Newborn babies have a lower risk of measles than older infants, owing to protective maternal antibodies, although in recent US outbreaks, maternal antibody protection was lower than expected.[1]

PROGNOSIS The World Health Organization estimated that in the year 2000, measles caused 777 000 deaths and 27.5 million disability adjusted life years.[8] **Disease in healthy people:** In developed countries, most prognostic data come from the pre-vaccination era and from subsequent outbreaks in non-vaccinated populations. In the USA, about 30% of reported measles cases involve complications of the disease. From 1989–1991 in the USA, measles resurgence among young children (< 5 years) who had not been immunised led to 55 622 cases with more than 11 000 hospital admissions and 125 deaths.[1] Measles complications include diarrhoea (8%), otitis media (7%), pneumonia (6%), death (0.1–0.2%), acute encephalitis (about 0.1% followed by death in 15% and permanent neurological damage in about 25%), seizures (with or without fever in 0.6–0.7%), idiopathic thrombocytopenia (1/6000 reported cases), and subacute sclerosing panencephalitis causing degeneration of the central nervous system and death 7 years after measles infection (range 1 month to 27 years; 0.5–1.0/100 000 reported cases).[1,9] Measles during pregnancy results in higher risk of premature labour, spontaneous abortion, and low birth weight infants. An association with birth defects remains uncertain.[1] **Disease in malnourished or immunocompromised people:** In malnourished or immunocompromised people, particularly those with vitamin A deficiency, measles case fatality can be as high as 25%. Worldwide, measles is a major cause of blindness and causes 5% of deaths in young children (< 5 years).[1,10]

AIMS OF INTERVENTION Preventing measles with minimum adverse effects.

OUTCOMES **Prevention, benefits:** Clinically apparent measles and measles related complications, including death. We have included a proxy outcome (seroconversion [see glossary, p 427]) because it is so highly correlated with vaccine efficacy.[11] **Prevention, harms:** Acute fever, febrile seizures, inflammatory bowel disease, developmental regression, autism, and clinical measles after seroconversion.

METHODS *Clinical Evidence* search and appraisal December 2002. The authors also searched World Health Organization, US Communicable Disease Control, and UK Public Health Laboratory Service websites, and hand searches of national and international policy documents. In the benefits section, we have included RCTs and stronger observational studies, given that RCTs have long been considered unethical for assessing the clinical efficacy of measles vaccines (see benefits, p 420). In the harms section, we have included RCTs and robust observational studies (see harms, p 422). In the comment section, we have included weaker studies (see comment, p 426). Unless otherwise specified, we have included only those studies of the combined measles, mumps, and rubella vaccine (see glossary, p 426) that used the Schwarz strain of the measles virus and only those studies of the monovalent measles vaccine (see glossary, p 426) that considered live attenuated strains of the virus, because of the relatively poor efficacy of killed-strain measles vaccines.

QUESTION **What are the effects of interventions to prevent measles infection?**

OPTION **MEASLES VACCINATION**

We found no RCTs comparing measles infection rates after the combined measles, mumps, and rubella vaccine versus placebo or versus monovalent vaccine alone. We found strong evidence from national population surveillance that combined measles, mumps, and rubella vacinnation and monovalent measles vaccination virtually eliminate risk of measles and measles complications. We found no evidence that measles, mumps, and rubella or live monovalent measles vaccines are associated with autism or inflammatory bowel disease. We found consistent evidence from RCTs and cohort studies that measles, mumps, and rubella and live monovalent measles vaccines are associated with small, similar risks of self limiting fever within 3 weeks of vaccination. Measles causes acute fever in 100% of infected children.

Benefits: **Monovalent measles vaccine or combined measles, mumps, and rubella (MMR) vaccine versus placebo or no vaccine: measles** See glossary, p 427. We found two early RCTs of monovalent measles vaccine versus placebo or no vaccine in the UK[12] and USA.[13] Both found efficacy rates of 95% or greater for vaccines using live attenuated Schwarz[12] and Edmonston[13] strains of the measles virus (Schwarz RCT: 9538 children received live vaccine, 16 239 unvaccinated; Edmonston RCT: 1308 live vaccine, 1271 placebo). We found no RCTs comparing the clinical effects of MMR versus no vaccine or placebo. Such studies are considered unethical because of previous evidence of the efficacy of measles vaccine and harms of measles infection. One large, retrospective cohort study of the entire US population from 1985–1992 compared measles infection rates in children who were vaccinated versus children whose parents had declined vaccination (17 390 cases from a vaccinated population of 51 264 140 to 52 377 192 from 1985–1992; 2827 cases from an unvaccinated population of 234 040 to 245 887 from 1985–1992).[14] The study did not state what proportion of vaccinated children received monovalent versus MMR vaccine, although MMR was already widely used in the USA by 1985. The study found that although overall measles incidence was low because of herd immunity (see glossary, p 426), vaccination reduced measles infection compared with no vaccination (RR unvaccinated *v* vaccinated 4–170, depending on age group and year of survey). One large, prospective cohort study followed up 9274 children who had been enrolled in a placebo controlled trial of live monovalent measles vaccine (see glossary, p 426) in 1964 (36 530 children aged 10 months to 2 years; Schwarz strain vaccine).[15] The cohort study found that by 1990, over a period of 15 years (12–27 years after the trial) and after controlling for subsequent vaccination in initial placebo groups, but not controlling for growing herd immunity after mass vaccination, measles incidence was higher in the unvaccinated group (AR 0.3/1000 person years with vaccine *v* 1/1000 person years with no vaccine; $P < 0.001$). **Monovalent measles vaccine or combined MMR vaccine versus placebo or no vaccine: seroconversion** We found two RCTs comparing seroconversion (see glossary, p 427) rates of MMR versus placebo.[16,17] The first compared MMR versus placebo in 282 previously non-immune children (92% of whom were ≤ 1 year old). At 8 weeks, almost all children receiving MMR seroconverted for measles, whereas none of the children receiving placebo seroconverted (measles seroconversion rate 99–100% with MMR, depending on vaccine batch used).[16] The second trial examined the MMR vaccine and seroconversion in 1481 children (1232 MMR, 249 placebo), of whom 446 in the vaccine group were naïve to measles, mumps, and rubella.[17] In this subgroup, seroconversion rates at 8 weeks approached 100%, whereas none of the previously non-immune placebo group seroconverted for measles. **Monovalent measles vaccine or combined MMR vaccine versus placebo or no vaccine: mortality** One systematic review (search date not stated, 10 cohort studies, 2 case control)[18] and one subsequent cohort study[19] examined effects of live monovalent measles vaccination on mortality. The review found that live, standard titre monovalent measles vaccination in seven developing countries reduced all-cause mortality by 30–80%, depending on follow up period and country.[18] The more recent study compared a group of children in Bangladesh vaccinated with live, Schwarz strain monovalent measles vaccine versus age matched, unvaccinated children (8135 matched pairs).[19] It found similar results (16 270 children aged 9–60 months; RR for death at 3 years' follow up vaccinated *v* unvaccinated 0.54, 95% CI 0.45 to 0.65). **Monovalent measles vaccine or combined MMR vaccine versus placebo or no vaccine: measles** We found many population based studies from different countries with different health care systems and different socioeconomic and demographic distributions. These studies have consistently found measles vaccination coverage to be associated with a steep decline in measles. One time series from the World Health Organization found a global decline in reported measles incidence (which underestimates true incidence) from about 4 500 000 a year in 1980 to about 1 000 000 a year in 2000.[20] The decline was associated with the rise in reported measles vaccination coverage from about 10% in 1980 to about 80% in 2000. One population based time series of measles incidence from Finland found that in a population of about 5 million people after the introduction of a live monovalent vaccination programme (1975–1981), the number of new measles cases each year fell from an average of 2074 cases in 1977–1981 to 44 cases in 1985. New cases declined to about zero by the mid-1990s. Shortly after introducing the MMR programme in Finland in 1982, rubella and mumps incidence also fell to about zero.[4] One cross-sectional study in a Brazilian city, which was repeated before and after a measles vaccination campaign in 1987 (8163 people, strain not stated) found that reported measles incidence fell from 222/100 000 in 1987 to 2.7/100 000 in 1988.[21] **MMR versus monovalent measles vaccine: measles** We found no RCTs comparing clinical effects of MMR versus monovalent vaccine in children of the same age. We found one RCT that compared live Schwarz strain monovalent measles vaccine given at 9 months of age followed by MMR at 15 months (442 children) versus MMR only (no prior vaccination) at 12 months (495 children).[22] Prevaccination measles seropositivity was higher in the younger, monovalent vaccine group, perhaps because of maternal antibody persistence (pre-vaccine, 8.1% seropositive in monovalent group *v* 1.4% in MMR group; $P < 0.0001$). After 60 months' follow up, measles infection rates were higher with monovalent vaccination followed by MMR compared with MMR alone (AR for infection 2.7% with monovalent plus MMR *v* 0% with MMR; ARR 2.7%; CI not stated; $P < 0.0001$); however, effects may be confounded by the different timing of the vaccinations. **MMR versus monovalent measles vaccine: seroconversion** We found two RCTs comparing measles seroconversion rates after live MMR versus Schwarz strain monovalent measles vaccine. The first trial (420 children with no clinical history of measles or mumps, mean age about 15 months) found similar seroconversion rates in both groups after 6 weeks (96.8% with monovalent measles *v* 92.6% with MMR).[23] The second RCT (319 children, mean age 13 months) also found similar seroconversion rates in both groups at 6 weeks (92% with Schwarz strain monovalent measles vaccine *v* 93% with MMR).[24]

Harms: **Acute fever and febrile convulsions:** We found one systematic review[25] and four RCTs[22–24,26] reporting fever due to vaccination in otherwise healthy children. Results should be interpreted in light of the 100% prevalence of acute fever in children with measles infection. The systematic review (search date 1998) reported that up to 5% of non-immune people develop moderate to high fever (≥ 38.6 °C) within 7–21 days of vaccination.[25] The first RCT (crossover design) compared the acute harms of MMR versus placebo in 1162 homozygous and heterozygous twins (460 children aged 1 year, of whom 1.3% had been previously vaccinated; 702 aged ≥ 2 years, 95% of whom had been previously vaccinated or experienced measles).[26] One member of each twin pair was randomly selected and allocated to MMR vaccination followed 3 weeks later by placebo, or vice versa. The other twin was allocated to the opposite combination. The trial found that among children aged 14–18 months, MMR was more likely to cause fever than placebo within 21 days (AR fever, 12% in MMR group *v* 4% in placebo group; OR for fever ≥ 39.5 °C 2.83, 95% CI 1.47 to 5.45; OR for fever ≥ 38.5 °C 3.28, 95% CI 2.23 to 4.82; OR for fever ≥ 37.5 °C 2.66, 95% CI 1.66 to 3.08). The second and third RCTs, which compared MMR versus Schwarz strain monovalent measles vaccine in infants with no history of measles, found no difference in fever rates between the two groups.[23,24] The fourth RCT compared Schwarz strain monovalent measles vaccine given at 9 months followed by MMR at 15 months versus MMR alone at 12 months.[22] It found similar rates of fever for monovalent measles vaccine and initial MMR, although results may be confounded by the age difference between the two groups (AR for fever 8.7% with monovalent vaccine *v* 11.2% with MMR; P value not provided). One retrospective cohort study in 679 942 children from four US health maintenance organisations found that children who had received MMR were more likely to experience febrile convulsions at 1–2 weeks after MMR than children of the same age who had not been vaccinated, although the estimated increase in absolute risk was small (RR for febrile seizure 8–14 days after vaccination 2.83, 95% CI 1.44 to 5.55; ARI of febrile seizure, estimated by comparison with background seizure risk in all children aged 12–24 months, 0.025%; NNH 4000; CI not provided).[27] However, the study found no increase in risk within the first week or from 2–4 weeks after vaccination (RR for first wk 1.73, 95% CI 0.72 to 4.15; RR for 15–30 days 0.97, 95% CI 0.49 to 1.95). Seven years' follow up of 543 children with febrile convulsions in the initial month of follow up (22 after MMR, 521 who had not been vaccinated) found no difference between MMR versus no vaccination for subsequent seizure. Similarly, among 271 children with febrile convulsion in one of the four participating health maintenance organisations, the study found no evidence that MMR vaccination before seizure increased risk of learning disability or developmental delay compared with no vaccination before seizure (RR after adjusting for age at first febrile seizure 0.56, 95% CI 0.07 to 4.20). We found one study that reported results of population based surveillance of harms of MMR in all 1.8 million people vaccinated over a 14 year period in Finland.[28] Surveillance relied on healthcare personnel to be aware of the surveillance programme and to report adverse events that they felt might be associated with MMR. Throughout the surveillance period, the programme was advertised in seminars, the media, and medical press. Acute reactions were more likely to have been reported than long term effects. The study found that fever was associated with MMR in 277 children (AR 0.02%). Children with fever that was not brought to the attention of health professionals would have escaped detection. Febrile seizure was reported in 52 cases (AR 0.003%), of which 28 cases could have been caused by MMR according to predefined clinical and serological criteria (AR 0.002%). **Developmental regression or autism:** The RCT comparing harms of MMR versus placebo found no evidence that MMR was associated with acute developmental regression (see glossary, p 426).[26] One large retrospective cohort study traced 537 303 children for 7 years (children born in Denmark between January 1991 and December 1998; 2 129 864 person years exposure).[29] The study found no association between MMR vaccination and autistic disorder of any kind (82% of population vaccinated; RR of autistic disorder in vaccinated *v* non-vaccinated children 0.92, 95% CI 0.68 to 1.24; RR of other autistic spectrum disorder in vaccinated *v* non-vaccinated children 0.83; 95% CI 0.65 to 1.07). The study also found no association between autistic spectrum disorder and age at time of vaccination (P = 0.23), time since vaccination (P = 0.42), or calendar date of vaccination (P = 0.06). Results remained unchanged by including children with autistic disorders due to fragile X syndrome, tuberous sclerosis, congenital rubella, or Angelman's syndrome. One previous systematic review of observational studies also found no association between MMR and autism.[30] The review included two large time series. Neither found evidence that MMR is associated with autism, but found that reported incidence of autism has been increasing independently of MMR coverage. The first study examined MMR vaccine coverage (see glossary, p 427) among children aged 14–17 months enrolled in Californian kindergartens (USA) and born between 1980 and 1994, and autism caseloads referred to the state developmental services department over the same period.[31] The study found that MMR coverage at 24 months rose slightly (from 72% in 1980 to 82% in 1994; 14% proportional rise); however, referral rates for new autism cases increased disproportionately in the same period (from 44/100 000 births in 1980 to 208/100 000 live births in 1994; 373% proportional rise). Referral rates to the department may not accurately reflect incidence of autistic syndromes. The second study, which took its data from a national UK general practice registry, found that the risk of autism among boys increased in the period 1988–1993, whereas MMR coverage remained almost constant at about 97% over the same period (AR of first diagnosis of autism aged 2–5 years 0.008%, 95% CI 0.004% to 0.014% for cohort born in 1988 *v* 0.029%, 95% CI 0.020% to 0.043% for cohort born in 1993).[32] A third, population based study identified 498 children diagnosed with autism born in eight health districts in the UK between 1979 and 1998.[33] The study found that the reported incidence of autism increased over this period. However, there was no step increase or change in the rate of increased incidence after the start of the MMR vaccination programme or after MMR coverage levelled off at almost 100%. The long term, population based passive surveillance study from Finland similarly reported no cases of developmental regression in 1.8 million people vaccinated with MMR.[28] It also reported no cases of autism in the long term, although the study may have limited reliability for detecting long term adverse effects. **Inflammatory**

bowel disease: We found one systematic review (search date 1998) of six large observational studies from different developed countries.[25] The review found no evidence of an association between inflammatory bowel disease and MMR or measles vaccines. We found three additional studies.[28,34,35] The first was a retrospective cohort study comparing rates of ulcerative colitis, Crohn's disease, and inflammatory bowel disease (assessed by postal questionnaire) in 7616 people who had received live monovalent measles vaccination versus those who had not received measles vaccination by the age of 5 years (mean age at vaccination 17.6 months, standard deviation 7.4 months). Participants were those available from an original population based cohort of all 16 000 children born in the first week of 1970 in the UK.[34] The study found no difference for risk of ulcerative colitis, Crohn's disease, or inflammatory bowel disease between people (aged 26 years at the time of the study) who had received monovalent measles vaccine and those who had not, whether or not the result was adjusted for sex, socioeconomic status, or crowding (AR for Crohn's disease 0.25% with vaccine *v* 0.31% without, adjusted OR 0.7, 95% CI 0.3 to 1.6; AR for ulcerative colitis 0.16% with vaccine *v* 0.27% without, adjusted OR 0.6, 95% CI 0.2 to 1.6; AR for inflammatory bowel disease 0.41% with vaccine *v* 0.58% without, adjusted OR 0.6, 95% CI 0.3 to 1.2). The second study (the long term, prospective population based passive surveillance study from Finland) reported no cases of inflammatory bowel disease associated with vaccination in 1.8 million people vaccinated with MMR followed up for 14 years.[28] The third was a case control study of 142 people with definite or probable inflammatory bowel disease from members of four US health maintenance organisations (67 people with ulcerative colitis and 75 with Crohn's disease).[35] Cases were identified by computerised search of electronic records and manual abstraction of medical records (from 1958–1989 for 3 organisations and from 1979–1989 for 1; people who were not organisation members between 6 months of age and disease onset were excluded). The study found that people with inflammatory bowel disease were not more likely to have received MMR than people without inflammatory bowel disease taken from the same health maintenance organisation and matched for sex and year of birth (OR for Crohn's disease 0.40, 95% CI 0.08 to 2.00; OR for ulcerative colitis 0.80, 95% CI 0.18 to 3.56; OR for all inflammatory bowel disease 0.59, 95% CI 0.21 to 1.69). The study similarly found no evidence of an association between all measles containing vaccines, Crohn's disease, ulcerative colitis, or all inflammatory bowel disease. **Measles risk after seroconversion:** One systematic review of cohort studies (search date 1995) examined risk of measles infection at least 21 days after vaccine induced seroconversion (monovalent or polyvalent vaccine).[11] It identified 10 studies that met inclusion criteria. In the subset of six cohort studies examining live vaccine, where vaccination status was cross checked against medical records, risk of clinical measles infection in children who had seroconverted after vaccination was about zero (0 infections from 2061 people exposed; CI not provided).

Measles

Comment: **Benefits:** Many case control studies conducted during measles outbreaks have found that live measles vaccination (monovalent or MMR) protects against infection, with protective efficacy of about 95% or higher. Given the evidence for benefit already described, we have not included further details of these studies. In addition, and although not the focus of this topic, it should be noted that the MMR vaccine also protects people from mumps and rubella, which cause serious complications in non-immune people (mumps causes orchitis, pancreatitis, meningoencephalitis, deafness, and congenital fetal abnormalities; congenital rubella infection causes deafness, blindness, heart defect, liver, spleen and brain damage, and stillbirth). **Harms:** In addition to the more reliable evidence described above, we found two case series. The first was a population based series of 473 children with childhood autism or atypical autism (see glossary, p 426) born between 1979 and 1998 and registered in five health districts in London, UK.[36] Of these children, 118 had documented evidence of developmental regression. The study found no trends for risk of developmental regression with respect to year of birth from 1979–1998, although MMR vaccination was introduced in 1988. The study found that MMR vaccination was just as likely to precede or follow documented parental concerns about development, suggesting that the temporal relation of vaccination and onset of developmental problems was not compatible with a causal association (443 children with autism in whom timing of first parental concerns was recorded; 26% vaccinated before parental concern about development *v* 26% vaccinated after parental concerns expressed; P = 0.83). The second series raised the question of a possible relation between MMR and developmental disorder in 12 children with bowel symptoms.[37] The series was retrospective (parents surveyed up to 8 years after vaccination), small, lacked a control group, and was selective in its sample. For these reasons, we found that the study does not establish MMR as a cause of inflammatory bowel disease, autism, or developmental regression, and that its hypothesis has been satisfactorily tested by scientifically reliable studies (see harms above).

GLOSSARY

Acute developmental regression Rapid loss of acquired developmental skills.

Atypical autism Atypical autism shares clinical features with autism but does not meet ICD-10 or DSM-IV diagnostic criteria.

Childhood autism ICD-10 or DSM-IV autism (comprising communication difficulties, problems with social interaction, and behavioural problems) in children aged younger than 3 years.

Combined measles, mumps, and rubella (MMR) vaccine Vaccine with components that aim to raise immunity to measles, mumps, and rubella infections. Contains live attenuated measles virus (Schwarz strain).

Herd immunity Background level of immunity in the community. A high level of herd immunity reduces risk of infection even in non-immune individuals, because there is no pool of at risk individuals who may transmit the infectious agent.

Live monovalent measles vaccine Commonly known as the single measles vaccine. Uses live, attenuated virus (most commonly Schwarz strain), and only to bring about measles immunity.

Seroconversion Development in the blood of specific antimeasles antibody. Seroconversion is a proxy for clinical efficacy.
Vaccine coverage Prevalence of vaccination in the community.

REFERENCES

1. Center for Disease Control. *Epidemiology and prevention of vaccine-preventable diseases*. Atlanta: CDC, 2000.
2. http://www.unicef.org/programme/health/document/meastrat.pdf (last accessed 20 Jan 03).
3. http:/www.who.int/vaccines-surveillance/graphics/htmls/meainc.htm (last accessed 20 Jan 03).
4. Peltola H, Heinonen P, Valle M, et al. The elimination of indigenous measles, mumps and rubella from Finland by a 12-year, two-dose vaccination program. *N Eng J Med* 1994;331:1397–1402.
5. Peltola H, Davidkin I, Valle M, et al. No measles in Finland. *Lancet* 1997;350:1364–1365.
6. de Quadros CA, Olive J, Hersh BS, et al. Measles elimination in the Americas: evolving strategies. *JAMA* 1996;275:224–229.
7. Pan American Health Organization. Surveillance in the Americas. *Weekly Bulletin* 1995;1.
8. World Health Report, 2001: Statistical annex. Geneva: WHO, 2001.
9. Miller E, Waight P, Farrington CP, et al. Idiopathic thrombocytopenic purpura and MMR vaccine. *Arch Dis Child* 2001;84:227–229.
10. http://www.who.int/child-adolescent-health/OVERVIEW/Child_Health/child_epidemiology.htm (last accessed 20 Jan 03).
11. Anders J, Jacobson R, Poland G, et al. Secondary failure rates of measles vaccines: a metaanalysis of published studies. *Pediatr Infect Dis J* 1996;15:62–66. Search date 1995; primary sources Medline (English language only) and hand searches of references cited in initial search and references cited within first generation references.
12. Measles Vaccination subcommittee of the Committee on Development of Vaccines and Immunisation Procedures. Clinical trial of live measles vaccine given alone and live vaccine preceded by killed vaccine. Fourth report to the Medical Research Council. *Lancet* 1977;2:571–575.
13. Guinee VF, Henderson DA, Casey HL, et al. Cooperative measles vaccine field trial. I. Clinical efficacy. *Pediatrics* 1966;37:649–665.
14. Salmon DA, Haber M, Gangarosa E, et al. Health consequences of religious and philosophical exemptions from immunization laws: individual and societal risk of measles. *JAMA* 1999;282:47–53.
15. Ramsay ME, Moffatt D, O'Connor M. Measles vaccine: a 27-year follow up. *Epidemiol Infect* 1994;112:409–412.
16. Bloom JL, Schiff GM, Graubarth H, et al. Evaluation of a trivalent measles, mumps, rubella vaccine in children. *J Pediatr* 1975;87:85–87.
17. Schwarz AJ, Jackson JE, Ehrenkranz J, et al. Clinical evaluation of a new measles–mumps–rubella trivalent vaccine. *Am J Dis Child* 1975;129:1408–1412.
18. Aaby P, Samb B, Simondon F, et al. Non-specific beneficial effect of measles immunisation: analysis of mortality studies from developing countries. *BMJ* 1995;311:481–485. Search date not stated; primary source Medline.
19. Koenig MA, Khan B, Wojtynak B. Impact of measles vaccination on childhood mortality in rural Bangladesh. *Bull World Health Organ* 1990;68:441–447.
20. http://www.who.int/vaccines-surveillance/graphics/htmls/IncMeas.htm (last accessed 20 Jan 03).
21. Pannuti CS, Moraes JC, Souza VA, et al. Measles antibody prevalence after mass immunization in Sao Paulo, Brazil. *Bull World Health Organ* 1991;69:557–560.
22. Ceyhan M, Kanra G, Erdem G, et al. Immunogenicity and efficacy of one dose measles–mumps–rubella (MMR) vaccine at twelve months of age as compared to monovalent measles vaccination at nine months followed by MMR revaccination at fifteen months of age. *Vaccine* 2001;19:4473–4478.
23. Edees S, Pullan CR, Hull D. A randomised single blind trial of a combined mumps measles rubella vaccine to evaluate serological response and reactions in the UK population. *Public Health* 1991;105:91–97.
24. Robertson CM, Bennet VJ, Jefferson N, et al. Serological evaluation of a measles, mumps, and rubella vaccine. *Arch Dis Child* 1988;63:612–616.
25. Duclos P, Ward BJ. Measles vaccines: a review of adverse events. *Drug Saf* 1998;6:435–454. Search date 1998; primary sources Stratton RS, Howe CJ, Johnston Jr RB. Adverse events associated with childhood vaccines: evidence bearing on causality. Washington DC: National Academy Press 1994 for papers published before 1994; for articles published after 1994 primary sources WHO Collaborating Centre for International Drug Monitoring Database, discussion groups, advisory committee documents, and other unspecified databases.
26. Virtanen M, Peltola H, Paunio M, et al. Day-to-day reactogenicity and the healthy vaccinee effect of measles–mumps–rubella vaccination. *Pediatrics* 2000;106:e62.
27. Barlow WE, Davis RL, Glasser JW. The risk of seizures after receipt of whole cell pertussins or measles mumps and rubella vaccine. *N Eng J Med* 2001;345:656–661.
28. Patja A, Davidkin I, Kurki T, et al. Serious adverse events after measles–mumps–rubella vaccination during a fourteen year prospective follow up. *Pediatr Infect Dis J* 2000;19:1127–1134.
29. Madsen KM, Hviid A, Vestergaard M, et al. A population-based study of measles, mumps, and rubella vaccination and autism. *New Engl J Med 2002*;347:1477–1482.
30. Institute of Medicine. *Immunization safety review: measles–mumps–rubella vaccine and autism.* Washington DC: National Academy Press, 2001.
31. Dales L, Hammer SJ, Smith N. Time trends in autism and in MMR immunization coverage in California. *JAMA* 2001;285:1183–1185.
32. Kaye JA, del Mar Melero-Montes M, Jick H. Mumps, measles, and rubella vaccine and the incidence of autism recorded by general practitioners: a time trend analysis. *BMJ* 2001;322:460–463.
33. Taylor B, Miller E, Farrington CP, et al. Autism and measles, mumps, and rubella vaccine: no epidemiological evidence for a causal association. *Lancet* 1999;353:2026–2029.
34. Morris DL, Montgomery SM, Thompson NP. Measles vaccination and inflammatory bowel disease: a National British Cohort study. *Am J Gastroenterol* 2000;95:3507–3512.

35. Davis RL, Kramarz P, Bohlke K, et al. Measles–mumps–rubella and other measles containing vaccines do not increase risk for inflammatory bowel disease: a case control study from the Vaccine Safety Datalink project. *Arch Pediatr Adolesc Med* 2001;155:354–359.
36. Taylor B, Miller E, Lingam R, et al. Measles, mumps, and rubella vaccination and bowel problems or developmental regression in children with autism: a population study. *BMJ* 2002;324:393–396.
37. Wakefield AJ, Murch SH, Anthony A, et al. Ileal–lymphoid–nodular hyperplasia, non-specific colitis, and pervasive developmental disorder in children. *Lancet* 1998;351:637–641.

Bazian Ltd
London
UK

Competing interests: None declared.

Migraine headache in children

Search date January 2003

Nick Barnes, Guy Millman, and Elizabeth James

QUESTIONS

INTERVENTIONS

See glossary, p 435

Key Messages

Treatment

- **Antiemetics; codeine phosphate; non-steroidal anti-inflammatory drugs; paracetamol; $5HT_1$ antagonists** We found insufficient evidence to compare these interventions with each other or with placebo in children with migraine headache.

Prevention

- **Stress management** We found limited evidence from one small RCT that self administered stress management improved headache severity and frequency compared with no stress management.
- **β Blockers** We found conflicting evidence from small RCTs about effects of β blockers compared with placebo in children with migraine headache.
- **Dietary manipulation; pizotifen; progressive muscle relaxation; thermal biofeedback** We found insufficient evidence about effects of these interventions to prevent migraine in children.

Migraine headache in children

DEFINITION Migraine is defined by the International Headache Society (IHS) as a recurrent headache that occurs with or without aura (see glossary, p 435) and lasts 2–48 hours.[1] It is usually unilateral in nature, pulsating in quality, of moderate or severe intensity, and is aggravated by routine physical activity. Nausea, vomiting, photophobia, and phonophobia are common accompanying symptoms (see table 1, p 436). This topic focuses on children younger than 18 years. Diagnostic criteria for children are broader than criteria for adults, allowing for a broader range of duration and a broader localisation of the pain (see table 1, p 436).[2] Diagnosis is difficult in young children, because the condition is defined by subjective symptoms. Studies that do not explicitly use criteria that are congruent with IHS diagnostic criteria (or revised IHS criteria in children under 15 years of age) have been excluded from this topic.

INCIDENCE/ PREVALENCE Migraine occurs in 3–10% of children,[3–7] and currently affects 50/1000 school age children in the UK and an estimated 7.8 million children in the European Union.[8] Studies in developed countries suggest that migraine is the most common diagnosis among children presenting with headache to a medical practitioner. It is rarely diagnosed in children under 2 years of age because of the symptom based definition, but increases steadily with age thereafter.[1,9,10] It affects boys and girls similarly before puberty, but after puberty girls are more likely to suffer from migraine.[4,6,10] See incidence/prevalence of migraine headache, p 1547.

AETIOLOGY/ RISK FACTORS The cause of migraine headaches is unknown. We found few reliable data identifying risk factors or quantifying their effects in children. Suggested risk factors include stress, foods, menses, and exercise in genetically predisposed children and adolescents.[10,11]

PROGNOSIS We found no reliable data about prognosis of childhood migraine headache diagnosed by IHS criteria. It has been suggested that more than half the children will have spontaneous remission after puberty.[10] It is believed that migraine that develops during adolescence tends to continue in adult life, although attacks tend to be less frequent and severe in later life.[12] We found one longitudinal study from Sweden (73 children with "pronounced" migraine and mean age onset 6 years) with over 40 years follow up, which predated the IHS criteria for migraine headache.[13] It found that migraine headaches had ceased before the age of 25 years in 23% of people. However, by the age of 50 years, more than 50% of people continued to have migraine headaches. We found no prospective data examining long term risks in children with migraine.

AIMS OF INTERVENTION To provide relief from symptoms; to prevent recurrent attacks in the long term, and to minimise the disruption of childhood activities, with minimal adverse effects.

OUTCOMES Pain scores (usually on visual analogue scales); migraine recurrence; functional indicators (such as time off school, behavioural scores, sleep scores, and sleep satisfaction); any adverse effects of treatment. Migraine index is a validated scale for measuring severity in adult migraine. Its validity in children is unclear.

METHODS *Clinical Evidence* search and appraisal January 2003.

QUESTION What are the effects of treatments for acute attacks of migraine headache in children? New

OPTION PARACETAMOL

We found no reliable RCTs addressing the effects of paracetamol (acetaminophen) in children or adolescents with migraine headache.

Benefits: We found no systematic review or reliable RCTs evaluating the effects of paracetamol (acetaminophen) compared with placebo or no treatment in children with migraine headache.

Harms: We found no evidence about adverse effects of licensed doses of paracetamol in children with migraine. See paracetamol poisoning for symptoms and treatment of paracetamol overdose, p 1664.

Comment: We found one three way crossover RCT (106 children) comparing paracetamol, ibuprofen, and placebo. The RCT had high withdrawal rates (17%) and did not report results before crossover.[14] This may have introduced bias due to continued treatment effects after crossover, and due to unequal withdrawals among groups.

OPTION NON-STEROIDAL ANTI-INFLAMMATORY DRUGS

We found no reliable RCTs assessing the effects of non-steroidal anti-inflammatory drugs in children and adolescents with migraine headache.

Benefits: We found no systematic review or reliable RCTs evaluating the effects of non-steroidal anti-inflammatory drugs in children with migraine headache.

Harms: We found no RCTs addressing harms of non-steroidal anti-inflammatory drugs in children or adolescents with migraine headache.

Comment: We found one three-way crossover RCT (106 children), but it was excluded because it had methodological flaws that compromised the validity of its results, including failure to report results before crossover.[14]

OPTION CODEINE PHOSPHATE

We found no systematic review or RCTs addressing the effects of codeine phosphate in children or adolescents with migraine headache.

Benefits: We found no systematic review or RCTs addressing the effects of codeine phosphate in children or adolescents with migraine headache.

Harms: We found no RCTs assessing the effects of codeine phosphate in children with migraine. Known adverse effects of codeine include nausea, vomiting, constipation, drowsiness, potential for respiratory depression in overdose, difficulty for micturition, and dry mouth.

Comment: None.

OPTION	$5HT_1$ ANTAGONISTS (E.G. TRIPTANS)

We found insufficient evidence about effects of oral or nasal $5HT_1$ antagonists in children and adolescents with migraine headache.

Benefits: **Versus placebo:** We found no systematic review. We found two RCTs.[15,16] The first RCT (653 children aged 12–17 years) compared three different doses of nasal sumatriptan (5, 10, or 20 mg) with placebo.[15] It found that nasal sumatriptan increased complete resolution compared with placebo at 2 hours, although the result was significant only for the lowest dose (74/118 [63%] with 20 mg; 85/133 [64%] with 10 mg; 84/128 [66%] with 5 mg; 69/131 [53%] with placebo; $P < 0.05$ for 5 mg *v* placebo, but not for other doses *v* placebo).[15] The second RCT (360 children aged 12–17 years) compared rizatriptan versus placebo.[16] It found no significant difference between rizatriptan and placebo for partial or complete pain relief at 2 hours (pain free: 48/149 [32%] with rizatriptan *v* 40/142 [28%] with placebo, $P = 0.47$; partial pain relief: 98/149 [66%] with rizatriptan *v* 80/142 [56%] with placebo, $P = 0.08$).[16]

Harms: The first RCT found that taste disturbance was more common with sumatriptan compared with placebo (2% with placebo *v* 19% with 5 mg *v* 30% with 10 mg *v* 26% with 20 mg).[15] However, it found no significant differences among treatments or placebo for other adverse effects. The second RCT found that nausea and somnolence were significantly more common with placebo than with rizatriptan.[16] It reported that one child taking rizatriptan developed transient jaundice and hyperglycaemia, which resolved within 1 week.

Comment: **Oral sumatriptan versus placebo:** We found one RCT, published in abstract form only.[17] It could not, therefore, be assessed adequately for reliability. A second double blind, placebo controlled, crossover RCT did not report results before crossover and had a high withdrawal rate (26%), and it has, therefore, been excluded.[18] **Nasal sumatriptan versus placebo:** We found one small crossover RCT (14 children aged 6.4–9.8 years).[19] However, it did not present results before crossover, and so has been excluded. **Rizatriptan versus placebo:** In the RCT comparing rizatriptan with placebo 360 children were originally enrolled. Of these, 64 children did not receive placebo or rizatriptan, the reasons for which were not stated. Seven children subsequently dropped out, although reasons for stopping treatment were not stated.

OPTION	ANTIEMETICS

We found no systematic review or RCTs of antiemetics in children with migraine headache.

Benefits: We found no systematic review or RCTs comparing antiemetics with placebo, no treatment, or other treatments in children with migraine headache.

Harms: We found no RCTs.

Comment: None.

QUESTION What are the effects of prophylaxis for migraine in children? New

OPTION β BLOCKERS

Three RCTs found conflicting evidence about the effects of β blockers compared with placebo in children with migraine headache.

Benefits: We found no systematic review. **Versus placebo:** We found three RCTs that compared propranolol with placebo.[20–22] The first RCT (double blind, crossover, 32 children aged 7–16 years) found that propranolol (60–120 mg/day divided in three doses) significantly increased perception of benefit compared with placebo during a 3 month period (report of "some benefit" before crossover: 13/13 [100%] with propranolol *v* 4/15 [27%] with placebo; $P < 0.001$).[20] However, reliability may be limited because 13% of people were lost to follow up. The second RCT (double blind, crossover, 53 children aged 9–15 years) compared propranolol 40–120 mg daily with placebo.[21] It found that propranolol significantly increased headache duration compared with placebo (results before crossover: mean duration of headache: 436 minutes with propranolol *v* 287 minutes with placebo, $P < 0.01$). The third RCT (double blind, crossover, 33 children aged 6–12 years) found no significant difference in the number of episodes of migraine between propranolol 3 mg/kg daily and placebo at 3 months (results before crossover: mean number of headaches 14.9 with propranolol *v* 13.3 with placebo, $P = 0.47$).[22] In five people in whom migraine was thought to be provoked by food, diet was restricted to avoid those foods (no details about type of foods reported). This may have confounded apparent treatment effects.

Harms: The first RCT reported insomnia in 2/13 (18%) children taking propranolol, but did not report on adverse effects in the placebo group.[20] The second RCT found no significant difference in adverse effects between placebo and propranolol (12 children affected in each group).[21] Adverse effects in both groups included abdominal pain, increased appetite, worsening of headaches, and fatigue. However, the trial was too small to yield reliable information about harms. The third trial did not report on adverse effects.[22] All RCTs probably lacked power to exclude clinically important differences.

Comment: None.

OPTION PIZOTIFEN

We found no reliable RCTs addressing the effects of pizotifen in children with migraine headache.

Benefits: We found no systematic review or reliable RCTs evaluating the effects of pizotifen in children with migraine headache.

Harms: We found no systematic review or RCTs that met International Headache Society (IHS) criteria for migraine (see comment below).

Comment: We found one RCT (47 children aged 7–14 years) comparing pizotifen with placebo.[23] It pre-dated the IHS diagnostic criteria for migraine and people in this study would not all fulfil the current IHS definition. The study has, therefore, been excluded. We found one further RCT comparing pizotifen with placebo.[24] It has only been published in abstract form and so we could not reliably review its methods.

OPTION DIETARY MANIPULATION

We found no reliable RCTs in children with migraine headache.

Benefits: We found no systematic review and no reliable RCTs of dietary manipulation (see glossary, p 435) in children with migraine headache.

Harms: We found no RCTs of dietary manipulation in children and adolescents with migraine headache.

Comment: We found one small RCT (39 children allocated to treatment), which attempted to investigate effects of excluding dietary vasoactive amines on morbidity related to migraine.[25] However, the study pre-dated the International Headache Society criteria for migraine and a large proportion (33%) of eligible children were excluded before randomisation. The study has, therefore, been excluded.

OPTION THERMAL BIOFEEDBACK

We found no reliable RCTs examining effects of thermal biofeedback (see glossary, p 435) in children with migraine headache.

Benefits: We found no systematic review and no reliable RCTs.

Harms: We found no reliable RCTs.

Comment: We found two RCTs with more than 10 people in each treatment arm.[26,27] However, the first had high loss to follow up (46%),[26] and the second was published only as a conference abstract.[27]

OPTION PROGRESSIVE MUSCLE RELAXATION

We found no RCTs examining effects of progressive muscle relaxation in children with migraine headache.

Benefits: We found no RCTs (see comment below).

Harms: We found no reliable RCTs.

Comment: We found one RCT (99 people aged 9–17 years), which compared progressive muscle relaxation (see glossary, p 435) with psychological counselling.[28] However, high loss to follow up (30%) precluded reliable conclusions.

OPTION STRESS MANAGEMENT

We found limited evidence from one small RCT that a self administered stress management programme improved headache severity and frequency compared with no stress management.

Benefits: We found no systematic review. We found one RCT (87 people, aged 11–18 years).[29] It found that a self administered stress management (see glossary, p 435) programme reduced headache severity and frequency compared with both a stress management programme delivered by the clinic, and with no stress management, at 1 month (16/24 [67%] improved with self administered treatment *v* 10/23 [44%] with treatment delivered by the clinic *v* 6/25 [24%] with no stress management; $P < 0.01$ for self administered treatment *v* no treatment).[29]

Harms: The RCTs did not report on harms.[29]

Comment: None.

GLOSSARY

Aura A premonitory sensation or warning experienced before the start of a migraine headache.

Dietary manipulation A change in diet aimed specifically at reducing or removing from the diet a foodstuff that is thought to provoke migraine headache.

Dietary vasoactive amines Dietary amines (protein subunits) that may have an effect on cerebral vascular tone.

Progressive muscle relaxation Volitional muscle relaxation aimed at altering the perception of symptoms such as headache.

Stress management Coping or relaxation strategies that aim to alter the perception of symptoms.

Thermal biofeedback A treatment in which an individual attempts to alter their skin temperature by responding to feedback about their skin temperature.

REFERENCES

1. Headache Classification Committee of the International Headache Society. Classification and diagnostic criteria for headache disorders, cranial neuralgias and facial pain. *Cephalalgia* 1988;8(suppl 7):1–96.
2. Winner P, Martinez W, Mate L, et al. Classification of pediatric migraine: proposed revisions to the IHS criteria. *Headache* 1995;35:407–410.
3. Hockaday JM, Barlow CF. Headache in children. In: Olesen J, Tfelt-Hansen P, Welch KMA, eds. *The headaches*. New York: Raven Press, 1993:795–808.
4. Bille B. Migraine in schoolchildren. *Acta Paediatr* 1962;51(suppl 136):1–151.
5. Goldstein M, Chen TC. The epidemiology of disabling headache. *Adv Neurol* 1982;33:377–390.
6. Abu-Arefeh I, Russell G. Prevalence of headache and migraine in schoolchildren. *BMJ* 1994;309:765–769.
7. Ueberall M. Sumatriptan in paediatric and adolescent migraine. *Cephalalgia* 2001;21(suppl 1):21–24.
8. Evers S. Drug treatment of migraine in children. A comparative review. *Paediatr Drugs* 1999;1:7–18.
9. Migraine. In: Behrman RE, Kliegman RM, Jenson HB, eds. *Nelson textbook of pediatrics.* 16th ed. Philadelphia: Saunders, 2000:1832–1834.
10. Amery WK, Vandenbergh V. What can precipitating factors teach us about the pathogenesis of migraine? *Headache* 1987;27:146–150.
11. Blau JN, Thavapalan M. Preventing migraine: a study of precipitating factors. *Headache* 1988;28:481–483.
12. Pearce JMS. Migraine. In: Weatherall DJ, Ledingham JGG, Warrell DA, eds. *Oxford textbook of medicine.* Oxford: Oxford University Press 1996:4024–4026.
13. Bille B. A 40-year follow-up of school children with migraine. *Cephalalgia* 1997;17:488–491.
14. Hamalainen ML, Hoppu K, Valkeila E, Santavuori P. Ibuprofen or acetaminophen for the acute treatment of migraine in children. *Neurology* 1997;48:103–107.
15. Winner P, Rothner AD, Saper J, et al. A randomized, double-blind, placebo-controlled study of sumatriptan nasal spray in the treatment of acute migraine in adolescents. *Pediatrics* 2000;106:989–997.
16. Winner P, Lewis D, Visser WH, et al. Rizatriptan 5 mg for the acute treatment of migraine in adolescents: a randomised, double-blind, placebo-controlled study. *Headache* 2002;42:49–55.
17. Korsgard AG. The tolerability, safety and efficacy of oral sumatriptan 50 mg and 100 mg for the acute treatment of migraine in adolescents. *Cephalalgia* 1995;15(suppl 16):99.
18. Hamalainen ML, Hoppu K, Santavuori P. Sumatriptan for migraine attacks in children: a randomized placebo-controlled study. Do children with migraine respond to oral sumatriptan differently from adults? *Neurology* 1997;48:1100–1103.
19. Ueberall MA, Wenzel D. Intranasal sumatriptan for the acute treatment of migraine in children. *Neurology* 1999;52:1507–1510.
20. Ludviggson J. Propranolol used in the prophylaxis of migraine in children. *Acta Neurol Scand* 1974;50:109–115.

Migraine headache in children

21. Forsythe WI, Gillies D, Sills MA. Propranolol ("Inderal") in the treatment of childhood migraine. *Dev Med Child Neurol* 1984;26:737–741.
22. Olness K, Macdonald JT, Uden DL. Comparison of self-hypnosis and propranolol in the treatment of juvenile classic migraine. *Pediatrics* 1987;79:593–597.
23. Gillies D, Sills M, Forsythe I. Pizotifen (Sanomigran) in childhood migraine. A double-blind controlled trial. *Eur Neurol* 1986;25:32–35.
24. Salmon MA. Pizotifen (BC.105. Sanomigran) in the prophylaxis of childhood migraine [abstract]. *Cephalalgia* 1985;5(suppl 3):178.
25. Salfield SAW, Wardley BL, Houlsby WT, et al. Controlled study of exclusion of dietary vasoactive amines in migraine. *Arch Dis Child* 1987;62:458–460.
26. Labbe EL, Williamson DA. Treatment of childhood migraine using autogenic feedback training. *J Consult Clin Psychol* 1984;52:968–976.
27. Andrasik F, Attanasio V, Blanchard EB, et al. Behavioural treatment of pediatric migraine headache. In: Andrasik F (Chair), Recent developments in the assessment and treatment of headache. Symposium conducted at the annual meeting of the Association for Advancement of Behaviour Therapy, Philadelphia, PA, 1984.
28. McGrath PJ, Humphreys P, Goodman JT, et al. Relaxation prophylaxis for childhood migraine: a randomised placebo-controlled trial. *Dev Med Child Neurol* 1988;30:626–631.
29. McGrath PJ, Humphreys P, Keene D, et al. The efficacy of a self-administered treatment for adolescent migraine. *Pain* 1992;49:321–324.

Nick Barnes
Specialist Registrar Paediatrics
John Radcliffe Hospital
Oxford
UK

Guy Millman
Specialist Registrar
Paediatric Neurology
Manchester Children's Hospital
Manchester
UK

Elizabeth James
General Practitioner
Didcot Health Centre
Didcot
UK

Competing interests: None declared.

TABLE 1 **International Headache Society criteria for migraine.[1] Text in parentheses indicates suggested revisions for children under 15 years of age.[2]**

At least 5 episodes **without aura** fulfilling **all** of criteria **1–3:**	**OR**	At least 2 episodes **with aura** fulfilling at least **three** of criteria **1–4:**
1. Headache lasting 1–48 hours		1. One or more fully reversible aua symtoms including focal cortical, brain stem dysfunction, or both
2. Headache meeting at least two of the following criteria: a) Unilaterial or bilateral (either frontal or temporal) distribution of pain b) Throbbing c) Moderate to sever intensity d) Aggravated by routine physical activity		2. At least one aura sympton that develops gradually over more than 4 minutes, or 2 or more symptons that occure in succession
3. At least one of the following sumptons while headache is present: a) Nausea, vomiting, or both b) Photophobia, phonophobia, or both		3. No aura symptoms lasting more than 60 minutes
		4. Headache follows aura within 60 minutes

Nosebleeds in children

Search date June 2003

Gerald McGarry

QUESTIONS

INTERVENTIONS

Key Messages

- **Antiseptic cream** One RCT found that chlorhexidine/neomycin cream reduced nosebleeds compared with no treatment at 8 weeks.
- **Antiseptic cream versus cautery** One small RCT found no significant difference in nosebleeds between chlorhexidine/neomycin cream and silver nitrate cautery at 8 weeks. However, the study may have lacked power to detect clinically important differences between treatments. Some children found the smell and taste of the antiseptic cream unpleasant. All children found cautery painful despite the use of local anaesthesia.
- **Cautery plus antiseptic cream** One small RCT found insufficient evidence about the effects of silver nitrate cautery plus chlorhexidine/neomycin cream compared with chlorhexidine/neomycin cream alone.
- **Cautery versus no treatment** We found no RCTs about the effects of this intervention.

DEFINITION Recurrent idiopathic epistaxis is recurrent, self limiting, nasal bleeding in children for which no specific cause is identified. There is no consensus on the frequency or severity of recurrences.

INCIDENCE/ PREVALENCE A cross-sectional study of 1218 children (aged 11–14 years) found that 9% had frequent episodes of epistaxis.[1] It is likely that only the most severe episodes are considered for treatment.

AETIOLOGY/ RISK FACTORS In children, most epistaxis occurs from the anterior part of the septum in the region of Little's area.[2] Initiating factors include local inflammation, mucosal drying, and local trauma (including nose picking).[2] Epistaxis caused by other specific local (e.g. tumours) or systemic factors (e.g. clotting disorders) is not considered here.

PROGNOSIS Recurrent epistaxis is less common in people over 14 years old, and many children "grow out" of this problem.

AIMS OF INTERVENTION To reduce the number and severity of epistaxis episodes; to minimise adverse effects of treatment.

OUTCOMES Number and severity of epistaxis episodes.

METHODS *Clinical Evidence* search and appraisal June 2003.

QUESTION **What are the effects of treatments for recurrent idiopathic epistaxis in children?**

OPTION **ANTISEPTIC CREAMS**

One RCT found that chlorhexidine/neomycin cream reduced nosebleeds compared with no treatment at 8 weeks. One small RCT found no significant difference in nosebleeds between chlorhexidine/neomycin cream and silver nitrate cautery at 8 weeks, although the study may have lacked power to detect a clinically important effect. Some children found the smell and taste of antiseptic cream unpleasant. All children found cautery painful, despite the use of local anaesthesia.

Benefits: We found no systematic review. **Versus no treatment:** We found one RCT (103 children aged 3–13 years with recurrent epistaxis for a mean 20 months, unblinded design) that compared antiseptic cream (chlorhexidine hydrochloride 0.1%, neomycin sulphate 3250 U/g) applied to both nostrils twice daily for 4 weeks versus no treatment.[3] It found that antiseptic cream significantly increased the proportion of children who had complete resolution of bleeding compared with no treatment at 8 weeks (no bleeding in past 4 weeks: 26/47 [55%] with antiseptic cream *v* 12/41 [29%] with no treatment; RR 0.53, 95% CI 0.31 to 0.91; NNT 4, 95% CI 3 to 9). **Versus cautery:** We found one small RCT (48 children aged 3–14 years with at least 1 episode of epistaxis during the previous 4 weeks and a "history of repeated epistaxis"), which compared antiseptic cream (chlorhexidine hydrochloride 0.1%, neomycin sulphate 3250 U/g) applied to both nostrils twice daily for 4 weeks versus silver nitrate cautery.[4] Cautery was undertaken in secondary care using silver nitrate applied on a stick to prominent vessels or bleeding points. The RCT found no significant difference in the proportion of children with complete resolution of bleeding at 8 weeks (no bleeding during the past 4 weeks: 12/24 [50%] with antiseptic cream *v* 13/24 [54%] with cautery; RR 0.92, 95% CI 0.54 to 1.59). It also found similar rates of partial success with antiseptic cream compared with cautery at 8 weeks (proportion of children with 50% reduction in number of bleeds during the past 4 weeks: 4/24 [16.6%] with antiseptic cream *v* 3/24 [12.5%] with cautery) and failure at 8 weeks (proportion of children with less than 50% reduction in number of bleeds in past 4 weeks: 7/24 [29%] with antiseptic cream *v* 6/24 [25%] with cautery). **Plus cautery:** See benefits of silver nitrate cautery, p 439.

Harms: The RCT comparing antiseptic cream with no treatment gave no information about adverse effects.[3] Some commercial antiseptic creams contain arachis (peanut) oil, and the RCT excluded all children with peanut allergies.[3] The RCT comparing antiseptic cream with cautery found no adverse reactions with antiseptic cream, but some children found the smell and taste unpleasant (no further data reported).[4] Chlorhexidine/neomycin cream may cause occasional skin reactions. All children undergoing cautery experienced pain, even with 5% cocaine as a local anaesthetic.[4]

Comment: See comment under silver nitrate cautery, p 439.

OPTION SILVER NITRATE CAUTERY

We found no RCTs comparing silver nitrate cautery with no treatment. One small RCT found no significant difference in nosebleeds between silver nitrate cautery and antiseptic cream at 8 weeks. One small RCT found insufficient evidence about the effects of silver nitrate cautery plus chlorhexidine/neomycin cream versus chlorhexidine/neomycin cream alone.

Benefits: We found no systematic review. **Versus no treatment:** We found no RCTs. **Versus antiseptic cream:** See benefits of antiseptic creams, p 438. **Plus antiseptic cream:** One RCT (40 adults, 24 children) compared once only silver nitrate cautery plus chlorhexidine hydrochloride 0.1%/neomycin sulphate 3250 U/g cream twice daily for 2 weeks versus antiseptic cream alone.[5] The RCT did not provide discrete results in children and included too few children to draw conclusions.

Harms: The RCT did not report harms.[5] Recognised complications of cautery include pain and septal perforation, although the incidence of septal perforation following unilateral cautery in children is not known (see harms of antiseptic creams, p 439).

Comment: Both RCTs involving silver nitrate cautery were undertaken in the context of secondary care.[4,5] Silver nitrate cautery is also used in primary care. It is unknown whether complication rates differ. Simultaneous bilateral cautery in children is not recommended because of an expected increased risk of perforation.

REFERENCES

1. Rodeghiero F, Castaman G, Dini E. Epidemiological investigation of the prevalence of von Willebrand's disease. *Blood* 1987;69:454–459.
2. Watkinson JC. Epistaxis. In: Kerr AG, Mackay IS, Bull TR, eds. *Scott-Brown's Otolaryngology, Volume 4 Rhinology*. Oxford: Butterworth-Heinemann, 1997;18:1–19.
3. Kubba H, MacAndie C, Botma M, et al. A prospective, single blind, randomized controlled trial of antiseptic cream for recurrent epistaxis in childhood. *Clin Otolaryngol* 2001;26:465–468.

4. Ruddy J, Proops DW, Pearman K, et al. Management of epistaxis in children. *Int J Paediatr Otorhinolaryngol* 1991;21:139–142.
5. Murthy P, Nilssen ELK, Rao S, et al. A randomised clinical trial of antiseptic nasal carrier cream and silver nitrate cautery in the treatment of recurrent anterior epistaxis. *Clin Otolaryngol* 1999;228–231.

Gerald McGarry
Consultant Otorhinolaryngologist
Honorary Clinical Senior Lecturer
Glasgow Royal Infirmary
Glasgow
UK

Competing interests: None declared.

The following previous contributors of this topic would also like to be acknowledged: Martin Burton, and Robert Walton.

Reducing pain during blood sampling in infants

Search date May 2003

Deborah Pritchard

QUESTIONS

INTERVENTIONS

See glossary, p 454

Key Messages

Reducing pain related distress during heel puncture

- **Holding (skin to skin) versus swaddling in term infants** RCTs found that holding reduced crying during heel puncture compared with swaddling in term infants.
- **Oral glucose** RCTs found that oral glucose reduced pain responses (particularly the duration of crying) in preterm and term infants compared with water or no treatment.

Reducing pain during blood sampling in infants

- **Oral sucrose** Systematic reviews and additional RCTs found good evidence in preterm infants and limited evidence in term infants that oral sucrose reduced pain responses (particularly the duration of crying) compared with water or no treatment. One RCT found that sucrose did not appear to increase the benefit of holding. Three RCTs in term infants found that sucrose plus pacifier was more effective than pacifier alone, although one RCT in preterm infants found no significant difference in pain score between a pacifier dipped in sucrose and pacifier alone. One RCT found insufficient evidence about the effects of oral sucrose compared with lidocaine–prilocaine emulsion in term infants undergoing heel puncture.
- **Other sweeteners** RCTs have found that other sweeteners (hydrogenated glucose or an artificial sweetener, 10 parts cyclamate and 1 part saccharin) reduce pain scores and the percentage of time spent crying in term infants compared with water.
- **Pacifiers** RCTs in term and preterm infants have found that pacifiers given before heel puncture reduce pain responses compared with no treatment.
- **Positioning (tucking arms and legs) in preterm infants** One RCT found limited evidence that pain responses were reduced by tucking the arms and legs into a mid-line flexed position during heel puncture.
- **Rocking** We found limited evidence that rocking reduces pain related stress compared with placebo.
- **Multiple doses of sweet solution** One small RCT found no significant difference in pain of heel puncture between multiple and single doses of sucrose.
- **Swaddling** One small RCT found no significant difference in pain responses from swaddling compared with no swaddling.
- **Breast milk or breast feeding** RCTs found no evidence that breast milk or breast feeding during heel puncture reduced pain responses or crying in neonates compared with water.
- **Prone position** One RCT found no significant difference in pain score between prone position and either side or supine position during heel puncture.
- **Topical anaesthetics** Systematic reviews and additional RCTs found no evidence of reduced pain responses, particularly crying, following heel puncture with topical anaesthetic (lidocaine, lidocaine–prilocaine emulsion, or tetracaine [amethocaine]) compared with placebo.
- **Warming** Two RCTs in term infants found no benefit of warming before heel puncture.

Reducing pain related distress during venepuncture

- **Breast feeding** One RCT found that breast feeding during venepuncture reduced pain responses compared with oral water or being held. The RCT found no significant difference in pain response between breast feeding and oral glucose.
- **Oral glucose** RCTs have found that oral glucose reduces pain responses (particularly the duration of crying) in term and preterm infants compared with water or no treatment. One RCT found no significant difference in pain scores between sucrose and glucose.
- **Oral sucrose** RCTs have found that oral sucrose reduces pain responses (particularly the duration of crying) in term and preterm infants compared with water or no treatment. One RCT found no significant difference in pain between sucrose and glucose.

- **Pacifiers** One RCT found that pacifiers reduced pain responses compared with water or no treatment in term infants undergoing venepuncture.
- **Topical anaesthetics** Four RCTs found limited evidence that lidocaine–prilocaine emulsion reduced pain responses to venepuncture compared with placebo. Two RCTs found that tetracaine (amethocaine) gel reduced pain and crying during venepuncture compared with placebo.
- **Other sweeteners** We found no RCTs of other sweeteners for venepuncture.

DEFINITION Methods of sampling blood in infants include heel puncture, venepuncture, and arterial puncture. Heel puncture involves lancing of the lateral aspect of the infant's heel, squeezing the heel, and collecting the pooled capillary blood. Venepuncture involves aspirating blood through a needle from a peripheral vein. Arterial blood sampling is not discussed in this review. RCTs in this review were performed in a hospital care setting and the evidence relates to preterm and ill infants who have multiple blood tests, rather than infants undergoing heel puncture tests for routine screening. The results therefore cannot be applied to routine screening heel puncture tests in healthy infants.

INCIDENCE/ PREVALENCE Almost every infant in the developed world undergoes heel puncture to screen for metabolic disorders (e.g. phenylketonuria). Many infants have repeated heel punctures or venepunctures to monitor blood glucose or haemoglobin. Preterm or ill neonates may undergo 1–21 heel punctures or venepunctures per day.[1–3] These punctures are likely to be painful. Heel punctures comprise 61–87% and venepunctures comprise 8–13% of the invasive procedures performed on ill infants. Analgesics are rarely given specifically for blood sampling procedures, but 5–19% of infants receive analgesia for other indications.[2,3] In one study, comfort measures were provided during 63% of venepunctures and 75% of heel punctures.[3]

AETIOLOGY/ RISK FACTORS Blood sampling in infants can be difficult to perform, particularly in preterm or ill infants. Young infants may have increased sensitivity and more prolonged responses to pain than older age groups.[4] Factors that may affect the infant's pain responses include post-conceptional age, previous pain experience, and procedural technique.

PROGNOSIS Pain caused by blood sampling is associated with acute behavioural and physiological deterioration.[4] Experience of pain during heel puncture seems to heighten pain responses during subsequent blood sampling.[5] Other adverse effects of blood sampling include bleeding, bruising, haematoma, and infection.

AIMS OF INTERVENTION To obtain an adequate blood sample with minimal pain for the infant and minimal adverse effects of treatments.

OUTCOMES We found no easily administered, widely accepted assessment of pain in infants. Where available, we have analysed the proportion of infants crying, or the duration of crying. Other pain related responses measured in the studies included facial expressions (the number of specific expressions, or the duration of those expressions), heart rate, and transcutaneous oxygen saturation levels. Studies used composite scales composed of behavioural and cardiorespiratory signs of pain related distress, or both, only some of which have been validated, such as the Premature Infant Pain

Profile (see glossary, p 454) scale. We have not pooled differences in pain related responses or for different pain scales. The assessment of pain is difficult in pre-verbal children. Pain assessment methods varied in the RCTs, and a validated scale was not always used. Some measurements (e.g. facial expression) are difficult to score objectively. In many RCTs, blinding was not possible (e.g. where pacifiers were used).

METHODS *Clinical Evidence* search and appraisal May 2003, and additional hand searches by contributors.

QUESTION **What are the effects of interventions to reduce pain related distress during heel puncture?**

OPTION **ORAL SWEET SOLUTIONS**

RCTs have found that oral sucrose, glucose, or other sweeteners reduce pain responses in preterm and term infants (particularly the duration of crying when given 2 minutes before blood sampling) compared with water or no treatment. Evidence for sucrose in term infants was more limited; less than half of the RCTs found an effect. One small RCT found no significant difference between multiple and single doses of sucrose in pain scores for heel puncture. We found no clear evidence that any one sugar is superior to the others. There was weak evidence that solutions of 24% or more were more effective. Three RCTs in term infants found that sucrose plus pacifier was more effective than pacifier alone, but one RCT found no effect in preterm infants.

Benefits: **Sucrose:** We found one systematic review (search date 2001,[6] 4 RCTs[7–10]) and three additional RCTs[11–13] comparing oral sucrose (0.05–2.00 mL of 7.5–70%) versus water or no treatment in preterm newborns. All seven RCTs found that sucrose (24–70%) significantly reduced pain responses and pain scores compared with water. Three of these seven RCTs also found that the time spent crying during the procedure and the total duration of crying was significantly reduced with sucrose (25% and 50%).[7,9,13] One RCT found no significant difference between 15% sucrose and water.[13] We found one systematic review (search date 2001,[6] 7 RCTs [9,10,14–18]) and 12 additional RCTs [11–13,19–28] comparing oral sucrose (0.05–2.00 mL of 7.5–70%) versus water or no treatment in term newborns. Eight of the 19 RCTs found that sucrose (12–70%) significantly reduced pain scores compared with water.[10,12,15,17,23–26] Eight of the 19 RCTs found that sucrose decreased the percentage of time spent crying compared with water.[14,15,17,19–21,24,28] Nine of the 19 RCTs found that sucrose significantly reduced crying time (mean or median differences 16–90 seconds).[9,16,18,22–27] Two of the 19 RCTs found a significant difference only for infants given 25–50% sucrose and not for those given lower concentrations.[13,16] One RCT used a low concentration of sucrose (2 mL of 7.5%), and found no significant difference in duration of crying.[29] **Sucrose plus pacifier:** We found three RCTs comparing a pacifier (see glossary, p 454) dipped in 12–24% sucrose or table sugar crystals versus pacifier dipped in water.[27,28,30] One RCT was in preterm infants.[30] It found no significant difference in pain responses (mean Premature Infant Pain

Profile [PIPP] score [see glossary, p 454]) between pacifier dipped in 12–24% sucrose or table sugar crystals and pacifier dipped in water.[30] Two RCTs were in term infants.[27,28] Both RCTs found that pacifier dipped in 12–24% sucrose or table sugar crystals reduced crying time compared with pacifier dipped in water.[27,28] **Sucrose plus holding:** We found one RCT (94 term infants) comparing sucrose, sucrose plus holding, holding with water, and water alone.[15] It found that pain scores and duration of crying decreased in the holding group compared with no holding and in the sucrose groups compared with no sucrose, but the differences were of borderline significance. There was no evidence of an interaction between sucrose and holding (P = 0.37). We found no RCTs in preterm infants. **Glucose:** We found four systematic reviews (search dates 1995,[31] 2001,[6] 1998,[32] 2000;[33] 2 RCTs [14,34]), three additional RCTs, and one subsequent RCT.[26,35–37] One of the additional RCTs (crossover, 17 infants) was in preterm infants.[35] It found that 10% glucose significantly reduced mean pain scores compared with no treatment. Two RCTs identified by the systematic reviews, two additional RCTs, and one subsequent RCT were in term infants.[14,26,34,35,37] All five RCTs compared glucose (1–2 mL of 10–33% solution) with water or no treatment before heel puncture.[14,26,34,35] Two RCTs found fewer infants cried with 30% glucose compared with water or no treatment.[34,35] One RCT found that 30% glucose significantly reduced crying time (75% decrease) compared with no treatment, but it found no significant difference in crying time (50% decrease) between 10% glucose and no treatment (50% decrease).[34] One RCT found no significant difference in mean crying time between 12% glucose and water.[14] One RCT found a significant reduction in pain scores with 33% glucose compared with no treatment.[37] One RCT found no significant difference in mean crying time or pain scores between 12.5% glucose and water (pain: mean PIPP score reduced by 2.5; P < 0.001).[26] **Glucose plus pacifier:** We found three RCTs comparing a pacifier dipped in 10–33% glucose versus no treatment, water, glucose alone, or pacifier alone.[26,36,37] One crossover RCT was in preterm infants.[36] It found that glucose plus pacifier significantly reduced the mean pain score compared with no treatment (glucose plus pacifier *v* no treatment: reduction in mean PIPP score 3.6 for glucose plus pacifier; P = 0.001).[36] Two RCTs were in term infants.[26,37] The RCTs found that glucose (12.5% and 33%, respectively) dipped pacifiers significantly reduced crying time and pain score compared with glucose alone, water, or no treatment.[26,37] **Other sweeteners:** We found three systematic reviews (search dates 1995,[31] 2001,[6] 1998;[32] 1 RCT[17]) and one additional RCT in term infants.[38] The RCT in the review found that hydrogenated glucose (see glossary, p 454) significantly decreased pain scores, duration of first cry, and percentage of time spent crying compared with water, but found no significant difference compared with sucrose.[17] The additional RCT (120 term infants) comparing an artificial sweetener (10 parts cyclamate and 1 part saccharin) with water found small but significant differences in percentage of time crying and pain scores.[38] We found no RCTs in preterm infants. **Concentration of glucose or sucrose:** We found two systematic reviews (search dates 2001[6] and 1998;[32] 1 RCT[34]) and six additional RCTs of the effects of glucose or sucrose concentration in heel puncture.[14,16,17,22,34,39] We found no RCTs solely in preterm infants. We found one RCT of 60 term and preterm infants.[34] It found no significant difference between 10% and 30% glucose in the duration of crying or in the proportion of babies who cried at all (no crying: 40% with 10% glucose *v* 53% with 30% glucose; $P > 0.05$). Three RCTs were in term infants.[14,16,17] One RCT (75 neonates) found that increasing concentrations of sucrose (2 mL of 12.5%, 25%, and 50%) produced significantly greater reductions in duration of crying.[16] The other two RCTs (56 infants) found no difference in duration of crying with different sucrose concentrations (2 mL of 25–50% or 12–25% sucrose).[14,17] **Multiple doses of sweeteners:** We found one RCT (32 preterm neonates, mean gestation 31 weeks), which compared a single dose (0.5 mL) of 24% sucrose 2 minutes before heel puncture versus three doses given 2 minutes before the procedure, immediately before the procedure, and during the procedure.[11] Pain scores measured at five points during the procedure were significantly different only at the latest time. We found no RCTs in term infants. **Sucrose versus glucose:** We found two RCTs (226 term infants undergoing heel puncture) comparing glucose versus sucrose.[22,26] One RCT found that 30% sucrose reduced crying time by a mean of 30 seconds compared with 30% glucose ($P = 0.006$).[22] The second RCT found no significant difference between 12.5% sucrose and 12.5% glucose.[26] We found no RCTs in preterm infants. **Sucrose versus breast milk:** We found one small RCT (20 term infants).[28] It found that sucrose plus pacifier significantly reduced the percentage of time crying compared with colostrum plus pacifier. We found no RCTs in preterm infants.

Harms: No adverse effects from oral sucrose or glucose administered to full term or preterm infants were reported in any of the RCTs. Transient choking and oxygen desaturation have been associated with the administration of oral sweeteners (directly into the mouth and when administered on a pacifier).[40] The safety of repeated oral administration of sucrose or glucose has not been adequately investigated. There is no evidence that repeated dosing with sweeteners leads to conditioning. Theoretical adverse effects include hyperglycaemia and necrotising enterocolitis.

Comment: There is concern that parents, impressed with the calming effect of sweeteners, may continue to use it at home. This could be harmful in high concentrations or repeated doses. Some studies were crossover RCTs, which may produce biased estimates of the effect of sucrose if neonates become habituated to pain or if the washout period between interventions is too short.[7,9,12] Only some RCTs reported adequate concealment of allocation.[7,8,11,15,23,35,39] In one study, it was uncertain whether infants were randomly allocated.[20] Most had blinded measurement of at least some of the pain responses, particularly crying, on the basis of independent audio or video tape recordings. One RCT had no blinded outcome assessment.[9] We found inadequate evidence about the benefits or harms of repeated administration of sucrose or glucose for repeated blood sampling.

OPTION BREAST MILK OR BREAST FEEDING

RCTs found no evidence that breast milk or breast feeding reduced pain responses or crying in neonates undergoing heel puncture compared with water. One RCT found no evidence that breast milk plus pacifier was more effective than pacifier alone. One RCT found that breast feeding reduced pain responses compared with swaddling in the cot.

Benefits: **Breast milk:** We found one systematic review (search date 1998,[32] 2 RCTs,[18,34] 126 preterm and term neonates undergoing heel puncture) and two subsequent RCTs (177 term infants)[25,38] comparing breast milk or colostrums (1–2 mL) versus water. None found a significant effect of breast milk on duration of crying[18,25,34,38] or proportion of infants not crying.[34] **Breast milk plus pacifier:** One RCT (20 term infants) found no significant difference between infants given a pacifier (see glossary, p 454) dipped in breast milk versus a pacifier dipped in water.[28] **Breast feeding:** One RCT compared term infants who were held and breast fed with infants given water or breast milk in their cot (62 term infants).[25] No significant effect was found for breast feeding compared with water or breast milk on the duration of crying. Another RCT (30 term infants) compared breast feeding with being swaddled in the cot.[41] Breast feeding decreased the duration of grimacing (mean 17.2 seconds in breastfed *v* 83.3 seconds in swaddled babies) and the duration of crying (mean 8.8 seconds breastfed *v* 72.7 seconds).

Harms: None reported.

Comment: Concealment of allocation was not clearly stated in any RCT. Assessment of pain responses was blind in two RCTs[25,38] and not clearly stated in two other RCTs.[18,34]

OPTION TOPICAL ANAESTHETICS

Systematic reviews and additional RCTs found no evidence of reduced pain responses, particularly crying, following heel puncture with topical anaesthetic (lidocaine, lidocaine–prilocaine emulsion, or tetracaine [amethocaine]) compared with placebo.

Benefits: **Lidocaine or lidocaine–prilocaine emulsion:** We found three systematic reviews (search dates 1996,[42] 1998,[32] and 1998;[43] 5 RCTs[44–48]) and one additional RCT,[1] comparing lidocaine or lidocaine–prilocaine emulsion versus placebo in neonates undergoing heel puncture. Treatments were usually given 30–60 minutes before heel puncture, with the exception of one RCT that randomised infants to eight application times (10–120 minutes before heel puncture).[47] The six RCTs used different assessments of pain responses. Three RCTs included 186 preterm neonates,[1,44,45] and three RCTs included 192 infants who were mainly term neonates.[46–48] None of the RCTs found a significant difference in pain scores between lidocaine or lidocaine–prilocaine emulsion and placebo. One RCT found no significant difference between lidocaine–prilocaine emulsion and placebo in the proportion of infants who cried during the procedure (54/56 [96%] *v* 52/54 [96%]).[47] **Tetracaine (amethocaine) versus placebo:** One RCT

(60 infants, median gestation 36 weeks, undergoing heel puncture using an automated device) found no significant difference between tetracaine and placebo in pain score or the proportion of infants who cried (20/30 [67%] with tetracaine *v* 13/29 [45%]; ARI +22%, 95% CI –4% to +47%).[49] **Topical anaesthetic versus sucrose:** We found no studies of topical anaesthetic versus sweet solutions for heel puncture. **Topical anaesthetic versus pacifiers:** We found no RCTs.

Harms: We found six RCTs (250 infants), which reported absence of adverse reactions to lidocaine–prilocaine emulsion or to placebo, or no difference in minor, transient local reactions.[1,46–48,50,51] One cohort study (500 neonates) found unusual cutaneous effects associated with lidocaine–prilocaine emulsion in four neonates under 32 weeks' gestation.[52] Methaemoglobinaemia can occur with the prilocaine constituent of lidocaine–prilocaine emulsion. Levels of methaemoglobin over 25–30% can cause clinical symptoms of hypoxia.[53] We found one systematic review (search date 1996, 12 RCTs or cohort studies, > 355 neonates)[42] and two subsequent RCTs (167 neonates)[1,53] of lidocaine–prilocaine emulsion for heel puncture, venepuncture, circumcision, or lumbar puncture. All but one of these studies found mean methaemoglobin levels less than 1.5% in neonates given lidocaine–prilocaine emulsion. The other RCT (47 preterm and term infants given lidocaine–prilocaine emulsion) found that the highest mean methaemoglobin levels (2.3%, range 0.6–6.2%) occurred after 15 days of repeated doses of lidocaine–prilocaine emulsion.[52] A systematic review found two case reports of neonates who were treated with oxygen at methaemoglobin levels of 12% and 16%.[42] No local skin reactions were seen after application of tetracaine or placebo in the 140 neonates studied.

Comment: Some of the studies reported adequate concealment of allocation.[51,54–56] Three RCTs used videotaped recordings of pain responses to blind assessors to the intervention.[50,51,54,55] In the other RCTs, although placebo ointment was used, pain responses were assessed by observers at the time of the procedure, rather than by scoring of video film. Deduction of treatment allocation may have been possible in the studies including lidocaine–prilocaine emulsion because of the smell and skin blanching caused by lidocaine–prilocaine emulsion. One study excluded 25% of children who had high behaviour scores before puncture, and presented results only for selected subgroups.[50] The findings of this study may be difficult to generalise.

OPTION PACIFIERS

Eight RCTs have found reduced pain responses in term and preterm infants given pacifiers compared with no treatment before heel puncture. Three RCTs found weak evidence that pacifiers dipped in sucrose reduced pain responses compared with pacifiers alone.

Benefits: **Pacifier alone:** We found one systematic review (search date 2001,[6] 1 RCT[30]) and seven additional RCTs comparing pacifiers (see glossary, p 454) versus no treatment (445 infants, of whom

271 were preterm).[24,30,36,57–60] Four of the RCTs were crossover trials.[30,36,57,58] Pacifiers were given 2–5 minutes before heel puncture. RCTs found that pacifiers significantly reduced pain responses[36,45,59] or the percentage of time spent in a distressed, fussy, or awake state compared with no pacifiers.[58,59] In the three RCTs in term infants, those given a pacifier cried for significantly less time,[24,57,60] spent less time in fussy or awake states,[60] or had reduced pain score.[57] However, reductions were not significant for all measures of pain; in one study grimacing was not significantly reduced by the pacifier[24] and, in another, the pain score was similar during the procedure but fell more quickly in babies given pacifiers.[57] **Pacifier plus multimodal sensory stimulation:** We found two RCTs.[36,37] They found that a pacifier plus multimodal sensory stimulation (pacifer plus glucose, massage, visual, and auditory stimulation) during heel puncture significantly reduced the pain score when compared with no treatment,[36] or pacifier alone, or glucose plus pacifier.[37] One RCT (crossover, 17 preterm infants) found a mean Premature Infant Pain Profile score (see glossary, p 454) reduction when compared with no pacifier (7.15; $P < 0.001$) and when compared with glucose plus pacifer, pacifier alone, or glucose alone (mean Premature Infant Pain Profile score reduction 2.6–4.55; $P < 0.01$ for each of the 3 comparisons).[36] Another RCT found that multimodal sensory stimulation was even more effective than glucose plus pacifier in reducing pain scores in term infants.[37] **Pacifiers plus sucrose:** See benefits of oral sweet solutions, p 444.

Harms: No adverse effects were reported in any of the studies. The use of pacifiers has been associated with transient choking and oxygen desaturation.

Comment: None of the studies explicitly defined the method of allocation to pacifier or no treatment. Three RCTs blinded assessors to the intervention by analysing audio tapes of crying during the procedure.[36,58,60] Measurement of pain responses on the basis of facial expressions were not blinded to the pacifiers or music intervention.

OPTION PHYSICAL CONTACT (HOLDING, ROCKING, POSITIONING, SWADDLING, WARMING, AND PRIOR HANDLING)

We found insufficient evidence from one small RCT about the effects of swaddling. Two RCTs have found that holding reduces crying during heel puncture compared with swaddling. One RCT found that sucrose did not appear to modify the effect of holding. We found limited evidence that rocking reduces pain related stress compared with placebo. One RCT found limited evidence that pain responses were reduced by tucking the arms and legs into a mid-line flexed position during heel puncture, or by avoiding stressful handling before heel puncture. One RCT found no significant difference in pain score between prone position and either side or supine position during heel puncture. Two RCTs found no effect of warming before heel puncture.

Benefits: **Swaddling versus no swaddling:** We found no systematic review but found one small crossover RCT (15 neonates).[61] It found no significant difference in facial expressions of pain or arousal state between swaddling immediately after heel puncture and no swaddling.[61] **Holding versus swaddling:** We found no systematic review but found two RCTs (124 term infants undergoing heel puncture).[15,62] One RCT (30 infants) compared holding the baby with skin to skin contact versus being swaddled in a crib.[62] It found that holding significantly reduced crying and grimacing compared with swaddling (proportion crying during procedure 8% *v* 45%; ARR 37%, CI not reported; NNT 3, 95% CI 2 to 13). **Rocking:** We found no systematic review but found two RCTs comparing rocking versus no intervention.[8,60] One RCT (44 preterm infants, 25–34 weeks' gestation) compared 0.05 mL water given before heel puncture versus simulated rocking using a respirator attached to an air mattress.[8] The study found no significant differences in facial expressions of pain. The other RCT (40 term neonates) compared no intervention with being held vertically and rocked by the examiner.[60] The study found that rocking reduced the duration of crying ($P = 0.05$) during the procedure and the risk of persistent crying (2/20 [10%] with rocking *v* 9/20 [45%] with no intervention; ARR 35%, CI 10% to 60%; NNT 3, 95% CI 2 to 10). **Positioning:** We found no systematic review but found four RCTs comparing positioning, swaddling, or stressful handling versus no intervention.[30,61,63,64] One crossover RCT (122 preterm infants, 25–34 weeks' gestation, undergoing heel puncture) compared prone position versus side or supine position.[30] The study found no significant difference in the mean pain score. Another RCT (crossover, 30 preterm neonates, 25–35 weeks' gestation) compared facilitative tucking during and after heel puncture (defined as the gentle containment of arms and legs in a flexed, mid-line position) versus no intervention.[63] The RCT found a significant reduction in the total crying time and time to quietening (mean cry duration 2.2 *v* 0.3 minutes; $P < 0.001$). The fourth RCT (48 mainly preterm infants, mean gestation < 35 weeks) compared handling (as if being prepared for a lumbar puncture) with avoidance of handling for 10 minutes prior to heel puncture.[64] The study found that prior handling increased facial expressions of pain, the proportion of time crying, and crying at all during the 2 minutes after heel puncture (21/21 [100%] handled babies cried *v* 21/27 [78%] non-handled babies; ARR +22%; CI –24% to +68%). **Warming:** We found one systematic review (search date 1998,[32] 1 RCT[65]) and one subsequent RCT.[66] The RCT identified by the review compared 57 term infants undergoing heel puncture on 80 occasions with an automated lancet with (41 infants) or without (40 infants) prior warming of the heel. The heel was warmed for 10 minutes with a gel pack at 40 °C. It found no significant difference in the proportion of infants who grimaced and cried between warming and not warming (14/41 [34%] *v* 10/40 [25%]; RR 1.4, 95% CI 0.7 to 2.7). Sampling time was slightly longer in the warmed heels (median time 44 seconds, interquartile range 25–62 seconds *v* 40 seconds, interquartile range 28–72 seconds), but the number of repeat punctures was slightly lower (5/41 [12%] *v* 8/40 [20%]; RR 0.6, 0.2 to 1.7). The subsequent RCT (100 preterm infants) found no significant difference in the crying time or number of repeated punctures after heel warming compared with no warming.[66]

Harms: No adverse events were reported for any of these interventions.

Comment: **Holding:** Assessment of crying was based on analysis of audio or videotape recordings and was blind to the sucrose intervention but not to holding.[15,62] Assessments based on facial expressions were not blind to the intervention. **Rocking:** The method of allocation to rocking or standard care was adequate in one study[8] and unclear in the other.[59] Both studies used blinded assessment of pain responses based on video[8] and audio tape[60] recordings. **Position, swaddling, and prior handling:** None of the studies explicitly reported the method of allocation to the interventions, and only the study comparing handling versus no handling assessed pain responses blind to the intervention.[64] **Warming:** The method of allocation was not reported and assessment of outcomes was not blind to the intervention.

QUESTION **What are the effects of interventions to reduce pain related distress during venepuncture?**

OPTION **ORAL SWEET SOLUTIONS**

RCTs have found that oral sucrose or glucose reduce pain responses (particularly the duration of crying) compared with water, topical anaesthetic or no treatment in term and preterm infants undergoing venepuncture. One RCT found that 25% glucose was more effective than 10% glucose. We found no RCTs of other sweetners.

Benefits: **Sucrose:** We found two systematic reviews (search dates 1995,[31] 2001;[6] 2 RCTs[39,67]) and one additional RCT.[68] One RCT (28 infants) in the review was in preterm infants.[67] It found that 24% sucrose reduced crying time compared with water but found no significant difference between 12% sucrose and water (20 infants: mean duration of crying 19 seconds with 24% sucrose *v* 73 seconds with water). One RCT identified by the review and the additional RCT were in term infants.[39,68] Both RCTs (201 infants) found that 24–30% sucrose significantly reduced the duration of crying and pain scores compared with water or no treatment. **Glucose:** We found four RCTs comparing 2 mL of 10–30% glucose versus water in infants undergoing venepuncture.[35,39,69,70] One RCT (60 infants) was in preterm infants.[69] It found that 25% glucose significantly reduced the duration of crying compared with water but found no significant difference between 10% glucose and water (mean duration of crying: 40.5 seconds [SD 38.98] with 25% glucose *v* 68.9 seconds [SD 44.15] with 10% glucose *v* 85.5 seconds [SD 44.1] with water). Three RCTs were in term infants.[35,39,70] The first RCT (60 infants) found that glucose significantly reduced pain scores compared with water but found no difference in the proportion of infants crying (46% with glucose *v* 39% with water).[35] The second RCT (75 infants) found significantly reduced median pain scores with glucose compared with water or no treatment (median pain score difference 2 [glucose 5, water 7], 95% CI 1 to 4; P = 0.005).[39] The third RCT (201 infants) compared 30% glucose plus placebo on the skin versus lidocaine–prilocaine topical anaesthetic cream plus oral water.[70] It found that glucose significantly improved Premature Infant Pain Profile (PIPP) score (see glossary, p 454) and duration of pain compared with topical anaesthetic cream (PIPP scores: 4.6 with glucose *v* 5.7 with anaesthetic cream, P = 0.0314; median duration of crying: 1 second with glucose *v* 18 seconds with topical anaesthetic, P < 0.001). It also found that glucose significantly reduced the proportion of infants thought to have pain (defined as PIPP > 6: 19.3% with glucose *v* 41.7% with anaesthetic cream, P = 0.0007). **Other sweeteners:** We found no RCTs of other sweeteners for venepuncture. **Concentration of glucose or sucrose:** One RCT found that 25% glucose significantly reduced the duration of crying compared with 10% glucose (40.5 seconds *v* 68.9 seconds).[69] **Sucrose versus glucose:** One RCT (150 term infants) found no significant difference between 30% sucrose and 30% glucose in pain scores.[39]

Harms: No adverse effects from oral sucrose or glucose administered to full term or preterm infants were reported in any of the RCTs. Transient choking and oxygen desaturation have been associated with the administration of oral sweeteners (directly into the mouth and when administered on a pacifier).[40] The safety of repeated oral administration of sucrose or glucose has not been adequately investigated. Theoretical adverse effects include hyperglycaemia and necrotising enterocolitis.

Comment: See comment under oral sweet solutions with heel puncture, p 446.

OPTION TOPICAL ANAESTHETICS

Four RCTs found limited evidence that lidocaine–prilocaine emulsion reduced pain responses to venepuncture compared with placebo. Two RCTs found that tetracaine (amethocaine) gel reduced pain and crying during venepuncture compared with placebo.

Benefits: **Lidocaine–prilocaine emulsion:** We found two systematic reviews (search dates 1996[42] and 1998;[32] 2 RCTs[54,71]) and two additional RCTs[50,51], which compared lidocaine–prilocaine emulsion versus placebo in infants undergoing venepuncture. One RCT (120 term infants) found that lidocaine–prilocaine emulsion significantly reduced the duration of crying and pain score at 15 seconds after venepuncture compared with placebo, but found no significant difference in pain score 60 seconds after venepuncture (median duration of crying: 12 seconds *v* 31 seconds; P < 0.05; pain score: Neonatal Facial Coding System score (see glossary, p 454) 287 *v* 374; P = 0.02).[54] The second RCT (60 children) found that 19/28 in the lidocaine–prilocaine emulsion group and 14/28 in the placebo group did not cry at all during the procedure.[71] The study did not measure duration of crying or pain score. The third RCT (41 infants and toddlers) found that lidocaine–prilocaine emulsion significantly reduced behavioural pain score compared with placebo (P < 0.01).[50] The fourth RCT (19 preterm infants) found no significant difference in pain or total duration of crying between lidocaine–prilocaine emulsion and placebo (pain assessed using Neonatal Facial Coding System score, mean difference 0, 95% CI −2.00 to +1.75; median difference in duration of crying: −22 seconds, 95% CI −96 seconds to +24 seconds).[51] **Tetracaine (amethocaine) versus placebo:** Two RCTs (80 preterm and term neonates undergoing venepuncture) found that tetracaine significantly reduced pain scores and the proportion who cried compared with placebo (4/19 [21%] with tetracaine *v* 15/20 [75%] with placebo; ARR 54%, 95% CI 2% to 80%; NNT 2, 95% CI 1 to 4).[55,56] **Topical anaesthetic versus sucrose:** We found one RCT (55 venepunctures in 51 term neonates), which compared lidocaine–prilocaine emulsion versus 24% sucrose versus lidocaine–prilocaine emulsion plus sucrose versus water.[68] Crying was taped and assessed blind to treatment. Lidocaine–prilocaine emulsion alone was reported to be less effective than sucrose alone or lidocaine–prilocaine emulsion plus sucrose, but analyses were not presented. **Topical anaesthetic versus oral glucose:** See oral sweet solutions, p 451. **Topical anaesthetic versus pacifiers:** We found no RCTs.

Harms: See harms under topical anaesthetics with heel puncture, p 448.

Comment: Some of the studies reported adequate concealment of allocation.[46,47,49] One RCT used videotaped recordings of pain responses to blind assessors to the intervention.[49]

OPTION PACIFIERS

One RCT found that pacifiers reduced pain responses compared with water or no treatment in term infants undergoing venepuncture.

Benefits: We found one RCT (100 term infants undergoing venepuncture) comparing a pacifier (see glossary, p 454) or a pacifier plus sucrose versus no treatment or 2 mL water orally in infants.[67] The study found a significant reduction in the pain score during the procedure (median difference in 10 point pain score 5 for pacifiers alone *v* water and 6 for pacifiers plus sucrose *v* water; $P < 0.0001$).

Harms: The RCT reported no adverse effects.[67] The use of pacifiers has been associated with transient choking and oxygen desaturation.

Comment: The RCT did not explicitly define the method of allocation to pacifier or no treatment.[67]

OPTION BREAST FEEDING New

One RCT found that breast feeding during venepuncture reduced pain responses compared with oral water or being held. The RCT found no significant difference in pain response between breast feeding and oral glucose

Benefits: We found no systematic reviews but we found one RCT.[72] The RCT (180 term infants) compared four treatments while the infant was held in its mother's arms during venepuncture: breast feeding, no intervention, sterile water, and 30% glucose plus pacifier. It found that breast feeding significantly reduced pain response compared with holding alone or sterile water (median premature infant pain profile score [see glossary, p 454]: 4.5 with breast feeding *v* 13 with holding *v* 12 with sterile water; $P < 0.0001$ for breast feeding *v* holding; $P < 0.0001$ for breast feeding *v* sterile water). It found no significant difference in pain response between breast feeding and glucose (median premature infant pain profile score 4.5 with breast feeding *v* 4 with glucose, $P = 0.28$).

Harms: The RCT found no adverse effects.[72]

Comment: Blinding was impossible in the RCT because of the nature of the interventions.[72]

GLOSSARY

Hydrogenated glucose syrup An aqueous solution of hydrogenated part hydrolysed starch composed of a mixture of mainly maltitol with sorbitol and hydrogenated oligosaccharides and polysaccharides. Preparations containing a minimum 98% maltitol are known as maltitol syrup.

Neonatal Facial Coding System (NFCS) score Facial coding system used to evaluate pain responses in full term and preterm infants. Presence or absence of six facial actions (e.g. eyes squeezed shut, deepening of the naso-labial furrow) is recorded.

Pacifier A device with a teat that a baby sucks on for comfort. Some pacifiers can deliver a liquid to the baby. Also known as a "dummy", "soother", or "plug" in some countries.

Premature Infant Pain Profile (PIPP) score A seven item composite scale that scores behavioural and cardiorespiratory pain responses coded 0 to 3 (maximum score 21).

Substantive changes

Oral sweet solutions (venepuncture) One RCT added;[70] conclusions unchanged.

REFERENCES

1. Stevens B, Johnston C, Taddio A, et al. Management of pain from heel lance with lidocaine–prilocaine (EMLA) cream: is it safe and efficacious in preterm infants? *J Dev Behav Pediatr* 1999;20:216–221.
2. Johnston CC, Collinge JM, Henderson SJ, et al. A cross-sectional survey of pain and pharmacological analgesia in Canadian neonatal intensive care units. *Clin J Pain* 1997;13:308–312.
3. Porter FL, Anand KJS. Epidemiology of pain in neonates. *Res Clin Forum* 1998;20:9–18.
4. Anand K, Stevens BJ, McGrath PJ. *Pain in neonates*. Amsterdam: Elsevier Science BV, 2000.
5. Taddio A, Gurguis MG, Koren G. Lidocaine-prilocaine cream versus tetracaine gel for procedural pain in children. *Ann Pharmacother* 2002;36:687–692.
6. Stevens B, Yamada J, Ohlsson A. Sucrose for analgesia in newborn infants undergoing painful procedures. In: The Cochrane Library, Issue 3, 2002. Oxford: Update Software. Search date 2001; primary sources Medline, Embase, Reference Update, Cochrane Library, and hand searches of personal files, bibliographies, recent neonatal and pain journals, and conference proceedings.
7. Bucher HU, Moser T, von Siebenthal K, et al. Sucrose reduces pain reaction to heel lancing in preterm infants: a placebo-controlled, randomized and masked study. *Pediatr Res* 1995;38:332–335.
8. Johnston CC, Stremler RL, Stevens BJ, et al. Effectiveness of oral sucrose and simulated rocking on pain response in preterm neonates. *Pain* 1997;72:193–199.
9. Ramenghi LA, Wood CM, Griffith GC, et al. Reduction of pain response in premature infants using intraoral sucrose. *Arch Dis Child Fetal Neonatal Ed* 1996;74:F126–F128.
10. Gibbins SA. Efficacy and safety of sucrose for procedural pain relief in preterm and term neonates. *Dissert Abstract Int* 2001;62–04B:1804.
11. Johnston CC, Stremler R, Horton L, et al. Effect of repeated doses of sucrose during heel stick procedure in preterm neonates. *Biol Neonate* 1999;75:160–166.
12. Mellah D, Gourrier E, Merbouche S, et al. Analgesia with saccharose during heel capillary prick. A randomized study in 37 newborns of over 33 weeks of amenorrhea. *Arch Pediatr* 1999;6:610–616 [in French].
13. Storm H, Fremming A. Food intake and oral sucrose in preterms prior to heel prick. *Acta Paediatr* 2002;91:555–560.
14. Abad Massanet F, Diaz Gomez NM, Domenech Martinez E, et al. Analgesic effect of oral sweet solution in newborns. *An Esp Pediatr* 1995;43:351–354.
15. Gormally S, Barr RG, Wertheim L, et al. Contact and nutrient caregiving effects on newborn infant pain responses. *Dev Med Child Neurol* 2001;43:28–38.
16. Haouari N, Wood C, Griffiths G, et al. The analgesic effect of sucrose in full term infants: a randomised controlled trial. *BMJ* 1995;310:1498–1500.
17. Ramenghi LA, Griffith GC, Wood CM, et al. Effect of non-sucrose sweet tasting solution on neonatal heel prick responses. *Arch Dis Child Fetal Neonatal Ed* 1996;74:F129–F131.
18. Ors R, Ozek E, Baysoy G, et al. Comparison of sucrose and human milk on pain response in newborns. *Eur J Pediatr* 1999;158:63–66.
19. Blass EM, Hoffmeyer LB. Sucrose as an analgesic for newborn infants. *Pediatrics* 1991;87:215–218.
20. Blass EM. Pain-reducing properties of sucrose in human newborns. *Chem Senses* 1995;20:29–35.

21. Blass EM. Milk-induced hypoalgesia in human newborns. *Pediatrics* 1997:99:825–829.
22. Isik U, Ozek E, Bilgen H, et al. Comparison of oral glucose and sucrose solutions on pain response in neonates. *J Pain* 2000;1:275–278.
23. Overgaard C, Knudsen A. Pain-relieving effect of sucrose in newborns during heel prick. *Biol Neonate* 1999;75:279–284.
24. Blass EM, Watt LB. Suckling- and sucrose-induced analgesia in human newborns. *Pain* 1999;83:611–623.
25. Bilgen H, Ozek E, Cebeci D, et al. Comparison of sucrose, expressed breast milk, and breast-feeding on the neonatal response to heel prick. *J Pain* 2001;2:301–305.
26. Akman I, Zek E, Bilgen H, et al. Sweet solutions and pacifiers for pain relief in newborn infants. *J Pain* 2002;3:199–202
27. Greenberg CS. A sugar-coated pacifier reduces procedural pain in newborns. *Pediatr Nurs* 2002;28:271–277.
28. Blass EM, Miller LW. Effects of colostrum in newborn humans: dissociation between analgesic and cardiac effects. *J Dev Behav Pediatr* 2001;22:385–390.
29. Rushforth JA, Levene MI. Effect of sucrose on crying in response to heel stab. *Arch Dis Child* 1993;69:388–389.
30. Stevens B, Johnston C, Franck L, et al. The efficacy of developmentally sensitive interventions and sucrose for relieving procedural pain in very low birth weight neonates. *Nurs Res* 1999;48:35–43.
31. Stevens B, Taddio A, Ohlsson A, et al. The efficacy of sucrose for relieving procedural pain in neonates: a systematic review and meta-analysis. *Acta Paediatr* 1997;86:837–842. Search date 1995; primary sources Medline, Embase, Reference Update, and hand searches of personal files, bibliographies, most recent neonatal and pain journals, and conference proceedings.
32. Ohlsson A, Taddio A, Jadad AR, et al. Evidence-based decision making, systematic reviews and the Cochrane collaboration: implications for neonatal analgesia. In: Anand K, Stevens B, McGrath PJ, eds. *Pain in Neonates*. Amsterdam: Elsevier Science BV, 2000:251–268. Search date 1998; primary sources Medline, Cochrane Library, hand searches of personal files, and reference lists.
33. Bauer K, Versmold H. Oral sugar solutions in pain therapy of neonates and premature infants. *Z Geburtshilfe Neonatol* 2001;205:80–85. Search date 2000; primary source PubMed.
34. Skogsdal Y, Eriksson M, Schollin J. Analgesia in newborns given oral glucose. *Acta Paediatr* 1997;86:217–220.
35. Eriksson M, Gradin M, Schollin J. Oral glucose and venepuncture reduce blood sampling pain in newborns. *Early Hum Dev* 1999;55:211–218.
36. Bellieni CV, Buonocore G, Nenci A, et al. Sensorial saturation: an effective analgesic tool for heel-prick in preterm infants: a prospective randomized trial. *Biol Neonate* 2001;80:15–18.
37. Bellieni CV, Bagnoli F, Perrone S, et al. Effect of multisensory stimulation on analgesia in term neonates: a randomized controlled trial. *Pediatr Res* 2002;51:460–463.
38. Bucher HU, Baumgartner R, Bucher N, et al. Artificial sweetener reduces nociceptive reaction in term newborn infants. *Early Hum Dev* 2000:59:51–60.
39. Carbajal R, Chauvet X, Couderc S, et al. Randomised trial of analgesic effects of sucrose, glucose, and pacifiers in term neonates. *BMJ* 1999;319:1393–1397.
40. Horitz N. Does oral glucose reduce the pain of neonatal procedure? *Arch Dis Child* 2002;80–81.
41. Gray L, Miller LW, Philipp BL, et al. Breastfeeding is analgesic in healthy newborns. *Pediatrics* 2002;109:590–593.
42. Taddio A, Ohlsson A, Einarson TR, et al. A systematic review of lidocaine–prilocaine cream (EMLA) in the treatment of acute pain in neonates. *Pediatrics* 1998;101:E1. Search date 1996; primary sources Medline, Embase, Reference Update, and hand searches of personal files and meeting proceedings.
43. Essink-Tjebbes CM, Hekster YA, Liem KD, et al. Topical use of local anesthetics in neonates. *Pharm World Sci* 1999;21:173–176. Search date 1998; primary source Medline.
44. Ramaioli F, Amice De D, Guzinska K, et al. EMLA cream and the premature infant [abstract]. *Int Monitor Reg Anaesthesia* 1993;59.
45. Stevens B, Johnston C, Taddio A, et al. *The safety and efficacy of EMLA for heel lance in premature neonates*. International Association for the Study of Pain, 8th World Congress on Pain, Vancouver, Canada 1996;239:181–182.
46. Rushforth JA, Griffiths G, Thorpe H, et al. Can topical lignocaine reduce behavioural response to heel prick? *Arch Dis Child Fetal Neonatal Ed* 1995;72:F49–F51.
47. Larsson BA, Jylli L, Lagercrantz H, et al. Does a local anaesthetic cream (EMLA) alleviate pain from heel-lancing in neonates? *Acta Anaesthesiol Scand* 1995;39:1028–1031.
48. Wester U. Analgesic effect of lidocaine ointment on intact skin in neonates. *Acta Paediatr* 1993;82:791.
49. Jain A, Rutter N, Ratnayaka M. Topical amethocaine gel for pain relief of heel prick blood sampling: a randomised double blind controlled trial. *Arch Dis Child Fetal Neonatal Ed* 2001;84:F56–F59.
50. Robieux I, Kumar R, Radhakrishnan S, et al. Assessing pain and analgesia with a lidocaine–prilocaine emulsion in infants and toddlers during venipuncture. *J Pediatr* 1991;118:971–973.
51. Acharya AB, Bustani PC, Phillips JD, et al. Randomised controlled trial of eutectic mixture of local anaesthetics cream for venepuncture in healthy preterm infants. *Arch Dis Child Fetal Neonatal Ed* 1998;78:F138–F142.
52. Gourrier E, Karoubi P, el Hanache A, et al. Use of EMLA cream in a department of neonatology. *Pain* 1996;68:431–434.
53. Brisman M, Ljung BM, Otterbom I, et al. Methaemoglobin formation after the use of EMLA cream in term neonates. *Acta Paediatr* 1998;87:1191–1194.
54. Larsson BA, Tannfeldt G, Lagercrantz H, et al. Alleviation of the pain of venepuncture in neonates. *Acta Paediatr* 1998;87:774–779.
55. Jain A, Rutter N. Does topical amethocaine gel reduce the pain of venepuncture in newborn infants? A randomised double blind controlled trial. *Arch Dis Child Fetal Neonatal Ed* 2000;83:F207–F210.
56. Moore J. No more tears: a randomized controlled double-blind trial of Amethocaine gel vs. placebo in the management of procedural pain in neonates. *J Adv Nurs* 2001;34:475–482.
57. Bo LK, Callaghan P. Soothing pain-elicited distress in Chinese neonates. *Pediatrics* 2000:105:E49.
58. Corbo MG, Mansi G, Stagni A, et al. Nonnutritive sucking during heelstick procedures decreases behavioral distress in the newborn infant. *Biol Neonate* 2000;77:162–167.

59. Field T, Goldson E. Pacifying effects of nonnutritive sucking on term and preterm neonates during heelstick procedures. *Pediatrics* 1984;74:1012–1015.
60. Campos RG. Rocking and pacifiers: two comforting interventions for heelstick pain. *Res Nurs Health* 1994;17:321–331.
61. Fearon I, Kisilevsky BS, Hains SMJ, et al. Swaddling after heel lance: age-specific effects on behavioural recovery in preterm infants. *J Dev Behav Pediatr* 1997;18:222–232.
62. Gray L, Watt L, Blass EM. Skin-to-skin contact is analgesic in healthy newborns. *Pediatrics* 2000;105(1):e14.
63. Corff KE, Seideman R, Venkataraman PS, et al. Facilitated tucking: a nonpharmacologic comfort measure for pain in preterm neonates. *J Obstet Gynecol Neonatal Nurs* 1995;24:143–147.
64. Porter FL, Wolf CM, Miller JP. The effect of handling and immobilization on the response to acute pain in newborn infants. *Pediatrics* 1998;102:1383–1389.
65. Barker DP, Willetts B, Cappendijk VC, et al. Capillary blood sampling: should the heel be warmed? *Arch Dis Child Fetal Neonatal Ed* 1996;74:F139–F140.
66. Janes M, Pinelli J, Landry S, et al. Comparison of capillary blood sampling using an automated incision device with and without warming the heel. *J Perinatol* 2002;22:154–158.
67. Abad F, Diaz NM, Domenech E, et al. Oral sweet solution reduces pain-related behaviour in preterm infants. *Acta Paediatr* 1996;85:854–858.
68. Abad F, Diaz-Gomez NM, Domenech E, et al. Oral sucrose compares favourably with lidocaine–prilocaine cream for pain relief during venepuncture in neonates. *Acta Paediatr* 2001;90:160–165.
69. Deshmukh LS, Udani RH. Analgesic effect of oral glucose in preterm infants during venipuncture: a double blind, randomized, controlled trial. *J Trop Pediatr* 2002;48:138–141.
70. Gradin M, Eriksson M, Holmqvist G, et al. Pain reduction at venepuncture in newborns: oral glucose compared with local anesthetic cream. *Pediatrics* 2002;110:1053–1057.
71. Lindh V, Wiklund U, Hakansson S. Assessment of the effect of EMLA during venipuncture in the newborn by analysis of heart rate variability. *Pain* 2000;86:247–254.
72. Carbajal R, Veerapen S, Couderc S, et al. Analgesic effect of breast feeding in term neonates: randomised controlled trial. *BMJ* 2003;326:13.

Deborah Pritchard
Medical Assessor (Paediatrics)
Medicines and Healthcare Products
Regulatory Agency
London
UK

Competing interests: None declared.

Sudden infant death syndrome

Search date March 2003

David Creery and Angelo Mikrogianakis

QUESTIONS

INTERVENTIONS

*Observational evidence only, RCTs unlikely to be conducted

See glossary, p 463

Key Messages

- **Advice to avoid prone sleeping** Several observational studies found that campaigns involving advice to encourage non-prone sleeping positions were followed by a reduced incidence of sudden infant death syndrome. RCTs are unlikely to be conducted.
- **Advice to avoid tobacco smoke exposure** Several observational studies found limited evidence that campaigns to reduce several risk factors for sudden infant death, which included tobacco smoke exposure, were followed by a reduced incidence of sudden infant death syndrome. RCTs are unlikely to be conducted.
- **Advice to avoid bed sharing** One observational study found that a campaign to reduce several risk factors for sudden infant death, which included advice to avoid bed sharing, was followed by a reduced incidence of sudden infant death syndrome. RCTs are unlikely to be conducted.
- **Advice to avoid over heating or over wrapping** Three observational studies found limited evidence that campaigns to reduce several risk factors for sudden infant death, which included over wrapping, were followed by a reduced incidence of sudden infant death syndrome. RCTs are unlikely to be conducted.
- **Advice to avoid soft sleeping surfaces** We found no evidence on the effects of avoiding soft sleeping surfaces in the prevention of sudden infant death syndrome.
- **Advice to breastfeed** One non-systematic review of observational studies and three additional observational studies found that campaigns to reduce several risk factors for sudden infant death, which included advice to breastfeed, were followed by a reduced incidence of sudden infant death syndrome. In some countries, however, incidence had begun to fall before the national advice campaigns. RCTs are unlikely to be conducted.

- **Advice to promote soother use** We found insufficient evidence on soother use in the prevention of sudden infant death syndrome.

DEFINITION Sudden infant death syndrome (SIDS) is the sudden death of an infant aged under 1 year that remains unexplained after review of the clinical history, examination of the scene of death, and postmortem.

INCIDENCE/ PREVALENCE The incidence of SIDS has varied over time and among nations (incidence per 1000 live births of SIDS in 1996: Netherlands 0.3, Japan 0.4, Canada 0.5, England and Wales 0.7, USA 0.8, and Australia 0.9).[1]

AETIOLOGY/ RISK FACTORS By definition, the cause of SIDS is not known. Observational studies have found an association between SIDS and several risk factors including prone sleeping (see glossary, p 463) position,[2,3] prenatal or postnatal exposure to tobacco smoke,[4] soft sleeping surfaces,[5,6] hyperthermia/over wrapping (see tables A, B, and C on web extra),[7,8] bed sharing (particularly with mothers who smoke),[9,10] lack of breastfeeding,[11,12] and soother (see glossary, p 463) use.[7,13]

PROGNOSIS Although by definition prognosis is not applicable for an affected infant, the incidence of SIDS is increased in the siblings of that infant.[14,15]

AIMS OF INTERVENTION To reduce the incidence of SIDS, with minimal adverse effects from interventions.

OUTCOMES Incidence of SIDS; adverse effects of interventions, measured directly or by quality of life questionnaires.

METHODS *Clinical Evidence* search and appraisal March 2003, including a search for observational studies.

QUESTION **What are the effects of interventions to reduce the risk of sudden infant death syndrome?**

OPTION **ADVICE TO AVOID PRONE SLEEPING**

One non-systematic review and 12 observational studies found that campaigns involving advice to encourage non-prone sleeping positions were followed by a reduced incidence of sudden infant death syndrome.

Benefits: We found no systematic review and no RCTs comparing advice to avoid prone sleeping (see glossary, p 463) positions versus no such advice (see comment below). **Observational studies after national advice campaigns:** We found one non-systematic review (3 observational studies, 1 of which has also been reported separately[16]),[12] and 12 additional observational studies after national advice campaigns (see comment below).[9,17–28] The review and additional observational studies describe eight campaigns that delivered advice to avoid prone positioning alone (see table 1, p 465),[17–19,21,22,24–26] and seven campaigns that provided advice to avoid a combination of different risk factors including prone positioning (see table 2, p 466).[9,12,16,20,23,27,28] The review and additional observational studies all found that the incidence of sudden infant death syndrome (SIDS) was reduced after the campaigns (see table 1, p 465 and table 2, p 466). One of the additional observational studies found that the incidence of prone positioning decreased significantly after the campaign (from 54% before campaign to 5% after campaign; $P < 0.001$).[27]

Harms: No increased frequency of adverse effects of non-prone positioning were reported in 13 observational studies of advice to avoid prone sleeping.[9,12,16–28] Two studies found no increase in the risk of inhaling vomitus associated with non-prone positioning.[26,29] Two observational studies have documented a temporal relationship between advice to avoid prone sleeping and an increase in the incidence of occipital plagiocephaly without synostosis (see glossary, p 463), whereas the incidence of other forms of plagiocephaly with synostosis remained constant.[30,31]

Comment: The review of SIDS risk factor reduction campaigns in Norway, Denmark, and Sweden reported that the campaign in Norway provided advice to avoid prone sleeping plus advice to avoid tobacco smoke exposure.[12] However, the original paper describing the Norwegian campaign reported that this campaign only provided advice to avoid prone sleeping.[16] One of the additional observational studies reported that the incidence of SIDS was declining before the campaign started, and hence the reduction attributable to advice provided by the campaign is not clear.[9,20] A second additional observational study did not report how advice was provided or exactly which SIDS risk factors were targeted, and it did not describe details of the advice given to avoid exposure to cigarette smoke (i.e. prenatally, postnatally, or both; maternal smoking alone or smoking by other household members as well).[23] A third additional observational study did not specify whether the advice to stop smoking was given to mothers or other family members and what advice was given regarding avoidance of over heating.[27] Systematic reviews of observational studies have found an association between prone sleeping position and an increased risk of SIDS, leading to the initiation of non-prone sleep campaigns in several countries.[2,3] RCTs investigating the effects of advice to avoid prone positioning may be considered unethical given the existing observational evidence; they would also be difficult to conduct given the extremely large units of randomisation required and the high level of pre-existing public awareness regarding the risks associated with prone positioning in sleep

OPTION ADVICE TO AVOID TOBACCO SMOKE EXPOSURE

One non-systematic review and four observational studies found limited evidence that campaigns to reduce several risk factors for sudden infant death, which included tobacco smoke exposure, were followed by a reduced incidence of sudden infant death syndrome.

Benefits: We found no systematic review and no RCTs comparing advice to avoid tobacco smoke exposure versus no such advice (see comment below). **Observational studies after national advice campaigns:** We found one non-systematic review (3 observational studies, 1 of which has also been reported separately[16]),[12] and four additional observational studies after national advice campaigns (see table 2, p 466).[9,20,23,27,28] The review and additional observational studies found that the campaigns were all followed by a reduced incidence of sudden infant death syndrome (SIDS) during the data collection periods (see table 2, p 466). However, the campaigns included advice in addition to avoiding tobacco smoke exposure, and in some countries the incidence of SIDS had started to fall before the campaign started (see comment under advice to avoid prone sleeping, p 459). The first additional observational study found that the population attributable risk (see glossary, p 463) of SIDS associated with maternal smoking alone was 44% (prevalence 19%; OR 5.17), and for maternal smoking plus bed sharing it was 33% (prevalence 5%; OR 11.1).[9,20] The third additional observational study found that the percentage of mothers not smoking during pregnancy increased significantly after the campaign (from 77% before campaign to 82% after campaign; $P < 0.01$).[27] The fourth additional observational study found that maternal smoking in Kanagawa province in Japan decreased from 9.4% to 0% after the campaign.[28]

Harms: None of the studies we found reported evidence on harms of a reduction in infant tobacco smoke exposure.

Comment: The SIDS reduction attributable to a reduction in maternal smoking is unclear. RCTs investigating the effects of advice to reduce infant tobacco smoke exposure would be difficult to conduct given the extremely large units of randomisation required and the high level of pre-existing public awareness regarding the risks associated with tobacco smoke exposure.

OPTION ADVICE TO AVOID SOFT SLEEPING SURFACES

We found no evidence on the effects of advice to avoid soft sleeping surfaces in the prevention of sudden infant death syndrome.

Benefits: We found no systematic review, RCTs, or observational studies of sufficient quality (see comment below).

Harms: None of the studies we found reported evidence on harms of advice to avoid soft sleeping surfaces.

Comment: RCTs investigating the effects of advice to avoid soft sleeping surfaces would be difficult to conduct given the extremely large units of randomisation required.

OPTION ADVICE TO AVOID OVER HEATING OR OVER WRAPPING

One non-systematic review and one observational study found limited evidence that campaigns to reduce several risk factors for sudden infant death, which included over wrapping, were followed by a reduced incidence of sudden infant death syndrome.

Benefits: We found no systematic review and no RCTs comparing advice to avoid overheating or over wrapping (see glossary, p 463) versus no such advice (see comment below). **Observational studies after national advice campaigns:** We found one non-systematic review

(3 observational studies, 1 of which has also been reported separately[16]),[12] and one additional observational study after national advice campaigns (see table 2, p 466).[27] Two of the national advice campaigns reported in the review and the additional observational study provided advice to avoid over heating or over wrapping plus advice to avoid other risk factors for sudden infant death syndrome (see comment under advice to avoid prone sleeping, p 459).[12,27] The third campaign reported by the review did not provide advice on over heating or over wrapping.[12,16] The review and additional observational study found that the campaigns were all followed by a reduction in the incidence of sudden infant death syndrome during the data collection periods (see table 2, p 466).

Harms: None of the studies we found reported evidence on harms of advice to avoid over heating or over wrapping.

Comment: RCTs investigating the effects of advice to avoid over heating or over wrapping would be difficult to conduct given the extremely large units of randomisation required.

OPTION ADVICE TO AVOID BED SHARING

One observational study found that a campaign to reduce several risk factors for sudden infant death, which included advice to avoid bed sharing, was followed by a reduced incidence of sudden infant death syndrome.

Benefits: We found no systematic review and no RCTs comparing advice to avoid bed sharing versus no advice (see comment below). **Observational studies after national advice campaigns:** We found one observational study, which reported the results of a national campaign that provided advice to avoid bed sharing, to avoid prone sleeping (see glossary, p 463), to avoid exposing infants to tobacco smoke from any source either during pregnancy or for the first year of life, and to breastfeed if possible (see comment below) (see table 2, p 466).[9,20] The observational study found that the incidence of sudden infant death syndrome reduced after the campaign (see table 2, p 466), and that the population attributable risk (see glossary, p 463) for sudden infant death syndrome associated with maternal smoking plus bed sharing was 33% (prevalence 5%; OR 11.1).

Harms: None of the studies we found reported evidence on harms associated with advice to avoid bed sharing.

Comment: The observational study reported that advice to avoid bed sharing was introduced after the main campaign had started.[9,20] The study also reported that the incidence of sudden infant death syndrome was declining before the campaign started, and hence the reduction attributable to advice provided by the campaign is not clear. RCTs investigating the effects of advice to avoid bed sharing would be difficult to conduct given the extremely large units of randomisation required.

OPTION ADVICE TO BREASTFEED

One non-systematic review and three observational studies found that campaigns to reduce several risk factors for sudden infant death, which included advice to breastfeed, were followed by a reduced incidence of sudden infant death syndrome.

Benefits: We found no systematic review and no RCTs comparing advice to encourage breastfeeding versus no such advice in order to reduce the incidence of sudden infant death syndrome (SIDS; see comment below). **Observational studies after national advice campaigns:** We found one non-systematic review (3 observational studies, 1 of which has also been reported separately[16]),[12] and three additional observational studies after national advice campaigns (see table 2, p 466).[9,20,27,28] The review and additional observational studies found that the campaigns were all followed by a reduced incidence of SIDS during the data collection periods (see table 2, p 466). However, the campaigns included advice other than advice to encourage breastfeeding, and in some countries the incidence of SIDS had started to fall before the campaign started (see comment under advice to avoid tobacco smoke exposure, p 460). The second additional observational study found that the incidence of no breastfeeding decreased significantly after the campaign (from 21% before campaign to 7% after campaign; $P < 0.001$).[27] The third additional observational study found that rates of breastfeeding only in Kanagawa province in Japan increased from 53.1% to 67.3% after the campaign.[28]

Harms: None of the studies we found reported evidence on harms of with advice to encourage breastfeeding.

Comment: RCTs investigating the effects of promotion of breastfeeding would be unethical given the evidence of benefits associated with breastfeeding.

OPTION ADVICE TO PROMOTE SOOTHER USE

We found insufficient evidence on soother use in the prevention of sudden infant death syndrome.

Benefits: We found no systematic review and no RCTs comparing advice to encourage use of a soother (see glossary, p 463) with no such advice to reduce the incidence of sudden infant death syndrome. **Observational studies after national advice campaigns:** We found no observational studies after national advice campaigns. **Other observational studies:** We found one systematic review (search date 2000) that identified four case control studies.[32] All four studies included in the review found an association between increased soother use and a reduced risk of sudden infant death syndrome, but none of the studies concluded that the association was causal.

Harms: The studies we found provided no evidence on harms of soother use.

Comment: RCTs investigating the effects of advice to promote soother use would be difficult to conduct given the extremely large units of randomisation required.

GLOSSARY

Occipital plagiocephaly with or without synostosis Flattening of the occipital bone with or without a malformation of the corresponding cranial suture line.
Over wrapping Wrapping/bundling of infants in excessive amounts of clothing or bedding to result in sweating, raised core temperatures, or both.
Population attributable risk A measure of the disease rate in exposed people compared with that in unexposed people, multiplied by the prevalence of exposure to the risk factor in the population.
Prone sleeping Sleeping on one's front.
Soother (dummy, pacifier) An object placed in the infant's mouth for the sole purpose of providing comfort.

Substantive changes

Advice to avoid prone sleeping One observational study added;[28] conclusions unchanged
Advice to avoid tobacco smoke exposure One observational study added;[28] conclusions unchanged.
Advice to breastfeed One observational study added;[28] conclusions unchanged.
Advice to promote soother use One systematic review of observational studies added;[32] conclusions unchanged.

REFERENCES

1. Canadian Bureau of Reproductive and Child Health/Laboratory Centre for Disease Control/Canadian Perinatal Surveillance System (CPSS); Fact sheet: http://www.hc-sc.gc.ca/hpb/lcdc/brch/factshts/sids_e.html (last accessed 10 June 2003).
2. Beal SM, Finch CF. An overview of retrospective case-control studies investigating the relationship between prone sleeping position and SIDS. *J Paediatr Child Health* 1991;27:334–339.
3. American Academy of Pediatrics AAP Task Force on Infant Positioning and SIDS. Positioning and SIDS. *Pediatrics* 1992;89(6 pt 1):1120–1126.
4. Anderson HR, Cook DG. Passive smoking and sudden infant death syndrome: review of the epidemiological evidence. *Thorax* 1997;52:1003–1009.
5. Mitchell EA, Thompson JM, Ford RP, et al. Sheepskin bedding and the sudden infant death syndrome. New Zealand Cot Death Study Group. *J Pediatr* 1998;133:701–704.
6. Ponsonby AL, Dwyer T, Gibbons LE, et al. Factors potentiating the risk of sudden infant death syndrome associated with the prone position. *N Engl J Med* 1993;329:377–382.
7. Fleming PJ, Blair PS, Bacon C, et al. Environment of infants during sleep and risk of the sudden infant death syndrome: results of the 1993–5 case-control study for confidential enquiry into stillbirths and deaths on infancy. Confidential Enquiry into Stillbirths and Deaths Regional Coordinators and Researchers. *BMJ* 1996;313:85–89.
8. Ponsonby AL, Dwyer T, Gibbons LE, et al. Thermal environment and sudden infant death syndrome: case-control study. *BMJ* 1992;304:277–282.
9. Mitchell EA, Tuohy PG, Brunt JM, et al. Risk factors for sudden infant death syndrome following the prevention campaign in New Zealand: a prospective study. *Pediatrics* 1997;100:835–840.
10. Scragg R, Mitchell EA, Taylor BJ, et al. Bed sharing, smoking, and alcohol in the sudden infant death syndrome. New Zealand Cot Death Study Group. *BMJ* 1993;307:1312–1318.
11. Mitchell EA, Taylor BJ, Ford RP, et al. Four modifiable and other major risk factors for cot death: the New Zealand study. *J Paediatr Child Health* 1992;28(suppl 1):S3–S8.
12. Wennergren G, Alm B, Oyen N, et al. The decline in the incidence of SIDS in Scandinavia and its relation to risk-intervention campaigns. Nordic Epidemiological SIDS Study. *Acta Paediatr* 1997;86:963–968.
13. L'Hoir MP, Engelberts AC, van Well GT, et al. Risk and preventive factors for cot death in The Netherlands, a low-incidence country. *Eur J Pediatr* 1998;157:681–688.
14. Oyen N, Skjaerven R, Irgens LM. Population-based recurrence risk of sudden infant death syndrome compared with other infant and fetal deaths. *Am J Epidemiol* 1996;144:300–305.
15. Guntheroth WG, Lohmann R, Spiers PS. Risk of sudden infant death syndrome in subsequent siblings. *J Pediatr* 1990;116:520–524.
16. Haaland K, Thoresen M. Crib death, sleeping position and temperature [in Norwegian]. *Tidsskr Nor Laegeforen* 1992;112:1466–1470.
17. Schellscheidt J, Ott A, Jorch G. Epidemiological features of sudden infant death after a German intervention campaign in 1992. *Eur J Pediatr* 1997;156:655–660.
18. Skadberg BT, Morild I, Markestad T. Abandoning prone sleeping: effect on the risk of sudden infant death syndrome. *J Pediatr* 1998;132:340–343.
19. Wigfield RE, Fleming PJ, Berry PJ, et al. Can the fall in Avon's sudden infant death rate be explained by changes in sleeping position? *BMJ* 1992;304:282–283.
20. Mitchell EA, Aley P, Eastwood J. The national cot death prevention program in New Zealand. *Aust J Public Health* 1992;16:158–161.

21. Markestad T, Skadberg B, Hordvik E, et al. Sleeping position and sudden infant death syndrome (SIDS): effect of an intervention programme to avoid prone sleeping. *Acta Paediatr* 1995;84:375–378.
22. Vege A, Rognum TO, Opdal SH. SIDS — changes in the epidemiological pattern in Eastern Norway 1984–1996. *Forensic Sci Int* 1998;93:155–166.
23. Adams EJ, Chavez GF, Steen D, et al. Changes in the epidemiologic profile of sudden infant death syndrome as rates decline among California infants: 1990–1995. *Pediatrics* 1998;102:1445–1451.
24. Mitchell EA, Ford RP, Taylor BJ, et al. Further evidence supporting a causal relationship between prone sleeping position and SIDS. *J Paediatr Child Health* 1992;28(suppl 1):S9–S12.
25. Dwyer T, Ponsonby AL, Blizzard L, et al. The contribution of changes in the prevalence of prone sleeping position to the decline in sudden infant death syndrome in Tasmania. *JAMA* 1995;273:783–789.
26. Spiers PS, Guntheroth WG. Recommendations to avoid the prone sleeping position and recent statistics for sudden infant death syndrome in the United States. *Arch Pediatr Adolesc Med* 1994;148:141–146.
27. Kiechl-Kohlendorfer U, Peglow UP, Kiechl S, et al. Epidemiology of sudden infant death syndrome (SIDS) in the Tyrol before and after an intervention campaign. *Wien Klin Wochenschr* 2001;113:27–32.
28. Sawaguchi T, Nishida H, Fukui F, Horiuchi T, Nelson EAS. Study on social responses (encouraging public awareness) to sudden infant death syndrome: evaluation of SIDS prevention campaigns. *Forensic Sci Int* 2002;130(suppl):S78–S80.
29. Malloy M. Trends in postneonatal aspiration deaths and reclassification of sudden infant death syndrome: impact of the "Back to Sleep" program. *Pediatrics* 2002;109:661–665.
30. Kane AA, Mitchell LE, Craven KP, et al. Observations on a recent increase in plagiocephaly without synostosis. *Pediatrics* 1996;97(6 pt 1):877–885.
31. Gonzalez de Dios J, Moya M, Jimenez L, et al. Increase in the incidence of occipital plagiocephaly. *Rev Neurol* 1998;27:782–784.
32. Zotter H, Kerbl R, Kurz R, Muller W. Pacifier use and sudden infant death syndrome: Should health professionals recommend pacifier use based on present knowledge. *Wien Klin Wochenschr* 2992;114:791–794. Search date 2000; primary sources Medline and Pubmed.

David Creery

Angelo Mikrogianakis

Children's Hospital of Eastern Ontario
Ottawa
Canada

Competing interests: None declared.

TABLE 1 **Observational studies after national campaigns providing advice to avoid prone sleeping positions (see text, p 458).**

Country/reference	Dissemination	SIDS incidence/1000 live births (95% CI) From	To	Number of infants	Risk of prone sleeping after campaign (95% CI)
Germany (West) North Rhine	Not specified	1.56	0.92	59 cases, 156 controls	OR 11.7 (5.3 to 26.2)
Westphalia[17]		2.17	1.33		
Norway[18]	Health professional education Media campaign	3.5 (2.64 to 4.36)	0.3 (0.05 to 0.54)	6 cases, 493 controls	OR 42.0 (5 to 390)
UK, Avon[19]	Maternal education Health professional education	3.5	1.7	32 cases, 70 controls, 152 population based controls	NA
Norway/Hordaland[21]	Health professional education Media campaign	3.5	1.6	30 cases, 123 controls	OR 11.3 (3.6 to 36.5)
Norway[22]	Health professional education Media campaign	2	0.6	200 cases	NA
New Zealand[24]	Maternal education Health professional education Media campaign	4	3.1	485 cases, 1800 controls	NA
Australia[25]	Maternal education Health professional education	3.8 (3.5 to 4.2)	1.5 (0.9 to 2.2)	449 cases	NA
USA[26]	Media campaign	2.36	2.02	233 cases	NA

NA, not available; SIDS, sudden infant death syndrome.

TABLE 2 **Observational studies after national campaigns providing advice to avoid several sudden infant death syndrome risk factors including prone sleeping positions (see text, p 458).**

Country/ year of start	Data collection	Advice to: *avoid* or [encourage]	Dissemination	SIDS incidence/ 1000 live births (95% CI)		Number of infants	Risk (95% CI)
				From	To		
Norway 1989[12,16]	1992–95	*prone sleeping*	Newspapers National media broadcasts Midwives Other healthcare professionals Presentation at a SIDS prevention conference	2.3	0.6	244 cases 869 controls	Adjusted OR prone sleeping 5.4 (2.8 to 10.5)
Denmark 1991[12]	1992–95	*prone sleeping* *tobacco smoke over wrapping*	Not described	1.6	0.2	244 cases 869 controls	Adjusted OR prone sleeping 5.4 (2.8 to 10.5)
Sweden 1992[12]	1992–95	*prone sleeping* *tobacco smoke over wrapping* [breast feeding]	Not described	1.0	0.4		

TABLE 2 continued

Country/ year of start	Data collection	Advice to: *avoid* or [encourage]	Dissemination	SIDS incidence/ 1000 live births (95% CI)		Number of infants	Risk (95% CI)
				From	To		
New Zealand 1990[9,20]	1991–93	*prone sleeping* *tobacco smoke*(any source; during pregnancy/first year of life) *bed sharing* [breast feeding]	Parents antenatal classes Postnatal wards Healthcare professionals Conferences Journals Public newspapers TV programmes	4.1	2.1	127 cases 922 controls	Not reported
California 1990–1995[23]		*prone sleeping* *cigarette smoking*	Public	2.69 (black infants) 1.04 (other infants)	2.15 (black infants) 0.61 (other infants)	3508 cases	Not reported
Austria 1994–1995[27]		*prone sleeping* *smoking* *over heating* [breast feeding]	Parents antenatal classes, maternity wards, routine health checks Public newspapers Radio/TV	1984–1994: 1.83	1995: 0.4 1996–1998 unchanged	160 cases	Not reported
Japan 1996[28]	1995 and 1998		Medical professional education Maternal education	0.44	0.33	Not reported	Not reported

SIDS, sudden infant death syndrome.

Urinary tract infection in children

Search date September 2002

James Larcombe

QUESTIONS

INTERVENTIONS

TREATMENT

Likely to be beneficial

Oral versus initial intravenous antibiotics 474

Unknown effectiveness

Immediate empirical versus delayed antibiotic treatment .471

Unlikely to be beneficial

Longer (7–14 days) versus shorter (2–4 days) courses of oral antibiotics (for non-recurrent lower urinary tract infections in the absence of renal tract abnormality) 472

Longer versus short courses of initial intravenous antibiotics .474

Likely to be ineffective or harmful

Prolonged delay in treatment (> 7 days)..............471

Single dose versus longer course (10 days) of oral amoxicillin .472

PREVENTION OF RECURRENCE

Likely to be beneficial

Immunotherapy............476

Prophylactic antibiotics 475

Unknown effectiveness

Surgical correction of moderate to severe bilateral vesicoureteric reflux (grades III–IV) with bilateral nephropathy 478

Unlikely to be beneficial

Surgical correction of minor functional anomalies 478

Surgical correction of moderate to severe vesicoureteric reflux with adequate glomerular filtration rate (similar benefits to medical management) 478

See glossary, p 479

Key Messages

Treatment of acute infection

- **Antibiotics versus placebo** Placebo controlled trials of antibiotics for symptomatic acute urinary tract infection in children are considered unethical.
- **Oral versus initial intravenous antibiotics** One RCT found no significant difference between oral cephalosporins alone and initial intravenous plus continued oral cephalosporins in duration of fever, reinfection, renal scarring, or extent of scarring in children aged 2 years or younger with first confirmed urinary tract infection. The RCT found weak evidence that, in children with grades III–IV reflux, renal scarring at 6 months may be more common with oral versus initial intravenous treatment.

- **Immediate empirical versus delayed antibiotic treatment** We found no RCTs on the effects of giving early empirical treatment versus awaiting the results of microscopy or culture in acute urinary tract infection in children. Retrospective analysis of one RCT found no significant difference in risk of renal scarring with antibiotic (cephalosporins) treatment within 24 hours versus 24 hours after the onset of fever in children under 2 years with urinary tract infections.
- **Longer (7–14 days) versus shorter (2–4 days) courses of oral antibiotics** One systematic review found no significant difference for longer (7–14 days) versus shorter courses (2–4 days) of the same antibiotic in cure rate at 7 days after treatment in children with no history of renal tract abnormality and judged not to have acute pyelonephritis.
- **Longer versus short courses of initial intravenous antibiotics** Two RCTs found no significant difference between long (7–10 days) and short (3 days) course of initial cephalosporins in renal scarring in children with acute pyelonephritis.
- **Prolonged delay in treatment (> 7 days)** We found no RCTs. Five retrospective studies found that medium to long term delays (4 days to 7 years) in treatment may be associated with an increased risk of renal scarring.
- **Single dose versus longer course (10 days) of oral amoxicillin** One systematic review has found that longer (10 days) versus single dose amoxicillin increases cure rate at 3–30 days after the start of treatment.

Prevention of recurrence

- **Immunotherapy** One systematic review in premature and low birth weight neonates has found that intravenous immunoglobulins reduce serious infections, including urinary tract infections, compared with placebo. One RCT in children with recurrent urinary tract infection found that adding pidotimod (an immunotherapeutic agent) reduced recurrence compared with adding placebo to antibiotic treatment.
- **Prophylactic antibiotics** One systematic review and an additional RCT found limited evidence that prophylactic antibiotics (co-trimoxazole, nitrofurantoin) reduced urinary tract infection recurrence in children compared with placebo or no treatment. One RCT found that nitrofurantoin significantly reduced recurrence of urinary tract infection over 6 months compared with trimethoprim. It also found that more children discontinued treatment with nitrofurantoin because of adverse effects. We found no RCTs evaluating the optimum duration of prophylactic antibiotics.
- **Surgical correction of moderate to severe bilateral vesicoureteric reflux (grades III–IV) with bilateral nephropathy** One small RCT found a steady, but not significant, decline in glomerular filtration rate over 10 years with medical treatment versus surgery in children with moderate to severe bilateral vesicoureteric reflux.
- **Surgical correction of minor functional anomalies** We found no RCTs. One observational study suggested that children with minor anomalies do not develop renal scarring and therefore may not benefit from surgery.
- **Surgical correction of moderate to severe vesicoureteric reflux with adequate glomerular filtration rate (similar benefits to medical management)** One systematic review and one subsequent RCT found that, although surgery abolished reflux, there was no significant difference between surgical and medical management (prophylactic antibiotic treatment) in preventing recurrence or complications from urinary tract infection after 6 months to 5 years in children with moderate to severe vesicoureteric reflux.

Urinary tract infection in children

DEFINITION Urinary tract infection (UTI) is defined by the presence of a pure growth of more than 10^5 colony forming units of bacteria per millilitre. Lower counts of bacteria may be clinically important, especially in boys and in specimens obtained by urinary catheter. Any growth of typical urinary pathogens is considered clinically important if obtained by suprapubic aspiration. In practice, three age ranges are usually considered on the basis of differential risk and different approaches to management: children under 1 year; young children (1–4, 5, or 7 years, depending on the information source); and older children (up to 12–16 years). Recurrent UTI is defined as a further infection by a new organism. Relapsing UTI is defined as a further infection with the same organism.

INCIDENCE/ PREVALENCE Boys are more susceptible before the age of 3 months; thereafter the incidence is substantially higher in girls. Estimates of the true incidence of UTI depend on rates of diagnosis and investigation. At least 8% of girls and 2% of boys will have a UTI in childhood.[1]

AETIOLOGY/ RISK FACTORS The normal urinary tract is sterile. Contamination by bowel flora may result in urinary infection if a virulent organism is involved or if the child is immunosuppressed. In neonates, infection may originate from other sources. *Escherichia coli* accounts for about three quarters of all pathogens. *Proteus* is more common in boys (about 30% of infections). Obstructive anomalies are found in 0–4% and vesicoureteric reflux in 8–40% of children being investigated for their first UTI.[2] Although vesicoureteric reflux is a major risk factor for adverse outcome, other as yet unidentified triggers may also need to be present.

PROGNOSIS After first infection, about half of girls have a further infection in the first year and three quarters within 2 years.[3] We found no figures for boys, but a review suggests that recurrences are common under 1 year of age, but rare subsequently.[4] Renal scarring occurs in 5–15% of children within 1–2 years of their first UTI, although 32–70% of these scars are noted at the time of initial assessment.[2] The incidence of renal scarring rises with each episode of infection in childhood.[5] Retrospective analysis of an RCT comparing oral versus intravenous antibiotics found that new renal scarring after a first UTI was more common in children with vesicoureteric reflux than in children without reflux (logistic regression model: AR of scarring 16/107 [15%] with reflux *v* 10/165 [6%] without reflux; RR 2.47, 95% CI 1.17 to 5.24).[6] A study (287 children with severe vesicoureteric reflux treated either medically or surgically for any UTI) evaluated the risk of renal scarring with serial DMSA scintigraphy (see glossary, p 479) over 5 years. It found that younger children (< 2 years) were at greater risk of renal scarring than older children regardless of treatment for the infection (AR for deterioration in DMSA scan over 5 years 21/86 [24%] for younger children *v* 27/201 [13%] for older children; RR 1.82, 95% CI 1.09 to 3.03).[7] Renal scarring is associated with future complications: poor renal growth, recurrent adult pyelonephritis (see glossary, p 480), impaired glomerular function, early hypertension, and end stage renal failure.[8–11] A combination of recurrent UTI, severe vesicoureteric reflux, and the presence of renal scarring at first presentation is associated with the worst prognosis. One prospective observational study assessed the persistence of scarring on DMSA scans in children with a first UTI.[12] Grading of scars was as follows: mild (< 25% kidney affected), moderate (25–50% kidney), and severe (> 50% kidney). The study found that vesicoureteric reflux was associated with more persistent scarring at 6 months (in children with severe scarring on initial scan, 7/8 [88%] with reflux had a persisting lesion *v* 1/7 [14%] without reflux; RR 6.13, 95% CI 0.98 to 38.00; in children with mild to moderate scarring on initial scan, 3/8 [38%] with reflux had persisting lesions *v* 5/31 [16%] without reflux; RR 2.70, 95% CI 0.81 to 9.10).[12] The study also found that vesicoureteric reflux was associated with a higher risk of pyelonephritis on the initial scan (RR for pyelonephritis with reflux *v* without 1.62, 95% CI 1.14 to 2.31).

AIMS OF INTERVENTION To relieve acute symptoms; to eliminate infection; and to prevent recurrence, renal damage, and long term complications.

OUTCOMES **Short term:** clinical symptoms and signs (dysuria, frequency, and fever); urine culture; incidence of new renal scars. **Long term:** incidence of recurrent infection; prevalence of renal scarring; renal size and growth; renal function; prevalence of hypertension and renal failure.

METHODS *Clinical Evidence* search and appraisal September 2002.

QUESTION What are the effects of treatment of acute urinary tract infection in children?

OPTION ANTIBIOTICS VERSUS PLACEBO

Placebo controlled trials of antibiotics for symptomatic acute urinary tract infections in children are considered unethical.

Benefits: We found no RCTs.

Harms: We found no RCTs.

Comment: Placebo controlled trials would be considered unethical because there is a strong consensus that antibiotics are likely to be beneficial. The improved response seen with longer versus very short courses of antibiotics is indirect evidence that antibiotics are likely to be more effective than no treatment.

OPTION IMMEDIATE EMPIRICAL VERSUS DELAYED ANTIBIOTIC TREATMENT

We found no RCTs on the effects of giving early empirical treatment versus awaiting the results of microscopy or culture in acute urinary tract infection in children. Retrospective analysis of one RCT found no significant difference in risk of renal scarring with antibiotic (cephalosporin) treatment within 24 hours versus 24 hours after the onset of fever in children under 2 years with urinary tract infections.

Benefits: We found no RCTs comparing immediate empirical treatment versus treatment delayed while awaiting the results of microscopy or culture. We found one RCT that compared oral cefixime for 14 days (double dose on day 1) versus intravenous cefotaxime for 3 days plus oral cefixime for 11 days for urinary tract infection in children under 2 years.[6] Retrospective analysis of its results found no evidence that children treated 24 hours after the onset of fever were at greater risk of renal scarring than children presenting within 24 hours (9/99 [9%] of children presenting before 24 hours developed scarring *v* 19/159 [12%] of children presenting later; RR 1.3, 95% CI 0.6 to 2.7; P = 0.29).

Harms: The RCT did not report on any adverse effects.[6]

Comment: Five retrospective observational studies found increased rates of scarring in children in whom diagnosis was delayed between 4 days (in acute urinary tract infection) to 7 years (when a child presented with chronic non-specific symptoms).[2]

OPTION LONGER VERSUS SHORT COURSES OF ORAL ANTIBIOTICS

Two systematic reviews found no significant difference between longer (7–14 days) and shorter courses (2–4 days) of antibiotics in cure rate or recurrence of urinary tract infection 10 days to 15 months after treatment. One systematic review found that single dose versus longer course (10 days) amoxicillin decreased cure rate at 3–30 days after the start of treatment. Two systematic reviews found no significant difference in cure rate between longer (7–14 days) and shorter courses (single dose to 4 days) of sulphonamides, such as co-trimoxazole.

Benefits: We found two systematic reviews that compared longer versus short course only of the same antibiotic.[13,14] Both reviews included the following antibiotics: amoxicillin, nitrofurantoin, trimethoprim/sulfadiazine, nalidixic acid, pivmecillinam, nitrofurantoin, amoxicillin/clavulanic acid, and cefuroxime. We found one systematic review (search date 2001, 17 RCTs) that compared longer versus shorter courses of any antibiotic.[15] **Versus single dose and short course:** The first review (search date 1999, 17 RCTs, children and adolescents aged < 18 years with uncomplicated cystitis) included single dose drug regimens.[13] It found that longer (≥ 5 days) versus short (≤ 4 days) courses of an antibiotic increased microbiological cure rate between 3 and 30 days after start of treatment (difference in cure rates 7.9%, 95% CI 2.1% to 13.8%).[13] However, studies were statistically heterogeneous and meta-analysis may not have been appropriate (P = 0.01). The review found that longer (10 days) versus single dose amoxicillin significantly increased microbiological cure rate between 3 and 30 days after enrolment (4 RCTs: difference in cure rate for longer *v* short course 13%, 95% CI 4% to 24%; NNT with longer course for cure 8, 95% CI 5 to 25; no statistical heterogeneity among studies in meta-analysis). However, it found no significant difference for longer (7–10 days) versus shorter course or single dose (≤ 3 days) co-trimoxazole for microbiological cure (6 RCTs: difference in cure rate for longer *v* short course +6.2%, 95% CI –3.7% to +16.2%). The second systematic review excluded single dose regimens.[14] The third systematic review similarly found that 7–14 day courses of any antibiotic significantly reduced treatment failure compared with single day or single dose regimens (RR 2.73, 95% CI 1.38 to 5.40).[15] Compared with any short course, including single day or single dose regimens, it found that longer courses significantly reduced treatment failure (RR 1.94, 95 CI 1.19 to 3.15).[15] **Versus short course, but not single dose or single day regimens:** The second review (search date 2001, 10 RCTs, 652 children and adolescents aged 3 months to 18 years with urinary tract infections [UTI] and asymptomatic infection) excluded antibiotic courses of less than 2 days' duration.[14] All studies in the review excluded children with known renal tract abnormalities or acute pyelonephritis (see glossary, p 480) and all included children with a history of recurrent UTI. The review found no significant difference for longer (7–14 days) versus short (2–4 days) antibiotic courses for microbiological cure within 7 days of treatment and no significant difference for UTI recurrence 10 days to 15 months after treatment (8 RCTs: RR of positive urine culture up to 7 days after treatment for longer *v* short courses 1.06, 95% CI 0.64 to 1.76; RR of UTI recurrence 10 days to 15 months after treatment for longer *v* shorter courses 1.01, 95% CI 0.77 to 1.33).[14] No significant heterogeneity was found among studies in the meta-analysis. The review found no significant difference between longer (7–14 days) versus short (2–4 days) course sulphonamides, such as co-trimoxazole, for persistence of UTI after treatment or recurrence of UTI 10 days to 15 months after treatment (6 RCTs, 233 children: RR of UTI at end of treatment 1.72, 95% CI 0.64 to 3.80; RR of recurrent UTI 1.04, 95% CI, 0.71 to 1.52).[14] The third review found no significant difference between 7–14 day courses and 3 day course of any antibiotic for treatment failure (RR 1.36, 95% CI 0.68 to 2.72).[15]

Harms: The first systematic review reported that dose related adverse effects, such as neutropenia with β-lactam antibiotics, seemed to increase in frequency with the length of administration.[13] The second systematic review found no significant difference with short versus longer courses for antibiotic resistant UTI (persistent resistant bacteriuria at the end of treatment: 1 RCT, RR 0.57, 95% CI 0.32 to 1.01; resistant recurrent UTI: 3 RCTs, RR 0.39, 95% CI 0.12 to 1.29).[14]

Comment: The studies included in the reviews differed in the lengths of treatment and antibiotics used, the definitions of cure, relapse, reinfection, and the diagnostic criteria for pyelonephritis or complicated UTI. Comparisons were made both for the whole group and for subgroups. In the first review, treatment groups were compared with fixed or random effects models, based on statistical analysis of the heterogeneity of the groups.[13] The second review included an unspecified number of children with asymptomatic bacteriuria.[14] The clinical importance of treating this group remains unclear. Several factors may reduce the generalisability of results to all children with lower UTI. First, the review only excluded children with acute pyelonephritis, which may not have excluded all cases of upper UTI. Second, all the RCTs in the second review included children with recurrent UTI, who have higher rates of treatment failure than children with no history of UTI.[14] Finally, many studies included in the reviews were in children attending outpatient departments and emergency rooms. Response to treatment may be lower in this group than in unselected populations.[15]

OPTION ORAL VERSUS INITIAL INTRAVENOUS ANTIBIOTICS

One RCT found no significant difference between oral cephalosporins alone and initial intravenous plus continued oral cephalosporins in duration of fever, reinfection rate, renal scarring, or extent of scarring in children aged 2 years or younger with first confirmed urinary tract infection. The RCT found weak evidence that in children with grades III–IV reflux, renal scarring at 6 months may be more common with oral versus initial intravenous treatment.

Benefits: We found one RCT (309 children, aged ≤ 2 years, fever > 38.2 °C, with a first urinary tract infection confirmed from catheter specimen) sufficiently powered to produce meaningful results. The RCT compared oral cefixime for 14 days (double dose on day 1) versus initial intravenous cefotaxime for 3 days plus 11 days of oral cefixime.[6] It found no significant difference between treatments in mean duration of fever (24.7 hours with oral treatment *v* 23.9 hours with initial iv treatment; P = 0.76), reinfection rate (132/153 [86%] with oral treatment *v* 134/153 [88%] with initial iv treatment; P = 0.28), incidence of renal scarring (intention to treat analysis: 15/153 [10%] with oral treatment [21 children not scanned and counted as having no scarring] *v* 11/153 [7%] with initial iv treatment [13 children not scanned]; P = 0.21), and mean extent of scarring (8% of renal parenchyma with oral treatment *v* 9% with initial iv treatment). The RCT found weak evidence from a post hoc subgroup analysis in children with grades III–IV (see glossary, p 480) reflux that renal scarring at 6 months may be more common with oral versus initial intravenous treatment (new renal scarring within 6 months: 8/24 [33%] after oral antibiotics *v* 1/22 [5%] after iv antibiotics; ARI 29%, 95% CI 8% to 49%; NNH 3, 95% CI 2 to 13).[6]

Harms: The RCT did not report on adverse effects.[6]

Comment: The trial excluded 3/309 children because investigators considered that the severity of symptoms in these children warranted intravenous treatment.[6]

OPTION LONGER VERSUS SHORT COURSES OF INITIAL INTRAVENOUS ANTIBIOTICS

Two RCTs in children with acute pyelonephritis found no significant difference between long (7–10 days) and short (3 days) course of initial intravenous cephalosporins in renal scarring in children with acute pyelonephritis.

Benefits: We found two RCTs comparing the effect of a long versus short course of initial intravenous antibiotics (ceftriaxone) on development of renal scarring in children with acute pyelonephritis (see glossary, p 480). One RCT (220 children aged 3 months to 16 years with positive urine culture and acute renal lesions on initial DMSA scintigraphy [see glossary, p 479]) compared a 10 day versus a 3 day course of initial intravenous ceftriaxone (50 mg/kg/day) followed by oral cefixime (4 mg/kg twice daily) to complete a 15 day course.[16] Scintigraphy was repeated after 3 months. Renal scars were defined as persistent or partially resolved changes in the same location as the lesions on the original DMSA scan. The RCT found no significant difference with a 10 day versus a 3 day course of initial intravenous antibiotic treatment in development of renal scarring at 3 months (AR 36/110 [33%] children with 10 day course *v* 40/110 [36%] children with 3 day course; RR 1.10; 95% CI 0.77 to 1.60). The development of renal scarring was unaffected by age, sex, duration of fever before treatment, degree of inflammation, presence of vesicoureteric reflux, or recruitment centre. The second RCT (92 children aged 6 weeks to 13 years, with a clinical diagnosis of acute pyelonephritis, positive urine culture, and abnormal DMSA scan) compared a 7 day versus a 3 day course of initial intravenous ceftizoxime followed by oral cefixime.[17] The DMSA scan was repeated after 6 months for detection of total or partial persistence of renal abnormalities. The RCT found no significant difference with a 3 day versus a 7 day course of initial intravenous antibiotic treatment on renal abnormalities at 6 months (11/44 [25%] children with 3 day course *v* 8/43 [19%] children with 7 day course; RR 1.34, 95% CI 0.60 to 3.01).

Harms: The two RCTs did not assess harms.[16,17]

Comment: Unlike the studies of long versus short courses of oral treatment and the study of oral versus intravenous antibiotics, there were few exclusions for severe presentation. In the larger study, 206 children failed to meet the strict entry criteria,[16] but there were then no further exclusions. Eleven of 103 children were excluded in the smaller study.[17]

QUESTION What are the effects of interventions to prevent recurrence?

OPTION PROPHYLACTIC ANTIBIOTICS

One systematic review and an additional RCT found limited evidence that prophylactic antibiotics (co-trimoxazole, nitrofurantoin) reduced urinary tract infection recurrence in children compared with placebo or no treatment. One RCT found that nitrofurantoin reduced recurrence of urinary tract infection over 6 months compared with trimethoprim. It also found that more children discontinued treatment with nitrofurantoin because of adverse effects. We found no RCTs evaluating the optimum duration of prophylactic antibiotics.

Benefits: **Versus no prophylaxis:** We found one systematic review (search date 2001)[18] and one additional RCT.[19] The systematic review (3 RCTs, 151 children aged < 18 years at risk of recurrent urinary tract infection [UTI] but without a renal tract abnormality or major neurological, urological, or muscular disease) compared the effects of antibiotics (nitrofurantoin, co-trimoxazole) versus placebo or no treatment on risk of recurrent UTI.[18] There was variation between the RCTs in the duration of antibiotic prophylaxis (10 weeks to 12 months) and method of concealment (see comment below). The review found that antibiotics versus placebo or no treatment significantly reduced the risk of recurrent UTI (RR 0.36, 95% CI 0.16 to 0.77).[18] The additional RCT (double blind, crossover trial, 18 girls [1 with vesicoureteric reflux], aged 3–13 years) found that antibiotics (nitrofurantoin) versus no antibiotics significantly reduced recurrent

UTI (2 episodes in 1 year with antibiotics *v* 35 episodes without antibiotics; $P < 0.01$); see comment below.[20] **Comparison of antibiotics:** We found one systematic review (search date 2001, 1 RCT) comparing nitrofurantoin versus trimethoprim.[18] It found that nitrofurantoin versus trimethoprim significantly reduced recurrence of UTI over 6 months (RR 0.48, 95% CI 0.25 to 0.92; NNT 5, 95% CI 3 to 33). **Duration of prophylaxis:** We found no RCTs evaluating the optimum length of prophylaxis even in children with vesicoureteric reflux (although 2 studies of prolonged acute treatment were identified).[21]

Harms: **Versus no prophylaxis:** No adverse effects were reported in the RCTs included in the systematic review.[18] The additional RCT found no adverse effects with nitrofurantoin.[19] **Comparison of antibiotics:** One RCT found that significantly more children discontinued treatment with nitrofurantoin versus trimethoprim because of adverse effects, including nausea, vomiting, or stomach ache (RR 3.17, 95% CI 1.36 to 7.37; NNH 5, 95% CI 3 to 13).[18] Potential harms include those of using long term antibiotics. One study found that although gastrointestinal flora were affected by treatment, *E coli* (cultured from rectal swabs from 70% of children) remained sensitive to the prophylactic antibiotic co-trimoxazole).[22] However, another study found that children who had recently received co-trimoxazole for 4 or more weeks were more likely to have resistant *E coli* isolates than those who had received no antibiotics (OR 23.4, 95% CI 12.0 to 47.6).[23]

Comment: The systematic review was thorough but the RCTs it identified had weak methods.[18] None of the RCTs included in the systematic review used intention to treat analyses. Only one had adequate concealment and one specified the outcome measures. The additional RCT was a crossover study that did not include a washout period and had a withdrawal rate of 20%. It did not report the results for the period before the crossover separately.[19] It may not be possible clinically to identify children who are at high risk of recurrent UTIs and long term damage.[24] Routine prophylaxis until the results of investigations are known may, therefore, be warranted, but we found no good evidence about the benefits or harms of antibiotic prophylaxis.

OPTION IMMUNOTHERAPY

One systematic review in premature and in low birth weight neonates has found that intravenous immunoglobulins reduce serious infections, including urinary tract infections, compared with placebo. One RCT in children with recurrent urinary tract infection found that adding pidotimod (an immunotherapeutic agent) reduced recurrence compared with adding placebo to antibiotic treatment.

Benefits: **Intravenous immunoglobulin:** We found one systematic review (search date 1997, 15 RCTs), which compared intravenous immunoglobulin (see glossary, p 479) prophylaxis with placebo or no treatment.[25] It found that intravenous immunoglobulin prophylaxis significantly reduced serious infections, including urinary tract infections (UTIs), in preterm and in low birth weight neonates (RR for all serious infections 0.80, 95% CI 0.68 to 0.94; NNT 24, 95% CI 15 to 83).[25] The dose varied from 120 mg/kg to 1 g/kg. The number of treatments varied from 1–7. The specific effect on UTIs was not reported. **Other immunotherapeutic agents:** We found one RCT (double blind, 60 children aged 2–8 years with recurrent UTI) comparing pidotimod versus placebo added to standard antibiotic treatment.[26] The study included a further 60 day phase, using half dose pidotimod versus half dose placebo. The RCT found that adding pidotimod significantly reduced relapse rates compared with adding placebo at 60 days (4/30 [13%] children with relapse with pidotimod *v* 13/30 [43%] children with placebo; $P < 0.05$).[26] An open pilot study (40 children) compared nitrofurantoin with an antigenic extract of *E coli*.[27] No significant difference was found between the two treatments during active treatment or during the subsequent 6 months.

Harms: Parenteral treatment can cause pain, and there is an unmeasured risk from the administration of human blood products.[25] **Intravenous immunoglobulin:** The systematic review found that prophylactic intravenous immunoglobulin was not associated with any short term serious adverse effects.[25] **Other immunotherapeutic agents:** In the RCT of pidotimod, the only adverse effects recorded were thought to be attributable to concomitant antibiotic treatment.[26] The open pilot study found no significant difference in withdrawal rates between the antigenic extract of *E coli* (1/22 [5%]) and nitrofurantoin (1/18 [6%]).[27]

Comment: **Intravenous immunoglobulin:** We found no evidence for or against the suggestion that preparations with specific antibodies against common pathogens are more beneficial.[28] The greatest benefits were noted in units with higher nosocomial infection (see glossary, p 479) rates. It remains unclear whether intravenous immunoglobin is only justified where infection control policies have failed to reduce the infection rate.[25] Preterm and low birth weight neonates might have greater immune deficiency than other neonates and might be expected to gain more from treatment with immunoglobulin. **Other immunotherapeutic agents:** We found one non-randomised, age matched study in 10 otherwise healthy girls (aged 5–11 years) with recurrent UTI who were given intramuscular injections of inactivated uropathogenic bacteria (Solco-Urovac preparation). It found that the girls who had received the inactivated uropathogenic bacteria had significantly reduced frequency of subsequent UTI compared with 10 other age matched girls with UTI who had not received the inactivated bacteria preparation.[29] This study is limited by its non-randomised design and small sample size. We found another study (40 children aged 3–12 years with recurrent UTI caused by *E coli* and no anatomical or functional impairments of the urinary tract) comparing prophylactic antibiotics (amoxicillin with clavulanic acid or cephalosporins) versus prophylactic antibiotics plus an immunomodulator with *E coli* antigens (Uro-Vaxom) for 3 months followed up for 3 months after the end of treatment.[30] The method of randomisation was not stated. The study found that urinary sIgA levels, initially low in both groups were significantly raised 3 months after the end of treatment in the active treatment group but not in the control group. It also found that antibiotics plus immunomodulator versus antibiotics alone reduced recurrences over 6 months (recurrences, 2/25 [8%] with antibiotics plus immunomodulator *v* 8/13 [61%] with antibiotics alone).[30]

OPTION SURGICAL CORRECTION FOR ANOMALIES OBSTRUCTING MICTURITION

We found no RCTs. One observational study suggested that children with minor anomalies do not develop renal scarring and therefore may not benefit from surgery.

Benefits: We found no systematic review or RCTs.

Harms: Potential harms include the usual risks of surgery.

Comment: One small prospective observational study (271 children) suggested that children with minor anomalies do not develop renal scarring and therefore may not benefit from surgery.[31] Renal scars were present in more children with moderate degrees of vesicoureteric reflux than in children with minor anomalies (8/20 [40%] with moderate degrees of vesicoureteric reflux *v* 0/6 [0%] with minor anomalies). In the presence of major anomalies, the prevention of urinary tract infections is not the prime motive of surgical intervention.

OPTION SURGICAL CORRECTION FOR VESICOURETERIC REFLUX

One systematic review and one subsequent RCT found that, although surgery abolished reflux, there was no significant difference between surgical and medical management (prophylactic antibiotic treatment) in preventing recurrence or complications from urinary tract infections after 6 months to 5 years in children with moderate to severe vesicoureteric reflux. One small RCT found a steady but not statistically significant decline in glomerular filtration rate over 10 years with medical treatment compared with surgery in children with moderate to severe bilateral vesicoureteric reflux.

Benefits: **Versus medical management:** We found one systematic review[32] and two subsequent RCTs.[33,34] The systematic review (search date 1988, 4 RCTs, 830 children with moderate to severe [grades III–V — see glossary, p 480] vesicoureteric reflux) compared surgical correction versus medical management (continuous prophylactic antibiotics).[32] It found that surgery abolished reflux, but found no significant differences in rates of subsequent urinary tract infection, renal function, incidence of new renal scars, hypertension, or end stage renal failure among groups over a period of 6 months to 5 years. The first subsequent RCT (132 children aged ≤ 10 years with grades III–V vesicoureteric reflux, glomerular filtration rate ≥ 70 mL/minute per 1.73 m^2) compared surgery versus medical management (prophylactic antibiotics) over 5 years. The RCT found no significant difference in development of new renal scarring with surgery versus medical management but found that surgery versus medical management reduced the incidence of pyelonephritis (see glossary, p 480) (pyelonephritis in 5/64 [8%] with surgery *v* 15/68

[22%] treated medically; ARR 14%, 95% CI 2% to 19%; RRR 65%, 95% CI 10% to 87%).[34] The second subsequent RCT (25 boys and 27 girls aged 1–12 years with bilateral vesicoureteric reflux [grades III–V] and bilateral nephropathy, glomerular filtration rate ≥ 20 mL/minute per 1.73 m^2) compared corrective surgery versus medical management (prophylactic antibiotics: co-trimoxazole, trimethoprim, or nitrofurantoin) over 4 years.[33] It found no significant difference in development of new scars between medical treatment versus corrective surgery after 4 years (AR 7/54 [13%] kidneys with medical treatment *v* 8/50 [16%] kidneys with corrective surgery; RR 0.81, 95% CI 0.32 to 2.07).[33] **Longer term outcome:** We found one RCT (25 boys and 27 girls aged 1–12 years with bilateral vesicoureteric reflux [grades III–V] and bilateral nephropathy) with 10 years' follow up.[33] It found a steady decline in glomerular filtration rate over 10 years in children on medical treatment versus surgery (see table 1, p 481). There was no statistically significant difference between medical treatment versus surgery, but the study was underpowered to detect a clinically important effect.

Harms: **Versus medical management:** The review gave no information on surgical complications, and none of the individual studies were designed to compare rates of adverse effects.[32] In one arm of the subsequent RCT, 7/9 children who had postoperative obstruction developed evidence of renal scarring on DMSA scintigraphy (see glossary, p 479). This may have negated an otherwise beneficial effect of surgery over medical management.[34]

Comment: **Versus medical management:** The best results were obtained by centres handling the greatest number of children.[35] Surgery is usually considered only in children with more severe vesicoureteric reflux (grades III–V), who are less likely to experience spontaneous resolution.[4,36] **Longer term outcome:** The RCT involving children with bilateral moderate to severe vesicoureteric reflux and nephropathy found that, over a period of 4 years, 20/54 (37%) kidneys of children in the medical group had spontaneous resolution to no, or minimal, vesicoureteric reflux (grades 0 or I) and 47/50 (94%) kidneys had uncomplicated corrections in the surgical group (ARI 57%, 95% CI 47% to 69%).[33] We found one prospective cohort study (226 children aged 5 days to 12 years who presented with urinary tract infection and were found to have grades III–IV vesicoureteric reflux) with follow up of 10–41 years.[8] It found that surgery was associated with a higher rate of resolution of reflux compared with medical treatment (AR of resolution from age 8–14 years on micturating cystourethrography: 29/33 [88%] with surgery *v* 134/193 [69%] treated medically; ARI 19%, 95% CI 6% to 31%). The study did not compare clinical outcomes.[8]

GLOSSARY

DMSA scintigraphy A scan following intravenous injection of a radioisotope solution, which is excreted by the kidneys. The scan yields information about the structure and function of the urinary tract.

Intravenous immunoglobulins Immunoglobulin preparations derived from donated human plasma containing antibodies prevalent in the general population.

Nosocomial infection Definitions vary but typically an infection arising at least 48–72 hours after admission to hospital. The infection may have been acquired from other people, hospital staff, the hospital environment, or from pre-existing subclinical infection.

Pyelonephritis Inflammation of the kidney and its pelvis because of bacterial infection.

Severity of vesicoureteric reflux:

Grade I Reflux into ureters only.

Grade II Reflux into ureters, pelvis, and calyces.

Grade III Mild to moderate dilatation or tortuosity of ureters and mild to moderate dilatation of pelvis, but little or no forniceal blunting.

Grade IV As grade III, but with complete obliteration of forniceal angles, yet maintenance of papillary impressions in calyces.

Grade V Gross dilatation of ureters, pelvis, and calyces, and papillary impressions in calyces obliterated.

Substantive changes

Longer versus short courses of oral antibiotics Two systematic reviews added;[14,15] conclusions amended.

REFERENCES

1. Hellstrom A, Hanson E, Hansson S, et al. Association between urinary symptoms at 7 years old and previous urinary tract infections. *Arch Dis Child* 1991;66:232–234.
2. Dick PT, Feldman W. Routine diagnostic imaging for childhood urinary tract infections: a systematic overview. *J Pediatr* 1996;128:15–22. Search date 1994; primary sources Medline, Current Contents, and hand searches of article bibliographies.
3. Smellie JM, Katz G, Gruneberg RN. Controlled trial of prophylactic treatment in childhood urinary tract infection. *Lancet* 1978;ii:175–178.
4. Jodal U, Hansson S, Hjalmas K. Medical or surgical management for children with vesico-ureteric reflux? *Acta Paediatr Suppl* 1999;431:53–61.
5. Jodal U. The natural history of bacteriuria in childhood. *Infect Dis Clin North Am* 1987;1:713–729.
6. Hoberman A, Wald ER, Hickey RW, et al. Oral versus initial intravenous therapy for urinary tract infections in young febrile children. *Pediatrics* 1999;104:79–86.
7. Piepsz A, Tamminen-Mobius T, Reiners C, et al. Five-year study of medical and surgical treatment in children with severe vesico-ureteric reflux dimercaptosuccinic acid findings. International Reflux Study Group in Europe. *Eur J Pediatr* 1998;157:753–758.
8. Smellie JM, Prescod NP, Shaw PJ, et al. Childhood reflux and urinary infection: a follow-up of 10–41 years in 226 adults. *Pediatr Nephrol* 1998;12:727–736.
9. Berg UB. Long-term follow-up of renal morphology and function in children with recurrent pyelonephritis. *J Urol* 1992;148:1715–1720.
10. Martinell J, Claeson I, Lidin-Janson G, et al. Urinary infection, reflux and renal scarring in females continuously followed for 13–38 years. *Pediatr Nephrol* 1995;9:131–136.
11. Jacobson S, Eklof O, Erikkson CG, et al. Development of hypertension and uraemia after pyelonephritis in childhood: 27 year follow up. *BMJ* 1989;299:703–706.
12. Biggi A, Dardanelli L, Cussino P, et al. Prognostic value of the acute DMSA scan in children with first urinary tract infection. *Pediatr Nephrol* 2001;16:800–804.
13. Tran D, Muchant DG, Aronoff SC. Short-course versus conventional length antimicrobial therapy for uncomplicated lower urinary tract infections in children: a meta-analysis of 1279 patients. *J Pediatr* 2001;139;93–99. Search date 1999; primary sources Medline, and eference lists of identified studies.
14. Michael M, Hodson EM, Craig JC, et al. Short compared with standard duration of antibiotic treatment for urinary tract infection: a systematic review of randomized controlled trials. *Arch Dis Child* 2002;87:118–123. Search date 2001; primary sources Medline, Embase, Cochrane Controlled Trials Register, and hand searches of reference lists and abstracts of scientific meetings. No language restrictions were applied.
15. Keren R, Chan E. A meta-analysis of randomized, controlled trials comparing short- and long-course antibiotic therapy for urinary tract infections in children. *Pediatrics* 2002;109:e70. Search date 2001; primary sources Medline, Cochrane Controlled Trials Register, hand searches of references, and contact with experts. Limited to English language published articles.
16. Benador D, Neuhaus TJ, Papazyan J-P, et al. Randomised controlled trial of three day versus 10 day intravenous antibiotics in acute pyelonephritis: effect on renal scarring. *Arch Dis Child* 2001;84;241–246.
17. Levtchenko E, Lahy C, Levy J, et al. Treatment of children with acute pyelonephritis: a prospective randomized study. *Paediatr Nephrol* 2001;16;878–884.
18. Williams GJ, Lee A, Craig JC. Long-term antibiotics for preventing recurrent urinary tract infection in children. In: The Cochrane Library, Issue 4, 2001. Oxford: Update Software. Search date 2001; primary sources Medline, Embase, Cochrane Controlled Trials Register, reference lists in reviews, and contact with experts.
19. Lohr JA, Nunley DH, Howards SS, et al. Prevention of recurrent urinary tract infections in girls. *Pediatrics* 1977;59:562–565.
20. Benador D, Benador N, Slozman D, et al. Are younger patients at higher risk of renal sequelae after pyelonephritis? *Lancet* 1997;349:17–19.
21. Garin EH, Campos A, Homsy Y. Primary vesico-ureteral reflux: a review of current concepts. *Pediatr Nephrol* 1998;12:249–256.
22. Smellie JM, Gruneberg RN, Leakey A, et al. Long term low dose co-trimoxazole in prophylaxis of childhood urinary tract infection: clinical aspects/bacteriological aspects. *BMJ* 1976;2:203–208.

23. Allen UD, MacDonald N, Fuite L, et al. Risk factors for resistance to "first-line" antimicrobials among urinary tract isolates of Escherichia coli in children. *CMAJ* 1999;160:1436–1440.
24. Greenfield SP, Ng M, Gran J. Experience with vesicoureteric reflux in children: clinical characteristics. *J Urol* 1997;158:574–577.
25. Ohlsson A, Lacy JB. Intravenous immunoglobulin for preventing infection in pre-term and/or low-birth-weight infants. In: The Cochrane Library, Issue 4, 2001. Oxford: Update Software. Search date 1997; primary sources Medline, Embase, Cochrane Library, Reference Update, Science Citation Index, and hand searches of reference lists of identified RCTs and personal files.
26. Clemente E, Solli R, Mei V, et al. Therapeutic efficacy and safety of pidotimod in the treatment of urinary tract infections in children. *Arzneim Forsh* 1994;44:1490–1494.
27. Lettgen B. Prevention of urinary tract infections in female children. *Curr Ther Res* 1996;57:464–475.
28. Weisman LE, Cruess DF, Fischer GW. Opsonic activity of commercially available standard intravenous immunoglobulin preparations. *Paediatr Inf Dis* J 1994;13:1122–1125.
29. Nayir A, Emre S, Sirin A, et al. The effects of vaccination with inactivated uropathogenic bacteria in recurrent urinary tract infections of children. *Vaccine* 1995;13:987–990.
30. Czerwionka-Szarflarska M, Pawlowska M. Uro-vaxom in the treatment of recurrent urinary tract infections in children. *Pediatria Polska* 1996;71:599–604.
31. Pylkannen J, Vilska J, Koskimies O. The value of childhood urinary tract infection in predicting renal injury. *Acta Paediatr Scand* 1981;70:879–883.
32. Shanon A, Feldman W. Methodological limitations in the literature on vesicoureteric reflux: a critical review. *J Pediatr* 1990;117:171–178. Search date 1988; primary source Medline.
33. Smellie JM, Barratt TM, Chantler C, et al. Medical versus surgical treatment in children with severe bilateral vesicoureteric reflux and bilateral nephropathy: a randomized controlled trial. *Lancet* 2001;357:1329–1333.
34. Weiss R, Duckett J, Spitzer A. Results of a randomized clinical trial of medical versus surgical management of infants and children with grades III and IV primary vesico-ureteral reflux (United States): the international reflux study in children. *J Urol* 1992;148:1667–1673.
35. Smellie JM. Commentary: management of children with severe vesicoureteral reflux. *J Urol* 1992;148:1676–1678.
36. Sciagra R, Materassi M, Rossi V, et al. Alternative approaches to the prognostic stratification of mild to moderate primary vesicoureteral reflux in children. *J Urol* 1996;155:2052–2056.

James Larcombe
General Practitioner, Sedgefield and
Regional Research Fellow
NHSE Northern and Yorkshire
Sedgefield
UK

Competing interests: None declared.

TABLE 1 **Average glomerular filtration rates in children with bilateral vesicoureteric reflux and bilateral nephropathy at the commencement of the study, at 4 years, and at 10 years after randomisation to medical or surgical management (see text, p 478).[33]**

Mean GFR (mL/min)	At entry	At 4 years	At 10 years
Medical management	72.4	70.2	68.3
Surgical management	71.7	73.7	74.1
Difference in change in GFR from entry (95% CI)	–	+7.1% (–6.4% to +20.6%)	+8.9% (–10.3% to +28.2%)

GFR, glomerular filtration rate.

Anal fissure

Search date September 2002

Marion Jonas and John Scholefield

QUESTIONS

INTERVENTIONS

To be covered in future updates
Nifedipine for chronic anal fissure
Treatments for acute anal fissure

See glossary, p 489

Key Messages

- **Anal advancement flap (as effective as internal anal sphincterotomy)** One RCT found no significant difference with lateral internal anal sphincterotomy versus anal advancement flap in patient satisfaction or fissure healing.
- **Anal stretch** One systematic review found no significant difference with internal anal sphincterotomy versus anal stretch in persistence of fissures, and that both procedures healed 70–95% of fissures. Anal stretch versus internal anal sphincterotomy significantly increased rates of flatus incontinence.
- **Botulinum A toxin-haemagglutinin complex (botulinum A toxin-hc)** One small RCT found that botulinum A toxin-hc versus placebo increased fissure healing after 2 months. One small RCT found that botulinum A toxin-hc versus topical glyceryl trinitrate (GTN) 0.2% significantly increased fissure healing rates after 2 months. Two RCTs found no significant difference with high dose versus low dose botulinum A toxin-hc in healing rates after 2–3 months.
- **Botulinum A toxin-haemagglutinin complex (botulinum A toxin-hc) plus nitrates** We found no RCTs comparing botulinum A toxin-hc plus nitrates versus placebo. One small RCT in people with anal fissures that had failed to heal with topical nitrates found that botulinum A toxin-hc plus topical isosorbide dinitrate three times daily versus botulinum A toxin-hc alone significantly increased fissure healing at 6 weeks, but found no significant difference at 8 or 12 weeks.
- **Diltiazem** We found no placebo controlled RCTs. One small RCT found no significant difference with oral diltiazem versus topical diltiazem in fissure healing after 8 weeks. One small RCT found no significant difference in healing rate between topical diltiazem versus topical GTN at 8 weeks.

- **Indoramin** One RCT found no significant difference with oral indoramin versus placebo in fissure healing after 6 weeks.
- **Internal anal sphincterotomy** One systematic review found no significant difference with internal anal sphincterotomy versus anal stretch in persistence of fissures, and that both procedures healed 70–95% of fissures. It found no significant difference with open versus closed internal sphincterotomy in persistence of fissures. Three RCTs have found that sphincterotomy significantly improved fissure healing compared with topical GTN after 6 weeks to 1 year.
- **Topical glyceryl trinitrate (GTN)** Two RCTs found that topical GTN versus placebo significantly increased fissure healing after 8 weeks. Two further RCTs found no significant difference in fissure healing after 4 weeks of treatment, although they may have lacked power to detect a clinically important benefit. Three RCTs have found that sphincterotomy significantly improved fissure healing compared with topical GTN after 6 weeks to 1 year. One systematic review found that botulinum A toxin-hc versus GTN significantly increased fissure healing after 2 months. One RCT found no significant difference with GTN ointment versus a GTN patch in fissure healing after 8 weeks. One RCT found no significant difference between topical GTN versus topical diltiazem in healing at 8 weeks.

DEFINITION Anal fissure is a split or tear in the lining of the distal anal canal. It is a painful condition often associated with fresh blood loss from the anus and perianal itching. **Acute anal fissures** have sharply demarcated, fresh mucosal edges, and often with granulation tissue at the base. **Chronic anal fissures** margins are indurated, there is less granulation tissue, and muscle fibres of the internal anal sphincter may be seen at the base. Fissures persisting for longer than 6 weeks are generally defined as chronic.

INCIDENCE/ PREVALENCE Anal fissures are common in all age groups, but we found no evidence to quantify incidence.

AETIOLOGY/ RISK FACTORS Low intake of dietary fibre may be a risk factor for the development of acute anal fissures.[1] People with anal fissure often have raised resting anal canal pressures with anal spasm.[2,3] Men and women are equally affected by anal fissures, and up to 11% of women develop anal fissures after childbirth.[4]

PROGNOSIS Placebo controlled studies found that 70–90% of untreated "chronic" fissures did not heal during the study.[5,6]

AIMS OF INTERVENTION To relieve symptoms (pain, bleeding, irritation); to heal the fissure; to minimise adverse effects of treatment.

OUTCOMES Number of people with fissure healing (intact anal mucosal lining); symptom score for intensity of symptoms of pain, bleeding, and irritation (typically a linear visual analogue scale that consists of an unmarked 100 mm horizontal line, the left end of which represents absence of symptoms and the right end represents the worst symptoms imaginable; a vertical mark is made across this line by the person with the fissure); number of people reporting adverse effects of treatment.

METHODS *Clinical Evidence* search and appraisal September 2002.

QUESTION What are the effects of treatments for chronic anal fissure?

OPTION TOPICAL GLYCERYL TRINITRATE

Two RCTs found that topical glyceryl trinitrate (GTN) versus placebo significantly increased fissure healing after 8 weeks. Two further RCTs found no significant difference in fissure healing after 4 weeks of treatment, although they may have lacked power to detect a clinically important benefit. Three RCTs have found that sphincterotomy significantly improved fissure healing compared with topical GTN after 6 weeks to 1 year. One small RCT found that botulinum A toxin-hc versus 6 weeks of treatment with GTN significantly increased fissure healing rates after 2 months. One RCT found no significant difference with GTN ointment versus a GTN patch in fissure healing after 8 weeks. One RCT found no significant difference in healing rates at 8 weeks with GTN versus topical diltiazem.

Benefits: **Versus placebo:** We found one systematic review (search date not stated, 4 RCTs, 312 people; no statistical pooling of data provided).[7] The first RCT (80 people) found that GTN (see glossary, p 489) versus placebo significantly increased the proportion of people with healed anal fissures (analysis not by intention to treat; 3 people excluded; 26/38 [68%] with GTN *v* 3/39 [8%] with placebo; RR 8.9, 95% CI 2.94 to 26.95), and significantly reduced median pain scores (pain scores measured using a linear analogue scale; median score 6.0; range 0–78 with GTN *v* median score 40.0; range 0–92 with placebo; $P < 0.05$) after 8 weeks of treatment.[5] The second RCT in the review compared three treatments: 0.2% GTN; escalating dose topical GTN (starting with 0.2% and increasing by 0.1% increments weekly to maximum 0.6%); and placebo.[6] It found that both GTN treatments combined versus placebo significantly increased anal fissure healing after 8 weeks of treatment and at follow up after 2 weeks (31/46 [67%] with GTN *v* 7/22 [32%] with placebo; RR 2.1, 95% CI 1.11 to 4.03), but found no significant difference in pain scores (measured using a linear analogue scale; $P = 0.04$).[6] The third RCT (43 people) identified by the review found no significant difference with GTN versus placebo in the proportion of people with healed anal fissures after 4 weeks of treatment (11/24 [46%] with GTN *v* 3/19 [16%] with placebo; RR 2.0, 95% CI 0.65 to 6.45), and did not provide comparative data between treatments for pain scores.[8] The fourth RCT identified by the review found no significant difference with GTN versus placebo in the proportion of people with healed anal fissures after 4 weeks of treatment (29/59 [49%] with GTN *v* 31/60 [52%] with placebo; RR 0.95, 95% CI 0.67 to 1.36), and did not provide comparative data between treatments for pain scores.[9] **Versus internal sphincterotomy:** See glossary, p 489. We found one systematic review (search date not stated, 1 RCT),[7] one additional RCT,[10] and one subsequent RCT.[11] The RCT (82 people with chronic anal fissures receiving stool softeners and fibre supplements) identified by the review found that internal sphincterotomy versus GTN ointment significantly improved fissure healing at 6 weeks (34/38 [89%] *v* 13/44 [30%]; ARI 60%, 95% CI 38% to 81%;

RR 3.0, 95% CI 1.9 to 4.8).[12] The additional RCT (49 people with chronic anal fissure of duration 4 months receiving a high fibre diet and a laxative) also found that internal sphincterotomy versus topical GTN (ointment [0.2%] or patch [10 mg]) significantly improved fissure healing at 1 year (24/37 [65%] with GTN *v* 11/12 [92%] with internal sphincterotomy; RR 0.71, 95% CI 0.53 to 0.95).[10] The subsequent RCT (60 people) found that internal sphincterotomy versus GTN ointment significantly increased the proportion of people with healed anal fissures at 8 weeks (26/27 [96%] *v* 20/33 [61%]; RR 1.6, 95% CI 1.20 to 2.11).[11] See also benefits of surgical treatments, p 488. **Versus botulinum A toxin-hc (see glossary, p 489):** See benefits of botulinum A toxin-haemagglutinin complex, p 486. **GTN ointment versus GTN patch:** We found one RCT (42 people), which found no significant difference with GTN ointment (0.2% applied twice daily) versus a GTN patch (10 mg/day) in fissure healing at 8 weeks (analysis not by intention to treat; 5 people excluded; 12/18 [67%] healed with GTN ointment *v* 12/19 [60%] with a GTN patch; RR 1.1, 95% CI 0.66 to 1.70).[10] **Versus topical diltiazem:** We found one RCT (72 people) which found no significant difference between GTN (0.2% ointment applied twice daily for 6–8 wks) versus topical diltiazem (2% cream applied twice daily for 6–8 wks) in healing at 8 weeks (25/29 [86%] with GTN *v* 24/31 [77%] with diltiazem; RR 0.69, 95% CI 0.39 to 1.22].[13]

Harms: **Versus placebo:** Topical GTN caused headaches in 29–72% of people compared to 21–27% with placebo.[5,6,8] **Versus diltiazem:** One RCT found that GTN versus diltiazem significantly increased the proportion of people who had overall adverse effects (21/29 [72%] with GTN *v* 13/31 [42%] people with diltiazem; RR 1.84, 95% CI 1.11 to 3.04). Headaches and gastrointestinal adverse effects were more common in people receiving GTN versus diltiazem (headaches: 17/29 [59%] with GTN *v* 8/31 [26%] with diltiazem; gastrointestinal effects: 9/29 [31%] with GTN *v* 3/31 [10%] with diltiazem).[13]

Comment: We found insufficient evidence about the optimal duration of topical GTN treatment. Recurrent fissures may occur after GTN treatment is discontinued.

OPTION DILTIAZEM

We found no placebo controlled RCTs. One RCT found no significant difference in healing rates between topical diltiazem and topical glyceryl trinitrate at 8 weeks. One small RCT found no significant difference with oral diltiazem versus topical diltiazem in fissure healing after 8 weeks.

Benefits: We found no systematic review. **Versus placebo:** We found no RCTs. **Topical diltiazem versus topical glyceryl trinitrate (GTN):** See benefits of topical GTN, p 484. **Oral versus topical diltiazem:** We found one RCT (50 people with chronic anal fissures), which found no significant difference with oral diltiazem (60 mg twice daily) versus 2% topical diltiazem gel (700 mg twice daily) in the proportion of people with healed fissures after 8 weeks treatment (9/24 [38%] with oral diltiazem *v* 17/26 [65%] with diltiazem gel; RR 0.57, 95% CI 0.32 to 1.03).[14]

Harms: **Oral versus topical diltiazem:** The RCT reported that oral diltiazem caused adverse effects in 8/24 (33%) people (nausea/vomiting in 3 people, headache in 2 people, rash in 2 people, altered sense of smell and taste in 1 person), and that topical diltiazem caused none of these adverse effects.[14]

Comment: We found insufficient evidence about the optimal duration of diltiazem treatment. The role of diltiazem in treating fissures previously failing to heal with GTN is also unclear.

OPTION INDORAMIN

One RCT found no significant difference with oral indoramin versus placebo in fissure healing after 6 weeks, but may have been too small to detect a clinically important difference.

Benefits: We found no systematic review. **Versus placebo:** We found one small RCT (23 people with chronic anal fissures), which found no significant difference with oral indoramin (20 mg twice daily) versus placebo in the proportion of people with healed fissures after 6 weeks (1/14 [7%] with indoramin *v* 2/9 [22%] with placebo; RR 0.3, 95% CI 0.03 to 3.05; see comment below).[15] The RCT did not provide comparative data between treatments for pain scores.

Harms: The RCT reported that indoramin caused adverse effects in 7/14 (50%) of people.[15]

Comment: The RCT was small and may have lacked adequate power to detect a clinically important difference. It found that the single fissure that healed with indoramin recurred after 3 months.[15]

OPTION BOTULINUM A TOXIN-HAEMAGGLUTININ COMPLEX (BOTULINUM A TOXIN-HC)

One small RCT found that botulinum A toxin-hc versus placebo significantly increased fissure healing rates after 2 months. One RCT found that botulinum A toxin-hc injection versus topical application of glyceryl trinitrate 0.2% increased fissure healing rates at 2 months. Two RCTs found no significant difference with high dose versus low dose botulinum A toxin-hc in healing rates after 2–3 months.

Benefits: **Versus placebo:** We found one systematic review (search date not stated, 1 RCT, 30 people with chronic idiopathic anal fissure).[7] The RCT identified by the review compared botulinum A toxin-hc (see glossary, p 489) (Botox preparation) versus placebo (saline) injection into the internal anal sphincter.[16] It found that botulinum A toxin-hc significantly increased healing rates (formation of a scar) after 2 months (11/15 [73%] with botulinum A toxin-hc *v* 2/15 [13%] with placebo; ARR 60%, 95% CI 25% to 95%; RR 5.5, 95% CI 1.5 to 21). **Versus topical glyceryl trinitrate (GTN):** We found one systematic review (search date not stated, 1 RCT, 50 people with chronic anal fissure).[7] The RCT identified by the review found that botulinum A toxin-hc injection (20 units Botox preparation) versus GTN 0.2% for 6 weeks significantly increased fissure healing rates at 2 months (96% with botulinum A toxin-hc *v* 60% with GTN; P = 0.005).[17] **Different doses of botulinum A toxin-hc:** We found no systematic review. We found two RCTs.[18,19] The first RCT

(50 people) found no significant difference with higher dose (40 units) versus lower dose (20 units) botulinum A toxin-hc (Dysport preparation) in healing rates at 3 months (20/25 [80%] with higher dose v 19/25 [76%] with lower dose; RR 1.1, 95% CI 0.78 to 1.41).[18] The second RCT (150 people) compared botulinum A toxin-hc (Botox preparation) 20 units plus retreatment with 30 units if the fissure persisted at 1 month (lower dose) versus botulinum A toxin-hc 30 units initially plus retreatment with 50 units if the fissure persisted (higher dose). It found that higher versus lower dose botulinum A toxin-hc increased healing rates at 1 month (65/75 [87%] with higher dose v 55/75 [73%] with lower dose; P = 0.04), but found no significant difference in healing rates at 2 months (72/75 [96%] healed with higher dose v 67/75 [89%] healed with lower dose; RRs and CI were not reported; P reported as non-significant).[19]

Harms: One RCT comparing different doses of botulinum A toxin-hc found flatus incontinence in 6% of people for less than 2 weeks, and faecal incontinence in 4% of people for 1 week.[18] One RCT found that mild flatus incontinence was more common with higher versus lower dose botulinum A toxin-hc at 2 weeks after injection (5/75 [7%] with higher dose v 0/75 [0%] with lower dose; RRs and CI were not reported).[19] Two RCTs reported no adverse effects associated with the use of botulinum A toxin-hc.[16,17] Earlier pilot studies have also reported complications associated with the use of botulinum A toxin-hc, including pain, bleeding, sepsis associated with injection, and faecal incontinence, in up to 7% of people.[20,21]

Comment: Recurrent fissures may occur after treatment is discontinued. We found one cross-sectional study (57 people with idiopathic anal fissure), which found that a higher dosage regimen (20 units Botox preparation) versus a lower dosage regimen (15 units Botox preparation) of botulinum A toxin-hc increased the proportion of people with healed fissures at 2 months (23/34 [68%] with high dose botulinum A toxin-hc v 10/23 [43%] with low dose botulinum A toxin-hc).[22]

OPTION BOTULINUM A TOXIN-HAEMAGGLUTININ COMPLEX (BOTULINUM A TOXIN-HC) PLUS NITRATES

We found no RCTs comparing botulinum A toxin-hc plus nitrates versus placebo. One small RCT found that botulinum A toxin-hc plus topical isosorbide dinitrate three times daily versus botulinum A toxin-hc alone significantly increased fissure healing at 6 weeks, but found no significant difference at 8 or 12 weeks.

Benefits: **Versus placebo:** We found no RCTs. **Versus topical isosorbide dinitrate:** We found no systematic review. One RCT (30 people with anal fissures that had not healed with topical isosorbide dinitrate alone) found that botulinum A toxin-hc injection (20 units) followed by three times daily application of topical isosorbide dinitrate (2.5 mg) versus botulinum A toxin-hc injection alone significantly increased the proportion of people with healed anal fissures at

6 weeks (10/15 [66%] with botulinum A toxin-hc plus isosorbide dinitrate v 3/15 [20%] with botulinum A toxin-hc alone; ARI 47%, 95% CI 11% to 82%; RR 3.3, 95% CI 1.14 to 9.75; NNT 3, 95% CI 2 to 5), but found no significant difference at 8 and 12 weeks after treatment.[23]

Harms: The RCT did not report on harms.[23] See also harms of botulinum A toxin-hc, p 487.

Comment: The RCT was small and may have lacked power to detect a statistically significant differences at 8 and 12 weeks.[23]

OPTION SURGICAL TREATMENTS

One systematic review found no significant difference with internal anal sphincterotomy versus anal stretch in persistence of fissures, and that both procedures healed 70–95% of fissures. It found no significant difference with open versus closed internal sphincterotomy in persistence of fissures. The review found that anal stretch versus internal anal sphincterotomy significantly increased rates of flatus incontinence. One systematic review, one additional RCT, and one subsequent RCT found conflicting results for topical glyceryl trinitrate versus internal sphincterotomy in fissure healing after 6–8 weeks. One RCT found no significant difference with lateral internal sphincterotomy versus anal advancement flap in patient satisfaction or fissure healing.

Benefits: **Internal anal sphincterotomy:** We found one systematic review (search date not stated; data pooled for end points of persistence of fissure and postoperative incontinence of flatus; 6 RCTs, 386 people), which compared internal anal sphincterotomy versus anal stretch (see glossary, p 489).[24] It found that both internal anal sphincterotomy and anal stretch healed 70–95% of fissures. The review found no significant difference with anal stretch versus internal anal sphincterotomy in persistence of fissures (6 RCTs; RR 1.16, 95% CI 0.65 to 2.08; see comment below), and no significant difference with open versus closed internal sphincterotomy in persistence of fissures (2 RCTs; RR 1.61, 95% CI 0.28 to 9.28; see comment below). See also benefits of topical glyceryl trinitrate, p 484. **Anal advancement flap surgery:** We found no systematic review. We found one RCT (40 people) which found no significant difference with lateral internal sphincterotomy versus anal advancement flap (see glossary, p 489) in patient satisfaction or fissure healing (20/20 [100%] fissures healed after sphincterotomy v 17/20 [85%] following an advancement flap; P = 0.12).[25]

Harms: **Anal stretch versus sphincterotomy:** The systematic review found that anal stretch versus internal anal sphincterotomy significantly increased rates of flatus incontinence (4 RCTs; RR 6.63, 95% CI 2.06 to 21.3; see comment below), but found no significant difference with open versus closed lateral internal sphincterotomy in the risk of postoperative flatus incontinence (2 RCTs; RR 0.79, 95% CI 0.29 to 2.13; see comment below).[24] **Anal sphincterotomy versus anal advancement flap:** See harms of anal stretch above for comparative harms. In a single RCT (40 people), no participant experienced incontinence after either anal sphincterotomy or after anal advancement flap.[23]

Comment: Only two outcomes were considered by the systematic review: persistence of the fissure and flatus incontinence.[24] Other outcomes (e.g. complications related to wound healing) may be relevant. The review reported that, in contrast to the evidence from randomised studies, observational studies found that anal stretch versus internal anal sphincterotomy significantly increased rates of non-healing in four retrospective studies (RR 1.89, 95% CI 1.28 to 2.81).[24] The possibility of lower rates of fissure healing with anal advancement flap than with anal sphincterotomy requires further investigation.

GLOSSARY

Anal advancement flap Edges of the fissure are excised and healthy anal mucosa is mobilised to cover the defect.

Anal stretch Traditionally index and middle fingers of each hand inserted into the anal canal and pulled in opposite directions, the stretch held for 1 minute.

Botulinum A toxin-haemagglutinin complex (botulinum A toxin-hc) A formulation of botulinum A toxin and haemagglutinin for injection. Different preparations are used at different doses for the same indication and the strength (in units) of one preparation may not be equivalent to that of another preparation labelled as containing the same number of units.

Internal anal sphincterotomy Incision in the internal anal sphincter either posteriorly or laterally, but more commonly laterally, and usually "tailored" to the length of the fissure.

Topical glyceryl trinitrate (GTN) Usually applied as 0.2–0.3% ointment.

REFERENCES

1. Jensen SL. Diet and other risk factors for fissure-in-ano. Prospective case control study. *Dis Colon Rectum* 1988;31:770–773.
2. Gibbons CP, Read NW. Anal hypertonia in fissures: cause or effect? *Br J Surgery* 1986;73:443–445.
3. Lund JN, Scholefield JH. Internal sphincter spasm in anal fissure. *Br J Surg* 1997;84:1723–1724.
4. Martin JD. Postpartum anal fissure. *Lancet* 1953;i:271–273.
5. Lund JN, Scholefield JH. A randomised, prospective, double-blind, placebo-controlled trial of glyceryl trinitrate ointment in the treatment of anal fissure. *Lancet* 1997;349:11–14.
6. Carapeti EA, Kamm MA, McDonald PJ, et al. Randomised controlled trial shows that glyceryl trinitrate heals anal fissures, higher doses are not more effective, and there is a high recurrence rate. *Gut* 1999;44:727–730.
7. Cook TA, Brading AF, Mortensen NJMcC. The pharmacology of the internal anal sphincter and new treatments of ano-rectal disorders. *Aliment Pharmacol Ther* 2001;15:887–898. Search date not stated; primary sources Medline and hand searches of reference lists from relevant papers.
8. Kennedy ML, Sowter S, Nguyen H, et al. Glyceryl trinitrate ointment for the treatment of chronic anal fissure: results of a placebo-controlled trial and long-term follow-up. *Dis Colon Rectum* 1999;42:1000–1006.
9. Altomare DF, Rinaldi M, Milito G, et al. Glyceryl trinitrate for chronic anal fissure: healing or headache? Results of a multicenter, randomized, placebo-controlled, double-blind trial. *Dis Colon Rectum* 2000;43:174–179; discussion 179–181.
10. Zuberi BF, Rajput MR, Abro H, et al. A randomized trial of glyceryl trinitrate ointment and nitroglycerin patch in healing of anal fissures. *Int J Colorectal Dis* 2000;15:243–245.
11. Evans J, Luck A, Hewett P. Glyceryl trinitrate vs. lateral sphincterotomy for chronic anal fissure: Prospective, randomized trial. *Dis Colon Rectum* 2001;44:93–97.
12. Richard CS, Gregoire R, Plewes EA, et al. Internal sphincterotomy is superior to topical nitroglycerin in the treatment of chronic anal fissure: results of a randomized, controlled trial by the Canadian Colorectal Surgical Trials Group. *Dis Colon Rectum* 2000;43:1048–1057; discussion 1057–1058.
13. Kocher HM, Steward M, Leather AJM, et al. Randomized clinical trial assessing the side-effects of glyceryl trinitrate and diltiazem hydrochloride in the treatment of chronic anal fissure. *Br J Surg* 2002;89:413–417.
14. Jonas M, Neal KR, Abercrombie JF, et al. A randomized trial of oral vs. topical diltiazem for chronic anal fissures. *Dis Colon Rectum* 2001;44:1074–1078.
15. Pitt J, Dawson PM, Hallan RI, et al. A double-blind randomized placebo-controlled trial of oral indoramin to treat chronic anal fissure. *Colorectal Dis* 2001;3:165–168.
16. Maria G, Cassetta E, Gui D, et al. A comparison of botulinum toxin and saline for the treatment of chronic anal fissure. *N Engl J Med* 1998;338:217–220.
17. Brisinda G, Maria G, Bentivoglio AR, et al. A comparison of injections of botulinum toxin and topical nitroglycerin ointment for the treatment of chronic anal fissure. *N Engl J Med* 1999;341:65–69.
18. Jost W, Schrank B. Chronic anal fissures treated with botulinum toxin injections: a dose-finding study with Dysport. *Colorectal Dis* 1999;1:26–29.
19. Brisindi G, Maria G, Sganga G, et al. Effectiveness of higher doses of botulinum toxin to induce healing in patients with chronic anal fissures. *Surgery* 2002;131:179–184.

20. Jost WH, Schanne S, Mlitz H, et al. Perianal thrombosis following injection therapy into the external anal sphincter using botulinum toxin. *Dis Colon Rectum* 1995;38:781.
21. Jost WH. One hundred cases of anal fissure treated with botulin toxin: early and long-term results. *Dis Colon Rectum* 1997;40:1029–1032.
22. Maria G, Brisinda G, Bentivoglio AR, et al. Botulinum toxin injections in the internal anal sphincter for the treatment of chronic anal fissure: long-term results after two different dosage regimens. *Ann Surg* 1998;228:664–669.
23. Lysy J, Israelit-Yatzkan Y, Sestiery-Ittah M, et al. Topical nitrates potentiate the effect of botulinum toxin in the treatment of patients with refractory anal fissure. *Gut* 2001;48:221–224.
24. Nelson R. Operative procedures for fissure in ano. In: The Cochrane Library, Issue 4, 2001. Oxford: Update Software. Search date not stated; primary sources Cochrane Library, Medline, the Internet, and hand searches of cited reference lists from included reports.
25. Leong AF, Seow-Choen F. Lateral sphincterotomy compared with anal advancement flap for chronic anal fissure. *Dis Colon Rectum* 1995;38:69–71.

Marion Jonas
Specialist Registrar, General Surgery

John Scholefield
Professor of Surgery

University of Nottingham
Nottingham
UK

Competing interests: MJ none declared. JS has received commercial funding for research and for attending symposia.

Appendicitis

Search date February 2003

John Simpson and William Speake

QUESTIONS

INTERVENTIONS

See glossary, p 497

Key Messages

Treatments

- **Adjuvant antibiotics** One systematic review and one subsequent RCT in children and adults with simple or complicated appendicitis undergoing appendicectomy have found that prophylactic antibiotics reduce wound infections and intra-abdominal abscesses compared with no antibiotics. Subgroup analysis from the systematic review has found that antibiotics reduce the number of wound infections in children with complicated appendicitis compared with no antibiotics. Subgroup analysis from the systematic review also found no significant difference in the number of wound infections between antibiotics and no antibiotics in children with simple appendicitis. One subsequent RCT in children with simple appendicitis found no significant difference with antibiotic prophylaxis compared with no antibiotic prophylaxis in wound infections, but the RCT may have been too small to exclude a clinically important difference.
- **Laparoscopic surgery versus open surgery (in children)** One systematic review has found that, in children, laparoscopic surgery reduced the number of wound infections and the length of hospital stay compared with open surgery, but found no significant difference in postoperative pain, time to mobilisation, or proportion of intra-abdominal abscesses.
- **Antibiotics versus surgery** We found no RCTs comparing antibiotics with placebo or no treatment. One small RCT in adults with suspected appendicitis found that conservative treatment with antibiotics reduced pain and morphine consumption for the first 10 days compared with appendicectomy. However, the RCT found that 35% of people were readmitted within 1 year with acute appendicitis after conservative management with antibiotics and subsequently had an appendicectomy.

- **Laparoscopic surgery versus open surgery (in adults)** One systematic review has found that laparoscopic surgery in adults reduces the number of wound infections, pain on the first postoperative day, duration of hospital stay, and time taken to return to work compared with open surgery. However, laparoscopic surgery increased postoperative intra-abdominal abscesses compared with open surgery.
- **Open surgery versus no treatment** We found no RCTs comparing surgery with no surgery.
- **Stump inversion at open appendicectomy** One RCT found no significant difference between stump inversion and simple ligation in wound infection, length of hospital stay, or intra-abdominal abscesses. Another RCT found that stump inversion increased wound infections compared with simple ligation, but found no significant difference between groups for intra-abdominal abscesses or length of hospital stay.

DEFINITION Acute appendicitis is acute inflammation of the vermiform appendix.

INCIDENCE/ PREVALENCE The incidence of acute appendicitis is falling, although the reason for this is unclear. The reported lifetime risk of appendicitis in the USA is 8.7% in men and 6.7% in women,[1] and there are about 60 000 cases reported annually in England and Wales. Appendicitis is the most common surgical emergency requiring operation.

AETIOLOGY/ RISK FACTORS The cause of appendicitis is uncertain although various theories exist. Most relate to luminal obstruction, which prevents escape of secretions and inevitably leads to a rise in intraluminal pressure within the appendix. This can lead to subsequent mucosal ischaemia, and the stasis provides an ideal environment for bacterial overgrowth. Potential causes of the obstruction are faecoliths, often because of constipation, lymphoid hyperplasia, or caecal carcinoma.[2]

PROGNOSIS The prognosis of untreated appendicitis is unknown, although spontaneous resolution has been reported in at least 1/13 (8%) episodes.[3] The recurrence of appendicitis after conservative management,[3,4] and recurrent abdominal symptoms in certain people,[5] suggests that chronic appendicitis and recurrent acute or subacute appendicitis may also exist.[6] The standard treatment for acute appendicitis is appendicectomy. RCTs comparing treatment with no treatment would be regarded as unethical. The mortality from acute appendicitis is less than 0.3%, rising to 1.7% after perforation.[7] The most common complication of appendicectomy is wound infection, occurring in 5–33% of cases.[8] Intra-abdominal abscess formation occurs less frequently in 2% of appendicectomies.[9] A perforated appendix in childhood does not appear to have subsequent negative consequences on female fertility.[10]

AIMS OF INTERVENTION To reduce pain; prevent postoperative infection; shorten hospital stay; and hasten return to normal activity.

OUTCOMES Wound infection rates; intra-abdominal infection rates; postoperative pain; return of bowel function; return to normal activity; mortality.

METHODS *Clinical Evidence* search and appraisal February 2003.

QUESTION What are the effects of medical treatment for acute appendicitis?

OPTION ANTIBIOTICS

We found no RCTs comparing antibiotics with placebo or no treatment. One small RCT in adults with suspected appendicitis found that conservative treatment with antibiotics reduced pain and morphine consumption for the first 10 days compared with appendicectomy. However, the RCT found that 35% of people were readmitted within 1 year with acute appendicitis after conservative management with antibiotics and subsequently had an appendicectomy.

Benefits: **Versus no treatment:** We found no systematic review and no RCTs comparing antibiotics versus placebo or no treatment. **Versus surgery:** We found one RCT (40 adults with suspected appendicitis), which compared antibiotic treatment (iv cefotaxime 2 g twice daily plus tinidazole 800 mg/day for 2 days followed by oral ofloxacin 200 mg twice daily plus tinidazole 500 mg twice daily for 8 days) with open appendicectomy.[4] It found that antibiotics significantly reduced pain in the period from 12 hours to 10 days after initiation of treatment compared with appendicectomy ($P < 0.01$; other data presented graphically) and significantly reduced morphine consumption ($P < 0.001$).

Harms: **Versus no treatment:** We found no systematic review and no RCTs. **Versus surgery:** The RCT (40 adults with suspected appendicitis) found that all people treated conservatively with antibiotics were discharged from hospital within 48 hours, except one who had surgery for generalised peritonitis after a perforation of the appendix 12 hours after randomisation to receive antibiotic treatment.[4] The RCT found that 7/20 (35%) people who received conservative management were readmitted with acute appendicitis and had an appendicectomy within 1 year (mean 7 months, range 3–12 months). The RCT found that there was one wound infection in the surgically treated group, and that no deaths occurred with either treatment.

Comment: Inclusion criteria for the RCT included typical symptoms and signs of acute appendicitis, positive findings on ultrasound, and raised neutrophil/C-reactive protein levels on blood assays.

QUESTION What are the effects of surgical treatment for acute appendicitis?

OPTION OPEN SURGERY

We found no systematic review or RCTs of open surgery compared with no treatment. One RCT in adults with suspected appendicitis found that conservative treatment with antibiotics reduced pain and morphine consumption during the period of 12 hours to 10 days after starting treatment compared with appendicectomy. However, it found that 35% of people were readmitted within 1 year with acute appendicitis after conservative management with antibiotics and subsequently had an appendicectomy.

Benefits: **Versus no treatment:** We found no systematic review or RCTs of open surgery versus no treatment. **Versus antibiotics:** See benefits of antibiotics, p 493.

Harms: **Versus no treatment:** We found no RCTs. **Versus antibiotics:** See harms of antibiotics, p 493.

Comment: An RCT that compares open surgery with no treatment is unlikely to be conducted.

OPTION LAPAROSCOPIC SURGERY VERSUS OPEN SURGERY

One systematic review has found that laparoscopic surgery in adults reduces the number of wound infections, pain on the first postoperative day, duration of hospital stay, and time taken to return to work compared with open surgery. However, laparoscopic surgery increased postoperative intra-abdominal abscesses compared with open surgery. The review found that, in children, laparoscopic surgery reduced the number of wound infections and the length of hospital stay compared with open surgery, but found no significant difference in postoperative pain, time to mobilisation, or proportion of intra-abdominal abscesses.

Benefits: We found one systematic review (search date 2002) comparing laparoscopic surgery versus open surgery.[11] **In adults:** The systematic review found that laparoscopic surgery significantly reduced the number of wound infections compared with open surgery but significantly increased the number of postoperative intra-abdominal abscesses (wound infections: 34 RCTs, 4324 adults; 86/2213 [4%] with laparoscopic surgery *v* 161/2111 [8%] with open surgery; OR 0.47, 95% CI 0.36 to 0.62; abscesses: 34 RCTs, 4373 adults; 41/2239 [2%] with laparoscopic surgery *v* 13/2134 [< 1%] with open surgery; OR 2.77, 95% CI 1.61 to 4.77).[11] The review also found that laparoscopic surgery significantly reduced pain on the first postoperative day compared with open surgery and reduced both the duration of hospital stay and the time taken to return to work (pain measured using a 100 mm visual analogue scale, a reduction of 8 mm, 95% CI 3 mm to 13 mm; difference in length of hospital stay of 0.7 days, 95% CI 0.4 days to 1.0 days; difference in time to return to work of 3 days, 95% CI 1 day to 5 days). **In children:** The systematic review (5 RCTs, 436 children aged 1–16 years) found that laparoscopic surgery significantly reduced the number of wound infections and the length of hospital stay compared with open surgery (wound infections: 5 RCTs, 436 children; OR 0.22, 95% CI 0.08 to 0.61; difference in hospital stay: 1 RCT, difference of –0.7 days, 95% CI –1.1 days to –0.3 days).[11] The review found no significant difference between laparoscopic surgery and open surgery for intra-abdominal abscesses, in postoperative pain and in the time to mobilisation (intra-abdominal abscesses: 5 RCTs, 436 children: 1/220 [0.45%] with laparoscopic appendicectomy *v* 1/216 [0.46%] with conventional appendicectomy; OR 1.00, 95% CI 0.06 to 16.50; postoperative pain, 2 RCTs, 124 children; difference in visual analogue scale –0.068 cm, 95% CI –0.797 cm to +0.660 cm; time to mobilisation, 1 RCT, 58 children; difference of –0.25 days, 95% CI –0.65 days to +0.15 days).

Harms: The review did not report any further data on harms.[11]

Comment: The systematic review included people with a clinical diagnosis of acute appendicitis and provided no information on preoperative imaging or the use of perioperative antibiotics.[11] Analyses were performed on an intention to treat basis. Studies reporting a negative appendicectomy rate of more than 50% were excluded. The number of trials looking specifically at paediatric practice is small and, as in the adult studies, not all outcomes were assessed in all trials. Most trials were unblinded and, in addition, heterogeneity was present in most analyses, although not for wound infections or intra-abdominal abscesses. The definition and reporting of additional operative or postoperative complications was inconsistent. One RCT included in the review subsequently presented results from a subset of 25 children aged 4 to 15 years with complicated appendix.[12] It found no significant difference between laparoscopic and open surgery in the length of hospital stay or time to return to normal activities. It found two major complications (one pelvic abscess and one entero-cutaneous fistula) in 13 people receiving laparoscopic surgery compared with no major complications in 12 people receiving open surgery.

OPTION STUMP INVERSION AT OPEN APPENDICECTOMY

One RCT found no significant difference between stump inversion and simple ligation in wound infection, length of hospital stay, or intra-abdominal abscesses. Another RCT found that stump inversion increased wound infections compared with simple ligation, but found no significant difference between groups for intra-abdominal abscesses or length of hospital stay.

Benefits: We found no systematic review but found two RCTs.[13,14] The first RCT (735 people aged 14–91 years with complicated or simple appendicitis — see glossary, p 497) compared double invagination (purse string with Z stitch, 374 people) versus simple ligation of the stump (361 people).[13] The RCT found no significance difference in wound infection between double invagination and simple ligation, length of hospital stay, or intra-abdominal abscesses (wound infection: 33/374 [8.8%] with double invagination *v* 30/361 [8.3%] with simple ligation; length of hospital stay: 4.6 days with double invagination *v* 4.9 days with simple ligation; intra-abdominal abscesses: 6/374 [1.6%] with double invagination *v* 2/361 [< 1%] with simple ligation). The second RCT (134 people aged 4–90 years) compared simple ligation versus double invagination.[14] The RCT found significantly higher incidence of wound infection with double invagination compared with simple ligation but found no significant difference for intra-abdominal abscesses or length of hospital stay (wound infection : 4/55 [7.3%] with double invagination *v* 0/79 [0%] with simple ligation, $P = 0.017$; abscesses: 1 in each group; length of hospital stay: median 5 days for both groups).

Harms: In the two RCTs,[13,14] postoperative adhesive ileus was seen more frequently in the double invagination groups (6/374 [1.6%] with double invagination *v* 1/361 [< 1%] with simple ligation, $P < 0.05$[13] and 1/55 [1.8%] with double invagination *v* 0/79 [0%] with simple ligation[14]). No other specific complications were documented.[13,14]

Comment: Potential explanations for increased complications after invagination are believed to be due to longer operative time. Two trials[13,14] both comment theoretically on the potential caecal distortion after invagination of the appendix stump, which has mimicked caecal cancer on subsequent contrast imaging — a further potential hazard of stump invagination.

QUESTION **What are the effects of adjuvant treatments for acute appendicitis?**

OPTION **ADJUVANT ANTIBIOTICS**

One systematic review and one subsequent RCT in children and adults with simple or complicated appendicitis undergoing appendicectomy have found that prophylactic antibiotics reduce wound infections and intra-abdominal abscesses compared with no antibiotics. Subgroup analysis from the systematic review has found that antibiotics reduce the number of wound infections in children with complicated appendicitis compared with no antibiotics. Subgroup analysis from the systematic review also found no significant difference in the number of wound infections between antibiotics and no antibiotics in children with simple appendicitis. One subsequent RCT in children with simple appendicitis found no significant difference with antibiotic prophylaxis compared with no antibiotic prophylaxis in wound infections, but the RCT may have been too small to exclude a clinically important difference.

Benefits: **Versus placebo or no treatment:** We found one systematic review (search date 2000, 44 RCTs or CCTs, 9298 adults and children having an appendicectomy with either simple appendicitis or complicated appendicitis — see glossary, p 497)[9] and one subsequent RCT, which compared antibiotic prophylaxis versus placebo or no prophylaxis.[15] The review found that perioperative systemic antibiotic prophylaxis significantly reduced wound infections and intra-abdominal abscesses compared with no antibiotic prophylaxis (wound infections, 20 RCTs/CCTs: 287/4326 [7%] with antibiotics *v* 632/4317 [15%] with no antibiotics; OR 0.32, 95% CI 0.24 to 0.42; see comment below; intra-abdominal abscesses, 8 RCTs/CCTs: 16/2211 [< 1%] with antibiotics *v* 39/2257 [2%] with no antibiotics; OR 0.35, 95% CI 0.13 to 0.91).[9] Subgroup analysis found that, in people with simple appendicitis, antibiotic prophylaxis significantly reduced wound infections and intra-abdominal abscesses compared with no antibiotics (wound infections: 26 RCTs/CCTs: 113/2610 [4%] with antibiotics *v* 286/2707 [11%] with no antibiotics; OR 0.37, 95% CI 0.30 to 0.46; intra-abdominal abscesses, 8 RCTs/CCTs: 9/1433 [< 1%] with antibiotics *v* 22/1535 [1%] with no antibiotics; OR 0.46, 95% CI 0.23 to 0.94). A subgroup analysis in people with complicated appendicitis found that antibiotic prophylaxis significantly reduced wound infections but found no significant difference in intra-abdominal abscesses (wound infections: 24 RCTs/CCTs: 121/645 [19%] with antibiotics *v* 175/507 [35%] with no antibiotics; OR 0.28, 95% CI 0.21 to 0.38; intra-abdominal abscesses, 3 RCTs/CCTs: 3/262 [1%] with antibiotics *v* 4/205 [2%] with no antibiotics; OR 0.54, 95% CI 0.12 to 2.43). The review also found no significant difference in wound infections between topical antibiotics and placebo (52/339 [15%] with topical antibiotics *v* 61/340 [18%] with placebo; OR 0.77, 95% CI 0.49 to 1.23). **In children:** The systematic review (7 RCTs, 987 children aged 0–15 years with either simple or complicated appendicitis) found no significant difference between perioperative systemic antibiotic prophylaxis and no antibiotic prophylaxis in wound infections or intra-abdominal abscesses (wound infections: 23/548 [4%] with antibiotics *v* 34/542 [6%] with no antibiotics; OR 0.64, 95% CI 0.37 to 1.10; intra-abdominal abscesses (1/142 [< 1%] with antibiotics *v* 5/141 [4%] with no antibiotics; OR 0.25, 95% CI 0.05 to 1.26; see comment below).[9] Subgroup analysis in children with simple appendicitis found no significant difference between treatments in wound infections, although in children with complicated appendicitis antibiotic prophylaxis significantly reduced wound infections (simple appendicitis, 3 RCTs/CCTs: 7/347 [2%] with antibiotics *v* 8/357 [2%] with no antibiotics; OR 0.92, 95% CI 0.33 to 2.57; complicated appendicitis, 3 RCTs/CCTs: 5/134 [4%] with antibiotics *v* 15/119 [13%] with no antibiotics; OR 0.31, 95% CI 0.12 to 0.77). The subsequent RCT (108 children with simple appendicitis) compared three treatments: no antibiotic, one antibiotic dose (1 g ceftriaxone), and 5 days of regular antibiotics (1 g/day ceftriaxone).[15] The RCT reported that only one wound infection occurred, and this was in a child who received no antibiotics (other numerical data not provided).

Harms: Several harms have been considered in the benefits section. The review and RCT did not report any further data on harms.[9,15]

Comment: The systematic review did not distinguish between antibiotic regimens or between different antibiotic drugs.[9] These issues are being addressed in a systematic review to be published in the future. There were limited numbers of children in the systematic review and RCT; therefore, the results may lack statistical power.[9,15] The review found insufficient data to provide subgroup analysis for numbers of intra-abdominal abscesses in children with either simple or complicated appendicitis.[9] The benefit of antibiotics for simple appendicitis in children is unclear. The review did not report on preoperative imaging studies.[9]

GLOSSARY

Complicated appendicitis Perforated or gangrenous appendicitis or the presence of a periappendicular abscess.

Simple appendicitis Clinically normal or inflamed appendix, in the absence of gangrene, perforation or abscess around the appendix.

REFERENCES

1. Addiss DG, Shaffer N, Fowler BS, et al. The epidemiology of appendicitis and appendectomy in the United States. *Am J Epidemiol* 1990;132:910–925.
2. Larner AJ. The aetiology of appendicitis. *Br J Hosp Med* 1988;39:540–542.
3. Cobben LP, de van Otterloo AM, Puylaert JB. Spontaneously resolving acute appendicitis: frequency and natural history in 60 patients. *Radiology* 2000;215:349–352.
4. Eriksson S, Granstrom L. Randomized controlled trial of appendicectomy versus antibiotic therapy for acute appendicitis. *Br J Surg* 1995;82:166–169.
5. Barber MD, McLaren J, Rainey JB. Recurrent appendicitis. *Br J Surg* 1997;84:110–112.
6. Mattei P, Sola JE, Yeo CJ. Chronic and recurrent appendicitis are uncommon entities often misdiagnosed. *J Am Coll Surg* 1994;178:385–389.
7. Velanovich V, Satava R. Balancing the normal appendectomy rate with the perforated

appendicitis rate: implications for quality assurance. *Am Surg* 1992;58:264–269.

8. Krukowski ZH, Irwin ST, Denholm S, et al. Preventing wound infection after appendicectomy: a review. *Br J Surg* 1988;75:1023–1033.
9. Andersen BR, Kallehave FL, Andersen HK. Antibiotics versus placebo for prevention of postoperative infection after appendectomy. In: The Cochrane Library, Issue 2, 2002. Oxford: Update Software. Search date 2000; primary sources Cochrane Controlled Trials Register, Medline, Embase, Cochrane Colorectal Cancer Group Specialised Register, and hand searches of reference lists of identified trials.
10. Andersson R, Lambe M, Bergstrom R. Fertility patterns after appendicectomy: historical cohort study. *BMJ* 1999;318:963–967.
11. Sauerland SR, Lefering R, Neugebauer EAM. Laparoscopic versus open surgery for suspected appendicitis. In: The Cochrane Library, Issue 2, 2002. Oxford: Update Software. Search date 2002; primary sources The Cochrane Library, Medline, Embase, Scisearch, and Biosis.
12. Lintula H, Kokki H, Vanamo K, et al. Laparoscopy in children with complicated appendicitis. *J Pediatr Surg* 37:1317–1320.
13. Engstrom L, Fenyo G. Appendicectomy: assessment of stump invagination versus simple ligation: a prospective, randomized trial. *Br J Surg* 1985;72:971–972.
14. Jacobs PP, Koeyers GF, Bruyninckx CM. [Simple ligation superior to inversion of the appendiceal stump; a prospective randomized study]. *Ned Tijdschr Geneeskd* 1992;136:1020–1023.
15. Gorecki WJ, Grochowski JA. Are antibiotics necessary in nonperforated appendicitis in children? A double blind randomised controlled trial. *Med Sci Monit* 2001;7:289–292.

John Simpson
MRC Fellow

William Speake
Specialist Registrar

Division of Gastrointestinal Surgery
University Hospital Nottingham
Nottingham
UK

Competing interests: None declared.

Colonic diverticular disease

Search date October 2002

John Simpson and Robin Spiller

QUESTIONS

INTERVENTIONS

See glossary, p 507

Key Messages

Treatment of uncomplicated diverticular disease

- **Bran and ispaghula husk** Two small RCTs found no consistent effect of bran or ispaghula husk versus placebo on symptom relief after 12–16 weeks.
- **Elective surgery** We found no RCTs of elective open or laparoscopic colonic resection.
- **Lactulose** One RCT found no significant difference with lactulose versus a high fibre diet in the number of people who considered themselves to be "much improved" after 12 weeks.
- **Methylcellulose** One small RCT found no significant difference with methylcellulose versus placebo in mean symptom score after 3 months.
- **Rifaximin (plus glucomannan *v* glucomannan alone)** One RCT found that oral rifaximin plus glucomannan versus glucomannan plus placebo significantly increases the proportion of people with uncomplicated diverticular disease who are symptom free after 12 months of treatment.

Treatment to prevent complications

- **Increased fibre intake** We found no RCTs of advice to consume a high fibre diet or of dietary fibre supplementation.

- **Mesalazine (after an attack of acute diverticulitis)** One RCT found that mesalazine reduced symptomatic recurrence compared with no treatment in people previously treated for an episode of acute diverticulitis, but was associated with abdominal pain.

Treatment of acute diverticulitis

- **Medical treatment** We found no RCTs of medical treatment versus placebo. One RCT comparing intravenous cefoxitin versus intravenous gentamicin plus intravenous clindamycin found no significant difference in rates of clinical cure. Observational studies in people with acute diverticulitis have found low mortality with medical treatment, but found that recurrence rates may be high.
- **Surgery (for diverticulitis complicated by generalised peritonitis)** We found no RCTs of surgery versus no surgery or versus medical treatment. One RCT comparing acute resection versus no acute resection (involving a transverse colostomy) of the sigmoid colon found no significant difference in mortality. A second RCT comparing primary versus secondary sigmoid colonic resection found no significant difference in mortality, but found that primary resection significantly reduced rates of postoperative peritonitis and emergency reoperation.

DEFINITION Colonic diverticula are mucosal out pouchings through the large bowel wall. They are often accompanied by structural changes (elastosis of the taenia coli, muscular thickening, and mucosal folding). They are usually multiple and occur most frequently in the sigmoid colon.

INCIDENCE/ PREVALENCE In the UK, the incidence of diverticulosis (see glossary, p 507) increases with age; about 5% of people are affected in their fifth decade of life and about 50% by their ninth decade.[1] Diverticulosis is common in developed countries, although there is a lower prevalence of diverticulosis in Western vegetarians consuming a diet high in roughage.[2] Diverticulosis is almost unknown in rural Africa and Asia.[3]

AETIOLOGY/ RISK FACTORS There is an association between low fibre diets and diverticulosis of the colon.[3] Prospective observational studies have found that both physical activity and a high fibre diet are associated with a lower risk of developing diverticular disease (see glossary, p 507).[4,5] One case control study found an association between the ingestion of non-steroidal anti-inflammatory drugs and the development of severe diverticular complications, including pericolic abscess, generalised peritonitis, bleeding, and fistula formation.[6] People in Japan, Singapore, and Thailand develop diverticula that mainly affect the right side of the colon.[7]

PROGNOSIS Symptoms will develop in 10–25% of people with diverticula at some point in their lives.[1] It is unclear why some people develop symptoms and some do not. Even after successful medical treatment of acute diverticulitis (see glossary, p 507) almost two thirds of people suffer recurrent pain in the lower abdomen.[8] Recurrent diverticulitis is observed in 7–42% of people with diverticular disease, and after recovery from the initial attack the calculated yearly risk of suffering a further episode is 3%.[9] About half of recurrences occur within 1 year of the initial episode and 90% occur within 5 years.[10] Complications of diverticular disease (perforation, obstruction, haemorrhage, and fistula formation) are each seen in about 5% of people with colonic diverticula when followed up for 10–30 years.[11] Intra-abdominal abscess formation may also occur.

AIMS OF INTERVENTION To reduce mortality, symptoms, and complications, with minimal adverse effects.

OUTCOMES Subjective gastrointestinal symptoms assessed by the use of validated questionnaires. Admission and readmission rates as a result of diverticular disease and its complications. Incidence of diverticulitis, haemorrhage, perforation, abscess, fistula formation, and mortality. Stool weight and transit time are surrogate outcomes.

METHODS *Clinical Evidence* search and appraisal October 2002.

QUESTION **What are the effects of treatments for uncomplicated diverticular disease?**

OPTION **BRAN AND ISPAGHULA HUSK**

Two RCTs in people with uncomplicated diverticular disease found no consistent effect of bran or ispaghula husk versus placebo on symptom relief after 12–16 weeks.

Benefits: **Versus placebo:** We found no systematic review, but found two RCTs of fibre supplements versus placebo.[12,13] The first RCT (76 people with uncomplicated diverticular disease (see glossary, p 507), no other gastrointestinal disorders, and no prior abdominal operations) compared three treatments: bran crispbread (6.99 g/day fibre); ispaghula husk drink (a bulk forming laxative; 9.04 g/day fibre); and placebo (2.34 g/day fibre).[12] It found no significant differences among treatments for pain score, lower bowel symptom score (combination of the pain score and sensation of incomplete emptying, straining, stool consistency, flatus, and aperients taken), or total symptom score (including nausea, vomiting, dyspepsia, belching, and abdominal distension; see comment below) after 16 weeks. The RCT also found that both active treatments versus placebo significantly reduced straining at stool (bran *v* placebo, $P < 0.01$; ispaghula husk *v* placebo, $P < 0.001$; CI not provided), increased wet stool weight (both active treatments *v* placebo, $P < 0.001$; CI not provided), and stool frequency (both active treatments *v* placebo, $P < 0.001$; CI not provided), and significantly softened the stools (both active treatments *v* placebo, $P < 0.001$; CI not provided) after 16 weeks. The second RCT (18 people with radiologically confirmed diverticula and no other colonic disorder) compared bran crispbread (6.7 g/day fibre) versus placebo crispbread (0.6 g/day fibre).[13] It found that bran crispbread significantly improved total symptom score (RR and CI not provided; $P < 0.002$) and pain score (RR and CI not provided; $P < 0.02$), but found no significant difference in the scores for bowel dysfunction (passage of excessive flatus, need to strain, frequency of evacuation, consistency of motion, presence of anal pain on defaecation, feeling of incomplete evacuation, presence of blood or mucus, use of laxatives) or dyspeptic symptoms (nausea, vomiting, heartburn, belching, and abdominal distension) after 3 months.

Harms: No significant adverse effects were reported in the RCTs.[12,13]

Comment: In the first RCT, 18/76 (24%) people withdrew from the trial and analysis of data was not by intention to treat.[12] The RCT did not specify the exact number of people receiving each treatment, precluding calculations of relative risk and confidence interval. People in both RCTs had been investigated to exclude coexisting abdominal pathology but the extent of the investigations was not stated.[12,13] Both studies were small in size, of short duration, and the difference in fibre content between control and treatment interventions was also small. Both treatment and control groups improved during the RCTs. One further RCT has been identified and is awaiting translation.[14]

OPTION METHYLCELLULOSE

One RCT in people with uncomplicated diverticular disease found no significant difference with methylcellulose versus placebo on mean symptom score after 3 months.

Benefits: We found no systematic review but found one RCT (30 people with symptomatic diverticular disease (see glossary, p 507) and no other gastrointestinal disease) that compared methylcellulose (500 mg twice daily) versus placebo.[15] It found no significant difference between treatments on mean symptom score after 3 months (see comment below; mean symptom score 13.0 with methylcellulose *v* 16.7 with placebo; difference in means –3.7, 95% CI –8.9 to +1.5).

Harms: None reported.

Comment: The RCT used a categorical scale for several different symptoms where 1 = mild and 6 = severe.[15] The score used to assess symptoms and signs was not described clearly, but included barium enema results. The RCT was small, of short duration, and both the methylcellulose and placebo treatments were associated with an improvement in symptom scores. Diverticular disease was confirmed by barium enema but the extent of any other investigations to exclude comorbidity was not stated.

OPTION LACTULOSE

One RCT in people with uncomplicated diverticular disease found no significant difference with lactulose versus a high fibre diet in the number of people who considered themselves to be "much improved" (not defined) after 12 weeks.

Benefits: We found no systematic review. **Versus placebo:** We found no RCTs. **Versus high fibre diet:** We found one RCT (43 people with diverticular disease (see glossary, p 507) and no other abdominal pathology) comparing lactulose (15 mL twice daily) versus a high fibre diet (30–40 g/day fibre).[16] It found no significant difference in the number of people who reported their symptoms to be much improved after 12 weeks (see comment below; 7/20 [35%] people with lactulose *v* 9/21 [43%] people with high fibre diet; RR 0.80, 95% CI 0.34 to 1.77).

Harms: The RCT found a non-significant increase in the risk of new symptoms with high fibre diet versus lactulose (12/21 [57%] people with high fibre diet *v* 9/20 [45%] people with lactulose; RR 1.30, 95% CI 0.70 to 2.34).[16] The symptoms were described as minor but no further details were provided. The RCT found that 2/20 (10%) people taking lactulose withdrew from the trial because of symptoms: one with abdominal pain and one with nausea.

Comment: Although "much improved" was used as an outcome by the RCT, this term was not defined clearly.[16] People were investigated to exclude coexisting abdominal pathology but the extent of the investigations was not stated.

OPTION ANTIBIOTICS (RIFAXIMIN)

One RCT in people with uncomplicated diverticular disease has found that rifaximin plus glucomannan versus glucomannan plus placebo significantly increases the number of people who are symptom free after 12 months of treatment.

Benefits: We found no systematic review but found one RCT.[17] The RCT (168 people with uncomplicated diverticular disease — see glossary, p 507) compared dietary fibre supplementation (glucomannan 2 g/day) plus oral rifaximin (see glossary, p 507) (400 mg twice daily) versus dietary fibre supplementation (glucomannan 2 g/day) plus placebo. Both treatments were given for 7 days each month for 1 year (see comment below). The RCT found that dietary fibre supplementation plus rifaximin significantly increased the number of people with no symptoms or only mild symptoms after 12 months of treatment (69% of people with rifaximin *v* 39% of people with placebo; P = 0.001; results presented graphically; absolute numbers not provided). The RCT found no significant difference between treatments in the severity of diarrhoea, tenesmus, or upper abdominal pain (absolute data and significance testing not provided).

Harms: The RCT did not report on harms.[17]

Comment: The RCT reported that 17/168 (10%) people did not complete the trial, although analysis was not by intention to treat.[17] For each treatment group, 2/84 (2%) people were withdrawn because of acute diverticulitis (see glossary, p 507)

OPTION ELECTIVE SURGERY

We found no RCTs of elective colonic resection (open or laparoscopic) in people with uncomplicated diverticular disease.

Benefits: We found no systematic review or RCTs.

Harms: We found no data on harms of elective surgery in people with diverticular disease (see glossary, p 507).

Comment: None.

QUESTION **What are the effects of treatments to prevent complications of diverticular disease?**

OPTION **ADVICE TO INCREASE FIBRE INTAKE**

We found no RCTs examining complication rates following advice to consume a high fibre diet or dietary fibre supplementation versus no advice or supplements.

Benefits: We found no systematic review and no RCTs.

Harms: We found no RCTs.

Comment: Fibre is often used with the aim of preventing complications in people with diverticular disease (see glossary, p 507) because observational studies have found that the disease is less frequent in populations with high fibre intake (see incidence and aetiology, p 500).

OPTION **MESALAZINE**

One RCT found that mesalazine reduced symptomatic recurrence compared with no treatment in people previously treated for an episode of acute diverticulitis, but was associated with abdominal pain.

Benefits: We found no systematic review. One RCT (166 people previously treated for an episode of mild/moderate diverticulitis) compared 8 weeks' treatment with oral mesalazine (400 mg twice daily) versus no treatment.[18] People in both groups had received intramuscular sulbactam-ampicillin (1.5 g twice daily) and oral rifaximin (see glossary, p 507) (400 mg twice daily) for 7 days before randomisation. The RCT found that mesalazine versus no treatment reduced symptomatic recurrence at 4 years (12/81 [15%] with mesalazine *v* 39/85 [46%] with no treatment; RR 0.32, 95% CI 0.18 to 0.57; NNT 4, 95% CI 3 to 6).[18]

Harms: The RCT found that abdominal pain was more common with mesalazine than placebo (13/81 [16%] with mesalazine *v* 4/85 [5%] with no treatment; RR 3.40, 95% CI 1.16 to 10.00; NNH 8, 95% CI 4 to 70).[18]

Comment: The recurrence of inflammation was diagnosed according to unspecified clinical and laboratory criteria.[18] Methods for determining symptom scores, including the assessment of pain, were not reported. Forty four people did not complete the study, but there was no difference in withdrawal rate between groups (3 people died; 9 people had a severe complication of diverticular disease [see glossary, p 507], and 33 were withdrawn because of poor adherence to treatment).[18]

QUESTION What are the effects of treatments for acute diverticulitis?

OPTION MEDICAL TREATMENT

We found no RCTs of medical treatment versus placebo. One RCT found no significant difference with intravenous cefoxitin versus intravenous gentamicin plus intravenous clindamycin in rates of clinical cure. Observational studies in people with acute diverticulitis have found low mortality with medical treatment but that recurrence rates may be high.

Benefits: We found no systematic review. **Versus placebo:** We found no RCTs. **Versus other medical treatments:** We found one RCT (51 people with a clinical diagnosis of acute diverticulitis (see glossary, p 507) who did not need immediate surgery) that compared intravenous cefoxitin (1–2 g every 6 h) versus intravenous gentamicin (1.7 mg/kg loading dose followed by 1.0–1.4 mg/kg every 8 h) plus intravenous clindamycin (total dose of 2400–2700 mg/day in 3 or 4 equal doses).[19] It found no significant difference in clinical cure rate (see comment below; 27/30 [90%] people with cefoxitin *v* 18/21 [86%] people with gentamicin plus clindamycin; RR 1.10, 95% CI 0.85 to 1.30).

Harms: In the RCT, toxicity (possibly antibiotic related) occurred with both treatments, although the numbers of people affected were not significantly different between treatments (2/30 [7%] people with cefoxitin *v* 3/21 [14%] people with gentamicin plus clindamycin; RR 0.47, 95% CI 0.09 to 2.56).[19]

Comment: Clinical cure was defined as complete resolution of symptoms and signs associated with diverticulitis plus discharge from hospital without recurrence for at least 6 weeks or plus having undergone an elective surgical procedure with primary anastomosis in the absence of colostomy without septic complications.[19] We found many observational studies of medical treatment for acute diverticulitis, with variable follow up periods (1–12 years), which consistently report low mortality (0–5%).[9,20–22] These observational trials also reported that 7–42% of people treated medically suffer recurrent episodes of acute diverticulitis.

OPTION SURGERY

One RCT in people with acute diverticulitis complicated by generalised peritonitis found no significant difference with acute sigmoid colonic resection versus no acute resection (involving a transverse colostomy) in mortality. Subgroup analysis found that, for people with purulent rather than faecal peritonitis, acute sigmoid colonic resection may increase mortality. A second RCT in people with acute diverticulitis complicated by generalised peritonitis found no significant difference with primary versus secondary sigmoid colonic resection in mortality, but found that primary sigmoid colonic resection significantly reduced rates of postoperative peritonitis and emergency reoperation.

Benefits: We found no systematic review. **Surgery versus placebo or medical treatment:** We found no RCTs. **Open surgery versus other types of open surgery:** We found two RCTs.[23,24] The first

RCT (62 people with diffuse peritonitis complicating perforated acute diverticulitis (see glossary, p 507) of the left colon; median age 72 years) compared acute sigmoid colonic resection (see glossary, p 507) versus no acute resection (acute transverse colostomy, suture, and omental covering of a visible perforation).[24] The RCT found no significant difference with acute sigmoid colonic resection versus no acute resection in mortality within 30 days (mortality: 8/31 [26%] with acute resection *v* 6/31 [19%] with no acute resection; RR 1.30, 95% CI 0.52 to 3.39). However, subgroup analysis of people with purulent peritonitis (46 people) found that acute sigmoid colonic resection versus no acute resection significantly increased postoperative mortality (6/25 [24%] people with acute resection *v* 0/21 [0%] people with no acute resection; ARI 24%, 95% CI 4.5% to 44%). Subgroup analysis of people with faecal peritonitis (16 people) found no significant difference with acute sigmoid colonic resection versus no acute resection in postoperative mortality (2/6 [33%] people with acute resection *v* 6/10 [60%] people with no acute resection; RR 0.60, 95% CI 0.16 to 1.92; see comment below). The second RCT (105 people with generalised peritonitis complicating sigmoid diverticulitis; mean age 66 years) compared primary versus secondary sigmoid colonic resection.[24] Primary resection involved surgical removal of the affected sigmoid colon plus either formation of an end colostomy, or formation of a primary colorectal anastomosis with or without a proximal defunctioning colostomy (see glossary, p 507). Secondary resection involved closing any visible bowel perforations initially plus the formation of a defunctioning colostomy. A second (definitive) procedure was then undertaken at a later date to perform a sigmoid colon resection plus a colorectal anastomosis with or without a defunctioning colostomy. The RCT found that primary versus secondary sigmoid colonic resection significantly reduced rates of postoperative peritonitis following the initial procedure (1/55 [2%] people with primary resection *v* 10/44 [23%] people with secondary resection; RR 0.09, 95% CI 0.01 to 0.70; NNT 5, 95% CI 3 to 12) and significantly reduced rates of emergency reoperation (2/55 [4%] people with primary resection *v* 9/48 [19%] people with secondary resection; RR 0.19, 95% CI 0.04 to 0.90; NNT 7, 95% CI 4 to 35). The RCT found no significant difference between treatments in mortality (13/55 [24%] people with primary resection *v* 9/48 [19%] people with secondary resection; RR 1.30, 95% CI 0.60 to 2.70; see comment below). **Open surgery versus laparoscopic surgery:** We found no RCTs.

Harms: The first RCT found no significant difference between treatments in rates of cardiopulmonary complications (13/31 [42%] with acute resection *v* 14/31 [45%] with no acute resection; RR 0.90, 95% CI 0.53 to 1.63), thromboembolism (3/31 [9.7%] with acute resection *v* 5/31 [16%] with no acute resection; RR 0.60, 95% CI 0.16 to 2.30), mental confusion (4/31 [13%] with acute resection *v* 4/31 [13%] with no acute resection; RR 1.00, 95% CI 0.27 to 3.65), or other complications (including wound dehiscence, wound infection but no dehiscence, intraperitoneal abscess formation, ileus, colocutaneous fistula, and revision of colostomy).[23] The second RCT found no significant difference between treatments in rates of wound complications (20/55 [36%] with primary resection *v* 23/48

[48%] with secondary resection; RR 0.80, 95% CI 0.48 to 1.20), rates of extra-abdominal septic complications (11/55 [20%] with primary resection *v* 12/48 [25%] with secondary resection; RR 0.80, 95% CI 0.39 to 1.65), or rates of extra-abdominal non-septic complications (26/55 [47%] with primary resection *v* 21/48 [44%] with secondary resection; RR 1.08, 95% CI 0.71 to 1.65).[24]

Comment: The first RCT was conducted in a single centre and took 14 years to recruit 62 people.[23] The second RCT was conducted in 17 centres and took 7 years to recruit 105 people.[24] Both studies were small and may have lacked power to detect a significant difference between treatments. The high complication rates reported are not unexpected in predominantly elderly people following a perforation of the large bowel. The wide spectrum of presentation and operative treatment options for acute complicated diverticulitis makes RCTs difficult to perform.

GLOSSARY

Acute diverticulitis This condition occurs when a diverticulum becomes acutely inflamed. There may be general symptoms and signs of infection (including fever and rapid heart rate) with or without local symptoms and signs (pain and localised tenderness, usually in the lower left abdomen, sometimes with a mass that can be felt on abdominal or rectal examination).

Acute sigmoid colonic resection Immediate resection of the sigmoid colon, involving end colostomy of the proximal bowel and creating a mucus fistula with the distal bowel or oversewing the rectal stump.

Defunctioning colostomy Stoma created to divert faecal flow.

Diverticular disease This term is used to describe diverticula associated with any symptoms.[25] Symptoms commonly include abdominal pain and alteration in bowel habit. Diverticular disease may be complicated by abscess formation, fistulae, perforation, obstruction, or haemorrhage.

Diverticulosis The presence of diverticula that are asymptomatic. Most people with sigmoid colonic diverticula have no symptoms.

Rifaximin A rifamycin antibacterial drug with antimicrobial actions similar to those of rifampicin. It is marketed predominantly in Italy.

REFERENCES

1. Parks TG. Natural history of diverticular disease of the colon. *Clin Gastroenterol* 1975;4:53–69.
2. Gear JS, Ware A, Fursdon P, et al. Symptomless diverticular disease and intake of dietary fibre. *Lancet* 1979;1:511–514.
3. Painter NS, Burkitt DP. Diverticular disease of the colon, a 20th century problem. *Clin Gastroenterol* 1975;4:3–21.
4. Aldoori WH, Giovannucci EL, Rimm EB, et al. Prospective study of physical activity and the risk of symptomatic diverticular disease in men. *Gut* 1995;36:276–282.
5. Aldoori WH, Giovannucci EL, Rimm EB, et al. A prospective study of diet and the risk of symptomatic diverticular disease in men. *Am J Clin Nutr* 1994;60:757–764.
6. Campbell K, Steele RJ. Non-steroidal anti-inflammatory drugs and complicated diverticular disease: a case-control study. *Br J Surg* 1991;78:190–191.
7. Sugihara K, Muto T, Morioka Y, et al. Diverticular disease of the colon in Japan. A review of 615 cases. *Dis Colon Rectum* 1984;27:531–537.
8. Munson KD, Hensien MA, Jacob LN, et al. Diverticulitis. A comprehensive follow-up. *Dis Colon Rectum* 1996;39:318–322.
9. Haglund U, Hellberg R, Johnsen C, et al. Complicated diverticular disease of the sigmoid colon. An analysis of short and long term outcome in 392 patients. *Ann Chir Gynaecol* 1979;68:41–46.
10. Parks TG, Connell AM. The outcome in 455 patients admitted for treatment of diverticular disease of the colon. *Br J Surg* 1970;57:775–778.
11. Boles RS, Jordon SM. The clinical significance of diverticulosis. *Gastroenterology* 1958;35:579–581.
12. Ornstein MH, Littlewood ER, Baird IM, et al. Are fibre supplements really necessary in diverticular disease of the colon? A controlled clinical trial. *BMJ* 1981;282:1353–1356.
13. Brodribb AJ. Treatment of symptomatic diverticular disease with a high-fibre diet. *Lancet* 1977;1:664–666.
14. Darnis F, Souillac P. Treatment of functional colonic diseases and colonic diverticulosis.

Comparative effects of bran and Kaologeais using a crossover method [in French]. *Med Chir Dig* 1980;9:435–437.

15. Hodgson WJ. The placebo effect. Is it important in diverticular disease? *Am J Gastroenterol* 1977;67:157–162.
16. Smits BJ, Whitehead AM, Prescott P. Lactulose in the treatment of symptomatic diverticular disease: a comparative study with high-fibre diet. *Br J Clin Pract* 1990;44:314–318.
17. Papi C, Ciaco A, Koch M, et al. Efficacy of rifaximin in the treatment of symptomatic diverticular disease of the colon. A multicentre double-blind placebo-controlled trial. *Aliment Pharmacol Ther* 1995;9:33–39.
18. Trespi E, Colla C, Panizza P, et al. Therapeutic and prophylactic role of mesalazine (5-ASA) in symptomatic diverticular disease of the colon. 4-year follow-up results. *Minerva gastroenterologica e dietologica* 1999;45: 245–252
19. Kellum JM, Sugerman HJ, Coppa GF, et al. Randomized, prospective comparison of cefoxitin and gentamicin–clindamycin in the treatment of acute colonic diverticulitis. *Clin Ther* 1992;14:376–384.
20. Larson DM, Masters SS, Spiro HM. Medical and surgical therapy in diverticular disease: a comparative study. *Gastroenterology* 1976;71:734–737.
21. Sarin S, Boulos PB. Long-term outcome of patients presenting with acute complications of diverticular disease. *Ann R Coll Surg Engl* 1994;76:117–120.
22. Farthmann EH, Ruckauer KD, Haring RU. Evidence-based surgery: diverticulitis — a surgical disease? *Langenbecks Arch Surg* 2000;385:143–151.
23. Kronborg O. Treatment of perforated sigmoid diverticulitis: a prospective randomised trial. *Br J Surg* 1993;80:505–507.
24. Zeitoun G, Laurent A, Rouffet F, et al, and the French Association for Surgical Research. Multicentre, randomized clinical trial of primary versus secondary sigmoid resection in generalized peritonitis complicating sigmoid diverticulitis. *Br J Surg* 2000;87:1366–1374.
25. Kohler L, Sauerland S, Neugebauer E. Diagnosis and treatment of diverticular disease: results of a consensus development conference. The Scientific Committee of the European Association for Endoscopic Surgery. *Surg Endosc* 1999;13:430–436.

John Simpson
Surgical Fellow

Robin Spiller
Professor of Gastroenterology

Division of Gastroenterology
University Hospital Nottingham
Nottingham
UK

Competing interests: None declared.

Colorectal cancer

Search date December 2002

Charles Maxwell-Armstrong and John Scholefield

QUESTIONS

INTERVENTIONS

Beneficial
Adjuvant chemotherapy 510

Likely to be beneficial
Routine intensive follow up . . .513

Trade off between benefits and harms
Preoperative radiotherapy 511

Unknown effectiveness
Total mesorectal excision 514

To be covered in future updates
Colonoscopic polypectomy
Immunotherapy
Liver resection for metastases
Specialist versus generalist surgical care
Surgery

See glossary, p 515

Key Messages

- **Adjuvant chemotherapy** Three systematic reviews and one subsequent RCT have found that adjuvant chemotherapy reduces mortality compared with surgery alone in people with Dukes' A, B, and C colorectal cancer. One RCT found that adding levamisole to adjuvant fluorouracil did not significantly reduce mortality or recurrence compared with adjuvant fluorouracil alone in people with Dukes' A, B, and C colorectal cancer. One RCT found that mortality and recurrence rates were similar with adjuvant fluorouracil plus high or low dose folinic acid in people with Dukes' A, B, and C colorectal cancer.
- **Routine intensive follow up** One systematic review and one subsequent RCT have found that intensive follow up increases survival compared with less intensive follow up in people treated surgically with curative intent.
- **Preoperative radiotherapy** Two systematic reviews and two subsequent RCTs found that adding preoperative radiotherapy to surgery is at least as effective as surgery alone for mortality and recurrence in people with rectal cancer. One RCT found no significant difference in mortality between preoperative and postoperative radiotherapy but preoperative radiotherapy reduced local tumour recurrence. One systematic review has found that preoperative radiotherapy increases early postoperative morbidity.
- **Total mesorectal excision** We found no RCTs of total mesorectal excision in people with rectal cancer. Observational studies suggest that total mesorectal excision may reduce the rate of local recurrence compared with conventional surgery.

DEFINITION Colorectal cancer is a malignant neoplasm arising from the lining (mucosa) of the large intestine (colon and rectum). Nearly two thirds of colorectal cancers occur in the rectum or sigmoid colon. Colorectal cancer may be categorised as A, B, or C Dukes' (see glossary, p 515).

INCIDENCE/ PREVALENCE Colorectal cancer is the third most common malignancy in the developed world. It accounts for about 20 000 deaths each year in the UK and 60 000 deaths each year in the USA. Although the incidence of, and mortality from, colorectal cancer has changed little over the past 40 years, the incidence of the disease has fallen recently in both the UK and the USA.[1,2] In the UK, about a quarter of people with colorectal cancer present with either intestinal obstruction or perforation.[3,4]

AETIOLOGY/ RISK FACTORS Colon cancer affects almost equal proportions of men and women, most commonly between the ages of 60 and 80 years. Rectal cancer is more common in men.[1] The pathogenesis of colorectal cancer involves genetic and environmental factors. The most important environmental factor is probably diet.[5]

PROGNOSIS Overall 5 year survival is about 50% and has not changed over the past 40 years. Disease specific mortality in both USA and UK cancer registries is decreasing but the reasons for this are unclear.[1,2] Surgery is undertaken with curative intent in over 80% of people, but about half experience cancer recurrence.

AIMS OF INTERVENTION To reduce morbidity (e.g. bowel obstruction or perforation) and mortality associated with the tumour; to minimise adverse effects of treatment (e.g. avoiding permanent stoma by restoring intestinal continuity); to maximise quality of life.

OUTCOMES Survival; proportion of people with permanent stoma; incidence of local recurrence; rates of metastasis; adverse effects of treatment; quality of life.

METHODS *Clinical Evidence* search and appraisal December 2002.

QUESTION **What are the effects of adjuvant chemotherapy in people with colorectal cancer?**

Three systematic reviews and one subsequent RCT have found that adjuvant chemotherapy reduces mortality compared with surgery alone in people with Dukes' A, B, and C colorectal cancer. One RCT found that adding levamisole to adjuvant fluorouracil did not significantly reduce mortality or recurrence rate compared with adjuvant fluorouracil alone in people with Dukes' A, B, and C colorectal cancer. One RCT found mortality and recurrence rates were similar with adjuvant fluorouracil plus high or low dose folinic acid in people with Dukes' A, B, and C colorectal cancer.

Benefits: **Versus placebo or no treatment:** We found three systematic reviews[6–8] and one subsequent RCT.[9] The first systematic review (search date 1993, 39 RCTs, 1673 people with Dukes' C colon cancer and 695 with Dukes' B or C rectal cancer [see glossary, p 515]) has found that adjuvant chemotherapy significantly reduces mortality after 5 years compared with surgery alone (OR 0.91, 95% CI 0.83 to 0.99).[6] The second systematic review (search date not stated, 10 RCTs, 3088 people with Dukes' A, B, or C colorectal cancer) compared 1 week of portal vein infusion of fluorouracil with or without mitomycin–C within 5–7 days of surgery versus no further treatment after surgery.[7] It found that portal vein infusion of fluorouracil significantly reduces mortality compared with surgery alone (absolute reduction in 5 year mortality 6%; P = 0.01). The third systematic review (search date not stated, 7 RCTs, 3437 people with Dukes' B or C colorectal cancer) compared adjuvant treatment with intravenous fluorouracil (plus leucovorin or levamisole) versus surgery alone.[8] It found that adjuvant fluorouracil based treatment significantly reduces mortality and significantly increases the number of people without recurrence at 5 years: 71% with fluorouracil based treatment *v* 64% with surgery alone; HR 0.76, 95% CI 0.68 to 0.85; recurrence free rate: 69% with fluorouracil based treatment *v* 58% with surgery alone; HR 0.68, 95% CI 0.60 to 0.76). The subsequent RCT (1029 people with Dukes' B or C colorectal cancer) compared adjuvant fluorouracil plus levamisole for 1 year versus surgery alone.[9] It found that adding fluorouracil and levamisole reduces mortality compared with surgery alone at 5 years (AR of survival 68% with fluorouracil based treatment *v* 58% with surgery alone; P = 0.007). **Fluorouracil plus levamisole versus fluorouracil alone:** We found one RCT (4927 people with Dukes' A, B, or C colorectal cancer and no residual disease after surgery), which compared chemotherapy with levamisole plus intravenous fluorouracil and folinic acid versus intravenous fluorouracil and folinic acid alone.[10] It found no significant difference in mortality or recurrence rate after 3 years (mortality: OR 1.10, 95% CI 1.00 to 1.22; recurrence: OR 1.00, 95% CI 0.97 to 1.13). **Low versus high dose folinic acid:** We found one RCT (4927 people with Dukes' A, B, or C colorectal cancer and no residual disease after surgery), which compared high dose folinic acid with low dose folinic acid in people given intravenous fluorouracil.[10] It found no significant difference in mortality or recurrence rate after 3 years (mortality: OR 1.04, 95% CI 0.94 to 1.15; recurrence: OR 1.00, 95% CI 0.91 to 1.09).

Harms: We found little good evidence on the harms of adjuvant chemotherapy in the treatment of colorectal cancer. In the first systematic review, the incidence of severe adverse effects (stomatitis, diarrhoea, nausea, and leukopenia) with fluorouracil and levamisole ranged from 10–30%, with life threatening toxicity occurring in about 5% of people.[6] For every 10 people treated, about three will experience an additional, severe adverse effect.[10,11]

Comment: In the UK, people aged over 75 years are not routinely considered for chemotherapy because of its potential toxicity, although we found no evidence to support or refute this policy.

QUESTION **What are the effects of preoperative radiotherapy in people with rectal cancer?**

Two systematic reviews and two subsequent RCTs found that adding preoperative radiotherapy to surgery is at least as effective as surgery alone for mortality and recurrence in people with rectal cancer. One RCT found no significant difference in mortality between preoperative and

postoperative radiotherapy. However, it found that preoperative radiotherapy reduces local tumour recurrence. One systematic review has found that preoperative radiotherapy increases early postoperative morbidity.

Benefits: **Versus surgery alone:** We found two systematic reviews[12,13] and two subsequent RCTs.[14,15] The first systematic review (search date 1999, 14 RCTs, 5974 people with rectal cancer) has found that preoperative radiotherapy significantly reduces mortality and local recurrence at 5 years compared with no preoperative radiotherapy (mortality: OR 0.84, 95% CI 0.72 to 0.98, NNT 25; local recurrence: 11 RCTs, 4494 people, OR 0.49, 95% CI 0.38 to 0.62, NNT 10).[12] It found no significant difference in risk of distant metastases at 5 years (OR 0.93, 95% CI 0.73 to 1.18). The second systematic review (search date not stated, 19 RCTs, 6623 people with rectal cancer) found no significant difference in annual death rates between preoperative radiotherapy and no preoperative radiotherapy (RR 0.94; P = 0.09; CI not reported).[13] The first subsequent RCT (1861 people) compared preoperative radiotherapy plus total mesorectal excision versus total mesorectal excision alone.[14] It found that radiotherapy did not reduce mortality or overall recurrence rate at 2 years (mortality: HR 1.02, 95% CI 0.83 to 1.25; recurrence: 16% with radiotherapy *v* 21% with surgery alone; HR 1.21, 95% CI 0.97 to 1.52). The second subsequent RCT (557 people) found no significant difference between radiotherapy and surgery in mortality or distant metastasis. However, the RCT found that radiotherapy significantly reduced local recurrence after 10 years compared with surgery (mortality: HR 0.87, 95% CI 0.71 to 1.08; distant metastasis: HR 0.97, 95% CI 0.73 to 1.28; local recurrence: 0.46, 95% CI 0.31 to 0.69).[15] **Versus postoperative radiotherapy:** We found one RCT (415 people with Dukes' [see glossary, p 515] B or C rectal carcinoma), which compared preoperative radiotherapy (25.5 Gy in 1 week) with postoperative radiotherapy (60.0 Gy over 7–8 weeks).[16] It found no significant difference in 5 year survival. However, it found that preoperative radiotherapy significantly reduces local tumour recurrence after 5 years (survival: P = 0.5; results presented graphically; absolute numbers not provided; local recurrence: 13% with preoperative *v* 22% with postoperative radiotherapy; RR 0.59, 95% CI 0.37 to 0.91; NNT 11, 95% CI 7 to 49).

Harms: **Versus surgery alone:** We found one systematic review (search date 1998, 19 RCTs, 5110 people) of harms associated with preoperative adjuvant radiotherapy.[17] It found that preoperative radiotherapy increased early postoperative morbidity and mortality. Early harms included diarrhoea, wound infections (20% with preoperative radiotherapy *v* 10% with surgery alone), bowel obstruction, cardiovascular problems, and pain. In people with low rectal tumours who underwent abdominoperineal excision, preoperative radiotherapy versus surgery alone increased the rate of perineal wound breakdown (20% *v* 10%). Two RCTs (1027 people) identified by the review found that preoperative radiotherapy compared with surgery alone significantly increased the risk of venous thromboembolism, fracture of the hip, intestinal obstruction, postoperative fistulae, cardiovascular events, and thrombotic events.[18] One observational study (171 people) found that preoperative radiotherapy increased bowel frequency and urgency, impairing social life in about 30% of people compared with surgery.[19] One RCT (1531 people) found that preoperative radiotherapy increased perioperative blood loss and perineal complications compared with surgery alone, but it found no significant difference in perioperative mortality (mean perioperative blood loss 100 mL greater with radiotherapy; perineal complication rate 29% *v* 18%; $P = 0.008$).[20] **Versus postoperative radiotherapy:** We found one systematic review (search date 1998, 9 RCTs) of harms associated with preoperative versus postoperative radiotherapy.[17] It found that postoperative radiotherapy increased anastomotic complications (breakdown and stricture formation) compared with preoperative radiotherapy.

Comment: There is limited evidence of modest improvement in survival following preoperative radiotherapy compared with surgery alone for rectal cancer. There is some evidence of an improvement in local recurrence but the risk of local recurrence for Dukes' A tumours is so low that preoperative radiotherapy is unlikely to provide much absolute benefit. There are unresolved issues about preoperative staging of rectal cancers and case selection for preoperative radiotherapy.

QUESTION **What are the effects of routine intensive follow up in people with colorectal cancer?**

One systematic review and one subsequent RCT has found that intensive follow up increases survival compared with less intensive follow up in people treated surgically with curative intent.

Benefits: We found one systematic review and one subsequent RCT.[21,22] The systematic review (search date 2001, 5 RCTs, 1342 people with colorectal cancer treated surgically with curative intent) found that intensive follow up significantly reduced all cause mortality and time to detection of recurrence, and increased detection rates for isolated local recurrence compared with control follow up (5 year mortality: 197/666 [30%] with intensive follow up *v* 247/676 [37%] with control follow up; RR 0.81, 95% CI 0.70 to 0.94; difference in mean time until detection of any recurrence with intensive *v* control follow up 8.5 months, 95% CI 7.6 months to 9.4 months, $P < 0.001$; RR for local recurrence, 3 RCTs: 1.61, 95% CI 1.12 to 2.32).[21] The subsequent RCT (358 people with no distant metastases treated surgically with curative intent alone) compared minimal surveillance versus a follow up programme guided by formal assessment of risk of recurrence (risk adapted follow up; see comment).[22] The RCT found that risk adapted follow up significantly improved overall survival at 5 years compared with minimal follow up (actuarial survival at 5 years in people at high risk: 50% with risk adapted follow up *v* 32% with minimal follow up, $P < 0.05$; in people at low risk: 80% with risk adapted follow up *v* 60% with minimal follow up, $P < 0.01$).[22]

Harms: We found no evidence about harms.

Comment: One RCT (212 people being followed up after treatment for colorectal cancer) included in the review found that follow up increased feelings of reassurance but not quality of life.[23] Most people in the trial said that they would still prefer follow up even if it did not lead to earlier detection of recurrence. Current follow up regimens are variable in frequency and intensity. We found no evidence on whether follow up should be stopped in elderly people (aged > 75 years), although many people with colorectal cancer are in this age group. The role of carcino-embryonic antigen monitoring is also uncertain. In the RCT assessing risk adapted follow up, rules for follow up in the risk adapted group depended on baseline risk factors.[22] People who had signs of recurrence underwent more sophisticated tests (flexible colonoscopy, barium enema, urography, computed tomography, and nuclear magnetic resonance). Within this group, people at high risk of recurrence underwent intensive follow up with clinical visits and carcino-embryonic antigen tests every 3 months for the first 24 months; every 4 months in year 3, and every 6 months in years 4 and 5. People at high risk also received abdominal and pelvic ultrasound every 6 months for the first 36 months and annually in years 4 and 5, and received chest x ray annually for 5 years. People at high risk and with rectal cancer also received rigid rectosigmoidoscopy. People at low risk of recurrence had low intensity follow up with clinical visits and carcino-embryonic antigen tests every 6 months for the first 24 months then annually in years 3 to 5; abdominal and pelvic ultrasound every 6 months for the first 24 months and annually thereafter, annual chest x ray and, in people with rectal cancer, rigid rectosigmoidoscopy annually for 2 years then every 2 years thereafter and annual chest x ray.

QUESTION What are the effects of total mesorectal excision in people with rectal cancer?

We found no RCTs of total mesorectal excision in people with rectal cancer. Observational studies suggest that total mesorectal excision may reduce the rate of local recurrence compared with conventional surgery.

Benefits: We found no systematic review or RCTs.

Harms: After total mesorectal excision (see glossary, p 515) more people experienced increased stool frequency compared with techniques leaving a rectal stump (median 4–5 daily *v* 1–2 daily). Observational studies have found that there is a higher incidence of anastomotic leakage with total mesorectal excision (11–15% *v* 8–10%).[24]

Comment: One observational study (441 people) compared local recurrence rates before and after the introduction of total mesorectal excision (see table 1, p 517).[25] It found that local recurrence rates 1 year after surgery fell after the introduction of total mesorectal excision (4% before total mesorectal excision *v* 9% after). Several other observational studies have found similar results (see table 1, p 517).[24,26,27] Total mesorectal excision requires coloanal anastomosis, which may be important in the surgical treatment of rectal cancer.[25,26,28] Many surgeons routinely use a temporary defunctioning stoma after total mesorectal excision in an attempt to reduce the clinical consequences of anastomotic leakage.[25]

GLOSSARY

Dukes' classification Dukes' original classification of the pathological stages of carcinoma of the colon and rectum includes three stages: A, limited to mucosa and submucosa; B, penetration of the entire bowel wall and serosa or pericolic fat; C, stages A and B, and invasion into the regional draining lymph node system.[29] More recently, stage D has been proposed to classify patients with advanced and widespread regional involvement (metastasis).

Total mesorectal excision Removal of the entire rectal mesentery along with the rectum by sharp dissection.

Substantive changes

Routine follow up One systematic review and one RCT added.[21,22] Intervention recategorised from Unknown effectiveness to Likely to be beneficial.

REFERENCES

1. Office of Population Censuses and Surveys. *Mortality statistics, cause, England and Wales 1993*. dh22. London: HMSO, 1995.
2. Miller BA, Ries LA, Hankey BF, et al. *Cancer statistics review 1973–1989*. Rockville, MD: National Institutes of Health, National Cancer Institute. Report No: NIH-NCI 92–2789.
3. Mella J, Biffen A, Radcliffe AG, et al. A population based on audit of colorectal cancer management in two United Kingdom health districts. *Br J Surg* 1997;84:1731–1736.
4. Scholefield JH, Robinson MHE, Mangham C, et al. Screening for colorectal cancer reduces emergency admissions. *Eur J Surg Oncol* 1998;24:47–50.
5. Kune G, ed. *Causes and control of colorectal cancer: a model for cancer prevention*. Boston: Kluwer Academic Publishers, 1996.
6. Dube S, Heyen F, Jenicek M. Adjuvant chemotherapy in colorectal carcinoma. Results of a meta analysis. *Dis Colon Rectum* 1997;40:35–41. Search date 1993; primary source Medline.
7. Liver Infusion Meta-analysis Group. Portal vein chemotherapy for colorectal cancer: a meta-analysis of 4000 patients in 10 studies. *J Natl Cancer Inst* 1997;89:497–505. Search date not stated; primary sources Medline, Cancerlit, Excerpta Medica, and hand searched books, journals, and registers of trials.
8. Sargent DJ, Goldberg RM, Jacobson SD, et al. A pooled analysis of adjuvant chemotherapy for resected colon cancer in elderly patients. *N Engl J Med* 2001;345:1091–1097. Search date not stated; primary sources Medline, bibliographies, and early trials leaders.
9. Taal BG, van Tinteren H, Zoetmulder FA, et al. Adjuvant 5FU plus levamisole in colonic or rectal cancer: improved survival in stage II and III. *Br J Cancer* 2001;85:1437–1443.
10. QUASAR Collaborative Group. Comparison of fluorouracil with additional levamisole, higher dose folinic acid or both as adjuvant chemotherapy for colorectal cancer: a randomised trial. *Lancet* 2000;355:1588–1596.
11. International Multicenter Pooled Analysis of Colon Cancer Trials (IMPACT) Investigators. Efficacy of adjuvant fluorouracil and folinic acid in colon cancer. *Lancet* 1995;345:939–944.
12. Camma C, Giunta M, Pagliaro L. Preoperative radiotherapy for resectable rectal cancer. A meta analysis. *JAMA* 2000:284:1008–1015. Search date 1999; primary sources Medline, Cancerlit, and hand searched reference lists. No company sponsorship stated.
13. Colorectal Cancer Collaborative Group. Adjuvant radiotherapy for rectal cancer: a systematic overview of 8507 patients from 22 randomised trials. *Lancet* 2001;358:1291–1304. Search date not stated; primary sources details not stated, based on the Early Breast Cancer Trialists' Collaborative Groups' methods who identified studies from: lists prepared by three international cancer research groups, hand searching meeting abstracts, consulting experts, and a computer aided literature search.
14. Kapiteijn E, Marijnen CA, Nagtegaal ID, et al. Preoperative radiotherapy combined with total mesorectal excision for resectable rectal cancer. *N Engl J Med* 2001;345:638–646.
15. Martling A, Holm T, Johansson H, et al. The Stockholm II trial on preoperative radiotherapy in rectal carcinoma: long-term follow-up of a population-based study. *Cancer* 2001;92:896–902.
16. Jansson-Frykholm G, Glimelius B, Pahlman L. Preoperative or postoperative irradiation in adenocarcinoma of the rectum. Final treatment results of a randomised trial and an evaluation of late secondary effects. *Dis Colon Rectum* 1993;36:564–572.
17. Ooi B, Tjandra J, Green M. Morbidities of adjuvant chemotherapy and radiotherapy for resectable rectal cancer: an overview. *Dis Colon Rectum* 1999;42:403–418. Search date 1998; primary source Medline.
18. Holm T, Singnomklao T, Rutqvist LE, et al. Adjuvant preoperative radiotherapy in patients with rectal carcinoma. Adverse effects during long term follow-up of two trials. *Cancer* 1996;78:968–976.
19. Dahlberg M, Glimelius B, Graf W, et al. Preoperative irradiation affects functional results after surgery for rectal cancer: results from a randomised study. *Dis Colon Rectum* 1998;41:543–549.
20. Marijnen CAM, Kapiteijn E, Van de Velde CJH, et al. Acute side effects and complications after short-term preoperative radiotherapy combined with total mesorectal excision in primary rectal cancer: report of a multicenter randomised trial. *J Clin Oncol* 2002;20:817–825.
21. Renehan AG, Egger M, Saunders MP, et al. Impact on survival of intensive follow up after curative resection for colorectal cancer: systematic review and meta-analysis of randomised trials. *BMJ* 2002;324:1–8. Search date 2001; primary sources Medline, Embase, Cancerlit, Cochrane Controlled Trials Register, abstracts of meetings, and Cochrane colorectal cancer group.
22. Secco GB, Fardelli R, Gianquinto D, et al. Efficacy and cost of risk-adapted follow-up in patients after

colorectal cancer surgery: a prospective, randomized and controlled trial. *Eur J Surg Oncol* 2002;28:418–423.
23. Stiggelbout AM, de Haes JCJM, Vree R, et al. Follow up of colorectal cancer patients: quality of life and attitudes towards follow up. *Br J Cancer* 1997;75:914–920.
24. Karanja ND, Corder AP, Bearn P, et al. Leakage from stapled low anastomosis after total mesorectal excision for carcinoma of the rectum. *Br J Surg* 1994;81:1224–1226.
25. McFarlane JK, Ryall RDH, Heald RJ. Mesorectal excision for rectal cancer. *Lancet* 1993;341:457–460.
26. Enker WE, Thaler HT, Cranor ML, et al. Total mesorectal excision in the operative treatment of carcinoma of the rectum. *J Am Coll Surg* 1995;181:335–346.
27. Singh S, Morgan MBF, Broughton M, et al. A ten-year prospective audit of outcome of surgical treatment for colorectal carcinoma. *Br J Surg* 1995;82:1486–1490.
28. Arbman G, Nilsson E, Hallbook O, et al. Local recurrence following total mesorectal excision for rectal cancer. *Br J Surg* 1996;83:375–379.
29. Dukes CE. The classification of cancer of the rectum. *J Pathol Bacteriol* 1932;35:323–332.

Charles Maxwell-Armstrong
Consultant Surgeon
Queens Medical Centre
Nottingham
UK

John Scholefield
Professor of Surgery
University Hospital
Nottingham
UK

Competing interests: None declared.

TABLE 1 Effects of total mesorectal excision: results of non-randomised studies (see text, p 513).

Ref	Dukes' stage (number of people)	Intervention	Recurrence at 5 years (95% CI)		RRR of death by 5 years (95% CI)	Incidence of anastomic leak
			Local	Overall		
24	B (88)	TME	5% (0% to 7.5%)	18% (10% to 25%)	78% (68% to 88%)	11% clinical
	C (73)					6.4% radiological
25	B (99) C (147)	TME	7.3%	23%	74%	NA
26	A, B, and C (158 in total)	TME	8%	24%	60%	10%
27	A (67)	TME	6% at 1 year	NA	NA	8% (57% stoma rate)
	B (89) C (100)	Non-TME	14% at 1 year			9% (15% stoma rate)

NA, not applicable; Ref, reference; TME, total mesorectal excision.

Gastro-oesophageal reflux disease

Search date November 2002

Paul Moayyedi, Brendan Delaney, and David Forman

QUESTIONS

INTERVENTIONS

Key Messages

Initial treatment

- **Antacids/alginates** Two RCTs found limited evidence that antacids versus placebo reduced symptom scores at 4–8 weeks, but found no significant difference in endoscopic healing. We found limited evidence on the effects of antacids versus H_2 receptor antagonists in people with oesophagitis. The first RCT found no significant difference between antacids versus cimetidine on endoscopic healing at 8 weeks. The second RCT found that antacids were significantly less effective for healing compared with ranitidine at 12 weeks.
- **H_2 receptor antagonists** One systematic review in people with oesophagitis found that H_2 receptor antagonists significantly increased healing compared with placebo, but reduced healing compared with proton pump inhibitors.
- **Lifestyle advice** RCTs found insufficient evidence on the effects of lifestyle measures for the treatment of reflux oesophagitis.
- **Motility stimulants** One RCT found that cisapride significantly increased endoscopic healing compared with placebo at 12 weeks. The use of cisapride has been restricted in some countries because of concerns about heart rhythm abnormalities. We found no RCTs of domperidone or metoclopramide.

Clin Evid 2003;10:518–534.

- **Proton pump inhibitors** One systematic review has found that proton pump inhibitors increased incidence of healing compared with placebo or H_2 receptor antagonists. One systematic review found that esomeprazole significantly increased healing at 4 weeks compared with omeprazole. RCTs have found no significant difference in clinical benefit among other proton pump inhibitors.

Maintenance treatment

- **Antacids/alginates** We found no RCTs on the effects of antacids/alginates on long term management of reflux oesophagitis.
- **H_2 receptor antagonists** One RCT found no significant difference between ranitidine versus placebo for relapse of oesophagitis at 6 months in people with previously healed reflux oesophagitis. RCTs have found that H_2 receptor antagonists are less effective than proton pump inhibitors for maintaining remission up to 12 months.
- **Laparoscopic surgery** One systematic review found no fully published RCTs comparing laparoscopic surgery versus medical treatment for maintenance treatment in people with gastro-oesophageal reflux disease and oesophagitis. Two RCTs found no significant difference between open and laparasopic fundoplication for remission at 3 months to 2 years. One RCT found that complication rates were lower with laparoscopic versus open surgery.
- **Lifestyle advice** We found no RCTs on the effects of lifestyle advice on long term management of reflux oesophagitis.
- **Motility stimulants** We found limited evidence on the effects of cisapride compared with placebo. Three RCTs found that cisapride compared with placebo improved maintenance of healing at 6–12 months. Two further RCTs found no evidence of a difference. However, they might have lacked power to detect a clinically important effect. We found no RCTs comparing other prokinetics versus placebo or each other in people with gastro-oesophageal reflux disease and oesophagitis. The use of cisapride has been restricted in some countries because of concerns about effects on heart rhythms.
- **Open surgery** RCTs have found that open Nissen fundoplication compared with medical treatment improved the endoscopic grade of oesophagitis in people with chronic gastro-oesophageal reflux disease and oesophagitis at between 3 and 38 months. However, longer term follow up from one of those RCTs found no significant difference in endoscopic appearance between surgery and medical treatment at 10 years. Two RCTs found no significant difference between open and laparoscopic fundoplication for remission at 3 months to 2 years. One RCT found that mortality was higher with open surgery compared with medical treatment. One RCT found that complication rates were higher with open versus laparoscopic surgery.
- **Proton pump inhibitors** RCTs have found that proton pump inhibitors compared with placebo or H_2 receptor antagonists increase remission rates in people with healed reflux oesophagitis at 6–18 months. RCTs have found that proton pump inhibitors compared with placebo or H_2 receptor antagonists increase remission rates in people with healed reflux oesophagitis at 6–18 months. One systematic review has found that standard dose lansoprazole (30 mg/day) was as effective as omeprazole (20 mg/day) for maintaining healing at 12 months. However, it found that lower dose lansoprazole (15 mg/day) was less effective than higher dose lansoprazole (30 mg/day), omeprazole, or esomeprazole for maintaining healing for up to 12 months.

DEFINITION Gastro-oesophageal reflux disease (GORD) is defined as reflux of gastroduodenal contents into the oesophagus causing symptoms that are sufficient to interfere with quality of life.[1] People with GORD often have symptoms of heartburn and acid regurgitation.[2] GORD can be classified according to results of upper gastrointestinal endoscopy. An endoscopy showing mucosal breaks in the distal oesophagus indicate the presence of oesophagitis, which is graded in severity from grade A (mucosal breaks of < 5 mm in the oesophagus) to grade D (circumferential breaks in the oesophageal mucosa).[1,3] Alternatively, severity may be graded according to the Savary–Miller classification (grade I: linear, non-confluent erosions to grade IV: severe ulceration or stricture).

INCIDENCE/ PREVALENCE Surveys from Europe and the USA suggest that 20–25% of the population have symptoms of GORD, and 7% have heartburn daily.[4,5] In primary care settings, about 25–40% of people with GORD have oesophagitis on endoscopy, but most have endoscopy negative reflux disease.[6]

AETIOLOGY/ RISK FACTORS We found no evidence of clear predictive factors for GORD. Obesity is reported to be a risk factor for GORD but epidemiological data are conflicting.[7,8] Smoking and alcohol are also thought to predispose to GORD, but observational data are limited.[8,9] It has been suggested that some foods, such as coffee, mints, dietary fat, onions, citrus fruits, or tomatoes, may predispose to GORD.[10] However, we found insufficient data on the role of these factors. We found limited evidence that drugs that relax the lower oesophageal sphincter, such as calcium channel blockers, may promote GORD.[11] Twin studies suggest that there may be a genetic predisposition to GORD.[9]

PROGNOSIS GORD is a chronic condition, with about 80% of people relapsing once medication is discontinued.[12] Many people therefore require long term medical treatment or surgery. Endoscopy negative reflux disease remains stable, with a minority of people developing oesophagitis over time.[13] However, people with severe oesophagitis may develop complications such as oesophageal stricture and Barrett's oesophagus.[1]

AIMS OF INTERVENTION To relieve reflux symptoms, increase healing rates, and reduce the complications of GORD, such as stricture formation; to improve quality of life; to minimise adverse effects of treatment.

OUTCOMES Frequency and severity of symptoms, quality of life. **GORD associated with reflux oesophagitis:** Healing rates (assessed endoscopically in people with oesophagitis), which have been shown to be closely associated with clinical outcomes.[14,15] pH measurement of reflux is an intermediate outcome that is often used in RCTs, but it is difficult to interpret clinically. We excluded RCTs based solely on this outcome.

METHODS *Clinical Evidence* search and appraisal November 2002.

QUESTION **What are the effects of interventions in the initial treatment of gastro-oesophageal reflux disease associated with oesophagitis?**

OPTION **LIFESTYLE ADVICE**

RCTs found insufficient evidence on the effects of lifestyle measures for the treatment of reflux oesophagitis.

Benefits: We found no systematic review. **Raising the head of the bed:** One RCT (71 people aged 22–77 years with endoscopically diagnosed gastro-oesophageal reflux [grade C]) compared raising the head of the bed (to produce a 10° slope) versus not raising the head of the bed in people additionally randomised to ranitidine (150 mg twice daily) versus placebo for 6 weeks.[16] It found that, in people taking placebo, raising the head of the bed increased participant reported improvement at 6 weeks (grading of improvement not specified; 10/17 [59%] with bed raised *v* 4/14 [29%] without; significance of individual comparisons not stated). The benefit of raising the head of the bed was increased in people taking ranitidine versus placebo (13/15 [87%] in those taking ranitidine *v* 10/17 [59%] in those receiving placebo; significance not stated). Endoscopic appearances were not significantly different among any of the four groups. **Weight loss:** One RCT (20 people with gastro-oesophageal reflux confirmed by 24 h pH measurement, mean body mass index 31.4 kg/m^2) compared a low calorie diet (430 kcal/day for the first 6 wks) plus advice and support for 6 months versus standard instructions about reflux disease and general advice to lose weight.[17] It found no significant difference between groups in symptoms or the number of episodes of reflux (analysis not by intention to treat; 19 people in analysis; no further data reported), but the study may have lacked power to detect a clinically important difference. **Reducing coffee intake; stopping smoking; reducing alcohol intake; reducing fatty food intake:** We found no RCTs on these lifestyle measures.

Harms: We found no RCTs.

Comment: None.

OPTION **ANTACIDS/ALGINATES**

Two RCTs found limited evidence that antacids compared with placebo reduced symptom scores at 4–8 weeks, but neither found a significant difference in endoscopic healing. We found limited evidence on the effects of antacids compared with H_2 receptor antagonists in people with oesophagitis. The first RCT found no significant difference between antacids compared with cimetidine in endoscopic healing at 8 weeks. The second RCT found that antacids were significantly less effective for heartburn symptoms compared with ranitidine at 12 weeks.

Benefits: We found no systematic review. **Versus placebo:** We found two RCTs.[18,19] The first RCT (91 people with gastro-oesophageal reflux disease and endoscopically confirmed oesophagitis grade A–C) compared antacids (1 tablet aluminium hydroxide/magnesium carbonate 1 h after meals and at bedtime) versus cimetidine (400 mg twice a day) versus placebo for 8 weeks.[18] It found that antacids versus placebo significantly reduced the number of days with reflux symptoms (5 days *v* 13 days; $P < 0.05$) and reduced the median symptom score (measured on a 100 mm visual analogue scale [100 mm = worst score]: 8 with antacids *v* 33 with placebo). However, it found no significant difference in endoscopic healing at 8 weeks (8/27 [30%] with antacids *v* 6/29 [21%] with placebo). The second RCT (32 people with gastro-oesophageal reflux disease and oesophagitis confirmed by pH monitoring and an acid perfusion test) compared antacids (15 mL doses of aluminium and magnesium hydroxide 7 times daily) versus placebo for 4 weeks.[19] Results of this RCT may be biased in favour of antacids because 11 people who had no heartburn symptoms after taking placebo for 1 week were eliminated from the analysis. It found no significant difference between antacids and placebo in the frequency or severity of reflux or in endoscopic healing at 4 weeks. **Versus H_2 receptor antagonists:** We found two RCTs.[18,19] The first RCT (91 people, described above) found no significant difference between antacids and cimetidine in endoscopic healing at 8 weeks (8/27 [30%] people taking antacids *v* 11/29 [38%] people taking cimetidine).[18] The second RCT (155 people with oesophagitis up to grade D) found that calcium carbonate (750 mg as needed) versus ranitidine (150 mg twice daily) significantly increased the frequency and severity of heartburn after 1 week (results presented graphically; $P < 0.05$).[20] Subgroup analysis in people with erosive oesophagitis of grade A or greater (73 people) found that calcium carbonate versus ranitidine significantly reduced the proportion of people with endoscopic healing at 12 weeks (10/35 [29%] with calcium carbonate *v* 21/38 [55%] with ranitidine; RR 0.52, 95% CI 0.28 to 0.94).

Harms: One of the RCTs (91 people) found that six people in the antacid group reported transient constipation after 4 weeks of treatment.[18] One RCT (32 people) found that antacids versus placebo caused significantly more gastrointestinal adverse effects, including diarrhoea, nausea, vomiting, occult blood in the stool, gas, constipation, and duodenal ulcer (12% with antacids *v* 3% with ranitidine; $P = 0.056$).[19] One person taking antacids developed a duodenal ulcer. The RCT also found that a smaller proportion of people had headache, dizziness, insomnia, malaise, fatigue, weakness, chills, and nervousness with antacids versus placebo (1% with antacids *v* 4% with ranitidine), but the difference was not significant ($P = 0.37$).

Comment: None.

OPTION MOTILITY STIMULANTS

One RCT found that cisapride significantly increased endoscopic healing compared with placebo at 12 weeks. The use of cisapride has been restricted in some countries because of concerns about heart rhythm abnormalities. We found no RCTs of domperidone or metoclopramide.

Benefits: We found one RCT (177 people with uncomplicated gastro-oesophageal reflux disease and oesophagitis) comparing cisapride (10 or 20 mg 4 times daily) versus placebo for 12 weeks.[21] It found that cisapride 20 mg compared with placebo significantly increased endoscopic healing of oesophagitis at 12 weeks. (Analysis not by intention to treat; 20 people excluded from analysis: 26/51 [51%] healed with cisapride 20 mg *v* 21/51 [41%] with 10 mg *v* 20/55 [36%] with placebo; $P < 0.05$; no further data reported.) We found no RCTs comparing metoclopramide or domperidone versus placebo or other prokinetic drugs.

Harms: In some countries, use of cisapride has been restricted because of concerns about heart rhythm abnormalities that are associated with sudden death.[22] The RCT found no significant difference between cisapride and placebo in any adverse effects.[21] Common adverse events included diarrhoea (16.4% cisapride 20 mg *v* 12.5% cisapride 10 mg *v* 8.3% placebo), headache (11.5% *v* 16.1% *v* 26.7%), and constipation (6.6% *v* 10.7% *v* 6.7%).

Comment: None.

OPTION H$_2$ RECEPTOR ANTAGONISTS

One systematic review in people with oesophagitis found that H$_2$ receptor antagonists significantly increased healing compared with placebo. It found that H$_2$ receptor antagonists significantly reduced healing compared with proton pump inhibitors.

Benefits: **Versus placebo:** We found one systematic review (search date not stated; 10 RCTs, 2171 people) comparing H$_2$ receptor antagonists versus placebo in people with oesophagitis.[23] It found that H$_2$ receptor antagonists versus placebo significantly decreased risk of persistent oesophagitis (time to outcome not stated: RR of oesophagitis persisting with H$_2$ receptor antagonists *v* placebo 0.79, 95% CI 0.72 to 0.87; NNT 6, 95% CI 5 to 10). **Versus proton pump inhibitors:** See benefits of proton pump inhibitors for initial treatment of gastro-oesophageal reflux disease, p 523.

Harms: The systematic review did not report on harms.[23]

Comment: A systematic review evaluating drug treatment in the short term management of oesophagitis is currently being conducted.[24]

OPTION PROTON PUMP INHIBITORS

One systematic review found that proton pump inhibitors increased the incidence of healing compared with placebo or H$_2$ receptor antagonists. One systematic review found that esomeprazole significantly increased healing at 4 weeks compared with omeprazole. RCTs have found no significant differences in clinical benefit among other proton pump inhibitors.

Benefits: **Versus placebo:** We found one systematic review (search date not stated; 4 RCTs, 380 people with gastro-oesophageal reflux disease and oesophagitis) comparing proton pump inhibitors versus placebo.[23] It found that proton pump inhibitors were more effective than placebo for preventing persistence of oesophagitis (RR 0.31,

95% CI 0.13 to 0.75; time to outcome not specified; NNT 2, 95% CI 1 to 5). **Versus H_2 receptor antagonists:** The same systematic review (search date not stated, 16 RCTs, 2321 people) found that proton pump inhibitors versus H_2 receptor antagonists significantly decreased persistent oesophagitis (RR 0.5, 95% CI 0.43 to 0.58; NNT 4, 95% CI 3 to 4; time to outcome not stated).[23] **Versus each other:** We found two systematic reviews (search dates 2000)[25,26] and three subsequent RCTs[27–29] comparing different proton pump inhibitors in people with reflux oesophagitis. The reviews found similar results, although results in the second review were reported more clearly and covered additional comparisons.[26] It found that esomeprazole (40 mg) versus omeprazole (20 mg once daily) significantly increased healing at 4 weeks (3 RCTs; healing rate 1814/2446 [74%] with esomeprazole *v* 1583/2431 [65%] with omeprazole; RR 1.14, 95% CI 1.10 to 1.18; NNT 13, 95% CI 9 to 17). The review found no significant difference between lansoprazole (30 mg) and omeprazole (20 mg) at 4 weeks (5 RCTs; healing rate 704/972 [72%] with lansoprazole v 692/979 [71%] with omeprazole; RR 1.02, 95% CI 0.97 to 1.08). The review found no significant difference between pantoprazole (40 mg) and omeprazole (20 mg) or between rabeprazole (20 mg) and omeprazole (20 mg) at 4 weeks (pantoprazole v omeprazole, 3 RCTs, healing rate: 388/574 [68%] with pantoprazole v 325/474 [69%] with omeprazole; RR 0.99, 95% CI 0.91 to 1.07; rabeprazole v omeprazole, healing rate: 81/100 [81%] with rabeprazole v 83/102 [81%] with omeprazole; RR 1.00, 95% CI 0.87 to 1.14).[26] The first subsequent RCT (328 people with grade I oesophagitis) comparing pantoprazole (20 mg once daily) versus omeprazole (20 mg once daily) found no significant difference between treatments in healing rate at 8 weeks or symptom relief at 4 weeks (symptom relief: 77% with pantoprazole *v* 84% with omeprazole; no further data reported; healing rates: 90% with pantoprazole *v* 95% with omeprazole; OR 0.62, 95% CI 0.34 to 1.13).[27] The second subsequent RCT (461 people with symptomatic grade I–IV oesophagitis) compared three interventions: omeprazole (20 mg/day modified release tablets); lansoprazole (30 mg/day); and pantoprazole (40 mg/day).[28] It found no significant difference between omeprazole and lansoprazole or pantoprazole in complete resolution of heartburn symptoms at 8 weeks (89% heartburn free with pantoprazole *v* 87% with omeprazole *v* 81% with lansoprazole; ARR for omeprazole *v* pantoprazole +2%, 90% CI –4.6% to +7.6%; ARI for omeprazole *v* lansoprazole +6%, 90% CI –0.8% to +12.8%). The third subsequent RCT (251 people with symptomatic grade II–III oesophagitis) found no significant difference between rabeprazole (20 mg/day) and omeprazole (40 mg/day) in complete relief of heartburn, regurgitation, or epigastric pain after 3 days (analysis not by intention to treat; relief of heartburn 99/118 [84%] with rabeprazole *v* 96/116 [83%] with omeprazole; ARI +1.1%, 95% CI –8.4% to +10.7%; no regurgitation 101/112 [90%] with rabeprazole *v* 102/115 [89%] with omeprazole; ARI +1.5%, 95% CI –6.5% to +9.5%; no epigastric pain 89/112 [80%] with rabeprazole *v* 99/115 [86%] with omeprazole; ARR +6.6%, 95% CI –3.2% to +16.4%).[29]

Harms: The systematic review gave no information on harms.[23] The subsequent RCT found similar rates of adverse events with pantoprazole and omeprazole (any adverse event: 57% with pantoprazole *v* 50% with omeprazole; severe adverse events: 10% *v* 13%; nausea 8% *v* 7%; diarrhoea 5% *v* 6%; headache 6% *v* 3%).[27]

Comment: A systematic review evaluating drug treatment in the short term management of oesophagitis is currently being conducted.[24]

QUESTION What are the effects of interventions in the maintenance treatment of reflux oesophagitis?

OPTION LIFESTYLE ADVICE

We found no RCTs on the effects of lifestyle advice on long term management of reflux oesophagitis.

Benefits: We found no systematic review or RCTs.

Harms: We found no RCTs.

Comment: None.

OPTION ANTACIDS/ALGINATES

We found no RCTs on the effects of antacids/alginates on long term management of reflux oesophagitis.

Benefits: We found no systematic review or RCTs.

Harms: See benefits of antacids/alginates for the initial treatment of gastro-oesophageal reflux disease, p 521.

Comment: None.

OPTION MOTILITY STIMULANTS

Three RCTs have found that cisapride compared with placebo improved maintenence of healing at 6–12 months. Two further RCTs found no evidence of a difference, but they might have lacked power to detect a clinically important effect. We found no RCTs comparing other prokinetics versus placebo or each other in people with gastro-oesophageal reflux disease and oesophagitis. The use of cisapride has been restricted in some countries because of concerns about effects on heart rhythms.

Benefits: We found no systematic review. We found five RCTs (1398 people) comparing cisapride (up to 40 mg/day) versus placebo for 6–12 months.[30–34] Two RCTs found no significant difference between treatments in endoscopic healing,[32,34] and three RCTs found that cisapride significantly increased healing (see table 1, p 532).[30,31,33] We found no RCTs comparing other prokinetic drugs versus placebo for maintanence treatment in people with gastro-oesophageal reflux disease and healed oesophagitis.

Harms: See motility stimulants for initial treatment of gastro-oesophageal reflux disease, p 523.

Comment: None.

OPTION **H_2 RECEPTOR ANTAGONISTS**

One RCT found no significant difference between ranitidine versus placebo for relapse of oesophagitis at 6 months in people with previously healed reflux oesophagitis. RCTs have found that H_2 antagonists are less effective than proton pump inhibitors for maintaining remission at up to 12 months.

Benefits: **Versus placebo:** We found no systematic review. We found one RCT (69 people with endoscopically healed oesophagitis) comparing ranitidine (150 mg at bedtime) versus placebo for 6 months.[35] It found no significant difference between ranitidine and placebo in relapse rates at 6 months (8 people excluded from analysis: 14/33 [42%] with ranitidine v 10/28 [36%] with placebo; CI and P value not stated). **Versus proton pump inhibitors:** See benefits of proton pump inhibitors for maintenance treatment in gastro-oesophageal reflux disease, p 526.

Harms: The RCT found that four people, all taking placebo, reported adverse effects (rashes, transient headache, transient parasthaeia).[35] RCTs have shown similar rates of adverse events between H_2 receptor antagonists and placebo.[36]

Comment: None.

OPTION **PROTON PUMP INHIBITORS**

RCTs have found that proton pump inhibitors compared with placebo or H_2 receptor antagonists increase remission rates in people with healed reflux oesophagitis at 6–18 months. One systematic review has found that standard dose lansoprazole (30 mg/day) was as effective as omeprazole (20 mg/day) for maintaining healing at 12 months. However, it found that lower dose lansoprazole (15 mg/day) was less effective than higher dose lansoprazole (30 mg/day), omeprazole, or esomeprazole for maintaining healing for up to 12 months.

Benefits: **Versus placebo:** We found one systematic review (search date 2000; 7 RCTs; 1320 people with healed oesophagitis),[25] four subsequent RCTs,[37–40] and one additional RCT.[41] The systematic review did not pool results.[25] All seven RCTs included in the review found that proton pump inhibitors (rabeprazole 10 or 20 mg/day; omeprazole 10 or 20 mg/day; lansoprazole 15 or 30 mg/day) versus placebo reduced relapse rate at 6 months (results reported graphically; RR about 0.1 to about 0.8). The subsequent and additional RCTs found similar results (see table 2, p 533). **Versus H_2 receptor antagonists:** We found one systematic review that compared proton pump inhibitors versus ranitidine (search date 2000, 5 RCTs, 638 people with healed oesophagitis)[25] and one additional RCT.[42] The systematic review did not pool results.[25] All five RCTs included in the review found that proton pump inhibitors (omeprazole 10 or 20 mg/day; lansoprazole 15 or 30 mg/day) reduced relapse rate compared with ranitidine at 6 months (results reported graphically: RR about 0.1 to about 0.6). The additional RCT (264 people with healed oesophagitis and no symptoms of gastro-oesophageal reflux) found that omeprazole (10 mg/day) versus ranitidine (150 mg twice daily) increased remission rate at 12 months (AR 68% with omeprazole v 39% with ranitidine; RR 1.43, 95% CI 1.26 to 1.57).[42] **Versus each other:** We found one systematic review (search date 2001, 12 RCTs),[43] one additional RCT,[44] and one subsequent RCT.[45] The review found that lansoprazole (15 mg/day) was less effective for maintaining healing than esomeprazole (20 mg/day), higher dose lansoprazole (30 mg/day), or omeprazole (20 mg/day) (esomeprazole 20 mg *v* lansoprazole 15 mg: 1 RCT, 1224 people, RR for maintaining healing at 6 months 1.09, 95% CI 1.02 to 1.17; lansoprazole 30 mg *v* lansoprazole 15 mg: 7 RCTs; 1505 people; RR at 12 months 1.12, 95% CI 1.05 to 1.18; omeprazole 20 mg *v* lansoprazole 15 mg: 1 RCT, 597 people, RR at 12 months 1.19, 95% CI 1.10 to 1.30).[43] However, the review found no significant difference between higher dose lansoprazole (30 mg/day) versus omeprazole (20 mg/day) for maintenance of healing at 12 months (2 RCTs; 859 people; RR 1.01, 95% CI 0.96 to 1.06). The additional RCT (243 people with healed oesophagitis) found no significant difference with rabeprazole (10 or 20 mg/day) versus omeprazole (20 mg/day) for relapse rates at 12 months (AR 5% with 10 mg rabeprazole, 4% with 20 mg rabeprazole, 5% with 20 mg omeprazole).[44] The subsequent RCT (137 people with healed grade I–III oesophagitis) found no significant difference between daily low dose lansoprazole (15 mg) versus alternate day full dose lansoprazole (30 mg) for oesophagitis recurrence at 6 months (AR 12.1% with daily low dose lansoprazole *v* 19.0% with alternate day full dose lansoprazole; OR 1.31; 95% CI 0.57 to 3.02).[45]

Harms: See benefits of proton pump inhibitors for initial treatment in gastro-oesophageal reflux disease, p 523.

Comment: Limited evidence from cohort studies and small RCTs has suggested that long term proton pump inhibitor treatment may be associated with atrophic gastritis in people with *Helicobacter pylori*.[46–48] Gastric atrophy is a risk factor for gastric cancer.[49] However, we found no reliable evidence of long term clinical effects of proton pump inhibitors on gastric cancer rates in people with gastro-oesophageal reflux disease and oesophagitis. One crossover RCT (233 people with upper gastrointestinal disorders; 214 with GORD, whose symptoms were controlled with proton pump inhibitors) compared 4 weeks treatment with omeprazole versus rabeprazole. Post-crossover analysis found that a similar proportion of people preferred each of the treatments over the other (data and P value for overall comparison not reported).[50]

OPTION OPEN SURGERY

RCTs have found that open Nissen fundoplication compared with medical treatment improves the endoscopic grade of oesophagitis in people with chronic gastro-oesophageal reflux disease and oesophagitis at between 3 and 38 months. However, longer term follow up from one of those RCTs found no significant difference in endoscopic appearance between surgery and medical treatment at 10 years. Two RCTs found no significant difference between open and laparasopic fundoplication for remission at 3 months to 2 years.

Benefits: **Versus medical treatment:** We found one systematic review (search date 1999, 4 RCTs, 518 people with chronic gastro-oesophageal reflux disease [GORD] and oesophagitis).[51] Three included RCTs compared open antireflux surgery versus antacids and H_2 receptor antagonists in people with severe or complicated GORD. All reported that surgery significantly reduced reflux and improved the endoscopic grade of oesophagitis versus medical treatment (see table 3, p 534). The fourth RCT compared open surgery versus omeprazole and found similar results but was only available in abstract form at the time of review. It has since been published in full (see table 3, p 534).[52] Ten years' follow up of one of the RCTs included in the review (239/247 people originally enrolled) found no significant difference in endoscopic appearance between open surgery and medical treatment (mean endoscopic grade 1.80 with surgery *v* 1.89 with medical treatment; P = 0.76).[53] **Open surgery versus laparoscopic surgery:** We found two RCTs.[54,55] The first RCT (148 people with persistent GORD and oesophagitis following medical treatment) found no significant difference between open and laparoscopic Nissen fundoplication in symptomatic remission at 3 months (35 people excluded from end point analysis: 98% remission with open surgery *v* 97% with laparoscopic surgery; reported as non-significant; no further data reported).[54] The second RCT (42 people with GORD) also found no clear difference in symptoms or endoscopically defined remission at 2 years with open versus laparoscopic Nissen fundoplication (analysis not by intention to treat; endoscopic remission: all people receiving laparoscopic surgery were in remission *v* all but 2 people with open surgery, number of people in analysis not stated; symptoms [4 people excluded from analysis]: 79% free of heartburn with laparascopic surgery *v* 58% with open surgery; 95% free of regurgitation in both groups; significance not assessed).[55]

Harms: **Versus medical treatment:** One RCT included in the review reported significantly higher mortality with surgery versus medical treatment (RR 1.57, 95% CI 1.01 to 2.46), mainly because of cardiovascular disease during long term follow up.[51] The systematic review reported that one included RCT found that open Nissen fundoplication versus medical treatment signficantly increased early satiety, inability to belch, and inability to vomit.[51] **Versus laparoscopic surgery:** The first RCT found that overall complication rate (including splenectomy, pneumothorax, subphrenic abscess, wound infection, cicatricial hernia) was higher with open versus laparoscopic Nissen fundoplication (6/57 [11%] people with laparoscopy *v* 10/46 [22%] with open Nissen fundoplication).[54] The second RCT did not report on operative complications.[55]

Comment: None.

OPTION LAPAROSCOPIC SURGERY

One systematic review identified no fully published RCTs comparing the effects of laparoscopic surgery versus medical treatment for maintenance treatment in people with gastro-oesophageal reflux disease and oesophagitis. Two RCTs found no significant difference with open versus laparasopic fundoplication in remission at 3 months to 2 years.

Benefits: **Laparoscopic surgery versus medical treatment:** We found one systematic review (search date 1999).[51] It identified no fully published RCTs that examined effects on symptoms or endoscopically defined healing (see comment below). **Laparoscopic surgery versus open surgery:** See benefits of open surgery, p 528.

Harms: **Versus medical treatment:** We found insufficient evidence to compare harms of laparoscopic surgery versus medical treatment. **Versus open surgery:** See harms of open surgery, p 528.

Comment: The review identified one RCT (90 people with severe gastro-oesophageal reflux disease for at least 6 months) that was published as an abstract only.[51] It found similar results for laparoscopic surgery versus proton pump inhibitors for quality of life at 3 months (scale not reported).

REFERENCES

1. Dent J, Brun J, Fendrick AM, et al. An evidence-based appraisal of reflux disease management: the Genval Workshop Report. *Gut* 1999;44(suppl 2):S1–S16.
2. Klauser AG, Schindlbeck NE, Muller-Lissner SA. Symptoms in gastro-oesophageal reflux disease. *Lancet* 1990;335:205–208.
3. Armstrong D, Bennett JR, Blum AL, et al. The endoscopic assessment of esophagitis: a progress report on observer agreement. *Gastroenterology* 1996;111:85–92.
4. Kay L, Jorgensen T. Epidemiology of upper dyspepsia in a random population. *Scand J Gastroenterol* 1994;29:1–6.
5. Isolauri J, Laippala P. Prevalence of symptoms suggestive of gastro-oesophageal reflux disease in an adult population. *Ann Med* 1995;27:67–70.
6. Armstrong D, Bennett JR, Blum AL, et al. The endoscopic assessment of esophagitis: a progress report on observer agreement. *Gastoenterology* 1996;111:85–92.
7. Lagergren J. Bergstrom R. Nyren O. No relation between body mass and gastro-oesophageal reflux symptoms in a Swedish population based study. *Gut* 2000;47:26–29.
8. Locke GR III, Talley NJ, Fett SL, et al. Risk factors associated with symptoms of gastroesophageal reflux. *Am J Med* 1999;106:642–649.
9. Romero Y, Cameron AJ, Locke GR III, et al. Familial aggregation of gastroesophageal reflux in patients with Barrett's esophagus and esophageal adenocarcinoma. *Gastroenterology* 1997;113:1449–1456.
10. Terry P, Lagergren J, Wolk A, et al. Reflux-inducing dietary factors and risk of adenocarcinoma of the esophagus and gastric cardia. *Nutr Cancer* 2000;38:186–191.
11. Lagergren J, Bergstrom R, Adami HO, et al. Association between medications that relax the lower esophageal sphincter and risk for esophageal adenocarcinoma. *Ann Intern Med* 2000;133:165–175.
12. Dent J, Yeomans ND, Mackinnon M, et al. Omeprazole v ranitidine for the prevention of relapse of reflux oesophagitis. A controlled double blind trial of their efficacy and safety. *Gut* 1994;35:590–598.
13. Trimble KC, Douglas S, Pryde A, et al. Clinical characteristics and natural history of symptomatic but not excess gastro-esophageal reflux. *Dig Dis Sci* 1995;40:1098–1104.
14. Hatlebakk JG, Berstad A. Prognostic factors for relapse of reflux oesophagitis and symptoms during 12 months of therapy with lansoprazole. *Aliment Pharmacol Ther* 1997;11:1093–1099.
15. Vakil NB, Shaker R, Johnson DA, et al. The new proton pump inhibitor esomeprazole is effective as a maintenance therapy in GERD patients with healed erosive oesophagitis: a 6-month, randomized, double-blind, placebo-controlled study of efficacy and safety. *Aliment Pharmacol Ther* 2001;15:927–935.
16. Harvey RF, Hadley N, Gill TR, et al. Effects of sleeping with the bed-head raised and of ranitidine in patients with severe peptic oesophagitis. *Lancet* 1987;2:1200–1203.
17. Kjellin A, Ramel S, Rossner S, et al. Gastroesophageal reflux in obese patients is not reduced by weight reduction. *Scand J Gastroenterol* 1996;31:1047–1051.
18. Farup PG, Weberg R, Berstad A, et al. Low-dose antacids versus 400mg cimetidine twice daily for reflux oesophagitis. *Scand J Gastroenterol* 1990;25:315–320.
19. Graham DY, Patterson DJ. Double-blind comparison of liquid antacid and placebo in the treatment of symptomatic reflux esophagitis. *Dig Dis Sci* 1983;28:559–563.
20. Earnest D, Robinson M, Rodriguez-Stanley S, et al. Managing heartburn at the "base" of the GERD "iceberg": effervescent ranitidine 150 mg bd provides faster and better heartburn relief than antacids. *Aliment Pharmacol Ther* 2000;14:911–918.
21. Richter JE, Long JF. Cisapride for gastrooesophageal reflux disease: a placebo-controlled, double-blind study. *Am J Gastroenterol* 1995;90:423–430.
22. Piquette RK. Torsade de pointes induced by cisapride/clarithromycin interaction. *Ann Pharmacother* 1999;33:22–26.
23. Delaney B, Moayyedi P. *Dyspepsia. Health Care Needs Assessment*, 4th ed. Stevens A, Raftery J (eds). NHS Executive, 2002 (in press). http://hcna.radcliffe-oxford.com/dyspepsia.htm (last accessed 17 February 2003). Search date not stated; primary sources are a recent systematic review funded by the NHS R&D HTA programme, three recently published Cochrane reviews, and abstracts of recently completed trials.
24. Preston C, Donnellan C, Moayyedi P. Medical treatments for the short term management of reflux oesophagitis (protocol for a Cochrane Review). In: The Cochrane Library, Issue 2, 2002. Oxford: Update Software.

25. Caro JJ, Salas M, Ward A. Healing and relapse rates in gastro-oesophageal reflux disease treated with the newer proton-pump inhibitors lansoprazole, rabeprazole and pantoprazole compared with omeprazole, ranitidine and placebo: evidence from randomized controlled trials. *Clin Ther* 2001;23:998–1017. Search date 2000; primary sources Medline and hand searches of reference lists
26. Edwards SJ, Lind T, Lundell L. Systematic review of proton pump inhibitors for the acute treatment of reflux oesophagitis. *Aliment Pharmacol Ther* 2001;15:1729–1736. Search date 2000; primary sources Medline, Embase, Biosis, and AstraZeneca internal database.
27. Bardhan KD, van Rensburg C. Comparable clinical efficacy and tolerability of 20 mg pantoprazole and 20 mg omeprazole in patients with grade I reflux oesophagitis. *Aliment Pharmacol Ther* 2001;15:1585–1591.
28. Mulder C, Westerveld B, Smit J, et al. A double blind, randomized comparison of omeprazole Multiple Unit Pellet System (MUPS) 20 mg, lansoprazole 30 mg and pantoprazole 40 mg in symptomatic reflux oesophagitis followed by 3 months of omeprazole MUPS maintenance treatment: a Dutch multicentre trial. *Eur J Gastroenterol Hepatol* 2002;14:649–656.
29. Holtmann G, Bytzer P, Metz M, et al. A randomized, double blind, comparative study of standard dose rabeprazole and high dose omeprazole in gastro-oesophageal reflux disease. *Aliment Pharmacol Ther* 2002:16;479–485.
30. Toussaint J, Gossuin A, Deruyttere M, et al. Healing and prevention of relapse of reflux oesophagitis by cisapride. *Gut* 1991;32:1280–1285.
31. Blum AL, Adami B, Bouzo MH, et al. Effect of cisapride on relapse of esophagitis. A multinational, placebo-controlled trail in patients healed with an antisecretory drug. *Dig Dis Sci* 1993;38:551–560.
32. McDougall NI, Watson RGP, Collins JSA, et al. Maintenance therapy with cisapride after healing of erosive oesophagitis: a double blind placebo controlled trial. *Aliment Pharmacol Ther* 1997;11:487–495.
33. Hatlebakk JG, Johnsson F, Vilien M, et al. The effect of cisapride in maintaining symptomatic remission in patients with gastro-oesophageal reflux disease. *Scand J Gastroenterol* 1997;32:1100–1106.
34. Tytgat GNJ, Hansen OJA, Carling L, et al. Effect of cisapride on relapse of reflux oesophagitis, healed with an antisecretory drug. *Scand J Gastroenterol* 1992;27:175–183.
35. Koelz HR, Birchler R, Bretholz A, et al. Healing and relapse of reflux esophagitis during treatment with ranitidine. *Gastroenterology* 1986;91:1198–1205.
36. Freston JW. Cimetidine. I. Developments, pharmacology, and efficacy. *Ann Intern Med* 1982;97:573–580.
37. Birbara C, Breiter J, Perdomo C, et al. Rabeprazole for the prevention of recurrent erosive or ulcerative gastro-oesophageal reflux disease. *Eur J Gastroenterol Hepatol* 2000;12:889–897.
38. Caos A, Moskovitz M, Dayal Y, et al. Rabeprazole for the prevention of pathological and symptomatic relapse of erosive or ulcerative gastroesophageal reflux disease. *Am J Gastroenterol* 2000;95:3081–3088.
39. Johnson DA, Benjamin SB, Vakil NB, et al. Esomeprazole once daily for 6 months is effective therapy for maintaining healed erosive esophagitis and for controlling gastroesophageal reflux symptoms: a randomised, double-blind, placebo-controlled study of efficacy and safety. *Am J Gastroenterol* 2001;96:27–34.
40. Vakil NB, Shaker R, Johnson DA, et al. The new proton pump inhibitor esomeprazole is effective as a maintenance therapy in GERD patients with healed erosive esophagitis: a 6-month randomized, double-blind, placebo-controlled study of efficacy and safety. *Aliment Pharmacol Ther* 2001;15:927–935.
41. Bardhan KD, Cherian P, Vaishnavi A, et al. Erosive oesophagitis: outcome of repeated long term maintenance treatment with low dose omeprazole 10 mg or placebo. *Gut* 1998;43:458–464.
42. Festen HPM, Schenk E, Tan G, et al. Omeprazole versus high-dose ranitidine in mild gastro-oesophageal reflux disease: short- and long-term treatment. *Am J Gastroenterol* 1999;94:931–936.
43. Edwards S, Lind T, Lundell L. Systematic review of proton pump inhibitors for the maintenance of healed reflux oesophagitis. *J Drug Assess* 2002;5:165–178. Search date 2001; primary sources Embase, Medline, and Astra Zeneca's internal database.
44. Thjodleifsson B, Beker JA, Dekkers C, et al. Rabeprazole versus omeprazole in preventing relapse of erosive or ulcerative gastroesophageal reflux disease. *Dig Dis Sci* 2000;45:845–853.
45. Baldi F, Morselli-Labate A, Cappiello R, et al. Daily low-dose versus alternate day full-dose lansoprazole in the maintenance treatment of reflux oesophagitis. *Am J Gastroenterol* 2002;97:1358–1364.
46. Kuipers EJ, Lundell L, Klinkenberg-Knol EC, et al. Atrophic gastritis and *Helicobacter pylori* infection in patients with reflux esophagitis treated with omeprazole or fundoplication. *N Engl J Med* 1996;334:1018–1022.
47. Eissele R, Brunner G, Simon B, et al. Gastric mucosa during treatment with lansoprazole: *Helicobacter pylori* is a risk factor for argyrophil cell hyperplasia. *Gastroenterology* 1997;112:707–717.
48. Lundell L, Miettinen P, Myrvold HE, et al. Lack of effect of acid suppression therapy on gastric atrophy. *Gastroenterology* 1999;117:319–326.
49. Uemura N, Okamoto S, Yamamoto S, et al. *Helicobacter pylori* infection and the development of gastric cancer. *N Engl J Med* 2001;345:784–789.
50. Johnson M, Guiford S, Libretto S et al . Patients have preferences: A multicentre, double-blind, crossover study comparing rabeprazole and omeprazole. *Curr Med Res Opin* 2002;18:303–310.
51. Allgood PC, Bachmann M. Medical or surgical treatment for chronic gastro-oesophageal reflux? A systematic review of published evidence of effectiveness. *Eur J Surg* 2000;166:713–721. Search date 1999; primary sources Medline, Embase, Science Citation Index, hand searches of eight key journals and reference lists, and authors and experts contacted.
52. Lundell L, Miettinen P, Myrvold HE, et al. Long-term management of gastro-oesophageal reflux disease with omeprazole or open antireflux surgery: results of a prospective randomised clinical trial. *Eur J Gastroenterol Hepatol* 2000;12:879–887.
53. Spechler SJ, Lee E, Ahnen D, et al. Long-term outcome of medical and surgical therapies for gastroesophageal reflux disease. *JAMA* 2001;285:2331–2338.

54. Bias JE, Bartelsman JFWM, Bonjer HJ, et al. Laparoscopic or conventional Nissen fundoplication for gastro-oeosophageal reflux disease: randomized clinical trial. *Lancet* 2000;355:170–174.

55. Heikkinen T-J, Haukipuro K, Bringman S, et al. Comparison of laparoscopic and open Nissen fundoplication 2 years after operation. *Surg Endosc* 2000;14:1019–1023.

Paul Moayyedi
Professor

Brendan Delaney
Dr

Department of Primary Care and General Practice
University of Birmingham Medical School
Birmingham
UK

David Forman
Professor
Upper Gastrointestinal and Pancreatic Diseases Cochrane Group
University Cochrane Group
University of Leeds
Leeds
UK

Competing interests: PM has received fees for speaking for Astra Zeneca and Wyeth Laboratories. PM has acted as an independent media advisor for Astra Zeneca. DF has received lecture fees and consultancy fees from Astra Zeneca and lecture fees from Wyeth and Takeda. BD has received fees for speaking at conferences and educational meetings from Astra Zeneca and Axlan.

TABLE 1 **Summary of RCTs comparing cisapride versus placebo for maintenance treatment in people with reflux oesophagitis (see text, p 525).**

Ref	Intervention	Number of people	Duration (months)	Remission with cisapride	Remission with placebo	RR for remaining in remission with cisapride *v* placebo (95 % CI)
30	Cisapride 10 mg twice daily	80 people with healed oesophagitis after cisapride 40 mg/day given for at least 8 wks	6	28/37 (76%)	25/43 (58%)	1.30 (0.95 to 1.79)
31	Cisapride 10 mg twice daily*	443 people with complete endoscopic resolution of active reflux oesophagitis after treatment with an acid antisecretory agent	12	98/149 (66%)	70/143 (49%)	1.35 (1.10 to 1.64)
32	Cisapride 20 mg/day	42 people with healed oesophagitis after omeprazole 20 mg twice daily for 8–14 wks	6	0/21 (0%)	4/21 (19%)	0.81 (0.66 to 1.00)
33	Cisapride 20 mg twice daily†	535 people without reflux or with mild reflux oesophagitis after 4–8 weeks treatment with either H^2 receptor antagonists or proton pump inhibitors	6	74/176 (42%)	65/184 (35%)	1.19 (0.92 to 1.54)
34	Cisapride 20 mg twice daily	298 people with oesophagitis	6	Absolute numbers not reported (55 %)	Absolute numbers not reported (79 %)	CI and P value not reported

*This trial also evaluated cisapride 20 mg at night with similar results to those with cisapride 10 mg twice daily.

†This trial also evaluated cisapride 20 mg daily with similar results to those with cisapride 20 mg twice daily.

Ref, reference. References 30 and 31 used oesophagitis recurrence as the main end point; references 32–34 used reflux symptom recurrence as the main end-point; data from reference 34 was estimated from life tables presented in the results section and is not actual data given in the papers.

TABLE 2 **Further RCTs comparing proton pump inhibitors with placebo for maintenance treatment in people with reflux oesophagitis (see text, p 526).**

Ref	Drug evaluated	Duration (months)	Remission in PPI arm	Remission in placebo arm	RR of remission with PPI *v* placebo (95% CI)
37	Rabeprazole 20 mg/day	12	80/93 (86%)	29/99 (29%)	2.94 (2.13 to 4.00)
38	Rabeprazole 20 mg/day	12	62/69 (90%)	20/70 (29%)	3.13 (2.17 to 4.55)
39	Esomeprazole 40 mg/day	6	77/82 (94%)	22/77 (29%)	3.33 (2.33 to 4.76)
40	Esomeprazole 40 mg/day	6	81/92 (88%)	27/94 (29%)	3.00 (2.22 to 4.17)
41	Omeprazole 10 mg/day*	18	66/130 (51%)	14/133 (11%)	5.00 (2.86 to 8.33)
37	Rabeprazole 10 mg/day*	12	72/93 (77%)	29/99 (29%)	2.63 (1.92 to 3.70)
38	Rabeprazole 10 mg/day*	12	51/70 (73%)	20/70 (29%)	2.56 (1.72 to 3.85)
39	Esomeprazole 20 mg/day*	6	76/82 (93%)	22/77 (29%)	3.23 (2.27 to 4.55)
40	Esomeprazole 20 mg/day*	6	77/98 (78%)	27/94 (29%)	2.70 (1.96 to 3.85)

*Maintenance dose.
PPI, proton pump inhibitor; Ref, reference.

TABLE 3 **Summary of RCTs comparing open antireflux surgery versus medical treatment for maintenance of remission in people with gastro-oesophageal reflux disease and oesophagitis (see text, p 527).**

Ref	Patient population	Intervention	Follow up (months)	Outcome assessed	Result
51	Adults with complicated GORD	88 antacids + ranitidine 77 continuous antacids + ranitidine 82 open Nissen fundoplication	12	Reduction in grade of oesophagitis at 12 months	Surgery significantly more effective than medical treatment (P 0.003; no further data reported)
51	Adults with severe GORD	16 antacids 10 Belsey–Mark IV repair 5 anterior fundoplication + Hills posterior gastropexy	38	Absence of reflux at 1 year using the acid perfusion test	11/15 (73%) with surgery *v* 3/16 (19%) with antacids (OR 11.9, 95% CI 2.1 to 65.2)
51	Adults with GORD and asthma	30 placebo 30 cimetidine 30 posterior gastropexy	3	pH testing for absence of reflux	Not intention to treat: 25/26 (96%) with surgery *v* 3/27 (11%) with control (OR 200, 95% CI 19.4 to 2059)
52	Adults with healed reflux oesophagitis	155 omeprazole 20 mg/day 155 open antireflux surgery	36	Endoscopic remission	Not intention to treat; 103/119 (87%) with surgery *v* 111/113 (83%) with omeprazole (OR not stated)

GORD, gastro-oesophageal reflux disease; Ref, reference.

Helicobacter pylori infection

Search date December 2002

Brendan Delaney, Paul Moayyedi, and David Forman

QUESTIONS

The effects of treatments for *Helicobacter pylori* in people with:

INTERVENTIONS

See glossary, p 546

Key Messages

- ***H pylori* eradication for healing and preventing recurrence of duodenal ulcer** Systematic reviews and one subsequent RCT have found that *H pylori* eradication increases ulcer healing at 6 weeks and reduces 1 year recurrence compared with acid suppression or antisecretory treatment. One systematic review found that *H pylori* eradication compared with ulcer healing alone, or compared with ulcer treatment plus subsequent acid suppression maintenance treatment, reduced the risk of rebleeding.

- ***H pylori* eradication for healing and preventing recurrence of gastric ulcer** One systematic review found no good evidence on endoscopic healing of gastric ulcers. One systematic review has found that *H pylori* eradication treatment, compared with antisecretory treatment, reduces recurrent ulcers at 1 year. Observational evidence identified by the review found that eradication treatment heals 83% of gastric ulcers within 6 weeks of starting treatment. We found no RCTs of *H pylori* eradication treatment on preventing complications of gastric ulcers.
- ***H pylori* eradication for non-ulcer dyspepsia** One systematic review in people with non-ulcer dyspepsia has found that *H pylori* eradication reduces dyspeptic symptoms compared with placebo at 3–12 months.
- ***H pylori* eradication rather than empirical acid suppression for uninvestiaged dyspepsia** One RCT found that *H pylori* eradication increased relief from dyspeptic symptoms compared with placebo after 1 year.
- ***H pylori* eradication rather than endoscopy in people with uninvestigated dyspepsia not at high risk of malignancy** One RCT has found that *H pylori* eradication increased relief from dyspeptic symptoms after 1 year compared with placebo. One systematic review and one subsequent RCT have found no significant difference between *H pylori* testing plus eradication compared with management based on initial endoscopy in dyspepsia after 1 year. The review found that *H pylori* testing plus eradication reduced the need for endoscopy compared with endoscopy based management.
- **Three day quadruple regimen (*v* 1 week triple regimen)** One RCT comparing a 3 day quadruple regimen compared with a 1 week triple regimen found no significant difference in *H pylori* eradication at 6 weeks, but found that people taking the 3 day quadruple regimen experienced fewer days of adverse effects.
- **Triple regimen (*v* dual regimen)** We found no systematic review or RCTs of the effects of dual regimen compared with triple regimens on dyspeptic symptom scores, proportion of individuals with symptoms, quality of life, or mortality. One systematic review has found that dual compared with triple regimens eradicate *H pylori* from fewer people.
- **Two week triple regimen (*v* 1 week triple regimen)** One systematic review found that 14 days treat ment with proton pump inhibitor based treatment increased *H pylori* cure rates compared with 7 days treatment.
- ***H pylori* eradication for gastric B cell lymphoma** We found no RCTs of *H pylori* eradication treatment in people with B cell gastric lymphoma. Observational studies found limited evidence that 60–93% of people with localised, low grade B cell lymphoma respond to *H pylori* eradication treatment possibly avoiding, or delaying, the need for radical surgery, radiotherapy, or chemotherapy.
- ***H pylori* eradication for prevention of gastric cancer (adenocarcinoma)** We found no RCTs of *H pylori* eradication in people at risk of gastric cancer. One RCT in people with gastric atrophy or intestinal metaplasia found that *H pylori* eradication increased the regression of high risk lesions compared with no eradication. We found consistent evidence from observational studies of an association between *H pylori* infection and increased risk of distal gastric adenocarcinoma.
- **One triple regimen versus another** We found no systematic review or RCTs of the effects of different triple regimens on symptoms, quality of life, or mortality. One systematic review has found that clarithromycin 500 mg twice daily compared with clarithromycin 250 mg twice daily plus a proton pump inhibitor plus amoxicillin increases *H pylori* eradication, but found no significant

difference between clarithromycin 500 mg twice daily and clarithromycin 250 mg twice daily plus a proton pump inhibitor plus metronidazole in *H pylori* eradication rates. Another systematic review has found that a triple regimen containing ranitidine bismuth plus clarithromycin plus metronidazole compared with a triple regimen containing ranitidine bismuth plus clarithromycin plus amoxicillin increases eradication at 5–7 days.

- ***H pylori* eradication in people with gastro-oesophageal reflux disease** One RCT in people with gastro-oesophageal reflux disease found no significant difference between *H pylori* eradication treatment and placebo in symptomatic relapse.

DEFINITION *Helicobacter pylori* is a Gram negative flagellated spiral bacterium found in the stomach. Infection with *H pylori* is predominantly acquired in childhood. The organism is associated with lifelong chronic gastritis and may cause other gastroduodenal disorders.[1]

INCIDENCE/ PREVALENCE *H pylori* prevalence rates vary with year of birth and social class in the developed world. Prevalence rates in many developed countries tend to be much higher (50–80%) in individuals born before 1950 compared with rates (< 20%) in individuals born more recently.[2] In many developing countries, the infection has a high prevalence (80–95%) irrespective of the period of birth.[3] Adult prevalence is believed to represent the persistence of a historically higher rate of infection acquired in childhood, rather than increasing acquisition of infection during life.

AETIOLOGY/ RISK FACTORS Overcrowded conditions associated with childhood poverty lead to increased transmission and higher prevalence rates. Adult reinfection rates are low — less than 1% a year.[3]

PROGNOSIS *H pylori* infection is believed to be causally related to the development of duodenal and gastric ulceration, gastric B cell lymphoma, and distal gastric cancer. About 15% of people infected with *H pylori* will develop a peptic ulcer, and 1% of people will develop gastric cancer during their lifetime.[4] *H pylori* infection is not associated with a specific type of dyspeptic symptom.

AIMS OF INTERVENTION Improvement in dyspeptic symptoms; reduction in peptic ulcer complications; reduced mortality from peptic ulcer complications of gastric cancer; improved quality of life.

OUTCOMES Dyspeptic symptom scores and proportion of people with symptoms; quality of life; mortality.

METHODS *Clinical Evidence* search and appraisal December 2002.

QUESTION **What are the effects of *H pylori* eradication treatment in people with a proven duodenal ulcer?**

Systematic reviews and one subsequent RCT have found that *H pylori* eradication compared with acid suppression or antisecretory treatment increases the proportion of ulcers healed at 6 weeks and reduces 1 year recurrence. One systematic review found that *H pylori* eradication compared with ulcer healing alone, or compared with ulcer treatment plus subsequent acid suppression maintenance treatment, reduced the risk of rebleeding.

Benefits: **Endoscopic healing:** We found two systematic reviews,[5,6] and one subsequent RCT,[7] of *H pylori* eradication treatment in people with proven duodenal ulcers. The first systematic review (search date 1995, 15 RCTs that directly compared treatments) found that triple regimens compared with antisecretory treatment (see glossary, p 546) increased duodenal ulcer healing rates.[5] Out of 16 trials (15 of them RCTs), 14 found higher healing rates with triple therapy compared with antisecretory drugs alone (the time to outcome varied, the review did not report how many RCTs found significant results, no meta-analysis was conducted, and results were presented graphically). The second systematic review (search date 1996, 7 RCTs conducted in the USA, 989 *H pylori* positive people with duodenal ulcer given dual regimen) assessed ulcer healing in people receiving *H pylori* eradication treatment.[6] It only included RCTs with endoscopic follow up for 6 months after treatment. It found that most duodenal ulcers were endoscopically healed 6 weeks after the start of eradication treatment (68%, 95% CI 65% to 71% with eradication treatment). The review provided no comparative information on the ulcer healing rate in people given control treatment. The subsequent RCT (277 people with active duodenal ulcer) compared eradication treatment (metronidazole plus amoxicillin [amoxycillin] plus omeprazole) for 2 weeks followed by omeprazole 20 mg until the ulcer had healed compared with omeprazole 20 mg twice daily until the ulcer had healed.[7] It found no significant difference between eradication treatment compared with omeprazole alone in healing of duodenal ulcer at 4 weeks (84% *v* 92%; P = 0.07). The RCT assessed the two groups for a further 2 years (see prevention of recurrence below).[7] **Prevention of recurrence:** We found one systematic review[5] and one subsequent RCT,[7] which compared the effects of eradication treatment with antisecretory drugs alone on ulcer recurrence 1 year after treatment. The systematic review (search date 1995, 20 RCTs) directly compared any type of eradication treatment with antisecretory treatment.[5] The review (20 RCTs) found that any type of eradication treatment compared with antisecretory treatment reduced ulcer recurrence at 1 year (128/1059 [12%] with eradication *v* 575/988 [58%] with control). In the subsequent RCT above, the 250 people whose ulcers had healed by 16 weeks entered the next phase of the study, which lasted 2 years.[7] In the first year, people in the omeprazole alone group were given omeprazole 20 mg and people receiving eradication treatment were given placebo. In the second year, both groups received no treatment and were observed. The RCT found no significant difference on intention to treat analysis in ulcer recurrence between eradication and omeprazole after 1 year (10/139 [7%] with eradication *v* 15/137 [11%] with omeprazole; RR 0.66, 95% CI 0.30 to 1.38). A completer analysis of the second year of observation alone (173 people) found that initial eradication treatment compared with initial omeprazole alone significantly reduced ulcer recurrence (5/86 [6%] with eradication *v* 39/87 [45%] with omeprazole; RR of recurrence 0.13, 95% CI 0.05 to 0.31; NNT 3, 95% CI 2 to 4) after 2 years. **Prevention of bleeding:** We found one systematic review (search date 2000, 4 RCTs, 262 people),[8] which compared *H pylori* eradication versus ulcer treatment alone or versus ulcer treatment plus subsequent acid suppression maintenance treatment. The review found that *H pylori* eradication compared with ulcer treatment alone significantly reduced the risk of rebleeding (6/133 [4.5%] with eradication *v* 28/129 [22%] with ulcer treatment alone; RR 0.24, 95% CI 0.11 to 0.53; NNT 6, 95% CI 4 to 11), and *H pylori* eradication compared with ulcer treatment plus acid suppression also significantly reduced the risk of rebleeding (4/257 [1.6%] with eradication *v* 12/213 [5.6%] with ulcer treatment plus acid suppression; RR 0.3, 95% CI 0.09 to 0.77; NNT 25, 95% CI 13 to 167). **Prevention of perforation or obstruction:** We found no systematic review and no RCTs.

Harms: One systematic review (search date 1995) found that minor adverse effects are common with bismuth (see glossary, p 546) (40% of people), metronidazole (39%), clarithromycin (22%), and tinidazole (7%).[9] Discontinuation of treatment because of severe adverse effects is rare (bismuth 4%, metronidazole 2%, clarithromycin 1%, and tinidazole < 1%).

Comment: We excluded analyses that grouped people by *H pylori* status at the end of the trial. Observational evidence from RCTs suggests that duodenal ulcer recurrence rates 1 year after treatment are lower in people with successful *H pylori* eradication treatment (in the review of US RCTs: 20%, 95% CI 14% to 26%, in people cured of *H pylori* *v* 56%, 95% CI 50% to 61%, for people remaining infected).[6] The recurrence rate in non-US trials was lower than the recurrence rate found in the US trials (6% for people cured of *H pylori*). The difference in recurrence rates between US and non-US studies may be explained partially by the marked loss to follow up in the US trials (9–41%). However, countries with low prevalence of *H pylori* infection also have a low prevalence of duodenal ulcers, but a greater proportion of those ulcers arise from causes other than *H pylori*; therefore, eradication may be less effective where *H pylori* prevalence is low. Poor adherence to *H pylori* eradication treatment and the use of less effective regimens may lead to increased antibiotic resistance in *H pylori*, but we found no direct evidence to support this. The harms of *H pylori* eradication treatment are mainly the minor short term effects of the antibiotics, particularly nausea from metronidazole or clarithromycin, and diarrhoea. Bismuth may turn the stools black.

QUESTION What are the effects of *H pylori* eradication treatment for people with a proven gastric ulcer?

One systematic review found no good evidence on endoscopic healing of gastric ulcers. One systematic review has found that *H pylori* eradication treatment compared with antisecretory treatment reduces recurrent ulcers at 1 year. The review found that, within 6 weeks of starting eradication treatment, 83% of gastric ulcers healed. We found no RCTs of *H pylori* eradication treatment on preventing complications of gastric ulcers.

Benefits: **Endoscopic healing:** We found one systematic review (search date 1995, 6 RCTs), which compared eradication treatment versus no eradication treatment but did not analyse endoscopic healing of gastric ulcers.[5] **Prevention of recurrence:** The systematic review found that *H pylori* eradication treatment compared with 4–6 weeks antisecretory treatment (see glossary, p 546) significantly reduced recurrent ulcers at 1 year (6 RCTs; RR 0.18, 95% CI 0.1 to 0.3; NNT 3, 95% CI 2 to 4).[5] **Prevention of complications:** We found no systematic review or RCTs.

Harms: See harms under effects of eradication treatment for *H pylori* in people with a proven duodenal ulcer, p 539.

Comment: We found one systematic review (search date 1995, 14 cohort studies of people with uncomplicated gastric ulcer), which analysed the *H pylori* eradication arm.[5] It found that, 6 weeks after the start of *H pylori* eradication treatment, 83% (95% CI 78% to 88%) of gastric ulcers were healed.

QUESTION What are the effects of *H pylori* eradication treatment in people with proven gastro-oesophageal reflux disease?

One RCT in people with gastro-oesophageal reflux disease found no significant difference between *H pylori* eradication treatment and placebo in symptomatic relapse.

Benefits: We found no systematic review but found one RCT (190 *H pylori* positive people with gastro-oesophageal reflux disease but no duodenal ulcer), which compared *H pylori* eradication treatment versus placebo. It found no significant difference in symptomatic relapse (83% in both groups; difference 0%, 95% CI –11% to +11%).[10]

Harms: We found insufficient evidence about the harms of *H pylori* eradication treatment in people with gastro-oesophageal reflux disease. Case control studies have found an increased risk of reflux symptoms after *H pylori* eradication.[11] However, discontinuation of acid suppression treatment after *H pylori* eradication might have unmasked symptoms of co-existing gastro-oesophageal reflux disease. Two RCTs in people with duodenal ulcer compared the effects of *H pylori* eradication treatment versus placebo on heartburn symptoms, but no analysis by intention to treat was reported.[12,13]

Comment: One RCT (2324 people from the general population who tested positive for *H pylori*) found no significant difference *between H pylori* eradication and placebo in reflux symptoms at 2 years.[14]

QUESTION What are the effects of *H pylori* eradication treatment in people with B cell lymphoma of the stomach?

We found no RCTs of *H pylori* eradication treatment in people with B cell gastric lymphoma. Observational studies found limited evidence that 60–93% of people with localised, low grade B cell lymphoma may respond to *H pylori* eradication treatment, possibly avoiding, or delaying the need for radical surgery, radiotherapy, or chemotherapy.

Benefits: We found no systematic review and no RCTs.

Harms: We found no RCTs.

Comment: Treatment options for primary gastric lymphoma include surgery, radiotherapy, chemotherapy, and *H pylori* eradication. We found no direct comparative studies. We found six prospective cohort studies of *H pylori* eradication in people with localised, low grade lymphomas.[15] Tumour regression occurred in 60–93% of people, but responses were sometimes delayed and some people relapsed within 1 year of treatment. A further uncontrolled study (28/34 people with gastric B cell lymphoma (see glossary, p 546) who were found to be *H pylori* positive and were given eradication treatment) found that 14/28 people (50%, 95% CI 31 to 69%) achieved complete remission at 18 months' follow up.[16]

QUESTION **What are the effects of *H pylori* eradication treatment on the risk of developing gastric cancer?**

We found no RCTs of *H pylori* eradication in people at risk of gastric cancer. One RCT in people with gastric atrophy or intestinal metaplasia found that *H pylori* eradication compared with no eradication increased the regression of high risk lesions. We found consistent evidence from case control studies of an association between *H pylori* infection and increased risk of distal gastric adenocarcinoma.

Benefits: **General population:** We found no systematic review and no RCTs of *H pylori* eradication treatment to prevent gastric cancer (adenocarcinoma). **In people at high risk of gastric cancer:** We found no systematic review and no RCTs of the effects of *H pylori* eradication on the development of gastric cancer in people at high risk. One RCT (852 people with gastric atrophy or intestinal metaplasia found at screening endoscopy) compared four treatments: *H pylori* eradication treatment; β carotene; ascorbic acid; and placebo.[17] It found that *H pylori* eradication treatment compared with no eradication treatment significantly increased lesion regression (calculated by multivariate modelling) for both atrophy (RR 4.8, 95% CI 1.6 to 14.2) and intestinal metaplasia (RR 3.1, 95% CI 1.0 to 9.3; no absolute numbers provided).

Harms: We found no RCTs in people at risk of gastric cancer.

Comment: We found one systematic review of nested case control studies (search date 1999, 12 studies, 1228 cases, 3406 controls).[18] In the absence of trial data, this is the best evidence of an association between *H pylori* infection and gastric cancer. The review found that, overall, there was a significant association between *H pylori* infection and the subsequent development of gastric cancer (OR 2.36, 95% CI 1.98 to 2.81). The review found no significant association between *H pylori* and cardia cancer (OR 0.99, 95% CI 0.72 to 1.35), but did find a significant association for non-cardia cancer (OR 2.97, 95% CI 2.34 to 3.77). Second, the review found a strong interaction with age and time from sample collection. *H pylori* does not colonise areas of cancer, intestinal metaplasia, or atrophy, and antibodies may be lost with increasing age. Prospective studies with a short time period between the collection of the serum sample and the development of the cancer, or retrospective studies, may underestimate the association. The review found a significant association between *H pylori* and non-cardia (distal) cancer where the time from sampling to cancer was more than 10 years (OR 5.93, 95% CI 3.41 to 10.3).

QUESTION **What are the effects of *H pylori* eradication treatment in people with proven non-ulcer dyspepsia?**

One systematic review in people with non-ulcer dyspepsia has found that *H pylori* eradication compared with placebo reduces dyspeptic symptoms at 3–12 months.

Benefits: We found one systematic review (search date 2000, 9 RCTs, 2541 people with non-ulcer dyspepsia), which found that *H pylori* eradication compared with placebo significantly improved recurrent dyspeptic symptoms at 3–12 months (AR of recurrent symptoms 896/1401 [64%] with eradication treatment *v* 820/1140 [72%] with placebo; RR 0.91, 95% CI 0.86 to 0.96; NNT 15, 95% CI 10 to 31).[19] Three RCTs (839 people) in the systematic review found no significant difference between *H pylori* eradication treatment compared with placebo on quality of life at 12 months (WMD −0.25, 95% CI −3.49 to +2.99).[19]

Harms: See harms under effects of eradication treatment for H pylori in people with a proven duodenal ulcer, p 539. We found two RCTs that assessed whether *H pylori* eradication treatment increases the prevalence of oesophagitis in people with non-ulcer dyspepsia.[20,21] They found no significant difference between *H pylori* eradication treatment and placebo in endoscopically assessed oesophagitis (5.7% with eradication treatment *v* 2.9% with placebo; ARI +2.8%, 95% CI −0.5% to +6.0%; RR 2.1, 95% CI 0.9 to 4.6). No trial evaluated individual dyspeptic symptoms, so the effect on reflux symptoms cannot be estimated separately from epigastric pain.

Comment: None.

QUESTION **What are the effects of *H pylori* eradication treatment in people with uninvestigated dyspepsia?**

One RCT has found that *H pylori* eradication compared with placebo increased relief from dyspeptic symptoms after 1 year. One systematic review in people not at high risk of gastro-intestinal malignancy and one subsequent RCT in people with uninvestigated dyspepsia have found no significant difference between *H pylori* testing plus eradication and management based on initial endoscopy in dyspepsia after 1 year. The review found that *H pylori* testing plus eradication compared with endoscopy based management reduced the proportion of people requiring endoscopy.

Benefits: ***H pylori* eradication versus placebo:** We found one RCT (294 people with dyspeptic symptoms and confirmed *H pylori* infection), which found that *H pylori* eradication compared with placebo significantly increased relief from dyspeptic symptoms at 1 year (61/145 [42%] *v* 80/149 [54%]; RR 0.78, 95% CI 0.61 to 0.99; NNT 9, 95% CI 5 to 554).[22] **Initial *H pylori* testing plus eradication versus management based on initial endoscopy:** We found one systematic review (search date 1999, 3 RCTs, 1366 people not considered to be at high risk of gastro-intestinal malignancy; see comment below), which compared *H pylori* testing plus eradication versus management based on initial endoscopy.[23] It found no significant difference between *H pylori* testing plus eradication and endoscopy based management in dyspepsia at 1 year (140/414 [34%] *v* 137/414 [33%]; RR 1.02, 95% CI 0.85 to 1.23). It found that *H pylori* testing plus eradication compared with endoscopy based management significantly reduced the proportion of people requiring endoscopy (169/500 [34%] at 2–6 weeks after eradication treatment *v* 486/489 [99%] with prompt endoscopy; RR 0.34, 95% CI 0.30 to 0.39). One subsequent RCT (708 people aged < 55 years referred for endoscopic investigation of dyspepsia by their primary care physician) found no significant difference between *H pylori* eradication and endoscopy in dyspeptic symptoms at 1 year (260/293 [89%] with *H pylori* eradication *v* 249/291 [86%] with endoscopy; RR 1.03, 95% CI 0.97 to 1.1).[24] Only 8.2% of people initially randomised to *H pylori* eradication had an endoscopy in the following year.

Harms: The systematic review gave no information on adverse effects.[23] Two of the RCTs in the review found that a small number of people given *H pylori* eradication treatment discontinued treatment because of short term adverse effects, which were not specified (14/104 [13%] people in the first RCT in the review[25] and 4/80 [5%] in the second RCT[26]).

Comment: The results of the systematic review may not be applicable to all people with dyspepsia. People with "alarm" symptoms (dysphagia, weight loss, jaundice, epigastric mass, or anaemia), or over the age of 55 years, with either continuous epigastric pain or first onset of symptoms in the previous year, may have a significant risk of upper gastrointestinal malignancy and may benefit from prompt endoscopy. Two of the RCTs in the review were conducted in a hospital setting and the third, conducted in primary care, is not yet published in full.[27] One of the RCTs in the review, conducted in a hospital setting, stipulated that all eligible people with dyspepsia who were consulting with a general medical practitioner should be included, but the other entered only routine referrals. The results of the review might not apply directly to primary care, where people with less severe dyspepsia might be treated and *H pylori* eradication rates might be lower, and the reassuring or anxiety provoking effect of specialist consultation might not be replicated.[23]

QUESTION **Do eradication treatments differ in their effects?**

OPTION **DUAL VERSUS TRIPLE REGIMENS**

We found no systematic review or RCTs of the effects of dual compared with triple regimens on dyspeptic symptom scores, proportion of individuals with symptoms, quality of life, or mortality. One systematic review has found that dual compared with triple regimens eradicate *H pylori* from fewer people.

Benefits: **Duodenal ulcer complication rates:** We found no systematic review and no RCTs. **Eradication rates:** We found one systematic review (search date 1995; 19 RCTs of omeprazole plus amoxicillin [amoxycillin] versus containing bismuth; 17 RCTs of dual regimens containing a proton pump inhibitor versus triple regimens [see glossary, p 546]).[9] No formal meta-analysis was performed, but dual regimens compared with triple regimens (two antibiotics plus either a proton pump inhibitor or bismuth) eradicated *H pylori* from fewer people (results presented graphically).

Harms: See harms under effects of eradication treatment for *H pylori* in people with a proven duodenal ulcer, p 537.

Comment: Many RCTs of *H pylori* eradication treatment have methodological problems, such as lack of a gold standard for defining cure, and many are published only as an abstract. A systematic review comparing eradication treatments for *H pylori* eradication is in progress.[27] Factors that might influence the choice of eradication treatment for an individual also include ease of adherence, potential harms, allergy or sensitivity, drug resistance, and cost.

OPTION DIFFERENT TRIPLE REGIMENS

We found no systematic review or RCTs of the effects of different triple regimens on dyspeptic symptom scores, proportion of individuals with symptoms, quality of life, or mortality. One systematic review has found that clarithromycin 500 mg twice daily compared with clarithromycin 250 mg twice daily plus a proton pump inhibitor plus amoxicillin increases *H pylori* eradication, but found no significant difference between clarithromycin 500 mg twice daily and clarithromycin 250 mg twice daily plus a proton pump inhibitor plus metronidazole in *H pylori* eradication rates. Another systematic review has found that a triple regimen containing ranitidine bismuth plus clarithromycin plus metronidazole compared with a triple regimen containing ranitidine bismuth plus clarithromycin plus amoxicillin increases eradication at 5–7 days.

Benefits: **Duodenal ulcer complication rates:** We found no systematic review and no direct comparison of the effect of different triple regimens (see glossary, p 546) on complication rates. **Eradication rates:** We found four systematic reviews comparing different triple regimens, two of which included indirect comparisons (see glossary, p 546) between RCTs.[9,28–30] The first systematic review (search date 1998, 4 RCTs with direct, head-to-head comparisons of eradication regimens) found that clarithromycin 500 mg twice daily compared with clarithromycin 250 mg twice daily in combination with a proton pump inhibitor (see glossary, p 546) and amoxicillin (amoxycillin) significantly increased *H pylori* eradication (90% with clarithromycin 500 mg *v* 80% with 250 mg; RR 0.89, 95% CI 0.81 to 0.97; NNT 11, 95% CI 6 to 38).[28] The review found no significant difference between clarithromycin 500 mg twice daily and clarithromycin 250 mg twice daily in combination with a proton pump inhibitor and metronidazole in eradication rates (89% with clarithromycin 500 mg twice daily *v* 87% with 250 mg twice daily; RR 0.98, 95% CI 0.93 to 1.04). The second systematic review (search date 2000, 8 RCTs, 1139 people with direct comparisons of eradication regimens) found that ranitidine bismuth (see glossary, p 546) 400 mg daily plus clarithromycin 250 mg plus metronidazole 400 mg twice daily compared with ranitidine 400 mg daily plus clarithromycin 500 mg twice daily plus amoxicillin 1000 mg twice daily significantly increased eradication at 5–7 days (499/565 [88%] *v* 467/574 [81%]; RR 1.09, 95% CI 1.03 to 1.14).[29] The limited evidence from two systematic reviews with indirect comparisons found the highest eradication rates (85–90%) with omeprazole (20 mg daily, or equivalent) plus a combination of two of the following: amoxicillin (1–1.5 g daily), metronidazole (1.2 g daily), or clarithromycin (500 mg daily) with metronidazole or 1 g daily with amoxicillin (see comment below).[9,28] **Antibiotic resistance:** We found one systematic review (search date 1995, 19 RCTs, 1006 people with metronidazole sensitive *H pylori*, 452 with metronidazole resistant *H pylori*)[9] and one subsequent RCT,[31] which assessed the efficacy of metronidazole (or other nitroimidazole) based triple and quadruple regimens with strains of *H pylori* that were resistant in the laboratory. The review found that nitroimidazole based regimens achieved *H pylori* eradication in significantly fewer people with strains showing nitroimidazole resistance in the laboratory than in people with sensitive strains (99%, 95% CI 97% to 100% eradication in people with sensitive strains *v* 69%, 95% CI 60% to 77% in people with resistant strains).[9] The subsequent RCT (33 people with a proven duodenal ulcer and *H pylori* infection, and primary metronidazole resistance, and 81 without resistance) found that metronidazole resistance decreased the *H pylori* eradication rate with omeprazole, metronidazole and clarithromycin from 77/81 (95.1%) without resistance to 25/33 (75.8%) with metronidazole resistance; RR 0.79, 95% CI 0.62 to 0.93).[31]

Harms: See harms under effects of eradication treatment for *H pylori* in people with a proven duodenal ulcer, p 539.

Comment: Indirect comparison is a weak form of evidence.[9,28] The characteristics of the people, settings, and procedures in the different RCTs may not be comparable. The systematic review assessing nitroimidazole resistance concluded that clinically important reduction of eradication rates is unlikely with a proportion of resistant strains below 15–25%.[9] Systematic reviews of *H pylori* eradication treatments are difficult to interpret (see dual versus triple regimens, p 543).

OPTION DURATION OF *H PYLORI* ERADICATION TREATMENT

One systematic review found that 14 days compared with 7 days treatment with proton pump inhibitor based triple regimens increased *H pylori* cure rates. One subsequent RCT comparing a 3 day quadruple regimen versus a 1 week triple regimen found no significant difference in *H pylori* eradication at 6 weeks, but found that people taking the 3 day quadruple regimen experienced fewer days of adverse effects.

Benefits: **Duodenal ulcer complication rates:** We found no systematic review and no RCTs. **Eradication rates:** We found one systematic review[32] and one subsequent RCT.[33] The review (search date 1999, 7 RCTs, 906 people) compared 14 days treatment with proton pump inhibitor based triple regimens (see glossary, p 546) versus 7 days treatment with proton pump inhibitor based triple regimens.[32] It found that 14 day treatment compared with 7 day treatment significantly increased *H pylori* cure rates (339/470 [72.1%] *v*

353/436 [81.0%]; RR 0.89, 95% CI 0.83 to 0.96; NNT 11, 95% CI 7 to 33). One subsequent RCT (118 people with active duodenal ulcer at endoscopy) compared a 3 day quadruple regimen (lansoprazole plus clarithromycin plus metronidazole plus bismuth subcitrate) versus a 7 day triple regimen (lansoprazole plus clarithromycin plus metronidazole).[33] It found no significant difference in *H pylori* eradication at 6 weeks (50/58 [86.2%] with 3 day quadruple regimen *v* 52/60 [86.7%] with 7 day triple regimen; RR 0.99, 95% CI 0.79 to 1.09).

Harms: See harms under effects of eradication treatment for H pylori in people with a proven duodenal ulcer, p 539. The RCT, comparing a 3 day quadruple regimen versus a 1 week triple regimen, found that people taking the 3 day regimen experienced significantly fewer days of bitter taste, bowel disturbance, malaise, and dark stools (mean 2.54 days with 3 day quadruple regimen *v* mean 4.58 days with 7 day triple regimen; $P < 0.001$).[33] The systematic review found insufficient data to report harms.[32]

Comment: The systematic review only considered regimens containing clarithromycin plus either metronidazole or amoxicillin.[32] The risk of failure of a 7 day regimen as opposed to a 14 day regimen in any particular individual will relate to the local prevalence of antibiotic resistance, as 14 day regimens may overcome resistance to one of the antibiotics used. As longer regimens cost more and have a longer duration of minor adverse effects, the balance between local failure rate and cost must be decided on the basis of locally validated data.

GLOSSARY

Antisecretory treatment A treatment that reduces the production of acid by the stomach. These may either be H_2 receptor antagonists or proton pump inhibitors.

Bismuth A compound containing bismuth, such as bismuth subsalicilate or ranitidine bismuth citrate.

Dual regimen *H pylori* eradication regimen consisting of two components.

Indirect comparisons Indirect comparisons combine the results for the same intervention across different RCTs and compare against the results for another intervention combined across different RCTs. This method loses the benefits of randomisation and increases the risk of confounding as the characteristics of the people, settings, and procedures in the different RCTs may not be comparable.

MALT "Mucosa-associated lymphoid tissue" is constitutionally found in the intestine but not in the stomach. MALT lymphoma is also known as B cell gastric lymphoma.

Proton pump inhibitor A drug that directly inhibits the mechanism within the stomach that secretes acid, such as esomeprazole, lansoprazole, omeprazole, or rabeprazole.

Triple regimen *H pylori* eradication regimen consisting of three components. The original "triple regimen" was bismuth subsalicilate, metronidazole, and either amoxicillin (amoxycillin) or tetracycline. Now the term usually applies to a proton pump inhibitor plus two antibiotics.

Substantive changes

***H pylori* eradication for non-ulcer dyspepsia** Evidence reinterpreted; intervention recategorised as Beneficial.

REFERENCES

1. Nguyen TN, Barkun AN, Fallone CA. Host determinants of *Helicobacter pylori* infection and its clinical outcome. *Helicobacter* 1999;4:185–197.
2. Harvey RF, Spence RW, Lane JA, et al. Relationship between the birth cohort pattern of *Helicobacter pylori* infection and the epidemiology of duodenal ulcer. *Q J Med* 2002;95:519–25.
3. Axon AT. *Helicobacter pylori* infection. *J Antimicrob Chemother* 1993;32(suppl A):61–68.
4. Graham DY. Can therapy ever be denied for *Helicobacter pylori* infection? *Gastroenterology* 1997;113:S113–S117.
5. Penston JG. Review article: clinical aspects of *Helicobacter pylori* eradication therapy in peptic ulcer disease. *Aliment Pharmacol Ther* 1996;10:469–486. Search date 1995; primary sources Medline and conference abstracts.
6. Laine L, Hopkins RJ, Girardi LS. Has the impact of *Helicobacter pylori* therapy on ulcer recurrence in the United States been overstated? A meta-analysis of rigorously designed trials. *Am J Gastroenterol* 1998;93:1409–1415. Search date 1996; primary sources Medline, conference abstracts, and pharmaceutical companies (US trials only).
7. Bytzer P, Aalykke C, Rune S, et al. Eradication of *Helicobacter pylori* compared with long-term acid suppression in duodenal ulcer disease. A randomised trial with 2-year follow up. *Scand J Gastroenterol* 2000;10:1023–1032.
8. Sharma VK, Sahai AV, Corder FA, et al. *Helicobacter pylori* eradication is superior to ulcer healing with or without maintenance therapy to prevent further ulcer haemorrhage. *Aliment Pharmacol Ther* 2001;15:1939–1947. Search date 2000; primary sources Medline and conference abstracts.
9. Penston JG, McColl KEL. Eradication of *Helicobacter pylori*: an objective assessment of current therapies. *Br J Clin Pharmacol* 1997;43:223–243. Search date 1995; primary sources Medline and conference abstracts.
10. Moayyedi P, Bardhan C, Young L, et al. *Helicobacter pylori* eradication does not exacerbate reflux symptoms in gastroesophageal reflux disease. *Gastroenterology* 2001;121:1120–1126.
11. Labenz J, Blum AL, Bayerdorffer E, et al. Curing *Helicobacter pylori* infection in patients with duodenal ulcer may provoke reflux esophagitis. *Gastroenterology* 1997;112:1442–1447.
12. Vakil N, Hahn B, McSorley D. Recurrent symptoms and gastro-oesophageal reflux disease in patients with duodenal ulcer treated for *Helicobacter pylori* infection. *Aliment Pharmacol Ther* 2000;14:45–51.
13. Fallone CA, Barkun AN, Friedman G, et al. Is *Helicobacter pylori* eradication associated with gastroesophageal reflux disease? *Am J Gastroenterol* 2000;95:914–920.
14. Moayyedi P, Feltbower R, Brown J, et al. Effect of population screening and treatment for *Helicobacter pylori* on dyspepsia and quality of life in the community: a randomised controlled trial. *Lancet* 2000;355:1665–1669.
15. Roher HD, Vereet PR, Wormer O, et al. *Helicobacter pylori* in the upper gastrointestinal tract: medical or surgical treatment of gastric lymphoma? *Langenbecks Arch Surg* 2000;385:97–105. Search date not stated; primary sources Medline and hand searches.
16. Steinbach G, Ford R, Glober G, et al. Antibiotic treatment of gastric lymphoma of mucosa-associated lymphoid tissue. An uncontrolled trial. *Ann Intern Med* 1999;131:88–95.
17. Correa P, Fontham ETH, Bravo JC, et al. Chemoprevention of gastric dysplasia: Randomized trial of antioxidant supplements and anti-*Helicobacter pylori* therapy. *J Natl Cancer Inst* 2000;92:1881–1888.
18. *Helicobacter* and Cancer Collaborative Group. Gastric cancer and *Helicobacter pylori*: a combined analysis of 12 case control studies nested within prospective cohorts. *Gut* 2001;49:347–353. Search date 1999; primary sources Medline and contact with investigators.
19. Soo S, Moayyedi P, Deeks J, et al. Eradication *Helicobacter pylori* for non-ulcer dyspepsia. In: The Cochrane Library, Issue 3, 2001. Oxford: Update Software. Search date 2000; primary sources Medline, Embase, Science Citation Index, conference abstracts, and survey of experts.
20. Blum AL, Talley NJ, O'Morain C, et al. Lack of effect of treating *Helicobacter pylori* infection in patients with nonulcer dyspepsia. *N Engl J Med* 1998;339:1875–1881.
21. Koelz HR, Arnold R, Stolte M, et al. Treatment of *Helicobacter pylori* (HP) does not improve symptoms of functional dyspepsia. *Gastroenterology* 1998;114:A182.
22. Chiba N, Veldhuyzen van Zanten SJO, Paul Sinclair, et al. Treating *Helicobacter pylori* infection in primary care patients with uninvestigated dyspepsia: the Canadian adult dyspepsia empiric treatment *Helicobacter pylori* positive (CADET-Hp) randomised controlled trial. *BMJ* 2002;324:1012.
23. Delaney BC, Innes MA, Deeks J, et al. Initial management strategies for dyspepsia. In: The Cochrane Library, Issue 3, 2001. Oxford: Update Software. Search date 1999; primary sources Medline, Embase, Science Citation Index, conference abstracts, and survey of experts.
24. McColl KEL, Murray LS, Gillen D, et al. Randomised trial of endoscopy with testing for *Helicobacter pylori* compared with non-invasive *H pylori* testing alone in the management of dyspepsia. *BMJ* 2002;324:999.
25. Lassen AT, Pedersen FM, Bytzer P, et al. *Helicobacter pylori* "test and eradicate" or prompt endoscopy for management of dyspeptic patients. A randomised controlled trial with one year follow-up. *Lancet* 2000;356:455–460.
26. Heaney A, Collins JSA, Watson RGP, et al. A prospective randomised trial of a "test and treat" policy versus endoscopy based management in young *Helicobacter pylori* positive patients with ulcer-like dyspepsia, referred to a hospital clinic. *Gut* 1999;45:186–190.
27. Forman D, Bazzoli F, Bennett C, et al. Therapies for the eradication of *Helicobater pylori*. Protocol for a Cochrane Review. In: The Cochrane Library, Issue 4, 2001. Oxford: Update Software.
28. Pipkin GA, Dixon JS, Williamson R, et al. Clarithromycin dual therapy regimens for eradication of *Helicobacter pylori*: a review. *Helicobacter* 1997;2:159–171. Search date 1997; primary sources Medline and conference abstracts.
29. Huang JQ, Hunt RH. The importance of clarithromycin dose in the management of *Helicobacter pylori* infection: a meta-analysis of triple therapies with a proton pump inhibitor, clarithromycin and amoxycillin or metronidazole. *Aliment Pharmacol Ther* 1999;13:719–729. Search date 1998; primary sources Medline and conference abstracts.

30. Janssen M, Van Oijen A, Verbeek A, et al. A systematic comparison of triple therapies for treatment of *Helicobacter pylori* infection with proton pump inhibitor/ranitidine bismuth citrate plus clarithromycin and either amoxicillin or a nitroimidazole. *Aliment Pharmacol Ther* 2001;15:613–624. Search date 2000; primary sources Medline and hand searches of reference lists and meetings abstracts.
31. Lind T, Peal MFU. The Mach 2 study: role of omeprazole in eradication of *Helicobacter pylori* with 1-week triple therapies. *Gastroenterology* 1999;116:248–253.
32. Calvet X, Garcia N, Lopez T, et al. A meta-analysis of short versus long therapy with a proton pump inhibitor, clarithromycin and either metronidazole or amoxycillin for treating *Helicobacter pylori* infection. *Aliment Pharmacol Ther* 200;14:603–609. Search date 1999; primary sources Medline and conference proceedings.
33. Wong B, Wang W, Wong W, et al. Three-day lansoprazole quadruple therapy for *Helicobacter pylori*-positive duodenal ulcers: a randomised controlled study. *Aliment Pharmacol Ther* 2001;15:843–849.

Brendan Delaney
Department of Primary Care and General Practice
University of Birmingham
Birmingham
UK

Paul Moayyedi
City Hospital NHS Trust
Birmingham
UK

David Forman
Cochrane Upper Gastrointestinal and Pancreatic Disease Collaborative Review Group
University of Leeds
Leeds
UK

Competing interests: BD has received fees for speaking at conferences and educational meetings from Astra Zeneca and Axlan. DF has received consulting fees from Astra Zeneca, Wyeth, and TAP-TAKEDA. PM has accepted fees for speaking from Astra Zeneca, Wyeth, Mareda, and Abbott laboratories.

Pancreatic cancer

Search date November 2002

Bazian Ltd

QUESTIONS

INTERVENTIONS

TREATMENTS IN PEOPLE WITH RESECTABLE PANCREATIC CANCER

Likely to be beneficial

Unknown effectiveness

To be covered in future updates

Adjuvant chemoimmunotherapy for resectable disease
Adjuvant chemoradiotherapy for resectable disease
Adjuvant local chemotherapy for resectable disease
Treatments for advanced disease

*RCTs comparing surgery versus no surgery may be considered unethical in people with pancreatic cancer that is considered suitable for complete tumour resection (see key messages below).

See glossary, p 554

Key Messages

- **Pylorus-preserving pancreaticoduodenectomy** Four small RCTs found no evidence that pylorus-preserving surgery improved overall quality of life or 5 year survival compared with classical Whipple's procedure. The studies may have lacked power to detect clinically important differences for these outcomes.
- **Surgery** We found no RCTs comparing surgery versus non-surgical treatment in people with resectable pancreatic cancer. Observational data provide limited evidence that surgery may reduce mortality compared with non-surgical treatment, although results may be confounded by differences in disease stage.
- **Systemic fluorouracil-based chemotherapy after resection** One RCT has found that adjuvant fluorouracil-based chemotherapy improves median survival compared with no adjuvant chemotherapy in people with resected pancreatic cancer. However, it found no evidence that fluorouracil improved 5 year survival, although the study may have lacked power to detect a difference. A second RCT did not directly compare chemotherapy alone versus no chemotherapy.

Pancreatic cancer

- **Systemic gemcitabine-based chemotherapy after resection** One systematic review found insufficient evidence about effects of adjuvant gemcitabine compared with no adjuvant chemotherapy in people with resected pancreatic cancer.

DEFINITION Primary adenocarcinoma of the pancreas. Other pancreatic malignancies, such as carcinoid tumour, are not considered in the present review. Pancreatic cancer is staged according to disease spread. Stage I disease is limited to the pancreas, duodenum, bile duct, or peri-pancreatic tissues, with no distant metastases or regional lymph node involvement. Stages II–IV describe disease that has spread more extensively or become metastatic. A pancreatic tumour is considered resectable if surgery aims to completely remove all cancerous tissue. Early stage tumours in the tail or body of the pancreas are more likely to be resectable than the more common, later stage cancers in the head of the pancreas. Other factors that influence resectability include proximity of the tumour to major blood vessels and perceived peri-operative risk. Symptoms include pain, jaundice, nausea, weight loss, loss of appetite, and symptoms of gastrointestinal obstruction and diabetes.

INCIDENCE/ PREVALENCE Pancreatic cancer is the eighth most frequent cancer in the UK.[1] Annual incidence in England and Wales is about 12/100 000. Prevalence is similar in males and females, with 5–10% presenting with resectable disease.[2] Pancreatic cancer is the fourth most common cause of cancer death in higher income countries, responsible for about 30 000 deaths each year in the US.[3]

AETIOLOGY/ RISK FACTORS Pancreatic cancer is more likely in people who smoke and have high alcohol intake. Dietary factors, such as lack of fruit and vegetables, are also reported risk factors.[4] One meta-analysis of observational studies found that people with diabetes mellitus of more than 5 years' duration are more likely to develop pancreatic cancer compared with the general population.[5] However, estimates of the magnitude of increased risk vary. Additional risk factors include pancreatitis and, in some cases, a family history.[1]

PROGNOSIS Prognosis is poor. One year survival is about 12%, with 5 year survival ranging from less than 1% in those with advanced cancer at presentation to 5% in those with early stage cancer at presentation.[1,6]

AIMS OF INTERVENTION Treatment in people with early stage (resectable) pancreatic cancer aims to improve survival and quality of life. In people with advanced pancreatic cancer, treatment aims to improve symptoms and quality of life.

OUTCOMES One year and 5 year survival; quality of life; symptoms; and adverse effects of treatment.

METHODS *Clinical Evidence* search and appraisal November 2002.

QUESTION What are effects of surgical treatments in people with pancreatic cancer that is considered suitable for complete tumour resection?

OPTION SURGERY

We found no RCTs comparing surgical versus non-surgical treatment in people with resectable pancreatic cancer. Observational data provide limited evidence that surgery may reduce mortality compared with non-surgical treatment, although results may be confounded by differences in disease stage.

Benefits: We found no RCTs comparing surgery alone versus non-surgical treatment in people with resectable (early stage) pancreatic cancer (see comment below).

Harms: We found no RCTs comparing harms of surgery versus harms of non-surgical or no treatment in people with resectable pancreatic cancer (see comment below).

Comment: RCTs comparing surgery versus non-surgical treatment may be considered unethical in people with tumours that are considered suitable for resection. One large cohort study (100 313 people with pancreatic cancer) found that people undergoing pancreatectomy lived longer than people not treated surgically (5 year survival, 23% with surgery *v* 5% without surgery).[7] However, results may be confounded by differences in disease stage between those undergoing surgery and those treated without surgery. Conventional surgery for pancreatic cancer is a radical procedure involving removal of the pancreas, duodenum, and gastric pylorus.

OPTION PYLORUS-PRESERVING SURGERY

Four small RCTs found no evidence that pylorus-preserving surgery improved overall quality of life or 5 year survival compared with classical Whipple's procedure in people with resectable tumours. The studies may have lacked power to detect clinically important differences for these outcomes.

Benefits: **Versus classical Whipple's procedure:** We found four RCTs.[8–11] The first RCT (38 people with resectable head of pancreas or peri-ampullary cancer) did not report on cancer recurrence, quality of life, or survival.[8] The second RCT (48 people with resectable head of pancreas or peri-ampullary cancer) found no difference between pylorus-preserving surgery and Whipple's procedure (see glossary, p 554) for global quality of life scores at 2–60 weeks (quality of life measured by 100 point EORTC-QLQ-30 score; results presented graphically, score in both groups about 50 preoperatively and 35 at 60 wks; $P > 0.05$).[9] The third RCT (40 people with head of pancreas or peri-ampullary cancer) found no significant difference between procedures for 5 year survival (20% with pylorus-preserving surgery *v* 13% with Whipple's). The study may have lacked power to detect a clinically important difference.[10] The fourth

RCT (77 people with head of pancreas or peri-ampullary cancer) similarly found no difference between techniques after a median follow up of 1.1 years (61 people included in analysis: median survival 24 months with pylorus-preserving surgery *v* 16 months with Whipple's; P = 0.29).[11]

Harms: The first RCT found no difference in peri-operative blood loss between pylorus-preserving and classical Whipple's surgery (mean blood loss 451 mL with pylorus-preserving surgery *v* 687 mL with Whipple's; P > 0.2; CI for difference not reported).[8] It also found no differences between treatments for peri-operative death (1 person with pylorus-preserving surgery *v* 0 with Whipple's); biliary leak (0 in both groups); pancreatitis (1 in both groups); wound infection (1 in both groups); cardiovascular events (0 with pylorus-preserving surgery *v* 1 with Whipple's); or upper gastrointestinal bleeding (0 with pylorus-preserving surgery *v* 1 with Whipple's). However, the RCT may have lacked power to exclude clinically important differences for these outcomes. Delayed gastric emptying was more common with pylorus-preserving surgery (6 people with pylorus-preserving surgery *v* 1 with Whipple's).[8] The second RCT also found that complication rates were similar in both groups (pylorus-preserving surgery *v* Whipple's; wound infection 3 *v* 4 people; pneumonia 2 *v* 3 people; peritonitis 1 in both groups; and sepsis 0 *v* 2 people).[9] The third RCT reported similar complications and frequencies to the other trials. Differences between procedures were not significant for any of these complications except gastric atony (6 people with pylorus-preserving surgery *v* 1 with Whipple's; P < 0.05).[10] The fourth RCT found no significant differences between the techniques for delayed gastric emptying (32% with pylorus-preserving surgery *v* 45% with Whipple's); fistula (2% *v* 3%); wound infection (7% *v* 8%); or peri-operative mortality (2.7% *v* 5%).[11]

Comment: The RCTs may have lacked power to detect clinically important differences between procedures.

QUESTION **What are effects of adjuvant treatments in people with resected pancreatic cancer?**

OPTION **ADJUVANT SYSTEMIC GEMCITABINE-BASED CHEMOTHERAPY**

One systematic review found insufficient evidence about the effects of adjuvant gemcitabine compared with no adjuvant chemotherapy in people with resected pancreatic cancer.

Benefits: **Versus no adjuvant chemotherapy:** We found one systematic review examining effects of gemcitabine-based chemotherapy in people with pancreatic cancer (search date 2000).[1] It identified no RCTs comparing adjuvant chemotherapy with gemcitabine alone versus no chemotherapy or placebo (see comment below).[1]

Harms: The systematic review identified two studies that assessed harms of gemcitabine from both controlled and uncontrolled clinical trials.[1] Both studies included people with non-pancreatic tumours. The studies found that gemcitabine was associated with the following grade 3–4 toxicities: anaemia (about 7%), leukopenia (about 9%), neutropenia (about 25%), and thrombocytopenia (5–7%).

Comment: The option described above excludes adjuvant gemcitabine combined with radiotherapy or immunotherapy.

OPTION ADJUVANT SYSTEMIC FLUOROURACIL-BASED CHEMOTHERAPY

One RCT has found that adjuvant fluorouracil-based chemotherapy improves median survival compared with no adjuvant chemotherapy in people with resected pancreatic cancer. However, it found no evidence that fluorouracil improved 5 year survival, although the study may have lacked power to detect a clinically important effect. A second RCT did not directly compare chemotherapy alone versus no chemotherapy.

Benefits: **Versus no adjuvant chemotherapy:** We found two RCTs comparing the effects of fluorouracil-based chemotherapy after successful surgical resection (no residual disease observed macroscopically or in the tumour resection margins).[12,13] The first RCT (multicentre trial in 61 people: 47 with resected pancreatic cancer and 14 with carcinoma of the papilla of Vater) compared chemotherapy (6 cycles of fluorouracil 500 mg/m^2, doxorubicin 40 mg/m^2, and mitomycin C 6 mg/m^2 once every 3 wks) versus no adjuvant chemotherapy. It found that chemotherapy significantly improved median survival compared with no adjuvant treatment (intention to treat analysis: median survival 23 months with chemotherapy *v* 11 months without; $P = 0.04$), but no difference for 5 year survival (4% with adjuvant chemotherapy *v* 8% without; $P = 0.10$; CI not reported). The study may have lacked power to detect clinically important differences in 5 year survival.[12] The second RCT (541 people with resected pancreatic cancer) compared four adjuvant strategies: chemotherapy (425 mg/m^2 fluorouracil plus folinic acid 20 mg/m^2); chemoradiotherapy; chemoradiotherapy plus the chemotherapy regimen; and observation only. It did not report results for chemotherapy alone versus no chemotherapy (see comment below).[13]

Harms: The first RCT reported that one person died of chemotherapy associated sepsis.[12] Other adverse effects of chemotherapy included non-fatal sepsis (4 people), alopecia (11 people), leukopenia $< 2.5 \times 10^9$/L white cells (occurred 5 times overall), cardiotoxicity (2 people), and nephrotoxicity (2 people). After 3 months, four people experienced nausea and vomiting with chemotherapy versus none in the control group.

Comment: The option described above excludes adjuvant fluorouracil combined with radiotherapy or immunotherapy. The first RCT included only people under 75 years old with high performance status (Karnofsky score > 60).[12] Six of 30 people allocated to chemotherapy received no chemotherapy and 17 did not complete all six cycles of therapy. The second RCT found that chemotherapy with or without chemoradiotherapy significantly improved survival compared with no chemotherapy (median survival 19.7 months with chemoradiotherapy *v* 14.0 months without chemoradiotherapy; HR 0.66, 95% CI 0.52 to 0.83).[13] It was not possible from this analysis to establish whether effects were due to chemotherapy or concomitant radiotherapy.

GLOSSARY

Whipple's procedure Radical surgery involving removal of the pancreas, duodenum, and gastric pylorus.

REFERENCES

1. Ward S, Morris E, Bansback N, et al. A rapid and systematic review of the clinical effectiveness and cost-effectiveness of gemcitabine for the treatment of pancreatic cancer. *Health Technol Assess* 2001;5:1–70. Search date 2000; primary sources Medline, Embase, Science Citation Index, Cochrane Library, NHS CRD, NHS EED, NHS HTA, Pubmed, OHE HEED, National and International Research Registers, contact with HTA agencies.
2. Maisey N, Chau I, Cunningham D, et al. Multicenter randomized Phase III trial comparing protracted venous infusion (PVI) fluorouracil (5-FU) with PVI 5-FU plus mitomycin in inoperable pancreatic cancer. *J Clin Oncol* 2002;14:3130–3136.
3. Jemal PA, Murray T, Samuels A. Cancer statistics, 2003. *CA Cancer J Clin* 2003;53:5–26.
4. Working Group on Diet and Cancer. Nutritional aspects of the development of cancer. (Committee on Medical Aspects of Food and Nutrition Policy; no. 48.) London: Department of Health, 1998.
5. Everhart, J, Wright, D. Diabetes mellitus as a risk factor for pancreatic cancer. A meta-analysis. *JAMA* 1995;273:1605–1609.
6. Bramhall SR, Allum WH, Jones AG, et al. Treatment and survival in 13,560 patients with pancreatic cancer: an epidemiological study in the West Midlands. *Br J Surg* 1995;82:111–115.
7. Sener SF, Fremgen A, Menck HR, et al. Pancreatic cancer: a report of treatment and survival trends for 100,313 patients diagnosed from 1985–1995, using the National Cancer Database. *J Am Coll Surg* 1999;189:1–7.
8. Lin PW, Lin YJ. Prospective randomized comparison between pylorus-preserving and standard pancreaticoduodenectomy. *Br J Surg* 1999;86:603–607.
9. Wenger F, Jacobi C, Haubold K, et al. Gastrointestinal quality of life after duodenopancreatectomy in pancreatic carcinoma. Preliminary results of a prospective randomized study: pancreatoduodenectomy or pylorus-preserving pancreatoduodenectomy. *Chirurg* 1999;70:1454–1459. [German]
10. Paquet K-J. Comparison of Whipple's pancreaticoduodenectomy with the pylorus-preserving pancreaticoduodenectomy — a prospectively controlled, randomized long-term trial. *Chirurg Gastroenterol* 1998;14:54–58.
11. Seiler C, Wagner M, Sadowski C, et al. Randomized prospective trial of pylorus-preserving vs. Classic duodenopancreatectomy (Whipple procedure): initial clinical results. *J Gastrointest Surg* 2000;4:443–452.
12. Bakkevold KE, Arnesjo B, Dahl O, et al. Adjuvant combination chemotherapy (AMF) following radical resection of carcinoma of the pancreas and papilla of Vater — results of a controlled, prospective, randomised multicentre study. *Eur J Cancer* 1993;29A:698–703.
13. Neoptolemos JP, Dunn JA, Stocken DD, et al. Adjuvant chemoradiotherapy and chemotherapy in resectable pancreatic cancer: a randomised controlled trial. *Lancet* 2001;358:1576–1585.

Bazian Ltd
London
UK

Competing interests: None declared.

Stomach cancer

Search date January 2003

Charles Bailey

QUESTIONS

INTERVENTIONS

Likely to be beneficial
Complete surgical resection* . .557
Subtotal gastrectomy (as effective as total gastrectomy) for resectable distal tumours . . .557

Unknown effectiveness
Adjuvant chemotherapy 561
Radical versus conservative lymphadenectomy 559

Likely to be ineffective or harmful
Removal of adjacent organs. . .559

To be covered in future updates
Addition of bacterial and fungal extracts to adjuvant chemotherapy
Adjuvant radiotherapy
Endoscopic mucosal resection for early gastric cancer
Regional chemotherapy

*Observational evidence only; RCTs unlikely to be conducted.

See glossary, p 563

Key Messages

- **Complete surgical resection** RCTs of complete surgical resection are unlikely to be conducted. Observational studies and multivariate analysis of RCTs have found a strong association between survival and complete resection of the primary tumour.
- **Subtotal gastrectomy (as effective as total gastrectomy) for resectable distal tumours** RCTs in people with primary tumours in the distal stomach have found no significant difference with total versus subtotal gastrectomy in 5 year survival or postoperative mortality.
- **Adjuvant chemotherapy** Systematic reviews and subsequent RCTs have found conflicting evidence that adjuvant chemotherapy increases survival compared with surgery alone. Two RCTs found that adjuvant chemotherapy increased postoperative complications. The size of any benefit remains uncertain, and many recent adjuvant chemotherapy regimens have not been evaluated fully in RCTs.
- **Radical versus conservative lymphadenectomy** Two large RCTs found no significant difference in 5 year survival rates between radical and conservative lymphadenectomy. However, confounding factors may have affected reliability of results, and we found conflicting data from subgroup analyses of prospective cohort studies.

- **Removal of adjacent organs** One RCT found no significant difference between radical gastrectomy plus splenectomy and radical gastrectomy alone in 5 year survival rates or postoperative mortality. The RCT found that radical gastrectomy plus splenectomy significantly increased the number of post-operative infections compared with radical gastrectomy alone. Retrospective analyses of observational studies and RCTs in people with stomach cancer found that removal of additional organs (spleen and distal pancreas) increased morbidity and mortality compared with no organ removal.

DEFINITION Stomach cancer is usually an adenocarcinoma arising in the stomach and includes tumours arising at or just below the gastro-oesophageal junction (type II and III junctional tumours). Tumours are staged according to degree of invasion and spread (see table 1, p 565). Only non-metastatic stomach cancers are considered in this topic.

INCIDENCE/ PREVALENCE The incidence of stomach cancer varies among countries and by sex (incidence per 100 000 population a year in Japanese men is about 80, Japanese women 30, British men 18, British women 10, white American men 11, white American women 7).[1] Incidence has declined dramatically in North America, Australia, and New Zealand since 1930, but the decline in Europe has been slower.[2] In the USA, stomach cancer remains relatively common among particular ethnic groups, especially Japanese–Americans and some Hispanic groups. The incidence of cancer of the proximal stomach and gastro-oesophageal junction is rising rapidly in many European populations and in North America.[3,4] The reasons for this are poorly understood.

AETIOLOGY/ RISK FACTORS Distal stomach cancer is strongly associated with lifelong infection with *Helicobacter pylori* and poor dietary intake of antioxidant vitamins (A, C, and E).[5,6] In Western Europe and North America, distal stomach cancer is associated with relative socioeconomic deprivation. Proximal stomach cancer is strongly associated with smoking (OR about 4),[7] and is probably associated with gastro-oesophageal reflux, obesity, high fat intake, and medium to high socioeconomic status.

PROGNOSIS Invasive stomach cancer (stages T2–T4) is fatal without surgery. Mean survival without treatment is less than 6 months from diagnosis.[8,9] Intramucosal or submucosal cancer (stage T1) may progress slowly to invasive cancer over several years.[10] In the USA, over 50% of people recently diagnosed with stomach cancer have regional lymph node metastasis or involvement of adjacent organs. The prognosis after macroscopically and microscopically complete resection (R0) is related strongly to disease stage (see glossary, p 563), particularly penetration of the serosa (stage T3) and lymph node involvement. Five year survival rates range from over 90% in intramucosal cancer to about 20% in people with stage T3N2 disease (see table 1, p 565). In Japan, the 5 year survival rate for people with advanced disease is reported to be about 50%, but the explanation for the difference remains unclear. Comparisons between Japanese and Western practice are confounded by factors such as age, fitness, and disease stage, as well as by tumour location, because many Western series include gastro-oesophageal junction adenocarcinoma with a much lower survival after surgery.

AIMS OF INTERVENTION To prevent progression; extend survival; and relieve symptoms, with minimal adverse effects.

OUTCOMES Survival; quality of life; adverse effects of treatment.

METHODS *Clinical Evidence* search and appraisal January 2003. Hand searches of conference proceedings and consultations with experts were used to identify relevant studies. In many instances, we have separated trials and results from different geographical areas, because of differences in baseline risk and demographics, and possible differences in response to treatments. However, the meaning of terms to describe such populations, such as "Western" and "Asian", were not clearly defined in many identified studies.

QUESTION What are the effects of radical versus conservative surgical resection?

OPTION COMPLETE VERSUS INCOMPLETE TUMOUR RESECTION

Observational studies and multivariate analysis of RCTs have found a strong association between survival and complete excision of the primary tumour.

Benefits: We found no systematic review or RCTs directly comparing complete versus incomplete tumour resection or positive versus clear microscopic resection margins (see comment below). Multivariate risk factor analysis of RCTs and retrospective cohort studies found that failure to achieve microscopically clear resection margins was associated with a poor outcome independently of other indicators of tumour spread and behaviour.[11–13]

Harms: We found no systematic review or RCTs.

Comment: Current consensus is that improving long term survival is best achieved by complete resection of the primary tumour with microscopic confirmation of clear resection margins ("curative" gastrectomy). We found two observational studies of surgery versus no surgery.[8,9] They found that people who did not undergo resection (generally those with the most advanced disease and highest comorbidity) had a near zero 5 year survival in all case series, and mean survival without treatment from time of diagnosis was found to be less than 6 months. In view of this evidence it is unlikely that an RCT of surgery versus no surgery or complete versus incomplete tumour removal would be carried out. In people with similar stage weight loss and performance status, macroscopically incomplete tumour resection (palliative gastrectomy) was associated with twice the survival time of non-resection and with better quality of life owing to relief of tumour symptoms.[14]

OPTION TOTAL VERSUS SUBTOTAL GASTRECTOMY FOR RESECTABLE DISTAL TUMOURS

Two RCTs in people with primary tumours in the distal stomach found no significant difference in 5 year survival or postoperative mortality between total and subtotal gastrectomy.

Benefits: We found no systematic review, but found two RCTs (787 people) comparing total versus subtotal (see glossary, p 563) gastrectomy.[15–18] Neither RCT used blinded allocation. **Five year survival:** The first RCT (648 people aged < 76 years with a resectable tumour and a macroscopic proximal margin of more than 6 cm) compared total versus subtotal gastrectomy.[15,16] All people involved in the RCT had a regional lymphadenectomy (D2). The RCT found no significant difference in the incidence of microscopic resection margin involvement or in 5 year survival (microscopic resection margin involvement: 15/315 [4.8%] with subtotal gastrectomy *v* 6/303 [2.0%] with total gastrectomy; ARI +2.8%, 95% CI –0.1% to +9.6%; Kaplan–Meier 5 year survival estimates 65% for subtotal *v* 62% for total gastrectomy; HR 0.89, 95% CI 0.68 to 1.17). Multivariate analysis found that after adjustment for covariates, the type of stomach surgery had no significant effect on 5 year survival (HR 1.01, 95% CI 0.76 to 1.33). The second RCT (169 people with potentially curable distal stomach cancer) compared total versus subtotal gastrectomy and found no significant difference in 5 year survival (48% in each group; CI not reported).[17,18] **Nutritional function and quality of life:** These outcomes were better with distal subtotal gastrectomy versus total gastrectomy.[19–22]

Harms: **Postoperative morbidity:** Morbidity included intra-abdominal sepsis, chest infections, wound sepsis, and fistulae. The first RCT found no significant difference between subtotal and total gastrectomy in postoperative morbidity or length of hospital stay (postoperative morbidity: 29/320 [9%] with subtotal gastrectomy *v* 40/304 [13%] with total gastrectomy; RR 0.67, 95% CI 0.44 to 1.08; hospital stay: 13.8 days for subtotal *v* 15.4 days for total gastrectomy).[15,16] The second RCT also found no significant difference in postoperative morbidity (32/93 [34%] for subtotal gastrectomy *v* 25/76 [32%] for total gastrectomy; RR 1.05, 95% CI 0.68 to 1.60).[17,18] **Postoperative mortality:** The first RCT found no significant difference in postoperative mortality (4/320 [1%] with subtotal gastrectomy *v* 7/304 [2%] with total gastrectomy; RR 0.54, 95% CI 0.16 to 1.84). The second RCT also found no significant difference in postoperative mortality (3/93 [3.2%] with subtotal gastrectomy *v* 1/76 [1.3%] with total gastrectomy; RR 2.45, 95% CI 0.26 to 23.01). Nearly all non-randomised studies that we identified reported higher mortality with total gastrectomy versus subtotal gastrectomy, but total gastrectomy tended to be performed in people with more extensive disease.

Comment: Infiltration of the proximal resection margin by microscopic tumour deposits is perceived as a problem in people with poorly differentiated "diffuse" cancer of the distal stomach undergoing distal subtotal gastrectomy. Some surgeons have therefore recommended total gastrectomy "de principe" (see glossary, p 563) for these tumours. The two RCTs have found similar survival after total and subtotal gastrectomy in people with primary tumours in the distal stomach.[15–18] Both RCTs recruited otherwise fit people, which may explain the low postoperative mortality. The lack of any evidence of survival benefit, and the poorer nutritional and quality of life outcomes, argue against total gastrectomy where subtotal distal gastrectomy is technically possible with an adequate margin.

OPTION REMOVAL OF ADJACENT ORGANS

One RCT found no significant difference between radical gastrectomy plus splenectomy and radical gastrectomy alone in 5 year survival rates or postoperative mortality. The RCT found that radical gastrectomy plus splenectomy significantly increased the number of postoperative infections compared with radical gastrectomy alone. Retrospective analyses of observational studies and RCTs in people with stomach cancer found that removal of additional organs (spleen and distal pancreas) increased morbidity and mortality compared with no organ removal.

Benefits: We found no systematic review. We found one RCT (187 people, aged 25–80 years), which compared radical (D2) gastrectomy plus splenectomy versus radical gastrectomy alone.[23] It found no significant difference in 5 year survival rates (42% with gastrectomy plus splenectomy *v* 36% with gastrectomy alone; $P > 0.5$; absolute numbers not provided).

Harms: The RCT (187 people) found that gastrectomy plus splenectomy versus radical gastrectomy alone significantly increased the number of postoperative infections (including fever > 38 °C, $P < 0.04$; pulmonary infections, $P < 0.008$; subphrenic abscesses, $P < 0.05$), but found no significant difference in postoperative mortality (4/90 [4%] with gastrectomy plus splenectomy *v* 3/97 [3%] with gastrectomy alone; RR 1.40, 95% CI 0.33 to 6.24).[23] Retrospective analyses of RCTs and cohort studies in which removal of the spleen and distal pancreas had been performed routinely during radical total (see glossary, p 563) gastrectomy (D2) (see table 2, p 566), and at the surgeon's discretion during non-radical total gastrectomy (D1), found that removal of the spleen or distal pancreas was associated with increased perioperative mortality (OR about 2) and no evidence of improved long term survival.[24,25]

Comment: Some advocates of radical surgery have suggested routine removal of the spleen and distal pancreas to ensure complete regional lymph node dissection during total gastrectomy. Current consensus is that removal of adjacent organs is justified only when necessary to ensure complete tumour removal, or when required because of trauma during surgery. An RCT has started in Japan to evaluate the role of splenectomy in total gastrectomy for proximal gastric cancer.[26]

OPTION RADICAL VERSUS CONSERVATIVE LYMPHADENECTOMY

Two large RCTs found no significant difference in 5 year survival rates between radical and conservative lymphadenectomy. However, confounding factors may have affected the reliability of results, and we found conflicting data from subgroup analyses of prospective cohort studies.

Benefits: **Radical (D2, D3) versus conservative lymphadenectomy (D1):** We found no systematic review but found four RCTs comparing radical (regional and local) removal of perigastric lymph nodes (see glossary, p 563) versus conservative (local) removal of lymph nodes.[27–30] The first RCT (711 people) found no significant difference in 5 year survival rates (45% with conservative lymphadenectomy *v* 47% with radical lymphadenectomy; ARR +2%, 95% CI –5.6% to +9.6%).[27] The second RCT (400 people) also found no significant difference in 5 year survival rates (35% with conservative lymphadenectomy *v* 33% with radical lymphadenectomy; HR 1.1, 95% CI 0.87 to 1.39).[28] The other two smaller RCTs (55 people[29] and 43 people[30]) did not report evaluable 5 year survival rates. Subgroup analysis from the second RCT found a possible advantage for D2 resection in people with stage II and IIIA disease (corresponding to T1N2M0, T2N1M0, T3N0M0, T2N2M0, T3N1M0, and T4N0M0), particularly in those people who did not have additional organ removal.[28] **Para-aortic (D4) versus regional and local (D3, D2) lymphadenectomy:** We found one small pilot study for an RCT (70 people with stomach cancer that had spread to the serosa or adjacent organs, T3 or T4) conducted in Japan, which compared removal of local, regional, and para-aortic lymph nodes with removal of only local and regional lymph nodes (see glossary, p 563).[31] This pilot study was too small to detect clinically important differences in survival.

Harms: The four RCTs comparing radical versus conservative lymphadenectomy found increased perioperative mortality with the more extensive operation.[27–30] The second RCT (400 people) found significantly higher mortality with D2 versus D1 resection (13% with D2 resection *v* 6% with D1 resection; $P < 0.04$).[28] In the first RCT (711 people), the difference in mortality nearly achieved significance (10% with D2 *v* 6% with D1; $P = 0.06$).[27] In both of these large RCTs the excess mortality may have been due to associated pancreatic and splenic removal, rather than the radical lymphadenectomy.[27,28]

Comment: The RCTs were conducted by surgeons with limited prior experience and training in D2 resection, and results may have been affected by both learning curve effects[32] and failure to apply the assigned treatment (contamination and non-compliance).[33] One large prospective cohort study (1654 people with gastric cancer) found no benefit from D2 resection (defined within this study as > 25 lymph nodes removed; 300 people) versus D1 resection (≤ 25 nodes removed; 1096 people) in the entire cohort of people with gastric cancer after 10 years' follow up. Subgroup analysis found that there may be a beneficial effect of D2 versus D1 resection in the subgroup of people with stage II tumours (230 people; RR of long term survival 1.8, 95% CI 1.3 to 2.7).[34] Cohort studies comparing radical versus conservative lymphadenectomy are affected by numerous biases, particularly selection bias, where surgeons reserve D2 surgery for younger or fitter people, or where recent D2 operations are compared with historical D1 controls; definition differences (in the meaning of "limited" and "extended"); and stage migration bias (see glossary, p 563). These biases make the interpretation of observational data difficult.

QUESTION **What are the effects of adjuvant chemotherapy?**

Systematic reviews and subsequent RCTs have found conflicting evidence that adjuvant chemotherapy increases survival compared with surgery alone. Two RCTs found that adjuvant chemotherapy increased postoperative complications. The size of any benefit remains uncertain, and many recent adjuvant chemotherapy regimens have not been evaluated fully in RCTs.

Benefits: **Adjuvant chemotherapy versus surgery alone:** We found four systematic reviews[35–38] and two subsequent RCTs,[39,40] which compared adjuvant chemotherapy (see glossary, p 563) versus surgery alone. The first review (search date 1991, 11 RCTs, 2096 people) found that adjuvant chemotherapy versus surgery alone reduced the risk of death by the end of follow up, but the result was not significant (OR 0.88, 95% CI 0.78 to 1.08).[35] This review was criticised for involving trials that included people with known residual tumour after surgery and trials that also included immunotherapy and intraperitoneal delivery of the adjuvant treatment. A subsequent update of the review found that adjuvant chemotherapy versus surgery alone significantly reduced the risk of death by the end of follow up (OR 0.82, 95% CI 0.68 to 0.97).[41] The second review (search date 1999, 13 RCTs, 1990 people in non-Asian countries) excluded trials of people with known residual tumour after surgery or that also included immunotherapy and intraperitoneal treatment.[36] The review found that adjuvant chemotherapy versus surgery alone significantly reduced the risk of death (595/979 [61%] with adjuvant chemotherapy *v* 660/1011 [65%] with surgery alone; RR 0.93, 95% CI 0.87 to 0.99; NNT 22, 95% CI 12 to 353). The third review (search date 2000, 20 RCTs, 3658 people; see comment below) included most of the RCTs from the first two reviews, but also included two subsequent RCTs.[37] It found that adjuvant chemotherapy versus surgery alone significantly reduced the risk of death (HR 0.82, 95% CI 0.75 to 0.89). The fourth systematic review (search date 1998, 60 RCTs plus 92 non-randomised studies; 12 367 people) found that adjuvant chemotherapy versus surgery alone significantly improved survival (21 RCTs, 3692 people; OR 0.84, 95% CI 0.74 to 0.96).[38] Subgroup analysis found that adjuvant chemotherapy versus surgery alone significantly improved survival in people from Asian countries (OR 0.58, 95% CI 0.44 to 0.76), but found no significant difference in people from Western countries (OR 0.96, 95% CI 0.83 to 1.12). The first subsequent RCT (137 people with gastric adenocarcinoma and positive lymph nodes) compared adjuvant chemotherapy versus surgery alone and found that adjuvant chemotherapy significantly increased median survival time (31 months, range 7 to > 60 months with adjuvant chemotherapy *v* 18 months, range 2 to > 60 months with surgery alone; $P < 0.01$; HR for death 1.96, 95% CI 1.32 to 2.92).[39] The second subsequent RCT (274 patients with gastric adenocarcinoma T3, T4 or N1, N2) found no significant difference between adjuvant chemotherapy and surgery alone in 5 year survival (overall survival: 52% with adjuvant chemotherapy *v* 48% with surgery alone; HR 0.93, 95% CI 0.65 to 1.34).[40]
Japanese RCTs: We found 10 Japanese RCTs comparing adjuvant chemotherapy versus surgery alone, most of which were included in

the systematic reviews. One recent RCT (579 people after curative gastrectomy for early cancer, stage T1 or T2) compared adjuvant chemotherapy (mitomycin, fluorouracil, uracil, tegafur) versus surgery alone.[42] It found no significant difference in cancer related mortality after a median follow up of 72 months (47/288 [16%] with adjuvant chemotherapy *v* 59/291 [20%] with surgery alone; OR 0.77, 95% CI 0.50 to 1.17). A second recent RCT (435 people with stage II or III cancer) compared surgery plus intraperitoneal chemotherapy (using cisplatin alone) versus surgery plus intraperitoneal chemotherapy (using cisplatin plus tegafur-uracil, an orally administered derivative of 5-fluorouracil) and found no significant difference in 3 year survival rates or disease free survival rates.[43] A third recent RCT (139 people) compared three groups: surgery plus hyperthermic intraperitoneal chemotherapy; surgery plus normothermic intraperitoneal chemotherapy; and surgery alone.[44] It found that surgery plus hyperthermic chemotherapy (mitomycin C plus cisplatin at 42 °C) versus surgery alone significantly increased overall 5 year survival rates ($P = 0.01$; result presented graphically), and that surgery plus hyperthermic chemotherapy versus surgery plus normothermic chemotherapy (mitomycin C plus cisplatin at 37 °C) also significantly increased overall 5 year survival rates ($P = 0.05$; result presented graphically). Subgroup analysis found that these results were consistent for people with advanced disease (T3 or node positive), but in people with less advanced disease (T2 or node negative) found no significant difference in overall 5 year survival rates. Of the seven older RCTs published before 1985, only one found a significant benefit for chemotherapy.[45] This RCT (120 people) compared three groups: adjuvant chemotherapy with mitomycin alone versus adjuvant chemotherapy with mitomycin plus cytarabine plus fluorouracil versus surgery alone. It found that adjuvant chemotherapy with mitomycin plus cytarabine plus fluorouracil versus both other treatments significantly improved survival. The other six RCTs found no significant difference between adjuvant chemotherapy versus surgery alone in survival.

Harms: Two RCTs reported toxicity (mainly nausea and vomiting) in 53% of people.[46,47] Serious toxicity was usually because of cardiac or cumulative haematological problems; treatment related mortality was 1–2%. We found no definitive evidence from completed studies to justify the concern that preoperative chemotherapy increases postoperative morbidity or mortality. Two RCTs found significant increases in some types of postoperative complications after intraperitoneal chemotherapy (pain, intra-abdominal sepsis without anastamotic leak, bleeding, and fistula formation),[48,49] but a more recent RCT in people from Japan found no such increase.[44]

Comment: The four systematic reviews included several trials in common.[35–38] Only published trials were included. All included trials were reported in English. There was no evidence of publication bias. No statistical heterogeneity of effects was found by the first two systematic reviews, but random effects meta-analysis was used, which may give a conservative estimate of the treatment effect.[35,36] The third systematic review is difficult to interpret.[37] Some of the results, included in the meta-analysis as if they were independent trials, seem to be duplicate versions of the same RCT.[50,51] This systematic review found significant heterogeneity between results of RCTs (P = 0.028), but a fixed effects model was used. These factors reduce confidence in the published estimate of effect. The significant effect observed by all four systematic reviews might indicate a small but real effect or alternatively the impact of undetected biases. It is also possible that certain subgroups of people may respond differently to other subgroups. Subgroup analysis in the second systematic review[36] suggested an effect only in RCTs in which at least two thirds of people had node positive disease, but the power was insufficient to draw definite conclusions and the result was not confirmed in the third systematic review.[37] Many more recent adjuvant chemotherapy regimens have not been evaluated fully in RCTs. Japanese adjuvant chemotherapy regimens often contain bacterial or fungal extracts. We found some evidence from one well designed RCT that addition of these substances to combined surgery and chemotherapy was associated with improved 5 year survival;[52] this will be reviewed in a future update. The analysis applied to only 19% of those randomised and may not be generalised to all people with inoperable gastric cancer. One further meta-analysis has been identified, which will be incorporated in this review at a subsequent update.[53] Preoperative superselective intra-arterial chemotherapy may not be available outside of specialist centres.

GLOSSARY

Adjuvant chemotherapy Treatment with cytotoxic drugs given in addition to surgery in an attempt to achieve cure.
Disease stage Surgical and microscopic assessment of the primary tumour. Microscopic spread to distant sites can be detected only by radical surgery, creating a potential bias.
Perigastric lymph nodes Lymph nodes that lie adjacent to the stomach.
Regional lymph nodes Lymph nodes that lie along the blood vessels that supply the stomach.
Stage migration bias Apparent increase in stage specific survival without influencing overall survival caused by recategorisation of the stage after removal of diseased lymph nodes.
Subtotal distal gastrectomy Removal of lower part (usually two thirds or four fifths) of the stomach.
Total gastrectomy Removal of the whole stomach.
Total gastrectomy "de principe" Total gastrectomy where it is not technically necessary to remove a distal tumour; this technique is used to minimise the risk of resection line involvement or later second cancer of the gastric stump.

Substantive changes

Adjuvant chemotherapy One RCT added;[40] conclusions unchanged.

REFERENCES

1. Whelan SL, Parkin DM, Masuyer E, eds. *Trends in cancer incidence and mortality* (IARC scientific publication no. 102). Lyon: IARC Scientific Publications, 1993.
2. Cancer Research Campaign. *Factsheet 18*. London: Cancer Research Campaign, 1993.
3. Powell J, McConkey CC. Increasing incidence of adenocarcinoma of the gastric cardia and adjacent sites. *Br J Cancer* 1990;62:440–443.
4. Devesa SS, Blot WJ, Fraumeni JF Jr. Changing patterns in the incidence of esophageal and gastric carcinoma in the United States. *Cancer* 1998;83:2049–2053.
5. EUROGAST study group. An international association between *Helicobacter pylori* infection and gastric cancer. *Lancet* 1993;341:1359–1362.

6. Buiatti E, Palli D, Decarli A, et al. A case-control study of gastric cancer and diet in Italy. II Association with nutrients. *Int J Cancer* 1990;45:896–901.
7. Rios-Castellanos E, Sitas F, Shepherd NA, et al. Changing pattern of gastric cancer in Oxfordshire. *Gut* 1992;33:1312–1317.
8. Boddie AW Jr, McMurtrey MJ, Giacco GG, et al. Palliative total gastrectomy and esophagogastrectomy: an evaluation. *Cancer* 1983;51:1195–2000.
9. McCulloch P. Should general surgeons treat gastric carcinoma? An audit of practice and results. *Br J Surg* 1994;81:417–420.
10. Kohli Y, Kawai K, Fujita S. Analytical studies of the growth of human gastric cancer. *J Clin Gastroenterol* 1981;3:129–133.
11. Maruyama K, Okabayashi K, Kinoshita T. Progress in gastric cancer surgery in Japan and its limits of radicality. *World J Surg* 1987;11:418–425.
12. Jakl RJ, Miholic J, Koller R, et al. Prognostic factors in adenocarcinoma of the cardia. *Am J Surg* 1995;169:316–319.
13. Allum WH, Hallissey MT, Kelly KA. Adjuvant chemotherapy in operable gastric cancer: 5 year follow-up of the first British Stomach Cancer Group trial. *Lancet* 1989;1:571–574.
14. Haugstvedt T. Benefits of resection in palliative surgery. *Dig Surgery* 1994;11:121–125.
15. Bozzetti F, Marubini E, Bonfanti G, et al. Total versus subtotal gastrectomy: surgical morbidity and mortality rates in a multicenter Italian randomized trial. *Ann Surg* 1997;226:613–620.
16. Bozzetti F, Marubini E, Bonfanti G, et al. Subtotal versus total gastrectomy for gastric cancer: five-year survival rates in a multicenter randomized Italian trial. *Ann Surg* 1999;230:170–178.
17. Gouzi JL, Huguier M, Fagniez PL, et al. Gastrectomie totale contre gastrectomie partielle pour adeno-cancer de l'antre. Une etude francaise prospective controlee. *Ann Chir* 1989;43:356–360.
18. Gouzi JL, Huguier M, Fagniez PL, et al. Total versus subtotal gastrectomy for adenocarcinoma of the gastric antrum. A French prospective controlled study. *Ann Surg* 1989;209:162–166.
19. Davies J, Johnston D, Sue-Ling H, et al. Total or subtotal gastrectomy for gastric carcinoma? A study of quality of life. *World J Surg* 1998;22:1048–1055.
20. Wu CW, Hsieh MC, Lo SS, et al. Quality of life of patients with gastric adenocarcinoma after curative gastrectomy. *World J Surg* 1997;21:777–782.
21. Svedlund J, Sullivan M, Liedman B, et al. Quality of life after gastrectomy for gastric carcinoma: controlled study of reconstructive procedures. *World J Surg* 1997;21:422–433.
22. Roder JD, Stein HJ, Eckel F, et al. Quality of life after total and subtotal gastrectomy for gastric carcinoma. *Dtsch Med Wochenschr* 1996;121:543–549.
23. Csendes A, Burdiles P, Rojas J, et al. A prospective randomised study comparing D2 total gastrectomy versus D2 total gastrectomy plus splenectomy in 187 patients with gastric carcinoma. *Surgery* 2002;131:401–407.
24. Bonenkamp JJ, Songun I, Hermans J, et al. Randomised comparison of morbidity after D1 and D2 dissection for gastric cancer in 996 Dutch patients. *Lancet* 1995;345:745–748.
25. Cuschieri A, Fayers P, Fielding J, et al. Postoperative morbidity and mortality after D1 and D2 resections for gastric cancer: preliminary results of the MRC randomised controlled surgical trial. *Lancet* 1996;347:995–999.
26. Sano T, Yamanoto S, Sasako M. Randomized controlled trial to evaluate splenectomy in total gastrectomy for proximal gastric cancer. *Jpn J Clin Oncol* 2002;32:363–364.
27. Bonenkamp JJ, Hermans J, Sasako M, et al. Extended lymph-node dissection for gastric cancer. Dutch Gastric Cancer Group. *N Engl J Med* 1999;340:908–914.
28. Cuschieri A, Weedon S, Fielding J, et al. Patient survival after D1 and D2 resections for gastric cancer: long-term results of the MRC randomised surgical trial. *Br J Cancer* 1999;79:1522–1530.
29. Robertson CS, Chung SC, Woods SD, et al. A prospective randomised trial comparing R1 subtotal gastrectomy with R3 total gastrectomy for antral cancer. *Ann Surg* 1994;220:176–182.
30. Dent DM, Madden MV, Price SK. Randomised comparison of R1 and R2 gastrectomy for gastric carcinoma. *Br J Surg* 1988;75:110–112.
31. Maeta M, Yamashiro H, Saito H, et al. A prospective pilot study of extended (D3) and superextended para-aortic lymphadenectomy (D4) in patients with T3 or T4 gastric cancer managed by total gastrectomy. *Surgery* 1999;125:325–331.
32. Parikh D, Chagla L, Johnson M, et al. D2 gastrectomy: lessons from a prospective audit of the learning curve. *Br J Surg* 1996;83:1595–1599.
33. Bunt AMG, Hermans J, Boon MC, et al. Evaluation of the extent of lymphadenectomy in a randomised trial of Western versus Japanese style surgery in gastric cancer. *J Clin Oncol* 1994;12:417–422.
34. Siewert JR, Bottcher K, Stein HJ, et al. Relevant prognostic factors in gastric cancer: ten-year results of the German Gastric Cancer Study. *Ann Surg* 1998;228:449–461.
35. Hermans J, Bonenkamp JJ, Ban MC, et al. Adjuvant therapy after curative resection for gastric cancer: a meta-analysis of randomised trials. *J Clin Oncol* 1993;11:1441–1447. Search date 1991; primary sources Medline and hand searched references.
36. Earle CC, Maroun JA. Adjuvant chemotherapy after curative resection for gastric cancer in non-Asian patients: revisiting a meta-analysis of randomised trials. *Eur J Cancer* 1999;35:1059–1064. Search date 1999; primary sources Medline and Cancerlit.
37. Mari E, Floriani I, Tinazzi A, et al. Efficacy of adjuvant chemotherapy after curative resection for gastric cancer: a meta-analysis of published randomised trials. A study of the GISCAD (Gruppo Italiano per lo Studio dei Carcinomi dell'Apparato Digerente). *Ann Oncol* 2000;11:837–843. Search date 2000; primary sources Medline, Embase, Cancerlit, and hand searched references.
38. Janunger KG, Hafstrom L, Nygren P, et al. A systematic overview of chemotherapy effects in gastric cancer. *Acta Oncol* 2001;40:309–326. Search date 1998; primary sources Medline, Cancerlit, and the Cochrane Library.
39. Neri B, Cini G, Andreoli F, et al. Randomized trial of adjuvant chemotherapy versus control after curative resection for gastric cancer: 5-year follow-up. *Br J Cancer* 2001;84:878–880.
40. Bajetta E, Buzzoni R, Mariani L, et al. Adjuvant chemotherapy in gastric cancer: 5-year results of a randomised study by the Italian Trials in Medical Oncology (ITMO) Group. *Ann Oncol* 2002;13:299–307.
41. Hermans J, Bonenkamp H. In reply [letter]. *J Clin Oncol* 1994;12:879–880.
42. Nakajima T, Nashimoto A, Kitamura M, et al. Adjuvant mitomycin and fluorouracil followed by oral uracil plus tegafur in serosa-negative gastric

cancer: a randomised trial. Gastric Cancer Surgical Study Group. *Lancet* 1999;354:273–277.
43. Yoshino K, Fujita M, Hirata K, et al. Interim report on JFMTC Study no. 21 on the effectiveness of UFT as an adjuvant therapy for semi-advanced cancer of the stomach. *Gan To Kagaku Ryoho* 2000;27:263–270.
44. Yonemura Y, De Aretxabala X, Fujimura T, et al. Intraoperative chemohyperthermic peritoneal perfusion as an adjuvant to gastric cancer: final results of a randomized controlled study. *Hepato-gastroenterology* 2001;48:1776–1782.
45. Nakajima T, Fukami A, Takagi K, et al. Adjuvant chemotherapy with mitomycin C and with a multi drug combination of mitomycin, fluoro-uracil and cytosine arabinoside, after curative resection of gastric cancer. *Jpn J Clin Oncol* 1990;10:187–194.
46. Coombes RC, Schein PS, Chilvers CE, et al. A randomised trial comparing adjuvant 5-fluoro-uracil, doxorubicin and mitomycin C with no treatment in operable gastric cancer. International Collaborative Cancer Group. *J Clin Oncol* 1990;8:1362–1369.
47. Hallissey MT, Dunn JA, Ward LC, et al. The second British Stomach Cancer Group trial of adjuvant radiotherapy or chemotherapy in advanced gastric cancer: 5 year follow-up. *Lancet* 1994;343:1309–1312.
48. Rosen HR, Jatzko G, Repse S, et al. Adjuvant intraperitoneal chemotherapy with carbon-adsorbed mitomycin in patients with gastric cancer: results of a randomized multicenter trial of the Austrian Working Group for Surgical Oncology. *J Clin Oncol* 1998;16:2733–2738.
49. Yu W, Whang I, Averbach A, et al. Morbidity and mortality of early postoperative intraperitoneal chemotherapy as adjuvant therapy for gastric cancer. *Am Surg* 1998;64:1104–1108.
50. Alcobendas F, Milla A, Estape J, et al. Mitomycin C as an adjuvant in resected gastric cancer. *Ann Surg* 1983;198:13–17.
51. Grau JJ, Estape J, Alcobendas F. Positive results of adjuvant mitomycin C in resected gastric cancer: a randomised trial on 134 patients. *Eur J Cancer* 1993;29A:340–342.
52. Nakazato H, Koike A, Saji S, et al. Efficacy of immunochemotherapy as adjuvant treatment after curative resection of gastric cancer. Study Group of Immunochemotherapy with PSK for Gastric Cancer. *Lancet* 1994;343:1122–1126.
53. Panzini I, Gianni L, Fattori P, et al. Adjuvant chemotherapy in gastric cancer: a meta-analysis of randomized trials and a comparison with previous meta-analyses. *Tumori* 2002;88:21–27.

Charles Bailey
Clinical Research Fellow
Department of Surgery, Oncology, and Technology
Imperial College
London
UK

Competing interests: None declared.

The following previous contributor of this topic would also like to be acknowledged: Peter McCulloch.

TABLE 1 **Staging of stomach cancer (see text, p 556).**

Stage	Description
T1	Involvement of mucosa +/– submucosa
T2	Involvement of muscularis propria
T3	Involvement of serosa but no spread to adjacent organs
T4	Involvement of adjacent organs
N0	No lymph node involvement
N1	Local (perigastric) nodes involved
N2	Regional nodes involved
N3	More distant intra-abdominal nodes involved
M0	No metastases
M1	Metastases

TABLE 2 **Different types of surgical resection for stomach cancer (see text, p 559).**

Resection	Description
R0	Removal of all detectable tumour, with a margin of healthy tissue confirmed microscopically: synonymous with "curative" resection.
R1	Incomplete removal, with histological evidence of cancer at the resection margin.
R2	Incomplete removal, with macroscopically obvious remnants of the main tumour: synonymous with "palliative" resection.
D1	Removal of all or part of the stomach, together with local (perigastric) nodes.
D2	Removal of all or part of the stomach, together with local and regional nodes, which lie along the branches of the coeliac axis.
D3/D4	More radical lymph node resection, including removal of para-aortic nodes and nodes within the small bowel mesentery.

Acute sinusitis

Search date January 2003

Kim Ah-See

QUESTIONS

INTERVENTIONS

See glossary, p 573

Key Messages

In people with clinically diagnosed acute sinusitis

- **Antibiotics** One RCT found no evidence that amoxicillin reduced or cured symptoms compared with placebo in people with clinically diagnosed acute sinusitis. It found that diarrhoea was more common with amoxicillin than with placebo.
- **Antihistamines; decongestants; steroids** We found no RCTs examining the effects of antihistamines, decongestants, or steroids in people with clinically diagnosed acute sinusitis.

In people with radiologically or bacteriologically confirmed acute sinusitis

- **Cefalosporins and macrolides** One systematic review in people with radiologically or bacteriologically confirmed acute sinusitis found no significant difference in clinical resolution between amoxicillin or amoxicillin–clavulanate and cefalosporins or macrolides. However, cefalosporins and macrolides caused fewer adverse effects than amoxicillin and amoxicillin–clavulanate. One RCT found no significant difference in clinical improvement or clinical cure between cefalosporins and azithromycin (a macrolide).

- **Amoxicillin and amoxicillin-clavulanate** One systematic review identified two RCTs in people with radiologically or bacteriologically confirmed acute maxillary sinusitis, which found that amoxicillin improved early clinical cure rate compared with placebo, but was associated with more frequent adverse effects, mainly gastrointestinal. One systematic review in people with radiologically or bacterological confirmed acute sinusitis found no significant difference in clinical resolution between amoxicillin or amoxicillin–clavulanate and cefalosporins or macrolides. However amoxicillin and amoxicillin-clavulanate caused more adverse effects.
- **Different dosages of antibiotics** One RCT in people with radiologically or bacteriologically confirmed acute sinusitis found no significant difference in clinical resolution rates or adverse events between two and three daily doses of cefaclor.
- **Long course antibiotic regimens** RCTs in people with confirmed acute sinusitis found no significant difference in clinical resolution rates between a 10 day course and 3–5 day courses of either co-trimoxazole or cefuroxime up to 3 weeks after treatment. One RCT found that adverse effects, which were mainly gastrointestinal, were more frequent with longer course cefuroxime than with shorter course cefuroxime.
- **Antihistamines; decongestants; steroids** We found no RCTs examining effects of antihistamines, decongestants, or steroids in people with radiologically or bacteriologically confirmed acute sinusitis.

DEFINITION Acute sinusitis is defined pathologically, by transient inflammation of the mucosal lining of the paranasal sinuses lasting less than 4 weeks. Clinically, it is characterised by nasal congestion, rhinorrhoea, facial pain, hyposmia (see glossary, p 573), sneezing, and, if more severe, additional malaise and fever. The diagnosis is usually made clinically (on the basis of history and examination, but without radiological or bacteriological investigation). Clinically diagnosed acute sinusitis is less likely to be due to bacterial infection than is acute sinusitis confirmed by radiological or bacteriological investigation.[1] In this chapter, we have excluded studies in children, in people with symptoms for more than 4 weeks (chronic sinusitis), and in people with symptoms following facial trauma. We have made it clear in each section whether we are dealing with clinically diagnosed acute sinusitis or acute sinusitis that has been confirmed by bacteriological or radiological investigation, because the effects of treatment may be different in these groups.

INCIDENCE/ PREVALENCE Each year in Europe, between 1% and 5% of adults are diagnosed with acute sinusitis by their general practitioner.[2] Extrapolated to the British population, this is estimated to cause 6 million restricted working days per year.[3,4] Most people with acute sinusitis are assessed and treated in a primary care setting. The prevalence varies according to whether diagnosis is made on clinical grounds or on the basis of radiological or bacteriological investigation.

AETIOLOGY/ RISK FACTORS One systematic review (search date 1998) reported that about 50% of people with a clinical diagnosis of acute sinusitis have bacterial sinus infection.[1] The usual pathogens in acute bacterial sinusitis are *Streptococcus pneumoniae* and *Haemophilus influenzae*, with occasional infection with *Moraxella catarrhalis*. Preceding viral upper respiratory tract infection is often the trigger for acute bacterial sinusitis,[5] with about 0.5% of common colds becoming complicated by the development of acute sinusitis.[6]

PROGNOSIS One meta-analysis of RCTs found that up to two thirds of people with acute sinusitis had spontaneous resolution of symptoms without active treatment.[7] One non-systematic review reported that people with acute sinusitis are at risk of chronic sinusitis and irreversible damage to the normal mucociliary mucosal surface.[8] One further non-systematic review reported rare life-threatening complications such as orbital cellulitis (see glossary, p 573) and meningitis following acute sinusitis.[9] However, we found no reliable data to quantify these risks.

AIMS OF INTERVENTION To relieve symptoms as quickly as possible, with minimal adverse effects.

OUTCOMES Symptom scores; time to self reported symptom resolution; time to clinical resolution (defined by examiner). In the identified studies, clinical improvement and clinical cure were often used as outcome measures. "Clinical improvement" was defined as improvement in clinical state as rated by the assessor or by the participant. "Clinical cure" was defined as resolution of symptoms as rated by assessor or participant.

METHODS *Clinical Evidence* search and appraisal January 2003 for the following interventions: topical or systemic decongestants; topical or systemic steroids; topical or systemic antihistamines; amoxicillin; amoxicillin–clavulanate; co-trimoxazole; cefalosporins; erythromycin; and azithromycin.

QUESTION **What are the effects of treatments in people with clinically diagnosed acute sinusitis?** New

OPTION **ANTIBIOTICS**

One RCT found no evidence that amoxicillin reduced or cured symptoms compared with placebo in people with clinically diagnosed acute sinusitis, who had not had radiological or bacteriological confirmation of disease. It found that diarrhoea was more common with amoxicillin than with placebo. We found no RCTs examining effects of other antibiotics (amoxicillin–clavulanate, co-trimoxazole, cefalosporins, azithromycin, and erythromycin) versus placebo.

Benefits: **Amoxicillin versus placebo:** We found one RCT in people with an exclusively clinical diagnosis of acute sinusitis, without reliance on radiological or bacteriological investigations.[10] The RCT (416 people in a primary care setting) compared amoxicillin 500 mg three times daily versus placebo for 10 days. It found no significant difference between amoxicillin and placebo in treatment success at the end of treatment (treatment success defined by absent or mild symptoms: 35% with amoxicillin group *v* 29% with placebo; RR 1.14, 95% CI 0.92 to 1.42). **Amoxicillin–clavulanate, co-trimoxazole, cefalosporins, azithromycin, or erythromycin versus placebo:** We found no RCTs.

Harms: **Amoxicillin versus placebo:** The RCT found that diarrhoea was significantly more common with amoxicillin than with placebo (29% with amoxicillin *v* 19% with placebo; RR 1.28, CI 1.05 to 1.57).[10]
Amoxicillin–clavulanate, co-trimoxazole, cefalosporins, azithromycin, or erythromycin versus placebo: We found no RCTs.

Comment: **Amoxicillin versus placebo:** The RCT may have lacked adequate follow up to detect clinically important differences between amoxicillin and placebo.

OPTION DECONGESTANTS, TOPICAL STEROIDS, AND ANTIHISTAMINES

We found no RCTs examining clinical effects of topical or systemic decongestants, topical steroids or antihistamines in people with clinically diagnosed acute sinusitis.

Benefits: **Decongestants:** We found no RCTs. **Topical steroids:** We found no RCTs. **Antihistamines:** We found no RCTs.

Harms: We found no RCTs.

Comment: None.

QUESTION What are the effects of antibiotics in people with radiologically or bacteriologically confirmed acute sinusitis? New

OPTION AMOXICILLIN AND AMOXICILLIN-CLAVULANATE

One systematic review identified two RCTs in people with radiologically or bacteriologically confirmed acute maxillary sinusitis, which found that amoxicillin improved early clinical cure rate compared with placebo, but was associated with more frequent adverse effects, mainly gastrointestinal. One systematic review in people with radiologically or bacterological confirmed acute sinusitis found no significant difference in clinical resolution between amoxicillin or amoxicillin–clavulanate and cefalosporins or macrolides. However amoxicillin and amoxicillin-clavulanate caused more adverse effects.

Benefits: **Amoxicillin versus placebo:** We found two systematic reviews (search date 1999, number of relevant RCTs not stated, 761 adults with acute uncomplicated sinusitis;[1] and search date 1998, 2 RCTs, 344 adults with acute sinusitis[11]). The review with the most recent search date did not report separately on effects of amoxicillin compared with placebo.[1] The earlier review found that 7–10 days of amoxicillin significantly increased complete symptom resolution compared with placebo (2 RCTs; OR 2.24, 95% CI 1.40 to 3.56).[11]
Amoxicillin–clavulanate versus placebo: The review with the most recent search date did not report separately on the effects of amoxicillin-clavulanate compared with placebo.[1] The earlier review found no RCTs.[11] We found no subsequent RCTs. **Versus cefalosporin and macrolides:** See cefalsoporins and macrolides, p 571.

Harms: **Amoxicillin versus placebo:** Both RCTs included in the earlier review[11] reported significantly greater adverse effects (mainly gastrointestinal) with antibiotic than with placebo (first RCT:[12] diarrhoea 47% with amoxicillin *v* 11% with placebo, P = 0.001; second RCT:[13] all adverse effects 28% with amoxicillin *v* 9% with placebo, P < 0.001). **Amoxicillin–clavulanate versus placebo:** We found no RCTs.

Comment: One of the RCTs that compared amoxicillin versus placebo was a three arm trial, which also examined effects of penicillin. We have not reported results in the penicillin group.

OPTION CEFALOSPORINS AND MACROLIDES

One systematic review in people with radiologically or bacteriologically confirmed acute sinusitis found no significant difference in clinical resolution between amoxicillin or amoxicillin–clavulanate and cefalosporins or macrolides. However, cefalosporins and macrolides caused fewer adverse effects than amoxicillin and amoxicillin–clavulanate. One RCT found no significant difference in clinical improvement or clinical cure between cefalosporins and azithromycin (a macrolide).

Benefits: **Versus placebo:** We found two systematic reviews (search dates 1999[1] and 1998[11]). The review with the most recent search date did not report seperately on the effects of these antibiotics compared with placebo.[1] The earlier review found no RCTs comparing these antibiotics versus placebo.[11] We found no subsequent RCTS. **Versus amoxicillin:** The earlier systematic review found 10 RCTs (1590 adults), which compared penicillin antibiotics (including amoxicillin) versus cefalosporins, macrolides, or minocycline in people with radiologically or bacteriologically confirmed acute maxillery sinusitis.[11] It found no significant difference in clinical resolution rate between newer non-penicillins and the other antibiotics (OR 0.85, 95% CI 0.70 to 1.08). **Versus amoxicillin–clavulanate:** The systematic review found 10 RCTs (3957 adults), which compared amoxicillin–clavulanate versus macrolides or cefalosporins.[11] It found no significant difference in clinical resolution rate between amoxicillin–clavulanate and the other antibiotics (OR 0.90, 95% CI 0.76 to 1.08). **Macrolides versus cefalosporins:** The systematic review[11] identified one RCT (496 people).[14] It found no significant difference between azithromycin (500 mg once daily for 3 days) and cefaclor (250 mg three times daily for 10 days) in clinical improvement or resolution of symptoms after 11–15 days (clinical improvement or clinical resolution: 228/245 [93%] with azithromycin *v* 233/241 [97%] with cefaclor; P value not reported).

Harms: **Versus placebo:** We found no RCTs. **Versus amoxicillin:**The systematic review found that the risk of stopping treatment due to adverse effects was lower with cefalosporins and macrolides than with penicillins (OR 0.54, 95% CI 0.29 to 1.00).[11] **Versus amoxicillin–clavulanate:** The systematic review found that the risk of stopping treatment due to adverse effects was lower with cefalosporins and macrolides than with amoxicillin-clavulunate (OR 0.37, 95% CI 0.26 to 0.52).[11]

Comment: None.

OPTION LONG COURSE ANTIBIOTIC REGIMENS

RCTs in people with confirmed acute sinusitis found no significant difference in clinical resolution rates between a 10 day course and 3–5 day courses of either co-trimoxazole or cefuroxime up to 3 weeks after treatment. One RCT found that adverse effects, which were mainly gastrointestinal, were more frequent with longer course cefuroxime than with shorter course cefuroxime.

Benefits: **Amoxicillin, amoxicillin–clavulanate, azithromycin, and erythromycin:** We found no RCTs comparing longer versus shorter courses of the same antibiotic. **Co-trimoxazole:** One RCT (80 people with confirmed sinusitis) found no significant difference in clinical resolution or improvement between a 10 day and a 3 day course of co-trimoxazole at 14 days follow up (AR for resolution or improvement about 76% in each group; CI not reported; P = 0.45).[15] **Cefalosporins:** One RCT (401 people with confirmed sinusitis) found no significant difference in clinical resolution rates between a 10 day and a 5 day course of cefuroxime 11–18 days after treatment (73% with 10 day course *v* 74% with 5 day course; ARR with shorter course +1%, 90% CI −7.5% to +8.5%).[2]

Harms: **Co-trimoxazole:** The RCT found no significant difference in adverse events between a 10 day and a 3 day course of co-trimoxazole (CI not reported; P = 0.2).[15] **Cefalosporins:** The RCT found that a larger proportion of people on the 10 day course of cefuroxime reported minor adverse effects, mainly gastrointestinal, compared with the 5 day course of cefuroxime (11.8% with 10 day course *v* 5.8% with 5 day course; significance not reported).[2]

Comment: None.

OPTION DIFFERENT DOSAGES OF ANTIBIOTICS

One RCT in people with radiologically or bacteriologically confirmed acute sinusitis found no significant difference in clinical resolution rates or adverse events between two and three daily doses of cefaclor.

Benefits: **Amoxicillin, amoxicillin–clavulanate, azithromycin, erythromycin, and co-trimoxazole:** We found no RCTs comparing different daily dosing regimens of the same antibiotic. **Cefalosporins:** One RCT (298 people with confirmed acute sinusitis) compared different daily dose regimens of the same cefalosporin.[16] It found no significant difference in clinical resolution rates between cefaclor 500 mg three times daily and cefaclor 750 mg twice daily at 14 days follow up (clinical resolution rate 95.7% with 500 mg three times daily *v* 97.3% with 750 mg twice daily; CI not reported; P = 0.333).

Harms: The RCT found no significant difference in adverse event rates between cefaclor 500 mg three times daily and cefaclor 750 mg twice daily (adverse event rate 24.7% with 750 mg three times daily *v* 32% with 500 mg twice daily; CI not reported; P = 0.162).[16]

Comment: None.

OPTION DECONGESTANTS, TOPICAL STEROIDS, AND ANTIHISTAMINES

We found no RCTs examining the effects of antihistamines, decongestants, or steroids in people with radiologically or bacteriologically confirmed acute sinusitis.

Benefits: **Decongestants:** We found no RCTs. **Topical steroids:** We found no RCTs. **Antihistamines:** We found no RCTs.

Harms: We found no RCTs.

Comment: None.

GLOSSARY

Hyposmia Reduced, not absent, sense of smell.
Orbital cellulitis Inflammation of the soft tissues in and around the eye socket.
Rhinorrhoea Discharge from the nasal cavity.

REFERENCES

1. Benninger MS, Sedory Holzer SE, Lau J. Diagnosis and treatment of uncomplicated acute bacterial rhinosinusitis: summary of the Agency for Health Care Policy and Research evidence-based report. *Otolaryngol Head Neck Surg* 2000;122:1–7. Search date 1999; primary sources Medline and bibliographies or retrieved articles.
2. Dubreuil C, Gehanno P, Goldstein F, et al. Treatment of acute maxillary sinusitis in adult outpatients: Comparison of a five versus ten day-course of cefuroxime axetil. *Med Malad Infect* 2001;31:70–78.
3. Kennedy DW. International conference on sinus terminology, staging, therapy. *Ann Otol Rhinol Laryngol* 1995;104:10.
4. Jones NS. Rhinosinusitis. In: *Statements of clinical effectiveness in otorhinolaryngology*. London British Association of Otorhinolaryngologists, Head and Neck Surgeons, 1998:21–31.
5. Henry DC, Moller DJ, Adelglass J, et al. Comparison of sparfloxacin and clarithromycin in the treatment of acute bacterial maxillary sinusitis. Sparfloxacin Multicenter AMS Study Group. *Clin Ther* 1999;21:340–352.
6. Low DE, Desrosiers M, McSherry J, et al. A practical guide for the diagnosis and treatment of acute sinusitis. *CMAJ* 1997;156(suppl 6):S1–S14.
7. de Ferranti SD, Ioannidis JP, Lau J, et al. Are amoxycillin and folate inhibitors as effective as other antibiotics for acute sinusitis? A meta-analysis. *BMJ* 1998;317:632–637.
8. Goodman GM, Slavin RG. Medical management in adults of chronic sinus disease. *Immunol Allergy Clin North Am* 1994;14:69–87.
9. Ramsey PG, Weymuller EA. Complications of bacterial infection of the ears, paranasal sinuses, and oropharynx in adults. *Emerg Med Clin North Am* 1985;3:143–160.
10. De Sutter AI, De Meyere MJ, Christiaens TC, et al. Does amoxixillin improve outcomes in patients with purulent rhinorrhea? A pragmatic randomized double-blind controlled trial in family practice. *J Fam Pract* 2002;51:317–23.
11. Williams JW, Aguilar C, Makela M, et al. Antibiotics for acute maxillary sinusitis (Cochrane Review). In: The Cochrane Library, Issue 3, 2002. Oxford: Update Software. Search date 1998; primary sources Medline, Embase, search of bibliographies of included studies, discussion with pharmaceutical companies.
12. Lindbaek M, Hjortdahl P, Johnsen ULH. Randomised, double blind, placebo controlled trial of penicillin V and amoxycillin in treatment of acute sinus infections in adults. *BMJ* 1996;313:325–329.
13. Van Buchem FL, Knottnerus JA, Schrijnemaekers VJJ, et al. Primary-care-based randomised placebo-controlled trial of antibiotic treatment in acute maxillary sinusitis. *Lancet* 1997;349:683–687.
14. O'Doherty B. An open comparative study of azithromycin versus cefaclor in the treatment of patients with upper respiratory tract infections. *J Antimicrob Chemother* 1996;37(suppl C):71–81.
15. Williams JW Jr, Holleman DR Jr, Samsa GP, et al. Randomized controlled trial of 3 vs 10 days of trimethoprim/sulfamethoxazole for acute maxillary sinusitis. *JAMA* 1995;273:1015–1021.
16. Turik M, Watkins M, Johns D Jr. Double-masked, randomized, parallel-group comparison of cefaclor AF and cefaclor in the treatment of acute bacterial sinusitis. *Curr Ther Res Clin Exp* 1997;58:227–239.

Kim Ah-See
Consultant Otolaryngologist-Head and Neck Surgeon
Aberdeen Royal Infirmary
Aberdeen
UK

Competing interests: None declared.

Chronic suppurative otitis media

Search date March 2003

Jose Acuin

QUESTIONS

INTERVENTIONS

To be covered in future updates
Management of cholesteatoma

Covered elsewhere in *Clinical Evidence*
See acute otitis media, p 301
See otitis media with effusion, p 612

See glossary, p 587

Key Messages

- We found no RCTs with long term follow up.

Adults

- **Topical antibiotics** We found no RCTs with long term follow up. Two RCTs found limited evidence that topical quinolone antibiotics improved otoscopic appearances compared with placebo in adults with chronic suppurative otitis media. Six RCTs found no clear evidence of clinically important differences among topical antibiotics in adults. One systematic review found that topical antibiotics were more effective than systemic antibiotics for reducing otoscopic features of chronic suppurative otitis media. One RCT found no significant effect of adding topical ceftizoxime to systemic ceftizoxime compared with systemic ceftizoxime alone. One RCT found no significant effect of preoperative topical antibiotics compared with no preoperative treatment in people undergoing tympanoplasty. Short term topical antibiotics have been associated with few adverse events in RCTs. Uncontrolled case studies have reported vestibular ototoxicity after topical non-quinolone antibiotics.
- **Ear cleansing (aural toilet)** We found no RCTs comparing ear cleansing versus no treatment.

- **Systemic antibiotics** We found insufficient evidence about the effects of systemic antibiotics compared with placebo, no treatment, or topical antiseptics. One systematic review found that systemic antibiotics were less effective than topical antibiotics in reducing otoscopic features of chronic suppurative otitis media. We found no evidence about long term treatment.
- **Topical antibiotics plus topical steroids** One systematic review found insufficient evidence from three RCTs about effects on symptoms of topical antibiotics plus topical steroids versus placebo or topical steroids alone.
- **Topical antiseptics** We found no RCTs comparing topical antiseptics versus placebo or no treatment. One RCT compared topical antiseptics plus ear cleansing under microscopic control versus topical antibiotics alone or versus oral antibiotics. It found no significant difference in the rate of persistent activity on otoscopy. However, the RCT was too small to exclude a clinically important difference.
- **Topical steroids** We found no RCTs comparing topical steroids versus placebo or no treatment.
- **Tympanoplasty with or without mastoidectomy** We found no RCTs comparing tympanoplasty with or without mastoidectomy versus no surgery for chronic suppurative otitis media without cholesteatoma.

Children

- **Ear cleansing** One systematic review found no significant difference in persistent otorrhoea or tympanic perforations with a simple form of ear cleansing versus no ear cleansing. However, a clinically important effect cannot be excluded.
- **Systemic antibiotics** RCTs found insufficient evidence about the effects of systemic antibiotics in children with chronic suppurative otitis media.
- **Topical antibiotics** We found no RCTs comparing topical antibiotics versus placebo.
- **Topical antibiotics plus topical steroids** We found insufficient evidence from small RCTs to compare topical antibiotics plus topical steroids versus cleansing only or topical antiseptics. We found no RCTs comparing topical antibiotics plus topical steroids versus either topical treatment alone.
- **Topical antiseptics** Two RCTs found no significant reduction in otorrhoea with topical antiseptics versus placebo after 2 weeks. One RCT found no significant difference in otorrhoea with topical antiseptics versus topical antibiotic plus steroid. However, the RCTs were too small to exclude a clinically important effect.
- **Topical steroids** We found no RCTs comparing topical steroids versus placebo.
- **Tympanoplasty with or without mastoidectomy** We found no RCTs comparing tympanoplasty with or without mastoidectomy versus no surgery for chronic suppurative otitis media without cholesteatoma.

DEFINITION Chronic suppurative otitis media is persistent inflammation of the middle ear or mastoid cavity. Synonyms include "chronic otitis media (without effusion)", chronic mastoiditis, and chronic tympanomastoiditis. Chronic suppurative otitis media is characterised by recurrent or persistent ear discharge (otorrhoea) over 2–6 weeks through a perforation of the tympanic membrane. Typical findings also include thickened granular middle ear mucosa, mucosal polyps, and cholesteatoma (see glossary, p 587) within the middle ear. Chronic suppurative otitis media is differentiated from chronic otitis media with effusion, in which there is an intact tympanic membrane with fluid in the middle ear but no active infection. Chronic suppurative otitis media does not include chronic perforations of the eardrum that are dry, or only occasionally discharge, and have no signs of active infection.

INCIDENCE/ PREVALENCE The worldwide prevalence of chronic suppurative otitis media is 65–330 million people. Between 39–200 million (60%) suffer from clinically significant hearing impairment. Otitis media was estimated to have caused 28 000 deaths and loss of over 2 million Disability Adjusted Life Years (see glossary, p 587) in 2000,[1] 94% of which were in developing countries. Most of these deaths were probably due to chronic suppurative otitis media because acute otitis media is a self limiting infection. Estimates of prevalence are shown in table A on web extra.[2–32]

AETIOLOGY/ RISK FACTORS Chronic suppurative otitis media is assumed to be a complication of acute otitis media, but the risk factors for chronic suppurative otitis media are not clear. Frequent upper respiratory tract infections and poor socioeconomic conditions (overcrowded housing,[33] hygiene, and nutrition) may be related to the development of chronic suppurative otitis media.[34,35] Improvement of housing, hygiene, and nutrition in Maori children was associated with a halving of the prevalence of chronic suppurative otitis media between 1978 and 1987.[36] See also acute otitis media, p 301.

PROGNOSIS Most children with chronic suppurative otitis media have mild to moderate hearing impairment (about 26–60 dB increase in hearing thresholds) based on surveys among children in Africa, Brazil,[37] India,[38] and Sierra Leone,[39] and among the general population in Thailand.[40] In many developing countries, chronic suppurative otitis media represents the most frequent cause of moderate hearing loss (40–60 dB).[41] Persistent hearing loss during the first 2 years of life may increase learning disabilities and poor scholastic performance.[42] Spread of infection may lead to life threatening complications such as intracranial infections and acute mastoiditis.[43] The frequency of serious complications fell from 20% in 1938 to 2.5% in 1948 and is currently estimated to be about 0.24% in Thailand and 1.8% in Africa. This is believed to be associated with increased use of antibiotic treatment, tympanoplasty, and mastoidectomy (see glossary, p 587).[44–46] Cholesteatoma is another serious complication that has been found in a variable proportion of people with chronic suppurative otitis media (range 0–60%).[47–50] In the West, the incidence of cholesteatoma is low (in 1993 in Finland the age standardised incidence of cholesteatoma was eight new cases per 100 000 population/year).[51]

AIMS OF INTERVENTION To improve symptoms of otorrhoea; heal perforations; improve hearing; and reduce complications, with minimum adverse effects of treatment.

OUTCOMES **Dichotomous variables:** Proportion of people with otorrhoea measured subjectively or by otoscopy; with tympanic perforation; hearing loss; intra- and extracranial complications; death; or adverse effects. The correlation between subjective cessation of otorrhoea and otoscopic findings was poor in one RCT.[52] Many RCTs used compound outcomes (e.g. otoscopic finding of otorrhoea or otoscopic finding of inflammation in the middle ear). **Continuous**

variables: Duration of otorrhoea free periods; severity of hearing loss. "Otoscopic activity" refers to appearances on otoscopy such as active discharge from the middle ear and inflammation of the middle ear mucosa.

METHODS *Clinical Evidence* search and appraisal March 2003. We found one systematic review (search date 1996, 24 RCTs, 1660 people) of treatments for chronic suppurative otitis media.[53] It did not analyse results for children and adults separately. We have excluded all studies that included both adults (aged ≥ 16) and children (aged ≤ 10),[54–57] or which failed to specify the age of participants.[58,59] The RCTs varied in their definitions of chronic suppurative otitis media and measurements of severity. All RCTs were brief (7 days to 3 weeks). Most had inadequate methods for us to draw reliable conclusions (see main text for descriptions). Participants with cholesteatoma were excluded from most, but not all, trials. All trials excluded people with impending serious complications.

QUESTION **What are the effects of treatments for chronic suppurative otitis media in adults?**

OPTION **EAR CLEANSING (AURAL TOILET)**

We found no RCTs of ear cleansing versus no treatment in adults.

Benefits: We found one systematic review (search date 1996), which found no RCTs in adults comparing ear cleansing (see glossary, p 587) versus no treatment.[53]

Harms: We found no RCTs.

Comment: Techniques of ear cleansing vary considerably. In Western countries, microsuction of the external and middle ear under microscopic control by a trained operator is the standard method of ear cleansing. Microscopic examination of the ear with ear cleansing is an important aspect of diagnosis of persistent otorrhoea. RCTs comparing ear cleansing versus no treatment would probably be considered unethical.

OPTION **TOPICAL ANTIBIOTICS**

We found no RCTs with long term follow up. Two RCTs found limited evidence that topical quinolone antibiotics improved otoscopic appearances compared with placebo in adults with chronic suppurative otitis media. Six RCTs found no clear evidence of clinically important differences among topical antibiotics in adults. One systematic review found that topical antibiotics were more effective than systemic antibiotics for reducing otoscopic features of chronic suppurative otitis media. One RCT found no significant effect of adding topical ceftizoxime to systemic ceftizoxime compared with systemic ceftizoxime alone. One RCT found no significant effect of preoperative topical antibiotics compared with no preoperative treatment in people undergoing tympanoplasty. Short term topical antibiotics have been associated with few adverse events in RCTs. Uncontrolled case studies have reported vestibular ototoxicity after topical non-quinolone antibiotics.

Benefits: **Versus placebo:** We found no systematic review but found two small RCTs in adults.[60,61] Both RCTs found that quinolone topical antibiotics improved otorrhoea compared with placebo, but both RCTs had weak methods. The first RCT (50 adults with chronic suppurative otitis media but no cholesteatoma [see glossary, p 587] in a hospital clinic in Thailand) found that, after 7 days, topical ciprofloxacin in 0.9% sodium chloride (5 drops 0.25 g/L 3 times/day for 7 days) significantly reduced persistent signs on otoscopic examination compared with topical 0.9% sodium chloride (3/19 [16%] had persistent signs with ciprofloxacin *v* 14/16 [88%] with 0.9% sodium chloride solution; RR 0.18, 95% CI 0.06 to 0.52; NNT 2, 95% CI 2 to 3).[60] The RCT lasted only 7 days, had 30% loss to follow up (15/50), and did not clearly describe the methods of randomisation and allocation concealment. The second RCT (51 adults with chronic suppurative otitis media without cholesteatoma in a hospital clinic in Israel; 60 ears) compared 3 weeks' treatment with topical ciprofloxacin versus topical tobramycin versus a dilute antiseptic solution (1% aluminium acetate), which was used as a placebo.[61] It found that ciprofloxacin significantly reduced the proportion of people with unimproved otorrhoea compared with diluted aluminium acetate (4/19 [21%] with ciprofloxacin *v* 10/17 [59%] with diluted aluminium acetate; OR 0.21, 95% CI 0.06 to 0.80; NNT 3, 95% CI 2 to 18). The RCT found that tobramycin did not significantly reduce otorrhoea compared with control (5/18 [28%] with tobramycin *v* 10/17 [59%] with control; OR 0.29, 95% CI 0.08 to 1.09). This RCT randomised people to treatments, but presented results in terms of number of ears. The 1% aluminium acetate may not have been an inert control (see topical antiseptics, p 580). **Versus each other:** We found one systematic review (search date 1996,[53] 4 RCTs, 406 adults) and two subsequent RCTs (see table 1, p 591).[61,66] Three RCTs found no clear difference between the otoscopic response with a topical quinolone (ciprofloxacin) and that with topical non-quinolones (gentamicin, tobramycin, and polymyxin–neomycin–hydrocortisone). The three RCTs comparing different topical non-quinolone antibiotics found no significant difference in the proportion of people who still had a wet ear on otoscopy at the end of treatment (see table 1, p 591).[67–69] **Versus systemic antibiotics:** See benefits of systemic antibiotics, p 581. **Versus topical antiseptics:** See benefits of topical antiseptics, p 580. **Added to systemic antibiotics:** We found one RCT (248 adults), which compared topical ceftizoxime (2 g/day) versus 0.9% sodium chloride solution among people who were given intramuscular ceftizoxime for 7 days.[70] It found no significant difference at the end of treatment between the two groups in terms of improvement of symptoms and otoscopic findings (improvement 96% with topical ceftizoxime *v* 93% with 0.9% sodium chloride; RR and CI not reported). **Added to non-antibiotic treatments:** We found one RCT (101 adults about to undergo tympanoplasty [see glossary, p 587]), which compared preoperative topical ofloxacin instilled for 10 minutes, preoperative topical ofloxacin instilled for 3 minutes, or no preoperative topical treatment.[71] It found no significant difference among groups for closure of tympanic perforations (28/33 with 10 minutes ofloxacin; 27/33 with 3 minutes ofloxacin; 31/35 with no treatment). However, the study may have lacked power to detect clinically important differences.

Harms: **Topical antibiotics versus placebo:** One systematic review found that adverse drug reaction rates in RCTs were low and did not vary appreciably among antibiotics.[53] The adverse events included *Candida* infections, dizziness, itching, stinging, and earache. One subsequent small RCT found no reported adverse events with topical ciprofloxacin used for 7 days in 19 ears.[60] Another subsequent RCT (322 people) found no significant difference in adverse event rate with topical ciprofloxacin versus topical polymyxin-B plus neomycin plus hydrocortisone (24/165 [15%] with ciprofloxacin *v* 12/153 [8%] with topical polymyxin-B plus neomycin plus hydrocortisone; RR 1.86, 95% CI 0.96 to 3.6).[66] Vertigo was reported by two people with topical ciprofloxacin and by none using topical polymyxin-B plus neomycin plus hydrocortisone. **Ototoxic effects of topical antibiotics:** We found one systematic review[53] and two subsequent RCTs[55,60] in adults and children, which examined hearing before and after topical antibiotics. The systematic review (search date 1996, 11 RCTs)[53] found negligible or no change in hearing after topical antibiotics. Three RCTs in adults and children[54,55,60] found no case of worsened hearing in those who were given topical ciprofloxacin or topical aminoglycoside. One RCT found deterioration of the audiogram in only one person with topical polymyxin-B plus neomycin plus hydrocortisone after 6–12 days (0/157 with topical ciprofloxacin *v* 1/138 with topical polymyxin-B plus neomycin plus hydrocortisone; OR 0.12, 95% CI 0.002 to 5.99).[66] The clinical importance of this difference is unclear.

Comment: There is consensus that topical antibiotics must be combined with thorough ear cleansing to be effective. We found no evidence about long term effects on complications. The comparative RCTs were small and their quality variable. We found no clear evidence from RCTs of ototoxicity from any topical antibiotic. Evidence about ototoxicity is based only on the assessment of audiograms after short term exposure to the antibiotics, and uncontrolled case studies have reported ototoxicity associated with some topical non-quinolone antibiotics for 7–120 days.[68,69,72] Most of the people in the observational studies had vestibular rather than cochlear symptoms, suggesting that the evidence from audiograms and hearing tests may not exclude ototoxicity. Most topical non-quinolone antibiotics have license restrictions against prolonged use, or use in people with perforation of the ear drum.

OPTION TOPICAL ANTIBIOTICS PLUS TOPICAL STEROIDS

We found no RCTs with long term follow up. Two small RCTs found that topical non-quinolone antibiotics plus topical steroid improved otoscopic appearances compared with placebo. One RCT found that topical non-quinolone antibiotic plus steroid improved otoscopic appearances compared with topical steroid alone. However, we are unable to draw reliable conclusions from this study.

Benefits: **Versus placebo:** We found one systematic review (search date 1996,[53] 2 RCTs,[52,73] 196 people, no pooling of results) of combined topical antibiotics plus steroid for 4–6 weeks compared with placebo. Both RCTs found that topical antibiotics plus steroid significantly reduced persistent otorrhoea compared with control. The first RCT (123 adults with chronic suppurative otitis media, no cholesteatoma, and no open mastoid cavity) found that significantly fewer people had otoscopically active otitis after treatment with gentamicin plus hydrocortisone than with placebo (appearance of active otitis: 33/64 [52%] people with treatment *v* 44/59 [75%] with placebo; OR 0.38, 95% CI 0.18 to 0.78).[52] Similar results were found in 42 other people who had an open mastoid cavity. The second RCT (31 adults) also found that gentamicin plus hydrocortisone reduced active otitis media on otoscopy compared with placebo at the end of 4 weeks of treatment (6/17 [35%] with treatment *v* 11/14 [79%] with placebo; OR 0.18, 95% CI 0.05 to 0.75).[73] **Versus topical steroid:** The systematic review[53] identified one RCT (64 adults),[67] which found that topical gentamicin plus hydrocortisone reduced the proportion of people with persistent activity on otoscopy compared with betametasone after 3 weeks of treatment (6/30 [20%] with gentamicin–hydrocortisone *v* 17/24 [71%] with betametasone; RR 0.28, 95% CI 0.13 to 0.60; NNT 2, 95% CI 2 to 4).

Harms: See harms under topical antibiotics, p 579.

Comment: See comment under topical antibiotics, p 579.

OPTION — TOPICAL ANTISEPTICS (ALUMINIUM ACETATE, BORAX, BORIC ACID, HYDROGEN PEROXIDE, IODINE POWDER)

We found no systematic review and no RCTs comparing topical antiseptics versus placebo or no treatment. One RCT in adults found no significant difference with topical antiseptics plus ear cleansing under microscopic control versus topical antibiotics or versus oral antibiotics. The RCT was too small to establish or exclude a clinically important effect from topical antiseptics in adults.

Benefits: **Versus placebo:** We found no systematic review and no RCT. **Versus topical antibiotics:** We found one systematic review (search date 1996,[53] 1 RCT,[74] 51 adults). The included RCT compared three treatments: topical antiseptics, topical antibiotics, and oral antibiotics.[74] It found no significant difference between topical antiseptics (boric acid and iodine powder plus ear cleansing [see glossary, p 587] under microscopic vision) and topical antibiotics (gentamicin or chloramphenicol) in persistent activity on otoscopy (13/20 [65%] with topical antiseptics *v* 15/18 [83%] with topical antibiotics; OR 0.40, 95% CI 0.10 to 1.66).[74] **Versus systemic antibiotics:** See benefits of systemic antibiotics, p 581.

Harms: Adverse effects included dizziness and local pain. The systematic review found negligible or no changes in hearing acuity after topical treatment.[53]

Comment: The available evidence from RCTs in adults is insufficient to establish or exclude a clinically important effect from topical antiseptics.

OPTION TOPICAL STEROIDS

We found no RCTs in adults comparing topical steroids versus placebo or no treatment.

Benefits: We found no systematic review or RCTs.

Harms: We found no systematic review or RCTs.

Comment: Topical steroids have been used in combination with topical antibiotics (see topical antibiotics, p 578).

OPTION SYSTEMIC ANTIBIOTICS

We found insufficient evidence about the effects of systemic antibiotics versus placebo, no treatment, or topical antiseptics. One systematic review found that systemic antibiotics were less effective than topical antibiotics in reducing otoscopic features of chronic suppurative otitis media. We found no evidence about long term treatment.

Benefits: **Versus placebo in people receiving no other treatment:** We found one systematic review (search date 1996), which found no RCTs investigating the effects of systemic antibiotics in adults receiving no other treatment.[53] **Versus topical antibiotics:** We found one systematic review (search date 1996,[53] 5 RCTs, 271 adults) (see table 2, p 592).[74–78] All RCTs found a better response with topical antibiotics than with systemic antibiotics. The topical antibiotics used were ofloxacin, ciprofloxacin, gentamicin, and chloramphenicol. The systemic antibiotics were oral cefalexin, cloxacillin, amoxicillin, ofloxacin, ciprofloxacin, co-amoxiclav, and intramuscular gentamicin. The systematic review found that, overall, topical antibiotics were more effective than systemic antibiotics at reducing otoscopic features of chronic suppurative otitis media by the end of the trials (34/153 [22%] with topical antibiotics *v* 77/138 [56%] with systemic antibiotics; OR 0.23, 95% CI 0.14 to 0.37). **Versus topical antiseptics:** We found one systematic review (search date 1996, 2 RCTs, 152 people).[53] The first RCT (51 adults) compared three treatments: oral antibiotics (cefalexin, flucloxacillin, cloxacillin, or amoxicillin according to bacterial sensitivity), topical antiseptics (boric acid and iodine powder plus ear cleansing [see glossary, p 587] under microscopic vision), and topical antibiotics (gentamicin or chloramphenicol).[74] It found no significant difference between oral antibiotics and topical antiseptics in the rate of persistent activity on otoscopy (8/13 [62%] with oral antibiotics *v* 13/20 [65%] with topical antiseptics *v* 15/18 [83%] with topical antibiotics; for oral antibiotic *v* topical antiseptic: OR 0.87, 95% CI 0.21 to 3.61). The second RCT (119 people with an age range from 11–79 years) found no significant difference between topical hydrogen peroxide or boric acid for 10–20 days versus various systemic antibiotics (choice based on sensitivity results, administered orally or intravenously) for otoscopically persistent discharge or inflamed mucosa at the end of treatment (33/71 [46%] with systemic antibiotic *v* 29/48 [60%] with topical antiseptic: OR 0.58, 95% CI 0.28 to 1.19). The confidence interval was too large to exclude a clinically important difference. **Systemic antibiotics versus other systemic antibiotics:** We found one systematic review (search date 1996,[53] 1 RCT, 75 adults) and one subsequent RCT (see comment below).[79] The RCT in the systematic review found no clear evidence of differences between oral ciprofloxacin (500 mg twice daily) and amoxicillin–clavulanate (500 mg 3 times daily) given for 5–10 days in persistent otoscopic activity at 3–4 weeks (16/40 [40%] with ciprofloxacin *v* 22/35 [63%] with amoxicillin–clavulanate; OR 0.41, 95% CI 0.16 to 1.00). The subsequent RCT (190 adults) found no significant difference between oral cefotiam hexetil and amoxicillin–clavulanate given for 10 days in persistent otoscopic abnormality after the end of treatment (37/94 [39%] with cefotiam *v* 33/94 [35%] with amoxicillin–clavulanate; OR 1.20, 95% CI 0.67 to 2.16).[79] **Added to other non-antibiotic treatments:** We found one systematic review (search date 1996,[53] 1 RCT,[80] 26 adults) comparing systemic antibiotics versus placebo in people receiving other forms of treatment. The RCT (26 adults having mastoidectomy/ tympanoplasty [see glossary, p 587]) found that intravenous ceftazidime (2 g 12 hours preoperatively and 1–2 g 8 hourly for 5 days postoperatively) reduced the proportion of people with otorrhoea on otoscopy or with positive *Pseudomonas aeruginosa* cultures at 2 months compared with no antibiotic (1/14 [7%] with iv ceftazidime *v* 7/12 [58%] with no antibiotic; OR 0.10, 95% CI 0.02 to 0.51).[80] Although randomisation was thorough, groups are likely to have been unbalanced for baseline severity, with more people in the antibiotic arm having only tympanoplasty. **Added to topical antibiotics:** We found one systematic review (search date 1996,[53] 2 RCTs,[75,80] 100 adults). The first included RCT found no significant difference in otorrhoea at 2 weeks with topical ciprofloxacin with and without oral ciprofloxacin given for 5–10 days (5/20 [25%] with oral ciprofloxacin *v* 3/20 [15%] with no oral ciprofloxacin; OR 1.84, 95% CI 0.40 to 8.49).[75] The second RCT found no significant difference in otorrhoea at the end of treatment with topical gentamicin–hydrocortisone (for 4 weeks) with and without oral metronidazole given for 2 weeks (6/14 [43%] with metronidazole *v* 6/16 [38%] without metronidazole; OR 1.24, 95% CI 0.29 to 5.23).[81] **Oral plus topical non-quinolone antibiotics versus topical quinolone antibiotics alone:** We found one RCT (80 adults, 89 ears),[82] which found that topical ofloxacin (0.3%) reduced the proportion of ears exhibiting persistent signs (ear pain, discharge, or inflammation on otoscopic examination) after 2 weeks compared with oral amoxicillin (amoxycillin) plus topical chloramphenicol (33% of ears with ofloxacin *v* 63% of ears with oral amoxicillin plus topical chloramphenicol; number of ears examined not stated; $P < 0.001$). The RCT randomised people but analysed the number of ears with persistent otorrhoea.

Harms: The systematic review found that adverse effects of systemic antibiotics include *Candida* infections, headache, nausea, and allergic reactions.[53] One RCT (80 adults) reported ototoxicity (defined as an elevation in bone conduction thresholds, speech reception thresholds of ≥5 dB, or both) with amoxicillin–chloramphenicol but not with ciprofloxacin (absolute numbers not stated).[82]

Comment: We found two further, recent RCTs comparing quinolone versus non-quinolone antibiotics; they are being translated and their results will be included in future *Clinical Evidence* updates.[83,84]

OPTION MASTOIDECTOMY AND/OR TYMPANOPLASTY

We found no RCTs comparing tympanoplasty with or without mastoidectomy versus no surgery in people with chronic suppurative otitis media and without cholesteatoma.

Benefits: We found no systematic review and no RCTs.

Harms: We found no RCTs.

Comment: We found many retrospective cohort studies. One of these (41 people with bilateral chronic suppurative otitis media operated on at one unit in Italy) compared hearing in ears that had previous tympanoplasty versus hearing in contralateral ears treated without surgery.[85] The hearing in both operated and non-operated ears progressively deteriorated, but the rate of decline was significantly slower in operated ears. Tympanoplasty can be combined with mastoidectomy (see glossary, p 587) when the possibility of restoring some functional hearing without jeopardising surgical clearance of the disease exists. Observational studies have found that the success of surgery depends on several factors: age, technical skill of the surgeon,[86] availability of remnant eardrum and ossicles,[87] and type of mastoidectomy performed. The success rate for sealing a tympanic perforation with a graft can be 90–95%. Hearing deficit may be corrected in about 50–70% of operated ears.[88–90]

QUESTION What are the effects of treatments for chronic suppurative otitis media in children?

OPTION EAR CLEANSING

One systematic review found insufficient evidence from two RCTs to compare a simple form of ear cleansing versus no ear cleansing in children with chronic suppurative otitis media.

Benefits: **Versus no treatment:** We found one systematic review (search 1996,[53] 2 RCTs,[91,92] 658 children), which found no significant difference in persistent otorrhoea or persistent ear drum perforation between a simple form of ear cleansing (see glossary, p 587) and no ear cleansing over 3–16 weeks (persisting otorrhoea, 2 RCTs; 125/170 [74%] with ear cleansing *v* 91/114 [80%] with no treatment; OR 0.63, 95% CI 0.36 to 1.12; persisting tympanic perforations, 1 RCT;[91] 125/144 [87%] *v* 63/73 [87%]; OR 1.04, 95% CI 0.46 to 2.38).

Harms: The review did not provide any evidence about the adverse effects of ear cleansing.

Comment: Techniques of ear cleansing vary considerably. In some countries, microsuction of the external and middle ear under microscopic control by a trained operator is a standard method of ear cleansing. In other countries, cleansing of the external auditory canal may be performed by parents, carers, or peers by dry mopping with cotton wool on orange sticks around four times daily. Both RCTs were performed in areas with a high prevalence of chronic suppurative otitis media (Solomon Islands[91] and Kenya[92]). The first RCT followed all the randomised children for 6 weeks but presented results as number of ears with persistent otorrhoea.[91] The second RCT randomised 145 schools but analysed the numbers of children with persistent otorrhoea.[92] It followed children for 16 weeks, but analysed results only for the 72% of the children who completed the RCT. Neither study described allocation concealment methods. In one RCT,[23] the randomisation process was described, but outcome assessors were not blinded to treatment allocation. The results of the meta-analysis in the systematic review[53] need to be approached with care because it combined results from the first RCT for the numbers of ears with persistent signs at 6 weeks with results from the second RCT for the number of children with persistent signs after 16 weeks. There was significant heterogeneity between the two RCTs in the effect of ear cleansing on otorrhoea ($P = 0.02$). Overall, we found no good evidence of benefit from simple ear cleansing, but the evidence is not strong enough to exclude a clinically important benefit.

OPTION TOPICAL ANTIBIOTICS

We found no RCTs about the effects of topical antibiotics in children with chronic suppurative otitis media.

Benefits: We found one systematic review (search date 1996, no RCTs exclusively in children) and no subsequent RCTs.[53]

Harms: We found insufficient evidence.[53]

Comment: We found no RCTs evaluating ototoxicity from any topical antibiotic. Evidence about ototoxicity is based only on the assessment of audiograms after short term exposure to the antibiotics, and uncontrolled case studies have reported ototoxicity associated with use of some topical non-quinolone antibiotics for 7–120 days.[93–95] Most of the people in the observational studies had vestibular rather than cochlear symptoms, suggesting that the evidence from audiograms and hearing tests may not exclude ototoxicity. Most topical non-quinolone antibiotics have license restrictions against prolonged use, or use in people with perforation of the eardrum.

OPTION TOPICAL ANTIBIOTICS PLUS TOPICAL STEROIDS

We found insufficient evidence from small RCTs to compare topical antibiotics plus topical steroids versus cleansing only or topical antiseptics. We found no RCTs comparing topical antibiotics plus topical steroids versus either topical treatment alone.

Benefits: **Versus placebo:** We found one systematic review (search date 1996,[53] 1 RCT,[91] 50 children, 67 ears) comparing combined topical antibiotics plus steroid (topical dexamethasone 0.05%, framycetin sulphate 0.5%, gramicidin 0.005%) versus ear cleansing (see glossary, p 587) only. The RCT found no significant difference between topical antibiotics plus steroid and ear cleansing only in the proportion of ears with unchanged otorrhoea on otoscopy after 6 weeks (17/41 [42%] with topical antibiotic plus steroid plus ear cleansing v 13/26 [50%] with ear cleansing alone; OR 0.71, 95% CI 0.27 to 1.90). **Versus topical antiseptics:** We found one systematic review (search date 1996,[53] 1 RCT,[91] 55 children, 73 ears), which found no significant difference between topical antiseptic (boric acid 2% in 20% alcohol, 3 drops to each ear, 4 times daily after ear cleansing) and topical antibiotic plus steroid (dexamethasone 0.05%, framycetin sulphate 0.5%, gramicidin 0.005%) in the proportion of ears with persistent otorrhoea (12/32 [38%] with topical antiseptic v 17/41 [41%] with topical antibiotic plus steroid; OR 0.85, 95% CI 0.33 to 2.17). **Versus topical steroid or topical antibiotics alone:** The systematic review found no RCTs.[53]

Harms: The RCTs did not provide any evidence about harms.[53]

Comment: One RCT[23] found no difference in effectiveness between topical antibiotics with steroids and ear cleansing alone. However, this study was small, did not report methods for allocation concealment and blinding, and randomised children but analysed ears. We found no RCTs or systematic reviews about long term effects on complications. See comment under topical antibiotics, p 584.

OPTION TOPICAL ANTISEPTICS (ALUMINIUM ACETATE, BORAX, BORIC ACID, HYDROGEN PEROXIDE, IODINE POWDER)

Two RCTs in children found no significant reduction of otorrhoea with topical antiseptics versus placebo. One RCT in children found no significant difference in otorrhoea between topical antiseptics and topical antibiotic plus steroid. The RCTs were too small to exclude a clinically important effect.

Benefits: **Versus placebo:** We found no systematic review but found two RCTs.[91,96] The first RCT (60 children with otorrhoea in a hospital clinic in South Africa, 67 ears) compared aluminium acetate solutions of varying concentrations (13% v 3.25% v 1.3%).[96] The most dilute solution was considered to be inactive. Results were obtained for 56 (84%) ears. The RCT found no significant difference in dry ears after 2 weeks (21/26 [81% of ears] with 13% aluminium acetate v 15/20 [75%] with a 3.25% aluminium acetate v 5/10 [50%] with 1.3% aluminium acetate; P = 0.18). The second RCT (43 children, 58 ears) found no significant difference between topical antiseptic (boric acid 2% in 20% alcohol, 3 drops to each ear, 4/day after ear cleansing [see glossary, p 587]) and ear cleansing alone in the proportion of children with unchanged otoscopic appearance after 6 weeks (12/32 [38%] with topical antiseptic v 13/26 [50%] with ear cleansing alone; OR 0.61, 95% CI 0.22 to 1.71).[91] **Versus topical antibiotic plus steroid:** See benefits of topical antibiotics plus topical steroids, p 584. **Versus systemic antibiotics:** See benefits of systemic antibiotics in children, p 586.

Harms: Adverse effects included dizziness and local pain. The systematic review found negligible or no changes in hearing acuity after topical treatment.[53]

Comment: We found small studies, which found no difference in the short term effects of topical antiseptics compared with systemic antibiotics (see systemic antibiotics, p 586). The available evidence is insufficient to establish or exclude a clinically important effect from topical antiseptics.

OPTION TOPICAL STEROIDS

We found no RCTs comparing topical steroids versus placebo or no treatment in children.

Benefits: We found no systematic review or RCTs.

Harms: We found no RCTs.

Comment: None.

OPTION SYSTEMIC ANTIBIOTICS

RCTs found insufficient evidence of the effects of systemic antibiotics in children with otitis media.

Benefits: **Versus placebo in children receiving no other treatment:** We found one systematic review (search date 1996),[53] which found no RCTs investigating the effects of systemic antibiotics in children receiving no other treatment. **Versus topical antibiotics:** We found one systematic review (search date 1996, no RCTs) and no subsequent RCTs.[53] **Versus topical antiseptics:** One systematic review (search date 1996) found no RCTs.[53] **Systemic antibiotics versus other systemic antibiotics:** We found one systematic review (search date 1996,[53] 1 RCT, 36 children) and one subsequent RCT.[97] The systematic review found no significant difference in otoscopic evidence of otorrhoea between intravenous mezlocillin and intravenous ceftazidime at the end of treatment (otoscopic evidence of otorrhoea: 0/17 [0%] with mezlocillin *v* 0/19 [0%] with ceftazidime).[53] The subsequent RCT (30 children) found no significant difference in success rates (complete disappearance of discharge) and days to disappearance between ceftazidime and aztreonam (disappearance of discharge: 84.6% with ceftazidime *v* 67% with aztreonam; P value reported as not significant; days to disappearance of discharge: 7.9 days with ceftazidime *v* 8.4 days with aztreonam).[97] **Added to non-antibiotic treatments:** We found one systematic review (search date 1996,[53] 1 RCT,[98] 33 children). The RCT (33 children having ear cleansing by suctioning and debridement for 1–2 weeks) found that intravenous antibiotic (mezlocillin or ceftazidime for 3–21 days) significantly reduced persistent otorrhoea detected at otoscopy after 6 months compared with no antibiotic (0/21 [0%] with iv antibiotic *v* 11/12 [92%]; OR 0.02, 95% CI 0.004 to 0.08). **Added to topical antibiotics:** We found one systematic review (search date 1996,[53] 1 RCT[91]). The RCT (62 children, 81 ears, all treated with ear cleansing plus drops containing dexamethasone 0.05%, framycetin sulphate 0.5%, gramicidin 0.005%) found no significant difference between oral clindamycin and no clindamycin (15 mg/kg daily) on the proportion of ears with unchanged otoscopic otorrhoea after 6 weeks (23/40 [58%] with clindamycin *v* 17/41 [41%] without clindamycin; OR 1.88, 95% CI 0.79 to 4.48).[91]

Harms: The systematic review found that (in all age groups) adverse effects of systemic antibiotics included *Candida* infections, headache, nausea, and allergic reactions.[53]

Comment: We found no clear evidence from RCTs that systemic antibiotics differ in their effectiveness. The studies in children found similar results to those in adults.

OPTION MASTOIDECTOMY AND/OR TYMPANOPLASTY

We found no RCTs in children comparing tympanoplasty with or without mastoidectomy versus no surgery for chronic suppurative otitis media without cholesteatoma.

Benefits: We found no systematic review and no RCTs.

Harms: We found no RCTs.

Comment: We found no evidence from RCTs, but found numerous retrospective observational studies. Tympanoplasty is often combined with mastoidectomy whenever the possibility of restoring some functional hearing without jeopardising surgical clearance of the disease exists. Observational studies have found that the success of surgery depends on several factors (age, technical skill of the surgeon,[99] presence of middle ear discharge,[100] type of mastoidectomy performed, and technique of middle ear construction[86]). Success rate for sealing a tympanic perforation with a graft can be 90–95%. Hearing deficit may be corrected in about 50–70% of operated ears.[88–90]

GLOSSARY

Cholesteatoma An accumulation of epithelial debris in the middle ear cavity that can arise congenitally or can be acquired. The tissue is probably derived from skin. It grows slowly but can erode and destroy adjacent structures (ossicles, the mastoid, the inner ear, or the bone leading to the intracranial cavity) potentially leading to persistent pain and otorrhoea, hearing loss, dizziness, facial nerve paralysis, and intracranial infection.

Disability Adjusted Life Year (DALY) A measure of the impact of a condition, designed to include the loss attributable to premature death and the loss caused by a disability of known duration and severity. One DALY is equivalent to the loss of 1 year of healthy life.

Ear cleansing Also known as aural toilet, this consists of mechanical removal of ear discharge and other debris from the ear canal and middle ear by mopping with cotton pledgets, wicking with gauze, flushing with sterile solution, or suctioning. This can be done with an otomicroscope or under direct vision with adequate illumination of the middle ear.

Mastoidectomy A general term used to describe various surgical procedures that are usually used to remove abnormal parts of the mastoid bone and surrounding structures, or to allow access to the middle ear.

Tympanoplasty A general term used to describe various surgical repairs of the eardrum or ossicles of the middle ear to improve hearing in people with conductive deafness.

REFERENCES

1. World Health Report, 2000. http://www.who.int/whr/2001/archives/2000/en/pdf/Annex4-en.pdf (last accessed 21 July 2003).
2. Bastos I, Reimer A, Ingvarsson L, et al. Chronic otitis media and hearing loss among school children in a refugee camp in Angola. *J Audiol Med* 1995;4:1–11.
3. Bastos I, Reimer A, Lundgren K. Chronic otitis media and hearing loss in otitis in urban schoolchildren in Angola — a prevalence study. *J Audiol Med* 1993;2:129–140.
4. Manni JJ. Lema PN. Otitis media in Dar es Salaam, Tanzania. *J Laryngol Otol* 1987;101:222–228.
5. Bastos I, Mallya J, Ingvarsson L, et al. Middle ear disease and hearing impairment in northern Tanzania. A prevalence study of schoolchildren in the Moshi and Monduli districts. *Int J Pediatr Otorhinolaryngol* 1995;32:1–12.
6. McPherson B, Holborow CA. A study of deafness in West Africa: the Gambian Hearing Health Project. *Int J Pediatr Otorhinolaryngol* 1985;10:115–135.
7. Pisacane A, Ruas I. Bacteriology of otitis media in Mozambique. *Lancet* 1982;1:1305.
8. Halama AR, Voogt GR, Musgrave GM. Prevalence of otitis media in children in a black rural community in Venda (South Africa). *Int J Pediatr Otorhinolaryngol* 1986;11:73–77.
9. Hatcher J, Smith A, Mackenzie I, et al. A prevalence study of ear problems in school children in Kiambu district, Kenya, May 1992. *Int J Pediatr Otorhinolaryngol* 1995;33:197–205.
10. Okeowo PA. Observations on the incidence of secretory otitis media in children. *J Trop Pediatr* 1985;31:295–298.
11. Bal I, Hatcher J. Results of Kenyan Prevalence Survey. *Her Net News* 1992;4:1–2. In Berman S. Otitis media in developing countries. *Pediatrics* 1996;1:126–130.
12. Cohen D, Tamir D. The prevalence of middle ear pathologies in Jerusalem school children. *Am J Otol* 1989;19:456–459.
13. Podoshin L, Fradis M, Ben-David Y, et al. Cholesteatoma: an epidemiologic study among members of kibbutzim in northern Israel. *Ann Otol Rhinol Laryngol* 1986;95:365–368.
14. Bafaqeeh SA, Zakzouk S, Muhaimed HA, et al. Relevant demographic factors and hearing impairment in Saudi children: epidemiological study. *J Laryngol Otol* 1994;108:294–298.
15. Noh KT, Kim CS. The changing pattern of otitis media in Korea. *Int J Pediatr Otorhinolaryngol* 1985;9:77–87.
16. Kim CS, Jung HW, Yoo KY. Prevalence and risk factors of chronic otitis media in Korea: results of a nation-wide survey. *Acta Otolaryngol* 1993;113:369–375.
17. Jacob A, Rupa V, Job A, et al. Hearing impairment and otitis media in a rural primary school in South India. *Int J Pediatr Otorhinolaryngol* 1997;39:133–138.
18. Elango S, Purohit GN, Hashim M, et al. Hearing loss and ear disorders in Malaysian school children. *Int J Pediatr Otorhinolaryngol* 1991;22:75–80.
19. Liming L, Weihua C, Fujie X. Disability among the elderly in China: analysis of the national sampling survey of disability in 1987. *Chin Med J* 1997;110:236–237.
20. Dang Hoang S, Nhan Trung S, Le T, et al. Prevalence of chronic otitis media in a randomly selected population sampled in two communities in Southern Vietnam. Proceedings of Copenhagen Otitis Media Conference, June 1–5, 1997;Abstr 13.
21. Garrett J, Stewart J. Hearing loss and otitis media in Guam: impact of professional services. *Asia Pac J Public Health* 1989;3:213–218.
22. Dever G, Stool S, Manning S, et al. Otitis oceania: middle ear disease in the Pacific basin. *Ann Otol Rhinol Laryngol* 1990;99(suppl 149):25–27.
23. Elango S, Purohit GN, Hashim M, et al. Hearing loss and ear disorders in Malaysian school children. *Int J Pediatr Otorhinolaryngol* 1991;22:75–80.
24. Eason R, Harding F, Nicholson R, et al. Chronic suppurative otitis media in the Solomon Islands: a prospective microbiological, audiometric and therapeutic survey. *N Z Med J* 1986;99:812–815.
25. Dever G, Stool S, Manning S, et al. Otitis oceania: middle ear disease in the Pacific basin. *Ann Otol Rhinol Laryngol* 1990;99(suppl 149):25–27.
26. Bastos I Reimer A, Andreasson L. Middle ear disease and hearing loss among urban children and orphans in Bauru, Brazil. A prevalence study. *J Audiol Med* 1994.
27. Browning GG, Gatehouse S. *The prevalence of middle ear disease in the adult British population. Clin Otolaryngol* 1992;17:317–321.
28. Alho OP, Jokinen K, Laitakari K, et al. Chronic suppurative otitis media and cholesteatoma. Vanishing diseases among Western populations? *Clin Otolaryngol* 1997;22:358–361.
29. Pedersen CB, Zachau-Christiansen B. Chronic otitis media and sequelae in the population of Greenland. *Scand J Soc Med* 1988;16:15–19.
30. Nelson SM, Berry RI. Ear disease and hearing loss among Navajo children — a mass survey. *Laryngoscope* 1994;94:316–323.
31. Canterbury D. Changes in hearing status of Alaskan natives. *Ann Otol Rhinol Laryngol* 1990;99(suppl):22–23.
32. Sunderman J, Dyer H. Chronic ear disease in Australian aborigines. *Med J Aust* 1984;140:708–711.
33. Homoe P. Otitis media in Greenland. Studies on historical, epidemiological, microbiological, and immunological aspects. *Int J Circumpolar Health* 2001;60(suppl 2):1–54.
34. Tos M. Sequelae of secretory otitis media and the relationship to chronic suppurative otitis media. *Ann Otol Rhino Laryngol* 1990;99:18–19.
35. Daly KA, Hunter LL, Levine SC, et al. Relationships between otitis media sequelae and age. *Laryngoscope* 1998;108:1306–1310.
36. New Zealand Health Technology Assessment Clearing House. Screening programmes for the detection of otitis media with effusion and conductive hearing loss in pre-school and new entrant school children: a critical appraisal of the literature (NZHTA REPORT 3). Christchurch, New Zealand, June 1998. http://nzhta.chmeds.ac.nz/screen.htm (last accessed 21 July 2003). Search date 1998; primary sources English language articles in Medline, Cinahl, HealthSTAR, Current Contents (combined files), Cochrane Library Database of Abstracts of Reviews of Effectiveness, NHS Economic Evaluation Database, New Zealand Bibliographic Network, New Zealand Ministry of Health publications, United States National Institute of Health publications, Catalogues of New Zealand medical libraries, and publications and current projects by the International Network of Agencies for Health Technology Assessment (INAHTA).

37. Bastos I. Otitis media and hearing loss among children in developing countries. Malmo: University of Malmo, 1994.
38. Jacob A, Rupa V, Job A, et al. Hearing impairment and otitis media in a rural primary school in south India. *Int J Pediatr Otorhinolaryngol* 1997;39:133–138.
39. Seely DR, Gloyd SS, Wright AD, et al. Hearing loss prevalence and risk factors among Sierra Leonean Children. *Arch Otolaryngol Head Neck Surg* 1995;121:853–858.
40. Antarasena S, Antarasena N, Lekagul S, et al. The epidemiology of deafness in Thailand. *Otolaryngol Head Neck Surg* 1988;3:9–13.
41. Muya EW, Owino O. *Special education in Africa: research abstracts*. Nairobi: UNESCO;1986.
42. Teele DW, Klein JO, Chase C, et al. Otitis media in infancy and intellectual ability, school achievement, speech, and language at age 7 years. Greater Boston Otitis Media Study Group. *J Infect Dis* 1990;162:685–694.
43. Osma U, Cureoglu S, Hosoglu S. The complications of chronic otitis media: report of 93 cases. *J Laryngol Otol* 2000;114:97–100.
44. Kenna M. Incidence and prevalence of complications of otitis media. *Ann Otol Rhinol Laryngol* 1990;99(suppl 149):38–39.
45. Berman S. Otitis media in developing countries. *Pediatrics* 1995;96:126–131.
46. Sorensen H. Antibiotics in suppurative otitis media. *Otolaryngol Clin North Am* 1977;10:45–50.
47. Mahoney JL. Mass management of otitis media in Zaire. *Laryngoscope* 1980;90:1200–1208.
48. Noh KT, Kim CS. The changing pattern of otitis media in Korea. *Int J Pediatr Otorhinolaryngol* 1985;9:77–87.
49. Nelson SM, Berry RI. Ear disease and hearing loss among Navajo children — a mass survey. *Laryngoscope* 1994;94:316–323.
50. Muhaimeid H, Zakzouk S, Bafaqeeh SA. Epidemiology of chronic suppurative otitis media in Saudi children. *Int J Pediatr Otorhinolaryngol* 1993;26:101–108.
51. Alho OP, Jokinen K, Laitakari K, et al. Chronic suppurative otitis media and cholesteatoma. Vanishing diseases among Western populations? *Clin Otolaryngol Allied Sci* 1997;22:358–361.
52. Browning GG, Gatehouse S, Calder IT. Medical management of active chronic otitis media: a controlled study. *J Laryngol Otol* 1988;102:491–495.
53. Acuin J, Smith A, Mackenzie I. Interventions for chronic suppurative otitis media. In: The Cochrane Library. Issue 4, 2001. Oxford: Update Software. Search date 1996; primary sources Medline, Hearing network database, handsearches, and experts.
54. Ozagar A, Koc A, Ciprut A, et al. Effects of topical otic preparations on hearing in chronic otitis media. *Otolaryngol Head Neck Surg* 1997;117:405–408.
55. De Miguel Martinez I, Vasallo M Jr, Ramos MA. Antimicrobial therapy in chronic suppurative otitis media. *Acta Otorrinolaringol Esp* 1999;50:15–19.
56. Rotimi V, Olabiyi D, Banjo T, et al. Randomised comparative efficacy of clindamycin, metronidazole, and lincomycin, plus gentamicin in chronic suppurative otitis media. *West Afr J Med* 1990;9:89–97.
57. Tutkun A, Ozagar A, Koc A, et al. Treatment of chronic ear disease — Topical ciprofloxacin vs topical gentamicin. *Arch Otolaryngol Head Neck Surg* 1995;121:1414–1416.
58. Tong MC, Woo JK, van Hasselt CA. A double-blind comparative study of ofloxacin otic drops versus neomycin-polymyxin B-hydrocortisone otic drops in the medical treatment of chronic suppurative otitis media. *J Laryngol Otol* 1996;110:309–314.
59. Clayton M, Osborne J, Rutherford D, et al. A double-blind, randomized, prospective trial of a topical antiseptic versus a topical antibiotic in the treatment of otorrhea. *Clin Otolaryngol* 1990;15:7–10.
60. Kasemsuwan L, Clongsuesuek P. A double blind, prospective trial of topical ciprofloxacin versus normal saline solution in the treatment of otorrhoea. *Clin Otolaryngol* 1997;22:44–46.
61. Fradis M, Brodsky A, Ben David J, et al. Chronic otitis media treated topically with ciprofloxacin or tobramycin. *Arch Otolaryngol Head Neck Surg* 1997;123:1057–1060.
62. Gyde MC, Randall RF. Comparative double-blind study of trimethoprim-sulfacetamide-polymyxin B and of gentamicine in the treatment of otorrhoea. *Ann Otolaryngol Chir Cervicofac* 1978;95:43–55.
63. Gyde M. A double-blind comparative study of trimethoprim-polymyxin B versus trimethoprim-sulfacetamide-polymyxin B otic solutions in the treatment of otorrhea. *J Laryngol Otol* 1981;95:251–259.
64. Gyde MC, Norris D, Kavalec EC. The weeping ear: clinical re-evaluation of treatment. *J Int Med Res* 1982;10:333–340.
65. Llorente J, Sabater F, Maristany M, et al. Multicenter comparative study of the effectiveness and tolerance of topical ciprofloxacine (0.3%) versus topical gentamicine (0.3%) in the treatment of chronic suppurative otitis media without cholesteatoma. *An Otorrinolaringol Ibero Am* 1995;5:521–533.
66. Miro N, Perello E, Casamitjana F, et al. Controlled multicenter study on chronic suppurative otitis media treated with topical applications of ciprofloxacin 0.2% solution in single-dose containers or combination of polymyxin B, neomycin, and hydrocortisone suspension. *Otolaryngol Head Neck Surg* 2000;23:617–623.
67. Crowther JA, Simpson D. Medical treatment of chronic otitis media: steroid or antibiotic with steroid ear-drops? *Clin Otolaryngol* 1991;6:142–144.
68. Marias J, Rutka JA. Ototoxicity and topical eardrops. *Clin Otolaryngol* 1998;23:360–367.
69. Leliever WC. Topical gentamicin-induced positional vertigo. *Otolaryngol Head Neck Surg* 1985;93:553–555.
70. Mira E, Benazzo M. Uso topico delle cefalosporine nel trattamento delle otiti medie purulente: valutazione della ceftizoxima (eposerin®). *Riv Ital Otorinolaringol Audiol Foniat* 1992;12:219–225.
71. Tong MC, Yue V, Ku PK, et al. Preoperative topical ofloxacin solution for tympanoplasty: a randomized, controlled study. *Otol Neurotol* 2002;23:18--20.
72. Longridge NS. Topical gentamicin vestibular toxicity. *J Otolaryngol* 1994;23:444–446.
73. Picozzi G, Browning G, Calder I. Controlled trial of gentamicin and hydrocortisone ear drops in the treatment of active chronic otitis media. *Clin Otolaryngol* 1983;8:367–368.
74. Browning G, Picozzi G, Calder I, et al. Controlled trial of medical treatment of active chronic otitis media. *BMJ* 1983;287:1024.
75. Esposito S, D'Errico G, Montanaro C. Topical and oral treatment of chronic otitis media with ciprofloxacin. *Arch Otolaryngol Head Neck Surg* 1990;116:557–559.
76. Esposito S, D'Errico G, Mantanaro C. Topical ciprofloxacin vs. intramuscular gentamicin for chronic otitis media. *Arch Otolaryngol Head Neck Surg* 1992;118:842–844.
77. Povedano Rodriguez V, Seco Pinero M, Jurado Ramos A, et al. Eficacia del ciprofloxacino topico

en el tratamiento de la otorrea cronica. *Acta Otorrinolaryngologica Española* 1995;46:15–18.
78. Yuen P, Lau S, Chau P, et al. Ofloxacin eardrop treatment for active chronic suppurative otitis media: prospective randomized study. *Am J Otol* 1994;15:670–673.
79. Cannoni M, Bonfils P, Sednaoui P, et al. Cefotiam hexetil versus amoxicillin/clavulanic acid for the treatment of chronic otitis media in adults. *Med Mal Infect* 1997;27:915–921.
80. Lildholdt T, Felding J, Juul A, et al. Efficacy of perioperative ceftazidime in the surgical treatment of chronic otitis media due to *Pseudomonas aeruginosa*. *Arch Otorhinolaryngol* 1986;243:167–169.
81. Picozzi G, Browning G, Calder I. Controlled trial of gentamicin and hydrocortisone ear drops with and without systemic metronidazole in the treatment of active chronic otitis media. *Clin Otolaryngol* 1984;9:305.
82. Supiyaphun P, Kerekhanjanarong V, Koranasophonepun J, et al. Comparison of ofloxacin otic solution with oral amoxycillin plus chloramphenicol ear drop in treatment of chronic suppurative otitis media with acute exacerbation. *J Med Assoc Thai* 2000;83:61–68.
83. Sanchez Gonzalez, Galindo T. An open, comparative study of treatment of chronic middle ear otitis with levofloxacine vs amoxycillin/clavulanate. *Invest Med Int* 2001;28:33–36.
84. Baba S, Ito H, Kinoshita H, et al. Comparative study of cefmetazole and cefazolin in the treatment of suppurative otitis media. *Jpn J Antibiot* 1982;35:1523–1552.
85. Colletti V, Fiorino FG, Indelicato T. Surgery vs natural course of chronic otitis media. Long term hearing evaluation. *Acta Otolaryngol* 1991;111:762–768.
86. Soldati D, Mudry A. Cholesteatoma in children: techniques and results. *Int J Pediatr Otorhinolaryngol* 2000;52:269–276.
87. Chang CC, Chen MK. Canal-wall-down tympanoplasty with mastoidectomy for advanced cholesteatoma. *J Otolaryngol* 2000;29:270–273.
88. Vartiainen E, Kansanen M. Tympanomastoidectomy for chronic otitis media without choleasteatoma. *Otolaryngol Head Neck Surg* 1992;106:230–234.
89. Mishiro Y, Sakagami M, Takahashi Y, et al. Tympanoplasty with and without mastoidectomy for non-cholesteatomatous chronic otitis media. *Eur Arch Otorhinolaryngol* 2001;258:13–15.
90. Berenholz LP, Rizer FM, Burkey JM, et al. Ossiculoplasty in canal wall down mastoidectomy. *Otolaryngol Head Neck Surg* 2000;123:30–33.
91. Eason R, Harding E, Nicholson R, et al. Chronic suppurative otitis media in the Solomon Islands: a prospective, microbiological, audiometric and therapeutic survey. *N Z Med J* 1986;99:812–815.
92. Smith A, Hatcher J, Mackenzie I, et al. Randomised controlled trial of treatment of chronic suppurative otitis media in Kenyan schoolchildren. *Lancet* 1996;348:1128–1133.
93. Marias J, Rutka JA. Ototoxicity and topical eardrops. *Clin Otolaryngol* 1998;23:360–367.
94. Leliever WC. Topical gentamicin-induced positional vertigo. *Otolaryngol Head Neck Surg* 1985;93:553–555.
95. Longridge NS. Topical gentamicin vestibular toxicity. *J Otolaryngol* 1994;23:444–446.
96. Thorp MA, Gardiner IB, Prescott CA. Burow's solution in the treatment of active mucosal chronic suppurative otitis media: determining an effective dilution. *J Laryngol Otol* 2000;114:432–436.
97. Somekh E, Cordova Z. Ceftazidime versus aztreonam in the treatment of pseudomonal chronic suppurative otitis media in children. *Scand J Infect Dis* 2000;32:197–199.
98. Fliss D, Dagan R, Houri Z, et al. Medical management of chronic suppurative otitis media without cholesteatoma in children. *J Pediatr* 1990;116:991–996.
99. Darrouzet V, Duclos JY, Portmann D, et al. Preference for the closed technique in the management of cholesteatoma of the middle ear in children: a retrospective study of 215 consecutive patients treated over 10 years. *Am J Otol* 2000;21:474–481.
100. Tos M, Stangerup SE, Orntoft S. Reasons for reperforation after tympanoplasty in children. *Acta Otolaryngol Suppl* 2000;543:143–146.

Jose Acuin
Associate Professor
De La Salle University
Health Sciences Campus
Dasmarinas Cavite
Philippines

Competing interests: None declared.

TABLE 1 RCTs of topical antibiotics versus each other (see text, p 578).

Ref	Population with CSOM (people/ears, age setting)	Comparison	Absolute results*	OR
Different topical non-quinolone antibiotics *v* each other				
62	Adults, 57 ears, France, Variable duration	Topical 0.3% gentamicin *v* topical trimethoprim-sulfacetamide-polymyxin B	4/30 (13%) 5/27(19%)	1.47 (0.36 to 6.03)
63	27 ears, France, 7–14 days	Topical trimethoprim-sulfacetamide-polymyxin B *v* topical trimethoprim-polymyxin B	4/13 (31%) 8/14 (57%)	0.36 (0.08 to 1.59)
64	14 adults, France, 30–40 years, 2 weeks	Topical 0.3% gentamicin *v* topical colistin-neomycin-hydrocortisone	1/8 (13%) 1/6 (17%)	0.73 (0.04 to 13.45)
Topical quinolone *v* topical non-quinolone antibiotics				
65	308 adults, Spain, 30 days	Topical 0.3% ciprofloxacin *v* topical 0.3% gentamicin	8/159 (5%) 9/149 (6%)	0.82 (0.31 to 2.19)
66	322 adults, 14–71 years, Spain, 6–12 days	Topical ciprofloxacin *v* topical polymyxin B-neomycin-hydrocortisone	22/168 (13%) 37/154 (24%)	0.48 (0.28 to 0.85) ITT 0.67 (0.30 to 1.51) on protocol
61	40 adults, Clinics in Israel, 3 weeks	Topical ciprofloxacin *v* topical tobramycin	10/19 (53%) 8/18 (44%)	1.38 (0.39 to 4.91)

*Outcomes for all RCTs are the proportion of people with wet ear on otoscopic examination and with negative culture, usually measured at the end of treatment. COSM, chronic suppurative otitis media; ITT, intention to treat analysis; OR, odds ratio; Ref, reference.

TABLE 2 RCTs of topical antibiotics versus systemic antibiotics (see text, p 581).

Ref	Population with chronic suppurative otitis media	Comparison	Persistent otorrhoea: Absolute results	Persistent otorrhoea: OR
74	Adults Scottish hospital clinic	Topical gentamicin or chloramphenicol *v* various systemic antibiotics	11/18 (61%) *v* 8/13 (62%)	0.98 (0.23 to 4.15)
75	60 adults 5–10 days	Topical ciprofloxacin *v* oral ciprofloxacin	3/20 (15%) *v* 12/20 (60%)	0.15 (0.04 to 0.54)
76	60 adults 5–10 days	Topical ciprofloxacin *v* im gentamicin	5/30 (17%) *v* 17/30 (57%)	0.15 (0.05 to 0.49)
77	60 adults 10 days	Topical ciprofloxacin *v* oral ciprofloxacin	5/30 (17%) *v* 15/30 50%)	0.23 (0.08 to 0.56)
78	60 adults 7 days	Topical ciprofloxacin *v* oral amoxicillin/clavulanate	7/30 (57%) *v* 20/30 (67%)	0.18 (0.07 to 0.49)

im, intramuscular; Ref, reference.

Menière's disease

Search date October 2002

Adrian James and Marc Thorp

QUESTIONS

INTERVENTIONS

See glossary, p 599

Key Messages

Treatments for acute attacks

- **Anticholinergics; benzodiazepines; betahistine** We found no RCTs on the effects of these interventions.

Prophylactic interventions

- **Betahistine (for hearing loss)** Four RCTs found no change in hearing as assessed by changes in pure tone audiograms with betahistine versus placebo. Two small RCTs in people with definite or possible Menière's disease found no significant difference with betahistine versus trimetazidine in hearing or tinnitus.
- **Betahistine (for vertigo or tinnitus)** Six RCTs found insufficient evidence about the effects of betahistine versus placebo on the frequency and severity of attacks of vertigo, tinnitus, and aural fullness. Two small RCTs in people with definite or possible Menière's disease found no significant difference with betahistine versus trimetazidine in hearing or tinnitus. One of these RCTs found that betahistine versus trimetazidine significantly decreased the proportion of people reporting that the intensity of vertigo was "substantially better or cured". The other RCT found no significant difference with betahistine versus trimetazidine in vertigo intensity.
- **Diuretics** One small crossover RCT in people with possible Menière's disease found no significant difference with triamterene plus hydrochlorothiazide versus placebo in change in hearing over 17 weeks, and found insufficient evidence on vertigo and tinnitus.

- **Lithium** Two small crossover RCTs in people with possible Menière's disease found no difference with lithium versus placebo in vertigo, tinnitus, aural fullness, or hearing, and found that lithium was associated with tremor, thirst, and polyuria in some people.
- **Trimetazidine** We found no RCTs comparing trimetazidine versus placebo to prevent attacks of Menière's disease. Two small RCTs in people with definite or possible Menière's disease found no significant difference with trimetazidine versus betahistine in hearing or tinnitus. One of these RCTs found that trimetazidine versus betahistine significantly increased the number of people reporting that the intensity of vertigo was "substantially better or cured". The other RCT found no significant difference with trimetazidine versus betahistine in vertigo intensity.
- **Dietary modification; psychological support; systemic aminoglycosides; vestibular rehabilitation** We found no RCTs on the effects of these interventions.

DEFINITION Menière's disease is characterised by recurrent episodes of spontaneous rotational vertigo and sensorineural hearing loss with tinnitus, and a feeling of fullness or pressure in the ear. It may be unilateral or bilateral. Acute episodes can occur in clusters of about 6–11 a year, although remission may last several months.[1] The diagnosis is made clinically.[2] It is important to distinguish Menière's disease from other types of vertigo that might occur independently with hearing loss and tinnitus, and respond differently to treatment (e.g. benign positional vertigo, acute labyrinthitis). Strict diagnostic criteria help to identify the condition. In this review, we applied the classification of the American Academy of Otolaryngology–Head and Neck Surgery to indicate the diagnostic rigour used in RCTs (see table 1, p 601).

INCIDENCE/ PREVALENCE Menière's disease is most common between 40–60 years of age, although younger people may be affected.[6,7] In Europe, the incidence is about 50–200/100 000 a year. A survey of general practitioner records of 27 365 people in the UK found an incidence of 43 affected people in a 1 year period (157/100 000).[8] Diagnostic criteria were not defined in this survey. A survey of over 8 million people in Sweden found an incidence of 46/100 000 a year with diagnosis strictly based on the triad of vertigo, hearing loss, and tinnitus.[9] From smaller studies, the incidence appears lower in Uganda[10] and higher in Japan (350/100 000, based on a national survey of hospital attendances during a single wk).[7]

AETIOLOGY/ RISK FACTORS Menière's disease is associated with endolymphatic hydrops (raised endolymph pressure in the membranous labyrinth of the inner ear),[11] but a causal relationship remains unproven.[12] Specific disorders associated with hydrops (such as temporal bone fracture, syphilis, hypothyroidism, Cogan's syndrome, and Mondini dysplasia — see glossary, p 599) can produce similar symptoms to Menière's disease.

PROGNOSIS Menière's disease is progressive, but fluctuates unpredictably. It is difficult to distinguish natural resolution from the effects of treatment. Significant improvement of vertigo is usually seen in the placebo arm of RCTs.[13,14] Acute attacks of vertigo often increase in frequency during the first few years after presentation then decrease in frequency in association with sustained deterioration in hearing.[6] In most people, vertiginous episodes eventually cease completely.[15] In one 20 year cohort study in 34 people, 28 (82%) people had at least moderate hearing loss (mean pure tone hearing loss > 50 dB)[1] and 16 (47%) developed bilateral disease. Symptoms other than hearing loss improve in 60–80% of people irrespective of treatment.[16]

AIMS OF INTERVENTION To prevent attacks of Menière's disease; to reduce the severity of vertigo in acute attacks; to relieve chronic symptoms of hearing loss and tinnitus; to improve quality of life, with minimum adverse effects of treatment.

OUTCOMES Frequency and severity of acute attacks of vertigo; hearing acuity; severity of tinnitus; sensation of aural fullness; functional impairment and quality of life; adverse effects of treatment.

METHODS *Clinical Evidence* search and appraisal October 2002. We excluded studies with loss to follow up of over 20%. We excluded RCTs that did not use American Academy of Otolaryngology–Head and Neck Surgery diagnostic criteria.[3–5]

QUESTION What are the effects of treatments for acute attacks?

OPTION ANTICHOLINERGIC DRUGS

We found no RCTs about the effects of anticholinergics for acute attacks of Menière's disease.

Benefits: We found no systematic review and no RCTs. We found one non-randomised trial (see comment below).[17]

Harms: The non-randomised trial gave no information on adverse effects.[17]

Comment: The non-randomised trial (37 people with definite Menière's disease) compared an anticholinergic (glycopyrrolate 2 mg twice daily as required) versus placebo for 4 weeks.[17] It found that glycopyrrolate versus placebo significantly reduced a symptom score based on a validated scale,[18] which included questions about the severity of vertigo and its impact on quality of life (Dizziness Handicap Inventory change from baseline to end of trial: 76 to 37 with glycopyrrolate *v* 73 to 75 with placebo; P < 0.001). The lack of randomisation means that this result should be interpreted with caution.

OPTION BENZODIAZEPINES

We found no RCTs about the effects of benzodiazepines for acute attacks of Menière's disease.

Benefits: We found no systematic review or RCTs.

Harms: We found no RCTs.

Comment: None.

OPTION BETAHISTINE

We found no RCTs about the effects of betahistine for acute attacks of Menière's disease.

Benefits: We found no systematic review or RCTs.

Harms: We found no RCTs.

Comment: One observational study held in 1940 found that intravenous histamine was associated with a reduced severity of acute attacks of Menière's disease.[19]

QUESTION What are the effects of prophylactic interventions for Menière's disease?

OPTION DIURETICS

One small crossover RCT in people with possible Menière's disease found no significant difference with triamterene plus hydrochlorothiazide versus placebo in change in hearing over 17 weeks, and found insufficient evidence on vertigo and tinnitus.

Benefits: We found no systematic review but found one crossover RCT (33 people with possible Menière's disease) of a diuretic (triamterene 50 mg plus hydrochlorothiazide 25 mg) versus placebo.[20] It found no significant audiological change in hearing over 17 weeks ($P > 0.2$).

Harms: The RCT gave no information on adverse effects.[20]

Comment: In the RCT, frequency of vertigo attacks was reduced and tinnitus was unchanged, but valid statistical analyses cannot be performed because only the mean of categorical data was presented.[20] An RCT of hydrochlorothiazide plus betahistine is being translated.[21]

OPTION TRIMETAZIDINE

We found no RCTs comparing trimetazidine versus placebo to prevent attacks of Menière's disease. Two small RCTs in people with definite or possible Menière's disease found no significant difference with trimetazidine versus betahistine in hearing or tinnitus. One of these RCTs found that trimetazidine versus betahistine significantly increased the proportion of people reporting that the intensity of vertigo was "substantially better or cured". The other RCT found no significant difference with trimetazidine versus betahistine in vertigo intensity.

Benefits: We found no systematic review. **Versus placebo:** We found no RCTs. **Versus betahistine:** We found two RCTs.[22,23] The first RCT (20 people with definite or probable Menière's disease) compared trimetazidine (20 mg three times daily) versus betahistine (8 mg three times daily) over 3 months.[22] It found no significant difference in hearing, tinnitus, aural fullness, or quality of life (RR for improved quality of life 1.0, 95% CI 0.34 to 2.93). Trimetazidine versus betahistine significantly increased the proportion of people reporting that the duration of vertigo was "substantially better or cured" (RR 1.8, 95% CI 1.0 to 3.2) or reporting that the intensity of vertigo was "substantially better or cured" (RR 1.7, 95% CI 1.0 to 2.8). Trimetazidine versus betahistine also improved the global impression of vertigo scale significantly more than betahistine, but it is not clear if this scale has been validated (RR 2.5, 95% CI 1.17 to 5.3).[22] The second RCT (45 people with possible Menière's disease) of trimetazidine (20 mg three times daily) versus betahistine (12 mg three times daily) over 2 months found no significant difference in hearing or tinnitus.[23] A beneficial effect of trimetazidine on vertigo intensity was reported, but is not confirmed by analysis of the available data (P = 0.23; 2 sided Fisher's exact test).[23]

Harms: No significant adverse effects were reported in the RCTs.[22,23]

Comment: None.

OPTION BETAHISTINE

Six RCTs found insufficient evidence about the effects of betahistine versus placebo on the frequency and severity of attacks of vertigo, tinnitus, and aural fullness. Four RCTs found no change in hearing as assessed by changes in pure tone audiograms with betahistine versus placebo. Two small RCTs in people with definite or possible Menière's disease found no significant difference with betahistine versus trimetazidine in hearing or tinnitus. One of these RCTs found that betahistine versus trimetazidine significantly decreased the number of people reporting that the intensity of vertigo was "substantially better or cured". The other RCT found no significant difference with betahistine versus trimetazidine in vertigo intensity.

Benefits: **Versus placebo:** We found one systematic review (search date 1999, 6 RCTs,[13,24–28] 162 people) of betahistine versus placebo in people with Menière's disease.[29] The review did not include a meta-analysis because of trial heterogeneity (see comment below).[29] The first RCT identified by the review (30 people with possible Menière's disease) found that after 6 weeks, betahistine (8 mg three times daily) versus placebo significantly reduced the severity of vertigo (P = 0.0001), tinnitus (P = 0.001), and aural fullness (P = 0.02).[24] The second RCT identified by the review (35 people with possible Menière's disease, crossover design) found that betahistine (24 mg three times daily in a slow release formulation) versus placebo for 16 weeks had no significant effect on tinnitus (P = 0.68) or aural fullness (P = 0.63).[13] Vertigo was not adequately assessed. The third RCT identified by the review (16/36 people had a possible diagnosis of Menière's disease) found that betahistine (18 mg twice daily) versus placebo for 2 weeks had no significant effect on the proportion of people reporting improved vertigo (RR 1.17, 95% CI 0.86 to 1.58) or tinnitus (RR 2.4, 95% CI 0.11 to 51.32).[25] The fourth RCT identified by the review (10 people with possible Menière's disease) found that betahistine (8 mg three times daily) versus placebo had no significant effect over 6–12 months on the number of people with improved vertigo (RR 5.0, 95% CI 0.3 to 84), tinnitus, or aural fullness.[26] None of the RCTs found any change in hearing as assessed by pure tone audiograms.[13,24–26] The remaining two RCTs identified by the review reported insufficient detail to confirm reliably that the participants had Menière's disease.[27,28] **Versus trimetazidine:** See benefits of trimetazidine, p 596.

Harms: None of the RCTs identified by the review reported any significant adverse effects.[24–28]

Comment: The systematic review reported "we found no trials with a low risk of methodological bias which used the highest level of diagnostic criteria and outcome measures".[29] It stated that the lack of diagnostic certainty made it inappropriate to combine results.[29] Crossover studies are difficult to interpret if used to evaluate the effects of treatments on conditions that fluctuate in intensity or if interventions have prolonged effects.[30] Menière's disease is not a stable condition and it is unknown if any effects of betahistine are prolonged. An RCT of hydrochlorothiazide plus betahistine is being translated.[21]

OPTION LITHIUM

Two small crossover RCTs in people with possible Menière's disease found no difference with lithium versus placebo in vertigo, tinnitus, aural fullness, or hearing, and found that lithium was associated with tremor, thirst, and polyuria in some people.

Benefits: We found no systematic review but found two crossover RCTs (50 people with possible Menière's disease) of lithium versus placebo.[31,32] They found no difference in vertigo, tinnitus, aural fullness, or hearing, but no analysable results were presented.

Harms: In the RCTs, serum lithium concentration was checked every 2 weeks to reduce the risk of adverse effects.[31,32] Two people withdrew from one RCT because of adverse effects from lithium (tremor, thirst, polyuria).[31]

Comment: The crossover RCT design may be inappropriate because Menière's disease is not stable and it is not clear that the lithium is free of any other effects.[31,32] Dosage was adjusted to maintain serum lithium concentration between 0.7–1.1 mmol/L.

OPTION DIETARY MODIFICATION

We found no RCTs about the effects of dietary modification in preventing attacks of Menière's disease.

Benefits: We found no systematic review or RCTs.

Harms: We found no RCTs.

Comment: It has been suggested that a low salt diet reduces endolymphatic pressure in endolymphatic hydrops,[33] but we found no RCTs.

OPTION SYSTEMIC AMINOGLYCOSIDES

We found no RCTs about the effects of systemic aminoglycosides in preventing attacks of Menière's disease.

Benefits: We found no systematic review or RCTs.

Harms: Systemic aminoglycosides have been reported to be associated with a risk of severe disruption of balance (including oscillopsia — see glossary, p 599) and sensorineural hearing loss.[34]

Comment: Aminoglycosides have been used in severe bilateral Menière's disease,[35–37] but we found no evidence from RCTs to support or to refute this.

OPTION PSYCHOLOGICAL SUPPORT

We found no RCTs about psychological support, such as reassurance, to prevent attacks of Menière's disease.

Benefits: We found no systematic review or RCTs.

Harms: We found no RCTs.

Comment: We found no good evidence about the effect of psychological support on Menière's disease. However, symptomatic improvement is seen with all treatments, including placebo[16,31] or being put on a waiting list for surgery.[38] Improvements noted after these types of psychological support have not been distinguished from improvements attributable to the natural history of Menière's disease.

OPTION VESTIBULAR REHABILITATION

We found no RCTs about the effects of vestibular rehabilitation exercises on Menière's disease.

Benefits: We found no systematic review or RCTs.

Harms: We found no RCTs.

Comment: Improvements noted after vestibular rehabilitation (see glossary, p 599) have not been distinguished from spontaneous improvement of Menière's disease.

GLOSSARY

Cogan's syndrome Episodic vertigo of the Menière's type, hearing loss, and interstitial keratitis, without syphilis.[5]

Mondini dysplasia A congenital deformity of the cochlea in which only the basal turns are present.

Oscillopsia A disabling disturbance of the vestibulo-ocular reflex, manifest as oscillating vision typically with head movement.

Vestibular rehabilitation Involves a series of exercises intended to improve the sense of balance through controlled movements of the head and body.[39] It is usually recommended for stable vestibular disorders.[40]

REFERENCES

1. Friberg U, Stahle J, Svedberg A. The natural course of Menière's disease. *Acta Otolaryngol Suppl* 1984;406:72–77.
2. Kitahara M. Concepts and diagnostic criteria of Menière's disease. In: Kitahara M, ed. *Menière's disease.* Tokyo: Springer-Verlag, 1990:3–12.
3. Alford BR. Menière's disease: criteria for diagnosis and evaluation of therapy for reporting. Report of subcommittee on equilibrium and its measurement. *Trans Am Acad Ophthalmol Otolaryngol* 1972;76:1462–1464.
4. Pearson BW, Brackmann DE. Committee on Hearing and Equilibrium guidelines for reporting treatment results in Menière's disease. *Otolaryngol Head Neck Surg* 1985;93:578–581.
5. Committee on Hearing and Equilibrium. Guidelines for the diagnosis and evaluation of therapy in Menière's disease. *Otolaryngol Head Neck Surg* 1995;113:181–185.
6. Moffat DA, Ballagh RH. Menière's disease. In: Kerr AG, Booth JB, eds. *Scott-Brown's otolaryngology.* 6th ed. Oxford: Butterworth-Heinemann, 1997:3/19/1–50.
7. Watanabe I. Incidence of Menière's disease, including some other epidemiological data. In: Oosterveld WJ, ed. *Menière's disease: a comprehensive appraisal.* Chichester: Wiley, 1983:9–23.

8. Cawthorne T, Hewlett AB. Menière's disease. *Proc Royal Soc Med* 1954;47:663–670.
9. Stahle J, Stahle C, Arenberg IK. Incidence of Menière's disease. *Arch Otolaryngol* 1978;104:99–102.
10. Nsamba C. A comparative study of the aetiology of vertigo in the African. *J Laryngol Otol* 1972;86:917–925.
11. Hallpike C, Cairns H. Observations on the pathology of Menière's syndrome. *J Laryngol Otol* 1938;53:625–655.
12. Ruckenstein MJ, Harrison RV. Cochlear pathology in Menière's disease. In: Harris JP, ed. *Menière's disease.* The Hague: Kugler Publications, 1999:195–202.
13. Schmidt JT, Huizing EH. The clinical drug trial in Menière's disease with emphasis on the effect of betahistine SR. *Acta Otolaryngol* 1992;497(suppl):1–189.
14. Moser M, Ranacher G, Wilmot TJ, et al. A double-blind clinical trial of hydroxyethylrutosides in Menière's disease. *J Laryngol Otol* 1984;98:265–272.
15. Silverstein H, Smouha E, Jones R. Natural history versus surgery for Menière's disease. *Otolaryngol Head Neck Surg* 1989;100:6–16.
16. Torok N. Old and new in Menière's disease. *Laryngoscope* 1977;87:1870–1877.
17. Storper IS, Spitzer JB, Scanlan M. Use of glycopyrrolate in the treatment of Menière's disease. *Laryngoscope* 1998;108:1442–1445.
18. Jacobson GP, Newman CW. The development of the Dizziness Handicap Inventory. *Arch Otolaryngol Head Neck Surg* 1990;116:424–427.
19. Sheldon CH, Horton BT. Treatment of Menière's disease with histamine administered intravenously. *Proceedings of the Staff Meetings of the Mayo Clinic* 1940;15:17–21.
20. van Deelen GW, Huizing EH. Use of a diuretic (Dyazide) in the treatment of Menière's disease. A double-blind cross-over placebo-controlled study. *ORL J Otorhinolaryngol Relat Spec* 1986;48:287–292.
21. Petermann W, Mulch G. Long-term therapy of Menière's disease. Comparison of the effects of betahistine dihydrochloride and hydrochlorothiazide [in German]. *Fortschr Medizin* 1982;100:431–435.
22. Kluyskens P, Lambert P, D'Hooge D. Trimetazidine contre betahistine dans le vertiges vestibulaires [in French]. *Ann Otolaryngol Chir Cervicofac* 1990;107(suppl 1):11–19.
23. Martini A, De Domenico F. Trimetazidine versus betahistine in Menière's disease. A double blind method [in French]. *Ann Otolaryngol Chir Cervicofac* 1990;107(suppl 1):20–27.
24. Salami A, Dellepiane M, Tinelle E, et al. Studio a doppia cecita' tra cloridrato di betaistina e placebo nel trattamento delle sindromi Menieriformi [in Italian]. *Valsalva* 1984;60:302–312.
25. Okamato K, Hazeyama F, Taira T, et al. Therapeutic results of betahistine in Menière's disease with statistical analysis. *Iryo* 1968;22:650–666.
26. Ricci V, Sittoni V, Nicora M. Valutazione terapeutica e tollerabilita del chloridrato di betaistina (Microser) in confronto a placebo nella malattia di Menière. *Riv Ital Ornitolog Audiolog Foniat* 1987;7:347–350.
27. Burkin A. Betahistine treatment of Menière's syndrome. *Clin Med* 1967;74:41–48.
28. Elia JC. Double-blind evaluation of a new treatment for Menière's syndrome. *JAMA* 1966;196:187–189.
29. James AL, Burton MJ. Betahistine for Menière's disease or syndrome. In: The Cochrane Library, Issue 3, 2002. Oxford: Update Software. Search date 1999; primary sources Cochrane Controlled Trials Register, Medline, Embase, Index Medicus, and hand searches of reference lists.
30. Fleiss JL. The crossover study. In: *The design and analysis of clinical experiments.* Chichester: Wiley, 1984.
31. Thomsen J, Bech P, Prytz S, et al. Menière's disease: lithium treatment (demonstration of placebo effect in a double blind cross-over trial). *Clin Otolaryngol* 1979;4:119–123.
32. Thomsen J, Bech P, Geisler A, et al. Lithium treatment of Menière's disease: results of a double-blind cross-over trial. *Acta Otolaryngol* 1976;82:294–296.
33. Furstenburg AC, Richardson G, Lathrop FD. Menière's disease. Addenda to medical therapy. *Arch Otolaryngol* 1941;34:1083–1092.
34. Balyan FR, Taibah A, De Donato G, et al. Titration streptomycin therapy in Menière's disease: long-term results. *Otolaryngol Head Neck Surg* 1998;118:261–266.
35. Wilson WR, Schuknecht HF. Update on the use of streptomycin therapy for Menière's disease. *Am J Otol* 1980;2:108–111.
36. Graham MD. Bilateral Menière's disease. Treatment with intramuscular titration streptomycin sulfate. *Otolaryngol Clin North Am* 1997;30:1097–1100.
37. Shea JJ, Ge X, Orchik DJ. Long-term results of low dose intramuscular streptomycin for Menière's disease. *Am J Otol* 1994;15:540–544.
38. Kerr AG, Toner JG. A new approach to surgery for Menière's disease: talking about surgery. *Clin Otolaryngol* 1998;23:263–264.
39. Dix MR. The rationale and technique of head exercises in the treatment of vertigo. *Acta Otorhinolaryngol Belg* 1979;33:370–384.
40. Clendaniel RA, Tucci DL. Vestibular rehabilitation strategies in Menière's disease. *Otolaryngol Clin North Am* 1997;30:1145–1158.

Adrian James
Department of Otolaryngology
Radcliffe Infirmary
Oxford
UK

Marc Thorp
Department of Otolaryngology
Corner Brook
Newfoundland
Canada

Competing interests: None declared.

TABLE 1 American Academy of Otolaryngology–Head and Neck Surgery definition of the certainty of diagnosis of Menière's disease (see text, p 594).[3–5]

Certain	Definite Menière's plus postmortem confirmation
Definite	Two or more episodes of vertigo* plus audiometrically confirmed sensorineural hearing loss plus tinnitus or aural fullness plus other causes excluded
Probable	One episode of vertigo* plus audiometrically confirmed sensorineural hearing loss plus tinnitus or aural fullness plus other causes excluded
Possible	Episodes of vertigo* with no hearing loss, or sensorineural hearing loss with dysequilibrium; other causes excluded

*Defined as spontaneous, rotational vertigo lasting more than 20 minutes.

Middle ear pain and trauma during air travel

Search date November 2002

Simon Janvrin

QUESTIONS

INTERVENTIONS

Key Messages

- **Oral decongestants in adults** One RCT in adult passengers with a history of ear pain during air travel found limited evidence that oral pseudoephedrine versus placebo significantly decreased barotrauma symptoms during air travel. One other RCT in adult passengers with a history of ear pain during air travel found limited evidence that oral pseudoephedrine versus placebo significantly decreased ear pain and hearing loss during air travel.
- **Oral decongestants in children** One small RCT in children up to the age of 6 years found no significant difference with oral pseudoephedrine versus placebo in ear pain at take off or landing.
- **Topical nasal decongestants** One small RCT in adults with a history of ear pain during air travel found no significant difference with oxymetazoline nasal spray versus placebo in symptoms of barotrauma.

DEFINITION The effects of air travel on the middle ear can include ear drum pain, vertigo, hearing loss, and ear drum perforation.

INCIDENCE/ PREVALENCE The prevalence of symptoms depends on the altitude, type of aircraft, and characteristics of the passengers. One point prevalence study found that 20% of adult and 40% of child passengers had negative pressure in the middle ear after flight, and that 10% of adults and 22% of children had auroscopic evidence of damage to the ear drum.[1] We found no data on the incidence of perforation, which seems to be extremely rare in commercial passengers.

AETIOLOGY/ RISK FACTORS During aircraft descent, the pressure in the middle ear drops relative to that in the ear canal. A narrow, inflamed, or poorly functioning Eustachian tube impedes the necessary influx of air. As the pressure difference between the middle and outer ear increases, the ear drum is pulled inward.

PROGNOSIS In most people symptoms resolve spontaneously. Experience in military aviation shows that most ear drum perforations will heal spontaneously.[2]

AIMS OF INTERVENTION To prevent ear pain and trauma during air travel.

OUTCOMES Incidence and severity of pain and hearing loss; incidence of perforation of ear drum.

METHODS *Clinical Evidence* search and appraisal November 2002.

QUESTION **What are the effects of preventive interventions?**

OPTION **ORAL DECONGESTANTS**

One RCT in adult passengers with a history of ear pain during air travel found limited evidence that oral pseudoephedrine versus placebo significantly decreased symptoms of barotrauma during air travel. One other RCT in adult passengers with a history of ear pain during air travel found limited evidence that oral pseudoephedrine versus placebo significantly decreased ear pain and hearing loss during air travel. One small RCT in children up to the age of 6 years found no significant difference with oral pseudoephedrine versus placebo in ear pain at take off or landing.

Benefits: We found no systematic review. We found three RCTs.[3–5] Two RCTs in adult passengers compared oral pseudoephedrine (120 mg given at least 30 mins before flight) versus placebo.[3,4] All people had a history of ear pain during air travel. Those with acute or chronic ear problems were excluded. Both RCTs assessed outcomes by a post-flight questionnaire returned by mail. The first RCT compared three treatments: oral pseudoephedrine; oxymetazoline nasal spray; or placebo.[3] The RCT found that pseudoephedrine versus placebo significantly decreased the proportion of people with symptoms of barotrauma (ear pain, blockage, hearing loss, dizziness/ vertigo, tinnitus: 34% [14/41] of people with pseudoephedrine *v* 71% [29/41] of people with placebo; RR 0.48, 95% CI 0.29 to 0.67).[3] The second RCT (190 adults) found that pseudoephedrine versus placebo significantly reduced ear pain (25/96 [26%] of people with pseudoephedrine v 43/94 [46%] of people with placebo; P = 0.007) and hearing loss (20/96 [21%] of people with pseudoephedrine v 38/94 [40%] of people with placebo; P = 0.006).[4] The third RCT (50 children up to the age of 6 years) compared oral pseudoephedrine versus placebo.[5] It found no significant difference in ear pain between children taking pseudoephedrine versus placebo at either take off or landing.

Harms: Adverse effects reported by the first RCT included drowsiness (4/41 [10%] with pseudoephedrine v 2/41 [5%] with placebo), dry mouth (4/41 [10%] v 1/41 [2%]), nasal irritation (1/41 [2%] v 0/41 [0%]), stomach upset (1/41 [2%] v 0/41 [0%]), and headache (0/41 [0%] v 1/41 [2%]).[3] The second RCT reported drowsiness (7.3% of people with pseudoephedrine v 2.2% of people with placebo) and nausea and dry mouth (4.2% v 4.3%).[4] The third RCT found more children taking pseudoephedrine were drowsy on take off compared with placebo (60% v 27%; P = 0.003).[5]

Comment: None.

OPTION TOPICAL NASAL DECONGESTANTS

One small RCT in adults with a history of ear pain during air travel found no significant difference with oxymetazoline nasal spray versus placebo in symptoms of barotrauma.

Benefits: We found no systematic review. We found one RCT in adults with a history of ear pain during air travel, which compared oxymetazoline nasal spray, oral pseudoephedrine, or placebo during air travel.[3] Outcomes were assessed by a post-flight questionnaire returned by mail. The RCT (83 people) found no significant difference in symptoms of barotrauma between oxymetazoline versus placebo (ear pain, blockage, hearing loss, dizziness/vertigo, tinnitus: 64% of people with oxymetazoline v 71% of people with placebo; P = 0.695).[3]

Harms: Adverse effects included nasal irritation (6/42 [14%] with oxymetazoline v 0/41 [0%] with placebo), drowsiness (1/42 [2%] v 2/41 [5%]), dry mouth (1/42 [2%] v 1/41 [2%]), stomach upset (1/42 [2%] v 0/41 [0%]), and headache (1/42 [2%] v 1/41 [2%]).[3]

Comment: The RCT may have been too small to rule out an effect of topical decongestants.

REFERENCES

1. Stangerup S-E, Tjernstrom O, Klokke M, et al. Point prevalence of barotitis in children and adults after flight, and the effect of autoinflation. *Aviat Space Environ Med* 1998;69:45–49.
2. O'Reilly BJ. Otorhinolaryngology. In: Ernsting J, Nicholson AN, Rainford DJ, eds. *Aviation Medicine*. 3rd edition. Oxford: Butterworth-Heinemann, 1999:319–336.
3. Jones JS, Sheffield W, White LJ, et al. A double-blind comparison between oral pseudoephedrine and topical oxymetazoline in the prevention of barotrauma during air travel. *Am J Emerg Med* 1998;16:262–264.
4. Csortan E, Jones J, Haan M, et al. Efficacy of pseudoephedrine for the prevention of barotrauma during air travel. *Ann Emerg Med* 1994;23:1324–1327.
5. Buchanan BJ, Hoagland J, Fischer PR. Pseudoephedrine and air travel-associated ear pain in children. *Arch Pediatr Adolesc Med* 1999;153:466–468.

Simon Janvrin
Civil Aviation Authority, West Sussex, UK

Competing interests: None declared.

Otitis externa

Search date November 2002

Daniel Hajioff

QUESTIONS

INTERVENTIONS

See glossary, p 611

Key Messages

Treatment of otitis externa

- **Topical aluminium acetate drops (as effective as topical anti-infective agents)** We found no RCTs that compared topical aluminium acetate versus placebo. One RCT found no significant difference in clinical cure between aluminium acetate drops and topical polymyxin–neomycin–hydrocortisone drops at 4 weeks.
- **Topical anti-infective agents (antibiotics or antifungals with or without steroids)** One RCT found that methylprednisolone–neomycin drops improved symptoms and signs compared with placebo at 28 days. Two RCTs found no significant difference in cure rate between topical quinolones and other topical anti-infective agents. One RCT found that triamcinolone–neomycin drops improved resolution rates compared with hydrocortisone–neomycin–polymyxin B drops. We found limited evidence from two RCTs that neomycin–dexamethasone–acetic acid spray improved clinical cure compared with topical anti-infective drops that did not contain acetic acid.
- **Topical steroids alone** One RCT found that topical budesonide improved symptoms and signs compared with placebo in people with mild to moderately severe otitis externa. One RCT found no significant difference in symptom scores between topical hydrocortisone and topical hydrocortisone butyrate after 1 week.
- **Oral antibiotics** We found no RCTs of oral antibiotics versus placebo or topical anti-infective agents.
- **Specialist aural toilet** We found no RCTs comparing specialist aural toilet versus no aural toilet. One RCT found no significant difference in clinical cure between an ear wick with anti-infective drops versus ribbon gauze impregnated with anti-infective ointment.

- **Oral antibiotics plus topical anti-infective agents (compared with topical anti-infective agents alone)** We found limited evidence from one RCT of no clinical effect of oral antibiotics plus topical anti-infective agents compared with topical anti-infective agents alone.

DEFINITION Otitis externa is inflammation, often with infection, of the external ear canal. This inflammation is usually generalised throughout the ear canal so it is often referred to as "diffuse otitis externa". The present topic excludes localised inflammations such as furuncles. Otitis externa has acute (< 6 weeks), chronic (> 3 months), and necrotising forms. Acute otitis externa may present as a single episode, or recur. It causes severe pain with aural discharge and associated hearing loss.[1] If the ear canal is visible, it appears red and inflamed. Chronic otitis externa may result in canal stenosis with associated hearing loss, for which it may be difficult to fit hearing aids. Necrotising otitis externa is defined by destruction of the temporal bone, usually in people with diabetes or in people who are immunocompromised. Necrotising otitis externa can be life-threatening.[2]

INCIDENCE/ PREVALENCE Otitis externa is common in all parts of the world. The incidence is not known precisely, but 10% of people are thought to have been affected at some time.[3] The condition affects children, but is more common in adults. It accounts for a large proportion of the workload of otolaryngology departments, but milder cases are often managed in primary care.[3]

AETIOLOGY/ RISK FACTORS Otitis externa may be associated with local or generalised eczema of the ear canal. It is more common in swimmers, in humid environments, in people with an absence of ear wax or narrow external ear canals, in hearing aid users, and after mechanical trauma.[4]

PROGNOSIS We found few reliable data. Many cases of otitis externa resolve spontaneously over several weeks or months. Acute episodes have a tendency to recur, although the risk of recurrence is unknown. Experience suggests that chronic inflammation affects a small proportion of people after a single episode of acute otitis externa, and may rarely lead to canal stenosis.[1] We found no reliable data about risks of necrotising otitis externa, although it is thought to be a complication that only affects people with diabetes or who are immunosuppressed.

AIMS OF INTERVENTION To improve or abolish symptoms, to prevent recurrence and complications with minimal adverse effects.

OUTCOMES Pain; discharge; hearing loss; prevention of recurrence; ability to use hearing aids; quality of life; "resolution" (resolution of all clinical manifestations including pain, hearing loss, discharge, and redness); adverse effects of treatment.

METHODS *Clinical Evidence* search and appraisal November 2002. We excluded studies with follow up of less than 80%. We excluded studies with follow up of less than 1 month, so that we could assess rates of sustained resolution and recurrence.

QUESTION What are the effects of empirical treatment? New

OPTION ORAL ANTIBIOTICS

We found no RCTs of oral antibiotics versus placebo or versus topical anti-infective agents. We found limited evidence from one RCT of no clinical effect of oral antibiotics plus topical anti-infective agents compared with topical anti-infective agents alone.

Benefits: We found no systematic review. **Oral antibiotics versus placebo:** We found no RCTs. **Oral antibiotics versus topical anti-infective agents:** We found no RCTs. **Oral antibiotics plus topical anti-infective agents versus topical anti-infective agents alone:** One double blind RCT (105 people with any severity of acute diffuse otitis externa on otoscopy) compared 5 days of oral co-trimoxazole versus placebo in a primary care setting.[5] Both groups received repeated applications of ointment containing triamcinolone, neomycin, and gramicidin and had suction of the external canal if discharge was present. The RCT found no significant difference between topical anti-infective agents plus oral cotrimoxazole versus topical anti-infective agents plus placebo in mean symptom and sign severity scores, duration of symptoms, or cure rate after treatment (improvement in score on scale ranging from 1 [no symptoms] to 5 [severe symptoms]: 0.72 with added oral co-trimoxazole *v* 0.69 with added placebo; $P > 0.4$; cure rates 18/47 [38%] with added oral co-trimoxazole *v* 21/53 [40%] with placebo; $P > 0.8$; mean duration of symptoms 3.1 days with added oral co-trimoxazole *v* 3.1 days with placebo, $P > 0.5$; no further data provided for any comparison).[5]

Harms: The RCT did not report on harms.[5]

Comment: None.

OPTION TOPICAL ANTI-INFECTIVE AGENTS

One RCT found that methylprednisolone–neomycin drops improved symptoms and signs compared with placebo at 28 days. Two RCTs found no significant difference in cure rate between topical quinolones and other topical anti-infective agents. One RCT found that triamcinolone–neomycin drops improved resolution rates compared with hydrocortisone–neomycin–polymyxin B drops. We found limited evidence from two RCTs that neomycin–dexamethasone–acetic acid spray improved clinical cure compared with topical anti-infective drops that did not contain acetic acid. We found insufficient evidence from one RCT about clinical effects of oral antibiotics plus topical anti-infective agents compared with topical anti-infective agents alone.

Benefits: We found no systematic review. **Topical anti-infective agents versus placebo:** One double blind RCT (40 people in secondary care with mild, moderate, or severe, acute or chronic diffuse otitis externa) compared methylprednisolone–neomycin drops versus placebo drops for 10 days.[6] All participants had "cleansing" of their external ear canals (details of cleansing not reported). The RCT found that methylprednisolone–neomycin drops improved symptoms compared with placebo at 28 days (11/20 [55%] reported "good" response with methylprednisolone–neomycin drops *v* 2/20 [10%] with placebo, $P < 0.001$; no further data provided) **Topical anti-infective agents versus oral antibiotics:** We found no RCTs. **Topical anti-infective agents alone versus oral antibiotics plus topical anti-infective agents:** See benefits of oral antibiotics, p 607. **Topical anti-infective agents versus each other:** We found four RCTs.[7–10] Three RCTs compared preparations containing a quinolone versus other agents.[7–9] The first, a double blind RCT (842 people with mild to severe acute diffuse otitis externa on otoscopy) compared ciprofloxacin drops with or without hydrocortisone versus polymyxin–neomycin–hydrocortisone drops in a primary care setting for 1 week.[7] Participants in both groups received suction or mopping of discharge if present. The RCT found no significant difference among treatments for improvement or resolution of signs and symptoms at 30 days (improvement or resolution: 222/239 [93%] with ciprofloxacin *v* 212/236 [90%] with ciprofloxacin–hydrocortisone *v* 198/228 [87%] with polymyxin–neomycin–hydrocortisone; $P > 0.5$ for each comparison). The second RCT (single blind, 601 people with any severity of acute diffuse otitis externa on otoscopy) compared ofloxacin drops versus neomycin–hydrocortisone–polymyxin B drops in a primary care setting for 10 days.[8] At 1 month, it found no significant difference between treatments for clinical or microbiological cure (clinical cure: 215/242 [89%] with ofloxacin *v* 206/232 [89%] with neomycin–hydrocortisone–polymyxin B drops, $P = 0.86$; no further data provided; microbiological cure: 85/93 [91%] with ofloxacin *v* 97/103 [94%] with neomycin–hydrocortisone–polymyxin B drops, $P = 0.77$; no further data provided). A third RCT is being translated and will be included in future updates of *Clinical Evidence*.[9] The fourth RCT (double blind, 55 people with moderate to severe acute or chronic diffuse otitis externa on otoscopy) compared drops containing hydrocortisone–neomycin sulphate and polymyxin B versus drops containing triamcinolone–neomycin undecenoate for 1 month or until resolution of all symptoms and signs.[10] The trial took place in a secondary care setting. All participants received microsuction of their ears if discharge was present. The RCT found that triamcinolone–neomycin drops significantly improved resolution rates compared with hydrocortisone–neomycin–polymyxin B drops at 1 month (resolution 27/34 [79%] with triamcinolone–neomycin *v* 10/21 [47%] with hydrocortisone–neomycin–polymyxin B; $P < 0.01$; no further data provided).[10] **Antibiotic–steroid–acetic acid spray versus antibiotic–steroid drops:** We found two RCTs. One single blind RCT (60 people with any severity of acute or chronic diffuse otitis externa on otoscopy) compared neomycin–dexamethasone–acetic acid spray versus framycetin–gramicidin–dexamethasone drops in a primary care setting for 10 days.[11] At 1 month, neomycin–dexamethasone–acetic acid spray significantly improved symptoms and signs compared with framycetin–gramicidin–dexamethasone drops (symptom free: 26/32 [81.3%] with neomycin–dexamethasone–acetic acid spray *v* 6/26 [23.1%] with framycetin–gramicidin–dexamethasone drops,

P < 0.0001; no further data provided; free of clinical signs: 17/32 [53.1%] with neomycin–dexamethasone–acetic acid spray *v* 10/28 [37.0%] with framycetin–gramicidin–dexamethasone drops, P < 0.05; no further data provided). A second non-blind RCT (187 people with any severity of acute or chronic diffuse otitis externa on otoscopy) compared neomycin–dexamethasone–acetic acid spray versus neomycin–hydrocortisone–polymyxin B drops in a primary care setting for 10 days.[12] It found no significant difference between treatments in the proportion of people with improved global symptom scores at 10 days and at 1 month (at 10 days: 86/91 [94.5%] improved with neomycin–dexamethasone–acetic acid spray *v* 79/85 [92.9%] with neomycin–hydrocortisone–polymyxin B drops, P > 0.5; no further data provided; at 1 month: 54/86 [62.8%] improved with neomycin–dexamethasone–acetic acid spray *v* 48/81 [59.3%] with neomycin–hydrocortisone–polymyxin B drops, P > 0.5; no further data provided).[12] However, compared with neomycin–hydrocortisone–polymyxin B drops, neomycin–dexamethasone–acetic acid spray increased the proportion of people considered to have "good" improvement in signs at 10 days (48/91 [52.7%] with neomycin–dexamethasone–acetic acid spray *v* 31/85 [36.5%] with neomycin–hydrocortisone–polymyxin B drops, P < 0.05; no further data provided).

Harms: One RCT found no significant difference between ofloxacin drops and neomycin–hydrocortisone–polymyxin B drops in rates of local pruritis, dizziness, or vertigo (local pruritis: 25/158 [15.8%] with ofloxacin *v* 18/156 [11.5%] with neomycin–hydrocortisone–polymyxin B; P = 0.33; dizziness or vertigo: 4/158 [2.5%] with ofloxacin *v* 2/156 [1.3%] with neomycin–hydrocortisone–polymyxin B; CI and P values not reported).[8] One RCT reported that 6/32 (18.8%) people taking neomycin–dexamethasone–acetic acid spray and 3/26 [11.5%] people taking framycetin–gramicidin–dexamethasone drops reported local stinging or burning in the first few days of treatment (significance not reported), which did not affect adherence.[11] The other RCTs did not report on harms.[7,9,10,12]

Comment: None.

OPTION TOPICAL STEROIDS ALONE

One RCT found that topical budesonide improved symptoms and signs compared with placebo in people with mild to moderately severe otitis externa. One RCT found no significant difference in symptom scores between topical hydrocortisone and topical hydrocortisone butyrate after 1 week.

Benefits: We found no systematic review. **Versus placebo:** We found one double blind RCT (60 people with mild or moderate acute or chronic diffuse otitis externa on otoscopy).[13] People with complete occlusion of the external ear canal were excluded. The RCT compared budesonide drops with placebo drops in a secondary care setting for 7 days.[13] Ear discharge was treated by suction in both groups. The RCT found that budesonide drops significantly improved symptoms and signs compared with placebo after 10 days (change from baseline in a global clinical score ranging from 0 [no symptoms/signs] to 3 [severe symptoms/signs]: –2.29 with budesonide *v* +0.23 with placebo; P = 0.001). **Versus topical anti-infective agents:** We found no RCTs. **Low versus high potency steroids:** One double blind RCT (55 people with any severity of acute or chronic diffuse otitis externa on otoscopy) compared low potency steroid drops (1% hydrocortisone) versus high potency steroid drops (hydrocortisone-17-α-butyrate) in a secondary care setting.[14] It found no significant difference between treatments in symptom scores after 1 week of treatment (score ranging from 0 [no symptoms] to 3 [severe symptoms] at 1 week: 0.84 with low potency steroid drops *v* 0.80 with high potency steroid drops; P > 0.2).[14]

Harms: The RCT comparing topical budesonide versus placebo found no significant difference in frequency of local or systemic adverse events (30% with budesonide *v* 27% with placebo).[13] The RCT comparing low versus high potency steroids did not report on harms.

Comment: None.

OPTION TOPICAL ALUMINIUM ACETATE

We found no RCTs that compared topical aluminium acetate versus placebo. One RCT found no significant difference in clinical cure between aluminium acetate drops and topical polymyxin–neomycin–hydrocortisone drops at 4 weeks.

Benefits: We found no systematic review. **Versus placebo:** We found no RCTs. **Versus topical anti-infective agents:** One RCT (126 people with any severity of acute diffuse otitis externa on otoscopy) compared aluminium acetate drops versus polymyxin–neomycin–hydrocortisone drops in a primary care setting for 14 days.[15] Participants in both groups had discharge removed if present (no further details of technique provided). The RCT found no significant difference in clinical cure rate or mean time to clinical resolution between treatments at 4 weeks (clinical cure rate: 59/65 [91%] with aluminium acetate *v* 49/61 [80%] with polymyxin–neomycin–hydrocortisone; P > 0.2; no further data provided; mean time to clinical resolution: 9.4 days with aluminium acetate *v* 11.1 days with polymyxin–neomycin–hydrocortisone; P > 0.2; no further data provided).

Harms: The RCT did not report on harms.[15]

Comment: None.

OPTION SPECIALIST AURAL TOILET

We found no RCTs comparing specialist aural toilet versus no aural toilet. One RCT found no significant difference in clinical cure between an ear wick with anti-infective drops versus ribbon gauze impregnated with anti-infective ointment.

Benefits: We found no systematic review. **Versus no aural toilet:** See glossary, p 611. We found no controlled trials. **Comparison ofdifferent types of aural toilet:** One RCT in a secondary care setting (94 people with moderate to severe acute diffuse otitis externa on otoscopy) compared an ear wick plus anti-infective drops (framycetin–gramicidin–dexamethasone or flumetasone) removed after 3 days versus ribbon gauze impregnated with anti-infective ointment (framycetin–gramicidin or triamcinolone–gramicidin–neomycin–nystatin) removed after 3 days.[16] It found no significant difference between treatments for resolution rates at 4 weeks (resolution defined as absence of symptoms and signs: 33/47 [70%] with ribbon gauze *v* 30/47 [64%] with ear wick; no further data provided; P = 0.58).

Harms: No adverse effects were reported.[16]

Comment: The results of studies may not be generalisable to settings where professionals have not been trained to provide specialist aural toilet.

GLOSSARY

Specialist aural toilet Aural toilet is usually performed in a secondary (specialist) setting and includes dry mopping of the ear canal or suction. These can be performed using a head light or microscope, which allows cleaning of the more medial areas of the ear canal.

REFERENCES

1. Agius AM, Pickles JM, Burch KL. A prospective study of otitis externa. *Clin Otolaryngol* 1992;17:150–154.
2. Doroghazi RM, Nadol JB, Hyslop NE, et al. Invasive external otitis. Report of 21 cases and review of the literature. *Am J Med* 1981;71:603–618.
3. Raza SA, Denholm SW, Wong JC. An audit of the management of otitis externa in an ENT casualty clinic. *J Laryngol Otol* 1995;109:130–133.
4. Hirsh BE. Infections of the external ear. *Am J Otolaryng* 1992;17:207.
5. Yelland MJ. The efficacy of oral cotrimoxazole in the treatment of otitis externa in general practice. *Med J Aust* 1993;158:697–699.
6. Cannon SJ, Grunwaldt E. Treatment of otitis externa with a tropical steroid–antibiotic combination. *Eye Ear Nose Throat Mon* 1967;46:1296–1302.
7. Pistorius B, Westberry K, Drehobl M, et al. Prospective, randomized, comparative trial of ciprofloxacin otic drops, with or without hydrocortisone, vs. polymyxin B–neomycin–hydrocortisone otic suspension in the treatment of acute diffuse otitis externa. *Infect Dis Clin Pract* 1999;8:387–395.
8. Jones RN, Milazzo J, Seidlin M. Ofloxacin otic solution for treatment of otitis externa in children and adults. *Arch Otolaryngol Head Neck Surg* 1997;123:1193–1200.
9. Sabater F, Maristany M, Mensa J, et al. Prospective double-blind randomized study of the efficacy and tolerance of topical ciprofloxacin vs topical gentamicin in the treatment of simple chronic otitis media and diffuse external otitis [in Spanish]. *Acta Otorrinolaringol Esp* 1996;47:217–220.
10. Worgan D. Treatment of otitis externa. Report of a clinical trial. *Practitioner* 1969;202:817–820.
11. Smith RB, Moodie J. A general practice study to compare the efficacy and tolerability of a spray ('Otomize') versus a standard drop formulation ('Sofradex') in the treatment of patients with otitis externa. *Curr Med Res Opin* 1990;12:12–18.
12. Smith RB, Moodie J. Comparative efficacy and tolerability of two antibacterial/anti-inflammatory formulations ('Otomize' spray and 'Otosporin' drops) in the treatment of otitis externa in general practice. *Curr Med Res Opin* 1990;11:661–667.
13. Jacobsson S, Karlsson G, Rigner P, et al. Clinical efficacy of budesonide in the treatment of eczematous external otitis. *Eur Arch Otorhinolaryngol* 1991;248:246–249.
14. Buch-Rasmussen A. Hydrocortisone alcoholic solution in eczematous external otitis. *J Int Med Res* 1979;7:449–451.
15. Lambert IJ. A comparison of the treatment of otitis externa with 'Otosporin' and aluminium acetate: a report from a services practice in Cyprus. *J R Coll Gen Pract* 1981;31:291–294.
16. Pond F, McCarty D, O'Leary S. Randomized trial on the treatment of oedematous acute otitis externa using ear wicks or ribbon gauze: clinical outcome and cost. *J Laryngol Otol* 2002;116:415–419.

Daniel Hajioff
Specialist Registrar
Department of Otolaryngology
Royal Free Hospital
London
UK

Competing interests: None declared.

Otitis media with effusion

Search date November 2002

Ian Williamson

QUESTIONS

INTERVENTIONS

Key Messages

- **Change in modifiable risk factors** We found no RCTs on the effects of avoiding risk factors such as passive smoking and bottle feeding in preventing otitis media with effusion.
- **Autoinflation with nasal balloon (short term benefit)** One systematic review has found that autoinflation with a nasal balloon significantly improves effusion compared with no treatment. Some children may find autoinflation difficult.
- **Antimicrobial drugs (possible short term benefit)** One systematic review found limited evidence that antimicrobial drugs significantly increased resolution of effusion at up to 1 month compared with placebo or no treatment. However, a subsequent systematic review found no significant difference between antimicrobial drugs and placebo. Timing to outcome of included RCTs was unclear. Adverse effects of antibiotics (mainly nausea, vomiting, and diarrhoea) have been reported in 2–32% of children.
- **Topical steroids** One small RCT found no significant difference between topical steroids alone and placebo for resolution of effusion. A second small RCT found limited evidence that topical steroids plus antibiotics improved short term symptoms as compared with antibiotics alone. It did not report on adverse events.

- **Mucolytics** One systematic review found no significant difference between 1–3 month courses of carbocisteine and placebo or no treatment in resolution of effusion. Three small RCTs of bromhexine versus placebo found conflicting results.
- **Antihistamines plus oral decongestants** One systematic review found no significant difference between antihistamines plus oral decongestants and placebo in clearance of effusion after 4 weeks.
- **Oral steroids** One systematic review found no significant difference between oral steroids and placebo in clearance of effusion after 2 weeks. It found limited evidence that oral steroids plus antibiotic improved resolution rates compared with antibiotic alone. Oral steroids may cause behavioural changes, increased appetite, and weight gain.
- **Grommets with or without adenoidectomy; other autoinflation devices; tonsillectomy** We found insufficient evidence on the effects of these interventions.

DEFINITION Otitis media with effusion (OME), or "glue ear", is serous or mucoid but not mucopurulent fluid in the middle ear. Children usually present with hearing loss and speech problems. In contrast to those with acute otitis media (see topic, p 301), children with OME do not suffer from acute ear pain, fever, or malaise. Hearing loss is usually mild and often identified when parents express concern regarding their child's behaviour, school performance, or language development.

INCIDENCE/ PREVALENCE One study in the UK found that, at any time, 5% of children aged 2–4 years have persistent (at least 3 months) bilateral hearing loss associated with OME. The prevalence declines considerably beyond age 6 years.[1] About 80% of children aged 10 years have been affected by OME at some time in the past. OME is the most common reason for referral for surgery in children in the UK. Middle ear effusions also occur infrequently in adults after upper respiratory tract infection or after air travel, and may persist for weeks or months after an episode of acute otitis media.[2]

AETIOLOGY/ RISK FACTORS Contributory factors include upper respiratory tract infection and narrow upper respiratory airways. Case control studies have identified risk factors, including age 6 years or younger at first onset, day care centre attendance, high number of siblings, low socioeconomic group, frequent upper respiratory tract infection, bottle feeding, and household smoking.[3,4] Most factors are associated with about twice the risk of developing OME.[5]

PROGNOSIS In 5% of preschool children, OME (identified by tympanometric screening) persists for at least 1 year.[6,7] One large cohort study (534 children) found that middle ear disease increased reported hearing difficulty at age 5 years (OR 1.44, 95% CI 1.18 to 1.76) and was associated with delayed language development in children up to age 10 years.[8]

AIMS OF INTERVENTION To improve hearing and wellbeing; to avoid poor behavioural, speech, and educational development; to prevent recurrent earache and otitis media.

OUTCOMES Resolution of effusion (both speed and completeness) assessed by otoscopy, tympanometry, or global clinical assessment; hearing impairment, assessed by audiometry or tympanometry (although the positive predictive value of these tests has been reported as low as 49%);[9] developmental and behavioural tests; language and speech development; adverse effects of treatment. Patient centred outcomes in children with OME (e.g. disability or quality of life) need further development and evaluation.

METHODS *Clinical Evidence* search and appraisal November 2002.

QUESTION What are the effects of preventive interventions?

OPTION MODIFYING RISK FACTORS

We found no RCTs that evaluated interventions to modify risk factors for otitis media with effusion, such as passive smoking and bottle feeding.

Benefits: We found no systematic review or RCTs of interventions aimed at modifying risk factors for otitis media with effusion.

Harms: We found insufficient data.

Comment: There is good epidemiological evidence that the risk of otitis media with effusion is increased by passive smoking,[3] bottle feeding,[4] low socioeconomic group, and exposure to a large number of other children.[9] Feasible preventive interventions may include strategies to reduce household smoking and encourage breast feeding.

QUESTION What are the effects of treatments?

OPTION ANTIMICROBIAL DRUGS

One systematic review found limited evidence that antibiotics improved short term outcomes. A second subsequent systematic review found no significant difference between antibiotics and placebo, but timing of outcome was unclear. Adverse effects with antibiotics (mainly nausea, vomiting, and diarrhoea) were reported in 2–32% of children.

Benefits: We found two systematic reviews.[9,10] The first systematic review (search date 1992, 10 RCTs, 1041 children with otitis media with effusion, age range not stated) compared antimicrobial drugs (amoxicillin [amoxycillin] with or without clavulanic acid, cefaclor, erythromycin, sulphisoxazole, sulfamethoxazole [suphamethoxazole], or trimethoprim) versus placebo or versus no treatment.[9] Treatment duration varied from 2–5 weeks. Follow up was from 10–60 days. At up to 1 month, resolution of effusion (assessed by pneumatic otoscopy, tympanometry, and audiometry) was significantly more likely with antimicrobial treatment (pooled ARR for non-resolution with antibiotics *v* placebo or no treatment 14%, 95% CI 4% to 24%; NNT 7). The second subsequent systematic review (search date 1997, 8 RCTs, 1292 children with otitis media with effusion, age range not stated) compared antibiotics versus placebo and found no significant difference in cure rate (cure rate 179/813 [22%] for antibiotics *v* 85/479 [18%] for placebo; ARI of cure +4.3%, 95% CI –0.1% to +8.6%).[10] The timing to outcomes of included RCTs was unclear. **Antibiotics plus corticosteroids:** See benefits of corticosteroids, p 615.

Harms: The systematic reviews did not report rates of adverse events in children on placebo or no treatment. Adverse events were frequent with antibiotics. For amoxicillin, diarrhoea was reported in 20–30% and rashes in 3–5% of children. For co-amoxiclav, diarrhoea was reported in 9%, nausea and vomiting in 4%, and skin rashes and urticaria in 3% of children.[9,11] For antibiotics overall, nausea and vomiting, diarrhoea, or both were reported in 2–32% of children, and cutaneous reactions in fewer than 5%.[11] Adherence to long courses of antibiotics was poor. Prescribing antibiotics for minor illness encouraged further consultations[12] and antibiotic resistance.[13]

Comment: The first systematic review included non-placebo controlled studies, and concerns have been raised about the studies included and methods used.[9] The second systematic review had some studies in common with the first review,[10] and the timing to outcomes was unclear. The systematic review included in previous *Clinical Evidence* updates has been excluded because the subsequent review eclipsed it,[10] and there were concerns about the inclusion of non-placebo controlled studies in the review.[14]

OPTION CORTICOSTEROIDS

One systematic review found no evidence on the long term effects of oral steroids compared with placebo in children with otitis media with effusion. It found limited evidence that oral steroids plus antibiotics improved resolution rates compared with antibiotics alone. One small RCT found no significant difference between topical steroids alone compared with placebo for resolution of effusion. A second small RCT found limited evidence that topical steroids plus antibiotics improved symptoms compared with antibiotics alone. Short courses of oral steroids can cause behavioural changes such as increased appetite and weight gain.

Benefits: We found one systematic review (search date 2002).[15] **Oral steroids versus placebo:** The systematic review identified three placebo controlled RCTs of oral steroids (either prednisone or dexamethasone) versus placebo (108 children with otitis media with effusion). Presence of effusion was assessed clinically by pneumatic otoscopy, tympanometry, and audiometry after 7–14 days of treatment. There was no significant difference in mean improvement at 2 weeks after treatment (AR of clearance compared with placebo +21%, 95% CI –3% to +44%). There were no available summary data beyond 8 weeks. **Oral corticosteroids plus antibiotic versus antibiotic alone:** The systematic review identified four RCTs (274 children) comparing antibiotic (cefixime, amoxycillin [amoxycillin], or sulfisoxazole) plus oral steroids (bethamethasone or prednisone) versus antibiotic alone.[15] Time to measurement of results varied from 1 week to 6 months. There was a significant difference in clearance rates with combined treatment compared with antibiotic alone (ARR for non-clearance *v* antibiotic alone at 2 weeks 32%, 95% CI 20% to 50%), but there was significant heterogeneity among studies (P < 0.01). **Topical steroids versus placebo:** The systematic review identified one RCT (45 children), which found no significant difference between intranasal dexamethasone and placebo for persistence of effusion at 3 weeks (OR 2.12, 95% CI 0.65 to 6.90).[16] **Topical steroids plus antibiotics:** The systematic review identified one RCT (59 children with chronic middle ear infection, ages 3–11 years), which found that intranasal steroids plus antibiotics compared with antibiotics plus placebo significantly reduced effusions at 4 and 8 weeks (CI not reported; P < 0.05).[17] It found that at 12 weeks intranasal steroids plus antibiotics significantly improved symptoms compared with antibiotics.

Harms: Short courses of oral steroids can cause behavioural changes, increased appetite, and weight gain. Idiosyncratic reactions have been reported, such as avascular necrosis of the femoral head and fatal varicella infections.

Comment: The trials were small. Use of secondary care populations weakens the applicability of results to primary care.

OPTION ANTIHISTAMINES AND DECONGESTANTS

One systematic review found no significant difference between antihistamines plus decongestants and placebo in clearance of effusion in children with otitis media with effusion after 4 weeks.

Benefits: We found one systematic review (search date 1992, 4 placebo controlled RCTs, 1202 infants and older children, age range not stated).[9] Treatment lasted for 4 weeks. Meta-analysis found no significant difference between antihistamine–decongestants and placebo in effusion clearance rate, as assessed by history, otoscopy, and tympanometry (hierarchical Bayes meta-analysis: change in probability –0.009, 95% CI –0.036 to +0.054).

Harms: Adverse effects of antihistamines include hyperactivity, insomnia, drowsiness, behavioural change, blood pressure variability, and seizures. One RCT in healthy volunteers found that decongestant nose drops given for 3 weeks or more led to iatrogenic rhinitis.[18]

Comment: The RCTs included clinically heterogeneous groups (e.g. infants and older children) and selected individuals from ambulatory care or waiting lists. There were too few children with allergies for subgroup analysis.

OPTION MUCOLYTICS

One systematic review found that 1–3 month courses of carbocisteine or carbocisteine lysine had no significant effect on resolution of effusion compared with placebo or no treatment. Three small RCTs found conflicting results on the effects of bromhexine.

Benefits: We found one systematic review (search date 1993, 6 RCTs, 428 children ages 3–11 years and 2 adults) comparing carbocisteine, carbocisteine lysine, or both, versus placebo or no treatment.[19]

Treatment lasted for 15–90 days. Meta-analysis found a greater frequency of complete resolution with mucolytics, but this did not quite reach significance (178 children; 80/81 [99%] with treatment v 54/98 [55%] with placebo; OR 2.25, 95% CI 0.97 to 5.22). Three small RCTs (155 children and 195 ears) comparing another mucolytic, namely bromhexine, versus placebo found conflicting results.[20–22]

Harms: The review gave no information on adverse effects.[19] Reported adverse effects of carbocisteine include gastric irritation, nausea, and rashes.

Comment: The RCTs were heterogeneous in their clinical outcomes and treatment duration.

OPTION AUTOINFLATION

One systematic review has found benefit from autoinflation using a nasal balloon, although some children may find autoinflation difficult. The value of other methods of autoinflation has not yet been adequately evaluated.

Benefits: We found one systematic review (search date not stated, 6 RCTs, age range not stated) comparing autoinflation versus no treatment.[23] Improvement was variously defined as being effusion free, improved tympanogram, or improvement in hearing. The RCTs assessing different treatment effects yielded different results. However, trials evaluating nasal balloons in children found a homogeneous effect size (3 RCTs, 386 children). Children treated with a purpose manufactured nasal balloon were more likely than control children to improve within 1 week to 3 months using tympanometric and audiometric criteria (OR 3.53, 95% CI 2.03 to 6.14).[23]

Harms: We found no reports of serious adverse effects.

Comment: The Eustachian tubes can be inflated by several methods, including blowing up a balloon through a plastic tube inserted into the nostril. In one RCT, 12% of children aged 3–10 years were unable to use the balloon.[24] Most trials appeared not to use intention to treat analysis, and beneficial effects were noted only when adherence was 70% or greater. The evidence is suboptimal because different methods were used, outcome assessments were not blinded, and follow up was short. Other methods of autoinflation (such as inflating a carnival blower through the nostril or forcible exhalation through the nostrils, with closed mouth, into an anaesthetic mask with a flowmeter attachment) have not been adequately evaluated.

OPTION SURGERY

We found no RCTs comparing surgery versus no treatment. One systematic review found limited evidence that surgery (insertion of grommets, adenoidectomy, or both) resulted in short term hearing gain. Grommets and adenoidectomy alone were similarly effective. One subsequent RCT found that grommets plus adenoidectomy was more effective than adenotonsillectomy or grommets either alone or combined. Three subsequent RCTs found no benefit in language development with grommets. We found no good evidence on the effects of tonsillectomy.

Otitis media with effusion

Benefits: We found one systematic review (search date 1992, 19 RCTs) of surgery in children with otitis media with effusion.[25] Nine RCTs reported the data per child (1508 children) and 10 reported data per ear (1452 children). None were placebo controlled, although some used children as their own controls. Outcomes were mean change in audiometry, tympanometry, and clinical and otoscopic evidence of otitis media with effusion. The review concluded that evidence for the effectiveness of surgical interventions was inconsistent. **Grommets:** The review reported a mean 12 dB improvement in hearing after insertion of grommets (CI not provided).[25] However, the authors concluded that this was difficult to interpret clinically. We found three subsequent RCTs.[26–28] The first RCT (187 children aged 16–24 months) compared treatment with ventilation tubes versus watchful waiting.[26] It found that verbal comprehension improved more in the children treated with ventilation tubes (significance not reported) and that expressive language improved more, by 1 month, in the children treated with ventilation tubes (significance not reported). However, the trial reported that the groups were not equivalent at baseline, with an initially higher level of educational development in children in the watchful waiting group. The second RCT (429 children aged ≤3 years) compared early versus delayed insertion of tympanostomy tubes.[27] It found no significant effect on language development measured on a range of scales. The third RCT (182 children, mean age 2.9 years) found that early insertion of bilateral grommets significantly reduced behavioural problems at 9 months compared with watchful waiting (24 withdrawals from watchful waiting, 8 from early surgery, no intention to treat analysis: Richman behaviour check list 25/84 [30%] *v* 31/66 [47%]; RR 0.63, 95% CI 0.30 to 0.96).[28] **Grommets plus adenoidectomy:** The review found that adenoidectomy gave little additional benefit over grommets alone in terms of mean hearing gain, which varied from 1.1–2.6 dB.[25] A subsequent RCT (228 children, ages 2–9 years) compared adenotonsillectomy or adenoidectomy (analysed together) versus neither procedure.[29] All children had a grommet inserted into one ear. Outcomes were mean audiometric change, and tympanometric and otoscopic clearance assessed over 6 months to 10 years after treatment. The trial found improved tympanometric and otoscopic clearance when combining adenoidectomy with grommets versus grommets alone or no surgery. Median duration of glue ear assessed tympanometrically was reduced from 7.8 years without treatment to 4.9 years with grommets, 4 years with adenoidectomy, and 2.8 years with adenoidectomy and grommets combined. The difference between duration for adenoidectomy alone and grommets alone was not significant (CI not reported; P = 0.2), but all other comparisons were significant. **Tonsillectomy:** The review found no good RCTs of tonsillectomy alone in otitis media with effusion.[25]

Harms: We found one systematic review (search date 1999), which found that transient otorrhoea was common postoperatively (7 studies, 1522 children: incidence 16%, 95% CI 14% to 18%) and later (23 studies, 5491 people: incidence 26%, 95% CI 25% to 27%).[30] Recurrent ear discharge was also common (7 studies, 1144 children: incidence 7.4%, 95% CI 6% to 9%) and often became chronic (3 studies, 451 children: incidence 3.8%, 95% CI 2% to 6%). A systematic review of observational and experimental studies (search date 1998) of the complications following grommet insertion found a reported prevalence of tympanosclerosis in 39–65% of ventilated ears as opposed to 0–10% of untreated ears.[31] Partial atrophy was noted in 16–73% of ears treated and in 5–31% of those untreated. Atelectasis ranged from 10–37% of ears treated as opposed to 1–20% of those untreated, and attic retraction between 10–52% and 29–40%, respectively. The average hearing loss associated with these abnormalities was less than 5 dB. **Adenoidectomy:** Deaths have been reported in 1/16 700–25 000 children when combined with tonsillectomy (no figures provided for adenoidectomy alone) and postoperative haemorrhage occurred in 0.5%.[32]

Comment: About half of children who have grommets inserted will undergo reinsertion within 5 years.[33] Resolution after surgery takes longer in younger children and in those whose parents smoke, irrespective of treatment.[28]

Substantive changes

Corticosteroids Systematic review updated;[15] conclusions unchanged.

REFERENCES

1. Williamson IG, Dunleavey J, Bain J, et al. The natural history of otitis media with effusion: a three year study of the incidence and prevalence of abnormal tympanograms in four SW Hampshire infant and first schools. *J Laryngol Otol* 1994;108:930–934.
2. Teele D, Klein J, Rosner B. Epidemiology of otitis media during the first seven years of life in children in greater Boston: a prospective, cohort study. *J Infect Dis* 1989;160:83–94.
3. Strachan DP, Cook DG. Health effects of passive smoking. 4. Passive smoking, middle ear disease and adenotonsillectomy in children. *Thorax* 1998;53:50–56. Search date 1997; primary sources Medline and Embase.
4. Paradise JL, Rockette HE, Colborn DK, et al. Otitis media in 2253 Pittsburgh area infants: prevalence and risk factors during the first two years of life. *Pediatrics* 1997;99:318–333.
5. Haggard M, Hughes E. *Objectives, values and methods of screening children's hearing — a review of the literature*. London: HMSO, 1991.
6. Zeilhuis GA, Rach GH, Broek PV. Screening for otitis media with effusion in pre-school children. *Lancet* 1989;1:311–314.
7. Fiellau-Nikolajsen M. Tympanometry in three year old children: prevalence and spontaneous course of MEE. *Ann Otol Rhinol Laryngol* 1980;89(Suppl 68):233–237.
8. Bennett KE, Haggard MP. Behaviour and cognitive outcomes in middle ear disease. *Arch Dis Child* 1999;80:28–35.
9. Stool SE, Berg SO, Berman S, et al. *Otitis media with effusion in young children: clinical practice guideline number 12.* AHCPR Publication 94–0622. Rockville, Maryland: Agency for Health Care Policy and Research, Public Health Service, United States Department of Health and Human Services, July, 1994. Search date 1992; primary sources online database of National Library of Medicine and 10 specialised bibliographic databases.
10. Cantekin EI, McGuire TW. Antibiotics are not effective for otitis media with effusion: reanalysis of meta-analysis. *Otorhinolaryngol Nova* 1998;8:214–222. Search date 1997; primary sources RCTs in refereed journals and proceedings published between 1980 and 1997 in English language publications.
11. Computerised clinical information system. Denver, Colorado: Micromedex Inc, June 1993.
12. Little P, Gould C, Williamson I, et al. Reattendance and complications in a randomised trial of prescribing strategies for sore throat: the medicalising effect of prescribing antibiotics. *BMJ* 1997;315:350–352.
13. Wise R, Hart T, Cars O, et al. Antimicrobial resistance is a major threat to public health [Editorial]. *BMJ* 1998;317:609–610.
14. Williams RL, Chalmers TC, Strange KC, et al. Use of antibiotics in preventing recurrent acute otitis media and in treating otitis media with effusion: a meta-analytic attempt to resolve the brouhaha. *JAMA* 1993;270:1344–1351. Search date 1993; primary sources Medline and Current Contents.
15. Butler CC, van der Voort JH. Oral or nasal steroids for hearing loss associated with otitis media with effusion in children. In: The Cochrane Library, Issue 4, 2002. Oxford: Update Software. Search date 2002; primary sources Cochrane Controlled Trials Register, Embase, and Medline.
16. Shapiro GG, Bierman CW, Furukuwa CT, et al. Treatment of persistent eustacian tube dysfunction with aerosolised nasal dexamethasone phosphate versus placebo. *Annals of Allergy* 1982;49:81–85.
17. Tracy TM, Demain JG, Hoffman KM, et al. Intranasal beclomethasone as an adjunct to treatment of chronic middle ear effusion. *Ann Allergy Asthma Immunol* 1998;80:198–206.
18. Graf P. Rhinitis medicamentosa: aspects of pathophysiology and treatment. *Eur J Allergy Clin Immunol* 1997;52(Suppl 40):28–34.
19. Pignataro O, Pignataro LD, Gallus G, et al. Otitis media with effusion and S-carboxymethylcysteine and/or its lysine salt: a critical overview. *Int J Pediatr Otorhinolaryngol* 1996;35:231–241. Search date 1993; primary sources Medline, Embase, and Biosis.

20. Van der Merwe J, Wagenfeld DJ. The negative effects of mucolytics in otitis media with effusion. *S Afr Med J* 1987;72:625–626.
21. Stewart IA, Guy AM, Allison RS, Thomson NJ. Bromhexine in the treatment of otitis media with effusion. *Clin Otolaryngol* 1985;10:145–149.
22. Roydhouse N. Bromhexine for otitis media with effusion. *N Z Med J* 1981;94:373–375.
23. Reidpath DD, Glasziou PP, Del Mar C. Systematic review of autoinflation for treatment of glue ear in children. *BMJ* 1999;318:1177–1178. Search date not stated; primary sources Medline, Cochrane Library, and pharmaceutical company database.
24. Blanshard JD, Maw AR, Bawden R. Conservative treatment of otitis media with effusion by autoinflation of the middle ear. *Clin Otolaryngol* 1993;18:188–192.
25. University of York. Centre for Reviews and Dissemination. 1992. The treatment of persistent glue ear in children. Effective Health Care 1(4). Search date 1992; primary sources BIDS, Medline, and Embase.
26. Rovers MM, Stratman H, Ingels K, et al. The effect of ventilation tubes on language development in infants with otitis media with effusion: a randomised trial. *Pediatrics* 2000;106:3–42.
27. Paradise J, Feldman HM, Campbell TF, et al. Effect of early or delayed insertion of tympanostomy tubes for persistent otitis media on developmental outcomes at the age of three years. *N Engl J Med* 2001;344:1179–1187.
28. Wilks J, Maw R, Peters TJ, et al. Randomised controlled trial of early surgery versus watchful waiting for glue ear: The effect on behavioural problems in pre-school children. *Clin Otol Allied Sci* 2000;25:209–214.
29. Maw R, Bawden R. Spontaneous resolution of severe chronic glue ear in children and the effect of adenoidectomy, tonsillectomy, and insertion of ventilation tubes. *BMJ* 1993;306:756–760.
30. Kay DJ, Nelson M, Rosenfeld RM. Meta-analysis of tympanostomy tube sequelae. *Otolaryngol Head Neck Surg* 2001;124:374–380. Search date 1999; primary sources Medline and hand searches.
31. Schilder AG. Assessment of complications of the conditions and of the treatment of otitis media with effusion. *Int J Pediatr Otolaryngol* 1999;49(Suppl 1):S247–S251. Search date 1998; primary sources not stated.
32. Yardley MP. Tonsillectomy, adenoidectomy and adenotonsillectomy; are they safe day case procedures. *J Laryngol Otol* 1992;106:299–300.
33. Maw AR. Development of tympanosclerosis in children with otitis media with effusion and ventilation tubes. *J Laryngol Otol* 1991;105:614–617.

Ian Williamson
Senior Lecturer in Primary Medical Care
The University of Southampton
Southampton
UK

Competing interests: None declared.

Seasonal allergic rhinitis

Search date January 2003

Aziz Sheikh, Sukhmeet Panesar, and Sangeeta Dhami

QUESTIONS

INTERVENTIONS

To be covered in future updates

Effects of prophylactic treatments: allergen avoidance; sodium cromoglycate; immunotherapy (intranasal, subcutaneous, and sublingual); homeopathy; anti-immunoglobulin E; and corticosteroids (intranasal and systemic).

Seasonal allergic rhinitis in children under 12 years of age.

See glossary, p 630

Key Messages

Quality of life

- **Oral fexofenadine** Three RCTs found that fexofenadine improved quality of life and rhinitis symptoms compared with placebo.
- **Oral leukotriene receptor antagonists** Two large RCTs found that oral montelukast improved quality of life compared with placebo.
- **Oral leukotriene receptor antagonists plus oral antihistamines** Two RCTs found that oral montelukast plus oral loratadine improved quality of life compared with loratadine alone or placebo.
- **Intranasal antihistamines; intranasal ipratropium bromide; oral decongestants; oral decongestants plus oral antihistamines; other oral antihistamines** We found no RCTs evaluating the effects of these interventions on quality of life.

Seasonal allergic rhinitis

Rhinitis symptoms

- **Intranasal levocabastine** RCTs found that intranasal levocabastine improved symptoms of seasonal allergic rhinitis compared with placebo.
- **Oral antihistamines (acrivastine, azatadine, brompheniramine, cetirizine, ebastine, fexofenadine, loratadine, or mizolastine)** Numerous RCTs have found that oral antihistamines (acrivastine, azatadine, brompheniramine, cetirizine, ebastine, loratadine, or mizolastine) improved rhinitis symptoms compared with placebo. Drowsiness, sedation, and somnolence were the most commonly reported adverse effects.
- **Oral pseudoephedrine plus oral antihistamines** RCTs have found that pseudoephedrine plus oral antihistamines (fexofenadine, acrivastine, cetirizine, terfenadine, triprolidine, loratadine, or azatadine) improved overall symptoms of seasonal allergic rhinitis compared with pseudoephedrine or oral antihistamine or placebo alone. The most common adverse effects reported with combination treatment were headache and insomnia.
- **Oral leukotriene receptor antagonists** Two large RCTs found that oral montelukast improved daytime nasal symptom score compared with placebo.
- **Oral leukotriene receptor antagonists plus oral antihistamines** Two RCTs found that oral montelukast plus oral loratadine improved nasal symptoms compared with placebo, although they found conflicting effects compared with single treatments.
- **Oral astemizole** RCTs have found that astemizole versus placebo improves rhinitis symptoms but astemizole has been associated with prolongation of the QTc interval, and may induce ventricular arrhythmias.
- **Oral terfenadine** RCTs have found conflicting results about effectiveness of terfenadine versus placebo on rhinitis symptoms. Terfenadine is associated with risk of fatal cardiac toxicity if used in conjunction with macrolide antibiotics, oral antifungal agents, or grapefruit juice.
- **Intranasal azelastine** RCTs have found conflicting results about effectiveness of intranasal azelastine versus placebo on symptoms of seasonal allergic rhinitis. Two small RCTs found no significant difference in nasal symptoms between intranasal antihistamines (azelastine, levocabastine) and oral antihistamines (cetirizine, terfenadine)
- **Intranasal ipratropium bromide** We found no systematic review or published RCTs.

DEFINITION Seasonal allergic rhinitis is a symptom complex that may affect several organ systems. Symptoms will typically consist of seasonal sneezing, nasal itching, nasal blockage, and watery nasal discharge.[1] Eye symptoms (red eyes, itchy eyes, and tearing) are common. Other symptoms may include peak seasonal coughing, wheezing, and shortness of breath, oral allergy syndrome (manifesting as an itchy swollen oropharynx on eating stoned fruits), and systemic symptoms such as tiredness, fever, a pressure sensation in the head, and itchiness. Confirming the presence of pollen hypersensitivity using objective allergy tests such as skin prick tests, detection of serum specific IgE, and nasal provocation challenge testing may improve diagnostic accuracy.

INCIDENCE/ PREVALENCE Seasonal allergic rhinitis is found throughout the world. Epidemiological evidence suggests that there is considerable geographical variation in its prevalence. Prevalence is highest in socioeconomically developed countries, where the condition may affect as much as 25% of the population.[2–4] Prevalence and severity are increasing. It is thought that improved living standards and reduced risk of childhood infections may lead to immune deviation of T helper cells in early life, which may increase susceptibility to seasonal allergic rhinitis (the so called "hygiene hypothesis").[5,6] Although people of all ages may be affected, the peak age of onset is adolescence.[7]

AETIOLOGY/ RISK FACTORS The symptoms of seasonal allergic rhinitis are caused by an IgE mediated type 1 hypersensitivity reaction to grass, tree, or weed pollen. Allergy to other seasonal aeroallergens such as fungal spores may also provoke symptoms. Typically, symptoms become worse during the relevant pollen season and in the open, when pollen exposure is increased. Risk factors include a personal or family history of atopy or other allergic disorders, male sex, birth order (increased risk being seen in first born), and small family size.[8,9]

PROGNOSIS Seasonal allergic rhinitis may impair quality of life, interfering with work, sleep, and recreational activities.[10] Other allergic problems such as asthma and eczema frequently coexist, adding to the impact of rhinitis.[11]

AIMS OF INTERVENTION Treatments for seasonal allergic rhinitis aim to minimise or eliminate symptoms, optimise quality of life, and reduce the risk of developing coexistent disease.

OUTCOMES We extracted data on the following outcomes: quality of life, days off school/work, rhinitis symptom scores (as described in studies), medication usage and medication usage scores (as defined in studies), and adverse effects. Although most of these outcome measures have face validity, few have been formally validated. Few studies used validated quality of life measures.

METHODS *Clinical Evidence* search and appraisal January 2003.

QUESTION **What are the effects of treatments for symptoms of seasonal allergic rhinitis?**

OPTION **ORAL ANTIHISTAMINES**

Three RCTs found that fexofenadine improved quality of life and rhinitis symptoms compared with placebo. RCTs have found that astemizole improves rhinitis symptoms compared with placebo, although astemizole has been associated with prolongation of the QTc interval, and may induce ventricular arrhythmias. RCTs have found conflicting results about the effectiveness of terfenadine versus placebo on rhinitis symptoms. Terfenadine is associated with risk of fatal cardiac toxicity if used with macrolide antibiotics, oral antifungal agents, or grapefruit juice. Numerous RCTs have found that other oral antihistamines (acrivastine, azatadine, brompheniramine, cetirizine, ebastine, loratadine, or mizolastine) improved rhinitis symptoms compared with placebo. Drowsiness, sedation, and somnolence were the most commonly reported adverse effects.

Benefits: We found no systematic review. We found numerous RCTs comparing oral antihistamines versus placebo or other antihistamines, but only three RCTs evaluated quality of life as an outcome measure.[12–14] Most of the RCTs used symptom scores to evaluate the effectiveness of oral antihistamines on rhinitis symptoms (see tables A, B, and C on web extra). **Acrivastine:** Three RCTs found that acrivastine (16–32 mg/day) significantly reduced rhinitis symptoms compared with placebo.[15–17] **Astemizole:** Eight RCTs found that astemizole (10 mg once daily or 10 or 25 mg once weekly) reduced overall symptoms compared with placebo.[18–25] One RCT did not specify either the dose of treatment or the frequency of its administration.[25] **Azatadine:** One small RCT (crossover, 38 people aged > 12 years with both asthma and rhinitis) found no significant difference in rhinitis symptoms between adding azatadine (1 mg twice daily) or placebo to the existing treatment regimen (not specified).[26] **Brompheniramine:** Two large RCTs comparing brompheniramine (8–24 mg/day) versus terfenadine (60–120 mg/day) or placebo found that brompheniramine significantly improved rhinitis symptoms compared with placebo.[27,28] **Cetirizine:** Six RCTs comparing cetirizine (10 mg/day) versus placebo found that cetirizine significantly improved rhinitis symptoms.[29–34] **Ebastine:** We found two RCTs comparing ebastine (10–40 mg/day) versus placebo,[35,36] and one RCT comparing ebastine (10 or 20 mg/day) versus loratadine (10 mg/day) or placebo.[37] All three RCTs found that ebastine significantly improved rhinitis symptoms compared with placebo. **Fexofenadine:** We found eight RCTs.[12–14,38–41] Three of these RCTs reported on quality of life. The first RCT (multicentre, 845 people aged 12–65 years with history of seasonal allergic rhinitis and positive skin test to an unspecified allergen) compared fexofenadine (120 or 180 mg/day) versus placebo over 2 weeks.[12] Outcomes were assessed with respect to quality of life (Rhinoconjunctivitis Quality of Life Questionnaire score — see glossary, p 630); work, classroom, and daily activity impairment (Work Productivity and Activity Impairment instrument — see glossary, p 631); and general health (SF-36 Health Survey — see glossary, p 631).The RCT found that fexofenadine significantly improved quality of life compared with placebo ($P \leq 0.006$) and reduced work and daily activity impairment ($P \leq 0.004$). The RCT found no significant difference in classroom impairment between fexofenadine and placebo. The second RCT (multicentre, 1948 people aged 11–68 years with 2 year history of seasonal allergic rhinitis and positive skin test to grass and tree allergens) also found that fexofenadine (120 mg/day) significantly improved quality of life compared with placebo ($P \leq 0.05$) and also reduced work impairment ($P \leq 0.05$).[13] The third RCT (multicentre, 688 people aged 12–75 years with a 2 year history of seasonal allergic rhinitis and a positive skin test for grass, tree pollen, or both) compared fexofenadine (120 mg/day) versus loratadine (10 mg/day) or placebo over 2 weeks.[14] It found that fexofenadine significantly improved quality of life compared with placebo ($P < 0.005$) and 24 hour reflective symptom scores compared with baseline ($P < 0.0001$). The remaining five RCTs did not report on quality of life.[38–41] All found that fexofenadine (80–240 mg/day) significantly improved rhinitis symptoms compared with placebo. **Loratadine/desloratadine:** Ten RCTs comparing loratadine versus placebo or other antihistamines (clemastine, mequitazine, terfenadine) found that loratadine reduced rhinitis symptom scores more than placebo.[42–51] One further RCT (337 people aged ≥ 12 years or with 2 year history of seasonal allergic rhinitis) found that, over 2 weeks, desloratadine (5 mg/day) reduced total rhinitis symptom score more than placebo ($P < 0.01$).[52] **Mizolastine:** Two RCTs found that mizolastine (10 or 15 mg/day) significantly reduced physician-rated overall symptom scores compared with placebo ($P < 0.005$), but found no significant difference between mizolastine 5 mg daily and placebo.[53,54] **Terfenadine:** We found 15 RCTs comparing terfenadine versus placebo or other antihistamines.[30,33,35,45–47,54–62] Eight of the RCTs found that terfenadine significantly reduced overall subject-rated symptom scores compared with placebo.[45–47,54–58] The seven other RCTs found no significant difference in subject-rated overall rhinitis symptom scores with terfenadine versus placebo.[30,33,35,59–62] **Other antihistamines:** We found no RCTs.

Harms: Most of the RCTs reported drowsiness, sedation, or somnolence as a common adverse effect (see tables A, B, and C on web extra). **Astemizole:** Astemizole has been associated with prolongation of the QTc interval, and thus has the potential to induce ventricular arrhythmias.[63] **Fexofenadine:** Two RCTs did not report specifically on any adverse effects.[12,13] One RCT found no significant difference in adverse effects between fexofenadine and placebo or loratadine.[14] **Desloratadine:** One RCT found no significant difference in adverse effects between desloratadine and placebo.[49] **Terfenadine:** Terfenadine is associated with risk of fatal cardiac toxicity if used in conjunction with macrolide antibiotics, oral antifungal agents, or grapefruit juice.[64] **Other antihistamines:** We found one cohort study (postmarketing surveillance of fexofenadine, acrivastine, cetirizine, and loratadine involving 43 363 people; the main outcome measure was sedation or drowsiness).[65] It found significantly higher incidence of sedation for acrivastine (OR 2.79, 95% CI 1.69 to 4.58; $P < 0.0001$) and cetirizine (OR 3.53, 95% CI 2.07 to 5.42; $P < 0.0001$) compared with loratadine, but found no difference between fexofenadine versus loratadine (OR 0.63, 95% CI 0.36 to 1.11; $P = 0.1$). No increase in risk of accident or injury was found with any of the four antihistamines.[65]

Comment: None.

OPTION INTRANASAL ANTIHISTAMINES

We found no systematic review or RCTs evaluating the effects of intranasal antihistamines on quality of life. One meta-analysis of 11 RCTs (10 unpublished) found that intranasal levocabastine improves symptoms of seasonal allergic rhinitis compared with placebo. Four RCTs found conflicting results on effectiveness of intranasal azelastine versus placebo on symptoms of seasonal allergic rhinitis. Two small RCTs found no significant difference in nasal symptoms between intranasal antihistamines (azelastine, levocabastine) and oral antihistamines (cetirizine, terfenadine).

Benefits: We found no systematic review or RCTs evaluating the effect of intranasal antihistamines on quality of life. **Levocabastine versus placebo:** We found one meta-analysis (11 RCTs, only 1 published study, total of 693 people, no significant heterogeneity found across individual studies) assessing global effectiveness of intranasal levocabastine versus placebo.[66] Global effectiveness was defined as response or no response of rhinitis symptoms to treatment, assessed by study investigators. The meta-analysis found that the global effectiveness of levocabastine was significantly better than placebo (pooled OR 2.30, 95% CI 1.70 to 3.11; $P < 0.001$). One of two additional levocabastine RCTs not included in the meta-analysis found that levocabastine significantly reduced subject rated rhinitis symptoms compared with placebo over a 4 week period ($P < 0.05$).[67] The second levocabastine trial was small (16 people).[68] It found no significant difference in symptoms between the active and placebo treated groups. **Azelastine versus placebo:** We found four RCTs comparing effects of azelastine versus placebo on rhinitis symptoms.[69–72] The first RCT (160 people aged 18–65 years with at least a 3 year history of seasonal allergic rhinitis) compared intranasal azelastine (1.12 mg/day) versus intranasal beclomethasone (0.4 mg/day) or placebo for 2 weeks.[69] Six symptoms (sneezing, nasal itching, rhinorrhoea, nasal stuffiness, eye itching, and watery eyes) were scored daily by the participants. The RCT found that azelastine significantly reduced subject rated rhinitis symptom scores compared with placebo ($P < 0.05$; summary data unavailable). The second RCT (multicentre, 262 people aged > 12 years with a history of seasonal allergic rhinitis for at least 2 years and positive skin test for unspecified seasonal allergens) compared intranasal azelastine (0.52–1.04 mg/day) versus oral chlorpheniramine (24 mg/day) versus placebo for 4 weeks.[70] Efficacy was measured as changes from baseline in total and major symptom complex severity scores. Symptoms included runny nose or sniffles; itchy nose; watery eyes; itchy eyes, ears, throat or palate; cough; postnasal drip; stuffiness; nose blows; and sneezes. The RCT found no significant difference between azelastine and placebo in total subject rated symptom scores 4 weeks after randomisation. The third RCT (30 people aged 18–53 years with 2 year history of seasonal allergic rhinitis and positive skin test to grass or Parietaria) found no significant difference between intranasal azelastine (0.28–0.56 mg/day) and placebo in symptoms scores (summary data or P value not provided).[71] The fourth RCT (99 people, aged 19–61 with at least a 1 year history of seasonal allergic rhinitis) found that azelastine decreased symptoms compared with placebo at 7 days, although statistical significance depended on how "response" was defined (decrease in total ocular and nasal scores by ≥ 50%, with fewer than 3 cetirizine rescue tablets in the first 7 days: 43% with azelastine *v* 30% on placebo [$P = 0.18$]; decrease of total ocular and nasal scores by ≥ 50% at day 7, with no cetirizine rescue tablets: 49% with azelastine *v* 28% with placebo [$P = 0.04$]).[72] **Intranasal versus oral antihistamines:** We found two small double blind RCTs comparing intranasal antihistamines with systemic antihistamines.[73,74] Both RCTs found no significant difference in nasal symptoms between intranasal antihistamines (azelastine, levocabastine) and oral antihistamines (cetirizine, terfenadine).

Harms: No serious adverse effects were reported in these trials. Frequency of adverse effects was similar in treatment and placebo arms. The most common adverse effects were sinusitis and headache.

Comment: **Intranasal versus oral antihistamines:** The two RCTs comparing topical with systemic antihistamines may have been underpowered to detect any significant difference between these two classes of treatment.[73,74]

OPTION ORAL DECONGESTANTS

We found no systematic review or RCTs evaluating the effect of oral decongestants on quality of life. RCTs have found that pseudoephedrine plus oral antihistamines (fexofenadine, acrivastine, cetirizine, terfenadine, triprolidine, loratadine, or azatadine) improved overall symptoms of seasonal allergic rhinitis compared with pseudoephedrine, oral antihistamine, or placebo. The most common adverse effects reported with combination treatment were headache and insomnia.

Benefits: We found no systematic review or RCTs evaluating the effect of oral decongestants on quality of life. We found no RCTs only comparing oral decongestants versus placebo. We found eight RCTs comparing the effects on rhinitis symptoms of oral decongestants plus oral antihistamines versus either decongestant alone, antihistamine alone, or placebo.[75–82] **Pseudoephedrine plus fexofenadine:** The first RCT (651 people aged 12–65 years with positive skin prick ragweed extract and clinical response to antihistamines) compared sustained release pseudoephedrine (120 mg twice daily) plus fexofenadine (60 mg twice daily) versus pseudoephedrine (120 mg twice daily) or fexofenadine (60 mg twice daily) for 2 weeks.[75] It found that pseudoephedrine plus fexofenadine reduced symptom scores for sneezing compared with pseudoephidrine ($P < 0.0001$); two or more of itchy nose, palate, or throat ($P = 0.002$); and itchy, watery, red eyes ($P = 0.0006$). Pseudoephedrine plus fexofenadine reduced nasal congestion scores compared with fexofenadine ($P = 0.0005$). **Pseudoephedrine plus acrivastine:** The second RCT (multicentre, double blind, 702 people aged ≥ 12 years with at least 2 year history of seasonal allergic rhinitis symptoms during the ragweed pollen season and a positive skin test for ragweed antigen) compared pseudoephedrine (60 mg/day) plus acrivastine (8 mg/day) versus pseudoephedrine (60 mg/day) or acrivastine (8 mg/day) or placebo for 2 weeks.[76] It found that pseudoephedrine plus acrivastine significantly reduced the mean nasal congestion scores compared with acrivastine alone ($P < 0.001$) and significantly improved the mean diary symptom scores from baseline when compared with acrivastine, pseudoephedrine, or placebo ($P < 0.01$). **Pseudoephedrine plus cetirizine:** The third RCT (687 people aged 12–65 years with history of pollen associated allergic rhinitis and positive skin test to unspecified seasonal allergens) compared sustained release pseudoephedrine (120 mg twice daily) plus cetirizine (5 mg twice daily) versus pseudoephedrine or cetirizine.[77] The main outcome measure was based on five symptoms (blocked nose, sneezing, runny nose, itchy nose, and itchy eyes) assessed by participants over the 2 week treatment period. The RCT found that pseudoephedrine plus cetirizine improved symptoms of sneezing, runny nose, itchy nose, and itchy eyes compared with pseudoephedrine or cetirizine (each outcome, $P < 0.001$) but not blocked nose. **Pseudoephedrine plus terfenadine:** The fourth RCT (41 people, pollen sensitivity status not provided) found that sustained release pseudoephedrine (120 mg twice daily) plus terfenadine (60 mg twice daily) versus terfenadine (60 mg twice daily) improved overall symptoms ($P < 0.05$) when assessed by both the physician and the participant.[78] **Pseudoephedrine plus triprolidine:** The fifth RCT (crossover, 40 people aged 22–47 years with clinical history of seasonal allergic rhinitis and positive skin test to mixed grasses, flowers, moulds, trees, house dust extract, and house dust mite) compared pseudoephedrine (60 mg 3 times daily) plus triprolidine (2.5 mg 3 times daily) versus pseudoephedrine alone, triprolidine alone, or placebo for 10 weeks.[79] Efficacy was measured with participant assessed symptom score. The RCT found that pseudoephedrine plus triprolidine gave the lowest sneezing, runny nose, and eye irritation score but pseudoephedrine alone gave the lowest blocked nose score. **Pseudoephedrine plus loratadine:** The sixth RCT (multicentre, 847 people aged 12–60 years with history of moderate or severe seasonal allergic rhinitis and positive skin test to ragweed and other prevalent seasonal allergens) compared pseudoephedrine (240 mg/day) plus loratadine (10 mg/day) versus pseudoephedrine alone, loratadine alone, or placebo for 2 weeks.[80] It found that pseudoephedrine plus loratadine or loratadine alone reduced total symptom scores ($P \leq 0.01$) compared with pseudoephedrine or placebo. The seventh RCT (multicentre, 435 people aged 12–60 years with history of moderate to severe symptoms of seasonal allergic rhinitis and positive skin test to unspecified allergens) compared modified release pseudoephedrine (120 mg twice daily) plus loratadine (5 mg twice daily) versus pseudoephedrine, loratadine, or placebo.[81] It found that pseudoephedrine plus loratadine versus either pseudoephedrine or placebo improved mean total symptom scores ($P < 0.05$). **Pseudoephedrine plus azatadine:** The eighth RCT (65 people aged 14–72 years with severe seasonal allergic rhinitis assessed by symptom scoring method) compared pseudoephedrine (60 mg twice daily) plus azatadine (1 mg twice daily) versus pseudoephedrine or placebo for 2 weeks.[82] It found that pseudoephedrine plus azatadine improved signs and symptoms of seasonal allergic rhinitis compared with placebo (74% people with pseudoephedrine plus azatadine *v* 29% people with placebo). **Other decongestants:** We found no RCTs.

Harms: The first RCT found no significant difference in the incidence of adverse effects between pseudoephedrine plus fexofenadine and pseudoephedrine alone.[75] It found that combination treatment increased adverse effects compared with fexofenadine alone ($P < 0.001$). Headache and insomnia were the most commonly reported adverse effects. The second RCT found a higher incidence of adverse effects (dry mouth, somnolence, nervousness, insomnia) with pseudoephedrine plus acrivastine compared with placebo.[76] The third RCT found no significant difference in the incidence of adverse effects between pseudoephedrine plus cetirizine and pseudoephedrine alone or cetirizine alone.[77] The fourth RCT did not compare the incidence of adverse effects between pseudoephedrine plus terfenadine versus terfenadine alone.[78] Terfenadine has been associated with serious adverse effects (see harms of oral antihistamines, p 625). The fifth RCT reported drowsiness with pseudoephedrine plus triprolidine and triprolidine alone.[79] Dry mouth was reported with combination treatment and pseudoephedrine alone. The sixth RCT found higher incidence of adverse effects (headache, dry mouth) with pseudoephedrine plus loratadine and pseudoephedrine alone compared with placebo ($P \leq 0.05$).[80] The seventh RCT found no significant difference in the incidence of adverse effects between pseudoephedrine plus loratadine and pseudoephedrine alone.[81] It found significantly higher incidence of adverse effects (insomnia, dry mouth) with the combination treatment compared with either loratadine alone or placebo ($P = 0.01$). The eighth RCT did not compare the incidence of adverse effects between pseudoephedrine plus azatadine versus placebo.[82]

Comment: None.

OPTION INTRANASAL IPRATROPIUM BROMIDE

We found no systematic review or fully published RCTs.

Benefits: We found no systematic review or fully published RCTs comparing intranasal ipratropium bromide versus placebo for seasonal allergic rhinitis (see comment below).

Harms: We found no systematic review or RCTs.

Comment: We found one RCT reported as an abstract only.[83] The RCT (429 people) compared intranasal ipratropium bromide (84 mg/nostril given 4 times daily) versus placebo for 3 weeks during the ragweed season. It found that ipratropium bromide versus placebo significantly reduced the severity ($P = 0.002$) and duration ($P = 0.008$) of rhinorrhoea during the 3 weeks of treatment. This benefit was maintained during periods of high pollen count. The RCT found no significant difference between ipratropium bromide and placebo for symptoms of nasal congestion, sneezing, or postnasal drip.

OPTION ORAL LEUKOTRIENE RECEPTOR ANTAGONISTS

RCTs have found that oral montelukast, with or without added antihistamines, improve symptoms and quality of life compared with placebo. Two RCTs found that oral montelukast plus oral loratadine improved quality of life compared with loratadine alone. The RCTs found conflicting evidence about effects on symptoms compared with loratadine alone.

Benefits: We found no systematic review. **Montelukast versus placebo:** We found two RCTs.[50,51] The first (1302 people aged 15–81 years with seasonal allergic rhinitis for at least 2 years) compared montelukast (10 mg/day), loratadine (10 mg/day), and placebo.[50] It found that montelukast significantly improved daytime nasal symptoms and quality of life compared with placebo (symptoms rated from 0 [none] to 3 [bothersome most of the time/very bothersome some of the time]; mean difference compared with placebo: –0.13, 95% CI –0.21 to –0.06; quality of life assessed by improvement in Rhinoconjunctivitis Quality of Life Questionnaire score [see glossary]: –0.89 with montelukast 630) v –0.65 with placebo; $P = 0.003$). One further RCT (907 people aged 15–82 years with seasonal allergic rhinitis for ≥ 2 years and positive skin test), carried out in the autumn, compared montelukast (10 mg/day), loratadine (10 mg/day), montelukast plus loratadine, and placebo.[51] Montelukast significantly improved daytime nasal symptom scores and quality of life compared with placebo (mean difference from baseline versus placebo: –0.23, 95% CI –0.35 to –0.11 compared with placebo; P < 0.001; difference in Rhinoconjunctivitis Quality of Life Questionnaire score: –1.09, 95% CI –1.26 to –0.92; P < 0.02). **Montelukast plus oral antihistamines:** We found two RCTs, both comparing montelukast (10 mg/day) plus loratadine (10 mg/day) versus montelukast (10 or 20 mg/day), loratadine (10 mg/day), or placebo for 2 weeks.[51,84] The first RCT (907 people aged 15–82 years with seasonal allergic rhinitis for ≥ 2 years and positive skin test) was carried out in the autumn.[51] It compared montelukast plus loratadine, montelukast alone, loratadine alone, and placebo. The RCT found that montelukast plus loratadine improved nasal symptom scores compared with placebo (–0.32, 95% CI –0.42 to –0.21; P < 0.001) but not compared with loratadine alone (–0.26, 95% CI –0.37 to –0.16). Combined treatment significantly improved Rhinoconjunctivitis Quality of Life Questionnaire score compared with placebo (–1.16, 95% CI –1.29 to –1.03; P < 0.001). However, improvements were not significantly greater than with montelukast alone (–1.09, 95% CI –1.26 to –0.92) or loratadine alone (–1.06, 95% CI –1.19 to –0.93). The second RCT (460 people aged 15–75 years with a clinical history of seasonal allergic rhinitis for at least 2 years and a positive skin test to at least 1 of 8 grass or tree pollens) compared montelukast (10 mg/day) plus loratadine (10 mg/day) versus montelukast (10 or 20 mg/day), loratadine (10 mg/day), or placebo for 2 weeks.[84] The primary outcome was daytime nasal symptoms score (average of congestion, rhinorrhoea, itching, and sneezing) recorded on a daily diary card; other outcomes included quality of life (Rhinoconjunctivitis Quality of Life Questionnaire). Efficacy was assessed as the average change from baseline over the 2 week treatment period. The RCT found that montelukast plus loratadine improved the daytime nasal symptoms score compared with placebo, montelukast alone or loratadine alone and improved quality of life compared with placebo (P < 0.05). The RCT found no significant difference in daytime nasal symptoms score with either montelukast alone or loratadine alone versus placebo. **Other oral leukotriene receptor antagonists:** We found no RCTs.

Harms: The RCTs found no significant difference in adverse effects among montelukast plus loratadine, montelukast alone, loratadine alone, and placebo.[50,51,84]

Comment: None.

GLOSSARY

Rhinoconjunctivitis Quality of Life Questionnaire is widely used in clinical trials to evaluate problems associated with rhinoconjunctivitis such as nose and eye symptoms by adults. It has 28 questions in seven domains (activity limitations, sleep problems, non-nasal/eye symptoms, practical problems, nose symptoms, eye symptoms, and emotional function) and is in both self administered and interviewer administered formats. People are asked to recall their experiences during the previous week and to give their responses on a seven point scale.[85]

SF-36 Health Survey includes one multi-item scale that assesses eight health concepts: limitations in physical activities because of health problems; limitations in social activities because of physical or emotional problems; limitations in usual role activities because of physical health problems; bodily pain; general mental health (psychological distress and wellbeing); limitations in usual role activities because of emotional problems; vitality (energy and fatigue); and general health perceptions. The survey was constructed for self administration by people aged 14 years or older, and for administration by a trained interviewer in person or by telephone.[86]

Work Productivity and Activity Impairment instrument is a questionnaire designed to measure work and activity impairment in adults during the previous 7 days. It is constructed for self administration or for use by interviewer in person or by telephone. The number of items varies between 6 and 9, depending on the version used.

Substantive changes

Oral antihistamines Three RCTs added;[49–51] conclusions unchanged.

Intranasal antihistamines One RCT added;[72] conclusions unchanged.

Oral leukotriene receptor antagonists Two RCTs added.[50,51] Oral leukotriene receptor antagonists recategorised from Unknown effectiveness to Likely to be beneficial.

REFERENCES

1. Lund VJ, Aaronsen D, Bousquet J, et al. International consensus report on the diagnosis and management of rhinitis. *Allergy* 1994;49:1–34.
2. The International Study of Asthma and Allergies in Childhood Steering Committee. Worldwide variation in prevalence of symptoms of asthma, allergic rhinoconjunctivitis, and atopic eczema: ISAAC. *Lancet* 1998;351:1225–1232.
3. Shamssain MH, Shamsian N. Prevalence and severity of asthma, rhinitis, and atopic eczema: the North East study. *Arch Dis Child* 1999;81:313–317.
4. Sibbald B, Rink E. Epidemiology of seasonal and perennial rhinitis; clinical presentation and medical history. *Thorax* 1991;46:895–901.
5. Fleming DM, Crombie DL. Prevalence of asthma and hay fever in England and Wales. *BMJ* 1987;294:279–283.
6. Durham SR. Summer hay fever. In: Durham SR, ed. ABC of allergies. London: BMJ Books, 1998:16–18.
7. Scadding GK, Church MK. Rhinitis. In: Holgate ST, Church MK, Lichtenstein LM, eds. Allergy 2nd ed. London: Mosby, 2001: 55–76.
8. Parikh A, Scadding GK. Seasonal allergic rhinitis. *BMJ* 1997;314:1392.
9. Ross AM, Fleming DM. Incidence of allergic rhinitis in general practice, 1981–92. *BMJ* 1994;308:897–900.
10. Blaiss MS. Quality of life in allergic rhinitis. *Ann Allergy Asthma Immunol* 1999;83:449–454.
11. Sheikh A. Asthma and coexistent disease. *Asthma Gen Pract* 1998;6:17–18.
12. Meltzer EO, Casale TB, Nathan RA, et al. Once-daily fexofenadine HCl improves quality of life and reduces work and activity impairment in patients with seasonal allergic rhinitis. *Ann Allergy Asthma Immunol* 1999;83:311–317.
13. Tanner LA, Reilly M, Meltzer EO, et al. Effect of fexofenadine HCl on quality of life and work, classroom, and daily activity impairment in patients with seasonal allergic rhinitis. *Am J Manag Care* 1999;5:S235–S247.
14. Van Cauwenberge P, Juniper EF, Albegger Almeida M, et al. Comparison of the efficacy, safety and quality of life provided by fexofenadine hydrochloride 120 mg, loratadine 10 mg and placebo administered once daily for the treatment of seasonal allergic rhinitis. *Clin Exp Allergy* 2000;30:891–899.
15. Leonhardt L, Gale NM, Gibbs TG. Placebo-controlled randomised evaluation of acrivastine in seasonal allergic rhinitis. *Acta Therap* 1988;14:241–248.
16. Bruno G, D'Amato G, Del Giacco GS, et al. Prolonged treatment with acrivastine for seasonal allergic rhinitis. *J Int Med Res* 1989;17:40B–46B.
17. Williams BO, Hull H, McSorley P, et al. Efficacy of acrivastine plus pseudoephedrine for symptomatic relief of seasonal allergic rhinitis due to mountain cedar. *Ann Allergy* 1996;76:432–438.
18. Franke W, Messinger D. Double-blind multicenter controlled clinical study comparing the efficacy of picumast dihydrochloride versus astemizole and placebo in patients with seasonal allergic rhinitis. *Drug Res* 1989;39:1360–1363.
19. Howarth PH, Emanuel MB, Holgate ST. Astemizole, a potent histamine H1-receptor antagonist: effect in allergic rhinoconjunctivitis, on antigen and histamine induced skin weal responses and relationship to serum levels. *Br J Clin Pharmacol* 1984;18:1–8.
20. Knight A. Astemizole — a new, non-sedating antihistamine for hayfever. *J Otolaryngol* 1985;14:85–88.
21. Oei HD. Double-blind comparison of loratadine (SCH 29851), astemizole, and placebo in hay fever with special regard to onset of action. *Ann Allergy* 1988;61:436–439.
22. Malmberg H, Holopainen E, Grahne B, et al. Astemizole in the treatment of hay fever. *Allergy* 1983;38:227–231.
23. Howarth PH, Holgate ST. Comparative trial of two non-sedative H1 antihistamines, terfenadine and astemizole, for hay fever. *Thorax* 1984;39:668–672.
24. Callier J, Engelen RF, Ianniello I, et al. Astemizole (R 43 512) in the treatment of hay fever. an international double-blind study comparing a weekly treatment (10 mg and 25 mg) with a placebo. *Curr Ther Res* 1981;29:24–35.
25. Sooknundun M, Kacker SK, Sundaram KR. Treatment of allergic rhinitis with a new long-acting H1 receptor antagonist: astemizole. *Ann Allergy* 1987;58:78–81.
26. Yan K, Harvey P, Pincus R. Trial of azatadine maleate (Zadine) in allergic asthma and rhinitis. *Clin Trials J* 1986;3:304–308.

27. Thoden WR, Druce HM, Furey SA, et al. Brompheniramine maleate: a double-blind, placebo-controlled comparison with terfenadine for symptoms of allergic rhinitis. *Am J Rhin* 1998;12:293–299.
28. Klein GL, Littlejohn T, Lockhart EA, et al. Brompheniramine, terfenadine, and placebo in allergic rhinitis. *Ann Allergy Asthma Immunol* 1996;77:365–370.
29. Ciprandi G, Passalacqua G, Mincarini M, et al. Continuous versus on demand treatment with cetirizine for allergic rhinitis. *Ann Allergy Asthma Immunol* 1997;79:507–511.
30. Ciprandi G, Tosca M, Ricca V, et al. Cetirizine treatment of rhinitis in children with pollen allergy: evidence of its antiallergic activity. *Clin Exp Allergy* 1997;27:1160–1166.
31. Grant JA, Nicodemus CF, Findlay SR, et al. Cetirizine in patients with seasonal rhinitis and concomitant asthma: prospective, randomized, placebo-controlled trial. *J Allergy Clin Immunol* 1995;95:923–932.
32. Lockey RF, Widlitz MD, Mitchell DQ, et al. Comparative study of cetirizine and terfenadine versus placebo in the symptomatic management of seasonal allergic rhinitis. *Ann Allergy Asthma Immunol* 1996;76:448–454.
33. Sabbah A, Daele J, Wade AG, et al. Comparison of the efficacy, safety and onset of action of mizolastine, cetirizine and placebo in the management of seasonal allergic rhinoconjunctivitis. *Ann Allergy Asthma Immunol* 1999;83:319–325.
34. Tarchalska-Krynska B, Zawisa E. Clinical assessment of cetirizine. *Polski Tygodnik Lekarski* 1990;45:123–126.
35. Ankier SI, Warrington SJ. A double-blind placebo-controlled study of the efficacy and tolerability of ebastine against hayfever in general practice patients. *J Int Med* 1989;226:453–458.
36. Storms WW. Clinical studies of the efficacy and tolerability of ebastine 10 or 20 mg once daily in the treatment of seasonal allergic rhinitis in the US. Adis International Limited. *Drugs* 1996;52:20–25
37. Ratner PH, Lim JC, Georges GC. Comparison of once-daily ebastine 20mg, ebastine 10mg, loratadine 10mg, and placebo in the treatment of seasonal allergic rhinitis. *J Allergy Clin Immunol* 2000;105:1101–1107.
38. Howarth PH, Stern MA, Roi L, et al. Double-blind, placebo-controlled study comparing the efficacy and safety of fexofenadine hydrochloride (120 and 180 mg once daily) and cetirizine in seasonal allergic rhinitis. *J Allergy Clin Immunol* 1999;104:927–933.
39. Bronsky EA, Falliers CJ, Kaiser HB, et al. Effectiveness and safety of fexofenadine, a new nonsedating H1-receptor antagonist, in the treatment of fall allergies. *Allergy Asthma Proc* 1998;19:135–141.
40. Casale TB, Andrade C, Qu R. Safety and efficacy of once-daily fexofenadine HCl in the treatment of autumn seasonal allergic rhinitis. *Allergy Asthma Proc* 1999;20:193–198.
41. Bernstein DI, Schoenwetter WF, Nathan RA, et al. Efficacy and safety of fexofenadine hydrochloride for treatment of seasonal allergic rhinitis. *Ann Allergy Asthma Immunol* 1997;79:443–448.
42. Gutkowski A, Bedard P, Del Carpio J, et al. Comparison of the efficacy and safety of loratadine, terfenadine, and placebo in the treatment of seasonal allergic rhinitis. *J Allergy Clin Immunol* 1988;81:902–907.
43. Del Carpio J, Kabbash L, Turenne Y, et al. Efficacy and safety of loratadine (10 mg once daily), terfenadine (60 mg twice daily), and placebo in the treatment of seasonal allergic rhinitis. *J Allergy Clin Immunol* 1989;84:741–746.
44. Bruttmann G, Pedrali P. Loratadine (SCH29851) 40 mg once daily versus terfenadine 60 mg twice daily in the treatment of seasonal allergic rhinitis. *J Int Med Res* 1987;15:63–70.
45. Irander K, Odkvist LM, Ohlander B. Treatment of hay fever with loratadine — a new non-sedating antihistamine. *Allergy* 1990;45:86–91.
46. Skassa-Brociek W, Bousquet J, Montes F, et al. Double-blind placebo-controlled study of loratadine, mequitazine, and placebo in the symptomatic treatment of seasonal allergic rhinitis. *J Allergy Clin Immunol* 1988;81:725–730.
47. Dockhorn RJ, Bergner A, Connell JT. Safety and efficacy of loratadine (Sch-29851): a new non-sedating antihistamine in seasonal allergic rhinitis. *Ann Allergy* 1987;58:407–411.
48. Horak F, Bruttmann G, Pedrali P, et al. A multicentric study of loratadine, terfenadine and placebo in patients with seasonal allergic rhinitis. *Arzneimittel-Forsch* 1988;38:124–128.
49. Berger WE, Schenkel EJ, Mansfield LE, and the Desloratadine Study group. Safety and efficacy of desloratadine 5mg in asthma patients with seasonal allergic rhinitis and nasal congestion. *Ann Allergy Asthma Immunol* 2002;89:485–491
50. Philip G, Malmstrom K, Hampel FC Jr, et al., for the Montelukast Spring Rhinitis Group. Montelukast for treating seasonal allergic rhinitis: a randomized, double-blind, placebo-controlled trial performed in the spring. *Clin Exp Allergy* 2002;32:1020–1028.
51. Nayak A, Philip G, Lu S, et al., and the Montelukast Fall Rhinitis Investigator Group. Efficacy and tolerability of montelukast alone or in combination with loratadine in seasonal allergic rhinitis: a multicenter, randomized, double-blind, placebo-controlled trial performed in the fall. *Ann Allergy Asthma Immunol* 2002;88592–600.
52. Meltzer EO, Prenner BM, Nayak A, Desloratadine Study Group. Efficacy and tolerability of once-daily 5mg desloratadine, an H-1 receptor antagonist with seasonal allergic rhinitis: assessment during the spring and fall seasons. *Clin Drug Invest* 2001;21:25–32.
53. Stern M, Blondin-Ertzbischoff P, Murrieta-Aguttes M, et al. Rapid and sustained efficacy of mizolastine 10 mg once daily in seasonal allergic rhinitis. *J Int Med Res* 1998;26:292–303.
54. Leynadier F, Bousquet J, Murrieta M, et al. Efficacy and safety of mizolastine in seasonal allergic rhinitis. The Rhinase Study Group. *Ann Allergy* 1996;76:163–168.
55. Boerner D, Metz K, Eberhardt R, et al. A placebo-controlled comparison of the efficacy and tolerability of picumast dihydrochloride and terfenadine in patients with seasonal allergic rhinitis. *Arzneimittel-Forsch* 1989;39:1356–1359.
56. Kagan G, Dabrowicki E, Huddlestone L. A double-blind trial of terfenadine and placebo in hay fever using a substitution technique for non-responders. *J Int Med Res* 1980;8:404–407.
57. Brandon ML, Weiner M. Clinical studies of terfenadine in seasonal allergic rhinitis. *Arzneimittel-Forsch* 1982;32:1204–1205.
58. Brooks CD, Karl KJ, Francom SF. Profile of ragweed hay fever symptom control with terfenadine started before or after symptoms are established. *Clin Exp Allergy* 1990;20:21–26.
59. Simpson RJ. Budesonide and terfenadine, separately and in combination, in the treatment of hay fever. *Ann Allergy* 1994;73:497–502.
60. Van Bavel J, Findlay SR, Hampel FC, et al. Intranasal fluticasone propionate is more effective than terfenadine tablets for seasonal allergic rhinitis. *Arch Int Med* 1994;154:2699–2704.

61. Bronsky EA, Dockhorn RJ, Meltzer EO, et al. Fluticasone propionate aqueous nasal spray compared with terfenadine tablets in the treatment of seasonal allergic rhinitis. *J Allergy Clin Immunol* 1996;97:915–921.
62. Darnell R, Pecoud A, Richards DH. A double-blind comparison of fluticasone propionate aqueous nasal spray, terfenadine tablets and placebo in the treatment of patients with seasonal allergic rhinitis to grass pollen. *Clin Exp Allergy* 1994;24:1144–1150.
63. Committee on Safety of Medicines. Astemizole (Hismanal): only available on prescription. Important new contraindications and interactions. http://www.mca.gov.uk (last accessed 9 June 2003).
64. Committee on Safety of Medicines. Terfenadine: Information for Doctors and Pharmacists, http://www.mca.gov.uk/aboutagency/regframework/csm/csmhome.htm (last accessed 9 June 2003).
65. Mann RD, Pearce GL, Dunn N, et al. Sedation with "non-sedating" antihistamines: four prescription-event monitoring studies in general practice. *BMJ* 2000;320:1184–1187.
66. Schuermans V, Lewi PJ, Gypen LM, et al. Meta-analysis of the global evaluation of levocabastine nasal spray versus placebo. *Drug Inf J* 1993;27:575–584.
67. Hampel FC, Martin BG, Dolen J, et al. Efficacy and safety of levocabastine nasal spray for seasonal allergic rhinitis *Am J Rhinology* 1999;13:55–62.
68. Di Lorenzo G, Gervasi F, Drago A, et al. Comparison of the effects of fluticasone propionate, aqueous nasal spray and levocabastine on inflammatory cells in nasal lavage and clinical activity during the pollen season in seasonal rhinitics. *Clin Exp Allergy* 1999;29:1367–1377.
69. Newson-Smith G, Powell M, Baehre M, et al. A placebo controlled study comparing the efficacy of intranasal azelastine and beclomethasone in the treatment of seasonal allergic rhinitis. *Eur Arch Otorhinolaryngol* 1997;254:236–241.
70. LaForce C, Dockhorn RJ, Prenner BM, et al. Safety and efficacy of azelastine nasal spray (Astelin NS) for seasonal allergic rhinitis: a 4-week comparative multicenter trial. *Ann Allergy Asthma Immunol* 1996;76:181–188.
71. Ciprandi G, Ricca V, Passalacqua G, et al. Seasonal rhinitis and azelastine: long- or short-term treatment? *J Allergy Clin Immunol* 1997;99:301–307.
72. Duarte C, Baĕhre M, Gharakhanian S, Leynadier F, and the French Azelastine Group. Treatment of severe seasonal rhinoconjunctivitis by a combination of azelastine nasal spray and eye drops: a double-blind, double-placebo study. *J Invest Allergol Clin Immunol* 2001;11:34–40.
73. Mosges R, Klimek L, Spaeth J, et al. Topical versus systemical treatment with antihistamines in seasonal allergic rhinitis. *Allergologi* 1995;18:145–150. [German]
74. Bahmer F, Ruprecht KW. Safety and efficacy of topical levocabastine compared with oral terfenadine. *Ann Allergy* 1994;72:429–434.
75. Sussman GL, Mason J, Compton D, et al. The efficacy and safety of fexofenadine HCl and pseudoephedrine alone and in combination in seasonal allergic rhinitis. *J Allergy Clin Immunol* 1999;104:100–106.
76. Dockhorn RJ, Williams BO, Sanders RL. Efficacy of acrivastine with pseudoephedrine in treatment of allergic rhinitis due to ragweed. *Ann Allergy Asthma Immunol* 1996;76:204–208.
77. Grosclaude M, Mees K, Pinelli ME, et al. Cetirizine and pseudoephedrine retard, given alone or in combination with seasonal allergic rhinitis. *Rhinology* 1997;35:67–73.
78. Panda NK, Mann SBS. Comparative efficacy and safety of terfenadine with pseudoephedrine and terfenadine alone in allergic rhinitis. *Otolaryngol Head Neck Surg* 1998;118:253–255.
79. Empey DW, Bye C, Hodder M, et al. A double-blind crossover trial of pseudoephedrine and triprolidine alone and in combination for the treatment of allergic rhinitis. *Ann Allergy* 1975;34:41–46.
80. Bronsky E, Boggs P, Findlay S, et al. Comparative efficacy and safety of a once-daily loratadine–pseudoephedrine combination versus its components alone and placebo in the management of seasonal allergic rhinitis. *J Allergy Clin Immunol* 1995;96:139–147.
81. Storms WW, Bodman SF, Nathan RA, et al. SCH 434: a new antihistamine/decongestant for seasonal allergic rhinitis. *J Allergy Clin Immunol* 1989;83:1083–1090.
82. Tarasido JC. Azatadine maleate/pseudoephedrine sulfate repetabs versus placebo in the treatment of severe allergic rhinitis. *J Int Med Res* 1980;8:391–394.
83. Busse W, Biondi R, Casale T, et al. Randomised double-blind, parallel placebo-controlled multi-centre trial of ipratropium bromide nasal spray 0.06% in patients with seasonal allergic rhinitis. *Ann Allergy Asthma Immunol* 1999;82:109. [Abstract]
84. Meltzer EO, Malmstrom K, Lu S, et al. Concomitant montelukast and loratadine as treatment for seasonal allergic rhinitis — a randomised placebo-controlled clinical trial. *J Allergy Clin Immunol* 2000;105:917–922.
85. Measurement of health related quality of life: adult rhinoconjunctivitis. http://www.qoltech.co.uk/Rhinocon.htm (last accessed 9 June 2003).
86. Ware JJ, Sherbourne CD. The MOS 36-item short-form health survey (SF-36). I. Conceptual framework and item selection. *Med Care* 1992;30:473–483.

Aziz Sheikh
Professor of Primary Care Research & Development
University of Edinburgh, Edinburgh, UK

Sukhmeet Panesar
Medical Student
Imperial College London, London, UK

Sangeeta Dhami
General Practitioner
GP Direct, Harrow, Middlesex, UK

Competing interests: None declared.

Tinnitus

Search date October 2002

Angus Waddell and Richard Canter

QUESTIONS

INTERVENTIONS

See glossary, p 642

Key Messages

- **Ginkgo biloba** One systematic review and one subsequent RCT found no significant difference between ginkgo biloba versus placebo in tinnitus symptoms.
- **Psychotherapy** One systematic review found insufficient evidence about cognitive behavioural treatment, relaxation therapy, counselling, education, hypnosis, biofeedback, or stress management compared with other or no treatment in people with chronic tinnitus.
- **Tocainide** One RCT found no significant difference with tocainide versus placebo in improving symptoms, but found evidence that tocainide caused significantly more adverse effects after 30 days' treatment.
- **Tricyclic antidepressants** One small RCT in people with depression and chronic tinnitus found that tricyclic antidepressants (nortriptyline) versus placebo significantly improved tinnitus related disability, audiometric tinnitus loudness matching, and symptoms of depression at 6 weeks, but found no significant difference in tinnitus severity. One small RCT in people with tinnitus but without depression found that a greater proportion of people rated themselves as improved with tricyclic antidepressants (amitriptyline) versus placebo at 6 weeks.
- **Acupuncture; antiepileptics; baclofen; benzodiazepines; cinnarizine; electromagnetic stimulation; hyperbaric oxygen; hypnosis; low power laser; nicotinamide; tinnitus masking devices; zinc** We found insufficient evidence about the effects of these interventions.

DEFINITION	Tinnitus is defined as the perception of sound, which does not arise from the external environment, from within the body (e.g. vascular sounds), or from auditory hallucinations related to mental illness. This review is concerned with chronic tinnitus, where tinnitus is the only, or the predominant, symptom in an affected person.
INCIDENCE/ PREVALENCE	Up to 18% of the general population in industrialised countries are mildly affected by chronic tinnitus, and 0.5% report tinnitus having a severe effect on their ability to lead a normal life.[1]
AETIOLOGY/ RISK FACTORS	Tinnitus may occur as an isolated idiopathic symptom or in association with any type of hearing loss. Tinnitus may be a particular feature of presbyacusis, noise induced hearing loss, Menière's disease (see glossary, p 642) (see Menière's disease, p 593), or the presence of an acoustic neuroma. In people with toxicity from aspirin or quinine, tinnitus can occur while hearing thresholds remain normal. Tinnitus is also associated with depression, although it may be unclear whether the tinnitus is a manifestation of the depressive illness or a factor contributing to its development.[2]
PROGNOSIS	Tinnitus may have an insidious onset, with a long delay before clinical presentation. It may persist for many years or decades, particularly when associated with a sensorineural hearing loss. In Menière's disease both the presence and intensity of tinnitus can fluctuate. Tinnitus may cause disruption of sleep patterns, an inability to concentrate, and depression.[3]
AIMS OF INTERVENTION	To reduce the loudness and intrusiveness of the tinnitus and to reduce its impact on daily life, with minimum adverse effects from treatment.
OUTCOMES	The number of people with resolution of tinnitus; tinnitus loudness (assessed by visual analogue scale, symptom scores, or by audiometric matching); impact of tinnitus measured by estimates of interference with activities of daily life or with emotional state.
METHODS	*Clinical Evidence* search and appraisal October 2002. We identified a few non-English language articles that require translation and, where appropriate, their results will be included in future *Clinical Evidence* updates.

QUESTION **What are the effects of treatments for chronic tinnitus?**

OPTION **TRICYCLIC ANTIDEPRESSANTS**

One RCT in people with depression and chronic tinnitus found that tricyclic antidepressants (nortriptyline) versus placebo significantly improved tinnitus related disability, audiometric tinnitus loudness matching, and symptoms of depression at 6 weeks, but found no significant difference in tinnitus severity. One small RCT in people with tinnitus but without depression found that a greater proportion of people rated themselves as improved with tricyclic antidepressants (amitriptyline) versus placebo at 6 weeks.

Benefits: **Versus placebo:** We found one systematic review (search date 1998, 1 RCT)[4] and one subsequent RCT.[5] The RCT included in the review (92 people with tinnitus and depression or depressive symptoms but no bipolar disorder or other mental health diagnosis) identified by the reviews found that nortriptyline (titrated to maintain therapeutic blood levels for depression) versus placebo significantly improved measures of depression, a tinnitus related disability score, and audiometric tinnitus loudness matching.[4] However, the RCT, found no significant difference in the proportion of people reporting overall improvement in tinnitus severity after 6 weeks (11 to 16 dB tinnitus loudness matching with nortriptyline *v* 19 to 18 dB with placebo; P = 0.006; 43% of people reported improved tinnitus severity with nortriptyline *v* 30% with placebo; P = 0.2; raw data not provided).[6] The subsequent RCT (37 people with no history of depression) found that a greater proportion of people rated themselves as "improved" with amitriptyline (50 mg/night for 1 wk followed by 100 mg/night for 5 wks) versus placebo after 6 weeks but found no significant difference between treatments in the frequency of occurrence of tinnitus (19/20 [95%] "improved" on amitriptyline *v* 2/17 [12%] with placebo; OR 8.1, 95% CI 5.6 to 10.6; no values were reported for tinnitus frequency).[5]

Harms: One RCT found mild sedation and dryness of the mouth lasting for 1–2 weeks but reported no major adverse effects.[5] Other studies have established that adverse effects of nortriptyline include dry mouth, blurred vision, and constipation (see harms of tricyclic antidepressants under depressive disorders, p 1121).

Comment: The subsequent RCT may have lacked power to detect clinically important effects on frequency of occurence of tinnitus.[5]

OPTION BENZODIAZEPINES

We found insufficient evidence about the effects of benzodiazepines.

Benefits: We found one systematic review (search date 1995, 1 RCT).[7] The RCT (40 people) identified by the review found that alprazolam (initially 0.5 mg/night) versus placebo significantly improved reported tinnitus severity after 12 weeks (13/17 [76%] improved with alprazolam *v* 1/19 [5%] with placebo; ARR 71%; RR 14.5, 95% CI 2.1 to 53), but interpretation of these results is difficult (see comment below).[8]

Harms: The RCT reported that two (10%) people receiving alprazolam withdrew from the trial because of excessive tiredness.[8] Long term use of benzodiazepines can lead to dependence (see harms of benzodiazepines under generalised anxiety disorder, p 1157).

Comment: The RCT used dose adjustment of alprazolam but no dose adjustment of placebo, potentially biasing the results because of a difference in the attention given to people in the two groups.[8] Another systematic review (search date 1998) found three other studies that used weaker methods; none of the studies provided evidence that benzodiazepines versus placebo improved symptoms of tinnitus.[4]

OPTION ANTIEPILEPTICS

One RCT found no significant difference between antiepileptics versus placebo for tinnitus severity at 30 days. However, the trial may have lacked power to detect a clinically important effect.

Benefits: We found one systematic review (search date 1995, 1 RCT)[7] and one subsequent RCT.[9] The RCT (48 people) identified by the review found no significant difference with carbamazepine (150 mg 3 times daily for 30 days) versus placebo on reported tinnitus severity after 30 days treatment (2/24 [8%] improved with carbamazepine *v* 3/24 [13%] with placebo; ARR 4.2%; RR 0.67, 95% CI 0.12 to 3.6).[10] The subsequent RCT (31 people) was a crossover trial comparing lamotrigine versus placebo.[9] However, it did not report results before the crossover (see comment below).[9]

Harms: The RCT identified by the review found that carbamazepine versus placebo significantly increased the number of people reporting adverse effects (including dizziness, nausea, and headaches; 25/34 [63%] with carbamazepine *v* 1/24 [4%] with placebo; RR 17.6, 95% CI 2.6 to 121; NNH 1, 95% CI 1 to 2).[5] The subsequent RCT did not report harms.[8]

Comment: A second systematic review (search date 1998) found four RCTs comparing antiepileptic treatment versus placebo.[4] All were appraised in the earlier review,[7] but were excluded from the review on methodological grounds. The subsequent RCT found no significant difference with lamotrigine (25 mg/day for 2 wks, 50 mg/day for 2 wks, and then 100 mg/day for 4 wks) versus placebo in tinnitus loudness or annoyance measured on a visual analogue scale (11/31 [35%] people improved with lamotrigine *v* 6/31 [19%] people with placebo; ARI 16%; RR 1.8, 95% CI 0.78 to 4.34).[9]

OPTION NICOTINAMIDE

One RCT found no significant difference between nicotinamide versus placebo for tinnitus severity at 30 days. However, the trial may have lacked power to detect a clinically important effect.

Benefits: We found one systematic review (search date 1998, 1 RCT).[4] The RCT (48 people) identified by the review found no significant difference with nicotinamide (70 mg 3 times daily for 30 days) versus placebo on subjective improvement after 30 days treatment (2/24 [8%] people improved with nicotinamide *v* 3/24 [13%] with placebo; ARR 4%; RR 0.7, 95% CI 0.1 to 3.6).[11]

Harms: The RCT found no significant difference with nicotinamide versus placebo in the number of people reporting headache (4/24 [16%] with nicotinamide *v* 1/24 [4%] with placebo; RR 4.0, 95% CI 0.5 to 33.2) or the number of people reporting dizziness (2/24 [8%] *v* 0/24 [0%]).[11]

Comment: None.

OPTION CINNARIZINE

One RCT found no significant difference between cinnarizine versus placebo for tinnitus severity. However, the trial may have lacked power to detect a clinically important effect.

Benefits: We found one systematic review (search date 1998, 1 RCT).[4] The RCT (30 people) identified by the review found no significant difference with cinnarizine (25 mg 3 times daily for 10 wks) versus placebo on reported subjective improvement (1/10 [10%] people improved with cinnarizine *v* 1/20 [5%] people with placebo; ARR 5%; RR 2.0, 95% CI 0.14 to 29; see comment below).[12]

Harms: The RCT did not report harms.[12]

Comment: The RCT did not specify the follow up period.[12]

OPTION ZINC

One RCT found no significant difference between zinc versus placebo for tinnitus severity at 8 weeks. However, the trial may have lacked power to detect a clinically important effect.

Benefits: We found one systematic review (search date 1998, 1 RCT).[4] The RCT (50 people) identified by the review found no significant difference with zinc (100 mg 3 times daily for 8 wks) versus placebo on reported tinnitus severity after 8 weeks treatment (2/23 [9%] people improved with zinc *v* 2/25 [8%] people with placebo; ARR 1%; RR 1.1, 95% CI 0.16 to 7).[13]

Harms: The RCT did not report harms.[13]

Comment: None.

OPTION BACLOFEN

One RCT found no significant difference between baclofen versus placebo for tinnitus severity. However, the trial may have lacked power to detect a clinically important effect.

Benefits: We found one systematic review (search date 1998, 1 RCT).[4] The RCT (63 people) identified by the review found no significant difference with baclofen (10 mg twice daily increasing to 30 mg twice daily for 3 wks) versus placebo on reported subjective improvement (3/31 [10%] improved with baclofen *v* 1/32 [3%] with placebo; ARR 7%; RR 3.1, 95% CI 0.34 to 28; see comment below).[14]

Harms: The RCT did not report harms.[14]

Comment: The RCT did not specify the follow up period.[14]

OPTION TOCAINIDE

One RCT found no significant difference with tocainide versus placebo in improving symptoms, but found evidence that tocainide caused significantly more adverse effects after 30 days' treatment.

Benefits: We found one systematic review (search date 1995, 2 RCTs).[7] The first RCT (40 people) identified by the review used a crossover design and did not give details of the washout period or the results before the crossover (see comment below).[15] The second RCT (48 people) identified by the review found no significant difference with tocainide (300 mg 3 times daily for 30 days) versus placebo on the proportion of people with improved symptoms after 30 days' treatment (1/24 [4%] with tocainide v 3/24 [13%] with control; ARR 8%; RR 0.33, 95% CI 0.04 to 3.0).[16]

Harms: The second RCT identified by the review found that tocainide versus placebo significantly increased adverse effects (11/24 [45.8%] v 2/24 [8.3%]; ARI 37%; RR 5.5, 95% CI 1.4 to 22.2; NNH 2, 95% CI 1 to 8).[16] The main adverse effects reported were rash (6/24 [25%] with tocainide v 1/24 [4%] with placebo), dizziness (3/24 [12%] with tocainide v 0/24 [0%] with placebo), and tremor (2/24 [8%] with tocainide v 0/24 [0%] with placebo).

Comment: The first RCT found no significant difference with oral tocainide (400 mg/day rising to 2.4 g/day for 4 wks) versus placebo in symptom scores (10/40 [25%] improved with tocainide v 4/40 [10%] with placebo; ARR 15%; RR 2.5, 95% CI 0.85 to 7.3).

OPTION ACUPUNCTURE

One systematic review found insufficient evidence about the effects of acupuncture.

Benefits: We found one systematic review (search date 1998, 6 studies, 185 people).[17] The review included one pseudo-randomised RCT,[18] two non-blinded RCTs,[12,19] two crossover RCTs,[20,21] and one blinded parallel group RCT.[22] All studies were small and brief. The blinded parallel group RCT (54 people) found no significant difference with acupuncture (25 sessions over 2 months) versus sham acupuncture (superficial penetration at random non-acupuncture points) in tinnitus loudness on a pooled visual analogue score (4% improvement with acupuncture v 1% deterioration with placebo).[22] The crossover RCTs did not report results before the crossover (see comment below).

Harms: The review did not report on adverse effects.[17]

Comment: The first crossover RCT identified by the review (14 people) found that acupuncture versus sham acupuncture significantly increased the number of people who reported a reduction in tinnitus loudness after one session of treatment (5/14 [36%] with acupuncture v 0/14 [0%] with sham acupuncture; $P = 0.05$).[20] The second crossover RCT (20 people) found no significant difference with acupuncture versus placebo on a pooled visual analogue score of subjective tinnitus severity after 3 weeks ($P = 0.22$).[21]

OPTION PSYCHOTHERAPY

One systematic review found insufficient evidence about effects of cognitive behavioural treatment, relaxation therapy, counselling, education, hypnosis, biofeedback, or stress management compared with other or no treatment in people with chronic tinnitus.

Benefits: We found one systematic review (search date 1998, 8 RCTs, 269 people) of different psychotherapeutic approaches (cognitive behavioural treatment, relaxation therapy, counselling, education/

information, hypnosis, biofeedback, and stress management).[23] We found no additional or subsequent RCTs. The review had important methodological problems (see comments below). It found significant reductions in subjective loudness and tinnitus annoyance for a combination of different psychotherapeutic approaches at 3 months or more post-treatment versus pre-treatment (SMD for subjective loudness 0.68, 95% CI 0.62 to 0.74; SMD for tinnitus annoyance 0.83, 95% CI 0.82 to 0.84).

Harms: The review did not report harms.[23]

Comment: Despite many studies on psychotherapeutic measures to treat tinnitus, the evidence for benefit remains limited. Many of the RCTs suffer from weak methods, high withdrawal rates, and pooled or surrogate outcome measures. The systematic review pooled study results across arms of trials, losing the benefits of randomisation and increasing the risk of bias. Pre-treatment to post-treatment effect sizes do not allow comparison of psychotherapy with no treatment or any other treatment.[23] The review did not report which interventions were used as control in the RCTs.

OPTION ELECTROMAGNETIC STIMULATION/EAR CANAL MAGNETS

We found insufficient evidence from four small RCTs about the effects of magnets and electromagnetic stimulation.

Benefits: **Electromagnetic stimulation:** We found no systematic review, but found three small RCTs (136 people) comparing electromagnetic stimulation versus placebo.[24–26] The first RCT (58 people) found that electromagnetic stimulation versus placebo significantly increased the number of people who had improved tinnitus (14/31 [45%] *v* 2/23 [9%]; RR 5.2, 95% CI 1.3 to 20.6; see comment below).[25] The second RCT (48 people) found no significant difference with electromagnetic stimulation versus placebo in tinnitus sensation levels after 1 week (6/24 [25%] *v* 6/24 [25%]; RR 0.4, 95% CI 0.38 to 2.66).[24] The third RCT (20 people; see comment below) used a crossover design and did not report results before the crossover.[26] **Magnets:** We found no systematic review but found one RCT (49 people).[27] The RCT found no significant difference with a simple ear canal magnet versus placebo on tinnitus symptoms after 4 weeks treatment (7/26 [27%] with magnet *v* 4/23 [17%] with placebo; RR 1.5, 95% CI 0.53 to 4.5).

Harms: The RCTs reported no adverse effects associated with electromagnetic stimulation.[24–26]

Comment: The first RCT, which did not specify the length of follow up, reported that 4/58 (7%) people withdrew from the trial and that the analysis was not by intention to treat.[25] The crossover RCT found no significant difference with electrical suppression versus a placebo device in reduction in tinnitus severity (2/20 [10%] active device *v* 4/20 [20%] with placebo device; P = NS).[26]

OPTION HYPNOSIS

One RCT found no significant difference between hypnosis versus counselling for symptom severity at 3 months. However, the trial may have lacked power to exclude clinically important effects.

Benefits: We found one systematic review (search date 1995)[7] and one additional RCT.[28] The review identified two studies, which were of insufficient quality for inclusion.[29,30] The additional RCT (92 people who were preselected to be suggestible to hypnosis) found no significant difference with three sessions teaching self hypnosis versus control (a single counselling session) on symptom severity scores after 3 months (24/44 [55%] improved with hypnosis *v* 23/42 [55%] with counselling; RR 1.0, 95% CI 0.68 to 1.46). The RCT also found no significant difference in the number of people reporting worsened tinnitus (11/44 [25%] with hypnosis *v* 14/42 [32%] with counselling; RR 0.8, 95% CI 0.4 to 1.5).

Harms: No adverse effects were reported.[7,28]

Comment: None.

OPTION LOW POWER LASER

One RCT found no significant difference between low power laser versus placebo for symptom severity at 1 month. However, the trial may have lacked power to exclude clinically important effects.

Benefits: We found no systematic review but found one RCT.[31] The RCT (49 people) found no significant difference with laser (50 mW directed towards the mastoid bone) versus placebo in the number of people with improved tinnitus symptoms after 1 month (2/25 [8%] with laser *v* 7/24 [29%] with placebo; RR 0.27, 95% CI 0.06 to 1.2).[31]

Harms: No adverse effects were reported.[31]

Comment: None.

OPTION TINNITUS MASKING DEVICES

We found insufficient evidence about the effects of tinnitus masking devices.

Benefits: **Masking devices versus no treatment:** We found one systematic review (search date 1998, 1 RCT).[4] The RCT (75 people with tinnitus but no hearing difficulties) compared two types of tinnitus masking device versus a non-blinded control group. It found that either type of masking device versus control significantly improved symptoms (chi squared analysis $P < 0.01$; no supporting data given).[32]

Harms: The systematic review and RCT did not report on harms.[4,32]

Comment: Masking devices have been widely prescribed but we could find no evidence to support their use.

OPTION GINKGO BILOBA

One systematic review and one subsequent RCT found no significant difference with ginkgo biloba versus placebo in tinnitus symptoms.

Benefits: We found one systematic review (search date 1998, 5 RCTs)[33] and one subsequent RCT.[34] The systematic review contained three RCTs of insufficient quality for inclusion in this review. Of the remaining two trials identified by the review, the first (crossover RCT, 20 people) found no significant difference with ginkgo biloba extract (29.2 mg/day for 2 wks) versus placebo in tinnitus symptoms (see comment below).[35] The second RCT (99 people) compared ginkgo biloba extract (120 mg/day for 12 wks) versus placebo.[36] The RCT found an improvement in measured tinnitus loudness from 42 dB to 39 dB with ginkgo biloba extract versus no improvement in the control group (significance not stated; additional numerical data not provided). The subsequent RCT (1121 people) compared ginkgo biloba (50 mg 3 times daily for 12 wks) versus placebo.[34] It found no significant difference in the number of people reporting subjective improvement after 12 weeks' treatment (34/360 [9.4%] with ginkgo biloba *v* 35/360 [9.7%] with placebo; ARI 0.3%, 95% CI –4.7% to 4.2%).

Harms: The subsequent RCT reported gastrointestinal upset (3%), dizziness (1%), and mouth dryness (1%) in both treatment and control groups.[34]

Comment: The crossover RCT identified by the review did not specify the length of follow up.[34]

OPTION HYPERBARIC OXYGEN

We found no systematic review or RCTs on the effects of hyperbaric oxygen for people with tinnitus.

Benefits: We found no systematic review or RCTs.

Harms: We found no evidence.

Comment: None.

GLOSSARY

Menière's disease A condition characterised by episodic vertigo, tinnitus, and sensorineural hearing loss.

REFERENCES

1. Coles RR. Epidemiology of tinnitus (1). *J Laryngol Otol* 1984;9(suppl):7–15.
2. Sullivan MD, Katon W, Dobie R, et al. Disabling tinnitus: association with affective disorder. *Gen Hosp Psychiatry* 1988;10:285–291.
3. Zoger S, Svedlund J, Holgers KM. Psychiatric disorders in tinnitus patients without severe hearing impairment: 24 month follow-up of patients at an audiological clinic. *Audiology* 2001;40:133–140.
4. Dobie RA. A review of randomized clinical trials in tinnitus. *Laryngoscope* 1999;109:1202–1211. Search date 1998; primary sources Medline and handsearches.
5. Bayar N, Boke B, Turan E, et al. Efficacy of amitriptyline in the treatment of subjective tinnitus. *J Otolaryngol* 2001;30:300–303.
6. Dobie RA, Sakai CS, Sullivan MD, et al. Antidepressant treatment of tinnitus patients: report of a randomized clinical trial and clinical prediction of benefit. *Am J Otol* 1993;14:18–23.
7. Schilter B, Jäger B, Heerman R, et al. Pharmacological and psychological treatment options in chronic subjective tinnitus: a meta-analysis of effective treatments. *HNO* 2000;48:589–597. Search date 1995; primary sources Medline, Psyindex, Psychlit, and handsearches including German, English, and French language papers.
8. Johnson RM, Brummett R, Schleuning A. Use of alprazolam for relief of tinnitus. A double-blind study. *Arch Otolaryngol Head Neck Surg* 1993;119:842–845.
9. Simpson JJ, Gilbert AM, Weiner GM, et al. The assessment of lamotrigine, an antiepileptic drug, in the treatment of tinnitus. *Am J Otol* 1999;20:627–631.
10. Hulshof JH, Vermeij P. The value of carbamazepine in the treatment of tinnitus. *ORL J Otorhinolaryngol Relat Spec* 1985;47:262–266.
11. Hulshof JH, Vermeij P. The effect of nicotinamide on tinnitus: a double-blind controlled study. *Clin Otolaryngol* 1987;12:211–214.
12. Podoshin L, Ben-David Y, Fradis M, et al. Idiopathic subjective tinnitus treated by biofeedback, acupuncture and drug therapy. *Ear Nose Throat J* 1991;70:284–289.
13. Paaske PB, Pedersen CB, Kjems G, et al. Zinc in the management of tinnitus. Placebo-controlled trial. *Ann Otol Rhinol Laryngol* 1991;100:647–649.

14. Westerberg BD, Roberson JB Jr, Stach BA. A double-blind placebo-controlled trial of baclofen in the treatment of tinnitus [see comments]. *Am J Otol* 1996;17:896–903.
15. Lenarz T. Treatment of tinnitus with lidocaine and tocainide. *Scand Audiol Suppl* 1986;26:49–51.
16. Hulshof JH, Vermeij P. The value of tocainide in the treatment of tinnitus. *Arch Otolaryngol* 1985;241:279–283.
17. Park J, White AR, Ernst E. Efficacy of acupuncture as a treatment for tinnitus: a systematic review. *Arch Otolaryngol Head Neck Surg* 2000;126:489–492. Search date 1998; primary sources Medline, Cochrane Controlled Trials Register, Embase, and Ciscom.
18. Axelsson A, Andersson S, Gu LD. Acupuncture in the management of tinnitus: a placebo-controlled study. *Audiology* 1994;33:351–360.
19. Furugard S, Hedin PJ, Eggertz A, et al. Acupuncture worth trying in severe tinnitus. *Lakartidningen* 1998;95:1922–1928.
20. Marks NJ, Emery P, Onisiphorou C. A controlled trial of acupuncture in tinnitus. *J Laryngol Otol* 1984;98:1103–1109.
21. Hansen PE, Hansen JH, Bentzen O. Acupuncture therapy of chronic unilateral tinnitus. A double-blind cross-over study. *Ugeskr Laeger* 1981;143:2888–2890.
22. Vilholm OJ, Moller K, Jorgensen K. Effect of traditional Chinese acupuncture on severe tinnitus: a double-blind, placebo-controlled, clinical investigation with open therapeutic control. *Br J Audiol* 1998;32:197–204.
23. Andersson G, Lyttkens L. A meta-analytic review of psychological treatments for tinnitus. *Br J Audiol* 1999;33:201–210. Search date 1998; primary sources Medline and psychological abstracts.
24. Fiedler SC, Pilkington H, Willatt DJ. Electromagnetic stimulation as a treatment of tinnitus: a further study. *Clin Otolaryngol* 1998;23:270.
25. Roland NJ, Hughes JB, Daley MB, et al. Electromagnetic stimulation as a treatment of tinnitus: a pilot study. *Clin Otolaryngol* 1993;18:278–281.
26. Dobie RA, Hoberg KE, Rees TS. Electrical tinnitus suppression: a double-blind crossover study. *Otolaryngol Head Neck Surg* 1986;95:319–333.
27. Coles R, Bradley P, Donaldson I, et al. A trial of tinnitus therapy with ear-canal magnets. *Clin Otolaryngol* 1991;16:371–372.
28. Mason JD, Rogerson DR, Butler JD. Client centred hypnotherapy in the management of tinnitus — is it better than counselling? *J Laryngol Otol* 1996;110:117–120.
29. Attias J, Shemesh Z, Sohmer H, et al. Comparison between self-hypnosis, masking and attentiveness for alleviation of chronic tinnitus. *Audiology* 1993;32:205–212.
30. Halama P. Erfahrungen mit der Hypnose-Therapie bei ambulaten Patienten, die unter Tinnitus leiden. Vergleichende Pilotstudie. *Experimental Klin Hypnose* 1992;8:49–69.
31. Mirz F, Zachariae R, Andersen SE, et al. The low-power laser in the treatment of tinnitus. *Clin Otolaryngol* 1999;24:346–354.
32. Stephens SDG, Corcoran AL. A controlled study of tinnitus masking. *Br J Audiol* 1985;19:159–167.
33. Ernst E, Stevinson C. Ginkgo biloba for tinnitus: a review. *Clin Otolaryngol* 1999;24:164–167. Search date 1998; primary sources Medline, Embase, The Cochrane Library, contact with manufacturers, and hand search of reference lists.
34. Drew S, Davies E. Effectiveness of ginkgo biloba in treating tinnitus: double blind, placebo controlled trial. *BMJ* 2001;322:73–75.
35. Holger K-M, Axelsson A, Pringle I. Ginkgo Biloba extract for the treatment of tinnitus. *Audiology* 1994;33:85–92.
36. Morgenstern C, Biermann E. Ginkgo-Spezialextrakt Egb 761 in der Behandlung des Tinnitus aurium. *Fortschr Med* 1997;115:7–11.

Angus Waddell
Southwest Training Scheme in Otolaryngology
University of Bristol
Bristol
UK

Richard Canter
Royal United Hospital NHS Trust and University of Bath
Bath
UK

Competing interests: None declared.

Tonsillitis

Search date August 2002

William McKerrow

QUESTIONS

INTERVENTIONS

Key Messages

- **Tonsillectomy versus antibiotics in adults** We found no RCTs evaluating tonsillectomy in adults.
- **Tonsillectomy versus antibiotics in children** Two systematic reviews found limited evidence that tonsillectomy may benefit some children with severe tonsillitis, but found insufficient evidence to compare surgical versus medical treatment. One subsequent RCT in less severely affected children found that surgery significantly reduced the frequency of tonsillitis compared with medical treatment over 3 years. The modest benefit may be outweighed by morbidity associated with the generation in populations with low incidence of tonsillitis.

DEFINITION Tonsillitis is infection of the parenchyma of the palatine tonsils. The definition of severe recurrent tonsillitis is arbitrary, but recent criteria have defined tonsillitis as five or more episodes of true tonsillitis a year, symptoms for at least a year, and episodes that are disabling and prevent normal functioning.[1]

INCIDENCE/ PREVALENCE Recurrent sore throat has an incidence in general practice in the UK of 100/1000 population a year.[2] Acute tonsillitis is more common in childhood.

AETIOLOGY/ RISK FACTORS Common bacterial pathogens include β haemolytic and other streptococci. Bacteria are cultured successfully only from a minority of people with tonsillitis. The role of viruses is uncertain.

PROGNOSIS We found no good data on the natural history of tonsillitis or recurrent sore throat in children or adults. Participants in RCTs who were randomised to medical treatment (courses of antibiotics as required) have shown a tendency towards improvement over time.[3,4] Recurrent severe tonsillitis results in significant morbidity, including time lost from school or work.

AIMS OF INTERVENTION To abolish tonsillitis; to reduce the frequency and severity of recurrent throat infections; to improve general wellbeing, behaviour, and educational achievement, with minimal adverse effects.

OUTCOMES Number and severity of episodes of tonsillitis or sore throat; requirement for antibiotics and analgesics; time off work or school; behaviour, school performance, general wellbeing; morbidity and mortality of surgery; and adverse effects of drugs.

METHODS *Clinical Evidence* search and appraisal August 2002

QUESTION **What are the effects of tonsillectomy in children and adults with severe tonsillitis?**

OPTION **TONSILLECTOMY VERSUS ANTIBIOTICS**

Two systematic reviews found limited evidence that tonsillectomy may benefit some children with severe tonsillitis, but found insufficient evidence to compare surgical versus medical treatment. One subsequent RCT in less severely affected children found that surgery significantly reduced the frequency of tonsillitis compared with medical treatment over 3 years. The modest benefit may be outweighed by morbidity associated with the generation in populations with low incidence of tonsillitis. We found no RCTs evaluating tonsillectomy in adults.

Benefits: We found two systematic reviews (search dates 1997[5] and 1998[6]) and one subsequent RCT.[7] **Children:** Both reviews identified the same two RCTs as being the only ones that met quality inclusion criteria.[3,4] The smaller RCT involved 91 children who fulfilled criteria for "severe tonsillitis" (7 episodes in the preceding year, or 5 episodes/year in the preceding 2 years, or 3 episodes/year in the preceding 3 years).[3] It compared three treatments: tonsillectomy alone (27 children); adenotonsillectomy (16 children); or intermittent courses of antibiotics as needed (48 children). Sixteen children were withdrawn from the non-surgical group by their parents and had surgery, and children who developed infections after surgery received antibiotics as necessary for each episode of infection. Secondary outcome measures, such as time off school, were also considered. The authors concluded that children undergoing tonsillectomy experienced significantly fewer throat infections than those on antibiotics, amounting to an average of three fewer throat infections in the first 2 years, but by the third year the difference was no longer significant. The larger RCT (246 "less severely affected children") is published only in abstract form.[4] Some children in this study also underwent adenoidectomy. The limited data available provide no evidence of a difference between surgical and medical treatment. The second review concluded that it was not possible to determine the effectiveness of tonsillectomy from these RCTs.[6] One subsequent RCT (328 children with a history of milder recurrent episodes of throat infection) evaluated the effects of tonsillectomy in two different populations by stratifying children according to their history and age. Children with no apparent indication for adenoidectomy (recurrent or persistent otitis media or obstructing adenoids) were randomised to tonsillectomy, adenotonsillectomy, or medical treatment (3 way trial, 177 children). Children with any apparent indication for adenoidectomy were randomised to adenotonsillectomy or medical treatment (2 way trial, 151 children). In both trials outcomes were significantly more favourable in children in the surgical group versus medical treatment (children without indication for adenoidectomy [3 way trial]; mean number of moderate or severe episodes per year during 3 years' follow up: 0.09 with tonsillectomy [$P = 0.002$] *v* 0.08 with adenotonsillectomy [$P = 0.003$] *v* 0.33 with control; in children with indication for adenotonsillectomy [2 way trial]: 0.07 with adenotonsillectomy *v* 0.28 with medical treatment; $P < 0.001$).[7] **Adults:** The reviews found no RCTs that evaluated tonsillectomy in adults with recurrent tonsillitis or sore throats. We found no RCTs addressing long term effects of tonsillectomy.

Harms: **Tonsillectomy:** The risks of tonsillectomy include those associated with general anaesthesia and those specific to the procedure (bleeding, pain, otalgia, and, rarely, nasopharyngeal stenosis). The double barrelled RCT[7] found that 16/203 (8%) of the children who had surgery suffered complications. One suffered anaesthetic induction trismus and possible incipient malignant hyperthermia; three children had intraoperative haemorrhage with one of them needing reintervention under anaesthesia; one child required a posterior nasopharyngeal pack and admission to intensive care. Seven children (3.4%) developed postoperative haemorrhage and five of these children were readmitted to hospital, one of them requiring transfusion. Mean duration of postoperative sore throat was 6.3 days (range 0–21 days).[7] The overall complication rate in the smaller RCT (91 children)[3] was 14% (all were "readily managed or self limiting") compared with 2–8% in one Scottish tonsillectomy audit.[8] Haemorrhage, either primary (in the immediate postoperative period) or secondary, occurred in 4% of children studied in the larger RCT[4] and fewer than 1% of children in the Scottish tonsillectomy audit.[8] **Antibiotics:** In the smaller RCT (91 children), erythematous rashes occurred in 4% of children in the non-surgical group while taking penicillin.[3] Other adverse effects of antibiotics include allergic reactions and the promotion of resistant bacteria.

One RCT found that, for people with milder episodes of sore throat, the prescribing of antibiotics compared with no initial prescription increased the proportion of people who returned to see their physician in the short term because of sore throat (716 people with sore throat and an abnormal physical sign; return rate 38% with initial antibiotics *v* 27% without; adjusted HR for return 1.39, 95% CI 1.03 to 1.89).[9] The double barrelled RCT found that rates of erythematous rash were similar in children from the surgical and control groups (4/190 [2%] in surgery groups *v* 3/138 [2%] in control groups).[7]

Comment: In the double barrelled RCT, 79% of the children allocated to tonsillectomy and 78.8% of those assigned to adenotonsillectomy had surgery within 90 days of the randomisation. In the control groups, 12/60 (20%) children in the three-way RCT and 19/78 (24%) in the two-way RCT eventually underwent surgery. Although a significant reduction was found in the mean number of episodes of throat illnesses with surgical interventions, rates of illness in control groups were low.[7] The authors of the RCT concluded that the benefits of surgery may outweigh the risks in populations with low incidence of illness such as the population of children included in the study.[7] **Background:** Tonsillectomy is one of the most frequently performed surgical procedures in the UK, particularly in children, and accounts for about 20% of all operations performed by otolaryngologists.[8] Adenoidectomy is now performed with tonsillectomy only when there is a specific indication to remove the adenoids as well as the tonsils. **Quality of the evidence:** In the smaller RCT[3] there were significant baseline differences between groups before treatment, and the authors pooled the results of tonsillectomy and adenotonsillectomy, making it impossible to assess the effectiveness of tonsillectomy alone. The subsequent RCT on less severely affected children[7] was designed and run at the same time as the other RCTs discussed,[3,4] but the authors did study tonsillectomy separately from adenoidectomy and the conclusions are more robust. **Gaps in the evidence:** We found no RCT that found improved general wellbeing, development, or behaviour despite suggestions that these are influenced by tonsillectomy.[8] **New techniques:** Diathermy tonsillectomy and adjuvant treatment[10] may reduce adverse effects and are currently being studied.

REFERENCES

1. Management of Sore Throat and Indications for Tonsillectomy. National Clinical Guideline No 34. Scottish Intercollegiate Guidelines Network, Royal College of Physicians, 9 Queen Street, Edinburgh EH2 1JQ.
2. Shvartzman P. Careful prescribing is beneficial. *BMJ* 1994;309:1101–1102.
3. Paradise JL, Bluestone CD, Bachman RZ, et al. Efficacy of tonsillectomy for recurrent throat infection in severely affected children. *N Engl J Med* 1984;310:674–683.
4. Paradise JL, Bluestone CD, Rogers KD, et al. Comparative efficacy of tonsillectomy for recurrent throat infection in more versus less severely affected children [abstract]. *Pediatric Res* 1992;31:126A.
5. Marshall T. A review of tonsillectomy for recurrent throat infection. *Br J Gen Pract* 1998;48:1331–1335. Search date 1997; primary sources Cochrane Library and Medline.
6. Burton MJ, Towler B, Glasziou P. Tonsillectomy versus non-surgical treatment for chronic/recurrent acute tonsillitis. In: The Cochrane Library, Issue 2, 2001. Oxford: Update Software. Search date 1998; primary sources Medline, Embase, Cochrane Controlled Trials Register, and hand searched references.
7. Paradise JL,Bluestone CD, Colborne DK, et al. Tonsillectomy and adenotonsillectomy for recurrent throat infection in moderately affected children. *Pediatrics* 2002;110:7–15.
8. Blair RL, McKerrow WS, Carter NW, et al. The Scottish tonsillectomy audit. *J Laryngol Otol* 1996;110(suppl 20):1–25.

9. Little P, Gould C, Williamson I, et al. Reattendance and complications in a randomised trial of prescribing strategies for sore throat: the medicalising effect of prescribing antibiotics. *BMJ* 1997;315:350–352.
10. Steward DL, Chung SJ. The role of adjuvant therapies and techniques in tonsillectomy. *Curr Opin Otolaryngol Head Neck Surg* 2000;8:186–192.

William McKerrow
Consultant Otolaryngologist
Raigmore Hospital
Inverness
UK

Competing interests: None declared.
The following previous contributors of this topic would also like to be acknowledged: Martin Burton.

Wax in ear

Search date April 2003

George Browning

QUESTIONS

INTERVENTIONS

*Although many practitioners consider these to be standard treatments, we found no RCTs of these interventions

See glossary, p 652

Key Messages

- **Ear syringing** There is consensus that ear syringing is effective but we found no RCTs comparing ear syringing versus no treatment or versus other treatment. Reported complications of ear syringing include otitis externa, perforation of the ear drum, damage to the skin of the external canal, tinnitus, pain, and vertigo.
- **Manual removal (other than ear syringing)** We found no RCTs about other mechanical methods of removing ear wax.
- **Wax softeners** One small RCT in people with impacted wax found that active treatment (with a proprietary softening agent, sodium bicarbonate, or sterile water) reduced the risk of persisting impaction after 5 days compared with no treatment, but found no significant difference among active treatments. Three RCTs found no consistent evidence that any one type of wax softener was superior to the others. RCTs found insufficient evidence to assess the effects of wax softeners prior to syringing.

Wax in ear

DEFINITION Ear wax is normal and becomes a problem only if it produces deafness, pain, or other aural symptoms. Ear wax may also need to be removed if it prevents inspection of the ear drum. The term "impacted" (see glossary, p 652) is used in different ways, and can merely imply the coexistence of wax obscuring the ear drum with symptoms in that ear.[1,2]

INCIDENCE/ PREVALENCE We found four surveys of the prevalence of impacted wax (see table 1, p 653).[3–6] The prevalence was higher in men than in women, in the elderly than in the young, and in people with intellectual impairment.[7] One survey found that 289 Scottish general practitioners each saw an average of nine people a month requesting removal of ear wax.[1]

AETIOLOGY/ RISK FACTORS Factors that prevent the normal extrusion of wax from the ear canal (e.g. wearing a hearing aid, using cotton buds) increase the chance of ear wax accumulating.

PROGNOSIS Most ear wax emerges from the external canal spontaneously. Without impaction or adherence to the drum, there is likely to be minimal, if any, hearing loss.

AIMS OF INTERVENTION To relieve symptoms or to allow examination by completely removing impacted wax or obstructing wax; and to soften impacted wax to ease mechanical removal.

OUTCOMES Proportion of people (or ears) with relief of hearing loss or discomfort; total removal of wax; proportion of people requiring further intervention to improve symptoms; ease of mechanical removal measured, for example, by the volume of water used to accomplish successful syringing.

METHODS *Clinical Evidence* search and appraisal April 2003.

QUESTION **What are the effects of methods to remove ear wax?**

OPTION **WAX SOFTENERS**

One small RCT in people with impacted wax found that active treatment (with a proprietary softening agent, sodium bicarbonate, or sterile water) reduced the risk of persisting impaction after 5 days compared with no treatment, but found no significant difference among active treatments. Three RCTs found no consistent evidence that any one type of wax softener was superior to the others. RCTs found insufficient evidence to assess the effects of wax softeners prior to syringing.

Benefits: We found no systematic review. **Versus placebo or no treatment:** We found one RCT (113 people with impacted wax [see glossary, p 652] in one or both ears) (see table 2, p 654).[2] Ears were randomly allocated to treatment by the nursing staff with sterile water, sodium bicarbonate, a proprietary softening agent (arachis oil/chlorobutanol/*p*-dichlorobenzene), or no treatment. Participants and nurses were blinded to the active treatment allocation. The people were recruited from a hospital for the elderly. People already using ear drops and people with other pathology of the ear canal or ear drum were excluded. Of those recruited, 13 left hospital and three died before completing the RCT. Analysis of the remaining 97 people (155 ears) found that the proportion of ears with persisting impaction was significantly reduced by any active form of treatment after 5 days compared with no treatment (AR: 26/38 [68%] ears with no treatment *v* 55/117 [47%] ears with any active treatment; RR 1.46, 95% CI 1.09 to 1.94; NNT 5, 95% CI 3 to 17).[2] It found no significant difference in wax clearance among active treatments (P value not reported).[2] **Versus other wax softeners:** We found six trials comparing wax softeners (see table 2, p 654).[2,8–12] Only three were RCTs,[2,11,12] the other trials did not state the allocation strategy or were quasi-randomised trials. The trials were conducted in a variety of settings. They varied in size from 35 people to 286 ears. The most common outcomes were a subjective assessment of the amount of wax remaining, the need for syringing, the perceived ease of syringing, or the result of syringing. The trials found no consistent evidence that any one type of wax softener was clinically superior to any other. **Prior to syringing:** We found four RCTs[13–16] and one quasi-randomised trial[17] comparing various wax softeners given prior to ear syringing. All had design deficiencies that could lead to bias. Two of the RCTs found differences in effectiveness among wax softeners, and the other RCTs two found no overall difference (see table 3, p 656). The quasi-randomised trial found no difference between water instilled for 15 minutes and oil instilled nightly for 3 days.[17]

Harms: Seven RCTs did not report complications or adverse effects. Two trials found single cases of irritation, itching, or buzzing.[8,9] One RCT found that the frequency of adverse effects was similar in people using arachis oil/chlorobutanol/*p*-dichlorobenzene versus a proprietary agent (Otocerol® — the composition of which was not stated — see table 2, p 654).[11]

Comment: We found no good evidence about the optimal duration of treatment. Most trials did not use rigorous methods of randomisation, and did not include control for degree of occlusion at randomisation. Many trials were sponsored by companies that manufactured only one of the products being tested, but the possibility of publication bias has not been assessed. The inclusion criteria for the RCTs were not always clear: many stated that the participants had impacted wax without defining how this was defined. The RCT that included a no treatment group found that 32% of ears with impacted wax showed spontaneous resolution after 5 days.[2]

OPTION MECHANICAL METHODS

We found no RCTs about mechanical methods of removing ear wax. There is consensus that ear syringing is effective but we found no RCTs comparing ear syringing versus no treatment or versus other treatment. Reported complications of ear syringing include otitis externa, perforation of the ear drum, damage to the skin of the external canal, tinnitus, pain, and vertigo.

Benefits: We found no systematic review and no RCTs comparing mechanical methods intended to remove ear wax versus no treatment or alternative treatment.

Wax in ear

Harms: One survey found that 38% of 274 general practitioners reported complications in people receiving syringing, including otitis externa, perforation of the ear drum, damage to the skin of the external canal, tinnitus, pain, and vertigo.[1] We found no study of the incidence of these complications, or the effect of training and experience. People may experience dizziness during syringing or when wax is removed by suction.

Comment: There is consensus that syringing is effective and that training can reduce complications, but we found no reliable evidence. Mechanical techniques other than syringing include manual removal under direct vision, with or without a microscope, using suction, probes, or forceps. These methods require specific training and access to appropriate equipment.

GLOSSARY

Impacted wax Wax that has been compressed in the ear canal, completely obstructing the lumen. In practice, many RCTs define impaction as the presence of symptoms associated with obstructing wax.

Obstructing wax Wax that obscures direct vision of the ear drum.

REFERENCES

1. Sharp JF, Wilson JA, Ross L, et al. Ear wax removal: a survey of current practice. *BMJ* 1990;301:1251–1252.
2. Keane EM, Wilson H, McGrane D, et al. Use of solvents to disperse ear wax. *Br J Clin Pract* 1995;49:7–12.
3. Kalantan KA, Abdulghani H, Al-Taweel AA, et al. Use of cotton tipped swab and cerumen impaction. *Ind J Otol* 1999;5:27–31.
4. Minja BM, Machemba A. Prevalence of otitis media, hearing impairment and cerumen impaction among school children in rural and urban Dar es Salaam, Tanzania. *Int J Pediatr Otorhinolaryngol* 1996;37:29–34.
5. Swart SM, Lemmer R, Parbhoo JN, et al. A survey of ear and hearing disorders amongst a representative sample of Grade 1 school children in Swaziland. *Int J Pediatr Otorhinolaryngol* 1995;32:23–34.
6. Lewis-Cullinan C, Janken JK. Effect of cerumen removal on the hearing ability of geriatric patients. *J Adv Nurs* 1990;15:594–600.
7. Brister F, Fullwood HL, Ripp T, et al. Incidence of occlusion due to impacted cerumen among mentally retarded adolescents. *Am J Ment Defic* 1990;15:594–600.
8. Dummer DS, Sutherland IA, Murray JA. A single-blind, randomized study to compare the efficacy of two ear drop preparations ("Andax" and "Cerumol") in the softening of ear wax. *Curr Med Res Opin* 1992;13:26–30.
9. Lyndon S, Roy P, Grillage MG, et al. A comparison of the efficacy of two ear drop preparations ("Aurax" and "Earex") in the softening and removal of impacted ear wax. *Curr Med Res Opin* 1992;13:21–25.
10. Fahmy S, Whitefield M. Multicentre clinical trial of Exterol as a cerumenolytic. *Br J Clin Pract* 1982;36:197–204.
11. Jaffe G, Grimshaw J. A multicentric clinical trial comparing Otocerol with Cerumol as cerumenolytics. *J Int Med Res* 1978;6:241–244.
12. Carr MM, Smith RL. Ceruminolytic efficacy in adults versus children. *J Otolaryngol* 2001;30:154–156.
13. Singer AJ, Sauris E, Viccellio AW. Ceruminolytic effects of docusate sodium: a randomized controlled trial. *Ann Emerg Med* 2000;36:228–232.
14. Amjad AH, Scheer AA. Clinical evaluation of cerumenolytic agents. *Eye Ear Nose Throat Mon* 1975;54:76–77.
15. Chaput de Saintonge DM, Johnstone CI. A clinical comparison of triethanolamine polypeptide oleate-condensate ear drops with olive oil for the removal of impacted wax. *Br J Clin Pract* 1973;27:454–455.
16. Fraser JG. The efficacy of wax solvents: *in vitro* studies and a clinical trial. *J Laryngol Otol* 1970;84:1055–1064.
17. Eekhof JA, de Bock GH, Le Cessie S, et al. A quasi-randomised controlled trial of water as a quick softening agent of persistent earwax in general practice. *Br J Gen Pract* 2001;51:635–637.

George Browning
Professor of Otorhinolaryngology
MRC Institute of Hearing Research
Glasgow
UK

Competing interests: None declared.

The following previous contributors of this topic would also like to be acknowledged: Martin Burton, Elizabeth Mogg.

TABLE 1 **Surveys of the prevalence of impacted wax in specified populations (see text, p 650).[3–6]**

Ref	Where	Who	% with impacted wax
3	Saudi Arabia	1278 people attending primary care centre (any reason)	25%
4	Tanzania	802 primary school children	16%
5	Swaziland	Infant school children	7%
6	USA	Hospitalised elderly people (not in intensive care)	35%

Ref, reference.

TABLE 2 Effects of wax softeners: results of comparative RCTs (see text, p 650).[2,8–12]

Ref	Wax softener	Administration	Selection characteristic; setting	Number of people (ears)	Randomisation; blinding	Outcome	Results	Adverse effects
2	(a) Arachis oil Chlorobutanol *p*-dichlorobenzene (Cerumol®) (b) Sodium bicarbonate (in glycerol) (c) Sterile water (d) Nothing	4 drops twice a day for 5 days	Impacted ear(s); hospital	113 recruited; 97 completed (155)	Randomisation (technique not described) Double blind (active treatments)	Residual wax; 3 tiered clinical rating scale	Treatment better than no treatment; persisting impaction: 55/117 with softeners *v* 26/38 with no treatment; no difference agents	None
8	(a) Ethyleneoxide-polyoxypropylene glycol Choline salicylate (b) Arachis oil Chlorobutanol *p*-dichlorobenzene (Cerumol®)		Impacted or hardened wax; general practice	50 (100)	Not stated; single blind	Wax amount, colour, and consistency; objective hearing; global impression of efficiency	No difference	Two irritation with (a); one itch, one buzzing with (b)
9	(a) Ethyleneoxide-polyoxypropylene glycol, Choline salicylate (b) Arachis oil Almond oil Rectified camphor oil	Drops to fill ear twice a day for 4 days	Symptoms requiring wax softener; general practice	36 (72)	Not stated; not blind	Need for syringing; ease of syringing; global impression of efficiency	(a) better than (b); easy removal: 37/38 *v* 19/30	One irritation with (b); one disliked smell
10	(a) 5% urea hydrogen peroxide in glycerol (b) Glycerol	5–10 drops twice a day for 1 week	Ear wax problems; ENT department	40 (80)	Alternation; double blind	Need for syringing; ease of syringing	(a) better than glycerol; success: 35/40 *v* 20/40	None

TABLE 2 continued

Ref	Wax softener	Administration	Selection characteristic; setting	Number of people (ears)	Randomisation; blinding	Outcome	Results	Adverse effects
10	(a) 5% urea hydrogen peroxide in glycerol (b) Arachis oil, Chlorobutanol, *p*-dichlorobenzene (Cerumol®)	5–10 drops twice a day for 1 week	Ear wax problems; ENT department	50 (100)	Alternation; double blind	Need for syringing; ease of syringing	(a) better than (b); success: 47/50 *v* 24/50	None
11	(a) 5% urea hydrogen peroxide in glycerol (b) Arachis oil, Chlorobutanol, *p*-dichlorobenzene, (Cerumol®)	5–10 drops twice a day for a week	Ear wax problems; general practice	160 (286)	Alternation; double blind	Need for syringing; ease of syringing	(a) better than (b); success: 146/157 *v* 93/129	None
11	(a) Otocerol® (b) Arachis oil, Chlorobutanol, *p*-dichlorobenzene (Cerumol®)	Three consecutive nights	For whom a wax softener would normally be prescribed; general practice	106 (not stated)	Random allocation; double blind	3 tiered clinical rating scale	No difference overall; 38/53 *v* 33/53	Pain; irritation; giddiness; smell (Otocerol® 7/53 Cerumol® 10/53)
12	(a) 10% aqueous sodium bicarbonate (b) 2.5% aqueous acetic acid	Daily applications for 14 days	Incidentally noted wax Paediatric and adult ENT departments	60 (138)	Randomisation strategy not stated; blind selection of bottles by the person. Observers blind	Otoscopic score of degree of wax	No difference in change in scores	Otalgia in 2/34 people on acetic acid.

ENT, ear, nose and throat; Ref, reference.

TABLE 3 **Effects of wax softeners prior to syringing: results of comparative RCTs (see text, p 650).[13–17]**

Ref	Wax softener	Administration	Selection characteristic; setting	Number of people (ears)	Randomisation; blind	Outcome	Results	Adverse effects
14	(a) Triethanolamine polypeptide oleate condensate (b) Carbamide peroxide	One dose 30 minutes before syringing	Hard or impacted wax; setting unclear	80 (not stated)	Random allocation; double blind	Result of syringing; 4 tiered clincal rating scale	(a) better than (b); success: 33/40 *v* 7/40 but (b) normally used as multiple installations	Not reported
15	(a) Triethanolamine polypeptide oleate condensate (b) Olive oil	One dose 20 minutes before syringing	Impacted wax suitable for syringing; hospital outpatient department	67 (not stated)	Random order; double blind	3 tiered clinical rating scale	No difference overall (20/32 *v* 21/35); (a) needed less water	None
13	(a) Triethylamine polypeptide (b) Docusate sodium (Waxol®)	One dose 15 minutes before syringing	Partial or totally accluding wax	50 (50)	Random order; not blind	Visualisation of tympanic membrane	(b) better than (a) (22/27 *v* 8/23)	None
17	(a) Water, cotton ear plug (b) Oil, cotton ear plug	(a) 15 minutes (b) nightly for 3 days	Persistent wax after five syringing attemps; general practice	130 (224)	Quasi-randomised (year of birth); not blind	Number of attemps needed to clear	No difference; however, statistical tests performed may have been inadequate	Not addressed
16	(a) Arachis oil Chlorobutanol *p*-dichlorobenzene (Cerumol®) (b) Docusate sodium (Waxsol®) (c) Olive oil *v* (d) Sodium bicarbonate (inglycerol)	Ear canal filled for 15 minutes, once daily every 3 days	Bilateral hard and occluding wax; geriatric hospital	124 (248)	Each participant was allocated (d) in one randomly chosen ear and treatment in the other ear. Double blind.	Failed forceful syringing	(a) better than (d), 1/24 *v* 5/24	Red canals

Ref, reference.

Foot ulcers and amputations in diabetes

Search date January 2003

Dereck Hunt and Hertzel Gerstein

QUESTIONS

INTERVENTIONS

See glossary, p 664

Key Messages

Preventive interventions

- **Screening and referral to foot care clinics (for major amputations in those at high risk)** One RCT found that a diabetes screening and protection programme (involving referral to a foot clinic) reduced the risk of major amputation compared with usual care after 2 years.
- **Education (for foot ulceration, serious foot lesions, amputation)** One systematic review found insufficient evidence about the effects of patient education for the prevention of foot complications.
- **Therapeutic footwear (for ulcer recurrence)** In people with diabetes and previous diabetic foot ulcer, one RCT found no significant difference in rates of foot ulceration between therapeutic footwear and usual footwear.

Treatments

- **Pressure off-loading with non-removable cast (for non-infected foot ulcer healing)** We found evidence that pressure off-loading with total contact casting or non-removable fibreglass casts improved non-infected diabetic foot ulcer healing compared with other treatments.
- **Human skin equivalent (for chronic neuropathic non-infected foot ulcer healing)** One RCT found that human skin equivalent increased ulcer healing rates compared with saline moistened gauze in people with chronic neuropathic non-infected foot ulcers.

Foot ulcers and amputations in diabetes

- **Systemic hyperbaric oxygen (for infected ulcers)** We found evidence that systemic hyperbaric oxygen plus usual care reduced the risk of foot amputation compared with usual care alone in people with severely infected foot ulcers.
- **Topical growth factors (for non-infected foot ulcer healing)** One systematic review found that topical growth factors increased healing rates compared with placebo in people with non-infected diabetic foot ulcers.
- **Cultured human dermis (for non-infected foot ulcer healing)** We found insufficient evidence of the effects of cultured human dermis on ulcer healing.
- **Pressure off-loading with felted foam versus pressure relief half shoe** We found insufficient evidence that a pressure off-loading felted foam dressing improved ulcer healing compared with a pressure relief half shoe.

DEFINITION Diabetic foot ulceration is full thickness penetration of the dermis of the foot in a person with diabetes. Ulcer severity is often classified using the Wagner system. Grade 1 ulcers are superficial ulcers involving the full skin thickness but no underlying tissues. Grade 2 ulcers are deeper, penetrating down to ligaments and muscle, but not involving bone or abscess formation. Grade 3 ulcers are deep ulcers with cellulitis or abscess formation, often complicated with osteomyelitis. Ulcers with localised gangrene are classified as grade 4 and those with extensive gangrene involving the entire foot are classified as grade 5.

INCIDENCE/ PREVALENCE Studies conducted in Australia, Finland, the UK, and the USA have reported the annual incidence of foot ulcers among people with diabetes as 2.5–10.7%, and the annual incidence of amputation as 0.25–1.8%.[1–10]

AETIOLOGY/ RISK FACTORS Long term risk factors for foot ulcers and amputation include duration of diabetes, poor glycaemic control, microvascular complications (retinopathy, nephropathy, and neuropathy) and peripheral vascular disease. The strongest predictors of foot complications are altered foot sensation, foot deformities, and previous foot ulcer or amputation.[1–10]

PROGNOSIS People with diabetes are at risk of foot ulcers, infections, and vascular insufficiency. Amputation is indicated if these are severe or do not improve with conservative treatment. As well as affecting quality of life, these complications account for a large proportion of the healthcare costs of diabetes. For people with healed diabetic foot ulcers, the 5 year cumulative rate of ulcer recurrence is 66% and of amputation is 12%.[11]

AIMS OF INTERVENTION To prevent diabetic foot complications, including ulcers and amputations; and to improve ulcer healing and prevent amputations where ulcers already exist, with minimum adverse effects.

OUTCOMES Rates of development or recurrence of foot ulcers or major foot lesions; rate of amputation (surgical removal of all or part of the lower extremity: minor amputations involve partial removal of a foot, including toe or forefoot resections; and major amputations are above or below knee amputations); time ulcers take to heal, or the proportion healed in a given period; rates of hospital admission; rates of foot infection; adverse effects of treatment.

METHODS *Clinical Evidence* search and appraisal January 2003.

QUESTION **What are the effects of preventive interventions?**

OPTION **SCREENING AND REFERRAL TO FOOT CARE CLINIC**

One RCT found that a diabetes screening and protection programme (involving referral to a foot clinic) reduced the risk of major amputation compared with usual care after 2 years.

Benefits: We found one systematic review (search date 1998, 1 RCT, 2002 people attending a general diabetes clinic).[12] The RCT compared a diabetes screening and protection programme versus usual care over 2 years.[13] People in the diabetes screening and protection programme were screened for deficits in pedal pulses, light touch, and vibration sensation. People with persistent abnormal findings were referred to the diabetic foot clinic if they had a history of foot ulcer, were found to have a low ankle-brachial index (< 0.75), or were noted to have foot deformities. The clinic provided podiatry and protective shoes as well as education regarding foot care. Usual care consisted of the normal follow up for people in the clinic, who could be referred to the foot care clinic if a healthcare professional requested this. The RCT found that the diabetes screening and protection programme reduced major amputation compared with usual care (AR 0.1% with the diabetes programme *v* 1.2% with usual care; ARR 1.1%, 95% CI 0.4% to 1.9%; NNT 91, 95% CI 53 to 250).

Harms: The RCT did not report adverse effects.[13]

Comment: None.

OPTION **THERAPEUTIC FOOTWEAR**

In people with diabetes and previous diabetic foot ulcer, one RCT found no significant difference in rates of foot ulceration between therapeutic footwear and usual footwear.

Benefits: We found one systematic review, which identified no RCTs (see comments).[12] We found one RCT (400 people with diabetes mellitus and previous foot ulcer but without severe deformity, mean age 62 years) comparing extra-depth and extra-width therapeutic shoes fitted with customised cork inserts versus therapeutic shoes fitted with polyurethane inserts versus usual footwear for 2 years.[14] The RCT found no significant difference in foot ulceration rates between therapeutic footwear and usual footwear (AR for foot ulceration 15% with cork insert *v* 14% with polyurethane insert *v* 17% with usual footwear; RR cork insert *v* usual footwear 0.88, 95% CI 0.51 to 1.52; RR polyurethane insert *v* usual footwear 0.85, 95% CI 0.48 to 1.48).

Harms: The RCT did not report adverse effects.[14]

Comment: The systematic review (search date 1998)[12] identified one non-randomised controlled trial.[15] The trial alternately allocated 69 people with a previous diabetic foot ulcer to either an intervention group (in which people received therapeutic shoes) or to a control group (in which people continued to wear their ordinary shoes).[15]

Therapeutic shoes were manufactured according to the Towey guidelines (super depth to fit customised insoles and toe deformities, and made with soft thermoformable leather along with semi-rocker soles). All participants received information on foot care and footwear. After 1 year, the trial found that wearing therapeutic shoes reduced ulcer recurrence compared with ordinary shoes (27% with therapeutic shoes *v* 58% with ordinary shoes; ARR 31%, 95% CI 7% to 55%; NNT 4, 95% CI 2 to 14). The trial did not report any adverse effects associated with therapeutic shoes. Alternate allocation increases the possibility of bias and confounding.

OPTION EDUCATION

One systematic review found insufficient evidence of the effects of education programmes for prevention of diabetic foot ulcers.

Benefits: We found one systematic review (search date 2001, three RCTs, one quasi randomised trial).[16] The first RCT in the review (352 people with diabetes attending 4 primary care teams, randomised by primary care team) compared structured care (a patient education session about foot care plus patient follow up reminders plus prompts to healthcare providers to examine feet and provide education) versus usual care (not described).[17] It found that structured care reduced "serious foot lesions" (based on the Seattle Wound Classification Scale [see glossary, p 664])[18] compared with controls after 12 months (OR 0.41, 95% CI 0.16 to 1.00). The second RCT in the review (266 people with diabetes attending primary care) compared foot care education (nine sessions on foot care and skin hygiene, diabetes, risk factors, diet, and weight management) versus usual care.[19] It found no significant difference in ulcer and amputation rates (combined) after 1.5 years (10/127 [8%] with foot care education *v* 16/139 [12%] with usual care; OR 0.66, 95% CI 0.30 to 1.49). The third RCT in the review (530 people with diabetes without any obvious need for foot care) compared education from a podiatrist (45 minute session covering footwear, hygiene, toenail cutting, emollient cream, avoiding risk, foot gymnastics, and preventive podiatric care) plus podiatric visits of 30–60 minutes' duration for 1 year versus written foot care instructions.[20,21] It found no significant difference in amputation and ulcer rates between foot education plus podiatric visits versus written foot care instructions and after 7 years (amputation rate: 1/267 with education plus podiatric visits *v* 0/263; P value undefined; ulcer rate: 0.6% with education plus podiatric visits *v* 0.6% with written instructions; P = 1.0) The quasi randomised trial in the review (227 people with diabetes, allocated according to social security number) compared a single 1 hour educational class about foot care versus routine diabetes education.[22] It found that the educational session reduced ulcer recurrences and major amputation after 2 years (ulcer recurrence: 4.5% for foot care education *v* 14.7% for routine education; RR 0.31, 95% CI 0.15 to 0.65; NNT 10, 95% CI 6 to 26; major amputation: 2.8% for foot care education *v* 10.2% for routine education; RR 0.28, 95% CI 0.11 to 0.70; NNT 14, 95% CI 8 to 50).

Harms: The systematic review did not report harms.[16]

Comment: The studies included in the systematic review were of poor methodological quality.[16] The flaws included the following: only one trial had blinded outcome assessment; one trial made no comment on loss to follow up; some studies offered no comment on concealment of randomisation in the studies; the trials did not use an intention to treat approach; and the eligibility criteria with respect to risk of ulceration were described adequately in only one trial.

QUESTION **What are the effects of treatments?**

OPTION **PRESSURE OFF-LOADING**

We found evidence that pressure off-loading with total contact casting or non-removable fibreglass casts improved healing of non-infected diabetic foot ulcers compared with other treatments. We found insufficient evidence that a pressure off-loading felted foam dressing improved ulcer healing compared with a pressure relief half shoe.

Benefits: We found one systematic review (search date 1998, one relevant RCT, 40 people with diabetes and plantar foot ulcers but no signs of infection or gangrene)[23] and three subsequent RCTs.[24–26] **Versus traditional dressing changes:** The RCT in the review compared total contact casting (see glossary, p 664) versus traditional dressing changes.[27] Casts were applied by an experienced physical therapist, changed after 5–7 days, and then every 2–3 weeks until healing occurred. Control participants were provided with accommodative footwear and crutches or a walker, and were instructed to complete wet to dry dressing changes 2–3 times daily. The RCT found that total contact casting significantly increased ulcer healing and reduced infection compared with traditional dressing changes (ulcer healing: 91% with total contact casting *v* 32% with traditional dressing; ARR 59%, 95% CI 31% to 87%; NNT 2, 95% CI 1 to 3; infection: 0/21 with total contact casting *v* 5/19 with traditional dressing; $P < 0.05$).[27] **Versus removable casts/shoes:** The first subsequent RCT (63 people with diabetes mellitus and non-infected neuropathic plantar foot ulcers) compared total contact casting versus a removable cast walker versus a half shoe.[24] All participants had weekly visits for wound care and debridements. The RCT found that total contact casting increased ulcer healing compared with removable cast walkers or half shoes after 12 weeks (89% with total contact casting *v* 61% with removable cast walker or half-shoe; ARR 28%, 95% CI 5% to 51%; NNT 4, 95% CI 2 to 19). The second subsequent RCT (50 people with diabetes mellitus and non-infected neuropathic plantar foot ulcers) compared non-removable fibreglass casts versus specialised cloth shoes with rigid soles and off-loading insoles over 30 days.[25] All participants had dressing changes every 2 days. It found that non-removable fibreglass casts improved ulcer healing compared with specialised cloth shoes (50% of ulcers healed with fibreglass casts *v* 21% with specialised cloth shoes; ARR 29%, 95% CI 1.4% to 57%; NNT 4, 95% CI 2 to 72). **Versus a pressure relief half shoe:** The third subsequent RCT (61 people with diabetes mellitus and a neuropathic plantar forefoot ulcer) compared pressure off-loading felted foam dressings versus a pressure relief half shoe over at least 10 weeks.[26] The RCT found no significant difference in time to ulcer healing (79.6 days with felted foam *v* 83.2 days with a half shoe, P = 0.61).

Harms: The RCT identified in the systematic review found that 3/21 (14%) people treated with total contact casting developed fungal infections requiring topical treatment. This did not prevent continued casting.[27] The other RCTs reported no adverse effects.[24–26]

Comment: Soft tissue infections and osteomyelitis are contraindications to total contact casting.

OPTION CULTURED HUMAN DERMIS

We found insufficient evidence of the effects of cultured human dermis on ulcer healing.

Benefits: We found one systematic review (search date 1998, 2 RCTs) comparing topical application of cultured human dermis substitute (see glossary, p 664) (weekly for 8 weeks) plus usual care versus usual care alone in people attending hospital outpatient clinics with diabetic foot ulcers with no signs of infection or severe vascular compromise.[23] All participants received wound debridement and were encouraged to avoid weight bearing on the affected limb. The review found no significant difference in ulcer healing at 12 weeks with cultured human dermis compared with control (+21% increase in ulcer healing with cultured human dermis compared with usual care at 12 weeks, 95% CI –13% to +36%).

Harms: One RCT identified by the systematic review found no significant difference between cultured human dermis and usual care in the rates of ulcer infections, and no effect on haematology or serum chemistry values or glycaemic control.[23] The other RCT found no significant differences in wound infection rates.

Comment: Cultured human dermis (Dermagraft) may not be widely available.

OPTION HUMAN SKIN EQUIVALENT

One RCT found that human skin equivalent increased ulcer healing compared with saline moistened gauze in people with chronic neuropathic non-infected foot ulceration.

Benefits: We found no systematic review. We found one RCT (208 people aged 18–80 years with diabetes mellitus and chronic neuropathic non-infected foot ulceration) comparing human skin equivalent (see glossary, p 664) (Graftskin applied weekly for a maximum of 5 weeks) versus saline moistened gauze (applied weekly).[28] It found that human skin equivalent improved ulcer healing compared with saline moistened gauze after 12 weeks (56% with human skin equivalent *v* 38% with saline moistened gauze; ARI 18%, 95% CI 5% to 33%; RR 1.5, 95% CI 1.1 to 2.0; NNT 6, 95% CI 3 to 20).

Harms: The RCT found no significant adverse effects.[28] Wound infections and cellulitis were equally frequent in both groups. Osteomyelitis and amputations were less frequent in people receiving human skin equivalent (osteomyelitis: 2.7% with human skin equivalent v 10.4% with saline moistened gauze; amputations: 6.3% with human skin equivalent v 15.6% with saline moistened gauze).

Comment: Human skin equivalent may not be widely available.

OPTION TOPICAL GROWTH FACTORS

One systematic review found that topical growth factors increased healing rates compared with placebo in people with non-infected diabetic foot ulcers.

Benefits: We found one systematic review (search date 1998, 6 RCTs) comparing four different topical growth factors (see glossary, p 664) versus placebo in people attending hospital outpatient clinics with diabetic foot ulcers who were free of signs of infection or severe vascular compromise. All participants received wound debridement and were encouraged to avoid weight bearing on the affected limb. The systematic review did not pool the results from the RCTs.[23] The first RCT (65 people) found that treatment with a topical growth factor (arginine–glycine–aspartic acid matrix) twice weekly for up to 10 weeks increased healing rates compared with placebo (AR for non-healing: 65% with matrix v 92% with placebo; ARR 27%, 95% CI 6% to 48%; NNT 4, 95% CI 2 to 15; P = 0.02).[29] The second RCT (118 people) found that treatment with platelet derived growth factors (30 µg/g once daily for up to 20 weeks) increased healing rates compared with placebo (AR for non-healing: 52% with platelet derived growth factors v 75% with placebo; ARR 23%, 95% CI 5% to 41%; NNT 5, 95% CI 3 to 14; P = 0.01).[30] The third RCT (382 people) found that platelet derived growth factors (100 µg/g once daily for up to 20 weeks) increased healing rates compared with placebo (AR for non-healing: 50% with platelet derived growth factors v 65% with placebo; ARR 15%, 95% CI 2% to 28%; NNT 7, 95% CI 4 to 42; P = 0.007).[31] The fourth RCT (13 people) found no significant difference in healing rates between thrombin induced human platelet derived growth factor (CT-102) applied twice weekly and placebo (complete healing: 5/7 with CT-102 v 1/6 with placebo; P value not reported).[32] The fifth RCT (81 people) found that CT-102 increased healing compared with placebo (non-healing: 20% with CT-102 v 71% with placebo; ARR 51%, 95% CI 19% to 84%; NNT 2, 95% CI 1 to 5; P = 0.01).[33] The sixth RCT (17 people) of recombinant growth factor found no significant difference in complete healing compared with placebo (complete healing: 3/9 [33%] with recombinant growth factor v 5/8 [63%] with placebo; P = 0.23).[34]

Harms: The systematic review reported no growth factor related adverse effects.[23]

Comment: These therapeutic agents are not widely available and may be expensive. There has been little long term follow up of people treated with these growth factors.

OPTION SYSTEMIC HYPERBARIC OXYGEN

We found limited evidence that systemic hyperbaric oxygen plus usual care reduced the risk of foot amputation compared with usual care alone in people with severely infected foot ulcers.

Benefits: We found one systematic review (search date 1998, 1 RCT)[23] and one additional RCT.[35] The RCT in the systematic review (70 people with severe infected diabetic foot ulcers with full thickness gangrene or abscess, or a large infected ulcer that had not healed after 30 days) compared systemic hyperbaric oxygen (see glossary, p 664) (daily 90 minute sessions at 2.2–2.5 atmospheres) plus usual care (aggressive debridement, broad spectrum iv antibiotics, revascularisation if indicated, and optimised glycaemic control) versus usual care alone.[36] After 10 weeks, systemic hyperbaric oxygen plus usual care reduced rates of major amputation compared with usual care alone (8.6% with systemic hyperbaric oxygen *v* 33% with usual care alone; RR 0.26, 95% CI 0.16 to 0.92; ARR 24%, 95% CI 4% to 45%; NNT 5, 95% CI 2 to 23). The additional RCT (30 people with chronic infected foot ulcers) compared usual care (including debridement, iv antibiotics, and optimised glycaemic control) versus usual care plus four treatments with systemic hyperbaric oxygen over 2 weeks.[35] It found no significant difference in the risk of major amputation (13.3% with systemic hyperbaric oxygen *v* 46.7% with usual care alone; ARR +33%, 95% CI –1.6% to +68%).

Harms: In one of the RCTs, two people developed symptoms of barotraumatic otitis, but this did not interrupt treatment.[36]

Comment: The additional RCT may have been too small to rule out a clinically important effect.

GLOSSARY

Cultured human dermis consists of neonatal fibroblasts cultured *in vitro* onto a bioabsorbable mesh to produce a living, metabolically active tissue containing normal dermal matrix proteins and cytokines.

Human skin equivalent consists of two allogenic layers containing human skin cells. One layer is formed by dermal cells (human fibroblasts) and the second layer is formed by epidermal cells. Human skin equivalent produces cytokines and growth factors involved in the skin healing process.

Pressure off-loading refers to the use of different techniques designed to minimise the amount of force applied to the ulcer site.

Systemic hyperbaric oxygen refers to exposing a patient to a high oxygen, high pressure environment designed to improve oxygen delivery to the ulcer site.

Topical growth factors are synthetically produced factors specifically designed to promote cellular proliferation or matrix production at an ulcer site.

Seattle wound classification system is used to standardise the description of diabetic foot ulcers. It has 10 categories from superficial wound (category 1) to deep wound involving infection and tissue necrosis (category 10).[18]

Total contact casting is the application of a layer of plaster over the foot and lower leg, designed to distribute pressure evenly over the entire plantar aspect of the foot to reduce exposure of plantar ulcers to pressure, even when the person is walking.

Substantive changes

Education One systematic review added;[16] conclusions unchanged.

Pressure off-loading with felted foam One RCT added (61 people);[26] it found no significant difference in time to ulcer healing between pressure off-loading felted foam dressings and a pressure relief half shoe. Conclusion: unknown effectiveness.

REFERENCES

1. Rith-Najarian SJ, Stolusky T, Gohdes DM. Identifying diabetic patients at high risk for lower-extremity amputation in a primary health care setting. *Diabetes Care* 1992;15:1386–1389.
2. Veves A, Murray HJ, Young MJ, et al. The risk of foot ulceration in diabetic patients with high foot pressure: a prospective study. *Diabetologia* 1992;35:660–663.
3. Young MJ, Breddy JL, Veves, et al. The prediction of diabetic neuropathic foot ulceration using vibration perception thresholds: a prospective study. *Diabetes Care* 1994;17:557–560.
4. Humphrey ARG, Dowse GK, Thoma K, et al. Diabetes and nontraumatic lower extremity amputations. Incidence, risk factors, and prevention: a 12 year follow-up study in Nauru. *Diabetes Care* 1996;19:710–714.
5. Lee JS, Lu M, Lee VS, et al. Lower-extremity amputation: incidence, risk factors, and mortality in the Oklahoma Indian diabetes study. *Diabetes* 1993;42:876–882.
6. Lehto S, Ronnemaa T, Pyorala K, et al. Risk factors predicting lower extremity amputations in patients with NIDDM. *Diabetes Care* 1996;19:607–612.
7. Moss SE, Klein R, Klein B. Long-term incidence of lower-extremity amputations in a diabetic population. *Arch Fam Med* 1996;5:391–398.
8. Nelson RG, Gohdes DM, Everhart JE, et al. Lower-extremity amputations in NIDDM: 12 year follow-up study in Pima Indians. *Diabetes Care* 1988;11:8–16.
9. Boyko ED, Ahroni JH, Stensel V, et al. A prospective study of risk factors for diabetic foot ulcer. The Seattle diabetic foot study. *Diabetes Care* 1999;22:1036–1042.
10. Abbott CA, Carrington AL, Ashe H, et al. The North-West Diabetes Foot Care Study: incidence of, and risk factors for, new diabetic foot ulceration in a community-based patient cohort. *Diabet Med* 2002;19:377–384.
11. Apelqvist J, Larsson J, Agardh CD. Long-term prognosis for diabetic patients with foot ulcers. *J Intern Med* 1993;233:485–491.
12. Mason J, O'Keeffe C, McIntosh A, et al. A systematic review of foot ulcer in patients with type 2 diabetes mellitus. I: prevention. *Diabet Med* 1999;16:801–812. Search date 1998; primary sources Cochrane Controlled Trials Register, Medline, Embase, Cinahl, Healthstar, Psychlit, Science Citation, Social Science Citation, Index to Scientific and Technical Conference Proceedings (ISI), HMIC database, and Sigle.
13. McCabe CJ, Stevenson RC, Dolan AM. Evaluation of a diabetic foot screening and protection programme. *Diabet Med* 1998;15:80–84.
14. Reiber GE, Smith DG, Wallace C, et al. Effect of therapeutic footwear on foot reulceration in patients with diabetes: a randomized controlled trial. *JAMA* 2002;287:2552–2558.
15. Uccioli L, Faglia E, Monticone G, et al. Manufactured shoes in the prevention of diabetic foot ulcers. *Diabetes Care* 1995;18:1376–1378.
16. Valk GD, Kriegsman DMW, Assendelft WJJ. Patient education for preventing diabetic foot ulceration. A systematic review. *Endocrinol Metab Clin N Am* 2002;31:633–658.
17. Litzelman DK, Slemenda CW, Langefeld CD, et al. Reduction of lower extremity clinical abnormalities in patients with non-insulin-dependent diabetes mellitus. *Ann Intern Med* 1993;119:36–41.
18. Pecoraro RE, Reiber GE. Classification of Wounds in Diabetic Amputees. *Wounds* 1990;2:65–73.
19. Bloomgarden ZT, Karmally W, Metzger MJ, et al. Randomized controlled trial of diabetic patient education: improved knowledge without improved metabolic status. *Diabetes Care* 1987;10:263–272.
20. Hamalainen H, Ronnemaa T, Toikka T, et al. Long-term effects of one year of intensified podiatric activities on foot-care knowledge and self-care habits in patients with diabetes. *Diabetes Education* 1998;24:734–740.
21. Ronnemaa T, Hamalainen H, Toikka T, et al. Evaluation of the impact of podiatrist care in the primary prevent of foot problems in diabetic subjects. *Diabetes Care* 1997;20:1833–1837.
22. Malone JM, Snyder M, Anderson G, et al. Prevention of amputation by diabetic education. *Am J Surg* 1989;158:520–524.
23. Mason J, O'Keeffe C, Hutchinson A, et al. A systematic review of foot ulcer in patients with type 2 diabetes mellitus. II: treatment. *Diabet Med* 1999;16:889–909. Search date 1998; primary sources Cochrane Controlled Trials Register, Medline, Embase, Cinahl, Healthstar, Psychlit, Science Citation, Social Science Citation, Index to Scientific and Technical Conference Proceedings (ISI), HMIC database, and Sigle.
24. Armstrong DG, Nguyen HC, Lavery LA, et al. Off-loading the diabetic foot wound: a randomized clinical trial. *Diabetes Care* 2001;24:1019–1022.
25. Caravaggi C, Faglia E, De Giglio R, et al. Effectiveness and safety of a nonremovable fiberglass off-bearing cast versus a therapeutic shoe in the treatment of neuropathic foot ulcers: a randomized study. *Diabetes Care* 2000;23:1746–1751.
26. Zimny S, Meyer MF, Schatz H, et al. Applied felted foam for plantar pressure relief is an efficient therapy in neuropathic diabetic foot ulcers. *Exp Clin Endocrinol Diabetes* 2002;110:325–328.
27. Mueller MJ, Diamond JE, Sinacore DR, et al. Total contact casting in treatment of diabetic planter ulcers. *Diabetes Care* 1989;12:384–388.
28. Veves A, Falanga V, Armstrong DG, et al. Graftskin, a human skin equivalent, is effective in the management of noninfected neuropathic diabetic foot ulcers: a prospective randomized multicenter clinical trial. *Diabetes Care* 2001;24:290–295.
29. Steed DL, Ricotta JJ, Prendergast JJ, et al. Promotion and acceleration of diabetic ulcer healing by arginine-glycine-aspartic acid (RGD) peptide matrix. *Diabetes Care* 1995;18:39–46.
30. Steed DL, and the Diabetic Ulcer Study Group. Clinical evaluation of recombinant human platelet-derived growth factor for the treatment of lower extremity diabetic ulcers. *J Vasc Surg* 1995;21:71–81.
31. Wieman TJ, Smiell JM, Su Y. Efficacy and safety of a topical gel formulation of recombinant human platelet-derived growth factor-BB (Becaplermin) in patients with chronic neuropathic diabetic ulcers. *Diabetes Care* 1998;21:822–827.
32. Steed D, Goslen J, Holloway G, et al. Randomized prospective double-blind trial in healing chronic diabetic foot ulcers. *Diabetes Care* 1992;15:1598–1604.

33. Holloway G, Steed D, DeMarco M, et al. A randomized controlled dose response trial of activated platelet supernatant, topical CT-102 in chronic, non-healing diabetic wounds. *Wounds* 1993;5:198–206.
34. Richard J, Richard C, Daures J, et al. Effect of topical basic fibroblast growth factor on the healing of chronic diabetic neuropathic ulcer of the foot. *Diabetes Care* 1995;18:64–69.
35. Doctor N, Pandya S, Supe A. Hyperbaric oxygen therapy in diabetic foot. *J Postgrad Med* 1992;38:112–114.
36. Faglia E, Favales F, Aldeghi A, et al. Adjunctive systemic hyperbaric oxygen therapy in treatment of severe prevalently ischemic diabetic foot ulcer. *Diabetes Care* 1996;19:1338–1343.

Dereck Hunt
Assistant Professor of Medicine

Hertzel Gerstein
Professor of Medicine

McMaster University
Hamilton, Ontario
Canada

Competing interests: None declared.

Glycaemic control in diabetes

Search date December 2002

Bazian Ltd

QUESTIONS

INTERVENTIONS

Key Messages

Intensive control of hyperglycaemia in people aged 13–75 years

- Large RCTs have found that diabetic complications increase with HbA1c concentrations above the non-diabetic range.
- One systematic review and large subsequent RCTs in people with type 1 or type 2 diabetes have found strong evidence that intensive versus conventional glycaemic control significantly reduces the development and progression of microvascular and neuropathic complications. A second systematic review has found that intensive versus conventional treatment is associated with a small reduction in cardiovascular risk.
- RCTs have found that intensive treatment increases the incidence of hypoglycaemia and weight gain, without adverse impact on neuropsychological function or quality of life.
- The benefit of intensive treatment is limited by the complications of advanced diabetes (such as blindness, end stage renal disease, or cardiovascular disease), major comorbidity, and reduced life expectancy.

Intensive control of hyperglycaemia in people with frequent severe hypoglycaemia

- The benefits of intensive treatment of hyperglycaemia are described above.
- It is difficult to weigh the benefit of reduced complications against the harm of increased hypoglycaemia. The risk of intensive treatment is increased by a history of severe hypoglycaemia or unawareness of hypoglycaemia, advanced autonomic neuropathy or cardiovascular disease, and impaired ability to detect or treat hypoglycaemia (such as altered mental state, immobility, or lack of social support). For people likely to have limited benefit or increased risk with intensive treatment, it may be more appropriate to negotiate less intensive goals for glycaemic management that reflect the person's self determined goals of care and willingness to make lifestyle modifications.

Glycaemic control in diabetes

DEFINITION Diabetes mellitus is a group of disorders characterised by hyperglycaemia (definitions vary slightly, one current US definition is fasting plasma glucose ≥ 7.0 mmol/L or ≥ 11.1 mmol/L 2 h after a 75 g oral glucose load, on 2 or more occasions). Intensive treatment is designed to achieve blood glucose values as close to the non-diabetic range as possible. The components of such treatment are education, counselling, monitoring, self management, and pharmacological treatment with insulin or oral antidiabetic agents to achieve specific glycaemic goals.

INCIDENCE/ PREVALENCE Diabetes is diagnosed in about 5% of adults aged 20 years or older in the USA.[1] A further 2.7% have undiagnosed diabetes on the basis of fasting glucose. The prevalence is similar in men and women, but diabetes is more common in some ethnic groups. The prevalence in people aged 40–74 years has increased over the past decade.

AETIOLOGY/ RISK FACTORS Diabetes results from deficient insulin secretion, decreased insulin action, or both. Many processes can be involved, from autoimmune destruction of the β cells of the pancreas to incompletely understood abnormalities that result in resistance to insulin action. Genetic factors are involved in both mechanisms. In type 1 diabetes there is an absolute deficiency of insulin. In type 2 diabetes, insulin resistance and an inability of the pancreas to compensate are involved. Hyperglycaemia without clinical symptoms but sufficient to cause tissue damage can be present for many years before diagnosis.

PROGNOSIS Severe hyperglycaemia causes numerous symptoms, including polyuria, polydipsia, weight loss, and blurred vision. Acute, life threatening consequences of diabetes are hyperglycaemia with ketoacidosis or the non-ketotic hyperosmolar syndrome. There is increased susceptibility to certain infections. Long term complications of diabetes include retinopathy (with potential loss of vision), nephropathy (leading to renal failure), peripheral neuropathy (increased risk of foot ulcers, amputation, and Charcot joints), autonomic neuropathy (cardiovascular, gastrointestinal, and genitourinary dysfunction), and greatly increased risk of atheroma affecting large vessels (macrovascular complications of stroke, myocardial infarction, or peripheral vascular disease). The physical, emotional, and social impact of diabetes and the demands of intensive treatment can also create problems for people with diabetes and their families. One systematic review (search date 1998) of observational studies in people with type 2 diabetes found a positive association between increased blood glucose concentration and mortality.[2] It found no minimum threshold level.

AIMS OF INTERVENTION To delay development and slow progression of microvascular, neuropathic, and cardiovascular complications of diabetes, while minimising adverse effects of treatment (hypoglycaemia and weight gain), and maximising quality of life.

OUTCOMES Quality of life; short term burden of treatment; long term clinical complications; risks and benefits of treatment. Both the development of complications in people who have previously been free of them, and the progression of complications. Scales of severity are used to detect disease progression (e.g. 19 step scales of diabetic retinopathy; normoalbuminuria, microalbuminuria, and albuminuria for nephropathy; absence or presence of clinical neuropathy).

METHODS *Clinical Evidence* search and appraisal December 2002.

QUESTION **What are the effects of intensive versus conventional glycaemic control?**

One systematic review and three subsequent RCTs in people with type 1 and type 2 diabetes have found that intensive treatment compared with conventional treatment reduces development and progression of microvascular and neuropathic complications. A second systematic review in people with type 1 diabetes and two additional RCTs in people with type 2 diabetes found no evidence that intensive treatment increased adverse cardiovascular outcomes. Intensive treatment reduces the number of macrovascular events, but has no significant effect on the number of people who develop macrovascular disease. Intensive treatment is associated with hypoglycaemia and weight gain, but does not seem adversely to affect neuropsychological function or quality of life.

Benefits: **Microvascular and neuropathic complications:** We found one systematic review (search date 1991, 16 small RCTs of type 1 diabetes),[3] and three subsequent long term RCTs.[4–6] The review and the RCTs all found that intensive treatment versus conventional treatment significantly reduced rates of retinopathy, nephropathy, and neuropathy (see table 1, p 675). In one large subsequent RCT (1441 people with type 1 diabetes), about half had no retinopathy and half had mild retinopathy at baseline.[4] At 6.5 years (the mean duration of the RCT), intensive treatment versus conventional treatment significantly reduced the progression of retinopathy and neuropathy. After a further 4 years, the benefit was maintained, regardless of whether people stayed in the groups to which they were initially randomised.[7] The difference in the median HbA1c concentration for people initially randomised to intensive or conventional care narrowed. After 6 years' follow up, people originally allocated to intensive treatment had lower rates of microalbuminuria and hypertension than those originally allocated to conventional treatment (microalbuminuria 4.5% with former intensive treatment *v* 12.3% with former conventional treatment, $P < 0.001$; hypertension 33% for former intensive treatment *v* 25% for former conventional treatment, $P < 0.001$).[8] However, another subsequent RCT compared a conventional dietary treatment policy with two different intensive treatment policies based on sulphonylurea and insulin (3867 people with newly diagnosed type 2 diabetes, age 25–65 years, fasting plasma glucose 6.1–15.0 mmol/L after 3 months' dietary treatment, no symptoms of hyperglycaemia, follow up 10 years).[6] HbA1c rose steadily in both groups. Intensive treatment was associated with a significant reduction in any diabetes related end point (40.9 *v* 46.0 events/1000 person years; RRR 12%, 95% CI 1% to 21%), but no significant effect on diabetes related deaths (10.4 *v* 11.5 deaths/1000 person years; RRR +10%, 95% CI −11% to +27%) or all cause mortality (17.9 *v* 18.9 deaths/1000 person years; RRR +6%, 95% CI −10% to +20%).

Secondary analysis found that intensive treatment was associated with a significant reduction in microvascular end points (8.6 *v* 11.4/1000 person years; RRR 25%, 95% CI 7% to 40%) compared with conventional treatment (see table 1, p 675).[6] **Cardiovascular outcomes:** We found one systematic review[9] and two additional RCTs.[5,6] The systematic review (search date 1996, 6 RCTs, 1731 people with type 1 diabetes followed for 2–8 years) found that intensive insulin treatment versus conventional treatment decreased the number of macrovascular events (OR 0.55, 95% CI 0.35 to 0.88), but had no significant effect on the number of people developing macrovascular disease (OR 0.72, 95% CI 0.44 to 1.17) or on macrovascular mortality (OR 0.91, 95% CI 0.31 to 2.65).[9] The additional RCTs included people with type 2 diabetes.[5,6] In the first RCT, the risk of major cerebrovascular, cardiovascular, and peripheral vascular events in the intensive treatment group was half that of the conventional treatment group (0.6 *v* 1.3 events/100 person years), but the event rate in this small trial was low and the results were not significant.[5] In the second RCT, intensive treatment versus conventional treatment was associated with a non-significant reduction in the risk of myocardial infarction (AR 387/2729 [14%] with intensive treatment *v* 186/1138 [16%] with conventional treatment; RRR +13%, 95% CI –2% to +27%), a non-significant increase in the risk of stroke (AR 148/2729 [5.4%] *v* 55/1138 [4.8%]; RRI +12%, 95% CI –17% to +51%), and a non-significant reduction in the risk of amputation or death from peripheral vascular disease (AR 29/2729 [1.1%] *v* 18/1138 [1.6%]; RRR +33%, 95% CI –20% to +63%).[6]

Harms: **Hypoglycaemia:** We found one systematic review[10] and three additional RCTs.[5,6,11] The systematic review (search date not stated, 14 RCTs with at least 6 months' follow up and monitoring of HbA1c, 2067 people with type 1 diabetes followed for 0.5–7.5 years) found that intensive treatment versus conventional treatment increased the median incidence of severe hypoglycaemia (7.9 episodes/100 person years for intensive *v* 4.6 episodes/100 person years for conventional treatment; OR 3.0, 95% CI 2.5 to 3.6).[10] The risk of severe hypoglycaemia was associated with the degree of HbA1c lowering in the intensive treatment groups ($P = 0.005$). The three additional RCTs included people with type 2 diabetes with lower baseline rates of hypoglycaemia. In the first RCT (110 people), there was no significant difference in rates of hypoglycaemia between groups.[5] In the second RCT (3867 people), the rates of major hypoglycaemic episodes per year were 0.7% with conventional treatment, 1.0% with chlorpropamide, 1.4% with glibenclamide, and 1.8% with insulin. People in the intensive treatment group had significantly more hypoglycaemic episodes than those in the conventional group ($P < 0.0001$).[6] In the third RCT (1704 overweight people), major hypoglycaemic episodes occurred in 0.6% of overweight people in the metformin treated group.[11] **Weight gain:** Four RCTs found more weight increase with intensive treatment than with standard treatment.[4–6,12] One RCT found weight remained stable in people with type 1 diabetes in the conventional treatment group, but body mass index increased by 5.8% in the intensive treatment group (95% CI not presented; $P < 0.01$).[12] In the second RCT (1441 people with type 1 diabetes) intensive treatment was associated with increased risk of developing a body weight more than 120% above the ideal (12.7 cases/100 person years with intensive treatment *v* 9.3 cases/100 person years with conventional treatment; RR 1.33). At 5 years, people treated intensively gained 4.6 kg more than people treated conventionally (CI not provided for weight data).[4] In the third RCT, the increase in body mass index from baseline to 6 years was not significant in either group (intensive treatment group 20.5–21.2 kg/m^2, conventional treatment group 20.3–21.9 kg/m^2).[5] In the fourth RCT, weight gain at 10 years was significantly higher in people with type 2 diabetes in the intensive treatment group compared with people in the conventional treatment group (mean difference 2.9 kg; $P < 0.001$), and people assigned insulin had a greater gain in weight (4.0 kg) than those assigned chlorpropamide (2.6 kg) or glibenclamide (1.7 kg).[6] We found one systematic review (search date 1996, 10 RCTs)[13] and one subsequent RCT[11] comparing metformin and sulphonylurea. Meta-analysis in the review found that sulphonylurea was associated with an increase in weight from baseline, and metformin with a decrease (difference 2.9 kg, 95% CI 1.1 kg to 4.4 kg). In the subsequent RCT, overweight participants randomly assigned to intensive blood glucose control with metformin had a similar change in body weight to the conventional treatment group, and less increase in mean body weight than people receiving intensive treatment with sulphonylureas or insulin.[11] **Neuropsychological impairment:** We found no systematic review on neuropsychological impairment, but found two RCTs.[14–17] One RCT (102 people) compared intensified with standard treatment in people with type 1 diabetes. It found no cognitive impairment associated with hypoglycaemia after 3 years.[14,15] The second RCT found that intensive treatment did not affect neuropsychological performance.[16] People who had repeated episodes of hypoglycaemia did not perform differently from people who did not have repeated episodes.[17] **Quality of life:** We found three RCTs that reported quality of life in people undergoing intensive versus conventional treatment.[18–20] Together, they suggested that quality of life is lowered by complications, but is not lowered directly by intensive versus conventional treatment. The first RCT (1441 people) found that intensive treatment did not reduce quality of life in people with type 1 diabetes.[18] Severe hypoglycaemia was not consistently associated with a subsequent increase in distress caused by symptoms or decline in the quality of life. However, in the primary prevention intensive treatment group, repeated severe hypoglycaemia (3 or more events resulting in coma or seizure) tended to increase the risk of distress caused by symptoms. The second RCT (77 adolescents with type 1 diabetes) found that behavioural intervention plus intensive diabetes management versus intensive diabetes management alone significantly improved quality of life, diabetes and medical self efficacy, and HbA1c after 1 year (7.5% *v* 8.5%; $P = 0.001$).[19] The behavioural intervention included six small group sessions and monthly follow up aimed at social problem solving, cognitive behaviour modification, and conflict resolution. The third RCT of intensive versus conventional treatment of type 2 diabetes assessed quality of life in two large cross-sectional samples at 8 and 11 years after randomisation (disease specific measures in 2431 people and generic measures in 3104 people), and also in a small cohort (diabetes specific quality of life measures in 374 people 6 months after randomisation and annually thereafter for 6 years).[20] The cross-sectional studies found no significant effect of intensive versus conventional treatment on scores for mood, cognitive mistakes, symptoms, work satisfaction, or general health. The longitudinal study also found no significant difference in quality of life scores other than a small increase in the number of symptoms in people allocated to conventional than to intensive treatment. In the cross-sectional studies, people who had macrovascular or microvascular complications in the past year had lower quality of life than people without complications. People treated with insulin who had two or more hypoglycaemic episodes during the previous year reported more tension, more overall mood disturbance, and less work satisfaction than those with no hypoglycaemic attacks (after adjusting for age, time from randomisation, systolic blood pressure, HbA1c, and sex). It was unclear whether frequent hypoglycaemic episodes affected quality of life, or whether people with certain personality traits or symptoms simply reported increased numbers of hypoglycaemic attacks.

Comment: We found one follow up study in people with type 1 diabetes 11.4 years after randomisation.[21] In people originally randomised to intensive treatment, it found that the fall in systolic blood pressure with upright posture (one measure of cardiovascular sympathetic dysfunction) and cardiovascular parasympathetic autonomic dysfunction (regardless of how it was measured) developed at a significantly slower pace.[21] We found one systematic review (search date 2000, 12 RCTs, 600 people with type 1 diabetes) that compared continuous subcutaneous insulin infusion with intensive insulin injections.[22] It found that continuous subcutaneous insulin infusion versus intensive insulin injections decreased mean blood glucose and glycated haemoglobin at 2.5–24 months (SMD: blood glucose 0.56, 95% CI 0.35 to 0.77, no significant heterogeneity; glycated haemoglobin 0.44, 95% CI 0.20 to 0.69, significant heterogeneity, $P = 0.07$).

QUESTION What is the optimum target blood glucose?

Large RCTs in people with type 1 and type 2 diabetes have found that development or progression of complications increases progressively as HbA1c increases above the non-diabetic range.

Benefits: We found no systematic review but found two large RCTs.[4,6] The first RCT (1441 people with type 1 diabetes) found that lower HbA1c was associated with a lower risk of complications.[4,23] The second RCT (3867 people with type 2 diabetes) found that, as concentrations of HbA1c were reduced, the risk of complications fell but the risk of hypoglycaemia increased.[6,20] A further analysis of the second RCT (3642 people who had HbA1c measured 3 months after the diagnosis of diabetes and who had complete data whether or not they were randomised in the trial) found that each 1% reduction in mean HbA1c was associated with reduced risk of any diabetes related microvascular or macrovascular event (RR 0.79, 95%

CI 0.76 to 0.83), diabetes related death (RR 0.79, 95% CI 0.73 to 0.85), all cause mortality (RR 0.86, 95% CI 0.81 to 0.91), microvascular complications (RR 0.63, 95% CI 0.59 to 0.67), and myocardial infarction (RR 0.86, 95% CI 0.79 to 0.92).[24] These prospective observational data suggested that there is no lower glycaemic threshold for the risk of complications; the better the glycaemic control, the lower the risk of complications. They also suggested that the rate of increase of risk for microvascular disease with hyperglycaemia is greater than that for macrovascular disease.

Harms: Both RCTs found that hypoglycaemia was increased by intensive treatment.[20,23]

Comment: It is difficult to weigh the benefit of reduced complications against the harm of increased hypoglycaemia. The balance between benefits and harms of intensive treatment in type 1 diabetes may be less favourable in children under 13 years or in older adults, and in people with repeated severe hypoglycaemia or unawareness of hypoglycaemia. Similarly, the balance between benefits and harms of intensive treatment in type 2 diabetes may be less favourable in people aged over 65 years or in those with longstanding diabetes. The benefit of intensive treatment is limited by the complications of advanced diabetes (such as blindness, end stage renal disease, or cardiovascular disease), major comorbidity, and reduced life expectancy. The risk of intensive treatment is increased by a history of severe hypoglycaemia or unawareness of hypoglycaemia, advanced autonomic neuropathy or cardiovascular disease, and impaired ability to detect or treat hypoglycaemia (such as altered mental state, immobility, or lack of social support). For people likely to have limited benefit or increased risk with intensive treatment, it may be more appropriate to negotiate less intensive goals for glycaemic management that reflect the person's self determined goals of care and willingness to make lifestyle modifications.

REFERENCES

1. Harris MI, Flegal KM, Cowie CC, et al. Prevalence of diabetes, impaired fasting glucose, and impaired glucose tolerance in US adults: the third national health and nutrition examination survey, 1988–1994. *Diabetes Care* 1998;2:518–524.
2. Groeneveld Y, Petri H, Hermans J, et al. Relationship between blood glucose level and mortality in type 2 diabetes mellitus: a systematic review. *Diabet Med* 1999;16:2–13. Search date 1998; primary source Medline.
3. Wang PH, Lau J, Chalmers TC. Meta-analysis of effects of intensive blood glucose control on late complications of type I diabetes. *Lancet* 1993;341:1306–1309. Search date 1991; primary source Medline.
4. The Diabetes Control and Complications Trial Research Group. The effect of intensive treatment of diabetes on the development and progression of long-term complications in insulin-dependent diabetes mellitus. *N Engl J Med* 1993;329:977–986.
5. Ohkubo Y, Kishikawa H, Arake E, et al. Intensive insulin therapy prevents the progression of diabetic microvascular complications in Japanese patients with non-insulin-dependent diabetes mellitus: a randomized prospective 6-year study. *Diabetes Res Clin Pract* 1995;28:103–117.
6. UK Prospective Diabetes Study Group. Intensive blood-glucose control with sulphonylureas or insulin compared with conventional treatment and risk of complications in patients with type 2 diabetes. *Lancet* 1998;352:837–853.
7. The DCCT/Epidemiology of Diabetes Interventions and Complications Research Group. Retinopathy and nephropathy in patients with type 1 diabetes four years after a trial of intensive therapy. *N Engl J Med* 2000;342:381–389.
8. Genuth S, Lipps J, Lorenzi G, et al. Effect of intensive therapy on the microvascular complications of type 1 diabetes mellitus. *JAMA* 2002;287:2563–2569.
9. Lawson ML, Gerstein HC, Tsui E, et al. Effect of intensive therapy on early macrovascular disease in young individuals with type 1 diabetes. *Diabetes Care* 1999;22:B35–B39. Search date 1996; primary sources Medline, Citation Index, reference lists, and personal files.
10. Egger M, Smith GD, Stettler C, et al. Risk of adverse effects of intensified treatment in insulin-dependent diabetes mellitus: a meta-analysis. *Diabet Med* 1997;14:919–928. Search date not stated; primary sources Medline, reference lists, and specialist journals.
11. UK Prospective Diabetes Study Group. Effect of intensive blood-glucose control with metformin on complications in overweight patients with type 2 diabetes. *Lancet* 1998;352:854–865.

12. Reichard P, Berglund B, Britz A, et al. Intensified conventional insulin treatment retards the microvascular complications of insulin-dependent diabetes mellitus (IDDM): the Stockholm diabetes intervention study (SDIS) after 5 years. *J Intern Med* 1991;30:101–108.
13. Johansen K. Efficacy of metformin in the treatment of NIDDM. *Diabetes Care* 1999;22:33–37. Search date 1996; primary sources current list of medical literature, Index Medicus, Medline, Embase, and hand searched references.
14. Reichard P, Nilsson BY, Rosenqvist U. The effect of long-term intensified insulin treatment on the development of microvascular complications of diabetes mellitus. *N Engl J Med* 1993;29:304–309.
15. Reichard P, Berglund A, Britz A, et al. Hypoglycaemic episodes during intensified insulin treatment: increased frequency but no effect on cognitive function. *J Intern Med* 1991;229:9–16.
16. The Diabetes Control and Complications Trial Research Group. Effects of intensive diabetes therapy on neuropsychological function in adults in the diabetes control and complications trial. *Ann Intern Med* 1996;124:379–388.
17. Austin EJ, Deary IJ. Effects of repeated hypoglycaemia on cognitive function. A psychometrically validated reanalysis of the diabetes control and complications trial data. *Diabetes Care* 1999;22:1273–1277.
18. The Diabetes Control and Complications Trial Research Group. Influence of intensive diabetes treatment on quality-of-life outcomes in the diabetes control and complications trial. *Diabetes Care* 1996;19:195–203.
19. Grey M, Boland EA, Davidson M, et al. Coping skills training for youth with diabetes mellitus has long-lasting effects on metabolic control and quality of life. *J Pediatr* 2000;137:107–113.
20. UK Prospective Diabetes Study Group. Quality of life in type 2 diabetic patients is affected by complications but not by intensive policies to improve blood glucose or blood pressure control (UKPDS 37). *Diabetes Care* 1999;22:1125–1136.
21. Reichard P, Jensen-Urstad K, Ericsson M, et al. Automonic neuropathy – a complication less pronounced in patients with type 1 diabetes mellitus who have lower blood glucose levels. *Diabet Med* 2000;17:860–866.
22. Pickup J, Mattock M, Kerry S. Glycaemic control with continuous subcutaneous insulin infusion compared with intensive insulin injections in patients with type 1 diabetes: meta-analysis of randomised controlled trials. *BMJ* 2002;324:1–6. Search date 2000; primary sources Medline, Embase, Cochrane database of controlled trials, authors' personal files, reviews, bibliographies, and contact with manufacturers of pump therapy, and INPUT a support group for people using pumps.
23. The Diabetes Control and Complications Trial Research Group. The absence of a glycaemic threshold for the development of long-term complications: the perspective of the diabetes control and complications trial. *Diabetes* 1996;45:1289–1298.
24. Stratton IM, Adler AI, Neil HAW, et al, on behalf of the UK Prospective Diabetes Study Group. Association of glycaemia with macrovascular and microvascular complications of type 2 diabetes (UKPDS 35): prospective observational study. *BMJ* 2000;321:405–412

Bazian Ltd
London
UK

Competing interests: None declared.

The following previous contributor of this topic would also like to be acknowledged: William Herman.

TABLE 1 **Risk (odds ratio) for development or progression of microvascular, nephropathic, and neuropathic complications with intensive versus conventional treatment. Odds ratio, number needed to treat, and confidence intervals were all calculated from data in papers (see text, p 669).**

	Systematic review[3]	**DCCT[4]**	**Kumamoto[5]**	**UKPDS[6]**
Studies	16 RCTs	RCT	RCT	RCT
Number of participants	ND	1441	110	3867
Type of diabetes	Type 1	Type 1	Type 2	Type 2*
Follow up	8–60 months	6.5 years	6 years	10 years
Change in HbA1c	1.4%	2.0%	2.0%	0.9%
Progression of retinopathy				
OR (95% CI)	0.49 (0.28 to 0.85)	0.39 (0.28 to 0.55)	0.25 (0.09 to 0.65)	0.66 (0.48 to 0.92)
NNT (95% CI) over duration of study	ND	5 (4 to 7)	4 (3 to 11)	10 (6 to 50)
Development of retinopathy				
OR (95% CI)	ND	0.22 (0.14 to 0.36)	ND	ND
NNT (95% CI) over duration of study	ND	6 (5 to 7)	ND	ND
Development or progression of nephropathy				
OR (95% CI)	0.34 (0.20 to 0.58)	0.50 (0.39 to 0.63)	0.26 (0.09 to 0.76)	0.54 (0.25 to 1.18)
NNT (95% CI) over duration of study	ND	7 (6 to 11)	5 (4 to 19)	ND
Development or progression of neuropathy				
OR (95% CI)	ND	0.36 (0.24 to 0.54)	ND	0.42 (0.23 to 0.78)
NNT (95% CI) over duration of study	ND	13 (11 to 18)	ND	5 (3 to 16)

*All participants had fasting plasma glucose > 6.0 mmol/L on two occasions: 93% had fasting plasma glucose ≥ 7.0 mmol/L (American Diabetes Association criterion) and 86% had fasting plasma glucose ≥ 7.8 mmol/L (World Health Organization criterion).
CI, confidence interval; ND, no data.

Obesity

Search date January 2003

David Arterburn

QUESTIONS

INTERVENTIONS

Key Messages

- **Diethylpropion** One systematic review found that diethylpropion promotes modest weight loss compared with placebo in healthy obese adults. We found two case reports describing pulmonary hypertension and psychosis with diethylpropion. We found insufficient evidence on weight regain and long term safety. A European Commission review concluded that a link between diethylpropion and heart and lung problems could not be excluded.
- **Fluoxetine** One systematic review found that fluoxetine promotes modest weight loss compared with placebo in healthy obese adults. We found insufficient evidence on weight regain and long term safety of fluoxetine in obesity. One systematic review of antidepressant treatment has found an association between selective serotonin reuptake inhibitors and uncommon but serious adverse events, including bradycardia, bleeding, granulocytopenia, seizures, hyponatraemia, hepatotoxicity, serotonin syndrome, and extrapyramidal effects.
- **Mazindol** One systematic review found that mazindol promotes modest weight loss compared with placebo in healthy obese adults. We found one case report of pulmonary hypertension diagnosed 1 year after stopping treatment with mazindol. We found one case series of mazindol in people with stable cardiac disease that reported cardiac events such as atrial fibrillation and syncope. We found insufficient evidence on weight regain and long term safety.

- **Orlistat** Systematic reviews and subsequent RCTs have found that, in addition to a low energy diet, orlistat modestly increases weight loss compared with placebo in healthy obese adults (body mass index 25–40 kg/m^2) and in obese people with diabetes, hyperlipidaemia, and hypertension. Adverse effects such as oily spotting from the rectum, flatulence, and faecal urgency occurred in a high proportion of people taking orlistat. We found insufficient evidence on weight regain and long term safety.
- **Phentermine** One systematic review found that phentermine promotes modest weight loss compared with placebo in healthy obese adults. We found insufficient evidence on weight regain and long term safety. A European Commission review concluded that a link between phentermine and heart and lung problems could not be excluded.
- **Sibutramine** A systematic review and RCTs have found that sibutramine promotes modest weight loss compared with placebo in healthy obese adults (body mass index 25–40 kg/m^2) and in obese people with diabetes and hypertension. One RCT has found that sibutramine is more effective than placebo for weight maintenance after weight loss in healthy, obese adults, but weight regain occurs when sibutramine is discontinued. Sibutramine was temporarily suspended from the market in Italy for use in obesity because of concerns about severe adverse reactions, including arrhythmias, hypertension, and two deaths resulting from cardiac arrest. Two RCTs found no difference in the incidence of valvular heart disease between sibutramine and placebo, although these trials may have been too small to detect clinically important differences.
- **Sibutramine plus orlistat (*v* sibutramine alone)** We found insufficient evidence about the effects of sibutramine plus orlistat and sibutramine alone.
- **Dexfenfluramine** One systematic review found that dexfenfluramine promotes weight loss compared with placebo in healthy obese adults. Dexfenfluramine has been associated with valvular heart disease and pulmonary hypertension.
- **Fenfluramine** One systematic review found that fenfluramine promotes modest weight loss compared with placebo in healthy obese adults. Fenfluramine has been associated with valvular heart disease and pulmonary hypertension.
- **Fenfluramine plus phentermine** One RCT found that fenfluramine plus phentermine promotes weight loss compared with placebo. The combination of fenfluramine plus phentermine has been associated with valvular heart disease and pulmonary hypertension.
- **Phenylpropanolamine** One systematic review found that phenylpropanolamine promotes modest weight loss compared with placebo in healthy obese adults. One case control study found that phenylpropanolamine increased risk of haemorrhagic stroke in the first 3 days of use.

DEFINITION Obesity is a chronic condition characterised by an excess of body fat. It is most often defined by the body mass index (BMI — see glossary, p 687), a mathematical formula that is highly correlated with body fat. BMI is weight in kilograms divided by height in metres squared (kg/m^2). Worldwide, people with BMIs between 25–30 kg/m^2 are categorised as overweight, and those with BMIs above 30 kg/m^2 are categorised as obese.[1,2] Nearly 5 million US adults used prescription weight loss medication between 1996 and 1998. A quarter of users were not overweight, suggesting that weight loss medication may be inappropriately used. This is thought to be especially the case among women, white people, and Hispanic people.[3] The National Institutes of Health has issued guidelines for obesity treatment, which indicate that all obese adults (BMI ≥ 30 kg/m²) and all adults with a BMI ≥ 27 kg/m² and concomitant risk factors or diseases are candidates for drug therapy.[1]

INCIDENCE/ PREVALENCE Obesity has increased steadily in many countries since 1900. In the UK in 2001, it was estimated that 21% of men and 24% of women were obese.[4] In the past decade alone, the prevalence of obesity in the USA has increased from 22.9% between 1988 and 1994, to 30.5% between 1999 and 2000.[5]

AETIOLOGY/ RISK FACTORS Obesity is the result of long term mismatches in energy balance where daily energy intake exceeds daily energy expenditure.[6] Energy balance is modulated by a myriad of factors, including metabolic rate, appetite, diet, and physical activity.[7] Although these factors are influenced by genetic traits, the increase in obesity prevalence in the past few decades cannot be explained by changes in the human gene pool, and is more often attributed to environmental changes that promote excessive food intake and discourage physical activity.[7,8] Obesity may also be induced by drugs (e.g. high dose glucocorticoids), or be secondary to a variety of neuroendocrine disorders such as Cushing's syndrome and polycystic ovary syndrome.[9]

PROGNOSIS Obesity is a risk factor for several chronic diseases, including hypertension, dyslipidaemia, diabetes, cardiovascular disease, sleep apnoea, osteoarthritis, and some cancers.[1] The relationship between increasing body weight and mortality is curvilinear, where the mortality rate is highest among adults with low body weight (BMI < 18.5 kg/m²) and among adults with the highest body weight (BMI > 35 kg/m²).[2] Results from five prospective cohort studies and 1991 national statistics suggest that the number of annual deaths attributable to obesity among US adults is about 280 000.[10] Obese adults also have more annual hospitalisations, more outpatient visits, higher prescription drug costs, and worse health related quality of life than normal weight adults.[11,12]

AIMS OF INTERVENTION To achieve realistic gradual weight loss, and prevent the morbidity and mortality associated with obesity, without undue adverse effects.

OUTCOMES We found no studies that used the primary outcomes of functional morbidity or mortality. Proxy measures include mean weight loss (kg), number of people losing 5% or more of baseline body weight, and number of people maintaining weight loss.

METHODS *Clinical Evidence* search and appraisal January 2003.

QUESTION **What are the effects of drug treatments in adults?**

OPTION **SIBUTRAMINE**

One systematic review and subsequent RCTs have found that that sibutramine promotes modest weight loss compared with placebo in healthy obese adults (body mass index 25–40 kg/m²) and in obese people with diabetes and hypertension. One RCT has found that sibutramine is

also more effective than placebo for weight maintenance after weight loss in healthy obese adults, but weight regain occurs when sibutramine is discontinued. Sibutramine was temporarily suspended from the market in Italy for use in obesity because of concerns about severe adverse reactions, including arrhythmias, hypertension, and two deaths resulting from cardiac arrest. Two RCTs found no difference in the incidence of valvular heart disease between sibutramine and placebo, although these trials may have lacked power to detect clinically important differences. One RCT found that sibutramine achieved greater weight loss than either orlistat or metformin. We found insufficient evidence about the effects of sibutramine plus orlistat versus sibutramine alone.

Benefits: **Versus placebo:** We found one systematic review (search date 2000, 11 RCTs),[13] and five subsequent RCTs[14–18] comparing sibutramine versus placebo. The systematic review pooled data for groups of RCTs with similar follow up.[13] The review found that sibutramine (10–20 mg daily) reduced weight more than placebo after 8 weeks (3 RCTs, 106 people, WMD –3.4 kg, 95% CI –4.22 kg to –2.58 kg).[13] The review also found that sibutramine (10–20 mg daily) achieved weight loss of 5% or greater more frequently than placebo after 6 months (2 RCTs, 207 people, RR for > 5% weight loss: sibutramine *v* placebo 2.1, 95% CI 1.7 to 2.6).[13] The first subsequent RCT (1001 healthy obese adults) compared intermittent sibutramine (15 mg daily for weeks 1–12, 19–30, and 37–48); continuous sibutramine (15 mg daily), and placebo for 48 weeks.[14] Only 79% of people completed this study. It found no significant difference between intermittent and continuous sibutramine: both regimens reduced weight more than placebo (–3.3 kg with intermittent sibutramine *v* –3.8 kg with continuous sibutramine *v* +0.2 kg with placebo; P < 0.001). The second subsequent RCT (184 healthy obese people) compared sibutramine (10 or 20 mg daily) versus placebo for 6 months.[17] It found that sibutramine significantly reduced weight compared with placebo (–9.3 kg with 10 mg sibutramine *v* –11.7 kg with 20 mg sibutramine *v* –4.6 kg with placebo; P < 0.001). The third and fourth subsequent RCTs compared sibutramine and placebo in obese adults with type 2 diabetes.[16,18] The third subsequent RCT (134 people) compared sibutramine 15 mg daily versus placebo for 6 months.[16] It found that sibutramine significantly reduced weight compared with placebo (–4.5 kg with sibutramine *v* –1.7 kg with placebo; P < 0.001). The fourth subsequent RCT (132 people) compared sibutramine (15 or 20 mg daily) versus placebo for 1 year.[18] Only 74% of people completed this study. It found that sibutramine significantly reduced weight compared with placebo (–5.5 kg with sibutramine 15 mg *v* –8.0 kg with sibutramine 20 mg *v* –1.7 kg with placebo; P < 0.001). The fifth subsequent RCT (605 healthy obese adults) compared sibutramine for weight maintenance versus placebo for 24 months.[15] People received sibutramine (10 mg daily) plus diet for 6 months. A total of 467 people with more than 5% weight loss were then randomly assigned to sibutramine (10–20 mg daily) or placebo for an additional 18 months. Only 56% of people completed the full 2 years of the study. The RCT found that a greater proportion of people maintained 80% or more of their original weight loss at 24 months with sibutramine compared with placebo (43% with sibutramine *v* 16% with placebo; P < 0.001). **Versus**

orlistat or metformin: We found one RCT (150 obese women) comparing sibutramine (20 mg daily); orlistat (120 mg 3 times daily), and metformin (850 mg twice daily) for 6 months.[19] All people were also instructed to follow a reduced calorie diet. The RCT found that sibutramine achieved greater weight loss than either orlistat or metformin (–13.0 kg with sibutramine *v* –8.0 kg with orlistat *v* –9.0 kg with metformin; P value for sibutramine versus orlistat < 0.0001; P value for sibutramine versus metformin < 0.0001). **Sibutramine plus orlistat**: We found one RCT (34 women who had completed 1 year of sibutramine plus lifestyle modification), which compared sibutramine (10–15 mg daily) plus orlistat (120 mg 3 times daily) versus sibutramine plus placebo for weight maintenance.[20] Only 76% of the women completed the study. Mean body weight did not change significantly in either group over a 16 week period (+0.1 kg with combined treatment *v* +0.5 kg with sibutramine plus placebo).

Harms: **Versus placebo:** We found no evidence about safety beyond 2 years of treatment. Common adverse effects were headache, dry mouth, anorexia, constipation, insomnia, rhinitis, and pharyngitis occurring in 10–30% of people taking sibutramine compared with 8–19% of people on placebo (significance of difference not provided).[13] Mean increases in systolic and diastolic blood pressure (1–3 mm Hg) and heart rate (4–5 beats/minute) have been reported in people taking sibutramine at doses of 5–20 mg daily.[13] We found two RCTs that reported the effects of sibutramine on heart valve function.[17,21] The first RCT (210 obese people) compared sibutramine versus placebo for 12 months.[21] It found no significant difference in the incidence of valvular disease between sibutramine and placebo (3/133 [2.3%] with sibutramine 15–20 mg daily *v* 2/77 [2.6%] with placebo; OR 0.87, 90% CI 0.19 to 3.97). The trial did not report on efficacy. The second RCT (184 healthy obese people) compared sibutramine 10 mg or 20 mg daily versus placebo.[17] It reported no change in valvular appearance on echocardiogram in any group (no statistical comparisons between or within groups reported). Sibutramine was temporarily suspended from the market in Italy in March 2002 in response to 50 reported adverse reactions, including seven severe adverse reactions (tachycardia, hypertension, and arrhythmia) and two deaths resulting from cardiac arrest. The Central European Committee for Proprietary Medicinal Products (CPMP) completed a review of sibutramine in June 2002, and concluded that the risk–benefit profile of sibutramine remains positive. To date, none of the other regulatory agencies, including the Medicines Control Agency, UK; the Food and Drug Administration, USA; Health, Canada; and the Therapeutics Goods Administration, Australia, have taken any regulatory actions against the drug.[22] **Versus orlistat or metformin:** One RCT reported dry mouth, insomnia, constipation, and hypertension with sibutramine, and abdominal discomfort with orlistat and metformin.[19] **Sibutramine plus orlistat:** One RCT reported that people who received sibutramine plus orlistat experienced more soft stools (50% with sibutramine plus orlistat *v* 9.1% with sibutramine alone), increased frequency of bowel movements (50% with sibutramine plus orlistat *v* 9.1% with sibutramine alone), oily evacuation (42.9% with sibutramine plus orlistat *v* 0% with sibutramine alone), and more faecal urgency (42.9% with sibutramine plus orlistat *v* 9.1% with sibutramine alone).[20]

Comment: Most of the RCTs provided concomitant dietary interventions, and about 25% also provided an exercise intervention. The RCTs examining incidence of heart valve dysfunction with sibutramine and placebo may have been too small to detect clinically important effects. Two RCTs (in three publications) provided information on weight regain after discontinuing sibutramine therapy.[15,23,24] A cross over study (82 people) found that people averaged 43% weight regain at 6 months after stopping sibutramine 10 mg daily.[23,24] The placebo arm of a 2 year weight maintenance study found that 115 people averaged 55% weight regain at 18 months after stopping sibutramine 10 mg daily.[15]

OPTION PHENTERMINE

One systematic review found that phentermine promotes modest weight loss compared with placebo in healthy obese adults. We found insufficient evidence on weight regain and long term safety. A European Commission review concluded that a link between phentermine and heart and lung problems could not be excluded.

Benefits: We found one systematic review (search date 1999, 6 relevant RCTs, 368 participants) comparing phentermine (15–30 mg daily) versus placebo in healthy obese adults, with mean follow up of 13.2 weeks (range 2–24 weeks).[25] The review found that phentermine produced significantly more weight loss than placebo (effect size = mean weight loss in treatment group minus mean weight loss in the control group divided by the pooled standard deviation for both groups: < 0.6 [information presented graphically]; difference in weight loss between phentermine and placebo in the six RCTs ranged from 0.6–6.0 kg). The review also compared phentermine versus other agents (diethylpropion, dexfenfluramine, fenfluramine, fluoxetine, mazindol, orlistat, phenylpropanolamine, and sibutramine) and found no significant difference in effect size between phentermine and the other agents (based on 95% CIs presented graphically).[25]

Harms: The systematic review did not make any comment on adverse effects.[25] Phentermine given alone has not been associated with valvular heart disease.[26] A European Commission review reported that, although no new safety problems were identified with phentermine, a link between phentermine and "heart and lung problems could not be totally excluded".[27]

Comment: Most of the people treated with phentermine received additional lifestyle treatment.[25] High withdrawal rates have been reported for phentermine.

OPTION MAZINDOL

One systematic review found that mazindol promotes modest weight loss compared with placebo in healthy obese adults. We found one case report of pulmonary hypertension diagnosed 1 year after stopping treatment with mazindol. We found one case series of mazindol in people with stable cardiac disease that reported cardiac events such as atrial fibrillation and syncope. We found insufficient evidence on weight regain and long term safety.

Benefits: We found one systematic review (search date 1999, 22 relevant RCTs, 906 participants) comparing mazindol (1–3 mg daily) versus placebo in healthy obese adults with mean follow up of 11 weeks (range 2–20 weeks).[25] The review found that mazindol produced significantly more weight loss than placebo (effect size = mean weight loss in treatment group minus mean weight loss in the control group divided by the pooled standard deviation for both groups: < 0.5; difference in weight loss between mazindol and placebo in the 22 RCTs ranged from 0.1–7.3 kg). The review also compared mazindol with other agents (diethylpropion, dexfenfluramine, fenfluramine, fluoxetine, orlistat, phenylpropanolamine, phentermine, and sibutramine) and found no significant difference in effect size between mazindol and the other agents (based on 95% CIs presented graphically) except sibutramine (effect size: 0.95) and fenfluramine (effect size: 0.85).[25]

Harms: The systematic review did not comment on adverse effects.[25] We found a single case report of pulmonary hypertension diagnosed 12 months after stopping mazindol that had been taken for 10 weeks.[28] One case series of mazindol in people with stable cardiac disease reported several cardiac events (3 episodes of atrial fibrillation and 2 of syncope in 15 people receiving mazindol for 12 weeks).[29] The frequency of serious adverse events with this agent remains unclear.

Comment: None.

OPTION DIETHYLPROPION

One systematic review found that diethylpropion promotes modest weight loss compared with placebo in healthy obese adults. We found two case reports describing pulmonary hypertension and psychosis with diethylpropion. We found insufficient evidence on weight regain and long term safety. A European Commission review concluded that a link between diethylpropion and heart and lung problems could not be excluded.

Benefits: We found one systematic review (search date 1999, 9 relevant RCTs, 353 people) comparing diethylpropion (75 mg daily) versus placebo in healthy obese adults with mean follow up of 17.6 weeks (range 6–52 weeks).[25] The review found that diethylpropion produced significantly more weight loss than placebo (effect size = mean weight loss in the treatment group minus the mean weight loss in the control group divided by the pooled standard deviation for both groups: < 0.55 [information presented graphically]; difference in weight loss between diethylpropion and placebo in the 9 RCTs ranged from 1.6–11.5 kg). The review also compared diethylpropion versus other agents (dexfenfluramine, fenfluramine, fluoxetine, mazindol, orlistat, phenylpropanolamine, phentermine, and sibutramine), and found no significant difference in effect size between diethylpropion and the other agents (based on 95% CIs presented graphically).[25]

Harms: The systematic review did not comment on adverse effects.[25] Case reports have described pulmonary hypertension and psychosis in users of diethylpropion.[30,31] The frequency of serious adverse events with this diethylpropion remains unclear. A European Commission review of the risks and benefits of diethylpropion concluded that randomised trials do not adequately show efficacy for weight loss.[27] Although no new safety problems were identified with diethylpropion, the Commission commented that a link between diethylpropion and "heart and lung problems could not be totally excluded".

Comment: None.

OPTION FLUOXETINE

One systematic review found that fluoxetine promotes modest weight loss compared with placebo in healthy obese adults. We found insufficient evidence on weight regain and long term safety of fluoxetine in obesity. One systematic review of antidepressant treatment has found an association between selective serotonin reuptake inhibitors and uncommon but serious adverse events, including bradycardia, bleeding, granulocytopenia, seizures, hyponatraemia, hepatotoxicity, serotonin syndrome, and extrapyramidal effects.

Benefits: We found one systematic review (search date 1999, 11 relevant RCTs, 1219 people) comparing fluoxetine (32.5–60.0 mg daily) versus placebo in healthy obese adults with mean follow up of 27.5 weeks (range 6–60 weeks).[25] The review found that fluoxetine produced significant weight loss compared with placebo (effect size = mean weight loss in the treatment group minus the mean weight loss in the control group divided by the pooled standard deviation for both groups: < 0.45 [information presented graphically]; difference in weight loss between fluoxetine and placebo in the 11 RCTs ranged from 0.2–7.4 kg). The review also compared fluoxetine versus other agents (diethylpropion, dexfenfluramine, fenfluramine, mazindol, orlistat, phenylpropanolamine, phentermine, and sibutramine) and found no significant difference in effect size between fluoxetine and the other agents (based on 95% CIs) except sibutramine (effect size: 0.95) and fenfluramine (effect size: 0.85).[25]

Harms: The systematic review did not comment on adverse effects.[25] One older systematic review (search date 1998) of antidepressant treatment found that selective serotonin reuptake inhibitors were associated with a 10–15% incidence of anxiety, diarrhoea, dry mouth, headache, and nausea. The review also found an association between selective serotonin reuptake inhibitors and uncommon but serious adverse events, including bradycardia, bleeding, granulocytopenia, seizures, hyponatraemia, hepatotoxicity, serotonin syndrome, and extrapyramidal effects (see glossary, p 687).[32]

Comment: None.

OPTION FENFLURAMINE, DEXFENFLURAMINE, OR FENFLURAMINE PLUS PHENTERMINE

One systematic review found that fenfluramine, dexfenfluramine, or fenfluramine plus phentermine promotes modest weight loss compared with placebo in healthy obese adults. Dexfenfluramine, fenfluramine, and fenfluramine plus phentermine have been associated with valvular heart disease and pulmonary hypertension.

Benefits: **Fenfluramine:** We found one systematic review (search date 1999, 14 relevant RCTs, 577 people) comparing fenfluramine (39–120 mg daily) versus placebo in healthy obese adults with mean follow up of 9.7 weeks (range 4–18 weeks).[25] The review found that fenfluramine produced significant weight loss (effect size = the mean weight loss in the treatment group minus the mean weight loss in the control group divided by the pooled standard deviation for both groups: > 0.85 [information presented graphically]; difference in weight loss between fenfluramine and placebo in the 14 RCTs ranged from 0.1–5.0 kg). The review found no significant difference in effect size between fenfluramine and the other agents (based on 95% CIs presented graphically) except sibutramine (effect size: 0.95). **Dexfenfluramine:** We found one systematic review (search date 1999, 14 relevant RCTs, 1269 people) comparing dexfenfluramine (30–130 mg daily) versus placebo in healthy obese adults with mean follow up of 30 weeks (range 4–56 weeks).[25] The review found that dexfenfluramine produced significantly more weight loss than placebo (effect size = the mean weight loss in the treatment group minus the mean weight loss in the control group divided by the pooled standard deviation for both groups: < 0.45 [information presented graphically]; difference in weight loss between dexfenfluramine and placebo in the 14 RCTs ranged from 0.2–10.0 kg). The review found no significant difference in effect size between dexfenfluramine and the other agents (based on 95% CIs presented graphically) except sibutramine (effect size: 0.95) and fenfluramine (effect size: 0.85). **Fenfluramine plus phentermine:** We found one RCT (121 people, 30–80% overweight), which found that phentermine (15 mg daily) plus fenfluramine (60 mg daily) reduced weight significantly more than placebo after treatment for 6 months (–14.3 kg with phentermine plus fenfluramine *v* –4.6 kg with placebo; mean difference –9.7 kg, 95% CI –12.0 to –7.4 kg). The trial found that weight loss ceased at 18 weeks of treatment; weight regain was noted after 60 weeks of treatment.[33]

Harms: **Dexfenfluramine, fenfluramine, fenfluramine plus phentermine:** These agents have been associated with valvular heart disease and primary pulmonary hypertension.[34,35] We found one systematic review examining harms of fenfluramine, dexfenfluramine, and the combination of fenfluramine or dexfenfluramine with phentermine (search date 2000, 9 observational studies, total 8778 people).[36] It found that overweight or obese people receiving fenfluramine, dexfenfluramine, and the combination of fenfluramine or dexfenfluramine with phentermine for more than 90 days were more likely to have valvular regurgitation than people not taking them (12.0% in people receiving fenfluramine, dexfenfluramine, and the combination of fenfluramine or dexfenfluramine with phentermine *v* 5.9% in people not taking them; OR 2.2, 95% CI 1.7 to 2.7). The review found no significant difference in prevalence of valvular regurgitation in people taking fenfluramine, dexfenfluramine and the combination of fenfluramine or dexfenfluramine with phentermine for less than 90 days and people not taking them (6.7% in people receiving these drugs *v* 5.8% in people not taking them; OR 1.4, 95% CI 0.8 to 2.4). One case control study (95 people with primary pulmonary hypertension and 355 matched controls) found a history of fenfluramine use was associated with increased risk of primary pulmonary hypertension (OR 6.3, 95% CI 3.0 to 13.2). The odds ratio was higher among people who had taken fenfluramine in the past year (OR 10.1, 95% CI 3.4 to 29.9), and among people treated for more than 3 months (OR 23.1, 95% CI 6.9 to 77.7).[37]

Comment: None.

OPTION PHENYLPROPANOLAMINE

One systematic review found that phenylpropanolamine promotes modest weight loss compared with placebo in healthy obese adults. One case control study found that phenylpropanolamine increased risk of haemorrhagic stroke in the first 3 days of use.

Benefits: We found one systematic review (search date 1999, 7 relevant RCTs, 321 people) comparing phenylpropanolamine (57–75 mg daily) versus placebo in healthy obese adults with mean follow up of 7.4 weeks (range 2–14 weeks).[25] The review found that phenylpropanolamine produced significant weight loss (effect size = the mean weight loss in the treatment group minus the mean weight loss in the control group divided by the pooled standard deviation for both groups: < 0.5 [information presented graphically]; difference in weight loss between phenylpropanolamine and placebo ranged from 0.3–2.0 kg). The review also compared phenylpropanolamine versus other agents (diethylpropion, dexfenfluramine, fenfluramine, fluoxetine, mazindol, orlistat, phentermine, and sibutramine), and found no significant difference in effect size between phenylpropanolamine and the other agents (based on 95% CIs presented graphically) except sibutramine (effect size: 0.95) and fenfluramine (effect size: 0.85).[25]

Harms: A case control study (men and women aged 18–49 years) found that phenylpropanolamine used as an appetite suppressant increased the risk of haemorrhagic stroke within the first 3 days of use (adjusted OR 15.9, lower confidence limit 2.04; P = 0.013). For the association between phenylpropanolamine in appetite suppressants and risk for haemorrhagic stroke among women, the adjusted odds ratio was 16.6 (lower confidence limit 2.2; P = 0.011).[38]

Comment: None.

OPTION ORLISTAT

Systematic reviews and subsequent RCTs have found that, in addition to a low energy diet, orlistat modestly increases weight loss compared with placebo in adults with obesity. Adverse effects such as oily spotting from the rectum, flatulence, and faecal urgency occurred in a high proportion of people taking orlistat. We found insufficient evidence on weight regain and long term safety.

Benefits: We found two systematic reviews (search dates 2000)[39,40] and two subsequent RCTs.[41,42] The most comprehensive of the reviews included 14 RCTs and pooled data for groups of RCTs with similar study designs.[40] Studies were excluded if they did not separately analyse people who were not overweight or obese. The 11 published RCTs in the systematic review (5124 adults with mean body mass index [see glossary, p 687] > 30 kg/m^2) found no significant difference in weight after 12 weeks between orlistat (50–60 mg 3 times daily) plus reduced calorie diet and placebo plus diet (2 RCTs: WMD −1.24 kg, 95% CI −2.65 kg to +0.16 kg).[40] However, higher dose orlistat (120 mg 3 times daily) was associated with greater weight loss than placebo at 12 weeks (1 RCT: mean weight loss 4.74 kg with orlistat *v* 2.98 kg with placebo; P = 0.001).[40] Two trials of 6 months duration were not included in the pooling. The first 6 month RCT (119 people) compared orlistat (120 mg 3 times daily) versus placebo. All people received an energy restricted diet. At 6 months, orlistat reduced weight more than placebo (mean weight loss: 10.75 kg with orlistat *v* 7.34 kg with placebo; P < 0.05).[43] The second 6 month RCT (605 people on a reduced energy diet) compared orlistat (30, 60, 120, or 240 mg 3 times daily) versus placebo. All doses of orlistat significantly increased weight loss at 6 months compared with placebo (weight loss from baseline: 6.5% with placebo *v* 8.5% with orlistat 30 mg; P value not reported; *v* 8.8% with orlistat 60 mg; P ≤ 0.002; *v* 9.8% with orlistat 120 mg; P ≤ 0.001; *v* 9.3% with orlistat 240 mg; P ≤ 0.001).[44] Pooled analysis of four trials with 1 year duration (2111 people) found that orlistat (120 mg 3 times daily) significantly reduced weight more than placebo (WMD for weight change with orlistat *v* placebo −2.90 kg, 95% CI −3.61 kg to −2.19 kg).[40] Two RCTs were not included in the 1 year pooled analysis. In these trials, 901 people were placed on a reduced energy diet and were also randomised to orlistat (120 mg 3 times daily) versus placebo. Both found that orlistat increased weight loss compared with placebo (AR > 10% weight loss from baseline at 1 year: 35% with orlistat *v* 21% with placebo; P = 0.02;[45] 30% with orlistat *v* 16% with placebo; P < 0.001[46]). The review found similar results at 2 years. Two trials examining change in body weight using orlistat (120 mg 3 times daily) or placebo for 2 years were pooled. People taking orlistat had significantly greater weight loss (WMD –3.19 kg, 95% CI –4.25 kg to –2.12 kg).[40] One included RCT compared effects of orlistat (30, 60, and 120 mg 3 times daily) versus placebo on weight regain after 6 months of diet plus exercise counselling.[40] It found that orlistat reduced weight regain compared with placebo ($P < 0.001$ for orlistat 120 mg *v* placebo).[47] We found two subsequent RCTs.[41,42] The first subsequent RCT (376 adults with type 2 diabetes, hypercholesterolaemia, or hypertension) found that dietary counselling plus orlistat (120 mg 3 times daily) significantly increased the proportion of people who lost 5% or more of their initial body weight compared with placebo (54% with orlistat *v* 41% with placebo; $P < 0.001$), but did not significantly increase weight reduction of 10% or more (AR 19% *v* 14.6%).[41] The second subsequent RCT (294 people with hypercholesterolaemia) compared orlistat (120 mg 3 times daily) versus placebo for 24 weeks. It found that orlistat significantly increased weight loss compared with placebo (mean weight loss: 4.66 kg with orlistat *v* 1.88 kg with placebo; $P < 0.001$).[42]

Harms: Gastrointestinal adverse events such as loose stools, increased defaecation, abdominal pain, nausea/vomiting, oily spotting from the rectum, flatulence, and faecal urgency were more common with orlistat than placebo (48–95% with orlistat 120 mg 3 times daily *v* 18–68% with placebo)[40–42] The review also found that orlistat was associated with lower serum levels of fat soluble vitamins, such that vitamin supplements were sometimes deemed necessary.[40]

Comment: We found five subsequent RCTs comparing orlistat versus placebo in obese adults that were excluded owing to high losses to follow up.[48–52] People in six of the seven trials in one systematic review were selected for participation after losing weight on a preliminary low calorie diet with placebo for 4–5 weeks before randomisation.[53] Because of the high rates of gastrointestinal adverse effects associated with orlistat, authors have queried whether blinded evaluation is possible. At the end of a "double blinded" 16 week trial, 22/26 people correctly identified their treatment group.[20]

GLOSSARY

Body mass index Expressed as weight in kilograms divided by height in metres squared (kg/m^2). In the USA and UK, individuals with body mass indexes of 25–30 kg/m^2 are considered overweight; those with body mass indexes above 30 kg/m^2 are considered obese.

Extrapyramidal effects Include acute dystonia, a parkinsonism-like syndrome, and akathisia.

Serotonin syndrome Clinical features include agitation, ataxia, diaphoresis, diarrhoea, fever, hyper-reflexia, myoclonus, shivering, and changes in mental status. The occurrence and severity of syndrome does not seem to be dose related.

Substantive changes

Sibutramine Two RCTs added;[17,21] conclusions unchanged.

Fenfluramine or dexfenfluramine One systematic review added;[36] conclusions unchanged.

REFERENCES

1. National Institutes of Health. *Clinical guidelines on the identification, evaluation, and treatment of overweight and obesity in adults: the Evidence Report.* Bethesda, Maryland: US Department of Health and Human Services, 1998.
2. World Health Organization. *Obesity: preventing and managing the global epidemic. Report of a WHO consultation.* WHO Technical Series: World Health Organization, 2000; No.894. Geneva.
3. Khan LK, Serdula MK, Bowman BA, et al. Use of prescription weight loss pills among U.S. adults in 1996–1998. *Ann Intern Med* 2001;134:282–286.
4. Obesity statistics. British Heart Foundation Statistics Website. Source: Health Survey for England 2001. Available at: http://www.dphpc.ox.ac.uk/bhfhprg/ (last accessed 12 August 2003).
5. Flegal KM, Carroll MD, Ogden CL, et al. Prevalence and trends in obesity among US adults, 1999–2000. *JAMA* 2002;288:1723–1727.
6. Schwartz MW, Woods SC, Porte D, et al. Central nervous system control of food intake. *Nature* 2000;404:661–671.
7. Weinsier RL, Hunter GR, Heini AF, et al. The etiology of obesity: relative contribution of metabolic factors, diet, and physical activity. *Am J Med* 1998;105:145–150.
8. French SA, Story M, Jeffery RW. Environmental influences on eating and physical activity. *Annu Rev Public Health* 2001;22:309–35.
9. Bray GA. Obesity: etiology. In: UpToDate, issue 8/1, 2000. Wellesley, Massachusetts: UpToDate Inc.
10. Allison DB, Fontaine KR, Manson JE, et al. Annual deaths attributable to obesity in the United States. *JAMA* 1999;282:1530–1538.
11. Quesenberry CP, Caan B, Jacobson A. Obesity, health services use, and health care costs among members of a health maintenance organization. *Arch Intern Med* 1998;158:466–472.
12. Kushner RF, Foster GD. Obesity and quality of life. *Nutrition* 2000;16:947–952.
13. University of York, NHS Centre for Reviews and Dissemination. A systematic review of the clinical effectiveness of sibutramine and orlistat in the management of obesity. York, UK: NHS Centre for Reviews and Dissemination, 2000. Search date 2000.
14. Wirth A, Krause J. Long-term weight loss with sibutramine: a randomized controlled trial. *JAMA* 2001;286:1331–1339.
15. James WP, Astrup A, Finer N, et al. Effect of sibutramine on weight maintenance after weight loss: a randomized trial. STORM Study Group. Sibutramine Trial of Obesity Reduction and Maintenance. *Lancet* 2000;356:2119–2125.
16. Serrano-Rios M, Melchionda N, Moreno-Carretero E. Role of sibutramine in the treatment of obese type 2 diabetic patients receiving sulphonylurea therapy. *Diabet Med* 2002;19:119–124.
17. Zannad F, Gille B, Grentzinger A, et al. Effects of sibutramine on ventricular dimensions and heart valves in obese patients during weight reduction. *Am Heart J* 2002;144:508–515.
18. McNulty SJ, Ur E, Williams G; Multicenter Sibutramine Study Group. A randomized trial of sibutramine in the management of obese type 2 diabetic patients treated with metformin. *Diabetes Care* 2003;26:125–131.
19. Gokcel A, Gumurdulu Y, Karakose H, et al. Evaluation of the safety and efficacy of sibutramine, orlistat, and metformin in the treatment of obesity. *Diabetes Obes Metab* 2002;4:49–55.
20. Wadden TA, Berkowitz RI, Womble LG, et al. Effects of sibutramine plus orlistat in obese women following 1 year of treatment by sibutramine alone: a placebo-controlled trial. *Obes Res* 2000;8:431–437.
21. Bach DS, Rissanen AM, Mendel CM, et al. Absence of cardiac valve dysfunction in obese patients treated with sibutramine. *Obes Res* 1999;7:363–369.
22. Health Sciences Authority. Centre for Pharmaceutical Administration. Drug Alerts. Updates Report on Sibutramine. Information page. http://www.hsa.gov.sg/hsa/CPA/CPA_pharma_drugalerts.htm#12(last accessed 3 September 2002).
23. Fanghanel G, Cortinas L, Sanchez-Reyes L, et al. A clinical trial of the use of sibutramine for the treatment of patients suffering essential obesity. *Int J Obes* 2000;24:144–150.
24. Fanghanel G, Cortinas L, Sanchez-Reyes L, et al. Second phase of a double-blind study clinical trial on sibutramine for the treatment of patients suffering from essential obesity: 6 months after treatment cross-over. *Int J Obes* 2001;25:741–747.
25. Haddock CK, Poston WSC, Dill PL, et al. Pharmacotherapy for obesity: a quantitative analysis of four decades of published randomized clinical trials. *Int J Obes* 2002;26:262–273. Search date 1999; primary sources Medline, PsychInfo, handsearching, and personal contact with individual authors.
26. Gaasch WH, Aurigemma GP. Valvular heart disease induced by anorectic drugs. In: UpToDate. 8/3. 2003. Wellesley, Massachusetts: UpToDate Inc.
27. Medicines Control Agency. Committee on Safety in Medicines. Important safety message: European withdrawal of anorectic agents/appetite suppressants: new legal developments, no new safety issues: licences for phentermine and amfepramone being withdrawn May 2001. Information page. http://www.mca.gov.uk/ourwork/monitorsafequalmed/safetymessages/anorectic.htm (last accessed 18 August 2003).
28. Hagiwara M, Tsuchida A, Hyakkoku M, et al. Delayed onset of pulmonary hypertension associated with an appetite suppressant, mazindol: a case report. *Jpn Circ* 2000;64:218–221.
29. Bradley MH, Blum NJ, Scheib RJ. Mazindol in obesity with known cardiac disease: a clinical evaluation. *J Int Med Res* 1974;2:347–349.
30. Thomas SH, Butt AY, Corris PA, et al. Appetite suppressants and primary pulmonary hypertension in the United Kingdom. *Br Heart J* 1995;74:660–663.
31. Little JD, Romans SE. Psychosis following readministration of diethylpropion: a possible role for kindling? *Int Clin Psychopharmacol* 1993;8:67–70.
32. Mulrow CD, Williams JW Jr, Trivedi M, et al. Treatment of depression: newer pharmacotherapies. *Psychopharmacol Bull* 1998;34:409–795. Search date 1998; primary sources the Cochrane Collaboration Depression, Anxiety and Neurosis (CCDAN) Review Group register of trials, and bibliographies of trial and review articles.

33. Weintraub M. Long term weight control study: the National Heart, Lung, and Blood Institute funded multimodal intervention study. *Clin Pharmacol Ther* 1992;51:581–646.
34. Poston WS, Foreyt JP. Scientific and legal issues in fenfluramine/dexfenfluramine litigation. *J Texas Med* 2000;96:48–56.
35. Connolly HM, Crary JL, McGoon MD, et al. Valvular heart disease associated with fenfluramine-phentermine. *N Engl J Med* 1997;337:581–588.
36. Sachdev M, Miller WC, Ryan T, et al. Effect of fenfluramine-derivative diet pills on cardiac valves: a meta-analysis of observational studies. *Am Heart J* 2002;144:1065–1073. Search date 2000; primary sources Medline, Current Contents, Cochrane Library, International Database of Pharmaceuticals, handsearching of identified articles and of conference proceedings published in selected journals, and contact with principal authors.
37. Abenhaim L, Moride Y, Brenot F, et al. Appetite-suppressant drugs and the risk of primary pulmonary hypertension. International primary pulmonary hypertension study group. *N Engl J Med* 1996;335:609–616.
38. Horwitz RI, Brass LM, Kernan WN, et al. Phenylpropanolamine and risk of hemorrhagic stroke: final report of the hemorrhagic stroke project. http://www.fda.gov/ohrms/dockets/ac/00/backgrd/3647b1_tab19.doc (last accessed 18 August 2003).
39. Lucas KH, Kaplan-Machlis B. Orlistat: a novel weight loss therapy. *Ann Pharmacother* 2001;35:314–328. Search date 2000; primary sources Medline, Roche Laboratories, organisational guidelines, National Institutes of Health and Food and Drug Administration web sites, Doctor's Guide online, and reference sections of published articles.
40. O'Meara S, Riemsma R, Shirran L, et al. A rapid and systematic review of the clinical effectiveness and cost-effectiveness of orlistat in the management of obesity. *Health Technol Assess* 2001;5:1–81. Search date 2000; primary sources Amed, Biosis, British Nursing Index, the Cochrane Library, Cinahl, Dare, DH-Data, EconLit, Embase, Health Management Information Service, HTA database, Index to Scientific and Technical Proceedings, King's Fund database, Medline, National Research Register, NEED, Health Economic Evaluations Database, Science Citation Index, Social Science Citation Index, Internet searches, reference lists of relevant reviews, and contact with the authors of conference abstracts.
41. Lindgarde F. The effect of orlistat on body weight and coronary heart disease risk profile in obese patients: the Swedish Multimorbidity Study. *J Intern Med* 2000;248:245–254.
42. Muls E, Kolanowski J, Scheen A, et al. The effects of orlistat on weight and on serum lipids in obese patients with hypercholesterolemia: a randomized, double-blind, placebo-controlled, multicentre study. *Int J Obes* 2001;25:1713–1721.
43. Micic D, Ivkovic-Lazar T, Dragojevic R, et al. Orlistat, a gastrointestinal lipase inhibitor, in therapy of obesity with concomitant hyperlipidemia. *Med Pregl* 1999;52:323–333.
44. Van Gaul LF, Broom JI, Enzi G, et al. Efficacy and tolerability of orlistat in the treatment of obesity: a 6-month dose-ranging study. *Eur J Clin Pharmacol* 1998;54:125–132.
45. Finer N, James WPT, Kopelman PG, et al. One-year treatment of obesity: a randomized, double-blind, placebo-controlled, multicentre study of orlistat, a gastrointestinal lipase inhibitor. *Int J Obes* 2000;24:306–313.
46. Sjostrom L, Rissanen A, Anderson T, et al. Randomised placebo-controlled trial of orlistat for weight loss and prevention of weight regain in obese patients. *Lancet* 1998;352:167–173.
47. Hill JO, Hauptman J, Anderson JW, et al. Orlistat, a lipase inhibitor, for weight maintenance after conventional dieting: a 1-y study. *Am J Clin Nutr* 1999 69:1108–1116.
48. Hanefeld M, Sachse G. The effects of orlistat on body weight and glycaemic control in overweight patients with type 2 diabetes: a randomized, placebo-controlled trial. *Diabetes Obes Metab* 2002; 4:415–423.
49. Kelley DE, et al. Clinical efficacy of orlistat therapy in overweight and obese patients with insulin-treated type 2 diabetes: a 1-year randomized controlled trial. *Diabetes Care* 2002;25:1033–1041.
50. Miles JM, et al. Effect of orlistat in overweight and obese patients with type 2 diabetes treated with metformin. *Diabetes Care* 2002;25:1123–1128.
51. Bakris G, et al. Orlistat improves blood pressure control in obese subjects with treated but inadequately controlled hypertension. *J Hypertens* 2002;20:2257–2267.
52. Broom I, Wilding J, Stott P, et al. Randomised trial of the effect of orlistat on body weight and cardiovascular disease risk profile in obese patients: UK multimorbidity study. *Int J Clin Pract* 2002; 56:494–499.
53. Anonymous. Orlistat: no hurry. *Can Fam Physician* 1999;45:2331–2351. Search date 1999; primary sources Medline, Embase, Reactions, the Cochrane Library, hand searches of international journals, the Prescribe Library, and clinical pharmacology reference texts, and personal contact with Produits Roche, the European Medicines Evaluation Agency, and Food and Drug Administration committees.

David Arterburn
Assistant Professor of Medicine
University of Cincinnati Institute for Health Policy and Health Services Research, and the Cincinnati Department of Veterans Affairs
Cincinnati
USA

Competing interests: None declared. The views expressed in this article are those of the authors and do not necessarily represent the views of the US Department of Veterans Affairs.

The following previous contributors of this topic would also like to be acknowledged: Polly Hitchcock-Noel and Cynthia Mulrow.

Prevention of cardiovascular events in diabetes

Search date December 2002

Janine Malcolm, Hilary Meggison, and Ronald Sigal

QUESTIONS

INTERVENTIONS

*No RCT but observational evidence suggests some benefit.

See glossary, p 711

Key Messages

Smoking cessation

- **Smoking cessation** We found no RCTs on promotion of smoking cessation. Observational evidence and extrapolation from evidence in people without diabetes suggest that promotion of smoking cessation is likely to reduce cardiovascular events.

Blood pressure

- **Antihypertensive treatment versus no antihypertensive treatment** One systematic review and RCTs have found that blood pressure lowering with antihypertensive agents in people with diabetes and hypertension reduces cardiovascular morbidity and mortality compared with no antihypertensive treatment.
- **Lower target blood pressures** Large RCTs including people with diabetes and hypertension have found that control of blood pressure to a target diastolic blood pressure of no more than 80 mm Hg or less reduces the risk of major cardiovascular events. One RCT in normotensive people with diabetes found that intensive blood pressure lowering reduced cerebral vascular accidents but found no significant difference in cardiovascular death, myocardial infarction, congestive heart failure, or all cause mortality.
- **Different antihypertensive drugs** Systematic reviews and RCTs have found that angiotensin converting enzyme inhibitors, diuretics, β blockers, and calcium channel blockers all reduce cardiovascular morbidity and mortality in people with diabetes and hypertension. However, there are differences in the types of adverse effects reported with different antihypertensive drugs. RCTs have found that people taking atenolol gained more weight than those taking captopril, an increase in risk of congestive heart failure with lisinopril compared with chlorthalidone, a higher frequency of headache with diltiazem compared with diuretics or β blockers, and a higher rate of withdrawal from treatment because of adverse effects with atenolol compared with losartan.

Dyslipidaemia

- **Statins versus placebo** One systematic review and RCTs have found that statins reduce cardiovascular morbidity and mortality compared with placebo.
- **Aggressive versus moderate lipid lowering with statins** One RCT found that, compared with usual care, treatment with atorvastatin to achieve a target low density lipoprotein (LDL) concentration below 2.6 mmol/L (< 100 mg/dL) reduces cardiovascular morbidity and mortality. Another RCT found no significant difference between a lower target LDL (1.55–2.20 mmol/L) using lovastatin, along with cholestyramine if necessary, and a moderate target LDL (3.36–3.62 mmol/L) in 4 year event rate for myocardial infarction and death.
- **Fibrates** One RCT found that gemfibrozil reduced cardiovascular events over 5 years compared with placebo whereas another smaller RCT found no significant difference. One RCT found that bezafibrate reduced cardiovascular events compared with placebo, whereas another RCT found no significant difference in myocardial infarction between fenofibrate and placebo.
- **Low versus standard statin dose in older people** One RCT found no significant difference in cardiovascular events between low dose pravastatin (5 mg/day) and standard dose pravastatin (10–20 mg/day) over 4 years.

Prevention of cardiovascular events in diabetes

Antiplatelet drugs

- **Clopidogrel** We found no RCTs comparing only clopidogrel versus placebo. One RCT in people with diabetes and with recent ischaemic stroke, myocardial infarction, or established peripheral arterial disease found no significant difference between clopidogrel and aspirin at 28 days in cardiovascular events. This RCT also found a lower proportion of people hospitalised for a bleeding event with clopidogrel than with aspirin.
- **Prophylactic aspirin** One systematic review and RCTs have found that prophylactic aspirin reduces cardiovascular morbidity and mortality compared with controls. One RCT found that aspirin increased non-fatal major bleeds and minor bleeds but not fatal bleeds compared with placebo. Another RCT found no increase in the risks of vitreous, retinal, gastrointestinal, or cerebral haemorrhage with aspirin compared with placebo.
- **Adding glycoprotein IIb/IIIa inhibitors to heparin in acute coronary syndromes** One RCT in people presenting with unstable angina or acute myocardial infarction without ST segment elevation found that addition of tirofiban (a glycoprotein IIb/IIIa inhibitor) to heparin reduced the composite outcome of death, myocardial infarction, or refractory ischaemia at 180 days compared with heparin alone. This RCT found no significant difference between tirofiban plus heparin and heparin alone in risk of bleeding in people already taking aspirin.
- **Adding clopidogrel to aspirin in acute coronary syndromes** One RCT in people presenting with unstable angina or non-Q-wave myocardial infarction and also taking aspirin found no significant reduction in cardiovascular events after 12 months with addition of clopidigrel compared with placebo. This RCT also found a higher proportion of major bleeds with addition of clopidogrel than with placebo.

Blood glucose control

- **Metformin versus diet alone in obese people** One RCT in obese people with type 2 diabetes found that intensive treatment with metformin compared with conventional treatment with diet alone reduced myocardial infarction but not stroke over 5 years. This RCT found no significant increase in major hypoglycaemic episodes in the metformin group compared with the diet only group.
- **Intensive versus conventional glycaemic control** Three RCTs found no significant difference in cardiovascular morbidity and mortality between intensive and conventional treatment for blood glucose control. These RCTs also found an increase in hypoglycaemic episodes and weight gain with intensive compared with conventional treatment.

Revascularisation

- **Coronary artery bypass graft (CABG) versus percutaneous transluminal coronary angioplasty (PTCA)** One large RCT in people with diabetes and multivessel coronary artery disease has found that CABG reduces mortality or myocardial infarction within 8 years compared with PTCA. Another smaller RCT found a non-significant reduction in mortality with CABG compared with PTCA at 4 years.
- **Stent plus glycoprotein IIb/IIIa inhibitors in people undergoing PTCA** RCTs in people with diabetes undergoing PTCA have found that the combination of stent and a glycoprotein IIb/IIIa inhibitor reduces cardiovascular morbidity and mortality compared with stent plus placebo.

- **CABG plus stent versus PTCA plus stent** One RCT in people with diabetes and multivessel coronary artery disease found no significant difference between CABG plus stent and PTCA plus stent in cardiovascular morbidity or mortality (to time of discharge). However, it found that CABG plus stent compared with PTCA plus stent in the short term increased cardiovascular risk at 1 year.
- **PTCA versus thrombolysis** We found no systematic review or RCTs comparing PTCA versus thrombolysis for prevention of cardiovascular events in people with diabetes.

DEFINITION **Diabetes mellitus:** See definition under glycaemic control in diabetes, p 667. **Cardiovascular disease:** Atherosclerotic disease of the heart and/or the coronary, cerebral, or peripheral vessels leading to clinical events such as acute myocardial infarction (see glossary, p 711), congestive heart failure, sudden cardiac death, stroke, gangrene, and/or need for revascularisation procedures. **Population:** In previous versions of *Clinical Evidence* we attempted to differentiate between primary and secondary prevention in this topic. However, in middle aged and older people with type 2 diabetes this distinction may not be clinically important. We are not aware of any intervention that has been shown to be effective in secondary prevention but ineffective in primary prevention, or vice versa, in people with diabetes. In most cases a large proportion of people with diabetes entered into cardiovascular disease prevention trials are middle aged and older with additional cardiovascular disease risk factors, and a large portion of these actually have undiagnosed cardiovascular disease.

INCIDENCE/ PREVALENCE Diabetes mellitus is a major risk factor for cardiovascular disease. In the USA, a survey of deaths in 1986 suggested that 60–75% of people with diabetes die from cardiovascular causes.[1] The annual incidence of cardiovascular disease is increased in people with diabetes (men: RR 2–3; women: RR 3–4, adjusted for age and other cardiovascular risk factors).[2] About 45% of middle aged and older white people with diabetes have evidence of coronary artery disease compared with about 25% of people without diabetes in the same populations. In a Finnish population based cohort study (1059 people with diabetes and 1373 people without diabetes, aged 45–64 years), the 7 year risk of acute myocardial infarction was as high in adults with diabetes without previous cardiac disease (20.2/100 person years) as it was in people without diabetes with previous cardiac disease (18.8/100 person years).[3]

AETIOLOGY/ RISK FACTORS Diabetes mellitus increases the risk of cardiovascular disease. Cardiovascular risk factors in people with diabetes include conventional risk factors (age, prior cardiovascular disease, cigarette smoking, hypertension, dyslipidaemia, sedentary lifestyle, family history of premature cardiovascular disease) and more diabetes specific risk factors (elevated urinary protein excretion, poor glycaemic control). Conventional risk factors for cardiovascular disease contribute to an increase in the relative risk of cardiovascular disease in people with diabetes to about the same extent as in those without diabetes (see aetiology under primary prevention, p 154). One prospective cohort study (164 women and 235 men with diabetes [mean age 65 years] and 437 women and 1099 men without diabetes [mean age 61 years] followed for mortality for a mean of 3.7 years following acute myocardial infarction) found that significantly more people with diabetes died compared with people without diabetes (116/399 [29%] *v* 204/1536 [13%]; RR 2.2, 95% CI 1.8 to 2.7).[4] It also found that the mortality risk after myocardial infarction associated with diabetes was higher for women than for men (adjusted HR 2.7, 95% CI 1.8 to 4.2 for women *v* 1.3, 95% CI 1 to 1.8 for men). Physical inactivity is a significant risk factor for cardiovascular events in both men and women. Another cohort study (5125 women with diabetes) found that participation in little (< 1 hour/week) or no physical activity compared with physical activity for at least 7 hours a week was associated with doubling of the risk of a cardiovascular event.[5] A third cohort study (1263 men with diabetes, mean follow up 12 years) found that low baseline cardiorespiratory fitness increased overall mortality compared with moderate or high fitness (RR 2.9, 95% CI 2.1 to 3.6), and overall mortality was higher in those reporting no recreational exercise in the previous 3 months than in those reporting any recreational physical activity in the same period (RR 1.8, 95% CI 1.3 to 2.5).[6] The absolute risk of cardiovascular disease is almost the same in women as in men with diabetes. Diabetes specific cardiovascular risk factors include the duration of diabetes during adulthood (the years of exposure to diabetes before age 20 years add little to the risk of cardiovascular disease); raised blood glucose concentrations (reflected in fasting blood glucose or HbA1c [see glossary, p 711]); and any degree of microalbuminuria (albuminuria 30–299 mg/24 hours).[7] People with diabetes and microalbuminuria have a higher risk of coronary morbidity and mortality than do people with normal levels of urinary albumin and a similar duration of diabetes (RR 2–3).[8,9] Clinical proteinuria increases the risk of mortality from cardiac events in people with type 2 diabetes (RR 2.61, 95% CI 1.99 to 3.43)[10] and type 1 diabetes (RR 9)[7,11,12] compared with people with the same type of diabetes who have normal albumin excretion. An epidemiological analysis of people with diabetes enrolled in the Heart Outcomes Prevention Evaluation cohort study (3498 people with diabetes and at least 1 other cardiovascular risk factor, age > 55 years, of whom 1140 [32%] had microalbuminuria at baseline; 5 years' follow up) found higher risk for major cardiovascular events in those with microalbuminuria (albumin : creatinine ratio [ACR] ≥ 2.0 mg/mmol) than in those without microalbuminuria (adjusted RR 1.97, 95% CI 1.68 to 2.31), and for all cause mortality (RR 2.15, 95% CI 1.78 to 2.60).[13] It also found an association between ACR and the risk of major cardiovascular events (ACR 0.22–0.57 mg/mmol: RR 0.85, 95% CI 0.63 to 1.14; ACR 0.58–1.62 mg/mmol: RR 1.11, 95% CI 0.86 to 1.43; ACR 1.62–1.99 mg/mmol: RR 1.89, 95% CI 1.52 to 2.36).

PROGNOSIS Diabetes mellitus increases the risk of mortality or serious morbidity after a coronary event (RR 1.5–3).[2,3,14,15] This excess risk is partly accounted for by increased prevalence of other cardiovascular risk factors in people with diabetes. A systematic review (search date 1998, 15 prospective cohort studies) found that, in people with diabetes admitted to hospital for acute myocardial infarction, "stress hyperglycaemia" was associated with significantly higher mortality in hospital compared with lower blood glucose levels

(RR 1.7, 95% CI 1.2 to 2.4).[16] One large prospective cohort study (91 285 men aged 40–84 years) found higher all cause and coronary heart disease mortality at 5 years' follow up in men with diabetes than in men without coronary artery disease or diabetes (age adjusted RR 3.3, 95% CI 2.6 to 4.1 in men with diabetes and without coronary artery disease *v* RR 2.3, 95% CI 2.0 to 2.6 in healthy people; RR 5.6, 95% CI 4.9 to 6.3 in men with coronary artery disease but without diabetes *v* RR 2.2, 95% CI 2.0 to 2.4 in healthy people; RR 12.0, 95% CI 9.9 to14.6 in men with both risk factors *v* RR 4.7, 95% CI 4.0 to 5.4 in healthy people).[17] Multivariate analysis did not materially alter these associations. Diabetes mellitus alone is associated with a twofold increase in risk for all cause death, with a threefold increase in risk of death from coronary heart disease, and, in people with pre-existing coronary heart disease, with a 12-fold increase in risk of death from coronary heart disease compared with people with neither risk factor.[17]

AIMS OF INTERVENTION To reduce mortality and morbidity from cardiovascular disease, with minimum adverse effects.

OUTCOMES Incidence of fatal or non-fatal acute myocardial infarction; congestive heart failure; sudden cardiac death; coronary revascularisation; stroke; gangrene; angiographic evidence of coronary, cerebral, vascular, or peripheral arterial stenosis.

METHODS *Clinical Evidence* search and appraisal December 2002. We searched for systematic reviews and RCTs with at least 10 confirmed clinical cardiovascular events among people with diabetes. Studies reporting only intermediate end points (e.g. regression of plaque on angiography, lipid changes) were not included. Most of the evidence comes from subgroup analyses of large RCTs that included people with diabetes. As with all subgroup analyses, and studies with small numbers, these results must be interpreted as suggestive rather than definitive.

QUESTION What are the effects of promoting smoking cessation in people with diabetes?

We found no RCTs on promotion of smoking cessation specifically in people with diabetes. Observational evidence and extrapolation from people without diabetes suggest that promotion of smoking cessation is likely to reduce cardiovascular events.

Benefits: We found no systematic review or RCTs on promotion of smoking cessation specifically in people with diabetes.

Harms: We found no RCTs.

Comment: Observational studies have found that cigarette smoking is associated with increased cardiovascular death in people with diabetes. Smoking cessation in people without diabetes has been found to be associated with reduced risk. People with diabetes are likely to benefit from smoking cessation at least as much as people who do not have diabetes but have other risk factors for cardiovascular events (see smoking cessation under secondary prevention of ischaemic cardiac events, p 188).

QUESTION **What are the effects of controlling blood pressure in people with diabetes?**

OPTION **ANTIHYPERTENSIVE TREATMENT VERSUS NO ANTIHYPERTENSIVE TREATMENT**

One systematic review and RCTs have found that, in people with diabetes and hypertension, blood pressure lowering with antihypertensive agents reduces cardiovascular morbidity and mortality compared with no antihypertensive treatment.

Benefits: We found two systematic reviews[18,19] and four subsequent RCTs.[20–23] The first systematic review (search date 1997) was withdrawn from the Cochrane Library and is currently being updated.[18] The second systematic review (search date not stated) found that, compared with controls, blood pressure lowering with antihypertensive agents significantly reduced mortality, but it found no significant effect on myocardial infarction (6 RCTs, 7572 people with diabetes with or without diagnosis of cardiovascular disease [CVD], aged > 50 years; mortality: 10 deaths/1000 person years in treatment arms *v* 19 deaths/1000 person years in control arms; RR 0.51, 95% CI 0.38 to 0.69; myocardial infarction: 14/1000 person years in treatment arms *v* 16/1000 person years in control arms; rate ratio 0.76, 96% CI 0.51 to 1.01).[19] The first subsequent RCT found that, compared with placebo, antihypertensive treatment with nitrendipine or enalapril with or without hydrochlorothiazide significantly reduced all cardiovascular events over a median of 2 years but it had no significant effect on overall mortality (1 RCT, 495 people with diabetes without a diagnosis of CVD, aged ≥ 60 years with blood pressure 165–220/< 95 mm Hg; all CVD events over median 2 years: 13/252 [5.2%] with antihypertensive treatment *v* 31/240 [12.9%] with placebo; ARR 8%, 95% CI 3% to 10%; RR 0.4, 95% CI 0.21 to 0.75; NNT 13, 95% CI 10 to 31; overall mortality: 16/252 [6.3%] with antihypertensive treatment *v* 26/240 [10.8%] with placebo; ARR +4.5%, 95% CI –0.7% to +7.4%; RR 0.59, 95% CI 0.32 to 1.06).[20] The second subsequent RCT found no significant difference between antihypertensive treatment with irbesartan or amlodipine and placebo in cardiovascular composite outcomes over 2.6 years (1 RCT, 1715 people with nephropathy due to type 2 diabetes and hypertension, aged 30–70 years; 138/579 [24%] with irbesartan *v* 144/569 [25%] with placebo; RR 0.91, 95% CI 0.72 to 1.14; 128/567 [23%] with amlodipine *v* 144/569 [25%] with placebo; RR 0.88, 95% CI 0.69 to 1.12; 138/579 [23%] with irbesartan *v* 158/567 [28%] with amlodipine; RR 1.03, 95% CI 0.81 to 1.31).[21] The third subsequent RCT found no significant difference between antihypertensive treatment with irbesartan and placebo in non-fatal cardiovascular events over 2 years (1 RCT, 590 people with type 2 diabetes, microalbuminuria, and hypertension, mean age 58 years; 8/194 [4.1%] with irbesartan *v* 17/201 [8.5%] with placebo; RR 0.49, 95% CI 0.22 to 1.10).[22] The fourth subsequent RCT found that, compared with placebo, antihypertensive treatment with ramipril significantly reduced major cardiovascular events and death from any cause over 4.5 years (1 RCT, 3 arm study, 9541 people aged

≥ 55 years with diabetes and additional CVD risk factors such as diagnosed coronary vascular disease, current smoker, hypercholesterolaemia, hypertension, or microalbuminuria; major cardiovascular event such as coronary vascular disease death, acute myocardial infarction, or stroke: 277/1808 [15.3%] with ramipril *v* 351/1769 [19.8%] with placebo; RR 0.75, 95% CI 0.64 to 0.88; ARR 4.5%; NNT 22, 95% CI 14 to 43; death from any cause: 196/1808 [10.8%] with ramipril *v* 248/1769 [14.0%] with placebo; RR 0.76, 95% CI 0.67 to 0.92; ARR 3.2%; NNT 32, 95% CI 19 to 98).[23] The relative effect of ramipril was present in all subgroups regardless of hypertensive status, microalbuminuria, type of diabetes, and nature of diabetes treatment (diet, oral agents, or insulin). The RCT also compared vitamin versus placebo and found no significant effect on morbidity or mortality.[23–25]

Harms: The systematic review[19] and first subsequent RCT[20] gave no information on adverse effects. The second subsequent RCT found a significantly higher incidence of hyperkalaemia resulting in discontinuation of treatment with irbesartan than with amlodipine or placebo (11/579 [1.9%] with irbesartan *v* 3/567 [0.5%] with amlodipine *v* 2/569 [0.4%] with placebo; P = 0.01 for both comparisons).[21] The third subsequent RCT stated that significantly more people had "serious adverse events" with irbesartan than with placebo but it did not state what they were (15.4% with irbesartan *v* 22.8% with placebo).[22] The fourth subsequent RCT found that cough was 5% more frequent with the angiotensin converting enzyme inhibitor (ramipril) than with placebo.[23]

Comment: None.

OPTION DIFFERENT ANTIHYPERTENSIVE DRUGS

Systematic reviews and RCTs have found that angiotensin converting enzyme inhibitors, diuretics, β blockers, and calcium channel blockers all reduce cardiovascular morbidity and mortality in people with diabetes and hypertension. However, there are differences in the types of adverse effects reported for different antihypertensive drugs. RCTs have found that people taking atenolol gained more weight than those taking captopril, an increase in risk of congestive heart failure with lisinopril compared with chlorthalidone, a higher frequency of headache with diltiazem than with diuretics or β blockers, and a higher rate of withdrawal from treatment because of adverse effects with atenolol than with losartan.

Benefits: We found one systematic review (search date 2000),[26] one subsequent RCT,[27] and two additional RCTs.[28,29] **Angiotensin converting enzyme (ACE) inhibitors versus calcium channel blockers:** One systematic review (search date 2000)[26] identified two RCTs comparing ACE inhibitors (fosinopril, enalapril) versus calcium channel blockers (amlodipine, nisoldipine) in people with diabetes without a diagnosis of cardiovascular disease (CVD).[30,31] The review found that ACE inhibitors significantly reduced combined cardiovascular events compared with calcium channel blockers, but it found no significant reduction in acute myocardial infarction (see glossary, p 711), stroke, or death in people with diabetes without a diagnosis of CVD (2 RCTs; combined cardiovascular events —

cardiovascular death, acute myocardial infarction, congestive heart failure, stroke, pulmonary infarction, angina: 34/424 [8%] with ACE inhibitors *v* 70/426 [16%] with calcium channel blockers; ARR 8%, 95% CI 4% to 13%; RR 0.49, 95% CI 0.33 to 0.72; NNT 13, 95% CI 7 to 25; death: 17/424 [4.0%] with ACE inhibitors *v* 22/426 [5.2%] with calcium channel blockers; ARR 1%; RR 0.78, 95% CI 0.42 to 1.44; acute myocardial infarction: 15/424 [4%] with ACE inhibitors *v* 38/426 [9%] with calcium channel blockers; ARR 5%, 95% CI 2% to 9%; RR 0.40, 95% CI 0.22 to 0.71; NNT 19, 95% CI 12 to 46; stroke: 11/424 [2.6%] with ACE inhibitors *v* 21/426 [4.9%] with calcium channel blockers; ARR 2.3%; RR 0.53, 95% CI 0.26 to 1.08).[30,31] The subsequent RCT compared ACE inhibitors (enalapril, lisinopril), calcium channel blockers (felodipine, isradipine), β blockers (atenolol, metoprolol, pindolol), and diuretics (hydrochlorothiazide plus amiloride).[27] It found that, compared with calcium channel blockers, ACE inhibitors significantly reduced fatal and non-fatal myocardial infarctions (1 RCT, 719 people with diabetes without a diagnosis of CVD, mean age 76 years, mean blood pressure 190/99 mm Hg; 17/235 [7%] *v* 32/231 [14%]; RR 0.51, 95% CI 0.28 to 0.92) but it found no significant difference between groups in the incidence of major cardiovascular events over 4 years (major cardiovascular events per 1000 person years: 64.2 with ACE inhibitors *v* 67.7 with calcium channel blockers *v* 75.0 with β blockers or diuretics). **ACE inhibitors versus β blockers:** One RCT[32] identified in a systematic review[26] found no significant difference between captopril and atenolol in number of cardiovascular events over 8.4 years (1 RCT, 758 people with diabetes without a diagnosis of CVD; cardiovascular events: 102/400 [25.5%] with captopril *v* 75/358 [20.9%] with atenolol; ARI +5%, 95% CI –1% to +11%; RR 1.22, 95% CI 0.94 to 1.58). **ACE inhibitors versus β blockers or diuretics**: One RCT[33] identified by the systematic review[26] found that, compared with diuretics or β blockers, captopril significantly reduced acute myocardial infarction, stroke, or death (1 RCT, 572 people with or without a diagnosis of CVD; acute myocardial infarction, stroke, or death: 46/263 [17.5%] with diuretics/β blockers *v* 35/309 [11.3%] with captopril; RR 0.65, 95% CI 0.43 to 0.97). **ACE inhibitors or calcium channel blockers versus diuretics:** One RCT found no significant difference between lisinopril or amlodipine and chlorthalidone in 6 year fatal cardiac heart disease, non-fatal myocardial infarction, fatal and non-fatal stroke, or all cause mortality (1 RCT, 12 063 people with diabetes and established hypertension, aged 55 years or older; primary outcome of non-fatal myocardial infarction plus coronary heart disease death: chlorthalidone versus lisinopril: RR 1.00, 95% CI 0.87 to 1.14; amlodipine versus chlorthalidone: RR 1.04, 95% CI 0.94 to 1.14; absolute numbers for the diabetic subgroup not provided, results presented graphically).[34] **Angiotensin II receptor antagonists versus β blockers:** One RCT found that, compared with atenolol, losartan significantly reduced composite cardiovascular outcomes over 4 years (1 RCT, 1195 people with diabetes with or without a diagnosis of CVD, aged 55–80 years; composite cardiovascular outcomes — mortality, stroke, and myocardial infarction: 103/586 [17.6%] with losartan *v* 139/609 [22.8%] with atenolol; RR 0.77, 95% CI 0.61 to 0.97;

NNT 19, 95% CI 11 to 142).[29] **Calcium channel blockers versus diuretics or β blockers:** One RCT found no significant difference between diltiazem and conventional antihypertensive treatment with diuretic, β blocker, or combination of the two in fatal or non-fatal stroke, myocardial infarction, and other cardiovascular death (1 RCT, 727 people with diabetes and diastolic pressure ≥100 mm Hg on two occasions, aged 50–74 years; fatal or non-fatal stroke, myocardial infarction, and other cardiovascular death: 44/351 [12.5%] with diltiazem *v* 44/376 [11.7%] with conventional treatment; RR 1.07, 95% CI 0.72 to 1.59.[35]

Harms: **ACE inhibitors versus calcium channel blockers:** One systematic review[26] and a subsequent RCT[27] gave no information on adverse effects. **ACE inhibitors versus β blockers:** One RCT identified in the systematic review found that people taking atenolol gained more weight than did those taking captopril (3.4 kg with atenolol *v* 1.6 kg with captopril; P = 0.02).[32] Over the first 4 years of the trial people allocated to atenolol had higher mean HbA1c (see glossary, p 711) (7.5% *v* 7.0%; P = 0.004), but no significant difference was found between groups over the subsequent 4 years. No significant difference was found between atenolol and captopril in rates of hypoglycaemia, lipid concentrations, tolerability, blood pressure lowering, or prevention of disease events. **ACE inhibitors versus β blockers or diuretics:** One RCT gave no information on adverse effects.[33] **ACE inhibitors or calcium channel blockers versus diuretics:** One RCT found an increased risk of congestive heart failure with lisinopril than with chlorthalidone (RR 1.22, 95% CI 1.05 to 1.42) and with amlodipine than with chlorthalidone (RR 1.42, 95% CI 1.23 to 1.64).[34] A previous report for this RCT described an increased risk of combined coronary vascular disease events with doxasazin than with chlorthalidone when these agents were used to treat hypertension (coronary heart disease death, non-fatal myocardial infarction, stroke, angina, coronary revascularization, congestive heart failure, and peripheral arterial disease: RR 1.24, 95% CI 1.12 to 1.38).[28] The doxazosin arm of the RCT was terminated because of this increase in risk.[28] **Angiotensin II receptor antagonists versus β blockers:** One RCT found that discontinuation of treatment because of adverse effects was less common with losartan than with atenolol (2/586 *v* 9/609; RR 0.23, 95% CI 0.05 to 1.06; P = 0.065).[29] Adverse events that occurred with significantly greater frequency with losartan than with atenolol were bradycardia (1% *v* 9%; P < 0.0001), cold extremities (4% *v* 6%; P < 0.0001), albuminuria (5% *v* 6%; P = 0.0002), hyperglycaemia (5% *v* 7%; P = 0.007), asthenia/fatigue (15% *v* 17%; P = 0.001), back pain (12% *v* 10%; P = 0.004), dyspnoea (10% *v* 14%; P < 0.0001), and lower extremity oedema (12% *v* 14%; P = 0.002).[29] **Calcium channel blockers versus diuretics or β blockers:** One RCT found significantly greater frequency of headache with diltiazem than with diuretics or β blockers (8.5% with diltiazem *v* 5.7% with diuretics or β blockers; P < 0.001).[35]

Comment: The evidence suggests that thiazide diuretics, β blockers, ACE inhibitors, and calcium channel blockers all significantly reduce cardiovascular events in people with diabetes. The results of one large RCT cast doubt on the conclusions of earlier, smaller studies suggesting that ACE inhibitors are superior to calcium channel blockers.[34] The RCT indicates that chlorthalidone is at least as effective as an ACE inhibitor as initial therapy for hypertension in terms of prevention of major cardiovascular events.[34] It is unclear whether ACE inhibitors and β blockers are equivalent. In most RCTs combination treatment with more than one agent was required to achieve target blood pressures. One large RCT found that the ACE inhibitor ramipril, which reduces urinary protein excretion, also reduced cardiovascular morbidity and mortality in older diabetic people with other cardiac risk factors.[23] The relative cardioprotective effect of the ACE inhibitor was present to the same extent in people with or without hypertension, and with or without microalbuminuria.

OPTION TARGET BLOOD PRESSURE

Large RCTs including people with diabetes and hypertension have found that tighter control of blood pressure to a target diastolic blood pressure of no more than 80 mm Hg or less reduces the risk of major cardiovascular events. One RCT in normotensive people with diabetes found that intensive blood pressure lowering reduced cerebral vascular accidents but found no significant difference in cardiovascular death, myocardial infarction, congestive heart failure, or all cause mortality.

Benefits: We found no systematic review but found three RCTs.[32,36–38] The first RCT found that, compared with moderate target blood pressure (BP; ≤ 180/105 mm Hg), tight target BP (≤ 150/85 mm Hg) significantly reduced fatal or non-fatal acute myocardial infarction (see glossary, p 711) and stroke, but it found no significant difference for peripheral vascular events over 8.4 years (1 RCT, 1148 people with hypertension managed with atenolol or captopril; fatal or non-fatal acute myocardial infarction: 107/758 [14%] with tight BP target *v* 83/390 [21%] with moderate BP target; RR 0.66, 95% CI 0.51 to 0.86, NNT 14, 95% CI 9 to 35; stroke: 38/758 [5.0%] with tight BP target *v* 34/390 [8.7%] with moderate BP target; RR 0.58, 95% CI 0.37 to 0.90; NNT 27, 95% CI 18 to 116; peripheral vascular events: 8/758 [1.1%] with tight BP target *v* 8/390 [2.1%] with moderate BP target; RR 0.52, 95% CI 0.195 to 1.36).[32,36] The second RCT found that the risk of major cardiovascular events was reduced by 50% over 3.8 years with a target diastolic BP of 80 mm Hg or less compared with a target BP of 90 mm Hg or less (1 multicentre RCT, 3 arm study, 1501 people with hypertension managed with felodipine, ACE inhibitors, β blockers, or diuretics; major cardiovascular events: 22/499 [4.4%] with target BP ≤ 80 mm Hg *v* 45/501 [9.0%] with target BP ≤ 90 mm Hg; RR 0.5, 95% CI 0.3 to 0.8; NNT 22, 95% CI 16 to 57).[37] The third RCT found a significantly lower incidence of cerebral vascular accidents with a target diastolic BP of 10 mm Hg below baseline compared with a target diastolic BP of 80–89 mm Hg over 5.3 years (1 RCT, 480 people with baseline BP < 140/90 mm Hg being managed with nisoldipine or enalapril; cerebral vascular accidents: 4/237 [1.7%] *v* 13/243 [5.4%]; OR 3.29, CI 1.06 to 10.25; NNT 27, 95% CI 14 to 255).[38] The RCT found no significant difference in cardiovascular death, myocardial infarction, congestive heart failure, or all cause mortality.

Harms: We found no good evidence of a threshold below which it is harmful to lower BP. One RCT found that a significantly greater proportion of people gained weight with atenolol than with captopril (mean weight gain over 9 years: 3.4 kg with atenolol *v* 1.6 kg with captopril; P = 0.02) but it found no significant difference in hypoglycaemia or weight gain with tight BP control (≤ 150/85 mm Hg) compared with moderate BP control (≤ 180/105 mm Hg).[32,36] The second RCT comparing tight versus moderate BP control did not provide information on adverse effects.[37] The third RCT in normotensive people gave no information on adverse effects.[38]

Comment: Aggressive lowering of BP in people with diabetes and hypertension reduces cardiovascular morbidity and mortality. In most trials combination treatment with more than one agent was required to achieve target BPs.

QUESTION **What are the effects of treating dyslipidaemia in people with diabetes?**

OPTION **FIBRATES**

One RCT found that gemfibrozil reduced cardiovascular events over 5 years compared with placebo, whereas another smaller RCT found no significant difference. One RCT found that bezafibrate reduced cardiovascular events compared with placebo, whereas another RCT found no significant difference in myocardial infarction between fenofibrate and placebo.

Benefits: We found one systematic review (search date 2000),[19] one additional RCT,[39] and one subsequent RCT.[40] One RCT identified by the systematic review found that gemfibrozil did not significantly reduce myocardial infarction or cardiac death over 5 years compared with placebo (1 RCT, 135 men aged 40–55 years with diabetes without a diagnosis of cardiovascular disease [CVD]: 2/59 [3.4%] events with gemfibrozil *v* 8/76 [10.5%] with placebo; ARR +7.1%, 95% CI −2.1% to +16.8%; RR 0.32, 95% CI 0.07 to 1.46).[41] The additional RCT (164 people aged 35–65 years with type 2 diabetes without a diagnosis of CVD) found that bezafibrate significantly reduced myocardial infarction or new ischaemic changes on electrocardiogram over 3 years compared with placebo (164 people aged 35–65 years with type 2 diabetes without a diagnosis of CVD)(5/64 [7.8%] events with bezafibrate *v* 16/64 [25%] events with placebo; ARR 17.2%, 95% CI 4.6% to 30.1%; RR 0.31, 95% CI 0.12 to 0.80; NNT 6, 95% CI 5 to 20).[39] Another RCT identified by the systematic review found that gemfibrozil 1200 mg daily significantly reduced coronary heart disease death or non-fatal acute myocardial infarction over 5 years compared with placebo (1 RCT, 627 people aged < 74 years with diabetes and a diagnosis of CVD: 88/309 [28%] events with gemfibrozil *v* 116/318 [36%] events with placebo; RR 0.78, 95% CI 0.62 to 0.98).[42] The subsequent RCT (418 people with diabetes and with or without CVD diagnosis, mean age 57 years) found no significant difference in the proportion of people who either had myocardial infarction or died after 39 months of treatment between fenofibrate 200 mg daily and placebo (15/207 [7.2%] events with fenofibrate *v* 21/211 [9.9%] events with placebo; ARR +2.7%, 95% CI –2.8% to +8.3%; RR 0.73, 95% CI 0.39 to 1.37).[40]

Harms: The systematic review (search date 2000)[19] and the additional RCT[39] provided no information on adverse effects. The subsequent RCT found no significant difference between fenofibrate and placebo in gallbladder symptoms (0.5% *v* 1.4%), liver toxicity (1.5% *v* 0%), muscle pain (0% *v* 0.5%), joint pain (3.4% *v* 2.5%), or cancer (2.4% v 3.3%).[40]

Comment: None.

OPTION STATINS

One systematic review and RCTs have found that statins reduce cardiovascular morbidity and mortality compared with placebo. One RCT found that treatment with atorvastatin to achieve a target low density lipoprotein below 2.6 mmol/L reduces cardiovascular morbidity and mortality compared with usual care. Another RCT found no significant difference between use of lovastatin, with cholestyramine if necessary, to achieve lower target low density lipoprotein of 1.55–2.20 mmol/L and a moderate target low density lipoprotein of 3.36–3.62 mmol/L in 4 year event rate for myocardial infarction and death. One RCT found no significant difference in cardiovascular events in older people with low dose pravastatin 5 mg daily and standard dose pravastatin 10–20 mg daily over 4 years.

Benefits: We found one systematic review (search date 2000)[19] and five subsequent RCTs.[43–47] **Versus placebo:** The systematic review found that pravastatin or simvastatin significantly reduced cardiovascular events over 6 years compared with placebo (3 RCTs,[48–50] 1570 people: 34 events with statins *v* 44 events with placebo per 1000 person years; RR 0.77, 95% CI 0.62 to 0.96; person years needed to treat 120, 95% CI 61 to 4856).[19] One RCT identified in the systematic review found no significant difference between lovastatin and placebo in myocardial infarction, unstable angina, or sudden cardiac death over 5 years (4/84 [4.8%] events with lovastatin *v* 6/71 [8.5%] events with placebo; ARR +3.7%, 95% CI –5.6% to +11.9%; RR 0.56, 95% CI 0.16 to 1.91).[51] The first subsequent RCT found that, compared with placebo, simvastatin significantly reduced all cause mortalilty, non-fatal myocardial infarction, coronary heart disease (CHD) death, total stroke, or any revascularisation over 5 years in people without a diagnosis of cardiovascular disease (CVD; 1 RCT, 3982 people aged 4–80 years with diabetes: 276/2006 [13.8%] events with simvastatin *v* 367/1976 [18.6%] events with placebo; ARR 4.8%; NNT 21, 95% CI 14 to 40; see comment below).[43] By the end of the study 38% of those allocated to placebo were taking a non-study statin. The RCT also found a similar risk reduction in people with diabetes and diagnosis of CHD (1 RCT, 1981 people: 325/972 [33.4%] events with simvastatin *v* 381/1009 [37.8%] events with placebo; ARR 4.3%; NNT 23, 95% CI 12 to 897).[43] The second subsequent RCT found that fluvastatin significantly reduced cardiac death, non-fatal myocardial infarction, and reintervention over 4 years compared with placebo (1 RCT, 202 people aged 18–80 years with diabetes and a diagnosis of CVD: 26/120 [21%] events with fluvastatin *v* 31/82 [37.8%] events with placebo; ARR 0.161, 95% CI 0.033 to 0.290; NNT 7, 95% CI 4 to 30).[44] The third subsequent RCT found no significant difference in cardiac death or non-fatal myocardial infarction between pravastatin 40 mg daily and placebo over 4.8 years (1 RCT, 3638 people aged ≥ 55 years with type 2 diabetes and additional CHD risk factors; CHD death plus non-fatal myocardial infarction: RR 0.89, 95% CI 0.71 to 1.10; absolute numbers not provided, results presented graphically).[45] Baseline low density lipoprotein (LDL) cholesterol was required to be in the range 3.1–4.9 mmol/L for people with no known CHD and 2.6–3.3 mmol/L for those with previously diagnosed CHD. Usual care could include lipid lowering agents at the primary care physician's discretion. **Aggressive versus moderate lipid lowering:** One RCT[52] identified by a systematic review[19] found no significant difference between aggressive lipid lowering and moderate lipid lowering in 4 year event rate for myocardial infarction and death (1 RCT, 116 people aged 21–74 years with type 2 diabetes and a diagnosis of CVD; 4 year event rate for death: 6.5 with aggressive lipid lowering *v* 9.6 with moderate lipid lowering; RR 0.67, 99% CI 0.12 to 3.75; 4 year event rate for myocardial infarction: 4.8 with aggressive lipid lowering *v* 11.6 with moderate lipid lowering; RR 0.40, 99% CI 0.07 to 2.47). The RCT used lovastatin and cholestyramine as necessary to achieve the targets for aggressive lipid lowering (LDL cholesterol of 1.55–2.20 mmol/L [60–85 mg/dL]) and moderate lipid lowering (LDL cholesterol of 3.36–3.62 mmol/L [130–140 mg/dL]). This RCT had limited power because of the small number of people enrolled who had diabetes.[52] A subsequent RCT found that, compared with usual care, treatment with atorvastatin to achieve a target LDL of below 2.6 mmol/L (< 100 mg/dL) significantly reduced the risk of all cause mortality, non-fatal myocardial infarction, unstable angina, congestive heart failure, revascularization, and stroke over 3 years (1 RCT, 313 people with a diagnosis of CVD, mean age 58 years: RRR 0.42; P = 0.0001; results presented graphically). The atorvastatin dose was titrated from 10 mg daily to a maximum of 80 mg daily to achieve a target LDL cholesterol of below 2.6 mmol/L. Usual care consisted of treatment by the family practitioner, which could include diet, exercise, weight loss, and/or drug treatment including lipid lowering agents; 14% of participants in the usual care group received any lipid lowering agents.[46] **Low versus standard statin dose in older people:** One subsequent RCT found no significant difference in cardiovascular events between low dose pravastatin 5 mg daily and standard dose pravastatin 10–20 mg daily over 4 years (1 RCT, 199 people aged > 60 years with diabetes: 17/104 events with low dose pravastatin *v* 15/95 events with standard dose pravastatin; ARR +0.006, 95% CI –0.097 to +0.108).[47]

Harms: **Versus placebo:** One systematic review (search date 2000) did not report on adverse effects.[19] The first subsequent RCT evaluated the effects of simvastatin compared with placebo on adverse outcomes other than cardiovascular events in people with diabetes.[43] The RCT found no significant difference between simvastatin and placebo for withdrawal from treatment because of elevated liver enzymes (48 [0.5%] *v* 35 [0.3%]) or muscle symptoms (49 [0.5%] *v* 50 [0.5%) or hospitalisation due to chronic obstructive pulmonary disease/asthma (132 [1.3%] *v* 150 [1.5%]). The second subsequent RCT conducted a safety analysis for fluvastatin compared with placebo in 1640 people. It found no significant difference between fluvastatin and placebo in the proportion of people withdrawing from treatement (174/822 [21%] with fluvastatin *v* 196/818 [24%] with placebo; RR 0.88, 95% CI 0.74 to 1.06).[44] The third subsequent RCT specifically stated that no data on adverse effects were collected.[45] **Aggressive versus moderate lipid lowering:** One RCT did not report any adverse events.[52] The subsequent RCT found no significant difference between atorvastatin and usual care in the proportion of people withdrawn from the study because of elevated liver enzymes.[46] **Low versus standard statin dose in older people:** One RCT comparing low versus standard pravastatin dose found no significant difference in adverse events between groups.[47]

Comment: We found one RCT that is of major importance.[43] The RCT is interesting because it was not necessary to have an abnormal lipid profile or prior vascular disease to be enrolled and it provides the first clear evidence that statin treatment is effective for primary prevention of CVD.[43] Most published RCTs with sufficient power to detect effects on cardiovascular events have enrolled comparatively few people with diabetes or have excluded them altogether. The available evidence is therefore based almost entirely on subgroup analyses of larger trials. Several large ongoing trials are evaluating the effects of fibrates in people with diabetes.

QUESTION What are the effects of antiplatelet drugs in people with diabetes?

OPTION PROPHYLACTIC ASPIRIN

One systematic review and RCTs have found that prophylactic aspirin reduces cardiovascular morbidity and mortality compared with controls. One RCT found that aspirin increased non-fatal major bleeds and minor bleeds but not fatal bleeds compared with placebo. Another RCT found no increase in the risks of vitreous, retinal, gastrointestinal, or cerebral haemorrhage with aspirin compared with placebo.

Benefits: We found one systematic review (search date 1990),[53] one additional RCT,[54] and two subsequent RCTs.[37,55] The systematic review found that antiplatelet treatement, mainly with aspirin, significantly reduced the risk of cardiovascular disease (CVD) related mortality and morbidity compared with controls (145 RCTs in people with a diagnosis of CVD; CVD mortality and morbidity: 415/2248 [19%] with antiplatelet treatment *v* 502/2254 [22%] with controls; RR 0.83, 95% CI 0.74 to 0.93).[53] The additional RCT found that aspirin significantly reduced the risk of acute myocardial infarction (see glossary, p 711) over 5 years compared with placebo (1 RCT, 533 male physicians with diabetes but no diagnosis of CVD: 11/275 [4%] with aspirin *v* 26/258 [10.1%] with placebo; RR 0.39,

95% CI 0.20 to 0.79; NNT 16, 95% CI 12 to 47).[54] The first subsequent RCT reported that, compared with placebo, aspirin reduced acute myocardial infarction to a similar degree in the subgroup of people with diabetes and in the overall trial population, but it did not specify the number of people with diabetes (1 RCT, 18 790 people aged 50–80 years with or without diabetes; RR 0.85, 95% CI 0.73 to 0.99).[37] The second subsequent RCT found that aspirin 650 mg daily significantly reduced fatal or non-fatal myocardial infarction but not stroke over 5 years compared with placebo (1 RCT, 3711 people; fatal or non-fatal myocardial infarction: 241/1856 [13%] with aspirin *v* 283/1855 [15%] with placebo; RR 0.851, 95% CI 0.726 to 0.998; NNT 44, 95% CI 22 to 3490; fatal or non-fatal stroke: 92/1856 [5%] with aspirin *v* 78/1855 [4%] with placebo; RR 1.179, 95% CI 0.878 to 1.583 [calculated by *Clinical Evidence*]).[55] **Versus clopidogrel:** See benefits of clopidogrel, p 706. **Aspirin plus clopidogrel:** See benefits of clopidogrel, p 706.

Harms: In the systematic review, doses of aspirin ranged from 75–1500 mg daily. Most RCTs used aspirin 75–325 mg daily.[53] Doses higher than 325 mg daily increased the risk of haemorrhagic adverse effects without improving preventive efficacy. No difference in efficacy or adverse effects was found in the dose range 75–325 mg. The additional RCT found no significant difference in adverse events between aspirin and placebo.[54] The first subsequent RCT found that aspirin significantly increased non-fatal major bleeds and minor bleeds but not fatal bleeds compared with placebo (non-fatal bleeds: 129/9399 [1.37%] *v* 70/9391 [0.75%]; RR 1.84, 95% CI 1.38 to 2.46; minor bleeds: 156/9399 [1.66%] *v* 87/9391 [0.93%]; RR 1.79, 95% CI 1.38 to 2.33; fatal bleeds: 7/9399 [0.07%] *v* 8/9391 [0.09%]; RR 0.87, 95% CI 0.32 to 2.41).[37] The second subsequent RCT found no significant increase with aspirin in the risks of vitreous, retinal, gastrointestinal, or cerebral haemorrhage compared with placebo.[55]

Comment: We found insufficient evidence to define precisely which people with diabetes should be treated with aspirin. The risk of CVD is very low before age 30 years; most white adults with diabetes aged over 30 years are at increased risk of CVD. Widely accepted contraindications to aspirin treatment include aspirin allergy, bleeding tendency, anticoagulant treatment, recent gastrointestinal bleeding, and clinically active liver disease.[56]

OPTION CLOPIDOGREL — New

We found no RCTs comparing only clopidogrel versus placebo. One RCT in people with diabetes and with recent ischaemic stroke, myocardial infarction, or established peripheral arterial disease found no significant difference between clopidogrel and aspirin at 28 days in cardiovascular events. This RCT also found a lower proportion of people hospitalised for a bleeding event with clopidogrel than with aspirin. One RCT in people presenting with unstable angina or non-Q-wave myocardial infarction and also taking aspirin found no significant reduction in cardiovascular events after 12 months with addition of clopidigrel compared with placebo. This RCT also found a higher proportion of major bleeds with clopidogrel than with placebo.

Prevention of cardiovascular events in diabetes

Benefits: **Versus placebo:** We found no RCTs comparing only clopidogrel versus placebo. **Versus aspirin:** One RCT in people in people with diabetes and with recent ischaemic stroke, myocardial infarction, or established peripheral arterial disease found no significant difference between clopidogrel and aspirin at 28 days in cardiovascular events (1 RCT, 3866 people, mean age 64 years; angina, vascular death, myocardial infarction, all cause stroke, and rehospitalization for ischaemic events: 299/1914 [15.6%] with clopidogrel *v* 345/1952 [17.7%] with aspirin; ARR +2.1%, 95% CI –0.3% to +4.4%; RR 0.88, 95% CI 0.77 to 1.02).[57] **Adding clopidogrel to aspirin:** One RCT in people presenting with unstable angina or non-Q-wave myocardial infarction and also taking aspirin found no significant reduction in cardiovascular events after 12 months with addition of clopidigrel compared with placebo (1 RCT, 2840 people with diabetes, mean age 64 years; cardiovascular death, non-fatal myocardial infarction, or stroke at 12 months: 200/1405 [16.7%] with clopidogrel *v* 240/1435 [14.2%] with placebo; RR 0.85, 95% CI 0.71 to 1.01).[58] Participants were randomised within 24 hours of an acute event and were given either given clopidigrel (300 mg bolus then 75 mg/day) plus aspirin (75–325 mg/day) or placebo plus aspirin.[58]

Harms: **Versus placebo:** One RCT found that a significantly lower proportion of people were hospitalised for a bleeding event with clopidogrel than with aspirin at 28 days (1 RCT, 3866 people, mean age 64 years; hospitalisation for a bleeding event: 34/1914 [1.8%] with clopidogrel *v* 55/1952 [2.8%] with aspirin; RRR 37.0%, 95% CI 3.8% to 58.7%; P = 0.031).[57] **Adding clopidogrel to aspirin:** One RCT in people presenting with unstable angina or non-Q-wave myocardial infarction and also taking aspirin found a significantly higher proportion of major bleeds with clopidogrel than with placebo (3.7% with clopidogrel *v* 2.7% with placebo; RR 1.38, 95% CI 1.13 to 1.67; P = 0.001).[58]

Comment: None.

OPTION GLYCOPROTEIN IIB/IIIA INHIBITORS

We found no RCTs comparing glycoprotein IIb/IIIa inhibitors versus no antiplatelet treatment. One RCT in people presenting with unstable angina or acute myocardial infarction without ST segment elevation found that the addition of tirofiban (a glycoprotein IIb/IIIa inhibitor) to heparin reduced the composite outcome of death, myocardial infarction, or refractory ischaemia at 180 days compared with heparin alone. This RCT found no significant difference between tirofiban plus heparin and heparin alone in risk of bleeding in people already taking aspirin.

Benefits: We found no RCTs comparing glycoprotein IIb/IIIa inhibitors versus no antiplatelet treatment. **Adding glycoprotein IIb/IIIa inhibitors to heparin:** One RCT, in people with diabetes presenting with unstable angina or acute myocardial infarction (see glossary, p 711) without ST segment elevation, found that addition of tirofiban (a glycoprotein IIb/IIIa inhibitor) to heparin compared with heparin alone significantly reduced the composite outcome of death, myocardial infarction, or refractory ischaemia at 180 days (1 RCT, 362 people already taking aspirin, mean age 65 years: 19/169 [11.2%] with tirofiban plus heparin *v* 37/193 [19.2%] with heparin alone; ARR 8.0%, 95% CI 0.7% to 15.3%; RR 0.586, 95% CI 0.351 to 0.980; P = 0.03; NNT 13, 95% CI 7 to 146).[59] **Adjunct to percutaneous coronary revascularisation:** See benefits of intracoronary stenting plus glycoprotein IIb/IIIa inhibitors, p 710.

Harms: **Adding glycoprotein IIb/IIIa inhibitors to heparin:** One RCT found no significant difference between tirofiban plus heparin and heparin alone in risk of bleeding in people already taking aspirin (9.5% with tirofiban plus heparin *v* 8.3% with heparin alone; RR 1.16, 95% CI 0.56 to 2.39).[59]

Comment: None.

QUESTION **What are the effects of blood glucose control in prevention of cardiovascular disease in people with diabetes?**

One RCT in obese people with type 2 diabetes found that intensive treatment with metformin compared with conventional treatment with diet alone reduced myocardial infarction but not stroke over 5 years. This RCT found no significant increase in major hypoglycaemic episodes in the metformin group compared with the diet only group. Three other RCTs found no significant difference in cardiovascular morbidity and mortality with intensive compared with conventional treatment for blood glucose control. These RCTs also found an increase in weight gain and hypoglycaemic episodes with intensive compared with conventional treatment.

Benefits: **We found no systematic review but found four RCTs.**[60–63] **Metformin versus diet alone in obese people:** One RCT in obese people with type 2 diabetes found that intensive treatment with metformin compared with conventional treatment with diet alone significantly reduced myocardial infarction but not stroke over 5 years (1 RCT, 753 people without a diagnosis of cardiovascular disease [CVD], mean age 53 years; myocardial infarction: 39/342 [11%] with metformin *v* 73/411 [18%] with diet alone; RR 0.61, 95% CI 0.41 to 0.89; stroke: 12/342 [3.5%] *v* 23/411 [5.6%] with diet alone; RR 0.59, 95% CI 0.29 to 1.18).[60] **Intensive versus conventional glycaemic control:** One RCT found no significant difference in major macrovascular events between intensive and conventional treatment over a mean of 6.5 years (1 RCT, 1441 people with type 1 diabetes but without a diagnosis of CVD, aged 13–39 years; major macrovascular events: 23/711 [3.2%] events with intensive treatment *v* 40/730 [5.5%] events with conventional treatment; ARR 2.2%; RR 0.59, 95% CI 0.32 to 1.1).[61] Major macrovascular events were defined as fatal or non-fatal myocardial infarction, sudden cardiac death, revascularisation procedure, angina with confirmed coronary artery disease, stroke, lower limb amputation, peripheral arterial events, and peripheral vascular disease. Conventional glycaemic control consisted of one or two daily injections of insulin without self adjustment of insulin dosage according to blood or urine glucose monitoring results. Intensive glycaemic control consisted of administration of three or more injections of insulin with the dosage adjusted according to self monitoring of blood glucose levels.[61] A second RCT found no significant difference between intensive and conventional glycaemic control in myocardial infarction or stroke over 5 years (1 RCT, 1138 people with type 2 diabetes but without a diagnosis of CVD, mean age 54 years; myocardial infarction: 387/2729 [14.2%] with intensive control *v* 186/1138 [16.3%] with conventional control; RR 0.84, 95% CI 0.71 to 1.00; $P = 0.052$; stroke: 148/2729 [5.4%] with intensive control *v* 55/1138 [4.8%] with conventional control; RR 1.11, 95% CI 0.81 to 1.51).[62] A third RCT found no significant difference between intensive insulin treatment with a stepped plan designed to achieve near normal blood sugar levels and standard once daily insulin injection in the rate of new cardiovascular events over 27 months (1 RCT, 153 men with type 2 diabetes, mean age 60 years, many of whom had previous cardiovascular events; new cardiovascular events: 24/75 [32%] with intensive treatment *v* 16/80 [20%] with standard treatment; RR 1.6, 95% CI 0.92 to 2.5).[63]

Harms: **Metformin versus diet alone in obese people:** One RCT found no significant increase in major hypoglycaemic episodes in the metformin group compared with the diet only group (0.6% *v* 0.7%).[60] **Intensive versus conventional glycaemic control:** One RCT found that weight gain and waist to hip ratio were significantly increased in the intensive treatment group compared with conventional treatment (weight gain: $P \leq 0.001$; waist to hip ratio: $P = 0.02$).[61] A second RCT found that intensive treatment significantly increased weight gain and hypoglycaemic episodes compared with conventional treatment ($P < 0.0001$).[62] A third RCT found significantly higher mild and moderate hypoglycaemic events with intensive treatment compared with conventional treatment (16.5 per patient per year with intensive treatment v 1.5 per patient year with conventional treatment; $P < 0.001$). However, it was noted that some hypoglycaemic episodes may not have been detected in the conventional treatment group because of less frequent measurement of blood glucose levels.[63]

Comment: The role of intensive glucose lowering in primary prevention of cardiovascular events remains unclear. However, such treatment clearly reduces the risk of microvascular disease and does not increase the risk of CVD. The potential of the first larger primary prevention RCT to demonstrate an effect of tighter glycaemic control was limited by the small difference achieved in median HbA1c (see glossary, p 711) between intensive and conventional treatment.[61,64] In contrast, in another primary prevention trial, a larger 1.9% difference in median HbA1c was achieved between groups, but the young age of the participants and consequent low incidence of cardiovascular events limited the power of the study to detect an effect of treatment on incidence of cardiovascular disease.[60,62] The RCT of insulin in type 2 diabetes included men with a high baseline risk of cardiovascular events and achieved a 2.1% absolute difference in HbA1c.[63] The RCT was small and the observed difference between groups could have arisen by chance.

QUESTION What are the effects of revascularisation procedures in people with diabetes?

OPTION CORONARY ARTERY BYPASS VERSUS PERCUTANEOUS TRANSLUMINAL ANGIOPLASTY

One large RCT in people with diabetes and multivessel coronary artery disease has found that coronary artery bypass graft (CABG) reduces mortality or myocardial infarction within 8 years compared with percutaneous transluminal coronary angioplasty (PTCA). Another smaller RCT found a non-significant reduction in mortality with CABG compared with PTCA at 4 years. One RCT in people with diabetes and multivessel coronary artery disease found no significant difference between CABG plus stent and PTCA plus stent in cardiovascular morbidity or mortality (to time of discharge). However, it found that CABG plus stent compared with PTCA plus stent in the short term increased cardiovascular risk at 1 year.

Benefits: We found no systematic review but found three RCTs[65–67] **Without stenting:** Two RCTs compared CABG versus PTCA, without stenting or a glycoprotein IIb/IIIa inhibitor.[65,66] The first RCT found that CABG significantly reduced the proportion of people who died or suffered Q wave myocardial infarction over a mean of 7.7 years compared with PTCA (1 RCT, 353 people with diabetes and 2 or 3 vessel coronary disease, mean age 62 years: 60/173 [34.7%] with CABG *v* 85/170 [50%] with PTCA; ARR 15%, 95% CI 5% to 26%; RR 0.69, 95% CI 0.54 to 0.89; NNT 7, 95% CI 4 to 20).[65] This survival benefit was confined to those receiving at least one internal mammary graft. The second RCT found no significant difference in mortality 4 years after CABG or PTCA (1 RCT, 125 people, mean age 61 years; mortality: 8/63 [12.5%] *v* 14/62 [22.6%]; RR 0.56, 95% CI 0.25 to 1.25; ARR +9.9%, 95% CI –3.4% to +23.1%).[66] **With stenting:** One RCT found no significant difference in people with diabetes treated with CABG or PTCA in short term risks (up to discharge) of composite end point of death, myocardial infarction, repeat CABG, and repeat PTCA (1 RCT, 208 with diabetes and 2 or 3 vessel coronary disease; composite outcome of death, myocardial infarction, repeat CABG, and repeat PTCA: 11/112 [9.8%] with PTCA *v* 9/96 [9.4%] with CABG; RR 1.05, 95% CI 0.45 to 2.42).[67]

Harms: **Without stenting:** One RCT found higher in-hospital mortality among people with diabetes (1.2% after CABG *v* 0.6% after PTCA) and myocardial infarction during the initial hospitalisation (5.8% after CABG *v* 1.8% after PTCA), but these differences were not found to be significant.[65] The second RCT did not report on harms.[66] **With stenting:** One RCT found a significant increase in risk of stroke with CABG compared with PTCA (4 with CABG *v* 0 with PTCA plus stent; P = 0.04). However, at 1 year the same RCT also found a significantly higher incidence of the composite end point with PTCA plus stenting (1 RCT, 208 with diabetes and 2 or 3 vessel coronary disease; composite outcome of death, myocardial infarction, repeat CABG, and repeat PTCA: 41/112 [36%] with PTCA plus stent *v* 15/96 [15.6%] with CABG; RR 2.34, 95% CI 1.38 to 3.96; NNH 5, 95% CI 4 to 11).[67]

Comment: None.

OPTION PERCUTANEOUS TRANSLUMINAL CORONARY ANGIOPLASTY VERSUS THROMBOLYSIS

We found no systematic review or RCTs comparing percutaneous transluminal coronary angioplasty versus thrombolysis for prevention of cardiovascular events in people with diabetes. One RCT, in people with diabetes presenting with an acute myocardial infarction, found no significant difference between percutaneous transluminal coronary angioplasty and thrombolysis with alteplase in single outcome of death or composite outcome of death, reinfarction, or disabling stroke at 30 days.

Benefits: We found no systematic review or RCTs comparing percutaneous transluminal coronary angioplasty (PTCA) versus thrombolysis for prevention of cardiovascular events in people with diabetes. **In people presenting with acute myocardial infarction:** One RCT found no significant difference between PTCA and thrombolysis with alteplase in single outcome of death or composite outcome of death, reinfarction, or disabling stroke at 30 days (1 RCT, 177 people with diabetes, mean age of 65 years, presenting with acute myocardial infarction [see glossary, p 711] within 12 hours of chest pain onset; single outcome of death: 8/99 [8.1%] after PTCA *v* 5/78 [6.4%] after alteplase; RR 1.26, 95% CI 0.43 to 3.71; composite outcome of death, reinfarction, or disabling stroke: 11/99 [11%] after PTCA *v* 13/78 [17%] after alteplase; RR 0.67, 95% CI 0.32 to 1.41).[68] The RCT found no significant difference in 30 day mortality among people with diabetes (8/99 [8.1%] after PTCA *v* 5/78 [6.4%] after alteplase).

Harms: **In people presenting with acute myocardial infarction:** One RCT did not report on adverse effects of PTCA and thrombolysis with alteplase.[68]

Comment: None.

OPTION INTRACORONARY STENTING PLUS GLYCOPROTEIN IIB/IIIA INHIBITORS

RCTs in people with diabetes undergoing percutaneous transluminal coronary angioplasty have found that the combination of stent and a glycoprotein IIb/IIIa inhibitor reduces cardiovascular morbidity and mortality compared with stent plus placebo.

Benefits: We found one non-systematic review of individual patient data[69] and two subsequent RCTS.[70,71] **Versus placebo:** The non-systematic review[69] pooled data from three placebo controlled trials of percutaneous coronary intervention: EPILOG,[72] EPISTENT,[73–75] and EPIC.[76] The non-systematic review found that, compared with placebo, abciximab (a glycoprotein IIb/IIIa inhibitor) significantly reduced overall mortality at 1 year (1462 people with diabetes, mean age 60.9 years; mortality: 22/888 [2.5%] with abciximab *v* 26/574 [4.5%] with placebo; 0.547, 95% CI 0.313 to 0.956; P = 0.03).[69] The first subsequent RCT found, that compared with placebo, eptifibatide (a glycoprotein IIb/IIIa inhibitor) significantly reduced the composite outcome of death or myocardial infarction but found no significant difference for single outcome of death at 1 year (1 RCT, 466 people with diabetes undergoing non-urgent coronary stent implantation, mean age 62 years; composite outcome of death or myocardial infarction: 18/232

[7.8%] with eptifibatide v 31/234 [13.4%] with placebo; HR 0.57, 95% CI 0.32 to 1.02; P = 0.001; single outcome of mortality: 3/232 [1.3%] with eptifibatide v 8/234 [3.5%] with placebo; HR 0.37, 95% CI 0.10 to 1.41; P = 0.28).[71] **Comparison of glycoprotein IIb/IIIa inhibitors:** The second subsequent RCT found no significant difference between tirofiban and abciximab in composite outcomes of death or myocardial infarction at 30 days and 6 months, or overall mortality at 1 year (1 RCT, 1117 people with diabetes undergoing percutaneous coronary interventions, mean age 62 years; composite outcomes of death or myocardial infarction: at 30 days 33/560 [5.9%] with tirofiban v 29/557 [5.2%] with abciximab; HR 1.14, 95% CI 0.69 to 1.87; P = 0.6; at 6 months 46/560 [8.2%] with tirofiban v 42/557 [7.5%] with abciximab; HR 1.09, 95% CI 0.72 to 1.65; P = 0.7; overall mortality at 1 year: 2.9% with tirofiban v 2.1% with abciximab; P = 0.4, absolute numbers not reported).[70]

Harms: **Versus placebo:** One non-systematic review of individual patient data found that there was slightly greater bleeding in people given abciximab than in those given placebo (4.3% v 3.0% for major bleeding; 6.9% v 6.3% for minor bleeding; 0% v 0.17% for intracranial haemorrhage). None of these differences were significant.[69] The subsequent RCT report on any adverse events associated with eptifibatide.[70] **Comparison of glycoprotein IIb/IIIa inhibitors:** One RCT found no significant difference between abciximab and tirofiban in major bleeding events (P = 0.725).[71]

Comment: For people with diabetes undergoing percutaneous procedures, the combination of stent and glycoprotein IIb/IIIa inhibitor reduces restenosis rates and serious morbidity. It is unclear whether these adjunctive treatments would reduce morbidity, mortality, and restenosis associated with percutaneous revascularisation procedures to the levels seen with coronary artery bypass grafting. The study comparing abciximab with tirofiban and the study comparing eptifibatide with placebo were both insufficiently powered to detect reductions in major cardiovascular events in the subgroups of people with diabetes.

GLOSSARY

Acute myocardial infarction is infarction that occurs when circulation to a region of the heart is obstructed and necrosis is occurring; clinical symptoms include severe pain, pallor, perspiration, nausea, dyspnoea, and dizziness. Myocardial infarction is gross necrosis of the myocardium as a result of interruption of blood supply usually caused by atherosclerosis of the coronary arteries; myocardial infarction without pain or other symptoms (silent infarction) is common in people with diabetes.

HbA1c The haemoglobin A1c test is the most common laboratory test of glycated haemoglobin (haemoglobin that has glucose irreversibly bound to it). HbA1c provides an indication of the "average" blood glucose over the preceding 3 months. The HbA1c is a weighted average over time of the blood glucose level; many different glucose profiles can produce the same level of HbA1c.

Substantive changes

Definition Clarification of population covered in this topic.

Different antihypertensive drugs Two RCTs added;[34,35] conclusions unchanged.

Statins Two RCTs added;[45,46] conclusions unchanged.

Intracoronary stenting plus glycoprotein IIb/IIIa inhibitors Two RCTs added;[70,71] conclusions unchanged.

REFERENCES

1. Geiss LS, Herman WH, Smith PJ. Mortality in non-insulin-dependent diabetes. In: Harris MI, ed. *Diabetes in America.* 2nd ed. Bethesda, MD: National Institutes of Health, 1995:233–255.
2. Wingard DL, Barrett-Connor E. Heart disease and diabetes. In: Harris MI, ed. *Diabetes in America.* 2nd ed. Bethesda, MD: National Institutes of Health, 1995:429–448.
3. Haffner SM, Lehto S, Ronnemaa T, et al. Mortality from coronary heart disease in subjects with type 2 diabetes and in nondiabetic subjects with and without prior myocardial infarction. *N Engl J Med* 1998;339:229–234.
4. Mukamai KJ, Nesto RW, Cohen MC, et al. Impact of diabetes on long-term survival after acute myocardial infarction. *Diabetes Care* 2001;24:1422–1427.
5. Hu FB, Stampfer MJ, Solomon C, et al. Physical activity and risk for cardiovascular events in diabetic women. *Ann Intern Med* 2001;134:96–105.
6. Wei M, Gibbons LW, Kampert JB, et al. Low cardiorespiratory fitness and physical inactivity as predictors of mortality in men with type 2 diabetes. *Ann Intern Med* 2000;132:605–611.
7. Krolewski AS, Warram JH, Freire MB. Epidemiology of late diabetic complications. A basis for the development and evaluation of preventive programs. *Endocrinol Metab Clin North Am* 1996;25:217–242.
8. Messent JW, Elliott TG, Hill RD, et al. Prognostic significance of microalbuminuria in insulin-dependent diabetes mellitus: a twenty-three year follow-up study. *Kidney Int* 1992;41:836–839.
9. Dinneen SF, Gerstein HC. The association of microalbuminuria and mortality in non-insulin-dependent diabetes mellitus: a systematic overview of the literature. *Arch Intern Med* 1997;157:1413–1418. Search date 1995; primary sources Medline, SciSearch, and hand searching of bibliographies.
10. Valmadrid CT, Klein R, Moss SE, et al. The risk of cardiovascular disease mortality associated with microalbuminuria and gross proteinuria in persons with older-onset diabetes mellitus. *Arch Intern Med* 2000;160:1093–1100.
11. Borch Johnsen K, Andersen PK, Deckert T. The effect of proteinuria on relative mortality in type 1 (insulin-dependent) diabetes mellitus. *Diabetologia* 1985;28:590–596.
12. Warram JH, Laffel LM, Ganda OP, et al. Coronary artery disease is the major determinant of excess mortality in patients with insulin-dependent diabetes mellitus and persistent proteinuria. *J Am Soc Nephrol* 1992;3(suppl 4):104–110.
13. Gerstein Hertzel C, Johannes FE, Qilong Yi, et al. Albuminuria and risk of cardiovascular events, death and heart failure in diabetic and nondiabetic individuals. *JAMA* 2001;286:421–426.
14. Behar S, Boyko V, Reicher-Reiss H, et al. Ten-year survival after acute myocardial infarction: comparison of patients with and without diabetes. SPRINT Study Group. Secondary Prevention Reinfarction Israeli Nifedipine Trial. *Am Heart J* 1997;133:290–296.
15. Mak KH, Moliterno DJ, Granger CB, et al. Influence of diabetes mellitus on clinical outcome in the thrombolytic era of acute myocardial infarction: GUSTO-I Investigators: global utilization of streptokinase and tissue plasminogen activator for occluded coronary arteries. *J Am Coll Cardiol* 1997;30:171–179.
16. Capes SE, Hunt D, Malmberg K, et al. Stress hyperglycaemia and increased risk of death after myocardial infarction in patients with and without diabetes: a systematic overview. *Lancet* 2000;355:773–778. Search date 1998; primary sources Medline, Science Citation Index, hand searches of bibliographies of relevant articles, and contact with experts in the field.
17. Lotufo PA, Gazziano M, Chae CU, et al. Diabetes and all-cause coronary heart disease mortality among US male physicians. *Arch Intern Med* 2001;161:242–247.
18. Fuller J, Stevens LK, Chaturvedi N, et al. Antihypertensive therapy in preventing cardiovascular complications in people with diabetes mellitus. In: The Cochrane Library, Issue 3, 2001. Oxford, Update Software. Search date not stated; primary sources Medline, Embase, and hand searches of specialist journals in cardiovascular disease, stroke, renal disease, and hypertension. Review subsequently withdrawn by The Cochrane Library and is currently being updated.
19. Huang ES, Meigs JB, Singer DE. The effect of interventions to prevent cardiovascular disease in patients with type 2 diabetes mellitus. *Am J Med* 2001;111:633–642. Search date 2000; primary sources Medline and reference lists.
20. Tuomilehto J, Rastenyte D, Birkenhäger WH, et al. Effects of calcium-channel blockade in older patients with diabetes and systolic hypertension. *N Engl J Med* 1999;340:677–684.
21. Lewis EJ, Hunsicker LG, et al. Renoprotective effect of the angiotensin receptor antagonist irbesartan in patients wit nephropathy due to type 2 diabetes. *N Engl J Med* 2001:345:851–860.
22. Parving HH, Lehnert H, et al. The effect of irbesartan on the development of diabetic nephropathy in patients with type 2 diabetes. *N Engl J Med* 2001;345:870–878.
23. Heart Outcomes Prevention Evaluation (HOPE) Study Investigators. Effects of ramipril on cardiovascular and microvascular outcomes in people with diabetes mellitus: results of the HOPE study and the MICRO-HOPE substudy. *Lancet* 2000;355:253–259.
24. Bosch J, Yusuf S, Pogue J, et al. Use of ramipril in preventing stroke: double blind randomized trial. *BMJ* 2002;324:699–702.
25. Lonn E, Roccaforte R, Yi Q, et al. Effect of long-term therapy with ramipril in high-risk women. *J Am Coll Cardiol* 2002;40:693–702.
26. Pahor M, Psaty BM, Alderman MH, et al. Therapeutic benefits of ACE inhibitors and other antihypertensive drugs in patients with type 2 diabetes. *Diabetes Care* 2000;23:888–892. Search date 2000; primary source Medline.
27. Lindholm LH, Hansson L, Ekbom T, et al. Comparison of antihypertensive treatment in preventing cardiovascular events in elderly diabetic patients: results from the Swedish trial in old patients with hypertension–2. *J Hypertens* 2000;18:1671–1675.
28. ALLHAT Collaborative Research Group. Major cardiovascular events in hypertensive patients randomised to doxazosin vs chlorthalidone: the antihypertensive and lipid-lowering treatment to prevent heart attack trial (ALLHAT). *JAMA* 2000;283:1967–1975.
29. Lindholm LH, Ibsen H, Dahlof B, et al. Cardiovascular morbidity and mortality in patients with diabetes in the Losartan Intervention for Endopoint reduction in hypertension study (LIFE): a randomized trial against atenolol. *Lancet* 2002;359:1004–1010.
30. Tatti P, Pahor M, Byington RP, et al. Outcome results of the Fosfinopril versus Amlodipine

Cardiovascular Events randomised Trial (FACET) in patients with hypertension and NIDDM. *Diabetes Care* 1998;21:597–603.
31. Estacio RO, Jeffers BW, Hiatt WR, et al. The effect of nisoldipine as compared with enalapril on cardiovascular events in patients with non-insulin-dependent diabetes and hypertension. *N Engl J Med* 1998;338:645–652.
32. UK Prospective Diabetes Study Group. Efficacy of atenolol and captopril in reducing risk of macrovascular and microvascular complications in type 2 diabetes: UKPDS 39. *BMJ* 1998;317:713–720.
33. Niskanen L, Hedner T, et al. Reduced cardiovascular morbidity and mortality in hypertensive diabetic patients on first line therapy with an ACE inhibitor compared with diuretic beta blocker based treatment regiment, a sub analysis of the captopril prevention project. *Diabetes Care* 2001;24:2091–2096.
34. ALLHAT Officers and Coordinators for the ALLHAT Collaborative Research Group. The Antihypertensive and Lipid-Lowering Treatment to Prevent Heart Attack Trial. Major outcomes in high-risk hypertensive patients randomized to angiotensin-converting enzyme inhibitor or calcium channel blocker vs diuretic: The Antihypertensive and Lipid-Lowering Treatment to Prevent Heart Attack Trial (ALLHAT). *JAMA* 2002;288:2981–2997.
35. Hansson L, Hedner T, Lund-Johansen P, et al. Randomized trial of effects of calcium antagonists compared with diuretics and beta-blockers on cardiovascular morbidity and mortality in hypertension: the Nordic Diltiazem (NORDIL) study. *Lancet* 2000;356:359–365.
36. UK Prospective Diabetes Study Group. Tight blood pressure control and risk of macrovascular and microvascular complications in type 2 diabetes: UKPDS 38. *BMJ* 1998;317:703–713.
37. Hansson L, Zanchetti A, Carruthers SG, et al. Effects of intensive blood-pressure lowering and low-dose aspirin in patients with hypertension: principal results of the Hypertension Optimal Treatment (HOT) randomised trial. *Lancet* 1998;351:1755–1762.
38. Schrier RW, Estacio RO, et al. Effects of aggressive blood pressure control in normotensive type 2 diabetic patients on albuminuria, retinopathy and strokes. *Kidney Int* 2002;6:1086–1097.
39. Elkeles RS, Diamond JR, Poulter C, et al. Cardiovascular outcomes in type 2 diabetes. A double-blind placebo-controlled study of bezafibrate: the St Mary's, Ealing, Northwick Park Diabetes Cardiovascular Disease Prevention (SENDCAP) Study. *Diabetes Care* 1998;21:641–648.
40. Diabetes Atherosclerosis Interventions Study Investigators. Effect of fenofibrate on progression of coronary-artery disease in type 2 diabetes: The Diabetes Atherosclerosis Interventions Study, a Randomized Study. *Lancet* 2001;357:905–910.
41. Koskinen P, Manttari M, Manninen V, et al. Coronary heart disease incidence in NIDDM patients in the Helsinki Heart Study. *Diabetes Care* 1992;15:820–825.
42. Rubins HB, Robins SJ, Collins D, et al. Gemfibrozil for the secondary prevention of coronary heart disease in men with low levels of high-density lipoprotein cholesterol. Veterans Affairs High-Density Lipoprotein Cholesterol Intervention Trial Study Group. *N Engl J Med* 1999;341:410–418.
43. Heart Protection Study Collaborative Group. MRC/BHF Heart Protection Study of cholesterol lowering with simvastatin in 20 536 high-risk individuals: a randomised placebo-controlled trial. *Lancet* 2002;360:7–22.
44. Serruys P, Feyter P, Macaya C, et al. Fluvastatin for the prevention of cardiac events following successful first percutaneous coronary intervention. *JAMA* 2002;287:3215–3222.
45. The ALLHAT officers and coordinators for the ALLHAT Collaborative research group. Major outcomes in moderately hypercholesterolemic, hypertensive patients randomized to pravastatin versus usual care. *JAMA* 2002;288:2998–3007.
46. Athyros V, Papageorgiou A, Mercouris B, et al. Treatment with atorvastatin to the National Cholesterol Educational Program goal versus "usual" care in secondary coronary heart disease prevention. The GREek Atorvastatin and Coronary-heart-disease Evaluation (GREACE) study. *Curr Med Res Opin* 2002;18:220–228.
47. Ito H, Yasuyoshi O, Yasuo O, et al. A comparison of low versus standard dose pravastatin therapy for the prevention of cardiovascular events in the elderly: the Pravastatin anti-atheroscelerosis trial in the elderly (PATE). *J Atheroscler Thromb* 2001;8:33–44.
48. Pyorala K, Pedersen TR, Kjekshus J, et al. Cholesterol lowering with simvastatin improves prognosis of diabetic patients with coronary heart disease. A subgroup analysis of the Scandinavian Simvastatin Survival Study (4S). *Diabetes Care* 1997;20:614–620.
49. The Long-term Intervention with Pravastatin in Ischemic Disease (LIPID) Study Program. Prevention of cardiovascular events and death with pravastatin in patients with coronary heart disease and a broad range of initial cholesterol levels. *N Engl J Med* 1998;339:1349–1357.
50. Sacks FM, Pfeffer MA, Moye LA, et al. The effect of pravastatin on coronary events after myocardial infarction in patients with average cholesterol levels. Cholesterol and Recurrent Events Trial investigators. *N Engl J Med* 1996;335:1001–1009.
51. Downs JR, Clearfield M, Weis S, et al. Primary prevention of acute coronary events with lovastatin in men and women with average cholesterol levels: results of AFCAPS/TexCAPS. Air Force/Texas Coronary Atherosclerosis Prevention Study. *JAMA* 1998;279:1615–1622.
52. Hoogwerf BJ, Waness A, et al. Effects of aggressive cholesterol lowering and low dose anticoagulation on clinical and angiographic outcomes in patients with diabetes. *Diabetes* 1999;48:1289–1294.
53. Collaborative overview of randomised trials of antiplatelet therapy–I: Prevention of death, myocardial infarction, and stroke by prolonged antiplatelet therapy in various categories of patients. Antiplatelet Trialists' Collaboration. *BMJ* 1994;308:81–106. Search date 1990; primary sources Medline, Current Contents, manual searches of journals, reference lists from clinical trials and review articles, and enquiry among colleagues and manufacturers of antiplatelet agents for unpublished studies.
54. Steering Committee of the Physicians' Health Study Research Group. Final report on the aspirin component of the ongoing Physicians' Health Study. *N Engl J Med* 1989;321:129–135.
55. ETDRS Investigators. Aspirin effects on mortality and morbidity in patients with diabetes mellitus. *JAMA* 1992;268:1292–1300.
56. American Diabetes Association. Aspirin therapy in diabetes. *Diabetes Care* 1997;20:1772–1773.

57. Bhatt DL, Marso SP, Hirsch AT, et al. Amplified benefit of clopidogrel versus aspirin in patients with diabetes mellitus. *Am J Cardiol* 2002;90:625–628.
58. The Clopidogrel in Unstable Angina to Prevent Recurrent Events Trial Investigators. Effects of clopidogrel in addition to aspirin in patients with acute coronary syndromes without ST-segment elevation. *N Engl J Med* 2001;345:494–502.
59. Theroux P, Alexander J, Pharand C, et al. Glycoprotein IIb/IIIa receptor blockade improves outcomes in diabetic patients presenting with unstable angina/Non-ST-elevation myocardial infarction results from the platelet receptor inhibitor in ischemic syndrome management in patients limited by unstable signs and symptoms. *Circulation* 2000;102:2466–2472.
60. UK Prospective Diabetes Study Group. Effect of intensive blood-glucose control with metformin on complications in overweight patients with type 2 diabetes (UKPDS 34). *Lancet* 1998;352:854–865.
61. DCCT Research Group. Effect of intensive diabetes management on macrovascular events andrisk factors in the Diabetes Control and Complications Trial. *Am J Cardiol* 1995;75:894–903.
62. UK Prospective Diabetes Study Group. Intensive blood-glucose control with sulphonylureas or insulin compared with conventional treatment and risk of complications in patients with type 2 diabetes (UKPDS 33). *Lancet* 1998;352:837–853.
63. Abraira C, Colwell J, Nuttall F, et al. Cardiovascular events and correlates in the Veterans Affairs Diabetes Feasibility Trial: Veterans Affairs Cooperative Study on glycemic control and complications in type II diabetes. *Arch Intern Med* 1997;157:181–188.
64. DCCT Research Group. The effect of intensive treatment of diabetes on the development and progression of long-term complications in insulin-dependent diabetes mellitus. *N Engl J Med* 1993;329:977–986.
65. The BARI Investigators. Seven-year outcome in the Bypass Angioplasty Revascularization Investigation (BARI) by treatment and diabetic status. *J Am Coll Cardiol* 2000;35:1122–1129.
66. Kurbaan AS, Bowker TJ, Ilsley CD, et al. Difference in the mortality of the CABRI diabetic and nondiabetic populations and its relation to coronary artery disease and the revascularization mode. *Am J Cardiol* 2001;87:947–950.
67. Abizaid A, Costa MA, et al. Clinical and economic impact of diabetes mellitus on percutaneous and surgical treatment of multivessel coronary disease patients indights form the arterial revascularization therapy study (ARTS) trial. Circulation 2001;104:533–538.
68. Hasdai D, Granger CB, Srivatsa S, et al. Diabetes mellitus and outcome after primary coronary angioplasty for acute myocardial infarction: lessons from the GUSTO-IIb angioplasty study. *J Am Coll Cardiol* 2000;35:1502–1512.
69. Bhatt DL, Marso SP, Lincoff AM, et al. Abciximab reduces mortality in diabetics following percutaneous coronary intervention. *J Am Coll Cardiol* 2000;35:922–928.
70. Roffi M, Moliterno D, Meier B, et al. Impact of different platelet glycoprotein IIb/IIIa receptor inhibitors among diabetic patients undergoing percutaneous coronary intervention. *Circulation* 2002;105:2730–2736.
71. Labinaz M, Madan M, O'Shea JO, et al. Comparison of one-year outcomes following coronary artery stenting in diabetic versus nondiabetic patients (from the Enhanced Suppression of the Platelet IIb/IIIa Receptor With Integrilin Therapy [ESPRIT] Trial). *Am J Cardiol* 2002;90;585–590.
72. Kleiman NS, Lincoff AM, Kereiakes DJ, et al. Diabetes mellitus, glycoprotein IIb/IIIa blockade, and heparin: evidence for a complex interaction in a multicenter trial. EPILOG Investigators. *Circulation* 1998;97:1912–1920.
73. Marso SP, Lincoff AM, Ellis SG, et al. Optimizing the percutaneous interventional outcomes for patients with diabetes mellitus: results of the EPISTENT (Evaluation of platelet IIb/IIIa inhibitor for stenting trial) diabetic substudy. *Circulation* 1999;100:2477–2484.
74. The EPISTENT Investigators. Randomised placebo-controlled and balloon-angioplasty-controlled trial to assess safety of coronary stenting with use of platelet glycoprotein-IIb/IIIa blockade. The EPISTENT Investigators. Evaluation of platelet IIb/IIIa inhibitor for stenting. *Lancet* 1998;352:87–92.
75. Topol EJ, Mark DB, Lincoff AM, et al. Outcomes at 1 year and economic implications of platelet glycoprotein IIb/IIIa blockade in patients undergoing coronary stenting: results from a multicentre randomised trial. EPISTENT Investigators. Evaluation of Platelet IIb/IIIa Inhibitor for Stenting. *Lancet* 1999;354:2019–2024. [Published erratum appears in *Lancet* 2000;355:1104].
76. The EPIC Investigation. Use of a monoclonal antibody directed against the platelet glycoprotein IIb/IIIa receptor in high-risk coronary angioplasty. *N Engl J Med* 1994;330:956–961.

Janine Malcolm
Clinical Scholar, Endocrinology and Metabolism

Hilary Meggison
Fellow, Endocrinology and Metabolism
Ottawa Hospital, Ottawa, Canada

Ronald Sigal
Associate Professor of Medicine and Human Kinetics
University of Ottawa, Ottawa, Canada

Competing interests: RS has received speaker's fees from Aventis (manufacturer of glyburide, metformin, glimepiride, ramipril, and insulin glargine), Novo Nordisk (manufacturer of insulin and repaglinide), and Pfizer (manufacturer of atorvastatin). He has received reimbursement for travel expenses from Bristol-Myers Squibb (manufacturer of pravastatin), Aventis, and Pfizer, and has received consulting fees from Pfizer. HM and JM none declared.

The following previous contributor of this topic would also like to be acknowledged: Marie-France Levac.

Primary hypothyroidism

Search date April 2003

Birte Nygaard

QUESTIONS

INTERVENTIONS

CLINICAL (OVERT) HYPOTHYROIDISM

Beneficial

Levothyroxine (L-thyroxine)* . . .717

Unknown effectiveness

Levothyroxine (L-thyroxine) plus liothyronine 718

SUBCLINICAL HYPOTHYROIDISM

Unknown effectiveness

Levothyroxine (L-thyroxine) 718

*No RCT evidence, but there is clinical consensus that levothyroxine is beneficial in clinical (overt) hypothyroidism. A placebo controlled trial would be considered unethical.

See glossary, p 720

Key Messages

Clinical (overt) hypothyroidism

- **Levothyroxine (L-thyroxine)** We found no RCTs comparing levothyroxine (L-thyroxine) versus placebo, although there is consensus that treatment is beneficial. Treating clinical (overt) hypothyroidism with thyroid hormone (levothyroxine; L-thyroxine) can induce hyperthyroidism and reduce bone mass in postmenopausal women and increase the risk of atrial fibrillation.
- **Levothyroxine (L-thyroxine) plus liothyronine** We found insufficient evidence about the effects of levothyroxine (L-thyroxine) plus liothyronine versus levothyroxine alone in people with clinical (overt) hypothyroidism. Thyroid hormone treatment can induce hyperthyroidism and reduce bone mass in postmenopausal women and increase the risk of atrial fibrillation.

Subclinical hypothyroidism

- **Levothyroxine (L-thyroxine)** One RCT in women with biochemically defined subclinical hypothyroidism found no significant difference between levothyroxine (L-thyroxine) and placebo for dry skin, cold intolerance, and constipation at 1 year. The RCT may, however, have lacked power to exclude a clinically important difference between treatments. Another RCT found no significant difference in health related quality of life scores between levothyroxine and placebo. One RCT found inconclusive results about the effect of levothyroxine versus placebo on cognitive function in people with subclinical hypothyroidism. One RCT found that levothyroxine improved left ventricular function at 6 months compared with placebo. Treating subclinical hypothyroidism with thyroid hormone can induce hyperthyroidism and reduce bone mass in postmenopausal women and increase the risk of atrial fibrillation.

Primary hypothyroidism

DEFINITION Hypothyroidism is characterised by low levels of blood thyroid hormone. **Clinical (overt) hypothyroidism** is diagnosed on the basis of characteristic clinical features consisting of mental slowing, depression, dementia, weight gain, constipation, dry skin, hair loss, cold intolerance, hoarse voice, irregular menstruation, infertility, muscle stiffness and pain, bradycardia, hypercholesterolaemia, combined with a raised blood level of thyroid stimulating hormone (TSH) (serum TSH levels > 12 mU/L), and a low serum thyroxine (T_4 — see glossary, p 720) level (serum T_4 < 60 nmol/L). **Subclinical hypothyroidism** is diagnosed when serum TSH is raised (serum TSH levels > 4 mU/L) but serum thyroxine is normal and there are no symptoms or signs, or only minor symptoms or signs, of thyroid dysfunction. **Primary hypothyroidism** is seen after destruction of the thyroid gland because of autoimmunity (the most common cause), or medical intervention such as surgery, radioiodine, and radiation. **Secondary hypothyroidism** is seen after pituitary or hypothalamic damage, and results in insufficient production of TSH. Secondary hypothyroidism is not covered in this review. **Euthyroid sick syndrome** is diagnosed when triiodothyronine (T_3 — see glossary, p 720) levels are low, serum thyroxine is low and TSH levels are normal or low. Euthyroid sick syndrome is not covered in this review.

INCIDENCE/ PREVALENCE Hypothyroidism is more common in women than in men (in the UK, female : male ratio of 6 : 1). One study (2779 people in the UK with a median age of 58 years) found the incidence of clinical (overt) hypothyroidism was 40/10 000 women per year and 6/10 000 men per year. The prevalence was 9.3% in women and 1.3% in men.[1] In areas with high iodine intake, the incidence of hypothyroidism can be higher than in areas with normal or low iodine intake. In Denmark, where there is moderate iodine insufficiency, the overall incidence of hypothyroidism is 1.4/10 000 per year increasing to 8/10 000 per year in people older than 70 years.[2] The incidence of subclinical hypothyroidism increases with age. Up to 10% of women over the age of 60 years have subclinical hypothyroidism (evaluated from data from the Netherlands and USA).[3,4]

AETIOLOGY/ RISK FACTORS Primary thyroid gland failure can occur as a result of chronic autoimmune thyroiditis, postradioactive iodine treatment, or thyroidectomy. Other causes include drug adverse effects (e.g. amiodarone and lithium), transient hypothyroidism due to silent thyroiditis, subacute thyroiditis, or postpartum thyroiditis.

PROGNOSIS Hypothyroidism results in mental slowing, depression, dementia, weight gain, constipation, dry skin, hair loss, cold intolerance, hoarse voice, irregular menstruation, infertility, muscle stiffness and pain, bradycardia, and hypercholesterolaemia. In people with subclinical hypothyroidism, the risk of developing overt hypothyroidism is described in the UK Whickham Survey (25 years' follow up; for women: OR 8, 95% CI 3 to 20; for men: OR 44, 95% CI 19 to 104; if both a raised TSH and positive antithyroid antibodies were present; for women: OR 38, 95% CI 22 to 65; for men: OR 173, 95% CI 81 to 370). For women, the survey found an annual risk of 4.3%/year (if both raised serum TSH and antithyroid antibodies were present), 2.6%/year (if raised serum TSH was present alone);

the minimum number of people with raised TSH and antithyroid antibodies who would need treating to prevent this progression to clinical (overt) hypothyroidism in one person over 5 years is 5–8.[1] **Cardiovascular disease:** A large cross-sectional study (25 862 people with serum TSH between 5.1–10 mU/L) found significantly higher mean total cholesterol concentrations in hypothyroid people compared with euthyroid people (5.8 *v* 5.6 mmol/L).[3] Another study (124 elderly women with subclinical hypothyroidism, 931 euthyroid women) found a significantly increased risk of myocardial infarction in women with subclinical hypothyroidism (OR 2.3, 95% CI 1.3 to 4.0) and for aortic atherosclerosis (OR 1.7, 95% CI 1.1 to 2.6).[4] **Mental health:** Subclinical hypothyroidism is associated with depression.[5] People with subclinical hypothyroidism may have depression that is refractory to both antidepressant drugs and thyroid hormone alone. Memory impairment, hysteria, anxiety, somatic complaints, and depressive features without depression have been described in people with subclinical hypothyroidism.[6]

AIMS OF INTERVENTION To eliminate the symptoms of hypothyroidism and maximise quality of life.

OUTCOMES Quality of life and neuropsychological impairments (evaluated by congestive function tests, memory tests, reaction time, self rating mood scales, and depression scores); cardiovascular disease (episodes of atrial fibrillation and ischaemic events); cardiac function (evaluated by echocardiography); changes in body composition (measured by osteodensitometry or bioimpedance measurements); prevention of progression from subclinical to overt hypothyroidism; adverse effects of treatments (bone mass, fracture rate, development of hyperthyroidism).

METHODS *Clinical Evidence* search and appraisal April 2003, with an additional manual search of reference lists.

QUESTION **What are the effects of treatments for clinical (overt) hypothyroidism?**

OPTION **LEVOTHYROXINE (L-THYROXINE) FOR CLINICAL (OVERT) HYPOTHYROIDISM**

We found no RCTs comparing levothyroxine (L-thyroxine) versus placebo, although there is consensus that treatment is beneficial. Treating clinical (overt) hypothyroidism with thyroid hormone (levothyroxine; L-thyroxine) can induce hyperthyroidism and reduce bone mass in postmenopausal women and increase the risk of atrial fibrillation.

Benefits: We found no RCTs comparing levothyroxine versus placebo in people with clinical hypothyroidism, although there is consensus that treatment is beneficial (see comment below).

Harms: We found no RCTs comparing levothyroxine versus placebo in people with clinical hypothyroidism. Over-treatment with levothyroxine may cause hyperthyroidism. **Fracture rate:** One longitudinal observational study (1180 people on levothyroxine followed for an average of 8.6 years) found no significant increase in fracture rate between levothyroxine and control.[7] **Bone mass:** We found one systematic review (search date not stated, 13 RCTs) in a total of 441 premenopausal women and 317 postmenopausal women.[8] All women had received prolonged levothyroxine treatment with reduced serum TSH concentration but normal T_4 and T_3 (see glossary, p 720) values. In premenopausal women (average age 40 years, treated with levothyroxine 164 µg/day for 8.5 years leading to suppressed serum TSH) the review found no significant difference between levothyroxine and control in bone mass after 8.5 years (2.7% less bone mass with levothyroxine *v* control; P reported as non significant). In postmenopausal women (average age 61.2 years, treated with levothyroxine 171 µg/day for 9.9 years leading to suppressed serum TSH), it found that levothyroxine significantly reduced bone mass compared with control after 9.9 years (bone mass 9.0% lower with levothyroxine than control, 95% CI 2.4% to 15.7%). **Atrial fibrillation:** One observational study found that in people aged over 60 years taking levothyroxine, a low serum TSH concentration (≤0.1 mU/L) was associated with an increased risk of atrial fibrillation (diagnosed by electrocardiogram) at 10 years (incidence of atrial fibrillation, 28% in people with low TSH *v* 11% in people with normal TSH values; RR 3.1, 95% CI 1.7 to 5.5).[9]

Comment: A placebo controlled trial would be considered unethical.

OPTION LEVOTHYROXINE (L-THYROXINE) PLUS LIOTHYRONINE FOR CLINICAL (OVERT) HYPOTHYROIDISM

We found insufficient evidence about the effects of levothyroxine (L-thyroxine) plus liothyronine versus levothyroxine alone in people with clinical (overt) hypothyroidism. Thyroid hormone treatment can induce hyperthyroidism and reduces bone mass in postmenopausal women and increase the risk of atrial fibrillation.

Benefits: We found no systematic review and no RCTs that met our inclusion criteria.

Harms: See harms of levothyroxine for clinical hypothyroidism, p 717.

Comment: We found two small crossover RCTs, which did not provide pre-crossover results.[10,11] The results reported in these RCTs are at risk of being confounded by the pre-crossover treatments. Therefore we excluded these studies.

QUESTION What are the effects of treatments for subclinical hypothyroidism?

OPTION LEVOTHYROXINE (L-THYROXINE) FOR SUBCLINICAL HYPOTHYROIDISM

One RCT in women with biochemically defined subclinical hypothyroidism found no significant difference between levothyroxine (L-thyroxine) and placebo for dry skin, cold intolerance, and constipation at 1 year. The RCT may, however, have lacked power to exclude a clinically important difference between treatments. Another RCT found no significant difference in health related quality of life scores between levothyroxine and placebo. One RCT found inconclusive results about the effect of levothyroxine versus placebo on cognitive function in people with

subclinical hypothyroidism. One RCT found that levothyroxine improved left ventricular function at 6 months compared with placebo. Treating subclinical hypothyroidism with thyroid hormone can induce hyperthyroidism and reduce bone mass in postmenopausal women and increase the risk of atrial fibrillation.

Benefits: We found no systematic review, but found four RCTs evaluating the effect of levothyroxine in people with subclinical hypothyroidism.[12–15] **General symptoms:** We found two RCTs.[12,14] The first RCT compared levothyroxine (50 μg/day) versus placebo in 33 women with increased thyroid stimulating hormone (TSH); normal serum thyroxine and normal free T_4 and T_3 (see glossary, p 720), and on average, two of the following symptoms: muscle cramps, dry skin, cold intolerance, fatigue, or constipation.[12] Physical examination revealed no signs of hypothyroidism, apart from dry or coarse skin, which was present in about 50% of women in each group. The RCT examined the effects of treatment on general symptoms (evaluated by a questionnaire in participants stating if they were feeling better, unchanged, or worse) for 1 year. It found no significant difference in overall symptom improvement between levothyroxine and placebo (8/17 [47%] people with levothyroxine *v* 3/16 [19%] people with placebo; $P = 0.14$, recalculated by *Clinical Evidence*).[12] The second RCT (40 women with increased TSH and normal T_4) compared levothyroxine versus placebo for 6 months. The RCT found no significant difference between levothyroxine and placebo in health related quality of life scores (Hospital Anxiety and Depression Scale and the 30-item General Health Questionnaire).[14] **Cognitive function:** We found one RCT (37 people, aged > 55 years, TSH >6.0 mU/L, normal T_4, T_3, and thyroxine binding globulin) comparing levothyroxine (25 μg/day for 4 weeks then 50 μg/day) versus placebo for 10 months. It found no significant difference between levothyroxine and placebo in any outcome except in one psychometric memory score, based on a battery of cognitive function tests evaluating memory.[13] No firm conclusions could be drawn from these findings. **Cardiac function:** We found one RCT (20 people with increased TSH, and normal T_4 and T_3 for least 1 year) which compared the effects of levothyroxine (50 μg/day) versus placebo on cardiac function for 1 year.[15] Cardiac function was evaluated by conventional two-dimensional Doppler echocardiography and ultrasonic videodensitometry. The RCT found that levothyroxine significantly improved left ventricular function compared with placebo at 6 months (increased isovolumic relaxation time, $P < 0.03$; peak A, $P < 0.01$; pre-ejection/ejection time ratio, $P < 0.03$; cyclic variation index, $P < 0.05$).[15]

Harms: One RCT did not report on adverse effects.[12] The second RCT found a significant worsening in anxiety scores with levothyroxine versus placebo ($P = 0.03$).[14] In the third RCT, 2/18 (11%) people taking levothyroxine withdrew because of complications (1 had increased angina and 1 had new onset atrial fibrillation).[13] The fourth RCT did not report on adverse effects.[15]

Comment: None.

GLOSSARY

T_3 is used as an abbreviation for endogenous tri-iodothyronine in medical and biochemical reports.

T_4 is used as an abbreviation for endogenous thyroxine in medical and biochemical reports.

REFERENCES

1. Vanderpump MP, Tunbridge WM, French JM, et al. The incidence of thyroid disorder in the community: a twenty-year follow-up of the Whickham survey. *Clin Endocriniol (Oxf)* 1995;43:55–68.
2. Laurberg P, Bülow Pedersen I, Pedersen KM, et al. Low incidence rate of overt hypothyroidism compared with hyperthyroidism in an area with moderately low iodine intake. *Thyroid* 1999;9:33–38.
3. Canaris GJ, Manowitz NR, Mayor G, et al. The Colorado thyroid disease prevalence study. *Arch Intern Med* 2000;160:526–533.
4. Hak AE, Pols HA, Visser TJ, et al. Subclinical hypothyroidism is an independent risk factor for atherosclerosis and myocardial infarction in elderly women: the Rotterdam Study. *Ann Intern Med* 2000;132:270–278.
5. Haggerty JJ, Stern RA, Mason GA, et al. Subclinical hypothyroidism: a modifiable risk factor for depression? *Am J Psychiatry* 1993;150:508–510.
6. Monzani F, Del Guerra P, Caraccio N, et al. Subclinical hypothyroidism: neurobehavioral features and beneficial effect of L-thyroxine treatment. *Clin Invest* 1993;71:367–371.
7. Leese GP, Jung RT, Guthrie C, et al. Morbidity in patients on L-thyroxine: a comparison of those with a normal TSH to those with a suppressed TSH. *Clin Endocrinol* 1992;37:500–503.
8. Faber J, Galløe AM. Changes in bone mass during prolonged subclinical hyperthyroidism due to L-thyroxine treatment: a meta-analysis. *Eur J Endocrinol* 1994;130:350–356. Search date not stated; primary sources Medline and hand searches of references from literature and abstracts published at international endocrinological meetings 1985–1992.
9. Sawin CT, Geller A, Wolf PA, et al. Low serum thyrotropin concentrations as a risk factor for atrial fibrillation in older persons. *N Engl J Med* 1994;331:1249–1252.
10. Bunevicius R, Kazanavicius G, Zalinkevicius R, et al. Effects of thyroxine as compared with thyroxine plus triiodothyronine in patients with hypothyroidism. *N Engl J Med* 1999;340:424–470.
11. Smith RN, Taylor SA, Massey JC. Controlled clinical trial of combined triiodothyronine and thyroxine in the treatment of hypothyroidism. *BMJ* 1970;4:145–148.
12. Cooper DS, Halpern R, Wood LC, et al. L-thyroxine therapy in subclinical hypothyroidism. *Ann Intern Med* 1984;101:18–24.
13. Jaeschke R, Guyatt G, Gerstein H, et al. Does treatment with L-thyroxine influence health status in middle-aged and older adults with subclinical hypothyroidism? *J Gen Intern Med* 1996;11:744–749.
14. Kong WM, Sheikh MH, Lumb PJ, et al. A 6-month randomized trial of thyroxine treatment in woman with mild subclinical hypothyroidism. *Am J Med* 2002;112:348–354.
15. Monzani F, Bello VD, Caraccio N, et al. Effect of levothyroxine on cardiac function and structure in subclinical hypothyroidism: a double blind placebo-controlled study. *J Clin Endocrinol Metab* 2001;86:1110–1115.

Birte Nygaard
University of Copenhagen
Copenhagen
Denmark

Competing interests: None declared.

The following previous contributor of this topic would also like to be acknowledged: Lars Kristensen

Acute anterior uveitis

Search date June 2003

André Curi, Kimble Matos, and Carlos Pavesio

QUESTIONS

INTERVENTIONS

To be covered in future updates

Mydriatics

Oral steroids

Slow taper of drug treatment

Subconjunctival steroid injection

Treatment of chronic iridocyclitis

See glossary, p 725

Key Messages

- **Topical non-steroidal anti-inflammatory drug eye drops** One RCT found no significant difference between non-steroidal anti-inflammatory drug and placebo eye drops in clinical cure rate after 21 days. Three RCTs found no significant difference between non-steroidal anti-inflammatory drugs and steroid eye drops in clinical cure rate after 14 or 21 days.
- **Topical steroid eye drops** One small RCT found no significant difference with steroid (betamethasone phosphate/clobetasone butyrate) eye drops compared with placebo eye drops in symptom severity after 14 or 21 days. Two RCTs found no significant difference between prednisolone and rimexolone, in the anterior chamber cell count (a marker of disease severity). One RCT found that prednisolone increased the proportion of people with fewer than five anterior chamber cells per examination field compared with loteprednol after 28 days. The results of a second RCT comparing prednisolone with loteprednol were difficult to interpret. RCTs found that rimexolone and loteprednol were less likely than prednisolone to be associated with increased intraocular pressure, although differences were not statistically significant. Three RCTs found no significant difference between steroid and non-steroidal anti-inflammatory drug eye drops in clinical cure rate after 14 or 21 days.

Acute anterior uveitis

DEFINITION Anterior uveitis is inflammation of the uveal tract, and includes iritis and iridocyclitis (see glossary, p 725). It can be classified according to its clinical course into acute or chronic anterior uveitis, or according to its clinical appearance into granulomatous or non-granulomatous anterior uveitis. Acute anterior uveitis is characterised by an extremely painful red eye, often associated with photophobia and occasionally with decreased visual acuity. Chronic anterior uveitis is defined as inflammation lasting over 6 weeks. It is usually asymptomatic, but many people have mild symptoms during exacerbations.

INCIDENCE/ PREVALENCE Acute anterior uveitis is rare with an annual incidence of 12/100 000 population.[1] It is particularly common in Finland (annual incidence 22.6/100 000 population, prevalence 68.7/100 000 population), probably owing to genetic factors such as the high frequency of HLA-B27 in the Finnish population.[2] It is equally common in men and women and more that 90% of cases occur in people older that 20 year of age.[2,3]

AETIOLOGY/ RISK FACTORS No cause is identified in 60–80% of people with acute anterior uveitis. Systemic disorders that may be associated with acute anterior uveitis include ankylosing spondylitis; Reiter's syndrome; juvenile chronic arthritis; Kawasaki syndrome; infectious uveitis; Behçet's syndrome; inflammatory bowel disease; interstitial nephritis; sarcoidosis; multiple sclerosis; Wegener's granulomatosis; Vogt-Koyanagi-Harada syndrome; and masquerade syndromes (see glossary, p 725). Acute anterior uveitis also occurs in association with HLA-B27 expression not linked to any systemic disease, and may also be the manifestation of an isolated eye disorder such as Fuchs' iridocyclitis, Posner-Schlossman syndrome, or Schwartz syndrome. Acute anterior uveitis may also occur after surgery or as an adverse drug or hypersensitivity reaction.[2,3]

PROGNOSIS Acute anterior uveitis is often self limiting, but we found no evidence about how often it resolves spontaneously, in which people, or over what length of time. Complications include posterior synechiae (see glossary, p 725), cataract, glaucoma, and chronic uveitis. In a study of 154 people (232 eyes) with acute anterior uveitis (119 people HLA-B27 positive), visual acuity was better than 20/60 in 209/232 (90%) eyes, 20/60 or worse in 23/232 (10%) eyes, including worse than 20/200 (classified as legally blind) in 11/232 (5%) eyes.[4]

AIMS OF INTERVENTION To reduce inflammation; to relieve pain; and to prevent complications and loss of visual acuity, with minimal adverse effects.

OUTCOMES Degree of inflammation using scores that register cell counts and flare in the anterior chamber; keratic precipitates; ciliary flush; and severity of symptoms (photophobia and pain). Scores include the number of anterior chamber cells per examination field — a clinical marker of disease severity.

METHODS *Clinical Evidence* search and appraisal June 2003.

QUESTION **What are the effects of topical anti-inflammatory eye drops?**

OPTION **TOPICAL STEROID EYE DROPS**

One small RCT found no significant difference with steroid (betamethasone phosphate/clobetasone butyrate) eye drops compared with placebo eye drops in symptom severity after 14 or 21 days. Two RCTs found no significant difference between prednisolone and rimexolone, in the anterior chamber cell count (a marker of disease severity). One RCT found that prednisolone increased the proportion of people with fewer than five anterior chamber cells per examination field compared with loteprednol after 28 days. The results of a second RCT comparing prednisolone with loteprednol were difficult to interpret. RCTs found that rimexolone and loteprednol were less likely than prednisolone to be associated with increased intraocular pressure, although differences were not statistically significant. RCTs found no significant difference between steroid and non-steroidal anti-inflammatory drug eye drops in clinical cure rate after 14 or 21 days.

Benefits: We found no systematic review. **Versus placebo:** We found one RCT (60 people) that compared three treatments: betamethasone phosphate 1% (2 drops every 2 hours), clobetasone butyrate 0.1% (2 drops every 2 hours), and placebo.[5] The RCT found no significant difference with steroid (betamethasone phosphate/clobetasone butyrate) compared with placebo eye drops in symptom severity after 14 or 21 days (results presented graphically; see comment below). **Versus each other:** We found two papers reporting four RCTs.[6,7] Two RCTs (183 people and 93 people) compared prednisolone 1% versus rimexolone 1% eye drops.[6] The larger RCT (183 people) found no significant difference in the number of anterior chamber cells per examination field after 28 days (see comment below; 0.4 cells per examination field with rimexolone *v* 0.2 cells per examination field with prednisolone, difference 0.2 cells per examination field, CI not reported; P = 0.16). The smaller RCT (83 people) also found no significant difference in the number of anterior chamber cells per examination field after 28 days (see comment below; 0.3 cells per examination field with rimexolone *v* 0.2 cells per examination field with prednisolone, difference 0.1 cells per examination field; CI not reported; P = 0.40).[6] Two RCTs (175 people and 70 people) compared prednisolone 1% versus loteprednol 0.5% eye drops.[7] The larger RCT (175 people) found that prednisolone significantly increased the proportion of people with fewer than five anterior chamber cells per examination field after 28 days compared with loteprednol (5 people lost to follow up; 77/89 [87%] with prednisolone *v* 58/81 [72%] with loteprednol; RR 1.20, 95% CI 1.03 to 1.42; NNT 7, 95% CI 4 to 35). The smaller RCT (70 people; see comment below) found more people had fewer than five anterior chamber cells per examination field with prednisolone compared with loteprednol but the difference was not significant.[7] **Versus topical non-steroidal anti-inflammatory drug eye drops:** See topical non-steroidal anti-inflammatory drug eye drops, p 724.

Harms: In the RCTs, adverse events were generally mild, resolved without treatment, and did not result in permanent damage.[5–7] In the smaller RCT comparing loteprednol versus prednisolone eye drops, 4/70 (6%) people were withdrawn because of adverse effects: cystoid macular oedema and ocular symptoms in the loteprednol group, and interstitial keratitis and increased age-related macular degeneration in the prednisolone group.[7] **Raised intraocular pressure:** The largest RCT found clinically significant increases in intraocular pressure (defined as > 10 mm Hg from baseline) more frequently with prednisolone versus rimexolone and with prednisolone versus loteprednol, although the differences were not statistically significant (11/94 [12%] people with prednisolone *v* 6/89 [7%] people with rimexolone; RR 1.7, 95% CI 0.7 to 4.5;[6] 6/91 [7%] people with prednisolone *v* 1/84 [1%] people with loteprednol; RR 5.5, 95% CI 0.7 to 45.0[7]). Widely known adverse effects of topical steroid eye drops include local irritation, hyperaemia, oedema, and blurred vision. Rarely, topical eye drops have been associated with glaucoma, cataract, and herpes simplex keratitis.

Comment: In the RCT comparing steroid eye drops versus placebo, 12/60 (20%) people did not complete the trial and analysis of data was not by intention to treat.[5] Of these, 4/12 (33%) people were withdrawn from the placebo group because of the severity of their anterior uveitis. The trial was too small to rule out any clinically important effect of topical steroids. In the RCTs comparing prednisolone versus rimexolone, people were excluded from analysis for a variety of reasons (23/183 [13%] in the larger RCT and 8/93 [9%] in the smaller RCT).[6] The smaller RCT of prednisolone versus loteprednol enrolled people in the USA and UK; however, it only reported results for the subgroup of people recruited from the USA.[7] This makes the results difficult to interpret. Topical steroids have been standard treatment for anterior uveitis since the early 1950s, especially for people with acute or severe uveitis.

OPTION TOPICAL NON-STEROIDAL ANTI-INFLAMMATORY DRUG EYE DROPS

One RCT found no significant difference between non-steroidal anti-inflammatory drug and placebo eye drops in clinical cure rate after 21 days. Three RCTs found no significant difference between non-steroidal anti-inflammatory drug and steroid eye drops in clinical cure rate after 14 or 21 days.

Benefits: We found no systematic review. **Versus placebo:** We found one RCT (100 people) that compared three treatments: non-steroidal anti-inflammatory drug (NSAID) (tolmetin 5%), steroid (prednisolone 0.5%), and placebo (sterile saline 0.9%) eye drops (see *v* topical steroids below).[8] People were asked to instil two drops every 2 hours during the waking period plus atropine 1% eye drops once daily. The RCT found no significant difference between NSAIDs and placebo eye drops in clinical cure rate after 21 days (15/32 [47%] with tolmetin *v* 16/32 [50%] with placebo; RR 0.9, 95% CI 0.6 to 1.6). **Versus topical steroids:** We found three RCTs.[8–10] The first

RCT (71 people) compared three treatments: prednisolone disodium phosphate 0.5%, betamethasone disodium phosphate 0.1%, and tolmetin sodium dihydrate 5%.[9] People were asked to instil one drop every 2 hours during the waking period, and all received atropine 1% eye drops once daily. The RCT found no significant difference between an NSAID (tolmetin sodium dihydrate) and steroid (prednisolone disodium phosphate/betamethasone disodium phosphate) eye drops in clinical cure rate after 21 days (see comment below; 12/21 [57%] people with tolmetin sodium dihydrate *v* 31/39 [79%] with prednisolone disodium phosphate/betamethasone disodium phosphate; RR 1.4, 95% CI 0.9 to 2.1).[9] The second RCT (49 people) compared NSAID eyedrops (indometacin [indomethacin] 0.1%) with steroid (dexamethasone 1%) eye drops given six times daily.[10] Most people (equal numbers in each group) also received atropine eye drops three times daily. The RCT found a lower proportion of people clinically cured after 14 days with indometacin but the difference was of borderline significance (see comment below; 12/25 [48%] people with indometacin *v* 18/24 [75%] people with dexamethasone; RR 0.6, 95% CI 0.4 to 1.0). The third RCT (100 people) compared three treatments: steroid (prednisolone 0.5%), NSAID (tolmetin 5%), and placebo eye drops (sterile saline 0.9%) (see *v* placebo above).[8] It found no significant difference between NSAIDs and steroid eye drops in clinical cure rate after 21 days (see comment below; 15/32 [47%] people with tolmetin *v* 22/32 [69%] people with prednisolone; RR 0.7, 95% CI 0.4 to 1.1).

Harms: See harms of topical steroid treatments, p 724. In the RCT comparing NSAID with steroid eye drops, 6/20 (30%) people receiving NSAID eye drops reported a transient stinging sensation in their eyes.[9] In the RCT comparing indometacin 0.1% with dexamethasone 1% eye drops, more people receiving indometacin reported eye irritation, although the difference was not significant (7/25 [28%] people with indometacin *v* 3/24 [13%] people with dexamethasone; RR 2.2, 95% CI 0.7 to 7.8).[10]

Comment: Two RCTs used "clinical cure" as an outcome measure, although neither defined this term.[8,9] The third RCT defined "clinical cure" as absence of clinical signs or symptoms suggestive of inflammation.[10] The RCT comparing NSAID with placebo eye drops reported that 6/71 (8%) people did not complete the trial,[8] and the first RCT comparing NSAID with steroid eye drops reported that 11/71 (15%) people did not complete the trial.[9] Neither of these RCTs analysed data by intention to treat.

GLOSSARY

Iridocyclitis Inflammation of both iris and ciliary body. Cells are present in the anterior chamber and in the vitreous.

Iritis Inflammation of the iris. Cells are seen in the anterior chamber but not in the vitreous.

Masquerade syndromes Comprise a group of disorders that occur with intraocular inflammation and are often misdiagnosed as a chronic idiopathic uveitis.

Posterior synechiae Adhesions between the iris and the lens capsule.

Acute anterior uveitis

REFERENCES

1. Darrel RW, Wagner HP, Kurland CT. Epidemiology of uveitis: incidence and prevalence in a small urban community. *Arch Ophthalmol* 1962;68:501–514.
2. Paivonsalo-Hietanen T, Tuominen J, Vaahtoranta-Lehtonen H, et al. Incidence and prevalence of different uveitis entities in Finland. *Acta Ophthalmol Scand* 1997;75:76–81.
3. Rosenbaum JT. Uveitis. An internist's view. *Arch Intern Med* 1989;149:1173–1176.
4. Linssen A, Meenken C. Outcomes of HLA-B27-positive and HLA-B27-negative acute anterior uveitis. *Am J Ophthalmol* 1995;120:351–361.
5. Dunne JA, Travers JP. Topical steroids in anterior uveitis. *Trans Ophthalmol Soc UK* 1979;99:481–484.
6. Foster CS, Alter G, DeBarge RL, et al. Efficacy and safety of rimexolone 1% ophthalmic suspension vs prednisolone acetate in the treatment of uveitis. *Am J Ophthalmol* 1996;122:171–182.
7. The Loteprednol Etabonate US Uveitis Study Group. Controlled evaluation of loteprednol etabonate and prednisolone acetate in the treatment of acute anterior uveitis. *Am J Ophthalmol* 1999;127:537–544.
8. Young BJ, Cunninghan WF, Akingbehin T. Double-masked controlled clinical trial of 5% tolmetin versus 0.5% prednisolone versus 0.9% saline in acute endogenous nongranulomatous anterior uveitis. *Br J Ophthalmol* 1982;66:389–391.
9. Dunne JA, Jacobs N, Morrison A, et al. Efficacy in anterior uveitis of two known steroids and topical tolmetin. *Br J Ophthalmol* 1985;69:120–125.
10. Sand BB, Krogh E. Topical indometacin, a prostaglandin inhibitor, in acute anterior uveitis. A controlled clinical trial of non-steroid versus steroid anti-inflammatory treatment. *Acta Ophthalmol* 1991;69:145–148.

André Curi
Clinical Research Fellow

Kimble Matos
Research Fellow

Carlos Pavesio
Consultant Ophthalmic Surgeon

Moorfields Eye Hospital
London
UK

Competing interests: None declared.

Age related macular degeneration

Search date November 2002

Jennifer Arnold and Shirley Sarks

QUESTIONS

INTERVENTIONS

See glossary, p 739

Key Messages

Prevention of progression

- **Antioxidant vitamin and zinc supplementation** One systematic review found modest evidence from one large RCT that, compared with placebo, antioxidant vitamins plus zinc supplements reduce the risk of progression to late age related macular degeneration over 6 years in people who already have moderate amounts of drusen, choroidal neovascularisation, or geographic atrophy in one eye.
- **Laser to drusen** We found insufficient evidence that drusen reduction by laser prevents late age related macular degeneration — choroidal neovascularisation or geographic atrophy. One RCT found that, compared with no laser treatment, laser treatment to eyes with high risk drusen significantly improved visual acuity after 2 years. A second RCT found that, compared with no laser treatment, visual acuity with laser treatment only improved in a subgroup of eyes with a reduction in the number of drusen of greater than 50%. It also found that, compared with no treatment, laser treatment increased the short term incidence of choroidal neovascularisation in eyes with unilateral (but not bilateral) drusen.

Age related macular degeneration

Treatment

- **Photodynamic treatment with verteporfin** Two RCTs in selected people with exudative age related macular degeneration found that, compared with placebo, photodynamic treatment with verteporfin reduced the risk of moderate and severe visual loss after 1–2 years. In the first RCT, subgroup analysis suggests the benefit is greatest in people with predominantly classic lesions on fluorescein angiography. In the second RCT, a more modest benefit was seen in the second year of treatment in people with only occult (no classic) lesions on fluorescein angiography. Both RCTs found that photodynamic treatment with verteporfin was associated with an initial loss of vision and photosensitive reactions in a small proportion of people.
- **Thermal laser photocoagulation** Four large RCTs in people with exudative age related macular degeneration and well demarcated lesions have found that, compared with no treatment, thermal laser photocoagulation decreases the rate of severe visual loss after 2–3 years and preserves contrast sensitivity. Choroidal neovascularisation recurs within 2 years in about half of those treated. Photocoagulation may reduce visual acuity initially.
- **Proton beam and scleral plaque radiotherapy** We found no RCTs.
- **Submacular surgery** We found insufficient evidence on the effects of submacular surgery. Case series have found that rates of recurrent choroidal neovascularisation are high, and there is a clinically important risk of ocular complications resulting in visual loss and a need for further surgical intervention.
- **External beam radiation** One large RCT found no significant difference between low dose external beam radiation and placebo in the proportion of people with exudative age related macular degeneration and moderate visual loss after 1 year. Smaller RCTs comparing both low and high dose external beam radiation versus placebo or no treatment found conflicting evidence. We found insufficient evidence on long term safety, although RCTs found no evidence of toxicity to the optic nerve or retina after 12–24 months.
- **Subcutaneous interferon alfa-2a** One large RCT found that, compared with placebo, subcutaneous interferon alfa-2a increased visual loss after 1 year, although the difference was not significant, and found evidence of serious ocular and systemic adverse effects.

DEFINITION Age related macular degeneration (AMD) (see glossary, p 739) has two forms in the late (sight threatening) stage: atrophic (or dry) AMD, characterised by geographic atrophy (see glossary, p 740); and exudative (or wet) AMD, characterised by choroidal neovascularisation (see glossary, p 739), which eventually causes a disciform scar.

INCIDENCE/ PREVALENCE AMD is a common cause of blindness registration in industrialised countries. Atrophic AMD is more common than the more sight threatening exudative AMD, affecting about 85% of people with AMD.[1] End stage (blinding) AMD is found in about 2% of all people aged over 50 years, and incidence rises with age (0.7–1.4% of people aged 65–75 years; 11–19% of people aged > 85 years).[2–4]

AETIOLOGY/ RISK FACTORS Proposed hypotheses for the cause of AMD involve vascular factors and oxidative damage coupled with genetic predisposition.[5] Age is the strongest risk factor. Ocular risk factors for the development of exudative AMD include the presence of soft drusen (see glossary, p 740), macular pigmentary change, and choroidal neovascularisation in the other eye. Systemic risk factors include hypertension, smoking, and a family history of AMD.[5–7] Hypertension, diet (especially intake of antioxidant micronutrients), and oestrogen use are suspected as aetiological agents, but this remains unproved.[5]

PROGNOSIS AMD impairs central vision, which is required for reading, driving, face recognition, and all fine visual tasks. **Atrophic AMD** progresses slowly over many years, and time to legal blindness (see glossary, p 740) is highly variable (usually about 5–10 years).[8,9] **Exudative AMD** is more often threatening to vision; 90% of people with severe visual loss owing to AMD have the exudative type. This condition usually manifests with a sudden worsening and distortion of central vision. A modelling exercise (derived primarily from cohort studies) found the risk of developing exudative AMD in people with bilateral soft drusen was 1–5% at 1 year and 13–18% at 3 years.[10] The observed 5 year rate in a population survey was 7%.[11] Most eyes (estimates vary from 60–90%) with exudative AMD progress to legal blindness and develop a central defect (scotoma) in the visual field.[12–15] Peripheral vision is preserved, allowing the person to be mobile and independent. The ability to read with visual aids depends on the size and density of the central scotoma and the degree to which the person retains sensitivity to contrast. Once exudative AMD has developed in one eye, the other eye is at high risk (cumulative estimated incidence: 10% at 1 year, 28% at 3 years, and 42% at 5 years).[16]

AIMS OF INTERVENTION To minimise loss of visual acuity and central vision; to preserve the ability to read with or without visual aids; to optimise quality of life; to minimise adverse effects of treatment.

OUTCOMES Visual acuity; rates of legal blindness; contrast sensitivity; quality of life; visual fields; rate of progression to late AMD; rate of adverse effects of treatment. Visual acuity is measured using special eye charts (logMar charts, usually the Early Treatment of Diabetic Retinopathy Study chart), although many studies do not specify which chart was used. Stable vision is usually defined as loss of two lines or less on the Early Treatment of Diabetic Retinopathy Study chart. Moderate and severe visual loss is defined as a loss of greater than three and six lines, respectively. Loss of vision to legal blindness (< 20/200) is also used as an outcome. A reading of 20/200 (or 6/60 in metric) on the Snellen chart means that a person can see at 20 feet (or 6 m) what a normally sighted person can see at 200 feet (or 60 m).

METHODS *Clinical Evidence* search and appraisal November 2002.

QUESTION What are the effects of interventions to prevent progression of age related macular degeneration?

OPTION ANTIOXIDANT VITAMIN AND MINERAL SUPPLEMENTS

New

One systematic review found modest evidence from one large RCT that, compared with placebo, antioxidant vitamins plus zinc supplements reduce the risk of progression to late age related macular degeneration over 6 years in people who already have moderate amounts of drusen, choroidal neovascularisation, or geographic atrophy in one eye.

Benefits: We found one systematic review (search date 2001, 7 RCTs, 4119 people).[17] Six of the trials reported were small with inconsistent results and these studies are not considered further. The large RCT identified by the review found that compared with placebo, antioxidants plus zinc supplements significantly reduced the proportion of people progressing to advanced age related macular degeneration (AMD) (see glossary, p 739) over 6.3 years (1 RCT, 3640 people aged 55–80 years; OR 0.72, 99% CI 0.52 to 0.98).[18] The RCT also found a significant reduction in moderate vision loss (see glossary, p 740) with antioxidants plus zinc supplements compared with placebo (OR 0.73, 99% CI 0.54 to 0.99). The RCT included people with signs of AMD (at least moderate drusen [see glossary, p 740] in both eyes or late AMD [choroidal neovascularisation or geographic atrophy — see glossary, p 740] in one eye) randomised to one of four treatment groups: placebo; zinc (total daily dose, zinc 80 mg plus copper 2 mg); antioxidants (total daily dose, vitamin C 500 mg plus vitamin E 400 IU plus beta-carotene 15 mg); or zinc plus antioxidants. Progression to advanced AMD was defined as the development of choroidal neovascularisation or geographic atrophy. Only 15/1063 people (5 year incidence rate 1.5%) with early AMD (moderate bilateral drusen) developed advanced AMD and the effect of supplementation compared with placebo was found to be higher when these people were excluded (antioxidants plus zinc OR 0.66, 99% CI 0.47 to 0.91; zinc alone OR 0.71, 99% CI 0.52 to 0.99; antioxidants alone OR 0.76, 99% CI 0.55 to 1.05).[18]

Harms: In the large RCT, 71% of people were taking 75% or more of their tablets at 5 years.[18] There was little evidence of harm in the large RCT although an increase in yellow skin discolouration was reported in people taking antioxidants (151/1823 [8.3%] with antioxidants *v* 108/1798 [6.0%] with placebo; OR 1.4, 95% CI 1.1 to 1.8; $P < 0.01$) and in admission to hospital for genitourinary complications in people taking zinc (134/1783 [7.5%] with zinc *v* 90/1838 [4.9%] with placebo; OR 1.6, 95% CI 1.2 to 2.1; $P < 0.01$). However, harmful effects of long term supplementation with the dosages used in the RCT cannot be ruled out.[18] High dose zinc supplementation may result in gastrointestinal intolerance. There is evidence from other (non-ophthalmic) studies suggesting potentially harmful effects of beta-carotene in smokers with an increased risk of lung cancer.[19,20]

Comment: The high dosages given in this study cannot be achieved by dietary intake alone. The study was conducted in relatively well nourished American people (57% of participants were supplementing with zinc or antioxidant vitamins before enrolment, and 67% took additional multivitamin supplements to recommended daily allowance levels during the study). Trials in other populations with other nutritional statuses are required. We found no evidence that people with no AMD or early signs of the disease (early drusen only) or established late AMD (choroidal neovascularisation or geographic atrophy) in both eyes benefit from antioxidant vitamin and zinc supplementation. An allied systematic review (search date 2002) found that there is no evidence that people without any signs of AMD should take antioxidant vitamins and mineral supplements to prevent or delay onset of the disease.[21] Results are awaited from four large ongoing studies in the USA and Australia that address this question.

OPTION LASER TO DRUSEN

One RCT found that, compared with no treatment, laser treatment improved visual acuity. A second RCT found no significant difference between laser treatment and no treatment in the number of eyes with an increased visual acuity of one line or more on the Early Treatment of Diabetic Retinopathy Study chart after 1 year. However, subgroup analysis found that visual acuity improved in eyes with a reduction of 50% or more in the number of drusen after laser treatment. It also found that, compared with no treatment, laser treatment increased the short term incidence of choroidal neovascularisation in eyes with unilateral (but not bilateral) drusen. We found insufficient evidence that laser induced drusen reduction results in a decreased incidence of late age related macular degeneration — choroidal neovascularisation or geographic atrophy.

Benefits: We found no systematic review. **Versus no treatment:** We found two RCTs.[22–24] The first RCT (229 eyes, 75 people with unilateral drusen [see glossary, p 740] and 77 people with bilateral drusen; see comment below) compared three treatments: diode laser (see glossary, p 740) treatment at a threshold level (visible burns; 56 eyes); diode laser treatment at a subthreshold level (invisible burns; 49 eyes); and no laser treatment (91 eyes).[22] It found that laser treatment at either level (threshold or subthreshold) versus no laser treatment significantly increased the number of eyes with improved visual acuity (defined as an improvement of ≥ 2 lines on the Early Treatment of Diabetic Retinopathy Study [ETDRS] chart) after 2 years (12/105 [11%] with laser treatment *v* 0/91 [0%] with no treatment; NNT 9, 95% CI 6 to 25). The RCT found no significant difference between threshold and subthreshold treatment in the number of eyes with improved visual acuity after 2 years (8/56 [14%] with threshold laser treatment *v* 4/49 [8%] with subthreshold treatment; RR 1.80, 95% CI 0.56 to 5.50). The second RCT (120 eyes with unilateral drusen, 312 eyes with bilateral drusen, 276 people; see comment below) compared argon-green laser versus no laser treatment.[23,24] It found no significant difference with laser treatment versus no treatment in the number of eyes with an increased visual acuity of one line or more on the ETDRS chart after 1 year (60/167 [36%] with laser treatment *v* 48/183 [26%] with no laser treatment; RR 1.40, 95% CI 1.00 to 1.88), and no significant difference in the number of eyes with decreased visual acuity of one line or more on the ETDRS chart after 1 year (44/167 [26%] with laser treatment *v* 65/183 [36%] with no laser treatment; RR 0.70, 95% CI 0.54 to 1.02). Subgroup analysis found that significantly more eyes with a reduction of 50% or more in the number of drusen versus eyes with less than 50% reduction in the number of drusen after laser treatment had an increase in visual acuity of one line or more on the ETDRS chart after 1 year (36/77 [48%] with ≥ 50% reduction *v* 24/90 [27%] with < 50% reduction; RR 1.80, 95% CI 1.16 to 2.66).

Harms: Macular laser treatment may induce choroidal neovascularisation (CNV) (see glossary, p 739) and retinal atrophy. The first RCT found no significant difference between threshold and non-threshold laser treatment in the number of eyes with CNV after 24 months (7/59 [12%] with threshold laser treatment *v* 4/49 [8%] with subthreshold laser treatment; RR 1.50, 95% CI 0.45 to 4.68).[22] In the second RCT, early analysis found that in the subgroup of people with unilateral drusen, argon-green laser compared with no laser treatment significantly increased the incidence of CNV (estimated 12 month incidence 10/59 [17%] with laser treatment *v* 2/61 [3%] with no laser treatment; $P < 0.05$; CI not provided; see comment below).[24] In the subgroup of people with bilateral drusen, the second RCT found no significant difference between laser treatment and no treatment in the estimated 12 month incidence of CNV (5% with laser treatment *v* 2% with no laser treatment; RR 2.00, 95% CI 0.37 to 11.00). All RCTs sought to minimise CNV by using low intensity and subthreshold lasers and by positioning laser burns at a distance (generally > 500 μm) from the fovea centre. Both RCTs found that laser induced retinal atrophy was uncommon, with 2/120 (2%) treated eyes affected in one study,[24] and 1/105 (1%) treated eyes affected in the other.[22]

Comment: The first RCT reported that 196/229 (86%) eyes completed 24 months' follow up, although it is not clear whether analysis of data was by intention to treat.[22] The second RCT ceased enrolment and treatment prematurely because of a higher incidence of CNV within the first 12 months in people receiving laser treatment with unilateral (but not with bilateral) drusen.[23,24] The second RCT reported that 351/432 (81%) eyes completed 12 months' follow up, although analysis of data was not by intention to treat and people with CNV were excluded.[23,24] We found no evidence of an effective treatment for the majority of people with exudative age related macular degeneration (see glossary, p 739). There is now considerable interest in preventive strategies for people with high risk drusen. One model estimates that a preventive measure of 10% efficacy in people with bilateral drusen would more than double the prevention of legal blindness (see glossary, p 740) relative to current treatment.[25] Other RCTs of laser to drusen are either ongoing[26] or planned.[22,23] We also found three small exploratory RCTs that were under powered but found similar results to the larger RCTs cited above.[27–29]

QUESTION **What are the effects of treatments for exudative age related macular degeneration?**

OPTION **THERMAL LASER PHOTOCOAGULATION**

Four large RCTs in people with well demarcated exudative age related macular degeneration have found that, compared with no treatment, thermal laser photocoagulation decreases the rate of severe visual loss after 2–5 years, although two RCTs found an initial loss of visual acuity. The RCTs found that choroidal neovascularisation recurs in about half of those treated within 2 years. Of four smaller RCTs, one found that, compared with no treatment, fovea sparing laser photocoagulation increased the proportion of eyes with improved or maintained visual acuity after 12 months, whereas the other three RCTs found no significant difference in occult choroidal neovascularisation between scatter (non-confluent) laser and no treatment. Three RCTs found no significant difference between two different wavelengths of laser photocoagulation in visual acuity after a maximum of 5 years.

Benefits: We found no systematic review. **Versus no treatment:** We found four large unblinded multicentre RCTs in selected populations with exudative age related macular degeneration comparing laser (see glossary, p 740) photocoagulation versus no treatment (see table 1, p 743).[12–15,30–32] We also found four smaller RCTs that included a wider range of people.[33–36] All four large RCTs found that laser treatment versus no treatment clinically and statistically reduced the risk of severe visual loss (defined as loss of ≥ 6 lines on the special eye chart) after 3 years' follow up. Participants differed in terms of the position of the choroidal neovascularisation (CNV) (see glossary, p 739) on the retina, whether far, near, or under the centre of fixation (extrafoveal,[12,14] juxtafoveal,[15,30] or subfoveal[13,31,32]). In the study of extrafoveal CNV, a significant reduction in severe visual loss with laser photocoagulation treatment compared with no treatment was found (either by intention to treat analysis or by treatment analysis), despite the fact that 22/117 (19%) eyes randomised to observation later received laser photocoagulation.[12,14] Reanalysis of data for people with juxtafoveal CNV found that the significant reduction in severe visual loss with laser photocoagulation treatment compared with no treatment after 3 years was limited to those people with pure classic CNV (no occult element) on fluorescein angiography (237/496 [48%] of randomised eyes; OR 2.2, 95% CI 1.4 to 3.4). The two RCTs in people with subfoveal CNV (new and recurrent disease) found a significant reduction in severe visual loss with laser photocoagulation treatment compared with no treatment despite an immediate loss of vision in the treated groups (loss of an average of 3 lines on the special eye chart).[13] Of the four smaller RCTs, one RCT (127 eyes) found that fovea sparing laser photocoagulation compared with no treatment significantly increased the number of eyes with improved or maintained visual acuity (defined as loss of < 3 lines on the Early Treatment of Diabetic Retinopathy Study chart) after 12 months (28/68 [41%] with laser treatment *v* 12/59 [20%] with no treatment; RR 2.00, 95% CI 1.13 to 3.61; NNT 5, 95% CI 3 to 16).[33] The other three

RCTs found no significant difference between scatter (non-confluent) laser and no treatment in occult CNV (see comment below).[34–36] **Different wavelengths:** We found three RCTs that compared two wavelengths of laser photocoagulation (krypton-red or argon-green [see glossary, p 740]) and each other for CNV in age related macular degeneration.[37,38] All three RCTs found no significant difference between krypton-red versus argon-green laser photocoagulation in visual acuity after a maximum of 5 years. **Versus submacular surgery:** See benefits of submacular surgery, p 736. **Effects in people with CNV identified by indocyanine green angiography:** We found no RCTs. Uncontrolled case series in selected people have reported good outcomes.

Harms: Laser destroys new vessels and surrounding retina, and the resultant scar causes a corresponding defect in the central visual field. If the laser is applied to subfoveal lesions, or if the laser burn spreads to the fovea, visual acuity will be impaired; two of the RCTs described immediate loss of visual acuity with laser treatment (an average loss of 3 lines on the special eye chart).[13,32] We found no evidence of other adverse effects.

Comment: Three of the four small RCTs comparing scatter laser photocoagulation versus no treatment were too small to rule out any significant treatment effect.[34–36] The benefits of laser photocoagulation depend on accurate, complete treatment requiring high quality angiography and trained, experienced practitioners.[12–15,30–32] The risk of immediate loss of visual acuity with laser photocoagulation may limit its acceptability.

OPTION RADIOTHERAPY

We found conflicting evidence of the effect of low dose external beam radiation compared with placebo or no treatment in people with exudative age related macular degeneration. Two large RCTs found no significant effect in the number of people with moderate vision loss, while a third found significant effect in mean number of lines of vision lost. Smaller RCTs comparing both low and high dose external beam radiation versus placebo or no treatment found conflicting evidence. We found no RCTs comparing proton beam versus scleral plaque radiotherapy. We found insufficient evidence on long term safety, although RCTs found no evidence of toxicity to the optic nerve or retina after 12–24 months.

Benefits: We found no systematic review. **Low dose external beam radiation:** We found three large[39–41] and two smaller RCTs.[42,43] The first large RCT found no significant difference in the proportion of people with moderate visual loss 1 year after receiving external beam radiation or placebo (1 RCT, 205 people with new subfoveal choroidal neovascularisation [CNV; see glossary, p 739]; 51% with radiotherapy treatment *v* 53% with placebo; P = 0.88; CI not provided; absolute numbers not available; see comment below).[39] No treatment benefit was detected for subgroups of people classified as having some classic CNV (83 people, 41 treated, 42 control) or occult only lesions (122 people, 60 treated, 62 control) on the basis of fluorescein angiography (occult lesions: 47% with radiotherapy treatment *v* 49% with placebo; P = 0.80; classic/mixed lesions: 58% with radiotherapy treatment *v* 58% with placebo; P = 0.47; CI not provided; absolute numbers not available). The external beam radiation group received eight fractions of 2 Gy/ fraction and placebo group received eight fractions of 0 Gy/fraction delivered to the macula. The second large RCT found no significant difference in the proportion of people with moderate or severe visual loss 1 or 2 years after receiving external beam radiation compared with observation (1 RCT, 203 people; moderate visual loss: 53/93 [57%] with external beam radiation *v* 52/91 [57%] with observation at 12 months, P = 0.91; 61/87 [70%] with external beam radiation *v* 71/87 [82%] with observation at 24 months, P = 0.08; severe visual loss: 26/93 [28%] with external beam radiation *v* 37/91 [41%] with observation at 12 months, P = 0.06; 31/87 [36%] with external beam radiation *v* 44/87 [51%] with observation at 24 months, P = 0.29).[40] The external beam radiation group received 12 Gy in six equal fractions. The third large RCT found that compared with placebo, two different dosages of external beam radiation significantly reduced the mean number of lines of vision lost at 18 months after treatment (1 RCT, 161 people; mean number of lines of vision lost at 18 months 1.73 with 8 Gy radiation *v* 3.23 with placebo [1 Gy], P = 0.011; 1.93 with 16 Gy *v* 3.23 with placebo [1 Gy], P = 0.05).[41] The two dosages of external beam radiation were given as 8 Gy in four fractions of 2 Gy and 16 Gy in four fractions of 4 Gy. The two smaller RCTs found conflicting evidence.[42,43] The first small RCT found no significant difference after 12 months between external beam radiation (7 fractions of 2 Gy/ fraction) and placebo (sham radiation) in visual acuity measured on an Early Treatment of Diabetic Retinopathy Study chart (1 RCT, 83 people; mean number of lines lost 4.14 with radiation treatment *v* 3.39 with placebo; P = 0.35; CI not provided) or in angiographic outcomes (lesion size/progression of CNV, see comment below).[42] The second small RCT found that compared with observation, external beam radiation significantly reduced mean visual loss after 2 years (1 RCT, 101 people; P < 0.0001; CI not provided; absolute numbers not available; visual acuity reported as logarithm of the minimum angle of resolution).[43] **High dose external beam radiation:** We found one RCT.[44] The RCT (74 people with new subfoveal CNV) compared external beam radiation (4 fractions of 6 Gy/fraction) delivered to the macula versus observation.[44] It found no significant difference between treatments in the number of people with moderate or severe visual loss (defined as losses of 3 or 6 lines on a special eye chart) after 12 months (absolute numbers not available; 32.0% with radiotherapy *v* 52.2% observation; AR −20%, 95% CI −44% to +4%). **Proton beam and scleral plaque radiotherapy:** We found no RCTs.

Harms: The five RCTs of low dose radiotherapy found no radiation related adverse events up to 24 months' follow up, although one study[40] noted decreased tear film production and stability in the treated group.[39–43] Radiotherapy is potentially toxic to the retina, optic nerve, lens, and lacrimal system, with toxic effects sometimes manifesting up to 2 years after treatment.[45] The biological effects of external beam radiation, both benefits and harms, depend on the dose in each fraction, the number of fractions delivered, and the time between each fraction. Total doses of up to 25 Gy, delivered in daily fractions of 2 Gy or less, are generally claimed not to cause damage to the retina or optic nerve. Uncontrolled pilot studies suggest that the main risks using the present dosing and delivery techniques are cataract formation (2/41 [5%] people in one series)[46] and transient dry eye symptoms (10/75 [13%] in a second case series).[47] One case series using total doses of 16–20 Gy in fraction sizes of 4–5 Gy found radiation toxicity of the optic nerve, retina, or choroid in 20/231 (9%) eyes after 12–24 months.[48] Another case series of proton beam radiation found radiation retinopathy in 11/27 (41%) eyes exposed to higher doses after 12 months.[49] A two centre case series of people treated with external beam radiation (5–10 fractions of 2 Gy/fraction) reported an abnormal choroidal vascular growth pattern associated with macular bleeding and exudation, and marked loss of visual acuity.[50] This change was detected in 12/95 (12%) people and 7/98 (7%) people after 3–12 months.

Comment: In the first RCT, we could not replicate the percentages presented in the paper from the raw data provided for cataract and dry eye symptom results.[39] In the second RCT, recruitment was ceased early (before the estimated sample size of 100 people had been reached) because of small differences in outcomes between groups at 1 year.[42] Results for the third RCT are only expressed as change in the mean vision, and percentages with moderate or severe vision loss (see glossary, p 740) are not given.[41] We also found one small exploratory RCT[51] that was under powered but found similar results to the larger RCT cited above.[44] Further RCTs are under way using both low and high dose external beam radiotherapy. Experience from pilot studies and case series suggests that, although higher radiation doses may be more effective in inducing regression of CNV, they carry an increased risk of sight threatening toxicity. RCTs with less than 2 years' follow up may miss important adverse effects.

OPTION SUBMACULAR SURGERY

We found insufficient evidence on the effects of submacular surgery. Case series have found that rates of recurrent choroidal neovascularisation are high, and there is a clinically significant risk of ocular complications resulting in visual loss and the potential need for further surgical intervention.

Benefits: We found no systematic review. **Versus no treatment:** We found no RCTs. **Versus laser photocoagulation:** We found no RCTs. We found one small exploratory under powered study that found no significant difference between submacular surgery (see glossary, p 740) and laser (see glossary, p 740) photocoagulation in the number of eyes with improved visual acuity after 2 years (70 people with recurrent subfoveal choroidal neovascularisation [see glossary, p 739] after previous laser photocoagulation treatment) defined as visual acuity better than or no more than 1 line worse than baseline as measured on a modified Bailey-Lovie chart (14/28 [50%] with surgery *v* 20/31 [65%] with laser treatment; RR 0.80, 95% CI 0.49 to 1.22).[52] **Versus alternative surgical techniques:** We found one RCT (80 eyes with exudative age related macular degeneration

[AMD; see glossary, p 739]) comparing submacular surgery plus subretinal injection of tissue plasminogen activator versus submacular surgery plus subretinal injection of a control solution (balanced salt solution).[53] It found no significant difference in the number of eyes with any visual improvement using an Early Treatment of Diabetic Retinopathy Study chart (5/40 [12%] with surgery plus tissue plasminogen activator *v* 6/40 [15%] with surgery plus control; RR 0.80, 95% CI 0.28 to 2.51) or with fluorescein angiographic evidence of active choroidal neovascularisation after 1 year (7/40 [18%] with surgery plus tissue plasminogen activator *v* 8/40 [20%] with surgery plus control; RR 0.90, 95% CI 0.35 to 2.18).

Harms: Submacular surgery may threaten vision itself or necessitate further surgical intervention. However, we found no information on the frequency of adverse events. The largest case series of people with AMD and non-AMD treated with submacular surgery reported cataract formation (in up to 40%), retinal detachment (5–8%), recurrent new vessel formation (18–35% within 12 months), and macular complications (haemorrhage and pucker; no rates provided).[54]

Comment: Most evidence for submacular surgery currently comes from small uncontrolled case series (< 50 people with AMD) with short follow up times, often including people with other types of macular degeneration. These series found that few people with AMD had improved vision with surgery.[45,54] Comparing results is difficult because of evolving surgical techniques, changes in outcome measures, and variations in follow up. Several large non-blinded RCTs are currently recruiting and will compare standardised surgical technique versus no treatment in new and haemorrhagic choroidal neovascularisation in people with AMD (S Bressler, personal communication, 1999). Other surgical techniques are being developed in volunteers, including macular translocation and retinal pigment epithelial transplantation, but these have yet to be evaluated formally.

OPTION SUBCUTANEOUS INTERFERON ALFA-2A

One large RCT found that, compared with placebo, subcutaneous interferon alfa-2a (an antiangiogenesis drug) increased visual loss, although the difference was not significant, and found evidence of serious ocular and systemic adverse effects.

Benefits: We found no systematic review. We found one RCT (481 people with subfoveal choroidal neovascularisation due to age related macular degeneration [see glossary, p 739]) comparing three doses of subcutaneous interferon alfa-2a (1.5, 3, and 6 million IU 3 times/week for 1 year) versus placebo.[54] It found that interferon alfa-2a at all doses increased the number of people with a reduction in visual acuity of at least three lines on a Snellen chart after 52 weeks compared with placebo, although the difference was not significant (see comment below; 142/286 [50%] with interferon alfa-2a *v* 40/105 [38%] with placebo; RR 1.20, 95% CI 0.90 to 1.62).[54]

Harms: Adverse effects of interferon alfa-2a were common and potentially severe in this RCT[54] and in other poorer quality RCTs. Effects included fatigue and influenza-like symptoms, gastrointestinal symptoms (including nausea, diarrhoea, and loss of appetite), and central and peripheral nervous system effects (including headaches and dizziness). Although at least one adverse event was reported in 90/105 (86%) people taking placebo, the proportion of people on active treatment who suffered adverse effects increased with dose, as did the severity of adverse effects. The RCT reported that 20/286 (7%) people receiving interferon alfa-2a developed interferon associated retinopathy (retinal haemorrhages or cotton wool spots).[55]

Comment: In the RCT, 90/481 (18%) of people did not complete the trial and analysis of data was not by intention to treat.[53] There is widespread interest in safe, effective antiangiogenesis drugs for prophylaxis in exudative age related macular degeneration. Several drugs are currently under preclinical and early phase clinical study. RCTs are currently investigating the use of intraocular or periocular steroids and antivascular endothelial growth factor.

OPTION PHOTODYNAMIC TREATMENT WITH VERTEPORFIN

Two RCTs in people with age related macular degeneration found that, compared with placebo, photodynamic treatment with verteporfin reduced the number of people with moderate or severe vision loss after 1–2 years. In the first RCT, subgroup analysis suggested the benefit is greatest in people with predominantly classic lesions on fluorescein angiography. Subgroup analysis in the second RCT suggested a more modest benefit in the second year of treatment in people with only occult (no classic) lesions on fluorescein angiography. Both RCTs found that photodynamic treatment with verteporfin was associated with an initial loss of vision and photosensitive reactions in a small number of people.

Benefits: We found one systematic review (search date 2000, 1 RCT, 609 people with new and recurrent subfoveal choroidal neovascularisation [CNV] due to age related macular degeneration [see glossary, p 739])[56] and one subsequent RCT.[57] The RCT included in the review compared photodynamic treatment with verteporfin (see glossary, p 740) (6 mg/m^2 body surface area) versus placebo (photodynamic treatment with 5% dextrose solution). Treatments were repeated as necessary every 3 months. Results were reported after 12 months[56] and, subsequently, after 24 months.[58] The RCT reported in the systematic review found that photodynamic treatment with verteporfin versus placebo significantly increased the number of people with stable vision after 12 months (defined as a loss of < 15 letters or 3 lines of vision on a special eye chart; 246/402 [61%] with photodynamic treatment with verteporfin *v* 96/207 [46%] with placebo; RR 1.30, 95% CI 1.12 to 1.56; NNT 7, 95% CI 5 to 15)[56] and after 24 months (213/402 [53%] with photodynamic treatment with verteporfin *v* 78/207 [38%] with placebo; RR 1.40, 95% CI 1.15 to 1.71; NNT 7, 95% CI 5 to 14).[58] Subgroup analysis found that benefit was greater in people with predominantly classic CNV (see glossary, p 740) lesions (94/159 [59%] with photodynamic treatment with verteporfin *v* 26/83 [31%] with placebo; RR 1.90, 95% CI 1.34 to 2.66) and greatest in people with only classic lesions (65/93 [70%] photodynamic treatment with verteporfin *v* 14/49 [29%] with placebo; RR 2.50, 95% CI 1.54 to 3.88) after 24 months. The subsequent RCT (339 people with occult or classic CNV due to age related macular degeneration; see comment below) found that photodynamic treatment with verteporfin (6 mg/m^2 body surface area) versus placebo (photodynamic treatment with 5% dextrose solution) significantly reduced the number of people with moderate vision loss (see glossary, p 740) (defined as a loss of ≥ 15 letters of vision on a special eye chart; 121/225 [54%] with photodynamic treatment with verteporfin *v* 76/114 [67%] with placebo; RR 0.80, 95% CI 0.68 to 0.96; NNT 8, 95% CI 5 to 39) and severe vision loss (see glossary, p 740) (defined as a loss of ≥ 30 letters of vision on a special eye chart; 67/225 [30%] with photodynamic treatment with verteporfin *v* 54/114 [47%] with placebo; RR 0.60, 95% CI 0.48 to 0.83; NNT 6, 95% CI 4 to 15) after 2 years.[57] Subgroup analysis of people with only occult CNV (no classic lesions) on fluorescein angiography (166/225 [74%] people receiving photodynamic treatment with verteporfin *v* 92/114 [81%] people receiving placebo) found that photodynamic treatment with verteporfin versus placebo significantly reduced the number of people with moderate vision loss (91/166 [55%] with photodynamic treatment with verteporfin *v* 63/92 [68%] with placebo; RR 0.80, 95% CI 0.70 to 0.97) and with severe vision loss (48/166 [29%] with photodynamic treatment with verteporfin *v* 43/92 [47%] with placebo; RR 0.60, 95% CI 0.45 to 0.86; see comment below) after 2 years.

Harms: Verteporfin is a photosensitive dye and care must be taken to avoid leakage into surrounding tissues during infusion and exposure to bright light soon after treatment. Advice in the study was to avoid light for 48 hours but some photosensitive reactions were observed in treated people after 3–5 days.[56] The treatment was well tolerated but was more likely than the control intervention to cause a transient decrease in vision, injection site reactions, photosensitivity, and infusion related low back pain. Severe loss of vision (> 20 letters or 4 lines on a special eye chart) was recorded in 3/402 people (< 1%) in the first RCT[56,58] and 10/225 people (4%) in the subsequent RCT[57] within 7 days of treatment, although some visual recovery occurred in most cases. The risk seems to be higher in people with occult and no classic CNV. The possibility of rare but severe adverse events remains.

Comment: The subsequent RCT included a subset of people with only occult and no classic CNV lesions.[57] Further analysis of this subgroup has suggested that the treatment effect recorded by the RCT may be influenced by baseline visual acuity and lesion size.[59]

GLOSSARY

Age related macular degeneration (AMD) Degenerative disease of the macula (centre of the retina): classified as early (marked by drusen and pigmentary change, and usually associated with normal vision) and late (choroidal neovascularisation and geographic atrophy, associated with a decrease in central vision). Age related maculopathy is an older term for early AMD.

Choroidal neovascularisation (CNV) New vessels in the choroid, classified by fluorescein angiography: in terms of its position in relation to the fovea — extrafoveal, juxtafoveal, or subfoveal; in terms of its appearance — classic (well defined) or occult (poorly defined); and in terms of its borders — well demarcated or poorly demarcated.

Age related macular degeneration

Drusen Small, yellow, bright objects, often near the macula, seen by ophthalmoscopy. They are located under the basement membrane of the retinal pigment epithelium. They are present in many older people with normal vision, but a greater number of large drusen indicate higher risk of subsequent loss of acuity from age related macular degeneration.
Geographic atrophy The end stage of atrophic age related macular degeneration with atrophy of the retina and inner choroidal layers at the macular leaving only the deep choroidal vessels visible.
Laser (diode, krypton, argon-green) Lasers used in ophthalmology that produce focused light of different specific wavelengths.
Legal blindness Visual acuity less than 20/200.
Moderate vision loss Loss of three or more lines of distance vision measured on a special eye chart, corresponding to a doubling of the visual angle.
Photodynamic treatment A two step procedure of intravenous infusion of a photosensitive dye followed by application of a non-thermal laser that activates the dye. The treatment aims to cause selective closure of the choroidal new vessels.
Predominantly classic choroidal neovascularisation Choroidal neovascularisation in which more than 50% of lesion area consists of classic choroidal neovascularisation on fluorescein angiography.
Severe vision loss Loss of six or more lines of distance vision measured on a special eye chart, corresponding to a quadrupling of the visual angle.
Submacular surgery Removal of haemorrhage, choroidal neovascularisation, or both after vitrectomy.
Verteporfin A photosensitive dye used in photodynamic treatment.

Substantive changes

Radiotherapy Two RCTs added;[40,41] conclusions unchanged.

REFERENCES

1. Bressler SB, Bressler NM, Fine SL. Age-related macular degeneration. *Surv Ophthalmol* 1988;32:375–413.
2. Klein R, Klein BEK, Linton KLP. Prevalence of age-related maculopathy: the Beaver Dam Eye Study. *Ophthalmology* 1992;99:933–943.
3. Vingerling JR, Dielemans I, Hofman A, et al. The prevalence of age-related maculopathy in the Rotterdam study. *Ophthalmology* 1995;102:205–210.
4. Mitchell P, Smith W, Attebo K, et al. Prevalence of age-related maculopathy in Australia. The Blue Mountains Eye Study. *Ophthalmology* 1995;102:1450–1460.
5. Evans JR. Risk factors for age-related macular degeneration. *Prog Retin Eye Res* 2001;20:227–253.
6. Pieramici DJ, Bressler SB. Age-related macular degeneration and risk factors for the development of choroidal neovascularization in the fellow eye. *Curr Opin Ophthalmol* 1998;9:38–46.
7. Smith W, Assink J, Klein R, et al. Risk factors for age-related macular degeneration: pooled findings from three continents. *Ophthalmology* 2001;108:697–704.
8. Maguire P, Vine AK. Geographic atrophy of the retinal pigment epithelium. *Am J Ophthalmol* 1986;102:621–625.
9. Sarks JP, Sarks SH, Killingsworth M. Evolution of geographic atrophy of the retinal pigment epithelium. *Eye* 1988;2:552–577.
10. Holz FG, Wolfensberger TJ, Piguet B, et al. Bilateral macular drusen in age-related macular degeneration: prognosis and risk factors. *Ophthalmology* 1994;101:1522–1528.
11. Klein R, Klein BEK, Jensen SC, et al. The five-year incidence and progression of age-related maculopathy. The Beaver Dam Eye study. *Ophthalmology* 1997;104:7–21.
12. Macular Photocoagulation Study Group. Argon laser photocoagulation for neovascular maculopathy: five-year results from randomized clinical trials. *Arch Ophthalmol* 1991;109:1109–1114.
13. Macular Photocoagulation Study Group. Laser photocoagulation of subfoveal neovascular lesions of age-related macular degeneration: updated findings from two clinical trials. *Arch Ophthalmol* 1993;111:1200–1209.
14. Macular Photocoagulation Study Group. Argon laser photocoagulation for neovascular maculopathy. Three-year results from randomized clinical trials. *Arch Ophthalmol* 1986;104:694–701.
15. Macular Photocoagulation Study Group. Laser photocoagulation for juxtafoveal choroidal neovascularisation. Five-year results from randomized clinical trials. *Arch Ophthalmol* 1994;112:500–509.
16. Macular Photocoagulation Study Group. Risk factors for choroidal neovascularisation secondary to age-related macular degeneration. Arch Ophthalmol 1997;115:741–747.
17. Evans JR. Antioxidant vitamin and mineral supplements for age-related macular degeneration (Cochrane Review). In: The Cochrane Library, Issue 4, 2002. Oxford: Update Software. Search date 2001; primary sources Medline, Embase, Cochrane Controlled Trials Register, Science

Citation Index, hand searches of reference lists of relevant trials, and personal communication with investigators of included studies.

18. Age-related Eye Disease Study Research Group. A randomised placebo-controlled clinical trial of high-dose supplementation with vitamins C and E, beta carotene, and zinc for age-related macular degeneration and vision loss: AREDS report no 8. *Arch Ophthalmol* 2001;119:1417–1436.
19. The Alpha-tocopherol, Beta Carotene Cancer Prevention Study Group. The effect of vitamin E and beta carotene on the incidence of lung cancer and other cancers in male smokers. *N Engl J Med* 1994;330:1029–1035.
20. Omenn GS, Goodman GE, Thornquist MD, et al. Effects of a combination of beta carotene and vitamin A on lung cancer and cardiovascular disease. *N Engl J Med* 1996;334:1150–1155.
21. Evans JR, Henshaw K. Antioxidant vitamin and mineral supplementation for preventing age-related macular degeneration (Cochrane Review). In: The Cochrane Library, Issue 4, 2002. Oxford: Update Software. Search date 2002; primary sources Medline, Embase, Cochrane Controlled Tirals Register, Science Citation Index, hand searches of reference lists of relevant trials, and personal communication with investigators and experts in the field.
22. Olk, RJ, Friberg TR, Stickney KL, et al. Therapeutic benefits of infrared (810 nm) diode laser macular grid photocoagulation in prophylactic treatment of nonexudative age-related macular degeneration: two-year results of a randomized pilot study. *Ophthalmology* 1999;106:2082–2090.
23. Ho CA, Maguire MG, Yoken J, et al. The Choroidal Neovascularization Prevention Trial research group. Laser-induced drusen reduction improves visual function at 1 year. *Ophthalmology* 1999;106:1367–1373.
24. The Choroidal Neovascularization Prevention Trial research group. Laser treatment in eyes with large drusen. Short-term effects seen in a pilot randomized clinical trial. *Ophthalmology* 1998;105:11–23.
25. Lanchoney DM, Maguire MG, Fine SL. A model of the incidence and consequences of choroidal neovascularisation secondary to age-related macular degeneration. Comparative effects of current treatment and potential prophylaxis on visual outcomes in high-risk patients. *Arch Ophthalmol* 1998;116:1045–1052.
26. Owens SL, Guymer RH, Gross-Jendroska M, et al. Fluorescein angiographic abnormalities after prophylactic macular photocoagulation for high-risk age-related maculopathy. *Am J Ophthalmol* 1999;127:681–687.
27. Little HL, Showman JM, Brown BW. A pilot randomized controlled study on the effect of laser photocoagulation of confluent soft macular drusen. *Ophthalmology* 1997;104:623–631.
28. Frennesson C, Nilsson SEG. Prophylactic laser treatment in early age-related maculopathy reduced the incidence of exudative complications. *Br J Ophthalmol* 1998;82:1169–1174.
29. Figueroa MS, Regueras A, Bertrand J, et al. Laser photocoagulation for macular soft drusen. Updated results. *Retina* 1997;17:378–384.
30. Macular Photocoagulation Study Group. Occult choroidal neovascularization. Influence on visual outcome in patients with age-related macular degeneration. *Arch Ophthalmol* 1996;114:400–412.
31. Macular Photocoagulation Study Group. Persistent and recurrent neovascularization after laser photocoagulation for subfoveal choroidal neovascularization of age-related macular degeneration. *Arch Ophthalmol* 1994;112:489–499.
32. Macular Photocoagulation Study Group. Visual outcome after laser photocoagulation for subfoveal choroidal neovascularization secondary to age-related macular degeneration. The influence of initial lesion size and initial visual acuity. *Arch Ophthalmol* 1994;112:480–488.
33. Coscas G, Soubrane G, Ramahefasolo C, et al. Perifoveal laser treatment for subfoveal choroidal new vessels in age-related macular degeneration. Results of a randomized clinical trial. *Arch Ophthalmol* 1991;109:1258–1265.
34. Bressler NM, Maguire MG, Murphy PL, et al. Macular scatter ("grid") laser treatment of poorly demarcated subfoveal choroidal neovascularisation in age-related macular degeneration. Results of a randomised pilot trial. *Arch Ophthalmol* 1996;114:1456–1464.
35. Arnold J, Algan M, Soubrane G, et al. Indirect scatter laser photocoagulation to subfoveal choroidal neovascularization in age-related macular degeneration. *Graefes Arch Clin Exp Ophthalmol* 1997;235:208–216.
36. Barondes MJ, Pagliarini S, Chisholm IH, et al. Controlled trial of laser photocoagulation of pigment epithelial detachments in the elderly: 4 year review. *Br J Ophthalmol* 1992;76:5–7.
37. Macular Photocoagulation Study Group. Evaluation of argon green vs krypton red laser for photocoagulation of subfoveal choroidal neovascularisation in the Macular Photocoagulation Study. *Arch Ophthalmol* 1994;112:1176–1184.
38. Willan AR, Cruess AF, Ballantyne M. Argon green vs krypton red laser photocoagulation for extrafoveal choroidal neovascularization secondary to age-related macular degeneration: 3-year results of a multicentre randomized trial. *Can J Ophthalmol* 1996;31:11–17.
39. The Radiation Therapy for Age-related Macular Degeneration (RAD) study group. A prospective randomized double-masked trial on radiation therapy for neovascular age-related macular degeneration (RAD) study. *Ophthalmology* 1999;106:2239–2247.
40. Hart PM, Chakravarthy U, Mackenzie G, et al. Visual outcomes in the subfoveal radiotherapy study: a randomized controlled trial of teletherapy for age-related macular degeneration. *Arch Ophthalmol* 2002;120:1029–1038.
41. Valmaggia C, Reis G, Ballinari P. Radiotherapy for subfoveal choroidal neovascularisation in age-related macular degeneration: a randomised clinical trial. *Am J Ophthalmol* 2002;133:521–529.
42. Marcus DM, Sheils W, Johnson MH, et al. External beam irradiation of subfoveal choroidal neovascularization complicating age-related macular degeneration: one-year results of a prospective, double-masked, randomized clinical trial. *Arch Ophthalmol* 2001;119:171–180.
43. Kobayashi H, Kobayashi K. Age-related macular degeneration: long-term results of radiotherapy for subfoveal neovascular membranes. *Am J Ophthalmol* 2000;130:617–635.
44. Bergink GJ, Hoyng CB, Van der Maazen RW, et al. A randomized controlled clinical trial on the efficacy of radiation therapy in the control of subfoveal choroidal neovascularization in age-related macular degeneration: radiation versus observation. *Graefes Arch Clin Exp Ophthalmol* 1998;236:321–325.
45. Ciulla TA, Danis RP, Harris A. Age-related macular degeneration: a review of experimental treatments. *Surv Ophthalmol* 1998;43:134–146.

46. Hart PM, Chakravarthy U, MacKenzie G, et al. Teletherapy for subfoveal choroidal neovascularisation of age-related macular degeneration: results of follow up in a non-randomised study. *Br J Ophthalmol* 1996;80:1046–1050.
47. Finger PT, Berson A, Sherr D, et al. Radiation therapy for subretinal neovascularization. *Ophthalmology* 1996;103:878–889.
48. Mauget-Faysse M, Chiquet C, Milea D, et al. Long term results of radiotherapy for subfoveal choroidal neovascularisation in age-related macular degeneration. *Br J Ophthalmol* 1999;83:923–928.
49. Flaxel CJ, Fridrichsen EJ, Osborn Smith J, et al. Proton beam irradiation of subfoveal choroidal neovascularisation in age-related macular degeneration. *Eye* 2000;14:155–164.
50. Spaide RF, Leys A, Herrmann-Delemazure B, et al. Radiation-associated choroidal neovasculopathy. *Ophthalmology* 1999;106:2254–2260.
51. Char DH, Irvine AI, Posner MD, et al. Randomized trial of radiation for age-related macular degeneration. *Am J Ophthalmol* 1999;127:574–578.
52. Submacular Surgery Trials Pilot Study Investigators. Submacular surgery trials randomized pilot trial of laser photocoagulation versus surgery for recurrent choroidal neovascularization secondary to age-related macular degeneration: I. Ophthalmic outcomes. Submacular surgery trials pilot study report number 1. *Am J Ophthalmol* 2000;130:387–407.
53. Lewis H, Van der Brug MS. Tissue plasminogen activator-assisted surgical excision of subfoveal choroidal neovascularization in age-related macular degeneration: a randomized, double-masked trial. *Ophthalmology* 1997;104:1847–1851.
54. Thomas MA, Dickinson JD, Melberg NS, et al. Visual results after surgical removal of subfoveal choroidal neovascular membranes. *Ophthalmology* 1994;101:1384–1396.
55. Pharmacological Therapy for Macular Degeneration study group. Interferon alfa-2a is ineffective for patients with choroidal neovascularization secondary to age-related macular degeneration: results of a prospective randomized placebo-controlled clinical trial. *Arch Ophthalmol* 1997;115:865–872.
56. Wormald R, Evans J, Smeeth L. Photodynamic therapy for neovascular age-related macular degeneration. In: The Cochrane Library, Issue 4, 2002. Oxford: Update Software. Search date 2000; primary sources Cochrane Controlled Trials Register, Cochrane Eyes and Vision Group Register, Medline, Embase, Science Citation Index, experts, and hand searched references.
57. Verteporfin In Photodynamic Therapy Study Group. Verteporfin therapy of subfoveal choroidal neovascularization in age-related macular degeneration: two-year results of a randomized clinical trial including lesions with occult with no classic choroidal neovascularization: verteporfin in photodynamic therapy report 2. *Am J Ophthalmol* 2001;131:541–560.
58. Treatment of age-related macular degeneration with photodynamic therapy (TAP) study group. Photodynamic therapy of subfoveal choroidal neovascularisation in age-related macular degeneration with verteporfin. Two-year results of 2 randomized clinical trials: TAP report 2. *Arch Ophthalmol* 2001;119:198–207.
59. Bressler NM. Verteporfin therapy of subfoveal choroidal neovascularization in age-related macular degeneration: two-year results of a randomized clinical trial including lesions with occult with no classic choroidal neovascularization-verteporfin in photodynamic therapy report 2. *Am J Ophthalmol* 2002;133:168–169.

Jennifer Arnold
Consultant Ophthalmologist
Marsden Eye Specialists
Parramatta, New South Wales
Australia

Shirley Sarks
Honorary Senior Research Associate
Prince of Wales Medical Research Institute
Randwick, New South Wales
Australia

Competing interests: JA was a clinical investigator in the study of photodynamic treatment using verteporfin, funded by Novartis/QLT, and has been supported by Novartis for attendance at conferences and symposia. SS none declared.

TABLE 1 **Laser photocoagulation of choroidal neovascularisation versus observation in exudative age related macular degeneration: results of Macular Photocoagulation Study Group RCTs (see text, p 733).**

Site of CNV (type of laser)	Number of eyes	Severe visual loss (6 or more lines)	Vision level treated *v* control	Rate of recurrence in treated eyes
Extrafoveal CNV (argon-blue-green)[12,14]	236	RR 1.5 at 6 months to 5 years; P = 0.001	≥ 20/40 at 3 years; 33% *v* 22%	54% at 5 years
Juxtafoveal CNV (krypton-red)[15,30]	496	RR 1.2 at 6 months to 5 years; P = 0.04	≥ 20/40 at 3 years; 13% *v* 7%	76% at 5 years (classic CNV only)
New subfoveal CNV (argon-green or krypton)[13,31,32]	373	20% treated *v* 37% control at 2 years; P < 0.01	> 20/200 at 4 years; 12% *v* 11%	44% at 3 years
Recurrent subfoveal CNV (argon-green or krypton)[13,31,32]	206	9% treated *v* 28% control at 2 years; P = 0.03	> 20/200 at 3 years; 25% *v* 12%	39% at 3 years

CNV, choroidal neovascularisation.

Bacterial conjunctivitis

Search date June 2003

Justine Smith

QUESTIONS

INTERVENTIONS

Key Messages

- **Antibiotic treatment in culture positive bacterial conjunctivitis** One systematic review has found that antibiotics (polymyxin–bacitracin, ciprofloxacin, or ofloxacin) increase rates of clinical and microbiological cure compared with placebo. Four RCTs found no significant difference among antibiotics in clinical or microbiological cure. One RCT found that fusidic acid increased clinical cure rate compared with chloramphenicol. One RCT found that topical netilmicin increased clinical cure rate compared with topical gentamicin. One RCT found that topical levofloxacin increased microbiological cure rate, but not clinical cure rate, compared with topical ofloxacin.
- **Empirical antibiotic treatment of suspected bacterial conjunctivitis** One systematic review found limited evidence from one RCT that topical norfloxacin increased rates of clinical and microbiological improvement or cure after 5 days compared with placebo. RCTs comparing different topical antibiotics versus each other found no significant difference in rates of clinical or microbiological cure. One RCT found no significant difference between topical polymyxin–bacitracin ointment and oral cefixime for clinical or microbiological improvement or cure.

DEFINITION Conjunctivitis is any inflammation of the conjunctiva, generally characterised by irritation, itching, foreign body sensation, and watering or discharge. Bacterial conjunctivitis may often be distinguished from other types of conjunctivitis by the presence of a yellow–white mucopurulent discharge. There is also usually a papillary reaction (small bumps with fibrovascular cores on the palpebral conjunctiva, appearing grossly as a fine velvety surface). Bacterial conjunctivitis is usually bilateral. This review covers non-gonococcal bacterial conjunctivitis.

INCIDENCE/ PREVALENCE We found no good evidence on the incidence or prevalence of bacterial conjunctivitis.

AETIOLOGY/ RISK FACTORS Conjunctivitis may be infectious (caused by bacteria or viruses) or allergic. In adults, bacterial conjunctivitis is less common than viral conjunctivitis, although estimates vary widely (viral conjunctivitis has been reported to account for 8–75% of acute conjunctivitis).[1–3] *Staphylococcus* species are the most common pathogens for bacterial conjunctivitis in adults, followed by *Streptococcus pneumoniae* and *Haemophilus influenzae*.[4,5] In children, bacterial conjunctivitis is more common than viral, and is mainly caused by *H influenzae*, *S pneumoniae*, and *Moraxella catarrhalis*.[6,7]

PROGNOSIS Most bacterial conjunctivitis is self limiting. One systematic review (search date 2001) found clinical cure or significant improvement with placebo within 2–5 days in 64% of people (99% CI 54% to 73%).[8] Some organisms cause corneal or systemic complications, or both. Otitis media may develop in 25% of children with *H influenzae* conjunctivitis,[9] and systemic meningitis may complicate primary meningococcal conjunctivitis in 18% of people.[10]

AIMS OF INTERVENTION To achieve rapid cure of inflammation, and to prevent complications, with minimum adverse effects of treatment.

OUTCOMES Time to cure or improvement. **Clinical signs/symptoms:** hyperaemia, discharge, papillae, follicles, chemosis, itching, pain, photophobia. Most studies used a numbered scale to grade signs and symptoms. Some studies also included evaluation by investigators and participants regarding success of treatment. **Culture results:** These are proxy outcomes usually expressed as the number of colonies, sometimes with reference to a threshold level. Results were often classified into categories such as eradication, reduction, persistence, and proliferation.

METHODS *Clinical Evidence* search and appraisal June 2003.

QUESTION **What are the effects of empirical treatment with antibiotics in adults and children with suspected bacterial conjunctivitis?**

One systematic review found limited evidence from one RCT that topical norfloxacin increased rates of clinical and microbiological improvement or cure after 5 days compared with placebo. RCTs comparing different topical antibiotics versus each other found no significant difference in rates of clinical or microbiological cure. One RCT found no significant difference between topical polymyxin–bacitracin ointment and oral cefixime for clinical or microbiological improvement or cure.

Benefits: **Versus placebo:** We found one systematic review (search date 2001, 1 RCT, 284 adults; 50% of participants were culture positive) comparing topical norfloxacin versus placebo (see table A on web extra).[8] It found that norfloxacin significantly increased rates of clinical and microbiological improvement or cure after 5 days compared with placebo (88%, 95% CI 81% to 93% with norfloxacin *v* 72%, 95% CI 63% to 79% with placebo; $P < 0.01$; see comment below). **Versus each other:** We found no systematic review but found 27 RCTs conducted in adults and children (see table A on web extra).[2,11–36] These RCTs found no significant difference between different topical antibiotics and each other in rates of clinical or microbiological cure. **Versus oral antibiotics:** We found one RCT (80 children).[37] It found no significant difference between polymyxin–bacitracin ointment plus oral placebo and topical placebo plus oral cefixime in clinical improvement or bacteriological failure rates (failure rate: 15/40 [37.5%] with cefixime *v* 7/40 [17.5%] with polymyxin–bacitracin; $P = 0.07$).

Harms: **Versus placebo:** One RCT identified by the review reported minor adverse events in 4.2% of people for norfloxacin compared with 7.1% for placebo (P value not reported).[5] One non-systematic review reported four cases of aplastic anaemia with topical chloramphenicol and three cases of Stevens–Johnson syndrome with topical sulphonamides.[38] However, the review did not report the number of people using these drugs, making it difficult to exclude other possible causes of aplastic anaemia. **Versus each other:** See table A on web extra.[2,11–36]

Comment: The placebo controlled RCT identified by the review did not assess the effect of topical antibiotics on antibiotic resistance.[5] Most other trials included children as well as adults, and the ratio of children to adults was usually not specified. The comparisons of lomefloxacin versus chloramphenicol and fusidic acid, the comparison of norfloxacin versus fusidic acid, and the comparison of tobramycin versus fusidic acid were single blind. One RCT found that a significantly greater proportion of participants rated topical tobramycin as more inconvenient than the viscous preparation of fusidic acid, because of a difference in the frequency of administration.[35] The RCT also found that adherence among children was significantly higher with fusidic acid.

QUESTION **What are the effects of topical antibiotics in adults and children with culture positive bacterial conjunctivitis?**

One systematic review has found that antibiotics (polymyxin–bacitracin, ciprofloxacin, or ofloxacin) increase rates of both clinical and microbiological cure compared with placebo. Four RCTs found no significant difference among antibiotics in clinical or microbiological cure. One RCT found that fusidic acid increased clinical cure rate compared with chloramphenicol. One RCT found that topical netilmicin increased clinical cure rate compared with topical gentamicin. One RCT found that topical levofloxacin increased microbiological cure rate, but not clinical cure rate, compared with topical ofloxacin.

Benefits: **Versus placebo:** We found one systematic review (search date 2000, 3 RCTs) in people with culture positive bacterial conjunctivitis, which compared antibiotics (polymyxin–bacitracin, ciprofloxacin, and ofloxacin) versus placebo (see table A on web extra).[8] The first RCT identified by the review (84 children with culture proven *H influenzae* and *S pneumoniae* bacterial conjunctivitis) found that topical polymyxin–bacitracin significantly increased clinical cure after 3–5 days compared with placebo but found no significant difference after 8–10 days (3–5 days: 62% with antibiotic *v* 28% with placebo; $P < 0.02$; 8–10 days: 91% with antibiotic *v* 72% with placebo; $P > 0.05$).[17] The RCT found that topical polymyxin–bacitracin significantly increased microbiological cure rates after both 3–5 days and 8–10 days compared with placebo. The second RCT (177 people, age not specified) found that ciprofloxacin significantly increased microbiological cure rates after 3 days compared with placebo (132/140 [94%] with antibiotic *v* 22/37 [59%] with placebo; RR 1.59, 95% CI 1.21 to 2.08).[18] The third RCT identified by the review, which compared antibiotics versus placebo, is published only in abstract form (see comment below).[19] **Versus each other:** We found no systematic review but found seven RCTs (see table A on web extra).[18,20–24,39] The first RCT (139 children) found that fusidic acid significantly increased clinical cure rate compared with chloramphenicol (85% with fusidic acid *v* 48% with chloramphenicol; $P < 0.0001$).[20] The second RCT (251 people) found no significant difference in reduction or eradication of bacteria between ciprofloxacin and tobramycin after 7 days (94.5% with ciprofloxacin *v* 91.9% with tobramycin; $P > 0.5$).[18] The third RCT (141 children) found no significant difference in clinical cure between ciprofloxacin and tobramycin (87% with ciprofloxacin *v* 90% with tobramycin; $P > 0.05$) or in microbiological cure rate (90% with ciprofloxacin *v* 84% with tobramycin; $P = 0.29$) after 7 days.[21] The fourth RCT (156 children) compared three treatments: trimethoprim–polymyxin, gentamicin, and sulfacetamide (sulphacetamide).[22] It found no significant difference in clinical cure rate between any of the treatments (84% with trimethoprim–polymyxin *v* 88% with gentamicin *v* 89% with sulfacetamide; $P > 0.1$) or in microbiological cure rate (83% with trimethoprim–polymyxin *v* 68% with gentamicin *v* 72% with sulfacetamide; $P > 0.1$) after 2–7 days. The fifth RCT (40 people) found no significant difference in symptom resolution between lomefloxacin and ofloxacin after 7 days (88% with lomefloxacin *v* 75% ofloxacin; $P < 0.08$).[23] The sixth RCT (121 people) found that topical netilmicin (0.3%) administered as one or two drops to affected eyes four times daily significantly increased clinical cure rate after both 5 and 10 days compared with 0.3% topical gentamicin ($P = 0.01$ after 5 days; $P = 0.001$ after 10 days; other results presented graphically).[24] The seventh RCT (423 adult and children entered, 208 included in per protocol analysis; see comment below) found that topical levofloxacin 0.5% for 5 days significantly increased microbiological cure rate but found no significant difference in clinical cure rate at 6–10 days compared with topical ofloxacin 0.3% (microbiological cure: 89% with levofloxacin *v* 80% with ofloxacin; $P = 0.034$; clinical cure: 76% with levofloxacin *v* 76% with ofloxacin; $P > 0.05$).[39]

Harms: **Versus each other:** The sixth RCT found no significant difference between topical netilmicin and topical gentamicin in the rate of adverse reactions (redness, itching, and burning).[24] The seventh RCT found no significant difference between topical levofloxacin and topical ofloxacin in treatment related adverse effects (15/207 [7.3%] ofloxacin *v* 10/206 [4.9%] with levofloxacin).[39] The following minor adverse effects of topical antibiotics compared with each other were reported in RCTs that included people with suspected bacterial conjunctivitis: punctuate epithelial erosions (35% for tobramycin *v* 20% for ciprofloxacin); bad taste (20% for norfloxacin *v* 6% for fusidic acid); stinging (50% for norfloxacin *v* 37% for fusidic acid); and burning (33% with gentamicin *v* 20% with lomefloxacin; 1.45% with levofloxacin *v* 0.97% with ofloxacin).[13,25,26,39]

Comment: One RCT included in the review (abstract only; 132 people, age not specified) found that ofloxacin significantly increased clinical and microbiological improvement after 2 days compared with placebo (64% with ofloxacin *v* 22% with placebo; $P < 0.001$).[19] In the seventh RCT (423 people entered) comparing antibiotics versus each other, 215 people were excluded from the per protocol analysis because of a negative baseline culture, missing postbaseline data, and violations of either entry criteria or protocol.[39] None of the RCTs addressed the effect on antibiotic resistance of using topical antibiotics in bacterial conjunctivitis, which would be of interest given the self limiting nature of the disease. The age of the study participants was not always specified and no RCTs reported any patient orientated outcomes or assessed rates of reinfection.

Substantive changes

Culture positive One RCT added;[39] conclusions unchanged.

REFERENCES

1. Wishart PK, James C, Wishart MS, et al. Prevalence of acute conjunctivitis caused by chlamydia, adenovirus, and herpes simplex virus in an ophthalmic casualty department. *Br J Ophthalmol* 1984;68:653–655.
2. Fitch CP, Rapoza PA, Owens S, et al. Epidemiology and diagnosis of acute conjunctivitis at an inner-city hospital. *Ophthalmology* 1989;96:1215–1220.
3. Woodland RM, Darougar S, Thaker U, et al. Causes of conjunctivitis and keratoconjunctivitis in Karachi, Pakistan. *Trans R Soc Trop Med Hygiene* 1992;86:317–320.
4. Seal DV, Barrett SP, McGill JI. Aetiology and treatment of acute bacterial infection of the external eye. *Br J Ophthalmol* 1982;66:357–360.
5. Miller IM, Wittreich J, Vogel R, et al, for the Norfloxacin-Placebo Ocular Study Group. The safety and efficacy of topical norfloxacin compared with placebo in the treatment of acute bacterial conjunctivitis. *Eur J Ophthalmol* 1992;2:58–66.
6. Gigliotti F, Williams WT, Hayden FG, et al. Etiology of acute conjunctivitis in children. *J Pediatr* 1981;98:531–536.
7. Weiss A, Brinser JH, Nazar-Stewart V. Acute conjunctivitis in childhood. *J Pediatr* 1993;122:10–14.
8. Sheikh A, Hurwitz B, Cave J. Antibiotics versus placebo for acute bacterial conjunctivitis. In: The Cochrane Library, Issue 2, 2003. Oxford: Update Software. Search date 2001; primary sources Cochrane Controlled Trials Register, Medline, bibliographies of identified trials, Science Citation Index, and personal contacts with investigators and pharmaceutical companies.
9. Bodor FF. Conjunctivitis-otitis media syndrome: more than meets the eye. *Contemp Pediatr* 1989;6:55–60.
10. Barquet N, Gasser I, Domingo P, et al. Primary meningococcal conjunctivitis: report of 21 patients and review. *Rev Infect Dis* 1990;12:838–847.
11. Kettenmeyer A, Jauch A, Boscher M, et al. A double-blind double-dummy multicenter equivalence study comparing topical lomefloxacin 0.3% twice daily with norfloxacin 0.3% four times daily in the treatment of acute bacterial conjunctivitis. *J Clin Res* 1998;1:75–86.
12. Agius-Fernandez A, Patterson A, Fsadni M, et al. Topical lomefloxacin versus topical chloramphenicol in the treatment of acute bacterial conjunctivitis. *Clin Drug Invest* 1998;15:263–269.
13. Montero J, Casado A, Perea E, et al. A double-blind double-dummy comparison of topical lomefloxacin 0.3% twice daily with topical gentamicin 0.3% four times daily in the treatment of acute bacterial conjunctivitis. *J Clin Res* 1998;1:29–39.
14. Adenis JP, Arrata M, Gastaud P, et al. Etude randomisee multicentrique acide fusidique gel ophtalmique et rifamycine collyre dans les conjonctivites aigues. *J Fr Ophtalmol* 1989;12:317–322.
15. Huerva V, Ascaso FJ, Latre B, et al. Tolerancia y eficacia de la tobramicina topica vs cloranfenicol

en el tratamiento de las conjunctivitis bacterianas. *Ciencia Pharmaceutica* 1991;1:221–224.
16. Gallenga PE, Lobefalo L, Colangelo L, et al. Topical lomefloxacin 0.3% twice daily versus tobramycin 0.3% in acute bacterial conjunctivitis: a multicenter double-blind phase III study. *Ophthalmologica* 1999;213:250–257.
17. Gigliotti G, Hendley JO, Morgan J, et al. Efficacy of topical antibiotic therapy in acute conjunctivitis in children. *J Pediatr* 1984;104:623–626.
18. Leibowitz HM. Antibacterial effectiveness of ciprofloxacin 0.3% ophthalmic solution in the treatment of bacterial conjunctivitis. *Am J Ophthalmol* 1991;112:29S–33S.
19. Ofloxacin Study Group III. A placebo-controlled clinical study of the fluoroquinolone ofloxacin in patients with external infection. *Invest Ophthalmol Vis Sci* 1990;31:572.
20. Van Bijsterveld OP, El Batawi Y, Sobhi FS, et al. Fusidic acid in infections of the external eye. *Infection* 1987;15:16–19.
21. Gross RD, Hoffman RO, Lindsay RN. A comparison of ciprofloxacin and tobramycin in bacterial conjunctivitis is children. *Clin Pediatr* 1997;36:435–444.
22. Lohr JA, Austin RD, Grossman M, et al. Comparison of three topical antimicrobials for acute bacterial conjunctivitis. *Pediatr Infect Dis J* 1988;7:626–629.
23. Tabbara KF, El-Sheik HF, Monowarul Islam SM, et al. Treatment of acute bacterial conjunctivitis with topical lomefloxacin 0.3% compared to topical ofloxacin 0.3%. *Eur J Ophthalmol* 1999; 9:269–275.
24. Papa V, Aragona P, Scuderi AC, et al. Treatment of acute bacterial conjunctivitis with topical netilmicin. *Cornea* 2002;21:43–47.
25. Alves MR, Kara JN. Evaluation of the clinical and microbiological efficacy of 0.3% ciprofloxacin drops and 0.3% tobramycin drops in the treatment of acute bacterial conjunctivitis. *Revista Brasiliera de Oftalmol* 1993;52:371–377.
26. Wall AR, Sinclair N, Adenis JP. Comparison of Fucithalmic (fusidic acid viscous eye drops 1%) and Noroxin (norfloxacin ophthalmic solution 0.3%) in the treatment of acute bacterial conjunctivitis. *J Clin Res* 1998;1:316–325.
27. Behrens-Baumann W, Quentin CD, Gibson JR, et al. Trimethoprim-polymyxin B sulphate ophthalmic ointment in the treatment of bacterial conjunctivitis: a double-blind study versus chloramphenicol ophthalmic ointment. *Curr Med Res Opin* 1988;11:227–231.
28. Van-Rensburg SF, Gibson JR, Harvey SG, Burke CA. Trimethoprim-polymyxin ophthalmic solution versus chloramphenicol ophthalmic solution in the treatment of bacterial conjunctivitis. *Pharmatherapeutica* 1982;3:274–277.
29. Gibson JR. Trimethoprim-polymyxin B ophthalmic solution in the treatment of presumptive bacterial conjunctivitis — a multicentre trial of its efficacy versus neomycin-polymyxin B-gramicidin and chloramphenicol ophthalmic solutions. *J Antimicrob Chemother* 1983;11:217–221.
30. Genee E, Schlechtweg C, Bauerreiss P, et al. Trimethoprim-polymyxin eye drops versus neomycin-polymyxin-gramicidin eye drops in the treatment of presumptive bacterial conjunctivitis — a double-blind study. *Ophthalmologica* 1982;184:92–96.
31. Malminiemi K, Kari O, Latvala M-L, et al. Topical lomefloxacin twice daily compared with fusidic acid in acute bacterial conjunctivitis. *Acta Ophthalmol Scand* 1996;74:280–284.
32. Carr WD. Comparison of Fucithalmic (fusidic acid viscous eye drops 1%) and Chloromycetin Redidrops (chloramphenicol eye drops 0.5%) in the treatment of acute bacterial conjunctivitis. *J Clin Res* 1998;1:403–411.
33. Horven I. Acute conjunctivitis. A comparison of fusidic acid viscous eye drops and chloramphenicol. *Acta Ophthalmol* 1993;71:165–168.
34. Hvidberg J. Fusidic acid in acute conjunctivitis. Single-blind, randomized comparison of fusidic acid and chloramphenicol viscous eye drops. *Acta Ophthalmol* 1987;65:43–47.
35. Jackson WB, Low DE, Dattani D, et al. Treatment of acute bacterial conjunctivitis: 1% fusidic acid viscous drops vs. 0.3% tobramycin drops. *Can J Ophthalmol* 2002;37:228–237.
36. Sinclair, Leigh DA. A comparison of fusidic acid viscous eye drops and chloramphenicol eye ointment in acute conjunctivitis. *Curr Ther Res* 1988;44:468–474.
37. Wald ER, Greenberg D, Hoberman A. Short term oral cefixime therapy for treatment of bacterial conjunctivitis. *Pediatr Infect Dis J* 2001;20:1039–1042.
38. Stern GA, Killingsworth DW. Complications of topical antimicrobial agents. *Int Ophthalmol Clin* 1989;29:137–142.
39. Schwab IR, Friedlaender M, McCulley J, et al, and the Levofloxacin Bacterial Conjunctivitis Active Control Study Group. A phase III clinical trial of 0.5% levofloxacin ophthalmic solution versus 0.3% ofloxacin ophthalmic solution for the treatment of bacterial conjunctivitis. *Ophthalmology* 2003;110:457–465.

Justine Smith
Assistant Professor of Ophthalmology
Casey Eye Institute
Oregon Health & Science University
Portland
USA

Competing interests: None declared.

Diabetic retinopathy

Search date September 2002

Simon Harding

QUESTIONS

INTERVENTIONS

DIABETIC RETINOPATHY

Beneficial

Control of diabetes (see glycaemic control in diabetes, p 667)

Control of hypertension (see primary prevention, p 154)

Macular photocoagulation in people with clinically significant macular oedema 754

Peripheral retinal laser photocoagulation in people with preproliferative *(moderate/severe non-proliferative)* retinopathy and maculopathy 752

Peripheral retinal laser photocoagulation in people with proliferative retinopathy 752

Smoking cessation (see primary prevention, p 154)

Likely to be beneficial

Grid photocoagulation to zones of retinal thickening in people with diabetic maculopathy 754

Unknown effectiveness

Macular photocoagulation in people with maculopathy but without clinically significant macular oedema 754

Peripheral retinal laser photocoagulation in people with background or preproliferative (*non-proliferative*) retinopathy without maculopathy 752

VITREOUS HAEMORRHAGE

Likely to be beneficial

Vitrectomy in people with severe vitreous haemorrhage and proliferative retinopathy (if performed early) 756

Unknown effectiveness

Vitrectomy in people with maculopathy 756

To be covered in future updates

Aspirin

Cataract surgery in diabetic retinopathy

Octreotide

Surgery for retinal detachment in diabetic retinopathy

Covered elsewhere in *Clinical Evidence*

Prevention of diabetic retinopathy (see glycaemic control in diabetes, p 667)

In this topic terms used in the UK are written in normal text, and visual acuities are presented in units of metres; where terms used in the USA are different they are written in italics and visual acuities are presented in units of feet (see table 1, p 758).

See glossary, p 756

Key Messages

Diabetic retinopathy

- **Control of diabetes** (see glycaemic control in diabetes, p 667).
- **Control of hypertension** (see primary prevention, p 154).

- **Grid photocoagulation to zones of retinal thickening in people with diabetic maculopathy** One RCT found a significant improvement in visual acuity in eyes treated with grid photocoagulation versus untreated eyes at 12 months and at 24 months. Photocoagulation versus no photocoagulation reduced the risk of moderate visual loss by 50–70%.
- **Macular photocoagulation in people with clinically significant macular oedema** One large RCT has found that laser photocoagulation to the macula versus no treatment reduces visual loss at 3 years in eyes with macular oedema and mild to moderate diabetic retinopathy, with some evidence of greater benefit in eyes with better vision. Subgroup analysis found that focal laser treatment was significantly more effective in reducing visual loss in eyes with clinically significant macular oedema, particularly in people in whom the centre of the macula was involved or imminently threatened.
- **Macular photocoagulation in people with maculopathy but without clinically significant macular oedema** We found no RCTs of macular photocoagulation in this population.
- **Peripheral retinal laser photocoagulation in people with background or preproliferative (*non-proliferative**) retinopathy without maculopathy** We found no RCTs in people with background or preproliferative retinopathy without maculopathy.
- **Peripheral retinal laser photocoagulation in people with preproliferative (*moderate/severe non-proliferative**) retinopathy and maculopathy** RCTs in eyes with preproliferative retinopathy and maculopathy have found that peripheral retinal photocoagulation versus no treatment significantly reduces the risk of severe visual loss at 5 years.
- **Peripheral retinal laser photocoagulation in people with proliferative retinopathy** RCTs have found that peripheral retinal photocoagulation versus no treatment significantly reduces the risk of severe visual loss at 2–3 years. One RCT in eyes with high risk proliferative diabetic retinopathy found that low intensity versus standard intensity argon laser significantly reduced vitreous haemorrhage and macular oedema. It found no significant difference between treatments for visual acuity, although it may have lacked power to detect clinically important effects.
- **Smoking cessation** (see primary prevention, p 154).

Vitreous haemorrhage

- **Vitrectomy in people with maculopathy** The role of vitrectomy in this population remains unclear.
- **Vitrectomy in people with severe vitreous haemorrhage and proliferative retinopathy (if performed early)** One RCT found that early versus deferred (for 1 year) vitrectomy significantly reduced visual loss at 1, 2, and 3 years in eyes with severe vitreous haemorrhage and proliferative retinopathy. Subgroup analysis found significant benefit in people with type 1 diabetes but not those with type 2.

*Terms in italics indicate US definitions

DEFINITION Diabetic retinopathy is characterised by varying degrees of microaneurysms, haemorrhages, exudates *(hard exudates)*, venous changes, new vessel formation, and retinal thickening. It can involve the peripheral retina or the macula, or both. The range of severity of retinopathy includes background *(mild non-proliferative)*, preproliferative *(moderate/severe non-proliferative)*, proliferative and advanced retinopathy (see glossary, p 756). Involvement of the macula can be focal, diffuse, ischaemic (see glossary, p 757), or mixed.

INCIDENCE/ PREVALENCE Diabetic eye disease is the most common cause of blindness in the UK, responsible for 12% of registrable blindness in people aged 16–64 years.[1]

AETIOLOGY/ RISK FACTORS Risk factors include age, duration and control of diabetes, raised blood pressure, and raised serum lipids.[2]

PROGNOSIS Natural history studies from the 1960s found that at least half of people with proliferative diabetic retinopathy progressed to Snellen visual acuity (see glossary, p 757) of less than 6/60 (*20/200*) within 3–5 years.[3–5] After 4 years' follow up, the rate of progression to less than 6/60 *(20/200)* visual acuity in the better eye was 1.5% in people with type 1 diabetes; 2.7% in people with non-insulin requiring type 2 diabetes, and 3.2% in people with insulin requiring type 2 diabetes.[6]

AIMS OF INTERVENTION To prevent visual disability, partial sight and blindness; to improve quality of life, with minimum adverse effects.

OUTCOMES Visual acuity (measured using a Snellen chart, unless otherwise stated). Incidence of visual disability (visual acuity 6/24 [*20/80*] or worse in the better eye), partial sight registration (visual acuity 6/60 [*20/200*] or worse in the better eye), and registrable blindness (visual acuity 3/60 [*10/200*] or worse in the better eye). Much of the published data used eyes as the unit of analysis rather than people. Significant loss of vision is often defined as loss of two or more Snellen lines of acuity (vision measured on standard Snellen chart) roughly equivalent to doubling of the visual angle (visual angle is the angle subtended at the eye of the smallest letter visible by that eye) — a measure used extensively in research.

METHODS *Clinical Evidence* search and appraisal September 2002. Additional papers were identified from manual searches. All trials with sufficient data to allow calculation of numbers needed to treat were included. Where no large trials were found, smaller, less detailed trials were included. Figures for numbers needed to treat and numbers needed to harm refer to the number of eyes rather than patients.

QUESTION What are the effects of treatment for diabetic retinopathy?

OPTION PERIPHERAL RETINAL LASER PHOTOCOAGULATION

RCTs have found that peripheral retinal photocoagulation versus no treatment reduces the risk of severe visual loss in eyes with preproliferative (*moderate/severe non-proliferative*) retinopathy and maculopathy; proliferative retinopathy, and early proliferative retinopathy with high risk characteristics. We found no RCTs in people with preproliferative (*moderate/severe non-proliferative*) retinopathy without maculopathy. We found no evidence that one type of laser is better than another. One RCT in eyes with high risk proliferative diabetic retinopathy

found that low intensity versus standard intensity argon laser significantly reduced vitreous haemorrhage and macular oedema, although the study may have lacked power to detect clinically important effects on visual acuity.

Benefits: **Peripheral photocoagulation versus no treatment:** We found no systematic review but found six RCTs[7–13] (see table 2, p 759) that recruited people with different grades of diabetic retinopathy, and compared different regimens of peripheral retinal photocoagulation versus no treatment or versus deferred treatment. Two RCTs recruited only people with proliferative diabetic retinopathy; both found that peripheral photocoagulation versus no treatment significantly reduced the risk of blindness after 2 or 3 years.[7,8] Two large RCTs recruited people with either preproliferative (see glossary, p 757) (*moderate/severe non-proliferative*) or proliferative retinopathy.[9,10,13] Both found that early photocoagulation versus no early photocoagulation decreased the risk of severe visual loss at 5 years, but in one of the RCTs, the rate of severe visual loss was low and the effect was not significant. A subgroup analysis[14] of one of these RCTs[10,13] found that the benefit was significant in people with type 2 diabetes and with severe preproliferative (*severe non-proliferative*) or early proliferative retinopathy without high risk characteristics (see glossary, p 756). The other two RCTs recruited only people with preproliferative (*moderate/severe non-proliferative*) diabetic retinopathy, but most of the people in these RCTs had diabetic maculopathy.[11,12] Both RCTs found that peripheral photocoagulation versus no treatment significantly reduced the risk of visual deterioration at 5 years. We found no RCTs of photocoagulation in people with preproliferative (*moderate/severe non-proliferative*) retinopathy who have not yet developed maculopathy. **Different types of laser:** We found no systematic review. A large multicentre RCT found no difference in effectiveness between krypton red and argon laser in the treatment of proliferative diabetic retinopathy with new vessels on the disc.[15] A smaller RCT compared argon versus double frequency YAG lasers in 42 eyes with proliferative diabetic retinopathy and found no difference in rates of regression of new vessels after mean follow up of 29 months.[16] **Low versus standard intensity laser:** We found one RCT (50 people; 65 eyes with high risk proliferative diabetic retinopathy) that compared low intensity argon laser (minimum energy to produce barely visible blanching of the epithelium, median 235 mW) versus standard intensity argon laser (median 450 mW).[17] It found no significant difference between treatments in visual acuity (mean visual acuity on logMAR chart [see glossary, p 757] 0.18 in eyes treated with low intensity laser *v* 0.27 in eyes treated with standard intensity laser, $P = 0.231$).

Harms: Adverse effects include loss of visual field and visual acuity,[16,18,19] increased glare,[20] reduced contrast[20,21] and colour sensitivity,[22] temporary choroidal effusion, anterior uveitis, worsening macular oedema, and pain during treatment. Most studies were too small to provide accurate estimates of the frequency of these adverse effects, and they probably overestimate the risks because they used old treatment protocols. In one RCT, using an argon treatment protocol that has since been modified in current practice, constriction of visual field to within 45° of fixation occurred in 5% of eyes

(NNH 20), constriction within 30° in 0%, and loss of vision by two or more Snellen lines in 3% (NNH 33).[9] **Fractionation:** One RCT found that adverse effects (including exudative retinal detachment, choroidal detachment, and angle closure) were reduced if photocoagulation was administered in multiple sessions spaced over time rather than in a single session.[23] **Different types of laser:** We found no clear evidence of different rates of complications with different lasers. Argon blue/green causes temporarily reduced colour sensation in treating surgeons. Dye laser[24] and orange laser (600 nm)[25] may be more painful than argon for peripheral retinal photocoagulation.[23] **Low versus standard intensity laser:** The RCT comparing low versus high intensity laser found that low intensity laser significantly reduced clinically significant macular oedema (see glossary, p 756) and vitreous haemorrhage (see glossary, p 757) compared with standard intensity laser, but found no significant difference for choroidal detachment or neurotrophic keratopathy (clinically significant macular oedema: 1 eye treated with low intensity laser *v* 7 with standard intensity, $P = 0.023$; vitreous haemorrhage: no eyes *v* 6 eyes, $P = 0.009$; choroidal detachment: no eyes *v* 3 eyes, $P = 0.103$; neurotrophic keratopathy: no eyes *v* 2 eyes, $P = 0.224$).[17]

Comment: Limited prospective observational data suggest that peripheral retinal photocoagulation should be repeated until there is evidence of regression.[25] We found no evidence that theoretical advantages with certain lasers are reflected in significant improvements in clinical outcomes. Studies of visual field loss do not consider field loss before laser photocoagulation; one study found significant field loss in people with diabetes before laser compared with people without diabetes ($P < 0.01$).[26] We found one meta-analysis[27] of photocoagulation versus no treatment for diabetic retinopathy; its results are difficult to interpret because it was not based on a published systematic review, it did not include the largest RCT,[10] and it included one RCT of macular photocoagulation.[28]

OPTION MACULAR LASER PHOTOCOAGULATION FOR MACULOPATHY

RCTs have found that laser photocoagulation to the macula versus no treatment reduces visual loss at 2–3 years in eyes with macular oedema and mild to moderate preproliferative *(moderate/severe non-proliferative)* diabetic retinopathy, with some evidence of greater benefit in eyes with better vision. Subgroup analysis in one large RCT found that focal laser treatment versus no treatment was significantly more effective in reducing visual loss in eyes with clinically significant macular oedema, particularly in people in whom the centre of the macula was involved or imminently threatened. Effects of photocoagulation in other categories of maculopathy remain unclear. We found no evidence that one type of laser is better than another in diabetic maculopathy.

Benefits: **Macular photocoagulation versus no treatment:** We found no systematic review. We found three RCTs comparing macular argon laser photocoagulation versus no treatment in eyes with maculopathy, two using focal treatment to micoraneurysms,[28–30] and one using a grid to zones of thickened retina.[31] **Focal treatment to**

microaneurysms: The first RCT (39 people with symmetrical macular oedema and preproliferative [*moderate/severe non-proliferative*] diabetic retinopathy — see glossary, p 757) found that fewer people had visual deterioration after 2 years with photocoagulation versus no treatment, but the difference was not significant (visual deterioration of 30 completers: 7/30 [23%] eyes with laser *v* 13/30 [43%] eyes with no treatment; RR 0.54, 95% CI 0.25 to 1.16).[28] The second and much larger RCT (2244 people with macular oedema plus mild to moderate retinopathy) compared focal laser treatment (see glossary, p 756) using an argon laser versus observation.[30] At 3 years, treatment significantly reduced the risk of moderate visual loss (RR 0.50; NNT 8, 95% CI 7 to 12). Subgroup analysis found that focal laser treatment was significantly more effective in eyes with clinically significant macular oedema (see glossary, p 756), particularly in people in whom the centre of the macula was involved or imminently threatened.[13,32] The benefit was less in eyes with less extensive macular oedema. However, this may have been because both groups had low rates of visual loss from baseline. **Grid laser to zones of retinal thickening:** A single RCT (160 eyes with diffuse maculopathy with or without clinically significant macular oedema) found significant improvement in visual acuity in treated compared with untreated eyes at 12 months (RR 0.14; NNT 4, 95% CI 3 to 8) and at 24 months (RR 0.22; NNT 3, 95% CI 2 to 6).[31] Photocoagulation reduced the risk of moderate visual loss (defined as a doubling of the visual angle, equivalent to loss of about two Snellen lines) by 50–70%.[30,31] **Different types of laser:** We found no systematic review. Several small RCTs have found no difference between argon, diode, krypton red, and dye lasers in people with maculopathy.

Harms: Uncontrolled studies reported that loss of contrast sensitivity and visual acuity occurred after direct application of the laser to the centre of the fovea. We found no accurate estimates of the frequency of adverse effects. **Focal treatment to microaneurysms:** The largest RCT found no significant difference in the frequency of immediate visual loss in treated compared with untreated participants.[30] One prospective observational study reported a 40% reduction in macular function in people undergoing focal argon paramacular treatment.[33] Other complications include laser damage to the centre of the fovea and induction of choroidal neovascularisation, but we found no reliable data on frequency. **Grid laser to zones of retinal thickening:** In the relevant RCT, paracentral grid like scotomas or haze were visible to most people treated with grid photocoagulation, but the data were insufficient to estimate the frequency of this effect.[31]

Comment: The benefits of laser photocoagulation are less notable in people with maculopathy than in those with proliferative retinopathy. RCTs are needed to compare efficacy and harm of focal and grid laser protocols (see glossary, p 756). We found no evidence that theoretical advantages of certain types of laser result in significant improvements in clinical outcomes.

Diabetic retinopathy

QUESTION What are the effects of treatments for vitreous haemorrhage?

OPTION VITRECTOMY

One RCT found that vitrectomy reduced visual loss if performed early in people with vitreous haemorrhage, especially in those with severe proliferative retinopathy. Its role in people with both vitreous haemorrhage and diabetic maculopathy remains unclear.

Benefits: We found no systematic review. **In retinopathy:** We found one RCT comparing early vitrectomy (see glossary, p 757) or deferral of vitrectomy for 1 year in 616 eyes with proliferative retinopathy and recent severe vitreous haemorrhage (see glossary, p 757) (reducing visual acuity to ≤2/60 [*5/200*]).[34] At 1, 2, and 3 years after treatment, eyes in the early treatment group were significantly more likely to have visual acuity of at least 6/12 (*20/40*) than those in the deferred treatment group (at 2 years: RR with vitrectomy *v* deferred vitrectomy for visual acuity < 6/12 0.84; ARR 10%; NNT 10, 95% CI 6 to 29). Subgroup analysis showed significant benefit in people with type 1 diabetes but not in those with type 2 diabetes. **In maculopathy:** We found no RCTs.

Harms: A retrospective study of 260 eyes treated with vitrectomy reported neovascular glaucoma in 6%, retinal detachment in 8%, and cataract in 27%.[35] Glaucoma was more likely in people with associated preoperative retinal detachment. In one RCT, the use of preoperative intravitreal tissue plasminogen activator failed to reduce the rate of complications in 56 patients undergoing vitrectomy for the complications of proliferative diabetic retinopathy.[36]

Comment: None.

GLOSSARY

Advanced retinopathy Retinopathy characterised by tractional retinal detachment (see below), vitreous haemorrhage obscuring fundus details, or both.

Background retinopathy *(mild non-proliferative)* Characterised by microaneurysms, small haemorrhages, and exudates *(hard exudates)*.

Clinically significant macular oedema Characterised by one or more of the following: retinal thickening at or within 500 μm of the centre of the fovea; exudates *(hard exudates)* at or within 500 μm of the centre of the fovea when accompanied by retinal thickening; one or more disc area(s) of thickening extending to within one disc diameter of the centre of the fovea. This is a clinical feature of maculopathy common to many eyes with maculopathy and indicates a significant threat to vision.

Diffuse exudative maculopathy Characterised by thickened oedematous retina at the fovea, often with cystic changes.

Focal exudative maculopathy Characterised by exudates *(hard exudates)* within one disc diameter of the centre of the fovea or circinate rings of exudates *(hard exudates)* within the macula.

Focal laser treatment Laser applied directly to microaneurysms.

Grid laser treatment Laser applied in a grid pattern to zones of retinal thickening and/or zones of capillary non-perfusion.

High risk characteristics (1) New vessels at the disc extending over at least a third of the disc area; and/or (2) new vessels at the disc extending over less than a third of the disc area or new vessels elsewhere extending over at least half of the disc area, both in the presence of vitreous or pre-retinal haemorrhage.

Ischaemic maculopathy Characterised by zones of capillary non-perfusion visible only on fluorescein angiography but often inferred from presence of deep blot haemorrhages within the fovea.

logMAR chart A tool for measuring visual acuity, similar to but more precise than a Snellen chart. The chart is typically read at 4 m and scored from the total number of letters read. A score of 1.0 is equivalent to Snellen acuity 6/60 and indicates that all 5 letters on the top line, but no others, were read. A score of 0.1 is equivalent to Snellen acuity 6/6.

Preproliferative retinopathy Mild, moderate, or severe *(moderate or severe non-proliferative)* depending on number/location of lesions; characterised by cotton wool spots, deep round haemorrhages, venous beading, loops and reduplication, and intraretinal microvascular anomalies.

Proliferative retinopathy Characterised by new vessels at the disc or elsewhere.

Snellen visual acuity The Snellen chart usually includes letters, numbers, or pictures printed in lines of decreasing size, which are read or identified from a fixed distance; distance visual acuity is usually measured from a distance of 6 m *(20 feet)*. The Snellen visual acuity is written as a fraction: 6/18 means that from 6 m away the best line that can be read is a line that could normally be read from a distance of 18 m away.

Tractional retinal detachment Fibrous scar tissue between the vitreous humour and retina pulls the retina away from the underlying retinal pigment epithelium. This type of retinal detachment is most common in the proliferative diabetic retinopathy.

Vitrectomy The vitreous is the normally clear gelatinous material that fills most of the inside of the eye. The vitreous can be affected by bleeding, inflammatory cells, debris, or scar tissue. Vitrectomy involves removal of the abnormal vitreous material.

Vitreous haemorrhage Bleeding into the vitreous of the eye from blood vessels arising from the retina.

REFERENCES

1. Evans J, Rooney C, Ashwood F, et al. Blindness and partial sight in England and Wales: April 1990–March 1991. *Health Trends* 1996;28:5–12.
2. Ebeling P, Koivisto VA. Occurrence and interrelationships of complications in insulin-dependent diabetes in Finland. *Acta Diabetol* 1997;34:33–38.
3. Beetham WP. Visual prognosis of proliferating diabetic retinopathy. *Br J Ophthalmol* 1963;47:611–619.
4. Caird FI, Burditt AF, Draper GJ. Diabetic retinopathy: a further study of prognosis for vision. *Diabetes* 1968;17:121–123.
5. Deckert T, Simonsen SE, Poulsen JE. Prognosis of proliferative retinopathy in juvenile diabetes. *Diabetes* 1967;10:728–733.
6. Klein R, Klein BEK, Moss SE. The Wisconsin epidemiologic study of diabetic retinopathy: an update. *Aust NZ J Ophthalmol* 1990;18:19–22.
7. British Multicentre Study Group. Proliferative diabetic retinopathy: treatment with xenon arc photocoagulation. *BMJ* 1977;i:739–741.
8. Hercules BL, Gayed II, Lucas SB, et al. Peripheral retinal ablation in the treatment of proliferative diabetic retinopathy: a three-year interim report of a randomised, controlled study using the argon laser. *Br J Ophthalmol* 1977;61:555–563.
9. Diabetic Retinopathy Study Research Group. DRS group 8: photocoagulation treatment of proliferative diabetic retinopathy. *Ophthalmology* 1981;88:583–600.
10. Flynn HW Jr, Chew EY, Simons BD, et al. Pars plana vitrectomy in the Early Treatment Diabetic Retinopathy Study. ETDRS report number 17. *Ophthalmology* 1992;99:1351–1357.
11. British Multicentre Study Group. Photocoagulation for diabetic maculopathy: a randomized controlled clinical trial using the xenon arc. *Diabetes 1983*;32:1010–1016.
12. Patz A, Schatz H, Berkow JW, et al. Macular edema — an overlooked complication of diabetic retinopathy. *Trans Am Acad Ophthalmol Otol* 1973;77:34–42.
13. Early Treatment Diabetic Retinopathy Study Research Group. Early photocoagulation for diabetic retinopathy: ETDRS report 9. *Ophthalmology* 1991;98:766–785.
14. Ferris F. Early photocoagulation in patients with either type I or type II diabetes. *Trans Am Ophthalmol Soc* 1996;94:505–537.
15. Bandello F, Brancato R, Lattanzio R, et al. Double-frequency Nd:YAG laser vs argon-green laser in the treatment of proliferative diabetic retinopathy: randomized study with long-term follow-up. *Lasers Surg Med* 1996;19:173–176.
16. Blankenship GW. A clinical comparison of central and peripheral argon laser panretinal photocoagulation for proliferative diabetic retinopathy. *Ophthalmology* 1988;95:170–177.
17. Bandello F, Brancato R, Menchini U, et al. Light panretinal photocoagulation (LPRP) versus classic

panretinal photocoagulation (CPRP) in proliferative diabetic retinopathy. *Semin Ophthalmol* 2001;16:12–18.
18. Pearson AR, Tanner V, Keightey SJ, et al. What effect does laser photocoagulation have on driving visual fields in diabetics? *Eye* 1998;12:64–68.
19. Theodossiadis GP. Central visual field changes after panretinal photocoagulation in proliferative diabetic retinopathy. *Ophthalmologica* 1990;201:71–78.
20. Mackie SW, Walsh G. Contrast and glare sensitivity in diabetic patients with and without pan-retinal photocoagulation. *Ophthalmic Physiol Opt* 1998;18:173–181.
21. Khosla PK, Rao V, Tewari HK, et al. Contrast sensitivity in diabetic retinopathy after panretinal photocoagulation. *Ophthalmic Surg* 1994;25:516–520.
22. Birch J, Hamilton AM. Xenon arc and argon laser photocoagulation in the treatment of diabetic disc neovascularization. Part 2: effect on colour vision. *Trans Ophthalmol Soc UK* 1981;101:93–99.
23. Doft BH. Single versus multiple treatment sessions of argon laser panretinal photocoagulation for proliferative diabetic retinopathy. *Ophthalmology* 1982;89:772–779.
24. Seiberth V, Schatanek S, Alexandridis E. Panretinal photocoagulation in diabetic retinopathy: argon versus dye laser coagulation. *Graefes Arch Clin Exp Ophthalmol* 1993;231:318–322.
25. Cordeiro MF, Stanford MR, Phillips PM, et al. Relationship of diabetic microvascular complications to outcome in panretinal photocoagulation treatment of proliferative diabetic retinopathy. *Eye* 1997;11:531–536.
26. Buckley S. Field loss after pan retinal photocoagulation with diode and argon lasers. *Doc Ophthalmol* 1992;82:317–322.
27. Duffy SW, Rohan TE, Altman DG. A method for combining matched and unmatched binary data: application to randomized, controlled trials of photocoagulation in the treatment of diabetic retinopathy. *Am J Epidemiol* 1989;130:371–378.
28. Blankenship GW. Diabetic macular edema and argon laser photocoagulation: a prospective randomized study. *Ophthalmology* 1979;86:69–75.
29. The Krypton Argon Regression Neovascularization Study Research Group. Randomized comparison of krypton versus argon scatter photocoagulation for diabetic disc neovascularization: the krypton argon regression neovascularization study report number 1. *Ophthalmology* 1993;100:1655–1664.
30. Early Treatment Diabetic Retinopathy Study Research Group. Photocoagulation for diabetic macular edema. *Arch Ophthalmol* 1985;103:1796–1806.
31. Olk RJ. Modified grid argon (blue–green) laser photocoagulation for diffuse diabetic macular edema. *Ophthalmology* 1986;93:938–950.
32. Anonymous. Focal photocoagulation treatment of diabetic macular edema: relationship of treatment effect to fluorescein angiographic and other retinal characteristics at baseline: ETDRS report 19. *Arch Ophthalmol* 1995;113:1144–1155.
33. Ciavarella P, Moretti G, Falsini B, et al. The pattern electroretinogram (PERG) after laser treatment of the peripheral or central retina. *Curr Eye Res* 1997;16:111–115.
34. Diabetic Retinopathy Vitrectomy Study Group. Early vitrectomy for severe vitreous hemorrhage in diabetic retinopathy. Four-year results of a randomized trial: diabetic retinopathy vitrectomy study report 5. *Arch Ophthalmol* 1990;108:958–964.
35. Sima P, Zoran T. Long-term results of vitreous surgery for proliferative diabetic retinopathy. *Doc Ophthalmol* 1994;87:223–232.
36. Le Mer Y, Korobelnik, JF, Morel C, et al. TPA-assisted vitrectomy for proliferative diabetic retinopathy: results of a double-masked, multicenter trial. *Retina* 1999;19:378–382.

Simon Harding
Consultant Ophthalmologist
St Paul's Eye Unit
Royal Liverpool University Hospital
Liverpool
UK

Competing interests: None declared.

TABLE 1 Equivalent UK and US terminology where different.

UK terminology	US terminology
Background retinopathy	*Mild non-proliferative retinopathy*
Preproliferative retinopathy	*Moderate non-proliferative retinopathy*
Severe preproliferative retinopathy	*Severe non-proliferative retinopathy*
Exudate	*Hard exudate*
Snellen visual acuity measured in metres (e.g. 6/24)	*Snellen visual acuity measured in feet (e.g. 20/80)*

TABLE 2 RCTs of peripheral photocoagulation versus no treatment in people with diabetic retinopathy (see text, p 752).

Ref	Number of people (eyes)	Degree of retinopathy*			Comparison	Outcome (at time)	Result* (analyses by number of eyes) (95% CI)
		Preproliferative (Non-proliferative)	Proliferative	Diabetic maculopathy			
7	100 (200)	No	All (bilateral)		Peripheral xenon arc *v* no treatment	Blindness by last assessment (mean around 2 years)	5/100 *v* 17/100 RR 0.29 (0.11 to 0.77) NNT 9 (5 to 31)
8	94 (188)	No	All (bilateral)		Peripheral argon laser *v* no treatment	Blindness (3 years)	7/94 (7%) *v* 36/94 (38%) RR 0.19 (0.09 to 0.41) NNT 3 (3 to 6)
9	1742 (3484)	Yes if bilateral	Yes	Yes	Peripheral + focal photocoagulation *v* no treatment	Severe visual loss (5 years)	90/650 (14%) *v* 171/519 (33%) RR 0.42 (0.34 to 0.53) NNT 6 (5 to 7)
13	3711 (7422)	Yes	Yes	Yes	Various early photocoagulation regimens *v* deferred photocoagulation	Severe visual loss (5 years)	2.6% *v* 3.7%† HR 0.77 (0.56 to 1.06)
10	As above	As above	As above	As above	As above	Vitrectomy rate‡ (5 years)	2.3% *v* 4.0%†

TABLE 2 continued

Ref	Number of people (eyes)	Degree of retinopathy*: Preproliferative (Non-proliferative)	Proliferative	Diabetic maculopathy	Comparison	Outcome (at time)	Result* (analyses by number of eyes) (95% CI)
7	100 (200)	No	All (bilateral)		Peripheral xenon arc *v* no treatment	Blindness by last assessment (mean around 2 years)	5/100 *v* 17/100 RR 0.29 (0.11 to 0.77) NNT 9 (5 to 31)
11	99 (198)	Yes	No	All	Peripheral xenon arc *v* no treatment	Visual deterioration (5 years)	19/60 (32%) *v* 39/60 (55%) RR 0.49 (0.32 to 0.74) NNT 3 (2 to 7)
12	63 (126)	Yes if bilateral	No	Yes	Peripheral laser *v* no treatment	Visual deterioration (26 months)	4/63 (6%) *v* 40/63 (63%) RR 0.10 (0.04 to 0.26) NNT 2 (2 to 3)

In these columns, a blank means that the RCT did not explicitly state if included people had that characteristic. "All": only people with that characteristic were included; "Yes": some people with that characteristic were included; "No": all people with that characteristic were explicitly excluded.
*Where necessary, relative risks were calculated by *Clinical Evidence* using absolute risks stated in each RCT.
†RCT reported percentages and did not provide absolute numbers. Hazard ratio taken from the published report based on Cox proportional hazards model.
‡The indication for vitrectomy changed halfway through the RCT. Initially vitrectomy was performed only after onset of severe visual loss. Later, it was performed 1–6 months after severe vitreous haemorrhage.

Glaucoma

Search date August 2002

Rajiv Shah and Richard Wormald

QUESTIONS

INTERVENTIONS

*No placebo controlled RCTs but strong consensus that treatments are effective.

See glossary, p 767

Key Messages

Primary open angle glaucoma

- **Laser trabeculoplasty (*v* medical treatment)** One RCT found that combined treatment with initial laser trabeculoplasty followed by medical treatment versus medical treatment alone significantly reduced intraocular pressure and deterioration in optic disc appearance, and significantly improved visual fields after a mean of 7 years.
- **Laser trabeculoplasty (*v* surgical treatment)** RCTs found that laser trabeculoplasty reduced intraocular pressures significantly less than surgical trabeculectomy, but found conflicting results for changes in visual acuity after 5–7 years.

- **Surgical trabeculectomy** RCTs found that surgical trabeculectomy versus medical treatment significantly reduced both visual field loss and intraocular pressures, but found no significant difference between treatments in visual acuity after about 5 years. RCTs found that surgical trabeculectomy versus laser trabeculoplasty significantly reduced intraocular pressure, but found mixed effects for changes in visual acuity after 5–7 years. Observational studies have found limited evidence that surgical trabeculectomy may reduce central vision.
- **Topical medical treatment** One systematic review found limited evidence that topical medical treatments versus placebo significantly reduced intraocular pressure after a minimum of 3 months, but found no significant difference between treatments in visual field loss on long term follow up. The systematic review did not clearly define the medical treatments involved.

Normal tension glaucoma

- **Medical treatments for lowering intraocular pressure in normal pressure glaucoma** One RCT found that surgical or medical treatment significantly reduced progression of visual field loss after 8 years.
- **Surgical treatments for lowering intraocular pressure in normal pressure glaucoma** One RCT found that surgical or medical treatment significantly reduced progression of visual field loss after 8 years. However, it found that surgery significantly increased cataract formation.

Acute angle closure glaucoma

- **Medical treatments of acute angle closure glaucoma** We found no placebo controlled RCTs, but strong consensus suggests that medical treatments are effective. One RCT found no significant difference in intraocular pressure after 2 hours with low dose pilocarpine versus an intensive pilocarpine regimen versus pilocarpine ocular inserts. We found no RCTs of other medical treatments.
- **Surgical treatments of acute angle closure glaucoma** We found no placebo controlled RCTs, but strong consensus suggests that surgical treatments are effective. One RCT found no significant difference with surgical iridectomy versus laser iridotomy in visual acuity or intraocular pressure after 3 years.

DEFINITION Glaucoma is a group of diseases characterised by progressive optic neuropathy. It is usually bilateral but asymmetric and may occur at any point within a wide range of intraocular pressures. All forms of glaucoma show optic nerve cupping with pallor associated with peripheral visual field loss. **Primary open angle glaucoma** occurs in people with an open drainage angle and no secondary identifiable cause. **Normal tension glaucoma** occurs in people with intraocular pressures that are consistently below 21 mm Hg (two standard deviations above the population mean). **Acute angle closure glaucoma** is a rapid and severe rise in intraocular pressure caused by physical obstruction of the anterior chamber drainage angle.

INCIDENCE/ PREVALENCE Glaucoma occurs in 1–2% of white people aged over 40 years, rising to 5% at 70 years. Primary open angle glaucoma accounts for two thirds of those affected, and normal tension glaucoma for about a quarter.[1,2] In black people glaucoma is more prevalent, presents at a younger age with higher intraocular pressures, is more difficult to control, and is the main irreversible cause of blindness.[1,3] Glaucoma related blindness is responsible for 8% of new blind registrations in the UK.[4]

AETIOLOGY/ RISK FACTORS The major risk factor for developing primary open angle glaucoma is raised intraocular pressure. Lesser risk factors include family history and ethnic origin. The relationship between systemic blood pressure and intraocular pressure may be an important determinant of blood flow to the optic nerve head and, as a consequence, may represent a risk factor for glaucoma.[5] Systemic hypotension, vasospasm (including Raynaud's disease and migraine), and a history of major blood loss have been reported as risk factors for normal tension glaucoma in hospital based studies. Risk factors for acute angle closure glaucoma include family history, female sex, being long sighted, and cataract. A recent systematic review failed to find any evidence supporting the theory that routine pupillary dilatation with short acting mydriatics was a risk factor for acute angle closure glaucoma.[6]

PROGNOSIS Advanced visual field loss is found in about 20% of people with primary open angle glaucoma at diagnosis,[7] and is an important risk factor for glaucoma related blindness.[8] Blindness results from gross loss of visual field or loss of central vision. Once early field defects have appeared, and where the intraocular pressure is greater than 30 mm Hg, untreated people may lose the remainder of the visual field in 3 years or less.[9] As the disease progresses, people with glaucoma have difficulty moving from a bright room to a darker room, and judging steps and kerbs. Progression of visual field loss is often slower in normal tension glaucoma. Acute angle glaucoma leads to rapid loss of vision, initially from corneal oedema and subsequently from ischaemic optic neuropathy.

AIMS OF INTERVENTION To prevent progression of visual field loss and to minimise adverse effects of treatment.

OUTCOMES Visual acuity; visual fields. Optic disc cupping and intraocular pressure are surrogate outcomes.

METHODS *Clinical Evidence* search and appraisal August 2002.

QUESTION **What are the effects of treatments for established primary open angle glaucoma?**

OPTION **TOPICAL MEDICAL TREATMENT**

One systematic review found limited evidence that topical medical treatments versus placebo significantly reduce intraocular pressure after a minimum of 3 months, but found no significant difference between treatments in visual field loss on long term follow up. The systematic review did not clearly define the medical treatments involved.

Benefits: We found one systematic review (search date 1991, 16 placebo controlled RCTs, 86 comparative RCTs, 5000 people).[10] **Intraocular pressure:** The review found that medical treatment versus placebo significantly reduced mean intraocular pressure after a minimum of 3 months (see comment below; 16 placebo controlled RCTs; mean reduction in intraocular pressure

4.9 mm Hg, 95% CI 2.5 mm Hg to 7.3 mm Hg). **Visual field loss:** The review found no significant difference with medical treatment versus placebo in visual field loss after long term follow up (see comment below; 3 RCTs, 302 people; pooled OR for any worsening of visual field loss 0.75, 95% CI 0.42 to 1.35).

Harms: Systemic adverse effects of topical treatments are uncommon but may be serious, including exacerbation of chronic obstructive airways disease after use of non-selective topical β blockers. Non-selective topical β blockers can also cause systemic hypotension and reduction in resting heart rate.[11]

Comment: We could not identify the types of participants, types of topical medical treatments, or the definition of long term follow up from the systematic review.[10] Two RCTs sponsored by the US National Institutes of Health are under way and have not yet reported any results: The Early Manifest Glaucoma Study and the Ocular Hypertension Treatment Study. The European Glaucoma Prevention Study is also due to present its findings soon.

OPTION LASER TRABECULOPLASTY

One RCT found that combined treatment with initial laser trabeculoplasty followed by medical treatment versus medical treatment alone significantly reduced intraocular pressure and deterioration in optic disc appearance, and significantly improved visual fields after a mean of 7 years. Two RCTs found that surgical trabeculectomy versus laser trabeculoplasty reduced intraocular pressures, but found conflicting results for changes in visual acuity.

Benefits: We found no systematic review, but found three RCTs.[12–14] **Versus medical treatment:** The first RCT (203 people) found that combined treatment (initial laser trabeculoplasty [see glossary, p 767] followed by medical treatment) versus medical treatment alone significantly reduced intraocular pressure (1.2 mm Hg greater reduction in intraocular pressure with combined treatment; $P = 0.001$; CI not provided), significantly improved visual fields (0.6 dB greater improvement with combined treatment; $P < 0.001$; CI not provided), and significantly reduced deterioration in optic disc appearance ($P = 0.005$; CI not provided) after a mean of 7 years.[12] **Versus surgical treatment:** See benefits of surgical trabeculectomy, p 765.

Harms: Adverse effects of laser trabeculoplasty are mild and include a transient rise in intraocular pressure (>5 mm Hg in 91/271 participants) and formation of peripheral anterior synechiae (see glossary, p 767) (in 93/271 participants).[12]

Comment: The first RCT was a multicentre trial with multiple observers, although it is not clear whether these observers were masked to the intervention.[12]

OPTION SURGICAL TRABECULECTOMY

Two RCTs found that surgical trabeculectomy versus medical treatment significantly reduced both visual field loss and intraocular pressures, but found no significant difference between treatments in visual acuity. Two

RCTs found that surgical trabeculectomy versus laser trabeculoplasty reduced intraocular pressure, but found mixed effects for changes in visual acuity. Observational studies have found a reduction in central vision with surgical trabeculectomy.

Benefits: We found no systematic review. **Versus medical treatment:** We found two RCTs.[13,15] One RCT (116 people) compared trabeculectomy (see glossary, p 767) (followed by medical treatment when indicated) versus medical treatment (followed by trabeculectomy when medical treatment failed).[15] It found no significant difference between treatments in visual acuity (P = 0.44; other results presented graphically; CI not provided), but found that trabeculectomy versus medical treatment significantly reduced visual field loss (P = 0.03; other results presented graphically; CI not provided) after a mean of 4.6 years. The second RCT (186 people) compared three treatments: medical treatment (pilocarpine ± timolol ± a sympathomimetic), laser trabeculoplasty (see glossary, p 767), and surgical trabeculectomy.[13] It found that surgical trabeculectomy versus both other treatments significantly reduced intraocular pressures (P = 0.0001; other results presented graphically; CI not provided), but found no significant difference between any of the treatments in visual acuity (results presented graphically) after 5 years. **Versus initial laser trabeculoplasty:** We found two RCTs.[13,14] One RCT (776 eyes with advanced glaucoma; 451 black people, 325 white people) compared surgical trabeculectomy versus laser trabeculoplasty as initial treatments.[14] Initial surgical trabeculectomy was followed by laser trabeculoplasty and repeat surgical trabeculectomy as required; initial laser trabeculoplasty was followed by surgical trabeculectomy as required. Subgroup analysis of the RCT found that in black people initial laser trabeculoplasty versus surgical trabeculectomy significantly improved vision (both visual acuity and visual field; P < 0.01; other results presented graphically; CI not provided), although in white people the RCT found no significant difference between treatments in vision (results presented graphically) after 7 years. The RCT also found that in both black people and white people surgical trabeculectomy versus laser trabeculoplasty reduced intraocular pressure (significance not reported and results presented graphically). The second RCT is described above.[13]

Harms: Surgical trabeculectomy is associated with a reduction in central vision. In one study, 83% of participants lost two lines of Snellen visual acuity.[16] One RCT in people with normal tension glaucoma has found that treatment, including trabeculectomy, versus no treatment significantly increased cataract formation after 8 years (see harms of lowering intraocular pressure in normal tension glaucoma, p 766).[17,18]

Comment: None.

QUESTION **What are the effects of lowering intraocular pressure in people with normal tension glaucoma?**

One RCT found that surgical and/or medical treatment significantly reduced progression of visual field loss after 8 years, but surgery significantly increased cataract formation.

Benefits: We found no systematic review. We found one RCT (140 eyes in 140 people), which compared treatment to reduce intraocular pressure by 30% (with drugs or trabeculectomy [see glossary, p 767], or both; 61 eyes) versus no treatment (79 eyes).[17] Progression of visual field loss was defined by deepening of an existing scotoma, a new or expanded field defect coming close to central vision, or a fresh scotoma in a previously normal part of the visual field. Optic disc changes were photographed and independently assessed by two ophthalmologists. The RCT found that treatment significantly reduced progression of visual field loss after 8 years (7/61 [12%] eyes with treatment *v* 28/79 [35%] eyes with no treatment; RR 0.32, 95% CI 0.15 to 0.70; NNT 5, 95% CI 3 to 9).

Harms: The RCT found that treatment (drugs ± trabeculectomy) versus no treatment significantly increased cataract formation after 8 years (23/61 [38%] with treatment *v* 11/79 [14%] with no treatment; RR 2.71, 95% CI 1.4 to 5.1; NNH 4, 95% CI 2 to 10).[17] Subgroup analysis found that the excess risk of cataract formation was confined to those people treated surgically ($P = 0.0001$; CI not provided). See harms of surgical trabeculectomy, p 766.

Comment: A companion paper[18] to the RCT[17] suggests that the favourable effect of intraocular pressure lowering treatment versus no treatment is evident only when the cataract inducing effect of trabeculectomy is removed. Not all cases of normal pressure glaucoma progress when untreated (40% at 5 years).[18]

QUESTION What are the effects of treatment for acute angle closure glaucoma?

OPTION MEDICAL TREATMENTS

We found no RCTs of pilocarpine versus placebo in acute angle closure glaucoma. One RCT found no significant difference between low dose pilocarpine versus an intensive pilocarpine regimen versus pilocarpine ocular inserts in intraocular pressure after 2 hours. We found no RCTs of other medical treatments for acute angle closure glaucoma.

Benefits: **Pilocarpine versus placebo:** We found no RCTs (see comment below). **Low dose pilocarpine versus intensive pilocarpine:** We found no systematic review, but found one RCT (77 eyes) that compared three groups: initial treatment with low dose pilocarpine (2% pilocarpine drops applied to the eye twice in 1 h); intensive pilocarpine (4% pilocarpine drops applied to the eye every 5 min for 1 h or longer); and pilocarpine ocular inserts (releasing 40 μg pilocarpine/h).[19] All of the people in the RCT also received treatment with intravenous acetazolamide (500 mg iv). The RCT reported no significant difference in intraocular pressures after 2 hours (further data and P value not provided).

Harms: The RCT reported that ocular inserts were associated with local discomfort (statistical data not provided).[19]

Comment: RCTs of pilocarpine versus placebo would be considered unethical. There is a strong consensus that medical treatments that involve pressure lowering drugs (especially those that can be given parenterally, such as iv acetazolamide) are effective in acute angle closure glaucoma. We found no evidence from RCTs to support this view.

OPTION SURGICAL IRIDECTOMY AND LASER IRIDOTOMY

One RCT found no significant difference with surgical iridectomy versus laser iridotomy in visual acuity or intraocular pressure after 3 years.

Benefits: **Surgical or laser procedure versus placebo:** We found no RCTs. **Surgical peripheral iridectomy versus Nd:YAG laser iridotomy:** We found no systematic review, but found one RCT (48 people with uniocular acute angle closure glaucoma) that compared peripheral iridectomy versus Nd:YAG laser iridotomy (see glossary, p 767).[20] It found no significant difference in visual acuity (0.30 logMAR units with peripheral iridectomy *v* 0.57 logMAR units with laser iridotomy; statistical data not provided) and no significant difference in intraocular pressure (intraocular pressure < 21 mm Hg: 15/21 [70%] with peripheral iridectomy *v* 19/27 [72%] with laser iridotomy; RR 1.02, 95% CI 0.71 to 1.46) after 3 years.

Harms: Surgical iridectomy (see glossary, p 767) involves an open operation on the eye, with risk of serious complications, including intraocular infection or haemorrhage. We found no published evidence quantifying these risks. Nd:YAG laser iridotomy is associated with haemorrhage from the iris, pressure spikes, and corneal oedema.[21] Nd:YAG and argon laser iridotomy can produce focal, non-progressive lens opacity.[22] In one RCT, iris haemorrhage was more common with the Nd:YAG laser but pupil distortion, iritis, and late blockage were more common with the argon laser.[23]

Comment: Management of acute angle closure glaucoma is aimed at restoring flow of aqueous humour to the anterior chamber angle and adjacent trabecular meshwork. One RCT found that the mean number of laser burns required to penetrate the iris was six with the Nd:YAG laser and 73 with the argon laser.[23]

GLOSSARY

Laser iridotomy Involves making a hole in the base of the iris (without opening the eye) using either an argon or Nd:YAG laser.

Laser trabeculoplasty Laser trabeculoplasty is performed with a laser, using a contact lens with an internal mirror, which allows focal burning of the pigmented trabecular meshwork.

Surgical iridectomy Opening the eye at the corneal limbus and removing a triangle of tissue from the base of the iris.

Synechiae Adhesions between the iris and surrounding structures, which can form following inflammation. Synechiae may form between the iris and the lens or between the iris and the inner surface of the cornea.

Trabeculectomy A microsurgical procedure in which a partial thickness trapdoor in the sclera is elevated at its junction with the cornea under the conjunctiva. Under the trapdoor, a small hole is fashioned from the sclera to the anterior chamber. This allows drainage of aqueous into the subconjunctival space. An iridectomy is performed at the site of the hole in the sclera.

REFERENCES

1. Sommer A, Tielsch JM, Katz J, et al. Relationship between intraocular pressure and primary open angle glaucoma among white and black Americans. *Arch Ophthalmol* 1991;109:1090–1095.
2. Coffey M, Reidy A, Wormald R, et al. The prevalence of glaucoma in the west of Ireland. *Br J Ophthalmol* 1993;77:17–21.
3. Leske MC, Connell AM, Wu SY, et al. Incidence of open-angle glaucoma: the Barbados Eye Studies. The Barbados Eye Studies Group. *Arch Ophthalmol* 2001;119:89–95.
4. Government Statistical Service. *Causes of blindness and partial sight amongst adults*. London: HMSO, 1988.
5. Tielsch JM, Katz J, Quigley HA, et al. Diabetes, intraocular pressure, and primary open-angle glaucoma in the Baltimore Eye Survey. *Ophthalmology* 1995;102:48–53.
6. Pandit RJ, Taylor R. Mydriasis and glaucoma: exploding the myth. A systematic review. *Diabet Med* 2000;17:693–699.
7. Sheldrick JH, Ng C, Austin DJ, et al. An analysis of referral routes and diagnostic accuracy in cases of suspected glaucoma. *Ophthalmic Epidemiol* 1994;1:31–38.
8. Fraser S, Bunce C, Wormald R, et al. Deprivation and late presentation of glaucoma: case-control study. *BMJ* 2001;322:639–643.
9. Jay JL, Murdoch JR. The rates of visual field loss in untreated primary open angle glaucoma. *Br J Ophthalmol* 1993;77:176–178.
10. Rossetti L, Marchetti I, Orzalesi N, et al. Randomised clinical trials on medical treatment of glaucoma: are they appropriate to guide clinical practice? *Arch Ophthalmol* 1993;111:96–103. Search date 1991; primary source Medline.
11. Diamond JP. Systemic adverse effects of topical ophthalmic agents: implications for older patients. *Drugs Aging* 1997;11:352–360.
12. Glaucoma Laser Trial Group. The glaucoma laser trial (GLT) and glaucoma laser trial follow-up study: results. *Am J Ophthalmol* 1995;120:718–731.
13. Migdal C, Gregory W, Hitchins R, et al. Long-term functional outcome after early surgery compared with laser and medicine in open angle glaucoma. *Ophthalmology* 1994;101:1651–1657.
14. The Advanced Glaucoma Intervention Study (AGIS): 4. Comparison of treatment outcomes within race. Seven year results. *Ophthalmology* 1998;105:1146–1164.
15. Jay JL, Allan D. The benefit of early trabeculectomy versus conventional management in primary open angle glaucoma relative to severity of disease. *Eye* 1989;3:528–535.
16. Costas UP, Smith M, Spaeth GL, et al. Loss of vision after trabeculectomy. *Ophthalmology* 1993;100:599–612.
17. Collaborative Normal-tension Glaucoma Study Group. Comparison of glaucomatous progression between untreated patients with normal-tension glaucoma and patients with therapeutically reduced intraocular pressure. *Am J Ophthalmol* 1998;126:487–497.
18. Collaborative Normal-tension Glaucoma Study Group. The effectiveness of intraocular pressure reduction in the treatment of normal-tension glaucoma. *Am J Ophthalmol* 1998;126:498–505.
19. Edwards RS. A comparative study of Ocusert Pilo 40, intensive pilocarpine and low-dose pilocarpine in the initial treatment of primary acute angle-closure glaucoma. *Curr Med Res Opin* 1997;13:501–509.
20. Fleck BW, Wright E, Fairley EA. A randomised prospective comparison of operative peripheral iridectomy and Nd:YAG laser iridotomy treatment of acute angle closure glaucoma: 3 year visual acuity and intraocular pressure control outcome. *Br J Ophthalmol* 1997;81:884–888.
21. Fleck BW, Dhillon B, Khanna V, et al. A randomised, prospective comparison of Nd:YAG laser iridotomy and operative peripheral iridectomy in fellow eyes. *Eye* 1991;5:315–321.
22. Pollack IP, Robin AL, Dragon DM, et al. Use of neodymium:YAG laser to create iridotomies in monkeys and humans. *Trans Am Ophthalmol Soc* 1984;82:307–328.
23. Moster MR, Schwartz LW, Spaeth GL, et al. Laser iridectomy. A controlled study comparing argon and neodymium:YAG. *Ophthalmology* 1986;93:20–24.

Rajiv Shah
Ophthalmic Surgeon
Australia

Richard Wormald
Consultant Ophthalmic Surgeon
Moorfields Eye Hospital
London
UK

Competing interests: RS none declared. RW has received honoraria for speaking and attending meetings from various pharmaceutical companies producing treatments for glaucoma including Alcon, Allergan, Menke amd Pharmacia.

The following previous contributors of this topic would also like to be acknowledged: Jeremy Diamond, Colm O'Brien.

Ocular herpes simplex

Search date December 2002

Nigel H Barker

QUESTIONS

INTERVENTIONS

See glossary, p 776

Key Messages

Treating epithelial keratitis

- **Debridement** One systematic review has found no significant difference between debridement and placebo in the proportion of people healed, but has found that debridement plus antiviral treatment versus debridement alone significantly increases the proportion of people healed after 7 and 14 days. "Healing" was not clearly defined.
- **Interferons** One systematic review has found that topical interferons (alpha or beta) significantly increase healing after 7 and 14 days compared with placebo. The review found no significant difference between a topical interferon and a topical antiviral agent in healing after 7 days, but found that a topical interferon significantly increased healing after 14 days. "Healing" was not clearly defined.
- **Topical antiviral agents** One systematic review has found that idoxuridine or vidarabine significantly increases healing after 14 days compared with placebo, and that trifluridine or aciclovir significantly increases healing compared with idoxuridine after 7 and 14 days. "Healing" was not clearly defined.

Ocular herpes simplex

Treating stromal keratitis

- **Oral aciclovir** One RCT in people receiving topical corticosteroids plus antiviral treatment found no significant difference between oral aciclovir versus placebo in rates of treatment failure at 16 weeks.
- **Topical corticosteroids** One RCT in people receiving topical antiviral treatment found that topical corticosteroids significantly reduced the progression and shortened the duration of stromal keratitis compared with placebo.

Preventing recurrence of epithelial or stromal ocular herpes simplex

- **Long term (1 year) oral aciclovir** One large RCT in people with at least one previous episode of epithelial or stromal keratitis found that long term oral aciclovir significantly reduced recurrence compared with placebo after 1 year.
- **Short term (3 wks) oral aciclovir** One RCT in people with epithelial keratitis receiving topical trifluridine found no significant difference between short term prophylaxis with oral aciclovir and placebo in the rate of stromal keratitis or iritis at 1 year.

Preventing ocular herpes simplex in people with corneal grafts

- **Oral aciclovir** One small RCT found limited evidence that prophylactic use of oral aciclovir significantly reduced recurrence and improved graft survival compared with placebo.

DEFINITION Ocular herpes simplex is usually caused by herpes simplex virus type 1 (HSV-1) but also occasionally by the type 2 virus (HSV-2). Ocular manifestations of HSV are varied and include blepharitis (inflammation of the eyelids), canalicular obstruction, conjunctivitis, epithelial keratitis, stromal keratitis (see glossary, p 776), iritis, and retinitis. HSV infections are classified as neonatal, primary (HSV in a person with no previous viral exposure), and recurrent (previous viral exposure with humoral and cellular immunity present).

INCIDENCE/ PREVALENCE Infections with HSV are usually acquired in early life. A US study found antibodies against HSV-1 in about 50% of people with high socioeconomic status and 80% of people with low socioeconomic status by the age of 30 years.[1] However, only about 20–25% of people with HSV antibodies had any history of clinical manifestations of ocular or cutaneous herpetic disease.[2] Ocular HSV is the most common cause of corneal blindness in high income countries and is the most common cause of unilateral corneal blindness in the world.[3] A 33 year study of the population of Rochester, Minnesota, found the annual incidence of new cases of ocular herpes simplex was 8.4/100 000 (95% CI 6.9 to 9.9) and the annual incidence of all episodes (new and recurrent) was 20.7/100 000 (95% CI 18.3 to 23.1).[4] The prevalence of ocular herpes was 149 cases/100 000 population (95% CI 115 to 183). Twelve per cent of people had bilateral disease.[4]

AETIOLOGY/ RISK FACTORS Epithelial keratitis results from productive, lytic viral infection of the corneal epithelial cells. Stromal keratitis and iritis are thought to result from a combination of viral infection and compromised immune mechanisms. Observational evidence (346 people with ocular HSV in the placebo arm of an RCT) found that the risk of developing stromal keratitis was 4% in people with no previous history of stromal keratitis (RR 1.0) compared with 32% (RR 10, 95% CI 4.32 to 23.38) with previous stromal keratitis, but that a history of epithelial keratitis was not a risk factor for recurrent epithelial keratitis.[5] Age, sex, ethnicity, and previous experience of non-ocular HSV disease were not associated with an increased risk of recurrence.[5]

PROGNOSIS HSV epithelial keratitis tends to resolve spontaneously within 1–2 weeks. In a trial of 271 people treated with topical trifluorothymidine and randomly assigned to receive either oral aciclovir or placebo, the epithelial lesion had resolved completely or was at least less than 1 mm after 1 week of treatment with placebo in 89% of people and after 2 weeks in 99% of people.[6] Stromal keratitis or iritis occurs in about 25% of people following epithelial keratitis.[7] The effects of HSV stromal keratitis include scarring, tissue destruction, neovascularisation, glaucoma, and persistent epithelial defects. Rate of recurrence of ocular herpes for people with one episode is 10% at 1 year, 23% at 2 years, and 50% at 10 years.[8] The risk of recurrent ocular HSV infection (epithelial or stromal) has also been found to increase with the number of previous episodes reported (2 or 3 previous episodes: RR 1.41, 95% CI 0.82 to 2.42; 4 or more previous episodes: RR 2.09, 95% CI 1.24 to 3.50).[5] Of corneal grafts performed in Australia over a 10 year period, 5% were in people with visual disability or with actual or impending corneal perforation following stromal ocular herpes simplex. The recurrence of HSV in a corneal graft has a major effect on graft survival. The Australian Corneal Graft Registry has found that, in corneal grafts performed for HSV keratitis, there was at least one HSV recurrence in 58% of corneal grafts that failed over a follow up period of 9 years.[9]

AIMS OF INTERVENTION To reduce the morbidity of HSV keratitis and iritis; to reduce the risk of recurrent disease after a first episode; to reduce the risk of recurrent disease; and to improve corneal graft survival after penetrating keratoplasty (see glossary, p 776).

OUTCOMES Healing time; severity and duration of symptoms; severity of complications; rates of recurrence; corneal graft survival.

METHODS *Clinical Evidence* search and appraisal December 2002.

QUESTION **What are the effects of treatments in people with epithelial ocular herpes simplex?**

OPTION **TOPICAL ANTIVIRAL AGENTS**

One systematic review has found that antiviral treatment (idoxuridine or vidarabine) significantly increases healing after 14 days compared with placebo. The review also found that either trifluridine or aciclovir significantly increases healing compared with idoxuridine after 7 and 14 days, but found no significant difference in healing with vidarabine compared with idoxuridine after 7 or 14 days. "Healing" was not clearly defined.

Benefits: We found one systematic review (search date 2000, 96 RCTs, 4991 people; see comment below).[10] **Versus placebo:** The review found that idoxuridine versus placebo significantly increased the healing after 7 days (10 RCTs; OR 4.05, 95% CI 2.60 to 6.30; see comment below) and after 14 days (2 RCTs; OR 4.17, 95% CI 1.33 to 13.00).[10] The review also compared vidarabine versus placebo and found no significant difference in healing after 7 days (numerical data not provided), but found that vidarabine significantly increased healing after 14 days (1 RCT; OR 5.40, 95% CI 1.42 to 20.5). **Versus each other:** The review found that trifluridine versus idoxuridine significantly increased healing after 7 days (3 RCTs; OR 4.74, 95% CI 2.52 to 8.91) and after 14 days (4 RCTs; OR 6.83, 95% CI 3.02 to 15.5).[10] The review also found that aciclovir versus idoxuridine significantly increased healing after 7 days (8 RCTs; OR 5.33, 95% CI 3.33 to 8.53) and after 14 days (11 RCTs; OR 3.71, 95% CI 2.27 to 6.08), but that there was no significant difference with vidarabine versus idoxuridine in healing after 7 days (3 RCTs; OR 1.24, 95% CI 0.72 to 2.00) or after 14 days (3 RCTs; OR 1.24, 95% CI 0.65 to 2.37). **Antiviral treatment plus physical debridement:** See benefits of debridement, p 772.

Harms: The review did not report harms.[10]

Comment: The outcome measure "healing" was not clearly defined.[10] It reported that the number of people involved in the comparison of vidarabine versus placebo was small, although it did not provide any absolute numbers.

OPTION DEBRIDEMENT

One systematic review has found no significant difference between debridement compared with placebo in healing after 7 or 14 days. The review found that debridement plus antiviral treatment significantly increased healing compared with debridement alone after both 7 and 14 days, and that debridement plus antiviral treatment significantly increased healing compared with antiviral treatment alone after 7 days but not after 14 days. "Healing" was not clearly defined.

Benefits: We found one systematic review (search date 2000, 96 RCTs, 4991 people).[10] **Debridement alone:** The review compared different types of physicochemical debridement versus placebo and found no significant difference in healing after 7 days (2 RCTs; OR 1.62, 95% CI 0.72 to 3.61; see comment below) or after 14 days (1 RCT; OR 2.12, 95% CI 0.38 to 12.0).[10] **Debridement plus antiviral treatment:** The review found that physicochemical debridement plus an antiviral agent significantly increased healing compared with physicochemical debridement alone after 7 days (7 RCTs; OR 2.08, 95% CI 1.17 to 3.71) and after 14 days (2 RCTs; OR 10.81, 95% CI 1.81 to 64.5).[10] The review also found that physicochemical debridement plus an antiviral agent significantly increased healing compared with antiviral treatment alone after 7 days (7 RCTs; OR 2.01, 95% CI 1.21 to 3.34), but found no significant difference in healing after 14 days (significance testing not provided). One RCT identified by the review compared debridement plus aciclovir versus debridement plus idoxuridine and found no significant difference in healing after 7 or 14 days (significance testing not provided).

Harms: The review reported that epithelial keratitis (see glossary, p 776) occurred in some people after physicochemical debridement alone (absolute numbers not provided), and limited the use of this treatment.[10]

Comment: The review found that all methods of debriding the corneal epithelium produced similar rates of re-epithelialisation.[10] The variety of treatments used in the review limits the applicability of the summary results. The review included "healed" as an outcome measure without clearly defining this term.

OPTION INTERFERONS

One systematic review has found that topical interferon significantly increases healing compared with placebo after both 7 and 14 days. The review found no significant difference between topical interferon versus a topical antiviral agent in healing after 7 days, but found that topical interferon significantly increased healing after 14 days. The review also found that topical interferon plus a topical antiviral agent significantly increased healing compared with a topical antiviral agent alone after 14 days. "Healing" was not clearly defined.

Benefits: We found one systematic review (search date 2000, 96 RCTs, 4991 people).[10] **Versus placebo:** The review found that topical interferons (alpha or beta) significantly increased healing after 7 days (3 RCTs; OR 2.09, 95% CI 1.15 to 3.81; see comment below) and after 14 days compared with placebo (2 RCTs; OR 3.43, 95% CI 1.30 to 9.02).[10] **Different concentrations:** One RCT identified by the review found no significant difference between low concentration interferon (< 1 MU/mL) and higher concentrations of interferon in healing after 7 days (1 RCT; OR 0.21, 95% CI 0.02 to 2.42).[10] The RCT may have been too small to exclude a clinically important difference. **Versus topical antivirals:** The review found no significant difference in healing after 7 days with topical interferon compared with topical antiviral agents (2 RCTs; OR 1.18, 95% CI 0.29 to 4.75), but found that topical interferon significantly increased healing compared with a topical antiviral agent after 14 days (3 RCTs; OR 3.48, 95% CI 1.06 to 11.4).[10] **Topical interferons plus antiviral agents:** The review found that topical interferon plus a topical antiviral agent significantly increased healing compared with a topical antiviral agent alone (usually trifluridine) after 7 days (8 RCTs; OR 13.3, 95% CI 7.41 to 23.9) but found no significant difference in healing after 14 days (5 RCTs; OR 2.62, 95% CI 0.91 to 7.57).[10]

Harms: The review did not report on harms.[10]

Comment: The outcome measure "healing" was not clearly defined.[10]

QUESTION What are the effects of treatments in people with stromal ocular herpes simplex?

OPTION TOPICAL CORTICOSTEROIDS

One RCT in people receiving topical antiviral treatment found that topical corticosteroids significantly reduced progression and shortened the duration of stromal keratitis compared with placebo.

Benefits: We found one RCT (106 people; see comment below) comparing topical prednisolone sodium phosphate (in decreasing concentrations over 10 wks) versus placebo.[11] All participants received topical trifluridine. It found that prednisolone significantly reduced the persistence or progression of stromal inflammation and shortened the duration of stromal keratitis (see glossary, p 776) compared with placebo (median 26 days with corticosteroid *v* median 72 days with placebo; difference in medians 46 days, 95% CI 14 to 58 days).

Harms: In the RCT, nine people in the steroid group reported adverse effects.[11] Four people developed dendritic epithelial keratitis (see glossary, p 776) and were removed from the trial. Four people developed toxic responses to trifluridine after week 5. These people were not withdrawn but the trifluridine was stopped. One person developed an epithelial defect and was withdrawn. Adverse events were reported in six people receiving placebo. All six were withdrawn from the study (1 person developed dendritic keratitis, 3 people developed an epithelial defect, and 2 people developed allergic conjunctivitis attributed to trifluorothymidine within the first 9 days of the trial).

Comment: The trial did not specify whether or not intention to treat analysis was performed.[11]

OPTION ORAL ACICLOVIR

One RCT in people receiving topical corticosteroids plus antiviral treatment found no significant difference between oral aciclovir compared with placebo in rates of treatment failure at 16 weeks.

Benefits: We found one RCT (104 people with herpes simplex virus stromal keratitis [see glossary, p 776] receiving concomitant topical corticosteroids and trifluridine) of oral aciclovir.[12] The primary outcome was time to treatment failure, defined as worsening or no improvement of stromal keratitis or an adverse event. The RCT found no significant difference between aciclovir compared with placebo in median time to treatment failure (84 days with aciclovir *v* 62 days with placebo; $P = 0.46$; CI not reported), and no significant difference in reported rates of treatment failure by week 16 (38/51 [75%] with aciclovir *v* 39/53 [74%] with placebo; RR 1.01, 95% CI 0.78 to 1.24).[12]

Harms: The RCT found that two people in the placebo group developed adverse effects attributed to trifluridine (epithelial keratopathy in 1 person and an allergic reaction in the other).[12] Other adverse effects reported included pneumonia with possible pulmonary embolus (1 person), congestive heart failure (1 person), diarrhoea (1 person), oedema of the lower extremities (1 person), and anaemia (1 person). Adverse reactions reported in the aciclovir group included toxicity to trifluorothymidine (1 person) and headache (1 person).

Comment: None.

QUESTION **What are the effects of interventions to prevent recurrence in people with epithelial or stromal ocular herpes simplex?**

OPTION **ORAL ACICLOVIR**

One large RCT in people with at least one previous episode of epithelial or stromal keratitis found that long term (1 year) oral aciclovir significantly reduced the risk of recurrences after 1 year compared with placebo. One RCT in people with epithelial keratitis receiving topical trifluridine found no significant difference between short term prophylaxis (3 wks) with oral aciclovir versus placebo in the rate of stromal keratitis or iritis at 1 year.

Benefits: We found no systematic review. We found two RCTs.[6,13] The first RCT (703 immunocompetent people aged ≥12 years who had epithelial or stromal ocular herpes simplex virus in one or both eyes within the preceding 12 months) compared oral aciclovir (400 mg twice daily for 1 year) versus placebo.[13] It found that aciclovir treatment significantly reduced the risk of any type of recurrence after 1 year (19% with aciclovir *v* 32% with placebo; RR 0.55, 95% CI 0.41 to 0.75). Prespecified subgroup analysis (337 people with at least 1 previous episode of stromal keratitis) found that aciclovir significantly reduced the risk of stromal keratitis (see glossary, p 776) compared with placebo, but only in people who had at least one prior episode (14% with aciclovir *v* 28% with placebo; RR 0.48, 95% CI 0.29 to 0.80). The RCT found no rebound in the rate of ocular herpes simplex virus in the 6 months after stopping treatment. The second RCT (287 people with epithelial keratitis (see glossary, p 776) all treated with topical trifluridine) compared a 3 week course of oral aciclovir versus placebo.[6] It found no significant difference in the rate of stromal keratitis or iritis (11% with aciclovir *v* 10% with placebo; RR 1.04, 95% CI 0.52 to 2.10), and no significant difference in the cumulative probability of developing stromal keratitis or iritis at 1 year of follow up (12% with aciclovir *v* 11% with placebo; P = 0.92; CI not reported).

Harms: One RCT found that adverse effects (mostly gastrointestinal problems) were uncommon and occurred with similar frequency in both groups.[13] Thirty two people (15 aciclovir *v* 17 placebo) discontinued treatment because of adverse effects. The most common adverse effect reported was gastrointestinal upset (7 aciclovir *v* 9 placebo).

Comment: None.

QUESTION **What are the effects of interventions to prevent recurrence in people with corneal grafts?**

OPTION **ORAL ACICLOVIR**

One small RCT found limited evidence that prophylactic use of oral aciclovir significantly reduced recurrences and improved graft survival compared with placebo.

Benefits: We found no systematic review. We found one small non-blinded RCT (22 people, 23 eyes, who had received keratoplasty [see glossary, p 776]), which compared oral aciclovir (800 or 1000 mg, 4 or 5 times orally daily, tapered during the first 12 months, for a maximum of 15 months) versus placebo.[14] Oral aciclovir was started before surgery or on the first day after surgery. The RCT found that oral aciclovir significantly reduced the number of recurrences of ocular herpes simplex compared with placebo after a mean follow up of 17 months in people receiving aciclovir and 21 months in those receiving placebo (0% with aciclovir *v* 44% with placebo; $P < 0.01$), and also that aciclovir versus usual care significantly reduced the number of eyes with graft failure (14% with aciclovir treated eyes *v* 56% with placebo; $P < 0.05$; CI not provided).

Harms: None reported.

Comment: None.

GLOSSARY

Epithelial keratitis Inflammation of the cells that form the surface layer of the cornea.

Keratoplasty A procedure in which diseased corneal tissue is removed and replaced by donor corneal material.

Stromal keratitis Inflammation of the middle layer of the cornea. The stroma forms 90% of the corneal substance. It lies between the epithelium and Bowman's membrane anteriorly and Desçemet's membrane and the endothelium posteriorly.

REFERENCES

1. Nahmias AJ, Lee FK, Beckman-Nahmias S. Sero-epidemiological and sociological patterns of herpes simplex virus infection in the world. *Scand J Infect Dis Suppl* 1990;69:19–36.
2. Kaufman HE, Rayfield MA, Gebhardt BM. Herpes simplex viral infections. In: Kaufman HE, Baron BA, McDonald MB, eds. *The Cornea*. 2nd ed. Woburn, MA: Butterworth-Heinemann, 1997.
3. Dawson CR, Togni B. Herpes simplex eye infections: clinical manifestations, pathogenesis, and management. *Surv Ophthalmol* 1976;21:121–135.
4. Liesegang TJ, Melton LJ III, Daly PJ, et al. Epidemiology of ocular herpes simplex. Incidence in Rochester, Minnesota, 1950 through 1982. *Arch Ophthalmol* 1989;107:1155–1159.
5. Herpetic Eye Disease Study Group. Predictors of recurrent herpes simplex virus keratitis. *Cornea* 2001;20:123–128.
6. The Herpetic Eye Disease Study Group. A controlled trial of oral acyclovir for the prevention of stromal keratitis or iritis in patients with herpes simplex virus epithelial keratitis. The Epithelial Keratitis Trial. *Arch Ophthalmol* 1997;115:703–712.
7. Wilhelmus KR, Coster DJ, Donovan HC, et al. Prognosis indicators of herpetic keratitis. Analysis of a five-year observation period after corneal ulceration. *Arch Ophthalmol* 1981;99:1578–1582.
8. Liesegang TJ. Epidemiology of ocular herpes simplex. Natural history in Rochester, Minnesota, 1950 through 1982. *Arch Ophthalmol* 1989;107:1160–1165.
9. Williams KA, Muehlberg SM, Lewis RF, et al. *The Australian Corneal Graft Registry:1996 Report*. Adelaide: Mercury Press, 1997.
10. Wilhelmus KR. Interventions for herpes simplex virus epithelial keratitis. In: The Cochrane Library, Issue 3, 2001. Oxford: Update Software. Search date 2000; primary sources Medline, Central, Embase, Index medicus, Excerpta Medica Ophthalmology, Cochrane Eyes and Vision Group specialised register, The Cochrane Controlled Trials Register, hand searching of reference lists of primary reports, review articles, and corneal textbooks, and conference proceedings pertaining to ocular virology.
11. Wilhelmus KR, Gee L, Hauck WW, et al. Herpetic Eye Disease Study. A controlled trial of topical corticosteroids for herpes simplex stromal keratitis. *Ophthalmology* 1994;101:1883–1895.
12. Barron BA, Gee L, Hauck WW, et al. Herpetic Eye Disease Study. A controlled trial of oral acyclovir for herpes simplex stromal keratitis. *Ophthalmology* 1994;101:1871–1882.
13. Herpetic Eye Disease Study Group. Acyclovir for the prevention of recurrent herpes simplex virus eye disease. *N Engl J Med* 1998;339:300–306.
14. Barney NP, Foster CS. A prospective randomized trial of oral acyclovir after penetrating keratoplasty for herpes simplex keratitis. *Cornea* 1994;13:232–236.

Nigel Barker
Consultant Ophthalmologist
Warrens Eye Centre, Manor Lodge, St Michael, Barbados

Competing interests: None declared.

Trachoma

Search date February 2003

Denise Mabey and Nicole Fraser-Hurt

QUESTIONS

INTERVENTIONS

See glossary, p 784

Key Messages

Interventions to prevent scarring trachoma by reducing active trachoma

- **Promotion of face washing plus topical tetracycline** One RCT found that promotion of face washing plus topical tetracycline reduced the rate of severe trachoma after 1 year compared with topical tetracycline alone, but found no significant difference in the overall rate of trachoma. However, the RCT may lack power to rule out a clinically important effect. One RCT found that face washing plus topical tetracycline reduced the proportion of children with trachoma after 3 months compared with no intervention.
- **Antibiotics (*v* placebo or no treatment)** One systematic review found insufficient evidence on the effects of antibiotics versus placebo or no treatment in active trachoma. However, RCTs were heterogeneous and the review may not exclude clinically important effects.
- **Face washing alone** One RCT found no significant difference between face washing alone and no intervention rate of trachoma in children after 3 months.
- **Oral azithromycin (*v* topical tetracycline)** One systematic review found insufficient evidence on the effects of oral azithromycin versus topical tetracycline in active trachoma. However, RCTs were heterogeneous and the review may not exclude clinically important effects.

Treatment of scarring trachoma

- **Bilamellar tarsal rotation or tarsal advance and rotation (*v* other eyelid surgery)** In people with major trichiasis, one RCT found limited evidence that bilamellar tarsal rotation increased operative success after 2 weeks compared with eversion splinting, tarsal advance, or tarsal grooving, but found no significant difference between bilamellar tarsal rotation and tarsal advance and rotation in operative success after 2 weeks. A second RCT found that bilamellar tarsal rotation increased operative success after 25 months compared with tarsal advance and rotation. In both RCTs, one experienced surgeon performed most of the operations. In people with minor trichiasis, one of the RCTs found that tarsal rotation increased operative success after 25 months compared with cryoablation or electrolysis. One further RCT reporting combined results for major and minor trichiasis found no significant difference in recurrence between bilamellar tarsal rotation and tarsal advance and lid margin rotation after 3 months, although there were more minor complications (lid notching and pyogenic granuloma) with the bilamellar procedure. In this RCT, the procedures were undertaken by less experienced surgeons under supervision.

DEFINITION **Active trachoma** is chronic inflammation of the conjunctiva caused by infection with *Chlamydia trachomatis*. The World Health Organization classification for active trachoma defines mild trachoma (grade TF) as the presence of five or more follicles in the upper tarsal conjunctiva of at least 0.5 mm in diameter. Severe trachoma (grade TI) is defined as pronounced inflammatory thickening of the upper tarsal conjunctiva that obscures more than half of the normal deep vessels. **Scarring trachoma** is caused by repeated active infection by *C trachomatis* in which the upper eyelid is shortened and distorted (entropion) and the lashes abrade the eye (trichiasis). Scarring can exist without entropion/trichiasis but if entropion/trichiasis is present, there will be scarring. Blindness results from corneal opacification, which is related to the degree of entropion/trichiasis.

INCIDENCE/ PREVALENCE Trachoma is the world's leading cause of preventable blindness and is second only to cataract as an overall cause of blindness.[1] Globally, active trachoma affects an estimated 150 million people, most of them children. About 5.5 million people are blind or at risk of blindness as a consequence. Trachoma is a disease of poverty regardless of geographical region. Scarring trachoma is prevalent in large regions of Africa, the Middle East, south west Asia, the Indian subcontinent, and Aboriginal communities in Australia, and there are also small foci in Central and South America.[1] In areas where trachoma is constantly present at high prevalence, active disease is found in more than 50% of preschool children and may have a prevalence as high as 60–90%.[2] The prevalence of active trachoma decreases with increasing age, with fewer than 5% of adults showing signs of active disease.[2] Although similar rates of active disease are observed in boys and girls, the later sequelae of trichiasis, entropion, and corneal opacification are more common in women than men.[2] As many as 75% of women and 50% of men over the age of 45 years may show signs of scarring disease.[3]

AETIOLOGY/ RISK FACTORS Active trachoma is associated with youth and close contact between people. Discharge from the eyes and nose may be a source of further reinfection.[4] Sharing a bedroom with someone who has active trachoma is a risk factor for infection.[5] Facial contact with flies is held to be associated with active trachoma, but studies reporting this relationship used weak methods.[6]

PROGNOSIS Corneal damage from trachoma is caused by multiple processes. Scarring may cause an inadequate tear film and a dry eye may be more susceptible to damage from inturned lashes, leading to corneal opacification. The prevalence of scarring and consequent blindness increases with age, and therefore, is most commonly seen in older adults.[7]

AIMS OF INTERVENTION To prevent active trachoma; to reduce the rate of progression to scarring; to relieve entropion and trichiasis in people with scarring trachoma; to minimise adverse effects of treatment.

OUTCOMES Rates of active trachoma; clinical signs of active trachoma using the World Health Organization grading scale; laboratory evidence of *C trachomatis* infection; eyelid position; degree of entropion/trichiasis. RCTs conducted before 1987 may use definitions of trachoma that differ from the present World Health Organization definition.

METHODS *Clinical Evidence* search and appraisal February 2003.

QUESTION **What are the effects of interventions to prevent scarring trachoma by reducing active trachoma?**

OPTION **PUBLIC HEALTH INTERVENTIONS**

One RCT found that promotion of face washing plus topical tetracycline reduced the rate of severe trachoma after 1 year compared with topical tetracycline alone, but found no significant difference in the overall rate of trachoma. However, the RCT may lack power to rule out a clinically important effect. One RCT found no significant difference between face washing alone and no intervention in children with trachoma after 3 months. The same RCT found that face washing plus topical tetracycline reduced the proportion of children with trachoma after 3 months compared with no intervention. Fly control using deltamethrin reduced the incidence of trachoma after 3 months compared with no intervention in a pilot study for an RCT.

Benefits: We found one systematic review[8] and one additional RCT.[9] The systematic review (search date 1999) identified three RCTs (see comment below) and one pilot study.[8] **Face washing with or without topical tetracycline:** The review identified one cluster RCT (1417 children aged 1–7 years in 6 villages) that compared promotion of face washing plus 30 days of daily topical tetracycline (ointment) versus 30 days of daily topical tetracycline alone.[10] It found that promoting face washing plus topical tetracycline significantly reduced the risk of severe trachoma after 1 year compared with topical tetracycline alone (OR for severe trachoma 0.62, 95% CI 0.40 to 0.97), but this reduction was not significant for all grades of trachoma combined (OR for any trachoma 0.81, 95% CI 0.42 to 1.59).[10] The RCT found that when all participants from intervention and control villages were pooled, children who had a sustained clean face were significantly less likely to have active trachoma than those who never had a clean face or had a clean face at only one follow up visit during the study period (OR 0.58, 95% CI 0.47 to 0.72).[10] The additional RCT (1143 children in 36 communities) compared three groups: daily face washing alone; daily face washing plus daily topical tetracycline (as drops for 1 week each month); and no intervention.[9] Face washing was performed by a teacher.

Trachoma was defined as the presence of at least one follicle or some papillae on the upper tarsal plate (this study predated the present World Health Organization definition of trachoma). Losses to follow up were included in the analysis as being trachoma positive. The RCT found no significant difference between face washing alone and no intervention in terms of the proportion of children with trachoma after 3 months (191/246 [78%] with face washing alone *v* 160/211 [76%] with no intervention; regression analysis, $P > 0.05$).[9] It also found that face washing plus tetracycline drops significantly reduced the proportion of children with trachoma after 3 months compared with no intervention (215/312 [69%] with face washing plus topical tetracycline *v* 160/211 [78%] with no intervention; regression analysis, $P < 0.05$).[9] **Fly control using insecticide:** The systematic review[8] identified one pilot study for an RCT (414 children < 10 years) that compared spraying of deltamethrin for 3 months versus no intervention in two pairs of villages.[6] One pair of villages received deltamethrin or no intervention in the wet season and the other pair received deltamethrin or no intervention in the dry season. There were a total of 191 children under 10 years of age in the control villages and 223 children in the intervention villages. The pilot study found that spraying of deltamethrin significantly reduced the number of new cases of trachoma (World Health Organization classification) after 3 months compared with no intervention (RR 0.25, 95% CI 0.09 to 0.64).[6]

Harms: The review and additional RCT did not report adverse effects.[8,9]

Comment: Cluster randomisation limits the power to detect differences between groups and interpretation of results for individual children.[6,9,10] Two RCTs identified by the systematic review compared antibiotics versus health education plus face washing. It was not possible to extract data relating to the health education and face washing interventions separately.[8] The additional RCT predates the simplified World Health Organization classification of trachoma, limiting applicability of the results.[9]

OPTION ANTIBIOTICS

One systematic review found insufficient evidence on the effects of antibiotics versus placebo or no treatment in active trachoma. The same review found insufficient evidence on oral azithromycin versus topical tetracycline in active trachoma, or on oral antibiotics other than azithromycin versus topical antibiotics in active trachoma. However, trials were heterogeneous and the review may not exclude clinically important effects.

Benefits: We found one systematic review (search date 2001; see comment below).[11] **Versus placebo or no treatment:** The review identified nine RCTs (8 reports; 2177 people) comparing topical or oral antibiotics versus control (no treatment, placebo, or a monthly vitamin tablet) (see table 1, p 786).[9,12–18] The review did not pool results because of statistical and clinical heterogeneity (see comment below).[11] At 3 months, six RCTs found that antibiotic significantly decreased the proportion of people with active trachoma compared with control ($P < 0.05$), whereas three RCTs found no significant difference in active trachoma between antibiotic and control.[11] At 12 months, three RCTs found that antibiotic significantly reduced the proportion of people with active trachoma compared with control ($P < 0.05$), whereas one RCT found no significant difference in active trachoma between antibiotic and control.[11] **Oral azithromycin versus topical tetracycline:** The review identified six RCTs (4 reports; 7666 people) comparing oral azithromycin versus topical tetracycline (see table 2, p 787).[19–22] The review did not pool results because of trial heterogeneity (see comment below).[11] At 3 months, two RCTs found that oral azithromycin significantly reduced the proportion of people with active trachoma compared with topical tetracycline ($P < 0.05$), whereas four RCTs found no significant difference in active trachoma between oral azithromycin and topical tetracycline.[11] At 12 months, two RCTs found that oral azithromycin significantly reduced the proportion of people with active trachoma compared with topical tetracycline ($P < 0.05$), whereas two RCTs found no significant difference in active trachoma between oral azithromycin and topical tetracycline.[11] **Oral antibiotics other than azithromycin versus topical antibiotics:** The review[11] identified three RCTs[13,15,17] of oral antibiotics other than oral azithromycin versus a topical antibiotic (see table 1, p 786). At 3 months, one RCT found that oral antibiotics significantly decreased the proportion of people with active trachoma compared with topical antibiotics ($P < 0.05$), whereas two RCTs found no significant difference in active trachoma between oral antibiotics and topical antibiotics.[11] At 12 months, three RCTs found no significant difference in active trachoma between oral antibiotics and topical antibiotics.[11]

Harms: The review did not report any harms.[11]

Comment: Outcomes were reported by the systematic review at 3 and 12 months.[11] As not all the RCTs collected outcomes at those times, the review reported as 3 months those outcomes measured by RCTs before 6 months, and as 12 months those outcomes measured by RCTs between 6 and 18 months.[11] Where more then one outcome was available, the nearest reported to 3 or 12 months was selected.[11] **Versus placebo or no treatment:** The RCTs were undertaken in various settings. Most were in children attending boarding schools.[11] The RCTs were all of moderate or poor quality and many lacked intention to treat analysis.[11] Antibiotic treatments included topical and oral doses. The review stated "no conclusions can be drawn on the effectiveness of antibiotic treatment for active trachoma but there is a suggestion of a reduction in the point prevalence of the relative risk for those treated with either oral or topical antibiotics."[11] **Oral azithromycin versus topical tetracycline:** Two of the RCTs included in the review were small and of low power.[20,21] The third cluster RCT compared mass treatment, in which people were treated irrespective of disease status and were randomly allocated by village.[21] Correlation analysis found some similarity between individuals within a cluster, limiting the validity of results. The review found no evidence regarding development of bacterial resistance.[11]

QUESTION What are the effects of surgical treatments for scarring trachoma (entropion and trichiasis)?

OPTION LID ROTATION SURGERY

In people with major trichiasis, one RCT found limited evidence that bilamellar tarsal rotation increased operative success after 2 weeks compared with eversion splinting, tarsal advance, or tarsal grooving, but found no significant difference between bilamellar tarsal rotation and tarsal advance and rotation in operative success after 2 weeks. A second RCT found that bilamellar tarsal rotation increased operative success after 25 months compared with tarsal advance and rotation. In both RCTs, one experienced surgeon performed most of the operations. In people with minor trichiasis, one of the RCTs found that tarsal rotation increased operative success after 25 months compared with cryoablation or electrolysis. One further RCT reporting combined results for major and minor trichiasis found no significant difference in recurrence between bilamellar tarsal rotation and tarsal advance and lid margin rotation after 3 months, although there were more minor complications (lid notching and pyogenic granuloma) with the bilamellar procedure. In this RCT, the operations were undertaken by less experienced surgeons under supervision.

Benefits: We found no systematic review but found three RCTs that compared surgical interventions versus each other.[23–25] In the first two RCTs, one experienced surgeon performed most of the operations.[23,24] In the third RCT, surgery was performed by second year ophthalmology residents who were trained in the techniques employed and supervised by an experienced consultant ophthalmic surgeon and senior resident.[25] The RCTs defined operative success as no lashes in contact with the globe in the primary position of gaze and complete lid closure with gentle voluntary effort. The first two RCTs reported outcomes by severity of trichiasis before surgery. The third RCT analysed combined results. **Major trichiasis:** See glossary, p 784. The first RCT (165 Omani villagers, 165 eyelids) compared five surgical techniques: bilamellar tarsal rotation; eversion splinting; tarsal advance; tarsal grooving; and tarsal advance and rotation (see glossary, p 784).[23] It found that bilamellar tarsal rotation significantly increased operative success after 2 weeks compared with eversion splinting, tarsal advance, and tarsal grooving (30/44 [68%] with tarsal rotation *v* 8/25 [32%] with eversion splinting; RR 2.13, 95% CI 1.16 to 3.91; 30/44 [68%] with tarsal rotation *v* 11/41 [27%] with tarsal advance; RR 2.5, 95% CI 1.5 to 4.4; 30/44 [68%] with tarsal rotation *v* 3/32 [9%] with tarsal grooving; RR 7.3, 95% CI 2.4 to 21.8), but found no significant difference between bilamellar tarsal rotation and tarsal advance and rotation in operative success after 2 weeks (30/44 [68%] with tarsal rotation *v* 10/23 [43%] with tarsal advance and rotation; RR 1.57, 95% CI 0.94 to 2.6). However, the trial was underpowered and lacked intention to treat analysis. The second RCT (Omani villagers, 200 eyelids) compared bilamellar tarsal rotation versus tarsal advance and rotation.[24] It found that tarsal rotation significantly increased operative success after 25 months compared with tarsal advance and rotation (HR for failure, tarsal advance and rotation *v* tarsal rotation 3.1, 95% CI 1.9 to 5.2). **Minor trichiasis:** See glossary, p 784. The second RCT (172 eyelids) compared three treatments: tarsal rotation, cryoablation, and electrolysis.[24] It found that tarsal rotation significantly increased operative success after 25 months compared with both other treatments (HR of failure, electrolysis *v* tarsal rotation 6.1, 95% CI 2.9 to 12.8; HR of failure, cryoablation *v* tarsal rotation 7.5, 95% CI 3.6 to 15.4). **Minor and major trichiasis:** The third RCT (153 Ethiopians, 256 eyelids) compared bilamellar tarsal rotation (Weis) versus tarsal advance and rotation (Trabut). In the bilamellar tarsal rotation group, 99/115 (86.1%) of procedures were reported as successful, 12/115 (10.4%) had recurrence, and 4/115 (3.5%) were over corrected after 3 months.[25] In the tarsal advance and rotation group, 107/122 (87.7%) of procedures were reported as successful, 15/122 (12.3%) had recurrence, and 0/122 (0%) were over corrected after 3 months.[25] The RCT reported no significant difference in recurrence between bilamellar tarsal rotation and tarsal advance and rotation after 3 months (P = 0.711).[25]

Harms: Adverse outcomes of interventions were corneal exposure, ulceration, phthisis bulbi (see glossary, p 784), and severe recurrent trichiasis.[23,26] In the first two RCTs that compared different surgical techniques versus each other, major trichiasis and defective closure were more common after eversion splinting, tarsal advance, and tarsal grooving than after bilamellar tarsal rotation and tarsal advance and rotation.[23,24] Cryoablation of the eyelashes can cause necrosis of the lid margin and corneal ulcers. In the RCT in which cryoablation was used it was the only procedure associated with onset of phthisis bulbi (2/57 cases).[24] The third RCT reported the non-serious complications of lid notching and pyogenic granuloma occurred significantly more frequently with the bilamellar procedure (absolute numbers not reported; P = 0.002).[25] No major harms were reported.[25] Further details of harms are summarised in table 3, p 788.

Comment: In the first two RCTs definitions of trichiasis and minor trichiasis are specific to these trials.[23,24] In both RCTs comparing surgical interventions, one experienced operator performed most of the surgery. The evidence of both benefits and harms may not be applicable to different operators, or where the quality of surgical equipment does not match those in the trials. We found one RCT (158 people with major trichiasis) looking at site of surgery that compared village versus health centre based tarsal rotation surgery for major trichiasis.[27] It found that attendance rates were not significantly different between interventions (57/86 [66%] with village based surgery *v* 32/72 [44%] with health centre based surgery; RR 1.5, 95% CI not provided). Problems with the unit of randomisation prevented the calculation of confidence limits for the relative risks stated. The RCT found that there was no significant difference between settings for operative success rate (defined as no evidence of trichiasis) after 3 months (intention to treat analysis by *Clinical Evidence*; 52/86 [60%] with village surgery *v* 30/72 [42%] with health centre surgery; RR 1.4, 95% CI not available).[27]

Trachoma

GLOSSARY

Bilamellar tarsal rotation The upper lid is cut full thickness horizontally in a line parallel and 3 mm from the eyelid margin and running from just lateral to the lacrimal punctum to the lateral canthus. Everting sutures are then placed through all layers of the lid to prevent the margin from turning inwards.
Eversion splinting The lid margin is split posterior to the lashes, the eversion of the anterior section is maintained by sutures tied over a roll of paraffin gauze.
Major trichiasis Lid closure complete; six or more lashes in contact with eyeball.
Minor trichiasis Lid closure complete; one to five lashes in contact with eyeball.
Phthisis bulbi A disorganised, shrunken eye that does not perceive light.
Tarsal advance The lid margin is split posterior to the lashes. The skin, lashes, and orbicularis are freed from the tarsal plate and retracted away from the cornea and are sutured back on to the tarsal plate, leaving a bare area of tarsus to act as the lid margin.
Tarsal advance and rotation The upper lid is everted over a speculum. The tarsal plate is fractured parallel to, and 3 mm from, the lid margin. In this operation the skin and orbicularis are not cut. The short portion of tarsal plate attached to the lid margin is then rotated through 180° and sutured into place to form the new lid margin.
Tarsal grooving A wedge of skin, orbicularis, and tarsus is removed parallel to the lid margin. Sutures through all layers act to evert the lid margin.

Substantive changes

Lid rotation surgery One RCT added;[25] tarsal advance and rotation categorised as Likely to be beneficial.

REFERENCES

1. Thylefors B, Negrel AD, Pararajasegaram R, et al. Global data on blindness. *Bull World Health Organ* 1995;73:115–121.
2. West SK, Munoz B, Turner VM, et al. The epidemiology of trachoma in central Tanzania. *Int J Epidemiol* 1991;20:1088–1092.
3. Courtright P, Sheppard J, Schachter J, et al. Trachoma and blindness in the Nile Delta: current patterns and projections for the future in the rural Egyptian population. *Br J Ophthalmol* 1989;73:536–540.
4. Bobo L, Munoz B, Viscidi R, et al. Diagnosis of *Chlamydia trachomatis* eye infection in Tanzania by polymerase chain reaction/enzyme immunoassay. *Lancet* 1991;338:847–850.
5. Bailey R, Osmond C, Mabey DCW, et al. Analysis of the household pattern of trachoma in a Gambian village using a Monte Carlo simulation procedure. *Int J Epidemiol* 1989;18:944–951.
6. Emerson PM, Lindsay SW, Walraven GE, et al. Effect of fly control on trachoma and diarrhoea. *Lancet* 1999;353:1401–1403.
7. Munoz B, West SK. Trachoma: the forgotten cause of blindness. *Epidemiol Rev* 1997;19:205–217.
8. Pruss A, Mariotti SP. Preventing trachoma through environmental sanitation: a review of the evidence base. *Bull World Health Organ* 2000;78:258–266. Search date 1999; primary sources Medline, Healthstar, and hand searches of reference lists and selected conference proceedings.
9. Peach H, Piper S, Devanesen D, et al. Trial of antibiotic drops for the prevention of trachoma in school-age Aboriginal children. *Annual Report Menzies School for Health Research* 1986;74–76.
10. West S, Munoz B, Lynch M, et al. Impact of facewashing on trachoma in Kongwa, Tanzania. *Lancet* 1995;345:155–158.
11. Mabey D, Fraser-Hurt N. Antibiotics for trachoma (Cochrane Review). In: The Cochrane Library, Issue 1, 2003. Oxford: Update Software. Search date 2001; primary sources Medline, Embase, Cinahl, Science Citation Index, Cochrane Controlled Trials Register, and personal contacts.
12. Attiah MA, el Kohly AM. Clinical assessment of the comparative effect of terramycin and GS 2989 in the mass treatment of trachoma. *Rev Int Trach Pathol Ocul Trop Subtrop Sante Publique* 1973;50:11–20.
13. Darougar S, Jones BR, Viswalingam N, et al. Family-based suppressive intermittent therapy of hyperendemic trachoma with topical oxytetracycline or oral doxycycline. *Br J Ophthalmol* 1980;64:291–295.
14. Dawson CR, Hanna L, Wood TR, et al. Controlled trials with trisulphapyrimidines in the treatment of chronic trachoma. *J Infect Dis* 1969;119:581–590.
15. Foster SO, Powers DK, Thygeson P. Trachoma therapy: a controlled study. *Am J Ophthalmol* 1966;61:451–455.
16. Hoshiwara I, Ostler HB, Hanna L, et al. Doxycycline treatment of chronic trachoma. *JAMA* 1973;224:220–223.
17. Shukla BR, Nema HV, Mathur JS, et al. Gantrisin and madribon in trachoma. *Br J Ophthalmol* 1966;50:218–221.
18. Woolridge RL, Cheng KH, Chang IH, et al. Failure of trachoma treatment with ophthalmic antibiotics and systemic sulphonamides used alone or in combination with trachoma vaccine. *Am J Ophthalmol* 1967;63(suppl):1577–1586.
19. Bowman RJC, Sillah A, Van Dehn C, et al. Operational comparison of single-dose azithromycin and topical tetracycline for trachoma. *Invest Ophthalmol Vis Sci* 2000;41:4074–4079.

20. Dawson CR, Schachter J, Sallam S, et al. A comparison of oral azithromycin with topical oxytetracycline/polymyxin for the treatment of trachoma in children. *Clin Infect Dis* 1997;24:363–368.
21. Schachter J, West SK, Mabey D, et al. Azithromycin in control of trachoma. *Lancet* 1999;354:630–635.
22. Tabbara KF, Abu el Asrar A, al Omar O, et al. Single-dose azithromycin in the treatment of trachoma. A randomized, controlled study. *Ophthalmology* 1996;103:842–846.
23. Reacher MH, Huber MJE, Canagaratnam R, et al. A trial of surgery for trichiasis of the upper lid from trachoma. *Br J Ophthalmol* 1990;74:109–113.
24. Reacher MH, Munoz B, Alghassany A, et al. A controlled trial of surgery for trachomatous trichiasis of the upper lid. *Arch Ophthalmol* 1992;110:667–674.
25. Adamu Y, Alemayehu W. A randomized clinical trial of the success rates of bilamellar tarsal rotation and tarsotomy for upper eyelid trachomatous trichiasis. *Ethiop Med J* 2002; 40:107–114.
26. Reacher MH, Taylor HR. The management of trachomatous trichiasis. *Rev Int Trach Pathol Ocul Trop Subtrop Sante Publique* 1990;67:233–262.
27. Bowman RJ, Soma OS, Alexander N, et al. Should trichiasis surgery be offered in the village? A community randomised trial of village vs. health centre-based surgery. *Trop Med Int Health* 2000;5:528–533.

Denise Mabey
Guy's and St Thomas' Hospital Trust
London
UK

Nicole Fraser-Hurt
Epiconsult Ltd
Nhlangano
Swaziland

Competing interests: None declared.

TABLE 1 **Interventions to prevent scarring trachoma by reducing active trachoma: RCTs of antibiotics compared with no treatment, placebo, or a monthly vitamin tablet in people with active trachoma (see text, p 780).**

Study	Treatment	Route	Dose	Duration	Comparison
9	Tetracycline	Topical	Not stated	Daily for 5 days a month for 3 months	No treatment
12	Tetracycline derivative GS2989	Topical	0.25%	Once every school day for 11 weeks	No treatment
12	Oxytetracycline	Topical	Not stated	Once every school day for 11 weeks	No treatment
13	Oxytetracycline	Topical	1%	Twice daily for 7 consecutive days every month for 12 months	Vitamin pills, orally, 1 dose every month for 12 months
13	Doxycycline	Oral	5 mg/kg	1 dose every month for 12 months	Vitamin pills, orally, 1 dose every month for 12 months
14	Trisulfapyrimidine	Oral	3.5 g/day	3 daily during 3 consecutive weeks	Lactose, orally, 3 daily for 3 weeks
14	Trisulfapyrimidine	Oral	3.5 g/day	3 daily during 3 consecutive weeks	Lactose, orally, 3 daily for 3 weeks
15	Sulfametopyridazine	Oral	0.5 g	Once daily for 5 consecutive days every week for 3 weeks	No treatment
15	Tetracycline	Topical	1%	3 times daily on 5 consecutive days every week for 6 weeks	No treatment
16	Doxycycline	Oral	2.5–4.0 mg/kg	Once daily for 5 consecutive days every week up to 28 doses in 40 days	Placebo once daily for 5 consecutive days every week up to 28 doses in 40 days
17	Sulfafurazole plus sulfadimethoxine	Topical plus oral	15%/100 mg/kg	Twice daily for 5 consecutive days every month for 5 months/biweekly for 5 months	No treatment
17	Sulfadimethoxine	Oral	100 mg/kg	Twice weekly or weekly dose for 5 months	No treatment
17	Sulfafurazole	Topical	15%	Twice daily for 5 consecutive days every month for 5 months	No treatment
18	Tetracycline	Topical	1%	Twice daily for 6 consecutive days every week for 6 weeks	No treatment

TABLE 2 **Interventions to prevent scarring trachoma by reducing active trachoma: RCTs comparing rates of active trachoma and bacteriological infection following oral azithromycin or topical tetracycline (see text, p 780).**

Study	Treatment	Dose	Duration	Comparison	Dose/duration
19	Azithromycin orally	20 mg/kg	1 dose	Topical tetracycline	Twice daily for 6 weeks
20	Azithromycin orally	20 mg/kg	1 dose, or 3 times 1 dose at weekly intervals, or 6 times 1 dose at 28 day intervals	1% topical oxytet/polymyxin plus oral placebo	Ointment once daily for 5 consecutive days monthly for 6 months
21	Azithromycin orally	20 mg/kg up to 1 g	Once a week for 3 weeks	1% topical oxytetracycline	Once daily for 6 weeks
	Women of childbearing age; erythromycin	500 mg twice daily or 250 mg four times daily	14 days	ND	ND
22	Azithromycin orally	20 mg/kg	1 dose	1% topical tetracycline	Twice daily for 5 consecutive days every week for 6 weeks

ND, no data.

TABLE 3 **Summary of harms following surgery for scarring trachoma (see text, p 783).**

	Bilamellar tarsal rotation	Tarsal advance and rotation	Eversion splinting	Tarsal advance	Tarsal grooving
Reference[24]					
Major trichiasis	4/150	4/101	ND	ND	ND
Defective closure	2/150	1/101	ND	ND	ND
Reference[25]					
Major trichiasis	9/86	13/81	ND	ND	ND
Minor trichiasis	3/29	2/41	ND	ND	ND
Over correction	4/115	0/122	ND	ND	ND
Reference[26]					
Major trichiasis	1/44	1/23	7/25	10/41	11/32
Defective closure	2/44	0/23	0/25	0/41	5/32

ND, no data.

HIV infection

Search date November 2002

David Wilkinson and Martin Talbot

QUESTIONS

INTERVENTIONS

PREVENTION

Beneficial

Early diagnosis and treatment of sexually transmitted diseases 791

Likely to be beneficial

Postexposure prophylaxis in healthcare workers* 792

Unknown effectiveness

Presumptive mass treatment of sexually transmitted diesases 792

TREATMENT

Beneficial

Three drug antiretroviral regimens .795

Trade off between benefits and harms

Two drug versus single drug antiretroviral regimens 793

Unknown effectiveness

Early versus delayed antiretroviral treatment with multidrug regimens...............796

*Based on observational studies and indirectly from RCTs in other settings

Covered elsewhere in *Clinical Evidence*

Preventing mother to child transmission (see HIV: mother to child transmission, p 799).

Prophylaxis against specific opportunistic infections (see HIV: opportunistic infections, p 809).

Key Messages

Prevention

- **Early diagnosis and treatment of sexually transmitted diseases (STDs)** One RCT has found that early diagnosis and treatment of STDs reduces the risk of acquiring HIV infection over 2 years.
- **Postexposure prophylaxis in healthcare workers** One case control study found limited evidence suggesting that postexposure prophylaxis with zidovudine may reduce the risk of HIV infection over 6 months. Evidence from other settings suggests that combining several antiretroviral drugs is likely to be more effective than zidovudine alone.
- **Presumptive mass treatment of STDs** One RCT found no difference with presumptive, mass treatment for STDs versus no treatment in the incidence of HIV over 20 months.

Treatment

- **Three drug antiretroviral regimens** One systematic review has found that three drug regimens are beneficial compared with two drug regimens. Some of the reviewed trials included a non-nucleoside reverse-transcriptase inhibitor as a third drug, and some a protease inhibitor.
- **Two drug versus single drug antiretroviral regimens** Large RCTs, with follow up of 1–3 years, have found that two drug regimens (zidovudine plus another nucleoside analogue or protease inhibitor drug) reduce the risk of new AIDS defining illnesses and death compared with zidovudine alone. Adverse events were common in all treatment groups.
- **Early versus delayed antiretroviral treatment** We found no RCTs evaluating early versus delayed treatment with two or three drug regimens. RCTs conducted when zidovudine was the only drug available found no difference between early versus delayed treatment in survival at 1 year.

DEFINITION HIV infection refers to infection with the human immunodeficiency virus type 1 or type 2. Clinically, this is characterised by a variable period (average around 8–10 years) of asymptomatic infection, followed by repeated episodes of illness of varying and increasing severity as immune function deteriorates. The type of illness varies greatly by country, availability of specific treatments for HIV, and prophylaxis for opportunistic infections.

INCIDENCE/ PREVALENCE Worldwide estimates suggest that, by December 1999, about 50 million people had been infected with HIV, about 16 million people had died as a result, and about 16 000 new HIV infections were occurring each day.[1] About 90% of HIV infections occur in the developing world.[1] Occupationally acquired HIV infection in healthcare workers has been documented in 95 definite and 191 possible cases, although this is likely to be an underestimate.[2]

AETIOLOGY/ RISK FACTORS The major risk factor for transmission of HIV is unprotected heterosexual or homosexual intercourse. Other risk factors include needlestick injury, sharing drug injecting equipment, and blood transfusion. An HIV infected woman may also transmit the virus to her baby. This has been reported in 15–30% of pregnant women with HIV infection. Not everyone who is exposed to HIV will become infected, although risk increases if exposure is repeated, at high dose, or through blood. There is at least a two to five times greater risk of HIV infection among people with sexually transmitted diseases.[3]

PROGNOSIS Without treatment, about half of people infected with HIV will become ill and die from AIDS over about 10 years. A meta-analysis of 13 cohort studies from Europe and the USA looked at 12 574 treatment naive people starting highly active antiretroviral therapy with a combination of at least three drugs.[4] During 24 310 person years of follow up, 1094 people developed AIDS or died. Baseline CD4 cell count and baseline HIV-1 viral load were associated with the probability of progression to AIDS or death. Other independent predictors of poorer outcome were advanced age, infection through injection drug use, and a previous diagnosis of AIDS. The CD4 cell count at initiation was the dominant prognostic factor in people starting highly active antiretroviral therapy. Genetic factors have been shown to affect response to antiretroviral treatment, but were not considered in the meta-analysis.[4]

AIMS OF INTERVENTION To reduce transmission of HIV; to prevent or delay the onset of AIDS, as manifested by opportunistic infections and cancers; to increase survival; to minimise loss of quality of life caused by inconvenience and adverse effects of current regimens.

OUTCOMES Incidence of HIV infection, new AIDS diseases, and adverse events; mortality; quality of life.

METHODS *Clinical Evidence* search and appraisal November 2002. In addition, we contacted experts in the field, and reviewed abstract books and CDs for conferences held since 1995. Trials were included if they were designed to detect differences in clinical end points. Where trials using clinical end points were unavailable, we included trials using surrogate markers known to denote higher risk of disease progression. Many trials of new treatments are of short duration, which may reflect the fact that many new drugs have only short term effects. We have included evidence on single and two drug antiretroviral regimens, because it may be useful in countries where three drug treatment is not widely available.

QUESTION What are the effects of preventative interventions?

OPTION EARLY DETECTION AND TREATMENT OF SEXUALLY TRANSMITTED DISEASES

One RCT has found that early diagnosis and treatment of sexually transmitted diseases reduces the incidence of HIV infection.

Benefits: We found no systematic review. One RCT randomised 12 communities in Tanzania (about 12 000 people) to intervention or no intervention.[5] Intervention consisted of diagnosis and treatment of sexually transmitted diseases (STDs) at a local health centre (within 90 minutes walking distance), provision of free condoms during the current STD episode, and health education by healthcare workers trained in STD case management. The RCT found that intervention reduced the risk of acquiring HIV over 2 years (RR 0.58, 95% CI 0.42 to 0.79).

Harms: Syndromic case management (treating people for the most likely causes of their symptoms and signs) may result in wrong or unnecessary treatment. The RCT gave no information on this.[5]

Comment: There is a clear biological mechanism for the synergistic effect of STDs on HIV transmission, and for STD control as an HIV control strategy. The inflammation associated with STDs increases HIV shedding in genital secretions, and treating STDs reduces this inflammation.[6] Syndromic management of STDs is more commonly used in resource limited settings. In resource limited settings a microbiological diagnosis is usually made, allowing specific treatment. The trial, randomised by the community and analysed by the individual, uses regression analysis in an attempt to overcome the associated cluster bias, but it is unclear whether this is successful.

OPTION PRESUMPTIVE SEXUALLY TRANSMITTED DISEASE TREATMENT

One RCT found no evidence of benefit from presumptive, mass treatment for sexually transmitted diseases.

Benefits: We found no systematic review. One RCT randomised 10 communities in Uganda (about 12 000 people) to intervention or no intervention.[7] Intervention consisted of treating all adults with several drugs for sexually transmitted diseases (STDs) every 10 months. Although prevalence of some STDs fell in intervention communities, there was no significant difference in the incidence of HIV between intervention and control communities over 20 months of follow up (incidence of HIV in both groups about 1.5/100 person years; RR intervention *v* control 0.97, 95% CI 0.81 to 1.16).

Harms: Mass treatment means that many uninfected people will be unnecessarily treated for STDs, exposing them to risks of adverse drug reactions and possibly of drug resistance. The RCT gave no information on this.[7]

Comment: The trial's negative finding has several possible explanations other than ineffectiveness of the intervention: a high incidence of symptomatic STDs between rounds of mass treatment; a low population risk for treatable STDs; and intense exposure to HIV. The trial, randomised by the community and analysed by the individual, uses regression analysis in an attempt to overcome the associated cluster bias, but it is unclear whether this is successful. As many as 80% of STDs are unrecognised or asymptomatic.[8]

QUESTION What are the effects of postexposure prophylaxis in healthcare workers?

One case control study found that, in people exposed to HIV, those who became infected were less likely to have received postexposure prophylaxis with zidovudine. Evidence from other settings suggests that combined treatment with several antiretroviral drugs is likely to be more effective than treatment with zidovudine alone.

Benefits: We found no systematic review or RCTs. **Zidovudine alone:** One case control study from the USA and France evaluated outcomes in 31 health workers who acquired HIV infection after occupational exposure, and outcomes in 679 controls who did not acquire HIV infection despite occupational exposure.[9] This study included people followed up for at least 6 months after exposure. HIV infection was less likely in people who received postexposure prophylaxis compared with those who did not (reduction in OR by 81%, 95% CI 43% to 94%). It found that the risk of seroconversion increased with severity of exposure; for example, a penetrating injury with a hollow, bloody needle carried the greatest risk. **Zidovudine plus other antiretroviral drugs:** We found no studies of postexposure prophylaxis using combinations of antiretroviral drugs.

Harms: Short term toxicity (including fatigue, nausea, and vomiting) and gastrointestinal discomfort have been reported by 50–75% of people taking zidovudine and caused 30% to discontinue postexposure prophylaxis.[10] Treatment studies suggest that the frequency of adverse effects is higher in people taking a combination of antiretroviral drugs (reported in 50–90%), which may reduce adherence to postexposure prophylaxis (24–36% discontinued). The risk of drug interactions is also increased. Severe adverse effects, including hepatitis and pancytopenia, have been reported in people taking combination postexposure prophylaxis, but the incidence is not known.

Comment: Case control studies are considered sufficient because experimental studies are hard to justify ethically, and are logistically difficult because of the low rate of seroconversion in exposed people. A summary of 25 studies (22 seroconversions in 6955 exposed people) found that the risk of HIV transmission after percutaneous exposure was 0.32% (95% CI 0.18% to 0.45%) and that the risk after mucocutaneous exposure was 0.03% (95% CI 0.006% to 0.19%).[2] Indirect evidence for postexposure prophylaxis comes from animal studies[9] and from a placebo controlled RCT of zidovudine in pregnant women,[11] which found reduced frequency of mother to child HIV transmission, presumed to be caused in part by postexposure prophylaxis. RCTs have found that combinations of two, three, or more antiretroviral drugs are more effective than single drug regimens in suppressing viral replication. There is also an unquantified risk that zidovudine alone may not prevent transmission of zidovudine resistant strains of HIV. This constitutes the rationale for combining antiretroviral drugs for postexposure prophylaxis.

QUESTION **What are the effects of different antiretroviral treatment regimens?**

OPTION **TWO DRUG VERSUS ONE DRUG ANTIRETROVIRAL REGIMENS**

Large RCTs, with follow up of 1–3 years, have found that two drug regimens (zidovudine plus another nucleoside analogue or protease inhibitor drug) reduce the risk of new AIDS defining illnesses and death compared with ziduvudine alone. Adverse events were common in all treatment groups.

Benefits: We found one systematic review (search date not stated, 6 RCTs, 7700 people),[12] two additional RCTs,[13,14] and one subsequent RCT[15] comparing two drug versus one drug regimens. The review compared zidovudine plus didanosine or zidovudine plus zalcitabine versus zidovudine alone.[12] Participants entered the trials with various stages of infection and were followed for an average of 29 months, during which time 2904 people developed progressive disease and 1850 died. The combined drug regimens significantly delayed disease progression compared with single drug regimens (RR for dieases progression with addition of didanosine 0.74, 95% CI 0.67 to 0.82; RR with addition of zalcitabine 0.86, 95% CI 0.78 to 0.94) and death (RR with addition of didanosine 0.72, 95%

CI 0.64 to 0.82; RR with addition of zalcitabine 0.87, 95% CI 0.77 to 0.98). After 3 years, the estimated percentages of people who were alive and without a new AIDS event were 53% for zidovudine plus didanosine versus 49% for zidovudine plus zalcitabine versus 44% for zidovudine alone; the percentages alive were 68% versus 63% versus 59%. The first additional RCT (940 people) comparing zalcitabine plus saquinavir (a protease inhibitor) versus either drug as monotherapy found that combination treatment significantly reduced clinical disease (RR 0.51, 95% CI 0.36 to 0.72) or death (RR 0.32, 95% CI 0.16 to 0.64) at 1 year.[13] The second additional RCT (1895 people with CD4 positive T cell counts 25–250/mm^3) found that adding lamivudine (a nucleoside analogue) to regimens containing zidovudine (zidovudine alone in 62%, zidovudine plus didanosine or zalcitabine in the rest) significantly reduced the risk of AIDS or death over about 1 year (HR 0.42, 95% CI 0.32 to 0.57).[14] The subsequent RCT (996 people who had never received antiretroviral treatment) compared zidovudine plus indinavir (a protease inhibitor) versus either zidovudine or indinavir alone.[15] It found that combination treatment significantly reduced the rate of progression to AIDS compared with zidovudine alone after a median follow up of 1 year (combination *v* zidovudine: RR 0.30, 95% CI 0.18 to 0.50). It found no significant difference between combination treatment versus indinavir alone (RR 0.77, 95% CI 0.72 to 2.32). We found one additional RCT, which was stopped prematurely because of low study size and power (see comment below).[16]

Harms: Adverse effects such as anaemia and neutropenia were common in all groups in all of the RCTs cited above. Up to a third of participants experienced a serious adverse event, with the highest rates in people with lower CD4 counts. Adverse events led to cessation of blind treatment in about a third of participants. The addition of didanosine to zidovudine versus zidovudine alone increased the risks of nausea (RR 1.8, 95% CI 1.1 to 2.9), abdominal pain (RR 1.6, 95% CI 1.0 to 2.7), and pancreatitis (RR 4.6, 95% CI 1.0 to 22.0). Addition of zalcitabine increased the risk of neuropathy (RR 2.2, 95% CI 1.4 to 3.6).[12] Addition of lamivudine did not significantly increase the rate of adverse events.[14] The subsequent RCT found that frequent adverse effects in all three treatment groups were abdominal pain, fever, asthenia/fatigue, and malaise.[15] Both indinavir alone and indinavir plus zidovudine versus zidovudine significantly increased the risk of kidney stone formation (40/332 [12%] with indinavir or indinavir plus zidovudine *v* 13/332 [4%] with zidovudine; RR 3.08, 95% CI 1.72 to 5.29; NNH 12, 95% CI 6 to 36). Overall, 2.9% of people permanently discontinued some or all of their study treatment because of adverse effects before an AIDS related clinical event.[17]

Comment: We found one RCT (256 people with HIV but not AIDS and with CD4 count 300–500/mm^3) comparing zidovudine plus zalcitabine versus zidovudine alone.[16] It found no significant difference between treatments for AIDS defining events after a median 634 days' follow up (10 AIDS events in total). However, clinically important differences could not be excluded because recruitment and follow up were terminated prematurely and the study size did not meet planned power requirements. Two drug regimens often allow substantial residual viral replication in an environment where drug resistant variants have selective advantage. Resistance to these drugs tends to develop over several months to years.[17] The relevance of this is not fully understood but prior use of, and measurable resistance to, nucleoside analogue reverse transcriptase inhibitors tends to be associated with poorer virological response to new regimens that include drugs of this class.[18–20]

OPTION THREE DRUG REGIMENS VERSUS TWO DRUG REGIMENS

One systematic review has found that three drug regimens are beneficial compared with two drug regimens. Some of the reviewed trials included a non-nucleoside reverse-transcriptase inhibitor as a third drug, and some a protease inhibitor.

Benefits: We found one systematic review (search date 2001, 54 RCTs, 4558 people) comparing different drug regimens.[21] The review identified 12 RCTs comparing three versus two drug regimens. It found that triple therapy significantly improved clinical outcomes compared with double therapy after less than 2 years of follow up (OR 0.6, 95% CI 0.5 to 0.8). The largest RCT identified by the review (3485 people with CD4 counts of 50–350/mm^3 who had never received zidovudine) compared zidovudine plus zalcitabine plus saquinavir versus zidovudine plus zalcitabine or zidovudine plus saquinavir.[22] It found that triple therapy significantly reduced the risk of AIDS or death (RR of AIDS or death 0.50; CI not reported; P = 0.0001). Health related quality of life did not change significantly over 48 weeks for individuals in the triple therapy group (change from baseline –0.4 points for physical health summary and + 1.4 for mental health summary); a deterioration occurred in both dual therapy groups (–2.5 and + 0.1, respectively, for zalcitabine plus saquinavir and –2.2 and + 0.3, respectively, for zidovudine plus saquinavir).[23]

Harms: In the included RCT, about 25% of people in each group had nausea, 10% diarrhoea, 10% vomiting, 10% headache, 4% abdominal pain, and 3% peripheral neuropathy.[22] There was no significant difference between people taking three versus two drugs in other adverse effects (fever, asthenia, anorexia, rash, pruritus, myalgia, insomnia, anaemia, buccal mucosa ulceration, and dyspepsia). The prevalence of clinical lipodystrophy in children is not yet reliably established. One trial in children comparing three versus two drug regimens, with the addition of nelfinavir, reported that the incidence of minor adverse events (vomiting, diarrhoea, cutaneous reaction, fever, and anaemia) were similar with nelfinavir and placebo groups per 100 child years (84.8 with nelfinavir, 84.4 with placebo; P = 0.26).[24] However, all diarrhoea events occurred in the nelfinavir group (P = 0.01).

Comment: Few of the trials used clinical end points. Longer term follow up of people taking protease inhibitors has found abnormal fat distribution, hyperglycaemia, and raised triglyceride and cholesterol concentrations. The clinical significance of these changes is uncertain. Many drugs interact with protease inhibitors because of inhibition of cytochrome P450. There is an urgent need for large RCTs in children. The relevance of lipodystrophy and other metabolic changes in growing children is uncertain. Treatment of children should, wherever possible, be undertaken by experts in paediatric HIV infection.

OPTION EARLY VERSUS DELAYED ANTIRETROVIRAL TREATMENT

One systematic review compared early versus delayed antiretroviral treatment, but the RCTs were all started when zidovudine was the only drug available. Overall, they found no significant difference in the risk of AIDS free survival or overall survival with extended follow up. We found no RCTs exploring this question with two or three drug regimens.

Benefits: We found one systematic review (search date not stated, 5 RCTs, 7722 people with asymptomatic HIV mainly with CD4 counts > 200/mm^3) comparing zidovudine given immediately versus zidovudine deferred until the early signs of AIDS.[25] It found that immediate treatment significantly increased AIDS free survival compared with deferred treatment at 1 year (78/4431 [1.76%] with immediate zidovudine *v* 131/3291 [3.98%] with deferred zidovudine; OR 0.52, 95% CI 0.39 to 0.68), but the difference was not significant at the end of the RCTs (median follow up of 50 months; 1026/4431 [23.2%] with immediate zidovudine *v* 882/3291 [26.8%] with deferred zidovudine; OR 0.96, 95% CI 0.87 to 1.05). Overall survival was similar in the two groups at 1 year (24/4431 [5.4%] with immediate zidovudine *v* 18/3291 [5.5%] with deferred zidovudine; OR 1.22, 95% CI 0.67 to 2.25) and at the end of the RCTs (734/4431 [16.6%] with immediate zidovudine *v* 617/3291 [18.7%] with deferred zidovudine; OR 1.04, 95% CI 0.93 to 1.16).

Harms: A meta-analysis presented pooled toxicity data in terms of events per 100 patient years.[26] In asymptomatic people, early treatment conferred a small but significant increase in the risk of anaemia (RR of haemoglobin < 8.0 g/dL; early *v* deferred treatment 2.1, 95% CI 1.1 to 4.1; AR 0.4 events per 100 person years). There was also a small increase in risk of neutropenia with early treatment (AR 1.1 events per 100 person years; CI not reported; P = 0.07). In symptomatic people, the excess incidence of severe anaemia probably reflected the high doses of zidovudine (1200–1500 mg/day; RR of severe anaemia, high *v* low dose 3.6, 95% CI 1.3 to 10). The authors advised that the toxicity results should be interpreted cautiously, because the results varied considerably.

Comment: No new trials on this question are ongoing. With three drug regimens, rates of AIDS and death are currently low and treatment is known to be beneficial up to and over a 2 year period (see three drug regimens, p 795). Many people feel sufficiently certain about when to start treatment — based on evidence about HIV pathogenesis, resistance, immune regeneration with treatment, and long term adverse effects — and so would not consider randomisation to immediate versus deferred treatment. Decisions on when to initiate multidrug treatment are currently based on our understanding of how HIV induces immune damage, the capacity for immune regeneration while on treatment, the toxicity and inconvenience of treatment, and the risk of resistance, rather than on results of RCTs.

Substantive changes

Three versus two drug regimens One systematic review added;[21] conclusions unchanged.

REFERENCES

1. United Nations AIDS website: http://www.unaids.org (last accessed 7 May 2003).
2. Public Health Laboratory Services. *Occupational transmission of HIV. Summary of published reports.* London: PHLS, December 1997.
3. Centres for Disease Control and Prevention. HIV prevention through early detection and treatment of other sexually transmitted diseases – United States. *MMWR Morb Mortal Wkly Rep* 1998;47:RR12.
4. Egger M, May M, Chene G, et al. Prognosis of HIV-1-infected patients starting highly active antiretrviral therapy: a collaborative analysis of prospective studies. *Lancet* 2002;360:119–128.
5. Grosskurth H, Mosha F, Todd J, et al. Impact of improved treatment of sexually transmitted diseases on HIV infection in rural Tanzania: randomised controlled trial. *Lancet* 1995;346:530–536.
6. Cohen MS, Hoffman IF, Royce RA, et al. Reduction of concentration of HIV-1 in semen after treatment of urethritis: implications for prevention of sexual transmission of HIV-1. *Lancet* 1997;349:1868–1873.
7. Wawer MJ, Sewankambo NK, Serwadda D, et al. Control of sexually transmitted diseases for AIDS prevention in Uganda: a randomised community trial. *Lancet* 1999;353:525–535.
8. Wilkinson D, Abdool Karim SS, Harrison A, et al. Unrecognised sexually transmitted infections in rural South African women: a hidden epidemic. *Bull World Health Organ* 1999;77:22–28.
9. Centers for Disease Control and Prevention. Public health service guidelines for the management of health-care worker exposures to HIV and recommendations for post exposure prophylaxis. *MMWR Morb Mortal Wkly Rep* 1998;47:RR7.
10. Cardo DM, Culver DH, Ciesielski CA, et al. Case-control study of HIV seroconversion in health care workers after percutaneous exposure. *N Engl J Med* 1997;337:1485–1490.
11. Connor EM, Sperling RS, Gelber R, et al. Reduction of maternal–infant transmission of human immunodeficiency virus type 1 with zidovudine treatment: paediatric AIDS clinical trials group protocol 076 study group. *N Engl J Med* 1994;331:1173–1180.
12. HIV Trialists' Collaborative Group. Zidovudine, didanosine, and zalcitabine in the treatment of HIV infection: meta-analyses of the randomised evidence. *Lancet* 1999;353:2014–2015. Search date not stated; primary sources Medline, hand searches of conference proceedings, and personal contact with investigators and pharmaceutical companies.
13. Haubrich R, Lalezari J, Follansbee SE, et al. Improved survival and reduced clinical progression in HIV-infected patients with advanced disease treated with saquinavir plus zalcitabine. *Antivir Ther* 1998;3:33–42.
14. CAESAR Co-ordinating Committee. Randomized trial of addition of lamivudine or lamivudine plus loviride to zidovudine-containing regimens for patients with HIV-1 infection: the CAESAR trial. *Lancet* 1997;349:1413–1421.
15. Lewi DS, Suleiman JM, Uip DE, et al. Randomized, double-blind trial comparing indinavir alone, zidovudine alone and indinavir plus zidovudine in antiretroviral therapy-naïve HIV-infected individuals with CD4 cells counts between 50 and 250/mm^3. *Rev Inst Med Trop Sao Paulo* 2000;42:27–36.
16. Moyle GJ, Bouza E, Antunes F, et al. Zidovudine monotherapy versus zidovudine plus zalcitabine combination therapy in HIV-positive persons with CD4 cell counts 300–500 cells/mm^3: a double-blind controlled trial. The M50003 Study Group Coordinating and Writing Committee. *Antivir Ther* 1997;2:229–236.
17. Brun-Vezinet F, Boucher C, Loveday C, et al. HIV-1 viral load, phenotype, and resistance in a subset of drug-naïve participants from the Delta trial. *Lancet* 1997;350:983–990.
18. D'Aquila RT, Johnson VA, Welles SL, et al. Zidovudine resistance and HIV-1 disease progression during antiretroviral therapy. *Ann Intern Med* 1995;122:401–408.
19. Ledergerber B, Egger M, Opravil M, et al. Clinical progression and virological failure on highly active antiretroviral therapy in HIV-1 patients: a prospective cohort study. *Lancet* 1999;353:863–868.
20. Staszewski S, Miller V, Sabin CA, et al. Virological response to protease inhibitor therapy in an HIV clinic cohort. *AIDS* 1999;13:367–373.
21. Jordan R, Gold L, Cummins C et al. Systematic review and meta-analysis of evidence for increasing numbers of drugs in antiretroviral therapy. *BMJ* 2002;324:757–760. Search date 2001; primary sources Medline, the Cochrane Library, Embase, CINAHL, PsychLIT, Healthstar, appropriate internet sites such as AIDSTRIALS, citation lists, and contact with pharmaceutical companies.
22. Stellbrink H-J, Hawkins D, Clumeck N, et al. Randomized, multicentre phase III study of saquinavir plus zidovudine plus zalcitabine in previously untreated or minimally pretreated HIV-infected patients. *Clin Drug Invest* 2000;20:295–307.
23. Revicki DA, Moyle G, Stellbrink HJ, et al. Quality of life outcomes of combination zalcitabine–zidovudine, saquinavir–zidovudine, and saquinavir–zalcitabine–zidovudine therapy for HIV-infected adults with CD4 cell counts between 50 and 350/mm^3. *AIDS* 1999;13:851–858.
24. Anonymous. PENTA comparison of dual nucleoside-analogue reverse transcriptase inhibitor regimens with and without nelfinavir in children with HIV-1 who have not previously been treated: the PENTA 5 randomised trial. *Lancet* 2002;359:733–740.
25. Darbyshire J, Foulkes M, Peto R, et al. Immediate versus deferred zidovudine (AZT) in asymptomatic or mildly symptomatic HIV infected adults. In: The Cochrane Library, Issue 4, 2000. Oxford: Update Software. Search date not stated; primary sources Medline, hand searches of conference abstracts, and contact with investigators and pharmaceutical companies.
26. Ioannidis JP, Cappelleri JC, Lau J, et al. Early or deferred zidovudine therapy in HIV-infected patients without an AIDS-defining illness: a meta-analysis. *Ann Intern Med* 1995;122:856–866. Search date 1994; primary sources Medline, AIDSLine, AIDSTrials, AIDSDrugs, CHEMID, hand searches of current contents, and international conferences on AIDS.

HIV infection

David Wilkinson
Professor
Pro Vice Chancellor and Vice President
Division of Health Sciences
University of South Australia
Adelaide
Australia

Martin Talbot
Consultant Physician in Genito-urinary Medicine/HIV and Director of Undergraduate Medical Education
Sheffield Teaching Hospitals
Sheffield
UK

Competing interests: None declared.

The following previous contributors of this topic would like to be acknowledged: Andrew Philips, Margaret Johnson, and Bazian Ltd.

HIV: mother to child transmission

Search date September 2002

Jimmy Volmink

QUESTIONS

INTERVENTIONS

See glossary, p 805

Key Messages

- **Antiretroviral drugs** One systematic review has found that zidovudine versus placebo significantly reduces the incidence of HIV infection in infants. One RCT has found that the longer versus shorter courses of zidovudine (long–long versus short–short courses) given to mother and infant significantly reduces the incidence of HIV in infants. One RCT has found that nevirapine versus zidovudine given to the mother and to her newborn significantly reduces the risk of HIV transmission. One RCT found no additional advantage in giving nevirapine to the mother and baby when transmission rates are already reduced by mothers receiving standard antiretroviral treatment. One RCT has found that zidovudine plus lamivudine versus placebo given in the antenatal and intrapartum period, or in the intrapartum and postpartum period, significantly reduces the risk of transmission of HIV.
- **Avoiding breast feeding** One RCT in women with HIV who had access to clean water and health education has found that formula feeding versus breast feeding significantly reduces the incidence of HIV in infants after 24 months without increasing infant mortality.
- **Elective caesarean section** One RCT found limited evidence that elective caesarean section versus vaginal delivery in women with HIV reduced the incidence of HIV in infants at 18 months.
- **Immunotherapy** One RCT found no significant difference in the incidence of HIV in infants of mothers taking hyperimmune globulin (HIVIG) versus immunoglobulin without HIV antibody (IVIG) in addition to a standard zidovudine regimen, but it may have been too small to exclude a clinically important difference.
- **Vaginal microbicides** We found insufficient evidence about the effects of vaginal microbicides on the transmission of HIV to infants.
- **Vitamin supplements** RCTs found no significant difference in the incidence of HIV at birth, 6 weeks, or 3 months in the infants of pregnant women given vitamin A or multivitamins versus placebo.

HIV: mother to child transmission

DEFINITION Mother to child transmission of HIV-1 (see glossary, p 805) infection can occur during pregnancy in the intrapartum period, or postnatally through breast feeding.[1] By contrast, HIV-2 (see glossary, p 805) is rarely transmitted from mother to child.[2] Infected children usually have no symptoms and signs of HIV at birth, but develop them over subsequent months or years.[3]

INCIDENCE/ PREVALENCE A review of 13 cohorts found that the risk of mother to child transmission of HIV without antiviral treatment is on average about 15–20% in Europe, 15–30% in the USA, and 25–35% in Africa.[4] The risk of transmission is estimated to be between 15 and 30% during pregnancy, with an additional risk of about 10–20% postpartum through breast feeding.[5] It has been estimated that 800 000 children below the age of 15 years were newly infected with HIV during 2001, bringing the total number of children with HIV/AIDS to 3 million worldwide.[6] Most of these children were infected from their mother and 90% live in sub-Saharan Africa.

AETIOLOGY/ RISK FACTORS Transmission of HIV to children is more likely if the mother has a high viral load.[1,7,8] Women with detectable viraemia (by p24 antigen or culture) have double the risk of transmitting HIV-1 to their infants than those who do not.[1] Breast feeding has also been shown in prospective studies to be a risk factor.[9,10] Other risk factors include sexually transmitted diseases, chorioamnionitis, prolonged rupture of membranes, and vaginal mode of delivery.[11–15]

PROGNOSIS About 25% of infants infected with HIV progress rapidly to AIDS or death in the first year. Some survive beyond 12 years of age.[3] One European study found a mortality of 15% in the first year of life and a mortality of 28% by the age of 5 years.[16] A recent report estimated the mortality attributable to HIV/AIDS in children under 5 years of age in sub-Saharan Africa after correcting for competing causes of mortality.[17] HIV accounted for 2% of deaths in 1990 rising significantly to almost 8% in 1999. Five countries (Botswana, Namibia, Swaziland, Zambia, and Zimbabwe) had rates of HIV attributable mortality in excess of 30/1000 in children under the age of 5 years.

AIMS OF INTERVENTION To reduce mother to child transmission of HIV and improve infant survival, with minimal adverse effects.

OUTCOMES HIV infection status of the child; infant morbidity and mortality; maternal morbidity and mortality; adverse effects of treatment.

METHODS *Clinical Evidence* search and appraisal September 2002.

QUESTION **What are the effects of measures to reduce mother to child transmission of HIV?**

OPTION **ANTIRETROVIRAL DRUGS**

One systematic review has found that zidovudine versus placebo significantly reduces the incidence of HIV in infants. One RCT has found that the longer versus shorter courses of zidovudine (long–long versus short–short courses) given to mother and infant significantly reduces the incidence of HIV in infants. One RCT has found that nevirapine versus zidovudine given to the mother and to her newborn significantly reduces

the risk of HIV transmission. One RCT found no additional advantage in giving nevirapine to the mother and baby when transmission rates are already reduced by mothers receiving standard antiretroviral treatment. One RCT has found that zidovudine plus lamivudine versus placebo given in the antenatal and intrapartum period, or in the intrapartum and postpartum period, significantly reduces the risk of transmission of HIV.

Benefits: **Zidovudine versus placebo:** We found one systematic review (search date 2001, 4 RCTs, 1585 women) that compared zidovudine versus placebo given to the mother before, during, or after labour (see table 1, p 808).[18] In one of the included RCTs, infants of mothers receiving zidovudine were also given zidovudine for 6 weeks after birth.[19] Meta-analysis found that zidovudine versus placebo significantly reduced the incidence of HIV in infants (AR 79/616 [13%] with zidovudine *v* 150/634 [24%]; RR 0.54, 95% CI 0.42 to 0.69). The results were still significant when the RCT of zidovudine that used the most intensive regimen[19] was excluded from the analysis (combined results for less intensive regimens *v* placebo: AR 70/495 [14%] *v* 119/507 [23%]; RR 0.60, 95% CI 0.46 to 0.79).[20–22] The effect of zidovudine versus placebo was similar in reducing the incidence of HIV in infants from breast feeding and non-breastfeeding mothers (breast feeding RR 0.62, 95% CI 0.46 to 0.85; non-breastfeeding RR 0.50, 95% CI 0.30 to 0.85). **Alternative zidovudine regimens:** One RCT (1437 women) compared four different zidovudine regimens; zidovudine was given to mothers from a specific time in gestation until delivery and to the infant until a specific age: "short–short" course (mother from 35 wks, infant for up to 3 days); "long–long" (mother from 28 wks, infant for up to 6 wks); "short–long" (mother from 35 wks, infant for up to 6 wks); and "long–short" (mother from 28 wks, infant for up to 3 days). The RCT found that a "long–long" course versus a "short–short" course significantly reduced the number of infants with HIV (AR 9/220 [4%] with long course *v* 24/229 [10%] with short course; RR 2.56, 95% CI 1.22 to 5.39). As the short–short regimen seemed not to reduce transmission of HIV it was discontinued at the first interim analysis. The trial found no significant difference between a "long–long" versus "short–long" (26/401 [7%] with "long–long" *v* 29/338 [9%] with "short–long" course; RR 1.32, 95% CI 0.80 to 2.20) or versus a "long–short" (26/401 [7%] with "long–long" *v* 16/340 [5%] with "long–short" course; RR 0.73, 95% CI 0.40 to 1.33).[23] **Nevirapine:** The systematic review[18] identified one unblinded RCT (626 women from a predominantly breastfeeding population in Uganda) that compared zidovudine versus nevirapine.[24] It found that nevirapine given to mothers as a single oral dose at the onset of labour and to infants as a single dose within 72 hours of birth versus zidovudine given orally to women during labour and to their newborns for 7 days after birth, significantly reduced the number of infants with HIV at 14–16 weeks (AR 37/246 [15%] with nevirapine *v* 65/250 [26%] with zidovudine; RR 0.58, 95% CI 0.40 to 0.83). However, an RCT of the same nevirapine regimen conducted in the USA, Europe, Brazil, and the Bahamas among 1506 non-breastfeeding women who were already receiving standard antiretroviral treatment found no additional benefit.[25] After 6 months' follow up, the transmission risk in the nevirapine versus placebo arm (AR 9/631 [1.4%] with addition of nevirapine v 10/617 [1.6%] with addition of placebo; ARR −0.2, 95% CI −1.5 to +1.2; RR 0.88, 95% CI 0.36 to 2.15). The trial was stopped early because it was considered unlikely that a clinically important effect could be detected given the low overall HIV transmission rate. Only 1270 (84.3%) women eventually received the study treatment. **Combination antiretroviral regimens:** One RCT (1797 predominantly breastfeeding women in South Africa, Uganda, and Tanzania) compared zidovudine plus lamivudine (3C) versus placebo.[26] This combination of antiretroviral drugs reduced the risk of HIV transmission at 6 weeks when administered in the antenatal (from 36 wks), intrapartum, and postpartum (to mother and baby for 1 wk) period (regimen A) (AR 16/281 [5.7%] with zidovudine plus lamivudine v 40/261 [15.3%] with placebo; RR 0.37, 95% CI 0.21 to 0.65; NNT 11, 95% CI 7 to 24) and during the intrapartum and postpartum period (regimen B) (AR 24/270 [8.9%] with zidovudine plus lamivudine v 40/261 [15.3%] with placebo; RR 0.58, 95% CI 0.36 to 0.94; NNT 16, 95% CI 9 to 126). The RCT found that zidovudine plus lamivudine given during the intrapartum period alone (regimen C) did not significantly affect the risk of transmission (AR 40/282 [14.2%] with zidovudine plus lamivudine v 40/261 [15.3%] with placebo; RR 0.93, 95% CI 0.62 to 1.40). Survival analysis found no significant difference in the incidence of HIV infection in infants at 18 months (regimen A: 14.9%; regimen B: 18.1%; regimen C: 20.0%; and placebo 22.2%). Infant mortality rates at 18 months were 10.1%, 14.2%, 12.8%, and 13.4%, respectively (P = 0.40).

Harms: **Zidovudine versus placebo:** The review found that intensive zidovudine versus placebo significantly increased the risk of neonatal haematological toxicity (RR 1.86, 95% CI 1.18 to 2.94; specific effects undefined), whereas no significant difference was found for less intensive regimens versus placebo (RR 0.77, 95% CI 0.44 to 1.35).[18] Infants who received the most intensive regimen and were followed for 18 months had mild reversible anaemia that resolved by 12 weeks of age.[27] The same trial in uninfected infants followed for a median of 4.2 years found no significant difference between zidovudine versus placebo in growth patterns, immunological parameters, or the occurrence of childhood cancers.[28] The RCT of combination antiretroviral treatment has reported no serious adverse drug reactions to date.[18] **Nevirapine:** The RCT of zidovudine versus nevirapine found no significant difference in serious adverse effects in mothers and infants (4.0% with zidovudine v 4.7% with nevirapine in mothers; 19.8% with zidovudine v 20.5% with nevirapine in infants up to 18 months of age).[28] In the multicentre RCT of nevirapine, adverse events were on the whole rare and similar in the two arms. Most commonly reported was severe "non-rash toxicity", especially anaemia, which was in most cases judged to be unrelated to the study medication (nevirapine v placebo: mothers 6.2% v 6.1%; babies 32.9% v 27.9%). **Alternative zidovudine regimens:** The RCT found that the rate of serious adverse events in mothers and infants was similar for all regimens. The rates of severe anaemia in infants were "long–long" (1%); "long–short" (0%); "short–long" (0.3%); and "short–short" (1.3%).[23] **Combination antiretroviral regimens:** One RCT found no difference in adverse effects between those receiving zidovudine plus lamivudine and those receiving placebo. For grade 3 and 4 laboratory events (before wk 6) the rates in mothers were: regimen A 9%, regimen B 6%, regimen C 7%, and placebo 8%; the corresponding rates in babies was 5% in each of the groups. Congenital abnormalities for the four groups were 7%, 8%, 6%, and 7%. The rates for neurological events (up to 18 months) in babies were 2%, 4%, 4%, and 3%.[26]

Comment: The RCT found that zidovudine plus lamivudine given during the intrapartum period alone did not significantly affect the risk of transmission (RR 1.01, 95% CI 0.74 to 1.38).

OPTION AVOIDING BREAST FEEDING

One RCT in women with HIV who had access to clean water and health education has found that formula feeding versus breast feeding significantly reduces the incidence of HIV in infants at 24 months without increasing mortality.

Benefits: We found no systematic review. We found one RCT (425 HIV-1 [see glossary, p 805] seropositive women with access to clean water and health education in Kenya) that found that formula feeding versus breast feeding significantly reduced the number of infants with HIV at 24 months. (AR 31/205 [15%] with formula feeding *v* 61/197 [31%] with breast feeding; RR 0.49, 95% CI 0.33 to 0.72; NNT 7, 95% CI 5 to 13).[28] Although infants were breast fed throughout the RCT duration, the greatest exposure to breast milk occurred during the first 6 months of life. The RCT found no significant difference in mortality at 24 months with breast feeding versus formula feeding (AR 39/204 [19%] with formula feeding *v* 45/197 [23%] with breast feeding; RR 0.84, 95% CI 0.57 to 1.23).[5]

Harms: The RCT did not report on adverse effects (see comment below).

Comment: In countries with high infant mortality, avoiding breast feeding may further increase infant morbidity and mortality through its effect on nutrition, immunity, maternal fertility, and birth spacing. Access to clean water and education when using formula feeds may explain the similar mortality in breast fed and formula fed infants.

OPTION ELECTIVE CAESAREAN SECTION

One RCT found limited evidence that elective caesarean section versus vaginal delivery significantly reduced the incidence of HIV in infants at 18 months.

Benefits: We found one systematic review (search date not stated, 1 RCT, 436 women) that compared elective caesarean section at 38 weeks versus vaginal delivery.[29] It found that caesarean section significantly reduced the number of infants with HIV at 18 months (AR 3/170 [3%] with caesarean section *v* 21/200 [11%] with vaginal delivery; RR 0.16, 95% CI 0.05 to 0.55; NNT 11, 95% CI 10 to 21).

Harms: No serious adverse effects were reported in either group. Postpartum fever was significantly more common in women having caesarean section versus vaginal delivery (15/225 [7%] with caesarean section *v* 2/183 [1%] with vaginal delivery; RR 6.1, 95% CI 1.5 to 22.0; NNH 18, 95% CI 16 to 50). Postpartum bleeding, intravascular coagulation, or severe anaemia occurred rarely in either group.

Comment: A total of 15% of the women withdrew from the trial or were lost to follow up. None of the women analysed breast fed, although this was not stated as specific exclusion criterion. More women who gave birth by caesarean section versus vaginal delivery had received zidovudine during pregnancy (70% with caesarean section *v* 58% with vaginal delivery); this means that the observed difference between groups may not have been exclusively due to the different delivery methods.

OPTION IMMUNOTHERAPY

One RCT found no significant difference in the incidence of HIV in infants of mothers taking HIV hyperimmune globulin versus immunoglobulin without HIV antibody in addition to a standard zidovudine regimen, but it may have been too small to exclude a clinically important difference.

Benefits: We found one systematic review (search date not stated, 1 RCT, 501 women) that compared HIV hyperimmune globulin (HIVIG) versus immunoglobulin without HIV antibody (IVIG) given to women during pregnancy, the intrapartum period, and to their infants at birth.[29] Women in both groups received a standard course of zidovudine and no infants were breast fed. The RCT found no significant difference in transmission of HIV between HIVIG versus IVIG regimens at 6 months of age (4.1% with HIVIG *v* 6.0% with IVIG; no CI available; P = 0.36).

Harms: The trial reported no significant adverse effects.[29]

Comment: The low overall transmission rate (5%) in this study was much lower than the anticipated rate of greater than 15% used to calculate the appropriate sample size. The trial is unable to exclude a clinically important effect of HIVIG on the number of children with HIV.[29]

OPTION VAGINAL MICROBICIDES

We found insufficient evidence about the effects of vaginal microbicides on the incidence of HIV in infants.

Benefits: We found one systematic review (search date 2002, 1 quasi-randomised trial, 898 women) that assessed the effectiveness of vaginal irrigation with chlorhexidine during labour for reducing the risk of transmission.[30] HIV-positive women at a hospital in Kenya were allocated to vaginal irrigation or no irrigation during alternate weeks.[31] The trial found no evidence of a lower rate of HIV transmission after vaginal cleansing versus no cleansing (AR 63/307 [20.5%] with vaginal cleansing *v* 64/295 [21.7%] without vaginal cleansing; RR 0.95, 95% CI 0.69 to 1.29).

Harms: The single quasi-randomised trial reported no adverse effects in mothers or infants.[30]

Comment: In the trial identified a true randomisation method was not used, concealment of allocation was inadequate, and the analysis did not take into account the effect of clustering. Caution is therefore warranted in interpreting the study findings.

OPTION VITAMIN SUPPLEMENTS

Two RCTs found that vitamin supplements versus placebo given to pregnant women had no significant effect on the incidence of HIV in their infants at birth, 6 weeks, or 3 months.

Benefits: We found a systematic review (search date 2002, 2 RCTs, 1813 women) comparing vitamin A supplementation versus placebo given during the antenatal and intrapartum period.[32] The first of these RCTs (1085 women with HIV-1 between 12 and 27 wks' gestation in Tanzania) compared vitamin A and/or multivitamin supplements (excluding vitamin A) versus placebo, using a factorial design. It found no significant difference in the number of infants with HIV in women taking multivitamins versus placebo (AR 31/191 [16%] with multivitamins *v* 28/179 [16%] with placebo; RR 1.04, 95% CI 0.65 to 1.66).[33] The second RCT (728 pregnant women with HIV in South Africa) compared vitamin A with placebo.[34] A meta-analysis included in the systematic review found no reduction in the risk of HIV transmission to infants of mothers receiving vitamin A versus placebo (AR 123/558 [22.0%] with vitamin A *v* 109/527 [20.7%] with placebo; RR 1.07, 95% CI 0.85 to 1.34).[32]

Harms: The meta-analysis[32] found no evidence of an effect of vitamin A versus placebo on the incidence of stillbirth (RR 1.06, 95% CI 0.65 to 1.75), preterm birth either less than 34 weeks (RR 0.87, 95% CI 0.59 to 1.29) or less than 37 weeks (RR 0.90, 95% CI 0.74 to 1.10), or low birth weight (< 2500 g) (RR 0.88, 95% CI 0.67 to 1.15).

Comment: The RCTs were performed because observational studies have found an association in pregnant women between transmission of HIV and low serum levels of vitamin A.[35]

GLOSSARY

Human immunodeficiency virus type 1 (HIV-1) is the most common cause of HIV disease throughout the world.

Human immunodeficiency virus type 2 (HIV-2) is predominantly found in West Africa and is more closely related to the simian immunodeficiency virus than to HIV-1.

REFERENCES

1. John GC, Kreiss J. Mother-to-child transmission of human immunodeficiency virus type 1. *Epidemiol Rev* 1996;18:149–157.
2. Adjorlolo-Johnson G, De Cock KM, Ekpini E, et al. Prospective comparison of mother-to-child transmission of HIV-1 and HIV-2 in Abidjan, Ivory Coast. *JAMA* 1994;272:462–466.
3. Peckham C, Gibb D. Mother-to-child transmission of the human immunodeficiency virus. *N Engl J Med* 1995;333:298–302.
4. The Working Group on MTCT of HIV. Rates of mother-to-child transmission of HIV-1 in Africa, America and Europe: results of 13 perinatal studies. *J Acquir Immune Defic Syndr* 1995;8:506–510.
5. Nduati R, John G, Mbori-Ngacha D, et al. Effect of breastfeeding and formula feeding on transmission of HIV-1: a randomized clinical trial. *JAMA* 2000;283:1167–1174.
6. Report of the global HIV/AIDS epidemic UNAIDS, Geneva 2002.

7. Mofenson LM. Epidemiology and determinants of vertical HIV transmission. *Semin Pediatr Infect Dis* 1994;5:252–256.
8. Khouri YF, McIntosh K, Cavacini L, et al. Vertical transmission of HIV-1: correlation with maternal viral load and plasma levels of CD4 binding site anti-gp 120 antibodies. *J Clin Invest* 1995;95:732–737.
9. Dunn DT, Newell ML, Ades AE, et al. Risk of human immunodeficiency virus type-1 transmission through breastfeeding. *Lancet* 1992;240:585–588.
10. Miotti PG, Taha ET, Newton I, et al. HIV transmission through breastfeeding: a study in Malawi. *JAMA* 1999;282:744–749.
11. UNAIDS (Joint United Nations Programme on HIV/AIDS). *Report of the global HIV/AIDS epidemic.* June 2000. Geneva: UNAIDS; 2000. UNAIDS/00.13E.
12. Nair P, Alger L, Hines S, et al. Maternal and neonatal characteristics associated with HIV infection in infants of seropositive women. *J Acquir Immune Defic Syndr* 1993;6:298–302.
13. Minkoff H, Burns DN, Landesman S, et al. The relationship of the duration of ruptured membranes to vertical transmission of human immunodeficiency virus. *Am J Obstet Gynecol* 1995;173:585–589.
14. European Collaborative Study. Risk factors for mother-to-child transmission of HIV-1. *Lancet* 1992;339:1007–1012.
15. Mofenson LM. A critical review of studies evaluating the relationship of mode of delivery to perinatal transmission of human immunodeficiency virus. *Pediatr Infect Dis J* 1995;14:169–176.
16. The European Collaborative Study. Natural history of vertically acquired human immunodeficiency virus-1 infection. *Pediatrics* 1994;94:815–819.
17. Walker N, Schwartlander B, Bryce J. Meeting international goals in child survival and HIV/AIDS. *Lancet* 2002. http://image.thelancet.com/extras/01art9188web.pdf (last accessed 07 Jan 2003).
18. Brocklehurst P, Volmink J. Antiretrovirals for reducing the risk of mother-to-child transmission of HIV infection (Cochrane Review). In:The Cochrane Library, Issue 3, 2002: Oxford: Update Software. Search date 2001; primary sources Cochrane Pregnancy and Childbirth Register of Controlled Trials, CCTR and Conference abstracts.
19. Connor EM, Sperling RS, Gelber RD, et al. Reduction of maternal-infant transmission of human immunodeficiency type 1 with zidovudine treatment. *N Engl J Med* 1994;311:1173–1180.
20. Shaffer N, Chuachoowong R, Mock PA, et al. Short-course zidovudine for perinatal HIV-1 transmission in Bangkok, Thailand: a randomised controlled trial. Bangkok Collaborative Perinatal HIV Transmission Study Group. *Lancet* 1999;353:773–780.
21. Wiktor SZ, Ekpini E, Karon JM, et al. Short-course oral zidovudine for prevention of mother-to-child transmission of HIV-1 in Abidjan, Cote d'Ivoire: a randomised trial. *Lancet* 1999;353:781–785.
22. Dabis F, Msellati P, Meda N, et al. Six-month efficacy, tolerance, and acceptability of a short regimen of oral zidovudine to reduce vertical transmission of HIV in breastfed children in Cote d'Ivoire and Burkina Faso: a double-blind placebo-controlled multicentre trial. DITRAME Study Group. Diminution de la Transmission Mere-Enfant. *Lancet* 1999;353:786–792.
23. Lallemant M, Jourdain G, Le Couer S, et al. A trial of shortened zidovudine regimens to prevent mother-to-child transmission of human immunodeficiency virus type 1. *N Engl J Med* 2000:343:982–991.
24. Guay LA, Musoke P, Fleming T, et al. Intrapartum and neonatal single-dose nevirapine compared with zidovudine for prevention of mother-to-child transmission of HIV-1 in Kampala, Uganda: HIVNET 012 randomised trial. *Lancet* 1999;354:795–802.
25. Dorenbaum A, Cunningham CK, Gelber RD, et al. Two-dose intrapartum/newborn nevirapine and standard antiretroviral therapy to reduce perinatal HIV transmission. A randomized trial. *JAMA* 2002;288:189–198.
26. The Petra study team. Efficacy of three short-course regimens of zidovudine and lamivudine in preventing early and late transmission of HIV-1 from mother to child in Tanzania, South Africa, and Uganda (Petra study): a randomised, double-blind, placebo-controlled trial. *Lancet* 2002;359:1178–86.
27. Sperling RS, Shapiro DE, McSherry GD, et al. Safety of the maternal-infant zidovudine regimen utilized in the Pediatric AIDS Clinical Trial Group 076 Study. *AIDS* 1998;12:1805–1813.
28. Culnane M, Fowler MG, Lee S, et al. Lack of long term effects of in utero exposure to zidovudine among uninfected children born to HIV-infected women. *JAMA* 1999;281:151–157.
29. Brocklehurst P. Interventions aimed at decreasing the risk of mother-to-child transmission of HIV infection. In: The Cochrane Library, Issue 3, 2000. Oxford: Update Software. Search date not stated; primary sources Cochrane Pregnancy and Childbirth Group Trials Register and Cochrane Controlled Trials Register.
30. Shey Wiysonge CU, Brocklehurst P, Sterne JAC. Vaginal disinfection during labour for reducing the risk of mother-to-child transmission of HIV infection (Cochrane Review). In: The Cochrane Library, Issue 3, 2002. Oxford: Update Software. Search date 2002; primary sources CTTR, Cochrane Pregnancy and Childbirth Register, Pubmed, Embase, Aidsline, Lilacs, Aidstrials, Aidsdrugs, Reference lists, Conference abstracts, contact with experts and pharmaceutical companies.
31. Gaillard P, Mwanyumba F, Verhofstede C, et al. Vaginal lavage with chlorhexidine during labour to reduce mother-to-child HIV transmission: clinical trial in Mombassa, Kenya. *AIDS* 2001;15:389–396.
32. Shey Wiysonge CU, Brocklehurst P, Sterne JAC. Vitamin A supplementation for reducing the risk of mother-to-child transmission of HIV infection (Cochrane Review). In: The Cochrane Library, Issue 3, 2002. Oxford: Update Software. Search date 2002: primary sources CTTR, Cochrane Pregnancy and Childbirth Register, Pubmed, Embase, Aidsline, Lilacs, Aidstrials, Aidsdrugs, Reference lists, Conference abstracts, contact with experts and pharmaceutical companies.
33. Fawzi WW, Msamanga G, Hunter D, et al. Randomized trial of vitamin supplements in relation to vertical transmission of HIV-1 in Tanzania. *J Acquir Immune Defic Syndr* 2000;23:246–254.
34. Coutsoudis A, Pillay K, Spooner E, et al. Randomized trial testing the effect of vitamin A supplementation on pregnancy outcomes and early, mother-to-child HIV-1 transmission in Durban, South Africa. *AIDS* 1999;13:1517–1524.
35. Fawzi WW, Hunter DJ. Vitamins in HIV disease progression and vertical transmission. *Epidemiology* 1998;9:457–466.

HIV: mother to child transmission

Jimmy Volmink
Professor and Chair of Primary Health Care
Faculty of Health Sciences
University of Cape Town
Cape Town
South Africa

Competing interests: None declared.

TABLE 1 **Placebo controlled trials of zidovudine to reduce mother to child transmission of HIV (see text, p 801).**

Ref	Participants	Maternal treatment	Infant treatment	Transmission rate	RR (95% CI)
Infants not breast fed					
19	477 women with confirmed HIV (60 centres in the USA and France)	*Antepartum* Orally 100 mg 5 times daily starting at 14–34 weeks' gestation *Intrapartum* 2 mg/kg iv over 1 hour then 1 mg/kg/hour until delivery	Orally 2 mg/kg every 6 hours for 6 weeks (given only to babies of mothers treated with ZDV)	At 18 months: placebo 26%, ZDV 8%	0.32 (0.18 to 0.59)
20	397 women with confirmed HIV-1 (2 centres in Bangkok and Thailand)	*Antepartum* Orally 300 mg twice daily from 36 weeks' gestation *Intrapartum* Orally 300 mg every 3 hours until delivery	Nil	At 6 months: placebo 19%, ZDV 9%	0.52 (0.30 to 0.85)
Infants breast fed					
21	280 women with confirmed HIV-1 (1 hospital in the Ivory Coast)	*Antepartum* Orally 300 mg twice daily from 36 weeks' gestation *Intrapartum* Orally 300 mg every 3 hours until delivery	Nil	At 3 months: placebo 25%, ZDV 16%	0.63 (0.38 to 1.05)
22	431 women with confirmed HIV-1 (Ivory Coast and Burkina Faso)	*Antepartum* Orally 250 or 300 mg twice daily from 36–38 weeks' gestation *Intrapartum* Orally single dose of 500 or 600 mg at onset of labour *Postpartum* Orally 250 or 300 mg twice daily for 7 days	Nil	At 6 months: placebo 28%, ZDV 18%	0.62 (0.40 to 0.95)

iv, intravenously; Ref, reference; ZDV, zidovudine.

HIV: prevention of opportunistic infections

Search date April 2003

John Ioannidis and David Wilkinson

QUESTIONS

INTERVENTIONS

HIV: prevention of opportunistic infections

See glossary, p 827

Key Messages

Prophylaxis for *P carinii* pneumonia (PCP) and toxoplasmosis

- **Trimethoprim/sulfamethoxazole (TMP/SMX—co-trimoxazole) for PCP** Systematic reviews have found that TMP/SMX reduces the incidence of PCP compared with placebo or pentamidine. Two systematic reviews have found that TMP/SMX reduced incidence of PCP compared with dapsone (with or without pyrimethamine), although only one of these reviews found that the reduction was significant. One systematic review and one subsequent RCT found no significant difference between high and low dose TMP/SMX for PCP prophylaxis, although adverse effects were more common with the higher dose.
- **Atovaquone (no difference from dapsone or aerosolised pentamidine for PCP in people intolerant of TMP/SMX)** We found no RCTs comparing atovaquone versus placebo. RCTs found no significant difference in the incidence of PCP with atovaquone compared with dapsone or aerosolised pentamidine, both of which are regarded as effective in people intolerant of TMP/SMX.
- **Azithromycin (for PCP)** One RCT has found that azithromycin, either alone or in combination with rifabutin, reduces the risk of PCP in people receiving standard PCP prophylaxis compared with rifabutin alone.

- **TMP/SMX (for toxoplasmosis)** One RCT found no significant difference between TMP/SMX and placebo for preventing toxoplasmosis. One systematic review has found no significant difference between TMP/SMX and dapsone (with or without pyrimethamine) for preventing toxoplasmosis.

Prophylaxis for tuberculosis

- **Tuberculosis prophylaxis versus placebo (in people with positive tuberculin test)** Systematic reviews have found that in people who are HIV and tuberculin skin test positive, antituberculosis prophylaxis reduces the frequency of tuberculosis compared with placebo over 2–3 years. The reviews found no evidence of benefit in people who are HIV positive but tuberculin skin test negative. One RCT found that the benefit of prophylaxis diminished with time after treatment was stopped.
- **Isoniazid for 6–12 months (*v* combination treatment for 2 months — similar benefits, fewer harms)** RCTs found no evidence of a difference in effectiveness between regimens using combinations of tuberculosis drugs for 2–3 months and those using isoniazid alone for 6–12 months. One RCT found that multidrug regimens increased the number of people with adverse reactions resulting in cessation of treatment.

***M avium* complex (MAC) prophylaxis (no previous MAC)**

- **Azithromycin** One RCT has found that azithromycin reduces the incidence of MAC compared with placebo.
- **Clarithromycin** One RCT has found that clarithromycin reduces the incidence of MAC compared with placebo.
- **Combination treatment (rifabutin plus either clarithromycin or azithromycin)** One RCT has found that rifabutin plus clarithromycin or clarithromycin alone reduces the incidence of MAC compared with rifabutin alone. One RCT has found that rifabutin plus azithromycin reduces the incidence of MAC compared with azithromycin alone or rifabutin alone at 1 year. One systematic review and two subsequent RCTs found that toxicity, including uveitis, was more common with combination therapy compared with clarithromycin or rifabutin alone.

MAC prophylaxis (previous MAC)

- **Clarithromycin, rifabutin, and ethambutol (*v* clarithromycin plus clofazimine)** One RCT found that clarithromycin, rifabutin and ethambutol reduced MAC relapse compared with clarithromycin plus clofazimine.
- **Ethambutol added to clarithromycin plus clofazimine** One RCT found that adding ethambutol to clarithromycin and clofazimine reduced MAC relapse compared with clarithromycin plus clofazimine.
- **Rifabutin added to clarithromycin plus ethambutol** One RCT found no significant difference in survival by adding rifabutin to clarithromycin plus ethambutol in people with previous MAC.
- **Clofazimine added to ethambutol plus clarithromycin (*v* clofazimine plus ethambutol)** One RCT found that adding clarithromycin to clofazimine and ethambutol was associated with higher mortality compared with clofazimine plus ethambutol.

Prophylaxis for cytomegalovirus (CMV), herpes simplex virus (HSV), and varicella zoster virus (VZV)

- **Aciclovir (for HSV and VZV)** One systematic review has found that aciclovir reduces HSV and

HIV: prevention of opportunistic infections

- **Oral ganciclovir (in people with severe CD4 depletion)** One RCT has found that oral ganciclovir reduces the incidence of CMV in people with severe CD4 depletion compared with placebo. It found that 25% of people taking ganciclovir developed severe neutropenia. A second RCT found no significant differences between treatments.
- **Famciclovir (for recurrent HSV)** One small RCT found that famciclovir reduced the rate of viral shedding compared with placebo, but provided insufficient evidence on the effect of famciclovir on HSV recurrence.
- **Valaciclovir (*v* aciclovir for CMV)** One RCT has found that valaciclovir versus aciclovir reduces the incidence of CMV, but may be associated with increased mortality.

Prophylaxis for fungal disease (no previous fungal disease)

- **Fluconazole or itraconazole** RCTs in people with advanced HIV disease have found that both fluconazole and itraconazole reduce the incidence of invasive fungal infections compared with placebo. One RCT found that fluconazole reduced the incidence of invasive fungal disease and mucocutaneous candidiasis compared with clotrimazole. One RCT found no difference between high and low dose fluconazole.

Prophylaxis for fungal disease (previous fungal disease)

- **Itraconazole (for *P marneffei*)** Two RCTs have found that itraconazole reduces the incidence of relapse of *P marneffei* infection and candidiasis compared with placebo.
- **Itraconazole (for histoplasmosis)** We found no RCTs.
- **Itraconazole (*v* fluconazole for maintenance treatment of cryptococcal meningitis)** One RCT found that itraconazole increased the risk of relapse of cryptococcal meningitis compared with fluconazole.

Discontinuation of prophylaxis in people on highly active antiretroviral treatment (HAART)

- **Discontinuing prophylaxis for MAC in people with CD4 > 100/mm^3 on HAART** Two RCTs in people taking HAART found that discontinuation of prophylaxis for MAC disease did not increase the incidence of MAC disease.
- **Discontinuing prophylaxis for PCP and toxoplasmosis in people with CD4 > 200/mm^3 on HAART** One systematic review of two unblinded RCTs in people taking HAART found that discontinuation of prophylaxis did not increase the incidence of PCP. Two unblinded RCTs found that discontinuation of prophylaxis did not increase the incidence of toxoplasmosis.
- **Discontinuing prophylaxis for CMV in people with CD4 > 100/mm^3 on HAART** We found insufficient evidence on the effects of discontinuation of maintenance treatment for CMV retinitis or other end organ disease in people taking HAART.

DEFINITION Opportunistic infections are intercurrent infections that occur in people infected with HIV. Prophylaxis aims to avoid either the first occurrence of these infections (primary prophylaxis) or their recurrence (secondary prophylaxis, maintenance treatment). This review includes *Pneumocystis carinii* pneumonia (PCP), *Toxoplasma gondii* encephalitis, *Mycobacterium tuberculosis*, *Mycobacterium avium* complex (MAC) disease, cytomegalovirus (CMV) disease (most often retinitis), infections from other herpesviruses (herpes simplex virus [HSV] and varicella zoster virus [VZV]), and invasive fungal disease (*Cryptococcus neoformans*, *Histoplasma capsulatum*, and *Penicillium marneffei* [see glossary, p 827]).

INCIDENCE/ PREVALENCE The incidence of opportunistic infections is high in people with immune impairment. Data available before the introduction of highly active antiretroviral treatment (HAART) suggest that, with a CD4 < 250/mm^3, the 2 year probability of developing an opportunistic infection is 40% for PCP, 22% for CMV, 18% for MAC, 6% for toxoplasmosis, and 5% for cryptococcal meningitis.[1] The introduction of HAART has reduced the rate of opportunistic infections. One cohort study found that the introduction of HAART decreased the incidence of PCP by 94%, CMV by 82%, and MAC by 64%, as presenting AIDS events. HAART decreased the incidence of events subsequent to the diagnosis of AIDS by 84% for PCP, 82% for CMV, and 97% for MAC.[2]

AETIOLOGY/ RISK FACTORS Opportunistic infections are caused by a wide array of pathogens and result from immune defects induced by HIV. The risk of developing opportunistic infections increases dramatically with progressive impairment of the immune system. Each opportunistic infection has a different threshold of immune impairment, beyond which the risk increases substantially.[1] Opportunistic pathogens may infect the immunocompromised host *de novo*, but usually they are simply reactivations of latent pathogens in such hosts.

PROGNOSIS Prognosis depends on the type of opportunistic infection. Even with treatment they may cause serious morbidity and mortality. Most deaths owing to HIV infection are caused by opportunistic infections.

AIMS OF INTERVENTION To prevent the occurrence and relapse of opportunistic infections; to discontinue unnecessary prophylaxis; to minimise adverse effects of prophylaxis and loss of quality of life.

OUTCOMES First occurrence and relapse of opportunistic infections and adverse effects of treatments. We have not considered neoplastic diseases associated with specific opportunistic infections.

METHODS *Clinical Evidence* search and appraisal April 2003. We also reviewed abstract books/CDs for the following conferences held between 1995 and early 2001: European Clinical AIDS, HIV Drug Treatment, Interscience Conferences on Antimicrobial Agents and Chemotherapy, National Conferences on Human Retroviruses and Opportunistic Infections, and World AIDS Conference. We placed emphasis on systematic reviews and RCTs published after 1993.

QUESTION **What are the effects of prophylaxis for *P carinii* pneumonia (PCP) and toxoplasmosis?**

John Ioannidis

OPTION **TRIMETHOPRIM/SULFAMETHOXAZOLE (TMP/SMX — CO-TRIMOXAZOLE)**

Systematic reviews have found that TMP/SMX (co-trimoxazole) is more effective than pentamidine or placebo at reducing the incidence of PCP. One RCT found no significant difference between TMP/SMX and placebo

for preventing PCP or toxoplasmosis. Two systematic reviews have found that TMP/SMX reduced incidence of PCP compared with dapsone (with or without pyrimethamine), although only one of these reviews found that the reduction was significant. One systematic review has found no difference between TMP/SMX and dapsone (with or without pyrimethamine) for incidence of toxoplasmosis. One systematic review and one subsequent RCT found no significant difference between high and low dose TMP/SMX for PCP prophylaxis, although adverse effects are more common with the higher dose.

Benefits: We found two systematic reviews (search dates 1995[3] and not stated[4]). **TMP/SMX versus placebo:** The first systematic review (35 RCTs) found that prophylaxis with TMP/SMX reduced the incidence of PCP more than placebo (RR 0.32, 95% CI 0.23 to 0.46). One subsequent RCT (545 people in sub-Saharan Africa with symptomatic disease; second or third clinical stage disease in the WHO staging system [see glossary, p 827]; regardless of CD4 cell count) comparing TMP/SMX with placebo found no significant difference in incidence of PCP or toxoplasmosis.[5] **TMP/SMX versus pentamidine:** The first systematic review found that TMP/SMX compared with aerosolised pentamidine significantly reduced the incidence of PCP (RR 0.58, 95% CI 0.45 to 0.75).[3] The second systematic review found no significant difference between TMP/SMX and aerosolised pentamidine for preventing toxoplasmosis (RR 0.78, 95% CI 0.55 to 1.11).[4] **TMP/SMX versus dapsone (with or without pyrimethamine):** The first systematic review found that TMP/SMX compared with dapsone (with or without pyrimethamine) reduced the incidence of PCP, but the result did not reach significance (RR 0.61, 95% CI 0.34 to 1.10).[3] The second review found that TMP/SMX was significantly more effective in preventing PCP than dapsone/pyrimethamine (RR 0.49, 95% CI 0.26 to 0.92).[4] It found no significant difference between TMP/SMX and dapsone/pyrimethamine in preventing toxoplasmosis (RR 1.17, 95% CI 0.68 to 2.04). **High versus low dose TMP/SMX:** The first systematic review found no significant difference in the rate of PCP infection between lower dose (160/800 mg 3 times/week or 80/400 mg/day) and higher dose (160/800 mg/day) TMP/SMX (failure rate per 100 person years was 1.6, 95% CI 0.9 to 2.5 with lower dose *v* 0.5, 95% CI 0 to 2.9 with higher dose; significance not reported).[3] One subsequent RCT (2625 people) also found no significant difference in the rate of PCP infection in people receiving TMP/SMX 160/800 mg daily compared with three times weekly (3.5 *v* 4.1 per 100 person years; $P = 0.16$).[6]

Harms: **TMP/SMX:** The first systematic review found that severe adverse effects (predominantly rash, fever, and haematological effects leading to discontinuation within 1 year) occurred in more people taking higher doses of TMP/SMX than in those taking lower doses (25% *v* 15%).[3] The RCT comparing high dose with low dose TMP/SMX found that discontinuation because of adverse effects was significantly more common in people taking high doses of TMP/SMX (RR 2.14; $P < 0.001$).[6] The RCT in sub-Saharan Africa found that people on TMP/SMX were less likely to suffer a serious event (death or hospital admission, irrespective of the cause) than those on placebo, regardless of their initial CD4 cell count (HR 0.57, 95% CI 0.43 to

0.75; P < 0.001).[5] Moderate neutropenia occurred more frequently with TMP/SMX (neutropenia AR 62/271 [23%] with TMP/SMX *v* 26/244 [10%] with placebo; RR 2.1, 95% 1.4 to 3.3; NNH 8, 95% CI 5 to 14). Two RCTs (largest 377 people) found that gradual initiation of TMP/SMX may improve tolerance of the regimen compared with abrupt initiation.[7,8] Two RCTs (238 people; 50 people) found no significant benefit from acetylcysteine in preventing TMP/SMX hypersensitivity reactions in HIV infected people.[9,10] **Dapsone:** The first systematic review found that adverse effects were more frequent with high doses than low doses of dapsone (29% *v* 12%).[3] A third systematic review (search date 1996, 16 trials, 4267 people) evaluating dapsone toxicity found no significant difference in mortality between dapsone and other prophylaxis (OR for mortality for dapsone *v* other prophylaxis 1.11, 95% CI 0.96 to 1.29).[11] **Pentamidine:** Bronchospasm occurred in 3% of people taking aerosolised pentamidine 300 mg monthly.[3]

Comment: **Concomitant coverage for toxoplasmosis:** Standard TMP/SMX prophylaxis or dapsone should offer adequate coverage for toxoplasmosis. Pentamidine has no intrinsic activity against *T gondii*. Toxoplasmosis risk is probably clinically meaningful only with CD4 < 100/mm³ and positive toxoplasma serology.[1] **Role of highly active antiretroviral treatment (HAART):** We found more than 50 RCTs on the prophylaxis of PCP and/or toxoplasmosis, but their results should be interpreted with caution because they were conducted mostly before the advent and widespread use of HAART. Although this is unlikely to affect the comparative results, HAART has resulted in a large decrease in the rate of PCP, toxoplasmosis, and other opportunistic infections; therefore, the absolute benefits of these prophylactic regimens are probably smaller when used with HAART. **Prophylaxis in Africa:** Beneficial effects of TMP/SMX in Africa may be largely because of prophylaxis for bacterial infections rather than PCP. The largest trial conducted in Africa found that TMP/SMX significantly reduced mortality and hospital admissions.[5] However, a smaller trial (100 people) found no significant effect on mortality or hospital admission, although it may have lacked power to detect a significant difference (HR for death or hospital admission 1.10, 95% CI 0.57 to 2.13).[12]

OPTION ATOVAQUONE IN TRIMETHOPRIM/SULFAMETHOXAZOLE (TMP/SMX — CO-TRIMOXAZOLE) INTOLERANT PEOPLE

We found no RCTs comparing atovaquone versus placebo. RCTs found no significant difference between atovaquone versus dapsone or aerosolised pentamidine in preventing PCP.

Benefits: We found no systematic review. **Versus placebo:** We found no RCTs. **Versus dapsone:** One RCT (1057 people intolerant of TMP/SMX, of whom 298 had a history of PCP) found no significant difference between atovaquone 1500 mg daily compared with dapsone 100 mg daily (15.7 *v* 18.4 cases of PCP per 100 person years; P = 0.20).[13] **Versus pentamidine:** One RCT (549 people intolerant of TMP/SMX) compared high dose with low dose atovaquone (1500 mg/day v 750 mg/day) with monthly aerosolised pentamidine (300 mg). It found no significant difference between the groups in the incidence of PCP (26% v 22% v 17%) or mortality (20% v 13% v 18%) after a median follow up of 11.3 months.[14]

Harms: The RCT comparing atovaquone with dapsone found that the overall risk of stopping treatment because of adverse effects was similar in the two arms (RR 0.94, 95% CI 0.74 to 1.19).[13] Atovaquone was stopped more frequently than dapsone in people who were receiving dapsone at baseline (RR 3.78, 95% CI 2.37 to 6.01), and less frequently in people not receiving dapsone at baseline (RR 0.42, 95% CI 0.30 to 0.58).

Comment: See role of highly active antiretroviral treatment in comment under TMP/SMX, p 815.

OPTION AZITHROMYCIN

One RCT has found that azithromycin, either alone or in combination with rifabutin, reduces the risk of PCP compared with rifabutin alone in people receiving standard PCP prophylaxis.

Benefits: We found no systematic review. **Versus placebo:** We found no RCTs. **Versus other drugs:** We found one RCT (693 people) that compared azithromycin, rifabutin, and both drugs in combination in people who were already receiving standard PCP prophylaxis. It found that azithromycin, either alone or in combination with rifabutin, reduced the relative risk of developing PCP by 45% when compared with rifabutin alone (P = 0.008).[15]

Harms: Gastrointestinal adverse effects are common with azithromycin, but they are usually mild and do not lead to stopping treatment. The addition of rifabutin significantly increased the risk of stopping treatment (RR 1.67; P = 0.03).[16]

Comment: See role of highly active antiretroviral treatment in comment under trimethoprim/sulfamethoxazole (co-trimoxazole), p 815. The low incidence of PCP infection in people taking highly active antiretroviral treatment means that the absolute benefit of prophylaxis is smaller.

QUESTION What are the effects of antituberculosis prophylaxis in people with HIV infection?

David Wilkinson

OPTION ANTITUBERCULOSIS PROPHYLACTIC REGIMENS VERSUS PLACEBO

Two systematic reviews have found that in people who are HIV and tuberculin skin test positive, antituberculosis prophylaxis reduces frequency of tuberculosis compared with placebo over 2–3 years. The reviews found no evidence of benefit in people who are HIV positive but tuberculin skin test negative. One RCT found that the benefit of prophylaxis diminished with time after treatment was stopped.

Benefits: We found two systematic reviews.[17,18] The first systematic review (search date 2000) identified seven RCTs in 4652 HIV positive adults from Haiti, Kenya, USA, Zambia, and Uganda.[17] All compared isoniazid (6–12 months) or combination treatment (3 months) with placebo. Mean follow up was 2–3 years, and the main outcomes, stratified by tuberculin skin test positivity, were tuberculosis (either microbiological or clinical) and death. Among tuberculin skin test positive adults, antituberculosis prophylaxis significantly reduced the incidence of tuberculosis (RR compared with placebo 0.24, 95% CI 0.14 to 0.40) and was associated with a non-significant reduction in the risk of death (RR compared with placebo 0.77, 95% CI 0.58 to 1.03). Among tuberculin skin test negative adults there was no significant difference in risk of tuberculosis (RR compared with placebo 0.87, 95% CI 0.56 to 1.36) or death (RR compared with placebo 1.07, 95% CI 0.88 to 1.30). The second review (search date not stated, 7 trials, 4529 people) compared isoniazid versus placebo only.[18] Among tuberculin skin test positive participants, the incidence of tuberculosis was significantly reduced (RR compared with placebo 0.40, 95% CI 0.24 to 0.65), but again there was no significant difference among tuberculin skin test negative participants (RR compared with placebo 0.84, 95% CI 0.54 to 1.30). This review found no evidence of any impact on mortality.[18] One of the RCTs included in the systematic reviews (1053 Zambian adults; 161 tuberculin skin test positive, 517 negative, the rest unknown) comparing isoniazid versus rifampicin plus pyrazinamide versus placebo for up to 6 months recently published results at 3 years' follow up.[19] Many people taking placebo were offered isoniazid after randomisation. Intention to treat analysis found that isoniazid or rifampicin plus pyrazinamide versus placebo significantly reduced the risk of tuberculosis at 2.5 years (cumulative AR not provided; RR 0.55, 95% CI 0.32 to 0.93), although the benefit diminished over this time. We found one subsequent RCT published as a letter (see comment below).[20]

Harms: Data on adverse drug reactions were not always stratified by tuberculin skin test positivity. In the first review there was a significant increase in adverse drug reactions requiring cessation of treatment with isoniazid compared with placebo (RR 1.75, 95% CI 1.23 to 2.47).[17] In the second review, the estimated RR was 1.36 (95% CI 1.00 to 1.86).[18]

Comment: Without prophylaxis, people who are HIV and tuberculin skin test positive have a 50% or more lifetime risk of developing tuberculosis compared with a 10% lifetime risk in people who are HIV positive but tuberculin skin test negative.[21] Clinical features of tuberculosis may be atypical in people with HIV infection and diagnosis may be more difficult, disease progression more rapid, and outcome worse. The subsequent RCT published as a letter (237 HIV positive Haitian adults with negative tuberculin skin test) found no significant difference between isoniazid (300 mg) versus no treatment in mortality, or the incidence of AIDS or tuberculosis at 1 year.[20]

OPTION DIFFERENT ANTITUBERCULOSIS PROPHYLACTIC REGIMENS

RCTs found no evidence of a difference in effectiveness between regimens using combinations of tuberculosis drugs for 2–3 months and those using isoniazid alone for 6–12 months. One RCT found that multidrug regimens increased the number of people with adverse reactions resulting in cessation of treatment.

Benefits: We found no systematic review. We found six RCTs.[19,22–26] Three RCTs (750, 1583, and 393 people) compared isoniazid versus rifampicin/pyrazinamide in people who were HIV and tuberculin skin test positive.[22–24] All found no significant difference in rates of tuberculosis. The fourth RCT (1564 HIV and tuberculin skin test positive people from Uganda) compared three treatments (isoniazid alone, isoniazid plus rifampicin and isoniazid, rifampicin, and pyrazinamide) versus placebo.[25] It reported comparisons between each regimen versus placebo, but did not directly compare different regimens against each other (see comment). The fifth RCT (133 adults, mixed tuberculin skin test positive and negative) comparing isoniazid for 12 months versus isoniazid plus rifampicin for 3 months found no significant difference in the incidence of tuberculosis (AR 4.2% with isoniazid *v* 2.1% with isoniazid plus rifampicin; RR 0.51, 95% CI 0.09 to 2.8).[26] The sixth RCT (1053 Zambian adults; 161 tuberculin skin test positive, 517 negative, the rest unknown) compared isoniazid for 6 months versus rifampicin plus pyrazinamide for 3 months versus placebo.[19] Many people in the placebo group were offered isoniazid after randomisation. Intention to treat analysis found no significant difference between isoniazid versus rifampicin plus pyrazinamide in the rate of tuberculosis at any time during a mean follow up of 3 years.

Harms: One RCT found that the proportion of people discontinuing treatment increased with the number of drugs given: isoniazid 1%, isoniazid plus rifampicin 2%, and all three drugs 6%.[23]

Comment: The fourth RCT compared each of three drug regimens versus placebo, but not versus each other.[25] It found that the risk of tuberculosis was significantly reduced with isoniazid alone (RR compared with placebo 0.33, 95% CI 0.14 to 0.77), and with isoniazid and rifampicin combined (RR compared with placebo 0.40, 95% CI 0.18 to 0.86). However, it found only a non-significant trend toward reduction with isoniazid, rifampicin, and pyrazinamide combined (RR compared with placebo 0.51, 95% CI 0.24 to 1.08). There is concern about emergence of rifampicin resistance if this drug is used in antituberculosis prophylaxis, although we found no reports of this. There is a theoretical risk that widespread, unsupervised use of isoniazid alone could promote resistance to this drug, although we found no evidence that this has happened.

QUESTION What are the effects of prophylaxis for disseminated *M avium* complex (MAC) disease for people without previous MAC disease?

John Ioannidis

OPTION AZITHROMYCIN

One RCT has found that azithromycin significantly reduces the incidence of MAC compared with placebo.

Benefits: We found no systematic review. One RCT (174 people with AIDS and CD4 < $100/mm^3$) found that azithromycin reduced the incidence of MAC more than placebo (11% *v* 25%; P = 0.004).[27]

Harms: Gastrointestinal adverse effects were more likely with azithromycin than with placebo (71/90 [79%] *v* 25/91 [28%]; NNH 2, CI not provided), but they were rarely severe enough to cause discontinuation of treatment (8% *v* 2% in the two arms; P = 0.14).[27]

Comment: Prospective cohort studies found that the risk of disseminated MAC disease increased substantially with a lower CD4 count and was clinically important only for CD4 < $50/mm^3$.[1] **Role of highly active antiretroviral treatment (HAART):** Most of the RCTs of MAC prophylaxis were conducted before the widespread use of HAART. HAART reduces the absolute risk of MAC infection. The absolute risk reduction of prophylactic regimens may be smaller when used in people treated with HAART.

OPTION CLARITHROMYCIN

One RCT has found that clarithromycin reduces the incidence of MAC compared with placebo.

Benefits: We found one systematic review (search date 1997) of prophylaxis and treatment of MAC.[28] It identified one RCT (682 people with advanced AIDS) that found that clarithromycin compared with placebo significantly reduced the incidence of MAC (6% *v* 16%; HR 0.31, 95% CI 0.18 to 0.53). It found no significant difference in the death rate (32% *v* 41%; HR 0.75; P = 0.026).[29]

Harms: Adverse effects led to discontinuation of treatment in slightly more people taking clarithromycin than placebo (8% *v* 6%; P = 0.45). More people taking clarithromycin suffered altered taste (11% *v* 2%) or rectal disorders (8% *v* 3%).[27]

Comment: Prospective cohort studies found that the risk of disseminated MAC disease increased substantially with a lower CD4 count and was clinically important only for CD4 < $50/mm^3$.[1] See role of highly active antiretroviral treatment in comment under azithromycin, p 816.

OPTION COMBINATION TREATMENT

One RCT has found that clarithromycin alone and clarithromycin plus rifabutin both reduce the incidence of MAC compared with rifabutin alone. One RCT found that azithromycin plus rifabutin reduced the incidence of

MAC compared with azithromycin alone or rifabutin alone. One systematic review and two subsequent RCTs found that toxicity, including uveitis, was more common with combination therapy than with clarithromycin or rifabutin alone.

Benefits: **Clarithromycin plus rifabutin:** We found no systematic review. One RCT (1178 people with AIDS) compared rifabutin versus clarithromycin versus clarithromycin plus rifabutin.[30] It found that the risk of MAC was significantly reduced in the clarithromycin alone group (RR 0.56 for clarithromycin *v* rifabutin; P = 0.005) and the combination group when compared with rifabutin alone (RR 0.43 for combination *v* rifabutin; P = 0.0003). There was no significant difference in the risk of MAC between the combination and clarithromycin arms (P = 0.36). **Azithromycin plus rifabutin:** One RCT (693 people) found that the combination of azithromycin plus rifabutin versus azithromycin alone or rifabutin alone significantly reduced the incidence of MAC at 1 year (15.3% with rifabutin *v* 7.6% for azithromycin *v* 2.8% with rifabutin plus azithromycin; P = 0.008 for rifabutin *v* azithromycin; P = 0.03 for combination *v* azithromycin).[16]

Harms: In one RCT, dose limiting toxicity was more likely with azithromycin plus rifabutin than with azithromycin alone (HR 1.67; P = 0.03).[16] In another RCT, adverse events occurred in 31% of people receiving the combination of clarithromycin and rifabutin compared with 16% on clarithromycin alone and 18% on rifabutin alone (P < 0.001).[28] Uveitis occurred in 42 people: 33 were on clarithromycin plus rifabutin, seven were on rifabutin alone, and two were on clarithromycin alone. **Uveitis:** We found one systematic review (search date 1994, 54 people with rifabutin associated uveitis).[31] It found that uveitis was dose dependent. It occurred from 2 weeks to more than 7 months after initiation of rifabutin treatment, and was more likely in people taking rifabutin and clarithromycin. In most people, uveitis resolved 1–2 months after discontinuation of rifabutin.

Comment: Prospective cohort studies found that the risk of disseminated MAC disease increased substantially with a lower CD4 count and was clinically important only for CD4 < 50/mm^3.[1] Clarithromycin may inhibit rifabutin metabolism; rifabutin may decrease levels of delavirdine and saquinavir. See role of highly active antiretroviral treatment in comment under azithromycin, p 816.

QUESTION **What are the effects of prophylaxis for disseminated *M avium* complex (MAC) disease for people with previous MAC disease?**

John Ioannidis

OPTION **COMBINATION TREATMENT**

One RCT found that adding ethambutol to clarithromycin and clofazimine reduced MAC relapse compared with clarithromycin plus clofazimine. One RCT found that adding clofazimine to clarithromycin and ethambutol was associated with higher mortality. One RCT found that clarithromycin,

rifabutin and ethambutol reduced MAC relapse compared with clarithromycin plus clofazimine. One RCT found no significant difference in survival by adding rifabutin to clarithromycin plus ethambutol.

Benefits: We found no systematic review but found four RCTs.[32–35] **Clarithromycin, clofazimine, and ethambutol versus clarithromycin and clofazimine:** The first RCT (95 people) found that the combination of clarithromycin 1000 mg daily, clofazimine, and ethambutol was associated with significantly fewer relapses of MAC than the combination of clarithromycin plus clofazimine without ethambutol (68% relapsed in 3 drug regimen *v* 12% in 2 drug regimen at 36 weeks; P = 0.004).[32] **Clarithromycin, clofazimine, and ethambutol versus clarithromycin and ethambutol:** The second RCT (106 people) found that the addition of clofazimine to clarithromycin and ethambutol did not improve clinical response and was associated with higher mortality (see harms below).[33] **Clarithromycin, rifabutin, and ethambutol versus clarithromycin and clofazimine:** The third RCT (144 people) found that the combination of clarithromycin, rifabutin, and ethambutol reduced the relapse rate of MAC compared with clarithromycin plus clofazimine.[34] **Clarithromycin and ethambutol versus rifabutin, clarithromycin, and ethambutol:** The fourth RCT (198 people) found no significant difference in survival between people taking clarithromycin plus ethambutol and people taking clarithromycin plus ethambutol plus rifabutin.[35]

Harms: The second RCT, which added clofazimine to clarithromycin plus rifabutin, found higher mortality in the clofazimine arm (62% with clofazimine *v* 38% without clofazimine; P = 0.012).[33] High doses of clarithromycin (1000 mg twice daily)[36,37] and clofazimine[33] increased mortality. One RCT (85 people) comparing clarithromycin 500 mg twice daily versus 1000 mg twice daily found that, after a median follow up of 4.5 months, more people died with the higher dose (17/40 [43%] with 1000 mg twice daily *v* 10/45 [22%] with 500 mg twice daily; ARI 20%, 95% CI 0.2% to 33%; NNH 5, 95% CI 3 to 470).[36] A similar difference was seen in another RCT (154 people).[37] Combinations of drugs may lead to increased toxicity. Optic neuropathy may occur with ethambutol, but has not been reported in RCTs in people with HIV, where the dose and symptoms were carefully monitored.[35,36]

Comment: The observed increased mortality associated with clofazimine and high doses of clarithromycin has led to avoidance of these drugs.

QUESTION **What are the effects of prophylaxis for cytomegalovirus (CMV), herpes simplex virus (HSV), and varicella zoster virus (VZV)?**

John Ioannidis

OPTION **GANCICLOVIR**

One RCT has found that oral ganciclovir reduces the incidence of CMV in people with severe CD4 depletion compared with placebo. It found that 25% of people who did not take ganciclovir developed severe neutropenia. A second RCT found no significant differences.

Benefits: We found no systematic review. **Versus placebo:** We found two RCTs.[38,39] The first RCT (725 people with a median CD4 count of 22/mm^3) found that oral ganciclovir halved the incidence of CMV compared with placebo (event rate 16% *v* 30%; P = 0.001).[38] The second RCT (994 HIV-1 infected people with CD4 < 100/mm^3 and CMV seropositivity) found no significant difference in the rate of CMV in people taking oral ganciclovir compared with placebo (event rates 13.1 *v* 14.6 per 100 person years; HR 0.92, 95% CI 0.65 to 1.27).[39] Both RCTs found no significant difference in overall mortality.

Harms: In the first RCT, severe neutropenia that required granulocyte colony stimulating factor was more common with ganciclovir versus placebo (24% *v* 9%).[38]

Comment: Differences in the results of RCTs may have arisen by chance or owing to protocol variability; for example, no baseline ophthalmologic examinations were performed in the second trial.[39] The low incidence of CMV disease in people taking highly active antiretroviral treatment, and the high rates of adverse events, means that the clinical value of oral ganciclovir in people who have not had active CMV disease is unclear.

OPTION ACICLOVIR AND VALACICLOVIR

One systematic review has found that aciclovir does not reduce the incidence of CMV disease, but reduces HSV and VZV infection and overall mortality in people at different clinical stages of HIV infection compared with placebo. One RCT found that valaciclovir reduced the incidence of CMV disease more than aciclovir, but non-significantly increased mortality.

Benefits: We found one systematic review of individual patient data (search date not stated, 8 RCTs) in people with HIV infection (ranging from asymptomatic infection to full-blown AIDS).[40] It found no significant difference in protection against CMV disease between aciclovir compared with no treatment or placebo. However, aciclovir significantly reduced overall mortality (RR 0.81; P = 0.04) and HSV and VZV infections (P < 0.001 for both).[40] One RCT (1227 CMV seropositive people with CD4 < 100/mm^3) compared valaciclovir, high dose aciclovir, and low dose aciclovir. It found increased mortality in the valaciclovir group, which did not reach statistical significance (P = 0.06).[41] The CMV rate was lower in the valaciclovir group than the aciclovir groups (12% *v* 18%; P = 0.03).

Harms: One RCT found that toxicity and early medication discontinuations were significantly more frequent in the valaciclovir arm (1 year discontinuation rate: 51% for valaciclovir *v* 46% for high dose aciclovir *v* 41% for low dose aciclovir).[39]

Comment: The survival benefit with aciclovir is unclear. The absolute risk reduction may be higher in people who have frequent HSV or VZV infections.

OPTION FAMCICLOVIR

One small RCT found that famciclovir reduced the rate of viral shedding compared with placebo, but provided insufficient evidence on the effect of famciclovir on HSV recurrence.

Benefits: We found no systematic review. One small crossover placebo controlled RCT (48 people) found that famciclovir suppressed HSV in people with frequent recurrences (HSV was isolated in 9/1071 famciclovir days *v* 122/1114 placebo days; $P < 0.001$).[42] Breakthrough reactivations on famciclovir were short lived and often asymptomatic.

Harms: Famciclovir was well tolerated, and the incidence of adverse effects was similar in both groups.

Comment: The conclusions of this study are difficult to interpret. The randomisation process allocated participants to groups, but the intention to treat analysis involved the number of days with symptoms rather than the number of participants who improved. There was no assessment of statistical significance of clinical outcomes. The trial's analysis is impeded by a high withdrawal rate.

QUESTION What are the effects of prophylaxis for invasive fungal disease in people without previous fungal disease?

John Ioannidis

OPTION AZOLES

RCTs in people with advanced HIV disease have found that both fluconazole and itraconazole reduce the incidence of invasive fungal infections compared with placebo. One RCT found that fluconazole reduced the incidence of invasive fungal disease and mucocutaneous candidiasis more than clotrimazole. One RCT found no difference between high and low dose fluconazole.

Benefits: We found no systematic review. **Fluconazole versus placebo:** One RCT (323 women with CD4 ≤ 300/mm^3) found that fluconazole versus placebo significantly reduced the incidence of candidiasis (44% *v* 58% suffered at least 1 episode of candidiasis; RR 0.56, 95% CI 0.41 to 0.77).[43] **Itraconazole versus placebo:** We found three RCTs.[44–46] The first RCT (295 people with advanced HIV disease) found that itraconazole reduced the incidence of invasive fungal infections ($P = 0.0007$).[44] It found no significant effect on recurrent or refractory candidiasis. The second RCT (129 people with CD4 cell count < 200/mm^3) also found that itraconazole reduced invasive fungal infections compared with placebo after a median of about 40 weeks (AR 1.6% with itraconazole *v* 16.7% with placebo; RR 0.1; $P = 0.003$; CI not stated).[45] In the third RCT (344 people with CD4 cell count < 300/mm^3), itraconazole did not significantly reduce invasive fungal infections compared with placebo (AR 5.9% with itraconazole *v* 7.0% with placebo; $P = 0.42$).[46] However, the study may have lacked power to detect clinically important differences. **High dose versus low dose fluconazole:** One RCT (636 people) compared fluconazole 200 mg daily with

400 mg once weekly and found no difference in the rate of invasive fungal infections over a follow up of 74 weeks (8% *v* 6%; ARR +2.2%, 95% CI –1.7% to +6.%).[47] However, the incidence of candidiasis was twice as common in people taking the weekly dose. **Fluconazole versus clotrimazole:** One RCT found that fluconazole reduced the incidence of invasive fungal disease and mucocutaneous candidal infections compared with clotrimazole (4% *v* 11%; hazard ratio 3.3, 95% CI 1.5 to 7.6).[48]

Harms: Congenital anomalies have occurred in a few children born to mothers receiving fluconazole. Itraconazole is embryotoxic and teratogenic in animals. Trials have therefore excluded pregnant women. Azoles may interact with antiretroviral regimens.[49] Azole drugs inhibit the metabolism of some drugs such as terfenadine. Theoretically they may increase the risk of sudden death because of ventricular tachycardia.

Comment: Azoles effectively reduce invasive fungal disease. Any absolute benefit is probably even lower in people treated with highly active antiretroviral treatment. Lack of evidence of any survival benefit, potential for complex drug interactions with current antiretroviral regimens, and potential for developing resistant fungal isolates means that there is doubt about routine antifungal prophylaxis in HIV infected people without previous invasive fungal disease.

QUESTION What are the effects of prophylaxis for invasive fungal disease in people with previous fungal disease?

John Ioannidis

OPTION AZOLES

Two RCTs found that itraconazole reduced the incidence of relapse of *P marneffei* infection and candidiasis compared with placebo. One RCT found that itraconazole increased the relapse of cryptococcal meningitis compared with fluconazole. We found no RCTs on intraconazole for histoplasmosis.

Benefits: We found no systematic review. **Itraconazole versus placebo:** One RCT (71 people with AIDS in Asia) found that itraconazole significantly reduced the relapse of *P marneffei* infection (see glossary, p 827) compared with placebo (0/36 [0%] *v* 20/35 [57%] relapsed within 1 year; $P < 0.001$).[50] A second RCT (44 people with HIV infection and candidiasis, treated with itraconazole 200 mg for 4 weeks before randomisation) compared prophylaxis with itraconazole versus placebo for 24 weeks. It found that itraconazole reduced relapse rates (5/24 [21%] with itraconazole *v* 14/20 [70%] with placebo; ARR 49%, 95% CI 19% to 64%; NNT 2, 95% CI 2 to 5) and increased the time interval before relapse occurred (median time to relapse: itraconazole 8.0 weeks *v* placebo 10.4 weeks; $P = 0.001$).[51] **Itraconazole versus fluconazole:** One RCT (108 people with HIV infection) found that fluconazole reduced relapses of successfully treated cryptococcal meningitis more than itraconazole (13/57 [23%] with itraconazole *v* 2/51 [4%] with fluconazole; ARR 19%, 95% CI 6.2% to 31.7%; RR 0.17, 95% CI 0.04 to 0.71; NNT 5, 95% CI 3 to 16).[52] The trial was stopped early because of the higher rate of relapse with itraconazole.

Harms: In one RCT, discontinuation of itraconazole occurred in two people because of skin rashes, one because of severe anaemia, and one because of gastrointestinal effects compared with none taking fluconazole.[52]

Comment: Recurrent infection is common in people with previous *C neoformans*, *H capsulatum*, and *P marneffei* infections. Lifelong maintenance may be needed in the presence of immune impairment.

QUESTION What are the effects of discontinuing prophylaxis against opportunistic pathogens in people on highly active antiretroviral treatment (HAART)?

John Ioannidis

OPTION DISCONTINUATION OF PROPHYLAXIS FOR *P CARINII* PNEUMONIA (PCP) AND TOXOPLASMOSIS IN PEOPLE WITH CD4 > 200/MM^3 ON HAART

One systematic review of two unblinded RCTs found that discontinuation of prophylaxis did not increase the incidence of PCP. Two unblinded RCTs found that discontinuation of prophylaxis did not increase the incidence of toxoplasmosis.

Benefits: **PCP:** We found one systematic review (search date 2001, 2 RCTs, 3584 people, two non-randomised controlled trials, and 10 studies with other designs) about the effects of discontinuing prophylaxis.[53] The review found a low incidence of PCP in people discontinuing both primary and secondary prophylaxis after a mean of 1.5 years (7/3035 [0.23%] with discontinuing primary prophylaxis and 1/549 [0.18%] discontinuing secondary prophylaxis; mean annual incidence over 1.5 years 0.23%, 95% CI 0.10% to 0.46%; no statistical heterogeneity among studies). Neither of the two RCTs identified in the review found any cases of PCP after discontinuation (first RCT: 587 people with satisfactory response to HAART, CD4 > 200/mm^3, and viral load < 5000 copies/mm^3 for > 3 months, AR for PCP or toxoplasma encephalitis at median 20 months 0%, whether or not prophylaxis continued;[54] second RCT: 708 people taking HAART, CD4 > 200/mm^3 for 3 months, AR for PCP at 6 months 0%).[55] **Toxoplasmosis:** We found two RCTs.[55,56] The first, which was included in the systematic review, found no cases of toxoplasma encephalitis at 6 months in people discontinuing prophylaxis (see PCP above).[55] The second RCT (302 people with a satisfactory response to HAART) compared discontinuation with continuation of toxoplasma prophylaxis.[56] After a median of 10 months it found no episodes of toxoplasma encephalitis in either group.

Harms: The systematic review found no direct harms from discontinuing prophylaxis.[53]

Comment: The risk of PCP may increase after discontinuing prophylaxis in people who do not respond to antiretroviral treatment. We found no direct evidence of the effects of different HAART regimens on the risk of PCP or toxoplasmosis. Antiretroviral regimens with different mechanisms of action may have different clinical effects on opportunistic infections and HIV disease progression, despite inducing satisfactory suppression of HIV-1 replication and adequate CD4 responses. Also, CD4 cell count is an incomplete marker of immune reconstitution. It is possible that people with the same CD4 count may have different immune deficits regarding control of PCP and other opportunistic pathogens. An extensive amount of research is being conducted on other parameters of immune reconstitution, but the clinical implications are uncertain at present. One decision analysis based on the systematic review suggested that, in the long term, discontinuation of PCP prophylaxis in people who respond to HAART should result in fewer PCP episodes and fewer prophylaxis related adverse effects.[53]

OPTION DISCONTINUATION OF PROPHYLAXIS FOR *M AVIUM* COMPLEX (MAC) DISEASE IN PEOPLE WITH CD4 > 100/MM^3 ON HAART

Two RCTs found that discontinuation of prophylaxis for MAC disease did not increase the incidence of MAC disease.

Benefits: We found no systematic review but we found two RCTs. The first RCT (520 people without previous MAC disease, with CD4 > 100/mm^3 in response to HAART) compared azithromycin with placebo.[57] There were no episodes of confirmed MAC disease in either group over a median follow up of 12 months. The second RCT (643 people with CD4 > 100/mm^3 in response to HAART) compared azithromycin 1200 mg once weekly versus placebo. Over a median follow up of 16 months there was no significant difference in the incidence of MAC between the groups (2/321 [0.62%] with placebo *v* 0/322 [0%] with azithromycin; difference +0.5 events per 100 person years, 95% CI –0.2 to +1.2 events per 100 person years).[58]

Harms: In both RCTs, adverse effects leading to discontinuation of treatment were more common with azithromycin than with placebo (7% *v* 1%, P = 0.002; 8% *v* 2%, P < 0.001).[57,58]

Comment: It is not clear whether different antiretroviral regimens have different clinical effects on opportunistic infections and on the need for specific prophylaxis.

OPTION DISCONTINUATION OF MAINTENANCE TREATMENT FOR CYTOMEGALOVIRUS (CMV) IN PEOPLE WITH A CD4 > 100/MM^3 ON HAART

We found insufficient evidence on the effects of discontinuation of maintenance treatment for CMV retinitis or other end organ disease.

Benefits: We found no systematic review or RCTs.

Harms: We found no evidence from systematic reviews or RCTs.

Comment: We found several small case series (see table 1, p 830).[59–68] Of the two studies with the longest follow-up, one found no relapses in 41 people after a mean of 20.4 months from discontinuing maintenance treatment[59] and the other found only 1 relapse among 36 people after a median follow up of 21 months from discontinuing treatment.[68] The relapse occurred in a person with immunological failure (CD4 62/mm^3). However, another study with mean follow up of 14.5 months found five (29%) relapses among 17 participants who withdrew from maintenance; all of them occurred after the CD4 cell count had dropped again to below 50/mm^3 (8 days/10 months after this event).[62] In one case series, 12/14 (86%) participants had evidence of immune reconstitution retinitis even before starting withdrawal of prophylaxis.[61] Worsening uveitis was associated with a substantial vision loss (> 3 lines) in three participants. It is difficult to conduct a RCT with adequate power to exclude modest differences in relapse rates. The observational evidence suggests that withdrawal of CMV maintenance treatment may be considered in selected people in whom CMV disease is in remission, CD4 > 100mm^3, and HIV replication remains suppressed. We found no clear evidence on whether CMV viral load should be considered in the decision to withdraw from maintenance. One small case series found that relapses were associated with a drop in the CD4 cell count.[62] However, we found no randomised or other reliable evidence about when to restart CMV maintenance treatment.

GLOSSARY

***Penicillium marneffei* infection** A common opportunistic infection in southeast Asia.

The WHO staging system for HIV infection and disease consists of a "clinical axis" that is represented by a sequential list of clinical conditions believed to have prognostic significance, which subdivides the course of HIV infection into four clinical stages; and a "laboratory axis" that subdivides each clinical stage into three strata according to CD4 cell count or total lymphocyte count.

REFERENCES

1. Gallant JE, Moore RD, Chaisson RE. Prophylaxis for opportunistic infections in patients with HIV infection. *Ann Intern Med* 1994;120:932–944.
2. Detels R, Tarwater P, Phair JP, et al. Effectiveness of potent antiretroviral therapies on the incidence of opportunistic infections before and after AIDS diagnosis. *AIDS* 2001;15:347–355.
3. Ioannidis JPA, Cappelleri JC, Skolnik PR, et al. A meta-analysis of the relative efficacy and toxicity of *Pneumocystis carinii* prophylactic regimens. *Arch Intern Med* 1996;156:177–188. Search date 1995; primary sources Medline and conference abstracts.
4. Bucher HC, Griffith L, Guyatt GH, et al. Meta-analysis of prophylactic treatments against *Pneumocystis carinii* pneumonia and toxoplasma encephalitis in HIV-infected patients. *J Acquir Immune Defic Syndr Hum Retrovirol* 1997;15:104–114. Search date not stated; primary sources Medline, Aidsline, Aidstrials, Aidsdrugs, screening the Proceedings of the International and European Conferences on AIDS, bibliographies of identified trials, and by contacting experts.
5. Anglaret X, Chene G, Attia A, et al. Early chemoprophylaxis with trimethroprim-sulphamethoxazole for HIV-1-infected adults in Abidjan, Cote d'Ivoire: a randomized trial. *Lancet* 1999;353:1463–1468.
6. El-Sadr W, Luskin-Hawk R, Yurik TM, et al. A randomized trial of daily and thrice weekly trimethoprim-sulfamethoxazole for the prevention of *Pneumocystis carinii* pneumonia in HIV-infected individuals. *Clin Infect Dis* 1999;29:775–783.
7. Leoung GS, Stanford JF, Giordano MF, et al. Trimethoprim-sulfamethoxazole (TMP-SMZ) dose escalation versus direct rechallenge for Pneumocystis carinii pneumonia prophylaxis in human immunodeficiency virus-infected patients with previous adverse reaction to TMP-SMZ. *J Infect Dis* 2001;184:992–997.
8. Para MF, Finkelstein D, Becker S, et al. Reduced toxicity with gradual initiation of trimethoprim-sulfamethoxazole for *Pneumocystis carinii* pneumonia. *J Acquir Immune Defic Syndr* 2000;24:337–343.
9. Walmsley SL, Khorasheh S, Singer J, et al. A randomized trial of N-acetylcysteine for prevention of trimethoprim-sulfamethoxazole hypersensitivity reactions in *Pneumocystis carinii* pneumonia prophylaxis (CTN057). Canadian HIV Trials Network 057 Study Group. *J Acquir Immune Defic Syndr Hum Retrovirol* 1998;19:498–505.
10. Akerlund B, Tynell E, Bratt G, et al. N-acetylcysteine treatment and the risk of toxic reactions to trimethoprim-sulphamethoxazole in primary *Pneumocystis carinii* prophylaxis in HIV-infected patients. *J Infect* 1997;35:143–147.
11. Saillour-Glenisson F, Chene G, Salmi LR, et al. Effect of dapsone on survival in HIV-infected patients: a meta-analysis. *Rev Epidemiol Sante Publique* 2000;48:17–30. Search date 1996; primary sources Medline, Aidstrials, Aidsdrugs, registries of clinical trials, abstracts from international AIDS conferences and infectious diseases meetings, and consultation with active experts.
12. Maynart M, Lievre L, Sow PS, et al. Primary prevention with cotrimoxazole for HIV-1-infected adults: results of the pilot study in Dakar, Senegal. *J Acquir Immune Defic Syndr* 2001;26:130–136.

13. El Sadr WM, Murphy RL, Yurik TM, et al. Atovaquone compared with dapsone for the prevention of *Pneumocystis carinii* pneumonia in patients with HIV infection who cannot tolerate trimethoprim, sulfonamides, or both. Community Programs for Clinical Research on AIDS and the AIDS Clinical Trials Group. *N Engl J Med* 1998;339:1889–1895.
14. Chan C, Montaner J, Lefebre EA, et al. Atovaquone suspension compared with aerosolized pentamidine for prevention of *Pneumocystis carinii* in human immunodeficiency virus-infected subjects intolerant of trimethoprim or sulfonamides. *J Infect Dis* 1999;180:369–376.
15. Dunne MW, Bozzette S, McCutchan JA, et al. Efficacy of azithromycin in prevention of *Pneumocystis carinii* pneumonia: a randomized trial. California Collaborative Treatment Group. *Lancet* 1999;354:891–895.
16. Havlir DV, Dube MP, Sattler FR, et al. Prophylaxis against disseminated *Mycobacterium avium* complex with weekly azithromycin, daily rifabutin, or both. California Collaborative Treatment Group. *N Engl J Med* 1996;335:392–398.
17. Wilkinson D. Drugs for preventing tuberculosis in HIV infected persons. In: The Cochrane Library, Issue 4, 2001. Oxford: Update Software. Search date 2000; primary sources Cochrane Infectious Diseases Group Trials Register, Cochrane Controlled Trials Register Issue 3, Embase, and hand searched references.
18. Bucher HC, Griffith LE, Guyatt GH, et al. Isoniazid prophylaxis for tuberculosis in HIV infection: a meta-analysis of randomised controlled trials. *AIDS* 1999;13:501–507. Search date not stated; primary sources Medline, Embase, CAB Health, Biosis, Health Star, IDIS Drug File, DHSS-Data, Medical Toxicology and Health, Drug Information, Aidsline, Aidstrial, Aidsdrug, Cochrane Controlled Trials Register, hand searched references, and conference proceedings.
19. Quigley MA, Mwinga A, Hosp M, et al. Long-term effect of preventive therapy for tuberculosis in a cohort of HIV infected Zambian adults. *AIDS* 2001;15:215–222.
20. Fitzgerald DW, Severe P, Joseph P, et al. No effect of isoniazid prophylaxis for purified protein derivative negative HIV-infected adults living in a country with endemic tuberculosis: results of a randomised trial. *J Acquir Immune Defic Syndr* 2001;28:305–307.
21. Selwyn PA, Hartel D, Lewis VA, et al. A prospective study of the risk of tuberculosis among intravenous drug users with human immunodeficiency virus infection. *N Engl J Med* 1989;320:545–550.
22. Halsey NA, Coberly JS, Desmormeaux J, et al. Randomised trial of isoniazid versus rifampicin and pyrazinamide for prevention of tuberculosis in HIV-1 infection. *Lancet* 1998;351:786–792.
23. Mwinga A, Hosp M, Godfrey-Fausset P, et al. Twice weekly tuberculosis preventive therapy in HIV infection in Zambia. *AIDS* 1998;12:2447–2457.
24. Gordin F, Chaisson RE, Matts JP, et al. Rifampin and pyrazinamide vs isoniazid for prevention of tuberculosis in HIV-infected persons: an international randomized trial. *JAMA* 2000;283:1445–1450.
25. Whalen CC, Johson JL, Okwera A, et al. A trial of three regimens to prevent tuberculosis in Ugandan adults with the human immunodeficiency virus. *N Engl Med* 1997;337:801–808.
26. Alfaro EM, Cuadra F, Solera J, et al. Assessment of two chemoprophylaxis regimens for tuberculosis in HIV-infected patients. *Med Clin* 2000;115:161–165.
27. Oldfield EC, Fessel WJ, Dunne MW, et al. Once weekly azithromycin therapy for prevention of *Mycobacterium avium* complex infection in patients with AIDS: a randomized, double-blind, placebo-controlled multicenter trial. *Clin Infect Dis* 1998;26:611–619.
28. Faris MA, Raasch RH, Hopfer RL, et al. Treatment and prophylaxis of disseminated *Mycobacterium avium* complex in HIV-infected individuals. *Ann Pharmacother* 1998;32:564–573. Search date 1997; primary sources Medline and Aidsline.
29. Pierce M, Crampton S, Henry D, et al. A randomized trial of clarithromycin as prophylaxis against disseminated *Mycobacterium avium* complex infection in patients with advanced immunodeficiency syndrome. *N Engl J Med* 1996;335:384–391.
30. Benson CA, Williams PL, Cohn DL, et al. Clarithromycin or rifabutin alone or in combination for primary prophylaxis of *Mycobacterium avium* complex disease in patients with AIDS: a randomized, double-blind, placebo-controlled trial. *J Infect Dis* 2000;181:1289–1297.
31. Tseng AL, Walmsley SL. Rifabutin-associated uveitis. *Ann Pharmacother* 1995;29:1149–1155. Search date 1994; primary sources Medline and hand searches of reference lists and conference abstracts.
32. Dube MP, Sattler FR, Torriani FJ, et al. A randomized evaluation of ethambutol for prevention of relapse and drug resistance during treatment of *Mycobacterium avium* complex bacteremia with clarithromycin-based combination therapy. *J Infect Dis* 1997;176:1225–1232.
33. Chaisson RE, Keiser P, Pierce M, et al. Clarithromycin and ethambutol with or without clofazimine for the treatment of bacteremic *Mycobacterium avium* complex disease in patients with HIV infection. *AIDS* 1997;11:311–317.
34. May T, Brel F, Beuscart C, et al. Comparison of combination therapy regimens for the treatment of human immunodeficiency virus-infected patients with disseminated bacteremia due to *Mycobacterium avium*. ANRS Trial 033 Curavium Group. Agence Nationale de Reserche sur le Sida. *Clin Infect Dis* 1997;25:621–629.
35. Gordin F, Sullam P, Shafran S, et al. A placebo-controlled trial of rifabutin added to a regimen of clarithromycin and ethambutol in the treatment of *M. avium* complex bacteremia. *Clin Infect Dis* 1999;28:1080–1085.
36. Cohn DL, Fisher EJ, Peng GT, et al. A prospective randomized trial of four three-drug regimens in the treatment of disseminated *Mycobacterium avium* complex disease in AIDS patients: excess mortality associated with high-dose clarithromycin. Terry Beirn Programs for Clinical Research on AIDS. *Clin Infect Dis* 1999;29:125–133.
37. Chaisson RE, Benson CA, Dube MP, et al. Clarithromycin therapy for bacteremic *Mycobacterium avium* complex disease: a randomized, double-blind, dose-ranging study in patients with AIDS. *Ann Intern Med* 1994;121:905–911.
38. Spector SA, McKinley GF, Lalezari JP, et al. Oral ganciclovir for the prevention of cytomegalovirus disease in persons with AIDS. Roche Cooperative Oral Ganciclovir Study Group. *N Engl J Med* 1996;334:1491–1497.
39. Brosgart CL, Louis TA, Hillman DW, et al. A randomized, placebo-controlled trial of the safety and efficacy of oral ganciclovir for prophylaxis of cytomegalovirus disease in HIV-infected individuals. Terry Beirn Community Programs for Clinical Research on AIDS. *AIDS* 1998;12:269–277.

40. Ioannidis JPA, Collier AC, Cooper DA, et al. Clinical efficacy of high-dose acyclovir in patients with human immunodeficiency virus infection: a meta-analysis of randomized individual patient data. *J Infect Dis* 1998;178:349–359. Search date not stated; primary sources Medline, abstract searching from major meetings, trial directories, and communication with experts, investigators of the identified trials, and industry researchers.
41. Feinberg JE, Hurwitz S, Cooper D, et al. A randomized, double-blind trial of valaciclovir prophylaxis for cytomegalovirus disease in patients with advanced human immunodeficiency virus infection. AIDS Clinical Trials Group Protocol 204/Glaxo Wellcome 123–014 International CMV Prophylaxis Study Group. *J Infect Dis* 1998;177:48–56.
42. Schacker T, Hu HL, Koelle DM, et al. Famciclovir for the suppression of symptomatic and asymptomatic herpes simplex virus reactivation in HIV-infected persons: a double-blind, placebo-controlled trial. *Ann Intern Med* 1998;128:21–28.
43. Schuman P, Capps L, Peng G, et al. Weekly fluconazole for the prevention of mucosal candidiasis in women with HIV infection: a randomized, double-blind, placebo-controlled trial. *Ann Intern Med* 1997;126:689–696.
44. McKinsey DS, Wheat LJ, Cloud GA, et al. Itraconazole prophylaxis for fungal infections in patients with advanced human immunodeficiency virus infection: randomized, placebo-controlled, double-blind study. National Institute of Allergy and Infectious diseases Mycoses Study Group. *Clin Infect Dis* 1999;28:1049–1056.
45. Chariyalertsak S, Supperatpinyo K, Sirisanthana T, et al. A controlled trial of itraconazole as primary prophylaxis for systemic fungal infections in patients with advanced human immunodeficiency virus infection in Thailand. *Clin Infect Dis* 2002;34:277–284.
46. Smith DE, Bell J, Johnson M, et al. A randomized, double-blind, placebo-controlled study of itraconazole capsules for the prevention of deep fungal infections in immunodeficient patients with HIV infection. *HIV Med* 2001;2:78–83.
47. Havlir DV, Dube MP, McCutchan JA, et al. Prophylaxis with weekly versus daily fluconazole for fungal infections in patients with AIDS. *Clin Infect Dis* 1998;27:253–256.
48. Powderly WG, Finkelstein DM, Feinberg J, et al. A randomized trial comparing fluconazole with clotrimazole troches for the prevention of fungal infections in patients with advanced human immunodeficiency virus infection. *N Engl J Med* 1995;332:700–705.
49. Tseng AL, Foisy MM. Management of drug interactions in patients with HIV. *Ann Pharmacother* 1997;31:1040–1058.
50. Supparatpinyo K, Perriens J, Nelson KE, et al. A controlled trial of itraconazole to prevent relapse of *Penicillium marneffei* infection in patients with the human immunodeficiency virus. *N Engl J Med* 1998;339:1739–1743.
51. Smith D, Midgley J, Gazzard B. A randomized, double-blind study of itraconazole versus placebo in the treatment and prevention of oral or oesophageal candidosis in patients with HIV infection. *Int J Clin Pract* 1999;53:349–352.
52. Saag MS, Cloud GA, Graybill JR, et al. A comparison of itraconazole versus fluconazole as maintenance therapy for AIDS-associated cryptococcal meningitis. *Clin Infect Dis* 1999;28:291–296.
53. Trikalinos TA, Ioannidis JPA. Discontinuation of *Pneumocystis carinii* prophylaxis in patients infected with human immunodeficiency virus: a meta-analysis and decision analysis. *Clin Infect dis* 2001;33:1901–1909. Search date 2001; primary sources Medline, Aidsline, Embase, and abstracts from major meetings.
54. Lopez Bernaldo de Quiros JC, Miro JM, Pena JM, et al. A randomized trial of the discontinuation of primary and secondary prophylaxis against *Pneumocystis carinii* pneumonia after highly active antiretroviral therapy in patients with HIV infection. *N Engl J Med* 2001;344:159–167.
55. Mussini C, Pezzotti P, Govoni A, et al. Discontinuation of primary prophylaxis for *Pneumocystis carinii* pneumonia and toxoplasmic encephalitis in human immunodeficiency virus type I-infected patients: the changes in opportunistic prophylaxis study. *J Infect Dis* 2000;181:1635–1642.
56. Miro JM, Lopez JC, Podzamczer D, et al, and the GESIDA 04/98B study group. Discontinuation of toxoplasmic encephalitis prophylaxis is safe in HIV-1 and *T. gondii* co-infected patients after immunological recovery with HAART. Preliminary results of the GESIDA 04/98B study. In: Abstracts of the 7th Conference on Retroviruses and Opportunistic Infections, Alexandria, Virginia: Foundation for Retrovirology and Human Health. Abstract no. 230.
57. El-Sadr WM, Burman WJ, Grant LB, et al. Discontinuation of prophylaxis for *Mycobacterium avium* complex disease in HIV-infected patients who have a response to antiretroviral therapy. *N Engl J Med* 2000;342:1085–1092.
58. Currier JS, Williams PL, Koletar SL, et al. Discontinuation of Mycobacterium avium complex prophylaxis in patients with antiretroviral therapy-induced increases in CD4+ cell count. A randomized, double-blind, placebo-controlled trial. *Ann Intern Med* 2000;133:493–503.
59. Curi AL, Muralha A, Muralha L, et al. Suspension of anticytomegalovirus maintenance therapy following immune recovery due to highly active antiretroviral therapy. *Br J Ophthalmol* 2001;85:471–473.
60. Jouan M, Saves M, Tubiana R, et al. Discontinuation of maintenance therapy for cytomegalovirus in HIV-infected patients receiving highly active antiretroviral therapy. RESTIMOP study team. *AIDS* 2001;15:23–31.
61. Whitcup SM, Fortin E, Lindblad AS, et al. Discontinuation of anticytomegalovirus therapy in patients with HIV infection and cytomegalovirus retinitis. *JAMA* 1999;282:1633–1637.
62. Torriani FJ, Freeman WR, MacDonald JC, et al. CMV retinitis recurs after stopping treatment in virological and immunological failure of potent antiretroviral therapy. *AIDS* 2000;14:173–180.
63. Postelmans L, Gerald M, Sommereijns B, et al. Discontinuation of maintenance therapy for CMV retinitis in AIDS patients on highly active antiretroviral therapy. *Ocul Immunol Inflamm* 1999;7:199–203.
64. Jabs DA, Bolton SG, Dunn JP, et al. Discontinuing anticytomegalovirus therapy in patients with immune reconstitution after combination therapy. *Am J Opthalmol* 1998;126:817–822.
65. Vrabec TR, Baldassano VF, Whitcup SM. Discontinuation of maintenance therapy in patients with quiescent cytomegalovirus retinitis and elevated CD4+ counts. *Ophthalmology* 1998;105:1259–1264.
66. McDonald JC, Torriani FJ, Morse LS, et al. Lack of reactivation of cytomegalovirus (CMV) retinitis after stopping CMV maintenance therapy in AIDS patients with sustained elevations in CD4 T cells in response to highly active antiretroviral therapy. *J Infect Dis* 1998;177:1182–1187.

67. Tural C, Romeu J, Sirera G, et al. Long-lasting remission of cytomegalovirus retinitis without maintenance therapy in human immunodeficiency virus-infected patients. *J Infect Dis* 1998;177:1080–1083.

68. Berenguer J, Gonzalez J, Pulido F, et al. Discontinuation of secondary prophylaxis in patients with cytomegalovirus retinitis who have responded to highly active antiretroviral therapy. *Clin Infect Dis* 2002;34:394–397.

John Ioannidis
Chairman
Department of Hygiene and Epidemiology
University of Ioannina School of Medicine
Ioannina
Greece

David Wilkinson
Pro Vice Chancellor and Vice President
Division of Health Sciences
University of South Australia
Adelaide
Australia

Competing interests: None declared.

The following previous contributors of this topic would also like to be acknowledged: Margaret Johnson and Andrew Phillips.

TABLE 1 **Observational studies of discontinuation of cytomegalovirus maintenance treatment in people with previous cytomegalovirus disease (see text, p 826).**

Ref	Criteria for discontinuation	Participants	Follow up (months)	Relapses
62*	CD4 >70	17	14.5 (mean)	5
63	CD4 ≥ 75	8	8 (median)	0
61	CD4 >150	14	16.4 (mean)	0
64	CD4 297 (median)	15	8 (median)	0
65	CD4 >100	8	11.4 (mean)	0
66*	CD4 183 (median)	11	5 (median)	0
67	CD4 >150 VL < 200/mL –ve CMV by PCR	7	9 (median)	0
59	CD4 > 143	41	20.4 (mean)	0
60	CD4 > 75 VL < 30 000/mL	48	11 (mean)	2
68	CD4 > 100 VL < 500 or CD4 >150 VL < 10 0000 copies/mL	36	21 (median)	1

Studies with more than five people are included. CD4 count is measured in cells/mm^3.
*McDonald et al[66] is an early report of the same study followed by the Torriani et al[62] report. All relapses in the latter report occurred in people who had already experienced a decrease of CD4 to < 50 cells/mm^3.
CMV, cytomegalovirus; PCR, polymerase chain reaction; Ref, reference; VL, viral load (HIV-1 RNA in plasma).

Chickenpox

Search date November 2002

George Swingler

QUESTIONS

INTERVENTIONS

See glossary, p 837

Key Messages

Prevention

- **Aciclovir in people with immunocompromise other than HIV** We found no RCTs.
- **High dose aciclovir (> 3200 mg/day) in people with HIV infection** One systematic review has found that high dose aciclovir (at least 3200 mg/day) significantly reduces the risk of clinical chickenpox and reduces all cause mortality over 22 months' treatment compared with placebo.
- **Live attenuated vaccine in healthy children** Two RCTs have found that live attenuated varicella vaccine significantly reduces clinical chickenpox compared with placebo, with no significant increase in adverse effects.
- **Live attenuated vaccine in healthy adults or immunocompromised people** We found no RCTs in immunocompromised people on the effects of live attenuated varicella vaccine.

- **Zoster immune globulin versus human serum globulin in healthy children** One small RCT in children exposed to a sibling with chickenpox found that zoster immune globulin significantly reduced the number of exposed children with clinical chickenpox at 20 days compared with human immune serum globulin.
- **Zoster immune globulin versus varicella zoster immune globulin in immunocompromised children** One RCT in immunocompromised children exposed to a sibling with chickenpox found no significant difference in clinical chickenpox with zoster immune globulin compared with varicella zoster immune globulin at 12 weeks.

Treatment

- **Intravenous aciclovir for treatment of chickenpox in children with malignancy** Two RCTs compared intravenous aciclovir versus placebo; one large RCT has found that aciclovir significantly reduces clinical deterioration, and the other small RCT found no significant difference in clinical deterioration.
- **Oral aciclovir in healthy people (given < 24 h of onset of the rash)** Two systematic reviews have found that oral aciclovir, compared with placebo, reduces the symptoms of chickenpox in healthy people.
- **Oral aciclovir in healthy people (given > 24 h after the onset of the rash)** One systematic review and one additional RCT have found that oral aciclovir given beyond 24 hours after onset of rash does not significantly reduce the symptoms of chickenpox compared with placebo.

DEFINITION Chickenpox is due to primary infection with varicella zoster virus. In healthy people it is usually a mild self limiting illness, characterised by low grade fever, malaise, and a generalised, itchy, vesicular rash.

INCIDENCE/ PREVALENCE Chickenpox is extremely contagious. Over 90% of unvaccinated people become infected, but infection occurs at different ages in different parts of the world: over 80% of people have been infected by the age of 10 years in the USA, UK, and Japan, and by the age of 30 years in India, Southeast Asia, and the West Indies.[1,2]

AETIOLOGY/ RISK FACTORS Chickenpox is caused by exposure to varicella zoster virus.

PROGNOSIS **Infants and children:** In healthy children the illness is usually mild and self limiting. In the USA, death rates in infants and children aged 1–14 years with chickenpox are about 7/100 000 and 1.4/100 000, respectively.[3] In Australia, mortality in children aged between 1 and 11 years with chickenpox is about 0.5–0.6/100 000, and in infants with chickenpox it is about 1.2/100 000.[4] Bacterial skin sepsis is the most common complication in children under 5 years of age, and acute cerebellar ataxia is the most common complication in older children; both cause hospital admission in 2–3/10 000 children.[5] **Adults:** Mortality in adults is higher, at about 31/100 000.[3] Varicella pneumonia is the most common complication, causing 20–30 hospital admissions/10 000 adults.[5] Activation of latent varicella zoster virus infection can cause herpes zoster, also known as shingles (see postherpetic neuralgia, p 942). **Cancer chemotherapy:** One case series (77 children with cancer and chickenpox) found that more children receiving chemotherapy versus those in remission developed progressive chickenpox with multiple organ involvement (19/60 [32%] *v* 0/17 [0%]) and more children died (4/60 [7%] v 0/17 [0%]).[6] **HIV infection:** One retrospective case series found that one in four children with HIV who acquired chickenpox in hospital developed pneumonia and 5% died.[7] In a retrospective cohort study (73 children with HIV and chickenpox), infection beyond 2 months occurred in 10 children (14%) and recurrent varicella zoster virus infections occurred in 38 children (55%).[8] Half of recurrent infections involved generalised rashes and the other half had zoster. **Newborns:** We found no cohort studies of untreated children with perinatal exposure to chickenpox. One cohort study (281 neonates receiving varicella zoster immune globulin [see glossary, p 837] because their mothers had developed a chickenpox rash during the month before or after delivery) found that 134 (48%) developed a chickenpox rash and 19 (14%) developed severe chickenpox.[9] Severe chickenpox occurred in neonates of mothers whose rash had started during the 7 days before delivery.

AIMS OF INTERVENTION To prevent clinical chickenpox (characterised by a rash); to reduce the duration of illness and complications of chickenpox.

OUTCOMES Development of clinical chickenpox; duration of illness (time to no new lesions, disappearance of fever); complications of chickenpox; mortality.

METHODS *Clinical Evidence* search and appraisal November 2002. All identified RCTs with English abstracts were reviewed.

QUESTION What are the effects of interventions to prevent chickenpox?

OPTION LIVE ATTENUATED VARICELLA VACCINE

Two RCTs identified by a systematic review have found that, live attenuated varicella vaccine significantly reduces chickenpox in healthy children compared with placebo, with no significant increase in adverse effects. We found no RCTs in healthy adults or immunocompromised people.

Benefits: We found one systematic review (search date 2000, 2 RCTs reporting clinical outcomes).[10] **In healthy children:** The first RCT (914 healthy children aged 1–14 years) found that live attenuated varicella vaccine significantly reduced clinical chickenpox at 9 months (0/468 [0%] with vaccine v 38/446 [8.5%] with placebo; OR 0.0, 95% CI 0.0 to 0.09)[11] and at 2 years (1/163 [1%] with vaccine v 21/161 [13%] with placebo; OR 0.05, 95% CI 0.01 to 0.35).[12] The second RCT (327 healthy children aged 10–30 months) also found that live attenuated varicella vaccine significantly reduced clinical chickenpox after a mean of 29 months (AR 5/166 [3.0%] with vaccine v 41/161 [25%] with placebo; RR 0.12, 95% CI 0.05 to 0.29).[13] **In healthy adults:** The review found no RCTs assessing clinical outcomes in healthy adults with chickenpox. **In immunocompromised people:** The review identified no RCTs assessing clinical outcomes in people receiving cancer chemotherapy, in people with HIV, or in those aged under 1 month or over 65 years.[10]

Harms: **In healthy people:** The second RCT found that the only reported adverse effect with varicella vaccine was a non-significant increase in varicella-like papules or vesicles (AR 5.4% with vaccine *v* 3.7% with placebo; RR 1.45, 95% CI 0.53 to 4.0).[10] No children had fever or constitutional symptoms. One postmarketing analysis of a database of 89 753 vaccinated adults and children found no associations with any rare serious adverse events.[14] Another analysis found that the rate of serious adverse events was 2.9/100 000 doses.[15] **In immunocompromised people:** One RCT reporting non-clinical outcomes found that, of 22 children vaccinated at the start of cancer chemotherapy, three (14%) developed mild maculopapular rashes and fever 16, 24, and 40 days after vaccination, and one had an isolated fever 7 days after vaccination.[16]

Comment: A new systematic review of vaccines for preventing varicella in children and adults is under way.[17]

OPTION ACICLOVIR

One systematic review in people with HIV infection, has found that high dose aciclovir significantly reduces the risk of clinical chickenpox and reduces all cause mortality over 22 months' treatment compared with placebo. We found no RCTs in people with other forms of immunocompromise.

Benefits: **In people with HIV:** We found one systematic review (search date not stated, 8 RCTs, 1792 people with different stages of HIV, median CD4 count 34–607/mm^3) comparing high dose aciclovir versus placebo.[18] Three of the RCTs were unpublished, including two pharmaceutical company trials. The review found that aciclovir (at least 3200 mg/day for up to 22 months) significantly reduced clinical chickenpox (AR 14/895 [2%] with aciclovir *v* 54/897 [6%] with placebo; OR 0.29, 95% CI 0.13 to 0.63; NNT 23, 95% CI 17 to 39). All cause mortality was also reduced (HR 0.78, 95% CI 0.65 to 0.93; OR 0.75, 95% CI 0.57 to 1.00). We found no RCTs of lower doses of aciclovir in people with HIV. **In other immunocompromised people:** We found no RCTs of aciclovir in people with other forms of immunocompromise.

Harms: The systematic review did not assess adverse effects (see harms under aciclovir for treatment, p 836).

Comment: None.

OPTION ZOSTER IMMUNE GLOBULIN

We found insufficient evidence to assess zoster immune globulin in healthy or immunocompromised adults. One small RCT in healthy children found that zoster immune globulin reduced the number of children with clinical chickenpox compared with immune serum globulin. We found no RCTs comparing zoster immune globulin versus varicella zoster immune globulin in healthy children. One RCT in immunocompromised children exposed to a sibling with chickenpox found no significant difference in clinical chickenpox at 12 weeks with zoster immune globulin compared with varicella zoster immune globulin.

Benefits: We found no systematic review. **Versus placebo:** We found no RCTs. **Versus immune serum globulin (ISG) in healthy children:** See glossary, p 837. We found one small RCT (12 healthy susceptible children exposed to a sibling with recent onset of chickenpox) comparing zoster immune globulin (ZIG) (see glossary, p 837) (2 mL/10 kg) versus ISG (2 mL/10 kg).[19] It found that ZIG significantly reduced the number of children with clinical chickenpox at 20 days (AR 0/6 [0%] *v* 6/6 [100%]; OR 0.0, 95% CI 0 to 0.28). **Versus ISG in immunocompromised children:** We found no RCTs. **Versus varicella zoster immune globulin (VZIG) in healthy children:** We found no RCTs. **Versus VZIG in immunocompromised children:** See glossary, p 837. We found one RCT (164 immunocompromised children, mostly with leukaemia, exposed to a sibling with chickenpox) comparing ZIG (1.25 mL/10 kg) versus VZIG (1.25 mL/10 kg).[20] It found no significant difference in the number of children with clinical chickenpox at 12 weeks (AR 31/88 [37%] with ZIG *v* 36/81 [44%] with VZIG; RR 0.84, 95% CI 0.58 to 1.22). A second RCT compared high dose VZIG (2.5 mL/10 kg) versus low dose VZIG (1.25 mL/10 kg).[20] It found no significant difference in the number of children with clinical chickenpox at 12 weeks (AR 19/40 [47.5%] with low dose *v* 22/46 [48%] with high dose; RR 1.00, 95% CI 0.61 to 1.65).

Harms: None of the RCTs assessed adverse effects.

Comment: The imprecise estimates might not exclude clinically important differences, especially in the comparison of high dose versus low dose VZIG.[20]

QUESTION What are the effects of treatments for chickenpox?

OPTION ACICLOVIR

Two systematic reviews have found that, oral aciclovir compared with placebo reduces the symptoms of chickenpox in healthy people. A systematic review and a subsequent RCT found an effect when given within 24 hours of onset of the rash, but found no significant difference if started after 24 hours. Two RCTs compared intravenous aciclovir versus placebo in children with cancer; one large RCT found that aciclovir significantly reduced clinical deterioration, whereas the other smaller RCT found no significant difference.

Benefits: **In healthy children:** We found one systematic review in children and adolescents[21] and one additional RCT in both children and adults.[22] The systematic review (search date 2002, 3 RCTs, 979 children) compared aciclovir versus placebo given within 24 hours of onset of rash in otherwise healthy children aged 0–18 years.[21] It did not perform a meta-analysis because of differences in age among participants. Two of the three RCTs included in the review found that aciclovir (20 mg/kg or 800 mg 4 times daily) significantly reduced the time to no new lesions (WMD 1.2 days, 95% CI 1.0 to 1.5 in the first RCT; WMD 1.1 days, 95% CI 0.5 to 1.8 in the second RCT). The remaining RCT found no significant difference in the time to new lesions with aciclovir (10–20 mg/kg) compared with placebo (WMD 0 days, 95% CI –0.5 to 0.5). The number of days to no fever was significantly reduced by aciclovir in all three RCTs (WMD 1.1 days, 95% CI 0.9 to 1.3; 1.0 days, 95% CI 0.5 to 1.5; and 1.3 days, 95% CI 0.6 to 2.0, respectively).[21] We found one additional RCT that included children, adolescents, and adults (77 people).[22] It found that aciclovir started on the second versus the third day of the rash significantly reduced the time to no new lesions in children (median 4 days *v* 5 days; P < 0.04) but found no significant difference in adolescents and adults. Earlier treatment significantly reduced the time to cessation of fever in adolescents (median 2–3 days *v* 3–4 days; P < 0.02) but not in children and adults. **In healthy adults:** We found one systematic review (search date 1997, 3 RCTs).[23] It did not perform a meta-analysis. The first RCT identified by the review (76 adults) compared early and late administration of aciclovir, (800 mg 5 times daily), versus placebo. It found that aciclovir given within 24 hours of the rash significantly reduced the maximum number of lesions and the time to full crusting of lesions compared with placebo, but found no difference in time to full crusting of lesions if aciclovir was given 24–72 hours after the rash. The two remaining RCTs (total of 168 healthy adults) compared aciclovir given more than 24 hours after the onset of the rash versus placebo. Neither found a significant difference in the time to no new lesions, and did not provide numerical information on the time to cessation of fever. We found one additional RCT that included children, adolescents, and adults (see in healthy children above).[22] **In immunocompromised children:** We found two placebo controlled RCTs of intravenous aciclovir in children with cancer receiving chemotherapy.[24,25] The largest RCT (50 children aged 1–14 years with chickenpox, 60% of whom had a rash for > 24 h) found that significantly fewer children receiving aciclovir (500 mg/m²), deteriorated clinically and were transferred to open aciclovir (1/25 [4%] with aciclovir *v* 12/25 [48%] with placebo; RR 0.08, 95% CI 0.01 to 0.59; NNT 3, 95% CI 2 to 4).[24] Analysis of the remaining children not moved to open aciclovir found that aciclovir significantly reduced the time to full crusting of lesions (mean 5.7 *v* 7.1 days on placebo; P < 0.013), but found no significant difference in cessation of fever. The second RCT (20 children, mean age 6.4 years) comparing aciclovir (500 mg/m²) versus placebo found no significant difference in the number of children who deteriorated clinically and were moved to open aciclovir (AR 1/8 [12.5%] with aciclovir *v* 5/12 [42%] with placebo; RR 0.30, 95% CI 0.04 to 2.1).[25] However, the RCT was too small to exclude a clinically important difference. **In immunocompromised adults:** We found no RCTs.

Harms: No serious harms were reported in any of the seven RCTs in healthy people, except for one child taking placebo who developed cerebellar ataxia. Of the three RCTs (total of 979 people) in the first review reporting possible adverse effects, none found significant differences between treatment and control groups, or unfavourable trends in children taking aciclovir.[21] Adverse effects assessed included gastrointestinal symptoms, leukopoenia, thrombocytopoenia, and abnormalities of liver enzymes.

Comment: The effect on the measured outcomes was small and of questionable clinical importance in healthy people who make an uneventful recovery without treatment. In the first RCT in immunocompromised children, the exclusion from the subsequent analysis of children taking placebo who deteriorated clinically means that the effect of placebo may have been overestimated.[24]

GLOSSARY

Immune serum globulin (ISG) Immunoglobulin prepared from pooled human plasma.
Varicella zoster immune globulin (VZIG) Prepared from units of donor plasma selected for high titres of antibodies to varicella zoster virus.
Zoster immune globulin (ZIG) Prepared from the plasma of donors convalescing from herpes zoster (sustainable supplies are difficult to obtain).

REFERENCES

1. Lee BW. Review of varicella zoster seroepidemiology in India and Southeast Asia. *Trop Med Int Health* 1998;3:886–890.
2. Garnett GP, Cox MJ, Bundy DA, et al. The age of infection with varicella-zoster virus in St Lucia, West Indies. *Epidemiol Infect* 1993;110:361–372.
3. Preblud SR. Varicella: complications and costs. *Pediatrics* 1986;78:728–735.
4. Scuffman PA, Lowin AV, Burgess MA. The cost effectiveness of varicella vaccine programs for Australia. *Vaccine* 1999;18:407–415.
5. Guess HA, Broughton DD, Melton LJ, et al. Population-based studies of varicella complications. *Pediatrics* 1986;78:723–727.
6. Feldman S, Hughes WT, Daniel CB. Varicella in children with cancer: seventy-seven cases. *Pediatrics* 1975;56:388–397.
7. Leibovitz E, Cooper D, Giurgiutiu D, et al. Varicella-zoster virus infection in Romanian children infected with the human immunodeficiency virus. *Pediatrics* 1993;92:838–842.
8. von Seidlein L, Gillette SG, Bryson Y, et al. Frequent recurrence and persistence of varicella-zoster virus infections in children infected with human immunodeficiency virus type 1. *J Pediatr* 1996;128:52–57.
9. Miller E, Cradock-Watson JE, Ridehalgh MK. Outcome in newborn babies given anti-varicella-zoster immunoglobulin after perinatal maternal infection with varicella-zoster virus. *Lancet* 1989;2:371–373.
10. Skull SA, Wang EE. Varicella vaccination: a critical review of the evidence. *Arch Dis Child* 2001;85:83–90. Search date 2000; primary sources Medline, Embase, The Cochrane Library, reference lists, the internet for position papers from health organisations, and vaccine product information.
11. Weibel RE, Neff BJ, Kuter BJ, et al. Live attenuated varicella virus vaccine. Efficacy trial in healthy children. *New Engl J Med* 1984;310:1409–1415.
12. Kuter BJ, Weibel RE, Guess HA, et al. Oka/Merck varicella vaccine in healthy children: final report of a 2-year efficacy study and 7-year follow-up studies. *Vaccine* 1991;9:643–647.
13. Varis T, Vesikari T. Efficacy of high-titer live attenuated varicella vaccine in healthy young children. *J Infect Dis* 1996;174:S330–S334.
14. Black S, Shinefield H, Ray P, et al. Postmarketing evaluation of the safety and effectiveness of varicella vaccine. *Pediatr Infect Dis J* 1999;18:1041–1046.
15. Wise RP, Salive ME, Braun MM, et al. Postlicensure safety surveillance for varicella vaccine. *JAMA* 2000;284:1271–1279.
16. Cristofani LM, Weinberg A, Peixoto V, et al. Administration of live attenuated varicella vaccine to children with cancer before starting chemotherapy. *Vaccine* 1991;9:873–876.
17. Coole L, Law B, McIntyre P. Vaccines for preventing varicella in children and adults. (Protocol for a Cochrane Review). In: The Cochrane Library, Issue 1, 2002. Oxford: Update Software.
18. Ioannidis JP, Collier AC, Cooper DA, et al. Clinical efficacy of high-dose aciclovir in patients with human immunodeficiency virus infection: a meta-analysis of randomized individual patient data. *J Infect Dis* 1998;178:349–359. Search date not stated; primary sources Medline, handsearching of abstracts from meetings, trial directories, and communication with experts.
19. Brunell PA, Ross A, Miller LH, et al. Prevention of varicella by zoster immune globulin. *N Engl J Med* 1969;280:1191–1194.
20. Zaia JA, Levin MJ, Preblud SR, et al. Evaluation of varicella-zoster immune globulin: protection of immunosuppressed children after household exposure to varicella. *J Infect Dis* 1983;147:737–743.
21. Klassen TP, Belseck EM, Wiebe N, et al. Acyclovir for treating varicella in otherwise healthy children and adolescents (Cochrane Review). In: The Cochrane Library, Issue 4, 2002. Oxford: Update Software. Search date 2002; primary sources Cochrane Controlled Trials Register, Medline, Embase, PubMed, handsearch of reference lists, and contact with authors and pharmaceutical companies.
22. Balfour HH Jr, Edelman CK, Anderson RS, et al. Controlled trial of acyclovir for chickenpox evaluating time of initiation and duration of therapy and viral resistance. *Pediatr Infect Dis J* 2001;20:919–926.
23. Alfandari S. Second question: antiviral treatment of varicella in adult or immunocompromised patients. *Medecine et Maladies Infectieuses* 1998;28:722–729. Search date 1997; primary sources Medline, Embase, and handsearches of reference lists and selected journals.
24. Nyerges G, Meszner Z, Gyarmati E, et al. Aciclovir prevents dissemination of varicella in immunocompromised children. *J Infect Dis* 1988;157:309–313.
25. Prober CG, Kirk LE, Keeney RE. Aciclovir therapy of chickenpox in immunosuppressed children: a collaborative study. *J Pediatr* 1982;101:622–625.

George Swingler
School of Child and Adolescent Health,
Red Cross Children's Hospital and the
University of Cape Town
Cape Town
South Africa

Competing interests: None declared.

The following previous contributor of this topic would also like to be acknowledged: Jimmy Volmink.

Congenital toxoplasmosis

Search date November 2002

Piero Olliaro

QUESTIONS

INTERVENTIONS

Unknown effectiveness

See glossary, p 841

Key Messages

- **Spiramycin and other antiparasitic drugs** Two systematic reviews of cohort studies in women who seroconvert during pregnancy found insufficient evidence on the effects of current antiparasitic treatment compared with no treatment on mother or baby.

Congenital toxoplasmosis

DEFINITION Toxoplasmosis is caused by the parasite *Toxoplasma gondii*. Infection is asymptomatic or unremarkable in immunocompetent individuals, but leads to a lifelong antibody response. During pregnancy, toxoplasmosis can be transmitted across the placenta and may cause intrauterine death, neonatal growth retardation, mental retardation, ocular defects, and blindness in later life. Congenital toxoplasmosis (confirmed infection of the fetus or newborn) can present at birth, either as subclinical disease, which may evolve with neurological or ophthalmological disease later in life, or as a disease of varying severity, ranging from mild ocular damage to severe mental retardation.

INCIDENCE/ PREVALENCE Reported rates of toxoplasma seroprevalence vary across and within countries, as well as over time. The risk of primary infection is highest in young people, including young women during pregnancy. We found no cohort studies describing annual seroconversion rates in women of childbearing age nor incidence of primary infection. One systematic review (search date 1996) identified 15 studies that reported rates of seroconversion in non-immune pregnant women ranging from 2.4–16/1000 in Europe and from 2–6/1000 in the USA.[1] France began screening for congenital toxoplasmosis in 1978, and during the period 1980–1995 the seroconversion rate during pregnancy in non-immune women was 4–5/1000.[2]

AETIOLOGY/ RISK FACTORS Toxoplasma infection is usually acquired by ingesting either sporocysts (from unwashed fruit or vegetables contaminated by cat faeces) or tissue cysts (from raw or undercooked meat). The risk of contracting toxoplasma infection varies with eating habits, contact with cats and other pets, and occupational exposure.

PROGNOSIS One systematic review of studies conducted from 1983–1996 found no population based prospective studies of the natural history of toxoplasma infection during pregnancy.[1] One systematic review (search date 1997) reported nine controlled, non-randomised studies, and found that untreated toxoplasmosis acquired during pregnancy was associated with infection rates in children of between 10–100%.[3] We found two European studies that correlated gestation at time of seroconversion with risk of transmission and severity of disease at birth.[4,5] Risk of transmission increased with gestational age at maternal seroconversion, reaching 70–90% for infections acquired after 30 weeks' gestation. In contrast, the risk of the infected infant developing clinical disease was highest when infection occurred early in pregnancy. The highest risk of early signs of disease (including chorioretinitis and hydrocephaly) was about 10%, and occurred with infection between 24 and 30 weeks' gestation.[5] Infants with untreated congenital toxoplasmosis and generalised neurological abnormalities at birth develop mental retardation, growth retardation, blindness or visual defects, seizures, and spasticity. Children with untreated subclinical infection at birth may have cognitive and motor deficits and visual defects or blindness, which may go undiagnosed for many years. One case control study (845 school children in Brazil) found mental retardation and retinochoroiditis to be significantly associated with positive toxoplasma serology (population attributable risk 6–9%).[6]

AIMS OF INTERVENTION To prevent transmission from mother to child, congenital infection, visual impairment, and neurological impairment in neonates and in later life, with minimum adverse effects.

OUTCOMES Incidence of spontaneous abortion, fetal infection, and overt neonatal disease (neurological and visual impairment); serological positivity in the newborn; adverse effects of treatment.

METHODS *Clinical Evidence* search and appraisal November 2002.

QUESTION **What are the effects on mother and baby of antiparasitic treatment in women found to be seropositive for toxoplasma during pregnancy?**

We found no reliable evidence on the effects of treating women who seroconvert during pregnancy.

Benefits: We found two systematic reviews (search dates 1997).[3,7] The first identified no RCTs.[3] The second review identified nine small cohort studies comparing treatments (spiramycin alone, pyrimethamine-sulphonamides, or a combination of the 2 treatments) versus no treatment.[7] One study of case series of women treated with spiramycin or spiramycin plus pyrimethamine–sulphonamide found no evidence of difference in outcomes (fetal infection, overt neonatal disease).[8] Comparing data from these studies was difficult because of different follow up periods.

Harms: Spiramycin and pyrimethamine–sulphonamides are reportedly well tolerated and non-teratogenic.[9] Sulpha drugs are known to carry a risk of kernicterus (see glossary, p 841) in the newborn and should be avoided if possible in the third trimester; there is also a risk of bone marrow suppression, which can be reduced through concomitant use of folic acid.[9]

Comment: We found that the quality of evidence was poor. Studies included in the systematic review were small and did not account for differences in gestation. Only two studies provided information about the control group and congenital infection was common in the treatment groups.[7] One decision analysis on screening and treatment for intrauterine toxoplasma infection has suggested that treatment may save the pregnancy without preventing infection in the neonate. This may lead to an increase in congenital disease.[10] Drug regimens of co-trimoxazole (trimethoprim plus sulfamethoxazole [sulphamethoxazole]), atovaquone, or fluoroquinolones, which are either used or are being tested for secondary prophylaxis of toxoplasmosis in immunocompromised people (particularly those with HIV infection), have not been studied in pregnancy because their reproductive toxicity has not been properly documented. Finally, optimal duration of follow up is not established, although the longer the children are observed the higher the incidence of sequelae.

GLOSSARY

Kernicterus Cerebral toxicity, caused by high levels of bilirubin in the neonate. Clinical effects include vomiting, lethargy, fever, and fits.

REFERENCES

1. Eskild A, Oxman A, Magnus P, et al. Screening for toxoplasmosis in pregnancy: what is the evidence of reducing a health problem? *J Med Screen* 1996;3:188–194. Search date 1996; primary sources Medline, Cochrane Pregnancy and Childbirth Database, and hand searched references.
2. Carme B, Tirard-Fleury V. Toxoplasmosis among pregnant women in France: seroprevalence, seroconversion and knowledge levels: trends 1965–1995. *Med Malad Infect* 1996;26:431–436.
3. Wallon M, Liou C, Garner P, et al. Congenital toxoplasmosis: systematic review of evidence of efficacy of treatment in pregnancy. *BMJ* 1999;318:1511–1514. Search date 1997; primary sources Medline, Embase, Pascal, Biological Abstracts, and personal communications.
4. Foulon W, Villena I, Stray-Pedersen B, et al. Treatment of toxoplasmosis during pregnancy: a multicenter study of impact on fetal transmission and children's sequelae at age 1 year. *Am J Obstet Gynecol* 1999;180:410–415.
5. Dunn D, Wallon M, Peyron F, et al. Mother-to-child transmission of toxoplasmosis: risk estimates for clinical counselling. *Lancet* 1999;353:1829–1833.
6. Caiaffa WT, Chiari CA, Figueiredo AR, et al. Toxoplasmosis and mental retardation: report of a case-control study. *Mem Inst Oswaldo Cruz* 1993;88:253–261.
7. Peyron F, Wallon M, Liou C, et al. Treatments for toxoplasmosis in pregnancy. In: The Cochrane Library, Issue 2, 2000. Oxford: Update Software. Search date 1997; primary sources Medline, Embase, Pascal, Biological Abstracts, and the Cochrane Controlled Trials Register.
8. Vergani P, Ghidini A, Ceruti P, et al. Congenital toxoplasmosis: efficacy of maternal treatment with spiramycin alone. *Am J Reprod Immunol* 1998;39:335–340.
9. Garland SM, O'Reilly MA. The risks and benefits of antimicrobial therapy in pregnancy. *Drug Saf* 1995;13:188–205.
10. Bader TJ, Macones GA, Asch DA. Prenatal screening for toxoplasmosis. *Obstet Gynecol* 1997;90:457–464.

Piero Olliaro
Scientist/Manager
UNDP/World Bank/WHO Special Programme for Research and Training in Tropical Diseases CDS/TDR/World Health Organization
Geneva
Switzerland

Competing interests: None declared.

Diarrhoea in adults

Search date October 2002

Guy de Bruyn

QUESTIONS

INTERVENTIONS

See glossary, p 849

Key Messages

- **Amino acid oral rehydration solution (ORS) (*v* standard ORS)** One small RCT has found that amino acid ORS versus standard ORS reduces the total volume and duration of diarrhoea.
- **Antimotility agents** RCTs have found that loperamide hydrochloride and loperamide oxide versus placebo significantly reduce the time to relief of symptoms, but frequently cause constipation. We found insufficient evidence about the effects of other antimotility agents.
- **Bicarbonate ORS (*v* standard ORS)** Two RCTs found no significant difference in the duration or volume of diarrhoea with bicarbonate ORS versus standard ORS. One RCT found no significant difference in total stool output or duration of diarrhoea with bicarbonate ORS versus an otherwise identical ORS in which the bicarbonate was replaced with chloride.
- **Empirical antibiotic treatment in community acquired diarrhoea** RCTs have found that ciprofloxacin versus placebo reduces the duration of community acquired diarrhoea by 1–2 days. RCTs found limited evidence that other antibiotics, except for lomefloxacin, reduced duration of diarrhoea compared with placebo. Adverse effects varied by agent.

Diarrhoea in adults

- **Empirical antibiotic treatment in travellers' diarrhoea** One systematic review and one additional RCT have found that empirical use of antibiotics versus placebo significantly increases cure rate at 3 and 6 days. Antibiotic treatment is associated in some people with prolonged presence of bacterial pathogens in the stool and development of resistant strains.
- **Reduced osmolarity ORS (*v* standard ORS)** Three RCTs comparing reduced osmolarity ORS versus standard ORS found a small and inconsistent effect on total volume of stool and duration of diarrhoea.
- **Rice based ORS (*v* standard ORS)** One systematic review has found that rice based ORS versus standard ORS significantly reduced the 24 hour stool volume.

DEFINITION Diarrhoea is watery or liquid stools, usually with an increase in stool weight above 200 g daily and an increase in daily stool frequency. This chapter covers empirical treatment of suspected infectious diarrhoea in adults.

INCIDENCE/ PREVALENCE An estimated 4000 million cases of diarrhoea occurred worldwide in 1996, resulting in 2.5 million deaths.[1] In the USA, the estimated incidence for infectious intestinal disease is 0.44 episodes per person a year (1 episode per person every 2.3 years), resulting in about one consultation with a doctor per person every 28 years.[2] A recent community study in the UK reported an incidence of 19 cases per 100 person years, of which 3.3 cases per 100 person years resulted in consultation with a general practitioner.[3] The epidemiology of travellers' diarrhoea (in people who have crossed a national boundary) is not well understood. Incidence is higher in travellers visiting developing countries, but it varies widely by location and season of travel.[4]

AETIOLOGY/ RISK FACTORS The cause of diarrhoea depends on geographic location, standards of food hygiene, sanitation, water supply, and season. Commonly identified causes of sporadic diarrhoea in adults in developed countries include *Campylobacter*, *Salmonella*, *Shigella*, *Escherichia coli*, *Yersinia*, protozoa, and viruses. No pathogens are identified in more than half of people with diarrhoea. In returning travellers, about 50% of episodes are caused by bacteria such as enterotoxigenic *E coli*, *Salmonella*, *Shigella*, *Campylobacter*, *Vibrio*, enteroadherent *E coli*, *Yersinia*, and *Aeromonas*.[5]

PROGNOSIS In developing countries, diarrhoea is reported to cause more deaths in children under 5 years of age than any other condition.[1] Few studies have examined which factors predict poor outcome in adults. In developed countries, death from infectious diarrhoea is rare, although serious complications, including severe dehydration and renal failure, can occur and may necessitate admission to hospital. Elderly people and those in long term care have an increased risk of death.[6]

AIMS OF INTERVENTION To reduce the infectious period, length of illness, risk of dehydration, risk of transmission to others, and rates of severe illness; and to prevent complications and death.

OUTCOMES Time from start of treatment to last loose stool; number of loose stools a day; stool volume; time to first formed stool; duration of diarrhoea; duration of excretion of organisms; presence of bacterial resistance; relief of cramps, nausea and vomiting; incidence of vomiting; incidence of severe illness; and rate of hospital admission.

METHODS *Clinical Evidence* search and appraisal October 2002.

QUESTION What are the effects of empirical antibiotic treatment in travellers' diarrhoea?

One systematic review and one additional RCT have found that empirical use of antibiotics versus placebo significantly increases the cure rate of travellers' diarrhoea. Antibiotic treatment is associated in some people with prolonged presence of bacterial pathogens in the stool and development of resistant strains.

Benefits: We found one systematic review[7] and one additional RCT.[8] The systematic review (search date 2000, 12 RCTs, 1474 people with travellers' diarrhoea, including students, package tourists, military personnel, and volunteers) compared empirical use of antibiotics versus placebo.[7] Antibiotics evaluated included aztreonam, bicozamycin, ciprofloxacin, co-trimoxazole (trimethoprim–sulfamethoxazole [sulphamethoxazole]), fleroxacin, norfloxacin, ofloxacin, and trimethoprim, which were given for durations varying from a single dose to 5 days. The review found that antibiotics versus placebo significantly increased the cure rate at 72 hours (defined as cessation of unformed stools or > 1 unformed stool/24 h without additional symptoms; OR 5.9, 95% CI 4.1 to 8.6). The additional RCT (598 people, 70% of whom had travelled recently) compared norfloxacin versus placebo. It found that norfloxacin versus placebo significantly increased the number of people cured after 6 days (34/46 [74%] with norfloxacin *v* 18/48 [38%] with placebo; RR 1.97, 95% CI 1.32 to 2.95).[8]

Harms: The systematic review found that adverse effects varied with each antibiotic and ranged in frequency from 2–18%.[7] Gastrointestinal symptoms (cramps, nausea, and anorexia), dermatological symptoms (rash), and respiratory symptoms (cough and sore throat) were most frequently reported. One small RCT included in the review found that significantly more people taking ciprofloxacin developed resistant isolates at 48 hours (ciprofloxacin *v* placebo; ARI 50%, 95% CI 15% to 85%).[7] Another RCT (181 adults with acute diarrhoea) reported three cases of continued excretion of *Shigella* in people taking trimethoprim–sulfamethoxazole versus one person taking placebo.[9] Two of these isolates became resistant to the drug, although the participants were clinically well.[7] Other RCTs found no post-treatment resistance or did not report it.[7] The additional RCT found that people with *Salmonella* infection treated with norfloxacin versus placebo had significantly prolonged excretion of *Salmonella* species (median time to clearance of *Salmonella* species from stools: 50 days with norfloxacin *v* 23 days with placebo; CI not provided).[8] In addition, 6/9 *Campylobacter* isolates obtained after treatment had developed resistance to norfloxacin.

Comment: Only 3/10 trials using the duration of diarrhoea as an outcome reported adequate statistical data for the duration of diarrhoea after initiation of treatment.[7] This limits the applicability of the results.

QUESTION What are the effects of empirical antibiotic treatment in community acquired diarrhoea?

RCTs have found that ciprofloxacin reduces the duration of community acquired diarrhoea by 1–2 days. RCTs found limited evidence that other antibiotics, except lomefloxacin, reduced duration of diarrhoea compared with placebo. Adverse effects varied by agent.

Benefits: We found no systematic review. We found 10 RCTs in nine reports (1848 people)[10–18] comparing one or more antibiotics with placebo (see table 1, p 851). RCTs were conducted in 13 sites in 12 countries. Five RCTs were conducted in developed countries and the remainder in developing countries. Eight RCTs evaluated quinolones, four evaluated trimethoprim–sulfamethoxazole, one evaluated clioquinol, and one evaluated nifuroxazide.[10–18] Entry criteria varied among the RCTs, and treatment duration ranged from a single dose to 5 days. Six RCTs found that antibiotics reduced illness duration or decreased the number of liquid stools at 48 hours,[12,13,15–18] whereas three RCTs found no reduction in duration of illness.[10,11,14] One RCT found reduced duration of diarrhoea for ciprofloxacin but not for trimethoprim–sulfamethoxazole.[13]

Harms: Adverse effects varied by agent. In one RCT (88 people) comparing lomefloxacin versus placebo, 33% of lomefloxacin treated people reported adverse effects compared with 3% taking placebo (ARI 31%, 95% CI 17% to 46%).[11] Two people taking lomefloxacin were withdrawn from the trial after developing anaphylactic reactions. In the same RCT, 18% of treated people developed isolates resistant to lomefloxacin. In the multicentre RCT (173 people with acute diarrhoea) of ciprofloxacin and trimethoprim–sulfamethoxazole, five people with *Campylobacter* isolated from stools (2 treated with ciprofloxacin, 3 treated with trimethoprim–sulfamethoxazole) developed isolates resistant to the treatment antibiotic.[15] In the largest RCT (508 adults), three deaths occurred (2 with fleroxacin *v* 1 with placebo).[16] Two of the deaths occurred from hypovolaemic shock (1 with fleroxacin *v* 1 with placebo).

Comment: The main pathogenic organisms found in each study varied and may partly explain variations in effect. Reported outcomes varied between trials, which precludes direct comparisons or summaries of treatment effect.

QUESTION What are the effects of oral rehydration for severe diarrhoea?

We found no RCTs of oral rehydration compared with placebo or no treatment. Numerous RCTs compared one type of rehydration with another. One small RCT comparing intravenous rehydration versus rehydration through a nasogastric tube found no difference in duration or volume of diarrhoea. One RCT comparing amino acid oral rehydration solution (ORS) versus standard ORS found that amino acid ORS reduced the total volume and duration of diarrhoea. One RCT found no significant

difference in total stool output or duration of diarrhoea with bicarbonate ORS versus chloride ORS. Two RCTs found no significant difference in the duration or volume of diarrhoea with bicarbonate ORS versus citrate ORS. Three RCTs found a small and inconsistent effect on total volume of stool and duration of diarrhoea with reduced osmolarity ORS versus standard ORS. One systematic review has found that rice based ORS versus standard ORS reduces the 24 hour stool volume.

Benefits: We found one systematic review and 10 additional RCTs of ORSs in severe diarrhoea (see table A on web extra).[19–29] **Versus no rehydration:** We found no systematic review or RCTs. RCTs of oral rehydration versus no rehydration would be considered unethical. **Versus intravenous rehydration:** We found no systematic review. We found one small RCT (20 adults with cholera and severe dehydration) comparing enteral rehydration through a nasogastric tube versus intravenous rehydration.[19] Both groups received initial intravenous fluids for up to 90 minutes. The RCT found no significant difference in the total duration of diarrhoea (44 h with iv fluids *v* 37 h with nasogastric fluids; difference +7 h, 95% CI –6 to +20 h), total volume of stool passed (8.2 L *v* 11 L; difference –2.9 L), or duration of *Vibrio* excretion (1.1 days *v* 1.4 days; difference 0.3 days, 95% CI 0 days to 1 day). **Amino acid ORS:** We found no systematic review. We found two RCTs (97 men,[20] 108 men[21]) comparing amino acid ORS versus ORS without amino acids. In the RCT with intravenous rehydration, amino acid ORS versus standard ORS (see glossary, p 849) was associated with a non-significant reduction in the total duration of diarrhoea and significantly reduced the total volume of stool.[20] **Bicarbonate ORS:** We found no systematic review. We found one small RCT (60 people with cholera and severe dehydration) comparing bicarbonate ORS versus an otherwise identical ORS in which the bicarbonate was replaced with chloride.[22] The RCT found no significant difference in total stool output or duration of diarrhoea. We found three RCTs (367 people) comparing standard/citrate versus bicarbonate ORS.[23–25] Two of the RCTs found no significant difference between treatments in the duration or volume of diarrhoea.[23,25] One RCT did not report on significance, although duration and volume of diarrhoea were worse with bicarbonate ORS.[24] **Reduced osmolarity ORS:** We found no systematic review. We found three RCTs, which found a small and inconsistent effect on total volume of stool and duration of diarrhoea.[26–28] **Rice based ORS:** We found one systematic review (search date 1998, 4 RCTs) in people with cholera and non-cholera diarrhoea.[29] The review found that, in adults with cholera, rice based ORS versus standard ORS significantly reduced the 24 hour stool volume (4 RCTs, WMD –51 mL/kg, 95% CI –66 mL/kg to –36 mL/kg). One RCT found that both rice based ORS and low sodium rice based ORS reduced stool output compared with standard ORS (4 L for rice based ORS *v* 5 L for standard ORS, $P < 0.02$; 3 L for low sodium rice based ORS *v* 5 L for standard ORS, $P < 0.05$).[28]

Harms: **Versus amino acid ORS:** One RCT (108 men) reported no episodes of hypernatraemia or hyponatraemia in people taking a modified ORS or standard ORS.[21] **Bicarbonate ORS:** One RCT (130 people with cholera) reported that more people taking citrate

ORS had an unpleasant taste than those taking bicarbonate ORS (29% of people v 13% of people).[24] In another RCT, 2/115 people taking an effervescent citrate ORS had an unpleasant taste (results not reported for bicarbonate ORS).[25] **Versus reduced osmolarity ORS:** Reduced osmolarity ORS significantly increased the risk of non-symptomatic hyponatraemia (OR 2.1, 95% CI 1.1 to 4.1).[26] In RCTs evaluating symptomatic hyponatraemia, no cases were reported.[26,27]

Comment: All people with cholera received antibiotic treatment in addition to fluid treatment. Oral tetracycline or doxycycline were widely used, and were initiated at varying intervals after the start of oral fluid treatment. Response to ORS in people with cholera may not be comparable to those with less severe forms of diarrhoea.

QUESTION What are the effects of antimotility agents for acute diarrhoea in adults?

RCTs have found that, in people with acute diarrhoea, loperamide hyrochloride and loperamide oxide versus placebo significantly reduce the time to relief of symptoms, but significantly increase constipation. We found insufficient evidence about the effects of other antimotility agents.

Benefits: We found no systematic review. **Difenoxin:** We found no RCTs of sufficient quality. **Diphenoxylate:** One RCT (152 adults with acute diarrhoea for < 24 h) comparing diphenoxylate–atropine versus placebo found that diphenoxylate significantly reduced the number of bowel actions in the 24 hours after treatment ($P = 0.05$).[30] The RCT found no significant difference in median time to last loose stool (25 h v 30 h; $P = 0.29$). **Lidamidine:** We found two RCTs comparing lidamidine (loading dose of 2–4 mg, then subsequent doses 6/h or as required) versus placebo.[31,32] The first RCT (30 adults with acute diarrhoea) found that lidamidine reduced the stool weight after 29 hours (435 g with lidamidine 4 mg v 364 g with lidamidine 2 mg v 576 g with placebo).[31] The second RCT (105 adults with acute diarrhoea) compared lidamidine versus loperamide versus placebo.[32] It found that lidamidine reduced the number of loose stools after 72 hours (8.5 stools v 3.9 stools; P values not provided). **Loperamide hydrochloride:** We found four RCTs comparing loperamide hydrochloride (loading dose of 4 mg, then 2 mg with each loose stool) versus placebo.[32–35] Two of the RCTs (409 people[33] and 261 people[34] with acute diarrhoea) found that loperamide significantly reduced the median time to complete relief of symptoms, which was defined as the time between taking the loading dose of loperamide and the time after which one pasty, watery, or loose stool was passed (189 people: 27 h with loperamide v 45 h with placebo, $P = 0.006$;[33] 123 people: 18 h with loperamide v 37 h with placebo, $P = 0.007$[34]). The third RCT (50 people) found that loperamide versus placebo significantly reduced the number of stools for the first 2 days, but subsequently the difference was not significant.[35] The fourth RCT (105 adults with acute diarrhoea) found no significant difference in the number of stools passed within 72 hours.[32] **Loperamide oxide:** We found five

RCTs (409 people,[33] 261 people,[34] 230 people,[36] 242 people,[37] 258 people[38] with acute diarrhoea) comparing loperamide oxide (loading dose 1–8 mg, followed by 0.5–4 mg with each loose stool) versus placebo. All RCTs found that loperamide oxide significantly reduced the time to complete relief of symptoms.

Harms: **Lidamidine:** Constipation occurred in one person taking lidamidine compared with no people taking placebo (1/35 [3%] *v* 0/35 [0%]).[32] **Loperamide hydrochloride:** Two RCTs (409 people[33] and 261 people[34]) found that constipation was significantly more frequent in people taking loperamide versus placebo (25% *v* 7%; ARI 18%, 95% CI 8% to 28%; NNH 5, 95% CI 3 to 12;[33] 22% *v* 10%; ARI 12%, 95% CI 5% to 29%; NNH 5, 95% CI 3 to 18[34]). **Loperamide oxide:** One RCT (409 people) found that significantly more people taking loperamide oxide had constipation (24% with loperamide oxide *v* 7% with placebo; ARI 17%, 95% CI 7% to 27%; NNH 5, 95% CI 3 to 14).[33] Another RCT (230 people) found that symptom scores for tiredness and sleepiness were significantly higher in people taking loperamide oxide 1 mg versus placebo ($P = 0.01$).[36]

Comment: The RCTs used different outcome measures, making it difficult to summarise and compare results.

GLOSSARY

Standard ORS An oral rehydration solution that includes citrate 10 mmol/L and glucose 111 mmol/L, and has an osmolarity of 311 mmol/L.

REFERENCES

1. *The World Health Report 1997*. Geneva: World Health Organization, 1997:14–22.
2. Garthwright WE, Archer DL, Kvenberg JE. Estimates of incidence and costs of intestinal infectious diseases in the United States. *Public Health Rep* 1988;103:107–115.
3. Wheeler JG, Sethi D, Cowden JM, et al. Study of infectious intestinal disease in England: rates in the community, presenting to general practice, and reported to national surveillance. *BMJ* 1999;318:1046–1050.
4. Cartwright RY, Chahed M. Foodborne diseases in travellers. *World Health Stat Q* 1997;50:102–110.
5. Jiang ZD, Lowe B, Vernekar MP, et al. Prevalence of enteric pathogens among international travelers with diarrhea acquired in Keyna (Mobasa), India (Goa), or Jamaica (Montego Bay). *J Infect Dis* 2002;185:497–502.
6. Lew JF, Glass RI, Gangarosa RE, et al. Diarrheal deaths in the United States 1979 through 1987. *JAMA* 1991;265:3280–3284.
7. De Bruyn G, Hahn S, Borwick A. Antibiotic treatment for travellers' diarrhoea (Cochrane Review). In: The Cochrane Library, Issue 3, 2002. Oxford: Update Software. Search date 2000; primary sources The Cochrane Collaboration Trials Register (Issue 3, 1998), Medline, Embase, and hand searching and contact with experts.
8. Wistrom J, Jertborn M, Ekwall E, et al. Empiric treatment of acute diarrheal disease with norfloxacin: a randomized, placebo-controlled study. Swedish Study Group. *Ann Intern Med* 1992;117:202–208.
9. Ericsson CD, Johnson PC, DuPont HL, et al. Ciprofloxacin or trimethoprim–sulfamethoxazole as initial therapy for travelers' diarrhea. *Ann Intern Med* 1987;106:216–220.
10. De la Cabada FJ, DuPont HL, Gyr K, et al. Antimicrobial therapy of bacterial diarrhea in adult residents of Mexico — lack of an effect. *Digestion* 1992;53:134–141.
11. Ellis-Pegler RB, Hyman LK, Ingram RJ, et al. A placebo controlled evaluation of lomefloxacin in the treatment of bacterial diarrhoea in the community. *J Antimicrob Chemother* 1995;36:259–263.
12. Pichler HE, Diridl G, Stickler K, et al. Clinical efficacy of ciprofloxacin compared with placebo in bacterial diarrhea. *Am J Med* 1987;82(suppl 4A):329–332.
13. Goodman LJ, Trenholme GM, Kaplan RL, et al. Empiric antimicrobial therapy of domestically acquired acute diarrhea in urban adults. *Arch Intern Med* 1990;150:541–546.
14. Noguerado A, Garcia-Polo I, Isasia T, et al. Early single dose therapy with ofloxacin for empirical treatment of acute gastroenteritis: a randomised, placebo-controlled double-blind clinical trial. *J Antimicrob Chemother* 1995;36:665–672.
15. Dryden MS, Gabb RJ, Wright SK. Empirical treatment of severe acute community-acquired gastroenteritis with ciprofloxacin. *Clin Infect Dis* 1996;22:1019–1025.
16. Butler T, Lolekha S, Rasidi C, et al. Treatment of acute bacterial diarrhea: a multicenter international trial comparing placebo with fleroxacin given as a single dose or once daily for 3 days. *Am J Med* 1993;94(3A):187S–194S.
17. Lolekha S, Patanachareon S, Thanangkul B, et al. Norfloxacin versus co-trimoxazole in the treatment

of acute bacterial diarrhoea: a placebo controlled study. *Scand J Infect Dis* 1988;56(suppl):35–45.
18. Bouree P, Chaput JC, Krainik F, et al. Double-blind controlled study of the efficacy of nifuroxazide versus placebo in the treatment of acute diarrhea in adults. *Gastroenterol Clin Biol* 1989;13:469–472.
19. Pierce NF, Sack RB, Mitra RC, et al. Replacement of water and electrolyte losses in cholera by an oral glucose-electrolyte solution. *Ann Intern Med* 1969;70:1173–1181.
20. Patra FC, Sack DA, Islam A, et al. Oral rehydration formula containing alanine and glucose for treatment of diarrhoea: a controlled trial. *BMJ* 1989;298:1353–1356.
21. Khin-Maung-U, Myo-Khin, Nyunt-Nyunt-Wai, et al. Comparison of glucose/electrolyte and maltodextrin/glycine/glycyl-glycine/electrolyte oral rehydration solutions in cholera and watery diarrhoea in adults. *Ann Trop Med Parasitol* 1991;85:645–650.
22. Sarker SA, Mahalanabis D. The presence of bicarbonate in oral rehydration solution does not influence fluid absorption in cholera. *Scand J Gastroenterol* 1995;30:242–245.
23. Mazumder RN, Nath SK, Ashraf H, et al. Oral rehydration solution containing trisodium citrate for treating severe diarrhoea: controlled clinical trial. *BMJ* 1991;302:88–89.
24. Hoffman SL, Moechtar MA, Simanjuntak CH, et al. Rehydration and maintenance therapy of cholera patients in Jakarta: citrate-based versus bicarbonate-based oral rehydration salt solution. *J Infect Dis* 1985;152:1159–1165.
25. Ahmed SM, Islam MR, Butler T. Effective treatment of diarrhoeal dehydration with an oral rehydration solution containing citrate. *Scand J Infect Dis* 1986;18:65–70.
26. Alam NH, Majumder RN, Fuchs GJ. Efficacy and safety of oral rehydration solution with reduced osmolarity in adults with cholera: a randomised double-blind clinical trial. *Lancet* 1999;354:296–299.
27. Faruque ASG, Mahalanabis D, Hamadani JD, et al. Reduced osmolarity oral rehydration salt in cholera. *Scand J Infect Dis* 1996;28:87–90.
28. Bhattacharya MK, Bhattacharya SK, Dutta D, et al. Efficacy of oral hyposmolar glucose-based and rice-based oral rehydration salt solutions in the treatment of cholera in adults. *Scand J Gastroenterol* 1998;33:159–163.
29. Fontaine O, Gore SM, Pierce NF. Rice-based oral rehydration solution for treating diarrhoea. In: The Cochrane Library, Issue 3, 2002. Oxford: Update Software. Search date 1998; primary sources Medline, Embase, Lilacs, Cochrane Controlled Trials Register, and Cochrane Infectious Diseases Group.
30. Lustman F, Walters EG, Shroff NE, et al. Diphenoxylate hydrochloride (Lomotil®) in the treatment of acute diarrhoea. *Br J Clin Pract* 1987;41:648–651.
31. Heredia Diaz JG, Alcantara I, Solis A. Evaluation of the safety and effectiveness of WHR-1142A in the treatment of non-specific acute diarrhea. *Rev Gastroenterol Mex* 1979;44:167–73 [in Spanish].
32. Heredia Diaz JG, Kajeyama Escobar ML. Double-blind evaluation of the effectiveness of lidamidine hydrochloride (WHR-1142A) vs. loperamide vs. placebo in the treatment of acute diarrhea. *Salud Publica Mex* 1981;23:483–491 [in Spanish].
33. Hughes IW. First line treatment in acute non-dysenteric diarrhoea: clinical comparison of loperamide oxide, loperamide and placebo. *Br J Clin Pract* 1995;49:181–185.
34. Van den Eynden B, Spaepen W. New approaches to the treatment of patients with acute, nonspecific diarrhea: a comparison of the effects of loperamide and loperamide oxide. *Curr Ther Res* 1995;56:1132–1141.
35. Van Loon FPL, Bennish ML, Speelman P, et al Double blind trial of loperamide for treating acute watery diarrhoea in expatriates in Bangladesh. *Gut* 1989;30:492–495.
36. Dettmer A. Loperamide oxide in the treatment of acute diarrhea in adults. *Clin Ther* 1994;16:972–980.
37. Dreverman JWM, Van der Poel AJM. Loperamide oxide in acute diarrhoea: a double-blind, placebo-controlled trial. *Aliment Pharmacol Ther* 1995;9:441–446.
38. Cardon E, Van Elsen J, Frascio M, et al. Gut-selective opiates: the effect of loperamide oxide in acute diarrhoea in adults. The Diarrhoea Trialists Group. *Eur J Clin Res* 1995;7:135–144.
39. Nalin DR, Cash RA, Rahman M, et al. Effect of glycine and glucose on sodium and water absorption in patients with cholera. *Gut* 1970;11:768–772.

Guy de Bruyn
Fellow in Program in Infectious Diseases
University of Washington and Fred
Hutchinson Cancer Research Centre
Seattle, Washington
USA

Competing interests: None declared.

TABLE 1 **Effects of empirical antibiotic treatment of community acquired diarrhoea: results of placebo controlled RCTs** **(see text, p 846).**

Intervention	Total number of participants	Mean duration of diarrhoea from start of treatment*		Difference between means (95% CI)†
		Placebo group	Intervention group	
Lomefloxacin 400 mg daily for 5 days [11]	84	3.2 days	4.4 days	+1.2 days (0.1 days to 2.5 days)
Ofloxacin 400 mg single dose [14]	117	3.4 days	2.5 days	–0.9 days (–1.8 days to 0.0 days)
Co-trimoxazole 800/160 mg bd for 3 days [10]	287	30.2 h	24.4 h	–5.8 h
Cloquinol 250 mg tds for 3 days [10]	287	30.2 h	25.5 h	–4.7 h
Enoxacin 400 mg bd for 5 days [10]	137	44.9 h	38.9 h	–6.0 h
Co-trimoxazole 160/800 mg bd for 5 days [10]	137	44.9 h	42.3 h	–2.6 h
Ciprofloxacin 500 mg bd for 5 days [12]	162	2.9 days	1.5 days	–1.4 days
Ciprofloxacin 500 mg bd for 5 days [13]	173	3.4 days	2.4 days	–1.0 day
Co-trimoxazole 160/800 mg bd for 5 days [13]	173	3.4 days	NA	NA
Ciprofloxacin 500 mg bd for 5 days [15]	85	4.6 days	2.2 days	–2.4 days
Nifuroxazide 400 mg bd for 5 days [18]	88	3.3 days	2.1 days	–1.2 days

*Two other RCTs [16,17] did not report mean duration of diarrhoea. †If available from published data.
bd, twice daily; h, hours; NA, not available from published data; tds, three times daily.

Hepatitis B

Search date February 2003

Kamran Siddiqi

QUESTIONS

INTERVENTIONS

See glossary, p 864

Key Messages

In countries with high endemicity

- **Universal immunisation of infants** One non-systematic review and three additional and subsequent RCTs have found that, in countries with high endemicity, universal immunisation of infants, using either recombinent or plasma derived vaccines, reduces acute hepatitis and development of chronic carrier state compared with placebo. One non-systematic review and four additional and subsequent RCTs have found that universal (both recombinant and plasma derived) hepatitis B immunisation in infants in countries with high endemicity, compared with placebo, reduces acute hepatitis and development of a chronic carrier state. The longest RCT found universal immunisation protected at 15 years. Two historical cohort studies found reduced secondary mortality from hepatocellular carcinoma in children born after the introduction of a universal plasma derived hepatitis immunisation program. One additional historical cohort study found a lower rate of related chronic liver disease, cirrhosis, and hepatocellular cancer after the introduction of a universal plasma derived immunisation program. Three non-systematic reviews and one RCT found only minor adverse reactions after recombinant hepatitis B immunisation. One cluster RCT found universal immunisation with first plasma and then recombinant vaccine reduced the development of chronic carrier state and acute hepatitis events compared with immunisation of high risk groups.

- **Selective immunisation of high risk individuals** The available evidence relates only to children born to HbsAg mothers. One non-systematic review of both plasma derived and recombinant vaccine in mainly observational studies and three RCTs of plasma hepatitis B immunisation compared with placebo or no treatment, found that immunisation prevents chronic carrier state in children born to HbsAg positive mothers. One RCT found minor adverse events with immunisation, the other RCTs did not report on adverse events. We found no good evidence in other high risk groups. One cluster RCT found that selective immunisation in high risk individuals was less effective than universal immunisation of infants in reducing the development of chronic carrier state and acute hepatitis events.

In countries with low endemicity

- **Selective immunisation of high risk individuals** One systematic review in countries with low endemicity found that plasma derived hepatitis B immunisation prevented acute hepatitis B and development of chronic carrier state in healthcare workers at high risk of exposure to bodily fluids. Three RCTs found that plasma derived hepatitis B immunisation prevented acute hepatitis B in homosexual men. One small RCT found no significant difference in hepatitis B events in heterosexual partners of infected people. Three RCTs of plasma derived immunisation in people on regular haemodialysis found potentially conflicting results. Two RCTs from France and Belgium found good protective efficacy against chronic carrier state. However, one large US based RCT found no good evidence of benefit. The systematic review of plasma derived vaccination found no significant difference between immunisation and placebo in the rate and severity of adverse events. One observational study showed a high prevalence of hepatitis B carrier state and low immunisation uptake in young homosexuals despite a national strategy to immunise high risk groups. We found insufficient evidence to compare the effectiveness of selective immunisation of high risk individuals with other strategies.
- **Universal immunisation of infants** One historical cohort study found a reduction in the prevalence of hepatitis B chronic carrier state following universal immunisation. We found insufficient evidence to compare its effectiveness with other strategies. Two cohort studies and surveillance data did not report any links between hepatitis B immunisation and serious adverse reactions.
- **Comparatic effectiveness of different strategies** We found no good systematic reviews, RCTs, or observational studies comparing the effectiveness of different immunisation strategies in countries with low endemicity.
- **Universal immunisation of adolescents** We found insufficient evidence to assess the effects of universal adolescent immunisation, or to compare its effectiveness with other strategies. One observational study suggests minor adverse effects following hepatitis B immunisation in this group.

DEFINITION Hepatitis B is a viral infectious disease with an incubation period of 40–160 days. Acute hepatitis B infection is characterised by anorexia, vague abdominal discomfort, nausea and vomiting, jaundice, and occasional fever. Illness is associated with deranged liver function tests (especially raised alanine transaminases) and presence of serological markers of acute hepatitis B infection (e.g. HbsAg [see glossary, p 864], antiHBc IgM).[1]

INCIDENCE/ PREVALENCE The incidence of acute hepatitis B and prevalence of its chronic carrier state (see glossary, p 864) varies widely across the globe. In areas with high endemicity (HbsAg prevalence ≥8%, e.g. South East Asia and Africa), more than half of the population becomes infected at some point in their lives.[2] In countries with low endemicity (HbsAg prevalence < 2%, e.g. North America, western Europe, Australia), most of the population do not become infected.[2] Nearly a third of the world population has been infected by hepatitis B at some point, and at least 350 million people (5–6% of world population) are currently chronic carriers of hepatitis B infection.[3]

AETIOLOGY/ RISK FACTORS In countries with high endemicity, most infections occur during childhood from an infected mother to her baby (vertical transmission) or from one child to another (horizontal transmission).[4] However, most hepatitis B infection in developed countries occurs later from either sexual activity, injection drug use, or occupational exposure. Less frequent causes of infection include household contact, regular haemodialysis, transmission from a health professional, and receipt of organs or other blood products.[5] The vaccination policy of a country is a large determinant of the risk of developing hepatitis B. Since the development of plasma derived hepatitis B vaccine in the early 1980s, subsequently replaced by recombinant vaccine (see glossary, p 864), many countries have adopted a policy of universal immunisation of all infants. On the basis of disease burden, the World Health Organization recommended that hepatitis B vaccine be incorporated into routine infant and childhood immunisation programmes in countries with high endemicity by 1995 and in all countries by 1997.[6] Despite this, in many countries with low endemicity, universal immunisation policy remains controversial and has still not been adopted.[7] Some of these countries have adopted a policy of selective immunisation of high risk individuals, others have adopted a universal adolescent immunisation policy.

PROGNOSIS Hepatitis B infection resolves in most cases after the acute infection. In the remainder, it may result in a number of serious sequelae. Massive hepatic necrosis occurs in 1% of people with acute viral hepatitis, leading to a serious and often fatal condition called acute fulminant hepatitis. Between 2 and 10% of those infected as adults become chronic carriers with hepatitis B surface antigen (HbsAg), persisting for longer than 6 months. Chronic carriage is more frequent in those infected as children, and reaches up to 90% in those infected during the perinatal period.[1] Between 20 and 25% of chronic carriers develop a progressive chronic liver disease. This progresses to the most important sequelae of hepatitis B infection, cirrhosis and hepatocellular carcinoma. These complications usually arise in older adults and are major causes of mortality in populations with high hepatitis B endemicity.[4] Observational studies suggest that, in these countries, almost 80% of chronic liver disease and cirrhosis is attributed to hepatitis B, and these complications lead to at least a million deaths every year.[2]

AIMS OF INTERVENTION To reduce the risk of acquiring hepatitis B infection in susceptible people, while minimising adverse effects of interventions.

OUTCOMES Incidence of acute hepatitis B; prevalence of chronic carrier state; chronic liver disease; cirrhosis and hepatocellular carcinoma secondary to hepatitis B; mortality secondary to hepatitis B infection and its chronic sequelae; adverse events.

METHODS *Clinical Evidence* search and appraisal February 2003, including a search for observational studies. Where there were no good RCT data for a given comparison or outcome, we included the best available observational data. Both plasma derived and recombinant vaccines were included.

QUESTION **What are the effects of immunisation in countries with high endemicity?** New

OPTION **UNIVERSAL IMMUNISATION OF INFANTS**

One non-systematic review and three additional and subsequent RCTs have found that in countries with high endemicity, universal immunisation of infants, using either recombinent or plasma derived vaccines, reduces acute hepatitis and development of a chronic cancer state compared with placebo. One non-systematic review and four additional and subsequent RCTs have found that universal (both recombinant and plasma derived) hepatitis B immunisation in infants in countries with high endemicity, compared with placebo, reduces acute hepatitis and development of a chronic carrier state. The longest RCT found universal immunisation protected at 15 years. Two historical cohort studies found reduced secondary mortality from hepatocellular carcinoma in children born after the introduction of a universal plasma derived hepatitis immunisation programme. One additional historical cohort study found a lower rate of related chronic liver disease, cirrhosis, and hepatocellular cancer after the introduction of a universal plasma derived immunisation programme. Three non-systematic reviews and one RCT found only minor adverse reactions after recombinant hepatitis B immunisation. One cluster RCT found universal immunisation with first plasma and then recombinant vaccine reduced the development of chronic carrier state and acute hepatitis events compared with immunisation of high risk groups.

Benefits: **Versus placebo or no immunisation:** We found one non-systematic review (search date 1989, 2 RCTs, 203 infants, aged less than 1 year),[8] two subsequent RCTs,[9–12] one additional RCT,[13] and three additional historical cohort studies,[14–16] comparing hepatitis B vaccine versus placebo. The review found that recombinant hepatitis B vaccine protected against development of the chronic carrier state at both 9 months after immunisation (protective efficacy [see glossary, p 864] 87%; 15/148 [10.1%] HbsAg positive in the intervention group) and 15 months (protective efficacy 96%; 2/55 [3.6%] HBsAg positive in the intervention group). Confidence limits and numbers of people in control group not reported. One subsequent RCT in the Gambia (1864 infants) compared four doses of hepatitis B vaccine (recombinant or plasma derived) given along with the WHO recommended Expanded Program Immunisation versus Expanded Program Immunisation only.[9,10] It found that hepatitis B vaccine plus Expanded Program Immunisation significantly protected against development of the chronic carrier state at 4 years after immunisation (protective efficacy 94%, 95% CI 84% to 98%; 4/720 [0.6%] HBsAg positive with intervention *v* 103/816 [13%] with placebo). It found the results were still significant after 9 years (protective efficacy 90%, 95% CI 79% to 95%; 4/677 [0.5%] HBsAg positive with intervention *v* 99/823 [12%] with placebo).

One subsequent RCT in China (649 children aged 3–36 months, with no serological markers for previous infection) compared three doses of plasma derived hepatitis B vaccine versus placebo.[11] It found that hepatitis B vaccine significantly protected children against development of the chronic carrier state at 5, 12, and 15 years after immunisation (5 year protective efficacy 100%, 0/152 [0%] HBsAg positive with immunisation *v* 24/190 [12.6%] with placebo, P < 0.001; 12 year protective efficacy 82.2%, 3/171 [1.8%] HBsAg positive with immunisation *v* 18/179 [10.1%] with placebo, P < 0.01; 15 year protective efficacy 88%, 1/52 [1.9%] HBsAg positive with immunisation *v* 9/154 [16.7%] with placebo, P < 0.01; CIs not reported). The second subsequent RCT, also in China (513 children aged 3–36 months, with no serological markers for previous infection) compared three doses of plasma derived hepatitis B vaccine versus placebo.[12] It found hepatitis B vaccine significantly protected children against development of the chronic carrier state at 12 years after immunisation (protective efficacy 92%; 1/167 [0.6%] HBsAg positive with immunisation *v* 14/183 [7.6%] with placebo; P < 0.0001, CI not reported). One additional RCT from Burundi (480 infants) compared the protective efficacy of a plasma derived hepatitis vaccine (see glossary, p 864) versus placebo 1 year after immunisation.[13] It found the vaccine significantly protected children from both acute hepatitis B events (see glossary, p 864) (efficacy 100%; event rates 0/59 [0%] with immunisation *v* 5/59 [8.5%] with placebo; P = 0.046) and development of chronic carrier state (efficacy 100%; carrier rates 0/59 [0%] with hepatitis B vaccine *v* 4/59 [6.8%] with placebo; statistics not reported). One additional historical cohort study in Taiwan estimated the incidence of hepatocellular carcinoma in three historical cohorts (children born during 1981–1986 [17 million], children born during 1987–1990 [14 million], and children born during 1991–1994 [14 million]) 5–13 years after immunisation with a plasma vaccine.[14] The average annual incidence of hepatocellular carcinoma was significantly reduced in children born after the introduction of universal immunisation (see glossary, p 864) in 1984 (0.7 per 100 000 [95% CI 0.65 to 0.78] in the 1981–1986 cohort, 0.57 per 100 000 [95% CI 0.48 to 0.62] in the 1987–1990 cohort, and 0.36 per 100 000 [95% CI 0.23 to 0.48] in the 1991–1994 cohort; P < 0.01 for comparison between before and after the 1990 cohorts). Mortality secondary to hepatocellular carcinoma was also reduced in the 1991–1994 cohort compared with the two other cohorts combined (incidence of hepatocellular deaths before July 1990 0.72 and after July 1990 0.33; RR 0.51; P < 0.001) (see comment below). The second additional historical cohort study (children aged 1–9 years) in Taiwan also found a lower hepatocellular carcinoma standardised mortality ratio following the vaccination programme with a plasma derived vaccine (1.25, 95% CI 0.70 to 2.25 in 1983 and 0.34, 95% CI 0.14 to 0.89 in 1993, comparative statistical results not reported).[15] This contrasted with no change in the adult standardised mortality ratio secondary to hepatocellular carcinoma during this period. The third additional historical cohort study (children, adolescents, and young people) assessed the impact of universal immunisation (initially with plasma and then with recombinant vaccine [see glossary, p 864]) on related chronic liver disease, cirrhosis, and hepatocellular carcinoma in a town in southern Italy.[16] It found a decline in the prevalence of chronic carrier state 15 years after starting the immunisation programme (prevalence of HBsAg 8.3% during 1978–1983 *v* 1% in 1997, $P < 0.001$). It also reported a reduction in the prevalence of related chronic liver disease, cirrhosis, and hepatocellular carcinoma, but no numerical data were provided. **Versus selective immunisation in high risk individuals:** We found one cluster RCT in Italy (2 towns with a population of about 60 000 each), which compared a universal immunisation strategy (all infants and adolescents) versus immunisation of high risk groups only (people living with chronic carriers, homosexual men, intravenous drug abusers, infants born to infected mothers, healthcare workers, commercial sex workers, people receiving transfusion and other blood products, people exposed to needle stick injuries, and people with chronic eczema and psoriasis).[17] It used plasma derived vaccine until 1987 and then recombinant vaccine. It found universal immunisation was associated with a bigger reduction in the incidence of hepatitis B (with universal immunisation, mean annual incidence of hepatitis B 63/100 000 during 1963–1990 and 3/100 000 during 1991–1993; with high risk group immunisation, mean annual incidence was 55/100 000 during 1963–1990 and 15/100 000 in 1991–1993). It also found universal immunisation was associated with lower prevalence of HBsAg positivity (13.4% in 1978 to 3% in 1993 with universal immunisation *v* 13.6% in 1978 to 7.4% with selective immunisation; statistical significance not reported).

Harms: **Versus placebo or no treatment:** The non-systematic review found that 10% of children (13 trials, 2096 enrolled) and 4% of neonates (11 trials, 1 187 enrolled) had adverse reactions following hepatitis B recombinant immunisation. Sore arm (8.5%) in children and mild fever (2.5%) in neonates were the two most commonly reported symptoms.[8] It found no serious adverse reactions. We found two other non-systematic reviews that assessed connective tissue disorders (see glossary, p 864) and recombinant vaccine.[18,19] The first review found two uncontrolled population based studies. The first study (166 757 children in New Zealand) of plasma derived vaccine found that arthritis or arthralgia occurred in less than 1 episode in 10 000 vaccines. The second study of plasma derived vaccine (43 618 people in Alaska) found that arthritis or arthralgia lasting more than 3 days occurred in less than 1 episode in 3000 vaccines.[18] It found weak evidence (case reports and case series) of a link between hepatitis B vaccine and serious connective tissue disorders. The second non-systematic review (search date 2000, number of studies not reported) found no evidence (from case series and case reports) of a causal link between systematic lupus erythrematosis and recombinant vaccine.[19] One RCT in Egypt (590 infants) compared the addition of three doses of hepatitis B vaccine (recombinant) plus routine immunisation starting at birth (group A) versus immunisation at 2 months (group B) versus routine immunisation only (group C).[20] It found infants who started hepatitis B immunisation at 2 months had a significantly higher proportion of minor adverse reaction compared with children immunised at birth or with routine immunisation alone (group A 5/178 [2.8%] had local reaction and 10/178 [5.6%] had fever *v* group B 12/167 [7.2%] had local reaction and 12/167 [7.2%] had fever *v* group C 3/191 [1.6%] had local reaction and 4/191 [2.1%] had fever; $P < 0.05$ for group B *v* A and C) after the first dose. It found no serious adverse reactions in any group. One RCT found that infants immunised from birth onwards suffer less frequent adverse reactions than infants who received their first dose at the age of 2 months.[20] The RCT used strict inclusion criteria excluding underweight children and those with other disorders. The trial claimed to have lost only 10% of participants at follow up, with none because of adverse effects, but did not say how this was assessed. None of the reviews, RCTs, or cohort studies in the benefits section reported on harms.[9–16] **Versus selective immunisation of high risk individuals:** The RCT did not report any adverse effects with either intervention.[17]

Comment: **Versus placebo or no treatment:** All RCTs mentioned in the Benefits section had high loss to follow up.[8–16] This proportion was particularly high in one 15 year long study (83%) in China.[11] However, sensitivity analysis in the RCT conducted in the Gambia found immunisation reduced incidence after 9 years even after taking the 31% loss to follow up into account.[10] One cohort study in Taiwan, which found reduced incidence and secondary mortality of hepatocellular carcinoma in vaccinated children compared with historical controls,[14] used at least three methods for validating their data, thereby reducing errors. The results were compared with the changes in another childhood cancer and adult hepatocellular carcinoma incidence restricting confounding by other factors. The study in Italy had possible misclassification bias as final diagnosis of hepatitis events were made only clinically by GPs and not validated.[16] **Versus selective immunisation of high risk indivudals:** The cluster RCT in the two towns in southern Italy was possibly exposed to cross contamination and the effects of migration.[17] Despite these possible limitations, the difference between the declines in the incidences of hepatitis was overwhelmingly supportive towards universal immunisation strategy.

OPTION SELECTIVE IMMUNISATION OF HIGH RISK INDIVIDUALS

One non-systematic review of mainly observational studies with both plasma derived and recombinant vaccine, and three RCTs of plasma derived hepatitis B immunisation, compared with placebo or no treatment, all found immunisation prevents chronic carrier state in children born to HbsAg positive mothers. One RCT found minor adverse events with immunisation; the other RCTs did not report on adverse events. We found no good evidence in other high-risk groups. One cluster RCT found that selective immunisation in high risk individuals was less effective than universal immunisation of infants in reducing the development of chronic carrier state and acute hepatitis events.

Benefits: **Versus placebo or no treatment:** We found one non-systematic review[21] and two additional RCTs.[22–24] The review (24 studies in infants; mainly individual, clinical, and epidemiological surveillance studies) assessed the protective efficacy of both plasma derived and recombination vaccine in neonates born to mothers infected with hepatitis B.[21] The review did not do a meta-analysis owing to differences in study design. However, it found consistently high protective efficacy for both types of vaccines compared with placebo or historical controls in a number of studies. One RCT in Hong Kong, included in the review (236 children), compared plasma derived vaccine in children born to HbeAg positive mothers versus placebo.[25] It randomised people into four groups; groups A, B, and C received hepatitis B vaccine at birth and at 1, 2, and 6 months. Group A also received seven monthly injections of hepatitis B immunoglobulin (HBIG), group B received one HBIG injection at birth, group D received placebo for both vaccine and HBIG, and group C received vaccine only. It found that vaccine significantly protected all groups compared with placebo at the end of 3 years (protective efficacy 87% in group A, 80% in group B, and 65% in group C, P < 0.0001; prevalence of HbsAg [see glossary, p 864] in group A 5/60 [8.3%], group B 9/64 [14%], group C 15/63 [24%], and group D 30/47 [64%]) versus the placebo group. It also found that groups receiving HBIG in addition to the vaccine had more protection than the group receiving vaccine only (P value not reported). The first additional RCT in Taiwan, compared plasma derived vaccine with or without HBIG versus no immunisation (group A vaccine alone, group B vaccine plus HBIGx1, group C vaccine plus HBIGx2, and group D no vaccine).[22] Infants receiving immunisation were more protected 6 months after immunisation against HBsAg compared with no immunisation in group D (HBsAg positives in group A 9/38 [23.7%]; efficacy 73.7%; P < 0.05, group B 4/36 [11.1%]; efficacy 87.7%; reported as non-significant, but P value not reported, group C 2/38 [5.3%] efficacy 94.1%; P < 0.05, and group D 26/29 [90%]). It also found that HBIG significantly increased protection compared with vaccine only. The second additional RCT, in China (208 children born to HBsAg positive mothers), compared two different brands of plasma derived vaccine with or without HBIG versus placebo in preventing the development of chronic carrier state (see glossary, p 864) (group A placebo, group B vaccine produced by an international company; group C vaccine produced locally, and group D local vaccine along with HBIG).[23,24] It found that children receiving international vaccine brand were significantly less likely to develop the chronic carrier state than children who received placebo or the local brand after 6 months (prevalence of HBsAg in group A 24/55 [47%], group B 3/55 [5.4%], group C 12/56 [21%], and group D 2/27 [7%]; protective efficacy 87% [P < 0.001] in group B, 51% [P < 0.03] in group C, and 83% [P < 0.003] in group D), and at 5 years (prevalence of HBsAg in group A 19/31[66%], group B 2/19 [11%] protective efficacy 72%, group C 4/20 [22%] protective efficacy 38%; and group D 2/11 [12%]; P values not reported). It found similar protective efficacy in group B (international brand) and D (addition of HBIG to the local vaccine) in preventing hepatitis B carrier state (CI or P values not reported). **Versus universal immunisation of infants:** See universal immunisation of infants, p 855.

Harms: **Versus placebo or no treatment:** In China, one RCT reported minor adverse reactions (5%, mainly irritability and rash) after immunisation of infants born to HbsAg positive mothers.[26] No further comparison with the control group was made. The other RCTs did not report on adverse events.[22–25] **Versus universal immunisation of infants:** See universal immunisation of infants, p 857.

Comment: **Versus placebo or no treatment:** Two RCTs were conducted in China. Only 55% of women eligible for the trial agreed to take part in one RCT, which might make the results not representative of the population.[26] The other RCT, which lasted for 10 years, lost 56% of participants during follow up at 9 years.[23,24] Although groups were similar at baseline, this can still lead to attrition bias. Two RCTs from Thailand and Hong Kong completed follow up of 87% (1 year) and 95% (3 years) of people initially recruited in the trial.[25,27] The Hong Kong RCT may have had an insufficient sample size to detect clinically significant differences between the individual groups during sub-analysis. One RCT in China (220 children born to HbsAg positive mothers) compared plasma derived vaccine against recombinant vaccine (see glossary, p 864) (group A plasma derived vaccine only, group B plasma derived vaccine with HBIG, group C recombinant vaccine 20 μg and group D recombinant vaccine 10 μg) in preventing the development of chronic carrier state.[26] It found that recombinant vaccine in either dose with or without HBIG provides more protection (protective efficacy (see glossary, p 864) and prevalence of HBsAg 51% and 12/49 [24.5%] in group A, 82.6% and 4/46 [8.7%] in group B, 92% and 2/50 [4%] in group C, and 87% and 3/49 [6.1%] in group D, respectively; no P values reported) against plasma derived vaccine after 12 months. **Versus universal immunisation of infants:** See universal immunisation of infants, p 858.

QUESTION **What are the effects of immunisation in countries with low endemicity?** New

OPTION **SELECTIVE IMMUNISATION OF HIGH RISK INDIVIDUALS**

One systematic review, in countries with low endemicity, found plasma derived hepatitis B immunisation prevented acute hepatitis B and development of chronic carrier state in healthcare workers at high risk of exposure to bodily fluids. Three RCTs found plasma derived hepatitis B immunisation prevented acute hepatitis B in homosexual men. One small RCT found no significant difference in hepatitis B events in heterosexual partners of infected people. Three RCTs of plasma derived immunisation in people on regular haemodialysis found potentially conflicting results. Two RCTs from France and Belgium found good protective efficacy against chronic carrier state. However, one large US based RCT found no good evidence of benefit. The systematic review of plasma derived vaccination found no significant difference between immunisation and placebo in the rate and severity of adverse events. One observational study showed a high prevalence of hepatitis B carrier state and low immunisation uptake in young homosexuals despite a national strategy to immunise high risk groups. We found insufficient evidence to compare the effectiveness of selective immunisation in high risk individuals with other strategies.

Benefits: **Versus placebo or no immunisation:** We found one systematic review (search date 2003, 4 RCTs, 2701 people) of plasma derived vaccines in healthcare workers.[28] It found vaccination significantly reduced hepatitis B compared with placebo (OR 0.33, 95% CI 0.21 to 0.53, NNT estimated between 7–145 depending on the baseline incidence of hepatitis B). Mean length of follow up was 14.5 months. We found three RCTs in homosexual men.[29–31] The first RCT (800 homosexual men in the Netherlands) compared immunisation with plasma derived vaccine versus placebo for 21.5 months.[29] It found that immunisation significantly reduced the incidence of acute hepatitis infections compared with placebo (17/397 [4.3%] *v* 56/403 [13.9%]; RR 0.31, 95% CI 0.18 to 0.52; NNT 11, 95% CI 8 to 18) among homosexual men. The second RCT (1083 homosexual men in the USA) compared hepatitis immunisation with plasma derived vaccine versus placebo.[30] It found that vaccine significantly protected against acute hepatitis B events (hepatitis B events 77/431 [21%] with placebo *v* 13/448 [2.7%] with immunisation; OR 55.12; $P < 0.0001$) and chronic carrier state (see glossary, p 864) (protective efficacy 87%; $P < 0.0001$; HbsAg positive 90/448 [23.5%] with placebo and 12/448 [2.7%] with immunisation; OR 71.6; CI not reported) at the end of 2 years. The third RCT (1402 homosexual men in the USA) compared hepatitis B immunisation with plasma derived vaccine versus placebo.[31] It found immunisation significantly prevented hepatitis B events 2 years after immunisation (hepatitis events 110/443 [21%] with placebo *v* 58/482 [9%] with immunisation; $P < 0.001$). We found one RCT (160 partners of infected people) that assessed the post-exposure prophylactic efficacy of hepatitis B immunisation among regular heterosexual partners of infected people.[32] It found no significant difference in the incidence of acute hepatitis events rate at 9 months (12/75 [16%] with immunisation and 13/71 [18.3%] with placebo; $P > 0.5$). We found three RCTs comparing hepatitis B immunisation versus placebo in people on haemodialysis.[33–35] The first RCT in France (138 people) found immunisation with plasma derived vaccine significantly reduced events 12 months after immunisation[33] (15/72 [21%] with vaccine group *v* 29/66 [45%] with placebo; $P < 0.02$). The second RCT in Belgium (401 people) of plasma derived vaccine found a large and significant reduction in the hepatitis B attack rates (7/197 [4%] with immunisation *v* 30/191 [18%] with placebo; protective efficacy 78%; $P = 0.00016$) with immunisation in the 435 days assessment.[34] However, one large RCT in the USA (1311 people) of plasma derived vaccine did not find any significant difference in the incidence of acute hepatitis B events (42/660 [6.4%] with immunisation *v* 35/651 [5.4%] placebo; $P > 0.05$) 2 years after immunisation.[35] **Versus universal immunisation:** We found no good systematic reviews, RCTs, or observational studies.

Harms: The systematic review of plasma derived hepatitis B immunisation in healthcare workers did not find any significant difference in incidence of adverse events (OR 1.13, 95% CI 0.95 to 1.35), severity of systemic adverse events (OR 1.60, 95% CI 0.64 to 4.04), or severity of local adverse events (OR 1.09, 95% CI 0.90 to 1.33) between vaccination and placebo.[28] The first RCT in homosexual men of plasma derived vaccine found no significant difference between the two groups (incidence of adverse events 24.3% in the intervention group, and 21.4% in the control group; difference not statistically significant; P values not reported).[30] The other two RCTs of plasma derived vaccine found a higher incidence of mild adverse reaction with immunisation compared with placebo.[29,31] One RCT found increased incidence of sore arm and dizziness after immunisation (8.9% and 2.6% with immunisation *v* 5.9% and 0.6% with placebo; $P < 0.001$) and the other RCT found a significant increase in sore arm (64% with sore arm in the vaccinated group *v* 45% in placebo after first dose; $P < 0.001$). One RCT in people receiving haemodialysis found a significantly higher incidence of adverse reactions with plasma derived vaccine immunisation compared with placebo (42% with immunisation *v* 22% with placebo; $P < 0.005$).[34] The other two RCTs in people receiving haemodialysis found no significant difference (3% *v* 9% in the French RCT and 13% *v* 14% in the US RCT).[33,35] None of these RCTs found any serious adverse reactions.

Comment: Both RCTs from the USA in homosexual men had high loss to follow up (19% and 25%) during 2 years, raising the possibility of bias.[30,31] The RCT from the Netherlands lost 4–4.8% of participants during follow up.[29] All three RCTs had comparable groups in both intervention and control arms. However, one cross sectional study from USA suggests poor uptake and high prevalence of chronic carrier state in this group despite a national high-risk immunisation programme (see glossary, p 864).[36] This may be an underestimate of the actual problem, as only 62% were approached out of all eligible men, and only 62% of these agreed to take part in the study. One RCT found no advantage in providing immunisation as a post-exposure prophylaxis to the regular partners of people infected with hepatitis B identified during their hospital admission for recent jaundice.[32] The RCT was able to recruit only 75% of the eligible partners, which might make the results unrepresentative. One cohort study found that hepatitis B vaccine provides protection against the development of chronic carrier state in residents of mentally handicap institutions up to 11 years. However, nearly 51% of participants did not complete follow up in this study. The US based RCT in people on haemodialysis lost 35% of participants during follow up as opposed to 15% in the French RCT, and less than 1% in the Belgian RCT. The US trial also had a low event rate in both placebo and intervention arms compared with the other two trials. This may be the reason for not detecting any significant difference between the two groups.

OPTION UNIVERSAL IMMUNISATION OF INFANTS

One historical cohort study found a reduction in the prevalence of hepatitis B chronic carrier state following universal immunisation. We found insufficient evidence to compare its effectiveness with other strategies. Two cohort studies and surveillance data did not report any links between hepatitis B immunisation and serious adverse reactions.

Benefits: **Versus placebo or no immunisation:** We found no RCTs conducted in countries with low endemicity of hepatitis B assessing the efficacy of universal immunisation. One historical cohort study in

Alaska (7 villages, 533 children aged up to 10 years) found a marked decline in the prevalence of chronic carrier state after the adoption of universal immunisation strategy (prevalence of HbsAg 3.1% during 1982–1987 and 0.0% during 1993–1994, statistical significance not reported).[37] **Versus other immunisation strategies:** We found no good systematic reviews, RCTs, or observational studies.

Harms: One retrospective cohort study in the USA (6515 children age < 6 years) of recombinant vaccine compared the incidence of adverse reactions in vaccinated versus unvaccinated children.[38] It found children who received hepatitis B immunisation had higher rates of arthritis, acute ear infection and pharyngitis compared with unvaccinated children (arthritis OR 5.91, 95% CI 1.05 to 33.14, acute ear infection OR 1.60, 95% CI 1.00 to 2.58, and pharyngitis OR 1.41, 95% CI 0.95 to 2.09). The results were adjusted for demographic differences, but absolute risk and exact number of events were not given. A second cohort study (conducted in the USA, 5655 children) of recombinant vaccine found no significant difference in the adverse events (27/3302 [0.8%] in vaccinated *v* 26/2353 [1.1%] unvaccinated, P = 0.28) reported to health services in the first 21 days after birth between vaccinated and unvaccinated children.[39] Fever, allergic reactions, seizures, or other neurological events were among the most common events in both groups. Post-marketing surveillance data in USA during 1991–1995 of recombinant vaccine found no unexpected adverse events in children given recombinant hepatitis B vaccine with or without other routine immunisation (no statistical analysis done).[40] It reported 18 neonatal deaths during 1991–1998 following hepatitis B immunisations,[41] but no causal link was established between these deaths and immunisation. Surveillance data from Italy (1991–2000) of recombinant vaccine reported 19 serious post-immunisation adverse events, none of which was linked to multiple sclerosis or any other serious neurological disease.[42] Surveillance data from US did not suggest any link between hepatitis B immunisation and neurological or other serious adverse reactions.[40,41]

Comment: The Alaskan study was only able to recruit 49% of children approached, which might make results unrepresentative.[37] Two studies (one cohort,[39] one case control[38]), both with a large sample size, found conflicting results. However, none reported any serious adverse reactions. Both studies did not validate their data from other sources. The case control study had a potential for non-response bias, as the responding cohort may not represent the population of interest. The cohort study analysed adverse events reported only to hospitals thereby probably underestimating actual events.

OPTION UNIVERSAL IMMUNISATION OF ADOLESCENTS

We found insufficient evidence to assess the effects of universal adolescent immunisation or to compare its effectiveness with other strategies. One observational study suggests minor adverse effects following hepatitis B immunisation in this group.

Benefits: We found no systematic reviews or RCTs assessing universal adolescent immunisation strategies.

Harms: One study from the routine post-marketing vaccine surveillance system in Canada (41 494 students age 11 years) found 69 adverse events.[43] The major categories were injection site reactions (23%), fainting (20%), and rashes (17%). There were four cases of arthritis and one instance of anaphylaxis. The study had no control group, which makes establishing causality difficult.

Comment: We found no strong evidence on the effects of the adolescent immunisation strategy adopted in many parts of the USA and Canada. Evaluation of adolescent immunisation schemes in Canada did not include the primary outcome measures adopted in this review.[44] Surveillance data from the USA and Canada have reported few serious adverse reactions. The results are based on self reported events and had no control group.[43]

GLOSSARY

Acute hepatitis B events Any acute illness with raised liver enzymes (ALT levels) and serological signs of acute hepatitis (HBsAg, antiHBc IgM).[45]
Chronic carrier state A person is considered a chronic carrier if the HBsAg has been persistently positive for more than 6 months.[45]
Connective tissue disorders These are multisystemic conditions secondary to an inflammatory response in the body against its own tissues resulting in damage and long term disability.[45]
Countries with high hepatitis B endemicity HBsAg prevalence 8% or higher.[36]
Countries with low hepatitis B endemicity HBsAg prevalence less than 2%.[46]
HBsAg Hepatitis B surface antigen is a serological marker on the surface of hepatitis B virus. It indicates acute or chronic hepatitis B infection.[46]
High risk immunisation strategy In this strategy hepatitis B vaccine is recommended in individuals and groups who are at high risk of hepatitis B because of their lifestyle, occupation, and other factors. These include close contact of a case or a carrier, babies born to infected mothers, parenteral drug misusers, individuals who change sexual partners frequently, homosexual or bisexual men, haemophilics, people on heamodialysis, healthcare workers, and residents of institutions for individuals with severe learning disabilities.[46]
Hepatitis vaccine Both types of vaccines (plasma derived vaccine rarely used now and yeast derived recombinant vaccine most commonly used).[46]
Recombinant vaccine It contains HBsAg absorbed on aluminium hydroxide adjuvant and is prepared from yeast cells using recombinant DNA technology.[1]
Protective efficacy $[(R_1 - R_2)/R_1] \times 100$ where R_1 is the incidence of event in control population and R_2 is the incidence of event in the immunised population.[26] This is the same as the relative risk reduction.
Universal immunisation strategy In this strategy, routine hepatitis B immunisation is carried out for either all infants or adolescents through a national programme.[46]

REFERENCES

1. Department of Health. *Immunisation against infectious disease*. London: HMSO, 1996.
2. Kane M. Global programme for control of hepatitis B infection. *Vaccine* 1995;13(suppl 1):47–49.
3. Margolis HS. Hepatitis B virus infection. *Bull World Health Organ* 1998;76(suppl 2):152–153.
4. Kao JH, Chen DS. Global control of hepatitis B virus infection. *Lancet Infect Dis* 2002;2:395–403.
5. Lee WM. Hepatitis B virus infection (comment). *N Engl J Med* 1997;337:1733–1745.
6. World Health Organization. Hepatits B Vaccine. *Wkly Epidemiol Rec* 1991;11.

7. Edmunds WJ. Universal or selective immunisation against hepatitis B virus in the United Kingdom? A review of recent cost-effectiveness studies. *Commun Dis Public Health* 1998;1:221–228.
8. Andre FE. Summary of safety and efficacy data on a yeast-derived hepatitis B vaccine. *Am J Med* 1989;87:14S–20S.
9. Fortuin M, Chotard J, Jack AD, et al. Efficacy of hepatitis B vaccine in the Gambian expanded programme on immunisation. *Lancet* 1993;341:1129–1131.
10. Viviani S, Jack A, Hall AJ, et al. Hepatitis B vaccination in infancy in The Gambia: protection against carriage at 9 years of age. *Vaccine* 1999;17:2946–2950.
11. Liao SS, Li RC, Li H, et al. Long-term efficacy of plasma-derived hepatitis B vaccine: A 15-year follow-up study among Chinese children. *Vaccine* 1999;17:2661–2666.
12. Liao SS, Li RC, Li H, et al. Long-term efficacy of plasma-derived hepatitis B vaccine among Chinese children: a 12-year follow-up study. *World J Gastroenterol* 1999;5:165–166.
13. Perrin J, Coursaget P, Ntareme F, et al. Hepatitis B immunization of newborns according to a two dose protocol. *Vaccine* 1986;4:241–244.
14. Chang MH, Chen CJ, Lai MS, et al. Universal hepatitis B vaccination in Taiwan and the incidence of hepatocellular carcinoma in children. Taiwan Childhood Hepatoma Study Group. *N Engl J Med* 1997;336:1855–1859.
15. Lee CL, Ko YC. Hepatitis B vaccination and hepatocellular carcinoma in Taiwan. *Pediatrics* 1997;99:351–353.
16. Da Villa G, Piccinino F, Scolastico C, et al. Long-term epidemiological survey of hepatitis B virus infection in a hyperendemic area (Afragola, southern Italy): results of a pilot vaccination project. *Res Virol* 1998;149:263–270.
17. Da Villa G, Picciottoc L, Elia S, et al. Hepatitis B vaccination: universal vaccination of newborn babies and children at 12 years of age versus high risk groups. A comparison in the field. *Vaccine* 1995;13:1240–1243.
18. Arkachaisri T. Serum sickness and hepatitis B vaccine including review of the literature. *J Med Assoc Thail* 2002;85(suppl 2):607–612.
19. Hanslik T, Vaillant JN, Audrain L, et al. Systemic lupus erythematosus and risk of hepatitis B vaccination: from level of evidence to prescription [in French]. *Rev Med Interne* 2000;21:785–790.
20. Bassily S, Kotkat A, Gray G, et al. Comparative study of the immunogenicity and safety of two dosing schedules of hepatitis B vaccine in neonates. *Am J Trop Med Hygiene* 1995;53:419–422.
21. Andre FE, Zuckerman AJ. Review: protective efficacy of hepatitis B vaccines in neonates. *Med Virol* 1994;44:144–151.
22. Lo KJ, Tsai YT, Lee SD. Combined passive and active immunization for interruption of perinatal transmission of hepatitis B virus in Taiwan. *Hepatogastroenterology* 1985;32:65–68.
23. Xu ZY, Liu CB, Francis DP, et al. Prevention of perinatal acquisition of hepatitis B virus carriage using vaccine: preliminary report of a randomized, double-blind placebo-controlled and comparative trial. *Pediatrics* 1985;76:713–718.
24. Xu ZY, Duan SC, Margolis HS, Purcell RH, et al. Long-term efficacy of active postexposure immunization of infants for prevention of hepatitis B virus infection. United States-People's Republic of China Study Group on Hepatitis B. *J Infect Dis* 1995;171:54–60.
25. Ip HMH, Wong VCW, Lelie PN, Kuhns MC, Reesink HW. Prevention of hepatitis B virus carrier state in infants according to maternal serum levels of HBV DNA. *Lancet* 1989;1:406–410.
26. Halliday ML, Kang LY, Rankin JG, et al. An efficacy trial of a mammalian cell-derived recombinant DNA hepatitis B vaccine in infants born to mothers positive for HBsAg, in Shanghai, China. *Int J Epidemiol* 1992;21:564en573.
27. Poovorawan Y, Sanpavat S, Pongpunglert W, et al. Long term efficacy of hepatitis B vaccine in infants born to hepatitis B e antigen-positive mothers. *Pediatr Infect Dis J* 1992;11:816–821.
28. Jefferson T, Demicheli V, Deeks J, et al. Vaccines for preventing hepatitis B in health-care workers. In: The Cochrane Library, Issue 1, 2003. Oxford: Update Software. Search date not stated; primary sources Medline, Embase, The Cochrane Library, hand search of *Vaccine*, hand search of reference lists, and contact with authors, researchers, and manufacturers.
29. Coutinho RA, Lelie N, Albrecht VL. Efficacy of a heat inactivated hepatitis B vaccine in male homosexuals: outcome of a placebo controlled double blind trial. *BMJ* 1983;286:1305–1308.
30. Szmuness W, Stevens CE, Zang EA, et al. A controlled clinical trial of the efficacy of the hepatitis B vaccine (Heptavax B): a final report. *Hepatology* 1981;1:377–385.
31. Francis DP, Hadler SC, Thompson SE, et al. The prevention of hepatitis B with vaccine. Report of the centers for disease control multi-center efficacy trial among homosexual men. *Ann Intern Med* 1982;97:362–366.
32. Roumeliotou-Karayannis A, Papaevangelou G, Tassopoulos N, et al. Post-exposure active immunoprophylaxis of spouses of acute viral hepatitis B patients. *Vaccine* 1985;3:31–34.
33. Crosnier J, Jungers P, Courouce AM. Randomised placebo-controlled trial of hepatitis B surface antigen vaccine in French haemodialysis units: II, Haemodialysis patients. *Lancet* 1981;1:797–800.
34. Desmyter J, Colaert J, De Groote G, et al. Efficacy of heat-inactivated hepatitis B vaccine in haemodialysis patients and staff. Double-blind placebo-controlled trial. *Lancet* 1983;2:1323–1328.
35. Stevens CE, Alter HJ, Taylor PE, et al. Hepatitis B vaccine in patients receiving hemodialysis. Immunogenicity and efficacy. *N Engl J Med* 1984;311:496–501.
36. MacKellar DA, Valleroy LA, Secura GM, et al. Two decades after vaccine license: hepatitis B immunization and infection among young men who have sex with men. *Am J Public Health* 2001;91:965–971.
37. Harpaz R, McMahon BJ, Margolis HS, et al. Elimination of new chronic hepatitis B virus infections: results of the Alaska immunization program. *J Infect Dis* 2000;181:413–418.
38. Fisher MA, Eklund SA, James SA, et al. Adverse events associated with hepatitis B vaccine in U.S. children less than six years of age, 1993 and 1994. *Ann Epidemiol* 2001;11:13–21.
39. Lewis E, Shinefield HR, Woodruff BA, et al. Safety of neonatal hepatitis B vaccine administration. *Pediatr Infect Dis J* 2001;20:1049–1054.
40. Niu MT, Davis DM, Ellenberg S. Recombinant hepatitis B vaccination of neonates and infants: emerging safety data from the Vaccine Adverse Event Reporting System. *Pediatr Infect Dis J* 1996;15:771–776.
41. Niu MT, Salive ME, Ellenberg SS. Neonatal deaths after hepatitis B vaccine: the vaccine adverse event reporting system, 1991–1998. *Arch Pediatr Adolesc Med* 1999;153:1279–1282.

42. Zanetti AR. Update on hepatitis B vaccination in Italy 10 years after its implementation. *Vaccine* 2001;19:2380–1283.
43. Dobson S, Scheifele D, Bell A. Assessment of a universal, school-based hepatitis B vaccination program (comment). *JAMA* 1995;274:1209–1213.
44. Bell A. Universal hepatitis B immunization: the British Columbia experience. *Vaccine* 1995;13:S77–S81.
45. Andreoli TE, Carpenter CCJ, Griggs RC, et al (eds). *Cecil essentials of medicine*. Philadelphia: WB Saunders company, 1993.
46. Chin JE (ed). *Control of communicable diseases*. Washington: American Public Health Association, 2000.

Kamran Siddiqi
Dr
Nuffield Institute for Health
Leeds
UK

Competing interests: None declared.

Influenza

Search date November 2002

Lucy Hansen

QUESTIONS

INTERVENTIONS

Key Messages

- **Oral amantadine for early treatment of influenza A in adults (duration of symptoms reduced)** One systematic review and three additional RCTs have found that oral amantadine reduces the duration of influenza A symptoms by about 1 day compared with placebo. We found insufficient evidence about adverse effects in this setting. We found no good evidence of benefit if amantadine is started more than 2 days after symptom onset.
- **Orally inhaled zanamivir for early treatment of influenza A and B in adults (duration of symptoms reduced)** One systematic review has found that orally inhaled zanamivir reduces the duration of influenza symptoms by about 1 day compared with placebo. Adverse effects were similar in people taking zanamivir and in people taking placebo. We found no good evidence of benefit if zanamivir is started more than 2 days after symptom onset.
- **Oral oseltamivir for early treatment of influenza A and B in adults (duration of symptoms reduced)** Two RCTs have found that oral oseltamivir reduces the duration of influenza symptoms by about 1 day compared with placebo. Oral oseltamivir increases the incidence of nausea and vomiting compared with placebo. We found no good evidence of benefit if oseltamivir is started more than 1.5 days after symptom onset.
- **Oral rimantadine for early treatment of influenza A in adults (duration of symptoms reduced)** One systematic review has found that oral rimantadine reduces the duration of influenza A symptoms by about 1 day compared with placebo. We found insufficient evidence about adverse effects in this setting. We found no good evidence of benefit if rimantadine is started more than 2 days after symptom onset.

- **All antivirals for preventing serious influenza complications** We found insufficient evidence about the effects of antiviral agents on reducing serious complications of influenza.

DEFINITION Influenza is caused by infection with influenza viruses. Uncomplicated influenza is characterised by the abrupt onset of fever, chills, non-productive cough, myalgias, headache, nasal congestion, sore throat, and fatigue.[1] Influenza is usually diagnosed clinically. Not all people infected with influenza viruses become symptomatic. People infected with other pathogens may have symptoms identical to those of influenza.[2] The percentage of infections resulting in clinical illness can vary from about 40–85%, depending on age and pre-existing immunity to the virus.[3] Influenza can be confirmed by viral culture, immunofluorescence staining, enzyme immunoassay, or rapid diagnostic testing of nasopharyngeal, nasal or throat swab specimens, or by serological testing of paired sera. Some rapid tests detect influenza A only, some detect and distinguish between influenza A and B, whereas others detect but do not distinguish between influenza A and B.

INCIDENCE/ PREVALENCE In temperate areas of the northern hemisphere, influenza activity typically peaks between late December and early March, whereas in temperate areas of the southern hemisphere influenza activity typically peaks between May and September. In tropical areas, influenza can occur throughout the year.[2] The annual incidence of influenza varies yearly, and depends partly on the underlying level of population immunity to circulating influenza viruses.[1] One localised study in the USA found that serological conversion with or without symptoms occurred in 10–20% a year, with the highest infection rates in people aged under 20 years.[4] Attack rates are higher in institutions and in areas of overcrowding.[5]

AETIOLOGY/ RISK FACTORS Influenza viruses are transmitted primarily from person to person through respiratory droplets disseminated during sneezing, coughing, and talking.[1,6]

PROGNOSIS The incubation period of influenza is 1–4 days and infected adults are usually contagious from the day before symptom onset until 5 days after symptom onset. The signs and symptoms of uncomplicated influenza usually resolve within a week, although cough and fatigue may persist.[1] Complications include otitis media, bacterial sinusitis, secondary bacterial pneumonia, and, less commonly, viral pneumonia and respiratory failure. Complications are also caused by exacerbation of underlying disease.[1,2] In the USA each year, over 110 000 admissions to hospital and about 20 000 deaths are related to influenza.[2] The risk of hospitalisation is highest in people 65 years or older, in very young children, and in those with chronic medical conditions.[1,7,8] Over 90% of influenza related deaths during recent seasonal epidemics in the USA have been in people 65 years or older.[1] During influenza pandemics, morbidity and mortality may be high in younger age groups.[1] Severe illness is more common with influenza A infections than with influenza B infections.[1]

AIMS OF INTERVENTION To reduce the duration and severity of influenza signs and symptoms, and the risk of complications, and to minimise adverse effects of treatment.

OUTCOMES Severity and duration of symptoms; frequency and severity of complications of influenza; adverse effects of treatment.

METHODS *Clinical Evidence* search and appraisal November 2002. The authors searched Medline (1966–2001; major MeSH topics: amantadine and influenza, rimantadine and influenza; keywords: zanamivir, 4-guanidino-Neu5Ac2en, GG167, oseltamivir, GS4104, and Ro64-0796). Meeting abstracts were used to identify unpublished studies of zanamivir and oseltamivir. We included only systematic reviews and double blind RCTs of treatment versus placebo for naturally occurring influenza. We excluded RCTs and reviews of chemoprophylaxis of influenza, experimentally induced influenza, and reviews that combined RCTs of more than one agent. We only assessed people with laboratory confirmed influenza. For amantadine and rimantadine, we included only RCTs of influenza A. For zanamivir and oseltamivir, we included studies of influenza A or B. For zanamivir, we included only RCTs of orally inhaled drug and excluded intranasal drops plus oral inhalation unless oral inhalation results were reported separately. For amantadine, rimantadine, and oseltamivir we included only RCTs of oral administration. We excluded RCTs primarily on children younger than 18 years, those that used an antipyretic rather than a placebo as control, RCTs in which the delay from symptom onset to starting treatment was unclear, and RCTs without quantitative measures of clinical effectiveness.

QUESTION **What are the effects of antiviral treatment of influenza in adults?**

OPTION **ORAL AMANTADINE**

One systematic review and additional RCTs have found that oral amantadine reduces the duration of influenza A symptoms by about 1 day compared with placebo. We found insufficient evidence to assess adverse effects in this setting.

Benefits: We found one systematic review (search date 1997, 7 RCTs, 531 otherwise healthy people)[9] and three additional RCTs[10–12] of oral amantadine (usually started within 48 hours of symptom onset) versus placebo for the treatment of influenza A (see table A on web extra). The review found that amantadine significantly reduced the duration of fever (temperature > 37.0 °C reduced by 1 day, 95% CI 0.7 days to 1.3 days). We found no RCTs of the effect of amantadine in preventing serious complications of influenza, such as pneumonia or exacerbation of chronic diseases. We found no RCTs of amantadine for treatment of influenza A in pregnant women, those with chronic disease, or in immunised people.

Harms: The review found no significant difference in the frequency of adverse effects between amantadine and placebo groups. However, the included RCTs contained little information about the relative adverse effects of amantadine compared with placebo when used for treatment of influenza A (see table A on web extra).[13–15] More evidence is available about the harms of amantadine when used for prophylaxis of influenza A (see comment below).

Comment: In vitro studies have found that amantadine has specific antiviral activity against influenza A but not influenza B viruses.[16] The RCTs used different outcome measures, and so summarising the results is difficult. Only one RCT examined amantadine in elderly people.[12] All RCTs considered only people with laboratory confirmed influenza A, and so the analyses were not by intention to treat. The proportion of influenza A isolates from the general population exhibiting resistance to amantadine has remained low.[17,18] Amantadine resistant influenza A viruses have not been found to be more virulent than non-resistant viruses.[2] The limited evidence from elderly and high risk groups makes it difficult to generalise results to these populations. A systematic review found that use of amantadine for prophylaxis of influenza A is associated with an increased incidence of gastrointestinal and central nervous system adverse effects compared with placebo.[9]

OPTION ORAL RIMANTADINE

One systematic review has found that oral rimantadine reduces the duration of influenza A symptoms by about 1 day compared with placebo. We found insufficient evidence about adverse effects in this setting.

Benefits: We found one systematic review (search date 1997, 3 RCTs, 104 otherwise healthy adults)[9] and one small additional RCT[19] of rimantadine (usually started within 48 hours of symptom onset) versus placebo for the treatment of influenza A (see table A on web extra). The review found that rimantadine significantly reduced the duration of fever compared with placebo (temperature > 37.0 °C reduced by 1.3 days, 95% CI 0.8 days to 1.8 days). We found no RCTs of rimantadine for treatment of influenza A in people over 65 years of age, in pregnant women, in those with chronic disease, or in immunised people. We found no RCTs of the effect of rimantadine in preventing serious complications of influenza, such as pneumonia or exacerbation of chronic diseases.

Harms: The review found insufficient evidence about the adverse effects of rimantadine compared with placebo in people with influenza A.[9] One non-systematic review (340 adults treated for influenza) of rimantadine versus placebo found that more people taking rimantadine had central nervous system symptoms, most commonly insomnia (10.8% *v* 8.6%; P value not provided); and gastrointestinal symptoms, most commonly abdominal pain and nausea (6.0% *v* 2.3%; P value not provided).[20] Additional evidence is available about adverse effects of rimantadine when used for prophylaxis of influenza A (see comment below).

Comment: In vitro studies have found that rimantadine has specific antiviral activity against influenza A but not influenza B viruses.[16] The RCTs used different outcome measures and so summarising results is difficult. Additional studies of rimantadine have been performed in Russia, but information in English is limited.[21] Viruses that are resistant to rimantadine show cross-resistance to amantadine, and *vice versa*.[17] Influenza A viruses resistant to rimantadine have not been found to be more virulent than non-resistant viruses.[2] The proportion of influenza A isolates from the general population exhibiting resistance to rimantadine (or amantadine) has remained low.[17,18] The limited evidence from elderly and high risk groups makes it difficult to generalise results to these populations. A systematic review found that use of rimantadine for prophylaxis of influenza A is associated with an increased incidence of gastrointestinal adverse effects compared with placebo.[9]

OPTION ORALLY INHALED ZANAMIVIR

One systematic review has found that orally inhaled zanamivir reduces the duration of influenza symptoms by about 1 day compared with placebo. Adverse effects were similar in people taking zanamivir and placebo.

Benefits: We found one systematic review (search date 2000, 5 RCTs, 1498 people with influenza)[22] and two additional RCTs (78 people with influenza)[23,24] that compared inhaled zanamivir (usually started within 48 hours of symptom onset) versus placebo (see table B on web extra). Some of the RCTs included small numbers of people aged 65 years or older, and people with chronic cardiac or respiratory illness.[24–27] **Symptoms in all people:** The review found that zanamivir significantly reduced the time to alleviation of symptoms (median time reduced by 1.4 days, 95% CI 0.8 days to 1.9 days) compared with placebo. One of the additional RCTs (27 people with influenza) found no significant difference between zanamivir and placebo in the time to alleviation of symptoms (median time reduced by 4.5 days, $P = 0.3$).[24] The other additional RCT (51 people with influenza) found that zanamivir reduced the time to alleviation of symptoms by 0.5 days (P value not provided) compared with placebo.[23] **Symptoms in high risk people:** The review performed a meta-analysis including one RCT (313 high risk people with influenza) and subgroups of people at high risk from four of the original RCTs (171 people).[28] It found no significant difference between zanamivir and placebo in the time to alleviation of symptoms (484 people; median time reduced by +1.67 days, 95% CI –0.02 to +3.37 days).[28] **Complications:** We found no fully published RCTs of the effect of zanamivir in preventing serious complications of influenza, such as pneumonia or exacerbation of chronic diseases.

Harms: Adverse effects were similar in people taking zanamivir compared with placebo (the inhaled lactose vehicle alone) (see table B on web extra).[22] Use of zanamivir has been associated with bronchospasm and worsening of underlying respiratory disease (see comment below).[29]

Comment: Zanamivir is administered as an orally inhaled powder. In vitro studies have found that zanamivir has antiviral activity against both influenza A and B viruses.[30] RCTs have predominantly included people with influenza A (≥ 85%). Because of the short period for which zanamivir has been available, and the lack of optimal assays to detect resistant strains, we found insufficient evidence to comment on the development of viral resistance to zanamivir.[2,31–36] We found one RCT (525 people with obstructive airways disease and influenza) published in abstract form only.[37] It found that zanamivir significantly reduced time to symptom resolution compared with placebo (median reduction with zanamivir *v* placebo 1.5 days; P = 0.009). We found some observational evidence that zanamivir is associated with bronchospasm and worsening of underlying respiratory disease.[29] However, the RCT published in abstract found a small but significant increase in morning and evening peak expiratory flow rate with zanamivir compared with placebo (morning peak expiratory flow rate 12.9 L/minute higher with zanamivir *v* placebo, P = 0.011; evening peak expiratory flow rate 13.1 L/minute higher, P = 0.007).[37] It found a non-significant reduction between zanamivir and placebo in complications needing antibiotics or a change in respiratory medication (ARR 58% with zanamivir *v* placebo, P = 0.064).

OPTION ORAL OSELTAMIVIR

Two RCTs have found that oral oseltamivir reduces the duration of influenza symptoms by about 1 day compared with placebo, but increases the incidence of nausea and vomiting.

Benefits: We found no systematic review of oseltamivir used to treat influenza. We found two RCTs that compared oseltamivir with placebo.[38,39] People in both RCTs were selected with a temperature of 38.0 °C or greater. Both RCTs found that oseltamivir (started within 36 hours of symptom onset) significantly reduced the duration of influenza symptoms by about 1 day compared with placebo (see table B on web extra). We found no RCTs of oseltamivir for influenza in people 65 years or older, in pregnant women, in people with chronic disease, or in vaccinated people. We found no RCTs of the effect of oseltamivir in preventing serious complications of influenza, such as pneumonia, or exacerbation of chronic diseases.

Harms: Nausea and vomiting were significantly more common in people receiving oseltamivir compared with placebo.[38,39]

Comment: Studies in mice and ferrets have found that oseltamivir has *in vitro* activity against both influenza A and B viruses.[40] The RCTs predominantly included people with influenza A (97%).[38,39] Because of the short period for which oseltamivir has been available, and the lack of optimal assays to detect resistant strains, we found insufficient evidence about viral resistance to oseltamivir.[2,32,36,41]

REFERENCES

1. Cox NJ, Fukuda K. Influenza. *Infect Dis Clin North Am* 1998;12:27–38.
2. Bridges CB, Fukuda K, Uyeki TM, et al. Prevention and control of influenza: recommendations of the Advisory Committee on Immunization Practices (ACIP). *MMWR Recomm Rep* 2002;51(RR-3):1–31.
3. Fox JP, Cooney MK, Hall CE, et al. Influenza virus infections in Seattle families, 1975–1979. II. Pattern of infection in invaded households and relation of age and prior antibody to occurrence of infection and related illness. *Am J Epidemiol* 1982;116:228–242.
4. Sullivan KM, Monto AS, Longini IM. Estimates of the US health impact of influenza. *Am J Public Health* 1993;83:1712–1716.
5. Kilbourne ED. *Influenza*. New York: Plenum Medical Book Co, 1987:269–270.
6. Tablan OC, Anderson LJ, Arden NH, et al. Hospital Infection Control Practices Advisory Committee. Guideline for prevention of nosocomial pneumonia. *Infect Control Hosp Epidemiol* 1994;15:587–604.
7. Neuzil KM, Mellen BG, Wright PF, et al. The effect of influenza on hospitalizations, outpatient visits, and courses of antibiotics in children. *N Engl J Med* 2000;342:225–231.
8. Izurieta HS, Thompson WW, Kramarz P, et al. Influenza and the rates of hospitalization for respiratory disease among infants and young children. *N Engl J Med* 2000;342:232–239.

9. Jefferson TO, Demicheli V, Deeks JJ, et al. Amantadine and rimantadine for preventing and treating influenza A in adults. In: The Cochrane Library, Issue 1, 2003. Oxford: Update Software. Search date 1997; primary sources Medline, Cochrane Controlled Trials Register, Embase, reviews of references of identified trials, and letters to manufacturers and authors.
10. Baker LM, Shock MP, Iezzoni DG. The therapeutic efficacy of Symmetrel (amantadine hydrochloride) in naturally occurring influenza A2 respiratory illness. *J Am Osteopath Assoc* 1969;68:1244–1250.
11. Galbraith AW, Schild AW, Schild GC, et al. The therapeutic effect of amantadine in influenza occurring during the winter of 1971–1972 assessed by double-blind study. *J R Coll Gen Pract* 1973;23:34–37.
12. Walters HE, Paulshock M. Therapeutic efficacy of amantadine HCl. *Mo Med* 1970;67:176–179.
13. Kitamoto O. Therapeutic effectiveness of amantadine hydrochloride in influenza A2: double-blind studies. *Jpn J Tuberc Chest Dis* 1968;15:17–26.
14. Kitamoto O. Therapeutic effectiveness of amantadine hydrochloride in naturally occurring Hong Kong influenza: double-blinded studies. *Jpn J Tuberc Chest Dis* 1971;17:1–7.
15. Van Voris LP, Betts RF, Hayden FG, et al. Successful treatment of naturally occurring influenza A/USSR/77 H1N1. *JAMA* 1981;245:1128–1131.
16. Tominack RL, Hayden FG. Rimantadine hydrochloride and amantadine hydrochloride use in influenza A virus infections. *Infect Dis Clin North Am* 1987;1:459–478.
17. Belshe RB, Burk B, Newman F, et al. Resistance of influenza A viruses to amantadine and rimantadine: results of one decade of surveillance. *J Infect Dis* 1989;159:430–435.
18. Ziegler T, Hemphill ML, Ziegler M-L, et al. Low incidence of rimantadine resistance in field isolates of influenza A viruses. *J Infect Dis* 1999;180:935–939.
19. Rabinovich S, Baldini JT, Bannister R. Treatment of influenza: the therapeutic efficacy of rimantadine HCl in a naturally occurring influenza A2 outbreak. *Am J Med Sci* 1969;257:328–335.
20. Soo W. Adverse effects of rimantadine: summary from clinical trials. *J Respir Dis* 1989;10(suppl.):S26–S31.
21. Zlydnikov DM, Kubar OI, Kovaleva TP, et al. Study of rimantadine in the USSR: a review of the literature. *Rev Infect Dis* 1981;3:408–421.
22. Burls A, Clark W, Stewart A, et al. *Zanamivir for the treatment of influenza in adults, West Midlands Development and Evaluation Service*. Birmingham, 2000. Report for the National Institute for Clinical Excellence (NICE). Available at http://www.nice.org.uk (last accessed 3 June 2003). Search date 2000; primary sources Cochrane Library, Medline, Embase, Science Citation Index, GlaxoSmithKline, Clinical Trials Register, hand searching of Scrip, FDA submissions and conference abstracts, and information submitted by GlaxoSmithKline to NICE.
23. Matsumoto K, Ogawa N, Nerome K, et al. Safety and efficacy of the neuraminidase inhibitor zanamivir in treating influenza virus infection in adults: results from Japan. *Antiviral Ther* 1999;4:61–68.
24. Boivin G, Goyette N, Hardy I, et al. Rapid antiviral effect of inhaled zanamivir in the treatment of naturally occurring influenza in otherwise healthy adults. *J Infect Dis* 2000;181:1471–1474.
25. The MIST (Management of Influenza in the Southern Hemisphere Trialists) Study Group. Randomized trial of efficacy and safety of inhaled zanamivir in treatment of influenza A and B infections. *Lancet* 1998;352:1877–1881.
26. Lalezari J, Klein T, Stapleton J, et al. The efficacy and safety of inhaled zanamivir in the treatment of influenza in otherwise healthy and "high risk" individuals in North America [abstract]. *J Antimicrob Chemother* 1999;44(suppl. A):42.
27. Makela MJ, Pauksens K, Rostila T, et al. Clinical efficacy and safety of the orally inhaled neuraminidase inhibitor zanamivir in the treatment of influenza: a randomized, double-blind, placebo-controlled European study. *J Infect* 2000;40:42–48.
28. National Institute for Clinical Excellence. *Zanamivir for the treatment of influenza in adults*. Supplement to the assessment report: 2000. Available at http://www.nice.org.uk (last accessed 3 Sept 2002).
29. Henney JE. Revised labeling for zanamivir. *JAMA* 2000;284:1234.
30. Woods JM, Bethell RC, Coates JAV, et al. 4-guanidino-2,4-dideoxy-2,3-dehydro-N-acetylneuraminic acid is a highly effective inhibitor of both the sialidase (neuraminidase) and growth of a wide range of influenza A and B viruses *in vitro*. *Antimicrob Agents Chemother* 1993;37:1473–1479.
31. Read RC. Letter to the Editor. *Lancet* 1999;353:668–669.
32. Tisdale M. Monitoring of viral susceptibility: new challenges with the development of influenza NA inhibitors. *Rev Med Virol* 2000;10:45–55.
33. Barnett JM, Cadman A, Gor D. Zanamivir susceptibility monitoring and characterization of influenza virus clinical isolates obtained during phase II clinical efficacy studies. *Antimicrob Agents Chemother* 2000;44:78–87.
34. Gubareva LV, Kaiser L, Brenner MK, et al. Evidence for zanamivir resistance in an immunocompromised child infected with influenza B virus. *J Infect Dis* 1998;178:1257–1262.
35. Gubareva LV, Webster RG, Hayden FG. Detection of influenza virus resistance to neuraminidase inhibitors by an enzyme inhibition assay. *Antiviral Res* 2002;53:47–61.
36. Zambon M, Hayden FG. Position statement: global neuraminidase inhibitor susceptibility network. *Antiviral Res* 2001;49:147–156.
37. Berger W, Stein WJ, Sharp SJ, Szymborski PG. Effect of inhaled zanamivir on pulmonary function and illness duration in asthma and/or chronic chronic obstructive pulmonary disease (COPD) patients with influenza. *Ann Allergy Asthma Immunol* 2001;86:85.
38. Treanor JJ, Hayden FG, Vrooman PS, et al. Efficacy and safety of the oral neuraminidase inhibitor oseltamivir in treating acute influenza: a randomized controlled trial. *JAMA* 2000;283:1016–1024.
39. Nicholson KG, Aoki FY, Osterhaus ADME, et al. Efficacy and safety of oseltamivir in treatment of acute influenza: a randomized controlled trial. *Lancet* 2000;355:1845–1850.
40. Mendel DB, Tai CY, Escarpe PA, et al. Oral administration of a prodrug of the influenza virus neuraminidase inhibitor GS4071 protects mice and ferrets against influenza infection. *Antimicrob Agents Chemother* 1998;42:640–646.
41. Gubareva LV, Webster RG, Hayden FG. Detection of influenza virus resistance to neuraminidase inhibitors by an enzyme inhibition assay. *Antiviral Res* 2002;53:47–61.

Lucy Hansen
Locum Consultant Physician with
Specialist interest in Immunology
Hairmyres Hospital
East Kilbride
UK

Competing interests: None declared.

The following previous contributors of this topic would also like to be acknowledged: Timothy Uyeki and Bazian Ltd.

Leprosy

Search date March 2003

Diana Lockwood

QUESTIONS

INTERVENTIONS

To be covered in future updates

Treatment of reactions

*Observational evidence only, RCTs unlikely to be conducted.

See glossary, p 881

Key Messages

Prevention

- **Bacillus Calmette Guerin (BCG) vaccine; BCG plus killed *Mycobacterium leprae*; ICRC vaccine; *Mycobacterium w* vaccine** One RCT evaluated four different vaccines and found that the largest effect was with ICRC vaccine and BCG plus killed *M leprae*, followed by BCG alone. The effectiveness of *Mycobacterium w* was only marginal. However, only for the vaccine BCG alone were the findings corroborated by large controlled clinical trials with long term follow up. Only one RCT reported on harms of vaccination; it found these to be minimal.

Treatment

- **Multidrug treatment for multibacillary leprosy** We found no reliable comparisons between multidrug treatment with rifampicin plus clofazimine plus dapsone versus dapsone alone, or versus dapsone plus rifampicin, in people with multibacillary leprosy. Observational studies found that multidrug treatment improved skin lesions and was associated with a low relapse rate. The evidence on the incidence of adverse effects is poor. Multidrug treatment was not compared with dapsone alone because rising dapsone resistance rates meant that it would have been unethical to do such a study. The same applies for multidrug treatment for paucibacillary leprosy below.

- **Multidrug treatment for paucibacillary leprosy** We found no reliable comparisons between multidrug treatment with dapsone plus rifampicin versus dapsone alone in people with paucibacillary leprosy. Observational studies found that multidrug treatment improved skin lesions and was associated with a low relapse rate. We found poor evidence on the incidence of adverse effects.
- **Multiple dose compared with single dose treatment for single skin lesion leprosy (both achieve high cure rates but multiple dose is likely to achieve higher)** One RCT found that multiple dose treatment with rifampicin monthly plus dapsone daily for 6 months achieved higher cure rates at 18 months than single dose treatment with rifampicin plus minocycline plus ofloxacin. Some improvement occurred in 99% of people in both groups. Adverse effects were similar with both regimens.

DEFINITION Leprosy is a chronic granulomatous disease caused by *Mycobacterium leprae*, primarily affecting the peripheral nerves and skin. The clinical picture depends on the individual's immune response to *M leprae*. At the tuberculoid end of the Ridley–Jopling scale, individuals have good cell mediated immunity and few skin lesions. At the lepromatous end of the scale, individuals have low reactivity for *M leprae*, causing uncontrolled bacterial spread and skin and mucosal infiltration. Peripheral nerve damage occurs across the spectrum. Nerve damage may occur before, during, or after treatment. Some patients have no nerve damage, others develop anaesthesia of the hands and feet, which puts them at risk of developing neuropathic injury. Weakness and paralysis of the small muscles of the hands, feet, and eyes puts patients at risk of developing deformity and contractures. Loss of the fingers and toes is due to repeated injury in a weak, anaesthetic limb. These visible deformities cause stigmatisation the world over. Classification is based on clinical appearance and bacterial index of lesions (see glossary, p 881). The World Health Organization field leprosy classification is based on the number of skin lesions: single lesion leprosy (1 lesion), paucibacillary leprosy (2–5 skin lesions), and multibacillary leprosy (see glossary, p 882) (> 5 skin lesions).[1]

INCIDENCE/ PREVALENCE Worldwide, about 720 000 new cases of leprosy are reported each year,[2] and about 2 million people have leprosy related disabilities. Six major endemic countries (India, Brazil, Myanmar, Madagascar, Nepal, and Mozambique) account for 88% of all new cases. Cohort studies show a peak of disease presentation between 10–20 years of age.[3] After puberty, there are twice as many male as female cases.

AETIOLOGY/ RISK FACTORS *M leprae* is discharged from the nasal mucosa of people with untreated lepromatous leprosy, and spreads, via the recipient's nasal mucosa, to infect their skin and nerves. It is a hardy organism and has been shown to survive outside human hosts in India for many months.[4] Risk factors for infection include household contact with a person with leprosy. We found no good evidence of an association with HIV infection, nutrition, and socioeconomic status.[5]

PROGNOSIS Complications of leprosy include nerve damage, immunological reactions, and bacillary infiltration. Without treatment, tuberculoid infection eventually resolves spontaneously. Most people with borderline tuberculoid and borderline lepromatous leprosy gradually develop lepromatous infection. Many people have peripheral nerve damage at the time of diagnosis, ranging from 15% in Bangladesh[6] to 55% in Ethiopia.[7] Immunological reactions can occur with or without antibiotic treatment. Further nerve damage occurs through immune mediated reactions (type 1) and neuritis (see glossary, p 882). Erythema nodosum leprosum (see glossary, p 882) (type 2 reaction) is an immune complex mediated reaction causing fever, malaise, and neuritis, which occurs in 20% of people with lepromatous leprosy and 5% with borderline lepromatous leprosy.[8] Secondary impairments (wounds, contractures, and digit resorption) occur in 33–56% of people with established nerve damage.[9] We found no recent information on mortality.

AIMS OF INTERVENTION **Prevention:** To prevent infection. **Treatment:** To treat infection and improve skin lesions; to prevent relapse and complications (nerve damage and erythema nodosum leprosum). Prevention of complications such as ulcers and deformity may improve the quality of life for the individual and help reduce the severe stigmatisation that still accompanies leprosy.

OUTCOMES **Prevention:** Incidence of leprosy **Treatment:** Clinical improvement, relapse rate, quality of life, adverse effects of treatment, and mortality.

METHODS *Clinical Evidence* search and appraisal March 2003, including a search for observational studies. The author identified additional references from hand searches of reference lists. RCTs of preventive interventions need a long follow up period as the incubation period can be 2–15 years, depending on disease type. We excluded trials with less than 2 years' follow up.

QUESTION What are the effects of interventions to prevent leprosy?

OPTION VACCINATION

One RCT evaluated four different vaccines and found that the largest effect was with ICRC vaccine and BCG plus killed *M leprae*, followed by BCG alone. The effectiveness of *Mycobacterium w* was only marginal. However, only for the BCG alone vaccine were the findings corroborated by large controlled clinical trials with long term follow up. Only one RCT reported on harms of vaccination; it found these to be minimal.

Benefits: We found no systematic review. **Different vaccines versus placebo:** We found one RCT carried out in a leprosy endemic area with clinical leprosy as the outcome measure (see table A on web extra).[10] The RCT (double blind, 171 400 healthy people in India aged 1–65 years, follow up for 6–7 years) compared four vaccines (ICRC vaccine [see glossary, p 882], 22 541 people; *Mycobacterium w* vaccine, 33 720 people; BCG, 38 213 people; and BCG plus killed *M leprae*, 38 229 people) versus normal saline (38 697 people). It included a statistical adjustment for the multiple comparisons against placebo. All four vaccines significantly reduced the incidence of leprosy compared with placebo. The most effective vaccines were ICRC vaccine (RRR 65.5%, 95% CI 48.0% to 77.0%) and BCG plus killed *M leprae* (RRR 64.0%, 95% CI 50.4% to

73.9%). BCG alone was also effective (RRR 34.1%, 95% CI 13.5% to 49.8%), whereas the significance of the effect of *Mycobacerium w* was marginal (RRR 25.7%, 95% CI 1.9% to 43.8%). **BCG versus no treatment or placebo:** In addition to the RCT mentioned above,[10] we found three controlled clinical trials comparing BCG alone versus placebo, carried out in leprosy endemic areas, with clinical leprosy as the outcome measure (see table A on web extra).[11–13] The controlled trials (in a total of over 39 000 children in Uganda, Myanmar, and Papua New Guinea) were quasi or non-randomised, but had longer follow up than the RCT (13–16 years). They found that BCG significantly reduced the incidence of leprosy. The degree of protection against leprosy varied between countries, with higher protection in Uganda than Myanmar. One of the trials also looked at mortality and found a significant reduction (442/2707 [16.3%] deaths from all causes with BCG *v* 489/2649 [18.5%] with saline; RR 0.89, 95% CI 0.79 to 0.99; NNT 47, 95% CI 24 to 997).[10,12] **BCG plus killed *M leprae* versus placebo:** In addition to the RCT mentioned above,[10] we found one further RCT carried out in leprosy endemic areas, with clinical leprosy as the outcome measure (see table A on web extra).[14] The RCT stratified people according to the presence of a BCG scar. Those with a scar or a possible scar (54 865 people) received either BCG, BCG plus killed *M leprae*, or placebo. This RCT (double blind, 121 020 healthy people in Malawi without history of previous leprosy or tuberculosis, severe malnutrition, or other severe illness, aged ≥ 3 months, follow up for 5–9 years) found that combined results for BCG and BCG plus killed *M leprae* significantly reduced the incidence of leprosy compared with placebo (combined analysis for BCG or BCG plus killed *M leprae* versus placebo; RR 0.51, 95% CI 0.26 to 0.99).[14] Those without a scar (66 155 people) received BCG or BCG plus killed *M leprae*. **ICRC vaccine versus placebo:** We found one RCT (see different vaccines *v* placebo above).[10] ***Mycobacterium w* versus placebo:** We found one RCT (see different vaccines *v* placebo above).[10] **Dose of vaccine:** The controlled trial performed in Myanmar compared two different concentrations of BCG vaccine versus no treatment.[13] The vaccine with the higher concentration of bacilli significantly reduced the incidence of leprosy over 14 years (3.8/1000 person years [see glossary, p 882] with BCG *v* 5.4/1000 person years for controls; RRR 30%, 95% CI 9–40%). The vaccine with the lower concentration of bacilli had no significant protective effect (5.0/1000 person years with BCG *v* 5.6/1000 person years; RRR +11%, 95% CI –3% to +23%). The RCT performed in Malawi found no significant differences between a higher and a standard dose of killed *M leprae*.[14]

Harms: The RCT conducted in India found that "fluctuant lymphadenitis" was minimal with all four vaccines used, and no other adverse effects were observed (numbers not reported).[10] The other trials did not report on harms.[11–14]

Comment: In the trial in Malawi, 7/82 people (9%) tested positive for HIV.[14] Eleven different batches of BCG were used. The number of people lost to follow up was high (26%), and the sample size may have been insufficient to rule out clinically important effects, given that there were multiple comparisons against placebo.[14]

QUESTION What are the effects of treatments for leprosy?

OPTION MULTIDRUG TREATMENT FOR PAUCIBACILLARY LEPROSY

We found no reliable comparison between multidrug treatment with dapsone plus rifampicin versus dapsone alone in people with paucibacillary leprosy, and RCTs would probably be unethical. Observational studies found that multidrug treatment improved skin lesions and was associated with a low relapse rate. The evidence on the incidence of adverse effects is poor.

Benefits: We found no systematic review or RCT (see comment below). We found seven observational studies assessing the affects of multidrug treatment (dapsone 100 mg/day plus rifampicin 600 mg monthly for 6 months), with follow up ranging from 6 months to 10 years (see table 1, p 884 and table 2, p 885).[15–22] The studies used different methods of assessment making it difficult to compare results. **Skin lesions:** Three cohort studies reported rates of resolution of skin lesions (see comment below) (see table 1, p 884).[15–17,19] One study (499 people) found that resolution of lesions occurred in 38% of people after 1 year;[16] another (50 people) found that resolution occurred in 8% of people after 6 months.[15] The number of people with lesions that were clinically active after treatment ranged from 2–44%.[15–17] **Nerve impairment:** Two studies reported rates of new or worsening nerve impairment (see table 1, p 884).[17,19] One (499 people) found that new disabilities occurred in 2.5% of people, and worsening of existing disabilities occurred in 3.3% after 4 years.[19] The other study (130 people) found that the visible disabilities (World Health Organization grade II — see glossary, p 882) increased from 4% at enrolment to 7% after 8–10 years' follow up.[17] **Relapse:** Six studies reported relapse rates over a 3–8 year follow up period (see table 2, p 885).[17–22] Rates ranged from 0% in Ethiopia[18] to 2.5% over 4 years in Malawi (see table 2, p 885).[19] The risk of relapse ranged from 0.66/1000 person years in China[22] to 6.5/1000 person years in Malawi.[19] (It is clinically difficult to differentiate relapse from reaction in paucibacillary leprosy — see glossary, p 882.)

Harms: None of the studies formally monitored adverse effects. In one study, hepatitis due to rifampicin occurred in 1/130 people (0.8%), but the method of diagnosis was not stated.[17] In another study 1/503 people (0.2%) suffered an "allergic reaction" to rifampicin and dapsone (details not reported).[16]

Comment: Because studies had shown that 30% of *M leprae* isolates were resistant to dapsone,[23] the World Health Organization introduced the combination of dapsone plus rifampicin urgently in 1982, without formal trials comparing it against dapsone.

OPTION MULTIDRUG TREATMENT FOR MULTIBACILLARY LEPROSY

We found no reliable comparisons between multidrug treatment with rifampicin plus clofazimine plus dapsone versus dapsone alone, or versus dapsone plus rifampicin, in people with multibacillary leprosy. Observational studies found that multidrug treatment improved skin lesions and was associated with a low relapse rate. The evidence on the incidence of adverse effects is poor.

Benefits: We found no systematic review or RCTs. We found six observational studies assessing the effects of multidrug treatment (monthly supervised rifampicin 600 mg and clofazimine 300 mg, plus daily unsupervised dapsone 100 mg and clofazimine 500 mg) for 24 months.[17,18,20,22,24,25] **Skin lesions:** One study in Thailand (53 people) found that 29% lesions were still active at 3 years (see table 3, p 885).[17] **Nerve impairment:** The study in Thailand found that the proportion of people with visible deformity (World Health Organization grade II — see glossary, p 882) increased from 8% at enrolment to 13% at 8–10 years' follow up.[17] **Relapse:** Six observational studies reported relapse rates (see table 4, p 886),[17,18,20,22,24,25] which varied from 0% (per 100 person years — see glossary, p 882) in Ethiopia to 20.4% in India. In the study conducted in India, the overall relapse rate was 20/260 (7.7%) over about 8 years (2.04/1000 person years), and 18/20 (90%) relapses were in people with a bacterial index (see glossary, p 881) greater than 4 at the start of treatment.[24]

Harms: Most studies did not report on adverse effects. Skin pigmentation may occur with clofazimine, which may be especially problematic in people with fair skin.

Comment: Only one study[24] stratified its results according to bacterial index. The World Health Organization study group on chemotherapy recommended that treatment be given for 24 months.[26] In 1998, the 7th Expert committee gave the option of reducing the length of treatment from 24 months to 12 months.[1] We found no controlled trial to support this recommendation. We found one RCT (93 people with untreated lepromatous leprosy), which compared dapsone 50 mg/day plus daily rifampicin 450 mg versus dapsone 50 mg/day plus monthly rifampicin 1200 mg for the first 6 months of treatment.[27] It found no significant difference in clinical improvement between daily versus monthly rifampicin (40/47 [85%] with daily rifampicin v 43/46 [91%]; RR 0.91, 95% CI 0.62 to 1.03). Adverse effects were more common with daily than with monthly rifampicin, causing discontinuation in 8.5% of people with daily rifampicin compared with 0% with monthly rifampicin.[27]

OPTION MULTIPLE DOSE VERSUS SINGLE DOSE TREATMENT FOR SINGLE SKIN LESIONS

One RCT found that multiple dose treatment with rifampicin monthly plus dapsone daily for 6 months achieved higher cure rates at 18 months than single dose treatment with rifampicin plus minocycline plus ofloxacin. Some improvement occurred in 99% of people in both groups. Adverse effects were similar with both regimens.

Benefits: We found no systematic review. We found one RCT (1483 people with single skin lesions typical of paucibacillary leprosy — see glossary, p 882; see comment below) comparing single dose treatment with rifampicin 600 mg plus ofloxacin 400 mg plus minocycline 100 mg versus multiple dose treatment with dapsone 100 mg /daily plus rifampicin 600 mg monthly for 6 months.[28] Outcomes measured at 18 months were based on a scoring system involving five measurements: disappearance of the lesion, reduction in hypopigmentation, reduction in the degree of infiltration, reduction in the size of the lesion, and improvement in sensation in the lesion. Treatment failure was defined as no change or an increase of the clinical score, and marked improvement was defined as a difference of 13 between the baseline and 18 month scores. The RCT found that multiple dose treatment significantly increased the proportion of people with marked improvement compared with single dose treatment (392/684 [57.3%] with multiple dose *v* 361/697 [51.8%] with single dose; P = 0.04), and with complete cure (374/684 [54.7%] *v* 327/697 [46.9%]; RR 1.17, 95% CI 1.05 to 1.28; NNT 13, 95% CI 8 to 40). There were 12 treatment failures (6 in each group), and 99.1% of people in both groups had some improvement by the end of the study.[28]

Harms: Allergic reactions (which were not specified) occurred in seven people (6 taking multiple dose *v* 1 taking single dose treatment), and gastrointestinal effects occurred in five people (2 taking multiple dose *v* 3 taking single dose treatment). There was no significant difference in the number of type 1 reactions (see glossary, p 882) (7/697 [1.0%] with single dose treatment *v* 3/684 [0.4%] with multiple dose; ARI +0.6%, 95% CI –0.2% to +3.4%).

Comment: The RCT did not specify its diagnostic criteria and did not confirm the clinical diagnosis. The follow up of only 18 months for people in the single dose group is short for detection of relapse. Some infections in this group would have resolved spontaneously, and the absence of a placebo control group means that the treatment effect cannot be estimated.[28] Single dose treatment has previously been assessed in people with paucibacillary leprosy. One RCT (622 people in Zaïre) compared two single dose regimens: rifampicin 40 mg/kg plus clofazimine 1200 mg versus rifampicin 40 mg/kg plus clofazimine 100 mg plus dapsone 100 mg plus ethionamide 500 mg. It found that the overall relapse rate was 20.4/1000 person years (see glossary, p 882), which was substantially higher than the relapse rate found for 6 months' treatment with dapsone plus rifampicin (see dapsone plus rifampicin, p 879), or rifampicin plus dapsone plus clofazimine (see rifampicin plus dapsone plus clofazimine, p 880). However, single dose treatment has operational advantages in the field, particularly when people live in remote areas and are unable to attend a clinic for several months.[29]

GLOSSARY

Bacteriological index A measure of the density of *M leprae* in the skin. Slit skin smears are made at several sites, the smears are stained and examined microscopically. The number of bacteria per high power field is scored on a logarithmic scale (0–6), and the index calculated by dividing the total score by the numbers of sites sampled.

Heaf grade 0 = 0–4 mm induration; 1 = 5–9; 2 = 10–14; 3 = 15–19; 4 = ≥20. A grade 3 or 4 test generally indicates infection with *M tuberculosis*, although the cut off point varies between countries.
ICRC vaccine A vaccine developed at the Indian Cancer Research Centre.
Multibacillary leprosy More than five skin lesions (WHO 1998, WHO expert committee on leprosy seventh report 874).
Neuritis Inflammation of a nerve presenting with any of the following: spontaneous nerve pain, paraesthesia, tenderness, sensory, motor, or autonomic impairment.
Paucibacillary leprosy Between two and five skin lesions.
Person years at risk The number of new cases of disease in a specified time period divided by the number of person years at risk during that period (average number at risk of relapse multiplied by the length of observation)
Single lesion leprosy One skin lesion.
Type 1 (reversal) reaction A delayed type hypersensitivity reaction occurring at sites of *M leprae* antigen. It presents with acutely inflamed skin lesions and acute neuritis (nerve tenderness with loss of function).
Type 2 reaction or Erythema Nodosum Leprosum (ENL) An immunological complication of multibacillary leprosy presenting with short lived and recurrent crops of tender erythematous subcutaneous nodules that may ulcerate. There may be signs of systemic involvement with fever, inflammation in lymph nodes, nerves, eyes, joints, testes, fingers, toes, or other organs.
World Health Organization disability grading These are simple gradings for use in the field, mainly for collection of general data regarding disabilities.[1] Grade 0 = no anaesthesia, no visible deformity or damage; Grade 1 = anaesthesia present, but no visible deformity or damage; Grade 2 = visible deformity or damage present.

REFERENCES

1. WHO Expert Committee on Leprosy. *World Health Organ Tech Rep Ser* 1988;768:1–51.
2. World Health Organization. Leprosy global situation. *Wkly Epidemiol Rec* 2002;77:1–8.
3. Fine PE. Leprosy: the epidemiology of a slow bacterium. *Epidemiol Rev* 1982;4:161–188.
4. Desikan KV, Sreevatsa. Extended studies on the viability of *Mycobacterium leprae* outside the human body. *Lepr Rev* 1995;66:287–295.
5. Lienhardt C, Kamate B, Jamet P, et al. Effect of HIV infection on leprosy: a three-year survey in Bamako, Mali. *Int J Lepr Other Mycobact Dis* 1996;64:383–391.
6. Croft RP, Richardus JH, Nicholls PG, et al. Nerve function impairment in leprosy: design, methodology, and intake status of a prospective cohort study of 2664 new leprosy cases in Bangladesh (The Bangladesh Acute Nerve Damage Study). *Lepr Rev* 1999;70:140–159.
7. Saunderson P, Gelore S, Desta K, et al. The pattern of leprosy-related neuropathy in the AMFES patients in Ethiopia: definitions, incidence, risk factors and outcome. *Lepr Rev* 2000;71:285–308.
8. Pfaltzgraff R, Ramu G. Clinical leprosy. In: Hastings R ed. *Leprosy*. Edinburgh: Churchill Livingstone, 1994:237–287.
9. van Brakel WH. Peripheral neuropathy in leprosy and its consequences. *Lepr Rev* 2000;71:S146–S153.
10. Gupte MD, Vallishayee RS, Anantharaman DS, et al. Comparative leprosy vaccine trial in south India. *Indian J Lepr* 1998;70:369–388.
11. Brown JA, Stone MM, Sutherland I. BCG vaccination of children against leprosy in Uganda: results at end of second follow-up. *BMJ* 1968;1:24–27.
12. Bagshawe A, Scott GC, Russell DA, et al. BCG vaccination in leprosy: final results of the trial in Karimui, Papua New Guinea, 1963–79. *Bull World Health Organ* 1989;67:389–399.
13. Lwin K, Sundaresan T, Gyi MM, et al. BCG vaccination of children against leprosy: fourteen-year findings of the trial in Burma. *Bull World Health Organ* 1985;63:1069–1078.
14. Karonga Prevention Trial Group. Randomised controlled trial of single BCG, repeated BCG, or combined BCG and killed *Mycobacterium leprae* vaccine for prevention of leprosy and tuberculosis in Malawi. *Lancet* 1996;348:17–24.
15. Kar PK, Arora PN, Ramasastry CV, et al. A clinicopathological study of multidrug therapy in borderline tuberculoid leprosy. *J Indian Med Assoc* 1994;92:336–337.
16. Boerrigter G, Ponnighaus JM, Fine PE. Preliminary appraisal of a WHO-recommended multiple drug regimen in paucibacillary leprosy patients in Malawi. *Int J Lepr Other Mycobact Dis* 1988;56:408–417.
17. Dasananjali K, Schreuder PA, Pirayavaraporn C. A study on the effectiveness and safety of the WHO/MDT regimen in the northeast of Thailand; a prospective study, 1984–1996. *Int J Lepr Other Mycobact Dis* 1997;65:28–36.
18. Gebre S, Saunderson P, Byass P. Relapses after fixed duration multiple drug therapy: the AMFES cohort. *Lepr Rev* 2000;71:325–331.
19. Boerrigter G, Ponnighaus JM, Fine PE, et al. Four-year follow-up results of a WHO-recommended multiple-drug regimen in paucibacillary leprosy patients in Malawi. *Int J Lepr Other Mycobact Dis* 1991;59:255–261.
20. Schreuder PA. The occurrence of reactions and impairments in leprosy: experience in the leprosy

control program of three provinces in northeastern Thailand, 1987–1995 [correction of 1978–1995]. I. Overview of the study. *Int J Lepr Other Mycobact Dis* 1998;66:149–158.
21. Chopra NK, Agarawal JS, Pandya PG. A study of relapse in paucibacillary leprosy in a multidrug therapy project, Baroda District, India. *Lepr Rev* 1990;61:157–162.
22. Li HY, Hu LF, Hauang WB, et al. Risk of relapse in leprosy after fixed duration multi-drug therapy. *Int J Lepr Other Mycobact Dis* 1997;65:238–245.
23. Ji B. Drug resistance in leprosy – a review. *Lepr Rev* 1985;56:265–278.
24. Girdhar BK, Girdhar A, Kumar A. Relapses in multibacillary leprosy patients: effect of length of therapy. *Lepr Rev* 2000;71:144–153.
25. Shaw IN, Natrajan MM, Rao GS, et al. Long-term follow up of multibacillary leprosy patients with high BI treated with WHO/MDT regimen for a fixed duration of two years. *Int J Lepr Other Mycobact Dis* 2000;68:405–409.
26. Chemotherapy of leprosy. Report of a WHO study group. WHO Technical Report Series, No 847, 1994
27. Yawalkar SJ, McDougall AC, Languillon J, et al. Once-monthly rifampicin plus daily dapsone in initial treatment of lepromatous leprosy. *Lancet* 1982;1:1199–1202.
28. Single-lesion Multicentre Trial Group. Efficacy of single-dose multidrug therapy for the treatment of single-lesion paucibacillary leprosy. *Indian J Leprosy* 1997;69:121en129.
29. Pattyn SR. A randomized clinical trial of two single-dose treatments for paucibacillary leprosy. *Lepr Rev* 1994;65:45–57.

Diana Lockwood
Consultant Leprologist
London School of Hygiene & Topical Medicine and The Hospital for Tropical Diseases
London
UK

Competing interests: None declared.

TABLE 1 **Dapsone plus rifampicin in paucibacillary leprosy: clinical outcomes** (see text, p 877).

Ref	Location	Cohort size	Follow up (years)	Skin lesions	Nerve impairment
16,19	Malawi	499	1[16] 4[19]	**At 1 year[16]** *Not evident:* 180/473 (38.0%)[16] *Visible but not active:* 282/473 (59.6%)[16] *Visible and active:* 11/473 (2.3%)[16]	**At 4 years[19]** *New disabilities:* 12/484 (2.5%)[16] *Worsening of existing disabilities:* 16/484 (3.3%)[16]
15	India	50	0.5	*Inactive:* 4/50 (8%) *Marked improvement:* 16/50 (32%) *Regression (active):* 22/50 (44%) *Increased activity:* 8/50 (16%)	No data
17	Thailand	130	8–10	*Clinically active after treatment:* 27/123 (22%)	*Grade 2 disability:* At enrolment, 4% At follow up, 7% (absolute numbers not provided)

Ref, reference.

TABLE 2 **Dapsone plus rifampicin in paucibacillary leprosy: relapse rates (see text, p 877).**

Ref	Location	Cohort size	Treatment	Follow up (years)	Relapse rate
20	Thailand	420	MDT	About 5	8/393 (2.0%) 4.1/1000 PYAR (estimated as timescale not definite)
19	Malawi	499	MDT	4	12/484 (2.5%) 6.5/1000 PYAR
21	India	11 095	MDT (723 people received a second course)	3	21/10 995 (0.19%) PYAR not calculable as relapse rate for people receiving two courses was not presented separately
22	China	878 (who had not previously received chemotherapy)	MDT	5	0.66/1000 PYAR
17	Thailand	124	MDT	Mean 8.2	2/112 [1.8%] 2.0/1000 PYAR
18	Ethiopia	246	MDT	Mean 4.1	0

MDT, multidrug treatment; PYAR, person-years at risk; Ref, reference.

TABLE 3 **Dapsone/rifampicin/clofazimine in multibacillary leprosy: clinical outcomes (see text, p 880).**

Reference	Location	Cohort size	Skin lesions	Nerve impairment
17	Thailand	53	Clinically active at about 3 years: 14/49 (29%)	Grade 2 disability: Start of treatment: 8% End of treatment: 13%

TABLE 4 **Dapsone/ rifampicin/clofazimine in multibacillary leprosy — relapse rates (see text, p 880).**

Ref	Location	Cohort size	Follow up (years)	Relapse rate
20	Thailand	220	3	2/198 (1.0%) 3.3/1000 PYAR
22	China	2318	10	0/1000 PYAR
17	Thailand	53 (12 with BI ≥ 5 at enrolment	8 (range 2–10)	0/1000 PYAR
18	Ethiopia	256 (57 people with BI > 4 at enrolment)	4.3 (range 0–8.6) 38% followed up for ≥ 5 years	0/1000 PYAR
24	India	260	Range 1–8	20/260 (7.6%) 20.4/1000 PYAR 18/20 (90%) with BI > 4 at enrolment
25	India	65	Range 1–8	1/46 (2.1%) 0.023/1000 PYAR

BI, bacterial index, PYAR, person years at risk; Ref, reference.

Lyme disease

Search date January 2003

Edward Hayes

QUESTIONS

INTERVENTIONS

Beneficial

Lyme disease vaccine in people exposed to North American strains of *Borrelia burgdorferi* 890

Prophylactic antibiotics after *Ixodes scapularis* tick bites in Lyme disease endemic areas in North America 891

Likely to be beneficial

*Cefotaxime (more effective than penicillin for late neurological Lyme disease) 894

*Cefotaxime (more effective than penicillin for Lyme arthritis) . .893

*Ceftriaxone (more effective than penicillin for Lyme arthritis) . .893

Doxycycline (as effective as amoxicillin plus probenecid for Lyme arthritis) 893

Penicillin (better than placebo for Lyme arthritis) 893

Unknown effectiveness

Ceftriaxone (in late neurological Lyme disease) 894

Lyme disease vaccine in Europe or Asia 890

Likely to be ineffective or harmful

Ceftriaxone plus doxycycline (in people with late neurological Lyme disease who had been previously treated) 894

*Based on subgroup analysis of RCTs

See glossary, p 895

Key Messages

Administration of Lyme disease vaccine

- **Lyme disease vaccine in people exposed to North American strains of *Borrelia burgdorferi*** One RCT has found that, compared with placebo, three doses of a vaccine (consisting of recombinant outer surface protein A [Osp–A] of *B burgdorferi* combined with adjuvant) reduces the incidence of Lyme disease in immunocompetent aged 15–70 years in Lyme disease endemic areas in North America.
- **Lyme disease vaccine in Europe or Asia** We found no RCTs about the effects of recombinant Osp–A vaccine in European or Asian populations. There is heterogeneity of the species that cause Lyme disease in Europe and Asia. The vaccine may not be as effective in European or Asian populations as it is in North American populations.

Prophylactic treatment of tick bite

- **Prophylactic antibiotics after *Ixodes scapularis* tick bites in Lyme disease endemic areas in North America** One systematic review in people with recognised *I scapularis* tick bites in the preceding 72 hours found that antibiotics reduced the risk of developing clinical Lyme disease compared with placebo, but the difference was not significant. One subsequent large RCT in people who had removed an attached *I scapularis* tick in the preceding 72 hours found that doxycycline reduced the proportion of people with erythema migrans at the site of the tick bite compared with placebo.

Treatment of Lyme arthritis

- **Cefotaxime (more effective than penicillin for Lyme arthritis)** One RCT found weak evidence from a small subgroup analysis of people with Lyme arthritis that cefotaxime increased the proportion of people with full recovery compared with penicillin.
- **Ceftriaxone (more effective than penicillin for Lyme arthritis)** One RCT found weak evidence from a small subgroup analysis of people with Lyme arthritis that ceftriaxone improved symptoms compared with penicillin.
- **Doxycycline (as effective as amoxicillin plus probenecid for Lyme arthritis)** One RCT in people with Lyme arthritis found no significant difference between doxycycline and amoxicillin plus probenecid in resolution of Lyme arthritis.
- **Penicillin (better than placebo for Lyme arthritis)** One RCT in people with Lyme arthritis has found that penicillin increases resolution of Lyme arthritis compared with placebo.

Treatment of late neurological Lyme disease

- **Cefotaxime (more effective than penicillin for late neurological Lyme disease)** One RCT found weak evidence from a small subgroup analysis of people with late Lyme disease that cefotaxime improved symptoms of neuropathy compared with penicillin.
- **Ceftriaxone (in late neurological Lyme disease)** One RCT found insufficient evidence from a small subgroup analysis in people with late neurological Lyme disease about effects of ceftriaxone and cefotaxime.
- **Ceftriaxone plus doxycycline (in people with late neurological Lyme disease who had been previously treated)** One RCT comparing ceftriaxone plus doxycycline versus placebo in people with previously treated Lyme disease and persistent neurological symptoms found no significant difference in health related quality of life at interim analysis at 180 days; therefore the RCT was terminated.

DEFINITION Lyme disease is an inflammatory illness resulting from infection with spirochetes of the *Borrelia burgdorferi* genospecies transmitted to humans by ticks. Some infected people have no symptoms. The characteristic manifestation of early Lyme disease is erythema migrans: a circular rash at the site of the infectious tick attachment that expands over a period of days to weeks in 80–90% of people with Lyme disease. Early disseminated infection may cause secondary erythema migrans, disease of the nervous system (facial palsy or other cranial neuropathies, meningitis, and radiculoneuritis), musculoskeletal disease (arthralgia), and, rarely, cardiac disease (myocarditis or transient atrioventricular block). Untreated or inadequately treated Lyme disease can cause late disseminated manifestations weeks to months after infection. These late manifestations include arthritis, polyneuropathy, and encephalopathy. Diagnosis of Lyme disease is based primarily on clinical findings and a high likelihood of exposure to infected ticks. Serological testing may be helpful in people with endemic exposure who have clinical findings consistent with later stage disseminated Lyme disease.

INCIDENCE/ PREVALENCE Lyme disease occurs in temperate regions of North America, Europe, and Asia. It is the most commonly reported vector borne disease in the USA, with over 16 000 cases reported a year.[1] Most cases occur in the north-eastern and north-central states, with a reported annual incidence in endemic states as high as 67.9/100 000 people.[1] In highly endemic communities, the incidence of Lyme disease may exceed 1000/100 000 people a year.[2] In some countries of Europe, the incidence of Lyme disease has been estimated to be over 100/100 000 people a year.[3] Foci of Lyme disease have been described in northern forested regions of Russia, in China, and in Japan.[4] Transmission cycles of *B burgdorferi* have not been described in tropical areas or in the southern hemisphere.[4]

AETIOLOGY/ RISK FACTORS Lyme disease is caused by infection with any of the *B burgdorferi* sensu lato genospecies. Virtually all cases of Lyme disease in North America are the result of infection with *B burgdorferi*. In Europe, Lyme disease may be caused by *B burgdorferi*, *B garinii*, or *B afzelii*. The infectious spirochetes are transmitted to humans through the bite of certain *Ixodes* ticks.[4] Humans who have frequent or prolonged exposure to the habitats of infected *Ixodes* ticks are at highest risk of acquiring Lyme disease. Individual risk depends on the likelihood of being bitten by infected tick vectors, which varies with the density of vector ticks in the environment, the prevalence of infection in ticks, and the extent of a person's contact with infected ticks. The risk of Lyme disease is often concentrated in focal areas. In the USA, risk is highest in certain counties within north-eastern and north-central states during the months of April to July.[2] People become infected when they engage in activities in wooded or bushy areas that are favourable habitats for ticks, and deer and rodent hosts.

PROGNOSIS Lyme disease is rarely fatal. Untreated Lyme arthritis resolves at a rate of 10–20% a year; over 90% of facial palsies due to Lyme disease resolve spontaneously, and most cases of Lyme carditis resolve without sequelae.[5] However, untreated Lyme disease can result in arthritis (50% of untreated people), meningitis or neuropathies (15% of untreated people), carditis (5–10% of untreated people with erythema migrans), and, rarely, encephalopathy.

AIMS OF INTERVENTION To prevent Lyme disease; to ameliorate or eliminate the symptoms of established Lyme disease; to reduce sequelae, with minimal adverse effects.

OUTCOMES **For prophylaxis:** incidence of Lyme disease, adverse events. **For treatment:** incidence, prevalence, or severity of symptoms and signs of short term manifestations; long term sequelae of infection; quality of life.

METHODS *Clinical Evidence* search and appraisal January 2003. Additional searches of author's files.

QUESTION **What are the effects of measures to prevent Lyme disease?**

OPTION **LYME DISEASE VACCINE**

One RCT has found that, compared with placebo, a vaccine (consisting of recombinant outer surface lipoprotein A of *B burgdorferi* combined with adjuvant) reduces the incidence of Lyme disease in immunocompetent adults aged 15–70 years in North America who are at high risk of Lyme disease. We found no RCTs about the effects of recombinant outer surface protein A vaccine in European or Asian populations. There is heterogeneity of the species that cause Lyme disease in Europe and Asia. The vaccine may not be as effective in European or Asian populations as it is in North American.

Benefits: We found no systematic review but found one RCT (10 936 people, aged 15–70 years, living in Lyme disease endemic areas in the USA) that compared a vaccine made of recombinant outer surface lipoprotein A (Osp–A) plus adjuvant (see glossary, p 895) versus placebo.[6] People in the RCT were self selected and were at high risk of Lyme disease. The RCT found that, compared with placebo, the vaccine significantly reduced laboratory confirmed Lyme disease after two doses in the first year (AR of developing Lyme disease 22/5469 [0.4%] with vaccine *v* 43/5467 [0.8%] with placebo; RR 0.51, 95% CI 0.31 to 0.85; NNT 260, 95% CI 146 to 1046). After a third dose 1 year later, it found a greater reduction of the incidence of laboratory confirmed Lyme disease (16/5469 [0.3%] with vaccine *v* 66/5467 [1.2%] with placebo; RR 0.24, 95% CI 0.14 to 0.42; NNT 110, 95% CI 80 to 167); asymptomatic infection was prevented completely (0/5469 [0%] with vaccine *v* 15/5467 [0.3%] with placebo; NNT 365, 95% CI 222 to 687).[6]

Harms: We found nine RCTs evaluating adverse effects of Osp–A vaccines.[6–14] No serious adverse events were found to be causally related to the vaccine in any of these trials. The results are summarised in table 1, p 897.

Comment: The rOsp–A vaccine is no longer commercially available. **Applicability of the evidence:** The absolute benefit of vaccination in the RCT was high (1 case of Lyme disease prevented for every 110 people vaccinated), which was partly because the people recruited into the RCT were self selected and had a very high incidence of Lyme disease in the untreated group.[6] If the risk of Lyme disease in the unvaccinated population was 100/100 000 people a year (comparable to the reported Lyme disease incidence in many endemic areas),[1,3] then about 1316 people would need to be vaccinated to prevent one case of Lyme disease. We found no evidence about the effects of this vaccine in Europe or Asia where a greater variety of *B burgdorferi* genospecies cause Lyme disease, and no clinical evidence of efficacy in children. The vaccine may not be as effective in European or Asian populations as it is in North

American. **Other RCTs:** One RCT evaluated the efficacy of recombinant Osp–A vaccine without adjuvant.[7] It found that the vaccine reduced the incidence of Lyme disease by 68% (95% CI 36% to 85%) after two doses in the first year. However, the criteria for confirming the diagnosis of Lyme disease were not defined clearly. Of 1734 suspected cases of Lyme disease in 2 years, only 499 were reviewed "in depth" by the Data and Safety Monitoring Board. The RCT reported an estimate of vaccine efficacy after a third dose of vaccine, but this dose was not part of the original RCT protocol, was given only to a subset of participants, and the criteria for selection of the subset who received the third dose were not specified. This RCT found that the efficacy of vaccine was highest in people aged less than 60 years, but results for this subgroup were not provided.[7]

OPTION PROPHYLACTIC TREATMENT OF TICK BITE

One systematic review in people with recognised *I scapularis* tick bites in the preceding 72 hours found that antibiotics reduced the risk of developing clinical Lyme disease compared with placebo, but the difference was not significant. One subsequent large RCT in people who had removed an attached *I scapularis* tick in the preceding 72 hours found that doxycycline reduced the proportion of people with erythema migrans at the site of the tick bite compared with placebo.

Benefits: We found one systematic review[15] and one subsequent RCT[16] comparing prophylactic antibiotics versus placebo for the treatment of tick bite (see table 2, p 899). The review (search date 1995, 3 RCTs,[17–19] 639 adults and children with recognised *I scapularis* tick bites in the preceding 72 hours; see comment below) found that prophylactic treatment with antibiotics (penicillin, amoxicillin [amoxycillin], and tetracycline were studied in the individual trials) reduced the risk of developing clinical Lyme disease (erythema migrans) compared with placebo, but the difference was not significant (0/308 [0%] with antibiotics *v* 4/292 [1.4%] with placebo; ARR 1.4%, 95% CI 0% to 3%; OR 0.0, 95% CI 0.0 to 1.5; P = 0.12).[15] The subsequent large RCT (482 people ≥ 12 years old who had removed an attached *I scapularis* tick in the preceding 72 hours; see comment below) compared doxycycline (200 mg as a single dose) versus placebo with 6 weeks' follow up.[16] It found that doxycycline significantly reduced the proportion of people with erythema migrans at the site of the tick bite compared with placebo (1/235 [0.4%] with doxycycline *v* 8/247 [3.2%] with placebo; ARR 2.8%, 95% CI 0.4% to 5.2%; NNT 36, 95% CI 20 to 250), and the proportion of people with any evidence of Lyme disease (erythema migrans at the site of the tick bite, or at other sites, or a viral-like illness with laboratory evidence of Lyme disease, 3/235 [1.3%] with doxycycline *v* 11/247 [4.5%] with placebo; ARR 3.2%, 95% CI 0.2% to 6.2%; NNT 31, 95% CI 16 to 500). Of 431 people who had serum samples tested at study entry and 3 and 6 weeks later, none had asymptomatic seroconversion for antibody to *B burgdorferi*. Erythema migrans at the site of the tick bite only occurred after the removed tick was in the nymph stage, was partially engorged, and was estimated to be attached for more than 72 hours. A subgroup analysis found that in people who removed partially engorged nymphal ticks, doxycycline significantly reduced erythema migrans at the site of the tick bite compared with placebo (AR 1/78 [1.3%] with doxycycline *v* 8/81 [9.9%] with placebo; ARR 8.6%, 95% CI 1.4% to 15.8%; NNT 12, 95% CI 7 to 71).[16]

Harms: One RCT in the review reported a rash with penicillin (AR 1/27 [4%] with penicillin *v* 0/29 [0%] with placebo), and another RCT reported a rash with amoxicillin (AR 2/205 [1%] with amoxicillin *v* 0/182 [0%] with placebo) (see table 2, p 899). The third RCT in the review reported no adverse effects among persons who had been treated with antibiotics. The RCT conducted after the review found that of the 309 people who recorded data on adverse events, significantly more people taking doxycycline had nausea or vomiting compared with placebo (33/156 [21.0%] with doxycycline *v* 6/153 [3.9%] with placebo; ARI 17.2%, 95% CI 9.8% to 24.6%; NNH 6, 95% CI 4 to 10).[16] It also reported abdominal discomfort (11/156 [7.1%] with doxycycline *v* 6/153 [3.9%] with placebo; P = 0.34), diarrhoea (6/156 [3.8%] with doxycycline *v* 6/153 [3.9%] with placebo; P = 0.79), and dizziness (4/156 [2.6%] with doxycycline *v* 1/153 [0.7%] with placebo; P = 0.37).[16]

Comment: The three RCTs included in the systematic review and the subsequent RCT were all conducted in Lyme disease endemic areas in North America.[15,16] There is a possibility that people treated with antibiotics for tick bite may not develop erythema migrans but could progress to late stages of Lyme disease. However, none of the people who were treated with antibiotics in the RCTs had asymptomatic infection with *B burgdorferi*, or developed late manifestations of Lyme disease during follow up (ranging from 6 weeks to up to 3 years). The most recent and largest RCT found that for a baseline risk of 1% for contracting Lyme disease in the control group, the number needed to treat for a single dose of doxycycline (200 mg) to prevent Lyme disease was 31.[16] The same RCT found that the number needed to harm for nausea or vomiting from this treatment was six; therefore, about five people would develop nausea or vomiting for every person in whom Lyme disease was prevented. People in the RCT with adult and/or non-engorged ticks did not develop Lyme disease, although Lyme disease can occur after the bite of an engorged adult tick. If treatment was limited to people with engorged nymphal ticks (NNT 12), then two people would develop nausea and less than one person would develop vomiting for every person in whom Lyme disease was prevented.

QUESTION What are the effects of antibiotic treatment for Lyme disease arthritis?

One RCT in people with Lyme arthritis has found that penicillin increases resolution of Lyme arthritis compared with placebo. Another RCT in people with Lyme arthritis found no significant difference between doxycycline and amoxicillin plus probenecid in resolution of Lyme arthritis. One RCT found weak evidence from a small subgroup analysis of people with Lyme arthritis that ceftriaxone improved symptoms compared with penicillin. One RCT found weak evidence from a small subgroup analysis of people with Lyme arthritis that cefotaxime increased the

proportion of people with full recovery compared with penicillin. Some people have developed symptoms of neuroborreliosis after oral antibiotic treatment of Lyme arthritis with concurrent neuroborreliosis.

Benefits: We found no systematic review. **People with Lyme arthritis:** We found two RCTs that selected people with Lyme disease arthritis and randomised them to different treatments.[20,21] The first RCT (40 people with Lyme disease arthritis) compared intramuscular benzathine penicillin versus saline placebo.[20] It found that penicillin significantly increased the proportion of people having complete resolution of the arthritis compared with placebo (AR 7/20 [35%] with penicillin *v* 0/20 [0%] with placebo; $P < 0.02$).[20] The second RCT (48 people with Lyme arthritis) compared oral doxycycline (100 mg twice daily for 30 days) versus oral amoxicillin (500 mg) plus probenecid (4 times daily for 30 days).[21] After 3 months, an intention to treat analysis found no significant difference in rates of arthritis resolution in both groups (AR 18/25 [72%] with doxycycline *v* 16/23 [70%] with amoxicillin plus probenecid; RR 1.04, 95% CI 0.72 to 1.49). In the doxycycline group, one person had recurrence of arthritis and another developed polyneuropathy after treatment. In the amoxicillin plus probenecid group, one person had recurrent arthritis, two developed polyneuropathy, and two developed encephalopathy. **Subgroup analyses of people with Lyme arthritis:** We found three other RCTs that recruited people with a variety of forms of late Lyme disease (including Lyme arthritis).[22–24] The first RCT (23 people with late Lyme disease, 70% with arthritis) compared ceftriaxone (2 g iv every 12 hours for 14 days) versus penicillin (4 MU iv every 4 hours for 10 days).[22] Ceftriaxone seemed to be more effective than penicillin, but the differences in rates of clinical improvement after 3 months were not significant (AR of improvement 12/13 [92%] with ceftriaxone *v* 5/10 [50%] with penicillin; RR 1.85, 95% CI 0.97 to 3.50). More of the subgroup of people with arthritis improved with ceftriaxone (AR 9/9 [100%] with ceftriaxone *v* 2/7 [29%] with penicillin; NNT 2, 95% CI 1 to 4). The second RCT (135 people with late Lyme disease, 73 with arthritis) compared cefotaxime (6 g/day for 8–10 days) versus penicillin G (20 MU/day for 8–19 days).[23] Two years after treatment, full recovery was significantly more frequent with cefotaxime compared with penicillin (AR 44/69 [64%] with cefotaxime *v* 25/66 [38%] with penicillin; RR 1.68, 95% CI 1.18 to 2.41; NNT 3, 95% CI 2 to 11). In the subgroup of people with arthritis, full recovery was also significantly increased by cefotaxime compared with penicillin (17/39 [44%] with cefotaxime *v* 4/34 [12%] with penicillin; RR 3.7, 95% CI 1.4 to 9.9; NNT 4, 95% CI 2 to 10). The third RCT (62 people with disseminated Lyme disease, 13 people with Lyme arthritis) did not report separate results for the subgroup with arthritis. It compared intravenous ceftriaxone followed by oral amoxicillin plus probenecid versus oral cefixime plus probenecid.[24]

Harms: Some people have developed symptoms of neuroborreliosis (see glossary, p 895) after oral antibiotic treatment of arthritis.[21] Jarisch-Herxheimer reactions (see glossary, p 895) have been described in people treated for late Lyme disease. One RCT reported symptoms suggestive of a mild Jarisch-Herxheimer reaction in 12/44 (27%) of people treated with ceftriaxone and 1/10 (10%) of people with penicillin,[22] and one RCT reported "Herxheimer-like" reactions in 20% of people treated with penicillin and 40.5% of people treated with cefotaxime.[23] Possible "Herxheimer-like" reactions, including fever, transient rash, and worsening of symptoms or cardiac arrhythmia, were reported in an unspecified number of people treated with cefixime and probenecid, and with ceftriaxone followed by amoxicillin.[24] No significant differences were found in the risk of developing a prolonged form of such reactions for people receiving ceftriaxone plus amoxicillin versus cefixime plus probenecid (18/30 [60%] with ceftriaxone plus amoxicillin treatment *v* 12/30 [40%] with cefixime plus probenecid; RR 1.50, 95% CI 0.88 to 2.54).[24] Other harms include those expected from the antibiotics. In RCTs including people with Lyme arthritis, the following adverse effects were reported: diarrhoea and skin rash with ceftriaxone;[22] shock and colitis with penicillin; anaphylaxis and colitis with cefotaxime;[23] rash and gastrointestinal effects with amoxicillin and probenecid;[21] diarrhoea and rash with cefixime; and nausea, diarrhoea, and rash with ceftriaxone followed by amoxicillin.[24]

Comment: Results of the RCTs that presented results for subgroups of people with Lyme arthritis should be interpreted with caution as people with arthritis were not randomly assigned to treatment groups. The RCTs were small, and the type, dose, and regimen of antibiotics used varied between trials. The enrolment criteria also varied between trials. Only one RCT had a placebo control.[20] The proportion of people who respond in comparative RCTs is difficult to interpret because, without a placebo comparison, it is unclear how many people would have improved without treatment.

QUESTION What are the effects of antibiotic treatments for late neurological Lyme disease?

One RCT comparing ceftriaxone plus doxycycline versus placebo in people with previously treated Lyme disease and persistent late neurological symptoms found no significant difference in health related quality of life at interim analysis at 180 days; therefore, the RCT was terminated. One RCT found weak evidence from a small subgroup analysis of people with late Lyme disease that cefotaxime improved symptoms of neuropathy compared with penicillin. One RCT found weak evidence from a small subgroup analysis in people with late neurological Lyme disease that there was no significant difference between ceftriaxone and cefotaxime in the proportion of people who were asymptomatic.

Benefits: We found no systematic review. **People with late neurological Lyme disease:** We found one RCT (129 people, 78 people seropositive for *B burgdorferi*, 51 people who were seronegative) comparing antibiotics (iv ceftriaxone 2 g/day for 30 days followed by oral doxycycline 100 mg twice daily for 60 days) versus placebo.[25] All participants had been previously treated for Lyme disease but had persistent symptoms including arthralgia, myalgia, neurocognitive changes, altered sensation, malaise, headache, and sleep disturbance. At 180 days, a planned interim analysis of 107 people found that the probability of finding a significant difference in health related quality of life (measured on the medical outcomes survey short form general health survey; SF-36) after full study enrolment was less than 5%, and the study was therefore terminated.[25] **Subgroup analyses in people with late neurological Lyme disease:** We found two comparative RCTs that reported results for people with late neurological Lyme disease.[23,26] The first RCT (135 people with late Lyme disease, 93 with neuropathy) compared cefotaxime (6 g/day for 8–10 days) versus penicillin G (20 MU/day for 8–19 days).[23] Two years after treatment, cefotaxime significantly increased complete recovery compared with penicillin (44/69 [64%] with cefotaxime *v* 25/66 [38%] with penicillin; RR 1.68, 95% CI 1.18 to 2.41). Similar results were reported for the subgroup with neuropathy (35/49 [71%] with cefotaxime *v* 20/44 [46%] with penicillin; RR 1.57, 95% CI 1.09 to 2.27). The second RCT (33 people with Lyme neuroborreliosis [see glossary, p 895] of varying duration) compared ceftriaxone (2 g iv/day for 10 days) versus cefotaxime (2 g iv every 8 hours for 10 days).[26] Some of the people treated with ceftriaxone were asymptomatic before treatment, and so were excluded from analysis (3/17). Of the remaining people, most (17/30) had disease duration of over 30 days at study entry, and some (8/30) had a duration over 60 days. The RCT found no significant difference between ceftriaxone and cefotaxime in the proportion of people who were asymptomatic after 8 months (8/14 [57%] with ceftriaxone *v* 9/16 [56%] with cefotaxime; RR 1.02, 95% CI 0.54 to 1.90).

Harms: See harms under treatments for Lyme disease arthritis, p 893. The RCT in people with previously treated Lyme disease found no significant difference in the overall rate of adverse events between the antibiotic and placebo groups. In the other clinical trials involving people with late neurological Lyme disease reported above, the following adverse effects were reported: shock and colitis with penicillin, and anaphylaxis and colitis with cefotaxime;[22] rash with cefotaxime, and fever, diarrhoea, and elevated liver enzymes with ceftriaxone.[26] One case control study found an association between biliary disease and ceftriaxone treatment of suspected late Lyme disease.[27]

Comment: The RCTs of previously untreated people either recruited people with late Lyme disease, some of whom had neurological manifestations, or people with Lyme neuroborreliosis, some of whom had late disease. Results presented for these subsets of study participants may be subject to undetected biases, because people with late neurological disease were not randomly assigned to treatment groups. None of these RCTs had a placebo treated control group. The antibiotics used in RCTs, as well as doses and schedules, varied between trials. The enrolment criteria also varied between trials.

GLOSSARY

Adjuvant A substance such as aluminium hydroxide included in a vaccine to enhance its effectiveness.

Jarisch-Herxheimer reaction An inflammatory reaction in tissues induced by antibiotic treatment of spirochetal diseases, and believed to be caused by an immunological reaction to the release of spirochetal antigens.

Neuroborreliosis Central or peripheral neuropathy resulting from infection with *Borrelia* sp spirochetes.

REFERENCES

1. Orloski KA, Hayes EB, Campbell GL, et al. Surveillance for Lyme disease — United States, 1992–1998. *MMWR Morb Mortal Wkly Rep* 2000;49(SS-3):1–11.
2. Centers for Disease Control. Recommendations for the use of Lyme disease vaccine: recommendations of the Advisory Committee on Immunization Practices (ACIP). *MMWR Morb Mortal Wkly Rep* 1999;48(RR-7):1–17, 21–25.
3. O'Connel S, Granstorm M, Gray JS, et al. Epidemiology of European Lyme borreliosis. *Zentralbl Bakteriol* 1998;287:229–240.
4. Dennis DT. Epidemiology, ecology, and prevention of Lyme disease. In: Rahn DW, Evans J, eds. *Lyme disease*. Philadelphia: American College of Physicians, 1998:7–34.
5. Rahn DW, Evans J, eds. *Lyme disease*. Philadelphia: American College of Physicians, 1998.
6. Steere AC, Sikand VJ, Meurice F, et al. Vaccination against Lyme disease with recombinant *Borrelia burgdorferi* outer-surface lipoprotein A with adjuvant. *N Engl J Med* 1998;339:209–215.
7. Sigal LH, Zahradnik JM, Lavin P, et al. A vaccine consisting of recombinant *Borrelia burgdorferi* outer-surface protein A to prevent Lyme disease. *N Engl J Med* 1998;339:216–222.
8. Feder HM, Beran J, Van Hoecke C, et al. Immunogenicity of a recombinant *Borrelia burgdorferi* outer surface protein A vaccine against Lyme disease in children. *J Pediatr* 1999;135:575–579.
9. Keller D, Koster FT, Marks DH, et al. Safety and immunogenicity of a recombinant outer surface protein A Lyme vaccine. *JAMA* 1994;271:1764–1768.
10. Van Hoecke C, Comberbach M, De Grave D, et al. Evaluation of the safety, reactogenicity and immunogenicity of three recombinant outer surface protein (OspA) Lyme vaccines in healthy adults. *Vaccine* 1996;14:1620–1626.
11. Beran J, De Clercq N, Dieussaert I, et al. Reactogenicity and immunogenicity of a Lyme disease vaccine in children 2–5 years old. *Clin Infec Dis* 2000;31:1504–1507.
12. Sikand VJ, Halsey N, Krause PJ, et al. Safety and immunogenicity of a recombinant *Borrelia burgdorferi* outer surface protein A vaccine against Lyme disease in health children and adolescents: a randomized controlled trial. *Pediatrics* 2001;108:123–128.
13. Van Hoecke C, Lebacq E, Beran J, et al. Alternative vaccination schedules (0, 1, and 6 months versus 0, 1, and 12 months) for a recombinant OspA Lyme disease vaccine. *Clin Infect Dis* 1999;28:1260–1264.
14. Schoen RT, Sikand VK, Caldwell MC, et al. Safety and immunogenicity profile of a recombinant outer-surface protein A Lyme disease vaccine: clinical trial of a 3-dose schedule at 0, 1, and 2 months. *Clin Ther* 22:315–325.
15. Warshafsky S, Nowakowski J, Nadelman RB, et al. Efficacy of antibiotic prophylaxis for prevention of Lyme disease. *J Gen Intern Med* 1996;11:329–333. Search date 1995; primary sources Medline and hand searches of reference lists for English language papers.
16. Nadelman RB, Nowakowski J, Fish D, et al. Prophylaxis with single-dose doxycycline for the prevention of Lyme disease after an *Ixodes scapularis* tick bite. *N Engl J Med* 2001;345:79–84.
17. Costello CM, Steere AC, Pinkerton RE, et al. A prospective study of tick bites in an endemic area for Lyme disease. *J Infect Dis* 1989;159:136–139.
18. Shapiro ED, Gerber MA, Holabird NB, et al. A controlled trial of antimicrobial prophylaxis for Lyme disease after deer-tick bites. *N Engl J Med* 1992;327:1769–1773.
19. Agre F, Schwartz R. The value of early treatment of deer tick bites for the prevention of Lyme disease. *Am J Dis Children* 1993;147:945–947.
20. Steere AC, Green J, Schoen RT, et al. Successful parenteral penicillin therapy of established Lyme arthritis. *N Engl J Med* 1985;312:869–874.
21. Steere AC, Levin RE, Molloy PJ, et al. Treatment of Lyme arthritis. *Arthritis Rheum* 1994;37:878–888.
22. Dattwyler RJ, Halperin JJ, Volkman DJ, et al. Treatment of late Lyme borreliosis — randomized comparison of ceftriaxone and penicillin. *Lancet* 1998;1:1191–1194.
23. Hassler D, Zoller M, Haude H-D, et al. Cefotaxime versus penicillin in the late stage of Lyme disease — prospective, randomized therapeutic study. *Infection* 1990;18:16–20.
24. Oksi J, Nikoskelainen J, Vijanen MK. Comparison of oral cefixime and intravenous ceftriaxone followed by oral amoxicillin in disseminated Lyme borreliosis. *Eur J Clin Microbiol Infect Dis* 1998;17:715–719.
25. Klempner MS, Hu LT, Evans J, et al. Two controlled trials of antibiotic treatment in patients with persistent symptoms and a history of Lyme disease. *N Engl J Med* 2001;345:85–92.
26. Pfister H-W, Preac-Mursic V, Wilske B, et al. Randomized comparison of ceftriaxone and cefotaxime in Lyme neuroborreliosis. *J Infect Dis* 1991;163:311–318.
27. Ettestad PJ, Campbell GL, Welbel SF, et al. Biliary complications in the treatment of unsubstantiated Lyme disease. *J Infect Dis* 1995;171:356–361.

Edward Hayes
Medical Epidemiologist
US Centers for Disease Control and Prevention
Fort Collins, Colorado
USA

Competing interests: None declared.

TABLE 1 **Adverse effects related to Lyme disease vaccine; results of RCTs (see text, p 890).[6–14]**

Ref	Study population	Regimen	Local effects	Systemic effects
Versus placebo comparisons				
6	10 936 people (15–70 years), 9998 evaluated for adverse effects	Osp–A 30 μg *v* placebo at 0, 1, and 12 months	Pain, redness, swelling: vaccine *v* placebo; all $P < 0.001$	**< 30 days** Myalgias, achiness, influenza-like illness, fever, chills (all $P < 0.001$) **> 30 days** Similar in both groups
12	4087 people (4–18 years)	Osp–A 30 μg *v* placebo at 0, 1, and 12 months	Pain, redness, swelling: vaccine *v* placebo; 78% *v* 55%; $P < 0.001$	Fever, fatigue, headache, rash, arthralgia: vaccine *v* placebo; 30% *v* 22%; $P < 0.001$
7	10 305 people (≥ 18 years)	Osp–A 30 μg *v* placebo at 0 and 1 month (7515 people had booster at 12 months)	Pain at injection site: vaccine *v* placebo *1st dose:* 0.3% *v* 0.04% *2nd dose:* 0.8% *v* 0.1% *3rd dose:* 1.5% *v* 0.2%	Musculoskeletal: vaccine *v* placebo *1st dose:* 6.4% *v* 1.3% *2nd dose:* 3.3% *v* 1.1% *3rd dose:* not stated
9	36 people (18–65 years)	Adjuvanted Osp–A 10 μg *v* unadjuvanted Osp–A 10 μg *v* placebo	Pain, tenderness, or both were more common with vaccine *v* placebo; small sample size	Small sample size
Dose versus dose comparisons				
11	91 children (2–5 years old)	Osp–A 15 μg *v* Osp–A 30 μg, both given at 0 and 1 month	Pain, redness, swelling: Osp–A 15 μg *v* Osp–A 30 μg; 77.2% *v* 77.8%; $P > 0.05$	Arthralgia, drowsiness, fever, irritability, rash: Osp–A 15 μg *v* Osp–A 30 μg; 47.8% *v* 38.9%; $P > 0.05$
8	250 children (5–15 years)	Osp–A 15 μg *v* Osp–A 30 μg, both with adjuvant and given at 0, 1, and 2 months	Redness, swelling, soreness: no significant difference between doses	Only significant difference was headache: Osp–A 15 μg *v* Osp–A 30 μg, 15% *v* 9%; $P < 0.008$

TABLE 1 continued

10	240 people (18–50 years)	Three formulations of the Osp–A vaccine	One or more of the symptoms of pain, redness, swelling, and induration occurred in up to 48.8% of people after any single dose	One or more of the symptoms of fever, headache, malaise, rash, arthralgia, were reported by ≤ 10.1% of people after any single dose
Different dosing schedules				
13	800 adults (15–50 years)	Osp–A vaccine given at 0, 1, and 6 months *v* at 0, 1, and 12 months	At least one local symptom occurred in 75% of people in each group	At least one systemic symptom occurred in 19% in both groups
14	956 adults (17–72 years)	Osp–A vaccine 30 μg given at 0, 1, and 12 months *v* at 0, 1, 2, and 12 months	Soreness was most common: in both groups 82.5% with 3 doses *v* 81.7% with 4 doses; NS	Fatigue was the most common symptom: 21.8% *v* 19.7%; NS. Arthralgia: 12.5% with 3 doses *v* 9.6% with 4 doses; P = 0.007

NS, not significant; ref, reference.

TABLE 2 Prophylactic treatment of tick bite with antibiotics; results of placebo controlled RCTs (see text, p 891).[16–19]

Ref	Population (all noticed tick bites < 72 hours prior to study enrolment)	Intervention	Number of people with any evidence of Lyme disease (antibiotic *v* placebo)	Adverse effects (antibiotic *v* placebo)
16	482 people aged ≥ 12 years	Doxycycline (200 mg single dose) versus placebo	3/235 (1%) *v* 11/247 (4%); ARR 3.2%, 95% CI 0.2% to 6.2%	Nausea: 24/156 (15.4%) *v* 4/153 (2.6%); ARI 12.8%, 95% CI 6.4% to 19.2%; NNH 8, 95% CI 6 to 16 Vomiting: 9/156 (5.8%) *v* 2/153 (1.3%); ARI 4.5%, 95% CI 0.3% to 8.6%; NNH 23, 95% CI 12 to 303)
17	68 people aged ≥ 5 years	Penicillin (250 mg qds for 10 days) versus placebo	0/32 (0%) *v* 1/36 (3%); ARR 2.8%, 95% CI –3.0% to +8.5%	Rash: 1/27 (4%) *v* 0/29 (0%)
18	372 people of any age	Amoxicillin (250 mg tds for 10 days) versus placebo	0/205 (0%) *v* 2/182 (1%); ARR 1.1%, 95% CI –0.3% to +2.5%	Rash possibly due to amoxicillin: 2/205 (1%) *v* 0/182 (0%)
19	184 people aged 3–19 years	Penicillin (250 mg qds for 10 days in people < 9 years) or tetracycline (250 mg qds for 10 days in people > 9 years) versus placebo	0/89 (0%) *v* 4/90 (4%); ARR 4.4%, 95% CI 0.1% to 8.8%	Hives reported in one person who received placebo

qds, four times daily; ref, reference; tds, three times daily.

Malaria in endemic areas

Search date October 2002

Aika Omari and Paul Garner

QUESTIONS

INTERVENTIONS

See glossary, p 909

Key Messages

Medical treatments for falciparum malaria

- **Artemether (*v* quinine)** Two systematic reviews and one subsequent RCT found no significant difference between artemether versus quinine for preventing death in people with severe malaria.
- **Chloroquine versus quinine** Two RCTs in children found no significant difference in mortality with chloroquine versus quinine. However, these RCTs were conducted in the Gambia between 1988 and 1994, when chloroquine resistance was uncommon.
- **Desferrioxamine mesylate** One systematic review found weak evidence that desferrioxamine mesylate versus placebo reduced the risk of persistent seizures in children with cerebral malaria. However, we were unable to draw reliable conclusions.
- **Dexamethasone** One systematic review has found no significant difference in mortality with dexamethasone versus placebo, but gastrointestinal bleeding and seizures were more common with dexamethasone.
- **Exchange blood transfusion** One systematic review has found no suitable RCTs.
- **High first dose quinine** One systematic review and one additional RCT found no significant difference in mortality between quinine regimens with high initial quinine dose versus no loading dose. The systematic review found that high first dose of quinine reduced parasite and fever clearance times compared with no loading dose.

- **Initial blood transfusion** One systematic review found no significant difference in deaths in clinically stable children who received an initial blood transfusion for malaria anaemia and found more adverse events.
- **Intramuscular versus intravenous quinine** One RCT in children found no significant difference with intramuscular versus intravenous quinine in recovery times or deaths in Kenya in 1990.
- **Quinine** We found no RCTs comparing quinine versus placebo or no treatment, but there is consensus that treatment is likely to be beneficial.
- **Rectal artemisinin (as effective as quinine)** One systematic review found no significant difference in mortality with rectal artemisinin versus quinine.
- **Sulfadoxine–pyrimethamine versus quinine** One RCT found that sulfadoxine–pyrimethamine versus quinine cleared parasites faster in children with complicated non-cerebral malaria in 1992–1994 in the Gambia, but found no significant difference in mortality.

DEFINITION Severe malaria is caused by the protozoan infection of red blood cells with *Plasmodium falciparum*. Clinically complicated malaria presents with life threatening conditions, which include coma, severe anaemia, renal failure, respiratory distress syndrome, hypoglycaemia, shock, spontaneous haemorrhage, and convulsions. The diagnosis of cerebral malaria should be considered where there is encephalopathy in the presence of malaria parasites. A strict definition of cerebral malaria requires the presence of unrousable coma, and no other cause of encephalopathy (e.g. hypoglycaemia, sedative drugs) in the presence of *P falciparum* infection.[1] This review does not currently include the treatment of malaria in pregnancy.

INCIDENCE/ PREVALENCE Malaria is a major health problem in the tropics with 300–500 million clinical cases occurring annually, and an estimated 1.1–2.7 million deaths each year as a result of severe malaria.[2] Over 90% of deaths occur in children below 5 years of age, mainly from cerebral malaria and anaemia.[2] In areas where malaria transmission is stable (endemic), those most at risk of acquiring severe malaria are children under 5 years old, because adults and older children have partial immunity that offers some protection. In areas where malaria transmission is unstable (non-endemic), severe malaria affects both adults and children. Non-immune travellers and migrants are also at risk from developing severe malaria.

AETIOLOGY/ RISK FACTORS Malaria is transmitted by the bite of infected female anopheline mosquitoes. Certain genes are associated with resistance to severe malaria. Human leukocyte antigens (HLA), namely HLA-Bw53 and HLA-DRB1*1302, protect against severe malaria. However, the associations of HLA antigens with severe malaria are limited to specific populations.[3,4] Haemoglobin S[3] and haemoglobin C[5] are also protective against severe malaria. Genes, such as the tumour necrosis factor gene have also been associated with an increased susceptibility to severe malaria (see aetiology under malaria: prevention in travellers, p 911).[6]

PROGNOSIS In children under 5 years of age with cerebral malaria, the estimated case fatality of treated malaria is 19%, although reported hospital case fatality may be as high as 10–40%.[1,7] Neurological sequelae persisting for more than 6 months occur in more than 2% of the survivors, and include ataxia, hemiplegia, speech disorders, behavioural disorders, epilepsy, and blindness. Severe malarial anaemia has a case fatality rate higher than 13%.[7] In adults, the mortality of cerebral malaria is 20%; this rises to 50% in pregnancy,[8] and neurological sequelae occur in about 3% of survivors.[8]

AIMS OF INTERVENTION To prevent death and cure the infection; to prevent long term disability; to minimise neurological sequelae resulting from cerebral malaria, with minimal adverse effects of treatment.

OUTCOMES Death; parasite clearance at day 7 or 14; parasite clearance time; fever clearance time (see glossary, p 909); time to walking and drinking; coma recovery time; neurological sequelae at follow up; adverse events.

METHODS *Clinical Evidence* search and appraisal October 2002. The World Health Organization criteria for severe malaria were applied to included RCTs.[1]

QUESTION What are the effects of medical treatments for complicated falciparum malaria in non-pregnant people?

OPTION QUININE VERSUS PLACEBO OR NO TREATMENT

Consensus statements recommend quinine for the treatment of severe falciparum malaria.

Benefits: We found no RCTs comparing quinine with placebo or no treatment.

Harms: We found two observational studies on hypoglycaemia secondary to hyperinsulinaemia induced by quinine. One study in people with severe malaria treated with quinine in Thailand found a correlation between plasma quinine and insulin levels during hypoglycaemic episodes ($P = 0.007$).[9] One prospective cohort study in Zaire (9 children and 19 adults) treated severe malaria with intravenous quinine (average dose 8.5 mg/kg base hourly). Nine people developed significant hypoglycaemia (glucose < 2.8 mmol/L), which was associated with inappropriately high plasma insulin levels.[10] It is not clear from these studies if hypoglycaemia was caused by malaria or by quinine administration.

Comment: RCTs of quinine versus placebo in severe malaria would be regarded as unethical. The use of quinine to treat severe malaria was established before modern trial methods were developed. In a case series in Singapore (1944–1945), 15 adults with acute severe malaria were treated with continuous intravenous quinine;[11] 13 recovered and two comatose people died. In a non-comparative study in Zaire (1987), intravenous quinine (10 mg/kg 8 hourly for 3 days) was given to 34 children (7 months to 13 years) with severe or moderate falciparum malaria (see glossary, p 909).[12] One child who was comatose on admission died. The mean parasite clearance time (see glossary, p 909) was 59.6 hours. The mean fever clearance time (see glossary, p 909) was 44.1 hours. Thirty three children were clinically well and had negative blood slides on day 7. Reviews[13,14] and consensus statements[1,15,16] recommend quinine for treating severe falciparum malaria, particularly in chloroquine resistant areas.

OPTION CHLOROQUINE VERSUS QUININE

Two RCTs in children found no significant difference in mortality with chloroquine versus quinine. However, these RCTs were conducted in the Gambia between 1988 and 1994, when chloroquine resistance was uncommon.

Benefits: We found no systematic review. We found two RCTs.[17,18] One RCT (50 children from the Gambia, age 1–10 years with severe malaria) compared intramuscular chloroquine (3.5 mg base/kg 6 hourly) versus intramuscular quinine (20 mg salt/kg immediately followed by 10 mg salt/kg 12 hourly) in 1988.[17] It found no significant difference in mortality (2/25 [8%] with chloroquine *v* 6/25 [24%] with quinine; RR 0.33, 95% CI 0.07 to 1.50) or fever resolution (37.7 h with chloroquine *v* 39.1 h with quinine; WMD –1.4 h, 95% CI –14.0 h to +11.2 h). Median time to full recovery from coma was 18 hours in both groups. Recovery time from prostration was similar in both groups (median time to standing: 42 h with chloroquine *v* 48 h with quinine). Recovery time to drinking was also similar in both groups (10 h with chloroquine *v* 11 h with quinine). The second RCT (92 Gambian children, aged 1–9 years) compared subcutaneous chloroquine (2.5 mg/kg 4 hourly) versus intramuscular quinine (10 mg/kg 8 hourly) in the treatment of complicated, non-cerebral malaria between 1992 and 1994.[18] One child in each group died. The fever clearance time (see glossary, p 909) was faster with chloroquine (median: 27 h [range 6–66 h] with chloroquine *v* 42 h [range 6–96 h] with quinine; P = 0.02).

Harms: In the first RCT, one child treated with chloroquine developed pruritus (chloroquine *v* quinine RR 3.00, 95% CI 0.13 to 70.30), whereas three children treated with quinine developed hypoglycaemia (chloroquine *v* quinine RR 0.14, 95% CI 0.01 to 2.63).[17]

Comment: The effects on mortality were inconclusive because of the small number of people in both trials. One RCT excluded participants with cerebral malaria who are an important group in children suffering from severe malaria.[18] Chloroquine resistance was documented in the second trial.[18] Chloroquine resistance has since become widespread in sub-Saharan Africa, resulting in more deaths and an increase in severe disease.[19]

OPTION SULFADOXINE–PYRIMETHAMINE VERSUS QUININE

One RCT found sulfadoxine–pyrimethamine cleared parasites faster than quinine in children with complicated non-cerebral malaria in 1992–1994 in the Gambia, but found no significant difference in mortality.

Benefits: We found no systematic review. We found one RCT (92 Gambian children aged 1–9 years with complicated, non-cerebral malaria, in 1992–1994) that compared intramuscular sulfadoxine–pyrimethamine (sulfadoxine 25 mg/kg plus pyrimethamine 1.25 mg/kg) versus intramuscular quinine (10 mg/kg 8 hourly) versus chloroquine.[18] It found no difference inmortality (2/36 [6%]

with sulfadoxine–pyrimethamine v 1/28 [4%] with quinine; RR 1.56, 95% CI 0.15 to 16.3). Sulfadoxine–pyrimethamine cleared parasites faster than quinine (median parasite clearance time (see glossary, p 909) 42 h [range 18–78 h] v 66 h [range 30–90 h]; P < 0.001).

Harms: One child treated with quinine developed an injection abscess (0/36 [0%] with sulfadoxine–pyrimethamine v 1/28 [3.6%] with quinine; RR 0.26, 95% CI 0.01 to 6.18).[18]

Comment: Children with cerebral malaria, who form an important subgroup of people with severe malaria, were excluded from this RCT. Resistance to sulfadoxine–pyrimethamine was documented in the Gambia in 1991.[18]

OPTION INTRAMUSCULAR VERSUS INTRAVENOUS QUININE

One RCT in children found no difference between intramuscular and intravenous quinine in treating severe malaria in Kenya in 1990.

Benefits: We found no systematic review. We found one RCT (59 children < 12 years old), which compared high dose intramuscular versus high dose intravenous quinine (20 mg salt/kg loading immediately followed by 10 mg salt/kg 12 hourly) versus standard dose intravenous quinine in severe falciparum malaria (see glossary, p 909) in Kenya (1989–1990).[20] The RCT found no significant difference in mortality (3/20 [15%] deaths with im quinine v 1/18 [5.6%] with iv quinine; RR 2.7, 95% CI 0.3 to 23.7), in mean parasite clearance time (see glossary, p 909) (57 h with im quinine v 58 h with iv quinine; WMD −1.0 h, 95% CI −12.2 h to +10.2 h), in mean recovery times to drinking (47 h with im quinine v 32 h with iv quinine; WMD +15 h, 95% CI −5.6 h to +35.6 h), or in mean recovery times to walking (98 h with im quinine v 96 h with iv quinine; WMD +2.0 h, 95% CI −24.5 h to +28.5 h).

Harms: Neurological sequelae were reported in two children in the intramuscular group, and one child in the intravenous group had transient neurological sequelae, which was not specified (2/20 [10%] with im quinine v 1/18 [5.6%] with iv quinine; RR 1.8, 95% CI 0.2 to 18.2).

Comment: Quinine concentration profiles were similar with both routes of administration, and peak concentrations were achieved soon after intramuscular injection. The sample size might have been insufficient to rule out important clinical differences.

OPTION HIGH FIRST DOSE OF QUININE VERSUS STANDARD DOSE QUININE

One systematic review and one additional RCT found no significant difference in mortality between quinine regimens with high initial quinine dose versus no loading dose. The systematic review found that high first dose of quinine reduced parasite and fever clearance times compared with no loading dose.

Benefits: We found one systematic review (search date 2002, 3 RCTs, 92 people)[21] and one additional RCT.[22] The systematic review found no significant difference in mortality for initial high dose quinine (20 mg salt/kg or 16 mg base/kg given im or iv) versus no loading dose, followed in both groups by standard dose quinine (2 RCTs, 2/35 [5.7%] died with high dose *v* 5/37 [13.5%] with standard dose; RR 0.43, 95% CI 0.09 to 2.15).[21] One of the included RCTs (39 children) found no significant difference for initial high dose versus no loading dose in mean time to recover consciousness (14 h with initial high dose *v* 13 h with standard dose; WMD +1.0 h, 95% CI –8.8 h to +10.8 h).[20] Parasite clearance time and fever clearance time (see glossary, p 909) were shorter for the initial high dose quinine group versus no loading dose (parasite clearance time: 2 RCTs, 67 people; WMD –7.4 h, 95% CI –13.2 h to –1.6 h; fever clearance time: 2 RCTs, 68 people, WMD –11.1 h, 95% CI –20.0 h to –2.2 h). The additional RCT (72 children aged 8 months to 15 years in Togo [1999–2000]) found no significant difference for initial high dose intravenous quinine regimen (20 mg quinine salt/kg over 4 h, then 10 mg quinine salt/kg 12 hourly) versus standard quinine regimen (15 mg salt/kg 12 hourly) in mortality (2/35 [6%] with initial high dose *v* 2/37 [5%] with standard dose; RR 1.06, 95% CI 0.16 to 7.1).[22] It found no significant difference between high initial dose versus standard dose quinine for recovery of consciousness or parasite clearance time (recovery of consciousness: 35.5 h with initial high dose *v* 28.6 h with standard dose, WMD +6.9 h, 95% CI –0.6 h to +14.4 h; time for 100% parasite clearance 48 h with high initial dose *v* 60 h with standard dose).

Harms: The systematic review found no significant difference between initial high dose of quinine versus no loading dose for rate of hypoglycaemia (2 RCTs, 4/35 [11%] hypoglycaemia with initial high dose *v* 3/37 [8%] with standard dose; RR 1.39, 95% CI 0.32 to 6.00).[21] One RCT (33 people) in the review found that initial high dose quinine versus no loading dose significantly increased transient partial hearing loss (10/17 [59%] *v* 3/16 [19%], RR 3.14, 95% CI 1.05 to 9.38).[23] One RCT (39 children) in the review found no significant difference between high initial dose of quinine and no loading dose in neurological sequelae (1/18 [6%] initial high dose *v* 2/21 [10%] standard dose; RR 0.58, 95% CI 0.06 to 5.91).[20]

Comment: The RCTs may have been too small to detect a clinically important difference.[20,22,23]

OPTION ARTEMETHER VERSUS QUININE

Two systematic reviews and one subsequent RCT found no significant difference between artemether versus quinine for preventing deaths in people with severe malaria.

Benefits: We found two systematic reviews[24,25] and one subsequent RCT.[26] The first review (search date not stated, 7 RCTs, 1919 adults and children) analysed individual participant data. It found no significant difference in mortality for intramuscular artemether versus intravenous or intramuscular quinine (im quinine in 1 RCT only) for severe falciparum malaria (see glossary, p 909) (mortality 136/961

[14%] with artemether v 164/958 [17%] with quinine, OR 0.80, 95% CI 0.62 to 1.02).[24] Parasite clearance was faster for artemether versus quinine (HR 0.62, 95% CI 0.56 to 0.69). The review found no significant difference in the speed of coma recovery, fever clearance time (see glossary, p 909), or neurological sequelae for artemether versus quinine (coma recovery with quinine HR 1.09, 95% CI 0.97 to 1.22; fever clearance with quinine HR 1.01, 95% CI 0.90 to 1.15; neurological sequelae 81/807 [10%] with artemether v 91/765 [12%] with quinine, OR 0.82, 95% CI 0.59 to 1.15). The second review (search date 1999, 11 RCTs, 2142 people) found a small significant reduction in mortality for intramuscular artemether versus intravenous quinine (OR 0.72, 95% CI 0.57 to 0.91). However, more rigorous analysis excluding three poorer quality RCTs found no significant difference for mortality (OR 0.79, 95% CI 0.59 to 1.05).[25] The review found no significant difference in neurological sequelae at recovery for artemether versus quinine (OR 0.8, 95% CI 0.52 to 1.25). The subsequent RCT (105 people aged 15–40 years with cerebral malaria in Bangladesh) compared intramuscular artemether (160 mg initially, then 80 mg/kg once daily) versus intravenous quinine (loading dose 20 mg/kg, then 10 mg/kg 8 hourly).[26] It found no significant difference in death for artemether versus quinine (9/51 [18%] with artemether v 10/54 [19%] with quinine; OR 0.94, 95% CI 0.35 to 2.55). Mean fever clearance time and coma recovery time were significantly longer for artemether versus quinine (fever clearance time 58 h with artemether v 47 h with quinine, WMD 11.0 h, 95% CI 1.6 h to 20.4 h; coma recovery time 74 h with artemether v 53 h with quinine, WMD 20.8 h, 95% CI 3.6 h to 38.0 h). There was no significant difference in mean parasite clearance time (see glossary, p 909) for artemether versus quinine (52 h with artemether v 61 h with quinine; WMD −8.6 h, 95% CI −22.5 h to +5.3 h).

Harms: Two systematic reviews and one subsequent RCT found no significant difference in neurological sequelae for artemether versus quinine (systematic reviews:[24,25] see benefits above; additional RCT:[26] 3/51 [6%] with artemether v 1/54 [2%] with quinine, RR 3.18, 95% CI 0.34 to 29.56). However, in the first meta-analysis, the combination of either death or neurological sequelae as an adverse outcome was lower for artemether versus quinine (OR 0.77, 95% CI 0.62 to 0.96; P = 0.02).[24]

Comment: We found a second subsequent RCT (52 people).[27] However, it was not clear whether participants had severe malaria and outcomes were poorly reported.

OPTION **RECTAL ARTEMISININ DERIVATIVES (ARTEMISININ OR ARTESUNATE) VERSUS QUININE**

One systematic review has found no significant difference in mortality between rectal artemisinin and quinine.

Benefits: We found one systematic review (search date 1999, 3 RCTs), which compared rectal artemisinin versus quinine in severe malaria.[25] Two RCTs were conducted in Vietnam and one in Ethiopia (1996–1997). Meta-analysis found lower mortality with artemisinin (3 RCTs, 9/87 [10%] with artemisinin v 16/98 [16%] with quinine;

RR 0.73, 95% CI 0.35 to 1.50) and quicker coma recovery time (2 RCTs, 59 people; WMD −9.0 h, 95% CI −19.7 h to +1.7 h), but the difference was not significant. Fever clearance time (see glossary, p 909) was not significantly different (no figures provided). We found no RCTs comparing rectal artesunate with quinine.

Harms: Artemisinin versus quinine significantly reduced the risk of hypoglycaemia in one trial (3/30 [10%] with artemisinin *v* 19/30 [63%] with quinine; RR 0.16, 95% CI 0.05 to 0.48).[28]

Comment: The World Health Organization is currently conducting a trial of prompt administration rectal artesunate for severe malaria by paramedical staff before referral to hospital (Olliaro P, personal communication, 2002).

OPTION DESFERRIOXAMINE MESYLATE

One systematic review found weak evidence that the risk of persistent seizures was reduced with desferrioxamine mesylate versus placebo.

Benefits: **Versus placebo:** We found one systematic review (search date 1998, 2 RCTs, 435 children > 6 years of age with cerebral malaria treated with quinine) of desferrioxamine mesylate (100 mg/kg/day iv for 72 h) versus placebo.[29] Both RCTs were conducted in Zambia (1990–1991). The review found no difference in overall mortality (39/217 [18%] with desferrioxamine *v* 28/218 [13%] with placebo; RR 1.40, 95% CI 0.89 to 2.18) but results were heterogeneous. The review found that desferrioxamine mesylate significantly reduced the risk of persistent seizures (93/168 [55.4%] with desferrioxamine *v* 115/166 [69.3%] with placebo; RR 0.80, 95% CI 0.67 to 0.95).

Harms: One RCT found no significant difference between desferrioxamine mesylate versus placebo for phlebitis (26/172 [15%] with desferrioxamine *v* 20/172 [12%] with placebo; RR 1.30, 95% CI 0.76 to 2.24) or recurrent hypoglycaemia (43/172 [25%] with desferrioxamine *v* 29/172 [17%] with placebo; RR 1.48, 95% CI 0.97 to 2.26).[30]

Comment: The trials were probably underpowered to detect a clinically significant difference in adverse events.

OPTION GLUCOCORTICOID DRUGS (DEXAMETHASONE)

One systematic review has found no significant difference in mortality between dexamethasone versus placebo, but gastrointestinal bleeding and seizures were more common with dexamethasone.

Benefits: **Versus placebo:** We found one systematic review (search date 1999, 2 RCTs, 143 people treated with quinine) of dexamethasone versus placebo over 48 hours.[31] One RCT was conducted in Indonesia and the other in Thailand. The review found no significant difference in mortality (14/71 [20%] with dexamethasone *v* 16/72 [25%] with placebo; RR 0.89, 95% CI 0.47 to 1.68). One RCT found a longer mean time between start of treatment and coma resolution with dexamethasone group (76 h with dexamethasone *v* 57 h with placebo; $P < 0.02$),[32] but the other RCT found no significant difference (83.4 h with dexamethasone *v* 80.0 h with placebo; WMD +3.4 h, 95% CI –31.3 h to +38.1 h).[33]

Harms: Gastrointestinal bleeding (7/71 [10%] with dexamethasone *v* 0/72 [0%] with placebo; RR 8.17, 95% CI 1.05 to 63.6) and seizures (11/71 [15.5%] with dexamethasone *v* 3/72 [4%] with placebo; RR 3.32, 95% CI 1.05 to 10.47) were significantly more common with dexamethasone.[31]

Comment: No effect of steroids on mortality was shown but the trial numbers are small. The effect of steroids on disability was not reported.

OPTION — INITIAL BLOOD TRANSFUSION FOR TREATING MALARIAL ANAEMIA

One systematic review has found no significant difference in mortality, but more adverse events among clinically stable children who receive an initial blood transfusion for malaria anaemia.

Benefits: We found one systematic review (search date 1999, 2 RCTs, 230 children).[34] One RCT compared initial blood transfusion versus conservative treatment in children for Tanzania and the other RCT compared blood transfusion versus iron supplements in children from the Gambia. Both trials excluded children who were clinically unstable with respiratory distress or signs of cardiac failure. Meta-analysis found fewer deaths in the transfused children but the difference was not significant (1/118 [1%] with transfusion *v* 3/112 [3%] with control; RR 0.41, 95% CI 0.06 to 2.70).

Harms: Coma and convulsions occurred more often after transfusion (8/118 [6.8%] with transfusion *v* 0/112 [0%] without transfusion; RR 8.6, 95% CI 1.1 to 66.0).[34] Seven of the eight adverse events occurred in one RCT. Meta-analysis combining deaths and severe adverse events found no significant difference between transfused and non-transfused people (8/118 [7%] with transfusion *v* 3/112 [3%] without transfusion; RR 2.5, 95% CI 0.7 to 9.3). Hepatitis B or HIV transmission were not reported.

Comment: Studies were small and loss to follow up was greater than 10%, both of which are both potential sources of bias. No results were available on adults. Significantly more children in the non-transfused group required transfusion in addition to the primary allocated intervention (1/118 [1%] with transfusion *v* 11/112 [10%] without transfusion; RR 0.12, 95% CI 0.02 to 0.68).[34]

OPTION — EXCHANGE BLOOD TRANSFUSION

One systematic review has found no RCTs.

Benefits: We found one systematic review (search date 2001).[35] It found no suitable RCTs in people with malaria. We found no additional RCTs that met our inclusion criteria (see comment below).

Harms: We found no good evidence.

Comment: We found one systematic review of case control studies[35] and one small RCT.[36] The review (search date 2001, 8 studies, 279 people) found no significant difference in mortality between exchange transfusion plus antimalarial drugs versus antimalarial drugs only (8 studies, OR for death 1.2, 95% CI 0.7 to 2.1).[36] Admission criteria for exchange transfusion varied in the included studies but generally parasitaemia was greater than 10%, and most people had failed to improve after 24 hours of antimalarial treatment. The methods and volumes used for exchange transfusion also varied. Those who received exchange blood transfusions had higher mean levels of parasitaemia before treatment began (26% with exchange transfusion *v* 11% with no exchange transfusion; $P < 0.05$) and fulfilled more World Health Organization criteria for the diagnosis of severe malaria (mean 3.6 with exchange transfusion *v* 2.8 with no exchange transfusion; $P = 0.03$). We excluded one RCT that compared exchange transfusion plus antimalarial drugs versus antimalarial drugs only because it included only eight people.[36]

GLOSSARY

Falciparum malaria Malaria resulting from an infection with *Plasmodium falciparum*, one of the four species of malaria parasites found in humans.

Fever clearance time The time between commencing treatment and the temperature returning back to normal.

Parasite clearance time (PCT) The time between commencing treatment and the first negative blood test. PCT 50 is the time taken for parasites to be reduced to 50% of first test value and PCT 90 is the time taken for parasites to be reduced to 10% of first test value.

Substantive changes

High first dose of quinine versus standard dose quinine One systematic review added;[21] conclusions unchanged.

High first dose of quinine versus standard dose quinine One RCT added;[22] conclusions unchanged.

Artemether versus quinine One RCT added;[27] conclusions unchanged.

Exchange transfusion One systematic review added;[35] conclusions unchanged.

REFERENCES

1. World Health Organization. Severe falciparum malaria. World Health Organization, Communicable Diseases Cluster. *Trans R Soc Trop Med Hyg* 2000;94:S1–S90.
2. World Health Organization. WHO Expert Committee on Malaria: Twentieth report. 1998 Geneva Switzerland. *World Health Organ Tech Rep Ser* 2000;892:i–v:1–74.
3. Hill AVS. Malaria resistance genes: a natural selection. *Trans R Soc Trop Med Hyg* 1992;86:225–226.
4. Hill AVS. Genetic susceptibility to malaria and other infectious diseases: from the MHC to the whole genome. *Parasitology* 1996;112:S75–S84.
5. Modiano D, Luoni G, Sirima BS, et al. Haemoglobin C protects against clinical *Plasmodium falciparum* malaria. *Nature* 2001;414:305–308.
6. McGuire W, Hill AV, Allsopp CE, et al. Variation in the TNF-alpha promoter region associated with susceptibility to cerebral malaria. *Nature* 1994;371:508–510.
7. Murphy SC, Breman JG. Gaps in the childhood malaria burden in Africa: cerebral malaria, neurological sequelae, anemia, respiratory distress, hypoglycemia, and complications of pregnancy. *Am J Trop Med Hyg* 2001;64:S57–S67.
8. White NJ. Malaria. In: Cook GC, ed. *Manson's tropical diseases*. 20th ed. London: WB Saunders 1996:1087–1164.
9. White N, Warrell D, Chanthavanich P, et al. Severe hypoglycemia and hyperinsulinemia in falciparum malaria. *N Engl J Med* 1983;309:61–66.
10. Okitolonda W, Delacollette C, Malengreau M, et al. High incidence of hypoglycaemia in African patients treated with intravenous quinine for severe malaria. *BMJ* 1987;295:716–718.
11. Strahan JH. Quinine by continuous intravenous drip in the treatment of acute falciparum malaria. *Trans R Soc Trop Med Hyg* 1948;41:669–76.
12. Greenberg AE, Nguyen-Dinh P, Davachi F, et al. Intravenous quinine therapy of hospitalized children with *Plasmodium falciparum* malaria in Kinshasa, Zaire. *Am J Trop Med Hyg* 1988;40:360–364.
13. Hall AP. The treatment of severe falciparum malaria. *Trans R Soc Trop Med Hyg* 1977;71:367–378.

14. Warrell DA. Treatment of severe malaria. *J R Soc Med* 1989;82(suppl 17):44–50.
15. World Health Organization. The use of antimalarial drugs. Report of a WHO Informal consultation, 13–17 November 2000 (WHO/CDS/RBM/2001.33). Geneva: World Health Organization, 2001.
16. Looareesuwan S, Olliaro P, White NJ, et al. Consensus recommendation on the treatment of malaria in Southeast Asia. *Southeast Asian J Trop Med Public Health* 1998;29:355–360.
17. White NJ, Waller D, Kwiatkowski D, et al. Open comparison of intramuscular chloroquine and quinine in children with severe chloroquine-sensitive falciparum malaria. *Lancet* 1989;2:1313–1316.
18. Giadom B, De Veer GE, van Hensbroek B, et al. A comparative study of parenteral chloroquine, quinine and pyrimethamine–sulfadoxine in the treatment of Gambian children with complicated, non-cerebral malaria. *Ann Trop Paediatr* 1996:16;85–91.
19. Nuwaha F. The challenge of chloroquine-resistant malaria in sub-Saharan Africa. *Health Policy Plan* 2001;16:1–12.
20. Pasvol G, Newton CRJC, Winstanley PA, et al. Quinine treatment of severe falciparum malaria in African children: a randomized comparison of three regimens. *Am J Trop Med Hyg* 1991;45:702–713.
21. Lesi A, Meremikwu M. High first dose quinine for treating severe malaria. In: The Cochrane Library, Issue 3, 2002. Oxford: Update Software. Search date 2002; primary sources Cochrane Infectious Diseases Group specialised trials register, Cochrane Controlled Trials Register, Medline, Embase, Lilacs, conference proceedings, researchers working in the field, and hand searches of references.
22. Assimadi JK, Gbadoé AD, Agbodjan-Djossou O, et al. Intravenous quinine treatment of cerebral malaria in African children: comparison of a loading dose regimen to a regimen without loading dose [French]. *Arch Pediatr* 2002;9:587–594.
23. Tombe M, Bhatt KM, Obel AOK. Quinine loading dose in severe falciparum malaria at Kenyatta National Hospital, Kenya. *East Afr Med J* 1992;69:670–674.
24. Artemether Quinine Meta-analysis Study Group. A meta-analysis using individual patient data of trials comparing artemether with quinine in the treatment of severe falciparum malaria. *Trans R Soc Trop Med Hyg* 2001;95:637–650. Search date not stated; primary sources Medline, Cochrane, and discussions with an international panel of malaria clinical investigators.
25. McIntosh HM, Olliaro P. Artemisinin derivatives for treating severe malaria. In: The Cochrane Library, Issue 3, 2001. Oxford: Update Software. Search date 1999; primary sources Cochrane Infectious Diseases Group Trials Register, Medline, Bids, Science Citation Index, Embase, African Index Medicus, Lilacs, hand searches of reference lists and conference abstracts, and contact with organisations and researchers in the field and pharmaceutical companies.
26. Faiz A, Rahman E, Hossain A, et al. A randomized controlled trial comparing artemether and quinine in the treatment of cerebral malaria in Bangladesh. *Ind J Malariol* 2001;38:9–18.
27. Singh NB, Bhagyabati Devi S, Singh TB, et al. Artemether vs quinine therapy in *Plasmodium falciparum* malaria in Manipur — a preliminary report. *J Communic Dis* 2001;33:83–87.
28. Birku Y, Makonnen E, Bjorkman A. Comparison of rectal artemisinin with intravenous quinine in the treatment of severe malaria in Ethiopia. *East Afr Med J* 1999;76:154–159.
29. Smith HJ, Meremikwu M. Iron chelating agents for treating malaria. In: The Cochrane Library, Issue 3, 2001. Oxford: Update Software. Search date 1998; primary sources Trials Register of the Cochrane Infectious Diseases Group, Cochrane Controlled Trials Register, Medline, Embase, and hand searches of reference lists.
30. Thuma PE, Mabeza GF, Biemba G, et al. Effect of iron chelation therapy on mortality in children with cerebral malaria. *Trans R Soc Trop Med Hyg* 1998;92:214–218.
31. Prasad K, Garner P. Steroids for treating cerebral malaria (Cochrane Review). In: The Cochrane Library, Issue 3, 2001. Oxford: Update Software. Search date 1999; primary sources Trials Register of the Cochrane Infectious Diseases Group and Cochrane Controlled Trials Register.
32. Warrell DA, Looareesuwan S, Warrell MJ, et al. Dexamethasone proves deleterious in cerebral malaria. A double-blind trial in 100 comatose patients. *N Engl J Med* 1982;306:313–319.
33. Hoffman SL, Rustama D, Punjabi NH, et al. High-dose dexamethasone in quinine-treated patients with cerebral malaria: a double-blind, placebo-controlled trial. *J Infect Dis* 1988;158:325–331.
34. Meremikwu M, Smith HJ. Blood transfusion for treating malarial anaemia. In: The Cochrane Library, Issue 3, 2001. Oxford: Update Software. Search date 1999; primary sources Trials Register of the Cochrane Infectious Diseases Group, Embase, African Index Medicus, Lilacs, hand searches of reference lists, and contact with experts.
35. Riddle MS, Jackson JL, Sanders JW, et al. Exchange transfusion and an adjunct therapy in severe *Plasmodium falciparum* malaria: a meta-analysis. *Clin Infect Dis* 2002:34:1192–1198. Search date 2001; primary sources Medline, Embase, Fedrip, and the Cochrane Database of Clinical Trials.
36. Saddler M, Barry M, Ternouth I, et al. Treatment of severe malaria by exchange transfusion [letter]. *N Engl J Med* 1990;322:58.

Aika Omari

Paul Garner
Professor of Medicine

Liverpool School of Tropical Medicine
Liverpool
UK

Competing interests: None declared.

Malaria: prevention in travellers

Search date November 2002

Ashley M Croft

QUESTIONS

INTERVENTIONS

Key Messages

- **Insecticide treated nets in adults** We found no RCTs in travellers. One systematic review in adult and child residents of malaria endemic settings found that insecticide treated nets reduce the number of mild episodes of malaria and reduce child mortality.

Malaria: prevention in travellers

- **Atovaquone plus proguanil in adults** One RCT in migrants with limited immunity found that atovaquone plus proguanil reduced the proportion of people with malaria compared with placebo. One RCT found no significant difference between atovaquone plus proguanil and chloroquine plus proguanil in preventing malaria. One RCT of atovaquone plus proguanil versus mefloquine found no cases of clinical malaria throughout the trial, but found a higher rate of neuropsychiatric harm with mefloquine compared with atovaquone plus proguanil.
- **Doxycycline in adults** One RCT in soldiers and one RCT in migrants with limited immunity found that doxycycline reduces the risk of malaria compared with placebo. One of the RCTs found that doxycycline was associated with nausea and vomiting, diarrhoea, cough, headache, and unspecified dermatological symptoms over 13 weeks.
- **Insecticide treated clothing in adults** Two RCTs in soldiers and refugee householders found that permethrin treated fabric (clothing or sheets) reduces the incidence of malaria.
- **Mefloquine in adults** One systematic review of one RCT in soldiers found that, compared with placebo, mefloquine had 100% protective efficacy. One RCT of mefloquine versus atovaquone plus proguanil found no cases of clinical malaria throughout the trial, but found a higher rate of neuropsychiatric harm with mefloquine compared with atovaquone plus proguanil.
- **Aerosol insecticides in adults** We found no RCTs on the effects of aerosol insecticides in preventing malaria in travellers. One large questionnaire survey in travellers found insufficient evidence on the effects of aerosol insecticides in preventing malaria. Two community RCTs in residents of malaria endemic areas found that indoor spraying of aerosol insecticides reduced clinical malaria.
- **Air conditioning and electric fans in adults** We found no RCTs on the effects of air conditioning or electric fans in preventing malaria in travellers. One large questionnaire survey found that air conditioning reduced the incidence of malaria. One small observational study found that electric ceiling fans reduced total catches of culicine mosquitos in indoor spaces but did not significantly reduce total catches of anopheline mosquitoes.
- **Chloroquine in adults** We found no RCTs on the effects of chloroquine in travellers. One RCT in Austrian workers residing in Nigeria found no significant difference between chloroquine and sulfadoxine plus pyrimethamine in the incidence of malaria after 6–22 months.
- **Chloroquine plus proguanil in adults** One RCT found no significant difference between chloroquine plus proguanil and chloroquine plus sulfadoxine plus pyrimethamine in the incidence of *Plasmodium falciparum* malaria. One RCT found no significant difference between chloroquine plus proguanil and proguanil alone in the incidence of *P falciparum* malaria. One RCT found no significant difference between chloroquine plus proguanil and atovaquone plus proguanil in preventing malaria.
- **Full length clothing in adults** We found no RCTs on the effects of full length clothing in preventing malaria in travellers. One large questionnaire survey in travellers found that wearing trousers and long sleeved shirts reduced the incidence of malaria.
- **Insecticide treated nets in pregnant travellers** We found no RCTs on the effects of insecticide treated nets in preventing malaria in pregnant travellers. One RCT of pregnant long term residents of a malaria endemic area found insufficient evidence on the effects of permethrin treated nets in preventing malaria.

- **Mosquito coils and vaporising mats in adults** We found no RCTs on the effects of coils and vaporising mats in preventing malaria in travellers. One RCT of coils and one observational study of pyrethroid vaporising mats found that these devices reduced numbers of mosquitoes in indoor spaces.
- **Pyrimethamine plus dapsone in adults** We found no RCTs in travellers. One RCT in Thai soldiers found insufficient evidence to compare pyrimethamine plus dapsone versus proguanil plus dapsone.
- **Smoke in adults** We found no RCTs on the effects of smoke in preventing malaria. One controlled clinical trial found that smoke repelled mosquitoes during the evening.
- **Topical (skin applied) insect repellents in adults** We found no RCTs on the effects of topical (skin applied) insect repellents in preventing malaria in travellers. One small crossover RCT found that DEET preparations protected against mosquito bites.
- **Vaccines** We found no RCTs in travellers. One systematic review of antimalaria vaccines in residents of malaria endemic areas found that the SPf66 vaccine reduces first attacks of malaria compared with placebo.
- **Amodiaquine in adults** We found no RCTs on the effects of amodiaquine in preventing malaria in travellers. We found limited observational evidence that amodiaquine may cause liver damage and hepatitis.
- **Doxycycline in children** We found no RCTs in child travellers on the use of doxycycline. Case reports in young children found adverse effects with doxycycline.
- **Sulfadoxine plus pyrimethamine in adults** One RCT found no significant difference between chloroquine plus proguanil and chloroquine plus sulfadoxine plus pyrimethamine in the incidence of *P falciparum* malaria. One retrospective observational study suggested that sulfadoxine plus pyrimethamine was associated with severe cutaneous reactions.
- **Topical (skin applied) insect repellents containing DEET in children** We found no RCTs on the effects of DEET in preventing malaria in child travellers. Case reports in young children found serious adverse effects with DEET.
- **Antimalaria drugs in airline pilots; antimalaria drugs in pregnant travellers; biological control measures in adults; insect electrocuters and ultrasonic buzzers in adults; insecticide treated clothing in pregnant travellers; mefloquine in children; topical (skin applied) insect repellents in pregnant travellers** We found no RCTs on the effects of these interventions.

DEFINITION Malaria is caused by a protozoan infection of red blood cells with one of four species of the genus *Plasmodium*: *P falciparum*, *P vivax*, *P ovale*, and *P malariae*.[1] Clinically, malaria may present in different ways but it is usually characterised by fever (which may be swinging), tachycardia, rigors, and sweating. Anaemia, hepatosplenomegaly, cerebral involvement, renal failure, and shock may occur.[2,3] Travellers are defined here as visitors from a malaria free area to a malaria endemic area, and who stay in the endemic area for less than 1 year.

INCIDENCE/ PREVALENCE Each year there are 300–500 million clinical cases of malaria. About 40% of the world's population is at risk of acquiring the disease.[2,3] Each year 25–30 million people from non-tropical countries visit malaria endemic areas, of whom 10 000–30 000 contract malaria.[4,5] Most RCTs of malaria prevention have been conducted in soldiers and travellers. The results of these trials may not be applicable to people such as refugees and migrants, who are likely to differ in their health status and in their susceptibility to disease and adverse drug effects.

AETIOLOGY/ RISK FACTORS Malaria is mainly a rural disease, requiring nearby standing water. It is transmitted by bites of infected female anopheline mosquitoes, mainly at dusk and during the night.[1,6–8] In cities, mosquito bites are usually from female culicine mosquitoes, which are not vectors of malaria.[9] Malaria is resurgent in most tropical countries and risk to travellers is increasing.[10] The sickle cell trait has been shown to convey some protection against malaria in non-immune carriers of that trait. Non-immune adults with the sickle cell trait who develop severe malaria have lower parasite densities, fewer complications (e.g. cerebral malaria), and a reduced mortality compared with adults without the trait.[11] There is little good evidence on the degree of protection afforded by the sickle cell trait.[12]

PROGNOSIS Ninety per cent of tourists and business travellers who contract malaria do not become ill until after they return home.[5] "Imported malaria" is easily treated if diagnosed promptly, and follows a serious course in only about 12% of people.[13,14] The most severe form is cerebral malaria, with a case fatality rate in adult travellers of 2–6%, mainly because of delays in diagnosis.[3,15]

AIMS OF INTERVENTION To reduce the risk of infection; to prevent illness and death, with minimal adverse effects of treatment.

OUTCOMES Rates of clinical malaria and death, and adverse effects of treatment. Proxy measures include numbers of mosquito bites and rates of mosquito catches in indoor areas. We found limited evidence linking numbers of mosquito bites and risk of malaria.[16]

METHODS *Clinical Evidence* search and appraisal November 2002. Additional hand searches by the author of his own files. Observational (non-RCT) data have been included in some sections where appropriate control studies are lacking or may be considered unethical.

QUESTION **What are the effects of non-drug preventive interventions in adult travellers?**

OPTION **AEROSOL INSECTICIDES IN ADULTS**

We found no RCTs on the effects of aerosol insecticides in preventing malaria in travellers. One large questionnaire survey in travellers found insufficient evidence on the effects of aerosol insecticides in preventing malaria. Two community RCTs in residents of malaria endemic areas found that indoor spraying of aerosol insecticides reduced clinical malaria.

Benefits: We found no systematic review or RCTs in travellers (see comment below). Two community RCTs found that indoor residual spraying of synthetic pyrethroids reduced clinical malaria in lifelong residents of malaria endemic areas.[17,18]

Harms: We found no reports of adverse effects.

Comment: One large questionnaire survey (89 617 European tourists returning from East Africa) found that commercially available personal aerosol insecticides did not significantly reduce the incidence of malaria (P = 0.55).[19] Historically, indoor residual spraying has not been recommended for short stay travellers, but we found no evidence to support this.

OPTION BIOLOGICAL CONTROL MEASURES IN ADULTS

We found no RCTs on the effects of biological control measures in preventing malaria in travellers.

Benefits: We found no systematic review or RCTs of biological control measures (see glossary, p 928) in preventing malaria in travellers (see comment below).

Harms: We found no evidence of harms.

Comment: One systematic review (search date 1997) identified two cohort studies based on mosquito counts. It found no evidence that growing the citrosa plant and encouraging natural predation of insects by erecting bird or bat houses reduced bites to humans from infected anopheline mosquitoes.[20] The only known way to reduce mosquito populations naturally is to eliminate sources of standing water, such as blocked gutters, tree stump holes, and discarded tyres, cans and bottles.[20]

OPTION AIR CONDITIONING AND ELECTRIC FANS IN ADULTS

We found no RCTs on the effects of air conditioning or electric fans in preventing malaria in travellers. One large questionnaire survey in travellers found that air conditioning reduced the incidence of malaria. One small observational study found that electric ceiling fans reduced total catches of culicine mosquitoes but did not significantly reduce total catches of anopheline mosquitoes in indoor spaces.

Benefits: We found no systematic review or RCTs (see comment below).

Harms: We found no evidence of harms.

Comment: One questionnaire survey of 89 617 European tourists returning from East Africa found that sleeping in an air conditioned room significantly reduced the incidence of malaria (P = 0.04).[19] One cohort study (6 experimental huts in villages in Pakistan) of various antimosquito interventions found that an electric ceiling fan run at high speed significantly reduced total catches of blood fed culicine mosquitoes ($P < 0.05$), but did not significantly reduce total catches of blood fed anopheline mosquitoes.[21] These studies support the finding that mosquitoes are reluctant to fly in windy conditions,[22] but suggest that anopheline mosquitoes are more tolerant of air turbulence than are culicine mosquitoes.

OPTION INSECT ELECTROCUTERS AND ULTRASONIC BUZZERS IN ADULTS

We found no RCTs on the effects of insect electrocuters and ultrasonic buzzers in preventing malaria.

Benefits: We found no systematic review and no RCTs with clinical malaria as an outcome.

Harms: We found no RCTs.

Comment: We found one non-randomised controlled trial (18 houses in Gabon) of a commercially available ultrasound emitting device. The trial lasted 6 weeks and used total mosquito catches as an outcome.[23] Most mosquitoes were culicine. It found no significant difference in mosquito catches between the ultrasound emitting device and a sham device (P = 0.48).[23] See comment under biological control measures in adults, p 915.

OPTION MOSQUITO COILS AND VAPORISING MATS IN ADULTS

We found no RCTs on the effects of coils and vaporising mats in preventing malaria in travellers. One RCT of coils and one observational study of pyrethroid vaporising mats found that these devices reduced numbers of mosquitoes in indoor spaces.

Benefits: We found no systematic review and no RCTs that used clinical malaria as an outcome. We found one RCT (18 houses in Malaysia) of various mosquito coil formulations versus no treatment.[24] It found that treated coils reduced populations of culicine mosquitoes by 75%.[24]

Harms: We found no evidence of harms.

Comment: One observational study of pyrethroid vaporising mats in six experimental huts in a Pakistan village setting found that the mats reduced total catches of blood fed mosquitoes by 56%.[21]

OPTION SMOKE IN ADULTS

We found no RCTs on the effects of smoke in preventing malaria in travellers. One controlled clinical trial found that smoke repelled mosquitoes during the evening.

Benefits: We found no systematic review and no RCTs of smoke in preventing malaria. We found one controlled clinical trial (see comment below).[25]

Harms: There may be an irritant and toxic effect of smoke on the eyes and respiratory system, but this effect was not quantified in the controlled clinical trial.[25]

Comment: One controlled clinical trial, in which five small fires were tended on five successive evenings in a village in Papua New Guinea, found a smoke specific and species specific effect from different types of smoke. Catches of one anopheline species were reduced by 84% by burning betelnut (95% CI 62% to 94%), 69% by burning ginger (95% CI 25% to 87%), and 66% by burning coconut husks (95% CI 17% to 86%).[25]

OPTION INSECTICIDE TREATED NETS IN ADULTS

We found no RCTs in travellers. One systematic review in adult and child residents of malaria endemic settings found that insecticide treated nets reduce the number of mild episodes of malaria and reduce child mortality.

Benefits: We found no systematic review and no RCTs in travellers. We found one systematic review (search date not stated) that identified 18 RCTs in malaria endemic settings (non-traveller children and adults).[26] It found that nets sprayed or impregnated with a pyrethroid insecticide such as permethrin versus no nets or untreated nets reduced the number of mild episodes of malaria (stable transmission area > 1 infective bite per person per year: insecticide treated nets *v* no nets: 2 RCTs, RRR 48%, 95% CI 41% to 54%; insecticide treated nets *v* untreated nets: 3 RCTs, RRR 39%, 95% CI 27% to 48%; see comment below) and child mortality (impregnated nets *v* no nets: 3 RCTs, RR 0.83, CI not reported; impregnated nets *v* untreated nets: 1 RCT, RR 0.77, CI not reported).[26] The review reported a summary risk difference of 5.6 deaths averted per 1000 children protected per year (4 RCTs, CI not reported).[26]

Harms: We found no evidence of harms.

Comment: In 7 RCTs randomisation and allocation were done by individual (or household), whereas in 11 RCTs it was done by group (household, zones within 1 village, hamlets, villages, or blocks of villages).[26] Reported CIs for protective efficacy are not corrected for cluster randomisation.[26] Permethrin remains active for about 4 months.[6] Although the analysis of insecticide treated nets was undertaken in non-traveller children and adults, the results may be generalisable to other groups such as travellers.

OPTION INSECTICIDE TREATED CLOTHING IN ADULTS

Two RCTs in soldiers and refugee householders found that permethrin treated fabric (clothing or sheets) reduces the incidence of malaria.

Benefits: We found no systematic review but found two RCTs.[27,28] The first RCT (172 male Colombian soldiers patrolling a malaria endemic area for a mean of 4.2 weeks) found that permethrin impregnated uniforms significantly reduced the incidence of malaria compared with non-impregnated uniforms (3/86 [3%] *v* 12/86 [13%]; RR 0.25, 95% CI 0.07 to 0.85).[27] The second RCT (102 refugee households in northwestern Pakistan) found that permethrin treated wraps and top sheets significantly reduced the risk of falciparum malaria compared with placebo (RR 0.56, 95% CI 0.41 to 0.78).[28]

Harms: The first RCT also included an analysis of permethrin impregnated uniforms versus non-impregnated uniforms in 286 soldiers patrolling a leishmaniasis endemic area for a mean 6.6 weeks.[27] It found that 2/229 (0.9%) participants wearing permethrin impregnated uniforms experienced irritation and itching. No comparative information was given for soldiers wearing non-impregnated uniforms.

Comment: In the first RCT, the entire uniform (hat, shirt, undershirt, trousers, socks) was treated with a single application of permethrin. All participants were instructed to wear the uniform continuously, day and night, with the sleeves rolled down. Each participant washed his own uniform two to three times during the study, using soap and water, but uniforms were not reimpregnated with permethrin. Topical (skin applied) insect repellents were not used. Trials in soldiers may not be generalisable to other travellers.

Malaria: prevention in travellers

OPTION FULL LENGTH CLOTHING IN ADULTS

We found no RCTs on the effects of full length clothing in preventing malaria in travellers. One large questionnaire survey in travellers found that wearing trousers and long sleeved shirts reduced the incidence of malaria.

Benefits: We found no systematic review or RCTs (see comment below). **Other lifestyle changes:** We found no studies (see comment below).

Harms: None.

Comment: We found one large questionnaire survey (89 617 European tourists returning from East Africa), which found that wearing long sleeved shirts and trousers significantly reduced the incidence of malaria ($P = 0.02$).[19] Lifestyle change implies not travelling to malaria endemic regions during the rainy season (when most malaria transmission occurs) and not going outdoors in the evening or at night. Travellers who take day trips from a malaria free city to a malaria endemic region may be at minimal risk if they return to the city before dusk.[29] Some authors suggest wearing long sleeved shirts and trousers at dusk and wearing light rather than dark colours, as insects prefer landing on dark surfaces.[9,29]

OPTION TOPICAL (SKIN APPLIED) INSECT REPELLENTS IN ADULTS

We found no RCTs on the effects of topical (skin applied) insect repellents in preventing malaria in travellers. One small crossover RCT found that DEET preparations protected against mosquito bites.

Benefits: We found no systematic review and no RCTs of the effects of topical (skin applied) repellents in preventing malaria in travellers. One small crossover RCT (4 people), involving successive random exposure to female culicine mosquitoes, compared six different controlled release preparations of DEET.[30] It found that all gave at least 95% protection against mosquito bites.[30] **Topical (skin applied) repellents plus insecticide treated clothing:** See insecticide treated clothing in adults, p 917.

Harms: We found a case series of systemic toxic reactions (confusion, irritability, insomnia) in US national park employees after repeated and prolonged use of DEET.[31] We found 14 case reports of contact urticaria and irritant contact dermatitis (mostly in soldiers) as a result of DEET.[19] The risk of absorption is especially high if DEET is left in the antecubital fossa overnight.[32] DEET also degrades certain plastics, such as in spectacle frames.[33]

Comment: DEET is a broad spectrum repellent effective against mosquitoes, biting flies, chiggers, fleas, and ticks, and has been used for over 40 years.[20] Although most authorities would recommend the use of topical (skin applied) repellents in malaria endemic areas, the only evidence comes from small RCTs with non-clinical outcomes. Larger RCTs are needed to compare DEET with other topical (skin applied) repellents and placebo in preventing malaria.

QUESTION What are the effects of drug prophylaxis in adult travellers?

OPTION CHLOROQUINE IN ADULTS

We found no RCTs in travellers on the effects of chloroquine. One RCT in Austrian workers residing in Nigeria found no significant difference between chloroquine and sulfadoxine plus pyrimethamine in the incidence of malaria after 6–22 months.

Benefits: We found no systematic review or RCTs in travellers. One RCT (173 Austrian industrial workers residing in Nigeria) found no significant difference between chloroquine and sulfadoxine plus pyrimethamine in the incidence of malaria after 6–22 months.[34]

Harms: The RCT found that chloroquine was associated with insomnia in 3/87 (3%) people.[35] Two people withdrew from the study because of adverse effects: one with skin rash and the other with visual disturbance. Retrospective questionnaire surveys have suggested that severe adverse effects are rare at prophylactic dosages.[35]

Comment: Alcohol consumption, other medication, and comorbidities can modify the effects of antimalaria drugs.[36,37] *P falciparum* resistance to chloroquine is now established in almost all malaria endemic regions of the world, although there are countries (principally in Central America and the Near East) where there has been no reported resistance as yet.

OPTION CHLOROQUINE PLUS PROGUANIL IN ADULTS

One RCT found no significant difference between chloroquine plus proguanil and chloroquine plus sulfadoxine plus pyrimethamine in the incidence of *P falciparum* malaria. One RCT found no significant difference between chloroquine plus proguanil and proguanil alone in the incidence of *P falciparum* malaria. One RCT found no significant difference between atovaquone plus proguanil and chloroquine plus proguanil in preventing malaria.

Benefits: We found no systematic review but found two RCTs. **Versus chloroquine plus sulfadoxine plus pyrimethamine:** One open label RCT (767 Scandinavian travellers to East Africa) comparing chloroquine plus proguanil versus chloroquine plus sulfadoxine plus pyrimethamine found no significant difference in rates of *P falciparum* malaria (4/384 [1%] *v* 3/383 [0.7%] travellers; RR 1.3, 95% CI 0.3 to 5.9).[38] **Versus proguanil alone:** One RCT in Dutch travellers to Africa found no significant difference between chloroquine 300 mg weekly plus proguanil 200 mg daily and proguanil alone in incidence of *P falciparum* malaria (risk per 100 person months: chloroquine plus proguanil 2.8, 95% CI 0.9 to 10.1 *v* proguanil alone 6.0, 95% CI 2.6 to 14.0).[39] **Versus atovaquone plus proguanil:** See benefits of atovaquone plus proguanil in adults, p 922.

Harms: In the RCT conducted in Scandinavian travellers, adverse effects associated with chloroquine plus proguanil were nausea (3%), diarrhoea (2%), and dizziness (1%).[38] One cohort study (470 British soldiers in Belize) found that the risk of mouth ulcers almost doubled with chloroquine plus proguanil compared with proguanil alone (P = 0.025).[40]

Comment: The incidence of confirmed *P falciparum* malaria in both trials was so low that a clinically important effect cannot be excluded.

OPTION DOXYCYCLINE IN ADULTS

One RCT in soldiers and one RCT in migrants with limited immunity found that doxycycline reduces the risk of malaria compared with placebo. One of the RCTs found that doxycycline was associated with nausea and vomiting, diarrhoea, cough, headache, and unspecified dermatological symptoms over 13 weeks. We found no evidence on long term safety.

Benefits: We found no systematic review but found two RCTs. The first RCT (136 Indonesian soldiers) compared doxycycline versus mefloquine versus placebo in a malaria endemic setting (see comment below).[41] It found that, in an area of drug resistance, doxycycline significantly reduced the risk of malaria compared with placebo (AR 1/67 [2%] with doxycycline *v* 53/69 [77%] with placebo; RR 0.02, 95% CI 0.003 to 0.14; NNT 2, 95% CI 2 to 2).[41] The second RCT (300 Indonesian migrants with limited immunity) comparing azithromycin versus doxycycline versus placebo found that doxycycline significantly reduced the incidence of malaria compared with placebo (2/75 [3%] cases of *P falciparum* malaria with doxycycline *v* 29/77 [38%] with placebo; RR 0.07, 95% CI 0.02 to 0.29; NNT 3, 95% CI 2 to 4; 1/75 [2%] cases of *P vivax* malaria with doxycycline *v* 27/77 [35%] with placebo; RR 0.04, 95% CI 0.01 to 0.28).[42]

Harms: The first RCT found that doxycycline was associated with gastrointestinal symptoms (including nausea and vomiting, abdominal pain, and diarrhoea) in 16/67 (24%) soldiers, unspecified dermatological problems in 22/67 (33%), cough in 21/67 (31%), and headache in 11/67 (16%) over 13 weeks.[41] One questionnaire survey (383 returned Australian travellers taking doxycycline) found that 40% reported nausea or vomiting, 12% reported diarrhoea, and 9% of female travellers reported vaginitis.[43] Evidence from case reports suggests that, in sunny conditions, up to 50% of travellers using doxycycline may experience photoallergic skin rash.[44]

Comment: Most drug trials in travellers have been in soldiers, and the results may not be generalisable to tourists or business travellers.[45,46] The first RCT was a three arm parallel RCT.[41] It compared mefloquine (68 people) versus doxycycline (67 people) versus placebo (69 people). Only the comparison of doxycycline versus placebo is included here.[41]

OPTION MEFLOQUINE IN ADULTS

One systematic review of one RCT in soldiers found that, compared with placebo, mefloquine had a protective efficacy of 100%. One RCT of mefloquine versus atovaquone plus proguanil found no cases of clinical malaria throughout the trial, but found a higher rate of neuropsychiatric harm with mefloquine compared with atovaquone plus proguanil.

Benefits: **Versus placebo:** We found one systematic review (search date 2000) that identified one RCT (203 Indonesian soldiers) comparing mefloquine versus doxycycline versus placebo in a malaria endemic setting (see comment below).[46] It found that, compared with placebo, mefloquine had a protective efficacy of 100%, 95% CI 93% to 100% (malaria cases: 0 in 202 person-months of exposure with mefloquine *v* 53 in 109 person-months of exposure with placebo).[46] **Versus atovaquone plus proguanil:** One RCT (976 people) comparing mefloquine versus atovaquone plus proguanil found no clinical cases of malaria among people included in the trial.[47]

Harms: The systematic review found no significant difference between mefloquine and alternative antimalaria prophylaxis (chloroquine or doxycycline) in withdrawal (29/863 [3%] with mefloquine *v* 20/798 [2%] with alternative prophylaxis; RR 1.32, 95% CI 0.75 to 2.31).[46] Commonly reported adverse effects associated with mefloquine were headache (16%), insomnia (15%), and fatigue (8%).[46] The review found over 500 case reports of mefloquine adverse effects, including four reports of death. These reports suggest that mefloquine is a potentially harmful drug for tourists and business travellers and requires more careful evaluation through an RCT in these groups.[46] One subsequent RCT (1013 non-immune tourists and business travellers) compared mefloquine plus placebo versus atovaquone plus proguanil plus placebo.[47] It found no significant difference in the risk of adverse events (313/493 [63.5%] with atovaquone plus proguanil *v* 324/483 [67.1%] with mefloquine; ARR +2.6%, 95% CI –3.4% to +8.5%). However, when adverse effects specifically attributable to the study drug were analysed, there were significantly more adverse effects caused by mefloquine than by atovaquone plus proguanil (204/483 [42%] with mefloquine *v* 149/493 [30%] with atovaquone plus proguanil; RR 1.40, 95% CI 1.18 to 1.66; NNH 9, 95% CI 6 to 17; see comment below). Specifically, mefloquine versus atovaquone plus proguanil increased the incidence of "strange or vivid dreams" (66/483 [14%] *v* 33/493 [7%]), insomnia (65/483 [13%] *v* 15/493 [3%]), dizziness or vertigo (43/483 [9%] *v* 11/493 [2%]), anxiety (18/483 [4%] *v* 3/493 [1%]), depression (17/483 [4%] *v* 3/493 [1%]), visual difficulties (16/483 [3%] *v* 8/493 [2%]), and headache (19/493 [4%] *v* 32/483 [7%]). Retrospective questionnaire surveys in tourists and business travellers found that sleep disturbance and psychosis were common.[47,48] One review of 74 dermatological case reports found that up to 30% of mefloquine users developed a maculopapular rash and 4–10% had pruritus.[49] Ten cohort studies in tourists found that more women than men experienced adverse effects (including dizziness, sleep disturbance, headache, diarrhoea, and nausea) with mefloquine.[43,48,50–57] One retrospective questionnaire survey of 93 668 European travellers to East Africa found that elderly travellers experienced fewer adverse reactions (not specified) with mefloquine than younger travellers ($P < 0.05$).[58] A review of 516 published case reports suggested that many of mefloquine's adverse effects could be explained as a posthepatic syndrome due to mefloquine use combined with concurrent insults to the liver (such as from alcohol, dehydration, an oral contraceptive pill, recreational drugs, and other liver damaging drugs), and that in some users mefloquine may also cause a symptomatic thyroid disturbance.[59]

Comment: Trials in soldiers may not be generalisable to other travellers. The RCT in Indonesian soldiers was a three arm parallel RCT. It compared mefloquine (68 people) versus doxycycline (67 people) versus placebo (69 people). Only the comparison of mefloquine versus placebo is included here.[46] The subsequent RCT of mefloquine versus atovaquone plus proguanil suggested a higher rate of adverse effects with mefloquine than in previous studies, but this RCT only reported adverse events that occurred after starting active treatment, which was 3 weeks earlier in the mefloquine group than in the atovaquone plus proguanil group.

OPTION ATOVAQUONE PLUS PROGUANIL IN ADULTS

One RCT in migrants with limited immunity found that atovaquone plus proguanil reduced the proportion of people with malaria compared with placebo. One RCT found no significant difference between atovaquone plus proguanil and chloroquine plus proguanil in preventing malaria in travellers. One RCT of mefloquine versus atovaquone plus proguanil found no cases of clinical malaria throughout the trial, but found a higher rate of neuropsychiatric harm with mefloquine compared with atovaquone plus proguanil.

Benefits: We found no systematic review, but found three RCTs.[47,60,61] **Versus placebo:** One RCT (299 Indonesian migrants with limited immunity) found that atovaquone plus proguanil significantly decreased the proportion of people with malaria compared with placebo (AR 3/150 [2%] with atovaquone plus proguanil *v* 37/149 [25%] with placebo; $P < 0.001$).[60] **Versus chloroquine plus proguanil:** One multicentre RCT (1083 travellers) comparing atovaquone plus proguanil versus chloroquine plus proguanil found no significant difference in the incidence of malaria (1/511 [0.2%] cases of *P ovale* malaria with atovaquone plus proguanil *v* 3/511 [0.6%] cases of *P falciparum* malaria with chloroquine plus proguanil; ARR 0.4%; RR 0.33, 95% CI 0.03 to 3.16).[61] **Versus mefloquine:** See benefits of mefloquine in adults, p 921.

Harms: **Versus placebo:** The RCT found that stomatitis ($P < 0.001$) and back pain ($P = 0.009$) occurred significantly more frequently in the atovaquone plus proguanil group, whereas abdominal pain ($P = 0.02$) and malaise ($P = 0.01$) occurred significantly more frequently with placebo (absolute numbers not given).[60] Most adverse events were described as mild or moderate. Four subjects had severe events that were possibly drug related (3 people with abdominal pain and 1 with skin rash).[60] **Versus chloroquine plus**

proguanil: The multicentre RCT in travellers found no significant difference between atovaquone plus proguanil versus chloroquine plus proguanil in one or more adverse events (311/351 [61%] with atovaquone plus proguanil *v* 329/511 [64%] with chloroquine plus proguanil; RR 0.95, 95% CI 0.85 to 1.04).[61] Common adverse effects were mainly gastrointestinal (atovaquone plus proguanil *v* chloroquine plus proguanil: diarrhoea 5% *v* 7%, mouth ulcers 4% *v* 5%, abdominal pain 3% *v* 6%, nausea 2% *v* 7%), neuropsychiatric (atovaquone plus proguanil *v* chloroquine plus proguanil: strange/vivid dreams 4% *v* 3%, dizziness 3% *v* 4%, insomnia 2% *v* 2%), and visual difficulties (2% *v* 2%).[61] **Versus mefloquine:** See harms of mefloquine in adults, p 921.

Comment: None.

OPTION AMODIAQUINE IN ADULTS

We found no RCTs on the effects of amodiaquine in preventing malaria in travellers. We found limited observational evidence that amodiaquine may cause liver damage and hepatitis.

Benefits: We found no RCTs in travellers.

Harms: One retrospective cohort study in 10 000 British travellers taking prophylactic amodiaquine reported severe neutropenia in about 1/2000 users.[62] We found 28 case reports describing liver damage or hepatitis in travellers who had taken amodiaquine to treat or prevent malaria.[63–68]

Comment: None.

OPTION PYRIMETHAMINE PLUS DAPSONE IN ADULTS

We found no RCTs in travellers. One RCT in Thai soldiers found insufficient evidence to compare pyrimethamine plus dapsone versus proguanil plus dapsone.

Benefits: We found no RCTs in travellers. One RCT in Thai soldiers comparing pyrimethamine plus dapsone versus proguanil plus dapsone found no significant difference in *P falciparum* infection rates over 40 days (10.3% with proguanil plus dapsone *v* 11.3% with pyrimethamine plus dapsone; results presented graphically, P value not reported) but found a significantly lower *P vivax* infection rate with proguanil plus dapsone compared with pyrimethamine plus dapsone (1.6% *v* 12.4%; results presented graphically, $P < 0.001$).[69]

Harms: The RCT in Thai soldiers found that fewer than 2% reported any drug related symptoms from pyrimethamine plus dapsone.[69] One retrospective cohort study in 15 000 Swedish travellers taking pyrimethamine plus dapsone reported agranulocytosis in about 1/2000 users.[70]

Comment: None.

OPTION SULFADOXINE PLUS PYRIMETHAMINE IN ADULTS

One RCT found no significant difference between chloroquine plus proguanil and chloroquine plus sulfadoxine plus pyrimethamine in the incidence of *P falciparum* malaria. One retrospective observational study suggested that sulfadoxine plus pyrimethamine was associated with severe cutaneous reactions.

Benefits: We found no RCTs of sulfadoxine plus pyrimethamine alone. We found one RCT of sulfadoxine plus pyrimethamine plus chloroquine versus chloroquine plus proguanil (see benefits of chloroquine plus proguanil in adults, p 919).

Harms: One retrospective observational study in 182 300 US travellers taking prophylactic sulfadoxine plus pyrimethamine reported severe cutaneous reactions (erythema multiforme, Stevens-Johnson syndrome, toxic epidermal necrolysis) in 1/5000–8000 users, with a mortality of about 1/11 000–25 000 users.[70]

Comment: None.

QUESTION What are the effects of antimalaria vaccines in travellers?

We found no RCTs in travellers of the effects of antimalaria vaccines. One systematic review of antimalaria vaccines in residents of malaria endemic areas found that the SPf66 vaccine reduces first attacks of malaria compared with placebo.

Benefits: We found no systematic review or RCTs of antimalaria vaccines in travellers. One systematic review (search date 1999, 13 RCTs) of antimalaria vaccines in residents of malaria endemic areas found that the SPf66 vaccine significantly reduced first attacks of *P falciparum* malaria compared with placebo (1039/3718 [28%] with SPf66 *v* 1108/3681 [30%] with placebo; RR 0.90, 95% CI 0.84 to 0.96).[71]

Harms: The systematic review found that, in all but one of the RCTs of the SPf66 vaccine, fewer than 10% of recipients reported a systemic reaction (fever, headache, gastric symptoms, muscle pain, dizziness), and fewer than 35% reported a local reaction (inflammation, nodules, pain, erythema, pruritus, induration, injection site warmth).[71] The remaining RCT found a larger proportion of local cutaneous reactions, although these resolved within 24 hours with symptomatic treatment. It also reported higher systemic reaction rates after vaccination (11–16%), although rates after placebo were also higher (10–13%). Surveillance was also more intense than in the other RCTs.

Comment: None.

QUESTION What are the effects of antimalaria interventions in child travellers?

OPTION TOPICAL (SKIN APPLIED) INSECT REPELLENTS CONTAINING DEET IN CHILDREN

We found no RCTs on the effects of DEET in preventing malaria in child travellers. Case reports in young children found serious adverse effects with DEET.

Benefits: We found no systematic review or RCTs.

Harms: We found 13 case reports of encephalopathic toxicity in children aged under 8 years after excessive use (not clearly defined) of topical (skin applied) insect repellents containing DEET.[72,73]

Comment: Infants and young children have thinner skin and greater surface area to mass ratio.[74] Some authors advise that ethylhexanediol should be issued as a topical (skin applied) insect repellent in preference to DEET in children aged 1–8 years;[75] however, we found insufficient evidence.

OPTION DOXYCYCLINE IN CHILDREN

We found no RCTs in child travellers on the use of doxycycline. Case reports in young children found adverse effects with doxycycline.

Benefits: We found no systematic review or RCTs.

Harms: Case reports have found that doxycycline inhibits bone growth and discolours teeth in children aged under 12 years.[9,35]

Comment: None.

OPTION MEFLOQUINE IN CHILDREN

We found no RCTs of the effects of mefloquine in preventing malaria in child travellers.

Benefits: We found no systematic review or RCTs.

Harms: Three RCTs in children and adults with symptomatic *P falciparum* malaria found that mefloquine was associated with less vomiting, nausea, anorexia, diarrhoea, and dizziness in children than in adults.[76–78]

Comment: None.

QUESTION What are the effects of antimalaria interventions in pregnant travellers?

OPTION INSECTICIDE TREATED NETS IN PREGNANT TRAVELLERS

We found no RCTs on the effects of insecticide treated nets in preventing malaria in pregnant travellers. One RCT of pregnant residents of a malaria endemic area found insufficient evidence on the effects of permethrin treated nets in preventing malaria.

Benefits: We found no systematic review or RCTs in pregnant travellers. We found one RCT (341 pregnant women living in Thailand, 3 sites in a malaria endemic area), which compared permethrin treated nets versus non-treated nets versus usual practice.[79] Two sites found no significant difference in the incidence of malaria with treated nets, whereas the third site found that treated nets significantly reduced the incidence of malaria.

Harms: We found no evidence relating to pregnant travellers. The RCT of permethrin treated nets in Thailand found no evidence of toxic effects to mother or fetus.[79]

Comment: Pregnant women are relatively immunosuppressed and are at greater risk of malaria than non-pregnant women.[80] Contracting malaria significantly increases the likelihood of losing the fetus.[81]

OPTION INSECTICIDE TREATED CLOTHING IN PREGNANT TRAVELLERS

We found no RCTs in pregnant travellers of the effects of impregnated clothing.

Benefits: We found no systematic review or RCTs.

Harms: We found little evidence relating to pregnant travellers. **Permethrin:** One RCT (341 pregnant women living in Thailand) of permethrin treated nets found no evidence of toxic effects to mother or fetus.[79] **DEET:** See harms of topical (skin applied) insect repellents in pregnant travellers, p 926.

Comment: Pregnant women are relatively immunosuppressed and are at greater risk of malaria than non-pregnant women.[80] Contracting malaria significantly increases the likelihood of losing the fetus.[81]

OPTION TOPICAL (SKIN APPLIED) INSECT REPELLENTS IN PREGNANT TRAVELLERS

We found no RCTs in pregnant travellers. It is unclear which topical (skin applied) insect repellents are safe in pregnancy.

Benefits: We found no systematic review or RCTs.

Harms: We found little evidence in pregnant travellers. **DEET:** We found one case report indicating an adverse fetal outcome (mental retardation, impaired sensorimotor coordination, craniofacial dysmorphology) in a child whose mother had applied DEET daily throughout her pregnancy.[82] One RCT in pregnant women (897 refugees in a Thai forest area of low malaria endemicity) comparing DEET (median dose 214.2 g per pregnancy) versus a cosmetic cream found no differences in weekly reporting of headache, dizziness, or nausea and vomiting. It also found no adverse effects on infant survival, growth, or development at either birth or 1 year (survival 95.2% with DEET *v* 94.0% without DEET, $P = 0.57$; mean weight at 1 year 7983 g with DEET *v* 7984 g without DEET).[83] Some animal studies have found that DEET crosses the placental barrier.[84] Animal studies of reproductive effects of DEET are inconclusive.[81,85]

Comment: The RCT in refugees reported that DEET significantly increased the number of women reporting skin warmth (359/449 [80%] with DEET *v* 258/448 [58%] with cosmetic cream; RR 1.39, 95% CI 1.27 to 1.52), although the clinical significance of this is unclear.[83] Pregnant women are relatively immunosuppressed and are at greater risk of malaria than non-pregnant women.[80] Contracting malaria significantly increases the likelihood of losing the fetus.[81] Some authors advise that only plant derived skin applied insect repellents are safe in pregnancy because of a potential risk of mutagenicity from DEET.[75] However, we found no evidence on the effects of alternative repellents.

OPTION ANTIMALARIA DRUGS IN PREGNANT TRAVELLERS

We found no RCTs on the effects of antimalaria drugs in pregnant travellers. We found insufficient evidence on the safety of chloroquine, doxycycline, and mefloquine in pregnancy.

Benefits: We found one systematic review (search date 2000), which identified no RCTs in pregnant travellers. It identified 15 RCTs of antimalaria drugs in pregnancy: all in residents of malaria endemic settings.[86] It found that antimalaria prophylaxis significantly reduced the number of women infected at least once compared with no prophylaxis (5/167 [3%] *v* 37/170 [22%]; RR 0.14, 95% CI 0.06 to 0.34) and significantly reduced the number of episodes of fever (22/119 [18%] with prophylaxis *v* 45/108 [42%] with no prophylaxis; RR 0.42, 95% CI 0.27 to 0.66). It found no significant difference between antimalaria prophylaxis and no prophylaxis in the number of perinatal deaths (66/1494 [4%] *v* 64/1426 [4%]; RR 1.02, 95% CI 0.73 to 1.43) or preterm births (17/182 [9%] with prophylaxis *v* 22/175 [12%] with no prophylaxis; RR 0.75, 95% CI 0.42 to 1.35), but found that antimalaria prophylaxis resulted in significantly higher birth weight in the infant compared with no prophylaxis (OR 0.53, 95% CI 0.32 to 0.81).[86]

Harms: **Chloroquine:** One RCT (1464 pregnant long term residents of Burkina Faso) gave no information on adverse effects.[87] **Doxycycline:** Case reports have found that doxycycline taken in pregnancy or while breast feeding may damage fetal or infant bones or teeth.[9,35] **Mefloquine:** One RCT (339 long term Thai residents) found that mefloquine versus placebo significantly increased the number of women reporting dizziness (28% with mefloquine *v* 14% with placebo; $P < 0.005$), but found no other significant adverse effects on the mother, the pregnancy, or on infant survival or development over 2 years' follow up.[88]

Comment: Pregnant women are relatively immunosuppressed and are at greater risk of malaria than non-pregnant women.[80] Contracting malaria significantly increases the likelihood of losing the fetus.[81] Mefloquine is secreted in small quantities in breast milk, but it is believed that levels are too low to harm infants.[35]

QUESTION What are the effects of antimalaria interventions in airline pilots?

OPTION ANTIMALARIA DRUGS IN AIRLINE PILOTS

We found no RCTs on the effects of antimalaria drugs in airline pilots.

Benefits: We found no systematic review or RCTs (see comment below).

Harms: **Doxycycline:** One retrospective questionnaire survey (28 Israeli pilots) found that 39% experienced adverse effects from doxycycline (abdominal pain 7/28, fatigue 5/28; see comment below).[89]
Mefloquine: One placebo controlled RCT of adverse effects (23 trainee commercial pilots) found no evidence that mefloquine significantly affected flying performance (mean total number of errors recorded by the instrument coordination analyser 12.6 with mefloquine *v* 11.7 with placebo).[90] One retrospective questionnaire survey (15 Israeli non-aviator aircrew) found that 13% experienced adverse effects from mefloquine (dizziness, nausea, and abdominal pain in 2/15, abdominal discomfort in 1/15; see comment below).[89]

Comment: One retrospective questionnaire survey (28 Israeli pilots taking doxycycline and 15 non-aviator crew taking mefloquine) found no cases of malaria at 4 weeks.[89]

GLOSSARY

Biological control measures Antimosquito interventions based on modifying the local flora or fauna.

Substantive changes

Atovaquone plus proguanil One RCT added;[60] recategorised as Likely to be beneficial.

REFERENCES

1. White NJ. Malaria. In: Cook GC, ed. *Manson's tropical diseases*. 20th ed. London: WB Saunders, 1996:1087–1164.
2. World Health Organization. *The world health report 1997. Conquering suffering, enriching humanity*. Geneva: WHO Office of Information, 1997.
3. Murphy GS, Oldfield EC. Falciparum malaria. *Infect Dis Clin North Am* 1996;10:747–755.
4. Kain KC, Keystone JS. Malaria in travelers. Epidemiology, disease and prevention. *Infect Dis Clin North Am* 1998;12:267–284.
5. World Health Organization. *International Travel and Health*. Geneva: WHO, 1999.
6. Winstanley P. Malaria: treatment. *J R Coll Physicians Lond* 1998;32:203–207.
7. Baudon D, Martet G. Paludisme et voyageurs: protection et information [in French]. *Med Trop (Mars)* 1997;57:497–500.
8. *Health information for international travel, 1996–97*. Atlanta: US Department of Health and Human Services, Public Health Service, Centers for Disease Control and Prevention, National Center for Infectious Diseases, Division of Quarantine; 1997 HHS Publication No 95:8280.
9. Bradley DJ, Warhurst DC. Guidelines for the prevention of malaria in travellers from the United Kingdom. *Commun Dis Rep CDR Rev* 1997;7:R137–R152.
10. Krogstad DJ. Malaria as a reemerging disease. *Epidemiol Rev* 1996;18:77–89.
11. Hill AVS. Malaria resistance genes: a natural selection. *Trans R Soc Trop Med Hyg* 1992;86:225–232.
12. Fleming AF. Haematological diseases in the tropics. In: Cook GC, ed. *Manson's tropical diseases*. 20th ed. London: WB Saunders, 1996:101–173.
13. Olsen VV. Basic considerations in connection with malaria prophylaxis [in Danish]. *Ugeskr Læger* 1998;160:2410–2411.
14. Miller SA, Bergman BP, Croft AM. Epidemiology of malaria in the British Army from 1982–1986. *J R Army Med Corps* 1999;145:20–22.
15. Dolmans WMV, van der Kaay HJ, Leentvaar-Kuijpers A, et al. Malariaprofylaxe: adviezen wederom aangepast. *Ned Tijdschr Geneeskd* 1996;140:892–893.
16. Beier JC, Oster CN, Onyango FK, et al. *Plasmodium falciparum* incidence relative to entomological inoculation rates at a site proposed for testing malaria vaccines in western Kenya. *Am J Trop Med Hyg* 1994;50;529–536.
17. Misra SP, Webber R, Lines J, et al. Spray versus treated nets using deltamethrin — a community randomized trial in India. *Trans R Soc Trop Med Hyg* 1999;93:456–457.
18. Rowland M, Mahmood P, Iqbal J, et al. Indoor residual spraying with alphacypermethrin controls malaria in Pakistan: a community-randomized trial. *Trop Med Int Health* 2000;5:472–481.
19. Schoepke A, Steffen R, Gratz N. Effectiveness of personal protection measures against mosquito

bites for malaria prophylaxis in travelers. *J Travel Med* 1998;128:931–940.
20. Fradin MS. Mosquitoes and mosquito repellents: a clinician's guide. *Ann Intern Med* 1998;128:931–940. Search date 1997; primary sources Medline, the Internet, the Extension Toxicology Network database, hand searches of reference lists, and contact with distributors of natural insect repellents.
21. Hewitt SE, Farhan M, Urhaman H, et al. Self-protection from malaria vectors in Pakistan: an evaluation of popular existing methods and appropriate new techniques in Afghan refugee communities. *Ann Trop Med Parasitol* 1996;90:337–344.
22. Service MW. *Mosquito ecology: field sampling methods*. 2nd ed. London: Chapman and Hall, 1993.
23. Sylla el-HK, Lell B, Krsmsner PG. A blinded, controlled trial of an ultrasound device as mosquito repellent. *Wein Klin Wochenschr* 2000;112:448–450.
24. Yap HH, Tan HT, Yahaya AM, et al. Field efficacy of mosquito coil formulations containing d-allethrin and d-transallethrin against indoor mosquitoes especially *Culex quinquefasciatus*. *Southeast Asian J Trop Med Public Health* 1990;21:558–563.
25. Vernède R, van Meer MMM, Aplers MP. Smoke as a form of personal protection against mosquitoes, a field study in Papua New Guinea. *Southeast Asian J Trop Med Public Health* 1994;25:771–775.
26. Lengeler C. Insecticide treated bednets and curtains for preventing malaria. In: The Cochrane Library, Issue 4, 2002. Oxford: Update Software. Search date not stated; primary sources Cochrane Infectious Diseases Group Trial Register, Medline, Embase, and hand searches of reference lists, relevant journals, and personal contact with funding agencies and manufacturers.
27. Soto J, Medina F, Dember N, Berman J. Efficacy of permethrin-impregnated uniforms in the prevention of malaria and leishmaniasis in Colombian soldiers. *Clin Infect Dis* 1995;21:599–602.
28. Rowland M, Durrani N, Hewitt S, et al. Permethrin-treated *chaddars* and top-sheets: appropriate technology for protection against malaria in Afghanistan and other complex emergencies. *Trans R Soc Trop Med Hyg* 1999;93:465–472.
29. Juckett G. Malaria prevention in travelers. *Am Fam Physician* 1999;59:2523–2530.
30. Gupta RK, Rutledge LC. Laboratory evaluation of controlled-release repellent formulations on human volunteers under three climatic regimens. *J Am Mosq Control Assoc* 1989;5:52–55.
31. McConnell R, Fidler AT, Chrislip D. Everglades National Park health hazard evaluation report. Cincinatti, Ohio: US Department of Health and Human Services, Public Health Service, 1986. NIOSH Health Hazard Evaluation Report No. HETA-83-085-1757.
32. Lamberg SI, Mulrennan JA. Bullous reaction to diethyl toluamide (DEET) resembling a blistering insect eruption. *Arch Dermatol* 1969;100:582–586.
33. Curtis CF, Townson H. Malaria: existing methods of vector control and molecular entomology. *Br Med Bull* 1998;54:311–325.
34. Stemberger H, Leimer R, Widermann G. Tolerability of long-term prophylaxis with Fansidar: a randomized double-blind study in Nigeria. *Acta Trop* 1984;41:391–399.
35. Petersen E. Malariaprofylakse. *Ugeskr Læger* 1997;159:2723–2730.
36. Gherardin T. Mefloquine as malaria prophylaxis. *Aust Fam Physician* 1999;28:310.
37. Schlagenhauf P. Mefloquine for malaria chemoprophylaxis 1992–1998: a review. *J Travel Med* 1999;6:122–133.
38. Fogh S, Schapira A, Bygbjerg IC, et al. Malaria chemoprophylaxis in travellers to east Africa: a comparative prospective study of chloroquine plus proguanil with chloroquine plus sulfadoxine-pyrimethamine. *BMJ* 1988;296:820–822.
39. Wetsteyn JCFM, de Geus A. Comparison of three regimens for malaria prophylaxis in travellers to east, central, and southern Africa. *BMJ* 1993;307:1041–1043.
40. Drysdale SF, Phillips-Howard PA, Behrens RH. Proguanil, chloroquine, and mouth ulcers. *Lancet* 1990;335:164.
41. Ohrt C, Richie TL, Widjaja H, et al. Mefloquine compared with doxycycline for the prophylaxis of malaria in Indonesian soldiers. A randomized, double-blind, placebo-controlled trial. *Ann Intern Med* 1997;126:963–972.
42. Taylor WR, Richie TL, Fryauff DJ, et al. Malaria prophylaxis using azithromycin: a double-blind, placebo-controlled trial in Irian Jaya, Indonesia. *Clin Infect Dis* 1999;28:74–81.
43. Phillips MA, Kass RB. User acceptability patterns for mefloquine and doxycycline malaria chemoprophylaxis. *J Travel Med* 1996;3:40–45.
44. Leutscher PDC. Malariaprofylakse. *Ugeskr Læger* 1997;159:4866–4867.
45. Anonymous. Mefloquine and malaria prophylaxis [letter]. *Drug Ther Bull* 1998;36:20–22.
46. Croft AMJ, Garner P. Mefloquine for preventing malaria in non-immune adult travellers. In: The Cochrane Library, Issue 4, 2002. Oxford: Update Software. Search date 2000; primary sources Cochrane Infectious Diseases Group Trial Register, Medline, Embase, Lilacs, Science Citation Index, hand searches of reference lists of articles, and personal contact with researchers in the subject of malaria chemoprophylaxis and drug companies.
47. Overbosch D, Schilthuis H, Bienzle U, et al. Atovaquone-proguanil versus mefloquine for malaria prophylaxis in nonimmune travelers: results from a randomized double-blind study. *Clin Infect Dis* 2001;33:1015–1021.
48. Barrett PJ, Emmins PD, Clarke PD, Bradley DJ. Comparison of adverse events associated with use of mefloquine and combinations of chloroquine and proguanil as antimalarial prophylaxis: postal and telephone survey of travellers. *BMJ* 1996;313:525–528.
49. Smith HR, Croft AM, Black MM. Dermatological adverse effects with the antimalarial drug mefloquine: a review of 74 published case reports. *Clin Exp Dermatol* 1999;24:249–254.
50. Weinke T, Trautmann M, Held T, et al. Neuropsychiatric side effects after the use of mefloquine. *Am J Trop Med Hyg* 1991;45:86–91.
51. Bem L, Kerr L, Stuerchler D. Mefloquine prophylaxis: an overview of spontaneous reports of severe psychiatric reactions and convulsions. *J Trop Med Hyg* 1992;95:167–169.
52. Huzly D, Schönfeld C, Beurle W, et al. Malaria chemoprophylaxis in German tourists: a prospective study on compliance and adverse reactions. *J Travel Med* 1996;3:148–155.
53. Schlagenhauf P, Steffen R, Lobel H, et al. Mefloquine tolerability during chemoprophylaxis: focus on adverse event assessments, stereochemistry and compliance. *Trop Med Int Health* 1996;1:485–494.
54. Handschin JC, Wall M, Steffen R, et al. Tolerability and effectiveness of malaria chemoprophylaxis with mefloquine or chloroquine with or without co-medication. *J Travel Med* 1997;4:121–127.
55. Van Riemsdijk MM, van der Klauw MM, van Heest JAC, et al. Neuro-psychiatric effects of antimalarials. *Eur J Clin Pharmacol* 1997;52:1–6.
56. Micheo C, Arias C, Rovira A. Adverse effects and compliance with mefloquine or

chloroquine + proguanil malaria chemoprophylaxis. *Proceedings of the Second European Conference on Travel Medicine*, Venice, Italy, 2000:29–31.
57. van Riemsdijk MM, Ditters JM, Sturkenboom MCJM, et al. Neuropsychiatric events during prophylactic use of mefloquine before travelling. *Eur J Clin Pharmacol* 2002;58:441–445.
58. Mittelholzer ML, Wall M, Steffen R, et al. Malaria prophylaxis in different age groups. *J Travel Med* 1996;4:219–223.
59. Croft AM, Herxheimer A. Adverse effects of the antimalaria drug, mefloquine: due to primary liver damage with secondary thyroid involvement? *BMC Public Health* 2002;2:6.
60. Ling J, Baird JK, Fryauff DJ, et al. Randomized, placebo-controlled trial of atovaquone/proguanil for the prevention of *Plasmodium falciparum* or *Plasmodium vivax* malaria among migrants to Papua, Indonesia. *Clin Infect Dis* 2002;35:825–833.
61. Hogh B, Clarke PD, Camus D, et al. Atovaquone-proguanil versus chloroquine-proguanil for malaria prophylaxis in non-immune travellers: a randomised, double-blind study. *Lancet* 2000;356:1888–1894.
62. Hatton CSR, Peto TEA, Bunch C, et al. Frequency of severe neutropenia associated with amodiaquine prophylaxis against malaria. *Lancet* 1986;1:411–414.
63. Neftel K, Woodtly W, Schmid M, et al. Amodiaquine induced agranulocytosis and liver damage. *BMJ* 1986;292:721–723.
64. Larrey D, Castot A, Pessayre D, et al. Amodiaquine-induced hepatitis. A report of seven cases. *Ann Intern Med* 1986;104:801–803.
65. Woodtli W, Vonmoos P, Siegrist P, et al. Amodiaquin-induzierte hepatitis mit leukopenie. *Schweiz Med Wochenschr* 1986;116:966–968.
66. Bernuau J, Larrey D, Campillo B, et al. Amodiaquine-induced fulminant hepatitis. *J Hepatol* 1988;6:109–112.
67. Charmot G, Goujon C. Hépatites mineures pouvant être duesà l'amodiaquine. *Bull Soc Pathol Exot* 1987;80:266–270.
68. Raymond JM, Dumas F, Baldit C, et al. Fatal acute hepatitis due to amodiaquine. *J Clin Gastroenterol* 1989;11:602–603.
69. Shanks GD, Edstein MD, Suriyamongkol V, et al. Malaria chemoprohylaxis using proguanil/dapsone combinations on the Thai-Cambodian border. *Am J Trop Med Hyg* 1992;46:6543–648.
70. Miller KD, Lobel HO, Satriale RF, et al. Severe cutaneous reactions among American travelers using pyrimethamine-sulfadoxine for malaria prophylaxis. *Am J Trop Med Hyg* 1986;35:451–458.
71. Graves P, Gelbland H. Vaccines for preventing malaria. In: The Cochrane Library, Issue 4, 2002. Oxford: Update Software. Search date 1999; primary sources Cochrane Infectious Diseases Group Trials Register, Cochrane Controlled Trial Register, Medline, Embase, hand searches of reference lists, and personal contact with organisations and researchers in the field.
72. Osimitz TG, Murphy JV. Neurological effects associated with use of the insect repellent *N,N*-diethyl-*m*-toluamide (DEET). *J Toxicol Clin Toxicol* 1997;35:435–441.
73. De Garbino JP, Laborde A. Toxicity of an insect repellent: *N,N*-diethyl-*m*-toluamide. *Vet Hum Toxicol* 1983;25:422–423.
74. Are insect repellents safe [editorial]? *Lancet* 1988;ii:610–611.
75. Bouchaud O, Longuet C, Coulaud JP. Prophylaxie du paludisme. *Rev Prat* 1998;48:279–286.
76. Smithuis FM, van Woensel JBM, Nordlander E, et al. Comparison of two mefloquine regimens for treatment of *Plasmodium falciparum* malaria on the northeastern Thai-Cambodian border. *Antimicrob Agents Chemother* 1993;37:1977–1981.
77. Ter Kuile FO, Dolan G, Nosten F, et al. Halofantrine versus mefloquine in treatment of multidrug-resistant falciparum malaria. *Lancet* 1993;341:1044–1049.
78. Luxemburger C, Price RN, Nosten F, et al. Mefloquine in infants and young children. *Ann Trop Paediatr* 1996;16:281–286.
79. Dolan G, ter Kuile FO, Jacoutot V, et al. Bed nets for the prevention of malaria and anaemia in pregnancy. *Trans R Soc Trop Med Hyg* 1993;87:620–626.
80. Suh KN, Keystone JS. Malaria prophylaxis in pregnancy and children. *Infect Dis Clin Pract* 1996;5:541–546.
81. Osimitz TG, Grothaus RH. The present safety assessment of DEET. *J Am Mosq Control Assoc* 1995;11:274–278.
82. Schaefer C, Peters PW. Intrauterine diethyltoluamide exposure and fetal outcome. *Reprod Toxicol* 1992;6:175–176.
83. McGready R, Hamilton KA, Simpson JA, et al. Safety of the insect repellent *N,N*-diethyl-*m*-toluamide (DEET) in pregnancy. *Am J Trop Med Hyg* 2001;65:285–289.
84. Blomquist L, Thorsell W. Distribution and fate of the insect repellent 14C-*N,N*-diethyl-*m*-toluamide in the animal body. II. Distribution and excretion after cutaneous application. *Acta Pharmacol Toxicol (Copenh)* 1977;41:235–243.
85. Samuel BU, Barry M. The pregnant traveler. *Infect Dis Clin North Am* 1998;12:325–354.
86. Garner P, Gülmezoglu AM. Prevention versus treatment for malaria in pregnant women. In: The Cochrane Library, Issue 4, 2002. Oxford: Update Software. Search date 2000; primary sources Cochrane Infectious Diseases Group Trial Register, Cochrane Controlled Trials Register, Medline, Embase, hand searches of reference lists, and personal contact with researchers.
87. Cot M, Roisin A, Barro D, et al. Effect of chloroquine chemoprophylaxis during pregnancy on birth weight: results of a randomized trial. *Am J Trop Med Hyg* 1992;46:21–27.
88. Nosten F, ter Kuile F, Maelankiri L, et al. Mefloquine prophylaxis prevents malaria during pregnancy: a double-blind, placebo-controlled study. *J Infect Dis* 1994;169:595–603.
89. Shamiss A, Atar E, Zohar L, Cain Y. Mefloquine versus doxycycline for malaria prophylaxis in intermittent exposure of Israeli Air Force aircrew in Rwanda. *Aviat Space Environ Med* 1996;67:872–873.
90. Schlagenhauf P, Lobel H, Steffen R, et al. Tolerance of mefloquine by Swissair trainee pilots. *Am J Trop Med Hyg* 1997;56:235–240.

Ashley M Croft
Director of Public Health
NATO Headquarters Rheindahlen, Mönchengladbach, Germany

Competing interests: None declared.

Meningococcal disease

Search date March 2003

Jailson B Correia and C A Hart

QUESTIONS

INTERVENTIONS

Likely to be beneficial

Antibiotics for throat carriage (reduce carriage but unknown effect on risk of disease) . . .933

Pre-admission parenteral penicillin in suspected cases*. 934

Prophylactic antibiotics in contacts* 933

To be covered in future updates

Hospital treatment of meningococcal disease

Vaccines (monovalent/multivalent, polysaccharide alone, or conjugate)

*Based on observational evidence. RCTs unlikely to be conducted

See glossary, p 935

Key Messages

- **Antibiotics for throat carriage (reduce carriage but unknown effect on risk of disease)** RCTs have found that antibiotics reduce throat carriage of meningococci compared with placebo. We found no evidence that eradicating throat carriage reduces the risk of meningococcal disease.
- **Pre-admission parenteral penicillin in suspected cases** We found no RCTs on the effects of pre-admission antibiotics in suspected cases. It is unlikely that RCTs will be performed because of the unpredictably rapid course of meningococcal disease in some people, the likely risks involved in delaying treatment, and the low risk of causing harm. Most observational studies suggest benefit with antibiotics, but at least one did not.
- **Prophylactic antibiotics in contacts** We found no RCTs on the effects of prophylactic antibiotics on the incidence of meningococcal disease among contacts. RCTs are unlikely to be performed because the intervention has few associated risks whereas meningococcal disease has high associated risks. Observational evidence suggests that antibiotics reduce the risk of meningococcal disease. We found no evidence regarding which contacts should be treated.

Meningococcal disease

DEFINITION Meningococcal disease is any clinical condition caused by *Neisseria meningitidis* (the meningococcus) groups A, B, C, W135, or other serogroups. These conditions include purulent conjunctivitis, septic arthritis, meningitis, and septicaemia (see glossary, p 935) with or without meningitis.

INCIDENCE/ PREVALENCE Meningococcal disease is sporadic in temperate countries, and is most commonly caused by group B or C meningococci. Annual incidence in Europe varies from fewer than 1 case/100 000 people in France, up to 4–5 cases/100 000 people in the UK and Spain, and in the USA it is 0.6–1.5/100 000 people.[1,2] Occasional outbreaks occur among close family contacts (see glossary, p 935), secondary school pupils, military recruits, and students living in halls of residence. Sub-Saharan Africa has regular epidemics in countries lying in the expanded "meningitis belt", reaching 500/ 100 000 people during epidemics, which are usually due to serogroup A, although recent outbreaks of serogroup W135 cause concern.[3–5]

AETIOLOGY/ RISK FACTORS The meningococcus colonises and infects healthy people and is transmitted by close contact, probably by exchange of upper respiratory tract secretions (see table 1, p 938).[6–14] Risk of transmission is greatest during the first week of contact.[9] Risk factors include crowding and exposure to cigarette smoke.[15] In the UK, children younger than 2 years have the highest incidence, with a second peak between ages 15–24 years. There is currently an increased incidence of meningococcal disease among university students, especially among those in their first term and living in catered accommodation,[16] although we found no accurate numerical estimate of risk from close contact in, for example, halls of residence. Close contacts of an index case have a much higher risk of infection than do people in the general population.[9,12,13] The risk of epidemic spread is higher with groups A and C meningococci than with group B meningococci.[6–8,10] It is not known what makes a meningococcus virulent. Certain clones tend to predominate at different times and in different groups. Carriage of meningococcus in the throat has been reported in 10–15% of people; recent acquisition of a virulent meningococcus is more likely to be associated with invasive disease.

PROGNOSIS Mortality is highest in infants and adolescents, and is related to disease presentation and availability of therapeutic resources. In developed countries case fatality rates have been around 19–25% for septicaemia, 10–12% for meningitis plus septicaemia, and less than 1% in meningitis alone, but an overall reduction in mortality was observed in recent years in people admitted to paediatric intensive care units.[17–21]

AIMS OF INTERVENTION To prevent disease in contacts; to prevent development of meningococcal disease and its complications.

OUTCOMES Rates of infection; rates of eradication of throat carriage; adverse effects of treatment; case–fatality; sequelae.

METHODS *Clinical Evidence* search and appraisal March 2003, including a search for observational studies. In addition, the authors drew from a collection of references from the pre-electronic data era and cross-references from relevant papers.

QUESTION **What are the effects of interventions to prevent meningococcal disease in contacts and carriers?**

OPTION **PROPHYLACTIC ANTIBIOTICS IN CONTACTS**

We found no RCTs on the effects of prophylactic antibiotics on the incidence of meningococcal disease among contacts. One observational study suggested that sulfadiazine reduced the risk of meningococcal disease over 8 weeks. We found no good evidence regarding which contacts should be treated.

Benefits: We found no systematic review and no RCTs examining the effect of prophylactic antibiotics in people in contact (see glossary, p 935) with someone with meningococcal disease (see comment below). **Rifampicin:** We found only anecdotal data. **Phenoxymethylpenicillin:** We found one retrospective study, but the results of that study cannot be generalised beyond the sample tested.[22] **Sulfadiazine:** One cohort study of soldiers in temporary troop camps in the 1940s compared the incidence of meningococcal disease in camps where sulfadiazine (sulphadiazine) was given to everyone after a meningococcal outbreak versus the incidence in camps where no prophylaxis was given.[23] The study reported a higher incidence of meningococcal disease in soldiers not given prophylaxis (approximate figures 17/9500 [0.18%] *v* 2/7000 [0.03%] over 8 weeks).

Harms: **Rifampicin:** No excess adverse effects compared with placebo were found in RCTs on eradicating throat carriage of meningococcal disease.[24,25] However, rifampicin is known to cause various adverse effects, including turning urine and contact lenses orange, and inducing hepatic microsomal enzymes, potentially rendering oral contraception ineffective. Rifampicin prophylaxis may be associated with emergence of resistant strains.[26] **Sulfadiazine:** One in 10 soldiers experienced minor adverse events, including headache, dizziness, tinnitus, and nausea.[23]

Comment: RCTs addressing this question are unlikely to be performed because the intervention has few associated risks whereas meningococcal disease has high associated risks. RCTs would also need to be large to find a difference in incidence of meningococcal disease. In the sulfadiazine cohort study, the two infected people in the treatment group only became infected after leaving the camp.[23]

OPTION **ANTIBIOTICS FOR THROAT CARRIAGE**

RCTs have found that antibiotics reduce throat carriage of meningococci compared with placebo. We found no evidence that eradicating throat carriage reduces the risk of meningococcal disease.

Benefits: We found no systematic review. **Incidence of disease:** We found no RCTs or observational studies that examined whether eradicating throat carriage (see glossary, p 935) of meningococcus reduces the risk of meningococcal disease. **Throat carriage:** We found five placebo controlled RCTs that examined the effect of antibiotics on carriage of meningococcus in the throat (see table 2, p 939).[24,25,27–29] All trials found that antibiotics (rifampicin, minocycline, or ciprofloxacin) achieved high rates of eradication (ranging from 90–97%), except one trial of rifampicin in students with heavy growth on culture, in which the rate of eradication was 73%.[24] Eradication rates on placebo ranged from 9–29%. We found seven RCTs that compared different antibiotic regimens (see table 3, p 940).[30–36] Three RCTs found no significant difference between rifampicin and minocycline, ciprofloxacin, or intramuscular ceftriaxone.[31,34,36] A fourth RCT randomised households to different treatments and found that intramuscular ceftriaxone increased eradication rates compared with rifampicin.[33] However, that trial used cluster randomisation, and therefore the results should be interpreted with caution. Another trial found no significant difference between oral azithromycin and rifampicin in eradicating meningococcal throat carriage.[35]

Harms: **Minocycline:** One RCT reported adverse effects (1 or more of nausea, anorexia, dizziness, and abdominal cramps) in 36% of participants.[31] **Rifampicin:** See harms of postexposure antibiotic prophylaxis, p 933. **Ciprofloxacin:** Trials of single dose prophylactic regimens reported no more adverse effects than with comparators or placebo.[28,29,34] Ciprofloxacin is contraindicated in pregnancy and in children because animal studies have indicated a possibility of articular cartilage damage in developing joints.[37] **Ceftriaxone:** Two trials of ceftriaxone found no significant adverse effects.[33,34] In one trial, 12% of participants complained of headache.[35] Ceftriaxone is given as a single intramuscular injection. **Azithromycin:** No serious or moderate adverse effects were reported, but nausea, abdominal pain, and headache of short duration were reported equally in the azithromycin and rifampicin treated groups.[35]

Comment: Eradicating meningococcal throat carriage is a well accepted surrogate for preventing meningococcal disease. It is unlikely that any RCT will be conducted on the efficacy of prophylactic antibiotics in preventing secondary community acquired meningococcal disease in household contacts because the number of participants required would be large.

QUESTION What are the effects of interventions to treat suspected cases before admission to hospital?

We found no RCTs on the effects of pre-admission parenteral penicillin in meningococcal disease. Most observational studies we found suggest benefit with antibiotics, but at least one found no benefit.

Benefits: We found seven observational studies on the effect of pre-admission parenteral penicillin in people of all ages with meningococcal disease (see table 4, p 941).[38–44] We also found two reports of pooled data from six of the observational studies.[47,48] The first report (3 English observational studies,[38–40] 487 people) found that antibiotics significantly reduced mortality (OR 2.61, 95% CI 1.04 to 7.18).[47] However, the second report (664 people; the same people in the English studies[38–40] plus partial data from a Danish cohort[45]) found no significant benefit with antibiotics (outcomes not specified; OR 0.82, 95% CI 0.43 to 1.56).[48]

Harms: It is difficult to differentiate people with early features of meningococcal disease from those with self limiting illnesses. According to more or less strict criteria for suspicion, between 28% and 89% of individuals receive parenteral penicillin unnecessarily.[49–52] One study of the harms of penicillin found that anaphylaxis occurred in about 0.04% of cases and that fatal anaphylaxis occurred in about 0.002% of cases.[53]

Comment: We found no studies about the relationship between early treatment with antibiotics and development of subsequent antibiotic resistance. Retrospective observational studies usually provide limited evidence for treatment interventions. In the case of pre-admission penicillin, no study was able to adjust adequately for clinical severity, stage of disease progression, or cointerventions such as earlier suspicion and referral (following media coverage and official recommendation). However, it is unlikely that RCTs on pre-admission antibiotics will be performed because of the unpredictably rapid course of disease in some people and the likely risks involved in delaying treatment, combined with a low risk of causing harm.

GLOSSARY

Carrier Individual in whom *N meningitidis* can be retrieved from nasopharynx by swabbing. Most carriers are asymptomatic and unaware of their carriage status.

Confirmed case Clinical diagnosis of meningitis, septicaemia or other invasive disease plus the finding of *N meningitidis* (culture, polymerase chain reaction, Gram staining) in normally sterile site or the presence of meningococcal antigen in blood, cerebrospinal fluid or urine.[54]

Contact Those recently exposed to an index case of meningococcal disease and who have a higher risk of developing the disease when compared with the general population (usually close, prolonged contact in the same household or direct contact with respiratory secretions).[54]

Meningitis (meningococcal) A case with clinical signs of meningitis (i.e. fever, headache, vomiting, nuchal rigidity) plus laboratory evidence of meningococcal infection, such as a positive blood or cerebrospinal fluid culture or polymerase chain reaction.[55]

Possible case Clinical diagnosis of meningitis or septicaemia or other invasive disease where the public health physician, in consultation with the physician and microbiologist, considers that diagnoses other than meningococcal disease are at least as likely.[54]

Probable case Clinical diagnosis of meningitis or septicaemia or other invasive disease where the public health physician, in consultation with the physician and microbiologist, considers that meningococcal infection is the most likely diagnosis.[54]

Septicaemia (meningococcal) A case with systemic signs and symptoms of infection (i.e. fever, malaise, patient "unwell") plus a skin rash, which can be purpuric (petechial, ecchymotic) or, less often, maculopapular. Laboratory provides evidence of meningococcal infection in the blood.

Suspected case Cases with early clinical signs of meningitis, septicaemia or both, where the health care worker (usually GP) suspects meningococcal aetiology.

Meningococcal disease

Substantive changes

Pre-admission parenteral penicillin Five observational studies added;[42,49–52] conclusions unchanged.

REFERENCES

1. Hubert B, Caugant DA. Recent changes in meningococcal disease in Europe. *Euro Surveill* 1997;2:69–71.
2. Centers for Disease Control. Summary of notifiable diseases United States, 1997. *MMWR Morb Mortal Wkly Rep* 1998;46:1–87.
3. Hart CA, Cuevas LE. Meningococcal disease in Africa. *Ann Trop Med Parasitol* 1997;91:777–785.
4. Molesworth AM, Thomson MC, Connor SJ, et al. Where is the meningitis belt? Defining an area at risk of epidemic meningitis in Africa. *Trans R Soc Trop Med Hyg* 2002;96:242–9.
5. World Health Organization. Emergence of W135 meningococcal disease. Report of a WHO consultation, Geneva 17–18 September 2001. Geneva: World Health Organization; 2002. http://www.who.int/csr/resources/publications/meningitis/whocdscrgar20021.pdf (last accessed 24 June 2003).
6. French MR. Epidemiological study of 383 cases of meningococcus meningitis in the city of Milwaukee, 1927–1928 and 1929. *Am J Public Health* 1931;21:130–137.
7. Pizzi M. A severe epidemic of meningococcus meningitis in 1941–1942, Chile. *Am J Public Health* 1944;34:231–239.
8. Lee WW. Epidemic meningitis in Indianapolis 1929–1930. *J Prev Med* 1931;5:203–210.
9. De Wals P, Herthoge L, Borlée-Grimée I, et al. Meningococcal disease in Belgium. Secondary attack rate among household, day-care nursery and pre-elementary school contacts. *J Infect* 1981;3(suppl 1):53–61.
10. Kaiser AB, Hennekens CH, Saslaw MS, et al. Seroepidemiology and chemoprophylaxis of disease due to sulphonamide resistant *Neisseria meningitidis* in a civilian population. *J Infect Dis* 1974;130:217–221.
11. Zangwill KM, Schuchat A, Riedo FX, et al. School-based clusters of meningococcal disease in the United States. *JAMA* 1997;277:389–395.
12. The Meningococcal Disease Surveillance Group. Meningococcal disease secondary attack rate and chemoprophylaxis in the United States. *JAMA* 1976;235:261–265.
13. Olcen P, Kjellander J, Danielson D, et al. Epidemiology of *Neisseria meningitidis*: prevalence and symptoms from the upper respiratory tract in family members to patients with meningococcal disease. *Scand J Infect Dis* 1981;13:105–109.
14. Hudson, PJ, Vogt PL, Heun EM, et al. Evidence for school transmission of *Neisseria meningitidis* during a Vermont outbreak. *Pediatr Infect Dis* 1986;5:213–217.
15. Stanwell-Smith RE, Stuart JM, Hughes AO, et al. Smoking, the environment and meningococcal disease: a case control study. *Epidemiol Infect* 1994;112:315–328.
16. Communicable Disease Surveillance Centre. Meningococcal disease in university students. *Commun Dis Rep CDR Wkly* 1998;8:49.
17. Andersen BM. Mortality in meningococcal infections. *Scand J Infect Dis* 1978;10:277–282.
18. Thomson APJ, Sills JA, Hart CA. Validation of the Glasgow meningococcal septicaemia prognostic score: a 10 year retrospective survey. *Crit Care Med* 1991;19:26–30.
19. Riordan FAI, Marzouk O, Thomson APJ, et al. The changing presentation of meningococcal disease. *Eur J Pediatr* 1995;154:472–474.
20. Booy R, Habibi P, Nadel S, et al. Reduction in case fatality rate from meningococcal disease associated with improved healthcare delivery. *Arch Dis Child* 2001;85:386–390.
21. Thorburn K, Baines P, Thomson A, et al. Mortality in severe meningococcal disease. *Arch Dis Child* 2001;85:382–385.
22. Hoiby EA, Moe PJ, Lystad A, et al. Phenoxymethyl-penicillin treatment of household contacts of meningococcal disease patients. *Antonie Van Leeuwenhoek* 1986;52:255–257.
23. Kuhns DW, Nelson CT, Feldman HA, et al. The prophylactic value of sulfadiazine in the control of meningococcic meningitis. *JAMA* 1943;123:335–339.
24. Deal WB, Sanders E. Efficacy of rifampicin in treatment of meningococcal carriers. *N Engl J Med* 1969;281:641–645.
25. Eickhoff TC. In vitro and in vivo studies of resistance to rifampicin in meningococci. *J Infect Dis* 1971;123:414–420.
26. Weidmer CE, Dunkel TB, Pettyjohn FS, et al. Effectiveness of rifampin in eradicating the meningococcal carrier state in a relatively closed population: emergence of resistant strains. *J Infect Dis* 1971;124:172–178.
27. Devine LF, Johnson DP, Hagerman CR, et al. The effect of minocycline on meningococcal nasopharyngeal carrier state in naval personnel. *Am J Epidemiol* 1971;93:337–345.
28. Renkonen OV, Sivonen A, Visakorpi R. Effect of ciproflaxacin on carrier rate of *Neisseria meningitidis* in army recruits in Finland. *Antimicrob Agents Chemother* 1987;31:962–963.
29. Dworzack DL, Sanders CC, Horowitz EA, et al. Evaluation of single dose ciprofloxacin in the eradication of *Neisseria meningitidis* from nasopharyngeal carriers. *Antimicrob Agents Chemother* 1988;32:1740–1741.
30. Artenstein MS, Lamson TH, Evans JR. Attempted prophylaxis against meningococcal infection using intramuscular penicillin. *Mil Med* 1967;132:1009–1011.
31. Guttler RB, Counts GW, Avent CK, et al. Effect of rifampicin and minocycline on meningococcal carrier rates. *J Infect Dis* 1971;124:199–205.
32. Blakebrough IS, Gilles HM. The effect of rifampicin on meningococcal carriage in family contacts in northern Nigeria. *J Infect* 1980;2:137–143.
33. Schwartz B, Al-Tobaiqi A, Al-Ruwais A, et al. Comparative efficacy of ceftriaxone and rifampicin in eradicating pharyngeal carriage of Group A *Neisseria meningitidis*. *Lancet* 1988;1:1239–1242.
34. Cuevas LE, Kazembe P, Mughogho GK, et al. Eradication of nasopharyngeal carriage of *Neisseria meningitidis* in children and adults in rural Africa: A comparison of ciprofloxacin and rifampicin. *J Infect Dis* 1995;171:728–731.
35. Girgis N, Sultan Y, Frenck RW Jr, et al. Azithromycin compared with rifampin for eradication of masopharyngeal colonization by *Neisseria meningitidis*. *Pediatr Infect Dis* J 1998;17:816–819.
36. Simmons G, Jones N, Calder L. Equivalence of ceftriaxone and rifampicin in eliminating

nasopharyngeal carriage of serogroup B *Neisseria meningitidis*. *J Antimicrob Chemother* 2000;45:909–911.
37. Schulter G. Ciprofloxacin: a review of its potential toxicologic effects. *Am J Med* 1987(suppl 4A);82:91–93.
38. Strang JR, Pugh EJ. Meningococcal infections: reducing the case fatality rate by giving penicillin before admission to hospital. *BMJ* 1992;305:141–143.
39. Cartwright K, Reilly S, White D, et al. Early treatment with parenteral penicillin in meningococcal disease. *BMJ* 1992;305:143–147.
40. Gossain S, Constantine CE, Webberley JM. Early parenteral penicillin in meningococcal disease. *BMJ* 1992;305:523–524.
41. Woodward CM, Jessop EG, Wale MCJ. Early management of meningococcal disease. *Commun Dis Rep CDR Rev* 1995;5:R135–R137.
42. Nørg rd B, Sørensen HT, Jensen ES, et al. Pre-hospital parenteral antibiotic treatment of meningococcal disease and case fatality: a Danish population-based cohort study. *J Infect* 2002;45:144–151.
43. Jefferies C, Lennon D, Stewart J, et al. Meningococcal disease in Auckland, July 1992 – June 1994. *N Z Med J* 1999;112:115–117.
44. Jolly K, Stewart G. Epidemiology and diagnosis of meningitis: results of a five-year prospective, population-based study. *Commun Dis Public Health* 2001;4:124–129.
45. Sorensen HT, Moller-Petersen J, Krarup HB, et al. Early treatment of meningococcal disease. *BMJ* 1992;305:774.
46. Sorensen HT, Nielsen GL, Schonheyder HC, et al. Outcome of pre-hospital antibiotic treatment of meningococcal disease. *J Clin Epidemiol* 1998;51:717–721.
47. Cartwright K, Strang J, Gossain S, et al. Early treatment of meningococcal disease [letter]. *BMJ* 1992;305:774.
48. Sorensen HT, Steffensen FH, Schonheyder HC, et al. Clinical management of meningococcal disease. Prospective international registration of patients may be needed. *BMJ* 1998;316:1016–1017.
49. Wells LC, Smith JC, Weston VC, et al. The child with a non-blanching rash: how likely is meningococcal disease? *Arch Dis Child* 2001;85:218–222.
50. Mandl KD, Stack AM, Fleisher GR. Incidence of bacteremia in infants and children with fever and petechiae. *J Pediatr* 1997;131:398–404.
51. Brogan PA, Raffles A. The management of fever and petechiae: making sense of rash decisions. *Arch Dis Child* 2000;83:506–507.
52. Nielsen HE, Andersen EA, Andersen J, et al. Diagnostic assessment of haemorrhagic rash and fever. *Arch Dis Child* 2001;85:160–165.
53. Idsoe O, Guthe T, Willcox RR, et al. Nature and extent of penicillin side-reactions, with particular reference to fatalities from anaphylactic shock. *Bull World Health Organ* 1968;38:159–188.
54. Public Health Laboratory Service Meningococcus Forum. Guidelines for public health management of meningococcal disease in the UK. *Commun Dis Public Health* 2002;5:187–204.
55. Hackett SJ, Carrol ED, Guiver M, et al. Improved case confirmation in meningococcal disease with whole blood Taqman PCR. *Arch Dis Child* 2002;86:449–452.

Jailson B Correia
Dr
Instituto Materno Infantil de Pernambuco
Recife
Brazil

C A Hart
Professor
Department of Medical Microbiology and
Genitourinary Medicine
University of Liverpool
Liverpool
UK

Competing interests: None declared.

TABLE 1 Risk of infection among contacts (see text, p 932).

Group of meningococcus	Setting	Risk
A	Household contacts in Milwaukee, USA[6]	AR 1100/100 000; RR not possible to estimate
	General population in Santiago province, Chile	Attack rate in general population 23–262/100 000 (1941 and 1942)
	Household contacts in Chile[7]	Attack rate in household contacts 250/100 000 (0.25%) over both years
	General population in Indianapolis, USA[8]	AR 4500/100 000; RR not possible to estimate
B	Household contacts in Belgium[9]	RR 1245*
	Nursery schools[9]	RR 23*
	Day care centres[9]	RR 76*
C	Household contacts from two lower socioeconomic groups Dade County, Florida, USA[10]	Attack rate in two communities 13/100 000 population. Attack rate in household contacts 5/85 (582/100 000)
Unspecified	School based clusters in USA. Predominant meningococcal types: 13 clusters of Gp C, 7 Gp B, 1 Gp Y, 1 GpC/W135 (impossible to distinguish)[11]	RR 2.3*
	Household contacts from several states in USA, meningococcus types B and C predominantly[12]	RR 500–800*
	Household contact in Norway. Meningococcus types A, B, and C predominantly[13]	RR up to 4000*
	Schools in Vermont. Predominant meningococcus type C[14]	OR 14.1 (95% CI 1.6 to 127)

*Compared with the risk in the general population.

TABLE 2 **Effect of antibiotics on throat carriage: results of placebo controlled RCTs(see text, p 934).**

Antibiotic	Group of meningococcus	Participants	Eradication		RR (95% CI)
			Treatment (%)	Placebo (%)	
Rifampicin (oral)[24]	B, X, Z	30 students with heavy growth on culture	11/15 (73)	2/15 (13)	5.5 (1.5 to 21)
Rifampicin (oral)[25]	B, C, Y, Z29 E, W 135, NT	76 airforce recruits	36/38* (95)	3/22‡ (14)	7.0 (5.8 to 8.1)
Minocycline (oral)[27]	Predominantly Y (63%)	149 naval recruits	37/41 (90)†	14/48 (29)§	3.1 (2.6 to 3.6)
Ciprofloxacin (oral)[28]	Non-groupable (61%), B (17.5%)	120 army recruits in Finland	54/56 (97) 5 second samples missing	7/53 (13) 6 second samples missing or not a carrier	7.3 (6.5 to 8.1)
Ciprofloxacin (oral)[29]	B (41%), Z (33%)	46 healthy volunteers	22/23 (96) (1 did not adhere to treatment)	2/22 (9)	10.5 (8.9 to 12.1)

*9 lost to follow up. †37 either did not have meningococci prior to treatment or did not provide a full set of cultures. ‡7 lost to follow up.
§23 either did not have meningococci prior to treatment or did not provide a full set of cultures.

TABLE 3 Effects of antibiotics on throat carriage: results of comparative RCTs (see text, p 934).

Antibiotic	Group of meningococcus	Participants	Rate of eradication (%)	RR (95% CI)
Phenoxymethylpenicillin (im)[30]	C (49%), B (33%), NG (17%)	Adults	41/118 (35)	No data
Erythromycin (oral)[30]	C	Adults	0/7 (0)	No data
Rifampicin (oral)[31]	B + C (31%), NG (69%)	Adults	43/51 (84)	0.89 (0.76 to 1.02)
Minocycline (oral)[31]	B + C (31%), NG (69%)	Adults	36/38 (95)	No data
Rifampicin (oral)[31]	A	Children	37/48 (77)	No data
Sulfadimidine (oral)[32]	A	Children	0/34 (0)	No data
Ceftriaxone (im)[33]	A	Adults and children	66/68 (97)	1.29 (1.10 to 1.49)
Rifampicin (oral)[33]	A	Adults and children	27/36 (75)	No data
Ceftriaxone (im)[34]	A	Adults and children	39/41 (95)	No data
Ciprofloxacin (oral)[34]	A	Adults and children	70/79 (89)	No data
Rifampicin (oral)[34]	A	Adults and children	85/88 (97)	No data
Azithromycin (oral)[35]	B (63%), A (37%)	Adults	56/60 (93)	No data
Rifampicin (oral)[35]	B (63%), A (37%)	Adults	56/59 (95)	No data
Ceftriaxone (im)[36]	B (54%), other serogroups (46%)	Adults and children	97/100 (97)	No data
Rifampicin (oral)[36]	B (51%), other serogroups (49%)	Adults and children	78/82 (95.1)	No data

im, intramuscular.

TABLE 4 **Effects of early (pre-admission) parenteral penicillin: results of observational studies (see text, p 934).**

Setting	Group of meningococcus	Participants	Parenteral penicillin (number of deaths/number of people [%])		RR (95% CI)
			Given	Not given	
District general hospital in Darlington, UK (from 1986–1991)[38]	NR	46 people admitted to hospital with confirmed, probable, and possible MD, all age groups (52% < 5 years of age)	0/13 (0)	8/33 (24.3)	Incalculable
Three health districts in south-west England, UK (from 1982–1991)[39]	Mostly B and C	340* confirmed, probable, and possible cases of MD, all age groups (36% < 5 years of age)	5/93 (5.4)	22/246 (8.9)	RR 0.6 (0.23 to 1.54)
Worcester health district, England, UK (1986–1992)[40]	NR	102† confirmed, probable, and possible cases of MD; age distribution not reported	1/23 (4.4)	11/79 (13.9)	RR 0.31 (0.04 to 2.29)
District hospital in Wessex, England, UK (1990–1993)[41]	NR	68 cases of MD, all age groups (44% < 5 years of age)	0/13 (0)	3/55 (5.5)	Not calculated
Counties of North Jutland and Aarhus, Denmark‡[42]	Mostly B (56%) and C (22%)	479 cases of MD seen by GPs before admission to hospital. All age groups.	9/77 (11.7)	26/402 (6.5)	Adjusted OR 2.4 (95% CI 1.0 to 5.6)§
Hospitals in Auckland, New Zealand (1992–1997)[43]‡‡	Predominantly B	106 confirmed or probable cases of MD, all age groups.	1/24 (4.2)	2/42 (4.9)	RR 0.85 (0.08 to 8.93)
Health district in England, UK (from 1994–1998)[44]‡‡	Mostly B (53%) and C (30%)	258†† confirmed, probable, and possible cases of MD; all age groups (49% < 5 years of age)	2/72 (2.8)	16/186 (8.6)	RR 0.32 (0.08 to 1.37)

*Number of individuals seen by their general practitioners (GPs) before admission; in one fatal case, there was no information on previous antibiotic use. †A total of 109 patients had their records reviewed, but seven were excluded from analysis because they had received oral penicillin. ‡Two previous partial series of 177 and 302 cases from the Danishhistorical cohort were reported in 1992[45] and 1998,[46] respectively, showing similar trends of excess mortality in the treated group. §Adjusted OR, multivariate analysis. ††The paper also reports meningitis of other aetiologies. Only those regarded as meningococcal disease are described here. ‡‡The only prospective studies found. Others in the table are retrospective.
CI, confidence interval; MD, meningococcal disease; NR, not reported.

Postherpetic neuralgia

Search date May 2003

David Wareham

QUESTIONS

INTERVENTIONS

Key Messages

Preventing postherpetic neuralgia

- **Aciclovir, famciclovir, valaciclovir, netivudine** One systematic review has found limited evidence from RCTs that aciclovir given for 7–10 days reduced pain at 1–3 months. One systematic review found that famciclovir reduces mean pain duration after acute herpes zoster compared with placebo. One RCT found that valaciclovir reduced the prevalence of postherpetic neuralgia at 6 months compared with aciclovir. One RCT found no significant difference in effectiveness between netivudine and aciclovir. One RCT found no significant difference between valaciclovir and famciclovir in the resolution of postherpetic neuralgia or in adverse effects over 7 days.
- **Amitriptyline** One small RCT found no significant difference between amitriptyline and placebo started within 48 hours of rash onset in the prevalence of postherpetic neuralgia at 6 months. The RCT may have lacked power to detect a clinically important difference.
- **Topical antiviral agents (idoxuridine) for pain at 6 months** One systematic review has found that idoxuridine increases short term pain relief in acute herpes zoster compared with placebo or oral aciclovir, but found no significant difference at 6 months.

- **Corticosteroids** Systematic reviews found conflicting evidence from RCTs about the effects of corticosteroids alone on postherpetic neuralgia. We found insufficient evidence from two RCTs about effects of high dose steroids plus antiviral agents. There is concern that corticosteroids may cause dissemination of herpes zoster.
- **Adenosine phosphate; amantadine; cimetidine; inosine pranobex; levodopa** RCTs found insufficient evidence on the effects of these interventions.

Treating established postherpetic neuralgia

- **Gabapentin** One systematic review has found that gabapentin reduces pain at 8 weeks compared with placebo.
- **Tricyclic antidepressants** One systematic review has found that tricyclic antidepressants increase pain relief in postherpetic neuralgia after 2–6 weeks compared with placebo.
- **Oral opioids (oxycodone, morphine, methadone)** We found no RCTs examining effects of morphine or methadone in people with postherpetic neuralgia. One small RCT found that oral oxycodone reduced pain after 4 weeks compared with placebo, but was associated with more adverse effects.
- **Topical counterirritants** Two systematic reviews and one small subsequent RCT found limited evidence that the topical counterirritant capsaicin improved pain relief in postherpetic neuralgia compared with placebo, but found that capsaicin may cause painful skin reactions.
- **Topical anaesthesia** We found insufficient evidence from three RCTs about the effects of lidocaine (lignocaine).
- **Tramadol** One small RCT found that tramadol reduced pain more than clomipramine after 6 weeks. However, we were unable to draw reliable conclusions from this small study.
- **Dextromethorphan** One systematic review and one subsequent RCT found no evidence that dextromethorphan was more effective than placebo or lorazepam after 3–6 weeks, but found that dextromethorphan was associated with sedation and ataxia at high doses.
- **Epidural morphine** One small RCT found that epidural morphine reduced pain by more than 50% compared with placebo but the reduction was not maintained beyond 36 hours. Epidural morphine caused intolerable opioid effects in 75% of people.

DEFINITION Postherpetic neuralgia is pain that sometimes follows resolution of acute herpes zoster and healing of the zoster rash. It can be severe, accompanied by itching, and follows the distribution of the original infection. Herpes zoster is an acute infection caused by activation of latent varicella zoster virus (human herpes virus 3) in people who have been rendered partially immune by a previous attack of chickenpox. Herpes zoster infects the sensory ganglia and their areas of innervation. It is characterised by pain along the distribution of the affected nerve, and crops of clustered vesicles over the area.

INCIDENCE/ PREVALENCE In a UK general practice survey of 3600–3800 people, the annual incidence of herpes zoster was 3.4/1000.[1] Incidence varied with age. Herpes zoster was relatively uncommon in people under the age of 50 years (< 2/1000 a year), but rose to 5–7/1000 a year in people aged 50–79 years, and 11/1000 in people aged 80 years or older. In a population based study of 590 cases in Rochester,

Minnesota, USA, the overall incidence was lower (1.5/1000) but there were similar increases in incidence with age.[2] Prevalence of postherpetic neuralgia depends on when it is measured after acute infection. There is no agreed time point for diagnosis.

AETIOLOGY/ RISK FACTORS The main risk factor for postherpetic neuralgia is increasing age. In a UK general practice study (involving 3600–3800 people, 321 cases of acute herpes zoster) there was little risk in those under the age of 50 years, but postherpetic neuralgia developed in over 20% of people who had had acute herpes zoster aged 60–65 years and in 34% aged over 80 years.[1] No other risk factor has been found to predict consistently which people with herpes zoster will experience continued pain. In a general practice study in Iceland (421 people followed for up to 7 years after an initial episode of herpes zoster), the risk of postherpetic neuralgia was 1.8% (95% CI 0.6% to 4.2%) for people under 60 years of age and the pain was mild in all cases.[2] The risk of severe pain after 3 months in people aged over 60 years was 1.7% (95% CI 0% to 6.2%).

PROGNOSIS About 2% of people with acute herpes zoster in the UK general practice survey had pain for more than 5 years.[1] Prevalence of pain falls as time elapses after the initial episode. Among 183 people aged over 60 years in the placebo arm of a UK trial, the prevalence of pain was 61% at 1 month, 24% at 3 months, and 13% at 6 months after acute infection.[3] In a more recent RCT, the prevalence of postherpetic pain in the placebo arm at 6 months was 35% in 72 people over 60 years of age.[4]

AIMS OF INTERVENTION To prevent or reduce postherpetic neuralgia by intervention during acute attack; to reduce the severity and duration of established postherpetic neuralgia, with minimal adverse effects of treatment.

OUTCOMES Prevalence of persistent pain 6 months after resolution of acute infection and healing of rash. We did not consider short term outcomes such as rash healing or pain reduction during the acute episode. It is difficult to assess the clinical significance of reported changes in "average pain"; therefore, we present data as dichotomous outcomes where possible (pain absent or greatly reduced, or pain persistent).

METHODS Our initial search was part of two systematic reviews of treatments for acute herpes zoster and postherpetic neuralgia on the basis of comprehensive searches of published and unpublished studies to 1993.[5,6] The details of the searches are described in the published reports. This search was updated by a *Clinical Evidence* search and appraisal in May 2003. Where reliable meta-analyses from systematic reviews were available, they were taken to be the most accurate estimates of treatment effectiveness. In trials, the most common time point chosen for assessing the prevalence of persistent pain was 6 months, which we use in this review unless otherwise specified.

QUESTION What are the effects of interventions during an acute attack of herpes zoster aimed at preventing postherpetic neuralgia?

OPTION ORAL ANTIVIRAL AGENTS (ACICLOVIR, FAMCICLOVIR, VALACICLOVIR, NETIVUDINE)

One systematic review has found limited evidence from RCTs that aciclovir given for 7–10 days reduced pain at 1–3 months. One systematic review has found that famciclovir reduces mean pain duration after acute herpes zoster compared with placebo. One RCT found that valaciclovir reduced the prevalence of postherpetic neuralgia at 6 months compared with aciclovir. One RCT found no significant difference in effectiveness between netivudine and aciclovir. One RCT found no significant difference between valaciclovir and famciclovir in the resolution of postherpetic neuralgia or in adverse effects over 7 days.

Benefits: **Aciclovir versus placebo:** We found one systematic review (search date 1998).[7] It included results from 6 RCTs comparing aciclovir alone versus placebo. It found important heterogeneity among studies making it difficult to summarise results. Meta-analysis was not conducted. The first RCT (376 people) compared aciclovir (4 g/day for 7 days) versus placebo. It found no significant difference between aciclovir and placebo for pain at 3 or 6 months (at 3 months AR for pain 24% in both groups; at 6 months AR 14% with aciclovir *v* 13% placebo; CI not reported in the review). The second RCT (187 people; aciclovir 4 g/day for 10 days) found that aciclovir significantly reduced pain compared with placebo at 1–3 months (AR for pain 4.2% with aciclovir *v* 16.7% with placebo; P = 0.012). However, it found no significant difference at 4–6 months (3.9% *v* 6.3%, CI not reported in the review). The third included RCT (83 people; aciclovir 4 g/day for 7 days) found that aciclovir significantly reduced pain at 3 months (AR 10% *v* 40%; P = 0.0082). The fourth RCT (46 people; aciclovir 4 g/day for 10 days) found that aciclovir significantly reduced pain at 3 months (7% *v* 38%; P = 0.05), but the difference was not significant at 6 months (5% with aciclovir *v* 26% with placebo; P = 0.07). The fifth RCT (65 people; aciclovir 2 g/day for 10 days) found no significant difference in pain between aciclovir and placebo (time to outcome and AR not stated in the review). The final included RCT (86 people; aciclovir 4 g/day for 7 or 14 days) found no significant difference between aciclovir and placebo for pain at 6 months (13% in both groups). **Famciclovir versus placebo:** We found one systematic review (search date 1998, 1 RCT, 419 people).[7] The multicentre RCT in the review compared two different doses of famciclovir in immunocompetent adults (age > 18 years) and defined duration of postherpetic neuralgia as time to pain resolution. It found that both doses of famciclovir significantly reduced the duration of pain after acute herpes zoster compared with placebo (median duration of pain with 500 mg [138 people] 63 days, with 750 mg [135 people] 61 days, with placebo [146 people] 119 days; CI not reported). **Aciclovir versus other antiviral agents:** We found one systematic review (search date 1998, 1 RCT, 1141 people).[7] The RCT in the review compared valaciclovir (a precursor of aciclovir) given three times daily for 7 or 14 days versus 7 days of aciclovir. When the results from the two valaciclovir regimens were combined, those treated with valaciclovir had a lower prevalence of pain at 6 months (AR 19.3% *v* 25.3%; RR 0.92; NNT 16, 95% CI 9 to 100). We found one double blind RCT comparing netivudine versus aciclovir (511 people), which found no significant difference in effectiveness between treatments.[8] **Addition of amitriptyline:** We found no systematic review or RCTs. **Valaciclovir versus famciclovir:** We found no systematic review. One RCT (597 immunocompetent people aged ≥ 50 years) compared valaciclovir (1 g 3 times daily) versus famciclovir (500 mg 3 times daily) started within 72 hours of appearance of the rash and given for 7 days.[9] It found no significant difference in postherpetic neuralgia (HR 1.01, 95% CI 0.82 to 1.24).

Harms: One previous systematic review (search date 1993) found that the most common adverse events reported with aciclovir were headache and nausea.[5] In placebo controlled trials, these effects occurred with similar frequency with treatment and placebo (headache 37% *v* 43%, nausea 13% *v* 14%). There were no major adverse events reported in the RCTs included in the systematic review.[5] In the RCTs, famciclovir, valaciclovir, and netivudine had similar safety profiles to aciclovir.[8,10,11] In the RCT comparing valaciclovir versus famciclovir the two drugs had similar safety profiles.[9]

Comment: We found no evidence on adherence, but it has been suggested that adherence to treatment may be better with the newer antiviral drugs because they are given one to three times daily compared with five times daily for aciclovir.

OPTION TOPICAL ANTIVIRAL AGENTS (IDOXURIDINE)

One systematic review has found that idoxuridine increases short term pain relief in acute herpes zoster compared with placebo or oral aciclovir, but found no significant difference at 6 months.

Benefits: We found one systematic review (search date 1993, 4 RCTs, 431 people).[5] **Versus placebo:** Three RCTs (242 people) compared topical idoxuridine versus placebo. Pooled results were not reported because of heterogeneity and poor quality of the trials. Two of the RCTs found that treatment during an acute attack significantly increased pain relief at 1 month, but none of the three RCTs found any significant difference at 6 months. **Versus aciclovir:** One RCT found that topical idoxuridine significantly increased pain relief at 1 month compared with oral aciclovir (OR 0.41, 95% CI 0.15 to 1.11), but found no significant difference in prevalence of pain at 6 months (RR 0.38, 95% CI 0.13 to 1.00).[12]

Harms: We found no reports of important adverse effects from idoxuridine. Application beneath dressings may be cumbersome.

Comment: None.

OPTION CORTICOSTEROIDS

Systematic reviews found conflicting evidence from RCTs about the effects of corticosteroids alone on postherpetic neuralgia. We found insufficient evidence from two RCTs about effects of high dose steroids plus antiviral agents. There is concern that corticosteroids may cause dissemination of herpes zoster.

Benefits: **Corticosteroids alone:** We found two systematic reviews (search dates 1993[5] and 1998[7]). The earlier review (search date 1993) included RCTs of corticosteroids with conflicting results and concluded that it was not possible to assess the effect of corticosteroids.[5] The more recent review (search date 1998) found similar results but identified one RCT (201 people) subsequent to the earlier review.[7] The RCT found no significant differences in pain at 3 or 6 months. **Corticosteroids plus aciclovir:** We found one systematic review (search date 1998, 2 RCTs, 608 people).[7] The first identified RCT (400 people) randomised people into four active treatment groups: 7 days of aciclovir (101 people); 7 days of aciclovir plus 21 days of prednisone (99 people); 21 days of aciclovir (101 people); or 21 days of aciclovir plus prednisone (99 people).[13] It found no significant differences in relief of postherpetic neuralgia. The second RCT (208 people) had a factorial design, randomising people to 21 days of aciclovir plus prednisone (60 mg initially, tapered over 3 weeks), prednisone plus placebo, aciclovir plus placebo, or two placebos.[14] Although there was evidence of short term benefit from prednisone, there was no significant effect on pain prevalence at 6 months after disease onset.

Harms: It is feared that corticosteroids might cause dissemination of herpes zoster. This effect was not reported in an RCT of prednisone in the earlier systematic review.[5] In the RCT of aciclovir plus prednisone, two people receiving prednisone plus aciclovir placebo and one receiving aciclovir plus prednisone placebo developed cutaneous dissemination of lesions (see harms of corticosteroids under rheumatoid arthritis, p 1454).[14]

Comment: None.

OPTION TRICYCLIC ANTIDEPRESSANTS (AMITRIPTYLINE)

One small RCT found no significant difference between amitriptyline and placebo started within 48 hours of rash onset in the prevalence of postherpetic neuralgia at 6 months. The RCT may have lacked power to detect a clinically important difference.

Benefits: We found one systematic review (search date 1998, 1 RCT, 90 people).[7] The RCT in the review (72 people aged > 60 years) found that amitriptyline 25 mg taken within 48 hours of rash onset (prescribed with or without antiviral agents, at the practitioner's discretion) and continued for 90 days reduced the prevalence of postherpetic neuralgia at 6 months compared with placebo, but the result did not reach significance (AR 16% *v* AR 35%; RR 0.45; ARR +0.19%, 95% CI −0.003% to +0.39%).[4]

Harms: The RCT did not report adverse effects.[4] In another RCT, amitriptyline was associated with adverse anticholinergic effects such as dry mouth, sedation, and urinary difficulties.[5]

Comment: Interpretation of the RCT is complicated because practitioners were allowed to decide whether an antiviral agent was prescribed as well as amitriptyline.[4] Blinding may also have been inadequate.

OPTION OTHER DRUG TREATMENTS

RCTs found insufficient evidence on the effects of other drug treatments in acute herpes zoster.

Benefits: We found one systematic review (search date 1993), which identified small, single RCTs of adenosine phosphate, amantadine, and levodopa.[5] The RCTs found limited evidence of short term benefit in treating herpes zoster. No benefit was found in small studies of cimetidine and inosine pranobex.[5]

Harms: We found no evidence.

Comment: None.

QUESTION What are the effects of interventions to relieve established postherpetic neuralgia after the rash has healed?

OPTION TRICYCLIC ANTIDEPRESSANTS

One systematic review has found that tricyclic antidepressants increase pain relief in postherpetic neuralgia after 2–6 weeks compared with placebo.

Benefits: We found two systematic reviews (search dates 1993[6] and 2000[15]). Three RCTs (216 people) comparing tricyclic antidepressants versus placebo were common to both reviews. Two of these RCTs compared amitriptyline versus placebo. The other RCT compared desipramine versus placebo. The first review pooled results and found that tricyclic antidepressants taken for 3–6 weeks significantly improved pain relief from postherpetic neuralgia at the end of the treatment period compared with placebo (OR for complete or large reduction in pain at end of treatment period 0.15, 95% CI 0.08 to 0.27).[6] The more recent review found one subsequent RCT that compared amitriptyline alone; amitriptyline plus fluphenazine; fluphenazine alone; and placebo.[15] However, it did not report results for amitriptyline alone compared with placebo.

Harms: Tricyclic antidepressants are associated with anticholinergic adverse effects. In one RCT, amitriptyline increased the following adverse effects compared with placebo: dry mouth (AR 62% *v* 40%), sedation (AR 62% *v* 40%), and urinary difficulties (AR 12% *v* $<$ 5%).[16] Syncope and heart block occurred in one person in a trial of desipramine in people with postherpetic neuralgia.[17]

Comment: The adverse effects of tricyclic antidepressants are dose related. Adverse effects may be less pronounced when treating postherpetic neuralgia rather than depression because lower doses are used. Treatments were not assessed for more than 8 weeks.

OPTION TOPICAL COUNTERIRRITANTS

Two systematic reviews and one small subsequent RCT found limited evidence that the topical counterirritant capsaicin improved pain relief in postherpetic neuralgia compared with placebo, but found that capsaicin may cause painful skin reactions.

Benefits: We found two systematic reviews (search date 1993[5] and 2000[15]) and one subsequent RCT.[18] Both reviews identified the same two placebo controlled RCTs. The first review (205 people) found that capsaicin significantly improved pain relief compared with placebo (OR for complete or greatly reduced pain 0.29, 95% CI 0.16 to 0.54).[5] The second review did not pool results, but reached the same conclusion. The subsequent RCT (31 people) found that capsaicin 0.025% was not effective.[18]

Harms: Reported local skin reactions included burning, stinging, and erythema. These effects tended to subside with time and frequency of use.[19]

Comment: The difficulty in blinding studies with capsaicin because of skin burning could have caused overestimation of benefit.

OPTION TOPICAL ANAESTHESIA

We found insufficient evidence from three RCTs about the effects of lidocaine (lignocaine).

Benefits: We found one systematic review (search date 2000, 2 RCTs with evaluation period > 24 hours, 204 people)[15] and one additional RCT.[20] The first trial included in the review (unpublished, 171 people) found no significant difference for pain relief between lidocaine patches and placebo after 3–4 weeks (pain score on 0–5 pain scale 2.6 for lidocaine *v* 2.1 for placebo).[15] The second RCT only recruited people who had responded to lidocaine patches (see comment below).[15] The additional RCT (35 people) found that lidocaine patches reduced average pain scores on a visual analogue scale over 12 hours compared with placebo.[20]

Harms: No systemic adverse effects were noted with lidocaine patches, and systemic absorption as determined by blood concentrations was minimal.[20]

Comment: One RCT included in the review only recruited people who had responded to lidocaine.[15] Results are therefore likely to be biased in favour of lidocaine. It found that lidocaine patches were more effective for pain relief than placebo.

OPTION GABAPENTIN

One systematic review has found that gabapentin reduces pain in postherpetic neuralgia at 8 weeks compared with placebo.

Benefits: We found one systematic review (search date not stated,[21] 2 multicentre RCTs[22,23]). Both RCTs assessed pain using an 11 point Likert scale. The first RCT identified by the review (229 people who remained on tricyclic antidepressants or opiates during the trial) found that gabapentin significantly reduced the proportion of people reporting pain after 8 weeks of treatment (no pain: 16% with gabapentin *v* 8% with placebo; pain much or moderately reduced: 43% with gabapentin *v* 12% with placebo; $P < 0.001$).[23] The second RCT identified by the review (334 people) found that gabapentin (1800 mg/day or 2400 mg/day in 3 divided doses) significantly reduced mean daily pain scores at 7 weeks compared with placebo (pain reduction with gabapentin 1800 mg *v* placebo: –18.8%, 95% CI –10.9% to –26.8%; pain reduction with gabapentin 2400 mg *v* placebo: – 18.7%, 95% CI –10.7% to –26.7%).[22]

Harms: The first RCT in the review[21] found that gabapentin increased adverse effects compared with placebo (somnolence: 7% *v* 5%; dizziness: 24% *v* 5%; ataxia: 7% *v* 0%; peripheral oedema: 10% *v* 3%; infection: 8% *v* 3%).[23] It found no significant difference in withdrawal rates due to adverse effects between gabapentin and placebo (13.3% with gabapentin *v* 9.5% with placebo). The second RCT in the review also found that gabapentin increased adverse effects compared with placebo (somnolence: 17% with 1800 mg *v* 20% with 2400 mg *v* 6% with placebo; dizziness: 31% *v* 33% *v* 10%; peripheral oedema: 5% *v* 11% *v* 0%).[22] This RCT found that gabapentin increased withdrawal rates due to adverse effect (13% with 1800 mg *v* 18% with 2400 mg *v* 6% with placebo).

Comment: None.

OPTION NARCOTIC ANALGESICS

We found no RCTs examining effects of morphine or methadone in people with postherpetic neuralgia. One small RCT found that oral oxycodone reduced pain after 4 weeks compared with placebo but was associated with more adverse effects. The review and one subsequent RCT found no evidence that dextromethorphan was more effective than placebo or lorazepam after 3–6 weeks, but found that dextromethorphan was associated with sedation and ataxia at high doses. One additional RCT found that epidural morphine reduced pain more than placebo over 36 hours, but was poorly tolerated because of adverse effects. The review found limited evidence from one RCT that tramadol reduced pain more than clomipramine after 6 weeks. However, we were unable to draw reliable conclusions from this small study.

Benefits: We found no RCTs examining effects of morphine or methadone. We found one systematic review (search date 2000, 3 RCTs, 103 people), one subsequent RCT, and one additional RCT not identified by the review.[15,24,25] The first RCT included in the review (a blinded crossover RCT; 50 people, 4 weeks on each treatment; comparing oxycodone *v* placebo) found that oxycodone significantly improved pain on a visual analogue scale after 4 weeks, but the data were not converted into a dichotomous outcome. However, it found that a greater proportion of people preferred oxycodone to placebo (67% *v* 11%).[15] A second, small, double blind, crossover RCT (18 people) found no evidence of pain relief from 6 weeks' treatment with dextromethorphan (a codeine analogue) compared with placebo.[15] The third included RCT (35 people) compared tramadol versus clomipramine with or without levomepromazine.[15] It found that tramadol improved pain relief compared with other treatments (after 6 weeks, AR for "good or excellent" pain relief 60% with tramadol *v* 45% with control; RR, CI and P values not reported in the review). The first subsequent crossover RCT (22 people) compared three treatments: dextromethorphan, memantine, and lorazepam.[24] It found no significant difference between dextromethorphan and lorazepam for pain score at 3 weeks (20 point pain Gracely score; mean difference between dextromethorphan and lorazepam –0.9, 95% CI –2.3 to +0.5). The additional, small, single blind, placebo controlled RCT found that epidural morphine reduced pain by more than 50% in a significantly greater proportion of people than placebo, but this was not sustained beyond 36 hours.[25]

Harms: The review found that oxycodone produced adverse effects such as constipation, nausea, and sedation with greater frequency than placebo (76% *v* 49%; RR 1.4, 95% CI 0.5 to 3.4).[15] High dose dextromethorphan produced sedation and ataxia, causing 5/18 (28%) people to stop treatment.[15] Epidural morphine produced intolerable opioid effects in 6/8 (75%) people treated.[25]

Comment: The studies were small and in the tramadol study, results may have been biased by the co-intervention (levomepromazine).

Substantive changes

Gabapentin One systematic review added;[21] conclusions unchanged.

REFERENCES

1. Hope-Simpson RE. Postherpetic neuralgia. *J R Coll Gen Pract* 1975;25:571–575.
2. Ragozzino MW, Melton J III, Kurland LT, et al. Population based study of herpes zoster and its sequelae. *Medicine* 1982;61:310–316.
3. Mckendrick MW, McGill JI, Wood MJ. Lack of effect of aciclovir on postherpetic neuralgia. *BMJ* 1989;298:431.
4. Bowsher D. The effects of pre-emptive treatment of postherpetic neuralgia with amitriptyline: a randomised, double-blind, placebo-controlled trial. *J Pain Symptom Manage* 1997;13:327–331.
5. Lancaster T, Silagy C, Gray S. Primary care management of acute herpes zoster: systematic review of evidence from randomised controlled trials. *Br J Gen Pract* 1995;45:39–45. Search date 1993; primary sources Medline, hand searched primary care journals, references from books, specialists, and makers of drugs in identified trials for published and unpublished data.
6. Volmink J, Lancaster T, Gray S, et al. Treatments for postherpetic neuralgia — a systematic review of randomised controlled trials. *Fam Pract* 1996;13:84–91. Search date 1993; primary sources Medline and Embase.
7. Alper BS, Lewis R. Does treatment of acute herpes zoster prevent or shorten postherpetic neuralgia? A systematic review of the literature. *J Fam Pract* 2000;49:255–264. Search date 1998; primary sources Medline, Cochrane Controlled Trials Register, hand searched reference lists, and web based searches.
8. Soltz-Szots J, Tyring S, Andersen PL, et al. A randomised controlled trial of aciclovir versus netivudine for treatment of herpes zoster. International zoster study group. *J Antimicrob Chemother* 1998;41:549–556.
9. Tyring SK, Beutner KR, Tucker BA, et al. Antiviral therapy for herpes zoster: Randomised, controlled clinical trial of valaciclovir and famciclovir therapy in immunocompetent patients aged 50 years and older. *Arch Fam Med* 2000;9:863–869.
10. Tyring S, Barbarash RA, Nahlik JE, et al. Famciclovir for the treatment of acute herpes zoster: effects on acute disease and postherpetic neuralgia. A randomised, double-blind, placebo-controlled trial. Collaborative famciclovir herpes zoster study group. *Ann Intern Med* 1995;123:89–96.
11. Beutner KR, Friedman DJ, Forszpaniak C, et al. Valaciclovir compared with aciclovir for improved therapy for herpes zoster in immunocompetent adults. *Antimicrob Agents Chemother* 1995;39:1546–1553.
12. Aliaga A, Armijo M, Camacho F, et al. A topical solution of 40% idoxuridine in dimethyl sulfoxide compared to oral aciclovir in the treatment of herpes zoster. A double-blind multicenter clinical trial [in Spanish]. *Med Clin (Barc)* 1992;98:245–249.
13. Wood MJ, Johnson RW, McKendrick MW, et al. A randomised trial of aciclovir for 7 days or 21 days with and without prednisolone for treatment of acute herpes zoster. *N Engl J Med* 1994;330:896–900.

14. Whitley RJ, Weiss H, Gnann JW Jr, et al. Aciclovir with and without prednisone for the treatment of herpes zoster. A randomized, placebo-controlled trial. The National Institute of Allergy and Infectious Diseases Collaborative Antiviral Study Group. *Ann Intern Med* 1996;125:376–383.
15. Alper BS, Lewis PR. Treatment of postherpetic neuralgia: a systematic review of the literature. *J Fam Pract* 2002;51:121–128. Search date 2000; primary sources Medline, Cochrane Controlled Trials Register, Current Contents, and a manual search of reference lists, contact with authors, experts, and the FDA website.
16. Max MB, Schafer SC, Culnane M, et al. Amitriptyline, but not lorazepam, relieves postherpetic neuralgia. *Neurology* 1988;38:1427–1432.
17. Kishore-Kumar R, Max MB, Schafer SC, et al. Desipramine relieves postherpetic neuralgia. *Clin Pharmacol Ther* 1990;47:305–312.
18. Torre-Mollindo F, Ferna A, Barreira R, et al. Local capsaicin 0.025% in the management of postherpetic neuralgia. *Rev Soc Esp Dolor* 2001;8:468–475.
19. Bernstein JE, Korman NJ, Bickers DR, et al. Topical capsaicin treatment of chronic postherpetic neuralgia. *J Am Acad Dermatol* 1989;21:265–270.
20. Rowbotham MC, Davies PS, Verkempinck C, et al. Lidocaine patch: double-blind controlled study of a new treatment method for postherpetic neuralgia. *Pain* 1996;65:39–44.
21. Backonja, M and Glanzman, RL. Gabapentin dosing for neuropathic pain: evidence from randomized, placebo-controlled trials. *Clin Ther* 2003;25:81–104. Search date not stated; primary sources PubMed, Medline, manufacturer of gabapentin, and clinical trial web sites.
22. Rice ASC, Maton S, Baronowski AP. Gabapentin in postherpetic neuralgia: A randomized, double blind, placebo controlled study. *Pain* 2001;94:215–224.
23. Rowbotham M, Harden N, Stacey B, et al. Gabapentin for the treatment of postherpetic neuralgia: a randomised controlled trial. *JAMA* 1998;280:1837–1842.
24. Sang CN, Booher S, Gilron I, et al. Dextromethorphan and memantine in painful diabetic neuropathy and postherpetic neuralgia: Efficacy and dose-response trials. *Anesthesiology* 2002;96:1053–1061.
25. Watt JW, Wiles JR, Bowsher DR. Epidural morphine for postherpetic neuralgia. *Anaesthesia* 1996;51:647–651.

David Wareham
Clinical Training Fellow & Honorary SpR in Medical Microbiology
Queen Mary University of London & Barts & The London NHS Trust
London
UK

Competing interests: DW has received funding to attend an overseas infectious disease conference from Pfizer, the manufacturer of gabapentin.

The following previous contributors of this topic would also like to be acknowledged: Tim Lancaster and John Yaphe.

Acute renal failure

Search date December 2002

John A Kellum, Martine Leblanc, and Ramesh Venkataraman

QUESTIONS

INTERVENTIONS

To be covered in future updates
Antibodies against adhesion molecules
Antioxidants
Endothelin receptor antagonists
Growth factors
Noradrenaline
Nutritional management

*We found insufficient evidence of effectiveness, but strong indirect evidence and historical controls suggest that failure or delay in hydration results in harm. The available evidence is strong enough to deem unethical RCTs that limit hydration.

See glossary, p 972

Key Messages

Preventing acute renal failure

- **Low osmolality contrast media (better than standard)** One systematic review comparing low osmolality contrast media with standard contrast media has found that the development of acute renal failure or need for dialysis are rare in people undertaking diagnostic tests with contrast media. However, nephrotoxicity (evaluated by serum creatinine) was less likely with low osmolality contrast media, especially in people with underlying renal impairments.
- **Fluids** We found no RCTs of fluids compared with no intervention to prevent acute renal failure. However, dehydration is an important risk factor for acute renal failure, and recommended volumes of fluid have little potential for harm. One RCT found that hydration with 0.9% sodium chloride intravenous infusion compared with 0.45% sodium chloride intravenous infusion reduced the incidence of contrast media associated nephropathy. One RCT found inconclusive evidence on the effects of inpatient compared with outpatient hydration regimens.
- **Single dose aminoglycosides (better than multiple doses of aminoglycosides)** One systematic review in people with fever and neutropenia and receiving antibiotics including aminoglycosides, found no significant difference in cure rates or nephrotoxicity between one single daily dose and multiple doses of aminoglycosides. One additional RCT found that in people with fever and requiring antibiotic treatment including aminoglycosides, a single daily dose of aminoglycoside reduced nephrotoxicity compared with multiple doses.
- **Acetylcysteine** Four RCTs found inconclusive evidence on the effects of *N*-acetylcysteine in preventing radiocontrast induced nephropathy.
- **Lipid formulations of amphotericin B (better than standard formulations)** We found no RCTs. Lipid formulations of amphotericin B seem to cause less nephrotoxicity compared with standard formulations, but direct comparisions of long term safety are lacking.
- **Fenoldopam** Three RCTs found insufficient evidence that fenoldopam is of benefit in the prevention of acute renal failure.
- **Mannitol** Small RCTs in people with traumatic rhabdomyolysis, or in people who had undergone coronary artery bypass, vascular, or biliary tract surgery, found that mannitol did not reduce acute renal failure compared with hydration alone. One RCT found that mannitol increased the risk of acute renal failure, compared with 0.9% sodium chloride infusion, but the difference was not significant.
- **Theophylline in acute renal failure induced by contrast media** RCTs found that theophylline does not prevent acute renal failure induced by contrast media compared with placebo when people are adequately hydrated. One RCT also found that theophylline did not prevent acute renal failure after coronary artery bypass surgery compared with placebo.
- **Calcium channel blockers for early allograft dysfunction** One large RCT found no significant difference between isradipine and placebo in reducing graft dysfunction in renal transplantation. We found no RCTs on the effects of calcium channel blockers in other forms of acute renal failure.

- **Dopamine** One systematic review and one subsequent RCT found that dopamine does not prevent the onset of acute renal failure, the need for dialysis, or death compared with placebo. One systematic review in people with sepsis found no evidence of harms. One RCT found insufficient evidence on the effects of combined dopamine and diltiazem in people undergoing cardiac surgery. Dopamine is associated with potentially serious side effects, such as extravasation necrosis, gangrene, and conduction abnormalities.
- **Loop diuretics** One systematic review found that loop diuretics compared with fluids alone do not prevent acute renal failure. One RCT in people with acute tubular necrosis induced by contrast media found that diuretics compared with 0.9% sodium chloride infusion increased acute renal failure. Another RCT found that diuretics compared with 0.9% sodium chloride infusion increased acute renal failure after cardiac surgery.
- **Natriuretic peptides** One large RCT found no significant difference in the prevention of acute renal failure induced by contrast media between natriuretic peptides and placebo. Subgroup analysis in another RCT found that atrial natriuretic peptide reduced dialysis free survival in non-oliguric people compared with placebo.

Treating acute renal failure in critically ill people

- **High dose continuous replacement renal therapy (better than low dose)** One RCT has found that high dose continuous renal replacement therapy (haemofiltration) significantly reduces mortality compared with standard dose therapy. A small prospective study found that intensive (daily) intermittent haemodialysis reduced mortality in people with acute renal failure compared with conventional alternate day haemodialysis. A subsequent small three arm RCT found no significant difference in survival at 28 days between early, low volume haemofiltration, early, high volume haemofiltration and late, low volume haemofiltration.
- **Combined diuretics and albumin; continuous versus bolus diuretics** We found insufficient evidence on the effects of these interventions.
- **Continuous versus intermittent renal replacement therapy** One systematic review of previously published randomised and observational studies compared intermittent with continuous renal replacement therapies and found no overall difference between therapies. However, it found a survival benefit with continuous renal replacement therapy when the analysis was restricted to the subgroup of studies comparing people with similar baseline severity of illness. Weaknesses in included studies preclude a definitive conclusion.
- **Synthetic dialysis membranes (better than cellulose based membranes)** Two systematic reviews found inconclusive evidence on the effects of synthetic based membranes on mortality in critically ill people with acute renal failure compared with cellulose based membranes.
- **Loop diurectics** RCTs in people with oliguric acute renal failure found no significant difference in renal recovery, number of days spent on dialysis, or mortality between loop diuretics and placebo. Loop diuretics have been associated with toxicity and low renal perfusion.
- **Dopamine** One systematic review found no significant difference in mortality or need for dialysis between dopamine and control. One additional RCT found that low dose dopamine did not reduce renal dysfunction compared with placebo. Dopamine has been associated with important adverse effects, including extravasation necrosis, gangrene, tachycardia, and conduction abnormalities.

- **Natriuretic peptides** RCTs found no significant difference between atrial natriuretic peptide, ularitide (urodilantin) and placebo in dialysis free survival in oliguric and non-oliguric people. One of the RCTs found that atrial natriuretic peptide may reduce survival in non-oliguric people.

DEFINITION Acute renal failure is characterised by abrupt and sustained decline in glomerular filtration rate (see glossary, p 973),[1] which leads to accumulation of urea and other chemicals in the blood. There is no clear consensus on a biochemical definition,[2] but most studies define it as a serum creatinine of 2–3 mg/dL (200–250 μmol/L), an elevation of more than 0.5 mg/dL (45 μmol/L) over a baseline creatinine below 2 mg/dL (170 μmol/L), or a twofold increase of baseline creatinine. "Severe" acute renal failure has been defined as a serum concentration of creatinine above 5.5 mg/dL (500 μmol/L) or as requiring renal replacement therapy. Acute renal failure is usually classified according to the location of the predominant primary pathology (prerenal, intrarenal, and postrenal failure). Critically ill people are unstable and at imminent risk of death, which usually implies that they need to be in, or have been admitted to, the intensive care unit.

INCIDENCE/ PREVALENCE Two prospective observational studies (2576 people) have found that established acute renal failure affects nearly 5% of people in hospital and as many as 15% of critically ill people, depending on the definitions used.[3,4]

AETIOLOGY/ RISK FACTORS **For acute renal failure prevention:** Risk factors for acute renal failure that are consistent across multiple causes include hypovolaemia; hypotension; sepsis; pre-existing renal, hepatic, or cardiac dysfunction; diabetes mellitus; and exposure to nephrotoxins (e.g. aminoglycosides, amphotericin, immunosuppressive agents, non-steroidal anti-inflammatory drugs, angiotensin converting enzyme inhibitors, iv contrast media) (see table 1, p 976). Isolated episodes of acute renal failure are rarely seen in critically ill people, but are usually part of multiple organ dysfunction syndromes (see glossary, p 973). Acute renal failure requiring dialysis is rarely seen in isolation (< 5% of people). The kidneys are often the first organs to fail.[10] In the perioperative setting, acute renal failure risk factors include prolonged aortic clamping, emergency rather than elective surgery, and use of higher volumes (> 100 mL) of intravenous contrast media. One study (3695 people) using multiple logistic regression identified the following independent risk factors: baseline creatinine clearance below 47 mL/minute (OR 1.20, 95% CI 1.12 to 1.30); diabetes (OR 5.5, 95% CI 1.4 to 21.0), and a marginal effect for doses of contrast media above 100 mL (OR 1.01, 95% CI 1.00 to 1.01). Mortality of people with acute renal failure requiring dialysis was 36% during hospitalisation.[11] **For acute renal failure in critically ill people:** Prerenal acute renal failure is caused by reduced blood flow to the kidney from renal artery disease, systematic hypotension, or maldistribution of blood flow. Intrarenal acute renal failure is caused by parenchymal injury (acute tubular necrosis, interstitial nephritis, embolic disease, glomerulonephritis, vasculitis, or small vessel disease). Postrenal acute renal failure is caused by urinary tract obstruction. Observational studies (in several hundred people from Europe, North

America, and west Africa with acute renal failure) found a prerenal cause in 40–80%, an intrarenal cause in 10–50%, and a post-renal cause in the remaining 10%.[12–17] Prerenal acute renal failure is the most common type of acute renal failure in people who are critically ill,[12,18] but acute renal failure in this context is usually part of multisystem failure, and most frequently because of acute tubular necrosis resulting from ischaemic or nephrotoxic injury, or both.[19,20]

PROGNOSIS One retrospective study (1347 people with acute renal failure) found that mortality was less than 15% in people with isolated acute renal failure.[21] One recent prospective study (> 700 people) found that, in people with acute renal failure, overall mortality and the need for dialysis was higher in an than in a non-intensive care unit (ICU) setting, despite no significant difference between the groups in mean maximal serum creatinine (need for dialysis 71% in ICU *v* 18% in non-ICU; $P < 0.001$; mortality 72% in the ICU *v* 32% in non-ICU settings; $P = 0.001$).[22]

AIMS OF INTERVENTION **Prevention:** To preserve renal function. **Critically ill people:** To prevent death; to prevent complications of acute renal failure (volume overload, acid–base disturbance, and electrolyte abnormalities); and to prevent the need for chronic dialysis, with minimum adverse effects.

OUTCOMES **Prevention:** Rates of acute renal failure, nephrotoxicity (see glossary, p 973), or both. Surrogate outcomes were limited to measurements of biochemical evidence of organ function (serum creatinine or creatinine clearance) after the intervention. Surrogate markers such as urine output or renal blood flow were not considered as evidence of effectiveness. **Critically ill people:** Rate of death; rate of renal recovery; adverse effects of treatment. Extent of natriuresis is a proxy outcome.

METHODS *Clinical Evidence* search and appraisal December 2002.

QUESTION **What are the effects of interventions to prevent acute renal failure in people at high risk?**

Ramesh Venkataraman, Martine Leblanc, and John A Kellum

OPTION **FLUIDS**

We found insufficient evidence on the effect of fluids in the prevention of acute renal failure compared with no intervention in people at high risk. However, dehydration is an important risk factor for acute renal failure, and recommended volumes of fluid have little potential of harm. One RCT found that hydration with 0.9% sodium chloride infusion reduced radiocontrast induced nephropathy compared with 0.45% sodium chloride. This effect was greater in women, people with diabetes, and individuals who received more than 250 mL of contrast. One RCT found inconclusive evidence on the effects of inpatient hydration regimens compared with outpatient hydration regimens.

Benefits: **Versus no treatment:** We found no RCTs comparing fluids with no intervention. RCTs have combined fluids (especially 0.45% sodium chloride infusion) with other active treatments. Comparisons between outcomes in these trials and historical untreated controls are difficult but suggest benefit from fluids.[23] In certain settings, such as traumatic rhabdomyolysis, early and aggressive fluid resuscitation has had dramatic benefits compared with historical controls.[24] **Versus other fluids:** We found one RCT (1620 people who had a coronary angiography), which compared 0.9% sodium chloride infusion and 0.45% sodium chloride in dextrose infusion in radiocontrast induced nephropathy.[25] Radiocontrast induced nephropathy was defined as an increase in serum creatinine of more than 0.5 mg/dL (45 μmol/L) within 48 hours. The RCT found that hydration with 0.9% sodium chloride infusion compared with 0.45% sodium chloride in dextrose infusion, significantly reduced radiocontrast induced nephropathy (0.7% with 0.9% sodium chloride infusion *v* 2% with 0.45% sodium chloride infusion; $P = 0.04$). Three pre-defined subsets of people (women, people with diabetes, and individuals receiving > 250 mL of the contrast) benefited the most from 0.9% sodium chloride infusion hydration. **Inpatient versus outpatient hydration regimens:** We found one RCT (36 people), which compared an inpatient hydration regimen (0.45% sodium chloride solution at 75 mL/hour intravenously for 12 hours before and after cardiac catheterisation) with an outpatient hydration regimen (1 L of clear liquids over 10 hours followed by 6 hours of iv hydration beginning just before contrast exposure) for the prevention of radiocontrast induced renal dysfunction.[26] The pre-defined primary end point was maximal change in creatinine up to 48 hours after cardiac catheterisation. No significant differences were found in the maximal changes in serum creatinine between groups (0.21 ± 0.38 mg/dL for inpatients *v* 0.12 ± 0.23 mg/dL for outpatients; $P > 0.05$, no additional data available). However, this study may be underpowered to rule out clinically important differences. The outpatient group also received more fluid volume.

Harms: The volumes of fluids recommended (e.g. 1 L) and the rates of infusion (generally < 500 mL/hour) have little potential for harm in most people. No significant differences were found in cardiac or peripheral vascular complications between hydration with 0.9% sodium chloride and 0.45% sodium chloride plus dextrose (cardiac complications: 5.3% with 0.9% sodium chloride *v* 6.4% with 0.45% sodium chloride plus dextrose; $P = 0.59$; peripheral vascular complications: 1.6% *v* 1.5%; $P = 0.93$).[25] The RCT comparing inpatient and outpatient hydration regimens did not report harms data.[26]

Comment: Hypovolaemia is a significant risk factor for acute renal failure. The provision of adequate maintenance fluids is considered important in preventing acute renal failure. Additional fluid loading may be useful because it assures adequate intravascular volume. It also stimulates urine output, theoretically limiting renal exposure time to higher concentrations of nephrotoxins.

OPTION LOOP DIURETICS

One systematic review has found that loop diuretics are not effective and may be harmful in preventing acute renal failure compared with fluids alone in people at high risk of acute renal failure. Two RCTs found that diuretics compared with 0.9% sodium chloride infusion seem to worsen outcome in acute tubular necrosis induced by contrast media and after cardiac surgery.

Benefits: We found one systematic review (search date 1997, 7 RCTs), which compared fluids alone with diuretics in people at risk of acute renal failure from various causes.[27] It found no evidence of improved survival, decreased incidence of acute renal failure, or need for dialysis associated with diuretics. The systematic review also assessed the efficacy of loop diuretics in the prevention of acute tubular necrosis (1 RCT, 121 people randomised to receive 1 mg/hour of furosemide or placebo immediately after major thoraco-abdominal or vascular surgery, and maintained during stay in the intensive care unit). It found no significant difference between furosemide and placebo in creatinine clearance. Both groups had significant reductions in creatinine clearance compared to baseline, but no differences were found between groups (reduction compared to baseline values: 83% with furosemide *v* 81% with placebo). The study did not address the use of loop diuretics given during the procedure.[28]

Harms: Diuretics seem to worsen outcomes in acute tubular necrosis induced by contrast media[23] and after cardiac surgery.[29] We found two RCTs addressing harms. The first RCT (78 people with chronic renal insufficiency who had a cardiac angiography, mean serum creatinine 2.1 ± 0.6 mg/dL or 186 ± 53 μmol/L) found that acute renal failure (defined as an increase in serum creatinine ≥ 0.5 mg/dL or 44 μmol/L at 48 hours) was significantly more likely to occur when people were treated with furosemide (frusemide) (10/25 [40%] with furosemide *v* 3/28 [11%] with 0.9% sodium chloride infusion; RR 3.73, 95% CI 1.16 to 12.10; NNH 4, 95% CI 2 to 17).[19] The second RCT found that furosemide compared with 0.9% sodium chloride was associated with the development of post-cardiac surgery acute renal failure (6/41 [15%] with furosemide *v* 0/40 [0%] with sodium chloride; NNH 6, 95% CI 3 to 34).[29]

Comment: The trials addressing harms[23,29] provided a three way comparison showing significant differences among the three groups ($P < 0.05$). Although they seem to have used the same control group for both comparisons, no adjustment or multiple comparisons were made.

OPTION MANNITOL

We found insufficient evidence from low powered RCTs assessing the effects of mannitol on the development of acute renal failure in people with traumatic rhabdomyolysis, or in people undergoing coronary artery bypass surgery or vascular or biliary tract surgery. One RCT found that mannitol increased the risk of acute renal failure compared with 0.9% sodium chloride, but the difference was not significant.

Benefits: We found no systematic review. Several small RCTs did not find a reduction in the incidence of acute renal failure with mannitol over hydration alone in a variety of conditions, including coronary artery bypass surgery,[30] traumatic rhabdomyolysis,[31] vascular,[32] or biliary tract surgery.[33] One trial comparing 0.9% sodium chloride, furosemide, and mannitol (78 people with chronic renal insufficiency who had a cardiac angiography, mean serum creatinine

2.1 ± 0.6 mg/dL or 186 ± 53 µmol/L) found that acute renal failure (defined as an increase in serum creatinine ≥ 0.5 mg/dL or 44 µmol/L at 48 hours) was more likely to occur in people treated with mannitol rather than with 0.9% sodium chloride, although the difference was not significant (see harms below).[23]

Harms: In acute renal failure induced by contrast media, mannitol was not associated with a significantly increased risk of acute renal failure compared with saline fluids (AR 7/25 [28%] with mannitol *v* 3/28 [11%] with 0.9% sodium chloride; RR 2.61, 95% CI 0.76 to 9.03), but the sample size was small and it was not possible to exclude harms.[23]

Comment: Mannitol is an intravascular volume expander and may also function as a free radical scavenger, as well as an osmotic diuretic. A trial addressing the effect of mannitol on renal function[23] provided a three way comparison showing significant differences among the three groups ($P < 0.05$). Although the same control group seems to have been used to compare both interventions, no adjustment was made for multiple comparisons.

OPTION DOPAMINE

We found good evidence that dopamine is ineffective in the prevention of acute renal failure compared with placebo in people at high risk of acute renal failure. We found insufficient evidence on the effects of combined dopamine and diltiazem in people undergoing cardiac surgery.

Benefits: We found one systematic review (search date 1999, 17 RCTs, 854 people)[34] and one subsequent large RCT[35] using dopamine for the prevention of acute renal failure. The meta-analysis was adequately powered and suggested that dopamine compared with placebo did not prevent mortality (11 RCTs, 508 people; 4.7% with dopamine *v* 5.6% with placebo; RR 0.83, 95% CI 0.39 to 1.77), onset of acute renal failure (11 RCTs, 511 people; 15.3% with dopamine *v* 19.5% with placebo; RR 0.79, 95% CI 0.54 to 1.13), or need for dialysis (10 RCTs, 618 people; 13.9% with dopamine *v* 16.5% with placebo; RR 0.89, 95% CI 0.66 to 1.21).[34] The subsequent RCT, which is the largest to date (328 critically ill people with signs of sepsis), evaluated dopamine in early renal dysfunction (see glossary, p 973). It found that dopamine compared with placebo had no significant effect on the development of acute renal failure (peak serum creatinine concentration during treatment was 2.7 ± 1.6 mg/dL [245 ± 144 µmol/L] in the dopamine group *v* 2.8 ± 1.6 mg/dL [249 ± 147 µmol/L] in the placebo group; $P = 0.93$), the requirement of dialysis (35/161 [22%] with dopamine *v* 40/163 [25%] with placebo; RR 0.89, 95% CI 0.58 to 1.30), intensive care unit length of stay (13 ± 14 days with dopamine *v* 14 ± 15 days with placebo; $P = 0.67$), hospital length of stay (29 ± 27 days with dopamine *v* 33 ± 39 days with placebo; $P = 0.29$), or mortality (69/161 [43%] with dopamine *v* 66/163 [40%] with placebo; RR 1.06, 95% CI 0.8 to 1.33).

Harms: One systematic review (search date 1997)[27] and one large RCT in people with sepsis[35] found no evidence on harms. Dopamine has known adverse effects, including extravasation necrosis, gangrene, tachycardia, headache, conduction abnormalities, and effects of prolactin. One four arm RCT (60 people undergoing coronary artery bypass grafting) compared dopamine, diltiazem and dopamine plus diltiazem with control (not specified). Drug administration (iv infusion rates 2 μg/kg/minute of diltiazem and 2 μg/kg/minute dopamine) was initiated 24 hours before surgery and continued for 72 hours after surgery.[36] Creatinine clearance (primary end point) was significantly higher in the combined diltiazem and dopamine group compared with the dopamine only, diltiazem only, and control groups 24 hours after surgery. However, this study is extremely underpowered, and the hydration status of the people was not controlled.

Comment: The increase in urine output associated with dopamine is often thought to be caused exclusively by the increase in renal blood flow and, therefore, it may be confused with evidence of benefit. However, dopamine also has a significant diuretic effect.

OPTION DOPAMINE 1 RECEPTOR AGONISTS (FENOLDOPAM)

We found limited evidence from three RCTs suggesting that fenoldopam may be of some benefit in maintaining renal perfusion and creatinine clearance, but found no evidence that it is effective in the prevention of acute renal failure. Fenoldapam may induce hypotension.

Benefits: We found three RCTs.[37–39] The first RCT (31 people undergoing elective coronary re-vascularisation) compared intravenous 0.1 μg/kg/minute fenoldopam with placebo (not described, presumably 0.9% sodium chloride). Mean creatinine clearance decreased in the placebo group from 107 ± 36 mL/minute to 71 ± 22 mL/minute ($P < 0.01$) and from 107 ± 36 to 79 ± 26 mL/minute ($P < 0.01$) for the 0–4 hour and 4–8 hour intervals, respectively, but not the fenoldopam group after separation from cardiopulmonary bypass. However, the clinical significance of this end point is not clear, comparisons were made within groups, and this study was underpowered to assess relevant clinical outcomes, such as need for dialysis. The second RCT,[38] evaluated the role of fenoldopam in preventing acute renal failure after aortic surgery in 28 people undergoing elective aortic surgery requiring infra-renal aortic cross clamping. People were randomised to intravenous 0.1 μg/kg/minute fenoldopam or placebo (not described) before skin incision and until release of the aortic clamp. On application of the aortic cross clamp, creatinine clearance decreased significantly in the placebo group (83 ± 20 mL/minute to 42 ± 29 mL/minute; $P < 0.01$) but not in the fenoldopam group. No comparisons were made between groups. This decrease persisted for at least 8 hours after release of cross clamp. Plasma creatinine concentration increased significantly from baseline on the first day after surgery in the placebo group (87 ± 12 mmol/L to 103 ± 28 mmol/L; $P < 0.01$) but not in the fenoldopam group. However, this study is small and the clinical significance of end point studied is unclear. The third RCT[39] randomised 45 people with chronic renal insufficiency (defined as creatinine level 2.0–5.0 mg/dL) and undergoing contrast angiography to hydration plus 0.1 μg/kg/minute fenoldopam mesylate or hydration with 0.45% sodium chloride. The primary end point was change in renal plasma flow 1 hour after contrast infusion. The secondary end point was incidence of radiocontrast induced nephropathy, defined as a 0.5 mg/dL or a 25% rise in serum creatinine level at 48 hours. Fenoldopam plus hydration significantly increased renal plasma flow 1 hour after angiography compared with hydration alone (+15.8% with fenoldapam plus hydration *v* –33.2% with hydration; $P < 0.05$). Fenoldapam also produced a non-significant reduction in radiocontrast induced nephropathy. Renal plasma flow is a surrogate outcome and the RCT was underpowered to find any significant difference in clinical outcomes. Drugs that have been shown to improve renal plasma flow may not improve clinical outcomes (e.g. dopamine).

Harms: Only one of these four RCTs reported data on potential harm from fenoldopam. The RCT found that fenoldopam, compared with sodium chloride, significantly lowered the mean arterial pressure within 30 minutes of the infusion and for the entire 4 hour infusion after angiography.[39]

Comment: There is conflicting evidence on the efficacy of fenoldopam in the prevention of radiocontrast induced nephropathy. Although small RCTs and one systematic review (search date 2000)[40] have shown that fenoldopam increases renal blood flow,[41] renal plasma flow[42] and creatinine clearance,[37] we found no evidence from RCTs that clinical outcomes are improved. Fenoldopam may cause hypotension and therefore it can potentially predispose to renal failure by reducing renal perfusion pressure.[43]

OPTION NATRIURETIC PEPTIDES

One large RCT found no significant difference in the prevention of acute renal failure induced by contrast media between natriuretic peptides and placebo. Subgroup analysis in another RCT found that atrial natriuretic peptide reduced dialysis free survival in non-oliguric people compared with placebo.

Benefits: We found no systematic review, but found one large RCT (247 people) comparing three different doses of atrial natriuretic peptide (0.01, 0.05, and 0.1 μg/kg/minute) with placebo in the prevention of acute renal failure induced by contrast media.[44] It found no difference in the incidence of acute renal failure between groups (19% with placebo *v* 23 % with 0.01 μg/kg/minute anaritide *v* 23% with 0.05 μg/kg/minute anaritide *v* 25% with 0.10 μg/kg/minute anaritide).

Harms: We found one RCT (504 people with early acute renal failure). It found worse dialysis free survival in a subgroup of people (378 non-oliguric people) when treated with atrial natriuretic peptide compared with placebo (survival rates 88/183 [48%] with atrial natriuretic peptide *v* 116/195 [59%] with placebo; RR 1.24, 95% CI 1.02 to 1.50; NNH 8, 95% CI 4 to 36).[45]

Comment: Natriuretic peptides (atrial natriuretic peptide and urodilantin) have also been evaluated in the treatment of acute renal failure (see benefits of natriuretic peptides, p 972).

OPTION THEOPHYLLINE

Three RCTs have found that, in people with adequate intravenous hydration, theophylline does not prevent radiocontrast induced nephropathy. One RCT found no significant reduction in renal impairment after elective coronary artery bypass surgery with theophylline.

Benefits: We found no systematic review. **Radiocontrast induced nephropathy:** We found three RCTs.[46–48] The first RCT (39 people receiving 100 mL of non-ionic low osmolar contrast media) found that glomerular filtration rates were unchanged with a pre-treatment dose of 5 mg/kg of intravenous theophylline (75 ± 26 mL/minute/1.72 m^2 *v* 78 ± 33 mL/minute/1.72 m^2) but decreased modestly without pretreatment (88 ± 40 mL/minute/1.72 m^2 *v* 75 ± 32 mL/minute/1.72 m^2; $P < 0.01$).[46] The second RCT (58 people receiving 40 mL of high-osmolar contrast medium) found that pre-treatment with 165 mg theophylline abolished the decline in glomerular filtration rates seen with placebo (107.5 ± 3.6 *v* 85.4 ± 3.8 mL/minute; $P < 0.001$). In people receiving placebo, radiocontrast agent induced a significant increase in plasma creatinine compared to baseline values (88.1 ± 2.7 *v* 113.4 ± 4.7 μmol/L; $P < 0.001$). Theophylline prevented this increase (89.2 ± 3.1 *v* 89.3 ± 3.5 μmol/L). In both the above RCTs, the hydration status of people receiving the radiocontrast agent was unclear. However, in a more recent prospective, double blind, randomised placebo-controlled study of 80 people with pre-existent mild to moderate renal insufficiency, the glomerular filtration rate was preserved with hydration alone. In the third RCT, serum creatinine concentration and creatinine clearance did not change significantly in either group. Two people in the theophylline group and one in the placebo group (5.7% *v* 3.4%) developed acute renal failure, defined as an increase of serum creatinine of at least 0.5 mg/dL. The administration of theophylline in addition to hydration did not bring any significant change in serum creatinine concentration or creatinine clearance).[48] **After coronary artery bypass grafting:** We found one small RCT (56 people with normal renal function), which compared theophylline (a bolus of 4 mg/kg and a subsequent continuous infusion of 0.25 mg/kg/hour for up to 96 hours) with 0.9% sodium chloride for prevention of renal impairment after elective coronary artery bypass surgery.[49] Renal impairment (defined as increase in serum creatinine of ≥ 0.4 mg/dL from the baseline at day 5 after surgery) was not significantly different between the groups (5/28 [18%] with theophylline *v* 4/28 [14%] with sodium chloride; $P > 0.05$), but the RCT may have been underpowered to rule out clinically important differences.

Harms: Theophylline has a narrow therapeutic index and known adverse effects (see harms of theophyllines under chronic obstructive pulmonary disease, p 1786). Harms were not reported in the above RCTs.[46–48]

Comment: We found no evidence of benefit from the use of theophylline in prevention or renal failure in any setting.

OPTION CALCIUM CHANNEL BLOCKERS

One RCT found that isradipine did not significantly reduce early allograft dysfunction in renal transplantation compared with placebo. We found no RCTs assessing the effects of calcium channel blockers in reducing other forms of acute renal failure.

Benefits: We found one RCT (210 people) comparing isradipine for renal allograft function after transplantation with placebo.[50] Median serum creatinine levels at 3 months (185 μmol/L with isradipine *v* 220 μmol/L with placebo; $P = 0.002$) and 12 months (141 μmol/L with isradipine *v* 158 μmol/L with placebo; $P = 0.021$) were significantly better in the isradipine group. However, there was no significant difference in the incidence of graft dysfunction (34/98 [35%] with isradipine *v* 44/112 [39%] with placebo; RR 1.13, 95% CI 0.79 to 1.62) or in the severity or duration (isradipine 9.1 days *v* placebo 9.3 days) of graft dysfunction.

Harms: As a class, calcium channel blockers are associated with hypotension and bradycardia as well as a number of less serious adverse effects. The incidence and nature of adverse effects varies between individual drugs (see harms of antihypertensive drug treatment, p 95).

Comment: None.

OPTION ACETYLCYSTEINE

Four RCTs found inconclusive evidence of the effects of *N*-acetylcysteine in preventing radiocontrast induced nephropathy.

Benefits: We found no systematic review but found four RCTs.[51–54] The first RCT (83 people with chronic renal insufficiency and undergoing computer tomography with contrast media) compared acetylcysteine with placebo to prevent acute renal failure induced by contrast media.[51] It found that the incidence of acute renal failure (defined as an increase in serum creatinine ≥ 0.5 mg/dL or 44 μmol/L at 48 hours) was significantly reduced (1/41 [2%] with acetylcysteine *v* 9/42 [21%] with placebo; RR 0.11, 95% CI 0.02 to 0.86; NNT 6, 95% CI 3 to 21).[51] The second RCT (54 people with chronic renal insufficiency defined as serum creatinine ≥ 1.4 mg/dL or calculated creatinine clearance < 50 mL/minute and requiring cardiac catheterisation with contrast media) evaluated twice daily doses of 600 mg of *N*-acetylcysteine diluted in 30 mL of ginger ale compared with placebo (not described, presumably ginger ale).[52] A total of four 600 mg doses were given, one before cardiac catheterisation and three after the procedure. Intravenous hydration and low osmolarity contrast agents were given to each person. The development of radiocontrast induced nephropathy was defined as a serum creatinine increase of ≥ 0.5 mg/dL or 25% above baseline 48 hours after catheterisation. Radiocontrast induced nephropathy was significantly reduced with *N*-acetylcysteine (2/25 [8%] with *N*-acetylcysteine *v* 13/29 [45%] with placebo; RR 0.21, 95% CI 0.06 to 0.8; $P < 0.001$). The third RCT (79 people undergoing cardiac angiography with serum creatinine > 1.7 mg/dL) evaluated the effects of intravenous hydration and 1200 mg of

N-acetylcysteine 1 hour before angiography plus a second dose 3 hours after the procedure compared with intravenous hydration and placebo.[53] The primary end point of this study was incidence of radiocontrast induced nephropathy defined as the increase of serum creatinine by 0.5 mg/dL from the baseline. No significant reduction in radiocontrast induced nephropathy was achieved with acetylcysteine (10/38 [26%] with *N*-acetylcysteine *v* 9/41 [22%] with placebo; $P > 0.05$; RR 1.4, 95% CI 0.6 to 3.1). The largest RCT we identified (183 people with renal impairment undergoing coronary, peripheral angiography/angioplasty, or both) compared hydration plus twice daily dose of 600 mg orally *N*-acetylcysteine with hydration using 0.45% sodium chloride.[54] Primary end point was incidence of radio contrast induced nephropathy defined as > 25% increase in the baseline serum creatinine level at 48 hours. A non-significant reduction in the incidence of radiocontrast induced nephropathy with *N*-acetylcysteine was found (6/92 [7%] with *N*-acetylcysteine *v* 10/91[11%] with hydration alone; $P > 0.05$; RR 0.59, 95% CI 0.23 to 1.57).

Harms: Acetylcysteine has been widely used to treat people with acetaminophen overdose, and has virtually no toxicity at therapeutic levels (see harms of paracetamol poisoning, p 1664). No data on harms were reported in the above RCTs.[51–54]

Comment: Radiocontrast induced nephropathy, defined as an increase in serum creatinine of 0.5 mg/dL from baseline after 48 hours, was the primary outcome from the above studies. The clinical significance of this outcome is unclear. None of the studies provided long term follow up, and all were underpowered to evaluate the effects of *N*-acetylcysteine in reducing dialysis or death rates. The timing of administration of *N*-acetylcysteine differed between RCTs. In the RCT with negative findings, *N*-acetylcysteine was given 1 hour before contrast agent,[53] whereas in the two positive RCTs[52,54] it was given 1 day before contrast agent.

OPTION SINGLE VERSUS MULTIPLE DOSES OF AMINOGLYCOSIDES

One systematic review in people with fever and neutropenia receiving antibiotic therapy including aminoglycosides found no significant differences in cure rates or nephrotoxicity with once versus thrice daily administration of the aminoglycoside. One good quality RCT found that single doses of aminoglycosides significantly reduced nephrotoxicity compared with multiple doses in people with fever and receiving antibiotic therapy including an aminoglycoside.

Benefits: We found one systematic review[55] and one additional RCT.[56] The systematic review (search date 1995, 4 RCTs, 803 people with fever and neutropenia, not limited to people in intensive care units) found equal antimicrobial efficacy (2 RCTs, 57 people RR 1.00, 95% CI 0.86 to 1.16), and similar clinical cure rates (4 RCTs, 961 episodes [see comment]; RR 0.97, 95% CI 0.91 to 1.05) and no difference in nephrotoxicity (see glossary, p 973) with single doses compared with multiple doses of aminoglycosides (3 RCTs, 718 episodes [see comment]; RR 0.78, 95% CI 0.31 to 1.94). One RCT not included in the review (85 people with fever), which was highlighted for its scientific rigour, compared once daily dose of gentamicin with three times daily doses of gentamicin. It found equal efficacy but significantly less incidence of nephrotoxicity with single dosing (2/40 [5%] with single dosing v 11/45 [24%]; RR 0.21, 95% CI 0.05 to 0.87; NNT 5, 95% CI 2 to 24).[56] Nephrotoxicity was defined as an increase in serum creatinine of 0.5 mg/dL (45 μmol/L) or more.

Harms: The review found no evidence of greater harm from once daily aminoglycoside dosing (see RR of nephrotoxicity in benefits section above).

Comment: The risk from aminoglycosides is highest in people with volume depletion, underlying renal, cardiac, or hepatic disease, or when combined with diuretics or other nephrotoxic agents (see glossary, p 973). Two studies included in the systematic review randomised episodes of infection, allowing for people to be included in more than one opportunity in the study.[59]

OPTION LIPID FORMULATIONS OF AMPHOTERICIN B VERSUS STANDARD FORMULATIONS

We found no RCTs. Lipid formulations of amphotericin B seem to cause less nephrotoxicity compared with standard formulations, but direct comparisons of long term safety are lacking.

Benefits: We found no systematic review and no RCTs.

Harms: We found no evidence of greater harms from lipid formulations of amphotericin B (see glossary, p 973). However, these formulations are still nephrotoxic and should be used with care.

Comment: A Phase II trial of a lipid formulation of amphotericin B (556 people) found an incidence of renal toxicity (defined by any increase in serum creatinine) of 24% (*v* 60–80% with standard formulation of amphotericin B). People with baseline serum creatinine in excess of 2.5 mg/dL (221 μmol/L) on standard amphotericin B showed a significant decrease in serum creatinine when transferred to the lipid formulation ($P < 0.001$).[57] One trial found that simply infusing amphotericin B in a lipid solution designed for parenteral nutrition did not result in any benefit and may be associated with pulmonary adverse effects.[58] Fluid loading can be useful in reducing the risk of acute renal failure from all nephrotoxins. Considerable variability may exist between individual lipid formulations of amphotericin B in terms of efficacy and safety.

OPTION LOW OSMOLALITY VERSUS STANDARD CONTRAST MEDIA

One systematic review has found that low osmolality contrast media are associated with less renal toxicity compared with standard osmolality contrast media. The benefit was greatest in people with pre-existing renal impairment (especially those with diabetes mellitus).

Benefits: We found one systematic review (search date 1991, 31 RCTs, 5146 people) comparing low osmolality contrast media (see glossary, p 973) with standard contrast media.[59] Overall, low osmolality contrast media did not influence the development of acute renal failure or need for dialysis (these are rare events), but there was less nephrotoxicity (see glossary, p 973) with low osmolality contrast media, measured by serum creatinine. The overall benefit was small for people without prior renal failure (20 RCTs, 2865 people; OR 0.75, 95% CI 0.52 to 1.10), and was greatest in people with underlying renal impairment (8 RCTs, 1418 people; OR 0.50, 95% CI 0.36 to 0.68).

Harms: We found no evidence of increased harms with low osmolality contrast media.

Comment: Low osmolality contrast media are more expensive than standard contrast media. Acute renal failure induced by contrast media usually occurs in people with diabetic nephropathy (incidence nearly 50%, varies with the degree of baseline renal function).

QUESTION What are the effects of treatments for critically ill people with acute renal failure?

Martine Leblanc, Ramesh Venkataraman, and John A Kellum

OPTION CONTINUOUS VERSUS INTERMITTENT RENAL REPLACEMENT THERAPY

One systemic review found insufficient evidence to conclude whether continuous renal replacement therapy is associated with improved outcomes compared with intermittent renal replacement therapy in critically ill people with acute renal failure.

Benefits: We found two systematic reviews.[60,61] The more recent systematic review included all previously published randomised and observational studies comparing intermittent to continuous renal replacement therapies (see glossary, p 973) (search date 1998, 13 studies, 3 RCTs, 1400 critically ill people with acute renal failure).[61] It found no significant difference in mortality (mortality with continuous *v* intermittent therapy; RR 0.93, 95% CI 0.79 to 1.09). Subgroup analysis, adjusting by baseline severity of illness, found a survival benefit with continuous renal replacement therapy (mortality; RR 0.48, 95% CI 0.34 to 0.69). A secondary analysis, including all studies and adjusting for study quality, found that continuous modalities significantly reduced mortality (RR 0.72, 95% CI 0.60 to 0.87).[61] The second systematic review (search date 1994, 15 observational studies, 1173 people)[60] has been eclipsed by the one described above.[61]

Harms: We found no good studies comparing the adverse effects of continuous renal replacement with intermittent renal replacement therapy (see glossary, p 973). The systematic reviews provided no data on harms.[60,61] Heparin is often used with intermittent and continuous renal replacement therapy, and may have adverse effects (see thromboembolism, p 273).[62] Hypotension is common with intermittent haemodialysis, whereas haemodynamic stability is better preserved with continuous renal replacement therapy.[63]

Comment: The evidence from the latest systematic review may be insufficient to draw conclusions regarding the preferred mode of renal replacement for critically ill people with acute renal failure. Only after adjusting for baseline severity, study quality, or both was the review able to show a benefit with continuous renal replacement therapies. The systematic review concluded that, although there is a suggestion of benefit with continuous renal replacement therapy, there was insufficient data to draw reliable conclusions.[61] A prospective multicentre epidemiologic survey (587 people in 28 intensive care units) found no significant difference in survival between continuous and intermittent renal replacement therapy.[64]

OPTION HIGH DOSE VERSUS LOW DOSE CONTINUOUS RENAL REPLACEMENT THERAPY

One RCT has found that high dose continuous renal replacement therapy (haemofiltration) reduces mortality compared with standard dose continuous renal replacement therapy. A small prospective study found that intensive (daily) intermittent haemodialysis reduced mortality in people with acute renal failure compared with conventional alternate day haemodialysis. A subsequent small three arm RCT found no significant difference in survival at 28 days between early, low volume haemofiltration, early, high volume haemofiltration, and late, low volume hemofiltration.

Benefits: We found no systematic review but found two RCTs.[65,66] The first RCT (425 people)[65] compared three doses of continuous replacement renal therapy (20, 35, and 45 mL/kg/hour of haemofiltration in post-dilution). Mortality was similar for the two high dose arms (60/139 [43%] with 35 mL/kg/hour v 59/140 [42%] with 45 mL/kg/hour), but was significantly higher in the low dose arm (86/146 [59%] with 20 mL/kg/hour). Survival time analysis was adjusted for three way comparison (combined RR 1.38, 95% CI 1.14 to 1.67; NNT 7, 95% CI 4 to 16).[65] The second, three arm RCT (106 severely ill people with oliguric acute renal failure recruited in two different centres) compared early, high volume haemofiltration (72–96 L/day), early, low volume haemofiltration (24–36 L/day), or late, low volume haemofiltration (24–36 L/day).[66] It found no significant difference in survival at 28 days between groups, but the study had low power to detect differences. Haemofiltration was started a mean of 7 hours after inclusion in the "early" groups and 42 hours after inclusion in the "late" group. No significant differences were found in survival at day 28 (26/35 [74%] with early, high volume, 24/35 [69%] with early, low volume, and 27/37 [73%] with late, low volume; $P > 0.05$ for two way and three way comparisons).

Harms: We found no evidence that the higher dialysis dose is associated with increased adverse effects (such as haemodynamic instability, intolerance, or bleeding). In a prospective study on daily intermittent haemodialysis,[67] there was no evidence of increased morbidity compared with alternate day dialysis. In particular, hypotension was less common with daily treatment. No data on harms were found in the above RCTs.[55,66]

Comment: There is no standard method to compare dialysis dosage between continuous and intermittent renal replacement therapies (see glossary, p 973), but urea kinetic modelling predicts that the doses used in this study would be impossible to achieve without continuous renal replacement therapy (see glossary, p 973).[68] In addition, the underlying mechanisms for solute removal are different based on the type of treatment applied (convection with haemofiltration compared with diffusion with haemodialysis). This makes comparisons of elimination of diverse solutes difficult. However, a recent, small, prospective study (160 people) has found that a higher dose of dialysis delivered as daily intermittent haemodialysis compared with alternate day haemodialysis sessions is associated with improved survival in people with acute renal failure (RR 0.59, 95% CI 0.39 to 91).[67] Although this study may have had low power to detect important differences and did not deliver the prescribed dialysis dose, it does support the concept that a dose–response relationship exists for dialysis in acute renal failure, and suggests that the traditional, end stage renal disease based dose recommendation may be too low.

OPTION **SYNTHETIC VERSUS CELLULOSE BASED DIALYSIS MEMBRANES**

Two systematic reviews found inconclusive evidence of the effects of synthetic versus cellulose based membranes on mortality in critically ill people with acute renal failure.

Benefits: We found two systematic reviews comparing synthetic and cellulose based dialysis membranes in critically ill people with all cause acute renal failure.[69,70] The first systematic review (search date 2000, 7 RCTs and controlled clinical trials, 722 people) found that synthetic membranes had similar effects on mortality among people with acute renal failure requiring in centre haemodialysis as cellulose based membranes (RR 0.92, 95% CI 0.76 to 1.13). Subgroup analysis revealed that synthetic membranes faired best against unsubstituted cellulose (RR 0.82, 95% CI 0.62 to 1.08), although the result was still not significant.[71] The second systematic review (search date 2000, 8 prospective trials providing survival data, data on recovery of renal function, or both, 867 people) found that synthetic membranes significantly increased survival rates (OR 1.37, 95% CI 1.02 to 1.83; $P = 0.03$) and showed a non-significant trend toward improved renal recovery (OR 1.23, 95% CI 0.90 to 1.68; $P = 0.18$). A sensitivity analysis performed by stratifying studies according to the type of membrane used in the control group found that the mortality reduction observed with synthetic membranes was evident when compared with unsubstituted cellulose, but not when compared with modified cellulose.[70]

Harms: Severe anaphylactoid reactions in people taking angiotensin converting enzyme inhibitors have been reported occasionally with certain synthetic biocompatible membranes (exact frequency unknown).[71]

Comment: Many of the RCTs included in both systematic reviews had methodological limitations, and all studies were underpowered. Differences in effect on outcomes seem most easily demonstrable when synthetic membranes are compared with unsubstituted cellulose.

Whether synthetic membranes are superior to modified cellulose (e.g. cellulose tri-acetate) remains controversial. However, no study has shown an advantage with any cellulose based membrane over synthetic membranes except that the former are generally less expensive.

OPTION DOPAMINE

One systematic review found no significant difference in mortality or need for dialysis between dopamine and control. One additional RCT found that low dose dopamine did not reduce renal dysfunction compared with placebo. Dopamine has been associated with important adverse effects, including extravasation necrosis, gangrene, tachycardia, and conduction abnormalities.

Benefits: We found one systematic review[34] and one additional RCT.[35] The systematic review (search date 1999, 58 trials, of which 17 were RCTs, 2149 people) found that, among the 24 studies reporting on clinical outcomes, dopamine produced no significant reduction in mortality (11 trials, 508 people, 4.7% with dopamine *v* 5.6% with control; RR 0.83, 95% CI 0.39 to 1.77) or need for dialysis with dopamine (10 trials, 618 people; 13.9% with dopamine *v* 16.5 with control; RR 0.89, 95% CI 0.66 to 1.21).[34] The additional RCT (multicentre, double blind, placebo controlled: 328 people with early renal dysfunction defined as oliguria [see glossary, p 973] or increase in serum creatinine) found that compared with placebo, low dose dopamine did not reduce mortality at discharge (69/161 [43%] with dopamine *v* 66/163 [41%] with placebo; RR 1.06, 95% CI 0.82 to 1.37).[35]

Harms: Dopamine has recognised adverse effects, including extravasation necrosis, gangrene, tachycardia, headache, conduction abnormalities, and effects of prolactin. We found no good evidence on harms in this setting. The systematic review and the RCT provided no data on harms.[34,35]

Comment: Studies using dopamine to prevent renal failure or to ameliorate progression have found no benefit (see prevention of acute renal failure, p 957). Studies evaluating the effectiveness of dopamine for the treatment of acute renal failure have focused on early renal dysfunction and have often included people with normal renal function who were at risk of acute renal failure.

OPTION LOOP DIURETICS

Two small RCTs found that loop diuretics had no significant effect on renal recovery, the number of days spent on dialysis, or mortality compared with placebo. The RCTs lacked power to exclude a clinically important effect, and included people from a non-intensive care unit setting. Loop diuretics have been associated with toxicity and low renal perfusion.

Benefits: We found no systematic review. We found two RCTs (66 and 58 people, respectively; some in intensive care units, proportion unknown) comparing intravenous furosemide with placebo in people with oliguric acute renal failure of various causes.[72,73] In the second RCT, all people received one dose of furosemide 1 g and were then randomised to continued treatment or placebo. Neither RCT found significant differences in renal recovery (first RCT 19/33 [58%] with furosemide *v* 22/33 [67%] with placebo; RR 0.86, 95% CI 0.50 to 1.20;[72] second RCT 10/28 [36%] with furosemide *v* 12/28 [43%] with placebo; RR 0.83, 95% CI 0.37 to 1.45)[73] or mortality. The RCTs lacked power to exclude a clinically important effect of loop diuretics on these outcomes.

Harms: Ototoxicity can occur with high doses of loop diuretics. No adverse effects were reported in the first trial.[74] Deafness occurred in two people in the second trial; both were randomised to furosemide. Hearing loss was permanent in one of these people.[73] Diuretics may reduce renal perfusion and add a pre-renal component to the renal failure, but the frequency of this event is uncertain.[75] See harms of loop diuretics, p 959.

Comment: None.

OPTION CONTINUOUS INFUSION VERSUS BOLUS INJECTION OF LOOP DIURETICS

We found no RCTs comparing continuous infusion with bolus injection of loop diuretics in critically ill people with acute renal failure.

Benefits: We found no systematic review and no RCTs in critically ill people with acute renal failure.

Harms: One small, crossover RCT (8 people with acute deterioration of chronic renal failure, mean creatinine clearance 0.28 mL/second) found that fewer people experienced myalgia when treated with continuous infusion than with bolus dosing of bumetanide (3/8 [38%] people with bolus dosing *v* 0/8 [0%] with continuous infusion).[76]

Comment: The small, crossover trial found that continuous infusion resulted in a net increase in sodium excretion over 24 hours (mean increase in sodium excretion 48 mmol/day, 95% CI 16 mmol/day to 60 mmol/day; P = 0.01).

OPTION INTRAVENOUS ALBUMIN SUPPLEMENTATION PLUS LOOP DIURETICS

We found no RCTs on the effects of adding intravenous albumin to loop diuretic treatment in critically ill people with acute renal failure.

Benefits: We found no systematic review and no RCTs evaluating clinical outcomes in critically ill people with acute renal failure.

Harms: We found insufficient evidence in people with acute renal failure. One systematic review (30 RCTs, 1419 people, most without acute renal failure) found that albumin increased the risk of death in unselected critically ill people (mortality 98/704 [14%] with albumin *v* 58/715 [8%] with control; RR 1.68, CI 1.26 to 2.23). All of the included trials were small and combined highly heterogeneous populations.[77]

Comment: One crossover RCT (9 people with nephrotic syndrome) compared three interventions: furosemide alone, furosemide plus albumin, and albumin alone.[78] It found that furosemide was superior to albumin alone, and furosemide plus albumin resulted in the greatest urine and sodium excretion. The clinical significance of this finding is unclear.

OPTION NATRIURETIC PEPTIDES

RCTs have found that both atrial natriuretic peptide and ularitide (urodilantin) are ineffective in treating acute renal failure in oliguric and non-oliguric people. Atrial natriuretic peptide may be harmful in non-oliguric people.

Benefits: We found no systematic review but found three RCTs.[45,79,80] One large RCT (504 people) found no overall difference in dialysis free survival with atrial natriuretic peptide compared with placebo in people with acute renal failure.[45] Pre-planned subgroup analysis suggested a possible benefit to people with oliguria (see glossary, p 973), and lower survival rates in non-oliguric people. However, a recent RCT (220 people)[79] in people with oliguric acute renal failure found no improvement in dialysis free survival with a 24 hour infusion of atrial natriuretic peptide compared with placebo. A third RCT compared ularitide ([urodilantin] a natriuretic peptide with less system haemodynamic effects) in a dose finding (5, 20, 40, or 80 ng/kg/minute ularitide), placebo controlled RCT (176 people). Ularitide did not reduce the requirement for dialysis (people who needed dialysis: 35% with 5 ng/kg/minute ularitide *v* 36% with 20 ng/kg/minute ularitide *v* 28% with 40 ng/kg/minute ularitide *v* 41% with 80 ng/kg/minute ularitide *v* 36% with placebo; P = NS).[80]

Harms: One RCT found that natriuretic peptide caused significant hypotension compared with placebo (95% with natriuretic peptide *v* 55% with placebo; $P < 0.01$). Also, atrial natriuretic peptide may be associated with a worse outcome in people with non-oliguric renal failure (dialysis free survival in 378 non-oliguric people was 48% with anaritide *v* 59% with placebo; $P = 0.03$).[79] See harms of natriuretic peptides, p 962.

Comment: We found no evidence of significant improvement of acute renal failure with atrial natriuretic peptide.

GLOSSARY

Biocompatible Artificial materials can induce an inflammatory response. This response can be humoral (including complement) or cellular. Synthetic dialysis membranes seem to produce less of an inflammatory response *in vitro* and are classified as more "biocompatible". By contrast, cellulose based membranes seem to be less biocompatible (cause more inflammation). When cellulose based membranes are rendered semi synthetic by modifications or substitution of materials like acetate, they may be become more biocompatible. We found no standards by which this comparison can be made.

Cellulose based Dialysis membranes may be made from cellulose. "Unsubstituted" cellulose has not undergone modification to attempt to improve biocompatibility. Synthetic membranes do not use cellulose.

Continuous renal replacement therapy Any extracorporeal blood purification treatment intended to substitute for impaired renal function over an extended period of time and applied for, or aimed at being applied for, 24 hours a day.
Early allograft dysfunction Renal dysfunction that occurs after renal transplantation, and which is usually secondary to ischaemic injury.
Early renal dysfunction An acute derangement in renal function that is still evolving.
Glomerular filtration rate The rate of elaboration of protein free plasma filtrate (ultrafiltration) across the walls of the glomerular capillaries.
Intermittent renal replacement therapy Renal support that is not, nor intended to be, continuous; usually prescribed for a period of 12 hours or less.
Lipid formulations of amphotericin B Complexes of amphotericin B and phospholipids or sterols. This reduces the toxicity of amphotericin B while preserving its antifungal activity.
Low osmolality contrast media Contrast media with osmolality less than 300 mOsm/L.
Multiple organ dysfunction syndrome A syndrome of progressive organ failure, affecting one organ after another and believed to be the result of persistent or recurrent infection or inflammation.
Nephrotoxic agents Any agent that has the potential to produce nephrotoxicity.
Nephrotoxicity Renal parenchymal damage manifested by a decline in glomerular filtration rate, tubular dysfunction, or both.
Oliguria Urine output less than 5 mL/kg daily.

Substantive changes

Fluids in prevention of acute renal failure One RCT added,[26] allowing for a new comparison to be made between inpatient and outpatient settings; categorisation unchanged.
Dopamine in prevention One RCT added;[36] conclusions unchanged.
Fenoldopam in prevention Three RCTs added;[37–39] conclusions unchanged.
Theophylline in prevention Two RCTs added, which assess the effects of radiocontrast induced nephropathy;[46,47] one new RCT assesses the effects after coronary bypass grafting;[49] conclusions unchanged.
Acetylcysteine Three RCTs added;[52–54] conclusions unchanged.
High dose versus low dose continuous renal replacement therapy in treatment One RCT added;[66] conclusions unchanged.
Dialysis membranes Two systematic reviews added;[69,70] these eclipse previous RCTs; conclusions have changed.

REFERENCES

1. Nissenson AR. Acute renal failure: definition and pathogenesis. *Kidney Int Suppl* 1998;66:7–10.
2. Bellomo R, Ronco C. The changing pattern of severe acute renal failure. *Nephrology* 1991;2:602–610.
3. Hou SH, Bushinsky DA, Wish JB, et al. Hospital-acquired renal insufficiency: a prospective study. *Am J Med* 1983;74:243–248.
4. Brivet FG, Kleinknecht DJ, Loirat P, et al. Acute renal failure in intensive care units — causes, outcomes and prognostic factors of hospital mortality: a prospective multicenter study. *Crit Care Med* 1996;24:192–198.
5. Wiecek A, Zeier M, Ritz E. Role of infection in the genesis of acute renal failure. *Nephrol Dial Transplant* 1994;9(suppl 4):40–44.
6. Myers BD, Moran SM. Hemodynamically mediated acute renal failure. *N Engl J Med* 1986;314:97–100.
7. Ward MM. Factors predictive of acute renal failure in rhabdomyolysis. *Arch Intern Med* 1988;148:1553–1557.
8. Kahlmeter G, Dahlager JI. Aminoglycoside toxicity — a review of clinical studies published between 1975 and 1982. *J Antimicrob Chemother* 1984;13(suppl A):9–22. Search date 1982; primary sources Medline, Toxline, and personal contact with pharmaceutical companies.
9. Butler WT, Bennett JE, Alling DW, et al. Nephrotoxicity of amphotericin B, early and late events in 81 patients. *Ann Intern Med* 1964;61:175–187.
10. Tran DD, Oe PL, De Fijter CWH, et al. Acute renal failure in patients with acute pancreatitis: prevalence, risk factors, and outcome. *Nephrol Dial Transplant* 1993;8:1079–1084.
11. McCullough PA, Wolyn R, Rocher LL, et al. Acute renal failure after coronary intervention: incidence, risk factors, and relationship to mortality. *Am J Med* 1997;103:368–375.

12. Thadhani R, Pascual M, Bonventre JV. Acute renal failure. *N Engl J Med* 1996;334:1448–1460.
13. Kleinknecht D. Epidemiology in acute renal failure in France today. In: Biari D, Neild G, eds. *Acute renal failure in intensive therapy unit*. Berlin: Springer-Verlag, 1990:13–21.
14. Coar D. Obstructive nephropathy. *Del Med J* 1991;63:743–749.
15. Kaufman J, Dhakal M, Patel B, et al. Community acquired acute renal failure. *Am J Kidney Dis* 1991;17:191–198.
16. Bamgboye EL, Mabayoje MO, Odutala TA, et al. Acute renal failure at the Lagos University Teaching Hospital. *Ren Fail* 1993;15:77–80.
17. Nolan CR, Anderson RJ. Hospital-acquired acute renal failure. *J Am Soc Nephrol* 1998;9:710–718.
18. Cantarovich F, Bodin L. Functional acute renal failure. In: Cantarovich F, Rangoonwala B, Verho M, eds. *Progress in acute renal failure*. Paris: Hoechst Marion Roussel, 1998:55–65.
19. Brezis M, Rosen S. Hypoxia of the renal medulla. Its implication for disease. *N Engl J Med* 1995;332:647–655.
20. Bonventre JV. Mechanisms of ischemic acute renal failure. *Kidney Int* 1993;43:1160–1178.
21. Turney JH, Marshall DH, Brownjohn AM, et al. The evolution of acute renal failure, 1956–1988. Q J Med 1990;74:83–104.
22. Liano F, Junco E, Pascual J, et al. The spectrum of acute renal failure in the intensive care unit compared to that seen in other settings. The Madrid Acute Renal Failure Study Group. *Kidney Int Suppl* 1998;53:16–24.
23. Solomon R, Werner C, Mann D, et al. Effects of saline, mannitol, and furosemide to prevent acute decreases in renal function induced by radiocontrast agents. *N Engl J Med* 1994;331:1416–1420.
24. Better OS, Stein JH. Early management of shock and prophylaxis of acute renal failure in traumatic rhabdomyolysis. *N Engl J Med* 1990;322:825–829.
25. Mueller C, Buerkle G, Buettner HJ, et al. Prevention of contrast media-associated nephropathy: randomized comparison of 2 hydration regimes in 1620 patients undergoing coronary angioplasty. *Arch Intern Med* 2002;162:329–336.
26. Taylor AJ, Hotchkiss D, Morse RW, et al. Preparation for angiography in renal dysfunction: a randomized trial of inpatient versus outpatient hydration protocols for cardiac catheterization in mild-to-moderate renal dysfunction. *Chest* 1998;114:1570–1574.
27. Kellum JA. The use of diuretics and dopamine in acute renal failure: a systematic review of the evidence. *Crit Care* 1997;1:53–59. Search date 1997; primary sources Medline and hand searches of bibliographies of relevant articles.
28. Hager B, Betschart M, Krapf R. Effect of postoperative intravenous loop diuretic on renal function after major surgery. *Schweiz Med Wochenschr* 1996;126:666–673.
29. Lassnigg A, Donner E, Grubhofer G, et al. Lack of renoprotective effects of dopamine and furosemide during cardiac surgery. *J Am Soc Nephrol* 2000;11:97–104.
30. Ip-Yam PC, Murphy S, Baines M, et al. Renal function and proteinuria after cardiopulmonary bypass: the effects of temperature and mannitol. *Anesth Analg* 1994;78:842–847.
31. Homsi E, Barreiro MF, Orlando JM, et al. Prophylaxis of acute renal failure in patients with rhabdomyolysis. *Ren Fail* 1997;19:283–288.
32. Beall AC, Holman MR, Morris GC, et al. Mannitol-induced osmotic diuresis during vascular surgery. *Arch Surg* 1963;86:34–42.
33. Gubern JM, Sancho JJ, Simo J, et al. A randomized trial on the effect of mannitol on postoperative renal function in patients with obstructive jaundice. *Surgery* 1988;103:39–44.
34. Kellum JA, Decker JM. The use of dopamine in acute renal failure: a meta-analysis. *Crit Care Med* 2001;29:1526–1531. Search date 1999; primary sources Medline and bibliographies of review articles.
35. Bellomo R, Chapman M, Finfer S, et al. Low-dose dopamine in patients with early renal dysfunction: a placebo-controlled randomised trial. Australian and New Zealand Intensive Care Society (ANZICS) Clinical Trials Group. *Lancet* 2000;356:2139–2143.
36. Yavuz S, Ayabakan N, Goncu MT, et al. Effect of combined dopamine and diltiazem on renal function after cardiac surgery. *Med Sci Monit* 2002;8:PI45–P1550.
37. Halpenny M, Lakshmi S, O'Donnell A, et al. Fenoldopam: renal and splanchnic effects in patients underoing coronary artery bypass grafting. *Anaesthesia* 2001;56:953–960.
38. Halpenny M, Rushe C, Breen P, et al. The effects of fenoldopam on renal function in patients undergoing elective aortic surgery. *Eur J Anesthesiol* 2002;19:32–39.
39. Tumlin JA, Wang A, Murray PT et al. Fenoldopam mesylate blocks reductions in renal plasma flow after radioccontrast dye infusion: a pilot trial in the prevention of contrast nephropathy. *Am Heart J* 2002;143:894–903.
40. Chu VL, Cheng GW. Fenoldopam in the prevention of contrast media-induced acute renal failure. *Ann Pharmacother* 2001;35:1278–1282. Search date 2000; primary source Medline.
41. Mathur VS, Swan SK, Lambrecht LJ, et al. The effects of fenoldopam, a selective dopamine receptor agonist, on systemic and renal hemodynamics in normotensive subjects. *Crit Care Med* 1999;27:1832–1837.
42. Tumlin JA, Wang A, Murray PT, et al. Fenoldopam mesylate blocks reductions in renal plasma flow after radiocontrast dye infusion: a pilot trial in the prevention of contrast nephropathy. *Am Heart J* 2002;143:894–903.
43. Mathur VS, Swan SK, Lambrecht LJ, et al. The effects of fenoldopam, a selective dopamine receptor agonist, on systemic and renal hemodynamics in normotensive subjects. *Crit Care Med* 1999;27:1832–1837.
44. Kurnik BR, Allgren RL, Genter FC, et al. Prospective study of atrial natriuretic peptide for the prevention of radiocontrast-induced nephropathy. *Am J Kidney Dis* 1998;31: 674–680.
45. Allgren RL, Marbury TC, Rahman SN, et al. Anaritide in ATN. Auriculin anaritide ARF study group. *N Engl J Med* 1997;336:828–834.
46. Erley CM, Duda SH, Schlepckow S, et al. Adenosine antagonist theophylline prevents the reduction of glomerular filtration rate after contrast media application. *Kidney Int* 1994;45:1425–1431.
47. Kolonko A, Wiecek A, Kokot F. The nonselective adenosine antagonist theophylline does prevent renal dysfunction induced by radiographic contrast agents. *J Nephrol* 1998;11:151–156.

48. Erley CM, Duda SH, Rehfuss D, et al. Prevention of radiocontrast-media-induced nephropathy in patients with pre-existing renal insufficiency by hydration in combination with the adenosine antagonist theophylline. *Nephrol Dial Transplant* 1999;14:1146–1149.
49. Kramer BK, Preuner J, Ebenburger A, et al. Lack of renoprotective effect of theophylline during aortocoronary bypass surgery. *Nephrol Dial Transplant* 2002;17:910–915.
50. Van Riemsdijk IC, Mulder PG, De Fijter JW, et al. Addition of Isradipine (lomir) results in a better renal function after kidney transplantation: a double-blind, randomized, placebo-controlled, multi-center study. *Transplantation* 2000;70:122–126.
51. Tepel M, Van der Giet M, Schwarzfeld C, et al. Prevention of radiographic-contrast-agent-induced reductions in renal function by acetylcysteine. *N Engl J Med* 2000;343:180–184.
52. Diaz-Sandoval LJ, Kosowsky BD, Losordo DW. Acetylcysteine to prevent angiography-related renal tissue injury (the APART trial). *Am J Cardiol* 2002;89:356–358.
53. Durham JD, Caputo C, Dokko J, et al. A randomized controlled trial of *N*-acetylcysteine to prevent contrast nephropathy in cardiac angiography. *Kidney Int* 2002;62:2202–2207.
54. Briguori C, Manganelli F, Scarpato P, et al. Acetylcysteine and contrast agent-associated nephropathy: *J Am Coll Cardiol* 2002;40:298–303.
55. Hatala R, Dinh TT, Cook DJ. Single daily dosing of aminoglycosides in immunocompromised adults: a systematic review. *Clin Infect Dis* 1997;24:810–815. Search date 1995; primary sources Medline, hand searches of selected infectious diseases journals and bibliographies of relevant articles, and personal contact with primary investigators of selected studies.
56. Prins JM, Buller HR, Kuijper EJ, et al. Once versus thrice daily gentamicin in patients with serious infections. *Lancet* 1993;341:335–339.
57. Walsh TJ, Hiemenz JW, Seibel NL, et al. Amphotericin B lipid complex for invasive fungal infections: analysis of safety and efficacy in 556 cases. *Clin Infect Dis* 1998;26:383–396.
58. Schoffski P, Freund M, Wunder R, et al. Safety and toxicity of amphotericin B in glucose 5% or intralipid 20% in neutropenic patients with pneumonia or fever of unknown origin: randomised study. *BMJ* 1998;317:379–384.
59. Barrett BJ, Carlisle EJ. Metaanalysis of the relative nephrotoxicity of high and low-osmolality iodinated contrast media. *Radiology* 1993;188:171–178. Search date 1991; primary sources Medline, Embase, hand searches of reference lists of selected articles, and personal contact with authors of selected primary studies and pharmaceutical companies manufacturing contrast media.
60. Jakob SM, Frey FJ, Uehlinger DE. Does continuous renal replacement therapy favourably influence the outcome of the patients? *Nephrol Dial Transplant* 1996;11:1250–1255. Search date 1994; primary sources not stated.
61. Kellum JA, Angus DC, Johnson JP, et al. Continuous versus intermittent renal replacement therapy: a meta-analysis. *Int Care Med* 2002;28:29–37. Search date 1998; primary sources Medline, meeting abstracts and bibliographies of review articles.
62. Ronco C. Continuous renal replacement therapies for the treatment of acute renal failure in intensive care patients. *Clin Nephrol* 1993;40:187–198.
63. Heering P, Morgera S, Schmitz FJ, et al. Cytokine removal and cardiovascular hemodynamics in septic patients with continuous venovenous hemofiltration. *Intensive Care Med* 1997;23:288–296.
64. Guerin C, Girard R, Selli JM, et al. Intermittent versus continuous renal replacement therapy for acute renal failure in intensive care units: Results from a multicenter prospective epidemiological survey. *Int Care Med* 2002;28:1411–1418.
65. Ronco C, Bellomo R, Homel P, et al. Effects of different doses in continuous veno-venous haemofiltration on outcomes of acute renal failure: a prospective randomised trial. *Lancet* 2000;356:26–30.
66. Bouman CSC, Oudemans-van Straaten HM, Tijssen JGP, et al. Effects of early high-volume continuous venovenous hemofiltration on survival and recovery of renal function in intensive care patients with acute renal failure: A prospective, randomized trial. *Crit Care Med* 2002;30:2205–2211.
67. Schiffl H, Lang SM, Fischer R. Daily hemodialysis and the outcome of acute renal failure. *N Engl J Med* 2002;346:305–310.
68. Gotch FA, Sargent JA, Keen ML. Whither goest Kt/V? *Kidney Int* 2000;58(suppl 76):3–18.
69. Jaber BL, Lau J, Schmid CH, et al. Effect of biocompatibility of hemodialysis membranes on mortality in acute renal failure: A meta-analysis. *Clinl Nephrol* 2002;57:274–282. Search date 2000; primary sources Medline, meeting abstracts and bibliographies of review articles.
70. Subramanian S, Venkataraman R, Kellum JA. Influence of dialysis membrane on outcomes in acute renal failure: A meta-analysis. *Kidney Int* 2002;62:1819–1823. Search date 2000; primary sources Medline, meeting abstracts and bibliographies of review articles.
71. Kammerl MC, Schaefer RM, Schweda F, et al. Extracorporal therapy with AN69 membranes in combination with ACE inhibition causing severe anaphylactoid reactions: still a current problem? *Clin Nephrol* 2000;53:486–488.
72. Kleinknecht D, Ganeval D, Gonzales-Duque LA, et al. Furosemide in acute oliguric renal failure. A controlled trial. *Nephron* 1976;17:51–58.
73. Brown CB, Ogg CS, Cameron JS. High dose furosemide in acute renal failure: a controlled trial. *Clin Nephrol* 1981;15:90–96.
74. Himmelfarb J, Tolkoff RN, Chandran P, et al. A multicenter comparison of dialysis membranes in the treatment of acute renal failure requiring dialysis. *J Am Soc Nephrol* 1998;9:257–266.
75. Kellum JA. Use of diuretics in the acute care setting. *Kidney Int* 1998;53(suppl 66):67–70.
76. Rudy DW, Voelker JR, Greene PK, et al. Loop diuretics for chronic renal insufficiency: a continuous infusion is more efficacious than bolus therapy. *Ann Intern Med* 1991;115:360–366.
77. The Albumin Reviewers. Human albumin solution for resuscitation and volume expansion in critically ill patients. In: The Cochrane Library, Issue 4, 2002. Oxford: Update Software. Search date 2001; primary sources The Cochrane Injuries Group Register, the Cochrane Library, Medline, Embase, Bids, Index to Scientific and Technical Proceedings, and hand searched references.
78. Fliser D, Zurbruggen I, Mutschler E, et al. Coadministration of albumin and furosemide in patients with the nephrotic syndrome. *Kidney Int* 1999;55:629–634.
79. Lewis J, Salem M, Chertow GM, et al. Atrial natriuretic factor in oliguric acute renal failure. Anaritide Acute Renal Failure study group. *Am J Kidney Dis* 2000;36:767–774.
80. Meyer M, Pfarr E, Schirmer G, et al. Therapeutic use of natriuretic peptide ularitide in acute renal failure. *Ren Fail* 1999;21:85–100.

Acute renal failure

John Kellum
Associate Professor
Department of Critical Care Medicine
University of Pittsburgh
Pittsburgh
USA

Martine Leblanc
Assistant Professor of Nephrology and Critical Care
Maisonneuve–Rosemont Hospital
University of Montreal
Montreal
Canada

Ramesh Venkataraman
Assistant Professor
Department of Critical Care Medicine
University of Pittsburgh
Pittsburgh
USA

Competing interests: JK has received compensation for lectures and consulting work for Gambro and Renal Tech. ML and RV none declared.

TABLE 1 **Selected risk factors for acute renal failure (ARF) (see text, p 956).**

Risk factor	Incidence of ARF	Comments
Sepsis	Unknown	Sepsis seems to be a contributing factor in as many as 43% of ARF cases[5]
Aortic clamping	Approaches 100% when > 60 minutes[6]	Refers to cross-clamping (no flow) above the renal arteries
Rhabdomyolysis	16.5%[7]	None
Aminoglycosides	8–26%[8]	None
Amphotericin	88% with > 5 g total dose[9]	60% overall incidence of nephrotoxicity

Benign prostatic hyperplasia

Search date November 2002

Robyn Webber

QUESTIONS

INTERVENTIONS

Key Messages

- **α Blockers** We found evidence that α blockers improve lower urinary tract symptoms compared with placebo. We found limited evidence that different α blockers have similar effects. We found limited evidence that α blockers improve symptoms more than 5α reductase inhibitors. We found no evidence comparing α blockers versus surgical treatment. We found limited evidence that α blockers and saw palmetto are equally effective in improving symptoms.
- **5α Reductase inhibitors** We found evidence that 5α reductase inhibitors improve symptoms and reduce complications compared with placebo. We found limited evidence that 5α reductase inhibitors were less effective at improving symptoms than α blockers. We found no evidence comparing 5α reductase inhibitors versus surgical treatment.
- **Saw palmetto plant extracts** One systematic review has found that saw palmetto improves symptoms compared with placebo. It found no significant difference in symptom scores between saw palmetto and finasteride. We found evidence of a similar improvement in symptom scores with saw palmetto or tamsulosin. We found evidence of no treatment advantage in combining saw palmetto with tamsulosin.
- **Transurethral microwave thermotherapy** We found evidence that transurethral microwave thermotherapy reduced symptoms compared with sham treatment. We found limited evidence that transurethral resection relieved short term symptoms better than thermotherapy. We found limited evidence that thermotherapy improved symptoms more than α blockers over 18 months.
- **Transurethral resection versus no surgery** We found evidence that transurethral resection reduced symptoms more than watchful waiting, and did not increase the risk of erectile dysfunction or incontinence.

- **β-Sitosterol plant extract** One systematic review found that β-sitosterol plant extract improved lower urinary tract symptoms compared with placebo in the short term.
- **Rye grass pollen extract** One systematic review found limited evidence that rye grass pollen extract increased self rated improvement and reduced nocturia in the short term compared with placebo. However, the review identified only two small RCTs, from which we were unable to draw reliable conclusions.
- **Transurethral resection versus less invasive surgical techniques** We found no evidence of a significant difference in symptoms between transurethral resection and transurethral incision or between transurethral resection and electrical vaporisation. We found limited evidence that transurethral resection improved symptoms more than visual laser ablation but that transurethral resection may be associated with a higher risk of blood transfusion.
- **Transurethral resection versus transurethral needle ablation** We found limited evidence that transurethral resection reduced symptoms compared with transurethral needle ablation, although transurethral needle ablation caused fewer adverse effects.

DEFINITION Benign prostatic hyperplasia is defined histologically. Clinically, it is characterised by lower urinary tract symptoms (urinary frequency, urgency, a weak and intermittent stream, needing to strain, a sense of incomplete emptying, and nocturia), and can lead to complications, including acute urinary retention.

INCIDENCE/ PREVALENCE Estimates of the prevalence of symptomatic benign prostatic hyperplasia range from 10–30% for men in their early 70s, depending on how benign prostatic hyperplasia is defined.[1]

AETIOLOGY/ RISK FACTORS The mechanisms by which benign prostatic hyperplasia causes symptoms and complications are unclear, although bladder outlet obstruction is an important factor.[2] The best documented risk factors are increasing age and functioning testes.[3]

PROGNOSIS Community and practice based studies suggest that men with lower urinary tract symptoms can expect slow progression of the symptoms.[4,5] However, symptoms can wax and wane without treatment. In men with symptoms of benign prostatic hyperplasia, rates of acute urinary retention range from 1–2% a year.[5–7]

AIMS OF INTERVENTION To reduce or alleviate lower urinary tract symptoms; to prevent complications; and to minimise adverse effects of treatment.

OUTCOMES Burden of lower urinary tract symptoms; rates of acute urinary retention and prostatectomy; risks of adverse effects of treatment; and self rated improvement. Symptoms are measured using the validated International Prostate Symptom Score (IPSS), which includes seven questions measuring symptoms on an overall scale of 0–35, with higher scores representing more frequent symptoms.[8] Older studies used a variety of symptom assessment instruments, which makes comparisons difficult.

METHODS This review was originally based on ongoing Medline searches and prospective journal hand searches by the Patient Outcomes Research Team for Prostatic Diseases (Agency for Health Care Policy and Research grant number HS0839). *Clinical Evidence* search and appraisal November 2002.

QUESTION What are the effects of medical treatments?

OPTION α BLOCKERS

We found evidence that α blockers improve lower urinary tract symptoms compared with placebo. We found limited evidence that different α blockers have similar effects. We found limited evidence that α blockers improved symptoms more than 5α reductase inhibitors. We found no evidence comparing α blockers versus surgical treatment. We found limited evidence that α blockers and saw palmetto are equally effective in improving symptoms.

Benefits: **Versus placebo:** We found four systematic reviews[9–12] and two subsequent RCTs.[13,14] Two systematic reviews examined the effects of any α blocker (search dates 1998, 21 RCTs;[9] and 1999, 24 RCTs[10]), one systematic review examined the effects of tamsulosin (search date 2000, 6 RCTs[11]), and one systematic review examined the effects of terazosin (search date 2001, 10 RCTs[12]). Most RCTs included in the first two reviews found a greater improvement in symptoms with α blockers than with placebo, but overall results were not reported (results presented graphically or in tabular form).[9,10] The largest RCT (2084 men) compared terazosin at doses of up to 10 mg daily for 1 year versus placebo. Treatment achieved significantly greater mean improvement in International Prostate Symptom Score (IPSS) (–7.6 points from baseline with terazosin *v* –3.7 with placebo; mean change, terazosin *v* placebo –3.9 points, 95% CI –5.5 points to –3.3 points).[15] One small RCT included in the reviews (81 men) found that sustained release alfuzosin (5 mg twice daily) for 48 hours increased the ability to pass urine after catheter removal in men catheterised for acute retention from 5–29%.[16] The third review found that tamsulosin (0.4 or 0.8 mg/day) improved symptoms and peak urine flow compared with placebo (WMD for mean change in Boyarsky Symptom Score [see glossary, p 991] for 0.4 mg tamsulosin *v* placebo –1.1 points, 95% CI –1.49 points to –0.72 points; for 0.8 mg tamsulosin *v* placebo –1.6 points, 95% CI –2.3 points to –1.0 points; WMD for change in peak urine flow from baseline for 0.4 mg tamsulosin 1.1 mL/second, 95% CI 0.59 mL/second to 1.51 mL/second; for 0.8 mg tamsulosin 1.1 mL/second, 95% CI 0.65 mL/second to 1.48 mL/second).[11] The fourth review found that terazosin improved the Boyarsky Symptom Score and the American Urological Association Symptom Index (AUASI — see glossary, p 991) compared with placebo at 4 to 52 weeks, but the statistical significance was not reported (mean improvement in Boyarsky Symptom Score in 4 RCTs 37% with terazosin *v* 15% with placebo, P value not reported; mean improvement in AUASI in 2 RCTs 38% for terazosin *v* 17% for placebo, P value not reported).[12] It also found that terazosin improved peak urinary flow rates compared with placebo, but the statistical significance was not reported (improvement 23% with terazosin *v* 11% with placebo, P value not reported). The first subsequent RCT (795 men) compared controlled released versus standard doxazosin versus placebo.[13] It found that more men had a reduction from baseline in IPSS of at least 30% with either formulation of doxazosin compared with placebo, but the statistical significance was not reported (74.7% with doxazosin *v* 73.5% with doxazosin controlled release *v* 53.5% with placebo; absolute figures and P value not reported). The second subsequent RCT (536 men) compared prolonged release alfuzosin 10 mg versus placebo, and prolonged release alfuzosin 15 mg versus placebo.[14] It found that alfuzosin 10 and 15 mg significantly improved symptoms compared with placebo (mean change in IPSS from baseline at end point –3.6 points with alfuzosin 10 mg *v* –3.4 points with alfuzosin 15 mg *v* –1.6 points with placebo; alfuzosin 10 mg *v* placebo, P = 0.001; alfuzosin 15 mg *v* placebo, P = 0.004). There was no significant difference in symptoms between 10 and 15 mg alfuzosin. **Versus each other:** We found two systematic reviews, one comparing tamsulosin with other α blockers (search date 2000, 5 RCTs)[11] and one comparing terazosin with other α blockers (search date 2001, 6 RCTs),[12] one additional RCT,[17] and two subsequent RCTs (reported in the same paper).[18] The first review did not pool results for comparisons between tamsulosin and all other α blockers combined.[11] It found no significant difference between tamsulosin 0.2 mg daily and terazosin 2–5 mg daily for improving IPSS and urine flow (4 RCTs; WMD for change in IPSS –0.72 points, 95% CI –2.54 points to +1.51 points; WMD for change in peak urine flow –0.26 mL/second, 95% CI –1.12 mL/second to +0.60 mL/second). It found no significant differences between tamsulosin and alfuzosin or prazosin (tamsulosin *v* alfuzosin: 1 RCT; improvement in Boyarsky Symptom Score about 40% in each group; increase in peak urine flow about 16% in each group; tamsulosin *v* prazosin: 1 RCT; improvement in IPSS 26% with tamsulosin *v* 38% with prazosin; improvement in peak urine flow 15% with tamsulosin *v* 27% with prazosin, P reported as not significant). The second review found no significant difference between terazosin and tamsulosin in IPPS scores or peak flow rates (3 RCTs: improvement in IPPS score 40% with terazosin *v* 41% with tamsulosin; WMD of IPPS score +0.72, 95% CI –1.51 to +2.93; increase in peak flow 25% with terazosin *v* 29% with tamsulosin; WMD +0.26%, 95% CI –0.60% to +1.12%).[12] It found no difference in Boyarsky Symptom Scores between terazosin and doxazosin, and no difference between terazosin and prazosin in IPPS scores (terazosin *v* doxazosin: 1 RCT; improvement in Boyarsky Symptom Score 38–47% with terazosin *v* 42% with doxazosin; P value not reported; terazosin *v* prazosin: 1 RCT; improvement in IPPS score 39% with terazosin *v* 38% with prazosin; P value not reported). The additional RCT (103 people) found no significant difference in reduction in Boyarsky Symptom Score between alfuzosin and prazosin at 21 days (change in score: –2.6 with alfuzosin *v* – 2.8 with prazosin; P value not reported).[17] The results of the two subsequent RCTs (total 1475 men) were combined in a meta-analysis.[18] It found no significant difference between standard and controlled release doxazosin for IPSS improvement from baseline (–7.9 points with controlled release *v* –8.0 points with standard; adjusted mean difference –0.1 points, 95% CI –0.5 points to +0.3 points).[18] **Versus 5α reductase inhibitors:** We found one systematic review (search date 2001, 1 relevant RCT, 1229 men)[12] and one additional RCT.[19] Both RCTs were of limited quality (see comment below). The RCT identified by the review compared terazosin versus finasteride versus both treatments combined.[20] It found that terazosin significantly reduced AUASI score compared with finasteride (mean change in AUASI score −6.1 with terazosin *v* −3.2 with finasteride; WMD −2.80, 95% CI −3.88 to −1.72; P < 0.001). There was no significant difference between finasteride plus terazosin and terazosin alone. The additional RCT (1051 men) compared alfuzosin versus finasteride versus both drugs combined over 6 months.[19] It found that alfuzosin significantly decreased the mean IPSS score from baseline compared with finasteride and found no significant difference between alfuzosin alone and alfuzosin plus finasteride. **Versus transurethral microwave thermotherapy:** See benefits of transurethral microwave thermotherapy, p 987. **Versus saw palmetto:** See benefits of saw palmetto plant extracts, p 989.

Harms: **Versus placebo:** One systematic review found that withdrawals attributed to adverse events were similar for alfuzosin, tamsulosin (0.4 mg dose), and placebo (results were presented graphically; significance not stated).[9] There was little observable difference in rates of dizziness between either alfuzosin or tamsulosin compared with placebo (results presented graphically; significance not stated). However, terazosin and doxazosin increased dizziness compared with placebo (results presented graphically; significance not stated). Both selective and less selective α blockers may be associated with abnormal ejaculation; the risk of abnormal ejaculation was higher with tamsulosin than placebo (4.5% with tamsulosin *v* 1.0% with placebo).[21] Another systematic review found no significant difference between tamsulosin and placebo for withdrawal due to adverse events (4 RCTs; RR 1.08, 95% CI 0.72 to 1.62).[11] However, it found that tamsulosin significantly increased abnormal ejaculation, rhinitis, and dizziness compared with placebo (abnormal ejaculation: 4 RCTs; AR 10.8% with tamsulosin *v* < 1% with placebo; RR 17.0, 95% CI 2.5 to 114.0; rhinitis: 4 RCTs; AR 11.2% with tamsulosin *v* 6% with placebo; RR 1.84, 95% CI 1.24 to 2.72; dizziness: 5 RCTs; AR 11.9% with tamsulosin *v* 7.8% with placebo; RR 1.50, 95% CI 1.13 to 1.98). Another systematic review found that terazosin significantly increased dizziness, asthenia, and postural hypotension compared with placebo (dizziness: 6 RCTs; RR 2.43, 95% CI 1.82 to 3.25; asthenia: 5 RCTs; RR 2.24, 95% CI 1.68 to 3.00; postural hypotension: 4 RCTs; RR 5.27, 95% CI 5.27 to 10.72).[12] It found no significant difference in discontinuation rates between terazosin and placebo (10 RCTs: 27% with terazosin *v* 34% with placebo; RR 0.94, 95% CI 0.76 to 1.17). Discontinuations due to adverse events were significantly higher with terazosin compared with placebo (6 RCTs: 229/1817 [12.6%] with terazosin *v* 140/1607 [8.7%] with placebo; RR 1.50, 95% CI 1.23 to 1.83). **Versus each other:** One systematic review found no significant difference between tamsulosin and a less selective α blocker, alfuzosin (1 RCT; dizziness 7%, asthenia 2%, and postural hypotension 2% of men in each group).[9] Another systematic review comparing tamsulosin versus other α blockers found that discontinuation of treatment due to adverse effects was less likely with tamsulosin 0.2 mg daily compared with terazosin (4 RCTs; RR 0.15, 95% CI 0.04 to 0.57).[11] Compared with alfuzosin or prazosin, tamsulosin 0.4 or 0.2 mg daily was associated with greater all cause withdrawal from treatment, although the differences were not significant (tamsulosin *v* alfuzosin: 1 RCT; RR for withdrawal 1.46, 95% CI 0.66 to 3.25; tamsulosin *v* prazosin: 1 RCT; RR for withdrawal 2.87, 95% CI 0.65 to 12.65).[11] The review found no significant difference between tamsulosin and alfuzosin for dizziness (1 RCT: AR 6.8% with tamsulosin *v* 7.3% with alfuzosin; RR 0.94, 95% CI 0.39 to 2.29), asthenia (1 RCT: AR 3% with tamsulosin *v* 1.6% with alfuzosin; RR 1.88, 95% CI 0.35 to 10.08), but a lower incidence of headache with alfuzosin (1 RCT: AR 7.6% with tamsulosin *v* 3.2% with alfuzosin; RR 2.35, 95% CI 0.76 to 7.29). The review also found that risk of abnormal ejaculation increased with increasing dose of tamsulosin (0% with 0.2 mg/day; 18% with 0.8 mg/day; significance not reported). Another systematic review found no significant difference in discontinuation rates between terazosin and either prazosin or doxazosin (terazosin *v* prazosin: 1 RCT; RR 3.93, CI 95% 0.92 to 16.72; terazosin *v* doxazosin: 1 RCT; RR 1.75, 95% CI 0.48 to 6.41).[12] The review found no significant difference between terazosin and alfuzosin in dizziness (1 RCT; 5.1% with terazosin *v* 0% with alfuzosin; RR 4.50, 95% CI 0.22 to 90.64). It found no significant difference in dizziness or headache between terazosin and doxazosin (dizziness: 1 RCT; 14.3% with terazosin *v* 4.5% with doxazosin; RR 3.14, 95% CI 0.35 to 27.88; headache: 1 RCT; 4.8% with terazosin *v* 4.5% with doxazosin; RR 1.05, 95% CI 0.07 to 15.69). **Versus 5α reductase inhibitors:** In the RCT comparing terazosin versus finasteride, dizziness, generalised weakness, rhinitis, and postural hypotension were more common with terazosin than finasteride (dizziness: 26% with terazosin *v* 8% with finasteride; generalised weakness: 14% with terazosin *v* 7% with finasteride; rhinitis: 7% with terazosin *v* 3% with finasteride; postural hypotension: 8% with terazosin *v* 2% with finasteride), whereas sexual dysfunction was more common in men taking finasteride (impotence: 9% with finasteride *v* 6% with terazosin).[20] **Versus saw palmetto:** See harms of saw palmetto plant extracts, p 989.

Comment: Men with severe symptoms can expect the largest absolute fall in their symptom scores with medical treatment.[15,22] Prazosin, terazosin, and doxazosin lower blood pressure and may be used to treat both hypertension and benign prostatic hyperplasia.[23] One RCT included in the review that compared α blockers is limited by its small sample size, low drug doses, and unclear methods of randomisation and blinding.[12]

OPTION 5α REDUCTASE INHIBITORS

We found evidence that 5α reductase inhibitors improve symptoms and reduce complications compared with placebo. We found limited evidence that 5α reductase inhibitors are less effective at improving symptoms than α blockers. We found no evidence comparing 5α reductase inhibitors versus surgical treatment.

Benefits: **Versus placebo:** We found one systematic review (search date 1999, 12 RCTs, 11 338 men)[10] and one subsequent RCT (generating numerous publications).[7,24–27] The systematic review did not include a meta-analysis.[10] Ten of the 12 RCTs in the review found that finasteride significantly reduced symptom scores compared with placebo. The first RCT in the review (2902 men) found that 5 mg finasteride significantly improved symptom score compared with placebo at 24 months (change in Boyarsky Symptom Score [see glossary, p 991]: –20% with finasteride v –13% with placebo; P < 0.001). The second RCT in the review (2112 men) found that 5 mg finasteride significantly improved symptom score compared with placebo at 12 months (change in American Urological Association Symptom Index [AUASI — see glossary, p 991] score: –26% with finasteride v –20% with placebo; P < 0.01). The third RCT in the review (496 men) found that 5 mg finasteride significantly improved symptom score compared with placebo at 12 months (change in Boyarsky Symptom Score: –20% with finasteride v –14% with placebo; P < 0.05). The fourth RCT in the review (472 men) found that 5 mg finasteride significantly improved symptom score compared with placebo at 24 months (change in Boyarsky Symptom Score: –13% with finasteride v –4% with placebo; P < 0.01). The fifth RCT in the review (707 men) found that 5 mg finasteride significantly improved symptom score compared with placebo at 24 months (change in Boyarsky Symptom Score: –15% with finasteride v +2% with placebo; P < 0.01). The sixth RCT in the review (895 men) found that 5 mg finasteride significantly improved symptom score compared with placebo at 12 months (change in Boyarsky Symptom Score: –26% with finasteride v –10% with placebo; P < 0.05). The seventh RCT in the review (46 men) found that 5 mg finasteride significantly improved symptom score compared with placebo at 6 months (change in AUASI score: –30% with finasteride v –12% with placebo; P < 0.05). The eighth RCT in the review (2760 men) found that 5 mg finasteride significantly improved symptom score compared with placebo (change in AUASI score: –17% with finasteride v –7% with placebo; P < 0.001). The ninth RCT in the review (99 men) found that 5 mg finasteride significantly improved symptom score compared with placebo at 12 months (change in AUASI score: –30% with finasteride v –10% with placebo; P < 0.05). The 10th RCT in the review (182 men) found that 5 mg finasteride significantly improved symptom score compared with placebo at 6 months (change in Boyarsky Symptom Score: –23% with finasteride v –9% with placebo; P = 0.05). The 11th RCT in the review (615 men) found no significant difference in symptom scores between 1–10 mg finasteride and placebo at 12 months (change in AUASI score: –20% with finasteride v –16% with placebo; P = 0.63). The 12th RCT in the review (52 men) found that finasteride improved symptom score at 3 months compared with placebo but the statistical significance was not reported in the review (change in AUASI score: –21% with finasteride v –19% with placebo). The subsequent RCT (3040 men) compared finasteride 5 mg daily versus placebo.[7] After 4 years, finasteride significantly reduced symptoms compared with placebo (difference in symptom score –1.6 points, 95% CI –2.5 points to –0.7 points [range of score 0–34 points]). It also found that finasteride significantly reduced the risk of acute urinary retention and prostatectomy compared with placebo (urinary retention 6.6% with finasteride v 2.8% with placebo; NNT 26, 95% CI 22 to 38; prostatectomy 8.3% with finasteride v 4.2% with placebo; NNT 24, 95% CI 19 to 37).

There was a greater effect among men with higher concentrations of prostate specific antigen at baseline (3.3–12.0 ng/mL), reflecting larger prostates (risk of either acute urinary retention or needing prostatectomy 19.9% with placebo *v* 8.3% with finasteride; NNT 8, 95% CI 7 to 11).[28] The RCT also found that, after 4 years, finasteride produced a larger fall in International Prostate Symptom Score compared with placebo. The fall was greater for men with prostate specific antigen levels greater than 1.3 ng/mL than for men with prostate specific antigen levels equal to or lower than 1.3 ng/mL.[24] **Versus α blockers:** See benefits of α blockers, p 979.

Harms: The systematic review found that finasteride increased adverse events in the first year compared with placebo.[10] The most common adverse events with finasteride in the first year were decreased libido, impotence, and ejaculatory dysfunction. The largest RCT (3168 men) found decreased libido, increased impotence, and increased ejaculatory dysfunction compared with placebo (decreased libido 4.0% *v* 2.8%; not significant; increased impotence 6.6% *v* 4.7%; significant; ejaculatory dysfunction 2.1% *v* 0.6%; significant; none of the P values reported). Another large RCT (2342 men) found decreased libido, increased impotence, and increased ejaculatory dysfunction compared with placebo (decreased libido 3.1% *v* 1.2%; significant; impotence 6.8% *v* 3.2%; significant; increased ejaculatory dysfunction 2.3% *v* 0.5%; significant; none of the P values reported). The large subsequent 4 year RCT (3040 men) found that, after the first year of treatment, there was no significant difference in decreased libido (2.6% *v* 2.6%) or impotence (5.1% *v* 5.1%) between finasteride and placebo, but there was still a slightly greater rate of ejaculation disorder (0.2% *v* 0.1%; significance not tested).[7] Although finasteride reduced concentrations of prostate specific antigen by a mean of 50% (individual responses were highly variable), its use for up to 4 years did not change the rate of detection of prostate cancer compared with placebo.[7] **Versus α blockers:** See harms of α blockers, p 981.

Comment: We found two non-systematic reviews comparing finasteride versus placebo.[28,29] The first non-systematic review (6 RCTs) found that finasteride significantly decreased symptom scores compared with placebo (difference in symptom score –0.9 points, 95% CI –1.2 points to –0.6 points [range of score 0–30 points]).[29] The benefit over placebo was greatest in men with larger prostates (≥ 40 g). The second non-systematic review (meta-analysis of 3 RCTs) found that finasteride reduced acute urinary retention requiring catheterisation after 2 years from 2.7% to 1.1%.[28] The meta-analysis also found that finasteride was significantly more effective than placebo in men with larger prostates at 1–2 years. However, the absolute difference in mean decrease of symptom score from baseline between men with the smallest and largest prostates was only about 1 point. The relative effectiveness of finasteride compared with placebo also seemed higher in men with slightly raised prostate specific antigen levels, and it is assumed that the higher prostate specific antigen is a proxy for a larger prostate.[24]

QUESTION What are the effects of surgical treatments?

OPTION TRANSURETHRAL RESECTION OF THE PROSTATE

We found evidence that transurethral resection reduced symptoms more than watchful waiting, and did not increase the risk of erectile dysfunction or incontinence. We found no evidence of a significant difference in symptoms between transurethral resection and transurethral incision or between transurethral resection and electrical vaporisation. We found limited evidence that transurethral resection improved symptoms more than visual laser ablation but that transurethral resection may be associated with a higher risk of blood transfusion.

Benefits: **Versus watchful waiting:** We found no systematic review. We found two RCTs comparing transurethral resection of the prostate (TURP) versus conservative treatment.[30,31] The first RCT (556 men with moderate symptoms of benign prostatic hyperplasia) compared TURP with watchful waiting.[30] It found that TURP improved symptoms compared with watchful waiting (90% with TURP *v* 39% with watchful waiting). After 5 years, the treatment failure rate was 10% with TURP compared with 21% with watchful waiting (NNT 9, 95% CI 7 to 17), and 36% of men assigned to watchful waiting had crossed over to surgery.[32] Treatment failure was defined as death, acute urinary retention, high residual urine volume, renal azotaemia, bladder stones, persistent incontinence, or a high symptom score. The major categories of treatment failure reduced by TURP were acute urinary retention, development of a large bladder residual (> 350 mL), and deterioration to a severe symptom level. The second RCT (223 men) had a shorter duration of follow up (7.5 months).[31] It found that TURP significantly improved the International Prostate Symptom Score (IPSS) compared with monitoring (difference in IPSS 10.4 points, 95% CI 8.5 points to 12.3 points). **Versus less invasive techniques:** We found three systematic reviews, each comparing TURP with a different less invasive technique,[33–35] one additional RCT,[36] and four subsequent RCTs.[37–40] The first systematic review (search date 1999, 9 RCTs) compared TURP versus transurethral incision.[33] Four of the included RCTs (243 men) examined symptom scores at 12 months and found no significant difference between TURP and transurethral incision (WMD +0.2 points, 95% CI –0.8 points to +1.1 points). The review found little good, long term evidence. The second systematic review (search date 1999, 5 RCTs) compared TURP versus visual laser ablation (4 RCTs, 331 men) or laser contact vaporisation (1 RCT, 28 men).[34] The review did not perform a meta-analysis. It found that TURP was more effective at reducing symptom score than visual laser ablation, but length of hospital stay was shorter with visual laser ablation. The largest RCT (151 men) found significantly better changes in symptom scores at 52 weeks' follow up with TURP (American Urological Association Symptom Index [see glossary, p 991] mean score reduced from 18.2 to 5.1 with TURP *v* from 18.1 to 7.7 with laser ablation). The review found no significant difference between TURP and laser contact vaporisation in symptom scores or quality of life at 12 months' follow up. The third systematic review (search date 1999, 5 RCTs, 454 men) compared TURP versus electrical vaporisation.[35] Meta-analysis of three RCTs found a greater improvement in symptom scores at 12–24 months with electrical vaporisation but the difference was not significant (figures reported as SMD +0.21, 95% CI –0.03 to +0.44). One of the RCTs reported a significant reduction in symptom score with electrical vaporisation and four found no significant difference. The additional RCT (120 men) compared holmium laser ablation versus TURP.[36] It found no significant difference in symptom scores at 1 year (American Urological Association Symptom Index: holmium 4.2 *v* TURP 4.8; P = 0.92). The first subsequent RCT (98 men) found that TURP reduced surgical re-treatment rates compared with laser ablation after 5 years (18/47 [38%] with visual laser ablation *v* 8/51 [16%] with TURP; P = 0.006).[37] The second subsequent RCT (148 men) found that TURP reduced surgical re-treatment rates with laser contact vaporisation after 3 years (13/72 [18%] with laser contact vaporisation *v* 7/76 [9%] with TURP; P value not reported).[38] The third and fourth subsequent RCTs compared TURP versus electrical vaporisation.[39,40] The third RCT (100 men) found no significant difference between treatments in symptoms at 3 months after treatment (mean IPSS decreased from 21.6 points to 5.0 points with TURP *v* from 19.4 points to 4.0 points with vaporisation; CI and P value for direct comparison not reported).[39] The fourth RCT (185 men) also found no significant difference between treatments for symptoms at 12 months (mean decrease in IPSS from baseline 12.8 points for TURP *v* 12.5 points for vaporisation; CI and P value not reported).[40] **Versus transurethral microwave thermotherapy and transurethral needle ablation:** See benefits of transurethral microwave thermotherapy, p 987 and benefits of transurethral needle ablation, p 988.

Harms: Analysis of administrative data found that mortality in the 30 days after TURP for benign prostatic hyperplasia ranged from 0.4% for men aged 65–69 years to 1.9% for men aged 80–84 years, and has fallen in recent years.[41] In one review of observational studies, TURP for benign prostatic hyperplasia was associated with immediate surgical complications in 12% of men, bleeding requiring intervention in 2%, erectile dysfunction in 14%, retrograde ejaculation in 74%, and incontinence in about 5%.[42–44] Analysis of claims data found a reoperation rate, implying need for retreatment, of about 1% a year.[41] However, in the only comparative trial, men randomised to prostatectomy did not seem to have a greater rate of erectile dysfunction or incontinence than men assigned to watchful waiting.[30,32] One systematic review found that visual laser ablation is associated with a lower risk of blood transfusion than TURP but a higher risk of urinary tract infection (blood transfusion: 0/145 [0%] with laser ablation *v* 15/146 [10%] with TURP; RR 0.09, 95% CI 0.02 to 0.47; urinary tract infection: RR 3.85, 95% CI 1.87 to 7.94; absolute figures not reported).[34] The largest RCT found fewer cases of blood transfusion with visual laser ablation compared with TURP (0/76 [0%] with laser ablation *v* 12/75 [16%] with TURP). The third systematic review found that TURP and electrical vaporisation had similar risks of blood transfusion, irritative symptoms, and urinary tract infections, although confidence intervals were large.[35] However, electrical vaporisation was associated with a significant increase in the risk of urinary retention (17.1% with electrical vaporisation *v* 3.8% with TURP; RR 3.64, 95% CI 1.68 to 7.92; absolute figures not reported) compared with TURP. One RCT (150 men) in the review reported more transient stress urinary incontinence with electrical vaporisation than with TURP (13/70 [19%] with electrical vaporisation *v* 0/80 [0%] with TURP). One of the subsequent RCTs (100 men) found that no-one having either TURP or electrical vaporisation required transfusion.[39] It also found no significant difference for rates of erectile dysfunction between the two groups (22% with TURP *v* 24% with vaporisation; P values and CI not reported). However, another subsequent RCT (185 men) found no significant difference between TURP and electrical vaporisation for rates of postoperative incontinence (6/92 [6.5%] with TURP *v* 5/93 [5.4%] with vaporisation; RR 1.2, 95% CI 0.4 to 3.8).[40] Rates of haemorrhage requiring blood transfusion and of urethral stricture were low in both groups and not significantly different (transfusion: 9/92 [9.8%] with TURP *v* 6/93 [6.5%] with vaporisation; RR 1.5, 95% CI 0.6 to 4.1; urethral stricture: 7/92 [7.6%] with TURP *v* 5/93 [5.4%] with vaporisation; RR 1.4, 95% CI 0.5 to 4.3). A further small RCT (340 men) examined sexual function after TURP, laser prostatectomy, and conservative management.[45] It found that TURP reduced the proportions with erectile dysfunction, reduced pain or discomfort on ejaculation, and increased ejaculatory dysfunction compared with conservative management (erectile dysfunction OR 0.37, 95% CI 0.19 to 0.74; pain or discomfort on ejaculation OR 0.06, 95% CI 0.007 to 0.49; ejaculatory dysfunction OR 3.27, 95% CI 1.69 to 6.35).

Comment: Rapid changes in techniques and few controlled trials with adequate follow up make comparisons between TURP and newer surgical techniques difficult. The second review reported that RCTs comparing TURP versus laser ablation were limited generally by small sample size, brief follow up, and lack of blinding.[34] The third review comparing TURP versus electrical vaporisation found that none of the RCTs were blinded or analysed by intention to treat, but four out of five RCTs had less than 10% loss to follow up.[35]

OPTION TRANSURETHRAL MICROWAVE THERMOTHERAPY

We found evidence that transurethral microwave thermotherapy reduced symptoms compared with sham treatment. We found limited evidence that transurethral resection relieved short term symptoms better than thermotherapy. We found limited evidence that thermotherapy improved symptoms more than α blockers over 18 months.

Benefits: **Versus sham treatment:** We found no systematic review. We found three RCTs comparing transurethral microwave thermotherapy (TUMT) versus sham treatment.[46–48] In the largest RCT (220 men), TUMT improved the International Prostate Symptom Score (IPSS) significantly more than sham treatment (5 points lower; $P < 0.05$).[46] In the second RCT (169 men), TUMT significantly improved IPSS more than sham treatment at 6 months ($P < 0.05$).[47] The third RCT (50 men) compared TUMT versus sham treatment. It found a greater reduction in Madsen symptom score (range 0–27, higher scores indicating worse symptoms) with TUMT compared with sham treatment (reduction in Madsen symptom score reduction 7.3 with TUMT *v* 3.9 with sham treatment; significance was not tested). **Versus transurethral resection of the prostate:** We found one systematic review[35] (search date 1999, 3 RCTs, 200 men) and one additional RCT comparing TUMT versus transurethral resection of the prostate (TURP).[49] In the systematic review, symptom improvement was significantly better with TURP in one RCT ($P < 0.05$) but not significantly different in the other two.[35] The additional RCT (147 men) found better symptomatic outcomes with TURP but the statistical significance was not reported (IPSS change *v* baseline at 1 year: 60% with TUMT *v* 85% with TURP).[49] **Versus α blockers:** We found one RCT (103 men).[50,51] It found that TUMT significantly improved symptoms at 6 and 18 months compared with terazosin (up to 10 mg/day; difference in IPSS at 18 months 35%; $P < 0.001$).

Harms: Adverse events associated with TUMT varied among trials, but included the need for catheterisation for more than 1 week (8% with TUMT *v* 2% with sham treatment),[47] persistent irritative symptoms (22% with TUMT *v* 8% with sham treatment),[46] haematuria (14% with TUMT *v* 1% with sham treatment),[46] and sexual dysfunction (mostly haematospermia and other ejaculatory abnormalities; 29% with TUMT *v* 1% with sham treatment).[46] In one RCT, retrograde ejaculation was substantially less common after TUMT compared with TURP (27% with TUMT *v* 74% with TURP).[52] The RCT (103 men) comparing TUMT versus α blockers found more adverse events in the α blocker group over the first 6 months (17 events between 52 men with α blockers *v* 7 events between 51 men with TUMT).[50,51] With α blockers, the most common adverse events were dizziness (7 cases) and asthenia (4 cases); in the TUMT group they were urinary tract infection (3 cases).

Comment: TUMT can be performed in an outpatient setting, and uses heat generated by a microwave antenna in the urethra to coagulate prostate tissue. The long term effects of TUMT have not been adequately evaluated in controlled studies. The systematic review reported that trials were limited by small sample size, short duration of follow up (maximum 30 months), and large loss to follow up.

OPTION TRANSURETHRAL NEEDLE ABLATION

We found limited evidence from one RCT that transurethral resection reduced symptoms compared with transurethral needle ablation, although transurethral needle ablation caused fewer adverse effects.

Benefits: We found no systematic review. **Versus transurethral resection:** We found one RCT (121 men) comparing transurethral resection of the prostate (TURP) versus transurethral needle ablation (TUNA).[53] The mean International Prostate Symptoms Score (IPSS) at 1 year was significantly lower with TURP than TUNA (IPSS 11.1 points with TUNA *v* 8.3 points with TURP; $P = 0.04$).

Harms: Compared with TURP, TUNA was associated with less retrograde ejaculation (38% with TURP *v* 0% with TUNA) and bleeding (100% with TURP *v* 32% with TUNA).[53]

Comment: TUNA can be performed in an outpatient setting, and uses radiofrequency energy through two intraprostatic electrodes to generate heat to coagulate prostate tissue. Anaesthesia requirements vary in reported studies. The long term effects of treatment have not been adequately evaluated.

QUESTION What are the effects of herbal treatments?

OPTION SAW PALMETTO PLANT EXTRACTS

One systematic review has found that saw palmetto improves symptoms compared with placebo. It found no significant difference in symptom scores between saw palmetto and finasteride. We found evidence of a similar improvement in symptom scores with saw palmetto or tamsulosin. We found evidence of no treatment advantage in combining saw palmetto with tamsulosin.

Benefits: We found one systematic review that included all saw palmetto preparations (search date 1997, 18 RCTs, 2939 men)[54] and two subsequent RCTs.[55,56] **Versus placebo:** The systematic review found that more men reported self rated improvement with saw palmetto compared with placebo (6 relevant RCTs: RR 1.7, 95% CI 1.2 to 2.4).[54] It found a significant reduction in nocturia with saw palmetto compared with placebo (10 RCTs: WMD 0.76 episodes/night, 95% CI 0.32 to 1.21). **Versus 5α reductase inhibitors:** The systematic review (2 relevant RCTs, 1440 men) found no significant difference in International Prostate Symptoms Score (IPSS) between finasteride and saw palmetto (WMD +0.37, 95% CI −0.44 to +1.19).[54] **Versus α blockers:** We found one RCT (704 men).[55] It found no significant difference between tamsulosin and saw palmetto in IPSS or maximum flow rate at 12 months (increase in maximum flow rate 1.8 mL/second with saw palmetto *v* 1.9 mL/second with tamsulosin, P value not significant).[55] **Plus α blocker:** We found one RCT (352 patients).[56] It found no significant difference in symptom score between tamsulosin and tamsulosin plus saw palmetto (improvement in IPPS score: 5.2 with tamsulosin *v* 6.0 with tamsulosin plus saw palmetto, P value not significant).

Harms: The systematic review found significantly higher withdrawal rates with saw palmetto compared with placebo (9% with saw palmetto *v* 7% with placebo; P = 0.02).[54] It found no significant difference in withdrawal rates between saw palmetto and finasteride (9% with saw palmetto *v* 11% with finasteride; P = 0.87). The risk of erectile dysfunction was similar with saw palmetto and placebo (1.1% with saw palmetto *v* 0.7% with placebo; P = 0.58). Erectile dysfunction rates were significantly lower with saw palmetto compared with finasteride (1.1% with saw palmetto *v* 4.9% with finasteride; P < 0.001).[54] In one RCT comparing saw palmetto and tamsulosin, a similar proportion of men withdrew because of adverse events (7.7% with saw palmetto *v* 8.2% with tamsulosin).[55] The risk of ejaculatory disorder was significantly less with saw palmetto than with tamsulosin (2/349 [0.6%] with saw palmetto *v* 15/354 [4.2%] with tamsulosin; P = 0.001).[55]

Comment: The RCTs included in the systematic reviews were short term and few used a validated symptom score. Different preparations, which may not be equivalent, are available directly to consumers without prescription in many countries.[54] The most recent RCT used a standardised preparation of saw palmetto.[55] There was no placebo arm in this trial.

OPTION β-SITOSTEROL PLANT EXTRACT

One systematic review has found that β-sitosterol plant extract improves lower urinary tract symptoms compared with placebo in the short term.

Benefits: **Versus placebo:** We found one systematic review (search date 1998, 4 RCTs, 519 men), which compared β-sitosterol versus placebo.[52] Trials lasted for 4–26 weeks. The review found that β-sitosterol significantly reduced the International Prostate Symptom Score (2 RCTs: WMD –4.9 points, 95% CI –6.3 points to –3.5 points).

Harms: Gastrointestinal adverse effects were more common with β-sitosterol than placebo (1.6% with β-sitosterol *v* 0% with placebo; significance not reported).[52] Impotence was also more common with β-sitosterol (0.5% β–sitosterol *v* 0% with placebo; significance not reported). Withdrawal rates were similar in both groups (7.8% with β-sitosterol *v* 8.0% with placebo; significance not reported).

Comment: The RCTs were limited by a short follow up period (maximum 26 weeks). Different preparations are available, which may be of variable content, making it difficult to generalise results.

OPTION RYE GRASS POLLEN EXTRACT

One systematic review found limited evidence that rye grass pollen extract increased self rated improvement and reduced nocturia compared with placebo in the short term. However, both RCTs included in the review were small and of short duration.

Benefits: **Versus placebo:** We found one systematic review (search date 1997, 2 RCTs, 163 men), which compared rye grass pollen extract versus placebo.[57] It found that pollen extract significantly increased self rated improvement and significantly reduced nocturia compared with placebo (proportion improved: 1 RCT, 60 men: 20/31 [65%] with pollen *v* 7/26 [27%] with placebo; RR 2.40, 95% CI 1.21 to 4.75; NNT 3, 95% CI 2 to 9; proportion with reduced nocturia: 2 RCTs, 50/79 [63%] with pollen *v* 23/74 [31%] with placebo; RR 2.05, 95% CI 1.41 to 3.99). However, the results should be interpreted with caution (see comment below).

Harms: The review found that nausea occurred in one man taking pollen extract (number in placebo group not stated).[57] Withdrawal rates were not significantly different (4.8% with pollen *v* 2.7% with placebo; P = 0.26).

Comment: Both RCTs were limited by small sample sizes and a short follow up period (12 and 24 weeks). Concealment of treatment allocation was unclear. The composition of the preparations was unknown, making it difficult to generalise results.

GLOSSARY

American Urological Association Symptom Index (AUASI) is a patient questionnaire that asks seven questions about the severity of symptoms (range 0–35). Mild symptoms score 0 to 7 points, moderate symptoms 8 to 19 points, and severe symptoms 20 to 35 points.

Boyarsky Symptom Score is a patient questionnaire that asks nine questions about severity of symptoms (range 0–27); no symptoms = 0, maximum severity = 27.

Substantive changes

α Blockers One systematic review added;[12] conclusions unchanged.

Transurethral resection of the prostate One RCT added;[45] conclusions unchanged.

Saw palmetto Two RCTs added;[55,56] conclusions unchanged.

REFERENCES

1. Bosch JL, Hop WC, Kirkels WJ, et al. Natural history of benign prostatic hyperplasia: appropriate case definition and estimation of its prevalence in the community. *Urology* 1995;46(suppl A):34–40.
2. Barry MJ, Adolfsson J, Batista JE, et al. Committee 6: measuring the symptoms and health impact of benign prostatic hyperplasia and its treatments. In: Denis L, Griffiths K, Khoury S, et al, eds. *Fourth International Consultation on BPH, Proceedings.* Plymouth, UK: Health Publication Ltd, 1998:265–321.
3. Oishi K, Boyle P, Barry MJ, et al. Committee 1: Epidemiology and natural history of benign prostatic hyperplasia. In: Denis L, Griffiths K, Khoury S, et al, eds. *Fourth International Consultation on BPH, Proceedings.* Plymouth, UK: Health Publication Ltd, 1998:23–59.
4. Jacobsen SJ, Girman CJ, Guess HA, et al. Natural history of prostatism: longitudinal changes in voiding symptoms in community dwelling men. *J Urol* 1996;155:595–600.
5. Barry MJ, Fowler FJ, Bin L, et al. The natural history of patients with benign prostatic hyperplasia as diagnosed by North American urologists. *J Urol* 1997;157:10–15.
6. Jacobsen S, Jacobson D, Girman C, et al. Natural history of prostatism: risk factors for acute urinary retention. *J Urol* 1997;158:481–487.
7. McConnell J, Bruskewitz R, Walsh P, et al. The effect of finasteride on the risk of acute urinary retention and the need for surgical treatment among men with benign prostatic hyperplasia. *N Engl J Med* 1998;338:557–563.
8. Barry MJ, Fowler FJ Jr, O'Leary MP, et al. The American Urological Association symptom index for benign prostatic hyperplasia. *J Urol* 1992;148:1549–1557.
9. Djavan B, Marberger M. A meta-analysis on the efficacy and tolerability of α1-adrenoceptor antagonists in patients with lower urinary tract symptoms suggestive of benign prostatic obstruction. *Eur Urol* 1999;36:1–13. Search date 1998; primary source Medline.
10. Clifford GM, Farmer RDT. Medical therapy for benign prostatic hyperplasia: a review of the literature. *Eur Urol* 2000;38:2–19. Search date 1999; primary sources Medline, Embase, and the Cochrane Library.
11. Wilt TJ, MacDonald R, Nelson D. Tamsulosin for treating lower urinary tract symptoms compatible with benign prostatic obstruction: a systematic review of efficacy and adverse effects. *J Urol* 2002;167:177–183. Search date 2000; primary sources Medline, Embase, The Cochrane Library, Cochrane prostatic Disease and Urologic Malignancies Group Trial Register, and hand searched reference lists.
12. Wilt TJ, Howe W, MacDonald R. Terazosin for treating symptomatic benign prostatic obstruction: a systematic review of efficacy and adverse effects. *BJU Int* 2002;89:214–225. Search date: 2001; primary sources Medline, Embase, Cochrane Library, the Prostatic Diseases and Urological Malignancies Group specialised register, and reference lists from previous reviews.
13. Andersen M, Dahlstrand C, Hoye K. Double-blind trial of the efficacy and tolerability of doxazosin in the gastrointestinal therapeutic system, doxazosin standard, and placebo in patients with benign prostatic hyperplasia. *Eur Urol* 2000;38:400–409.
14. Roehrborn CG. Efficacy and safety of once-daily alfuzosin in the treatment of lower urinary tract symptoms and clinical benign prostatic hyperplasia: a randomized, placebo-controlled trial. *Urology* 2001;58:953–959.
15. Roehrborn CG, Oesterling JE, Auerbach S, et al. The Hytrin community assessment trial study: a one-year study of terazosin versus placebo in the treatment of men with symptomatic benign prostatic hyperplasia. *Urology* 1996;47:159–168.
16. McNeil SA, Daruwala PD, Mitchell IDC, et al. Sustained-release alfuzosin and trial without catheter after acute urinary retention: a prospective placebo-controlled trial. *BJU Int* 1999;84:622–627.
17. Buzelin JM, Herbert M, Blondin P, et al. Alpha-blocking treatment with alfuzosin in symptomatic benign prostatic hyperplasia: comparative study with prazosin. *Br J Urol* 1993;72:922–927.
18. Kirby RS, Andersen M, Gratzke P, et al. A combined analysis of double-blind trials of the efficacy and tolerability of doxazosin-gastrointestinal therapeutic system, doxazosin standard and placebo in patients with benign prostatic hyperplasia. *BJU Int* 2001;87:192–200.
19. Debruyne FMJ, Jardin A, Colloi D, et al. Sustained-release alfuzosin, finasteride and the combination of both in the treatment of benign prostatic hyperplasia. *Eur Urol* 1998;34:169–175.
20. Lepor H, Williford WO, Barry MJ, et al. The efficacy of terazosin, finasteride, or both in benign prostatic hyperplasia. Veterans' Affairs cooperative studies benign prostatic hyperplasia study group. *N Engl J Med* 1996;335:533–539.

21. Hofner K, Claes H, De Reijke TM, et al. Tamsulosin 0.4 mg once daily: effect on sexual function in patients with lower urinary tract symptoms suggestive of benign prostatic obstruction. *Eur Urol* 1999;36:335–341.
22. Mobley D, Dias N, Levenstein M. Effects of doxazosin in patients with mild, intermediate, and severe benign prostatic hyperplasia. *Clin Ther* 1998;20:101–109.
23. Kaplan S, Kaplan N. Alpha-blockade: monotherapy for hypertension and benign prostatic hyperplasia. *Urology* 1996;48:541–550.
24. Roehrborn CG, Boyle P, Bergner D, et al. Serum prostate specific antigen and prostate volume predict long-term changes in symptoms and flow rate: results of a four-year, randomised trial comparing finasteride and placebo. *Urology* 1999:54;663–669.
25. Roehrborn CG, McConnell JD, Lieber M, et al. Serum prostate-specific antigen concentration is a powerful predictor of acute urinary retention and the need for surgery in men with clinical benign prostatic hyperplasia. *Urology* 1999;53:473–480.
26. Roehrborn CG, Bruskewitz R, Nickel GC, et al. Urinary retention in patients with BPH treated with finasteride or placebo over 4 years. *Eur Urol* 2000;37:528–536.
27. Kaplan S, Garvin D, Gilhooly P, et al. Impact of baseline symptom severity on future risk of benign prostatic hyperplasia-related outcomes and long-term response to finasteride. *Urology* 2000;56:610–616.
28. Andersen J, Nickel J, Marshall V, et al. Finasteride significantly reduces acute urinary retention and need for surgery in patients with symptomatic benign prostatic hyperplasia. *Urology* 1997;49:839–845.
29. Boyle P, Gould AL, Roehrborn CG. Prostate volume predicts outcome of treatment of benign prostatic hyperplasia with finasteride: meta-analysis of randomized clinical trials. *Urology* 1996;48:398–405.
30. Wasson J, Reda D, Bruskewitz R, et al. A comparison of transurethral surgery with watchful waiting for moderate symptoms of benign prostatic hyperplasia. *N Engl J Med* 1995;332:75–79.
31. Donovan JL, Peters T, Neal DE, et al. A randomized trial comparing transurethral resection of the prostate, laser therapy and conservative treatment of men with symptoms associated with benign prostatic enlargement: the ClasP study. *J Urol* 2000;164:65–70.
32. Flanigan RC, Reda DC, Wasson JH, et al. Five year outcome of surgical resection and watchful waiting for men with moderately symptomatic benign prostatic hyperplasia: a Department of Veterans' Affairs cooperative study. *J Urol* 1998;160:12–17.
33. Yang Q, Peters TJ, Donovan JL, et al. Transurethral incision compared with transurethral resection of the prostate for bladder outlet obstruction: a systematic review and meta-analysis of randomized controlled trials. *J Urol* 2001;165:1526–1532. Search date 1999; primary sources Medline, Embase, ISI, the Cochrane Library, and Cochrane Prostatic Diseases and Urologic Cancers Group Trial Register.
34. Wheelahan J, Scott NA, Cartmill R, et al. Minimally invasive laser techniques for prostatectomy: a systematic review. *BJU Int* 2000;86:805–815. Search date 1999; primary sources Medline, Embase, Current Contents, and the Cochrane Library.
35. Wheelahan J, Scott NA, Cartmill R, et al. Minimally invasive non-laser thermal techniques for prostatectomy: a systematic review. *BJU Int* 2000;86:977–988. Search date 1999; primary sources Medline, Embase, Current Contents, and the Cochrane Library.
36. Gilling PJ, Mackey M, Cresswell M, et al. Holmium laser versus transurethral resection of the prostate: a randomized prospective trial with 1-year followup. *J Urol* 1999;162:1640–1644.
37. McAllister WJ, Absalom MJ, Mir K, et al. Does endoscopic laser ablation of the prostate stand the test of time? Five-year results test results from a multicentre randomised controlled trial of endoscopic laser ablation against transurethral resection of the prostate. *BJU Int* 2000;85:437–439.
38. Keoghane SR, Lawrence KC, Gray AM, et al. A double-blind randomized controlled trial and economic evaluation of transurethral resection vs contact laser vaporization for benign prostatic enlargement: a 3-year follow-up. *BJU Int* 2000;85:74–78.
39. Kupeli S, Yilmaz E, Soygur T, et al. Randomized study of transurethral resection of the prostate and combined transurethral resection and vaporization of the prostate as a therapeutic alternative in men with benign prostatic hyperplasia. *J Endourol* 2001;15:317–321.
40. Helke C, Manseck A, Hakenberg OW, et al. Is transurethral vaporesection of the prostate better than standard transurethral resection? *Eur Urol* 2001;39:551–557.
41. Lu-Yao GL, Barry MJ, Chang CH, et al. Transurethral resection of the prostate among Medicare beneficiaries in the United States: time trends and outcomes. *Urology* 1994;44:692–698.
42. McConnell JD, Barry MJ, Bruskewitz RC, et al. *Direct treatment outcomes — complications. Benign prostatic hyperplasia: diagnosis and treatment.* Clinical Practice Guideline, Number 8. Rockville, Maryland: Agency for Health Care Policy and Research, Public Health Service, US Department of Health and Human Services, 1994:91–98.
43. McConnell JD, Barry MJ, Bruskewitz RC, et al. *Direct treatment outcomes — sexual dysfunction. Benign prostatic hyperplasia: diagnosis and treatment.* Clinical Practice Guideline, Number 8. Rockville, Maryland: Agency for Health Care Policy and Research, Public Health Service, US Department of Health and Human Services, 1994:99–103.
44. McConnell JD, Barry MJ, Bruskewitz RC, et al. *Direct treatment outcomes — urinary incontinence. Benign prostatic hyperplasia: diagnosis and treatment.* Clinical Practice Guideline, Number 8. Rockville, Maryland: Agency for Health Care Policy and Research, Public Health Service, US Department of Health and Human Services, 1994:105–106.
45. Brookes ST, Donovan JL, Peters TJ, et al. Sexual dysfunction in men after treatment for lower urinary tract symptoms: evidence from randomized controlled trial. *BMJ* 2002;324:1059–1064.
46. Roehrborn C, Preminger G, Newhall P, et al. Microwave thermotherapy for benign prostatic hyperplasia with the Dornier Urowave: results of a randomized, double-blind, multicenter, sham-controlled trial. *Urology* 1998;51:19–28.
47. Larson T, Blute M, Bruskewitz R, et al. A high-efficiency microwave thermoablation system for the treatment of benign prostatic hyperplasia: results of a randomized, sham-controlled, prospective, double-blind, multicenter clinical trial. *Urology* 1998;51:731–742.

48. De la Rosette J, De Wildt M, Alivizatos G, et al. Transurethral microwave thermotherapy (TUMT) in benign prostatic hyperplasia: placebo versus TUMT. *Urology* 1994;44:58–63.
49. Francisca EA, D'Ancona FC, Meuleman EJ, et al. Sexual function following high energy microwave thermotherapy: results of a randomized controlled study comparing transurethral microwave thermotherapy to transurethral prostatic resection. *J Urol* 1999;161:486–490.
50. Djavan B, Roehrborn CG, Shariat S, et al. Prospective randomized comparison of high energy transurethral microwave thermotherapy versus alpha blocker treatment of patients with benign prostatic hyperplasia. *J Urol* 1999;161:139–143.
51. Djavan B, Seitz C, Roehrborn C, et al. Targeted transurethral microwave thermotherapy versus alpha-blockade in benign prostatic hyperplasia: outcomes at 18 months. *Urology* 2001;57:66–70.
52. Wilt TJ, Macdonald R, Ishani A. Beta-sitosterol for the treatment of benign prostatic hyperplasia: a systematic review. *BJU Int* 1999;83:976–983. Search date 1998; primary sources Medline, Embase, Phytodok, and the Cochrane Library.
53. Bruskewitz R, Issa M, Roehrborn C, et al. A prospective, randomized 1-year clinical trial comparing transurethral needle ablation to transurethral resection of the prostate for the treatment of symptomatic benign prostatic hyperplasia. *J Urol* 1998;159:1588–1594.
54. Wilt T, Ishani A, Stark G, et al. Serenoa repens for benign prostatic hyperplasia. In: The Cochrane Library, Issue 2, 2002. Oxford: Update Software. Search date 1997; primary sources Medline, Embase, Phytodok, and the Cochrane Library.
55. DeBruyne F, Koch G, Boyle P, et al. Comparison of a phytotherapeutic agent (Permixon) with an α blocker (Tamsulosin) in the treatment of benign prostatic hyperplasia: a 1-year randomized international study. *Eur Urol* 2002;41:497–507.
56. Glemain P, Coulange C, Billebaud T, et al. Tamsulosine avec ou sans Serenoa repens dans l'hypertrophie bénigne de la prostate: l'essai OCOS [in French]. *Prog Urol* 2002;12:395–403.
57. Macdonald R, Ishani A, Rutks I, et al. A systematic review of Cernilton for the treatment of benign prostatic hyperplasia. *BJU Int* 2000;85:836–841. Search date 1997; primary sources Embase and the Cochrane Library. Additional Medline search 1998.

Robyn Webber
Consultant Urologist
Hairmyres Hospital
East Kilbride
Scotland

Competing interests: RW has been reimbursed by MSD, the manufacturers of finasteride, for attending several conferences.

The following previous contributors of this topic would like to be acknowledged: Michael Barry and Claus Roehrborn.

Chronic prostatitis

Search date February 2003

Jeffrey Stern and Anthony Schaeffer

QUESTIONS

INTERVENTIONS

CHRONIC BACTERIAL PROSTATITIS

Likely to be beneficial

α Blockers (when added to antimicrobials) 997

Unknown effectiveness

Local injection of antimicrobials 997
Oral antimicrobial drugs 996
Radical prostatectomy 998
Transurethral resection 998

CHRONIC ABACTERIAL PROSTATITIS

Unknown effectiveness

α Blockers 998
5α Reductase inhibitors 999
Allopurinol 1000
Anti-inflammatory medications 999
Biofeedback 1001
Prostatic massage 1001
Sitz bath 1001
Transurethral microwave thermotherapy 1000

Key Messages

In men with chronic bacterial prostatitis

- **α Blockers (when added to antimicrobials)** We found no RCTs comparing α blockers versus placebo or no treatment. We found limited evidence from one RCT suggesting that adding α blockers to antimicrobials may improve symptoms and reduce recurrence compared with antimicrobials alone.
- **Local injection of antimicrobials** We found no RCTs comparing local injection of antimicrobials versus placebo or no treatment. One small RCT found that anal submucosal injection of amikacin improved symptom scores and bacterial eradication rates at 3 months compared with intramuscular amikacin.
- **Oral antimicrobial drugs** We found no placebo controlled RCTs. One RCT found no significant difference between lomefloxacin and ciprofloxacin in rates of clinical success or bacteriological cure at 6 months. We found no other RCTs of the effects of oral antimicrobial drugs. Retrospective observational studies reported cure rates of 0–88% depending on the drug used and the duration of treatment.
- **Radical prostatectomy; transurethral resection** We found no RCTs on the effects of these interventions.

In men with chronic abacterial prostatitis

- **α Blockers** One systematic review found limited evidence from two small RCTs that α blockers may improve maximal flow time and pain compared with placebo. However, we were unable to draw reliable conclusions from these small studies.

- **5α Reductase inhibitors** One systematic review of one small RCT found insufficient evidence about the effects of 5α reductase inhibitors compared with placebo in men with chronic abacterial prostatitis.
- **Allopurinol** We found insufficient evidence from one small RCT about the effects of allopurinol compared with placebo in men with chronic abacterial prostatitis.
- **Anti-inflammatory medications** We found insufficient evidence about the effects of anti-inflammatory medications compared with placebo or no treatment in men with chronic abacterial prostatitis.
- **Transurethral microwave thermotherapy** One systematic review found limited evidence from one small RCT suggesting that transurethral microwave thermotherapy may significantly improve quality of life at 3 months, and symptoms over 21 months, compared with sham treatment. However, we were unable to draw reliable conclusions from this one small study.
- **Biofeedback; prostatic massage; Sitz bath** We found no good evidence on these interventions.

DEFINITION **Chronic bacterial prostatitis** is characterised by a positive culture of expressed prostatic secretions. It can be symptomatic (recurrent urinary tract infection, or suprapubic, lower back, or perineal pain), asymptomatic, or associated with minimal urgency, frequency, and dysuria. **Chronic abacterial prostatitis** is characterised by pelvic or perineal pain, often associated with urinary urgency, nocturia, weak urinary stream, frequency, dysuria, hesitancy, dribbling after micturition, interrupted flow, and inflammation (white cells) in prostatic secretions. Symptoms can also include suprapubic, scrotal, testicular, penile, or lower back pain or discomfort, known as prostodynia, in the absence of bacteria in prostatic secretions.

INCIDENCE/ PREVALENCE One US community based study (58 955 visits by men ≥ 18 years to office based physicians) estimated that 9% of men have a diagnosis of chronic prostatitis at any one time.[1] Another study found that, of men with genitourinary symptoms, 8% presenting to urologists and 1% presenting to primary care physicians are diagnosed with chronic prostatitis.[2] Most cases of chronic prostatitis are abacterial. Acute bacterial prostatitis, although easy to diagnose, is rare.

AETIOLOGY/ RISK FACTORS Organisms commonly implicated in bacterial prostatitis include *Escherichia coli*, other Gram negative Enterobacteriaceae, occasionally *Pseudomonas* species, and rarely Gram positive enterococci. The cause of abacterial prostatitis is unclear, but autoimmunity could be involved.[3]

PROGNOSIS One recent study found that chronic abacterial prostatitis had an impact on quality of life similar to that from angina, Crohn's disease, or a previous myocardial infarction.[4]

AIMS OF INTERVENTION To relieve symptoms and eliminate infection where present, with minimum adverse effects.

OUTCOMES Symptom improvement (symptom scores, bother scores); quality of life; urodynamics; rates of bacteriological cure (clearance of previously documented organisms from prostatic secretions).

METHODS *Clinical Evidence* search and appraisal February 2003.

QUESTION What are the effects of treatments for chronic bacterial prostatitis?

OPTION ORAL ANTIMICROBIAL DRUGS

We found no RCTs comparing oral antimicrobial drugs versus placebo or no treatment. One RCT found no significant difference between lomefloxacin and ciprofloxacin in rates of clinical success or bacteriological cure at 6 months. Retrospective observational studies report cure rates of 0–88% depending on the drug used and the duration of treatment.

Benefits: **Versus placebo or no antmicrobials:** We found no systematic reviews or RCTs. **Oral antimicrobials versus each other:** We found no systematic reviews but we found one RCT (182 men), which compared lomefloxacin (400 mg daily) versus ciprofloxacin (500 mg twice daily) for 4 weeks.[5] It found no significant difference between lomefloxacin and ciprofloxacin in rates of clinical success or bacteriological cure after 6 months (clinical success: 61/93 [81.3%] with lomefloxacin *v* 64/89 [88.9%] with ciprofloxacin; difference −7.6%, 95% CI −23.6% to +6%; biological eradication: 49/93 [62.8%] with lomefloxacin *v* 54/89 [72.0%] with ciprofloxacin; difference −9.2%, 95% CI −26% to +6%). Clinical success was defined as clinical cure (baseline symptoms completely resolved) or improvement (symptoms improved but not completely resolved).

Harms: The RCT (182 men) comparing lomefloxacin with ciprofloxacin found that the most common adverse effects with both treatments were gastrointestinal disorders (5/93 [5%] with lomefloxacin *v* 8/89 [9%] with ciprofloxacin; P value not reported). Adverse effects caused the premature withdrawal of 5/93 [5%] on lomefloxacin compared with 4/89 [4%] on ciprofloxacin.

Comment: We found data from an observational series about the cure rates of different antibiotics. These data do not compare effects of antimicrobials versus placebo, no treatment or other treatment. **Trimethoprim–sulfamethoxazole:** One non-systematic review identified eight retrospective case series in 1140 men with bacteriologically confirmed prostatitis treated with trimethoprim–sulfamethoxazole (sulphamethoxazole) (160 mg/800 mg twice daily for 10–140 days).[6] The studies reported cure rates of 0–71%. Over 30% of men were cured when treated for at least 90 days. The review did not report adverse effects. **Quinolones:** One review summarised three retrospective case series in 106 men treated with norfloxacin (400 mg twice daily for 10, 28, and 174 days).[7] The studies reported cure rates of 64–88%. We also found six retrospective case series in 141 men treated with ciprofloxacin (250–500 mg twice daily for 14–259 days), with cure rates of 60–75%. **Amoxicillin/clavulanic acid and clindamycin:** One case series included 50 men who were resistant to empirical treatment with quinolone. The expressed prostatic secretions from 24 of these men exhibited high colony counts of Gram positive and Gram negative anaerobic bacteria, either alone (18 men) or in combination with aerobic bacteria (6 men). After treatment with either amoxicillin (amoxycillin)/clavulanic acid or clindamycin for 3–6 weeks, all men had a decrease or total elimination of symptoms and no anaerobic bacteria were detected in prostatic secretions.[8] Higher cure rates with quinolones may be explained by greater penetration into the prostate.[9] We reviewed only studies that used standard methods to localise infection to the prostate.[10]

OPTION LOCAL INJECTION OF ANTIMICROBIALS

We found no RCTs comparing local injection of antimicrobials versus placebo or no treatment. One small RCT found that anal submucosal injection of amikacin improved symptom scores and bacterial eradication rates at 3 months compared with intramuscular amikacin.

Benefits: We found no placebo controlled RCTs. We found one small RCT (50 men with prostatic secretions sensitive to amikacin), which compared anal submucosal injection of amikacin 400 mg versus intramuscular amikacin 400 mg daily for 10 days.[11] It found that anal submucosal injection of amikacin significantly improved NIH–PSI score (see glossary, p 1001) and significantly increased bacteriological cure rates compared with intramuscular amikacin at 3 months (NIH–PSI: 9.0 with submucosal injection *v* 22.5 with intramuscular injection; $P < 0.05$; negative bacterial culture: 28/30 [93%] with submucosal injection *v* 7/20 [35%] with intramuscular; $P < 0.05$).

Harms: The RCT comparing anal submucosal and intramuscular amikacin found no obvious adverse effects other than the passage of slightly blood stained faeces in 3/30 [10%] men after the first anal submucosal injection.[11] Infection is a theoretical risk of this invasive procedure.

Comment: One small cohort study (24 men with refractory chronic bacterial prostatitis) found that eradication of infection was eventually achieved after an unstated period in 15 men with gentamicin (160 mg) plus cefazolin (cephazolin) (3 g) injected directly into the prostate through the perineum.[12]

OPTION α BLOCKERS

We found no RCTs comparing α blockers alone versus placebo or no treatment. We found limited evidence from one RCT suggesting that adding α blockers to antimicrobials may improve symptoms and reduce recurrence compared with antimicrobials alone.

Benefits: We found no systematic review. We found no RCTs comparing α blockers versus placebo. We found one RCT (64 men with bacterial prostatitis; mean age 48 years) of α blockers (either 1–2 mg terazosin daily, 2.5 mg terazosin daily, or 2.5 mg alfuzosin once or twice daily) plus antimicrobials versus antimicrobials alone.[13] It found that α blockers plus antimicrobials significantly increased symptomatic improvement and significantly reduced recurrence rates compared with antimicrobials alone (recurrence rates assessed by culture of expressed prostatic secretion; $P = 0.02$; no RR or CI reported; 5 people withdrew from treatment).

Harms: No adverse effects of α blockers were reported in this study.[13]

Comment: None.

OPTION TRANSURETHRAL RESECTION

We found no RCTs on the effects of transurethral resection.

Benefits: We found no systematic review, RCTs, or prospective cohort studies.

Harms: One RCT in men with benign prostatic hypertrophy found no difference in the incidence of impotence or urinary incontinence with transurethral resection or watchful waiting.[14]

Comment: One retrospective study reported 40–50% cure rates in 50 men with chronic prostatitis treated with transurethral resection. However, proof of bacterial prostatitis was not obtained in many men.[15]

OPTION RADICAL PROSTATECTOMY

We found no RCTs on the effects of radical prostatectomy.

Benefits: We found no systematic review or RCTs.

Harms: Case series found that radical prostatectomy can cause impotence (9–75% depending upon age)[16] and varying degrees of urinary stress incontinence (8%).[17] Other potential harms include those associated with any open surgery.

Comment: We found one report of radical prostatectomy in two young men whose refractory bacterial prostatitis caused relapsing haemolytic crises.[18]

QUESTION What are the effects of treatments for chronic abacterial prostatitis?

OPTION α BLOCKERS

One systematic review found limited evidence from two small RCTs that α blockers may improve maximal flow time and pain compared with placebo. However, we were unable to draw reliable conclusions from these small studies.

Benefits: We found one systematic review (search date 1999, 2 RCTs, 50 men).[19] The first RCT (20 people) identified by the review compared alfuzosin (2.5 mg three times daily) versus placebo. It found a significant improvement in maximal flow time with alfuzosin (with 15.4 mL/second to 20.3 mL/second alfuzosin *v* 13.9 mL/second to 15.6 mL/second with placebo; $P = 0.01$; RR not reported).[20] It found no significant difference in other outcomes (insufficient information was presented to assess comparative effects on symptom scores). The second RCT (30 people) identified by the review found that pain after prostatic massage significantly improved with α blockers (phenoxybenzamine 10 mg twice daily) versus placebo (at 6 weeks; $P < 0.05$).

Harms: The first RCT reported a transient decrease in systolic blood pressure in four people and a slight decrease in libido in two people all treated with alfuzosin.[19]

Comment: None.

OPTION 5α REDUCTASE INHIBITORS

One systematic review of one small RCT found insufficient evidence on the effects of 5α reductase inhibitors compared with placebo in men with chronic abacterial prostatitis.

Benefits: We found one systematic review (search date 1999, 1 RCT, 41 men), which compared finasteride versus placebo.[19] The RCT found that, although symptom scores decreased significantly with finasteride after 1 year, there was no significant difference in pain between finasteride and placebo.[21] The RCT was small and had low power (31/41 [75%] of men were allocated to finasteride *v* 10/41 [25%] of men to placebo).

Harms: Three people treated with finasteride reported partial impotence compared with none in the placebo group.[21]

Comment: Finasteride is known to decrease prostate volume (as it did in this study; $P < 0.03$), but it is unclear how this relates to symptoms of prostatitis.[21]

OPTION ANTI-INFLAMMATORY MEDICATIONS

We found insufficient evidence about the effects of anti-inflammatory medications compared with placebo or no treatment in men with chronic abacterial prostatitis.

Benefits: We found one systematic review (search date 1999, 1 RCT, 30 men).[19] The included RCT compared pentosan polysulfate sodium (100 mg twice daily) versus placebo. Outcomes included symptom changes by physician rating, symptom score, and uroflowmetry. The RCT found no significant difference in either physician rated improvement (pentosan polysulfate sodium group 7/10 [70%] improved *v* placebo 5/14 [36%] improved; RR 2.0, 95% CI 0.87 to 4.4) or in local symptom scores (pentosan polysulfate sodium 5/10 [50%] improved *v* placebo 6/14 [43%] improved; RR 1.2, 95% CI 0.5 to 2.8).[22] Six people were excluded from the analysis for non-compliance or having bacterial prostatitis (analysis was not intention to treat). The RCT may have been too small to rule out important clinical differences.

Harms: Two people given pentosan polysulfate sodium reported diarrhoea. No people treated with placebo developed gastrointestinal adverse symptoms.

Comment: "Physician rated improvement" is not an objective measurement. There was no significant difference between experimental and control groups with other, more objective and standardised, outcomes.

OPTION TRANSURETHRAL MICROWAVE THERMOTHERAPY

One systematic review found limited evidence from one small RCT suggesting that transurethral microwave thermotherapy may significantly improve quality of life at 3 months and symptoms over 21 months compared with sham treatment. However, we were unable to draw reliable conclusions from this one small study.

Benefits: We found one systematic review (search date 1999,[19] 1 double blind RCT,[23] 20 men). The included RCT compared transurethral microwave thermotherapy versus sham treatment.[23] It found a significant improvement in quality of life at 3 months with thermotherapy compared with sham treatment (scale 0–10; quality of life improved from 4.4 to 3.0 with transurethral microwave thermotherapy *v* unchanged at 5.2 with sham treatment; $P < 0.05$). Significantly more men had improvement of a subjective global assessment by more than 50% over a mean of 21 months with thermotherapy compared with sham treatment (7/10 [70%] *v* 1/10 [10%]; RR 7, 95% CI 1 to 47; NNT 2, 95% CI 2 to 6). The review found no good evidence on the effects of thermotherapy on cure or recurrence rate.

Harms: Four men complained of transient (resolved in 3 weeks) adverse reactions, including haematuria (2 men), urinary tract infection, impotence, urinary retention, urinary incontinence, and premature ejaculation (each occurring in 1 man).[23] However, the RCT did not report if the men with adverse events were treated with active treatment or sham treatment.

Comment: Thermotherapy caused persistent elevation of leucocytes in the prostatic fluid, which could indicate tissue damage.

OPTION ALLOPURINOL

We found insufficient evidence from one small RCT about the effects of allopurinol compared with placebo in men with chronic abacterial prostatitis.

Benefits: We found one systematic review (search date 2000,[24] 1 RCT,[25] 54 men). The RCT compared treatment with allopurinol (600 mg daily), allopurinol (300 mg daily), and placebo. Thirty four men (63%) completed the study, which lasted 240 days. All recorded data were used in the analysis. The RCT found allopurinol significantly reduced the "degree of discomfort" score (pretreatment score = 0; score –1.1 with allopurinol *v* placebo –0.2 with placebo; $P = 0.02$).[25]

Harms: None of the men receiving allopurinol reported any significant adverse events, but the RCT did not explain what constitutes a significant adverse event; 55% of people on placebo and 68% of people on allopurinol completed the trial.[25]

Comment: The symptom score was not validated and the high withdrawal rate makes the results difficult to interpret.[25]

OPTION PROSTATIC MASSAGE

We found no RCTs on the effects of prostatic massage.

Benefits: We found no systematic review or RCTs.

Harms: We found no good evidence.

Comment: None.

OPTION SITZ BATHS

We found no RCTs on the effects of Sitz baths.

Benefits: We found no systematic review or RCTs.

Harms: We found no good evidence.

Comment: None.

OPTION BIOFEEDBACK

We found no RCTs on the effects of biofeedback.

Benefits: We found no systematic review or RCTs.

Harms: We found no good evidence.

Comment: None.

GLOSSARY

NIH–CPSI (National Institute of Health–Chronic Prostatis Symptom Index). Includes nine items across three domains: pain (4 items; 0–21); urinary symptoms (2 items; 0–10), and quality of life impact (3 items; 0–12). In all domains, higher scores indicate worse outcomes.

Substantive changes

Oral antimicrobial drugs One RCT added;[5] conclusions unchanged.
Local injection of antimicrobials One RCT added;[11] conclusions unchanged.

REFERENCES

1. Roberts RO, Lieber MM, Rhodes T, et al. Prevalence of a physician-assigned diagnosis of prostatitis: the Olmsted County study of urinary symptoms and health status among men. *Urology* 1998;51:578–584.
2. Collins MM, Stafford, RS, O'Leary MP, et al. How common is prostatitis? A national survey of physician visits. *J Urol* 1998;159:1224–1228.
3. Alexander RB, Brady F, Ponniah S. Autoimmune prostatitis: evidence of T cell reactivity with normal prostatic proteins. *Urology* 1997;50:893–899.
4. Wenninger K, Heiman JR, Rothman I, et al. Sickness impact of chronic nonbacterial prostatitis and its correlates. *J Urol* 1996;155:965–968.
5. Naber KG. Lomefloxacin versus ciprofloxacin in the treatment of chronic bacterial prostatitis. *Int J Antimicrob Agents* 2002;20:18–27.
6. Hanus PM, Danzinger LH. Treatment of chronic bacterial prostatitis. *Clin Pharm* 1984;3:49–55.
7. Naber KG, Sorgel F, Kees F, et al. Norfloxacin concentration in prostatic adenoma tissue (patients) and in prostatic fluid in patients and volunteers. 15th International Congress of Chemotherapy, Landsberg. In: Weidner N, Madsen PO, Schiefer HG, eds. *Prostatitis: etiopathology, diagnosis and therapy.* New York: Springer Verlag, 1987.
8. Szoke I, Torok L, Dosa E, et al. The possible role of anaerobic bacteria in chronic prostatitis. *Int J Androl* 1998;21:163–168.
9. Cox CE. Ofloxacin in the management of complicated urinary tract infections, including prostatitis. *Am J Med* 1980;87(suppl 6c):61–68.
10. Meares EM, Stamey TA. Bacteriologic localization patterns in bacterial prostatitis and urethritis. *Invest Urol* 1968;5:492–518.
11. Hu W-L, Zhong S-Z, He H-X. Treatment of chronic bacterial prostatitis with amikacin through anal submucosal injection. *Asian J Androl* 2002;4:163–167.
12. Baret L, Leonare A. Chronic bacterial prostatitis: 10 years of experience with local antibiotics. *J Urol* 1998;140:755–757.
13. Barbalias GA, Nikiforidis G, Liatsikos EN. Alpha-blockers for the treatment of chronic prostatitis in combination with antibiotics. *J Urol* 1998;159:883–887.

14. Wasson JH, Reda DJ, Bruskewitz RC, et al. A comparison of transurethral surgery with watchful waiting for moderate symptoms of benign prostatic hyperplasia. *N Engl J Med* 1995;332:75–79.
15. Smart CJ, Jenkins JD, Lloyd RS. The painful prostate. *Br J Urol* 1975;47:861–869.
16. Quinlan DM, Epstein JI, Carter BS, et al. Sexual function following radical prostatectomy: influence of preservation of neurovascular bundles. *J Urol* 1991;145:998–1002.
17. Steiner MS, Morton RA, Walsh PC. Impact of radical prostatectomy on urinary continence. *J Urol* 1991;145:512–515.
18. Davis BE, Weigel JW. Adenocarcinoma of the prostate discovered in 2 young patients following total prostatovesiculectomy for refractory prostatitis. *J Urol* 1990;144:744–745.
19. Collins M, MacDonald R, Wilt T. Diagnosis and treatment of chronic abacterial prostatitis: a systematic review. *Ann Intern Med* 2000;133:367–368. Search date 1999; primary sources Medline, Cochrane Library, hand searches of bibliographies, and contact with an expert.
20. de la Rosette JJ, Karthaus HF, van Kerrebroeck PE, et al. Research in "prostatitis syndromes": the use of alfuzosin (a new alpha 1-receptor-blocking agent) in patients mainly presenting with micturition complaints of an irritative nature and confirmed urodynamic abnormalities. *Eur Urol* 1992;22:222–227.
21. Leskinen M, Lukkarinen O, Marttila T. Effects of finasteride in patients with inflammatory chronic pelvic pain syndrome: a double-blind, placebo-controlled, pilot study. *Urology* 1999;53:502–505.
22. Wédren H. Effects of sodium pentosanpolysulphate on symptoms related to chronic non-bacterial prostatitis. *Scand J Urol Nephrol* 1987;21:81–88.
23. Nickel J, Sorensen R. Transurethral microwave thermotherapy for nonbacterial prostatitis: a randomized double-blind sham controlled study using new prostatitis specific assessment questionnaires. *J Urol* 1996;155:1950–1955.
24. McNaughton Collins M, MacDonald R, Wilt T. Interventions for chronic abacterial prostatitis. In: The Cochrane Library, Issue 2, 2002. Oxford: Update Software. Search date 2000; primary sources Medline, The Cochrane Library, hand searches of bibliographies of identified articles and reviews, and contact with an expert.
25. Persson B, Ronquist G, Ekblom M. Ameliorative effect of allopurinol on nonbacterial prostatitis: a parallel double-blind controlled study. *J Urol* 1996;155:961–964.

Anthony Schaeffer
Professor and Chair

Jeffrey Stern

Department of Urology
Northwestern University Medical School
Chicago
USA

Competing interests: None declared.

Erectile dysfunction

Search date December 2002

Robyn Webber

QUESTIONS

INTERVENTIONS

See glossary, p 1010

Key Messages

- **Intracavernosal alprostadil** One large RCT found that intracavernosal alprostadil increased the chances of a satisfactory erection compared with placebo.
- **Intraurethral alprostadil (in men who had responded to a single test dose)** One large RCT (in men who had previously responded to alprostadil) found limited evidence that intraurethral alprostadil (prostaglandin E1) increased the chances of successful sexual intercourse and at least one orgasm over 3 months compared with placebo. About a third of men suffered penile ache. We found no direct comparisons of intraurethral alprostadil versus either intracavernosal alprostadil or oral drug treatments.
- **Sildenafil** One systematic review and six subsequent RCTs found that sildenafil improved erections and increased rates of successful intercourse compared with placebo. Adverse effects, including headaches, flushing, and dyspepsia, are reported in up to a quarter of men. Deaths have been reported in men on concomitant treatment with oral nitrates.
- **Yohimbine** One systematic review has found that yohimbine improves self reported sexual function and penile rigidity at 2–10 weeks compared with placebo. Transient adverse effects are reported in up to a third of men.
- **Topical alprostadil** Two quasi randomised trials found limited evidence that topical alprostadil increased the number of men with erections sufficient for intercourse compared with placebo but was commonly associated with skin irritation.
- **L-arginine** One small RCT found no significant difference in sexual function between L-arginine and placebo, but it may have been too small to exclude a clinically important difference.
- **Penile prostheses** We found no RCTs of penile prostheses in men with erectile dysfunction.

Clin Evid 2003;10:1003–1011.

- **Trazodone** One small RCT found no significant difference in erections or libido between trazodone and placebo, but it may have been too small to exclude a clinically important difference.
- **Vacuum devices** Vacuum devices have not been adequately assessed in RCTs. One small RCT found limited evidence that they were as effective as intracavernosal alprostadil (prostaglandin E1) injections for rigidity but not for orgasm.

DEFINITION Erectile dysfunction has largely replaced the term "impotence". It is defined as the persistent inability to obtain or maintain sufficient rigidity of the penis to allow satisfactory sexual performance.

INCIDENCE/ PREVALENCE We found little good epidemiological information, but one cross sectional study found that age is the variable most strongly associated with erectile dysfunction, and that up to 30 million men in the USA may be affected.[1] Even among men in their 40s, nearly 40% report at least occasional difficulty obtaining or maintaining erection, whereas this approaches 70% in 70 year olds.

AETIOLOGY/ RISK FACTORS It is now believed that about 80% of cases of erectile dysfunction have an organic cause, the rest being psychogenic in origin. Risk factors include increasing age, smoking, and obesity. Erectile problems fall into three categories: failure to initiate; failure to fill, caused by insufficient arterial inflow into the penis to allow engorgement and tumescence because of vascular insufficiency; and failure to store because of veno-occlusive dysfunction. Erectile dysfunction is a recognised side effect of a wide variety of pharmaceutical agents.

PROGNOSIS We found no good evidence on prognosis in untreated organic erectile dysfunction.

AIMS OF INTERVENTION To restore satisfactory erections, with minimal adverse effects.

OUTCOMES Patient and partner self reports of satisfaction and sexual function; objective tests of penile rigidity; adverse effects of treatment.

METHODS *Clinical Evidence* search and appraisal December 2002.

QUESTION What are the effects of treatments?

OPTION YOHIMBINE

One systematic review has found that yohimbine improves self reported sexual function and penile rigidity at 2–10 weeks compared with placebo. Transient adverse effects are reported in up to a third of men.

Benefits: **Versus placebo:** We found one systematic review (search date 1997, 7 RCTs, 11–100 men with erectile dysfunction, defined variously as organic, psychogenic, and of unknown cause) comparing yohimbine versus placebo.[2] Duration of treatment ranged from 2–10 weeks, and outcomes varied from self reported change in sexual function to objective tests of penile rigidity. The RCTs found positive responses in significantly more men taking yohimbine than in those taking placebo (34–73% *v* 9–45%; OR 3.85, 95% CI 2.22

to 6.67; absolute numbers not reported). One subsequent placebo controlled, crossover trial (22 men, randomisation not mentioned) comparing yohimbine single daily dose 100 mg for 30 days versus placebo found no significant difference between treatments in erectile function.[3]

Harms: The review found that adverse events were reported in 10–30% of men receiving yohimbine compared with 5–16% with placebo (significance not reported) and were generally mild, including agitation, anxiety, headache, mild increase in blood pressure, increased urinary output, and gastrointestinal upset.[2] In the small subsequent trial no men discontinued treatment.[3]

Comment: The end points in some of these trials were subjective and of questionable validity. The subsequent trial did not make clear whether it was randomised.[3]

OPTION SILDENAFIL

One systematic review and six subsequent RCTs found that sildenafil improved erections and increased rates of successful intercourse compared with placebo. Adverse effects, including headaches, flushing, and dyspepsia, are reported in up to a quarter of men. Deaths have been reported in men on concomitant treatment with oral nitrates.

Benefits: We found one systematic review (search date 2000, 27 RCTs)[4] and six subsequent RCTs.[5–10] **In men with any cause of erectile dysfunction:** The systematic review found that, in trials evaluating flexible "as needed" dosing (14 RCTs, 2283 men with any cause of erectile dysfunction), sildenafil significantly increased the proportion of men who experienced at least one episode of successful intercourse compared with placebo (2283 men; 83% with sildenafil *v* 45% with placebo; RRI 1.8, 95% CI 1.7 to 1.9). In trials evaluating fixed doses of sildenafil (6 RCTs), efficacy was slightly higher on higher doses (> 50 mg) and less effective on a low dose (< 25 mg). The six subsequent RCTs compared 12 weeks of treatment with sildenafil 25–100 mg versus placebo. The first subsequent RCT (236 men) compared sildenafil (25–100 mg taken as needed before attempted intercourse) versus placebo.[5] After 12 weeks of treatment, sildenafil significantly improved sexual function (questions 3 and 4 of the International Index of Erectile Dysfunction [see glossary, p 1010]) and rate of successful intercourse attempts compared with placebo (mean improvement on question 3: 1.87 points with sildenafil *v* 0.68 points with placebo, $P < 0.0001$; mean improvement on question 4: 2.12 points with sildenafil *v* 0.86 points with placebo, $P < 0.0001$; rate of successful intercourse attempts: 62% with sildenafil *v* 30% with placebo, $P < 0.0001$). The second subsequent RCT (152 men with erectile dysfunction and depressive symptoms) compared 12 weeks of treatment with sildenafil versus placebo.[6] It found that sildenafil significantly improved self reported improvement in erections, self reported improvement in ability to have intercourse, and improvement in sexual function (90% reported improvement in erections with sildenafil *v* 11% with placebo, P value not reported; 89% reported improvement in ability to have sexual intercourse with sildenafil *v*

13% with placebo, P value not reported; P < 0.001 in favour of sildenafil for difference in scores for questions 3 and 4 of the International Index of Erectile Dysfunction). The third subsequent RCT (247 men) found that sildenafil (25–100 mg) significantly improved the primary outcomes of participant and partner rated ability to achieve and maintain erection and satisfaction with intercourse compared with placebo at 12 weeks (questions 3, 4, and 7 of the International Index of Erectile Dysfunction; P < 0.001 for all comparisons).[7] The fourth subsequent RCT (141 men) found significantly greater improvement in self reported sexual function with sildenafil compared with placebo at 12 weeks (improved scores on the International Index of Erectile Function questionnaire [IIEF]: 66% with sildenafil *v* 15% with placebo for frequency of penetration; 78% with sildenafil *v* 21% for ability to maintain erection after penetration; P < 0.0001 for both comparisons).[8] The fifth subsequent RCT (214 men) found that mean scores for all questions on the IIEF were significantly higher with sildenafil compared with placebo (P < 0.0001).[9] Men reported an improvement in both frequency of penetration (P < 0.0001) and the ability to maintain erections after penetration (P < 0.0001). The sixth subsequent RCT (158 men) found that significantly more men taking sildenafil reported improved erection (77% with sildenafil *v* 46% with placebo, P < 0.001) and successful attempts at intercourse (65% with sildenafil *v* 35% with placebo, P < 0.05).[10] **In men with diabetes:** The more recent systematic review included two RCTs restricted to men with diabetes, and 14 trials (551 men) providing subgroup analysis in men with diabetes.[4] Based on subgroup analysis, the review found that significantly more men experienced successful intercourse with sildenafil compared with placebo (44% with sildenafil *v* 16% with placebo; WMD 26.9, 95% CI 19.9 to 33.9) and experienced successful erections (63% with sildenafil *v* 19% with placebo; RRI 3, 95% CI 2.5 to 3.7). We found one additional placebo controlled RCT (219 men).[11] It found that sildenafil (25–100 mg) improved participant rated improvement in erections and score on questions 3 and 4 of the International Index of Erectile Dysfunction after 12 weeks (64.6% had improved erections with sildenafil *v* 10.5% with placebo; 95% CI presented graphically, P < 0.0001; mean improvement in question 3 score: 3.42 with sildenafil *v* 1.86 with placebo; mean improvement in question 4 score: 3.35 with sildenafil *v* 1.84 with placebo; P < 0.0001 for both comparisons). **In men with spinal cord injury:** The more recent systematic review included two RCTs (203 men) restricted to men with spinal cord injury.[4] It found that more men experienced improved erections with sildenafil (83% with sildenafil *v* 12% with placebo; RRI 7.2, 95% CI 4.7 to 10.9).

Harms: The more recent systematic review found that, in a subset of 14 flexible dose trials (3780 men), 48% of those randomised to sildenafil reported at least one adverse effect compared with 36% of men taking placebo (RRI 1.4, 95% CI 1.3 to 1.6). Adverse effects included headache (11% with sildenafil *v* 4% with placebo), flushing (12% *v* 2%), dyspepsia (5% *v* 1%), and visual disturbance (3% *v* 0.8%).[4] One RCT (236 men with any cause of erectile dysfunction) found that sildenafil was associated with facial flushing (25.2%), dizziness (6.7%), headache (5.9%), and palpitations (3.4%).[5] A second RCT found that headache, flushing, dyspepsia, and abnormal perception of colour or brightness were more common with sildenafil than placebo (20% *v* 6% for headache; 15% *v* 0% for dyspepsia; 15% *v* 1% for flushing; 8% *v* 1% for abnormal vision).[6] A third RCT found similar results.[7] Another study reported specifically on adverse effects of sildenafil.[12] It summarised results from a series of RCTs (4274 men aged 19–87 years with erectile dysfunction owing to a range of causes for > 6 months and a mean of 5 years). All men were treated for up to 6 months, and 2199 received further open label treatment for up to 1 year. It found more adverse events with sildenafil than with placebo, including headache (16% *v* 4%; significance not reported), flushing (10% *v* 1%; significance not reported), and dyspepsia (7% *v* 2%; significance not reported). Similar proportions in both groups discontinued treatment (about 2.4%).[12] An important contraindication to prescribing sildenafil is concomitant use of oral nitrates. This combination results in precipitous hypotension. One small RCT (105 men) evaluated the cardiovascular effects of sildenafil during exercise in men with coronary heart disease.[13] It found no effect on symptoms, presence, and extent of ischaemia induced by exercise. By 1999, about 60 deaths had been reported to the US Food and Drug Administration in men who had been prescribed sildenafil, but it is not known whether any of the deaths were directly attributable to the drug. Long term (> 1 year) safety of sildenafil is unknown. One of the RCTs in men with psychogenic or mixed aetiology erectile dysfunction found that adverse effects were mild and transient.[14]

Comment: None.

OPTION L-ARGININE

One small RCT found no significant difference in sexual function between L-arginine and placebo, but it may have been too small to exclude a clinically important difference.

Benefits: We found no systematic review. We found one small RCT (50 men with erectile dysfunction) comparing high dose L-arginine (5 g/day given orally) versus placebo.[15] It found no significant difference in sexual function between L-arginine and placebo, although the power of the study was not adequate to rule out a clinically important difference (sexual function improved in 9/29 [31%] men with L-arginine *v* 2/17 [12%] with placebo; RR 2.6, 95% CI 0.6 to 10.8).

Harms: The trial reported decreases in systolic or diastolic blood pressure, or both, although this caused no systemic effects and required no drug interruptions. The trial found some "fluctuation in heart rate", which was described as clinically insignificant.

Comment: Nausea, vomiting, diarrhoea, headache, flushing, and numbness have been reported after the administration of L-arginine, although none of the men in this study reported any such complaints.

OPTION TRAZODONE

One small RCT found no significant difference in erections or libido with trazodone compared with placebo, but it may have been too small to exclude a clinically important difference.

Benefits: We found no systematic review. One small crossover RCT (48 men with erectile dysfunction, washout period 3 weeks) compared trazodone versus placebo.[16] Men were treated with either trazodone (50 mg) or placebo at bedtime for 3 months. It found no evidence that trazodone improved erections or libido (improved erections reported by 19% with trazodone *v* 24% with placebo; CI and P value not reported, described as NS; improved libido reported by 35% with trazodone *v* 20% with placebo; CI and P value not reported, described as NS).

Harms: The trial reported drowsiness (31% of men), dry mouth (1%), and fatigue (19%) with trazodone. Comparative rates for trazodone versus placebo were not available.

Comment: None.

OPTION INTRAURETHRAL ALPROSTADIL

One large RCT (in men who had previously responded to alprostadil) found limited evidence that intraurethral alprostadil (prostaglandin E1) increased the chances of successful sexual intercourse and at least one orgasm over 3 months compared with placebo. About a third of men suffered penile ache. We found no direct comparisons of intraurethral alprostadil with either intracavernosal alprostadil or oral drug treatments.

Benefits: We found no systematic review. We found one RCT (996 men aged 27–88 years who had previously responded to intraurethral alprostadil) comparing alprostadil versus placebo.[17] It found that those given alprostadil were more likely to report having successful sexual intercourse over 3 months (65% with alprostadil *v* 19% with placebo; $P < 0.001$) and at least one orgasm (64% with alprostadil *v* 24% with placebo; $P < 0.001$). Subsequent RCTs, published only in abstract form, found slightly lower increased rates of satisfactory erections of 30–48% with alprostadil.

Harms: The most common adverse effect was mild to moderate penile ache, occurring in about a third of men during clinic testing (36%). In total 36/1511 (2.4%) withdrew from the trial because of it.[17] We found no reports of priapism, penile fibrosis, or other serious adverse events.

Comment: The RCT preselected men who had a good response to alprostadil before randomisation. This will tend to increase the size of the effect compared with placebo.

OPTION INTRACAVERNOSAL ALPROSTADIL

One large RCT found that intracavernosal injection of alprostadil (prostaglandin E1) increased the chances of a satisfactory erection compared with placebo. We found no direct comparisons of intracavernosal alprostadil versus either intraurethral or oral drug

treatments. One small RCT found limited evidence that vacuum devices were as effective as intracavernosal alprostadil injections for rigidity but not for orgasm.

Benefits: We found no systematic review. We found one large multicentre trial (1128 men of whom 300 were randomly assigned with all causes of erectile dysfunction, but excluding heavy smokers and men with uncontrolled hypertension or diabetes) comparing 2.5, 5, 10, or 20 μg alprostadil versus placebo.[18] Injections were given and outcome was assessed by an investigator or research nurse. None of the 59 men who received placebo had a response. There were significant differences in clinical evaluation with all the doses of alprostadil compared with placebo and a significant dose–response relationship. **Versus vacuum devices:** One crossover RCT (50 men with erectile dysfunction, 44 of whom completed the study) compared intracavernosal self injections of alprostadil versus vacuum devices.[19] Outcome was assessed by a questionnaire given to men and their partners after 15 uses for each device, and couples were followed for 18–24 months. There was no significant difference in the ability to achieve an erection suitable for intercourse. However, the ability to attain orgasm was significantly better with alprostadil ($P < 0.05$). On a scale of 1 to 10, overall satisfaction was significantly better when using alprostadil, both for men (6.5 with alprostadil *v* 5.4 with vacuum device; $P < 0.05$) and partners (6.5 with alprostadil *v* 5.1 with vacuum device; $P < 0.05$). Younger men (< 60 years) and those with shorter duration of erectile dysfunction (< 12 months) favoured alprostadil ($P < 0.05$).

Harms: Penile pain was reported by a half of the men in the multicentre trial, and priapism (prolonged erection for > 4 hours) by 1%.[18] There was no significant difference in the frequency of adverse events between vacuum devices and alprostadil.[19]

Comment: Most men can be taught to inject themselves using small gauge needles. In the RCT comparing injections and vacuum devices, 80% of the 44 couples who completed the study were still using one or other treatment after 18–24 months.[19]

OPTION TOPICAL ALPROSTADIL

Two quasi randomised trials found limited evidence that topical alprostadil increased the number of men with erections sufficient for intercourse compared with placebo but was commonly associated with skin irritation.

Benefits: We found no systematic review. We found two quasi randomised trials (see comment below).[20,21] The first single blind trial (48 men with erectile dysfunction owing to organic, psychogenic, or mixed causes) compared topical alprostadil versus placebo.[20] Men were assigned in sequential order to either 0.5, 1, or 2.5 mg alprostadil gel (36 men) or placebo (12 men). One dose of alprostadil or placebo gel was applied to the glans and shaft of the penis and washed off after 3 hours. Alprostadil significantly increased the proportion of men who achieved an erection sufficient for intercourse compared with placebo (25/36 [69%] with alprostadil *v* 2/12 [17%] with placebo; RR 4.2, 95% CI 1.8 to 5.5; NNT 2, 95% CI 1 to

8). The second RCT (62 men) compared alprostadil topically applied only to the glans of the penis in a clinic setting versus placebo. It found significantly more men reported an erection deemed sufficient for penetration with alprostadil compared with placebo (12/31 [39%] v 2/29 [7%]; RR 5.6, 95% CI 1.4 to 23.0; NNT 3, 95% CI 2 to 9).[21]

Harms: Men receiving alprostadil to the glans and shaft of the penis were more likely to have skin irritation than those on placebo (100% on 0.5 mg dose v 67% on placebo; no P value provided). Irritation was more severe with alprostadil than with placebo (measured by mean irritation score ranging from 0–2; 1.75 with 0.5 mg dose v 0.67 with placebo; $P < 0.0013$).[20] In the trial in which alprostadil was applied to the glans only, significantly greater erythema was reported with alprostadil than with placebo ($P < 0.001$; absolute figures not reported).[21] Severe erythema was reported by 3% of men.

Comment: Allocation of men in both trials was sequential and may mean that the groups were systematically different; the characteristics of each group were not reported.[20,21]

OPTION VACUUM DEVICES

Vacuum devices have not been adequately assessed in RCTs. One small RCT found limited evidence that they were as effective as intracavernosal alprostadil (prostaglandin E1) injections for rigidity but not for orgasm.

Benefits: **Versus placebo:** We found no systematic review and no RCTs. **Versus intracavernosal injections:** See benefits of intracavernosal alprostadil, p 1009.

Harms: We found insufficient evidence.

Comment: Vacuum devices may be less popular than injections because only the distal portion of the penis becomes firm, but they are presumed to be safe.[19]

OPTION PENILE PROSTHESES

We found no RCTs of penile prostheses in men with erectile dysfunction. Use of penile prostheses is usually considered only after less invasive treatments have failed.

Benefits: We found no RCTs. Anecdotal evidence suggests that patient satisfaction may be high, but we found no good studies.

Harms: One recent study found the morbidity of penile prostheses to be 9% (surgical revision 7%, mechanical failure 2.5%). Infection rates were between 2% and 7%.[22]

Comment: Use of penile prostheses is usually considered only after less invasive treatments have failed.

GLOSSARY

Questions 3 and 4 of the International Index of Erectile Function The questions have been validated for assessing the effects of sildenafil on sexual function. The questions ask "over the past 4 weeks, when you have attempted sexual intercourse, how often were you able to penetrate (enter) your partner?", and "over the past 4 weeks, during sexual intercourse, how often were you able to maintain your erection after you have penetrated (entered) your partner?" Questions are answered on a six point scale.

Substantive changes

Sildenafil One systematic review[4] and three RCTs[8–10] added; conclusions unchanged.

REFERENCES

1. Feldman HA, Goldstein I, Dimitrios GH, et al. Impotence and its medical and psychosocial correlates: results of the Massachusetts male aging study. *J Urol* 1994;151:54–61.
2. Ernst E, Pittler MH. Yohimbine for erectile dysfunction: a systemic review and meta-analysis of randomized clinical trials. *J Urol* 1998;159:433–436. Search date 1997; primary sources Medline, Embase, The Cochrane Library, and hand searched references.
3. Teloken C, Rhoden EL, Sogari P, et al. Therapeutic effects of high dose yohimbine hydrochloride on organic erectile dysfunction. *J Urol* 1998;159:122–124.
4. Fink HA, MacDonald R, Rutks IR, et al. Sildenafil for male erectile dysfunction. A systematic review and meta-analysis. *Arch Intern Med* 2002;162:1349–1360. Search date 2000; primary sources Medline, Health-STAR, Current Contents, Cochrane Library, review of bibliographies of retrieved trials and review articles, and a hand search of urology journals and national meeting abstracts.
5. Chen KK, Hsieh JT, Huang ST, et al. ASSESS-3: a randomised, double-blind, flexible-dose clinical trial of the efficacy and safety of oral sildenafil in the treatment of men with erectile dysfunction in Taiwan. *Int J Impot Res* 2001;13:221–229.
6. Seidman SN, Roose SP, Menza MA, et al. Treatment of erectile dysfunction in men with depressive symptoms: results of a placebo-controlled trial with sildenafil citrate. *Am J Psychiatry* 2001;158:1623–1630.
7. Lewis R, Bennett CJ, Borkon WD, et al. Patient and partner satisfaction with Viagra (sildenafil citrate) treatment as determined by the Erectile Dysfunction Inventory of Treatment Satisfaction Questionnaire. *Urology* 2001;57:960–965.
8. Becher E, Tejada NA, Gomez R et al. Sildenafil citrate (Viagra) in the treatment of men with erectile dysfunction in southern Latin America: A double blind, randomized, placebo-controlled, parallel-group, multicenter, flexible-dose escalation study. *Int J Impot Res* 2002;14(suppl):33–41.
9. Glina S, Bertero E, Claro J, et al. Efficacy and safety of flexible dose oral sildenafil citrate (Viagra) in the treatment of erectile dysfunction in Brazilian and Mexican men. *Int J Impot Res* 2002;14(suppl): 27–32.
10. Gomez F, Davila H, Costa A, et al. Efficacy and safety of oral sildenafil citrate (Viagra) in the treatment of male erectile dysfunction in Colombia, Ecuador, and Venezuela: a double-blind, multicenter, placebo-controlled study. *Int J Impot Res* 2002;14(suppl):42–47.
11. Boulton AJ, Selam JL, Sweeney M, et al. Sildenafil citrate for the treatment of erectile dysfunction in men with Type II diabetes mellitus. *Diabetologia* 2001;44:1296–1301.
12. Morales A, Gingell C, Collins M, et al. Clinical safety of oral sildenafil citrate (Viagra) in the treatment of erectile dysfunction. *Int J Impot Res* 1998;10:69–74.
13. Arruda-Olson AM, Mahoney DW, Nehra DW et al. Cardiovascular effects of sildenafil during exercise in men with known or probable coronary artery disease: a randomized crossover trial. *JAMA* 2002; 287: 719–725.
14. Olsson AM, Speakman MJ, Dinsmore WW, et al. Sildenafil citrate (Viagra) is effective and well tolerated for treating erectile dysfunction of psychogenic or mixed aetiology. *Int J Clin Pract* 2000;54:561–566.
15. Chen J, Wollman Y, Chernichovsky T, et al. Effect of oral administration of high-dose nitric oxide donor L-arginine in men with organic erectile dysfunction: results of a double-blind randomized placebo-controlled study. *BJU Int* 1999;83:269–273.
16. Costabile RA, Spevak M. Oral trazodone is not effective therapy for erectile dysfunction: a double blind placebo-controlled trial. *J Urol* 1999;161:1819–1822.
17. Padma-Nathan H, Hellstrom WJ, Kaiser FE, et al, for the Medicated Urethral System for Erection (MUSE) Study Group. Treatment of men with erectile dysfunction with transurethral alprostadil. *N Engl J Med* 1997;336:1–7.
18. PGE1 Study Group. Prospective, multicenter trials of efficacy and safety of intracavernosal alprostadil (prostaglandin E1) sterile powder in men with erectile dysfunction. *N Engl J Med* 1996;334:873–877.
19. Soderdahl DW, Thrasher JB, Hansberry KL, et al. Intracavernosal drug induced erection therapy vs external vacuum device in the treatment of erectile dysfunction. *Br J Urol* 1997;79:952–957.
20. McVary KT, Polepalle S, Riggi S, et al. Topical prostaglandin E1 SEPA gel for the treatment of erectile dysfunction. *J Urol* 1999;162:726–730.
21. Goldstein I, Payton TR, Schechter PJ. A double blind placebo controlled efficacy and safety study of topical gel formulation of 1% alprostadil (Topiglan) for the in office treatment of erectile dysfunction. *Urology* 2001;57:301–305.
22. Goldstein I, Newman L, Baum N, et al. Safety and efficacy outcome of Mentor α 1 inflatable penile prosthesis implantation for impotence treatment. *J Urol* 1997;157:833–839.

Robyn Webber
Consultant Urological Surgeon
Hairmyres Hospital
East Kilbride
Scotland

Competing interests: The author has received funding from Pfizer to attend several educational meetings.

The following previous contributors of this topic would also like to be acknowledged: Michael O'Leary and Bazian Ltd.

Prostate cancer (metastatic)

Search date September 2002

M Dror Michaelson, Matthew R Smith, and James A Talcott

QUESTIONS

INTERVENTIONS

*Categorisation based on observational evidence; RCTs unlikely to be conducted.

See glossary, p 1020

Key Messages

In men with metastatic prostate cancer

- **Androgen deprivation** We found limited evidence from RCTs suggesting that androgen deprivation reduced mortality compared with no initial treatment. One non-systematic review of RCTs found that orchidectomy, diethylstilbestrol, and gonadorelin analogues initially improved symptoms and objective signs of disease in most men, but found no evidence of a difference between different types of androgen deprivation.
- **Combined androgen blockade (androgen deprivation and antiandrogen) versus androgen deprivation alone** Systematic reviews found limited evidence of a 2–5% improvement in 5 year survival associated with combined androgen blockade (androgen deprivation plus a non-steroidal antiandrogen) compared with androgen deprivation alone.
- **Intermittent androgen deprivation** We found no RCTs comparing long term effects of intermittent androgen deprivation versus those of continuous androgen deprivation on mortality, morbidity, or quality of life.

- **Deferred androgen deprivation without surveillance** One systematic review found limited evidence of a small survival advantage at 10 years for immediate androgen deprivation therapy with gonadorelin analogues or orchidectomy in men with advanced, asymptomatic prostate cancer. There was no significant change in overall survival at 1, 2, or 5 years. The risk of major complications is increased in men whose treatment is deferred until disease progression.

In men with symptomatic androgen independent metastatic prostate cancer

- **Chemotherapy (palliation but no evidence of an effect on survival)** RCTs found limited evidence that chemotherapy with some new agents plus corticosteroids reduced pain, lengthened palliation, and improved quality of life, but found no improvement in overall survival compared with corticosteroids alone. Earlier RCTs failed to demonstrate any benefit of chemotherapy in men with metastatic prostate cancer.
- **External beam radiation (palliation but no evidence of an effect on survival)** We found no RCTs comparing external beam radiation with palliative treatments other than radionuclides. Observational evidence suggests that complete pain relief is avoided in about a quarter of people, and placebo controlled RCTs would probably be considered unethical.
- **Radionuclides (palliation but no clear evidence of an effect on survival)** One systematic review found one small RCT in men with symptomatic bone metastases, which found no significant difference in survival between external beam radiation plus placebo and external beam radiation plus strontium-89. However, strontium-89 significantly reduced the number of new sites of pain. One small subsequent RCT in men with painful bone metastases found that samarium-153 significantly reduced pain scores compared with placebo. A second small subsequent RCT, in a selected population, found an improvement in survival with strontium-89 compared with placebo, but the results are difficult to generalise.
- **Bisphosphonates** One systematic review of two RCTs found insufficient evidence about the effects of bisphosphonates.

DEFINITION See prostate cancer (non-metastatic), p 1023. Androgen independent metastatic disease is defined as disease that progresses despite androgen deprivation.

INCIDENCE/ PREVALENCE See prostate cancer (non-metastatic), p 1023.

AETIOLOGY/ RISK FACTORS See prostate cancer (non-metastatic), p 1023.

PROGNOSIS Prostate cancer metastasises predominantly to bone. Metastatic prostate cancer can result in pain, weakness, paralysis, and death.

AIMS OF INTERVENTION To reduce mortality and disability; to control symptoms and maximise quality of life; and to minimise adverse effects of treatment.

OUTCOMES Survival; response in terms of symptoms and signs; quality of life; adverse effects of treatment.

METHODS *Clinical Evidence* search and appraisal September 2002.

Prostate cancer (metastatic)

QUESTION What are the effects of treatment for men with metastatic prostate cancer?

OPTION ANDROGEN DEPRIVATION

We found limited evidence from RCTs suggesting that androgen deprivation reduced mortality compared with no initial treatment. One systematic review and one subsequent RCT found no evidence of a difference in effectiveness between different methods of androgen deprivation (orchidectomy, diethylstilbestrol, and gonadorelin analogues).

Benefits: **Versus no initial treatment:** We found no systematic review or recent RCTs comparing androgen deprivation (see glossary, p 1020) versus no initial treatment. Three RCTs (about 4000 men with all stages of prostate cancer) performed between 1959 and 1975 compared androgen deprivation (diethylstilbestrol [stilboestrol], orchidectomy [see glossary, p 1020], or oestrogens) versus no initial treatment. They found no difference in overall survival. Reanalysis of updated data from these RCTs found a modest survival advantage with androgen deprivation.[1] The report did not provide statistical details. **Different types of androgen deprivation:** We found one systematic review[2] and one subsequent RCT.[3] The systematic review (search date 1998, 24 RCTs, > 6600 men with metastatic prostate cancer) found no significant differences between treatment groups in overall progression free survival, time to progression, or overall survival in the most of the trials.[2] It found no significant differences in 2 year survival between orchidectomy and the gonadorelin analogues leuprolide or goserelin acetate (HR 1.26, 95% CI 0.91 to 1.39), diethylstilbestrol (HR 0.98, 95% CI 0.76 to 1.27), or non-steroidal antiandrogen (see glossary, p 1020) monotherapy (HR 1.22, 95% CI 0.99 to 1.50). One large subsequent RCT (915 men with advanced prostate cancer stage T0–4, M1; see table 1 in prostate cancer non-metastatic, p 1023) compared parenteral oestrogen versus total androgen ablation (orchidectomy or triptorelin).[3] It found no significant difference in mortality at follow up (mortality at 18 months' median follow up 266/458 [58%] with oestrogen *v* 269/457 [59%] with total androgen ablation; RR 0.99, 95% 0.89 to 1.10).

Harms: All forms of androgen deprivation are known to be associated with vasomotor flushing, loss of libido, gynaecomastia, weight gain, osteoporosis, and loss of muscle mass; we found insufficient prospective frequency data for these adverse effects. One RCT (915 men with metastatic prostate cancer) found that androgen deprivation by orchidectomy, or by combination of gonadotrophin releasing hormone analogue with an antiandrogen, induces significantly more hot flushes than polyestradiol phosphate (1 or more flushes, 336/452 [74.3%] *v* 135/449 [30.1%]; RR 2.5, 95% CI 2.1 to 2.9; NNH 3, 95% CI 2 to 3).[4] Diethylstilbestrol is associated with an increased risk of cardiovascular events, gastric irritation, and allergic reactions, and for these reasons is not used routinely.[1] Orchidectomy has cosmetic and potential psychological consequences. Gonadorelin analogues may cause an initial clinical flare owing to transient increases in androgen levels.

Comment: Androgen deprivation therapy has been used as the standard of care for men with metastatic disease because of the frequency and duration of effect; therefore, there are no contemporary randomised trials with a no treatment arm. The lack of apparent benefit in earlier trials[1] was probably because of the high cardiovascular event rate associated with high dose diethylstilbestrol.

OPTION IMMEDIATE VERSUS DEFERRED ANDROGEN DEPRIVATION

One systematic review found limited evidence of a small survival advantage at 10 years for immediate androgen deprivation therapy in men with advanced, asymptomatic prostate cancer. There was no significant change in overall survival at 1, 2, or 5 years. The risk of major complications is increased in men whose treatment is deferred until disease progression.

Benefits: We found one systematic review (search date 2001, 4 RCTs, 2167 men with locally advanced prostate cancer or asymptomatic metastases), which compared immediate versus deferred androgen deprivation (see glossary, p 1020) therapy.[5] Outcome measures were overall survival, progression free survival, and complications due to prostate cancer at 1, 2, 5, and 10 years. The review found a significant improvement in overall survival only at 10 years, favouring the immediate therapy group (at 1 year: OR 1.16, 95% CI 0.90 to 1.49; at 2 years: OR 1.08, 95% CI 0.89 to 1.33; at 5 years: 1.19, 95% CI 0.95 to 1.50; and at 10 years: 1.50, 95% CI 1.04 to 2.16). Progression free survival was consistently better in all studies in the immediate therapy group, but disease specific survival was not significantly different at any point. One large RCT included in the review reported complications due to disease progression. It found an approximate halving of the risk of major complications, including spinal cord compression (9/469 [1.9%] with immediate treatment *v* 23/465 [4.9%] with deferred treatment; $P < 0.025$), ureteric obstruction (33/469 [7%] with immediate treatment *v* 55/465 [12%] with deferred treatment: $P < 0.025$), extraskeletal metastases (37/469 [7.9%] with immediate treatment *v* 55/465 [12%] with deferred treatment; $P < 0.05$), and a non-significant reduction in pathological fractures (11/469 [2.3%] with immediate treatment *v* 21/465 [4.5%] with deferred treatment; $P > 0.05$).[6] The trial did not make clear the time interval over which outcomes were recorded, although this seemed to be at least 10 years.

Harms: We found no systematic review or RCTs with prospective data on adverse effects of immediate compared with deferred androgen deprivation in men with metastatic prostate cancer. Adverse effects of immediate therapy were not analysed in the systematic review. However, adverse events reported in one trial were much more common in the immediate treatment arm (OR 5.66, 95% CI 2.76 to 11.62).[5]

Comment: The systematic review included two RCTs published in the 1970s, and the remaining two in 1997 and 1999. Treatments received and indications varied between RCTs.[5] Androgen deprivation therapy may be offered at an earlier stage of disease than that considered for participants in the systematic review.

OPTION COMBINED ANDROGEN BLOCKADE (ANDROGEN DEPRIVATION AND ANTIANDROGEN)

Systematic reviews found limited evidence of a 2–5% improvement in 5 year survival associated with combined androgen blockade (androgen deprivation plus a non-steroidal antiandrogen) compared with androgen deprivation alone.

Benefits: We found two systematic reviews.[7,8] The first and largest systematic review (search date not stated, 27 RCTs, 8275 men, most of whom had stage D2 disease [see table 1 in non-metastatic prostate cancer, p 1023]) compared different methods of androgen deprivation (orchidectomy, flutamide, gonadorelin analogue, or a combination of these [see glossary, p 1020]) versus androgen deprivation alone. It found no clearly significant difference in mortality (72.4% with androgen deprivation alone *v* 70.4% with combined blockage; RR 0.96, 95% CI 0.94 to 1.00). Exclusion of seven trials (1784 men) of cyproterone acetate found a small reduction in mortality from combined androgen blockade, p 0 (20 RCTs, 6491 men: 75.3% with androgen deprivation alone *v* 72.4% combined with non-steroidal antiandrogens (see glossary, p 1020); ARR 2.9%; P = 0.005). The second systematic review (search date 1998, 21 RCTs, 6871 men) compared androgen deprivation alone (orchidectomy or gonadorelin analogues) versus androgen deprivation combined with steroidal or non-steroidal antiandrogens (cyproterone, nilutamide, and flutamide).[8] Overall, the review found a significant improvement in 5 year survival in men receiving combined androgen blockade (HR 0.871, 95% CI 0.805 to 0.942). No significant differences were seen at 1 or 2 years' follow up. Five years' follow up was only provided in 10 of the 21 RCTs.

Harms: The most recent review did not report on adverse events.[8] An overlapping, earlier systematic review of 6320 men in 20 RCTs found that, compared with monotherapy (androgen deprivation alone), combined androgen blockade using non-steroidal antiandrogens increased the risk of diarrhoea (10% with combined antiandrogen blockade *v* 2% with monotherapy), gastrointestinal pain (7% with combined antiandrogen blockade *v* 2% with monotherapy), and non-specific ophthalmologic events (29% with combined antiandrogen blockade *v* 5% with monotherapy).[9] Flutamide is also associated with a higher rate of anaemia (8% *v* 5%).[4]

Comment: The authors of the most recent overview note the need for quality of life data, given the modest survival benefit and the potential for toxicity.[8]

OPTION INTERMITTENT VERSUS CONTINUOUS ANDROGEN DEPRIVATION

We found insufficient evidence on the effects of intermittent androgen deprivation in men with metastatic prostate cancer.

Benefits: We found no systematic review and no RCTs assessing the long term effects of intermittent androgen deprivation on mortality, morbidity, or quality of life.

Harms: We found insufficient evidence to assess harms.

Comment: None.

QUESTION **What are the effects of treatments for men with symptomatic androgen independent metastatic disease?**

OPTION **CHEMOTHERAPY**

RCTs found limited evidence that chemotherapy with some new agents (mitoxantrone or suramin) plus corticosteroids reduced pain, lengthened palliation, and improved quality of life, but found no improvement in overall survival compared with corticosteroids alone. Earlier RCTs failed to demonstrate any benefit of chemotherapy in men with metastatic prostate cancer.

Benefits: We found no systematic review. Multiple earlier RCTs found no benefit in men with metastatic prostate cancer of various chemotherapy drugs, including mitomycin C, cyclophosphamide, doxorubicin, methotrexate, 5-fluorouracil, or estramustine phosphate (EMP).[10–14] In the largest of these studies, 419 men with untreated metastatic or locally advanced prostate cancer were randomised to orchiectomy (see glossary, p 1020) alone versus orchiectomy plus EMP.[12] There was no difference between groups in overall survival or time to progression. Subgroup analyses demonstrated no benefit in the group of men with metastatic disease, but did demonstrate significant delay in time to progression in younger patients (aged < 73 years). An earlier study randomised 319 men to androgen deprivation therapy, combination of androgen deprivation therapy and chemotherapy (cyclophosphamide plus 5-fluorouracil), or EMP alone.[10] It found no significant differences between the groups in progression free or overall survival. However, we found three more recent RCTs demonstrating benefit of newer chemotherapy agents in men with advanced prostate cancer.[15–17] The first of these (161 men with symptomatic androgen independent metastatic prostate cancer) compared mitoxantrone plus prednisone versus prednisone alone.[15] Men taking placebo were crossed over to mitoxantrone at disease progression or if not responding at 6 weeks. It found that men receiving chemotherapy were significantly more likely to experience pain reduction (29% with chemotherapy plus prednisone *v* 12% with prednisone alone; $P = 0.01$), enjoy longer pain relief (43 *v* 18 weeks; $P < 0.0001$), and show improvements in quality of life. It found no significant difference in overall survival. The comparison was done before crossover. The second unblinded RCT (242 men) compared mitoxantrone plus hydrocortisone versus hydrocortisone alone.[16] Men were allowed alternative chemotherapy after disease progression. It found no significant difference in survival (median duration 12.3 months with mitoxantrone plus hydrocortisone *v* 12.6 months with hydrocortisone; $P = 0.77$). However, pain and analgesic use were significantly reduced after chemotherapy. The third RCT (458 men with prostate cancer and painful bone metastases) compared suramin plus hydrocortisone versus placebo plus hydrocortisone.[17] Men on placebo were allowed to cross over to suramin at disease progression. It found that chemotherapy reduced pain (pain response 43% *v* 28%; P = 0.01). It found no significant effect on survival (median survival 286 days with suramin *v* 279 days with placebo; reported as non-significant, statistics not reported).

Harms: The RCTs reported no treatment related deaths. There were nine episodes of febrile neutropenia (World Health Organization grade 3 or 4) among 130 men treated with 796 courses of mitoxantrone.[17] Five men experienced cardiac arrhythmias or decreased left ventricular ejection fraction, including two who developed congestive heart failure. A higher incidence of nausea and cardiovascular events was observed in men receiving EMP plus orchiectomy compared with orchiectomy alone.[12]

Comment: The crossover design in the recent chemotherapy trials reduced the contrast between treatment arms and increased the study size in order to find small survival benefits, as most people allocated to placebo eventually received chemotherapy. Early, unpublished clinical trials have suggested high response rates for taxane based chemotherapy, and an intergroup RCT comparing it with established regimens is ongoing.

OPTION EXTERNAL BEAM RADIATION THERAPY

We found no RCTs comparing external beam radiation versus palliative treatments other than radionuclides. Observational evidence suggests complete pain relief in about a quarter of people, and placebo controlled RCTs would probably be considered unethical. A systematic review of one RCT in men with symptomatic bone metastases found no difference in survival between external beam radiation and strontium-89; however, strontium-89 was associated with significantly fewer new sites of pain and reduced need for additional radiotherapy. One systematic review found no significant differences in pain relief between different radiation treatment fraction schedules and doses.

Benefits: **Versus no treatment or placebo:** We found one systematic review (search date 1996, no RCTs), which found no RCTs comparing external beam radiation versus no treatment or placebo.[18] We found no additional RCTs (see comment below). Eleven observational studies of 1486 people found complete pain relief in 368/1373 (27%) of people and at least 50% pain relief in 628/1486 (42%) of people treated with external beam radiotherapy (see comment below). **External beam versus radionuclides:** We found one systematic review (search date 1996, 1 RCT, 284 men).[18] The RCT (305 men) compared external beam radiation versus strontium-89.[19] It found that strontium-89 was associated with significantly fewer new sites of pain (P < 0.05), and significantly reduced the need for additional radiotherapy (P < 0.04). However, it found no significant difference in survival (median survival 33 weeks with strontium-89 *v* 28 weeks with radiotherapy; P = 0.10).[19] **Different schedules and doses:** We found one systematic review (search date 1996, 9 RCTs, 1486 men with symptomatic bone metastases from a variety of malignancies).[18] The RCTs compared different radiation treatment fractionation schedules and doses of external beam radiation. It found minimal differences in pain relief between different fractionation schedules and doses.

Harms: The systematic review reported that adverse event reporting was poor.[18]

Comment: In men with painful bone metastases, it would be considered unethical to compare external beam radiation versus placebo or no treatment. It is reasonable to consider the effectiveness of no treatment to be zero, as spontaneous remission has not been described in bone metastases from prostate cancer.

OPTION RADIONUCLIDE THERAPY

One systematic review found one small RCT in men with symptomatic bone metastases, which found no difference in survival between external beam radiation plus placebo and external beam radiation plus strontium-89. However, strontium-89 significantly reduced the number of new sites of pain. One small subsequent RCT in men with painful bone metastases found that samarium-153 significantly reduced pain scores compared with placebo. A second small subsequent RCT in a selected population found an improvement in survival with strontium-89 compared with placebo, but the results are difficult to generalise.

Benefits: **Versus other palliative treatments:** We found one systematic review (search date 1996, 1 RCT, 126 men)[18] and two subsequent RCTs.[20,21] The RCT in the systematic review (126 men) compared external beam radiation plus strontium-89 versus external beam radiation plus placebo.[22] Although the RCT found no significant difference in overall survival or symptom relief, strontium-89 significantly reduced the number of new sites of pain ($P < 0.02$) and significantly reduced analgesic requirement (17% stopped taking analgesics with radionuclide *v* 2% on placebo; $P < 0.05$). The first subsequent RCT (118 people with painful bone metastases from multiple primaries) compared samarium-153 lexidronam 0.5 mCi/kg versus samarium-153 lexidronam 1 mCi/kg versus placebo over 4 weeks.[21] It found that samarium-153 1 mCi/kg significantly reduced pain scores compared with placebo at weeks 1–4 ($P < 0.034$). Samarium-153 0.5 mCi/kg reduced pain scores significantly more than placebo at week 1 ($P = 0.044$) but not at other weeks ($P > 0.078$). The second subsequent RCT (72 men with androgen independent, metastatic prostate cancer who had initially responded to "induction" chemotherapy with ketoconazole and doxorubicin alternating with estramustine and vinblastine) compared maintenance chemotherapy (doxorubicin) with and without strontium-89.[20] From follow up of 67 people to death, it was estimated that strontium-89 significantly increased median overall survival (27.7 months with chemotherapy plus strontium-89 *v* 16.8 months with chemotherapy alone; $P < 0.002$) and significantly increased time to progression (13.9 months with chemotherapy plus strontium-89 *v* 7.0 months with chemotherapy alone; $P < 0.0001$) (see comment below). **Versus external beam radiation:** See external beam versus radionuclides under benefits of external beam radiation therapy, p 1018.

Harms: Strontium-89 was associated with thrombocytopenia (World Health Organization grade 3 or 4) in 7–33% of men and leukopenia (World Health Organization grade 3 or 4) in 3–12% of men.[18,23] Other radionuclides with selective bone localisation have similar rates of haematological toxicity. There was no significant difference between treatment schedules and doses of external beam radiation in rates of nausea, vomiting, or diarrhoea.[24]

Comment: One RCT[23] included in previous versions of *Clinical Evidence* was removed because of its small size and weak methods. The results of the second subsequent RCT are difficult to generalise because a selected population was used, and participants reacted favourably to a particular chemotherapy regimen.[20]

OPTION BISPHOSPHONATES

One systematic review of two RCTs found insufficient evidence about the effects of bisphosphonates compared with no treatment.

Benefits: One systematic review (search date not stated, 2 RCTs, 156 men with prostate cancer and symptomatic bone metastases) found no reduction in bone pain with bisphosphonates compared with no bisphosphonates.[25]

Harms: The systematic review identified 18 RCTs of bisphosphonates in men with bone metastases from a variety of cancers.[25] No RCT reported major toxicity. Treatment with pamidronate was associated with increased frequency of anterior uveitis and episcleritis.[25]

Comment: Both RCTs in the systematic review[25] had weak methods; one did not use a pain scale, whereas the other assessed etidronate, a bisphosphonate that is pharmacologically unsuitable for treating bone metastases. One RCT found potential benefit of pamidronate in preventing bone loss in men receiving androgen deprivation therapy, but it was not designed to assess effect on disease progression.

GLOSSARY

Androgen deprivation Orchiectomy, gonadorelin analogue (leuprolide or goserelin), or estrogenic treatment.

Antiandrogen Androgen receptor blockers such as flutamide, nilutamide or bicalutamide.

Combined androgen blockade A combination of gonadorelin analogues or orchiectomy (androgen deprivation therapy) plus an androgen receptor blocker (antiandrogen).

Orchidectomy Also known as orchiectomy, meaning surgical removal of the testicles.

Substantive changes

Immediate versus deferred androgen deprivation One new systematic review added,[5] eclipsing previous RCTs; conclusions unchanged.
Combined androgen blockade (androgen deprivation and antiandrogen) One systematic review added;[8] conclusions unchanged.
Chemotherapy in androgen independent cancer Five RCTs added;[10–14] conclusions unchanged.

REFERENCES

1. Byar DP, Corle DK. Hormone therapy for prostate cancer: results of the Veterans Administration Cooperative Urologic Research Group studies. *NCI Monogr* 1988;7:165–170.
2. Seidenfeld J, Samson DJ, Hasselblad V, et al. Single-therapy androgen suppression in men with advanced prostate cancer: a systematic review and meta-analysis. *Ann Intern Med* 2000;132:566–577. Search date 1998; primary sources Medline, Cancerlit, Embase, The Cochrane Library, and Current Contents.
3. Hedlund PO, Henriksson P. Parenteral estrogen versus total androgen ablation in the treatment of advanced prostate carcinoma: effects on overall survival and cardiovascular mortality. *Urology* 2000;55:328–332.
4. Spetz A, Hammar M, Lindberg B, et al. Prospective evaluation of hot flashes during treatment with parenteral estrogen or complete androgen ablation for metastatic carcinoma of the prostate. *J Urol* 2001;166:517–520.
5. Nair B, Wilt T, MacDonald R, et al. Early versus deferred androgen suppression in the treatment of advnaced prostatic cancer. In: The Cochrane Library, Issue 3, 2002. Oxford: Update Software. Search date 2001; primary sources Medline, Cancerlit, Embase, Cochrane Controlled Trials Register, VA Cochrane Prostate Disease and Urologic Cancer Register, and Current Contents.
6. Medical Research Council Prostate Cancer Working Party Investigators Group. Immediate versus deferred treatment for advanced prostatic cancer: initial results of the Medical Research Council trial. *Br J Urol* 1997;79:235–246.
7. Prostate Cancer Clinical Trialists' Collaborative Group. Maximum androgen blockade in advanced prostate cancer: an overview of the randomized trials. *Lancet* 2000;355:1491–1498. Search date not stated; primary sources computerised literature search, proceedings of congresses, contacts with authors, trial groups, and pharmaceutical industry.
8. Samson DJ, Seidenfeld J, Schmitt B, et al. Systematic review and meta-analysis of monotherapy compared with combined androgen blockade for patients with advanced prostate carcinoma. *Cancer* 2002;95:361. Search date 1998; primary sources Medline, Embase, Cancerlit, Cochrane databases, and Current Contents.
9. Schmitt B, Wilt TJ, Schellhammer PF, et al. Combined androgen blockade with non-steroidal antiandrogens for advanced prostate cancer: a systematic review. *Urology* 2001;57:727–732. Search date not stated; primary sources Blue Cross and Blue Shield Association's Technology Evaluation Center data set, Cochrane Controlled Trials Register, Cochrane Central Register, and the Veterans Administration Cochrane Prostate Disease and Urologic Malignancy Register.
10. Murphy GP, Huben RP, Priore R. Results of another trial of chemotherapy with and without hormones in patients with newly diagnosed metastatic prostate cancer. *Urology* 1986;28:36.
11. Saxman S, Ansari R, Drasga R, et al. Phase III trial of cyclophosphamide versus cyclophosphamide, doxorubicin, and methotrexate in hormone-refractory prostatic cancer: A Hoosier Oncology Group study. *Cancer* 1992;70:2488.
12. Janknegt RA, Boon TA, Van De Beek C, et al Combined hormono/chemotherapy as primary treatment for metastatic prostate cancer: A randomized, multicenter study of orchiectomy alone versus orchiectomy plus estramustine phosphate. *Urology* 1997;49:411.
13. Fontana D, Bertetto O, Fasolis G, et al. Randomized comparison of goserelin acetate versus mitomycin C plus goserelin acetate in previously untreated prostate cancer patients with bone metastases. *Tumori* 1998;84:39.
14. De Reijke TM, Keuppens, FI, Whelan P, et al. Orchiectomy and orchiectomy plus mitomycin C for metastatic prostate cancer in patients with poor prognosis: the final results of a European Organization for Research in Cancer Therapy Genitourinary Group Trila. *J Urol* 1999;162:1658.
15. Tannock IF, Osoba D, Stockler MR, et al. Chemotherapy with mitoxantrone plus prednisone or prednisone alone for symptomatic hormone-resistant prostate cancer: a Canadian randomized trial with palliative end points. *J Clin Oncol* 1996;14:1756–1764.
16. Kantoff PW, Halabi S, Conaway M, et al. Hydrocortisone with or without mitoxantrone in men with hormone-refractory prostate cancer: results of the Cancer and Leukemia Group B 9182 Study. *J Clin Oncol* 1999;17:2506–2513.
17. Small EJ, Marshall E, Reyno L, et al. Suramin therapy for patients with symptomatic hormone-refractory prostate cancer: results of a randomised phase III trial comparing suramin plus hydrocortisone to placebo plus hydrocortisone. *J Clin Oncol* 2000;18:1440–1450.
18. McQuay HJ, Carroll D, Moore RA. Radiotherapy for painful bone metastases: a systematic review. *Clin Oncol* 1997;9:150–154. Search date 1996; primary sources Medline, the Oxford Pain Relief database, Embase, Cochrane Library, and reference lists.
19. Quilty PM, Kirk D, Bolger JJ, et al. A comparison of the palliative effects of strontium-89 and external beam radiotherapy in metastatic prostate cancer. *Radiother Oncol* 1994;31:33–40.
20. Tu S, Millikan RE, Mengistu B, et al. Bone-targeted therapy for advanced androgen-independent carcinoma of the prostate: a randomized Phase II trial. *Lancet* 2001;357:336–341.
21. Serafini AN, Houston SJ, Resche I, et al. Palliation of pain associated with metastatic bone cancer using samarium-153 lexidronam: a double-blind placebo-controlled clinical trial. *J Clin Oncol* 1998;16:1574–1581.
22. Porter AT, McEwan AJ, Powe JE, et al. Results of a randomized Phase-III trial to evaluate the efficacy of strontium-89 adjuvant to local field external

beam irradiation in the management of endocrine resistant metastatic prostate cancer. *Int J Radiat Oncol Biol Phys* 1993;25:805–813.

23. Maxon HR, Schroder LE, Hertzberg VS, et al. Rhenium-186(Sn)HEDP for treatment of painful osseous metastases: results of a double-blind crossover comparison with placebo. *J Nucl Med* 1991;32:1877–1881.
24. Robinson RG, Preston DF, Schiefelbein M, et al. Strontium 89 therapy for the palliation of pain due to osseous metastases. *JAMA* 1995;274:420–424. Search date 1994; primary source Medline.
25. Bloomfield DJ. Should bisphosphonates be part of the standard therapy of patients with multiple myeloma or bone metastases from other cancers? An evidence-based review. *J Clin Oncol* 1998;16:1218–1225. Search date not stated; primary sources Medline, hand search of major cancer journals, reference lists, and contact with experts.

M Dror Michaelson
Instructor in Medicine

Matthew R Smith
Assistant Professor of Medicine

Massachusetts General Hospital
Boston
USA

James A Talcott
Assistant Professor of Medicine
Harvard Medical School
Boston
USA

Competing interests: None declared.

The following previous contributor of this topic would also like to be acknowledged: Philip Kantoff.

Prostate cancer (non-metastatic)

Search date February 2003

Timothy Wilt

QUESTIONS

INTERVENTIONS

See glossary, p 1036

Key Messages

Clinically localised prostate cancer

- **Radical prostatectomy** Two RCTs found no significant difference in death from any cause between radical prostatectomy and watchful waiting in men with clinically detected disease after median follow up of 6.2 and 23 years. The larger of the RCTs found that radical prostatectomy reduced death due to prostate cancer and metastases at 6 years compared with watchful waiting. Two small RCTs found that radical prostatectomy reduced the risk of treatment failure compared with external beam radiation. Radical prostatectomy carries the risks of major surgery and of sexual and urinary dysfunction.
- **Watchful waiting** Two RCTs found no significant difference in overall survival between watchful waiting and radical prostatectomy in men with clinically detected disease after median follow up of 6 and 23 years. The larger RCT found that radical prostatectomy reduced death rates due to prostate cancer and metastases at 6 years compared with watchful waiting. One RCT found that radical prostatectomy increased erectile dysfunction compared with watchful waiting but found no significant difference in quality of life after 12 months.

Prostate cancer (non-metastatic)

- **Androgen suppression** We found no RCTs of early androgen suppression on length or quality of life in men with asymptomatic, clinically localised prostate cancer. One RCT identified by a systematic review found limited evidence that oestrogen decreased prostate cancer related deaths compared with watchful waiting. It found no significant difference in overall survival. One preliminary report of three large ongoing RCTs in men with localised or locally advanced prostate cancer found that bicalutamide plus standard care reduced rates of radiological progression and bone metastases at 2–3 years compared with standard care alone. There was no significant difference between treatments in overall survival.
- **External beam radiation** We found no RCTs comparing external beam radiation versus watchful waiting. Two RCTs found that external beam radiation increased the risk of treatment failure compared with radical prostatectomy. Two small RCTs found no significant difference between conformal radiotherapy and conventional radiotherapy in overall survival or tumour control at 3–5 years. One systematic review found limited evidence that conformal radiotherapy with dose escalation reduced acute and late treatment related morbidity compared with conventional radiotherapy for men with T1 or T2 low or intermediate risk prostate cancer.
- **Androgen suppression in asymptomatic men with raised prostate specific antigen concentrations after early treatment; brachytherapy; cryosurgery** We found no RCTs on the effects of these interventions.

Locally advanced prostate cancer

- **Immediate androgen suppression after radical prostatectomy and pelvic lymphadenectomy in men with node positive prostate cancer (compared with radical prostatectomy and deferred androgen suppression)** One small RCT in men with node positive prostate cancer found that immediate androgen suppression compared with deferred androgen suppression after radical prostatectomy and pelvic lymphadenectomy reduced mortality over a median of 7 years' follow up.
- **Androgen suppression initiated at diagnosis** RCTs found no significant difference in overall survival between androgen suppression with bicalutamide and no androgen suppression in men with localised or locally advanced prostate cancer at 2–10 years. The RCTs found that bicalutamide reduced objective progression compared with no bicalutamide. One systematic review found that early androgen suppression increased survival at 10 years compared with deferred treatment in men with locally advanced prostate cancer but found no significant difference in survival at 5 years. One RCT found limited evidence that immediate androgen suppression reduced complications compared with deferred androgen suppression.
- **Early androgen suppression plus external beam radiation (compared with radiation and deferred androgen suppression)** RCTs found limited evidence that androgen suppression initiated at diagnosis plus external beam radiation improved long term survival compared with radiation alone or radiation plus deferred androgen suppression. One RCT found limited evidence that immediate androgen suppression reduced complications compared with deferred androgen suppression.

DEFINITION Prostatic cancer is staged according to two systems: the tumour, node, metastasis (TNM) classification system and the American urologic staging system (see table 1, p 1038). Non-metastatic prostate cancer can be divided into clinically localised disease and locally advanced disease. Clinically localised disease is prostate cancer thought, after clinical examination, to be confined to the prostate gland. Locally advanced disease is prostate cancer that has spread outside the capsule of the prostate gland but has not yet spread to other organs. Metastatic disease is prostate cancer that has spread outside the prostate gland to either local, regional, or systemic lymph nodes, seminal vesicles, or to other body organs (e.g. bone, liver, brain) and is not connected to the prostate gland. We consider clinically localised and locally advanced disease here. Metastatic disease is covered in a separate chapter (see prostate cancer [metastatic], p 1012).

INCIDENCE/ PREVALENCE Prostate cancer is the sixth most common cancer in the world and the third most common cancer in men. In 2000, an estimated 513 000 new cases of prostate cancer were diagnosed and about 250 000 deaths were attributed to prostate cancers worldwide. Prostate cancer is uncommon under the age of 50 years. About 85% of men with prostate cancer are diagnosed after the age of 65 years. Autopsy studies suggest that the prevalence of subclinical prostate cancer is high at all ages: 30% for men aged 30–39 years, 50% for men aged 50–59 years, and more than 75% for men older than 85 years. Incidence varies widely by ethnic group and around the world. The highest rates occur in men of black ethnic group living in the USA and the lowest among men living in China.[1]

AETIOLOGY/ RISK FACTORS Risk factors for prostate cancer include increasing age, family history of prostate cancer, black ethnic group, and possibly higher dietary consumption of fat and meat, low intake of lycopene (from tomato products), low intake of fruit, and high dietary calcium. In the USA, black men have about a 60% higher incidence than white men.[2] The prostate cancer incidence for black men living in the USA is about 90/100 000 in men aged less than 65 years and about 1300/100 000 in men aged 65–74 years. For white men, incidence is about 44/100 000 in men aged less than 65 years and 900/100 000 in men aged 65–74 years.[2]

PROGNOSIS The chance that men with well to moderately differentiated, palpable, clinically localised prostate cancer will remain free of symptomatic progression is 70% at 5 years and 40% at 10 years.[3] The risk of symptomatic disease progression is higher in men with poorly differentiated prostate cancer.[4] One retrospective analysis of a large surgical series in men with clinically localised prostate cancer found that the median time from the increase in prostate specific antigen (PSA) concentration to the development of metastatic disease was 8 years.[5] Time to PSA progression, PSA doubling time, and Gleason score (see glossary, p 1036) were predictive of the probability and time to development of metastatic disease. Once men developed metastatic disease, the median actuarial time to death was less than 5 years.[5] Morbidity from local or regional disease progression includes haematuria, bladder obstruction, and lower extremity oedema. The age adjusted prostate cancer specific mortality in the USA for all men aged 65 years and older has decreased by about 15% (244 deaths/100 000 to 207 deaths/100 000) from 1991–1997. The reasons for this are unclear, although inaccurate death certification, PSA screening, and earlier, more intensive treatment, including radical prostatectomy (see glossary, p 1036), radiotherapy, and androgen suppression (see glossary, p 1036), have been suggested. However, regions of the USA and Canada where PSA testing and early treatment are more common have similar prostate cancer mortality to regions with lower testing and early treatment rates.[6] Similarly, countries with low rates of PSA testing and treatment, such as the UK, have similar age adjusted prostate cancer mortality to countries with high rates of testing and treatment, such as the USA.[7]

AIMS OF INTERVENTION To prevent premature death and disability, and to minimise adverse effects of treatment.

OUTCOMES Survival; development of metastatic disease; development of symptomatic local or regional disease progression; time to progression; response in terms of symptoms and signs; quality of life; adverse effects of treatment. Where clinical outcomes are not available, surrogate outcomes have been used (PSA concentration; Gleason score for histological grade).

METHODS *Clinical Evidence* search and appraisal February 2003. Additional author search: Cochrane Library and Medline to 2001 for systematic reviews and RCTs, and using the search strategy of the Department of Veterans' Affairs Coordinating Center for the Cochrane Review Group on Prostatic Diseases.

QUESTION **What are the effects of treatments for clinically localised prostate cancer?**

OPTION **WATCHFUL WAITING**

Two RCTs found no significant difference in overall survival between watchful waiting and radical prostatectomy in men with clinically detected disease after median follow up of 6 and 23 years. One RCT found that radical prostatectomy reduced death due to prostate cancer and reduced metastases at 6 years compared with watchful waiting. One RCT found that radical prostatectomy increased erectile dysfunction compared with watchful waiting but found no significant difference in quality of life after 4 years.

Benefits: **Versus radical prostatectomy:** See benefits of radical prostatectomy, p 1027. **Versus early androgen suppression:** See glossary, p 1036. See benefits of androgen suppression, p 1031.

Harms: **Versus radical prostatectomy:** See harms of radical prostatectomy, p 1028. **Versus early androgen suppression:** See harms of androgen suppression, p 1032.

Comment: We found two large cohort studies, which found that, in men with clinically detected localised prostate cancer managed with watchful waiting, 15 year disease specific survival was 80% — ranging from 95% for well differentiated to 30% for poorly differentiated cancers.[10,11] However, most men with newly diagnosed prostate cancer are now detected by prostate specific antigen (PSA) testing. There is about a 10–15 year lead time between the detection of cancers by raised PSA concentrations and clinical detection by digital rectal examination or the development of symptoms.[12] This means that outcomes are likely to be similar in men with palpable tumours who are followed for 15 years and men whose tumours are detected because of raised PSA concentrations who are followed for 25–30 years (lead time bias). Therefore, compared with men with clinically detected prostate cancer, any benefit in men with PSA detected tumours (if it exists) is likely to be of smaller magnitude and require a longer period of time to occur. Until better information is available to guide treatment selection men have to weigh the potential but unproved risks and benefits of various treatment options. For example, men treated with watchful waiting may avoid the risks of surgery and may have similar overall survival and quality of life compared with men treated with other interventions. However, they do not have the opportunity to have their cancer removed or "definitively" treated with radiotherapy. This could potentially result in disease progression, disability, and premature death. Preliminary results from one RCT indicate that, on average, 25 men with clinically detected prostate cancer would need to be treated with surgery to prevent one death attributed to prostate cancer over a 6 year time period, without evidence that this would improve length or quality of life.[9] People should balance the potential risks and benefits of various treatment options.

OPTION RADICAL PROSTATECTOMY

Two RCTs found no significant difference in death from any cause between radical prostatectomy and watchful waiting in men with clinically detected disease after median follow up of 6.2 and 23 years. The larger of the RCTs found that radical prostatectomy reduced death due to prostate cancer and metastases at 6 years compared with watchful waiting. Two small RCTs found that that radical prostatectomy reduced the risk of treatment failure compared with external beam radiation. Radical prostatectomy carries the risks of major surgery and of sexual and urinary dysfunction.

Benefits: **Versus watchful waiting:** We found one systematic review (search date 2002, 2 RCTs) that compared radical prostatectomy (see glossary, p 1036) versus watchful waiting in men with clinically localised prostate cancer.[8] The first RCT in the review (142 men) found no significant difference in survival after median follow up of 23 years (range 19–27 years) between radical prostatectomy and watchful waiting (median survival 10.6 years with prostatectomy *v* 8 years with watchful waiting; CI not reported).[13] Analysis was not by intention to treat, treatment groups were not comparable at baseline for important prognostic factors, and the RCT is likely to have been too small to exclude a clinically important difference between groups. The second RCT in the review (695 men with newly diagnosed prostate cancer, clinical stage T1b, T1c, or T2) found that radical prostatectomy significantly reduced death due to prostate cancer after a median of 6.2 years follow up compared with watchful waiting.[9] There was no significant difference in overall death rates (death due to prostate cancer: 16/374 [4.6%] with surgery *v* 31/348 [8.9%] with watchful waiting; HR 0.50, 95% CI 0.27 to 0.91; distant metastases: HR 0.63, 95% CI 0.41 to 0.96; death from any cause: 53/347 [15.3%] with surgery *v* 62/348 [17.8%] with watchful waiting; HR 0.83, 95% CI 0.57 to 1.20). **Versus external beam radiation:** We found one systematic review (search date 2002, 1 RCT)[8] and one additional RCT.[14] The

Prostate cancer (non-metastatic)

RCT in the review (95 men with either localised or locally advanced cancer) found that radical prostatectomy significantly increased prostate cancer specific survival after 5 years compared with external beam radiation (96.6% with prostatectomy *v* 84.6% with radiation, P = 0.02).[8] The additional RCT (106 men with clinically localised prostate cancer) found that radical prostatectomy significantly reduced treatment failure, primarily defined as a positive bone scan, compared with external beam radiation (4/41 [9.8%] treatment failures with prostatectomy *v* 17/56 [30.4%] with radiation; RR 0.32, 95% CI 0.12 to 0.88; NNT 5, 95% CI 3 to 25).[14]

Harms: One RCT (376 men with localised prostate cancer, 326 men followed up) compared self reported adverse effects and quality of life in men treated with radical prostatectomy and watchful waiting.[15] It found that radical prostatectomy increased erectile dysfunction and urinary leakage at 12 months or more after surgery compared with watchful waiting but reduced symptoms of urinary obstruction (erectile dysfunction: 80% with radical prostatectomy *v* 45% with watchful waiting; urinary leakage: 49% with surgery *v* 21% with watchful waiting; weak urinary stream: 28% with surgery *v* 44% with watchful waiting). The RCT found no significant difference between radical prostatectomy and watchful waiting in bowel function, anxiety, depression, wellbeing, or subjective quality of life (distress from bowel symptoms: 5/159 [3%] with surgery *v* 10/156 [6%] with watchful waiting; low or moderate psychological wellbeing: 35% with surgery *v* 36% with watchful waiting; low or moderate quality of life: 40% with surgery *v* 45% with watchful waiting). One systematic review found that 12 months after radical prostatectomy 20–70% of men reported reduced sexual function and 15–50% reported urinary problems.[8] Fatal complications have been reported in 0.5–1.0% of men treated with radical prostatectomy and may exceed 2% in men aged 75 years and older.[16] Nearly 8% of men older than 65 years suffered major cardiopulmonary complications within 30 days of operation. The incidence of other adverse effects of surgery was over 80% for sexual dysfunction, 30% for urinary incontinence requiring pads or clamps to control wetness, 18% for urethral stricture, 3% for total urinary incontinence, 5% for faecal incontinence, and 1% for bowel injury requiring surgical repair.[17–20]

Comment: Both RCTs of radical prostatectomy took place before the advent of tests for prostate specific antigen.[13,14] Radical prostatectomy may benefit selected groups of men with localised prostate cancer, particularly younger men with higher grade tumours, but the RCTs did not look for this effect. The available evidence suggests that in most men the benefits of radical prostatectomy in quality adjusted life expectancy are at best small and sensitive to individual preferences.[21] A non-randomised study examining a population based, self administered survey of men aged over 65 years in the USA found no differences in general health related quality of life between radical prostatectomy, radiation, or watchful waiting.[22] We are aware of two further ongoing trials comparing radical prostatectomy versus watchful waiting.[23,24] Any benefit of radical prostatectomy in men with prostate specific antigen detected tumours is likely to be of smaller magnitude and require a longer period of time to occur than clinically detected tumours. People should balance the potential risks and benefits of various treatment options.

OPTION **EXTERNAL BEAM RADIATION**

We found no RCTs comparing external beam radiation versus watchful waiting. Two RCTs found that external beam radiation increased the risk of treatment failure compared with radical prostatectomy. Two small RCTs found no significant difference between conformal radiotherapy and conventional radiotherapy in overall survival or tumour control at 3–5 years. One systematic review found limited evidence that conformal radiotherapy with dose escalation reduced acute and late treatment related morbidity compared with conventional radiotherapy for men with T1 or T2 low or intermediate risk prostate cancer.

Benefits: **Versus watchful waiting:** We found no RCTs. **Versus radical prostatectomy:** See glossary, p 1036. See benefits of radical prostatectomy, p 1027.[14] **Conformal versus conventional radiotherapy:** We found one systematic review (search date 2001, 1 RCT)[25] and one additional RCT that compared conformal radiotherapy (see glossary, p 1036) versus conventional radiotherapy.[26] The RCT identified by the review (301 men with T1 or T2, low or intermediate risk prostate cancer) found no significant difference in overall survival at 5 years between conformal radiotherapy and conventional radiotherapy when used as sole treatment, but survival was greater with conformal treatment (69% with conventional *v* 79% with conformal, P = 0.06).[25] The additional RCT (225 men with non-metastatic prostate cancer T1–T4, N0, or M0) did not report on survival, but found no significant difference in tumour control (measured by prostate specific antigen [PSA] level) between treatments after a median follow up of 3.6 years.[26]

Harms: One systematic review (search date 2002) found that 20–40% of men with no prior erectile dysfunction who received external beam radiation developed dysfunction after 12–24 months.[8] One survey of men treated with external beam radiation found that 7% wore pads to control wetness, 23–32% were impotent, and 10% reported problems with bowel dysfunction.[27] Treatment related mortality was less than 0.5%.[17] External beam radiation requires that men return for daily outpatient treatment for up to 6 weeks. **Versus radical prostatectomy:** One systematic review (search date 2002, 1 meta-analysis of 40 non-randomised studies published before 1995) found that radiation increased the probability of retaining sexual function compared with radical prostatectomy (69% with radiotherapy *v* 42% with prostatectomy).[8] **Conventional versus conformal radiotherapy:** We found one systematic review (search date 2001, 3 RCTs reporting on toxicity).[25] Two of the three RCTs found that conformal radiotherapy (without an increase in dose) reduced acute toxicity compared with conventional radiotherapy. The third RCT found no significant difference in acute toxicity between conformal radiotherapy (with dose escalation) and conventional radiotherapy. Two of the three RCTs in the review reporting on chronic adverse effects (> 1 year after treatment) found no significant difference between an increased dose of conformal radiotherapy and conventional radiotherapy but the third RCT reporting on chronic adverse effects found that conventional radiotherapy significantly increased radiation induced proctitis and rectal bleeding compared with the same dose of conformal radiotherapy (proctitis ≥ grade 1 radiation and oncology grade 56% with conventional *v* 36% with conformal, P = 0.004; rectal bleeding ≥ grade 2 radiation and oncology grade 3% with conventional *v* 12% with conformal, P = 0.01).

Comment: Up to 30% of men with clinically localised prostate cancer treated with radiotherapy still have positive biopsies 2–3 years after treatment.[28] One retrospective, non-randomised, multicentre pooled analysis estimated overall survival at 5 years at 85%, disease specific survival at 95%, and freedom from biochemical failure (as defined by raised PSA) at 66%.[29] Estimated 5 year rates of no biochemical recurrence according to PSA concentrations before treatment and Gleason scores (see glossary, p 1036) ranged from 81% for pretreatment PSA less than 10 ng/mL to 29% for PSA of 20 ng/mL or more, and a Gleason score from 7–10.

OPTION BRACHYTHERAPY

A systematic review found no RCTs of brachytherapy in men with clinically localised prostate cancer.

Benefits: We found one systematic review (search date 2002), which identified no RCTs comparing brachytherapy (see glossary, p 1036) alone or in combination with other treatments (androgen suppression [see glossary, p 1036] or radiation).[8]

Harms: The systematic review reported that 36% of men had some erectile dysfunction, 2–12% had some urinary symptoms (including urinary incontinence in 7%), and 18% had some bowel dysfunction 1 year after treatment.[8] However the review stated that these figures came from poor quality studies and should be interpreted with caution.

Comment: We found two older systematic reviews that have not been presented in the benefits section (search date 1999).[30,31] One systematic review[30] identified 13 case series and three cohort studies (2 retrospective, 1 prospective) and we found one additional retrospective cohort study.[32] The studies used proxy outcomes (evidence of disease measured by prostate specific antigen [PSA] testing).[30,32] Results varied considerably from one series to another and were highly dependent on tumour stage, grade, and pretreatment serum PSA levels. Results in men with T1 or T2 tumours, Gleason score (see glossary, p 1036) of 6 or lower, and serum PSA level of 10 ng/mL or less were similar to those from case series of people having a radical prostatectomy (see glossary, p 1036). The additional cohort study (1872 men) found that in low risk men (stage T1c, stage T2, PSA concentration ≤ 10 ng/mL, and Gleason score ≤ 6) the chance of a high PSA concentration at 5 years was similar whether they were treated with radiation or brachytherapy implant (with or without preceding androgen suppression) or with radical prostatectomy.[32] Men at intermediate or high risk (Gleason score > 6 or PSA > 10 ng/mL) were more likely to have high PSA concentration at 5 years with brachytherapy than with radical prostatectomy (RR of high PSA in men at intermediate risk 3.1, 95% CI 1.5 to 6.1; RR in men at high risk 3.0, 95% CI 1.8 to 5.0).[32] RCTs comparing brachytherapy versus radical prostatectomy are ongoing (Wilt T, personal communication, 2000).

OPTION CRYOSURGERY

We found no RCTs of cryotherapy in men with clinically localised prostate cancer.

Benefits: We found no systematic review or RCTs.

Harms: Complications reported in case series include impotence (65%), transient scrotal oedema (10%), sloughed urethral tissue (3%), urethral stricture (1%), incontinence, urethrorectal fistula, and prostatic abscess (1%).[33]

Comment: One ongoing trial is comparing cryosurgery versus radiation (Wilt T, personal communication, 2000).

OPTION ANDROGEN SUPPRESSION

We found no RCTs of early androgen suppression on length or quality of life in men with asymptomatic, clinically localised prostate cancer. One RCT identified by a systematic review found limited evidence that oestrogen decreased prostate cancer related deaths compared with watchful waiting but it found no significant difference in overall survival. One preliminary report of three large ongoing RCTs in men with localised or locally advanced prostate cancer found that bicalutamide plus standard care reduced rates of radiological progression and bone metastases at 2–3 years compared with standard care alone but there was no significant difference between treatments in overall survival.

Benefits: We found no RCTs of primary treatment with early androgen suppression (see glossary, p 1036) in the absence of symptoms on length or quality of life in men with clinically localised prostate cancer. **Versus watchful waiting:** We found one systematic review (search date 2002, 1 RCT) in men with clinically localised prostate cancer.[8] The RCT identified by the review (285 men) compared three treatments: oestrogen, estramustine, and watchful waiting.[8] It found that oestrogen significantly reduced prostate cancer specific deaths compared with watchful waiting (prostate cancer related deaths: 12% with oestrogen *v* 28% with watchful waiting; $P = 0.03$). It found no significant difference between treatments in overall survival (overall survival: 47% with oestrogen *v* 40% with deferred treatment; $P = 0.48$). The RCT was methodologically flawed (see comment below). **Plus standard care versus standard care alone:** We found one preliminary report of three ongoing RCTs (8113 men with localised or locally advanced prostate cancer T1–T4, Nx/N, M0) comparing bicalutamide 150 mg daily plus standard care versus standard care alone.[1] Standard care included radical prostatectomy (see glossary, p 1036), radiotherapy, and watchful waiting. The meta-analysis in the report found that bicalutamide plus standard care significantly reduced rates of radiological progression and bone metastases at 2–3 years compared with standard care alone (progression: 363/4052 [9.0%] with bicalutamide plus standard care *v* 595/4061 [14.7%] with standard care alone; HR 0.58, 95% CI 0.51 to 0.66; $P < 0.0001$; bone metastases: 214 events with bicalutamide plus standard care *v* 321 events with standard care alone; RR 0.67, 95% CI 0.56 to 0.79). There was no significant difference between treatments in overall survival (overall survival: HR 0.93, 95% CI 0.79 to 1.11).[1]

Harms: See harms of androgen suppression in men with locally advanced prostate cancer, p 1034. One preliminary report of three ongoing RCTs (8113 men with localised or locally advanced prostate cancer) found that bicalutamide plus standard care increased gynaecomastia, breast pain, asthenia, impotence, and hot flushes compared with standard care alone but the statistical significance of differences was not reported (gynaecomastia 66% with bicalutamide plus standard care *v* 8% with standard care alone; breast pain 73% with bicalutamide plus standard care *v* 7% with standard care alone; asthenia 10% with bicalutamide plus standard care *v* 7% with standard care alone; impotence 9% with bicalutamide plus standard care *v* 6% with standard care alone; hot flushes 9% with bicalutamide plus standard care *v* 5% with standard care alone).[1] The systematic review found that androgen deprivation treatment with luteinising hormone releasing hormone agonist reduced sexual function in 40–70% and led to breast swelling in 5–25%, and hot flushes in 50–60%.[8]

Comment: One RCT identified by the systematic review compared oestrogen with deferred treatment. It was not analysed on an intention to treat basis, 24% were excluded or withdrew, treatment groups were not comparable at baseline, and there was a high cardiovascular mortality in the oestrogen group.[8] We found one additional RCT, which is awaiting translation.[34]

QUESTION **In men who have received primary treatment and remain asymptomatic, should androgen suppression be offered when raised concentrations of prostate specific antigens are detected?**

We found no RCTs of initiating androgen suppression when prostate specific antigen rises or persists after primary treatment.

Benefits: We found one systematic review (search date 1998), which identified no RCTs.[35]

Harms: See harms of androgen suppression in men with locally advanced prostate cancer, p 1034.

Comment: In the USA, clinicians often monitor blood concentrations of prostate specific antigen and offer androgen suppression (see glossary, p 1036) when these rise.[35] Consequently, more men with persistent disease are considered for androgen suppression and treatment is initiated earlier in the natural course of the disease. RCTs are needed to evaluate the effectiveness of this approach and of intermittent treatment, in which androgen suppression is initiated when prostate specific antigen rises after primary treatment and discontinued when the antigen concentrations return to the lowest level.[35]

QUESTION **What are the effects of treatments for locally advanced prostate cancer?**

OPTION **ANDROGEN SUPPRESSION**

RCTs found no significant difference in overall survival between androgen suppression with bicalutamide and no androgen suppression in men with localised or locally advanced prostate cancer after 2–10 years. The RCTs

found that bicalutamide reduced radiological progression compared with no bicalutamide. One systematic review found that early androgen treatment increased survival at 10 years compared with deferred treatment in men with locally advanced prostate cancer. It found no significant difference in survival at 5 years. One RCT found limited evidence that immediate androgen suppression reduced complications compared with deferred androgen suppression.

Benefits: **Versus no androgen suppression:** We found one preliminary report of three ongoing RCTs[1] and one reanalysis of three RCTs performed between 1960 and 1975.[36] The three ongoing RCTs (8113 men with localised or locally advanced prostate cancer T1–T4, Nx/N, M0) compared bicalutamide 150 mg once daily plus standard care with standard care alone.[1] Standard care included radical prostatectomy (see glossary, p 1036), radiotherapy, and watchful waiting. Meta-analysis found that bicalutamide plus standard care significantly reduced radiological progression and bone metastases after 2–3 years compared with standard care alone (progression: 363/4052 [9.0%] with bicalutamide plus standard care *v* 595/4061 [14.7%] with standard care alone; HR 0.58, 95% CI 0.51 to 0.66; $P < 0.0001$; bone metastases: 214 events with bicalutamide plus standard care *v* 321 events with standard care alone; RR 0.67, 95% CI 0.56 to 0.79). There was no significant difference between treatments in overall survival (overall survival: HR 0.93, 95% CI 0.79 to 1.11).[1] The three earlier RCTs (about 4000 men with all stages of newly diagnosed prostate cancer) compared androgen suppression (see glossary, p 1036) (diethylstilbestrol [stilboestrol], orchidectomy, or oestrogens) versus no initial treatment.[36] They found no significant difference in overall survival. Reanalysis of updated data (published 1988) from these RCTs provided limited evidence of a modest survival advantage with androgen suppression, particularly in younger people with more advanced disease.[36]
Immediate (initiated at diagnosis) versus deferred androgen suppression: We found one systematic review (search date 2001, 4 RCTs, 2167 men with locally advanced prostate cancer).[37] All RCTs included in the review were conducted before prostate specific antigen testing was introduced. Each RCT used different methods of androgen suppression and had different requirements for initiation of treatment. It found no significant difference in overall survival at 1, 2, or 5 years with early compared with deferred androgen suppression (3 RCTs, 1307 men, at 1 year 88% with early *v* 86% with deferred; RR 1.04, 95% CI 0.99 to 1.09; at 2 years 73% with early *v* 71% with deferred; RR 1.05, 95% CI 0.97 to 1.12; at 5 years 44% with early *v* 37% with deferred; RR 1.08, 95% CI 0.96 to 1.22). However, it found that early treatment significantly increased survival at 10 years compared with deferred treatment (18% with early *v* 12% with deferred; OR 1.50, 95% CI 1.04 to 2.16). The most recent of the RCTs[38] identified by the review (938 men with stage C [locally advanced] or stage D [asymptomatic metastatic] disease) was not included in the meta-analysis (see comment below). It found that in men with stage C disease, immediate androgen suppression significantly improved survival compared with deferred treatment (survival benefit measured by survival curve; $P = 0.02$; CI not

reported). The RCT found that in people with stage C disease, immediate androgen suppression was associated with a non-significant lower risk of major complications, such as pathological fractures compared with deferred treatment (3/256 [1.2%] with immediate v 6/244 [2.5%] with deferred; RR 0.48, 95% CI 0.12 to 1.90), ureteric obstruction (22/256 [8.6%] with immediate v 28/244 [11.5%] with deferred; RR 0.75, 95% CI 0.44 to 1.30), and extraskeletal metastases (17/256 [6.6%] with immediate v 26/244 [10.7%] with deferred; RR 0.62, 95% CI 0.35 to 1.10). Analysis including all participants found a significant reduction for combined results of pathological fracture and cord compression (RR 0.48, 95% CI 0.28 to 0.79). The RCT did not make clear the time interval over which outcomes were recorded, although this seemed to be at least 10 years.[38] One additional RCT in men with cancers of different stages found that bicalutamide significantly improved disease free progression at 2.6 years compared with placebo.[39] See benefits of androgen suppression under effects of treating clinically localised prostate cancer, p 1031.

Harms: Adverse events were not well reported in the review.[37] Earlier initiation of androgen suppression means longer exposure to adverse effects, which include osteoporosis, weight gain, hot flushes (10–60%), loss of muscle mass, gynaecomastia (5–10%), impotence (10–30%), and loss of libido (5–30%).[35] These adverse effects are particularly important in the treatment of men with long life expectancy or younger men with lower grade cancers. The review did not report on quality of life. See harms of androgen suppression under effects of treating clinically localised prostate cancer, p 1032.

Comment: The RCTs conducted in the 1960s and 1970s[35] included men who were older and had more advanced cancers than those in the more recent RCT.[38] The most recent RCT[38] will be included in the meta-analysis of the systematic review[37] in future updates of the Cochrane Library. RCTs are needed to evaluate the effectiveness of androgen suppression before surgery when disease extends beyond the capsule.

OPTION ANDROGEN SUPPRESSION PLUS EXTERNAL BEAM RADIATION VERSUS EXTERNAL BEAM RADIATION ALONE

RCTs found limited evidence that androgen suppression initiated at diagnosis plus external beam radiation improved long term survival compared with radiation alone or radiation plus deferred androgen suppression. One RCT found limited evidence that immediate androgen suppression reduced complications compared with deferred androgen suppression.

Benefits: We found one systematic review (search date 1998, 4 RCTs, 1565 men)[35] and one additional RCT.[40] The review compared early versus deferred androgen suppression (see glossary, p 1036) in men receiving external beam radiation.[35] Early androgen suppression was initiated at the same time as radiation treatment for locally advanced, or asymptomatic but clinically evident, metastatic prostate cancer, and was continued until the development of hormone refractory disease. The deferred group received radiation treatment alone, with androgen suppression initiated only in those in whom the disease progressed. The systematic review found that early androgen suppression significantly improved overall 5 year survival compared with deferred treatment (percentage surviving at 5 years 76.5% with early *v* 68.2% with deferred; ARR 8.3%; HR 0.63, 95% CI 0.48 to 0.83; NNT at 5 years 12).[35] Long term follow up of one of the RCTs included in the review (476 men, stages T2–T4, with or without pelvic lymph node involvement) found that more people survived with early androgen suppression at 8 years compared with deferred treatment, but the difference was not significant (53% with early *v* 44% with deferred; P = 0.1). There was a significant improvement in disease free survival (33% with early *v* 21% with deferred; P = 0.004) and in the incidence of distant metastases (34% with early *v* 45% with deferred; P = 0.04).[41] The additional RCT (277 men with advanced localised prostate cancer; T2–T4, M0, with and without nodal disease) compared three treatments: orchidectomy alone, radiotherapy alone, or radiotherapy in addition to orchidectomy.[40] It found no significant difference in overall survival or need for further treatment for local disease progression between the three treatment groups (data presented graphically; P value not reported), but it is likely to have been underpowered to detect a clinically important difference.

Harms: The review reported adverse effects of androgen suppression (see harms of androgen suppression for the treatment of men with locally advanced prostate cancer, p 1034).[35] In the additional RCT, adverse effects associated with radiotherapy included bowel symptoms (19%), urinary symptoms including transient frequency (8%), bowel and urinary complications (1%), rectal bleeding necessitating blood transfusion (2%), and radiation proctitis (1%), which was a contributory factor in two deaths. It found that the predominant adverse effect after orchidectomy was hot flushes (15%).[40]

Comment: We found no evidence from RCTs of external beam radiation alone in men with locally advanced prostate cancer.

OPTION ANDROGEN SUPPRESSION AFTER RADICAL PROSTATECTOMY AND PELVIC LYMPHADENECTOMY

One small RCT in men with node positive prostate cancer found that immediate androgen suppression compared with deferred androgen suppression after radical prostatectomy and pelvic lymphadenectomy reduced mortality over a median of 7 years' follow up.

Benefits: We found one RCT (98 men who had had a radical prostatectomy [see glossary, p 1036] and pelvic lymphadenectomy for nodal metastases) comparing immediate androgen suppression (see glossary, p 1036) (with either goserelin or bilateral orchidectomy) versus androgen suppression deferred until disease progression.[42] It found that androgen suppression significantly reduced mortality in the long term compared with watchful waiting (median follow up 7.1 years; mortality 7/47 [14.9%] with androgen suppression *v* 18/51 [35.3%] with watchful waiting; ARR 20.4%; RR 0.42, 95% CI 0.19 to 0.92; NNT 4, 95% CI 3 to 33), and resulted in a higher proportion of men with undetectable prostate specific antigen (P < 0.001).

Harms: The RCT found that, compared with deferred androgen suppression, immediate androgen suppression caused more haematological effects (15% with immediate *v* 4% with deferred), gastrointestinal effects (25% with immediate *v* 6% with deferred), non-specific genitourinary effects (48% with immediate *v* 12% with deferred), hot flushes (56% with immediate *v* 0% with deferred), and weight gain (18% with immediate *v* 2% with deferred).[42]

Comment: None.

GLOSSARY

Androgen suppression Monotherapy uses a single drug or surgical procedure for androgen suppression. Methods include orchidectomy (removal of both testes), diethylstilbestrol, luteinising hormone releasing hormone agonist injections, or non-steroidal antiandrogens. Combined androgen blockade uses the addition of a non-steroidal antiandrogen to standard androgen suppression monotherapy with orchidectomy, diethylstilbestrol, or luteinising hormone releasing hormone agonist injection.

Brachytherapy Radiotherapy where the sources of ionising radiation are radioactive implants, many of which are permanently inserted directly into the prostate gland.

Conformal radiotherapy Three dimensional radiotherapy planning systems and methods to match the radiation treatment to irregular tumour volumes.

Gleason score A number from 1–10 with 1 being the most well differentiated and 10 being the most poorly differentiated tumour or a histological examination.

Radical prostatectomy Surgical removal of the prostate with its capsule, seminal vesicles, ductus deferens, some pelvic fasciae, and sometimes pelvic lymph nodes; performed through either the retropubic or the perineal route.

Substantive changes

Radical prostatectomy in localised prostate cancer One systematic review[8] and one RCT added;[15] option recategorised from Unknown effectiveness to Trade-off between benefits and harms.

External beam radiation in localised prostate cancer Two systematic reviews added;[8,25] conclusions unchanged.

Brachytherapy in localised prostate cancer One systematic review added;[8] conclusions unchanged.

Androgen suppression in localised prostate cancer One systematic review[8] and a report of three RCTs added;[1] conclusions unchanged.

Watchful waiting in localised prostate cancer One systematic review[8] and two RCTs added;[9,15] conclusions unchanged.

REFERENCES

1. See WA, Wirth MP, McLeod DG et al. Bicalutamide as immediate therapy either alone or as adjuvant to standard care of patients with localized or locally advanced prostate cancer: first analysis of the early prostate cancer program. *J Urol* 2002;168:429–435.
2. Stanford JL, Stephenson RA, Coyle LM, et al. Prostate Cancer Trends 1973–1995, SEER Program, National Cancer Institute. NIH Pub. No. 99–4543. Bethesda, MD, 1999.
3. Adolfsson J, Steineck G, Hedund P. Deferred treatment of clinically localized low-grade prostate cancer: actual 10-year and projected 15-year follow-up of the Karolinska series. *Urology* 1997;50:722–726.
4. Johansson J-E, Holmberg L, Johansson S, et al. Fifteen-year survival in prostate cancer: prospective, population-based study in Sweden. *JAMA* 1997;277:467–471.
5. Pound CR, Partin AW, Eisenberger MA, et al. Natural history of progression after PSA elevation following radical prostatectomy. *JAMA* 1999;281:1591–1597.
6. Lu-Yao G, Albertsen PC, Stanford JL et al. Natural experiment examining impact of aggressive screening and treatment on prostate cancer mortality in two fixed cohorts from Seattle area and Connecticut. *BMJ* 2002;325:740.
7. Frankel S, Smith GD, Donovan J, et al. Screening for prostate cancer. *Lancet* 2003;361:1122–1128.
8. Harris RP, Lohr KN, Beck R, et al. *Screening for prostate cancer*. Systematic Evidence Review no. 16. Rockville, MD: Agency for Healthcare Research and Quality, 2001. Available online at http://www.ahrq.gov/clinic/serfiles.htm (last accessed 16 September 2003).

9. Holmberg L, Bill-Axelson A, Helgesen F et al. A randomized trial comparing radical prostatectomy with watchful waiting in early prostate cancer. *N Engl J Med* 2002;347:781–789.
10. Albertsen PC, Hanley JA, Gleason DF, et al. Competing risk analysis of men aged 55 to 74 years at diagnosis managed conservatively for clinically localized prostate cancer. *JAMA* 1998;280:975–980.
11. Lu-Yao GL, Yao S. Population-based study of long-term survival in patients with clinically localised prostate cancer. *Lancet* 1997;349:906–910.
12. Gann PH, Hennekens CH, Stampfer MJ. A prospective evaluation of plasma prostate-specific antigen for detection of prostatic cancer. *JAMA* 1995;273:289–294.
13. Iversen P, Madsen PO, Corle DK. Radical prostatectomy versus expectant treatment for early carcinoma of the prostate: 23 year follow-up of a prospective randomized study. *Scand J Urol Nephrol* 1995;172(suppl):65–72.
14. Paulson DF, Lin GH, Hinshaw W, et al. Radical surgery versus radiotherapy for adenocarcinoma of the prostate. *J Urol* 1982;128:502–504.
15. Steineck G, Helgesen Adolfsson J, et al. Quality of life after radical prostatectomy or watchful waiting. *N Engl J Med* 2002;347:790–796.
16. Lu-Yao GL, McLerran D, Wasson JH. An assessment of radical prostatectomy: time trends, geographic variation, and outcomes. *JAMA* 1993;269:2633–2636.
17. Middleton RG, Thompson IM, Austenfeld MS, et al. Prostate cancer clinical guidelines panel summary report on the management of clinically localized prostate cancer. *J Urol* 1995;154:2144–2148. Search date 1993; primary source Medline.
18. Anonymous. Screening for prostate cancer. *Ann Intern Med* 1997;126:480–484.
19. Fowler FJ, Barry MJ, Lu-Yao G, et al. Patient-reported complications and follow-up treatment after radical prostatectomy: the national Medicare experience 1988–1990 (updated June 1993). *Urology* 1993;42:622–629.
20. Bishoff JT, Motley G, Optenberg SA, et al. Incidence of fecal and urinary incontinence following radical perineal and retropubic prostatectomy in a national population. *J Urol* 1998;160:454–458.
21. Fleming C, Wasson J, Albertsen PC, et al. A decision analysis of alternative strategies for clinically localized prostate cancer. *JAMA* 1993;269:2650–2658.
22. Litwin MS, Hays RD, Fink A, et al. Quality-of-life outcomes in men treated for localized prostate cancer. *JAMA* 1995;273:129–135.
23. Wilt TJ, Brawer MK. The prostate cancer intervention versus observation trial. *Oncology* 1997;11:1133–1139.
24. Norlen BJ. Swedish randomized trial of radical prostatectomy versus watchful waiting. *Can J Oncol* 1994;4(suppl 1):38–42.
25. Brundage M, Lukka H, Crook J, et al. The use of conformal radiotherapy and the selection of radiation dose in T1 or T2 low or intermediate risk prostate cancer – a systematic review. *Radiother Oncol* 2002;64:239–250. Search date 2001; primary sources Medline, Cancerlit, proceedings of the *American Society of Clinical Oncology* and the *American Society for Therapeutic Radiology and Oncology*, personal files, and bibliographies of identified articles and reviews.
26. Dearnaley DP, Khoo VS, Norman AR, et al. Comparison of radiation side-effects of conformal and conventional radiotherapy in prostate cancer: a randomized trial. *Lancet* 1999;353:267–272.
27. Fowler FJ, Barry MJ, Lu-Yao G, et al. Outcomes of external beam radiation therapy for prostate cancer: a study of Medicare beneficiaries in three surveillance, epidemiology, and end results areas. *J Clin Oncol* 1996;14:2258–2265.
28. Crook J, Perry G, Robertson S, et al. Routine prostate biopsies: results for 225 patients. *Urology* 1995;45:624–632.
29. Shipley WU, Thames HD, Sandler HM, et al. Radiation therapy for clinically localized prostate cancer. A multi-institutional pooled analysis. *JAMA* 1999;281:1598–1604.
30. Crook J, Lukka H, Klotz L, et al. Systematic overview of the evidence for brachytherapy in clinically localized prostate cancer. *Can Med Assoc J* 2001;164:975–981. Search date 1999; primary sources Medline and Cancerlit.
31. Wills F, Hailey D. Brachytherapy for prostate cancer. Edmonton, AB, Canada: The Alberta Heritage Foundation for Medical Research. *Health Technol Assess* 1999:1–65. Search date 1999; primary sources The Cochrane Library, Medline, Healthstar, Cancerlit, Embase, Cinahl, hand searches of reference lists, and internet searches.
32. Talcott JA, Clark JC, Stark P, et al. Long term complications of brachytherapy for early prostate cancer. A survey of treated patients. American Society of Clinical Oncology Annual Meeting 1999; Abstract 1196.
33. Littrup PJ, Mody A, Sparschu RA. Prostate cryosurgery complications. *Semin Int Radiol* 1994;11:226–230.
34. Rauchenwald M. First results of the early prostate cancer program study. *J Urol Urogynakol* 2001;8:21–27.
35. Agency for Health Care Policy and Research. Relative effectiveness and cost-effectiveness of methods of androgen suppression in the treatment of advanced prostatic cancer. Summary. Rockville, MD: Agency for Health Care Policy and Research, 1999. (Evidence Report/Technology Assessment: No 4.) http://www.ahcpr.gov/clinic/epcsums/prossumm.htm (last accessed 10 July 2003). Search date 1998; primary sources Medline, Cancerlit, Embase, Current Contents, and Cochrane Library.
36. Byar DP, Corle DK. Hormone treatment for prostate cancer: results of the Veterans' Administration cooperative urologic research group studies. *NCI Monograph* 1988;7:165–170.
37. Nair B, Wilt T, MacDonald, R, et al. Early versus deferred androgen suppression in the treatment of advanced prostatic cancer. In: The Cochrane Library, Issue 2, 2002. Oxford: Update Software. Search date 2001; primary sources Medline, Embase, Cancerlit, Cochrane Library, VA Cochrane Prostate Disease register, and hand searches of bibliographies.
38. The Medical Research Council Prostate Cancer Working Party Investigators Group. Immediate versus deferred treatment for advanced prostatic cancer: initial results of the Medical Research Council trial. *Br J Urol* 1997;79:235–246.
39. Wirth M, Tyrrell C, Wallace M, et al. Bicalutamide (Casodex) 150 mg as immediate therapy in patients with localized or locally advanced prostate cancer significantly reduces the risk of disease progression. *Urology* 2001;58:146–150.
40. Fellows GJ, Clark PB, Beynon LL, et al. Treatment of advanced localised prostatic cancer by orchiectomy, radiotherapy, or combined treatment. *Br J Urol* 1992:70;304–309.

41. Pilepich M, Winter M, Madhu J, et al. Phase III Radiation Therapy Oncology Group (RTOG) trial 86–10 of androgen deprivation adjuvant to definitive radiotherapy in locally advanced carcinoma of the prostate. *Int J Radiat Oncol Biol Phys* 2001;50:1243–1252.
42. Messing EM, Manola J, Sarodsy M, et al. Immediate hormonal therapy compared with observation after radical prostatectomy and pelvic lymphadenectomy in men with node-positive prostate cancer. *N Engl J Med* 1999;341:1781–1789.

Timothy Wilt
Professor of Medicine
VA Coordinating Center for the Cochrane Review Group in Prostate Diseases and Urologic Malignancies and the Center for Chronic Diseases Outcomes Research
Minneapolis VA Hospital, Minneapolis, MN, USA

Competing interests: None declared.

The following previous contributor of this topic would also like to be acknowledged: Michael Brawer.

TABLE 1 **Prostatic cancer staging systems (see text, p 1024).**

Tumour, node, metastasis (TNM) classification system	
Tumour	
T0	Clinically unsuspected
T1	Clinically inapparent (not palpable or visible by imaging)
T2	Tumour confined within prostate
T3	Tumour outside capsule or extension into vesicle
T4	Tumour fixed to other tissue
Nodes	
N0	No evidence of involvement of regional nodes
N1	Involvement of regional nodes
Metastases	
M0	No evidence of distant metastases
M1	Evidence of distant metastases
American urologic staging system	
Stage A	No palpable tumour
Stage B	Tumour confined to the prostate gland
Stage C	Extracapsular extension
Stage D	Metastatic prostate cancer
Stage D1	Pelvic lymph node metastases
Stage D2	Distant metastases

Anorexia nervosa

Search date August 2002

Janet Treasure and Ulrike Schmidt

QUESTIONS

INTERVENTIONS

See glossary, p 1048

Key Messages

- **Cisapride** One small RCT found no significant difference with cisapride versus placebo in weight gain at 8 weeks. Use of cisapride has been restrictmany countries because of concern about cardiac irregularities, including ventricular tachycardia, torsades de pointes, and sudden death.
- **Cyproheptadine** Three small RCTs found no significant difference with cyproheptadine versus placebo in weight gain.
- **Inpatient versus outpatient treatment setting (in people not so severely ill as to warrant emergency intervention)** Limited evidence from one small RCT found no significant difference between outpatient treatment and inpatient treatment for increasing weight and improving Morgan Russell scale global scores at 1, 2, and 5 years in people who did not need emergency intervention.
- **Neuroleptic drugs that increase the QT interval** We found no RCTs. The QT interval may be prolonged in people with anorexia nervosa, and many neuroleptic drugs (haloperidol, pimozide, sertindole, thioridazine, chlorpromazine, and others) also increase the QT interval. Prolongation of the QT interval may be associated with increased risk of ventricular tachycardia, torsades de pointes, and sudden death.
- **Oestrogen treatment (for prevention of fractures)** We found no good evidence about the effects of hormonal treatment on fracture rates in people with anorexia. One small RCT found no significant effect of oestrogen versus no treatment on bone mineral density in people with anorexia.

- **Psychotherapies** We found insufficient evidence from small RCTs to compare psychotherapies versus dietary counselling or versus each other. One small RCT found limited evidence that focal analytical therapy or family therapy versus usual treatment significantly increased the number of people recovered or improved as assessed by the Morgan Russell scale at 1 year.
- **Selective serotonin reuptake inhibitors (fluoxetine)** We found insufficient evidence from two small RCTs to compare fluoxetine versus placebo in people with anorexia.
- **Tricyclic antidepressants** Two small RCTs found no evidence of benefit with amitriptyline compared with placebo. They found that amitriptyline was associated with more adverse effects, such as palpitations, dry mouth, and blurred vision.
- **Zinc** One small RCT found limited evidence that zinc may improve daily body mass index gain compared with placebo in people managed in an inpatient setting. However, we were unable to draw firm conclusions.

DEFINITION Anorexia nervosa is characterised by a refusal to maintain weight at or above a minimally normal weight (< 85% of expected weight for age and height, or body mass index [see glossary, p 1048] < 17.5 kg/m^2), or a failure to show the expected weight gain during growth. In association with this there is often an intense fear of gaining weight, preoccupation with weight, denial of the current low weight and its adverse impact on health, and amenorrhoea. Two subtypes of anorexia nervosa, binge–purge and restricting, have been defined.[1]

INCIDENCE/ PREVALENCE A mean incidence in the general population of 19/100 000 a year in females and 2/100 000 a year in males has been estimated from 12 cumulative studies.[2] The highest rate was in female teenagers (age 13–19 years), where there were 50.8 cases/100 000 a year. A large cohort study of Swedish school children (4291 people, aged 16 years) were screened by weighing and subsequent interview, and the prevalence of anorexia nervosa cases (defined using DSM-III and DSM-III-R criteria) was found to be 7/1000 for girls and 1/1000 for boys.[3] Little is know of the incidence or prevalence in Asia, South America, or Africa.

AETIOLOGY/ RISK FACTORS Anorexia nervosa has been related to family, biological, social, and cultural factors. Studies have found that anorexia nervosa is associated with a family history of anorexia nervosa (HR 11.4, 95% CI 1.1 to 89.0), of bulimia nervosa (adjusted HR 3.5, 95% CI 1.1 to 14.0),[4] depression, generalised anxiety disorder, obsessive compulsive disorder, or obsessive compulsive personality disorder (adjusted RR 3.6, 95% CI 1.6 to 8.0).[5] A twin study suggested that anorexia nervosa may be related to genetic factors but it was unable to estimate reliably the contribution of non-shared environmental factors.[6] Specific aspects of childhood temperament thought to be related include perfectionism, negative self evaluation, and extreme compliance.[7] Perinatal factors include prematurity (OR 3.2, 95% CI 1.6 to 6.2), particularly if the baby was small for gestational age (OR 5.7, 95% CI 1.4 to 4.1).

PROGNOSIS One prospective study followed up 51 people with teenage-onset anorexia nervosa, about half of whom received no or minimal treatment (< 8 sessions). After 10 years, 14/51 people (27%) had a persistent eating disorder, three (6%) had ongoing anorexia nervosa, and six (12%) had experienced a period of bulimia nervosa. People with anorexia nervosa were significantly more likely to have an affective disorder than controls matched for sex, age, and school (lifetime risk of affective disorder 96% in people with anorexia *v* 23% with controls, ARI 73%, 95% CI 60% to 85%). Obsessive compulsive disorder was, similarly, significantly more likely in people with anorexia nervosa (30%) compared with controls (10%) (ARI 20%, 95% CI 10% to 41%). However, in 35% of people with obsessive compulsive disorder and anorexia nervosa, obsessive compulsive disorder preceded the anorexia. About half of all participants continued to have poor psychosocial functioning at 10 years (assessed using the Morgan Russell scale (see glossary, p 1048) and Global Assessment of Functioning Scale).[8] A summary of treatment studies (68 studies published between 1953 and 1989, 3104 people, length of follow up 1–33 years) found that 43% of people recover completely (range 7–86%), 36% improve (range 1–69%), 20% develop a chronic eating disorder (range 0–43%), and 5% die from anorexia nervosa (range 0–21%).[9] Favourable prognostic factors include an early age at onset and a short interval between onset of symptoms and the beginning of treatment. Unfavourable prognostic factors include vomiting, bulimia, profound weight loss, chronicity, and a history of premorbid developmental or clinical abnormalities. The all cause standardised mortality ratio of eating disorders (anorexia nervosa and bulimia nervosa) has been estimated at 538, about three times higher than other psychiatric illnesses.[10] The average annual risk of mortality was 0.59% a year in females in 10 eating disorder populations (1322 people) with a minimum follow up of 6 years.[11] The mortality risk was higher for people with lower weight and with older age at presentation. Young women with anorexia nervosa are at an increased risk of fractures later in life.[12]

AIMS OF INTERVENTION To restore physical health (weight within the normal range and no sequelae of starvation, e.g. regular menstruation, normal bone mass), normal patterns of eating and attitudes towards weight and shape, and no additional psychiatric comorbidity (e.g. depression, anxiety, obsessive compulsive disorder); to reduce the impact of the illness on social functioning and quality of life.

OUTCOMES The most widely used measure of outcome is the Morgan Russell scale,[13] which includes nutritional status, menstrual function, mental state, and sexual and social adjustment. Biological outcome criteria alone such as weight (body mass index or in relation to matched population weight) and menstrual function are used infrequently as outcome measures. RCTs do not usually have sufficient power or long enough follow up periods to examine mortality. Other validated outcome measures include eating symptom measures.[14–17] Bone mass density is included as a proxy outcome for fracture risk.

METHODS *Clinical Evidence* search and appraisal August 2002 and hand searches of reference lists of identified reviews. To be included, an RCT had to have at least 30 people and follow up greater than 75%. Results from each of the identified trials were extracted independently by the two reviewers. Any disagreements were discussed until a consensus was reached.

QUESTION **What are the effects of treatments in anorexia nervosa?**

OPTION **PSYCHOTHERAPY**

We found insufficient evidence from small RCTs to compare psychotherapies versus dietary counselling or versus each other. One small RCT found limited evidence that focal analytical therapy or family therapy versus usual treatment significantly increased the number of people recovered or improved as assessed by the Morgan Russell scale at 1 year.

Benefits: **Versus treatment as usual or dietary counselling:** We found no systematic review. We found three small RCTs of limited quality that compared different psychotherapies versus dietary counselling (see glossary, p 1048) or treatment as usual (see table A on web extra). All three RCTs were carried out in an outpatient setting in people with a late age of onset and long duration of illness.[18–20] The largest RCT found significant improvements in weight gain for some psychotherapies versus treatment as usual and for the number of people classified as recovered.[18] The second RCT found a significant improvement for cognitive therapy versus baseline.[20] All people treated with dietary counselling either did not take up or withdrew from treatment and refused release of their results, making it impossible to compare the two groups. The third RCT found no difference in outcomes between the groups.[19] **Versus each other:** We found six small RCTs of limited quality that compared different psychotherapies. Three of these were undertaken in an outpatient setting[21–23] in people with an early age of onset and short illness duration. Two of the RCTs were carried out in an outpatient setting in people with a later age of onset and longer duration of illness.[18,24] One RCT included people with early and late onset anorexia nervosa and with long and short duration of illness (see table A on web extra).[25,26] None of the RCTs found an overall significant difference between different psychotherapies.

Harms: The acceptability of the treatment varied among RCTs. Failure to take up treatment ranged from 0–30% and withdrawal from treatment ranged from 0–70% among RCTs but this may have been caused by different methods of case ascertainment (see table A on web extra). The proportion of people admitted for inpatient treatment (see glossary, p 1048) also varied among RCTs, ranging from 0–36%. One death was attributed to anorexia nervosa in the control group in one outpatient RCT with a 1 year follow up.[18] Three deaths attributed to anorexia nervosa occurred in the 5 year follow up period of one inpatient based RCT.[26]

Comment: All the RCTs were small and had limited power to detect clinically important differences if they existed. The amount of therapeutic input varied considerably among and within the RCTs. There was variation in methods of recruitment, reporting of key results (e.g. withdrawal rates), and the description of participants' characteristics and selection. The people in the inpatient RCT covered a broad range of severity.[25]

OPTION **TRICYCLIC ANTIDEPRESSANTS**

Two small RCTs found no evidence of benefit with amitriptyline compared with placebo. They found that amitriptyline was associated with more adverse events, such as palpitations, dry mouth, and blurred vision.

Benefits: We found no systematic review. We found two small RCTs.[27,28] The first RCT (43 people with early onset and short duration anorexia nervosa, mean age 16.6 years, mean 27% below average weight, mean duration of anorexia nervosa 1.5 years) in two units (5 outpatients) compared amitriptyline versus placebo.[28] Participants could also receive various kinds of psychotherapy (see glossary, p 1048). Eighteen people refused to participate and were used as a third comparison group. The RCT found no significant difference between the groups on any of the outcome scales measured at 5 weeks (> 50% improvement in global response 1/11 [9%] with amitriptyline *v* 1/14 [7%] with placebo; RR 1.2, 95% CI 0.1 to 16.7). The second RCT (72 women, mean age 20.6 years, mean 2.9 years' duration) compared amitriptyline, cyproheptadine, and placebo.[28] The drug treatment had no significant effect on treatment efficiency — that is, the reciprocal of days to reach target weight, multiplied by 90 (a dummy figure of 120 was used if people failed to reach target weight). See benefits under cyproheptadine, p 1045.[28]

Harms: Adverse events more common with amitriptyline included increased perspiration (2/11 [18%] with amitriptyline *v* 0/14 [0%] with placebo), drowsiness (6/11 [55%] with amitriptyline *v* 0/14 [0%] with placebo), dry mouth (4/11 [36%] with amitriptyline *v* 2/14 [14%] with placebo), blurred vision (1/11 [9%] with amitriptyline *v* 0/14 [0%] with placebo), urinary retention (1/11 [9%] with amitriptyline *v* 0/14 [0%] with placebo), hypotension (2/11 [18%] with amitriptyline *v* 0/14 [0%] with placebo), and leukopenia (1/11 [9%] with amitriptyline *v* 0/14 [0%] with placebo). Adverse events more common with placebo included palpitations (0/11 [0%] with amitriptyline *v* 1/14 [7%] with placebo) and dizziness (0/11 [0%] with amitriptyline *v* 2/14 [14%] with placebo). The QT interval may be prolonged in people with anorexia nervosa[29] and tricyclic antidepressants (amitriptyline, protriptyline, nortriptyline, doxepin, and maprotiline) also increase the QT interval.[30–32] In an observational study (495 people with mental illness and 101 healthy controls) an increased risk of QTc was seen with tricyclic use, adjusting for age and other drug use (adjusted OR 2.6, 95% CI 1.2 to 5.6).[33] The RCT of amitriptyline versus placebo found more adverse effects with amitriptyline than placebo. General harms of tricyclic antidepressants are described in the section on depression (see depressive disorders, p 1121).

Comment: The RCTs were both of short duration. Prolongation of the QT interval may be associated with increased risk of ventricular tachycardia, torsades de pointes, and sudden death.[31,32] It is not clear if people in the second amitriptyline RCT also received psychotherapy.[28]

OPTION SELECTIVE SEROTONIN REUPTAKE INHIBITORS

We found insufficient evidence from two small RCTs to compare fluoxetine versus placebo in people with anorexia.

Benefits: We found two small RCTs.[34,35] The first RCT (33 women; mean age 26.2 years; mean body mass index (see glossary, p 1048) 15.0 kg/m^2; mean duration of anorexia nervosa 8.0 years) compared fluoxetine 60 mg versus placebo for the duration (mean 36 days) of inpatient treatment (see glossary, p 1048), which included individual and group psychotherapy (see glossary, p 1048).[34] There were two early withdrawals from the fluoxetine group. The RCT found no significant differences in weight gain, eating symptoms, or depressive symptoms between the groups. The second RCT (39 women, binge–purge type anorexia excluded, mean age about 22 years, mean duration of anorexia nervosa 4–7 years) compared fluoxetine (starting dosage 20 mg/day) versus placebo for 1 year. All women had been discharged from hospital after weight gain (minimum weight restoration was 75% of average body weight). Women were allowed additional psychotherapy. Women who had substantial and incapacitating symptoms were encouraged to withdraw from the study. Withdrawal rates were too high to draw reliable conclusions about effects, although withdrawal rate was significantly lower with fluoxetine versus placebo (6/16 [37%] with fluoxetine *v* 16/19 [84%] with placebo; RR 0.45, 95% CI 0.23 to 0.86).[35]

Harms: General harms of selective serotonin reuptake inhibitors are described in the section on depression (see depressive disorders, p 1121).

Comment: In the second RCT, four further women were excluded from the analysis. Three became aware of the treatment and one stopped taking medication before the end of 30 days.[35]

OPTION NEUROLEPTIC MEDICATION

We found no good evidence.

Benefits: We found no systematic review and no RCTs.

Harms: General harms of neuroleptic drugs are described in the section on schizophrenia (see schizophrenia, p 1208). The QT interval may be prolonged in people with anorexia nervosa[29,30] and many neuroleptic drugs (haloperidol, pimozide, sertindole, thioridazine, chlorpromazine, and others) may also increase the QT interval.[31,32] An observational study (495 people with mental illness and 101 healthy controls) found an increased risk of QTc with high and very high dose neuroleptic use after adjusting for age and other drug use (high dose: adjusted OR 3.4, 95% CI 1.2 to 10.1; very high dose: adjusted OR 5.6, 95% CI 1.6 to 19.3).[33]

Comment: Prolongation of the QT interval may be associated with increased risk of ventricular tachycardia, torsades de pointes, and sudden death.[31,32]

OPTION ZINC

One small RCT found limited evidence that zinc may improve daily body mass index gain compared with placebo in people managed in an inpatient setting.

Benefits: We found no systematic review. We found one RCT (54 people aged > 15 years, mean body mass index (see glossary, p 1048) 15.8 kg/m^2, mean duration of anorexia nervosa 3.7 years, admitted to 2 eating disorder units), which compared 100 mg zinc gluconate versus placebo.[36] All but three of the people had normal zinc levels before treatment. Treatment was continued until the individual had gained 10% of weight over the admission weight on two consecutive weeks. Ten people in the zinc group and nine in the placebo group did not complete the study. The RCT found a significant difference in rate of body mass index gain/day (0.079 with zinc *v* 0.039 with placebo; $P = 0.03$).[36]

Harms: None reported.

Comment: The rationale for zinc supplements in people with normal zinc levels is unclear.

OPTION CYPROHEPTADINE

One RCT in an outpatient setting and two RCTs in inpatient settings found no significant difference between cyproheptadine and placebo for weight gain.

Benefits: We found no systematic review. We found three small RCTs. The first RCT (24 women in an outpatient setting) compared cyproheptadine versus placebo.[37] It found no significant difference in response to treatment after 2 months. The second RCT (81 women in 3 specialised inpatient units) compared cyproheptadine versus placebo, and behaviour therapy versus no behaviour therapy.[38] The effect of behaviour therapy was not reported. There were no significant differences in weight gain between the cyproheptadine and placebo groups. The third RCT (72 women, mean age 20.6 years, mean 77% of target weight, mean duration of anorexia 2.9 years, at 2 specialised inpatient units) compared amitriptyline (up to a maximum of 160 mg) versus cyproheptadine (up to a maximum of 32 mg) versus placebo.[28] It found no significant difference between cyproheptadine and placebo for rate of weight gain (measured as a reciprocal function of the time to reach target weight).

Harms: No harms were reported in the first two RCTs.[37,38] In the third RCT, on both day 7 and day 21, placebo exceeded the amitriptyline group in number of physical adverse events rated moderate or severe. Adverse effects were less frequent with cyproheptadine. No one had to be withdrawn from the protocol because of adverse effects.[28]

Comment: All three RCTs were of short duration.

OPTION INPATIENT VERSUS OUTPATIENT TREATMENT SETTING IN ANOREXIA NERVOSA

Limited evidence from one small RCT found no significant difference between outpatient treatment and inpatient treatment for increasing weight and improving Morgan Russell scale global scores at 1, 2, and 5 years in people who did not need emergency intervention.

Benefits: We found one systematic review (search date 1999) comparing inpatient treatment (see glossary, p 1048) with outpatient care.[39] The review identified one RCT, which had a 5 year follow up.[40,41] Ninety people referred with anorexia nervosa (mean age 22 years, weight loss 26% of matched population mean weight, mean duration 3.2 years) were randomised to four treatment groups: inpatient treatment, outpatient treatment (individual and family therapy), outpatient group therapy, and assessment interview only. Assessors were not blind to treatment allocation. Adherence to allocated treatment (defined as accepting allocation and at least 1 attendance at a treatment group or individual treatment session) differed significantly among groups: inpatient treatment 18/30 (60%), outpatient treatment (individual and family therapy) 18/20 (90%), outpatient group psychotherapy (see glossary, p 1048) 17/20 (85%), and assessment interview only 20/20 (100%). Treatment adherence differed significantly between outpatient and inpatient treatment (RR 1.5, 95% CI 1.1 to 2.0). Average acceptance of treatment also varied among groups (20 wks inpatient treatment, 9 outpatient sessions, and 5 group sessions). In the assessment interview only group, six people had no treatment of any kind in the first year and the others had treatment elsewhere (6 had inpatient treatment, 5 had outpatient hospital treatment, and 3 had at least weekly contact with their general practitioners). Six people in this group spent almost the entire year in treatment. There were no significant differences in mean weight or in the Morgan Russell scale (see glossary, p 1048) global scores among any of the four groups at 1, 2, and 5 years. The proportion of people with a good outcome with inpatient treatment was 5/29 (17%) at 2 years and 9/27 (33%) at 5 years; with outpatient treatment (individual and family therapy) 4/20 (20%) at 2 years and 8/17 (47%) at 5 years; with outpatient group psychotherapy 5/19 (26%) at 2 years and 10/19 (53%) at 5 years; and with assessment interview only 2/20 (10%) at 2 years and 6/19 (32%) at 5 years.

Harms: One person died from anorexia nervosa between the assessment and the start of outpatient group treatment, and one of the people allocated to inpatient treatment died from anorexia nervosa by 5 years.[40,41]

Comment: The systematic review[39] was unable to draw meaningful conclusions from numerous case series because participant characteristics, treatments, mortality, and outcomes varied widely. People admitted for inpatient treatment had a lower mean weight than those treated as outpatients. One subsequent observational study (355 people with anorexia nervosa; 169 of whom had bulimic type anorexia; mean age 25 years; mean duration of illness 5.7 years; 75% available for 2.5 years' follow up) found that benefits of longer intervention were greater in people with longer duration of illness.[42] People with a shorter duration of illness had a higher likelihood of good outcome with briefer inpatient treatment. Median duration of inpatient treatment was 11.6 weeks for anorexia nervosa and 10.6 weeks for bulimia nervosa.

OPTION CISAPRIDE

One small RCT found no significant difference with cisapride versus placebo in weight gain at 8 weeks. Use of cisapride has been restricted in many countries because of concern about cardiac irregularities, including ventricular tachycardia, torsades de pointes, and sudden death.

Benefits: We found no systematic review. We found one small RCT (34 inpatients aged 18–40 years at 2 hospitals; mean duration 2.7 years; body mass index (see glossary, p 1048) 15.1 kg/m^2) comparing cisapride (30 mg) versus placebo for 8 weeks.[43] The trial found no difference in weight gain (5.1 kg with cisapride *v* 5.7 kg with placebo; $P > 0.05$).

Harms: No adverse events were noted in this RCT. The QT interval in anorexia nervosa is prolonged even in the absence of medication. Therefore, cisapride, which may prolong the QT interval, is not recommended in anorexia nervosa. Use of cisapride has been restricted in many countries because of concern about cardiac irregularities, including ventricular tachycardia, torsades de pointes, and sudden death.[31,32]

Comment: Five people withdrew from the RCT and were not included in the analysis.

QUESTION What are the effects of interventions to prevent or treat complications of anorexia nervosa?

OPTION HORMONAL TREATMENT

We found no good evidence about the effects of hormonal treatment on fracture rates in people with anorexia. One small RCT found no significant effect of oestrogen versus no treatment on bone mineral density.

Benefits: We found no systematic review. We found one RCT (48 women, mean age 23.7 years, mean duration of anorexia nervosa 4.0 years) of hormone replacement therapy (conjugated oestrogens 0.625 mg on days 1–25 of each month plus medroxyprogesterone 5 mg on days 16–25) versus an oral contraceptive containing 35 µg ethinyl oestradiol versus no medication over 6 months.[44] All women maintained a calcium intake of 1500 mg using oral calcium carbonate. Spinal bone mineral density was measured at 6 monthly intervals. There was no significant difference in the final bone density at follow up of 0.5–3.0 years.

Harms: Three women withdrew from the oestrogen treatment; two because of adverse effects, and one because she had left the country. One woman who was in the control group was unwilling to return for further testing.

Comment: Improvements in bone mineral density may not reduce fracture risk.

Anorexia nervosa

GLOSSARY

Body mass index Weight (kg) divided by height (m) squared.

Dietary counselling Dieticians with experience of eating disorders discuss diet, mood, and daily behaviours.

Family therapy Treatment that includes members of the family of origin or the constituted family, and that addresses the eating disorder as a problem of family life.

Inpatient treatment This has been regarded as the standard approach to the management of anorexia nervosa.[45] One of the key components of inpatient treatment is refeeding, which is achieved through structured, supervised meals. Psychotherapy (of a variety of different types) and pharmacotherapy are included in many programmes.

Morgan Russell scale A widely used measure of outcome for anorexia nervosa that consists of two scores: an average outcome score and a general outcome score. The average outcome score is based on the outcome in five areas: nutritional status, menstrual function, mental state, sexual adjustment, and socioeconomic status.

Psychotherapy Different types of psychological treatments given individually or in groups are included here. These use psychodynamic, cognitive behavioural, or supportive techniques, or combinations of these.

REFERENCES

1. American Psychiatric Association. *Diagnostic and statistical manual of mental disorders (DSM-IV)*. 4th ed. Washington DC: APA, 1994.
2. Pawluck DE, Gorey KM. Secular trends in the incidence of anorexia nervosa: integrative review of population-based studies. *Int J Eat Disord* 1998;23:347–352.
3. Rastam M, Gillberg C, Garton M. Anorexia nervosa in a Swedish urban region. A population-based study. *Br J Psychiatry* 1989;155:642–646.
4. Strober M, Freeman R, Lampert C, et al. Controlled family study of anorexia nervosa and bulimia nervosa: evidence of shared liability and transmission of partial syndromes. *Am J Psychiatry* 2000;157;393–401.
5. Lilenfeld LR, Kaye WH, Greeno CG, et al. A controlled family study of anorexia nervosa and bulimia nervosa: psychiatric disorders in first-degree relatives and effects of proband comorbidity. *Arch Gen Psychiatry* 1998;55:603–610.
6. Wade TD, Bulik CM, Neale M, et al. Anorexia nervosa and major depression: shared genetic and environmental risk factors. *Am J Psychiatry* 2000;157:469–471.
7. Fairburn CG, Cooper Z, Doll HA, et al. Risk factors for anorexia nervosa: three integrated case-control comparisons. *Arch Gen Psychiatry* 1999;56:468–476.
8. Wentz E, Gillberg C, Gillberg IC, et al. Ten-year follow-up of adolescent-onset anorexia nervosa: psychiatric disorders and overall functioning scales. *J Child Psychol Psychiatry* 2001;42:613–622.
9. Steinhausen, H-C. The course and outcome of anorexia nervosa. In: Brownell K, Fairburn CG, eds. *Eating disorders and obesity: a comprehensive handbook*. New York: Guilford Press, 1995:234–237.
10. Harri, EC, Barraclough B. Excess mortality of mental disorder. *Br J Psychiatry* 1998;173:11–53.
11. Nielsen S, Møller-Madsen S, Isager T, et al. Standardized mortality in eating disorders: a quantitative summary of previously published and new evidence. *J Psychosom Res* 1998;44:413–434.
12. Lucas A, Melton L, Crowson C, et al. Long term fracture risk among women with anorexia nervosa: a population-based cohort study. *Mayo Clin Proc* 1999;74:972–977.
13. Morgan HG, Russell GF. Value of family background and clinical features as predictors of long-term outcome in anorexia nervosa: four-year follow-up study of 41 patients. *Psychol Med* 1975;5:355–371.
14. Cooper Z, Fairburn CG. The Eating Disorders Examination. A semi-structured interview for the assessment of the specific psychopathology of eating disorders. *Int J Eat Disord* 1987;6:1–8.
15. Garner DM. *Eating Disorder Inventory-2 (EDI-2): professional manual*. Odessa FL: Psychological Assessment Resources Inc, 1991.
16. Garner DM, Garfinkel PE. The eating attitudes test: an index of the symptoms of anorexia nervosa. *Psychol Med* 1979;9:273–279.
17. Henderson M, Freeman CPL. A self-rating scale for bulimia: the 'BITE'. *Br J Psychiatry* 1987;150:18–24.
18. Dare C, Eisler I, Russell G, et al. Psychological therapies for adult patients with anorexia nervosa: a randomised controlled trial of outpatient treatments. *Br J Psychiatry* 2001;178:216–221.
19. Hall A, Crisp AH. Brief psychotherapy in the treatment of anorexia nervosa. Outcome at one year. *Br J Psychiatry* 1987;151:185–191.
20. Serfaty MA. Cognitive therapy versus dietary counselling in the outpatient treatment of anorexia nervosa: effects of the treatment phase. *Eur Eat Dis Rev* 1999;7:334–350.
21. Eisler I, Dare C, Hodes M, et al. Family therapy for adolescent anorexia nervosa: the results of a controlled comparison of two family interventions. *J Child Psychol Psychiatry* 2000;41:727–736.
22. Robin AL, Siegel PT, Moye AW, et al. A controlled comparison of family versus individual therapy for adolescents with anorexia nervosa. *J Am Acad Child Adolesc Psychiatry* 1999;38:1482–1489.
23. Wallin U, Kronvall P, Majewski ML. Body awareness therapy in teenage anorexia nervosa: outcome after 2 years. *Eur Eat Dis Rev* 2000;8:19–30.
24. Treasure JL, Todd G, Brolly M, et al. A pilot study of a randomized trial of cognitive analytical therapy

vs educational behavioral therapy for adult anorexia nervosa. *Behav Res Ther* 1995;33:363–367.
25. Russell GFM, Szmukler G, Dare C, et al. An evaluation of family therapy in anorexia nervosa and bulimia nervosa. *Arch Gen Psychiatry* 1987;44:1047–1056.
26. Eisler I, Dare C, Russell GFM, et al. Family and individual therapy in anorexia nervosa. A 5-year follow-up. *Arch Gen Psychiatry* 1997;54:1025–1030.
27. Biederman J, Herzog DB, Rivinus TM, et al. Amitriptyline in the treatment of anorexia nervosa: a double-blind, placebo-controlled study. *J Clin Psychopharmacol* 1985;5:10–16.
28. Halmi KA, Eckert E, LaDu TJ, et al. Anorexia nervosa. Treatment efficacy of cyproheptadine and amitriptyline. *Arch Gen Psychiatry* 1986;43:177–181.
29. Ackerman MJ. The long QT syndrome: ion channel diseases of the heart. *Mayo Clin Proc* 1998;73:250–269.
30. Becker A, Grinspoon SK, Klibanski A, et al. Current concepts: eating disorders. *N Engl J Med* 1999;340:1092–1098.
31. Yap Y, Camm J. Risk of torsades de pointes with non-cardiac drugs: doctors need to be aware that many drugs can cause QT prolongation. *BMJ* 2000;320:1158–1159.
32. Sheridan DJ. Drug-induced proarrhythmic effects: assessment of changes in QT interval. *Br J Clin Pharmacol* 2000;50:297–302.
33. Reilly JG, Ayis SA, Ferrier IN, et al. QTc interval abnormalities and psychotropic drug therapy in psychiatric patients. *Lancet* 2000;355:1048–1052.
34. Attia E, Haiman C, Walsh BT, et al. Does fluoxetine augment the inpatient treatment of anorexia nervosa? *Am J Psychiatry* 1998;155:548–551.
35. Kaye WH, Nagata T, Weltzin TE, et al. Double-blind placebo-controlled administration of fluoxetine in restricting- and restricting-purging-type anorexia nervosa. *Soc Biol Psych* 2001;49:644–652.
36. Birmingham CL, Goldner EM, Bakan R. Controlled trial of zinc supplementation in anorexia nervosa. *Int J Eat Disord* 1994;15:251–255.
37. Vigersky RA, Loriaux L. The effect of cyproheptadine in anorexia nervosa: a double blind trial. In: Vigersky RA, ed. *Anorexia nervosa.* New York: Raven Press, 1977:349–356.
38. Goldberg SC, Halmi KA, Eckert RC, et al. Cyproheptadine in anorexia nervosa. *Br J Psychiatry* 1979;134:67–70.
39. West Midlands Development and Evaluation Service. *In-patient versus out-patient care for eating disorders.* DPHE 1999 Report No 17. Birmingham: University of Birmingham, 1999. Search date 1999; primary sources Medline, Psychlit, The Cochrane Library, variety of internet sites, and hand searches of relevant editions of relevant journals and references from identified articles.
40. Crisp AH, Norton K, Gowers S, et al. A controlled study of the effect of therapies aimed at adolescent and family psychopathology in anorexia nervosa. *Br J Psychiatry* 1991;159:325–333.
41. Gowers S, Norton K, Halek C, et al. Outcome of outpatient psychotherapy in a random allocation treatment study of anorexia nervosa. *Int J Eat Disord* 1994;15:65–177.
42. Kächele H for the study group MZ-ESS. Eine multizentrische Studie zu Aufwand und Erfolg bei psychodynamischer Therapie von Eβstörungen. *Psychother Med Psychol (Stuttg)* 1999;49:100–108.
43. Szmukler GI, Young GP, Miller G, et al. A controlled trial of cisapride in anorexia nervosa. *Int J Eat Disord* 1995;17:347–357.
44. Klibanski A, Biller BMK, Schoenfeld DA, et al. The effects of estrogen administration on trabecular bone loss in young women with anorexia nervosa. *J Clin Endocrinol Metab* 1995;80:898–904.
45. American Psychiatric Association. Practice guideline for the treatment of patients with eating disorders (revision). *Am J Psychiatry* 2000;157(suppl 1):1–39.

Janet Treasure
Psychiatrist
Institute of Psychiatry
Kings College London
London
UK

Ulrike Schmidt
Psychiatrist
South London and Maudsley NHS Trust
London
UK

Competing interests: None declared.

Bipolar disorder

Search date April 2002

John Geddes

QUESTIONS

INTERVENTIONS

See glossary, p 1067

Key Messages

Mania

- **Lithium** One RCT in people with bipolar type I disorder experiencing a manic episode found that lithium increased the proportion of people who responded after 3–4 weeks compared with placebo. One systematic review found that lithium increased the proportion of people who had remission of manic symptoms at 3 weeks compared with chlorpromazine, and found no significant difference in symptoms at 3–6 weeks between lithium and haloperidol, olanzapine, valproate, lamotrigine, or clonazepam. One RCT found that lithium was less effective than risperidone in reducing manic symptoms at 4 weeks.

Lithium can cause a range of adverse effects. The RCTs provided insufficient evidence about how the adverse effects of lithium compared with those of other antipsychotic drugs.

- **Olanzapine** One systematic review in people with bipolar type I disorder found that olanzapine increased the proportion of people who responded at 3–6 weeks compared with placebo, both as monotherapy and as add on therapy to lithium or valproate, and found no significant difference in symptoms at 28 days between olanzapine and lithium. RCTs found that olanzapine was more effective in reducing symptoms than valproate, but was also more likely to cause adverse effects such as sedation and weight gain. The acceptability of olanzapine may be limited by weight gain.
- **Valproate** One systematic review in people with bipolar type I disorder experiencing a manic episode found that valproate increased the proportion of people who responded over 3 weeks compared with placebo. It found no significant difference in response at 1–6 weeks between valproate and lithium, haloperidol, or carbamazepine. It found that valproate was less effective in reducing manic symptoms than olanzapine, but was also less likely to cause adverse effects such as sedation and weight gain.
- **Carbamazepine** RCTs in people with bipolar type I disorder experiencing a manic episode found no significant difference in manic symptoms at 4–6 weeks between carbamazepine and lithium or valproate.
- **Clonazepam** We found no RCTs comparing clonazepam versus placebo in people with bipolar mania. RCTs in people with bipolar type I disorder experiencing a manic episode suggest that clonazepam may be as effective as lithium in improving manic symptoms at 1–4 weeks.
- **Haloperidol** We found no RCTs comparing haloperidol versus placebo in people with bipolar mania. RCTs in people with bipolar type I disorder experiencing a manic episode found no significant difference in manic symptoms at 1–3 weeks between haloperidol and lithium or valproate, although haloperidol was associated with more extrapyramidal adverse effects and sedation than valproate.
- **Risperidone** We found no RCTs comparing risperidone versus placebo in people with bipolar mania. One RCT in people with bipolar type I disorder experiencing a manic episode found that risperidone reduced manic symptoms at 4 weeks compared with lithium. It gave no information on adverse effects.
- **Chlorpromazine** One very small RCT in people with mania found limited evidence that chlorpromazine may improve manic symptoms over 7 weeks more than placebo or imipramine. One systematic review found that fewer people had remission of symptoms at 3 weeks with chlorpromazine than with lithium.
- **Lamotrigine** We found no RCTs comparing lamotrigine versus placebo in people with bipolar mania. One RCT in people with bipolar type I disorder experiencing a manic episode found no significant difference in manic symptoms at 4 weeks between lamotrigine and lithium.

Bipolar depression

- **Lamotrigine** One RCT in people with bipolar type I disorder experiencing a major depressive episode found that lamotrigine increased the proportion of people who responded over 7 weeks compared with placebo.

Bipolar disorder

- **Antidepressants** Systematic reviews found that antidepressants improved depressive symptoms at the end of the trial (unspecified) compared with placebo. They found limited evidence that selective serotonin reuptake inhibitors were more effective than tricyclic antidepressants, and found no significant difference in symptoms between monoamine oxidase inhibitors and tricyclic antidepressants or between selective serotonin reuptake inhibitors and serotonin noradrenaline reuptake inhibitors. The reviews provided insufficient evidence to assess whether antidepressants induce bipolar mania.
- **Carbamazepine; lithium** One systematic review identified no RCTs of sufficient quality to assess these treatments in people with bipolar depression.
- **Psychological treatments; valproate** We found no RCTs of these treatments in people with bipolar depression.

Preventing relapse of mania or bipolar depression

- **Lithium** RCTs have found that lithium reduces relapse over 2 years compared versus placebo, and have found no significant difference in relapse between lithium and valproate, carbamazepine, or lamotrigine.
- **Carbamazepine** We found no RCTs comparing carbamazepine versus placebo in preventing relapse. One systematic review found no significant difference between carbamazepine and lithium in the proportion of people who relapsed over 1–3 years.
- **Education to recognise symptoms of relapse** One RCT found limited evidence that an educational programme to recognise symptoms of relapse reduced manic relapse over 18 months, but that it may increase depressive episodes.
- **Lamotrigine (bipolar depressive episodes)** Three RCTs have found that lamotrigine reduces relapse compared with placebo. However, secondary analyses in two of the RCTs suggested that lamotrigine protected against depressive relapse, but not manic relapse. RCTs have found no significant difference between lamotrigine and lithium in the proportion of people who relapse.
- **Valproate** One RCT found that valproate reduced relapse over 12 months compared with placebo. One systematic review found no significant difference between lithium and valproate in relapse over 12 months.
- **Antidepressant drugs** One systematic review provided insufficient evidence to assess antidepressants in preventing relapse of bipolar disorder.
- **Family focused psychoeducation** One RCT found that 21 sessions of family focused psychoeducation reduced relapse over 12 months compared with two family sessions plus crisis management.

DEFINITION Bipolar disorder (bipolar affective disorder, manic depressive disorder) is characterised by marked mood swings between mania (mood elevation) and bipolar depression that cause significant personal distress or social dysfunction, and are not caused by drugs or known physical disorder. **Bipolar type I disorder** is diagnosed when episodes of depression are interspersed with mania or mixed episodes. **Bipolar type II disorder** is diagnosed when depression is interspersed with less severe episodes of elevated mood that do not lead to dysfunction or disability (hypomania). Bipolar disorder has been subdivided in several further ways (see table 1, p 1069).[1]

INCIDENCE/ PREVALENCE One 1996 cross-national community based study (38 000 people) found lifetime prevalence rates of bipolar disorder ranging from 0.3% in Taiwan to 1.5% in New Zealand.[2] It found that men and women were at similar risk, and that the age at first onset ranged from 19–29 years (average of 6 years earlier than first onset of major depression).

AETIOLOGY/ RISK FACTORS The cause of bipolar disorder is uncertain, although family and twin studies suggest a genetic basis.[3] The lifetime risk of bipolar disorder is increased in first degree relatives of a person with bipolar disorder (40–70% for a monozygotic twin; 5–10% for other first degree relatives). If the first episode of mania occurs in an older adult, it may be secondary mania due to underlying medical or substance induced factors.[4]

PROGNOSIS Bipolar disorder is a recurring illness and one of the leading causes of worldwide disability, especially in the 15–44 year age group.[5] One 4 year inception cohort study (173 people treated for a first episode of mania or mixed affective disorder) found that 93% of people no longer met criteria for mania at 2 years (median time to recover from a syndrome 4.6 weeks), but that only 36% had recovered to premorbid function.[6] It found that 40% of people had a recurrent manic (20%) or depressive (20%) episode within 2 years of recovering from the first episode. A meta-analysis, comparing observed suicide expected rates of suicide in an age and sex matched sample of the general population, found that the lifetime prevalence of suicide was about 2%, or 15 times greater than expected, in people with bipolar disorder.[7]

AIMS OF INTERVENTION To alleviate mania and bipolar depressive symptoms; to prevent relapse (see glossary, p 1067) and suicide; to optimise social and occupational functioning; and to improve quality of life, with minimal adverse effects of treatment.

OUTCOMES Level of symptoms on rating scales (completed by clinician, patient, or both); proportion of people with clinically important response to treatment; time to remission; quality of life scores; social and occupational functioning scores; relapse; hospital admission; rates of suicide; frequency of adverse events; and clinical trial withdrawal rates. Commonly used instruments for assessing symptoms include the Young Mania Rating Scale, which rates 11 manic symptoms with a total score of 0–60; the Schedule for Affective Disorders Change Mania Sub Scale, which rates 18 manic items with a total score of 10–65; and the Hamilton Depression Rating Scale, which has both a 17 and a 21 item version. On these scales, a clinically important response to treatment is usually defined as a > 50% reduction in score from baseline.[8] A person is usually considered to be in remission if, at the end of trial, they score ≤ 12 on the Young Mania Rating Scale and ≤ 8 on the Hamilton Depression Rating Scale.[8] Quality of life is assessed by scales such as the SF-36, and social and occupational functioning on scales such as the Clinical Global Impression Scale.

METHODS *Clinical Evidence* search and appraisal April 2002, including a search for observational studies on adverse effects of treatments. The author also performed a search for systematic reviews in the Cochrane Library, Issue 3, 2003.

QUESTION What are the effects of treatments in mania? New

OPTION LITHIUM

One RCT in people with bipolar type I disorder experiencing a manic episode found that lithium increased the proportion of people who responded after 3–4 weeks compared with placebo. One systematic review found that lithium increased the proportion of people who had remission of manic symptoms at 3 weeks compared with chlorpromazine, and found no significant difference in symptoms at 3–6 weeks between lithium and haloperidol, olanzapine, valproate, lamotrigine, or clonazepam. One RCT found that lithium was less effective than risperidone in reducing manic symptoms at 4 weeks. Lithium can cause a range of adverse effects. The RCTs provided insufficient evidence about how the adverse effects of lithium compared with those of other antipsychotic drugs.

Benefits: **Versus placebo:** We found one systematic review (search date 1999, 1 RCT, 179 people with bipolar type I disorder).[9] The RCT compared three treatments: lithium (36 people); valproate (69 people); and placebo (74 people). It found that lithium significantly increased the proportion of people who responded after 3–4 weeks compared with placebo (response defined as ≥ 50% improvement in mania score on the Schedule for Affective Disorders and Schizophrenia-Change [SADS-C]; 18/36 [50%] with lithium *v* 19/74 [27%] with placebo; RR 1.95, 95% CI 1.17 to 3.23; NNT 5, 95% CI 3 to 20). **Versus chlorpromazine:** We found one systematic review (search date 1999, 4 RCTs, 114 people with bipolar type 1 disorder).[9] It found that lithium significantly increased the proportion of people who had remission of symptoms at 3 weeks compared with chlorpromazine (remission not defined, 3 RCTs that assessed outcomes at 3 weeks: 23/57 [40%] with lithium *v* 7/57 [12%] with chlorpromazine; RR 1.96, 95% CI 1.02 to 3.77; NNT 4, 95% CI 3 to 9). **Versus haloperidol:** We found one systematic review (search date 1999, 2 RCTs, 50 people with bipolar type I disorder).[9] It found no significant difference between haloperidol and lithium in symptom scores at 3 weeks (assessed by the Brief Psychiatric Rating Scale [BPRS]: effect size –2.14, 95% CI –6.57 to +2.30). **Versus risperidone:** We found one systematic review (search date 1999, 1 RCT, 54 people with bipolar type I disorder).[9] It found that risperidone was significantly more effective than lithium in improving symptom severity score at 4 weeks (assessed by BPRS: effect size –2.79, 95% CI –4.22 to –1.36). **Versus olanzapine:** We found no systematic review but found one RCT (30 people with bipolar type I disorder).[10] It found no significant difference between lithium and olanzapine in Young Mania Rating Scale [YMRS] score at 28 days (13.2 with lithium *v* 10.2 with olanzapine; P = 0.315). **Versus valproate:** We found one systematic review (search date 2002, 3 RCTs, 158 people with bipolar type 1 disorder).[8] It found no significant difference between valproate and lithium in the proportion of people who failed to respond over 3–6 weeks (response defined as 50% reduction in mania score on the YMRS or the SADS-C; 45/97 [46%] with valproate *v* 26/61 [43%] with lithium; RR 1.05, 95% CI 0.74 to 1.50). **Versus**

carbamazepine: We found one systematic review (search date 1999, 3 RCTs, 176 people with bipolar type I disorder).[9] The review could not perform a meta-analysis of all three RCTs because of differences in outcomes assessed. The first RCT (105 people) found no significant difference in the proportion of people who responded over 4 weeks between lithium and carbamazepine (15/54 [28%] with lithium *v* 14/51 [27%] with carbamazepine; RR 1.01, 95% CI 0.54 to 1.88). The other two RCTs (71 people) found no significant difference in global severity of symptoms over 4 weeks between lithium and carbamazepine (assessed by Clinical Global Impression [CGI] scores: effect size +0.44, 95% CI –0.78 to +1.67).[9] **Versus lamotrigine:** We found no systematic review but found one RCT (30 people with bipolar type I disorder).[11] It found no significant difference between lithium and lamotrigine in YMRS scores at 4 weeks (mean 13.2 with lithium *v* 14.3 with lamotrigine; reported as non-significant; no further data reported). **Versus clonazepam:** We found one systematic review (search date 1999, 2 RCTs, 52 people with bipolar type I disorder).[9] The review could not perform a meta-analysis because the RCTs assessed different outcomes. The first RCT (12 people) found limited evidence that clonezepam improved some measures of mania more than lithium after 10 days treatment (mean motor activity score 1.8 with clonazepam *v* 2.8 with lithium; mean logorrhoea score 2.2 with clonazepam *v* 2.9 with lithium; CI not reported). The second RCT (40 people, unblinded) found no significant difference between lithium and clonezepam in symptom severity at 4 weeks assessed by BPRS (mean score 6.27 with lithium *v* 7.79 with clonazepam) or global severity of symptoms assessed by CGI Scale (mean score 2.07 with lithium *v* 1.68 with clonazepam; reported as non-significant, CI not reported) after 4 weeks.

Harms: **Versus placebo:** The RCT identified by the review found that lithium significantly increased the proportion of people who had adverse effects compared with placebo (33/36 [92%] with lithium *v* 58/74 [78%] with placebo; RR 1.17, 95% CI 1.00 to 1.37; NNH 8, 95% CI 4 to 334).[9] Adverse effects were not specified. **Versus chlorpromazine:** The review gave no information on adverse effects.[9] **Versus haloperidol:** The review gave no information on adverse effects.[9] **Versus risperidone:** The review gave no information on adverse effects.[9] **Versus olanzapine:** The RCT found no extrapyramidal adverse effects associated with lithium or olanzapine.[10] **Versus valproate:** The review found that valproate significantly reduced the proportion of people who had fever compared with lithium (1 RCT 1/69 [1%] with valproate *v* 5/36 [14%] with lithium; RR 0.10, 95% CI 0.01 to 0.86), but found no significant difference in the rates of other adverse events.[8] **Versus carbamazepine:** The review found no significant difference in adverse effects between lithium and carbamazepine (2 RCTs: 27/73 [37%] with lithium *v* 35/66 [53%] with carbamazepine; RR 0.71, 95% CI 0.49 to 1.02).[9] **Versus lamotrigine:** The RCT found no significant difference in adverse effects between lithium and lamotrigine, but it is likely to have been too small to detect a clinically important difference.[11] One person taking lithium withdrew because of a seizure and one person taking lamotrigine withdrew because of aggravation of diabetes. **Versus clonazepam:** The review gave no information on adverse effects.[9]

Comment: None.

OPTION VALPROATE

One systematic review in people with bipolar type I disorder experiencing a manic episode found that valproate increased the proportion of people who responded over 3 weeks compared with placebo. It found no significant difference in response at 1–6 weeks between valproate and lithium, haloperidol, or carbamazepine. It found that valproate was less effective in reducing manic symptoms than olanzapine, but was also less likely to cause adverse effects such as sedation and weight gain.

Benefits: **Versus placebo:** We found one systematic review (search date 2002, 3 RCTs, 316 people with bipolar type I disorder).[8] It found that valproate significantly increased the proportion of people who responded over 3 weeks compared with placebo (response defined as 50% reduction in mania score on the Young Mania Rating Scale [YMRS] or the Schedule for Affective Disorders and Schizophrenia-Change [SADS-C]; proportion of people who failed to respond: 66/155 [42%] with valproate *v* 111/161 [69%] with placebo; RR of failing to respond 0.62, 95% CI 0.51 to 0.77).[8] **Versus lithium:** See benefits of lithium, p 1054. **Versus haloperidol:** We found one systematic review (search date 2002, 1 RCT, 36 people with bipolar type I disorder).[8] The RCT found no significant difference in the proportion of patients who failed to respond over 6 days between valproate and haloperidol (11/21 [52%] with valproate *v* 10/15 [67%] with lithium; RR 0.79, 95% CI 0.46 to 1.35). **Versus olanzapine:** We found one systematic review (search date 2002, 2 RCTs, 363 people with bipolar type I disorder).[8] It found that people taking olanzapine had greater symptom reductions at the end of the trial (unspecified) than those taking valproate (symptoms assessed by the YMRS: WMD 2.81, 95% CI 0.83 to 4.79). One of the RCTs (251 people) found that olanzapine significantly increased the proportion of people who responded at the end of the trial (unspecified) compared with valproate (response defined as 50% reduction in YMRS; proportion of people who failed to respond: 77/123 [63%] with valproate *v* 57/125 [46%] with olanzapine; RR of failing to respond 1.27, 95% CI 0.99 to 1.62). **Versus carbamazepine:** We found one systematic review (2 RCTs, 59 people with bipolar type I disorder), which found no significant difference between valproate and carbamazepine in the proportion of people who failed to respond at 4–6 weeks (response defined with 50% reduction in mania score on the YMRS or the SADS-C; 11/30 [37%] with valproate *v* 16/29 [55%] carbamazepine; RR 0.66, 95% CI 0.38 to 1.16).[8]

Harms: **Versus placebo:** The review found no significant difference between valproate and placebo in the proportion of people who withdrew from the trial because of adverse effects (9/158 [6%] with valproate v 5/163 [3%] with placebo; RR 1.95, 95% CI 0.66 to 5.71), but found that people taking valproate were significantly more likely to suffer from dizziness (13/138 [9%] with valproate v 4/141 [3%] with placebo; RR 3.17, 95% CI 1.13 to 8.88).[8] No other adverse effects were more commonly reported with valproate than with placebo. **Versus lithium:** See harms of lithium, p 1055. **Versus haloperidol:** The RCT found that valproate caused significantly fewer extrapyramidal adverse effects compared with haloperidol (0/21 [0%] with valproate v 8/15 [53%] with haloperidol; RR 0.04, 95% CI 0.00 to 0.69), dry mouth (1/21 [5%] with valproate v 3/15 [20%] with haloperidol; RR 0.24, 95% CI 0.03 to 2.07), and was less likely to cause sedation than haloperidol (1/21 [5%] with valproate v 4/15 [27%] with haloperidol; RR 0.18, 95% CI 0.02 to 1.44).[8] **Versus olanzapine:** The review found no significant difference between valproate and olanzapine in the proportion of patients who withdrew because of adverse events (1 RCT: 9/126 [7%] with valproate v 12/125 [10%] with olanzapine; RR 0.74, 95% CI 0.33 to 1.70) or had movement disorders (akathisia: WMD –0.02, 95% CI –0.27 to +0.23; abnormal involuntary movement: WMD –0.17, 95% CI –0.62 to +0.28).[8] It found that valproate caused significantly more nausea than olanzapine (1 RCT: 36/126 [28%] with valproate v 13/125 [10%] with olanzapine; RR 2.75, 95% CI 1.53 to 4.93), but caused less increased appetite (1 RCT: 3/126 [2%] with valproate v 15/125 [12%] with olanzapine; RR 0.20, 95% CI 0.06 to 0.67), weight gain (WMD –2.14 kg, 95% CI –2.65 kg to –1.62 kg), dry mouth (8/126 [6%] with valproate v 42/125 [34%] with olanzapine; RR 0.19, 95% CI 0.09 to 0.39), and sedation (2 RCTs: 44/189 [23%] with valproate v 76/182 [42%] with olanzapine; RR 0.55, 95% CI 0.41 to 0.76). **Versus carbamazepine:** One RCT (28 people) assessed adverse effects.[8] It found no significant difference in adverse effects between valproate and carbamazepine, but it is likely to have been underpowered to detect a clinically important difference.

Comment: None.

OPTION CHLORPROMAZINE

One very small RCT in people with mania found limited evidence that chlorpromazine may improve manic symptoms over 7 weeks compared with placebo or imipramine. One systematic review found that fewer people had remission of symptoms at 3 weeks with chlorpromazine than with lithium.

Benefits: **Versus placebo:** We found one non-systematic review, which identified one very small RCT (13 people with mania) comparing three treatments: chlorpromazine, imipramine, and placebo.[12] It found that chlorpromazine significantly improved global outcome at 7 weeks compared with imipramine or placebo (assessed on a scale from –9 to +9 where +9 = improvement: +6.1 with chlorpromazine v +2.0 with imipramine v –2.8 with placebo; reported as significant; no further data reported). **Versus lithium:** See benefits of lithium, p 1054.

Harms: **Versus placebo:** The non-systematic review gave no information on adverse effects.[12] **Versus lithium:** See harms of lithium, p 1055.

Comment: The evidence for older antipsychotic drugs is sparse and there are currently no systematic reviews available. The drugs are, however, widely used in mania.

OPTION HALOPERIDOL

We found no RCTs comparing haloperidol versus placebo in people with bipolar mania. RCTs in people with bipolar type I disorder experiencing a manic episode found no significant difference in manic symptoms at 1–3 weeks between haloperidol and lithium or valproate, although haloperidol was associated with more extrapyramidal adverse effects and sedation than valproate.

Benefits: **Versus placebo:** We found no systematic review and no RCTs comparing haloperidol versus placebo. **Versus lithium:** See benefits of lithium, p 1054. **Versus valproate:** See benefits of valproate, p 1056.

Harms: **Versus placebo:** We found no RCTs. **Versus lithium:** See harms of lithium, p 1055. **Versus valproate:** See harms of valproate, p 1056.

Comment: The evidence for older antipsychotics is sparse and there are currently no systematic reviews available. The drugs are, however, widely used in bipolar mania.

OPTION RISPERIDONE

We found no RCTs comparing risperidone versus placebo in people with bipolar mania. One RCT in people with bipolar type I disorder experiencing a manic episode found that risperidone reduced manic symptoms at 4 weeks compared with lithium. It gave no information on adverse effects.

Benefits: **Versus placebo:** We found no systematic review and no RCTs. **Versus lithium:** See benefits of lithium, p 1054.

Harms: **Versus placebo:** We found no RCTs. **Versus lithium:** See harms of lithium, p 1055.

Comment: None.

OPTION OLANZAPINE

One systematic review in people with bipolar type I disorder found that olanzapine increased the proportion of people who responded at 3–6 weeks compared with placebo, both as monotherapy and as add on therapy to lithium or valproate, and found no significant difference in symptoms at 28 days between olanzapine and lithium. RCTs found that olanzapine was more effective in reducing symptoms than valproate, but was also more likely to cause adverse effects such as sedation and weight gain. The acceptability of olanzapine may be limited by weight gain.

Benefits: **Versus placebo:** We found one systematic review (search date 2002, 6 RCTs, 1422 people with bipolar type I disorder).[13] It found that olanzapine significantly increased the proportion of people who responded over 3–4 weeks compared with placebo (response defined as 50% reduction in mania score on the Young Mania Rating Scale; 2 RCTs: proportion who failed to respond 56/125 [45%] with olanzapine *v* 89/129 [69%] with placebo; RR of failing to respond 0.64, 95% CI 0.52 to 0.81). It also found that adding olanzapine to lithium or valproate significantly increased the proportion of people who responded at 6 weeks compared with placebo (1 RCT; proportion who failed to respond: 80/229 [35%] with olanzapine *v* 64/115 [56%] with placebo; RR of failing to respond 0.63, 95% CI 0.49 to 0.80). **Versus lithium:** See benefits of lithium, p 1054. **Versus valproate:** See benefits of valproate, p 1056.

Harms: The review found that olanzapine, both as monotherapy and as add-on therapy to lithium or valproate, caused significantly more weight gain than placebo (3 RCTs, 581 people: WMD 2.27 kg, 95% CI 1.56 kg to 2.99 kg).[13] It found no significant difference in movement disorders between olanzapine and placebo (measured on the Barnes Akathisia Scale; 2 RCTs, 246 people: WMD –0.13, 95% CI –0.32 to +0.06), but found that olanzapine significantly increased somnolence (162/354 [46%] with olanzapine *v* 48/244 [20%] with placebo; RR 2.13, 95% CI 1.62 to 2.79), dry mouth (100/354 [28%] *v* 18/244 [7%]; RR 3.64, 95% CI 2.24 to 5.91), dizziness (54/354 [15%] *v* 16/244 [6%]; RR 2.37, 95% CI 1.39 to 4.04), muscle weakness (61/354 [17%] *v* 23/244 [9%]; RR 1.69, 95% CI 1.09 to 2.64), increased appetite (54/229 [23%] *v* 9/115 [8%]; RR 3.01, 95% CI 1.54 to 5.88), and speech disorder (15/229 [6%] with olanzapine *v* 1/115 [0.9%] with placebo; RR 7.53, 95% CI 1.01 to 56.32).**Versus lithium:** See harms of lithium, p 1055. **Versus valproate:** See harms of valproate, p 1056.

Comment: None.

OPTION CARBAMAZEPINE

RCTs in people with bipolar type I disorder experiencing a manic episode found no significant difference in manic symptoms at 4–6 weeks between carbamazepine and lithium or valproate.

Benefits: **Versus placebo:** We found no RCTs. **Versus lithium:** See benefits of lithium, p 1054. **Versus valproate:** See benefits of valproate, p 1056.

Harms: **Versus placebo:** We found no RCTs. **Versus lithium:** See harms of lithium, p 1055. **Versus valproate:** See harms of valproate, p 1056.

Comment: None.

OPTION LAMOTRIGINE

We found no RCTs comparing lamotrigine versus placebo in people with bipolar mania. One RCT in people with bipolar type I disorder experiencing a manic episode found no significant difference in manic symptoms at 4 weeks between lamotrigine and lithium.

Benefits: **Versus placebo:** We found no systematic review or RCTs comparing lamotrigine versus placebo in people with bipolar mania. **Versus lithium:** See benefits of lithium, p 1054.

Harms: **Versus placebo:** We found no RCTs. **Versus lithium:** See harms of lithium, p 1055.

Comment: None.

OPTION CLONAZEPAM

We found no RCTs comparing clonazepam versus placebo in people with bipolar mania. RCTs in people with bipolar type I disorder experiencing a manic episode suggest that clonazepam may be as effective as lithium in improving manic symptoms at 1–4 weeks.

Benefits: **Versus placebo:** We found no systematic review or RCTs comparing clonazepam versus placebo in people with bipolar mania. **Versus lithium:** See harms of lithium, p 1055.

Harms: **Versus placebo:** We found no RCTs. **Versus lithium:** See harms of lithium, p 1055.

Comment: None.

QUESTION What are the effects of treatments in bipolar depression? New

OPTION PSYCHOLOGICAL TREATMENTS

We found no RCTs of psychological treatments in people with bipolar depression.

Benefits: We found no systematic review or RCTs in people with bipolar depression (see comment below).

Harms: We found no RCTs.

Comment: We found no RCTs of psychological interventions in bipolar depression. It is unclear if it is reasonable to extrapolate from the evidence for treatments for unipolar depression. It is likely that specific interventions will have some effect, but RCTs are needed to estimate the size of any benefits and harms of these treatments. (See depressive disorders in adults, p 1121.)

OPTION ANTIDEPRESSANTS

Systematic reviews found that antidepressants improved depressive symptoms at the end of the trial (unspecified) compared with placebo. They found limited evidence that selective serotonin reupdate inhibitors were more effective that tricyclic antidepressants, and found no significant difference in symptoms between monoamine oxidase inhibitors and tricyclic antidepressants or between selective serotonin reuptake inhibitors and serotonin noradrenaline reuptake inhibitors. The reviews provided insufficient evidence to assess whether antidepressants induce bipolar mania.

Benefits: We found two systematic reviews of antipressents in people with bipolar depression or mixed unipolar/bipolar depression.[14,15] **Versus placebo:** The first review (search date not reported, 12 RCTs; 732 people with depressive disorder or mixed episode disorder with at least one previous episode of mania), published only as an abstract, found that people taking antidepressants (tricyclic antidepressants [TCAs], selective serotonin reuptake inhibitors [SSRIs], selective noradrenaline reuptake inhibitors [SNRIs], or monoamine oxidase inhibitors [MAOIs]) were significantly less likely to fail to respond to treatment at the end of the trial (unspecified) than people taking placebo (302 people: 87/180 [48%] *v* 92/122 [75%]; OR 0.30, 95% CI 0.18 to 0.48; NNT 4, 95% CI 3 to 7).[14] **Versus each other:** The first review found no significant difference between SSRIs and TCAs in the proportion of people who responded to treatment at the end of the trial (unspecified), although people taking SSRIs were less likely to fail to respond (31/65 [48%] *v* 44/69 [64%]; OR 0.53, 95% CI 0.27 to 1.04).[14] It also found no significant difference in the proportion of people who responded at the end of the trial (unspecified) between MAOIs and TCAs (54/109 [49%] *v* 54/103 [52%]; OR 0.89, 95% CI 0.52 to 1.52) or between SSRIs and SNRIs (19/34 [56%] *v* 21/35 [60%]; OR 0.85, 95% CI 0.33 to 2.17). The second review (search date 2000; 6 RCTs; 422 people with bipolar depression, 190 people with unipolar depression, about 25% taking lithium, carbamazepine, or valproate) also found similar responses to treatment among antidepressants, but did not quantify its conclusions.[15] **Versus adding lithium or valproate:** We found one small RCT (27 people with mania or bipolar depression receiving lithium or valproate), which compared the addition of paroxetine versus the addition of a second dose of lithium or valproate. It found no significant difference between groups in depressive or manic symptoms over 6 weeks (results presented graphically).[16]

Harms: **Versus each other:** The first review found that SSRIs were significantly less likely to induce mania than TCAs (OR 0.14, 95% CI 0.02 to 0.81).[14] The second review also concluded that tricyclic drugs were more likely to induce mania than other antidepressants, but did not quantify its conclusions.[15]

Comment: A systematic review of antidepressants in bipolar depression is in progress.[17] The evidence for treatment of unipolar depression (see depressive disorders in adults, p 1121) is believed to be applicable, although the efficacy of the treatments may be different, and specific adverse effects such as antidepressant induced mania should be considered.

OPTION LITHIUM

One systematic review identified no RCTs of sufficient quality to assess lithium in people with bipolar depression.

Benefits: We found one systematic review (search date 2000), which identified no RCTs of sufficient quality in people with bipolar depression (see comment below).[15]

Harms: We found no good RCTs.

Comment: The review identified one crossover trial in people with depression (52 people, 40 with bipolar depression).[15] Participants were randomised to 2 weeks of lithium and then crossed over to 6 days of placebo. The trial found that lithium improved symptoms in 32/40 (80%) people over 2 weeks, and that 12/32 (38%) of these relapsed when taking placebo. It found limited evidence that lithium did not induce more manic switching (see glossary, p 1067) than placebo in bipolar depression.[15]

OPTION CARBAMAZEPINE

One systematic review identified no RCTs of sufficient quality to assess carbamazepine in people with bipolar depression.

Benefits: We found one systematic review (search date 2000), which identified no RCTs of sufficient quality in people with bipolar depression (see comment below).[15]

Harms: We found no good RCTs.

Comment: The review identified one crossover trial in people with depression (35 people, 24 with bipolar depression).[15] Participants were randomised to placebo before and after being crossed over to carbamazepine over 45 days. The trial found that carbamazepine improved symptoms in 62% of people over a mean 45 days. It found limited evidence that lithium did not induce more manic switching (see glossary, p 1067) than placebo in bipolar depression.

OPTION VALPROATE

We found no RCTs of valproate in people with bipolar depression.

Benefits: We found no systematic review or RCTs of valproate in people with bipolar depression.

Harms: We found no RCTs.

Comment: None.

OPTION LAMOTRIGINE

One RCT in people with bipolar type I disorder experiencing a depressive episode found that lamotrigine increased the proportion of people who responded over 7 weeks compared with placebo.

Benefits: We found one systematic review (search date 2000),[15] which identified one RCT (195 people aged 19–75 years with bipolar type 1 disorder experiencing a major depressive episode).[18] The RCT compared three treatments: lamotrigine 200 mg daily, lamotrigine 50 mg daily, and placebo.[18] It found no significant difference between lamotrigine and placebo in Hamilton Depression Rating Scale score over 7 weeks, but found that lamotrigine 200 mg daily significantly improved Mongometry–Asberg Depression Rating Scale score (mean reduction −13.3 with lamotrigine *v* −7.8 with placebo; $P < 0.05$) and increased the proportion of people who responded to treatment (measured by Clinical Global Impression Scale scores: mean change 2.6 with lamotrigine *v* 3.3 with placebo; $P < 0.05$).

Harms: The RCT found that significantly more people had headache with lamotrigine compared with placebo (20/63 [32%] with lamotrigine 200 mg v 11/65 [17%]; $P < 0.05$).[18]

Comment: None.

QUESTION What are the effects of interventions to prevent relapse of mania or bipolar depression? New

OPTION PSYCHOLOGICAL TREATMENTS

One RCT found limited evidence that an educational programme to recognise symptoms of relapse reduced manic relapse over 18 months, but that it may increase depressive episodes. Another RCT found that 21 sessions of family focused psychoeducation reduced relapse over 12 months compared with two family sessions plus crisis management.

Benefits: **Education to recognise symptoms of relapse:** We found one RCT (69 outpatients with bipolar disorder who had relapsed in the previous year) comparing an educational programme to recognise symptoms of relapse (see glossary, p 1067) versus treatment as usual over 18 months.[19] It found that people in the educational programme were significantly less likely to suffer a manic relapse over 18 months compared with people receiving usual care (9/33 [27%] with educational programme v 20/35 [57%] with usual care; RR 0.48, 95% CI 0.25 to 0.86; NNT 4; 95% CI 2 to 16), but may have been more likely to suffer from a depressive episode (18/33 [55%] with educational programme v 13/35 [37%] with usual care; RR 1.47, 95% CI 0.87 to 2.54), although the difference was not significant. It found that, compared with usual care, the educational programme significantly improved social function from baseline at 18 months (measured on a 4 point scale assessing 8 areas of social activity where 0 is fair/good performance and 4 inability to carry out function; mean difference in score 1.97, 95% CI 0.71 to 3.23).[19] **Family focused psychoeducation:** We found one RCT (101 people with bipolar disorder who had recently recovered from an acute episode recruited from inpatient and outpatient facilities, all taking antipsychotic drugs) comparing 21 sessions of family focused pyschoeducation versus two family sessions plus crisis management over 12 months.[20] Family focused psychoeducation involved education about the symptoms, causes and treatment of bipolar disorder, education to recognise symptoms of relapse, preparation of a relapse prevention plan, and training in problem solving and communication skills. Crisis management involved emergency counselling sessions as needed, with a minimum of a monthly telephone call. The RCT found that family focused psychoeducation significantly reduced the proportion of people who relapsed over 12 months compared with family session plus crisis management (HR 1.47, CI not reported; P = 0.42).

Harms: **Education to recognise symptoms of relapse:** The RCT found that, compared with usual care, education may increase depressive relapse; (see benefits above). **Family focused psychoeducation:** The RCT gave no information on harms.[20]

Comment: None.

OPTION **LITHIUM**

RCTs have found that lithium reduces relapse over 2 years compared with placebo, and have found no significant difference in relapse between lithium and valproate, carbamazepine, or lamotrigine.

Benefits: **Versus placebo:** We found three systematic reviews in people with bipolar disorder, unipolar disorder, or mixed unipolar/bipolar disorder,[21–23] and two subsequent RCTs.[24,25] The first review (search date not reported, 9 RCTs, 825 people with bipolar or unipolar disorder) found that lithium reduced the risk of relapse (see glossary, p 1067) by 41% at up to 2 years compared with placebo (3 RCTs, 412 people with bipolar disorder: relapse as defined in the trial [including hospital admission or requiring additional medication]; 73/202 [36%] with lithium *v* 128/210 [61%] with placebo; RR 0.59, 95% CI 0.48 to 0.73).[21] The review found no significant difference between lithium and placebo in the proportion of people with bipolar or unipolar disorder who committed suicide, but it is likely to have been underpowered to detect a clinically important difference (4 RCTs, 0/186 [0%] *v* 2/189 [1%]; RR 0.32, 95% CI 0.03 to 2.98). The second review (search date not reported, 15 RCTs, including 8 identified by the first review, 558 people with bipolar disorder) found that, in people with bipolar disorder, there was an average 48% decrease in the absolute risk of relapse by the end of the trial (unspecified) with lithium compared with placebo.[22] The third review (search date 2000, 3 RCTs identified by the first review, 19 observational studies) assessed the effect of long term lithium treatment on suicide rates.[23] It found that people with bipolar or unipolar disorder treated with lithium had lower suicide rates compared with untreated people (159 *v* 876 deaths per 100 000 patient years of treatment; RR 8.85, 95% CI 4.12 to 19.1). Two subsequent RCTs (647 people aged 18 years or over with bipolar type I or type II disorder who had recently recovered from a manic or depressive/hypomanic episode and remained stable after an 8–16 week run in, during which they began taking lamotrigine and withdrew other psychotropic drugs), compared three treatments: lithium, lamotrigine, and placebo over 76 weeks.[24,25] Both RCTs found that, compared with placebo, lithium significantly increased the time to requirement of additional intervention for a manic or a depressive episode (median time to additional medication 24–42 weeks with lithium *v* 12–13 weeks with placebo: P = 0.05 in both RCTs). Secondary analyses in the RCTs suggested that lithium protected against manic but not depressive relapse. **Versus valproate:** We found one systematic review (search date not reported), which identified one RCT (372 people) comparing three treatments: lithium, valproate, and placebo.[26] It found no significant difference between lithium and valproate in relapse at 12 months (relapse defined as withdrawal due to episode of bipolar disorder; 12/187 [6%] *v* 9/91 [10%]; RR 0.8, 95% CI 0.5 to 1.2), but it is likely to have been too small to detect a clinically important difference. **Versus carbamazepine:** We found one systematic review (search date not reported, 10 RCTs, 572 people with unipolar or bipolar disorder) comparing lithium versus carbamazepine.[22] It found no significant difference between lithium and carbamazepine in the proportion of people who relapsed over 1–3 years (60% with lithium *v* 55% with carbamazepine; reported as non-significant; no further data reported; see comment below). **Versus lamotrigine:** We found no systematic review but found two RCTs comparing three treatments: lithium, lamotrigine, and placebo.[24,25] Both RCTs (647 people with bipolar type I or type II disorder who had recently recovered from a manic or depressive/hypomanic episode and remained stable after an 8–16 week run in, during which they began taking lamotrigine and withdrew other psychotropic drugs) found no significant difference between lithium and lamotrigine in the time to requirement of additional intervention for a mood episode (median time to additional medication 24–42 weeks with lithium *v* 20–29 weeks with lamotrigine: $P > 0.05$ in both RCTs). Secondary analysis in one of the RCTs suggested that lithium may significantly reduce manic relapse compared with lamotrigine ($P = 0.092$).[25]

Harms: **Versus placebo:** The first review found that significantly more people had overall adverse effects (not specified) with lithium than with placebo (160/233 [69%] with lithium *v* 112/225 [50%] with placebo; RR 1.4, 95% CI 1.2 to 1.6), and that lithium may increase hypothyroidism (7/158 [4%] with lithium *v* 0/152 [0%] with lithium; RR 5.1, 95% CI 0.9 to 27.7).[21] **Versus valproate:** The review found that valproate was significantly more likely than lithium to cause sedation (1 RCT: 78/187 [42%] with valproate *v* 24/91 [26%] with lithium; RR 1.6, 95% CI 1.1 to 2.3) and infection (1 RCT: 51/187 [27%] with valproate *v* 12/91 [13%] with lithium; RR 2.1, 95% CI 1.2 to 3.7), but significantly less likely to cause polyuria (15/187 [8%] with valproate *v* 17/91 [19%] with lithium; RR 0.4, 95% CI 0.2 to 0.8), thirst (11/187 [6%] with valproate *v* 14/91 [15%]; RR 0.4, 95% CI 0.2 to 0.8), and possibly diarrhoea (65/187 [35%] with valproate *v* 42/91 [46%] with lithium; RR 0.75, 95% 0.6 to 1.0).[26] **Versus carbamazepine:** The review gave no information on adverse effects.[22] One RCT (144 people with bipolar disorder) identified by the review found that, although more people taking carbamazepine than taking lithium withdrew from the trials (9/70 [13%] with carbamazepine *v* 4/74 [5%] with lithium; reported as non-significant; no further data reported), a significantly higher proportion of people taking lithium compared with carbamazepine had "slight or moderate" adverse effects over 2.5 years (61% *v* 21%; $P < 0.001$).[27] **Versus lamotrigine:** The first RCT found that lithium caused significantly fewer headaches than lamotrigine (4% *v* 20%; $P = 0.02$) but more diarrhoea (28% *v* 5%, $P = 0.002$).[24] The second RCT gave no information on adverse effects.[25]

Comment: **Versus carbamazepine:** The results of the review should be interpreted with caution as it combined trials of unipolar and bipolar disorder.[22]

OPTION VALPROATE

One RCT found that valproate reduced relapse over 12 months compared with placebo. One systematic review found no significant difference between lithium and valproate in relapse over 12 months.

Benefits: **Versus placebo:** We found one systematic review (search date not reported, 1 RCT, 372 people with bipolar disorder) comparing three treatments: valproate, lithium, and placebo.[26] It found that lithium significantly reduced relapse (see glossary, p 1067) over 12 months compared with placebo (relapse defined as withdrawal because of an episode of bipolar disorder; 45/187 [24%] with valproate *v* 36/94 [38%] with placebo; RR 0.6, 95% CI 0.4 to 0.9), but found no significant difference in time to relapse (P = 0.33; no further data reported). **Versus lithium:** See benefits of lithium, p 1064.

Harms: **Versus placebo:** The review found that valproate was significantly more likely than placebo to cause tremor (RR 3.2, 95% CI 1.9 to 5.6); weight gain (RR 2.9, 95% 1.3 to 6.2); alopecia (RR 2.4, 95% CI 1.1 to 5.7), and nausea (RR 1.37, 95% CI 1.0 to 1.9).[26] **Versus lithium:** See harms of lithium, p 1065.

Comment: None.

OPTION CARBAMAZEPINE

We found no RCTs comparing carbamazepine versus placebo in preventing relapse, but one systematic review found no significant difference between carbamazepine and lithium in the proportion of people who relapsed over 1–3 years.

Benefits: **Versus placebo:** We found no systematic review or RCTs comparing carbamazepine versus placebo in preventing relapse (see glossary, p 1067). **Versus lithium:** See benefits of lithium, p 1064.

Harms: **Versus placebo:** We found no RCTs. **Versus lithium:** See benefits of lithium, p 1064.

Comment: A systematic review of the effects of carbamazepine in preventing relapse is in progress.[28]

OPTION LAMOTRIGINE

Three RCTs have found that lamotrigine reduces relapse compared with placebo. However, secondary analyses in two of the RCTs suggested that lamotrigine protected against depressive relapse, but not manic relapse. RCTs have found no significant difference between lamotrigine and lithium in the proportion of people who relapse.

Benefits: **Versus placebo:** We found no systematic review but found three RCTs.[24,25,29] Two RCTs (647 people aged 18 years or over with bipolar type I or type II disorder who had recently recovered from a manic episode or depressive/hypomanic episode and remained stable after 8–16 weeks during which they began taking lamotrigine and withdrew other psychotropic drugs) compared three treatments over 76 weeks: lamotrigine, lithium, and placebo (see comment below).[24,25] Both RCTs found that, compared with placebo, lamotrigine significantly increased the time to requiring additional medication for a manic or bipolar depressive episode (median time to additional medication 20–29 weeks with lamotrigine *v* 12–13 weeks with placebo; P = 0.05 in both RCTs). Secondary analyses suggested that lamotrigine reduced depressive but not manic relapse (see glossary, p 1067).[24,25] The third RCT (182 people with rapid cycling bipolar disorder (see table 1, p 1069) found no significant difference between lamotrigine and placebo in the time to requiring additional medication (P = 0.177, results presented graphically).[29] **Versus lithium** See benefits of lithium, p 1064.

Harms: **Versus placebo:** The RCTs gave no information on adverse effects.[24,25] The third RCT found no significant difference between lamotrigine and placebo in the proportion of people who had adverse effects, including nausea and headache (67% with lamotrigine *v* 68% with placebo, reported as non-significant, CI not reported).[29] **Versus lithium** See benefits of lithium, p 1064.

Comment: The first RCT is published only as an abstract.[24]

OPTION ANTIDEPRESSANTS

One systematic review provided insufficient evidence to assess antidepressants in preventing relapse of bipolar disorder.

Benefits: We found one systematic review (search date 2000; 4 RCTs, 258 people with bipolar type I or type II disorder) comparing tricyclic antidepressants with placebo or lithium.[30] The review did not perform a meta-analysis. It provided a narrative overview of the studies and found no clear evidence that tricyclic antidepressants reduce relapse (see glossary, p 1067) over 1–2 years compared with placebo. It suggested that tricyclic antidepressants may be less effective in preventing relapse over 1–2 years than lithium.

Harms: The review suggested that antidepressants may induce mood instability or manic episodes.[30]

Comment: None.

GLOSSARY

Manic switching involves onset of a manic episode shortly after treatment for a depressive episode. It may be more likely after treatment with antidepressants.

Relapse A return of symptoms to the extent that the disorder again meets criteria for the full syndromes. In practice, patients with bipolar disorder learn to recognise early warning signs and begin treatment before criteria are met. For this reason, relapse is often pragmatically defined as the need for drug treatment due to re-emergence of depressive or manic symptoms.

REFERENCES

1. American Psychiatric Association. *Diagnostic and statistical manual of mental disorders,* 4th ed. Washington, D.C.: American Psychiatric Association, 1994.
2. Weissman MM, Bland RC, Canino GJ, et al. Cross-national epidemiology of major depression and bipolar disorder. *JAMA* 1996;276:293–299.
3. Müller-Oerlinghausen B, Berghöfer A, Bauer M. Bipolar disorder. *Lancet* 2002;359:241–247.
4. Tohen M, Shulman KI, Satlin A. First-episode mania in late life. *Am J Psychiatry* 1994;151:130–132.
5. Murray CJ, Lopez AD. Global mortality, disability, and the contribution of risk factors: Global Burden of Disease Study. *Lancet* 1997;349:1436–1442.
6. Tohen M, Hennen J, Zarate C, et al. Harvard first episodes project: predictors of recovery and relapse. *Bipolar Disord* 2002;4(suppl 1):135–136.
7. Harris EC, Barraclough B. Suicide as an outcome for mental disorders. A meta-analysis. *Br J Psychiatry* 1997;170:205–208.
8. Macritchie K, Geddes JR, Scott J, et al. Valproate for acute affective episodes in bipolar disorder. In: The Cochrane Library, Issue 3, 2003. Oxford: Update Software. Search date 2002; primary sources Cochrane Collaboration Depression, Anxiety and Neurosis Review Group Controlled Trials Register, Cochrane Controlled Trials Register and hand searches of reference lists of relevant papers and textbooks and personal contact with authors of trials, experts and pharmaceutical companies.
9. Poolsup N, Li Wan Po A, de Oliveira IR. Systematic overview of lithium treatment in acute mania. *J Clin Pharm Ther* 2000;25:139–156. Search date 1999; primary sources Medline, Embase, Science Citation Index, the Cochrane Library and hand searches of reference lists of identified RCTs and reviews.
10. Berk M, Ichim M, Brook S. Olanzapine compared to lithium in mania: a double-blind randomized controlled trial. *Int Clin Psychopharmacol* 1999;14:339–343.
11. Ichim L, Berk M, Brook S. Lamotrigine compared with lithium in mania: a double-blind randomized controlled trial. *Ann Clin Psychiatry* 2000;12:5–10.
12. McElroy SL, Keck PE. Pharmacologic agents for the treatment of acute bipolar mania. *Biol Psychiatry* 2000;48:539–557.
13. Rendell JM, Gijsman HJ, Keck P, et al. Olanzapine alone or in combination for acute mania. In: The Cochrane Library, Issue 3, 2003. Oxford: Update

Software. Search date 2002; primary sources The Cochrane Collaboration Depression, Anxiety and Neurosis Controlled Trials Register, The Cochrane Central Register of Controlled Trials, EMBASE, MEDLINE, CINAHL, and PsycINFO.
14. Gijsman HJ, Geddes JR, Rendell JM, et al. Systematic review of antidepressants for bipolar depression [abstract]. *J Psychopharmacol* 2001;15(suppl):A19. Search date not reported; primary sources Cochrane Collaboration Depression Anxiety and Neurosis Controlled Trials Register.
15. Nolen WA, Bloemkolk D. Treatment of bipolar depression: a review of the literature and a suggestion for an algorithm. *Neuropsychobiology* 2000;42(suppl 1):11–17. Search date 2000; primary sources Medline and hand searches of reference lists and recent congress abstracts books.
16. Young LT, Joffe RT, Robb JC, et al. Double-blind comparison of addition of a second mood stabilizer versus an antidepressant to an initial mood stabilizer for treatment of people with bipolar depression. *Am J Psychiatry* 2000;157:124–126.
17. Gijsman HJ, Rendell J, Geddes J, et al. Antidepressants for bipolar depression (protocol for a Cochrane Review). In: The Cochrane Library, Issue 3, 2003. Oxford: Update Software.
18. Calabrese JR, Bowden CL, Sachs GS, et al. A double-blind placebo controlled study of lamotrigine monotherapy in outpatients with bipolar 1 depression. *J Clin Psychiatry* 1999;60:79–88.
19. Perry A, Tarrier N, Morriss R, McCarthy E, Limb K. Randomised controlled trial of efficacy of teaching patients with bipolar disorder to identify early symptoms of relapse and obtain treatment. *BMJ* 1999;318:149–153.
20. Miklowitz DJ, Simoneau TL, George EL, et al. Family-focused treatment of bipolar disorder: 1-year effects of a psychoeducational program in conjunction with pharmacotherapy. *Biol Psychiatry* 2000;48:582–592.
21. Burgess S, Geddes J, Hawton K, et al. Lithium for maintenance treatment of mood disorders. In: The Cochrane Library, Issue 3, 2003. Oxford: Update Software. Search date not reported; primary sources Cochrane Collaboration Depression, Anxiety and Neurosis Review Group Specialised Register, Cochrane Controlled Trials Register and hand searches of reference lists of relevant papers, major textbooks of mood disorder and the journals Lithium and Lithium Therapy Monographs and personal communication with authors, other experts in the field and pharmaceutical companies.
22. Davis JM, Janicak PG, Hogan DM. Mood stabilizers in the prevention of recurrent affective disorders: a meta-analysis. *Acta Psychiatr Scand 1999;*100:406–417. Search date not reported; primary sources Medline, PsychLit, Pubmed and hand searches of reference lists of identified studies and personal communication with colleagues.
23. Tondo L, Hennen J, Baldessarini RJ. Lower suicide risk with long-term lithium treatment in major affective illness: a meta-analysis. *Acta Psychiatrica Scand* 2001;104:163–172. Search date 2000; primary sources Medline, Current Contents, PsychLit, Pubmed and hand searches of reference lists of relevant publications and contents lists and/or indices of leading international psychiatric research journals and personal communication with colleagues who have done research in the field.
24. Bowden CL, Calabrese JR, Sachs G, et al. A placebo-controlled 18-month trial of lamotrigine and lithium maintenance treatment in recently manic or hypomanic patients with bipolar 1 disorder. *Arch Gen Pshychiatry* 2003;60:392–400.
25. Bowden CL, Ghaemi N, Gyulai, et al. Lamotrigine delays mood episodes in recently depressed bipolar 1 patients. Am Psychiatr Assoc 2002.
26. Macritchie KAN, Geddes JR, Scott J, et al. Valproic acid, valproate and valproate semisodium in the maintenance treatment of bipolar disorder. In: The Cochrane Library, Issue 3, 2003. Oxford: Update Software. Search date not reported; primary sources Cochrane Collaboration Depression, Anxiety and Neurosis Review Group Specialised Register, Cochrane Controlled Trials Register, Embase, Medline, Lilacs, PsychLit, Psyndex and hand searches of reference lists of relevant papers, major textbooks on mood disorder, Comprehensive Psychiatry and relevant conference proceedings and personal communication with authors, other experts and pharmaceutical companies.
27. Greil W, Ludwig–Mayerhofer W, Erazo N, et al. Lithium versus carbamazepine in the maintenance treatment of bipolar disorders: a randomised study. *J Affect Disord* 43:151–161.
28. Bandeira CA, Lima MS, Geddes J, et al. Carbamazepine for bipolar affective disorders (protocol for a Cochrane Review). In: The Cochrane Library, Issue 3, 2003. Oxford: Update Software.
29. Calabrese, JR Suppes, T, Bowden, CL, et al. A double-blind, placebo-controlled, prophylaxis study of lamotrigine in rapid-cycling bipolar disorder. Lamictal 614 Study Group. *J Clin Psychiatry* 2000;61:841–850.
30. Ghaemi SN, Lenox MS, Baldessarini RJ. Effectiveness and safety of long-term antidepressant treatment in bipolar disorder. *J Clin Psychiatry* 2001;62:565–569. Search date 2000; primary sources Medline, HealthStar, Current Contents, PsychInfo and hand searches of bibliographies of identified reports and recent reviews.

John Geddes
Department of Psychiatry
University of Oxford
Oxford
UK

Competing interests: Sanofi-Synthelabo have donated supplies of Depakote and to the BALANCE trial, of which JG is the principal investigator.

TABLE 1 **DSM-IV classification of bipolar disorders (see text, p 1052). Reprinted with permission from Elsevier (Müller-Oerlinghausen B, Berghöfer A, Bauer M Bipolar Disorder Lancet 2002; 359: 241–47).[1]**

DSM IV Category	Criteria	Course specifiers and examples
Bipolar I disorder	One or more manic or mixed episodes, usually accompanied by one or more major depressive episodes	To describe current (or most recent episode): mild, moderate, severe without psychotic features; severe with psychotic features; in partial or full remission; with catatonic features; with postpartum onset To describe current (or most recent) major depressive episode: chronic; with melancholic features; with atypical features
		To describe pattern of episodes: with or without full interepisode recovery; with seasonal pattern; with rapid cycling (> 4 episodes in previous 12 months)
Bipolar II disorder	Recurrent major depressive episodes with one or more hypomanic (milder than manic) episodes	To describe current (or most recent episode): hypomanic; depressed To describe current (or most recent) major depressive episode and pattern of episodes: see bipolar I disorder
Cyclothymic disorder	Chronic (> 2 years), fluctuating mood disturbance involving numerous periods of mild hypomanic and depressive symptoms that do not meet criteria for a major depressive episode	Over 2 years any symptom free intervals last no longer than 2 months
Bipolar disorder (not otherwise specified)	Disorders with bipolar features that do not meet criteria for any specific bipolar disorder	Examples: very rapid cycling (over days); recurrent hypomanias without depressive symptoms; indeterminate whether primary or secondary (due to a general medical condition or substance abuse)

Bulimia nervosa

Search date December 2002

Phillipa Hay and Josue Bacaltchuk

QUESTIONS

INTERVENTIONS

See glossary, p 1080

Key Messages

Antidepressants

- **Antidepressant medication (tricyclic antidepressants, monoamine oxidase inhibitors, and fluoxetine)** Systematic reviews and one subsequent RCT have found short term reduction in bulimic symptoms with tricyclic antidepressants, monoamine oxidase inhibitors, and fluoxetine. A further subsequent RCT found no significant difference in symptoms between moclobemide and placebo. One systematic review and one subsequent RCT found no significant difference in symptoms with antidepressants versus cognitive behavioural therapy.
- **Other antidepressants (venlafaxine, mirtazapine, and reboxetine)** We found no RCTs on the effects of venlafaxine, mirtazapine, and reboxetine.
- **Selective serotonin reuptake inhibitors (other than fluoxetine)** We found no good evidence on selective serotonin reuptake inhibitors other than fluoxetine.
- **Antidepressants as maintenance** We found insufficient evidence to assess the effects of antidepresssants for maintenance.

Psychotherapy

- **Cognitive behavioural therapy** One systematic review has found that cognitive behavioural therapy compared with remaining on a waiting list reduces specific symptoms of bulimia nervosa and improves non-specific symptoms such as depression. One systematic review found cognitive behavioural therapy compared with other psychotherapies improved abstinence from binge eating and depression scores at the end of treatment. One RCT in the review found that cognitive behavioural therapy compared with interpersonal psychotherapy reduced binge eating in the short term, but there was no significant difference in the longer term. One systematic review and one subsequent RCT found no significant difference in symptoms with cognitive behavioural therapy compared with antidepressants.

- **Other psychotherapies** One systematic review has found that non-cognitive behavioural psychotherapy increases abstinence from binge eating compared with waiting list controls. The systematic review found that the combined result for four specific psychotherapies, other than cognitive behavioural therapy, reduced bulimic symptoms compared with specified control psychotherapies, but the review included RCTs with weak methods, and the result was significant in only one of the four individual results. One systematic review found cognitive behavioural therapy compared with other psychotherapies improved abstinence from binge eating and depression scores at the end of treatment. One RCT in the review found that cognitive behavioural therapy compared with interpersonal psychotherapy reduced binge eating in the short term, but there was no significant difference in the longer term.

Combination treatment

- **Combination treatment (antidepressants plus psychotherapy)** One systematic review and one subsequent RCT found no significant difference between combination treatment (antidepressants plus psychotherapy) and antidepressants alone in binge frequency, depressive symptoms, and remission rates. The systematic review found that, compared with psychotherapy alone, combination treatment improved short term remission, but there was no significant difference in binge frequency and depressive symptoms. The systematic review found that combination treatment was with psychotherapy were associated with higher withdrawal rates compared with psychotherapy alone. One subsequent RCT of cognitive behavioural therapy in a self help form plus fluoxetine found limited evidence that combined treatment reduced bulimic symptoms compared with cognitive behavioural therapy alone. A second subsequent RCT found no significant difference in symptoms between group based CBT, fluoxetine, and their combination.

DEFINITION Bulimia nervosa (see glossary, p 1080) is an intense preoccupation with body weight and shape, with regular episodes of uncontrolled overeating of large amounts of food (binge eating — see glossary, p 1080) associated with use of extreme methods to counteract the feared effects of overeating. If a person also meets the diagnostic criteria for anorexia nervosa, then the diagnosis of anorexia nervosa takes precedence.[1] Bulimia nervosa can be difficult to identify because of extreme secrecy about binge eating and purgative behaviour. Weight may be normal but there is often a history of anorexia nervosa or restrictive dieting. Some people alternate between anorexia nervosa and bulimia nervosa. Some RCTs included participants with subthreshhold bulimia nervosa or a related eating disorder, binge eating disorder. Where possible, only results relevant to bulimia nervosa are reported in this review.

INCIDENCE/ PREVALENCE In community based studies, the prevalence of bulimia nervosa is between 0.5% and 1.0% in young women, with an even social class distribution.[2–4] About 90% of people diagnosed with bulimia nervosa re women. The numbers presenting with bulimia nervosa in idustrialised countries increased during the decade that followed its recognition in e late 1970s and "a cohort effect" is reported in community surveys,[2,5,6] implying an increase in incidence. The prevalence of eating disorders such as bulimia nervosa is lower in non-industrialised populations,[7] and varies across ethnic groups. African-American women have a lower rate of restrictive dieting than white American women, but have a similar rate of recurrent binge eating.[8]

AETIOLOGY/ RISK FACTORS Young women from the developed world who restrict their dietary intake are at greatest risk of developing bulimia nervosa and other eating disorders. One community based case control study compared 102 people with bulimia nervosa with 204 healthy controls and found higher rates of the following in people with the eating disorder: obesity, mood disorder, sexual and physical abuse, parental obesity, substance misuse, low self esteem, perfectionism, disturbed family dynamics, parental weight/shape concern, and early menarche.[9] Compared with a control group of 102 women who had other psychiatric disorders, women with bulimia nervosa had higher rates of parental problems and obesity.

PROGNOSIS A 10 year follow up study (50 people with bulimia nervosa from a trial of mianserin treatment) found that 52% had fully recovered, and only 9% continued to experience full symptoms of bulimia nervosa.[10] A larger study (222 people from a trial of antidepressants and structured, intensive group psychotherapy) found that, after a mean follow up of 11.5 years, 11% still met criteria for bulimia nervosa, whereas 70% were in full or partial remission.[11] Short term studies found similar results: about 50% of people made a full recovery, 30% made a partial recovery, and 20% continued to be symptomatic.[12] There are few consistent predictors of longer term outcome. Good prognosis has been associated with shorter illness duration, a younger age of onset, higher social class, and a family history of alcohol abuse.[10] Poor prognosis has been associated with a history of substance misuse,[13] premorbid and paternal obesity,[14] and, in some studies, personality disorder.[15–18] One study (102 people) of the natural course of bulimia nervosa found that 31% still had the disorder at 15 months and 15% at 5 years.[19] Only 28% received treatment during the follow up period. In an evaluation of response to cognitive behavioural therapy, early progress (by session 6) best predicted outcome.[20] A subsequent systematic review of the outcome literature found no consistent evidence to support early intervention and a better prognosis.[21]

AIMS OF INTERVENTION To reduce symptoms of bulimia nervosa; to improve general psychiatric symptoms; to improve social functioning and quality of life.

OUTCOMES Frequency of binge eating, abstinence from binge eating, frequency of behaviours to reduce weight and counter the effects of binge eating, severity of extreme weight and shape preoccupation, severity of general psychiatric symptoms, severity of depression, improvement in social and adaptive functioning, remission rates, relapse rates, and withdrawal rates.

METHODS *Clinical Evidence* search and appraisal December 2002 and hand search of reference lists from identified reviews.

QUESTION What are the effects of treatments for bulimia nervosa in adults?

OPTION COGNITIVE BEHAVIOURAL THERAPY

One systematic review has found that cognitive behavioural therapy compared with remaining on a waiting list reduces specific symptoms of bulimia nervosa and improves non-specific symptoms such as depression. One systematic review found cognitive behavioural therapy compared with other psychotherapies improved abstinence from binge eating and depression scores at the end of treatment. One RCT in the review found that cognitive behavioural therapy compared with interpersonal psychotherapy reduced binge eating in the short term, but there was no significant difference in the longer term. One systematic review and one subsequent RCT found no significant difference in symptoms with cognitive behavioural therapy compared with antidepressants.

Benefits: We found one systematic review (search date 2002, 34 RCTs).[22] It included RCTs of other binge eating disorders, although most studies were of people with bulimia nervosa (see glossary, p 1080) (18 RCTs in people with bulimia nervosa characterised by purging behaviour).[22] The review reported data separately for bulimia nervosa and other disorders of binge eating. Unless otherwise specified, results reported here refer only to analyses of people with bulimia nervosa. **Versus waiting list controls:** One systematic review (search date 2002; individual analyses included a maximum of 10 RCTs and 735 people) found that cognitive behavioural therapy (CBT — see glossary, p 1080) compared with remaining on a waiting list significantly increased the proportion of people abstaining from binge eating at the end of the trial (3 RCTs; RR 0.62, 95% CI 0.47 to 0.83), significantly reduced mean bulimic symptom scores (6 RCTs; SMD −0.85, 95% CI −1.14 to −0.57), and mean depression scores (3 RCTs; SMD −1.13, 95% CI −1.60 to −0.67).[22] It found no significant difference, in a mixed population, between CBT and remaining on the waiting list in weight at the end of treatment (3 RCTs, 1 with bulimia nervosa participants; SMD +0.12, 95% CI −0.23 to +0.46, 135 people). The review found insufficient evidence about other outcomes, such as social functioning. **Versus placebo medication:** One subsequent RCT (91 people) found no significant difference in efficacy between unguided manual based self help CBT and placebo medication.[23] **Versus other psychotherapies:** See table 1, p 1083. The systematic review (search date 2002) found that CBT compared with other psychotherapies significantly improved abstinence from binge eating (6 RCTs, 448 people; RR 0.78, 95% CI 0.70 to 0.87) and depression scores at the end of treatment (6 RCTs, 206 people; SMD −0.66, 95% CI −0.94 to −0.37).[22] For all RCTs (including both binge eating disorder and bulimia nervosa participants) CBT plus exposure therapy (see glossary, p 1080) was not significantly more effective than CBT alone (3 RCTs, 168 people; RR for abstinence from binge eating 0.87, 95% CI 0.65 to 1.16). Depression scores were significantly lower at the end of treatment with CBT plus exposure therapy compared with CBT alone (4 RCTs, 145 people; SMD 0.45, 95% CI 0.11 to 0.79). CBT in a full or less intensive form was not significantly superior to CBT in a pure self help form (see glossary, p 1081) (5 RCTs, 264 people; RR 0.92, 95% CI 0.82 to 1.03). One RCT included in the review (220 people) compared classic CBT versus interpersonal psychotherapy (see glossary, p 1080) for bulimia nervosa that involved purging.[24] It found that CBT significantly improved abstinence from binge eating at the end of treatment (19 individual sessions conducted ≥ 20 weeks; intention to treat analysis; 29% with CBT *v* 6% with interpersonal psychotherapy; $P < 0.01$). However, the difference was not significant at 4, 8, and 12 months of follow up, with improvement in both groups from baseline. We found one subsequent RCT (125 people with bulimia nervosa), which compared four sessions of CBT versus motivational enhancement therapy (see glossary, p 1080).[25] It found no significant differences between CBT and motivational enhancement therapy in engaging participants or the chance of achieving a clinically significant reduction in binge frequency (17/25 [68%] *v* 23/43 [53%]; RR 1.3, 95% CI 0.9 to 1.9). However, results were reported only on the first 4 weeks of treatment, which was prior to all people receiving a further 8 weeks of individual or group CBT. **Versus antidepressants:** See benefits of antidepressants, p 1076. **Versus combination treatment:** See benefits of combination treatment, p 1079.

Harms: The systematic review (search date 2002) found that the RCTs did not report details of adverse effects.[22] It found no significant difference in completion rates between interventions,[22] suggesting no major difference in acceptability. However, it could not exclude infrequent serious adverse effects.[22] An observational study found that group psychotherapy offered very soon after presentation was sometimes perceived as threatening.[10]

Comment: We found a second systematic review in German, which is awaiting translation, and may be included in a future *Clinical Evidence* update.[26] One systematic review (search date 2002)[22] defined CBT as psychotherapy that uses the techniques and models specified by Wilson and Fairburn,[27] but it did not specify the number of sessions or specialist expertise (classical CBT for bulimia nervosa specifies 19 individual sessions over 20 weeks conducted by trained therapists[27]). Effect sizes for CBT were large, but over 50% of people were still binge eating at the end of treatment.[22] Further research is needed to evaluate the specific and non-specific effects of CBT and other psychotherapies, to explore individual characteristics (such as readiness to change) that may predict response, and to explore the long term effects of treatment. Waiting list or delayed treatment control groups are subject to bias because it is not possible to "blind" someone to the knowledge they are not in the active treatment group. It is difficult to interpret the clinical importance of the statistically significant changes in depression scores. Further limitations are that the quality of trials was variable (e.g. 57% were not blinded).[22] Sample sizes were often small. None of the studies measured harms rigorously. Two further analyses[28,29] found limited observational evidence that motivation and compliance factors may influence outcomes. One study[28] performed additional analyses in an RCT of CBT versus interpersonal psychotherapy.[24] It found that "stage of change", or psychological motivation and greater readiness to change, was not related to non-completion, but was associated with a good outcome in those who completed interpersonal psychotherapy. The second RCT examined the effects of compliance on outcome in 62 people randomised to guided self help or to full CBT for 16 weeks.[29] At 6 months' follow up, but not the end of treatment, binge eating abstinence rates were greater in those who had completed two or more of the CBT exercises (P = 0.04; CI not reported). Stricter inclusion criteria in the review removed previously included RCTs in people with binge eating disorders other than bulimia nervosa.[22] **Versus antidepressants:** See antidepressants, p 1076.

OPTION OTHER PSYCHOTHERAPIES

One systematic review has found that non-cognitive behavioural psychotherapy increases abstinence from binge eating compared with waiting list controls. The systematic review found that the combined result for four specific psychotherapies, other than cognitive behavioural therapy, reduced bulimic symptoms compared with specified control psychotherapies. However, the review included RCTs with weak methods, and the result was significant in only one of the four individual results. One systematic review found cognitive behavioural therapy compared with other psychotherapies improved abstinence from binge eating and depression scores at the end of treatment. One RCT in the review found that CBT compared with interpersonal psychotherapy reduced binge eating in the short term, but there was no significant difference in the longer term.

Benefits: **Versus waiting list controls:** We found one systematic review (search date 2002),[22] which also included studies of other binge eating (see glossary, p 1080) syndromes. It found that, for bulimia nervosa (see glossary, p 1080) participants only, non-cognitive behavioural psychotherapies (e.g. hypnobehavioural therapy and interpersonal psychotherapy — see glossary, p 1080) compared with waiting list control significantly increased abstinence from binge eating (3 RCTs, 124 people; RR 0.67, 95% CI 0.55 to 0.81) and reduced the number of people who did not achieve remission (4 RCTs, 162 people; RR 0.63, 95% CI 0.53 to 0.75). **Versus a control therapy:** The systematic review included four RCTs in which psychotherapies other than cognitive behavioural therapy were compared with a control therapy.[22] One compared nutritional counselling with stress management; one compared guided imagery with self monitoring; one was a three-armed RCT comparing self psychology (the active treatment), cognitive orientation (see glossary, p 1080), and a control nutritional counselling therapy, and the fourth compared interpersonal psychotherapy with behavioural therapy alone. The combined results for psychotherapy, for participants with bulimia nervosa, significantly reduced bulimic symptoms compared with a control treatment (4 RCTs, 163 people; SMD –0.64 95% CI –1.00 to –0.29).[22] However, in only one trial was the ndividual result significant. **Versus antidepressants:** See antidepressants, p 1076. **Versus cognitive behavioural therapy:** See benefits of cognitive behavioural therapy, p 1073. **Versus combination treatment:** See combination treatment, p 1078. We found one subsequent RCT, which is awaiting translation.[30]

Harms: The systematic review (search date 2002) found that the RCTs did not report details of adverse effects.[22] It found no significant difference in completion rates between interventions,[22] suggesting no major difference in acceptability. However, it could not exclude infrequent serious adverse effects.[22] An observational study found that group psychotherapy offered very soon after presentation was sometimes perceived as threatening.[10] Non-cognitive behavioural psychotherapies include a large number of options, and it remains unclear which therapies are most effective.

Comment: The quality of trials was variable, few were blinded, sample sizes were small, and none of the studies measured harms rigorously (see comment under cognitive behavioural therapy, p 1074). Waiting list or delayed treatment control groups are subject to bias because it is not possible to "blind" someone to the knowledge they are not in the active treatment group. Stricter inclusion criteria in the review removed previously included RCTs in people with binge eating disorders other than bulimia nervosa.[22]

OPTION ANTIDEPRESSANTS

Systematic reviews and one subsequent RCT have found short term reduction in bulimic symptoms with tricyclic antidepressants, monoamine oxidase inhibitors, and fluoxetine. A further subsequent RCT found no significant difference in symptoms between moclobemide and placebo. One systematic review and one subsequent RCT found no significant difference in symptoms or relapse rates with antidepressants versus cognitive behavioural therapy. One systematic review and one subsequent RCT found no significant difference between combination treatment (antidepressants plus psychotherapy) and antidepressants alone in binge frequency, depressive symptoms, and remission rates. We found no RCTs on the effects of venlafaxine, mirtazapine, and reboxetine. We found no good evidence on selective serotonin reuptake inhibitors other than fluoxetine. We found insufficient evidence to assess the effects of antidepresssants for maintenance.

Benefits: We found two systematic reviews (search date 2001[31] and 2000[32]), three additional RCTs of longer term maintenance (not primary treatment studies),[33–35] and one subsequent RCT.[36] **Versus placebo:** We found one systematic review comparing antidepressants with placebo.[31] It found that antidepressants reduced bulimic symptoms.[31] The review (search date 2001; antidepressants were imipramine [5 RCTs], amitriptyline [1 RCT], desipramine [5 RCTs], phenelzine [2 RCTs], isocarboxazid [1 RCT], brofaromine [1 RCT], fluoxetine [5 RCTs], mianserin [1 RCT], bupropion [1 RCT], and trazodone [1 RCT]) found significantly more frequent short term remission of bulimic episodes with antidepressants (9 RCTs, 777 people, 20% *v* 8% with placebo; pooled RR 0.87, 95% CI 0.81 to 0.93).[31] The review found no significant difference in effect between different classes of antidepressants, but there were too few RCTs to exclude a clinically important difference (see table 2, p 1084). Most RCTs were of tricyclic antidepressants or monoamine oxidase inhibitors; fluoxetine was the only selective serotonin reuptake inhibitor included in the reviews.[31] The first subsequent, four armed RCT (91 women) compared fluoxetine 60 mg daily, placebo, self help cognitive behavioural therapy manual, and fluoxetine plus a self help manual.[23] It found a significantly greater reduction with fluoxetine compared with placebo in vomiting and binge eating symptoms at week 4 ($P < 0.05$). Remission rates after a 16 week treatment period with fluoxetine were 16%, and were not reported for placebo. The second subsequent RCT (78 women with bulimia nervosa [see glossary, p 1080]) compared moclobemide (a reversible monoamine oxidase inhibitor) 600 mg daily versus placebo.[36] It reported no significant differences in weekly binge and vomiting episodes, Hamilton depression scores, and scores on three self report measures of eating disorder symptoms between those randomised to active drug or placebo, among the 52 women who completed the RCT. It was not possible to provide quantified results, as insufficient data were provided. Remission rates were not reported. We found no RCTs on the effects of other selective serotonin reuptake inhibitors (sertraline, paroxetine, and citalopram), venlafaxine, mirtazapine, and reboxetine. **Versus psychotherapy:** We found one systematic review (search date 2000, 5 RCTs) of antidepressants versus psychotherapy (all CBT RCTs) and one subsequent RCT.[32,37] We found another trial comparing fluoxetine with psychotherapy, which is awaiting translation.[38] The systematic review found no significant difference in remission rates, bulimic symptom severity (4 RCTs), or depression symptom severity at the end of the trials (3 RCTs).[32] A subsequent RCT (53 people) compared three treatments: group based CBT, fluoxetine 60 mg daily, and CBT plus fluoxetine.[37] Completer only analysis found no significant differences in 1 month abstinence from binge eating at the end of treatment (5/19 with CBT *v* 2/16 with fluoxetine; RR 2.11, 95% CI 0.47 to 9.43) or in 1 month absence from self induced vomiting (7/19 with CBT, 1/16 with fluoxetine; RR 5.9, 95% CI 0.81 to 42.99).[37] **Versus combination treatment:** See combination treatment, p 1078. **Antidepressants as maintenance:** We found two small RCTs of maintenance treatment.[33,34] The first very small RCT (9 people who had responded well to despiramine over the previous 24 weeks) compared continuation of desipramine versus placebo.[33] It found no significant difference between treatments (relapse: 1/5 [20%] with desipramine *v* 2/4 [50%] with placebo; RR 0.4, 95% CI 0.1 to 3.0). The second very small RCT (9 women who had responded well to imipramine over the previous 10 weeks) compared continuation of imipramine versus placebo.[34] It found no significant difference in relapse (relapse: 2/3 [67%] with imipramine *v* 5/6 [83%] with placebo; RR 0.8, 95% CI 0.3 to 1.9).[34]

Harms: One systematic review (search date 2000) found that withdrawal significantly increased with antidepressants compared with psychotherapy (4 RCTs, 189 people; AR 40% *v* 18%; RR 2.18, 95% CI 1.09 to 4.35).[32] One subsequent RCT (53 people) found no significant difference in withdrawals with fluoxetine compared with

CBT and with combined treatment (42% with CBT, 25% with fluoxetine; RR 1.68, 95% CI 0.62 to 4.57; and 33% with combined treatment; RR 1.33, 95% CI 0.46 to 3.89).[37] The authors thought this might be due to cultural differences because psychotherapy is rarely offered as part of a treatment trial in Germany. A second systematic review (search date 2001) found significantly increased withdrawal in people taking antidepressants compared with placebo (12 RCTs, 1123 people, 10.5% with any antidepressant *v* 5.1% with placebo; RR 1.83, 95% CI 1.13 to 2.95; NNH 7, 95% CI 4 to 18).[31] It found no significant difference in withdrawal due to adverse effects between and within classes of antidepressants. It found that withdrawal due to any cause was more likely with tricyclic antidepressants than with placebo (6 RCTs, 277 people, 29% with tricyclic *v* 14% with placebo; RR 1.93, 95% CI 1.15 to 3.25), but was more likely with placebo than with selective serotonin reuptake inhibitors (3 RCTs, 706 people, 37% with a selective serotonin reuptake inhibitor *v* 40% with placebo; RR 0.83, 95% CI 0.68 to 0.99). We found one RCT examining specific adverse effects. One found significant increases in reclining and standing blood pulse rate, lying systolic and diastolic blood pressure, and greater orthostatic effects on blood pressure with desipramine versus placebo.[39] Cardiovascular changes were well tolerated and few people withdrew because of these effects. Meta-analyses of two double blind RCTs of fluoxetine versus placebo found no significant difference in the incidence of suicidal acts or ideation in people treated with fluoxetine versus placebo.[40] However, the overall incidence of events was low (suicide attempts 1.2%, none fatal; emergent suicidal ideation 3.1%). The third subsequent RCT did not report on withdrawal or adverse events.[23]

Comment: We found no consistent predictors of response to treatment. We found no good evidence for the efficacy of other selective serotonin reuptake inhibitors apart from fluoxetine or the "newer" antidepressants venlafaxine, reboxetine, and mirtazapine. One review commented on the lack of follow up.[31] The second subsequent RCT found no differences between active and placebo groups in withdrawal rates because of adverse events, and no changes in blood pressure in those on moclobemide despite reports in food diaries of a high consumption of tyramine-containing foods.[36] The RCTs of maintenance both made multiple randomisations and compared a number of different groups. This meant that there were very few people in the groups for maintenance treatment.

OPTION COMBINATION TREATMENT

One systematic review and one subsequent RCT found no significant difference between combination treatment (antidepressants plus psychotherapy) and antidepressants alone in binge frequency, depressive symptoms, and remission rates. The systematic review found that, compared with psychotherapy alone, combination treatment improved short term remission, but there was no significant difference in binge frequency and depressive symptoms. The systematic review found that combination treatment with psychotherapy was associated with higher withdrawal rates compared with psychotherapy alone. One subsequent RCT of cognitive behavioural therapy in a self help form plus fluoxetine

found limited evidence that combined treatment reduced bulimic symptoms compared with cognitive behavioural therapy alone. A second subsequent RCT found no significant difference in symptoms between group based CBT, fluoxetine, and their combination.

Benefits: **Versus antidepressants alone:** We found one systematic review (search date 2000, 7 RCTs, 247 people)[32] and one subsequent RCT comparing combination treatment (antidepressants plus psychotherapy) versus antidepressants alone.[37] The systematic review found that combination treatment compared with antidepressants alone did not significantly improve binge frequency, depressive symptoms, and short term remission rates, although outcomes were better with combination treatment (binge frequency 4 RCTs; SMD +0.34, 95% CI –0.05 to +0.73; depressive symptoms 3 RCTs; SMD +0.24, 95% CI –0.14 to +0.62; short term remission rates 4 RCTs, 141 people, 42% with combined treatment *v* 23% with antidepressants alone; RR 1.40, 95% CI 0.98 to 1.99).[32] The subsequent RCT (53 people) compared three treatments: group based cognitive behavioural therapy (CBT); fluoxetine 60 mg daily; and CBT plus fluoxetine (see option, p 1076).[37] Completer only analysis found no significant difference in 1 month abstinence from binge eating (2/16 with fluoxetine *v* 3/18 with combination; RR 1.05, 95% CI 0.80 to 1.30) or in 1 month abstinence from self induced vomiting (1/16 with fluoxetine *v* 1/18 with combination; RR 0.99, 95% CI 0.84 to 1.18). **Versus psychotherapy alone:** We found one systematic review (search date 2000, 7 RCTs, 343 people)[32] and two subsequent RCTs comparing combination treatment (antidepressants plus psychotherapy) versus antidepressants alone.[23,37] The systematic review found that combination treatment compared with psychotherapy alone significantly increased short term remission (6 RCTs, 257 people, 49% *v* 36%; RR 1.21, 95% CI 1.02 to 1.45) but found no significant difference in depressive symptoms or in frequency of binge eating (see glossary, p 1080) (6 RCTs; SMD +0.12, 95% CI –0.21 to +0.46).[32] The first subsequent RCT found that people who received both the self help manual and fluoxetine 60 mg daily had the greatest reduction in bulimic symptoms compared with those in the placebo, fluoxetine, or self help only arms, but significance was not reported.[23] Remission rates did not differ significantly across the three active treatment arms. The second subsequent RCT (53 people) compared three treatments: group based CBT; fluoxetine 60 mg daily; and CBT plus fluoxetine.[37] Completer only analysis found no significant difference in 1 month abstinence from binge eating (5/19 with CBT *v* 3/18 with combination; RR 1.58, 95% CI 0.44 to 5.67), or in 1 month abstinence from self induced vomiting (7/19 with CBT *v* 1/18 with combination; RR 6.63, 95% CI 0.90 to 48.69).

Harms: The review found no significant difference in withdrawal rates between combination treatment and antidepressants alone (4 RCTs, 196 people, 34% with combination treatment *v* 41% with antidepressants alone; RR 1.19, 95% CI 0.69 to 2.05).[32] Withdrawal rates were significantly lower with psychotherapy alone compared with combination treatments (6 RCTs, 295 people, 16% *v* 30%; RR 0.57, 95% CI 0.38 to 0.88).[32] The subsequent RCT[37] did not find higher non-completion rates when CBT was combined with fluoxetine.

Comment: Modest effect sizes in these analyses may be clinically relevant, but the small number and size of trials limit conclusions.

GLOSSARY

Binge eating Modified from DSM-IV.[1] Eating, in a discrete period (e.g. hours), a large amount of food, accompanied by a lack of control over eating during the episode.

Bulimia nervosa The American Psychiatric Association DSM-IV[1] criteria include recurrent episodes of binge eating; recurrent inappropriate compensatory behaviour to prevent weight gain; frequency of binge eating and inappropriate compensatory behaviour both, on average, at least twice a week for 3 months; self evaluation unduly influenced by body shape and weight; and disturbance occurring not exclusively during episodes of anorexia nervosa. Types of bulimia nervosa, modified from DSM-IV[1], are purging: using self induced vomiting, laxatives, diuretics, or enemas; non-purging: fasting, exercise, but not vomiting or other abuse as for the purging type. Many studies however evaluate efficacy for samples that may include participants with subthreshold bulimia nervosa or binge eating disorder. Where possible, only data of bulimia nervosa participants are reported in this review.

Cognitive behavioural therapy In bulimia nervosa this uses three overlapping phases. Phase one aims to educate the person about bulimia nervosa. People are helped to increase regularity of eating, and resist urge to binge or purge. Phase two introduces procedures to reduce dietary restraint (e.g. broadening food choices). In addition, cognitive procedures supplemented by behavioural experiments are used to identify and correct dysfunctional attitudes and beliefs, and avoidance behaviours. Phase three is the maintenance phase. Relapse prevention strategies are used to prepare for possible future set backs.[41]

Cognitive orientation therapy The cognitive orientation theory aims to generate a systematic procedure for exploring the meaning of a behaviour around themes, such as avoidance of certain emotions. Therapy for modifying behaviour focuses on systematically changing beliefs related to themes, not beliefs referring directly to eating behaviour. No attempt is made to persuade the people that their beliefs are incorrect or maladapative.[42]

Dialectical behaviour therapy A type of behavioural therapy that views emotional dysregulation as the core problem in bulimia nervosa, with binge eating and purging understood as attempts to influence, change, or control painful emotional states. Patients are taught a repertoire of skills to replace dysfunctional behaviours.[43]

Exposure therapy In bulimia nervosa this is a modification of the exposure and response prevention therapy developed for obsessive compulsive disorder. It involves exposure to food, for example, and then psychological prevention strategies to control weight behaviour, such as vomiting after eating until the urge or compulsion to vomit has receded.[44]

Hypnobehavioural psychotherapy Uses a combination of behavioural techniques, such as self monitoring to change maladaptive eating disorders, and hypnotic techniques to reinforce and encourage behaviour change.

Interpersonal psychotherapy In bulimia nervosa, this is a three phase treatment. Phase one analyses in detail the interpersonal context of the eating disorder. This leads to the formulation of an interpersonal problem area, which forms the focus of the second stage, which is aimed at helping the person make interpersonal changes. Phase three is devoted to the person's progress and an exploration of ways to handle future interpersonal difficulties. At no stage is attention paid to eating habits or body attitudes.[24]

Motivational enhancement therapy (MET) This is based on a model of change ith focus on stages of change. Stages of change represent constellations of intentions and behaviours through which individuals pass as they move from having a problem to doing something to resolve it. People in "precontemplation" show no intention to change. People in "contemplation" acknowledge they have a problem and are thinking about change, but have not yet made a commitment to change. People in the third "action" stage are actively engaged in overcoming their problem, and people in "maintenance" work to prevent relapse. Transition from one stage to the next is sequential, but not linear. The aim of MET is to help people move from earlier stages into "action, utilising cognitive and emotional strategies". There is an emphasis on the therapeutic alliance. With precontemplators, the therapist explores perceived positive and negative aspects of their behaviours. Open-ended questions are used to elicit client expression, and reflective paraphrase is used to reinforce key points of motivation. During a session following structured assessment, most of the time is devoted to explaining feedback to the client. Later in MET, attention is devoted to developing and consolidating a change plan.[45]

Pure self help cognitive behavioural therapy A modified form of cognitive behavioural therapy, in which a treatment manual is provided for people to proceed with treatment on their own, or with support from a non-professional. "Guided self help" usually implies that the support person may or may not have some professional training, but is usually not a specialist in eating disorders.

Self psychology therapy This approaches bulimia nervosa as a specific case of the pathology of the self. The treated person cannot rely on people to fulfil their needs such as self esteem. They rely instead on a substance, food, to fulfil personal needs. Therapy progresses when the people move to rely on humans, starting with the therapist.[42]

Substantive changes

Cognitive behavioural therapy One updated systematic review added.[22] Stricter inclusion criteria removed previously included RCTs in people with binge eating disorders other than bulimia nervosa. It found that cognitive behavioural therapy compared with other psychotherapies significantly improved abstinence from binge eating and depression. One subsequent RCT added;[37] conclusions unchanged. Other conclusions unchanged.

Other psychotherapies One updated systematic review added.[22] It found that cognitive behavioural therapy compared with other psychotherapies significantly improved abstinence from binge eating and depression.

Antidepressants Two updated systematic reviews.[31,32] One subsequent RCT added;[36] conclusions unchanged.

Combination treatment One updated systematic review added.[32] The review now finds no significant difference between combination treatment and antidepressants alone in binge frequency and depressive symptoms; categorisation unchanged. One subsequent RCT added;[37] conclusions unchanged.

REFERENCES

1. American Psychiatric Association. *Diagnostic and statistical manual of mental disorders* 4th ed. Washington DC: American Psychiatric Press, 1994.
2. Bushnell JA, Wells JE, Hornblow AR, et al. Prevalence of three bulimic syndromes in the general population. *Psychol Med* 1990;20:671–680.
3. Garfinkel PE, Lin B, Goering P, et al. Bulimia nervosa in a Canadian community sample: prevalence, co-morbidity, early experiences and psychosocial functioning. *Am J Psychiatry* 1995;152:1052–1058.
4. Gard MCE, Freeman CP. The dismantling of a myth: a review of eating disorders and socioeconomic status. *Int J Eat Disord* 199;20:1–12.
5. Hall A, Hay PJ. Eating disorder patient referrals from a population region 1977–1986. *Psychol Med* 1991;21:697–701.
6. Kendler KS, Maclean C, Neale M, et al. The genetic epidemiology of bulimia nervosa. *Am J Psychiatry* 1991;148:1627–167.
7. Choudry IY, Mumford DB. A pilot study of eating disorders in Mirpur (Pakistan) using an Urdu version of the Eating Attitude Test. *Int J Eat Disord* 1992;11:243–251.
8. Striegel-Moore RH, Wifley DE, Caldwell MB, et al. Weight-related attitudes and behaviors of women who diet to lose weight: a comparison for black dieters and white dieters. *Obes Res* 1996;4:109–116.
9. Fairburn CG, Welch SL, Doll HA, et al. Risk factors for bulimia nervosa: a community-based case-control study. *Arch Gen Psychiatry* 1997;54:509–517.
10. Collings S, King M. Ten year follow-up of 50 patients with bulimia nervosa. *Br J Psychiatry* 1994;164:80–87.

11. Keel PK, Mitchell JE, Davis TL, et al. Long-term impact of treatment in women diagnosed with bulimia nervosa *Int J Eat Disord* 2002;31:151–158.
12. Keel PK, Mitchell JE. Outcome in bulimia nervosa. *Am J Psychiatry* 1997;154:313–321.
13. Keel PK, Mitchell JE, Miller KB, et al. Long-term outcome of bulimia nervosa. *Arch Gen Psychiatry* 1999;56:63–69.
14. Fairburn CG, Norman PA, Welch SL, et al. A prospective study of outcome in bulimia nervosa and the long-term effects of three psychological treatments. *Arch Gen Psychiatry* 1995;52:304–312.
15. Coker S, Vize C, Wade T, et al. Patients with bulimia nervosa who fail to engage in cognitive behaviour therapy. *Int J Eat Disord* 1993;13:35–40.
16. Fahy TA, Russell GFM. Outcome and prognostic variables in bulimia. *Int J Eat Disord* 1993;14:135–146.
17. Rossiter EM, Agras WS, Telch CF, et al. Cluster B personality disorder characteristics predict outcome in the treatment of bulimia nervosa. *Int J Eat Disord* 1993;13:349–358.
18. Johnson C, Tobin DL, Dennis A. Differences in treatment outcome between borderline and nonborderline bulimics at 1-year follow-up. *Int J Eat Disord* 1990;9:617–627.
19. Fairburn C, Cooper Z, Doll H, et al. The natural course of bulimia nervosa and binge eating disorder in young women. *Arch Gen Psychiatry* 2000:57:659–665.
20. Agras WS, Crow SJ, Halmi KA, et al. Outcome predictors for the cognitive behavior treatment of bulimia nervosa: data from a multisite study. *Am J Psychiatry* 2000;157:1302–1308.
21. Reas DL, Schoemaker C, Zipfel S, et al. Prognostic value of duration of illness and early intervention in bulimia nervosa: a systematic review of the outcome literature. *Int J Eat Disord* 2001;30:1–10. Search date 1999; primary sources; not stated.
22. Hay PJ, Bacaltchuk J. Psychotherapy for bulimia nervosa and binging. In: The Cochrane Library, Issue 1, 2003. Oxford: Update Software. Search date 2002; primary sources Medline, Extramed, Embase, Psychlit, Current Contents, Lilacs, Scisearch, The Cochrane Controlled Trials Register 1997, The Cochrane Collaboration Depression and Anxiety Trials Register, hand search of *Int J Eat Disord* since its first issue, citation lists in identified studies and reviews, and personal contacts.
23. Mitchell JE, Fletcher L, Hanson K, et al. The relative efficacy of fluoxetine and manual-based self-help in the treatment of outpatients with bulimia nervosa. *J Clin Psychopharmacol* 2001;21:298–304.
24. Agras WS, Walsh BT, Fairburn CG, et al. A multicenter comparison of cognitive-behavioral therapy and interpersonal psychotherapy. *Arch Gen Psychiatry* 2000; 54:459–465.
25. Treasure JL, Katzman M, Schmidt U, et al. Engagement and outcome in the treatment of bulimia nervosa: first phase of a sequential design comparing motivation enhancement therapy and cognitive behavioural therapy. *Behav Res Ther* 1999;37:405–418.
26. Leichsenring von F Zur. Wirksamkeit tiefenpsychologisch fundierter und psychodynamischer Therapie. Eine ubersicht unter berucksichtigung von kriterien der evidence-based medicine. *Z Psychosom Med Psychother* 2002;48:139–162.
27. Wilson GT, Fairburn CG. Treatments for eating disorders. In: Nathan PE, Gorman JM, eds. *A Guide to Treatments that Work. New York*: Oxford University Press, 1998:501–530.
28. Wolk SL, Devlin MJ. Stage of change as a predictor of response to psychotherapy for bulimia nervosa. *Int J Eat Disord* 2001;30:96–100.
29. Thiels C, Schmidt U, Troop N, et al. Compliance with a self-care manual in guided self-change for bulimia nervosa. *Eur Eat Disord Rev* 2001;9:115–122.
30. Eizaguirre E, et al. Un ensayo controlado de intervenciones familiares en trastornos alimentarios *An Psiquiatria (Madrid)* [in Spanish] 2000;16:322–336.
31. Bacaltchuk J, Hay P. Antidepressants versus placebo for people with bulimia nervosa. In: The Cochrane Library Issue 1, 2003. Oxford: Update Software. Search date 2001; primary sources Medline, Extramed, Embase, Psychlit, Current Contents, Lilacs, Scisearch, The Cochrane Controlled Trials Register, The Cochrane Collaboration Depression and Anxiety Trials Register, hand search of citation lists in identified studies and reviews, and personal contact.
32. Bacaltchuk J, Hay P. Antidepressants versus psychological treatments and their combination for people bulimia nervosa (Cochrane Review). Cochrane Library Issue 1, 2003. Oxford: Update Software. Search date 2000; primary sources Medline, Extramed, Embase, Psychlit, Current Contents, Lilacs, Scisearch, Cochrane Controlled Trials Register, Cochrane Collaboration Depression and Anxiety Trials Register, hand search of *Int J Eat Disord* since its first issue, citation lists of identified studies and reviews, and personal contacts.
33. Walsh BT, Hadigan CM, Devlin MJ, et al. Long-term outcome of antidepressant treatment for bulimia nervosa. *Am J Psychiatry* 1991;148:1206–1212.
34. Pyle RL, Mitchell JE, Eckert ED, et al. Maintenance treatment and 6-month outcome for bulimic patients who respond to initial treatment. *Am J Psychiatry* 1990;147:871–875.
35. Agras WS, Rossiter EM, Arnow B, et al. One-year follow-up of psychosocial and pharmacologic treatments for bulimia nervosa. *J Clin Psychiatry* 1994;55:179–183.
36. Carruba MO, Cuzzolaro M, Riva L, et al. Efficacy and tolerability of moclobemide in bulimia nervosa: a placebo-controlled trial. *Int Clin Psychopharmacol* 2001;16:27–32.
37. Jacobi C, Dahme B, Dittman R Cognitive-behavioural, fluoxetine and combined treatment for bulimia nervosa: short- and long-term results. *Eur Eat Disord* 2002;10:179–198.
38. Campanelli M. Cecinella confronto tra gli effetti della terapia farmacologica con fluoxetine e las psicoterapia nel trattamento della bulimia nervosa [in Italian]. *Minerva Psichiatr* 2002 43(suppl 1):1–24.
39. Walsh BT, Hadigan CM, Wong LM. Increased pulse and blood pressure associated with desipramine treatment of bulimia nervosa. *J Clin Psychopharmacol* 1992;12:163–168.
40. Wheadon DE, Rampey AH, Thompson VL, et al. Lack of association between fluoxetine and suicidality in bulimia nervosa. *J Clin Psychiatry* 1992;53:235–241.
41. Fairburn CG, Marcus MD, Wilson GT. Cognitive-behavioral therapy for binge eating and bulimia nervosa: a comprehensive treatment manual. In :Fairburn CG, Wilson GT, eds. *Binge eating: nature, Assessment, and Treatment.* New York: Guilford Press, 1993:361–404.

42. Bachar E, Latzer Y, Kreitler S, et al. Empirical comparison of two psychological therapies. Self psychology and cognitive orientation in the treatment of anorexia and bulimia. *J Psychother Pract Res* 1999;8:115–128.
43. Safer DL, Telch CF, Agras WS. Dialectical behavior therapy for bulimia nervosa. *Am J Psychiatry* 2001;158:632–634.
44. Leitenberg H, Rosen J, Gross J, et al. Exposure plus response-prevention treatment of bulimia nervosa. *J Consult Clin Psychol* 1988;56:535–541.
45. Schmidt U, Treasure J, eds. *Clinician's guide to getting better bit(e) by bit(e)*. Hove: Psychology Press, 1997.

Phillipa Hay
Psychiatrist
University of Adelaide, Adelaide, Australia

Josue Bacaltchuk
Psychiatrist
Federal University of Sao Paulo, Sao Paulo, Brazil

Competing interests: PH has received reimbursement for attending symposia from Solvay Pharmaceuticals, Bristol-Myers Squibb, and Pfizer Pharmaceuticals, and for educational training of family doctors from Bristol-Myers Squibb, Pfizer Pharmaceuticals, and Lundbeck, and has been funded by Jansenn-Cilag to attend symposia. JB none declared.

TABLE 1 **Comparison of remission rates between cognitive behaviour therapy or other active psychotherapy and comparison group (see text, p 1073).[22]**

Comparison	Number of RCTs	Number of people	Absolute remission rates	RR of not remitting (95% CI)
CBT *v* waiting list	3	122	43% *v* 5%	0.62 (0.47 to 0.83)
CBT *v* other psychotherapy	6	448	37% *v* 20%	0.78 (0.70 to 0.87)
CBT-M *v* other psychotherapy	3	316	33% v 16%	0.81 (0.69 to 0.95)
Other psychotherapy *v* waiting list	3	124	37% *v* 3%	0.67 (0.55 to 0.81)

CBT, cognitive behavioural therapy (broadly definied); CBT-M, cognitive behavourial therapy — manualised.[44]

TABLE 2 **Comparison of remission rates between active drug and placebo by class of antidepressant (see text, p 1077).[31]**

Class: drug(s)	Number of RCTs	Number of people	Absolute remission rates	RR (95% CI)
TCA: desipramine, imipramine	3	132	21% *v* 9%	0.90 (0.79 to 1.04)
SSRI: fluoxetine	2	420	19% *v* 11%	0.91 (0.83 to 0.99)
MAOI: phenylzine, isocarboxacid	2	98	24% *v* 6%	0.81 (0.68 to 0.96)
Other: bupropion, trazodone	2	127	17% *v* 8%	0.86 (0.76 to 0.94)

MAOI, monoamine oxidase inhibitor; SSRI, selective serotonin reuptake inhibitor; TCA, tricyclic antidepressant.

Deliberate self harm

Search date April 2003

G Mustafa Soomro

QUESTIONS

INTERVENTIONS

See glossary, p 1095

Key Messages

- We found little RCT evidence for any intervention in people with deliberate self harm. Most RCTs and meta-analyses of small RCTs are likely to have been underpowered to detect clinically important outcomes of interventions.
- **Continuity of care** One systematic review of one RCT found limited evidence that follow up after hospital treatment with the same compared with a different therapist may increase repetition of deliberate self harm over 3 months, although this may be explained by a higher level of risk factors for repetition in the group receiving same therapist follow up, despite randomisation.
- **Dialectal behaviour therapy** One RCT found limited and equivocal evidence that dialectical behaviour therapy may reduce the proportion of people who repeat deliberate self harm over 12 months compared with usual care.
- **Emergency card** One systematic review found no significant difference in the proportion of people who repeated deliberate self harm over 12 months between emergency card (allowing emergency admission or contact with a doctor) and usual care.
- **Flupentixol depot injection** One small RCT found that flupentixol depot injection reduced the proportion of people who repeated deliberate self harm over 6 months compared with placebo. However, we were unable to draw reliable conclusions from this small study. Typical antipsychotics such as flupentixol are associated with a wide range of adverse effects.
- **Hospital admission** One RCT found no significant difference between hospital admission and immediate discharge in the proportion of people who repeated deliberate self harm over 16 weeks, but it is likely to have been too small to exclude a clinically important difference.

- **Intensive outpatient follow up plus outreach** One systematic review found no significant difference in the proportion of people who repeated deliberate self harm over 4–12 months between intensive intervention plus outreach and usual care.
- **Mianserin** RCTs provided insufficient evidence to assess mianserin.
- **Nurse led case management** One RCT found no significant difference between nurse led case management and usual care in the proportion of people who were admitted to emergency departments for episodes of deliberate self harm over 12 months.
- **Paroxetine** One RCT in people with deliberate self harm receiving psychotherapy found no significant difference between paroxetine and placebo in the proportion of people who repeated self harm over 12 months. It found that paroxetine increased diarrhoea and tremor compared with placebo.
- **Problem solving therapy** One systematic review of small RCTs found no significant difference between problem solving therapy and usual care in the proportion of people who repeated deliberate self harm over 6–12 months. Another systematic review found that problem solving therapy reduced depression, anxiety, and hopelessness, and improved problems compared with usual care.
- **Psychodynamic interpersonal therapy** One RCT found that psychodynamic interpersonal therapy for 4 weeks reduced repetition of deliberate self harm, depression, and suicidal ideation over 6 months compared with usual care. However, we were unable to draw reliable conclusions from one RCT.
- **Same number of therapy sessions given over long term versus over short term** One systematic review of one RCT found no significant difference in the proportion of people who repeated deliberate self harm at 12 months with therapy given over 3 months compared with 12 months.
- **Telephone contact** One RCT found no significant difference between telephone contact at 4 and 8 months and usual care in repetition of deliberate self harm, global functioning, and suicidal ideation over 12 months.
- **General practice based guidelines** One large cluster randomised trial comparing the use of general practitioner guidelines for management of deliberate self harm versus usual care found no significant difference in the proportion of people who repeated deliberate self harm over 12 months or in the time to repetition of self harm.

DEFINITION Deliberate self harm is an acute non-fatal act of self harm carried out deliberately in the form of an acute episode of behaviour by an individual with variable motivation.[1] The intention to end life may be absent or present to a variable degree. Other terms used to describe this phenomenon are "attempted suicide" and "parasuicide". The terms are not entirely satisfactory. Common methods of deliberate self harm include self cutting and self poisoning, such as overdosing on medicines. Some acts of deliberate self harm are characterised by high suicidal intent, meticulous planning (including precautions against being found out), and severe lethality. Other acts of deliberate self harm are characterised by no or low intention of suicide, lack of planning and concealing of the act, and low lethality of the method used. The related term of "suicide" is defined as an act with a fatal outcome that is deliberately initiated and performed by the person with the knowledge or expectation of its fatal outcome.[1] This review focuses on recent deliberate self harm as the main presenting problem and excludes RCTs in which deliberate self harm is assessed as an outcome associated with other disorders, such as depression or borderline personality disorder. Deliberate self harm is not defined in the *Diagnostic and statistical manual of mental disorders* (DSM IV)[2] or the *International classification of mental and behavioural disorders* (ICD-10).[3]

INCIDENCE/ PREVALENCE Based on data from 16 European countries between 1989–1992, the lifetime prevalence of deliberate self harm in people treated in hospital and other medical facilities, including general practice settings, is estimated at about 3% for women and 2% for men.[4] Over the last 50 years there has been a rise in the incidence of deliberate self harm in the UK.[4] A reasonable current estimate is about 400/100 000 population a year.[5] In two community studies in the USA, 3–5% of responders said that they had made an attempt at deliberate self harm at some time.[6] Self poisoning using organophosphates is particularly common in developing countries.[7] A large hospital (catering for 900 000 people) in Sri Lanka, reported 2559 adult hospital admissions and 41% occupancy of medical intensive care beds for deliberate self harm with organophosphates over 2 years.[8] An international survey using representative community samples of adults (aged 18–64 years) reported lifetime prevalence of self reported suicide attempts of 3.82% in Canada, 5.93% in Puerto Rico, 4.95% in France, 3.44% in West Germany, 0.72% in Lebanon, 0.75% in Taiwan, 3.2% in Korea, and 4.43% in New Zealand.[6]

AETIOLOGY/ RISK FACTORS Familial, biological, and psychosocial factors may contribute to deliberate self harm. Evidence for genetic factors includes a higher risk of familial suicide and greater concordance in monozygotic than dizygotic twins for deliberate self harm and suicide.[9] Evidence for biological factors includes reduced cerebrospinal fluid 5-hydroxyindole acetic acid (5-HIAA) levels and blunted prolactin response to fenfluramine challenge test, indicating a reduction in the function of serotonin in the central nervous system.[10] People who deliberately self harm also show traits of impulsiveness and aggression, inflexible and impulsive cognitive style, and impaired decision making and problem solving (see glossary, p 1095).[11] Deliberate self harm is more likely in women, young adults, and people who are single or divorced, of low education level, unemployed, disabled, or suffering from a psychiatric disorder[12] particularly depression,[13] substance misuse,[14] borderline and antisocial personality disorders,[15] severe anxiety disorders,[16] and physical illness.[17]

PROGNOSIS Suicide is highest during the first year after deliberate self harm.[18] One systematic review found median rates of repetition of deliberate self harm of 16.0% (interquartile range [IQR] 12.0% to 25.0%) within the first year, 21.0% (IQR 12.0% to 30.0%) within 1–4 years, and 23% (IQR 11% to 32%) within 4 years or longer. It found median mortality from suicide after deliberate self harm of 1.8% (IQR 0.8% to 2.6%) within the first year, 3.0% (IQR 2.0% to 4.4%) within 1–4 years, 3.4% (IQR 2.5% to 6.0%) within 5–10 years, and 6.7% (IQR 5.0% to 11.0%) within 9 years or longer.[18] Repetition of deliberate self harm is more likely in people aged 25–49 years, who are unemployed, divorced, from lower social class, or who suffer from substance misuse, depression, hopelessness, powerlessness, personality disorders, have unstable living conditions or live alone, have a criminal record, previous psychiatric treatment, a history of stressful traumatic life events, or a history of coming from broken home or of family violence.[12] Factors associated with risk of suicide after deliberate self harm are age over 45 years, male sex, being unemployed, retired, separated, divorced, or widowed, living alone, poor physical health, psychiatric disorder (particularly depression, alcoholism, schizophrenia, and sociopathic personality disorder), high suicidal intent in current episode including leaving a written note, violent method used in current episode, and history of deliberate self harm.[19]

AIMS OF INTERVENTION To reduce repetition of deliberate self harm, desire to self harm, to prevent suicide, and improve social functioning and quality of life, with minimal adverse effects.

OUTCOMES Repetition of deliberate self harm, occurrence of suicide, admission to hospital, improvement in underlying psychiatric symptoms, improvement in coping, quality of life, and adverse effects. Some of the validated scales used for assessing psychiatric symptoms and deliberate self harm are: Symptom Checklist-90 (SCL-90), a self administered rating scale for assessing nine areas of psychopathology (somatisation, obsessive-compulsive, interpersonal sensitivity, depression, anxiety, hostility, phobic-anxiety, paranoid ideation, and psychoticism),[20–22] Beck Depression Inventory (a 21 item self administered Likert scale for measuring severity of depression),[23] Hospital Anxiety Depression Scale (a self administered 14 item Likert scale for measuring depression and anxiety),[24] Beck Scale for Suicidal Ideation (a 21-item self administered Likert scale covering thoughts and plans about suicide and aims at assessing the risk of a later suicide attempt),[25] Beck Hopelessness Scale (a 20 item true-false self administered items and aims at assessing hopelessness about the future),[26] and Global Severity Index (GSI; a mean of all items in SCL-90).[21]

METHODS *Clinical Evidence* search and appraisal April 2003.

QUESTION **What are the effects of treatments for deliberate self harm in adults?** New

OPTION **PAROXETINE**

One RCT in people with deliberate self harm receiving psychotherapy found no significant difference between paroxetine and placebo in the proportion of people who repeated self harm over 12 months. It found that paroxetine increased diarrhoea and tremor compared with placebo.

Benefits: We found one systematic review (search date 1999),[27] which identified one RCT[28] (91 outpatients who had previously been admitted to hospital for deliberate self harm, without current depression, receiving psychotherapy) comparing paroxetine 40 mg daily versus placebo for 12 months. It found no significant difference between paroxetine and placebo in the proportion of people repeating deliberate self harm over 12 months (15/46 [33%] with paroxetine *v* 21/45 [47%] with placebo; RR 0.70, 95% CI 0.40 to 1.18).

Harms: The RCT found that, compared with placebo, paroxetine significantly increased the proportion of people with diarrhoea (10/46 [22%] with paroxetine *v* 1/45 [2%] with placebo; P = 0.007), tremor (8/46 [17%] with paroxetine *v* 1/46 [2%] with control; P = 0.03), and delayed orgasm (9/46 [19%] with paroxetine *v* 0/45 [0%] with placebo; P = 0.003).[28] It also found that paroxetine was associated with large bruises in two people.

Comment: The review did not report any other outcomes.[27]

OPTION MIANSERIN

RCTs provided insufficient evidence to assess mianserin.

Benefits: We found one systematic review (search date 1999),[27] which identified two RCTs.[29,30] The first RCT (38 people with borderline or histrionic personality disorder and a history of deliberate self harm, admitted to hospital after an episode of self harm) identified by the review found no significant difference between mianserin 30 mg daily and placebo in the proportion of people who repeated deliberate self harm over 6 months' treatment (8/17 [47%] with mianserin *v* 12/21 [57%] with placebo; RR 0.82, 95% CI 0.44 to 1.54), but it is likely to have been too small to detect a clinically important difference.[29] The second RCT (114 people admitted to hospital after deliberate self poisoning, history of deliberate self harm not stated) identified by the review compared mianserin 30–60 mg daily or nomifensine 75–150 mg daily versus placebo for 6 weeks' treatment (see comment below).[30] The RCT did not compare mianserin alone versus placebo. It found no significant difference between mianserin or nomifensine and placebo in the proportion of people who repeated deliberate self harm over 12 weeks (16/76 [21%] with mianserin or nomifensine *v* 5/38 [13%] with placebo; RR 1.60, 95% CI 0.63 to 4.04), but it is likely to have been too small to detect a clinically important difference.

Harms: The review[27] and RCTs[29,30] gave no information on adverse effects.

Comment: The review did not report any other outcomes.[27] Nomifensine was withdrawn worldwide in the 1980s because of association with immune haemolytic anaemia.[30]

OPTION FLUPENTIXOL DEPOT INJECTION

One small RCT found that flupentixol depot injection reduced the proportion of people who repeated deliberate self harm over 6 months compared with placebo. However, we were unable to draw reliable conclusions from this small study. Typical antipsychotics such as flupentixol are associated with a wide range of adverse effects.

Benefits: We found one systematic review (search date 1999), which identified one RCT (30 people with a history of deliberate self harm) comparing flupentixol decanoate (20 mg im once every 4 weeks) versus placebo for 6 months.[27] It found that flupentixol significantly reduced the proportion of people who repeated deliberate self harm over 6 months compared with placebo (3/14 [21%] with flupentixol *v* 12/16 [75%] with placebo; RR 0.29, 95% CI 0.10 to 0.81).

Harms: The review gave no information on adverse effects (see comment below).[27]

Comment: We found insufficient evidence about the adverse effects of flupentixol in people with deliberate self harm. Typical antipsychotics such as flupentixol are associated with a wide range of adverse effects.[31] The review did not investigate other outcomes.[27]

OPTION PROBLEM SOLVING THERAPY

One systematic review of small RCTs found no significant difference between problem solving therapy and usual care in the proportion of people who repeated deliberate self harm over 6–12 months. Another systematic review found that problem solving therapy reduced depression, anxiety, and hopelessness, and improved problems compared with usual care.

Benefits: We found one systematic review (search date 1999)[27] that assessed the effects of problem solving therapy (see glossary, p 1095) on repetition of deliberate self harm and one systematic review (search date not stated)[32] that assessed the effects of problem solving therapy on depression, anxiety, and hopelessness. The first review identified five RCTs (571 people) comparing problem solving therapy versus usual care (standard care [from psychiatrist, community psychiatric nurse, or social worker], marital counselling, or general practitioner counselling).[27] Four of the RCTs were in people who had been admitted to hospital for deliberate self poisoning and included people with both a history of deliberate self harm and experiencing their first episode; one RCT was in people admitted to hospital after deliberate self harm who had self harmed at least once before in the previous year. The duration of interventions for four RCTs was 2–8 sessions, and for one RCT 3 months; follow up ranged from 6–12 months. The review found no significant difference between problem solving therapy and usual care in the proportion of people who repeated deliberate self harm over 6–12 months (45/290 [15%] with problem solving therapy *v* 54/281 [19%] with usual care; RR 0.77, 95% CI 0.55 to 1.08).[27] The second review (6 RCTs, including 5 identified by the first review) found that, compared with usual care, problem solving therapy significantly reduced depression (assessed by Beck Depression Inventory and Hospital Anxiety Depression Scale, 4 RCTs, 158 people, SMD –0.36 95% CI –0.61 to –0.11) and hopelessness (assessed by Beck Hopelessness Scale, 3 RCTs, 63 people; WMD –2.97 95% CI –4.81 to –1.13) and "improved problems" (2 RCTs, 211 people; OR 2.31, 95% CI 1.29 to 4.13; see comment below).[32]

Harms: The reviews gave no information on adverse effects.[27,32]

Comment: The second review did not state how improvement in problems was assessed.[32] The reviews did not assess other outcomes.[27,32]

OPTION DIALECTICAL BEHAVIOUR THERAPY

One RCT found limited and equivocal evidence that dialectical behaviour therapy may reduce the proportion of people who repeat deliberate self harm over 12 months compared with usual care.

Benefits: We found one systematic review (search date 1999)[27] which identified one RCT (39 women with borderline personality disorder and a history of deliberate self harm who had self harmed in the previous 8 weeks) comparing dialectical behaviour therapy (see glossary, p 1095) versus usual care (alternative therapy referrals). It found that dialectical behaviour therapy significantly reduced the proportion who repeated deliberate self harm over 1 year compared with usual care (5/19 [26%] with dialectical behaviour therapy *v* 12/20 [60%] with usual care; OR 0.24, 95% CI 0.06 to 0.93; see comment below).

Harms: The review gave no information on adverse effects.[27]

Comment: The results of the RCT are sensitive to the method of statistical calculation used; calculation of relative risk renders the difference between dialectical behaviour therapy and usual care non-significant (RR 0.44, 95% CI 0.19 to 1.01).[27] The review did not assess other outcomes.

OPTION CONTINUITY OF CARE

One RCT found limited evidence that follow up after hospital treatment with the same compared with a different therapist may increase repetition of deliberate self harm over 3 months, although this may be explained by a higher level of risk factors for repetition in the group receiving same therapist follow up, despite randomisation.

Benefits: We found one systematic review (search date 1999), which identified one RCT (141 people with a history of deliberate self harm who had been admitted to hospital for 3 day crisis intervention [see glossary, p 1095] after an episode of self harm) comparing follow up by the same therapist who assessed them in hospital versus different therapist follow up.[27] All participants also received a "motivational interview [see glossary, p 1095], letter, and assessment of motivation towards therapy". It found that follow up by the same therapist significantly increased the proportion of people who repeated deliberate self harm over 3 months compared with different therapist follow up (12/68 [18%] with same therapist *v* 4/73 [5%] with different therapist; RR 3.22, 95% CI 1.09 to 9.51; see comment below).

Harms: The review gave no information on adverse effects.[27]

Comment: The authors commented that the increase in deliberate self harm in people who had continuity of care may have been because of a higher prevalence of risk factors (unspecified) for repetition in the same therapist group despite randomisation.[27] The review and RCTs did not assess other outcomes.

OPTION SAME NUMBER OF SESSIONS OF THERAPY GIVEN OVER LONG TERM VERSUS OVER SHORT TERM

One systematic review of one RCT found no significant difference in the proportion of people who repeated deliberate self harm over 12 months with therapy given over 3 months compared with 12 months.

Benefits: We found one systematic review (search date 1999, 1 RCT, 80 people with deliberate self harm and a history of deliberate self harm) comparing 12 sessions of therapy given over 12 months versus the same number of session given over 3 months (see comment below).[27] It found no significant difference between longer and shorter duration of therapy in the proportion of people who repeated deliberate self harm over 12 months (9/40 [22%] with longer therapy *v* 9/40 [22%] with shorter therapy; RR 1.00, 95% 0.44 to 2.26).

Harms: The review gave no information on adverse effects.[27]

Comment: The RCT did not specify what type of therapy participants received.[27] The review did not assess other outcomes.

OPTION PSYCHODYNAMIC INTERPERSONAL THERAPY

One RCT found that, compared with usual care, psychodynamic interpersonal therapy for 4 weeks reduced repetition of deliberate self harm, depression, and suicidal ideation over 6 months. However, we were unable to draw reliable conclusions from one RCT.

Benefits: We found no systematic review. We found one RCT (119 people admitted to hospital after deliberate self poisoning, 60% with a history of "deliberate self harm") that compared psychodynamic interpersonal therapy (see glossary, p 1095) versus usual care (referral to usual services) for 4 weeks.[33] It found that, compared with usual care, brief psychodynamic interpersonal therapy significantly reduced repetition of deliberate self harm at 6 months (5/58 [9%] with psychodynamic interpersonal therapy *v* 17/61 [28%] with usual care; $P = 0.009$). It also found that brief psychodynamic interpersonal therapy significantly reduced depression (measured by Beck Depression Inventory, mean difference in score with interpersonal therapy *v* usual care –5.0, 95% CI –9.7 to –0.3) and suicidal ideation (measured by Beck Scale for Suicidal Ideation, mean difference in score –4.9, 95% CI –8.2 to –1.6).

Harms: The RCT gave no information on adverse effects.[33]

Comment: The RCT did not assess other outcomes.[33]

OPTION INTENSIVE OUTPATIENT FOLLOW UP PLUS OUTREACH

One systematic review found no significant difference in the proportion of people who repeated deliberate self harm over 4–12 months between outreach plus intensive intervention and usual care.

Benefits: We found one systematic review (search date 1999, 6 RCTs, 1161 people admitted to hospital after deliberate self harm, 30–100% with a history of deliberate self harm) comparing intensive intervention plus outreach versus usual care over 3–12 months.[27] Intensive outpatient follow up plus outreach varied but usually involved in person or phone contact of the person in the community, including encouragement to attend health services. Usual care involved treatment by various professionals, not involving outreach. It found no significant difference between intensive intervention plus outreach and usual care in the proportion of people who repeated deliberate self harm over 4–12 months (92/580 [16%] with intensive intervention *v* 107/581 [18%] with usual care; RR 0.87, 95% CI 0.68 to 1.12).

Harms: The review gave no information on adverse effects.[27]

Comment: The review did not assess other outcomes.[27]

OPTION EMERGENCY CARD

One systematic review found no significant difference in the proportion of people who repeated deliberate self harm over 12 months between emergency card (allowing emergency admission or contact with a doctor) and usual care.

Benefits: We found one systematic review (search date 1999, 2 RCTs, 1 RCT in 212 adults admitted to hospital after their first episode of deliberate self harm, 1 RCT in 105 children admitted to hospital after deliberate self harm, history of self harm not stated).[27] It compared emergency card (indicating that a doctor was available and how to contact them or allowing readmission to a paediatric hospital ward) versus usual care (referral to and treatment from usual inpatient, outpatient, or primary care services as appropriate). It found no significant difference in the proportion of people who repeated deliberate self harm over 12 months between emergency card and usual care (8/148 [5%] with emergency card *v* 19/169 [11%] with usual care; RR 0.48, 95% CI 0.22 to 1.07; see comment below).

Harms: The review gave no information on adverse effects.[27]

Comment: The review pooled results from RCTs of heterogeneous populations (adults and children) to try to increase the power of its meta-analysis but it may not be appropriate to pool results in such different groups.[27] The review did not assess other outcomes.

OPTION HOSPITAL ADMISSION

One RCT found no significant difference between hospital admission and immediate discharge in the proportion of people who repeated deliberate self harm over 16 weeks, but it is likely to have been underpowered to detect a clinically important difference.

Benefits: We found one systematic review (search date 1999) which identified one RCT (77 people).[27] The RCT found no significant difference between hospital admission for a median of 17 hours and immediate discharge in the proportion of people who repeated deliberate self harm over 16 weeks (3/38 [8%] with hospital admission *v* 4/39 [10%] with immediate discharge; RR 0.77, 95% CI 0.18 to 3.21), but it is likely to have been underpowered to detect a clinically important difference.

Harms: The review gave no information on adverse effects.[27]

Comment: The review did not assess other outcomes.[27]

OPTION GENERAL PRACTICE BASED GUIDELINES

One large cluster randomised trial comparing the use of general practitioner guidelines for management of deliberate self harm versus usual care found no significant difference in the proportion of people who repeated deliberate self harm over 12 months or in the time to repetition of self harm.

Benefits: We found no systematic review. We found one cluster randomised trial (98 general practices, 2084 people who had attended hospital emergency departments after deliberate self harm, 11–14 with a recent recorded history of deliberate self harm).[34] It compared inviting people for consultation with their general practitioner who followed guidelines for managing self harm versus usual care (provided by general practitioner or referral to mental health or other services as appropriate). It found no significant difference between use of guidelines and usual care in repetition of deliberate self harm (211/964 [22%] with guidelines *v* 189/968 [20%] with usual care; OR 1.17, 95% CI 0.94 to 1.47), mean repeat episodes per person (mean 0.48 with guidelines *v* 0.37 with usual care; incident rate ratio 1.24, 95% CI 0.92 to 1.68), and mean days to first episode of self harm (mean 105 with guidelines *v* 110 with usual care; HR 1.15, 95% CI 0.94 to 1.42).

Harms: The RCT gave no information on adverse effects.[34]

Comment: The RCT did not assess other outcomes.[34]

OPTION NURSE LED CASE MANAGEMENT

One RCT found no significant difference between nurse led case management and usual care in the proportion of people who were admitted to emergency departments for episodes of deliberate self harm over 12 months.

Benefits: We found no systematic review. We found one RCT (467 people who had attended hospital emergency departments after deliberate self harm, 47% with a history of deliberate self harm) comparing nurse led case management (see glossary, p 1095) versus usual care (triage, psychiatric assessment, and inpatient care if appropriate) for 12 months.[35] It found no significant difference between groups in rates of readmission to hospital as a result of deliberate self harm over 12 months (19/220 [9%] with nurse led case management *v* 25/247 [10%] with usual care; OR 0.84, 95% CI 0.45 to 1.57).

Harms: The RCT gave no information on adverse effects.[35]

Comment: The RCT did not assess other outcomes.[35]

OPTION TELEPHONE CONTACT

One RCT found no significant difference between telephone contact at 4 and 8 months and usual care in repetition of deliberate self harm, global functioning, and suicidal ideation over 12 months.

Benefits: We found one RCT (216 people admitted to hospital after deliberate self harm, 51–54% with a history of deliberate self harm) that compared telephone contact at 4 and 8 months aimed at increasing motivation versus usual care (undefined).[36] It found no significant difference between telephone contact and usual care in the proportion of people repeating deliberate self harm over 12 months (14/83 [17%] with telephone contact *v* 15/89 [17%] with usual care; reported as non-significant, CI not reported; results not intention to treat, 19% lost to follow up). It found similar rates in overall functioning between telephone contact and usual care (assessed by Global Assessment of Functioning Scale: mean score 61.4 with telephone contact *v* 58.6 with usual care; CI not reported). It also found similar scores on the scale for suicidal ideation (mean score 5.8 with telephone contact group *v* 4.0 with usual care; CI not reported) and on the Symptom Checklist-90 scale at 12 months (mean score 0.82 with telephone contact group *v* 0.88 with usual care; CI not reported).

Harms: The RCT gave no information on adverse effects.[36]

Comment: None.

GLOSSARY

Case management Involves a case manager managing an individual's care including comprehensive assessment of their needs, development of individualised package of care, the arrangement of access to services, monitoring of quality of services provided, and long term flexible support.

Crisis intervention Involves short term help with current and acute difficult life events using variety of counselling, problem solving, and practical measures.

Dialectical behaviour therapy Is a multimodal cognitive behaviour therapy used particularly in the treatment of people with borderline personality disorder who repeatedly engage in deliberate self harm. It involves helping to replace extremes of emotions and behaviour with behaviour that is a moderate synthesis of extremes.

Motivational interviewing Uses principles of motivational psychology and is aimed at helping people to change and engage in demanding treatments.

Problem solving therapy Uses a set of sequential steps in solving problems and aims at minimising negative emotion and maximising identification, evaluation, and implementation of optimal solutions.

Psychodynamic interpersonal therapy Is a psychotherapeutic intervention aimed at improving interpersonal problems using the model developed by Hobson.

REFERENCES

1. Gelder M, Mayou R, Cowen P. *Shorter oxford textbook of psychiatry*. Oxford: Oxford University Press, 2001.
2. American Psychiatric Association. *Diagnostic and statistical manual of mental disorders*, 4th ed. Washington, DC: American Psychiatric Association, 1994.
3. World Health Organization. *The ICD-10 classification of mental and behavioural disorders*. Geneva: World Health Organization, 1992.
4. Schmidtke A, Bille-Brahe U, DeLeo D, et al. Attempted suicide Europe: rates, trends and sociodemographic characteristics of suicide attempters during the period 1989–1992. Results of the WHO/EURO Multicentre Study on Parasuicide. *Acta Psychiatr Scand* 1996;93:327–338.
5. The University of York. NHS Centre for Reviews and Dissemination. 1998. Deliberate self harm. *Effective Health Care* 4:1–12.
6. Weissman MM, Bland RC, Canino GJ, et al. Prevalence of suicide ideation and suicide attempts in nine countries. *Psychol Med* 1999;29:9–17.
7. Eddleston M. Patterns and problems of deliberate self-poisoning in the developing world. *QJM* 2000;93:715–731.
8. Eddleston M, Sheriff MH, Hawton K. Deliberate self harm in Sri Lanka: an overlooked tragedy in the developing world. *BMJ* 1998;317:133–135.
9. Roy A, Nielsen D, Rylander G, et al. Genetics of suicidal behaviour. In: Hawton K, van Heeringen K, eds. *International handbook of suicide and attempted suicide*. Chichester: Wiley, 2000: 209–221.

10. Traskman-Bendz L, Mann JJ. Biological aspects of suicidal behaviour. In: Hawton K, van Heeringen K, eds. *International handbook of suicide and attempted suicide*. Chichester: Wiley, 2000: 65–78.
11. Williams JMG, Pollock LR. The psychology of suicidal behaviour. In: Hawton K, van Heeringen K, eds. *International handbook of suicide and attempted suicide*. Chichester: Wiley, 2000: 79–93.
12. Kerkhof AJFM. Attempted suicide: trends and patterns. In: Hawton K, van Heeringen K, eds. *International handbook of suicide and attempted suicide*. Chichester: Wiley, 2000: 49–64.
13. Lonnqvist JK. Psychiatric aspects of suicidal behaviour: depression. In: Hawton K, van Heeringen K, eds. *International handbook of suicide and attempted suicide*. Chichester: Wiley, 2000: 107–120.
14. Murphy GE. Psychiatric aspects of suicidal behaviour: substance abuse. In: Hawton K, van Heeringen K, eds. *International handbook of suicide and attempted suicide*. Chichester: Wiley, 2000: 135–146.
15. Linehan MM, Rizvi SL, Welch SS, et al. Psychiatric aspects of suicidal behaviour: personality disorder. In: Hawton K, van Heeringen K, eds. *International handbook of suicide and attempted suicide*. Chichester: Wiley, 2000: 147–178.
16. Allgulander C. Psychiatric aspects of suicidal behaviour: anxiety disorders. In: Hawton K, van Heeringen K, eds. *International handbook of suicide and attempted suicide*. Chichester: Wiley, 2000: 179–192.
17. Stenager EN, Stenager E. Physical illness and suicidal behaviour. In: Hawton K, van Heeringen K, eds. *International handbook of suicide and attempted suicide*. Chichester: Wiley, 2000: 405–420.
18. Owens D, Horrocks J, House A. Fatal and non-fatal repetition of self-harm. Systematic review. *Br J Psychiatry* 2002;181:193–199.
19. Hawton K. Treatment of suicide attempters and prevention of suicide and attempted suicide. In: Gelder MG, Lopez-Ibor JJ Jr, Andreasen NC, eds. *New Oxford textbook of psychiatry*. Oxford: Oxford University Press, 2000: 1050–1059.
20. Bridges K, Goldberg D. Self-administered scales of neurotic symptoms. In: Thompson C, ed. *The instruments of psychiatric research*. London: Wiley, 1989: 157–176.
21. Derogatis LR. Symptom Checklist-90-Revised (SCL-90-R). In: American Psychiatric Association, eds. *Handbook of psychiatric measures*. Washington, DC: American Psychiatric Association, 2000: 81–84.
22. Thompson C. Anxiety. In: Thompson C, ed. *The instruments of psychiatric research*. London: Wiley, 1989: 127–156.
23. Beck A, Steer A. Beck Depression Inventory (BDI). In: American Psychiatric Association, eds. *Handbook of psychiatric measures*. Washington, DC: American Psychiatric Association, 2000: 519–523.
24. Snaith RP, Zigmond AS. Hospital Anxiety and Depression Scale (HADS). In: American Psychiatric Association, eds. *Handbook of psychiatric measures*. Washington, DC: American Psychiatric Association, 2000:547–548.
25. Beck A, Kovacs M, Weissman A. Beck Scale for Suicidal Ideation (BSS). In: American Psychiatric Association, eds. *Handbook of psychiatric measures*. Washington, DC: American Psychiatric Association, 2000:264–266.
26. Beck A, Weissman A, Lester D, et al. Beck Hopelessness Scale (BHS). In: American Psychiatric Association, eds. *Handbook of psychiatric measures*. Washington, DC: American Psychiatric Association, 2000:268–270.
27. Hawton K, Townsend E, Arensman E, et al. Psychosocial and pharmacological treatments for deliberate self harm. In: The Cochrane Library, Issue 2, 2003. Oxford, Update Software. Search date 1999; primary sources Medline, PsychLit, Embase, Cochrane Controlled Trials Register, hand searches of 10 relevant journals, reference lists of relevant papers, and personal contact with trialists and other experts in the field.
28. Verkes RJ, Van der Mast RC, Hengeveld MW, et al. Reduction by paroxetine of suicidal behavior in patients with repeated suicide attempts but not major depression. *Am J Psychiatry* 1998;155:543–547.
29. Montgomery SA, Roy D, Montgomery DB. The prevention of recurrent suicidal acts. *Br J Clin Pharmacol* 1983;15:183S–188S.
30. Lasser KE, Alan PD, Woolhandler SJ, et al. Timing of new black box warnings and withdrawals for prescription medications. *JAMA* 2002;287:2215–2220.
31. British Medical Association and Royal Pharmaceutical Society of Great Britain. *British national formulary*. London: British Medical Association and Royal Pharmaceutical Society of Great Britain, 2002.
32. Townsend E, Hawton K, Altman DG, et al. The efficacy of problem-solving treatments after deliberate self-harm: meta-analysis of randomized controlled trials with respect to depression, hopelessness and improvement in problems. *Psychol Med* 2001;31:979–988. Search date not stated; primary sources Embase, PyschLit, Medline, Cochrane Controlled Trials Register, Cochrane Depression, Anxiety and Neurosis Review Group Trials Register, and hand searches of worldwide literature on deliberate self harm.
33. Guthrie E, Kapur N, Mackway-Jones K, et al. Randomised controlled trial of brief psychological intervention after deliberate self poisoning. *BMJ* 2001;323:135–138.
34. Bennewith O, Stocks N, Gunnell D, et al. General practice based intervention to prevent repeat episodes of deliberate self harm: cluster randomised controlled trial. *BMJ* 2002;324:1254–1257.
35. Clarke T, Baker P, Watts CJ, et al. Self-harm in adults: a randomised controlled trial of nurse-led case management versus routine care only. *J Mental Health* 2002;11:167–176.
36. Cedereke M, Monti K, Ojehagen A. Telephone contact with patients in the year after a suicide attempt: does it affect treatment attendance and outcome? A randomised controlled study. *Eur Psychiatry* 2002;17:82–91.

G Mustafa Soomro
Honorary Research Fellow
Section of Community Psychiatry
St George's Hospital Medical School, London, UK

Competing interests: None declared

Dementia

Search date October 2002

James Warner, Rob Butler, and Pramod Prabhakaran

QUESTIONS

INTERVENTIONS

See glossary, p 1116

Key Messages

- People in dementia RCTs are often not representative of people in routine settings. Few RCTs are conducted in primary care and few are conducted in people with types of dementia other than Alzheimer's disease.

Cognitive symptoms

- **Donepezil** One systematic review and two subsequent RCTs have found that donepezil compared with placebo improves cognitive function and global clinical state at up to 52 weeks in people with mild to moderate Alzheimer's disease. The review found no significant difference in patient rated quality of life at 12 or 24 weeks between donepezil and placebo. One RCT in people with mild to moderate Alzheimer's disease found no significant difference in cognitive function at 12 weeks between donepezil and rivastigmine, although significantly fewer people taking donepezil withdrew from the trial for any cause.
- **Galantamine** RCTs identified by a systematic review, and one additional RCT, have found that galantamine improves cognitive function compared with placebo in people with Alzheimer's disease or vascular dementia.
- **Ginkgo biloba** RCTs found limited evidence that ginkgo biloba improved cognitive function compared with placebo in people with Alzheimer's disease.

- **Lecithin** Small, poor RCTs identified by a systematic review provided insufficient evidence to assess lecithin in people with Alzheimer's disease.
- **Music therapy** Poor studies identified by a systematic review provided insufficient evidence to assess music therapy.
- **Nicotine** One systematic review found no RCTs of adequate quality on the effects of nicotine.
- **Non-steroidal anti-inflammatory drugs** One RCT in people with Alzheimer's disease found no significant difference in cognitive function after 25 weeks' treatment with diclofenac plus misoprostol compared with placebo. Another RCT in people with Alzheimer's disease found that indometacin (indomethacin) improved cognitive function after 6 months' treatment compared with placebo.
- **Oestrogen (in women)** One systematic review has found that, in women with mild to moderate Alzheimer's disease, oestrogen improves cognition over 7–12 months' treatment compared with no oestrogen.
- **Physostigmine** One systematic review in people with Alzheimer's disease found limited evidence that slow release physostigmine improved cognitive function compared with placebo, but adverse effects, including nausea, vomiting, diarrhoea, dizziness, and stomach pain, were common.
- **Reality orientation** One systematic review of small RCTs found that reality orientation improved cognitive function compared with no treatment in people with various types of dementia.
- **Reminiscence therapy** One systematic review provided insufficient evidence to assess reminiscence therapy.
- **Rivastigmine** One systematic review and one additional RCT have found that rivastigmine improves cognitive function compared with placebo in people with Alzheimer's disease or Lewy body dementia, but adverse effects such as nausea, vomiting, and anorexia are common. Subgroup analysis from one RCT in people with Alzheimer's disease suggests that people with vascular risk factors may respond better to rivastigmine than those without. One RCT in people with mild to moderate Alzheimer's disease found no significant difference in cognitive function at 12 weeks between donepezil and rivastigmine, although rivastigmine significantly increased the proportion of people who withdrew from the trial for any cause.
- **Selegiline** One systematic review has found that, in people with mild to moderate Alzheimer's disease, selegiline improves cognitive function, behavioural disturbance, and mood compared with placebo, but has found no significant difference in global clinical state.
- **Tacrine** Systematic reviews found limited evidence that tacrine improved cognitive function and global state in Alzheimer's disease compared with placebo, but adverse effects, including nausea and vomiting, diarrhoea, anorexia, and abdominal pain, were common.
- **Vitamin E** One RCT in people with moderate to severe Alzheimer's disease found no significant difference in cognitive function after 2 years' treatment with vitamin E compared with placebo. However, it found that vitamin E reduced mortality, institutionalisation, loss of ability to perform activities of daily living, and the proportion of people who developed severe dementia.

Behavioural and psychological symptoms

- **Carbamazepine** One RCT found that carbamazepine reduced agitation and aggression compared with placebo in people with various types of dementia.

- **Cholinesterase inhibitors** One RCT in people with mild to moderate Alzheimer's disease found no significant difference in psychiatric symptoms at 3 months between galantamine and placebo, but another RCT found that galantamine significantly improved psychiatric symptoms at 6 months compared with placebo. One RCT in people with moderate to severe Alzheimer's disease found that donepezil significantly improved functional and behavioural symptoms at 24 weeks compared with placebo, but another RCT in people with mild to moderate Alzheimer's disease found no significant difference in psychiatric symptoms at 24 weeks between donepezil and placebo.
- **Haloperidol** One systematic review in people with various types of dementia found no significant difference in agitation between haloperidol and placebo, but found limited evidence that haloperidol may reduce aggression.
- **Olanzapine** One RCT in people with Alzheimer's disease found that olanzapine (5–10 mg daily) reduced agitation, hallucinations, and delusions compared with placebo.
- **Reality orientation** One systematic review of small RCTs found that reality orientation significantly improved behaviour compared with no treatment in people with various types of dementia.
- **Risperidone** One RCT in people with moderate to severe dementia, including Alzheimer's disease and vascular dementia, found that risperidone significantly improved behavioural and psychological symptoms over 12 weeks compared with placebo, but another RCT in people with severe dementia and agitation found no significant difference in symptoms over 13 weeks.
- **Sodium valproate** One RCT found that sodium valproate reduced agitation over 6 weeks in people with dementia, but another RCT found no significant difference in aggressive behaviour over 8 weeks between sodium valproate and placebo.
- **Trazodone** One RCT in people with Alzheimer's disease found no significant difference between trazodone and haloperidol in reducing agitation. Another RCT in people with dementia plus agitated behaviour found no significant difference in agitation among trazodone, haloperidol, behavioural management techniques, and placebo. The RCTs may have been too small to exclude a clinically important difference.

DEFINITION **Dementia** is characterised by chronic, global, non-reversible impairment of cerebral function. It usually results in loss of memory (initially of recent events), loss of executive function (such as the ability to make decisions or sequence complex tasks), and changes in personality. **Alzheimer's disease** is a type of dementia characterised by an insidious onset and slow deterioration, and involves speech, motor, personality, and executive function impairment. It should be diagnosed after other systemic, psychiatric, and neurological causes of dementia have been excluded clinically and by laboratory investigation. **Vascular dementia** is multi-infarct dementia involving a stepwise deterioration of executive function with or without language and motor dysfunction occurring as a result of cerebral arterial occlusion. It usually occurs in the presence of vascular risk factors (diabetes, hypertension, and smoking). Characteristically, it has a more sudden onset and stepwise progression than Alzheimer's disease. **Lewy body dementia** is a type of dementia involving insidious impairment of executive functions with (1) Parkinsonism, (2) visual hallucinations, and (3) fluctuating cognitive abilities and increased risk of falls or autonomic failure.[1,2]

Careful clinical examination of people with mild to moderate dementia, and the use of established diagnostic criteria, has an antemortem positive predictive value of 70–90% compared with the gold standard of postmortem diagnosis.[3,4]

INCIDENCE/ PREVALENCE About 6% of people aged over 65 years and 30% of people aged over 90 years have some form of dementia.[5] Dementia is rare before the age of 60 years. Alzheimer's disease and vascular dementia (including mixed dementia) are each estimated to account for 35–50% of dementia, and Lewy body dementia is estimated to account for up to 20% of dementia in the elderly, varying with geographical, cultural, and racial factors.[1,5–10]

AETIOLOGY/ RISK FACTORS **Alzheimer's disease:** The cause of Alzheimer's disease is unclear. A key pathological process is deposition of abnormal amyloid in the central nervous system.[11] Most people with the relatively rare condition of early onset Alzheimer's disease (before age 60 years) show an autosomal dominant inheritance due to mutations on presenelin or amyloid precursor protein genes. Several genes (*APP*, *PS-1*, and *PS-2*) have been identified. Later onset dementia is sometimes clustered in families, but specific gene mutations have not been identified. Head injury, Down's syndrome, and lower premorbid intellect may be risk factors for Alzheimer's disease. **Vascular dementia** is related to cardiovascular risk factors, such as smoking, hypertension, and diabetes. **Lewy body dementia:** The aetiology of Lewy body dementia is unknown. Brain acetylcholine activity is reduced in many forms of dementia, and the level of reduction correlates with cognitive impairment. Many treatments for Alzheimer's disease enhance cholinergic activity.[1,6]

PROGNOSIS **Alzheimer's disease:** Alzheimer's disease usually has an insidious onset with progressive reduction in cerebral function. Diagnosis is difficult in the early stages. Average life expectancy after diagnosis is 7–10 years.[10] **Lewy body dementia:** People with Lewy body dementia have an average life expectancy of around 6 years after diagnosis.[5] Behavioural problems, depression, and psychotic symptoms are common in all types of dementia.[12,13] Eventually, most people with dementia find it difficult to perform simple tasks without help.

AIMS OF INTERVENTION To improve cognitive function (memory, orientation, attention, and concentration); to reduce behavioural and psychological symptoms (wandering, aggression, anxiety, depression, and psychosis); to improve quality of life for both the individual and carer, with minimum adverse effects.

OUTCOMES **Cognitive symptoms and global assessment of function:** Quality of life of the person with dementia and their carer (rarely used in clinical trials). Comprehensive scales of cognitive function (e.g. Alzheimer's Disease Assessment Scale cognitive subscale [ADAS-cog], 70-point scale, lower scores indicate better function;[14] Mini Mental State Examination, 30-point scale, higher scores indicate better function[15] Clinical Dementia Rating Scale [CDR], 3-point scale assessing 6 cognitive and functional parameters, higher scores indicate worse function;[16] Alzheimer's Disease Functional Assessment and Change Scale [ADFACS], 7 point scale, higher scores indicate worse function[16]). ADAS-cog is more sensitive than

Mini Mental State Examination, but neither scale directly reflects outcomes important to people with dementia or their carers. A 7 point change in the ADAS-cog has been regarded as clinically important. Measures of global state (e.g. clinician interview based impression of change with caregiver input scale, Clinician's Interview Based Impression of Change-Plus, 7 points scale). **Behavioural and psychological symptoms:** Measures of psychiatric symptoms (e.g. Neuropsychiatric Inventory, 12-item caregiver rated scale, maximum score 144, higher scores indicate greater difficulties; Dementia Mood Assessment Scale and Brief Psychiatric Rating Scale, which use lower scores to signify improved symptoms; Behave-AD scale, scores 0–75, lower scores indicate better function). Time to institutionalisation or death are rarely reported because of the short duration of most trials.[16] Functional measures include the Disability Assessment for Dementia, a 40-item scale assessing 10 domains of function[17] and the Instrumental Activities of Daily Living Scale, maximum score 14 (higher scores indicate better function).[18]

METHODS *Clinical Evidence* search and appraisal October 2002. Dementia is often considered to have two domains of symptoms: cognitive impairment and non-cognitive symptoms (behavioural and psychological symptoms). We have separated the evidence into these two domains because they are often therapeutic targets at different stages of dementia and many RCTs focus on one or other domain of symptoms. In many RCTs, missing data were managed using "last observation carried forward", which does not account for the tendency of people with dementia to deteriorate with time. These RCTs may overestimate the benefit derived from interventions, especially when there are higher withdrawal rates in the intervention arm compared with controls. We found few RCTs in people with types of dementia other than Alzheimer's disease.

QUESTION What are the effects of treatments on cognitive symptoms of dementia?

OPTION DONEPEZIL

One systematic review and two subsequent RCT have found that donepezil compared with placebo improves cognitive function and global clinical state at up to 52 weeks in people with mild to moderate Alzheimer's disease. The review found no significant difference in patient rated quality of life at 12 or 24 weeks between donepezil and placebo. One RCT in people with mild to moderate Alzheimer's disease found no significant difference in cognitive function at 12 weeks between donepezil and rivastigmine, although significantly fewer people taking donepezil withdrew from the trial for any cause.

Benefits: **Versus placebo:** We found one systematic review[19] and three subsequent RCTs in people with Alzheimer's disease (see comment below).[20–22] The systematic review (search date 2000) identified eight RCTs of 12, 24, and 52 weeks' duration (2664 people with mild to moderate Alzheimer's disease) comparing donepezil versus placebo.[19] Five RCTs identified by the review reported results using the Alzheimer's Disease Assessment Scale cognitive subscale

(ADAS-cog) or the Clinician's Interview Based Impression of Change-Plus (CIBIC-Plus). The review found that donepezil (10 mg daily) significantly improved cognitive function (measured by ADAS-cog scores) at 12 and 24 weeks compared with placebo (see table 1, p 1120), and significantly improved global clinical state at 24 weeks (CIBIC-Plus score unchanged or worse: 5 RCTs, 799 people; 295/390 [76%] with donepezil *v* 356/409 [87%] with placebo; OR for improvement in CIBIC-Plus score 2.1, 95% 1.3 to 3.6), but found no significant difference in patient rated quality of life at 12 or 24 weeks (at 24 wks: WMD +2.79, 95% CI –2.56 to +8.14).[19] An unblinded extension of one of the RCTs identified by the review observed 133 people taking donepezil (3–10 mg daily) for up to 240 weeks.[23] It found that improved cognitive function compared with baseline was present for 38 weeks in people taking domepezil, and throughout the period of observation cognitive function remained above the level estimated had people not been treated. The first subsequent RCT (24 wks, 290 people with more severe Alzheimer's disease aged 48–92 years, Mini Mental State Examination [MMSE] score 5 to 17) compared donepezil (5–10 mg daily) versus placebo.[20] It found that donepezil significantly improved CIBIC-Plus scores at 24 weeks compared with placebo (mean difference 0.54, no 95% CI provided, results presented graphically; NNT 5, 95% CI 4 to 10 for improved or no change on CIBIC-Plus).[20] The second subsequent RCT (431 people with mild to moderate Alzheimer's disease aged 49–94 years, MMSE score 12–20) compared donepezil (10 mg daily) versus placebo for 1 year. It found that donepezil delayed the median time to "clinically evident functional decline" by 5 months compared with placebo (median 357 days with donepezil *v* 208 days with placebo; CI not provided). It found that a significantly higher proportion of people had no "clinically evident functional decline" at 1 year with donepezil compared with placebo (no functional decline: 123/207 [59%] with donepezil *v* 92/208 [44%] with placebo; NNT 7, 95% CI 5 to 17). **Versus rivastigmine:** We found one open label RCT (111 people with mild to moderate Alzheimer's disease, MMSE score 10–26) comparing donepezil (5– 10mg daily) versus rivastigmine (1.5–6 mg twice daily). It found no significant difference in cognitive function at 12 weeks between donepezil and rivastigmine (assessed by clinicians blind to intervention; mean difference in ADAS-cog –0.15, 95% CI –1.47 to +1.71).[22]

Harms: Adverse effects common to all cholinesterase inhibitors include anorexia, nausea, vomiting, and diarrhoea. **Versus placebo:** The RCTs identified by the review found that donepezil was associated with nausea, vomiting, and diarrhoea, which tended to be mild and transient.[19] The review found no difference between donepezil and placebo in the proportion of people who withdrew for any cause (27% with 10 mg donepezil *v* 20% with 5 mg *v* 21% with placebo).[19] Long term follow up of people taking donepezil (≤ 10 mg; open label extension) found that 86% experienced at least one adverse effect, often occurring later in the study. Common adverse events included agitation (24%), pain (20%), insomnia (11%), and diarrhoea (9%).[23] The first subsequent RCT found no significant difference between donepezil and placebo in the proportion of people who experienced any adverse event over 24 weeks (120/144 [83%] *v*

117/146 [80%]; RR 1.04, 95% CI 0.93 to 1.16).[20] **Versus rivastigmine:** The RCT found that fewer people had at least one adverse event with donepezil than with rivastigmine, but the difference was not significant (24/56 [43%] with donepezil *v* 32/55 [58%] with rivastigmine; RR 0.74, 95% CI 0.51 to 1.07). It found that, compared with rivastigmine, donepezil significantly reduced the proportion of people who withdrew from the trial for any cause (6/56 [11%] with donepezil *v* 17/55 [31%] with rivastigmine; RR of withdrawal 0.35, 95% CI 0.15 to 0.81; NNH 5, 95% CI 3 to 20).[22]

Comment: In the second subsequent RCT, "clinically evident functional decline" was defined as a decline of at least one point on the Alzheimer's Disease Functional Assessment and Change Scale or an increase of at least one point on the Clinical Dementia Rating Scale. Donepezil is taken once daily; this is a potential advantage over other cholinesterase inhibitors for people with dementia. Improvement usually starts within 2–4 months of starting donepezil. Open label studies should be interpreted with caution but do suggest that the effect of continued treatment is sustained in the long term.[23] We found no RCTs of donepezil in people with Lewy body or vascular dementia.

OPTION GALANTAMINE

RCTs identified by a systematic review, and one additional RCT, have found that galantamine improves cognitive function compared with placebo in people with Alzheimer's disease or vascular dementia.

Benefits: We found one systematic review (search date 2002, 7 RCTs)[24] in people with mild to moderate Alzheimer's disease and one additional RCT in people with vascular dementia (see comment below).[25] The review found that galantamine (12 mg or 16 mg twice daily) significantly improved cognitive function compared with placebo (measured by Alzheimer's Disease Assessment Scale cognitive subscale [ADAS-cog] score) over 6 months and improved global status (Clinician's Interview Based Impression of Change [CIBIC] Plus score unchanged or improved: galantamine 12 mg twice daily, 3 RCTs 339/508 [67%] with galantamine *v* 286/567 [50%] with placebo OR for improvement in CIBIC-Plus score 2.0, 95% CI 1.5 to 2.5; galantamine 16 mg twice daily, 3 RCTs 233/459 [51%] with galantamine *v* 212/568 [37%] with placebo; OR for improvement in CIBIC-Plus score 1.9, 95% CI 1.4 to 2.5) (see table 1, p 1120). The additional RCT (592 people with vascular dementia or Alzheimer's disease plus cerebrovascular disease) compared galantamine 24 mg daily (396 people) versus placebo (196 people) for 6 months.[25] It found that galantamine significantly improved cognitive function from baseline at 6 months compared with placebo (4 point improvement in ADAS-cog: 35% with galantamine *v* 22% with placebo; NNT 8, 95% CI 5 to 17). It also found that galantamine significantly improved global clinical state at 6 months compared with placebo (CIBIC score "improved" or "no change": 74% with galantamine *v* 59% with placebo; NNT for "no deterioration" 7, 95% CI 5 to 15).[25]

Harms: Adverse effects common to all cholinesterase inhibitors include anorexia, nausea, vomiting, and diarrhoea. The review in people with Alzheimer's disease found that adverse effects over 6 months were more frequent with larger doses of galantamine, including nausea (42% with galantamine 16 mg twice daily *v* 25% with placebo) and vomiting (21% with galantamine 16 mg twice daily *v* 7% with placebo). It also found that higher doses of galantamine increased the proportion of people who discontinued treatment because of adverse effects over 6 months (27% with galantamine 16 mg twice daily *v* 15% with galantamine 12 mg twice daily *v* 8% with placebo).[24] The additional RCT comparing galantamine versus placebo in people with vascular dementia found that more people taking galantamine withdrew because of adverse effects (20% with galantamine *v* 8% with placebo).[25]

Comment: We found no RCTs of galantamine in people with Lewy body dementia.

OPTION RIVASTIGMINE

One systematic review and one additional RCT have found that rivastigmine improves cognitive function in people with Alzheimer's disease or Lewy body dementia compared with placebo, but adverse effects such as nausea, vomiting, and anorexia are common. Subgroup analysis from one RCT in people with Alzheimer's disease suggests that people with vascular risk factors may respond better to rivastigmine than those without. One RCT in people with mild to moderate Alzheimer's disease found no significant difference in cognitive function at 12 weeks between donepezil and rivastigmine, although rivastigmine significantly increased the proportion of people who withdrew from the trial for any cause.

Benefits: **Versus placebo:** We found one systematic review (search date 2000, 4 RCTs, 12 or 26 wks' duration, 3370 people with mild to moderate Alzheimer's disease)[26] (see table 1, p 1120) and one additional RCT[27] in people with Lewy body dementia (see comment below). The review found that, over 26 weeks, rivastigmine (6–12 mg twice daily) produced small but significant improvements in cognitive function compared with placebo in people with Alzheimer's disease (Alzheimer's Disease Assessment Scale cognitive subscale [ADAS-cog]: 4 RCTs; 1917 people WMD –2.1, 95% CI –2.7 to –1.5; Mini Mental State Examination: WMD 0.8, 95% CI 0.5 to 1.1) and global clinical state (Clinician's Interview Based Impression of Change [CIBIC] score unchanged or worse: 4 RCTs, 715/973 [73%] *v* 675/839 [80%] with placebo; OR for improvement in CIBIC score 1.5, 95% CI 1.2 to 1.8). Quality of life results were not provided. A subgroup analysis of an RCT identified by the review[26] (699 people with Alzheimer's disease) comparing rivastigmine 1–4 mg daily or 6–12 mg daily versus placebo over 26 weeks found that people with vascular risk factors responded better than those without (mean ADAS-cog difference –2.3).[28] The additional RCT (120 people with Lewy body dementia) found that rivastigmine (dose titrated to 6 mg twice daily) significantly improved a computerised psychometric measure of cognitive function at 20 weeks compared with placebo (intention to treat analysis; P = 0.05; no further data provided) and improved a global measure of behavioural function (NNT for at least 30% improvement on Neuropsychiatric Inventory score 3, 95% CI 2 to 6).[27] **Versus donepezil:** We found one RCT comparing rivastigmine versus donepezil (see donepezil, p 1101).[22]

Harms: Adverse effects common to all cholinesterase inhibitors include anorexia, nausea, vomiting, and diarrhoea. The systematic review in people with Alzheimer's disease found that rivastigmine increased the proportion of people who discontinued treatment compared with placebo (35% with 6–12 mg rivastigmine *v* 18% with 1–4 mg rivastigmine *v* 17% with placebo).[26] The RCT in people with Lewy body dementia found that rivastigmine increased the proportion of people who had nausea compared with placebo (37% *v* 22%), vomiting (25% *v* 15%), anorexia (19% *v* 10%), and somnolence (9% *v* 5%; no further data provided).[27]

Comment: We found no RCTs of rivastigmine in people with vascular dementia.

OPTION PHYSOSTIGMINE

One systematic review in people with Alzheimer's disease found limited evidence that slow release physostigmine improved cognitive function compared with placebo but adverse effects, including nausea, vomiting, diarrhoea, dizziness, and stomach pain, were common.

Benefits: We found one systematic review (search date 2000, 15 RCTs) comparing physostigmine versus placebo in people mild to severe Alzheimer's disease (see comment below).[26] The RCTs differed widely in the preparations of physostigmine used, and most had weak reporting methods so the review could not perform a meta-analysis. Four were small trials of intravenous physostigmine, which did not report quantitative results. Seven were small trials (131 people, 6 crossover design) of standard oral preparation. The crossover trials did not provide precrossover results. One RCT (16 people) found no significant difference in cognition between oral physostigmine and placebo but it is likely to have been too small to exclude a clinically important difference. Four RCTs (1456 people) used controlled release preparations, but three of these reported results only for people who responded to physostigmine in a prestudy titration phase (see comment below). One RCT (170 people) found that physostigmine (27 mg daily) improved cognition after 12 weeks compared with placebo (Alzheimer's Disease Assessment Scale cognitive subscale: –2.0, 95% CI –3.6 to –0.5) but did not significantly improve activities of daily living or Clinician Based Impression of Change.

Harms: Common adverse effects of physostigmine include nausea, vomiting, diarrhoea, dizziness, and stomach pain. In RCTs that randomised all people with Alzheimer's disease rather than selecting those who tolerated and responded to physostigmine, withdrawals were more common with physostigmine (234/358 [65%] with physostigmine *v* 31/117 [26%] with placebo; OR 4.80, 95% CI 3.17 to 7.33).[29]

Comment: We found no RCTs of physostigmine in people with Lewy body or vascular dementia. Physostigmine is a sympathomimetic drug and has a very short half life. Screening out non-responders to a drug before the trial is likely to overestimate its effectiveness.

OPTION TACRINE

Two systematic reviews found limited evidence that tacrine improved cognitive function and global state in Alzheimer's disease compared with placebo, but adverse effects, including nausea and vomiting, diarrhoea, anorexia, and abdominal pain, were common.

Benefits: We found two systematic reviews comparing tacrine versus placebo in people with Alzheimer's disease (search date not stated, 12 RCTs, 1984 people;[30] search date 1997, 21 RCTs, including 12 RCTs identified by the first review, 3555 people;[31] see comment below). Various doses of tacrine were used in the RCTs, and the duration of treatment varied from 3–36 weeks. The first review found that tacrine significantly increased the proportion of people with overall clinical improvement compared with placebo (OR 1.58, 95% CI 1.18 to 2.11) and improved cognition (Mini Mental State Examination at 12 wks: SMD 0.77, 95% CI 0.35 to 1.20; Alzheimer's Disease Assessment Scale cognitive subscale at 12 wks: SMD –2.7, 95% CI –1.36 to –2.78).[30] A subsequent subgroup analysis indicated that the five non-industry sponsored studies found no significant effect between tacrine and placebo, but most (6/7) manufacturer supported studies found clinical benefit (1 RCT could not be located for inclusion in the subgroup analysis).[32]

Harms: One RCT identified by the review found that withdrawals because of adverse events were common (OR for withdrawal 3.6, 95% CI 2.8 to 4.7)[30] and were more likely with higher doses (265/479 [55%] with high dose tacrine *v* 20/184 [11%] with placebo; RR 5.1, 95% CI 3.3 to 7.7; NNH 3, 95% CI 2 to 3), and reversible elevation of liver enzymes was found in 133/265 (50%) of people taking tacrine.[33] Common adverse events included nausea and vomiting (35% with 160 mg daily), diarrhoea (18%), anorexia (12%), and abdominal pain (9%).

Comment: The quality of tacrine trials was generally poor.[30,31] We found no RCTs of tacrine in people with Lewy body or vascular dementia.

OPTION LECITHIN

Small, poor RCTs identified by a systematic review provided insufficient evidence to assess lecithin in people with Alzheimer's disease.

Benefits: We found one systematic review (search date 2000, 10 RCTs, 256 people with Alzheimer's disease) comparing lecithin versus placebo (see comment below).[34] It found no significant improvement in cognition, functional performance, quality of life, or global impression between lecithin and placebo (see comment below).[34] One RCT identified by the review (90 people with "Parkinsonian dementia"), which may have included people with Lewy body dementia, found no benefit from lecithin compared with placebo.

Harms: The review found that adverse effects were more common with lecithin (41% with lecithin *v* 10% with placebo; OR 6.0, 95% CI 1.5 to 24).[34] The specific nature of the adverse effects was not stated.

Comment: One RCT (included in the systematic review)[34] comparing lecithin versus placebo in people with minimal cognitive impairment found that some components of cognition were significantly better in the placebo group. Most studies of lecithin were small and weak. Meta-analysis in the systematic review was hampered by diverse outcome criteria. We found no RCTs of lecithin in people with Lewy body or vascular dementia.

OPTION NICOTINE

We found one systematic review, which found no RCTs of adequate quality in people with dementia.

Benefits: One systematic review (search date 2001) found no RCTs of adequate quality.[35]

Harms: We found no RCTs.

Comment: None.

OPTION NON-STEROIDAL ANTI-INFLAMMATORY DRUGS

One RCT in people with Alzheimer's disease found no significant difference in cognitive function after 25 weeks' treatment with diclofenac plus misoprostol compared with placebo. Another RCT in people with Alzheimer's disease found that indometacin improved cognitive function after 6 months' treatment compared with placebo.

Benefits: We found two RCTs in people with Alzheimer's disease (see comment below).[36,37] The first RCT (41 people with Alzheimer's disease) found no significant difference in cognitive function after 25 weeks' treatment with diclofenac plus misoprostol compared with placebo (Alzheimer's Disease Assessment Scale cognitive subscale [ADAS-cog] score: mean difference +1.14, 95% CI –2.9 to +5.2) or global status (Clinician's Interview Based Impression of Change score: +0.24, 95% CI –0.26 to +0.74).[36] The second RCT (44 people with mild to moderate Alzheimer's disease) found that indometacin (indomethacin) (≤ 150 mg daily) for 6 months significantly improved cognitive function compared with placebo (Mini Mental State Examination and ADAS-cog score; inadequately described results for only 28/44 completers).[37]

Harms: See non-steroidal anti-inflammatory drugs, p 1393. In one RCT,[36] more people withdrew by week 25 with diclofenac plus misoprostol than with placebo (12 [50%] *v* 2 [12%]). No serious drug related adverse events were reported.[36] In the RCT of indometacin, 21% of people on indometacin withdrew because of gastrointestinal symptoms.[37]

Comment: We found one systematic review of aspirin for vascular dementia (search date 2000), which identified no RCTs.[38] Earlier versions of a systematic review of aspirin in vascular dementia included one RCT (70 people), which was subsequently removed because of inadequate quality, including a lack of placebo control.[38] We found no RCTs of lecithin in people with Lewy body dementia.

OPTION OESTROGEN

One systematic review has found that, in women with mild to moderate Alzheimer's disease, oestrogen improves cognition over 7 weeks to 12 months' treatment compared with no oestrogen.

Benefits: We found one systematic review (search date 2000, 8 RCTs, 313 women with mild to moderate Alzheimer's disease aged over 56 years) comparing oestrogen (0.625–1.25 mg daily) versus no oestrogen for 7 weeks to 12 months (see comment below).[39] The review found that oestrogen improved cognitive function compared with no oestrogen (5 RCTs, Mini Mental State Examination: WMD 2.3, 95% CI 1.7 to 3.4).

Harms: There is concern that oestrogen treatment may increase the risk of developing breast cancer and cardiovascular events (see harms of hormone replacement therapy under secondary prevention of ischaemic cardiac events, p 188).

Comment: Most RCTs in the review were small and heterogeneity may have distorted the results of the meta-analysis. We found no RCTs of oestrogen in people with Lewy body or vascular dementia. A meta-analysis of 14 observational studies (5990 people, length of follow up not stated) found that hormone replacement therapy is associated with a lower risk of developing dementia (dementia in 13% with HRT *v* 21% with controls; RR 0.56, 95% CI 0.46 to 0.68).[39] Observational studies provide only indirect evidence; the observed association may be explained by confounders (e.g. educational level, lifestyle factors).

OPTION SELEGILINE

One systematic review has found that, in people with mild to moderate Alzheimer's disease, selegiline improves cognitive function, behavioural disturbance, and mood compared with placebo, but has found no significant difference in global clinical state.

Benefits: We found one systematic review (search date not stated, 15 RCTs) comparing selegiline versus placebo in people with mild to moderate Alzheimer's disease (average number of people 50, typical duration of treatment 3 months; see comment below).[40] Analysis of pooled results found that selegiline improved several outcome measures: cognitive function scores (measured by several parameters: 4 RCTs, 160 people; SMD –0.56, 95% CI –0.88 to –0.24), mood score (Dementia Mood Assessment Scale: 1 RCT, 20 people; SMD –1.14, 95% CI –2.11 to –0.18), and behavioural symptom score (Brief Psychiatric Rating Scale: 3 RCTs, 98 people; SMD –0.53, 95% CI –0.94 to –0.12). The review found no significant difference in global clinical state between selegiline and placebo (4 RCTs, 94 people; SMD –0.11, 95% CI –0.49 to +0.27).

Harms: The RCTs identified by the review found no difference in adverse effects (anxiety, agitation, dizziness, nausea, dyspepsia) between selegiline and placebo.[40]

Comment: The trials used a variety of outcomes, making comparison with other treatments difficult. We found no RCTs of selegiline in people with Lewy body or vascular dementia.

OPTION GINKGO BILOBA

RCTs found limited evidence that ginkgo biloba may improve cognitive function compared with placebo in people with Alzheimer's disease or vascular dementia.

Benefits: We found one systematic review (search date 2002, 33 RCTs) comparing ginkgo biloba versus placebo in people with cognitive impairment, Alzheimer's disease, or vascular dementia (see comment below).[41] Trial duration ranged from 3–53 weeks, doses and preparations of ginkgo biloba varied widely, and diverse outcomes were assessed, making results difficult to synthesise.[41] The review stated that it was unable to provide intention to treat analyses as most RCTs provided only completer analyses. It found that ginkgo biloba at any dose significantly improved cognition over 24 weeks (cognition assessed by a variety of validated scales: 5 RCTs, 3 of which were in people with Alzheimer's disease or vascular dementia [757 people]; results presented as SMD; P = 0.008). The review included two large RCTs in people with Alzheimer's disease or vascular dementia. The first large RCT (216 people with mild to moderate Alzheimer's disease or vascular dementia) found that ginkgo biloba (≥ 200 mg daily) significantly increased the proportion of people who were rated as improved at 24 weeks (completer analysis: improvement in Clinician's Interview Based Impression of Change [criteria for improvement not defined] 57/79 [72%] *v* 42/77 [55%] with placebo; RR 1.32, 95% CI 1.03 to 1.69). The second large RCT (327 people, 236 people with Alzheimer's disease) provided an intention to treat analysis (see table 1, p 1120).[42] It found that, in people with Alzheimer's disease, ginkgo biloba significantly improved cognition (intention to treat analysis for people with Alzheimer's disease, change in Alzheimer's Disease Assessment Scale cognitive subscale score: –1.7, 95% CI –3.1 to –0.20; NNT for 4 point change in ADAS-cog: 8, 95% CI 5 to 50) and care giver assessed improvement over 26 weeks compared with placebo (change in Geriatric Evaluation by Relative's Rating Instrument score: –0.16, 95% CI –0.25 to –0.06), but did not significantly improve the mean Clinician's Global Impression of Change score (change in score: +0.1, 95% CI –0.1 to +0.2).[42] The RCT had a high withdrawal rate; 137/309 (44%) people withdrew from the trial.

Harms: The review found no significant difference between ginkgo biloba and placebo in the proportion of people who had at least one adverse effect (adverse effects not specified: 117/591 [19.7%] with ginkgo *v* 59/471 [12.5%] with placebo; RR 0.95, 95% CI 0.72 to 1.26).

Comment: Many of the RCTs in the review included people with memory and cognitive impairment other than dementia so the results of the meta-analysis may not be fully generalisable to people with

Alzheimer's disease or vascular dementia. We found no RCTs of ginkgo biloba in people with Lewy body dementia. Preparations of ginkgo biloba available over the counter differ in terms of purity and concentration of active ingredients compared with high purity extract (EGb 761) used in most RCTs.

OPTION VITAMIN E

One RCT in people with moderate to severe Alzheimer's disease found no significant difference in cognitive function between vitamin E and placebo after 2 years' treatment, but found that vitamin E reduced mortality, institutionalisation, loss of ability to perform activities of daily living, and the proportion of people who developed severe dementia.

Benefits: We found one systematic review (search date 2000, 1 multicentre RCT, 169 people with moderate to severe Alzheimer's disease; see comment below).[43] The RCT compared four treatments: vitamin E (α-tocopherol; 2000 IU daily); selegiline; vitamin E plus selegiline; or placebo.[44] It found that no significant difference in cognitive function with high dose vitamin E alone for 2 years compared with placebo (measured by the cognitive portion of the Alzheimer's Disease Assessment Scale: mean change in score 8.3 with vitamin E *v* 6.7 with placebo; reported as non-significant; no further details reported; see comment below). It found that vitamin E significantly increased event free survival compared with placebo (defined as death, or survival until institutionalisation, loss of ability to perform activities of daily living, or severe dementia [clinical dementia rating of 3]; OR 0.49, 95% CI 0.25 to 0.96).[44]

Harms: The RCT found no significant difference in adverse effects between placebo and vitamin E.[44] Other studies have found weak evidence of associations between high dose vitamin E and bowel irritation, headache, muscular weakness, visual complaints, vaginal bleeding, bruising, thrombophlebitis, deterioration of angina pectoris, worsening of diabetes, syncope, and dizziness.[45] A few case reports have created concern that vitamin E may increase the risk of haemorrhagic stroke.

Comment: The groups in the RCT identified by the review were not matched evenly at baseline: the placebo group had a higher mean Mini Mental State Examination score, and these baseline scores were a significant predictor of outcome.[44] Attempts to correct for this imbalance suggested that vitamin E might increase mean survival, but the need for statistical adjustments weakens the strength of this conclusion. We found no RCTs of vitamin E in people with Lewy body or vascular dementia.

OPTION MUSIC THERAPY

Poor studies identified by a systematic review provided insufficient evidence to assess music therapy.

Benefits: We found one systematic review of music therapy (search date 1998, 21 studies, 336 people with various types of dementia).[46] It included studies with weak methods and found that music therapy significantly improved cognitive and behavioural outcomes compared with control interventions (mean effect size 0.79, 95% CI 0.62 to 0.95; see comment below). Significant effects were noted with different types of music therapy (active *v* passive, taped *v* live).

Harms: The systematic review gave no information on harms.[46]

Comment: The primary studies lacked adequate controls, had potential for bias, used diverse interventions, and used inadequate outcome measures. Although one meta-analysis found significant benefits for music therapy on pooling the results of many studies, further high quality studies are needed to clarify whether the results are explained by a true effect or by bias. A previous Cochrane systematic review has been withdrawn.[47]

OPTION REALITY ORIENTATION

One systematic review of small RCTs found that reality orientation improved cognitive function compared with no treatment in people with various types of dementia.

Benefits: We found one systematic review (search date 2000, 6 RCTs, 125 people with various types of dementia).[48] The RCTs compared reality orientation (see glossary, p 1116) versus no treatment and used different measures of cognition. The review found that reality orientation significantly improved cognitive function score compared with no treatment (SMD −0.59, 95% CI −0.95 to −0.22). No separate analysis was done for specific types of dementia.

Harms: The RCTs gave no information on adverse effects.[48]

Comment: The RCTs did not use standardised interventions or outcomes.[48]

OPTION REMINISCENCE THERAPY

RCTs provided insufficient evidence to assess reminiscence therapy.

Benefits: We found one systematic review of reminiscence therapy (see glossary, p 1116; search date 2000, 2 RCTs, 42 people).[49] Analysis of pooled data was hindered by poor trial methods, diverse outcomes, and no separation of data for different types of dementia.

Harms: We found no RCTs.

Comment: None.

QUESTION What are the effects of treatments on behavioural and psychological symptoms of dementia?

OPTION ANTIPSYCHOTICS

One systematic review in people with various types of dementia found no significant difference in agitation between haloperidol and placebo, but found that haloperidol may reduce aggression. One RCT in people with moderate to severe dementia, including Alzheimer's disease and vascular

dementia, found that risperidone significantly improved behavioural and psychological symptoms over 12 weeks compared with placebo, but another RCT in people with severe dementia and agitation found no significant difference in symptoms over 13 weeks. One RCT in people with Alzheimer's disease found that olanzapine reduced agitation, hallucinations, and delusions compared with placebo. RCTs have found no significant difference in efficacy between different antipsychotics. Two RCTs in people with dementia found no significant difference in agitation between trazodone and haloperidol, but may have been too small to exclude a clinically important difference.

Benefits: **Antipsychotics (various) versus placebo:** We found one systematic review comparing antipsychotics versus placebo (search date 1995, 7 RCTs, 4–12 wks' duration, 294 people with various types of dementia and behavioural problems).[50] It assessed a variety of antipsychotics, including haloperidol (2 RCTs). The other antipsychotics assessed (acetophenazine, loxapine, trifluoperazine, thiothixene) are no longer commonly used. It found that antipsychotics significantly increased the proportion of people who improved compared with placebo (61% with antipsychotics *v* 34% with placebo; $P < 0.001$).[50] **Haloperidol versus placebo:** We found one systematic review of haloperidol for agitation in various types of dementia, including Alzheimer's disease and vascular dementia (search date 2000, 5 RCTs, none of which were included in the older review).[51] It found no significant difference in agitation at 6–16 weeks between haloperidol and placebo (change in symptoms from baseline measured by the Cohen-Mansfield Agitation Inventory or the psychomotor score of the Behavioural Symptoms Scale for Dementia; WMD –0.48, 95% CI –1.43 to +0.53). However, it found that haloperidol significantly reduced aggression from baseline at 3–6 weeks compared with placebo (2 RCTs, 240 people: WMD –1.11, 95% CI –2.02 to –0.11).[51] **Haloperidol versus trazodone:** We found two RCTs (see antidepressants, p 1115). **Risperidone versus placebo:** We found two RCTs.[52,53] The first RCT (double blind, 625 people with moderate to severe dementia plus behavioural and psychological symptoms, 73% with Alzheimer's disease, mean age 83 years, 68% women) compared risperidone versus placebo over 12 weeks.[52] A response was defined as a reduction of at least 50% in the Behave-AD scale. It found that risperidone (1 and 2 mg daily) significantly improved the chance of responding over 12 weeks compared with placebo (45% with risperidone 1 mg *v* 33% with placebo *v* 50% with risperidone 2 mg; for risperidone 1 mg *v* placebo NNT 9, 95% CI 5 to 100; for risperidone 2 mg *v* placebo NNT 6, 95% CI 4 to 17). Gender and the type of dementia did not significantly affect the results. The second RCT (344 people with agitation and severe dementia, 67% with Alzheimer's, 26% with vascular dementia, mean age 81 years, 56% women) compared adjusted doses of risperidone (mean dose 1.1 mg) versus placebo or haloperidol (mean dose 1.2 mg) over 13 weeks for the treatment of behavioural symptoms.[53] A response was defined as a reduction of at least 30% in the Behave-AD scale. It found no significant difference in the proportion of people who responded over 13 weeks between risperidone and placebo (37/68 [54%] with risperidone *v* 35/74 [47%] with placebo; ARI +7%, 95% CI –9% to +23%; see below for risperidone *v* haloperidol).

Olanzapine versus placebo: We found one RCT (double blind, 6 wks' duration, 206 elderly US nursing home residents with Alzheimer's disease [177 people] or Lewy body dementia [29 people] plus psychotic or behavioural symptoms).[53] The RCT compared olanzapine (given as a fixed dose of 5, 10, or 15 mg daily) versus placebo. Agitation, hallucinations, and delusions were improved by the two lower doses but not by the highest dose of olanzapine compared with placebo (subscale of the Neuropsychiatric Inventory [nursing home version]: –7.6 with olanzapine 5 mg *v* –6.1 with olanzapine 10 mg *v* –4.9 with olanzapine 15 mg *v* –3.7 with placebo). **Comparisons between antipsychotics:** The review (search date 1995) identified eleven RCTs comparing different antipsychotics.[50] It found no significant difference in efficacy among haloperidol, diazepam, thioridazene, loxapine, or oxazepam.[50] One subsequent RCT comparing adjusted doses of risperidone versus haloperidol or placebo found no significant difference in the proportion of people who responded over 13 weeks between risperidone and haloperidol.[53] A response was defined as a reduction of at least 30% in the Behave-AD scale.

Harms: **Antipsychotics (various) versus placebo:** One systematic review (search date 1995) found that antipsychotics significantly increased adverse effects, including sedation (21%), movement disorders (13%), and orthostatic hypotension (8%) compared with placebo ($P < 0.01$)[50] However, it found no significant difference between antipsychotics and placebo in the proportion of people who withdrew from the trial ($P = 0.50$).[50] One study (2 year prospective, longitudinal, 71 people with dementia) found that the mean decline in cognitive scores in 16 people who took antipsychotics was twice that of people who did not (expanded Mini Mental State Examination 21 *v* 9; $P = 0.002$).[54] **Risperidone versus placebo:** The first RCT found that discontinuation because of adverse events was more common with high dose risperidone than with low dose risperidone or placebo (16% with 1 mg risperidone *v* 24% with 2 mg *v* 12% with placebo *v* 8% with 0.5 mg).[52] **Olanzapine versus placebo:** The RCT found that olanzapine increased sedation (25% with 5 mg olanazapine *v* 26% with 10 mg *v* 36% with 15 mg *v* 6% with placebo) and gait disturbance compared with placebo (20% with 5 mg olanzapine *v* 14% with 10 mg *v* 17% with 15 mg *v* 2% with placebo).[55] **Comparisons between antipsychotics:** In the RCT comparing risperidone versus placebo or haloperidol, about 18% of people withdrew because of adverse effects from each of the three arms.[53] Extrapyramidal adverse effects were more common in people receiving haloperidol than placebo (22% with haloperidol *v* 15% with risperidone *v* 11% with placebo).

Comment: High response rates with placebo indicate that many behavioural problems resolve spontaneously in the short term. Most people with dementia are sensitive to adverse effects from antipsychotics, especially sedation and extrapyramidal symptoms. People with Lewy body dementia are particularly sensitive to these adverse effects,[56] suggesting that antipsychotics have a poor balance of benefits and harms in people with Lewy body dementia. More studies are needed to determine whether newer atypical antipsychotics have a better ratio of benefits to harms than older antipsychotics.

OPTION ANTIEPILEPTIC DRUGS

One RCT found that carbamazepine significantly reduced agitation and aggression compared with placebo in people with agitation and dementia. One RCT found that sodium valproate reduced agitation over 6 weeks in people with dementia, but another RCT found no significant difference in aggressive behaviour over 8 weeks between sodium valproate and placebo. We found no RCTs about other antiepileptic drugs.

Benefits: We found no systematic review. **Carbamazepine:** We found one RCT (single blind, 51 nursing home patients with agitation and Alzheimer's disease, vascular dementia or mixed Alzheimer's disease and vascular dementia, 6 wks' duration) comparing carbamazepine (individualised doses; modal dose 300 mg; mean serum level 5.3 μg/mL) versus placebo.[57] It found that carbamazepine significantly improved a measure of agitation and aggression (mean total Brief Psychiatric Rating Scale score: 7.7 with carbamazepine *v* 0.9 with placebo) and a measure of global status compared with placebo (Clinical Global Impressions rating: 77% with carbamazepine *v* 21% with placebo). **Sodium valproate:** We found two RCTs.[58,59] The first RCT (single blind, 56 people with Alzheimer's disease or vascular dementia in nursing homes, 6 wks' duration) compared sodium valproate versus placebo.[58] It found that when several covariates were taken into account, sodium valproate significantly improved agitation and aggression compared with placebo (measured by Brief Psychiatric Rating Scale score; P = 0.05 only after adjustment) and a measure of global status (Clinical Global Impressions rating: 68% with sodium valproate *v* 52% with placebo; P = 0.06). The second RCT (43 people with various types of dementia plus behavioural problems, crossover design) comparing sodium valproate (480 mg daily) versus placebo for 3 weeks found no significant difference in aggressive behaviour over 8 weeks after crossover (mean change in Social Dysfunction and Agression Scale-9 score –0.72 with valproate *v* –0.72 with placebo; P = 0.99).[59]

Harms: **Carbamazepine:** The RCT found that adverse effects were significantly more common with carbamazepine than with placebo (16/27 [59%] with carbazepine *v* 7/24 [29%] with placebo; P = 0.003). These were considered clinically significant in two cases: 1 person with tics, 1 with ataxia. Carbamazepine in the elderly may cause cardiac toxicity. **Sodium valproate:** The first RCT found that adverse effects, generally rated as mild, were significantly more common with sodium valproate than with placebo (68% with sodium valproate *v* 33% with placebo; P = 0.003).[58] See epilepsy, p 1508.

Comment: The need to perform adjustments for covariates in the second RCT weakens the strength of the findings.

OPTION ANTIDEPRESSANTS

One RCT in people with dementia found no significant difference in agitation between trazodone and haloperidol. Another RCT in people with Alzheimer's disease and agitated behaviour found no significant difference in outcomes among trazodone, haloperidol, behaviour management techniques, and placebo. The RCTs may have been too small to exclude a clinically important difference.

Benefits: We found no systematic review but found two RCTs.[60,61] The first RCT (double blind, 28 elderly people with agitated behaviour associated with Alzheimer's disease, vascular dementia or mixed Alzheimer's disease and vascular dementia, 9 wks' duration) compared trazodone (50–250 mg daily) versus haloperidol (1–5 mg daily).[60] It found no significant difference in agitation between the groups, but the trial was too small to exclude a clinically important difference. The second RCT (double blind, 149 people with Alzheimer's disease and agitated behaviours, 16 wks' duration) compared four treatments: haloperidol (mean dose 1.1 mg daily); trazodone (mean dose 200 mg daily); behaviour management techniques; or placebo.[61] It found no significant difference in outcome (Alzheimer's Disease Co-operative Study Clinical Global Impression of Change) between the four interventions, but it may have been too small to exclude a clinically important difference.

Harms: In the first RCT, adverse effects were more common in the group treated with haloperidol than trazodone.[60] In the second RCT no significant differences in adverse events were seen between the trazodone group and the placebo group.[61] Priapism has been reported with trazodone, occurring in about 1/10 000 people.

Comment: The RCTs were too small to exclude clinically important differences between the interventions.[60,61]

OPTION CHOLINESTERASE INHIBITORS

RCTs provided inconclusive evidence about the effects of donepezil or galantamine compared with placebo on behavioural and psychiatric symptoms in people with mild to moderate Alzheimer's disease.

Benefits: **Donepezil:** We found no systematic review but found two RCTs.[20,62] The first RCT (290 people with moderate to severe Alzheimer's disease aged 48–92 years, Mini Mental State Examination [MMSE] score 5–17) compared donepezil (5–10 mg daily) versus placebo.[20] It found that donepezil significantly improved functional and behavioural symptoms at 24 weeks compared with placebo (Disability Assessment for Dementia score; mean difference 8.23, no 95% CI provided; $P < 0.001$; Neuropsychiatric Inventory score; mean difference 5.64, no 95% CI provided; $P < 0.0001$). The second RCT (208 people with mild to moderate Alzheimer's disease, at least 1 symptom on the Neuropsychiatric Inventory Nursing Home version and living in a nursing home) found no significant difference in psychiatric symptoms after 24 weeks of treatment between donepezil and placebo (change in mean Neuropsychiatric Inventory Nursing Home version scores –4.9 with donepezil *v* –2.3 with placebo; reported as non-significant; no further data provided).[62] **Galantamine:** We found one systematic review (search date 2002), which identified two RCTs that assessed the effects of galantamine on behavioural and psychological symptoms.[24] A meta-analysis was not performed because of differences in length of follow up between the trials. Both trials used the Neuropsychiatric Inventory (NPI); scores range from 0–120, reduction indicates improvement. The first RCT (386 people with mild to moderate Alzheimer's disease; MMSE score 10–22) found no significant difference in psychiatric symptoms at 3 months between galantamine (12–16 mg twice daily) and placebo (mean reduction in NPI score: –0.30 with galantamine *v* +0.50 with placebo; WMD –0.80, 95% CI –2.67 to +1.07). The second RCT (978 people with mild to moderate Alzheimer's disease; MMSE score 12–24) found that galantamine (16 mg daily) significantly reduced psychiatric symptoms at 6 months compared with placebo (mean reduction in NPI score –0.10 with galantamine *v* +2.00 with placebo; WMD –2.10, 95% CI –4.04 to –0.16), but found no significant difference with galantamine (8 mg daily or 24 mg daily).[24]

Harms: See harms of donepezil, p 1102 and galantamine, p 1104.

Comment: Cholinesterase inhibitors improve cognitive function and are well tolerated in older people.

OPTION REALITY ORIENTATION

One systematic review found that reality orientation improved behaviour compared with no treatment in people with various types of dementia.

Benefits: We found one systematic review (search date 2000, 6 RCTs, 125 people with various types of dementia).[48] It found that reality orientation significantly improved behavioural symptom score compared with no treatment (SMD –0.66, 95% CI –1.27 to –0.05). No separate analysis was done for specific types of dementia.

Harms: The RCTs gave no information on adverse effects.[48]

Comment: The RCTs did not use standardised interventions or outcomes.[48]

GLOSSARY

Reality orientation Involves presenting information that is designed to reorient a person in time, place, or person. It may range in intensity from a board giving details of the day, date, and season, to staff reorienting a patient at each contact.

Reminiscence therapy Involves encouraging people to talk about the past in order to enable past experiences to be brought into consciousness. It relies on remote memory, which is relatively well preserved in mild to moderate dementia.

REFERENCES

1. van Duijn CM. Epidemiology of the dementia: recent developments and new approaches. *J Neurol Neurosurg Psychiatry* 1996;60:478–488.
2. McKeith IG, Galasko D, Kosaka K, et al. Consensus guidelines for the clinical and pathological diagnosis of dementia with Lewy bodies (DLB): report of the consortium on DLB International workshop. *Neurology* 1996;47:1113–1124.
3. Rasmusson DX, Brandt J, Steele C, et al. Accuracy of clinical diagnosis of Alzheimer disease and clinical features of patients with non-Alzheimer's disease neuropathology. *Alzheimer Dis Assoc Disord* 1996;10:180–188.
4. Verghese J, Crystal HA, Dickson DW, et al. Validity of clinical criteria for the diagnosis of dementia with Lewy bodies. *Neurology* 1999;53:1974–1982.
5. Lobo A, Launer LJ, Fratiglioni L, et al. Prevalence of dementia and major subtypes in Europe: a collaborative study of population-based cohorts. *Neurology* 2000;54:S4–S9.
6. Farrer L. Intercontinental epidemiology of Alzheimer's disease: a global approach to bad gene hunting. *JAMA* 2001;285:796–798.
7. Skoog I. A population-based study of dementia in 85 year olds. *N Engl J Med* 1993;328:153–158.

8. McKeith IG. Clinical Lewy body syndromes. *Ann N Y Acad Sci* 2000;920:1–8.
9. Inkeda M, Hokoishi K, Maki N, et al. Increased prevalence of vascular dementia in Japan: a community-based epidemiological study. *Neurology* 2001;57:839–844.
10. McKeith I. The differential diagnosis of dementia. In: Burns A, Levy R, eds. *Dementia*. 1st ed. London: Chapman and Hall, 1994:39–57.
11. Hardy J. Molecular classification of Alzheimer's disease. *Lancet* 1991;1:1342–1343.
12. Eastwood R, Reisberg B. Mood and behaviour. In: Panisset M, Stern Y, Gauthier S, eds. *Clinical diagnosis and management of Alzheimer's disease*. 1st ed. London: Dunitz, 1996:175–189.
13. Absher JR, Cummings JL. Cognitive and noncognitive aspects of dementia syndromes. In: Burns A, Levy R, eds. *Dementia*. 1st ed. London: Chapman and Hall, 1994:59–76.
14. Rosen WG, Mohs RC, Davis KL. A new rating scale for Alzheimer's disease. *Am J Psychiatry* 1984;141:1356–1364.
15. Folstein MF, Folstein SE, McHugh PR. Mini Mental State: a practical method for grading the cognitive state of patients for the clinician. *J Psychiatr Res* 1975;12:189–198.
16. Burns A, Lawlor B, Craig S. Assessment scales in old age psychiatry. London: Martin Dunitz. 1998.
17. Gelinas I, Gauthier L, McIntyre M, et al. Development of a functional measure for persons with Alzheimer's disease: the Disability Assessment of Dementia. *Am J Occupat Ther* 1999;53:471–481.
18. Lawton MP, Brody EM. Assessment of older people: self-maintaining and instrumental activities of daily living. *Gerontologist* 1969;9:179–186.
19. Birks JS, Melzer D, Beppu H. Donepezil for mild and moderate Alzheimer's disease. In: The Cochrane Library, Issue 4, 2002. Oxford: Update Software. Search date 2000; primary sources Cochrane Dementia and Cognitive Impairment Group Specialized Register of Clinical Trials, Medline, Psychlit, Embase, the Donepezil Study Group, and Eisai Inc.
20. Feldman H, Gauthier S, Hecker J, et al. A 24-week, randomized, double blind study of donepezil in moderate to severe Alzheimer's disease. *Neurology* 2001;57:613–620.
21. Mohs, RC, Doody, RS, Morris, JC, et al, and Study Group. A 1-year, placebo-controlled preservation of function survival study of donepezil in AD patients. *Neurology* 2001;57:481–488.
22. Wilkinson DG. Passmore AP. Bullock R. et al. A multinational, randomised, 12-week, comparative study of donepezil and rivastigmine in patients with mild to moderate Alzheimer's disease. *Int J Clin Pract* 2002;56:441–446.
23. Rogers SL, Doody RS, Pratt RD, et al. Long term efficacy and safety of donepezil in the treatment of Alzheimer's disease: final analysis of a US multicentre open-label study. *Eur Neuropsychopharmacol* 2000;10:195–203.
24. Olin J, Schneider L. Olin J, et al. Galantamine for Alzheimer's disease. In: The Cochrane Library, Issue 4, 2002. Oxford: Update Software. Search date 2002; primary sources Cochrane Dementia Group Specialized Register of Clinical Trials, Cochrane Controlled Trials Register, Embase, Medline, Psychlit, Combined Health Information Database, National Research Register, Alzheimer's Disease Education and Referral Centre Clinical Database, Biomed (Biomedicine and Health), GlaxoWellcome Clinical Trials Register, National Institutes of Health Clinical Trials Databases, Current Controlled Trials, Dissertation Abstracts, Index to UK Theses, hand searched reference lists, and additional information collected from an unpublished investigational brochure for galantamine.
25. Erkinjuntti T, Kurz A, Gauthier S, et al. Efficacy of galantamine in probable vascular dementia and Alzheimer's disease combined with cerebrovascular disease: a randomised trial. *Lancet* 2002;359:1283–1290.
26. Birks J, Iakovidou V, Tsolaki M, et al. Rivastigmine for Alzheimer's disease. In: The Cochrane Library, Issue 4, 2002. Oxford: Update Software. Search date 2000; primary sources Cochrane Controlled Trials Register, Cochrane Dementia Group Specialized Register of Clinical Trials, Medline, Embase, Psychlit, Cinahl, and hand searches of geriatric and dementia journals and conference abstracts.
27. McKeith I, Del Ser T, Spano P, et al. Efficacy of rivastigmine in dementia with Lewy bodies: a randomised, double-blind, placebo-controlled international study. *Lancet* 2000;356:2031–2036.
28. Kumar V, Anand R, Messina J, et al. An efficacy and safety analysis of Exelon in Alzheimer's disease patients with concurrent vascular risk factors. *Eur J Neurol* 2000;7:159–169.
29. Coelho F, Filho JM, Birks J. Physostigmine for Alzheimer's disease. In: The Cochrane Library, Issue 1, 2002. Oxford: Update Software. Search date 2000; primary sources the Cochrane Dementia Group Specialized Register of Clinical Trials and pharmaceutical companies.
30. Qizilbash N, Whitehead A, Higgins J, et al. Cholinesterase inhibition for Alzheimer disease. *JAMA* 1998;280:1777–1782. Search date not stated; primary sources Cochrane Dementia Group Registry of Clinical Trials, trial investigators, and Parke-Davis Pharmaceuticals.
31. Arrieta JR, Artalejo FR. Methodology, results and quality of clinical trials of tacrine in the treatment of Alzheimer's disease: a systematic review of the literature. *Age Ageing* 1998;27:161–179. Search date 1997; primary sources Cochrane Library and Medline.
32. Koepp R, Miles SH. Meta-analysis of tacrine for Alzheimer's disease: the influence of industry sponsors. *JAMA* 1999;281:2287–2288.
33. Knapp MJ, Knopman DS, Solomon PR, et al. A 30-week randomized controlled trial of high-dose tacrine in patients with Alzheimer's disease. The Tacrine Study Group. *JAMA* 1994;271:985–991.
34. Higgins JPT, Flicker L. Lecithin for dementia and cognitive impairment. In: The Cochrane Library, Issue 4, 2002. Oxford: Update Software. Search date 2000; primary sources Cochrane Dementia and Cognitive Impairment Group Specialized Register of Clinical Trials, Medline, Embase, Psychlit, ISI, Current Contents, and hand searched reference lists and textbooks.
35. López-Arrieta JM, Rodr guez JL, Sanz F. Efficacy and safety of nicotine on Alzheimer's disease patients. In: The Cochrane Library, Issue 4, 2002. Oxford: Update Software. Search date 2001; primary source Cochrane Dementia Group Specialized Register of Clinical Trials.
36. Scharf S, Mander A, Ugoni A, et al. A double-blind, placebo-controlled trial of diclofenac/misoprostol in Alzheimer's disease. *Neurology* 1999;53:197–201.
37. Rogers J, Kirby LC, Hempleman SR, et al. Clinical trial of indomethacin in Alzheimer's disease. *Neurology* 1993;43:1609–1611.
38. Williams PS, Spector A, Orrell M, et al. Aspirin for vascular dementia. In: The Cochrane Library, Issue 4, 2002. Oxford: Update Software. Search date 2000; primary sources Medline, Cochrane Library Trials Register, Embase, Cinahl, Psychlit, Amed,

Sigle, National Research Register, hand searched reference lists, and contact with specialists.
39. Hogervorst E, Williams J, Budge M, et al. The nature of the effect of female gonadal hormone replacement therapy on cognitive function in post-menopausal women: a meta-analysis. *Neuroscience* 2000;101:485–512. Search date 2000; primary sources Medline, Embase, Psychlit, and hand searches of reference lists.
40. Birks J, Flicker L. Selegiline for Alzheimer's disease. In: The Cochrane Library, Issue 4, 2002. Oxford: Update Software. Search date not stated, review amended 1998; primary source Cochrane Dementia and Cognitive Impairment Group Register of Clinical Trials.
41. Birks J, Grimley Evans J, Van Dongen M. Ginkgo biloba for cognitive Impairment and dementia In: The Cochrane Library, Issue 4, 2002. Oxford, Update Software. Search date 2002; primary source Cochrane Dementia and Cognitive Impairment Group Specialised Register of Controlled Clinical Trials.
42. Le Bars P, Katz MM, Berman N, et al. A placebo-controlled, double-blind, randomised trial of an extract of Ginkgo biloba for dementia. *JAMA* 1997;278:1327–1332.
43. Tabet N, Birks J, Grimley Evans J. Vitamin E for Alzheimer's disease. In: The Cochrane Library, Issue 4, 2002. Oxford: Update Software. Search date 2000; primary sources Cochrane Dementia and Cognitive Impairment Group Specialized Register of Clinical Trials
44. Sano M, Ernesto C, Thomas RG, et al. A controlled trial of selegiline, α-tocopherol, or both as treatment for Alzheimer's disease. *N Engl J Med* 1997;336:1216–1222.
45. Myers DG, Maloley PA, Weeks D. Safety of antioxidant vitamins. *Arch Intern Med* 1996;156:925–935.
46. Koger SM, Chaplin K, Brotons M. Is music therapy an effective intervention for dementia? A meta-analytic review of the literature. *J Music Ther* 1999;36:2–15. Search date 1998; primary sources Medline, Psychlit, and hand searched reference lists.
47. Koger SM, Brotons M. Music therapy for dementia symptoms. In: Cochrane Library, Issue 4, 2002. Oxford: Update Software. Search date 2000; primary sources Medline, Cochrane Dementia and Cognitive Improvement Group Trials Register, Embase, Cinahl, and Psychlit.
48. Spector A, Orrell M, Davies S, et al. Reality orientation for dementia. In: The Cochrane Library, Issue 4, 2002. Oxford: Update Software. Search date 2000; primary sources Medline, Psychlit, Embase, Cochrane Database of Systematic Reviews, Omni, Bids, Dissertation Abstracts International, Sigle, plus internet searching of HealthWeb, Mental Health Infosources, American Psychiatric Association, Internet Mental Health, Mental Health Net, NHS Confederation, and hand searching of specialist journals.
49. Spector A, Orrell M. Reminiscence therapy for dementia. In: The Cochrane Library, Issue 4, 2002. Oxford: Update Software. Search date 2000; primary sources Cochrane Controlled Trials Register, Medline, Psychlit, Embase, Omni, Bids, Dissertation Abstracts International, Sigle, reference lists of relevant articles, internet sites, and hand searching of specialist journals.
50. Lanctot KL, Best TS, Mittmann N, et al. Efficacy and safety of neuroleptics in behavioural disorders associated with dementia. *J Clin Psychiatry* 1998;59:550–561. Search date 1995; primary sources Medline and hand search of references.
51. Lonergan E, Luxenberg J, Colford J. Haloperidol for agitation in dementia. In: The Cochrane Library, Issue 4, 2002. Oxford: Update Software. Search date 2000; primary sources Cochrane Controlled Trials Register, Cochrane Dementia Group Specialized Register of Clinical Trials, Medline, Embase, Psychlit, Cinahl, and Glaxo-Wellcome Trials database.
52. Katz IR, Jeste DV, Mintzer JE, et al. Comparison of risperidone and placebo for psychosis and behavioural disturbances associated with dementia: a randomized double-blind trial. *J Clin Psychiatry* 1999;60:107–115.
53. De Deyn PP, Rabheru K, Rasmussen A, et al. A randomized trial of risperidone, placebo, and haloperidol for behavioural symptoms of dementia. *Neurology* 1999;53:946–955.
54. McShane R, Keene J, Gedling K, et al. Do neuroleptic drugs hasten cognitive decline in dementia? Prospective study with necropsy follow up. *BMJ* 1997;314:266–269.
55. Street JS, Clark WS, Gannon KS, et al. Olanzapine treatment of psychotic and behavioural symptoms in patients with Alzheimer's disease in nursing care facilities: a double-blind, randomised, placebo-controlled trial. *Arch Gen Psychiatry* 2000;57:968–976.
56. McKeith IG. Dementia with Lewy Bodies. *Br J Psychiatry* 2002;180:144–147.
57. Tariot PN, Erb R, Podgorski CA, et al. Efficacy and tolerability of carbamazepine for agitation and aggression in dementia. *Am J Psychiatry* 1998;155:54–61.
58. Porsteinsson AOP, Tariot PN, Erb R, et al. Placebo-controlled study of divalproex sodium for agitation in dementia. *Am J Geriatr Psychiatry* 2001;9:58–66.
59. Sival RC, Haffmans PMJ, Jansen PAF, et al. Sodium valproate in the treatment of aggressive behaviour in patients with dementia — a randomised placebo controlled clinical trial. *Int J Geriatr Psychiatry* 2002;17:579–585.
60. Sultzer DL, Gray KF, Gunay I, et al. A double-blind comparison of trazodone and haloperidol for treatment of agitation in patients with dementia. *Am J Geriatr Psychiatry* 1997;5:60–69.
61. Teri L, Logsdon RG, Peskind E, et al. Treatment of agitation in AD: a randomised, placebo-controlled clinical trial. *Neurology* 2000;55:1271–1278.
62. Taroit PN, Cummings JL, Katz IR, et al. A randomized double blind placebo controlled study of the efficacy and safety of donepezil in patients with Alzheimer's disease in the nursing home setting. *J Am Geriatr Soc* 2001;49:1590–1599.

James Warner
Senior Lecturer/Consultant in Old Age Psychiatry
Imperial College
London
UK

Rob Butler
Honorary Senior Lecturer in Psychiatry
and Consultant in Old Age Psychiatry
University of Auckland and Waitemata
Health
Auckland
New Zealand

Pramod Prabhakaran
Specialist Registrar
CNWL Mental Health Trust
London
UK

Competing interests: JW has been reimbursed by Novartis, the manufacturer of rivastigmine, for conference attendance and has received speaker fees from Janssen Pharmaceuticals for educational events. RB has been reimbursed by Novartis for conference attendance. PP none declared.

TABLE 1 **Effects of donepezil, galantamine, and rivastigmine compared with placebo (see text, p 1102).**

Drug	Dose (mg)	Duration (weeks)	Difference in ADAS-cog	NNT for at least 4 point change in ADAS-cog	OR for global improvement	OR for all cause withdrawal	Ref
Donepezil	10 od	24	–2.9 (–3.7 to –2.2)	N/A	2.1 (1.3 to 3.6)	1.4 (1.0 to 1.8)	19
Galantamine	12 bd	24	–3.3 (–3.9 to –2.7)	7 (4 to 10)	1.9 (1.4 to 2.5)	2.1 (1.5 to 2.9)	24
(observed case analysis)	16 bd	24	–3.3 (–4.1 to –2.4)	5 (5 to 12)	2.0 (1.6 to 2.5)	3.3 (2.5 to 4.3)	24
Rivastigmine	6–12 bd	28	–2.0 (–0.49 to –3.60)	17 (12 to 34)	1.5 (1.2 to 1.8)	2.4 (2.0 to 3.0)	27
Gingko biloba (completer analysis)	120 od	52	–1.7 (–3.2 to –0.2)	8 (5 to 50)	N/A	N/A	41

Results are intention to treat unless stated. bd, twice daily; od, once daily; N/A, not applicable; Ref, reference.

Depressive disorders

Search date July 2002

John Geddes, Rob Butler, and Simon Hatcher

QUESTIONS

INTERVENTIONS

Beneficial

Cognitive therapy (in mild to moderate depression) 1133

Continuation treatment with antidepressant drugs (reduces risk of relapse in mild to moderate depression) 1137

Electroconvulsive therapy (in severe depression) 1132

Interpersonal psychotherapy (in mild to moderate depression) 1133

Prescription antidepressant drugs (tricyclic and heterocyclic antidepressants, monoamine oxidase inhibitors, selective serotonin reuptake inhibitors and related drugs) in mild to moderate and severe depression 1125

Likely to be beneficial

Care pathways (in mild to moderate depression) 1129

Combining prescription antidepressant drugs and psychological treatment (in mild to moderate and severe depression) 1134

Non-directive counselling (in mild to moderate depression) . . 1133

Problem solving treatment (in mild to moderate depression) . . 1133

St John's Wort (in mild to moderate depression) 1130

Unknown effectiveness

Befriending (in mild to moderate depression) 1137

Bibliotherapy (in mild to moderate depression) 1136

Care pathways versus usual care for long term outcomes (in mild to moderate depression) . . 1138

Cognitive therapy versus antidepressants for long term outcomes (in mild to moderate depression) 1138

Exercise (in mild to moderate depression) 1136

Psychological treatments (cognitive therapy, interpersonal psychotherapy, problem solving treatment) in severe depression 1133

To be covered in future updates

Behaviour therapy

See glossary, p 1139

Key Messages

- We found no reliable direct evidence that one type of treatment (drug or non-drug) is superior to another in improving symptoms of depression. However, we found strong evidence that some treatments are effective, whereas the effectiveness of others remains uncertain. Of the interventions examined, prescription antidepressant drugs and electroconvulsive therapy are the only treatments for which there is good evidence of effectiveness in severe and psychotic depressive disorders. We found no RCTs comparing drug and non-drug treatments in severe depressive disorders.

- **Befriending (in mild to moderate depression)** One small RCT provided insufficient evidence to assess befriending.
- **Bibliotherapy (in mild to moderate depression)** One systematic review of RCTs in younger and older adults recruited by advertisement found limited evidence that bibliotherapy may reduce mild depressive symptoms compared with waiting list control or standard care. Another systematic review in people with combined anxiety and depression, anxiety, or chronic fatigue found that bibliotherapy may improve symptoms over 2–6 months compared with standard care. It is unclear whether people in the RCTs identified by the reviews are clinically representative of people with depressive disorders.
- **Care pathways (in mild to moderate depression)** Five RCTs in people aged over 18 years found that the effectiveness of antidepressant treatment may be improved by several approaches, including collaborative working between primary care clinicians and psychiatrists plus intensive patient education, case management, telephone support, and relapse prevention programmes. One RCT found that a clinical practice guideline and practice based education did not improve either detection or outcome of depression compared with usual care.
- **Care pathways versus usual care for long term outcomes (in mild to moderate depression)** One RCT found that a multifaceted "quality improvement programme" significantly improved symptoms and increased the proportion of people who returned to work over 1 year compared with usual care, but found no significant difference in outcomes at 2 years.
- **Cognitive therapy (in mild to moderate depression)** One systematic review in younger and older adults has found that cognitive therapy significantly improves the symptoms of depression compared with no treatment.
- **Cognitive therapy versus antidepressants for long term outcomes (in mild to moderate depression)** One systematic review and one additional RCT in younger and older adults found limited evidence by combining relapse rates across different RCTs that cognitive therapy may reduce the risk of relapse over 1–2 years compared with antidepressants.
- **Combining prescription antidepressant drugs and psychological treatment (in mild to moderate and severe depression)** One non-systematic review of RCTs in people aged 18–80 years has found that, in people with severe depression, adding drug treatment to interpersonal psychotherapy or to cognitive therapy compared with either psychological treatment alone improves symptoms, but found no significant difference in symptoms in people with mild to moderate depression. Subsequent RCTs in younger and older adults with mild to moderate depression have found that combining antidepressants plus psychotherapy improves symptoms significantly more than either antidepressants or psychotherapy alone. One RCT in older adults with mild to moderate depression found that cognitive behavioural therapy plus desipramine improved symptoms significantly more than desipramine alone.
- **Continuation drug treatment in mild to moderate depression (reduces risk of relapse in mild to moderate depression)** One systematic review and subsequent RCTs in younger and older adults have found that continuation treatment with antidepressant drugs compared with placebo for 4–6 months after recovery significantly reduces the risk of relapse. One RCT in people aged over 60 years has found that continuation treatment with dosulepin (dothiepin) significantly reduces the risk of relapse over 2 years compared with placebo.

- **Electroconvulsive therapy (in severe depression)** Two systematic reviews and additional RCTs in people aged over 16 years have found that electroconvulsive therapy significantly improves symptoms in severe depression compared with simulated electroconvulsive therapy.
- **Exercise (in mild to moderate depression)** One systematic review found limited evidence from poor RCTs that exercise may improve symptoms compared with placebo, and may be as effective as cognitive therapy or antidepressants.
- **Interpersonal psychotherapy (in mild to moderate depression)** One large RCT has found that interpersonal psychotherapy significantly improves rates of recovery from depression after 16 weeks compared with antidepressants or standard care.
- **Non-directive counselling (in mild to moderate depression)** One systematic review in people aged over 18 years with recent onset psychological problems, including depression, found that brief, non-directive counselling significantly reduced symptom scores in the short term (< 6 months) compared with usual care, but found no significant difference in scores in the long term (> 6 months).
- **Prescription antidepressant drugs (in mild to moderate and severe depression)** Systematic reviews in people aged 16 years or over have found that antidepressant drugs are effective in acute treatment of all grades of depressive disorders compared with placebo. Systematic reviews have found no significant difference in outcomes with different kinds of antidepressant drug. One systematic review in people aged 55 years or over with all grades of depressive disorder has found that tricyclic antidepressants, selective serotonin reuptake inhibitors, or monoamine oxidase inhibitors significantly reduce the proportion of people who fail to recover over 26–49 days compared with placebo. We found no specific evidence on adverse effects in older adults. However, the drugs differ in their adverse event profiles.
  - **Monoamine oxidase inhibitors** One systematic review found that monoamine oxidase inhibitors were less effective than tricyclic antidepressants in people with severe depressive disorders, but may be more effective in atypical depressive disorders with biological features such as increased sleep, increased appetite, mood reactivity, and rejection sensitivity.
  - **Selective serotonin reuptake inhibitors and related drugs** One systematic review found that selective serotonin reuptake inhibitors were associated with a lower rate of adverse effects compared with tricyclic antidepressants, but the difference was small. Another systematic review and one retrospective cohort study found no strong evidence that fluoxetine was associated with increased risk of suicide compared with tricyclic antidepressants or placebo. One RCT and observational data suggest that abrupt withdrawal of selective serotonin reuptake inhibitors is associated with symptoms including dizziness, nausea, paraesthesia, headache, and vertigo, and that these symptoms are more likely with drugs with a short half life, such as paroxetine.
  - **Tricyclic antidepressants** One systematic review found that tricyclic antidepressants were associated with higher rates of adverse effects compared with selective serotonin reuptake inhibitors, but the difference was small.

Depressive disorders

- **Problem solving treatment (in mild to moderate depression)** RCTs have found that problem solving treatment significantly improves symptoms over 3–6 months compared with placebo or control, and have found no significant difference in symptoms between problem solving treatment and drug treatment.
- **Psychological treatments (cognitive therapy, interpersonal psychotherapy, and problem solving treatment) in severe depression** RCTs found insufficient evidence to assess psychological treatments in severe depression.
- **St John's Wort (in mild to moderate depression)** Systematic reviews in people with mild to moderate depressive disorders have found that St John's Wort (*Hypericum perforatum*) significantly improves depressive symptoms over 4–12 weeks compared with placebo, and have found no significant difference in symptoms with St John's Wort versus prescription antidepressant drugs. The results of the reviews should be interpreted with caution because the RCTs did not use standardised preparations of St John's Wort, and doses of antidepressants varied. One subsequent RCT in people aged over 18 years with major depressive disorder found no significant difference in depressive symptoms at 8 weeks between a standardised preparation of St John's Wort and placebo or sertraline, but it is likely to have been underpowered to detect a clinically important difference between groups.

DEFINITION **Depressive disorders** are characterised by persistent low mood, loss of interest and enjoyment, and reduced energy. They often impair day to day functioning. Most of the RCTs assessed in this review classify depression using the *Diagnostic and statistical manual of mental disorders* (DSM IV)[1] or the *International classification of mental and behavioural disorders* (ICD-10).[2] DSM IV divides depression into major depressive disorder or dysthymic disorder. **Major depressive disorder** is characterised by one or more major depressive episodes (i.e. at least 2 wks of depressed mood or loss of interest accompanied by at least 4 additional symptoms of depression). **Dysthymic disorder** is characterised by at least 2 years of depressed mood for more days than not, accompanied by additional symptoms that do not reach the criteria for major depressive disorder.[1] ICD-10 divides depression into mild to moderate or severe depressive episodes.[2] **Mild to moderate depression** is characterised by depressive symptoms and some functional impairment. **Severe depression** is characterised by additional agitation or psychomotor retardation with marked somatic symptoms.[2] In this review, we use both DSM IV and ICD-10 classifications, but treatments are considered to have been assessed in severe depression if the RCT included inpatients. **Older adults:** Older adults are generally defined as people aged 65 years or older. However, some of the RCTs of older people in this review included people aged 55 years or over. The presentation of depression in older adults may be atypical: low mood may be masked and anxiety or memory impairment may be the principal presenting symptoms. Dementia should be considered in the differential diagnosis of depression in older adults.[3]

INCIDENCE/ PREVALENCE Depressive disorders are common, with a prevalence of major depression between 5% and 10% of people seen in primary care settings.[4] Two to three times as many people may have depressive symptoms but do not meet DSM IV criteria for major depression.

Women are affected twice as often as men. Depressive disorders are the fourth most important cause of disability worldwide and they are expected to become the second most important cause by the year 2020.[5,6] **Older adults:** Between 10% and 15% of older people have depressive symptoms, although major depression is relatively rare in older adults.[7]

AETIOLOGY/ RISK FACTORS The causes are uncertain but include both childhood events and current psychosocial adversity.

PROGNOSIS About half of people suffering a first episode of major depressive disorder experience further symptoms in the next 10 years.[8] **Older adults:** One systematic review (search date 1996, 12 prospective cohort studies, 1268 people, mean age 60 years) found that the prognosis may be especially poor in elderly people with a chronic or relapsing course of depression.[9] Another systematic review (search date 1999, 23 prospective cohort studies in people aged ≥ 65 years, including 5 identified by the first review) found that depression in older people was associated with increased mortality (15 studies; pooled OR 1.73, 95% CI 1.53 to 1.95).[10]

AIMS OF INTERVENTION To improve mood, social and occupational functioning, and quality of life; to reduce morbidity and mortality; to prevent recurrence of depressive disorder; and to minimise adverse effects of treatment.

OUTCOMES Depressive symptoms rated by the depressed person and clinician; social functioning; occupational functioning; quality of life; admission to hospital; rates of self harm; relapse of depressive symptoms; rates of adverse events. Trials often use continuous scales to measure depressive symptoms (such as the Hamilton Depression Rating Scale and the Beck Depression Inventory). **Older adults:** The Hamilton Depression Rating Scale is not ideal for older people because it includes several somatic items that may be positive in older people who are not depressed. It has been the most widely used scale, although specific scales for elderly people (such as the Geriatric Depression Scale) avoid somatic items.

METHODS The contributors conducted a validated search for systematic reviews and RCTs between May and September 1998 from the Cochrane Database of Systematic Reviews and the Database of Abstracts of Reviews of Effectiveness, *Best Evidence* and *Evidence-Based Mental Health*, Medline, Psychlit, and Embase. Studies were included by using epidemiological criteria and relevance to the clinical question. A *Clinical Evidence* search and appraisal was conducted in July 2002, including a search for data on depression in older adults. In this review, studies are included under the heading older adults if they specifically included people aged over 55 years.

QUESTION **What are the effects of treatments?**

OPTION **PRESCRIPTION ANTIDEPRESSANT DRUGS**

Systematic reviews in people aged 16 years or over have found that antidepressant drugs (monoamine oxidase inhibitors, selective serotonin reuptake inhibitors, or tricyclic antidepressants) improve symptoms in

acute treatment of all grades of depressive disorder compared with placebo. Two systematic reviews have found no significant difference in outcomes with different kinds of antidepressant drug, although one systematic review found that monoamine oxidase inhibitors were less effective than tricyclic antidepressants in people with severe depressive disorders, but may be more effective in atypical depressive disorders with reversed biological features such as increased sleep, increased appetite, mood reactivity, and rejection sensitivity. Systematic reviews have found that antidepressant drugs differ in their adverse event profiles. One systematic review has found that selective serotonin reuptake inhibitors were associated with fewer adverse effects compared with tricyclic antidepressants, but the difference was small. Another systematic review and one retrospective cohort study found no strong evidence that fluoxetine was associated with increased risk of suicide compared with tricyclic antidepressants or placebo. One RCT and observational data suggest that abrupt withdrawal of selective serotonin reuptake inhibitors is associated with symptoms including dizziness and rhinitis, and that these symptoms are more likely with drugs with a short half life, such as paroxetine. One systematic review in people aged 55 years or over with all grades of depressive disorder has found that tricyclic antidepressants, selective serotonin reuptake inhibitors, or monoamine oxidase inhibitors significantly reduce the proportion of people who fail to recover over 26–49 days compared with placebo. We found no specific evidence on adverse effects in older adults.

Benefits: **Antidepressants versus placebo:** We found three systematic reviews.[11,12,13] The first review (search date 1995, 49 RCTs in people aged 18–70 years with mild to moderate or severe depressive disorders) included five RCTs in people admitted to hospital (probably with severe depressive disorders), 40 RCTs in a setting outside hospital, one in both settings, and three that did not specify the setting.[11] All RCTs identified by the review were of least 4 weeks' duration and included three way comparisons, including two antidepressant drugs (monoamine oxidase inhibitors [MAOIs], selective serotonin reuptake inhibitors [SSRIs], or tricyclic antidepressants [TCAs]) and placebo. The review only included RCTs that measured improvement in depressive symptoms using validated scales such as the Hamilton Depression Rating Scale and Montgomery-Asberg Depression Rating Scale. It found that the mean effect size (see glossary, p 1139) for change in score with antidepressants versus placebo was 0.5, which means that 69% of people taking placebo had worse outcomes than the average person taking antidepressants (see comment below).[11] The second review (search date 1997, 15 RCTs, 1871 people aged ≥ 18 years) compared antidepressants (SSRIs, TCAs, MAOIs, amisulpride, amineptine, or ritanserin) versus placebo in people with dysthymia (chronic mild depressive disorders).[12] It found that antidepressants versus placebo significantly increased the proportion of people who responded to treatment at 4–12 weeks (response defined as a 50% decrease in Hamilton Depression Rating Scale score or scoring 1 or 2 on item 2 of the Clinical Global Impression Score; RR 1.9, 95% CI 1.6 to 2.3; NNT 4, 95% CI 3 to 5). The third systematic review (search date 1998, 18 RCTs, 838 people aged > 18 years with depression and a physical illness [e.g. cancer, cardiovascular disorders, diabetes]) found that antidepressants versus placebo significantly reduced the proportion of people who failed to recover over 4–12 weeks (177/366 [48%] with antidepressant *v* 229/325 [70%] with placebo; RR 0.68, 95% CI 0.60 to 0.77; NNT 4, 95% CI 3 to 7).[13] People allocated to antidepressants were more likely to withdraw from the study than were those on placebo (NNH 10, 95% CI 5 to 43). **In older adults; antidepressants versus placebo:** We found one systematic review (search date 2000, 17 RCTs, 1326 people aged ≥ 55 years with mild to moderate or severe depression) comparing antidepressants versus placebo.[14] It found that TCAs, SSRIs, or MAOIs versus placebo significantly reduced the proportion of people who failed to recover over 26–49 days (125/245 [51%] with TCAs *v* 167/223 [75%] with placebo: RR 0.68, 95% CI 0.59 to 0.68, NNT 4, 95% CI 4 to 5; 261/365 [72%] with SSRIs *v* 310/372 [83%] with placebo: RR 0.86, 95% CI 0.79 to 0.93, NNT 9, 95% CI 9 to 10; 34/58 [59%] with MAOIs *v* 57/63 [90%] with placebo: RR 0.64, 95% CI 0.50 to 0.81, NNT 4, 95% CI 3 to 4).[14] **TCAs versus SSRIs:** We found three systematic reviews (search dates 1999,[15] 1997,[16] and 1998[17]) and one subsequent RCT[18] in people with mild to moderate or severe depression comparing SSRIs versus TCAs. The reviews found no significant difference in overall effectiveness between TCAs and SSRIs.[15,16] The second review (search date 1997, 95 RCTs, 10 533 people aged 18–80 years) found that SSRIs may be slightly more acceptable overall than TCAs, as measured by the number of people who withdrew from clinical trials for any cause (RR of withdrawal 0.88, 95% CI 0.83 to 0.93; NNH 26, 95% CI 18 to 46).[16] The third systematic review (search date 1998, 28 RCTs, 5940 people aged ≥ 18 years) compared the efficacy of newer antidepressants versus placebo or versus older antidepressants in primary care.[17] The average response rate was 63% for newer agents, 35% for placebo, and 60% for TCAs (RR for SSRIs versus placebo 1.6, 95% CI 1.2 to 2.1). The subsequent RCT (152 people with major depression) compared adherence on dosulepin (dothiepin) versus fluoxetine over 12 weeks and found no significant difference between the drugs.[18] However, the RCT was probably underpowered to detect a clinically important difference. **MAOIs versus TCAs:** We found one systematic review (search date not stated, 55 RCTs) comparing MAOIs versus TCAs in several subgroups of people with depression aged 18–80 years.[19] It found that MAOIs were less effective than TCAs in people with severe depressive disorders but may be more effective in atypical depressive disorders (depressive disorders with reversed biological features, e.g. increased sleep, increased appetite, mood reactivity, and rejection sensitivity). **Antidepressants plus benzodiazepines:** We found one systematic review (search date 1999, 8 RCTs, 679 people aged 18–65 years, 1 RCT in people aged 20–73 years with major depression) comparing combination treatment with antidepressants plus benzodiazepines versus antidepressants alone.[20] It found that combination treatment versus antidepressants alone was significantly more likely to produce a response within 1 week (RR of > 50% reduction on symptom rating scale 1.64, 95% CI 1.19 to 2.27), although this difference was not apparent at 6 weeks.

Harms: **Common adverse events with TCAs versus SSRIs:** One systematic review (search date 1996) compared adverse events with TCAs versus SSRIs in people aged 18 years or over with all severities of depression (see table 1, p 1143).[21] **Adverse effects with different SSRIs:** One large cohort study of people receiving four different SSRIs (fluvoxamine [983 people], fluoxetine [692 people], sertraline [734 people], and paroxetine [13 741 people]) in UK primary care found that reports of common adverse events (nausea/vomiting, malaise/lassitude, dizziness, and headache/migraine) varied between SSRIs (fluvoxamine 78/1000 participant months; fluoxetine 23/1000 participant months; RR *v* fluvoxamine 0.29, 95% CI 0.27 to 0.32; paroxetine 28/1000 participant months; RR 0.35, 95% CI 0.33 to 0.37; sertraline 21/1000 participant months; RR 0.26, 95% CI 0.25 to 0.28).[22] Only 52% of people responded to the questionnaire, although this response rate was similar for all four drugs. A study of spontaneous reports to the UK Committee on Safety of Medicines found no difference in safety profiles between the same four SSRIs.[23] **Suicide with TCAs versus SSRIs:** One systematic review (search date not stated, which included RCTs completed by December 1989) pooled data from 17 double blind RCTs in people with depressive disorders aged 12–90 years comparing a TCA (731 people) versus fluoxetine (1765 people) or versus placebo (569 people).[24] It found no significant difference in the rate of suicidal acts between the groups (TCAs 0.4%, fluoxetine 0.3%, and placebo 0.2%), but development of suicidal ideation was less frequent in the fluoxetine group (1% fluoxetine *v* 3% placebo, P = 0.04; and *v* 4% TCAs, P = 0.001). One historical cohort study followed 172 598 people who had at least one prescription for 1/10 antidepressants during the study period in general practice in the UK.[25] The risk of suicide was higher in people who received fluoxetine (19/10 000 person years, 95% CI 9 to 34) than in those receiving dosulepin (RR of suicide *v* dosulepin 2.1, 95% CI 1.1 to 4.1). In a nested case controlled subanalysis in people with no history of suicidal behaviour or previous antidepressant prescription, the risk remained the same, although the confidence interval broadened to make the result non-significant (RR 2.1, 95% CI 0.6 to 7.9). Although the apparent association may be because of residual confounding, there remains uncertainty about the possible association between fluoxetine and suicide. However, any absolute increase in risk is unlikely to be large. **Withdrawal effects with SSRIs:** We found one RCT in people aged 18 years or over (average age 30–40 years) comparing abrupt discontinuation of fluoxetine (96 people) versus continued treatment (299 people) in people who had been taking the drug for 12 weeks.[26] Abrupt discontinuation was associated with increased dizziness (7% *v* 1%), dysmenorrhoea (3% *v* 0%), rhinitis (10% *v* 3%), and somnolence (4% *v* 0%). However, there was a high withdrawal rate in this study because of the return of symptoms of depression (39%), so these may be underestimates of the true rate of withdrawal symptoms. Between 1987 and 1995 the rate of spontaneous reports of suspected withdrawal reactions per million defined daily doses to the World Health Organization Collaborating Centre for International Drug Monitoring was higher for paroxetine than for sertraline and fluoxetine.[27] The most common withdrawal effects were dizziness, nausea, paraesthesia, headache, and vertigo. **MAOIs versus TCAs:** The systematic review found that MAOIs were associated with a similar level of overall adverse effects as were TCAs.[19] Adverse effects associated with MAOIs included hypotension, dizziness, mydriasis, piloerection, oedema, tremor, anorgasmia, and insomnia. **During pregnancy:** One systematic review (search date 1999) assessing the risk of fetal harm of antidepressants in pregnancy found four small prospective studies published since 1993.[28] No evidence of increased risk was found, although the risk of adverse effects cannot be excluded. Decreased birth weights of infants exposed to fluoxetine during the third trimester were identified in one study, and direct drug effects and withdrawal syndromes were identified in some neonates. **In older adults:** We found no specific evidence on adverse effects in older adults.

Comment: **Antidepressants versus placebo:** The first review found that results were sensitive to the diagnostic criteria used; the mean effect size for antidepressants was 0.5 in those RCTs in which depressive disorders were diagnosed according to standard criteria (mainly *Diagnostic and statistical manual of mental disorders*, 3rd edition, revised) and 0.4 in those RCTs that did not use objective diagnostic criteria.[11] **In older adults:** The systematic review of antidepressants versus placebo in older people was limited by the diversity of populations included and by the brevity of the studies.[13] The reviewers recommended at least 6 weeks of antidepressant treatment in elderly people to achieve optimal effect. A systematic review is under way to examine adverse effects in elderly people. Metabolic and physical changes with age mean that older people may be more prone to adverse effects such as falls. Because older people often take more medications, they may be at greater risk of drug interactions.

OPTION CARE PATHWAYS

Five RCTs in people aged over 18 years found that the effectiveness of antidepressant treatment may be improved by several approaches, including collaborative working between primary care clinicians and psychiatrists plus intensive patient education, case management, telephone support, and relapse prevention programmes. One RCT found that a clinical practice guideline and practice based education did not improve either detection or outcome of depression compared with usual care.

Benefits: We found no systematic review but found six RCTs.[29–34] **Collaborative working between primary care clinicians and psychiatrists plus intensive patient education:** The first RCT (217 people aged 19–76 years with mild to moderate or major depression in primary care in the USA) found that, compared with standard treatment (including antidepressants), the addition of a multifaceted programme, including collaborative working between primary care physician and psychiatrist plus intensive patient education, improved outcomes over 12 months.[29] Improvement in depressive symptoms assessed using the Symptom Checklist-90 was significant only in the subgroup of people with major depressive disorder (91 people; AR of clinical response of > 50% reduction in symptom checklist 74% *v* 44% with standard treatment; NNT 4, 95% CI 3 to 10).[29] **Care management:** The second RCT (613 people, mean age 46 years) in a Health Maintenance Organization in Seattle (USA) compared three interventions: usual care (antidepressants), usual care plus feedback (in which doctors received a detailed report on each person at 8 and 16 wks after randomisation), or usual care plus feedback plus care management (in which the care manager assessed people with depression by telephone at 8 and 16 wks, doctors received a detailed report, and care managers facilitated the follow up).[30] It found that feedback plus care management versus usual care significantly increased the proportion of people with a clinically important reduction in depressive symptoms at 6 months after randomisation (about 56% of people with care management *v* 40% with usual care [results presented graphically]; OR 2.22, 95% CI 1.31 to 3.75). **Clinical practice guideline and practice based education:** The third RCT (cluster randomised, based in UK primary care, people aged over 16 years) compared the effects of a clinical practice guideline and practice based education versus usual care.[31] It found that the intervention did not improve either detection or outcome of depression. **Telephone support:** The fourth RCT (302 people with major depressive disorder or dysthymia aged 19–90 years) compared usual physician care (selective serotonin reuptake inhibitor [SSRI]; 117 people), usual care plus nurse telehealth (SSRI plus 12–14 telephone support calls during 16 wks of treatment; 62 people), or usual care plus telehealth plus peer support (123 people).[32] Nurse telehealth versus usual clinician care significantly increased the proportion of people with a 50% reduction in symptoms at 6 months (57% with nurse telehealth *v* 38% with usual care; NNT 6, 95% CI 4 to 18). **Relapse prevention programme:** The fifth RCT (386 people aged > 18 with recurrent major depression or dysthymia who had largely recovered after 8 wks of antidepressant treatment) compared a relapse prevention programme (2 primary care visits and 3 telephone calls) versus usual care for 1 year.[33] It found that relapse prevention versus usual care significantly improved depressive symptoms over 1 year (results presented graphically; P = 0.04) but found no significant difference in relapse rates (35% in both groups). **Multifaceted quality improvement programme:** The sixth RCT compared a multifaceted "quality improvement programme" including antidepressants plus psychotherapy or plus cognitive behavioural therapy (see glossary, p 1139) versus usual care and assessed outcomes at 1 and 2 years (see which treatments are most effective at improving long term outcome, p 1138).[34] **Older adults:** We found no systematic review or RCTs specifically in older adults.

Harms: The RCTs gave no information about adverse effects.[29–34]

Comment: None.

OPTION **ST JOHN'S WORT (*HYPERICUM PERFORATUM*)**

Two systematic reviews in people with mild to moderate depressive disorders have found that St John's Wort (*H perforatum*) significantly improves depressive symptoms over 4–12 weeks compared with placebo,

and have found no significant difference in symptoms between St John's Wort and prescription antidepressant drugs. The results of the reviews should be interpreted with caution because the RCTs did not use standardised preparations of St John's Wort, and doses of antidepressants varied. One subsequent RCT in people aged over 18 years major depressive disorder found no significant difference in depressive symptoms at 8 weeks between a standardised preparation of St John's Wort and placebo or sertraline, but it is likely to have been underpowered to detect a clinically important difference between groups.

Benefits: We found two systematic reviews[35,36] and one subsequent RCT.[37] The first review (search date 1998) identified 17 RCTs (1168 people aged > 18 years with mild to moderate depression) comparing St John's Wort versus placebo (16 RCTs using single preparations of hypericum, and 1 RCT using combinations of hypericum and 4 other plant extracts; see comment below).[35] It also identified 10 RCTs (1123 people) comparing St John's Wort versus other antidepressants or sedative drugs (8 RCTs using single preparations of hypericum, and 2 RCTs using combinations of hypericum and valeriana). It found that *H perforatum* preparations versus placebo significantly increased the proportion of people who responded over 4–12 weeks (response defined as a Hamilton Depression Rating Scale score of < 10 or < 50% of baseline score; 267/465 [57%] with hypericum *v* 122/485 [25%] with placebo; RR 2.47, 95% CI 1.69 to 3.61), and found no significant difference in the proportion of people who responded with St John's Wort versus antidepressants or sedatives (177/352 [50%] with single preparations of hypericum *v* 176/339 [52%] with placebo; 88/130 [68%] *v* 66/132 [50%]; RR 1.01, 95% CI 0.87 to 1.16; combinations RR 1.52, 95% CI 0.78 to 2.94). The second review (search date 2000, 23 RCTs, 2776 people with mild to moderate depression) included 14 RCTs identified by the first review, but applied different inclusion criteria for RCTs and excluded 13 of the RCTs included in the first review.[36] It identified 14 RCTs (1336 people) comparing St John's Wort versus placebo and nine RCTs (1394 people) comparing St John's Wort versus other antidepressants. It found that St John's Wort versus placebo significantly increased the proportion of people who responded over 4–8 weeks (390/690 [57%] *v* 184/646 [28%]; RR 1.98, 95% CI 1.49 to 2.62), but found no significant difference in depressive symptoms over 4–6 weeks with St John's Wort versus other antidepressants (422/694 [61%] *v* 423/700 [60%]; RR 1.00, 95% CI 0.91 to 1.11). These results did not change when only RCTs that met stricter methodological treatment were combined (6 RCTs; St John's Wort *v* placebo: 153/257 [60%] *v* 79/232 [34%]; RR 1.77, 95% CI 1.16 to 2.70; St John's Wort *v* other antidepressants: 260/440 [59%] *v* 261/468 [56%]; RR 1.04, 95% CI 0.94 to 1.15). The subsequent RCT (340 people aged over 18 years with major depressive disorder defined as a total score of ≥ 20 on the Hamilton Depression Rating Scale) compared St. John's Wort (standardised extract, hypericin 0.12%–0.28%, 900–1500 mg/day) versus placebo or sertraline (50–100 mg/day).[37] It found no significant difference in the proportion of people who responded at 8 weeks with St John's Wort compared with placebo (response defined as Clinical Global Impression Score of 1 [very much improved] or 2 [much improved] or a Hamilton Depression Rating Scale score of < 8: 24% with St John's Wort v 32% with placebo v 25% with sertraline; P = 0.21 for St John's Wort v placebo; P for St John's Wort v sertraline not stated). The RCT is likely to have been underpowered to detect a clinically important difference between groups.[37] **Older adults:** We found no systematic review or RCTs specifically in older adults.

Harms: We found three systematic reviews that assessed adverse effects associated with St John's Wort.[35,36,38] The first review (search date 1998) found that adverse events were poorly reported in the trials.[35] Adverse effects were reported by 26% of people taking St John's Wort versus 45% of people taking standard antidepressants (RR 0.57, 95% CI 0.47 to 0.69), and by 15% of people taking combinations of hypericum and valeriana versus 27% taking amitriptyline or desipramine (RR 0.49, 95% CI 0.23 to 1.04). The second systematic review (search date 2000) found no significant difference in the proportion of people who had adverse effects (including gastrointestinal effects, headaches, restlessness, and fatigue) with St John's Wort versus placebo (43/236 [18%] v 29/177 [16%]; RR 1.04, 95% CI 0.68 to 1.58), and found that St John's Wort versus antidepressants significantly reduced the proportion of people with adverse effects (260/440 [59%] v 261/448 [58%]; RR 0.59, 95% CI 0.52 to 0.71).[36] The third systematic review (search date 1997) included RCTs and observational surveillance studies after marketing of St John's Wort.[38] It found that the most common adverse effects of St John's Wort in the included studies were gastrointestinal symptoms, dizziness/confusion, tiredness/sedation, and dry mouth, although all occurred less frequently than on conventional drugs. Findings from observational studies were consistent with these results. Photosensitivity is theoretically possible; however, only two cases have been reported.

Comment: The results of the systematic reviews must be interpreted with caution because the preparations and doses of *H perforatum* and types and doses of antidepressants varied widely.[35,36] More RCTs are needed using standardised preparations. Interactions with other drugs are possible and should be considered.

OPTION ELECTROCONVULSIVE THERAPY

Two systematic reviews and additional RCTs in people aged over 16 years have found that electroconvulsive therapy significantly improves symptoms in severe depression compared with simulated electroconvulsive therapy.

Benefits: We found two systematic reviews,[39,40] three additional RCTs,[41–43] and two subsequent RCTs.[44,45] The first review (search date not stated, 6 RCTs published between 1960 and 1978, 205 people with severe depressive disorder, age range not stated) compared electroconvulsive therapy (ECT) versus simulated ECT (in which people received everything but electric stimulation; see comment below).[39] It found that people given real versus simulated ECT were significantly more likely to respond to treatment (response defined as global clinical state or a "clinically significant" difference in scores on depressive scales such as the Hamilton Depression Rating Scale: 73/109 [67%] *v* 33/96 [34%]; pooled RR 1.95, 95% CI 1.43 to 2.65; NNT 3, 95% CI 2 to 5; calculated by the author from data in the article). The second review (search date 1998, which included 11 additional RCTs published between 1987 and 1998) also found good evidence for the beneficial effects of ECT, but did not quantify its conclusions.[40] The results of the additional and subsequent RCTs are consistent with the findings of the review.[41–45] **Older adults:** We found no systematic review or RCTs specifically in older adults.

Harms: The systematic reviews gave no information on adverse effects,[39,40] and we found no good evidence about possible adverse cognitive effects of ECT. However, people often complain of memory impairment after ECT. One of the main difficulties in studying the association between memory impairment and ECT is that depressive disorders also lead to cognitive impairment that usually improves during the course of treatment. For this reason, most of the small studies in this area find an average improvement in memory in people treated with ECT. This does not rule out the possibility of more subtle, subjective memory impairment secondary to ECT. Adverse memory effects may vary according to the dose and electrode location.

Comment: Because ECT may be unacceptable to some people and because it is a short term treatment, there is consensus that it should normally be reserved for people who cannot tolerate or have not responded to drug treatment, although it may be useful when a rapid response is required.

OPTION PSYCHOLOGICAL TREATMENTS

One systematic review in younger and older adults with mild to moderate depression has found that cognitive therapy significantly improves symptoms compared with no treatment. One systematic review in people aged over 18 years with recent onset psychological problems, including depression, found that brief, non-directive counselling significantly reduced symptom scores in the short term (< 6 months) compared with usual care, but found no significant difference in scores in the long term (> 6 months). RCTs in younger and older adults with mild to moderate depression found that problem solving treatment or interpersonal psychotherapy significantly improved depressive symptoms in the short term compared with placebo, and found no significant difference in symptoms with problem solving treatment or interpersonal psychotherapy compared with antidepressant treatment. RCTs found insufficient evidence to assess the relative efficacy of drug and non-drug treatment in severe depression. One systematic review in people aged over 55 years with mild to moderate depression found no significant difference in symptoms between psychological treatments (such as cognitive therapy or cognitive behaviour therapy) and no treatment. However, it also found no significant difference in symptoms between psychological treatments and similar but non-specific attention. This review was based on a small number of RCTs, the populations varied (although most were community samples), and many of the studies were short term. RCTs found limited evidence about the effects of psychological treatments in severe depression.

Benefits: The evidence comparing psychological treatments versus drug or no treatment is summarised in table 2 (see table 2, p 1144).[46–50] RCTs found insufficient evidence to assess the relative efficacy of drug and non-drug treatment in severe depression (see comment below). **Older adults:** We found one systematic review (search date 1995, 14 small RCTs, < 24 people, age > 55 years in an outpatient or community setting) of pharmacological and psychological treatments.[51] It found four RCTs in older adults that compared psychological treatments versus no treatment. None of the RCTs found a significant difference between treatment and no treatment, measured on the Hamilton Depression Rating Scale. It also found six RCTs comparing different psychological treatments. Five of six comparisons of "rational" treatments (such as cognitive therapy or cognitive behavioural therapy (see glossary, p 1139)) versus no treatment in older adults found significant benefit with treatment. Combined, the "rational" treatments performed significantly better than no treatment (mean difference in the Hamilton Depression Rating Scale score −7.3, 95% CI −10.1 to −4.4), but were not significantly different from the "non-specific attention" control. None of the RCTs found significant differences in effectiveness between psychological treatments.

Harms: The systematic review and RCTs gave no information on adverse effects.[46–50]

Comment: Large RCTs are needed in more representative people in a range of clinical settings, including primary care. Because of varying exclusion criteria, the generalisability of the studies is questionable (see table 2, p 1144). Other factors to be considered when psychological treatments are compared with drug treatment include whether serum concentrations of drugs reach therapeutic concentrations, whether changes in medication are allowed (reflecting standard clinical practice), and whether studies reflect the natural course of depressive disorders. It is difficult to conduct studies of psychological treatments for severe depression because of the ethics surrounding withholding a proved treatment (antidepressant drugs) in a group of people at risk of self harm or neglect.[52]

OPTION PSYCHOLOGICAL TREATMENTS PLUS PRESCRIPTION ANTIDEPRESSANT DRUGS

One non-systematic review of RCTs in people aged 18–80 years has found that, in people with severe depression, adding drug treatment to interpersonal psychotherapy or to cognitive therapy compared with either psychological treatment alone improves symptoms, but found no significant difference in symptoms in people with mild to moderate depression. Subsequent RCTs in younger and older adults with mild to moderate depression have found that combining antidepressants plus psychotherapy improves symptoms significantly more than either antidepressants or psychotherapy alone. One RCT in older adults with mild to moderate depression found that cognitive behavioural therapy plus desipramine improved symptoms significantly more than desipramine alone.

Benefits: We found no systematic review, but found one non-systematic review[52] and two subsequent RCTs.[53,54] The non-systematic review (6 RCTs, 595 people aged 18–80 years with major depression) found that, in more severe depressive disorders, antidepressants plus interpersonal psychotherapy (see glossary, p 1139) or plus cognitive therapy (see glossary, p 1139) significantly increased the proportion of people who responded after 16 weeks of treatment compared with interpersonal psychotherapy or cognitive therapy alone (response defined as 4 wks with Hamilton Depression Rating Scale score < 7; $P = 0.001$).[52] It found no advantage in combining antidepressants and specific psychological treatments in mild to moderate depressive disorders ($P = 0.10$). The first subsequent RCT (681 adults with chronic depressive disorder, mean age 43 years) compared three interventions: nefazodone alone, cognitive behavioural therapy (see glossary, p 1139) alone, or nefazodone plus cognitive behavioural therapy.[53] It found that combined treatment significantly improved the proportion of people with a clinical response compared with either treatment alone (defined as at least 50% reduction in Hamilton Depression Rating Scale score and a score of ≤ 15; 152/226 [67%] with combined treatment *v* 92/220 [42%] with nefazodone alone *v* 90/226 [40%] with psychotherapy alone; combined treatment *v* either single intervention; $P < 0.001$; NNT 5, 95% CI 3 to 6). The second subsequent RCT (167 people with a major depressive episode) compared antidepressants (fluoxetine, amitriptyline, or moclobemide) plus short term psychodynamic supportive psychotherapy (see glossary, p 1140) versus antidepressants alone (see comment below).[54] It found that combined treatment versus antidepressants significantly increased the proportion of people who had improved after 24 weeks (improvement defined as Hamilton Depression Rating Scale score of ≤ 7, Clinical Global Impression score of 1 or 2, Symptom Checklist-90 or Quality of Life Depression Scale score of at least 1 standard deviation from baseline; mean success rate 41% *v* 59%; NNT 5, 95% CI 3 to 11). **Older adults:** We found one RCT (102 people aged > 60 years with major depressive disorder) that compared three interventions: desipramine plus cognitive behavioural therapy; desipramine alone; or cognitive behavioural therapy alone.[55] It found that all three groups showed a significant reduction in symptoms from baseline as assessed using the Hamilton Depression Rating Scale after 16–20 weeks of treatment (reduction of 0.20 with desipramine, 0.36 with cognitive behavioural therapy, and 0.41 with combined treatments; $P < 0.05$ for all comparisons). It found that combined treatments versus desipramine alone significantly improved symptoms over 16–20 weeks ($P < 0.05$). It found no significant difference among the three groups in the proportion of people who withdrew for any cause (desipramine 34%, cognitive behavioural therapy 23%, and combined treatments 33%; $P = 0.52$).

Harms: The non-systematic review and RCTs gave no information on adverse effects.[52–55]

Comment: A systematic review is needed to address this question. In the second subsequent RCT, 38/167 people initially randomised refused the proposed treatment: 27/84 (32%) of people offered antidepressants and 11/83 (13%) of people offered combined treatment.[54] This makes the results of the RCT very difficult to interpret.

OPTION EXERCISE

One systematic review found limited evidence from poor RCTs that exercise may improve symptoms compared with placebo, and may be as effective as cognitive therapy. One poor RCT in older adults identified by the review found limited evidence that exercise may be as effective as antidepressants in improving symptoms and may reduce relapse over 10 months.

Benefits: We found one systematic review (search date 1999, 14 RCTs, 851 people).[56] It found limited evidence that exercise versus no treatment may improve symptoms and found that exercise may be as effective as cognitive therapy (see glossary, p 1139). However, it suggested that these results were inconclusive because of methodological problems in all of the RCTs; randomisation was adequately concealed in only three of the RCTs, intention to treat analysis was undertaken in only two, and assessment of outcome was blinded in only one of the RCTs. **Older adults:** The systematic review[56] identified one RCT (156 people with major depression, mean age 57 years) comparing aerobic exercise, sertraline hydrochloride (a selective serotonin reuptake inhibitor), and combined treatment for 16 weeks.[57] It found that the proportion of people who recovered (those no longer meeting criteria for depression or with a Hamilton Depression Rating Scale score < 8) was not significantly different across the treatment groups (60% with exercise *v* 69% with sertraline *v* 66% with combined treatments). A 10 month follow up of this RCT found lower rates of relapse with exercise versus medication (30% with exercise *v* 52% with sertraline *v* 55% with combined treatment).[58] However, about half of the people in the medication group engaged in exercise during follow up, making it difficult to draw firm conclusions about effects of exercise. The clinical importance of the observed difference at 10 months remains unclear.

Harms: The review gave no information about adverse effects.[56]

Comment: There is a need for a well designed RCT of the effects of exercise in people with all grades of depression assessing clinical outcomes over an adequate time period.

OPTION BIBLIOTHERAPY

One systematic review of RCTs in younger and older adults recruited by advertisement found limited evidence that bibliotherapy may reduce mild depressive symptoms compared with waiting list control or standard care. Another systematic review in people with combined anxiety and depression, anxiety, or chronic fatigue found that bibliotherapy may improve symptoms over 2–6 months compared with standard care. It is unclear whether people in the RCTs identified by the reviews are clinically representative of people with depressive disorders.

Benefits: **Younger and older adults:** We found two systematic reviews (search date not stated[59] and search date 1999[60]). The first review identified six small short term RCTs of bibliotherapy (see glossary, p 1139) versus waiting list control in 273 people (described as adults in 4 RCTs and elderly in 2 RCTs; no age range provided) recruited by advertisement through the media and probably with only mild depression (see comment below).[59] The mean effect size (see glossary, p 1139) of bibliotherapy was 0.82 (95% CI 0.50 to 1.15). This means that 79% of people in the waiting list control group had a worse outcome than the average person in the bibliotherapy group. The second systematic review identified eight randomised and non-randomised trials in younger and older people, but only one of them included people with depression.[60] It found that, in people with combined anxiety and depression, anxiety, or chronic fatigue, bibliotherapy may improve symptoms over 2–6 months compared with standard care. The RCT identified by the second review that included people with depression found that bibliotherapy versus standard care significantly improved symptoms of anxiety over 4 weeks as assessed using the Hamilton Depression Rating Scale, but found no significant difference in symptoms of depression at 4 or 12 weeks. **Older adults:** We found no systematic review or RCTs specifically in older adults.

Harms: None reported.

Comment: The review did not clearly describe the characteristics of the people in the RCTs it identified, and it is unclear whether people were receiving interventions in addition to bibliotherapy.[59] Further RCTs are needed in clinically representative groups.

OPTION BEFRIENDING

One small RCT provided insufficient evidence to assess befriending.

Benefits: We found one small RCT (86 women with chronic depression, aged > 18 years, primarily aged 25–40 years, based in London, UK) of befriending (see glossary, p 1139) versus waiting list control.[61] Initial identification was by postal screening of women registered with, but not attending, primary care. It found that befriending versus waiting list control significantly increased the proportion of women with remission of symptoms at 13 months (65% with befriending *v* 39% with control; $P < 0.05$; NNT 4, 95% CI 2 to 18). **Older adults:** We found no systematic review or RCTs specifically in older adults.

Harms: The RCT gave no information on harms.[61]

Comment: In the RCT, 14% of women in the befriending group were taking antidepressants and 12% of women in the waiting list control group.[61] Fewer than half of the women screened by post were interested in befriending as a treatment option.

QUESTION What are the effects of continuation treatment with antidepressant drugs?

One systematic review and subsequent RCTs in younger and older adults have found that continuation treatment with antidepressant drugs compared with placebo for 4–6 months after recovery significantly reduces the risk of relapse. One RCT in people aged over 60 years has found that continuation treatment with dosulepin significantly reduces the risk of relapse over 2 years compared with placebo.

Benefits: We found one systematic review (search date not stated, 6 RCTs, 312 people, age range not stated).[62] It found that continuation of antidepressant medication versus placebo for 4–6 months after acute treatment reduced the relapse rate by nearly half (RR 0.6, 95% CI 0.4 to 0.7). Several more recent RCTs confirmed this reduction in risk of early relapse with continuing antidepressant treatment for 6–12 months after acute treatment. **Older adults:** We found one RCT (69 people aged > 60 years with mild to moderate or severe depression who had recovered sufficiently and consented to enter a 2 year trial of continuation treatment (see glossary, p 1139)), which compared dosulepin (dothiepin) versus placebo.[63] It found that dosulepin versus placebo reduced the risk of relapse over 2 years by 55% (RR 0.45, 95% CI 0.22 to 0.96).

Harms: Adverse effects seem to be similar to those reported in trials of acute treatment.

Comment: We found no adequate systematic review of maintenance treatment (see glossary, p 1140), but several RCTs have found that maintenance treatment reduced recurrence compared with placebo in recurrent depressive disorder. However, they all have problems with their methods (e.g. high withdrawal rates)[64] and will be considered in future *Clinical Evidence* updates. A systematic review of antidepressant treatment duration is in progress.[65]

QUESTION Which treatments are most effective at improving long term outcome (≥ 1 year)?

One systematic review and one additional RCT in younger and older adults found limited evidence by combining relapse rates across different RCTs that cognitive therapy may reduce the risk of relapse over 1–2 years compared with antidepressants. One RCT found that a multifaceted "quality improvement programme" significantly improved symptoms and increased the proportion of people who returned to work over 1 year compared with usual care, but found no significant difference in outcomes at 2 years.

Benefits: **Cognitive therapy versus antidepressants:** We found one systematic review (search date not stated) comparing cognitive therapy (see glossary, p 1139) versus antidepressants in people with mainly mild to moderate depressive disorders.[46] The review identified eight small RCTs (261 people, mean age 39.3 years) that assessed long term (1–2 year) relapse rates after treatment had stopped. Relapse was defined as a return of depressive symptoms (Beck Depression Inventory Score > 16) at 6–9 months after a 2 month remission. It found limited evidence by combining relapse rates across different RCTs that, overall, 30% of people treated with cognitive therapy relapsed compared with 60% of those treated with either antidepressants or antidepressants plus cognitive therapy. We found one small additional RCT (40 people) comparing cognitive therapy versus normal clinical management (antidepressants) for residual depressive symptoms in people who had responded to antidepressants. It also found that, at 2 years, fewer people relapsed with cognitive therapy than with antidepressants.[66] **Care pathways versus usual care:** One RCT (1356 people aged > 18 years with mild to moderate or major depression in 46 primary care clinics in US Health Maintenance Organizations) compared a multifaceted "quality improvement programme" (including antidepressants plus psychotherapy or plus cognitive behavioural therapy (see glossary, p 1139)) versus usual care (including mailed practice guidelines).[34] It found that the quality improvement programme versus usual care significantly increased the proportion of people who improved on continuous depression rating scales over 1 year. It found that, among people initially employed, 90% of people in the quality improvement programme worked at 1 year versus 85% of the people receiving usual care (P = 0.05). For people initially not working, there was no difference in employment rates at 12 months with quality improvement versus usual care (17% *v* 18%). A 2 year follow up of this RCT found no significant difference in outcomes with quality improvement versus usual care.[67] **Older adults:** We found no systematic review or RCTs specifically in older adults.

Harms: See harms of prescription antidepressant drugs, p 1128.

Comment: The review did not present information on the proportion of people who recovered and continued to remain well after 2 years.[46] The largest RCT identified by the review found that only a fifth of people remained well over 18 months' follow up, and that there were no significant differences between interpersonal psychotherapy (see glossary, p 1139), cognitive therapy, or drug treatment.[46] It is possible that different people respond to different treatments. Further large scale comparative studies are needed of the long term effectiveness of treatments in people with all severities of depressive disorders.

GLOSSARY

Befriending Consists of a befriender meeting the person to talk and socialise for at least 1 hour a week, acting as a friend.

Bibliotherapy Advising people to read written material such as *Feeling good: the new mood therapy* by David Burns (New York: New American Library, 1980).

Brief, non-directive counselling Helping people to express feelings and clarify thoughts and difficulties; therapists suggest alternative understandings and do not give direct advice but try to encourage people to solve their own problems.

Cognitive behavioural therapy Brief (20 sessions over 12–16 wks) structured treatment, incorporating elements of cognitive therapy and behavioural therapy. Behavioural therapy is based on learning theory and concentrates on changing behaviour.

Cognitive therapy Brief (20 sessions over 12–16 wks) structured treatment aimed at changing the dysfunctional beliefs and negative automatic thoughts that characterise depressive disorders. It requires a highly trained therapist.[68]

Continuation treatment Continuation of treatment after successful resolution of a depressive episode to prevent relapse.

Effect size This expresses the degree of overlap between the range of scores in the control and experimental groups. The effect size can be used to estimate the proportion of people in the control group who had a poorer outcome than the average person in the experimental group; a proportion of 50% indicates that the treatment has no effect.

Interpersonal psychotherapy Standardised form of brief psychotherapy (usually 12–16 weekly sessions) primarily intended for outpatients with unipolar non-psychotic depressive disorders. It focuses on improving the person's interpersonal functioning and identifying the problems associated with the onset of the depressive episode.[69]

Maintenance treatment Long term treatment of recurrent depressive disorder to prevent the recurrence of further depressive episodes.

Problem solving treatment Consists of three stages: (1) identifying the main problems for the person; (2) generating solutions; and (3) trying out the solutions. Potentially briefer and simpler than cognitive therapy and may be feasible in primary care.[48]

Psychodynamic supportive psychotherapy Aims to facilitate change by detecting and resolving underlying psychological conflicts. The treatment aims to be less challenging by incorporating supportive elements.

REFERENCES

1. American Psychiatric Association. *Diagnostic and statistical manual of mental disorders*, 4th ed. Washington, DC: American Psychiatric Association, 1994.
2. World Health Organization. *The ICD-10 classification of mental and behavioural disorders*. Geneva: World Health Organization, 1992.
3. Rosenstein, Leslie D. Differential diagnosis of the major progressive dementias and depression in middle and late adulthood: a summary of the literature of the early 1990s. *Neuropsychol Rev* 1998;8:109–167.
4. Katon W, Schulberg H. Epidemiology of depression in primary care. *Gen Hosp Psychiatry* 1992;14:237–247.
5. Murray CJ, Lopez AD. Regional patterns of disability-free life expectancy and disability-adjusted life expectancy: global burden of disease study. *Lancet* 1997;349:1347–1352.
6. Murray CJ, Lopez AD. Alternative projections of mortality and disability by cause 1990–2020: global burden of disease study. *Lancet* 1997;349:1498–1504.
7. Beekman ATF, Copeland JRM, Prince MJ. Review of community prevalence of depression in later life. *Br J Psychiatry* 1999;174:307–311.
8. Judd LL, Akiskal HS, Maser JD, et al. A prospective 12 year study of subsyndromal and syndromal depressive symptoms in unipolar major depressive disorders. *Arch Gen Psychiatry* 1988;55:694–700.
9. Cole MG, Bellavance F, Mansour A. Prognosis of depression in elderly community and primary care populations: a systematic review and meta-analysis. *Am J Psychiatry* 1999;156:1182–1189. Search date 1996; primary sources Medline 1981–1996, Psychinfo 1984–1996, and hand searches of the bibliographies of relevant articles.
10. Saz P, Dewey ME. Depression, depressive symptoms and mortality in persons aged 65 and older living in the community: a systematic review of the literature. *Int J Geriatr Psychiatry* 2001;16:622–630. Search date 1999; primary sources Embase, Medline, personal files, and hand searches of reference lists.
11. Joffe R, Sokolov S, Streiner D. Antidepressant treatment of depression: a meta-analysis. *Can J Psychiatry* 1996;41:613–616. Search date 1995; primary source Medline.
12. Lima MS, Moncrieff J. Drugs versus placebo for dysthymia. In: Cochrane Library, Issue 2, 2002. Oxford: Update Software. Search date 1997; primary sources Biological Abstracts, Medline, Psychlit, Embase, Lilacs, Cochrane Library, personal communication, conference abstracts, unpublished trials from the pharmaceutical industry, and book chapters on the treatment of depression.
13. Gill D, Hatcher S. Antidepressants for depression in medical illness. In: The Cochrane Library, Issue 2, 2002. Oxford: Update Software. Search date 1998; primary sources Medline, Cochrane Library Trials Register, Cochrane Depression and Neurosis Group Trials Register, and hand searches of two journals and reference lists.
14. Wilson K, Mottram P, Sivanranthan A, et al. Antidepressant versus placebo for the depressed elderly. In: The Cochrane Library, Issue 2, 2002. Oxford: Update Software. Search date 2000; primary sources Psychlit, Medline, Embase, Cinahl, Cochrane Controlled Trials register, CCDAN trials register, and hand searches.
15. Geddes JR, Freemantle N, Mason J, et al. Selective serotonin reuptake inhibitors (SSRIs) for depression. In: The Cochrane Library, Issue 2, 2002. Oxford: Update Software. Search date 1999; primary sources Medline, Embase, Cochrane Group Register of Controlled Trials, hand searches of reference lists of all located studies, and contact with manufacturers.
16. Anderson IM. Selective serotonin reuptake inhibitors versus tricyclic antidepressants: a meta-analysis of efficacy and tolerability. *J Affect Disord* 2000;58:19–36. Search date 1997; primary sources Medline, and hand searches of reference lists of meta-analyses and reviews.
17. Mulrow CD, Williams JW, Chiqueete E, et al. Efficacy of newer medications for treating depression in primary care people. *Am Med J* 2000;108:54–64. Search date 1998; primary sources Cochrane Depression Anxiety and Neurosis Group Specialised Register of Clinical Trials, hand searches of trials and 46 pertinent meta-analyses, and consultation with experts.
18. Thompson C, Peveler RC, Stephenson D, et al. Compliance with antidepressant medication in the treatment of major depressive disorder in primary care: a randomized comparison of fluoxetine and a tricyclic antidepressant. *Am J Psychiatry* 2000;157:338–343.
19. Thase ME, Trivedi MH, Rush AJ. MAOIs in the contemporary treatment of depression. *Neuropsychopharmacology* 1995;12:185–219. Search date not stated; primary sources Medline and Psychological Abstracts.
20. Furukawa TA, Streiner DL, Young LT. Antidepressant and benzodiazepine for major depression. In: The Cochrane Library, Issue 2, 2002. Oxford: Update Software. Search date 1999; primary sources Medline, Embase, International Pharmaceutical Abstracts, Biological Abstracts, LILACS, Psychlit, Cochrane Library, Cochrane Depression, Anxiety and Neurosis Group Trial Register, SciSearch, hand searches of reference lists, and personal contacts.
21. Trindade E, Menon D. *Selective serotonin reuptake inhibitors (SSRIs) for major depression. Part I. Evaluation of the clinical literature*. Ottawa: Canadian Coordinating Office for Health Technology Assessment, 1997 August Report 3E. *Evidence-Based Mental Health* 1998;1:50. Search date 1996; primary sources Medline, Embase, Psychinfo, International Pharmaceutical

Abstracts, Pascal, Health Planning and Administration, Mental Health Abstracts, Pharmacoeconomics and Outcomes News, Current Contents databases, scanning bibliographies of retrieved articles, hand searching of journals, and consulting researchers.

22. Mackay FJ, Dunn NR, Wilton LV, et al. A comparison of fluvoxamine, fluoxetine, sertraline and paroxetine examined by observational cohort studies. *Pharmacoepidemiol Drug Safety* 1997;6:235–246.
23. Price JS, Waller PC, Wood SM, et al. A comparison of the post marketing safety of four selective serotonin reuptake inhibitors including the investigation of symptoms occurring on withdrawal. *Br J Clin Pharmacol* 1996;42:757–763.
24. Beasley CM Jr, Dornseif BE, Bosomworth JC, et al. Fluoxetine and suicide: a meta-analysis of controlled trials of treatment for depression. *BMJ* 1991;303: 685–692. Search date not stated, but included trials that had been completed/analysed by December 1989; primary sources not given in detail but based on clinical report form data from trials and data from the Drug Experience Network Database.
25. Jick SS, Dean AD, Jick H. Antidepressants and suicide. *BMJ* 1995;310:215–218.
26. Zajecka J, Fawcett J, Amsterdam J, et al. Safety of abrupt discontinuation of fluoxetine: a randomised, placebo controlled study. *J Clin Psychopharmacol* 1998;18:193–197.
27. Stahl MM, Lindquist M, Pettersson M, et al. Withdrawal reactions with selective serotonin reuptake inhibitors as reported to the WHO system. *Eur J Clin Pharmacol* 1997;53:163–169.
28. Wisner KL, Gelenberg AJ, Leonard H, et al. Pharmacologic treatment of depression during pregnancy. *JAMA* 1999;282:1264–1269. Search date 1999; primary sources Medline, Healthstar, hand searches of bibliographies of review articles, and discussions with investigators in the field.
29. Katon W, Von Korff M, Lin E, et al. Collaborative management to achieve treatment guidelines: impact on depression in primary care. *JAMA* 1995;273:1026–1031.
30. Simon GE, Vonkorff M, Rutter C, et al. Randomised trial of monitoring, feedback, and management of care by telephone to improve treatment of depression in primary care. *BMJ* 2000;320:550–554.
31. Thompson C, Kinmonth AL, Stevens L, et al. Effects of a clinical-practice guideline and practice-based education on detection and outcome of depression in primary care: Hampshire Depression Project randomised controlled trial. *Lancet* 2000;355:185–191.
32. Hunkeler EM, Meresman JF, Hargreaves WA, et al. Efficacy of nurse telehealth care and peer support in augmenting treatment of depression in primary care. *Arch Fam Med* 2000;9:700–708.
33. Katon W, Rutter C, Ludman EJ, et al. A randomized trial of relapse prevention of depression in primary care. *Arch Gen Psychiatry* 2001;58:241–247.
34. Wells KB, Sherbourne C, Schoenbaum M, et al. Impact of disseminating quality improvement programs for depression in managed primary care: a randomized controlled trial. *JAMA* 2000;283:212–220.
35. Linde K, Mulrow CD. St John's Wort for depression. In: The Cochrane Library, Issue 2, 2002. Oxford: Update Software. Search date 1998; primary sources Medline, Embase, Psychlit, Psychindex, specialised databases: Cochrane Complementary Medicine Field, Cochrane Depression and Neurosis CRG, Phytodok, hand searches of references of pertinent articles, and contact with manufacturers, and researchers.
36. Whiskey A, Werneke U, Taylor D. A systematic review and meta-analysis of *Hypericum perforatum* in depression: a comprehensive clinical review. *Int Clin Psychopharmacol* 2001;16:239–252. Search date 2000; primary sources (in English or German) Medline, Embase, and hand searched references of primary studies.
37. Davidson JRT, Gadde KM, Fairbank JA. Effect of *Hypericum perforatum* (St John's wort) in major depressive disorder: a randomized controlled trial. *JAMA* 2002;287:1807–1814.
38. Ernst E, Rand JI, Barnes J, et al. Adverse effects profile of the herbal antidepressant St John Wort (*Hypericum perforatum L*). *Eur J Clin Pharmacol* 1998;54:589–594. Search date 1997; primary sources AMED, Cochrane Library 1997 Issue 2, Embase, Medline, hand searched reference lists, contacted WHO Collaborating Centre for International Drug Monitoring, UK Committee on Safety of Medicines, and German Bundesinstitut für Arzneimittel und Medizinproducte plus 12 German manufacturers of hypericum products.
39. Janicak PG, Davis JM, Gibbons RD, et al. Efficacy of ECT: a meta-analysis. *Am J Psychiatry* 1985;142:297–302. Search date not stated; primary source Medline.
40. Wijeratne C, Halliday GS, Lyndon RW. The present status of electroconvulsive therapy: a systematic review. *Med J Austr* 1999;171:250–254. Search date 1998; primary source Medline.
41. Johnstone EC, Deakin JF, Lawler P, et al. The Northwick Park electroconvulsive therapy trial. *Lancet* 1980;1:1317–1320.
42. Brandon S, Cowley P, McDonald C, et al. Electroconvulsive therapy: results in depressive illness from the Leicestershire trial. *BMJ* 1984;288:22–25.
43. Gregory S, Shawcross CR, Gill D. The Nottingham ECT study. A double-blind comparison of bilateral, unilateral and simulated ECT in depressive illness. *Br J Psychiatry* 1985;146:520–524.
44. Vaughan McCall W, Reboussin DM, Weiner RD, et al. Titrated moderately suprathreshold vs fixed high-dose right unilateral electroconvulsive therapy. *Arch Gen Psychiatry* 2000;57:438–444.
45. Sackeim HA, Prudic J, Devanand DP, et al. A prospective, randomized, double-blind comparison of bilateral and right unilateral electroconvulsive therapy at different stimulus intensities. *Arch Gen Psychiatry* 2000;57:425–434.
46. Gloaguen V, Cottraux J, Cucherat M, et al. A meta-analysis of the effects of cognitive therapy in depressed people 1998. *J Affect Disord* 1998;49:59–72. Search date not stated; primary sources Medline, Embase, references in books and papers, previous reviews and meta-analyses, abstracts from congress presentations, and preprints sent by authors.
47. Elkin I, Shea MT, Watkins JT, et al. National Institute of Mental Health treatment of depression collaborative research program: general effectiveness of treatments. *Arch Gen Psychiatry* 1989;46:971–982.
48. Mynors-Wallis LM, Gath DH, Lloyd-Thomas AR, et al. Randomised controlled trial comparing problem solving treatment with amitriptyline and placebo for major depression in primary care. *BMJ* 1995;310:441–445.
49. Dowrick C, Dunn G, Ayuso-Mateos JL, et al. Problem solving treatment and group psychoeducation for depression: multicentre randomised controlled trial. *BMJ* 2000;321:1450–1454.

50. Bower P, Rowland N, Mellor Clark J, et al. Effectiveness and cost effectiveness of counselling in primary care. In: The Cochrane Library, Issue 2, 2002. Oxford: Update Software. Search date 2001; primary sources Medline, Embase, Psychlit, Cinahl, Cochrane Controlled Trials Register, CCDAN trials register, personal contact with experts and CCDAN members, search of unpublished sources (clinical trials, books, dissertations, agency reports, etc.), and hand searches of one journal and reference lists.
51. McCusker J, Cole M, Keller E, et al. Effectiveness of treatments of depression in older ambulatory people. *Arch Intern Med* 1998;158:705–712. Search date 1995; primary sources Medline, Psychinfo, and hand searches of references.
52. Thase ME, Greenhouse JB, Frank E, et al. Treatment of major depression with psychotherapy or psychotherapy — pharmacotherapy combinations. *Arch Gen Psychiatry* 1997;54:1009–1015. Pooled results of six research protocols conducted 1982–1992 at the Mental Health Clinical Research Center, University of Pittsburgh School of Medicine.
53. Keller MB, McCullough JP, Klein DN, et al. A comparison of nefazodone, the cognitive behavioral-analysis system of psychotherapy, and their combination for the treatment of chronic depression. *N Engl J Med* 2000;342:1462–1470.
54. De Jonghe F, Kool S, van Aalst G, Dekker J, Peen J. Combining psychotherapy and antidepressants in the treatment of depression. *J Affect Disord* 2001;64:217–229.
55. Thompson LW, Coon DW, Gallagher-Thompson D, Sommer BR, Koin D. Comparison of desipramine and cognitive behavioural therapy in the treatment of elderly outpatients with mild-to-moderate depression. *Am J Geriatr Psychiatry* 2001;9:225–240.
56. Lawlor DA, Hopker SW. The effectiveness of exercise as an intervention in the management of depression: systematic review and meta-regression analysis of randomised controlled trials. *BMJ* 2001;322:763–767. Search date 1999; primary sources Medline, Embase, Sports Discus, Psychlit, Cochrane Library, and hand searches of reference lists and nine journals.
57. Blumenthal JA, Babyak MA, Moore KA, et al. Effects of exercise training on older people with major depression. *Arch Intern Med* 1999;159:2349–2356.
58. Babyak M, Blumenthal JA, Herman S, et al. Exercise treatment for major depression: maintenance of therapeutic benefit at 10 months. *Psychosom Med* 2000;62:633–638.
59. Cuijpers P. Bibliotherapy in unipolar depression: a meta-analysis. *J Behav Ther Exp Psychiatry* 1997;28:139–147. Search date not stated; primary sources Psychlit, Psychinfo, and Medline.
60. Bower P, Richards D, Lovell K. The clinical and cost-effectiveness of self-help treatments for anxiety and depressive disorders in primary care: a systematic review. *Br J Gen Pract* 2001;51:838–845. Search date 1999; primary sources Psychinfo, Medline, Embase, Cinahl, Cochrane Library, Counselling in Primary Care Counsel.lit database, National Research Register, personal contact with researchers, hand searches of reference lists and two journals.
61. Harris T, Brown GW, Robinson R. Befriending as an intervention for chronic depression among women in an inner city: randomised controlled trial. *Br J Psychiatry* 1999;174:219–224.
62. Loonen AJ, Peer PG, Zwanikken GJ. Continuation and maintenance therapy with antidepressive agents: meta-analysis of research. *Pharm Week Sci* 1991;13:167–175. Search date not stated; primary sources references of textbooks and review articles, Medline, Embase, and review of reference lists of primary studies.
63. Old age depression interest group. How long should the elderly take antidepressants? A double-blind placebo-controlled study of continuation/prophylaxis therapy with dothiepin. *Br J Psychiatry* 1993;162:175–182.
64. Keller MB, Kocsis JH, Thase ME, et al. Maintenance phase efficacy of sertraline for chronic depression: a randomized controlled trial. *JAMA* 1998;280:1665–1672.
65. Carney S, Geddes J, Davies D, et al. Antidepressants treatment duration for depressive disorder (protocol). In: The Cochrane Library, Issue 4, 2001. Oxford: Update Software.
66. Fava GA, Rafanelli C, Grandi S, et al. Prevention of recurrent depression with cognitive behavioral therapy: preliminary findings. *Arch Gen Psychiatry* 1998;55:816–820.
67. Sherbourne CD, Wells KB, Duan N, et al. Long term effectiveness of disseminating quality improvement for depression in primary care. *Arch Gen Psychiatry* 2001;58:696–703.
68. Haaga DAF, Beck AT. Cognitive therapy. In: Paykel ES, ed. *Handbook of affective disorders.* Edinburgh: Churchill Livingstone, 1992:511–523.
69. Klerman GL, Weissman H. Interpersonal psychotherapy. In: Paykel ES, ed. *Handbook of affective disorders.* Edinburgh: Churchill Livingstone, 1992:501–510.

John Geddes
Professor of Epidemiological Psychiatry
University of Oxford
Oxford
UK

Rob Butler
Honorary Senior Lecturer in Psychiatry/Consultant in Old Age Psychiatry
University of Auckland and Waitemata Health

Simon Hatcher
Senior Lecturer in Psychiatry/Honorary
Consultant in Liaison Psychiatry
University of Auckland
Auckland
New Zealand

Competing interests: RB has been reimbursed by Novartis for attending a conference. JG and SH none declared.

The following previous contributors of this topic would also like to be acknowledged: James Warner.

TABLE 1 **Adverse events (% of people) with selective serotonin reuptake inhibitors versus tricyclic antidepressants (see text, p 1128).[21]**

Adverse effects	SSRI event rates (%)	TCA event rates (%)
Dry mouth	21	55
Constipation	10	22
Dizziness	13	23
Nausea	22	12
Diarrhoea	13	5
Anxiety	13	7
Agitation	14	8
Insomnia	12	7
Nervousness	15	11
Headache	17	14

SSRI, selective serotonin reuptake inhibitors; TCA, tricyclic antidepressants.

TABLE 2 **Effects of specific psychological treatments for depressive disorders (see text, p 1134).**

Intervention	Evidence	Benefits	Harms	Disadvantages
Cognitive therapy	1 SR (48 RCTs of psychological therapies [2765 people, mean age 39.3 y] mainly outpatients in secondary care; therefore, probably with mild to moderate depression; people with psychotic or bipolar symptoms were excluded); 20 RCTs compared CT with waiting list or placebo and 17 compared it with drug treatment[46]	79% of people receiving placebo were more symptomatic than the average person receiving CT ($P < 0.0001$).[43] 65% of people receiving CT were less symptomatic than the average person treated with antidepressant drugs ($P < 0.0001$)[46]	No harms reported	Requires extensive training. Limited availability. RCTs in primary care suggest limited acceptability to some people
Interpersonal psychotherapy	No SR. 1 large RCT (people with mild to moderate depression, mean age 35 y) compared interpersonal psychotherapy *v* either drug treatment, CT, or placebo plus clinical management for 16 wks[47]	Rates of recovery from depression: interpersonal psychotherapy (43%; NNT 5, 95% CI 3 to 19), imipramine (42%; NNT 5, 95% CI 3 to 22), placebo clinical management (21%)[47]	No harms reported	Requires extensive training. Limited availability
Problem solving therapy	No SR. 1 large RCT (452 people aged 18–65 y with mild to moderate depression or adjustment disorders) compared PS, group treatment, and control.[49] 1 RCT (91 people aged 18–65 y with mild to moderate depression) compared problem solving, placebo, and amitriptyline[48]	PS *v* control significantly increased the proportion of people who were not depressed at 6 mo, but no significant difference at 1 y.[49] PS *v* placebo significantly improved symptoms at 12 wks, and no significant difference in symptoms with PS *v* amitriptyline[48]	No harms reported	Requires some training. Limited availability
Non-directive counselling	1 SR (7 RCTs, 772 people aged over 18 y with recent onset psychological problems, including depression in UK primary care) compared counselling *v* standard physician care[50]	Counselling *v* standard care significantly improved symptons in the short term (1–6 mo; WMD –2.03, 95% CI –3.82 to –0.24), but no significant difference in the long term (> 6 mo; WMD –0.03, 95% CI –0.39 to +0.32)[50]	No harms reported	Requires some training. Limited availability

CT, cognitive therapy; mo, month; PS, problem solving; SR, systematic review; y, year.

Domestic violence

Search date November 2002

Joanne Klevens and Laura Sadowski

QUESTIONS

INTERVENTIONS

See glossary, p 1154

Key Messages

- **Advocacy** One RCT and one non-randomised controlled trial found a reduction in reabuse with advocacy compared with no treatment. The RCT also found an improvement in women's quality of life with advocacy compared with no treatment. A controlled trial conducted in pregnant Hispanic women combining counselling with mentoring (similar to advocacy) found no significant differences in reabuse rates compared with a resource card, but found a small reduction in abuse when compared with unlimited counselling. A small RCT and a non-randomised controlled trial found no effects of advocacy on the reoccurrence of abuse but reported increased use of intimate partner violence services and resources by women assigned to advocates.
- **Cognitive behaviour orientated counselling** One controlled trial found cognitive behaviour orientated therapy to be better than non-specific support in improving women's assertiveness and reducing exposure to abuse.
- **Couple counselling** One RCT and one non-randomised controlled trial comparing gender specific counselling versus couples counselling found a reduction in levels of physical aggression. In addition, the non-randomised controlled trial found reductions in psychological aggression and depression in wives compared with baseline values. No differences were found between treatments. One controlled trial found no significant difference between group and individual couple counselling on reduction in physical violence or on psychological wellbeing.
- **Grief resolution orientated counselling** One controlled trial found grief resolution orientated counselling to be better than feminist orientated counselling in improving self esteem and self efficacy.

Domestic violence

- **Peer support groups** We found no systematic reviews or controlled trials on the effect of peer support groups.
- **Safety planning** We found no comparisons of safety planning in isolation versus other types of interventions. One controlled trial conducted in pregnant women that included safety planning along with advocacy, counselling, and a brochure found a decrease in spouse abuse and an increase in safety behaviours among the women receiving the intervention compared with women receiving a wallet sized card with information on community resources.
- **Shelters for women engaged in help seeking behaviour** We found evidence from a comparative cohort study on the utility of shelters but only in women who engage in other types of help seeking behaviour.
- **Unspecified orientation of counselling** Two controlled trials and one comparative cohort study found no effect of counselling compared with no treatment on medical care utilisation rates, reported exposure to violence and threats of violence, or depression, anxiety, and self esteem.

DEFINITION Domestic violence, also called intimate partner violence, is actual or threatened physical or sexual violence, or emotional or psychological abuse (including coercive tactics) by a current or former spouse or dating partner (including same sex partners).[1] Other terms commonly used to describe intimate partner violence include domestic violence or abuse, spouse abuse, marital violence, and battering.

INCIDENCE/ PREVALENCE Between 10% and 69% of women participating in population based surveys in 48 countries from around the world reported being physically assaulted by a partner during their lifetime.[2] Rates of assault by a partner are 4.3 times higher among women than men.[3] Nearly 25% of surveyed women in the USA reported being physically and/or sexually assaulted by a current or former partner at some time during their lives and 1.5% were victimised during the previous 12 months.[3] Rates of violence against pregnant women range from 0.9% to 20%.[4] Between 11.7–24.5% of women in prenatal clinics[5–8] and 5.5–17% of women in primary or ambulatory care reported being abused by a partner in the past year.[9–12]

AETIOLOGY/ RISK FACTORS A recent systematic review found that physical domestic violence in women is associated with lower levels of education and unemployment, low family income, marital discord, and with the partner's lower level of occupation, childhood experiences of abuse, witnessing interparental violence, higher levels of anger, depression, heavy or problem drinking, drug use, jealousy, and lack of assertiveness with spouse.[13] A similar review of research on psychological aggression found that the few demographic and psychological variables assessed either were inconsistently associated with psychological domestic violence or were found to be associated with psychological domestic violence in studies with serious methodological limitations.[14]

PROGNOSIS There are few prospective studies documenting the course of domestic violence and its outcomes. Cross-sectional surveys suggest that domestic violence is a repetitive event for at least two thirds of women.[15,16] Among black and Hispanic people persistence of domestic violence appears to be dependent on initial severity.[17] For all ethnic groups, half of those reporting moderate domestic violence have remission, but for people of black or Hispanic origin reporting severe domestic violence only a third reach remission. A case control study conducted in middle class working women found that, compared with non-abused women, women abused by their partners during the previous 9 years were significantly more likely to have or report headaches (48% *v* 35%), back pain (40% *v* 25%), sexually transmitted diseases (6% *v* 2%), vaginal bleeding (17% *v* 6%), vaginal infections (30% *v* 21%), pelvic pain (17% *v* 9%), painful intercourse (13% *v* 7%), urinary tract infections (22% *v* 12%), appetite loss (9% *v* 3%), digestive problems (35% *v* 19%), abdominal pain (22% *v* 11%), and facial injuries (8% *v* 1%).[18] After adjusting for age, race, insurance status, and cigarette smoking, a cross-sectional survey found that women experiencing psychological abuse are also more likely to report poor physical and mental health, disability preventing work, arthritis, chronic pain, migraine and other frequent headaches, sexually transmitted infections, chronic pelvic pain, stomach ulcers, spastic colon, frequent indigestion, diarrhoea, or constipation (see table 1, p 1156).[19]

AIMS OF INTERVENTION To improve quality of life, and psychological and physical wellbeing; to reduce risk of physical and mental illness, injury, or death.

OUTCOMES Self reported rates of domestic violence, mortality, non-fatal injuries, gynaecological and reproductive/obstetrical complications (e.g. chronic pelvic pain, miscarriage, recurrent vaginal infections), chronic disorders that may have a psychosomatic component (e.g. chronic pain, sleep or eating disorders, hypertension), and psychological conditions (e.g. depression, suicide, substance abuse, anxiety, low self esteem, low self efficacy, or poor assertiveness) associated with intimate partner violence, as well as quality of life, physical and functional status, and adverse effects of treatment. Utilisation of domestic violence services was also considered as an intermediate outcome. Scales frequently used were the Severity of Violence Against Women Scale, Spielberger's 20 item State-Trait Anxiety Inventory, Hudson's Index of Self-esteem, Self-efficacy Scale, Modified Conflict Tactics Scale, Beck Depression Inventory, and Index of Spouse Abuse Scale (see glossary, p 1154).

METHODS *Clinical Evidence* search and appraisal November 2002. *Clinical Evidence* searched Medline from 1966, Embase from 1980, PsycINFO from 1985, ASSIA from 1987, Cinahl from 1982, MIDIRS from 1990; Cochrane Library 2002 issue 4 and TRIP database; and identified systematic reviews, RCTs, other controlled trials, and observational studies using the following search terms: intimate partner violence, domestic violence, battered women, woman abuse, woman battering, family violence, husband to wife violence, marital violence, battered wives, conjugal violence, spouse abuse, violence against women, and abused women; and prevention, treatment, or intervention. We excluded public education, system level interventions, civil protection orders, screening for domestic violence or protocols focusing on identification of domestic violence victims, as well as interventions targeting only men (e.g. batterer treatment). Couple interventions were included only if women participated regularly in the intervention and reoccurrence of violence or other outcomes among women were measured. Given the paucity of studies, none were excluded because of methodological limitations; however, when high non-participation, attrition, or high rates of loss to follow up were found, these are mentioned in the comments sections.

QUESTION **What are the effects of interventions initiated by health care professionals, aimed at female victims of domestic violence, on the risk of reoccurrence?** New

OPTION **INDIVIDUAL, COUPLE, OR GROUP COUNSELLING**

Two controlled trials and one comparative cohort study found no effect of counselling compared with no treatment on medical care utilisation rates, reported exposure to violence and threats of violence, or depression, state anxiety, and self esteem. One controlled trial found grief resolution orientated counselling to be better than feminist orientated counselling in improving self esteem and self efficacy. One controlled trial found cognitive behaviour orientated therapy to be better than non-specific support in improving women's assertiveness and reducing exposure to abuse. One RCT and one controlled trial reported reductions in subsequent exposure to violence among couples in gender specific or couple therapy, with no differences between these two types of counselling.

Benefits: **Versus no treatment:** We found three systematic reviews (search dates 1997[20] and 2001[21,22]), which between them identified one cohort study[23] and one controlled trial.[24] We found one additional controlled trial.[25] The cohort study (117 women), conducted in Sweden, evaluated an intervention comprising emergency room counselling (see glossary, p 1154) by a social worker and psychiatrist, overnight hospital stay even if not warranted by injuries, counselling after release, and referrals to social and legal services offered to women self identified as battered.[23] Women receiving counselling had similar rates of utilisation of somatic and psychiatric care during the 5 year period after treatment to those of women who declined treatment or withdrew. No numbers or distribution of types of services were reported. The controlled trial identified by the systematic reviews (290 pregnant Hispanic women) evaluated three interventions: unlimited counselling, unlimited counselling plus a mentor, or a wallet sized resource card.[24] Clinics were assigned randomly (see comment). Women in all three groups reported a decrease in levels of violence and threats of violence at follow up 2 months post partum, which was sustained through follow up at 6, 12, and 18 months. In neither counselling group was there a significantly different finding compared with the resource card group (mean on the Severity of Violence Against Women Scale [see glossary, p 1155]: 34.7 for counselling plus mentor *v* 39.5 for unlimited counselling only *v* 38.2 for resource card; see note below for explanation of this score). Physical violence and threats of violence scores remained consistently lower at each follow up for the counselling plus mentor group (but not reaching statistical significance), whereas scores for women in the counselling only group were consistently higher than those in the resource card group. The additional controlled trial (33 women in two shelters in

South Korea) compared a problem solving/empowerment group intervention versus no intervention.[25] Anxiety proneness scores (measured using Spielberger's 20 item State-Trait Anxiety Inventory [see glossary, p 1155]) decreased significantly in the intervention group compared with the control group (size of change from pre-test to post-test: –11.81 *v* –0.35; $P < 0.01$), but there were no significant differences between groups in current levels of anxiety (–9.88 *v* –9.35; $P = 0.91$), self esteem (measured using Rosenberg's Self-esteem Scale [see glossary, p 1154]: 1.56 *v* 1.29; $P = 0.84$), or depression (measured using the CES-D [see glossary, p 1154]: –13.31 *v* –5.76; $P = 0.13$). **Grief orientated counselling versus feminist orientated counselling:** We found one systematic review (search date 2001, 1 controlled trial, 20 women)[22] and one additional controlled trial.[26] In the quasi-randomised trial, women requesting counselling at a battered women's programme were alternately allocated to grief resolution or feminist orientated individual counselling for 8 weeks.[27] Women in both groups improved based on pre–post evaluation with Hudson's Index of Self-esteem (see glossary, p 1154) and a Self-efficacy Scale (see glossary, p 1155). Pre–post score differences were statistically significant only for women in the grief resolution orientated group for both self esteem (66.9 *v* 53.5; $P < 0.01$) and self efficacy (63.3 *v* 74.7; $P < 0.01$), whereas women in the feminist orientated group showed no significant changes between pre- and post-intervention scores (self esteem: 45.7 *v* 39.5; self efficacy: 68.4 *v* 77.7). Differences between treatments were not reported. The additional controlled trial (20 women in Colombia, aged 19–50) compared 20 twice weekly 3 hour sessions of cognitive behavioural treatment versus non-structured support group.[26] Two women in the cognitive behavioural therapy group and four in the non-structured support group reported new episodes of domestic violence after the intervention began. Levels of assertiveness improved significantly in the intervention group (from pre- to post-intervention; $P < 0.05$), whereas in the control group they did not. Differences between treatments were not reported. **Group counselling versus individual couple counselling:** One systematic review (search date 1997) identified one controlled trial (68 couples).[20] It found no difference between group and individual couple intervention in reduction in physical violence or in psychological wellbeing. Withdrawal rates were higher in the group programme. **Gender specific versus couple counselling:** We identified one RCT[28] and one non-randomised controlled trial (124 couples) comparing gender specific counselling versus couple counselling.[29] In the RCT, 49 couples who indicated a desire to remain in their current relationship were randomly assigned to gender specific counselling or couple counselling.[28] There were no differences in victims' reports of subsequent physical violence at 6 month follow up for 26 (62%) of the couples (reports: 8.3% among couple therapy participants *v* 7.1% for gender specific therapy; $P = 0.91$). In the non-randomised controlled trial volunteer married and intact couples who reported at least two acts of husband to wife physical aggression (75 couples), excluding couples with alcohol dependence, mental disease, or who reported severe injuries or women who feared their partner, were alternately assigned to couple therapy or gender specific therapy.[29] The past year prevalence of husband to wife physical aggression was reduced from 100% before treatment to 74% after treatment ($P < 0.01$) in both groups, based on the Modified Conflict Tactics Scale (see glossary, p 1154). With both treatments there were significant decreases from pre-treatment scores to 1 year follow up in husband to wife psychological aggression (93.37 to 44.79; $P < 0.005$) and mild (19.31 to 8.63; $P < 0.001$) and severe physical aggression (3.34 to 1.71; $P < 0.05$), as well as wives' depression on the Beck Depression Inventory (see glossary, p 1154) (12.39 to 8.79; $P < 0.005$), with no differences between treatments. Women in couples group therapy reported that physical aggression resulted from content discussed in 2% of the sessions, with no differences between treatments.

Harms: No harms were reported for individual or group counselling. However, a potential harm of any intervention targeting victims of domestic violence is escalation of violence as a result of reprisal. Qualitative assessment of weekly reports did not support the belief that women who received couple counselling were placed in any further danger than those who attended individual therapy.[28]

Comment: It is unclear whether the controlled trial was an RCT because the allocation method is not described.[24] Rotating assignment to groups may have increased the possibility of contamination across groups. In the quasi-randomised trial comparing grief orientated versus feminist orientated counseling, the scoring range is unclear and the authors do not indicate whether the original 14 point Lickert scale was used.[27] The trial done in South Korea comparing a group problem solving/empowering intervention versus no intervention had high withdrawal rates (47% in group intervention *v* 43% in the no intervention group).[25] In the second trial comparing gender specific interventions versus couple intervention, two thirds of eligible couples declined to participate.[29] In addition, 67% of the participants withdrew at the start or dropped out during treatment or before follow up.

OPTION ADVOCACY

One RCT and one non-randomised controlled trial reported a reduction in reabuse with advocacy compared with no treatment. The RCT also found an improvement in women's quality of life with advocacy, compared with no treatment. A controlled trial conducted in pregnant Hispanic women combining counselling with mentoring (similar to advocacy) found no differences in reabuse rates compared with a resource card, but found a small reduction compared with unlimited counselling. A small RCT and a non-randomised controlled trial found no effect of advocacy on reoccurrence of abuse but reported increased use of domestic violence services and resources by women assigned to advocates.

Benefits: We found one systematic review (search date 1997, 2 controlled trials, 187 women) of interventions to prevent violence against women that compared advocacy versus usual services for women exiting shelters (see glossary, p 1155).[20] One controlled trial included in the review did not report reabuse rates in this publication but corresponds to the initial analyses of a longer study which will be reported in future *Clinical Evidence* updates. The other study, a small RCT, found no association between use of advocacy services and cessation of violence, but women in the advocacy groups of both studies felt better able to access resources. **Versus no treatment:** We found one RCT[30] and two non-randomised controlled trials.[31,32] The RCT allocated 278 battered women leaving shelter stay either to a trainee advocate or to a control group.[30] Advocates worked with participants for about 6.4 hours each week over a 10 week period. Follow up at 6, 12, 18, and 24 months indicated overall significant reductions in psychological abuse and increases in quality of life compared with baseline. No changes compared with baseline were found for depression. No significant differences between groups were found for psychological abuse or depression, but a significant improvement was found for quality of life between groups (P = 0.01). Reabuse was significantly reduced at 24 months in the advocate compared with the no-advocate group (76% women with advocate *v* 89% women in the no-advocate group; P < 0.01). The first non-randomised controlled trial, based in emergency departments, compared a consecutive group of women (222 women who had sustained injuries from intimate partner violence) agreeing to meet with an advocate for 1.5 hours (57% of those approached) versus a consecutive sample of women identified in the emergency department before there was an advocate.[31] Shelter use was greater in women with advocates than in the control group (28% *v* 11%; P = 0.003). Use of shelter based counselling (see glossary, p 1154) was also greater in women with advocates (15% *v* 1%; P < 0.001). There was no change in repeated police calls (25% *v* 35%; P = 0.14), full orders of protection (9% *v* 6%; P = 0.58), or repeat emergency department visits for intimate partner violence (11% *v* 8%; P = 0.63). The second non-randomised controlled trial (81 women seeking temporary restraining orders with incomes below the poverty line and access to a telephone, who had no obvious mental disorder, were not already represented by an attorney, or receiving extensive violence related resources) allocated 22 women to law school advocates and 59 to standard court services without an advocate.[32] Women assisted by advocates reported less physical reabuse (5% *v* 25%) and psychological reabuse (10% *v* 47%) compared with women receiving standard court services at 6 months' follow up. **Versus counselling:** We found one systematic review (search date 2001, 1 controlled trial, 290 pregnant Hispanic women).[22] The controlled trial compared unlimited counselling plus a mentor (who might be considered to have acted as an advocate) versus unlimited counselling only versus a resource card.[24] Participants in all three groups reported a reduction in levels of violence and threats of violence at follow up 2 months postpartum. Although women receiving unlimited counselling plus mentoring reported less physical violence than women receiving unlimited counselling only (mean on the Severity of Violence Against Women Scale [see glossary, p 1155] adjusted for entry scores: 34.7 *v* 39.5; P < 0.05), neither of these interventions had significantly different results compared with women receiving only a resource card. There were no differences at 6, 12, or 18 month follow up assessments.

Harms: No harms were reported. However, a potential harm for any intervention targeting victims of domestic violence is escalation of violence as a result of reprisal.

Comment: In the controlled trial based in emergency departments repeat emergency visits and police calls were used as proxy measures for reabuse.[31] These may only capture the most serious types of violence. In addition, only 60% of women in the advocacy group consented to police report follow up. In the second controlled trial (81 women below the poverty line), 41% of those approached did not consent to participate.[32] An additional 13% did not appear for their first appointment. Assignment to the intervention group was based on women's acceptance of free legal representation from a law student. The trial included in the systematic review[20] and the RCT[30] evaluated the effect of advocacy for women exiting shelters, and the controlled trial involving women below the poverty line utilised law school advocates in a legal setting (interventions not available in a health care setting).[32] Although referral to an advocate (usually available at community based intimate partner violence services) at any time was considered an intervention to which a health care professional could potentially refer a victim, the extent to which the effectiveness of these interventions for women exiting shelter or women seeking restraining orders can be generalised to women in other conditions is unknown.

OPTION EMERGENCY SHELTER

Limited evidence from one cohort study found a reduced incidence of violence in the weeks following shelter stay for women choosing to use the shelter when they were also engaged in other types of help seeking behaviour compared with women not choosing to stay at the shelter. Women choosing to stay at the shelter who had not sought help elsewhere experienced an increase in violence.

Benefits: We found one systematic review (search date 1997, 1 cohort study, 243 women).[20] In the cohort study, women who spontaneously went to a shelter (see glossary, p 1155) and women sent by the prosecutors' offices constituted the sampling frame.[33] Women voluntarily choosing to stay at the shelter were compared with women not choosing shelter stay. Stay ranged from 1–30 days. The study found that women choosing shelter and not seeking any other help were more likely to experience new episodes of violence during the 6 weeks after leaving the shelter compared with those who did not choose to stay at the shelter (OR 1.8; $P = 0.13$, after adjusting for initial risk of violence, days outside the shelter, and attrition). However, for women who engaged in at least one other type of help seeking behaviour the odds of experiencing new violence was reduced when shelters were used compared with non-use (OR 0.6; $P < 0.05$), suggesting that shelter stay is only effective when women utilise other resources.

Harms: Violence increased among women staying at shelters who had not sought other types of help.[33] However, women choosing shelters had previously experienced twice as much violence as those not choosing shelters.

Comment: Conclusions must be drawn carefully from this study because losses to follow up were 36%.[33] In the study help seeking behaviour was defined as the number of distinct kinds of help seeking actions taken during the 6 months before the baseline interview and included previous shelter stay, calling the police, trying to get a restraining order, seeking criminal justice prosecution, seeking counselling, and trying to get help from legal aid or a private attorney.[20]

OPTION PEER SUPPORT GROUPS

We found no systematic reviews, RCTs, non-randomised controlled trials, or cohort studies of peer support groups in women experiencing domestic violence.

Benefits: We found no RCTs, non-randomised controlled trials, or cohort studies of peer support groups (see glossary, p 1154) in women experiencing domestic violence.

Harms: We found no RCTs, non-randomised controlled trials, or cohort studies.

Comment: None.

OPTION SAFETY PLANNING

We found no controlled trials of safety planning alone. A controlled trial, in which pregnant women received three sessions helping them make a safety plan along with providing information on available resources and how to file criminal charges or apply for a protection order, found reduced spouse abuse at 6 and 12 months and increased use of safety behaviours at 12 months in women in the intervention group.

Benefits: We found no controlled trials of safety planning (see glossary, p 1154) alone. We found one systematic review (search date 2001, 1 non-randomised trial).[21] In the non-randomised trial, 199 pregnant women attending public prenatal clinics who had been physically or sexually assaulted in the past year by their partner were recruited consecutively first into the control group to receive standard prenatal care (67 women) and then into the safety planning group (132 women).[34] Women in the control group received a wallet sized resource card with information on community resources. In the safety planning group trained nurses helped participants to prepare a safety plan and provided them with information on applying for legal protection orders and filing for criminal charges, as well as community resource phone numbers. This information was provided during three evenly spaced sessions throughout pregnancy and was reinforced with a brochure at the end of each session. After adjusting for entry levels of violence, women in the safety planning group reported less ongoing physical and non-physical abuse on the Index of Spouse Abuse Scale (see glossary, p 1154) at 12 months (37.6 *v* 56.9; $P = 0.007$), and fewer threats and instances of actual violence on the Severity of Violence Against Women Scale (see glossary, p 1155) at 6 months (threats score 27.3 *v* 33.4; actual violence 33.1 *v* 35.9) and 12 months (threats score 27.0 *v* 33.6; actual violence 32.6 *v* 37.1) compared with women in the control group ($P = 0.052$), although it is unclear to which comparison the statistical test refers to. At 12 months the safety planning group had used significantly more relevant safety behaviours than women in the control group ($P < 0.001$).

Harms: None reported. However, a potential harm for any intervention targeting victims of domestic violence is escalation of violence as a result of reprisal.

Comment: In this study, the intervention group was recruited during prenatal care whereas the comparison group was recruited postpartum.[34] The influence of different periods of recruitment on recall of abuse was not explored.

GLOSSARY

Advocacy involves providing information to a clients on her legal, medical, and financial options; facilitating her access to and utilisation of community resources such as shelters, counselling, and protection orders; accessing and mobilising her natural support networks; assisting in goal setting and making choices; validating her feelings of being victimised; and providing emotional support.[6]

Beck Depression Inventory in its short version has 13 items. Scores above 4 indicate increasing levels of depression.

CES-D (Centers for Epidemiological Studies Depression) Scale Twenty item 4 point Lickert scale, with scores that range from 0 to 60. Higher scores indicate more symptoms of depression.

Counselling usually involves professional guidance in solving a client's problems. Counselling services tend to focus on providing information versus the use of psychological techniques. However, counselling, as employed in one of the controlled trials referred to above,[25] may also include referral to services and assistance in accessing these services (overlapping with advocacy).

Hudson's Index of Self-esteem Scores vary from 0 to 100. Higher scores indicate lower self esteem.

Index of Spouse Abuse Scale is a 30 item, self report scale measuring the frequency with which respondents have experienced 11 types of physical abuse and 19 types of non-physical abuse inflicted by a male partner. In scoring the measure, items are weighted differentially based on severity. Scores range from 0–100 on each subscale, with high scores indicating high frequency of severe abuse and low scores indicating relative absence of abuse.

Modified Conflict Tactics Scale The Modified Conflict Tactics Scale (CTS2) has 78 items measuring the frequency (on an 8 point scale from never to more than 20 times) with which partners engage in psychological and physical attacks on each other.

Peer support groups Sometimes facilitated by a professional, peer support groups are hypothesised to help women exposed to domestic violence by reducing social isolation (risk factor for or effect of domestic violence) and providing encouragement and support, for example by allowing women to see that they are not alone in their experience and that there are available alternatives to changing their situation.

Rosenberg's Self-esteem Scale A 10 item scale with a four point response format resulting in a score range of 10 to 40, with higher scores representing higher self steem.

Safety planning helps participants to identify behaviours that might signal increased danger and prepare, ahead of time, codes of communication with family or friends, as well as needed documents, keys, and clothing should a quick exit become necessary.

Self-efficacy Scale Scores on the original 23 item scale vary from 14 to 322, with a mean of 230 ± 39. Higher scores indicate higher self efficacy.[27]

Severity of Violence Against Women Scale Scores on the physical violence component range from 27 to 108, where 27 would equal never being exposed to any of the behaviours and 108 would equal being exposed many times to all of the behaviours in the inventory.

Shelters provide housing, food, and clothing, usually for 30–90 days, to victims and their children under 12 who leave their abuser. Many shelters also offer individual or group therapy or counselling, advocacy, child care, job training, and assistance in finding transitional housing.

Spielberger's 20 item State-Trait Anxiety Inventory Scores range from 20 to 80, where 20 equals not feeling like that at all (state anxiety) or ever (trait anxiety) and 80 would equal feeling like that very much (state anxiety) or always (trait anxiety).

REFERENCES

1. National Center for Injury Prevention and Control. *Injury fact book 2001–2002*. Atlanta, GA: Centers for Disease Control and Prevention, 2001.
2. Krug EG, Dahlberg LL, Mercy JA, et al. *World report on violence and health*. Geneva: World Health Organization, 2002.
3. Tjaden P, Thoennes N. *Full report of the prevalence, incidence, and consequences of violence against women*. Washington, DC: National Institute of Justice, 2000.
4. Gazmarian JA, Lazorick S, Spitz AM, et al. Prevalence of violence against pregnant women. *JAMA* 1996;275:1915–1920.
5. Savona-Ventura C, Savona-Ventura M, Dregsted-Nielsen S, et al. Domestic abuse in a central Meditarranean pregnant population. *Eur J Obstet Gynecol Reprod Biol* 2001;98:3–8.
6. Purwar MB, Jeyaseelan L, Varhadpande U, et al. Survey of physical abuse during pregnancy GMCH, Nagpur, India. *J Obstret Gynaecol Res* 1999;25:165–171.
7. Lueng WC, Lueng TW, Lam YY, et al. The prevalence of domestic violence against pregnant women in a Chinese community. *Int J Gynaecol Obstret* 1999;66:23–30.
8. Hedin LW, Grimstad H, Moller A, et al. Prevalne of physical and sexual abuse before and during pregnany among Swedish couples. *Acta Obstet Gynecol Scand* 1999;78:310–315.
9. Bauer H, Rodriguez MA, Perez-Stable EJ. Prevalence and determinants of intimate partner abuse among public hospital primary care patients. *J Gen Intern Med* 2000;15:811–817.
10. Richardson J, Coid J, Petruckevitch A, et al. Identifying domestic violence: cross-sectional study in primary care. *BMJ* 2002;324:271–277.
11. McCauley J, Kern DE, Kolodner K, et al. The "battering syndrome": prevalence and clinical characteristics of domestic violence in primary care internal medicine practices. *Ann Intern Med* 1995;123:737–746.
12. Gin NE, Ruker L, Frayne S, et al. Prevalence of domestic violence among patients in three ambulatory care internal medicine clinics. *J Gen Intern Med* 1991;6:317–322.
13. Schumacher JA, Felbau-Kohn S, Smith-Slep AM, et al. Risk factors for male to female physical abuse. *Aggression Violent Behav* 2001;6:281–352.
14. Schumacher JA, Smith-Slep AM, Heyman RE. Risk factors for male-to female psychological abuse. *Aggression Violent Behav* 2001;6:255–268.
15. Gelles RJ. *Intimate violence in families*, 3rd ed. Thousand Oaks, California: Sage, 1997.
16. Rand MR, Saltzman LE. The nature and extent of recurring intimate partner violence against women in the United States. *J Comp Fam Stud* 2003;34:137–149.
17. Caetano R. Stability and change in intimate partner violence and drinking among white, black, and Hispanic couples over a 5-year interval. *Alcoholism Clin Exp Res* 2003;27:295–297.
18. Campbell J, Jones AS, Dienemann J, et al. Intimate partner violence and physical health consequences. *Arch Intern Med* 2002;162:1157–1163.
19. Coker AL, Smith PH, Bethea L, et al. Physical health consequences of physical and psychological intimate partner violence. *Arch Fam Med* 2000;9:451–457.
20. Chalk R, King PA (ed). *Violence in families. assessing prevention and treatment programs*. Washington, DC: National Academy Press, 1998. Search date 1997; primary sources National Criminal Justice Reference Section, National Child Abuse and Neglect Data System, Medline, Legal Resource Index, Criminal Justice Periodical Index, ERIC, Social SciSearch, PsychINFO, Dissertation Abstracts Online, A-V Online, PAIS Online, IAC Business, ARTS, US Political Science Documents, British Education Index, Ageline, Religion Index, Public Opinion Online, National Center on Child Abuse and Neglect Clearinghouse, Family Violence and Sexual Assault Institute, National Clearinghouse for the Defense of Battered Women, National Resource enter on Domestic Violence, Family Violence Prevention Fund.
21. Ramsay J, Richardson J, Carter Y, et al. Should health professionals screen women for domestic violence? Systematic review. *BMJ* 2002;325:314–327. Search date 2001; primary sources Medline, Embase, Cinahl.
22. Centre for Clinical Effectiveness. *Is therapy/counseling/group work more effective than no treatment for women who are victims of domestic violence*? Melbourne: Southern Health/Monash Institute of Public Health, 2001. Search date 2001; primary sources Cochrane Library, Best Evidence, Medline, Cinahl, Current Contents, Premedline, PsychINFO, SocioFile, Journals OVID, National Guideline Clearinghouse, Australasian Medical Index.
23. Bergman B, Brismar B. A 5-year follow-up of 117 battered women. *Am J Public Health* 1991;81:1486–1489.
24. McFarlane J, Soeken K, Wiist W. An evaluation of interventions to decrease intimate partner violence to pregnant women. *Public Health Nursing* 2000;17:443–451.

Domestic violence

25. Kim S, Kim J. The effects of group intervention for battered women in Korea. *Arch Psychiatr Nursing* 2001;15:257–264.
26. Laverde DI. [Efectos del tratamiento cognoscitivo conductual en el maltrato f sico en la pareja] Effects of cognitive-behavioural therapy in controlling wife abuse. *Revista de Analisis del Comportamieno* 1987;3:193–200.
27. Mancoske RJ, Standifer D, Cauley C. The effectiveness of brief counseling services for battered women. *Res Social Work Pract* 1994;4:53–63.
28. Brannen SJ, Rubin A. Comparing the effectiveness of gender-specific and couples groups in court-mandated spouse abuse treatment program. *Res Social Work Pract* 1996;6:405–424.
29. O'Leary KD, Heyman RE, Neidig PH. Treatment of wife abuse: a comparison of gender-specific and conjoint approaches. *Behav Ther* 1999;30:475–505.
30. Sullivan CM, Bybee DI. Reducing violence using community based advocacy for women with abusive partners. *J Consult Clin Psychol* 1999;67:43–53.
31. Muelleman RL, Feighny KM. Effects of an emergency department-based advocacy program for battered women on community resource utilisation. *Ann Emerg Med* 1999;33:62–66.
32. Bell ME, Goodman LA. Supporting battered women involved with the court system: an evaluation of a law school-based advocacy intervention. *Violence Women* 2001;7:1377–1404.
33. Berk RD, Newton PJ, Berk SF. What a difference a day makes: an empirical study of the impact of shelters for battered women. *J Marriage Fam* 1986;48:481–490.
34. Parker B, McFarlane J, Soeken K, et al. Testing an intervention to prevent further abuse to pregnant women. *Res Nursing Health* 1999;22:59–66.

Joanne Klevens
Epidemiologist
Centers for Disease Control, National Center for Injury Prevention and Control, Division of Violence Prevention
Atlanta
USA

Laura Sadowski
Co-Director/Associate Professor
Collaborative Research Unit, Cook County Hospital/Department of Internal Medicine, Rush Medical College
Chicago
USA

Competing interests: None declared.

TABLE 1 Risks for reported conditions in women experiencing psychological abuse (see text, p 1147).[19]

Complaint	RR (95% CI)
Poor physical health	1.69 (1.20 to 2.29)
Poor mental health	1.74 (1.07 to 2.73)
Disability preventing work	1.49 (1.06 to 2.14)
Arthritis	1.67 (0.20 to 2.22)
Chronic pain	1.91 (1.49 to 2.36)
Migraine	1.54 (1.16 to 1.93)
Other frequent headaches	1.41 (1.05 to 1.82)
Sexually transmitted infections	1.82 (1.19 to 2.68)
Chronic pelvic pain	1.62 (1.03 to 2.48)
Stomach ulcers	1.72 (1.02 to 2.84)
Spastic colon	3.62 (1.63 to 7.50)
Frequent indigestion, diarrhoea, or constipation	1.30 (1.03 to 1.63)

Generalised anxiety disorder

Search date October 2002

Christopher Gale and Mark Oakley-Browne

QUESTIONS

INTERVENTIONS

See glossary, p 1169

Key Messages

- **Abecarnil** RCTs found conflicting evidence of the effects of abecarnil versus placebo in improving symptoms.
- **Antipsychotic drugs** We found limited evidence from one RCT that trifluoperazine significantly reduced anxiety compared with placebo after 4 weeks, but caused more drowsiness, extrapyramidal reactions, and other movement disorders.
- **Applied relaxation** We found no RCTs of applied relaxation versus placebo or no treatment. One RCT found no significant difference in symptoms at 13 weeks for applied relaxation versus cognitive behaviour therapy.
- **Benzodiazepines** One systematic review and one subsequent RCT found limited evidence that benzodiazepines versus placebo reduced symptoms over 2–9 weeks. However, RCTs and observational studies found that benzodiazepines increased the risk of dependence, sedation, industrial accidents, and road traffic accidents. One non-systematic review found that, if used in late pregnancy or while breast feeding, benzodiazepines may cause adverse effects in neonates. One RCT found no significant difference in symptoms of anxiety with sustained release alprazolam versus bromazepam, and another RCT found no significant difference in overall symptoms with mexazolam versus alprazolam. Limited evidence from RCTs found no significant difference in symptoms over 6–8 weeks with benzodiazepines versus buspirone, abecarnil, or antidepressants. One systematic review of poor quality RCTs found insufficient evidence about the effects of long term treatment with benzodiazepines.
- **β Blockers** We found no RCTs on the effects of β blockers.

Generalised anxiety disorder

- **Buspirone** RCTs have found that buspirone significantly improves symptoms compared with placebo over 4–9 weeks. RCTs found no significant difference in symptoms over 6–8 weeks for buspirone versus antidepressants, diazepam, or hydroxyzine, but the studies may have lacked power to detect clinically important differences among treatments.
- **Certain antidepressants (imipramine, opipramol, paroxetine, trazodone, venlafaxine)** One systematic review and four additional RCTs have found that antidepressants (imipramine, opipramol, paroxetine, trazodone, and venlafaxine) versus placebo significantly improve symptoms over 4–8 weeks. RCTs found no significant difference among these antidepressants or between antidepressants and benzodiazepines or buspirone. RCTs and observational studies have found that antidepressants are associated with sedation, dizziness, nausea, falls, and sexual dysfunction.
- **Cognitive therapy** Two systematic reviews have found limited evidence that cognitive behavioural therapy, using a combination of interventions, such as exposure, relaxation, and cognitive restructuring, improves anxiety and depression over 4–12 weeks compared with waiting list control, anxiety management training alone, relaxation training alone, or non-directive psychotherapy. Two subsequent RCTs found no significant difference in symptoms for cognitive therapy versus applied relaxation at 13 weeks and 24 months.
- **Hydroxyzine** Two RCTs compared hydroxyzine versus placebo and found different results. After about 1 month, one RCT found that hydroxyzine versus placebo significantly improved symptoms of anxiety, but the other found no significant difference between treatments. One further RCT found no significant difference for hydroxyzine versus buspirone after 28 days. We found no RCTs of longer term treatment.
- **Kava** One systematic review in people with anxiety, including generalised anxiety disorder, found that kava significantly reduced symptoms of anxiety compared with placebo over 4 weeks. Observational evidence suggests that kava may be associated with hepatotoxicity.

DEFINITION Generalised anxiety disorder (GAD) is defined as excessive worry and tension about every day events and problems, on most days, for at least 6 months, to the point where the person experiences distress or has marked difficulty in performing day-to-day tasks.[1] It may be characterised by the following symptoms and signs: increased motor tension (fatigability, trembling, restlessness, and muscle tension); autonomic hyperactivity (shortness of breath, rapid heart rate, dry mouth, cold hands, and dizziness); and increased vigilance and scanning (feeling keyed up, increased startling, and impaired concentration), but not panic attacks.[1] One non-systematic review of epidemiological and clinical studies found marked reduction of quality of life and psychosocial functioning in people with anxiety disorders (including GAD).[2] It also found that people with GAD have low overall life satisfaction and some impairment in ability to fulfil roles, social tasks, or both.[2]

INCIDENCE/ PREVALENCE One overview found that the prevalence of GAD among adults in the community is 1.5–3.0%.[3] It found that 3–5% of adults have had GAD in the past year and 4–7% have had GAD during their life. One non-systematic review identified the US National Comorbidity Survey, which found that over 90% of people diagnosed with GAD had a co-morbid diagnosis, including dysthymia (22%), depression (39–69%), somatisation, other anxiety disorders, bipolar disorder, or substance abuse.[4] The reliability of the measures used to diagnose GAD in epidemiological studies is unsatisfactory.[5,6] One US study, with explicit diagnostic criteria (DSM-III-R), estimated that 5% of people will develop GAD at some time during their lives.[6] A recent cohort study of people with depressive and anxiety disorders found that 49% of people initially diagnosed with GAD retained this diagnosis over 2 years.[7] One non-systematic review found that the incidence of GAD in men is only half the incidence in women.[8] One non-systematic review of seven epidemiological studies found reduced prevalence of anxiety disorders in older people.[9] Another non-systematic review of 20 observational studies in younger and older adults suggested that autonomic arousal to stressful tasks is decreased in older people, and that older people become accustomed to stressful tasks more quickly than younger people.[10]

AETIOLOGY/ RISK FACTORS One community study and a clinical study have found that GAD is associated with an increase in the number of minor stressors, independent of demographic factors,[11,12] but this finding was common in people with other diagnoses in the clinical population.[7] One non-systematic review (5 case control studies) of psychological sequelae to civilian trauma found that rates of GAD reported in four of the five studies were increased significantly compared with a control population (rate ratio 3.3, 95% CI 2.0 to 5.5).[13] One systematic review (search date 1997) of cross-sectional studies found that bullying (or peer victimisation) was associated with a significant increase in the incidence of GAD (effect size 0.21).[14] One systematic review (search date not stated) of the genetic epidemiology of anxiety disorders (including GAD) identified two family studies and three twin studies.[15] The family studies (45 index cases, 225 first degree relatives) found a significant association between GAD in the index cases and in their first degree relatives (OR 6.1, 95% CI 2.5 to 14.9). The twin studies (13 305 people) estimated that 32% (95% CI 24% to 39%) of the variance to liability to GAD was explained by genetic factors.[15]

PROGNOSIS One systematic review found that 25% of adults with GAD will be in full remission after 2 years, and 38% will have a remission after 5 years.[3]

AIMS OF INTERVENTION To reduce symptoms of anxiety; to minimise disruption of day-to-day functioning; and to improve quality of life, with minimum adverse effects.

OUTCOMES Severity of symptoms and effects on quality of life, as measured by symptom scores: usually the HAM-A, State-Trait Anxiety Inventory, or Clinical Global Impression Symptom Scores. Where numbers needed to treat are given, these represent the number of people requiring treatment within a given time period (usually 6–12 wks) for one additional person to achieve a certain improvement in symptom score. The method for obtaining numbers needed to treat was not standardised across studies. Some used a reduction by, for example, 20 points in the HAM-A as a response, others defined a response as a reduction, for example, by 50% of the premorbid score. We have not attempted to standardise methods, but instead have used the response rates reported in each study to calculate numbers needed to treat. Similarly, we have calculated numbers needed to harm from original trial data.

METHODS *Clinical Evidence* search and appraisal October 2002. Recent changes in diagnostic classification make it hard to compare older studies with more recent ones. In the earlier classification system (DSM-III-R) the diagnosis was made only in the absence of other psychiatric disorders. In current systems (DSM-IV and ICD-10), GAD can be diagnosed in the presence of any comorbid condition. All drug studies were short term — at most 12 weeks.

QUESTION What are the effects of treatments?

OPTION COGNITIVE THERAPY

Two systematic reviews have found that cognitive behavioural therapy, using a combination of interventions such as exposure, relaxation, and cognitive restructuring, improves anxiety and depression over 4–12 weeks compared with waiting list control, anxiety management training alone, relaxation training alone, or non-directive psychotherapy. Two subsequent RCTs found no significant difference in symptoms for cognitive therapy versus applied relaxation at 13 weeks and 24 months.

Benefits: We found two systematic reviews[16,17] and two subsequent RCTs[18,19] comparing cognitive therapy (see glossary, p 1169) versus waiting list control (no treatment) or versus other psychotherapies. The first systematic review (search date 1996, 13 RCTs, 722 people, 60% women) compared 22 cognitive behavioural therapies (see glossary, p 1169), which involved (alone or in combination) cognitive restructuring, relaxation training, exposure, and systematic desensitisation versus control (remaining on a waiting list, anxiety management training, relaxation training, and non-directive psychotherapy).[16] The review found that cognitive behavioural therapies versus control significantly improved symptoms over 4–12 weeks (effect size for anxiety 0.70, 95% CI 0.57 to 0.83 and for depression 0.77, 95% CI 0.64 to 0.90; dichotomous data not available). The second systematic review (search date not stated, 5 RCTs, 313 people) included three RCTs identified by the first review.[17] It found that cognitive behavioural therapies (including relaxation, cognitive therapy, cognitive behavioural therapy, analytical psychotherapy, and anxiety management training [alone or in combination]) versus waiting list control were associated with an improvement in symptoms (median effect size 0.9; CI not provided).[17] The first subsequent RCT (36 people aged 18–60 years with generalised anxiety disorder [GAD]) found no significant difference for 12 weekly sessions of cognitive therapy versus applied relaxation (see glossary, p 1169) in the proportion of people who responded after 13 weeks (response defined as improvement to score 3 or 4 on Cognitive Global Impression Scale, 10/18 [56%] with cognitive therapy *v* 8/15 [53%] with applied relaxation; ARR −2%, 95% CI −33% to +29%; RR 1.04, 95% CI 0.55 to 1.95).[18] The second subsequent RCT (76 people with GAD, 69 people completed) found no significant difference between 15 weekly sessions of cognitive therapy, applied relaxation, and a combination of these methods in the number of people not meeting criteria for GAD immediately after treatment and at 24 months (percentage of people without GAD at follow up: 8.7% in each group immediately after treatment; 14.3% with cognitive therapy *v* 19.1% with applied relaxation *v* 19.1% with combination of treatments at 24 months; P not reported).[19]

Harms: The reviews and subsequent RCTs gave no information on harms.[16–20]

Comment: A third systematic review (search date 1998, 6 RCTs comparing cognitive therapy with a variety of other psychological treatments, 404 people) did not compare treatments directly.[21] It reanalysed the raw data from individual RCTs to calculate the proportion of people who experienced a clinically significant improvement in symptoms after treatment and maintained that improvement for 6 months (see comment below). It found limited evidence that more people given individual cognitive therapy maintained recovery after 6 months than those given psychotherapies other than applied relaxation (individual cognitive therapy 41%, applied relaxation 52%, non-directive treatment 19%, group cognitive therapy 18%, group behaviour therapy 12%, individual behaviour therapy 18%, and analytical psychotherapy 0%; P values not provided).[21] Many of the RCTs were small and were not analysed on an intention to treat basis. Many of the RCTs identified by the reviews used the State-Trait Anxiety Inventory, which covers a restricted range of symptoms and may not satisfactorily reflect treatment outcomes in GAD.[16,17,21]

OPTION APPLIED RELAXATION

We found no RCTs of applied relaxation versus placebo or no treatment. One RCT found no significant difference in symptoms at 13 weeks for applied relaxation versus cognitive behavioural therapy.

Benefits: **Versus placebo or no treatment:** We found no systematic review or RCTs. **Versus other psychological treatments:** We found no systematic review but found one RCT[18] (see benefits of cognitive therapy, p 1160).

Harms: The RCT gave no information on harms.[18]

Comment: We found one systematic review (search date 1998, 6 RCTs comparing cognitive therapy (see glossary, p 1169) with a variety of other psychological treatments, 404 people), which did not compare treatments directly (see comment of cognitive therapy, p 1161).[21]

OPTION BENZODIAZEPINES

One systematic review and one subsequent RCT found limited evidence that benzodiazepines versus placebo reduced symptoms over 2–9 weeks. However, RCTs and observational studies found that benzodiazepines increased the risk of dependence, sedation, industrial accidents, and road traffic accidents. One non-systematic review found that, if used in

late pregnancy or while breast feeding, benzodiazepines may cause adverse effects in neonates. One RCT found no significant difference in symptoms of anxiety with sustained release alprazolam versus bromazepam, and another RCT found no significant difference in overall symptoms with mexazolam versus alprazolam. Limited evidence from RCTs found no significant difference in symptoms over 6–8 weeks with benzodiazepines versus buspirone, abecarnil, or antidepressants. One systematic review of poor quality RCTs found insufficient evidence about the effects of long term treatment with benzodiazepines.

Benefits: **Versus placebo:** We found one systematic review (search date 1996, 17 RCTs, 2044 people)[16] and one subsequent RCT.[22] The review found that benzodiazepines versus placebo were associated with a better response over 2–9 weeks (pooled mean effect size 0.70; CI not provided). The subsequent RCT (310 people) compared three interventions: diazepam (15–35 mg/day), abecarnil (7.5–17.5 mg/day), and placebo.[22] It found that diazepam versus placebo significantly increased the proportion of people with moderate improvement on the Clinical Global Impression scores at 6 weeks (73% with diazepam *v* 56% with placebo; $P < 0.01$).[22] **Versus each other:** The systematic review did not compare different benzodiazepines directly.[16] One subsequent RCT (121 people) compared sustained release alprazolam versus bromazepam and found no significant difference in Hamilton Anxiety Scale scores or Clinical Global Impression scores over 5 weeks (results presented graphically).[23] A second subsequent RCT (64 people) comparing mexazolam versus alprazolam found no significant difference in the proportion of people who had "highly improved" or "moderately improved" Clinical Global Impression scores at 3 weeks (98% with "highly improved" *v* 87% "moderately improved"; $P > 0.05$; results presented graphically).[24] **Long term treatment:** We found one systematic review (search date 1998, 8 RCTs, any benzodiazepine medication, > 2 months' duration).[25] It found that the weak methods of the RCTs identified prevent firm conclusions being made.[25] **Versus buspirone:** See benefits of buspirone, p 1163. **Versus abecarnil:** See benefits of abecarnil, p 1165. **Versus antidepressants:** See benefits of antidepressants, p 1166.

Harms: **Sedation and dependence:** Benzodiazepines have been found to cause impairment in attention, concentration, and short term memory. One RCT identified by the review found an increased rate of drowsiness (71% with diazepam *v* 13% with placebo; $P = 0.001$) and dizziness (29% with diazepam *v* 11% with placebo; $P = 0.001$).[16] Sedation can interfere with concomitant psychotherapy. One non-systematic review of the harms of benzodiazepines found that rebound anxiety on withdrawal has been reported in 15–30% of participants.[26] It also found that there is a high risk of substance abuse and dependence with benzodiazepines. **Memory:** Thirty one people with agoraphobia/panic disorder in an RCT of 8 weeks' alprazolam versus placebo were reviewed after 3.5 years.[27] Five people were still taking benzodiazepines and had significant impairment in memory tasks.[27] There was no significant difference in memory performance between those who had been in the placebo group and those who had been given alprazolam but were no longer taking the drug. **Road traffic**

accidents: We found one systematic review (search date 1997) examining the relation between benzodiazepines and road traffic accidents.[28] In the case control studies, the odds ratio for death or emergency medical treatment in those who had taken benzodiazepines compared with those who had not taken them ranged from 1.45–2.40. The odds ratio increased with higher doses and more recent intake. In the police and emergency ward studies, benzodiazepine use was a factor in 1–65% of accidents (usually 5–10%). In two studies in which participants had blood alcohol concentrations under the legal limit, benzodiazepines were found in 43% and 65% of people. For drivers over 65 years of age, the risk of being involved in reported road traffic accidents was higher if they had taken longer acting and larger quantities of benzodiazepines. These results are from case control studies and are, therefore, subject to confounding. **Pregnancy and breast feeding:** One systematic review (search date 1997) of 23 case series and reports found no association between cleft lip and palate and benzodiazepines in the first trimester of pregnancy.[29] However, one non-systematic review found that benzodiazepines taken in late pregnancy are associated with neonatal hypotonia and withdrawal syndrome.[30] Benzodiazepines are secreted in breast milk, and there have been reports of sedation and hypothermia in infants.[31] **Other:** One non-systematic industry funded review of eight RCTs of benzodiazepines versus placebo or buspirone found that recent use of benzodiazepines limited the effectiveness of buspirone in people with generalised anxiety disorder. [31]

Comment: All of the RCTs assessing benzodiazepines were short term (at most 12 wks).[16,23,24]

OPTION BUSPIRONE

RCTs have found that buspirone significantly improves symptoms compared with placebo over 4–9 weeks. RCTs found no significant difference in symptoms over 6–8 weeks for buspirone versus antidepressants, diazepam, or hydroxyzine, but the studies may have lacked power to detect clinically important differences.

Benefits: **Versus placebo:** We found one systematic review (search date 1996, 8 RCTs)[16] and two subsequent RCTs.[32,33] The systematic review found that buspirone versus placebo was associated with a greater response over 4–9 weeks (pooled mean effect size 0.39; CI not provided, withdrawal rate 17%).[16] The first subsequent RCT (162 people) of buspirone versus placebo found similar results (55% with buspirone *v* 35% with placebo; $P < 0.05$).[32] The second subsequent RCT (365 people) compared four interventions: buspirone (30 mg/day), venlafaxine (75 mg/day), venlafaxine (150 mg/day), and placebo over 8 weeks (see benefits of antidepressants, p 1166).[33] It found that buspirone versus placebo significantly increased the proportion of people who responded after 8 weeks of treatment (response defined as score of 1 or 2 on the Clinical Global Impression Scale; 52/95 [55%] with buspirone *v* 38/98 [39%] with placebo; $P = 0.03$).[33] **Versus benzodiazepines:** One large RCT (240 people) identified by the review[16] compared buspirone versus diazepam versus placebo.[34] It found no significant difference in the proportion of people who responded over 6 weeks with buspirone versus diazepam (response defined as ≥ 40% reduction in Hamilton Anxiety Scale score; 61% with diazepam *v* 54% with buspirone; P values not provided).[34] **Versus antidepressants:** See benefits of antidepressants, p 1166. **Versus hydroxyzine:** See benefits of hydroxyzine, p 1164.

Harms: **Sedation and dependence:** One RCT found that buspirone versus placebo significantly increased the proportion of people with nausea (27/80 [34%] with buspirone *v* 11/82 [13%] with placebo; RR 2.5, 95% CI 1.3 to 4.7; NNH 5, 95% CI 4 to 14), dizziness (51/80 [64%] with buspirone *v* 10/82 [12%] with placebo; RR 5.2, 95% CI 2.9 to 9.6; NNH 2, 95% CI 2 to 3), and somnolence (15/80 [19%] with buspirone *v* 6/82 [7%] with placebo; RR 2.6, 95% CI 1.0 to 6.3; NNH 9, 95% CI 5 to 104).[32] The RCT found no significant difference in the number of people reporting any adverse effect with buspirone versus diazepam (49% with buspirone *v* 63% with diazepam). Diazepam was associated with more fatigue and weakness compared with buspirone but less headache and dizziness. **Pregnancy and breast feeding:** We found no evidence.

Comment: We found one non-systematic review (8 RCTs, 520 people) that was sponsored by pharmaceutical companies and had been included in regulatory submissions for buspirone.[35] It found that buspirone versus placebo significantly increased the proportion of people "much or very much improved" as rated by their physician (54% with buspirone *v* 28% with placebo; P ≤ 0.001). A second non-systematic industry funded review (8 RCTs) of benzodiazepines versus placebo or buspirone found that recent use of benzodiazepines limited the effectiveness of buspirone in people with generalised anxiety disorder.[31]

OPTION HYDROXYZINE

Two RCTs compared hydroxyzine versus placebo and found different results. One RCT found that hydroxyzine versus placebo significantly improved symptoms of anxiety after 4 weeks. The second RCT found no significant difference in the proportion of people with improved symptoms of anxiety at 35 days with hydroxyzine versus placebo. One RCT found no significant difference for hydroxyzine versus buspirone after 28 days.

Benefits: **Versus placebo:** We found one non-systematic review (2 RCTs, 354 people).[36] We found no additional RCTs. The first RCT (110 people) identified by the review found a significantly greater improvement in Hamilton Anxiety Scale scores after 4 weeks with hydroxyzine (50 mg/day) versus placebo (results presented graphically). The second RCT (244 people entered, 213 people analysed) identified by the review compared hydroxyzine versus buspirone versus placebo for 28 days (followed by placebo in all groups for 7 days). It found no significant difference in the proportion of people with a Hamilton Anxiety Scale score reduction of 50% or greater at 35 days with hydroxyzine (50 mg/day) versus placebo (30/71 [42%] with hydroxyzine *v* 20/70 [29%] with placebo; ARR +14%, 95% CI −2% to +29%; RR 1.50, 95% CI 0.93 to 2.23; not intention to treat).[36] **Versus buspirone:** The second RCT identified by the non-systematic review also found no significant difference for hydroxyzine versus buspirone on the number of people with a Hamilton Anxiety Scale score reduction of 50% or greater after 28 days (30/71 [42%] with hydroxyzine *v* 26/72 [36%] with buspirone; RR 1.20, 95% CI 0.78 to 1.80; ARR +5%, 95% CI −11% to +21%).[36]

Harms: The second RCT (244 people) identified by the review found that hydroxyzine versus placebo increased somnolence (AR 10% with hydroxyzine *v* 0% with placebo) and headaches (AR 6% with hydroxyzine *v* 1% with placebo) compared with placebo.[36] Overall adverse effects were reported in 40% of people taking hydroxyzine versus 38% taking buspirone versus 28% taking placebo.

Comment: None.

OPTION ABECARNIL

One RCT found no significant difference in symptoms at 6 weeks with abecarnil versus placebo or versus diazepam. However, one smaller RCT found limited evidence that low dose abecarnil versus placebo significantly improved symptoms.

Benefits: We found no systematic review, but found two multicentre RCTs.[22,37] The first RCT (310 people) compared three interventions: abecarnil (7.5–17.5 mg/day), diazepam (15–35 mg/day), and placebo.[22] It found no significant difference with abecarnil versus placebo or versus diazepam for moderate improvement on the Clinical Global Impression scores at 6 weeks (AR for moderate improvement 62% with abecarnil *v* 56% with placebo; $P < 0.031$; 62% with abecarnil *v* 73% with diazepam; P value not provided).[22] A second RCT (129 people) compared 3 weeks of treatment with abecarnil (3–9, 7.5–15, and 15–30 mg/day) versus placebo.[37] Within each group the dose was escalated from the minimum to the maximum over the length of the trial. It found that abecarnil (3–9 mg/day) versus placebo significantly improved symptoms (outcome 50% reduction in Hamilton Anxiety Scale score 19/31 [61%] with abecarnil *v* 8/26 [31%] with placebo; $P = 0.05$), but found no significant difference in symptoms with higher doses of abecarnil versus placebo.[37] Results were not calculated by intention to treat (12/34 [35%] people withdrew with abecarnil 15–30 mg/day *v* 4/35 [11%] with abecarnil 7.5–15 mg/day *v* 1/32 [3%] with abecarnil 3–9 mg/day *v* 2/28 [7%] with placebo).

Harms: The second RCT found that abecarnil (3–9 mg/day) versus placebo significantly increased fatigue (4/32 [13%] with abecarnil *v* 0/28 [0%] with placebo; NNH 3, 95% CI 3 to 7) and equilibrium loss (2/32 [6%] with abecarnil *v* 0/28 [0%] with placebo; NNH 7, 95% CI 4 to 14).[37] Abercarnil versus placebo was also associated with more drowsiness (10/32 [31%] with abecarnil *v* 4/28 [14%] with placebo; RR 2.12, 95% CI 0.77 to 6.21). Higher doses were associated with more adverse effects (62% of people taking abecarnil 15–30 mg experienced at least 1 adverse effect *v* 51% of people taking abecarnil 7.5–15 mg *v* 22% with abecarnil 3–9 mg *v* 21% with placebo).[37]

Comment: None.

OPTION ANTIDEPRESSANTS

One systematic review and four additional RCTs have found that antidepressants (imipramine, opipramol, paroxetine, trazodone, and venlafaxine) versus placebo significantly improve symptoms over 4–8 weeks. RCTs found no significant difference among these antidepressants or between antidepressants and benzodiazepines or buspirone. RCTs and observational studies have found that antidepressants are associated with sedation, dizziness, nausea, falls, and sexual dysfunction.

Benefits: **Versus placebo or versus each other:** We found one systematic review (search date 2000, 4 RCTs with evaluable data, 787 people)[38] and four additional RCTs.[16,39–42] The review found that antidepressants (imipramine, trazodone, venlafaxine) versus placebo increased short term response rates (RR for no response to treatment with antidepressant *v* placebo 0.66, 95% CI 0.58 to 0.74).[38] The first additional RCT (230 people) compared four interventions: two antidepressants (imipramine and trazodone), placebo, and diazepam.[39] It found that both antidepressants versus placebo significantly increased participant assessed global improvement at the end of 8 weeks of treatment, but that imipramine and trazodone were not significantly different from each other (AR for improvement 73% with imipramine *v* 67% with trazodone *v* 39% with placebo). The results were not intention to treat (18/58 [31%] people withdrew with imipramine, 22/61 [36%] with trazodone, 18/56 [32%] with diazepam, and 20/55 [36%] with placebo).[39] The second additional RCT (318 people) compared opipramol (a tricyclic antidepressant with minimal serotonin reuptake blocking properties) versus placebo or versus alprazolam over 28 days. It found that opipramol versus placebo significantly increased response rate after 28 days (response defined as Clinical Global Impression score of < 2; 63/100 [63%] with opipramol *v* 50/107 [47%] with placebo; RR 1.35, 95% CI 1.05 to 1.69; NNT 7; 95% CI 1 to 26), but found no significant difference between opipramol versus alprazolam for response rate (63/100 [63%] with opipramol *v* 67/105 [64%] with alprazolam; RR 1.01, 95% CI 0.79 to 1.25).[40] The third additional RCT (324 people) found that paroxetine versus placebo significantly increased response rate after 8 weeks (response defined as a score of 1 or 2 on the Clinical Global Impression Scale; 100/161 [62%] with paroxetine *v* 77/163 [47%] with placebo; RR 1.31, 95% CI 1.07 to 1.61; NNT 6, 95% CI 4 to 24).[41] The fourth additional RCT (541 people) compared venlafaxine at three different doses (35, 75, or 150 mg/day) versus placebo.[42] It found that venlafaxine (75 or 150 mg) versus placebo significantly increased response rate at week 24 (response defined as 50% reduction in Hamilton Anxiety Scale score or Clinical Global Impression score of 1 or 2; results presented graphically; P < 0.001 for both doses). **Versus benzodiazepines:** We found no systematic review, but found two RCTs.[39,43] The first RCT (230 people) compared variable doses of four drugs: imipramine, trazodone, placebo, and diazepam.[39] It found no significant difference in participant assessed global improvement at the end of 8 weeks' treatment with antidepressants versus diazepam (73% of people improved with imipramine v 67% with trazodone v 66% with diazepam). The results were not intention to treat (18/58 [31%] people withdrew with imipramine, 22/61 [36%] with trazodone, 18/56 [32%] with diazepam, and 20/55 [36%] with placebo).[39] The second RCT (81 people) compared paroxetine, imipramine, and 2'-chlordesmethyldiazepam for 8 weeks.[43] Paroxetine and imipramine significantly improved anxiety scores compared with 2'-chlordesmethyldiazepam (mean Hamilton Anxiety Scale after 8 wks: 11.1 with paroxetine, 10.8 with imipramine, 12.9 with 2'-chlordesmethyldiazepam; P = 0.05). **Versus buspirone:** We found no systematic review. One RCT (365 people) compared venlafaxine at two different doses (75 or 150 mg/day) versus buspirone (30 mg/day) versus placebo over 8 weeks. It found no significant difference in response rate after 8 weeks' treatment with venlafaxine versus buspirone (response defined as Clinical Global Impression score of 1 or 2; 54/87 [62%] with venlafaxine 75 mg v 44/89 [49%] with 150 mg venlafaxine v 52/95 [55%] with buspirone; P values not provided).[33]

Harms: **Common adverse effects:** One RCT found sedation, confusion, dry mouth, and constipation with both imipramine and trazodone.[39] RCTs reported nausea, somnolence, dry mouth, sweating, constipation, anorexia, and sexual dysfunction with venlafaxine. One of the RCTs included in the review found that 26% of people taking venlafaxine and 17% of people taking placebo withdrew because of adverse effects.[44] Most of the adverse effects (apart from dizziness and sexual dysfunction) decreased over 6 months in those who continued to take the medication. There have been case reports of nausea in people taking paroxetine.[45] **Overdose:** In a series of 239 coroner directed necropsies from 1970–1989, tricyclic antidepressants were considered to be a causal factor in 12% of deaths and hypnosedatives (primarily benzodiazepines and excluding barbiturates) in 8% of deaths.[43] **Accidental poisoning:** Tricyclic antidepressants are a major cause of accidental poisoning.[46] A study estimated that there was one death for every 44 children admitted to hospital after ingestion of tricyclic antidepressants.[47] **Hyponatraemia:** One case series reported 736 incidents of hyponatraemia in people taking selective serotonin reuptake inhibitors; 83% of episodes were in hospital inpatients aged over 65 years.[48] It is not possible to establish causation from this type of data. **Falls:** One retrospective cohort study (2428 elderly residents of nursing homes) found an increased risk of falls in new users of antidepressants (665 people taking tricyclic antidepressants; adjusted RR 2.0, 95% CI 1.8 to 2.2; 612 people taking selective serotonin reuptake inhibitors; adjusted RR 1.8, 95% CI 1.6 to 2.0; and 304 people taking trazodone; adjusted RR 1.2, 95% CI 1.0 to 1.4).[49] The increased rate of falls persisted through the first 180 days of treatment and beyond. One case control study (8239 people aged ≥ 66 years, treated in hospital for hip fracture) found an increased risk of hip fracture in those taking antidepressants (adjusted OR, selective serotonin reuptake inhibitors 2.4, 95% CI 2.0 to 2.7; secondary amine tricyclic antidepressants such as nortriptyline 2.2, 95% CI 1.8 to 2.8; and tertiary amine tricyclic antidepressants such as amitriptyline 1.5, 95% CI 1.3 to 1.7).[50] This study could not control for confounding factors; people taking antidepressants may be at increased risk of hip fracture for other reasons. **In pregnancy:** We found no reports of harmful effects in pregnancy. One case control study found no evidence that imipramine or fluoxetine increased the rate of malformations in pregnancy.[51] **Sexual dysfunction:** A survey (1022 people mostly suffering from depression; 610 women) of people using antidepressants with previously acceptable sexual function has reported the incidence of sexual dysfunction to be 71% for paroxetine, 67% for venlafaxine, and 63% for fluvaxamine.[52]

Comment: None.

OPTION ANTIPSYCHOTIC DRUGS

One RCT found that trifluoperazine significantly reduced anxiety compared with placebo after 4 weeks, but caused more drowsiness, extrapyramidal reactions, and other movement disorders.

Benefits: We found no systematic review. We found one RCT (415 people) comparing 4 weeks of trifluoperazine treatment (2–6 mg/day) versus placebo.[53] It found that trifluoperazine versus placebo significantly reduced the total score on the Hamilton Anxiety Scale (difference 14 points; $P < 0.001$).

Harms: The RCT reported more cases of drowsiness (43% with trifluoperazine *v* 25% with placebo) and extrapyramidal reactions and movement disorders (17% with trifluoperazine *v* 8% with placebo) with trifluoperazine versus placebo.[53] A cohort study found that in the longer term, rates of tardive dyskinesia are increased if is treatment is frequently interrupted.[54]

Comment: None.

OPTION β BLOCKERS

We found no RCTs assessing β blockers in people with generalised anxiety disorder.

Benefits: We found no systematic review or RCTs.

Harms: We found no good evidence.

Comment: None.

OPTION KAVA

One systematic review in people with anxiety disorders, including generalised anxiety disorder, found that kava significantly reduced symptoms of anxiety compared with placebo over 4 weeks. Observational evidence suggests that kava may be associated with hepatotoxicity.

Benefits: **Versus placebo:** We found one systematic review (search date 1998, 7 RCTs, 377 people with anxiety disorders, proportion of people with generalised anxiety disorder not specified).[55] The review found that kava versus placebo significantly reduced Hamilton Anxiety Scores over 4 weeks (3 RCTs; 198 people; WMD 9.69, 95% CI 3.54 to 15.83).[55]

Harms: We found one systematic review (search date 2000, 30 papers including 9 clinical trials).[56] Adverse effects in the clinical trials were gastrointestinal symptoms, tiredness, restlessness, tremor, and headache. Post-marketing surveillance (4049 adults taking 150 mg/day kava extract) found an adverse reaction rate of 1.5% (61/4094). Case reports included five cases of dermatological reactions, four cases of acute dyskinesias, nine cases of liver damage, and one case of myoglobulinuria (the incidence of these adverse effects was not reported). One case was found where kava may have interacted with alprazolam, leading to decreased in level of consciousness.[56]

Comment: There have been concerns that kava may cause liver damage.[57]

GLOSSARY

Applied relaxation A technique involving training in relaxation techniques and self monitoring of symptoms without challenging beliefs.

Cognitive behavioural therapy Brief (20 sessions over 12–16 wks) structured treatment incorporating elements of cognitive therapy and behavioural therapy. Behavioural therapy is based on learning theory and concentrates on changing behaviour.

Cognitive therapy Brief (20 sessions over 12–16 wks) structured treatment aimed at identifying anxiety associated thoughts and beliefs, changing over monitoring of physical symptoms, and minimising the catastophising that characterises generalised anxiety disorder. This is combined with relaxation, exercise, and testing the validity of beliefs in real life situations. It requires a highly trained therapist.

REFERENCES

1. American Psychiatric Association. *Diagnostic and statistical manual of mental disorders*, 4th ed. Washington, DC: American Psychiatric Association, 1994.
2. Mendlowicz MV, Stein MB. Quality of life in individuals with anxiety disorders. *Am J Psychiatry* 2000;157:669–682.
3. Kessler RD Wittchen HU. Patterns and correlates of generalized anxiety disorder in community samples. *J Clin Psychiatry* 2002;63(suppl 8):4–10.
4. Stein D. Comorbidity in generalised anxiety disorder: impact and implications. *J Clin Psychiatry* 2001;62(suppl 11):29–34 [review].
5. Judd LL, Kessler RC, Paulus MP, et al. Comorbidity as a fundamental feature of generalised anxiety disorders: results from the national comorbidity study (NCS). *Acta Psychiatry Scand* 1998;98(suppl 393):6–11.
6. Andrews G, Peters L, Guzman AM, et al. A comparison of two structured diagnostic interviews: CIDI and SCAN. *Aust N Z J Psychiatry* 1995;29:124–132.
7. Kessler RC, McGonagle KA, Zhao S, et al. Lifetime and 12-month prevalence of DSM-III-R psychiatric disorders in the United States: results from the national comorbidity survey. *Arch Gen Psychiatry* 1994;51:8–19.
8. Seivewright N, Tyrer P, Ferguson B, et al. Longitudinal study of the influence of life events and personality status on diagnostic change in three neurotic disorders. *Depression Anx* 2000;11:105–113.
9. Pigott T. Gender differences in the epidemiology and treatment of anxiety disorders. *J Clin Psychiatry* 1999;60(suppl 18):4–15.
10. Jorm AF. Does old age reduce the risk of anxiety and depression? A review of epidemiological studies across the adult life span. *Psychol Med* 2000;30:11–22.
11. Lau AW, Edelstein BA, Larkin KT. Psychophysiological arousal in older adults: a critical review. *Clin Psychol Rev* 2001;21:609–630 [review].
12. Brantley PJ, Mehan DJ Jr, Ames SC, et al. Minor stressors and generalised anxiety disorders among low income patients attending primary care clinics. *J Nerv Ment Dis* 1999;187:435–440.
13. Brown ES, Fulton MK, Wilkeson A, et al. The psychiatric sequelae of civilian trauma. *Comp Psychiatry* 2000;41:19–23.
14. Hawker DSJ, Boulton MJ. Twenty years' research on peer victimisation and psychosocial maladjustment: a meta-analytic review of cross-sectional studies. *J Child Psychol Psychiatr* 2000;41:441–445. Search date 1997; primary sources Psychlit, Social Science Citation Index, OCLC Firstsearch and hand searches of relevant journals, bibliographies and reviews, reference lists of relevant articles, and book chapters and personal contact with authors.
15. Hettema JM, Neale MC, Kendler KS. A review and meta-analysis of the genetic epidemiology of anxiety disorders. *Am J Psychiatry* 2001;158:1568–1578. Search date not stated; primary source Medline.
16. Gould RA, Otto MW, Pollack MH, et al. Cognitive behavioural and pharmacological treatment of generalised anxiety disorder: a preliminary meta-analysis. *Behav Res Ther* 1997;28:285–305. Search date 1996; primary

sources Psychlit, Medline, examination of reference lists, and unpublished articles presented at national conferences.

17. Western D, Morrison K. A multidimensional meta-analysis of treatments for depression, panic and generalized anxiety disorder: an empirical examination of the status of empirically supported therapies. *J Consult Clin Psychol* 2001;69:875–889. Search date not stated but only included studies published 1990–1999; primary sources hand searches of 10 journals and psychological abstracts.
18. Ost L, Breitholts E. Applied relaxation vs. cognitive therapy in the treatment of generalized anxiety disorder. *Behav Res Ther* 2000;38:777–790.
19. Borkovec TD, Newman MG, Pincus AL. A component analysis of cognitive-behavioural therapy for generalized anxiety disorder and the role of interpersonal process. *J Consult Clin Psychology* 2002;20:288–298.
20. Barrowclough C, King P, Russell E, et al. A randomized trial of effectiveness of cognitive-behavioural therapy and supportive counselling for anxiety disorders in older adults. *J Consult Clin Psychol* 2001:69;756–762.
21. Fisher PL, Durham RC. Recovery rates in generalized anxiety disorder following psychological therapy: an analysis of clinically significant change in the STAI-T across outcome studies since 1990. *Psychol Med* 1999;29:1425–1434. Search date 1998; primary sources Medline, Psychlit, and Cochrane Controlled Trials Register.
22. Rickels K, DeMartinis N, Aufdembrinke B. A double-blind, placebo controlled trial of abecarnil and diazepam in the treatment of patients with generalized anxiety disorder. *J Clin Psychopharmacol* 2000:20:12–18.
23. Figueira ML. Alprazolam SR in the treatment of generalised anxiety: a multicentre controlled study with bromazepam. *Hum Psychother* 1999;14:171–177.
24. Vaz-Serra A, Figuerra L, Bessa-Peixoto A, et al. Mexazolam and alprazolam in the treatment of generalized anxiety disorder. *Clin Drug Invest* 2001;21:257–263.
25. Mahe V, Balogh A. Long-term pharmacological treatment of generalized anxiety disorder. *Int Clin Psychopharmacol* 2000;15:99–105. Search date 1998; primary sources Medline, Biosis, and Embase.
26. Tyrer P. Current problems with the benzodiazepines. In: Wheatly D, ed. *The anxiolytic jungle: where next?* Chichester: Wiley, 1990:23–47.
27. Kilic C, Curran HV, Noshirvani H, et al. Long-term effects of alprazolam on memory: a 3.5 year follow-up of agoraphobia/panic patients. *Psychol Med* 1999;29:225–231.
28. Thomas RE. Benzodiazepine use and motor vehicle accidents. Systematic review of reported association. *Can Fam Physician* 1998;44:799–808. Search date 1997; primary source Medline.
29. Dolovich LR, Addis A, Regis Vaillancourt JD, et al. Benzodiazepine use in pregnancy and major malformations of oral cleft: meta-analysis of cohort and case-control studies. *BMJ* 1998;317:839–843. Search date 1997; primary sources Medline, Embase, Reprotox, and references of included studies and review articles.
30. Bernstein JG. *Handbook of drug therapy in psychiatry*, 3rd ed. St Louis, Missouri: Mosby Year Book, 1995:401.
31. DeMartinis N, Rynn M, Rickels K, et al. Prior benzodiazepine use and buspirone response in the treatment of generalized anxiety disorder. *J Clin Psychiatry* 2000;61:91–94.
32. Sramek JJ, Transman M, Suri A, et al. Efficacy of buspirone in generalized anxiety disorder with coexisting mild depressive symptoms. *J Clin Psychiatry* 1996;57:287–291.
33. Davidson JR, DuPont RL, Hedges D, et al. Efficacy, safety and tolerability of venlafaxine extended release and buspirone in outpatients with generalised anxiety disorder. *J Clin Psychiatry* 1999;60:528–535.
34. Rickels K, Weisman K, Norstad N, et al. Buspirone and diazepam in anxiety: a controlled study. *J Clin Psychiatry* 1982;12:81–86.
35. Gammans RE, Stringfellow JC, Hvisdos AJ, et al. Use of buspirone in patients with generalized anxiety disorder and coexisting depressive symptoms: a meta-analysis of eight randomized, controlled trials. *Pharmacopsychiatry* 1992;25:193–201.
36. Lader M, Anxiolytic effect of hydroxyzine: a double-blind trial versus placebo and buspirone. *Hum Psychopharmacol Clin Exp* 1999:14;S94–S102.
37. Ballenger JC, McDonald S, Noyes R, et al. The first double-blind, placebo-controlled trial of a partial benzodiazepine agonist, abecarnil (ZK 112–119) in generalised anxiety disorder. *Adv Biochem Psychopharmacol* 1992;47:431–447.
38. Kapczinski F, Schmitt R, Lima MS The use of antidepressants for generalized anxiety disorder. In: The Cochrane Library, Issue 2, 2002. Oxford: Update Software. Search date 2000; primary sources CCDAN and CSG Controlled Trials Register, Medline, Lilacs, reference searching, personal communication, conference abstracts, pharmaceutical industry, and book chapters on the treatment of generalised anxiety disorder.
39. Rickels K, Downing R, Schweizer E, et al. Antidepressants for the treatment of generalised anxiety disorder: a placebo-controlled comparison of imipramine, trazodone and diazepam. *Arch Gen Psychiatry* 1993;50:884–895.
40. Moller HJ, Volz HP, Reimann IW, et al. Opipramol for the treatment of generalised anxiety disorder: a placebo-controlled trial including an alprazolam-treated group. *J Clin Psychopharmacol* 2001;21:51–65.
41. Pollack MH, Zaninelli R, Goddard A, et al. Paroxetine in the treatment of generalized anxiety disorder: results of a placebo-controlled, flexible-dosage trial. *J Clin Psychiatry* 2001;62:350–357.
42. Allgulander C, Hackett D, Salinas E. Venlafaxine extended release (ER) in the treatment of generalised anxiety disorder: twenty-four week placebo-controlled dose-ranging study. *Br J Psychiatry* 2001;179:15–22.
43. Dukes PD, Robinson GM, Thomson KJ, et al. Wellington coroner autopsy cases 1970–89: acute deaths due to drugs, alcohol and poisons. *N Z Med J* 1992;105:25–27. (Published erratum appears in *N Z Med J* 1992;105:135.)
44. Gelenberg A, Lydiard R, Rudolph R, et al. Efficacy of venlafaxine extended releases capsules in nondepressed outpatients with generalized anxiety disorder: a 6-month randomized controlled trial. *JAMA* 2000;283:3082–3088.
45. Rocca P, Fonzo V, Scotta M, et al. Paroxetine efficacy in the treatment of generalized anxiety disorder. *Acta Psychiatr Scand* 1997:95:444–450.
46. Kerr GW, McGuffie AC, Wilkie S. Tricyclic antidepressant overdose: a review. *Emerg Med J* 2001;18:236–241.

47. Pearn J, Nixon J, Ansford A, et al. Accidental poisoning in childhood: five year urban population study with 15 year analysis of fatality. *BMJ* 1984;288:44–46.
48. Lui BA, Mitmann N, Knowles SR, et al. Hyponatremia and the syndrome of inappropriate secretion of antidiuretic hormone associated with the use of selective serotonin reuptake inhibitors: a review of spontaneous reports. *Can Med Assoc J* 1995;155:519–527.
49. Thapa PB, Gideon P, Cost TW, et al. Antidepressants and the risk of falls among nursing home residents. *N Engl J Med* 1998;339:875–882.
50. Liu B, Anderson G, Mittmann N, et al. Use of selective serotonin-reuptake inhibitors of tricyclic antidepressants and risk of hip fractures in elderly people. *Lancet* 1998;351:1303–1307.
51. Kulin NA, Pastuszak A, Koren G. Are the new SSRIs safe for pregnant women? *Can Fam Physician* 1998;44;2081–2083.
52. Montejo AL, Llorca G, Izquierdo JA, et al. Incidence of sexual dysfunction associated with antidepressant agents: a prospective multicentre study of 1022 outpatients. *J Clin Psychiatry* 2000;62(suppl 3):10–21.
53. Mendels J, Krajewski TF, Huffer V, et al. Effective short-term treatment of generalized anxiety with trifluoperazine. *J Clin Psychiatry* 1986;47:170–174.
54. Van Harten PN, Hoek HW, Matroos GE, et al. Intermittent neuroleptic treatment and risk of tardive dyskinesia: Curacao extrapyramidal syndromes study III. *Am J Psychiatry* 1998;155:565–567.
55. Pittler MH, Ernst E. Kava extract for treating anxiety. In: The Cochrane Library, Issue 1, 2002. Oxford: Update Software. Search date 1998; primary sources Medline, Embase, Biosis, Amed, Ciscom, Cochrane Library, hand searches of references, personal files, and contact with manufacturers of kava preparations and experts.
56. Stevenson C, Huntley A, Ernst E. A systematic review of the safety of Kava extract in the treatment of anxiety. *Drug Saf* 2002;25;251–256. Search date 2000; primary sources Medline, Embase, Amed, Cochrane Library, reference lists, departmental files, contact with colleagues in herbal medicine, World Health Organization, USA Food and Drug Administration, UK Committee on Safety of Medicines, German Bundesinstitut fur Arzneimittel und Medizinprodukte, and 10 manufacturers of kava preparations.
57. National Center for Complimentary and Alternative Medicine. Consumer Advisory. Kava linked to liver damage. Internet 2003 [cited February 10]; http://www.nccam.nih.gov/health/alerts/kava/index.htm (last accessed 5March 2003).

Christopher Gale
Consultant Psychiatrist, Clinical Senior Lecturer
Faculty of Medicine and Health Sciences
University of Auckland
Auckland
New Zealand

Mark Oakley-Browne
Professor of Rural Psychiatry
University of Monash
Victoria
Australia

Competing interests: CG has been funded to attend conferences by Eli Lilly and Jansen Pharmaceuticals. MOB has been paid by GlaxoSmithKline, the manufacturer of Aropax (paroxetine) for contributing to educational sessions for general practitioners. MOB has also been reimbursed by Pfizer for attending a conference.

Obsessive compulsive disorder

Search date January 2003

G Mustafa Soomro

QUESTIONS

INTERVENTIONS

See glossary, p 1183

Key Messages

Initial treatment

- **Behavioural therapy** We found no RCTs comparing behavioural therapy versus no treatment. One systematic review and subsequent RCTs have found that behavioural therapy improves symptoms compared with relaxation. The review and one subsequent RCT found no significant difference in symptoms over 4–13 weeks between behavioural therapy and cognitive therapy. One subsequent RCT found limited evidence that group behavioural therapy improved symptoms after 12 weeks compared with group cognitive therapy.
- **Cognitive therapy** We found no RCTs comparing cognitive therapy versus no treatment. One systematic review and one subsequent RCT found no significant difference in symptoms over 4–13 weeks between behavioural therapy and cognitive therapy. Another subsequent RCT found limited evidence that group cognitive therapy was less effective in reducing symptoms over 12 weeks than group behavioural therapy.

- **Serotonin reuptake inhibitors (citalopram, clomipramine, fluoxetine, fluvoxamine, paroxetine, sertraline)** RCTs have found that selective and non-selective serotonin reuptake inhibitors (citalopram, clomipramine, fluoxetine, fluvoxamine, paroxetine) reduce symptoms compared with placebo. Two systematic reviews found inconsistent results about the effects of sertraline compared with placebo. RCTs have found that selective and non-selective serotonin reuptake inhibitors (citalopram, clomipramine, fluoxetine, fluvoxamine, paroxetine, sertraline) reduce symptoms compared with tricyclic antidepressants or monoamine oxidase inhibitors. RCTs have found no consistent evidence of a difference in efficacy among serotonin reuptake inhibitors, but have found that the non-selective serotonin reuptake inhibitor clomipramine is associated with more adverse effects than selective serotonin reuptake inhibitors.
- **Behavioural or cognitive therapy plus selective and non-selective serotonin reuptake inhibitors (compared with behavioural or cognitive therapy alone)** RCTs provided insufficient evidence to assess the effects of adding serotonin reuptake inhibitors to behavioural or cognitive therapy.
- **Electroconvulsive therapy** We found no RCTs of electroconvulsive therapy in people with obsessive compulsive disorder.
- **Venlafaxine** One RCT provided insufficient evidence to compare venlafaxine versus clomipramine.

Maintenance treatment

- **Optimum duration of treatment with selective and non-selective serotonin reuptake inhibitors** RCTs provided insufficient evidence to define the optimum duration of treatment with serotonin reuptake inhibitors.

In people who do not respond to selective and non-selective serotonin reuptake inhibitors

- **Addition of antipsychotics in people who have not responded to serotonin reuptake inhibitors** Three small RCTs in people unresponsive to serotonin reuptake inhibitors found that the addition of antipsychotics improved symptoms compared with placebo.

DEFINITION Obsessive compulsive disorder involves obsessions and/or compulsions that are not caused by drugs or a physical disorder, and which cause significant personal distress or social dysfunction.[1,2] The disorder may have a chronic or an episodic course (see glossary, p 1183). **Obsessions** are recurrent and persistent ideas, images, or impulses that cause pronounced anxiety and that the person perceives to be self produced. **Compulsions** are repetitive behaviours or mental acts performed in response to obsessions or according to certain rules, which are aimed at reducing distress or preventing certain imagined dreaded events. People with obsessive compulsive disorder may have insight into their condition, in that obsessions and compulsions are usually recognised and resisted. There are minor differences in the criteria for obsessive compulsive disorder between the third, revised third, and fourth editions of the *Diagnostic and Statistical Manual:* DSM-III, DSM-III-R, and DSM-IV[1] and *The ICD-10 classification of mental and behavioural disorders.*[2]

INCIDENCE/ PREVALENCE One national, community based survey of obsessive compulsive disorder in the UK (1993, 10 000 people) found that 1% of men and 1.5% of women reported symptoms in the past month.[3] A survey in the USA (18 500 people) found a lifetime prevalence of obsessive compulsive disorder of between 1.9 and 3.3% in 1984.[4] An international study found a lifetime prevalence of 3% in Canada, 3.1% in Puerto Rico, 0.3–0.9% in Taiwan, and 2.2% in New Zealand.[3]

AETIOLOGY/ RISK FACTORS The aetiology of obsessive compulsive disorder is uncertain. Behavioural, cognitive, genetic, and neurobiological factors have been implicated.[5–11] Risk factors include a family history of obsessive compulsive disorder, being single (which could be a consequence of the disorder), and belonging to a higher socioeconomic class.[12]

PROGNOSIS One study (144 people followed for a mean of 47 years) found that an episodic course of obsessive compulsive disorder was more common during the initial years (about 1–9 years), but a chronic course was more common afterwards.[13] Over time, the study found that 39–48% of people had symptomatic improvement. A 1 year prospective cohort study found 46% of people had an episodic course and 54% had a chronic course.[14]

AIMS OF INTERVENTION To improve symptoms, and to reduce the impact of illness on social functioning and quality of life, with minimal adverse effects of treatment.

OUTCOMES Severity of symptoms; social functioning; and adverse effects of treatment. Commonly used instruments for measuring symptoms include the Hamilton Anxiety Rating scale; the Hamilton Depression Rating scale; and the Yale-Brown obsessive compulsive scale, which is observer rated and well validated.[15–17] Most trials use a 25% reduction in Yale-Brown scale scores from baseline as indicative of clinically important improvement, but some studies use a 35% reduction.[17]

METHODS *Clinical Evidence* search and appraisal January 2003.

QUESTION What are the effects of initial treatments in adults?

OPTION SEROTONIN REUPTAKE INHIBITORS (CITALOPRAM, CLOMIPRAMINE, FLUOXETINE, FLUVOXAMINE, PAROXETINE, SERTRALINE) AND VENLAFAXINE

RCTs have found that selective and non-selective serotonin reuptake inhibitors (citalopram, clomipramine, fluoxetine, fluvoxamine, paroxetine) reduce symptoms compared with placebo. Two systematic reviews found inconsistent results about the effects of sertraline compared with placebo. RCTs have found that selective and non-selective serotonin reuptake inhibitors (citalopram, clomipramine, fluoxetine, fluvoxamine, paroxetine, sertraline) reduce symptoms compared with tricyclic antidepressants or monoamine oxidase inhibitors. One RCT found no significant difference in symptoms between clomipramine and venlafaxine, but it is likely to have been underpowered to detect a clinically important difference. RCTs have found no consistent evidence of a difference in efficacy among serotonin reuptake inhibitors, but have found that the non-selective serotonin reuptake inhibitor clomipramine is associated with more adverse effects than selective serotonin reuptake inhibitors.

Benefits: **Versus placebo:** We found two systematic reviews (search dates 1994[18] and not stated[19]) and two subsequent RCTs.[20,21] All found that selective and non-selective serotonin reuptake inhibitors (citalopram, clomipramine, fluoxetine, fluvoxamine, paroxetine) significantly improved symptoms compared with placebo (see table 1, p 1186; see comment below).[18–21] One of the reviews found that sertraline significantly improved symptoms compared with placebo[18] and the other review found no significant difference in symptoms.[19] **Versus each other:** We found two systematic reviews[18,19] and five subsequent RCTs.[22–26] All found no significant difference in symptoms between different selective and non-selective serotonin reuptake inhibitors.[18,19,22–26] The first review (search date 1994, 85 people, 3 RCTs) found no significant difference in symptoms among clomipramine, fluoxetine and fluvoxamine (SMD –0.04, 95% CI –0.43 to +0.35).[18] The second review (search date not stated) found no significant difference in symptoms between clomipramine and fluvoxamine (4 RCTs, including 2 RCTs from the first review; change in Yale-Brown scale score; SMD +1.23, 95% CI –1.11 to +3.56).[19] It also found no significant difference in symptoms between clomipramine and fluoxetine (1 RCT, not included in the first review, 55 people; change in Yale-Brown scale score; SMD +1.40, 95% CI –5.74 to +2.94) or clomipramine and paroxetine (1 RCT not included in the first review, 300 people; change in Yale-Brown scale score; SMD 0.00, 95% CI –1.94 to +1.94).[19] The first subsequent RCT (170 people) found that sertraline significantly reduced symptoms compared with clomipramine (8% greater mean reduction in Yale-Brown scale score, P = 0.036; see comment below).[22] The second subsequent RCT (133 people) found no significant difference in symptoms between clomipramine and fluvoxamine (change in Yale-Brown scale score, 12.6 with clomipramine *v* 12.3 with fluvoxamine; reported as non-significant, no further data reported).[23] The third subsequent RCT (227 people, double blind) found no significant difference between clomipramine (150–300 mg) and fluvoxamine (150–300 mg) and in severity of symptoms after 10 weeks (mean reduction in Yale-Brown score about 12 in both groups; P value not reported; proportion of people achieving at least 35% reduction in Yale-Brown score 65% with clomipramine *v* 62% with fluvoxamine, reported as non-significant).[24] The fourth subsequent RCT (150 people) compared sertraline (50–200 mg) versus fluoxetine (20–80 mg). It found similar symptom severity at 24 weeks between sertraline and fluoxetine (reduction in Yale-Brown score 9.6 points with sertraline *v* 9.7 points with fluoxetine, CI not reported).[25] The fifth subsequent RCT (30 people, observer blinded) compared three interventions: fluvoxamine, paroxetine, and citalopram. It found no significant difference in symptoms among drugs, but was too small to exclude a clinically important difference.[26] **Versus other antidepressants:** We found one systematic review[18] and three subsequent RCTs.[27–29] The review[18] and two of the subsequent RCTs[27,28] found that serotonin reuptake inhibitors significantly improved symptoms compared with tricyclic antidepressants or monoamine oxidase inhibitors. The other subsequent RCT found no significant difference in symptoms between clomipramine and venlafaxine, but it is likely to have been underpowered to detect a clinically important difference between treatments.[29] The systematic review (search date 1994, 7 RCTs, 147 people with obsessive compulsive disorder, including 67 children/adolescents) found that, compared with tricyclic antidepressants (desipramine, imipramine, nortripytyline) or monoamine oxidase inhibitors (clorgiline, phenelzine), clomipramine significantly reduced symptoms (SMD 0.65, 95% CI 0.36 to 0.92).[18] The first subsequent RCT (54 people) compared three interventions: fluoxetine, phenelzine (a monoamine oxidase inhibitor), and placebo.[27] It found that fluoxetine significantly reduced symptoms over 10 weeks compared with phenelzine or placebo (mean reduction in Yale-Brown scale score 2.8 with fluoxetine *v* 1.7 with phenelzine *v* 0.2 with placebo; $P < 0.05$ for fluoxetine *v* either comparison).[27] The second subsequent RCT (164 people with concurrent obsessive compulsive disorder and major depressive disorder) found that sertraline significantly increased the proportion of people who had a clinically important reduction in obsessive compulsive symptoms compared with desipramine (> 40% improvement on Yale-Brown scale 38/79 [48%] with sertraline *v* 26/85 [31%] with desipramine, $P = 0.01$) and significantly increased the proportion of people with remission of depressive symptoms (< 7 on Hamilton Depression Rating Scale 39/79 [49%] with sertraline *v* 30/85 [35%] with desipramine, $P = 0.04$).[28] The third subsequent RCT (73 people) compared clomipramine (150–225 mg daily, 47 people) versus venlafaxine (225–350 mg daily, 26 people).[29] It found no significant difference between clomipramine and venlafaxine in response at 12 weeks (response defined as ≥ 35% reduction in Yale-Brown scale score and CGI score of ≥ 2; 9/25 [36%] *v* 20/40 [50%]; RR 1.39, 95% CI 0.76 to 2.55). **Versus behavioural therapy:** We found one systematic review (search date 1997, number of studies and people not stated).[30] It found no significant difference in symptoms among serotonin reuptake inhibitors, behavioural therapy, and placebo, but these conclusions must be treated with caution as the review made indirect comparisons of effect sizes (standardised mean differences).[30] **Plus behavioural or cognitive therapy:** See behavioural or cognitive therapy plus serotonin reuptake inhibitors, p 1180.

Harms: **Versus placebo:** One systematic review (search date 1995, 16 RCTs) found that serotonin reuptake inhibitors significantly increased overall adverse effects (unspecified) compared with placebo (RRI *v* placebo: 54% with clomipramine, 11% with fluoxetine, 19% with fluvoxamine, and 27% with sertraline).[31] The systematic reviews gave no information on adverse effects.[18,19] The first subsequent RCT found that fluoxetine significantly increased tremor ($P < 0.001$), dry mouth ($P < 0.001$), and nausea ($P < 0.01$) compared with placebo (absolute numbers presented graphically).[20] The second subsequent RCT found that citalopram significantly increased nausea, insomnia, fatigue, sweating, dry mouth, and ejaculatory failure compared with placebo ($P < 0.05$).[21] **Versus each other:** The systematic reviews gave no information on adverse effects.[18,19] Three subsequent RCTs found that clomipramine increased adverse effects compared with selective serotonin reuptake inhibitors[22–24] and one subsequent RCT[25] found no significant difference in adverse effects between the selective serotonin reuptake inhibitors sertraline and fluoxetine. The first subsequent RCT (170 people) found that significantly more people withdrew because of adverse effects with clomipramine than with sertraline ($P < 0.05$).[22] Clomipramine was associated with dry mouth, nausea, tremor, anxiety, and constipation, whereas sertraline was associated with nausea and diarrhoea. The second subsequent RCT (133 people) found that clomipramine significantly increased dry mouth (38% *v* 10%) and constipation (26% *v* 10%) compared with fluvoxamine ($P < 0.05$).[23] The third subsequent RCT comparing clomipramine versus fluvoxamine (227 people) found that more people stopped clomipramine prematurely (16% withdrew with clomipramine *v* 8% with fluvoxamine; CI not reported), and found that clomipramine significantly increased the proportion of people who had anticholinergic adverse effects (dry mouth 43% with clomipramine *v* 10% with fluvoxamine; constipation 25% *v* 9%; tremor 22% *v* 9%; and dizziness 18% *v* 7%; $P = 0.05$ for frequency of all anticholinergic adverse effects with clomipramine *v* fluvoxamine).[24] The fourth subsequent RCT found no significant difference in adverse effects between sertraline and fluoxetine.[25] The fifth subsequent RCT gave no information on adverse effects.[26] One systematic review (search date 1997) of controlled and uncontrolled studies found that the withdrawal rate because of adverse effects was 11% with clomipramine, 10% with fluoxetine, 13% with fluvoxamine, 9% with sertraline, and 11% with paroxetine.[30] One non-systematic review of three prospective cohort studies and five surveys found that fluoxetine during pregnancy did not increase the risk of spontaneous abortion or major malformation (numerical values not provided).[32] The review included one prospective cohort study (174 people) and three surveys that found similar outcomes with other selective serotonin reuptake inhibitors (sertraline, paroxetine, and fluvoxamine). One prospective cohort study of 55 preschool children exposed to fluoxetine *in utero* found no significant difference from unexposed children in global IQ, language, or behaviour. It included no information on long term harms for the other selective serotonin reuptake inhibitors. The non-systematic review of effects in pregnancy did not describe how articles were selected.[32] **Versus other antidepressants:** The systematic review gave no information on adverse effects.[18] The second subsequent RCT (164 people) found that significantly more people discontinued treatment because of adverse effects with desipramine than with sertraline (26% *v* 10%; $P = 0.009$).[28] The third subsequent RCT (73 people) found that significantly more people had overall adverse effects with clomipramine than with venlafaxine (43/47 [92%] with clomipramine *v* 16/26 [62%] with venlafaxine; $P = 0.002$).[29] It found that, compared with venlafaxine, clomipramine significantly increased the proportion who had dry mouth (16/47 [34%] with clomipramine *v* 3/26 [12%] with venlafaxine; $P = 0.036$) and constipation (17/47 [36%] *v* 2/26 [8%]; $P = 0.008$). One systematic review comparing the harms of selective serotonin reuptake inhibitors versus tricyclic antidepressants found that selective serotonin reuptake inhibitors were associated with fewer anticholinergic adverse effects but more nausea, diarrhoea, anxiety, agitation, insomnia, and headache.[33]

Comment: The reviews found heterogeneity in the selection of participants and duration of treatment in the RCTs identified; the first review[18] found that this heterogeneity reached significance in RCTs comparing clomipramine versus placebo. Two RCTs comparing clomipramine versus placebo in the first review included 73 children, but the review did not analyse these RCTs separately.[18] Some RCTs identified by the reviews included people with depression associated with obsessive compulsive disorder. The first systematic review performed a subgroup analysis in people with obsessive compulsive disorder without depression and found that, compared with placebo, clomipramine reduced symptoms of obsessive compulsive disorder in people without depression (5 RCTs, 594 people, SMD 1.37, 95% CI 1.19 to 1.55).[18] This suggests that the effect of serotonin reuptake inhibitors on obsessive compulsive symptoms is independent of their effect on symptoms of depression. In the first subsequent RCT comparing sertraline versus clomipramine, people taking clomipramine received very low doses (median 90 mg daily). This makes the results of the RCT difficult to interpret. **Factors predicting outcome:** Four RCTs found that people who did not respond to serotonin reuptake inhibitors had younger age of onset, longer duration of the condition, higher frequency of symptoms, coexisting personality disorders, and a greater likelihood of previous hospital admission. Predictors of good response were older age of onset, history of remissions, no previous drug treatment, more severe obsessive compulsive disorder, and either high or low score on the Hamilton Depression Rating Scale.[34–37] Two cohort studies of people with obsessive compulsive disorder found that poor response to serotonin reuptake inhibitors was predicted by concomitant schizotypal personality disorder, by tic disorder (see glossary, p 1183), and also by severe obsessive compulsive disorder with cleaning rituals (OR 4.9, 95% CI 1.1 to 21.2).[38,39]

OPTION BEHAVIOURAL THERAPY

We found no RCTs comparing behavioural therapy versus no treatment. One systematic review and subsequent RCTs have found that behavioural therapy reduces symptoms compared with relaxation. The review and one subsequent RCT found no significant difference in symptoms over 4–13 weeks between behavioural therapy and cognitive therapy. Another subsequent RCT found limited evidence that group behavioural therapy may reduce symptoms over 12 weeks compared with group cognitive therapy.

Benefits: **Versus no treatment:** We found no systematic review or RCTs. **Versus relaxation:** We found one systematic review (search date 1995, 2 RCTs, 121 people) that found that behavioural therapy (see glossary, p 1183) significantly reduced symptoms over 4–16 weeks' treatment compared with relaxation (SMD 1.18, CI not reported; $P < 0.01$).[31] One subsequent RCT (218 people with DSM-IV obsessive compulsive disorder, 49% of whom were also taking a serotonin reuptake inhibitor) compared three treatments: behavioural therapy guided by a computer, behavioural therapy guided by a clinician, and relaxation.[40] It found that both types of behavioural therapy significantly improved Yale-Brown score after 10 weeks' treatment compared with relaxation (mean reduction 5.6

with computer guided behavioural therapy *v* 8.0 with clinician guided behavioural therapy *v* 1.7 with relaxation; P = 0.001 for relaxation *v* either type of behavioural therapy; P = 0.035 for clinician guided *v* computer guided behavioural therapy; analysis not by intention to treat).[40] **Versus cognitive therapy:** We found one systematic review[31] and two subsequent RCTs.[41,42] The systematic review (search date 1995, 4 RCTs, 92 people) found no significant difference in symptoms over 4–16 weeks between behavioural therapy and cognitive therapy (see glossary, p 1183) (SMD –0.19; reported as P > 0.05, no further data reported).[31] The first subsequent RCT (76 people) found no significant difference between group behavioural therapy (exposure with response prevention) and group cognitive behavioural therapy in recovery (defined as ≥6 point Yale Brown scale reduction and score ≤12) immediately after 12 weeks' treatment (AR 12/32 [38%] with behavioural therapy *v* 5/31 [16%] with cognitive therapy; P = 0.09), but found that behavioural therapy significantly improved recovery at 3 months' follow up compared with cognitive therapy (AR 14/31 [45%] with behavioural therapy *v* 4/31 [13%] with cognitive therapy; P = 0.01; analysis not by intention to treat). The second subsequent RCT (63 people) found no significant difference between behavioural therapy and cognitive therapy in the proportion of people achieving at least 25% improvement in Yale-Brown score after 16 weeks' treatment (OR 0.7, 95% CI 0.2 to 2.0).[42] **Plus serotonin reuptake inhibitors:** See behavioural therapy or cognitive therapy plus serotonin reuptake inhibitors, p 1180.

Harms: We found no evidence from RCTs or cohort studies of adverse effects from behavioural therapy. Case reports have described unbearable and unacceptable anxiety in some people receiving behavioural therapy.

Comment: **Factors predicting outcome:** We found two RCTs of behavioural therapy (total 96 people, duration 2.5 months and 32 weeks) and two retrospective cohort studies (total 346 people, duration 1 year and 11 weeks) that assessed factors predicting outcome.[43–46] These found poorer outcome to be predicted by initial severity, depression, longer duration, poorer motivation, and dissatisfaction with the therapeutic relationship. Good outcome was predicted by early adherence to "exposure homework" (that is, tasks to be carried out outside regular therapy sessions involving contact with anxiety provoking situations), employment, living with one's family, no previous treatment, having fear of contamination, overt ritualistic behaviour, and absence of depression.[43–45] Good outcome for women was predicted by having a co-therapist (someone, usually related to the woman concerned, who is enlisted to help with treatment outside regular treatment sessions; OR 19.5, 95% CI 2.7 to 139).[46] Two systematic reviews of drug, behavioural, cognitive, and combination treatments for obsessive compulsive disorder are being prepared. **Maintenance of improvement:** A prospective follow up (20 people with obsessive compulsive disorder, specific diagnostic criteria not provided) after a 6 month RCT of behavioural therapy found that 79% maintained improvement in obsessive compulsive symptoms at 2 years' follow up.[47] A prospective non-inception cohort study of behavioural therapy in 21 people with obsessive compulsive disorder (specific diagnostic criteria not provided) found that, after 2 weeks of treatment, 68–79% maintained complete or much improvement in symptoms at 3 months' follow up.[48] In both RCTs, some people received additional behavioural therapy during follow up.

OPTION COGNITIVE THERAPY

We found no RCTs comparing cognitive therapy versus no treatment. One systematic review and one subsequent RCT found no significant difference in symptoms over 4–13 weeks between behavioural therapy and cognitive therapy. Another subsequent RCT found limited evidence that group behavioural therapy reduced symptoms over 12 weeks compared with group cognitive therapy.

Benefits: **Versus no treatment:** We found no systematic review or RCTs. **Versus behavioural therapy:** See behavioural therapy, p 1178. **Plus serotonin reuptake inhibitors:** See behavioural therapy or cognitive therapy plus serotonin reuptake inhibitors, p 1180.

Harms: We found no evidence from RCTs or cohort studies of adverse effects from cognitive therapy.

Comment: None.

OPTION BEHAVIOURAL OR COGNITIVE THERAPY PLUS SELECTIVE AND NON-SELECTIVE SEROTONIN REUPTAKE INHIBITORS

RCTs provided insufficient evidence to assess the effects of adding serotonin reuptake inhibitors to behavioural or cognitive therapy.

Benefits: We found one systematic review[30] and two subsequent RCTs.[49,50] The systematic review (search date 1997, 77 studies, number of people not stated) did not make direct comparisons between treatments.[30] It included all types of study with the exception of case control studies. In indirect comparisons, it found similar reductions in symptoms with behavioural therapy alone versus placebo, behavioural therapy plus serotonin reuptake inhibitors (clomipramine, fluoxetine, fluvoxamine, paroxetine, or sertraline) versus placebo, and serotonin reuptake inhibitors alone versus placebo. One subsequent RCT (99 people in an outpatient setting) compared four interventions: behavioural therapy, cognitive therapy, behavioural therapy plus fluvoxamine (a selective serotonin reuptake inhibitor), and cognitive therapy plus fluvoxamine. It found no significant difference among interventions in symptoms after 16 weeks' treatment (mean reduction in Yale-Brown scale score 17.1 with behavioural therapy *v* 13.5 with cognitive therapy *v* 12.6 with behavioural therapy plus fluvoxamine *v* 15.6 with cognitive therapy plus fluvoxamine, reported as non-significant, no further data reported).[49] Another subsequent RCT (49 people in a hospital setting) found that behavioural therapy plus fluvoxamine significantly increased the proportion of people with improved symptoms after 9 weeks' treatment compared with behavioural therapy plus pill placebo (number of people with > 35% reduction of Yale-Brown score 21/24 [88%] *v* 15/25 [60%]; RR 1.46, 95% CI 1.02 to 2.08).[50]

Harms: We found no evidence from RCTs or cohort studies of adverse effects from behavioural therapy. Case reports have described unbearable and unacceptable anxiety in some people receiving behavioural therapy (see glossary, p 1183).

Comment: None.

OPTION ELECTROCONVULSIVE THERAPY

We found no RCTs of electroconvulsive therapy in people with obsessive compulsive disorder.

Benefits: We found no systematic review or RCTs.

Harms: We found no RCTs.

Comment: People with obsessive compulsive disorder who also have depression may be treated with electroconvulsive therapy. The evidence for the effects of electroconvulsive therapy in depression is summarised elsewhere in *Clinical Evidence* (see depressive disorders in adults, p 1121).

QUESTION What is the optimum duration of maintenance treatment with selective and non-selective serotonin reuptake inhibitors?

RCTs provided insufficient evidence to define the optimum duration of treatment with serotonin reuptake inhibitors.

Benefits: We found insufficient evidence to define the optimum duration of treatment with serotonin reuptake inhibitors. Most RCTs last only 10–12 weeks.[51] We found two RCTs that assessed maintenance of serotonin reuptake inhibitors for 1 year in people who had responded to treatment.[52,53] The first RCT (70 people who had responded to a 20 week course of fluoxetine) found no significant difference between maintenance of fluoxetine and replacement by placebo for 1 year in relapse rate over 1 year (21% with fluoxetine *v* 32% with placebo; P = 0.137).[52] The second RCT compared sertraline versus placebo in 223 people with obsessive compulsive disorder, who had all previously responded to 1 year's treatment with sertraline (response defined as at least 25% reduction in Yale-Brown score from baseline).[53] People continuing on sertraline were prescribed their previous dose (mean 183 mg). The RCT found that, compared with placebo, sertraline significantly reduced the proportion of people who withdrew because of relapse or insufficient clinical response over 24 weeks (9% with sertraline *v* 24% with placebo; P = 0.006). It found that sertraline reduced the proportion of people who had worsening of symptoms compared with placebo (12% with sertraline *v* 35% with placebo; P = 0.001), but found no significant difference in relapse rate over 24 weeks (2.7% with sertraline *v* 4.4% with placebo; P = 0.34).[53]

Harms: The first RCT found no significant difference between fluoxetine and placebo in overall adverse effects (reported as non-significant, adverse effects not specified, absolute numbers and CI not reported) or in the proportion of people who withdrew from the trial for any cause over 52 weeks (16/36 with fluoxetine [44%] *v* 23/35

[66%] with placebo; P = 0.072).[52] The second RCT found that upper respiratory infection, headache, and malaise were reported in ≥ 10% of people taking sertraline and that people taking placebo had dizziness and depression (no further data reported).[53] It found that fewer people taking sertraline withdrew because of adverse effects than people taking placebo (5/109 [5%] *v* 12/114 [11%]; P value not reported).

Comment: One prospective, 1 year study found further improvement after a 40 week open label extension of the study, with continuing adverse effects.[54] One observational study found that 16/18 (89%) people relapsed within 7 weeks of replacing clomipramine with placebo treatment.[55]

QUESTION What are the effects of treatments in adults who have not responded to initial treatment with serotonin reuptake inhibitors?

OPTION COMBINED ANTIPSYCHOTICS AND SEROTONIN REUPTAKE INHIBITORS

Three small RCTs in people unresponsive to serotonin reuptake inhibitors found that the addition of antipsychotics improved symptoms compared with placebo.

Benefits: We found no systematic review, but found three small RCTs that assessed combined antipsychotics and serotonin reuptake inhibitors in people who did not respond to serotonin reuptake inhibitors alone.[56–58] The first RCT (34 people with obsessive compulsive disorder who had not responded to 8 weeks' treatment with fluvoxamine) compared fluvoxamine (a selective serotonin reuptake inhibitor) plus haloperidol (an antipsychotic; maximum dose of haloperidol 10 mg/day) versus fluvoxamine plus placebo.[56] It found that fluvoxamine plus haloperidol significantly increased the proportion of people who met two out of three different response criteria compared with fluvoxamine plus placebo (11/17 [65%] *v* 0/17 [0%]; NNT 2, 95% CI 2 to 3; P < 0.0002). The second RCT (36 people with obsessive compulsive disorder who did not respond to 12 weeks of serotonin reuptake inhibitor) found that, compared with addition of placebo, addition of 6 weeks of risperidone (an antipsychotic) to the prior serotonin reuptake inhibitor significantly reduced symptoms of obsessive compulsive disorder (reduction in the Yale-Brown scale 36% *v* 9%; P = 0.001), depression (reduction in the Hamilton Depression Rating Scale 35% *v* 20%; P = 0.002), and anxiety (reduction in the Hamilton Anxiety Rating Scale 31% *v* 12%; P = 0.007).[57] People taking risperidone were more likely to have met two of the response criteria (8/18 [44%] with serotonin reuptake inhibitor plus risperidone *v* 0/15 [0%] with serotonin reuptake inhibitor plus placebo; NNT 2, 95% CI 2 to 3; P < 0.005). The third RCT (27 people who had been resistant to 3 months' treatment with fluoxetine, fluvoxamine, or clomipramine in an open label trial) compared a serotonin reuptake inhibitor plus quetiapine (an atypical antipsychotic 50–200 mg daily) versus a serotonin reuptake inhibitor plus placebo for 8 weeks.[58] People received the same serotonin reuptake inhibitors in the RCT as they had in the open label phase of the study. The RCT found that a serotonin reuptake inhibitor plus quetiapine significantly increased the proportion of people who responded compared with a serotonin reuptake inhibitor plus placebo (response defined as 30% or greater reduction in the Yale-Brown scale; 10/14 [71%] v 0/14 [0%]; $P < 0.0001$).

Harms: Extrapyramidal adverse effects are common with haloperidol, which can also cause prolactinaemia. The RCT of serotonin reuptake inhibitors plus risperidone found that sedation, restlessness, increased appetite, dry mouth, or tinnitus were experienced by at least 10% of people taking serotonin reuptake inhibitors plus risperidone and that blurred vision, excessive perspiration, headache, increased appetite, lightheadedness, restlessness, and sedation were experienced by at least 10% of people taking placebo.[57] Risperidone is commonly associated with hypotension and prolactinaemia. The RCT of serotonin reuptake inhibitors plus quetiapine found that people taking a serotonin reuptake inhibitor plus quetiapine had nausea (6/14), sedation (3/14), and dizziness (1/14), and people taking a serotonin reuptake inhibitor plus placebo had sedation (2/13), headache (1/13), and nervousness (1/13).[58]

Comment: None.

GLOSSARY

Behavioural therapy Consists of exposure to the anxiety provoking stimuli and prevention of ritualistic behaviour (engaging in compulsions).
Chronic Continuous course of obsessive compulsive disorder without periods of remission since first onset.
Cognitive therapy Aims to correct distorted thoughts (such as exaggerated sense of harm and personal responsibility) by Socratic questioning, logical reasoning, and hypothesis testing.
Episodic Episodic course of obsessive compulsive disorder with periods of remission since first onset.
Schizotypal personality disorder Characterised by discomfort in close relationships, cognitive and perceptual distortions, and eccentric behaviour.
Tic disorder Characterised by motor tics, vocal tics, or both.

Substantive changes

Serotonin reuptake inhibitors (citalopram, clomipramine, fluoxetine, fluvoxamine, paroxetine, sertraline) and venlafaxine One systematic review[19] and one subsequent RCT added;[29] conclusions unchanged.
Combined antipsychotics and serotonin reuptake inhibitors in people who have not responded to serotonin reuptake inhibitors One RCT added;[58] conclusions unchanged.

REFERENCES

1. American Psychiatric Association. *Diagnostic and statistical manual of mental disorders,* 4th ed. Washington, DC: APA, 1994:669–673.
2. World Health Organization. *The ICD-10 classification of mental and behavioural disorders*. Geneva: World Health Organization, 1992.
3. New3 Bebbington PE. Epidemiology of obsessive–compulsive disorder. *Br J Psychiatry* 1998;35(suppl.):2–6.
4. Karno M, Golding JM, Sorenson SB, et al. The epidemiology of obsessive–compulsive disorder in five US communities. *Arch Gen Psychiatry* 1988;45:1094–1099.
5. Baer L, Minichiello WE. Behavior therapy for obsessive–compulsive disorder. In: Jenike MA, Baer L, Minichiello WE, eds. *Obsessive–compulsive disorders*. St Louis: Mosby, 1998: 337–367.
6. Steketee GS, Frost RO, Rheaume J, et al. Cognitive theory and treatment of obsessive–compulsive disorder. In: Jenike MA, Baer L, Minichiello WE, eds. *Obsessive–compulsive disorders*. St Louis: Mosby, 1998: 368–399.
7. Alsobrook JP, Pauls DL. The genetics of obsessive–compulsive disorder. In: Jenike MA, Baer L, Minichiello WE, eds. *Obsessive–compulsive disorders*. St Louis: Mosby, 1998: 276–288.

8. Rauch SL, Whalen PJ, Dougherty D, et al. Neurobiologic models of obsessive compulsive disorder. In: Jenike MA, Baer L, Minichiello WE, eds. *Obsessive–compulsive disorders*. St Louis: Mosby, 1998: 222–253.
9. Delgado PL, Moreno FA. Different roles for serotonin in anti-obsessional drug action and the pathophysiology of obsessive–compulsive disorder. *Br J Psychiatry* 1998;35(suppl.):21–25.
10. Saxena S, Brody AL, Schwartz JM, et al. Neuroimaging and frontal–subcortical circuitry in obsessive–compulsive disorder. *Br J Psychiatry* 1998;35(suppl.):26–37.
11. Rauch SL, Baxter LR Jr. Neuroimaging in obsessive–compulsive disorder and related disorders. In: Jenike MA, Baer L, Minichiello WE, eds. *Obsessive–compulsive disorders*. St Louis: Mosby, 1998: 289–317.
12. Yaryura-Tobias JA, Neziroglu FA. *Obsessive-compulsive disorder spectrum*. Washington, DC: American Psychiatric Press, Inc., 1997.
13. Skoog G, Skoog I. A 40-year follow up of patients with obsessive–compulsive disorder. *Arch Gen Psychiatry* 1999;56:121–127.
14. Ravizza L, Maina G, Bogetto F. Episodic and chronic obsessive–compulsive disorder. *Depress Anxiety* 1997;6:154–158.
15. Goodman WK, Price LH, Rasmussen SA, et al. The Yale-Brown obsessive compulsive scale. I. Development, use, and reliability. *Arch Gen Psychiatry* 1989;46:1006–1011.
16. Goodman WK, Price LH, Rasmussen SA, et al. The Yale-Brown obsessive compulsive scale. II. Validity. *Arch Gen Psychiatry* 1989;46:1012–1016.
17. Goodman WK, Price LH. Rating scales for obsessive–compulsive disorder. In: Jenike MA, Baer L, Minichiello WE, eds. *Obsessive–compulsive disorders*. St Louis: Mosby, 1998: 97–117.
18. Piccinelli M, Pini S, Bellantuono C, et al. Efficacy of drug treatment in obsessive–compulsive disorder. A meta-analytic review. *Br J Psychiatry* 1995;166:424–443. Search dates 1994; primary sources Medline and Excerpta Medica-Psychiatry.
19. Ackerman DL, Greenland S. Multivariate meta-analysis of controlled drug studies for obsessive-compulsive disorder. *J Clin Psychopharmacol* 2002;22:309–317. Search date not reported; primary sources Medline, Psycinfo, and hand searches of bibliographies of published reviews and previous meta-analyses.
20. Tollefson GD, Rampey AH, Potvin JH, et al. A multicenter investigation of fixed-dose fluoxetine in the treatment of obsessive–compulsive disorder. *Arch Gen Psychiatry* 1994;51:559–567.
21. Montgomery SA, Kasper S, Stein DJ, et al. Citalopram 20 mg, 40 mg and 60 mg are all effective and well tolerated compared with placebo in obsessive-compulsive disorder. *Int Clin Psychopharmacol* 2001;16:75–86.
22. Bisserbe JC, Lane RM, Flament MF. A double blind comparison of sertraline and clomipramine in outpatients with obsessive–compulsive disorder. *Eur Psychiatry* 1997;12:82–93.
23. Mundo E, Maina G, Uslenghi C. Multicentre, double-blind, comparison of fluvoxamine and clomipramine in the treatment of obsessive–compulsive disorder. *Int Clin Psychopharmacol* 2000;15:69–76.
24. Mundo E, Rouillon F, Figuera L, et al. Fluvoxamine in obsessive-compulsive disorder: Similar efficacy but superior tolerability in comparison with clomipramine. *Hum Psychopharmacol* 2001;16:461–468.
25. Bergeron R, Ravindran AV, Chaput Y, et al. Sertraline and fluoxetine treatment of obsessive-compulsive disorder: Results of a double-blind, 6-month treatment study. *J Clin Psychopharmacol* 2002;22:148–154.
26. Mundo E, Bianchi L, Bellodi L. Efficacy of fluvoxamine, paroxetine, and citalopram in the treatment of obsessive–compulsive disorder: a single-blind study. *J Clin Psychopharmacol* 1997;17:267–271.
27. Jenike MA, Baer L, Minichiello WE, et al. Placebo-controlled trial of fluoxetine and phenelzine for obsessive–compulsive disorder. *Am J Psychiatry* 1997;154:1261–1264.
28. Hoehn-Saric R, Ninan P, Black DW, et al. Multicenter double-blind comparison of sertraline and desipramine for concurrent obsessive–compulsive and major depressive disorders. *Arch Gen Psychiatry* 2000;57:76–82.
29. Albert U, Aguglia E, Maina G, et al. Venlafaxine versus clomipramine in the treatment of obsessive-compulsive disorder: A preliminary single-blind, 12-week, controlled study. *J Clin Psychiatry* 2002;63:1004–1009.
30. Kobak KA, Greist JH, Jefferson JW, et al. Behavioral versus pharmacological treatments of obsessive compulsive disorder: a meta-analysis. *Psychopharmacology (Berl)* 1998;136:205–216. Search date 1997; primary sources Medline, PsycINFO, Dissertations, and Abstracts International databases.
31. Abramowitz JS. Effectiveness of psychological and pharmacological treatments for obsessive–compulsive disorder: a quantitative review. *J Consult Clin Psychol* 1997;65:44–52. Search date 1995; primary sources Medline and PsycLIT.
32. Goldstein DJ, Sundell K. A review of safety of selective serotonin reuptake inhibitors during pregnancy. *Hum Psychopharmacol Clin Exp* 1999;14:319–324.
33. Trindade E, Menon D. Selective serotonin reuptake inhibitors differ from tricyclic antidepressants in adverse events (Abstract). Selective serotonin reuptake inhibitors for major depression. Part 1. Evaluation of clinical literature. Ottawa: Canadian Coordinating Office for Health Technology Assessment, August 1997 Report 3E. *Evid Based Ment Health* 1998;1:50.
34. Ravizza L, Barzega G, Bellino S, et al. Predictors of drug treatment response in obsessive–compulsive disorder. *J Clin Psychiatry* 1995;56:368–373.
35. Cavedini P, Erzegovesi S, Ronchi P, et al. Predictive value of obsessive–compulsive personality disorder in antiobsessional pharmacological treatment. *Eur Neuropsychopharmacol* 1997;7:45–49.
36. Ackerman DL, Greenland S, Bystritsky A. Clinical characteristics of response to fluoxetine treatment of obsessive–compulsive disorder. *J Clin Psychopharmacol* 1998;18:185–192.
37. Ackerman DL, Greenland S, Bystritsky A, et al. Predictors of treatment response in obsessive–compulsive disorder: multivariate analyses from a multicenter trial of clomipramine. *J Clin Psychopharmacol* 1994;14:247–254.
38. Mundo E, Erzegovesi S, Bellodi L. Follow up of obsessive–compulsive patients treated with proserotonergic agents (letter). *J Clin Psychopharmacol* 1995;15:288–289.
39. Alarcon RD, Libb JW, Spitler D. A predictive study of obsessive–compulsive disorder response to clomipramine. *J Clin Psychopharmacol* 1993;13:210–213.
40. Greist JH, Marks IM, Baer L, et al. Behavior therapy for obsessive-compulsive disorder guided by a computer or by a clinician compared with relaxation as a control. *J Clin Psychiatry* 2002;63:138–145.

41. McLean PD, Whittal ML, Thordarson DS, et al. Cognitive versus behavior therapy in the group treatment of obsessive-compulsive disorder. *J Consult Clin Psychol* 2001;69:205–214.
42. Cottraux J, Note I, Yao SN, et al. A randomized controlled trial of cognitive therapy versus intensive behavior therapy in obsessive compulsive disorder. *Psychother Psychosom* 2001;70:288–297.
43. Keijsers GP, Hoogduin CA, Schaap CP. Predictors of treatment outcome in the behavioural treatment of obsessive–compulsive disorder. *Br J Psychiatry* 1994;165:781–786.
44. De Araujo LA, Ito LM, Marks IM. Early compliance and other factors predicting outcome of exposure for obsessive–compulsive disorder. *Br J Psychiatry* 1996;169:747–752.
45. Buchanan AW, Meng KS, Marks IM. What predicts improvement and compliance during the behavioral treatment of obsessive compulsive disorder? *Anxiety* 1996;2:22–27.
46. Castle DJ, Deale A, Marks IM, et al. Obsessive–compulsive disorder: prediction of outcome from behavioural psychotherapy. *Acta Psychiatr Scand* 1994;89:393–398.
47. Marks IM, Hodgson R, Rachman S. Treatment of chronic obsessive–compulsive neurosis by in-vivo exposure. A two-year follow up and issues in treatment. *Br J Psychiatry* 1975;127:349–364.
48. Foa EB, Goldstein A. Continuous exposure and complete response prevention in obsessive–compulsive neurosis. *Behav Ther* 1978;9:821–829.
49. van Balkom AJ, de Haan E, van Oppen P, et al. Cognitive and behavioral therapies alone versus in combination with fluvoxamine in the treatment of obsessive compulsive disorder. *J Nerv Ment Dis* 1998;186:492–499.
50. Hohagen F, Winkelmann G, Rasche-Ruchle H, et al. Combination of behaviour therapy with fluvoxamine in comparison with behaviour therapy and placebo. Results of a multicentre study. *Br J Psychiatry* 1998;35(suppl.):71–78.
51. Rauch SL, Jenike MA. Pharmacological treatment of obsessive compulsive disorder. In: Nathan PE, Gorman JM, eds. *Treatments that work*. New York: Oxford University Press, 1998:359–376.
52. Romano S, Goodman W, Tamura R, et al. Long-term treatment of obsessive-compulsive disorder after an acute response: a comparison of fluoxetine versus placebo. *J Clin Psychopharmacol* 2001;21:46–52.
53. Koran LM, Hackett E, Rubin A, et al. Efficacy of sertraline in the long-term treatment of obsessive-compulsive disorder. *Am J Psychiatry* 2002;159:88–95.
54. Rasmussen S, Hackett E, DuBoff E, et al. A 2-year study of sertraline in the treatment of obsessive–compulsive disorder. *Int Clin Psychopharmacol* 1997;12:309–316.
55. Pato MT, Zohar-Kadouch R, Zohar J, et al. Return of symptoms after discontinuation of clomipramine in patients with obsessive–compulsive disorder. *Am J Psychiatry* 1988;145:1521–1525.
56. McDougle CJ, Goodman WK, Leckman JF, et al. Haloperidol addition in fluvoxamine-refractory obsessive-compulsive disorder. A double-blind, placebo-controlled study in patients with and without tics. *Arch Gen Psychiatry* 1994;51:302–308.
57. McDougle CJ, Epperson CN, Pelton GH, et al. A double-blind, placebo-controlled study of risperidone addition in serotonin reuptake inhibitor-refractory obsessive-compulsive disorder. *Arch Gen Psychiatry* 2000;57:794–801.
58. Atmaca M, Kuloglu M, Tezcan E, et al.. Quetiapine augmentation in patients with treatment resistant obsessive-compulsive disorder: a single-blind, placebo-controlled study. *Int Clin Psychopharmacol* 2002;17:115–119.

G Mustafa Soomro
Honorary Research Fellow
Section of Community Psychiatry
St George's Hospital Medical School
London
UK

Competing interests: None declared.

TABLE 1 **Serotonin reuptake inhibitors (clomipramine, citalopram, fluoxetine, fluvoxamine, paroxetine, sertraline) versus placebo.**

	Total no of RCTs identified	Systematic review (95% CI)[18]	Systematic review (95% CI)[19]	Subsequent RCT[20]	Subsequent RCT[21]
Clomipramine	11	9 RCTs; 668 people	7 RCTs; 808 people		
Symptom improvement *v* placebo*		SMD 1.31 (1.15 to 1.47)	SMD –8.19 (–10.53 to –5.85)		
Citalopram	1				401 people
Symptom improvement *v* placebo†					AR 57% with citalopram 20 mg *v* 52% with 40 mg v 65% with 60 mg *v* 36.6% with placebo; NNT for 20 mg citalopram *v* placebo 5, 95% CI 3 to 14.
Fluoxetine	5	1 RCT; 287 people	3 RCTs; 329 people	350 people	
Symptom improvement *v* placebo*		SMD 0.57 (0.33 to 0.81)	SMD –1.61 (–2.18 to –1.04)	Mean reduction in score 4.6 with fluoxetine 20 mg, 5.5 with 40 mg, 6.5 with 60 mg *v* 0.9 with placebo ($P < 0.001$ for all doses *v* placebo)	

TABLE 1 continued

	Total no of RCTs identified	Systematic review (95% CI)[18]	Systematic review (95% CI)[19]	Subsequent RCT[20]	Subsequent RCT[21]
Fluvoxamine	5	SMD 0.57 (0.37 to 0.77)	SMD –4.84 (–7.78 to –1.83)		
Paroxetine	1		1 RCT; 300 people		
Symptom improvement *v* placebo*			SMD –3.00 (–4.91 to –1.09)		
Sertraline	4	3 RCTs; 270 people	4 RCTs; 598 people		
Symptom improvement *m* placebo*		SMD 0.52 (0.27 to 0.77)	SMD–2.47 (–6.13 to +1.20 [NS])		

*Symptoms assessed by Yale–Brown score; † > 25% reduction in Yale–Brown scale score. NS, non-significant.

Panic disorder

Search date January 2003

Shailesh Kumar and Mark Oakley-Browne

QUESTIONS

INTERVENTIONS

See glossary, p 1194

Key Messages

- **Selective serotonin reuptake inhibitors** Systematic reviews and one additional RCT have found that selective serotonin reuptake inhibitors improve symptoms in panic disorder compared with placebo. One subsequent RCT found that discontinuation of sertraline in people with a good response increased exacerbation of symptoms. A second subsequent RCT that found paroxetine plus cognitive behavioural therapy improved symptoms compared with placebo plus cognitive behavioural therapy.
- **Tricyclic antidepressants (imipramine)** One systematic review, one subsequent RCT and one additional RCT have found that imipramine improves symptoms compared with placebo. One subsequent RCT found that imipramine reduced relapse rates over 12 months.
- **Benzodiazepines** One systematic review and one additional RCT have found that alprazolam reduces the number of panic attacks and improves symptoms compared with placebo. However, benzodiazepines are associated with a wide range of adverse effects both during and after treatment.
- **Buspirone** We found insufficient evidence to assess the effects of buspirone compared with placebo.
- **Monoamine oxidase inhibitors** We found no RCTs on the effects of monoamine oxidase inhibitors.

DEFINITION A panic attack is a period in which there is sudden onset of intense apprehension, fearfulness, or terror often associated with feelings of impending doom. Panic disorder occurs when there are recurrent, unpredictable attacks followed by at least 1 month of persistent concern about having another panic attack, worry about the possible implications or consequences of the panic attacks, or a significant behavioural change related to the attacks.[1] The term panic disorder excludes panic attacks attributable to the direct physiological effects of a general medical condition, substance, or another mental disorder. Panic disorder is sometimes categorised as with or without agoraphobia.[1] Alternative categorisations focus on phobic anxiety disorders and specify agoraphobia with or without panic disorder.[2]

INCIDENCE/ PREVALENCE Panic disorder often starts at around 20 years of age (between late adolescence and the mid-30s).[3] Lifetime prevalence is 1–3%, and panic disorder is more common in women than in men.[4] An Australian community study found 1 month prevalence rates for panic disorder (with or without agoraphobia) of 0.4% using International Classification of Diseases (ICD)-10 diagnostic criteria and of 0.5% using Diagnostic and Statistical Manual (DSM)-IV diagnostic criteria.[5]

AETIOLOGY/ RISK FACTORS Stressful life events tend to precede the onset of panic disorder,[6,7] although a negative interpretation of these events in addition to their occurrence has been suggested as an important causal factor.[8] Panic disorder is associated with major depression,[9] social phobia, generalised anxiety disorder, obsessive compulsive disorder,[10] and a substantial risk of drug and alcohol abuse.[11] It is also associated with avoidant, histrionic, and dependent personality disorders.[10]

PROGNOSIS The severity of symptoms in people with panic disorder fluctuates considerably, with periods of no attacks, or only mild attacks with few symptoms, being common. There is often a long delay between the initial onset of symptoms and presentation for treatment. Recurrent attacks may continue for several years, especially if associated with agoraphobia. Reduced social or occupational functioning varies among people with panic disorder and is worse in people with associated agoraphobia. Panic disorder is also associated with an increased rate of attempted, but unsuccessful, suicide.[12] One study analysing RCT and systematic review data found that co-existence of anxiety and depressive features adversely affects treatment response at 12 years compared with panic disorder alone.[13]

AIMS OF INTERVENTION To reduce the severity and frequency of panic attacks, phobic avoidance, and anticipatory anxiety; to improve social and occupational functioning, with minimal adverse effects of treatment.

OUTCOMES Measures of panic attacks, agoraphobia, and associated disability (self reported and clinician rated, before and after treatment, and longer term) using general scales or specific scales for panic disorder (e.g. the panic and agoraphobia scale, the mobility inventory for agoraphobia).

METHODS *Clinical Evidence* search and appraisal January 2003. Studies with follow up periods of less than 6 months were excluded.

QUESTION **What are the effects of drug treatments for panic disorder?**

OPTION **TRICYCLIC ANTIDEPRESSANTS**

One systematic review, one subsequent RCT and one additional RCT have found that imipramine improves symptoms in people with panic disorder compared with placebo. One subsequent RCT found that imipramine reduced relapse rates after 12 months in people with panic disorder.

Benefits: We found one systematic review,[14] one additional RCT,[15] and two subsequent RCTs.[16,17] The systematic review (search date not stated, 27 RCTs, 2348 people) compared imipramine, selective serotonin reuptake inhibitors (paroxetine, fluvoxamine, zimelidine, and clomipramine; see comment below) and alprazolam versus placebo and versus each other (see benefits of selective serotonin reuptake inhibitors, p 1191 and benzodiazepines, p 1193).[14] It found that imipramine compared with placebo significantly increased the proportion of people judged to have improved ($P < 0.0001$; see comment below). The additional RCT (181 people with panic disorder with or without agoraphobia) compared three treatments: oral imipramine (maximum dose 225 mg; see comment below), oral alprazolam (maximum dose 10 mg; see comment below), and placebo (see benefits of benzodiazepines, p 1193).[15] It found that imipramine compared with placebo reduced the number of panic attacks after 8 months (results presented graphically, significance not calculated). The first subsequent RCT (56 adults with panic disorder and agoraphobia in stable remission after 24 weeks' treatment with oral imipramine) comparing oral imipramine 2.25 mg/kg daily with placebo found that significantly fewer people taking imipramine relapsed after 12 months (see comment below; 1/29 [3%] with imipramine *v* 10/27 [37%] with placebo; RR 0.09, 95% CI 0.01 to 0.68; NNT 5, 95% CI 3 to 14).[16] The second subsequent RCT (312 people) compared five groups: oral imipramine (maximum dose 300 mg/day; see comment below), cognitive behavioural therapy (see glossary, p 1194), placebo, cognitive behavioural therapy plus oral imipramine (maximum dose 300 mg/day; see comment below), and cognitive behavioural therapy plus placebo.[17] It found that imipramine compared with placebo significantly increased the proportion of people judged to have responded using the panic disorder severity scale after 6 months (38% response rate with imipramine *v* 13% response rate with placebo; absolute numbers not provided; $P = 0.02$).

Harms: Adverse effects associated with imipramine treatment included blurred vision, tachycardia, palpitations, blood pressure changes, insomnia, nervousness, malaise, dizziness, headache, nausea, vomiting, and reduced appetite (see harms of prescription antidepressant drugs under depressive disorders, p 1121).[15,18]

Comment: The review included clomipramine as a serotonin reuptake inhibitor. This drug is also often described as a tricyclic antidepressant.[14] The review used improvement as an outcome measure without a clear definition of this term. In the additional RCT and the second subsequent RCT, flexible dosing was used according to tolerance and therapeutic need.[15,17] In the subsequent RCT comparing imipramine versus placebo, relapse rate was not clearly defined.[16]

OPTION SELECTIVE SEROTONIN REUPTAKE INHIBITORS

Systematic reviews and one additional RCT have found that selective serotonin reuptake inhibitors improve symptoms compared with placebo in panic disorder. One subsequent RCT found that discontinuation of sertraline in people with a good response increased exacerbation of symptoms. A second subsequent RCT found that paroxetine plus cognitive behavioural therapy improved symptoms compared with placebo plus cognitive behavioural therapy.

Benefits: We found two systematic reviews (see benefits of tricyclic antidepressants, p 1190 and benzodiazepines, p 1193),[14,19] one additional RCT,[20] and two subsequent RCTs.[21,22] The first systematic review (search date not stated, 27 RCTs, 2348 people) found that selective serotonin reuptake inhibitors (paroxetine, fluvoxamine, zimelidine, and clomipramine; see comment below) significantly increased the proportion of people who improved compared with placebo ($P < 0.0001$; see comment below).[14] The second systematic review (search date not stated, 12 RCTs, 1741 people) only reported combined results as an effect size against placebo (effect size 0.55), and did not report statistical significance.[19] The additional RCT (279 people) compared five groups: oral citalopram 10 or 15 mg daily, oral citalopram 20 or 30 mg daily, oral citalopram 40 or 60 mg daily, oral clomipramine 60 or 90 mg daily, and placebo.[20] It found that citalopram (at all doses) compared with placebo significantly increased the proportion of people who responded (defined as no panic attacks and either no episodic increases in anxiety or only slight increases in anxiety precipitated by definite events or activities) after 12 months (citalopram 10 or 15 mg/day *v* placebo, $P = 0.05$; citalopram 20 or 30 mg/day *v* placebo, $P = 0.001$; citalopram 40 or 60 mg/day *v* placebo, $P = 0.003$; results presented graphically). The first subsequent RCT (182 people who had responded to open label sertraline for 52 weeks) compared double blind placebo (discontinuation of sertraline) versus sertraline for 28 weeks.[21] It found significantly more people on placebo had exacerbation of symptoms (33% with placebo *v* 13% with sertraline; $P = 0.005$; CI not available). The second subsequent RCT (43 people with panic disorder with or without agoraphobia who had been unsuccessfully treated with 15 sessions of manual guided cognitive behavioural therapy [see glossary, p 1194] alone) compared paroxetine 40 mg plus cognitive behavioural therapy versus placebo plus cognitive behavioural therapy (see comment below).[22] Success was defined as no panic attacks for a

2 week period or achieving cut-off scores or lower on panic disorder scales. It found combined treatment significantly increased success (12/19 [63%] with combined treatment v 5/19 [26%] with placebo plus cognitive behavioural therapy; RR 2.4, 95% CI 1.1 to 5.6; NNT 3, 95% CI 2 to 21).

Harms: The additional RCT reported that harms associated with citalopram included headache, tremor, dry mouth, and somnolence (see harms of prescription antidepressant drugs under depressive disorders, p 1121).[20] The first subsequent RCT found the highest incidence of adverse events with sertraline in the first 12 weeks of the study and tolerability seemed to improve with time.[21] The most common adverse events over the 52 weeks trial period were headache, malaise, insomnia, upper respiratory infection, diarrhoea, nausea, and dizziness. The second subsequent RCT did not report on adverse events.[22]

Comment: The first review included clomipramine as a selective serotonin reuptake inhibitor, although this drug is often described as a tricyclic antidepressant.[14] It also included the selective serotonin reuptake inhibitor zimelidine, which is rarely used these days. In addition, the review used improvement as an outcome measure without defining this term clearly. In the additional RCT, only just over half of people (28/54 [52%]) completed the trial; analysis was by intention to treat and people who withdrew from the trial were counted as treatment failures.[20] The RCT used flexible dosing according to tolerance and therapeutic need. Selective serotonin reuptake inhibitors can cause initial increased anxiety, which can exacerbate a tendency to focus on internal sensations and to avoid situations that trigger these sensations (catastrophise somatic sensations). Education about this event is likely to improve adherence with medication. The second systematic review found smaller RCTs were associated with larger effect sizes suggesting the possibility of publication bias.[19] The second subsequent RCT only used 8 weeks of medication as opposed to a more common 12 weeks, it only used clinician rated outcomes, and most people in both the placebo and paroxetine groups guessed correctly which treatment they had been allocated (62% with placebo *v* 79% with paroxetine).[22]

OPTION MONOAMINE OXIDASE INHIBITORS

We found no RCTs on the effects of monoamine oxidase inhibitors in panic disorder.

Benefits: We found no systematic review and no RCTs.

Harms: We found no evidence of harms associated specifically with the use of monoamine oxidase inhibitors in the long term treatment of panic disorder.

Comment: Our search strategy excluded studies with follow up of less than 6 months.

OPTION BUSPIRONE

We found insufficient evidence to assess the effects of buspirone in people with panic disorder.

Benefits: We found no systematic review but found two RCTs.[23,24] The first RCT (48 people) compared oral buspirone (maximum 60 mg/day) plus cognitive behavioural therapy (see glossary, p 1194) versus placebo plus cognitive behavioural therapy for 16 weeks.[23] It found that oral buspirone plus cognitive behavioural therapy significantly improved self rated panic and agoraphobia scores after 1 year (using a 90 point symptom scale where each symptom was graded from 0 = not present to 4 = severe; $P = 0.03$; absolute numbers not provided).[23] The second RCT (41 people with panic disorder and agoraphobia) compared 16 weeks of oral buspirone 30 mg daily plus cognitive behavioural therapy versus 16 weeks of placebo plus cognitive behavioural therapy.[24] It found no significant difference in the proportion of people who had a reduction of at least 50% in their agoraphobic symptoms after 68 weeks (44% with buspirone plus cognitive behavioural therapy *v* 68% with placebo plus cognitive behavioural therapy; absolute numbers of people not provided).

Harms: The RCTs did not report harms (see harms of buspirone under generalised anxiety disorder, p 1157).

Comment: The first RCT used a flexible dosing regimen with maximum dose adjustment according to tolerance and therapeutic need.[23]

OPTION BENZODIAZEPINES

One systematic review and one additional RCT have found that alprazolam reduces the number of panic attacks and improves symptoms compared with placebo in people with panic disorder. Benzodiazepines are associated with a wide range of adverse effects both during and after treatment.

Benefits: We found one systematic review (search date not stated, 27 RCTs, 2348 people; see benefits of tricyclic antidepressants, p 1190 and selective serotonin reuptake inhibitors, p 1191),[14] and one additional RCT.[15] The review found that alprazolam compared with placebo significantly increased the proportion of people judged to have improved ($P < 0.0001$; see comment below).[14] The additional RCT (181 people with panic disorder with or without agoraphobia) compared three treatments: oral alprazolam (maximum 10 mg/day; see comment below), oral imipramine (maximum 225 mg/day; see comment below), and placebo (see benefits of tricyclic antidepressants, p 1190 and selective serotonin reuptake inhibitors, p 1191).[15] It found that alprazolam compared with placebo was associated with fewer panic attacks after 8 months (results presented graphically; significance not calculated).

Harms: The systematic review did not report harms.[14] Adverse effects associated with alprazolam include sedation, insomnia, memory lapses, nervousness, irritability, dry mouth, tremor, impaired coordination, constipation, urinary retention, altered libido, and altered appetite (see harms of benzodiazepines under generalised anxiety disorder, p 1157).[15] We found one non-systematic review of the effects of benzodiazepines in anxiety disorder in people with a history of substance abuse or dependence.[25] The review reported that the mortality of long term benzodiazepine users was no higher than matched controls. It reported that the most pronounced adverse effects followed sudden withdrawal and included tinnitus, paraesthesia, vision disturbance, depersonalisation, seizures, withdrawal psychosis, and persistent discontinuation syndrome.

Comment: The review used improvement as an outcome measure without clearly defining this term.[14] The additional RCT used flexible dosing according to tolerance and therapeutic need.[15] Many RCTs of psychological and pharmacological treatments (even those not involving benzodiazepines) allowed people to receive small amounts of anxiolytic drugs during the study because benzodiazepine abuse is quite prevalent in people who suffer from panic disorder.

GLOSSARY

Cognitive behavioural therapy Brief structured treatment using relaxation and exposure procedures, and aimed at changing dysfunctional beliefs and negative automatic thoughts (typically 20 sessions over 12–16 weeks).

Substantive changes

Selective serotonin reuptake inhibitors One RCT added.[22] It found that paroxetine plus cognitive behavioural therapy improved symptoms more than placebo plus cognitive behavioural therapy.

REFERENCES

1. American Psychiatric Association. *Diagnostic and statistical manual of mental disorders*, 4th ed. Washington, DC: American Psychiatric Association, 1994.
2. World Health Organization. *The ICD-10 classification of mental and behavioural disorders*. Geneva: World Health Organization, 1992.
3. Robins LN, Regier DA, eds. *Psychiatric disorders in America: the epidemiologic catchment area study*. New York: Free Press, 1991.
4. Weissman MM, Bland MB, Canino GJ, et al. The cross-national epidemiology of panic disorder. *Arch Gen Psychiatry* 1997;54:305–309.
5. Andrews G, Henderson S, Hall W. Prevalence, comorbidity, disability and service utilisation. Overview of the Australian National Mental Health Survey. *Br J Psychiatry* 2001;178:145–153.
6. Last CG, Barlow DH, O'Brien GT. Precipitants of agoraphobia: role of stressful life events. *Psychol Rep* 1984;54:567–570.
7. De Loof C, Zandbergen H, Lousberg T, et al. The role of life events in the onset of panic disorder. *Behav Res Ther* 1989;27:461–463.
8. Rapee RM, Mattick RP, Murrell E. Impact of life events on subjects with panic disorder and on comparison subjects. *Am J Psychiatry* 1990;147:640–644.
9. Hirschfield RMA. Panic disorder: diagnosis, epidemiology and clinical course. *J Clin Psychiatry* 1996;57:3–8.
10. Andrews G, Creamer M, Crino R, et al. *The treatment of anxiety disorders*. Cambridge: Cambridge University Press, 1994.
11. Page AC, Andrews G. Do specific anxiety disorders show specific drug problems? *Aust N Z J Psychiatry* 1996;30:410–414.
12. Gorman JM, Coplan JD. Comorbidity of depression and panic disorder. *J Clin Psychiatry* 1996;57:34–41.
13. Tyrer P, Seivewright H, Simmonds S, et al. Prospective studies of cothymia (mixed anxiety-depression): how do they inform clinical practice? *Eur Arch Psychiatry Clin Neurosci* 2001;251:II53–II56.
14. Boyer W. Serotonin uptake inhibitors are superior to imipramine and alprazolam in alleviating panic attacks: a meta-analysis. *Int Clin Psychopharmacol* 1995;10:45–49. Search date not stated; primary sources Medline, Embase, Psychlit, and sponsoring agencies of two trials contacted for supplementary statistical information.
15. Curtis GC, Massana J, Udina C, et al. Maintenance drug therapy of panic disorder. *J Psychiatr Res* 1993;27:127–142.
16. Mavissakalian MR, Perel JM. Long-term maintenance and discontinuation of imipramine therapy in panic disorder with agoraphobia. *Arch Gen Psychiatry* 1999;56:821–827.
17. Barlow DH, Gorman J, Shear MK, et al. Cognitive-behavioral therapy, imipramine, or their combination for panic disorder: a randomized controlled trial. *JAMA* 2000;283:2529–2536.
18. Cassano GB, Toni C, Petracca A, et al. Adverse effects associated with the short-term treatment of panic disorder with imipramine, alprazolam or placebo. *Eur Neuropsychopharmacol* 1994;4:47–53.
19. Otto M, Tuby K, Gould R, et al. An effect-size analysis of the relative efficacy and tolerability of serotonin selective reuptake inhibitors for panic disorder. *Am J Psychiatry* 2001;158:1989–1992. Search date not stated; primary sources Medline, Psychlit, and hand searches of references.
20. Lepola UM, Wade AG, Leinonen EV, et al. A controlled, prospective, 1-year trial of citalopram in the treatment of panic disorder. *J Clin Psychiatry* 1998;59:528–534.
21. Rapaport M, Wolkow R, Rubin A, et al. Sertraline treatment of panic disorder: results of a long term study. *Acta Psych Scand* 2001;104:289–298.
22. Kampman M, Keijsers GP, Hoogduin CA, et al. A randomized, double-blind, placebo-controlled study of the effects of adjunctive paroxetine in panic disorder patients unsuccessfully treated with

cognitive-behavioral therapy alone. *J Clin Psychiatry* 2002;63:772–777.

23. Bouvard M, Mollard E, Guerin J, et al. Study and course of the psychological profile in 77 patients expressing panic disorder with agoraphobia after cognitive behaviour therapy with or without buspirone. *Psychother Psychosom* 1997;66:27–32.
24. Cottraux J, Note ID, Cungi C, et al. A controlled study of cognitive behaviour therapy with buspirone or placebo in panic disorder with agoraphobia. *Br J Psychiatry* 1995;167:635–641.
25. Posternak M, Mueller T. Assessing the risks and benefits of benzodiazepines for anxiety disorders in patients with a history of substance abuse or dependence. *Am J Addict* 2001;10:48–68.

Shailesh Kumar
Division of Psychiatry
Auckland Medical School
Auckland
New Zealand

Mark Oakley-Browne
Professor of Rural Psychiatry
Monash University
Gippsland, Victoria
Australia

Competing interests: SK was reimbursed by Eli-Lilly, the manufacturers of Prozac (fluoxetine), for attending several conferences. MOB has been paid by GlaxoSmithKline for contributing to educational sessions for general practitioners. The programme topic was "the recognition and management of generalised anxiety disorder". MOB has received reimbursement from Pfizer for attending a symposium.

Post-traumatic stress disorder

Search date September 2002

Jonathan Bisson

QUESTIONS

INTERVENTIONS

See glossary, p 1205

Key Messages

Prevention

- **Multiple episode cognitive behavioural therapy in all people exposed to a traumatic event** One RCT in bus drivers who had been attacked in the past 5 months found that cognitive behavioural therapy significantly improved measures of anxiety and intrusive symptoms at 6 months compared with usual care, but found no significant difference in measures of depression or avoidance symptoms. Another RCT comparing cognitive behavioural therapy versus standard care in people who had been exposed to a traumatic event in the past 5–12 months found no significant difference in overall symptoms of post-traumatic stress disorder at 6 months.

- **Multiple episode cognitive behavioural therapy in people with acute stress disorder** Two small RCTs in people with acute stress disorder after a traumatic event (accident or non-sexual assault) found that five sessions of cognitive behavioural therapy significantly reduces the proportion of people with post-traumatic stress disorder after 6 months compared with supportive counselling.
- **Multiple episode memory restructuring** One RCT provided insufficient evidence to assess memory restructuring compared with supportive care in people exposed to a traumatic event in the past 24 hours.
- **Multiple episode trauma support** Two RCTs provided insufficient evidence to assess collaborative care interventions involving emotional, social, and practical support in people exposed to a traumatic event in the past 1 day to 1 week.
- **Single episode psychological interventions ("debriefing") in all people exposed to a traumatic event** RCTs in people who had been exposed to a traumatic event in the previous month found no significant difference between a single session of psychological debriefing and no debriefing in the incidence of post-traumatic stress disorder at 3 months or 1 year.

Treatment

- **Cognitive behavioural therapy** RCTs have found that cognitive behavioural therapy significantly improves post-traumatic stress disorder symptoms, anxiety, and depression compared with no treatment or supportive counselling.
- **Eye movement desensitisation and reprocessing** RCTs have found that eye movement desensitisation and reprocessing improves symptoms compared with waiting list control or relaxation treatment. Two RCTs found no significant difference in symptoms between eye movement desensitisation and reprocessing compared with exposure therapy.
- **Fluoxetine** Two RCTs found that fluoxetine may reduce symptoms at 3 months compared with placebo.
- **Paroxetine** One systematic review and subsequent RCTs found that paroxetine reduced symptoms at 3 months compared with placebo.
- **Sertraline** One systematic review and subsequent RCTs found that sertraline significantly reduced symptoms at 3–7 months compared with placebo.
- **Affect management; drama therapy; hypnotherapy; inpatient programmes; other drug treatments (brofaromine, amitriptyline, lamotrigine, imipramine, phenelzine, nefazodone, carbamazepine, antipychotics, benzodiazepines); psychodynamic psychotherapy; supportive counselling** We found insufficient evidence about the effects of these interventions in improving symptoms.

DEFINITION Post-traumatic stress disorder (PTSD) can occur after a major traumatic event. Symptoms include upsetting thoughts and nightmares about the traumatic event, avoidance behaviour, numbing of general responsiveness, increased irritability, and hypervigilance for at least 1 month.[1] Acute stress disorder occurs within the first month after a major traumatic event and requires the presence of symptoms for at least 2 days. It is similar to PTSD but more dissociative symptoms are required to make the diagnosis.

INCIDENCE/ PREVALENCE	One large cross-sectional study in the USA found that 1/10 women and 1/20 men experience PTSD at some stage in their lives.[2]
AETIOLOGY/ RISK FACTORS	Risk factors include major trauma, such as rape, a history of psychiatric disorders, acute distress and depression after the trauma, lack of social support, and personality factors (such as neuroticism).[3]
PROGNOSIS	One large cross-sectional study in the USA found that over a third of sufferers continued to satisfy the criteria for a diagnosis of PTSD 6 years after diagnosis.[2] However, cross-sectional studies provide weak evidence about prognosis.
AIMS OF INTERVENTION	To reduce initial distress after a traumatic event; to prevent PTSD and other psychiatric disorders; to reduce levels of distress in the long term; to improve function and quality of life.
OUTCOMES	Presence or absence of PTSD and severity of symptoms assessed by continuous measures. Continuous measures for assessing changes in symptoms include impact of event scale and clinician administered PTSD scale; symptoms assessed include anxiety, depression, intrusion, and avoidance. Changes in continuous measures are often expressed as effect sizes. It is difficult to interpret effect sizes in terms of clinical importance rather than statistical significance. Some categorise effect sizes of less than 0.5 as small; 0.5–0.8 as medium; and greater than 0.8 as large.
METHODS	*Clinical Evidence* search and appraisal September 2002.

QUESTION What are the effects of preventive psychological interventions?

The evidence about the effects of preventive psychological interventions in preventing post-traumatic stress disorder (PTSD) is generally poor and inconclusive. RCTs in people who had been exposed to a traumatic event in the past month found no significant difference between a single debriefing session and no debriefing in the incidence of PTSD at 3 months or 1 year. Two RCTs in people with acute stress disorder after a traumatic event (road traffic accident or non-sexual assault) found that five sessions of either cognitive behavioural therapy or prolonged exposure significantly reduced the proportion of people with PTSD after 6 months compared with supportive counselling. One RCT in bus drivers who had been attacked in the past 5 months found that cognitive behavioural therapy significantly improved measures of anxiety and intrusive symptoms at 6 months compared with usual care, but found no significant difference in measures of depression or avoidance symptoms. Another RCT comparing cognitive behavioural therapy versus standard care in people who had been exposed to a traumatic event in the past 5–12 months found no significant difference in overall symptoms of PTSD at 6 months. RCTs provided insufficient evidence to assess collaborative care interventions involving emotional, social, and practical support, or memory restructuring in people exposed to a traumatic event in the past 1 day to 1 week.

Benefits: **Single episode intervention:** We found one systematic review (search date 2001, 11 RCTs, 1759 people)[4] and one subsequent RCT[5] comparing early (within 1 month) single episode interventions ("debriefing") versus no intervention. The RCTs in the review used psychological debriefing (see glossary, p 1205) or similar techniques after traumatic events. The review found that debriefing was associated with an increase in the risk of PTSD at 3 months and 1 year, although the difference was not significant (OR at 3 months 1.1, 95% CI 0.6 to 2.5; OR at 12 months 2.0, 95% CI 0.9 to 4.5).[4] The subsequent RCT (77 people who had been robbed) compared early group debriefing (within 10 h) versus delayed group debriefing (after > 48 h).[5] Early debriefing significantly reduced symptom severity measured on the Post-traumatic Stress Diagnostic Scale at 2 weeks compared with delayed debriefing (mean score 6.94 with early debriefing *v* 33.10 with delayed debriefing; P < 0.001). **Multiple episode intervention:** We found no systematic review but found seven RCTs.[6–12] The first RCT (24 people with acute stress disorder 2 wks after a road traffic accident or industrial accident) compared five sessions of cognitive behavioural therapy versus five sessions of supportive counselling (see glossary, p 1205).[6] It found that cognitive behavioural therapy significantly reduced the proportion of people who met PTSD diagnostic criteria immediately after treatment compared with supportive counselling (AR 8% with cognitive behavioural therapy *v* 83% with supportive counselling; P < 0.001) and at 6 months (AR 17% with cognitive behavioural therapy *v* 67% with supportive counselling; P < 0.05). The second RCT (45 survivors of road traffic accidents or non-sexual assault with acute stress disorder) compared three treatments: five 90 minute sessions of prolonged exposure (see glossary, p 1205) therapy; prolonged exposure therapy plus anxiety management; or supportive counselling.[7] It found that, immediately after completion of treatment, both prolonged exposure alone and prolonged exposure plus anxiety management significantly reduced rates of PTSD compared with supportive counselling (AR 2/14 [14%] with prolonged exposure *v* 9/16 [56%] with prolonged exposure plus anxiety management *v* 3/15 [20%] with supportive counselling; P < 0.05 for either group *v* supportive counselling). The differences remained significant at 6 months' follow up (AR 2/13 [15%] with prolonged exposure *v* 3/13 [23%] with anxiety management *v* 10/15 [67%] with supportive counselling; P < 0.05 for each group *v* supportive counselling). The third RCT (151 people who had been involved in a road traffic accident in the past 12 months) compared 3–6 sessions of educational and cognitive behavioural therapy techniques versus no psychological intervention.[8] The RCT found that people in the treatment group had a significantly higher baseline risk of PTSD compared with the no intervention group, which makes the results difficult to interpret. The RCT found no significant difference between groups in rates of PTSD at 6 months. The fourth RCT (132 bus drivers who had been attacked in the past 5 months) comparing 1–6 sessions of cognitive behavioural therapy versus standard care found that cognitive behavioural therapy significantly improved measures of anxiety and intrusive symptoms at 6 months, but found no significant difference in measures of depression or avoidance symptoms.[9] The fifth RCT (70 people who had been admitted to hospital after a road traffic accident in the past wk) compared three treatments: social work intervention (emotional, practical, and social support for 2–10 h in the first 3 months); immediate review (a single debriefing intervention); and no intervention.[10] It found that the social work intervention significantly reduced the risk of a poor outcome (based on traumatic neurosis symptoms) compared with immediate review, although both interventions reduced the risk of a poor outcome compared with no intervention (AR for a poor outcome 30% with social work *v* 60% with immediate review *v* 87% with no intervention; ARR for social work *v* no intervention 57%, NNT 2; ARR for immediate review *v* no intervention 27%, NNT 4; CIs not provided; $P < 0.001$ for either intervention group *v* no intervention; $P < 0.05$ for comparison between the intervention groups). The sixth RCT (34 survivors of road traffic accidents or assault in the past 24 h) compared a 4 month collaborative care (see glossary, p 1205) intervention (emotional, practical, and social support from a trauma support specialist) versus no intervention.[11] After 4 months, the risk of developing PTSD was lower with collaborative care than with no intervention, but the difference was not significant (AR for PTSD 17% with collaborative care *v* 43% with no intervention; CI not provided; $P > 0.1$). The RCT might have lacked power to exclude a clinically important difference between treatments. The seventh RCT (17 survivors of a road traffic accident in the past 24–48 h) compared two sessions of memory structuring versus supportive listening (see glossary, p 1205).[12] It found that memory structuring significantly reduced mean scores on the PTSD scale at 3 months compared with supportive listening (mean score 8.1 with memory structuring *v* 18.5 with supportive listening; $P < 0.05$).[12]

Harms: **Single episode intervention:** Two RCTs included in the systematic review found an increased risk of subsequent psychological problems in people receiving the intervention.[4] However, initial traumatic exposure had been higher in these people. **Multiple episode intervention:** The RCTs gave no information on adverse effects.[6–12]

Comment: The systematic review of single episode debriefing found that the overall quality of RCTs was poor.[4] Problems included lack of blinding, failure to state loss to follow up, and lack of intention to treat analysis despite high withdrawal rates. These method problems are also apparent in the multiple episode intervention RCTs. The third multiple episode psychological treatment RCT included multiple types of intervention (help, information, support, and reality testing/confrontation) in the treatment group.[8]

QUESTION What are the effects of psychological treatments?

Small RCTs have found that specific psychological treatments, including cognitive behavioural therapy, psychodynamic psychotherapy, and eye movement desensitisation and reprocessing, improve symptoms of post-traumatic stress disorder compared with supportive counselling, relaxation treatment, or no treatment. RCTs provided insufficient evidence to assess affect management, group therapy, psychodynamic psychotherapy, eclectic psychotherapy, or interapy. We found no RCTs of drama therapy or inpatient treatment programmes.

Benefits: **Cognitive behavioural therapy:** We found one systematic review (search date not stated)[13] and four subsequent RCTs of cognitive behavioural therapy (see glossary, p 1205).[14–17] The review compared a range of specific psychological treatments versus supportive counselling (see glossary, p 1205) or no treatment. It identified

17 RCTs (690 people), including 6 RCTs (232 people) of cognitive behavioural therapy. All RCTs identified by the review found that psychological treatments were associated with a greater improvement in immediate outcome (using a composite score of post-traumatic stress disorder [PTSD] symptoms, anxiety, and depression) compared with supportive counselling or no treatment (17 RCTs, 690 people: overall effect size immediately after treatment 0.54; CI not provided). The difference was still evident at 1 year (overall effect size from 12 RCTs with long term follow up 0.53; CI not provided). The first subsequent RCT (87 people) compared exposure, cognitive therapy, or both, versus relaxation treatment (see glossary, p 1205).[14] It found that all cognitive behavioural therapies reduced symptoms of PTSD more than relaxation treatment, immediately and at 3 months (53 people evaluated; no intention to treat analysis performed). The second subsequent RCT (72 people) found no significant difference in symptoms at 1 year between 16 1-hour sessions of imaginal exposure therapy (see glossary, p 1205) and cognitive therapy (results not intention to treat; 54 people analysed; effect size 0.88 with imaginal exposure *v* 1.06 with cognitive therapy; reported as non-significant). It found that overall 21/54 (39%) of people continued to suffer from PTSD at 1 year.[15] The third subsequent RCT (168 female victims of sexual assault or childhood sexual abuse with PTSD and chronic nightmares) compared three sessions of imagery rehearsal therapy (see glossary, p 1205) versus no treatment over 5 weeks.[16] It found that imagery rehearsal therapy significantly improved PTSD symptoms at 3 or 6 months compared with no treatment (AR for symptoms improving by at least one level of clinical severity 65% with imagery rehearsal *v* 31% with no treatment; ARR 34%; NNT 3, CI not provided; $P < 0.001$). The fourth subsequent RCT (171 female victims of sexual assault) compared three treatments: cognitive processing therapy; prolonged exposure (see glossary, p 1205); or minimal attention (telephone call every 2 wks) for 6 weeks.[17] It found that, immediately after treatment, both cognitive processing and prolonged exposure significantly reduced rates of PTSD compared with minimal attention (AR for PTSD 33/62 [53%] with cognitive processing *v* 33/62 [53%] with prolonged exposure *v* 1/45 [2%] with minimal attention; $P < 0.001$ for both interventions *v* placebo). **Psychodynamic psychotherapy:** The systematic review of a range of psychological treatments[13] identified one RCT (112 people) that compared four interventions: psychodynamic psychotherapy, exposure therapy, hypnotherapy (see glossary, p 1205), and waiting list control.[18] It found that symptoms were improved from baseline significantly more within all active groups compared with waiting list control. However, the trial did not test the significance of comparative results. **Eye movement desensitisation and reprocessing:** We found one systematic review (search date 2000), which identified 9 RCTs (number of people not stated) in people with PTSD.[19] It found that eye movement desensitisation and reprocessing (EMDR) (see glossary, p 1205) was significantly more effective than no treatment in reducing symptoms of PTSD (effect size 0.39, CI not stated; $P < 0.05$). However, it found no significant difference between EMDR and cognitive behavioural

therapy/exposure therapy (effect size for EMDR *v* cognitive behavioural therapy/exposure therapy –0.44, CI not stated; reported as non-significant) or between EMDR with eye movements and EMDR without eye movements (effect size 0.22, CI not stated; reported as non-significant). **Affect management:** We found no systematic review, but found one RCT (48 women) comparing 15 weeks of affect management (see glossary, p 1205) treatment (in addition to drug treatment) versus waiting list control.[20] It found that control of PTSD and dissociative symptoms was greater with affect management. **Group therapy:** We found no systematic review but found one RCT (55 female survivors of childhood sexual abuse with PTSD) comparing three treatments: trauma focused group therapy; present focused group therapy (see glossary, p 1205); or waiting list control.[21] Group therapy was undertaken in 90 minute sessions for 24 weeks. The RCT found that either type of group therapy significantly improved symptoms of dissociation and sexual abuse trauma ($P < 0.05$ for both outcomes) compared with waiting list control, but found no significant difference in overall symptoms (symptoms assessed using the Trauma Symptom Checklist 40: mean difference in score 8.1 with group therapy *v* 3.8 with wait list control; reported as non-significant; no further data provided). The RCT prospectively defined three groups, but combined results for both active treatment groups in its analysis. This makes the results difficult to interpret. It is likely to have been underpowered to detect a clinically important difference between groups. **Eclectic psychotherapy:** We found no systematic review but found one RCT (42 police officers) comparing brief eclectic psychotherapy (combining components of cognitive behavioural therapy and psychodynamic psychotherapy) versus waiting list control over 16 sessions of treatment.[22] It found that eclectic psychotherapy significantly reduced the proportion of people with PTSD immediately after treatment (AR for PTSD 9% with eclectic psychotherapy *v* 50% with waiting list control; $P < 0.01$) and at 3 months (AR 4% with eclectic psychotherapy *v* 65% with waiting list control; $P < 0.01$). **Interapy:** We found no systematic review but found one RCT (25 people) that compared interapy (see glossary, p 1205) versus waiting list control for 5 weeks.[23] It found that, at 5 weeks, interapy significantly improved intrusive symptom score from baseline compared with waiting list control (mean reduction 11.0 with interapy *v* 3.6 with waiting list control; $P < 0.04$) and reduced avoidance score (mean reduction 9.6 with interapy *v* 2.9 with waiting list control; $P < 0.03$). **Drama therapy:** See glossary, p 1205. We found no RCTs. **Inpatient treatment programmes:** We found no RCTs.

Harms: The systematic reviews[13,19] and subsequent RCTs[14–18,20,22,23] gave no information on adverse effects. Overall, cognitive behavioural therapy seems well tolerated. However, there have been case reports of worsening symptoms in some people receiving imaginal flooding (see glossary, p 1205), leading to calls for caution when evaluating people for treatment.[24] The RCT of affect management treatment had a high withdrawal rate (31%), specific drug treatments were not stated, and the analysis was not by intention to treat.

Comment: None.

QUESTION What are the effects of drug treatments?

One systematic review and subsequent RCTs have found that sertraline or paroxetine reduces symptoms at 3–7 months compared with placebo. RCTs found more limited evidence from the systematic review and one subsequent RCT that fluoxetine may reduce symptoms at 3 months compared with placebo. RCTs found insufficient evidence about brofaromine, amitriptyline, lamotrigine, imipramine, phenelzine, nefazodone, carbamazepine, antipsychotics, and benzodiazepines.

Benefits: **Antidepressant drugs:** We found one systematic review (search date 1999, 15 RCTs, 9 with sufficient data for inclusion in the meta-analysis, 868 people) of antidepressant drugs for post-traumatic stress disorder (PTSD), which used the Clinical Global Impressions (CGI) scale change item or close equivalent as the primary outcome measure.[25] The review found that the proportion of non-responders at 1–3.5 months was significantly lower with antidepressants than with placebo (response defined as CGI score of 1 [very much improved] or 2 [much improved]; RR 0.72, 95% CI 0.64 to 0.83). Two RCTs identified by the review assessed sertraline (42 people: OR 0.44, 95% CI 0.12 to 1.60; 183 people: OR 0.44, 95% CI 0.24 to 0.78), one paroxetine (280 people: OR 0.64, 95% CI 0.40 to 1.02), one fluoxetine (53 people: OR 0.30, 95% CI 0.09 to 1.02), two brofaromine (114 people: OR 0.94, 95% CI 0.45 to 1.99; 64 people: OR 0.40, 95% CI 0.15 to 1.08), one amitriptyline (40 people: OR 0.41, 95% CI 0.12 to 1.42), one lamotrigine (14 people: OR 0.39, 95% CI 0.04 to 3.71), and one imipramine or phenelzine (imipramine, 41 people: OR 0.23, 95% CI 0.07 to 0.78; phenelzine, 37 people: OR 0.21, 95% CI 0.06 to 0.73). We also found seven subsequent RCTs: six placebo controlled RCTs (3 evaluating sertraline,[26–28] 2 evaluating paroxetine,[29,30] and 1 evaluating fluoxetine[31]) and one RCT comparing sertraline versus nefazodone.[32] All but one subsequent RCT found improved symptoms with antidepressant treatment. The first subsequent RCT (208 people) found that sertraline (50–200 mg/day) significantly reduced symptoms at 12 weeks compared with placebo (mean reduction in PTSD symptom score on the clinician administered PTSD scale –33.0 with sertraline *v* –26.2 with placebo; $P = 0.04$).[26] The second subsequent RCT (96 people who had previously responded to sertraline for acute treatment of PTSD) found that sertraline significantly reduced PTSD relapse after 28 weeks compared with placebo (AR 5% with sertraline *v* 26% with placebo; ARR 21%; NNT 5; CI not provided; $P < 0.02$).[27] The third subsequent RCT (42 veteran male soldiers) found no significant difference between sertraline (50–200 mg/day) and placebo in symptoms of PTSD after 10 weeks of treatment (mean reduction in clinician administered PTSD score –18.7 with sertraline *v* –13.5 with placebo; $P = 0.53$; see comment below).[28] The fourth subsequent RCT (307 people) found that paroxetine 20–50 mg daily significantly increased response rate at 12 weeks compared with placebo (response defined as "very much improved" or "much improved" on the CGI scale; AR 59% with paroxetine *v* 38% with control; ARR 21%; NNT 5; CIs not provided; $P = 0.008$).[29] The fifth subsequent RCT (551 people) found that paroxetine 20 or 40 mg daily significantly improved response rate (using the same definition) at 12 weeks compared with placebo (AR for response 62% with 20 mg paroxetine *v* 54% with 40 mg paroxetine *v* 37% with placebo; $P < 0.001$ for both paroxetine groups compared with placebo).[30] The sixth subsequent RCT (301 people, primarily male soldiers) found that fluoxetine 50–80 mg daily significantly improved symptoms compared with placebo after 12 weeks treatment (mean reduction in clinician administered PTSD score −34.6 with fluoxetine *v* −29.6 with placebo; $P = 0.021$).[31] The seventh subsequent RCT comparing sertraline 50–100 mg daily versus nefazodone 200–400 mg daily found no significant difference in symptoms at 5 months (mean total eight item PTSD scale [TOP-8] score 5.23 with sertraline *v* 4.35 with nefazodone; $P = 0.36$).[32] However, the results of that RCT should be interpreted with caution because, despite randomisation, people taking sertraline had significantly higher baseline TOP-8 scores than people taking nefazodone. **Carbamazepine:** We found no RCTs. **Antipsychotic drugs:** We found no RCTs. **Benzodiazepines:** We found one RCT, which was not included in the systematic review above because of insufficient data.[25]

Harms: **Antidepressant drugs:** The systematic review gave no information on adverse effects, although it found no significant difference between antidepressants and placebo in the proportion of people who withdrew for any cause (7 RCTs; 712 people; RR 0.85, 95% CI 0.63 to 1.14).[25] The first subsequent RCT found that, compared with placebo, sertraline significantly increased insomnia (35% with sertraline *v* 22% with placebo; $P = 0.04$), diarrhoea (28% *v* 11%; $P = 0.003$), and nausea (23% *v* 11%; $P = 0.03$), and decreased appetite (12% with sertraline *v* 1% with placebo; $P = 0.001$).[26] The fourth subsequent RCT comparing paroxetine versus placebo found that adverse effects with an incidence of at least 10% and twice that of placebo were nausea (19.2% with paroxetine *v* 8.3% with placebo), somnolence (17.2% *v* 3.8%), dry mouth (13.9% *v* 4.5%), asthenia (13.2% *v* 5.2%), and abnormal ejaculation (11.8% *v* 3.7%).[29] One RCT (65 people) assessing the harms of fluoxetine in people with PTSD found that fluoxetine was associated with significantly higher rates of nausea, diarrhoea, and thirst compared with placebo ($P < 0.05$ for all outcomes).[33] Known adverse effects of antidepressants include possible hypertensive crisis with monoamine oxidase inhibitors (and also a need for dietary restriction), anticholinergic effects with tricyclic antidepressants, and nausea and headache with selective serotonin reuptake inhibitors (see harms of prescription antidepressant drugs under depressive disorders, p 1121). **Benzodiazepines:** Known adverse effects include dependency (see harms of benzodiazepines under generalised anxiety disorder, p 1157).

Comment: Small trial sizes and different populations make it difficult to compare results. The veteran soldiers in the third subsequent RCT evaluating sertraline had higher baseline clinician administered PTSD scores (mean baseline score 94.3) than people in the other RCTs of sertraline (mean baseline score about 74); this may explain the lack of significant improvement in symptoms between sertraline and placebo.[28]

GLOSSARY

Affect management A type of group treatment focusing on regulation of mood.

Cognitive behavioural therapy Covers a variety of techniques. *Imaginal exposure* entails exposure to a detailed account or image of what happened. *Real life exposure* involves confronting real life situations that have become associated with the trauma and cause fear and distress. *Cognitive therapy* entails challenging distorted thoughts about the trauma, the self, and the world. *Imaginal flooding* involves the intense reliving of the traumatic experience. *Memory structuring* involves listening to and clarifying the individual's narrative and structuring it for them to repeat to friends and family. *Stress inoculation* entails instruction in coping skills and some cognitive techniques such as restructuring. *Prolonged exposure* entails repeated exposure to memories of the trauma, and to non-dangerous real life situations that are avoided because of trauma related fear. *Supportive listening* involves actively listening to the individual's narrative and clarifying factual, sensory, and affective details.

Cognitive processing therapy Includes elements of cognitive therapy and writing and reading about the traumatic event.

Collaborative care Entails counselling, liaison, and coordination of care after discharge.

Drama therapy Entails using drama as a form of expression and communication.

Eye movement desensitisation and reprocessing (EMDR) Entails asking the person to focus on the traumatic event, a negative cognition associated with it, and the associated emotions.[34] The person is then asked to follow the therapist's finger as it moves from side to side.

Hypnotherapy Entails hypnosis to allow people to work through the traumatic event.

Imagery rehearsal therapy Involves encouraging participants to practice pleasant imagery exercises and employ cognitive behavioural tools to deal with unpleasant images.

Interapy A protocol driven treatment delivered through the internet, which includes psychoeducation and cognitive reappraisal. For further information, see http://www.interapy.nl.

Present focused group therapy A group intervention that involves identifying and modifying patterns of behaviour that have arisen from their past traumatic experience.

Psychodynamic psychotherapy Entails analysis of defence mechanisms, interpretations, and pre-trauma experiences.

Psychological debriefing A technique that entails detailed consideration of the traumatic event and the normalisation of psychological reactions.

Relaxation treatment A technique involving imagination of relaxing situations to induce muscular and mental relaxation.

Supportive counselling A non-directive intervention dealing with current issues rather than the trauma itself.

Trauma focused group therapy A group intervention that involves reconstructing a past traumatic event, identifying and modifying negative self images associated with it, and integrating memories of the event into the individual's conscious awareness of self and others.

REFERENCES

1. American Psychiatric Association. *Diagnostic and statistical manual of mental disorders*. 4th ed. Washington: APA, 1994.
2. Kessler RC, Sonnega A, Bromet E, et al. Posttraumatic stress disorder in the national comorbidity survey. *Arch Gen Psychiatry* 1995;52:1048–1060.
3. O'Brien S. *Traumatic events and mental health*. Cambridge: Cambridge University Press, 1998.
4. Rose S, Bisson J, Wessely S. Psychological debriefing for preventing post traumatic stress disorder (PTSD). In: The Cochrane Library, Issue 3, 2002. Oxford: Update Software. Search date 2001; primary sources Medline, Embase,

PsychLit, Pilots, Biosis, Pascal, Occupational Safety and Health, Sociofile, Cinahl, Psycinfo, Psyndex, Sigle, Lilacs, Cochrane Controlled Clinical Trials, National Research Register, hand search of Journal of Traumatic Stress, and contact with leading researchers.
5. Campfield KM, Hills AM. Effect of timing of critical incident stress debriefing (CISD) on posttraumatic symptoms. *J Traum Stress* 2001;14:327–340.
6. Bryant RA, Harvey AG, Basten C, et al. Treatment of acute stress disorder: a comparison of cognitive behavioural therapy and supportive counselling. *J Consult Clin Psychol* 1998;66:862–866.
7. Bryant RA, Sackville T, Dang ST, et al. Treating acute stress disorder: an evaluation of cognitive behavior therapy and supportive counselling techniques. *Am J Psychiatry* 1999;156:1780–1786.
8. Brom D, Kleber RJ, Hofman MC. Victims of traffic accidents: incidence and prevention of post-traumatic stress disorder. *J Clin Psychol* 1993;49:131–140.
9. Andre C, Lelord F, Legeron P, et al. Controlled study of outcomes after 6 months to early intervention of bus driver victims of aggression [in French]. *Encephale* 1997;23:65–71.
10. Bordow S, Porritt D. An experimental evaluation of crisis intervention. *Soc Sci Med* 1979;13A:251–256.
11. Zatzick DF, Roy-Byrne P, Russo JE, et al. Collaborative interventions for physically injured trauma survivors: a pilot randomized effectiveness trial. *Gen Hosp Psychiatry* 2001;23:114–123.
12. Gidron Y, Gal R, Freedman S, et al. Translating research findings to PTSD prevention: results of a randomised controlled pilot study. *J Trauma Stress* 2001;14:773–780.
13. Sherman JJ. Effects of psychotherapeutic treatments for PTSD: a meta-analysis of controlled clinical trials. *J Trauma Stress* 1998;11:413–436. Search date not stated; primary sources Psychlit, Eric, Medline, Cinahl, Dissertation Abstracts, and Pilots Traumatic Stress Database.
14. Marks I, Lovell K, Noshirvani H, et al. Treatment of posttraumatic stress disorder by exposure and/or cognitive restructuring: a controlled study. *Arch Gen Psychiatry* 1998;55:317–325.
15. Tarrier N, Sommerfield C, Pilgrim H, et al. Cognitive therapy or imaginal exposure in the treatment of post-traumatic stress disorder. *Br J Psychiatry* 1999;175:571–575.
16. Krakow B, Hollifield M, Johnston L, et al. Imagery rehearsal therapy for chronic nightmares in sexual assault survivors with posttraumatic stress disorder: a randomized controlled trial. *JAMA* 2001;286:537–545.
17. Resick A, Nishith P, Weaver TL, et al. A comparison of cognitive-processing therapy with prolonged exposure and a waiting condition for the treatment of chronic posttraumatic stress disorder in female rape victims. *J Consult Clin Psychol* 2002;70:867–879.
18. Brom D, Kleber RJ, Defares PB. Brief psychotherapy of posttraumatic stress disorders. *J Consult Clin Psychol* 1989;57:607–612.
19. Davidson PR, Parker KC. Eye movement desensitisation and reprocessing (EMDR): a meta-analysis. *J Consult Clin Psychol* 2001;69:305–316. Medline and Psychinfo searched between 1988 and April 2000, and Current Contents searched from 1997 to March 2000, plus reference lists from articles found in these searches.
20. Zlotnick C, Shea T, Rosen K, et al. An affect-management group for women with posttraumatic stress disorder and histories of childhood sexual abuse. *J Trauma Stress* 1997;10:425–436.
21. Classen C, Koopman C, Nevill-Manning K, et al. A preliminary report comparing trauma-focused and present-focused group therapy against a wait-listed condition among childhood sexual abuse survivors with PTSD. *J Aggress Maltreat Trauma* 2001;4:265–288.
22. Gersons BPR, Carlier IVE, Lamberts RD, et al. Randomised clinical trial of brief eclectic psychotherapy for police officers with posttraumatic stress disorder. *J Trauma Stress* 2000;13:333–348.
23. Lange A, Van de Ven JP, Schrieken B, et al. Interapy: treatment of posttraumatic stress through the Internet: a controlled trial. *J Behav Ther Exp Psychiatry* 2001;32:73–90.
24. Pitman RK, Altman B, Greenwald E, et al. Psychiatric complications during flooding therapy for posttraumatic stress disorder. *J Clin Psychiatry* 1991;52:17–20.
25. Stein DJ, Zungu-Dirwayi N, Van der Linden GJ, et al. Pharmacotherapy for posttraumatic stress disorder. In: The Cochrane Library, Issue 3, 2002. Oxford: Update Software. Search date 1999; primary sources Medline, Psychlit, Pilots Traumatic Stress Database, Dissertation Abstracts, trials register of the Cochrane Depression, Anxiety and Neurosis Controlled Group, hand searches of reference lists, and personal contact with post-traumatic stress disorder researchers and pharmaceutical companies.
26. Davidson JR, Rothbaum BO, van der Kolk BA, et al. Multicenter, double blind comparison of sertraline and placebo in the treatment of posttraumatic stress disorder. *Arch Gen Psychiatry* 2001;58:485–492.
27. Davidson J, Pearlstein T, Londborg P, et al. Efficacy of sertraline in preventing relapse of posttraumatic stress disorder: results of a 28-week double-blind, placebo-controlled study. *Am J Psychiatry* 2001;158:1974–1981.
28. Zohar J, Amital D, Miodownik C. Double-blind placebo-controlled pilot study of sertraline in military veterans with posttraumatic stress disorder. *J Clin Psychopharmacol* 2002;22:190–195.
29. Tucker P, Zaninelli R, Yehuda R, et al. Paroxetine in the treatment of chronic posttraumatic stress disorder: results of a placebo-controlled, flexible-dosage trial. *J Clin Psychiatry* 2001;62:860–868.
30. Marshall RD, Beebe KL, Oldham M, et al. Efficacy and safety of paroxetine treatment for chronic PTSD: a fixed-dose, placebo-controlled study. *Am J Psychiatry* 2001;158:1982–1988.
31. Martenyi F, Brown EB, Zhang H, et al. Fluoxetine versus placebo in posttraumatic stress disorder. *J Clin Psychiatry* 2002;63:199–206.
32. Saygin MZ, Sungur MZ, Sabol EU, et al. Nefazodone versus sertraline in treatment of posttraumatic stress disorder. *Bull Clin Psychopharmacol* 2002;12:1–5.
33. Barnett SD, Tharwani HM, Hertzberg MA, et al. Tolerability of fluoxetine in posttraumatic stress disorder. *Prog Neuropsychopharmacol Biol Psychiatry* 2002;26:363–367.
34. Shapiro F. Eye movement desensitisation: a new treatment for post-traumatic stress disorder. *J Behav Ther Exp Psychiatry* 1989;20:211–217.

Post-traumatic stress disorder

Jonathan Bisson
Consultant Liaison Psychiatrist
Cardiff and Vale NHS Trust
Cardiff
UK

Competing interests: None declared.

Schizophrenia

Search date December 2002

Zia Nadeem, Andrew McIntosh, and Stephen Lawrie

QUESTIONS

INTERVENTIONS

See glossary, p 1233

Key Messages

- Most evidence is from systematic reviews of RCTs that report disparate outcomes. There is a need for larger RCTs, over longer periods, with well designed end points, including standardised, validated symptom scales. No intervention has been found to consistently reduce negative symptoms.

- **Continuation of antipsychotic drugs for 6–9 months after an acute episode to reduce relapse rates** Systematic reviews have found that continuing antipsychotic drugs for at least 6 months after an acute episode reduces relapse rates compared with no treatment or placebo, and that some benefit of continuing antipsychotics is apparent for up to 2 years.
- **Multiple session family interventions to reduce relapse rates** One systematic review found that multiple session family interventions reduced relapse rates at 12 months compared with usual care, single session family interventions, or psychoeducational interventions.
- **Psychoeducational interventions to reduce relapse rates** One systematic review has found that psychoeducation reduces relapse rates at 9–18 months compared with a control intervention.
- **Behavioural therapy to improve adherence** One RCT found that behavioural interventions improved adherence to antipsychotic medication over 3 months compared with usual treatment. Two RCTs found limited evidence that behavioural interventions may improve adherence more than psychoeducational therapy.
- **Compliance therapy to improve adherence** Two RCTs found limited evidence that compliance therapy may increase adherence to antipsychotic drugs at 6 and 18 months compared with non-specific counselling.
- **Psychoeducational interventions to improve adherence** One systematic review found limited evidence that psychoeducation improved adherence to antipsychotic medication compared with usual care. Two RCTs found limited evidence that psychoeducational may improve adherence less than behavioural therapy.
- **Chlorpromazine** One systematic review has found that, compared with placebo, chlorpromazine reduces the proportion of people who have no improvement, or have marked or worse severity of illness at 6 months on a psychiatrist rated scale. The review found that chlorpromazine caused more adverse effects, such as sedation, acute dystonia, and parkinsonism, than placebo.
- **Clozapine** Two systematic reviews found that clozapine improved symptoms over 4–10 weeks compared with standard antipsychotic drugs. However, RCTs found that clozapine may be associated with blood dyscrasias. Three systematic reviews of small RCTs provided insufficient evidence to compare clozapine versus other new antipsychotic drugs. One systematic review in people resistant to standard treatment found that clozapine improved symptoms after 12 weeks and after 2 years compared with standard antipsychotic drugs. RCTs provided insufficient evidence to compare clozapine versus other newer antipsychotics in people resistant to standard antipsychotic drugs.
- **Depot bromperidol decanoate** RCTs found no significant difference in the proportion of people who needed additional medication, left the trial early, or had movement disorders over 6–12 months between depot bromperidol decanoate and haloperidol or fluphenazine decanoate.
- **Depot haloperidol decanoate** One systematic review of one small RCT found no significant difference in global clinical state at 4 months between depot haloperidol decanoate and oral haloperidol, but it may have been too small to exclude a clinically important difference. Haloperidol is associated with acute dystonia, akathisia, and parkinsonism.
- **Haloperidol** One systematic review has found that haloperidol increases physician rated global improvement at 6 and 24 weeks compared with placebo but is associated with acute dystonia, akathisia, and parkinsonism.

- **Thioridazine** One systematic review has found that thioridazine improves global mental state over 3–12 months compared with placebo.
- **Cognitive behavioural therapy to reduce relapse rates** Limited evidence from a systematic review of two RCTs found no significant difference in relapse rates between cognitive behavioural therapy plus standard care and standard care alone.
- **Multiple session family interventions to improve adherence** One systematic review found that "compliance with medication" over 9–24 months was higher in people who received multiple family interventions compared with usual care, single family interventions, or psychoeducational interventions, but the difference did not quite reach significance.
- **Perazine** RCTs provided insufficient evidence to assess perazine.
- **Social skills training to reduce relapse rates** One systematic review of small RCTs provided insufficient evidence to assess social skills training.
- **Amisulpride; loxapine; molindone; olanzapine; pimozide; quetiapine; risperidone; sulpiride; ziprasidone; zotepine** Systematic reviews have found that these newer antipsychotic drugs are as effective in improving symptoms as standard antipsychotic drugs, and have different profiles of adverse effects.

DEFINITION Schizophrenia is characterised by the positive symptoms (see glossary, p 1233) of auditory hallucinations, delusions, and thought disorder, and by the negative symptoms (see glossary, p 1233) of demotivation, self neglect, and reduced emotion.[1] People are defined as being resistant to standard antipsychotic drugs if, over the preceding 5 years, they have not had a clinically important improvement in symptoms after 2–3 regimens of treatment with standard antipsychotic drugs for at least 6 weeks (from at least 2 classes at doses equivalent to or greater than 1000 mg/day chlorpromazine) and they have had no period of good functioning.[2,3] Approximately 30% (10–45%) of people with schizophrenia meet these criteria.[3]

INCIDENCE/ PREVALENCE Onset of symptoms typically occurs in early adult life (average age 25 years) and is earlier in men than in women.[4,5] Prevalence worldwide is 2–4/1000. One in 100 people will develop schizophrenia in their lifetime.

AETIOLOGY/ RISK FACTORS Risk factors include a family history (although no major genes have been identified), obstetric complications, developmental difficulties, central nervous system infections in childhood, cannabis use, and acute life events.[4] The precise contributions of these factors and ways in which they may interact are unclear.

PROGNOSIS About three quarters of people suffer recurrent relapse and continued disability, although the proportion of people who improved significantly increased after the mid-1950s (mean 48.5% from 1956–1985 *v* 35.4% from 1895–1956).[6] Outcome may be worse in people with insidious onset and delayed initial treatment, social isolation, or a strong family history; in people living in industrialised countries; in men; and in people who misuse drugs.[5] Drug treatment is generally successful in treating positive symptoms, but up to a third of people derive little benefit and negative symptoms are notoriously difficult to treat. About half of people with schizophrenia do not adhere to treatment in the short term. The figure is even higher in the longer term.[7]

AIMS OF INTERVENTION To relieve symptoms and to improve quality of life, with minimal adverse effects of treatment.

OUTCOMES Severity of positive and negative symptoms; global clinical improvement; global clinical impression (a composite measure of symptoms and everyday functioning); rate of relapse; adherence to treatment; adverse effects of treatment.

METHODS *Clinical Evidence* search and appraisal December 2002. Most RCTs were small, short term, with high withdrawal rates, and employed many different outcome measures.[8] There were a large number of good systematic reviews. Therefore, if possible, we focused primarily on systematic reviews and included only the outcomes that we thought were the most clinically relevant. Because each treatment is associated with different benefits and harms, we used estimates of global effectiveness if they were available. We searched for placebo controlled RCTs of standard antipsychotic medication and comparative RCTs of newer antipsychotic drugs.

QUESTION What are the effects of drug treatments?

OPTION CHLORPROMAZINE

One systematic review has found that, compared with placebo, chlorpromazine reduces the proportion of people who have no improvement, or marked or worse severity of illness at 6 months on a psychiatrist rated scale. The review found that chlorpromazine caused more adverse effects, such as sedation, acute dystonia, and parkinsonism, than placebo.

Benefits: **Versus placebo:** We found one systematic review (search date 1999, 45 RCTs, 3116 people, mean dose 511 mg/day, range 25–2000 mg/day).[9] It found that, compared with placebo, chlorpromazine significantly reduced the proportion of people who had no improvement on a psychiatrist rated global impression scale at 6 months (13 RCTs; 583/921 [63%] with chlorpromazine *v* 609/790 [77%] with placebo; RR of failing to improve 0.72, 95% CI 0.62 to 0.83; NNT 7, 95% CI 5 to 10) and significantly reduced the proportion of people who had marked or worse severity of illness on a psychiatrist rated scale at 1 week to 6 months (5 RCTs; 323/493 [66%] with chlorpromazine *v* 231/285 [81%] with placebo; RR of increased severity of illness 0.77, 95% CI 0.71 to 0.84; NNT 5, 95% CI 4 to 8).

Harms: **Versus placebo:** The systematic review found that, compared with placebo, chlorpromazine caused significantly higher rates of sedation (218/698 [31%] with chlorpromazine *v* 65/490 [13%] with placebo; RR 2.4, 95% CI 1.7 to 3.3; NNH 6, 95% CI 4 to 8), acute dystonia (28/439 [6%] with chlorpromazine *v* 5/234 [2%] with placebo; RR 3.1, 95% CI 1.3 to 7.6; NNH 24, 95% CI 14 to 77), parkinsonism (123/723 [17%] with chlorpromazine *v* 40/542 [7%]

with placebo; RR 2.6, 95% CI 1.2 to 5.4; NNH 10, 95% CI 8 to 16), weight gain (31/75 [41%] with chlorpromazine *v* 7/90 [8%] with placebo; RR 4.4, 95% CI 2.1 to 9.0; NNH 3, 95% CI 2 to 5), skin photosensitivity (81/496 [16%] with chlorpromazine *v* 9/303 [3%] with placebo; RR 5.2, 95% CI 3 to 10; NNH 7, 95% CI 6 to 10), dizziness caused by hypotension (112/688 [16%] with chlorpromazine *v* 38/504 [7%] with placebo; RR 1.9, 95% CI 1.3 to 2.6; NNH 12, 95% CI 8 to 20), and dry mouth (32/473 [7%] with chlorpromazine *v* 4/283 [1%] with placebo; RR 4.0, 95% CI 1.6 to 10.0; NNH 19, 95% CI 12 to 37).[9] Chlorpromazine was also associated with higher rates of seizures (19/450 [4%] with chlorpromazine *v* 4/245 [2%] with placebo; RR 2.4, 95% CI 0.4 to 16) and blood dyscrasias (10/207 [5%] with chlorpromazine *v* 2/187 [1%] with placebo; RR 2.0, 95% CI 0.7 to 6.0), although the differences did not reach significance. We found no long term data on the risk of tardive dyskinesia or the rare but potentially fatal neuroleptic malignant syndrome. Despite the frequent adverse effects, the review found that people taking chlorpromazine were more likely to stay in RCTs in both the short and the medium term than people taking placebo.

Comment: The review did not categorise symptoms as positive or negative because this information was rarely available from included RCTs.[9] It found significant heterogeneity among RCTs, but found that the analysis of global improvement over 9 weeks to 6 months remained significant after removal of the heterogeneous RCTs (RR 0.65, 95% CI 0.5 to 0.9).

OPTION HALOPERIDOL

One systematic review has found that haloperidol increases the proportion of people with psychiatrist rated global improvement at 6 and 24 weeks compared with placebo, but is associated with acute dystonia, akathisia, and parkinsonism.

Benefits: **Versus placebo:** We found one systematic review (search date 1998, 20 RCTs, 1001 people).[10] It found that haloperidol (over a wide range of doses) significantly increased psychiatrist rated global improvement at 6 weeks (3 RCTs, 159 people; 61/88 [69%] with haloperidol *v* 23/71 [32%] with placebo; RR 2.3, 95% CI 1.7 to 3.3; NNT 3, 95% CI 2 to 5) and at 24 weeks (8 RCTs; 72/163 [44%] *v* 21/150 [14%]; RR 3.5, 95% CI 2.3 to 5.6; NNT 3, 95% CI 3 to 5) compared with placebo.

Harms: **Versus placebo:** The systematic review found that, compared with placebo, haloperidol significantly increased the risk of acute dystonia (2 RCTs; RR 4.7, 95% CI 1.7 to 44; NNH 5, 95% CI 3 to 9), akathisia (3 RCTs: RR 6.5, 95% CI 1.5 to 28; NNH 6, 95% CI 4 to 14), and parkinsonism (4 RCTs; RR 8.9, 95% CI 2.6 to 31; NNH 3, 95% CI 2 to 5).[10] People taking haloperidol were significantly more likely to be treated with anticholinergic drugs than people taking placebo (4 RCTs; RR 4.9, 95% CI 1.01 to 24; NNH 2, 95% CI 1 to 3).

Comment: The median size of RCTs in the review was 38 people, but the quality of the RCTs was higher than average for schizophrenia trials.[10] Although the dose range was very wide, most RCTs used 4–20 mg daily and adjusted dose according to need. The review found evidence of publication bias for the 6–24 months global outcome ratings.[10]

OPTION THIORIDAZINE

One systematic review has found that thioridazine improves global mental state over 3–12 months compared with placebo.

Benefits: **Versus placebo:** We found one systematic review (search date 1999, 11 RCTs, 560 people).[11] It found that thioridazine significantly reduced the proportion of people who were "no better or worse" in global clinical impression at 3–12 months compared with placebo (5 RCTs; 27/84 [32%] with thioridazine *v* 57/81 [70%] with placebo; RR 0.5, 95% CI 0.37 to 0.68; NNT 3, 95% CI 3 to 5).

Harms: **Versus placebo:** The review found no significant difference in adverse effects between thioridazine and placebo, but may have lacked power to detect a clinically important difference.[11]

Comment: None.

OPTION DEPOT BROMPERIDOL DECANOATE

RCTs found no significant difference in the proportion of people who needed additional medication, left the trial early, or had movement disorders over 6–12 months between depot bromperidol decanoate and haloperidol or fluphenazine decanoate.

Benefits: **Versus standard antipsychotic drugs:** One systematic review (search date 1999, 3 RCTs, 97 people) found no significant difference between depot bromperidol and haloperidol or fluphenazine decanoate in the proportion of people who needed additional antipsychotics or benzodiazepines over 6–12 months (19/48 [39%] with bromperidol *v* 18/49 [37%] with haloperidol or fluphenazine; RR 1.08, 95% CI 0.68 to 1.70) or who left the trial early (10/48 [21%] with bromperidol *v* 5/49 [10%] with haloperidol or fluphenazine; RR 1.92, 95% CI 0.80 to 4.60).[12]

Harms: **Versus standard antipsychotic drugs:** The review found no significant difference in movement disorders over 6–12 months between bromperidol and haloperidol or fluphenazine (2 RCTs: 16/38 [42%] with bromperidol *v* 22/39 [56%] with haloperidol or fluphenazine; RR 0.74, 95% CI 0.47 to 1.17).[12]

Comment: None.

OPTION DEPOT HALOPERIDOL DECANOATE

One systematic review of one small RCT found no significant difference in global clinical state at 4 months between depot haloperidol decanoate and oral haloperidol, but it may have been too small to exclude a clinically important difference. Haloperidol is associated with acute dystonia, akathisia, and parkinsonism.

Benefits: **Versus standard antipsychotic drugs:** We found one systematic review (search date 1998) that identified one small RCT (22 people) comparing depot haloperidol versus oral haloperidol.[13] It found no significant difference in the proportion of people with "no improvement" in global clinical impression at 4 months (8/11 [73%] with depot haloperidol *v* 9/11 [82%] with oral haloperidol; RR of no improvement 0.89, 95% CI 0.56 to 1.40). The RCT may have been too small to detect a clinically important difference.

Harms: **Versus standard antipsychotic drugs:** The RCT found no significant difference between depot and oral haloperidol in the proportion of people who needed anticholinergic drugs for movement disorders (3/11 [27%] with depot haloperidol *v* 1/11 [9%] with oral haloperidol; RR 3.00, 95% CI 0.37 to 24.58).[13] Also see harms of haloperidol, p 1212.

Comment: Depot injection is believed to ensure adherence, but we found no evidence from RCTs to support this.

OPTION CLOZAPINE

One systematic review found that clozapine improved symptoms over 4–10 weeks compared with standard antipsychotic drugs. However, RCTs found that clozapine may be associated with blood dyscrasias. One systematic review of small RCTs provided insufficient evidence to compare clozapine versus other newer antipsychotic drugs.

Benefits: **Versus standard antipsychotic drugs:** We found one systematic review (search date 1999, 31 RCTs, 2589 people), which compared clozapine versus standard antipsychotic drugs, such as chlorpromazine and haloperidol.[14] It found that clozapine significantly reduced the proportion of people with no clinical improvement over 4–10 weeks compared with standard antipsychotic drugs (14 RCTs; 267/561 [48%] with clozapine *v* 377/570 [66%] with standard antipsychotics; RR of no important improvement 0.75, 95% CI 0.66 to 0.84). This means that, on average, six people will need to be treated for one to improve (NNT 6, 95% CI 5 to 7). The review found that, despite the requirement for regular blood tests, significantly fewer people withdrew from treatment with clozapine over 7–24 months compared with standard antipsychotic drugs (111/750 [15%] with clozapine *v* 140/763 [18%] with standard antipsychotics; RR 0.76, 95% CI 0.66 to 0.92). **Versus other new antipsychotic drugs:** We found one systematic review (search date 1999, 8 RCTs, 795 people).[15] Five of the RCTs identified by the review were in people with treatment resistant schizophrenia (see benefits of clozapine in people who are resistant to standard antipsychotic drugs, p 1229).

Harms: **Versus standard antipsychotic drugs:** The review found that, compared with standard antipsychotic drugs, clozapine was significantly more likely to cause hypersalivation (351/699 [50%] with clozapine *v* 161/720 [22%] with standard antipsychotics; RR 2.23, 95% CI 1.95 to 2.57; NNH 3, 95% CI 3 to 4), increased temperature (129/560 [23%] with clozapine *v* 86/587 [15%] with standard antipsychotics; RR 1.57, 95% CI 1.27 to 1.98; NNH 11,

95% CI 7 to 25), and sedation (392/751 [52%] with clozapine v 332/776 [43%] with standard antipsychotics; RR 1.23, 95% CI 1.13 to 1.34; NNH 10, 95% CI 6 to 22), but that it was less likely to cause dry mouth (40/397 [10%] with clozapine v 111/402 [28%] with standard antipsychotics; RR 0.36, 95% CI 0.26 to 0.51; NNT 6, 95% CI 4 to 8) and extrapyramidal adverse effects (202/614 [33%] with clozapine v 304/621 [49%] with standard antipsychotics; RR 0.67, 95% CI 0.58 to 0.77; NNT 6, 95% CI 5 to 9).[14] A large case series found leucopenia in 3% of 99 502 people taking clozapine over 5 years.[16] However, it found that monitoring white cell (neutrophil) counts was associated with a lower rate of cases of agranulocytosis in people taking clozapine (382 v 995; AR 0.38% v 1%) and deaths (12 v 149).[16] The review found that clozapine significantly increased blood problems, including leucopenia and neutropenia compared with standard antipsychotic drugs (24/637 [4%] with clozapine v 12/656 [2%] with standard antipsychotics; RR 1.85, 95% CI 0.99 to 3.47).[14] We found one systematic review (search date 1996, 12 RCTs, all included in the first review) that performed a meta-regression analysis combining results with various new antipsychotic drugs and comparing them with results with haloperidol.[17] It found that the difference in withdrawal rates did not persist after controlling for dose of haloperidol.

Comment: Some of the benefits of clozapine were more apparent in the long term, depending on which drug was used for comparison in the RCTs.

OPTION AMISULPRIDE

Three systematic reviews found limited evidence that amisulpride may improve symptoms more than standard antipsychotic drugs, although one of the reviews suggested that effects may be attributable to differences in dose. The reviews found that extrapyramidal adverse effects were less likely with amisulpride than with standard antipsychotic drugs. RCTs found no significant difference in symptoms between amisulpride and olanzapine or risperidone.

Benefits: **Versus standard antipsychotic drugs**: We found three systematic reviews.[17–19] The first systematic review (search date 2000) identified four RCTs (651 people), which compared amisulpride versus a standard antipsychotic (haloperidol [3 RCTs] or flupentixol [1 RCT]), and used the Clinical Global Impression scale to assess outcomes.[18] It found that amisulpride significantly reduced the proportion of people who were less than "much improved" in global clinical impression compared with standard antipsychotic drugs (107/324 [33%] with amisulpride v 163/327 [50%] with standard antipsychotics; RR of failing to improve 0.66, 95% CI 0.55 to 0.80; NNT 6, 95% CI 5 to 11). It also found that amisulpride significantly reduced the proportion of people who left the study early (14 RCTs; 282/881 [32%] with amisulpride v 242/631 [38%] with standard antipsychotics; RR 0.72, 95% CI 0.62 to 0.83; NNT 9, 95% CI 7 to 16). The second systematic review (search date 1998, 4 RCTs, including 2 RCTs identified by the first review, duration 4–6 weeks, 683 people) compared amisulpride versus standard antipsychotic drugs, usually haloperidol.[17] It is unclear whether allocation concealment was adequately performed in all included RCTs. It found that symptom reduction was greater with amisulpride than with standard antipsychotic drugs (standardised effect size –0.35, 95% CI –0.52 to –0.18), indicating that about 64% (95% CI 57% to 70%) of people do worse with standard antipsychotic drugs than with amisulpride. It also found that, compared with standard antipsychotic drugs, amisulpride significantly reduced the proportion of people who withdrew from the trial (NNH 9, 95% CI 5 to 22). All four short term RCTs identified by the review included people randomised to relatively high doses of amisulpride (estimated equivalent to 20 mg haloperidol), which may have exaggerated results in favour of amisulpride.[17] The review performed a meta-regression analysis and found that, after adjustment for dose differences in standard antipsychotics (usually haloperidol or chlorpromazine), newer antipsychotic drugs (amisulpride, olanzapine, quetiapine, risperidone) lose their therapeutic advantage over standard antipsychotic drugs. Meta-regression was not available for amisulpride alone. The third systematic review (11 RCTs, 6 of which were included in the first or second review) found that amisulpride improved Brief Psychiatric Rating Scale (BPRS) scores compared with haloperidol or flupentixol (mean effect size 0.11; CI not stated; no further data provided).[19] It also found that people taking amisulpride were less likely to withdraw from the study early. **Versus olanzapine:** We found no systematic review but found one RCT (377 people) comparing amisulpride versus olanzapine for 2 months' treatment.[20] It found no significant difference in symptoms at 2 months assessed by BPRS score (mean reduction 17.6 with amisulpride *v* 16.3 with olanzapine; reported as non-significant; CI not stated). **Versus risperidone:** The first review identified one RCT (228 people), which found no significant difference between amisulpride and risperidone in BPRS symptom scores.[18]

Harms: **Versus standard antipsychotic drugs:** The first review found that, compared with standard antipsychotic drugs, amisulpride significantly reduced the proportion of people who had at least one adverse effect (6 RCTs; 261/373 [70%] with amisulpride *v* 308/378 [81%] with standard antipsychotics; RR 0.85, 95% CI 0.79 to 0.92; NNT 9, 95% 5% CI 6 to 17).[18] It also found that people taking amisulpride were significantly less likely to experience at least one extrapyramidal symptom (7 RCTs; 161/383 [42%] with amisulpride *v* 234/388 [60%] with standard antipsychotics; RR 0.68, 95% CI 0.60 to 0.79; NNT 5, 95% CI 4 to 8). The second review found that movement disorders, measured by the Simpson Angus scale, were significantly less frequent with amisulpride compared with standard antipsychotic drugs (SMD –0.44, 95% CI –0.26 to –0.61).[17] The reduction in extrapyramidal adverse effects remained significant despite adjustment for dose differences in standard antipsychotics.[17] The third systematic review found that people taking amisulpride experienced fewer movement disorders than people taking standard antipsychotic drugs.[19] It found that amisulpride significantly reduced the use of antiparkinsonian medication compared with standard antipsychotic drugs (effect size 0.25, 95% CI 0.17 to 0.32). **Versus olanzapine:** The RCT found that significantly fewer people had clinically important weight gain (more than 7% total body weight) with amisulpride than with olanzapine

(27/189 [14%] with amisulpride v 48/188 [25%] with olanzapine; P = 0.007).[20] **Versus risperidone:** The RCT identified by the first review found no significant difference in adverse effects, extrapyramidal symptoms, or withdrawal rate between amisulpride and risperidone.[18]

Comment: None.

OPTION LOXAPINE

One systematic review comparing loxapine versus standard antipsychotic drugs found no significant difference in global improvement or adverse effects.

Benefits: **Versus standard antipsychotic drugs:** We found one systematic review (search date 1999, 22 RCTs, 1073 people), which compared loxapine (dose range 25–250 mg/day) versus standard antipsychotic drugs, primarily chlorpromazine.[21] It found no significant difference in clinical global improvement between loxapine and standard antipsychotic drugs (9 RCTs; 59/206 [29%] with loxapine v 65/205 [32%] with standard antipsychotics; RR of no improvement 0.82, 95% CI 0.52 to 1.31).

Harms: The review found no significant difference in adverse effects between loxapine and standard antipsychotic drugs (11 RCTs; 164/255 [64%] with loxapine v 166/251 [66%] with standard antipsychotics; RR 0.90, 95% CI 0.57 to 1.41).[21]

Comment: All of the RCTs identified by the review were conducted in the USA or India and none lasted longer than 12 weeks.[21]

OPTION MOLINDONE

One systematic review found no significant difference in global clinical improvement or in the proportion of people who had adverse effects over 4–12 weeks between molindone and standard antipsychotic drugs.

Benefits: **Versus standard antipsychotic drugs:** We found one systematic review (search date 1999, 9 RCTs, 4 CCTs, 150 people) comparing molindone versus standard antipsychotic drugs, primarily haloperidol or chlorpromazine.[22] It found no significant difference between molindone and standard antipsychotic drugs in global clinical improvement over 4–12 weeks as assessed by a physician (4 RCTs; 25/84 [29.8%] with molindone v 20/66 [30.3%] with standard antipsychotics; RR of no improvement 1.10, 95% CI 0.68 to 1.78).

Harms: **Versus standard antipsychotic drugs:** The review found no significant difference between molindone and standard antipsychotic drugs in movement disorders (rigidity, tremor, akasthesia, use of antiparkinsonian medication) or in the proportion of people who had adverse effects (2 RCTs, 1 CCT; 24/42 [57%] with molindone v 25/42 [59%] with standard antipsychotics; RR 0.96, 95% CI 0.73 to 1.27).[22] One RCT identified by the review found that significantly more people taking molindone compared with standard antipsychotic drugs experienced confusion (9/14 [64%] with molindone v 6/30 [20%] with standard antipsychotics; RR 3.21, 95% CI 1.42 to 7.26). The review also found that significantly more people had weight loss with molindone than with standard antipsychotic drugs (2 RCTs; 12/30 [40%] with molindone *v* 4/30 [13%] with standard antipsychotics; RR 2.78, 95% CI 1.10 to 6.99) and that fewer people had weight gain with molindone than with standard antipsychotic drugs (2 RCTs; 4/30 [13%] with molindone *v* 11/30 [37%] with standard antipsychotics; RR 0.39, 95% CI 0.95 to 1.00).

Comment: None.

OPTION OLANZAPINE

Systematic reviews found limited evidence that olanzapine may improve symptoms more than standard antipsychotic drugs and good evidence that olanzapine has fewer adverse effects, although one of the reviews suggested that effects may be attributable to differences in dose. Systematic reviews found no clear difference in symptoms or adverse effects among olanzapine, amisulpride, risperidone, and clozapine.

Benefits: **Versus standard antipsychotic drugs:** We found three systematic reviews.[17,23,24] The first review (search date 1999, 15 RCTs, 3282 people) compared olanzapine versus standard antipsychotic drugs, usually haloperidol.[23] It found no significant difference in psychotic symptoms over 6–8 weeks between olanzapine (2.5–25 mg/day) and standard antipsychotic drugs (4 RCTs; 1056/1926 [55%] with olanzapine *v* 596/852 [70%] with standard antipsychotics; RR for no important response [defined as a 40% reduction on any scale] 0.90, 95% CI 0.76 to 1.06). The second review (search date 1998, 4 RCTs, all included in the first review, 2846 people) performed a meta-regression analysis comparing newer versus standard antipsychotics, which adjusted for dose of standard antipsychotic (see benefits of amisulpride, p 1215).[17] Meta-regression analysis was not available for olanzapine alone. The third review (search date 1998, 3 RCTs, all included in the previous review, 2606 people) also found no significant difference in the mean change on a combined rating of positive and negative symptoms (Positive and Negative Syndrome Scale [PANSS]) between olanzapine and haloperidol.[24] However, it conducted a subsequent meta-regression analysis to control for confounding variables (e.g. age and duration of illness, among others) and found limited evidence that olanzapine significantly improved mean PANSS rating scale score compared with standard antipsychotics (WMD –5.9, 95% CI –11.1 to –0.6). The meta-regression analysis did not appear to take account of the dose of haloperidol.[24] **Versus clozapine:** See benefits of clozapine, p 1214. **Versus amisulpride:** See benefits of amisulpride, p 1215. **Versus risperidone:** We found two systematic reviews[25,26] and one subsequent RCT.[27] The first review (search date 1999, 3 RCTs) found that olanzapine improved mean PANSS scores at 28–30 weeks compared with risperidone (2 RCTs, 392 people; WMD 7.5 points, 95% CI 2.9 to 12.0 on a scale of 210 points), although it found no significant difference at 54 weeks (1 RCT, 435 people; WMD 6.1, 95% CI 1.9 to 10.3).[25] Olanzapine was also associated with significantly fewer withdrawals for any cause at 28–30 weeks than risperidone (2 RCTs; 85/204 [42%] with olanzapine *v* 109/200 [54%]

with risperidone; RR 0.76, 95% CI 0.62 to 0.94).[25] The second review (search review 2000, 2 RCTs, including 1 RCT identified by the first review) found similar results but did not quantify its conclusions.[26] The subsequent RCT (377 people) found no significant difference between olanzapine and risperidone in the proportion of people who responded at 8 weeks (response defined as a < 20% reduction in PANSS score: 48% with olanzapine *v* 51% with risperidone; reported as non-significant; no further data provided).[27]

Harms: **Versus standard antipsychotic drugs:** The first review found no significant difference between olanzapine and standard antipsychotic drugs in the proportion of people who withdrew from the trial for any cause at 4–8 weeks (9 RCTs; 744/2068 [36%] with olanzapine *v* 464/952 [49%] with standard antipsychotics; RR 0.85, 95% CI 0.65 to 1.10) or at 1 year (4 RCTs; 1577/1905 [83%] *v* 748/833 [90%]; RR 0.90, 95% CI 0.75 to 1.08).[23] It found that, compared with standard antipsychotic drugs, olanzapine significantly reduced the proportion of people who required anticholinergic drugs for extrapyramidal adverse effects (293/1884 [15%] with olanzapine *v* 401/810 [49%] with standard antipsychotics; RR 0.26, 95% CI 0.17 to 0.40) and caused significantly less nausea (174/1576 [11%] with olanzapine *v* 117/771 [15%] with standard antipsychotics; RR 0.74, 95% CI 0.59 to 0.92; NNT 25, 95% CI 14 to 85), vomiting (97/1336 [7%] with olanzapine *v* 81/660 [12%] with standard antipsychotics; RR 0.59, 95% CI 0.45 to 0.78; NNT 20, 95% CI 12 to 46), or drowsiness (443/1576 [28%] with olanzapine *v* 268/771 [34%] with standard antipsychotics; RR 0.82, 95% CI 0.72 to 0.92; NNT 15, 95% CI 9 to 38). Olanzapine was associated with a significantly greater increase in appetite (1 RCT; 343/1336 [26%] with olanzapine *v* 103/660 [16%] with standard antipsychotics; RR 1.65, 95% CI 1.35 to 2.01; NNH 10, 95% CI 7 to 15) and weight gain than standard antipsychotic drugs.[23] The second review found that fewer people withdrew from the trial with olanzapine than with haloperidol, but the difference did not persist after adjustment for dose.[17] It found that dystonia and akathisia were significantly less frequent with olanzapine than with haloperidol, even after adjustment for dose (ARR for dystonia with olanzapine *v* haloperidol 14%, 95% CI 11% to 17%; ARR for akathisia with olanzapine *v* haloperidol 4.8%, 95% CI 3.1% to 6.5%). Olanzapine was associated with a 12% (95% CI 8% to 15%) increase in excessive appetite compared with haloperidol.[17]
Versus clozapine: See harms of clozapine, p 1214. **Versus amisulpride:** See harms of amisulpride, p 1216. **Versus risperidone:** The first review found that olanzapine was associated with significantly fewer extrapyramidal adverse effects compared with risperidone (1 RCT; 32/172 [19%] with olanzapine *v* 52/167 [31%] with risperidone; RR 0.60, 95% CI 0.41 to 0.88; NNT 8, 95% CI 5 to 28), less parkinsonism (1 RCT; 22/172 [13%] with olanzapine *v* 37/167 [22%] with risperidone; RR 0.58, 95% CI 0.37 to 0.94; NNT 11, 95% CI 6 to 77), and less need for antiparkinsonian medication (1 RCT; 34/172 [20%] with olanzapine *v* 55/167 [33%] with risperidone; RR 0.60, 95% CI 0.41 to 0.87; NNT 8, 95% CI 4 to 25).[25] People taking olanzapine had greater weight gain, but the difference was not significant either at 28–30 weeks (2 RCTs: WMD

+2.86, 95% CI –0.68 to +6.34) or at 54 weeks (WMD +3.56, 95% CI –0.20 to +6.90). The second review found similar results but did not perform a meta-analysis.[26] The subsequent RCT found no significant difference between olanzapine and risperidone in severity of extrapyramidal adverse effects, need for anticholinergics, or withdrawals from the trial.[27] Fewer people on risperidone experienced clinically important weight gain (AR for ≥ 7% weight gain 27.3% with olanzapine *v* 11.6% with risperidone).

Comment: **Versus standard antipsychotic drugs:** The results of the reviews are dominated by one large multicentre RCT reported by drug company employees.[17,23,24] Benefits seem to be highest at a dose of 15 mg daily, and higher doses may be associated with more harms. Results depended on the statistical test used, and their reliability may be compromised by heterogeneity.

OPTION PERAZINE

Two weak RCTs found no significant difference in global clinical impression over 28 days between perazine and haloperidol. Two RCTs provided insufficient evidence to assess perazine compared with zotepine, and one RCT found no significant difference in mental state at 28 days between perazine and amisulpride. Three RCTs found no significant difference in extrapyramidal effects over 28 days between perazine and zotepine or amisulpride.

Benefits: **Versus standard antipsychotic drugs:** We found one systematic review (search date 2001), which identified two RCTs (71 people) comparing perazine versus haloperidol.[28] It could not perform a meta-analysis because of poor reporting in one of the RCTs. One of the RCTs (32 people) found no significant difference between perazine and haloperidol in the proportion of people who were "no better or worse" in global clinical impression at 28 days (8/17 [47%] with perazine *v* 6/15 [60%] with haloperidol; RR 1.18, 95% CI 0.53 to 2.62). **Versus other new antipsychotic drugs:** The review identified two RCTs comparing perazine versus zotepine.[28] It could not perform a meta-analysis because of methodological differences between the RCTs. The first RCT (34 people) found that perazine was significantly less effective than zotepine in improving symptoms as assessed by mean Brief Psychiatric Rating Scale score at 28 days (WMD 7.9, 95% CI 1.1 to 14.7). The second RCT (40 people), which used a different method to calculate mean Brief Psychiatric Rating Scale score, found that perazine was significantly more effective than zotepine in improving symptoms at the end of the trial (trial duration not specified: WMD –0.4, 95% –0.7 to –0.1). One RCT identified by the review found no significant difference between perazine and amisulpride in the proportion of people whose mental state was "no better or worse" at 28 days (4/15 [27%] with perazine *v* 3/15 [20%] with amisulpride; RR 1.33, 95% CI 0.36 to 4.97).[28]

Harms: **Versus standard antipsychotic drugs:** The review gave no information about the adverse effects of perazine compared with haloperidol.[28] **Versus other new antipsychotic drugs:** The review (3 RCTs) found no significant difference between perazine and zotepine or amisulpride in the risk of akathesia (3/56 [5%] with perazine v 10/55 [18%] with zotepine or amisulpride; RR 0.30, 95% CI 0.09 to 1.00), dyskinesia (1/56 [2%] v 3/55 [5%]; RR 0.42, 95% CI 0.06 to 2.74), or parkinsonism over 28 days (10/41 [24%] with perazine v 8/40 [20%] with zotepine or amisulpride; RR 1.22, 95% CI 0.54 to 2.78).[28]

Comment: None.

OPTION PIMOZIDE

One systematic review comparing pimozide versus standard antipsychotic drugs found no significant difference in global clinical impression, and found that pimozide decreased sedation but increased tremor. It found no overall difference in cardiovascular adverse effects such as rise or fall in blood pressure or dizziness between pimozide and standard antipsychotic drugs.

Benefits: **Versus standard antipsychotic drugs:** We found one systematic review (search date 1999) comparing pimozide (mean dose 7.5 mg/day, range 1–75 mg/day) versus standard antipsychotic drugs, including chlorpromazine, haloperidol, fluphenazine, and carpipramine.[29] It found no significant difference in global clinical impression between pimozide and standard antipsychotics at 1–3 months (3 RCTs; 18/50 [36%] with pimozide v 22/50 [44%] with standard antipsychotics; RR 0.82, 95% CI 0.52 to 1.29) or at 4–6 months (6 RCTs; 57/104 [55%] with pimozide v 55/102 [54%] with standard antipsychotics; RR 1.01, 95% CI 0.80 to 1.28).

Harms: **Versus standard antipsychotic drugs:** The review found that, over 1–3 months, pimozide caused significantly less sedation than standard antipsychotic drugs (53/117 [45%] with pimozide v 68/115 [59%] with standard antipsychotics; RR 0.77, 95% CI 0.61 to 0.98; NNT 7, 95% CI 4 to 61), but that it was more likely to cause tremor (43/97 [44%] with pimozide v 27/95 [28%] with standard antipsychotics; RR 1.57, 95 CI 1.07 to 2.29; NNH 6, 95% CI 3 to 44).[29] It found similar cardiovascular symptoms such as rise or fall in blood pressure and dizziness between pimozide and standard antipsychotic drugs. There was little usable ECG data. One RCT in the review found no significant difference in ECG changes between pimozide and standard antipsychotic drugs, but it may have been too small to detect a clinically important difference (2/28 [7%] with pimozide v 3/28 [11%] with standard antipsychotics; RR 0.67, 95% CI 0.1 to 3.7).

Comment: Sudden death has been reported in a number of people taking pimozide at doses over 20 mg daily, but we found no evidence from RCTs that pimozide is more likely to cause sudden death than other antipsychotic drugs.[29] The manufacturer recommends periodic ECG monitoring in all people taking more than 16 mg daily pimozide and avoidance of other drugs known to prolong the QT interval on an ECG or cause electrolyte disturbances (other antipsychotic drugs, antihistamines, antidepressants, and diuretics).

OPTION QUETIAPINE

Three systematic reviews comparing quetiapine versus standard antipsychotic drugs found no significant difference in symptoms, but two of the reviews found that quetiapine reduced akathisia, parkinsonism, and the proportion of people who left the trial early.

Benefits: **Versus standard antipsychotic drugs:** We found two systematic reviews.[17,30] The first review (search date 2000, 7 RCTs) compared quetiapine (50–800 mg/day) versus standard antipsychotic drugs (usually haloperidol).[30] It found no significant difference in mental state over 6 weeks between quetiapine and standard antipsychotic drugs (Brief Psychiatric Rating Scale or Positive and Negative Syndrome Scale score not improved, 4 RCTs; 367/723 [51%] with quetiapine *v* 283/524 [54%] with standard antipsychotics; RR 0.91, 95% CI 0.73 to 1.13). The second review (search date 1998, 2 RCTs, both included in the first review, 511 people) performed a meta-regression analysis comparing newer versus standard antipsychotics, which adjusted for dose of standard antipsychotic (see benefits of amisulpride, p 1215).[17] Meta-regression was not available for quetiapine alone.

Harms: **Versus standard antipsychotic drugs:** The first review found that, compared with standard antipsychotic drugs, quetiapine was associated with significantly fewer people leaving trials early for any cause over 6 weeks (6 RCTs; 334/913 [36.5%] with quetiapine *v* 254/711 [35.7%] with standard antipsychotics; RR 0.86, 95% CI 0.75 to 0.98), less dystonia (3 RCTs; 4/580 [0.69%] with quetiapine *v* 19/379 [5%] with standard antipsychotics; RR 0.24, 95% CI 0.04 to 0.49), less akathisia (3 RCTs; 19/580 [3%] with quetiapine *v* 68/379 [18%] with standard antipsychotics; RR 0.24, 95% CI 0.15 to 0.38), and less parkinsonism (2 RCTs; 31/479 [6%] with quetiapine *v* 92/279 [33%] with standard antipsychotics; RR 0.22, 95% CI 0.15 to 0.33), but more dry mouth (2 RCTs: 31/322 [10%] with quetiapine *v* 11/327 [3%] with standard antipsychotics; RR 2.85, 95% CI 1.46 to 5.57).[30]

Comment: The RCTs in the review had substantial withdrawal rates and did not conduct intention to treat analyses.[30]

OPTION RISPERIDONE

Systematic reviews found limited evidence that risperidone may improve symptoms more than standard antipsychotic drugs (mainly haloperidol) and found good evidence that, at lower doses, risperidone has fewer adverse effects, although one of the reviews suggested that effects may be attributable to differences in dose. Systematic reviews found no significant difference in symptoms between risperidone and other new antipsychotic drugs.

Benefits: **Versus standard antipsychotic drugs:** We found three systematic reviews[17,24,31] and one additional RCT.[32] The first review (search date 1997, 14 RCTs, 3401 people) found that, at 12 weeks, risperidone (mean dose range 6.1–12 mg/day) significantly increased the proportion of people who had "clinical improvement" compared with standard antipsychotic drugs, usually haloperidol.[31]

"Clinical improvement" was variably defined but usually as a 20% reduction in symptoms (11 RCTs; 894/2088 [43%] with risperidone *v* 482/893 [54%] with standard antipsychotics; RR of no clinical improvement 0.81, 95% CI 0.75 to 0.88; NNT 10, 95% CI 7 to 16). The review did not find significant heterogeneity among RCTs. The second review (search date 1998, 8 RCTs, all included in the first review) found "substantial heterogeneity" among six RCTs of 4–12 weeks' treatment.[17] It found that risperidone improved symptom scores over 12 months compared with standard antipsychotic drugs (2 RCTs; WMD –0.40, 95% CI –0.27 to –0.54, indicating that about 66% of people taking standard antipsychotics had worse composite symptom scores than with risperidone). Meta-regression analysis suggested that this difference did not persist after controlling for dose of standard antipsychotic (see benefits of amisulpride, p 1215). The third review (search date 1998, 11 RCTs, including 8 identified by the first review, 1208 people) found that risperidone significantly improved negative and positive symptoms, as measured using the Positive and Negative Syndrome Scale, compared with haloperidol (WMD –8.3, 95% CI –13.8 to –2.7).[24] The additional RCT (99 people) comparing a range of doses of risperidone versus haloperidol found no significant difference in the proportion of people who responded over 8 weeks (response defined as ≥20% reduction in Positive and Negative Syndrome Scale; reported as non-significant; results presented graphically).[32] **Versus olanzapine:** See benefits of olanzapine, p 1218. **Versus amisulpride:** See benefits of amisulpride, p 1215. **Versus clozapine:** See benefits of clozapine, p 1214.

Harms: **Versus standard antipsychotic drugs:** The first review found no significant difference between risperidone and standard antipsychotic drugs in the proportion of people who withdrew from treatment because of adverse effects (139/1585 [9%] with risperidone *v* 70/591 [12%] with standard antipsychotics; RR 0.78, 95% CI 0.58 to 1.05).[31] It found that, compared with people taking standard antipsyschotic drugs, people taking risperidone developed significantly fewer extrapyramidal effects (347/1728 [20%] with risperidone *v* 234/551 [42%] with standard antipsychotics; RR 0.63, 95% CI 0.55 to 0.72; NNT 5, 95% CI 5 to 10), required less antiparkinsonian medication (444/1810 [24%] with risperidone *v* 274/626 [44%] with standard antipsychotics; RR 0.64, 95% CI 0.57 to 0.73; NNT 7, 95% CI 5 to 10), and were less likely to develop daytime somnolence (481/1509 [32%] with risperidone *v* 197/589 [33%] with standard antipsychotics; RR 0.87, 95% CI 0.76 to 0.99; NNT 22, 95% CI 11 to 500). However, it found that risperidone was associated with significantly more weight gain than standard antipsychotics (398/1290 [31%] with risperidone *v* 71/362 [20%] with standard antipsychotics; RR 1.37, 95% CI 1.10 to 1.71; NNH 13, 95% CI 8 to 36). The second review found no significant difference between risperidone and haloperidol in the proportion of people who withdrew from treatment, but found that risperidone reduced symptoms of dystonia (WMD –0.26, 95% CI –0.39 to –0.12), parkinsonism (WMD –0.39, 95% CI –0.51 to –0.27), and dyskinesia (WMD –0.16, 95% CI –0.28 to –0.04).[17] Differences persisted after controlling for dose. The third review found that, compared with haloperidol, risperidone significantly reduced the proportion of people who required medication for extrapyramidal side effects (OR 0.42, 95% CI 0.19 to 0.96; absolute numbers presented graphically).[24] The additional RCT found no significant difference in the rate of overall adverse effects between risperidone and haloperidol.[32] **Versus olanzapine:** See harms of olanzapine, p 1219 **Versus amisulpride:** See harms of amisulpride, p 1216. **Versus clozapine:** See harms of clozapine, p 1214.

Comment: The first review found evidence of publication bias.[31] Sensitivity analyses found that benefits in clinical improvement and continuing treatment of risperidone compared with standard antipsychotic drugs were no longer significant if RCTs using more than 10 mg haloperidol daily were excluded. This could be because of loss of power. Exclusion of the higher dosage RCTs did not remove the difference in rate of extrapyramidal adverse effects.[31]

OPTION SULPIRIDE

One systematic review found no significant difference in global clinical impression over 4–10 weeks between sulpiride and standard antipsychotic drugs. The review found that the use of antiparkinson drugs over 4–10 weeks was less frequent with sulpiride compared with standard antipsychotic drugs.

Benefits: **Versus standard antipsychotic drugs:** One systematic review (search date 1998, 7 RCTs, 366 people) found no significant difference in the proportion of people who had no improvement in global clinical impression over 4–10 weeks between sulpiride and standard antipsychotic drugs, usually haloperidol chlorpromazine, or perphenazine (74/248 [30%] with sulpiride *v* 96/266 [36%] with standard antipsychotics; RR of no important improvement 0.82, 95% CI 0.64 to 1.05).[33]

Harms: **Versus standard antipsychotic drugs:** The review found that the use of antiparkinson drugs over 4–10 weeks was significantly less frequent with sulpiride compared with standard antipsychotic drugs (84/253 [33%] *v* 115/258 [44%]; RR 0.73, 95% CI 0.59 to 0.90).[33]

Comment: The review stated that the other two RCTs it identified reported improvement in mental state with sulpiride compared with placebo, but that no raw data could be obtained because of poor reporting in the RCTs.[33] Observational evidence and clinical experience suggest that sulpiride may be associated with galactorrhoea, but RCT data did not quantify the risk.[34]

OPTION ZIPRASIDONE

One systematic review found no significant difference in mental state improvement between ziprasidone and haloperidol, and found that ziprasidone reduced akathisia and acute dystonia but increased nausea and vomiting.

Benefits: **Versus standard antipsychotic drugs:** We found one systematic review comparing ziprasidone versus standard antipsychotic drugs.[35] The review (search date 1999, 4 RCTs, 690 people) identified one RCT (301 people) that provided sufficient data to assess clinically important improvement in mental state (≥ 20% reduction in Positive and Negative Syndrome Scale score). It found no significant difference in mental state between ziprasidone and haloperidol (95/148 [64%] with ziprasidone *v* 114/153 [74%] with haloperidol; RR of no important improvement in mental state 0.86, 95% CI 0.74 to 1.00).

Harms: **Versus standard antipsychotic drugs:** The review found no clear difference in overall adverse effects between ziprasidone and haloperidol.[35] It found that, compared with haloperidol, ziprasidone was significantly less likely to cause akathisia over 1 week (2 RCTs; 19/296 [6%] with ziprasidone *v* 27/142 [19%] with haloperidol; RR 0.34, 95% CI 0.20 to 0.59; NNH 8, 95% CI 5 to 18) and over 28 weeks (1 RCT; 7/148 [5%] with ziprasidone *v* 25/153 [16%] with haloperidol; RR 0.3, 95% CI 0.1 to 0.7; NNH 9, 95% CI 5 to 21), and that it was less likely to cause acute dystonia over 1 week (2 RCTs; 13/296 [4%] with ziprasidone *v* 15/142 [10%] with haloperidol; RR 0.42, 95% CI 0.20 to 0.85; NNH 16, 95% CI 9 to 166). Ziprasidone was associated with significantly more nausea and vomiting both over 1 week (59/206 [29%] with ziprasidone *v* 8/100 [8%] with haloperidol; RR 3.58, 95% CI 1.78 to 7.20; NNH 5, 95% CI 4 to 8) and over 28 weeks (1 RCT; 31/148 [21%] with ziprasidone *v* 15/153 [10%] with haloperidol; RR 2.14, 95% CI 1.20 to 3.79; NNH 9, 95% CI 5 to 33) compared with haloperidol.

Comment: The duration of RCTs in the review was less than 6 weeks.[35] Most RCTs reported a withdrawal rate of over 20% and no RCT clearly described adequate precautions for the blinding of treatment allocation.

OPTION ZOTEPINE

One systematic review found weak evidence that zotepine increased the proportion of people with a clinically important improvement in symptoms compared with standard antipsychotic drugs, and reduced akasthesia, dystonia, and rigidity. This finding was not robust because removal of a single RCT from the analysis meant that the difference between zotepine and standard antipsychotics was no longer significant.

Benefits: **Versus standard antipsychotic drugs:** We found one systematic review (search date 1999, 8 RCTs, 356 people) comparing zotepine (75–450 mg/day) versus standard antipsychotic drugs, usually haloperidol.[36] It found that zotepine was significantly more likely than standard antipsychotic drugs to bring about "clinically important improvement" at 4–12 weeks, as defined by a pre-stated cut off point on the Brief Psychiatric Rating Scale (4 RCTs; 89/179 [50%] with zotepine *v* 62/177 [35%] with standard antipsychotics; RR 1.25, 95% CI 1.1 to 1.4; NNT 7, 95% CI 4 to 22; see comment below).

Harms: The review found that, compared with standard antipsychotic drugs, zotepine caused significantly less akathisia (67/199 [34%] with zotepine *v* 91/197 [46%] with standard antipsychotics; RR 0.73, 95% CI 0.58 to 0.93; NNT 8, 95% CI 5 to 34), dystonia (7/35 [20%] with zotepine *v* 15/35 [43%] with standard antipsychotics;

RR 0.47, 95% CI 0.24 to 0.93; NNT 4, 95% CI 2 to 56), and rigidity (19/83 [23%] with zotepine *v* 30/81 [37%] with standard antipsychotics; RR 0.63, 95% CI 0.40 to 0.98; NNT 7, 95% CI 4 to 360).[36] Two RCTs found abnormal ECG results in people taking zotepine, but few additional details were given.

Comment: All but one RCT identified by the review were of 12 weeks' or less duration and all were conducted in Europe.[36] Only one RCT favoured zotepine over standard antipsychotic drugs, and removal of this RCT from the analysis renders the results non-significant.

QUESTION Which interventions reduce relapse rates?

OPTION CONTINUED TREATMENT WITH ANTIPSYCHOTIC DRUGS

Systematic reviews have found that continuing antipsychotic drugs for at least 6 months after an acute episode reduces relapse rates compared with no treatment or placebo, and that some benefit of continuing antipsychotics is apparent for up to 2 years. Eight systematic reviews found no significant difference in relapse rates among antipsychotic drugs. One systematic review found that clozapine reduces relapse rates over 12 weeks compared with standard antipsychotic drugs. Another review found that fewer people taking depot zuclopenthixol decanoate relapsed over 12 weeks to 1 year compared with people taking other depot preparations. A third review found that bromperidol increased the proportion of people who relapsed compared with haloperidol or fluphenazine. One additional RCT found that risperidone reduced relapse over 2.2 years compared with haloperidol.

Benefits: **Versus no treatment or placebo:** We found three systematic reviews.[9,10,37] The first review (search date not stated, 66 studies, 4365 people taking antipsychotic drugs, mean dose 630 mg chlorpromazine equivalents daily, mean follow up of 6.3 months) included 29 controlled trials with a mean follow up of 9.7 months (see comment below).[37] It found that continuing compared with withdrawing antipsychotic drugs significantly reduced the proportion of people who relapsed (28 controlled studies, 2448 people; 16% with continued treatment *v* 51% with withdrawing treatment; ARR 35%, 95% CI 33% to 38%; NNT 3, 95% CI 3 to 4). Over time, the relapse rate in people maintained on antipsychotic treatment approached that in those withdrawn from treatment, but was still lower in those on treatment at 2 years. The second review (search date 1997, 5 RCTs, 2 included in the first review) found that continuing chlorpromazine significantly reduced relapse rates over 6–24 months compared with placebo (3 RCTs; 106/264 [40%] with chlorpromazine *v* 176/248 [71%] with placebo; RR 0.57, 95% CI 0.48 to 0.67; NNT 3, 95% CI 3 to 4).[9] The third review (search date 1998, 2 RCTs, neither included in the previous reviews, 70 people currently in remission) compared haloperidol versus placebo over 1 year.[10] It found that haloperidol significantly reduced relapse over 1 year compared with placebo (32/47 [68%] with haloperidol *v* 23/23 [100%] with placebo; RR 0.67, 95% CI 0.54 to 0.83, NNT 4, 95% CI 2 to 7). **Choice of drug:** We found 11 systematic reviews[12–14,23,29,38-43] and one additional RCT[44] evaluating the effects of newer versus older antipsychotics, newer antipsychotics versus each other, and oral versus intramuscular administration of antibiotics on relapse rates (see table 1, p 1237). Eight reviews found no significant difference between antipsychotics in relapse rates,[13,23,29,38–42] but in two of the reviews[23,29] the number of people studied was too small to rule out a clinically important difference. A ninth review (search date 1998) found that clozapine significantly reduced relapse rates over 12 weeks compared with standard antipsychotics (19 RCTs; RR 0.6, 95% CI 0.5 to 0.8).[14] A tenth review (search date 1998) found that significantly fewer people taking depot zuclopenthixol decanoate relapsed over 12 weeks to 1 year compared with people taking other depot preparations (3 RCTs; 296 people: RR 0.7, 95% CI 0.6 to 1.0; NNT 9, 95% CI 5 to 53).[43] An eleventh review (search date 1999) found that bromperidol significantly increased the proportion of people who relapsed compared with haloperidol or fluphenazine (2 RCTs; RR 3.92, 95% CI 1.05 to 14.6; NNH 5, 95% CI 3 to 28).[12] The additional RCT (365 people) found that risperidone versus haloperidol significantly reduced relapse over 2.2 years (NNT 5, 95% CI 4 to 10).[44]

Harms: **Versus no treatment or placebo:** The first review found that mild transient nausea, malaise, sweating, vomiting, insomnia, and dyskinesia were reported in an unspecified number of people after sudden drug cessation, but were usually acceptable with gradual dose reduction.[37] The other reviews gave no information on adverse effects of continuing treatment with antipsychotic drugs.[9,10] **Choice of drug:** The review comparing different depot antipsychotic drugs found that the annual incidence of tardive dyskinesia was 5%.[43]

Comment: In the systematic review of continued treatment versus withdrawal of treatment, meta-analysis of the 29 controlled trials gave similar results to those obtained when all 66 studies were included.[37] A commentary of the review suggested that it was weakened because all RCT results were used rather than weighted comparisons, no length of time was given since the last acute episode, and no distinction was made between people experiencing a first episode and those with chronic illness.[45] Some clinicians use depot antipsychotic drugs in selected people to ensure adherence to medication. We found no evidence from RCTs to support this practice.

OPTION COGNITIVE BEHAVIOURAL THERAPY

Limited evidence from a systematic review of two RCTs found no significant difference in relapse rates between cognitive behavioural therapy plus standard care and standard care alone.

Benefits: We found one systematic review (search date 2001), which identified two RCTs (123 people) comparing the effects of cognitive behavioural therapy plus standard care versus standard care alone on relapse rates.[46] Both RCTs identified by the review incorporated challenging key beliefs, problem solving, and enhancement of coping. The review found no significant difference between cognitive behavioural therapy plus standard care and standard care alone in relapse or readmission to hospital over 10 weeks (1 RCT; 0/33 [0%] with cognitive behavioural therapy plus standard care *v* 4/28 [14%] with standard care alone; RR 0.09, 95% CI 0.01 to 1.69) or over 9–24 months (2 RCTs; 36/63 [57%] with cognitive behavioural therapy plus standard care *v* 31/60 [52%] with standard care alone; RR 1.13, 95% CI 0.82 to 1.56).[46]

Harms: The systematic review gave no information on harms.[46]

Comment: None.

OPTION FAMILY INTERVENTIONS

One systematic review found that multiple session family interventions reduced relapse rates at 12 months compared with usual care, single session family interventions, or psychoeducational interventions.

Benefits: We found one systematic review (search date 1999) that compared multiple family interventions versus usual care, single family interventions, or psychoeducational interventions.[47] Family interventions consisted mainly of education about the illness and training in problem solving over at least six weekly sessions. The review found that multiple family interventions significantly reduced relapse rates at 12 months compared with other interventions (11 RCTs, 729 people; OR 0.52, 95% CI 0.31 to 0.89; absolute numbers not provided). On average, eight families would have to be treated to avoid one additional relapse (and likely hospitalisation) at 12 months in the family member with schizophrenia (NNT 8, 95% CI 6 to 18).[47]

Harms: The review gave no information on harms.[47]

Comment: These results may overestimate the effect of family interventions because of the difficulty of blinding people and investigators.[47] Although no harms were reported, illness education could possibly have adverse consequences on morale and outlook. The mechanism for the effects of family intervention remains unclear. It is thought to work by reducing "expressed emotion" (hostility and criticism) in relatives of people with schizophrenia. The time consuming nature of this intervention, which must normally take place at evenings or weekends, can limit its availability. It cannot be applied to people who have little contact with home based carers.

OPTION PSYCHOEDUCATIONAL INTERVENTIONS

One systematic review has found that psychoeducation reduces relapse rates at 9–18 months compared with usual care.

Benefits: **Versus usual treatment:** We found one systematic review (search date 2002), which identified one RCT of a brief individual intervention (10 sessions or less), six RCTs of brief group psychoeducational interventions, and four RCTs of standard length group psychoeducational interventions (11 sessions or more).[48] It found that standard length group psychoeducational interventions were significantly more effective than usual care in preventing relapse without readmission over 9–18 months (2 RCTs; 14/57 [24%] with psychoeducation *v* 24/57 [42%] with usual care; RR 0.58, 95% CI 0.34 to

0.99). It also found that brief group psychoeducational interventions were significantly more effective than usual care in preventing relapse or readmission over 1 year (5 RCTs; 153/326 [47%] with psychoeducation v 162/296 [55%] with usual care; RR 0.85, 95% CI 0.74 to 0.98; NNT 12, CI 6 to 83). The review found that any form of psychoeducation significantly reduced relapse with or without readmission to hospital over 9–18 months compared with usual care (6 RCTs; 176/383[46%] with psychoeducation v 192/337 [57%] with usual care; RR 0.78, 95% CI 0.62 to 0.98; NNT 9, 95% CI 6 to 22; see comment below).

Harms: The systematic review gave no information on harms.[48]

Comment: The systematic review found few good RCTs.[48] There was significant heterogeneity of both interventions and outcomes.

OPTION SOCIAL SKILLS TRAINING

One systematic review of small RCTs provided insufficient evidence to assess social skills training.

Benefits: We found one systematic review (search date not stated 1999), which identified nine RCTs (471 people) comparing the effect of social skills training versus standard care or psychoeducational interventions on relapse rates.[49] It found no significant difference in relapse rates over 1 year of treatment between social skills training and other interventions (4 RCTs, 125 people; OR 0.74, 95% CI 0.43 to 1.29; absolute numbers not provided), but found that social skills training reduced relapse over 2 years of treatment (2 RCTs, 264 people; OR 3.03, 95% CI 1.11 to 8.33; absolute numbers not provided).

Harms: The review gave no information on harms.[49]

Comment: None.

QUESTION Which interventions are effective in people who are resistant to standard antipsychotic drugs?

Systematic reviews in people resistant to standard antipsychotic drugs found that clozapine or olanzapine improved symptoms after 12 weeks and after 2 years compared with standard antipsychotic drugs. RCTs provided insufficient evidence to compare newer antipsychotics in people resistant to standard antipsychotic drugs.

Benefits: **Clozapine versus standard antipsychotic drugs:** We found one systematic review (search date 1999, 6 RCTs) comparing clozapine versus standard antipsychotic drugs in people who were resistant to standard treatment.[14] It found that, compared with standard antipsychotic drugs, clozapine significantly increased the proportion of people who improved at 6–12 weeks (4 RCTs, 370 people; RR for no improvement compared with standard antipsychotic drugs 0.7, 95% CI 0.6 to 0.8) and at 12–24 months (2 RCTs, 648 people; RR 0.8, 95% CI 0.6 to 1.0). It found no difference in relapse rates at 12 weeks. **Clozapine versus other new antipsychotic drugs:** We found one systematic review (search date 1988, 8 RCTs, 5 in people with treatment resistant schizophrenia, 595 people), which compared clozapine versus olanzapine, risperidone, and zotepine.[15] It found no significant difference between clozapine and other new antipsychotics in global clinical impression (Clinical Global Impression [CGI] score: WMD −0.09, 95% CI −0.34 to +0.15) or mental state (Brief Psychiatric Rating Scale or Positive and Negative Syndrome Scale < 20% improved: 83/173 [48%] with clozapine *v* 81/178 [45%] with olanzapine or risperidone; RR 1.05, 95% CI 0.84 to 1.32). However, the number of people studied was too small to rule out a clinically important difference. **Olanzapine versus standard antipsychotic drugs:** One systematic review (search date 1999, 1 RCT, 84 people) found no significant difference in psychotic symptoms over 8 weeks between olanzapine (25 mg/day) and chlorpromazine (39/42 [93%] with olanzapine *v* 42/42 [0%]; RR for no important response defined as a 40% reduction on the CGI scale 0.93, 95% CI 0.85 to 1.01).[23] The RCT is likely to have been too small to exclude a clinically important difference. **Olanzapine versus other new antipsychotic drugs:** We found one systematic review (search date 1999, 1 RCT, 180 people) comparing olanzapine versus clozapine, which found no significant difference in psychotic symptoms over 8 weeks (45/90 [50%] with olanzapine *v* 55/90 [0%] with clozapine; RR for no important response [defined as a 40% reduction on the CGI scale] 0.82, 95% CI 0.63 to 1.07).[23] The RCT is likely to have been too small to exclude a clinically important difference. **Other interventions:** We found no RCTs examining the effects of other interventions in people resistant to standard treatment.

Harms: **Clozapine versus standard antipsychotic drugs:** See harms of clozapine, p 1214. **Clozapine versus other new antipsychotic drugs:** The review found that, compared with other new antipsychotic drugs (mainly olanzapine and risperidone), clozapine was significantly less likely to cause extrapyramidal adverse effects (305 people; RR 0.3, 95% CI 0.1 to 0.6; NNT 6, 95% CI 4 to 9).[15] It also found that clozapine may be less likely to cause dry mouth and more likely to cause fatigue, nausea, dizziness, hypersalivation, and hypersomnia than other new antipsychotic drugs, but these findings were from one or at most two RCTs. It found that people taking clozapine tended to be more satisfied with their treatment than those taking other new antipsychotic drugs, but also tended to withdraw from RCTs more often. It found no significant difference in rates of blood dyscrasias between clozapine and other new antipsychotic drugs, but the number of people studied was too small (558) to rule out a clinically important difference.[15]

Comment: Some RCTs in the reviews included people who were partial responders to neuroleptic drugs and people unable to take some neuroleptic medication because of adverse effects.[14,15,23] The reviews did not specify the duration of treatment resistant illness of the participants in the RCTs. RCTs are underway to clarify the mode of action of cognitive behavioural therapy and establish its effects in people who are resistant to standard treatments.

QUESTION **Which interventions improve adherence to antipsychotic medication?**

OPTION **BEHAVIOURAL THERAPY**

One RCT found that behavioural interventions improved adherence to antipsychotic medication compared with usual treatment. Two RCTs found limited evidence that behavioural interventions may improve adherence more than psychoeducational therapy.

Benefits: We found no systematic review. **Versus usual treatment:** We found one RCT (36 men).[50] The behavioural training method comprised being told the importance of adhering to antipsychotic medication and instructions on how to take medication. Each participant was given a self monitoring spiral calendar, which featured a dated slip of paper for each dose of antipsychotic. Adherence was estimated by pill counts (see comment below). After 3 months fewer people had high pill adherence after usual treatment compared with behaviour therapy (figures not provided). **Versus psychoeducational therapy:** See benefits of psychoeducational interventions, p 1232.

Harms: None reported.

Comment: Assessing adherence by pill count has potential confounders in that people may throw pills away.[50]

OPTION **COMPLIANCE THERAPY**

Two RCTs found limited evidence that compliance therapy may increase adherence to antipsychotic drugs at 6 and 18 months compared with non-specific counselling.

Benefits: We found no systematic review, but found two RCTs.[51,52] The first RCT (47 people with acute psychoses, most of whom fulfilled criteria for schizophrenia or had been admitted with the first episode of a psychotic illness) compared compliance therapy (see glossary, p 1233) versus supportive counselling.[51] It found that, compared with non-specific counselling, compliance therapy significantly increased the proportion of people with improved adherence at 4–6 weeks (improved adherence defined as a score ≥ 5 on a scale from 1–7, where 1 is complete refusal and 7 active participation, ready acceptance, and taking some responsibility for adhering to antipsychotic medication; OR 6.3, 95% CI 1.6 to 24.6) and at 6 month follow up (OR 5.2, 95% CI 1.5 to 18.3; absolute numbers not provided; see comment below).[51] The second RCT (74 people with acute psychoses, most of whom fulfilled criteria for schizophrenia and had been admitted to hospital with relapse of symptoms) found that compliance therapy significantly improved compliance over 18 months measured on a 7 point scale of medication adherence compared with non-specific counselling (mean difference 1.4, 95% CI 0.9 to 1.6).[52]

Harms: The RCTs gave no information on harms.[51,52]

Comment: Other trials have examined the potential benefits of compliance therapy but either did not employ a standardised measure of adherence or did not assess adherence in a blind fashion. In the first RCT, about a third of each group did not complete the RCT, and missing data are estimated from the mean scores in each group.[51]

OPTION FAMILY INTERVENTIONS

One systematic review found that "compliance with medication" over 9–24 months was higher in people who received multiple family interventions compared with usual care, single family interventions, or psychoeducational interventions, but the difference did not quite reach significance.

Benefits: We found one systematic review (search date 1999) that compared multiple family interventions versus usual care, single family interventions, or psychoeducational interventions.[47] Family interventions consisted mainly of education about the illness and training in problem solving over at least six weekly sessions. The review found that "compliance with medication" over 9–24 months was higher in people who received multiple family interventions compared with other interventions, but the difference did not quite reach significance (5 RCTs, 393 people; OR 0.63, 95% CI 0.40 to 1.01; no further data provided).[47]

Harms: The review gave no information on harms.[47]

Comment: Although no harms were reported, illness education could possibly have adverse consequences on morale and outlook. The mechanism for the effects of family intervention remains unclear. It is thought to work by reducing "expressed emotion" (hostility and criticism) in relatives of people with schizophrenia. The time consuming nature of this intervention, which must normally take place at evenings or weekends, can limit its availability. It cannot be applied to people who have little contact with home based carers.

OPTION PSYCHOEDUCATIONAL INTERVENTIONS

One systematic review found limited evidence that psychoeducation improved adherence to antipsychotic medication compared with usual care. Two RCTs found limited evidence that psychoeducation may improve adherence less than behavioural therapy.

Benefits: **Versus usual treatment:** We found one systematic review (search date 2002), which identified four RCTs that assessed adherence with medication.[48] The RCTs compared individual or group psychoeducation of either standard length (11 sessions or more) or brief length (10 sessions or less) versus usual care. The first RCT (67 people) found no significant difference in adherence between brief individual psychoeducation and usual care measure on a continuous scale of medication compliance. The second RCT (82 people) found no significant difference in adherence over 18 months between standard length group interventions and usual care. However, two further RCTs identified by the review comparing brief group psychoeducational interventions versus control suggested that psychoeducation was more effective in improving adherence. The third

RCT (236 people) found that a brief group psychoeducational intervention significantly improved adherence compared with control (measured on a continuous scale of "medication concordance"; WMD −0.4, 95% CI −0.6 to −0.2). The fourth RCT (46 people) comparing a brief psychoeducational intervention versus usual care found limited evidence that psychoeducational interventions may improve adherence over 1 year (mean number of non-compliant episodes 0.38 with psychoeducation *v* 1.14 with usual care).[48]

Versus behavioural therapy: We found two RCTs.[50,53] The first RCT (36 men) compared three interventions: psychoeducation, behavioural therapy, or usual treatment.[50] The behavioural training method comprised being told the importance of complying with antipsychotic medication and instructions on how to take medication. Each participant was given a self monitoring spiral calendar, which featured a dated slip of paper for each dose of antipsychotic. Adherence was estimated by pill counts (see comment below). The RCT found that, after 3 months, fewer people had high pill adherence after psychoeducation compared with behavioural therapy, but the difference was not significant (3/11 [27%] with psychoeducation *v* 8/11 [72%] with behavioural therapy had pill adherence scores of 80% measured by pill counts; RR of high pill adherence score 0.37, 95% CI 0.13 to 1.05). The RCT is likely to have been too small to detect a clinically important difference.[50] The second RCT (39 people) compared a psychoeducational intervention, a behavioural intervention given individually, and a behavioural intervention involving the person with schizophrenia and their family.[53] The individual behavioural intervention consisted of specific written guidelines, and oral instructions given to people to use a pill box consisting of 28 compartments for every medication occasion during a week. The behavioural intervention, when given to the individual and their family, contained additional instructions for the family members to compliment the person with schizophrenia for taking their prescribed medication. The primary outcome measure was pill count at 2 months (see comment below). The RCT found that medication adherence was significantly more likely with behavioural interventions than with psychoeducation (> 90% adherence at 2 months, 25/26 [96%] with behavioural interventions *v* 6/13 [46%] with psychoeducation; RR 2.08, 95% CI 1.15 to 3.77, NNT 2, 95% CI 2 to 5).

Harms: None reported.

Comment: Assessing adherence by pill count has potential confounders in that people may throw pills away.[50,53] Each psychoeducational intervention varied in the protocol used and few employed the same outcome measurements.

GLOSSARY

Compliance therapy A treatment based on cognitive behavioural therapy and motivational interviewing techniques with a view to improving adherence to medication.

Negative symptoms This generally refers to qualities that are abnormal by their absence (e.g. loss of drive, motivation, and self care).

Positive symptoms This refers to symptoms that characterise the onset or relapse of schizophrenia, usually hallucinations and delusions, but sometimes including thought disorder.

Schizophrenia

Substantive changes

Amisulpride One RCT found no significant difference in symptoms at 2 months between amisulpride and olanzapine.[20]

Olanzapine One systematic review added;[26] conclusions unchanged.

Family interventions to reduce relapse rates One systematic review added;[47] conclusions unchanged.

Social skills training to reduce relapse rates One systematic review added;[49] conclusions unchanged.

Family interventions to improve adherence One systematic review added;[47] conclusions unchanged.

REFERENCES

1. Andreasen NC. Symptoms, signs and diagnosis of schizophrenia. *Lancet* 1995;346:477–481.
2. Kane JM, Honigfeld G, Singer J, et al. Clozapine for the treatment-resistant schizophrenic. *Arch Gen Psychiatry* 1988;45:789–796.
3. Meltzer HY. Treatment-resistant schizophrenia: the role of clozapine. *Curr Med Res Opin* 1997;14:1–20.
4. Cannon M, Jones P. Neuroepidemiology: schizophrenia. *J Neurol Neurosurg Psychiatry* 1996;61:604–613.
5. Jablensky A, Sartorius N, Ernberg G, et al. Schizophrenia: manifestations, incidence and course in different cultures. A World Health Organisation ten-country study. *Psychol Med* 1992;monograph supplement 20:1–97.
6. Hegarty JD, Baldessarini RJ, Tohen M, et al. One hundred years of schizophrenia: a meta-analysis of the outcome literature. *Am J Psychiatry* 1994;151:1409–1416.
7. Johnstone EC. Schizophrenia: problems in clinical practice. *Lancet* 1993; 341:536–538.
8. Thornley B, Adams C. Content and quality of 2000 controlled trials in schizophrenia over 50 years. *BMJ* 1998;317:1181–1184. Search date 1997; primary sources hand searching of conference proceedings, Biological Abstracts, Cinahl, The Cochrane Library, Embase, Lilacs, Psychlit, Pstndex, Medline, and Sociofile.
9. Thornley B, Adams CE, Awad G. Chlorpromazine versus placebo for those with schizophrenia. In: The Cochrane Library, Issue 2, 2002. Oxford: Update Software. Search date 1999; primary sources Biological Abstracts, Embase, Medline, Psychlit, SciSearch, Cochrane Library, Cochrane Schizophrenia Group's Register, hand searches of reference lists, and personal contact with pharmaceutical companies and authors of trials.
10. Joy CB, Adams CE, Lawrie SM. Haloperidol versus placebo for schizophrenia. In: The Cochrane Library, Issue 2, 2002. Oxford: Update Software. Search date 1998; primary sources Biological Abstracts, Cinahl, The Cochrane Schizophrenia Group's Register, Embase, Medline, Psychlit, SciSearch, hand searches of references, and contact with authors of trials and pharmaceutical companies.
11. Sultana A, Reilly J, Fenton M. Thioridazine for schizophrenia. In: The Cochrane Library, Issue 2, 2002. Oxford: Update Software. Search date 1999; primary sources Biological Abstracts, Cinahl, The Cochrane Library, The Cochrane Schizophrenia Group's Register, Embase, Medline, Psychlit, Sociofile, reference lists, pharmaceutical companies, and authors of trials.
12. Quraishi S, David A, Adams, CE. Depot bromperidol decanoate for schizophrenia. In: The Cochrane Library, Issue 2, 2002. Search date 1999; primary sources Biological Abstracts, Cochrane Library, Cochrane Schizophrenia Group's Register, Embase, Medline, PsycLIT, hand searches of reference lists and personal contact with Janssen Cilag.
13. Quraishi S, David A. Depot haloperidol decanoate for schizophrenia. In: The Cochrane Library, Issue 2, 2002. Oxford: Update Software. Search date 1998; primary sources Biological Abstracts, Embase, Medline, Psychlit, SciSearch, The Cochrane Library, reference lists, authors of studies, and pharmaceutical companies.
14. Wahlbeck K, Cheine M, Essali MA. Clozapine versus typical neuroleptic medication for schizophrenia. In: The Cochrane Library, Issue 2, 2002. Oxford: Update Software. Search date 1999; primary sources Biological Abstracts, Cochrane Schizophrenia Group's Register, Cochrane Library, Embase, Lilacs, Medline, Psychlit, SciSearch Science Citation Index, hand searches of reference lists, and personal communication with pharmaceutical companies.
15. Tuunainen A, Gilbody SM. Newer atypical antipsychotic medication versus clozapine for schizophrenia. In: The Cochrane Library, Issue 2, 2002. Oxford: Update Software. Search date 1998; primary sources Biological Abstracts, Cochrane Schizophrenia Group's Register, Cochrane Library, Embase, Lilacs, Medline, Psychlit, hand searches of reference lists, and personal contact with authors of trials and pharmaceutical companies.
16. Honigfeld G, Arellano F, Sethi J, et al. Reducing clozapine-related morbidity and mortality: five years experience of the clozaril national registry. *J Clin Psychiatry* 1998;59(suppl 3):3–7.
17. Geddes J, Freemantle N, Harrison P, et al, for the National Schizophrenia Development Group. Atypical antipsychotics in the treatment of schizophrenia: systematic review and meta-regression analysis. *BMJ* 2000;321:1371–1377. Search date 1998; primary sources Medline, Embase, Psychlit, and Cochrane Controlled Trials Register.
18. Mota Neto JIS, Lima MS, Soares BGO. Amisulpride for schizophrenia. In: The Cochrane Library, Issue 2, 2002. Oxford: Update Software. Search date 2000, Biological Abstracts Cinahl, Cochrane Library, Cochrane Schizophrenia Group's Register, Embase, Lilacs, Medline, Psyclit, Science Citation Index, hand searches of reference lists and personal contact with the manufacturer of amisulpride.
19. Leucht S, Pitschel-Walz G, Engel RR, et al. Amisulpride, an unusual "atypical" antipsychotic: a meta-analysis of randomized controlled trials. *Am J Psychiatry* 2002;159:177–179. Search date 2000; primary sources Medline, Current Contents, hand searches of reference lists and personal contact with the manufacturer of amisupride.
20. Martin S, Ljo H, Peuskens J, et al. A double blind, randomised comparative trial of amisulpiride

versus olanzapine in the treatment of schizophrenia: short term results at two months. *Curr Med Res Opin* 2002;18:355–362.

21. Fenton M, Murphy B, Wood J, et al. Loxapine for schizophrenia. In: The Cochrane Library, Issue 2, 2002. Oxford: Update Software. Search date 1999; primary sources Biological Abstracts, The Cochrane Library, The Cochrane Schizophrenia Group's Register, Embase, Lilacs, Psyndex, Psychlit, and hand searches of reference lists.
22. Bagnall AM, Fenton M, Lewis R, et al. Molindone for schizophrenia and severe mental illness. In: The Cochrane Library, Issue 2, 2002. Oxford: Update Software. Search date 1999; primary sources Biological Abstracts, The Cochrane Library, The Cochrane Schizophrenia Group's Register, Cinahl, Embase, Psychlit, pharmaceutical databases, hand searches of reference lists, and personal contact with authors of trials.
23. Duggan L, Fenton M, Dardennes RM, et al. Olanzapine for schizophrenia. In: The Cochrane Library, Issue 2, 2002. Oxford: Update Software. Search date 1999; primary sources Biological Abstracts, Embase, Medline, Psychlit, Cochrane Library, hand searches of reference lists and conference abstracts, and personal communication with authors of trials and pharmaceutical companies.
24. Peuskens J, de Hert M, Jones, M. The clinical value of risperidone and olanzapine: a meta-analysis of efficacy and safety. *Int J Psych Clin Prac* 2001;5:170–187. Search date 1998, primary sources Medline, Embase, Psychlit 1991–1998.
25. Gilbody SM, Bagnall AM, Duggan L, et al. Risperidone versus other atypical antipsychotic medication for schizophrenia. In: The Cochrane Library, Issue 2, 2002. Oxford: Update Software. Search date 1999; primary sources Biological Abstracts, Cochrane Library, Cochrane Schizophrenia Group's Register, Embase, Medline, Lilacs, Psyindex, Psychlit, pharmaceutical databases on the Dialog Corporation Datastar and Dialog services, hand search of reference lists, and contact with pharmaceutical companies and authors of trials.
26. De Rossi M, Donda P, Bellantuono C. Efficacy and tolerability of olanzapine: a critical review of the international literature. *Rivista di Psichiatria* 2001;36:183–203.
27. Conley RR, Mahmoud R. A randomized double-blind study of risperidone and olanzapine in the treatment of schizophrenia or schizoaffective disorder. *Am J Psychiatry* 2001;158:765–774.
28. Leucht S, Hartung B. Perazine for schizophrenia. In: The Cochrane Library, Issue 2, 2002. Search date 2001; primary sources Cochrane Schizophrenia Group's register (January 2001), Biological Abstracts, CINAHL, The Cochrane Library, Embase, Medline, Psyclit, Lilacs, Psyndex, Sociological Abstracts, Sociofile, hand searches of reference lists and personal contact with pharmaceutical companies and authors.
29. Sultana A, McMonagle T. Pimozide for schizophrenia or related psychoses. In: The Cochrane Library, Issue 2, 2002. Oxford: Update Software. Search date 1999; primary sources Biological Abstracts, The Cochrane Schizophrenia Group's Register, Embase, Janssen-Cilag UK's register of studies, Medline, hand searches of reference lists, and personal contact with pharmaceutical companies.
30. Srisurapanont M, Disayavanish C, Taimkaew K. Quetiapine for schizophrenia. In: The Cochrane Library, Issue 2, 2002. Oxford: Update Software. Search date 2000; primary sources Biological Abstracts, Embase, Medline, Psychlit, The Cochrane Library, Cinahl, Sigle, Sociofile, hand searches of journals, and personal communication with authors of studies and pharmaceutical companies.
31. Kennedy E, Song F, Hunter R, et al. Risperidone versus typical antipsychotic medication for schizophrenia. In: The Cochrane Library, Issue 2, 2002. Oxford: Update Software. Search date 1997; primary sources Biological Abstracts, The Cochrane Trials Register, Embase, Medline, Psychlit, hand searches of reference lists, and personal communication with pharmaceutical companies.
32. Lopez Ibor JJ, Ayuso JL, Gutierrez M, et al. Risperidone in the treatment of chronic schizophrenia: multicenter study comparative to haloperidol. *Actas Luso Esp Neurol Psiquiatr Cienc Afines* 1996;24:165–172.
33. Soares BGO, Fenton M, Chue P. Sulpiride for schizophrenia. In: The Cochrane Library, Issue 2, 2002. Oxford: Update Software. Search date 1998; primary sources Biological Abstracts, Cinahl, Cochrane Schizophrenia Group's Register, The Cochrane Library, Embase, Medline, Psychlit, Sigle, and Sociofile.
34. Harnryd C, Bjerkenstedt L, Bjork K, et al. Clinical evaluation of sulpiride in schizophrenic patients — a double-blind comparison with chlorpromazine. *Acta Psych Scand.* 1984;311:7–30.
35. Bagnall AM, Lewis RA, Leitner ML, et al. Ziprasidone for schizophrenia and severe mental illness. In: The Cochrane Library, Issue 2, 2002. Oxford: Update Software. Search date 1999; primary sources Biological Abstracts, The Cochrane Library, The Cochrane Schizophrenia Group's Register, Embase, Lilacs, Psyndex, Psychlit, pharmaceutical databases, hand searches of reference lists, and personal contact with authors of trials.
36. Fenton M, Morris F, De Silva P, et al. Zotepine for schizophrenia. In: The Cochrane Library, Issue 2, 2002. Oxford: Update Software. Search date 1999; primary sources Biological Abstracts, The Cochrane Library, The Cochrane Schizophrenia Group's Register, Embase, Dialog Corporation Datastar service, Medline, Psychlit, hand searches of reference lists, and personal contact with authors of trials and pharmaceutical companies.
37. Gilbert PL, Harris MJ, McAdams LA, et al. Neuroleptic withdrawal in schizophrenic people: a review of the literature. *Arch Gen Psychiatry* 1995;52:173–188. Search date not stated; primary source Medline.
38. Quraishi S, David A. Depot pipothiazine palmitate and undeclynate for schizophrenia. In: The Cochrane Library, Issue 2, 2002. Oxford: Update Software. Search date 1998; primary sources Biological Abstracts, Cochrane Library, Cochrane Schizophrenia Group's Register, Embase, Medline, Psychlit, hand searches of reference lists, and personal communication with pharmaceutical companies.
39. Adams CE, Eisenbruch M. Depot fluphenazine versus oral fluphenazine for those with schizophrenia. In: The Cochrane Library, Issue 2, 2002. Oxford: Update Software. Search date 1995; primary sources Biological Abstracts, The Cochrane Library, Cochrane Schizophrenia Group's Register, Embase, Medline, Psychlit, Science Citation Index, hand searches of reference lists, and personal communication with pharmaceutical companies.
40. Quraishi S, David A. Depot flupenthixol decanoate for schizophrenia or similar psychotic disorders. In: The Cochrane Library, Issue 2, 2002. Oxford:

Update Software. Search date 1998; primary sources Biological Abstracts, The Cochrane Library, Cochrane Schizophrenia Group's Register, Embase, Medline, Psychlit, SciSearch, references, and personal communication with authors of trials and pharmaceutical companies.
41. Quraishi S, David A. Depot fluspirilene for schizophrenia. In: The Cochrane Library, Issue 2, 2002. Oxford: Update Software. Search date 1998; primary sources Biological Abstracts, The Cochrane Library, The Cochrane Schizophrenia Group's Register, Embase, Medline, Psychlit, and hand searches of reference lists.
42. Quraishi S, David A. Depot perphenazine decanoate and enanthate for schizophrenia. In: The Cochrane Library, Issue 2, 2002. Oxford: Update Software. Search date 1998; primary sources Biological Abstracts, The Cochrane Library, The Cochrane Schizophrenia Group's Register, Embase, Medline, Psychlit, hand searches of reference lists, and personal communication with pharmaceutical companies.
43. Coutinho E, Fenton M, Quraishi S. Zuclopenthixol decanoate for schizophrenia and other serious mental illnesses. In: The Cochrane Library, Issue 2, 2002. Oxford: Update Software. Search date 1998; primary sources Biological Abstracts, Cinhal, The Cochrane Library, The Cochrane Schizophrenia Group's Register, Embase, Medline, and Psychlit. References of all eligible studies were searched for further trials. The manufacturer of zuclopenthixol was contacted.
44. Csernansky JG, Mahmoud R, Brenner R; The Risperidone-USA-79 Study Group. A comparison of risperidone and haloperidol for the prevention of relapse in patients with schizophrenia. *New Engl J Med* 2002;346:1:16–22.
45. Jeste D, Gilbert P, McAdams L, et al. Considering neuroleptic maintenance and taper on a continuum: need for an individual rather than dogmatic approach. *Arch Gen Psychiatry* 1995;52:209–212.
46. Cormac I, Jones C, Campbell C. Cognitive behavioural therapy for schizophrenia. In: The Cochrane Library, Issue 2, 2002. Oxford: Update Software. Search date 2001, primary sources Biological Abstracts, Cochrane Schizophrenia Group's Register, Cinahl, The Cochrane Library, Medline, Embase, Psychlit, Sigle, Sociofile, reference lists of articles, and personal communication with authors of trials.
47. Pilling S, Bebbington P, Kuipers E, et al. Psychological treatments in schizophrenia: I. Meta-analysis of family interventions and cognitive behaviour therapy. *Psychol Med* 2002;32:763–782.
48. Pekkala E, Merinder L. Psychoeducation for schizophrenia. In: The Cochrane Library, Issue 2, 2002. Oxford: Update Software. Search date 2002; primary sources Cinahl, The Cochrane Library, Cochrane Schizophrenia Group's Register, Embase, Medline, Psychlit, Sociofile, hand searched reference lists, and personal contact with authors.
49. Pilling S, Bebbington P, Kuipers E, et al. Psychological treatments in schizophrenia: II. Meta-analysis of randomised controlled trials of social skills training and cognitive remediation. *Psychol Med* 2002;32:783–791.
50. Boczkowski JA, Zeichner A, DeSanto N. Neuroleptic compliance among chronic schizophrenic outpeople: an intervention outcome report. *J Consult Clin Psychol* 1985;53:666–671.
51. Kemp R, Kirov G, Everitt B, et al. Randomised controlled trial of compliance therapy. 18-month follow-up. *Br J Psychiatry* 1998;172:413–419.
52. Kemp R, Hayward P, Applewhaite G, et al. Compliance therapy in psychotic people: randomised controlled trial. *BMJ* 1996;312:345–349.
53. Azrin NH, Teichner G. Evaluation of an instructional program for improving medication compliance for chronically mentally ill outpatients. *Behaviour Res Ther* 1998;36:849–861.

Zia Nadeem
Research Fellow
Department of Psychiatry

Andrew McIntosh
Lecturer in Psychiatry
Department of Psychiatry

Stephen Lawrie
Senior Clinical Research Fellow and
Honorary Consultant Psychiatrist

University of Edinburgh
UK

Competing interests: SL has been paid for speaking about critical appraisal by employees of the manufacturers of olanzapine, quetiapine, risperidone, and ziprasidone, and has been paid to speak about the management of schizophrenia by employees of the manufacturers of amisulpiride, olanzapine, risperidone, and clozapine. AM and ZN none declared.

TABLE 1 **Continued treatment with antipsychotic drugs: choice of drugs (see text, p 1227).**

Review	Search date	Number of RCTs	Comparisons	Main Conclusion
39	1995	6	Oral *v* depot fluphenazine	No significant difference
13	1998	7	Haloperidol decanoate *v* other depots	No significant difference
40	1999	8	Flupenthixol decanoate *v* other depots	No significant difference
38	1999	7	Pipotiazine (pipothiazine) palmitate *v* other depots	No significant difference
38	1999	2	Pipotiazine (pipothiazine) palmitate *v* oral antipsychotics	No significant difference
41	1999	1	Fluspirilene decanoate *v* oral chlorpromazine	No significant difference
41	1999	3	Fluspirilene decanoate *v* other depots	No significant difference
42	1999	1	Perphenazine enanthate *v* clopenthixol decanoate	No significant difference
29	2000	11	Pimozide *v* standard antipsychotics	No significant difference
23	1999	1	Olanzapine *v* standard antipsychotics	No significant difference
43	1998	3	Zuclopenthixol decanoate *v* other depots	People taking zuclopenthixol had lower relapse rates over 12 weeks to 1 year
14	1999	19	Clozapine *v* standard antipsychotics	Relapse rates up to 12 weeks were lower with clozapine
12	1999	2	Bromperidol *v* haloperidol or fluphenazine	Relapse rates over 6–12 months were lower with haloperidol or fluphenazine

Acute gout

Search date December 2002

Martin Underwood

QUESTIONS

INTERVENTIONS

Key Messages

Treatment of acute gout

- **Non-steroidal anti-inflammatory drugs** We found limited evidence from one RCT that tenoxicam reduced short term pain and tenderness in acute gout compared with placebo. However, we were unable to draw reliable conclusions from this small study. We found no evidence of the effects of other non-steroidal anti-inflammatory drugs compared with placebo in acute gout. We found insufficient evidence on the relative benefits and harms of different non-steroidal anti-inflammatory drugs.
- **Oral colchicine** We found limited evidence from one small RCT that colchicine improved pain in acute gout. However, we were unable to draw reliable conclusions from this small study.
- **Intra-articular corticosteroids; oral corticosteroids; parenteral corticosteroids** We found no evidence on the effects of intra-articular, parenteral, or oral corticosteroids for acute gout.

Prevention of recurrent gout

- **Advice to reduce alcohol intake; advice to reduce dietary intake of purines; allopurinol; benzbromarone; colchicine; probenecid; sulphinpyrazone; weight reduction advice** We found insufficient evidence on effects of these treatments to prevent attacks of recurrent gout.

 Clin Evid 2003;10:1238–1246.

DEFINITION Gout is a syndrome caused by deposition of urate crystals.[1] It typically presents as an acute monoarthritis of rapid onset. The first metatarsal phalangeal joint is the most commonly affected joint (podagra). Acute gout also affects other joints: joints in the foot, ankle, knee, wrist, finger, and elbow are the most frequently affected. Crystal deposits (tophi) may develop around hands, feet, elbows, and ears. The diagnosis is usually made clinically. The American College of Rheumatology (ACR) criteria for diagnosing gout are a) characteristic urate crystals in joint fluid, b) a tophus proved to contain urate crystals, or c) the presence of six or more defined clinical laboratory and x ray phenomena (see table 1, p 1246).[2] We have included studies of people meeting the ACR classification criteria for acute gout and studies that used other criteria or where the diagnosis was made clinically.

INCIDENCE/ PREVALENCE Prevalence data from general practice records suggest that gout is more common in older people and men.[3] In people aged 65–74 years in the UK, the prevalence is about 50/1000 in men and about 9/1000 in women.[3] The annual incidence of gout in the USA is 1.6/1000 men and 0.3/1000 for women aged over 50 years.[4] Gout may be more common in some non-white ethnic groups. Cohort studies of male former medical students found the annual incidence of gout to be 3.1/1000 person-years in black people and 1.8/1000 person-years in white people. After correcting for incident hypertension, the relative risk of gout was 1.3 (95% CI 0.77 to 2.19).[5]

AETIOLOGY/ RISK FACTORS Urate crystals form when serum urate concentration exceeds 0.42 mmol/L.[6] Serum urate concentration is the principal risk factor for a first attack of gout,[7] although the concentration may be normal in 40% of people if measured during an attack of gout.[6,8–10] A cohort study of 2046 men followed for about 15 years found that the annual incidence is about 0.4% in men with a urate concentration of 0.42–0.47 mmol/L, rising to 4.3% when serum urate concentration is 0.45–0.59 mmol/L.[11] A 5 year longitudinal study of 223 asymptomatic men with hyperuricaemia estimated 5 year cumulative incidence of gout to be 10.8% for those with baseline serum urate of 0.42–0.47 mmol/L, 27.7% for baseline urate 0.48–0.53 mmol/L, and 61.1% for baseline urate levels of 0.54 mmol/L or more.[7] The study found that a 0.6 mmol/L difference in baseline serum urate increased the odds of an acute attack of gout by a factor of 1.8 (OR adjusted for other risk factors for gout: 1.84, 95% CI 1.24 to 2.72). It also found that alcohol and diuretics were risk factors for gout (adjusted OR for any alcohol intake *v* no alcohol intake: 3.45, 95% CI 1.58 to 7.56; adjusted OR for diuretics *v* no diuretics: OR 6.55, 95% CI 2.98 to 14.35). Other suggested risk factors for gout include obesity, insulin resistance, dyslipidaemia, hypertension, and cardiovascular disorders.[12,13]

PROGNOSIS We found few reliable data about prognosis or complications of acute gout. One study of untreated acute gout found that 3/11 (27%) people with podagra experienced spontaneous resolution after 7 days.[14] A case series of 614 people with gout who had not had treatment to reduce urate levels and could recall the interval between first and second attacks reported recurrence rates of 62%

after 1 year, 78% after 2 years, and 84% by 3 years.[15] An analysis of two prospective cohort studies of 371 black and 1181 white male former medical students followed up for about 30 years found no significant difference in risk of coronary heart disease in men who had developed gout compared with men who had not (RR 0.85, 95% CI 0.40 to 1.81).[16]

AIMS OF INTERVENTION **For acute attacks:** to reduce the severity and duration of pain, loss of function, with minimal adverse effects of treatment. **For prevention:** to reduce the frequency and the severity of any acute episodes, and minimise the adverse effects of interventions.

OUTCOMES **For acute attacks:** severity of symptoms (pain scores, proportion of people with improved symptoms), adverse effects of treatment. **For prevention (over 6 months):** number of recurrent episodes a year, severity of recurrent episodes a year, adverse effects of treatment.

METHODS *Clinical Evidence* search and appraisal December 2002, hand searches of selected references. Only papers with 6 months or longer of follow up were included for prevention of recurrent gout. We excluded studies that were non-randomised, had 10 or fewer people in each treatment arm, had more than 20% loss to follow up, were crossover trials that did not present results before crossover, were not fully published (e.g. abstracts of conference proceedings, which could not be appraised for quality), or which reported only non-clinical outcomes such as serum urate levels.

QUESTION What are the effects of treatments for acute gout? New

OPTION NON-STEROIDAL ANTI-INFLAMMATORY DRUGS

We found limited evidence from one RCT that tenoxicam reduced short term pain and tenderness in acute gout compared with placebo. However, we were unable to draw reliable conclusions from this small study. We found no evidence of the effects of other non-steroidal anti-inflammatory drugs compared with placebo in acute gout. We found insufficient evidence on the relative benefits and harms of different non-steroidal anti-inflammatory drugs.

Benefits: **Versus placebo:** We found no systematic review. We found one RCT (30 people aged 21–70 years with acute gout of the knee, ankle, wrist, big toe, or elbow) that compared tenoxicam 40 mg once daily versus placebo.[17] It found that tenoxicam significantly reduced pain and tenderness compared with placebo after 1 day (pain improved by ≥ 50%: 10/15 [67%] with tenoxicam *v* 4/15 [26%] with placebo; $P < 0.05$; tenderness improved by ≥ 50%: 6/15 [40%] with tenoxicam *v* 1/15 [7%] with placebo; $P < 0.05$; pain on mobilisation improved ≥ 50%: 4/15 [27%] with tenoxicam *v* 1/15 [7%] with placebo; $P < 0.05$). However, it found no significant difference between tenoxicam and placebo in physician rated efficacy after 4 days (physician rated efficacy "good or excellent": 7/15 [47%] with tenoxicam *v* 4/15 [26%] with placebo; P value not provided).[17] **Versus each other:** We found no systematic review. We found six RCTs.[18–23] The first RCT (150 men with acute gout for < 24 hours, mean age 49 years) was an equivalence study, which compared indometacin ([indomethacin] 50 mg 3 times daily) versus etoricoxib (120 mg once daily).[18] It found indometacin and etoricoxib had equivalent effects on pain (measured on a 5 point Likert scale) after 2–5 days (difference +0.11, 95% CI –0.14 to +0.35; equivalence pre-specified as ±0.5). The second RCT (93 people with acute gout) compared indometacin (200 mg for 1 day in divided doses followed by a reducing regimen for 28 days) versus azapropazone (600 mg 3 times daily for 4 days followed by 600 mg twice daily for 28 days).[19] It found no significant difference in the proportion of people who reported that the treatment "suited them" after 4 days (35/47 [74%] with indometacin *v* 40/46 [87%] with azapropazone; P value quoted as "not significant"). The third RCT (61 people with acute gout aged 18–75 years) compared etodolac 300 mg twice daily versus naproxen 500 mg twice daily.[20] It found no significant difference in pain score (range 0–5, higher scores indicating worse pain) after 2, 4, or 7 days (mean pain score at 2 days: 2.6 with etodolac *v* 2.8 with naproxen; P value quoted as "not significant"; mean pain score at 4 days: 1.8 with etodolac *v* 2.0 with naproxen; P value quoted as "not significant"; mean improvement in pain score at 8 days: 1.4 with etodolac *v* 1.4 with naproxen; P value quoted as "not significant"). The fourth RCT (60 people with acute gout aged 18–75 years) compared etodolac 300 mg twice daily versus naproxen 500 mg twice daily.[21] It found no significant difference in pain between etodolac and naproxen after 1, 2, 4, and 7 days (results presented graphically, no AR or P value provided). The fifth RCT (59 people with acute gout for < 48 hours, aged 35–88 years) compared indometacin (up to 225 mg for 1 day in divided doses followed by 50 mg 3 times daily) versus ketoprofen (450 mg in divided doses for 1 day followed by 100 mg 3 times daily).[22] It found no significant difference in pain score between indometacin and ketoprofen (range 0–3, higher scores indicating worse pain) after 2, 5, or 8 days (mean pain score at 2 days: 0.9 with indometacin *v* 1.1 with ketoprofen; P value quoted as "not significant"; mean pain score at 5 days: 0.8 with indometacin *v* 1.3 with ketoprofen; P value quoted as "not significant"; mean pain score at 8 days: 0.3 with indometacin *v* 0.4 with ketoprofen; P value quoted as "not significant"). The sixth RCT (29 people with acute gout) compared indometacin (50 mg 4 times daily for 4 days followed by 25 mg 4 times daily for 5 days) versus flurbiprofen (100 mg 4 times daily for 1 day followed by 50 mg 4 times daily for 5 days).[23] It found no significant difference between indometacin and flurbiprofen in the proportion of people with improved pain at rest after 2 days (proportion with improved pain at rest: 11/12 [92%] with indometacin *v* 11/12 [92%] with flurbiprofen; P value not provided). **Versus other treatments:** We found no RCTs.

Harms: The harms of non-steroidal anti-inflammatory drugs are considered in detail elsewhere in *Clinical Evidence* (see non-steroidal anti-inflammatory drugs, p 1393) and include gastrointestinal ulceration and haemorrhage. The first RCT found that indometacin produced significantly more adverse events than etoricoxib (proportion with adverse events: 17/75 [23%] with etoricoxib *v* 35/75 [47%] with indometacin; P = 0.003).[18] No differences in important adverse event rates were found when indometacin was compared with ketoprofen,[22] azapropazone,[19] or flurbiprofen.[23] Neither study comparing etodolac versus naproxen reported any important adverse events.[20,21]

Comment: **Versus placebo:** The RCT comparing tenoxicam versus placebo[17] conducted many significance tests and no adjustment was reported for this. **Versus each other:** Phenylbutazone and indometacin were established as treatments for acute gout based on uncontrolled studies. Only the comparison between etoricoxib and indometacin was powered to show equivalence in efficacy between the two compounds tested.[18] Although the RCTs found no significant differences in effectiveness between different non-steroidal anti-inflammatory drugs, they may have lacked power to show differences or establish equivalence. Etoricoxib may be a useful alternative to conventional non-steroidal anti-inflammatory drugs for people at high risk of gastrointestinal adverse effects. We found five RCTs that compared phenylbutazone with other non-steroidal anti-inflammatory drugs. These have not been considered further because phenylbutazone for gout has been restricted in many countries because it can cause aplastic anaemia and other serious adverse effects.[24]

OPTION CORTICOSTEROIDS

We found insufficient evidence on the effects of parenteral, oral, or intra-articular corticosteroids for acute gout.

Benefits: We found no systematic review or RCTs.

Harms: We found insufficient evidence in people with gout. Potential harms of oral corticosteroids are covered elsewhere in *Clinical Evidence* (see rheumatoid arthritis, p 1454 and asthma, p 1757).

Comment: None.

OPTION ORAL COLCHICINE

We found limited evidence from one small RCT that colchicine improved pain in acute gout. However, we were unable to draw reliable conclusions from this small study.

Benefits: **Versus placebo:** We found no systematic review. We found one small RCT (43 hospital inpatients with acute gout confirmed by synovial fluid examination, aged 55–91 years; 40/43 were men) that compared colchicine (1 mg followed by 0.5 mg every 2 hours as tolerated or until complete response) versus placebo.[25] It found that colchicine reduced pain compared with placebo after 48 hours (proportion with ≥50% improvement in pain: 73% with colchicine *v* 36% with placebo; $P < 0.05$).

Harms: The RCT found that all the people taking colchicine experienced diarrhoea or vomiting within about 24 hours; 5/22 [23%] people taking placebo developed nausea.[25] The 50% improvement in pain occurred before diarrhoea and vomiting in 9/22 (40%), after the onset of diarrhoea and vomiting in 12/22 (55%), and at the same time in one.

Comment: Colchicine has been used since antiquity to treat acute gout. There is a large number of observational studies that support its use. Although it seems efficacious, narrow benefit to toxicity ratio limits its use for acute gout.[26]

QUESTION What are the effects of treatments to prevent acute gout in people with prior episodes? New

OPTION COLCHICINE

We found insufficient evidence on the effects of colchicine in preventing attacks of gout in people with prior episodes.

Benefits: We found no systematic review or RCTs.

Harms: We found no RCTs.

Comment: None.

OPTION WEIGHT REDUCTION ADVICE

We found insufficient evidence on the effects of advice to reduce weight to prevent gout attacks.

Benefits: We found no systematic review or RCTs.

Harms: We found no RCTs.

Comment: None.

OPTION ADVICE TO REDUCE ALCOHOL INTAKE

We found insufficient evidence on the effects of advice to reduce alcohol intake to prevent gout attacks.

Benefits: We found no systematic review or RCTs.

Harms: We found no RCTs.

Comment: None.

OPTION ADVICE TO REDUCE DIETARY INTAKE OF PURINES

We found insufficient evidence on the effects of advice to reduce dietary intake of purines to prevent gout attacks.

Benefits: We found no systematic review or RCTs.

Harms: We found no RCTs.

Comment: None.

OPTION ALLOPURINOL

We found insufficient evidence on the effects of allopurinol to prevent gout attacks.

Benefits: We found no systematic review or RCTs.

Harms: We found no RCTs.

Comment: None.

OPTION PROBENECID

We found insufficient evidence on the effects of probenecid to prevent gout attacks.

Benefits: We found no systematic review or RCTs (see comment below).

Harms: We found no RCTs.

Comment: We found one quasi-randomised trial (37 men with a history of gout, aged 27–78 years) that compared probenecid 1–2 g daily versus allopurinol 300–600 mg daily.[27] Treatment allocation was by the last digit of the hospital number. Both groups took prophylactic colchicine for the first few months of treatment. The trial found no significant difference between probenecid and allopurinol for recurrence after a mean follow up of 18.6 months (recurrence free: 8/17 [47%] with probenecid *v* 9/20 [45%]; no P value provided). However, results may have been biased by non-random treatment allocation and because five people allocated to probenecid received sulphinpyrazone instead.

OPTION SULPHINPYRAZONE

We found insufficient evidence on the effects of sulphinpyrazone to prevent gout attacks.

Benefits: We found no systematic review or RCTs.

Harms: We found no RCTs.

Comment: None.

OPTION BENZBROMARONE

We found insufficient evidence on the effects of benzbromarone to prevent gout attacks.

Benefits: We found no systematic review or RCTs.

Harms: We found no RCTs.

Comment: None.

REFERENCES

1. Emmerson BT. The management of gout. *N Engl J Med* 1996;334:445–451.
2. Wallace SL, Robinson H, Masi AT, et al. Preliminary criteria for the classification of the acute arthritis of primary gout. *Arthritis Rheum* 1977;20:895–900.
3. Harris CM, Lloyd DC, Lewis J. The prevalence and prophylaxis of gout in England. *J Clin Epidemiol* 1995;48:1153–1158.
4. Abbott RD, Brand FN, Kannel WB, et al. Gout and coronary heart disease: the Framingham Study. *J Clin Epidemiol* 1988;41:237–242.
5. Hochberg MC, Thomas J, Thomas DJ, et al. Racial differences in the incidence of gout. The role of hypertension. *Arthritis Rheum* 1995;38:628–632.
6. McGill NW. Gout and other crystal-associated arthropathies. *Baillieres Best Pract Res Clin Rheumatol* 2000;14:445–460.
7. Lin KC, Lin HY, Chou P. The interaction between uric acid level and other risk factors on the development of gout among asymptomatic hyperuricemic men in a prospective study. *J Rheumatol* 2000;27:1501–1505.
8. Schlesinger N, Baker DG, Schumacher HR Jr. Serum urate during bouts of acute gouty arthritis. *J Rheumatol* 1997;24:2265–2266.
9. Logan JA, Morrison E, McGill PE. Serum uric acid in acute gout. *Ann Rheum Dis* 1997;56:696–697.
10. Stewart OJ, Silman AJ. Review of UK data on the rheumatic diseases – 4. Gout. *Br J Rheumatol* 1990;29:485–488.
11. Campion EW, Glynn RJ, DeLabry LO. Asymptomatic hyperuricemia. Risks and consequences in the Normative Aging Study. *Am J Med* 1987;82:421–426.

12. Culleton BF. Uric acid and cardiovascular disease: a renal-cardiac relationship? *Curr Opin Nephrol Hypertens* 2001;10:371–375.
13. Bryan E. Are gout and increased uric acid levels risk factors for cardiac disease? Centre for Clinical Effectiveness, Monash University. 2002. http://www.med.monash.edu.au/healthservices/cce/evidence/pdf/b.805.pdf (last accessed 18 July 2003).
14. Bellamy N, Downie WW, Buchanan WW. Observations on spontaneous improvement in patients with podagra: implications for therapeutic trials of non-steroidal anti-inflammatory drugs. *Br J Clin Pharmacol* 1987;24:33–36.
15. Yu TF, Gutman AB. Efficacy of colchiciner prophylaxis in gout. *Ann Intern Med* 1961;55:179–192.
16. Gelber AC, Klag MJ, Mead LA, et al. Gout and risk for subsequent coronary heart disease. The Meharry-Hopkins Study. *Arch Intern Med* 1997;157:1436–1440.
17. Garcia de la Torre I. Estudio doble-ciego paralelo, comparativo con tenoxicam vs placebo en artritis gotosa aguda [Spanish, Double-blind parallel study comparing tenoxicam and placebo in acute gouty arthritis]. *Invet Med Int* 1987;14:92–97.
18. Schumacher HR Jr, Boice JA, Daikh DI, et al. Randomised double blind trial of etoricoxib and indometacin in treatment of acute gouty arthritis. *BMJ* 2002;324:1488–1492.
19. Fraser RC, Davis RH, Walker FS. Comparative trial of azapropazone and indomethacin plus allopurinol in acute gout and hyperuricaemia. *J R Coll Gen Pract* 1987;37:409–411.
20. Maccagno A, Di Giorgio E, Romanowicz A. Effectiveness of etodolac ("Lodine") compared with naproxen in patients with acute gout. *Curr Med Res Opin* 1991;12:423–429.
21. Lederman R. A double-blind comparison of Etodolac (Lodine™) and high doses of naproxen in the treatment of acute gout. *Adv Ther* 1990;7:344–354.
22. Altman RD, Honig S, Levin JM, et al. Ketoprofen versus indomethacin in patients with acute gouty arthritis: a multicenter, double blind comparative study. *J Rheumatol* 1988;15:1422–1426.
23. Lomen PL, Turner LF, Lamborn KR, et al. Flurbiprofen in the treatment of acute gout. A comparison with indomethacin. *Am J Med* 1986;80:134–139.
24. Non-steroidal anti-inflammatory drugs. In: Royal Pharmaceutical Society of Great Britain, eds. *British National Formulary.* Wallingford: Pharmaceutical Press, 2003: 478–506.
25. Ahern MJ, Reid C, Gordon TP, et al. Does colchicine work? The results of the first controlled study in acute gout. *Aust N Z J Med* 1987;17:301–304.
26. Schlesinger N, Schumacher HR Jr. Gout: can management be improved? *Curr Opin Rheumatol* 2001;13:240–244.
27. Scott JT. Comparison of allopurinol and probenecid. *Ann Rheum Dis* 1966;25:623–626.

Martin Underwood
Professor of General Practice
Institute of Community Health Sciences
Barts and the London, Queen Mary's
School of Medicine and Dentistry
Queen Mary, University of London
London
UK

Competing interests: MU has received speaker fees from Pfizer, the manufacturers of valdecoxib and celecoxib and from Menarini Pharmaceuticals, the manufacturers of Ketoprofen and Dexketoprofen. His salary is provided by NHS Research and Development. MU is a current or recent applicant on research projects funded in excess of £100,000 by NHS Health Technology Assessment Programme, Arthritis Research Campaign and UK Medical Council.

TABLE 1 **American College of Rheumatology criteria for acute gout (patients must fulfill six or more criteria; see text, p 1239).[2]**

1	More than one attack of acute arthritis
2	Maximum inflammation developed within 1 day
3	Monoarthritis attack
4	Redness observed over joints
5	First metatarsophalangeal joint painful or swollen
6	Unilateral first metatarsophalangeal joint attack
7	Unilateral tarsal joint attack
8	Tophus (proved or suspected)
9	Hyperuricaemia
10	Asymmetric swelling within a joint on x ray film
11	Subcortical cysts without erosions on x ray film
12	Monosodium urate monohydrate microcrystals in joint fluid during an attack
13	Joint culture negative for organism during attack

Ankle sprain

Search date November 2002

Peter Struijs and Gino Kerkhoffs

QUESTIONS

INTERVENTIONS

See glossary, p 1256

Key Messages

- **Functional treatment** One systematic review and one subsequent RCT found limited evidence that functional treatment reduced the risk of the ankle giving way compared with minimal treatment. One systematic review found that, compared with immobilisation, functional treatment improved seven outcomes at either short (up to 6 weeks), intermediate (6 weeks to 1 year), or long term (over 1 year) follow up. However, effects seemed to be less marked at long term follow up, or if only results from high quality trials were analysed. Another systematic review found that, compared with immobilisation, functional treatment resulted in less persistent subjective instability but no significant difference in pain. Two systematic reviews found insufficient evidence to compare functional treatment versus surgery. One systematic review and three additional RCTs provided insufficient evidence to compare different functional treatments.
- **Immobilisation** One systematic review found that, compared with functional treatment, immobilisation was associated with less improvement in seven outcomes at either short (up to 6 weeks), intermediate (6 weeks to 1 year), or long term (over 1 year) follow up. However, effects were less marked at long term follow up, or if only results from high quality trials were analysed. Another systematic review found that, compared with functional treatment immobilisation was less effective at reducing systematic instability, but found no significant difference in pain. One systematic review found no significant difference between immobilisation and surgery in pain or subjective instability. One systematic review found insufficient evidence to compare immobilisation versus physiotherapy.
- **Surgery** One systematic review found no significant difference between surgery and immobilisation in pain or subjective instability. One systematic review found insufficient evidence to compare surgery versus functional treatment. One systematic review found insufficient evidence to compare surgery versus conservative treatment (immobilisation or functional treatment).

- **Diathermy** One systematic review found insufficient evidence on the effects of diathermy versus placebo on walking ability and reduction in swelling.
- **Homeopathic ointment** One systematic review of one small RCT found limited evidence that homeopathic ointment improved outcome on a "composite criteria" of treatment success compared with placebo.
- **Cold pack compression** Two RCTs found no significant difference in symptoms between cold pack placement and placebo or control. One RCT found less oedema with cold pack placement compared with heat or a contrast bath at 3–5 days after injury.
- **Ultrasound** One systematic review found no significant difference between ultrasound and sham ultrasound in the general improvement of symptoms or the ability to walk or bear weight at 7 days. Three RCTs provided insufficient evidence to compare ultrasound versus other treatments.

DEFINITION Ankle sprain is an injury of the lateral ligament complex of the ankle joint. Such injury can range from mild to severe and is graded on the basis of severity.[1–5] Grade I is a mild stretching of the ligament complex without joint instability; grade II is a partial rupture of the ligament complex with mild instability of the joint (such as isolated rupture of the anterior talofibular ligament); grade III involves complete rupture of the ligament complex with instability of the joint.

INCIDENCE/ PREVALENCE Ankle sprain is a common problem in acute medical care, occurring at a rate of about one injury/10 000 population/day.[6] Injuries of the lateral ligament complex of the ankle form a quarter of all sports injuries.[6]

AETIOLOGY/ RISK FACTORS The usual mechanism of injury is inversion and adduction (usually referred to as supination) of the plantar flexed foot. Predisposing factors are a history of ankle sprains and specific malalignment, like crus varum and pes cavo-varus.

PROGNOSIS Some sports (e.g. basketball, football/soccer, and volleyball) are associated with a particularly high incidence of ankle injuries. Pain is the most frequent residual problem, often localised on the medial side of the ankle.[4] Other residual complaints include mechanical instability, intermittent swelling, and stiffness. People with more extensive cartilage damage have a higher incidence of residual complaints.[4] Long term cartilage damage can lead to degenerative changes, especially if there is persistent or recurrent instability. Every further sprain has the potential to add new damage.

AIMS OF INTERVENTION To reduce swelling and pain; to restore the stability of the ankle joint.

OUTCOMES Return to pre-injury level of sports; return to pre-injury level of work; pain; swelling; subjective instability; objective instability; recurrent injury; ankle mobility; complications; patient satisfaction.

METHODS *Clinical Evidence* search and appraisal November 2002.

QUESTION What are the effects of treatment strategies for acute ankle ligament ruptures?

OPTION IMMOBILISATION

One systematic review found that, compared with functional treatment, immobilisation was associated with less improvement in seven outcomes at either short (up to 6 weeks), intermediate (6 weeks to 1 year), or long term (over 1 year) follow up. However, effects were less marked at long term follow up, or if only results from high quality trials were analysed. Another systematic review found that, compared with functional treatment immobilisation was less effective at reducing systematic instability, but found no significant difference in pain. One systematic review found no significant difference between immobilisation and surgery in pain or subjective instability. One systematic review found insufficient evidence to compare immobilisation versus physiotherapy.

Benefits: We found five systematic reviews (search dates 1993,[7] 1994,[8] 1998,[9] and 2000[10,11]). **Versus functional treatment:** We found four systematic reviews.[7–10] The first systematic review (search date 2000, 21 RCTs, 2184 people) included any inpatient, outpatient, or home based intervention programme that comprised immobilisation (see glossary, p 1256) with or without a plaster cast.[10] It included any trials comparing immobilisation versus either another type or duration of immobilisation or a functional treatment (see glossary, p 1256) for injuries to the lateral ligament complex of the ankle, and it reported outcomes at short, intermediate, or long term follow up (see comment below). The review analysed a variety of different forms of functional treatment, including strapping, bracing, use of an orthosis, tubigrips, bandages, elastic bandages, and special shoes for at least 5 weeks. It found that functional treatment significantly improved seven outcomes measured at different follow up times compared with immobilisation. At short term follow up, it found that functional treatment significantly reduced the proportion of people with persistent swelling compared with immobilisation (3 RCTs; RR 1.7, 95% CI 1.2 to 2.6) and significantly decreased the proportion of people not returning to work (2 RCTs; RR 5.75, 95% CI 1.01 to 32.71). At intermediate term follow up, it found that immobilisation significantly increased objective instability, as assessed with stress x ray, compared with functional treatment (1 RCT; WMD 2.6°, 95% CI 1.2° to 4.0°) and found that significantly more people were satisfied with functional treatment compared with immobilisation (2 RCTs; RR 4.2, 95% CI 1.1 to 16.1). At long term follow up, it found that, compared with immobilisation functional treatment significantly decreased the proportion of people not returning to sports (5 RCTs; RR 1.9, 95% CI 1.2 to 2.9), the time taken to return to work (6 RCTs; WMD 8.2 days, 95% CI 6.3 to 10.2), and the time taken to return to sports (3 RCTs; WMD 4.9 days, 95% CI 1.5 to 8.3). At longer term follow up, differences in outcomes for persistent swelling, objective instability, proportion of people not returning to work, and patient satisfaction were no longer significant. A subgroup analysis using only 11 "high quality" RCTs (defined as scoring 50% or above on a recognised quality evaluation tool) found only one significant difference between groups: that functional treatment significantly reduced the time taken to return to work compared with immobilisation (2 RCTs; WMD 12.9 days, 95% CI 7.1 days to 18.7 days). The second review (search date 1998) found that functional treatment significantly reduced persistent subjective instability compared with immobilisation (5 RCTs; RR 0.6, 95% CI 0.4 to 0.8; AR and timescale not reported), but found no significant difference between functional treatment and immobilisation in pain (5 RCTs; RR 0.8, 95% CI 0.5 to 1.2; AR not reported).[9] The review included a variety of different forms of functional treatment, including strapping, bracing, use of an orthosis, elastic wrapping, special shoes for at least 5 weeks, and short term (up to 3 weeks) cast immobilisation. The other two reviews were narrative in character and no data were pooled.[7,8] **Versus surgery:** We found two systematic reviews (search date 1998, 9 RCTs, 694 people;[9] search date 2000, 17 RCTs, 1950 people[11]). The first review compared surgery versus any conservative treatment (including both immobilisation and functional treatments) for acute injuries to the lateral ligament complex of the ankle.[11] It included 12 RCTs comparing surgery versus immobilisation alone (see comment below). It found that surgery significantly reduced the proportion of people who did not return to sports compared with immobilisation (3 RCTs; RR 0.48, 95% CI 0.31 to 0.76) and who had objective instability (6 RCTs; RR 0.35, 95% CI 0.21 to 0.60). It found no significant difference between surgery and immobilisation in recurrence (8 RCTs; RR 0.86, 95% CI 0.63 to 1.18), pain (8 RCTs; RR 0.64, 95% CI 0.33 to 1.23), subjective instability (8 RCTs; RR 0.77, 95% CI 0.43 to 1.37), or swelling (9 RCTs; RR 0.67, 95% CI 0.38 to 1.18). The second review compared operative treatment followed by 6 weeks of cast treatment versus 6 weeks of cast treatment alone.[9] It found no significant difference in pain (5 RCTs; RR 1.1, 95% CI 0.6 to 2.1; AR not reported) or subjective instability (5 RCTs; RR 1.0, 95% CI 0.7 to 1.4; AR not reported). **Versus physiotherapy:** One systematic review identified one RCT but was unable to calculate outcomes because of insufficient data.[10] **Different forms of immobilisation:** One systematic review identified two RCTs.[10] The first RCT found that a semirigid cast significantly reduced the time taken to return to work compared with a rigid cast (WMD 3.8 days, 95% CI 1.16 days to 6.44 days), but found no significant difference in pain, swelling, or objective instability at short term follow up. The review was unable to calculate outcomes from the second RCT because of insufficient data.

Harms: Two RCTs found fewer cases of deep venous thrombosis after cast immobilisation than after surgery (deep venous thrombosis: 2/47 [4%] after cast immobilisation *v* 3/34 [9%] after surgery;[12] 0/33 [0%] after cast immobilisation *v* 1/32 [3%] after surgery[11]), and one RCT found an equal occurrence of deep vein thrombosis in both groups (1/50 [2%] after cast immobilisation *v* 1/50 [2%] after surgery[11]). Other RCTs did not specifically address harms. Other known harms of immobilisation include pain and impairment in activities of daily living.[12]

Comment: **Versus functional treatment:** In the first systematic review, follow up periods for outcome measures were categorised as short term (within 6 weeks of randomisation), intermediate term (6 weeks to 1 year), or long term (1 to 2 years after treatment).[10] The review excluded trials that focused on the treatment of chronic instability or post-surgical treatment unless such injuries occurred in under 10% of the whole study population. The second systematic review did not provide absolute figures.[9] The different treatment modalities included as functional treatment in the reviews make it difficult to draw definitive conclusions on individual forms of functional treatment compared with immobilisation. **Versus surgery:** The first systematic review noted that all included RCTs had methodological flaws, and there was insufficient evidence to determine the relative effectiveness of surgical and conservative treatment (see comment under surgery, p 1254).[11]

OPTION FUNCTIONAL TREATMENT

One systematic review and one subsequent RCT found limited evidence that functional treatment reduced the risk of the ankle giving way compared with minimal treatment. One systematic review found that, compared with immobilisation, functional treatment improved seven outcomes at either short (up to 6 weeks), intermediate (6 weeks to 1 year), or long term (over 1 year) follow up. However, effects were to be less marked at long term follow up, or if only results from high quality trials were analysed. Another systematic review found that, compared with immobilisation, functional treatment decreased persistent subjective instability, but found no significant difference in pain. Two systematic reviews found insufficient evidence to compare functional treatment versus surgery. One systematic review and three additional RCTs provided insufficient evidence to compare different functional treatments.

Benefits: We found six systematic reviews (search dates 1993,[7] 1994,[8] 1998,[9] and 2000[10,11,13] and four additional RCTs[14–17]) comparing functional treatment (see glossary, p 1256) as a treatment strategy. **Versus minimal treatment:** We found two systematic reviews[8,9] and one subsequent RCT.[14] The first systematic review (search date 1998, 3 RCTs, 214 people) compared functional treatment versus a minimal treatment policy.[9] It found that functional treatment significantly reduced the risk of the ankle giving way (RR 0.34, 95% CI 0.17 to 0.71). Although pain scores were better with functional treatment, the difference was not significant (RR 0.53, 95% CI 0.27 to 1.02). The second systematic review was narrative in character and no data were pooled.[8] The subsequent RCT (30 people with subacute or chronic ankle sprain without gross mechanical instability) compared the mortise separation adjustment (see glossary, p 1256) versus detuned ultrasound.[14] It found that mobilisation significantly reduced pain, increased ankle range of motion, and improved ankle function at 1 month (results presented graphically). **Versus immobilisation:** See benefits of immobilisation, p 1249. **Versus surgery:** We found four systematic reviews (search dates 1993,[7] 1994,[8] 1998,[9] and 2000[11]). The first review (search date 2000, 17 RCTs, 1950 people) compared any surgical treatment versus any conservative treatment (including both immobilisation and functional treatments) for acute injuries to the lateral ligament complex of the ankle.[11] It included eight RCTs comparing surgery versus functional treatment alone (see comment below). The review found no significant difference between surgery and functional treatment in return to sports (2 RCTs; RR 0.6, 95% CI 0.3 to 1.3), recurrence (5 RCTs; RR 1.2, 95% CI 0.8 to 1.8), pain (5 RCTs; RR 1.0, 95% CI 0.7 to 1.6), subjective instability (5 RCTs; RR 0.9, 95% CI 0.7 to 1.3), objective instability (4 RCTs; RR 0.6, 95% CI 0.3 to 1.2), and swelling (5 RCTs; RR 0.9, 95% CI 0.6 to 1.5; see comment below). The second systematic review (search date 1998, 7 RCTs, 914 people) included only people with rupture of the lateral ankle ligament.[9] It did not specify the kinds of surgery included within the RCTs. It found that surgery significantly reduced long term subjective instability compared with functional treatment (7 RCTs; RR 0.2, 95% CI 0.2 to 0.3; AR not reported), but found no significant difference in long term pain (6 RCTs; RR 0.5, 95% CI 0.2 to 1.5; AR not reported). The other two reviews were narrative in character and no data were pooled.[7,8]

Different types of functional treatment: We found one systematic review[13] and three additional RCTs.[15–17] The review (search date 2000, 9 RCTs, 892 people) compared four types of functional treatment (elastic bandage, tape, lace-up ankle support, and semirigid ankle support) and included RCTs comparing two different types of functional treatments in people with an acute injury to the lateral ligament complex of the ankle. It reported outcomes at short, intermediate, and long term follow up (see comment below). At short term follow up, it found that lace-up ankle support significantly reduced persistent swelling compared with semirigid ankle support (1 RCT; RR 4.2, 95% CI 1.3 to 14), elastic bandage (1 RCT; RR 5.5, 95% CI 1.7 to 17.8), and tape (1 RCT; RR 4.1, 95% CI 1.2 to 13.7), and that a semirigid ankle support significantly reduced the proportion of people with subjective instability compared with an elastic bandage (1 RCT; RR 8, 95% CI 1.03 to 62.07). It found no significant differences between different types of functional treatments at intermediate or long term follow up. It found that a semirigid ankle support significantly reduced the time taken to return to work compared with an elastic bandage (2 RCTs; WMD 4.2 days, 95% CI 2.4 days to 6.0 days) and the time taken to return to sports (1 RCT; WMD 9.6 days, 95% CI 6.3 days to 12.8 days). It found no other significant differences in outcomes between treatments (see comment below).[13] The first additional RCT (61 people without previous fractures in the ankle joint or clinically demonstrable ankle instability; mean follow up of 230 days) found that elastic bandage plus propriocepsis training reduced the risk of recurrent sprains compared with elastic bandage alone (RR 0.46, 95% CI 0.2 to 1.0).[16] Thirteen people withdrew from the RCT and were not included in the analysis. The remaining two additional RCTs found no significant differences in outcomes between treatments.[15,17] One RCT (116 people with all grades of ankle sprain) compared a semirigid device versus tape and found similar rates of recurrent sprains (recurrent sprains were found in 4% *v* 0%).[15] The other RCT (119 people not requiring surgery, treated within 24 hours of injury) compared two types of tape treatment with follow up of 5–7 days and found similar outcomes between groups (short term pain 8% *v* 5%; swelling 58% *v* 47%; limited range of movement 36% *v* 47%).[17]

Harms: Allergic reactions and skin problems have been recorded with tape.[18] In the systematic review comparing different functional treatments, tape treatment resulted in significantly more complications compared with elastic bandage (2 RCTs; 0/104 [0%] with elastic bandage *v* 8/104 [8%] with tape; RR 0.11, 95% CI 0.01 to 0.86).[13] The majority of these complications were skin problems (absolute numbers with skin problems not reported).[13]

Comment: The older systematic reviews did not perform meta-analysis and included people with different severity of ankle sprain.[7,8] **Versus surgery:** The most recent review noted that all included RCTs had methodological flaws, and there was insufficient evidence to determine the relative effectiveness of surgical and conservative treatment (see comment under surgery, p 1254).[11] The second systematic review presented results only as relative risks, which does not allow assessment of the number of people who benefited.[9] It also categorised short term cast use as a functional treatment. **Different types of functional treatment:** The systematic review reported follow up periods for outcome measures as short term (within 6 weeks of treatment), intermediate term (6 weeks to 1 year), or long term (1 to 2 years after treatment).[13] It noted that definitive conclusions were hampered by the variety of treatments used and the inconsistency of reported follow up times, and no definite conclusions concerning the optimal functional treatment strategy could be drawn.[13]

OPTION SURGERY

One systematic review found no significant difference between surgery and immobilisation in pain or subjective instability. Other systematic reviews found insufficient evidence to compare surgery versus functional treatment or versus conservative treatment (including both immobilisation and functional treatment).

Benefits: We found four systematic reviews (search dates 1993,[7] 1994,[8] 1998,[9] and 2000[11]). **Versus immobilisation:** See benefits of immobilisation, p 1249. **Versus functional treatment:** See benefits of functional treatment, p 1251. **Versus conservative (immobilisation and functional) treatment:** One systematic review (search date 2000, 17 RCTs, 1950 people) compared surgery versus conservative treatment (including both immobilisation and functional treatments) for acute injuries to the lateral ligament complex of the ankle.[11] Significant results were often not robust to sensitivity analysis (see comment below). When data from one quasi randomised trial was excluded, the review found that surgery significantly decreased the proportion of people with objective instability compared with conservative treatment (4 RCTs; RR 0.4, 95% CI 0.2 to 0.7) and surgery significantly increased the proportion of people with ankle stiffness compared with conservative treatment (2 RCTs; RR 1.9, 95% CI 1.2 to 3.1), but found no significant difference between groups in recurrence (10 RCTs; RR 0.96, 95% CI 0.7 to 1.2), pain on activity (8 RCTs; RR 0.9, 95% CI 0.7 to 1.2), swelling (9 RCTs; RR 0.83, 95% CI 0.6 to 1.1), or people not returning to sports (3 RCTs; RR 0.7, 95% CI 0.4 to 1.2; see comment below).[11]

Harms: Neurological injuries, infections, bleeding, osteoarthritis, and death are known harms of surgery.[12,19,20] Two RCTs found fewer cases of deep venous thrombosis after cast immobilisation (see glossary, p 1256) than with surgery (deep venous thrombosis: 2/47 [4%] after cast immobilisation *v* 3/34 [9%] after surgery;[12] 0/33 [0%] after cast immobilisation *v* 1/32 [3%] after surgery[11]) and one RCT found an equal occurrence of deep vein thrombosis in both groups (1/50 [2%] after cast immobilisation *v* 1/50 [2%] after surgery[11]). Other RCTs have found dysaesthesia (see glossary, p 1256) in 4–12% of all people after surgery.[21–26] Wound necrosis after surgery was reported in two RCTs (2/73 [3%] with surgery;[24] 3/45 [7%] with surgery[25]). Tenderness of the scar was reported by six RCTs after surgical intervention, occurring in between 2–19% of people.[22,23,26–29]

Comment: The systematic review comparing surgery versus conservative treatment noted that all RCTs had methodological flaws.[11] Data for pooling for individual outcomes were available for a maximum of 11 trials, and quality assessment ranged from 6 to 13 out of a possible 22 using a recognised quality evaluation tool.[11] Included trials were often heterogeneous, and significant results were often sensitive to the method of analysis used (random or fixed effects meta-analysis) or when data from quasi randomised trials were excluded. The review concluded that "there is insufficient evidence available from randomised controlled trials to determine the relative effectiveness of surgical and conservative treatment for acute injuries of the lateral ligament complex of the ankle."[11]

OPTION ULTRASOUND

One systematic review found no significant difference between ultrasound and sham ultrasound in the general improvement of symptoms or the ability to walk or bear weight at 7 days. Three RCTs provided insufficient evidence to compare ultrasound versus other treatments.

Benefits: We found one systematic review (search date 2001, 5 RCTs, 572 people; see comment below).[30] **Versus placebo:** Four RCTs in the review compared ultrasound versus a sham ultrasound treatment.[30] None of the RCTs demonstrated a significant difference for any outcome measure. The review found no significant difference in general improvement between ultrasound and sham ultrasound at 7 days (3 RCTs; 121/169 [72%] with ultrasound *v* 116/172 [68%] with sham ultrasound; RR 1.04, 95% CI 0.92 to 1.17). It found no significant difference in functional disability (the ability to walk or bear weight) between ultrasound and sham ultrasound at 7 days (2 RCTs; 69/95 [73%] with ultrasound *v* 61/92 [66%] with sham ultrasound; RR 1.09, 95% CI 0.92 to 1.30).[30] **Versus other treatments:** Three RCTs in the review compared ultrasound versus other treatment modalities.[30] The largest RCT (72 people in the smallest group) compared ultrasound plus placebo gel, ultrasound plus felbinac gel, and sham ultrasound plus felbinac gel over about 7 days. The comparison between ultrasound and felbinac gel resulted in small and non-significant differences. The second RCT (20 people in the smallest group) compared ultrasound versus electrotherapy. It found no significant difference in swelling, ability to walk, and recovery. The third low quality RCT (40 people in the smallest group) compared ultrasound versus immobilisation (see glossary, p 1256) with elastoplast over 2 weeks' follow up. It found no significant difference in the proportion of people who recovered with ultrasound compared with immobilisation after 7 days (46% ultrasound *v* 27% immobilisation; ARR +19%, 95% CI –2% to +40%) but found a significant difference after 14 days (86% ultrasound *v* 59% immobilisation; ARR 27%, 95% CI 8% to 46%).

Harms: Two included RCTs addressed adverse reactions.[31,32] One RCT found none.[31] The systematic review reported that in the other RCT 8/73 (11%) people in the ultrasound group (plus placebo gel) reported 11 non-serious adverse reactions, including gastro-intestinal events and skin reactions, and in one person treatment was discontinued because of skin reactions and the person was withdrawn from the RCT.[32]

Comment: In the review, the quality of four of the included RCTs was described as "modest" and one as "good".[30] The review reported RCTs in which pain, swelling, and/or functional disability due to an acute ankle sprain was present, and in which at least one group was treated with active ultrasound therapy. All the RCTs included followed people for less than 4 weeks.

OPTION COLD PACK COMPRESSION

Two RCTs found no significant difference in symptoms between cold pack placement and placebo or control. One RCT found less oedema with cold pack placement compared with heat or a contrast bath at 3–5 days after injury.

Benefits: We found one systematic review (search date 1994, 3 RCTs, 203 people).[8] The first RCT (143 people) identified by the review compared cryotherapy versus placebo (simulated) therapy.[33] The second RCT (30 people) identified by the review compared ice treatment plus physiotherapy versus no ice plus physiotherapy.[34] In both RCTs, no significant differences were found. The third RCT (30 people) identified by the review found significantly less oedema with cold than with heat or a contrast bath (see comment below) at 3–5 days after injury ($P < 0.05$).[35]

Harms: None of the RCTs addressed harms from cold pack placement.

Comment: The systematic review was narrative in character and no data were pooled.[8] The systematic review did not report the grade of injuries. In the third RCT, the injured ankle in the contrast bath group was submerged in warm water for three minutes and then in cold water for one minute. This was continued until the ankle had been given five heat and four cold treatments beginning and ending with heat.[35]

OPTION DIATHERMY

One systematic review found insufficient evidence on the effects of diathermy versus placebo on walking ability and reduction in swelling.

Benefits: We found one systematic review (search date 1994, 5 RCTs, 490 people).[8] The review included a range of severity of ankle sprains but excluded the most severe injuries (avulsion and osteochondral fractures). The largest high quality RCT (300 people with time from injury to treatment of 4 days or less) compared two forms of pulsating shortwave treatment versus placebo.[36] The RCT found that high frequency electromagnetic pulsing significantly improved walking ability more quickly compared with placebo ($P < 0.01$). The difference was not significant with low frequency electromagnetic pulsing. However, low frequency pulsing significantly reduced swelling compared with placebo, but there was no significant difference between the high frequency group compared with placebo (change in circumference of ankle with high frequency 4.5 mm *v* low frequency 5.0 mm *v* placebo 2.6 mm; $P < 0.01$ for low frequency *v* placebo). A second RCT (50 people) found that pulsating shortwave diathermy significantly reduced oedema compared with placebo ($P < 0.01$).[37] The other RCTs (73, 37, and 30 people) found no significant differences for pain, oedema, or range of motion compared with placebo.[38–40] The first of these presented results as graphs.[38] From these RCTs the grades of injuries were not clear. No other outcome measures were reported and no results were pooled.

Harms: No evidence of any harm was reported.

Comment: None.

OPTION **HOMEOPATHIC OINTMENT**

One systematic review of one small RCT found limited evidence that homeopathic ointment improved outcome based on a "composite criteria" of treatment success compared with placebo.

Benefits: We found one systematic review (search date 1998),[41] which included one small RCT in German (69 people with acute ankle sprains).[42] The review found that people treated with a homeopathic ointment had a significantly better outcome based on a "composite criteria of treatment success" compared with people treated with placebo. The review did not provide specific numerical results or timescale of outcome measurement but described a P value of 0.028.[41] People initially randomised in the RCT and losses to follow up were not reported.

Harms: Harms were not addressed in the review.

Comment: The RCT included in the systematic review will be translated and further details included in future *Clinical Evidence* updates.

GLOSSARY

Dysaesthesia Decreased sensitivity of the skin for stimuli.

Functional treatment Diverse functional treatments have been used. The main differences are the type of external device applied for treatment. The supports can be divided according to rigidity into elastic bandage, tape, lace-up ankle support, and semirigid ankle support. Proprioceptis training (to enhance joint stability) has also been used.

Immobilisation Limiting the mobility of a joint complex to zero degrees.

Mortise separation adjustment An adjustment technique involving special manual manipulation of the foot and ankle.[14]

Substantive changes

Immobilisation Two systematic reviews added;[10,11] conclusions unchanged.
Functional treatment Three systematic reviews added;[10,11,13] conclusions unchanged.
Surgery One systematic review added;[11] conclusions unchanged

REFERENCES

1. Bernett P, Schirmann A. Sportverletzungen des sprunggelenkes. *Unfallheilkunde* 1979;82:155–160.
2. Lassiter TE, Malone TR, Garret WE. Injuries to the lateral ligaments of the ankle. *Orthop Clin North Am* 1989;20:629–640.
3. Marti RK. Bagatelletsels van de voet. 56–61. 1982. Capita selecta, *Reuma Wereldwijd*.
4. Van Dijk CN, Bossuyt PM, Marti RK. Medial ankle pain after lateral ligament rupture. *J Bone Joint Surg Br* 1996;78:562–567.
5. Watson-Jones R. *Fractures and joint injuries*. London: Churchill Livingstone, 1976.
6. Katcherian DA. Treatment of Freiberg's disease. *Orthop Clin North Am* 1994;25:69–81.
7. Shrier I. Treatment of lateral collateral ligament sprains of the ankle: a critical appraisal of the literature. *Clin J Sport Med* 1995;5:187–195. Search date 1993; primary sources hand searches of bibliographies and reference lists.
8. Ogilvie-Harris DJ, Gilbart M. Treatment modalities for soft tissue injuries of the ankle: a critical review. *Clin J Sport Med* 1995;5:175–186. Search date 1994; primary sources Medline and Excerpta Medica.
9. Pijnenburg AC, Van Dijk CN, Bossuyt PM, et al. Treatment of ruptures of the lateral ankle ligaments: a meta-analysis. *J Bone Joint Surg Am* 2000;82:761–773. Search date 1998; primary sources Cochrane, Medline, Embase, hand searches of references from the published reviews, and personal contact with authors.
10. Kerkhoffs GMMJ, Rowe BH, Assendelft WJJ, et al. Immobilisation and functional treatment for acute lateral ankle ligament injuries in adults (Cochrane Review). In: The Cochrane Library, Issue 4, 2002. Oxford: Update Software. Search date 2000; primary sources Cochrane Musculoskeletal Injuries Group specialised register, Cochrane Controlled Trials Register, Medline, Embase, and hand searches of reference lists of articles and personal contact with organisations (Medical Departments of the Dutch Defence Forces and the Royal Dutch Football Association) and researchers in the field.
11. Kerkhoffs GMMJ, Handoll HHG, de Bie R, et al. Surgical versus conservative treatment for acute injuries of the lateral ligament complex of the ankle in adults (Cochrane Review). In: The Cochrane Library, Issue 1, 2003. Oxford: Update Software. Search date 2000; primary sources Cochrane Musculoskeletal Injuries Group specialised register, Cochrane Controlled Trials Register, Medline, Embase, Biosis, Current Contents, and hand searches of reference lists of articles and personal contact with organisations and researchers in the field.
12. Korkala O, Rusanen M, Jokipii P, et al. A prospective study of the treatment of severe tears of the lateral ligament of the ankle. *Int Orthop* 1987;11:13–17.
13. Kerkhoffs GMMJ, Struijs PAA, Marti RK, et al. Different functional treatment strategies for acute lateral ankle ligament injuries in adults (Cochrane Review). In: The Cochrane Library, Issue 1, 2003. Oxford: Update Software. Search date 2000; primary sources Cochrane Musculoskeletal Injuries Group specialised register, Cochrane Controlled Trials Register, Medline, Embase, Biosis, Current Contents, and hand searches of reference lists of articles and personal contact with organisations (Medical Departments of the Dutch Defence Forces and the Royal Dutch Football Association) and researchers in the field.
14. Pellow JE, Brantingham JW. The efficacy of adjusting the ankle in the treatment of subacute and chronic grade I and Grade II ankle inversion sprains. *J Manipulative Physiol Ther* 2001;24:17–24.
15. Johannes EJ, Sukul DM, Spruit PJ, et al. Controlled trial of a semi-rigid bandage ('Scotchrap') in patients with ankle ligament lesions. *Curr Med Res Opin* 1993;13:154–162.
16. Wester JU, Jespersen SM, Nielsen KD, et al. Wobble board training after partial sprains of the lateral ligaments of the ankle: a prospective randomized study. *J Orthop Sports Phys Ther* 1996;23:332–336.
17. Viljakka T, Rokkanen P. The treatment of ankle sprain by bandaging and antiphlogistic drugs. *Ann Chir Gynaecol* 1983;72:66–70.
18. Zeegers AVCM. Supination injury of the ankle joint [thesis]. Utrecht: University of Utrecht, The Netherlands, 1995.
19. Biegler M, Lang A, Ritter J. Comparative study on the effectiveness of early functional treatment using special shoes following surgery of ruptures of fibular ligaments [German]. *Unfallchirurg* 1985;88:113–117.
20. Sommer HM, Schreiber H. Early functional conservative therapy of fresh fibular capsular ligament rupture from the socioeconomic viewpoint. *Sportverletz Sportschaden* 1993;7:40–46.
21. Zwipp H, Hoffmann R, Thermann H, et al. Rupture of the ankle ligaments. *Int Orthop* 1991;15:245–249.
22. Evans GA, Hardcastle P, Frenyo AD. Acute rupture of the lateral ligament of the ankle. To suture or not to suture? *J Bone Joint Surg Br* 1984;66:209–212.
23. Delfosse P, Lafontaine D, Hardy D, et al. Rupture of the ankle ligaments: to repair or not to repair? Preliminary results of a randomized study [Abstract]. 6th Congress of the European Society of Sports Traumatology, Knee Surgery and Arthroscopy 1994;S66.
24. Povacz P, Salzburg F, Unger SF, et al. A randomized, prospective study of operative and non-operative treatment of injuries of the fibular collateral ligaments of the ankle. *J Bone Joint Surg Am* 1998;80:345–351.
25. Prins JG. Diagnosis and treatment of injury to the lateral ligament of the ankle: a comparative clinical study. *Acta Chir Scand Suppl* 1978;486:3–139.
26. Brostrom L. Sprained ankles V. Treatment and prognosis in recent ligament ruptures. *Acta Chir Scand* 1966;132:537–550.
27. Niedermann A, Andersen A, Bryde Andersen S, et al. Rupture of the lateral ligaments of the ankle: operation or plaster cast? *Acta Orthop Scand* 1981;52:579–587.
28. Klein J, Schreckenberger C, Roddecker K, et al. Operative or conservative treatment of recent

rupture of the fibular ligament in the ankle. A randomized clinical trial. *Unfallchirurg* 1988;91:154–160.

29. Van den Hoogenband CR, Van Moppes FI. Diagnostic and therapeutic aspects of inversion trauma of the ankle joint [thesis]. Maastricht: University of Maastricht, 1982.
30. Van der Windt DAWM, Van der Heijden GJMG, Van den Berg SGM, et al. Ultrasound therapy for acute ankle sprains (Cochrane Review). In: The Cochrane Library, Issue 1, 2003. Oxford: Update Software. Search date 2001; primary sources Cochrane Musculoskeletal Injuries Group specialised register, Cochrane Controlled Trials Register, Cochrane Rehabilitation and Related Therapies Field database, Medline, Embase, Cinahl, PEDro — the Physiotherapy Evidence Database, and hand searches of reference lists of articles and personal contact with colleagues.
31. Nyanzi CS, Langridge J, Heyworth JR, et al. Randomized controlled study of ultrasound therapy in the management of acute lateral ligament sprains of the ankle joint. *Clin Rehabil* 1999;13:16–22.
32. Oakland C. A comparison of the efficacy of the topical NSAID felbinac and ultrasound in the treatment of acute ankle injuries. *Br J Clin Res* 1993;4:89–96.
33. Sloan JP, Hain R, Pownall R. Clinical benefits of early cold therapy in accident and emergency following ankle sprain. *Arch Emerg Med* 1989;6:1–6.
34. Laba E, Roestenburg M. Clinical evaluation of ice therapy for acute ankle sprain injuries. *NZ J Physiother* 1989;17:7–9.
35. Cote DJ, Prentice WEJ, Hooker DN, et al. Comparison of three treatment procedures for minimizing ankle sprain swelling. *Physical Ther* 1988;68:1072–1076.
36. Pasila M, Visuri T, Sundholm A. Pulsating shortwave diathermy: value in treatment of recent ankle and foot sprains. *Arch Phys Med Rehabil* 1978;59:383–386.
37. Pennington GM, Danley DL, Sumko MH, et al. Pulsed, non-thermal, high-frequency electromagnetic energy (DIAPULSE) in the treatment of grade I and grade II ankle sprains. *Mil Med* 1993;158:101–404.
38. Barker AT, Barlow PS, Porter J, et al. A double-blind clinical trial of low power pulsed shortwave therapy in the treatment of a soft tissue injury. *Physiotherapy* 1985;71:500–504.
39. McGill SN. The effects of pulsed shortwave therapy on lateral ligament sprain of the ankle. *NZ J Physiother* 1988;16:21–24.
40. Michlovitz S, Smith W, Watkins M. Ice and high voltage pulsed stimulation in treatment of acute lateral ankle sprains. *J Orthop Sports Phys Ther* 1988;9:301–304.
41. Cucherat M, Haugh MC, Gooch M, et al. Evidence of clinical efficacy of homeopathy: a meta-analysis of clinical trials. *Eur J Clin Pharmacol* 2000;56:27–33. Search date 1998; primary sources Medline, Embase, Biosis, PsychInfo, Cinahl, British Library Stock Alert Service, SIGLE, AMED and hand searches of homeopathy journals, conference abstracts, references provided by colleagues, reference lists of selected papers, and personal contact with pharmaceutical companies.
42. Zell R, Connert WD, Mau J, et al. Treatment of acute sprains of the ankle joint. Double-blind study assessing the effectiveness of a homeopathic ointment preparation [German]. *Fortschr Med* 1988;106:96–100.

Peter Struijs

Gino Kerkhoffs

Academic Medical Center
Amsterdam
The Netherlands

Competing interests: None declared.

Bunions

Search date January 2003

Jill Ferrari

QUESTIONS

INTERVENTIONS

Likely to be beneficial

Chevron osteotomy (compared with no treatment or with orthoses) 1263

Different methods of bone fixation 1266

Unknown effectiveness

Chevron osteotomy (compared with proximal osteotomy). 1263

Chevron osteotomy plus adductor tenotomy 1263

Chevron osteotomy plus Akin osteotomy 1263

Continuous passive motion . .1267

Early weight bearing 1268

Keller's arthroplasty. 1262

Night splints 1262

Orthoses to treat hallux valgus in adults 1261

Slipper casts. 1268

Unlikely to be beneficial

Orthoses to prevent hallux valgus in high risk adults. 1261

Likely to be ineffective or harmful

Antipronatory orthoses in children 1261

See glossary, p 1268

Key Messages

- **Chevron osteotomy (compared with no treatment or with orthoses)** One RCT found that chevron osteotomy improved outcomes compared with orthoses or no treatment after 1 year.
- **Different methods of bone fixation** We found limited evidence on the effects of different methods of bone fixation. One small RCT found that screw fixation plus early weight bearing reduced time to return to work and social activity compared with suture fixation and later weight bearing.
- **Chevron osteotomy (compared with proximal osteotomy)** We found conflicting evidence on the effects of chevron osteotomy compared with proximal osteotomy.
- **Chevron osteotomy plus adductor tenotomy** We found no evidence that adductor tenotomy plus chevron osteotomy improved outcomes compared with chevron osteotomy alone.
- **Chevron osteotomy plus Akin osteotomy** We found insufficient evidence to compare effects of chevron osteotomy plus Akin osteotomy versus Akin osteotomy plus distal soft tissue reconstruction.
- **Continuous passive motion** One systematic review found insufficient evidence on the effects of continuous passive motion.
- **Early weight bearing** One systematic review has found insufficient evidence on the effects of early weight bearing.

- **Keller's arthroplasty** One systematic review found insufficient evidence on the effects of Keller's arthroplasty compared with other types of operation.
- **Night splints** We found insufficient evidence about the effects of night splints compared with other treatments.
- **Orthoses to treat hallux valgus in adults** We found limited evidence that orthoses reduced pain intensity compared with no treatment.
- **Slipper casts** One RCT found insufficient evidence on the effects of plaster slipper casts.
- **Orthoses to prevent hallux valgus in high risk adults** One RCT in men with rheumatoid arthritis found no significant difference between orthoses and no treatment in rates of development of hallux valgus after 3 years.
- **Antipronatory orthoses in children** One RCT in children found limited evidence that antipronatory orthoses increased deterioration in metatarsophalangeal joint angles after 3 years compared with no treatment.

DEFINITION **Hallux valgus** is a deformity of the great toe whereby the hallux (great toe) moves towards the second toe, overlying it in severe cases. This movement of the hallux is described as abduction (movement away from the midline of the body) and it is usually accompanied by some rotation of the toe so that the nail is facing the midline of the body (valgus rotation). With the deformity, the metatarsal head becomes more prominent and the metatarsal is said to be in an adducted position as it moves towards the midline of the body.[1] Radiological criteria for hallux valgus vary, but a commonly accepted criterion is to measure the angle formed between the metatarsal and the abducted hallux. This is called the metatarsophalangeal joint angle or hallux abductus angle and it is considered abnormal when it is greater than 14.5°.[2] **Bunion** is the lay term used to describe a prominent and often inflamed metatarsal head and overlying bursa. Symptoms include pain, limitation in walking, and problems with wearing normal shoes.

INCIDENCE/PREVALENCE The prevalence of hallux valgus varies in different populations. In a recent study of 6000 UK school children aged 9–10 years, 2.5% had clinical evidence of hallux valgus, and 2% met both clinical and radiological criteria for hallux valgus. An earlier study found hallux valgus in 48% of adults.[2] Differences in prevalence may result from different methods of measurement, varying age groups, or different diagnostic criteria (e.g. metatarsal joint angle > 10° or > 15°).[3]

AETIOLOGY/RISK FACTORS Nearly all population studies have found that hallux valgus is more common in women. Footwear may contribute to the deformity, but studies comparing people who wear shoes with those who do not have found contradictory results. Hypermobility of the first ray (see glossary, p 1269) and excessive foot pronation are associated with hallux valgus.[4]

PROGNOSIS We found no studies that looked at progression of hallux valgus. Progression of deformity and symptoms is rapid in some people, others remain asymptomatic. One study found that hallux valgus is often unilateral initially, but usually progresses to bilateral deformity.[2]

AIMS OF INTERVENTION To reduce symptoms and deformity, with minimum adverse effects.

OUTCOMES Hallux abductus/metatarsophalangeal joint angle. Intermetatarsal joint angle. Range of motion of the first metatarsophalangeal joint (the total range of both dorsiflexion and plantarflexion). Incidence of complications such as infection; reoperation; non-union; avascular necrosis; pain; general satisfaction and satisfaction with appearance; requirement for specialist or extra-width footwear; proportion of people with mobility problems; time to healing; development of transfer lesions (see glossary, p 1269); and adverse effects of treatment.

METHODS *Clinical Evidence* search and appraisal January 2003. An electronic search using a strategy developed by the Cochrane Musculoskeletal Injuries Group was undertaken to March 2003 and a hand search of podiatry journals to March 2003.

QUESTION What are the effects of conservative treatments?

OPTION ORTHOSES

We found insufficient evidence that antipronatory orthoses prevented hallux valgus in children and adults with rheumatoid arthritis. We found limited evidence that orthoses reduced pain in people with hallux valgus.

Benefits: We found no systematic review. We found three RCTs.[2,5,6] **In children:** One RCT comparing antipronatory orthoses (see glossary, p 1268) versus no treatment screened 6000 UK school children aged 9–10 years.[2] On the basis of a clinical examination, 150 children were selected for x ray examination and 122 of these children (13% of whom were boys) found to have metatarsophalangeal joint angles greater than 14.5° in one or both feet were subsequently included in the trial (see comment below). The RCT found that the metatarsophalangeal joint angles deteriorated both with orthoses and with no treatment, and found that the deterioration was greater in children treated with orthoses although this difference was not significant after 3 years (no direct statistical comparisons provided).[2] **In adults:** We found one RCT (102 men with rheumatoid arthritis, but without hallux valgus; see comment below) that compared orthoses versus no treatment to prevent the development of hallux valgus.[5] The RCT found no significant difference between treatments in the proportion of people who developed hallux valgus after 3 years (5/50 [10%] for adults with orthoses *v* 12/48 [25%] with no treatment; RR 0.4, 95% CI 0.2 to 1.1). We found one RCT (209 adults with hallux valgus) which compared three treatments: chevron osteotomy (see glossary, p 1268); orthoses; and no treatment (see benefits of chevron osteotomy, p 1263).[6] The RCT found that orthoses significantly reduced pain intensity after 6 months compared with no treatment (pain intensity on visual analogue scale with range 0 [no pain] to 100 [unbearable pain]: 36 with orthoses *v* 45 with no treatment; difference adjusted for baseline characteristics –14, 95% CI –22 to –6), but found no significant difference in pain intensity after 12 months (pain intensity on visual analogue scale with range 0 [no pain] to 100 [unbearable pain]: 40 with orthoses *v* 40 with no treatment; difference adjusted for baseline characteristics –6, 95%

CI –15 to +3). The RCT also found that orthoses significantly improved global assessment compared with no treatment but found no significant difference in satisfaction or functional assessment scores (AOFAS — see glossary, p 1268) after 12 months (proportion with improved global assessment: 46% with orthoses v 24% with no treatment, RR [adjusted for baseline characteristics] 0.38, 95% CI 0.18 to 0.78; satisfaction on visual analogue scale with range 0 [totally unsatisfied] to 100 [totally satisfied]: 70 with orthoses v 61 with no treatment; difference adjusted for baseline characteristics +9, 95% CI –1 to +20; AOFAS score: 64 with orthosis v 66 with no treatment, difference adjusted for baseline characteristics 0, 95% CI –4 to +5.) It also found no significant difference between orthoses and no treatment in the duration of the pain, ability to work, and cosmetic disturbance.[6]

Harms: The RCT in children did not report on harms.[2] The RCT in men with rheumatoid arthritis reported that orthoses caused mild discomfort in a small number of cases.[5]

Comment: The use of antipronatory orthoses in children is questionable because earlier studies have found that hallux valgus in children is not related to pronation but arises from positional changes in the first ray (see glossary, p 1269).[7] The first RCT reported that 29/122 (25%) children (mainly from the control group) were lost to follow up.[2] The RCT in people with rheumatoid arthritis included only men, although both rheumatoid arthritis and hallux valgus are more common in women.[5] This may limit the applicability of the results.

OPTION NIGHT SPLINTS

We found insufficient evidence about the effects of night splints compared with other treatments.

Benefits: We found no RCTs that compared night splints with no treatment.

Harms: We found no RCTs.

Comment: None.

QUESTION What are the effects of surgery?

OPTION KELLER'S ARTHROPLASTY

One systematic review found insufficient evidence on the effects of Keller's arthroplasty compared with other types of operation.

Benefits: **Versus no treatment:** We found no RCTs. **Versus distal osteotomy:** We found one systematic review (search date 1998, 3 relevant RCTs; see comment below)[8] that included one RCT (29 people) comparing distal metatarsal osteotomy versus Keller's arthroplasty (see glossary, p 1269).[9] The RCT found that osteotomy significantly improved both intermetatarsal angle and range of movement compared with Keller's arthroplasty but found no significant difference in proportion with unresolved pain or dissatisfaction after 3 years (intermetatarsal angle: 12.0° with Keller's arthroplasty v 7.0° with distal osteotomy (see glossary, p 1269); difference

–5.0°, 95% CI –8.9° to –1.1°; reduction in range of movement: 14.0° with Keller's arthroplasty v 1.0° with distal osteotomy; difference: 13.0°, 95% CI 5.0° to 21.1°; proportion with unresolved pain: 4/14 [29%] with Keller's arthroplasty v 4/15 [27%] with distal osteotomy; OR 0.91, 95% CI 0.18 to 4.64; proportion dissatisfied: 4/14 [29%] with Keller's arthroplasty v 4/15 [27%] with distal osteotomy; OR 0.91, 95% CI 0.18 to 4.64). **Versus arthrodesis:** The second RCT included in the review (81 people) found that Keller's arthroplasty significantly reduced the proportion of people with reduced mobility compared with arthrodesis. It found no significant difference in proportion with unresolved pain or dissatisfaction after 2 years (proportion with reduced mobility: 4/44 [9%] with Keller's arthrodesis v 11/37 [30%] with arthrodesis; OR 4.23, 95% CI 1.22 to 14.71; proportion with unresolved pain: 5/44 [11%] with Keller's osteotomy v 4/37 [11%] with osteotomy; OR 0.95, 95% CI 0.23 to 3.81; proportion dissatisfied: 11/44 [25%] with Keller's osteotomy v 10/37 [27%] with arthrodesis; OR 1.11, 95% CI 0.41 to 3.01).[10] **Plus joint distraction:** The third RCT included in the review found that a Kirschner wire (see glossary, p 1269) to distract the joint during healing after Keller's arthroplasty significantly improved subjective assessment scores for symptoms compared with Keller's arthroplasty with no wire use ($P < 0.05$), but found no significant difference in the hallux abductus angle, pain, or movement after a minimum of 1 year (hallux valgus angle: 21° for both groups, no P value provided; pain: no data provided; movement: no data provided).[11]

Harms: The review did not report any specific complications associated with any of the procedures. Reduced toe function has been described after Keller's procedure.[8] The systematic review reported high levels of patient dissatisfaction (up to 33%) in most trials.[8]

Comment: Most of the people included in the review having surgery were under 50 years of age and were followed up for no more than 3 years.[8] Longer term outcomes remain unclear. Many of the RCTs reported results for numbers of feet, and did not always report standard deviations of the results. The systematic review analysed the results by numbers of people.[8]

OPTION CHEVRON OSTEOTOMY

We found evidence that chevron osteotomy improved outcomes compared with orthoses or no treatment after 1 year. We found conflicting evidence on the effects of chevron osteotomy compared with proximal osteotomy. We found no evidence that adductor tenotomy plus chevron osteotomy improved outcomes compared with chevron osteotomy alone. We found limited evidence that Akin osteotomy plus chevron osteotomy improved outcomes after 1 year compared with Akin osteotomy plus distal soft tissue reconstruction.

Benefits: **Versus no treatment or versus orthoses:** We found one systematic review (search date 1998, no relevant RCTs)[8] and one subsequent RCT.[6] The subsequent RCT (209 adults) compared three treatments: chevron osteotomy (see glossary, p 1268); orthoses; and no treatment (see benefits of orthoses, p 1261).[6] It found that chevron osteotomy significantly reduced pain intensity and significantly improved cosmetic appearance and functional status compared with no treatment. It found no significant difference in the ability to work after 1 year (pain intensity on a visual analogue score range 0 [no pain] to 100 [unbearable pain]: 23 with chevron osteotomy *v* 40 with no treatment, difference adjusted for baseline characteristics –19, 95% CI –28 to –10; cosmetic appearance on a 7 point scale ranging from 0 [no cosmetic disturbance] to 6 [maximal cosmetic disturbance]: 1.9 with chevron osteotomy *v* 2.8 with no treatment, difference adjusted for baseline characteristics: –1.2, 95% CI –1.8 to –0.6; functional status (AOFAS — see glossary, p 1268): 75 with chevron osteotomy *v* 66 with no treatment, difference adjusted for baseline characteristics 11, 95% CI 7 to 16; ability to work on a visual analogue scale from 0 [total inability to work] to 100 [maximal working ability]: 89 with chevron osteotomy *v* 83 with no treatment, difference adjusted for baseline characteristics +4, 95% CI –3 to +11). The RCT also found that chevron osteotomy significantly reduced pain intensity and significantly improved cosmetic appearance and functional status compared with orthoses but found no significant difference in the ability to work after 1 year (pain intensity on a visual analogue score ranging from 0 [no pain] to 100 [unbearable pain]: 23 with chevron osteotomy *v* 40 with orthosis, difference adjusted for baseline characteristics –14, 95% CI –22 to –5; cosmetic appearance on a 7 point scale ranging from 0 [no cosmetic disturbance] to 6 [maximal cosmetic disturbance]: 1.9 with chevron osteotomy *v* 2.6 with orthosis, difference adjusted for baseline characteristics –1.4, 95% CI –2.1 to –0.8; functional status [AOFAS]: 75 with chevron osteotomy *v* 64 with orthosis, difference adjusted for baseline characteristics 11, 95% CI 7 to 15; ability to work on a visual analogue scale from 0 [total inability to work] to 100 [maximal working ability]: 89 with chevron osteotomy *v* 81 with orthosis, difference adjusted for baseline characteristics 6, 95% CI 0 to 13). **Versus proximal osteotomy:** We found one systematic review (search date 1998, 3 relevant RCTs, 205 people). [8] The first RCT (66 people) included in the review found no significant difference between proximal chevron osteotomy and proximal crescentic osteotomy in the hallux abductus angle, intermetatarsal angle, transfer lesions (see glossary, p 1269), or functional assessment score (AOFAS) after 22 months.[12] It found that proximal chevron osteotomy significantly reduced healing time compared with proximal crescentic osteotomy ($P < 0.001$) and significantly reduced postoperative dorsiflexion at the healed site ($P = 0.005$). The second RCT (68 people) included in the review found that chevron osteotomy significantly improved the hallux abductus and intermetatarsal angle compared with proximal osteotomy. It found no significant difference in pain, satisfaction, problems with footwear, or mobility after 2 years (hallux abductus angle: 25.0° with chevron osteotomy *v* 20.0° with proximal osteotomy; difference 5.0°, 95% CI 0.5° to 9.5°; intermetatarsal angle: 13.0° with chevron osteotomy *v* 10.0° with proximal osteotomy; difference 3.0°, 95% CI 1.0° to 5.0°).[13] The third RCT (51 people) included in the review found that Wilson osteotomy (see glossary, p 1269) significantly improved the hallux abductus angle compared with chevron osteotomy but found no significant difference in problems with footwear or mobility after 38 months (hallux abductus angle: 25.7° with chevron osteotomy *v* 13.3° with Wilson osteotomy; difference +12.4°, 95% CI +7.5° to +17.5°; footwear problems: 8/24 [33%] with chevron osteotomy *v* 3/26 [12%] with Wilson osteotomy; OR 0.26, 95% CI 0.06 to 1.14; limited walking: 5/24 [21%] with chevron osteotomy *v* 4/26 [15%] with Wilson osteotomy; OR 0.69, 95% CI 0.16 to 2.95).[14] **Plus adductor tenotomy:** We found one systematic review (search date 1998, 1 relevant RCT, 84 people).[8] The RCT included in the review found no significant difference in hallux abductus angle, range of motion, pain, patient satisfaction, people requiring special footwear, and mobility between chevron osteotomy plus adductor tenotomy and chevron osteotomy alone (final hallux abductus angle: 20.2° with chevron osteotomy plus adductor tenotomy *v* 23.5° with chevron osteotomy alone; mean difference –3.3°; 95% CI –8.63° to +2.03°; range of motion: 69° with chevron osteotomy plus adductor tenotomy *v* 67° with chevron osteotomy alone; mean difference +2°, 95% CI –2.7° to +6.73°; people remaining in pain: 8/38 [21%] with chevron osteotomy plus adductor tenotomy *v* 6/46 [13%] with chevron osteotomy alone; OR 1.78, 95% CI 0.56 to 5.67; people remaining dissatisfied: 10/38 [26%] with chevron osteotomy plus adductor tenotomy *v* 7/46 [15%] with chevron osteotomy alone; OR 1.99, 95% CI 0.68 to 5.87; people requiring special footwear: 2/38 [5%] with chevron osteotomy plus adductor tenotomy *v* 7/46 [15%] with chevron osteotomy alone; OR 0.31, 95% CI 0.06 to 1.59; people with reduced mobility: 1/38 [3%] with chevron osteotomy plus adductor tenotomy *v* 1/46 [2%] with chevron osteotomy alone; OR 1.22, 95% CI 0.07 to 20.12).[15] **Plus Akin osteotomy:** We found one RCT (23 people; see comment below) comparing Akin osteotomy (see glossary, p 1268) plus chevron osteotomy versus Akin osteotomy plus distal soft tissue reconstruction (DSTR) (see glossary, p 1269).[16] It found no significant difference in hallux abductus angle, intermetatarsal angle, or range of toe motion between the two treatment options after a minimum of 1 year (hallux abductus angle: 12.5° with chevron osteotomy plus Akin osteotomy *v* 17° with DSTR plus Akin osteotomy; mean difference +4.5°; 95% CI –5.77° to +14.72°; intermetatarsal angle: 7° with chevron osteotomy plus Akin osteotomy *v* 10° with DSTR plus Akin osteotomy; mean difference +3°; 95% CI –1.45° to +7.45°; range of toe motion: mean difference –3°; 95% CI –12.07° to +6.07°).

Harms: Complications were reported by most of the RCTs. The RCT comparing chevron osteotomy, orthoses, and no treatment reported complications in 4/71 (6%) people undergoing chevron osteotomy (complications consisted of one wound infection, one stress fracture, one episode of nerve damage, and one recurrence of deformity).[6] The RCT reported no complications associated with orthoses. The second RCT comparing proximal crescentic osteotomy with proximal chevron osteotomy found one case of delayed wound healing in the chevron group and two cases in the proximal osteotomy group. Eight further people experienced complications, though the authors did not state which group they belonged to.[12] The RCT comparing proximal osteotomy and chevron osteotomy reported one wound infection and two stress fractures in people undergoing chevron osteotomy and 11 complications in people undergoing proximal osteotomy, consisting mostly of pain in other areas of the forefoot (metatarsalgia).[13] The RCT comparing Wilson osteotomy with chevron osteotomy found no significant difference in the proportion with complications (11/26 [42%] with Wilson osteotomy *v* 9/24 [38%] with chevron osteotomy; RR 1.30, 95% CI 0.57 to 2.24).[14] Complications included swelling, over correction, slow healing, and recurrence of bunion. Transfer pain (see glossary, p 1269) and lesions were recurring problems in both groups. The RCT found that although Wilson osteotomy resulted in a significantly shortened metatarsal compared with chevron osteotomy (P = 0.02), with metatarsal dorsiflexion in 20% of people, this change in position did not correlate with development of new corns, callous, or pain. In the RCT that compared chevron osteotomy plus adductor tenotomy with chevron osteotomy alone, about 25% of both groups remained dissatisfied during follow up.[15] This may be related to greater postoperative reduction in the circumference of the ball of the foot; the RCT found that the ball circumference of dissatisfied people was significantly greater than that of satisfied people (P = 0.005). The RCT comparing Akin osteotomy plus chevron osteotomy with Akin osteotomy plus distal soft tissue reconstruction reported two complications with Akin osteotomy plus chevron osteotomy (one non-union and one where a transfer lesion developed resulting in further surgery), one complication with Akin osteotomy plus distal soft tissue reconstruction (nerve damage in the great toe).[16]

Comment: None of the RCTs included long term follow up. The RCT comparing chevron osteotomy plus Akin osteotomy with Akin osteotomy plus distal soft tissue reconstruction was poorly randomised and seems to be a subset of data from a larger RCT.[16]

OPTION DIFFERENT METHODS OF BONE FIXATION

We found limited evidence about the effects of different methods of bone fixation. One small RCT found that screw fixation plus early weight bearing reduced time to return to work and social activity compared with suture fixation and later weight bearing.

Benefits: We found no systematic review. We found two RCTs comparing different methods of bone fixation after Mitchell's osteotomy (see glossary, p 1269).[17,18] The first RCT (28 people, 39 feet; see comment below) found no significant difference between a standard method of fixation and absorbable pin fixation in clinical outcomes (range of movement: 61.2° with standard fixation *v* 69.2° with absorbable pin fixation; mean difference +8.0°, 95% CI –7.3° to +23.6°; people remaining in pain on walking: 1/17 [5.9%] with standard fixation *v* 2/21 [9.5%] absorbable pin fixation; P = 0.58; people with marked walking limitation: 1/17 [5.9%] with standard fixation *v* 1/21 [4.8%] with absorbable pin fixation; P = 0.24; people dissatisfied with cosmetic appearance: 1/17 [5.9%] with standard fixation *v* 3/21 [14.3%] with absorbable pin fixation; P = 0.38) or radiological outcomes (hallux abductus angle: 15.8° with standard fixation *v* 18.2° with absorbable pin fixation; mean difference +2.4°, 95% CI –4.81° to +9.61°; intermetatarsal angle:

9.1° with standard fixation *v* 9.4° with absorbable pin fixation; mean difference +0.3°, 95% CI −1.77° to +2.37°) after a mean follow up of 11 months (range 2–24 months).[17] The second RCT (30 people) compared screw fixation followed by early weight bearing in a plaster shoe versus vicryl suture fixation followed by 6 weeks of non-weight bearing in a plaster boot.[18] It found that screw fixation followed by early weight bearing in a plaster shoe significantly reduced time taken to return to social activities (mean 2.9 weeks with screw fixation *v* 5.7 weeks with suture fixation; $P < 0.001$) and time taken to return to work (mean 4.9 weeks with screw fixation *v* 8.7 weeks with suture fixation; $P < 0.001$), but found no significant difference in clinical and radiological outcomes after 6 months (hallux abductus angle: 10.8° with suture fixation *v* 12° with screw fixation; mean difference +1.2°, 95% CI −2.35° to +4.75°; inter-metatarsal angle: 9.1° with suture fixation *v* 10.7° with screw fixation; mean difference +1.6°, 95% CI −0.56 to +3.76).[18]

Harms: The first RCT (28 people, 39 feet) reported more complications with standard compared with pin fixation, although the difference was not significant (14/17 [82%] feet *v* 16/22 [73%] feet; RR 1.13, 95% CI 0.81 to 1.59).[17] These included recurrence of deformity (3/17 [18%] feet *v* 2/22 [9%] feet), problems primarily resulting in pain (5/17 [29%] feet *v* 6/22 [27%] feet), and continued swelling (3/17 [18%] feet *v* 0/22 [0%] feet). In the RCT (30 people) of screw fixation compared with suture fixation, 2/15 (13%) people had the screw removed because of pain.[18] The RCT reported that superficial infection occurred in three people overall (2 with screw fixation *v* 1 with suture fixation) and also found that fixation followed by early weight bearing in a plaster shoe significantly increased metatarsophalangeal joint stiffness after both 3 and 6 months.

Comment: Applicability of the results from the first RCT may be limited as people were used as the unit of randomisation and feet as the unit of statistical analysis.[17]

QUESTION What are the effects of postoperative care?

OPTION CONTINUOUS PASSIVE MOTION

One systematic review found insufficient evidence on the effects of continuous passive motion.

Benefits: We found one systematic review (search date 1998, 1 relevant RCT, 39 people).[8] The RCT included in the review found no significant difference in the range of motion or time taken to return to normal footwear between continuous passive motion plus physiotherapy versus physiotherapy alone (range of motion: 9.3° with continuous passive motion plus physiotherapy *v* 2.6° with physiotherapy alone; mean difference −6.7°, 95% CI −13.6° to +0.3°; time to return to normal footwear: no AR provided; $P < 0.01$).

Harms: No complications were reported by the RCT.[8]

Comment: None.

OPTION EARLY WEIGHT BEARING

One systematic review found insufficient evidence on the effects of early weight bearing.

Benefits: We found one systematic review (search date 1998, 1 relevant RCT, 56 people).[8] The RCT compared early weight bearing (initial weight bearing in a cast from 2–4 weeks after the operation) with late weight bearing (initial weight bearing 4 weeks after the operation).[8] It found no significant difference in rates of non-union at the site of arthrodesis (1/29 [3%] with early weight bearing *v* 2/27 [7%] with late weight bearing; RR 0.46, 95% CI 0.05 to 4.85).

Harms: See benefits above.

Comment: The only outcome assessed by the RCT was non-union at the site of arthrodesis.[8]

OPTION SLIPPER CASTS

One RCT found insufficient evidence on the effects of plaster slipper casts.

Benefits: We found no systematic review, but found one RCT (54 feet), which compared plaster slipper cast versus crepe bandage after a Wilson osteotomy (see glossary, p 1269).[19] Cast and dressings were changed 12 days after surgery and then kept on for a further 4 weeks. The RCT found no significant difference in hallux valgus angle, range of movement, or time to return to normal activities (hallux valgus angle: 19.4° with plaster slipper *v* 17.9° with crepe bandage; mean difference –1.5°, 95% CI –4.47° to +1.47°; range of movement: 48.9° with plaster slipper *v* 44.2° with crepe bandage; mean difference –4.7°, 95% CI –10.51° to +1.11°; return to normal activities: 6.2 weeks with plaster slipper *v* 6.6 weeks with crepe bandage; significance not reported).

Harms: The RCT reported that one failed union occurred with crepe bandaging versus none with plaster slipper cast treatment, and that two people receiving plaster slipper cast treatment developed superficial wound infections.[19]

Comment: The RCT was small and could not exclude clinically important differences between the groups.[19]

GLOSSARY

Akin osteotomy A procedure involving resection of the medial prominence of the first metatarsal head and a medial wedge osteotomy of the proximal phalanx of the great toe.

Antipronatory orthoses Insoles designed to reduce the amount of in-roll or flattening of the foot during gait.

AOFAS score American Orthopaedic Foot and Ankle Society functional assessment score, ranging from 0 to 100, higher scores indicating better functional ability.

Chevron osteotomy A v-shaped wedge of bone is removed from the distal end of the metatarsal shaft, allowing the metatarsal head to be realigned on the shaft.

Distal osteotomy A cut is made in the neck of the metatarsal so that the head of the metatarsal can be realigned on the shaft.

Distal soft tissue reconstruction A procedure involving the release of various ligaments, the capsule, and tendons around the first metatarsophalangeal joint.

First ray The first metatarsal and medial cuneiform function as a single unit called the first ray.

Keller's arthroplasty A procedure involving removal of the medial side of the metatarsal head and straight resection of the base of the proximal phalanx.

Kirschner wire A thin but rigid wire that is used to fix bone fragments. It is passed through drilled channels in the bone (sometimes called a K-wire).

Mitchell's osteotomy A distal metatarsal osteotomy whereby an incomplete osteotomy is performed perpendicular to the long axis of the bone. The distal portion is moved laterally and fixed in position. This results in shortening of the bone.

Proximal chevron osteotomy Removal of a v-shaped wedge of bone from the base of the metatarsal shaft followed by displacement and fixation of the distal portion of bone.

Proximal crescentic osteotomy A curved cut is made across the base of the metatarsal shaft. The distal portion of bone is slid across the proximal end of bone and fixed in a corrected position.

Transfer lesions Areas of corns or callus that develop when the weight bearing forces are transferred from one area of the foot to another.

Transfer pain Refers to pain that occurs in another area of the foot after surgery. It usually occurs in the second/third metatarsal heads after the surgeon has altered the first metatarsal head.

Wilson osteotomy A double oblique cut is made in the distal portion of the metatarsal shaft and the metatarsal head is slid into a corrected position.

REFERENCES

1. Dykyj D. Pathological anatomy of hallux abducto valgus. *Clin Podiatr Med Surg* 1989;6:1–15.
2. Kilmartin TE, Barrington RL, Wallace WA. A controlled prospective trial of a foot orthosis for juvenile hallux valgus. *J Bone Joint Surg Br* 1994;76:210–214.
3. Morris JB, Brash LF, Hird MD. Chiropodial survey of geriatric and psychiatric hospital in-patients – Angus District. *Chiropodist* 1980;April:128–139.
4. LaPorta G, Melillo T, Olinsky D. X-ray evaluation of hallux abducto valgus deformity. *J Am Podiatr Med Assoc* 1974;64:544–566.
5. Budiman-Mak E, Conrad KJ, Roach KE, et al. Can orthoses prevent hallux valgus deformity in rheumatoid arthritis? A randomised clinical trial. *J Clin Rheumatol* 1995;1:313–321.
6. Torkki M, Malmivaara A, Seitsalo S, et al. Surgery vs orthosis vs watchful waiting for hallux valgus. A randomized controlled trial. *JAMA* 2001;285:2474–2480.
7. Juriansz AM. Conservative treatment of hallux valgus: a randomised controlled trial of a hallux valgus night splint. MSc Thesis 1996: Faculty of Science, King's College London.
8. Ferrari J, Higgins JPT, William RL. Interventions for treating hallux valgus (abductovalgus) and bunions. In: The Cochrane Library, Issue 3, 2001. Oxford: Update Software. Search date 1998; primary sources Medline, Embase, Cinahl, Amed, Cochrane Controlled Trials Register, Cochrane Musculoskeletal Injuries Trials Register, bibliographies of identified trials, and hand searches of podiatry journals.
9. Turnbull T, Grange W. A comparison of Keller's arthroplasty and distal metatarsal osteotomy in the treatment of adult hallux valgus. *J Bone Joint Surgery Br* 1986;68:132–137.
10. O'Doherty PD, Lowrie IG, Magnussen PA, et al. The management of the painful first metatarsophalangeal joint in the older patient. Arthrodesis or Keller's arthroplasty? *J Bone Joint Surgery Br* 1990;72:839–842.
11. Sherman KP, Douglas DL, Benson MK. Keller's arthroplasty: is distraction useful? A prospective trial. *J Bone Joint Surgery Br* 1984;66:765–769.
12. Easley ME, Kiebzak GM, Davis WH, et al. Prospective, randomized comparison of proximal crescentric and proximal chevron osteotomies for correction of hallux valgus deformity. *Foot Ankle Int* 1996;17:307–316.
13. Resch S, Stenstrom A, Jonsson K, et al. Results after chevron osteotomy and proximal osteotomy for hallux valgus: a prospective, randomised study. *Foot* 1993;3:99–104.
14. Klosok IK, Pring DJ, Jessop JH, et al. Chevron or Wilson metatarsal osteotomy for hallux valgus. A prospective randomised trial. *J Bone Joint Surg Br* 1993;75:825–829.
15. Resch S, Stenstrom A, Reynisson K, et al. Chevron osteotomy for hallux valgus not improved by additional adductor tenotomy. A prospective, randomised study of 84 patients. *Acta Orthop Scand* 1994;65:541–544.
16. Basile A, Battaglia A, Campi A. Comparison of chevron-Akin osteotomy and distal soft tissue reconstruction-Akin osteotomy for correction of mild hallux valgus. *Foot Ankle Surg* 2000;6:155–163.
17. Prior TD, Grace DL, MacLean JB, et al. Correction of hallux abductovalgus by Mitchell's osteotomy: comparing standard fixation methods with absorbable polydioxanone pins. *Foot* 1997;7:121–125.

18. Calder JDF, Hollingdale JP, Pearse MF. Screw versus suture fixation of Mitchell's osteotomy. A prospective randomised study. *J Bone Joint Surg Br* 1999;81:621–624.

19. Meek RMD, Anderson EG. Plaster slipper versus crepe bandage after Wilson's osteotomy for hallux valgus. Foot 1999;9:138–141.

Jill Ferrari
Department of Podiatry
University College London
London
UK

Competing interests: None declared.

Carpal tunnel syndrome

Search date September 2002

Shawn Marshall

QUESTIONS

INTERVENTIONS

See glossary, p 1286

Key Messages

- **Diuretics** One small RCT found no significant difference with trichlormethiazide versus placebo in mean global symptom score after 2 or 4 weeks. One RCT found no significant difference with bendrofluazide versus placebo in the proportion of people with no improvement in symptoms after 4 weeks.
- **Endoscopic carpal tunnel release versus open carpal tunnel release** We found no RCTs comparing surgery versus placebo. One systematic review and subsequent RCTs found no clear evidence of a difference in symptoms with endoscopic carpal tunnel release versus open carpal tunnel release up to 12 months after the operation. RCTs found conflicting evidence on differences in the time taken to return to work between endoscopic carpal tunnel release versus open carpal tunnel release. Harms resulting from endoscopic carpal tunnel release and open carpal tunnel release vary between RCTs. One systematic review comparing the interventions suggests that endoscopic carpal tunnel release may cause more transient nerve problems whereas open carpal tunnel release may cause more wound problems.
- **Internal neurolysis in conjunction with open carpal tunnel release** Three RCTs found no significant difference with open carpal tunnel release alone versus open carpal tunnel release plus internal neurolysis in symptoms.

- **Local corticosteroid injection (short term)** Two RCTs found local corticosteroid injection (methylprednisolone, hydrocortisone) versus placebo or no treatment significantly improved symptoms after 4–6 weeks. One small RCT found that local betamethasone injection versus betamethasone injection into the deltoid significantly improved symptoms after 1 month. One RCT found no significant difference with local methylprednisolone injection versus oral prednisolone in symptoms after 2 weeks, but found that local methylprednisolone injection versus oral prednisolone significantly improved symptoms after 8 and 12 weeks. One small RCT found that local methylprednisolone injection versus helium neon laser significantly improved symptoms after 20 days, but found no significant difference in symptoms between the two groups after 6 months. One small RCT found no significant difference with local methylprednisolone injection versus non-steroidal anti-inflammatory plus nocturnal neutral angle wrist splints in symptoms after 2 or 8 weeks.
- **Nerve and tendon gliding exercises** One small RCT found no significant difference with nerve and tendon gliding exercises plus neutral angle wrist splint versus neutral angle wrist splint alone in mean symptom severity score or mean functional status score assessed 8 weeks after the end of the treatment.
- **Non-steroidal anti-inflammatory drugs** One small RCT found no significant difference with tenoxicam versus placebo in mean global symptom score after 2 or 4 weeks. One RCT found no significant difference in symptom severity scores with ibuprofen plus nocturnal wrist splint versus chiropractic manipulation plus ultrasound plus nocturnal wrist splint after 9 weeks.
- **Oral corticosteroids (short term)** One small RCT found that oral prednisone versus placebo significantly improved the mean global symptom score after 2 weeks, but not after 4 or 8 weeks. One small RCT found that oral prednisolone versus placebo significantly improved the mean global symptom score after 2 and 4 weeks. One small RCT found that oral prednisolone versus placebo significantly improved the median global symptom score after 2 and 8 weeks. One RCT found no significant difference with local methylprednisolone injection versus oral prednisolone in symptoms after 2 weeks, but found that local methylprednisolone injection versus oral prednisolone significantly improved symptoms after 8 and 12 weeks.
- **Pyridoxine** One very small RCT found a similar improvement in symptoms with pyridoxine versus placebo or no treatment after 10 weeks. The RCT may have been too small to detect a clinically important difference between treatments. One small RCT found no significant difference with pyridoxine versus placebo in nocturnal pain, numbness, or tingling after 12 weeks.
- **Surgery versus placebo or non-surgical intervention** We found no RCTs comparing surgery versus placebo. One very small RCT found limited evidence that surgical section of the anterior carpal ligament versus splinting of the hand, wrist, and arm for 1 month increased the proportion of people with clinical improvement after 1 year.
- **Therapeutic ultrasound** One RCT found ultrasound versus placebo significantly increased the proportion of wrists with satisfactory improvement or complete remission of symptoms after 6 months. One RCT found no significant difference in mean symptom severity with high intensity or low intensity ultrasound versus placebo after 2 weeks. One RCT found no significant difference in symptom severity scores with ibuprofen plus nocturnal wrist splint versus chiropractic manipulation plus ultrasound plus nocturnal wrist splint after 9 weeks.

- **Wrist splints** One RCT found a significant improvement in symptoms after 2 and 4 weeks with a nocturnal hand brace versus no treatment. RCTs found no significant difference in symptoms with neutral angle versus 20° extension wrist splinting, or with full time versus night time only neutral angle wrist splinting.
- **Wrist splints after carpal tunnel release surgery** Two RCTs in people after carpal tunnel release surgery found no significant difference with wrist splinting versus no splinting in median grip strength or in the number of people who considered themselves "cured". Another RCT found that splinting versus no splinting significantly increased pain at 1 month and the number of days taken to return to work.
- **Local corticosteroid injection (long term); oral corticosteroids (long term)** We found no RCTs on the effects of these interventions.

DEFINITION Carpal tunnel syndrome is a neuropathy caused by compression of the median nerve within the carpal tunnel.[1] Classical symptoms of carpal tunnel syndrome include numbness, tingling, burning, or pain in at least two of the three digits supplied by the median nerve (i.e. the thumb, index, and middle fingers).[2] The American Academy of Neurology has described diagnostic criteria (see glossary, p 1286) that rely on a combination of symptoms and physical examination findings.[3] Other diagnostic criteria include results from electrophysiological studies.[2]

INCIDENCE/ PREVALENCE A general population survey in Rochester, Minnesota, found the age adjusted incidence of carpal tunnel syndrome to be 105 (95% CI 99 to 112) cases per 100 000 person years.[4,5] Age adjusted incidence rates were 52 (95% CI 45 to 59) cases for men and 149 (95% CI 138 to 159) cases for women per 100 000 person years. The study found incidence rates increased from 88 (95% CI 75 to 101) cases per 100 000 person years in 1961–1965 to 125 (95% CI 112 to 138) cases per 100 000 person years in 1976–1980. Incidence rates of carpal tunnel syndrome increased with age for men, whereas for women they peaked between the ages of 45–54 years. A general population survey in the Netherlands found prevalence to be 1% for men and 7% for women.[6] A more comprehensive study in southern Sweden found the general population prevalence for carpal tunnel syndrome was 3% (95% CI 2% to 3%).[7] As in other studies, the overall prevalence in women was higher than in men (male to female ratio 1 : 1.4); however, among older people, the prevalence in women was almost four times that in men (age group 65–74 years: men 1%, 95% CI 0% to 4%; women 5%, 95% CI 3% to 8%).

AETIOLOGY/ RISK FACTORS Most cases of carpal tunnel syndrome have no easily identifiable cause (idiopathic).[4] Secondary causes of carpal tunnel syndrome include the following: space occupying lesions (tumours, hypertrophic synovial tissue, fracture callus, and osteophytes); metabolic and physiological (pregnancy, hypothyroidism, rheumatoid arthritis); infections; neuropathies (associated with diabetes mellitus or alcoholism); and familial disorders.[4] One case control study found that risk factors in the general population included repetitive activities requiring wrist extension or flexion, obesity, very rapid dieting, shorter height, hysterectomy without oopherectomy, and recent menopause.[8]

PROGNOSIS One observational study (carpal tunnel syndrome defined by symptoms and electrophysiological study results) found that 34% of people with idiopathic carpal tunnel syndrome without treatment had complete resolution of symptoms (remission) within 6 months of diagnosis.[9] Remission rates were higher for younger age groups, for women versus men, and for pregnant versus non-pregnant women. A more recent observational study of untreated idiopathic carpal tunnel syndrome also demonstrated that symptoms may spontaneously resolve in some people. The main positive prognostic indicators were short duration of symptoms and young age, whereas bilateral symptoms and a positive Phalen's test were indicators of a poorer prognosis.[10]

AIMS OF INTERVENTION To improve symptoms and reduce the physical signs of carpal tunnel syndrome; to prevent progression and loss of hand function secondary to carpal tunnel syndrome; to minimise loss of time from work.

OUTCOMES Clinical improvement of symptoms and reduction in physical signs; hand function; time to return to work.

METHODS *Clinical Evidence* search and appraisal September 2002.

QUESTION **What are the effects of drug treatment?**

OPTION **ORAL CORTICOSTEROIDS**

One small RCT found that oral prednisone versus placebo significantly improved the mean global symptom score after 2 weeks, but not after 4 or 8 weeks. One small RCT found that oral prednisolone versus placebo significantly improved the mean global symptom score after 2 and 4 weeks. One small RCT found that oral prednisolone versus placebo significantly improved the median global symptom score after 2 and 8 weeks. We found no RCTs that measured the effects of oral corticosteroids on symptoms long term. One RCT found no significant difference with local methylprednisolone injection versus oral prednisolone in symptoms after 2 weeks, but found that local methylprednisolone injection versus oral prednisolone significantly improved symptoms after 8 and 12 weeks.

Benefits: **Versus placebo:** We found one systematic review (search date 2000),[11] which included two RCTs[12,13] and found one subsequent RCT.[14] The systematic review did not pool data.[11] The first RCT (15 people) included in the review compared oral prednisone (20 mg daily for the first wk followed by 10 mg daily for the second wk) versus placebo.[12] The RCT found that prednisone significantly improved symptoms based on the mean Global Symptom Score (GSS) (see glossary, p 1286) compared with placebo at 2 weeks' follow up, but significance was not maintained at 4 or 8 weeks' follow up (results presented graphically; CI not provided). The second RCT (91 people) included in the review compared four treatments: oral prednisolone (20 mg daily for 2 wks followed by 10 mg daily for another 2 wks); an oral slow release non-steroidal anti-inflammatory drug (tenoxicam 20 mg daily); an oral diuretic (trichlormethiazide 2 mg daily); and placebo (see comment below).[13] It found that prednisolone (26 people) versus placebo (23 people) significantly reduced the mean GSS after 2 weeks (difference in mean GSS –6.6, 95% CI –10.4 to –2.8) and after 4 weeks (–10.8, 95% CI –15.0 to –6.7). The subsequent RCT (36 people) compared oral prednisolone (25 mg daily for 10 days) versus placebo.[14] The RCT found that prednisolone versus placebo significantly reduced the median GSS after 2 weeks (difference in median GSS –6, 95% CI –11 to –1) and after 8 weeks (difference in median GSS –6, 95% CI –11 to 0). **Versus injected corticosteroids:** We found one systematic review[15] that included one RCT (60 people)[16] comparing a single local corticosteroid injection (methylprednisolone 15 mg) plus oral placebo versus oral corticosteroid (prednisolone 25 mg daily for 10 days) plus placebo injection. The review found no significant difference in the mean GSS with local methylprednisolone injection versus oral prednisolone after 2 weeks (WMD –4.2, 95% CI –8.7 to +0.3), but found a significant improvement with local methylprednisolone injection versus oral prednisolone after 8 weeks (WMD –7.2, 95% CI –11.5 to –2.9) and 12 weeks (WMD –7.0, 95% CI –11.6 to –2.4).[15]

Harms: In the first RCT comparing oral prednisone versus placebo, three people in each group reported adverse effects, although none of these people discontinued their treatment.[12] In the prednisone group, one person with diabetes reported mild hyperglycaemia, whereas other reported symptoms included nausea, abdominal discomfort, constipation, and altered taste sensation. Symptoms in the placebo group included nausea, abdominal discomfort, constipation, insomnia, headache, dysuria, and burning nostrils. In the second RCT comparing oral prednisolone versus placebo adverse effects reported included nausea and epigastric pain (nausea: 3/23 [13%] of people with prednisolone *v* 1/16 [6%] of people with placebo; epigastric pain: 2/23 [9%] *v* 2/16 [12%]).[13] The subsequent RCT did not report adverse events.[14] The RCT comparing local corticosteroid injection versus oral corticosteroid reported nine side effects in the oral prednisolone and placebo injection group: bloating (2 people), insomnia (2 people), polyphagia (3 people), and injection pain (2 people).[15] The RCT reported two people had injection pain in the local corticosteroid injection group. Common adverse reactions to oral corticosteroids include nausea, anxiety, acne, menstrual irregularities, insomnia, headaches, and mood swings. More serious adverse reactions include peptic ulcer, steroid psychosis, osteoporosis, and adrenal insufficiency.[17]

Comment: The RCT comparing oral prednisolone versus placebo reported that 18/91 (20%) people did not complete the trial, although analysis of data was not by intention to treat.[13]

OPTION NON-STEROIDAL ANTI-INFLAMMATORY DRUGS

One small RCT found no significant difference with tenoxicam versus placebo in mean global symptom score after 2 or 4 weeks. One RCT found no significant difference in symptom severity scores with ibuprofen plus nocturnal wrist splint versus chiropractic manipulation plus ultrasound plus nocturnal wrist splint after 9 weeks.

Benefits: **Versus placebo:** We found one systematic review (search date 2000),[11] which included one RCT.[13] The RCT (91 people) included in the review compared four treatments: prednisolone; an oral slow release non-steroidal anti-inflammatory drug (NSAID) (tenoxicam 20 mg daily for 4 wks); trichlormethiazide; and placebo (see the benefits and comment under oral corticosteroids, p 1274).[13] It found that tenoxicam (18 people) versus placebo (16 people) did not significantly alter mean Global Symptom Score (see glossary, p 1286) after 2 weeks (difference in mean Global Symptom Score +3.1, 95% CI −1.4 to +7.6) or after 4 weeks (+3.2, 95% CI −1.7 to +8.1). **Versus other treatments:** We found one systematic review (search date 2000),[11] which included one RCT.[18] The RCT (91 people, age 21–45 years) included in the review compared an oral NSAID (ibuprofen 800 mg 3 times daily for 1 wk, then twice daily for 1 wk, and then as needed for 7 wks) plus nocturnal wrist splints versus chiropractic manipulation (3 sessions/wk for 2 wks, then 2 sessions/wk for 3 wks, then 1 session/wk for 4 wks) plus ultrasound treatments (1.0–1.5 W/cm^2 for 5 min) plus nocturnal wrist splints.[18] The RCT found no significant difference between treatments in symptom severity after 9 weeks (difference in mean symptom severity score for NSAID group *v* non-NSAID group −2.4, 95% CI −7.5 to +2.7; see comment below).[18]

Harms: The RCT comparing tenoxicam versus placebo reported nausea (3/18 [17%] of people with tenoxicam *v* 1/16 [6%] of people with placebo) and epigastric pain (3/18 [17%] *v* 2/16 [12%]).[13] The RCT comparing ibuprofen plus wrist splints versus chiropractic manipulation plus ultrasound plus wrist splints reported 10/46 (22%) people taking ibuprofen reported acute gastrointestinal intolerance, headache, and nausea.[18] Of these 10 people, 5/46 (11%) withdrew from the medication and 5/46 (11%) continued to take ibuprofen with an additional liquid antacid (see NSAIDs topic, p 1393). One person reported a sore neck after chiropractic manipulation.[18]

Comment: The RCT comparing ibuprofen plus wrist splints versus chiropractic manipulation plus ultrasound plus wrist splints used a numerical scoring system to grade symptom severity (0 = no symptoms; 16 = severe symptoms).[18]

OPTION DIURETICS

One small RCT found no significant difference with trichlormethiazide versus placebo in mean global symptom score after 2 or 4 weeks. One RCT found no significant difference with bendrofluazide versus placebo in the proportion of people with no improvement in symptoms after 4 weeks.

Benefits: We found one systematic review (search date 2000),[11] which included two RCTs.[13,19] The review did not pool data. The first RCT (91 people) included in the review compared four treatments: prednisolone; a non-steroidal anti-inflammatory drug; an oral diuretic (trichlormethiazide 2 mg daily for 4 wks); and placebo (see benefits and comment under oral corticosteroids, p 1274).[13] It found that trichlormethiazide (16 people) versus placebo (16 people) did not significantly alter mean Global Symptom Score (see glossary, p 1286) after either 2 weeks (difference in mean Global Symptom Score +0.7, 95% CI –3.0 to +4.4) or after 4 weeks (+0.8, –3.2 to +4.8).[13] The second RCT (48 people, 81 hands) included in the review compared bendrofluazide 5 mg daily for 4 weeks versus placebo.[19] It found no significant difference with bendrofluazide versus placebo the proportion of people with "no improvement in symptoms at all" after 4 weeks (no improvement at all: 54% of people with bendrofluazide *v* 50% of people with placebo; difference +4%, 95% CI –18% to +25%; see comment below).[11]

Harms: The first RCT reported epigastric pain in 2/16 (12%) people with diuretic versus 2/16 (12%) people with placebo.[13] The second RCT reported one person "felt unwell in a nonspecific way" on bendrofluazide and was withdrawn from the study.[19]

Comment: The RCT comparing bendrofluazide versus placebo used a numerical score from 0 to 5 to assess the degree of improvement in symptoms reported by people (0 = no improvement at all; 5 = full recovery).[19]

OPTION PYRIDOXINE

One very small RCT found a similar improvement in symptoms with pyridoxine versus placebo or no treatment after 10 weeks. The RCT may have been too small to detect a clinically important difference between treatments. One small RCT found no significant difference with pyridoxine versus placebo in nocturnal pain, numbness, or tingling after 12 weeks.

Benefits: We found one systematic review (search date 2000),[11] which included two RCTs.[20,21] The review did not pool data.[11] The first RCT (15 people) included in the review compared oral pyridoxine (200 mg daily); placebo (dextrose pill); and no treatment.[21] The RCT found a similar improvement in symptoms with pyridoxine versus placebo or no treatment after 10 weeks (symptoms improved: 3/6 [50%] with pyridoxine *v* 4/5 [80%] with placebo *v* 3/4 [75%] with no treatment; no statistical analysis reported; see comment below).[21] The second RCT (35 people) included in the review compared oral pyridoxine (200 mg daily) versus placebo.[20] The RCT found no significant difference with pyridoxine versus placebo in nocturnal pain, numbness, or tingling after 12 weeks (reported as not significant; P values not provided).[20]

Harms: Neither RCT reported harms.[20,21] Common adverse reactions associated with pyridoxine include numbness, paraesthesia, and an unsteady gait.[17]

Comment: The first RCT did not specify which symptoms were assessed nor how changes were scored.[21] The RCT may have been too small to detect a clinically important difference between treatments.[21] The second RCT used an unvalidated 4-point questionnaire with discrete numerical scoring of symptom severity (0 = no symptoms; 4 = severe symptoms).[20]

OPTION LOCAL CORTICOSTEROID INJECTION

Two RCTs found local corticosteroid injection (methylprednisolone, hydrocortisone) versus placebo or no treatment significantly improved symptoms after 4–6 weeks. One small RCT found that local betamethasone injection versus betamethasone injection into the deltoid significantly improved symptoms after 1 month. One RCT found no significant difference with local methylprednisolone injection versus oral prednisolone in symptoms after 2 weeks, but found that local methylprednisolone injection versus oral prednisolone significantly improved symptoms after 8 and 12 weeks. One small RCT found that local methylprednisolone injection versus helium neon laser significantly improved symptoms after 20 days, but found no significant difference in symptoms between the two groups after 6 months. One small RCT found no significant difference with local methylprednisolone injection versus non-steroidal anti-inflammatory plus nocturnal neutral angle wrist splints in symptoms after 2 or 8 weeks. We found no RCTs that assessed long term outcomes.

Benefits: We found one systematic review (search date 2002, 5 RCTs, 220 people)[15] and one additional RCT.[22] **Versus placebo or no treatment:** The systematic review included one RCT, which compared local injection of methylprednisolone (40 mg) versus local placebo injection.[23] The review found that local methylprednisolone injection versus placebo injection significantly improved symptom severity after 1 month (clinical improvement: 23/30 [77%] with methylprednisolone injection *v* 6/30 [20%] with placebo injection; RR 3.8, 95% CI 1.82 to 8.05; see comment below).[15] The additional RCT compared three treatments: local injection of low dose hydrocortisone (25 mg); local injection of high dose hydrocortisone (100 mg); and no injection.[22] It found significant improvement after 6 weeks in the number of people with improved symptoms with both doses of hydrocortisone versus no injection (see comment below; 21/32 [66%] with low dose hydrocortisone *v* 1/20 [5%] with no injection; RR 13.1, 95% CI 1.9 to 90.1; NNT 2, 95% CI 2 to 3; 20/32 [63%] with high dose hydrocortisone *v* 1/20 [5%] with no injection; RR 12.5, 95% CI 1.8 to 86.0; NNT 2, 95% CI 2 to 4). The RCT found no significant difference after 6 weeks in the number of people with improvement with low dose versus high dose hydrocortisone (21/32 [66%] with low dose hydrocortisone *v* 20/32 [63%] with high dose hydrocortisone; RR 1.0, 95% CI 0.7 to 1.5). **Versus systemic steroids:** The systematic review included two RCTs.[16,24] The first RCT included in the review compared local injection of betamethasone (1.5 mg) plus placebo (saline) injection into the deltoid muscle versus local placebo injection plus betamethasone (1.5 mg) injection into the deltoid muscle.[24] The review found that local betamethasone injection versus systemic betamethasone injection significantly improved symptom severity after 1 month (clinical improvement: 9/18 [50%] with local injection *v* 3/19 [16%] with systemic injection; RR 3.17, 95% CI 1.02 to 9.87; see comment below).[15] The second RCT included in the review compared a single local corticosteroid injection plus oral placebo versus oral corticosteroid plus placebo injection.[16] See benefits of oral corticosteroids, p 1274. **Versus helium neon laser:** The systematic review included one RCT, which compared local injection of methylprednisolone (20 mg) at baseline and 10 days later versus helium neon laser treatments given daily (3000 Hz for 20 min sessions, for an unstated number of days).[15] The review found that local injection of methylprednisolone versus helium neon laser significantly improved symptoms after 20 days (RR 0.27, 95% CI 0.09 to 0.83) but found no significant difference between the groups in symptoms after 6 months (RR 0.76, 95% CI 0.48 to 1.21).[15] **Versus oral non-steroidal anti-inflammatory plus neutral angle wrist splint:** The systematic review included one small RCT (23 people), which compared a local injection of methylprednisolone (40 mg), 4 cm proximal to the wrist crease, versus acemetacin (120 mg/day) plus neutral angle wrist splints worn at night.[15] The review found no significant difference with methylprednisolone injection versus non-steroidal anti-inflammatory plus nocturnal splints in symptoms measured by the symptom severity scale at 2 weeks (WMD 0.00, 95% CI –0.64 to +0.64) or 8 weeks (WMD 0.10, 95% CI –0.33 to +0.53).[15]

Harms: The systematic review did not report adverse events.[15] The RCT comparing local corticosteroid injection versus oral corticosteroid reported nine side effects in the oral prednisolone plus placebo injection group: bloating (2 people), insomnia (2 people), polyphagia (3 people), and injection pain (2 people).[16] The RCT reported two people had injection pain in the local corticosteroid injection group. Known serious adverse effects of local corticosteroid injection into the carpal tunnel include tendon rupture and injection into the median nerve.[25]

Comment: Two RCTs included in the systematic review only defined clinical outcomes loosely using a subjective ordinal ranking scale and neither RCT specified the magnitude of symptomatic improvement or the changes in specific symptoms.[23,24] The RCT comparing hydrocortisone injection versus placebo reported the number of people who scored their symptoms as "better" or "much better", but these terms were not quantified and changes in individual symptoms were not described.[22]

QUESTION What are the effects of non-drug treatment?

OPTION WRIST SPLINTS

One RCT found a significant improvement in symptoms after 2 and 4 weeks with a nocturnal hand brace versus no treatment. RCTs found no significant difference in symptoms with neutral angle versus 20° extension wrist splinting, or with full time versus night time only neutral angle wrist splinting.

Benefits: **Versus no treatment:** We found one RCT (83 people) that compared a nocturnal hand brace worn for 4 weeks versus no treatment.[26] It found a significant improvement with nocturnal hand brace versus no treatment in symptoms measured by the Boston Carpal Tunnel Symptom Questionnaire at 2 weeks (–1.03, 95% CI –1.98 to –0.08) and 4 weeks (–1.07, 95% CI –2.01 to –0.13). **Versus other treatments:** We found no RCTs. **Versus different**

splinting regimens: We found one systematic review (search date 1997, 1 RCT)[27] and one subsequent RCT.[28] The RCT in the review (59 people, 90 wrists) compared neutral angle wrist splinting versus wrist splinting in 20° extension (see comment below).[29] It found no significant difference after 2 weeks' follow up in the number of people who reported some degree of improvement in their symptoms (40/45 [89%] with neutral angle splinting *v* 38/45 [84%] with extension splinting; RR 1.1, 95% CI 0.9 to 1.2). The subsequent RCT (24 people) compared full time (day and night) wear of neutral angle wrist splints versus night time only wear. It found no significant difference after 6 weeks in mean symptom severity score (see comment below; difference in mean symptom severity score +0.1, 95% CI –0.3 to +0.5).[28]

Harms: In the RCT comparing nocturnal hand brace to no treatment, four people in the hand brace group experienced transient paraesthesias after the hand brace was removed.[26] Harms were not reported by the other RCTs.

Comment: The RCT in the systematic review graded improvement in symptoms as "none", "some", "a lot", or "complete"; however, individual symptoms and the method for grading changes in symptoms were not described.[29] The subsequent RCT used a validated numerical scale to assess changes in symptom severity.[28] The use of a night time splint was complete or nearly complete in 85% of people allocated to night time splinting only, but 23% of the people reported limited additional daytime use. Complete or nearly complete daytime wear was reported by only 27% of people allocated to full time wear. More men than women were included in the trial than would have been expected from the usual sex distribution of carpal tunnel syndrome.

OPTION NERVE AND TENDON GLIDING EXERCISES

One small RCT found no significant difference with nerve and tendon gliding exercises plus neutral angle wrist splint versus neutral angle wrist splint alone in mean symptom severity score or mean functional status score assessed 8 weeks after the end of the treatment.

Benefits: We found no systematic review but found one RCT.[30] The RCT (28 people, 36 wrists) compared nerve gliding and tendon gliding exercises (see glossary, p 1286) plus a custom made neutral angle wrist splint versus a wrist splint alone. The nerve and tendon gliding exercises were undertaken five times per day for 4 weeks, and people were instructed to wear the neutral angle wrist splints all night and during the day as much as possible for 4 weeks. The RCT found no significant difference with nerve and tendon gliding exercises plus neutral angle wrist splint versus neutral angle wrist splint alone in mean Symptom Severity score (P = 0.2) or mean Functional Status score (P = 0.5) at 8 weeks after the end of the treatment (see comment below).[30] The RCT found a significant improvement for pinch strength with exercise compared with wrist splint alone (P = 0.026) but found no significant difference in other physical examination parameters (grip strength, Phalen's sign, or Tinel's sign; see comment below).

Harms: The RCT did not report adverse events.[30]

Comment: The Symptom Severity Scale has 11 items concerning pain, nocturnal symptoms, numbness, tingling, and weakness; the Functional Status Scale measures eight items including difficulty in writing, buttoning clothes, opening jars, holding a book, gripping a telephone handle, household chores, carrying of grocery bags, bathing, and dressing.[30] Phalen's sign was performed by full flexion of the wrist for 60 seconds with the test recorded positive if paresthesia was experienced in at least one of three radial digits.[30] Tinel's sign was performed by percussing the median nerve at the wrist with the test recorded positive if paresthesia was experienced in at least one of three radial digits.[30]

OPTION THERAPEUTIC ULTRASOUND

One RCT found ultrasound versus placebo significantly increased the proportion of wrists with satisfactory improvement or complete remission of symptoms after 6 months. One RCT found no significant difference in mean symptom severity with high intensity or low intensity ultrasound versus placebo after 2 weeks. One RCT found no significant difference in symptom severity scores with ibuprofen plus nocturnal wrist splint versus chiropractic manipulation plus ultrasound plus nocturnal wrist splint after 9 weeks.

Benefits: **Versus placebo:** We found one systematic review (search date 2000),[11] which included two RCTs.[31,32] The review did not pool data.[11] The first RCT (45 people, 90 wrists) included in the review compared ultrasound (15 min, 5 times weekly for 2 wks followed by twice weekly for 5 wks at an intensity of 1.0 W/cm^2) versus placebo.[32] The dominant wrist was randomly allocated to ultrasound or placebo and the contralateral wrist was allocated to the other treatment. The RCT found at 6 months that significantly more wrists receiving ultrasound treatment had satisfactory improvement or complete remission of symptoms (22/30 [73%] wrists with ultrasound *v* 6/30 [20%] wrists with placebo; RR 3.7, 95% CI 1.7 to 7.7; NNT 2, 95% CI 2 to 4; see comment below).[32] The second RCT (18 women, 30 wrists) included in the review compared three groups: low intensity ultrasound (0.8 W/cm^2); high intensity ultrasound (1.5 W/cm^2); and placebo.[31] Each treatment was performed for 5 minutes, five times a week for 2 weeks. The RCT found no significant difference between low and high intensity ultrasound treatments or between either ultrasound treatment and placebo in mean symptom severity graded on a visual analogue scale at 2 weeks (mean difference with high intensity ultrasound *v* placebo −1.1, 95% CI −3.0 to +0.9; mean difference with low intensity ultrasound *v* placebo −0.4, 95% CI −2.5 to +1.6; mean difference with high intensity ultrasound *v* low intensity ultrasound −0.7, 95% CI −2.4 to +0.9).[31] **Plus chiropractic manipulation plus nocturnal wrist splint:** We found one systematic review,[11] which included one RCT[18] comparing ultrasound plus chiropractic manipulation plus nocturnal wrist splint versus ibuprofen plus wrist splint (see NSAIDs option, p 1276).

Harms: The RCT comparing ultrasound plus chiropractic manipulation plus wrist splint versus ibuprofen plus wrist splint found 10/46 (22%) people taking ibuprofen reported acute gastrointestinal intolerance, headache, and nausea.[18] Of these 10 people, 5/46 (11%) withdrew from the medication and 5/46 (11%) continued to take ibuprofen with an additional liquid antacid (see NSAIDs topic, p 1393). One person reported a sore neck after chiropractic manipulation.[18]

Comment: In the first RCT, 15/45 (33%) people did not complete the trial and analysis of data was not by intention to treat.[32] The RCT used "satisfactory improvement" and "complete remission" as outcome measures, although these terms were not clearly defined. The RCT comparing ultrasound plus chiropractic manipulation plus wrist splint versus ibuprofen plus wrist splint used a numerical scoring system to grade symptom severity (0 = no symptoms; 16 = severe symptoms).[18]

QUESTION What are the effects of surgical treatment?

OPTION SURGERY

We found no RCTs comparing surgery versus placebo. One very small RCT found limited evidence that surgical section of the anterior carpal ligament versus splinting of the hand, wrist, and arm for one month increased the proportion of people with clinical improvement after 1 year. One systematic review and subsequent RCTs found no clear evidence of a difference in symptoms with endoscopic carpal tunnel release versus open carpal tunnel release up to 12 months after the operation. RCTs found conflicting evidence on differences in the time taken to return to work between endoscopic carpal tunnel release versus open carpal tunnel release. Harms resulting from endoscopic carpal tunnel release and open carpal tunnel release vary between RCTs. One systematic review comparing the interventions suggests that endoscopic carpal tunnel release may cause more transient nerve problems whereas open carpal tunnel release may cause more wound problems.

Benefits: We found two systematic reviews (search date 2000, 14 RCTS, 1179 people;[33] search date 2001, 1 RCT, 22 women[34]) and one non-systematic review (search date 1997, 4 RCTs, 1394 people).[35] **Surgery versus placebo or non-surgical intervention:** We found no RCTs comparing surgery versus placebo. We found one systematic review, which included one very small RCT (22 women, symptoms ranging from 1 month to 20 years) comparing open surgical section of the anterior carpal ligament versus splinting of the hand, wrist, and arm for 1 month.[34] The review found surgical section of the anterior carpal ligament versus splinting of the hand, wrist, and arm significantly increased the proportion of people with clinical improvement after 1 year (clinical improvement: 10/11 [91%] with surgery v 2/11 [18%] with splinting; RR 5, 95% CI 1.4 to 17.8; see comment below).[34] **Endoscopic versus open carpal tunnel release:** We found one systematic review (search date 2000, 7 RCTS, 739 people; see comment below)[33] and two subsequent RCTs.[36,37] The systematic review included three "high quality" RCTs and four "low quality" RCTs comparing endoscopic carpal tunnel release versus open carpal tunnel release.[33] The systematic review included three RCTs that assessed effects on symptoms after 3 months.[33] It found no significant difference in symptoms after 3 months with endoscopic versus open carpal tunnel release (reported as improvement in paraesthesia, numbness in 99% with endoscopic carpal tunnel release *v* 98% with open carpal tunnel release after 12 wks, difference +1%, 95% CI –3 to +5% in 1 RCT; reported as "no significant difference" in pain after 3 months in 1 RCT; reported as "no significant difference" in symptom severity score after 3 months in 1 RCT; P values not provided).[33] The systematic review included one RCT that evaluated effects on symptoms after 6 months and 12 months. It found no significant difference in pain with endoscopic versus open carpal tunnel release after 6 months and 12 months (reported as "no significant difference"; P value not provided).[33] The first subsequent small RCT (26 men) found that tingling sensations and severity of night time numbness were improved in the endoscopic versus the open carpal tunnel release group at 2 weeks, but were no longer significantly different by 4 weeks (P values not provided).[37] It found endoscopic versus open carpal tunnel release significantly improved the severity of night time hand or wrist pain after 4 weeks (P value not provided).[37] The second subsequent RCT (25 people with bilateral carpal tunnel syndrome) randomly assigned one wrist to undergo endoscopic release, at which time the contralateral wrist on the same person was assigned to undergo open release.[36] All operations in the RCT were carried out by the same surgeon. The RCT found no significant difference with endoscopic versus open carpal tunnel release in hand function, grip strength, or sensation assessed at 6, 12, 26, or 52 weeks after the operation (reported as not significant; results presented graphically; P value not provided).[36] The RCT found no significant difference with endoscopic versus open carpal tunnel release in people's satisfaction with either procedure assessed over the same period (reported as not significant; results presented graphically; P value not provided).[36] Four RCTs included in the systematic review found a significant decrease in the time taken to return to work and/or activities of daily living with endoscopic carpal tunnel release versus open carpal tunnel release (endoscopic carpal tunnel release *v* open carpal tunnel release: reported as median 14 days *v* 28 days, P < 0.05 in 1 RCT; mean 24 days *v* 42 days, P < 0.05 in 1 RCT; mean 14 days *v* 39 days, P < 0.05 in 1 RCT; mean 20 days *v* 30 days, P < 0.05 in 1 RCT), whereas three RCTs included in the review found no significant difference (endoscopic carpal tunnel release *v* open carpal tunnel release: reported as mean 17 days *v* 19 days, "no significant difference" in 1 RCT; reported as more than 4 wks absence from work 16% *v* 13%, difference 3%, 95% CI –7% to +4% in 1 RCT; reported as time to return to work 17 days *v* 17 days, "no significant difference" in 1 RCT; P value not provided).[33]

Harms: **Surgery versus placebo or non surgical intervention:** None reported.[34] **Endoscopic versus open carpal tunnel release:** All seven RCTs included in the systematic review reported complications.[33] For endoscopic carpal tunnel release complications reported included partial transection of superficial palmar arch, digital nerve contusion, ulnar nerve neurapraxia (see glossary, p 1287), wound haematoma, four conversion to the open procedure, transient neurapraxia, three transient numbness on radial side of ring finger, ulnar nerve paraesthesia, incomplete release, increased numbness in fingertips, subcutaneous heamatoma, loss of strength and mobility in wrist, and algodystrophy. For open carpal tunnel release, complications reported included painful hypertrophic scar, reflex sympathetic dystrophy, prolonged wound secretion, wound infection, scar tethering, five scar hypertrophy, two loss of strength, and swollen/stiff fingers. The systematic review stated "it seems that endoscopic carpal tunnel release gives more transient nerve problems (e.g. neurapraxia, numbness, paraesthesia) and open carpal tunnel release more wound problems (e.g. infection, hypertrophic scar, scar tenderness)".[33] The subsequent RCT reported persisting wound pain (1 wrist) with endoscopic release, and persisting symptoms and signs of carpal tunnel syndrome (1 wrist), superficial sensory nerve injury (1 wrist), and persisting wound pain (1 wrist) with open release.[36] Harms resulting from endoscopic and open carpal tunnel release vary between RCTs, although rates of complications for both procedures are generally low.[37–44]

Comment: **Surgery versus placebo or non surgical intervention:** The RCT was not blinded, and there was no information on baseline clinical and electrophysiological status of the two groups.[34] The method of randomisation was not described.[34] **Endoscopic versus open carpal tunnel release:** Meta-analysis in the systematic review was not undertaken as the data could not be pooled.[33] Endoscopic release techniques vary between RCTs, which may account for some of the variation in complication rates.[35]

OPTION INTERNAL NEUROLYSIS IN CONJUNCTION WITH OPEN CARPAL TUNNEL RELEASE

Three RCTs found no significant difference with open carpal tunnel release alone versus open carpal tunnel release plus internal neurolysis in symptoms.

Benefits: We found one systematic review (search date 2000, 3 RCTs, 148 people; see comment below),[33] which included three RCTs, comparing open carpal tunnel release alone versus open carpal tunnel release plus internal neurolysis (see glossary, p 1286).[45–47] The first RCT (59 people, 63 wrists) found no significant difference between treatments in the proportion of people reporting relief from all or the majority of their symptoms after 12 months (28/32 [88%] with open carpal tunnel release alone *v* 25/31 [81%] with open carpal tunnel release plus internal neurolysis; RR 1.1, 95% CI 0.9 to 1.3).[45] The second RCT (48 people, 48 wrists) found no significant difference between treatments in the proportion of people who reported complete relief of symptoms after 6 months (23/24 [96%] with open carpal tunnel release alone *v* 23/24 [96%] with open carpal tunnel release plus internal neurolysis; RR 1.0, 95% CI 0.9 to 1.1).[47] The third RCT (41 people, 47 wrists with severe carpal tunnel syndrome; see comment below) found no significant difference between treatments in the proportion of wrists with a good (resolution of pain, improvement in sensory deficit, and no surgical complications) or excellent (resolution of pain, resolution of sensory deficit, and no surgical complications) clinical response (15/23 [65%] wrists with open carpal tunnel release alone *v* 16/24 [67%] wrists with open carpal tunnel release plus internal neurolysis; RR 1.0, 95% CI 0.6 to 1.5).[46]

Harms: The first and second RCTs did not report harms.[45,47] The third RCT (41 people, 47 wrists) found no significant difference between treatments in the proportion of wrists with persistent incisional pain, which was the most common complication reported in the trial (3/23 [13%] of wrists with open carpal tunnel release alone *v* 4/24 [17%] of wrists with open carpal tunnel release plus internal neurolysis; RR 0.8, 95% CI 0.2 to 3.1).[46] Other complications included 4% (1/24) wrists with hand swelling, 4% (1/24) wrists with adhesive capsulitis (see glossary, p 1286) in the open carpal tunnel release plus internal neurolysis group, and 4% (1/23) wrists with causalgia in the open carpal tunnel release alone group.

Comment: Meta-analysis in the systematic review was not undertaken as the data could not be pooled.[33] The third RCT defined severe carpal tunnel syndrome as including thenar atrophy, a fixed sensory deficit, or both, in addition to the more common symptoms and signs associated with the syndrome.[45]

QUESTION What are the effects of postoperative treatment?

OPTION WRIST SPLINTS AFTER CARPAL TUNNEL RELEASE SURGERY

Two RCTs in people after carpal tunnel release surgery found no significant difference with wrist splinting versus no splinting in median grip strength or in the number of people who considered themselves "cured". Another RCT found that splinting versus no splinting significantly increased pain at 1 month and the number of days taken to return to work.

Benefits: **Versus unrestricted range of motion:** We found no systematic review. We found three RCTs.[48–50] The first RCT (74 people, 82 wrists) compared rigid wrist splinting for 4 weeks after surgery versus no splinting plus advice to mobilise the affected wrist or wrists.[48] It found no significant difference between treatments in median grip strength (as a percentage of median preoperative grip strength: unsplinted 78%, 95% CI 70% to 86% *v* splinted 76%, 95% CI, 71% to 85%). The second RCT (47 people, 51 wrists) compared rigid wrist splinting for 2 weeks after surgery versus no splinting.[49] It found no significant difference in the number of people who considered themselves "cured" at follow up (see comment below; 12/26 [46%] with splinting *v* 8/17 [47%] with no splinting; RR 1.0, 95% CI 0.5 to 1.9). The third RCT (50 people, 50 wrists) compared rigid wrist splinting for 2 weeks after surgery versus no splinting.[50] It found that the average number of days taken to return to work was significantly lower in the unsplinted group (17 days with no splinting *v* 27 days with splinting; P = 0.005; RR and CI not provided). **Versus bulky dressings:** We found one systematic review (search date 1997) comparing wrist splinting versus bulky dressings after carpal tunnel decompression.[27] It found no RCTs.

Harms: The first RCT found no significant difference between treatments in the number of people reporting scar pain after 6 months (6/37 [16%] with splinting *v* 6/44 [14%] with no splinting; RR 1.2, 95% CI 0.4 to 3.4).[48] The second RCT reported complications for one person in the unsplinted group who had persistent symptoms and required reoperation.[49] The third RCT reported that pillar pain (see glossary, p 1286) was increased at 1 months' follow up for the splinted group (P = 0.02), as was scar tenderness (P = 0.04), although subjective scores for pain were not significantly different between treatments at 3 or 6 months after surgery (data not available).[50]

Comment: In the second RCT, although the term "cured" was used as an outcome measure, its meaning was not defined in the context of the trial and the length of follow up was not specified.[48] The RCT found that 7/47 (15%) people were lost to follow up. Analysis of data was not by intention to treat. The RCTs were too small to exclude the possibility of a clinically important increase in the risk of some complications (e.g. transient ulnar nerve injury) with splinting compared with no splinting.

GLOSSARY

Adhesive capsulitis A condition in which the joint capsule becomes contracted and thickened causing restriction in the range of movement.

American Academy of Neurology diagnostic criteria[3] The likelihood of carpal tunnel syndrome increases with the number of standard symptoms and provocative factors. Symptoms include dull aching discomfort in the hand, forearm or upper arm; paraesthesia in the hand; weakness or clumsiness of the hand; dry skin, swelling, or colour changes in the hand; or occurrence of any of these symptoms in the distribution of the median nerve. Provocative factors include sleep, sustained arm or hand positions, or repetitive actions of the hand or wrist. Relieving factors include changes in hand posture and shaking the hand. Physical examination may be normal, or symptoms may be elicited by tapping or direct pressure over the median nerve at the wrist or with forced flexion or extension of the wrist. Physical signs include sensory loss in the median nerve distribution; weakness or atrophy in the thenar muscles; and dry skin on the thumb, index, or middle fingers. Electromyography and nerve conduction studies can confirm, but not exclude, the diagnosis of carpal tunnel syndrome.

Global Symptom Score The numerical sum of five common carpal tunnel syndrome symptoms (pain, numbness, paresthesia, weakness/clumsiness, and nocturnal wakening), which are each rated from 0 (no symptoms) to 10 (severe symptoms).[12,13]

Internal neurolysis Decompression within the nerve accomplished by performing an epineurotomy and then dividing the nerve into multiple fascicular groups.[46]

Nerve gliding exercises Exercise therapy directed at restoring and maximising excursion of the median nerve through the carpal tunnel.[51]

Pillar pain Pain at the radial or ulnar border of the carpal tunnel.

Tendon gliding exercises Exercise therapy directed at restoring and maximising excursion of the finger flexor tendons through the carpal tunnel.[51]

Ulnar neurapraxia Failure of nerve conduction of the ulnar nerve, usually reversible, due to metabolic or microstructural abnormalities without disruption of the axon.

REFERENCES

1. Rozmaryn LM. Carpal tunnel syndrome: a comprehensive review. *Curr Opin Orthop* 1997;8:33–43.
2. Rempel D, Evanoff B, Amadio PC, et al. Consensus criteria for the classification of carpal tunnel syndrome in epidemiologic studies. *Am J Public Health* 1998;88:1447–1451.
3. Anonymous. Practice parameter for carpal tunnel syndrome (summary statement). Report of the Quality Standards Subcommittee of the American Academy of Neurology. *Neurology* 1993;43:2406–2409.
4. von Schroeder H, Botte MJ. Carpal tunnel syndrome. *Hand Clin* 1996;12:643–655.
5. Stevens JC, Sun S, Beard CM, et al. Carpal tunnel syndrome in Rochester, Minnesota, 1961 to 1980. *Neurology* 1988;38:134–138.
6. Dumitru D. *Textbook of Electrodiagnostic Medicine.* Hanley and Belfus, eds. Philadelphia: Mosby Publications, 1995.
7. Atroshi I, Gummesson C, Johnsson R, et al. Prevalence of carpal tunnel syndrome in a general population. *JAMA* 1999;282:153–158.
8. De Krom MCTF, Kester A, Knipschild P, et al. Risk factors for carpal tunnel syndrome. *Am J Epidemiol* 1990;132:1102–1110.
9. Fatami T, Kobayashi A, Utika T, et al. Carpal tunnel syndrome; its natural history. *Hand Surgery* 1997;2:129–130.
10. Padua L, Padua R, Aprile I, et al. Multiperspective follow-up of untreated carpal tunnel syndrome. A multicenter study. *Neurology* 2001;56:1459–1466.
11. Gerritsen AAM, de Krom MCTFM, Struijs MA, et al. Conservative treatment options for carpal tunnel syndrome: a systematic review of randomised controlled trials. *J Neurol* 2002;249:272–280. Search date 2000; primary sources Medline, Embase, Cochrane Controlled Trials Register, and hand searched references.
12. Herskovitz S, Berger AR, Lipton RB. Low-dose, short-term oral prednisone in the treatment of carpal tunnel syndrome. *Neurology* 1995;45:1923–1925.
13. Chang MH, Chiang HT, Lee SS, et al. Oral drug of choice in carpal tunnel syndrome. *Neurology* 1998;51:390–393.
14. Hiu ACF, Wong SM, Wong KS, et al. Oral steroid in the treatment of carpal tunnel syndrome. *Ann Rheum Dis* 2001;60:813–814.
15. Marshall S, Tardif G, Ashworth N. Local corticosteroid injection for carpal tunnel syndrome. In: Cochrane Library, Issue 4, 2002. Oxford: Update Software. Search date 2002; primary sources Cochrane Neuromuscular Disease Group Register, Medline, Embase, and Cinahl. No company sponsorship declared.
16. Wong SM, Hui ACF, Tang A, et al. Local vs systemic corticosteroids in the treatment of carpal tunnel syndrome. *Neurology* 2001;56:1565–1567.
17. Canadian Pharmacists Association. *Compendium of Pharmaceuticals and Specialties 2000.* Ottawa: Canadian Pharmacists Association, 2000.
18. Davis TP, Hulbert JR, Kassak KM, et al. Comparative efficacy of conservative medical and chiropractic treatments for carpal tunnel syndrome: a randomized clinical trial. *J Manipulative Physiol Ther* 1998;21:317–326.
19. Pal B, Mangion P, Hossain MA, et al. Should diuretics be prescribed for idiopathic carpal tunnel syndrome? Results of a controlled trial. *Clin Rehab* 1988;2:299–301.
20. Spooner GR, Desai HB, Angel JF, et al. Using pyridoxine to treat carpal tunnel syndrome. Randomized control trial. *Can Fam Physician* 1993;39:2122–2127.
21. Stransky M, Rubin A, Lava NS, et al. Treatment of carpal tunnel syndrome with vitamin B6: a double-blind study. *South Med J* 1989;82:841–842.
22. O'Gradaigh D, Merry P. Corticosteroid injection for the treatment of carpal tunnel syndrome. *Ann Rheum Dis* 2000;59:918–919.
23. Dammers JW, Veering MM, Vermeulen M, et al. Injection with methylprednisolone proximal to the carpal tunnel: randomized double blind trial. *BMJ* 1999;319:884–886.
24. Ozdogan H, Yazici H. The efficacy of local steroid injections in idiopathic carpal tunnel syndrome: a double-blind study. *Br J Rheumatol* 1984;23:272–275.
25. Babu SR, Britton JM. The role of steroid injection in the management of carpal tunnel syndrome. *J Orthop Rheumatol* 1994;7:59–60.
26. Manente G, Torrieri F, Di Blasio F, et al. An innovative hand brace for carpal tunnel syndrome: a randomised controlled trial. *Muscle Nerve* 2001;24:1020–1025.
27. Feuerstein M, Burrell LM, Miller VI, et al. Clinical management of carpal tunnel syndrome: a 12-year review of outcomes. *Am J Ind Med* 1999;35:232–245. Search date 1997; primary sources Medline, Cinahl, Psychlit, and Nioshtic. No company sponsorship declared.
28. Walker WC, Metzler M, Cifu DX, et al. Neutral wrist splinting in carpal tunnel syndrome: a comparison of night-only versus full-time wear instructions. *Arch Phys Med Rehabil* 2000;81:424–429.
29. Burke TD, Burke MM, Stewart GW, et al. Splinting for carpal tunnel syndrome: In search of the optimal angle. *Arch Phys Med Rehabil* 1994;75:1241–1244.
30. Akalin E, El O, Peker O, et al. Treatment of carpal tunnel syndrome with nerve and tendon gliding exercises. *Am J Phys Med Rehabil* 2002;81:108–113.
31. Oztas O, Turan B, Bora I, et al. Ultrasound therapy effect in carpal tunnel syndrome. *Arch Phys Med Rehabil* 1998;79:1540–1544.
32. Ebenbichler GR, Resch KL, Nicolakis P, et al. Ultrasound treatment for treating the carpal tunnel syndrome: randomised "sham" controlled trial. *BMJ* 1998;316:730–735.
33. Gerritsen AA, Uitdehaag BMJ, van Geldere D, et al. Systematic review of randomised clinical trials of surgical treatment for carpal tunnel syndrome. *Br J Surg* 2001;88:1285–1295. Search date 2000; primary sources Medline, Embase, the Cochrane Controlled Trials Register, reference lists of retrieved studies.
34. Verdugo RJ, Salinas RS, Castillo J, et al. Surgical versus non–surgical treatment for carpal tunnel syndrome. In: The Cochrane Library, Issue 3, 2002. Oxford: Update Software. Search date 2001; primary sources Medline, Embase, Lilacs, hand searched references, and contact with authors.

35. Jimenez DF, Gibbs SR, Clapper AT. Endoscopic treatment of carpal tunnel syndrome: a critical review [see comments]. *J Neurosurg* 1998;88:817–826. Search date 1997; primary sources not stated.
36. Ferdinand RD, MacLean JGB. Endoscopic versus open carpal tunnel release in bilateral carpal tunnel syndrome. A prospective, randomised, blinded assessment. *J Bone Joint Surg* 2002;84–B:375–379.
37. Mackenzie DJ, Hainer R, Wheatley MJ. Early recovery after endoscopic vs. short-incision open carpal tunnel release. *Ann Plastic Surg* 2000;44:601–604.
38. Hoefnagels WAJ, Van Kleef JGF, Mastenbroek GGA, et al. Surgical treatment of the carpal tunnel syndrome: Endoscopic or classical (open) surgery? A prospective randomised study. *Ned Tijdschr Geneeskd* 1997;141:878–882.
39. Benedetti RB, Sennwald G. Endoscopic decompression of the median nerve by the technique of Agee: A prospective study in comparison with the open decompression. *Handchir Mikrochir Plast Chir* 1996;28:151–155.
40. Stark B, Engkvist-Lofmark C. Carpal tunnel syndrome. Endoscopic release or conventional surgery. *Handchir Mikrochir Plast Chir* 1996;28:128–132.
41. Herren DB. Complications after endoscopic carpal tunnel decompression. *Z Unfallchir Versicherungsmed* 1994;87:120–127.
42. Brown RA, Gelberman RH, Seiler III, et al. Carpal tunnel release. A prospective, randomized assessment of open and endoscopic methods. *J Bone Joint Surg Am* 1993;75:1265–1275.
43. Erdmann MWH. Endoscopic carpal tunnel decompression. *J Hand Surg* 1994;19:5–13.
44. Agee JM, McCarroll J, Tortosa RD, et al. Endoscopic release of the carpal tunnel: a randomized prospective multicenter study. *J Hand Surg* 1992;17:987–995.
45. Mackinnon SE, McCabe S, Murray JF, et al. Internal neurolysis fails to improve the results of primary carpal tunnel decompression. *J Hand Surg Am* 1991;16:211–218.
46. Lowry WE Jr, Follender AB. Interfascicular neurolysis in the severe carpal tunnel syndrome. A prospective, randomized, double-blind, controlled study. *Clin Orthop* 1988;227:251–254.
47. Holmgren-Larsson H, Leszniewski W, Linden U et al. Internal neurolysis or ligament division only in carpal tunnel syndrome — results of a randomized study. *Acta Neurochir (Wien)* 1985;74:118–121.
48. Finsen V, Andersen K, Russwurm H. No advantage from splinting the wrist after open carpal tunnel release. A randomized study of 82 wrists. *Acta Orthop Scand* 1999;70:288–292.
49. Bury TF, Akelman E, Weiss AP. Prospective, randomized trial of splinting after carpal tunnel release. *Ann Plastic Surg* 1995;35:19–22.
50. Cook AC, Szabo RM, Birkholz SW, et al. Early mobilization following carpal tunnel release. A prospective randomized study. *J Hand Surg Br* 1995;20:228–230.
51. Rozmaryn LM, Dovelle S, Rothman ER, et al. Nerve and tendon gliding exercises and the conservative management of carpal tunnel syndrome. *J Hand Ther* 1998;11:171–179.

Shawn Marshall
Assistant Professor
University of Ottawa
Ottawa
Canada

Competing interests: None declared.

Chronic fatigue syndrome

Search date March 2003

Steven Reid, Trudie Chalder, Anthony Cleare, Matthew Hotopf, and Simon Wessely

QUESTIONS

INTERVENTIONS

Key Messages

- **Cognitive behavioural therapy** One systematic review found that cognitive behavioural therapy administered by highly skilled therapists in specialist centres improved quality of life and physical functioning compared with standard medical care or relaxation therapy. One additional multicentre RCT found that cognitive behavioural therapy administered by less experienced therapists may also be effective compared with guided support groups or no interventions.
- **Graded aerobic exercise** RCTs have found that a graded aerobic exercise programme improves measures of fatigue and physical functioning compared with flexibility and relaxation training or general advice. One RCT has found that an educational package to encourage graded exercise improved measures of physical functioning, fatigue, mood, and sleep at 1 year compared with written information alone.
- **Dietary supplements** One small RCT found no significant difference between a nutritional supplement (containing multivitamins, minerals, and coenzymes) and placebo in fatigue severity or functional impairment at 10 weeks.
- **Evening primrose oil** One small RCT found no significant difference between evening primrose oil and placebo in depression scores at 3 months.
- **Magnesium (intramuscular)** One small RCT found that intramuscular magnesium injections improved symptoms at 6 weeks compared with placebo. However, we were unable to draw reliable conclusions from this small study.
- **Antidepressants; corticosteroids; oral nicotinamide adenine dinucleotide** RCTs found insufficient evidence about the effects of these interventions in people with chronic fatigue syndrome.

- **Immunotherapy** Small RCTs found limited evidence that immunoglobulin G modestly improved physical functioning and fatigue at 3–6 months compared with placebo, but it was associated with considerable adverse effects. Small RCTs found insufficient evidence on the effects of interferon alfa or aciclovir compared with placebo. One RCT found that staphylococcus toxoid improved symptoms at six months compared with placebo, although it is associated with local reaction and could cause anaphylaxis.
- **Prolonged rest** We found no RCTs on the effects of prolonged rest. Indirect observational evidence in healthy volunteers and in people recovering from a viral illness suggests that prolonged rest may perpetuate or worsen fatigue and symptoms.

DEFINITION Chronic fatigue syndrome (CFS) is characterised by severe, disabling fatigue and other symptoms, including musculoskeletal pain, sleep disturbance, impaired concentration, and headaches. Two widely used definitions of CFS, from the US Centers for Disease Control and Prevention[1] and from Oxford, UK,[2] were developed as operational criteria for research (see table 1, p 1303). There are important differences between these definitions. The UK criteria insist upon the presence of mental fatigue, whereas the US criteria include a requirement for several physical symptoms, reflecting the belief that CFS has an underlying immunological or infective pathology.

INCIDENCE/ PREVALENCE Community and primary care based studies have reported the prevalence of CFS to be 0–3%, depending on the criteria used.[3,4] Systematic population surveys have found similar prevalences of CFS in people of different socioeconomic status and in all ethnic groups.[4,5]

AETIOLOGY/ RISK FACTORS The cause of CFS is poorly understood. Women are at higher risk than men (RR 1.3–1.7 depending on diagnostic criteria used).[6]

PROGNOSIS Studies have focused on people attending specialist clinics. A systematic review of studies of prognosis (search date 1996) found that children with CFS had better outcomes than adults: 54–94% of children showed definite improvement (after up to 6 years' follow up), whereas 20–50% of adults showed some improvement in the medium term and only 6% returned to premorbid levels of functioning.[7] Despite the considerable burden of morbidity associated with CFS, we found no evidence of increased mortality. The systematic review found that outcome was influenced by the presence of psychiatric disorders (depression and anxiety) and beliefs about causation and treatment.[7]

AIMS OF INTERVENTION To reduce levels of fatigue and associated symptoms, to increase levels of activity, and to improve quality of life.

OUTCOMES Severity of symptoms and their effects on physical function and quality of life. These outcomes are measured in several different ways: the medical outcomes survey short form general health survey (SF-36),[8] a rating scale measuring limitation of physical functioning caused by ill health (score range 0–100, where 0 = limited in all activities and 100 = able to carry out vigorous activities); the Karnofsky scale,[9] a modified questionnaire originally developed for the rating of quality of life in people undergoing chemotherapy for malignancy; the Beck Depression Inventory,[10] a checklist for quantifying depressive symptoms; the sickness impact profile,[11] a measure of the influence of symptoms on social and physical functioning; the Chalder fatigue scale,[12] a rating scale measuring subjective fatigue (score range 0–11, where scores ≥ 4 = excessive fatigue); the clinical global impression scale,[13] a validated measure of overall change compared with baseline at study onset, with seven possible scores from "very much worse" (score 7) to "very much better" (score 1); the checklist individual strength fatigue subscale (score range 8 (no fatigue at all) to 56 (maximally fatigued)[14]; and self reported severity of symptoms and levels of activity, the Nottingham health profile[15] contains questions in six categories: energy, pain perception, sleep patterns, sense of social isolation, emotional reactions, and physical mobility (weighted scores give maximum 100 for answer yes to all questions, and minimum 0 for someone with no complaints).

METHODS *Clinical Evidence* search and appraisal March 2003.

QUESTION **What are the effects of treatments?**

OPTION **ANTIDEPRESSANTS**

RCTs found insufficient evidence about the effects of antidepressants in people with chronic fatigue syndrome.

Benefits: We found one systematic review (search date 2000), which did not report quantified results.[16] **Fluoxetine:** The review identified two RCTs.[17,18] The first RCT (107 depressed and non-depressed people with chronic fatigue syndrome [CFS]) compared fluoxetine versus placebo for 8 weeks.[17] It found that fluoxetine significantly improved the Beck Depression Inventory compared with placebo (mean difference between fluoxetine and placebo in improvement in Beck Depression Inventory –0.19, 95% CI –0.35 to –0.02), but the difference may not be clinically important. It found no significant difference between fluoxetine and placebo in the sickness impact profile (mean difference between fluoxetine and placebo measured by fatigue subscale of Checklist Individual Strength –0.16, 95% CI –0.64 to +0.31).[19] The second RCT (136 people with CFS) compared four groups: fluoxetine plus graded exercise; drug placebo plus graded exercise; fluoxetine plus general advice to exercise; and drug placebo plus general advice to exercise. It found no significant difference in the level of fatigue, although modest improvements in measures of depression were seen at 12 weeks (Hospital Anxiety and Depression scale, mean change 1.1, 95% CI 0.03 to 2.2).[18,20] **Phenelzine:** The review identified one RCT.[16,21] The RCT (30 people with CFS) compared phenelzine versus placebo, using a modified Karnofsky scale and other outcome measures (including functional status questionnaire, profile of mood states, Centres for Epidemiological Study of Depression fatigue severity scale, and symptom severity checklist).[20] This study concluded that there was a pattern of improvement across several measures (significance tests for individual measures not carried out). **Moclobemide:** The review identified one RCT but did not report quantified results.[16,22] The RCT (90 people with CFS) compared moclobemide (450–600 mg daily) versus placebo.[22] It found that moclobemide was associated with a non-significant increase in subjectively reported global improvement (moclobemide 24/47 [51%] v placebo 14/43 [33%]; OR 2.16, 95% CI 0.9 to 5.1), and a non-significant improvement in the clinician rated Karnofsky scale. **Sertraline versus clomipramine:** We found one RCT comparing sertraline versus clomipramine in people with CFS.[23] It found no significant difference between sertraline and clomipramine. There was no placebo group, which makes it difficult to draw useful conclusions.

Harms: **Fluoxetine:** One RCT assessed separately the symptoms (which could be attributed to either CFS or to known adverse effects of fluoxetine) before starting treatment, after 2 weeks, after 6 weeks, and at the end of treatment (week 8). It found that fluoxetine increased complaints of tremor and perspiration compared with placebo at 8 weeks (tremor: $P = 0.006$; perspiration: $P = 0.008$).[16] It found no significant difference between fluoxetine and placebo at 2 and 6 weeks. It found that fluoxetine increased withdrawal due to adverse effects (9/54 [17%] v 2/53 [4%]).[17] The second RCT also found increased withdrawal rates with fluoxetine (24/68 people [36%] with fluoxetine withdrew v 16/69 people [24%] with placebo).[18] **Phenelzine:** Three of 15 people (20%) who took phenelzine withdrew because of adverse effects compared with none who took placebo.[21] **Sertraline versus clomipramine:** The RCT provided no information on adverse effects.[23]

Comment: Clinical trials were performed in specialist clinics. **Fluoxetine:** The first RCT[17] used a shorter duration of treatment and studied people with a longer duration of illness compared with the second RCT.[18]

OPTION CORTICOSTEROIDS

Four RCTs found insufficient evidence about the effects of corticosteroids compared with placebo in people with chronic fatigue syndrome.

Benefits: We found one systematic review (search date 2000), which did not report quantified results.[16] **Fludrocortisone:** The systematic review[16] identified two RCTs.[24,25] The first large RCT (100 people with chronic fatigue syndrome [CFS] and neurally mediated hypotension) compared fludrocortisone (titrated to 0.1 mg daily) versus placebo for 9 weeks. It found no significant difference on a self rated global scale of "wellness" (recorded improvement of ≥ 15 points: fludrocortisone 14% v placebo 10%; $P = 0.76$; raw data not provided).[24] The second randomised crossover trial (20 people), which measured change in symptom severity (visual analogue scale of symptoms from 0–10 corresponding to "no problem" to "could not be worse") and functional status (using the SF-36) for 6 weeks. It found no significant difference between fludrocortisone and placebo.[25] **Hydrocortisone:** The review identified two RCTs.[16,26,27] The first RCT (65 people) compared hydrocortisone (25–35 mg daily) versus placebo for 12 weeks. It found that hydrocortisone significantly improved a self rated scale of "wellness" (recorded improvement of ≥ 5 points: hydrocortisone 53% v placebo 29%; $P = 0.04$). Other self rating scales did not show significant benefit (Beck Depression Inventory: hydrocortisone –2.1 v placebo –0.4,

P = 0.17; activity scale: hydrocortisone 0.3 *v* placebo 0.7, P = 0.32; sickness impact profile: hydrocortisone –2.5 *v* placebo –2.2; P = 0.85).[26] The second RCT (32 people, crossover design) compared a lower dose of hydrocortisone (5 or 10 mg daily) versus placebo for 1 month. It found that hydrocortisone improved fatigue in the short term compared with placebo (self report fatigue scale: hydrocortisone 28% *v* placebo 9%; results before crossover not provided).[27]

Harms: **Fludrocortisone:** In the first RCT, fludrocortisone increased withdrawal rates due to adverse events compared with placebo (12/50 [24%] *v* 4/50 [8%]; RR 3, 95% CI 1.04 to 8.67; NNT 6, 95% CI 3 to 8).[24] Four people withdrew from the trial because of worsening symptoms.[25] **Hydrocortisone:** One RCT (25–35 mg daily doses of hydrocortisone) found that 12 people (40%) experienced adrenal suppression (assessed by measuring cortisol levels).[26] Another RCT (5 or 10 mg daily doses of hydrocortisone) reported minor adverse effects in up to 10% of participants. Three people on hydrocortisone had exacerbation of acne and nervousness, and one person on placebo had an episode of fainting.[27]

Comment: The RCTs used different reasons for their choice of active treatment. The use of fludrocortisone, a mineralocorticoid, was based on the hypothesis that CFS is associated with neurally mediated hypotension.[28] The use of hydrocortisone, a glucocorticoid, in the other RCTs was based on evidence of underactivity of the hypothalamic–pituitary–adrenocortical axis in some people with CFS.[29] Any benefit from low dose glucocorticoids seems to be short lived, and higher doses are associated with adverse effects.

OPTION ORAL NICOTINAMIDE ADENINE DINUCLEOTIDE

One small RCT found insufficient evidence about the effects of oral nicotinamide adenine dinucleotide compared with placebo in people with chronic fatigue syndrome.

Benefits: We found one systematic review (search date 2000), which did not report quantified results.[16] It identified one poor quality randomised crossover trial (35 people), which compared nicotinamide adenine dinucleotide (10 mg daily) with placebo for 4 weeks.[30] Of the 35 people, two were excluded for non-compliance and seven were excluded for using psychotropic drugs. It found that nicotinamide adenine dinucleotide significantly improved scores on a self devised 50 item symptom rating scale compared with placebo (8/26 people [30%] attained a 10% improvement with nicotinamide adenine dinucleotide *v* 2/26 people [8%] with placebo; P < 0.05, calculated by authors).

Harms: Minor adverse effects (loss of appetite, dyspepsia and flatulence) were reported on active treatment but did not lead to cessation of treatment.[30]

Comment: The RCT had a number of problems with its methods, including the use of inappropriate statistical analyses, the inappropriate exclusion of people from the analysis, and lack of numerical data preventing independent analysis of the published results.[31]

OPTION EXERCISE

RCTs have found that a graded aerobic exercise programme improves measures of fatigue and physical functioning compared with flexibility training and relaxation training or general advice. One RCT found that an educational package to encourage graded exercise improved measures of physical functioning, fatigue, mood, and sleep at 1 year compared with written information alone.

Benefits: We found one systematic review (search date 2000), which did not report quantified results.[16] **Graded aerobic exercise:** The review identified two RCTs.[18,32] One RCT (66 people) compared graded aerobic exercise (active intervention) versus flexibility and relaxation training (control intervention) over 12 weeks.[32] All participants undertook individual weekly sessions supervised by an exercise physiologist. The aerobic exercise group built up their level of activity to 30 minutes of exercise a day (walking, cycling, swimming up to a maximum oxygen consumption of 60% of V_{O_2}max). People in the flexibility and relaxation training group were taught stretching and relaxation techniques (maximum 30 minutes daily, 5 days/week) and were specifically told to avoid any extra physical activities. It found that Aerobic exercise increased reports of feeling "better" or "very much better" and improved physical fatigue and physical functioning compared with control (clinical global impression scale: 52% *v* 27%, P = 0.04; Chalder fatigue scale: –8.4 *v* –3.1, P = 0.004; SF-36 scale: 20.5 *v* 8.0, P = 0.01). The second RCT (136 people) compared four groups (graded aerobic exercise plus fluoxetine; graded aerobic exercise plus drug placebo; general advice plus fluoxetine; general advice plus drug placebo) over 24 weeks.[18] The graded exercise groups were given specific advice to undertake preferred aerobic exercise (such as walking, jogging, swimming, or cycling) for 20 minutes three times a week up to an energy expenditure of 75% of V_{O_2}max. The general advice (exercise placebo) groups were not given any specific advice on frequency, intensity, or duration of aerobic activity they should be undertaking. It found that Graded exercise reduced fatigue at 26 weeks compared with general advice (Chalder fatigue scale < 4: 12/67 [18%] *v* 4/69 [6%]; RR 3.1, 95% CI 1.05 to 9.10; NNT 9, 95% CI 5 to 91). **Educational intervention:** The review[16] identified one RCT (148 people).[33] The RCT compared three types of educational interventions to encourage graded exercise with written information only (control group).[33] The participants in the three educational intervention groups received two treatment sessions, two telephone follow ups, and an educational package that provided an explanation of symptoms and encouraged home based exercise. One group received seven additional follow up telephone calls and another received seven additional face to face sessions over 4 months. People in the written information group received advice and an information booklet that encouraged graded activity but gave no explanation for the symptoms. The RCT found that the educational interventions improved physical functioning, fatigue, mood, sleep, and disability (self reported) compared with written information only. The RCT found no significant difference between the educational interventions (mean for 3 educational intervention groups *v* written information, SF-36 subscale: ≥ 25 or an increase of ≥ 10, 1 year after randomisation, 69% *v* 6%, $P < 0.001$; Chalder fatigue scale: 3 *v* 10, $P < 0.001$; Hospital Anxiety and Depression scale: depression 4 *v* 10, $P < 0.001$; anxiety 7 *v* 10, $P < 0.01$).

Harms: None of the RCTs reported data on adverse effects, and we found no evidence that exercise is harmful in people with chronic fatigue syndrome. The second aerobic exercise RCT found no significant difference in withdrawal rates between exercise and no exercise (25/68 [37%] with exercise *v* 15/69 [22%] without exercise; RR 1.7, 95% CI 0.98 to 2.9).[18] The reasons for the withdrawals from the graded exercise groups were not stated.

Comment: Experience suggests that symptoms of chronic fatigue syndrome may be exacerbated by overly ambitious or overly hasty attempts at exercise.

OPTION PROLONGED REST

We found no RCTs on the effects of prolonged rest. Indirect observational evidence in healthy volunteers and in people recovering from a viral illness suggests that prolonged rest may perpetuate or worsen fatigue and symptoms.

Benefits: We found no systematic review or RCTs of prolonged rest in people with chronic fatigue syndrome.

Harms: We found no direct evidence of harmful effects of rest in people with chronic fatigue syndrome. We found observational evidence, which suggested that prolonged inactivity may perpetuate or worsen fatigue and is associated with symptoms in both healthy volunteers[34] and people recovering from viral illness.[35]

Comment: It is not clear that evidence from people recovering from viral illness can be extrapolated to people with chronic fatigue syndrome.

OPTION DIETARY SUPPLEMENTS New

One small RCT found no significant difference between a nutritional supplement (containing multivitamins, minerals, and coenzymes) and placebo in fatigue severity or functional impairment at 10 weeks.

Benefits: We found one RCT (53 people who fulfilled US Centers for Disease Control and Prevention criteria for chronic fatigue syndrome with high fatigue severity and high disability scores; duration of illness ranged from 2 to 12 years) that compared a polynutrient supplement (containing several vitamins, minerals and coenzymes, taken twice daily) versus placebo for 10 weeks.[36] It found no significant difference between treatment in fatigue severity or functional impairment (change in Checklist Individual Strength fatigue subscale from baseline to 10 weeks: 51.4 to 48.6 with supplements *v* 51.3 to 48.2 with placebo; difference 2.16, 95% CI −4.30 to +4.39; Sickness Impact Scale < 750 at 10 weeks: 4% with supplements *v* 12% with placebo).

Harms: Three people (11%) on active treatment withdrew because of nausea.[36]

Comment: The RCT may have been too small to detect a clinically important difference.[36]

OPTION MAGNESIUM

One small RCT found that intramuscular magnesium injections improved symptoms at 6 weeks compared with placebo. However, we were unable to draw reliable conclusions from this small study.

Benefits: We found one systematic review (search date 2000), which did not report quantified results.[16] The review identified one RCT (32 people with chronic fatigue syndrome, but not magnesium deficiency; see comment), which compared weekly intramuscular injections of magnesium sulphate 50% versus placebo (water for injection) for 6 weeks.[37] It found that magnesium improved overall benefit, energy, pain, and emotional reactions compared with placebo (overall benefit: 12/15 [80%] *v* 3/17 [18%]; RR 4.5, 95% CI 1.6 to 13.1; NNT 2, 95% CI 2 to 4; energy $P = 0.002$; pain: $P = 0.001$; and emotional reactions: $P = 0.013$).

Harms: The RCT reported no adverse effects.

Comment: In the RCT, plasma and whole blood magnesium were normal and only the red blood cell concentrations of magnesium were slightly lower than the normal range.[37] Three subsequent case control studies have not found a deficiency of magnesium in people with chronic fatigue syndrome.[38–40] In these three studies, magnesium was in the normal range and no different from controls without chronic fatigue syndrome. However, none of the studies state how the normal range was established, so it is difficult to say if they are equivalent.

OPTION EVENING PRIMROSE OIL

One small RCT found no significant difference between evening primrose oil and placebo in depression scores at 3 months.

Benefits: We found one systematic review (search date 2000), which did not report quantified results.[16] The review identified one RCT (50 people with chronic fatigue syndrome according to Oxford, UK, diagnostic criteria), which compared evening primrose oil (4 g daily) with placebo for 3 months.[41] It found no significant difference between treatments in depression scores (Beck Depression Inventory), physical symptoms, or participant assessment (at 3 months 46% were improved with placebo *v* 29% with evening primrose oil; $P = 0.09$; figures were not presented in a manner that allowed RR with CI to be calculated).

Harms: The RCT reported no adverse effects.

Comment: One RCT (63 people) compared evening primrose oil (4 g daily) versus placebo in people with a diagnosis of postviral fatigue syndrome.[42] This diagnosis was made on the basis of overwhelming fatigue, myalgia, and depression, which had been present for at least 1 year, and all had been preceded by a febrile illness. At 3 months, 33/39 (85%) of the people on active treatment had improved compared with 4/24 (17%) on placebo — a significant benefit ($P < 0.0001$). The difference in outcome may be partly explained by participant selection: the study in people with chronic fatigue syndrome used currently accepted diagnostic criteria.[41] Also, whereas the RCT in people with postviral fatigue syndrome used liquid paraffin as a placebo,[42] the chronic fatigue syndrome RCT used sunflower oil, which is better tolerated and less likely to affect the placebo response adversely.[41]

OPTION IMMUNOTHERAPY

Small RCTs found limited evidence that immunoglobulin G modestly improved physical functioning and fatigue at 3–6 months compared with placebo, but it was associated with considerable adverse effects. Small RCTs found insufficient evidence on the effects of interferon alfa or aciclovir compared with placebo. One RCT found that staphylococcus toxoid improved symptoms at six months compared with placebo, although it is associated with local reaction and could cause anaphylaxis.

Benefits: We found one systematic review (search date 2000), which did not report quantified results.[16] **Immunoglobulin G:** The review identified four relevant RCTs comparing immunoglobulin G versus placebo for 6 months.[43–46] The first RCT (30 people) compared monthly intravenous injections of immunoglobulin G (1 g/kg) versus placebo (albumin).[43] After 6 months, no large differences were found in measures of fatigue (self reported symptom severity) or in physical and social functioning (SF-36). It found that placebo significantly improved social function compared with immunoglobulin G (dichotomous figures not reported). The second RCT (49 people) compared monthly intravenous immunoglobulin G (2 g/kg) with intravenous placebo (a maltose solution) for 3 months.[44] It found that immunoglobulin G significantly increased the proportion of people who improved in terms of a physician rated assessment of symptoms and disability compared with placebo (10/23 [44%] *v* 3/26 [11%]; $P = 0.03$). The third RCT (99 adults) compared three doses of immunoglobulin G (0.5, 1, or 2 g/kg) versus placebo (albumin).[45] It found no significant difference in quality of life, scores on visual analogue scales, or changes in hours spent in non-sedentary activities. The fourth RCT (71 adolescents aged 11–18 years) compared immunoglobulin G (1 g/kg) with placebo (a solution of maltose plus albumin).[46] Three infusions were given 1 month apart. The RCT found that immunoglobulin G significantly improved mean functional outcome (assessed using the mean of clinician ratings from four areas of the participants' activities) compared with placebo (proportion of people who achieved improvement of ≥ 25% at 6 months: 26/36 [52%] with immunoglobin *v* 15/34 [31%] with placebo, RR 1.6, 95% CI 1.1 to 2.5). However, both groups showed significant improvements from baseline, which continued to the 6 month assessment after treatment. **Other treatments:** We found one systematic review (search date 2000)[16] and one subsequent RCT.[47] The review identified two RCTs (30 people) comparing interferon alfa with placebo.[48,49] The first RCT identified by the review only found treatment benefit on subgroup analysis of people with isolated natural killer cell dysfunction.[48] The second randomised crossover trial identified by the review did not present results in a manner that allowed clear interpretation of treatment effect.[49] Other RCTs in the review found no significant difference between placebo and aciclovir,[50] dialysable leucocyte extract (in a factorial design with cognitive behavioural therapy),[51] or terfenadine.[52] The subsequent RCT (100 women who met both the ACS criteria for fibromyalgia and the US Centers for Disease Control and Prevention criteria for chronic fatigue syndrome and had functional impairment > 6 months) compared weekly subcutaneous injections of staphylococcus toxoid (dose increased weekly from 0.1 to 1.0 mL, followed by 1.0 mL doses every 4 weeks) versus placebo.[47] It found that staphylococcus toxoid significantly improved the clinical global impression of change scale at 26 weeks compared with placebo (minimally improved, much improved or very much improved: 32/49 [65%] with toxoid *v* 9/49 [18%] with placebo; $P < 0.001$).

Harms: **Immunoglobulin G:** In the first RCT, adverse effects judged to be worse than pretreatment symptoms in either group included gastrointestinal complaints (18 people), headaches (23 people), arthralgia (6 people), and worsening fatigue. Of these symptoms, only headaches differed significantly between the groups (immunoglobulin G 14/15 [93%] *v* placebo 9/15 [60%]). Six participants (3 immunoglobulin G, 3 placebo) were considered to have major adverse effects. Adverse events by treatment group were only reported for headache.[43] **Other treatments:** In the RCT comparing interferon alfa 2/13 (15%) people taking active treatment developed neutropenia.[48] The RCT comparing staphylococcus toxoid with placebo found no significant difference in reported adverse effects, excluding local reactions (13/49[26%] with toxoid *v* 7/49 [14% with placebo, $P = 0.14$).[47] All those receiving the toxoid had a local reaction at the injection site.

Comment: **Immunoglobulin G:** The first two RCTs differed in that the second used twice the dose of immunoglobulin G, did not require participants to fulfil the operational criteria (similar but not identical to US Centers for Disease Control and Prevention criteria) for chronic fatigue syndrome, and made no assessments of them during the study, instead waiting until 3 months after completion.[44] **Other treatments:** Terfenadine, particularly at high blood concentrations, is associated with rare hazardous cardiac arrhythmias.[53] The RCT that compared staphylococcus toxoid with placebo only included women who also had a diagnosis of fibromyalgia.[47]

OPTION COGNITIVE BEHAVIOURAL THERAPY

One systematic review found that cognitive behavioural therapy administered by highly skilled therapists in specialist centres improved quality of life and physical functioning compared with standard medical care or relaxation therapy. One additional multicentre RCT found that cognitive behavioural therapy administered by less experienced therapists may also be effective compared with guided support groups or no interventions.

Benefits: We found two systematic reviews (search dates 1998[54] and 2000[16]). The first review[54] identified three RCTs that met the reviewers' inclusion criteria (all participants fulfilled accepted diagnostic criteria for chronic fatigue syndrome [CFS] and the trials used adequate randomisation and controls).[51,55,56] The second review identified one additional RCT that met inclusion criteria, but the review did not report quantified results.[17,57] The first RCT (90 people with CFS according to Australian diagnostic criteria that are similar to US Centers for Disease Control and Prevention [CDC] criteria) identified by the reviews evaluated cognitive behavioural therapy (CBT) and immunological therapy (dialysable leucocyte extract) using a factorial design.[51] Cognitive behavioural therapy was given every 2 weeks for six sessions of 30–60 minutes each, and people were encouraged to exercise at home and feel less helpless. The comparison group received standard medical care. The trial found no significant difference in quality of life measures (Karnofsky scale and symptom report on a visual analogue scale) between CBT and standard medical care. The second RCT (60 people with CFS according to Oxford, UK, diagnostic criteria) identified by the reviews compared CBT with normal general practice care in people attending a secondary care centre.[56] It found that CBT significantly improved quality of life (Karnofsky scale) at 12 months compared with those receiving standard medical care (final score > 80: 22/30 [73%] with CBT *v* 8/30 [27%] with placebo; RR 2.75, 95% CI 1.54 to 5.32; NNT 3, 95% CI 2 to 5). The active treatment consisted of a cognitive behavioural assessment, followed by 16 weekly sessions of behavioural experiments, problem solving activity, and re-evaluation of thoughts and beliefs that inhibited a return to normal functioning. The third RCT (60 people with CFS according to CDC diagnostic criteria in people attending a secondary care centre) identified by the reviews compared CBT with relaxation therapy.[55] It found that CBT significantly improvement physical functioning compared with relaxation therapy (improvement based on predefined absolute or relative increases in the SF-36 score: 19/30 [63%] with CBT *v* 5/30 [17%] with relaxation; RR 3.7, 95% CI 2.37 to 6.31; NNT 3, 95% CI 1 to 7). Improvement continued over 6–12 months' follow up. Cognitive behavioural therapy was given in 13 weekly sessions. A 5 year follow up study of 53 (88%) of the original participants found that more people rated themselves as "much improved" or "very much improved" with CBT compared with relaxation therapy (17/25 [68%] with CBT *v* 10/28 [36%] with relaxation therapy; RR 1.9, 95% CI 1.1 to 3.4; NNT 4, 95% CI 2 to 19).[58] More people treated with CBT met the authors' criteria for complete recovery at 5 years, but the difference was not significant (17/31 [55%] with CBT *v* 7/22 [32%] with relaxation therapy; RR 1.7, 95% CI 0.9 to 3.4). The additional multicentre RCT identified by the second review (278 people with CFS according to CDC criteria) compared CBT, guided support groups, or no intervention.[57] The CBT consisted of 16 sessions over 8 months administered by 13 therapists with no previous experience of treating CFS. The guided support groups were similar to CBT in terms of treatment schedule, with the participants receiving non-directive support from a social worker. At 8 months' follow up, the RCT found that more people in the CBT group met the criteria for clinical improvement for fatigue severity (checklist individual strength) and self reported improvement in fatigue compared with the guided support and no treatment groups (fatigue severity: CBT *v* support group, 27/83 [33%] *v* 10/80 [13%], RR 2.6, 95% CI 1.3 to 5.0; CBT *v* no intervention 27/83 [33%] *v* 8/62 [13%], RR 2.5, 95% CI 1.2 to 5.2; self reported improvement: CBT *v* support group 42/74 [57%] *v* 12/71 [17%], RR 3.4, 95% CI 1.9 to 5.8; CBT *v* no intervention 42/74 [57%] *v* 23/78 [30%], RR 1.9, 95% CI 1.3 to 2.9). The results were not corrected for multiple comparisons.

Harms: No harmful effects were reported.

Comment: The effectiveness of CBT for CFS outside of specialist settings has been questioned. The results of the multicentre RCT suggest that cognitive behavioural therapy may be effective when administered by less experienced therapists with adequate supervision. The trial had a high withdrawal rate (25% after 8 months), especially in the CBT and guided support groups. Although the presented confidence intervals are not adjusted for multiple comparisons, the results would remain significant after any reasonable adjustment. The authors commented that the results were similar after intention to treat analysis, but these results were not presented.[57] A randomised trial that comparing CBT and non-directive counselling found that both interventions were of benefit in the management of people who consulted their family doctor because of fatigue symptoms.[59] In this study, 28% of the sample conformed to CDC criteria for CFS.

Substantive changes

Immunotherapy One RCT added;[47] conclusions unchanged.

REFERENCES

1. Fukuda K, Straus S, Hickie I, et al. The chronic fatigue syndrome: a comprehensive approach to its definition and study. *Ann Intern Med* 1994;121:953–959.
2. Sharpe M, Archard LC, Banatvala JE. A report — chronic fatigue syndrome: guidelines for research. *J R Soc Med* 1991;84:118–121.
3. Wessely S, Chalder T, Hirsch S, et al. The prevalence and morbidity of chronic fatigue and chronic fatigue syndrome: a prospective primary care study. *Am J Public Health* 1997;87:1449–1455.
4. Steele L, Dobbins JG, Fukuda K, et al. The epidemiology of chronic fatigue in San Francisco. *Am J Med* 1998;105(suppl 3A):83–90.
5. Lawrie SM, Pelosi AJ. Chronic fatigue syndrome in the community: prevalence and associations. *Br J Psychiatry* 1995;166:793–797.
6. Wessely S. The epidemiology of chronic fatigue syndrome. *Epidemiol Rev* 1995;17:139–151.
7. Joyce J, Hotopf M, Wessely S. The prognosis of chronic fatigue and chronic fatigue syndrome: a systematic review. *QJM* 1997;90:223–233. Search date 1996; primary sources Medline, Embase, Current Contents, and Psychlit.
8. Stewart AD, Hays RD, Ware JE. The MOS short-form general health survey. *Med Care* 1988;26:724–732.
9. Karnofsky DA, Burchenal JH, MacLeod CM. *The clinical evaluation of chemotherapeutic agents in cancer.* New York: Columbia University Press; 1949:191–206.
10. Beck AT, Ward CH, Mendelson M, et al. An inventory for measuring depression. *Arch Gen Psychiatry* 1961;4:561–571.
11. Bergner M, Bobbit RA, Carter WB, et al. The sickness impact profile: development and final revision of a health status measure. *Med Care* 1981;19:787–805.
12. Chalder T, Berelowitz C, Pawlikowska T. Development of a fatigue scale. *J Psychosom Res* 1993;37:147–154.
13. Guy W. *ECDEU assessment manual for psychopharmacology*. Rockville: National Institute of Mental Health, 1976:218–222.
14. Vercoulen JH, Swanink CM, Fennis JF, et al. Dimensional assessment of chronic fatigue syndrome. *J Psychosom Res* 1994;38:383–392.
15. Hunt SM, McEwen J, McKenna SP. Measuring health status: a new tool for clinicians and epidemiologists. *J Roy Coll Gen Prac* 1985,35:185–188.
16. Whiting P, Bagnall A-M, Sowden A, et al. Interventions for the treatment and management of chronic fatigue syndrome: A systematic review. *JAMA* 2001;286:1360–1368. Search date 2000; primary sources Medline, Embase, Psychlit, ERIC, Current Contents, Internet searches, bibliographies from the retrieved references, individuals and organisations through a website dedicated to the review, and members of advisory panels.

17. Vercoulen J, Swanink C, Zitman F. Randomised, double-blind, placebo-controlled study of fluoxetine in chronic fatigue syndrome. *Lancet* 1996;347:858–861.
18. Wearden AJ, Morriss RK, Mullis R, et al. Randomised, double-blind, placebo controlled treatment trial of fluoxetine and a graded exercise programme for chronic fatigue syndrome. *Br J Psychiatry* 1998;172:485–490.
19. Vercoulen JHMM, Swanink CMA, Galama JMD, et al. Dimensional assessment of chronic fatigue syndrome. *J Psychosom Res* 1994;38:383–392.
20. Zigmond AS, Snaith RP. The Hospital Anxiety and Depression Scale (HAD). *Acta Psychiatr Scand* 1983;67:361–370.
21. Natelson BH, Cheu J, Pareja J, et al. Randomised, double blind, controlled placebo-phase in trial of low dose phenelzine in the chronic fatigue syndrome. *Psychopharmacology* 1996;124:226–230.
22. Hickie IB, Wilson AJ, Murray Wright J, et al. A randomized, double-blind, placebo-controlled trial of moclobemide in patients with chronic fatigue syndrome. *J Clin Psychiatry* 2000;61:643–648.
23. Behan PO, Hannifah H. 5-HT reuptake inhibitors in CFS. *J Immunol Immunopharmacol* 1995;15:66–69.
24. Rowe PC, Calkins H, DeBusk K, et al. Fludrocortisone acetate to treat neurally mediated hypotension in chronic fatigue syndrome. *JAMA* 2001;285:52–59.
25. Peterson PK, Pheley A, Schroeppel J, et al. A preliminary placebo-controlled crossover trial of fludrocortisone for chronic fatigue syndrome. *Arch Intern Med* 1998;158:908–914.
26. McKenzie R, O'Fallon A, Dale J, et al. Low-dose hydrocortisone for treatment of chronic fatigue syndrome. *JAMA* 1998;280:1061–1066.
27. Cleare AJ, Heap E, Malhi G, et al. Low-dose hydrocortisone in chronic fatigue syndrome: a randomised crossover trial. *Lancet* 1999;353:455–458.
28. Bou-Holaigah I, Rowe P, Kan J, et al. The relationship between neurally mediated hypotension and the chronic fatigue syndrome. *JAMA* 1995;274:961–967.
29. Demitrack M, Dale J, Straus S, et al. Evidence for impaired activation of the hypothalamic-pituitary-adrenal axis in patients with chronic fatigue syndrome. *J Clin Endocrinol Metab* 1991;73:1224–1234.
30. Forsyth LM, Preuss HG, MacDowell AL, et al. Therapeutic effects of oral NADH on the symptoms of patients with chronic fatigue syndrome. *Ann Allergy Asthma Immunol* 1999;82:185–191.
31. Colquhoun D, Senn S. Re: Therapeutic effects of oral NADH on the symptoms of patients with chronic fatigue syndrome. *Ann Allergy Asthma Immunol* 2000;84:639–640.
32. Fulcher KY, White PD. A randomised controlled trial of graded exercise therapy in patients with the chronic fatigue syndrome. *BMJ* 1997;314:1647–1652.
33. Powell P, Bentall RP, Nye FJ, et al. Randomised controlled trial of patient education to encourage graded exercise in chronic fatigue syndrome. *BMJ* 2001;322:387–390.
34. Sandler H, Vernikos J. *Inactivity: physiological effects.* London: Academic Press, 1986.
35. Dalrymple W. Infectious mononucleosis: 2. Relation of bed rest and activity to prognosis. *Postgrad Med* 1961;35:345–349.
36. Brouwers FM, van der Werf S, Bleijenberg G, et al. The effect of a polynutrient supplement on fatigue and physical activity of patients with chronic fatigue syndrome: a double-blind randomized controlled trial. *QJM* 2002;95:677–683.
37. Cox IM, Campbell MJ, Dowson D. Red blood cell magnesium and chronic fatigue syndrome. *Lancet* 1991;337:757–760.
38. Clague JE, Edwards RHT, Jackson MJ. Intravenous magnesium loading in chronic fatigue syndrome. *Lancet* 1992;340:124–125.
39. Hinds G, Bell NP, McMaster D, et al. Normal red cell magnesium concentrations and magnesium loading tests in patients with chronic fatigue syndrome. *Ann Clin Biochem* 1994;31:459–461.
40. Swanink CM, Vercoulen JH, Bleijenberg G, et al. Chronic fatigue syndrome: a clinical and laboratory study with a well matched control group. *J Intern Med* 1995;237:499–506.
41. Warren G, McKendrick M, Peet M. The role of essential fatty acids in chronic fatigue syndrome. *Acta Neurol Scand* 1999;99:112–116.
42. Behan PO, Behan WMH, Horrobin D. Effect of high doses of essential fatty acids on the postviral fatigue syndrome. *Acta Neurol Scand* 1990;82:209–216.
43. Peterson PK, Shepard J, Macres M, et al. A controlled trial of intravenous immunoglobulin G in chronic fatigue syndrome. *Am J Med* 1990;89:554–560.
44. Lloyd A, Hickie I, Wakefield D, et al. A double-blind, placebo-controlled trial of intravenous immunoglobulin therapy in patients with chronic fatigue syndrome. *Am J Med* 1990;89:561–568.
45. Vollmer-Conna U, Hickie I, Hadzi-Pavlovic D, et al. Intravenous immunoglobulin is ineffective in the treatment of patients with chronic fatigue syndrome. *Am J Med* 1997;103:38–43.
46. Rowe KS. Double-blind randomized controlled trial to assess the efficacy of intravenous gammaglobulin for the management of chronic fatigue syndrome in adolescents. *J Psychiatr Res* 1997;31:133–147.
47. Zachrisson O, Regland B, Jahreskog M, et al. Treatment with staphylococcus toxoid in fibromyalgia/chronic fatigue syndrome – a randomised controlled trial. *Eur J Pain* 2002;6:455–466.
48. See DM, Tilles JG. Alpha interferon treatment of patients with chronic fatigue syndrome. *Immunol Invest* 1996;25:153–164.
49. Brook M, Bannister B, Weir W. Interferon-alpha therapy for patients with chronic fatigue syndrome. *J Infect Dis* 1993;168:791–792.
50. Straus SE, Dale JK, Tobi M, et al. Acyclovir treatment of the chronic fatigue syndrome. Lack of efficacy in a placebo-controlled trial. *N Engl J Med* 1988;319:1692–1698.
51. Lloyd A, Hickie I, Boughton R, et al. Immunologic and psychological therapy for patients with chronic fatigue syndrome. *Am J Med* 1993;94:197–203.
52. Steinberg P, McNutt BE, Marshall P, et al. Double-blind placebo-controlled study of efficacy of oral terfenadine in the treatment of chronic fatigue syndrome. *J Allergy Clin Immunol* 1996;97:119–126.
53. Medicines Control Agency (UK). *Current Problems in Pharmacovigilance*, Volume 23, September 1997.
54. Price JR, Couper J. Cognitive behaviour therapy for CFS. In: The Cochrane Library, Issue 2. Oxford: Update Software, 2002. Search date 1998; primary sources Medline, Embase, Biological Abstracts, Sigle, Index to Theses of Great Britain and Ireland, Index to Scientific and Technical Proceedings, Science Citation Index, Trials Register of the Depression, Anxiety and Neurosis Group, citation lists, and personal contacts.

55. Deale A, Chalder T, Marks I, et al. Cognitive behaviour therapy for chronic fatigue syndrome: a randomized controlled trial. *Am J Psychiatry* 1997;154:408–414.
56. Sharpe M, Hawton K, Simkin S, et al. Cognitive behaviour therapy for chronic fatigue syndrome: a randomized controlled trial. *BMJ* 1996;312:22–26.
57. Prins JB, Bleijenberg G, Bazelmans E, et al. Cognitive behaviour therapy for chronic fatigue syndrome: a multicentre randomised controlled trial. *Lancet* 2001;357:841–847.
58. Deale A, Husain K, Chalder T, et al. Long-term outcome of cognitive behaviour therapy versus relaxation therapy for chronic fatigue syndrome: a 5-year follow-up study. *Am J Psychiatry* 2001;158:2038–2042.
59. Ridsdale L, Godfrey E, Chalder T, et al. Chronic fatigue in general practice: is counselling as good as cognitive behaviour therapy? A UK randomised trial. *Br J Gen Pract* 2001;51:19–24.

Steven Reid
Consultant Liaison Psychiatrist
St Mary's Hospital
London
UK

Trudie Chalder
Reader

Anthony Cleare
Senior Lecturer

Matthew Hotopf
Reader

Simon Wessely
Professor of Epidemiological and Liaison Psychiatry

Guy's, King's and St Thomas' School of Medicine and Institute of Psychiatry
London
UK

Competing interests: None declared.

TABLE 1 **Diagnostic criteria for chronic fatigue syndrome (see text, p 1290).**

CDC 1994[1]	Oxford, UK[2]
Clinically evaluated, medically unexplained fatigue of at least 6 months' duration that is:	Severe, disabling fatigue of at least 6 months' duration that:
– of new onset	– affects both physical and mental functioning
– not a result of ongoing exertion	– was present for more than 50% of the time
– not substantially alleviated by rest	
– a substantial reduction in previous levels of activity	
The occurrence of four or more of the following symptoms:	Other symptoms, particularly myalgia, sleep, and mood disturbance, may be present.
– subjective memory impairment	
– tender lymph nodes	
– muscle pain	
– joint pain	
– headache	
– unrefreshing sleep	
– postexertional malaise (> 24 hours)	
Exclusion criteria	
– Active, unresolved, or suspected disease likely to cause fatigue	– Active, unresolved, or suspect disease likely to cause fatigue
– Psychotic, melancholic, or bipolar depression (but not uncomplicated major depression)	– Psychotic, melancholic, or bipolar depression (but not uncomplicated major depression)
– Psychotic disorders	– Psychotic disorders
– Dementia	– Dementia
– Anorexia or bulimia nervosa	– Anorexia or bulimia nervosa
– Alcohol or other substance misuse	
– Severe obesity	

CDC, US Centers for Disease Control and Prevention.

Fracture prevention in postmenopausal women

Search date May 2003

Olivier Bruyere, John Edwards, and Jean-Yves Reginster

QUESTIONS

INTERVENTIONS

To be covered in future updates
Effects of dietary intervention
Effects of helmets
Effects of joint and limb pads
Prevention of pathological fractures
Raloxifene

See glossary, p 1319

Key Messages

- **Alendronate** Two systematic reviews in postmenopausal women have found that alendronate reduces vertebral and non-vertebral fractures compared with placebo.
- **Risedronate** One systematic review in postmenopausal women has found that risedronate reduces vertebral and non-vertebral fractures compared with placebo.
- **Calcitonin** One systematic review in postmenopausal women found that calcitonin reduced vertebral fractures compared with placebo, but found no significant difference between calcitonin and placebo in non-vertebral fractures.
- **Calcium plus vitamin D** One large RCT in women aged 69–106 years living in nursing homes found that calcium plus vitamin D3 reduced hip fractures and non-vertebral fractures over 18 months to 3 years compared with placebo. One smaller RCT in women and men aged 65 years or older found that calcium plus vitamin D3 reduced non-vertebral fractures compared with placebo, but found no significant difference in hip fractures. One smaller RCT in postmenopausal women found no significant difference between calcium plus vitamin D3 and placebo in hip fracture after 2 years. The two smaller

RCTs may have lacked power to exclude a clinically important difference. One systematic review in postmenopausal women reporting a combined analysis (for vitamin D alone and vitamin D plus calcium) found that standard or hydroxylated vitamin D with or without calcium reduced vertebral fractures compared with control, but found no significant difference between groups in non-vertebral fractures.

- **Etidronate** One systematic review in postmenopausal women found that etidronate reduced vertebral fractures over 2 years compared with control (placebo, calcium, or calcium plus vitamin D), but found no significant difference in non-vertebral fractures.
- **Hip protectors** One systematic review in elderly residents of nursing homes and one subsequent RCT found that hip protectors reduced hip fractures over 9–19 months compared with no hip protectors, whereas four other subsequent RCTs found no significant difference in hip fractures between groups. One other subsequent RCT in men and women aged over 65 years in institutional care found that a multifactorial intervention (including staff education, environmental manipulation, exercise, walking aids, drug regimen reviews, and hip protectors for those considered at higher risk) reduced hip fractures over 34 weeks compared with usual care. RCTs found no significant difference between hip protectors and no hip protectors in the occurrence of pelvic fractures.
- **Pamidronate** One RCT in men and postmenopausal women found that pamidronate reduced new vertebral fractures after 3 years compared with placebo. One small RCT in postmenopausal women found no significant difference between pamidronate and placebo in vertebral fracture rate, but it was too small to exclude a clinically important difference.
- **Environmental manipulation** We found no RCTs assessing environmental manipulation alone. One RCT in men and women aged over 70 years found no significant difference in new fractures over 4 years between health visitor care (aimed at assessing nutritional deficiencies, reducing smoking and alcohol intake, improving muscle tone and fitness, assessing medical conditions, use of medication, improving home environment such as lighting) and control. Another RCT in men and women aged over 65 years in institutional care found that a multifactorial intervention (including staff education, environmental manipulation, exercise, walking aids, drug regimen reviews, and hip protectors for those considered at higher risk) reduced hip fractures over 34 weeks compared with usual care.
- **Exercise** Three RCTs found no significant difference in falls resulting in fracture over 1 year between exercise (advice to walk briskly three times weekly or balance and strength exercises plus walking) and control. One small RCT in postmenopausal women found no significant difference between a 2 year back strengthening exercise programme and usual care in vertebral fractures over 10 years. Another RCT in men and women aged over 65 years in institutional care found that a multifactorial intervention (including staff education, environmental manipulation, exercise, walking aids, drug regimen reviews, and hip protectors for those considered at higher risk) reduced hip fractures over 34 weeks compared with usual care.
- **Calcium alone** One systematic review in postmenopausal women found no significant difference between calcium supplementation and placebo in vertebral or non-vertebral fractures.

Fracture prevention in postmenopausal women

- **Vitamin D alone** One large RCT in postmenopausal women and two large RCTs in postmenopausal women and men found no significant difference between vitamin D3 and placebo in hip fractures or non-vertebral fractures. One systematic review found limited evidence from two small RCTs in postmenopausal women that calcitriol reduced vertebral fractures over 3 years compared with placebo.
- **Hormone replacement therapy** We found insufficient evidence of benefit, but reliable evidence of harm. One systematic review in postmenopausal women found that hormone replacement therapy reduced vertebral fractures compared with control. However, another systematic review and one subsequent RCT in postmenopausal women found no significant difference in vertebral fractures. Two systematic reviews and two subsequent RCTs provided insufficient evidence on the effects of hormone replacement therapy on non-vertebral fractures. One large RCT of oestrogen plus progestin versus placebo for primary prevention of coronary heart disease in healthy postmenopausal women was stopped because hormonal treatment increased risks of invasive breast cancer, coronary events, stroke, and pulmonary embolism.

DEFINITION This topic covers interventions to prevent fractures in postmenopausal women. Fractures may be symptomatic or asymptomatic. A fracture is a break or disruption of bone or cartilage. Symptoms and signs may include immobility, pain, tenderness, numbness, bruising, joint deformity, joint swelling, limb deformity, and limb shortening.[1] Diagnosis is usually based on a typical clinical picture combined with results from an appropriate imaging technique. Usually in trials dealing with osteoporosis, menopause is considered to be present 12 months after the last menstruation.

INCIDENCE/ PREVALENCE The lifetime risk of fracture in white women is 20% for the spine, 15% for the wrist, and 18% for the hip.[2] The incidence of postmenopausal fracture increases with age.[3] One observational study found that age specific incidence rates for postmenopausal fracture of the hip increased exponentially beyond the age of 50 years.[4]

AETIOLOGY/ RISK FACTORS Fractures usually arise from trauma. General risk factors include those associated with an increased risks of falling (such as ataxia, drug and alcohol intake, loose carpets), age, osteoporosis, bony metastases, and other bone disorders. Postmenopausal women are at increased risk of fracture because of hormonal bone loss. Risk factors for fractures in postmenopausal women include increasing age, low body mass index, time since menopause, alcohol consumption, smoking, some endocrine diseases, such as hyperparathyroidism or thyroid disease, and steroid use, among others.

PROGNOSIS Fractures may result in pain, short or long term disability, haemorrhage, thromboembolic disease (see thromboembolism, p 273), shock, and death. Vertebral fractures are associated with pain, physical impairment, muscular atrophy, changes in body shape, loss of physical function, and lower quality of life.[5] About 20% of women die in the first year after a hip fracture, representing an increase in mortality of 12–20% compared with women of similar age and no hip fracture. Half of elderly women who had been independent become partly dependent after hip fracture. A third become totally dependent.

AIMS OF INTERVENTION To prevent fractures, with minimal adverse effects from treatment.

OUTCOMES Incidence of hip, wrist, non-vertebral and vertebral fractures (we have not reported intermediate outcomes such as bone mineral density data).

METHODS *Clinical Evidence* search and appraisal May 2003. We also hand searched journals of bone diseases and carried out manual searches using the bibliographies of review articles published after 1985. Some of the RCTs identified provide results generalised to fracture per person/year or overall fractures. These results provide an idea of the group effect of an intervention, but not of its effects on the incidence of fracture in an individual. Data on multiple fractures in one person clearly differ from data on multiple people experiencing a single fracture. Regulatory authorities and scientific groups have recommended that the results of studies evaluating new interventions are expressed in terms of the proportion of people experiencing new fractures.[6] This topic examines fracture prevention in postmenopausal women. However, we have included RCTs undertaken in people outside this group (men, premenopausal women) in some sections as results from these trials may be generalisable to postmenopausal women.

QUESTION What are the effects of treatments to prevent fractures in postmenopausal women?

OPTION BISPHOSPHONATES

Olivier Bruyere and Jean-Yves Reginster

Two systematic reviews in postmenopausal women have found that alendronate reduces vertebral and non-vertebral fractures compared with placebo. One systematic review in postmenopausal women found that etidronate reduced vertebral fractures over 2 years compared with control (placebo, calcium, or calcium plus vitamin D), but found no significant difference in non-vertebral fractures. One RCT in men and postmenopausal women found that pamidronate reduced new vertebral fractures after 3 years compared with placebo. One small RCT in postmenopausal women found no significant difference between pamidronate and placebo in vertebral fracture rate after 2 years, but it was too small to exclude a clinically important difference. One systematic review in postmenopausal women has found that risedronate reduces vertebral and non-vertebral fractures compared with placebo.

Benefits: **Alendronate:** We found two systematic reviews.[7,8] The first systematic review (search date 1999, 11 RCTs, 12 855 postmenopausal women) included RCTs that randomised postmenopausal women to alendronate or placebo and had a follow up of at least 1 year.[7] It found that alendronate (5 mg or more) significantly reduced vertebral fractures compared with placebo (8 RCTs, 9360 women; RR 0.52, 95% CI 0.43 to 0.65). It also found that alendronate (10 mg or more) significantly reduced non-vertebral fractures compared with placebo (6 RCTs, 3723 women; RR 0.51, 95% CI 0.38 to 0.69). The review did not state how fractures were diagnosed. The second systematic review (search date 1998, 7 RCTs, 10 287 postmenopausal women aged 39–85 years) found that, compared with placebo, alendronate significantly reduced vertebral fractures (fractures confirmed radiologically; 4 RCTs; RR 0.54, 95% CI 0.45 to 0.66) and non-vertebral fractures (6 RCTs; RR 0.81, 95% CI 0.72 to 0.92).[8] It found that fewer people had hip fractures over 1–4 years, but the difference was not significant (3 RCTs; RR 0.64, 95% CI 0.40 to 1.01; results presented graphically). **Etidronate:** We found one systematic review (search date 1998, 13 RCTs, 1010 postmenopausal women) comparing etidronate versus placebo, calcium, or calcium plus vitamin D.[9] It found that etidronate significantly reduced vertebral fractures over 2 years compared with control (9 RCTs: 32/538 [6%] *v* 54/538 [10%]; RR 0.60, 95% CI 0.41 to 0.88), but found no significant difference in non-vertebral fractures (7 RCTs: 48/433 [11%] *v* 49/434 [11%]; RR 0.98, 95% CI 0.68 to 1.42). The review did not describe clearly how fractures were diagnosed. **Pamidronate:** We found no systematic review but found two RCTs comparing pamidronate (150 mg/day) versus placebo.[10,11] The first RCT (23 men and 78 postmenopausal women) found that pamidronate significantly reduced new radiologically confirmed vertebral fractures after 3 years compared with placebo (5/46 [11%] with pamidronate *v* 15/45 [33%] with placebo; RR 0.33, 95% CI 0.14 to 0.77).[10] The second RCT (48 postmenopausal women) found no significant difference after 2 years between pamidronate and placebo in vertebral fractures (fractures confirmed radiologically; 13/100 person years with pamidronate *v* 24/100 person years with control; P = 0.07; see methods, p 1307).[11] However, it was too small to exclude a clinically important difference. **Risedronate:** We found one systematic review (search date 2000, 8 RCTs, 14 832 postmenopausal women), which included placebo controlled trials of risedronate in postmenopausal women (defined as > 6 months postmenopausal) with a follow up of at least 1 year.[12] The review found that risedronate (2.5 mg or more) significantly reduced vertebral fractures compared with placebo (5 RCTs, 2604 women; RR 0.64, 95% CI 0.54 to 0.77). It also found that risedronate (2.5 mg or more) significantly reduced non-vertebral fractures compared with placebo (7 RCTs, 12 958 women; RR 0.73, 95% CI 0.61 to 0.87). The review did not state how fractures were diagnosed.

Harms: **Alendronate:** Observational evidence suggests that oral alendronate is associated with oesophageal erosions and ulcerative oesophagitis. However, one RCT[13] identified by the second review[8] (in which people took alendronate with 180–240 mL water on rising in the morning and remained upright for at least 30 minutes after swallowing the tablet and until they had eaten something) found no significant difference in oesophagitis with alendronate compared with placebo. **Risedronate:** One observational study found limited evidence suggesting that the gastrointestinal safety of risedronate seems to be in the same range as alendronate.[14]

Comment: **Risedronate:** The systematic review noted that the major methodological weakness of included RCTs was loss to follow up, which was over 20% in most RCTs and over 35% in the largest RCT.[12] However, it noted the magnitude of the treatment effect was unrelated to loss to follow up.[12] **Pamidronate:** Although one of the RCTs included both men and women at risk of hip fracture,[10] it is likely that the results are generalisable to postmenopausal women.

OPTION CALCIUM AND VITAMIN D ALONE OR IN COMBINATION

Olivier Bruyere and Jean-Yves Reginster

One systematic review in postmenopausal women found no significant difference between calcium supplementation and placebo in vertebral or non-vertebral fractures. One large RCT in postmenopausal women and two large RCTs in postmenopausal women and men found no significant difference between vitamin D3 and placebo in hip fractures or non-vertebral fractures. One systematic review found limited evidence from two small RCTs in postmenopausal women that calcitriol reduced vertebral fractures over 3 years compared with placebo. One systematic review in postmenopausal women reporting a combined analysis (for vitamin D alone and Vitamin D plus calcium) found that standard or hydroxylated vitamin D with or without calcium reduced vertebral fractures compared with control, but found no significant difference between groups in non-vertebral fractures. One large RCT in women aged 69–106 years living in nursing homes found that calcium plus vitamin D3 reduced hip fractures and non-vertebral fractures over 18 months to 3 years compared with placebo. One smaller RCT in women and men aged 65 years or older found that calcium plus vitamin D3 reduced non-vertebral fractures compared with placebo, but found no significant difference in hip fractures. One smaller RCT in postmenopausal women found no significant difference between calcium plus vitamin D3 and placebo in hip fracture after 2 years. The two smaller RCTs may have lacked power to exclude a clinically important difference.

Benefits: **Calcium versus placebo:** We found one systematic review (search date 1998, 15 RCTs, 1806 postmenopausal women), which included trials of calcium supplementation in women older than 45 years with an absence of menses for a minimum of 6 months.[15] It found no significant difference between calcium and placebo in vertebral fractures (5 RCTs, 576 women; RR 0.77, 95% CI 0.54 to 1.09). It also found no significant difference between calcium and placebo in non-vertebral fractures (2 RCTs, 222 women; RR 0.86, 95% CI 0.43 to 1.72). It noted that the two RCTs reporting non-vertebral fractures had very few events, and the pooled confidence intervals were therefore wide (absolute numbers not reported). **Vitamin D3 versus placebo:** We found one systematic review (search date 2000, 1 RCT)[16] and two subsequent RCTs.[17,18] The RCT identified by the review (2578 people; 1916 women, 662 men, age 70 years or older, living at home; see comment below) found no significant difference between vitamin D3 and placebo in hip fracture (confirmed by clinical assessment and x ray films; 58/1284 [4.5%] *v* 48/1280 [3.7%]; RR 1.20, 95% CI 0.83 to 1.75), or any non-vertebral fracture over 3 years (135/1284 [11%] *v* 122/1280 [10%]; RR 1.10 95% CI 0.87 to 1.39).[16] The first subsequent RCT (1144 people resident in nursing homes; mean age 85 years; 75% were women) found no significant difference between vitamin D3 (10 μg/day) and placebo in hip fracture or any non-vertebral fracture (fractures confirmed by hospital discharge letter or x ray film) after 2 years' treatment (hip fracture: 50/569 [8.8%] with vitamin D *v* 47/575 [8.2%] with placebo; RR 1.09, 95% CI 0.73 to 1.63; non-vertebral fracture: 69/569 [12.1%] with vitamin D *v* 76/575 [13.2%] with placebo; RR 0.92, 95% CI 0.66 to 1.27).[17] The second subsequent RCT (2686 people; 2037 men and 649 women; age 65–85 years) reported separate results for men and women in the trial.[18] In women, it found no significant difference between vitamin D3 and placebo in first fractures at any site after 5 years (42/326 [13%] with vitamin D3 *v* 58/323 [18%] with placebo; RR 0.68, 95% CI 0.46 to 1.01). In women, it also found no significant difference between vitamin D3 and placebo in first hip fractures after 5 years (10/326 [3%] with vitamin D3 *v* 10/323 [3%] with placebo; RR 0.98, 95% CI 0.41 to 2.36) or vertebral fractures (4/326 [1%] with vitamin D3 *v* 6/323 [2%] with placebo; RR 0.65, 95% CI 0.18 to 2.3). **Vitamin D analogue (calcitriol) versus placebo:** The systematic review[16] also identified two small RCTs (68 women aged ≥54 years) comparing calcitriol (1,25 dihydroxy vitamin D) versus placebo. It found that calcitriol significantly reduced new vertebral fractures over 3 years compared with placebo (fractures confirmed radiologically; 8/34 [23%] with calcitriol *v* 17/34 [50%] with placebo; RR 0.49, 95% CI 0.25 to 0.95). **Calcium plus vitamin D3 versus placebo:** We found one systematic review (search date 2000, 2 RCTs, 3715 people)[16] and one subsequent RCT.[19] One of the RCTs identified by the review (3270 mobile elderly women, aged 69–106 years, living in nursing homes) found that, compared with placebo, calcium plus vitamin D3 significantly reduced hip fractures (80/1387 [6%] with calcium plus vitamin D3 *v* 110/1403 [8%] with placebo; RR 0.74, 95% CI 0.60 to 0.91) and all non-vertebral fractures (160/1387 [11%] with calcium plus vitamin D3 *v* 215/1403 [15%] with placebo; RR 0.75, 95% CI 0.62 to 0.91) over 18 months. This difference remained significant after 3 years of treatment (hip fracture: 137/1176 [12%] with calcium plus vitamin D3 *v* 178/1127 [16%] with placebo; RR 0.74, 95% CI 0.60 to 0.91; all non-vertebral fracture: 255/1176 [22%] with calcium plus vitamin D3 *v* 308/1127 [27%] with placebo; RR 0.72, 95% CI 0.60 to 0.84). The review did not state how fractures were diagnosed.[16] The other RCT identified by the review (246 women, 199 men, aged 65 years or older, living at home; see comment below) found no significant difference between calcium plus vitamin D3 and placebo in hip fractures over 3 years (0/187 [0%] *v* 1/202 [0.5%]; RR 0.36, 95% CI 0.01 to 8.78), but was underpowered to exclude a clinically important difference. It found that calcium plus vitamin D reduced overall non-vertebral fractures compared with placebo (11/187 [6%] with calcium plus vitamin D *v* 26/202 [13%] with placebo; RR 0.46, 95% CI 0.23 to 0.90). Fractures were diagnosed by self report, interview, and validation from case records.[16] The subsequent RCT (583 women in institutional care, mean age 85 years, range 64–99 years) found no significant difference between calcium plus vitamin D3 and placebo in hip fracture at 2 years (27/393 [6.9%] with calcium plus vitamin D *v* 21/190 [11.1%] with placebo; RR for placebo *v* calcium plus vitamin D 1.69, 95% CI 0.96 to 3.00).[19] **Standard or hydroxylated vitamin D alone or with calcium versus control (placebo or calcium):** We found one systematic review (search date 1999, 25 RCTs, 8124 postmenopausal women; see comment below), which included RCTs of standard or hydroxylated vitamin D with or without calcium supplementation in women older than 45 years with an absence of menses for a minimum of 6 months and a follow up of at least 1 year.[20] It analysed combined results for RCTs that used vitamin D alone or vitamin D plus calcium. It found that standard or hydroxylated vitamin D with or without calcium significantly reduced vertebral fractures compared with control (8 RCTs, 1130 women; RR 0.63, 95% CI 0.45 to 0.88). It found no significant difference between standard or hydroxylated vitamin D with or without calcium and control in the occurrence of non-vertebral fractures (6 RCTs, 6187 women; RR 0.77, 95% CI 0.57 to 1.04).

Harms: **Vitamin D3 or vitamin D analogue (calcitriol) versus placebo or calcium:** The systematic review found that vitamin D or vitamin D analogues compared with placebo or calcium increased hypercalcaemia (5 RCTs, 1009 people; 22/498 [4.4%] with vitamin D or vitamin D analogues *v* 18/511 [3.5%] with placebo or calcium; RR 1.71, 95% CI 1.01 to 2.89).[16]

Comment: Although some RCTs included both men and women at risk of hip fracture, it is likely that the results are generalisable to postmenopausal women.[16,17] The review that compared vitamin D alone or plus calcium versus control noted that inferences from the results of its analysis were limited by the variability of study designs, weaknesses in the primary study methods (including lack of blinding in many studies), the paucity of data, and the inconsistency of results of included RCTs.[20]

OPTION CALCITONIN

Olivier Bruyere and Jean-Yves Reginster

One systematic review in postmenopausal women found that calcitonin reduced vertebral fractures compared with placebo, but found no significant difference between calcitonin and placebo in non-vertebral fractures.

Benefits: We found two systematic reviews.[21,22] The first systematic review (search date 2000, 30 RCTs, 3993 postmenopausal women) included trials of at least 1 year duration, which compared calcitonin versus placebo or calcium and/or vitamin D in postmenopausal women.[21] It found that calcitonin significantly reduced vertebral fractures compared with placebo (4 RCTs, 1404 women; RR 0.46, 95% CI 0.25 to 0.87; see comment below). It found no significant difference between calcitonin and placebo in non-vertebral fractures (3 RCTs, 1481 women; RR 0.52, 95% CI 0.22 to 1.23). The second systematic review (search date 1996, 14 RCTs, 7 RCTs in perimenopausal women with crush fractures or osteoporosis, 7 RCTs in men and women with osteoporosis or taking corticosteroids, 1309 people, exact proportions of women and men not specified; see comment below) compared calcitonin (salcatonin) versus placebo, no treatment, calcium, or calcium plus vitamin D (see comment below).[22] It included three RCTs identified by the first systematic review. It found that fewer people developed vertebral or non-vertebral fractures with calcitonin compared with no calcitonin, but the difference was not significant (vertebral fractures: 166/1190 [14%] people with calcitonin *v* 96/554 [17%] with no calcitonin; RR 0.80, 95% CI 0.64 to 1.01; non-vertebral fractures: RR 0.48, 95% CI 0.20 to 1.15; no further data provided). The review did not state how fractures were diagnosed.

Harms: The first systematic review found the relative risk for headache from one included RCT was 0.57 (95% CI 0.34 to 0.93) and that for climacteric symptoms from another included RCT was 0.20 (95% CI 0.05 to 0.77).[21] It noted that, in general, included trials were poor in their reporting of adverse events. The second systematic review gave no information on harms.[22]

Comment: The first systematic review suggested caution in interpreting the magnitude of the effect of calcitonin in the pooled estimates.[21] The pooled estimate for vertebral fractures was based on three small RCTs and a fourth larger RCT with a large variability in results between them. Losses to follow up were 18.7%, 21%, 45%, and 59.3% in the four RCTs.[21] Similar issues were raised in the pooled estimate for non-vertebral fractures.[21] The second systematic review commented that its conclusions are limited because many of the RCTs identified did not report the occurrence of fractures, were not double blinded, and only two of the RCTs identified were of over 2 years' duration.[22]

OPTION ENVIRONMENTAL MANIPULATION

John Edwards

We found no RCTs assessing environmental manipulation alone. One RCT in men and women aged over 70 years found no significant difference in new fractures over 4 years between health visitor care (aimed at assessing nutritional deficiencies, reducing smoking and alcohol intake, improving muscle tone and fitness, assessing medical conditions, use of medication, improving home environment such as lighting) and control. Another RCT in men and women aged over 65 years in institutional care found that a multifactorial intervention (including staff education, environmental manipulation, exercise, walking aids, drug regimen reviews, and hip protectors for those considered at higher risk) reduced hip fractures over 34 weeks compared with usual care.

Benefits: We found no systematic review and no RCTs assessing environmental manipulation (see glossary, p 1319) alone. We found one RCT (674 men and women, age > 70 years) comparing health visitor care (aimed at assessing nutritional deficiencies, reducing smoking and alcohol intake, improving muscle tone and fitness, assessing medical conditions and use of medication, and improving home environment, such as lighting) versus control (not specified).[23] It found no significant difference between health visitor care and control in new fractures over 4 years (16/350 [4.5%] with health visitor care *v* 14/324 [4.3%] with control; RR 1.06, 95% CI 0.52 to 2.13). The RCT did not state how fractures were diagnosed. We found one further RCT assessing a multifactorial intervention (including an environmental manipulation component — see benefits of hip protectors, p 1314).[24]

Harms: The RCT examining health visitor care gave no information on harms.[23]

Comment: Although the RCT examining health visitor care included both men and women at risk of hip fracture, it is likely that the results are generalisable to postmenopausal women.[23]

OPTION EXERCISE

John Edwards

Three RCTs found no significant difference in falls resulting in fracture over 1 year between exercise (advice to walk briskly three times weekly or balance and strength exercises plus walking) and control. One small RCT in postmenopausal women found no significant difference between a 2 year back strengthening exercise programme and usual care in vertebral fractures over 10 years. Another RCT in men and women aged over 65 years in institutional care found that a multifactorial intervention (including staff education, environmental manipulation, exercise, walking aids, drug regimen reviews, and hip protectors for those considered at higher risk) reduced hip fractures over 34 weeks compared with usual care.

Benefits: We found one systematic review (search date 2001, 3 RCTs comparing exercise versus control in preventing falls resulting in fracture)[25] and one subsequent RCT.[26] The review did not perform a meta-analysis because of the heterogeneity of methods and interventions among trials.[25] The first RCT identified by the review (165 postmenopausal women living in the community who had fractured an upper limb in the previous 2 years) compared advice to walk briskly for up to 40 minutes three times weekly versus advice to carry out upper limb exercises. It found no significant difference between groups in falls resulting in fracture after 1 year (2/81 [2%] with brisk walking *v* 3/84 [4%] with upper limb exercises; RR 0.69, 95% CI 0.12 to 4.03). The second RCT identified by the review (77 women and 22 men, aged > 65 years, living in the community; see comment below) compared a home based exercise programme (balance and strength exercises plus walking) versus no exercise programme for 14 weeks. It found no significant difference between groups in falls resulting in fracture over 44 weeks (1/45 [2%] with exercise *v* 0/48 [0%] with no exercise; RR 3.20, 95% CI 0.13 to 76.48). The third RCT (162 women, 78 men, aged > 75 years; see comment below) found no significant difference in falls resulting in fracture over 1 year with a home exercise programme (balance and strength exercises plus walking) compared with usual care (2/121 [2%] with home exercise *v* 7/119 [6%] with usual care; RR 0.28, 95% CI 0.06 to 1.33). The review did not state how fractures were diagnosed in the RCTs.[25] The subsequent RCT (65 postmenopausal women) compared a programme of back muscle strengthening exercises versus usual care for 2 years.[26] It found no significant difference in vertebral fractures at 10 years between strengthening exercises and usual care (fractures confirmed radiologically; 3/27 [11.1%] with exercise *v* 7/23 [30.4%] with usual care; P = 0.85). We found one further RCT assessing a multifactorial intervention (including an exercise component — see benefits of hip protectors, p 1314).[24]

Harms: One of the RCTs found that brisk walking significantly increased the number of falls compared with control (15.0/100 person years, 95% CI 1.4/100 person years to 29.0/100 person years — see methods, p 1307).[25] This result should be interpreted with caution as reporting of falls is subject to recall bias.

Comment: Most of the RCTs identified by the review examined falls rather than fractures as the main outcome of interest.[25]

OPTION HIP PROTECTORS

John Edwards

One systematic review in elderly residents of nursing homes and one subsequent RCT found that hip protectors reduced hip fractures over 9–19 months compared with no hip protectors, whereas four other subsequent RCTs found no significant difference in hip fractures between groups. One other subsequent RCT in men and women aged over 65 years in institutional care found that a multifactorial intervention (including staff education, environmental manipulation, exercise, walking aids, drug regimen reviews, and hip protectors for those considered at higher risk) reduced hip fractures over 34 weeks compared with usual care. RCTs found no significant difference between hip protectors and no hip protectors in the occurrence of pelvic fractures.

Benefits: **Hip fractures:** We found one systematic review[27] and six subsequent RCTs.[24,28–32] The systematic review (search date 2000) identified six RCTs (3412 people, predominantly women; see comment below) assessing the effects of hip protectors versus no hip protectors on hip fractures.[27] It could not perform a meta-analysis of all of the RCTs because some of the RCTs used cluster randomisation and others randomised individuals. In the RCTs that randomised individuals, the review found that hip protectors significantly reduced hip fractures over 9–19 months compared with no hip protectors (3 RCTs, 202 people, 90–100% women in 2 RCTs, proportion of women and men not stated in 1 RCT; 4/111 [4%] *v* 15/91 [16%]; RR 0.22, 95% CI 0.09 to 0.57). The review did not state how fractures were diagnosed.[27] The first subsequent RCT (164 women, mean age 83 years) found that hip protectors significantly reduced hip fractures over about 1 year compared with control (1/88 [1%] *v* 8/76 [10%]; RR 0.11, 95% CI 0.01 to 0.84).[28] The RCT did not state how fractures were diagnosed. The second subsequent RCT (64 women and 8 men in a nursing home, age 71–96 years) found no significant difference between hip protectors and no hip protectors in hip fractures over 1 year (1/36 [3%] *v* 7/36 [19%]; RR 0.14, 95% CI 0.02 to 1.10), but it was too small to exclude a clinically important difference (see comment below).[29] The RCT did not state how hip fractures were diagnosed. The third subsequent RCT (174 women aged ≥ 75 years) found no significant difference in hip fractures between hip protectors and no hip protectors at 18 months (8/86 [9.3%] with hip protectors *v* 7/88 [8.0%] without; RR 1.17, 95% CI 0.44 to 3.08).[30] It may have lacked power to exclude a clinically important difference. The RCT did not state how hip fractures were diagnosed. The fourth subsequent RCT was a cluster randomised trial (439 men and women resident in institutional care, aged ≥ 65 years, 72% women).[24] It compared a multifactorial intervention (including staff education, environmental manipulation [see glossary, p 1319], exercise, walking aids, drug regimen reviews, and hip protectors for those considered at higher risk) versus usual care for 34 weeks. It found that the multifactorial intervention significantly reduced hip fractures over 34 weeks compared with usual care (3/188 [1.6%] with active intervention *v* 12/196 [6.1%] with usual care; RR 0.26, 95% CI 0.07 to 0.91). The RCT did not state how hip fractures were diagnosed. It was not clear which components of the intervention were responsible for reported effects. The fifth subsequent RCT was a cluster randomised trial (49 nursing homes, 942 residents aged 70 years or older, of which 813 were women, at "high risk" of falling; see comment below), which compared education (structured education of staff about hip protectors who then taught residents) plus the provision of free hip protectors versus usual care (brief information about hip protectors to the study co-ordinator and two hip protectors provided for demonstration purposes).[31] It found no significant difference between groups in the proportion of people with hip fractures after 15 months (21/459 [5%] people with intervention *v* 39/483 [8%] with usual care; RR 0.57, CI not reported; absolute risk difference −3.5%, 95% CI −7.3% to +0.3%). The sixth subsequent RCT (561 people of which 501 were women, age 70 years or over, living in sheltered housing or residential or nursing homes, at "high risk" of falls) found no significant difference in the occurrence of first hip fractures between provision of hip protector plus education (on bone health and risk factors for falls) and education alone (hip fracture: 18/276 [6%] with hip protector plus education *v* 19/285 [7%] with education alone; RR 0.98, 95% CI 0.52 to 1.82; see comment below).[32] **Pelvic fractures:** The systematic review identified three RCTs.[27] It could not perform a meta-analysis because of different trial methods. All three RCTs included men and women (see comment below). The first RCT (1801 people aged > 75 years, about 80% women) identified by the review found no significant difference in pelvic fractures over a mean 11–15 months between hip protectors and no hip protectors (2/653 [0.3%] with hip protectors *v* 12/1148 [1%] with no hip protectors; RR 0.29, 95% CI 0.07 to 1.31). The second RCT identified by the review (665 people aged > 69 years living in a nursing home, 70% women) found no significant difference in pelvic fractures over 11 months (0/247 [0%] with hip protectors *v* 2/418 [0.5%] with no hip protectors; RR 0.34, 95% CI 0.02 to 7.01). The third RCT identified by the review (64 men and 8 women, aged 71–96 years living in a nursing home) found no significant difference between hip protectors and no hip protectors in pelvic fractures over 12 months, but it may have been too small to exclude a clinically important difference (0/36 [0%] with hip protectors *v* 2/36 [5%] with no hip protectors; RR 0.20, 95% CI 0.01 to 4.03). The review did not state how fractures were diagnosed in the RCTs.[27] One subsequent RCT (174 women aged ≥75 years) found no significant difference in pelvic fractures at 18 months between hip protectors and no hip protectors (2/86 [2.3%] with hip protectors *v* 2/88 [2.3%] with no hip protectors; RR 1.02, 95% CI 0.15 to 7.10; not stated whether fractures were radiologically confirmed).[30] However, the RCT may have lacked power to exclude a clinically important difference. Another subsequent RCT (561 people of whom 501 were women, age 70 years or over, living in sheltered housing or residential or nursing homes, at "high risk" of falls) found no significant difference in pelvic fractures between provision of hip protector plus education (on bone health and risk factors for falls) and education alone (pelvic fractures: 2/276 [0.7%] with hip protector plus education *v* 3/285 [1%] with education alone; RR 0.69, 95% CI 0.12 to 4.09; see comment below).[32] It did not state whether pelvic fractures were radiologically confirmed.

Harms: **Non-hip or non-pelvic fractures and injuries:** One of the RCTs identified by the review (665 people) found no significant difference between hip protectors and no hip protectors in non-hip fractures over 11 months (15/247 [6.1%] with hip protectors *v* 25/418 [6.0%] with no hip protectors; RR 1.02, 95% CI 0.55 to 1.89).[27] Another small RCT identified by the review found no significant difference in non-hip fractures between hip protectors and no hip protectors (2/35 [5.7%] with hip protectors *v* 0/24 [0%] with no hip protectors; RR 3.47, 95% CI 0.17 to 69.27). A third RCT identified by the review (1801 people) also found no significant difference in the proportion of people with lower limb or other non-hip fractures over a mean of 11–15 months between hip protectors and no hip protectors (23/653 [3.5%] with hip protectors *v* 59/1148 [5.1%] with no hip protectors; RR 0.69, 95% CI 0.43 to 1.10). The first subsequent RCT found no significant difference in non-hip fractures over a mean 377 days between hip protectors and no hip protectors (2/88 [2.3%] with hip protectors *v* 0/76 [0%] with no hip protectors).[28] Another RCT found no significant difference in non-hip and non-pelvic fractures after 18 months (4/86 [4.7%] with hip protectors *v* 2/88 [4.5%] with no hip protectors; RR 1.02, 95% CI 0.26 to 3.96), but it may have been too small to exclude a clinically important difference.[30] One cluster randomised RCT found no significant difference between hip protectors plus education and usual care in non-hip fractures (35/459 [8%] with intervention *v* 32/483 [7%] with usual care; absolute risk difference +1%, 95% CI −4% to +6%; see comment below).[31] One RCT found no significant difference in non-hip non-pelvic fractures between hip protector plus education and education alone (14/276 [5%] with intervention *v* 11/285 [4%] with education alone; RR 1.31, 95% CI 0.61 to 2.84; see comment below).[32] **Falls:** One of the RCTs identified by the review found that hip protectors increased the proportion of people who fell on the hip compared with no hip protectors, but the difference was not significant (8/101 [7.9%] *v* 1/40 [2.5%]; RR 3.17, 95% CI 0.41 to 24.5).[27] The first subsequent RCT found no significant difference in the proportion of people sustaining one or more falls over about 1 year (40/88 [45%] *v* 28/76 [37%]; RR 1.23, 95% CI 0.85 to 1.79).[28] The other five RCTs identified by the review[27] and the second subsequent RCT[29] found a similar incidence of falls with hip protectors compared with no hip protectors, but gave no information on the proportion of people who fell. These results should be interpreted with caution as reporting of falls is subject to recall bias. **Mortality:** One RCT identified by the review found no significant difference in mortality over 12 months between hip protectors and no hip protectors (6/36 [17%] with hip protectors *v* 8/36 [22%] with no hip protectors; RR 0.75, 95% CI 0.29 to

1.94).[27] The first subsequent RCT also found no significant difference in mortality between hip protectors and no hip protectors but it may have been too small to exclude a clinically important difference (6/88 [7%] with hip protectors v 8/76 [10%] with no hip protectors; RR 0.65, 95% CI 0.23 to 1.78).[28] **Hospital admission:** One of the RCTs identified by the review found no significant difference between hip protectors and no hip protectors in the proportion of people permanently hospitalised over 12 months (10/36 [28%] with hip protectors v 9/36 [25%] with no hip protectors; RR 1.11, 95% CI 0.51 to 2.41).[27] The first subsequent RCT found no significant difference in the proportion of people who were hospitalised for reasons other than fracture over a mean of 377 days, but it may have been too small to exclude a clinically important difference (10/88 [11%] with hip protectors v 9/76 [12%] with no hip protectors; RR 0.96, 95% CI 0.41 to 2.24).[28]

Comment: Much of the evidence is taken from RCTs that included both men and women at risk of hip fracture. However, it is likely that the results are generalisable to postmenopausal women.[24,27] The results of the second subsequent RCT should be interpreted with caution as 60% of people who entered the trial were lost to follow up.[29] The RCT had protocol violations as three people were allocated to the hip protector group after randomisation when people initially randomised to hip protectors refused to wear them.[29] The fifth subsequent RCT may have been underpowered and included the possibility of selection bias.[31] The sixth subsequent RCT had methodological problems in that it was found *post hoc* to be underpowered and so the study period was extended from 52 weeks to a mean of 69.6 weeks to increase the total burden of fractures and hence the power of the study.[32]

OPTION HORMONE REPLACEMENT THERAPY

We found insufficient evidence of benefit, but reliable evidence of harm. One systematic review in postmenopausal women found that hormone replacement therapy reduced vertebral fractures compared with control. However, another systematic review and one subsequent RCT in postmenopausal women found no significant difference in vertebral fractures. Two systematic reviews and two subsequent RCTs provided insufficient evidence on the effects of hormone replacement therapy on non-vertebral fractures. One large RCT of oestrogen plus progestin versus placebo for primary prevention of coronary heart disease in healthy postmenopausal women was stopped because hormonal treatment increased risks of invasive breast cancer, coronary events, stroke, and pulmonary embolism.

Benefits: **Vertebral fractures:** We found two systematic reviews[33,34] and one subsequent RCT.[35] The first systematic review (search date 2001, 13 RCTs, mean age 48–73 years) included RCTs of postmenopausal women who were healthy, or who also had coronary artery disease, a vertebral fracture, or established osteoporosis.[33] It included RCTs that compared hormone replacement therapy (HRT) with placebo, calcium with or without vitamin D, or no treatment, with a follow up of at least 1 year. It found that HRT significantly reduced the incidence of vertebral fractures compared with control

(13 RCTs; 42/3507 [1.2%] with HRT *v* 63/3216 [2%] with control; RR 0.67, 95% CI 0.45 to 0.98). The second systematic review (search date 1999) included RCTs that evaluated HRT in postmenopausal women.[34] The HRT could be given in conjunction with a calcium and vitamin D supplement provided the comparison group received the same supplement, and the follow up was at least 1 year. It excluded three RCTs included in the first systematic review[33] on methodological grounds.[34] It found no significant difference between HRT and control in the incidence of vertebral fractures (5 RCTs, 3385 women; RR 0.66, 95% CI 0.41 to 1.07). The subsequent RCT (16 608 postmenopausal women, age 50–79 years) found that HRT (oestrogen plus progestin) significantly reduced vertebral fractures compared with placebo (HR 0.66, 95% CI 0.44 to 0.98).[35] However, after adjustment for multiple statistical testing as outlined in the monitoring plan, the difference between groups was no longer statistically significant (HR 0.66, 95% CI 0.32 to 1.34). **Non-vertebral fractures:** We found two systematic reviews[34,36] and two subsequent RCTs[35,37] comparing HRT versus placebo, no treatment, calcium, or calcium plus vitamin D. The first review (search date 2000, 22 RCTs, 8774 women) found that HRT compared with placebo, no treatment, calcium, or calcium plus vitamin D significantly reduced the proportion of women with non-vertebral fractures after 1–10 years' follow up (258/4929 [5%] *v* 307/3845 [8%]; RR 0.73, 95% CI 0.56 to 0.94).[36] This reduction remained significant in women taking HRT who had a mean age younger than 60 years (14 RCTs: RR 0.67, 95% CI 0.46 to 0.98; no further data provided). When RCTs in women with a mean age of 60 years or older were analysed, the review found no significant difference in non-vertebral fractures between HRT and placebo (8 RCTs: RR 0.88, 95% CI 0.71 to 1.08; no further data provided).[36] The second review (search date 1999) found no significant difference between HRT and control in non-vertebral fractures (6 RCTs, 5383 postmenopausal women; RR 0.87, 95% CI 0.71 to 1.08).[34] One large subsequent RCT (2763 postmenopausal women aged < 80 years) found no significant difference between HRT and placebo in hip fractures (fractures confirmed radiologically; 14/1380 [1.0%] with HRT *v* 13/1383 [0.9%] with placebo; RR 1.1, 95% CI 0.5 to 2.3) or wrist fracture (29/1380 [2.1] with HRT *v* 29/1383 [2.0] with placebo; RR 1.0, 95% CI 0.6 to 1.7), but it may have been too small to exclude a clinically important difference because the outcomes of interest were rare.[37] The second subsequent RCT (16 608 healthy postmenopausal women aged 50–79 years) compared oestrogen plus progestin versus placebo.[35] It found that HRT significantly reduced hip fractures after a mean 5.2 years' follow up compared with placebo (fractures confirmed radiologically; 44/8506 [0.52%] with HRT *v* 62/8102 [0.77%] with placebo; RR of hip fracture 0.66, 95% CI 0.45 to 0.98). However, after adjustment for multiple significance testing as specified in the monitoring plan, the difference was no longer significant (RR 0.66, 95% CI 0.33 to 1.33).

Harms: In one of the RCTs identified by the review assessing non-vertebral fractures, 96/464 women (21%) withdrew from the trial, and more women withdrew from the HRT groups than from the non-HRT groups (72/232 [31%] women *v* 24/232 [10%]; RR 3.0, 95%

CI 2.0 to 4.6).[38] The most common reasons cited for withdrawal were menstrual disorders and headache. The second subsequent RCT comparing oestrogen plus progestin versus placebo as a primary prevention strategy for coronary heart disease in healthy postmenopausal women was stopped after 5.2 years' follow up because of increased risk of invasive breast cancer, coronary events, stroke, and pulmonary embolism among women receiving HRT compared with placebo (invasive breast cancer: 166/8506 [2.0%] with HRT *v* 124/8102 [1.5%] with placebo; RR 1.3, 95% CI 1.0 to 1.6; coronary events: 164/8506 [1.9%] with HRT *v* 122/8102 [1.5%] with placebo; RR 1.3, 95% CI 1.0 to 1.6; stroke: 127/8506 [1.5%] with HRT *v* 85/8102 [1.1%] with placebo; RR 1.4, 95% CI 1.1 to 1.9; pulmonary embolism: 70/8506 [0.8%] with HRT *v* 31/8102 [0.4%] with placebo; RR 2.1, 95% CI 1.4 to 3.3).[35] See also HRT under secondary prevention of ischaemic cardiac events, p 188.

Comment: In the second RCT identified by the review assessing non-vertebral fractures,[36] the use of multiple treatment groups without the correct statistical analyses limits the validity of the study results.[38] In the subsequent large RCT (2763 postmenopausal women aged < 80 years), prevention of fractures was a secondary outcome, the primary outcome was the secondary prevention of coronary heart disease.[37] In addition to the RCTs described, we found many observational studies with conflicting results.[2,39–45] One non-systematic review of 11 observational studies found a reduced risk of hip fracture in women taking oestrogen compared with non-users.[2] A prospective cohort study (9704 women, age ≥ 65 years) found a significant reduction in radiologically confirmed hip fractures with oral oestrogen only in women who started HRT within 5 years of menopause and who used it continuously thereafter.[42] Other observational studies found similar fracture rates with HRT compared with no HRT.[46] We found no observational studies that detected an increased risk of fracture with HRT. Several observational studies found that only 8–20% of women continued HRT for at least 3 years.[47,48]

GLOSSARY

Environmental manipulation This involves the restructuring of a person's environment to remove hazards and reduce the risk of falling or of a fall resulting in fracture.

Substantive changes

Alendronate One systematic review added;[7] conclusions unchanged.

Risedronate One systematic review added;[12] risedronate recategorised as Beneficial.

Calcium versus placebo One systematic review added;[15] conclusions unchanged.

Vitamin D3 One RCT added;[18] conclusions unchanged.

Standard or hydroxylated vitamin D alone or with calcium versus control (placebo or calcium) One systematic review added;[20] calcium plus vitamin D recategorised as Likely to be beneficial.

Calcitonin One systematic review added;[21] recategorised as Likely to be beneficial.

Hip protectors Two RCTs added;[31,32] recategorised as Likely to be beneficial.

Hormone replacement therapy Two systematic reviews added;[33,34] conclusions unchanged.

Fracture prevention in postmenopausal women

REFERENCES

1. Cooper C. The crippling consequences of fracture and their impact on quality of life. *Am J Med* 1997;103:12–19.
2. Grady D, Rubin S, Petitti D, et al. Hormone therapy to prevent disease and prolong life in postmenopausal women. *Ann Intern Med* 1992;117:1016–1037.
3. Riggs BL, Melton LJ. Involutional osteoporosis. *N Engl J Med* 1986;314:1676–1686.
4. Kiel DP, Felson DT, Andresson JJ, et al. Hip fracture and the use of estrogens in postmenopausal women. *N Engl J Med* 1987;317:1169–1174.
5. Leidig-Bruckner G, Minne HW, Schlaich C, et al. Clinical grading of spinal osteoporosis: quality of life components and spinal deformity in women with chronic low back pain and women with vertebral osteoporosis. *J Bone Miner Res* 1997;12:663–675.
6. Reginster JY, Jones EA, Kaufman JM, et al (on behalf of the GREES). Recommendations for the registration of new chemical entities used in the prevention and treatment of osteoporosis. *Calcif Tissue Int* 1995;57:247–250.
7. Cranney A, Wells G, Willan A, et al. II. Meta-analysis of alendronate for the treatment of postmenopausal women. *Endocr Rev* 2002;23:508–516. Search date 1999; primary sources Medline, Embase, Current Contents, the Cochrane Controlled trials registry, citations of relevant articles, and the proceedings of international meetings.
8. Arboleya LR, Morales A, Fiter J. Effect of alendronate on bone mineral density and incidence of fractures in postmenopausal women with osteoporosis. A meta-analysis of published studies. *Med Clin* 2000;114:79–84. Search date 1998; primary sources Medline and Embase.
9. Crannney A, Welch V, Adachi JD, et al. Etidronate for treating and preventing postmenopausal osteoporosis. In: The Cochrane Library, Issue 2, 2003. Oxford: Update Software. Search date 1998; primary sources Medline, Healthstar, Embase, Current Contents, hand searches of conference abstracts, citations of relevant articles, the proceedings of international osteoporosis meetings, and contact with osteoporosis investigators to identify additional studies, primary authors, and pharmaceutical industry sources for unpublished data.
10. Brumsen C, Papapoulos SE, Lips P, et al. Daily oral pamidronate in women and men with osteoporosis: a 3-year randomized placebo-controlled clinical trial with a 2-year open extension. *J Bone Miner Res* 2002;17:1057–1064.
11. Reid IR, Wattie DJ, Evans MC, et al. Continuous therapy with pamidronate, a potent bisphosphonate, in postmenopausal osteoporosis. *J Clin Endocrinol Metab* 1994;79:1595–1599.
12. Cranney A, Tugwell P, Adachi J, et al. III. Meta-analysis of risedronate for the treatment of postmenopausal osteoporosis. *Endocr Rev* 2002;23:517–523. Search date 2000; primary sources Medline, citations of relevant articles, and the proceedings of international osteoporosis meetings.
13. Black DM, Cummings SR, Karpf DB, et al. Randomised trial of the effect of alendronate on the risk of fracture in women with existing vertebral fractures. *Lancet* 1996;348:1535–1541.
14. Lanza F, Schwartz H, Sahba B, et al. An endoscopic comparison of the effects of alendronate and risedronate on upper gastrointestinal mucosae. *Am J Gastroenterol* 2000;95:3112–3117.
15. Shea B, Wells G, Cranney A, et al. VII. Meta-analysis of calcium supplementation for the prevention of postmenopausal osteoporosis. *Endocr Rev* 2002;23:552–559. Search date 1998; primary sources Medline, Embase, the Cochrane Controlled Register, citations of relevant articles, proceedings of international meetings, contact with osteoporosis investigators and primary authors.
16. Gillespsie WJ, Avenell A, Henry DA, et al. Vitamin D and vitamin D analogues for preventing fractures associated with involutional and post-menopausal osteoporosis. In: The Cochrane Library, Issue 2, 2003. Oxford: Update Software. Search date 2000; primary sources Medline, Embase, Cinahl, Lilacs, Cabnar, Biosis, Healthstar, Current Contents, The Cochrane Database of Systematic Reviews, the Cochrane Musculoskeletal Injuries Group trials register, and bibliographies of identified trials and reviews.
17. Meyer HE, Smedshaug GB, Kvaavik E, et al. Can vitamin D supplementation reduce the risk of fracture in the elderly? A randomized controlled trial. *J Bone Miner Res* 2002;17:709–715.
18. Trivedi DP, Doll R, Khaw KT. Effect of four monthly oral vitamin D3 (cholecalciferol) supplementation on fractures and mortality in men and women living in the community: randomised double blind controlled trial. *BMJ* 2003;326:469–472.
19. Chapuy MC, Pamphile R, Paris E, et al. Combined calcium and vitamin D3 supplementation in elderly women: confirmation of reversal of secondary hyperparathyroidism and hip fracture risk: the Decalyos II study. *Osteoporos Int* 2002;13:257–264.
20. Papadimitropoulos E, Wells G, Shea B, et al. VIII: Meta-analysis of the efficacy of vitamin D treatment in preventing osteoporosis in postmenopausal women. *Endocr Rev* 2002;23:560–569. Search date 1999; primary sources Medline, Embase, citations of relevant articles, proceedings of international meetings, contact with osteoporosis investigators and primary authors
21. Cranney A, Tugwell P, Zytaruk N, et al. VI. Meta-analysis of calcitonin for the treatment of postmenopausal osteoporosis. *Endocr Rev* 2002;23:540–551. Search date 2000; primary sources Medline, Embase, citations of relevant articles, proceedings of international osteoporosis meetings, contact with osteoporosis investigators and primary authors.
22. Kanis JA, McCloskey EV. Effect of calcitonin on vertebral and other fractures. *QJM* 1999;92:143–149. Search date 1996; primary sources Medline, conference proceedings, and reference lists of various review articles and books.
23. Vetter NJ, Lewis PA, Ford D. Can health visitors prevent fractures in elderly people? *BMJ* 1992;304:888–890.
24. Jensen J, Lundin-Olsen L, Nyberg L, et al. Fall and injury prevention in older people living in residential care facilities. *Ann Intern Med* 2002;136:733–741.
25. Gillespie LD, Gillespie WJ, Robertson MC, et al. Interventions for preventing falls in elderly people. In: The Cochrane Library, Issue 2, 2003. Oxford: Update Software. Search date 2001; primary sources Cochrane Musculoskeletal Group specialised register, Cochrane Controlled Trials Register, Medline, Embase, Cinahl, The National

Research Register, Current Controlled Trials, reference lists of articles, and contact with researchers in the field.

26. Sinaki M, Itol E, Wahner HW. Stronger back muscles reduce the incidence of vertebral fractures: a prospective 10 year follow-up of postmenopausal women. *Bone* 2002;30:836–841.
27. Parker MJ, Gillespie LD, Gillespie WJ. Hip protectors for preventing hip fractures in the elderly. In: The Cochrane Library, Issue 2, 2003. Oxford: Update Software. Search date 2000; primary sources the Cochrane Musculoskeletal Injuries Group specialised register, Cochrane Controlled Trials Register, Medline, Embase, Cinahl, and reference lists of relevant articles.
28. Harada A, Mizuno M, Takemura M, et al. Hip fracture prevention trial using hip protectors in Japanese nursing homes. *Osteoporos Int* 2001;12:215–221.
29. Jäntti P, Aho H, Mäki-Jokela P. Turvahousut lonkanseudun murtumien ehkäisyssä. [Protector pants in the prevention of hip fractures.] *Suomen Lääkärilehti* 1996;51:3387–3389.
30. Cameron ID, Venman J, Kurrle SE, et al. Hip protectors in aged-care facilities: a randomized trial of use by individual higher-risk residents. *Age Ageing* 2001;30:477–481.
31. Meyer G, Warnke A, Bender R, et al. Effect on hip fractures of increased use of hip protectors in nursing homes: cluster randomised controlled trial. *BMJ* 2003;326:76–80.
32. van Schoor NM, Smit JH, Twisk JWR, et al. Prevention of hip fractures by external hip protectors: a randomised controlled trial. *JAMA* 2003;289:1957–1962.
33. Torgerson DJ, Bell-Syer SEM. Hormone replacement therapy and prevention of vertebral fractures: a meta-analysis of randomised trials. *BMC Musculoskelet Disord* 2001;2:7. Search date 2001; primary sources Medline, Embase, Science Citation Index, Cochrane Controlled Trials Register, reference lists of systematic reviews, and contact with authors, researchers in the field, and pharmaceutical companies.
34. Wells G, Tugwell P, Shea B, et al. V. Meta-analysis of the efficacy of hormone replacement therapy in treating and preventing osteoporosis in postmenopausal women. *Endocr Rev* 2002;23:529–539. Search date 1999; primary sources Medline, Embase, the Cochrane Controlled Register, citations of relevant articles, proceedings of international meetings, contact with osteoporosis investigators and primary authors.
35. Writing group for the Women's Health Initiative Investigators. Risk and benefits of estrogen plus progestin in healthy postmenopausal women. Principal results from the Women's Health Initiative randomized controlled trial. *JAMA* 2002;288:321–333.
36. Torgerson DJ, Bell-Syer SEM. Hormone replacement therapy and prevention of nonvertebral fractures. A meta-analysis of randomized trials. *JAMA* 2001;285:2891–2897. Search date 2000; primary sources Medline, Embase, Science Citation Index, Cochrane Controlled Trials Register, reference lists of systematic reviews, and contact with authors, researchers in the field, and pharmaceutical companies.
37. Cauley JA, Black DM, Barrett-Connor, et al. Effects of hormone replacement therapy on clinical fractures and height loss: the heart and estrogen/progestin replacement study (HERS). *Am J Med* 2001;110:442–450.
38. Komulainen M, Kröger H, Tuppurainen M, et al. HRT and vitamin D in prevention of non-vertebral fractures in postmenopausal women; a 5 year randomized trial. *Maturitas* 1998;31:45–54.
39. Ettinger B, Genant H, Cann C. Long-term estrogen replacement therapy prevents bone loss and fractures. *Ann Intern Med* 1985;102:319–324.
40. Maxim P, Ettinger B, Spitalny M. Fracture protection provided by long-term estrogen treatment. *Osteoporos Int* 1995;5:23–29.
41. Kanis J, Johnell O, Gullberg B, et al. Evidence for efficacy of drugs affecting bone metabolism in preventing hip fracture. *BMJ* 1992;305:1124–1128.
42. Cauley J, Seeley D, Ensrud K, et al. Estrogen replacement therapy and fractures in older women. *Ann Intern Med* 1995;122:9–16.
43. Michaëlsson K, Baron J, Farahmand B, et al. Hormone replacement therapy and risk of hip fracture: population based case-control study. *BMJ* 1998;316:1858–1863.
44. Michaëlsson K, Baron J, Johnell O, et al. Variation in the efficacy of hormone replacement therapy in the prevention of hip fracture. *Osteoporos Int* 1998;8:540–546.
45. Nguyen T, Jones G, Sambrook N, et al. Effects of estrogen exposure and reproductive factors on bone mineral density and osteoporotic fractures. *J Clin Endocrin Metab* 1995;80:2709–2714.
46. Kiel D, Baron J, Anderson J, et al. Smoking eliminates the protective effect of oral estrogens on the risk for hip fracture among women. *Ann Intern Med* 1992;116:716–721.
47. Ettinger B, Li D, Lein R. Continuation of postmenopausal hormone replacement therapy: comparison of cyclic versus continuous combined schedules. *Menopause* 1996;3:185–189.
48. Groeneveld F, Bareman F, Barentsen R, et al. Duration of hormonal replacement therapy in general practice: a follow up study. *Maturitas* 1998;29:125–131.

Olivier Bruyere
Research Fellow
WHO Collaborating Center for Public Health Aspects of Osteoarticular Disease
Liege
Belgium

John Edwards
General Practitioner
Wolstanton Medical Centre
Newcastle-under-Lyme
UK

Jean-Yves Reginster
Professor of Epidemiology and Public Health
Bone and Cartilage Metabolism Unit
University of Liege
Liege
Belgium

Competing interests: OB and JE none declared. JR has participated in several preclinical and clinical trials, reviewed and consulted scientific documentation, has been an author of publications, and has chaired and spoken at scientific meetings for the following companies: Asahi, Bayer, Boehringer Ingelheim, Chiesi, Eli Lilly, Hoechst-Marion-Roussel, Hologic, Hybritech, Igea, Johnson & Johnson, Merck Sharp & Dohme, Negma, Organon, Pfizer, Pharmascience, Procter & Gamble Pharmaceuticals, Rotta Research, Sanofi, Servier, SmithKline Beecham, Teva, Therabel, Tosse, Byk, UCB, and Will Pharma.

Herniated lumbar disc

Search date December 2002

Jo Jordan, Tamara Shawver Morgan, and James Weinstein

QUESTIONS

INTERVENTIONS

Covered elsewhere in *Clinical Evidence*
Non-specific acute low back pain, p 1343 and chronic low back pain, p 1359.

See glossary, p 1333

Key Messages

- **Microdiscectomy (as effective as standard discectomy)** We found no RCTs comparing microdiscectomy and conservative treatment. Three RCTs found no significant difference in clinical outcomes between microdiscectomy and standard discectomy. One RCT found no significant difference in satisfaction or pain between video-assisted arthroscopic microdiscectomy and standard discectomy at about 30 months, although postoperative recovery was slower with standard discectomy. We found conflicting evidence on the effects of automated percutaneous discectomy compared with microdiscectomy.
- **Spinal manipulation** One RCT in people with sciatica caused by disc herniation found that after 2 weeks, spinal manipulation increased perceived improvement compared with placebo. A second RCT found no significant difference in improvement between spinal manipulation, manual traction, exercise, and corsets after 1 month. A third RCT found that spinal manipulation significantly increased the proportion of people with improved symptoms compared with traction.
- **Standard discectomy** One RCT found that standard discectomy increased self reported improvement at 1 year, but not at 4 and 10 years, compared with conservative treatment (physiotherapy). Three RCTs found no significant differences in clinical outcomes between standard discectomy and microdiscectomy. Adverse effects were similar with both procedures.

Herniated lumbar disc

- **Advice to stay active** One systematic review of conservative treatments found no RCTs on advice to stay active.
- **Automated percutaneous discectomy** We found no RCTs comparing automated percutaneous discectomy versus either conservative treatment or standard discectomy. We found conflicting evidence on the clinical effects of automated percutaneous discectomy compared with microdiscectomy.
- **Bed rest** One systematic review of conservative treatment found no RCTs on bed rest in people with symptomatic herniated discs.
- **Epidural corticosteroid injections** One systematic review found limited evidence that epidural steroid injections increased global improvement compared with placebo. However, one subsequent RCT found no significant difference between epidural steroid injections plus conservative treatment compared with conservative treatment alone in pain, mobility, or return to work at 6 months.
- **Heat or ice** One systematic review identified no RCTs of heat or ice for sciatica caused by lumbar disc herniation.
- **Massage** One systematic review identified no RCTs of massage in symptomatic lumbar disc herniation.
- **Non-steroidal anti-inflammatory drugs** One systematic review found no significant difference in overall improvement between non-steroidal anti-inflammatory drugs and placebo in people with sciatica caused by disc herniation.
- **Analgesics; antidepressants; laser discectomy; muscle relaxants** We found no systematic review or RCTs on these interventions for treatment of symptomatic herniated lumbar disc.

DEFINITION Herniated lumbar disc is a displacement of disc material (nucleus pulposus or annulus fibrosis) beyond the intervertebral disc space.[1] The diagnosis can be confirmed by radiological examination; however, magnetic resonance imaging findings of herniated disc are not always accompanied by clinical symptoms.[2,3] This review covers treatment of people who have clinical symptoms relating to confirmed or suspected disc herniation. It does not include treatment of people with spinal cord compression or people with cauda equina syndrome (see glossary, p 1333), which often requires emergency intervention. The management of non-specific acute low back pain, p 1343 and chronic low back pain, p 1359 are covered elsewhere in *Clinical Evidence*.

INCIDENCE/ PREVALENCE The prevalence of symptomatic herniated lumbar disc is around 1–3% in Finland and Italy, depending on age and sex.[4] The highest prevalence is among people aged 30–50 years,[5] with a male : female ratio of 2 : 1.[6] In people aged between 25 and 55 years, about 95% of herniated discs occur at the L4–L5 level; in people over 55 years of age, disc herniation is more common above the L4–L5 level.[7,8]

AETIOLOGY/ RISK FACTORS Radiographical evidence of disc herniation does not reliably predict low back pain in the future or correlate with symptoms; 19–27% of people without symptoms have disc herniation on imaging.[2,9] Risk factors for disc herniation include smoking (OR 1.7, 95% CI 1.0 to 2.5), weight bearing sports, and certain work activities such as repeated lifting (lifting objects < 11.3 kg, < 25 times daily while twisting body, knees not bent, OR 7.2, 95% CI 2.0 to 25.8; lifting objects < 11.3 kg, < 25 times daily while twisting body, knees bent, OR 1.9, 95% CI 0.8 to 4.8). Driving motor vehicles is also associated with increased risk (OR 1.7, 95% CI 0.2 to 2.7, depending on the vehicle model).[6,10,11] This may be because the resonant frequency of the spine is similar to that of certain vehicles.

PROGNOSIS The natural history of disc herniation is difficult to determine because most people take some form of treatment for their back pain, and a formal diagnosis is not always made.[6] Clinical improvement is usual in most people, and only about 10% of people still have sufficient pain after 6 weeks to consider surgery. Sequential magnetic resonance images have shown that the herniated portion of the disc tends to regress over time, with partial to complete resolution after 6 months in two thirds of people.[12]

AIMS OF INTERVENTION To relieve pain; increase mobility and function; and improve quality of life.

OUTCOMES **Primary outcomes:** pain, function, or mobility; individuals' perceived overall improvement; quality of life; and adverse effects of treatment. **Secondary outcomes:** return to work; use of analgesia; and duration of hospitalisation.

METHODS *Clinical Evidence* search and appraisal December 2002. The authors searched AMED and PEDro in January 2003.

QUESTION What are the effects of oral drug treatments?

OPTION NON-STEROIDAL ANTI-INFLAMMATORY DRUGS

One systematic review found no significant difference in overall improvement between non-steroidal anti-inflammatory drugs and placebo in people with sciatica caused by disc herniation.

Benefits: **Versus placebo:** We found one systematic review of medical treatments for sciatica caused by disc herniation (search date 1998, 3 RCTs, 321 people).[13] The RCTs compared non-steroidal anti-inflammatory drugs (NSAIDs) (piroxicam 40 mg daily for 2 days or 20 mg daily for 12 days; indometacin [indomethacin] 75–100 mg 3 times daily; phenylbutazone 1200 mg daily for 3 days or 600 mg daily for 2 days) versus placebo. The review found no significant difference between NSAIDs and placebo in global improvement at 5–30 days (pooled AR for improvement in pain 80/172 [46.5%] *v* 57/149 [38.3%]; OR for global improvement 0.99, 95% CI 0.6 to 1.7; see comment below).

Harms: The systematic review did not report the adverse effects of NSAIDs. NSAIDs may cause gastrointestinal complications (see NSAIDs topic, p 1393).

Comment: The absolute numbers in the RCTs relate to the outcomes of improvement in pain (3 RCTs) and return to work (1 RCT).[13] However, the meta-analysis used the outcome measure of global improvement. The relationship between these measures is unclear.

OPTION ANALGESICS

We found no systematic review or RCTs of analgesics to treat symptomatic herniated lumbar disc.

Benefits: We found no systematic review or RCTs.

Harms: We found no systematic review or RCTs.

Comment: None.

OPTION ANTIDEPRESSANTS

We found no systematic review or RCTs of antidepressants to treat symptomatic herniated lumbar disc.

Benefits: We found no systematic review or RCTs.

Harms: We found no systematic review or RCTs.

Comment: None.

OPTION MUSCLE RELAXANTS

We found no systematic review or RCTs of muscle relaxants to treat herniated lumbar disc.

Benefits: We found no systematic review or RCTs that assessed the effectiveness of muscle relaxants in people with herniated lumbar disc.

Harms: We found no systematic review or RCTs.

Comment: None.

OPTION EPIDURAL CORTICOSTEROID INJECTIONS

One systematic review found limited evidence that epidural steroid injections increased global improvement compared with placebo. One subsequent RCT found no significant difference between epidural steroid injections plus conservative treatment compared with conservative treatment alone in pain, mobility, or return to work at 6 months.

Benefits: We found one systematic review of medical treatments for sciatica caused by disc herniation (search date 1998, 4 RCTs of epidural steroids, 265 people)[13] and one subsequent RCT.[14] The review compared four different doses of epidural steroid injections (8 mL methylprednisolone 80 mg; 2 mL methylprednisolone 80 mg; 10 mL methylprednisolone 80 mg; and 2 mL methylprednisolone acetate 80 mg) versus placebo (saline or lidocaine [lignocaine] 2 mL) after follow up periods of 2, 21, and 30 days.[13] The review found limited evidence that epidural steroids increased participant perceived global improvement (which was not defined) compared with placebo. The result was of borderline significance (73/160 [45.6%] with steroid *v* 56/172 [32.5%] with placebo; OR 2.2, 95% CI 1.0 to 4.7). The subsequent RCT (36 people with disc herniation confirmed by magnetic resonance imaging) compared epidural steroids (3 injections of methylprednisolone 100 mg in 10 mL bupivacaine 0.25% during the first 14 days of hospitalisation) plus conservative non-operative treatment versus conservative treatment alone.[14] Conservative treatment involved initial bed rest and analgesia followed by graded rehabilitation (hydrotherapy, electroanalgesia, postural exercise classes) followed by physiotherapy. It found no significant difference in mean pain scores at 6 weeks and 6 months measured on a visual analogue scale (at 6 months, 32.9 [range 0–85] with steroids *v* 39.2 [range 0–100] with conservative treatment). There were no significant differences in mean mobility scores (Hannover Functional Ability Questionnaire: 61.8 [range 25–88] with steroids *v* 57.2 [range 13–100]), in the number of people who had back surgery (2/17 [12%] with steroids *v* 4/19 [21%]; RR 0.56, 95% CI 0.09 to 2.17), or in people returning to work within 6 months (15/17 [88%] with steroids *v* 14/19 [74%]; RR 1.19, 95% CI 0.75 to 1.33).

Harms: No serious adverse effects were reported in the RCTs included in the systematic review, although 26 people complained of transient headache or transient increase in sciatic pain.[13] The subsequent RCT did not report adverse effects of epidural injections.[14]

Comment: None.

QUESTION What are the effects of non-drug treatments?

OPTION BED REST

One systematic review of conservative treatment found no RCTs of bed rest for symptomatic herniated discs.

Benefits: We found one systematic review (search date 1998) of conservative treatments for sciatica caused by disc herniation, which identified no RCTs of bed rest for treatment of symptomatic herniated discs.[13] We found no subsequent RCTs.

Harms: We found no systematic review or RCTs.

Comment: None.

OPTION ADVICE TO STAY ACTIVE

One systematic review of conservative treatments for sciatica caused by lumbar disc herniation found no RCTs of advice to stay active.

Benefits: We found one systematic review (search date 1998) of conservative treatments for sciatica caused by disc herniation, which found no RCTs of advice to stay active.[13] We found no subsequent RCTs.

Harms: We found no RCTs.

Comment: None.

OPTION MASSAGE

One systematic review identified no RCTs of massage in people with symptomatic lumbar disc herniation.

Benefits: We found one systematic review (search date 1998) of conservative treatments for sciatica caused by disc herniation, which found no RCTs of massage.[13] We found no subsequent RCTs.

Harms: We found no systematic review or RCTs.

Comment: None.

OPTION HEAT AND ICE

One systematic review identified no RCTs of heat or ice for sciatica caused by lumbar disc herniation.

Benefits: We found one systematic review (search date 1998) of conservative treatments for sciatica caused by disc herniation, which identified no RCTs on the use of heat or ice for herniated lumbar discs.[13] We found no subsequent RCTs.

Harms: We found no systematic review or RCTs.

Comment: None.

OPTION SPINAL MANIPULATION

One RCT in people with sciatica caused by disc herniation found that after 2 weeks, spinal manipulation increased perceived improvement compared with a placebo of infrequent infrared heat. A second RCT found no significant difference in improvement between spinal manipulation, manual traction, exercise, and corsets after 1 month. A third RCT found that spinal manipulation significantly increased the proportion of people with improved symptoms compared with traction.

Benefits: We found two systematic reviews[13,15] and one subsequent RCT.[16] The first systematic review (search date 1998), which did not perform meta-analysis, identified two RCTs of spinal manipulation for sciatica caused by disc herniation.[13] The second systematic review (search date not stated) identified no RCTs.[15] The first RCT (207 people) included in the review compared spinal manipulation (every day if necessary) versus placebo (infrared heat 3 times weekly).[13] It found that spinal manipulation increased overall self-perceived improvement at 2 weeks compared with placebo (98/123 [80%] *v* 56/84 [67%]; RR 1.19, 95% CI 1.01 to 1.32; NNT 8, 95% CI 5 to 109).[13] The second included RCT (322 people) compared four interventions: spinal manipulation, manual traction, exercise, and corsets, in a factorial design.[13] It found no significant difference among treatments in overall self-perceived improvement after 28 days (quantified results not available). The subsequent RCT (112 people with symptomatic herniated lumbar disc) compared pulling and turning manipulation versus traction.[16] It found that significantly more people were "improved" (absence of lumbar pain, improvement in lumbar functional movement) or "cured" (absence of lumbar pain, straight leg raising of > 70°, ability to return to work) with spinal manipulation compared with traction (54/62 [87.1%] with manipulation *v* 33/50 [66%] with traction; RR 1.32, 95% CI 1.06 to 1.65; NNT 5, 95% CI 4 to 16; timescale not stated).

Harms: The first systematic review did not report adverse effects.[13] The second systematic review identified one review of 135 case reports of serious complications after spinal manipulation published between 1950 and 1980.[15] However, the frequency of these effects was not certain. The case review attributed these complications to cervical manipulation, misdiagnosis, presence of coagulation dyscrasias, presence of herniated nucleus pulposus, or improper techniques. The subsequent RCT found that two out of 60 people receiving traction had syncope; no adverse effects were reported in people receiving manipulation.[16] We found a third systematic review (search date 2001, 5 prospective observational studies).[17] The largest study included in the review (4712 treatments in 1058 people undergoing both cervical and lumbar spinal manipulations) found that the most common reaction was local discomfort (53%), followed by headache (12%); tiredness (11%); radiating discomfort (10%); dizziness (5%); nausea (4%); hot skin (2%); and other complaints (2%). The incidence of serious adverse effects is reported as rare, and is estimated from published case series and reports to occur in one in 1–2 million treatments. The most common of these serious effects were cerebrovascular accidents (the total number of people undergoing manipulations was not reported and the rate of this adverse effect cannot be estimated). However, it is difficult to assess whether such events are directly related to treatment

Comment: In the third review, which examined risks, the percentages include both cervical and lumbar spinal manipulations, which may overestimate the effect of lumbar spinal manipulations.[17] The authors of the review advise caution in interpreting these results, as they are speculative and based on assumptions about the numbers of manipulations performed and unreported cases. More reliable data are needed on the incidence of specific risks.

QUESTION What are the effects of surgery?

OPTION STANDARD DISCECTOMY

One RCT found that standard discectomy increased self reported improvement at 1 year, but not at 4 and 10 years, compared with conservative treatment (physiotherapy). Three RCTs found no significant differences in clinical outcomes between standard discectomy and microdiscectomy. Adverse effects were similar with both procedures.

Benefits: **Versus conservative treatment:** Two systematic reviews (search dates 1997[18] and not stated[19]) included the same RCT (126 people with symptomatic L5/S1 disc herniation), which compared standard discectomy (see glossary, p 1333) versus conservative treatment (6 weeks of physiotherapy).[20] Each participant assessed and graded their improvement in terms of pain and function into four categories: "good" (completely satisfied), "fair", "poor", and "bad" (completely incapacitated for work because of pain). The RCT found that discectomy significantly increased the number of people reporting their improvement as "good" after 1 year compared with conservative treatment (intention to treat analysis: 39/60 [65%]

with surgery *v* 24/66 [36.4%] with conservative treatment; RR 1.79, 95% CI 1.30 to 2.18; NNT 3, 95% CI 2 to 9). However, at 4 and 10 years, there was no significant difference in the same outcome (at 4 years, AR for "good" improvement: 40/60 [66.7%] with surgery *v* 34/66 [51.5%] with conservative treatment; RR 1.29, 95% CI 0.96 to 1.56; at 10 years: 35/60 [58.3%] *v* 37/66 [56.1%]; RR 1.04, 95% CI 0.73 to 1.32). **Versus microdiscectomy:** One systematic review (search date 1997) identified three RCTs (219 people) comparing standard discectomy versus microdiscectomy (see glossary, p 1333).[18] Meta-analysis was not performed because outcomes were not comparable. The first RCT in the review (60 people with lumbar disc herniation) found no significant difference between standard discectomy and microdiscectomy in the number of people who rated their operative outcome as "good", "almost recovered", or "totally recovered" at 1 year (intention to treat analysis: 26/30 [87%] with standard discectomy *v* 24/30 [80%] with microdiscectomy; RR 1.08, 95% CI 0.78 to 1.20).[21] There was also no difference between treatments in the change in preoperative and postoperative pain scores (visual analogue scale; P value not provided) or in the duration of time taken to return to work (both 10 weeks). The second RCT in the review (79 people with lumbar disc herniation) also found no significant differences between microdiscectomy and standard discectomy in pain in the legs or back (visual analogue scale, not specified) or in analgesia use at any point during the 6 week follow up (absolute numbers not provided).[22] The third RCT (80 people) also found that clinical outcomes and duration of sick leave were similar at 15 months, but the review did not provide further details.[18]

Harms: **Versus conservative treatment:** The RCT included in both systematic reviews did not report on complications of standard discectomy.[20] **Versus microdiscectomy:** One systematic review reported that there was no significant difference between standard discectomy and microdiscectomy in perioperative bleeding, duration of stay, or scar tissue (numbers not provided).[18] The first RCT included in the review reported one person in each group with a nerve root tear and, of the people undergoing microdiscectomy, one had a dural leak and one had suspected discitis.[21] The second RCT included in the review did not report on the complications of either procedure.[22] Complication rates were reported inconsistently in studies, making it difficult to combine results to produce overall rates. Rates of complications for all types of discectomy have been compiled (see table 1, p 1335).[19]

Comment: The RCT of standard discectomy versus conservative treatment had considerable crossover between the two treatment groups. Of 66 people randomised to receive conservative treatment, 17 received surgery; of 60 people randomised to receive surgery, one refused the operation.[20] The results presented above are based on an intention to treat analysis. One systematic review of published reports (search date not stated) found 99 cases of vascular complications following lumbar disc surgery since 1965.[23] Reported risk factors for vascular complications included: previous disc or abdominal surgery leaving adhesions; chronic disc pathology from disruption or degeneration of anterior annulus fibrosus and anterior longitudinal ligament or peridiscal fibrosis; improper positioning of the patient; retroperitoneal vessels and operated disc in close proximity; and vertebral anomalies, such as hypertrophic spurs compressing vessels during operation. The systematic review did not state out of how many operations the 99 complications arose from, therefore we can not estimate the incidence of adverse vascular events from discectomy.[23]

OPTION MICRODISCECTOMY

We found no RCTs comparing microdiscectomy and conservative treatment. Three RCTs found no significant difference in clinical outcomes between microdiscectomy and standard discectomy. One RCT found no significant difference in self reported satisfaction or pain score between video-assisted arthroscopic microdiscectomy and standard discectomy after about 30 months, although postoperative recovery was slower with standard discectomy. We found conflicting evidence on the effects of automated percutaneous discectomy compared with microdiscectomy.

Benefits: We found no systematic review. **Versus conservative treatment:** We found no RCTs. **Versus standard discectomy:** See benefits of standard discectomy, p 1329. (See glossary, p 1333). **Video-assisted arthroscopic microdiscectomy versus standard discectomy:** We found one RCT (60 people with proven lumbar disc herniation and associated radiculopathy after failed conservative treatment).[24] It found no significant difference between video-assisted arthroscopic discectomy and standard discectomy in the number of people who were "very satisfied" on a 4 point satisfaction scale after about 31 months (22/30 [73%] with microdiscectomy [see glossary, p 1333] *v* 20/30 [67%] with standard discectomy; RR 1.10, 95% CI 0.71 to 1.34). There was also no significant difference in mean pain score (visual analogue scale from 0 [no pain] to 10 [severe and incapacitating pain]: 1.9 with standard discectomy *v* 1.2 with microdiscectomy). However, the mean duration of postoperative recovery was almost twice as long with open surgery as with microdiscectomy (49 days *v* 27 days; P value not stated). **Versus automated percutaneous discectomy:** See benefits of automated percutaneous discectomy, p 1332. (See glossary, p 1333).

Harms: **Video-assisted arthroscopic microdiscectomy versus open discectomy:** The RCT reported that one person undergoing open discectomy had leakage of spinal fluid from the dural sac 2 weeks after the operation.[24] No other postoperative complications or neurovascular injuries were observed in either the standard discectomy or the microdiscectomy groups. Complication rates were reported inconsistently in studies, making it difficult to combine results to produce overall rates. Rates of complications for all types of discectomy have been compiled (see table 1, p 1335).[19]

Comment: None.

OPTION AUTOMATED PERCUTANEOUS DISCECTOMY

We found no RCTs comparing automated percutaneous discectomy with either conservative treatment or standard discectomy. We found conflicting evidence on the clinical effects of automated percutaneous discectomy compared with microdiscectomy.

Benefits: **Versus conservative treatment:** We found no systematic review or RCTs. **Versus standard discectomy:** One systematic review (search date not stated) identified no RCTs comparing automated percutaneous discectomy (APD) versus standard discectomy (see glossary, p 1333).[19] **Versus microdiscectomy:** One systematic review (search date 1997) identified two RCTs that were not directly comparable because there were differences in the equipment used.[18] One RCT (71 people with radiographical confirmation of disc herniation) was stopped prematurely, after an interim analysis at 6 months found that APD was associated with significantly lower success rate than microdiscectomy (see glossary, p 1333) (overall outcome was classified as "success" or "failure" by the clinician and a masked observer [details not stated]: 9/31 [29%] with APD *v* 32/40 [80%] with microdisectomy; $P < 0.001$; CI not provided).[25] However, the other RCT (40 people with radiographical confirmation of disc herniation) reported similar improvements in the composite clinical score with APD versus microdiscectomy (scale 0–10, including back and leg pain, and sensory and motor deficit) at 2 years (preoperative scores: 4.55 with APD *v* 4.2 in microdiscectomy group; scores at 2 years: 8.23 with APD *v* 7.67 with microdiscectomy).[26] More people in the APD group rated their surgical outcomes as "excellent" or "good" than did those in the microdiscectomy group 2 years after surgery (14/20 [70%] with APD *v* 11/20 [55%] with microdiscectomy; $P = 0.33$).

Harms: The systematic review found that reoperations for recurrent or persistent disc herniations at the same level as the initial operations were reported more frequently with APD compared with either microdiscectomy or standard discectomy (APD 83%, 95% CI 76% to 88% *v* microdiscectomy 64%, 95% CI 48% to 78% *v* standard discectomy 49%, 95% CI 38% to 60%).[19] The first RCT did not report adverse effects.[25] The second RCT reported that no complications had occurred with APD, but did not comment on whether there had been any complications in the microdiscectomy group.[26] The mean duration of postoperative recovery was longer in people who had microdiscectomy compared with those who underwent APD (mean weeks of postoperative recovery [range]: 22.9 weeks [4 weeks to 1 year] for the microdiscectomy group *v* 7.7 weeks [1–26 weeks] for APD). Complication rates were reported inconsistently in studies, making it difficult to combine results to produce overall rates. Rates of complications for all types of discectomy have been compiled (see table 1, p 1335).[19]

Comment: None.

OPTION LASER DISCECTOMY

Systematic reviews found no RCTs on the effects of laser discectomy on disc herniations.

Benefits: Three systematic reviews (search dates 1997,[18] not stated,[19] and 2000[27]) found no RCTs on the effectiveness of laser discectomy.

Harms: We found no RCTs.

Comment: None.

GLOSSARY

Automated percutaneous discectomy Techniques using minimal skin incisions (generally several, all less than 3–5 mm) to allow small instruments to be inserted, using radiography to visualise these instruments, and using extensions for the surgeon to reach the operative site without having to dissect tissues.
Cauda equina A collection of spinal roots descending from the lower part of the spinal cord, which occupy the vertebral canal below the spinal cord.
Cauda equina syndrome Compression of the cauda equina causing symptoms, including changes in perineal sensation (saddle anaesthesia), and loss of sphincter control.
Laser discectomy The surgeon places a laser through a delivery device that has been directed under radiographic control to the disc, and removes the disc material using the laser. It uses many of the same techniques used in automated percutaneous discectomy.
Microdiscectomy Removal of protruding disc material, using an operating microscope to guide surgery.
Standard discectomy Surgical removal, in part or whole, of an intervertebral disc, generally with loop magnification (i.e. eyepieces).

Substantive changes

Spinal manipulation One systematic review added;[17] conclusions unchanged.

REFERENCES

1. Fardon DF, Milette PC. Nomenclature and classification of lumbar disc pathology: recommendations of the Combined Task Forces of the North American Spine Society, American Society of Spine Radiology, and American Society of Neuroradiology. *Spine* 2001;26:E93–E113.
2. Boden SD. The use of radiographic imaging studies in the evaluation of patients who have degenerative disorders of the lumbar spine. *J Bone Joint Surg Am* 1996; 78:114–125.
3. Borenstein DG, O'Mara JW Jr, Boden SD, et al. The value of magnetic resonance imaging of the lumbar spine to predict low-back pain in asymptomatic subjects. *J Bone Joint Surg Am* 2001;83-A(9):1306–1311.
4. Andersson G. Epidemiology of spinal disorders. In: Frymoyer JW, Ducker TB, Hadler NM, et al. eds. *The adult spine: principles and practice*. New York, NY: Raven Press, 1997:93–141.
5. Heliovaara M. *Epidemiology of sciatica and herniated lumbar intervertebral disc*. Helsinki, Finland: The Social Insurance Institution, 1988.
6. Postacchini F, Cinotti G. Etiopathogenesis. In: Postacchini F, ed. *Lumbar disc herniation*. New York: Spring-Verlag/Wien, 1999.
7. Friberg S, Hirsch C. Anatomical and clinical studies on lumbar disc degeneration. *Acta Orthop Scand* 1949;19:222–242.
8. Schultz A, Andersson G, Ortengren R, et al. Loads on the lumbar spine. *J Bone Joint Surg Am* 1982;64:713–720.
9. Jensen MC, Brant-Zawadzki MN, Obuchowski N, et al. Magnetic resonance imaging of the lumbar spine in people without back pain. *N Engl J Med* 1994;331:69–73.
10. Kelsey JL, Githens P, O'Connor T, et al. Acute prolapsed lumbar intervertebral disc: an epidemiologic study with special reference to driving automobiles and cigarette smoking. *Spine* 1984;9:608–613.
11. Pedrini-Mille A, Weinstein JN, Found ME, et al. Stimulation of dorsal root ganglia and degradation of rabbit annulus fibrosus. *Spine* 1990;15:1252–1256.
12. Deyo RA, Weinstein JN. Low back pain. *N Engl J Med* 2001;344:365–370.
13. Vroomen PC, de Krom MC, Slofstra PD, et al. Conservative treatment of sciatica: a systematic review. *J Spinal Disord* 2000;13:463–469. Search date 1998; primary sources Medline and Embase/Excerpta Medica.
14. Buchner M, Zeifang F, Brocai DR, et al. Epidural corticosteroid injection in the conservative management of sciatica. *Clin Orthop* 2000;375:149–156.
15. Shekelle PG, Adams AH, Chassin MR, et al. Spinal manipulation for low-back pain. *Ann Intern Med* 1992;117:590–598. Search date not stated; primary sources Medline and Index Medicus 1952 onwards, reference lists, and consulted experts.
16. Liu J, Zhang S. Treatment of protrusion of lumbar intervertebral disc by pulling and turning manipulations. *J Tradit Chin Med* 2000;20:195–197.
17. Stevinson C, Ernst E. Risks associated with spinal manipulation. *Am J Med* 2002;112:566–570. Search date 2001; primary sources Medline, Embase, Cochrane Library, authors' files, experts consulted, and reference lists.
18. Gibson JN, Grant IC, Waddell G. Surgery for lumbar disc prolapse. In: The Cochrane Library,

Issue 1, 2002. Oxford: Update Software. Search date 1997; primary sources Medline, Embase, Biosis, dissertation abstracts, Index to UK Theses, Cochrane Controlled Trials Register, reference lists, personal bibliographies, and hand searched *Spine* 1975–1997.

19. Hoffman RM, Wheeler KJ, Deyo RA. Surgery for herniated lumbar discs: a literature synthesis. *J Gen Intern Med* 1993;8:487–496. Search date not stated; primary sources Medline, reference lists, book bibliographies, and colleagues' files.
20. Weber H. Lumbar disc herniation: a controlled, prospective study with ten years of observation. *Spine* 1983;8:131–140.
21. Tullberg T, Isacson J, Weidenhielm L. Does microscopic removal of lumber disc herniation lead to better results than the standard procedure? Results of a one-year randomized study. *Spine* 1993;18:24–27.
22. Henriksen L, Schmidt V, Eskesen V, et al. A controlled study of microsurgery versus standard lumbar discectomy. *Br J Neurosurg* 1996;10:289–293.
23. Papadoulas S, Konstantinou D, Kourea HP, et al. Vascular injury complicating lumbar disc surgery. A systematic review. *Eur J Vasc Endovasc Surg* 2002;24:189–195. Search date not stated; primary source Medline 1965 onwards.
24. Hermantin FU, Peters T, Quartararo L, et al. A prospective, randomized study comparing the results of open discectomy with those of video-assisted arthroscopic microdiscectomy. *J Bone Joint Surg Am* 1999;81:958–965.
25. Chatterjee S, Foy PM, Findlay GF. Report of a controlled clinical trial comparing automated percutaneous lumbar discectomy and microdiscectomy in the treatment of contained lumbar disc herniation. *Spine* 1995;20:734–738.
26. Mayer HM, Brock M. Percutaneous endoscopic discectomy: surgical technique and preliminary results compared to microdiscectomy. *J Neurosurg* 1993;78:216–225.
27. Boult M, Fraser RD, Jones N, et al. Percutaneous endoscopic laser discectomy. *Aust N Z J Surg* 2000;70:475–479. Search date 2000; primary sources Medline, Current Contents, Embase, and The Cochrane Library.

Jo Jordan
Systematic Reviewer
The Chartered Society of Physiotherapy
London
UK

Tamara Shawver Morgan
Research Associate
Dartmouth Medical School
Hanover, NH
USA

James Weinstein
Chair of Orthopaedics, Dartmouth Medical School; Director, The Spine Center and the Center for Shared Decision-Making, Dartmouth-Hitchcock Medical Center; Co-Director, Dartmouth Clinical Trials Center
Dartmouth Medical School
Hanover, NH
USA

Competing interests: None declared.

TABLE 1 Reported complications from surgical procedures (see text, p 1330).[19]

Complications	Standard discectomy		Microdiscectomy		Percutaneous discectomy	
	Mean (% [95% CI])	Studies (n)*	Mean (% [95% CI])	Studies (n)*	Mean (% [95% CI])	Studies (n)*
Operative mortality	0.15 (0.09–0.24)	25	0.06 (0.01–0.42)	8	–	3
Total wound infections	1.97 (1.97–2.93)	25	1.77 (0.92–3.37)	16	–	2
Deep wound infections	0.34 (0.23–0.50)	17	0.06 (0.01–0.23)	8	–	2
Discitis	1.39 (0.97–2.01)	25	0.67 (0.44–1.02)	20	1.43 (0.42–4.78)	8
Dural tear	3.65 (1.99–6.65)	17	3.67 (2.03–6.58)	16	0.00	2
Total nerve root injuries	3.45 (2.21–5.36)	8	0.84 (0.24–2.92)	12	0.30 (0.11–0.79)	6
Permanent nerve root injuries	0.78 (0.42–1.45)	10	0.06 (0.00–0.26)	8	–	6
Thrombophlebitis	1.55 (0.78–1.30)	13	0.82 (0.49–1.35)	4	Not reported	0
Pulmonary emboli	0.56 (0.29–1.07)	14	0.44 (0.20–0.98)	5	Not reported	0
Meningitis	0.30 (0.15–0.60)	5	Not reported	0	Not reported	0
Cauda equina syndrome	0.22 (0.13–0.39)	3	Not reported	0	Not reported	0
Psoas haematoma	Not reported	0	Not reported	0	4.65 (1.17–15.5)	5
Transfusions	0.70 (0.19–2.58)	6	0.17 (0.08–0.39)	11	Not reported	0

*81 studies were included; 2 RCTs, 7 non-randomised controlled trials, 10 case control studies and 62 case series.

Leg cramps

Search date October 2002

Gavin Young

QUESTIONS

INTERVENTIONS

See glossary, p 1341

Key Messages

Idiopathic leg cramps

- **Quinine** One systematic review has found that quinine reduces the frequency of nocturnal leg cramp attacks compared with placebo over 4 weeks.
- **Quinine plus theophylline** One small RCT found limited evidence that quinine plus theophylline reduced the number of nights affected by leg cramps compared with quinine alone over 2 weeks.
- **Analgesics; antiepileptic drugs; compression hosiery** We found no RCTs on the effects of these interventions on idiopathic leg cramps.
- **Vitamin E** One small RCT found no significant difference between vitamin E and placebo in the number of nights disturbed by leg cramps.

Leg cramps in pregnancy

- **Magnesium salts** One systematic review identified one small RCT in pregnant women, which found that magnesium tablets (primarily magnesium lactate, magnesium citrate) reduced leg cramps compared with placebo after 3 weeks.
- **Calcium salts** One systematic review identified two RCTs that compared calcium versus placebo or no treatment, which found conflicting results.

- **Multivitamins and mineral supplements** One systematic review identified one small RCT in pregnant women, which found no significant difference between a multivitamin plus mineral tablet and placebo in leg cramps in the ninth month of pregnancy.
- **Sodium chloride** One systematic review found insufficient evidence about the effects of sodium chloride on leg cramps in pregnancy.

DEFINITION Leg cramps are involuntary, localised, and usually painful skeletal muscle contractions, which commonly affect calf muscles. Leg cramps typically occur at night and usually last only seconds to minutes. Leg cramps may be idiopathic (see glossary, p 1341) or related to a definable process or disease such as pregnancy, renal dialysis, or venous insufficiency.

INCIDENCE/ PREVALENCE Leg cramps are common and their incidence increases with age. About half of the people attending a general medicine clinic have had leg cramps within 1 month of their visit, and over two thirds of people over 50 years of age have experienced leg cramps.[1]

AETIOLOGY/ RISK FACTORS Very little is known about the causes of leg cramps. Risk factors include pregnancy, exercise, salt depletion, renal dialysis, electrolyte imbalances, peripheral vascular disease (both venous and arterial), peripheral nerve injury, polyneuropathies, motor neuron disease, muscle diseases, and certain drugs. Other causes of calf pain include trauma, deep venous thrombosis (see thromboembolism, p 273), and ruptured Baker's cyst (see glossary, p 1341).

PROGNOSIS Leg cramps may cause severe pain and sleep disturbance, both of which are distressing.

AIMS OF INTERVENTION To reduce the number and the severity of attacks of cramp, with minimal adverse effects of treatment.

OUTCOMES Number of attacks; severity of attacks; number of disturbed nights.

METHODS *Clinical Evidence* search and appraisal October 2002.

QUESTION What are the effects of treatments for idiopathic leg cramps?

OPTION COMPRESSION HOSIERY

We found no RCTs on the effects of compression hosiery in people with idiopathic leg cramps.

Benefits: We found no systematic review or RCTs.

Harms: We found no evidence on harms related to compression hosiery in people with idiopathic leg cramps (see glossary, p 1341) (see compression under prevention and treatment of venous leg ulcers, p 2225).

Comment: None.

OPTION QUININE

One systematic review has found that quinine reduces the frequency of nocturnal leg cramps compared with placebo over 4 weeks.

Benefits: We found one systematic review (search date 1997, 8 RCTs, 659 people).[2] Meta-analysis found that quinine significantly reduced the frequency of nocturnal leg cramps compared with placebo over a 4 week period (absolute reduction of 2.90 cramps/month with quinine *v* placebo, 95% CI 0.20 to 5.54; RR not available).

Harms: Adverse effects of quinine include headache, digestive disorders, tinnitus, fever, blurred vision, dizziness, and pruritus.[2] In the systematic review, tinnitus was significantly more common with quinine than placebo (20/659 [3.0%] with quinine *v* 7/659 [1.1%] with placebo; RR 2.86, 95% CI 1.22 to 6.71; NNH 50, 95% CI 27 to 230). Elevated quinine levels may cause cinchonism (see glossary, p 1341) — a syndrome that includes nausea, vomiting, tinnitus, and deafness.[3]

Comment: The systematic review excluded two RCTs because of a lack of individual participant data. Both of these RCTs found that quinine reduced leg cramps compared with placebo. We found no evidence about the optimal dose of quinine or length of treatment.

OPTION QUININE PLUS THEOPHYLLINE

One small RCT found limited evidence that quinine plus theophylline reduced nocturnal leg cramps compared with quinine alone over 2 weeks.

Benefits: We found no systematic review. We found one RCT (164 people), which compared quinine plus theophylline versus quinine alone for 2 weeks.[4] Baseline rates of leg cramp were measured for 1 week before randomisation, when all people received placebo (single blind). Among 126 people who completed at least 4 days' treatment in the 2 week period, quinine plus theophylline was rated as "good" or "very good" significantly more often than quinine alone or placebo (34/39 [87%] with quinine plus theophylline *v* 28/45 [62%] with quinine *v* 17/42 [40%] with placebo; $P < 0.001$ for quinine plus theophylline *v* either comparison; see comment below). After 2 weeks of treatment, theophylline plus quinine significantly reduced the mean number of nights affected by cramp compared with quinine alone (from 4.7 nights to 1.1 nights with theophylline plus quinine *v* from 4.8 nights to 2.2 nights with quinine alone; $P = 0.009$).

Harms: Six people reported adverse effects while taking placebo in the week before randomisation (nausea and vomiting in 2 people, nausea, heartburn, depression, bitter aftertaste). Three people reported adverse effects with quinine (nausea and vomiting, bloating and tenesmus, and nausea alone), resulting in two people withdrawing from the study. Four people had adverse effects with quinine plus theophylline (fall in blood pressure and dizziness, nausea in 2 cases, palpitations and tinnitus) and all four withdrew from the study.

Comment: The results of the RCT should be treated with caution as it did not specify criteria to categorise outcomes as "good" or "very good" and pooled the results only for people who received treatment for at least 4 out of 14 days (126 people out of 164 enrolled) without using an intention to treat analysis.

OPTION **VITAMIN E**

One small RCT found no significant difference between vitamin E and placebo in nocturnal leg cramps.

Benefits: We found no systematic review. We found one crossover RCT (27 men), which compared vitamin E versus placebo.[5] It found no significant difference between treatments in the median number of nights with leg cramps (15 nights with vitamin E *v* 13 nights with placebo; $P > 0.05$).

Harms: Adverse effects were reported as similar in the vitamin E and placebo groups, but no details were provided.[5]

Comment: None.

OPTION **ANALGESICS**

We found no RCTs on the effects of analgesics on idiopathic leg cramps.

Benefits: We found no systematic review or RCTs.

Harms: We found no RCTs.

Comment: None.

OPTION **ANTIEPILEPTIC DRUGS**

We found no RCTs on the effects of antiepileptic drugs on idiopathic leg cramps.

Benefits: We found no systematic review or RCTs.

Harms: Harms associated with the use of antiepileptic drugs are well described (see epilepsy, p 1508).

Comment: None.

QUESTION **What are the effects of treatments for leg cramps in pregnancy?**

OPTION **MAGNESIUM SALTS**

One systematic review identified one small RCT in pregnant women, which found that magnesium tablets (primarily magnesium lactate, magnesium citrate) reduced leg cramps compared with placebo after 3 weeks.

Benefits: We found one systematic review (search date 2001,[6] 1 RCT,[7] 73 pregnant women 22–36 weeks' gestation), which compared chewable magnesium tablets (primarily magnesium lactate, magnesium citrate) versus chewable placebo tablets (primarily sorbitol, fructose–dextrose) given for 3 weeks. The review found that magnesium significantly reduced persistence of leg cramps compared with placebo after 3 weeks' treatment (23/34 [68%] with magnesium *v* 33/35 [94%] with placebo; OR 0.18, 95% CI 0.05 to 0.60;

see comment below).[6] The RCT found that magnesium decreased the proportion of women who rated themselves "unchanged" or "worse" compared with placebo ("unchanged": 7/34 [21%] with magnesium *v* 16/35 [46%] with placebo; "worse": 0/34 [0%] with magnesium *v* 5/35 [14%] with placebo).[7]

Harms: Adverse effects (mainly slight nausea) were described as infrequent in both groups.[6] One woman in the placebo group discontinued treatment because of severe nausea.[6]

Comment: The RCT did not describe the method of randomisation, and symptoms were assessed after 3 weeks of treatment with no further follow up.[6]

OPTION MULTIVITAMINS AND MINERAL SUPPLEMENTS

One systematic review identified one small RCT in pregnant women, which found no significant difference between multivitamin plus mineral tablet and placebo in leg cramps in the ninth month of pregnancy.

Benefits: We found one systematic review (search date 2001,[6] 1 RCT,[8] 62 pregnant women), which compared a multivitamin plus mineral tablet (containing 12 different ingredients; see comment below) versus placebo (no details provided). Supplements were given from 3 months' gestation. The review found no significant difference between multivitamin plus mineral and placebo in persistence of leg cramps in the ninth month of pregnancy (AR for persistence 2/11 [18%] with multivitamin plus mineral *v* 10/18 [56%] with placebo; OR 0.23, 95% CI 0.05 to 1.01).[6]

Harms: The RCT found that 4% of women had adverse effects (nausea, vomiting, diarrhoea). It is not clear which treatment these women were taking.[8]

Comment: This small RCT was primarily undertaken to examine the effects of a multivitamin plus mineral supplement on zinc and copper levels during pregnancy.[8] In total, 29/62 (48%) of women were assessed for cramp at 9 months' gestation.[6] The high dropout rate is not explained. The supplement contained: zinc gluconate, copper gluconate, iron gluconate, magnesium lactate, chromium chloride, ascorbic acid, thiamine nitrate, riboflavin (riboflavine), pyridoxal chlorhydrate, folic acid, cyanocobalamin, and α-tocopheral acetate.[6]

OPTION SODIUM CHLORIDE

One systematic review found insufficient evidence about the effects of sodium chloride in pregnant women with leg cramps.

Benefits: We found one systematic review (search date 2001),[6] which included one controlled clinical trial[9] published in 1947 (see comment below).

Harms: We found no RCTs.

Comment: The controlled clinical trial was of poor quality. Initially, sodium chloride and calcium lactate were given to alternate participants.[9] It was then decided, based on the difference between the results of the two treatments, to also use two further control groups (saccharin and no treatment).[9] The dose of sodium chloride changed during the course of the study.[6]

OPTION CALCIUM SALTS

One systematic review identified two RCTs that compared calcium versus placebo or no treatment, which found conflicting results.

Benefits: We found one systematic review (search date 2001),[6] which included two RCTs[10,11] and one controlled clinical trial (see comment below). The first RCT (42 pregnant women) included in the review found that calcium (calcium gluconate, lactate, and carbonate) significantly improved leg cramps compared with no treatment (AR for lack of improvement in cramps 2/21 [10%] with calcium *v* 18/21 [86%] with no treatment; OR 0.05, 95% CI 0.02 to 0.17).[6] The second RCT (60 pregnant women) included in the review found no significant difference in leg cramps with calcium (calcium gluconate, lactate, and carbonate) compared with vitamin C (AR for lack of improvement in cramps 11/30 [37%] with calcium *v* 8/30 [27%] with vitamin C; OR 1.58, 95% CI 0.54 to 4.63; see comment below).[6]

Harms: The RCTs did not report harms.[6]

Comment: The controlled clinical trial identified by the review was of poor quality (see comment under sodium chloride, p 1341). There was a marked difference in the response of the control group in the two included RCTs. In the first RCT, 18/21 (86%) women with no treatment had no improvement in cramps.[10] In the second RCT, 8/30 (27%) women with vitamin C had no improvement.[11]

GLOSSARY

Baker's cyst A cyst or out pouching that occurs in the lining of the knee joint. Rupture of the cyst may be associated with calf pain.

Cinchonism Adverse effects caused by quinine and other derivatives of cinchona bark. It usually presents with nausea, vomiting, headache, tinnitus, deafness, vertigo, and visual disturbances.

Idiopathic leg cramps Leg cramps of unknown cause. The term is used in this review to distinguish the most common type of leg cramps from leg cramps in people who are receiving dialysis, have venous insufficiency, or are pregnant.

REFERENCES

1. Hall AJ. Cramp and salt balance in ordinary life. *Lancet* 1947;3:231–233.
2. Man-Son-Hing M, Wells G, Lau A. Quinine for nocturnal leg cramps: a meta-analysis including unpublished data. *J Gen Intern Med* 1998;13:600–606. Search date 1997; primary sources Medline, Embase, Current Contents, and contact with authorities.
3. McGee SR. Muscle cramps. *Arch Intern Med* 1990;150:511–518.
4. Gorlich HD, Gablez VE, Steinberg HW. Treatment of recurrent nocturnal leg cramps. A multicentric double blind, placebo controlled comparison between the combination of quinine and theophylline ethylene diamine and quinine. *Arzneimittelforschung* 1991;41:167–175.
5. Connolly PS, Shirley EA, Wasson JH, et al. Treatment of nocturnal leg cramps: a crossover trial of quinine vs vitamin E. *Arch Intern Med* 1992;152:1877–1880.
6. Young GL, Jewell D. Interventions for leg cramps in pregnancy (Cochrane Review). In: The Cochrane Library, Issue 3, 2002. Oxford: Update Software.

Search date 2001; primary sources Cochrane Pregnancy and Childbirth Group trials register.
7. Dahle LO, Berg G, Hammar M, et al. The effect of oral magnesium substitution on pregnancy-induced leg cramps. *Am J Obstet Gynecol* 1995;173:175–180.
8. Thauvin E, Fusselier M, Arnaud J, et al. Effects of a multivitamin mineral supplement on zinc and copper status during pregnancy. *Biol Trace Elem Res* 1992;32:405–414.
9. Robinson M. Cramps in pregnancy. *J Obstet Gynaecol Br Commonw* 1947;54:826–829.
10. Hammar M, Larsson L, Tegler L. Calcium treatment of leg cramps in pregnancy. *Acta Obstet Gynecol Scand* 1981;60:345–347.
11. Hammar M, Berg G, Solheim F, et al. Calcium and magnesium status in pregnant women. A comparison between treatment with calcium and vitamin C in pregnant women with leg cramps. *Int J Vitam Nutr Res* 1987;57:179–183.

Gavin Young
General Practitioner
Temple Sowerby Surgery
Penrith
UK

Competing interests: None declared.

Low back pain and sciatica (acute)

Search date February 2003

Maurits van Tulder and Bart Koes

QUESTIONS

INTERVENTIONS

See glossary, p 1355

Key Messages

- **Advice to stay active** Two systematic reviews and one subsequent RCT found that advice to stay active increased the rate of recovery, reduced pain, reduced disability, and reduced time spent off work compared with advice to rest in bed or bed rest.
- **Non-steroidal anti-inflammatory drugs** One systematic review and one additional RCT have found that non-steroidal anti-inflammatory drugs increased overall improvement after 1 week and reduced the need for additional analgesics compared with placebo. One systematic review and additional RCTs have found no significant difference among non-steroidal anti-inflammatory drugs or between non-steroidal anti-inflammatory drugs and other treatments (paracetamol, opioids, muscle relaxants, and non-drug treatments) in pain relief.
- **Behavioural therapy** One RCT found that cognitive behavioural therapy reduced acute low back pain and disability compared with traditional care or electromyographic biofeedback.

- **Multidisciplinary treatment programmes (for subacute low back pain)** We found no RCTs in people with acute low back pain. One systematic review in people with subacute low back pain found limited evidence that multidisciplinary treatment, including a workplace visit, reduced sick leave compared with usual care.
- **Muscle relaxants** Systematic reviews have found that muscle relaxants improve symptoms (including pain and muscle tension) and increase mobility compared with placebo, but found no significant difference in outcomes among muscle relaxants. Adverse effects in people using muscle relaxants were common and included dependency, drowsiness, and dizziness.
- **Acupuncture** We found no RCTs of acupuncture specifically in people with acute low back pain.
- **Analgesics (paracetamol, opioids)** We found no placebo controlled RCTs. Systematic reviews have found no consistent difference between analgesics and non-steroidal anti-inflammatory drugs in reducing pain.
- **Back schools** One systematic review found limited evidence that back schools increased rates of recovery and reduced sick leave compared with placebo in the short term. The review found no significant difference in outcomes between back school and physiotherapy, and found that back school increased pain and sick leave compared with McKenzie exercises.
- **Epidural steroid injections** One RCT found that epidural steroids increased the proportion of people who were pain free compared with subcutaneous lidocaine (lignocaine) injections after 3 months. A second RCT found no significant difference in the proportion of people cured or improved between epidural steroids and epidural saline, epidural bupivacaine, or dry needling.
- **Lumbar supports** We found no RCTs on the effects of lumbar supports.
- **Massage** One systematic review found insufficient evidence from one RCT about the effects of massage compared with spinal manipulation or electrical stimulation.
- **Spinal manipulation** Systematic reviews found conflicting evidence on the effects of spinal manipulation.
- **Traction** RCTs found conflicting evidence on the effects of traction.
- **Back exercises** Systematic reviews and additional RCTs have found either no significant difference between back exercises and conservative or inactive treatments in pain or disability, or have found that back exercises increase pain or disability.
- **Bed rest** Systematic reviews have found that bed rest could be worse than no treatment, advice to stay active, back exercises, physiotherapy, spinal manipulation, or non-steroidal anti-inflammatory drugs. One systematic review has found that adverse effects of bed rest include joint stiffness, muscle wasting, loss of bone mineral density, pressure sores, and venous thromboembolism.
- **Colchicine; electromyographic biofeedback; temperature treatments (short wave diathermy, ultrasound, ice, heat); transcutaneous electrical nerve stimulation** We found insufficient evidence on the effects of these interventions.

DEFINITION Low back pain is pain, muscle tension, or stiffness localised below the costal margin and above the inferior gluteal folds, with or without leg pain (sciatica — see glossary, p 1356),[1] and is defined as acute when it persists for less than 12 weeks.[2] Non-specific low back pain is low back pain not attributed to a recognisable pathology (such as infection, tumour, osteoporosis, rheumatoid arthritis, fracture, or inflammation).[1] This review excludes low back pain or sciatica with symptoms or signs at presentation that suggest a specific underlying condition.

INCIDENCE/ PREVALENCE Over 70% of people in developed countries will experience low back pain at some time in their lives.[3] Each year, 15–45% of adults suffer low back pain, and 1/20 (5%) people present to hospital with a new episode. Low back pain is most common between the ages of 35–55 years.[3]

AETIOLOGY/ RISK FACTORS Symptoms, pathology, and radiological appearances are poorly correlated. Pain is non-specific in about 85% of people. About 4% of people with low back pain in primary care have compression fractures and about 1% have a tumour. The prevalence of prolapsed intervertebral disc is about 1–3%.[3] Ankylosing spondylitis and spinal infections are less common.[4] Risk factors for the development of back pain include heavy physical work, frequent bending, twisting, lifting, and prolonged static postures. Psychosocial risk factors include anxiety, depression, and mental stress at work.[3,5]

PROGNOSIS Acute low back pain is usually self limiting (90% of people recover within 6 weeks), although 2–7% develop chronic pain. One study found recurrent pain accounted for 75–85% of absenteeism from work.[6]

AIMS OF INTERVENTION To relieve pain; to improve function; to develop coping strategies for pain, with minimal adverse effects from treatment; and to prevent the development of chronic back pain (see definition of low back pain [chronic], p 1359).[2,7]

OUTCOMES Pain intensity (visual analogue or numerical rating scale); overall improvement (self reported or observed); back pain specific functional status (such as Roland Morris questionnaire, Oswestry questionnaire); impact on employment (days of sick leave, number of people returned to work); medication use; intervention specific outcomes (such as coping and pain behaviour for behavioural treatment, strength and flexibility for exercise, depression for antidepressants, and muscle spasm for muscle relaxants and electromyographic biofeedback [see glossary, p 1355]).

METHODS *Clinical Evidence* search and appraisal February 2003. In addition, the authors searched Medline (1966 to December 1998), Embase (1980 to September 1998), and Psychlit (1984 to December 1998), using the search strategy recommended by the Cochrane Back Review Group.[8] Most earlier RCTs of treatments for low back pain were small (< 50 people/intervention group; range 9–169 people/intervention group), short term (mostly < 6 months' follow up), and of low overall quality. Problems included lack of power, no description of randomisation procedure, incomplete analysis with failure to account for people who withdrew from trials, and lack of blinding.[9] The quality of many recent RCTs is higher.

QUESTION What are the effects of oral drug treatments?

OPTION ANALGESICS (PARACETAMOL, OPIOIDS)

Systematic reviews have found no consistent difference between analgesics and non-steroidal anti-inflammatory drugs for pain, but have found that electroacupuncture or ultrasound improves pain relief compared with analgesics.

Benefits: We found two systematic reviews (search dates not stated[2] and 1995;[9] no placebo controlled RCTs; 6 comparative RCTs; no statistical pooling of data provided). **Versus non-steroidal anti-inflammatory drugs:** The reviews identified two RCTs (110 people), which found no significant difference between meptazinol (an opioid) and paracetamol or diflunisal (a non-steroidal anti-inflammatory drug [NSAID]) in pain relief.[2,9] A third RCT (219 people) identified by the reviews found that paracetamol increased pain relief compared with mefenamic acid (a NSAID).[2,9] **Versus non-drug treatments:** The reviews identified one RCT (40 people), which found that electroacupuncture (see glossary, p 1355) increased pain relief compared with paracetamol after 6 weeks, and one RCT (73 people), which found that ultrasound treatment significantly increased the proportion of people who were pain free after 4 weeks compared with analgesics.[2,9]

Harms: See paracetamol (acetaminophen) poisoning, p 1664. RCTs have found adverse effects (constipation and drowsiness) with analgesics in about 50% of people. One systematic review (search date 1995) found that combinations of paracetamol plus weak opioids increased the risk of adverse effects compared with paracetamol alone (single dose studies OR 1.1, 95% CI 0.8 to 1.5; multiple dose studies OR 2.5, 95% CI 1.5 to 4.2).[10]

Comment: None.

OPTION COLCHICINE

One RCT found insufficient evidence on the effects of colchicine.

Benefits: We found one systematic review (search date not stated, 1 RCT, 27 people), which found no significant difference between oral colchicine and placebo in outcomes, although the RCT identified by the review was too small to rule out a clinically important difference.[2]

Harms: The review reported gastrointestinal irritation and skin problems in about 33% of people taking colchicine.[2] Other adverse effects included chemical cellulitis and agranulocytosis.[11]

Comment: The review identified two further RCTs, which did not distinguish between acute and chronic low back pain.[2]

OPTION MUSCLE RELAXANTS

Systematic reviews have found that muscle relaxants improve symptoms (including pain and muscle tension) and increase mobility compared with placebo, but found no significant difference among muscle relaxants in outcomes. The reviews found that adverse effects in people using muscle relaxants are common and include dependency, drowsiness, and dizziness.

Benefits: We found three systematic reviews (search date not stated;[2] search date 1995,[9] 14 RCTs, 1160 people, no statistical pooling of data provided; search date 1999,[12] 11 RCTs). **Versus placebo:** The first two reviews identified nine RCTs (762 people), which compared a range of muscle relaxants (tizanidine, cyclobenzaprine, dantrolene, carisoprodol, baclofen, orphenadrine, or diazepam) versus placebo.[2,9] Seven of these RCTs found that muscle relaxants reduced pain and muscle tension and increased mobility compared with placebo. The remaining two RCTs found no significant difference in outcomes. The third review identified 11 RCTs comparing cyclobenzaprine versus placebo (2297 people with acute back or neck pain and muscle spasm).[12] The review did not pool results. Of eight included RCTs (1359 people) that reported a global measure of symptom improvement, six found that cyclobenzaprine significantly improved a global symptom measure compared with placebo (follow up 8–21 days). However, the clinical importance of these results is unclear. **Versus each other:** The first two reviews identified three RCTs (236 people), which found no significant difference among muscle relaxants (cyclobenzaprine, carisoprodol, and diazepam) in pain intensity, although two of the RCTs found that cyclobenzaprine or carisoprodol significantly increased overall improvement compared with diazepam.[2,9]

Harms: The reviews found that adverse effects included drowsiness or dizziness in up to 70% of people and a risk of dependency even after 1 week. More people experienced one or more adverse events with muscle relaxants compared with placebo (68% of people with baclofen *v* 30% of people with placebo).[2,9] One RCT identified by the reviews found that chlormezanone significantly increased adverse effects compared with methocarbamol (dyspepsia and drowsiness; 14/52 [27%] with chlormezanone *v* 6/55 [11%] with methocarbamol; RR 2.50, 95% CI 1.02 to 5.93; NNH 6, 95% CI 3 to 90).[2,9] One systematic review found that adverse reactions were significantly more common with cyclobenzaprine compared with placebo (53% with cyclobenzaprine *v* 28% with placebo; $P < 0.002$).[12] The most common adverse effects with cyclobenzaprine were drowsiness (20%), dry mouth (8%), and dizziness (7%).

Comment: None.

OPTION NON-STEROIDAL ANTI-INFLAMMATORY DRUGS

One systematic review and one additional RCT have found that non-steroidal anti-inflammatory drugs increased overall improvement after 1 week and reduced the proportion of people requiring additional analgesics compared with placebo. One systematic review and additional

RCTs have found no significant difference among non-steroidal anti-inflammatory drugs or between non-steroidal anti-inflammatory drugs and other treatments (paracetamol, opioids, muscle relaxants, and non-drug treatments) in pain relief.

Benefits: We found one systematic review (search date 1998, 45 RCTs, statistical pooling only for non-steroidal anti-inflammatory drugs [NSAIDs] *v* placebo)[13] and three additional RCTs.[14–16] **NSAIDs versus placebo:** The review identified nine RCTs, which found that NSAIDs increased the proportion of people experiencing global improvement compared with placebo after 1 week (pooled OR 2.0, 95% CI 1.4 to 3.0), and reduced the proportion of people requiring additional analgesics (pooled OR 0.64, 95% CI 0.45 to 0.91).[13] The review identified four RCTs (313 people), which found no significant difference between NSAIDs and placebo in relief of sciatica (see glossary, p 1356). The additional RCT (532 people) found that oral meloxicam (7.5 or 15.0 mg) increased pain relief compared with placebo after 3 and 7 days.[17] **Versus each other:** The review identified 18 RCTs (1982 people), which found no significant difference among NSAIDs in outcomes.[13] One additional RCT (104 people) found that nimesulide versus ibuprofen improved functional status, but found no significant difference in pain relief after 10 days.[14] A second additional RCT (489 people) found no significant difference between meloxicam and diclofenac in pain relief.[17] **Versus paracetamol:** The review identified two RCTs (93 people), which found no significant difference between mefenamic acid and paracetamol in recovery rates, and one RCT (60 people), which found that mefenamic acid increased pain relief compared with paracetamol.[13] The review identified one RCT (60 people), which found that mefenamic acid improved pain relief compared with dextropropoxyphene plus paracetamol. **Versus muscle relaxants plus opioid analgesics:** The review identified five RCTs (399 people), which found no significant difference between NSAIDs and muscle relaxants plus opioids in pain relief or overall improvement.[13] **Versus non-drug treatments:** The review identified three RCTs (461 people).[13] The first RCT (110 people) found that NSAIDs improved range of movement compared with bed rest, although the second RCT (241 people) found no significant difference between treatments in range of movement. Two RCTs (354 people) comparing NSAIDs versus physiotherapy or spinal manipulation found no significant difference in pain relief or improvement in mobility. **Versus NSAIDs plus adjuvant treatment:** The review identified three RCTs (232 people), which found no significant difference between NSAIDs alone and NSAIDs plus muscle relaxants in outcomes.[13] One RCT identified by the review,[13] and one additional RCT[18] found no significant difference between NSAIDs and versus NSAIDs plus vitamin B combinations in pain relief, although one of the RCTs found that NSAIDs alone reduced the proportion of people returning to work after 1 week compared with NSAIDs plus vitamin B combinations (78% of people with combination treatment *v* 35% with NSAIDs alone).

Harms: NSAIDs may cause gastrointestinal complications (see non-steroidal anti-inflammatory drugs, p 1393). One systematic review of harms of NSAIDs found that ibuprofen and diclofenac had the lowest gastrointestinal complication rate mainly because of the low doses used in practice (pooled OR for adverse effects versus placebo 1.30, 95% CI 0.91 to 1.80).[19] RCTs have found no significant difference with nimesulide versus ibuprofen, or with meloxicam versus diclofenac in adverse effects.

Comment: None.

QUESTION What are the effects of local injections?

OPTION EPIDURAL STEROID INJECTIONS

One systematic review has identified one RCT, which found that epidural steroids increased the proportion of people who were pain free after 3 months compared with subcutaneous lidocaine (lignocaine) injections. The review identified a second RCT, which found no significant difference between epidural steroids and epidural saline, epidural bupivacaine, or dry needling in the proportion of people cured or improved.

Benefits: We found one systematic review (search date 1998, 2 RCTs).[20] The first included RCT (57 people with acute low back pain and sciatica — see glossary, p 1356) found no significant difference between epidural steroids and subcutaneous lidocaine injections in pain relief after 1 month, but found that epidural steroids increased the proportion of people who were pain free after 3 months. The second RCT (63 people) compared four treatments: epidural steroids, epidural saline, epidural bupivacaine, and dry needling. It found no difference between any of the treatments in the proportion of people improved or cured.

Harms: Adverse effects were infrequent and included headache, fever, subdural penetration, and, more rarely, epidural abscess and respiratory depression.[20]

Comment: None.

QUESTION What are the effects of non-drug treatments?

OPTION ADVICE TO STAY ACTIVE

Two systematic reviews and subsequent RCTs found that advice to stay active (with or without other treatments) reduced disability, pain, and time spent off work compared with bed rest (with or without other treatments).

Benefits: We found one systematic review that compared advice to stay active alone versus advice to rest in bed or bed rest (search date 1998, 4 RCTs, 491 people with acute back pain or sciatica [see glossary, p 1356], no statistical pooling of data).[21] A second systematic review compared advice to stay active with or without other treatments versus those other treatments alone (search date not stated, 6 RCTs, 1957 people).[22] The first review identified two high quality RCTs.[21] The first RCT (186 people with acute low back pain) found that advice to stay active versus advice to rest in bed for 2 days significantly improved functional status and reduced sick leave after 3 weeks (weighted mean improvement in Oswestry questionnaire score for advice to remain active *v* bed rest 4.4, 95% CI 0.6 to 8.2; weighted mean reduction for days of sick leave for advice to remain active *v* bed rest 4.5 days, 95% CI 1.4 days to 7.6 days). However, the trial found no significant difference in pain intensity between groups after 3 weeks. The second RCT (183 people with sciatica) found no significant difference between advice to stay active and advice to rest in bed for 14 days in pain intensity, recovery, or duration of sick leave after 3 weeks (results not quantified in review). The second review similarly found that advice to stay active significantly reduced sick leave and reduced chronic disability compared with traditional medical treatment (analgesics as required, advice to rest, and "let pain be your guide") (see benefits of bed rest, p 1351).[22] We found two subsequent RCTs. The first subsequent RCT (457 people) found that advice to stay active significantly increased rates of recovery, reduced pain, and reduced disability compared with no advice.[23] The second subsequent RCT (278 people) found no significant differences in pain intensity and functional disability between normal activity and bed rest after 1 month (intensity of pain measured on visual analogue scale [0 = no pain and 100 = extreme unbearable pain]: 10.2 mm with normal activity *v* 13.7 mm with bed rest; difference +3.5 mm; 97.5% CI –2.6 mm to +0.5 mm; functional disability measured on the Eifel index, a French version of the Roland–Morris questionnaire [range 0–24]; at 1 month: 2.47 with normal activity *v* 3.3 with bed rest; difference –0.82; 99% CI –2.55 to +0.50). However, the second subsequent RCT found normal activity significantly reduced sick leave compared with bed rest up to day 5 (52% with advice to stay active *v* 86% with bed rest; $P < 0.0001$).[23]

Harms: The reviews and subsequent RCT did not report harms.[21,22,24]

Comment: Limitations in methods preclude meaningful quantification of effect sizes. Advice to stay active was provided either as a single treatment or in combination with other interventions such as back schools, a graded activity programme, or behavioural counselling. The two lower quality RCTs included in the first review were reported to have moderate to high risk of bias.[21] The first did not measure pain at follow up. The second found that 48 hours of strict bed rest significantly improved pain compared with advice to stay active (time to outcome and further details not reported in review).

OPTION BACK SCHOOLS

One systematic review found limited evidence that back schools increased rates of recovery and reduced sick leave compared with placebo in the short term. The review found no significant difference between back school and physiotherapy in outcomes and found that back school exercises increased pain and sick leave compared with McKenzie exercises.

Benefits: We found one systematic review (search date 1997, 3 RCTs, no statistical pooling of data provided).[25] The first included RCT (145 people), which found that back schools (short wave diathermy at lowest intensity) increased rates of recovery and reduced sick leave compared with placebo in the short term. The second included RCT (142 people) found no significant difference between back schools and physiotherapy in short term and long term outcomes. The third included RCT (100 people) found that ongoing McKenzie exercises (see glossary, p 1356) reduced pain and sick leave compared with one 45 minute session of back school for up to 5 years.

Harms: The review did not report harms.[25]

Comment: None.

OPTION BED REST

Systematic reviews have found no evidence that bed rest is better, but have found evidence that it could be worse than no treatment, advice to stay active, back exercises, physiotherapy, spinal manipulation, or non-steroidal anti-inflammatory drugs. One systematic review has found that adverse effects of bed rest include joint stiffness, muscle wasting, loss of bone mineral density, pressure sores, and venous thromboembolism.

Benefits: We found six systematic reviews (search date not stated, 4 RCTs;[2] search date 1995, 4 RCTs;[7] search date 1995, 6 RCTs;[9] search date 1999, 9 RCTs;[26] search date not stated, 10 RCTs;[22] search date not stated, 5 RCTs;[27] no statistical pooling provided). **Versus no treatment:** The reviews identified five RCTs (663 people), which compared bed rest versus no treatment and found either no significant difference between treatments or that no treatment improved outcomes compared with bed rest.[2,7,9,22,26,27] **Versus different lengths of bed rest:** The reviews identified two RCTs (254 people), which found no significant difference in outcomes with 7 days versus 2–4 days of bed rest.[2,7,9,22,26,27] **Versus other interventions:** The reviews identified five RCTs (921 people), which compared bed rest versus other interventions (advice to stay active, back exercises, physiotherapy, spinal manipulation, or non-steroidal anti-inflammatory drugs).[2,7,9,22,26,27] They found either no significant difference in outcomes (pain, recovery rate, time to return to daily activities, and sick leave) or an improvement in outcomes with the comparative interventions. The most recent systematic review found no significant difference between bed rest and advice to stay active in pain intensity after 3 weeks.[26]

Harms: One systematic review found that adverse effects of bed rest included joint stiffness, muscle wasting, loss of bone mineral density, pressure sores, and venous thromboembolism (see thromboembolism, p 273).[22]

Comment: None.

OPTION BEHAVIOURAL THERAPY

One RCT found that cognitive behavioural therapy reduced acute low back pain and disability compared with traditional care or electromyographic biofeedback.

Benefits: We found four systematic reviews (search dates not stated,[2] 1995,[7,9] and 1994;[28] no statistical pooling of data provided) and one subsequent RCT.[29] The reviews identified one RCT (107 people), which found that cognitive behavioural therapy (see glossary, p 1355) versus traditional care (analgesics plus back exercises until pain had subsided) reduced pain and perceived disability after 9–12 months. The additional RCT (50 people with acute low back pain and sciatica) found that risk factor based cognitive behavioural therapy versus electromyographic biofeedback (see glossary, p 1355) increased pain relief.[29]

Harms: The reviews and subsequent RCT did not report on harms.[2,7,9,28,29]

Comment: None.

OPTION ELECTROMYOGRAPHIC BIOFEEDBACK

We found insufficient evidence on electromyographic biofeedback.

Benefits: We found one RCT (50 people with acute low back pain and sciatica — see glossary, p 1356), which found that risk factor based cognitive behavioural therapy versus electromyographic biofeedback (see glossary, p 1355) improved pain relief.[29]

Harms: The RCT did not report on harms.[29]

Comment: None.

OPTION EXERCISE/BACK EXERCISES

Systematic reviews and additional RCTs have found either no significant difference between back exercises and conservative or inactive treatments in pain or disability, or have found that back exercises increase pain or disability.

Benefits: We found five systematic reviews (search dates not stated,[2] 1995,[7,9,30] and 1999;[31] no statistical pooling of data provided) and two additional RCTs.[17,32] The most recent review identified eight RCTs (1149 people), which compared specific back exercises (flexion, extension, aerobic, or strengthening programmes such as McKenzie exercises [see glossary, p 1356]) versus other conservative treatments (usual care by general practitioner, continuation of ordinary activities, bed rest, manipulation, non-steroidal anti-inflammatory drugs, mini back school, or short wave diathermy).[31] Seven of these RCTs found either no difference between treatments or that back exercises increased pain intensity and disability. The eighth RCT found that back exercises versus a mini back school improved pain and return to work. The review identified four RCTs (888 people) comparing back exercises versus inactive treatments (bed rest, educational booklet, and placebo ultrasound).[31] It found no significant difference between back exercises and inactive treatment in pain relief, global improvement, or functional status. The first additional RCT (66 people) found that endurance training back exercises increased improvement in functioning and pain relief after 3 weeks compared with no treatment, but found no significant difference in functioning or pain after 6 weeks.[17] The second additional RCT (41 people) found no significant difference between advice, minimal bed rest, or analgesics versus the same treatment plus specific, localised exercise of the multifidus muscle in pain and disability.[32]

Harms: The reviews and additional RCTs did not report harms.[2,7,9,17,30–32]

Comment: None.

OPTION LUMBAR SUPPORTS

We found no RCTs on the effects of lumbar supports.

Benefits: We found no systematic review or RCTs specifically in people with acute low back pain.

Harms: Harms associated with prolonged lumbar support use include decreased strength of the trunk musculature, a false sense of security, heat, skin irritation, and general discomfort.[2]

Comment: None.

OPTION MULTIDISCIPLINARY TREATMENT PROGRAMMES (FOR SUBACUTE LOW BACK PAIN)

We found no RCTs in people with acute back pain. However, one systematic review in people with subacute low back pain found limited evidence that multidisciplinary treatment including a workplace visit reduced sick leave compared with usual care.

Benefits: We found no RCTs specifically in people with acute back pain. We found one systematic review (search date 1998, 2 RCTs, 233 people with subacute low back pain), which found that multidisciplinary treatment (see glossary, p 1356), including a workplace visit, reduces sick leave compared with usual care.[33]

Harms: The review did not report harms.[33]

Comment: None.

OPTION TEMPERATURE TREATMENTS (SHORT WAVE DIATHERMY, ULTRASOUND, ICE, AND HEAT)

Two systematic reviews identified no RCTs on the effects of temperature treatments.

Benefits: We found two systematic reviews (search date not stated[2] and 1992[34]), which found no RCTs.

Harms: The reviews did not report harms.[2,34]

Comment: None.

OPTION MASSAGE

One systematic review found insufficient evidence from one RCT about the effects of massage compared with spinal manipulation or electrical stimulation.

Benefits: We found one systematic review (search date 2001, 1 RCT).[35] It identified one RCT (90 people), which compared massage (see glossary, p 1355) versus spinal manipulation or electrical stimulation and found no significant difference in pain relief, functional status, or mobility.[35]

Harms: The review gave no information on harms.[35]

Comment: None.

OPTION SPINAL MANIPULATION

Systematic reviews found conflicting evidence on the effects of spinal manipulation.

Benefits: We found six systematic reviews (search dates not stated,[2,36] 1995;[7,9,37] and 1997;[38] 18 RCTs; no statistical pooling of data provided). **Versus placebo:** The reviews identified five RCTs (383 people) comparing spinal manipulation versus placebo.[2,7,9,36–38] Two RCTs found that manipulation increased pain relief after 3 weeks, two RCTs found no significant difference in pain relief, and one RCT found that manipulation increased rates of recovery. **Versus other treatments:** The reviews identified 12 RCTs (899 people) comparing spinal manipulation versus other treatments (short wave diathermy, massage [see glossary, p 1355], exercises, back school, or drug treatment). Four of the reviews found that the results of these RCTs were conflicting.[2,7,9,37] The fifth review (7 RCTs, 731 people) found that spinal manipulation significantly increased recovery after 2–3 weeks (NNT 5, 95% CI 4 to 14).[36] The sixth review found limited evidence that spinal manipulation improved outcomes.[38]

Harms: In the RCTs that used a trained therapist to select people and perform spinal manipulation, the risk of serious complications was low (estimated risk: vertebrobasilar strokes 1/20 000–1/1 000 000 people; cauda equina syndrome < 1/1 000 000 people).[39]

Comment: Current guidelines do not advise spinal manipulation in people with severe or progressive neurological deficit.[2,11]

OPTION TRACTION

RCTs found conflicting evidence on the effects of traction.

Benefits: We found three systematic reviews (search dates 1995[7,9] and 1992[40]). The reviews identified two RCTs (225 people), which compared traction versus bed rest plus corset or infrared treatment. One RCT found that traction significantly increased overall improvement compared with both other treatments after 1 and 3 weeks, but the second RCT found no significant difference in overall improvement after 2 weeks.

Harms: The reviews did not report on harms.[7,9,40] Potential adverse effects include debilitation, loss of muscle tone, bone demineralisation, and thrombophlebitis.[2]

Comment: Of 16 RCTs identified, 12 RCTs (921 people) did not distinguish between acute and chronic low back pain, or included people with back pain of specific cause.[7,9,40–42]

OPTION — TRANSCUTANEOUS ELECTRICAL NERVE STIMULATION

We found no RCTs about effects of transcutaneous electrical nerve stimulation in people with acute back pain.

Benefits: We found no systematic reviews or RCTs specifically in people with acute low back pain.

Harms: We found no RCTs in people with acute low back pain.

Comment: None.

OPTION — ACUPUNCTURE

We found no RCTs of acupuncture specifically in people with acute low back pain.

Benefits: We found two systematic reviews (search dates 1996; see comment below), which found no RCTs of acupuncture (see glossary, p 1355) in people with acute low back pain.[43,44]

Harms: One systematic review (search date 1996) found that serious, rare, adverse effects included infections (HIV, hepatitis, bacterial endocarditis) and visceral trauma (pneumothorax, cardiac tamponade).[45]

Comment: Three RCTs identified by the systematic reviews combined acute and chronic low back pain and two RCTs did not specify the duration of symptoms. One RCT included people with back and neck pain.[43,44]

GLOSSARY

Acupuncture Needle puncture of the skin at traditional "meridian" acupuncture points. Modern acupuncturists also use non-meridian points and trigger points (tender sites occurring in the most painful areas). The needles may be stimulated manually or electrically. Placebo acupuncture is needling of traditionally unimportant sites or non-stimulation of the needles once placed.

Cognitive behavioural therapy This aims to identify and modify people's understanding of their pain and disability using cognitive restructuring techniques (such as imagery and attention diversion) or by modifying maladaptive thoughts, feelings, and beliefs.

Electroacupuncture Non-penetrative electrical stimulation of classical acupuncture points with low amplitude, pulsed electrical current.

Electromyographic biofeedback A person receives external feedback of their own electromyogram (using visual or auditory scales), and uses this to learn how to control the electromyogram and hence the tension within their own muscles. Electromyogram biofeedback for low back pain aims to relax the paraspinal muscles.

Massage Massage is manipulation of soft tissues (i.e. muscle and fascia) using the hands or a mechanical device, to promote circulation and relaxation of muscle spasm or tension. Different types of soft tissue massage include Shiatsu, Swedish, friction, trigger point, or neuromuscular massage.

Low back pain and sciatica (acute)

McKenzie exercises Extension exercises that use self generated stresses and forces to centralise pain from the legs and buttocks to the lower back. This method emphasises self care.

Multidisciplinary treatment Intensive physical and psychosocial training by a team (e.g. a physician, physiotherapist, psychologist, social worker, and occupational therapist). Training is usually given in groups and does not involve passive physiotherapy.

Sciatica Pain that radiates from the back into the buttock or leg and may also be used to describe pain anywhere along the course of the sciatic nerve.

Substantive changes

Advice to stay active One subsequent RCT added;[23] conclusions unchanged.

REFERENCES

1. Van der Heijden GJMG, Bouter LM, Terpstra-Lindeman E. De effectiviteit van tractie bij lage rugklachten. De resultaten van een pilotstudy. *Ned T Fysiotherapie* 1991;101:37–43.
2. Bigos S, Bowyer O, Braen G, et al. Acute low back problems in adults. Clinical Practice Guideline no. 14. AHCPR Publication No. 95–0642. Rockville MD: Agency for Health Care Policy and Research, Public Health Service, US, Department of Health and Human Services. December 1994. Search date not stated; primary sources The Quebec Task Force on Spinal Disorders Review to 1984, search carried out by National Library of Medicine from 1984, and references from expert panel.
3. Andersson GBJ. The epidemiology of spinal disorders. In: Frymoyer JW, ed. *The adult spine: principles and practice*. 2nd ed. New York: Raven Press, 1997:93–141.
4. Deyo RA, Rainville J, Kent DL. What can the history and physical examination tell us about low back pain? *JAMA* 1992;268:760–765.
5. Bongers PM, de Winter CR, Kompier MA, et al. Psychosocial factors at work and musculoskeletal disease. *Scand J Work Environ Health* 1993;19:297–312.
6. Frymoyer JW. Back pain and sciatica. *N Engl J Med* 1988;318:291–300.
7. Evans G, Richards S. *Low back pain: an evaluation of therapeutic interventions.* Bristol: Health Care Evaluation Unit, University of Bristol, 1996. Search date 1995; primary sources Medline, Embase, A-Med, Psychlit, and hand searches of references.
8. Van Tulder MW, Assendelft WJJ, Koes BW, et al, and the Editorial Board of the Cochrane Collaboration Back Review Group. Method guidelines for systematic reviews in the Cochrane Collaboration back review group for spinal disorders. *Spine* 1997;22:2323–2330.
9. Van Tulder MW, Koes BW, Bouter LM. Conservative treatment of acute and chronic nonspecific low back pain: a systematic review of randomized controlled trials of the most common interventions. *Spine* 1997;22:2128–2156. Search date 1995; primary sources Medline, Embase, Psychlit, and hand searches of references.
10. De Craen AJM, Di Giulio G, Lampe-Schoenmaeckers AJEM, et al. Analgesic efficacy and safety of paracetamol–codeine combinations versus paracetamol alone: a systematic review. *BMJ* 1996;313:321–325. Search date 1995; primary sources Medline, Embase, International Pharmaceutical Abstracts, Biosis, contact with pharmaceutical companies, and hand searches of references.
11. Waddell G, Feder G, McIntosh A, et al. *Low back pain evidence review.* London: Royal College of General Practitioners, 1999. Search date 1999; primary sources Medline, Embase, Science Citation Index, Social Sciences Citation Index, correspondence with experts and researchers, and hand searches of references.
12. Browning R, Jackson JF, O'Malley PG. Cyclobenzaprine and back pain. *Arch Intern Med* 2001;161:1613–1620. Search date 1999; primary sources Medline, Psychlit, Cinahl, Embase, Aidsline, Healthstar, Cancerlit, Microdex, and pharmaceutical companies.
13. Van Tulder MW, Scholten RJPM, Koes BW, et al. Non-steroidal anti-inflammatory drugs (NSAIDs) for non-specific low back pain. In: The Cochrane Library, Issue 1, 2003. Oxford: Update Software. Search date 1998; primary sources Medline, Embase, Cochrane Controlled Trials Register, and hand searches of references.
14. Pohjolainen T, Jekunen A, Autio L, et al. Treatment of acute low back pain with the COX-2 selective anti-inflammatory drug nimesulide: results of a randomised, double-blind comparative trial versus ibuprofen. *Spine* 2000;25:1579–1585.
15. Laws D. Double blind parallel group investigation in general practice of the efficacy and tolerability of acemetacin, in comparison with diclofenac, in patients suffering with acute low back pain. *Br J Clin Res* 1994;5:55–64.
16. Chok B, Lee R, Latimer J, et al. Endurance training of the trunk extensor muscles in people with subacute low back pain. *Phys Ther* 1999;79:1032–1042.
17. Dreiser RL, LeParc JM, Velicitat P, et al. Oral meloxicam is effective in acute sciatica: two randomised, double-blind trials versus placebo or diclofenac. *Inflamm Res* 2001;1:S17–S23.
18. Bruggemann G, Koehler CO, Koch EM. Results of a double-blind study of diclofenac + vitamin B1, B6, B12 versus diclofenac in patients with acute pain of the lumbar vertebrae: a multicenter study. *Klinische Wochenschrift* 1990;68:116–120.
19. Henry D, Lim LLY, Rodriguez LAG, et al. Variability in risk of gastrointestinal complications with individual non-steroidal anti-inflammatory drugs: results of a collaborative meta-analysis. *BMJ* 1996;312:1563–1566. Search date 1994; primary sources Medline, contact with study authors, and hand searches of references.
20. Koes BW, Scholten RJPM, Mens JMA, et al. Epidural steroid injections for low back pain and sciatica: an updated systematic review of randomized clinical trials. *Pain Digest* 1999;9:241–247. Search date 1998; primary sources Medline and hand searches of relevant publications.
21. Hilde G, Hagen KB, Jamtvedt G, et al. Advice to stay active as a single treatment for low back pain and sciatica (Cochrane Review). In: The Cochrane

Library, Issue 1, 2003. Oxford: Update Software. Search date 1998; primary sources Medline, Embase, Sport, Cochrane Controlled Trials Register, Musculoskeletal Group's trials register, and Scisearch.

22. Waddell G, Feder G, Lewis M. Systematic reviews of bed rest and advice to stay active for acute low back pain. *Br J Gen Pract* 1997;47:647–652. Search date not stated; primary sources Medline, contacted recently published authors and pharmaceutical companies, and hand searches of references.
23. Rozenberg S, Delval C, Rezvani Y, et al. Bed rest or normal activity for patients with acute low back pain: a randomized controlled trial. *Spine* 2002;27:1487–1493.
24. Hagen EM, Eriksen HR, Ursin H. Does early intervention with a light mobilization program reduce long-term sick leave for low back pain? *Spine* 2000;25:1973–1976.
25. Van Tulder MW, Esmail R, Bombardier C, et al. Back schools for non-specific low back pain. In: The Cochrane Library, Issue 1, 2003. Oxford: Update Software. Search date 1997; primary sources Medline, Embase, and hand searches of references.
26. Hagen KB, Hilde G, Jamtvedt G, et al. Bed rest for acute low back pain and sciatica (Cochrane Review). In: The Cochrane Library, Issue 1, 2003. Oxford: Update Software. Search date 1999; primary sources Cochrane Musculoskeletal Group's trials register, Cochrane Controlled Trials Register, Cochrane Library, Medline, Embase, Sport, Scisearch, and hand searches of reference lists and personal contact with the authors of included articles.
27. Koes BW, van den Hoogen HMM. Efficacy of bed rest and orthoses of low back pain. A review of randomized clinical trials. *Eur J Phys Med Rehabil* 1994;4:86–93. Search date not stated; primary sources Medline and hand searches of references.
28. Turner JA. Educational and behavioral interventions for back pain in primary care. *Spine* 1996;21:2851–2859. Search date 1994; primary sources Medline, Psychlit, hand searches, and inquiries to pharmaceutical companies, and expert researchers in the field.
29. Hasenbring M, Ulrich HW, Hartmann M, et al. The efficacy of a risk factor-based cognitive behavioral intervention and electromyographic biofeedback in patients with acute sciatic pain: an attempt to prevent chronicity. *Spine* 1999;24:2525–2535.
30. Faas A. Exercises: which ones are worth trying, for which patients and when? *Spine* 1996;21:2874–2879. Search date 1995; primary source Medline.
31. van Tulder MW, Malmivaara A, Esmail R, et al. Exercise therapy for non-specific low back pain. In: The Cochrane Library, Issue 1, 2003. Oxford: Update Software. Search date 1999; primary sources Medline, Psychlit, Cochrane Controlled Trials Register, Embase, and hand searches of reference lists.
32. Hides JA, Richardson CA, Jull GA. Multifidus muscle recovery is not automatic after resolution of acute first episode low back pain. *Spine* 1996;21:2763–2769.
33. Karjalainen K, Malmivaara A, van Tulder M, et al. Multidisciplinary biopsychosocial rehabilitation for subacute low back pain among working age adults. In: The Cochrane Library, Issue 1, 2003. Oxford: Update Software. Search date 1998; primary sources Medline, Embase, Psychlit, Cochrane Register of Controlled Clinical Trials, Science Citation Index, hand searches of reference lists, and personal contact with experts.
34. Gam AN, Johannsen F. Ultrasound therapy in musculoskeletal disorders: a meta-analysis. *Pain* 1995;63:85–91. Search date 1992; primary sources Index Medicus, Medline, and hand searches of references.
35. Furlan AD, Brosseau L, Imamura M, et al. Massage for low back pain. In: The Cochrane Library, Issue 1, 2003. Oxford: Update Software. Search date 2001; primary sources Medline, Embase, Cochrane Controlled Trials Register, Healthstar, Cinahl, Dissertation Abstracts, hand searches of references, and contact with content experts and massage associations.
36. Shekelle PG, Adams AH, Chassin MR, et al. Spinal manipulation for low back pain. *Ann Intern Med* 1992;117:590–598. Search date not stated; primary sources Medline, Index Medicus, contacted experts, and hand searches of references.
37. Koes BW, Assendelft WJJ, van der Heijden GJMG, et al. Spinal manipulation for low back pain. An updated systematic review of randomized clinical trials. *Spine* 1996;21:2860–2871. Search date 1995; primary sources Medline and hand searches of references.
38. Mohseni-Bandpei MA, Stephenson R, Richardson B. Spinal manipulation in the treatment of low back pain: a review of the literature with particular emphasis on randomized controlled trials. *Phys Ther Rev* 1998;3:185–194. Search date 1997; primary sources Medline, Cinahl, and Bids.
39. Assendelft WJJ, Bouter LM, Knipschild PG. Complications of spinal manipulation: a comprehensive review of the literature. *J Fam Pract* 1996;42:475–480.
40. Van der Heijden GJMG, Beurskens AJHM, Koes BW, et al. The efficacy of traction for back and neck pain: a systematic, blinded review of randomized clinical trial methods. *Phys Ther* 1995;75:93–104. Search date 1992; primary sources Medline, Embase, Index to Chiropractic Literature, Physiotherapy Index, and hand searches of non-indexed journals.
41. Ljunggren E, Weber H, Larssen S. Autotraction versus manual traction in patients with prolapsed lumbar intervertebral discs. *Scand J Rehabil Med* 1984;16:117–124.
42. Werners R, Pynsent PB, Bulstrode CJK. Randomized trial comparing interferential therapy with motorized lumbar traction and massage in the management of low back pain in a primary care setting. *Spine* 1999;24:1579–1584.
43. Ernst E, White AR. Acupuncture for back pain. A meta-analysis of randomized controlled trials. *Arch Intern Med* 1998;158:2235–2241. Search date 1996; primary sources Medline, Cochrane Controlled Trials Register, Ciscom, contacted authors and experts, and hand searches of references.
44. Van Tulder MW, Cherkin DC, Berman B, et al. Acupuncture in low back pain. In: The Cochrane Library, Issue 1, 2003. Oxford: Update Software. Search date 1996; primary sources Medline, Embase, Cochrane Complementary Medicine Field trials register, Cochrane Controlled Trials Register, Science Citation Index, and hand searches of references.
45. Ernst E, White A. Life-threatening adverse reactions after acupuncture? A systematic review. *Pain* 1997;71:123–126. Search date 1996; primary sources Medline, Ciscom, other specialised databases, contacted experts, and hand searches of references.

Low back pain and sciatica (acute)

Maurits van Tulder
Institute for Research in Extramural Medicine
Vrije Universiteit Medical Centre
Amsterdam
The Netherlands

Bart Koes
Department of General Practice
Erasmus University
Rotterdam
The Netherlands

Competing interests: None declared.

Low back pain and sciatica (chronic)

Search date February 2003

Maurits van Tulder and Bart Koes

QUESTIONS

INTERVENTIONS

See glossary, p 1373

Key Messages

- **Exercise** Systematic reviews and additional RCTs have found that exercise improves pain and functional status compared with usual care. RCTs found conflicting evidence on the effects of different types of exercise, or exercise compared with inactive treatments.
- **Intensive multidisciplinary treatment programmes** One systematic review has found that intensive multidisciplinary biopsychosocial rehabilitation with functional restoration reduces pain and improves function compared with inpatient or outpatient non-multidisciplinary treatments or usual care. The review found no significant difference between less intensive multidisciplinary treatments and non-multidisciplinary treatment or usual care in pain or function.
- **Analgesics** One RCT found that tramadol decreased pain and functional status compared with placebo. A second RCT found that paracetamol increased the proportion of people who rated the treatment as good or excellent compared with diflunisal.

- **Back schools in occupational settings versus no treatment** One systematic review has found that, in occupational settings, back schools improve pain and reduce disability compared with no treatment. Systematic reviews and one subsequent RCT found conflicting evidence on the effects of back schools compared with other treatments.
- **Behavioural therapy** Systematic reviews have found that behavioural therapy reduces pain and improves functional status and behavioural outcomes compared with no treatment, placebo, or waiting list control. Systematic reviews found no significant difference in functional status, pain, or behavioural outcomes between different types of behavioural therapy, and found conflicting results with behavioural therapy compared with other treatments.
- **Massage versus other treatments** One systematic review found that massage combined with exercises and education is more effective than inert treatment. The review found conflicting evidence about the effects of massage compared with other treatments.
- **Non-steroidal anti-inflammatory drugs** One RCT found that naproxen increased pain relief compared with placebo. One systematic review and additional RCTs found no significant difference with non-steroidal anti-inflammatory drugs compared with each other for symptom outcomes. Two RCTs found conflicting evidence on the effects of non-steroidal anti-inflammatory drugs compared with other analgesics.
- **Trigger point and ligamentous injections** One systematic review found limited evidence that steroid plus local anaesthetic injection of trigger points increased pain relief compared with local anaesthetic injection alone, and that phenol increased pain relief compared with saline injection of the lumbar interspinal ligament.
- **Acupuncture** We found conflicting evidence from two systematic reviews and two subsequent RCTs about the effects of acupuncture compared with placebo or no treatment. One systematic review and one subsequent RCT have found that acupuncture reduces pain intensity and increases overall improvement compared with transcutaneous electrical nerve stimulation.
- **Antidepressants** One systematic review and additional RCTs have found that antidepressants significantly increase pain relief compared with placebo. However, they found no consistent difference in functioning or depression. Additional RCTs found conflicting results on pain relief with antidepressants compared with each other or analgesics.
- **Electromyographic biofeedback** One systematic review found no difference in pain relief or functional status between electromyographic biofeedback and placebo or waiting list control, but found conflicting results on the effects of electromyographic biofeedback compared with other treatments.
- **Epidural steroid injections** One systematic review found no significant difference between epidural steroid injections and placebo in pain relief after 6 weeks or 6 months.
- **Lumbar supports** We found insufficient evidence on the effects of lumbar supports.
- **Muscle relaxants** We found insufficient evidence about the benefits of muscle relaxants. One RCT found that adverse effects in people using muscle relaxants are common and include dependency, drowsiness, and dizziness.
- **Physical conditioning programmes** One systematic review has found that physical conditioning programmes with a cognitive behavioural approach plus physical training for workers with back pain reduced sick days but not the risk of being off work at 12 months compared with general practitioner care.

- **Spinal manipulation** We found five systematic reviews, which identified 13 RCTs. One of the reviews found that spinal manipulation improved outcomes compared with placebo; one concluded that improvements in pain and disability scores were too small to be clinically worthwhile, and the other three were conflicting.
- **Transcutaneous electrical nerve stimulation** One systematic review found no significant difference in pain relief between transcutaneous electrical nerve stimulation and sham stimulation.
- **Facet joint injections** One systematic review found no significant difference in pain relief between facet joint injections and placebo or facet joint nerve blocks.
- **Traction** One systematic review and two additional RCTs found no significant difference between traction and placebo or between traction plus massage and interferential treatment in pain relief or functional status.

DEFINITION Low back pain is pain, muscle tension, or stiffness localised below the costal margin and above the inferior gluteal folds, with or without leg pain (sciatica — see glossary, p 1374),[1] and is defined as chronic when it persists for 12 weeks or more (see definition of low back pain and sciatica [acute], p 1343).[2] Non-specific low back pain is low back pain not attributed to a recognisable pathology (such as infection, tumour, osteoporosis, rheumatoid arthritis, fracture, or inflammation).[1] This review excludes low back pain or sciatica with symptoms or signs at presentation that suggest a specific underlying condition.

INCIDENCE/ PREVALENCE Over 70% of people in developed countries will experience low back pain at some time in their lives.[3] Each year, 15–45% of adults suffer low back pain, and 1/20 people present to hospital with a new episode. About 2–7% of patients with acute low back pain will go on to become chronic. Low back pain is most common between the ages of 35–55 years.[3]

AETIOLOGY/ RISK FACTORS Symptoms, pathology, and radiological appearances are poorly correlated. Pain is non-specific in about 85% of people. About 4% of people with low back pain in primary care have compression fractures and about 1% have a tumour. The prevalence of prolapsed intervertebral disc is about 1–3%.[3] Ankylosing spondylitis and spinal infections are less common.[4] Risk factors for the development of back pain include heavy physical work, frequent bending, twisting, lifting, and prolonged static postures. Psychosocial risk factors include anxiety, depression, and mental stress at work.[3,5] Having a previous history of low back pain and a longer duration of the present episode are significant risk factors for chronicity. A recently published systematic review of prospective cohort studies found that some psychological factors (distress, depressive mood, and somatisation) are associated with an increased risk of chronic low back pain.[6] Individual and workplace factors have also been reported to be associated with the transition to chronic low back pain.[7]

PROGNOSIS Generally, the clinical course of an episode of low back pain seems to be favourable, and most pain will resolve within 2 weeks. Back pain among primary care patients typically has a recurrent course characterised by variation and change, rather than an acute, self limiting course.[8] Most back pain patients will have experienced a previous episode, and acute attacks often occur as exacerbations of chronic low back pain. In general, recurrences will occur more frequently and be more severe if patients had frequent or long lasting low back pain complaints in the past. The course of sick leave due to low back pain is similarly favourable. One study reported that 67% of patients with sick leave due to low back pain will have returned to work within a week, and 90% within 2 months. However, the longer the period of sick leave the less likely the return to work becomes. Less than half of the low back pain patients who have been off work for 6 months will return to work. After 2 years of work absenteeism, the chance to return to work is virtually zero.[9]

AIMS OF INTERVENTION To relieve pain; to improve function; to develop coping strategies for pain, with minimal adverse effects from treatment.[2,10]

OUTCOMES Pain intensity (visual analogue or numerical rating scale); overall improvement (self reported or observed); back pain specific functional status (such as Roland Morris questionnaire, Oswestry questionnaire); impact on employment (days of sick leave, number of people returned to work); medication use; intervention specific outcomes (such as coping and pain behaviour for behavioural treatment, strength, and flexibility for exercise, depression [in people with depression and low back pain] for antidepressants, and muscle spasm for muscle relaxants and electromyographic biofeedback — see glossary, p 1373).

METHODS *Clinical Evidence* search and appraisal February 2003. The authors also searched Medline (1966 to December 1998), Embase (1980 to September 1998), and Psychlit (1984 to December 1998), using the search strategy recommended by the Cochrane Back Review Group.[11] Most of the earlier RCTs of treatments for low back pain were small (< 50 people/intervention group; range 9–169), short term (mostly < 6 months' follow up), and of low overall quality. Problems included lack of power, no description of randomisation procedure, incomplete analysis with failure to account for people who withdrew from trials, and lack of blinding.[12] The quality of the methods used by many recent RCTs is higher.

QUESTION What are the effects of oral drug treatments?

OPTION ANALGESICS (PARACETAMOL, OPIOIDS)

One RCT found that tramadol decreased pain and increased functional status compared with placebo. One RCT found no significant difference between paracetomol and diflusinal in the proportion of people who rated the treatment as good or excellent. Two RCTs found no significant difference in pain relief between non-steroidal anti-inflammatory drugs and an opioid analgesic.

Benefits: **Analgesics versus placebo:** One RCT (254 people) found that tramadol (an opioid) decreased pain and improved functional status compared with placebo.[13] **Analgesics versus non-steroidal anti-inflammatory drugs:** See non-steroidal anti-inflammatory drugs, p 1393.

Harms: RCTs found adverse effects (constipation and drowsiness) with analgesics in about 50% of people. One systematic review (search date 1995) comparing combinations of paracetamol plus weak opioids versus paracetamol alone found that combination treatment increased the risk of adverse effects (single dose studies OR 1.1, 95% CI 0.8 to 1.5; multiple dose studies OR 2.5, 95% CI 1.5 to 4.2).[14]

Comment: None.

OPTION ANTIDEPRESSANTS

One systematic review and additional RCTs have found that antidepressants versus placebo significantly increase pain relief, but found no consistent difference in functioning or depression. One RCT found that maproteline increased pain relief compared with paroxetine.

Benefits: We found one systematic review (search date 2000)[15] and six additional RCTs (2 RCTs in people with low back pain and depression; 2 RCTs in people with low back pain without depression; 2 RCTs did not report whether people were depressed).[16–21] **Versus placebo:** The review found that antidepressants significantly increased pain relief compared with placebo (SMD 0.41, 95% CI 0.22 to 0.61), but found no significant difference in functioning (SMD +0.24, 95% CI –0.21 to +0.69).[15] The six additional RCTs compared an antidepressant (imipramine, amitriptyline, trazodone, nortriptyline, doxepin, maprotiline, paroxetine, or clomipramine) with placebo and reported on depression. Most found no difference in depression, although two RCTs[17,19] found that an antidepressant significantly reduced depression compared with placebo. **Versus each other:** One RCT (67 people) found that maprotiline significantly increased pain relief compared with paroxetine (mean decrease on 0–20 scale: 5.41 with maprotiline *v* 2.34 with paroxetine).[20]

Harms: Adverse effects of antidepressants included dry mouth, drowsiness, constipation, urinary retention, orthostatic hypotension, and mania.[2] One RCT found that the prevalence of dry mouth, insomnia, sedation, and orthostatic symptoms was 60–80% with tricyclic antidepressants.[16] However, rates were only slightly lower in the placebo group and none of the differences were significant.

Comment: None.

OPTION MUSCLE RELAXANTS

One systematic review found insufficient evidence from one RCT about the effects of muscle relaxants. The included RCT found that adverse effects are common and include dependency, drowsiness, and dizziness.

Benefits: We found one systematic review (search date 1995, 1 RCT).[12] The RCT (50 people) identified by the review found that tetrazepam increased overall improvement and reduced pain after 10 days compared with placebo (64% with tetrazepam *v* 29% with placebo of people).[12]

Harms: The review found that adverse effects of muscle relaxants included drowsiness or dizziness in up to 70% of people and a risk of dependency even after 1 week.[12]

Comment: None.

OPTION NON-STEROIDAL ANTI-INFLAMMATORY DRUGS

One small RCT found that naproxen increased pain relief compared with placebo. One systematic review and additional RCTs found no significant differences in symptoms between different non-steroidal anti-inflammatory drugs. One RCT identified by the review found no significant difference between diflunisal and paracetamol in the proportion of people who rated the treatment as good or excellent. Two RCTs found no significant difference in pain relief between non-steroidal anti-inflammatory drugs and an opioid analgesic.

Benefits: We found one systematic review (search date 1998)[22] and two additional RCTs.[23,24] **Versus placebo:** One RCT (37 people) identified by the review found that naproxen increased pain relief compared with placebo.[22] **Versus each other:** Four RCTs (453 people) identified by the review found no significant difference between different non-steroidal anti-inflammatory drugs for symptoms.[22] The first additional RCT (196 people) found no significant difference between nimesulide and diclofenac in pain or functioning.[23] **Versus analgesics:** One RCT (29 people) identified by the review found no significant difference between diflunisal and paracetamol in the proportion of people rating their treatment as good or excellent at 4 weeks (10/16 [62%] *v* 4/12 [33%]; RR 1.87, 95% CI 0.77 to 4.55; calculated by *Clinical Evidence*).[22] However, the study may have lacked power to exclude a clinically significant difference. A second RCT (155 people) identified by the review found no difference between a parenteral non-steroidal anti-inflammatory drug and a parenteral opioid in pain relief.[22] One additional RCT (155 people) found no significant difference between ketorolac and meperidine in outcomes.[24]

Harms: Non-steroidal anti-inflammatory drugs may cause gastrointestinal complications (see non-steroidal anti-inflammatory drugs, p 1393). RCTs in people with acute and chronic back pain have found that ibuprofen and diclofenac have the lowest gastrointestinal complication rate mainly because of the low doses used in practice (pooled OR for adverse effects *v* placebo 1.30, 95% CI 0.91 to 1.80).[2,25,26] The first additional RCT found that nimesulide has a similarly low rate of gastrointestinal adverse effects as diclofenac.[23]

Comment: None.

QUESTION What are the effects of local injections?

OPTION EPIDURAL STEROID INJECTIONS

One systematic review found no significant difference between epidural steroid injections and placebo in pain relief after 6 weeks or 6 months.

Benefits: **Versus placebo:** We found one systematic review (search date 1996, 4 RCTs, 302 people) comparing epidural steroid injections versus placebo.[27] It found no significant difference in pain relief after 6 weeks (pooled RR 0.93, 95% CI 0.79 to 1.09) or 6 months (pooled RR 0.92, 95% CI 0.76 to 1.11).[27]

Harms: The review found that adverse events were infrequent.[27] These included headache, fever, subdural penetration, and, more rarely, epidural abscess and respiratory depression.

Comment: RCTs identified by the review were generally small (range 22–73 people), and included people with a variety of conditions (chronic low back pain with and without sciatica [see glossary, p 1374], sciatica alone, lumbar radicular pain syndrome, and post-laminectomy pain syndrome).

OPTION FACET JOINT INJECTIONS

One systematic review found no significant difference in pain relief between facet joint injections and placebo or facet joint nerve blocks.

Benefits: We found one systematic review (search date 1996, 3 RCTs, no statistical pooling of data).[27] Two RCTs (206 people) identified by the review found no significant difference in pain relief, disability, and flexibility between intra-articular corticosteroid and placebo (intra-articular saline) injections after 1, 3, or 6 months.[27] The third RCT (86 people) identified by the review found no significant difference in pain relief between facet joint injections and facet joint nerve blocks after 2 weeks, 1 month, or 3 months.[27]

Harms: The review found that adverse effects included pain at injection site, infection, haemorrhage, neurological damage, and chemical meningitis.[27]

Comment: Two RCTs from the review[27] did not distinguish between acute and chronic pain and have not been included in this review.

OPTION TRIGGER POINT AND LIGAMENTOUS INJECTIONS

One systematic review found limited evidence that steroid plus local anaesthetic injection of trigger points increased pain relief compared with local anaesthetic injection alone and that phenol increased pain relief compared with saline injection of the lumbar interspinal ligament.

Benefits: We found one systematic review (search date not stated, 2 RCTs, 138 people).[2] The first RCT (57 people) identified by the review found that trigger point injection using steroid (methylprednisolone or triamcinolone) plus lidocaine increased the number of people with complete relief of pain compared with lidocaine alone after 3 months (60–80% with steroid plus lidocaine *v* 20% with lidocaine alone).[2] The other RCT (81 people) identified by the review found that dextrose–glycerine–phenol increased pain relief compared with saline injection into the lumbar interspinal ligament after 1, 3, and 6 months.[2]

Harms: The review found that potential harms included nerve or other tissue damage, infection, and haemorrhage.[2]

Comment: None.

QUESTION What are the effects of non-drug treatments?

OPTION BACK SCHOOLS

One systematic review has found that, in occupational settings, back schools improve pain and reduce disability compared with no treatment. Systematic reviews and one subsequent RCT found conflicting evidence on the effects of back schools compared with other treatments.

Benefits: We found two systematic reviews (search date 1997, 14 RCTs, no statistical pooling of data;[28] search date 2000, 18 RCTs[29]) and one subsequent RCT.[30] Five RCTs (880 people) identified by the first review found that intensive back school programmes (see glossary, p 1373) in an occupational setting improved pain and reduced disability compared with no treatment. They found no difference in outcomes compared with other treatments (physiotherapy, callisthenics group training, or usual care).[28] Six RCTs (529 people) identified by the first review and the subsequent RCT compared back schools versus no treatment, waiting list control, or short wave diathermy. Four of these RCTs found that back schools improved outcomes in the short term;[28] two of these RCTs found no difference in the short term, and the remaining two RCTs found no difference in the long term.[28,30] Five RCTs (861 people) identified by the first review found that back schools increased pain relief and reduced disability compared with manipulation, non-steroidal anti-inflammatory drugs, or physiotherapy exercises after 6 months, but found no significant difference after 1 year.[28] The second systematic review found that back schools significantly increased pain relief after 3 months compared with no treatment or any other treatment, but found no difference in outcomes in the long term (see comment below).[29]

Harms: The reviews and subsequent RCT did not report on harms.[28–30]

Comment: The second review, which combined randomised and non-randomised studies, compared back schools, no treatment, and other active treatments in the same meta-analysis, and did not take the methods of the studies into account.[29]

OPTION BEHAVIOURAL THERAPY

Systematic reviews have found that behavioural therapy reduces pain and improves functional status and behavioural outcomes compared with no treatment, placebo, or waiting list control. Systematic reviews found no significant difference in functional status, pain, or behavioural outcomes between different types of behavioural therapy, and found conflicting results with behavioural therapy compared with other treatments.

Benefits: We found five systematic reviews (search dates not stated,[2] 1995,[10,12] 1994,[31] and 1999;[32] 20 RCTs, no statistical pooling of data). **Versus placebo, no treatment, or waiting list control:** Eleven RCTs (1223 people) identified by the reviews found that behavioural therapy compared with no treatment, placebo, or waiting list control, reduced pain intensity and improved functional status and behavioural outcomes.[2,10,12,31,32] **Different types of behavioural therapy versus each other:** The reviews identified nine RCTs (308 people), which found no significant difference between different types of behavioural therapy (cognitive behavioural therapy, operant behavioural treatments, and respondent behavioural treatment — see glossary, p 1373) in functional status, pain, or behavioural outcomes (including anxiety, depression, pain behaviour, and coping).[2,10,12,31,32] **Versus other treatments:** Two RCTs (202 people) identified by the reviews found that behavioural therapy increased the proportion of people who had returned to work after 12 weeks compared with traditional care (rest, analgesics, or physiotherapy) or back exercises, but found no difference in pain or depression after 6 months or 12 months.[2,10,12,31,32] Six RCTs (343 people) identified by the reviews comparing behavioural therapy plus other treatments (physiotherapy and back education, multidisciplinary treatment [see glossary, p 1374] programmes, inpatient pain management programmes, and back exercises) found that behavioural therapy plus the other treatments improved functional status in the short term compared with other treatments alone, but found no difference in pain or behavioural outcomes.[2,10,12,31,32]

Harms: The reviews did not report on harms.[2,10,12,31,32]

Comment: None.

OPTION ELECTROMYOGRAPHIC BIOFEEDBACK

One systematic review found no difference in pain relief or functional status between electromyographic biofeedback and placebo or waiting list control, but found conflicting results on the effects of electromyographic biofeedback compared with other treatments.

Benefits: We found one systematic review (search date 1995, 5 RCTs, 168 people, no statistical pooling of data).[12] **Versus placebo or waiting list control:** Three RCTs (102 people) identified by the review found no difference with electromyographic biofeedback (see glossary, p 1373) compared with placebo or waiting list control in pain relief or functional status.[12] **Versus other treatments:** Two RCTs (30 people) identified by the review found conflicting results with electromyographic biofeedback compared with progressive relaxation training in outcomes.[12] One RCT (30 people) identified by the review found no difference between rehabilitation programmes plus biofeedback versus biofeedback alone in pain or range of movement.[12]

Harms: The review did not report on harms.[12]

Comment: None.

OPTION EXERCISE

Systematic reviews and additional RCTs have found that exercise improves pain and functional status compared with usual care. RCTs found conflicting evidence on the effects of different types of exercise, or exercise compared with inactive treatments.

Benefits: We found five systematic reviews (search date not stated,[2] 1995,[10,12,33] and 1999;[34] 23 RCTs, 2240 people; no statistical pooling of data) and 14 additional RCTs.[35–48] **Versus inactive treatment:** Six RCTs (587 people) identified by one review compared exercise versus inactive treatments (hot packs plus rest, semi-hot packs plus sham traction, waiting list control, transcutaneous electrical nerve stimulation [TENS], sham TENS, detuned ultrasound, or short wave diathermy).[34] Three of these RCTs found that exercise increased overall improvement, whereas the remaining three RCTs found no significant difference in overall improvement. One additional small RCT (59 people) found that active rehabilitation consisting of 24 exercise sessions during 12 weeks improved pain intensity and functional disability compared with inactive treatments.[40] **Versus other treatments:** Nine RCTs (1020 people) identified by the reviews compared exercise with other treatments.[2,10,12,33,34] Three of these RCTs found no significant difference between exercise and conventional physiotherapy in pain, functional status, overall improvement, or return to work. One RCT found that exercise (as part of a combined physiotherapy programme) improved pain, functional status, and return to work compared with usual care by the general practitioner.[49] Three RCTs found that exercise improved both pain and functional status compared with back school education (see glossary, p 1373) plus early morning lumbar flexion control. One additional RCT (132 people) found that a full time, intensive 3 week multidisciplinary programme improved ability to work (but not return to work) and disability after 4 and 24 months, and improved pain relief after 4 months compared with exercise or exercise plus psychological pain management.[35,36] A second additional RCT (109 people) found no significant difference between exercise and massage (see glossary, p 1373) in pain and disability 4 weeks after the end of treatment.[37] **Versus each other:** One additional RCT (148 people) found no significant difference between active physiotherapy and muscle reconditioning with training devices and low impact aerobics in pain intensity after 6 months and 1 year, but found that muscle reconditioning and aerobic exercises reduced disability after 6 and 12 months compared with active physiotherapy.[42–45] A second additional RCT found that a combined exercise and motivation programme reduced pain and improved disability after 4 and 12 months compared with exercises alone.[39] **Extension exercises (including McKenzie exercises):** See glossary, p 1373. Three RCTs (153 people) identified by one review compared extension versus flexion back exercises.[34] Two of these RCTs found no significant difference in pain intensity, and the third RCT found that extension exercises reduced global improvement compared with flexion exercises. A subsequent RCT (60 patients) found no significant difference between extension exercises and whole body vibration exercises in pain intensity (VAS scale 0–10) and disability (Pain disability Index 0–70, where 0 = no limitation and 70 = most severe limitation) during 12 weeks of treatment and after 6 months (pain intensity: data not shown; change in pain disability index: from 20.3 at baseline to 10.5 after treatment with extension *v* 20.7 at baseline to 11.6 after treatment with vibration).[50] **Strengthening exercises:** Nine RCTs (899 people) identified by the reviews found no significant difference between strengthening exercises and other types of exercise in outcomes, and found conflicting evidence on strengthening exercises compared with inactive treatment.[2,10,12,33,34] **Stabilisation exercises:** One additional RCT (44 people with spondylolysis and spondylolisthesis) found that a 10 week specific stabilising exercise programme reduced pain intensity and functional disability after 30 months compared with usual care.[48] **Postural exercises (Mensendieck/Cesar):** One additional RCT (77 people who had just finished treatment for their last episode of back pain) found that a Mensendieck exercise (see glossary, p 1373) group treatment for 13 weeks reduced recurrences of back pain compared with usual care, but found no significant differences in sick leave, pain, or functioning after 1 and 3 years.[46,47] A second additional RCT (222 people) found that Cesar therapy (see glossary, p 1373) increased overall improvement after 3 and 6 months compared with usual care by the general practitioner, but found no significant difference after 1 year.[38] **Group exercises:** One additional RCT (109 people) found no significant differences between individual and group exercises in pain and disability 4 weeks after the end of treatment.[37]

Harms: The reviews and RCTs did not report on harms.

Comment: One additional study compared an intensive training programme versus home exercises versus control in people with both acute and chronic low back pain. Randomisation was only successful for home exercise versus control.[41]

OPTION LUMBAR SUPPORTS

We found insufficient evidence on the effects of lumbar supports.

Benefits: We found one systematic review (search date 1999, 1 RCT).[51] The RCT (19 people) identified by the review found that a lumbar corset plus a synthetic support improved symptom severity and functional disability compared with lumbar corset without synthetic support.[51]

Harms: The review did not report on harms.[51] Harms associated with prolonged lumbar support use include decreased strength of the trunk musculature, a false sense of security, heat, skin irritation, and general discomfort.

Comment: Five RCTs (1200 people) identified by the review did not differentiate between acute and chronic pain.[51]

OPTION MULTIDISCIPLINARY TREATMENT PROGRAMMES

One systematic review has found that intensive multidisciplinary biopsychosocial rehabilitation with functional restoration reduces pain and improves function compared with inpatient or outpatient non-multidisciplinary treatments or usual care. The review found no significant difference between less intensive multidisciplinary treatments and non-multidisciplinary treatment or usual care in pain or function.

Benefits: We found one systematic review (search date 1998, 10 RCTs, 1964 people),[52] which compared multidisciplinary treatment (see glossary, p 1374) versus a control treatment. The review found that intensive multidisciplinary biopsychosocial rehabilitation with functional restoration reduced pain and improved function compared with inpatient or outpatient non-multidisciplinary treatments or usual care.[52] The review found no significant difference between less intensive outpatient multidisciplinary treatments and non-multidisciplinary outpatient treatment or usual care in pain or function.[52]

Harms: The review did not report on harms.[52]

Comment: We found one RCT (195 people) that compared three treatments: extensive multidisciplinary treatment; light multidisciplinary treatment, and usual care. There was no overall analysis according to treatment allocation. However, subgroup analysis found that men returned to work more quickly with light multidisciplinary treatment than with usual care. It found no significant differences between extensive multidisciplinary treatment and usual care in men and no significant differences between any two interventions in women.[53]

OPTION PHYSICAL CONDITIONING PROGRAMMES New

One systematic review has found that physical conditioning programs with a cognitive behavioural approach plus physical training for workers with back pain reduced sick days but not risk of being off work at 12 months compared with general practitioner care.

Benefits: We found one systematic review of physical conditioning programmes compared with other treatments in adults with work disability related to back pain (search date 2000, 16 relevant RCTs).[54] The programmes were heterogeneous, all involving a cognitive behavioural approach plus a range of types of physical training (including aerobics, muscle strength and endurance training, and co-ordination training) given by a physiotherapist or a multidisciplinary team. The interventions varied in length from one session only to 1 hour per week for 18 months, most lasting between 3 and 6 weeks. The review found that physical conditioning programmes reduced the number of sick days compared with general practitioner advice or care after 12 months (2 RCTs, average reduction in sick days 45, 95% CI 3 to 88). There was no significant difference between physical conditioning programmes and general practitioner advice or care in the proportion of people off work at 12 months (physicial conditioning *v* general practitioner care: OR 0.8, 95% CI 0.58 to 1.09).[54]

Harms: The review did not report on harms.[54]

Comment: None.

OPTION MASSAGE

One systematic review found that massage combined with exercises and education is more effective than inert treatment. The review found conflicting evidence about the effects of massage compared with other treatments.

Benefits: We found one systematic review (search date 2001; 9 RCTs, 891 people; no statistical pooling of data; see comment below).[55] The review included one RCT, which found that massage combined with exercises and education is more effective than inert treatment (sham laser). The other eight RCTs included in the review compared massage with other treatments and found conflicting results.

Harms: The review did not report on harms.[55]

Comment: Problems with control group selection in the included RCTs limit the usefulness of their results.[55]

OPTION SPINAL MANIPULATION

We found five systematic reviews, which identified 13 RCTs. One of the reviews found that spinal manipulation improved outcomes compared with placebo; another review concluded that improvements in pain intensity and disability scores were not clinically worthwhile; and three reviews found that the results of the RCTs were conflicting.

Benefits: We found five systematic reviews (search dates 1995,[10,12,56] 2001,[57] and not stated[58]). Four RCTs (514 people) identified by the reviews compared manipulation versus placebo, and nine RCTs (597 people) identified by the reviews compared manipulation versus conservative treatments (usual care, short wave diathermy, massage, exercises, back schools [see glossary, p 1373], and drug treatment). Three of the reviews found that the results of included RCTs were conflicting.[10,56,58] The fourth review (5 RCTs, 543 people) found that spinal manipulation improved outcomes compared with placebo.[12] The fifth review found that spinal manipulation did not produce clinically worthwhile decreases in pain intensity scores compared with sham treatment or non-steroidal anti-inflammatory drugs, and no clinically worthwhile reductions in disability compared with non-steroidal anti-inflammatory drugs.[57]

Harms: In the RCTs identified by the reviews that used a trained therapist to select people and perform spinal manipulation, the risk of serious complications was low (estimated risk: vertebrobasilar strokes 1/20 000 to 1/1 000 000 people; cauda equina syndrome < 1/1 000 000 people).[10,12,56,58]

Comment: Current guidelines do not advise spinal manipulation in people with severe or progressive neurological deficit.[2,58]

OPTION TRACTION

One systematic review and two additional RCTs found no significant difference between traction and placebo or between traction plus massage and interferential treatment in pain relief or functional status.

Benefits: We found one systematic review (search date 1995, 1 RCT)[10] and two additional RCTs.[59,60] Two RCTs (176 people) found no significant difference between traction and placebo in global improvement, pain relief, or functional status after 5–9 weeks.[10,61] The second additional RCT (152 people) found no significant difference between lumbar traction plus massage and interferential treatment (see glossary, p 1373) in pain relief or improvement of disability 3 weeks and 4 months after the end of treatment.[59]

Harms: The review and additional RCTs did not report on harms.[10,59,60] Potential adverse effects include debilitation, loss of muscle tone, bone demineralisation, and thrombophlebitis.[2]

Comment: None.

OPTION TRANSCUTANEOUS ELECTRICAL NERVE STIMULATION

One systematic review found no significant difference in pain relief between transcutaneous electrical nerve stimulation and sham stimulation.

Benefits: We found one systematic review (search date 2000, 5 RCTs, 421 people).[61] It found no significant difference between transcutaneous electrical nerve stimulation and sham stimulation in pain measured using a visual analogue scale (3 RCTs, 171 people; pooled standardised mean difference –0.21, 95% CI –0.51 to +0.1).[61]

Harms: The review did not report on harms.[61]

Comment: None.

OPTION ACUPUNCTURE

We found conflicting evidence from two systematic reviews and two subsequent RCTs about the effects of acupuncture compared with placebo or no treatment. One systematic review and one subsequent RCT have found that acupuncture reduces pain intensity and increases overall improvement compared with transcutaneous electrical nerve stimulation

Benefits: We found two systematic reviews (search dates 1996, 12 RCTs; see comment below)[62,63] and three subsequent RCTs.[64–66] The reviews identified seven RCTs (380 people) comparing acupuncture (see glossary, p 1373) versus no treatment, placebo acupuncture, waiting list control, or transcutaneous electrical nerve stimulation.[62,63] One review found no significant difference between acupuncture and placebo acupuncture or no treatment in clinical outcomes.[63] The second review found that acupuncture increased overall improvement compared with control interventions (OR 2.3, 95% CI 1.3 to 4.1), but found no significant difference between acupuncture and placebo acupuncture in outcomes (OR 1.4, 95% CI 0.8 to 2.3).[62] The first subsequent RCT (60 people) found that acupuncture significantly reduced pain intensity and the number of analgesic tablets consumed a week compared with transcutaneous electrical nerve stimulation.[64] The second RCT (50 people) compared three treatments: manual acupuncture, electroacupuncture, and mock transcutaneous electrical nerve stimulation (placebo).[65] It found that manual and electroacupuncture significantly increased overall clinical improvement after 1 month compared with placebo (judged subjectively by investigator blinded to treatment allocation; 16/34 [47%] with acupuncture *v* 2/16 [13%] with placebo, $P < 0.05$; CI not reported). The third RCT (131 people) compared three treatments: acupuncture, sham acupuncture, and no treatment.[66] It found that acupuncture significantly reduced pain intensity and disability after 3 months, and disability after 9 months compared with control intervention. It found no significant difference between acupuncture and sham acupuncture for pain intensity and disability 9 months after the end of treatment (improvement in 10 cm visual analogue pain score 1.7 for acupuncture *v* 1.8 for sham acupuncture; improvement in 70 point pain disability index 9.0 for acupuncture *v* 8.5 for sham acupuncture).

Harms: One systematic review found that serious and rare adverse effects included infections (HIV, hepatitis, bacterial endocarditis) and visceral trauma (pneumothorax, cardiac tamponade).[63]

Comment: Three RCTs identified by the systematic reviews combined acute and chronic low back pain and two RCTs did not specify the duration of symptoms.[62,63] One RCT identified by the reviews included people with back and neck pain.[62,63]

GLOSSARY

Acupuncture Acupuncture is needle puncture of the skin at traditional "meridian" acupuncture points. Modern acupuncturists also use non-meridian points and trigger points (tender sites occurring in the most painful areas). The needles may be stimulated manually or electrically. Placebo acupuncture is needling of traditionally unimportant sites or non-stimulation of the needles once placed.

Back school Back school techniques vary widely, but essentially consist of repeated sessions of instruction about anatomy and function of the back and isometric exercises to strengthen the back.

Cesar therapy Cesar therapy is based on the hypothesis that there is an association between postural and movement deficiencies and back pain. The treatment aims to initiate a learning process aimed at correction of postural and movement deficiencies.

Cognitive behavioural therapy Cognitive behavioural therapy aims to identify and modify peoples understanding of their pain and disability using cognitive restructuring techniques (such as imagery and attention diversion) or by modifying maladaptive thoughts, feelings, and beliefs.

Electromyographic biofeedback With electromyographic biofeedback, a person receives external feedback of their own electromyogram (using visual or auditory scales), and uses this to learn how to control the electromyogram and hence the tension within their own muscles. Electromyogram biofeedback for low back pain aims to relax the paraspinal muscles.

Interferential therapy Interferential therapy is a low frequency current treatment that uses two medium frequency currents which "interfere" with each other to produce a beat frequency that the body recognises as a low frequency energy source. It is used as treatment for disorders in which inflammation is supposed to be a problem, such as back pain, osteoarthritis, rheumatoid arthritis, muscular pain/strain, and sports injuries.

Massage Massage is manipulation of soft tissues (i.e. muscle and fascia) using the hands or a mechanical device, to promote circulation and relaxation of muscle spasm or tension. Different types of soft tissue massage include Shiatsu, Swedish, friction, trigger point, or neuromuscular massage.

McKenzie exercises McKenzie exercises use self generated stresses and forces to centralise pain from the legs and buttocks to the lower back. This method emphasises self care.

Mensendieck therapy The Mensendieck approach combines postural exercises and education, emphasising "learning by doing". It is based on the assumption that human beings, through insight and guidance, can take responsibility for their own health and thus avoid the consequences of functional disability. Mensendieck therapy has been used for decades in the Netherlands and Scandinavia.

Multidisciplinary treatment Multidisciplinary treatment is intensive physical and psychosocial training by a team (e.g. a physician, physiotherapist, psychologist, social worker, and occupational therapist). Training is usually given in groups and does not involve passive physiotherapy.

Operant behavioural treatments Operant behavioural treatments include positive reinforcement of healthy behaviours and consequent withdrawal of attention from pain behaviours, time contingent instead of pain contingent pain management, and spouse involvement, while undergoing a programme aimed at increasing exercise tolerance towards a preset goal.

Respondent behavioural treatment Respondent behavioural treatment aims to modify physiological responses directly (e.g. reducing muscle tension by explaining the relation between tension and pain, and using relaxation techniques).

Sciatica Pain that radiates from the back into the buttock or leg and is most commonly caused by prolapse of an intervertebral disk; the term may also be used to describe pain anywhere along the course of the sciatic nerve.

Substantive changes

Exercise as part of a combined physiotherapy programme One RCT added;[49] conclusions unchanged.

Extension exercises versus whole body vibration exercises One RCT added;[50] conclusions unchanged

Spinal manipulation One systematic review added;[57] conclusions unchanged.

REFERENCES

1. Van der Heijden GJMG, Bouter LM, Terpstra-Lindeman E. De effectiviteit van tractie bij lage rugklachten. De resultaten van een pilotstudy. *Ned T Fysiotherapie* 1991;101:37–43.
2. Bigos S, Bowyer O, Braen G, et al. *Acute low back problems in adults*. Clinical Practice Guideline no. 14. AHCPR Publication No. 95–0642. Rockville MD: Agency for Health Care Policy and Research, Public Health Service, US, Department of Health and Human Services. December 1994. Search date not stated; primary sources The Quebec Task Force on Spinal Disorders Review to 1984, search carried out by National Library of Medicine from 1984, and references from expert panel.
3. Andersson GBJ. The epidemiology of spinal disorders. In: Frymoyer JW, ed. *The adult spine: principles and practice*. 2nd ed. New York: Raven Press, 1997:93–141.
4. Deyo RA, Rainville J, Kent DL. What can the history and physical examination tell us about low back pain? *JAMA* 1992;268:760–765.
5. Bongers PM, de Winter CR, Kompier MA, et al. Psychosocial factors at work and musculoskeletal disease. *Scand J Work Environ Health* 1993;19:297–312.
6. Pincus T, Burton AK, Vogel S, et al. A systematic review of psychological factors as predictors of chronicity/disability in prospective cohorts of low back pain. *Spine* 2002;27:E109–E120.
7. Fransen M, Woodward M, Norton R, et al. Risk factors associated with the transition from acute to chronic occupational back pain. *Spine* 2002;27:92–98.
8. Von Korff M, Saunders K. The course of back pain in primary care. *Spine*. 1996;21:2833–2837.
9. Waddell G. The clinical course of low back pain. In: *The back pain revolution*. Edinburgh: Churchill Livingstone, 1998:103–117.
10. Evans G, Richards S. *Low back pain: an evaluation of therapeutic interventions*. Bristol: Health Care Evaluation Unit, University of Bristol, 1996. Search date 1995; primary sources Medline, Embase, A-Med, Psychlit, and hand searches of references.
11. Van Tulder MW, Assendelft WJJ, Koes BW, et al. Method guidelines for systematic reviews in the Cochrane Collaboration Back Review Group for spinal disorders. *Spine* 1997;22:2323–2330.
12. Van Tulder MW, Koes BW, Bouter LM. Conservative treatment of acute and chronic nonspecific low back pain: a systematic review of randomized controlled trials of the most common interventions. *Spine* 1997;22:2128–2156. Search date 1995; primary sources Medline, Embase, Psychlit, and hand searches of references.
13. Schnitzer TJ, Gray WL, Paster RZ, et al. Efficacy of tramadol in treatment of chronic low back pain. *J Rheumatol* 2000;27:772–778.
14. De Craen AJM, Di Giulio G, Lampe-Schoenmaeckers AJEM, et al. Analgesic efficacy and safety of paracetamol–codeine combinations versus paracetamol alone: a systematic review. *BMJ* 1996;313:321–325. Search date 1995; primary sources Medline, Embase, International Pharmaceutical Abstracts, Biosis, contact with pharmaceutical companies, and hand searches of references.
15. Salerno SM, Browning R, Jackson JL. The effect of antidepressant treatment in chronic back pain: a meta-analysis. *Arch Intern Med* 2002;162:19–24. Search date 2000; primary sources Medline, Psychlit, Cinahl, Embase, Aidsline, Healthstar, Cancerlit, Cochrane Library, Micromedex, Federal Research in Progress databases, and reference lists of articles.
16. Atkinson JH, Slater MA, Williams RA, et al. A placebo-controlled randomized clinical trial of nortriptyline for chronic low back pain. *Pain* 1998;76:287–296.
17. Hameroff SR, Cork RC, Scherer K, et al. Doxepin effects on chronic pain, depression and plasma opioids. *J Clin Psychiatry* 1982;43:22–27.

18. Hameroff SR, Weiss JL, Lerman JC, et al. Doxepin's effects on chronic pain and depression: a controlled study. *J Clin Psychiatry* 1984;45:47–52.
19. Treves R, Montane de la Roque P, Dumond JJ, et al. Prospective study of the analgesic action of clomipramine versus placebo in refractory low back pain and sciatica (68 cases). [in French]. *Rev Rhum Mal Osteoartic* 1991;58:549–552.
20. Atkinson JH, Slater MA, Wahlgren DR, et al. Effects of noradrenergic and serotonergic antidepressants on chronic low back pain intensity. *Pain* 1999;83:137–145.
21. Dickens C, Jayson M, Sutton C, et al. The relationship between pain and depression in a trial using paroxetine in sufferers of chronic low back pain. *Psychosomatics* 2000;41:490–499.
22. Van Tulder MW, Scholten RJPM, Koes BW, et al. Non-steroidal anti-inflammatory drugs for low back pain. In: The Cochrane Library, Issue 2, 2002. Oxford: Update Software. Search date 1998; primary sources Medline, Embase, Cochrane Controlled Trials Register, and hand searches of reference lists from relevant papers.
23. Famaey JP, Bruhwyler J, Vandekerckhove K, et al. Open controlled randomised multicenter comparison of nimesulide and diclofenac in the treatment of subacute and chronic low back pain. *J Drug Assess* 1998;1:349–368.
24. Veenema KR, Leahey N, Schneider S. Ketorolac versus meperidine: ED treatment of severe musculoskeletal low back pain. *Am J Emerg Med* 2000;18:404–407.
25. Waddell G, Feder G, McIntosh A, et al. *Low back pain evidence review.* London: Royal College of General Practitioners, 1996. Search date 1996; primary sources Medline, Embase, Science Citation Index, Social Sciences Citation Index, correspondence with experts and researchers, and hand searches of references.
26. Watts RW, Silagy CA. A meta-analysis on the efficacy of epidural corticosteroids in the treatment of sciatica. *Anaesth Intensive Care* 1995;23:564–569. Search date not stated; primary sources Medline, hand searches from published reviews and clinical trials, and personal contact with published authors in the field and the pharmaceutical manufacturer.
27. Nelemans PJ, de Bie RA, de Vet HCW, et al. Injection therapy for subacute and chronic benign low back pain. In: The Cochrane Library, Issue 3, 2002. Oxford: Update Software. Search date 1996; primary sources Medline, Embase, and hand searches of reference lists.
28. Van Tulder MW, Esmail R, Bombardier C, et al. Back schools for non-specific low back pain. In: The Cochrane Library, Issue 1, 2003. Oxford: Update Software. Search date 1997; primary sources Medline, Embase, and hand searches of references.
29. Maier-Riehle B, Härter M. The effects of back schools: a meta-analysis. *Int J Rehab Res* 2001;24:199–206. Search date 2000; primary sources Medline, Psychlit, Psyindex, and hand searches of reference lists from relevant publications.
30. Dalichau S, Scheele K, Perrey RM, et al. Ultraschallgestützte Haltungs-und Bewegungsanalyse der Lendenwirbelsaüle zum Nachweis der Wirksamkeit einer Rückenschule [in German]. *Zentralbl Arbeitsmed* 1999;49:148–156.
31. Turner JA. Educational and behavioral interventions for back pain in primary care. *Spine* 1996;21:2851–2859. Search date 1994; primary sources Medline, Psychlit, hand searches, and inquiries to pharmaceutical companies and expert researchers in the field.
32. Van Tulder MW, Ostelo R, Vlaeyen JWS, et al. Behavioural treatment for chronic low back pain. In: The Cochrane Library, Issue 3, 2002. Oxford: Update Software. Search date 1999; primary sources Medline, Psychlit, Cochrane Controlled Trials Register, Embase, and hand searches of reference lists.
33. Faas A. Exercises: which ones are worth trying, for which patients and when? *Spine* 1996;21:2874–2879. Search date 1995; primary source Medline.
34. Van Tulder MW, Malmivaara A, Esmail R, et al. Exercise therapy for non-specific low back pain. In: The Cochrane Library, Issue 3, 2002. Oxford: Update Software. Search date 1999; primary sources Medline, Psychlit, Cochrane Controlled Trials Register, Embase, and hand searches of reference lists.
35. Bendix AF, Bendix T, Ostenfeld S, et al. Active treatment programs for patients with chronic low back pain: a prospective, randomized, observer-blinded study. *Eur Spine J* 1995;4:148–152.
36. Bendix AF, Bendix T, Labriola M, et al. Functional restoration for chronic low back pain: two-year follow-up of two randomized clinical trials. *Spine* 1998;23:717–725.
37. Franke A, Gebauer S, Franke K, Brockow T. Acupuncture massage vs Swedish massage and individual exercise vs group exercise in low back pain sufferers–a randomized controlled clinical trial in a 2 x 2 factorial design. [German] *Forsch Komplementarmed Klass Naturheilkd* 2000;7:286–293.
38. Hildebrandt VH, Proper KI, van den Berg R, et al. Cesar therapy is temporarily more effective in patients with chronic low back pain than the standard treatment by family practitioner: randomized, controlled and blinded clinical trial with 1 year follow-up. [Dutch]. *Nederlands Tijdschrift voor Geneeskunde* 2000;144:2258–2264.
39. Friedrich M, Gittler G, Halberstadt Y, et al. Combined exercise and motivation program: effect on the compliance and level of disability of patients with chronic low back pain: a randomized controlled trial. *Arch Phys Med Rehabil* 1998;79:475–487.
40. Kankaanpaa M, Taimela S, Airaksinen O, et al. The efficacy of active rehabilitation in chronic low back pain. Effect on pain intensity, self-experienced disability, and lumbar fatigability. *Spine* 1999;24:1034–1042.
41. Kuukkanen T, Malkia E. Effects of a three-month therapeutic exercise programme on flexibility in subjects with low back pain. *Physiother Res Int* 2000;5:46–61.
42. Mannion AF, Muntener M, Taimela S, et al. A randomized clinical trial of three active therapies for chronic low back pain. *Spine* 1999;24:2435–2448.
43. Mannion AF, Muntener M, Taimela S, et al. Comparison of three active therapies for chronic low back pain: results of a randomized clinical trial with one-year follow-up. *Rheumatology* 2001;40:772–778.
44. Mannion AF, Junge A, Taimela S, et al. Active therapy for chronic low back pain: part 3. Factors influencing self-rated disability and its change following therapy. *Spine* 2001;26:920–929.
45. Mannion AF, Taimela S, Muntener M, et al. Active therapy for chronic low back pain part 1. Effects on back muscle activation, fatigability, and strength. *Spine* 2001;26:897–908.

46. Soukup MG, Glomsrod B, Lonn JH, et al. The effect of a Mensendieck exercise program as secondary prophylaxis for recurrent low back pain. A randomized, controlled trial with 12-month follow-up. *Spine* 1999;24:1585–1591.
47. Soukup MG, Lonn J, Glomsrod B, et al. Exercises and education as secondary prevention for recurrent low back pain. *Physiother Res Int* 2001;6:27–39.
48. O'Sullivan PB, Twomey LT, Allison GT. Evaluation of specific stabilizing exercise in the treatment of chronic low back pain with radiologic diagnosis of spondylolysis or spondylolisthesis. *Spine* 1997;24:2959–2967.
49. Moseley, L. Combined physiotherapy and education is efficacious for chronic low back pain. *Aust J Physiother* 2002;48:297–302.
50. Rittweger J, Just K, Kautzsch K, Reeg P, Felsenberg D. Treatment of chronic lower back pain with lumbar extension and whole-body vibration exercise: a randomized controlled trial. *Spine* 2002; 27:1829–1834.
51. Van Tulder MW, Jellema P, van Poppel MNM, et al. Lumbar supports for prevention and treatment of low back pain. In: The Cochrane Library, Issue 1, 2003. Oxford: Update Software. Search date 1999; primary sources Medline, Cinahl, Current Contents, Cochrane Controlled Trials Register, Embase, Science Citation Index, and hand searches of reference lists.
52. Guzman J, Esmail R, Karjalainen K, et al. Multidisciplinary rehabilitation for chronic low back pain: systematic review. *BMJ* 2001;322:1511–1516. Search date 1998; primary sources Medline, Embase, Psychlit, Cinahl, Healthstar, Cochrane Library, citation tracking, and personal contact with content experts.
53. Skouen JS, Grasdal AL. Haldorsen EMH, et al. Relative cost-effectiveness of extensive and light multidisciplinary treatment programs versus treatment as usual for patients with chronic low back pain on long-term sick leave. *Spine* 2002;27:901–910.
54. Schonstein E, Kenny DT, Keating J, Koes BW. Work conditioning, work hardening and functional restoration for workers with back and neck pain. In: The Cochrane Library, Issue 1, 2003. Oxford: Update Software. Search date 2000; primary sources Medline, Embase, Cinahl, Biomedical Collection I to IV; Psychinfo, Pedro, Cochrane Controlled Trials Register, hand searches of reference lists of identified studies, and personal communication with the Cochrane Collaboration Back Group and domain experts.
55. Furlan AD, Brosseau L, Welch V, et al. Massage for low back pain. In: The Cochrane Library, Issue 1, 2003. Oxford: Update Software. Search date 2001; primary sources Medline, Embase, Cochrane Controlled Trials Register, Healthstar, Cinahl, Dissertation Abstracts, and hand searches of reference lists and contact with content experts and massage associations.
56. Koes BW, Assendelft WJJ, van der Heijden GJMG, et al. Spinal manipulation for low back pain. An updated systematic review of randomized clinical trials. *Spine* 1996;21:2860–2871. Search date 1995; primary sources Medline and hand searches of references.
57. Ferreira ML, Ferreira PH, Latimer J, et al. Does spinal manipulative therapy help people with chronic low back pain? *Aust J Physiother* 2002;48:277–284. Search date 2001; primary sources Embase, Cinahl, Medline, Pedro, and hand searches of the reference lists of all relevant previous systematic reviews.
58. Shekelle PG, Adams AH, Chassin MR, et al. Spinal manipulation for low back pain. *Ann Intern Med* 1992;117:590–598. Search date not stated; primary sources Medline, Index Medicus, contact with experts, and hand searches of references.
59. Werners R, Pynsent PB, Bulstrode CJK. Randomized trial comparing interferential therapy with motorized lumbar traction and massage in the management of low back pain in a primary care setting. *Spine* 1999;24:1579–1584
60. Ljunggren E, Weber H, Larssen S. Autotraction versus manual traction in patients with prolapsed lumbar intervertebral discs. *Scand J Rehabil Med* 1984;16:117–124.
61. Milne S, Welch V, Brosseau L, et al. Transcutaneous electrical nerve stimulation (TENS) for chronic low back pain. In: The Cochrane Library, Issue 1, 2003. Oxford: Update Software. Search date 2000; primary sources Medline, Embase, Pedro, Cochrane Controlled Trials Register, hand searches of bibliographic references, reference lists, Current Contents, abstracts in specialised journals, conference proceedings, and personal contact with co-ordinating offices of the trials registries of the Cochrane Field of Physical and Related Therapies and Cochrane Musculoskeletal Group and content experts.
62. Ernst E, White AR. Acupuncture for back pain. A meta-analysis of randomized controlled trials. *Arch Intern Med* 1998;158:2235–2241. Search date 1996; primary sources Medline, Cochrane Controlled Trials Register, Ciscom, contacted authors and experts, and hand searches of references.
63. Van Tulder MW, Cherkin DC, Berman B, et al. Acupuncture in low back pain. In: The Cochrane Library, Issue 1, 2003. Oxford: Update Software. Search date 1996; primary sources Medline, Embase, Cochrane Complementary Medicine Field trials register, Cochrane Controlled Trials Register, Science Citation Index, and hand searches of references.
64. Grant DJ, Bishop-Miller J, Winchester DM, et al. A randomized comparative trial of acupuncture versus transcutaneous electrical nerve stimulation for chronic back pain in the elderly. *Pain* 1999;82:9–13.
65. Carlsson CPO, Sjölund BH. Acupuncture for chronic low back pain: a randomized placebo-controlled study with long-term follow-up. *Clin J Pain* 2001;17:296–305.
66. Leibing E, Leonhardt U, Köster G, et al. Acupuncture treatment of chronic low back pain — a randomized, blinded, placebo-controlled trial with 9-month follow-up. *Pain* 2002;96:189–196.

Maurits van Tulder
Institute for Research in Extramural Medicine
Vrije Universiteit Medical Centre
Amsterdam
The Netherlands

Bart Koes
Department of General Practice
Erasmus University
Rotterdam
The Netherlands

Competing interests: None declared.

Neck pain

Search date January 2003

Allan Binder

QUESTIONS

INTERVENTIONS

See glossary, p 1390

Key Messages

Uncomplicated neck pain

- **Physical treatments (active physiotherapy, pulsed electromagnetic field treatment)** Systematic reviews and RCTs have found that active physiotherapy reduces pain compared with passive treatment, and that exercise reduces pain compared with stress management. It found limited evidence that pulsed electromagnetic field treatment reduced pain compared with sham treatment.

- **Drug treatments (analgesics, non-steroidal anti-inflammatory drugs, antidepressants, or muscle relaxants)** We found insufficient evidence on the effects of analgesics, non-steroidal anti-inflammatory drugs, antidepressants, or muscle relaxants for neck pain, although they are widely used. Several drugs used to treat neck pain are associated with well documented adverse effects.
- **Manual treatments (mobilisation and manipulation)** We found insufficient evidence about the effects of manipulation or mobilisation compared with other or no treatment in people with neck pain.
- **Multidisciplinary (multimodal) treatment** We found insufficient evidence from RCTs to compare effects of multimodal cognitive behavioural therapy with other treatments in people with uncomplicated neck pain.
- **Physical treatments (heat or cold, traction, biofeedback, spray and stretch, acupuncture, laser)** Systematic reviews found insufficient evidence about the effects of these physical treatments.
- **Soft collars or special pillows** We found no reliable evidence on the effects of soft collars or special pillows in people with non-specific neck pain.
- **Patient education** Three RCTs found no significant difference between patient education (advice or group instruction) with or without analgesics and no treatment, placebo, or usual care.

Acute whiplash

- **Early mobilisation** Systematic reviews and subsequent RCTs found limited evidence that early mobilisation reduced pain compared with immobilisation or rest plus a collar.
- **Early return to normal activity** Systematic reviews and subsequent RCTs found limited evidence that advice to "act as usual" plus anti-inflammatory drugs improved mild symptoms compared with immobilisation plus 14 days' sick leave.
- **Electrotherapy** One small RCT found limited evidence that electromagnetic field treatment reduced pain after 4 weeks but not after 3 months compared with sham treatment.
- **Multimodal treatment** One RCT found that multimodal treatment reduced pain at the end of treatment and after 6 months compared with physical treatment.

Chronic whiplash

- **Percutaneous radiofrequency neurotomy** One RCT found limited evidence that percutaneous radiofrequency neurotomy reduced pain compared with a sham procedure after 27 weeks.
- **Physiotherapy (*v* multimodal treatment)** One RCT found no significant difference between physiotherapy alone and multimodal treatment in disability, pain, or range of movement at the end of treatment or at 3 months.

Neck pain with radiculopathy

- **Drug treatments (epidural steroid injections, analgesics, non-steroidal anti-inflammatory drugs, or muscle relaxants)** We found no evidence about the effects of epidural steroid injections, analgesics, non-steroidal anti-inflammatory drugs, or muscle relaxants.
- **Surgery versus conservative treatment** One RCT found no significant difference between surgery and conservative treatment in symptoms after 1 year.

DEFINITION In this topic we have differentiated uncomplicated neck pain from whiplash, although many studies, particularly in people with chronic pain (duration more than 3 months), do not specify which types of participants are included. Most studies of acute pain (duration less than 3 months) are confined to whiplash. We have included under radiculopathy those studies involving people with predominantly radicular symptoms arising in the cervical spine. Neck pain often occurs in combination with limited movement and poorly defined neurological symptoms affecting the upper limbs. The pain can be severe and intractable, and can occur with radiculopathy or myelopathy.

INCIDENCE/ PREVALENCE About two thirds of people will experience neck pain at some time in their lives.[1,2] Prevalence is highest in middle age. In the UK about 15% of hospital based physiotherapy and in Canada 30% of chiropractic referrals are for neck pain.[3,4] In The Netherlands neck pain contributes up to 2% of general practitioner consultations.[5]

AETIOLOGY/ RISK FACTORS Most uncomplicated neck pain is associated with poor posture, anxiety and depression, neck strain, occupational injuries, or sporting injuries. With chronic pain, mechanical and degenerative factors (often referred to as cervical spondylosis) are more likely. Some neck pain results from soft tissue trauma, most typically seen in whiplash injuries. Rarely disc prolapse and inflammatory, infective, or malignant conditions affect the cervical spine and present with neck pain with or without neurological features.

PROGNOSIS Neck pain usually resolves within days or weeks but can recur or become chronic. In some industries, neck related disorders account for as much time off work as low back pain (see low back pain and sciatica [acute], p 1343).[6] The percentage of people in whom neck pain becomes chronic depends on the cause but is thought to be about 10%,[1] similar to low back pain. Neck pain causes severe disability in 5% of affected people.[2] **Whiplash:** Whiplash injuries were more likely to cause disability; up to 40% of sufferers reported symptoms even after 15 years' follow up.[7] Factors associated with a poorer outcome after whiplash are not well defined.[8] The incidence of chronic disability after whiplash varies among countries, although reasons for this variation are unclear.[9]

AIMS OF INTERVENTION To recover from acute episode within 4 weeks; to maintain activities of daily living and reduce absenteeism from work; to prevent development of long term symptoms.

OUTCOMES Pain; range of movement; function; adverse effects of treatment; return to work; level of disability (Neck Disability Index).[10]

METHODS *Clinical Evidence* search and appraisal January 2003. We also searched the following databases: Chirolars (now called Mantis) for English language articles from 1966 to November 1999; Bioethicsline (1973–1997); Cumulative Index to Nursing and Allied Health (Cinahl) (1982–1997); and Current Contents (1994–1997). Criteria for assessment of RCTs were based on a 100 point scale, including study population, interventions, effects, and data presentation and analysis.[11]

QUESTION **What are the effects of treatments for people with uncomplicated neck pain without severe neurological deficit?**

OPTION **PHYSICAL TREATMENTS**

Systematic reviews and RCTs have found that active physiotherapy reduces pain compared with passive treatment, and that exercise reduces pain compared with stress management. It found limited evidence that pulsed electromagnetic field treatment reduced pain compared with sham treatment. Systematic reviews found insufficient evidence about the effects of other physical treatments (heat or cold, traction, biofeedback, spray and stretch, acupuncture, and laser).

Benefits: We found six systematic reviews[12–17] and five subsequent RCTs (published in 6 articles).[18–23] Three of the systematic reviews considered all physical treatment modalities,[12,13,17] and the other three considered traction only,[14] or acupuncture only.[15,16] **All physical modalities:** The first systematic review (search date 1993, 13 RCTs, 760 people with neck pain but without neurological deficit) found no significant benefit from any of the following physical treatments: heat or cold, traction, electrotherapy (pulsing electromagnetic field or transcutaneous electrical nerve stimulation), biofeedback, spray and stretch, acupuncture, or laser.[12] The second systematic review (search date 1995, 17 RCTs, 1202 people) found possible benefit from active physiotherapy and pulsed electromagnetic field treatment, but not for traction, acupuncture, or other physical treatments.[13] The third systematic review (search date 2000, 7 CCTs/RCTs, 507 people with chronic neck pain) found some evidence of benefit for proprioceptive and strengthening exercise based on two low quality studies,[24,25] but no evidence that thermotherapy, massage, biofeedback, traction, ultrasound, transcutaneous electrical nerve stimulation, or combined rehabilitation interventions improved symptoms.[17] **Exercise:** One RCT (47 people) included in two reviews[12,13] found that active physiotherapy, including exercise (for 60 minutes each visit; mean 13 visits) significantly reduced pain immediately after treatment compared with passive treatment (heat, massage, and light stretching for 20 minutes each visit; mean 10 visits; $P < 0.05$).[26] Four subsequent RCTs (in 5 published articles) examined the effects of exercises.[18,19,21–23] The first subsequent RCT (103 women with work related neck pain) compared three exercise regimens (strength training, endurance training, and coordination exercises) versus stress management over 10 weeks.[18] It found that exercise significantly reduced pain compared with stress management ($P < 0.05$), but found no significant difference between any of the exercise programmes versus each other. It found no significant differences in neck pain between the different exercise regimens and stress management or versus each other after 3 years' follow up (AR for neck pain: 47% with strength training *v* 50% with endurance training *v* 58% with coordination exercises *v* 39% with stress management; no individual P values reported for each treatment *v* stress management). The second RCT compared three groups: strengthening exercises plus manipulation; strengthening exercises alone; and manipulation alone.[19] The third RCT compared intensive training, mobilisation physiotherapy, and manipulation (see benefits of manual treatments: mobilisation and manipulation, p 1382).[21,22] The fourth subsequent RCT (77 people) found no significant difference in pain intensity between general exercise, McKenzie treatment (see glossary, p 1390), and low power ultrasound (control) after 4 weeks of treatment and at 12 months (pain intensity after treatment measured on a 100 mm visual analogue scale [0 mm = no pain; 100 mm = unbearable pain]: 27 mm with general exercise *v* 19 mm with McKenzie treatment *v* 21 mm with control treatment; significance not stated; pain intensity at 12 months: 30 mm with general exercise *v* 26 mm with McKenzie treatment *v* 25 mm with control treatment; P value not reported).[23] However, it found that McKenzie treatment significantly reduced pain intensity compared with control treatment at 6 months (21 mm with McKenzie treatment *v* 27 mm with control treatment; $P < 0.05$). **Traction:** The fourth systematic review (search date 1992, 3 RCTs, 639 people) compared traction versus a range of alternative treatments, including heat, mobilisation, exercise, no treatment, collar, and analgesics.[14] The review found no consistent difference between traction and any of the other treatments in pain. **Pulsed electromagnetic field treatment:** One RCT included in the second review (81 people with neck pain and radiographic evidence of cervical osteoarthritis and 86 people with osteoarthritis of the knee with symptoms for at least 1 year; see comment below) compared true versus sham pulsed electromagnetic field treatment.[27] It found that, in people with chronic neck pain, pulsed electromagnetic field treatment significantly reduced pain ($P < 0.04$) and pain on passive motion ($P = 0.03$), but found no significant difference between treatments in difficulty with activities of daily living, tenderness, self assessment of improvement, or physicians' global assessment after 18 episodes of treatment. The RCT also found that active versus sham pulsed electromagnetic field treatment significantly increased the number of people who had improved in at least three of six variables (57/82 [70%] with active treatment *v* 37/82 [45%] with sham treatment; RR 1.54, 95% CI 1.21 to 1.80; NNT 4, 95% CI 3 to 11). This benefit was sustained up to 1 month (see comment below). **Acupuncture:** Two systematic reviews (search dates 1998, 13 RCTs) compared needle or laser acupuncture versus several different control procedures (sham treatments, diazepam, and physiotherapy) and found no consistent differences between treatments.[15,16] One subsequent RCT (177 people with chronic neck pain mainly because of fibromyalgia or whiplash) compared three groups: acupuncture, massage, and sham laser acupuncture.[20] It found no significant difference between acupuncture and sham laser acupuncture after 1 week (difference in pain score on a 100 point visual analogue scale: acupuncture *v* sham laser acupuncture +6.9 points, 95% CI –5.0 points to +18.9 points; $P = 0.33$), but found that acupuncture significantly reduced motion related pain after 1 week compared with massage (acupuncture reduced pain by 16.3 points more than massage on a 100 point visual analogue scale, 95% CI 4.4 points to 28.3 points; $P = 0.005$). The RCT found no significant difference between treatments after 3 months.

Harms: We found no good data on harms. The incidence of serious adverse events seems to be low for all physical treatments considered.

Comment: Although randomisation was properly conducted, baseline characteristics of treated and placebo groups were, by chance, different in the RCT comparing true versus sham pulsed electromagnetic field treatment.[27] People allocated to active treatment had higher pain scores, more tenderness, and more difficulty with the activities of daily living than the placebo group. The analysis in the RCT was based on changes from the baseline value, and it is not known how much of the observed effect was caused by bias introduced by the baseline differences.

OPTION MANUAL TREATMENTS: MOBILISATION AND MANIPULATION

We found insufficient evidence about the effects of manipulation or mobilisation compared with other or no treatment in people with neck pain.

Benefits: We found four systematic reviews (search dates 1990,[11] 1993,[28] 1995,[29] and 1995[13]), one additional RCT,[30] and three subsequent RCTs,[21,22,31] which assessed mobilisation and manipulation (see glossary, p 1390). Four reviews found that mobilisation or manipulation improved symptoms compared with a variety of control procedures.[11,13,28,29] **Mobilisation or manipulation:** One RCT (included in two reviews;[28,29] 256 people with chronic neck and back pain, 64 having chronic neck pain alone) compared four treatments: manual treatment (mobilisation, manipulation, or both); physical treatment (heat, electrotherapy, ultrasound, shortwave diathermy); usual medical care (analgesics, advice, home exercise, and bed rest); and placebo (detuned shortwave diathermy or ultrasound).[32] It found that manual treatment significantly improved outcomes after 12 months compared with all of the other treatments (statistical analysis specifically for people with neck pain was not provided). However, it was not possible to compare directly the effects of the two manual treatments, and more people received manipulation. **Mobilisation:** One RCT (included in all 4 systematic reviews; 30 people with acute pain who were all given a collar and allowed to take analgesics) found no significant difference in pain with mobilisation (10 people) compared with transcutaneous electrical nerve stimulation (10 people) or compared with control (10 people).[33] However, the trial may have lacked power to detect a clinically significant difference. One other RCT (included in two reviews;[28,29] 63 people) found that mobilisation plus analgesia significantly reduced pain compared with less active physiotherapy plus analgesia after 1 month (83% of the mobilisation group improved v 60% of the physiotherapy group; $P < 0.05$) but not thereafter.[34] **Manipulation:** One of the reviews performed a meta-analysis (3 RCTs, 155 people with chronic pain)[32,35,36] of manipulation compared with other treatments (diazepam, anti-inflammatory drugs, usual medical care).[29] It found no significant difference in improved outcomes between manipulation and other treatments (+12.6 mm on a 100 mm visual analogue scale, 95% CI –0.15 mm to +25.5 mm).[29] **Mobilisation versus**

manipulation: The additional RCT (100 people with mainly chronic neck pain) compared a single mobilisation treatment versus a single manipulation treatment.[30] It found no significant difference between treatments in the proportion of people reporting immediate improvement in pain (69% with mobilisation *v* 85% with manipulation; RR of improvement in pain with manipulation compared with mobilisation 1.23; P = 0.16 after adjusting for pre-treatment differences between groups). The RCT found that people in the manipulation group had improved range of movement, but the result was not significant (5.1° with manipulation *v* 3.9° with mobilisation; P = 0.5 [*t*-test]). The first subsequent RCT (119 people with chronic neck pain) compared three treatments: mobilisation physiotherapy, manipulation, and intensive training.[22] It found no significant difference in pain between groups by the end of treatment (P = 0.44) or after 12 months, although pain score improved from baseline in both groups (median pain score on a 30 point scale improved from 12 to 6 with intensive training or mobilisation *v* from 13 to 6 with manipulation). The second subsequent RCT (336 patients with chronic neck pain) found no significant difference in average pain, severe pain (average and severe pain measured on a 0–10 point index: 0 = no pain; 10 = unbearable pain), and neck disability scores (neck disability index measured on a 0–50 point index: 0 = no disability; 50 = most severe disability) between a variable number of chiropractic mobilisations and a variable number of manipulations after 6 months (severe pain difference from manipulation *v* mobilisation: –0.02 points; 95% CI –0.69 points to +0.65 points; average pain from manipulation *v* mobilisation: +0.010 points; 95% CI –0.52 points to +0.54 points; difference in neck disability scores: +0.46 points; 95 CI –0.89 points to +1.82 points).[31] **Manipulation plus exercise:** The third subsequent RCT (191 people with chronic neck pain who received a home exercise programme and were able to use proprietary medication) compared three treatments: strengthening exercises plus manipulation (combined treatment); strengthening exercises alone; and manipulation alone.[21] The duration of each treatment episode was the same. It found that strengthening exercises plus manipulation significantly improved participant satisfaction compared with both other treatments alone (P = 0.03), and significantly improved objective strength and range of movement compared with manipulation alone after 11 weeks (P < 0.05). The RCT also found that both the combined treatment and the strengthening exercises alone significantly improved pain (P = 0.02) and patient satisfaction (P = 0.002) compared with manipulation alone after 1 year, although it found no significant differences between treatments in health status, neck disability, or medication use. Two year follow up to this study (data available for 145/178 [76%] of original participants) found that manipulation alone significantly increased participant rated pain compared with manipulation plus exercise and exercise alone (P = 0.05 for manipulation *v* manipulation plus exercise; P = 0.02 for manipulation *v* exercise alone).[37] It found no significant differences in neck disability and general health status among the three groups.

Harms: **Mobilisation:** We found occasional reports of increased pain, but no serious adverse effects or deaths. **Manipulation:** The estimated risk from case reports of cerebrovascular accident is 1–3/million manipulations,[38] and of all serious adverse effects (such as death or disc herniation) is 5–10/10 million manipulations.[29] A non-systematic review of reported cases of injury attributable to manipulation of the cervical spine identified 116 articles published between 1925 and 1997 with 177 cases of injury. The most frequently reported injuries involved arterial dissection or spasm, lesions of the brain stem, and Wallenberg's syndrome (see glossary, p 1390); death occurred in 32 (18%) of the cases. However, the method of data collection and analysis makes it impossible to assess the frequency of complications with this treatment.[39]

Comment: In one RCT, only 336 of 960 eligible people agreed to participate.[31] This may reduce the external validity of the study. We found one systematic review examining mobilisation and manipulation for mechanical neck disorders. It included people with many types of neck pain, including uncomplicated pain, whiplash and neck pain with radiculopathy, and reported that trials were clinically heterogeneous. However, it did not provide a subgroup analysis in people with uncomplicated neck pain.[40] Across all of the people in the review, it reported that results were inconclusive.

OPTION MULTIDISCIPLINARY (MULTIMODAL) TREATMENT

We found insufficient evidence from RCTs to compare the effects of multimodal cognitive behavioural therapy with other treatments in people with uncomplicated neck pain.

Benefits: We found one systematic review (search date 1998, 1 RCT, 66 people)[41] and two subsequent RCTs in people with chronic neck pain.[42,43] The RCT included in the systematic review found no significant difference in time off work or physical function between multimodal cognitive behavioural therapy (administered directly by a psychologist) and exercise plus behavioural modification (with a psychologist acting as an advisor to other therapists) after 6 months.[41] The first subsequent RCT (76 people) compared three treatments: multimodal treatment (which emphasised exercise, relaxation, and behavioural support), supervised home exercises, and a recommendation to exercise.[42] It found that both supervised multimodal training and supervised exercise significantly reduced pain compared with a recommendation to exercise at 3 months (improvement in pain score from baseline on 10 cm visual analogue scale, 29 mm with multimodal treatment *v* 28 mm with supervised exercise *v* 12 mm with exercise recommendation; multimodal treatment or supervised exercise *v* exercise recommendation, $P < 0.001$), but it found no significant difference between treatments in pain after 12 months (individual data were not provided in the paper). The second subsequent RCT (243 people with chronic spinal pain) compared three treatments: multimodal cognitive behavioural therapy (6 sessions), an educational pamphlet, and a more extensive information programme.[43] It found no significant difference among treatments in pain but found that multimodal cognitive behavioural therapy significantly reduced time off work compared with an educational pamphlet (AR for sick leave of > 30 days in 6 months, 1% with multimodal cognitive behavioural therapy *v* 10% with educational pamphlets; RR 10; $P < 0.05$).[43]

Harms: None reported.

Comment: None.

OPTION PATIENT EDUCATION

We found insufficient evidence from three RCTs about the effects of patient education (advice or group instruction) with or without analgesics compared with no treatment, placebo, or usual care.

Benefits: We found three RCTs.[44–46] The first RCT (282 nursing aides with neck, shoulder, or back pain) compared three groups: an individualised education and exercise programme, stress management, and no intervention. It found no significant difference in pain between the groups immediately after treatment, or at 12 and 18 months (people with improved pain at 12 months: 8/41 with individualised education *v* 19/57 with stress management *v* 18/57 with no intervention; P value not reported).[44] The second RCT (79 hospital secretaries with chronic neck pain) compared three treatments: group instruction (traditional neck), neck school plus individual advice, and usual care.[45] It found no significant differences in neck movement or sick leave between groups (no data reported). The third RCT (93 people) found no significant difference between individualised education plus analgesic drugs/anti-inflammatory drugs and placebo (no data available).[46]

Harms: None reported.

Comment: We found one systematic review, which examined patient education for mechanical neck disorders; this has been withdrawn from the Cochrane Library because it is now considered out of date. It has therefore been excluded from this topic.

OPTION SOFT COLLARS AND SPECIAL PILLOWS

We found no reliable evidence on the effects of soft collars or special pillows in people with non-specific neck pain.

Benefits: **Soft collars:** We found no systematic reviews or RCTs. **Special pillows:** We found no reliable RCTs (see comment).

Harms: None reported.

Comment: We found one crossover RCT (41 people with chronic neck pain), which found that a water based pillow significantly reduced morning pain and improved quality of sleep compared with both a roll type pillow and a standard pillow ($P < 0.01$).[47] However, results in each group may have been confounded by pre-crossover treatment.

OPTION DRUG TREATMENTS (ANALGESICS, NON-STEROIDAL ANTI-INFLAMMATORY DRUGS, ANTIDEPRESSANTS, OR MUSCLE RELAXANTS)

We found insufficient evidence on the effects of analgesics, non-steroidal anti-inflammatory drugs, antidepressants, or muscle relaxants for neck pain, although they are widely used. Several drugs used to treat neck pain are associated with well documented adverse effects.

Benefits: We found two systematic reviews (search dates 1993[8,28] and one subsequent RCT[41]). **Simple analgesics (paracetamol, opioids) and oral non-steroidal anti-inflammatory drugs:** The reviews found no RCTs. **Antidepressants:** The reviews found no RCTs in people with uncomplicated neck pain (see comment). **Muscle relaxants and benzodiazepines:** We found one systematic review (2 RCTs, 159 people with chronic neck or back pain with acute spasm), which compared three treatments: cyclobenzaprine, diazepam, and placebo.[28] Both RCTs identified by the review found that cyclobenzaprine significantly improved symptoms compared with diazepam and placebo after 2 weeks ($P < 0.05$ in each study), but measured and follow up pain data could not be extracted.[48,49] Applicability of results may be limited in people with uncomplicated neck pain because people with other musculoskeletal disorders were included in the studies. The subsequent RCT (157 people with chronic neck pain) found that eperisone significantly improved pain control compared with placebo after 6 weeks ($P < 0.05$).[50]

Harms: **Simple analgesics (paracetamol and opioids):** We found no reports of harm from simple analgesics. **Oral non-steroidal anti-inflammatory drugs:** See harms of non-steroidal anti-inflammatory drugs, p 1393. One systematic review found no direct comparisons of harms of manipulation and non-steroidal anti-inflammatory drugs.[38] Calculations based on indirect comparisons found that the risk of a harm with non-steroidal anti-inflammatory drugs was considerably greater than for manipulation. **Antidepressants:** The reviews found no RCTs (see harms of antidepressants under generalised anxiety disorder, p 1157). **Muscle relaxants and benzodiazepines:** The RCTs found minor adverse effects, including weakness, dizziness, drowsiness, and gastrointestinal problems occurring in 4% of people treated with muscle relaxants (see harms of benzodiazepines under generalised anxiety disorder, p 1157).

Comment: Applicability of results in people with uncomplicated neck pain may be limited, because many of the RCTs included people with other musculoskeletal disorders, including back pain and acute whiplash.

QUESTION What are the effects of treatments for acute whiplash injury?

Systematic reviews and subsequent RCTs found limited evidence that early mobilisation reduced pain compared with immobilisation or rest plus a collar, that multimodal treatment reduced pain compared with physical treatment, and that electromagnetic field treatment reduced pain compared with sham treatment. The studies found that advice to "act as usual" plus anti-inflammatory drugs improved mild symptoms compared

with immobilisation plus 14 days' sick leave. One RCT found no significant difference between different home exercise programmes in pain or disability. We found no RCTs of drug treatments in acute whiplash injury.

Benefits: We found three systematic reviews of treatment for acute whiplash injury (search dates 1993,[8,28] 1998,[51] and three subsequent RCTs[52–54]). The reviews highlighted the paucity of evidence on all treatment modalities.[8,28,51] **Early mobilisation versus immobilisation or less active treatment:** The first review (search date 1993, 2 RCTs, 165 people)[8] plus two subsequent RCTs (104 people)[52,53] compared five treatments: early mobilisation physiotherapy, immobilisation, analgesics, rest, and education. The review found that early mobilisation significantly increased pain relief and improved range of movement after 4 and 8 weeks ($P < 0.01$). The first subsequent RCT, comparing early mobilisation versus immobilisation, found no significant difference in recovery after 12 weeks (see comment below).[52] The second subsequent RCT (97 people) found that active mobilisation significantly improved symptoms compared with rest plus a neck collar ($P < 0.001$), but only if started immediately after injury.[53] A 2 week delay resulted in no significant difference between treatments after 6 months. **Early resumption of normal activity versus immobilisation plus rest:** One RCT included in the second review (201 people presenting to an emergency department with acute whiplash)[51] compared advice to "act as usual" plus anti-inflammatory drugs versus immobilisation plus 14 days' sick leave.[55] It found that advice to "act as usual" plus anti-inflammatory drugs improved symptoms (including pain during daily activities, neck stiffness, memory, concentration, and headache) after 6 months, but found no significant difference between treatments in objective variables such as neck range and length of sick leave. The RCT also found no significant difference in severe symptoms after 6 months (11% with advice to "act as usual" *v* 15% with immobilisation; RR 0.75, 95% CI 0.08 to 1.42). **Home exercise programmes:** We found one RCT (59 people), which compared two home mobilisation regimens (a regular exercise treatment regimen or instructions to perform an additional isometric exercise at least 3 times a day) versus each other.[54] It found no significant difference between treatments in disability or pain after 3 or 6 months. **Electrotherapy:** One RCT (40 people with acute whiplash who all received analgesia and a neck collar) included in two reviews compared active pulsing electromagnetic field treatment versus sham pulsing electromagnetic field treatment.[56] It found that active pulsing electromagnetic field treatment significantly reduced pain after 4 weeks ($P < 0.05$), but not after 3 months compared with sham treatment. **Multimodal treatment:** One RCT (60 people) included in one of the reviews compared multimodal treatment (postural training, psychological support, eye fixation exercises, and manual treatment) versus physical treatment (electrical, sonic, ultrasound, and transcutaneous electrical nerve stimulation).[57] It found that multimodal treatment significantly reduced pain by the end of treatment ($P < 0.05$) and after 1 and 6 months ($P < 0.001$). The RCT also found that multimodal treatment reduced the time taken to return to work. **Drug treatments:** One systematic review found no RCTs.[51]

Harms: The reviews and RCTs did not consistently report adverse effects, although one trial has found that early mobilisation physiotherapy is not always well tolerated.[58]

Comment: In the first subsequent RCT comparing early mobilisation versus immobilisation, although early mobilisation led to early benefits in pain relief and movement, at 12 weeks' follow up there was no difference compared with use of a collar.[52] Only the 40% of people most severely affected by whiplash were included in the RCT comparing home exercise programmes, which may have led to a poorer outcome than that seen in practice.[54] The management of acute whiplash injury remains controversial and needs further investigation. We found one systematic review examining mobilisation and manipulation for mechanical neck disorders.[40] It included people with many types of neck pain, including uncomplicated pain, whiplash, and neck pain with radiculopathy, and reported that trials were clinically heterogeneous. However, it did not provide a subgroup analysis in people with whiplash. Across all of the people in the review, it reported that results were inconclusive.

QUESTION What are the effects of treatments for chronic whiplash injury?

One RCT found limited evidence that percutaneous radiofrequency neurotomy reduced pain compared with sham treatment after 27 weeks. A second RCT found no significant difference between physiotherapy alone and multimodal treatment in disability, pain, or range of movement at the end of treatment or at 3 months.

Benefits: We found one systematic review of treatment of chronic whiplash injury (search date 1993, 1 RCT, 24 people with chronic whiplash),[8] and one subsequent RCT.[59] The RCT identified in the review (24 people with chronic whiplash) found that neurotomy significantly increased the proportion of people who were free from pain compared with placebo after 27 weeks (58% with active treatment *v* 8% with placebo; ARR 50%, 95% CI 3% to 85%; NNT 2, 95% CI 1 to 29), and that neurotomy significantly increased the median time taken for more than half of the pain to return (263 days with radiofrequency neurotomy *v* 8 days with a sham treatment; $P = 0.04$).[60] The subsequent RCT (33 people with chronic whiplash) compared physiotherapy alone versus multimodal treatment (physiotherapy combined with cognitive behavioural therapy; see comment below).[59] It found no significant differences between treatments in disability, pain, or range of movement at the end of treatment or at 3 months. However, significantly more people treated with multimodal treatment were satisfied with pain control at the end of treatment and their ability to perform activities at 3 months ($P < 0.05$).

Harms: The RCTs did not report on adverse effects.[59,60]

Comment: Few RCTs have considered treatment for chronic whiplash and many people with whiplash are included in general RCTs of chronic mechanical neck pain. Limitations of the RCT comparing physiotherapy versus multimodal treatment include its small size, and the difference in time spent with the therapist in the two groups.[59]

QUESTION What are the effects of treatments for neck pain with radiculopathy?

OPTION SURGERY VERSUS CONSERVATIVE TREATMENT

One RCT found no significant difference between surgery and conservative treatment in symptoms after 1 year.

Benefits: We found one systematic review (search date 2000, 1 RCT).[61] One non-blinded RCT included in the review (81 people with severe radicular symptoms for at least 3 months; see comment below) compared surgery versus conservative treatment (physiotherapy or immobilisation in a neck collar).[62] It found no significant difference between treatments in symptoms after 1 year (mean visual analogue scale change: +30 mm with surgery *v* +39 mm with physiotherapy; mean difference –9 mm, 95% CI –23.4 mm to +5.4 mm).

Harms: The RCT did not report adverse effects.[62]

Comment: In the RCT, the number of people with prolapsed intervertebral disc was not stated.[62] The RCT reported that people who did not improve between 3 and 12 months were given additional treatments: one person in the physiotherapy group and five in the collar group underwent surgery; eight people in the surgery group underwent a second operation; and 12 people in the surgery group and 11 in the collar group received physiotherapy. The RCT also reported that 41% of people had a high anxiety score and 31% of people had a high depression score, which correlated with pain intensity after but not before treatment. At 1 year, 20% of people were depressed, which suggests that treatment should aim to improve both physical and psychological symptoms.[63] Conservative treatment needs further assessment, particularly in people considered to be poor risk candidates for surgery.

OPTION DRUG TREATMENTS (EPIDURAL STEROID INJECTIONS, ANALGESICS, NON-STEROIDAL ANTI-INFLAMMATORY DRUGS, OR MUSCLE RELAXANTS)

We found no evidence about the effects of epidural steroid injections, analgesics, non-steroidal anti-inflammatory drugs, or muscle relaxants.

Benefits: **Periradicular, cervical epidural steroid injections, or both:** We found no systematic review or RCTs. **Simple analgesics (paracetamol and opioids) and oral non-steroidal anti-inflammatory drugs:** We found no systematic review or RCTs. **Antidepressants:** We found no systematic review or RCTs. **Muscle relaxants and benzodiazepines:** We found no systematic review or RCTs.

Harms: **Periradicular, cervical epidural steroid injections, or both:** Case reports have documented occasional complications, such as infection or bleeding after cervical epidural injection. The incidence of adverse events after different cervical injection techniques is unknown.

Comment: None.

GLOSSARY

Manipulation The use of short or long lever high velocity thrusts directed at one or more of the cervical spine joints that does not involve anaesthesia or instrumentation.

McKenzie treatment Consists of comprehensive mechanical evaluation to assess the effect of repetitive movements, static positioning, or both, on the patient's symptoms. This mechanical diagnosis is meant to enable the physiotherapist to develop a mechanical treatment strategy aimed not only at resolving the patient's current symptoms, but also at long-term prevention of recurrence.

Mobilisation Any manual treatment to improve joint function that does not involve high velocity movement, anaesthesia, or instrumentation.

Wallenberg's syndrome (lateral medullary syndrome) Infarction of the dorsolateral aspect of the medulla oblongata. Manifestations may include loss of pain and temperature sensation in the same side of the face and opposite side of the body.

Substantive changes

Physical treatments One RCT[23] and longer term follow up[19] of an existing RCT added; conclusions unchanged.

Manual treatments (mobilisation and manipulation) One RCT[31] and longer term follow up[37] of an existing RCT added; intervention recategorised from Likely to be beneficial to Unknown effectiveness.

REFERENCES

1. Mäkelä M, Heliövaara M, Sievers K, et al. Prevalence, determinants, and consequences of chronic neck pain in Finland. *Am J Epidemiol* 1991;134:1356–1367.
2. Cote P, Cassidy D, Carroll L. The Saskatchewan health and back pain survey: the prevalence of neck pain and related disability in Saskatchewan adults. *Spine* 1998;23:1689–1698.
3. Hackett GI, Hudson MF, Wylie JB, et al. Evaluation of the efficacy and acceptability to patients of a physiotherapist working in a health centre. *BMJ* 1987;294:24–26.
4. Waalen D, White P, Waalen J. Demographic and clinical characteristics of chiropractic patients: a 5-year study of patients treated at the Canadian Memorial Chiropractic College. *J Can Chiropract Assoc* 1994;38:75–82.
5. Lamberts H, Brouwer H, Groen AJM, et al. Het transitiemodel in de huisartspraktijk. *Huisart Wet* 1987;30:105–113.
6. Kvarnstrom S. Occurrence of musculoskeletal disorders in a manufacturing industry with special attention to occupational shoulder disorders. *Scand J Rehabil Med Suppl* 1983;8:1–114.
7. Squires B, Gargan MF, Bannister GC. Soft-tissue injuries of the cervical spine: 15 year follow-up. *J Bone Joint Surg Br* 1996;78:955–957.
8. Spitzer WO, Skovron ML, Salmi LR, et al. Scientific monograph of the Quebec Task Force on whiplash-associated disorders: redefining "whiplash" and its management. *Spine* 1995;20(suppl 8):1–73. Search date 1993; primary sources Medline, TRIS, NTIS, personal contacts, and Task Force reference lists.
9. Ferrari R, Russell AS. Epidemiology of whiplash: an international dilemma. *Ann Rheum Dis* 1999;58:1–5.
10. Vernon H, Mior S. The neck disability index: a study of reliability and validity. *J Manipulative Physiol Ther* 1991;14:409–415.
11. Koes BW, Assendelft WJ, Van der Heijden GJ, et al. Spinal manipulation and mobilisation for back and neck pain: a blinded review. *BMJ* 1991;303:1298–1303. Search date 1990; primary source Medline.
12. Gross AR, Aker PD, Goldsmith CH, et al. Physical medicine modalities for mechanical neck disorders. In: The Cochrane Library, Issue 2, 2002. Oxford: Update Software. Search date 1993; primary sources Medline, Embase, Chirolars, Index to Chiropractic Literature, Cinahl, and Science Citation Index.
13. Kjellman GV, Skargren EI, Oberg BE. A critical analysis of randomised clinical trials on neck pain and treatment efficacy. A review of the literature. *Scand J Rehabil Med* 1999;31:139–152. Search date 1995; primary sources Medline, Cinahl, and hand searches of reference lists.
14. Van der Heijden GJ, Beurskens AJ, Koes BW, et al. The efficacy of traction for back and neck pain: a systematic, blinded review of randomized clinical trial methods. *Phys Ther* 1995;75:93–104. Search date 1992; primary sources Medline, Embase, Index to Chiropractic Literature, and Physiotherapy Index.
15. White AR, Ernst E. A systematic review of randomized controlled trials of acupuncture for neck pain. *Rheumatology* 1999;38:143–147. Search date 1998; primary sources Medline, Embase, Cochrane Library, and CISCOM (a database specialising in complementary medicine).
16. Smith LA, Oldman AD, McQuay HJ, et al. Teasing apart quality and validity in systematic reviews: an example from acupuncture trials in chronic neck and back pain. *Pain* 2000;86:119–132. Search date 1998; primary sources Medline, Embase, Cinahl, Psychlit, Cochrane Library, Oxford Pain Relief Database, and hand searches of reference lists.
17. Philadelphia Panel. Evidence-based clinical practice guidelines on selected rehabilitation interventions for neck pain. *Phys Ther* 2001;81:1701–1717. Search date 2000, primary sources Medline, Embase, Current

Contents, Cinahl, Cochrane Controlled Trials Register, Cochrane Field of Rehab and Related Therapies, Cochrane Musculoskeletal Group and PEDro.
18. Waling K, Sundelin G, Ahlgren C, et al. Perceived pain before and after three exercise programs – a controlled clinical trial of women with work-related trapezius myalgia. *Pain* 2000;85:201–207.
19. Waling K, Jaörvholm B, Sundelin G. Effects of training on female trapezius myalgia: an intervention study with a 3-year follow-up period. *Spine* 2002;27:789–796.
20. Irnich D, Behrens N, Molzen H, et al. Randomised trial of acupuncture compared with conventional massage and "sham" laser acupuncture for treatment of chronic neck pain. *BMJ* 2001;322:1574–1578.
21. Bronfort G, Evans R, Nelson B, et al. A randomized clinical trial of exercise and spinal manipulation for patients with chronic neck pain. *Spine* 2001;26:788–797.
22. Jordan A, Bendix T, Nielsen H, et al. Intensive training, physiotherapy, or manipulation for patients with chronic neck pain. A prospective, single-blinded, randomized clinical trial. *Spine* 1998;23:311–319.
23. Kjellman G, Oöberg B. A randomized clinical trial comparing general exercise, McKenzie treatment and a control group in patients with neck pain. *J Rehabil Med* 2002;34:183–190.
24. Goldie I, Landquist A. Evaluation of the effects of different forms of physiotherapy in cervical pain. *Scand J Rehabil Med* 1970;2:117–121.
25. Revel M, Minguet M, Gregory P, et al. Changes in cervicocephalic kinesthesia after a proprioceptive rehabilitation program in patients with neck pain: a randomised controlled study. *Arch Phys Med Rehabil* 1994;75:895–899.
26. Levoska S, Keinänen-Kiukaanniemi S. Active or passive physiotherapy for occupational cervicobrachial disorders? A comparison of two treatment methods with a 1-year follow-up. *Arch Phys Med Rehabil* 1993;74:425–430.
27. Trock DH, Bollet AJ, Markoll R. The effect of pulsed electromagnetic fields in the treatment of osteoarthritis of the knee and cervical spine. Report of randomized double-blind placebo controlled trials. *J Rheumatol* 1994;21:1903–1911.
28. Aker PD, Gross AR, Goldsmith CH, et al. Conservative management of mechanical neck pain: systematic overview and meta-analysis. *BMJ* 1996;313:1291–1296. Search date 1993; primary sources Medlars, Embase, Cinahl, and Chirolars.
29. Hurwitz EL, Aker PD, Adams AH, et al. Manipulation and mobilization of the cervical spine: a systematic review of the literature. *Spine* 1996;21:1746–1760. Search date 1995; primary sources Medline, Embase, Chirolars, and Cinahl.
30. Cassidy JD, Lopes AA, Yong-Hing K. The immediate effect of manipulation versus mobilization on pain and range of motion in the cervical spine: a randomised controlled trial. *J Manipulative Physiol Ther* 1992;15:570–575.
31. Hurwitz EL, Morgenstern H, Harber P, et al. A randomized trial of chiropractic manipulation and mobilization for patients with neck pain: clinical outcomes from the UCLA neck-pain study. *Am J Public Health* 2002;92:1634–1641.
32. Koes BW, Bouter LM, Van Mameren H, et al. Randomised clinical trial of manipulative therapy and physiotherapy for persistent back and neck complaints: results of one year follow up. *BMJ* 1992;304:601–605.
33. Nordemar R, Thörner C. Treatment of acute cervical pain: a comparative group study. *Pain* 1981;10:93–101.
34. Brodin H. Cervical pain and mobilization. *Manipulative Med* 1985;2:18–22.
35. Sloop PR, Smith DS, Goldenberg E, et al. Manipulation for chronic neck pain: a double-blind controlled study. *Spine* 1982;7:532–535.
36. Howe DH, Newcombe RG, Wade MT. Manipulation of the cervical spine: a pilot study. *J R Coll Gen Pract* 1983;33:574–579.
37. Evans R, Bronfort G, Nelson B, et al. Two-year follow-up of a randomized clinical trial of spinal manipulation and two types of exercise for patients with chronic neck pain. *Spine* 2002;27:2383–2389.
38. Dabbs V, Lauretti WJ. A risk assessment of cervical manipulation vs NSAIDS for the treatment of neck pain. *J Manipulative Physiol Ther* 1995;18:530–536.
39. Di Fabio RP. Manipulation of the cervical spine: risks and benefits. *Phys Ther* 1999;79:50–65.
40. Gross AK, Hondras M, Goldsmith C, et al. Manual therapy for mechanical neck disorders: a systematic review. *Man Ther* 2002;7:131–149. Search date 1998; primary sources Medline, Embase, Mantis, Cinahl, Index chiropractic literature, and Cochrane Controlled Trials Register.
41. Karjalainen K, Malmivaara A, Van Tulder M, et al. Multidisciplinary biopsychosocial rehabilitation for neck and shoulder pain among working age adults: a systematic review within the framework of the Cochrane Collaboration Back Review Group. *Spine* 2001;26:174–181. Search date 1998; primary sources Medline, Psychlit, Embase, and Cochrane.
42. Taimela S, Takala EP, Asklof T, et al. Active treatment of chronic neck pain: a prospective randomized intervention. *Spine* 2000;25:1021–1027.
43. Linton SJ, Andersson MA. Can chronic disability be prevented? A randomized trial of a cognitive-behaviour intervention and two forms of information for patients with spinal pain. *Spine* 2000:21:2825–2831.
44. Horneij E, Hemborg B, Jensen I, et al. No significant differences between intervention programmes on neck, shoulder and low back pain: a prospective randomized study among home-care personnel. *J Rehabil Med* 2001;33:170–176.
45. Kamwendo K, Linton SJ. A controlled study of the effect of neck school in medical secretaries. *Scand J Rehabil Med* 1991:23:143–152.
46. Koes BW. *Efficacy of manual therapy for back and neck complaints.* [Thesis]. den Haag: Cip-Gegevens Koninklijke Bibliotheek, 1992.
47. Lavin RA, Pappagallo M, Kuhlemeier KV. Cervical pain: a comparison of three pillows. *Arch Phys Med Rehabil* 1997;78:193–198.
48. Basmajian JV. Cyclobenzaprine hydrochloride effect on skeletal muscle spasm in the lumbar region and neck: two double-blind controlled clinical and laboratory studies. *Arch Phys Med Rehabil* 1978;59:58–63.
49. Bercel NA. Cyclobenzaprine in the treatment of skeletal muscle spasm in osteoarthritis of the cervical and lumbar spine. *Curr Ther Res* 1977;22:462–468.
50. Bose K. The efficacy and safety of eperisone in patients with cervical spondylosis: results of a randomised double-blind placebo-controlled trial. *Meth Find Exp Clin Pharmacol* 1999:21:209–213.
51. Verhagen AP, Peeters GG, de Bie RA, et al. Conservative treatment for whiplash. In: The Cochrane Library, Issue 2, 2002. Oxford: Update

Software. Search date 1998; primary sources Medline, Embase, Cinahl, Psychlit, and Cochrane Controlled Trials Register.
52. Bonk AD, Ferrari R, Giebel GD, et al. Prospective, randomized, controlled study of activity versus collar, and the natural history for whiplash injury, in Germany. *J Musculoskel Pain* 2000;8:123–132.
53. Rosenfeld M, Gunnarsson R, Borenstein P. Early intervention in whiplash-associated disorders: a comparison of two treatment protocols. *Spine* 2000;25:1782–1787.
54. Söderlund A, Olerud C, Lindberg P. Acute whiplash-associated disorders (WAD): the effects of early mobilization and prognostic factors in long-term symptomatology. *Clin Rehab* 2000;14:457–467.
55. Borchgrevink GE, Kaasa A, McDonagh D, et al. Acute treatment of whiplash neck sprain injuries: a randomised trial of treatment during the first 14 days after a car accident. *Spine* 1998;23:25–31.
56. Foley-Nolan D, Moore K, Codd M, et al. Low energy high frequency pulsed electromagnetic therapy for acute whiplash injuries. A double blind randomised controlled study. *Scand J Rehabil Med* 1992;24:51–59.
57. Provinciali L, Baroni M, Illuminati L, et al. Multimodal treatment to prevent the late whiplash syndrome. *Scand J Rehabil Med* 1996;28:105–111.
58. Pennie BH, Agambar LJ. Whiplash injuries: a trial of early management. *J Bone Joint Surg Br* 1990;72:277–279.
59. Söderlund A, Lindberg P. Cognitive behavioural components in physiotherapy management of chronic whiplash associated disorders (WAD) — a randomised group study. *Physiother Theory Pract* 2001;17:229–238.
60. Lord SM, Barnsley L, Wallis BJ, et al. Percutaneous radio-frequency neurotomy for chronic cervical zygapophyseal-joint pain. *N Engl J Med*. 1996;335:1721–1726.
61. Fouyas IP, Statham PF, Sandercock PA, et al. Surgery for cervical radiculomyelopathy. The Cochrane Library, Issue 2, 2001. Oxford: Update Software. Search date 2000; primary sources Medline, Embase, and Cochrane Controlled Trials Register.
62. Persson LC, Carlsson CA, Carlsson JY. Long-lasting cervical radicular pain managed with surgery, physiotherapy, or a cervical collar: a prospective randomised study. *Spine* 1997;22:751–758.
63. Persson LCG, Lilja A. Pain, coping, emotional state and physical function in patients with chronic radicular neck pain. A comparison between patients treated with surgery, physiotherapy or neck collar — a blinded, prospective randomized study. *Disabil Rehabil* 2001;23:325–335.

Allan Binder
Consultant Rheumatologist
Lister Hospital
Stevenage
UK

Competing interests: None declared.

Non-steroidal anti-inflammatory drugs

Search date September 2002

Peter C Gøtzsche

QUESTIONS

INTERVENTIONS

See glossary, p 1400

Key Messages

Differences between non-steroidal anti-inflammatory drugs (NSAIDs)

- **Choice between different NSAIDs** Systematic reviews have found no important differences in benefits among different NSAIDs or doses, but found differences in harms related to choice and dose of NSAID.
- **NSAIDs in increased doses** Systematic reviews have found that benefits of NSAIDs increase towards a maximum value at high doses. Recommended doses are close to creating the maximum benefit. In contrast, three systematic reviews found no ceiling for adverse effects, which increased in an approximately linear fashion with dose.

Preventing gastrointestinal adverse effects

- **H_2 blockers in people who cannot avoid NSAIDs** One systematic review in people who had taken NSAIDs for 3 months has found that double doses of H_2 blockers versus placebo significantly reduce the development of endoscopically diagnosed gastric and duodenal ulcers. One RCT found that omeprazole versus ranitidine in double doses significantly increased remission after 6 months. One RCT with a high withdrawal and exclusion rate found weak evidence that misoprostol versus ranitidine in doubles doses significantly reduced the number of people with gastric ulcers.

- **Misoprostol in people who cannot avoid NSAIDs** One systematic review in people who had taken NSAIDs for at least 3 months has found that misoprostol versus placebo significantly reduces the development of gastric or duodenal ulcers. One additional RCT in people with rheumatoid arthritis taking NSAIDs found that misoprostol versus placebo significantly reduced the incidence of serious upper gastrointestinal complications, such as perforation, gastric outlet obstruction, or bleeding over 6 months. Subgroup analysis found a greater absolute effect in people at high risk. RCTs have found that misoprostol versus placebo significantly increases gastrointestinal adverse events, such as diarrhoea and abdominal pain. One RCT found that more people with ulcers who had improved with either omeprazole or misoprostol, and who were then re-randomised to treatment with omeprazole or misoprostol, remained in remission with omeprazole versus misoprostol.
- **Omeprazole in people who cannot avoid NSAIDs** One systematic review in people who had taken NSAIDs for at least 3 months has found that omeprazole versus placebo significantly reduces the incidence of endoscopically diagnosed gastric and duodenal ulcers.

Topical NSAIDs

- **Topical NSAIDs in acute and chronic pain conditions** One systematic review in people with acute and chronic pain conditions has found that topical NSAIDs versus placebo significantly reduce pain.
- **Topical versus systemic NSAIDs or alternative analgesics** One systematic review found no high quality RCTs of topical NSAIDs versus oral forms of the same NSAID, or versus paracetamol.

DEFINITION Non-steroidal anti-inflammatory drugs (NSAIDs) have anti-inflammatory, analgesic, and antipyretic effects, and inhibit platelet aggregation. The drugs have no documented effect on the course of musculoskeletal diseases, such as rheumatoid arthritis and osteoarthritis.

INCIDENCE/ PREVALENCE NSAIDs are widely used. Almost 10% of people in the Netherlands used a non-aspirin NSAID in 1987, and the overall use was 11 defined daily doses (see glossary, p 1400) per 1000 population per day.[1] In Australia in 1994, overall use was 35 defined daily doses per 1000 population per day, with 36% of the people receiving NSAIDs for osteoarthritis, 42% for sprain and strain or low back pain, and 4% for rheumatoid arthritis; 35% were aged over 60 years.[2]

AIMS OF INTERVENTION To reduce symptoms in rheumatic disorders; to avoid severe gastrointestinal adverse effects.

OUTCOMES **Primary outcomes:** pain intensity; personal preference for one drug over another; global efficacy; clinically significant gastrointestinal complications. **Secondary outcomes:** number of tender joints; perforation; gastrointestinal haemorrhage; dyspepsia; and ulcer detected by routine endoscopy.

METHODS *Clinical Evidence* search and appraisal September 2002. More than 100 systematic reviews and thousands of RCTs have compared various NSAIDs. Many RCTs are unpublished or published in sources that are not indexed in publicly available databases. The quality of the RCTs is variable and bias is common, both in the design and analysis of the RCTs, to such an extent that one systematic review identified false significant findings favouring new drugs over control drugs in 6% of RCTs.[3] We included only large RCTs that provided clinically important information not already covered in the systematic reviews. We have favoured systematic reviews that have not been sponsored or authored by industry, as bias in such reviews has been repeatedly demonstrated, but may be difficult to detect.[4] For example, it is easy seemingly to follow the rules for systematic reviews and yet adopt inclusion and exclusion criteria that omit inconvenient studies. It is hard to find a systematic review sponsored by, or coauthored by, industry that concludes that the company's product is not better than those of its competitors.

QUESTION **Are there any important differences between available non-steroidal anti-inflammatory drugs (NSAIDs)?**

Systematic reviews have found no important differences in benefit between different NSAIDs or doses, but found differences in toxicity related to increased doses and to the nature of the NSAID itself. We found no large double blind RCTs comparing an NSAID with paracetamol in acute musculoskeletal syndromes. We found no evidence that NSAIDs are more effective than simple analgesics.

Benefits: **Rheumatoid arthritis:** We found two systematic reviews[5,6] and one subsequent RCT.[7] The first systematic review (search date 1985, 37 crossover RCTs, 1416 people) compared indometacin (indomethacin), an old drug, with 10 newer NSAIDs in people treated for a median of 2 weeks with each drug.[5] Four of the RCTs included a placebo period and one RCT compared four drugs. It found that only 5% more people (95% CI 0% to 10%) preferred the newer NSAID to indometacin. The second systematic review (search date 1988, 6440 people, 88 RCTs comparing 2 NSAIDs and 27 RCTs comparing an NSAID with placebo) found no significant differences in the number of tender joints improved between 17 different NSAIDs.[6] The subsequent RCT (1149 people) compared three doses of the cyclo-oxygenase 2 (COX-2) inhibitor celecoxib versus naproxen 1 g.[7] It found fewer endoscopically detected ulcers (5% *v* 26%; ARR 21%, 95% CI 13% to 29%). Only one of the ulcers was clinically significant and only 7/692 (1%) people taking celecoxib and 5/225 (2%) people taking naproxen withdrew because of gastrointestinal adverse effects.[7] **Osteoarthritis:** Two systematic reviews (search dates 1994[8] and 1996[9]) found no clear differences between various NSAIDs used to treat osteoarthritis of the hip (39 RCTs)[8] or the knee (16 RCTs).[9] One prespecified meta-analysis (8 RCTs, 5435 people) of rofecoxib versus other NSAIDs found a lower cumulative incidence over 12 months of clinically significant gastrointestinal adverse events with rofecoxib (1% *v* 2%; RR 0.51, 95% CI 0.26 to 1.00).[10] Fewer people taking rofecoxib withdrew because of gastrointestinal adverse effects (118/3357 [4%] *v* 75/1564 [5%]; ARR 1%; RR 0.73, 95% CI 0.55 to 0.97; NNT with rofecoxib *v* other NSAIDs to avoid 1 additional withdrawal because of gastrointestinal adverse effects 78, 95% CI 46 to 790). **Acute musculoskeletal syndromes:** We found two systematic reviews, which identified generally poor quality RCTs.[11,12] The first systematic review (search date 1998, 17 RCTs for shoulder pain) was inconclusive (see

NSAIDs under osteoarthritis, p 1402).[12] The second systematic review (search date 1993, 84 RCTs, 32 025 people with soft tissue injuries of the ankle) was unable to pool data to perform a statistical analysis of the different forms of treatment.[11] **Dose response relation:** One systematic review (search date 1985; 19 RCTs in which participants were randomised to more than 1 dose of 9 different NSAIDs) found a dose response relation that saturated at high doses.[13] This and another systematic review (search date 1992, 1545 people)[14] found that the recommended dosages were close to providing a ceiling effect.[13,14] The review of 115 RCTs found no significant differences between various doses of drugs;[6] 10/21 RCTs of ibuprofen had used a daily dosage of 1200 mg or less.[6]

Harms: **Versus placebo:** One systematic review (search date not stated, 100 RCTs, 12 853 people) found a non-significant tendency towards a higher rate of haemorrhage (ARI for NSAIDs *v* placebo +0.7%, 95% CI –0.1% to +1.5%) and proven ulcer (ARI for NSAIDs *v* placebo +0.05%, 95% CI –0.01% to +0.11%) with NSAIDs compared with placebo.[15] Mean treatment duration was short (2 months).[15] For 40 aspirin RCTs (22 234 people, mean treatment duration 1 year) the review found an increased risk of haemorrhage (ARI 0.6%, 95% CI 0.2% to 1.0%) and for proven ulcer (ARI 0.6%, 95% CI 0% to 1.2%).[15] The number needed to harm was in the range 100–1000. One systematic review (search date 1990, 38 placebo controlled RCTs) found that NSAIDs raised mean blood pressure by 5.0 mm Hg (95% CI 1.2 mm Hg to 8.7 mm Hg).[16] **Versus other NSAIDs:** One meta-analysis of 11 case control studies and one cohort study found that ibuprofen was significantly less toxic than other NSAIDs. The 11 comparator drugs were associated with a increase in risk of serious upper gastrointestinal complications (range RR 1.6 to 9.2-fold).[17] Cyclo-oxygenase 2 (COX-2) inhibitors were associated with less gastrointestinal toxicity than older NSAIDs, but the clinical significance is not clear (see benefits above).[7,10] One systematic review found that COX-2 inhibitors were associated with more serious thrombotic cardiovascular events than older NSAIDs.[18] The difference was significant for rofecoxib versus naproxen (RR 2.38, 95% CI 1.39 to 4.00; ARI 0.6%, 95% CI 0% to 1%), but for celecoxib versus ibuprofen or diclofenac the difference was not statistically significant (figures presented graphically). However, an indirect comparison in a meta-analysis of thrombosis prevention found a significant increase in the annual rate of myocardial infarction between both rofecoxib and celecoxib versus placebo (0.74% for rofecoxib *v* 0.80% for celecoxib *v* 0.52% for placebo; $P < 0.05$ for both comparisons), which suggests that there may be a class effect. **Dose response relation:** Three systematic reviews (search dates 1992[14,19] and 1994[17]) found no ceiling effect for adverse effects; the incidence of adverse effects increased in an approximately linear fashion with dose.

Comment: Important differences in adverse effects seem to exist between different NSAIDs. In contrast, the beneficial effects of NSAIDs seem similar. People's preferences for particular drugs have not been replicated and could, therefore, be because of chance or natural fluctuations in disease activity.[20,21] The evidence suggests that if the NSAID is unsatisfactory, switching to another NSAID will not solve the problem.[20,21] Likewise, doubling the dose of an NSAID leads to only a small increase in effect, which may not be clinically relevant. In acute musculoskeletal problems it is doubtful whether NSAIDs have any clinically relevant anti-inflammatory effect; we found no large double blind RCT comparing an NSAID with paracetamol. Paracetamol has been studied in osteoarthritis, where it had much the same effect as ibuprofen or naproxen (see simple analgesics v NSAIDs under osteoarthritis, p 1402).

QUESTION **What are the effects of co-treatments to reduce the risk of gastrointestinal adverse effects of non-steroidal anti-inflammatory drugs (NSAIDs)?**

One systematic review in people who had taken NSAIDs for 3 months has found that double doses of H_2 blockers versus placebo significantly reduce the development of endoscopically diagnosed gastric and duodenal ulcers. One RCT found that omeprazole versus H_2 blockers significantly increased remission after 6 months. One RCT with a high withdrawal and exclusion rate found weak evidence that misoprostol versus H_2 blockers significantly reduced the number of people with gastric ulcers. One systematic review in people who had taken NSAIDs for at least 3 months has found that misoprostol versus placebo significantly reduces the development of gastric or duodenal ulcers. One additional RCT in people with rheumatoid arthritis taking NSAIDs found that misoprostol versus placebo significantly reduced the incidence of serious upper gastrointestinal complications, such as perforation, gastric outlet obstruction, or bleeding over 6 months. Subgroup analysis found a greater absolute effect in people at high risk. RCTs have found that misoprostol versus placebo significantly increases gastrointestinal adverse effects such as diarrhoea and abdominal pain. One RCT found that more people with ulcers who had improved with treatment with either omeprazole or misoprostol and then re-randomised remained in remission with omeprazole versus misoprostol. One systematic review in people who had taken NSAIDs for at least 3 months has found that omeprazole versus placebo significantly reduces the incidence of endoscopically diagnosed gastric and duodenal ulcers.

Benefits: We found one systematic review.[22] **Misoprostol versus placebo:** The systematic review (search date 2000, 9 RCTs, 3329 people) included people who had received NSAIDs for at least 3 months and where ulcers were detected by routine endoscopy.[22] Misoprostol reduced the development of endoscopic ulcers compared with placebo (61/1620 [4%] *v* 221/1709 [13%]; ARR 10%, 95% CI 9% to 12% for gastric ulcer; and 46/1301 [4%] with misoprostol *v* 85/1394 [6%] with placebo; ARR 4%, 95% CI 2% to 5% for duodenal ulcer). Indirect comparisons of different RCTs suggested a dose response relationship (P = 0.006) for gastric ulcers in the dose range 400–800 µg. One additional 6 month RCT (8843 people with rheumatoid arthritis, mean age 68 years, all treated with NSAIDs) with clinically relevant outcomes compared misoprostol (800 µg daily) versus placebo.[23] Serious upper gastrointestinal complications (such as perforation, gastric outlet obstruction, or bleeding detected by clinical symptoms or investigation) were reduced by misoprostol compared with placebo (25/4404 [0.6%] with misoprostol v 42/4439 [1.0%] with placebo; ARR 0.4%; NNT 265, 95% CI 133 to 6965).[23] The risk of serious upper gastrointestinal complications was approximately doubled for people over 75 years old, and for those with a history of peptic ulcer, bleeding, or cardiovascular disease. People with all four risk factors had an absolute risk of 9% for a major complication in 6 months, corresponding to a number needed to treat with misoprostol rather than placebo of 28 people. **H_2 blockers versus placebo:** The systematic review included five RCTs with 1005 people who had received NSAIDs for at least 3 months.[22] Double doses (see glossary, p 1400) of H_2 blockers significantly reduced the development of endoscopic ulcers compared with placebo (17/151 [11%] v 38/147 [26%]; ARR 14%, 95% CI 6% to 23% for gastric ulcer; and 5/151 [3%] v 20/147 [14%]; ARR 10%, 95% CI 4% to 17% for duodenal ulcers). **Omeprazole versus placebo:** The systematic review included three RCTs with 774 people who had received NSAIDs for at least 3 months.[22] Omeprazole versus placebo reduced the development of ulcers detected of endoscopy (ARR 13%, 95% CI 8% to 18% for gastric ulcer; ARR 9%, 95% CI 5% to 12% for duodenal ulcer). **Misoprostol versus omeprazole:** We found one RCT (935 people treated with NSAIDs who had ulcers or more than 10 erosions at endoscopy). Treatment success was defined as fewer than five erosions at each site, no ulcers, and not more than mild dyspepsia.[24] At 8 weeks, treatment was successful in 76% of people given omeprazole (20 mg daily), 75% given omeprazole (40 mg daily), and 71% given misoprostol (800 µg daily). A total of 732 people in whom treatment was successful were re-randomised to maintenance treatment for 6 months. A higher percentage of people remained in remission with omeprazole (20 mg) than with misoprostol (400 µg) (61% v 48% [raw data not available]), and with either drug than with placebo (27% in remission with placebo; ARR for omeprazole v placebo 34%, 95% CI 25% to 43%; NNT 3; ARR for misoprostol v placebo 21%, 95% CI 12% to 30%; NNT 5). **Omeprazole versus H_2 blockers:** In a similarly designed RCT (541 people), treatment was successful in 80% given omeprazole (20 mg), 79% given omeprazole (40 mg), and 63% given ranitidine (300 mg daily).[25] The estimated proportions in remission after 6 months were 72% with omeprazole (20 mg) and 59% with ranitidine (300 mg) (ARR for omeprazole v ranitidine 13%, 95% CI 4% to 22%; NNT 8). **Misoprostol versus H_2 blockers:** One 8 week RCT (538 people with NSAID related upper gastrointestinal pain without endoscopic evidence of ulcers) compared misoprostol (800 µg) versus ranitidine (300 mg daily).[26] A third of the people were excluded from analysis because of problems with adherence and missing endoscopic examinations. Gastric ulcers at least 3 mm in diameter were found in 1% of people taking misoprostol and in 6% of people taking ranitidine (ARR for misoprostol v ranitidine 5%, 95% CI 2% to 9%; NNT 20). Duodenal ulcer rate was 1% with both drugs.

Harms: In one of the large RCTs, significantly more people receiving misoprostol than placebo withdrew from the study because of adverse events, primarily diarrhoea and abdominal pain (1210/4404 [27%] v 896/4439 [20%]; ARI 7%; RR 1.36, 95% CI 1.26 to 1.47;

NNH 14, 95% CI 12 to 19).[23] There was no significant difference in the number of deaths (17/4404 [0.4%] deaths in the misoprostol group *v* 21/4439 [0.5%] in the placebo group; ARR 0.1%; RR 0.82, 95% CI 0.43 to 1.55). One person on placebo died as a direct result of gastrointestinal toxicity. Few adverse events were reported in the RCT comparing omeprazole with ranitidine. Treatment discontinuations (all causes) occurred in 10% of people taking omeprazole (20 mg), 10% taking omeprazole (40 mg), and 14% taking ranitidine.[25] In the RCT comparing misoprostol with ranitidine, adverse events (mostly gastrointestinal) occurred in 77% of people taking misoprostol and 66% taking ranitidine, with withdrawal rates of 13% on misoprostol and 7% on ranitidine (ARR for withdrawal ranitidine *v* misoprostol 6%, 95% CI 1% to 11%; NNT 17).[26]

Comment: The clinical relevance of these findings is doubtful. The only RCT that used clinically relevant outcomes found little difference between active drug and placebo, except for people at high risk.[23] The rate of ulcers was more than 10 times higher in the studies where the investigators looked for them with regular endoscopy than in earlier RCTs of NSAIDs.[16] These ulcers were sometimes defined as endoscopic lesions with a size of only 3 mm, sometimes as any lesion of an unequivocal depth, and sometimes no definition was provided at all.

QUESTION What are the effects of topical non-steroidal anti-inflammatory drugs (NSAIDs)?

One systematic review has found that topical NSAIDs versus placebo are effective in acute pain conditions and chronic pain conditions. We found no high quality RCTs of topical versus oral formulations of the same drug, and found no direct comparisons of topical NSAIDs versus paracetamol.

Benefits: **Versus placebo:** We found one systematic review (search date 1996, 86 RCTs, 10 160 people) that primarily compared a topical NSAID with placebo[27] and one additional RCT.[28] The review was partly sponsored by two manufacturers. Many RCTs of acute pain conditions (soft tissue trauma, strains, and sprains) were small; in 37 RCTs, the average number of actively treated people was 32 and the effect declined significantly with sample size. In seven RCTs with more than 80 people per group, the number of people that would need to be treated for one extra good outcome was five (RR 1.6, 95% CI 1.3 to 1.9; NNT 5, 95% CI 4 to 6). A good outcome included patient global judgement; pain on movement; spontaneous pain; and physician global judgement. In 12 RCTs on chronic pain conditions (osteoarthritis, tendinitis), the number of people that would need to be treated for one extra good outcome was four (RR 2.0, 95% CI 1.5 to 2.7; NNT 4, 95% CI 3 to 4). The additional RCT (116 people with osteoarthritis of the hip or knee) compared copper salicylate gel versus placebo applied to the forearm.[28] It found no significant difference in effect (22% *v* 21% of participants reported good effect). **Versus oral NSAIDs:** Five RCTs in the systematic review compared topical versus oral NSAIDs, but they all had inadequate design and power.[27] We found no high quality RCT comparing the same NSAID given orally and topically (see effects of topical agents under osteoarthritis, p 1402). **Versus paracetamol:** We found no RCTs.

Harms: In the systematic review, local adverse effects occurred in 3% of people in both groups and systemic adverse events in 1%.[27] In the additional RCT, more people receiving copper salicylate gel reported adverse reactions, most commonly skin reactions (any adverse event 48/58 [83%] with copper salicylate gel *v* 29/56 [52%] with placebo; RR 1.6, 95% CI 1.2 to 2.1; NNH 4, 95% CI 3 to 7), and more people withdrew from the RCT because of these reactions (10/58 [17%] *v* 1/58 [2%]; ARR 13%; RR 10, 95% CI 1.3 to 75.6; NNH 6, 95% CI 3 to 20).[28]

Comment: Sample size bias hampers the interpretation of the available RCTs. We found no high quality RCTs comparing topical versus systemic administration of the same NSAID, and no RCTs comparing a topical NSAID with paracetamol.

GLOSSARY

Defined daily dose The assumed average daily dose for the main indication of a specified drug. The defined daily dose per 1000 population per day is an estimate of the proportion of that population receiving treatment with that drug.

Double doses Twice the defined daily dose.

REFERENCES

1. Leufkens HG, Ameling CB, Hekster YA, et al. Utilization patterns of non-steroidal anti-inflammatory drugs in an open Dutch population. *Pharm Weekbl Sci* 1990;12:97–103.
2. McManus P, Primrose JG, Henry DA, et al. Pattern of non-steroidal anti-inflammatory drug use in Australia 1990–1994. A report from the drug utilization sub-committee of the pharmaceutical benefits advisory committee. *Med J Aust* 1996;164:589–592.
3. Gøtzsche PC. Methodology and overt and hidden bias in reports of 196 double-blind trials of nonsteroidal anti-inflammatory drugs in rheumatoid arthritis (published erratum appears in *Control Clin Trials* 1989;10:356). *Control Clin Trials* 1989;10:31–56. Search date 1985; primary source Medline.
4. Smith GD, Matthias E. Meta-analysis: unresolved issues and future developments. *BMJ* 1998;316:221–225.
5. Gøtzsche PC. Patients' preference in indomethacin trials: an overview. *Lancet* 1989;i:88–91. Search date 1985; primary sources Medline, personal contact with companies that marketed proprietary products, and hand searched reference lists of collected articles.
6. Gøtzsche PC. Meta-analysis of NSAIDs: contribution of drugs, doses, trial designs, and meta-analytic techniques. *Scand J Rheumatol* 1993;22:255–260. Search date 1988; primary source Medline.
7. Simon LS, Weaver AL, Graham DY, et al. Anti-inflammatory and upper gastrointestinal effects of celecoxib in rheumatoid arthritis. *JAMA* 1999;282:1921–1928.
8. Towheed T, Shea B, Wells G, et al. Analgesia and non-aspirin, non-steroidal anti-inflammatory drugs in osteoarthritis of the hip. In: The Cochrane Library, Issue 3, 2002. Oxford: Update Software. Search date 1994; primary sources Cochrane Controlled Trials Register, Medline, and hand searched references.
9. Watson MC, Brookes ST, Kirwan JR, et al. Non-aspirin, non-steroidal anti-inflammatory drugs for treating osteoarthritis of the knee. In: The Cochrane Library, Issue 3, 2002. Oxford: Update Software. Search date 1996; primary sources Medline and Embase.
10. Langman MJ, Jensen DM, Watson DG, et al. Adverse upper gastrointestinal effects of rofecoxib compared with NSAIDs. *JAMA* 1999;282:1929–1933.
11. Ogilvie Harris DJ, Gilbart M. Treatment modalities for soft tissue injuries of the ankle: a critical review. *Clin J Sport Med* 1995;5:175–186. Search date 1993; primary sources Medline and Embase.
12. Green S, Buchbinder R, Glazier R, et al. Interventions for shoulder pain. In: The Cochrane Library, Issue 3, 2002. Oxford: Update Software. Search date 1998; primary sources Cochrane Musculoskeletal Group Trials Register, Cochrane Controlled Trials Register, Medline, Embase, Cinahl, and Science Citation Index.
13. Gøtzsche PC. Review of dose-response studies of NSAIDs in rheumatoid arthritis. *Dan Med Bull* 1989;36:395–399. Search date 1985; primary sources Medline, hand searches of reference lists, and contact with companies marketing proproctary preparations.
14. Eisenberg E, Berkey CS, Carr DB, et al. Efficacy and safety of nonsteroidal antiinflammatory drugs for cancer pain: a meta-analysis. *J Clin Oncol* 1994;12:2756–2765. Search date 1992; primary source Medline.
15. Chalmers TC, Berrier J, Hewitt P, et al. Meta-analysis of randomized controlled trials as a method of estimating rare complications of non-steroidal anti-inflammatory drug therapy. *Aliment Pharmacol Ther* 1988;2(suppl. 1):9–26. Search date not stated; primary source Medline.
16. Johnson AG, Nguyen TV, Day RO. Do nonsteroidal anti-inflammatory drugs affect blood pressure? A meta-analysis. *Ann Intern Med* 1994;121:289–300. Search date 1990; primary sources Medline, Embase, Biosis, Diagenes, Science Citation Abstracts, International Pharmaceutical Abstracts, IOWA Drug Information Service, Combined Health Informatics Database, and hand searched bibliographies, text books, and reference lists.

17. Henry D, Lim LL, Garcia Rodriguez LA, et al. Variability in risk of gastrointestinal complications with individual non-steroidal anti-inflammatory drugs: results of a collaborative meta-analysis. *BMJ* 1996;312:1563–1566. Search date 1994; primary source Medline.
18. Mukherjee D, Nissen SE, Topol EJ. Risk of cardiovascular events associated with selective COX-2 inhibitors. *JAMA* 2001;286:954–959. Search date 2001; primary sources Medline, the internet, and review of relevant submissions to the US Food and Drug Administration by pharmaceutical companies.
19. Cappelleri JC, Lau J, Kupelnick B, et al. Efficacy and safety of different aspirin dosages on vascular diseases in high-risk patients. A metaregression analysis. *Online J Curr Clin Trials* 1995;Doc No 174. Search date 1992; primary sources Medline and Current Contents.
20. Huskisson EC, Woolf DL, Balme HW, et al. Four new anti-inflammatory drugs: responses and variations. *BMJ* 1976;i:1048–1049.
21. Cooperating Clinics Committee of the American Rheumatism Association. A seven-day variability study of 499 patients with peripheral rheumatoid arthritis. *Arthritis Rheum* 1965;8:302–334.
22. Rostom A, Wells G, Tugwell P, et al. Prevention of chronic NSAID induced upper gastrointestinal toxicity. In: The Cochrane Library, Issue 3, 2002. Oxford: Update Software. Search date 2000; primary sources Medline, Current Contents, Embase, Cochrane Controlled Trials Register, hand searched conference proceedings, and personal contact with experts and companies.
23. Silverstein FE, Graham DY, Senior JR, et al. Misoprostol reduces serious gastrointestinal complications in patients with rheumatoid arthritis receiving nonsteroidal anti-inflammatory drugs. A randomized, double-blind, placebo-controlled trial. *Ann Intern Med* 1995;123:241–249.
24. Hawkey CJ, Karrasch JA, Szczepanski L, et al. Omeprazole compared with misoprostol for ulcers associated with nonsteroidal antiinflammatory drugs. Omeprazole versus misoprostol for NSAID-induced ulcer management (OMNIUM) study group. *N Engl J Med* 1998;338:727–734.
25. Yeomans ND, Tulassay Z, Juhasz L, et al. A comparison of omeprazole with ranitidine for ulcers associated with nonsteroidal antiinflammatory drugs. Acid suppression trial: ranitidine versus omeprazole for NSAID associated ulcer treatment (ASTRONAUT) study group. *N Engl J Med* 1998;338:719–726.
26. Raskin JB, White RH, Jaszewski R, et al. Misoprostol and ranitidine in the prevention of NSAID-induced ulcers: a prospective, double-blind, multicenter study. *Am J Gastroenterol* 1996;91:223–227.
27. Moore RA, Tramer MR, Carroll D, et al. Quantitative systematic review of topically applied non-steroidal anti-inflammatory drugs. *BMJ* 1998;316:333–338. Search date 1996; primary sources Medline, Embase, Oxford Pain Relief Database 1950–1994, contact with pharmaceutical companies, and hand searched references.
28. Shackel NA, Day RO, Kellett B, et al. Copper-salicylate gel for pain relief in osteoarthritis: a randomised controlled trial. *Med J Aust* 1997;167:134–136.

Peter Gøtzsche
Director
The Nordic Cochrane Centre
Copenhagen
Denmark

Competing interests: None declared.

Osteoarthritis

Search date November 2002

David Scott, Claire Smith, Stefan Lohmander, and Jiri Chard

QUESTIONS

INTERVENTIONS

To be covered in future updates
Other surgical interventions for osteoarthritis, including washout of the joint

See glossary, p 1424

Key Messages

- **Hip replacement** One systematic review of RCTs and observational studies has found that hip replacement is effective for at least 10 years.
- **Knee replacement** Systematic reviews of observational studies have found that knee replacement is effective in relieving pain and improving function. One RCT found limited evidence that unicompartmental knee replacement is more effective than tricompartmental replacement at 5 years' follow up. One systematic review of observational studies found better outcomes with unicompartmental knee operations compared with bicompartmental operations.

- **Oral non-steroidal anti-inflammatory drugs (NSAIDs) (short term pain relief)** Systematic reviews have found that NSAIDs reduce short term pain in osteoarthritis compared with placebo. NSAIDs are associated with an increased risk of gastrointestinal haemorrhage. RCTs provided insufficient evidence to compare the effects of oral versus topical NSAIDs. RCTs found no good evidence that simple analgesics, such as paracetamol (acetaminophen), are significantly different from NSAIDs in pain relief. Concerns exist relating to trial quality and commercial bias.
- **Simple oral analgesics (short term pain relief)** Systematic reviews in people with osteoarthritis of the hip or knee found limited evidence that simple analgesics, such as paracetamol, reduced pain compared with placebo. RCTs found no good evidence that simple analgesics, such as paracetamol (acetaminophen), are significantly different from NSAIDs in pain relief.
- **Topical agents (short term pain relief)** One systematic review and RCTs have found that topical agents containing NSAIDs reduce pain compared with placebo. One systematic review found that systemic adverse events were no more common than with placebo. RCTs provided insufficient evidence to compare the effects of oral versus topical NSAIDs. We found no RCTs comparing topical agents versus other local treatments such as heat or cold packs. RCTs found limited evidence that capsaicin improved pain compared with placebo.
- **Exercise (pain relief and improved function)** Systematic reviews and subsequent RCTs have found that exercise and physical therapy reduce pain and disability in people with hip or knee osteoarthritis, although many of the RCTs were limited by poor methods and reporting.
- **Intra-articular glucocorticoid injections of the knee (short term pain relief)** One systematic review and one subsequent RCT found limited evidence that intra-articular glucocorticoids reduced pain for 1–4 weeks compared with placebo.
- **Intra-articular hyaluronan injections of the knee** One systematic review and RCTs found limited evidence that hyaluronan reduced pain for 1–6 months compared with placebo.
- **Osteotomy** We found no RCTs comparing osteotomy versus conservative treatment. Two RCTs found similar functional outcomes with osteotomy compared with knee replacement. Two RCTs provided insufficient evidence on the effects of different types of osteotomy.
- **Physical aids** RCTs in people with knee osteoarthritis found limited evidence that joint bracing or taping may improve disease specific quality of life and symptoms compared with control treatment. RCTs provided insufficient evidence to compare the effects of different insoles.
- **Chondroitin** One systematic review and RCTs provided insufficient evidence on the effects of chondroitin in people with osteoarthritis.
- **Education** RCTs provided insufficient evidence to assess the effects of education and behavioural change in people with hip or knee osteoarthritis.
- **Glucosamine** Systematic reviews and subsequent RCTs found limited evidence that glucosamine improved symptoms compared with placebo, but publication bias and poor trial quality makes the results difficult to interpret.
- **Glucosamine plus chondroitin** We found no RCTs of glucosamine plus chondroitin alone. RCTs found limited evidence that glucosamine plus chondroitin plus manganese ascorbate improved disease severity scores compared with placebo.

- **Hip replacement (who is most likely to benefit)** We found no RCTs. One systematic review of observational studies has suggested younger age (< 45 years), older age (> 75 years), and weight over 70 kg may be associated with worse outcomes in terms of pain relief and function after hip replacement. One cohort study found that younger people were at greater risk of revision, whereas another study found lower rates of implant survival in obese people.
- **Intra-articular injections of the knee other than glucocorticoid or hyaluronan** We found insufficient evidence on the effects of other intra-articular treatments, such as radioactive isotopes, glycosaminoglycan polysulphuric acid, orgotein, and morphine.
- **Knee replacement (who is most likely to benefit)** We found no RCTs. We found insufficient evidence from observational studies on the effects of obesity on knee replacement outcomes. We found limited evidence from observational studies that knee replacement is effective in elderly people.
- **Oral NSAIDs in older people and people at risk of renal disease or peptic ulceration** Studies have found that NSAIDs increased the risk of renal or gastrointestinal damage in older people with osteoarthritis, particularly those with intercurrent disease.
- **Simple oral analgesics in people with existing liver damage** Observational evidence suggests that lower doses of paracetamol may cause liver damage in people with liver disease.

DEFINITION Osteoarthritis is a heterogeneous condition for which the prevalence, risk factors, clinical manifestations, and prognosis vary according to the joints affected. It most commonly affects hands, knees, hips, and spinal apophyseal joints. It is usually defined by pathological or radiological criteria rather than clinical features, and is characterised by focal areas of damage to the cartilage surfaces of synovial joints, associated with remodelling of the underlying bone and mild synovitis. When severe, there is characteristic joint space narrowing and osteophyte formation, with visible subchondral bone changes on radiography.

INCIDENCE/ PREVALENCE Osteoarthritis is a common and important cause of pain and disability in older adults.[1,2] Radiographic features are practically universal in at least some joints in people aged over 60 years, but significant clinical disease probably affects 10–20% of people. Knee disease is about twice as prevalent as hip disease in people aged over 60 years (about 10% *v* 5%).[3,4]

AETIOLOGY/ RISK FACTORS The main initiating factors are abnormalities in joint shape or injury. Genetic factors are probably implicated.

PROGNOSIS The natural history of osteoarthritis is poorly understood. Only a minority of people with clinical disease of the hip or knee joint progress to requiring surgery.

AIMS OF INTERVENTION To reduce pain, stiffness, and disability; to limit the risk of progressive joint damage; to improve quality of life, with minimal adverse effects.

OUTCOMES Frequency and severity of joint pain (particularly activity related pain and night pain); stiffness; functional impairment and disability; quality of life; perioperative complications (infection, bleeding, venous thromboembolism, and death); prosthesis survival and the need for revision surgery; a global knee rating scale that includes measures of pain, function, and range of movement; a modified Knee Society score;[5] the Western Ontario and McMaster osteoarthritis (WOMAC) scale;[6–8] the Lequesne Index;[9] the Arthritis Self-Efficacy (ASE); the Multidimensional Health Assessment Questionnaire (MDHAQ); the Brief Pain Inventory (BPI) questionnaire; the British Orthopedic Association (BOA) score.

METHODS *Clinical Evidence* search and appraisal November 2002. Additional hand searches by the authors of their own files. Observational (non-RCT) data have been included in some sections where appropriate control studies are lacking or may be considered unethical.

QUESTION What are the effects of treatments?

OPTION EXERCISE AND PHYSICAL THERAPY

Systematic reviews and subsequent RCTs have found that exercise and physical therapy reduce pain and disability in people with hip or knee osteoarthritis, although many of the RCTs were limited by weak methods and poor reporting.

Benefits: We found four systematic reviews,[10–13] one subsequent non-systematic review,[14] and 10 subsequent RCTs[15–24] of exercise in people with osteoarthritis of the knee or hip. A variety of therapies were included in the reviews, including aerobic exercise, strengthening exercise, stretching exercise, functional training, and range of motion exercise, among others. In the first systematic review (search date 1997, 11 RCTs, osteoarthritis of knee or hip), most of the included trials compared exercise therapy versus placebo or no treatment.[10] It concluded that exercise regimens were beneficial but that more evidence was needed (see table 1, p 1430). The second systematic review (search date 1993) of non-medicinal and non-invasive treatments for hip and knee osteoarthritis included trials that compared exercise therapy versus stretching and strengthening, diathermy, or routine care.[11] It concluded that, of seven modalities reviewed, exercise had the strongest evidence of benefit. The third systematic review (search date 1994) of exercises for osteoarthritis of the knee found only three admissible RCTs.[12] The review concluded that, despite a favourable impression, the evidence currently available was inadequate. The fourth systematic review (search date 2000) of selected rehabilitation interventions for knee pain concluded that therapeutic exercise (compared in RCTs with untreated control or usual care) or transcutaneous electrical nerve stimulation (compared in RCTs with placebo) were both beneficial for knee osteoarthritis.[13] The non-systematic review identified 13 RCTs comparing exercise to a variety of other interventions, including education, usual care, subtherapeutic ultrasound, sham electrical stimulation, and control (not specified).[14] The review found that there was small to moderate beneficial effects for pain and function from use of strengthening exercise, aerobic exercise interventions, or both. The first subsequent RCT (24 obese people with osteoarthritis, body mass index ≥ 28 kg/m^2) compared an exercise plus weight loss diet versus an exercise programme alone.[15] It found no significant differences in 6 month pain or function scores (no figures reported). The second subsequent RCT

(179 people with osteoarthritis, average age 74 years) found that a progressive home based exercise programme plus non-steroidal anti-inflammatory medication was significantly better than non-steroidal anti-inflammatory medication alone for pain (Western Ontario and McMaster osteoarthritis [WOMAC — see glossary, p 1425] pain subscale; P = 0.003), physical activity (WOMAC physical activity subscale; P = 0.006), pain at rest (visual analogue scale [VAS]; P = 0.02), and pain when walking (VAS; P = 0.002).[16] The third subsequent RCT (105 people) compared an education plus exercise package versus no intervention over 6 months.[17] It found that pain and quality of life were significantly improved at 6 weeks with the programme compared with no intervention, but the difference was not significant at 6 months (Impact of Rheumatic Disease on General Health and Lifestyle pain scale, in which a lower score is an improvement: change at 6 weeks, –0.4 with treatment *v* +1.2 with control, P = 0.045; at 6 months +0.2 with treatment *v* +0.6 with control, P = NS). The fourth subsequent RCT (126 people) compared personal exercise treatment; small group exercise treatment; and no treatment.[18] Pre-specified analysis combined the results from the two exercise groups and found a significant effect on pain after 8 weeks of treatment compared with no treatment (exercise *v* no treatment, P < 0.01; change in WOMAC pain scale: 10.6, 95% CI 6.3 to 15.0 with exercise *v* –1.5, 95% CI –5.5 to +2.4 with no treatment) and functional improvement (WOMAC function scale: 7.7, 95% CI 4.2 to 11.2 with exercise *v* –0.1, 95% CI –3.9 to +3.7 with no treatment). It found no significant difference between individual and group exercise treatment.[18] The fifth subsequent RCT (201 people) compared physiotherapist provided exercise versus standard care (patient education and drug treatment from their general medical practitioner if required).[19] Study inclusion criteria were American College of Rheumatology defined osteoarthritis of the hip or knee. Exclusion criteria included exercise treatment within the previous 6 months, problems on fewer than 10 out of 30 days, age under 40 or over 85 years, and indication for hip or knee replacement. It found that exercise significantly improved pain at 12 and 24 weeks compared with standard care (measured on a VAS in which 0 mm = no pain, 100 mm = very severe pain: difference at 12 weeks –17.0, 95% CI –23.6 to –10.4; difference at 24 weeks –11.5, 95% CI –19.7 to –3.3) but not at 36 weeks (difference at 36 weeks –6.6, 95% CI –14.7 to +1.6). Observed disability was determined by studying videos of performance of a series of standardised tests. A total disability score was calculated from five measures: 5 metres walking time, stand to sit time, stand to recline time, and levels of caution and rigidity during the performance of the tasks. It found no significant differences between groups (–0.19, 95% CI –0.38 to –0.01 at 12 weeks; –0.09, 95% CI –0.30 to +0.12 at 24 weeks; –0.10, 95% CI –0.31 to +0.11 at 36 weeks). The RCT suggested decreasing benefit over time may have been because of falling compliance.[19] The sixth subsequent RCT (250 people aged 60 years or above) compared aerobic exercise, resistance exercise, and education (including discussions and social gatherings).[20] Inclusion criteria included pain in knees on most days, difficulty with one of a range of daily activities (e.g. walking,

climbing stairs, shopping, cleaning, self-care activities), and radiographic evidence of knee osteoarthritis. It found that, compared with the education group, the exercise groups had significantly lower risks of loss of activities of daily living for both exercise groups compared with education (RR 0.57, 95% CI 0.38 to 0.85), for the resistance exercise group compared with education (RR 0.60, 95% CI 0.38 to 0.97), and for the aerobic exercise group compared with education (RR 0.53, 95% CI 0.33 to 0.85). The seventh subsequent RCT (69 people) compared physiotherapist led exercise versus no exercise.[21] The results presented were for a subgroup of people who reported osteoarthritis symptoms who were part of a larger RCT (299 people) examining the impact of exercise on sedentary older people. It found no significant difference at 12 months using the WOMAC scale. The eighth subsequent RCT (316 people with knee osteoarthritis, aged 60 years or over) compared four groups over 18 months: exercise alone; dietary weight loss alone; exercise plus dietary weight loss; and a healthy lifestyle control group (which included group presentations and talks on topics concerning osteoarthritis, obesity, and exercise).[22] Inclusion criteria included a body mass index of 28 kg/m^2 or more, knee pain on most days, a sedentary activity pattern, and difficulty in one of a range of daily activities (e.g. walking, climbing stairs, bending, kneeling, house cleaning, self care activities) and radiographic evidence of tibio-femoral osteoarthritis. The RCT found no significant difference among groups in a composite mental health score of the SF-36 after 18 months. It found that exercise plus dietary weight loss significantly improved a composite physical health score of the SF-36 compared with the healthy lifestyle control ($P < 0.01$; absolute numbers not reported), and exercise plus dietary weight loss or exercise alone significantly improved peoples' satisfaction with physical function compared with the healthy lifestyle control (either treatment *v* healthy lifestyle, $P < 0.01$; absolute numbers not reported). The RCT found that exercise alone, dietary weight loss alone, or exercise plus dietary weight loss all significantly improved peoples' satisfaction with their own appearance compared with the healthy lifestyle control (any treatment *v* healthy lifestyle, $P < 0.01$; absolute numbers not reported).[22] The ninth subsequent RCT (102 people with knee osteoarthritis) compared three groups: isometric resistance training; dynamic resistance training; and control (no intervention).[23] In both training groups, strength exercises for the legs were completed three times a week for 16 weeks. Inclusion criteria included a score of five or more on the WOMAC pain subscale and physician validated knee pain. Exclusion criteria included knee pain other than osteoarthritis and contraindications to exercise. The RCT found no significant difference in the WOMAC stiffness subscale within or among groups. The RCT found that the WOMAC functional limitations scale declined significantly from baseline in the dynamic resistance group ($P < 0.05$), but not in the isometric resistance or control groups. It found that the dynamic and isometric resistance groups reported similar significant declines from baseline in the time to perform functional tasks (time to get down to the floor, to get up off the floor, to go up 27 stairs, to go down 27 stairs) and the WOMAC pain subscale ($P < 0.05$), whereas the control group did not differ significantly over the duration of the study.[23] The 10th subsequent RCT (23 people aged 41–75 years with knee osteoarthrits) compared three groups: concentric isokinetic resistance training; combined concentric–eccentric isokinetic resistance training; and control (no training).[24] Inclusion criteria included bilateral osteoarthritis grade 2 or 3 as judged by Kellgren and Lawrence criteria. Exclusion criteria included health problems that might pose a risk during training. The RCT found that both training groups significantly increased functional capacity after 8 weeks compared with control (either training group *v* control, $P < 0.01$) and significantly decreased pain (either training group *v* control, $P < 0.01$). Functional capacity measurement included walking, standing, rising from a chair, stair climbing, and descending stairs.[24]

Harms: The reviews and RCTs did not report on adverse events.[10–20,22–24]

Comment: Many of the RCTs are limited by methodological and reporting issues. However, the most recent systematic review concluded that there was good evidence of benefit from therapeutic exercise or transcutaneous electrical nerve stimulation in knee osteoarthritis.

OPTION EDUCATION AND BEHAVIOURAL CHANGE

RCTs provided insufficient evidence to assess the effects of education and behavioural change in people with hip or knee osteoarthritis.

Benefits: We found one systematic review[25] and four subsequent RCTs.[26–29] The systematic review (search date 1993) included 10 controlled trials (see comment below) of education over 2–48 weeks.[25] Effect sizes associated with education were not significant for pain (WMD +0.16, 95% CI –0.69 to +1.02) or disability (WMD 0, 95% CI –0.61 to +0.61). The first subsequent RCT (211 people with osteoarthritis of the knee) compared self care education versus attention only education (see glossary, p 1424) over 1 year.[26] The self care education group improved more for both pain and disability. At both 4 and 12 months, there was a significant difference for function and pain with self care education compared with attention only education. The second subsequent RCT (252 people) assessed methods to improve adherence to treatment plans.[27] The RCT compared a targeted education programme versus an information pack, both delivered through a computer over 8 weeks. The targeted education programme explained the nature of the medication, side effects and benefits one might expect, the importance of the person in making decisions about the appropriateness of the medication, and other practical advice. The RCT found no significant difference in quality of life, pain, or disability between groups. The targeted education programme significantly improved stiffness compared with controls (effect size –0.63, 95% CI –0.81 to –0.45 *v* –0.39, 95% CI –0.53 to –0.25).[27] The third subsequent RCT (113 people) compared an isokinetic exercise regimen versus generic information lectures given by health professionals over 12 weeks.[28] It found no significant difference in leg strength, pain, or function between the groups. The fourth subsequent RCT (544 people with all types of arthritis) compared an education programme versus a waiting list control.[29] The intervention consisted of six weekly meetings, each lasting about 2 hours. The meetings involved providing information on arthritis, self management, exercise, cognitive symptom management, dealing with depression, nutrition, communication with family and health professionals, and contracting. Inclusion criteria were age greater than 18 years, and arthritis confirmed by a general medical practitioner. It found significant differences in favour of the intervention group at 4 months for pain (Arthritis Self-Efficacy Scale [see glossary, p 1424]: 2.65, 99% CI 0.85 to 4.44), fatigue (visual analogue scale [VAS] score: 0.48, 99% CI −1 to 0.04, P = 0.020), anxiety (Hamilton Depression Rating Scale [HAD]: −0.59, 99% CI −1.2 to +0.03, P = 0.014), and depression (HAD scale: −0.86, 99% CI −1.46 to −0.26), but found no significant difference between groups in the Health Assessment Questionnaire (P = 0.351) or VAS pain (P = 0.707).[29]

Harms: The review and subsequent RCTs did not report on adverse events.[25–29]

Comment: We found few well designed RCTs, and the participants in many RCTs were not representative of those in the general population. Studies of individual education in the systematic review also included biofeedback, exercises, and social support.[25] The systematic review did not state whether the controlled trials were RCTs.[25] One trial, which found a large improvement for pain and disability, was excluded from the analysis because its results were so different from the others.[25] It also included exercise in the intervention. The remaining nine trials had no significant heterogeneity of results.

OPTION PHYSICAL AIDS

RCTs in people with knee osteoarthritis found limited evidence that joint bracing or taping may improve disease specific quality of life and symptoms compared with control treatment. RCTs provided insufficient evidence to compare the effects of different insoles.

Benefits: We found no systematic reviews. We found five RCTs on physical aids.[30–34] **Joint bracing or taping:** The first RCT (119 people) compared two forms of valgus knee bracing (neoprene sleeve and unloader brace) versus control. It found that, compared with control, both the knee brace groups significantly improved disease specific quality of life (P = 0.001) and function (P < 0.001). It found no significant difference between Western Ontario and McMaster osteoarthritis (WOMAC) (see glossary, p 1425) scores for the two braces (P = 0.062).[30] The second small RCT (14 people) found that taping of the knee was associated with a reduction in pain compared with control (difference in mean pain score between neutral *v* medical taping 15.5, 95% CI 2.4 to 28.6; figures as presented in original paper, units not clear; differences in pain score between neutral and lateral taping −8, 95% CI −22.5 to +6.5; figures as presented in original paper, units not clear).[31] **Insoles:** The third RCT (90 women, age > 45 years, and with American College of Rheumatology (ACR) diagnosed osteoarthritis, but not congenital foot problems, fused joints, foot deformity, or limitations of range of motion) compared a strapped insole versus an inserted insole.[32] Both groups were also given indometacin (indomethacin)

(30 mg) twice daily. The RCT did not test the significance of differences between groups. It found that the Lequesne Index (see glossary, p 1424) significantly improved in both groups from baseline (strapped insole group, from mean 11.1 to 8.2, P = 0.006 *v* inserted insole group, from 10.1 to 8.8, P = 0.009), but pain significantly decreased only for the strapped insole group (visual analogue scale [VAS] mean 43.4 to 21.3, P = 0.041 *v* 42.3 to 46.5, P value not reported). The fourth RCT (156 people) compared laterally elevated insoles versus neutral insoles.[33] Study inclusion criteria included ACR defined osteoarthritis, age 18 years or more, pain on daily basis for at least 1 month, pain of greater than 3 on 10 cm VAS after physical activity, evidence of medial femorotibial osteoarthritis on radiograph, functional class of less than IV on Steinbrocker score, and greater or similar reduction in lateral than medial joint space. Exclusion criteria included secondary knee or hip osteoarthritis, hallux deformity of foot, advanced arthropathy of the hindfoot, any disease treated with insoles in previous 6 months, tibial osteotomy in previous 5 years, joint lavage in previous 3 months, intra-articular corticosteroid injection in previous month, and a change in osteoarthritis drug treatment within the previous week. The RCT included people with a range of osteoarthritis severity. No subgroup analysis was specified. At 6 months, the RCT found that the results of the WOMAC subscales showed no significant difference between groups for pain (percentage improved 19.5% with laterally wedged insoles *v* 21.6% with neutrally wedged insoles; P = 0.84), for stiffness (percentage improved 19.5% *v* 25.7%; P = 0.44), and for function (12.2% *v* 13.5%; P = 0.82). Reported compliance with the treatments was 88% for elevated insoles and 74.3% for the neutral insoles at 6 months.[33] The fifth RCT (71 women) compared insoles with subtalar strapping to insoles with talonavicular strapping over 8 weeks.[34] Both groups were also given acemetacin. Inclusion criteria included medial knee pain that met ACR criteria for a diagnosis of knee osteoathritis. Exclusion criteria included joint space narrowing, patellofemoral osteophytosis seen on lateral view, or lateral tibiofemoral compartment osteophytosis seen on anteroposterior view. The RCT did not test the significance of differences between groups. It found that in the subtalar strapping group, the femorotibial angle with insole use (179.0° ± 4.8°) was reduced by an average of –3.2° ± 2.7° with respect to without insole use. In the talonavicular strapping group, the femorotibial angle (180.2° ± 5.2°) differed by –0.4° ± 1.1° when compared with prior to insole use.[34]

Harms: The third RCT reported that adverse events were more common in the strapped insole group (13%) than in the inserted insole group (2%, significance not reported).[32] In the strapped insole group, three people complained of popliteal pain, two complained of back pain, and one reported foot sole pain. One person complained of foot sole pain in the inserted insole group. In no cases was the adverse effect so serious that the participant stopped wearing the insole.

Comment: None.

OPTION SIMPLE ORAL ANALGESICS

Systematic reviews in people with osteoarthritis of the hip or knee found limited evidence that simple analgesics, such as paracetamol, reduced pain compared with placebo. Observational evidence suggests that lower doses of paracetamol (acetaminophen) may cause liver damage in people with liver disease. RCTs found no good evidence that simple analgesics, such as paracetamol, are significantly different from non-steroidal anti-inflammatory drugs in pain relief.

Benefits: We found two systematic reviews, one evaluating simple analgesics in osteoarthritis of the hip (search date 1994, 3 RCTs)[35] and one evaluating simple analgesics in osteoarthritis of the knee (search date 1994).[36] The reviews found limited evidence that simple analgesics were effective in controlling pain associated with osteoarthritis compared with placebo. The only placebo controlled RCT included in the knee review (25 people with osteoarthritis of the knee)[36] found that, compared with placebo, paracetamol was superior for short term pain relief (improvement in pain at rest: 73% of knees with paracetamol *v* 5% of knees with control; P = 0.0001) and global responses (improved global response: 18/22 [82%] with paracetamol *v* 1/22 [5%] with control; RR 18.0, 95% CI 6.9 to 22.0; NNT 1, 95% CI 1 to 4).[37] **Versus oral non-steroidal anti-inflammatory drugs (NSAIDs):** We found two systematic reviews (search date 1994,[35] 1 RCT; and search date 1994,[36] 5 RCTs[38–42]), one additional study,[43] and one subsequent RCT.[44] The systematic reviews found no evidence for the superiority of NSAIDs over simple analgesics. One RCT (178 people with knee osteoarthritis) in the review compared naproxen versus paracetamol over 2 years.[38] The RCT found no significant difference in effects. Another RCT (184 people with osteoarthritis) in the review compared two doses of ibuprofen versus paracetamol.[39] It found no significant differences between the three groups. One subsequent study of 20 crossover trials of one person each ("n of 1" trials) compared paracetamol versus diclofenac.[43] It concluded that, although some people's pain was adequately controlled by paracetamol alone, others responded better to a NSAID. The subsequent crossover RCT (227 people) compared paracetamol (acetaminophen) versus diclofenac plus misoprostol over a 6 week period.[44] Inclusion criteria were age over 40 years, Kellgren and Lawrence grade 2–4 osteoarthritis, and visual analogue scale (VAS) score pain of greater than or equal to 30 mm. Exclusion criteria were severe comorbidities and hypersensitivity to test drugs. It found, compared with paracetamol, significantly better results with diclofenac plus misoprostol on the primary outcome of the Western Ontario and McMaster osteoarthritis score (see glossary, p 1425) for the target joint (difference –7.75; P < 0.001), and the Multidimensional Health Assessment Questionnaire pain score (difference –14.6; P < 0.001). Pre-specified subgroup analysis found the difference on the primary outcome measures increased with disease severity.

Harms: Liver damage results from overdose of paracetamol, or at lower doses in people with existing liver damage.[45] See paracetamol poisoning, p 1664. **Versus oral NSAIDs:** See harms of NSAIDs, p 1412. The subsequent RCT of paracetamol versus diclofenac plus misoprostol found that paracetamol was associated with fewer adverse effects (P = 0.046) and gastrointestinal events (P = 0.006). The subgroup analysis did not examine the number of adverse effects.[44]

Comment: None.

OPTION ORAL NON-STEROIDAL ANTI-INFLAMMATORY DRUGS

Systematic reviews have found that non-steroidal anti-inflammatory drugs (NSAIDs) reduce short term pain in osteoarthritis compared with placebo (see NSAIDs, p 1393). NSAIDs are associated with an increased risk of gastrointestinal haemorrhage. RCTs provided insufficient evidence to compare the effects of oral versus topical NSAIDs. RCTs found no good evidence that simple analgesics, such as paracetamol (acetaminophen), are significantly different from NSAIDs in pain relief. Studies have found that NSAIDs increased the risk of renal or gastrointestinal damage in older people with osteoarthritis, particularly those with intercurrent disease. Concerns exist relating to trial quality and commercial bias.

Benefits: We found three systematic reviews of analgesic and anti-inflammatory treatment in osteoarthritis of the hip (search date 1994, 14 RCTs)[35] and knee (search date 1996, 16 RCTs;[46] search date 1994, 45 RCTs[36]). The reviews found that NSAIDs were effective at reducing short term pain compared with placebo. We identified hundreds of RCTs comparing NSAIDs versus other NSAIDs or placebo for treatment of osteoarthritis. Most of these trials found benefit from using NSAIDs to treat osteoarthritis. **Versus topical NSAIDs:** See benefits of topical agents, p 1415. **Versus simple oral analgesics:** See benefits of simple oral analgesics, p 1411.

Harms: One RCT (812 people with osteoarthritis of the knee) found that indometacin (indomethacin) may accelerate joint damage in osteoarthritis.[47] A high withdrawal rate made the results difficult to interpret. Studies have found a risk with NSAIDs of gastrointestinal or renal damage in older people with osteoarthritis, particularly those with intercurrent disease.[48,49] Case control studies of several thousand people suggest that the odds ratio of gastrointestinal haemorrhage when taking any NSAID is about 4–5, the risk increasing with certain drugs and with increased doses.[49,50] A meta-analysis (search date 1994) ranked the risk from different drugs and found it to be dose dependent (see table 2, p 1430).[51] We found insufficient evidence about the gastrointestinal effects of cyclo-oxygenase-2 inhibitors versus traditional NSAIDs to calculate the comparative risk for more recently introduced NSAIDs (see differences between NSAIDs under NSAIDs, p 1393). **Versus simple oral analgesics:** See harms of simple oral analgesics, p 1411.

Comment: Despite the many studies of NSAID use in osteoarthritis, the evidence we found on efficacy remains poor and difficult to generalise. Most RCTs suffer from weak methods, including short duration; exclusion of older people, those with intercurrent disease, or those at risk of gastrointestinal and other drug complications; variable outcome measures; comparison of one drug versus another rather than versus placebo; and funding bias.[52,53] In the absence of clear evidence of the superiority of one type of treatment or product, other considerations such as safety (particularly the risk of gastrointestinal bleeding with NSAIDs) and cost should determine the choice of drug (see NSAIDs, p 1393).

OPTION GLUCOSAMINE

Systematic reviews and subsequent RCTs found limited evidence that glucosamine improved symptoms compared with placebo, but publication bias and poor trial quality makes the results difficult to interpret.

Benefits: We found two systematic reviews[54,55] and five subsequent RCTs.[56–60] The first review (search date 1999, 6 RCTs of glucosamine, 911 people) found a significant effect of glucosamine on symptoms, but it reported that publication bias and trial quality made the results difficult to interpret.[54] The second review (search date 1999, 16 RCTs, 2029 people) of glucosamine versus placebo found that glucosamine significantly reduced pain compared with placebo (7 RCTs; summary random effects SMD of glucosamine *v* placebo 1.40, 95% CI 0.65 to 2.14).[55] It found four RCTs comparing glucosamine versus a non-steroidal anti-inflammatory drug (NSAID). Three of the RCTs reported on pain, and these all found greater pain reduction with glucosamine than with an NSAID (see comment below).[55] The first subsequent RCT (98 people) compared glucosamine (500 mg 3 times daily) versus placebo over a 60 day period.[56] It found no significant difference in resting pain (P = 0.66) or walking pain (P = 0.69). The second subsequent RCT (212 people) compared glucosamine (1500 mg sulphate once daily) versus placebo over 3 years.[57] It found glucosamine significantly improved symptoms (Western Ontario and McMaster osteoarthritis [WOMAC — see glossary, p 1425] scale mean difference in symptoms at 3 years 21.6%, 95% CI 3.5% to 39.6%). The third subsequent RCT (202 people) compared glucosamine sulphate versus placebo over 3 years.[59] Inclusion criteria included diagnosis of knee osteoarthritis of the medial femorotibial compartment based on American College of Rheumatology criteria, and Lequesne index (see glossary, p 1424) score of at least 4 points. Exclusion criteria included clinically significant articular and rheumatic diseases other than osteoarthritis, evidence of rapid progression, Lequesne index score over 12 points, or systemic or intra-articular corticosteroid therapy within 3 months. The RCT found that glucosamine significantly reduced mean joint space narrowing measured by radiography after 3 years compared with placebo (difference in means: 0.23 mm, 95% CI 0.09 mm to 0.37 mm), and glucosamine significantly improved pain and function after 3 years compared with placebo (difference in means; Lequesne index: 0.91, 95% CI 0.34 to 1.5; WOMAC total scale: 3.1, 95% CI 0.77 to 5.5; WOMAC pain subscale: 0.7, 95% CI 0.06 to 1.3; WOMAC function subscale: 2.1, 95% CI 0.28 to 3.9; WOMAC stiffness subscale: 0.42, 95% CI 0.09 to 0.75).[59] The fourth subsequent RCT (80 people aged 42–94 years) compared glucosamine sulphate versus placebo over 6 months.[60] Inclusion criteria included radiologically defined, symptomatic osteoarthritis of at least one knee and discomfort for most days in the previous 3 months. People were excluded if they had prosthetic material in both knees, had previously taken glucosamine, or had recently received injections or an arthroscopic washout of the index knee. The RCT found no significant difference between glucosamine and placebo in symptoms (global pain, pain on movement, pain at rest, McGill affective, McGill sensory, WOMAC pain, function, and stiffness subscales). It found that glucosamine significantly increased knee flexion compared with placebo (mean difference: 13°, 95% CI 23.1° to 2.0°), but noted that the difference was small and could have been due to measurement error.[60] The fifth subsequent RCT (45 people) compared glucosamine sulphate versus ibuprofen for osteoarthritis of the temporomandibular joint.[58] Inclusion criteria included pain intensity greater than three on visual analogue scale, degenerative joint disease not as a result of trauma, infection or general joint/muscle disease, no history of intra-articular joint injections, no previous use of glucosamine or chondroitin sulphate and, if using an occlusal splint, it must have been for at least 3 months. It found significant differences in favour of glucosamine at 90 days for functional pain, on the Brief Pain Inventory (see glossary, p 1425), and paracetamol (acetaminophen) use between 90 and 120 days (for all results $P < 0.05$).

Harms: The second systematic review reported that the safety profile of glucosamine in the 16 RCTs was excellent.[55] Out of the nearly 1000 people randomised to glucosamine treatment in the RCTs, 14 were withdrawn because of toxicity (comparative figures not reported), but it found insufficient evidence on long term tolerance.

Comment: We were unable to replicate the review's calculation of an effect size for glucosamine compared with an NSAID.[55] The first review reported that there was likely to be some benefit from glucosamine, but the evidence did not allow us to estimate confidently the size of the effect.[55]

OPTION CHONDROITIN SULPHATE

One systematic review and RCTs provided insufficient evidence on the effects of chondroitin in people with osteoarthritis.

Benefits: We found one systematic review (search date 1999),[54] one subsequent RCT,[61] and one additional RCT.[62] The review reported that trial quality and publication bias probably had a major effect on results, making them difficult to interpret.[54] The subsequent RCT (130 people) found no significant difference between chondroitin sulphate (1 g/day) compared with placebo over 6 months on the Lequesne Index (see glossary, p 1424) ($P = 0.12$).[61] The additional RCT (146 men) compared chondroitin sulphate (400 mg 3 times daily) versus diclofenac sodium (50 mg 3 times daily) over 6 months.[62] At the end of the first month, diclofenac was significantly better than chondroitin measured on the Lequesne Index ($P < 0.001$) but, by day 60, the chondroitin group was significantly better than the diclofenac group ($P < 0.01$), and people in the diclofenac group were taking placebo by this period, whereas the chondroitin group were still on active treatment (see comment below).

Harms: The review did not report harms.[54]

Comment: During the first month, people in the non-steroidal anti-inflammatory drug group were treated with diclofenac and placebo, but from months 2 to 3 they were given placebo only. People in the chondroitin group were given chondroitin and placebo for the first month and then from months 2 to 3 they received chondroitin only.[62]

OPTION GLUCOSAMINE PLUS CHONDROITIN

We found no RCTs of glucosamine plus chondroitin alone. RCTs found limited evidence that glucosamine plus chondroitin plus manganese ascorbate improved disease severity scores compared with placebo.

Benefits: We found no RCTs of glucosamine plus chondroitin alone versus placebo. We found two RCTs[63,64] of glucosamine plus chondroitin plus manganese ascorbate (see comment below).

Harms: The second RCT found no significant difference in adverse effects between glucosamine plus chondroitin plus manganese versus placebo (17% with intervention *v* 19% with placebo).[64]

Comment: The first RCT (34 people) compared a combination of glucosamine plus chondroitin plus manganese ascorbate versus placebo. It found significant improvement in disease score (–16.3%; P = 0.05), self assessment (–0.89; P < 0.05), and visual analogue scale pain score (–26.6%; P < 0.05).[63] The second RCT (93 people) compared a combination of glucosamine plus chondroitin plus manganese versus placebo over 6 months.[64] It found no overall significant difference in the number of people achieving a 25% improvement on the Western Ontario and McMaster osteoarthritis (WOMAC) or Lequesne Indexes (see glossary, p 1424). Pre-specified subgroup analysis of mild and moderate cases found a significant difference in the response rates for WOMAC scores (58% *v* 28%; P = 0.04) but not in the Lequesne Index. Subgroup analysis of severe cases found no significant difference in response rates for either the WOMAC or Lequesne Index.

OPTION TOPICAL AGENTS

One systematic review and RCTs have found that topical agents containing non-steroidal anti-inflammatory drugs (NSAIDs) reduce pain compared with placebo. One systematic review found that systemic adverse events were no more common with topical NSAIDs than with placebo. RCTs provided insufficient evidence to compare the effects of oral versus topical NSAIDs. We found no RCTs comparing topical agents versus other local treatments such as heat or cold packs. RCTs found limited evidence that capsaicin improved pain compared with placebo.

Benefits: **Topical NSAIDs versus placebo:** See NSAIDs, p 1393. We found one systematic review (search date 1996, 86 trials),[65] three subsequent RCTs, and one additional RCT comparing topically applied agents containing NSAIDs versus placebo.[66–69] The systematic review found that these agents reduced pain compared with placebo (RR for relief of chronic musculoskeletal pain because of osteoarthritis and tendinitis 2.0, 95% CI 1.5 to 2.7).[65] The additional RCT (70 people with mild knee osteoarthritis) showed a significant improvement (measured by Western Ontario and McMaster osteoarthritis [WOMAC — see glossary, p 1425]) in the treatment group receiving diclofenac gel compared with the control group receiving vehicle gel (P = 0.05).[67] One subsequent RCT (119 people with osteoarthritis) found better pain relief with a topical NSAID (diclofenac–hyaluronan gel) compared with placebo gel, but the difference was not significant (P = 0.057).[66] The second subsequent RCT (237 people) compared eltenac gel (3 g 3 times daily) at 0.1%, 0.3%, and 1.0% concentrations or placebo gel over a 6 week period.[68] It found no significant difference between any of the treatment groups compared with placebo for pain (differences on a global pain scale eltenac 0.1% *v* placebo –6.1, 90% CI –20.5 to +8.2; eltenac 1.0% *v* placebo –10.8, 90% CI –25.3 to +3.6). The third subsequent RCT (100 people) compared 5% ibuprofen cream versus placebo cream over 7 days.[69] Inclusion criteria included age 45–70 years, primary knee osteoarthritis according to American College of Rheumatology criteria, and a total score of 5–13 on the Lequesne index (see glossary, p 1424). Exclusion criteria included secondary osteoarthritis, obesity, or chronic painful disease of the hip or ankle joint. Response was defined by reduced pain on movement measured by a difference of ≥ 20 mm from baseline on a 100 mm visual analogue scale (VAS). The RCT found that ibuprofen cream significantly increased response compared with placebo (response: 32/50 [64%] with ibuprofen *v* 15/50 [30%] with placebo; P = 0.000615). It found that ibuprofen cream significantly improved pain and disability compared with placebo (VAS pain on motion: –12.2 mm, 95% CI –17.9 mm to –6.6 mm; VAS pain at rest: –12.2 mm, 95% CI –17.3 mm to –7.1 mm; VAS pain on pressure: –7.5 mm, 95% CI –13.5 mm to –1.5 mm; Lequesne index: –1.6, 95% CI –13.5 to –1.5).[69] **Topical NSAIDs versus oral NSAIDs:** We found no RCT comparing the same NSAID given orally and topically. One good quality RCT (included in the review) in 235 people with mild osteoarthritis of the knee compared topical piroxicam gel versus oral ibuprofen (1200 mg/day) and found no significant difference in pain relief between the two groups (good or excellent relief in 60% *v* 64%; P = 0.56).[70] A second RCT (321 people with osteoarthritis of the fingers) compared diclofenac emulgel plus placebo versus placebo gel plus ibuprofen.[71] It found no significant difference in pain but fewer people withdrew on the gel (5 on active gel *v* 16 with active tablet). **Capsaicin:** One non-systematic meta-analysis of three RCTs of topically applied capsaicin found that capsaicin cream reduced pain compared with placebo (OR 4.4, 95% CI 2.8 to 6.9; dichotomous outcome not defined).[72] One subsequent RCT (70 people with osteoarthritis) compared 0.025% capsaicin cream versus non-medicated cream.[73] Active treatment resulted in significantly greater pain reduction than placebo (no quantified estimates of benefit available). A second subsequent RCT (200 people) compared topical capsaicin; glyceryl trinitrate; topical capsaicin plus glyceryl trinitrate; and placebo gel.[74] It found that pain scores were significantly reduced from baseline with topical capsaicin, glyceryl trinitrate, and topical capsaicin plus glyceryl trinitrate, but not for placebo gel;

direct statistical comparisons of the different treatments was not performed. **Versus other local treatments:** We found no systematic review or RCTs comparing agents containing NSAIDs or capsaicin with simple rubefacients (see glossary, p 1425) or local applications such as hot packs.

Harms: The main adverse effect of topical treatment is local skin irritation; systemic adverse effects were no more common than with placebo.[65] We found no reports of gastric or renal problems.

Comment: The evidence is poor, with most studies being short term, including a mixture of patient groups, and comparing different agents with no placebo control. The RCT comparing topical versus oral NSAIDs did not use the same drug so it is difficult to disentangle the effects of this and the different routes of administration.[68]

OPTION INTRA-ARTICULAR INJECTION OF THE KNEE

One systematic review and one subsequent RCT found limited evidence that intra-articular glucocorticoids reduced pain for 1–4 weeks compared with placebo. One systematic review, and RCTs found limited evidence that intra-articular hyaluronan reduced pain for 1–6 months compared with placebo. We found insufficient evidence on the effects of other intra-articular treatments.

Benefits: **Glucocorticoids:** We found one systematic review (search date not stated, 10 RCTs)[75] and one subsequent RCT.[76] The systematic review found that intra-articular injection of glucocorticoids into the knee (1 trial used 4 injections, the rest used single injections) provided a little additional pain relief compared with placebo (not defined).[75] Pain reduction lasted from 1 week to 1 month. The subsequent RCT (89 people randomised to 4 groups) evaluated a single injection with 24 weeks' follow up.[76] It found a short term benefit (1–4 weeks) of the steroid injection compared with placebo (saline) for both pain and for a functional index. **Hyaluronan:** We found one systematic review (search date not stated),[75] two subsequent non-systematic reviews,[77,78] and four additional RCTs.[79–82] The systematic review identified 10 RCTs of hyaluronan in the knee joint.[75] Treatment consisted of several injections of high molecular weight hyaluronan complexes over several weeks. The review found slightly greater benefit with the injections than with placebo at 1–6 months after treatment. The non-systematic reviews identified four additional RCTs not in the systematic review.[77,78] The first RCT (495 people) compared hyaluronan versus placebo injections (once weekly for 5 weeks) or oral naproxen with follow up to 26 weeks.[83] It found a significant difference in walking pain in favour of hyaluronan compared with placebo (8.8 mm on a 100 mm visual analogue scale [VAS] score; $P = 0.005$). It also found a significant difference in the number of people pain free or with only slight pain with hyaluronate compared with placebo (38.9% *v* 33.1%; $P = 0.04$). About a third (162/495 [33%]) of people, however, did not complete the RCT, and results were not by intention to treat. The second RCT (90 people) found a significant difference between hyaluronan compared with 6-methylprednisolone (1 injection weekly for 5 weeks) over a

60 day period for pain reduction ($P = 0.003$).[84] The third RCT (52 people) found no significant difference between hyaluronan and placebo injection (1 injection weekly for 5 weeks) over 26 weeks.[85] The fourth RCT (110 people) compared hyaluronate versus placebo injections (4 injections over a 3 week period) with 52 weeks' follow up.[85] At 3 weeks, it found a significant difference in pain after exercise ($P = 0.026$) and function ($P = 0.027$), although no difference in pain at rest ($P = 0.16$). At 1 year, there was only a significant difference in functional improvement ($P = 0.046$). The first additional RCT (36 people) compared five administrations of hyaluronic acid versus saline solution.[79] It found no significant difference in pain at day 35, but by day 90 there was significant differences in favour of hyaluronic acid for spontaneous pain ($P < 0.05$), pain on pressure ($P < 0.05$), and pain on movement ($P < 0.05$). However, the RCT entered the same four people into the trial twice, making the results difficult to interpret. The second additional RCT (100 people) found, compared with placebo, a significant benefit on the Lequense Index with hyaluronan at 5 weeks ($P = 0.03$) and 4 months ($P = 0.04$).[80] The third additional RCT (120 people) compared four treatments: hyaluronate injection (2 mL at 10 mg/mL) plus placebo tablets; placebo injection (2 mL of saline) plus non-steroidal anti-inflammatory drugs (NSAIDs); hyaluronate injection plus NSAIDs; and placebo injection plus placebo tablets.[81] People were graded 1–3 on Altman radiographic scale (0 mild to 3 severe). Exclusion criteria were exhibiting non-osteoarthritis arthritis, NSAID intolerance, peptic ulcer disease, avian allergy, consumption of herbal osteoarthritis products (glucosamine), and intra-articular injections of hyaluronan or corticosteroid in previous 6 months. The population characteristics were mean age 65.5 years, mean osteoarthritis grade 2.2, and mean chronic disease score 1. The results showed that on the VAS Western Ontario and McMaster osteoarthritis (WOMAC) pain scale (see glossary, p 1425) and disability scale, all the active group treatments showed significant reductions compared with baseline at week 4 ($P < 0.05$). However, all groups, including the placebo group, showed significant reductions compared with baseline on the VAS WOMAC stiffness scale at week 4 ($P < 0.05$). The statistical significance of differences between treatments was not tested.[81] The fourth additional RCT (43 people aged 55–78 years with bilateral knee osteoarthritis) compared hyaluronic acid injection versus no treatment.[82] One knee was randomly allocated to treatment, the other knee acted as control. Inclusion entry criteria included radiographic changes equivalent to Kellgren stage II–III bilaterally, and Lequesne scores (see glossary, p 1424) to vary by no more than ±2 points in the total value in both knees. Exclusion criteria included neurological deficits in the lower extremities, other diseases (e.g. joint infections, crystalline arthritis, recent arthroscopic surgery), and recent intra-articular injections of the knee. Compared with baseline, the injection group showed a significant decrease in the Lequesne score and VAS scores for pain at rest and pain on weight bearing, and an improvement in the isokinetic peak torque of the knee extensors and flexors ($P < 0.01$). The RCT found no significant difference in these outcomes compared with baseline in the control group. It found evaluation of the total work of the knee

flexors and extensors showed a significant difference between the treatment and control group ($P < 0.01$).[82] **Other intra-articular treatments:** Several other intra-articular treatments exist, but we found insufficient evidence on their effects. Treatments include radioactive isotopes, glycosaminoglycan polysulphuric acid, orgotein, and morphine.[4,86,87]

Harms: We found no reports of serious adverse effects. Localised discomfort after injection is common. A theoretical risk of infection exists, but we found no evidence of this.

Comment: There is little evidence of whether simple aspiration of the knee would be as effective as injection.

OPTION OSTEOTOMY

We found no RCTs comparing osteotomy versus conservative treatment. Two RCTs found similar functional outcomes with osteotomy compared with knee replacement. Two RCTs provided insufficient evidence on the effects of different types of osteotomy.

Benefits: **Versus conservative treatment:** We found no systematic reviews. We found no RCTs (see comment below). **Versus other surgical techniques:** We found four RCTs of osteotomy compared with other surgical treatments.[88–91] Subgroup analysis from one RCT (100 people randomised aged 55–70 years with medial osteoarthritis of the knee, grades I–III according to Ahlback's classification, with knee symptoms [mainly pain] regarded as justifying surgical treatment, but not with impairment of hips or ankles; subgroup analysis on 59 people with strictly unilateral knee pain) compared high tibial osteotomy versus unicompartmental prosthetic knee replacement (UKA).[89] Assessment was before, and 1 year after, surgery. It found an overall clinical improvement from baseline on the British Orthopaedic Association score (see glossary, p 1425), pain during walking, and the ability to ascend and descend steps, but the range of knee flexion and the isokinetic thigh muscle torque remained unchanged after 1 year with both osteotomy and UKA. On comparing treatments after 1 year, it found no significant difference between osteotomy and UKA, but walking outcomes were non-significantly better with UKA. The second RCT (60 people) compared high tibial osteotomy versus unicompartmental joint replacement.[88] The inclusion criteria were medial unicompartmental osteoarthritis, age over 60 years, varus malalignment < 10°, flexion contraction < 15°, and ligament instability < 2nd degree. It found no significant difference at latest follow up (range 7–10 years) in knee scores (mean scores of 76 [range 29–100] with osteotomy *v* 74 [range 31–94] with unicompartmental joint replacement using the Knee Society Clinical Rating System; higher scores represent a worse outcome; $P = 0.77$). It found no significant difference in functional score (mean functional score 71 [0 –100] with osteotomy *v* 59 [0–100] with unicompartmental joint replacement; $P = 0.22$). The third RCT (46 people with knee osteoarthritis, 50 operations) compared closed-wedge high tibial osteotomy (HTO) versus an open-wedge procedure based on hemicallotasis technique (HCO).[90] People with medial osteoarthritis of the knee of

Ahlback grade 1–3 were included. The RCT found no significant difference in the median hip–knee–ankle (HKA) angle between the two procedures after 2 years (median HKA angle: 182°, range 174° to 192° with HTO *v* 182°, range 179° to 189° with HCO; P = 0.3).[90] It found no significant difference between the two procedures in the Hospital for Special Surgery, Lysholm, and Wallgren-Tegner activity scores, and the Nottingham Health Profile questionnaire after 2 years. The RCT found that HCO significantly reduced hospital stay compared with closed-wedge HTO (P < 0.001), and significantly reduced convalescence period (P = 0.01).[90] The fourth RCT (63 people aged 49–74 years) compared two-level Mittelmeier osteotomy with lateral closed-wedge high tibial osteotomy using the AO/ASIF L-plate.[91] Inclusion criteria included that people were employed primarily in agriculture and had unicompartmental medial degenerative varus osteoarthritis with no previous history of knee surgery. Exclusion criteria included post-traumatic and rheumatic arthritis, knee extension deficit > 20°, range of motion < 60°, and two-compartment femorotibial arthritis. The RCT found that satisfactory results, using a recognised knee rating system, were similar in both groups (rated as "satisfactory results"; 5 years: 90% with Mittelmeier osteotomy *v* 91% with lateral closed-wedge HTO; 9 years: 70% *v* 73%; 12 years: 54% *v* 57%; differences reported as not statistically significant). After 1 year, the RCT found similar rates of satisfaction in both groups (people "very satisfied" or "satisfied": 91.4% with Mittelmeier osteotomy *v* 96.3% with lateral closed-wedge HTO). On longer term follow up, the RCT found similar rates of satisfaction between the two groups (people reporting "symptoms had improved"; 5 years: 91% with Mittelmeier osteotomy *v* 96% with lateral closed-wedge HTO; 7 years: 89% *v* 93%; 12 years: 66% *v* 68%; differences reported as not statistically significant). It found that 89% of people in each group returned to their previous agricultural activity within 8–12 months.[91]

Harms: The third RCT reported complications in four people in the HTO group resulting in changes in the HKA angle.[90] One person underwent revision surgery and was treated with antibiotics for deep infection. Closed reduction was carried on a second person and a cast maintained for 66 days. A third person was found to have an increased valgus angle 10 weeks after the operation by which time the osteotomy was considered healed. Closed reduction was carried out on a fourth person and the leg was immobilised in plaster for 59 days. This person developed lymphoedema below the knee and was still receiving lymph therapy twice a week at 2 years. Clinical scores at follow up were reported as good to excellent in one person, and fair to good in the remaining three people. In the HCO group, one person was admitted for 2 days with pain. There were no signs of any other complications. The RCT found 18 pin-track infections (classified as grade 1 to 2) in 15 people, which equals a rate of pin infection of 18%. The infections were localised to the tibial metaphysis in 14 people.[90] The fourth RCT reported non-fatal pulmonary embolism (1 person with Mittelmeier osteotomy *v* 0 with lateral closed-wedge HTO), deep vein thrombosis (2 *v* 2), superficial infection (0 *v* 1), skin necrosis (0 *v* 1), subcutaneous haematoma (2 *v* 1), transient peroneal nerve palsy (1 *v* 0), delayed union (2 *v* 0), pseudarthrosis (1 *v* 1), mechanical failure of hardware (1 *v* 1), enclosed sural nerve in fibula callus (1 *v* 1), and absorption of tibial tuberosity (1 *v* 0).[91] We found no evidence about harms in the other studies.

Comment: We also identified 18 observational studies. Of the observational studies, only one compared osteotomy with another technique (osteotomy *v* UKA). It found UKA had better results than osteotomy and that these results were sustained over long periods.[92] The other observational studies found that osteotomy was effective in subgroups with appropriate site of osteoarthritis, severity of disease, and degree of physical activity.

OPTION TOTAL HIP REPLACEMENT

One systematic review of RCTs and observational studies has found that hip replacement is effective for at least 10 years.

Benefits: We found two systematic reviews.[93,94] In the first systematic review (search date 1995, 17 RCTs, 61 observational studies of hip replacements) the mean ages of people in the trials ranged from 43–71 years.[73] The review found that at least 70% of people without prosthetic failure were rated "good/excellent" for pain and function at 10 years' follow up (see comment below). A second systematic review (search date 1995) identified 11 RCTs and 180 observational studies comparing different prostheses.[94] It found wide variations in outcome, with primary evidence too weak to draw valid conclusions.

Harms: **Death:** We found one systematic review (search date 1995).[95] It pooled data from 130 000 people who had undergone hip replacement and had not received thromboprophylaxis, and found that the rate of fatal pulmonary embolism was 0.1–0.2% and overall mortality was 0.3–0.4%. One retrospective cohort study (11 607 hip replacements) found mortality to be higher in the first 3 months after surgery than in the subsequent 9 months.[96] **Revision and infection:** Two high quality observational studies found that the risk of a revision operation was about 1% per annum, ranging from 0.2–2.0%.[93,97] Most studies found that revisions were not required until at least 10 years after implantation. One large study of a patient register in Sweden found that cumulative 10 year proportion of hip replacements that were revised due to infection fell to less that 0.5% between 1978 and 1990. It also found that after the immediate postoperative period, aseptic loosening accounted for about 80% of all requirements for replacement or revision surgery.[98] Observational studies found that the initial results of revision surgery were only slightly worse than primary surgery but the prostheses deteriorated more quickly.[99–101] One prospective cohort study (39 543 people) on the Norwegian Hip Replacement register found a lower standardised mortality ratio (0.81) for people who had undergone total hip replacement at mean follow up of 5.2 years (range 0–10.4 years).[102]

Comment: One poor quality narrative review of 20 mainly small uncontrolled studies evaluated self assessed quality of life (at least 2 out of the following factors: physical, social, emotional, economic, and overall satisfaction).[103] It found that improvement in non-physical measures occurred most often within 3 months. Benefit was sustained for up to 5 years after surgery. We found no longer term evidence. Most studies did not distinguish between hip replacement for osteoarthritis and hip replacement for other reasons, which may confound data for osteoarthritis. Outcome of hip replacement for osteoarthritis differs significantly from that for other conditions (e.g. hip fracture in the very elderly and frail, or replacement for rheumatoid arthritis). Hundreds of additional uncontrolled observational studies are available. These studies generally find that hip replacement is effective and beneficial. One recent observational study using the Swedish National Total Hip Arthroplasty register (1056 randomly selected people who had not had revision surgery) found that 10 years after surgery people usually had good health (based on SF-36 measures).[104]

OPTION KNEE REPLACEMENT

Systematic reviews of observational studies have found that knee replacement is effective in relieving pain and improving function. One subsequent RCT found limited evidence that unicompartmental knee replacement is more effective than tricompartmental knee replacement at 5 years' follow up. One systematic review of observational studies found better outcomes with unicompartmental compared with bicompartmental operations.

Benefits: We found one systematic review of tricompartmental prostheses (search date 1992)[105] and one systematic review of bicompartmental and unicompartmental prostheses (search date 1992).[106] **Tricompartmental prostheses:** The review identified 154 studies (4 RCTs, 130 cohort studies, 20 others) of 37 different tricompartmental prostheses in 9879 people (63% with osteoarthritis, mean follow up of 4.1 years).[105] Good or excellent outcomes were reported in 89% of people (improved function 5 years after surgery; pain relief after 5 years; mortality rate at 30 days and at 1 year; thromboembolism by 30 days after surgery; no failure of knee prosthesis). **Bicompartmental prostheses:** The review identified no RCTs but found 18 cohort studies (884 people).[106] The review found that bicompartmental prostheses were effective (based on a global knee rating scale that includes pain, function, and range of movement). **Unicompartmental prostheses:** The review identified no RCTs but 46 cohort studies (2391 people).[106] We found one subsequent RCT.[107] The review found that both unicompartmental and bicompartmental procedures were effective (based on a global knee rating scale that includes measures of pain, function, and range of movement), with better outcomes from unicompartmental operations, particularly since 1987.[106] The subsequent RCT (92 people) found that unicompartmental knee replacement is more effective than tricompartmental knee replacement at 5 years' follow up.[107] Pain relief was good in both groups, but the number of knees able to flex 120° or more was significantly higher in people treated with unicompartmental replacement ($P < 0.001$), and there were more excellent results (90–100 on the Bristol Knee Score) in this group (34/45 [76%] *v* 26/46 [57%]; RR 1.3, 95% CI 0.99 to 1.8).[107] **Quality of life:** Two observational studies published since the review found improvement in quality of life after all forms of knee replacement.[108,109] The first found that knee replacement improved function (measured by Western Ontario and McMaster osteoarthritis, from 58.2 before surgery to 18.4 at time of survey).[108] The second, a cross-sectional community survey, found that more people had moderate to severe pain (assessed using a modified Knee Society score) before surgery (361/487 [74%]) than 1 or more years afterwards (100/487 [21%]).[109]

Harms: **Death:** In one 6 year cohort of 338 736 US Medicare patients, the death rate within 30 days of hospital admission for total knee replacement was 2147 (0.63%).[110] The same cohort study reported a mean mortality of 1.5% per annum (no comparative data available). One observational study (208 people) found no significant increase in the risk of death after knee arthroplasty for women (standardised mortality ratio 1.03, 95% CI 0.76 to 1.37) or men (standardised mortality ratio 1.14, 95% CI 0.68 to 1.80) after a mean follow up of 6 years (range 0–20 years).[111] **Thrombosis:** We found three studies that reported rates of venous thrombosis.[94,112,113] They found that about 24% of people who had a total knee replacement developed a deep vein thrombosis. **Revision and infection:** This is the main long term risk. The first review found a revision rate of 3.8% during 4.1 years' follow up after tricompartmental replacements.[105] The second review found a revision rate of 9.2% over 4.6 years for unicompartmental prostheses and 7.2% over 3.6 years for bicompartmental prostheses.[106] Large patient register based studies in Sweden found that the cumulative 10 year risk for revision surgery because of infection had fallen to less than 1%.[98] Most implant revision surgery was because of aseptic loosening. For unicompartmental osteoarthritis, unicompartmental knee replacement was an effective alternative to total knee replacement.[114,115] **Postoperative pain:** This was rarely recorded, but seemed to be absent or mild in most people. **Wound infection:** We found no good evidence on the frequency of wound infections. One large retrospective cohort study found lower complication rates in centres with a higher volume of procedures.[116]

Comment: We found hundreds of observational studies that reported the time to prosthesis failure or revision surgery, but less evidence on patient related outcomes. The evidence suggests that benefits and harms of knee replacement now seem to be similar to that of hip replacement.

QUESTION Which people are most likely to benefit from hip replacement?

We found no RCTs. One systematic review of observational studies has suggested younger age (< 45 years), older age (> 75 years), and weight over 70 kg may be associated with worse outcomes in terms of pain relief and function after hip replacement. One cohort study found that younger people were at greater risk of revision, whereas another study found lower rates of implant survival in obese people.

Benefits: We found no RCTs (see comment below).

Harms: **Revision and infection:** One Swedish cohort study found that younger people and people doing heavy physical work were at greater risk of revision.[97] Another study found lower rates of long term survival of the implant in obese people.[99]

Comment: One systematic review (search date not stated) identified 40 observational studies (number of people not stated) relating individual characteristics to outcome after hip replacement.[117] It found that the following factors predicted better outcomes in terms of pain relief and function: age 45–75 years; weight less than 70 kg; good social support; higher educational level; and less preoperative morbidity. **Obesity:** One prospective cohort study (176 people) found no difference in the quality of life after a primary hip replacement between the non-obese and moderately obese either at 1 or 3 years, but the study reported no results in people with a body mass index greater than 40 kg/m^2.[118] **Age:** We found a few large observational studies. They found conflicting evidence, which suggested that older people had good self reported outcomes in terms of pain and function, but spent longer in hospital, needed more rehabilitation, and experienced more perioperative complications.[103,119–125] Consensus groups have reported from Sweden, the USA, Canada, and New Zealand.[126–129] Constant pain, particularly night or rest pain, with or without substantial functional impairment, were the generally agreed criteria for joint replacement (see table 3, p 1430). In practice, most surgeons prefer to have radiographic evidence of joint damage as well.

QUESTION Which people are most likely to benefit from knee replacement?

We found no RCTs. We found insufficient evidence from observational studies on the effects of obesity on knee replacement outcomes. We found limited evidence from observational studies that knee replacement is effective in elderly people.

Benefits: We found no RCTs (see comment below).

Harms: None found.

Comment: **Obesity:** We found insufficient evidence from observational studies on the effects of obesity on outcome of knee replacement.[130–133] **Age:** We found limited evidence from observational studies suggesting that knee replacement is effective in elderly people.[125,134,135]

GLOSSARY

Arthritis Self-Efficacy (ASE) The ASE consists of two subscales, one for pain (5 items) and one for other symptoms (6 items). Within each subscale, each item is scored from 0 (very uncertain) to 10 (very certain). Scores are summed across the items for each subscale, producing scores of 5–50 for pain and 6–60 for other symptoms.

Attention only education Information about arthritis but no guidance on self treatment.

Lequesne Index This includes the measurement of pain (5 questions), walking distance (1 question), and activities of daily living (4 questions), with versions available for the hip and knee. Scores for each question are added together to provide a combined disease severity score. Scores of 1–4 are classified as mild osteoarthritis, 5–7 moderate, 8–10 severe, 11–13 very severe, and 14 as extremely severe osteoarthritis.[9]

Modified Knee Society score This instrument combines three different domains (pain, function, and joint status) into a single score (patient function [i.e. walking ability and stair climbing] accounts for about 50% of the total score, with pain and joint status [i.e. stability and deformity] each accounting for about 25%).[5]

Rubefacient An agent that produces mild irritation and redness of the skin.

Self care education Individualised arthritis self care instruction based on patients' needs assessment.

The Brief Pain Inventory (BPI) questionnaire (validated) This measures pain intensity and effect (interference) on quality of life. Intensity (worst and least pain in the last week, average pain, pain right now) are recorded on numerical scales from 0 (no pain) to 10 (pain as bad as you can imagine). The effect of the pain are recorded in terms of how much it interferes with general activity, mood, walking ability, normal work, relations with others, sleep, and enjoyment of life, recorded on a numerical scale from 0 (does not interfere) to 10 (completely interferes).

The British Orthopedic Association (BOA) score This is used as clinical evaluation and has a maximum score of 39 points.

Western Ontario and McMaster osteoarthritis (WOMAC) scale This is a validated instrument for assessing lower limb (hip and knee) osteoarthritis and is sensitive to change. It is a self assessment questionnaire and includes questions on pain, stiffness, and physical function (such as walking ability). WOMAC is disease specific but not intervention specific; it can be used to assess any intervention in osteoarthritis.[6–8]

Substantive changes

Exercise and physical therapy Three RCTs added;[22–24] conclusions unchanged.

Physical aids One RCT added;[34] conclusions unchanged.

Glucosamine Two RCTs added;[59,60] conclusions unchanged.

Topical agents One RCT added;[69] conclusions unchanged.

Intra-articular injection of the knee One RCT added;[82] conclusions unchanged.

Osteotomy Two RCTs added;[90,91] conclusions unchanged.

REFERENCES

1. Petersson IF. Occurrence of osteoarthritis of the peripheral joints in European populations. *Ann Rheum Dis* 1996;55:659–661.
2. Felson DT. Epidemiology of hip and knee osteoarthritis. *Epidemiol Rev* 1988;10:1–28.
3. Gaffney KL. Intra-articular triamcinolone hexacetonide in knee osteoarthritis: factors influencing the clinical response. *Ann Rheum Dis* 1995;54:379–381.
4. Pavelka JKS. Glycosaminoglycan polysulfuric acid (GAGPS) in osteoarthritis of the knee. *Osteoarthritis Cartilage* 1995;3:15–23.
5. Insall JN, Dorr LD, Scott RD, et al. Rationale of the Knee Society clinical rating system. *Clin Orthopaed Rel Res* 1988;248:13–14.
6. Bellamy N, Buchanan WW, Goldsmith CH, et al. Validation study of WOMAC: a health status instrument for measuring clinically important patient relevant outcomes to antirheumatic drug therapy in patients with osteoarthritis of the hip or knee. *J Rheumatol* 1988;15:1833–1840.
7. Dougados M, Devogelaer JP, Annefeldt M, et al. Recommendations for the registration of drugs used in the treatment of osteoarthritis. *Ann Rheum Dis* 1996;55:552–557.
8. Altman R, Brandt K, Hochberg M, et al. Design and conduct of clinical trials in patients with osteoarthritis: recommendations from a task force of the Osteoarthritis Research Society. *Osteoarthritis Cartilage* 1996;4:217–243.
9. Lequesne M, Mery C, Samson M, et al. Indexes of severity for osteoarthritis of the hip and knee. *Scand J Rheumatol* 1987;65(suppl):85–89.
10. Van Baar ME, Assendelft WJ, Dekker J, et al. Effectiveness of exercise therapy in patients with osteoarthritis of the hip or knee: a systematic review of randomized clinical trials. *Arthritis Rheum* 1999;42:1361–1369. Search date 1997; primary sources Medline, Embase, Cinahl, and Cochrane Controlled Trials Register.
11. Puett DW, Griffin MR. Published trials of non-medicinal and non-invasive therapies for hip and knee osteoarthritis. *Ann Intern Med* 1994;121:133–140. Search date 1993; primary source Medline.
12. La Mantia K, Marks R. The efficacy of aerobic exercises for treating osteoarthritis of the knee. *NZ J Physiother* 1995;23:23–30. Search date 1994; primary sources Medline, Cinahl, hand searched references, and personal contacts.
13. Tugwell P. Philadelphia panel evidence-based clinical practice guidelines on selected rehabilitation interventions for knee pain. *Phys Ther* 2001;81:1675–1700. Search date 2000; primary sources Medline, Embase, Current Contents, Cinahl, the Cochrane Controlled Trials

Register, the Cochrane Field of Rehabilitation and Related Therapies, the Cochrane Musculoskeletal Group Register, the Physiotherapy Evidence Database (PEDro), reference lists of included studies, and contact with experts in the field.
14. Baker K, McAlindon TE. Exercise for knee osteoarthritis. *Curr Opin Rheumatol* 2000;12:456–463.
15. Messier SP, Loeser RF, Mitchell MN, et al. Exercise and weight loss in obese older adults with knee osteoarthritis: a preliminary study. *J Am Geriatr Soc* 2000;48:1062–1072.
16. Petrella RJ, Bartha C. Home based exercise therapy for older patients with knee osteoarthritis: a randomized clinical trial. *J Rheumatol* 2000;27:2215–2221.
17. Hopman-Rock M, Westhoff MH. The effects of a health educational and exercise program for older adults with osteoarthritis for the hip or knee. *J Rheumatol* 2000;27:1947–1954.
18. Fransen M, Crosbie J, Edmonds J. Physical therapy is effective for patients with osteoarthritis of the knee: a randomized controlled clinical trial. *J Rheumatol* 2001;28:156–164.
19. Van Baar ME, Dekker J, Oostendorp RA, et al. Effectiveness of exercise in patients with osteoarthritis of hip or knee: nine months' follow up. *Ann Rheum Dis* 2001;60:1123–1130.
20. Penninx BWJH, Messier SP, Rejeski WJ, et al. Physical exercise and the prevention of disability in activities of daily living in older persons with osteoarthritis. *Arch Intern Med* 2001;161:2309–2316.
21. Halbert J, Crotty M, Weller D, et al. Primary care-based physical activity programs: Effectiveness in sedentary older patients with osteoarthritis symptoms. *Arth Rheum Arth Care Res* 2001;45:228–234.
22. Rejeski WJ, Focht BC, Messier SP, et al. Obese, older adults with knee osteoarthritis: weight loss, exercise, and quality of life. *Health Psychol* 2002;21:419–426.
23. Topp R, Woolley S, Hornyak J, et al. The effect of dynamic versus isometric resistance training on pain and functioning among adults with osteoarthritis of the knee. *Arch Phys Med Rehabil* 2002;83: 1187–1195.
24. G r H, Cakfin N, Akova B, et al. Concentric versus combined concentric-eccentric isokinetic training: effects on functional capacity and symptoms in patients with osteoarthrosis of the knee. *Arch Phys Med Rehabil* 2002;83:308–316.
25. Superio-Cabuslay E, Ward MM, Lorig KR. Patient education interventions in osteoarthritis and rheumatoid arthritis: a meta-analytic comparison with non-steroidal anti-inflammatory drug treatment. *Arthritis Care Res* 1996;9:292–301. Search date 1993; primary sources Medline and hand searched references.
26. Mazzuca SA, Brandt KD, Katz BP, et al. Effects of self-care education on the health status of inner-city patients with osteoarthritis of the knee. *Arthritis Rheum* 1997;40:1466–1474.
27. Edworthy SM, Devins GM. Improving medication adherence through patient education distinguishing between appropriate and inappropriate utilization. Patient Education Study Group. *J Rheumatol* 1999;26:1793–1801.
28. Maurer BT, Stern AG, Kinossian B, et al. Osteoarthritis of the knee: isokinetic quadriceps exercise versus and educational intervention. *Arch Phys Med Rehabil* 1999;80:1293–1299.
29. Barlow JH, Turner AP, Wright CC. A randomized controlled study of the Arthritis Self-Management Programme in the UK. *Health Educ Res* 2000;15:665–680.
30. Kirkley A, Websterbogaert S, Litchfield R, et al. The effect of bracing on varus gonarthrosis. *J Bone Joint Surg* 1999;81:539–548.
31. Cushnaghan J, McCarthy C, Dieppe P. Taping the patella medially: a new treatment for osteoarthritis of the knee-joint. *BMJ* 1994;308:753–755.
32. Toda Y, Segal N, Kato A, et al. Effect of a novel insole on the subtalar joint of patients with medial compartment osteoarthritis of the knee. *J Rheumatol* 2001;28:2705–2710.
33. Maillefert JF, Hudry C, Baron G, et al. Laterally elevated wedged insoles in the treatment of medial knee osteoarthritis: a prospective randomized controlled study. *Osteoarthritis Cartilage* 2001;9:738–745.
34. Toda Y, Segal N, Kato A, et al. Correlation between body composition and efficacy of lateral wedged insoles for medial compartment osteoarthritis of the knee. *J Rheumatol* 2002;29:541–545.
35. Towheed T, Shea B, Wells G, et al. Analgesia and non-aspirin, non-steroidal anti-inflammatory drugs for osteoarthritis of the hip. In: The Cochrane Library, Issue 4, 2002. Oxford: Update Software. Search date 1994; primary sources Medline, Cochrane Library, and Controlled Clinical Trials Register.
36. Towheed TE, Hochberg MC. A systematic review of randomized controlled trials of pharmacological therapy in osteoarthritis of the knee, with an emphasis on trial methodology. *Semin Arthritis Rheum* 1997;26:755–770. Search date 1994; primary sources Medline and hand searched references.
37. Amadio P, Cummings DM. Evaluation of acetaminophen in the management of osteoarthritis of the knee. *Curr Ther Res Clin Exp* 1983;34:59–66.
38. Williams HJ, Ward JR, Egger MJ, et al. Comparison of naproxen and acetaminophen in a 2-year study of treatment of osteoarthritis of the knee. *Arthritis Rheum* 1993;36:1196–1206.
39. Bradley JD, Brandt KD, Katz BP, et al. Comparison of an anti-inflammatory dose of ibuprofen, an analgesic dose of ibuprofen, and acetaminophen in the treatment of patients with osteoarthritis of the knee. *N Engl J Med* 1991;325:87–91.
40. Solomon I, Abrams G. Orudis in the management of osteoarthritis of the knee. *S Afr Med J* 1974;48:1526–1529.
41. Muller F, Gosling J, Erdman G. A comparison of tolemetin with aspirin in the treatment of osteoarthritis of the knee. *S Afr Med J* 1977;51:794–796.
42. Valtonen EJ. Clinical comparison of fenbufen and aspirin in osteoarthritis. *Scand J Rheumatol* 1979;27:3–7.
43. March L, Irwig L, Schwarz J, et al. N of 1 trials comparing non-steroidal anti-inflammatory drug with paracetamol in osteoarthritis. *BMJ* 1993;309:1041–1046.
44. Pincus T, Koch GG, Sokka T, et al. A randomized, double-blind, crossover clinical trial of diclofenac plus misoprostol versus acetaminophen in patients with osteoarthritis of the hip or knee. *Arthritis Rheum* 2001;44:1587–1598.
45. Zimmerman HJ, Ishak KG. General aspects of drug induced liver disease. *Gastroenterol Clin North Am* 1995;24:739–757.
46. Watson MC, Brookes ST, Kirwan JR, et al. Osteoarthritis: the comparative efficacy of non-aspirin non-steroidal anti-inflammatory drugs for the management of osteoarthritis of the knee. In: The Cochrane Library, Issue 4, 2002. Oxford: Update Software. Search date 1996; primary sources Medline, BIDS, and Embase.

47. Huskisson EC, Berry H, Gishen P, et al. Effects of anti-inflammatory drugs on the progression of osteoarthritis of the knee. *J Rheumatol* 1995;22;1941–1946.
48. Giovanni G, Giovanni P. Do non-steroidal anti-inflammatory drugs and COX-2 selective inhibitors have different renal effects? *J Nephrol* 2002;15:480–488.
49. Langman MJ. Non-steroidal anti-inflammatory drugs and peptic ulcer. *Hepatogastroenterology* 1992;39(suppl 1):37–39.
50. Garcia Rodriguez LA, Williams R, Derby LE, et al. Acute liver injury associated with non-steroidal anti-inflammatory drugs and the role of risk factors. *Arch Intern Med* 1994;154:311–316.
51. Henry D, Lim LL, Garcia Rodriguez LA, et al. Variability in risk of gastrointestinal complications with individual non-steroidal anti-inflammatory drugs: results of a collaborative meta-analysis. *BMJ* 1996;312:1563–1566.
52. Brandt KD. Nonsurgical management of osteoarthritis, with an emphasis on nonpharmacologic measures. *Arch Fam Med* 1995;4:1057–1064.
53. Wollheim FA. Current pharmacological treatment of osteoarthritis. *Drugs* 1996;52(suppl 3):27–38.
54. McAlindon TE, LaValley MP, Gulin JP, et al. Glucosamine and chondroitin for treatment of osteoarthritis: a systematic quality assessment and meta-analysis. *JAMA* 2000;283:1469–1475. Search date 1999; primary sources Medline, Cochrane Controlled Trials Register, and hand searches of review articles, manuscripts, and supplements from rheumatology and osteoarthritis journals, and contact with content experts, study authors, and manufacturers of glucosamine or chondroitin.
55. Towheed TE, Anastassiades TP, Shea B, et al. Glucosamine therapy for treating osteoarthritis. In: The Cochrane Library, Issue 4, 2002. Oxford: Update Software. Search date 1999; primary sources Medline, Embase, Current Contents, Cochrane Controlled Trials Register, and hand searches of reference lists and personal contact with experts.
56. Rindone JP, Hiller D, Collacott E, et al. Randomized, controlled trial of glucosamine for treating osteoarthritis of the knee. *West J Med* 2000;172:91–94.
57. Thie NMR, Prasad NG, Major PW. Evaluation of glucosamine sulfate compared to ibuprofen for the treatment of temporomandibular joint osteoarthritis: A randomized double blind controlled 3 month clinical trial. *J Rheumatol* 2001;28:1347–1355.
58. Reginster JY, Deroisy R, Rovati LC, et al. Long-term effects of glucosamine sulphate on osteoarthritis progression: a randomised, placebo-controlled clinical trial. *Lancet* 2001;357:251–256.
59. Pavelka_ K, Gatterova_ J, Olejarova_ M, et al. Glucosamine sulfate use and delay of progression of knee osteoarthritis: a 3 year, randomized, placebo-controlled, double-blind study. *Arch Intern Med* 2002;162:2113–2123.
60. Hughes R, Carr A. A randomized, double-blind, placebo-controlled trial of glucosamine sulphate as an analgesic in osteoarthritis of the knee. *Rheumatology* 2002;41:279–284.
61. Mazieres B, Combe B, Phan Van A, et al. Chondroitin sulfate in osteoarthritis of the knee: a prospective, double blind, placebo controlled multicenter clinical study. *J Rheumatol* 2001;28:173–181.
62. Morreale P, Manopulo R, Galati M, et al. Comparison of the antiinflammatory efficacy of chondroitin sulfate and diclofenac sodium in patients with knee osteoarthritis. *J Rheumatol* 1996;23:1385–1391.
63. Leffler CT, Philippi AF, Leffler SG, et al. Glucosamine, chondroitin, and manganese ascorbate for degenerative joint disease of the knee or low back: a randomized, double-blind, placebo-controlled pilot study. *Mil Med* 1999;164:85–91.
64. Das A Jr, Hammad TA. Efficacy of a combination of FCHG49 glucosamine hydrochloride, TRH122 low molecular weight sodium chondroitin sulfate and manganese ascorbate in the management of knee osteoarthritis. *Osteoarthritis Cartilage* 2000;8:343–350.
65. Moore RA, Tramer MR, Carroll D, et al. Quantitative systematic review of topically applied non-steroidal anti-inflammatory drugs. *BMJ* 1998;316:333–338. Search date 1996; primary sources Embase, Medline, Oxford Pain Relief Database, hand searched references, and librarians and medical directors of 12 pharmaceutical companies asked for reports of their products.
66. Roth SH. A controlled clinical investigation of 3% diclofenac/2.5% sodium hyaluronate topical gel in the treatment of uncontrolled pain in chronic oral NSAID users with osteoarthritis. *Int J Tissue React* 1995;17:129–132.
67. Grace D, Rogers J, Skeith K, et al. Topical diclofenac versus placebo: a double blind, randomized clinical trial in patients with osteoarthritis of the knee. *J Rheumatol* 1999;26:2659–2663.
68. Ottillinger B, Michel BA, Pavelka K, et al. Efficacy and safety of eltenac gel in the treatment of knee osteoarthritis. *Osteoarthritis Cartilage* 2001;9:273–280.
69. Rovensky J, Micekova D, Gubzova Z, et al. Treatment of knee osteoarthritis with a topical non-steroidal antiinflammatory drug. Results of a randomized, double-blind, placebo-controlled study on the efficacy and safety of a 5% ibuprofen cream. *Drugs Exp Clin Res* 2001;27:209–221.
70. Dickson DJ. A double-blind evaluation of topical piroxicam gel with oral ibuprofen in osteoarthritis of the knee. *Curr Ther Res Clin Exp* 1991;49:199–207.
71. Zacher J, Burger K, Färber L, et al. Topical diclofenac versus oral ibuprofen: a double blind, randomized clinical trial to demonstrate efficacy and tolerability in patients with activated osteoarthritis of the finger joints (Heberden and/or Bouchard arthritis). *Aktuelle Rheumatologie* 2001;26:7–14.
72. Zhang WY, Po ALW. The effectiveness of topically applied capsaicin: a meta-analysis. *Eur J Clin Pharmacol* 1994;46:517–522. Search date 1994; primary sources BIDS, Medline, and hand searches of relevant published references.
73. Deal CL, Schnitzer TJ, Lipstein E, et al. Treatment of arthritis with topical capsaicin: a double-blind trial. *Clin Ther* 1991;13:383–395.
74. Weidenhielm L, Olsson E, Brostrom LA, et al. Improvement in gait one year after surgery for knee osteoarthrosis: a comparison between high tibial osteotomy and prosthetic replacement in a prospective randomized study. *Scand J Rehabil Med* 1993;25:25–31.
75. Kirwan JRR. Intra-articular therapy in osteoarthritis. *Baillieres Clin Rheumatol* 1997;11:769–794. Search date not stated; RCTs cited from 1958 to 1996; primary sources Medline and Embase.
76. Ravaud P, Moulinier L, Giraudeau B, et al. Effects of joint lavage and steroid injection in patients

with osteoarthritis of the knee: results of a multicenter, randomized, controlled trial. *Arthritis Rheum* 1999;42:475–482.

77. Altman RD. Intra-articular sodium hyaluronate in osteoarthritis of the knee. *Semin Arthrit Rheum* 2000;30:11–18.
78. Hochberg MC. Role of intra-articular hyaluronic acid preparations in medical management of osteoarthritis of the knee. *Semin Arthrit Rheum* 2000;30:2–10.
79. Formiguera SSE. Intra-articular hyaluronic acid in the treatment osteoarthritis of the knee: a short term study. *Eur J Rheumatol Inflamm* 1995;15:33–38.
80. Petrella RJ, DiSilvestro MD, Hildebrand C. Effects of hyaluronate sodium on pain and physical functioning in osteoarthritis of the knee — a randomized, double-blind, placebo-controlled clinical trial. *Arch Intern Med* 2002;162:292–298.
81. Huskisson EC, Donnelly S. Hyaluronic acid in the treatment of osteoarthritis of the knee. *Rheumatology* 1999;38:602–607.
82. Miltner O, Schneider U, Siebert CH, et al. Efficacy of intraarticular hyaluronic acid in patients with osteoarthritis: a prospective clinical trial. *Osteoarthritis Cartilage* 2002;10:680–686.
83. Altman R, Moskowitz R. Intraarticular sodium hyaluronate in the treatment of patients with osteoarthritis of the knee: a randomized clinical trial. *J Rheumatol* 1998;25:2203–2212.
84. Pietogrande V, Turchetto L. Hyaluronic-acid versus methylprednisolone intra-articularly injected for treatment of osteoarthritis of the knee. *Curr Ther Res Clin Exp* 1991;50:691–701.
85. Dougados M, Nguyen M, Listrat V, et al. High molecular weight sodium hyaluronate (hyalectin) in osteoarthritis of the knee: a 1 year placebo-controlled trial. *Osteoarthritis Cartilage* 1993;1:97–103.
86. McIlwain HSJ. Intra-articular orgotein in osteoarthritis of the knee: a placebo-controlled efficacy, safety, and dosage comparison. *Am J Med* 1989;87:295–300.
87. Likar RS. Intraarticular morphine analgesia in chronic pain patients with osteoarthritis. *Anesth Analg* 1997;84:1313–1317.
88. Stukenborg-Colsman C, Wirth CJ, Lazovic D, et al. High tibial osteotomy versus unicompartmental joint replacement in unicompartmental knee joint osteoarthritis: 7–10-year follow-up prospective randomised study. *Knee* 2001;8:187–194.
89. Broughton NS, Newman JH, Baily RAJ. Unicompartmental replacement and high tibial osteotomy for osteoarthritis of the knee. A comparative study after 5–10 years follow up. *J Bone Joint Surg* 1986;68:447–452.
90. Magyar G, Ahl TL, Vibe P, et al. Open-wedge osteotomy by hemicallotasis or the closed-wedge technique for osteoarthritis of the knee. A randomised study of 50 operations. *J Bone Joint Surg* 1999; 81:444–448.
91. Korovessis P, Katsoudas G, Salonikides P, et al. Medium and long term results of high tibial osteotomy for varus gonarthrosis in an agricultural population. *Orthopedics* 1999;22:729–735.
92. McCleane G. The analgesic efficacy of topical capsaicin is enhanced by glyceryl trinitrate in painful osteoarthritis: a randomized, double blind, placebo controlled study. *Eur J Pain* 2000;4:355–360.
93. Faulkner A, Kennedy LG, Baxter K, et al. Effectiveness of hip prostheses in primary total hip replacement: a critical review of evidence and an economic model. *Health Technol Assess* 1998;2:1–33. Search date 1995; primary sources Embase, Medline, and in-house database on epidemiology and service provision for total hip replacement.
94. Murray DW, Britton AR, Bulstrode CJ. Thromboprophylaxis and death after total hip replacement. *J Bone Joint Surg Br* 1996;78:863–870. Search date 1995; primary source Medline.
95. Seagroatt V, Soon Tan H, Goldacre M, et al. Elective total hip replacement: incidence, emergency readmission rate, and postoperative mortality. *BMJ* 1991;303:1431–1435.
96. Chang RW, Pellissier JM, Hazen GB. A cost-effectiveness analysis of total hip arthroplasty for osteoarthritis of the hip. *JAMA* 1996;275:858–865.
97. Malchau H, Herberts P, Ahnfelt L. Prognosis of total hip replacement in Sweden. Follow up of 92 675 operations performed 1978–1990. *Acta Orthop Scand* 1993;64:497–506.
98. Robinson AH, Palmer CR, Villar RN. Is revision as good as primary hip replacement? A comparison of quality of life. *J Bone Joint Surg Br* 1999;81:42–45.
99. Espehaug B, Havelin LI, Engesaeter LB, et al. Patient-related risk-factors for early revision of total hip replacements. A population register-based case-control study of 674 revised hips. *Acta Orthop Scand* 1997;68:207–215.
100. Johnsson R, Franzen H, Nilsson LT. Combined survivorship and multivariate analyses of revisions in 799 hip prostheses. A 10 to 20-year review of mechanical loosening. *J Bone Joint Surg Br* 1994;76:439–443.
101. Lie SA, Engesaeter LB, Havelin LI, et al. Mortality after total hip replacement: 0–10-year follow-up of 39 543 patients in the Norwegian Arthroplasty Register. *Acta Orthop Scand* 2000;71:19–27.
102. Fitzpatrick R, Shortall E, Sculpher M, et al. Primary total hip replacement surgery: a systematic review of outcomes and modelling of cost-effectiveness associated with different prostheses. *Health Technol Assess* 1998;2:1–64. Search date 1995; primary sources Medline and hand searched references.
103. Towheed TE, Hochberg MC. Health-related quality of life after total hip replacement. *Semin Arthrit Rheum* 1996;26:483–491.
104. Soderman P, Malchau H, Herberts P. Outcome after total hip arthroplasty. Part I. General health evaluation in relation to definition of failure in the Swedish National Total Hip Arthroplasty register. *Acta Orthop Scand* 2000;71:354–359.
105. Callahan CM, Drake BG, Heck DA, et al. Patient outcomes following tricompartmental total knee replacement: a meta-analysis. *JAMA* 1994;271:1349–1357. Search date 1992; primary sources Medlars and hand searched references.
106. Callahan CM, Drake BG, Heck DA, et al. Patient outcomes following unicompartmental or bicompartmental knee arthroplasty: a meta-analysis. *J Arthroplasty* 1995;10:141–150. Search date 1992; primary sources Medlars and hand searched references.
107. Newman JH, Ackroyd CE, Shah NA. Unicompartmental or total knee replacement? Five-year results of a prospective, randomised trial of 102 osteoarthritic knees with unicompartmental arthritis. *J Bone Joint Surg* 1998;80:862–865.
108. Kiebzak GM, Vain PA, Gregory AM, et al. SF-36 general health status survey to determine patient satisfaction at short-term follow up after total hip and knee arthroplasty. *J South Orthop Assoc* 1997;6:169–172.

109. Hawker G, Wright J, Coyte P, et al. Health related quality of life after knee replacement. *J Bone Joint Surg* 1998;80:163–173.
110. Freund DA. *Assessing and improving outcomes: total knee replacement: patient outcomes research team (PORT): final report.* Maryland: Agency for Health Care Policy and Research, 1997.
111. Bohm P, Holy T, Pietsch-Breitfeld B, et al. Mortality after total knee arthroplasty in patients with osteoarthrosis and rheumatoid arthritis. *Arch Orthop Trauma Surg* 2000;120:75–78.
112. Kim YH. The incidence of deep vein thrombosis after cementless and cemented knee replacement. *J Bone Joint Surg Br* 1990;72:779–783.
113. Fauno P, Suomalained O, Rehnberg V, et al. Prophylaxis for the prevention of venous thromboembolism after total knee arthroplasty. *J Bone Joint Surg Am* 1994;76:1814–1818.
114. Knutson K, Lewold S, Robertsson O, et al. The Swedish knee arthroplasty register. A nation-wide study of 30 003 knees. *Acta Orthop Scand* 1994;65:375–386.
115. Robertsson O, Borgquist L, Knutson K, et al. Use of unicompartmental instead of tricompartmental prostheses for unicompartmental arthrosis of the knee is a cost-effective alternative. 15 437 primary tricompartmental prostheses were compared with 10 624 primary medical or lateral unicompartmental prostheses. *Acta Orthop Scand* 1999;70:170–175.
116. Norton EC, Garfinkel SA, McQuay LJ, et al. The effect of hospital volume on the in-hospital complication rate in knee replacement patients. *Health Serv Res* 1998;33:1191–1210.
117. Young NL, Cheah D, Waddell JP, et al. Patient characteristics that affect the outcome of total hip arthroplasty: a review. *Can J Surg* 1998;41:188–195. Search date not stated; primary sources Medline and hand search of references.
118. Chan CL, Villar RN. Obesity and quality of life after primary hip arthroplasty. *J Bone Joint Surg Br* 1996;78:78–81.
119. Espehaug B, Havelin LI, Engesaeter LB, et al. Patient satisfaction and function after primary and revision total hip replacement. *Clin Orthop* 1998;351:135–148.
120. Garellick G, Malchau H, Herberts P, et al. Life expectancy and cost utility after total hip replacement. *Clin Orthop* 1998;346:141–151.
121. Brander VA, Malhotra S, Jet J, et al. Outcome of hip and knee arthroplasty in persons aged 80 years and older. *Clin Orthop* 1997;345:67–78.
122. Levy RN, Levy CM, Snyder J, et al. Outcome and long-term results following total hip replacement in elderly patients. *Clin Orthop* 1995;316:25–30.
123. Boettcher WG. Total hip arthroplasties in the elderly — morbidity, mortality, and cost-effectiveness. *Clin Orthop* 1992;274:30–34.
124. Jones AC, Voaklander DC, Johnston DWC, et al. The effect of age on pain, function, and quality of life after total hip and knee arthroplasty. *Arch Intern Med* 2001;161:454–460.
125. Braeken AM, Lochaas-Gerlach JA, et al. Determinants of 6–12 month postoperative functional status and pain after elective total hip replacement. *Int J Qual Health Care* 1997;9:413–418.
126. Swedish website: http://www.sos.se/sosmenye.htm (last accessed 19 August 2003).
127. National Institutes of Health. Total hip replacement. NIH consensus development panel on total hip replacement. *JAMA* 1995;273:1950–1956.
128. Naylor CD, Williams JI. Primary hip and knee replacement surgery: Ontario criteria for case selection and surgical priority. *Qual Health Care* 1996;5:20–30.
129. Hardorn DC, Holmes AC. The New Zealand priority criteria project. *BMJ* 1997;31:131–134.
130. Donnell ST, Neyret P, Dejour H, et al. The effect of age on the quality of life after knee replacement. *Knee* 1998;5:125–112.
131. De Leeuw JM, Villar RN. Obesity and quality of life after primary total knee replacement. *Knee* 1998;5:119–23.
132. Lubitz R, Dittus R, Robinson R, et al. Effects of severe obesity on health status 2 years after knee replacement. *J Gen Intern Med* 1996;11:145.
133. Winiarsky R, Barth P, Lotke P. Total knee arthroplasty in morbidly obese patients. *J Bone Joint Surg Am* 1998;80;1770–1774.
134. Ettinger WH Jr, Burns R, Messier SP, et al. A randomized trial comparing aerobic exercise and resistance exercise with a health education program in older adults with knee osteoarthritis. The fitness arthritis and seniors trial (FAST). *JAMA* 1997;277:25–31.
135. Laskin RS. Total knee replacement in patients older than 85 years. *Clin Orthop* 1999;367:43–49.

David Scott
Professor

Claire Smith
Research Fellow

King's College London Medical School
London
UK

Stefan Lohmander
Professor
Department of Orthopaedics
Lund University
Lund
Sweden

Jiri Chard
Research Associate
MRC Health Services Research Collaboration
University of Bristol
Bristol
UK

Competing interests: None declared.

The following previous contributor of this topic would also like to be acknowledged: Alex Faulkner.

TABLE 1 **Effect sizes (95% CI) of exercise in osteoarthritis of the knee and hip: results of the three highest quality RCTs identified in a systematic review (see text, p 1405).[10]**

RCT	Pain	Observed disability
1	0.31 (0.28 to 0.34)	0.31 (0.28 to 0.34)
2	0.47 (0.44 to 0.50)	0.89 (0.85 to 0.93)
3	0.58 (0.54 to 0.62)	0.28 (0.24 to 0.32)

Effectiveness of exercise therapy in patients with osteoarthritis of the hip or knee: a systematic review of randomized clinical trials, Van Baar ME, Assendelft WJ, Dekker J et al, Arthritis Rheum, Copyright © 1999, American College of Rheumatology. Reproduced with permission of John Wiley & Sons, Inc.

TABLE 2 **Estimated relative risk of gastrointestinal adverse effects with the use of individual NSAIDs (pooled data from 12 studies) (see text, p 1412).[51]**

Drug	Pooled RR	95% CI for pooled RR
Ibuprofen (low dose)*	1.0	ND
Fenoprofen	1.6	1.0 to 2.5
Aspirin	1.6	1.3 to 2.0
Diclofenac	1.8	1.4 to 2.3
Sulindac	2.1	1.6 to 2.7
Diflunisal	2.2	1.2 to 4.1
Naproxen	2.2	1.7 to 2.9
Indomethacin	2.4	1.9 to 3.1
Tometin	3.0	1.8 to 4.9
Piroxicam	3.8	2.7 to 5.2
Ketoprofen	4.2	2.7 to 6.4
Azapropazone	9.2	4.0 to 21.0

*Comparative data used low dose ibuprofen as the reference control for calculating the relative risk of other drugs.
ND, no data; NSAIDs, non-steroidal anti-inflammatory drugs.

TABLE 3 **Summary of New Zealand priority criteria for joint replacement (see text, p 1424).[129]**

Severity is scored out of a possible 100 on the basis of:

Pain: severity 0–20; duration 0–20
Function: walking difficulty 0–10; other 0–10
Joint damage: pain on passive movement 0–10; other/x ray 0–10
Other: other joints 0–10; work, care giving, independence 0–10

Plantar heel pain and fasciitis

Search date January 2003

Fay Crawford

QUESTIONS

INTERVENTIONS

See glossary, p 1442

Key Messages

- **Corticosteroid injection plus local anaesthesia versus local anaesthetic injection alone (short term)** One RCT found that prednisolone plus lidocaine injection reduced pain compared with lidocaine alone after 1 month. Observational studies have found a high rate of plantar fascia rupture and other complications associated with corticosteroid injections, which may lead to chronic disability in some people.
- **Casted orthoses (custom made insoles)** We found no RCTs on the effects of orthoses compared with placebo or no treatment. One systematic review and three RCTs found limited and conflicting evidence about the effects of orthoses compared with corticosteroids, corticosteroids plus local anaesthesia, or other physical supports.
- **Corticosteroid injection plus local anaesthesia versus heel pads (short term)** One RCT found that triamcinolone plus lidocaine injection improved pain compared with heel pad after 1 month. One small RCT found no significant

difference in pain between triamcinolone plus lidocaine injection and heel pad at 1, 2, or 12 weeks. One RCT found no significant difference in pain between dexamethasone plus local anaesthetic injection plus oral etodolac and heel pads plus paracetamol at 3 months. Observational studies have found a high rate of plantar fascia rupture and other complications associated with corticosteroid injections, which may lead to chronic disability in some people.

- **Corticosteroid injection plus local anaesthetic injection versus placebo (short term)** One systematic review identified no RCTs comparing corticosteroid injection plus local anaesthesia versus placebo.
- **Corticosteroid injection versus placebo (short term)** We found no RCTs comparing short term effects of corticosteroid injection alone and placebo.
- **Extracorporeal shock wave therapy** We found insufficient evidence from four small RCTs about effects of extracorporeal shock wave therapy compared with placebo. Two RCTs found limited evidence that high dose extracorporeal shock wave therapy reduced pain and walking scores compared with low dose therapy. However, the clinical importance of these effects is not clear.
- **Heel pads and heel cups** We found no RCTs on the effects of heel pads and heel cups compared with placebo or no treatment. One systematic review and subsequent RCTs found limited and conflicting evidence on the effects of heel pads and heel cups compared with other treatment modalities.
- **Lasers** One small RCT identified by a systematic review found no significant difference between laser treatment and placebo.
- **Local anaesthetic injection** We found no RCTs on the effects of local anaesthesia compared with placebo or no treatment. One RCT found that prednisolone plus lidocaine injection reduced pain compared with lidocaine alone after 1 month, although the difference was not significant after 3 or 6 months.
- **Night splints** One RCT found no significant difference in pain between a night splint and no splint after 3 months.
- **Stretching** We found no RCTs comparing stretching versus no treatment in people with heel pain. We found insufficient evidence from two RCTs to compare stretching versus stretching plus custom made orthoses, or to compare different types of stretching in people with heel pain.
- **Surgery** One systematic review found no RCTs of surgery for heel pain.
- **Ultrasound** One systematic review of one small RCT found no significant difference in pain between ultrasound and sham ultrasound.
- **Corticosteroid injection plus local anaesthesia versus heel pads (medium to long term)** One RCT found no significant difference in pain between triamcinolone plus lidocaine injection and heel pad after 24 weeks. One RCT found no significant difference in pain between dexamethasone plus local anaesthetic injection plus oral etodolac and heel pads plus paracetamol at 3 months. Observational studies have found a high rate of plantar fascia rupture and other complications associated with corticosteroid injections, which may lead to chronic disability in some people.
- **Corticosteroid injection plus local anaesthesia versus local anaesthetic injection alone (medium to long term)** One RCT found no significant difference in pain between prednisolone plus lidocaine injection and lidocaine alone after 3 or 6 months. Observational studies have found a high rate of plantar fascia rupture and other complications associated with corticosteroid injections, which may lead to chronic disability in some people.

- **Corticosteroid injection plus local anaesthetic injection versus placebo (medium to long term)** One systematic review identified no RCTs comparing corticosteroid plus local anaesthetic injection versus placebo. Observational studies have found a high rate of plantar fascia rupture and other complications associated with corticosteroid injections, which may lead to chronic disability in some people.
- **Corticosteroid injection versus placebo (medium to long term)** We found insufficient evidence from one RCT about clinical effects of corticosteroid injection versus placebo. Observational studies have found a high rate of plantar fascia rupture and other complications associated with corticosteroid injections, which may lead to chronic disability in some people.

DEFINITION Plantar heel pain is soreness or tenderness of the heel. It often radiates from the central part of the heel pad or the medial tubercle of the calcaneum, but may extend along the plantar fascia into the medial longitudinal arch of the foot. Severity may range from an irritation at the origin of the plantar fascia, which is noticeable on rising after rest, to an incapacitating pain. This review excludes clinically evident underlying disorders, for example, infection, calcaneal fracture, and calcaneal nerve entrapment, which may be distinguished clinically — a calcaneal fracture may present after trauma, and calcaneal nerve entrapment gives rise to shooting pains and feelings of "pins and needles" on the medial aspect of the heel.

INCIDENCE/ PREVALENCE The incidence and prevalence of plantar heel pain is uncertain. Plantar heel pain primarily affects those in mid to late life.[1]

AETIOLOGY/ RISK FACTORS Unknown.

PROGNOSIS One systematic review (search date 1997) found that almost all of the included trials reported an improvement in discomfort regardless of the intervention received (including placebo), suggesting that the condition is at least partially self limiting.[1] A telephone survey of 100 people treated conservatively (average follow up 47 months) found that 82 people had resolution of symptoms, 15 had continued symptoms but no limitations of activity or work, and three had continued symptoms that limited activity or changed work status.[2] Thirty one people said that they would have seriously considered surgical treatment at the time medical attention was sought. The three people still affected had bilateral symptoms but no other clear risk factors.

AIMS OF INTERVENTION To reduce pain and immobility, with minimal adverse effects.

OUTCOMES Pain reduction (often measured using visual analogue scales); walking distance.

METHODS *Clinical Evidence* search and appraisal January 2003.

QUESTION **What are the effects of treatments for plantar heel pain?**

OPTION **CORTICOSTEROID INJECTIONS**

We found insufficient evidence from one long-term RCT about clinical effects of corticosteroid injection versus placebo. Observational studies have found a high rate of plantar fascia rupture and other complications associated with corticosteroid injections, which may lead to chronic disability in some people.

Benefits: We found one systematic review (search date 1997).[1] **Versus placebo or no treatment:** The review found one small RCT (19 people with 22 heels with recalcitrant heel pain but not arthritis) comparing corticosteroid (hydrocortisone acetate 25 mg) injection with saline injection.[1] Both groups were also given a sponge heel pad (see glossary, p 1442). It found no significant difference between hydrocortisone and placebo in the proportion of heels with no relief of pain assessed between 6–18 months after the injection (3/13 [23%] heels *v* 4/9 [44%] heels; RR 0.52, 95% CI 0.15 to 1.79). **Versus orthoses:** The review found no RCTs. **Versus pads:** The review found no RCTs. **Versus pain medication alone:** The review found no RCTs. **Corticosteroid injection plus local anaesthesia:** See benefits of corticosteroid injections plus local anaesthesia, p 1435.

Harms: The RCT identified by the review gave no information on harms.[1] Corticosteroid injections can be painful. Complications observed from local corticosteroid injection throughout the body include infection, subcutaneous fat atrophy, skin pigmentation changes, fascial rupture, peripheral nerve injury, and muscle damage among others.[3] Observational studies have reported rupture of the plantar fascia in people receiving corticosteroid injections.[4,5] One study reported a 10% incidence of rupture among 122 injected heels.[5] A second study examined 37 people with a presumptive diagnosis of plantar fascia rupture, all of whom had had plantar fasciitis and all of whom had previously been treated with corticosteroid injection.[4] History revealed that in 13/37 (35%) people the rupture had been a sudden event, whereas in the remainder it seemed to be gradual. The study reported that most had resolution of symptoms, but this often took 6–12 months to occur.[4] Rupture may relieve the original heel pain, but may cause arch and mid-foot strain, lateral plantar nerve dysfunction, stress fracture, deformity, and swelling, all of which may persist.

Comment: The evidence from observational studies makes it difficult to define the clinical importance of rupture of the plantar fascia.

OPTION **LOCAL ANAESTHETIC INJECTION**

We found no RCTs comparing local anaesthesia versus placebo or no treatment. One RCT found that prednisolone plus lidocaine injection reduced pain scores compared with lidocaine alone after 1 month. However, the clinical importance of this result is unclear and the difference was not significant after 3 or 6 months.

Benefits: We found one systematic review (search date 1997).[1] **Versus placebo or no treatment:** The review found no RCTs.[1] **Versus corticosteroids plus local anaesthetic:** The review found no RCTs. We found one subsequent RCT (see benefits of corticosteroids plus local anaesthesia, p 1435), which found a short term benefit with lidocaine plus prednisolone injection compared with lidocaine injection alone.[6]

Harms: See harms of corticosteroid injections plus local anaesthetic, p 1437.

Comment: Epinephrine (adrenaline) is not recommended in local anaesthetics for procedures that involve the appendages because of the risk of ischaemic necrosis.[7]

OPTION CORTICOSTEROID INJECTIONS PLUS LOCAL ANAESTHESIA

One systematic review identified no RCTs comparing corticosteroid injections plus local anaesthesia versus placebo. One RCT found no significant difference in pain between prednisolone plus lidocaine injection and lidocaine alone after 3 or 6 months. Observational studies have found a high rate of plantar fascia rupture and other complications associated with corticosteroid injections, which may lead to chronic disability in some people.

Benefits: We found one systematic review (search date 1997), which included RCTs of injected corticosteroid plus local anaesthetic compared with various other treatments.[1] **Versus placebo or no treatment:** The review found no RCTs. **Versus heel pads:** The review found two RCTs.[1] The first RCT (80 people) in the review included people with pain on the plantar aspect of the heel but excluded people on anti-inflammatory medication, people who had a corticosteroid injection during the past 6 months, people with rheumatoid arthritis, and people with pain that radiated along the plantar fascia more distally. It compared three treatments: a heel pad (see glossary, p 1442) alone; an injection alone (triamcinolone hexacetonide 20 mg plus 2% lidocaine [lignocaine]), and injection plus heel pad. Analysis was not by intention to treat, and four people (5%) were lost to follow up. The RCT found that, after 1 month, the greatest improvement in pain was in people who received the injection alone (22 people), with the least improvement in people who had the pad alone (26 people) (100 mm visual analogue scale: injection alone *v* pad alone, mean difference –45 mm, 95% CI –59 mm to –31 mm). At 24 weeks, there was greater pain reduction with the injection alone versus the pad alone, but the difference was not significant (85% with injection alone *v* 75% with pad alone). The second RCT (17 people) in the review compared triamcinolone 20 mg plus 2% lidocaine injection versus a prefabricated silicone type heel pad. Although more people improved after treatment with the heel pad (66% with heel pad *v* 33% with injection at 12 weeks), the difference in pain was not significant at 1, 2, or 12 weeks. **Corticosteroid injection plus local anaesthesia plus non-steroidal anti-inflammatory drugs versus heel pad:** The review found no RCTs.[1] We found one subsequent RCT that included 103 people with plantar heel tenderness, a history of pain upon rising in the morning (first step pain), and no history of trauma in the previous 3 months.[8] Analysis was not by intention to treat and 18 people were lost to follow up. It compared three interventions: non-steroidal anti-inflammatory drugs plus three corticosteroid plus local anaesthetic injections into the heel (anti-inflammatory, 35 people), heel pads plus paracetamol (acetaminophen) as required (accommodative, 33 people), and a heel pad before fitting of custom made orthoses (see glossary, p 1442) (mechanical, 35 people). The anti-inflammatory regimen consisted of etodolac 600 mg and 0.5 mL dexamethasone sodium phosphate 4 mg/mL plus 1 mL of 0.5% bupivacaine hydrochloride without adrenaline (epinephrine). If there was no response, 0.2 mL of dexamethasone acetate 16 mg/mL injection was added cumulatively to the second (2 week) and third (4 week) injections. The RCT found that the anti-inflammatory regimen slightly reduced pain compared with the accommodative regimen at 3 months, but the difference was not significant (10 cm visual analogue scale: mean difference –1.2 cm, 95% CI –2.8 cm to +0.4 cm).[8] **Corticosteroid injection plus local anaesthesia plus non-steroidal anti-inflammatory drugs versus heel pad plus orthoses:** The review found no RCTs.[1] We found one subsequent RCT comparing an anti-inflammatory regimen versus a mechanical regimen.[8] At 3 months, it found that both the anti-inflammatory regimen and heel pads plus orthoses (mechanical regimen) improved pain, but the difference was not significant (10 cm visual analogue scale: mean difference –1 cm, 95% CI –2.5 cm to +0.5 cm). **Versus orthoses alone:** The review found no RCTs.[1] **Versus local anaesthetic alone:** The review found no RCTs.[1] We found one subsequent RCT (106 heels).[6] It compared a single injection of 1 mL prednisolone acetate 25 mg/mL plus 1 mL lidocaine hydrochloride 2% versus 2 mL lidocaine hydrochloride 2% alone. It found that the combined injection slightly improved pain score at 1 month, although the clinical importance of this result is unclear (10 cm visual analogue scale: mean difference –0.8 cm, 95% CI –1.5 cm to –0.2 cm), but no significant difference in pain thereafter (3 months: mean difference +0.1 cm, 95% CI –1.2 cm to +1.3 cm; and 6 months: +0.5 cm, 95% CI –0.8 cm to +1.7 cm). **Versus corticosteroid alone:** The review found no RCTs. **Versus corticosteroid plus local anaesthetic plus pad:** The review found one RCT (80 people).[1] It found that heel pad plus injection (triamcinolone hexacetonide 20 mg plus 2% lidocaine) significantly worsened pain score compared with injection alone 1 month after treatment, although the clinical importance of these results is unclear (100 mm visual analogue scale: mean difference 1.60 cm, 95% CI 0.07 cm to 3.12 cm).[1] However, at 24 weeks, people treated with pad plus injection versus injection alone had less pain, but this was not significant (94% with pad plus injection *v* 85% with injection alone). **Corticosteroid plus local anaesthetic plus pad versus pad alone:** The review found one RCT (80 people).[1] It found a significantly better response with injection (triamcinolone hexacetonide 20 mg plus 2% lidocaine) plus pad versus pad alone at 4 weeks (10 cm visual analogue scale: mean difference –2.9 cm, 95% CI

−4.4 cm to −1.4 cm) and 12 weeks, but not at 24 weeks (10 cm visual analogue scale: mean difference −1.07 cm, 95% CI −2.55 cm to +0.41 cm; AR for pain reduction 94% with injection plus pad *v* 75% with pad alone). However, the clinical importance of these results is unclear.

Harms: In one RCT, participants' heels were injected through the medial aspect of the heel pad. Half of the 106 participants were given a tibial nerve block and half received local injection only. The trial found no significant difference between these groups in pain at time of injection.[6] The other RCTs did not report on harms. See also harms of corticosteroid injections, p 1434.

Comment: The RCTs had many flaws (lack of intention to treat analysis, lack of power, high withdrawal rates, and lack of placebo control). Limitations of the available evidence make the use of corticosteroid injections in heel pain difficult to categorise in terms of benefits and harms. Heterogeneity of interventions prevented data pooling. A survey of UK rheumatologists found that corticosteroid injections are the most common treatment of heel pain and are used by 98% of UK rheumatologists (Crawford F, personal communication, 2000), confirming the results of similar surveys.[3] We found evidence from two observational studies of high rates of moderately severe harms from this treatment (see harms of corticosteroid injections, p 1434). This is also consistent with evidence about harms of corticosteroid injections in other areas.[3] These harms are particularly relevant because the evidence of benefit is poor, and spontaneous resolution of symptoms is common.

OPTION STRETCHING EXERCISES New

We found insufficient evidence to compare stretching versus no treatment, versus stretching plus custom made orthoses, or to compare different types of stretching in people with heel pain.

Benefits: **Versus no treatment:** We found no systematic review or RCTs. **Versus orthoses plus stretching:** We found one RCT comparing stretching exercises alone versus custom made orthoses (see glossary, p 1442) plus stretching exercises.[9] It found no significant difference in pain improvement at 8 weeks (100 mm visual analogue scale: difference −3.2 mm, 95% CI −17.4 mm to +11.0 mm; see comment below). **Sustained versus intermittent stretching:** We found one RCT (94 people with heel pain).[10] All participants stretched their Achilles' tendon by hanging the heel from a step while keeping the knee straight and, for those with flat foot arches, inverting the foot. People assigned to sustained stretching performed this exercise for 3 minutes, three times daily, for at least 4 months. People assigned to intermittent stretching performed this exercise in two daily sessions, with each session consisting of five repetitions of this manoeuvre, each of which was held for 20 seconds. The RCT found no significant difference between sustained and intermittent stretching in foot and ankle pain scores after 4 months (pain score not further described; P = 0.31).[10]

Harms: The RCTs did not report on harms.

Comment: Subgroup analysis in the RCT comparing orthoses plus stretching versus heel pads plus stretching found that, among people who stood for more than 8 hours daily, a greater reduction in pain was achieved with stretching alone than with customised insoles.[9] It found no significant difference in people who stood for less than 8 hours daily. This hypothesis requires testing as the primary outcome in an RCT. Only half of the participants in this subgroup analysis responded to the pain questionnaire.

OPTION CASTED ORTHOSES (CUSTOM MADE INSOLES)

We found no RCTs on the effects of orthoses versus placebo or no treatment. One systematic review and three RCTs found limited and conflicting evidence about the effects of orthoses versus corticosteroids, corticosteroids plus local anaesthesia, or other physical supports.

Benefits: We found one systematic review (search date 1997).[1] **Versus placebo or no treatment:** The review found no RCTs. **Orthoses plus heel pad versus steroid plus pain medication:** The review found no RCTs. We found one subsequent RCT, which found no significant difference in pain improvement (see benefits of corticosteroid injections plus local anaesthesia, p 1435).[8] **Orthoses plus heel pad versus heel pad plus pain medication:** The review found no RCTs. We found one RCT of a heel pad (see glossary, p 1442) applied for 4 weeks before fitting of a custom made orthosis (see glossary, p 1442) heel pad (28 people) versus a viscoelastic heel pad plus paracetamol as required (26 people).[8] It found a significantly better pain reduction with pad plus orthoses versus pad plus paracetamol (10 cm visual analogue scale: difference –2.2 cm, 95% CI –3.8 cm to –0.5 cm). **Orthoses plus stretching versus heel pad plus stretching:** The review found no RCTs. We found one subsequent RCT (236 people, 5 groups) in people with maximal tenderness over the medial calcaneal tuberosity for which they had received no previous treatment.[9] People with systemic disease, sciatica, or local nerve entrapment were excluded. The RCT compared customised orthoses plus stretching exercises versus prefabricated shoe inserts made from three different materials (silicone, felt, and rubber) plus stretching exercises (Achilles and plantar fascial stretching for 10 minutes twice daily). It found significantly less pain at 8 weeks in people who were assigned to prefabricated inserts (results combined) versus orthoses ($P = 0.007$). **Orthoses plus stretching versus stretching alone:** See benefits of stretching exercises, p 1437.

Harms: No RCTs reported on harms.

Comment: We found one RCT comparing heel pads versus custom made orthoses;[11] however, there was a significant difference in weight between the groups at baseline (19 lb [8.6 kg]) and weight was associated with severity of heel pain. This makes the results difficult to interpret.

OPTION HEEL PADS AND HEEL CUPS

We found no RCTs on the effects of heel pads and heel cups compared with placebo or no treatment. One systematic review and subsequent RCTs found limited and conflicting evidence on the effects of heel pads and heel cups compared with other treatment modalities.

Benefits: We found one systematic review (search date 1997),[1] which included RCTs of heel pads and heel cups (see glossary, p 1442) compared with various treatments. **Versus placebo or no treatment:** The review found no RCTs.[1] **Versus corticosteroid injection:** The review found no RCTs. **Versus corticosteroid injections plus local anaesthesia:** The review found two RCTs and we found one subsequent RCT, neither of which found evidence of a significant long term benefit (see benefits of corticosteroids plus pain medication versus heel pads, p 1435). **Versus corticosteroid injection plus pain medication:** We found one RCT, which found no significant difference in pain improvement between corticosteroid injection plus non-steroidal anti-inflammatory drugs and pads plus paracetamol (see benefits of corticosteroids plus local anaesthesia, p 1435).[8] **Versus custom made orthoses:** See glossary, p 1442. The review found one RCT[1] and we found one subsequent RCT.[8] They found conflicting evidence on improvement in pain (see benefits of casted orthoses custom made insoles, p 1438). **Heel pad plus corticosteroid injection plus local anaesthetic versus corticosteroid plus local anaesthetic:** The review found one RCT.[1] It found a short term benefit with the corticosteroid plus local anaesthetic injection alone (see benefits of corticosteroids plus local anaesthesia, p 1435).

Harms: None of the RCTs reported harms.

Comment: Heel cups and heel pads can be made from several different materials, but rubber, viscoelastic, and silicone can be bought as prefabricated shoe inserts. Podiatrists or orthotists sometimes use felt and foam to construct heel pads. We found one additional RCT of heel pads versus orthoses but the results were difficult to interpret. See comment of casted orthoses (custom made insoles), p 1438.[11]

OPTION EXTRACORPOREAL SHOCK WAVE THERAPY

Four small RCTs provided insufficient evidence to assess extracorporeal shock wave therapy compared with placebo. Two RCTs found limited evidence that high dose extracorporeal shock wave therapy reduced pain and walking scores compared with low dose therapy. However, the clinical importance of these effects is unclear.

Benefits: **Versus placebo:** We found one systematic review (search date 1997)[1] and three subsequent RCTs of extracorporeal shock wave therapy (ESWT — see glossary, p 1442).[12–14] The review found one single blind RCT (36 people with recalcitrant heel pain), which compared 1000 impulses (0.06 mJ/mm²) versus placebo (sham ESWT) three times at weekly intervals. It found that pain on manual pressure and pain free walking ability were significantly improved at

6 weeks ($P < 0.005$). Six people withdrew from the trial, and analysis was not intention to treat. The first subsequent RCT (260 people with recalcitrant heel pain) compared ESWT for a total of 1500 pulses at 18 kV versus sham treatment.[12] It found that more people reported improved pain after 12 weeks (improvement of ≥ 50% and ≥ 4 cm on a 10 cm visual analogue scale), but the difference did not reach significance (71/119 [60%] with ESWT *v* 56/116 [48%] with sham treatment; RR 1.24, 95% CI 0.97 to 1.57; results recalculated by *Clinical Evidence*). It also found slightly improved self assessed activity with ESWT, but it was not possible to calculate significance. The second subsequent RCT (166 people with plantar fasciitis) similarly found no significant difference in overall pain between ultrasound guided ESWT (1000 mJ/mm^2 weekly for 3 weeks) and placebo at 12 weeks after treatment (mean difference in score measured with 100 mm visual analogue scale [0 mm = no pain; 100 mm = maximal pain]; ESWT *v* placebo: +0.6 mm, 95% CI –10.3 mm to +11.5 mm).[13] The third subsequent RCT (32 people with recalcitrant heel pain) compared 1000 impulses of ESWT at 0.8 mJ/mm^2 versus placebo.[14] It found that ESWT significantly reduced rest pain compared with placebo at 48 weeks (mean score on 10 cm visual analogue scale [0 cm = no pain, 10 cm = maximal pain]: 0.7 cm with ESWT *v* 1.8 cm with placebo; $P = 0.01$). It also found that ESWT improved exercise tolerance (with footwear) compared with placebo at 48 weeks (proportion of people who could walk for longer than 60 minutes: 15/17 [88%] with ESWT *v* 8/15 [53%] with placebo; significance not stated). **Different doses:** The review identified one non-blinded RCT[1] and we found one additional RCT.[15] The RCT in the review (119 people) compared 1000 impulses versus 10 impulses of 0.08 mJ/mm^2 in people with recalcitrant heel pain. All treatments were given three times at weekly intervals. It found greater improvements in pressure pain between weeks 0–12 with the higher dose (100 mm visual analogue scale: mean difference –47 mm, 95% CI –54 mm to –40 mm). A supplementary report of outcomes from 78/119 (66%) of the original people in the RCT found significantly less pain on manual pressure with high dose compared with low dose ESWT after 5 years (100 mm visual analogue scale: mean difference –20 mm, 95% CI –28 mm to –11 mm).[16] The additional RCT (50 people) compared 3 x 500 impulses of ESWT versus 3 x 100 impulses (both at intensity 0.08 mJ/mm^2) in people with recalcitrant heel pain.[15] It found no significant difference in pain on pressure at 6 weeks (10 cm visual analogue scale: mean difference –0.4 cm, 95% CI –2.0 cm to +1.2 cm) or at 12 weeks (mean difference –1.4 cm, 95% CI –3.0 cm to +0.2 cm). It also found no significant difference in walking pain at 6 weeks (mean difference –0.8 cm, 95% CI –2.4 cm to +0.7 cm) or at 12 weeks (mean difference –0.9 cm, 95% CI –2.5 cm to +0.7 cm). Self reported walking pain at 12 months suggested a marginal long term benefit from higher doses of ESWT (10 cm visual analogue scale: mean difference –2.0 cm, 95% CI –3.7 cm to –0.2 cm).

Harms: ESWT without local anaesthetic can be painful. One of the RCTs reported a sensation of heat and numbness in one person receiving ESWT and a burning sensation in the heel and ankle in one person receiving placebo. One person receiving ESWT reported bruising.[13]

Comment: All trial participants had recalcitrant heel pain. Availability of ESWT is limited. Pain associated with ESWT and differences in procedures mean the single blinding in the first placebo controlled RCT was probably not maintained.[1] The large RCT reported a large increase in the number of people not using pain medications with ESWT (measured as any use between weeks 10 and 12; 70% with ESWT *v* 35% with sham treatment).[12] We found one small RCT reported in abstract only (37 people with recalcitrant heel pain). It found a non-significant reduction in pain associated with ESWT at 1500 pulses at 3 Hz versus sham treatment at 2 months (100 mm visual analogue scale: mean difference –15 mm, 95% CI –45 mm to +15 mm).[17]

OPTION SURGERY

One systematic review found no RCTs of surgery for heel pain.

Benefits: We found one systematic review (search date 1997),[1] which identified no RCTs of surgery for heel pain.

Harms: We found no RCTs.

Comment: The systematic review identified many observational studies of surgery for chronically painful heels.[1] One of the largest observational studies (76 people) compared postoperative complication rates after endoscopic fasciotomy versus traditional plantar fasciotomy.[18] It found that serious complications (recurrent pain, neuritis, infection) were less common in people treated with endoscopic fasciotomy versus traditional surgery (serious incidents per procedure: 11/66 [17%] with endoscopic fasciotomy *v* 9/26 [35%] with traditional surgery).

OPTION LASERS

One small RCT identified by a systematic review found no significant difference between laser treatment and placebo.

Benefits: One systematic review (search date 1997) included one small RCT (32 people) of laser treatment compared with placebo (treatment with a disabled laser) in people with pain of at least 1 months' duration; tenderness to pressure at the origin of the plantar fascia; on the mid-anterior inferior border of the calcaneus; and sharp shooting, localised, or both inferior foot pain made worse with activity or on rising in the morning.[1] It found no evidence of a significant effect.

Harms: The RCT reported that 96% of people had no adverse effects, and the rest (4%) reported a "mild sensation" during or after treatment.[1]

Comment: None.

OPTION ULTRASOUND

One systematic review of one small RCT found no significant difference in pain between ultrasound and sham ultrasound.

Benefits: One systematic review (search date 1997) included one small RCT in 19 people (7 with bilateral heel pain) of eight treatments of true ultrasound compared with the same number of applications of sham ultrasound.[1] Inclusion criteria were pain radiating from the medial tubercle of the calcaneum in response to both pressure and weight bearing first thing in the morning. It found no significant difference in pain between ultrasound and sham ultrasound (10 cm visual analogue scale; mean difference +0.1 cm, 95% CI –1.8 cm to +2.1 cm).[1]

Harms: The RCT did not assess harms.[1]

Comment: None.

OPTION NIGHT SPLINTS

One RCT found no significant difference in pain between a night splint and no splint after 3 months.

Benefits: One systematic review (search date 1997) found no good quality trials.[1] We found two subsequent RCTs.[19,20] The first RCT included 116 people with recalcitrant heel pain.[19] All participants received ankle dorsiflexion exercises and piroxicam (20 mg/day for 30 days), with or without a night splint that dorsiflexed the ankle joint by 5°. In people with bilateral complaints, only the most symptomatic foot was studied. The night splint was worn for 3 months. The RCT found no evidence of an effect on pain with night splinting compared with no splinting (RR 1.0, 95% CI 0.8 to 1.3).[19] The second RCT (255 people) compared custom made orthoses (see glossary, p 1442) versus night splints. The results were difficult to interpret because there was a large difference in withdrawals between the groups (26% with night splints *v* 7% with orthoses), and we were not able to report intention to treat analysis.[20]

Harms: The RCTs did not assess harms.[19,20]

Comment: The first RCT only studied the most symptomatic foot because of potential inconvenience and poor compliance from wearing two night splints simultaneously.[19]

GLOSSARY

Custom made orthoses Made from polyurethene or similar material to a negative cast of a person's foot.

Extracorporeal shock wave therapy (ESWT) Shock waves are pulsed acoustic waves that dissipate mechanical energy at the interface of two substances with different acoustic impedance.

Heel cups Prefabricated rubber heel cups (firmer than viscoelastic heel pads) that extend up the sides of the heel and enclose the fibro fatty heel pad.

Heel pads Prefabricated viscoelastic heel pads made of malleable material.

Substantive changes

Extracorporeal shock wave therapy Two RCTs added;[13,14] conclusions unchanged.

REFERENCES

1. Crawford F, Atkins D, Edwards J. Interventions for treating plantar heel pain (Cochrane Review). In: The Cochrane Library, Issue 1, 2003. Oxford: Update Software. Search date 1997; primary sources Medline, Embase, the Cochrane Library, hand searches of *The Foot*, *The Chiropodist* (later *Journal of British Podiatric Medicine*), and *British Journal of Podiatric Medicine*. In addition, investigators in the field were contacted to identify unpublished data or research in progress. Non-English language reports were excluded from the review.
2. Wolgin M, Cook C, Graham C, et al. Conservative treatment of plantar heel pain: long term follow up. *Foot Ankle Int* 1994;15:97–102.
3. Fadale PD, Wiggins MD. Corticosteroid injections: their use and abuse. *J Am Acad Orthop Surg* 1994;2:133–140.
4. Sellman JR. Plantar fascial rupture associated with corticosteroid injection. *Foot Ankle Int* 1994;15:376–381.
5. Acevedo JI, Beskin JL. Complications of plantar fascial rupture associated with steroid injection. *Foot Ankle Int* 1998;19:91–97.
6. Crawford F, Atkins D, Young P, et al. Steroid injection for heel pain: evidence of short term effectiveness. A randomised controlled trial. *Rheumatology* 1999;38:974–977.
7. McCauley WA, Gerace RV, Scilley C. Treatment of accidental digital injection of epinephrine. *Ann Emerg Med* 1991;6:665–668.
8. Lynch DM, Goforth WP, Martin JE, et al. Conservative treatment of plantar fasciitis. A prospective study. *J Am Podiatr Assoc* 1998;88:375–380.
9. Pfeffer G, Bacchetti P, Deland J, et al. Comparison of custom and prefabricated orthoses in the initial treatment of proximal plantar fasciitis. *Foot Ankle Int* 1999;20:214–221.
10. Porter D, Barrill E, Oneacre K, et al. The effects of duration and frequency of Achilles tendon stretching on dorsiflexion and outcome in painful heel syndrome: a randomized, blinded, controlled study. *Foot Ankle Int* 2002;23:619–624.
11. Turlik M, Donatelli T, Veremis M. A comparison of shoe inserts in relieving mechanical heel pain. *Foot* 1999;9:84–87.
12. Odgen J, Alvarex R, Levitt R, et al. Shock wave therapy for chronic proximal plantar fasciitis. *Clin Orthop Related Res* 2001;1:47–59.
13. Buchbinder R, Ptasnik R, Gordon J, et al. Ultrasound-guided extra corporeal shock wave therapy for plantar fasciitis. A randomized controlled trial. *JAMA* 2002;288:1364–1372.
14. Abt T, Hopfenmukker W, Mellerowicz H. Shock wave therapy for recalcitrant plantar fasciitis with heel spur: a prospective randomized placebo-controlled double-blind study [In German]. *Z Orthop* 2002;140:548–554.
15. Krischeck O, Rompe JD, Herbsthrofer B, et al. Symptomatic low-energy shockwave therapy in heel pain and radiologically detected plantar heel spur [in German]. *Z Orthop Ihre Grenzgeb* 1998;136:169–174.
16. Rompe JD, Schoellner C, Nafe B. Evaluation of low-energy extracorporeal shock wave application for treatment of chronic plantar fasciitis. *J Bone Joint Surg Br* 2002; 84A:335–341.
17. Speed CA, Nichols DW, Burnett SP, et al. Extracorporeal shock wave therapy (ESWT) in plantar fasciitis. A pilot double blind randomised placebo controlled study [abstract]. *Rheumatology* 2000;39(suppl 123):230.
18. Kinley S, Frascone S, Calderone D, et al. Endoscopic plantar fasciotomy versus traditional heel spur surgery: a prospective study. *J Foot Ankle Surg* 1993;32:595–603.
19. Probe RA, Baca M, Adams R, et al. Night splint treatment for plantar fasciitis. *Clin Orthop* 1999;368:191–195.
20. Martin J, Hosch J, Goforth W, et al. Mechanical treatment of plantar fasciitis. A prospective study. *J Am Pod Med Assoc* 2001;91:55–62.

Fay Crawford
Senior Research Fellow
Dental Health Services Research Unit
Dundee
UK

Competing interests: None declared.

Raynaud's (primary)

Search date February 2003

Janet Pope

QUESTIONS

INTERVENTIONS

Key Messages

- **Nifedipine** Six RCTs found that nifedipine reduced the frequency and severity of attacks over 4–12 weeks compared with placebo, and was rated by participants as more effective than placebo in improving overall symptoms. The RCTs found that nifedipine was associated with higher rates of adverse effects compared with placebo, including flushing, headache, oedema, and tachycardia.
- **Amlodipine; diltiazem; moxisylyte (thymoxamine)** We found no good RCTs of these interventions.
- **Inositol nicotinate; naftidrofuryl oxalate; nicardipine; prazosin** RCTs provided insufficient evidence to assess these interventions.

DEFINITION Raynaud's phenomenon is episodic vasospasm of the peripheral arteries, causing pallor followed by cyanosis and redness with pain and sometimes paraesthesia, and, rarely, ulceration of the fingers and toes (and in some cases of the ears or nose). Primary or idiopathic Raynaud's phenomenon (Raynaud's disease) occurs without an underlying disease. Secondary Raynaud's phenomenon (Raynaud's syndrome) occurs in association with an underlying disease — usually connective tissue disorders such as scleroderma, systemic lupus erythematosus, rheumatoid arthritis, or polymyositis. This review excludes secondary Raynaud's phenomenon.

INCIDENCE/ PREVALENCE The prevalence of primary Raynaud's phenomenon varies by gender, country, and exposure to workplace vibration. One large US cohort study (4182 people) found symptoms in 9.6% of women and 8.1% of men, of whom 81% had primary Raynaud's phenomenon.[1] Smaller cohort studies in Spain have estimated the prevalence of Raynaud's phenomenon to be 3.7–4.0%, of which 90% is primary Raynaud's phenomenon.[2,3] One cohort study in Japan (332 men, 731 women) found symptoms of primary Raynaud's phenomenon in 3.4% of women and 3.0% of men.[4]

AETIOLOGY/ RISK FACTORS The aetiology of primary Raynaud's phenomenon is unknown.[5] There is evidence for genetic predisposition,[6,7] most likely in those people with early onset Raynaud's phenomenon (aged < 40 years).[8] One prospective observational study (424 people with Raynaud's phenomenon) found that 73% of sufferers first developed symptoms before age 40 years.[8] Women are more at risk than men (OR 3.0, 95% CI 1.2 to 7.8, in 1 US case control study [235 people]).[9] The other known risk factor is occupational exposure to vibration from tools (symptoms developed in about 8% with exposure *v* 2.7% with no exposure in 2 cohorts from Japan).[10,11] People who are obese may be less at risk.[9] Symptoms are often worsened by cold or emotion.

PROGNOSIS Attacks may last from several minutes to a few hours. One systematic review (search date 1996, 10 prospective observational studies, 639 people with primary Raynaud's phenomenon) found that only 13% of long term sufferers later manifested an underlying disorder such as scleroderma.[12]

AIMS OF INTERVENTION To reduce the number and severity of attacks; to prevent tissue damage; to minimise adverse effects of treatment.

OUTCOMES Frequency and severity of symptoms (as assessed by patient diary); severity assessed by visual analogue scales, Likert scales, or the Raynaud's Condition Score;[13] rates, size, and healing of digital ulceration.

METHODS *Clinical Evidence* search and appraisal February 2003. We found no systematic review. Many RCTs included people with both primary and secondary Raynaud's phenomenon. We excluded RCTs in which less than 50% of people had primary Raynaud's phenomenon or where the type of Raynaud's was unclear. We also excluded RCTs in which attacks were experimentally induced (e.g. by dipping the hands in cold water) or which did not assess clinical outcomes.

Some RCTs compared changes in symptoms from baseline within each treatment group rather than directly comparing outcomes between treatment groups. These have been described in the comment sections.

QUESTION **What are the effects of treatments for primary Raynaud's phenomenon?**

OPTION **NIFEDIPINE**

Six RCTs found that nifedipine reduced the frequency and severity of attacks over 4–12 weeks compared with placebo, and was rated by participants as more effective than placebo in improving overall symptoms. The RCTs found that nifedipine was associated with higher rates of adverse effects compared with placebo, including flushing, headache, oedema, and tachycardia.

Benefits: **Versus placebo:** We found six RCTs comparing nifedipine versus placebo (457 people, 451 with primary Raynaud's phenomenon, 2 parallel, 4 crossover trials) (see table 1, p 1452).[14–19] All RCTs found that nifedipine significantly reduced the mean frequency of attacks over 4–12 weeks compared with placebo.[14–19] One RCT found that nifedipine reduced the mean grade of the most severe attack over 4 weeks compared with placebo,[18] but another RCT found no significant difference in the mean severity of attacks over 6 weeks.[15] Three RCTs found that a significantly higher proportion of people rated nifedipine as more effective than placebo in improving overall symptoms.[14,15,19]

Harms: Five RCTs found higher rates of adverse effects with nifedipine.[14–17,19] The first RCT found that significantly more people taking nifedipine compared with placebo had oedema (24% with nifedipine *v* 0% with placebo; $P < 0.01$) or flushing (8% with nifedipine *v* 0% with placebo; $P < 0.01$).[14] Two people taking nifedipine had tachycardia. The second RCT found that 10/22 (45%) people taking nifedipine 10 mg, 16/22 (72%) people taking nifedipine 20 mg, and 6/22 (27%) people taking placebo had adverse effects (CI not stated).[15] The third RCT found no significant difference between nifedipine and placebo in the overall incidence of adverse effects, but found that nifedipine significantly increased the risk of palpitations (7/18 [38.8%] with nifedipine *v* 1/18 [5.5%] with placebo; $P < 0.05$).[16] The fourth RCT found that significantly more people had adverse effects, including headaches, flushing, and ankle swelling over 8 weeks after crossover with nifedipine compared with placebo (14/23 [61%] with nifedipine *v* 2/23 [9%] with placebo; $P = 0.05$).[17] The fifth RCT found that 16/21 (76%) people had adverse effects with nifedipine, but did not report adverse effects with placebo.[18] The sixth RCT (34 people) found that more people had adverse effects, including flushing, headache, and oedema, with nifedipine over 12 weeks after crossover compared with placebo (26/34 [76%] with nifedipine *v* 5/34 [15%] with placebo; P value not stated).[19]

Comment: One of the RCTs included six people with secondary Raynaud's phenomenon.[19]

OPTION NICARDIPINE

One RCT found that nicardipine decreased the frequency of Raynaud's attacks over 8 weeks after crossover compared with placebo, but found no significant difference in the severity of attacks. Another RCT found no significant difference in frequency, severity, or duration of attacks with nicardipine compared with placebo, but it is likely to have been too small to exclude a clinically important difference in outcomes.

Benefits: We found two RCTs.[20,21] The first RCT (69 people with primary Raynaud's, crossover design, outcomes assessed after crossover; see comment below) found that nicardipine significantly decreased the frequency of attacks over 8 weeks compared with placebo (attacks/week: 4.9 with nicardipine *v* 5.8 with placebo; mean difference 0.9, 95% CI 0 to 2.2; P = 0.02) and reduced overall disability (measured on a visual analogue scale of 10 cm where 0 represented no disability; mean 2.6 with nicardipine *v* 3.3 with placebo; P = 0.018), but found no significant difference in the severity of attacks (measured on a scale of 1–4 where 1 represented mild and 4 highly severe; 1.36 with nicardipine *v* 1.55 with placebo; mean difference in severity 0.2, 95% CI 0 to 0.4; P reported as non-significant; no further data provided).[20] The second RCT (25 people, 16 with primary Raynaud's phenomenon, crossover design, outcomes assessed after crossover; see comment below) found no significant difference in frequency, severity, or duration of attacks at 6 weeks between nicardipine 30 mg twice daily and placebo (analysis in 16 people with primary Raynaud's; mean frequency 4.4 attacks/day with nicardipine *v* 4.4 attacks/day with placebo; mean severity of attacks on a 10 point scale where 0 represented no pain; 3.5 with nicardipine *v* 3.7 with placebo; mean duration of attacks 13 minutes with nicardipine *v* 11 minutes with placebo; reported as non-significant for all outcomes; no further data provided).[21] The RCT is likely to have been too small to exclude a clinically important difference in outcomes.

Harms: The first RCT found that 7/69 (10%) people withdrew from the trial because of adverse effects: five people while taking nicardipine and two while taking placebo.[20] In the second RCT, three people withdrew because of adverse effects (including flushing, headache, and palpitations), two while taking nicardipine, and one while taking placebo.[21]

Comment: The second RCT included nine people with secondary Raynaud's phenomenon.[21] The results of the crossover trials should be viewed with caution as no precrossover results were available and results may not allow for confounding factors such as inadequate washout and the naturally variable course of Raynaud's phenomenon.[20,21]

OPTION AMLODIPINE

We found no good RCTs.

Benefits: We found no RCTs that provided between group comparisons of amlodipine versus placebo (see comment below).

Harms: We found no good RCTs (see comment below).

Comment: We found one RCT that presented within group comparisons of changes in outcomes from baseline (24 people, 15 with primary Raynaud's phenomenon, crossover design, outcomes assessed after crossover).[22] It found that amlodipine significantly reduced the number of acute attacks a week from baseline at 7 weeks (from 11.8 attacks/week at baseline to 8.6 attacks/week after treatment; P < 0.001) and reduced the severity of attacks from baseline (from a discomfort score of 7.8 at baseline to 5.1 after treatment). However, the RCT did not assess the significance of the difference in frequency and severity of attacks between groups. It found that amlodipine was associated with ankle oedema (55% of people taking amlodipine *v* 0% of people taking placebo), flushing, and headaches compared with placebo (10–20% with amlodipine *v* 0% with placebo).[22] The RCT included people with secondary Raynaud's phenomenon, so results may not be applicable in people with primary Raynaud's phenomenon.

OPTION DILTIAZEM

We found no good RCTs.

Benefits: We found no good RCTs (see comment below).

Harms: We found no good RCTs (see comment below).

Comment: One crossover RCT (30 people, 19 with primary Raynaud's phenomenon, outcomes assessed after crossover) found that diltiazem significantly reduced the number of attacks compared with placebo (mean reduction in attacks from baseline 22.9/month with diltiazem *v* 4.6/month with placebo; P = 0.01) and reduced duration of attacks (mean reduction from baseline 444 minutes/month with diltiazem *v* 160 minutes/month with placebo; P < 0.01) over 8 weeks.[23] The results of this RCT should be interpreted with caution as it reported comparisons from baseline, thus removing the benefits of randomisation, and the results are not intention to treat (8/30 [27%] withdrew from the trial). Two people withdrew from the trial because of adverse effects (rash or headache) while taking diltiazem. The RCT included people with secondary Raynaud's phenomenon, so results may not be fully applicable in people with primary Raynaud's phenomenon.

OPTION NAFTIDROFURYL OXALATE

One RCT found that, compared with placebo, naftidrofuryl oxalate reduced the duration and intensity of Raynaud's attacks over 2 months and reduced the impact of attacks on daily activities.

Benefits: We found one RCT (102 people, 87 with primary Raynaud's phenomenon) comparing naftidrofuryl oxalate 600 mg daily versus placebo for 2 months.[24] It found that, over 2 months, naftidrofuryl oxalate significantly reduced the duration of attacks (measured as pain for < 15 minutes, for 15–30 minutes, or for > 30 minutes; overall P < 0.05; people who had pain for < 15 minutes; 28/51 [55%] with naftidrofuryl *v* 17/45 [38%] with placebo; P value not stated), intensity of attacks (measured as no pain, mild pain, strong pain; overall P < 0.001; people who had no pain 13/50 [26%] with naftidrofuryl v 3/49 [6%] with placebo; P value for this comparison not stated), and reduced the impact of attacks on daily activities compared with placebo (measured as no impact, weak impact, important impact; overall P < 0.05; people for whom Raynaud's had no impact on daily life 16/51 [31%] with naftidrofuryl v 8/49 [16%] with placebo; P value not stated) over 2 months.[24]

Harms: The RCT found no adverse effects associated with naftidrofuryl oxalate.[24]

Comment: The RCT included people with secondary Raynaud's phenomenon, so results may not be applicable in people with primary Raynaud's phenomenon.[24]

OPTION INOSITOL NICOTINATE

Two RCTs provided insufficient evidence to assess inositol nicotinate.

Benefits: We found two RCTs.[25,26] The first RCT (23 people with primary Raynaud's phenomenon) compared inositol nicotinate (4 g daily) versus placebo for 84 days during the winter.[25] It found that, compared with placebo, people taking inositol nicotinate had fewer and shorter attacks over 84 days, but the difference was not significant (P reported as non-significant; no further data provided). The RCT is likely to have been too small to exclude a clinically important difference.[25] The second RCT (65 people, 54 with primary Raynaud's phenomenon) found that, compared with placebo, more people taking inositol nicotinate 2 g twice daily improved over 12 weeks (as measured by a 5 point scale from 0 [no problem] to 5 [very severe]), but the difference was not significant (19/34 [56%] people scored 0–1 with inositol v 11/33 [33%] with placebo; RR 1.58, 95% CI 0.90 to 2.76; calculated from data in the paper; see comment below).[26]

Harms: The first RCT found no adverse effects associated with inositol nicotinate.[25] In the second RCT, three people taking inositol nicotinate withdrew from the trial because of gastrointestinal disturbance or dizziness compared with one person taking placebo.[26]

Comment: The second RCT included people with secondary Raynaud's phenomenon, so results may not be fully applicable in people with primary Raynaud's phenomenon.[26]

OPTION PRAZOSIN

One small crossover RCT found no clear evidence of benefit from prazosin. It found that prazosin reduced the number and duration of attacks over 6 weeks after crossover compared with placebo, but found no significant difference in the severity of attacks.

Benefits: We found one RCT (24 people, 14 with primary Raynaud's phenomenon, crossover design, outcomes assessed after crossover; see comment below) comparing prazosin (1 mg twice daily) versus placebo.[27] It found that, compared with placebo, prazosin significantly reduced the mean number of attacks over 6 weeks after crossover (attacks/day; 2.5 with prazosin v 4.1 with placebo;

P = 0.003) and reduced duration of attacks (21.9 minutes with prazosin *v* 29.9 minutes with placebo; P = 0.02), but found no difference in the severity of attacks (measured on a 10 point scale where 0 represented no pain; 4.1 with prazosin *v* 4.8 with placebo; P = 0.11).

Harms: The RCT found that 50% of people taking prazosin had adverse effects, including dizziness and palpitations, compared with 29% of people taking placebo.[27]

Comment: The results of the RCT should be viewed with caution as no precrossover results were available and results may not allow for confounding factors such as inadequate washout and the naturally variable course of Raynaud's phenomenon.[27] The RCT included people with secondary Raynaud's phenomenon, so results may not be fully applicable in people with primary Raynaud's phenomenon.

OPTION MOXISYLYTE (THYMOXAMINE)

We found no good RCTs of moxisylyte (thymoxamine).

Benefits: We found no RCTs of moxisylyte that assessed clinical outcomes.

Harms: We found no good RCTs.

Comment: None.

REFERENCES

1. Brand FN, Larson MG, Kannel WB, et al. The occurrence of Raynaud's phenomenon in a general population: the Framingham Study. *Vasc Med* 1997;2:296–301.
2. Rodriguez Garcia JL, Sabin Ruiz J. [Raynaud's phenomenon.] *Rev Clin Esp* 1989;184:311–321.
3. Riera G, Vilardell M, Vaque J, et al. Prevalence of Raynaud's phenomenon in a healthy Spanish population. *J Rheumatol* 1993;20:66–69.
4. Inaba R, Maeda M, Fujita S, et al. Prevalence of Raynaud's phenomenon and specific clinical signs related to progressive systemic sclerosis in the general population of Japan. *Int J Dermatol* 1993;32:652–655.
5. Wigley FM. Raynaud's phenomenon. *Curr Opin Rheumatol* 1993;5:773–784.
6. Smyth AE, Hughes AE, Bruce IN, et al. A case-control study of candidate vasoactive mediator genes in primary Raynaud's phenomenon. *Rheumatology (Oxford)* 1999;38:1094–1098.
7. Freedman RR, Mayes MD. Familial aggregation of primary Raynaud's disease. *Arthritis Rheum* 1996;39:1189–1191.
8. Planchon B, Pistorius Ma, Beurrier P, et al. Primary Raynaud's phenomenon. Age of onset and pathogenesis in a prospective study of 424 patients. *Angiology* 1994;45:677–686.
9. Keil JE, Maricq HR, Weinrich MC, et al. Demographic, social and clinical correlates of Raynaud phenomenon. *Int J Epidemiol* 1991;20:221–224.
10. Komura Y, Yoshida H, Nagata C, et al. [Differences in the prevalences of Raynaud's phenomenon in general; populations living in a mountain area and in a plain area.] *Nippon Koshu Eisei Zasshi* 1992;39:421–427.
11. Mirbod SM, Inaba R, Iwata H. A study on the vibration-dose limit for Japanese workers exposed to hand-arm vibration. *Ind Health* 1992;30:1–22.
12. Spencer-Green G. Outcomes in primary Raynaud phenomenon: a meta-analysis of the frequency, rates, and predictors of transition to secondary diseases. *Arch Intern Med* 1998;158:595–600. Search date 1996; primary sources Medline and hand searches of bibliographies of articles retrieved.
13. Merkel PA, Herlyn K, Martin RW, et al. Measuring disease activity and functional status in patients with scleroderma and Raynaud's phenomenon. *Arthritis Rheum* 2002;46:2410–2420.
14. Raynaud's Treatment Study Investigators. Comparison of sustained-release nifedipine and temperature biofeedback for treatment of primary Raynaud phenomenon. Results from a randomized clinical trial with 1-year follow-up. *Arch Intern Med* 2000;160:1101–1108.
15. Challenor VF, Waller DG, Hayward RA, et al. Vibrotactile sensation and response to nifedipine dose titration in primary Raynaud's phenomenon. *Angiology* 1989;40:122–128.
16. Sarkozi J, Bookman AA, Mahon W, et al. Nifedipine in the treatment of idiopathic Raynaud's syndrome. *J Rheumatol* 1986;13:331–336.
17. Corbin DO, Wood DA, Macintyre CC, et al. A randomized double blind cross-over trial of nifedipine in the treatment of primary Raynaud's phenomenon. *Eur Heart J* 1986;7:165–170.
18. Gjorup T, Kelbaek H, Hartling OJ, et al. Controlled double-blind trial of the clinical effect of nifedipine in the treatment of idiopathic Raynaud's phenomenon. *Am Heart J* 1986;111:742–745.
19. Waller DG, Challenor VF, Francis DA, et al. Clinical and rheological effects of nifedipine in Raynaud's phenomenon. *Br J Clin Pharmacol* 1986;22:449–454.
20. French Cooperative Multicenter Group for Raynaud Phenomenon. Controlled multicenter double-blind

trial of nicardipine in the treatment of primary Raynaud phenomenon. *Am Heart J* 1991;122:352–355.

21. Wollershiem H, Thien T. Double-blind placebo-controlled crossover study of oral nicardipine in the treatment of Raynaud's phenomenon. *J Cardiovasc Pharmacol* 1991;18:813–818.
22. La Civita L, Pitaro N, Rossi M, et al. Amlodipine in the treatment of Raynaud's phenomenon. A double-blind placebo-controlled crossover study. *Clin Drug Invest* 1997;13:126–131.
23. Rhedda A, McCans J, Willan AR, et al. A double blind controlled crossover randomized trial of diltiazem in Raynaud's phenomenon. *J Rheumatol* 1985;12:724–727.
24. Davinroy M, Mosnier M. Double-blind clinical-evaluation of naftidrofuryl in Raynaud's phenomenon. [French]. *Sem Hop Paris* 1993;69:1322–1326.
25. Sunderland GT, Belch JJF, Sturrock RD, et al. A double blind randomised placebo controlled trial of Hexopal in primary Raynaud's disease. *Clin Rheumatol* 1988;7:46–49.
26. Murphy R. The effect of inositol nicotinate (Hexopal) in patients with Raynaud phenomenon — a placebo-controlled study. *Clin Trials J* 1985;22:521–529.
27. Wollershiem H, Thien T, Fennis J, et al. Double-blind, placebo-controlled study of prazosin in Raynaud's phenomenon. *Clin Pharmacol Ther* 1986;40:219–225.

Janet Pope
Rheumatologist
St Joseph's Health Care
Rheumatology Centre
London, Ontario
Canada

Competing interests: None declared.

TABLE 1 RCTs comparing nifedipine versus placebo in people with primary Raynaud's phenomenon (see text, p 1446).[14–19]

Ref	Intervention	Number of people	RCT design	Time to outcome (weeks)	Results	Comment
14	Nifedipine (30 mg/day for 2 weeks, adjusted to daily, twice daily, or 0 depending on adverse effects) *v* placebo, biofeedback, or sham biofeedback for 1 year	313 people with primary Raynaud's	Parallel	56	**Frequency of attacks:** mean attacks/day 0.07 with nifedipine *v* 0.21 with placebo; $P < 0.001$ **Subjective assessment:** 51/70 (73%) people rated themselves as "improved" with nifedipine *v* 54/164 (33%) with placebo; $P < 0.001$	**Frequency:** attacks defined as the person reporting a Raynaud's episode at least 30 minutes after a previously recorded diary entry and indicating a corresponding code consistent with a true Raynaud's attack **Subjective assessment:** results not intention to treat; withdrawals not stated
15	Nifedipine (10 mg twice daily for 3 weeks, then 20 mg twice daily for 3 weeks) *v* placebo	22 people with primary Raynaud's	Crossover	6	**Frequency of attacks:** mean attacks/week 4.4 with nifedipine *v* 7.3 with placebo; $P < 0.01$ **Severity of attacks:** mean severity 1.7 with nifedipine *v* 1.9 with placebo; P reported as non-significant **Subjective assessment:** 12/22 (54%) people rated nifedipine *v* placebo as more effective; $P < 0.01$	**Severity:** measured on a scale of 1–3, where 1 represented mild, 2 moderate, and 3 severe attack **Subjective assessment:** measured on a 5 point scale
16	Nifedipine (10 mg 3 times daily increased to 20 mg 3 times daily after 5 weeks if no improvement) *v* placebo for 10 weeks	39 people with primary Raynaud's	Parallel	10	**Frequency of attacks:** mean reduction in frequency of attacks/week 48% with nifedipine *v* 25% with placebo; $P < 0.05$	No direct comparison of nifedipine *v* placebo; results are based on comparing changes in outcomes in each group before and after treatment

TABLE 1 continued

Ref	Intervention	Number of people	RCT design	Time to outcome (weeks)	Results	Comment
17	Nifedipine (5 mg 3 times daily for 1 week followed by 10 mg 3 times daily for 1 week and 15 mg 3 times daily for 2 weeks) *v* placebo	23 women with primary Raynaud's	Crossover	8	**Frequency of attacks:** median number of attacks/week in final 2 weeks of treatment after crossover 2.3 with nifedipine *v* 5.0 with placebo; $P < 0.01$	No precrossover results available*
18	Nifedipine (20 mg twice daily for 1 week followed by 40 mg twice daily for 1 week if no adverse effects, *v* placebo	26 people with primary Raynaud's	Crossover	4	**Frequency of attacks:** mean number of attacks/day after crossover: range 0–3.64 with nifedipine v 0.57–5.71 with placebo; $P < 0.01$ **Severity of attacks:** mean grade of the most severe attack: range 0–7.00 with nifedipine *v* 1.00–8.14 with placebo; $P < 0.01$	**Severity:** measured on a scale of 0–10 where 0 represented minimum and 10 maximum severity. No precrossover results available*
19	Nifedipine (20 mg twice daily for 8 weeks) *v* placebo (2 weeks washout between each 4 weeks of treatment)	34 people; 28 with primary Raynaud's	Crossover	12	**Frequency of attacks:** mean number of attacks/week after crossover 7.5 with nifedipine *v* 10.0 with placebo; $P < 0.001$ **Subjective assessment:** 20/29 (69%) rated nifedipine *v* placebo as more effective; $P < 0.001$	**Subjective assessment:** measured on a 5 point scale. No precrossover results available.* Included people with secondary Raynaud's phenomenon, so results may not be fully applicable in people with primary Raynaud's phenomenon

*Results after crossover may not allow for confounding factors such as inadequate washout and the naturally variable course of Raynaud's phenomenon.

Rheumatoid arthritis

Search date July 2002

Paul Emery and Maria Suarez-Almazor

QUESTIONS

INTERVENTIONS

See glossary, p 1473

Key Messages

- **Antimalarials** One systematic review has found that hydroxychloroquine reduces disease activity and joint inflammation compared with placebo in people with rheumatoid arthritis. We found insufficient evidence about effects on functional status. One systematic review found no consistent difference in effectiveness between antimalarials and other disease modifying antirheumatic drugs.
- **Auranofin (less effective than other disease modifying antirheumatic drugs)** One systematic review has found that auranofin (oral gold) versus placebo reduces disease activity and joint inflammation, but found no evidence on radiological progression or long term functional status. Limited evidence from RCTs suggests that auranofin is less effective than disease modifying antirheumatic drugs.
- **Azathioprine** One systematic review has found that azathioprine versus placebo reduces disease activity in the short term (16 weeks to 6 months). We found no evidence on radiological progression or long term functional status. A high level of toxicity limits the usefulness of azathioprine.

- **Ciclosporin** One systematic review has found that ciclosporin for a minimum of 4 months significantly reduces disease activity and joint inflammation, improves functional status, and may decrease the rate of radiological progression compared with methotrexate. One RCT found no significant difference between ciclosporin and parenteral gold for radiological joint damage or self assessment of change in disease activity at 36 months. A high frequency of toxicity limits the usefulness of ciclosporin.
- **Cyclophosphamide** One systematic review has found that cyclophosphamide significantly reduces disease activity and joint inflammation compared with placebo at 6 months. It may also reduce the rate of radiological progression, but evidence was limited. We found no evidence of its effect on long term functional status. Severe toxicity limits the usefulness of ciclosporin.
- **Early intervention with disease modifying antirheumatic drugs** One systematic review and one additional RCT found that introducing disease modifying antirheumatic drugs early (oral gold, intramuscular gold, hydroxychloroquine, methotrexate, minocycline) significantly improved radiological progression, swollen joint counts, and quality of life scores at 12–60 months compared with delayed treatment.
- **Leflunomide (long term safety unclear)** One systematic review has found that leflunomide versus placebo reduces disease activity and joint inflammation, improves functional status and health related quality of life, and decreases radiological progression. We found no good evidence on long term adverse effects. We found no consistent evidence of a difference in clinical efficacy between leflunomide and methotrexate or sulfasalazine.
- **Long term low dose oral corticosteroids** One systematic review and one subsequent RCT have found that low dose oral corticosteroids for at least 3 months significantly reduces pain, joint inflammation, and functional status compared with placebo. However, long term use is associated with considerable adverse effects.
- **Methotrexate** One systematic review has found that methotrexate reduces joint inflammation and radiological progression and improves functional status compared with placebo in people with rheumatoid arthritis. One systematic review and subsequent RCTs have found no consistent differences in efficacy between methotrexate versus leflunomide, parenteral gold, or etanercept.
- **Minocycline** RCTs have found that minocycline improves control of disease activity compared with placebo. We found no RCTs comparing minocycline versus other disease modifying antirheumatic drugs.
- **Parenteral gold** One systematic review has found that parenteral gold reduces disease activity and joint inflammation, and slows radiological progression compared with placebo in people with rheumatoid arthritis. We found no evidence on long term functional status. One systematic review and one RCT both indicate increased withdrawals because of toxicity. RCTs found no significant differences in clinical efficacy between parenteral gold versus methotrexate or ciclosporin at 1–3 years.
- **Penicillamine** One systematic review has found that penicillamine reduces disease activity and joint inflammation compared with placebo at 4–6 months. We found no evidence about effects of penicillamine on radiological progression or long term functional status. One systematic review has found no consistent difference between penicillamine versus other disease modifying antirheumatic drugs. Common and potentially serious adverse effects limit the usefulness of penicillamine.

Rheumatoid arthritis

- **Short term low dose oral corticosteroids** One systematic review has found that low dose oral corticosteroids for several weeks significantly reduces disease activity and joint inflammation compared with placebo.
- **Sulfasalazine** Systematic reviews have found that sulfasalazine versus placebo for 6 months significantly reduces disease activity and joint inflammation. We found inadequate evidence about effects on radiological progression and functional status. One systematic review found no consistent differences between sulfasalazine and other disease modifying antirheumatic drugs. Another systematic review of observational studies and RCTs found that over 5 years people were less likely to continue sulfasalazine than methotrexate.
- **Treatment with several disease modifying antirheumatic drugs combined** One systematic review and subsequent RCTs have found that combining certain disease modifying antirheumatic drugs is more effective than using individual drugs alone. However, the balance between benefit and harm varies among combinations.
- **Tumour necrosis factor antagonists (long term safety unclear)** RCTs have found that tumour necrosis factor antibodies (etanercept and infliximab) significantly improve symptoms, and reduce long term disease activity and joint inflammation compared with placebo. One RCT found no significant difference between etanercept and methotrexate for quality of life at 1 year. Short term toxicity is relatively low, but long term safety is less clear.

DEFINITION Rheumatoid arthritis is a chronic inflammatory disorder. It is characterised by a chronic polyarthritis that primarily affects the peripheral joints and related periarticular tissues. It usually starts as an insidious symmetric polyarthritis, often with non-specific systemic symptoms. Diagnostic criteria include arthritis lasting longer than 6 weeks (although evidence suggests that 12 wks is more specific), positive rheumatoid factor, and radiological damage.[1]

INCIDENCE/ PREVALENCE Prevalence ranges from 0.5–1.5% of the population in industrialised countries.[2,3] Rheumatoid arthritis occurs more frequently in women than men (ratio 2.5 : 1).[2,3] The annual incidence in women was recently estimated at 36/100 000 and in men at 14/100 000.[3]

AETIOLOGY/ RISK FACTORS The evidence suggests that the cause is multifactorial in people with genetic susceptibility.[4]

PROGNOSIS The course of rheumatoid arthritis is variable and unpredictable. Some people experience flares and remissions, and others a progressive course. Over the years, structural damage occurs, leading to articular deformities and functional impairment. About half of people will be unable to work within 10 years.[5] Rheumatoid arthritis shortens life expectancy.[6]

AIMS OF INTERVENTION To relieve symptoms; to improve physical function and slow/arrest progression of structural damage, resulting in improvement in quality of life; to minimise adverse effects of treatment.

OUTCOMES It is now a standard procedure to use composite outcome measures that include subjective and objective measures as well as functional measures. The American College of Rheumatology (ACR) has validated criteria for improvement. ACR20 criteria specify a 20% reduction in swollen and tender joints and 20% improvement in at least three of the following: pain, function, patient and physician global assessments, and acute phase reactants. ACR50 criteria uses a 50% and ACR70 criteria use a 70% improvement in the same parameters. RCTs of many new treatments, such as biological agents, use these aggregate indices as primary end points.[7] However, these are relative improvements and give no indication of the final state of the person. Consequently, in clinical practice the disease activity score is used more commonly. This uses similar measures but yields an absolute level of disease activity. A high level of disease activity indicates a need for treatment and low levels indicate a remission. Radiological progression is assessed in many RCTs by reference to standardised radiographs. Two scores are commonly used: the Sharp Score (see glossary, p 1473), which measures erosion and joint space narrowing separately; and the Larsen score. The Sharp Score is increasingly used because of its greater sensitivity to change. Most reviews reported results as standardised mean differences, but these have not been included because of difficulties in interpreting clinical relevance. Many small trials that found no significant difference between drugs may have lacked power to detect clinically important differences.

METHODS *Clinical Evidence* search and appraisal July 2002.

QUESTION **What are the effects of disease modifying antirheumatic drugs?**

OPTION **METHOTREXATE**

One systematic review has found that methotrexate is more effective than placebo in reducing joint inflammation and radiological progression, and in improving functional status in people with rheumatoid arthritis. One systematic review and subsequent RCTs have found no consistent differences in efficacy between methotrexate versus leflunomide, parenteral gold, or etanercept.

Benefits: **Versus placebo:** We found one systematic review (search date 1997, 5 RCTs, 321 people enrolled, 219 analysed) of low dose methotrexate for 12–18 weeks (usually < 20 mg/wk) versus placebo.[8] It found a significant improvement for methotrexate versus placebo in the number of swollen and tender joints, pain score, physician and patient global assessment, and functional status (all results presented as standardised weighted differences; significant heterogeneity was found for all outcomes except tender or swollen joint counts).[8] We found two subsequent RCTs of methotrexate versus leflunomide versus placebo, which found similar results.[9,10]

Versus other disease modifying antirheumatic drugs: We found one systematic review (search date 1990, 9 methotrexate treatment arms with 274 people)[11] of comparative RCTs and four subsequent RCTs.[9,10–13] The review found no consistent difference in effectiveness between methotrexate and other disease modifying antirheumatic drugs (antimalarials, auranofin, injectable gold, D-penicillamine, sulfasalazine, and azathioprine) using efficacy/toxicity trade-off plots but did not compare efficacy within RCTs directly. The first subsequent RCT (483 people) found that methotrexate was not significantly different from leflunomide over 1 year (see benefits of leflunomide, p 1466).[9] The second large subsequent RCT (999 people) found that leflunomide improved outcomes less than methotrexate (see benefits of leflunomide, p 1466).[10] The third subsequent RCT (141 people from a socially deprived Scottish community) found no significant difference between low dose methotrexate (median weekly dose 10 mg) versus parenteral gold over 48 weeks (see benefits of parenteral gold, p 1461).[12] The fourth subsequent RCT (174 people with active erosive disease > 4 months) found no significant difference between parenteral gold and intramuscular methotrexate for radiographic scores and number of erosive joints, but did not report any clinical outcomes.[13]

Harms: One systematic review (search date 1997, 5 RCTs, 161 people) of methotrexate versus placebo found that more people on methotrexate withdrew because of adverse effects (22% with methotrexate *v* 7% with placebo).[8] The adverse effects were mainly liver enzyme abnormalities (AR for liver abnormalities: 11% with methotrexate *v* 2.6% with placebo; ARI 9%; RR 4.5, 95% CI 1.6 to 11.0; NNH 11, 95% CI 4 to 65). Other common adverse effects were mucocutaneous, gastrointestinal, or haematological complaints. A systematic review of pancytopenia identified 99 cases, with risk factors being renal failure and co-administration of trimethoprim–sulfamethoxazole (sulphamethoxazole) and salazosulphapyridine. Pulmonary toxicity, hepatic fibrosis, and infections occur occasionally, even at the low dosages usually used in rheumatoid arthritis. Another systematic review (search date 1996) found that concurrent administration of folic acid decreased the risk of gastrointestinal and mucocutaneous adverse effects (AR 51% with folic acid *v* 83% without folic acid; ARR 33%, 95% CI 14% to 51%; NNT 3, 95% CI 2 to 7) with no adverse impact on the efficacy of methotrexate.[14] Although some studies reported an increased risk of tumours with methotrexate, results have not been consistent.[15] One systematic review (search date 1997) of observational studies and RCTs compared withdrawal rates over 60 months.[16] It found that methotrexate was associated with a higher rate of staying on treatment (36%) versus sulfasalazine (22%) and versus parenteral gold (23%). It found the lowest rate of withdrawals because of adverse effects with methotrexate (35%) versus parenteral gold (64%) and versus sulfasalazine (52%). It found no significant difference in withdrawal rates between observational studies and RCTs over 24 months. The subsequent RCT (141 people) of parenteral gold versus low dose methotrexate found that significantly more people withdrew because of adverse effects with gold (31/72 [43%] with parenteral gold *v* 13/69 [19%] with methotrexate; RR 2.3, 95% CI 1.3 to 4.0).[12]

Comment: One systematic review (search date 1991) of observational studies comparing effects of methotrexate versus other disease modifying antirheumatic drugs on radiological progression found a significant benefit from methotrexate only when compared with azathioprine (P = 0.049; CI not provided).[17] It found no significant difference between methotrexate and parenteral gold (results not provided). Systematic reviews included in previous *Clinical Evidence* updates have been removed because they were eclipsed by more recent or reliable reviews, because they did not directly answer our question, or because they were only available in abstract form.[18–20]

OPTION ANTIMALARIALS

One systematic review has found that hydroxychloroquine versus placebo reduces disease activity and joint inflammation in people with rheumatoid arthritis. We found insufficient evidence about effects on functional status. One systematic review found no consistent difference in effectiveness between antimalarials and other disease modifying antirheumatic drugs.

Benefits: **Versus placebo:** We found one systematic review (search date 2000, 4 RCTs of hydroxychloroquine given for 6–12 months, 592 people).[21] It found a significant improvement for hydroxychloroquine versus placebo in the number of swollen and tender joints, pain score, physician and patient global assessment (results presented as standardised weighted differences; no significant heterogeneity was found for any outcome). One RCT (119 people) assessed functional status and found no significant difference for hydroxychloroquine versus placebo. **Versus other disease modifying antirheumatic drugs:** We found one systematic review (search date 1990, 11 antimalarial treatment arms with 314 people).[11] It found no significant difference between antimalarials and other disease modifying antirheumatic drugs (methotrexate, auranofin, injectable gold, D-penicillamine, sulfasalazine, and azathioprine) using efficacy/toxicity trade off plots but did not compare efficacy within RCTs directly. Individual RCTs found no consistent advantage for any one drug, although some found better results with penicillamine and sulfasalazine than with antimalarials. **Hydroxychloroquine versus chloroquine:** We found no RCTs that compared chloroquine versus hydroxychloroquine adequately. One older RCT included both drugs but did not report a direct comparison.[22]

Harms: The systematic review (search date 1997, 4 placebo controlled RCTs) found no significant difference in the number of withdrawals because of adverse effects.[21] **Ocular toxicity:** No participants discontinued treatment because of ocular adverse effects, and mild toxicity was reported in only one person.[21] One long term retrospective observational study (97 people) found that more people receiving chloroquine alone versus hydroxychloroquine developed retinopathy (6/31 [19.4%] with chloroquine *v* 0/66 [0%] with hydroxychloroquine).[23] We found no good evidence on the optimal frequency for eye examinations; expert opinion ranges from every 6 months to 2 years. **Non-ocular adverse effects:** One RCT found that the most common non-ocular adverse effects were gastrointestinal disturbances, occurring in about 25% of people.[24] Skin reactions and renal abnormalities occur occasionally. Mild neurological abnormalities include non-specific symptoms such as vertigo and blurred vision. Cardiomyopathy and severe neurological disease are extremely rare. **Withdrawals:** One systematic review (search date 1997) of RCTs and observational studies found that over 2 years people with rheumatoid arthritis were more likely to continue on methotrexate than on antimalarials, but were more likely to continue on antimalarials than on parenteral gold or sulfasalazine.[16] Most people discontinued treatment because of lack of efficacy. One 5 year RCT (541 people) compared hydroxychloroquine versus penicillamine versus parenteral gold versus auranofin.[25] It found that at 5 years, a significantly greater proportion of people continued to take penicillamine (53%) than hydroxychloroquine (30%), although similar proportions continued parenteral gold (34%) and auranofin (31%).

Comment: Older RCTs of chloroquine versus placebo (not included in the systematic review because of weak methods) found a beneficial effect.

OPTION SULFASALAZINE

Systematic reviews have found that sulfasalazine is more effective than placebo in reducing disease activity and joint inflammation. We found inadequate evidence on radiological progression and functional status. One systematic review found no consistent difference in effectiveness between sulfasalazine and other disease modifying antirheumatic drugs. Another systematic review of observational studies and RCTs found that over 5 years people were less likely to continue sulfasalazine than methotrexate.

Benefits: **Versus placebo:** We found one systematic review[26] and one subsequent RCT.[27] The review (search date 1998, 8 RCTs, 903 people) of sulfasalazine versus placebo found better results with sulfasalazine on all outcome measures (decrease in number of swollen joints: 51% with sulfasalazine *v* 26% with placebo; $P < 0.0001$; CI not provided).[26] The subsequent RCT found that sulfasalazine (133 people) versus placebo (92 people) significantly improved patient and physician global assessment ($P < 0.001$).[27]
Versus other disease modifying antirheumatic drugs: We found one systematic review (search date 1998, 2 RCTs, 120 people)[26] and three additional RCTs[27–29] of sulfasalazine versus other disease modifying antirheumatic drugs. The systematic review found no significant difference between sulfasalazine versus hydroxychloroquine in number of swollen joints (improvement 37% with sulfasalazine *v* 28% with hydroxychloroquine; $P = 0.38$; CI not provided) or erythrocyte sedimentation rate (decreased by 43% with sulfasalazine *v* 26% with hydroxychloroquine; $P = 0.10$). One additional RCT (60 people) comparing sulfasalazine versus hydroxychloroquine found that sulfasalazine was significantly better in controlling radiological damage, although progression occurred with both drugs (median erosion scores at wk 48: 16 with hydroxychloroquine *v* 5 with sulfasalazine; $P < 0.02$; CI not provided).[28] However, hydroxychloroquine was given at a lower dose than is usually recommended. One subsequent RCT (358 people over 24 wks) of sulfasalazine versus leflunomide versus placebo found no significant difference between sulfasalazine and leflunomide in tender joint count, swollen joint count, or pain (on a visual analogue scale, see benefits of leflunomide, p 1466).[27] One RCT (200 people) comparing sulfasalazine versus penicillamine found significantly better functional status with sulfasalazine after 12 years.[29] However, differences were small, and many people had changed treatment or died during the 12 years.

Harms: Common adverse effects included gastrointestinal discomfort, rash, and liver enzyme abnormalities.[30] More serious haematological or hepatic toxicity was uncommon. Reversible leucopenia or agranulocytosis was observed occasionally. Treatment was discontinued for adverse effects less often than with other disease modifying antirheumatic drugs, with the exception of antimalarials. One systematic review (search date 1997) found that the proportion of people who remained on the same treatment over 5 years was lower with sulfasalazine than with methotrexate, but was the same as with parenteral gold.[16] More people withdrew because of adverse effects with parenteral gold than with sulfasalazine but less withdrew with methotrexate.

Comment: None.

OPTION PARENTERAL GOLD

One systematic review has found that parenteral gold versus placebo reduces disease activity and joint inflammation, and slows radiological progression in people with rheumatoid arthritis. We found no evidence on long term functional status. One systematic review and an RCT both indicate increased withdrawals because of toxicity. RCTs found no significant differences in clinical efficacy between parenteral gold versus methotrexate or ciclosporin at 1–3 years.

Benefits: **Versus placebo:** We found one systematic review (search date 1997, 4 RCTs, 415 people) of parenteral gold for 6 months versus placebo.[31] It found significant improvement in the number of swollen joints, patient and physician global assessments, and erythrocyte sedimentation rate (outcomes reported as effect size differences; $P < 0.05$ for all outcomes, CI not provided). Functional status was not evaluated. **Versus other disease modifying antirheumatic drugs:** We found one systematic review (search date 1990, 28 gold treatment arms with 648 people)[27] and two subsequent RCTs.[12,32] The review found no consistent differences between parenteral gold and other disease modifying antirheumatic drugs (antimalarials, methotrexate, auranofin, D-penicillamine, sulfasalazine, azathioprine) using efficacy/toxicity trade-off plots but did not directly compare efficacy within RCTs. The first subsequent RCT (141 people) found no significant difference between parenteral gold versus methotrexate in modified Paulus 50% response, disease inactivation rates, Health Assessment Questionnaire score, or global wellbeing at 48 weeks (modified Paulus 50% response 8/72 [11%] with parenteral gold *v* 15/69 [22%] with methotrexate, $P = 0.069$; disease inactivation rates 18% with parenteral gold *v* 6% with methotrexate, P not provided; Health Assessment Questionnaire score 1.9 for both treatments; global wellbeing "good" or "very good" 24% for both groups).[13] The second subsequent RCT (278 people with early active and severe rheumatoid arthritis) found no significant difference for parenteral gold versus ciclosporin in radiological joint damage or self assessment of change in disease activity at 36 months (change from baseline using Larsen Dale joint damage score 13.9 with parenteral gold *v* 15.5 with ciclosporin, $P = 0.52$; proportion considering disease much better 49% with parenteral gold *v* 55% with ciclosporin, P not provided).[32]

Harms: The systematic review (search date 1997, 4 RCTs, 309 people) of parenteral gold versus placebo found that more people receiving parenteral gold discontinued treatment because of adverse effects, including dermatitis, stomatitis, proteinuria, and haematological changes (withdrawals because of adverse events with parenteral gold 66/223 [30%] *v* with placebo 29/192 [15%]; RR 1.9; 95% CI 1.3 to 2.8).[31] Life threatening reactions such as aplastic anaemia, although rare, necessitate close monitoring. The subsequent RCT found that more people withdrew with parenteral gold because of toxicity (43% with parenteral gold *v* 19% with methotrexate).[12] One systematic review (search date 1997) found that the proportion of people who remained on the same treatment rates over 5 years were lower with sulfasalazine than with methotrexate but the same as with parenteral gold.[16] More people withdrew because of adverse effects on parenteral gold than with sulfasalazine or methotrexate (see harms of methotrexate, p 1458). One RCT found fewer serious adverse effects with gold versus ciclosporin (5/76 [6%] with parenteral gold *v* 12/84 [14%] with ciclosporin, P not provided).[32]

Comment: Use of parenteral gold is limited mainly by toxicity but also by the need for parental administration/frequent toxicity monitoring.

OPTION AURANOFIN (ORAL GOLD)

One systematic review has found that auranofin (oral gold) versus placebo reduces disease activity and joint inflammation, but found no evidence on radiological progression or long term functional status. Limited evidence from RCTs suggests that auranofin is less effective than other disease modifying antirheumatic drugs.

Benefits: **Versus placebo:** We found one systematic review (search dates 1998, 9 RCTs, 1049 people).[33] It found significantly better results with auranofin for tender joints, swollen joint scores, pain (improved by 4.68, scale 0–100), and erythrocyte sedimentation rate (fell by 9.9 mm). **Versus other disease modifying antirheumatic drugs:** We found one systematic review (search date 1990, 26 auranofin treatment arms with 1500 people)[11] and one subsequent RCT.[34] The review found that auranofin was significantly less effective than other disease modifying antirheumatic drugs (antimalarials, methotrexate, D-penicillamine, sulfasalazine, azathioprine) using efficacy/toxicity trade-off plots but did not compare efficacy within RCTs directly.[11] One subsequent RCT (200 people) of auranofin versus sulfasalazine found that people were more than twice as likely to continue with sulfasalazine than with auranofin (people continuing treatment over 5 years: 31% with sulfasalazine *v* 15% with auranofin; $P < 0.05$; CI not provided).[34]

Harms: The review found that the most common adverse effects of auranofin were gastrointestinal (OR compared with placebo 3.0, 95% CI 1.4 to 6.5), particularly diarrhoea (OR 3.0, 95% CI 1.3 to 7.1).[33] It found that withdrawals because of haematological or renal effects were rare (1% each). A review of adverse effects found that serious adverse effects, such as those associated with parenteral gold, were rare with auranofin (participants developing serious organ specific toxicity < 0.5%; blood 0.2%, renal 0.1%, lung 0.1%, and hepatic 0.4%).[35]

Comment: The lack of good comparative efficacy results means that auranofin is now used rarely.

OPTION MINOCYCLINE

Three RCTs have found that minocycline versus placebo improves control of disease activity in people with rheumatoid arthritis. We found no RCTs versus other disease modifying antirheumatic drugs.

Benefits: **Versus placebo:** We found no systematic review. We found three RCTs of minocycline versus placebo.[36–38] They found that minocycline improved control of disease activity. The largest RCT (219 people) compared minocycline versus placebo over 48 weeks.[36] It found that a greater proportion of people had improvement in swollen joints (54% with minocycline *v* 39% with placebo; P < 0.03; CI not provided) and joint tenderness (56% with minocycline *v* 41% with placebo; P < 0.03; CI not provided). The second RCT (80 people) compared minocycline versus placebo over 24 weeks.[37] It found a significant improvement on a multivariate joint analysis of clinical and laboratory outcomes (P < 0.05; CI not provided). The third RCT found that minocycline versus placebo at least halved the proportion of people who did not improve (3/23 [13%] with minocycline *v* 11/20 [55%] with placebo; ARR 42%, 95% CI 15% to 52%; RR 0.24, 95% CI 0.06 to 0.73; NNT 2, 95% CI 2 to 7).[38] **Versus other disease modifying antirheumatic drugs:** We found no RCTs.

Harms: The largest RCT reported adverse reactions including nausea (AR at 26 wks 50% with minocycline *v* 13% with placebo), dyspepsia, dizziness (AR 40% with minocycline *v* 15% with placebo), and skin pigmentation.[36] Other important but less frequent reactions include hepatitis and drug induced systemic lupus erythematosus.

Comment: The magnitude of the beneficial effects of minocycline seems moderate, and similar to that observed with antimalarials or sulfasalazine. However, we found no direct comparisons with other disease modifying antirheumatic drugs.

OPTION PENICILLAMINE

One systematic review has found that penicillamine versus placebo reduces disease activity and joint inflammation at 4–6 months. We found no evidence of its effect on radiological progression or long term functional status. One systematic review has found no consistent difference between penicillamine versus other disease modifying antirheumatic drugs. Common and potentially serious adverse effects limit its usefulness.

Benefits: **Versus placebo:** We found one systematic review (search date 2000, 6 RCTs, 683 people).[39] It found that moderate (500–1000 mg/day) and high (≥ 1000 mg/day) dose penicillamine versus placebo significantly reduced the number of swollen joints and erythrocyte sedimentation rate and improved the global physician score at 4–6 months (results presented as pooled effect sizes). **Versus other disease modifying antirheumatic drugs:** We found one systematic review (search date 1990, 79 RCTs, 6518 people, 22 treatment arms using penicillamine, 583 people completing the trials).[11] It found no consistent differences in effectiveness between penicillamine and other drugs, although some trials found penicillamine to be superior to antimalarials.

Harms: Adverse effects were common and sometimes serious. Reactions included mucocutaneous reactions, altered taste, gastrointestinal reactions, proteinuria, haematological effects, myositis, and autoimmune induced disease. The most frequent adverse effects responsible for D-penicillamine discontinuation were (all doses combined) haematological: 6.6%; mucosal/cutaneous: 4.9%, impaired/loss of taste 4.7%; renal: 4.1%; and gastrointestinal: 2.3%. The review reported more withdrawals because of adverse reactions with low dose penicillamine (10/87 [11.5%] with penicillamine 125–500 mg/day *v* 3/52 [5.8%] with placebo; RR 2.0, 95% CI 0.6 to 6.9), with medium dose penicillamine (46/220 [20.1%] penicillamine 500–1000 mg/day *v* 17/195 [8.7%] with placebo; RR 2.4, 95% CI 1.4 to 4.1), and with high dose penicillamine (29/118 [24.6%] with penicillamine ≥ 1000 mg/day *v* 6/117 [5.1%] with placebo; RR 4.5, 95% CI 2.0 to 10.0).[39]

Comment: The use of penicillamine is limited by the frequency of serious adverse effects. Observational studies found that most people discontinued the drug within the first 2 years of treatment.[40–43] Use of this drug is declining.

OPTION AZATHIOPRINE

One systematic review has found that azathioprine versus placebo reduces disease activity at 16 weeks to 6 months. We found no evidence on radiological progression or long term functional status. We found no evidence that it is superior to other disease modifying antirheumatic drugs. A high level of toxicity limits its usefulness.

Benefits: **Versus placebo:** We found one systematic review (search date 2000, 3 RCTs, 81 people).[44] It found that azathioprine versus placebo significantly improved the tender joint score at 16 weeks to 6 months (results presented as weighted mean difference). No other outcome was reported by all trials. **Versus other drug modifying antirheumatic drugs:** We found two systematic reviews (search dates 1990[11] and 1988[19]). They found limited evidence that azathioprine had less effect than most other disease modifying antirheumatic drugs, but about the same as that of antimalarials.

Harms: The review found that people on azathioprine were significantly more likely to withdraw than were those on placebo (RR 4.6, 95% CI 1.2 to 17.9).[44] The most common adverse reactions were gastrointestinal (5/34 [15%] with azathioprine *v* 0/30 [0%] with placebo; RR 5.3, 95% CI 0.7 to 42.0), mucocutaneous (4/15 [26%] with azathioprine *v* 1/13 [7.7%] with placebo; RR 3.5, 95% CI 0.4 to 27), and haematological disturbances (3/34 [9%] with azathioprine *v* 0/30 [0%] with placebo; RR 3.5, 95% CI 0.4 to 30.0). Serious haematological adverse reactions included leucopenia. The review reported that longer term observational studies found that azathioprine was associated with increased risk of liver function abnormalities, infection, and cancer (quantified results not provided).

Comment: Because of its toxicity profile, azathioprine tends to be reserved for people who have not responded to other disease modifying antirheumatic drugs.

OPTION CYCLOPHOSPHAMIDE

One systematic review has found that cyclophosphamide is more effective than placebo in reducing disease activity and joint inflammation in people with rheumatoid arthritis. We found limited evidence that it reduced the rate of radiological progression. We found no evidence of its effect on long term functional status. Severe toxicity limits its usefulness.

Benefits: **Versus placebo:** We found one systematic review (search date 2000, 2 RCTs of cyclophosphamide given for 6 months, 70 people).[45] Meta-analysis found significant reduction in number of tender and swollen joints versus placebo. One RCT reported radiological progression, which seemed to be delayed in the cyclophosphamide group. We found no evidence of its effect on functional status.

Harms: The review reported adverse effects including nausea or vomiting (58%), alopecia (26%), dysuria (26%), and amenorrhoea (comparative figures not provided).[45] Severe reactions include leucopenia, thrombocytopenia, anaemia, and haemorrhagic cystitis. People on cyclophosphamide were at increased risk of infections such as herpes zoster. One long term (20 years) observational study reported that prolonged use has been associated with increased risk of cancer, in particular bladder cancer.[46]

Comment: Because of its cytotoxic effects, cyclophosphamide is usually reserved for people who have not responded to other disease modifying antirheumatic drugs. Another related drug, chlorambucil, has also been used in people with severe rheumatoid arthritis that is unresponsive to other disease modifying antirheumatic drugs.

OPTION CICLOSPORIN

One systematic review has found that, compared with methotrexate, ciclosporin reduces disease activity and joint inflammation, improves functional status, and may decrease the rate of radiological progression. A high frequency of toxicity limits its usefulness. One RCT found no significant difference between ciclosporin versus parenteral gold for radiological joint damage or self assessment of change in disease activity at 36 months.

Benefits: **Versus placebo:** We found one systematic review (search date 1997, 3 RCTs of ciclosporin [cyclosporin] given for a minimum of 4 months, 318 people).[47] It found significant improvement in the number of tender and swollen joints, and in pain and functional status. It found limited evidence that radiological progression was also reduced. **Versus parenteral gold**: See benefits of parenteral gold, p 1461.

Harms: The review reported that ciclosporin was associated with adverse effects including gum hyperplasia (9/98 [9.1%] with ciclosporin *v* 0/98 [0%] with placebo; RR 10, 95% CI 1.3 to 77.0), paraesthesia (22/159 [13.8%] with ciclosporin *v* 10/159 [6.3%] with placebo; RR 2.2, 95% CI 1.1 to 4.5), nausea (41/159 [25.8%] with ciclosporin *v* 22/159 [13.8%] with placebo; RR 1.9, 95% CI 1.2 to 3.0), headache (10/61 [16.4%] with ciclosporin *v* 3/61 [4.9%] with placebo; RR 3.30, 95% CI 0.96 to 11.50), and tremor (41/133 [30.8%] with ciclosporin *v* 8/133 [6.0%] with placebo; RR 5.1, 95% CI 2.5 to 10.5).[47] **Renal toxicity:** People may develop nephropathy, which can be irreversible, and hypertension. One RCT found that ciclosporin reduced renal function after 36 months (creatinine clearance reduced by 16% from baseline).[32] Three months after ciclosporin was stopped, renal function remained reduced (creatinine clearance continued to be 16% below baseline). **Other adverse reactions:** Dyspepsia, hypertrichosis, gingival hyperplasia, and hepatotoxicity. It has been suggested that ciclosporin may be associated with increased risk of infections and tumours.

Comment: Ciclosporin is usually reserved for people with severe disease or those who do not respond to other less toxic disease modifying antirheumatic drugs.

OPTION LEFLUNOMIDE

One systematic review has found that leflunomide versus placebo reduces disease activity and joint inflammation, improves functional status and health related quality of life, and decreases radiological progression. We found no good evidence on long term adverse effects. We found no consistent evidence of a difference in clinical efficacy between leflunomide and methotrexate or sulfasalazine.

Benefits: **Versus placebo:** We found one systematic review (search date 1999, 3 RCTs, 1242 people) of leflunomide versus placebo.[48] It found that leflunomide improved quality of life and radiological progression. The first RCT (402 people with active rheumatoid disease) compared leflunomide (5, 10, or 25 mg/day) versus placebo.[49] Leflunomide (10 and 25 mg/day) was significantly more effective than placebo in reducing the number of swollen joints (–20 with leflunomide 10 mg *v* –20 with leflunomide 25 mg *v* –13 with placebo; P < 0.05; CI not provided). The second RCT (358 people) compared leflunomide versus placebo versus sulfasalazine.[27] It found a significant reduction at 6 months in the number of swollen joints with versus placebo (44% with leflunomide *v* 21% with placebo; P < 0.0001; CI not provided). The third RCT (482 people) compared leflunomide versus methotrexate versus placebo over 24 months.[50,51] Because of the high withdrawal rate with placebo, only

12 month comparison with placebo was reported. It found that 20% improvement (ACR20 criteria) was achieved by 52% with leflunomide versus 26% with placebo; ACR50 response criteria were achieved by 34% with leflunomide, 23% with methotrexate, and 8% with placebo ($P \leq 0.001$; CI not provided). Radiological progression was reduced in people receiving leflunomide compared with placebo. It found significant improvements in the quality of life with leflunomide.[51] **Versus other disease modifying antirheumatic drugs:** We found three RCTs.[9,10,27] One RCT (266 people) found no significant difference for leflunomide versus sulfasalazine in the proportion of people achieving ACR20 criteria at 24 weeks (71/133 [55%] for leflunomide *v* 74/133 [56%] for sulfasalazine).[27] A second RCT (483 people) compared methotrexate versus leflunomide versus placebo.[9] It found no significant difference between methotrexate and leflunomide at 1 year (ACR ≥ 20%: 52% with leflunomide *v* 46% with methotrexate; P and CI not provided) or at 2 years. The third RCT (999 people) comparing leflunomide versus methotrexate found that at 1 year, leflunomide was significantly less effective than methotrexate in reducing the numbers of tender joints (reduction 9.7 with methotrexate *v* 8.3 with leflunomide), swollen joints (reduction 9.0 with methotrexate *v* 6.8 with leflunomide) and improving patient and physician global assessments ($P < 0.05$ for all outcomes).[10] At 2 years, radiological disease progression was significantly less with methotrexate, but there was no significant difference in tender joint count and patient global assessment.

Harms: In one of the RCTs (358 people), adverse effects included diarrhoea (17% with leflunomide *v* 5% with placebo), nausea (10% with leflunomide *v* 7% with placebo), rash (10% with leflunomide *v* 4% with placebo), alopecia (8% with leflunomide *v* 2% with placebo), and liver enzyme abnormalities (2% with leflunomide *v* 1% with placebo); significance was not reported.[27] In the second RCT adverse events included diarrhoea (34% with leflunomide *v* 17% with placebo), nausea (21% with leflunomide *v* 19% with placebo), alopecia (10% with leflunomide *v* 1% with placebo), and hypertension (11% with leflunomide *v* 5% with placebo).[9] Adverse reactions were observed more frequently in the study comparing leflunomide with methotrexate, but the rate of serious adverse events was similar for all three groups (methotrexate, leflunomide, and placebo).[9] We found no evidence on long term adverse effects.

Comment: Leflunomide is a new drug, which seems to be as effective as other disease modifying antirheumatic drugs over 12 months but with different adverse events. Longer term observational studies are being performed.

QUESTION **What are the effects of combining disease modifying antirheumatic drugs?**

One systematic review and subsequent RCTs have found that combining certain disease modifying antirheumatic drugs is more effective than using individual drugs alone. However, the balance between benefits and harm varies among combinations.

Benefits: We found one systematic review (search date 1997, 20 RCTs, 1956 people),[52] eight subsequent RCTs,[53–60] and one long term follow up of one of these RCTs.[61] The review concluded that many combinations of disease modifying antirheumatic drugs (DMARDs) may be useful. Some RCTs included in the systematic review did not find significant differences between combinations of different agents and monotherapy.[52] Nine of the RCTs (1240 people) compared methotrexate plus another DMARD versus methotrexate or the other DMARD alone. A wide range of other DMARDs was included. The review found that methotrexate combined with most other DMARDs was more beneficial than treatment with a single drug.[52] The subsequent RCTs found that combinations of different agents (antimalarials, sulfasalazine, methotrexate, ciclosporin, steroids) have a greater beneficial effect than monotherapy.[53–58,61] Five year follow up of one of the RCTs found that combination DMARD treatment significantly improved Sharp Damage Score (see glossary, p 1473) compared with sulfasalazine alone after 56 weeks of treatment (difference in score 3.0, 95% CI 0.2 to 5.8, P = 0.03).[54,61] However, it found no significant difference for functional ability (change in Health Assessment Questionnaire score 0, 95% CI –0.04 to +0.04). The seventh RCT (195 people with rheumatoid arthritis for < 2 years) found that a combination of DMARDs (sulfasalazine, methotrexate, hydroxychloroquine) plus prednisolone versus single DMARD (initially sulfasalazine 500 mg twice daily) with or without low dose prednisolone significantly increased remission rates at 2 years (165 people analysed; remission defined by ACR criteria: 33/79 [42%] in remission with combination *v* 15/86 [17%] with single treatment; P = 0.001).[59] The eighth RCT (171 people with disease duration > 6 months) found that methotrexate plus hydroxychloroquine plus sulfasalazine increased ACR20 response rates compared with either methotrexate plus hydroxychloroquine or methotrexate plus sulfasalazine at 2 years (ACR20 response 45/58 [78%] with triple combination *v* 35/58 [60%] with methotrexate + hydroxychloroquine *v* 27/55 [49%] with methotrexate + sulfasalazine; P = 0.002 for first comparison, P = 0.05 for second comparison).[60] Concurrent treatment with corticosteroids was permitted.

Harms: Toxicity of combination treatments depends on the drugs used with monitoring as for the most toxic part of the combination. The adverse effects of combination treatments may be greater than the sum of individual treatments because of potential interactions.

Comment: An additional meta-analysis (search date 1992) pooled data from RCTs comparing single versus combination drug treatments.[62] However, the analysis did not provide adequate data on specific combinations. We found no evidence that any one or more DMARD combination treatments are more effective than any one of the other combination treatments.

QUESTION **When should disease modifying antirheumatic drugs be introduced?**

One systematic review and one additional RCT found that introducing disease modifying antirheumatic drugs early (oral gold, intramuscular gold, hydroxychloroquine, methotrexate, minocycline) significantly improved radiological progression, swollen joint counts, and quality of life scores at 12 to 60 months compared with delayed treatment.

Benefits: We found one systematic review (search date not stated, 3 RCTs, 336 people)[63] and one additional RCT.[64] The review did not pool data. The first small RCT identified by the review (23 people) found that early intramuscular gold versus 6 or 12 month delay significantly reduced radiological progression at 6 and 12 months.[63] The second included RCT (137 people enrolled, 75 people analysed) found that early oral gold versus placebo for 2 years significantly reduced swollen joint counts, Health Assessment Questionnaire scores, and radiological progression at 60 months.[65] The third RCT in the review (238 people with recently diagnosed rheumatoid arthritis) found that early intramuscular gold, hydroxychloroquine, or methotrexate versus delayed treatment significantly reduced swollen and tender joints, Health Assessment Questionnaire scores, erythrocyte sedimentation rate, and pain at 12 months but it found no significant difference in radiological progression between early and delayed treatment.[66] The additional RCT (38 people with disease for < 1 year) compared minocycline versus placebo.[64] All participants were given disease modifying antirheumatic drugs at the end of the 3 month study. After 4 years of follow up, eight people who originally received minocycline were in remission versus one in the placebo group ($P = 0.02$; CI not provided). The need for disease modifying antirheumatic drugs at 4 years was also reduced in the minocycline group.

Harms: There is concern that people left with active inflammation developed irreversible harm.

Comment: About 10% of people with rheumatoid arthritis experience a short illness that resolves and remains largely quiescent. Early treatment may expose them to adverse effects unnecessarily. The early introduction of disease modifying antirheumatic drugs requires an accurate diagnosis of rheumatoid arthritis. We are aware of one systematic review subsequent to our search date, which will be included in the next *Clinical Evidence* update.[67]

QUESTION **What are the effects of low dose oral corticosteroids?**

Two systematic reviews and one subsequent RCT have found benefit from both short and longer term treatment (> 3 months) with low dose oral corticosteroids. Short term treatment reduces disease activity and joint inflammation. Longer term treatment may reduce radiological progression while treatment continues. However, long term use is associated with considerable adverse effects.

Benefits: **Versus placebo or non-steroidal anti-inflammatory drugs:** We found two systematic reviews[68,69] and one subsequent RCT.[70] The first review (search date 1997, 10 RCTs, 402 people) compared short term treatment with low dose prednisolone (15 mg/day for several wks) versus placebo or non-steroidal anti-inflammatory drugs.[68] It found that, in the short term, prednisolone had a greater effect than placebo or non-steroidal anti-inflammatory drugs for controlling disease activity. Prednisolone versus placebo improved pain, grip strength, and joint tenderness (WMD for the number of tender joints –12, 95% CI –18 to –6). The second review (search date 1998, 7 RCTs, 508 people) evaluated longer term treatment with corticosteroids (for at least 3 months).[69] It found that longer term treatment with prednisolone was superior to placebo (WMD for tender joints –0.37, 95% CI –0.59 to –0.14; swollen joints –0.41, 95% CI –0.67 to –0.16; pain –0.43, 95% CI –0.74 to –0.12; and functional status –0.57, 95% CI –0.92 to –0.22). The review also found that prednisolone was comparable to aspirin or chloroquine. One RCT (128 people) included in the review evaluated radiological damage.[71] It found a significant decrease in the rate of progression in people treated with prednisolone (7.5 mg/day) versus placebo over 2 years. One follow up study of people in this RCT found that joint destruction resumed after discontinuing prednisolone.[72] The subsequent RCT (81 people with early previously untreated rheumatoid arthritis) found no significant difference between prednisolone (10 mg/day) versus placebo in functional disability, early morning stiffness, general wellbeing, and joint swelling at 2 years (change from baseline in functional disability assessed using Dutch version of Health Assessment Questionnaire: 0.1 with prednisolone *v* 0 with placebo, $P > 0.2$; early morning stiffness –43 min with prednisolone *v* –28 min with placebo, $P > 0.2$; general wellbeing using visual analogue scale –1 with prednisolone *v* 0 with placebo, $P > 0.2$; 28 point score for tenderness –2 with prednisolone *v* 0 with placebo, $P > 0.2$). It found that prednisolone versus placebo significantly reduced radiological damage and joint tenderness at 2 years (change from baseline: radiological damage using Sharp Damage Score (see glossary, p 1473) 16 with prednisolone *v* 29 with placebo, $P = 0.007$; 28 point score for swelling –2 with prednisolone *v* 0 with placebo, $P = 0.01$).[70] **Versus chloroquine:** One systematic review (search date 1998, 1 RCT, 56 people with rheumatoid arthritis diagnosed at age ≥ 60 years) found no significant difference between oral prednisolone and chloroquine in improving disease activity.[69]

Harms: Serious long term adverse effects of corticosteroids include hypertension, diabetes, osteoporosis, infections, gastrointestinal ulcers, obesity, and hirsutism. Observational studies of people with rheumatoid arthritis have suggested that mortality may be increased by long term treatment with steroids.[72] However, many of those studies included people receiving dosages greater than 7.5 mg daily, which are higher than those recommended currently. One systematic review found that bone loss was limited when lower dosages were prescribed.[73] One RCT found that mean body weight increased significantly from baseline to 2 years with prednisolone and there was an increase in the new vertebral fracture rate for prednisolone versus placebo ($P = 0.001$ for weight gain; vertebral fracture 5/40 [12.5%] with prednisolone *v* 2/41 [4.9%] with placebo, P not provided).[70]

Comment: The decision to give oral corticosteroids should balance the potential for increased comorbidity, which is affected by individual risk factors, and the potential improvement in disease activity. One RCT found that dose loading for 6 weeks at a higher dose than that usually recommended when initiating treatment with hydroxychloroquine increased the clinical response.[75] One case-control study (410 people with rheumatoid arthritis) found that vertebral deformities were significantly more common in people taking corticosteroids (mean dose 7 mg/day) than people not taking corticosteroids, but found no significant difference after adjusting for concomitant medication and functional capacity (deformities 52/205 [25%] with corticosteroids *v* 26/205 [13%] with no corticosteroids; unadjusted OR 2.34, 95% CI 1.39 to 3.93; adjusted OR 1.56, 95% CI 0.81 to 2.99).[76]

QUESTION What are the effects of biological agents?

OPTION TUMOUR NECROSIS FACTOR ANTIBODIES

Several RCTs have found that tumour necrosis factor antibodies (etanercept and infliximab) versus placebo improve symptoms, and reduce long term disease activity and joint inflammation. One RCT found no significant difference between etanercept and methotrexate for quality of life at 1 year. Short term toxicity is relatively low, but long term safety less clear. Problems have been identified with reactivation of demyelinating disease and tuberculosis.

Benefits: **Etanercept:** We found two 6 month placebo controlled RCTs and one RCT that compared etanercept versus methotrexate.[77–79] One RCT (234 people who had failed to respond to other disease modifying antirheumatic drugs) compared two doses of etanercept (10 and 25 mg both given twice weekly) versus placebo.[77] More people improved by at least 20% (ACR20 criteria) with etanercept (25 mg) than with the lower dose or with placebo (59% with high dose etanercept *v* 51% with low dose etanercept *v* 11% with placebo: 10 mg *v* placebo, $P < 0.001$; 25 mg *v* placebo, $P < 0.001$; 25 mg *v* 10 mg, $P = 0.2$; CI not provided). Improvement by at least 50% (ACR50 criteria) was found in 40% of people with high dose etanercept, in 24% with low dose etanercept, and in 5% with placebo (10 mg *v* placebo; $P < 0.001$; 25 mg *v* placebo; $P < 0.001$; 25 mg *v* 10 mg; $P = 0.032$; CI not provided). The RCT also found that etanercept improved functional status (measured by disability index; $P < 0.05$) and quality of life (measured by general health status; $P < 0.05$). The second RCT (89 people with inadequate response to methotrexate) compared etanercept (25 mg/wk) versus placebo.[78] People were allowed to continue methotrexate. More people achieved ACR20 criteria with etanercept than with placebo (71% with etanercept *v* 27% with placebo; $P < 0.001$; CI not provided). A 12 month RCT (632 people with early rheumatoid arthritis) compared methotrexate versus two doses of etanercept (10 and 25 mg both given twice weekly).[79] It found significantly more people achieved ACR20, ACR50, and ACR70 responses with etanercept (25 mg) versus methotrexate at 6 months. By 12 months there was no significant difference in ACR response rate (72% with etanercept *v* 65% with methotrexate; P = 0.16; CI not provided). The higher dose etanercept was significantly better than the lower dose in terms of ACR20, ACR50, and ACR70 response at 12 months (P < 0.03 for all comparisons). One double blind RCT (424 people with rheumatoid arthritis for < 3 years) found no significant difference between etanercept (25 mg sc twice weekly) versus oral methotrexate (rapidly escalating to 20 mg/wk) for health related quality of life at 52 weeks (SF-36 physical scale, mean improvement 10.7 points with etanercept *v* 9.6 points with methotrexate, P = 0.84; SF-36 mental scale, mean improvement 3.6 points with etanercept *v* 4.1 points with methotrexate, P = 0.39; health related quality of life, mean improvement 0.73 points with etanercept *v* 0.76 points with methotrexate, P = 0.46).[80] **Infliximab:** We found three placebo controlled RCTs.[81–83] The first RCT (73 people) compared infliximab (1 mg/kg) versus infliximab (10 mg/kg) versus placebo over 4 weeks.[81] More people experienced at least 20% improvement in the 10 mg/kg group (79%) than in the 1 mg/kg group (44%) or in the placebo group (placebo *v* 1 mg/kg, P = 0.008; placebo *v* 10 mg/kg, P < 0.0001).[79] A second RCT (101 people) compared 1, 3, or 10 mg/kg infliximab with or without methotrexate versus placebo. It found a greater improvement with 3 or 10 mg/kg infliximab versus placebo (ACR20 improvement: 60% in people taking 3 or 10 mg/kg infliximab *v* 15% in people taking placebo).[82] A third large multicentre RCT (428 people with active disease not responsive to methotrexate) compared five groups over 7 months: placebo versus infliximab at 3 or 10 mg/kg, given every 4 or 8 weeks.[83] All continued to receive methotrexate. ACR20 criteria were reached by 50–58% who received infliximab/methotrexate and by 20% of the methotrexate/placebo group. ACR50 was attained by 26–31% of the people receiving infliximab and by 5% in the placebo group (P < 0.001; CI not provided). Longer term results at 54 weeks found that all infliximab groups improved versus placebo in terms of ACR20, ACR50, and ACR70 criteria (all results P < 0.05; CI not provided).[84]

Harms: **Etanercept:** The most common adverse effect was mild injection site reaction (42–49% in the treated group *v* 7–13% in the placebo group). One report of placebo controlled trials (349 people on etanercept *v* 152 people on placebo) found that injection site reactions were significantly more common for etanercept versus placebo (7.73 events/patient years with etanercept *v* 0.62 events/patient years with placebo, P < 0.001).[85] Other adverse effects included upper respiratory symptoms or infections, headache, and diarrhoea. Autoantibodies to double stranded DNA developed in 5–9% of the treated group. Less than 1% of people developed malignancies or infections in the 6 month trials. Reactivation of demyelinating disease has been described. **Infliximab:** In the RCTs, common adverse reactions were upper respiratory infections, headache, diarrhoea, and abdominal pain. Reactions during or immediately after the injection (headache, nausea, urticaria) were also observed in the placebo groups, but were more frequent with infliximab. Antibodies to double stranded DNA were found in about 16% of people taking infliximab. The rates of serious adverse effects in treated and placebo groups were not significantly different, but there was insufficient power to detect clinically important differences. Worldwide, over 150 cases of reactivation of tuberculosis have been documented, and people should be screened for previous tuberculosis before treatment (Emery P, personal communication, 2002).

Comment: One indirect comparison of treatment arms in previous RCTs (349 people on etanercept *v* 152 people on placebo) found that injection site reactions were significantly more common for etanercept versus placebo (7.73 events/person years with etanercept *v* 0.62 event/person years with placebo, $P < 0.001$).[85] We found one non-English language review of tumour necrosis factor alpha inhibitors; it will be translated and, if relevant, included in future *Clinical Evidence* updates.[86] These drugs are generally restricted to people who have failed conventional disease modifying antirheumatic drugs and are used in secondary care. The effects on disease activity occurred within weeks, unlike other disease modifying antirheumatic drugs that may take several months to have an effect.

GLOSSARY

Sharp damage score Assesses radiological damage by measuring erosions and joint space narrowing in 44 different joints and reporting an aggregated score ranging from 0 to 448.

REFERENCES

1. Arnett FC, Edworthy SM, Bloch DA, et al. The American Rheumatism Association 1987 revised criteria for the classification of rheumatoid arthritis. *Arthritis Rheum* 1987;31:315–324.
2. Lawrence RC, Helmick CG, Arnett FC, et al. Estimates of the prevalence of arthritis and selected musculoskeletal disorders in the United States. *Arthritis Rheum* 1998;41:778–781.
3. Symmons DP, Barrett EM, Bankhead CR, et al. The incidence of rheumatoid arthritis in the United Kingdom: results from the Norfolk Arthritis Register. *Br J Rheumatol* 1994;33:735–739.
4. Winchester R, Dwyer E, Rose S. The genetic basis of rheumatoid arthritis: the shared epitope hypothesis. *Rheum Dis Clin North Am* 1992;18:761–783.
5. Yelin E, Henke C, Epstein W. The work dynamics of the person with rheumatoid arthritis. *Arthritis Rheum* 1987;30:507–512.
6. Mutru O, Laakso M, Isomäki H, et al. Ten year mortality and causes of death in patients with rheumatoid arthritis. *BMJ* 1985;290:1797–1799.
7. Felson DT, Anderson JJ, Boers M, et al. American College of Rheumatology preliminary definition of improvement in rheumatoid arthritis. *Arthritis Rheum* 1995;38:727–735.
8. Suarez-Almazor ME, Belseck E, Shea B, et al. Methotrexate for rheumatoid arthritis. In: The Cochrane Library, Issue 3, 2000. Oxford: Update Software. Search date 1997; primary sources Medline, Embase, Cochrane Controlled Trials Register, and hand searches of reference lists.
9. Strand V, Cohen S, Schiff M, et al. Treatment of active rheumatoid arthritis with leflunomide compared with placebo or methotrexate. *Arch Intern Med* 1999;159:2542–2550.
10. Emery P, Breedveld FC, Lemmel EM, et al. A comparison of the efficacy and safety of leflunomide and methotrexate for the treatment of rheumatoid arthritis. *Rheumatology* 2000;39:655–665.
11. Felson DT, Anderson JJ, Meenan RF. Use of short-term efficacy/toxicity trade-offs to select second-line drugs in rheumatoid arthritis: a meta-analysis of published clinical trials. *Arthritis Rheum* 1992;35:1117–1125. Search date 1990; primary sources Medline and hand searches of two key journals and reference lists.
12. Hamilton J, McInnes I, Thomson E, et al. Comparative study of intramuscular gold and methotrexate in a rheumatoid arthritis population from a socially deprived area. *Ann Rheum Dis* 2001;60:566–572.
13. Rau R, Herborn G, Menninger H, et al. Radiographic outcome after three years of patients with early erosive rheumatoid arthritis treated with intramuscular methotrexate or parenteral gold. Extension of a one-year double-blind study in 174 patients. *Rheumatology* 2002;41:196–204.
14. Ortiz Z, Shea B, Suarez-Almazor ME, et al. The efficacy of folic acid and folinic acid in reducing methotrexate gastrointestinal toxicity in rheumatoid arthritis: a meta-analysis of randomised controlled clinical trials. *J Rheumatol* 1998;25;36–43. Search date 1996; primary sources Medline, hand searches of bibliographic references, Current Contents, and abstracts selected from rheumatology meetings and journals.
15. Beauparlant P, Papp K, Haroui B. The incidence of cancer associated with the treatment of rheumatoid arthritis. *Semin Arthritis Rheum* 1999;29:145–148.
16. Maetzel A, Wong A, Strand V, et al. Meta-analysis of treatment termination rates among rheumatoid arthritis patients receiving disease-modifying anti-rheumatic drugs. *Rheumatology* 2000;39:975–981. Search date 1997; primary sources Medline and Embase.
17. Alarcon GS, Lopez-Mendez A, Walter J, et al. Radiographic evidence of disease progression in methotrexate treated and nonmethotrexate

disease modifying antirheumatic drug treated rheumatoid arthritis patients: a meta-analysis. *J Rheumatol* 1992;19:1868–1873. Search date 1991; primary sources Medline and hand searches of bibliographies and meetings abstract of the American College of Rheumatology 1988–1991.

18. Felson DT, Anderson JJ, Meenan RF. The comparative efficacy and toxicity of second-line drugs in rheumatoid arthritis: results of two meta-analyses. *Arthritis Rheum* 1990;33:1449–1461. Search date 1989; primary sources Medline, and hand searches of two key journals and reference lists.
19. Gotzsche PC, Podenphant J, Olesen M, et al. Meta-analysis of second-line antirheumatic drugs: sample size bias and uncertain benefit. *J Clin Epidemiol* 1992;45:587–594. Search date 1988; primary source Medline, hand searches of reference lists, and drug companies contacted for unpublished trials.
20. Suarez-Almazor ME, Belseck E, Wells G, et al. Meta-analyses of placebo controlled trials of disease-modifying antirheumatic drugs (DMARD) for the treatment of rheumatoid arthritis (RA). *Arthritis Rheum* 1998;41:S153. Search date not stated; primary sources Medline and Embase.
21. Suarez-Almazor ME, Belseck E, Shea B, et al. Antimalarials for rheumatoid arthritis. In: The Cochrane Library, Issue 2, 2002. Oxford: Update Software. Search date 2000; primary sources Medline, Embase, Cochrane Controlled Trials Register, and hand searches of reference lists.
22. Scull E. Chloroquine and hydroxychloroquine therapy in rheumatoid arthritis. *Arthritis Rheum* 1962;5:30–36.
23. Finbloom DS, Silver K, Newsome DA, et al. Comparison of hydroxychloroquine and chloroquine use and the development of retinal toxicity. *J Rheumatol* 1985;12:692–694.
24. The Hera Study Group. A randomized trial of hydroxychloroquine in early rheumatoid arthritis: the Hera study. *Am J Med* 1995;156–158.
25. Jessop JD, O'Sullivan MM, Lewis PA, et al. A long-term five-year randomized controlled trial of hydroxychloroquine, sodium aurothiomalate, auranofin and penicillamine in the treatment of patients with rheumatoid arthritis. *Br J Rheumatol* 1998;37:992–1002.
26. Weinblatt ME, Reda D, Henderson W, et al. Sulfasalazine treatment for rheumatoid arthritis: a metaanalysis of 15 randomized trials. *J Rheumatol* 1999;26:2123–2130. Search date 1998; primary sources Medline, Excerpta Medica, and Derwent Drug File.
27. Smolen JS, Kalden JR, Scott, DL, et al. Efficacy and safety of leflunomide compared with placebo and sulfasalazine in active rheumatoid arthritis: a double-blind, randomised, multicentre. Trial. *Lancet* 1999;353:259–266.
28. Van der Heijde DM, van Riel PL, Nuver-Zwart IH, et al. Effects of hydroxychloroquine and sulfasalazine on progression of joint damage in rheumatoid arthritis. *Lancet* 1989;1:1036–1038.
29. Capell HA, Maiden N, Madhok R, et al. Intention-to-treat analysis of 200 patients with rheumatoid arthritis 12 years after random allocation to either sulfasalazine or penicillamine. *J Rheumatol* 1998;25:1880–1886.
30. Suarez-Almazor ME, Belseck E, Shea B, et al. Sulfasalazine for rheumatoid arthritis. In: The Cochrane Library, Issue 3, 2000. Oxford: Update Software. Search date 1997; primary sources Medline, Embase, Cochrane Controlled Trials Register, and hand searches of reference lists.
31. Clark P, Tugwell P, Bennet K, et al. Injectable gold for rheumatoid arthritis. In: The Cochrane Library, Issue 2, 2002. Oxford: Update Software. Search date 1997; primary sources Medline and hand searches of reference lists and bibliographies in selected textbooks.
32. Kvein TK, Zeidler HK, Hannonone P, et al. Long term efficacy and safety of cyclosporin versus parenteral gold in early rheumatoid arthritis: a three year study of radiographic progression, renal function, and arterial hypertension. *Ann Rheum Dis* 2002:61:511–516.
33. Suarez-Almazor ME, Spooner CH, Belseck E, et al. Auranofin versus placebo in rheumatoid arthritis. In: The Cochrane Library, Issue 4, 2000. Oxford: Update Software. Search date 1998; primary sources Medline, Embase, Cochrane Controlled Trials Register, and hand searches of reference lists of retrieved articles.
34. McEntegart A, Porter D, Capell HA, et al. Sulfasalazine has a better efficacy/toxicity profile than auranofin — evidence from a 5 year prospective randomized trial. *J Rheumatol* 1996;23:1887–1890.
35. Singh G, Fieis JF, Williams CA, et al. Toxicity profiles of disease modifying antirheumatic drugs in rheumatoid arthritis. *J Rheumatol* 1991;18:188–194.
36. Kloppenburg M, Breedveld FC, Terwiel JP, et al. Minocycline in active rheumatoid arthritis: a double-blind, placebo-controlled trial. *Arthritis Rheum* 1994;37:629–636.
37. Tilley BC, Alarcon GS, Heyse SP, et al. Minocycline in rheumatoid arthritis: a 48-week, double-blind, placebo-controlled trial. MIRA trial group. *Ann Intern Med* 1995;122:81–89.
38. O'Dell JR, Haire CE, Palmer W, et al. Treatment of early rheumatoid arthritis with minocycline or placebo: results of a randomized, double-blind, placebo-controlled trial. *Arthritis Rheum* 1997;40:842–848.
39. Suarez-Almazor ME, Spooner C, Belseck E. Penicillamine for rheumatoid arthritis. In: The Cochrane Library, Issue 3, 2000. Oxford: Update Software. Search date 2000; primary sources Cochrane Musculoskeletal Group's Trials Register, Cochrane Controlled Trials Register, Medline, Embase, and hand searches of reference lists of trials retrieved.
40. Wolfe F, Hawley DJ, Cathey MA. Termination of slow acting anti-rheumatic therapy in rheumatoid arthritis: a 14 year prospective evaluation of 1017 starts. *J Rheumatol* 1990;17:994–1002.
41. Pincus T, Marcum SB, Callahan LF. Long-term drug therapy for rheumatoid arthritis in seven rheumatology private practices: II. Second line drugs and prednisone. *J Rheumatol* 1992;19:1885–1894.
42. Fries JF, Williams CA, Ramey D, et al. The relative toxicity of disease-modifying antirheumatic drugs. *Arthritis Rheum* 1993;36:297–306.
43. Suarez-Almazor ME, Soskolne CL, Saunders LD, et al. Use of second-line drugs in the treatment of rheumatoid arthritis in Edmonton, Alberta: patterns of prescription and long-term effectiveness. *J Rheumatol* 1995;22:836–843.
44. Suarez-Almazor ME, Spooner C, Bekseck E. Azathioprine for rheumatoid arthritis. In: The Cochrane Library, Issue 2, 2002. Oxford: Update Software. Search date 2000; primary sources Cochrane Musculoskeletal Group's Trials Register, Cochrane Controlled Trials Register, Medline, Embase, and hand searches of reference lists of trials retrieved.
45. Suarez-Almazor ME, Belseck E, Shea B, et al. Cyclophosphamide for rheumatoid arthritis. In: The Cochrane Library, Issue 3, 2000. Oxford: Update Software. Search date 2000; primary sources

Cochrane Controlled Trials Register, Medline, Embase, and hand searches of reference lists.

46. Radis CD, Kahl LE, Baker GL, et al. Effects of cyclophosphamide on the development of malignancy and on long-term survival of patients with rheumatoid arthritis. A 20-year follow up study. *Arthritis Rheum* 1995;38:1120–1127.
47. Wells G, Haguenauer D, Shea B, et al. Cyclosporin for rheumatoid arthritis. In: The Cochrane Library, Issue 3, 2000. Oxford: Update Software. Search date 1997; primary sources Medline, hand searches of reference lists and consultation with experts.
48. Hewitson PJ, DeBroe S, McBride A, et al. Leflunomide and rheumatoid arthritis: a systematic review of effectiveness, safety and cost implications. *J Clin Pharm Ther* 2000;25:295–302. Search date 1999; primary sources Medline, Embase, the Cochrane Library, Econlit, HMIC (Dhdata), HMIC (Helmis), HMIC (King's Fund Database), and Best Evidence3.
49. Mladenovic V, Domljan Z, Rozman B, et al. Safety and effectiveness of leflunomide in the treatment of patients with active rheumatoid arthritis. *Arthritis Rheum* 1995;38:1595–1603.
50. Cohen S, Cannon G, Schiff M, et al. Two-year, blinded, randomized, controlled trial of treatment of active rheumatoid arthritis with leflunomide compared with methotrexate. Utilization of Leflunomide in the Treatment of Rheumatoid Arthritis Trial Investigator Group. *Arthritis Rheum* 2001;44:1984–1992.
51. Strand V, Tugwell P, Bombardier C, et al. Function and health-related quality of life: results from a randomized controlled trial of leflunomide versus methotrexate or placebo in patients with active rheumatoid arthritis. *Arthritis Rheum* 1999;42:1870–1878.
52. Verhoeven AC, Boers M, Tugwell P. Combination therapy in rheumatoid arthritis: updated systematic review. *Br J Rheumatol* 1998;37:612–619. Search date 1997; primary sources Medline and hand searches of article bibliographies.
53. Van den Borne BE, Landewe RB, Goei HS, et al. Combination therapy in recent onset rheumatoid arthritis: a randomized double blind trial of the addition of low dose cyclosporin to patients treated with low dose chloroquine. *J Rheumatol* 1998;25:1493–1498.
54. Boers M, Verhoeven AC, Markusse HM, et al. Randomised comparison of combined step-down prednisolone, methotrexate and sulfasalazine with sulfasalazine alone in early rheumatoid arthritis. *Lancet* 1997;350:309–318.
55. Mottonen T, Hannonen P, Leirisalo-Repo M, et al. Comparison of combination therapy with single-drug therapy in early rheumatoid arthritis: a randomised trial. FIN-RACo trial group. *Lancet* 1999;353:1568–1573.
56. Calguneri M, Pay S, Caliskaner Z, et al. Combination therapy versus monotherapy for the treatment of patients with rheumatoid arthritis. *Clin Exp Rheumatol* 1999;17:699–704.
57. O'Dell JR, Haire CE, Erikson N, et al. Treatment of rheumatoid arthritis with methotrexate alone, sulfasalazine and hydroxychloroquine, or a combination of all three medications. *N Engl J Med* 1996; 334:1287–1291.
58. Proudman S, Conaghan P, Richardson C, et al. Treatment of poor-prognosis early rheumatoid arthritis: a randomized study of treatment with methotrexate, cyclosporin A, and intra-articular corticosteroids compared with sulfasalazine alone. *Arthritis Rheum* 2000;43:1809–1819.
59. Mottonen T, Hannonen P, Korpela M, et al. Delay to institution of therapy and induction of remission using single-drug or combination-disease-modifying antirheumatic drug therapy in early rheumatoid arthritis. *Arthritis Rheum* 2002;46:894–898.
60. O'Dell JR, Leff R, Paulsen G, et al. Treatment of rheumatoid arthritis with methotrexate and hydroxychloroquine, methotrexate and sulphasalazine or a combination of the three medications. *Arthritis Rheum* 2002;46:1164–1170.
61. Landewe RBM, Boers M, Verhoeven AC, et al. Cobra Combination therapy in patients with early rheumatoid arthritis. *Arthritis Rheum* 2002:46:347–356.
62. Felson DT, Anderson JJ, Meenan RF. The efficacy and toxicity of combination therapy in rheumatoid arthritis: a meta-analysis. *Arthritis Rheum* 1994;37:1487–1491. Search date 1992; primary sources Medline, and hand searches of five international rheumatology journals and abstracts of rheumatology society meetings.
63. Emery P, Breedveld FC, Dougados M, et al. Early referral recommendation for newly diagnosed rheumatoid arthritis: evidence based development of a clinical guide. *Ann Rheum Dis* 2002;61:290–297. Search date not stated; primary sources Medline and Current Contents.
64. O'Dell JR, Paulsen G, Haire CE, et al. Treatment of early seropositive rheumatoid arthritis with minocycline: four-year follow up of a double blind, placebo-controlled trial. *Arthritis Rheum* 1999;42:1691–1695.
65. Egsmose C, Lund B, Borg G, et al. Patients with rheumatoid arthritis benefit from early second line therapy: 5 year follow up of a prospective double blind placebo controlled study. *J Rheumatol* 1995;22:2208–2213.
66. Van Der Heide A, Jacobs JWG, Bijlsma JWJ, et al. The effectiveness of early treatment with "second-line" antirheumatic drugs: a randomized, controlled trial. *Ann Intern Med* 1996;124:699–707.
67. Quinn M, Conaghan P, Emery P. The therapeutic approach of early intervention for rheumatoid arthritis: what is the evidence? *Rheumatology* 2001;40:1211–1220.
68. Gotzsche PC, Johansen HK. Meta-analysis of short term low dose prednisolone versus placebo and non-steroidal anti-inflammatory drugs in rheumatoid arthritis. *BMJ* 1998;316:811–818. Search date 1997; primary sources Medline, Cochrane Controlled Trials Register, and hand searches of reference lists.
69. Criswell LA, Saag KG, Sems KM, et al. Moderate-term low dose corticosteroids for rheumatoid arthritis. In: The Cochrane Library, Issue 3, 2000. Oxford: Update Software. Search date 1998; primary sources Medline and hand searches of selected journals.
70. Van Everdingen AA, Jacobs JWG, Van Reesema DRS, et al. Low-dose prednisolone therapy for patients with early active rheumatoid arthritis: clinical efficacy, disease-modifying properties, and side-effects. *Ann Intern Med* 2002:136:1–12.
71. Kirwan JR. Arthritis and Rheumatism Council low dose glucocorticoid study group: the effect of glucocorticoids on joint destruction in rheumatoid arthritis. *N Engl J Med* 1995;333:142–146.
72. Hickling P, Jacoby RK, Kirwan JR, et al. Joint destruction after glucocorticoids are withdrawn in early rheumatoid arthritis. *Br J Rheumatol* 1998;37:930–936.
73. Wolfe F, Mitchell DM, Sibley JT, et al. The mortality of rheumatoid arthritis. *Arthritis Rheum* 1994;37:481–494.
74. Verhoeven AC, Boers M. Limited bone loss due to corticosteroids: a systematic review of prospective

studies in rheumatoid arthritis and other diseases. *J Rheumatol* 1997;24:1495–1503. Search date 1995; primary source Medline.
75. Furst DE, Lindsley H, Baethge B, et al. Dose-loading with hydroxychloroquine improves the rate of response in early, active rheumatoid arthritis: a randomized, double-blind six-week trial with eighteen-week extension. *Arthritis Rheum* 1999;42:357–365.
76. De Nijs, Jacobs RNJ, Bijlsma JWG, et al. Prevalence of vertebral deformities and symptomatic fracture in corticosteroid treated patients with rheumatoid arthritis. *Rheumatology* 2001;40:1375–1383.
77. Moreland LW, Schiff MH, Baumgartner SW, et al. Etanercept therapy in rheumatoid arthritis. A randomized, controlled trial. *Ann Intern Med* 1999;130:478–486.
78. Weinblatt ME, Kremer JM, Bankhurst AD, et al. A trial of etanercept, a recombinant tumor necrosis factor receptor: Fc fusion protein, in patients with rheumatoid arthritis receiving methotrexate. *N Engl J Med* 1999;340:253–259.
79. Bathon J, Martin R, Fleischmann R, et al. A comparison of etanercept and methotrexate in patients with early rheumatoid arthritis. *N Engl J Med* 2000;343:1586–1593.
80. Kosinski M, Kujawski SC, Martin R, et al. Health-related quality of life in early rheumatoid arthritis: impact of disease and treatment response. *Am J Manag Care* 2002;8:231–240.
81. Elliott MJ, Maini RN, Feldmann M, et al. Randomised double-blind comparison of chimeric monoclonal antibody to tumour necrosis factor alpha (cA2) versus placebo in rheumatoid arthritis. *Lancet* 1994;344:1105–1110.
82. Maini RN, Breedveld FC, Kalden JR, et al. Therapeutic efficacy of multiple intravenous infusions of anti-tumor necrosis factor α monoclonal antibody combined with low-dose weekly methotrexate in rheumatoid arthritis. *Arthritis Rheum* 1998;41:1552–1563.
83. Maini RN, St Clair EW, Breedweld F, et al. Infliximab (chimeric anti-tumour necrosis factor α monoclonal antibody) versus placebo in rheumatoid arthritis patients receiving concomitant methotrexate: a randomized Phase III trial. ATTRACT study group. *Lancet* 1999;354:1932–1939.
84. Lipsky P, van der Heijde D, St Claire W, et al. Infliximab and methotrexate in the treatment of rheumatoid arthritis. *N Engl J Med* 2000;343:1594–1602.
85. Moreland LW, Cohen SB, Baumgartner SW, et al. Long term safety and efficacy of etanercept in patients with rheumatoid arthritis. *J Rheumatol* 2001;28:1238–1244.
86. Reneses S, Pestana L. Systematic review of clinical trials on the treatment of rheumatoid arthritis with tumour necrosis factor alpha inhibitors [in French]. *Med Clin (Barc)* 2001;116:620–628.

Paul Emery
ARC Professor Head of Academic Unit of Musculoskeletal disease
University of Leeds
Leeds
UK

Maria Suarez-Almazor
Associate Professor of Medicine
Baylor College of Medicine
Houston, TX
USA

Competing interests: PE has undertaken lectures and consulting work for Pharmacia, Aventis, Schering-Plough and Wyeth.

Shoulder pain

Search date October 2002

Cathy Speed and Brian Hazleman

QUESTIONS

INTERVENTIONS

See glossary, p 1490

Key Messages

- Shoulder pain is not a specific diagnosis. Well designed, double blind RCTs of specific interventions in specific shoulder disorders are needed.
- Systematic reviews have found RCTs mostly with poor methods, and pronounced heterogeneity of study populations and outcome measures.
- We found insufficient evidence on the effects of most interventions in people with non-specific shoulder pain.
- **Arthroscopic laser subacromial decompression** One systematic review found no RCTs on arthroscopic subacromial decompression.
- **Electrical stimulation** One RCT found no significant difference in pain between electrical stimulation versus control. However, the study may have lacked power to detect clinically important differences.
- **Extracorporeal shock wave therapy** We found mixed results from three RCTs. The first RCT found that one or two sessions of high energy extracorporeal shock wave therapy versus placebo improved pain and function in people with calcific tendinitis. However, two further RCTs in people with rotator cuff tendinosis found no significant difference for extracorporeal shock wave therapy versus sham treatment for pain or function at 3–6 months.

- **Intra-articular corticosteroid injection** One small RCT found no significant difference for intra-articular triamcinolone versus saline in pain score, change in mobility, or function at 3 weeks. One small RCT found no significant difference for intra-articular methylprednisolone plus lidocaine (lignocaine) versus lidocaine alone in pain or shoulder motion at 24 weeks. The RCTs were small and may have lacked power to detect clinically important differences.
- **Intra-articular guanethidine** We found no systematic review or RCTs of intra-articular guanethidine in people with non-arthritic shoulder pain.
- **Laser treatment** We found mixed results from four small RCTs that compared laser treatment versus placebo in shoulder pain. Two short term RCTs found that laser improved recovery rate and pain compared with placebo at 2–4 weeks. However, two longer term RCTs found no significant difference in pain or recovery rate at 8–12 weeks.
- **Multidisciplinary biopsychosocial rehabilitation** One systematic review found no good quality RCTs of multidisciplinary biopsychosocial rehabilitation in people with shoulder pain.
- **Oral corticosteroids** Two small RCTs found no evidence of reduced pain or improved abduction with oral corticosteroids versus placebo or versus no treatment at 4–8 months. Adverse effects of corticosteroids are well documented (see rheumatoid arthritis, p 1454 and asthma, p 1757).
- **Oral non-steroidal anti-inflammatory drugs** We found insufficient evidence from one systematic review and one additional RCT to draw firm conclusions about effects of oral non-steroidal anti-inflammatory drugs versus placebo in people with non-specific shoulder pain.
- **Phonophoresis** We found no RCTs solely in people with shoulder pain.
- **Physiotherapy (exercises and manual treatments)** One systematic review has found insufficient evidence about effects of physiotherapy alone versus no treatment or advice to exercise in people with shoulder pain.
- **Subacromial corticosteroid injection** We found no RCTs comparing subacromial injection of steroids versus placebo. We found insufficient evidence from two small RCTs to compare clinical effects of corticosteroid plus lidocaine versus lidocaine alone in people with rotator cuff tendinitis. One small RCT found limited evidence that intra-articular plus subacromial corticosteroid injections versus intra-articular and subacromial lidocaine alone increased remission rates at 4 weeks.
- **Surgery/forced manipulation** We found no placebo controlled RCTs. One small RCT found that forced manipulation plus intra-articular hydrocortisone injection versus intra-articular hydrocortisone injection alone increased recovery rate at 3 months.
- **Transdermal glyceryl trinitrate** We found no reliable RCTs.
- **Ultrasound** One systematic review and two subsequent RCTs found no clinically important difference in pain, abduction, or quality of life with ultrasound versus sham treatment or no treatment.
- **Ice; paracetamol or opiates; topical or intra-articular non-steroidal anti-inflammatory drugs** We found no RCTs about these interventions.

DEFINITION Shoulder pain arises in or around the shoulder from the glenohumeral, acromioclavicular, sternoclavicular, "subacromial", and scapulothoracic articulations, and surrounding soft tissues. Regardless of the disorder, pain is the most common reason for consulting a practitioner. In adhesive capsulitis (frozen shoulder), pain is associated with pronounced restriction of movement. For most shoulder disorders, diagnosis is based on clinical features with imaging studies playing a role in some people. Post-stroke shoulder pain is not addressed in this topic.

INCIDENCE/ PREVALENCE Each year in primary care in the UK, about 1% of adults aged over 45 years present with a new episode of shoulder pain.[1] Prevalence is uncertain, with estimates from 4–20%.[2–6] One community survey (392 people) found a 1 month prevalence of shoulder pain of 34%.[7] A second community survey (644 people aged ≥ 70 years) reported a point prevalence of 21%, with a higher frequency in women than men (25% *v* 17%).[8] Seventy per cent of cases involved the rotator cuff. One survey of 134 people in a community based rheumatology clinic found that 65% of cases were rotator cuff lesions; 11% were caused by localised tenderness in the pericapsular musculature; 10% acromioclavicular joint pain; 3% glenohumeral joint arthritis; and 5% were referred pain from the neck.[9] One survey found that in adults, the annual incidence of frozen shoulder was about 2%, with those aged 40–70 years most commonly affected.[10] The age distribution of specific shoulder disorders in the community is unknown.

AETIOLOGY/ RISK FACTORS Rotator cuff disorders are associated with excessive overloading, instability of the glenohumeral and acromioclavicular joints, muscle imbalance, adverse anatomical features (narrow coracoacromial arch and a hooked acromion), cuff degeneration with aging, ischaemia, and musculoskeletal diseases that result in wasting of the cuff muscles.[11–14] Risk factors for frozen shoulder include female sex, older age, shoulder trauma, surgery, diabetes, cardiorespiratory disorders, cerebrovascular events, thyroid disease, and hemiplegia.[10,15,16] Arthritis of the glenohumeral joint can occur in numerous forms, including primary and secondary osteoarthritis, rheumatoid arthritis, and crystal arthritides.[11]

PROGNOSIS One survey in an elderly community found that most people with shoulder pain were still affected 3 years after the initial survey.[17] One prospective cohort study of 122 people in primary care found that 25% of people with shoulder pain reported previous episodes and 49% reported full recovery at 18 months' follow up.[18]

AIMS OF INTERVENTION To reduce pain and to improve range of movement and function, with minimal adverse effects.

OUTCOMES Pain scores (overall score, on activity, at night, at rest, during the day, analgesia count); range of movement measures; assessment of overall severity (self assessed or by blinded assessor); functional score; global improvement scores (self assessed or by blinded assessor); tenderness; strength; stiffness; and adverse effects of treatment. The shoulder pain and disability index is a validated shoulder related pain and disability questionnaire.[19–24] Other validated participant rated disability scores have been developed.[20]

METHODS *Clinical Evidence* search and appraisal October 2002. We found some articles that were not published in English; these articles are being translated and, if appropriate, will be included in future updates.

QUESTION **What are the effects of treatments on shoulder pain?**

OPTION **ORAL NON-STEROIDAL ANTI-INFLAMMATORY DRUGS**

We found insufficient evidence from one systematic review and one additional RCT to draw firm conclusions about effects of oral non-steroidal anti-inflammatory drugs versus placebo in people with non-specific shoulder pain.

Benefits: **Versus placebo:** We found one systematic review (search date 1998, 4 small RCTs, 151 people with shoulder pain for more than 72 h)[25] and one additional RCT.[26] The review pooled results from RCTs that reported sufficient data (90 people with rotator cuff tendinitis) and found no significant reduction of pain and no significant improvement of abduction between oral non-steroidal anti-inflammatory drugs (NSAIDs — diclofenac, naproxen) versus placebo after 4 weeks (pain: visual analogue scale, WMD +3%, 95% CI –19% to +25% where positive values represent deterioration; abduction: WMD +26°, 95% CI –9° to +61° where positive values represent improvement).[27,28] The additional RCT (69 people with acute shoulder pain of less than 96 h duration) found that oral flurbiprofen (300 mg daily) versus placebo for 14 days improved pain relief judged by the investigator (global assessment by investigator: 30/35 [86%] improved with NSAID *v* 19/32 [59%] with placebo; ARR 26%, CI 5% to 46%; NNT 4, 95% CI 3 to 20).[26]

Harms: Withdrawal because of adverse events occurred in fewer than 10% of people in non-randomised comparative studies, but in up to 20% of people in RCTs. Adverse events were mostly gastrointestinal symptoms, skin rash, headache, or dizziness. The review found no evidence that the incidence or nature of adverse effects varied among NSAIDs (naproxen, diclofenac, flurbiprofen, indometacin [indomethacin], diclofenac, etodolac, ibuprofen, fentiazac, phenylbutazone, piroxicam). We found no systematic review of the adverse effects of cyclo-oxygenase type II selective agents in people with shoulder pain (see differences between NSAIDs under the NSAIDs topic, p 1393).

Comment: Evidence about the effects of NSAIDs in shoulder disorders is limited by the lack of standardised approaches: diverse disorders have been considered under the universal term shoulder pain, different types of NSAIDs were used, and outcome measures and follow up periods vary among RCTs.

OPTION **TOPICAL NON-STEROIDAL ANTI-INFLAMMATORY DRUGS**

We found no RCTs about the effects of topical non-steroidal anti-inflammatory drugs specifically in shoulder pain.

Benefits: We found no systematic review or RCTs of topical non-steroidal anti-inflammatory drugs specifically in people with shoulder pain.

Harms: We found no systematic review or RCTs specifically in people with shoulder pain.

Comment: See topical non-steroidal anti-inflammatory drugs under osteoarthritis, p 1402.

OPTION INTRA-ARTICULAR NON-STEROIDAL ANTI-INFLAMMATORY DRUGS

We found no systematic review or RCTs evaluating intra-articular injection of non-steroidal anti-inflammatory drugs.

Benefits: We found no systematic review or RCTs evaluating intra-articular injection of non-steroidal anti-inflammatory drugs.

Harms: We found no RCTs.

Comment: None.

OPTION PARACETAMOL OR OPIATES

We found no RCTs evaluating paracetamol or opiates in people with shoulder pain.

Benefits: We found no systematic review or RCTs evaluating paracetamol or opiates in people with shoulder pain.

Harms: We found no RCTs.

Comment: None.

OPTION SUBACROMIAL CORTICOSTEROID INJECTIONS

We found no RCTs comparing subacromial injection of steroids versus placebo. We found insufficient evidence from two small RCTs to compare clinical effects of corticosteroid plus lidocaine versus lidocaine alone in people with rotator cuff tendinitis. One small RCT found limited evidence that intra-articular plus subacromial corticosteroid injections versus intra-articular and subacromial lidocaine (lignocaine) alone increased remission rates at 4 weeks.

Benefits: **Versus placebo:** We found no RCTs. **Plus lidocaine versus lidocaine alone:** We found one systematic review (search date 1998, 1 RCT, 50 people with rotator cuff tendinitis)[25] and one additional RCT.[29] The RCT identified by the review compared three treatments: subacromial injection with triamcinolone plus lidocaine (1 mL of 80 mg/mL trimacinolone plus 2 mL of 0.5% lidocaine) versus subacromial lidocaine injection (3 mL of 0.5%) versus oral diclofenac plus subacromial lidocaine injection (diclofenac 50 mg 3 times daily plus 3 mL of 0.5% lidocaine).[27] After 4 weeks, it found that subacromial injection with triamcinolone plus lidocaine versus lidocaine alone significantly improved abduction, but there was no significant difference in pain (improved abduction: WMD 35°, 95% CI 14° to 55°; reduction in pain: WMD +7%, 95% CI –33% to +47%). It also found that subacromial injection with triamcinolone plus lidocaine versus lidocaine alone increased clinical response rates at 4 weeks (response defined as improvement in a combination of overall pain severity score, range of active abduction, and limitation of function: 70% for triamcinolone plus lidocaine *v* 0% for lidocaine alone; $P < 0.001$). The additional RCT (55 people with rotator cuff tendinitis) found no significant difference between subacromial methylprednisolone (40 mg) plus lidocaine (1 mL of 1%) versus lidocaine alone for pain or remission rate at 12 weeks (pain using visual analogue scale 0–30: median pain improved by 8 points with active treatment *v* 8 points with placebo; P value not stated; remission defined as score of 0 on pain, active abduction, flexion, and external rotation: 32% in remission with corticosteroids *v* 26% with placebo; P value not stated).[29] **Combined intra-articular and subacromial corticosteroid injections versus placebo:** We found one systematic review (search date 1998, 1 RCT).[25] The RCT (100 people with pain or tenderness over supraspinatus during preceding 3 months) compared four treatments: intra-articular and subacromial triamcinolone plus lidocaine plus oral naproxen; intra-articular and subacromial triamcinolone plus lidocaine; intra-articular and subacromial lidocaine plus oral naproxen; and intra-articular and subacromial lidocaine.[28] It found that intra-articular and subacromial triamcinolone plus lidocaine increased remission rates compared with lidocaine alone at 4 weeks (remission defined as a perfect score in active abduction, pain and limitation of function: 28% for triamcinolone *v* 8% for placebo; P value not stated).[28]

Harms: The RCT included in the review (50 people with rotator cuff tendinitis) found no adverse effects with subacromial corticosteroid plus lidocaine versus lidocaine alone apart from mild discomfort.[27] Another RCT (50 people with rotator cuff tendinitis receiving treatments of interest) found similar adverse events with subacromial and intra-articular corticosteroid injection versus subacromial and intra-articular lidocaine alone (3/25 [12%, mild gastrointestinal symptoms; pityriasis rosea 2 days after the injection; increased frequency of urination] with corticosteroid injection *v* 3/25 [12%, mild gastrointestinal symptoms; diarrhoea; vasovagal reaction] with lidocaine injection).[28]

Comment: Range of movement is not a satisfactory surrogate measure of function. We found no evidence on the accuracy of placement of subacromial injections.

OPTION INTRA-ARTICULAR CORTICOSTEROID INJECTIONS

One small RCT found no significant difference for intra-articular triamcinolone versus saline in pain score, change in mobility, or function at 3 weeks. One small RCT found no significant difference for intra-articular methylprednisolone plus lidocaine versus lidocaine alone in pain or shoulder motion at 24 weeks. The RCTs were small and may have lacked power to detect clinically important differences.

Benefits: **Versus placebo:** We found no systematic review but found one RCT (37 people), which compared three injections of intra-articular triamcinolone versus saline.[30] It found no significant difference between triamcinolone and saline for pain score, change in mobility, or function at 3 weeks (visual analogue pain score 2.3 with triamcinolone *v* 0.2 with saline; median difference +1.9, 95% CI –0.1 to +3.0).[30] **Plus lidocaine (lignocaine) versus lidocaine alone:** We found one systematic review (search date 1998, 1 RCT, 48 people with frozen shoulder).[25] The RCT identified by the review compared four treatments: intra-articular methylprednisolone plus lidocaine versus intra-articular lidocaine versus intra-bursal methylprednisolone plus lidocaine versus intra-bursal lidocaine.[31] It found no significant difference for intra-articular methylprednisolone plus lidocaine versus lidocaine alone in mean pain score or total degrees of shoulder motion at 24 weeks (pain on 6 point pain scale [0 = no pain; 5 = most severe]: improvement of about 1 in point both groups [absolute score about 3 in both groups]; P > 0.05; shoulder motion: improvement of about 50° in both groups [absolute range of movement about 350° in both groups]; P > 0.05).[31] **Combined intra-articular and subacromial corticosteroid injections versus placebo:** See sub-acromial corticosteroid injection, p 1481.

Harms: Intra-articular injections are rarely associated with infection (estimated at 1/14 000 to 1/50 000 injections).[32,33] An acute self limited synovitis was reported in up to 2% of people. Prevalence of tendon rupture, including rupture of the bicipital tendon and rotator cuff, was reported at fewer than 1% of people after local injection of corticosteroids.[32] Subcutaneous fat necrosis or skin atrophy was found in fewer than 1%. Corticosteroid arthropathy and osteonecrosis were rare (< 0.8%) and seem to affect mostly weight bearing joints.[27] One RCT of corticosteroid injection versus physiotherapy in painful stiff shoulders reported more facial flushing (9/52 [17%] people treated with corticosteroid injections *v* 1/56 [2%] treated with physiotherapy) and more new menstrual irregularities (6/52 [12%] people treated with local corticosteroid injections *v* 0/56 [0%] after physiotherapy).[34] One small RCT found similar adverse reaction rates for triamcinolone versus saline injection (13/18 [72%] with triamcinolone *v* 12/19 [53%] with saline).[30]

Comment: Few RCTs of interventions in shoulder pain used high quality methods. One case control study found that clinical outcome correlated with accuracy of injection.[35] Another case control study found that only 10% of intra-articular injections were placed correctly even by experienced operators.[36] Confirmation of injection accuracy can be obtained with fluoroscopy or ultrasound. **Different doses:** We found one RCT (57 people with frozen shoulder).[37] It found that higher dose (40 mg) versus lower dose (10 mg) triamcinolone injection significantly reduced pain after 6 weeks (change on 100 mm visual analogue scale: 31 mm with low dose *v* 49 mm with high dose; no CI available; P < 0.01), movement restriction, and self rated functional impairment (change on 4 point ordinal scale: 0.7 with low dose *v* 1.3 with high dose; no CI available; P = 0.03), but did not significantly improve sleep disturbance. The RCT found no significant difference in any outcome after 6 months.

OPTION ORAL CORTICOSTEROIDS

Two small RCTs found no evidence of reduced pain or improved abduction with oral corticosteroids versus placebo. Adverse effects of corticosteroids are well documented.

Benefits: **Versus placebo:** We found no systematic review but found one RCT (32 people with frozen shoulder) that compared oral corticosteroids (cortisone acetate, 200 mg a day for first 3 days, 100 mg up to day 14 then 12.5 mg every 2 days up to 4 wks) versus placebo.[38] It found no evidence that oral corticosteroids reduced pain more than placebo after 18 weeks, but inter-group comparisons were not reported (mean improvement of 4 point rating scale [0 = no pain, 3 = severe pain]: from 1.4 at baseline to 0.5 with oral corticosteroids v 1.4 at baseline to 0.6 with placebo; P values not stated) or improved abduction (mean range of abduction from 75° at baseline to 154° with oral corticosteroids v 82° at baseline to 153° with placebo; no CI available; P values not stated).[38] **Plus home exercise versus home exercise alone:** We found one small RCT (40 people with frozen shoulder).[39] People in both groups also took non-salicylate analgesics and diazepam (5 mg) at night as needed. It found no significant difference for oral corticosteroids (10 mg for 4 wks and 5 mg for a further 2 wks) plus advice on home pendular exercises versus advice alone for pain or range of motion at 8 months (no figures available).[39]

Harms: Adverse effect of corticosteroids are well documented (see rheumatoid arthritis, p 1454 and asthma, p 1757). One RCT (40 people with frozen shoulder) reported mild indigestion in two people, which settled after reducing the dose of oral corticosteroids below 10 mg.[39] No other adverse events were reported. The other RCT did not report adverse events.[38]

Comment: None.

OPTION **PHYSIOTHERAPY (MANUAL TREATMENT AND EXERCISES)**

One systematic review has found insufficient evidence about effects of physiotherapy alone versus no treatment or advice alone in people with shoulder pain.

Benefits: **Versus no treatment:** We found one systematic review (search date 1998,[25] 1 RCT,[40] 19 people) of Maitland mobilisation (see glossary, p 1490) versus no treatment for frozen shoulder. The small RCT identified by the review compared four treatments: methylprednisolone acetate (20 mg) plus lidocaine (lignocaine) (1%); physiotherapy alone; ice pack alone and advice to do pendular home exercises.[40] It found no significant difference among treatments for pain at 3 months (no figures available).

Harms: One RCT of physiotherapy versus corticosteroid injection in people with painful stiff shoulders found frequent adverse effects in both groups (32/57 [56%] with physiotherapy *v* 30/57 [53%] with corticosteroid injection). After physiotherapy, these effects lasted longer than 2 days in 13% of people.[34] Fever during treatment was found in 1% of people and local skin irritation in 2% of people; 4% of people reported tingling, radiation of pain down the arm, or slight swelling after treatment.

Comment: Studies on the effects of physiotherapy in shoulder disorders are limited by the lack of standardised approaches. Diverse disorders are considered under the universal term shoulder pain, diverse forms of physiotherapy have been evaluated, and outcome measures and follow up periods vary.

OPTION **ULTRASOUND**

One systematic review and two subsequent RCTs found no clinically important difference in pain, abduction, or quality of life with ultrasound versus no treatment.

Benefits: We found one systematic review[41] and two subsequent RCTs.[42,43] The systematic review (search date 1997, 5 RCTs, 136 people) compared ultrasound versus placebo (sham ultrasound) and versus no treatment for shoulder disorders.[41] Clinical heterogeneity and insufficient description of outcome measures precluded pooling of results, but none of the individual RCTs found evidence of a clinically important effect of ultrasound versus placebo after 4–6 weeks. The first subsequent RCT (180 people with shoulder disorders who had failed to respond to 6 sessions of exercise) compared, in a blinded two by two factorial design, pulsed ultrasound versus dummy ultrasound, and bipolar interferential electrotherapy versus dummy electrotherapy.[42] It also included an additional control group that received no active or dummy treatments (39 people received only pulsed ultrasound and 68 received either no treatment or two dummy treatments). After 6 weeks, ultrasound was not significantly associated with improvement on a 7 point Likert scale (improvement occurred in 7/35 [20%] with no treatment *v* 19/73 [26%] with active ultrasound *v* 14/72 [19%] with dummy ultrasound; ARR for failure to improve with ultrasound *v* control treatments +6%, 95% CI −5% to +22%). Follow up at 12 months found no significant effect of ultrasound versus control treatments on the people reporting substantial improvement in functional status, pain, or range of movement. The second subsequent RCT (63 people, 70 shoulders) randomised shoulders, not people, to pulsed ultrasound (frequency 890 Hz; intensity 2.5 W/cm^2; pulsed mode 1 : 4) or an indistinguishable sham treatment over the area of calcification.[43] The first 15 treatments were given daily (5 times weekly) and the remainder three times weekly for 3 weeks. The treating therapist was blind to treatment allocation. Nine people (9 shoulders) did not complete the treatment: three in the ultrasound group and six in the sham group, two in the latter because of pain. The RCT found no significant difference between ultrasound versus sham treatment in pain or quality of life scores at 9 months (improvement in 15 point pain score 5.7 points with ultrasound *v* 4.0 points with sham, P = 0.23; improvement in 10 cm visual analogue quality of life score 2.4 cm with ultrasound *v* 1.9 cm with sham, P = 0.52).[43]

Harms: The systematic review and RCTs did not report on adverse events.[40–42]

Comment: In most RCTs, with the exception of the most recent,[42] there was considerable heterogeneity of the groups, interventions, and follow up duration among the RCTs. It is not clear if ultrasound machines were always adequately calibrated before use.

OPTION LASER TREATMENT

We found different results from four small RCTs that compared laser treatment versus placebo in shoulder pain. Two short term RCTs found that laser improved recovery rate and pain compared with placebo at 2–4 weeks. However, two longer term RCTs found no significant difference in pain or recovery rate at 8–12 weeks.

Benefits: We found no systematic review but found four placebo controlled RCTs.[44–47] The first RCT (35 people) found no significant difference between continuous irradiation laser versus dummy laser (10 min sessions, twice weekly for 8 wks) for pain or abduction at 8 weeks (pain on 10 cm visual analogue scale: improved by 3.6 cm with laser *v* 1.2 cm with placebo; P = 0.34; range of movement improved by 36° with laser *v* 29° with placebo; P = 0.23).[44] The second RCT (91 people) found that recovery rate was higher with laser than placebo at 1 month (42/47 [89%] *v* 18/44 [41%]; ARR 48%, 95% CI 31% to 65%).[45] The third RCT (20 people with rotator cuff tendinitis) found that low level infrared laser (5 mins 3 times weekly for 2 wks) versus dummy laser treatment reduced pain after 2 weeks (mean score difference 2.5%, 95% CI 2.0% to 3.0%).[46] The fourth RCT (24 people with supraspinatus tendinitis) found no significant difference for low level laser (9 treatments over a 3 wk period) versus placebo in shoulder pain at 12 weeks (no figures available).[47]

Harms: We found no evidence on harms.

Comment: The quality of studies on the effects of laser treatment in shoulder disorders is limited by the lack of standardised approaches.

OPTION ELECTRICAL STIMULATION

One RCT found no significant difference in pain between electrical stimulation versus control. However, the study may have lacked power to detect clinically important differences.

Benefits: **Versus control:** We found no systematic review but found two RCTs.[42,48] One RCT (180 people with shoulder disorders not improved by 6 exercise sessions) compared electrical stimulation (bipolar interferential electrical stimulation (see glossary, p 1490)) versus dummy electrical stimulation, and pulsed ultrasound versus dummy ultrasound in a blinded two by two factorial design (see benefits of ultrasound, p 1485).[42] After 6 weeks, it found no significant difference in the proportion of people who reported a "large improvement" (AR 17/73 [23%] with electrical stimulation *v* 16/72 [22%] with control; ARR +1%, 95% CI –13% to +15%). The second RCT (29 people with rotator cuff tendinitis not cured by corticosteroid injection) compared electrical stimulation induced by pulsed electromagnetic fields (5–9 h/day for 4 wks) versus placebo, but it did not report the number of people symptomless after 4 weeks.[48]

Harms: We found no evidence on harms.

Comment: The quality of studies on the effects of electrical treatments in shoulder disorders is limited by the lack of standardised approaches. We found no good evidence that different forms of electrical stimulation produce different effects.

OPTION ICE

We found no good evidence about the effects of ice.

Benefits: We found no systematic review or RCTs.

Harms: We found no evidence on harms.

Comment: None.

OPTION INTRA-ARTICULAR GUANETHIDINE

We found no systematic review or RCTs of intra-articular guanethidine in people with non-arthritic shoulder pain.

Benefits: We found no systematic review or RCTs of intra-articular guanethidine in people with non-arthritic shoulder pain (see comment below).

Harms: We found no RCTs.

Comment: We found one RCT (18 people with resistant shoulder pain, including 6 people with rheumatoid arthritis, 5 with osteoarthritis, 5 with frozen shoulder, 1 with rotator cuff tendinitis, and 1 with psoriatic arthritis) comparing intra-articular guanethidine versus intra-articular saline.[49] It found that guanethidine reduced pain more than placebo after 8 weeks (mean improvement on a 10 cm visual analogue scale: 36% with guanethidine *v* 16% with placebo; $P < 0.05$), but no significant change in range of movement (mean range of abduction 53° at baseline and 52° at 8 wks with guanethidine *v* 57° at baseline and 56° at 8 wks with placebo; no CI available).

OPTION TRANSDERMAL GLYCERYL TRINITRATE

We found no reliable RCTs.

Benefits: We found no systematic review but found one small RCT (20 people with supraspinatus tendinitis) of local transdermal glyceryl trinitrate versus placebo.[50] The RCT did not report direct comparisons between the treatment and placebo groups (see comment below).

Harms: Headaches were reported in 20% of the treatment group 24 hours after the treatment was started (no comparative figures available).[50]

Comment: The RCT[50] found a significant decrease when comparing pain scores 24 hours after glyceryl trinitrate with pain scores measured at baseline (mean pain intensities with active treatment measured on a 0–10 analogue scale: 7.1 at baseline; 4.5 at 24 h, $P < 0.001$; 2.0 at 48 h, $P < 0.001$). Changes in the placebo group were not reported. Relief was maintained after 15 days (figures not available). Mean duration of pain was also significantly reduced with active treatment (figures not available). Mean mobility (assessor rated 4 point scale) significantly improved with active treatment (2.0 at baseline *v* 0.1 at 5 days; P < 0.0001), but not with placebo (1.2 at baseline *v* 1.2 at 15 days). The significance figures quoted are not direct comparisons. Significance figures for treatment versus placebo were not stated.

OPTION PHONOPHORESIS

We found no RCTs solely in people with shoulder pain.

Benefits: **Versus placebo or sham phonophoresis:** See glossary, p 1490. We found no RCTs solely in people with shoulder pain (see comment below). **Phonophoresis alone versus other treatment:** We found no RCTs.

Harms: Adverse effects were not reported.

Comment: One RCT (24 people, 13 with rotator cuff tendinitis, 1 with biceps tendinitis, 1 triceps tendinitis, 9 with knee tendinitis) compared active phonophoresis (see glossary, p 1490) using topical dexamethasone, lidocaine (lignocaine), and aqueous gel versus placebo phonophoresis using aqueous gel only (5 sessions over 5–10 days). It found no significant difference in perceived pain (visual analogue scale [0 cm = no pain, 10 cm = extreme pain]; pain changed from 2.4 cm to 1.3 cm with active treatment *v* from 2.6 cm to 1.5 cm with placebo; not significant, but P value not stated). It found no significant effect for tenderness (localised force needed to elicit pain: 198 g, 95% CI 164 g to 235 g at session 1 to 204 g, 95% CI 170 g to 238 g at session 5 with active phonophoresis *v* 196 g, 95% CI 153 g to 235 g at session 1 to 249 g, 95% CI 221 g to 275 g at session 5 with placebo phonophoresis).[51]

OPTION EXTRACORPOREAL SHOCK WAVE THERAPY

Three RCTs compared extracorporeal shock wave therapy versus sham treatment or no treatment and found different results. One RCT found that one or two sessions of high energy extracorporeal shock wave therapy versus placebo improved pain and function in people with calcific tendinitis. One RCT found no significant difference for extracorporeal shock wave therapy versus sham treatment in shoulder pain or night pain at 3 or 6 months in people with non-calcifying rotator cuff tendinosis. One RCT found no significant difference for extracorporeal shock wave therapy versus sham treatment in shoulder function or pain at 12 weeks in people with chronic suprapinatus tendinosis. The RCTs were small and may have lacked power to detect a clinically important difference.

Benefits: We found no systematic review but found three RCTs.[52–54] The first RCT (115 people with calcific tendinitis) compared three different extracorporeal shock wave therapy regimens (low energy treatment in a single session *v* a single high energy session *v* 2 high energy sessions 1 wk apart) versus no treatment.[52] It found that high energy treatment increased subjective improvement of pain compared with low energy treatment or placebo at 3 months (81 people analysed; AR for improvement 14/20 [70%] with 2 high energy sessions *v* 12/20 [60%] with 1 high energy session *v* 6/21 [29%]

with low energy treatment v 0/20 [0%] with placebo; NNT 2 for high energy treatment compared with placebo, 95% CI 1 to 21 for single session and 1–14 for 2 session treatment). It also found that high energy treatment versus placebo significantly improved a combined measure of pain and function in activities of daily living (the Constant score difference; $P < 0.0001$). The second RCT (74 people with chronic non-calcifying rotator cuff tendinitis) found no significant difference for extracorporeal shock wave therapy (1500 pulses at 0.12 mJ/mm) versus sham treatment (3 sessions at monthly intervals) in shoulder pain or night pain at 3 or 6 months (improvement of 50% from baseline for shock wave therapy versus sham at 3 months on SPAD index (see glossary, p 1490): OR 1.760, 95% CI 0.081 to 0.710; night pain OR 0.94, 95% CI 0.65 to 1.36).[53] The third RCT (40 people with chronic supraspinatus tendinosis, 38 analysed) found no significant difference for extracorporeal shock wave therapy (6000 pulses at 0.11 mJ/mm) versus sham treatment (2 sessions weekly for 3 wks) in function or pain at 12 weeks (difference treatment v control: pain at rest on 10 point visual analogue scale +1.4, 95% CI –1.0 to +3.9; pain during activity on 10 point scale: +2.5, 95% CI –0.81 to +3.33).[54]

Harms: High intensity extracorporeal shock wave therapy can be painful during treatment. Small haematomas were reported in the first RCT, but the incidence was not stated and they could have been related to subcutaneous infiltration of local anaesthetic before treatment.[52]

Comment: The first RCT found no significant difference for two sessions versus a single session of extracorporeal shock wave therapy for continued pain (91 people analysed; 23/49 [47%] with 2 sessions v 23/42 [55%] with 1 session; RR of continued pain 0.85, 95% CI 0.50 to 1.23).[52] The mechanism of action of extracorporeal shock wave therapy remains unclear. There was radiological disappearance or disintegration of calcium deposits in a significantly greater proportion of people who received high energy treatment than placebo; 77% of those receiving two sessions of treatment had radiological disappearance or disintegration of calcium deposits after 6 months compared with 47% who had one session ($P = 0.05$).[52] Technical factors and the dosing regime of shockwave administration are likely to be important to clinical outcome.

OPTION SURGERY/FORCED MANIPULATION

We found no placebo controlled RCTs. One small RCT found that forced manipulation plus intra-articular hydrocortisone injection versus intra-articular hydrocortisone injection alone increased recovery rate at 3 months.

Benefits: **Versus placebo:** We found no systematic review and no RCTs. **Forced manipulation plus intra-articular hydrocortisone injection versus intra-articular hydrocortisone injection alone:** We found one RCT (30 people with frozen shoulder).[55] It found that forced manipulation under sedation plus intra-articular hydrocortisone injection alone increased recovery rates compared with intra-articular hydrocortisone injection at 3 months (recovery defined as no disability: 7/15 [47%] with forced manipulations v 2/15 [13%] with control; ARI 33%, 95% CI 1% to 65%).[55]

Shoulder pain

Harms: The RCT did not report adverse effects.[55]

Comment: There is a need for RCTs of specific surgical interventions in people with shoulder pain.

OPTION MULTIDISCIPLINARY BIOPSYCHOSOCIAL REHABILITATION

One systematic review found no good quality RCTs in people with shoulder pain of multidisciplinary biopsychosocial rehabilitation.

Benefits: We found one systematic review (search date 1998).[56] It found no good quality RCTs solely in people with shoulder pain of multidisciplinary biopsychosocial rehabilitation (see glossary, p 1490) versus usual treatment (see comment below).

Harms: The review found no reliable RCTs.[56]

Comment: The systematic review found one low quality RCT (70 people aged 20–55 years) in people with chronic neck and shoulder pain).[56] Co-interventions were not avoided, blinding of therapists was not specified, analysis was not by intention to treat, and treatment groups were dissimilar at baseline. It found no significant difference for multidisciplinary biopsychosocial rehabilitation versus usual treatment. The rehabilitation combined physiotherapy with psychological, behavioural, and educational interventions.

OPTION ARTHROSCOPIC LASER SUBACROMIAL DECOMPRESSION

One systematic review found no RCTs about arthroscopic subacromial decompression with a holmium:YAG laser.

Benefits: We found one systematic review (search date 2000) of arthroscopic subacromial decompression with holmium:YAG laser for people with shoulder pain due to impingement syndrome.[57] It identified no RCTs.

Harms: We found no evidence of harms.

Comment: None.

GLOSSARY

Interferential electrical stimulation Typically a high frequency current (4000 Hz) amplitude modulated at a lower frequency (60–100 Hz) given in bursts of 4 seconds and repeated for up to 15 minutes.

Maitland mobilisation A graded system of manipulations and exercises intended to increase mobility of specific joints.

Multidisciplinary biopsychosocial rehabilitation Combined physical, social, and psychological rehabilitation.

Phonophoresis The application of topical medication followed by ultrasound to the same area; the theory being that the ultrasound energy drives the medication through the skin.

SPAD index A self administered instrument for measuring pain (5 items) and disability (8 items).

REFERENCES

1. Royal College of General Practitioners; Office of Populations, Censuses and Surveys. Third National Morbidity Survey in General Practice, 1980–1981; Department of Health and Social Security, series MB5 No 1. London: HMSO.
2. Bergunnud H, Lindgarde F, Nilsson B, et al. Shoulder pain in middle age. *Clin Orthop* 1988;231:234–238.
3. McCormack RR, Inman RD, Wells A, et al. Prevalence of tendinitis and related disorders of the upper extremity in a manufacturing workforce. *J Rheumatol* 1990;17:958–964.
4. Allander E. Prevalence, incidence and remission rates of some common rheumatic diseases or syndromes. *Scand J Rheumatol* 1974;3:145–153.
5. Badley EM, Tennant A. Changing profile of joint disorders with age: findings from a postal survey of the population of Calderdale, West Yorkshire, UK. *Ann Rheum Dis* 1992;51:366–371.
6. Andersson HI, Ejlertsson G, Leden I, et al. Chronic pain in a geographically defined general population: studies of differences in age, gender, social class and pain localisation. *Clin J Pain* 1993;9:174–182.
7. Pope DP, Croft PR, Pritchard CM, et al. The frequency of restricted range of movement in individuals with self-reported shoulder pain: results from a population-based survey. *Br J Rheumatol* 1996:35;1137–1141.
8. Chard M, Hazleman R, Hazleman BL, et al. Shoulder disorders in the elderly: a community survey. *Arthritis Rheum* 1991;34:766–769.
9. Vecchio-P, Kavanagh R, Hazleman BL, et al. Shoulder pain in a community-based rheumatology clinic. *Br J Rheumatol* 1995;34:440–442.
10. Lundberg B. The frozen shoulder. *Acta Orthop Scand* 1969:suppl 119.
11. Riordan J, Dieppe PA. Arthritis of the glenohumeral joint. *Baillieres Clin Rheumatol* 1989;3:607–626.
12. Bonutti PM, Hawkins RJ. Rotator cuff disorders. *Baillieres Clin Rheumatol* 1989;3:535–550.
13. Jobe FW, Kvitne RS. Shoulder pain in the overhand or throwing athlete: the relationship of anterior instability and rotator cuff impingement. *Orthop Rev* 1989;18:963–975.
14. Soslowsky LJ, An CH, Johnston SP, et al. Geometric and mechanical properties of the coracoacromial ligament and their relationship to rotator cuff disease. *Clin Orthop* 1994;304:10–17.
15. Nash P, Hazleman BL. Frozen shoulder. *Baillieres Clin Rheumatol* 1989;3:551–566.
16. Wohlgethan JR. Frozen shoulder in hyperthyroidism. *Arthritis Rheum* 1987;30:936–939.
17. Vecchio PC, Kavanagh RT, Hazleman BL, et al. Community survey of shoulder disorders in the elderly to assess the natural history and effects of treatment. *Ann Rheumatol Dis* 1995;54:152–154.
18. Croft P, Pope D, Silman A. The clinical course of shoulder pain: prospective cohort study in primary care. *BMJ* 1996;313:601–602.
19. Roach KE, Budiman-Mak E, Songsiridej N, et al. Development of a shoulder pain and disability index. *Arthritis Care Res* 1991;4:143–149.
20. Croft P, Pope D, Zonca M, et al. Measurement of shoulder related disability: results of a validation study. *Ann Rheum Dis* 1994;53:525–528.
21. Beaton DE, Richards RR. Measuring function of the shoulder. A cross-sectional comparison of five questionnaires. *J Bone Joint Surg Am* 1996;78;882–890.
22. Gerber C. Integrated scoring systems for the functional assessment of the shoulder. In: Matsen III FA, Fu EH, Hawkins RJ, eds. *The shoulder: a balance of mobility and stability.* Rosemont, Illinois, US: The American Academy of Orthopaedic Surgeons, 1993:531–550.
23. Richards RR, An KN, Bigliani LU, et al. A standardised method for the assessment of shoulder function. *J Shoulder Elbow Surg* 1994;3:347–352.
24. L'Insalata JC, Warren RF, Cohen SF, et al. A self-administered questionnaire for assessment of symptoms and function of the shoulder. *J Bone Joint Surg* 1997;79:738–748.
25. Green S, Buchbinder R, Glazier R, et al. Interventions for shoulder pain. In: The Cochrane Library, Issue 3, 2001. Oxford: Update Software. Search date 1998; primary sources Cochrane Musculoskeletal Group trials register, Cochrane Controlled Trials Register, Medline, Embase, Cinahl, and Science Citation Index, and hand searches of major textbooks, bibliographies of relevant literature, the fugitive literature, and the subject indices of relevant journals.
26. Mena HR, Lomen PL, Turner LF, et al. Treatment of acute shoulder syndrome with flurbiprofen. *Am J Med* 1986;80:141–144.
27. Adejabo AO, Nash P, Hazleman BL. A prospective blind dummy placebo controlled study comparing triamcinolone hexacetonide injection with oral diclofenac 50 mg tds in patients with rotator cuff tendinitis. *J Rheumatol* 1990;17:1207–1210.
28. Petri M, Dobrow R, Neiman R, et al. Randomised double blind, placebo controlled study of the treatment of the painful shoulder. *Arthritis Rheum* 1987;30:1040–1045.
29. Vecchio PC, Hazleman BL, King RH. A double-blind trial comparing subacromial methylprednisolone and lignocaine in acute rotator cuff tendinitis. *Br J Rheumatol* 1993;32:743–745.
30. Snels IA, Beckerman H, Twisk JW, et al. Effect of triamcinolone acetonide injections on hemiplegic shoulder pain: a randomized clinical trial. *Stroke* 2000;31:2396–2401
31. Rizk T, Pinals R, Talaiver A. Corticosteroid injections in adhesive capsulitis: investigation of their value and site. *Arch Phys Med* 1991;72:20–22.
32. Gray RG, Gottlieb NL. Intra-articular corticosteroids. An updated assessment. *Clin Orth* 1983;177:235–263.
33. Hollander JL. The use of intra-articular hydrocortisone, its analogues, and its higher esters in arthritis. *Md Med J* 1970;61:511.
34. Van der Windt DA, Koes BW, Deville W, et al. Effectiveness of corticosteroid injections versus physiotherapy for treatment of painful stiff shoulder in primary care: randomised trial. *BMJ* 1998;317:1292–1296.
35. Eustace JA, Brophy DP, Gibney RP, et al. Comparison of the accuracy of steroid placement with clinical outcome in patients with shoulder symptoms. *Ann Rheum Dis* 1997;56:59–63.
36. Jones A, Regan M, Ledingham J, et al. Importance of placement of intra-articular steroid injections. *BMJ* 1993;307:1329–1330.
37. De Jong BA, Dahmen R, Hogeweg JA, et al. Intra-articular triamcinolone acetonide injection in patients with capsulitis of the shoulder: a comparative study of two dose regimens. *Clin Rehabil* 1998;12:211–215.
38. Blockey N, Wright J. Oral cortisone therapy in periarthritis of the shoulder. *BMJ* 1954;i:1455–1457.

39. Binder A, Hazleman BL, Parr G, et al. A controlled study of oral prednisolone in frozen shoulder. *Br J Rheum* 1986;25:288–292.
40. Bulgen D, Binder A, Hazleman B, et al. Frozen shoulder: prospective clinical study with an evaluation of three treatment regimes. *Ann Rheum Dis* 1984;43:353–360.
41. Van der Windt DAWM, Van der Heijden GJMG, Van der Berg SGM, et al. Ultrasound therapy for musculoskeletal disorders: a systematic review. *Pain* 1999;81:257–271. Search date 1997; primary sources Medline, Embase, and Cochrane Database of Randomised Clinical Trials.
42. Van der Heijden GJMG, Leffers P, Wolters PJMC, et al. No effect of bipolar interferential electrotherapy and pulsed ultrasound for soft tissue shoulder disorders: a randomised controlled trial. *Ann Rheum Dis* 1999;58:530–540.
43. Ebenbichler GR, Erdogmus CB, Resch KL, et al. Ultrasound therapy for calcific tendinitis of the shoulder. *N Engl J Med* 1999;340:1533–1588.
44. Vecchio P, Cave C, King V, et al. A double blind study of the effectiveness of low level laser treatment of rotator cuff tendinitis. *Br J Rheumatol* 1993;32:740–742.
45. Gudmundssen J, Vikne J. Laser treatment for epicondylitis humeri and rotator cuff syndrome. *Nord Tidskr Idrettsmed* 1987;2:6–15.
46. England S, Farrell A, Coppock J, et al. Low laser therapy of shoulder tendinitis. *Scand J Rheumatol* 1989;18:427–443.
47. Saunders L. The efficacy of low level laser therapy in supraspinatus tendinitis. *Clin Rehabil* 1995;9:126–134.
48. Binder A, Parr G, Hazleman B. Pulsed electromagnetic field therapy of persistent rotator cuff tendinitis. *Lancet* 1984;1:695–698.
49. Gado I, Emery P. Intra-articular guanethidine injection for resistant shoulder pain: a preliminary double blind study of a novel approach. *Ann Rheum Dis* 1996;55:199–201.
50. Berrazueta JR, Losada A, Poveda J, et al. Successful treatment of shoulder pain syndrome due to supraspinatus tendinitis with transdermal nitroglycerin. A double blind study. *Pain* 1996;66:63–67.
51. Penderghest CE, Kimura IF, Gulick DT. Double-blind clinical efficacy study of pulsed phonophoresis on perceived pain associated with symptomatic tendinitis. *J Sport Rehab* 1998;7:9–19.
52. Loew M, Daecke W, Kusnierczak D, et al. Shock-wave therapy is effective for chronic calcifying tendinitis of the shoulder. *J Bone Joint Surg Br* 1999;81:863–867.
53. Speed CA, Richards C, Nichols D, et al. Extracorporeal shock-wave therapy for tendinitis of the rotator cuff. A double-blind, randomised, controlled trial. *J Bone Joint Surg* 2002;84:509–512.
54. Schmitt J, Haake M, Tosche A, et al. Low-energy extracorporeal shock-wave treatment for tendinitis of the supraspinatus. *J Bone Joint Surg* 2001;83:873–876.
55. Thomas D, Williams R, Smith D. The frozen shoulder. A review of manipulative treatment. *Rheumatol Rehab* 1980;19:173–179.
56. Karjalainen K, Malmivaara A, van Tulder M, et al. Multidisciplinary biopsychosocial rehabilitation for neck and shoulder pain among working age adults. In: The Cochrane Library, Issue 3, 2001. Oxford: Update Software. Search date 1998; primary sources Medline, Embase, Cochrane Library, Medic (Finnish medical database), Science Citation Index, and hand searches of reference lists and contact with 24 experts in the field of rehabilitation.
57. Boult M, Wicks M, Watson DI, et al. Arthroscopic Subacromial Decompression with a holmium : YAG laser: review of the literature. *ANZ J Surg* 2001;71:172–177. Search date 2000; primary sources Medline, Embase, Current Contents, and The Cochrane Library.

Cathy Speed
Rheumatologist/Director of Sports and Exercise Medicine Unit

Brian Hazleman
Senior Consultant

Addenbrooke's Hospital
Cambridge
UK

Competing interests: None declared.

Tennis elbow

Search date August 2002

Willem Assendelft, Sally Green, Rachelle Buchbinder, Peter Struijs, and Nynke Smidt

QUESTIONS

INTERVENTIONS

See glossary, p 1502

Key Messages

- **Acupuncture** One systematic review and one subsequent RCT found insufficient evidence to assess the effects of acupuncture (either needle or laser).
- **Corticosteroid injections** We found one systematic review and two subsequent RCTs of corticosteroid injections, which found limited evidence of a short term improvement in symptoms with steroid injections versus placebo, a local anaesthetic, elbow strapping, or physiotherapy. It found no good evidence on long term effects of corticosteroids versus placebo or local anaesthetic. It found no evidence of a difference with corticosteroid injection versus mobilisation plus massage or versus elbow strapping in overall improvement at 1 year. However, one RCT identified by the review found significantly greater improvement in symptoms with physiotherapy versus an injection at 26 and 52 weeks. The review found limited evidence of greater self perceived improvement at 4 weeks with corticosteroid injection versus an oral non-steroidal anti-inflammatory drug (NSAID), but found greater improvement in pain at 26 weeks with an oral non-steroidal anti-inflammatory drug.
- **Exercise and mobilisation** One systematic review found limited evidence of a better outcome with exercise versus ultrasound plus friction massage at 8 weeks.
- **Extra-corporeal shock wave therapy** One systematic review found conflicting evidence from two RCTs of the effects on symptoms of extra-corporeal shock wave therapy versus sham treatment.
- **Non-steroidal anti-inflammatory drugs for longer term pain relief** We found insufficient evidence to assess the longer term effects of oral or topical non-steroidal anti-inflammatory drugs.

- **Oral non-steroidal anti-inflammatory drugs** One systematic review found limited evidence of a short term improvement in pain and function with an oral non-steroidal anti-inflammatory drug versus placebo. The review found limited evidence that fewer people receiving an oral non-steroidal anti-inflammatory drug versus a corticosteroid injection had self perceived improvement at 4 weeks, but found that an oral non-steroidal anti-inflammatory drug significantly reduced pain at 26 weeks. We found insufficient evidence to assess the longer term effects of oral or topical non-steroidal anti-inflammatory drugs.
- **Orthoses** One systematic review found insufficient evidence about the effects of orthoses (braces).
- **Surgery** One systematic review found no RCTs of surgical treatment for tennis elbow.
- **Topical non-steroidal anti-inflammatory drugs for short term pain relief** One systematic review has found that topical non-steroidal anti-inflammatory drugs versus placebo significantly improve pain in the short term. Minor adverse effects have been reported. We found no RCTs comparing oral versus topical non-steroidal anti-inflammatory drugs.

DEFINITION Tennis elbow has many analogous terms, including lateral elbow pain, lateral epicondylitis, rowing elbow, tendonitis of the common extensor origin, and peritendonitis of the elbow. Tennis elbow is characterised by pain and tenderness over the lateral epicondyle of the humerus and pain on resisted dorsi-flexion of the wrist, middle finger, or both. For the purposes of this review, tennis elbow is restricted to lateral elbow pain or lateral epicondylitis.

INCIDENCE/ PREVALENCE Lateral elbow pain is common (population prevalence 1–3%).[1] Peak incidence is 40–50 years, and for women of 42–46 years of age the incidence increases to 10%.[2,3] The incidence of lateral elbow pain in general practice is 4–7/1000 people a year.[3–5]

AETIOLOGY/ RISK FACTORS Tennis elbow is considered to be an overload injury, typically after minor and often unrecognised trauma of the extensor muscles of the forearm. Despite the title tennis elbow, tennis is a direct cause in only 5% of those with epicondylitis.[6]

PROGNOSIS Although lateral elbow pain is generally self limiting, in a minority of people symptoms persist for 18 months to 2 years and in some cases for much longer.[7] The cost is therefore high, both in terms of lost productivity and healthcare use. In a general practice trial of an expectant waiting policy, 80% of the people with elbow pain of already greater than 4 weeks' duration were recovered after 1 year.[8]

AIMS OF INTERVENTION To reduce lateral elbow pain and improve function.

OUTCOMES Pain at rest, with activities and resisted movements (visual analogue scale or Likert scale); function (validated disability questionnaire, includes 30 point Disabilities of the Arm, Shoulder, and Hand questionnaire, or visual analogue scale or Likert scale); quality of life (validated questionnaire); grip strength (dynamometer); return to work, normal activities, or both; overall participant reported improvement; adverse effects (participant or researcher report);

Roles-Maudsley subjective pain score where 1 = excellent, no pain, full movement, full activity; 2 = good, occasional discomfort, full movement and full activity; 3 = fair, some discomfort after prolonged activity; and 4 = poor, pain limiting activities.

METHODS *Clinical Evidence* search and appraisal August 2002. Studies were included based on the criteria: all randomised and quasi-RCTs of any of the listed interventions in (1) people older than 16 years of age; (2) lateral elbow pain for greater than 3 weeks' duration; (3) no history of significant trauma or systemic inflammatory conditions such as rheumatoid arthritis; and (4) studies of various soft tissue diseases and pain due to tendinitis at all sites, were included provided that the lateral elbow pain results were presented separately or that greater than 90% of people had lateral elbow pain.

QUESTION **What are the effects of treatments for reducing pain and improving function in tennis elbow (lateral epicondylitis)?**

OPTION **ACUPUNCTURE**

Sally E Green and Rachelle Buchbinder

One systematic review and one subsequent RCT found insufficient evidence to assess the effects of acupuncture (either needle or laser).

Benefits: We found one systematic review (search date 2001, 4 RCTs, 239 people with tennis elbow defined as lateral elbow pain aggravated by wrist and finger dorsiflexion)[9] and one subsequent RCT.[10] The review found that, because of problems with methods of the included trials (particularly small populations, uncertain allocation concealment, and substantial loss to follow up) and clinical differences between trials, results could not be combined in a meta-analysis. The first RCT (48 people) comparing needle acupuncture versus sham acupuncture (with needles not inserted) found significantly longer pain relief with acupuncture (WMD 18.8 h, 95% CI 10.1 to 27.5) and a significantly increased proportion of people with greater than or equal to 50% reduction in pain after one treatment (19/24 [79%] with acupuncture *v* 6/24 [25%] with sham treatment; RR 3.2, 95% 1.5 to 6.5).[11] The second RCT found needle acupuncture versus sham treatment significantly increased the proportion of people with a self reported good or excellent result (22/44 [50%] with needle acupuncture *v* 8/38 [21%] with sham treatment; RR 2.4, 95% CI 1.2 to 4.7) after 10 treatments. However, it found no significant differences in the longer term (after 3 or 12 months).[12] The third RCT compared laser (see glossary, p 1502) acupuncture versus sham treatment. It found no significant difference in participant report of no improvement or worse (after 10 sessions: 13/23 [56.5%] with laser *v* 9/26 [34.6%] with sham treatment, RR 1.36, 95% CI 0.48 to 3.86; at 3 months: 0.38, 95% CI 0.09 to 1.69; after 12 months: 3.47, 95% CI 0.15 to 80.36). The fourth RCT found no significant difference in cure rate (method of defining cure not defined) between vitamin B12 injection plus acupuncture versus vitamin B12 injection alone (risk of cure with B12 injection alone: RR 0.44, 95% CI 0.15 to 1.29). The subsequent RCT (45 people) compared 10 treatments of acupuncture versus sham acupuncture.[10] It found significantly greater reductions in pain intensity and functional impairment with acupuncture versus sham treatment at 2 weeks (on 30 mm visual analogue scale pain improved by 8.43 with acupuncture *v* 4.89 with sham treatment, $P < 0.05$; Disabilities of the Arm, Shoulder, and Hand questionnaire improved by 23.70 with acupuncture *v* 8.54 with sham treatment, $P < 0.05$). At 2 months, only the difference for functional impairment was significant. We found no RCT on the effect of acupuncture on quality of life, strength, or return to work.

Harms: The RCTs identified by the review did not report on adverse events.[9]

Comment: Although statistically significant, an increase of 18 hours in pain relief after needle acupuncture may not be clinically important.[9]

OPTION ORTHOSES (BRACING)

Willem JJ Assendelft and Peter AA Struijs

One systematic review found insufficient evidence about the effects of orthoses (braces).

Benefits: We found one systematic review (search date 1999).[13] Results were not pooled because of large heterogeneity among trials. **Versus placebo or no treatment:** The review identified no RCTs.[13] We found no subsequent RCTs. **Versus corticosteroid injections:** The review found two RCTs comparing orthoses versus corticosteroid injections.[13] The first RCT (16 people) compared an orthotic device versus corticosteroid injections. It found no significant difference in short term improvement in pain (improvement: 27.1 with corticosteroid *v* 13.6 with orthotic device; 100 mm visual analogue score difference +13.5, 95% CI −4.6 to +31.6).[13] The second RCT (70 people, 4 treatment groups) found that corticosteroid injection versus a splint or elbow band significantly increased the proportion of people having a good or excellent self reported outcome at 2 weeks (AR 34/37 [92%] pooled results for splint and elbow band group *v* 6/19 [32%] with injection; RR 2.9; 95% CI 1.8 to 5.7); however, the difference was not significant in the medium or long term (6 months: 19/37 [51%] *v* 14/19 [74%]; RR 0.7, 95% CI 0.46 to 1.05; 12 months: 22/37 [59%] *v* 13/19 [68%]; RR 0.9, 95% CI 0.6 to 1.03).[13] **Versus physiotherapy:** The review found one RCT (84 people) comparing an elbow support versus an unspecified physical therapy.[13] It found no significant difference in short term self reported satisfaction (23/49 [47%] with elbow support *v* 16/35 [46%] with unspecified physical therapy; RR 1.03; 95% CI 0.64 to 1.64). This study had insufficient information to assess pain improvement. It also had a withdrawal rate of 30% and results seem to be completor analysis. **Versus non-steroidal anti-inflammatory cream:** The review found 1 RCT (17 people) comparing a non-steroidal anti-inflammatory cream (AI cream; details of cream not provided in review) versus an elbow strap.[13] It found greater short term pain reduction with AI cream (WMD [scale not specified] 0.38, 95% CI 0.02 to 0.70).

Harms: The systematic review did not report on harms.[13]

Comment: The review reported that validity scores for the RCTs ranged from low to medium.[13] The review identified three RCTs comparing adding an orthotic device to corticosteroid injections or ultrasound. All three RCTs reported only short term results and there was insufficient data or too low power to indicate the effect of orthoses.

OPTION CORTICOSTEROID INJECTIONS

Willem JJ Assendelft and Nynke Smidt

One systematic review and two subsequent RCTs of corticosteroid injections found limited evidence of a short term improvement in symptoms with steroid injections versus placebo, a local anaesthetic, elbow strapping, or physiotherapy. It found no good evidence on long term effects of corticosteroids versus placebo or local anaesthetic. It found no evidence of a difference with corticosteroid injection versus mobilisation plus massage or elbow strapping in overall improvement at 1 year. However, one RCT identified by the review found significantly greater improvement in symptoms with physiotherapy versus an injection at 26 and 52 weeks. The review found limited evidence of greater self perceived improvement at 4 weeks with corticosteroid injections versus an oral non-steroidal anti-inflammatory drug, but found greater improvement in pain at 26 weeks with an oral non-steroidal anti-inflammatory drug.

Benefits: We found one systematic review (search date 1999)[14] and two subsequent RCTs.[15,16] **Versus placebo or no treatment:** The review identified two RCTs comparing steroid injection (1 mL methylprednisolone acetate) versus saline solution. The first RCT (29 people in smallest group) found a significantly lower chance of short term (not specified) global improvement with the placebo (RR 0.11, 95% CI 0.04 to 0.33). The RCT did not measure pain or grip strength. The second RCT (10 people in smallest group) found no significant difference in short term pain, global improvement, or grip strength. We found one subsequent RCT (39 people with symptoms > 4 wks) of corticosteroid injection versus a control injection.[15] All people received rehabilitation. It found that cotricosteroid injection significantly improved pain on a visual analogue scale from 8 weeks to 6 months (100 point visual analogue scale improvement: 24.3 with steroid injection *v* 8.9 with control injection; P = 0.04; CI not available). It found no significant difference in other pain outcomes or grip strength. We found one subsequent RCT (59 people in smallest group) of a corticosteroid injection versus no treatment versus physiotherapy.[16] It found corticosteroid injection versus no treatment significantly improved mean "main complaint" and functional disability at 3 and 6 weeks (at 6 wk mean difference in "main complaint" 24%, 95% CI 14% to 35%). It found no significant difference at 12, 26, and 52 weeks, and the mean was non-significantly worse with steroid injection at 26 and 52 weeks (at 52 wk mean difference in "main complaint" –9%, 95% CI –19% to +2%). **Versus local anaesthetic:** The review identified three RCTs comparing corticosteroid injections versus local anaesthetic alone.[14] Two RCTs (18 and 35 people in smallest groups) found an improvement in short term (4 wks; follow up not stated) global improvement with corticosteroid injections (1 mL hydrocortisone acetate 25 mg and 1 mL methylprednisolone acetate 10 mg), but data could not be pooled because of heterogeneity. The third small RCT (7 people smallest group) only reported medium term results. It found no significant difference in global improvement at 9–17 weeks (chance of not getting a good outcome: RR 0.97, 95% CI 0.41 to 2.32). **Versus elbow support:** See benefits of orthoses, p 1496. **Versus physiotherapies:** The review identified two RCTs

(53 and 12 people in smallest group) comparing corticosteroid injections (1 mL triamcinolone acetate 1% plus 1 mL lidocaine [lignocaine]) versus physiotherapies, and we found one additional RCT.[16] The first RCT (53 people in smallest group) found a significantly lower chance of an overall improvement with friction massage and a manipulation technique versus steroid injection (RR 0.45, 95% CI 0.29 to 0.69), and improvement in pain and grip strength. At 52 weeks, there was no significant difference for any outcome. The review was unable to report measured results for the second RCT. The additional RCT (59 people in smallest group) compared a corticosteroid injection versus no treatment versus physiotherapy (see *v* placebo or no treatment above).[16] It found injection versus physiotherapy (consisting of 9 sessions of ultrasound, deep friction massage, and exercise programme over 6 wk) significantly improved the "main complaint" and functional disability at 3 and 6 weeks (at 6 wks mean difference in "main complaint" 20%, 95% CI 10% to 31%). However, there was no significant difference at 12 weeks, and at 26 and 52 weeks physiotherapy versus injection significantly improved the "main complaint" (at 52 wks mean difference in "main complaint" 15%, 95% CI 5% to 25%). **Versus non-steroidal anti-inflammatory drugs:** See oral non-steroidal anti-inflammatory drugs versus corticosteroids, p 1499. We found no RCTs on the effect of corticosteroid injections on quality of life or return to work.

Harms: The review (8 RCTs) found no significant difference in adverse events between corticosteroid injections and control interventions (including facial flushes, post-injection pain, and local skin atrophy).[14] However, the review did not report measured results.

Comment: The review found that in the longer term there was a high rate of improvement in all groups.[14] It found that in general the quality of the methods of RCTs was poor to modest. The review provided the number of people in the smallest group for each trial rather than the total number of people in the trial. The corticosteroid suspensions used in these trials were methylprednisolone (2 RCTs), triamcinolone (4 RCTs), betamethasone (2 RCTs), hydrocortisone (5 RCTs), and dexamethasone (1 RCT). In one RCT, two different substances were used. The RCTs with longer term results of corticosteroid versus non-steroidal anti-inflammatory drugs and versus physiotherapy suggested that a steroid injection improved outcomes in the short term but increased recurrences in the medium term.

OPTION NON-STEROIDAL ANTI-INFLAMMATORY DRUGS

Sally E Green and Rachelle Buchbinder

One systematic review has found that topical non-steroidal anti-inflammatory drugs (NSAIDs) versus placebo significantly improve pain in the short term. Minor adverse effects have been reported. We found no RCTs comparing oral versus topical NSAIDs. One systematic review found limited evidence of a short term improvement in pain and function with an oral NSAID versus placebo. We found insufficient evidence to assess the longer term effects of NSAIDs. One systematic

review found limited evidence that fewer people receiving an oral NSAID versus a corticosteroid injection had self perceived improvement at 4 weeks, but found that an oral NSAID significantly reduced pain at 26 weeks.

Benefits: **Topical non-steroidal anti-inflammatory drugs versus placebo:** We found one systematic review (search date 2001, 3 RCTs, 130 people).[17] It found that topical non-steroidal anti-inflammatory drugs (NSAIDs) improved pain at up to 4 weeks significantly more than placebo (WMD –1.88, –2.54 to –1.21; scale 0 [no pain] to 10 [maximum pain]) and significantly reduced participant opinion of no benefit (2 RCTs; RR 0.39, 0.23 to 0.66). Inclusion of unblinded trials did not significantly change the results. It found no significant differences between topical NSAIDs and placebo for grip strength (reported as non-significant, further data not provided), or range of motion (RR for limitation of movement 1.01, 95% CI 0.80 to 1.28). It found an improvement in doctor's opinion of effect (RR for poor opinion of effect 0.61, 95% CI 0.37 to 0.99), and in tenderness with NSAIDs versus placebo, which just reached significance (RR for tenderness 0.83, 95% CI 0.70 to 0.99). The topical NSAIDs used were diclofenac (2 RCTs) and benzydamine (1 RCT). **Oral NSAIDs versus placebo:** We found one systematic review (search date 2001, 2 RCTs).[17] The RCTs were not pooled because one reported means and standard deviations and the other medians and ranges. One RCT of diclofenac versus placebo found limited evidence of a short term benefit in pain and function (WMD –13.9, 95% CI –23.2 to –4.6 on 100 point scale), but did not assess long term results. The second RCT found no significant difference in pain over 28 days (median [range] pain score at 4 wks, 4 [2–6] with naproxen *v* 3.5 [2–6] with placebo), or at 6 months or at 1 year (median [range] pain at 6 months: 1 [0–3] with NSAIDs *v* 1 [0–2.2] with placebo; at 12 months: 0 [0–2] with NSAIDs *v* 0 [0–2] with placebo), or for function (at 6 months: 0 [0–2.75] with NSAIDs *v* 0.5 [0–2] with placebo; at 12 months: 1 [0–1] with NSAIDs *v* 0 [0–0] with placebo). **Oral NSAIDs versus corticosteroid injection:** We found one systematic review (search date 2001, 3 RCTs).[17] Only two RCTs were included in the meta-analysis because of incomplete reporting of results. The first of these RCTs compared 20 mg methylprednisolone plus lidocaine versus 500 mg naproxen, and the second compared 6 mg betamethasone plus prilocaine plus placebo tablets versus 500 mg naproxen (initial high dose, then 250 mg). Meta-analysis of self reported perception of benefit found a significant difference in favour of injection at 4 weeks (RR of participant perceived benefit of injection 3.06, 95% CI 1.55 to 6.06). One RCT was not included in the meta-analysis because of skewed data; it found less functional limitation at 4 weeks in the injection group (median [range] 0 [0–2] with injection *v* 3 [1–5] with NSAIDs). The greater benefit of injection versus naproxen was only found in the short term. The largest RCT (53 people in smallest group) found significantly greater chance of improvement in pain at 26 weeks with a NSAID (RR 1.71, 95% CI 1.17 to 2.51). It found no significant difference in grip strength and results were not reported for global improvement. We found no RCTs investigating the effect of NSAIDs (either topical or oral) on return to work or quality of life.

Harms: **Topical NSAIDs:** One RCT found a significantly increased risk of any adverse event with NSAIDs versus placebo (RR 2.26, 95% CI 1.04 to 4.94).[18] Adverse effects were mild and no one was withdrawn from the study. Adverse effects reported in the published trials were foul breath and minor skin irritation. **Oral NSAIDs:** One trial of oral NSAIDs found an increased risk of abdominal pain (RR 3.17, 95% CI 1.35 to 7.41) and diarrhoea (RR 1.92, 95% CI 1.08 to 3.14). One systematic review (search date 1994, 12 RCTs of NSAIDs in a variety of disorders)[19] found the overall relative risk of complications from oral NSAIDs was 3.0–5.0. Adverse effects were predominantly gastrointestinal. See important differences between available NSAIDs under the NSAIDs topic, p 1393.

Comment: Both topical and oral NSAIDs may provide short term relief of pain in tennis elbow, although topical NSAIDs may be associated with less adverse effects. Further placebo controlled and comparative trials of oral versus topical NSAIDs would help clarify the effects of NSAIDs in the treatment of tennis elbow. Few trials used intention to treat analysis, and the sample size of most was small (populations range from 18–128 people for trials included in the meta-analysis).

OPTION EXERCISE AND MOBILISATION

Willem JJ Assendelft and Nynke Smidt

We found limited evidence from one systematic review of a better outcome with exercise versus ultrasound plus friction massage.

Benefits: We found one systematic review (search date 1999, 1 RCT, 19 people).[20] It found one small RCT, which found a significant improvement in symptoms at 8 weeks with exercise versus ultrasound plus friction massage (SMD –0.95, 95% CI –1.64 to –0.26). Four other RCTs were either of poor validity or provided insufficient data on relevant outcome measures.

Harms: In the systematic review no harms were described.[20]

Comment: None.

OPTION EXTRA-CORPOREAL SHOCK WAVE THERAPY

Rachelle Buchbinder and Sally E Green

One systematic review found conflicting evidence from two RCTs about the effects of extra-corporeal shock wave therapy versus sham treatment.

Benefits: We found one systematic review (search date 2001, 2 RCT, 286 people).[21] Both RCTs included similar study populations (mean age 41.9–46.9 years, slightly more women) with chronic symptoms (mean duration 21.9–27.6 months) who had not improved on at least 6 months of conservative treatment, including non-steroidal anti-inflammatory drugs, injections, brace or taping, casting, and physiotherapy. The frequency, doses, and technique of extra-corporeal shock wave therapy (ESWT) application were similar in both trials. In one RCT, the active treatment consisted of 1000 impulses of 0.08 mJ/mm^2 of ESWT at weekly intervals for 3 weeks.[21] The second RCT used "low energy" ESWT with 2000 pulses under local anaesthesia (3 mL mepivacaine 1%) at weekly intervals for 3 weeks using device dependent energy flux density ED+ between 0.07 and 0.09 mJ/mm^2.[21] The review found no significant difference in the risk of treatment failure (defined as Roles-Maudsley subjective pain score of 4) with ESWT versus placebo (6 wks; RR 0.40, 95% CI, 0.08 to 1.91, 1year: RR 0.44, 95% CI, 0.09 to 2.17 at 1 year). After 6 weeks, it found no significant improvement in pain at rest (WMD pain out of 100, –11.4, 95% CI –26.1 to +3.3), pain with resisted wrist extension (WMD pain out of 100, –16.2, 95% CI –47.8 to +15.4), or pain with resisted middle finger extension (WMD pain out of 100, –20.5, 95% CI –56.6 to +15.6). Combined longer term results (1 measured at 12 wks and 1 at 24 wks) found no significant difference in improvement of pain at rest (WMD pain out of 100, –14.7, 95% CI –35.4 to +6.1), pain with resisted wrist extension (WMD pain out of 100, –14.70, 95% CI –43.4 to +14.0), and pain with resisted middle finger extension (WMD pain out of 100, –21.1, 95% CI –58.3 to +16.1). The effect of ESWT on function, quality of life, and return to work was not reported. The effect of ESWT on grip strength was reported in both trials but the results were difficult to interpret in one RCT. The other RCT found no difference in improvement in grip strength between groups at 6 weeks, 12 weeks, or 1 year.

Harms: One RCT in the review did not report adverse events.[21] The other RCT reported significantly more adverse effects in the EWST group compared with placebo (OR 4.3, 95% CI 2.9 to 6.3). However, there were no treatment discontinuations or dosage adjustments related to adverse effects. The most frequently reported adverse effects in the ESWT treated group were transitory reddening of the skin (21.1% with ESWT *v* 4.7% with placebo); pains (4.8% with ESWT *v* 1.7% with placebo); and petechiae, bleeding, or haematomas (4.5% with ESWT *v* 1.7% with placebo). Migraine occurred in four people and syncope in three people after ESWT compared with no people treated with placebo.

Comment: Two placebo controlled trials of ESWT for chronic lateral elbow pain have yielded conflicting results.[21] When data from both trials are pooled, the benefits observed in the first trial are no longer apparent. This RCT, which found a significant improvement, had uncertain allocation concealment and no analysis of early withdrawals (15/115 [13%]). Further well designed trials are needed to clarify whether ESWT is of value for lateral elbow pain.

OPTION SURGERY

Rachelle Buchbinder and Sally E Green

One systematic review found no RCTs of surgical treatment.

Benefits: We found one systematic review (search date 2001), which identified no RCTs.[22] We found no subsequent RCTs.

Harms: We found no RCTs.

Comment: Various open and percutaneous operations for lateral elbow pain have been described based upon the surgeon's concept of the pathological entity. The most commonly described surgical procedures involve excision of abnormal tissue (comprising microscopic degeneration, rupture, or both, and immature repairative tissue) within the origin of extensor carpi radialis brevis, release of the extensor carpi radialis brevis from the lateral epicondyle region, or both. Additional procedures include release of the anterior capsule, removal of inflamed synovial folds, resection of a third of the orbicular ligament, debridement of articular damage, release of the posterior interosseous nerve, denervation of the lateral epicondyle, denervation of the radiohumeral joint, and excision of a radio-humeral bursa.[23–35]

GLOSSARY

Laser A source of light with a narrow, almost monochromatic, coherent light bundle. It contains a relative high energy intensity.

REFERENCES

1. Allander E. Prevalence, incidence and remission rates of some common rheumatic diseases and syndromes. *Scand J Rheumatol* 1974;3:145–153.
2. Chard MD, Hazleman BL. Tennis elbow – a reappraisal. *Br J Rheumatol* 1989;28:186–190.
3. Verhaar J. Tennis elbow: anatomical, epidemiological and therapeutic aspects. *Int Orthop* 1994;18:263–267.
4. Hamilton P. The prevalence of humeral epicondylitis: a survey in general practice. *J R Coll Gen Pract* 1986;36:464–465.
5. Kivi P. The etiology and conservative treatment of lateral epicondylitis. *Scand J Rehabil Med* 1983;15:37–41.
6. Murtagh J. Tennis elbow. *Aust Fam Physician* 1988;17:90,91,94,95.
7. Hudak P, Cole D, Haines T. Understanding prognosis to improve rehabilitation: the example of lateral elbow pain. *Arch Phys Rehabil* 1996;77:568–593.
8. Smidt N, van der Windt DAWM, Assendelft WJJ, et al. Corticosteroid injections for lateral epicondylitis are superior to physiotherapy and a wait and see policy at short-term follow-up, but inferior at long-term follow-up: results from a randomised controlled trial. *Lancet* 2002;359:657–662.
9. Green S, Buchbinder R, Barnsley L, et al. Acupuncture for lateral elbow pain. In: The Cochrane Library, Issue 3, 2002. Oxford: Update Software. Search date 2001; primary sources Medline, Cinahl, Embase, Scisearch, Cochrane Controlled Trials Register, and Cochrane Musculoskeletal Review Group Specialised Trial Database.
10. Fink M, Wolkenstein E, Karst M, et al. Acupuncture in chronic epicondylitis: a randomized controlled trial. *Rheumatology* 2002;41:205–209.
11. Molsberger A, Hille E. The analgesic effect of acupuncture in chronic tennis elbow pain. *Br J Rheumatol* 1994;33:1162–1165.
12. Haker E, Lundberg T. Acupuncture treatment in epicondylalgia: a comparative study of two acupuncture techniques. *Clin J Pain* 1990;6:221–226.
13. Struijs PAA, Smidt N, Arola H, et al. Orthotic devices for the treatment of tennis elbow. In: The Cochrane Library, Issue 3, 2002. Oxford: Update Software. Search date 1999; primary sources Medline, Embase, Cinahl, Cochrane Controlled Trials Register, Current Contents, hand searches of reference lists from all retrieved articles, and personal contact with subject experts.
14. Smidt N, Assendelft WJJ, van der Windt DAWM, et al. Corticosteroid injections for lateral epicondylitis: a systematic review. *Pain* 2002;96:23–40. Search date 1999; primary sources Medline, Embase, Cinahl, Cochrane Controlled Trials Register, Current Contents, Cochrane Rehabilitation and Related Therapies Field Trials Register, and hand searches of references from retrieved articles.
15. Newcomber K, Laskowski E, Idank D, et al. Corticosteroid injection in early treatment of lateral epicondylitis. *Clin J Sport Med* 2001;11:214–222.
16. Smidt N, van der Windt D, Assendelft W, et al. Corticosteroid injections, physiotherapy, or a wait-and-see policy for lateral epicondylitis: a randomised controlled trial. *Lancet* 2002;359:657–662.
17. Green S, Buchbinder R, Barnsley L, et al. Non-steroidal anti-inflammatory drugs (NSAIDs) for treating lateral elbow pain in adults. In: The Cochrane Library, Issue 3, 2002. Oxford: Update Software. Search date 2001; primary sources Medline, Cinahl, Embase, Scisearch, Cochrane Musculoskeletal Review Group Specialised Trials Register, and Cochrane Controlled Trials Register.
18. Percy E, Carson J. The use of DMSO in tennis elbow and rotator cuff tendonitis: a double blind study. *Med Sci Sports Exerc* 1981;13:215–219.
19. Rodriguez LAG. Nonsteroidal antiinflammatory drugs, ulcers and risk: a collaborative meta-analysis. *Semin Arthritis Rheum* 1997;26:16–20. Search date 1994; primary sources Medline, hand searches of bibliographies of previous meta-analyses, and personal contact with authors of relevant studies.
20. Smidt N. Chapter 2. In: Smidt N. *Conservative treatments for tennis elbow in primary care* [thesis]. Waseningen: Ponsen and Looijen BV, 2001. Search date 1999; primary sources Medline, Embase, Cinahl, Cochrane Controlled Trials Register, Current Contents, Cochrane Rehabilitation and Related Therapies Field Trials Register, and hand searches of references from retrieved articles.
21. Buchbinder R, Green S, White M, et al. Shock wave therapy for lateral elbow pain. In: The Cochrane Library, Issue 3, 2002. Oxford: Update Software. Search date 2001; primary sources of Medline, Cinahl, Embase, Scisearch, Cochrane Controlled Trials Registrar, and Cochrane Musculoskeletal Review Group Specialised Trials Database.
22. Buchbinder R, Green S, Bell S, et al. Surgery for lateral elbow pain. In: The Cochrane Library, Issue 3, 2002. Oxford: Update Software. Search date 2001; primary sources Medline, Cinahl, Embase,

Scisearch, Cochrane Controlled Trials Registrar, and Cochrane Musculoskeletal Review Group Specialised Trials Database.
23. Bosworth DM. Surgical treatment of tennis elbow. A follow-up study. *J Bone Joint Surg Am* 1965;47:1533–1536.
24. Boyd HB, McLeod HC Jr. Tennis elbow. *J Bone Joint Surg Am* 1973;55:1183–1187.
25. Calvert PT, Macpherson IS, Allum RL, et al. Simple lateral release in treatment of tennis elbow. *J R Soc Med* 1985;78:912–915.
26. Coonrad RW, Hooper WR. Tennis elbow: its course, natural history, conservative and surgical management. *J Bone Joint Surg Am* 1973;55:1177–1182.
27. Friden J, Lieber R. Physiological consequences of surgical lengthening of extensor carpi radialis brevis muscle–tendon junction for tennis elbow. *J Hand Surg Am* 1994;19A:269–274.
28. Goldberg EJ, Abraham E, Siegel I. The surgical treatment of chronic lateral humeral epicondylitis by common extensor release. *Clin Orthop* 1988;233:208–212.
29. Kaplan EB. Treatment of tennis elbow (epicondylitis) by denervation. *J Bone Joint Surg Am* 1959;41:147–151.
30. Nirschl RP, Pettrone FA. The surgical treatment of lateral epicondylitis. *J Bone Joint Surg Am* 1979;61:832–839.
31. Posch JN, Goldberg VM, Larrey R. Extensor fasciotomy for tennis elbow: a long term follow-up study. *Clin Orthop* 1978;135:179–182.
32. Verhaar J, Walenkamp G, Kester A, et al. Lateral extensor release for tennis elbow. A prospective long-term follow-up study. *J Bone Joint Surg Am* 1993;75:1034–1043.
33. Wilhelm A. Tennis elbow: treatment of resistant cases by denervation. *J Hand Surg Br* 1996;21:523–533.
34. Wittenberg RH, Schaal S, Muhr G. Surgical treatment of persistent elbow epicondylitis. *Clin Orthop* 1992;278:73–80.
35. Yerger B, Turner T. Percutaneous extensor tenotomy for chronic tennis elbow. *Orthopedics* 1985;8:1261–1263.

Willem Assendelft
Head of Department of Guideline Development and Research Policy
Dutch College of General Practitioners
Utrecht
The Netherlands

Sally Green
Senior Lecturer
Institute of Health Services Research
Monash University
Melbourne
Australia

Rachelle Buchbinder
Director
Department of Clinical Epidemiology
Cabrini Hospital and Monash University
Department of Epidemiology and Preventive Medicine
Melbourne
Australia

Peter Struijs
Academic Medical Center
Amsterdam
The Netherlands

Nynke Smidt
Institute for Research in Extramural Medicine
Amsterdam
The Netherlands

Competing interests: The authors of this piece are the authors of the Cochrane Reviews from which most of the evidence is drawn. WA has supervised and PS has conducted a trial sponsored by Bauerfeind, a manufacturer of orthoses. RB, SG, and NS none declared.

Bell's palsy

Search date November 2002

Rodrigo Salinas

QUESTIONS

INTERVENTIONS

See glossary, p 1507

Key Messages

- **Antiviral treatment** Two systematic reviews found no RCTs of aciclovir versus placebo. One RCT found limited evidence that aciclovir plus prednisone improved facial function compared with prednisone alone after 4 months.
- **Corticosteroids** One systematic review found no clear evidence that corticosteroid improved the recovery of facial motor function or cosmetically disabling sequelae compared with placebo after 6 months.
- **Facial nerve decompression surgery** One systematic review identified no RCTs of facial nerve decompression.

DEFINITION Bell's palsy is an acute, unilateral paresis or paralysis of the face in a pattern consistent with peripheral facial nerve dysfunction, without detectable causes.[1] Additional symptoms may include pain in or behind the ear, numbness in the affected side of the face, impaired tolerance to ordinary levels of noise, and disturbed taste on the anterior part of the tongue.[2–5]

INCIDENCE/ PREVALENCE The incidence is about 23/100 000 people a year, or about 1/60–70 people in a lifetime.[6] Bell's palsy affects men and women more or less equally, with a peak incidence between the ages of 10 and 40 years. It occurs with equal frequency on the right and left sides of the face.[7]

AETIOLOGY/ RISK FACTORS The cause is unclear. Viral infection, ischaemia, autoimmune inflammatory disorders, and heredity factors have been proposed as underlying causes.[2,8,9] A viral cause has gained popularity since the isolation of the herpes simplex virus-1 genome from facial nerve endoneurial fluid in people with Bell's palsy.[10]

PROGNOSIS More than two thirds of people with Bell's palsy achieve full spontaneous recovery. The largest series of people with Bell's palsy who received no specific treatment (1011 people) found the first signs of improvement within 3 weeks of onset in 85% of people.[11] For the other 15%, some improvement occurred 3–6 months later. The same series found that 71% of people recovered normal function of the face, 13% had insignificant sequelae, and the remaining 16% had permanently diminished function, with contracture of facial muscles and synkinesis (see glossary, p 1507). These figures are roughly similar to those of other series of people receiving no specific treatment for Bell's palsy.[7,8,12]

AIMS OF INTERVENTION To maximise recovery of facial function; to reduce the risk of complications, with minimum adverse effects.

OUTCOMES Grade of recovery of motor function of the face; presence of sequelae (motor synkinesis, autonomic dysfunction, hemifacial spasm); time to full recovery.

METHODS *Clinical Evidence* search and appraisal November 2002. Trials used different scoring systems for reporting outcomes.

QUESTION **What are the effects of treatments in adults and children?**

OPTION **CORTICOSTEROIDS**

One systematic review found no clear evidence that corticosteroid improved the recovery of facial motor function or cosmetically disabling sequelae compared with control after 6 months.

Benefits: **Versus placebo or no specific treatment:** We found one systematic review (search date 2000, 3 RCTs, 117 people).[13] In the review, one RCT (26 people aged 12–76 years) compared cortisone acetate versus placebo, one RCT (51 people, ages not specified) compared prednisone plus vitamins versus vitamins alone, and one

RCT (42 children aged 24–74 months) compared methylprednisolone versus no specific treatment. The review found no significant difference between corticosteroid (cortisone acetate, prednisone, methylprednisolone) and control in the number of people with incomplete recovery of facial motor function after 6 months (3 RCTs: 13/59 [22%] of people with corticosteroid *v* 15/58 [26%] of people with control; RR 0.86, 95% CI 0.47 to 1.59). When data from two quasi-randomised trials found by the review[12,14] were added to the pooled estimate, the result remained non-significant (RR 0.69, 95% CI 0.42 to 1.16; absolute numbers not provided; see comment below). The review also found no significant difference between corticosteroid and control in the number of people with cosmetically disabling sequelae after 6 months (8/59 [14%] of people with corticosteroid *v* 9/58 [16%] of people with control; RR 0.86, 95% CI 0.38 to 1.98). When data from two quasi-randomised trials found by the review[12,14] were added to the pooled estimate, the result remained non-significant (RR 0.82, 95% CI 0.39 to 1.73; absolute numbers not provided). **Versus aciclovir:** See benefits of antiviral treatment, p 1506.

Harms: No adverse effects were reported in the trials.

Comment: Of the two quasi-randomised trials identified by the review, one compared corticosteroids (preparation not stated) versus supportive therapy only, and used alternation in matched participants as the method of allocation.[12] The other compared dexamethasone versus placebo, and used allocation according to the day of admission.[14]

OPTION ANTIVIRAL TREATMENT

Two systematic reviews found no RCTs of aciclovir versus placebo. One RCT found limited evidence that aciclovir plus prednisone improved facial function compared with prednisone alone after 4 months.

Benefits: We found two systematic reviews (search date 2000, 2 RCTs, 200 people;[15] search date 2000, 3 RCTs, 230 people[16]). Neither review found RCTs of aciclovir versus placebo. Both included the same RCT (119 people) of aciclovir (400 mg 5 times daily for 10 days) plus prednisone versus prednisone alone (see comment below). The first review found that aciclovir plus prednisone versus prednisone alone significantly decreased the number of people with incomplete recovery of facial function (measured using a facial function scoring system) after 4 months (4/53 [8%] of people with aciclovir plus steroid had moderate or moderately severe dysfunction *v* 11/46 [24%] with steroid alone; RR 0.32, 95% CI 0.11 to 0.92; see comment below).[15]

Harms: The RCT reported mild to moderate gastrointestinal complaints, which did not require treatment. No numbers were reported.[15]

Comment: In the RCT, 20/119 (17%) of people enrolled in the trial were lost to follow up. It is not clear to which treatment group these belonged. Results were calculated from the 99/119 (83%) of people who completed the trial. The systematic reviews identified two further RCTs of aciclovir that were not of sufficient quality.

OPTION FACIAL NERVE DECOMPRESSION SURGERY

One systematic review found no RCTs of facial nerve decompression surgery for people with Bell's palsy.

Benefits: We found one systematic review (search date 2000), which found no RCTs of facial nerve decompression surgery for people with Bell's palsy.[16]

Harms: The systematic review found reports of permanent unilateral deafness in four non-randomised prospective studies of facial nerve decompression in people with Bell's palsy.[16] One study of people with complete facial palsy undergoing facial nerve decompression found that 4/41 (10%) people had conductive deafness and 2/41 (5%) people had perceptive deafness after 1 year.[12]

Comment: None.

GLOSSARY

Synkinesis Involuntary movement accompanying a voluntary movement.

REFERENCES

1. Niparko JK, Mattox DE. Bell's palsy and herpes zoster oticus. In: Johnson RT, Griffin JW, eds. *Current therapy in neurologic disease*. St Louis: Mosby, 1993;355–361.
2. Burgess LPA, Capt MC, Yim DWS, et al. Bell's palsy: the steroid controversy revisited. *Laryngoscope* 1984;94:1472–1476.
3. Knox GW. Treatment controversy in Bell's palsy. *Arch Otolaryngol Head Neck Surg* 1998;124:821–824.
4. May M, Klein SR, Taylor FH. Idiopathic (Bell's) facial palsy: natural history defies steroid or surgical treatment. *Laryngoscope* 1985;95:406–409.
5. Rowland LP. Treatment of Bell's palsy. *N Engl J Med* 1972;287:1298–1299.
6. Victor M, Martin J. Disorders of the cranial nerves. In: Isselbacher KJ, et al. eds. *Harrison's principles of internal medicine* 13th ed. New York: McGraw-Hill, 1994:2347–2352.
7. Prescott CAJ. Idiopathic facial nerve palsy. *J Laryngol Otol* 1988;102:403–407.
8. Adour KK. Diagnosis and management of facial paralysis. *N Engl J Med* 1982;307:348–351.
9. Lorber B. Are all diseases infectious? *Ann Intern Med* 1996;125:844–851.
10. Murakami S, Mizobuchi M, Nakashiro Y, et al. Bell palsy and herpes simplex virus: identification of viral DNA in endoneurial fluid and muscle. *Ann Intern Med* 1996;124:27–30.
11. Peitersen E. The natural history of Bell's palsy. *Am J Otol* 1982;4:107–111.
12. Brown JS. Bell's palsy: a 5 year review of 174 consecutive cases: an attempted double blind study. *Laryngoscope* 1982;92:1369–1373.
13. Salinas RA, Alvarez G, Alvarez MI, et al. Corticosteroids for Bell's palsy (idiopathic facial paralysis) (Cochrane Review). In: The Cochrane Library, Issue 1, 2002. Oxford: Update Software. Search date 2000; primary sources Cochrane Neuromuscular Disease Group register, Medline, Embase, Lilacs, hand searches of reference lists, and personal contact with experts.
14. Akpinar S, Boga M, Yardim M. Akut periferik fasiyel paralizi olgularinda steroid tedavisinin plasebo ile oranlanmasi [Steroid versus placebo treatments in cases of acute peripheral facial paralysis]. *Bulletin of Gulhane Military Medical Academy* 1979;21:45–51.
15. Sipe J, Dunn L. Aciclovir for Bell's palsy (idiopathic facial paralysis) (Cochrane Review). In: The Cochrane Library, Issue 1, 2001. Oxford: Update Software. Search date 2000; primary sources Cochrane neuromuscular disease group register, Medline, Embase, Lilacs hand searches of reference lists, and personal contact with authors and experts.
16. Grogan PM, Gronseth GS. Practice parameter: steroids, acyclovir, and surgery for Bell's palsy (an evidence-based review). *Neurology* 2001;56:830–836. Search date 2000; primary source Medline and hand searches of reference lists.

Rodrigo Salinas
Ministry of Health
Santiago
Chile

Competing interests: None declared.

Epilepsy

Search date March 2003

Anthony Marson and Sridharan Ramaratnam

QUESTIONS

INTERVENTIONS

Beneficial

Addition of second line drugs (gabapentin, levetiracetam, lamotrigine, oxcarbazepine, tiagabine, topiramate, vigabatrin, or zonisamide) for drug resistant partial epilepsy 1514
Antiepileptic monotherapy in generalised epilepsy* 1513
Antiepileptic monotherapy in partial epilepsy*. 1511

Likely to be beneficial

Educational programmes 1518

Trade off between benefits and harms

Antiepileptic drug withdrawal for people in remission 1515
Antiepileptic drugs after a single seizure 1510

Unknown effectiveness

Biofeedback 1516
Cognitive behavioural therapy.1517
Family counselling. 1520
Relaxation plus behavioural modification therapy. 1519
Relaxation therapy 1515
Yoga 1516

To be covered in future updates

Treatment of drug resistant generalised epilepsy

*We found no placebo controlled RCTs. However, widespread consensus holds that these drugs are effective.

See glossary, p 1520

Key Messages

- **Addition of second line drugs for drug resistant partial epilepsy** Systematic reviews in people with drug resistant partial epilepsy have found that adding gabapentin, levetiracetam, lamotrigine, oxcarbazepine, tiagabine, topiramate, vigabatrin, or zonisamide to usual treatment reduces seizure frequency compared with adding placebo. The reviews have found that adding any of the drugs increases the frequency of adverse effects compared with adding placebo. We found no good evidence from RCTs on which to base a choice among drugs.

- **Antiepileptic monotherapy in generalised epilepsy** We found no placebo controlled trials of the main antiepileptic drugs (carbamazepine, phenobarbital, phenytoin, sodium valproate), but widespread consensus holds that these drugs are effective. Systematic reviews found no good evidence on which to base a choice among these drugs in terms of seizure control.
- **Antiepileptic monotherapy in partial epilepsy** We found no placebo controlled RCTs of the main antiepileptic drugs (carbamazepine, phenobarbital, phenytoin, sodium valproate) used as monotherapy in people with partial epilepsy, but widespread consensus holds that these drugs are effective. Systematic reviews found no reliable evidence on which to base a choice among drugs in terms of seizure control. Systematic reviews have found that phenobarbital is more likely to be withdrawn than phenytoin or carbamazepine and that phenytoin is more likely to be withdrawn than carbamazepine.
- **Educational programmes** One RCT found that a 2 day education programme reduced seizure frequency at 6 months compared with waiting list control, although it found no significant difference in health related quality of life. Two RCTs found that an educational package improved knowledge and understanding of epilepsy, adjustment to epilepsy, and psychosocial functioning compared with control.
- **Antiepileptic drug withdrawal for people in remission** One systematic review of observational studies and one RCT have found that antiepileptic drug withdrawal for people in remission is associated with a higher risk of seizure recurrence than is continued treatment. Clinical predictors of relapse after drug withdrawal include age, seizure type, number of antiepileptic drugs being taken, whether seizures have occurred since antiepileptic drugs were started, and the period of remission before drug withdrawal.
- **Antiepileptic drugs after a single seizure** RCTs have found that immediate treatment of a single seizure with antiepileptic drugs reduces seizure recurrence at 2 years compared with no treatment. However, we found no evidence that treatment alters long term prognosis. Long term antiepileptic drug treatment is potentially harmful.
- **Cognitive behavioural therapy** We found insufficient evidence about the effects of cognitive behavioural therapy in people with epilepsy from two small RCTs.
- **Family counselling** We found insufficient evidence on family counselling from one small RCT that employed weak methods.
- **Relaxation plus behavioural modification therapy** RCTs found insufficient evidence about the effects of combined relaxation and behavioural modification on seizures.
- **Biofeedback; relaxation therapy; yoga** Systematic reviews found insufficient evidence on the effects of these interventions.

DEFINITION Epilepsy is a group of disorders rather than a single disease. Seizures can be classified by type as partial (categorised as simple partial, complex partial, and secondary generalised tonic clonic seizures), or generalised (categorised as generalised tonic clonic, absence, myoclonic, tonic, and atonic seizures).[1] See glossary, p 1520.

INCIDENCE/ PREVALENCE Epilepsy is common, with an estimated prevalence in the developed world of 5–10/1000, and an annual incidence of 50/100 000 people.[2] About 3% of people will be given a diagnosis of epilepsy at some time in their lives.[3]

AETIOLOGY/ RISK FACTORS Epilepsy can also be classified by cause.[1] Idiopathic generalised epilepsies (such as juvenile myoclonic epilepsy or childhood absence epilepsy) are largely genetic. Symptomatic epilepsies result from a known cerebral abnormality; for example, temporal lobe epilepsy may result from a congenital defect, mesial temporal sclerosis, or a tumour. Cryptogenic epilepsies are those that cannot be classified as idiopathic or symptomatic and in which no causative factor has been identified, but is suspected.

PROGNOSIS For most people with epilepsy the prognosis is good. About 70% go into remission, defined as being seizure free for 5 years on or off treatment. This leaves 20–30% who develop chronic epilepsy, which is often treated with multiple antiepileptic drugs.[4] About 60% of untreated people have no further seizures in the 2 years after their first seizure.[5]

AIMS OF INTERVENTION To reduce the risk of subsequent seizures and to improve the prognosis of the seizure disorder; in people in remission, to withdraw antiepileptic drugs without causing seizure recurrence; to minimise adverse effects of treatment.

OUTCOMES For treatment after a single seizure: time to subsequent seizures, time to achieve remission, proportion achieving remission. For treatment of newly diagnosed epilepsy: retention on allocated treatment or time to withdrawal of allocated treatment, time to remission, time to first seizure after treatment. For treatment of drug resistant epilepsy: percentage reduction in seizure frequency, proportion of responders (response defined as ≥ 50% reduction in seizure frequency). For drug withdrawal: time to seizure recurrence. Improvement in quality of life; reduction in anxiety, depression, and fear of seizures; coping or adjustment to epilepsy (assessed by validated measures).

METHODS *Clinical Evidence* search and appraisal for systematic reviews March 2003, and additional searches for RCTs by the contributors.

QUESTION Should single seizures be treated?

RCTs have found that treatment of a single seizure with antiepileptic drugs reduces seizure recurrence at 2 years compared with no treatment. However, we found no evidence that treatment alters long term prognosis. Long term antiepileptic drug treatment is potentially harmful.

Benefits: We found no systematic review. We found three RCTs, the largest of which (419 people, 42% women, 28% aged ≤ 16 years, 66% aged 16–60 years, 6% aged ≥ 60 years) compared immediate treatment after a first unprovoked seizure versus no immediate treatment.[6] People were randomised within 7 days of their first tonic clonic seizure (see glossary, p 1521). Longer term follow up of the RCT found that there were half as many second seizures with immediate treatment compared with no treatment at 2 years (HR 0.36, 95% CI 0.24 to 0.53).[7] However, it found no significant difference in the proportion of people achieving a 2 year remission in seizures (AR 60% v 68%; RR 0.82, 95% CI 0.64 to 1.03; RR adjusted for time of starting treatment 0.96, 95% CI 0.77 to 1.22).[7]

Harms: The RCT gave no information on adverse effects of antiepileptic drugs.[6,7] However, these are well known and include idiosyncratic reactions, teratogenesis, and cognitive effects.

Comment: One systematic review of prospective observational studies (search date not stated, about 2500 people, 30% receiving treatment) concluded that, within 2 years of their first seizure, 40% (95% CI 37% to 43%) of people have further seizures.[5] The RCT was too small to rule out the possibility that treating a first seizure alters the long term prognosis of epilepsy.[6,7]

QUESTION What are the effects of monotherapy in newly diagnosed partial epilepsy?

We found no placebo controlled RCTs of the main antiepileptic drugs (carbamazepine, phenobarbital, phenytoin, sodium valproate) used as monotherapy in people with partial epilepsy, but widespread consensus holds that these drugs are effective. Systematic reviews found no reliable evidence on which to base a choice among drugs in terms of seizure control. Systematic reviews have found that phenobarbital is more likely to be withdrawn than phenytoin or carbamazepine and that phenytoin is more likely to be withdrawn than carbamazepine.

Benefits: We found no systematic reviews or RCTs comparing antiepileptic drugs versus placebo or no treatment (see comment below). We found five systematic reviews that compared antiepileptic drugs versus each other.[8–12] **Sodium valproate versus carbamazepine:** The first systematic review (search date 1999, 5 RCTs, 1265 people, of whom 830 had partial epilepsy and 395 had generalised epilepsy, age 3–83 years, follow up < 5 years) compared sodium valproate versus carbamazepine.[8] The systematic review included a meta-analysis of the subgroup of people with partial epilepsy (with results expressed as HRs; HR > 1 for an event that is more likely with sodium valproate). It found no significant difference for treatment withdrawal between sodium valproate and carbamazepine (HR 1.00, 95% CI 0.79 to 1.26). Sodium valproate decreased 12 month remission compared with carbamazepine and significantly increased risk of first seizure (remission: HR 0.82, 95% CI 0.67 to 1.00; first seizure: HR 1.22, 95% CI 1.04 to 1.44). A test for statistical interaction was performed and was significant for time to first seizure but not for time to 12 month remission. These subgroup analyses must therefore be treated with caution. **Sodium valproate versus phenytoin:** The second systematic review (search date 2000, 5 RCTs, 250 people with partial epilepsy, and 419 with generalised epilepsy, age 3–95, follow up < 5 years) compared sodium valproate versus phenytoin.[9] It included a meta-analysis in people with partial epilepsy (with results expressed as HRs; HR > 1 for an event that is more likely with phenytoin). It found no significant difference in treatment withdrawal, 12 month remission, or first seizure (treatment withdrawal: HR 1.23, 95% CI 0.77 to 1.98; 12 month remission: HR 1.02, 95% CI 0.68 to 1.54; first seizure: HR 0.81, 95% CI 0.59 to 1.11). **Phenobarbital versus phenytoin:** The third systematic review (search date 1998, 3 RCTs, 599 people with partial or generalised epilepsy, age 3–77 years) compared phenobarbital versus phenytoin.[10] Results were expressed as HRs (HR > 1 for an event more likely with phenobarbital), but it did not undertake subgroup analyses for people with partial or generalised epilepsy. Overall, it found no significant difference in 12 month remission or first seizure (12 month remission: HR 0.93, 95% CI 0.70 to 1.23; first seizure: HR 0.84, 95% CI 0.68 to 1.05). It found that treatment withdrawal was greater with phenobarbital than with phenytoin, presumably because it was less well tolerated (HR 1.62, 95% CI 1.22 to 2.14). **Carbamazepine versus phenobarbital:** The fourth systematic review (search date 2002, 4 RCTs, 680 people, of whom 523 had partial epilepsy) compared carbamazepine versus phenobarbital.[11] Results were expressed as HRs (HR > 1 for an event more likely on phenobarbital). For people with partial epilepsy it found that phenobarbital was significantly more likely to be withdrawn than carbamazepine (HR 1.60, 95% CI 1.18 to 2.17). It found no significant difference in remission during the next 12 months (HR 1.03, 95% CI 0.72 to 1.49), but it found that phenobarbital significantly increased time to first seizure compared with carbamazepine (HR 0.71, 95% CI 0.55 to 0.91). **Carbamazepine versus phenytoin:** The fifth systematic review (search 2002, 3 RCTs, 552 adults and children, of whom 431 had partial epilepsy) compared carbamazepine versus phenytoin.[12] The review did not present results separately for people with partial epilepsy (see comment below).

Harms: Two RCTs found similar prevalence of adverse effects with carbamazepine and sodium valproate.[13,14] Rashes occurred more often with carbamazepine than with sodium valproate (11% *v* 1.7%, P < 0.05; 6.3% *v* 3.4%, NS). Weight gain was more common with sodium valproate (12% *v* 1.1%, P < 0.05; 10% *v* 3.9%, NS), usually after at least 3 months of treatment. Other adverse events with carbamazepine included dizziness (6.7% *v* 2.9%, NS; 6.3% *v* 0.8%, P < 0.05), headaches (6.1% *v* 3.4%), ataxia (2.2% *v* 0%), somnolence (20% *v* 9.3%, P < 0.05), fatigue (10% *v* 5.1%, NS), diplopia (3.9% *v* 0%, NS), and insomnia (3.9% *v* 0%, NS). Other drug related adverse events with sodium valproate were tremor (5.2% *v* 1.7%, NS), alopecia (2.9% *v* 0.6%, NS; 4.2% *v* 1.6%, NS), and appetite increase (2.3% *v* 0%, NS; 9.3% *v* 0%, P < 0.01). Treatment was withdrawn because of adverse events in 9% of people taking sodium valproate compared with 18% taking carbamazepine (18 *v* 15 people).[13,14]

Comment: Placebo controlled trials of these drugs would now be considered unethical. The meta-analysis provides weak evidence in support of the consensus view to use carbamazepine as the drug of choice in people with partial epilepsy.[8] The systematic review comparing carbamazepine versus phenytoin did not present results separately for people with generalised epilepsy and people with partial epilepsy.[12] Overall, however, it found no significant difference between carbamazepine and phenytoin for treatment withdrawal, first seizure, or 12 month remission (treatment withdrawal: HR 0.97, 95% CI 0.74 to 1.28; first seizure: HR 0.91, 95% CI 0.74 to 1.12; time to 12 month remission: HR 1.00, 95% CI 0.78 to 1.29).

QUESTION What are the effects of monotherapy in newly diagnosed generalised epilepsy (generalised tonic clonic seizures with or without other generalised seizure types)?

We found no placebo controlled trials of the main antiepileptic drugs (carbamazepine, phenobarbital, phenytoin, sodium valproate) used as monotherapy in people with generalised epilepsy, but widespread consensus holds that these drugs are effective. Systematic reviews found no evidence on which to base a choice among drugs in terms of seizure control.

Benefits: **Versus placebo:** We found no systematic review or RCTs comparing antiepileptic drugs versus placebo. We found four systematic reviews that compared different antiepileptic drugs.[8,9,11,12] The first two reviews were of RCTs that recruited people if they had generalised onset tonic clonic seizures (see glossary, p 1521) with or without other generalised seizure types (e.g. absence or myoclonus).[8,9] **Carbamazepine versus sodium valproate:** The first systematic review compared carbamazepine versus sodium valproate (search date 1999, 5 RCTs, 4 of the RCTs included 395 people with generalised epilepsy, age 3–79 years, follow up < 5 years).[8] Results were expressed as HRs (HR > 1 indicates that an event is more likely with sodium valproate). A meta-analysis of the generalised epilepsy subgroup found no significant difference between sodium valproate and carbamazepine for treatment withdrawal (HR 0.89, 95% CI 0.62 to 1.29), 12 month remission (HR 0.96, 95% CI 0.75 to 1.24), or first seizure (HR 0.86, 95% CI 0.68 to 1.67; see comment below). **Phenytoin versus sodium valproate:** The second systematic review compared phenytoin and sodium valproate (search date 2000, 5 RCTs, 419 people aged 3–95 years with generalised epilepsy).[9] Results were expressed as HRs (HR > 1 indicates that an event is more likely with phenytoin). A meta-analysis of the generalised epilepsy subgroup found no significant difference between sodium valproate and phenytoin for time to treatment withdrawal, 12 month remission, or first seizure (treatment withdrawal: HR 0.98, 95% CI 0.60 to 1.58; 12 month remission: HR 1.06, 95% CI 0.71 to 1.57; first seizure: HR 1.03, 95% CI 0.77 to 1.39; see comment below). **Carbamazepine versus phenobarbital:** The third systematic review (search date 2002, 4 RCTs, 680 people, of whom 157 had generalised epilepsy) compared carbamazepine versus phenobarbital.[11] Subgroup analysis in people with a generalized epilepsy found no significant differences for first seizure, 12 month remission, or treatment withdrawal (first seizure: HR 0.61, 95% CI 0.36 to 1.03; 12 month remission: HR 0.61, 95% CI 0.36 to 1.03; treatment withdrawal: HR 1.78, 95% CI 0.87 to 3.62). **Carbamazepine versus phenytoin:** The fourth systematic review (search 2002, 3 RCTs, 552 people, of whom 121 had generalized epilepsy) compared carbamazepine versus phenytoin.[12] It did not present results separately for people with generalised epilepsy (see comment under effects of monotherapy in newly diagnosed partial epilepsy, p 1512).

Harms: See harms under effects of monotherapy in newly diagnosed partial epilepsy, p 1512.

Comment: Although no difference was found in the systematic reviews between sodium valproate and either carbamazepine or phenytoin, the confidence intervals are wide and these results do not establish equivalence of sodium valproate and carbamazepine or phenytoin.[8,9] Also, the age distribution of people classified as having generalised epilepsy suggests errors in the classification of epilepsy type. Failure of the RCTs to document generalised seizures other than tonic clonic seizures is an important limitation. The meta-analysis does not provide evidence to support or refute the use of sodium valproate for people with generalised tonic clonic seizures as part of generalised epilepsy.

QUESTION Does the addition of second line drugs benefit people with drug resistant partial epilepsy?

Systematic reviews in people with drug resistant partial epilepsy have found that adding gabapentin, levetiracetam, lamotrigine, oxcarbazepine, tiagabine, topiramate, vigabatrin, or zonisamide to usual treatment reduces seizure frequency compared with adding placebo. The reviews have found that adding any of the drugs increases the frequency of adverse effects compared with adding placebo. We found no good evidence from RCTs on which to base a choice among drugs.

Benefits: We found eight systematic reviews that compared the addition of active drugs versus placebo in people who have not responded to usual drug treatment.[15–22] **Gabapentin versus placebo:** One systematic review (search date 2002, 5 RCTs, 997 people) found that adding gabapentin to usual treatment significantly reduced seizure frequency compared with adding placebo (see table 1, p 1524).[15] **Levetiracetam versus placebo:** One systematic review (search date 2003, 4 RCTs, 1023 people) found that adding levetiracetam to usual treatment significantly reduced seizure frequency compared with adding placebo (see table 2, p 1525).[16] **Lamotrigine versus placebo:** One systematic review (search date 2002, 11 RCTs, 1243 people) found that adding of lamotrigine to usual treatment significantly reduced seizure frequency compared with adding placebo (see table 2, p 1525).[17] **Oxcarbazepine versus placebo:** One systematic review (search date 2002, 2 RCTs, 961 adults and children) found that adding oxcarbazepine to usual treatment significantly reduced seizure frequency compared with adding placebo (see table 2, p 1525).[18] **Tiagabine versus placebo:** One systematic review (search date 2002, 3 RCTs, 769 people) found that adding tiagabine to usual treatment significantly reduced seizure frequency compared with adding placebo (see table 2, p 1525).[22] **Topiramate versus placebo:** One systematic review (search date 2002, 6 RCTs, 743 people) found that adding topiramate to usual treatment significantly reduced seizure frequency compared with adding placebo (see table 1, p 1524).[20] **Vigabatrin versus placebo:** One systematic review (search date 1995, 4 RCTs, 495 people) found that adding vigabatrin to usual treatment significantly reduced seizure frequency compared with adding placebo (see table 1, p 1524).[19] **Zonisamide versus placebo:** One systematic review (search date 2002, 3 RCTs, 499 people) found that adding zonisamide to usual treatment significantly reduced seizure frequency compared with adding placebo (see table 2, p 1525).[21]

Harms: Adverse effects and treatment withdrawal were more frequent with additional treatment than with placebo (see table 1, p 1524 and table 2, p 1525).[15,20] Lamotrigine is associated with a rash, which may be avoided by slower titration of the drug. Vigabatrin causes concentric visual field abnormalities in about 40% of people, which are probably irreversible.[23]

Comment: Few RCTs have compared these drugs directly with each other. Because of the irreversible visual field abnormalities associated with vigabatrin, the consensus view among neurologists is not to recommend this drug.

QUESTION Which people in remission from seizures are at risk of relapse on withdrawal of drug treatment?

One RCT in people who had been seizure free for at least 2 years found that further seizures were more likely if people stopped treatment than if they continued antiepileptic medication. Observational studies have found that nearly a third of people will relapse within 2 years if antiepileptic drugs are withdrawn. Clinical predictors of relapse after drug withdrawal include age, seizure type, number of antiepileptic drugs being taken, whether seizures have occurred since antiepileptic drugs were started, and the period of remission before drug withdrawal.

Benefits: One large RCT (1013 people who had been seizure free for > 2 years) compared continued antiepileptic treatment with slow antiepileptic drug withdrawal.[24,25] At 2 years, 78% of people who continued treatment remained seizure free compared with 59% in the withdrawal group. There were no significant differences in psychosocial outcomes between groups. Risk reductions with 95% confidence intervals for the main factors predicting recurrence of seizures are tabulated (see table 3, p 1526).[24] One systematic review of observational studies (search date not stated) found that, at 2 years, 29% (95% CI 24% to 34%) of people in remission from all types of epilepsy would relapse if antiepileptic drugs were withdrawn.[26]

Harms: Sixteen people died during the trial, 10 in the continued treatment group and six in the withdrawal group.[25] Only two deaths were attributed to epilepsy, and both of these occurred in people randomised to continued treatment.

Comment: People with a seizure recurrence were less likely to be in paid employment at 2 years.[24,25]

QUESTION What are the effects of behavioural and psychological treatments for people with epilepsy?

OPTION RELAXATION THERAPY

One systematic review found insufficient evidence about the effects of relaxation therapy compared with control in people with epilepsy.

Benefits: **Seizure frequency:** We found one systematic review (search date 2002,[27] 3 small unblinded controlled trials,[28–30] 50 people, including 32 women). The trials used weak methods (see comment below). Two of the studies found a non-significant reduction in seizure frequency with relaxation therapy (see glossary, p 1521) compared with no relaxation therapy, and one study found a significantly reduced seizure frequency. The weak methods preclude reliable conclusions.

Harms: The RCTs gave no information on adverse effects.[28–30]

Comment: All three trials used weak methods.[28–30] The treatment allocation methods were strict alternation,[30] alternation in blocks of five,[29] or were not stated.[28] The baseline seizure frequency varied considerably among the allocated groups in all of the trials. In one trial, two people in the treatment group had new antiepileptic medication added during the study period and one of these had a greater than 50% reduction in seizure frequency; another person discontinued antiepileptic medication.[29] Antiepileptic drug treatment was also adjusted during the trial, making it difficult to conclude whether the observed results were because of changes in drug treatment or because of the intervention. The trial duration and follow up was short. The possibility of publication bias cannot be excluded. The effects of relaxation therapy remain unclear.

OPTION YOGA

We found insufficient evidence from one systematic review about effects of yoga in people with epilepsy.

Benefits: **Seizure frequency:** We found one systematic review (search date 2002,[31] 1 quasi randomised trial,[32] 32 people). The RCT compared sahaja yoga (10 people) versus control (sham yoga 10 people, no intervention 12 people). The trial found that yoga reduced seizure frequency compared with control but it used weak methods, which precludes reliable conclusions.

Harms: The trial gave no information on adverse effects.[32]

Comment: The baseline seizure frequency and duration varied among the groups, making results difficult to interpret.[32]

OPTION BIOFEEDBACK

We found insufficient evidence from one systematic review about the effects of electroencephalographic feedback.

Benefits: **Seizure frequency:** We found one systematic review (search date 2002,[27] 1 controlled trial,[33] 24 people with uncontrolled epilepsy) of electroencephalographic (EEG) biofeedback (see glossary, p 1520) compared with control treatment. The trial compared three treatments: EEG biofeedback, sham (non-contingent) feedback, and no intervention (8 people in each group). It found a significant reduction in seizure frequency compared with the baseline frequency in people given biofeedback (median seizure reduction with biofeedback 61%; $P < 0.005$ *v* baseline; see comment below).

Harms: The trial gave no information on harms.[33]

Comment: The RCT did not provide data about seizure frequency in the control group.[33] We were therefore unable to compare the EEG biofeedback and control groups. The RCT did not report the number of people who had greater than 50% reduction in seizure frequency. The study was not blinded and the randomisation method is not clear. The duration of follow up was only 6 weeks. The evidence is insufficient to draw reliable conclusions about the effects of EEG biofeedback.

OPTION COGNITIVE BEHAVIOURAL TREATMENT

We found insufficient evidence about the effects of cognitive behavioural therapy in people with epilepsy. One small RCT found no significant difference in seizure frequency between group cognitive behavioural treatment and control treatment. The RCT found no significant improvement in psychosocial function. Another small RCT found that cognitive behavioural treatment improved a depression score in people with epilepsy plus depressed mood compared with control treatment.

Benefits: **Seizure frequency:** We found one systematic review (search date 2002)[27] that found one RCT (30 people)[34] comparing cognitive behavioural therapy (see glossary, p 1520) versus control treatment. The RCT found no significant difference between cognitive behavioural therapy and control treatment in seizure frequency, but the RCT was too small to exclude a clinically important difference. **Psychosocial functioning:** The RCT included in the review found no significant differences between cognitive behavioural therapy and control treatments in various psychological scales, such as the Washington Psycho Social Inventory, the Minnesota Multiphasic Inventory, and the Beck Depression Inventory (see glossary, p 1520).[34] Another RCT (15 people with epilepsy and depression) found that cognitive behavioural therapy significantly reduced depression and self reported anxiety or anger, and significantly increased involvement in social activities compared with control treatment.[35] The RCT did not report seizure frequencies, or specify the intervention given to controls or the concomitant antidepressant treatment.

Harms: The trial gave no information on harms.[34]

Comment: The method of randomisation concealment is not known for these small RCTs.[34,35] Publication bias cannot be excluded. The evidence is insufficient to define the effects of cognitive behavioural therapy on people with epilepsy.

OPTION EDUCATIONAL PROGRAMMES

One RCT found that a 2 day education programme reduced seizure frequency at 6 months compared with waiting list control, although it found no significant difference in health related quality of life. Two RCTs found that an educational package improved knowledge and understanding of epilepsy, adjustment to epilepsy, and psychosocial functioning compared with control.

Benefits: We found one systematic review (search date 2002,[27] 2 RCTs[36,37]) and one subsequent RCT.[38] **Seizure frequency:** The two RCTs included in the review did not report on seizure frequency.[36,37] The subsequent RCT (242 people) found that a 2 day educational programme significantly reduced seizure frequency at 6 months compared with waiting list control (proportion of people with at least 2 point reduction in seizure frequency on a 6 point scale [0 = no seizures in last 6 months, 5 = at least one seizure daily]: 19% with education *v* 7.2% with control; P value not reported).[38] However, the clinical importance of this effect is unclear. **Psychosocial functioning:** One RCT included in the review (100 adults with epilepsy) found that a specific 2 day educational programme significantly improved responses to a 50 item true/false questionnaire compared with control intervention (overall understanding of epilepsy, significant decrease in fear of seizures, significant decrease in hazardous medical self management) and significantly improved compliance with current medication (demonstrated by serum antiepileptic drug levels).[36] The second RCT included in the review (252 children with epilepsy aged 7–14 years) found that a child centred, family focused educational programme significantly improved questionnaire responses compared with control intervention (knowledge about what to do during a seizure, purpose of the electroencephalographic [see glossary, p 1520] examination, and minimal restriction in activities), increased the proportion of children likely to participate in normal activities, improved perceived academic and social competencies of the children, and reduced the anxiety of parents (see comment below).[37] The subsequent RCT found that a 2 day educational programme had no significant effect on SF-36 questionnaire scores (see glossary, p 1521) 6 months after the programme compared with waiting list control (SF-36 mental health component score 43.7 with educational package *v* 42.5 with control, P value not stated; SF-36 physical component score 50.4 with educational package *v* 52.0 with control, P value not stated).[38] Scales validated using the study population revealed significant improvement in epilepsy knowledge and coping with epilepsy.

Harms: None reported.

Comment: In one RCT, randomisation was by random number assignment, but only a proportion of medical records were available to the authors (65% in the experimental group *v* 47% of controls).[36] In the other

RCT the method of randomisation was not stated.[37] A minority of the people in the first RCT actively participated in the interventions (23/50 in the treatment group *v* 20/50 in the control group) or completed the study (20/50 in the treatment group *v* 18/50 in the control group).[36] In the subsequent RCT, the method of randomisation was not stated, and among 383 patients randomised 242 (113 in the treatment group and 119 in control group) completed the study.[38]

OPTION RELAXATION PLUS BEHAVIOURAL MODIFICATION THERAPY

Two RCTs found insufficient evidence about the effects of combined relaxation and behavioural modification treatment on seizures. One of the RCTs found that the intervention improved anxiety and adjustment compared with control.

Benefits: **Seizure frequency:** We found one systematic review[27] (search date 2002) that identified two RCTs of relaxation plus behaviour therapy versus control.[39,40] The first small RCT (18 children with uncontrolled epilepsy) compared three interventions for 6 weeks: behaviour modification (broad spectrum behaviour modification programme, which included teaching of symptom discrimination, relaxation, and countermeasure techniques to interrupt and abort seizures during early cues of the onset of a seizure); attention control (non-directive discussion around and experience of seizures, other people's reactions to seizures, and current problems); and control (usual care).[39] Both active treatments were given in six 1 hour sessions. It found that behaviour modification significantly reduced the median seizure index (the product of the seizure frequency and the seizure duration in seconds) compared with baseline after 1 year and that the median seizure index was increased compared with baseline in the control groups after 1 year. Long term follow up of the RCT found that behaviour modification significantly reduced the median seizure index after 8 years.[41] The RCT did not report actual values for these observations, so comparison of groups is not possible. The second RCT (150 adults with uncontrolled epilepsy) compared Jacobson's muscle relaxation plus behavioural therapy versus control treatment.[40] It reported separately the mean seizure frequencies for each seizure type but did not specify the number in each category. It reported separately the mean seizure frequencies for those people with fewer than 20 seizures and those with more than 20 seizures per month at baseline. We were unable to analyse these results in a meaningful way. **Psychological outcomes:** The second RCT found that relaxation plus behavioural modification significantly improved anxiety (Spielberger's self assessment questionnaire for trait and state anxiety; $P < 0.01$), and home, health, social, and emotional adjustment compared with control (assessed by adjustment inventory; P values not reported).[40]

Harms: The RCTs gave no information on harms.[39,40]

Comment: The randomisation method was not stated for one study and was by alternate allocation in the other. The seizure index reported in one study is not an ideal outcome measure.[39] One of the RCTs recruited only 18 children and the groups would not be expected to be balanced for baseline characteristics.[39] It is possible that the results of the psychological interventions on psychosocial functioning may depend on the baseline personality of the persons included in the study, and their education and intelligence.

OPTION FAMILY COUNSELLING

We found insufficient evidence on family counselling from one small RCT that employed weak methods.

Benefits: We found no systematic review but found one small RCT (36 people with epilepsy and job loss) that compared three interventions: family therapy (no detailed description but it appears that the family was present for discussion of problems for a mean of 7.8 sessions); one family session (in which information about the seizure profile was given); and usual care (vocational assistance in obtaining a job with no follow up other than site visit).[42] It did not report seizure frequencies, but found a significantly improved psychosocial inventory score with family therapy (Washington Psycho Social Inventory [see glossary, p 1521], 27 completers: improved perceived acceptance by family, emotional adjustment, interpersonal adjustment, adjustment to seizures, and overall psychosocial function). It found a trend toward improvement in job stability.

Harms: The study did not report harms.[42]

Comment: The method of concealment of randomisation was not described in the RCT.[42] Nine of the 36 people did not complete the study and withdrawal was uneven across the groups (2 with family therapy, 6 with 1 family session, 1 with no intervention). The available evidence is insufficient to define the effects of family counselling.

GLOSSARY

Absence seizure Previously known as "petit mal". Brief episodes of unconsciousness with vacant staring, sometimes with fluttering of the eyelids, as if "daydreaming". People with absence seizure do not fall to the ground and generally have a rapid recovery. The condition is rare in adults.

Atonic seizure Momentary loss of limb muscle tone causing sudden falling to the ground or drooping of the head.

Beck Depression Inventory Standardised scale to assess depression.

Cognitive behavioural therapy A broad category of interventions designed to identify and control stress and minimise its effects, often by using intellectual experience to correct damaging thoughts and behaviour.

Complex partial seizure Consciousness is impaired and memory of the episode is distorted, but the person may not collapse. The person may exhibit automatic behaviours ("automatisms", such as chewing, scratching the head, undressing). Complex partial seizures can spread to the rest of the brain to become a secondary generalised tonic clonic seizure (see below). The electrical abnormality commonly starts in the temporal lobes.

Electroencephalographic (EEG) biofeedback A technique of making EEG activity apparent to a person, who is then taught to produce certain EEG waves that are believed to increase the threshold for seizures.

Minnesota Multiphasic Personality Inventory (MMPI) A battery of standardised tests to assess personality (psychopathology).

Myoclonic seizure Sudden, symmetrical, shock like limb movements with or without loss of consciousness.

Relaxation therapy Techniques to train people to control muscle tension.

SF-36 score A scale that assesses health related quality of life across eight domains: limitations in physical activities (physical component); limitations in social activities; limitations in usual role activities due to physical problems; pain; psychological distress and wellbeing (mental health component); limitations in usual role activities because of emotional problems; energy and fatigue; and general health perceptions.

Simple partial seizure Electrical activity confined to one localised part of the brain causing symptoms and signs that depend on the part of the brain affected. The person remains conscious and fully aware.

Tonic clonic seizure Also known as a convulsion or "grand mal" attack. The person will become stiff (tonic) and collapse, and have generalised jerking (clonic) movements. Breathing might stop and the bladder might empty. Generalised jerking movements lasting typically for a few minutes are followed by relaxation and deep unconsciousness, before the person slowly comes round. People are often tired and confused, and may remember nothing. Tonic clonic seizures may follow simple partial or complex partial seizures (see above), where they are classified as secondary generalised tonic clonic seizures. Tonic clonic seizures occurring without warning and in the context of generalised epilepsy are classified as generalised tonic clonic seizures.

Tonic seizure Stiffening of the whole body with or without loss of consciousness.

Washington Psycho Social Inventory (WPSI) A standardised battery of tests to assess adjustment in various spheres (measure of psychosocial difficulties) in people with epilepsy.

Substantive changes

Partial epilepsy; monotherapy Two systematic reviews added;[11,12] conclusions unchanged.

Generalised epilepsy; monotherapy Two systematic reviews added;[11,12] conclusions unchanged.

REFERENCES

1. Commission on classification and terminology of the international league against epilepsy. Proposal for revised classification of epilepsies and epileptic syndromes. *Epilepsia* 1989;30:389–399.
2. Hauser AW, Annegers JF, Kurland LT. Incidence of epilepsy and unprovoked seizures in Rochester, Minnesota 1935–84. *Epilepsia* 1993;34:453–468.
3. Hauser WA, Kurland LT. The epidemiology of epilepsy in Rochester, Minnesota, 1935 through 1967. *Epilepsia* 1975;16:1–66.
4. Cockerell OC, Johnson AL, Sander JW, et al. Remission of epilepsy: results from the national general practice study of epilepsy. *Lancet* 1995;346:140–144.
5. Berg AT, Shinnar S. The risk of seizure recurrence following a first unprovoked seizure: a quantitative review. *Neurology* 1991;41:965–972. Search date not stated; primary sources Cumulated Index Medicus, and bibliographies of relevant papers.
6. First Seizure Trial Group (FIRST Group). Randomized clinical trial on the efficacy of antiepileptic drugs in reducing the risk of relapse after a first unprovoked tonic clonic seizure. *Neurology* 1993;43:478–483.
7. Musicco M, Beghi E, Solari A, et al, for the FIRST group. Treatment of first tonic clonic seizure does not improve the prognosis of epilepsy. *Neurology* 1997;49:991–998.
8. Marson AG, Williamson PR, Hutton JL, et al.; on behalf of the epilepsy monotherapy trialists. Carbamazepine versus valproate monotherapy for epilepsy. In: The Cochrane Library, Issue 1, 2003. Oxford: Update Software. Search date 1999; primary sources Medline, Cochrane Library, Cochrane Epilepsy Group Trials Register and personal contact with the drug manufacturers and investigators of the relevant trials found.
9. Tudur Smith C, Marson AG, Williamson PR. Phenytoin versus valproate monotherapy for partial onset seizures and generalized onset tonic-clonic seizures. In: The Cochrane Library, Issue 1, 2003. Oxford: Update Software. Search date 2000; primary sources Cochrane Epilepsy Group trial register, Medline and hand searches of the journals Epilepsia, Epilepsy Research and Acta Neurologica Scandinavica and personal contact with the drug manufacturers and original investigators of relevant trials.
10. Taylor S, Tudur Smith C, Williamson PR, et al. Phenobarbitone versus phenytoin monotherapy for partial onset seizures and generalized onset tonic-clonic seizures. In: The Cochrane Library, Issue 1, 2003. Oxford: Update Software. Search date 1998; primary sources Medline, Cochrane Controlled Trials Register and hand searches of the journals Epilepsia, Epilepsy Research and Acta

Neurologica Scandinavica and personal contact with the pharmaceutical industry and researchers in the field.

11. Tudur Smith C, Marson AG, Williamson PR. Carbamazepine versus phenobarbitone monotherapy for epilepsy (Cochrane Review). In: The Cochrane Library, Issue 1, 2003. Oxford: Update Software. Search date 2002; primary sources Cochrane Epilepsy Group trial register, Cochrane Controlled Trials Register, Medline, Embase, hand searches and personal contact with trial investigators and manufactures of carbamazepine.
12. Tudur Smith C, Marson AG, Clough HE, et al. Carbamazepine versus phenytoin monotherapy for epilepsy (Cochrane Review). In: The Cochrane Library, Issue 1, 2003. Oxford: Update Software. Search date 2002; primary sources Cochrane Epilepsy Group trial register, Cochrane Controlled Trials Register, Medline, Embase, hand searches and personal contact with trial investigators and manufactures of carbamazepine.
13. Mattson RH, Cramer JA, Collins JF. A comparison of valproate with carbamazepine for the treatment of complex partial seizures and secondarily generalized tonic-clonic seizures in adults. The Department of Veterans Affairs Epilepsy Cooperative Study No. 264 Group. *N Engl J Med* 1992;10:327:765–771.
14. Richens A, Davidson DL, Cartlidge NE, et al. A multicentre comparative trial of sodium valproate and carbamazepine in adult onset epilepsy: adult EPITEG collaborative group. *J Neurol Neurosurg Psychiatry* 1994;57:682–687.
15. Marson AG, Kadir ZA, Hutton JL, et al. Gabapentin add-on for drug-resistant partial epilepsy. In: The Cochrane Library, Issue 1, 2003. Oxford: Update Software. Search date 2002; primary sources Cochrane Epilepsy Group trials register, Cochrane Controlled Trials Register and hand searches of reference lists of articles and personal contact with the manufacturers of gabapentin and experts in the field.
16. Chaisewikul R, Privitera MD, Hutton JL, et al. Levetiracetam add-on for drug-resistant localization related (partial) epilepsy. In: The Cochrane Library, Issue 1, 2003. Oxford: Update Software. Search date 2003; primary sources Cochrane Epilepsy Group trials register, Cochrane Controlled Trials Register and personal contact with the manufacturers of levetiracetam) and experts in the field.
17. Ramaratnam S, Marson AG, Baker GA. Lamotrigine add-on for drug-resistant partial epilepsy. In: The Cochrane Library, Issue 1, 2003. Oxford: Update Software. Search date 2002; primary sources Cochrane Epilepsy Group trials register, Cochrane Controlled Trials Register, Medline and hand searches of reference lists of articles and personal contact with the manufacturers of lamotrigine.
18. Castillo S, Schmidt DB, White S. Oxcarbazepine add-on for drug-resistant partial epilepsy. In: The Cochrane Library, Issue 1, 2003. Oxford: Update Software. Search date 2002; primary sources Cochrane Epilepsy Group trials register, Cochrane Controlled Trials Register, Medline and hand searches of reference lists of articles and personal contact with the manufacturers of oxcarbazepine and experts in the field.
19. Marson AG, Kadir ZA, Hutton JL, et al. The new antiepileptic drugs: a systematic review of their efficacy and tolerability. *Epilepsia* 1997;38:859–880. Search date 1995; primary sources Medline, hand search of key journals, and contacting pharmaceutical companies.
20. Jette NJ, Marson AG, Hutton JL. Topiramate add-on for drug-resistant partial epilepsy. In: The Cochrane Library, Issue 1, 2003. Oxford: Update Software. Search date 2003; primary sources Cochrane Epilepsy Group specialized register, Cochrane Controlled Trials Register and personal contact with the manufacturers of topiramate and experts in the field.
21. Chadwick DW, Marson AG. Zonisamide add-on for drug-resistant partial epilepsy. In: The Cochrane Library, Issue 1, 2003. Oxford: Update Software. Search date 2002; primary sources Cochrane Epilepsy Group trial register, Cochrane Controlled Trials Register and personal contact with the manufacturers/licensees of zonisamide and experts in the field.
22. Pereira J, Marson AG, Hutton JL. Tiagabine add-on for drug-resistant partial epilepsy. In: The Cochrane Library, Issue 1, 2003. Oxford: Update Software. Search date 2002; primary sources Cochrane Epilepsy Group trials register, Cochrane Controlled Trials Register, Medline, and personal contact with the manufacturers of tiagabine and experts in the field.
23. Kalviainen R, Nousiainen I, Mantyjarvi M, et al. Vigabatrin, a gabaergic antiepileptic drug, causes concentric visual field defects. *Neurology* 1999;53:922–926.
24. Medical Research Council Antiepileptic Drug Withdrawal Study Group. Prognostic index for recurrence of seizures after remission of epilepsy. *BMJ* 1993;306:1374–1378.
25. Medical Research Council Antiepileptic Drug Withdrawal Study Group. Randomised study of antiepileptic drug withdrawal in patients in remission. *Lancet* 1991;337:1175–1180.
26. Berg AT, Shinnar S. Relapse following discontinuation of antiepileptic drugs. *Neurology* 1994;44:601–608. Search date not stated; primary sources Index Medicus and bibliographies of relevant papers.
27. Ramaratnam S, Baker GA, Goldstein L. Psychological treatments for epilepsy. In: The Cochrane Library, Issue 1, 2003. Oxford: Update Software. Search date 2002; primary sources Cochrane Epilepsy Group trial register, Cochrane Controlled Trials Register, Medline and hand searches of reference lists from identified publications.
28. Dahl J, Melin L, Lund L. Effects of a contingent relaxation treatment program on adults with refractory epileptic seizures. *Epilepsia* 1987;28:125–132.
29. Puskarich CA, Whitman S, Dell J, et al. Controlled examination of effects of progressive relaxation training on seizure reduction. *Epilepsia* 1992;33:675–680.
30. Rousseau A, Hermann B, Whitman S. Effects of progressive relaxation on epilepsy: Analysis of a series of cases. *Psychol Rep* 1985;57:1203–1212.
31. Ramaratnam S, Sridharan K. Yoga for epilepsy. In: The Cochrane Library, Issue 1, 2003. Oxford: Update Software. Search date 2002; primary sources Cochrane Epilepsy Group trial register, Cochrane Controlled Trials Register, Medline, Registries of the Research Council for Complimentary Medicine and hand searches of references of identified studies and personal contact with experts in the field.
32. Panjwani U, Selvamurthy W, Singh SH, et al. Effect of sahaja yoga practice on seizure control and EEG changes in patients of epilepsy. *Ind J Med Res* 1996;103:165–172.

33. Lantz DL, Sterman MB. Neuropsychological assessment of subjects with uncontrolled epilepsy: effects of EEG feedback training. *Epilepsia* 1988;29:163–171.
34. Tan SY Bruni J. Cognitive behavior therapy with adult patients with epilepsy: a controlled outcome study. *Epilepsia* 1986;27:225–233.
35. Davis GR, Armstrong HE Jr, Donovan DM, et al. Cognitive-behavioral treatment of depressed affect among epileptics: preliminary findings. *Journal of Clinical Psychology*. 1984;40:930–935
36. Helgeson DC, Mittan R, Tan SY, et al. Sepulveda epilepsy education: the efficacy of a psychoeducational treatment program in treating medical and psychosocial aspects of epilepsy. *Epilepsia* 1990;31:75–82.
37. Lewis MA, Salas I, De La Sota A, et al. Randomized trial of a program to enhance the competencies of children with epilepsy. *Epilepsia* 1990;31:101–109.
38. May TW, Pifflin M. The efficacy of an educations treatment program for patients with epilepsy (MOSES): results of a controlled, randomized study. *Epilepsia* 2002;43:539–549.
39. Dahl J, Melin L, Brorson LO, et al. Effects of a broad-spectrum behavior modification treatment program on children with refractory epileptic seizures. *Epilepsia*. 1985; 26: 303–309.
40. Sultana SM. *A study on the psychological factors and the effect of psychological treatment in intractable epilepsy*. PhD Thesis, University of Madras, India 1987.
41. Dahl J, Brorson LO, Melin L. Effects of a broad-spectrum behavioral medicine treatment program on children with refractory epileptic seizures: an 8-year follow-up. *Epilepsia* 1992;33:98–102.
42. Earl WL. Job stability and family counseling. *Epilepsia* 1986;27:215–219.

Anthony Marson
Lecturer in Neurology
University of Liverpool
Liverpool
UK

Sridharan Ramaratnam
Senior Consultant Neurologist
Apollo Hospitals
Chennai (Madras)
India

Competing interests: AM has been paid for speaking at meetings by Johnson and Johnson, manufacturers of topiramate, and by Janssen-Cilag, Sanofi, and GlaxoSmithKline for attending conferences. SR none declared

TABLE 1 **Effects of additional drug treatment in people not responding to usual treatment: results of systematic reviews (see text, p 1514).**

Drug	Daily dose (mg)	Percentage responding (95% CI)*	RR treatment withdrawal (95% CI)	RR adverse effects with CI (95% unless otherwise stated)	Comment
Gabapentin	**Adults only**				
	Placebo	9.9 (7.2 to 13.5)	1.4 (0.8 to 2.5)	Dizziness 2.25 (1.3 to 4)	5 RCTs (1 in children, 4 in adults)
	600	14.4 (12.0 to 17.3)		Fatigue 2.25 (1.1 to 4.6)	Efficacy increased with
	900	17.3 (14.6 to 20.3)		Somnolence 2.04 (1.2 to 3.4)	increasing dose. No plateauing
	1200	20.6 (17.1 to 24.6)			of response, so doses tested
	1800	28.5 (21.5 to 36.7)			may not have been optimal
	Adults and children		**Adults and children**	**Adults and children**	
	600–1800	RR 1.81 (1.32 to 2.49)	1.04 (0.71 to 1.52)	Dizziness 2.19 (1.24 to 3.89) Fatigue 2.30 (1.11 to 4.75) Somnolence 1.91 (1.20 to 3.05)	
Topiramate	Placebo 200	11.7 (8.7 to 15.7)	2.06 (1.38 to 3.08)	Ataxia 1.95 (99% CI 1.04 to 3.65)	9 RCTs
	400–1000	26.8 (15.8 to 41.3)		Dizziness 1.55 (99% CI 1.07 to 2.24)	
		46.5 (42.5 to 50.5)		Fatigue 2.21 (99% CI 1.42 to 3.45)	
				Somnolence 2.26 (99% CI 1.48 to 3.46)	
				Difficulty thinking 5.54 (99% CI 2.34 to 13.12)	
Vigabatrin (adults)	Placebo	13.8 (9.7 to 19.2)	2.95 (1.25 to 7.00)	No adverse effects significantly more frequent but 40% develop concentric visual field abnormalities[23]	3 RCTs
	1000 or 2000	22.8 (14.5 to 34.9)			
	3000 or 6000	45.9 (39.5 to 52.5)			

Results show percentage responding at particular daily doses, but results for treatment withdrawal and adverse effects are calculated for all doses.
*50% reduction in seizure frequency.

TABLE 2 **Effects of additional drug treatment in people not responding to usual treatment: results of systematic reviews (see text, p 1514).**

Drug	Daily dose (mg)	Percentage responding (95% CI)*	RR treatment withdrawal (95% CI)	RR adverse effects (95% CI)	Comment
Levetiracetam (adults)	1000–3000	3.78 (2.62 to 5.44)	1.21 (0.88 to 1.66)	Dizziness 2.50 (1.16 to 5.41) Infection 1.76 (1.03 to 3.02)	4 RCTs. Results of regression models with CI (95% unless otherwise stated) do not provide reliable estimates for a response to individual doses.
Lamotrigine (adults)	200–500	2.32 (1.67 to 3.23)	1.10 (0.81 to 1.50)	Ataxia 3.23 (1.93 to 5.42) Diplopia 3.47 (1.91 to 6.31) Dizziness 2.05 (1.52 to 2.78) Nausea 1.76 (1.18 to 2.64)	11 RCTs
Oxcarbazepine (adults and children)	600–2400	2.51 (1.88 to 3.33)	1.72 (1.35 to 2.18)	Ataxia 3.54 (1.75 to 7.13) Dizziness 2.87 (1.82 to 4.52) Fatigue 1.81 (1.00 to 3.29) Nausea 3.09 (1.74 to 5.49) Somnolence 2.36 (1.54 to 3.62) Diplopia 7.25 (3.12 to 16.80)	2 RCTs
Tiagabine	16–56	RR 3.67 (2.30 to 5.86)	1.81 (1.25 to 2.62)	Dizziness 1.69 (99% CI 1.13 to 2.51)	3 RCTs. Results of regression models do not provide accurate estimates for a response to individual doses
Zonisamide	400	2.46 (1.61 to 3.76)	1.64 (1.02 to 2.62)	Ataxia 4.50 (99% CI 1.05 to 19.22) Somnolence 1.91 (99% CI 1.08 to 3.38) Aggitation/irritability 2.37 (99% CI 1.00 to 5.64) Anorexia 3.00 (99% CI 1.31 to 6.88)	3 RCTs

*50% reduction in seizure frequency. All results are calculated for all doses.

TABLE 3 **Relative risks of seizure recurrence within 2 years of treatment withdrawal, according to prognostic variable (see text, p 1515).[24,25]**

Prognostic variable	RR (95% CI) of seizure recurrence within 2 years
Age < 16 years	1.8 (1.3 to 2.4)
Tonic clonic seizures	1.6 (1.1 to 2.2)
Myoclonus	1.8 (1.1 to 3.0)
Treatment with more than one antiepileptic drug	1.9 (1.4 to 2.4)
Seizures since antiepileptic drugs were started	1.6 (1.2 to 2.1)
Any electroencephalographic abnormality	1.3 (1.0 to 1.8)

Risk of recurrence also declined as the seizure free period increased, but in a complex manner.

Essential tremor

Search date September 2002

Joaquim Ferreira and Cristina Sampaio

QUESTIONS

INTERVENTIONS

See glossary, p 1536

Key Messages

- **All treatment options (long term)** We found no RCTs that reported the long term effects of drug treatments for essential tremor.
- **β Blockers other than propranolol (atenolol, sotalol)** Small RCTs found weak evidence that sotalol or atenolol versus placebo significantly improved symptoms and self evaluated measures of tremor at 5 days to 4 weeks. However, we were unable to draw reliable conclusions about effects.
- **Benzodiazepines** Two small short term RCTs found weak evidence that alprazolam may improve tremor and function compared with placebo. However, we were unable to draw reliable conclusions about effects. We found insufficient evidence to compare effects of clonazepam versus placebo. Adverse effects with benzodiazepines, including sedation and cognitive and behavioural effects, have been well described for other conditions (see panic disorder, p 1188).
- **Botulinum A toxin–haemagglutinin complex (evidence for short term only)** RCTs comparing botulinum A toxin–haemagglutinin complex versus placebo found short term improvement of clinical rating scales, but no consistent improvement of motor task performance or functional disability. Hand weakness, which is dose dependent and transient, is a frequent adverse effect.

Essential tremor

- **Calcium channel blockers (nicardipine, nimodipine)** Poor quality RCTs found insufficient evidence about the effects of dihydropyridine calcium channel blockers versus placebo.
- **Carbonic anhydrase inhibitors** Two RCTs found no evidence of benefit with carbonic anhydrase inhibitors compared with placebo.
- **Clonidine** One RCT found no significant difference between clonidine and placebo for clinical improvement. However, the study may have lacked power to detect clinically important differences.
- **Flunarizine** One small RCT found weak evidence that flunarizine versus placebo may improve symptoms after 1 month of treatment.
- **Gabapentin** Small crossover RCTs found insufficient evidence about the effects of gabapentin versus placebo.
- **Isoniazid** One RCT found no significant difference with isoniazid versus placebo in clinical score. However, the study may have lacked power to detect clinically important differences.
- **Phenobarbital (evidence for short term only)** One small RCT found limited evidence that phenobarbital versus placebo significantly improved tremor scores at 5 weeks. However, two further RCTs found no significant difference between phenobarbital and placebo. Phenobarbital is associated with depression and cognitive and behavioural adverse effects.
- **Primidone (evidence for short term only)** Three small, short term RCTs found limited evidence that primidone versus placebo improved tremor and functional ability. We found no long term RCTs. Primidone is associated with depression and cognitive and behavioural adverse effects.
- **Propranolol (evidence for short term only)** Small RCTs have found that propranolol versus placebo significantly improves short term clinical scores, tremor amplitude, and symptom severity for up to 6 weeks.
- **Topiramate** One RCT found that topiramate improved observer rated tremor score but was associated with more adverse effects compared with placebo. The clinical importance of the difference in tremor score is uncertain.

DEFINITION Tremor is a rhythmic, mechanical oscillation of at least one body region. The term essential tremor is used when there is either a persistent bilateral tremor of hands and forearms, or an isolated tremor of the head without abnormal posturing, and when there is no evidence that the tremor arises from another identifiable or separately named cause. The diagnosis is not made if there are abnormal neurological signs, known causes of enhanced physiological tremor, a history or signs of psychogenic tremor, sudden change in severity, primary orthostatic tremor, isolated voice tremor, isolated position specific or task specific tremors, and isolated tongue, chin, or leg tremor.[1]

INCIDENCE/ PREVALENCE Essential tremor is one of the most common movement disorders throughout the world, with a prevalence of 0.4–3.9% in the general population.[2]

AETIOLOGY/ RISK FACTORS Essential tremor is sometimes inherited with an autosomal dominant pattern. About 40% of people with essential tremor have no family history. Alcohol ingestion provides symptomatic benefit in 50–70% of people.[3]

PROGNOSIS Essential tremor is a persistent and progressive condition. It usually begins during young adulthood and the severity of the tremor increases slowly. Only a small proportion of people with essential tremor seek medical advice, but the proportion in different surveys varies from 0.5–11%.[2] Most people with essential tremor are only mildly affected. However, most of the people who seek medical care are disabled to some extent, and most are socially handicapped by the tremor.[4] A quarter of people receiving medical care for the tremor change jobs or retire because of essential tremor induced disability.[3,5]

AIMS OF INTERVENTION To reduce tremor; to minimise disability and social embarrassment; to improve quality of life, with minimal adverse effects from treatment.

OUTCOMES Severity of symptoms and disability measured by clinical rating scales or patient self evaluation. Clinical rating scales are often composite scores that grade tremor amplitude in each body segment in specific postures or tasks. Few scales have been formally validated. Tremorgraphic recordings are reported in many trials but they are proxy outcomes that have been included in this review only when clinical outcomes were not available.

METHODS *Clinical Evidence* search and appraisal September 2002. We excluded single dose studies and RCTs lasting under 1 week.

QUESTION **What are the effects of drug treatments in people with essential tremor of the hand?**

OPTION **PROPRANOLOL**

Several small RCTs have found that propranolol (60–240 mg) versus placebo for 1 month improves short term clinical scores, tremor amplitude, and self evaluation of severity. We found no RCTs of the long term effects of propranolol in essential tremor.

Benefits: **Propranolol versus placebo:** We found no systematic review but found 10 small (10–24 people), brief (up to 6 wks) RCTs, many of which had a crossover design.[6–15] One RCT[11] compared propranolol versus metoprolol versus placebo, and another RCT[15] compared propranolol versus pindolol versus placebo (see β blockers other than propranolol, p 1530). Seven of the nine RCTs evaluated clinical outcomes, including self evaluations of severity.[6–8,11–14] Propranolol (60–160 mg/day) versus placebo significantly increased the proportion of people categorised as "responders". The precise definition of responder varied among the RCTs, but the results were similar (22/23 [96%] with propranolol *v* 5/23 [22%] with placebo, ARR 69%, 95% CI 49% to 89%, NNT 2, no CI available;[6] ARR 80%, 95% CI 69% to 91%, NNT 2, no CI available;[7] ARR 64%, 95% CI 33% to 95%, NNT 2, 95% CI 2 to 4;[8] AR 10/16 [63%] with propranolol *v* 5/16 [31%] with placebo, ARR 32%, 95% CI 17% to 47%, NNT 4, 95% CI 2 to 6[14]). Six RCTs found that propranolol versus placebo significantly improved symptom scores ($P < 0.05$).[7,8,11–14]

Harms: Withdrawals (mainly because of fatigue and bradycardia) were rare (e.g. 1/10 [10%] people in 1 RCT).[8] Depression, diarrhoea, breathlessness, sedation, blurred vision, and sexual problems were each reported in fewer than 5% of people taking propranolol.

Comment: We found no RCTs on the long term effects of propranolol in essential tremor. All trials were analysed as "on treatment" rather than by intention to treat, and this may have biased results. Accelerometry is a proxy outcome that was reported in six of the RCTs. All six accelerometry results were in favour of propranolol, but there is an inconsistent relationship between accelerometry and clinical measures of effectiveness. People with congestive heart failure, second degree heart block, asthma, severe allergy, and insulin dependent diabetes were generally excluded from the RCTs. All the studies were small. The possibility of publication bias has not been excluded.

OPTION β BLOCKERS OTHER THAN PROPRANOLOL

Four small, brief RCTs found weak evidence that sotalol and atenolol improved symptoms in people with essential hand tremor. We found no adequate evidence comparing propranolol with other β blockers.

Benefits: **β Blockers other than propranolol versus placebo:** We found no systematic review, but found five small (9–24 people) brief (5 days to 4 wks) RCTs of different β blockers (sotalol, atenolol, metoprolol, nadolol, pindolol) versus placebo.[12,15–18] Two RCTs selected participants known to be responders or non-responders to propranolol.[12,17] The RCTs found limited evidence that both sotalol and atenolol versus placebo reduced symptom scores ($P < 0.02$),[12] and that sotalol versus placebo improved self evaluated measures of tremor ($P < 0.05$).[18] A small RCT of nadolol versus placebo found significant results only with a subgroup analysis.[17] The fourth crossover RCT (24 people) compared propranolol versus atenolol versus placebo. It found atenolol versus placebo improved accelerometer readings.[16] A crossover RCT of propranolol (120 mg/day) versus pindolol (30 mg/day) versus placebo found that pindolol versus placebo significantly worsened accelerometer recordings (see glossary, p 1536) ($P < 0.05$).[15] **β Blockers other than propranolol versus propranolol:** We found no systematic review but found three small (14–24 participants) crossover, double blind RCTs.[11,15,16] The first RCT compared propranolol (120–240 mg/day) versus metoprolol (150–300 mg/day) versus placebo.[11] The RCT reported three outcomes: a composite clinical score, self evaluation, and accelerometer records. Propranolol (120 mg) versus metoprolol (150 mg) significantly improved clinical scores ($P < 0.05$) and self assessment ($P < 0.01$). Propranolol (240 mg) versus metoprolol (300 mg) significantly improved self assessment ($P < 0.05$). Propranolol was statistically superior to placebo ($P < 0.05$), but metoprolol was not. The second RCT compared propranolol versus atenolol versus placebo. It found no significant difference between propranolol and atenolol in accelerometer readings, but more people preferred propranolol to atenolol (12/24

[50%] v 1/24 [4%]).[16] The third crossover RCT (24 people) compared propranolol (120 mg/day) versus pindolol (30 mg/day) versus placebo. It found that pindolol versus propranolol significantly worsened accelerometer recorded tremor amplitude ($P < 0.005$).[15]

Harms: See harms of propranolol, p 1530.

Comment: We found no long term RCTs. People with congestive heart failure, second degree heart block, asthma, severe allergy, and insulin dependent diabetes were generally excluded from the RCTs. All the studies were small. The possibility of publication bias has not been excluded. The weak evidence suggests but does not confirm that β blockers other than propranolol improve essential hand tremor compared with placebo.

OPTION BARBITURATES

Three small, short term RCTs found limited evidence that primidone versus placebo improved tremor and functional ability. One small, short term RCT found that phenobarbital versus placebo improved tremor scores, although two further RCTs found no significant difference between phenobarbital and placebo. We found no long term RCTs.

Benefits: We found no systematic reviews. **Primidone versus placebo:** We found three crossover RCTs.[19–21] All were small (8–22 people) and brief (2–5 wks). The first RCT compared primidone (up to 750 mg/day) versus phenobarbital (phenobarbitone) (up to 150 mg/day) versus placebo.[19] Primidone versus placebo significantly improved a clinical score and self evaluation of tremor ($P < 0.05$). In the second RCT (22 people), primidone (up to 750 mg/day) versus placebo significantly improved clinical scores ($P < 0.02$), functional tests ($P < 0.01$), and self evaluation ($P < 0.01$). Only 16/22 (73%) people completed the trial.[20] The third RCT (22 people) compared primidone (up to 750 mg/day, mean dose 402 mg) versus alprazolam versus acetazolamide versus placebo.[21] It found that primidone improved function compared with placebo after 4 weeks (observer rated score based on ability to write, feed and function socially [0 = normal, 11 = unable to keep pencil on paper, needs help to feed, and no social activity]; 5.2 with primidone v 7.8 with placebo; P value not provided). **Phenobarbital versus placebo:** We found three RCTs.[13,19,22] One crossover RCT (12 people) found that phenobarbital (120 mg/day) versus placebo significantly improved accelerometer recordings (see glossary, p 1536) ($P < 0.01$), symptom rating scale ($P < 0.05$) after 5 weeks, but found no significant differences for handwriting tests or self evaluation of tremor.[21] More people responded (decrease in tremor score ≥ 15%) to phenobarbital than to placebo (11/11 [100%] with phenobarbital v 6/11 [55%] with placebo; ARR 45%, 95% CI 15% to 75%; NNT 3, 95% CI 2 to 7). The second RCT (17 people; 12 completed the study) compared propranolol (1.7 mg/kg/day) versus phenobarbital (1.25 mg/kg/day) versus placebo.[13] Phenobarbital versus placebo produced no significant differences in a clinical tremor score or functional tests.[13] The third RCT (8 people) found no significant difference between phenobarbital and placebo.[19]

Harms: **Primidone:** In one RCT, 5/12 people taking primidone withdrew because of adverse effects (first dose acute toxic reaction, sedation, daytime sleepiness, tiredness, and depression).[20] In another RCT, 8/24 people receiving primidone discontinued treatment because of adverse effects, including nausea, ataxia, dizziness, or confusion.[21] **Other barbiturates:** Both primidone (metabolised to phenobarbital) and phenobarbital are associated with depression and cognitive and behavioural effects (particularly in children, elderly people, and people with neuropsychiatric problems). See epilepsy, p 1508.

Comment: The RCTs were short term, small, and many randomised people did not complete the trials. We found no long term RCTs.

OPTION BENZODIAZEPINES

Two small short term RCTs found weak evidence that alprazolam may improve tremor and function compared with placebo. However, we were unable to draw reliable conclusions about effects. We found insufficient evidence to compare effects of clonazepam versus placebo.

Benefits: We found no systematic review. We found three RCTs.[21,23,24] **Clonazepam versus placebo:** We found one RCT (15 people), which found no significant differences for any outcome.[23] However, nine people withdrew during an open run-in period with clonazepam, so only six entered the double blind phase. **Alprazolam versus placebo:** We found two RCTs.[21,24] The first RCT (24 people) found that alprazolam (up to 3 mg/day) improved observer rated global impression versus placebo, but found no significant difference in clinical scores, functional tests, or self evaluation of tremor.[24] The second RCT (22 people) compared alprazolam (up to 1.5 mg/day, mean dose 0.75 mg) versus acetazolamide versus primidone versus placebo.[21] It found that alprazolam improved function compared with placebo after 4 weeks (observer rated score based on ability to write, feed and function socially [0 = normal, 11 = unable to keep pencil on paper, needs help to feed, and no social activity]; 6.0 with alprazolam *v* 7.8 with placebo; P value not provided).

Harms: We found no data addressing harms of benzodiazepines specifically in populations with essential tremor. Adverse effects with benzodiazepines, including sedation and cognitive and behavioural effects, have been well described for other conditions (see panic disorder, p 1188).

Comment: None.

OPTION CARBONIC ANHYDRASE INHIBITORS

Two RCTs found no evidence of benefit with methazolamide or acetazolamide compared with placebo.

Benefits: We found no systematic review. **Methazolamide versus placebo:** We found one crossover RCT (25 people), which found methazolamide (up to 300 mg/day) versus placebo did not significantly improve clinical score, functional tasks, or self evaluation (7/18

[39%] improved with methazolamide *v* 4/18 [22%] with placebo; ARR +16%, 95% CI −15% to +45%).[25] **Acetazolamide versus placebo:** We found one RCT (22 people) comparing acetazolamide (up to 750 mg/day, mean dose 562 mg) versus alprazolam versus primidone versus placebo.[21] It found that acetazolamide did not significantly improve function compared with placebo after 4 weeks (observer rated score based on ability to write, feed and function socially [0 = normal, 11 = unable to keep pencil on paper, needs help to feed, and no social activity]; 7.3 with acetazolamide *v* 7.8 with placebo; P value not provided).

Harms: The methazolamide RCT did not report adverse effects.[25] In the acetazolamide RCT, 3/19 people receiving acetazolamide complained of tolerable paraesthesias.[21]

Comment: The RCTs were small. In the first RCT, the results were analysed on treatment rather than by intention to treat.[25] Seven people withdrew from the trial.

OPTION DIHYDROPYRIDINE CALCIUM CHANNEL BLOCKERS

Poor quality RCTs found insufficient evidence about the effects of dihydropyridine calcium channel blockers versus placebo.

Benefits: We found no systematic review. **Nicardipine versus placebo:** We found two RCTs.[26,27] One double blind, crossover RCT (11 people) found that nicardipine versus placebo produced no significant differences in accelerometer recordings (see glossary, p 1536) after 1 month.[26] No clinical outcomes were assessed. Another crossover RCT (14 people) compared nicardipine (1 mg/kg/day) for 1 month versus propranolol (160 mg/day) for 1 month versus placebo.[28] Both nicardipine and propranolol versus placebo improved a symptom score. **Nimodipine versus placebo:** We found one double blind, crossover RCT (15 people), which found that nimodipine (90 mg/day) versus placebo produced no significant difference in clinical scores after 2 weeks of treatment (ARR +20%, 95% CI −15% to +55%).[27]

Harms: Nicardipine and nimodipine can provoke or aggravate heart failure. They are associated with dizziness, flushing, peripheral oedema, lethargy, headache, and fatigue. Adverse gastrointestinal effects (nausea/vomiting, loss of appetite, constipation, weight gain, thirst, indigestion, or altered taste) are reported by 1–3% of people. Abnormalities of laboratory tests (liver function tests) have been observed, usually within 1–8 weeks after starting treatment.

Comment: The RCTs were small, brief, and used crossover design. The possibility of publication bias has not been excluded. The evidence is too weak to assess the role of calcium channel blockers in essential hand tremor.

OPTION FLUNARIZINE

One small RCT found weak evidence that flunarizine compared with placebo may reduce the symptoms of essential hand tremor.

Benefits: We found no systematic review. **Flunarizine versus placebo:** We found one crossover RCT (17 people), which found that flunarizine (10 mg/day) significantly improved clinical scores and tremor amplitude after 1 month of treatment (P = 0.0006) compared with placebo.[29] Most of the people who completed the study were considered improved with flunarizine (13/15 [87%]), but the number improving with placebo was not reported.[9]

Harms: Flunarizine is associated with adverse neuropsychiatric effects, and with the development of parkinsonism and other movement disorders.[30–33]

Comment: The RCT was small and brief. The evidence is inconclusive.

OPTION CLONIDINE

One RCT found no improvement of essential hand tremor with clonidine versus placebo. However, the study lacked power to rule out a clinically important difference.

Benefits: **Versus placebo:** We found no systematic review. One small, short term crossover RCT (10 people) of clonidine (up to 0.6 mg/day) versus placebo found no significant difference in the number of people who improved (1/10 [10%] with clonidine *v* 1/10 [10%] with placebo).[34]

Harms: The RCT did not look for adverse effects. Clonidine has been associated in other studies with sedation, lethargy, drowsiness, constipation, dry mouth, headache, dizziness, fatigue, and weakness.

Comment: None.

OPTION ISONIAZID

One RCT found no benefit with isoniazid versus placebo in essential hand tremor. However, the study may have lacked power to detect a clinically important difference.

Benefits: We found no systematic review. **Versus placebo:** We found one small, brief, crossover RCT (15 people, 11 with essential tremor) of isoniazid (up to 1200 mg/day) versus placebo.[35] No significant differences were found in clinical scores or in accelerometer recordings (see glossary, p 1536).

Harms: In other studies, isoniazid has been associated with hepatotoxicity and peripheral neuropathy.

Comment: None.

OPTION GABAPENTIN

Three small, brief RCTs found inconsistent evidence about the effects of gabapentin in essential hand tremor

Benefits: We found no systematic review. **Versus placebo:** We found three small crossover RCTs (16–25 people).[14,36,37] The first RCT of gabapentin (1800 mg/day) versus placebo found no significant differences in clinical scores, activities of daily living, or self evaluation.[36] The second RCT compared gabapentin (up to 1200 mg/day) versus propranolol (up to 120 mg/day) versus placebo. Compared with placebo, gabapentin improved response rate (10/16 [63%] responded with gabapentin v 5/16 [31%] with placebo; ARR 32%, 95% CI 17% to 47%; NNT 4, 95% CI 2 to 6), clinical scores ($P < 0.05$), disability ($P < 0.01$), self evaluation ($P < 0.006$), and accelerometer recordings (see glossary, p 1536) ($P < 0.05$).[14] The third RCT (25 people) compared gabapentin (1800 mg/day) versus gabapentin (3600 mg/day) versus placebo. The RCT found no significant differences with high versus low doses of gabapentin in the 20 people who completed the trial. Gabapentin (at either dose) versus placebo significantly improved participants' global assessments ($P < 0.05$), water pouring scores ($P < 0.05$), and scores of activities of daily living ($P < 0.005$). The RCT did not report hand tremor scores. It found no significant differences between gabapentin and placebo in accelerometry scores, spirographs, or investigator global impression scores.[37]

Harms: The RCTs reported fatigue, drowsiness, nausea, dizziness, and decreased libido in people taking gabapentin.[14,36,37] See epilepsy, p 1508.

Comment: The results of the three RCTs are contradictory. It is unclear whether the difference arose by chance or whether confounding variables, such as prior use of antitremor medications, baseline severity, or assessment rating scales, explain the difference.

OPTION BOTULINUM A TOXIN–HAEMAGGLUTININ COMPLEX

Two RCTs of botulinum A toxin–haemagglutinin complex versus placebo in essential hand tremor found short term improvement on clinical rating scales but no consistent improvement on motor tasks or functional disability. We found no RCTs addressing long term benefits or harms.

Benefits: We found no systematic review. We found two RCTs.[38,39] The first RCT (25 people with essential hand tremor unresponsive to medical treatment)[38] compared botulinum A toxin–haemagglutinin complex versus placebo. Botulinum toxin (50 U) was injected in forearm muscles and repeated if necessary after 1 month (100 U). A successful response to the first injection was more likely with the botulinum toxin than with placebo (12/13 [92%] with botulinum toxin v 1/12 [8%] with placebo). After 4 weeks, mild to moderate improvement was more likely with botulinum toxin (75% with botulinum toxin v 27% with placebo; ARR 48%, 95% CI 30% to 66%; NNT 3, 95% CI 2 to 4). Clinical scores were significantly improved by botulinum toxin versus placebo ($P < 0.05$), but functional tests and accelerometer recordings (see glossary, p 1536) were not significantly different. The second RCT (133 people with essential tremor of the hand by the Tremor Investigation Group criteria, 16 wks' follow up) compared single injections of low dose botulinum A toxin–haemagglutinin complex (50 U) versus high dose botulinum A toxin–haemagglutinin complex (100 U) versus placebo into the wrist flexors and extensors. Postural tremor on clinical rating scales was significantly improved after 12 weeks with low dose (P = 0.004) and by high dose (P = 0.0003) botulinum toxin type A. Both botulinum toxin doses did not significantly improve kinetic tremor, motor task performance, or functional disability.[39]

Harms: The main adverse effect of botulinum A toxin–haemagglutinin complex is dose dependent transient hand weakness.

Comment: None.

OPTION TOPIRAMATE

One RCT found that topiramate improved observer rated tremor score but was associated with more adverse effects compared with placebo. The clinical importance of the difference in tremor score is uncertain.

Benefits: We found no systematic review. We found one crossover RCT (24 people with tremor of hand, head, or voice), which compared topiramate (400 mg/day or maximum tolerated dose; mean dose 333 mg/day) versus placebo.[40] It found that topiramate improved observer rated tremor score compared with placebo after 2 weeks (tremor score improvement 0.88/12 *v* 0.15/12; P = 0.015).

Harms: Nine out of the 24 people withdrew from the RCT; six because of adverse effects (5 with topiramate, 1 with placebo).[40] The most common adverse effects with topiramate were appetite suppression, weight loss, and paraesthesias (see epilepsy, p 1508).

Comment: The RCT did not report tremor scores specifically for the hand. However, 23 of the 24 patients had hand tremor and only four patients had tremor in other locations. The primary outcome was based on observer rated tremor assessment with a non-validated scale developed by Fahn et al.[41] The clinical relevance of the difference is uncertain.

GLOSSARY

Accelerometer recording Recording of the movements from a body segment to allow measurement of frequency and amplitude of a tremor.

REFERENCES

1. Deuschl G, Bain P, Brin M, et al. Consensus statement of the Movement Disorder Society on Tremor. *Mov Disord* 1998;13(suppl 3):2–23.
2. Louis ED, Ottman R, Hauser WA. How common is the most common adult movement disorder? Estimates the prevalence of essential tremor throughout the world. *Mov Disord* 1988;13:803–808.
3. Koller WC, Busenbark K, Miner K. The relationship of essential tremor to other movement disorders: report on 678 patients. Essential Tremor Study Group. *Ann Neurol* 1994;35:717–723.
4. Auff E, Doppelbauer A, Fertl E. Essential tremor: functional disability vs. subjective impairment. *J Neural Transm Suppl* 1991;33:105–110.
5. Bain PG, Findley LJ, Thompson PD, et al. A study of hereditary essential tremor. *Brain* 1994;117:805–824.
6. Winkler GF, Young RR. Efficacy of chronic propranolol therapy in action tremors of the familial, senile or essential varieties. *N Engl J Med* 1974;290:984–988.
7. Tolosa ES, Loewenson RB. Essential tremor: treatment with propranolol. *Neurology* 1975;25:1041–1044.
8. Morgan MH, Hewer RL, Cooper R. Effect of the beta adrenergic blocking agent propranolol on essential tremor. *J Neurol Neurosurg Psychiatry* 1973;36:618–624.
9. Calzetti S, Findley LJ, Perucca E, et al. The response of essential tremor to propranolol evaluation of clinical variables governing its efficacy on prolonged administration. *J Neurol Neurosurg Psychiatry* 1983;46:393–398.
10. Cleeves L, Findley LJ. Propranolol and propranolol-LA in essential tremor: a double blind comparative study. *J Neurol Neurosurg Psychiatry* 1988;51:379–384.
11. Calzetti S, Findley LJ, Perucca E, et al. Controlled study of metoprolol and propranolol during prolonged administration in people with essential tremor. *J Neurol Neurosurg Psychiatry* 1982;45:893–897.
12. Jefferson D, Jenner P, Marsden CD. Beta-adrenoreceptor antagonists in essential tremor. *J Neurol Neurosurg Psychiatry* 1979;42:904–909.

13. Baruzzi A, Procaccianti G, Martinelli P, et al. Phenobarbitone and propranolol in essential tremor: a double-blind controlled clinical trial. *Neurology* 1983;33:296–300.
14. Gironell A, Kulisevsky J, Barbanoj M, et al. A randomised placebo-controlled comparative trial of gabapentin and propranolol in essential tremor. *Arch Neurol* 1999;56:475–480.
15. Teravainen H, Larsen A, Fogelholm R. Comparison between the effects of pindolol and propranolol on essential tremor. *Neurology* 1977;27:439–442.
16. Larsen TA, Teravainen H, Calne DB. Atenolol vs. propranolol in essential tremor. A controlled, quantitative study. *Acta Neurol Scand* 1982;66:547–554.
17. Koller WC. Nadolol in essential tremor. *Neurology* 1983;33:1076–1077.
18. Leigh PN, Jefferson D, Twomey A, et al. Beta-adrenoreceptor mechanisms in essential tremor; a double-blind placebo controlled trial of metoprolol, sotalol and atenolol. *J Neurol Neurosurg Psychiatry* 1983;46:710–715.
19. Sasso E, Perucca E, Calzetti S. Double-blind comparison of primidone and phenobarbitone in essential tremor. *Neurology* 1988;38:808–810.
20. Findley LJ, Cleeves L, Calzetti S. Primidone in essential tremor of the hands and head: a double-blind controlled clinical study. *J Neurol Neurosurg Psychiatry* 1985;48:911–915.
21. Gunal DI, Afsar N, Bekiroglu N, et al. New alternative agents in essential tremor therapy: double-blind placebo-controlled study of alprazolam and acetazolamide. *Neurol Sci* 2000;21:315–317.
22. Findley LJ, Cleeves L. Phenobarbitone in essential tremor. *Neurology* 1985;35:1784–1787.
23. Thompson C, Lang A, Parkes JD, et al. A double-blind trial of clonazepam in benign essential tremor. *Clin Neuropharmacol* 1984;7:83–88.
24. Huber SJ, Paulson GW. Efficacy of alprazolam for essential tremor. *Neurology* 1988;38:241–243.
25. Busenbark K, Pahwa R, Hubble J, et al. Double-blind controlled study of methazolamide in treatment of essential tremor. *Neurology* 1993;43:1045–1047.
26. Garcia-Ruiz PJ, Garcia-de-Yebenes-Prous J, Jimenez-Jimenez J. Effect of nicardipine on essential tremor: brief report. *Clin Neuropharmacol* 1993;16:456–459.
27. Biary N, Bahou Y, Sofi MA, et al. The effect of nimodipine on essential tremor. *Neurology* 1995;45:1523–1525.
28. Jimenez-Jimenez FJ, Garcia-Ruiz PJ, Cabrera-Valdivia F. Nicardipine versus propranolol in essential tremor. *Acta Neurol (Napoli)* 1994;16:184–188.
29. Biary N, Deeb S, Langenberg P. The effect of flunarizine in essential tremor. *Neurology* 1991;41:311–312.
30. Micheli FE, Pardal MM, Giannaula R, et al. Movement disorders and depression due to flunarizine and cinnarizine. *Mov Disord* 1989;4:139–146.
31. Capella D, Laporte JR, Castel JM, et al. Parkinsonism, tremor, and depression induced by cinnarizine and flunarizine. *BMJ* 1988;297:722–723.
32. Chouza C, Scaramelli A, Caamano JL, et al. Parkinsonism, tardive dyskinesia, akathisia and depression induced by flunarizine. *Lancet* 1986;1:1303–1304.
33. Micheli F, Pardal MF, Gatto M. Flunarizine and cinnarizine induced extrapyramidal reactions. *Neurology* 1987;37:881–884.
34. Koller W, Herbster G, Cone S. Clonidine in the treatment of essential tremor. *Mov Disord* 1986;4:235–237.
35. Hallett M, Ravitis J, Dubinsky RM, et al. A double-blind trial of isoniazid for essential tremor and other action tremors. *Mov Disord* 1991;6:253–256.
36. Pahwa R, Lyons K, Hubble JP, et al. Double-blind controlled trial of gabapentin in essential tremor. *Mov Disord* 1998;13:465–467.
37. Ondo W, Hunter C, Vuong KD, et al. Gabapentin for essential tremor: a multiple-dose, double-blind, placebo-controlled trial. *Mov Disord* 2000;15:678–682.
38. Jankovic J, Schwartz K, Clemence W, et al. A randomised, double-blind, placebo-controlled study to evaluate botulinum toxin type A in essential hand tremor. *Mov Disord* 1996;11:250–256.
39. Brin MF, Lyons KE, Doucette J, et al. A randomized, double masked, controlled trial of botulinum toxin type A in essential hand tremor. *Neurology* 2001;56:1523–1528.
40. Connor G. A double-blind placebo-controlled trial of topiramate treatment for essential tremor. *Neurology* 2002;59:132–134
41. Fahn SE, Tolosa E, Marin C. Clinical rating scale for tremor. In: Jankovic J, Tolosa E, eds. Parkinson's disease and movement disorders, 2nd ed. Baltimore: Williams & Wilkins, 1988:225–234.

Joaquim Ferreira
Neurologist

Cristina Sampaio
Assistant Professor

Instituto de Farmacologia e Terapêutica Geral Lisbon School of Medicine
University of Lisbon, Lisbon, Portugal

Competing interests: CS has accepted reimbursement for attending symposia, fees for speaking, fees for organising education, and funds for a member of staff from Allergan (Botox) and IPSEN (Dysport). JF has been paid by Allergen (Botox) and IPSEN (Dysport) for running educational programmes. JF declares involvement in the design and conduct of multiple clinical trials testing antiparkinsonian, antidystonic, and antiepileptic drugs developed by multiple companies. He declares no previous or present participation in trials in the field of tremor.

Headache (chronic tension-type)

Search date February 2003

Peter J Goadsby

QUESTIONS

INTERVENTIONS

To be covered in future updates

Other pharmacological treatments, including antiepileptic drugs
Treatment in children and adolescents

See glossary, p 1544

Key Messages

- We found only limited evidence about the treatment of chronic tension-type headache.
- **Amitriptyline (only short term evidence)** One systematic review and three small, short duration RCTs have found that amitriptyline reduces duration and frequency of chronic tension-type headache compared with placebo.
- **Cognitive behavioural therapy** One systematic review of three small RCTs and one subsequent RCT found limited evidence that cognitive behavioural therapy reduced symptoms at 6 months compared with no treatment.
- **Acupuncture** We found insufficient evidence from heterogeneous RCTs about effects of acupuncture compared with placebo in people with episodic or chronic tension-type headache. Many of the RCTs were of poor quality. Some of the RCTs may have lacked power to exclude a clinically important effect.
- **Benzodiazepines** Two RCTs found insufficient evidence about the effects of benzodiazepines compared with placebo or other treatments. Benzodiazepines are commonly associated with adverse effects if taken regularly.
- **Regular acute pain relief medication** We found no RCTs. We found insufficient evidence from one non-systematic review of observational studies about benefits of common analgesics in people with chronic tension-type headache. It found that sustained and frequent use of some analgesics was associated with chronic headache and reduced the effectiveness of prophylactic treatment.
- **Botulinum toxin; relaxation and electromyographic biofeedback therapy; serotonin reuptake inhibitors; tricyclic antidepressants other than amitriptyline** We found insufficient evidence about the effects of these interventions.

DEFINITION The 1988 International Headache Society criteria for chronic tension-type headache (CTTH) are headaches on 15 or more days a month (180 days/year) for at least 6 months; pain that is bilateral, pressing, or tightening in quality, of mild or moderate intensity, which does not prohibit activities and is not aggravated by routine physical activity; presence of no more than one additional clinical feature (nausea, photophobia, or phonophobia) and no vomiting.[1] CTTH is distinguished from chronic daily headache, which is simply a descriptive term for any headache type that occurs for 15 days or more a month that may be due to CTTH as well as migraine or analgesic associated headache.[2] In contrast to CTTH, episodic tension-type headache can last for 30 minutes to 7 days and occurs for fewer than 180 days a year. Terms based on assumed mechanisms (muscle contraction headache, tension headache) are not operationally defined. Old studies that used these terms may have included people with many different types of headache. The greatest obstacle to studying tension-type headache is the lack of any single proved specific or reliable, clinical, or biological defining characteristic of the disorder.

INCIDENCE/ PREVALENCE The prevalence of chronic daily headache from a survey of the general population in the USA was 4.1%. Half of sufferers met the International Headache Society criteria for CTTH.[3] In a survey of 2500 undergraduate students in the USA, the prevalence of CTTH was 2%.[4] The prevalence of CTTH was 2.5% in a Danish population based survey of 975 individuals.[5] One community based survey in Singapore (2096 people from the general population) found that prevalence was 1.8% in females and 0.9% in males.[6]

AETIOLOGY/ RISK FACTORS Tension type headache is more prevalent in women (65% of cases in one survey).[7] Symptoms begin before the age of 10 years in 15% of people with CTTH. Prevalence declines with age.[8] There is a family history of some form of headache in 40% of people with CTTH,[9] although a twin study found that risk of CTTH was similar for identical and non-identical twins.[10]

PROGNOSIS The prevalence of CTTH declines with age.[8]

AIMS OF INTERVENTION To reduce frequency, severity, and duration of headache, with minimal adverse effects from treatment.

OUTCOMES Headache frequency, intensity, and duration.

METHODS *Clinical Evidence* search and appraisal February 2003.

QUESTION **What are the effects of treatments for chronic tension-type headache?**

OPTION **REGULAR ACUTE PAIN RELIEF MEDICATION**

We found no RCTs. We found insufficient evidence from one non-systematic review of observational studies about effects of common analgesics in people with chronic tension-type headache. It found that sustained frequent use of some analgesics was associated with chronic headache and reduced effectiveness of prophylactic treatment.

Benefits: We found no RCTs but found one non-systematic review of 29 observational studies (2612 people), which found no evidence of benefits of common analgesia for chronic tension-type headache.[11]

Harms: We found no RCTs but found one non-systematic review of 29 observational studies (2612 people), which found that sustained frequent use (2–3 times/week) of some common analgesics in people with episodic headache was associated with chronic headache and reduced effectiveness of prophylactic treatment.[11] Many, but not all people improved over 1–6 months after withdrawal of the acute relief medication (73% of 1101 people, not all of whom had chronic tension-type headache).

Comment: Observational studies are difficult to interpret.

OPTION BENZODIAZEPINES

Two RCTs found insufficient evidence about any benefits of benzodiazepines versus placebo or other treatments that might outweigh the harms associated with regular use.

Benefits: We found no systematic review but found two RCTs.[12,13] One small RCT (16 people) found that diazepam versus placebo produced modest improvement over 12 weeks.[12] The dose of diazepam was not stated, and the International Headache Society criteria were not used. The other RCT, a crossover study (62 people), compared alprazolam (250 µg three times daily) versus placebo over 16 weeks, and also found a modest short term improvement ($P < 0.05$).[13] Fourteen people withdrew from the trial at various stages, and six of those withdrew before the trial started. It was not reported whether analysis was by intention to treat.

Harms: The harms of benzodiazepines found in studies for other indications include increased risk of motor vehicle accidents, falls and fractures, fatal poisonings, depression, dependency, decline in functional status, cognitive decline, confusion, bizarre behaviour, and amnesia.[14]

Comment: None.

OPTION SEROTONIN REUPTAKE INHIBITORS

We found insufficient evidence from two RCTs about effects of serotonin reuptake inhibitors compared with placebo or other treatments.

Benefits: We found two RCTs.[15,16] The first RCT (50 people) compared sertraline versus placebo.[15] It found no significant difference in symptoms (measured by headache frequency or headache index, a combined measure of frequency, severity, and duration of pain; quantitative data for between-group comparison and P value not reported). The second RCT compared serotonin reuptake inhibitors versus tricyclic antidepressants or placebo.[16] It found no significant benefit from citalopram versus placebo in headache duration, frequency, or severity. It found that amitriptyline significantly improved headache duration, frequency, and severity compared with citalopram (see table 1, p 1546).

Harms: One small cohort study found that four of eight people taking fluvoxamine had transient nausea, two complained of anorexia, and three complained of irritability.[19] The RCT comparing sertraline versus placebo reported nausea in six people taking sertraline and four taking placebo (no further data provided).[15]

Comment: One cohort study found significant benefit from fluvoxamine, but the people recruited were not randomised and those responding to placebo were excluded from the study.[19]

OPTION TRICYCLIC ANTIDEPRESSANTS

We found one systematic review and three small, short duration RCTs that found benefit from amitriptyline versus placebo for treating chronic tension-type headache.

Benefits: **Tricyclic antidepressants versus placebo:** We found one systematic review[20] (search date 1994, 1 RCT[21]) and three subsequent RCTs[16–18] of amitriptyline versus placebo (dosage range 10–150 mg; treatment duration 4–32 weeks). All four RCTs[16–18,21] found that amitriptyline significantly improved headache duration and frequency in people with moderate to severe, properly defined chronic tension-type headache. See table A on web extra.[1,22–25]

Harms: One RCT (53 people) found increased rates of dry mouth (54% with amitriptyline 75 mg/day *v* 17% with placebo; $P < 0.05$), drowsiness (62% with amitriptyline *v* 27% with placebo; $P < 0.05$), and weight gain (16% with amitriptyline *v* 0% with placebo; $P > 0.05$).[17] Similar results have been found in other studies for amitriptyline[16] and other tricyclic antidepressants.[19,22]

Comment: Most recent RCTs were small, short term, and used different outcome measures. Observational data were difficult to interpret. For example, one cohort study excluded those responding to placebo before the trial.[19] The trials finding benefit from amitriptyline were of short duration. Currently, they only reliably apply to people with properly defined, moderate to severe chronic tension headache, rather than to people with milder forms of headache. It is not clear whether benzodiazepines alone might contribute to daily headache. The modest benefit found in two small RCTs is unlikely to outweigh the risk of dependence with prolonged use.

OPTION RELAXATION AND ELECTROMYOGRAPHIC BIOFEEDBACK

We found insufficient evidence that electromyographic biofeedback or relaxation are effective.

Benefits: We found two systematic reviews (search dates 1994[20] and not stated[26]), which did not distinguish between RCTs and observational studies. Appraisal of the papers within the reviews identified 10 relevant RCTs (see table B on web extra).[27–36] We found one subsequent RCT.[4] The RCTs were generally of low quality, and included a variety of different electromyographic biofeedback and relaxation (see glossary, p 1544) techniques. Clear conclusions could not be drawn. One larger RCT included people with chronic tension headache and migraine and did not provide intention to treat analysis.[18]

Harms: The identified studies did not report adverse effects of electromyographic biofeedback or relaxation.

Comment: Relaxation and electromyographic biofeedback require additional trained staff and are time consuming.

OPTION COGNITIVE BEHAVIOURAL THERAPY

One systematic review of three small RCTs and one subsequent RCT have found limited evidence that cognitive behavioural therapy versus no treatment reduced the intensity of chronic tension-type headache.

Benefits: **Versus placebo:** We found one systematic review[20] and one subsequent RCT.[15] The systematic review (search date 1994, 3 small RCTs) found greater improvement with cognitive behavioural therapy than with no treatment, sham treatment, or no usual care.[20] The subsequent RCT (203 adults with chronic tension-type headache [CTTH]) compared cognitive behavioural therapy (relaxation [see glossary, p 1544] and cognitive coping) versus antidepressant (amitriptyline up to 100 mg/day or nortriptyline up to 75 mg/day) versus combined cognitive therapy plus antidepressant versus placebo.[18] It found that cognitive behavioural therapy versus placebo significantly reduced the headache index score after 6 months (WMD 0.79 U, 95% CI 0.30 U to 1.28 U), but found a non-significant increase in the frequency of clinically important improvement (at least 50% reduction in headache index score: 17/49 [35%] with cognitive behavioural therapy *v* 14/48 [29%] with placebo; RR 1.19, 95% CI 0.66 to 2.13). **Versus another treatment:** The review found nine additional comparative studies of relaxation or electromyographic biofeedback therapy (see glossary, p 1544) or both versus either cognitive therapy alone (2 studies) or in combination with relaxation or electromyographic biofeedback therapy (7 studies).[20] Results were inconclusive. **Versus antidepressants:** We found no systematic review but found one RCT (203 adults with CTTH)[18] comparing cognitive behavioural therapy (and cognitive coping) versus antidepressant (amitriptyline up to 100 mg/day or nortriptyline up to 75 mg/day) versus combined cognitive therapy plus antidepressant. It found no difference between cognitive behavioural therapy versus antidepressant treatment in either the headache index score after 6 months (score is the mean of pain ratings [0–10 scale] recorded by participants in a daily diary 4 times daily [higher scores represent more severe pain]; WMD –0.13 U, 95% CI –0.61 U to +0.35 U) or in the frequency of clinically important improvement after 6 months (at least 50% reduction in headache index score: 17/49 [35%] with cognitive behavioural therapy *v* 20/53 [38%] with antidepressant; RR 0.92, 95% CI 0.55 to 1.54).

Harms: The identified studies did not report any adverse effects of cognitive behavioural therapy.

Comment: The studies in the systematic review were small and had as few as five people in each group. Although the RCT found that the headache index score was reduced, it found no convincing reduction in the number of people who had a clinically important response. The evidence is too limited to define the role of cognitive therapy in CTTH.

OPTION ACUPUNCTURE

We found insufficient evidence from heterogeneous RCTs to compare acupuncture versus placebo in people with episodic or chronic tension-type headache. Many of the RCTs were of poor quality and some may have lacked power to exclude a clinically important effect.

Benefits: We found two systematic reviews.[37,38] The first systematic review (search date 1998, 6 RCTs, 182 people) found important heterogeneity among studies, making it difficult to summarise the results. A meta-analysis found no significant difference in response rates (defined as > 33% index reduction); however, this only included two RCTs (48 people, 17/24 [71%] with acupuncture *v* 11/24 [46%] with sham acupuncture; RR 1.49, 95% CI 0.96 to 2.03).[37] The meta-analysis might have had insufficient power to find clinically important differences. The second systematic review (search date 1998, 4 RCTs, 91 people) found insufficient evidence comparing the effectiveness of acupuncture versus placebo. The summary of results of the heterogeneous RCTs was not clear enough to allow appropriate meta-analysis.[38] A subsequent small RCT (47 people with chronic tension-type headache, 21 people with episodic headache) compared acupuncture versus sham, non-penetrative acupuncture.[39] Two treatments were given weekly over 5 weeks. The RCT found no significant differences with acupuncture versus sham in headache frequency immediately after treatment (mean 13.1 days/month with acupuncture *v* 16.6 days/month with sham) or at 5 months after the end of the treatment (mean 16.7 days/month with acupuncture *v* 17.2 days/month with sham). It also found no significant differences in pain intensity, as measured using a visual analogue scale.

Harms: Adverse effects were not reported.[37–39]

Comment: Many of the RCTs were of poor quality. Some may have lacked power to exclude a clinically important effect.

OPTION BOTULINUM TOXIN

We found insufficient evidence from three small RCTs about effects of botulinum toxin compared with placebo in people with chronic tension-type headache.

Benefits: We found no systematic review but found three double blind RCTs that compared pericranial intramuscular injection of botulinum toxin type A versus placebo in people with chronic tension-type headache.[40,41] The first RCT (59 people) found no significant difference between treatments in pain relief 8 weeks after treatment (> 25% pain relief at 8 weeks: 54% with botulinum *v* 38% with placebo; CI not reported; P > 0.05).[40] The second, smaller RCT (21 people) also found no significant differences between botulinum versus placebo for headache intensity, duration, and frequency at 4, 8, and 12 weeks (pain on 10 point visual analogue score [10 = most severe pain] about 6 for both groups at baseline; at 12 weeks pain score about 5 for botulinum toxin *v* about 4.5 for placebo; results presented graphically).[41] The third RCT (37 people) found that botulinum toxin A improved headache score more than placebo (AR for at least 25% improvement: 13/22 [59%] with botulinum *v* 2/15 [13%] with placebo; statistical significance not stated).[42]

Harms: The first RCT found no significant difference between treatments.[40] After 4 weeks, the following symptoms were noted: vertigo (2 with botulinum *v* 1 person with placebo) and pain at injection site (3 with botulinum *v* 1 person with placebo). By 8 weeks, the symptoms had resolved. Botulinum toxin may be associated with facial weakness, difficulty with swallowing, and disturbed local sensation. Adverse effects were not reported in the second RCT.[41] The third RCT found no significant difference in adverse events between botulinum toxin A and placebo (statistical analysis not presented).[42] The complaints reported were muscle cramps, flu-like symptoms, and subjective feelings of weakness in the neck muscles.

Comment: The RCTs were too small to exclude a clinically important difference between botulinum and placebo.

GLOSSARY

Electromyographic biofeedback Feedback of the amplified electromyographic signal from forehead and neck muscles through earphones or a loudspeaker to enable people to reduce the amount of muscle contraction.

Relaxation Includes Jacobson's progressive relaxation exercises, meditation, passive relaxation, autogenic training, and functional relaxation.[41]

Substantive changes

Serotonin reuptake inhibitors One RCT added;[15] conclusions unchanged.

Botulinum toxin One RCT added;[42] conclusions unchanged.

REFERENCES

1. Headache Classification Committee of the International Headache Society. Classification and diagnostic criteria for headache disorders, cranial neuralgias and facial pain. *Cephalalgia* 1988;8:1–96.
2. Silberstein SD, Lipton RB, Sliwinski M. Classification of daily and near-daily headaches: field trial of revised IHS criteria. *Neurology* 1996;47:871–875.
3. Schwartz BS, Stewart WF, Simon D, et al. Epidemiology of tension-type headache. *JAMA* 1998;279:381–383.
4. Rokicki LA, Semenchuk EM, Bruehl S, et al. An examination of the validity of the HIS classification system for migraine and tension-type headache in the college student population. *Headache* 1999;39:720–727.
5. Rasmussen BK, Jensen R, Olesen J. A population-based analysis of the diagnostic criteria of the International Headache Society. *Cephalalgia* 1991;11:129–134.
6. Ho KH, Ong BK. A community-based study of headache diagnosis and prevalence in Singapore. *Cephalalgia* 2003;23:6–13.
7. Friedman AP, von Storch TJC, Merritt HH. Migraine and tension headaches: a clinical study of two thousand cases. *Neurology* 1954;4:773–788.
8. Lance JW, Curran DA, Anthony M. Investigations into the mechanism and treatment of chronic headache. *Med J Aust* 1965;2:909–914.
9. Russell MB, Ostergaard S, Bendtsen L, et al. Familial occurrence of chronic tension-type headache. *Cephalalgia* 1999;19:207–210.
10. Svensson DA, Ekbom K, Larsson B, et al. Lifetime prevalence and characteristics of recurrent primary headaches in a population-based sample of Swedish twins. *Headache* 2002;42:754–765.
11. Diener H-C, Tfelt-Hansen P. Headache associated with chronic use of substances. In: Oleson J, Tfelt-Hansen P, Welch KMA, eds. *The headaches*. New York: Raven, 1993:721–727.
12. Paiva T, Nunes JS, Moreira A, et al. Effects of frontalis EMG biofeedback and diazepam in the treatment of tension headache. *Headache* 1982;22:216–220.
13. Shukla R, Nag D, Ahuja RC. Alprazolam in chronic tension-type headache. *J Assoc Physician India* 1996;44:641–644.
14. Holbrook AM, Crowther R, Lotter A, et al. The diagnosis and management of insomnia in clinical practice: a practical evidence-based approach. *CMAJ* 2000;162:216–220.
15. Singh NN, Misra S. Sertraline in chronic tension-type headache. *J Assoc Physicians India* 2002;50:873–878.
16. Bendtsen L, Jensen R, Olesen J. A non-selective (amitriptyline), but not a selective (citalopram), serotonin reuptake inhibitor is effective in the prophylactic treatment of chronic tension-type headache. *J Neurol Neurosurg Psychiatry* 1996;61:285–290.

17. Gobel H, Hamouz V, Hansen C, et al. Chronic tension-type headache: amitriptyline reduces clinical headache-duration and experimental pain sensitivity but does not alter pericranial muscle activity readings. *Pain* 1994;59:241–249.
18. Holroyd KA, O'Donnell FJ, Lipchik GL, et al. Management of chronic tension-type headache with tricyclic antidepressant medication, stress management therapy, and their combination: a randomized controlled trial. *JAMA* 2001;285:2208–2215.
19. Manna V, Bolino F, Di Cicco L. Chronic tension-type headache, mood depression and serotonin: therapeutic effects of fluvoxamine and mianserine. *Headache* 1994;34:44–49.
20. Bogaards MC, Moniek M, ter Kuile M. Treatment of recurrent tension-type headache: a meta-analytic review. *Clin J Pain* 1994;10:174–190. Search date 1994; primary sources Compact Cambridge, Psychlit, and reference lists of relevant articles.
21. Diamond S, Baltes BJ. Chronic tension headache treated with amitriptyline: a double-blind study. *Headache* 1971;11:110–116.
22. Fogelholm R, Murros K. Maprotiline in chronic tension headache: a double-blind cross-over study. *Headache* 1985;25:273–275.
23. Langemark M, Loldrup D, Bech P, et al. Clomipramine and mianserin in the treatment of chronic tension headache. A double-blind, controlled study. *Headache* 1990;30:118–121.
24. Pfaffenrath V, Essen D, Islet H, et al. Amitriptyline versus amitriptyline-*N*-oxide versus placebo in the treatment of chronic tension-type headache: a multi-centre randomised parallel-group double-blind study. *Cephalalgia* 1991;11:329–330.
25. Lance JW. *Mechanism and management of headache*. London: Butterworth, 1973.
26. Holroyd KA, Penzien DB. Client variables and the behavioural treatment of recurrent tension headache: a meta-analytic review. *J Behav Med* 1986;9:515–536. Search date not stated; primary sources Eric, Medlars, Psycinfo, Psycalert, and hand searches of key journals, book reviews, and conference proceedings.
27. Loew T, Sohn R, Martus P, et al. Functional relaxation as a somatopsychotherapeutic intervention: a prospective controlled study. *Altern Ther Health Med* 2000;6:70–75.
28. Reich B. Non-invasive treatment of vascular and muscle contraction headache: a comparative longitudinal clinical study. *Headache* 1988;29:34–41.
29. Andrasik F, Holroyd K. A test of specific and nonspecific effects in the biofeedback treatment of tension headache. *J Consult Clin Psychol* 1980;48:575–586.
30. Blanchard E, Appelbaum K, Guarnieri P, et al. Placebo-controlled evaluation of abbreviated progressive muscle relaxation combined with cognitive therapy in the treatment of tension headache. *J Consult Clin Psychol* 1990;58:210–215.
31. Blanchard E, Andrasik F, Appelbaum K, et al. The efficacy and cost-effectiveness of minimal-therapist-contact non-drug treatment of chronic migraine and tension headache. *Headache* 1985;25:214–220.
32. Bruhn P, Olesen J, Melgaard B. Controlled trial of EMG feedback in muscle contraction feedback. *Ann Neurol* 1979;6:34–36.
33. Collett L, Cottrauz J, Juenet C. GSR feedback and Schultz relaxation in tension headaches: a comparative study. *Pain* 1986;25:205–213.
34. Gada M. A comparative study of efficacy of EMG biofeedback and progressive muscular relaxation in tension headache. *Indian J Psychiat* 1984;26:121–127.
35. Holroyd K, Andrasik F, Westbrook T. Cognitive control of tension headache. *Cognitive Ther Res* 1977;1:121–133.
36. Larsson B, Carlsson J. A school-based, nurse-administered relaxation training for children with chronic tension-type headache. *J Pediatr Psychol* 1996;21:603–614.
37. Melchart D, Linde K, Fischer P, et al. Acupuncture for recurrent headaches: a systematic review of randomized controlled trials. *Cephalalgia* 1999;19:779–786. Search date 1998; primary sources Medline, Embase, Cochrane Field for Complementary Medicine database, Cochrane Controlled Trials Register, and hand searches of individual trial collections or private databases and bibliographies of articles obtained.
38. Vernon H, McDermaid CS, Hagino C. Systematic review of randomized clinical trials of complementary/alternative therapies in the treatment of tension-type and cervicogenic headache. *Complement Ther Med* 1999;7:142–155. Search date 1998; primary sources Medline, Psychlnfo, Cinahl, and hand searches of citations and reference lists from other systematic reviews.
39. Karst M, Reinhard M, Thum P, et al. Needle acupuncture in tension-type headache: a randomized, placebo-controlled study. *Cephalalgia* 2001;21:637–642.
40. Schmitt WJ, Slowey E, Fravi N, et al. Effect of botulinum toxin A injections in the treatment of chronic tension-type headache: a double-blind, placebo-controlled trial. *Headache* 2001;41:658–664.
41. Rollnik JD, Tanneberger O, Schubert M, et al. Treatment of tension-type headache with botulinum toxin type A: a double-blind, placebo-controlled study. *Headache* 2000;40:300–305.
42. Smuts JA, Baker MK, Smuts HM, et al. Prophylactic treatment of chronic tension-type headache using botulinum toxin type A. *Eur J Neurol* 1999;6:S99–S102.

Peter J Goadsby
Professor of Clinical Neurology
Institute of Neurology
London
UK

Competing interests: None declared.

The following previous contributor of this topic would also like to be acknowledged: Anish Bahra.

TABLE 1 **RCTs evaluating the efficacy of tricyclic antidepressants in the treatment of chronic tension-type headache, including one comparative study with serotonin reuptake inhibitors (see text, p 1540).**

Ref	Drug	Number of people	CTTH definition	Analgesic overuse excluded	Total duration and type of study	Outcome	Effect of drug compared with placebo
17	Amitriptyline 75 mg *v* placebo	53	IHS criteria[1]	Yes	6 week; parallel group	Reduction in mean daily headache duration	At 6 weeks, pain reduced by 3.2 hours/day with amitriptyline *v* 0.28 hours/day with placebo ($P < 0.01$)
16	Amitriptyline 75 mg *v* citalopram 20 mg *v* placebo	34	IHS criteria[1]	Yes	32 week; crossover	Reduction in the product of headache duration and intensity	With amitriptyline: reduced analgesic intake ($P = 0.01$), headache duration, and frequency ($P = 0.002$), but no difference in headache intensity With citalopram: no difference in headache duration, frequency, or severity
18	Amitriptyline or nortriptyline *v* stress management *v* placebo	150	IHS criteria[1]	Yes	8 months total	Reduction in mean pain scores from daily diary	Antidepressant and stress management both superior to placebo

CTTH, chronic tension-type headache; IHS, International Headache Society; Ref, reference.

Migraine headache

Search date December 2002

Luis E Morillo

QUESTIONS

INTERVENTIONS

To be covered in future updates
Effects of non-drug treatments for migraine headache
Effects of prophylactic treatments for migraine headache

See glossary, p 1562

Key Messages

- **Eletriptan** One systematic review and subsequent RCTs have found that eletriptan increases headache relief compared with placebo. Two RCTs found that eletriptan increased headache relief compared with sumatriptan.
- **Naratriptan** Four RCTs have found that naratriptan increases headache relief at 4 hours compared with placebo. One RCT comparing naratriptan versus sumatriptan found no significant difference in headache recurrence.
- **Rizatriptan** One systematic review and subsequent RCTs have found that rizatriptan improves headache relief compared with placebo.
- **Salicylates** RCTs have found that oral or intravenous lysine acetylsalicylic acid (alone or in combination with metoclopramide) and oral aspirin (alone or in combination with metoclopramide, paracetamol, or caffeine) increase headache relief compared with placebo. One RCT found no significant difference between aspirin and paracetamol plus codeine in headache relief, although both were more effective than placebo. One RCT found no significant difference between aspirin plus metoclopramide and sumatriptan in headache relief.
- **Sumatriptan** RCTs have found that subcutaneous, oral, or intranasal sumatriptan increases headache relief compared with placebo. RCTs found no significant difference in headache relief between sumatriptan and aspirin plus metoclopramide, tolfenamic acid, or zolmitriptan. RCTs found that oral or nasal sumatriptan increased headache relief compared with oral or nasal ergotamine. One RCT found no significant difference between sumatriptan and naratriptan in headache recurrence.
- **Zolmitriptan** Three large RCTs have found that oral zolmitriptan increases headache relief compared with placebo. Two RCTs found no significant difference between zolmitriptan and sumatriptan in headache relief.

Migraine headache

- **Diclofenac** RCTs found that oral or intramuscular diclofenac improved headache symptoms compared with placebo. One RCT found that intramuscular diclofenac improved migraine symptoms compared with intramuscular paracetamol.
- **Ergotamine** One systematic review found limited evidence from four RCTs that ergotamine or ergotamine plus caffeine improved headache relief compared with placebo. RCTs found that ergotamine (or its derivatives, with or without caffeine and cyclizine) was less effective for migraine symptoms than sumatriptan, and limited evidence that it was less effective than naproxen. One overview of harms suggested that ergotamine increased nausea and vomiting compared with placebo.
- **Ibuprofen** Five RCTs found that ibuprofen improved migraine symptoms compared with placebo.
- **Naproxen** Three small RCTs found that naproxen reduced migraine symptoms compared with placebo. Two RCTs found that naproxen reduced symptoms compared with ergotamine (with or without caffeine plus cyclizine). However, one further RCT found no significant difference between naproxen and ergotamine in pain relief after 1 hour.
- **Tolfenamic acid** RCTs found limited evidence that tolfenamic acid improved duration and severity of headache compared with placebo. RCTs found no significant difference in symptoms between tolfenamic acid and sumatriptan or paracetamol.

DEFINITION Migraine is a primary headache disorder manifesting as recurring attacks usually lasting for 4–72 hours and involving pain of moderate to severe intensity, often with nausea, sometimes vomiting, and/or sensitivity to light, sound, and other sensory stimuli. The 1988 International Headache Society criteria (see glossary, p 1562) include separate criteria for migraine with and migraine without associated aura.[1] Unless stated otherwise, RCTs used International Headache Society criteria for migraine with or without aura.

INCIDENCE/ PREVALENCE Migraine is common worldwide. Prevalence has been reported to be 5–25% in women and 2–10% in men. Overall, the highest incidence for migraine without aura has been reported between the ages of 10 and 11 years (10/1000 person years). The peak incidence of migraine without aura in males is between ages 10 and 11 years (10/1000 person years) and in females between ages 14 and 17 years (19/1000 person years).[2] The incidence of migraine with aura peaks in males at around age 5 years (7/1000 person years) and in females at around age 12–13 years (14/1000 person years).[2] Female prevalence of migraine with or without aura has a declining trend after age 45–50 years.

AETIOLOGY/ RISK FACTORS Data from independent representative samples from Canada,[3,4] the USA,[5,6] several countries in Latin America,[7] several countries in Europe,[8–11] Hong Kong,[12] and Japan[13] demonstrate a female to male predominance and a peak in middle aged women. Migraine has been reported to be 50% more likely in people with a family history of migraine.[14]

PROGNOSIS Acute migraine is self limiting and only rarely results in permanent neurological complications. Chronic recurrent migraine may cause disability through pain, and may affect daily functioning and quality of life.

AIMS OF INTERVENTION	To reduce frequency of migraine, intensity of accompanying symptoms, and duration of headache, with minimal adverse effects.
OUTCOMES	Headache relief or being pain free (see glossary, p 1562) at different times after medication. Pain relief at specific post-dose times. Table A on web extra specifies those RCTs in which 2 hour or 4 hour headache relief outcome is reported as the preferred clinical outcome measure.[15–36] In this review, headache relief is reported at 2 hours unless expressed otherwise. Some RCTs include the need for rescue medication and headache recurrence (see glossary, p 1562) as outcome measures.
METHODS	*Clinical Evidence* search and appraisal December 2002.

QUESTION **What are the effects of drug treatments for acute migraine?**

OPTION **SALICYLATES**

RCTs have found that oral or intravenous lysine acetylsalicylic acid (alone or in combination with metoclopramide) or oral aspirin (alone or in combination with metoclopramide, paracetamol, or caffeine) increase headache relief compared with placebo. One RCT found no significant difference between aspirin and paracetamol plus codeine in headache relief, although both were more effective than placebo. One RCT found no significant difference between aspirin plus metoclopramide and sumatriptan in headache relief.

Benefits: We found no systematic review but found 10 RCTs.[15–20,37–40] **Oral lysine acetylsalicylate (L-ASA):** One RCT (266 people, 475 migraine attacks) found that oral L-ASA 1620 mg plus metoclopramide 10 mg significantly increased headache relief (see glossary, p 1562) compared with placebo (AR 56% with L-ASA *v* 28% with placebo; RR 2.0, 95% CI 1.6 to 2.5).[15] A second RCT compared three treatments: oral L-ASA 1620 mg plus metoclopramide 10 mg, oral sumatriptan 100 mg, and placebo.[16] It found that L-ASA plus metoclopramide significantly increased headache relief compared with placebo (AR 57% with L-ASA *v* 24% with placebo; RR 2.4, 95% CI 1.7 to 3.3). The difference between active treatment groups was not significant (AR 57% with L-ASA *v* 54% with sumatriptan; P = 0.50). **Intravenous L-ASA:** One RCT (278 people) compared three treatments: L-ASA 1800 mg intravenously, sumatriptan 6 mg subcutaneously, and placebo.[17] It found that both L-ASA and sumatriptan significantly increased headache relief compared with placebo, and that sumatriptan significantly increased headache relief compared with L-ASA (AR 74% with L-ASA *v* 91% with sumatriptan *v* 24% with placebo; RR for L-ASA *v* placebo 3.1, 95% CI 1.8 to 5.4; RR for L-ASA *v* sumatriptan 0.8, 95% CI 0.7 to 0.9). A second, smaller, crossover RCT (112 attacks in 56 people) compared L-ASA 1000 mg intravenously versus ergotamine 0.5 mg subcutaneously.[37] It found no significant difference between groups in pain intensity score on a visual analogue scale. **Effervescent aspirin:** One crossover RCT (120 people) compared effervescent aspirin 650 mg with and without metoclopramide 10 mg versus placebo.[38] At 2 hours aspirin with or without metoclopramide reduced headache significantly more than placebo (P < 0.001). A second RCT (374 people) compared effervescent aspirin 1000 mg versus placebo.[20] It found that aspirin significantly increased headache relief compared with placebo (AR 55% with aspirin *v* 37%; RR 1.5, 95% CI 1.2 to 1.9). **Dispersible aspirin:** One crossover RCT (101 people with migraine, 73 of whom received both treatments) compared mouth dispersible aspirin 900 mg versus placebo in two consecutive attacks.[40] It found that aspirin significantly increased headache relief at 2 hours compared with placebo, and significantly reduced need for rescue medication (see glossary, p 1562) (AR for headache relief 48% with aspirin *v* 19% with placebo; P = 0.0005; difference in need for rescue medication: P < 0.01). **Other combinations:** One large RCT (1357 people with non-disabling migraine) compared oral paracetamol 250 mg plus aspirin 250 mg plus caffeine 65 mg versus placebo.[19] Combination treatment improved headache relief compared with placebo (AR 59% with the combination *v* 33% with placebo; RR 1.8, 95% CI 1.6 to 2.1). A second, crossover RCT (198 people treated for 3 consecutive migraine attacks) found no significant difference in headache relief between aspirin 1000 mg orally and paracetamol 400 mg plus codeine 25 mg.[39] However, both improved headache relief compared with placebo (P = 0.0003 for aspirin and P = 0.0002 with paracetamol plus codeine). **Aspirin versus sumatriptan:** One RCT (358 people) found no significant difference between oral aspirin 900 mg plus metoclopramide 10 mg and oral sumatriptan 100 mg in headache relief at 2 hours (AR 45% with aspirin plus metoclopramide *v* 56% with sumatriptan; P = 0.078).[18] **Versus tolfenamic acid:** See benefits of tolfenamic acid, p 1554.

Harms: One RCT reported adverse effects related to L-ASA in 2%, to sumatriptan in 15%, and to placebo in 2% of people treated.[17] In this trial, severe harms were related to L-ASA in 3%, to sumatriptan in 5%, and to the placebo control group in 2% of people treated. Another trial reported premature withdrawal of treatment in 2% with placebo, 1% with L-ASA, and 3% with sumatriptan.[16] The most frequently reported harms for L-ASA were somnolence, abdominal pain, nausea or vomiting, fatigue, and headache. The RCT comparing the combination of paracetamol, aspirin, and caffeine versus placebo reported no serious adverse effects.[19]

Comment: None.

OPTION DICLOFENAC

RCTs found that oral or intramuscular diclofenac improved headache symptoms compared with placebo. One RCT found that intramuscular diclofenac improved migraine symptoms compared with intramuscular paracetamol.

Benefits: We found no systematic review. **Versus placebo:** We found three RCTs of oral diclofenac[21,41,42] and one RCT of intramuscular diclofenac.[43] The first RCT (170 people) found that diclofenac compared with placebo significantly improved treatment success (defined at 2 hours as a visual analogue scale score below 10 mm or headache duration of less than 2 hours without need for rescue medication [see glossary, p 1562] within this period: AR 27% with diclofenac *v* 19% with placebo; RR 1.5, 95% CI 1.0 to 2.2).[41] The second RCT (72 people) found that diclofenac 50 mg or 100 mg significantly increased headache relief (see glossary, p 1562) compared with placebo (AR 39% with 50 mg *v* 44% with 100 mg *v* 22% with placebo; RR diclofenac 50 mg *v* placebo 1.8, 95% CI 1.0 to 3.1; RR diclofenac 100 mg *v* placebo 1.9, 95% CI 1.1 to 3.3).[21] The RCT found no significant difference between 50 mg and 100 mg doses of diclofenac, but found that diclofenac 100 mg significantly reduced need for rescue medication compared with placebo (AR 37% *v* 58%; RR 0.64, 95% CI 0.44 to 0.93). The third RCT (120 people with migraine with or without aura) compared 75 mg intramuscular diclofenac versus placebo.[43] At 1 hour, it found that diclofenac improved headache relief and reduced need for rescue medication compared with placebo in people with and without aura (headache relief in people without aura: AR 43.3% with diclofenac *v* 16.7% with placebo, $P < 0.01$; headache relief in people with aura: AR 50% with diclofenac *v* 13.3% with placebo, $P < 0.01$; rescue medication in people without aura: 20% with diclofenac *v* 50% with placebo, $P < 0.05$; rescue medication in people with aura: 11% with diclofenac *v* 42% with placebo, $P < 0.05$). The fourth RCT (156 people meeting International Headache Society criteria [see glossary, p 1562] for migraine with or without aura) compared three treatments: diclofenac potassium 50 or 100 mg, oral sumatriptan 100 mg, and placebo.[42] The trial found that diclofenac significantly reduced headache pain (measured on a visual analogue scale) at 2 hours compared with placebo ($P < 0.001$). **Versus sumatriptan**: The RCT comparing diclofenac, sumatriptan, and placebo found no significant difference between either dose of diclofenac and sumatriptan.[42] **Versus paracetamol:** One RCT (86 people) compared intramuscular diclofenac 75 mg versus intramuscular paracetamol in people with paroxysmal headaches accompanied by at least two of the following features: unilateral pain, nausea, visual and limb symptoms, and positive family history.[44] The trial found that diclofenac increased the proportion of people with partial relief of overall migraine symptoms (intensity and duration) within 35 minutes compared with paracetamol (AR 89% with diclofenac *v* 17% with paracetamol; RR 4.9, 95% CI 2.5 to 9.8).

Harms: In one RCT (72 people), 33% of people reported one or more adverse effects during one or more attacks.[21] Most adverse effects were rated as mild or moderate (gastrointestinal complaints were the most common, followed by tiredness and fatigue), but 12% of people rated adverse experiences as severe. In another RCT (170 people), 14% of people reported at least one side effect, with gastrointestinal effects being the most common (50%).[41] Only three people withdrew because of gastrointestinal symptoms. See non-steroidal anti-inflammatory drugs, p 1393.

Comment: None.

OPTION IBUPROFEN

Five RCTs found that ibuprofen improved migraine symptoms compared with placebo.

Benefits: **Versus placebo:** We found no systematic review but found five RCTs comparing ibuprofen versus placebo.[22,45–48] The first RCT (729 people) found that oral ibuprofen (400 mg and 600 mg in gel formulation) significantly improved headache relief (see glossary, p 1562) compared with placebo (AR 72% with 400 mg *v* 72% with 600 mg *v* 50% with placebo; ibuprofen 400 mg *v* placebo RR 1.4, 95% CI 1.2 to 1.7; ibuprofen 600 mg *v* placebo RR 1.4, 95% CI 1.2 to 1.7).[22] It found no significant difference in the need for rescue medication (see glossary, p 1562). The second RCT (25 people, 146 migraines) found that ibuprofen significantly improved migraine index (see glossary, p 1562) (25 ± 28 *v* 46 ± 27; $P = 0.0014$) and reduced the need for rescue medication 4 hours after treatment (26% *v* 56%; $P = 0.007$) compared with placebo.[45] The third RCT (40 people with common and classic migraine, 345 migraines) compared ibuprofen 800–1200 mg orally versus placebo.[46] The trial found that with ibuprofen significantly more attacks were rated as mild compared with placebo ($P < 0.001$) and significantly fewer attacks were rated as moderate ($P < 0.05$) or severe ($P < 0.05$). It also found that ibuprofen reduced the need for rescue medication compared with placebo (AR 22% *v* 81%; RR 0.27, 95% CI 0.20 to 0.36). One RCT (660 people with headache intensity not requiring bed rest or inhibiting daily activities in more than 50% of attacks) compared ibuprofen 200 mg or 400 mg versus placebo with a follow up of 6 hours.[47] It found that ibuprofen significantly increased headache relief at 2 hours compared with placebo (AR 41.7% with ibuprofen 400 mg *v* 40.8% with ibuprofen 200 mg *v* 28.1% with placebo; $P = 0.006$ for both doses *v* placebo). The fifth RCT (40 people) compared an ibuprofen arginine preparation (400 mg orally) versus placebo.[48] It found that more people taking ibuprofen arginine versus placebo achieved "considerable" or "complete" relief within 2 hours (51% *v* 7%; $P < 0.01$). Fewer people taking ibuprofen arginine needed rescue medication (31% *v* 48%) but no statistical analysis was performed.

Harms: One RCT did not report adverse effects.[46] Another RCT reported pain and stomach discomfort in 12% of people on treatment, which was not considered serious.[45] Another reported no significant difference in adverse events among treatment groups, and no serious adverse events.[47] See non-steroidal anti-inflammatory drugs, p 1393.

Comment: None.

OPTION NAPROXEN

Three small RCTs found that naproxen reduced migraine symptoms compared with placebo. Two RCTs found that naproxen reduced symptoms compared with ergotamine (with or without caffeine plus cyclizine). However, one further RCT found no significant difference between naproxen and ergotamine in pain relief after 1 hour.

Benefits: We found no systematic review. **Versus placebo:** We found one crossover RCT (37 people with classic or common migraine) comparing oral naproxen 750–1250 mg versus placebo.[49] It found that naproxen significantly reduced headache intensity (see glossary, p 1562) (P = 0.047), but it found no significant difference in need for rescue medication (see glossary, p 1562) (absolute numbers not provided; P = 0.13). Headache intensity was defined as follows: none = symptoms absent; mild = symptoms present but not influencing work or recreational activities; moderate = symptoms reducing ability to carry out work or recreational activities; or severe = symptoms hindering work or recreational activities completely. A second crossover RCT (40 people with common or classic migraine) comparing naproxen 750–1000 mg versus placebo found that naproxen reduced overall pain intensity (rated as mild, moderate, or severe; P = 0.011; time of evaluation not stated).[50] The need for rescue medication after 2 hours was also significantly lower for naproxen (AR 47% v 72%; P = 0.002; insufficient data for RR calculation). A third RCT compared three treatments: naproxen, ergotamine, and placebo.[51] It found that naproxen significantly increased pain relief compared with ergotamine at 1 hour after the first dose (P = 0.032). **Versus ergotamine:** We found three RCTs, which compared oral naproxen 750–1750 mg versus ergotamine 2–4 mg alone or with caffeine 91.5 mg plus cyclizine chlorhydrate 50 mg.[51–53] The first RCT (114 people) found that naproxen significantly reduced migraine intensity (rated as mild, moderate, severe, or incapacitating) compared with ergotamine plus caffeine plus cyclizine (P = 0.014), but found no significant difference in need for rescue medication.[52] The second RCT (37 people with classic or common migraine) compared naproxen versus ergotamine.[53] In this trial, 47% of people were reported to have terminated the study prematurely. The trial found that naproxen significantly reduced migraine intensity (rated as none, mild, moderate, or severe) compared with ergotamine (P = 0.04), but found no significant difference in need for rescue medication (23% v 29%). The third RCT (41 people) compared three treatments: naproxen, ergotamine, and placebo.[51] It found no significant difference in pain relief at 1 hour after the first dose between naproxen and ergotamine (P = 0.65).

Harms: In the first RCT, adverse effects were reported in 5/32 people taking naproxen; four had stomach pain and dyspepsia, and one withdrew from the trial because of severe stomach pain.[49] One RCT comparing naproxen versus ergotamine found that vomiting was more frequent with ergotamine (34% v 10%; P = 0.0083), and more people taking ergotamine withdrew because of severe symptoms (diarrhoea, vomiting, dizziness, nausea, shivering, sweating) compared with those taking naproxen (8% v 2%).[51] In another RCT, more people taking naproxen versus ergotamine discontinued medication (6/19 [32%] v 2/17 [12%]).[53] One RCT found that more people taking ergotamine versus naproxen had severe adverse effects (8/48 v 1/48), and two people taking ergotamine withdrew from the study.[52] See non-steroidal anti-inflammatory drugs, p 1393.

Comment: None of the RCTs used the International Headache Society criteria (see glossary, p 1562) to identify cases.

OPTION TOLFENAMIC ACID

RCTs found limited evidence that tolfenamic acid improved duration and severity of headache compared with placebo. RCTs found no significant difference in symptoms between tolfenamic acid and sumatriptan or paracetamol.

Benefits: We found no systematic review. **Versus placebo or sumatriptan:** One RCT (141 people, 289 migraine attacks) compared three treatments: tolfenamic acid 200 mg, sumatriptan 100 mg, and placebo.[23] The trial found that tolfenamic acid significantly increased headache relief (see glossary, p 1562) compared with placebo (AR 77% *v* 29%; RR 2.6, 95% CI 1.5 to 4.2), but found no significant difference between tolfenamic acid and sumatriptan. The use of rescue medication (see glossary, p 1562) was not significantly different between any of the three arms. **Versus placebo or acetylsalicylic acid or ergotamine:** One crossover RCT (20 women with common or classic migraine, 160 migraines) compared tolfenamic acid 200 mg, acetylsalicylic acid 500 mg, and ergotamine 1 mg versus placebo.[54] The RCT found that tolfenamic acid significantly reduced the duration of attacks compared with placebo ($P < 0.001$; time of evaluation not stated). The mean duration of attack was shortest with tolfenamic acid compared with the other treatments, but this was not significantly shorter than the mean duration of attack with the other drugs (P values not reported). The need for rescue medication after 2 hours was not significantly different. **Versus paracetamol:** One RCT (149 people with common or classic migraine) compared tolfenamic acid 400 mg versus paracetamol 1000 mg.[55] It found no significant difference between treatments in headache intensity, adverse effects, strength, effect duration, or need for additional medication after 3 hours of test medication. **Combination preparations:** One crossover RCT (49 people with common or classic migraine, 482 migraines) compared tolfenamic acid alone or in combination with either caffeine or metoclopramide versus placebo.[56] The trial found that tolfenamic acid, either alone or in combination, significantly reduced headache intensity (measured on a scale of no, slight, moderate, or severe symptoms) compared with placebo. All combinations of tolfenamic acid versus placebo significantly reduced the need for rescue medication ($P < 0.01$).

Harms: In one RCT comparing tolfenamic acid versus sumatriptan, the frequency of adverse effects was similar (30% *v* 41%).[51] See non-steroidal anti-inflammatory drugs, p 1393.

Comment: None.

OPTION ERGOTAMINE

One systematic review found limited evidence from four RCTs that ergotamine or ergotamine plus caffeine improved headache relief compared with placebo. RCTs found that ergotamine (or its derivatives, with or without caffeine and cyclizine) was less effective for migraine symptoms than sumatriptan, and limited evidence that it was less effective than naproxen. One overview of harms suggested that ergotamine increased nausea and vomiting compared with placebo.

Benefits: **Versus placebo:** We found one systematic review (search date 1991, 7 RCTs, 588 people).[57] Ergotamine was administered orally at doses between 1 mg and 6 mg. Ergotamine was given alone in three RCTs, combined with caffeine in three RCTs, and combined with alkaloids and barbiturates in one RCT. The RCT of ergotamine plus alkaloids plus barbiturates was not evaluable. None of the trials used International Headache Society criteria (see glossary, p 1562) for participant inclusion, and defined responders according to a variety of 3-point to 10-point scales. Two RCTs identified by the review found that ergotamine alone significantly increased headache relief compared with placebo ($P < 0.01$ in 1 RCT; reported as "significant" in the other RCT; P value not reported) and one RCT found that ergotamine alone significantly reduced the duration of attacks compared with placebo ($P < 0.001$). Two RCTs identified by the review found a similar use of rescue medication (see glossary, p 1562) with ergotamine alone and with placebo (P value not reported; no further data provided). Two RCTs identified by the review measuring migraine associated nausea or vomiting found similar results with ergotamine alone and with placebo (P value not reported). One RCT identified by the review found that ergotamine plus caffeine significantly increased headache relief (reported as "significant"; P value not reported) compared with placebo, but another RCT found no significant difference (P value not reported). The RCTs comparing ergotamine plus caffeine versus placebo did not assess duration of attack. Two RCTs identified by the review found that ergotamine plus caffeine significantly reduced need for rescue medication ($P < 0.05$ in 1 RCT; reported as "significant" in the other, P value not reported). Two RCTs identified by the review measuring nausea or vomiting found that placebo reduced these symptoms compared with ergotamine plus caffeine (no statistical analysis reported). **Versus sumatriptan:** One RCT (580 people) compared oral ergotamine 2 mg plus oral caffeine 100 mg versus oral sumatriptan 100 mg.[58] The trial found that ergotamine plus caffeine significantly improved headache relief (see glossary, p 1562) compared with sumatriptan (AR 48% *v* 66%; RR 0.73, 95% CI 0.62 to 0.85; $P < 0.001$). Significantly more people required rescue medication with ergotamine than with sumatriptan (AR 44% *v* 24%; RR 1.82, 95% CI 1.38 to 2.39). A second RCT (crossover design; 368 people treating two attacks) compared dihydroergotamine nasal spray (1 or 2 mg) versus sumatriptan nasal spray (20 mg).[59] It found that sumatriptan significantly increased headache relief at 1 hour and at 2 hours, and significantly reduced nausea at 1 hour compared with dihydroergotamine (headache relief at 1 hour: 53% with sumatriptan *v* 41% with sumatriptan, $P < 0.001$; headache relief at 2 hours, $P = 0.003$; relief of nausea at 1 hour: 64% with sumatriptan *v* 40% with dihydroergotamine, $P = 0.006$). However, the RCT found no significant differences between treatments with respect to relief from vomiting, photophobia, or phonophobia. **Plus metoclopramide:** One RCT (24 women with common or classic migraine, 176 migraines) found no significant difference between ergotamine alone and ergotamine plus metoclopramide in headache intensity (see glossary, p 1562) (measured on a 3-point scale as more than usual, usual, or less than usual) or need for rescue medication.[60]

Versus naproxen: See benefits of naproxen, p 1553.

Harms: In the systematic review comparing ergotamine versus placebo, two RCTs measuring nausea and vomiting found that ergotamine alone increased nausea and vomiting compared with placebo (no statistical analysis reported), and two RCTs found that ergotamine plus caffeine increased nausea and vomiting compared with placebo (no statistical analysis conducted).[57] We found one overview of the safety of dihydroergotamine mesylate (DHE) and ergotamine tartrate.[61] This overview identified two trials (24 and 311 people, respectively), which found that adverse effects with intramuscular DHE occurred in fewer than 10% of people (with leg cramps and pain at the injection site being most common) and that harms resolved within 1 hour. Three RCTs in the overview found that nausea and vomiting were the most common adverse effects, which subsided within 15 minutes. In another open trial (300 people), 32% of people taking DHE complained of nausea. Post-marketing surveillance studies have reported ischaemic complications, nausea, vomiting, seizures, cardiac and non-cardiac vascular disorders such as vasospasm and infarction, liver abnormalities, leg pain, chest pain, hypertensive crisis, injection site reactions, head and shoulder pain, and paraesthesia. Treatment related phenomena were reported in fewer than 4% of people receiving intranasal DHE. A bitter or unpleasant taste was reported by 2%. Dizziness and muscle pain were reported by fewer than 1%. Discontinuation of treatment occurred in 1% of people included in the RCTs. Worsening of baseline nausea or vomiting was suggested in five out of seven RCTs comparing acute administration of ergotamine tartrate versus placebo. Single case reports of less common adverse effects include abdominal discomfort, numbness or tingling of fingers or toes, ischaemic complications, swollen fingers, and leg cramps. With chronic use in excessive doses, ischaemic neuropathy, anorectal ulcers following suppository use, habituation, and overuse headaches have been reported.[61] In the RCT comparing sumatriptan versus dihydroergotamine nasal sprays, the incidence of adverse events was similar (around 10%) in both treatment groups after the first dose. The most common were disturbance of taste after sumatriptan, and nasal or sinus symptoms such as congestion, irritation, and rhinitis after dihydroergotamine. These were reported as being mild and self limiting.[59]

Comment: None.

OPTION ELETRIPTAN

One systematic review and subsequent RCTs have found that eletriptan increases headache relief compared with placebo. Two RCTs found that eletriptan increased headache relief compared with sumatriptan.

Benefits: We found one systematic review (search date 2000; 6 unpublished RCTs made available by the manufacturer; 4705 people) comparing eletriptan 20 mg, 40 mg, and 80 mg versus placebo.[24] It found that all doses of eletriptan significantly improved headache relief (see glossary, p 1562) compared with placebo (RR for 20 mg dose *v* placebo 2.0, 95% CI 1.6 to 2.6; RR for 40 mg *v* placebo 2.4, 95% CI 2.1 to 2.7; RR for 80 mg *v* placebo 2.5, 95% CI 2.2 to 2.9). We found three subsequent RCTs.[25,62,63] The first subsequent RCT (857 people) compared five treatments: eletriptan 20 mg, 40 mg, and 80 mg; 100 mg sumatriptan; and placebo.[25] It found that eletriptan significantly increased headache relief compared with placebo (AR for improved pain: 24% with placebo, 54% with eletriptan 20 mg, 65% with eletriptan 40 mg, 77% with eletriptan 80 mg; RR for eletriptan 20 mg *v* placebo 2.3, 95% CI 1.6 to 3.2; RR for eletriptan 40 mg *v* placebo RR 2.7, 95% CI 1.9 to 3.8; RR for eletriptan 80 mg *v* placebo 3.2, 95% CI 2.3 to 4.5). It also found that eletriptan 80 mg significantly increased headache relief compared with sumatriptan 100 mg (AR for improved pain: 77% with eletriptan 80 mg *v* 55% with sumatriptan 100 mg; RR 1.4, 95% CI 1.2 to 1.7). The second subsequent RCT (1008 people) compared two doses of eletriptan (40 mg and 80 mg), two doses of sumatriptan (50 mg and 100 mg), and placebo.[62] At 2 hours it found that both doses of eletriptan significantly increased headache relief compared with placebo or sumatriptan at 2 hours (AR 25/80 [31%] with placebo, 108/169 [64%] with 40 mg eletriptan, 107/160 [67%] with 80 mg eletriptan, 88/176 [50%] with 50 mg sumatriptan, 85/160 [53%] with 100 mg sumatriptan; $P < 0.0001$ for eletriptan 40 mg *v* placebo; $P < 0.0001$ for eletriptan 80 mg *v* placebo; $P < 0.01$ for either dose eletriptan *v* sumatriptan 50 mg; $P < 0.05$ for either dose eletriptan *v* sumatriptan 100 mg). The third subsequent RCT (1153 people) compared eletriptan 40 mg or 80 mg versus placebo.[63] It found that eletriptan increased the chance of headache relief at 2 hours compared with placebo (AR for headache relief: 62% with eletriptan 40 mg, 65% with eletriptan 80 mg, and 19% with placebo; $P < 0.0001$ for either dose of eletriptan *v* placebo).

Harms: In the first RCT, dizziness and fatigue were the only adverse effects that were significantly more common in people taking eletriptan than in those on placebo.[24] The first RCT found a dose response relationship for minor and major harms (see glossary, p 1562) for eletriptan (RR for major harm: 20 mg eletriptan *v* placebo 0.7, 95% CI 0.2 to 2.6; 40 mg *v* placebo 0.6, 95% CI 0.3 to 1.6; 80 mg *v* placebo 1.1, 95% CI 0.5 to 2.4; RR for minor harm: 80 mg eletriptan *v* placebo 2.0, 95% CI 1.6 to 2.6; 40 mg *v* placebo 1.5, 95% CI 1.2 to 1.9).[24] The RCT of two doses of eletriptan and sumatriptan reported a similar rate of adverse events (asthenia, nausea, dizziness, somnolence, chest symptoms, sweating, and withdrawal due to adverse effects) in each treatment group.[62] The third subsequent RCT found a dose response relationship for some adverse effects after the first attack with oral eletriptan (e.g. asthenia: 1.7% with placebo, 6.6% with oral eletriptan 40 mg, 11.7% with eletriptan 80 mg).[63]

Comment: None.

OPTION NARATRIPTAN

Four RCTs have found that naratriptan increases headache relief at 4 hours compared with placebo. One RCT comparing naratriptan versus sumatriptan found no significant difference in headache recurrence.

Benefits: We found no systematic review. **Versus placebo:** We found four RCTs.[26,27,64,65] The first RCT (613 people) compared naratriptan 2.5 mg, 1 mg, 0.25 mg, and 0.1 mg versus placebo.[65] It found that higher doses of naratriptan significantly increased headache relief (see glossary, p 1562) at 4 hours compared with placebo in a dose responsive manner (AR 60% with 2.5 mg naratriptan, 50% with 1 mg naratriptan, 35% with 0.25 mg naratriptan, 32% with 0.1 mg, and 34% with placebo; $P < 0.05$ for naratriptan 2.5 mg and 1 mg *v* placebo). Higher doses of naratriptan significantly increased the chance of being pain free (see glossary, p 1562) at 4 hours compared with placebo (33% with 2.5 mg naratriptan, 27% with 1 mg naratriptan, and 20% with placebo; $P = 0.031$ for both doses *v* placebo). The second RCT (643 people) found that naratriptan or sumatriptan significantly increased the proportion of people with headache relief at 4 hours compared with placebo (63% with naratriptan *v* 80% with sumatriptan *v* 31% with placebo; $P < 0.05$).[26] A third crossover RCT (740 people) compared naratriptan 2.5 mg, 1 mg, and 0.25 mg versus placebo.[27] This trial found that naratriptan 2.5 mg versus placebo was the most effective dose at producing headache relief at 4 hours (AR 68% *v* 33%; $P < 0.001$; insufficient data for RR calculation). Naratriptan 2.5 mg significantly reduced the need for rescue medication (see glossary, p 1562) after 4 hours (AR 52% *v* 26%; $P < 0.001$; insufficient data for RR calculation). Headache recurrence (see glossary, p 1562) within 24 hours of initial dosing occurred in fewer people taking naratriptan 2.5 mg than in those on placebo (27% *v* 36%; significance not stated). In a fourth RCT, a subgroup of 206 people with a poor response to sumatriptan 50 mg in a first attack were randomised 1 week later to either naratriptan 2.5 mg orally or placebo.[64] Naratriptan significantly increased headache relief at 2 hours (AR 25% with naratriptan *v* 10% with placebo; RR 2.5, 95% CI 1.3 to 4.7) and at 4 hours (AR 41% *v* 19%; RR 2.2, 95% CI 1.4 to 3.5) compared with placebo. **Versus sumatriptan:** One RCT comparing naratriptan 2.5 mg orally versus sumatriptan 100 mg orally found no significant difference in headache recurrence.[66]

Harms: In the crossover RCT (643 people) adverse effects occurred in fewer than 1% of people, with no difference between naratriptan and placebo.[27] The most common adverse effects reported were nausea or vomiting, which could not be differentiated as being caused by naratriptan or being a part of the symptoms accompanying migraine. Blood pressure changes, haemorrhage, bradycardia, tachyarrhythmias, extrasystoles, palpitations, and heart murmurs after the first dose of 2.5 mg naratriptan were reported by 1% of people. Thirteen people withdrew from the study; one (migraine exacerbation) was considered to be related to the administration of naratriptan and five were possibly related. No significant association between dose variation and adverse effects was found. Similar adverse effects were reported in another RCT but were more common (21% with naratriptan 2.5 mg orally v 23% with placebo; significance not stated).[26] The RCT comparing two doses of naratriptan with placebo found similar incidences of adverse events in all groups.[65]

Comment: Naratriptan or a different triptan in a second attack may be beneficial in people responding poorly to sumatriptan in a first attack, but this requires confirmation in further RCTs.

OPTION RIZATRIPTAN

One systematic review and subsequent RCTs have found that rizatriptan improves headache relief compared with placebo.

Benefits: We found one systematic review (search date 2000, 7 RCTs, 3528 people) comparing rizatriptan versus placebo.[28] A meta-analysis in the systematic review found that rizatriptan 5 mg and 10 mg versus placebo significantly increased headache relief (see glossary, p 1562) (AR 59% with 5 mg v 68% with 10 mg v 31% with placebo; RR of rizatriptan 5 mg v placebo 1.8, 95% CI 1.6 to 2.0; RR of rizatriptan 10 mg v placebo 2.2, 95% CI 2.0 to 2.5). One crossover RCT excluded from the meta-analysis above (1538 people) compared oral rizatriptan 5–10 mg or oral sumatriptan 25–50 mg versus placebo.[67] It found that rizatriptan 5 mg significantly increased headache relief compared with placebo (AR 68% with rizatriptan 5 mg v 68% with sumatriptan 50 mg v 38% with placebo; $P < 0.05$; insufficient data for RR calculation). Fewer people taking rizatriptan versus placebo needed rescue medication (see glossary, p 1562) (19% v 45%; $P < 0.05$). Another RCT (727 people) comparing rizatriptan 10 mg versus zolmitriptan 2.5 mg versus placebo found no significant difference in the proportion of people who had headache relief between rizatripan and zolmitriptan ($P = 0.23$). However, both treatments were superior to placebo in headache relief (AR rizatriptan 71%, AR zolmitriptan 67%, AR placebo 30%; either treatment v placebo, $P < 0.05$).[30]

Harms: The most frequently and consistently reported adverse effects in the RCTs include dizziness, somnolence, nausea, and fatigue.[28–30,67–69] In at least one RCT, these adverse effects were shown to have a dose dependent occurrence.[68]

Comment: None.

OPTION SUMATRIPTAN

RCTs have found that subcutaneous, oral, or intranasal sumatriptan increases headache relief compared with placebo. RCTs found no significant difference in headache relief between sumatriptan and aspirin plus metoclopramide, tolfenamic acid, or zolmitriptan. RCTs found that oral or nasal sumatriptan increased headache relief compared with oral or nasal ergotamine. One RCT found no significant difference between sumatriptan and naratriptan in headache recurrence.

Benefits: We found one systematic review (search date 1997, 26 reports on 30 RCTs, 7437 people) comparing different preparations of sumatriptan versus placebo.[31] **Subcutaneous sumatriptan:** The review found that subcutaneous sumatriptan 6 mg significantly increased headache relief (see glossary, p 1562) at 1 hour compared with placebo (12 RCTs, 3127 people; 69% *v* 19%; RR 3.7, 95% CI 3.3 to 4.2).[31] **Oral sumatriptan:** The review found that oral sumatriptan 100 mg significantly increased headache relief compared with placebo (12 RCTs, 2890 people; 58% *v* 25%; RR 2.3, 95% CI 2.1 to 2.6).[31] Subsequent RCTs compared oral sumatriptan 50 mg versus placebo in the treatment of one migraine attack in 485 people[32] and three consecutive attacks in 1003 people.[70] Sumatriptan significantly increased the proportion of people with headache relief after 2 hours in people with one attack, and after 4 hours in people with three attacks. A further subsequent RCT (1008 people) compared two doses of eletriptan (40 mg and 80 mg), two doses of sumatriptan (50 mg and 100 mg), and placebo.[62] At 2 hours it found that both doses of sumatriptan significantly increased headache relief compared with placebo ($P < 0.01$ for either dose of sumatriptan *v* placebo). **Intranasal sumatriptan:** The review found that intranasal sumatriptan 20 mg significantly increased headache relief compared with placebo (6 RCTs, 1420 people; 61% *v* 30%; RR 2.1, 95% CI 1.8 to 2.4).[31] One additional crossover RCT (246 people with up to 12 migraines) comparing subcutaneous sumatriptan 6 mg versus usual headache treatment (49% combinations, 24% ergotamine, 19% non-steroidal anti-inflammatory drugs, 7% dihydroergotamine) found that sumatriptan significantly improved headache relief (78% *v* 34%; $P < 0.001$).[33] In three additional RCTs (2475 people) intranasal sumatriptan significantly increased headache relief compared with placebo (60–64% with sumatriptan *v* 25–35% with placebo).[71–73] **Versus aspirin plus metoclopramide:** See benefits of salicylates, p 1549. **Versus tolfenamic acid:** See benefits of tolfenamic acid, p 1554. **Versus ergotamine:** See benefits of ergotamine, p 1555. **Versus naratriptan:** See benefits of naratriptan, p 1558. **Versus zolmitriptan:** See benefits of zolmitriptan, p 1561. **Versus eletriptan:** See benefits of eletriptan, p 1556. **Versus ergotamine derivatives:** See benefits of ergotamine, p 1555.

Harms: One non-systematic review reported that common adverse effects with sumatriptan included sensations of pressure, tightness, heaviness, and tingling affecting any part of the body, and that 3–5% of these symptoms can occur in the chest region.[74] The review found no association between sumatriptan and reported deaths. **Subcutaneous sumatriptan:** In one systematic review (search date 1997), 7/12 RCTs found that more people taking subcutaneous sumatriptan 6 mg than on placebo reported adverse effects (65% *v* 32%; OR 4, 95% CI 3 to 5).[31] **Oral sumatriptan:** In the same review, 9/12 RCTs found that more people taking oral sumatriptan 100 mg than on placebo reported adverse effects (36% *v* 24%; OR 1.72, 95% CI 1.48 to 2.08).[31]

Comment: There is a consensus that sumatriptan should not be used in people with ischaemic heart disease or concomitantly with ergotamine.

OPTION ZOLMITRIPTAN

Three large RCTs have found that oral zolmitriptan increases headache relief compared with placebo. Two RCTs found no significant difference between zolmitriptan and sumatriptan in headache relief.

Benefits: We found no systematic review. **Versus placebo:** We found three RCTs.[34,35,75] The first RCT (1144 people) compared oral zolmitriptan 1 mg, 2.5 mg, 5 mg, and 10 mg versus placebo.[34] The trial found that zolmitriptan 2.5 mg significantly increased the proportion of people with headache relief (see glossary, p 1562) (AR 65% *v* 34%; RR 1.9, 95% CI 1.5 to 2.5). Zolmitriptan reduced the proportion of people needing rescue medication (see glossary, p 1562) (AR 38% with zolmitriptan *v* 65% with placebo; RR 0.6, 95% CI 0.5 to 0.7). The second RCT (327 people) compared oral zolmitriptan 2.5 mg versus placebo.[35] It found that zolmitriptan significantly increased headache relief (AR 62% *v* 36%; RR 1.7, 95% CI 1.3 to 2.3) and reduced the proportion of people needing rescue medication (AR 43% *v* 67%; RR 0.6, 95% CI 0.5 to 0.8). The third RCT (734 people randomised in each of three attacks) compared zolmitriptan 2.5 mg versus placebo for the first attack, zolmitriptan 5 mg versus placebo for the second attack, and zolmitriptan 2.5 mg versus placebo for the third attack.[75] It found that either dose of zolmitriptan significantly increased headache relief compared with placebo at 2 hours (58.9% with zolmitriptan 2.5 mg *v* 34.6% with placebo, $P < 0.001$; 62.1% with zolmitriptan 5 mg *v* 36.0% with placebo, $P < 0.001$). **Versus sumatriptan:** We found two RCTs.[36,76] In the first RCT (1522 people), up to six consecutive attacks were treated with zolimtriptan 2.5 mg (500 people, 2671 attacks), zolmitriptan 5 mg (514 people, 2744 attacks), or sumatriptan 50 mg (508 people, 2693 attacks).[76] The RCT found no significant difference among groups for headache relief at 2 hours (AR 62.9% with zolmitriptan 2.5 mg, 65.7% with zolmitriptan 5 mg, 66.6% with sumatriptan 50 mg). The second RCT (1445 people) compared zolmitriptan 2.5–5 mg versus oral sumatriptan 25–50 mg.[36] The trial found no significant difference in headache relief between treatments at any dose. **Stratified care versus step care:** One RCT (835 people) randomised people into three arms.[77] The first arm, named "stratified care", randomised people with low disability scores to aspirin 800–1000 mg plus metoclopramide 10 mg, and people with higher disability scores to zolmitriptan 2.5 mg. The second arm, named "step care", involved treating initial attacks with aspirin plus metoclopramide and then switching to zolmitriptan 2.5 mg for the remaining two to three attacks. The third arm involved "step care within attacks", whereby all attacks were initially treated with aspirin plus metoclopramide, and non-responders were given zolmitriptan after 2 hours. It found that stratified care versus either of the step care groups significantly increased the proportion of people with headache relief (AR 53% with stratified care *v* 40% with step care *v* 36% with step care within attacks; RR stratified care *v* step care 1.3, 95% CI 1.1 to 1.7; stratified care *v* step care within attacks 1.4, 95% CI 1.2 to 1.7).

Harms: The first RCT found a dose response effect with zolmitriptan, with fewer adverse effects reported with lower doses than with higher doses (39% with 1 mg, 44% with 2.5 mg, 58% with 5 mg, and 67% with 10 mg).[34] More than 4% of people reported nausea, dizziness, somnolence, paraesthesia, fatigue, warm sensation, and tightness of throat or chest. The third RCT of zolmitripan versus placebo found that adverse events were more common with zolmitriptan than with placebo (42% of patients experienced at least one), but none of these were severe.[75] One RCT comparing zolmitriptan versus sumatriptan found no significant differences between treatments in adverse events.[76]

Comment: None.

GLOSSARY

Headache intensity Mild: normal activity allowed. Moderate: disturbing, but not prohibiting normal activity; bed rest not necessary. Severe: normal activity discontinued; bed rest may be necessary.

Headache recurrence In responders, change in headache intensity (see above) from mild/none to moderate/severe within 24 hours of study medication initial dose.

Headache relief Change in headache intensity (see above) score from severe/moderate to mild/none.

International Headache Society criteria (1988) *Migraine without aura (common migraine)* is defined as five or more headache attacks lasting for 4–72 hours with accompanying symptoms of either nausea/vomiting and/or phonophobia and photophobia. Pain should comply with at least two of the following four characteristics: unilateral, throbbing, moderate to severe intensity, and increase with physical activity. For *migraine with aura (classic migraine)*, two or more headache attacks are required that comply with three of the following four characteristics: one or more fully reversible aura symptom indicating focal cerebral cortical and/or brainstem dysfunction; at least one aura symptom developing gradually over more than 4 minutes or two or more symptoms occurring in succession; no aura symptom should last more than 1 hour; and headache follows aura with a pain free (see below) interval of less than 60 minutes. In both migraine with and without aura, secondary causes of headache should be excluded; if any structural damage is found, then it should not explain headache characteristics. Less stringent criteria for migraine without aura can be used. In clinical practice, the so called borderline migraine can be diagnosed when one of the above criteria is not met. International Headache Society criteria were not developed with the intention of identifying potential responders to different medications.

Major and minor harm Major harm is defined as death, serious illness, or any adverse effect of sufficient severity to cause withdrawal from the study. Minor harm is defined as any adverse effect that does not fulfil the criteria for a major harm.

Migraine index Pain scale for migraine resulting from duration times intensity of migraine where intensity is classified as 0 = none, 1 = mild, 2 = moderate, and 3 = severe.

Pain free Change in headache intensity (see above) score from severe/moderate to none.

Rescue medication Additional medications different to study medication permitted in non-responders, usually limited to the habitual medications a person uses to treat their migraine headache.

Substantive changes

Salicylates One RCT added;[40] conclusions unchanged.

Diclofenac One RCT added;[43] conclusions unchanged.

Ibuprofen One RCT added;[47] conclusions unchanged.
Ergotamine One RCT added;[59] conclusions unchanged.
Eletriptan Two RCTs added;[62,63] conclusions unchanged.
Naratriptan One RCT added;[65] conclusions unchanged.
Sumatriptan One RCT added;[62] conclusions unchanged.
Zolmitriptan Two RCTs added;[75,76] conclusions unchanged.

REFERENCES

1. Headache Classification Committee of the International Headache Society. Classification and diagnostic criteria for headache disorders, cranial neuralgias and face pain. *Cephalalgia* 1988;8:12–96.
2. Stewart W, Linet M, Celentano D, et al. Age and sex specific incidence rates of migraine with and without visual aura. *Am J Epidemiol* 1991;134:1111–1120.
3. O'Brien B, Goerre R, Streiner D. Prevalence of migraine headache in Canada: a population based survey. *Int J Epidemiol* 1994;23:1020–1026.
4. Pryse-Phillips W, Findlay H, Tugwell P, et al. A Canadian population survey on the clinical, epidemiological and societal impact if migraine and tension type headache. *Can J Neurol Sci* 1992;19:333–339.
5. Stewart W, Lipton R, Celentano D, et al. Prevalence of migraine headache in the United States. *JAMA* 1992;267:64–69.
6. Kryst S, Scherl E. A population based survey of social and personal impact of headache. *Headache* 1994;34:344–350.
7. Morillo L, Sanin L, Takeuchi Y, et al. Headache in Latin America: a multination population-based survey. *Neurology* 2001;56(suppl 3):A454.
8. Bank J, Marton S. Hungarian migraine epidemiology. *Headache* 2000;40:164–169.
9. Henry P, Michel P, Brochet B, et al. A nationwide survey of migraine in France: prevalence and clinical features. *Cephalalgia* 1992;12:229–237.
10. Rasmussen B, Jensen R, Schroll, et al. Epidemiology of headache in a general population: a prevalence study. *J Clin Epidemiol* 1991;44:1147–1157.
11. Steiner T, Stewart W, Kolodner K, et al. Epidemiology of migraine in England. *Cephalalgia* 1999;19:305.
12. Cheung RTF. Prevalence of migraine, tension type headache and other headaches in Hong Kong. *Headache* 2000;40:473–479.
13. Sakai F, Igarashi H. Prevalence of migraine in Japan: a nationwide survey. *Cephalalgia* 1997;17:15–22.
14. Stewart W, Staffa J, Lipton R, et al. Familial risk of migraine: a population based study. *Ann Neurol* 1997;41:166–172.
15. Chabriat H, Joire J, Danchot J, et al. Combined oral lysine acetylsalicylate and metoclopramide in the acute treatment of migraine: a multicentre double-blind placebo-controlled study. *Cephalalgia* 2001;14:297–300.
16. Tfelt-Hansen P, Henry P, Mulder L, et al. The effectiveness of combined oral lysine acetylsalicylate and metoclopramide compared with oral sumatriptan for migraine. *Lancet* 1995;346:923–926.
17. Deiner H. Efficacy and safety of intravenous acetylsalicylic acid lysinate compared to subcutaneous sumatriptan and parenteral placebo in the acute treatment of migraine: a double-blind, double-dummy, randomized, multicenter, parallel group study. The ASASUMAMIG Study Group. *Cephalalgia* 1999;19:581–588.
18. The Oral Sumatriptan and Aspirin plus Metoclopramide Comparative Study Group. A study to compare oral sumatriptan with oral aspirin plus metoclopramide in the acute treatment of migraine. *Eur Neurol* 1992;32:177–184.
19. Lipton R, Stewart W, Ryan RJ, et al. Efficacy and safety of paracetamol, aspirin, and caffeine in alleviating migraine headache pain: three double-blind, randomized, placebo-controlled trials. *Arch Neurol* 1998;55:210–217.
20. Lange R, Schwarz JA, Hohn M. Acetylsalicylic acid effervescent 1000 mg (aspirin) in acute migraine attacks; a multicentre, randomized, double-blind, single dose, placebo-controlled parallel group study. *Cephalalgia* 2000;20:663–667.
21. Dahlof C, Bjorkman R. Diclofenac-K (50 and 100 mg) and placebo in the acute treatment of migraine. *Cephalalgia* 1993;13:117–123.
22. Kellstein D, Lipton R, Geetha R, et al. Evaluation of a novel solubilized formulation of ibuprofen in the treatment of migraine headache: a randomized, double-blind, placebo-controlled, dose-ranging study. *Cephalalgia* 2000;20:233–243.
23. Myllyla V, Havanka H, Herrala L, et al. Tolfenamic acid rapid release versus sumatriptan in the acute treatment of migraine: comparable effect in a double-blind, randomized, controlled, parallel-group study. *Headache* 1998;38:201–207.
24. Smith LA, Oldman AD, McQuay HJ, et al. Eletriptan for acute migraine. In: The Cochrane Library, Issue 1, 2002. Oxford: Update Software. Search date 2000; primary sources data from all phase III randomised placebo controlled trials were made available by the manufacturer, Pfizer Inc. To date, these trials comprise the only data on eletriptan relevant to this review in a published or unpublished form; thus searches of electronic databases for further trials of eletriptan were not conducted.
25. Goadsby PJ, Ferrari MD, Olesen J, et al, for the Eletriptan Steering Committee. Eletriptan in acute migraine: a double-blind, placebo-controlled comparison to sumatriptan. *Neurology* 2000;54:156–163.
26. Havanka H, Dahlof C, Pop P, et al. Efficacy of naratriptan tablets in the acute treatment of migraine: a dose-ranging study. *Clin Ther* 2000;22:970–980.
27. Mathew N, Asgharnejad M, Peykamian M, et al. Naratriptan is effective and well tolerated in the acute treatment of migraine. Results of a double-blind, placebo-controlled, crossover study. *Neurology* 1997;49:1485–1490.
28. Oldman Ad, Smith LA, McQuay HJ, et al. Rizatriptan for acute migraine. In: The Cochrane Library, Issue 1, 2002. Oxford: Update Software. Search date 2000; primary sources Medline, Embase, Cochrane Library Issue 3 2000, and Oxford Pain Relief Database.
29. Kramer M, Matzura-Wolfe D, Polis A, et al. A placebo-controlled crossover study of rizatriptan in the treatment of multiple migraine attacks. Rizatriptan Multiple Attack Study Group. *Neurology* 1998;51:773–781.

30. Pascual J, Vega P, Deiner H-C, et al. Comparison of rizatriptan 10 mg vs. zolmitriptan 2.5 mg in the acute treatment of migraine. *Cephalalgia* 2000;20:455–461.
31. Tfelt-Hansen P. Efficacy and harms of subcutaneous, oral, and intranasal sumatriptan used for migraine treatment: a systematic review based on number needed to treat. *Cephalalgia* 2001;18:532–538. Search date 1997; primary sources Medline and hand searches of *Arch Neurol*, *Neurology*, *Headache*, and *Cephalalgia* from 1990.
32. Savani N, Brautaset NJ, Reunanen M, et al. A double-blind placebo-controlled study assessing the efficacy and tolerability of 50 mg sumatriptan tablets in the acute treatment of migraine. Sumatriptan Tablets S2CM07 Study Group. *Int J Clin Pract Suppl* 1999;105:7–15.
33. Boureau F, Chazot G, Emile J, et al. Comparison of subcutaneous sumatriptan with usual acute treatments for migraine. French Sumatriptan Study Group. *Eur Neurol* 1995;35:264–269.
34. Rapoport A, Ramadan N, Adelman J, et al. Optimizing the dose of zolmitriptan (Zomig, 311C90) for the acute treatment of migraine. A multicenter, double-blind, placebo-controlled, dose range-finding study. *Neurology* 1997;49:1210–1218.
35. Solomon G, Cady R, Klappew J, et al. Clinical efficacy and tolerability of 2.5 mg zolmitriptan for the acute treatment of migraine. *Neurology* 1997;49:1219–1225.
36. Gallagher R, Dennidh G, Spierings E, et al. A comparative trial of zolmitriptan and sumatriptan for the acute oral treatment of migraine. *Headache* 2000;40:119–128.
37. Limmroth V, May A, Diener H. Lysine-acetylsalicylic acid in acute migraine attacks. *Eur Neurol* 1999;41:88–93.
38. Tfelt-Hansen P, Olesen J. Effervescent metoclopramide and aspirin (Migravess) versus effervescent aspirin or placebo for migraine attacks: a double-blind study. *Cephalalgia* 1984;4:107–111.
39. Boureau F, Joubert JM, Lasserre V, et al. Double-blind comparison of an paracetamol 400 mg-codeine 25 mg combination versus aspirin 1000 mg and placebo in acute migraine attack. *Cephalalgia* 1994;14:156–161.
40. MacGregor EA, Dowson A, Davies PTG. Mouth-dispersible aspirin in the treatment of migraine:a placebo-controlled study. *Headache* 2002;42:249–259.
41. Massiou H, Serrurier D, Lasserre O, et al. Effectiveness of oral diclofenac in the acute treatment of common migraine attacks: a double-blind study versus placebo. *Cephalalgia* 1991;11:59–63.
42. The Diclofenac-K/Sumatriptan Migraine Study Group. Acute treatment of migraine attacks: efficacy and safety of nonsteroidal anti-inflammatory drug, diclofenac-potassium in comparison to oral sumatriptan and placebo. *Cephalalgia* 1999;19:232–240.
43. Bigal ME, Bordini CA, Speciali JG. Intramuscular diclofenac in the acute treatment of migraine: a double-blind placebo controlled study [in Portuguese]. *Arq Neuropsiquiatr* 2002;60:410–415.
44. Karachalios G, Fotiadou A, Chrisikos N, et al. Treatment of acute migraine attack with diclofenac sodium: a double blind study. *Headache* 1992;32:98–100.
45. Kloster R, Nestvold K, Vilming S. A double-blind study of ibuprofen versus placebo in the treatment of acute migraine attacks. *Cephalalgia* 1992;12:169–171.
46. Havanka-Kanniainen H. Treatment of acute migraine attack: ibuprofen and placebo compared. *Headache* 1989;29:507–509.
47. Codispoti JR, Prior MJ, Fu M, et al. Efficacy of non-prescription doses of ibuprofen in treating migraine headache. A randomized clinical trial. *Headache* 2001;41:665–679.
48. Sandrini G, Franchini S, Lanfranchi S, et al. Effectiveness of ibuprofen-arginine in the treatment of acute migraine attacks. *Int J Clin Pharmacol Res* 1998;18:145–150.
49. Andersson P, Hinge H, Johansen O, et al. Double-blind study of naproxen v placebo in the treatment of acute migraine attacks. *Cephalalgia* 1989;9:29–32.
50. Nestvold K, Kloster R, Partinen M, et al. Treatment of acute migraine attack: naproxen and placebo compared. *Cephalalgia* 1985;5:115–119.
51. Sargent J, Baumel B, Peters K, et al. Aborting a migraine attack: naproxen v ergotamine plus caffeine. *Headache* 1988;28:263–266.
52. Pradalier A, Rancurel G, Dordain G, et al. Acute migraine attack therapy: comparison of naproxen sodium and an ergotamine tartrate compound. *Cephalalgia* 1985;5:107–112.
53. Treves T, Streiffler M, Korczyn A. Naproxen sodium versus ergotamine tartrate in the treatment of acute migraine attacks. *Headache* 1992;32:280–282.
54. Hakkarainen H, Vapaatalo H, Gothoni G, et al. Tolfenamic acid is as effective as ergotamine during migraine attacks. *Lancet* 1979;2:326–328.
55. Norrelund N, Christiansen L, Plantener S. Tolfenamic acid versus paracetamol in migraine attacks. A double-blind study in general practice. *Ugeskr Laeger* 1989;151:2436–2438.
56. Tokola R, Kangasniemi P, Neuvonen P, et al. Tolfenamic acid, metoclopramide, caffeine and their combinations in the treatment of migraine attacks. *Cephalalgia* 1984;4:253–263.
57. Dahlof C. Placebo-controlled clinical trials with ergotamine in the acute treatment of migraine. *Cephalalgia* 1993;13:166–171. Search date 1991; primary sources Medline, Embase, and hand searched reference lists.
58. Multinational Oral Sumatriptan Cafergot Comparative Study Group. A randomized, double-blind comparison of sumatriptan and Cafergot in the acute treatment of migraine. *Eur Neurol* 1991;31:314–322.
59. Bourea F, Kappos L, Schoenen J, Esperanca P, Ashford E. A clinical comparison of sumatriptan nasal spray and dihydroergotamine nasal spray in the acute treatment of migraine. *Int J Clin Pract* 2000;54:281–286.
60. Hakkarainen H. Ergotamine vs. metoclopramide vs. their combination in acute migraine attacks. *Headache* 1982;22:10–12.
61. Lipton R. Ergotamine tartrate and dihydroergotamine mesylate: safety profiles. *Headache* 1997;37:S33–41.
62. Sandrini G, Farkkila M, Gurgess G, et al. Eletriptan versus ssumatriptan: a double-blind, multiple migraine attack study. *Neurology* 2002;59:1210–1217.
63. Stark R, Dahlos C, Haughie S, et al. Efficacy, safety and tolerability of oral eletriptan in the acute treatment of migraine: results of a phase III, multicentre, placebo controlled study across three attacks. *Cephalalgia* 2002;22:23–32.
64. Stark S, Spierings E, McNeal S, et al. Naratriptan efficacy in migraineurs who respond poorly to oral sumatriptan. *Headache* 2000;40:513–520.
65. Klassen A, Elkind A, Asgharejad M, et al. Naratriptan is effective and well tolerated in the

acute treatment of migraine. Results of a double-blind, placebo-controlled, parallel-group study. *Headache* 1997;37:640–645.
66. Gobel H, Winter P, Boswell D, et al. Comparison of naratriptan and sumatriptan in recurrence-prone migraine patients. *Clin Ther* 2000;22:981–989.
67. Goldstein J, Ryan R, Jaing K, et al. Crossover comparison of rizatriptan 5 mg and 10 mg versus sumatriptan 25 mg and 50 mg in migraine. *Headache* 1998;38:737–747.
68. Teall J, Tuchman M, Cutler N, et al. Rizatriptan (MAXALT) for the acute treatment of migraine and migraine recurrence. A placebo-controlled, outpatient study. *Headache* 1998;38:281–287.
69. Tfelt-Hansen P, Teall J, Rodriguez F, et al. Oral rizatriptan versus oral sumatriptan: a direct comparison study in the acute treatment of migraine. *Headache* 1998;38:748–755.
70. Pfaffenrath V, Cunin G, Sjonell G, et al. Efficacy and safety of sumatriptan tablets (25 mg, 50 mg, and 100 mg) in the acute treatment of migraine: defining the optimum doses of oral sumatriptan. *Headache* 1998;38:184–190.
71. Peikert A, Becker WJ, Ashford EA, et al. Sumatriptan nasal spray: a dose-ranging study in the acute treatment of migraine. *Eur J Neurol* 1999;6:43–49.
72. Diamond S, Elkind A, Jackson RT, et al. Multiple-attack efficacy and tolerability of sumatriptan nasal spray in the treatment of migraine. *Arch Fam Med* 1998;7:234–240.
73. Ryan R, Elkind A, Baker CC, et al. Sumatriptan nasal spray for the acute treatment of migraine. Results of two clinical studies. *Neurology* 1997;49:1225–1230.
74. Ensink F. The efficacy of sumatriptan in the acute treatment of migraine. *Headache Q* 1995;6:280–292.
75. Ryan RE Jr, Diamond S, Giammarco RAM, et al. Efficacy of zolmitriptan at early time-points for the acute treatment of migraine and treatment of recurrence: a randomized, placebo-controlled trial. *CNS Drugs* 2000;13:215–226.
76. Gruffyd-Jones K, Kies B, Middleton A, et al. Zolmitriptan versus sumatriptan for the acute oral treatment of migraine: a randomized, double-blind, international study. *Eur J Neurol* 2001;8:237–245.
77. Lipton RB, Stewart WF, Stone AM, et al. Stratified care vs step care strategies for migraine: the Disability in Strategies of Care (DISC) study: a randomized trial. *JAMA* 2000;284:2599–2605.

Luis E Morillo
Associate Professor
Javeriana University
Faculty of Medicine, Department of Neurosciences, Neurology Unit and Clinical Epidemiology and Biostatistics Unit
Bogota
Colombia

Competing interests: None declared.

Multiple sclerosis

Search date March 2003

Mike Boggild and Helen Ford

QUESTIONS

INTERVENTIONS

Key Messages

Reducing relapse rates and disability

- We found no evidence from RCTs that any treatment alters long term outcome in multiple sclerosis.
- **Glatiramer acetate** One RCT in people with relapsing and remitting multiple sclerosis found that, compared with placebo, glatiramer acetate reduced relapse rates over 2 years, but had no effect on disability. We found no good quality RCTs in people with secondary progressive multiple sclerosis.

- **Interferon beta** Two RCTs in people experiencing a first demyelinating event found that interferon beta-1a decreased the risk of conversion to clinically definite multiple sclerosis over 2–3 years compared with placebo. One systematic review in people with active relapsing remitting multiple sclerosis found limited evidence that, compared with placebo, interferon beta-1a/b reduced exacerbations and disease progression over 2 years. One subsequent RCT in people with relapsing remitting multiple sclerosis found that interferon beta-1b reduced the proportion of people with relapse over 2 years compared with interferon beta-1a. We found conflicting evidence from three RCTs about the effects of interferon beta on disease progression in people with secondary progressive multiple sclerosis.
- **Azathioprine** One systematic review in people with relapsing and remitting or progressive multiple sclerosis comparing azathioprine versus placebo or no treatment found a modest reduction in relapse rates over 2 years, but no evidence of a difference in disability. However, we were unable to draw reliable conclusions because of clinical heterogeneity among included RCTs.
- **Intravenous immunoglobulin** One RCT in people with relapsing and remitting multiple sclerosis found limited evidence from baseline comparisons that intravenous immunoglobulin may reduce disability over 2 years compared with placebo. However, the clinical importance of this difference is unclear. We found no good quality RCTs in people with secondary progressive multiple sclerosis.
- **Methotrexate** We found insufficient evidence from one small RCT about the effects of methotrexate in people with multiple sclerosis.
- **Mitoxantrone** One RCT in people with worsening, relapsing, remitting, or progressive multiple sclerosis found that mitoxantrone reduced progression of disability compared with placebo. One small RCT in people with active multiple sclerosis found limited evidence that mitoxantrone plus methylprednisolone reduced relapse compared with methylprednisolone alone. However, mitoxantrone is associated with leukopenia, menstrual disorders, and arrhythmia.

Treating acute relapses

- **Corticosteroids (methylprednisolone or corticotrophin)** One systematic review in people with multiple sclerosis requiring treatment for acute exacerbations has found that corticosteroids (methylprednisolone or corticotrophin) improves symptoms compared with placebo within the first 5 weeks of treatment. The optimal dose, route, and duration of treatment are unclear.
- **Plasma exchange** One small RCT provided insufficient evidence to assess plasma exchange in people with acute relapses of multiple sclerosis.

Fatigue

- **Amantadine** We found insufficient evidence from one systematic review of poor quality RCTs about the effects of amantadine in people with multiple sclerosis.
- **Behaviour modification** We found no RCTs on the effects of behavioural modification treatment in people with multiple sclerosis related fatigue.
- **Exercise** We found insufficient evidence from two RCTs about the effects of exercise in people with multiple sclerosis related fatigue.
- **Pemoline** One systematic review found no significant difference in the self reporting of fatigue with pemoline compared with placebo.

Spasticity

- **Botulinum toxin** We found insufficient evidence from one small RCT about the effects of botulinum toxin on functional outcomes in people with spasticity due to multiple sclerosis.
- **Intrathecal baclofen** One small crossover RCT provided insufficient evidence to assess functional effects of intrathecal baclofen.
- **Oral drug treatments** One systematic review found insufficient evidence about the effects of oral drugs on functional outcomes in people with spasticity due to multiple sclerosis. RCTs provided insufficient evidence to assess other oral drug treatments.
- **Physiotherapy** We found insufficient evidence from two small RCTs about the effects of physiotherapy. One of the RCTs found limited evidence that twice weekly hospital or home based physiotherapy for 8 weeks briefly improved mobility compared with no physiotherapy. The other, in people with progressive multiple sclerosis, found no significant difference between early versus delayed physiotherapy in mobility or activities of daily living.

Multidisciplinary care

- **Inpatient rehabilitation** Two small RCTs provided insufficient evidence to assess the effectiveness of inpatient rehabilitation. Both RCTs found short term benefit, but no reduction in neurological impairment. Longer term effects are uncertain.
- **Outpatient rehabilitation** One small RCT provided insufficient evidence to assess the effectiveness of outpatient rehabilitation.

DEFINITION Multiple sclerosis is a chronic inflammatory disease of the central nervous system. Diagnosis requires evidence of lesions that are separated in both time and space, and the exclusion of other inflammatory, structural, or hereditary conditions that might give a similar clinical picture. The disease takes three main forms: relapsing and remitting multiple sclerosis, characterised by episodes of neurological dysfunction interspersed with periods of stability; primary progressive multiple sclerosis, where progressive neurological disability occurs from the outset; and secondary progressive multiple sclerosis, where progressive neurological disability occurs later in the course of the disease.

INCIDENCE/ PREVALENCE Prevalence varies with geography and racial group; it is highest in white populations in temperate regions.[1] In Europe and North America, prevalence is 1/800 people, with an annual incidence of 2–10/100 000, making multiple sclerosis the most common cause of neurological disability in young adults. Age of onset is broad, peaking between 20 and 40 years.[2]

AETIOLOGY/ RISK FACTORS The cause remains unclear, although current evidence suggests that multiple sclerosis is an autoimmune disorder of the central nervous system resulting from an environmental stimulus in genetically susceptible individuals. Multiple sclerosis is currently regarded as a single disorder with clinical variants, but there is some evidence that it may consist of several related disorders with distinct immunological, pathological, and genetic features.[1,3]

PROGNOSIS In 90% of people, early disease is relapsing and remitting. Although some people follow a relatively benign course over many years, most develop secondary progressive disease, usually 6–10 years after onset. In 10% of people, initial disease is primary progressive. Apart from a minority of people with "aggressive" multiple sclerosis, life expectancy is not greatly affected and the disease course is often of more than 30 years' duration.

AIMS OF INTERVENTION To prevent or delay disability; to improve function; to alleviate symptoms of spasticity; to prevent complications (contractures, pressure sores); to optimise quality of life.

OUTCOMES Neurological disability, spasticity, fatigue, general health, relapse rate, and quality of life. **Neurological disability:** In clinical trials, disability in multiple sclerosis is usually measured using the disease specific Expanded Disability Status Scale, which ranges from 0 (no disability) to 10 (death from multiple sclerosis) in half point increments.[4] Lower scores (0–4) reflect specific neurological impairments and disability; higher scores reflect reducing levels of mobility (4–7) and upper limb and bulbar function (7–9.5). The scale is non-linear and has been criticised for indicating change poorly, for emphasising neurological examination and mobility, and for failing to reflect other disabilities (e.g. fatigue, sexual disability). Some timed outcomes include ambulation (time taken to walk a specified short distance), the nine-hole peg test (time taken to place some pegs into holes in a block), and the box and block test (time taken to transfer blocks between boxes). **Sustained disease progression:** This is reported when an increase in disability from either disease progression or incomplete recovery from relapse is sustained for 3 or 6 months. A relapse that resolves within this time period constitutes non-sustained progression. **Spasticity:** A variety of clinical measures are used, the most common being the Ashworth Scale, which scores muscle tone on a scale of 0–4, with 0 representing normal tone and 4 severe spasticity. For the purposes of this review, the Ashworth Scale was considered to represent an appropriate clinical outcome and was selected over other outcome measures for spasticity (e.g. neurophysiological measures, examination ratings) that represent proxy clinical outcomes. **General health:** Attempts have been made to customise generic health status scales, but these scales have not been widely used.[5]

METHODS *Clinical Evidence* search and appraisal March 2003. We included only trials focusing on clinical outcomes (disability, relapses, and symptoms).

QUESTION **What are the effects of interventions aimed at reducing relapse rates and disability?**

OPTION **INTERFERON BETA**

Two RCTs in people experiencing a first demyelinating event found that interferon beta-1a decreased the risk of conversion to clinically definite multiple sclerosis over 2–3 years compared with placebo. One systematic review in people with active relapsing remitting multiple sclerosis found limited evidence that, compared with placebo, interferon beta-1a/b reduced exacerbations and disease progression over 2 years. One subsequent RCT in people with relapsing remitting multiple sclerosis found that interferon beta-1b reduced the proportion of people with

relapse over 2 years compared with interferon beta-1a. We found conflicting evidence from three RCTs about the effects of interferon beta on disease progression in people with secondary progressive multiple sclerosis.

Benefits: **First demyelinating event:** We found two placebo controlled RCTs examining the effects of interferon beta-1a in people experiencing a first demyelinating event with evidence of subclinical demyelination on magnetic resonance imaging of the brain.[6,7] Both RCTs found that interferon beta-1a significantly reduced the risk of a second clinical event and, therefore, of conversion to a definite diagnosis of multiple sclerosis. The first RCT (383 people) found that interferon beta-1a significantly decreased the risk of conversion to clinically definite multiple sclerosis after 3 years compared with placebo (cumulative probability of conversion to clinically definite multiple sclerosis: 35% with interferon beta-1a *v* 50% with placebo; HR 0.56, 95% CI 0.38 to 0.81).[6] The second RCT (308 people) found that interferon beta-1a significantly decreased the proportion of people with clinically definite multiple sclerosis after 2 years compared with placebo (52/154 [34%] with interferon beta-1a *v* 69/154 [45%] with placebo; OR 0.61, 95% CI 0.37 to 0.99).[7] **Relapsing and remitting multiple sclerosis:** We found one systematic review (search date 2000, 1215 people), which identified seven RCTs comparing interferon beta-1a/b versus placebo in people with active relapsing remitting multiple sclerosis (2 relapses in previous 2 or 3 years).[8] The systematic review found that, over 2 years, interferon significantly reduced the risk of exacerbations and disease progression (3 RCTs, 919 people, RR for exacerbation 0.80, 95% CI 0.73 to 0.88; RR for disease progression, defined as 1 point progression on the Expanded Disability Status Scale sustained over 3 or 6 months 0.69, 95% CI 0.55 to 0.87). The review found results for exacerbation or disease progression were not significant if a sensitivity analysis assumed that all people lost to follow up had exacerbation or experienced disease progression (worst case scenario).[8] One subsequent RCT (188 people with relapsing remitting multiple sclerosis) compared interferon beta-1b (250 μg given on alternate days) versus interferon beta-1a (30 μg given once weekly).[9] Over 2 years, the proportion of people remaining relapse free was significantly higher with interferon beta-1b given on alternate days than with interferon beta-1a given once a week (relapse free: 49/96 [51%] with interferon beta-1b *v* 33/92 [36%] with interferon beta-1a; RR of relapse 0.76, 95% CI 0.59 to 0.99). Analysis was by intention to treat. Investigators were not blinded to treatment allocation. **Secondary progressive multiple sclerosis:** We found three RCTs.[10–12] The first RCT (718 people) compared interferon beta-1b (8 MIU on alternate days) versus placebo in people with secondary progressive multiple sclerosis and an Expanded Disability Status Scale score of 3.0–6.5.[10] After a median of 30 months' follow up, the trial found that interferon delayed sustained progression of disability (measured by the Expanded Disability Status Scale) by 9–12 months, reduced risk of progression, and reduced risk of being wheelchair bound (OR for confirmed progression 0.65, 95% CI 0.52 to 0.83; NNT to prevent 1 additional person becoming wheelchair bound 13, 95% CI 8 to 49). The treatment effect was apparent in people of all levels of baseline disability. There was a large number of withdrawals from each group (27% placebo and 25% interferon), and no data on quality of life were reported. The second RCT (618 people) compared subcutaneous interferon beta-1a (22 or 44 µg, 3 times weekly) versus placebo.[11] It found no significant difference for confirmed progression of disability, although interferon reduced risk of relapse compared with placebo (HR for progression of disability 0.83, 95% CI 0.65 to 1.07; AR for relapse in 1 year 50% with interferon *v* 71% with placebo; $P < 0.001$). The third RCT (436 people) found no significant difference in Expanded Disability Status Scale between interferon beta (60 µg once weekly) and placebo after 2 years.[12] However, Expanded Disability Status Scale was a secondary outcome measure. The RCT also found that interferon beta reduced progression compared with placebo after 2 years (progression measured by Multiple Sclerosis Functional Composite score comprising a 25-foot timed walk, nine-hole peg test, and the paced auditory serial addition test; difference between groups $P = 0.033$). However, this outcome has not been assessed in other RCTs and its clinical importance is uncertain.

Harms: The RCTs did not report any major adverse effects.[10,13–15] Mild to moderate effects included early flu-like symptoms (50% of people) and, rarely, leukopenia and asymptomatic elevation of transaminases. Injection site reactions occurred with subcutaneous administration in 80% of people. The RCT comparing interferon beta-1b versus interferon beta-1a found that most adverse events (flu-like syndrome, fever, fatigue, increased liver enzymes) were most frequent during the first months of treatment and reduced in frequency after the first 6 months.[9] Frequency of adverse events was similar in both groups. However, local skin reactions occurred more frequently in the interferon beta-1b group with one case of skin necrosis that caused treatment withdrawal.[9]

Comment: None.

OPTION GLATIRAMER ACETATE

One RCT in people with relapsing and remitting multiple sclerosis found that, compared with placebo, glatiramer acetate reduced relapse rates over 2 years, but found no effect on disability. We found no good quality RCTs in people with secondary progressive multiple sclerosis.

Benefits: We found no systematic review. **Relapsing and remitting multiple sclerosis:** We found one RCT (251 people, Expanded Disability Status Scale 0–5) comparing glatiramer acetate versus placebo.[16] The RCT found that glatiramer acetate (copolymer 1) 20 mg daily significantly reduced relapse rates over 2 years compared with placebo (mean relapse rate over 24 months: 1.19 with glatiramer acetate *v* 1.68 with placebo; ARR 29%; $P = 0.007$). It found no significant effect on disability. **Secondary progressive multiple sclerosis:** We found no good quality RCTs.

Harms: A self limiting allergic type reaction (flushing, chest tightness, and anxiety) lasting up to 30 minutes was reported by 15% of people on active treatment on at least one occasion (maximum 7 reactions).[16]

Comment: None.

OPTION INTRAVENOUS IMMUNOGLOBULIN

One RCT in people with relapsing and remitting multiple sclerosis found limited evidence from baseline comparisons that intravenous immunoglobulin may reduce disability scores over 2 years compared with placebo. However, the clinical importance of this difference is unclear. We found no good quality RCTs in people with secondary progressive multiple sclerosis.

Benefits: We found no systematic review. **Relapsing and remitting multiple sclerosis:** We found one RCT (150 people with relapsing and remitting multiple sclerosis) comparing intravenous immunoglobulin 0.2 g/kg monthly versus placebo.[17] Treatment was for a maximum of 2 years, but average duration was 21 months. It found that the level of disability significantly decreased from baseline in the experimental group (change in Expanded Disability Status Scale –0.23, 95% CI –0.43 to –0.03) compared with no significant change from baseline in the placebo group (change in Expanded Disability Status Scale +0.12, 95% CI –0.13 to +0.37).[17] The RCT found that the between group difference in the mean change of the Expanded Disability Status Scale was significant (P = 0.008). The RCT did not report the time to development of sustained progression of disability. **Secondary progressive multiple sclerosis:** We found no RCTs meeting our quality criteria.

Harms: No significant adverse effects were reported.[17] However, higher doses of intravenous immunoglobulin have been associated with aseptic meningitis and other systemic reactions.[18]

Comment: The reduction in disability score with intravenous immunoglobulin was modest. The clinical importance of this small effect is unclear.

OPTION AZATHIOPRINE

One systematic review in people with relapsing and remitting or progressive multiple sclerosis comparing azathioprine versus placebo or no treatment found a modest reduction in relapse rates over 2 years, but no evidence of a difference in disability. However, we were unable to draw reliable conclusions because of clinical heterogeneity among included RCTs.

Benefits: We found one systematic review of azathioprine (search date 1989, 7 RCTs, 793 people with relapsing and remitting multiple sclerosis or progressive multiple sclerosis).[19] The systematic review found that azathioprine significantly reduced the relapse rate at 2 years compared with placebo or no treatment (5 RCTs; OR of remaining relapse free 2.04, 95% CI 1.42 to 2.93) and reduced disability scores but the difference did not quite reach significance (4 RCTs; Expanded Disability Status Scale mean score difference –0.22, 95% CI –0.43 to +0.003).

Harms: About 10% of people were unable to tolerate therapeutic doses of azathioprine. Well documented adverse effects include hepatotoxicity and bone marrow suppression.[19] There are concerns about long term cancer risk.[20] In one large RCT, 21% of people on azathioprine withdrew after 1 year compared with 12% on placebo.[20]

Comment: The methods used in the multiple sclerosis trials have improved, making it hard to compare older and more recent RCTs. Trials in the systematic review included people with different categories of multiple sclerosis and used different definitions of relapse.[21] We were therefore unable to draw reliable conclusions about the effects of azathioprine.

OPTION METHOTREXATE

We found insufficient evidence from one small RCT about the effects of methotrexate in people with multiple sclerosis.

Benefits: We found no systematic review. We found one RCT (60 people with primary or secondary progressive multiple sclerosis) comparing low dose methotrexate (7.5 mg weekly) versus placebo.[22] The RCT found that methotrexate significantly reduced the risk of progression compared with placebo (ARR 31%; P = 0.01), defined by a composite outcome measure, including Expanded Disability Status Scale, ambulation, nine-hole peg test, and box and block test. However, the clinical importance of these results is unclear (see comment below).

Harms: No major toxicity was reported in the RCT, but bone marrow suppression and hepatotoxicity can occur with low dose methotrexate; regular monitoring is advised.[22]

Comment: The findings of the RCT mainly reflected changes in upper limb function.[22] RCTs of other drugs have not used composite outcome measures, which makes comparisons difficult. Relative risks for treatment failure were not reported.

OPTION MITOXANTRONE

One RCT in people with worsening, relapsing, remitting, or progressive multiple sclerosis found that mitoxantrone reduced progression of disability compared with placebo. One small RCT in people with active multiple sclerosis found limited evidence that mitoxantrone plus methylprednisolone reduced relapse compared with methylprednisolone alone. However, mitoxantrone is associated with leukopenia, menstrual disorders, and arrhythmia.

Benefits: We found no systematic review. We found two RCTs.[23,24] The first RCT studied 194 people with worsening relapsing, remitting, or secondary progressive multiple sclerosis and an Expanded Disability Status Scale of 3.0–6.0.[23] It compared mitoxantrone (5 mg/m^2 or 12 mg/m^2 intravenously every 3 months) versus placebo for 24 months. It found that the higher dose of mitoxantrone improved disability compared with placebo after 24 months (mean change in the Expanded Disability Status Scale from baseline: –0.13 with 12 mg/m^2 mitoxantrone *v* 0.23 with placebo; difference between groups 0.24, 95% CI 0.04 to 0.44). The RCT reported that lower dose mitoxantrone also improved disability compared with placebo (P = 0.01; no further data provided). A second, smaller unblinded RCT (42 people with active multiple sclerosis) compared monthly intravenous mitoxantrone (20 mg) plus methylprednisolone (1 g) versus methylprednisolone alone.[24] It found that, compared with methylprednisolone alone, mitoxantrone plus methylprednisolone significantly reduced disease activity after 6 months (as assessed by appearance on magnetic resonance imaging) and significantly lowered annual clinical relapse rates (mitoxantrone plus methylprednisolone 0.7 *v* methylprednisolone alone 3.0; $P < 0.01$).[24]

Harms: The major risk is dose related cardiotoxicity, but this is rare at the doses used in multiple sclerosis (see comment below). Leukopenia, nausea, and amenorrhoea are commonly reported.[25] The RCT comparing higher and lower dose mitoxantrone versus placebo found that nausea, alopecia, urinary tract infection, menstrual disorder, leukopenia, and arrhythmia were more common with the higher dose of mitoxantrone than with placebo (nausea: 20% with placebo *v* 76% with higher dose mitoxantrone; alopecia: 31% *v* 61%; urinary tract infection: 13% *v* 32%; menstrual disorder: 26% *v* 61%; leukopenia: 0% *v* 19%; arrhythmia: 8% *v* 18%).[23]

Comment: One retrospective case series of 1378 people with multiple sclerosis treated with mitroxantrone reported two cases of cardiotoxicity[26] and one case of acute leukaemia.[27]

QUESTION What are the effects of treatments for acute relapse?

OPTION CORTICOSTEROIDS

One systematic review in people with multiple sclerosis requiring treatment for acute exacerbations has found that corticosteroids (methylprednisolone or corticotrophin) improves symptoms compared with placebo within 5 weeks of treatment. The optimal dose, route, and duration of treatment are unclear.

Benefits: We found one systematic review (search date 1999, 377 people with multiple sclerosis requiring treatment for acute exacerbations, 4 RCTs of methylprednisolone, 2 RCTs of corticotrophin *v* placebo).[28] The systematic review found that, compared with placebo, methylprednisolone or corticotrophin significantly reduced the proportion of people whose symptoms were worse or unimproved within 5 weeks of treatment (5 RCTs; worse or unimproved within 5 weeks from randomisation: 63/175 [36%] with methylprednisolone or corticotrophin *v* 94/155 [60%] with placebo; OR 0.37, 95% CI 0.24 to 0.57). A small subgroup analysis using an indirect comparison suggested no difference between 5 days and 15 days of treatment with methylprednisolone.[28] One of the included RCTs (51 people) found no difference between oral methylprednisolone and placebo in the prevention of new relapses or in disability after 1 year.

Harms: Gastrointestinal symptoms and psychic disorders were significantly more common in people receiving oral high dose methylprednisolone than in people receiving placebo.[28] Weight gain and oedema were significantly more frequent in people receiving corticotrophin than in people receiving placebo.[28]

Comment: None.

OPTION **PLASMA EXCHANGE**

One small RCT provided insufficient evidence to assess plasma exchange in people with acute relapses of multiple sclerosis.

Benefits: We found no systematic review. We found one small, double blind, crossover RCT comparing plasma exchange versus sham treatment in people with acute relapses of multiple sclerosis (12 people) or other demyelinating disease (10 people; see comment below).[29] It found moderate or greater improvement in neurological disability in people receiving plasma exchange compared with sham treatment (8/19 [42%] with plasma exchange *v* 1/17 [6%] with sham treatment; ARI 36%, 95% CI 1% to 81%; RR 7.2, 95% CI 1.2 to 15; NNT 3, 95% CI 1 to 68).[29]

Harms: The RCT reported no major adverse effects.[29]

Comment: At the time of randomisation, all people had failed to respond to standard doses of intravenous corticosteroids and were within 3 months of onset of the acute deficit.[29]

QUESTION **What are the effects of treatments for fatigue?**

OPTION **AMANTADINE**

We found insufficient evidence from one systematic review of poor quality RCTs about the effects of amantadine in people with multiple sclerosis.

Benefits: We found one systematic review (search date 1999).[30] The review found one parallel and three crossover RCTs (236 people with multiple sclerosis; see comment below). It found limited evidence favouring amantadine compared with placebo. However, there were important methodological weaknesses in the included RCTs (see comment below). The parallel RCT included in the review found that amantadine significantly improved fatigue measured by "preferred treatment 2 weeks after end of trial", and "MS-specific Fatigue Scale" ($P < 0.05$), but found no significant difference measured by "preferred treatment at the end of trial", "Fatigue Severity Scale", or "Rand Index of Vitality".[30] The three crossover RCTs included in the review found different results with different measures of fatigue. One RCT found amantadine significantly improved fatigue measured by "effects on most affected activity VAS", "effects on activities of daily living", "response over previous period", and "preferred treatment" ($P < 0.05$), but not by "effects on fatigue VAS"; one found amantadine significantly improved fatigue measured by "preferred treatment" ($P < 0.05$); and one found amantadine significantly improved fatigue measured by "preferred treatment" ($P < 0.05$), but not by "fatigue; daily ratings; point scale 1–5".[30]

Harms: The review reported that there were no important differences in adverse effects between amantadine and placebo.[30]

Comment: The RCTs used a variety of methods to assess fatigue, and the significance of the results was sensitive to the scales or measures used.[30] The systematic review stated that all the RCTs were open to bias (arising from lack of clarity about the randomisation methods, blinding, incompleteness of follow up, and difficulties with interpretation of crossover RCTs). It found insufficient evidence about the effects of amantadine on the quality of life of people with multiple sclerosis.

OPTION PEMOLINE

One systematic review of poor quality RCTs found no significant difference in fatigue with pemoline compared with placebo.

Benefits: We found one systematic review (search date 1999).[30] It found one parallel and one crossover RCT (126 people with multiple sclerosis). The review found no significant difference with pemoline in the self reporting of fatigue compared with placebo.

Harms: The review found more reports of adverse effects (sleep disturbance, nausea, mood change, palpitations, irritability, insomnia, anorexia) with pemoline than with placebo.[30]

Comment: The RCTs used a variety of methods to assess fatigue, and the significance of the results was sensitive to the scales or measures used.[30] The systematic review stated that all the RCTs were open to bias (arising from lack of clarity about the randomisation methods, blinding, incompleteness of follow up, and difficulties with interpretation of crossover RCTs).[30]

OPTION BEHAVIOURAL MODIFICATION TREATMENT

We found no RCTs on the effects of behavioural modification treatment in people with multiple sclerosis related fatigue.

Benefits: We found no systematic reviews or RCTs.

Harms: We found no RCTs.

Comment: None.

OPTION EXERCISE

We found insufficient evidence from two RCTs about the effects of exercise in people with multiple sclerosis related fatigue.

Benefits: We found no systematic review. We identified two RCTs.[31,32] The first RCT (46 people, Expanded Disability Status Scale 0–6) compared 15 weeks of aerobic training versus no exercise.[31] Using a scale that measures mental and physical fatigue, the RCT found a significant reduction in fatigue at 10 weeks but not after completion of the exercise programme. A different scale that measured only physical fatigue remained unchanged in both groups of people. The RCT found significant improvements in other measures of emotional behaviour and quality of life (Profile of Mood States depression and anger score, Sickness Impact profile scores). The second RCT (26 people with clinically definite multiple sclerosis taking part in an inpatient rehabilitation programme, Expanded Disability Status

Scale 1–6.5) compared adding aerobic exercise training (five supervised training sessions/week for 3–4 weeks) to the usual rehabilitation programme versus the usual rehabilitation programme alone.[32] The RCT did not compare the two groups directly. Its results were expressed as changes from baseline within each group before and after intervention using a recognised fatigue severity scale. The RCT found no significant change in fatigue from baseline in either group.

Harms: None reported.

Comment: People with moderate disability or severe fatigue may have difficulty adhering to an aerobic exercise programme.

QUESTION What are the effects of treatments for spasticity?

OPTION PHYSIOTHERAPY

We found insufficient evidence from two small RCTs about the effects of physiotherapy. One of the RCTs found limited evidence that twice weekly hospital or home based physiotherapy for 8 weeks briefly improved mobility compared with no physiotherapy. The other, in people with progressive multiple sclerosis, found no significant difference between early versus delayed physiotherapy in mobility or activities of daily living.

Benefits: We found no systematic review. One single blind crossover RCT (40 people) comparing hospital based or home based physiotherapy (45 minutes, twice weekly for 8 weeks) versus no physiotherapy found significantly improved mobility assessed 1 week after treatment (hospital physiotherapy *v* no physiotherapy: Rivermead mobility index increased by 1.4 units, 95% CI 0.6 units to 2.1 units, $P < 0.001$; home physiotherapy *v* no physiotherapy: Rivermead mobility index increased by 1.5 units, 95% CI 0.7 units to 2.2 units, $P < 0.001$).[33] The treatment effect was short lived, being largely lost 8 weeks after treatment. One unblinded RCT (45 people with progressive multiple sclerosis) compared early versus delayed physiotherapy (9 weeks of inpatient treatment).[34] It found no significant difference in mobility (timed walk, Rivermead mobility index) or activities of daily living. It found treated people reported reduced mobility related stress ($P < 0.001$).

Harms: None reported.

Comment: None.

OPTION ORAL DRUG TREATMENT

One systematic review found insufficient evidence about the effects of oral drugs on functional outcomes in people with spasticity due to multiple sclerosis. RCTs provided insufficient evidence to assess other oral drug treatments.

Benefits: We found one systematic review (search date 2001, 36 RCTs of duration > 7 days).[35] Of these, only 13 RCTs used an appropriate outcome measure (the Ashworth score). **Oral baclofen versus placebo:** The systematic review identified one crossover RCT that used the Ashworth score.[36] The RCT (30 people) used baclofen (20 mg) with or without an exercise programme and found significant benefit from exercise plus baclofen compared with placebo.[35] It found no significant effect of exercise alone compared with placebo. **Dantrolene versus placebo:** The review found no RCTs that used a validated outcome measure.[35] **Tizanidine versus placebo:** The review identified two RCTs that used the Ashworth score. One RCT (220 people, tizanidine 2–36 mg/day) found no significant difference in Ashworth score but found that tizanidine reduced self reported clonus and spasm.[37] The other RCT (187 people, tizanidine 24–36 mg/day) found that tizanidine significantly reduced muscle tone, although it found no impact on mobility related activities of daily living.[38] **Baclofen versus tizanidine:** Seven RCTs comparing baclofen and tizanidine were identified, three of which used the Ashworth score. No significant differences on this or unvalidated measures of spasticity were found with baclofen and tizanidine. No other comparative RCTs used validated outcome measures.[35]

Harms: Comparative RCTs of baclofen and tizanidine found similar levels of adverse effects (including muscle weakness, sedation, and dry mouth), but tizanidine may be less likely than baclofen to cause muscle weakness.[39]

Comment: The review concluded that the absolute and comparative efficacy of antispasmodic drugs in multiple sclerosis is poorly documented.[35] The major difficulty in planning and designing future RCTs is the lack of a functionally relevant, well validated measure of spasticity.

OPTION INTRATHECAL BACLOFEN

One small crossover RCT provided insufficient evidence to assess functional effects of intrathecal baclofen.

Benefits: We found no systematic review. We found one small crossover RCT comparing intrathecal baclofen versus intrathecal saline (19 non-ambulant people with multiple sclerosis or spinal cord injury and with spasticity resistant to oral baclofen).[40] Baclofen significantly reduced spasticity and spasm frequency. Average Ashworth scores fell from 4.0 at baseline to 1.2 after 3 days of treatment ($P < 0.0001$), with scores for all people improving from baseline.[40]

Harms: Potential problems include pump failure, infection, and, rarely, baclofen overdose.

Comment: We found no evidence about intrathecal baclofen in ambulant people.

OPTION BOTULINUM TOXIN

We found insufficient evidence from one small RCT about the effects of botulinum toxin on functional outcomes in people with spasticity due to multiple sclerosis.

Benefits: We found no systematic review but found one RCT.[41] The RCT (74 people) compared three different doses of intramuscular botulinum toxin (500, 1000, or 1500 units) versus placebo for the treatment of hip adductor spasticity in multiple sclerosis.[41] The RCT did not examine functional outcomes. It found that the 1500 unit dose (17 people) compared with placebo (16 people) significantly improved maximum distance between the knees at 4 weeks ($P = 0.02$).[41] The 1000 unit (20 people) and 1500 unit (17 people) doses improved median hygiene scores from baseline at 4 weeks.

Harms: Botulinum toxin can cause local weakness. Adverse events were reported in 55% of all people with botulinum toxin compared with 63% of all people with placebo.[41] The most frequent were hypertonia (22% of all people with botulinum toxin *v* 25% of all people with placebo), weakness of non-injected muscles (14% *v* 6%), fatigue (7% *v* 13%), urinary tract infection (5% *v* 19%), headache (5% *v* 13%), micturition frequency (5% *v* 13%), back pain (5% *v* 0%), and diarrhoea (5% *v* 0%).[41] Twice as many adverse events were reported by the 1500 unit group (mean 2.7/person) compared with the 500 unit group (mean 1.1/person) and the 1000 unit group (mean 1.2/person).[41] Six people had serious adverse events (2 with botulinum toxin, 4 with placebo). The events (hospital admissions with diarrhoea, multiple infections, bowel spasticity, gastroparesis, pulmonary embolism, and blocked catheter) were considered to be unrelated to the study medication.[41]

Comment: None.

QUESTION What are the effects of multidisciplinary management?

OPTION INPATIENT REHABILITATION

Two small RCTs provided insufficient evidence to assess the effectiveness of inpatient rehabilitation. Both RCTs found short term benefit, but no reduction in neurological impairment. Longer term effects are uncertain.

Benefits: We found no systematic review but found two RCTs.[42,43] The first RCT compared brief inpatient rehabilitation (average 25 days) versus remaining on the waiting list (non-treatment control group) in 66 people with progressive multiple sclerosis who were selected as "good candidates" for rehabilitation.[42] Rehabilitation significantly improved disability at 6 weeks assessed by the functional independence measure ($P < 0.001$) and the London Handicap Scale ($P < 0.01$), despite unchanged levels of neurological impairment (Expanded Disability Status Scale). Benefit persisted for up to 9 months. The second RCT compared 3 weeks of inpatient rehabilitation versus exercises at home in 50 ambulant people with multiple sclerosis (Expanded Disability Status Scale 3–7).[43] The RCT found improvements in disability, assessed by the functional independence measure ($P < 0.004$), which persisted at 9 but not at 15 weeks' follow up.

Harms: None reported.

Comment: None.

OPTION OUTPATIENT REHABILITATION

One small RCT provided insufficient evidence to assess the effectiveness of outpatient rehabilitation.

Benefits: We found no systematic review. We found one RCT comparing outpatient rehabilitation (5 hours/week for 1 year) versus remaining on the waiting list (non-treatment control group) in 46 people with progressive multiple sclerosis. Rehabilitation reduced the frequency of fatigue (effect size –0.27) and multiple sclerosis symptoms (effect size –0.32), despite no significant change in neurological impairment in either group.[44]

Harms: None reported.

Comment: Future trials need to record effects on disability and quality of life as well as impairment.

Substantive changes

Interferon beta One RCT added;[12] conclusions unchanged.
Mitoxantrone One RCT added;[23] intervention re-categorised from Unknown effectiveness to Trade off between benefits and harms.
Glatiramer acetate Evidence re-appraised; interventions re-categorised from Unknown effectiveness to Likely to be beneficial.

REFERENCES

1. Compston A. Genetic epidemiology of multiple sclerosis. *J Neurol Neurosurg Psychiatry* 1997;62:553–561.
2. Weinshenker BG, Bass B, Rice GPA, et al. The natural history of multiple sclerosis: a geographically based study. 1. Clinical course and disability. *Brain* 1989;112:133–146.
3. Lucchinetti CF, Bruck W, Rodriguez M, et al. Distinct patterns of multiple sclerosis pathology indicates heterogeneity in pathogenesis. *Brain Pathol* 1996;6:259–274.
4. Kurtzke JF. Rating neurological impairment in multiple sclerosis: an Expanded Disability Status Scale (EDSS). *Neurology* 1983;33:1444–1452.
5. Vickrey BG, Hays RD, Genovese BJ, et al. Comparison of a generic to disease-targeted health-related quality-of-life measures for multiple sclerosis. *J Clin Epidemiol* 1997;50:557–569.
6. Jacobs LD, Beck RW, Simon JH, et al. Intramuscular interferon beta-1a therapy initiated during a first demyelinating event in multiple sclerosis. *N Engl J Med* 2000;343:898–904.
7. Comi G, Fillipi M, Barkhof F, et al. Effect of early interferon treatment on conversion to definite multiple sclerosis: a randomised study. *Lancet* 2001;357:1576–1582.
8. Rice GA, Incorvaia B, Munari L, et al. Interferon in relapsing-remitting multiple sclerosis. In: The Cochrane Library, Issue 2, 2002. Search date 2000; primary sources Medline, Embase, hand searches of reference lists, and personal contact with researchers and pharmaceutical companies.
9. Durelli L, Verdun E, Barbero P, et al. Every-other-day interferon beta-1b versus once weekly interferon beta-1a for multiple sclerosis: results of a 2 year prospective randomised multicentre study (INCOMIN). *Lancet* 2002;359:1453–1460.
10. Kappos L, Polman C, Pozzilli C, et al. Placebo-controlled multicentre randomised trial of interferon beta-1b in treatment of secondary progressive multiple sclerosis. *Lancet* 1998;352:1491–1497.
11. King J, McLeod J, Gonsette RE, et al. Randomised controlled trial of interferon beta-1a in secondary progressive MS: clinical results. *Neurology* 2001;56:1496–1504.
12. Cohen JA, Cutter GR, Fischer JS, et al. Benefit of interferon beta-1a on MSFC progression in secondary progressive MS. *Neurology* 2002;59:679–687.
13. Ebers GC, Rice G, Lesaux J, et al. Randomised double-blind placebo-controlled study of interferon beta-1a in relapsing/remitting multiple sclerosis. *Lancet* 1998;352:1498–1504.
14. Duquette P, Girard M, Despault L, et al. Interferon beta-1b is effective in relapsing–remitting multiple sclerosis. Clinical results of a multicenter, randomised, double-blind, placebo-controlled trial. *Neurology* 1993;43:655–661.
15. Jacobs LD, Cookfair DL, Rudick RA, et al. Intramuscular interferon beta-1a for disease progression in relapsing multiple sclerosis. *Ann Neurol* 1996;39:285–294.
16. Johnson KP, Brooks BR, Cohen JA, et al. Copolymer-1 reduces relapse rate and improves disability in relapsing-remitting multiple sclerosis: results of a Phase III multicenter, double-blind, placebo-controlled trial. *Neurology* 1995;45:1268–1276.
17. Fazekas F, Deisenhammer F, Strasser-Fuchs S, et al. Randomised placebo-controlled trial of monthly intravenous immunoglobulin therapy in relapsing–remitting multiple sclerosis. *Lancet* 1997;349:589–593.
18. Stangel M, Hartung HP, Marx P, et al. Side-effects of high-dose intravenous immunoglobulins. *Clin Neuropharmacol* 1997;20:385–393.
19. Yudkin PL, Ellison GW, Ghezzi A, et al. Overview of azathioprine treatment in multiple sclerosis. *Lancet* 1991;338:1051–1055. Search date 1989; primary sources Medline and hand searches of references.

20. Confavreux C, Saddier P, Grimaud J, et al. Risk of cancer from azathioprine therapy in multiple sclerosis: a case-control study. *Neurology* 1996;46:1607–1612.
21. Hughes RAC. Double-masked trial of azathioprine in multiple-sclerosis. *Lancet* 1988;2:179–183.
22. Goodkin DE, Rudick RA, VanderBrug Medendorp S, et al. Low-dose (7.5 mg) oral methotrexate reduces the rate of progression in chronic progressive multiple sclerosis. *Ann Neurol* 1995;37:30–40.
23. Hartung H, Gonsette R, Konig N, et al. Mitoxantrone in progressive multiple sclerosis: a placebo-controlled, double blind, randomised, multicentre trial. *Lancet* 2002;360:2018–2025.
24. Edan G, Miller D, Clanet M, et al. Therapeutic effect of mitoxantrone combined with methylprednisolone in multiple sclerosis: a randomised multicentre study of active disease using MRI and clinical criteria. *J Neurol Neurosurg Psychiatry* 1997;62:112–118.
25. MacDonald M, Posner LE, Dukart G, et al. A review of the acute and chronic toxicity of mitoxantrone. *Future Trends Chemother* 1985;6:443–450.
26. Ghalie RG, Edan G, Laurent M, et al. Cardiac adverse events associated with mitoxantrone (novantrone) therapy in patients with MS. *Neurology* 2002;59:909–913.
27. Ghalie RG, Mauch E, Edan G, et al. A study of therapy-related acute leukaemia after Mitoxantrone therapy for multiple sclerosis. *Mult Scler* 2002;8:441–445.
28. Filippini G, Brusaferri F, Sibley WA, et al. Corticosteroids or ACTH for acute exacerbations in multiple sclerosis. In: The Cochrane Library, Issue 2, 2002. Oxford: Update Software. Search date 1999; primary sources Medline, Cochrane Controlled Trials Register, hand searches of reference lists, main neurology journals, conference abstracts, dissertations, and personal contact with researchers and manufacturers.
29. Weinshenker BG, O'Brien PC, Petterson TM, et al. A randomised trial of plasma exchange in acute central nervous system inflammatory demyelinating disease. *Neurology* 1999;46:878–886.
30. Branas P, Jordan R, Fry-Smith A, et al. Treatments for fatigue in multiple sclerosis: a rapid and systematic review. The National Coordinating Centre for Health Technology Assessment (NCCHTA). 13665278. *Health Technol Assess* 2000;4:27:1–73. Search date 1999; primary sources Medline, Embase, hand searches of reference lists, and personal contact with experts.
31. Petajan JH, Gappmaier E, White AT, et al. Impact of aerobic training on fitness and quality of life in multiple sclerosis. *Ann Neurol* 1996;39:432–441.
32. Mostert S, Kesselring J. Effects of a short-term exercise training program on aerobic fitness, fatigue, health perception and activity level of subjects with multiple sclerosis. *Mult Scler* 2002;8:161–168.
33. Wiles CM, Newcombe RG, Fuller KJ, et al. Controlled randomised crossover trial of the effects of physiotherapy on mobility in chronic multiple sclerosis. *J Neurol Neurosurg Psychiatry* 2001;70:174–179.
34. Fuller KJ, Dawson K, Wiles CM. Physiotherapy in chronic multiple sclerosis: a controlled trial. *Clin Rehabil* 1996;10:195–204.
35. Shakespeare DT, Young CA, Boggild M. Anti-spasticity agents for multiple sclerosis (Cochrane Review). In: The Cochrane Library, Issue 2, 2002. Search date 2001; primary sources Medline, Cochrane Controlled Trials Register, Cochrane MS Review Group Specialised Trial Registry, National Health Service National Research Register, Medical Research Council Clinical Trials Directory, hand searches of reference lists, main neurology journals, conference abstracts, dissertations, and personal contact with researchers and manufacturers.
36. Brar S, Smith MB, Nelson LM, et al. Evaluation of treatment protocols on minimal to moderate spasticity in multiple sclerosis. *Arch Phys Med Rehabil* 1991;72:186–189.
37. Smith C, Birnbaum G, Carter JL, et al. Tizanidine treatment of spasticity caused by multiple sclerosis: results of a double-blind, placebo-controlled trial. *Neurology* 1994;44:34–42.
38. Barnes MP, Bates D, Corston RN, et al. A double-blind, placebo-controlled trial of tizanidine in the treatment of spasticity caused by multiple sclerosis. *Neurology* 1994;44:S70–S78.
39. Groves L, Shellenberger MK, Davis CS. Tizanidine treatment of spasticity: a meta-analysis of controlled, double-blind, comparative studies with baclofen and diazepam. *Adv Ther* 1998;15:241–251. Search date not stated; primary source records of Sandoz (now Novartis).
40. Penn RD, Savoy SM, Corcos D, et al. Intrathecal baclofen for severe spinal spasticity. *N Engl J Med* 1989;320:1517–1521.
41. Hyman N, Barnes M, Bhakta B, et al. Botulinum toxin (Dysport) treatment of hip adductor spasticity in multiple sclerosis: a prospective, randomised, double-blind, placebo controlled, dose ranging study. *J Neurol Neurosurg Psychiatry* 2000;68:707–712.
42. Freeman JA, Langdon DW, Hobart JC, et al. The impact of inpatient rehabilitation on progressive multiple sclerosis. *Ann Neurol* 1997;42:236–244.
43. Solari A, Fillipini G, Gasco P, et al. Physical rehabilitation has a positive effect on disability in multiple sclerosis patients. *Neurology* 1999;52:57–62.
44. Di Fabio RP, Soderberg J, Choi T, et al. Extended outpatient rehabilitation: its influence on symptom frequency, fatigue and functional status for persons with progressive multiple sclerosis. *Arch Phys Med Rehabil* 1998;79:141–146.

Mike Boggild
Consultant Neurologist
The Walton Centre for Neurology and Neurosurgery, Liverpool, UK

Helen Ford
Consultant Neurologist
St James's Hospital, Leeds, UK

Competing interests: MB has received financial support for attending scientific meetings from Biogen, Serono Pharmaceuticals, and Teva Pharmaceuticals, and has organised educational sessions for Serono. HF has received financial support for attending scientific meetings by Serono and Biogen, and for speaking at meetings by Scherise and Biogen.

Parkinson's disease

Search date December 2002

Carl Clarke and A Peter Moore

QUESTIONS

INTERVENTIONS

See glossary, p 1595

Key Messages

- **Selegiline in people with early disease** RCTs have found that selegiline improves the symptoms of Parkinson's disease and delays the need for levodopa compared with placebo. One of these RCTs found weak evidence of increased mortality in people treated with selegiline.
- **Dopamine agonists plus levodopa in people with a fluctuating response to levodopa*** Systematic reviews in people with later stage disease taking levodopa have found that adjuvant dopamine agonists reduce "off" time, improve motor impairments and activities of daily living, and reduce levodopa dose, but increase dopaminergic adverse effects and dyskinesias.

- **Dopamine agonists plus levodopa* versus levodopa alone in people with early disease** One systematic review and subsequent RCTs have found that dopamine agonist treatment plus levodopa reduces dyskinesia compared with levodopa alone. However, some of the RCTs found that dopamine agonist plus levodopa led to greater motor impairments and disability compared with levodopa alone.
- **Dopamine agonists versus levodopa* in people with early disease** One systematic review and one subsequent RCT have found that dopamine agonist monotherapy reduces the incidence of dyskinesias and fluctuations in motor response compared with levodopa monotherapy.
- **Levodopa* in people with early disease** We found no placebo controlled RCTs, although experience suggests that levodopa improves motor function, but that dyskinesias and fluctuations in motor response are related to long term levodopa treatment and are irreversible.
- **Pallidal surgery in people with later disease** One systematic review found limited evidence that unilateral pallidotomy improved motor examination and activities of daily living compared with medical treatment. One RCT found insufficient evidence to assess the effects of pallidotomy versus deep brain stimulation. We found no systematic review or RCTs comparing pallidal deep brain stimulation versus medical treatment. One small RCT found insufficient evidence to assess the effects of pallidal deep brain stimulation versus subthalamic deep brain stimulation. There is a high incidence of adverse effects with pallidotomy.
- **Subthalamic surgery in people with later disease** One systematic review found no RCTs comparing subthalamic surgery versus medical treatment. One small RCT comparing subthalamic deep brain stimulation versus pallidal deep brain stimulation found no significant difference in motor scores.
- **Thalamic surgery in people with later disease** One systematic review identified no RCTs comparing thalamic surgery versus medical treatment. One RCT found that thalamic deep brain stimulation versus thalamotomy improved functional status and caused fewer adverse effects. Case series found that thalamotomy was associated with permanent complications, including speech disturbance, apraxia, and death in 14–23% of people.
- **Modified release levodopa (*v* immediate release levodopa*) in people with early disease *RCTs found no significant difference with modified versus immediate release levodopa in motor complications or disease control after 5 years.***
- **Occupational therapy in people with later disease; physiotherapy in people with later disease; speech and language therapy for speech disturbance in people with later disease; swallowing therapy for dysphagia in people with later disease** Systematic reviews of poor quality RCTs found insufficient evidence about the effects of these interventions.

*We have used the term "levodopa" to refer to a combination of levodopa and a peripheral decarboxylase inhibitor.

DEFINITION Idiopathic Parkinson's disease is an age related neurodegenerative disorder, associated with a combination of asymmetric bradykinesia, hypokinesia, and rigidity, sometimes combined with rest tremor and postural changes. Clinical diagnostic criteria have a sensitivity of 80% and specificity of 30% compared with the gold standard of diagnosis at autopsy.[1] The primary pathology is progressive loss of cells producing the neurotransmitter dopamine from the substantia nigra in the brainstem. Treatment aims to replace or compensate for the lost dopamine. A good response to treatment supports, but does not confirm, the diagnosis. Several other catecholaminergic neurotransmitter systems are also affected in Parkinson's disease. There is no consistent definition of early and late stage Parkinson's disease. In this review, we consider people with early stage disease to be those who have not yet developed motor complications associated with long term levodopa treatment (such as dyskinesias [see glossary, p 1595] and "on/off" fluctuations). Late stage Parkinson's disease is taken to mean that motor complications of long term levodopa treatment are present.

INCIDENCE/ PREVALENCE Parkinson's disease occurs worldwide with equal incidence in both sexes. In 5–10% of people who develop Parkinson's disease it appears before the age of 40 years (young onset), with a mean age of onset of about 65 years. Overall age adjusted prevalence is 1% worldwide and 1.6% in Europe, rising from 0.6% at age 60–64 years to 3.5% at age 85–89 years.[2,3]

AETIOLOGY/ RISK FACTORS The cause is unknown. Parkinson's disease may represent different conditions with a final common pathway. People may be affected differently by a combination of genetic and environmental factors (viruses, toxins, 1-methyl-4-phenyl-1,2,3,6-tetrahydropyridine, well water, vitamin E, and smoking).[4–7] First degree relatives of affected people may have twice the risk of developing Parkinson's disease (17% chance of developing the condition in their lifetime) compared with people in the general population.[8–10] However, purely genetic varieties probably affect a small minority of people with Parkinson's disease.[11,12] The parkin gene on chromosome 6 may be associated with Parkinson's disease in families with at least one member with young onset Parkinson's disease, and multiple genetic factors, including the tau gene on chromosome 17q21, may be involved in idiopathic late onset disease.[13,14]

PROGNOSIS Parkinson's disease is currently incurable. Disability is progressive and associated with increased mortality (RR of death compared with matched control populations ranges from 1.6 to 3.0).[15] Treatment can reduce symptoms and slow progression but rarely achieves complete control. The question of whether treatment reduces mortality remains controversial.[16] Levodopa seemed to reduce mortality in the UK for 5 years after its introduction, before a "catch up" effect was noted and overall mortality rose toward previous levels. This suggested a limited prolongation of life.[17] An Australian cohort study followed 130 people treated for 10 years.[18] The standardised mortality ratio was 1.58 ($P < 0.001$). At 10 years, 25% had been admitted to a nursing home and only four were still employed. The mean duration of disease until death was 9.1 years. In a similar Italian cohort study conducted over 8 years, the relative risk of death for affected people versus healthy controls was 2.3 (95% CI 1.60 to 3.39).[19] Age at initial census date was the main predictor of outcome (for people aged < 75 years: RR of death 1.80, 95% CI 1.04 to 3.11; for people aged > 75 years: RR of death 5.61, 95% CI 2.13 to 14.80).

AIMS OF INTERVENTION To improve symptoms and quality of life; to slow disease progression; to limit short and long term adverse effects of treatment, such as motor fluctuations (see glossary, p 1595).

OUTCOMES Disease severity; severity of drug induced symptoms or signs; rate of progression of symptoms; need for levodopa or other treatment; adverse effects of treatment; withdrawals from treatment; and quality of life measures. There are no universal scales, but commonly used scales are the Unified Parkinson's Disease Rating Score (UPDRS) (see glossary, p 1595), the Hoehn and Yahr disability staging scale, Webster scale, the Core Assessment Programme for Intracerebral Transplantation,[20,21] the Parkinson's Disease Quality of Life questionnaire,[22] and the Parkinson's Disease Quality of Life questionnaire 39.[23]

METHODS *Clinical Evidence* search and appraisal December 2002. Unless stated otherwise, we have used the term "levodopa" to refer to a combination of levodopa and a peripheral dopa decarboxylase inhibitor.

QUESTION **What are the effects of drug treatments in people with early Parkinson's disease?**

OPTION **SELEGILINE**

RCTs have found that selegiline improves the symptoms of Parkinson's disease and delays the need for levodopa compared with placebo. One of these RCTs found weak evidence of increased mortality in people treated with selegiline.

Benefits: We found no systematic review. **Versus placebo:** We found nine RCTs comparing selegiline versus placebo in people with early Parkinson's disease.[24–32] The first RCT (54 people) found that selegiline delayed the need for levodopa compared with placebo (549 days to levodopa with selegiline *v* 312 days to levodopa with placebo; P < 0.002).[24] The second RCT (800 people) found that selegiline delayed the need for levodopa compared with placebo for 9 months (HR 0.50 for requiring levodopa in each time period, 95% CI 0.41 to 0.62).[28] The third RCT (101 people newly diagnosed with Parkinson's disease) found that selegiline significantly improved total Unified Parkinson's Disease Rating Scale (UPDRS) (see glossary, p 1595) score after 12 months of treatment and 2 months of washout compared with placebo (P < 0.001; CI not stated).[29] The fourth RCT (782 people) found no significant difference between selegiline and placebo in disability scores after 4 years (P = 0.95; CI not stated).[30] The fifth RCT (116 people) found that selegiline significantly reduced the number of people who required an increase in levodopa of 50% or more compared with placebo (50% with selegiline *v* 74% with placebo; P = 0.03; CI not stated).[31] The sixth RCT (163 people) found that selegiline significantly improved motor function after 5 years compared with placebo (UPDRS motor score 16.6 with selegiline *v* 23.8 with placebo; P < 0.01).[32] The seventh RCT (157 people) found that selegiline significantly delayed the need for levodopa compared with placebo (12.7 months with selegiline *v* 8.6 months with placebo; P = 0.028).[25] The eighth RCT (93 people) found that selegiline significantly improved overall function and motor function scores compared with placebo, but found no significant difference in activities of daily living scores at 3 months (measured by UPDRS; results presented graphically; total UPDRS, P = 0.008; motor score, P = 0.03; activity of daily living score P = 0.08).[26] The final RCT (44 people) found that selegiline delayed the need to start levodopa compared with placebo (median time to levodopa 545 days with selegiline *v* 372 days with placebo; P = 0.03).[27] **Versus other drugs:** We found one RCT (475 people) that compared selegiline versus levodopa, bromocriptine, and lisuride.[33] It did not report separate statistical differences for selegiline versus each of the other drugs. It found that decline in functional ability was smaller with selegiline than with all other drugs after a mean of 2 months (mean decline in UPDRS daily living score 1.4 with selegiline *v* 2.5 with levodopa *v* 1.9 with bromocriptine *v* 2.6 with lisuride; comparison between selegiline and all other treatments P = 0.03). However, the trial found no significant difference in decline in motor function between selegiline and other treatments (decline in UPDRS motor score 2.4 with selegiline *v* 3.4 with levodopa *v* 2.3 with bromocriptine *v* 3.2 with lisuride; P not stated).[33]

Harms: One non-systematic review (5 RCTs, 589 people) found no significant difference between selegiline and placebo in mortality at 2.5–4.0 years (15% with selegiline *v* 6% with placebo; HR 1.02, 95% CI 0.44 to 2.37).[34] One large RCT found no significant difference between selegiline and placebo in mortality at 35 months (no further data provided).[35] Another RCT found that selegiline versus placebo significantly increased mortality at interim analysis after 5.6 years' follow up (HR 1.57, 95% CI 1.07 to 2.31); the selegiline arm of the trial was terminated early.[30] Updated analysis (including blinded assessment of cause specific mortality) found that the increase in mortality did not quite reach significance (HR 1.30, 95% CI 0.99 to 1.72).[36,37] One retrospective observational study in 12 621 people who had taken an antiparkinsonian drug (excluding those also taking antipsychotic drugs) found increased mortality in people prescribed selegiline, but the increase was of borderline significance (ARI 11%, 95% CI 0% to 23%).[38]

Comment: One RCT (163 people) found that there was no deterioration in symptoms on withdrawal of selegiline after 5 years.[32] This could indicate that it was ineffective. Other studies of early selegiline treatment were either too small or too short to reach a conclusion.[34] A systematic review and a large RCT are under way (Clarke C, personal communication, 2003). The RCT comparing selegiline versus other drugs did not report statistical differences between effects of selegiline and each of the other drugs. The clinical importance of the results is, therefore, unclear.

OPTION MODIFIED RELEASE LEVODOPA

Two RCTs in people with early Parkinson's disease found no significant difference between modified and immediate release levodopa (see methods, p 1585) in motor complications or disease control after 5 years.

Benefits: We found no systematic review but found two RCTs.[39,40] The first RCT (134 people with early Parkinson's disease) compared modified versus immediate release co-beneldopa.[39] It found no significant difference in the incidence of dyskinesia (see glossary, p 1595) at 5 years (41% with modified release *v* 34% with immediate release; RR 1.21, 95% CI 0.59 to 1.92), motor fluctuations (see glossary, p 1595) (59% with modified release *v* 57% with immediate release; RR 1.03, 95% CI 0.60 to 1.39), motor impairment, or activities of daily living. The second RCT (618 people with early Parkinson's disease) compared modified versus immediate release co-careldopa.[40] It found no significant difference in dyskinesia or motor fluctuations measured by diary data at 5 years (22% of people taking modified release *v* 21% of people taking immediate release) but found that modified versus immediate release co-careldopa significantly improved activities of daily living (scores at 5 years; P = 0.03; CI not stated).

Harms: The RCT of co-careldopa found that immediate versus modified release significantly increased withdrawals because of nausea (P = 0.007; CI not stated).[40]

Comment: The RCT comparing modified versus immediate release co-beneldopa with a 5 year follow up had a withdrawal rate of about 50%.[39]

OPTION DOPAMINE AGONISTS VERSUS LEVODOPA IN EARLY DISEASE

Experience suggests that levodopa improves motor function, but that dyskinesias and fluctuations in motor response are related to long term levodopa treatment and are irreversible. One systematic review and one subsequent RCT have found that dopamine agonist monotherapy reduces the incidence of dyskinesias and fluctuations in motor response compared with levodopa monotherapy.

Benefits: We found one systematic review (search date 1999, 6 RCTs)[41] and one subsequent RCT.[42] The review compared bromocriptine versus levodopa (see methods, p 1585).[41] It found that bromocriptine delayed motor complications and dyskinesias (see glossary, p 1595), but did not report effects on disability or motor impairment. The subsequent RCT (294 people), which was published as an abstract, found that pergolide significantly reduced the proportion of people experiencing one or more motor complications compared with levodopa at 3 years (16% with pergolide *v* 33% with levodopa; P < 0.004; CI not stated).[42] Motor UPRDS scores were worse in the pergolide group.

Harms: The RCT comparing pergolide versus levodopa found that significantly more people in the pergolide group withdrew from treatment (18% with pergolide *v* 10% with levodopa; P < 0.05; CI not stated).[42]

Comment: Experience suggests that levodopa improves motor function, but that dyskinesias and fluctuations in motor response are related to long term levodopa treatment and are irreversible. A large UK based

RCT is examining quality of life and health economic outcomes of agonist monotherapy in people likely to develop motor complications (Clarke C, personal communication, 2003). A multicentre North American study is investigating the effect of levodopa on dopaminergic cell death.[43]

OPTION DOPAMINE AGONISTS PLUS RESCUE LEVODOPA VERSUS LEVODOPA ALONE IN EARLY DISEASE

Experience suggests that levodopa improves motor function, but that dyskinesias and fluctuations in motor response are related to long term levodopa treatment and are irreversible. One systematic review and subsequent RCTs have found that dopamine agonist treatment plus levodopa reduces dyskinesia compared with levodopa alone. However, some of the RCTs found that levodopa alone improved motor impairments and disability compared with dopamine agonist plus levodopa. One subsequent RCT found no significant difference between lisuride (lysuride) plus levodopa and levodopa alone in motor complications at 5 years.

Benefits: We found one systematic review (search date 2001, 8 RCTs)[44] and five subsequent RCTs.[45–49] The review compared bromocriptine plus levodopa versus levodopa alone and found a trend toward reduced dyskinesia (see glossary, p 1595) with combination treatment but no difference in duration of "off" time (see glossary, p 1595) (no further data provided).[44] The review did not report effects on disability or motor impairment. The first subsequent RCT (268 people) found that ropinirole plus rescue levodopa if needed significantly reduced dyskinesias compared with levodopa alone after 5 years (20% with ropinirole *v* 45% with levodopa; RR 0.44, 95% CI 0.31 to 0.64).[45] It found no significant difference in disability after 5 years (Unified Parkinson's Disease Rating Scale [see glossary, p 1595], activities of daily living scale) and a small increase in motor impairments with ropinirole. The second subsequent RCT (301 people) found that pramipexole plus rescue levodopa significantly reduced all motor complications compared with levodopa alone at 2 years (28% with pramipexole plus rescue levodopa *v* 51% with levodopa alone; HR 0.45, 95% CI 0.30 to 0.66).[46] Improvements in UPDRS motor and activities of daily living scores were greater in the levodopa group. The third subsequent RCT (419 people), which was published as an abstract, compared cabergoline plus rescue levodopa versus levodopa alone.[47] It found that cabergoline significantly reduced motor complications compared with levodopa at 5 years (22% with cabergoline *v* 34% with levodopa; $P < 0.05$; CI not stated). Activities of daily living scores were worse with cabergoline. The fourth subsequent RCT (90 people, unblinded), comparing lisuride plus rescue levodopa versus levodopa alone, found fewer motor complications in the lisuride group after 4 years, although total Parkinsonian disability was worse with lisuride alone compared with levodopa alone (dyskinesia: 64% with levodopa *v* 0% with lisuride; $P < 0.05$; 19% with levodopa + lisuride; $P < 0.001$ compared with levodopa alone; 20% with lisuride + levodopa; $P < 0.01$ compared with levodopa alone; improvement in Columbia University Rating Scale score 33 with lisuride v 25 with levodopa; P not stated).[48] The fifth subsequent RCT (82 people, partially blinded) found no significant difference between lisuride plus levodopa and levodopa alone in motor complications after 5 years (UPDRS 4 subscore change 0.49 to 0.96 with levodopa alone v 0.32 to 0.73 with levodopa plus lisuride; P reported as non-significant).[49]

Harms: The RCT comparing ropinirole versus levodopa found that adverse events, including nausea, vomiting, dizziness, confusion, hallucinations, and delusions, were similar in both treatment groups.[45] The RCT comparing pramipexole plus rescue levodopa versus levodopa alone found that pramipexole significantly increased somnolence ($P = 0.003$) and hallucinations ($P = 0.03$; CIs not stated).[46]

Comment: Experience suggests that levodopa improves motor function, but that dyskinesias and fluctuations in motor response are related to long term levodopa treatment and are irreversible. The subsequent RCTs with 5 years of follow up had withdrawal rates of about 50%.[45,47,49] In the RCT comparing lisuride plus levodopa versus levodopa alone, the doses used were low.[48] We found no direct comparisons of individual dopamine agonists (see comment under dopamine agonists versus levodopa in early disease, p 1587).

QUESTION **What are the effects of adding a dopamine agonist in people with a fluctuating response to levodopa?**

Systematic reviews have found that, in people taking levodopa, certain dopamine agonists significantly reduce "off" time, improve motor impairment and activities of daily living, and reduce requirement for levodopa, but increase dopaminergic adverse effects and dyskinesia.

Benefits: **Versus placebo:** We found six systematic reviews.[50–55] The first review (search date 1998, 7 RCTs, 396 people with later Parkinson's disease taking levodopa) compared adjuvant bromocriptine versus placebo.[50] Heterogeneity in trial design and outcomes made it impossible to draw reliable conclusions. The second review (search date 1998) comparing lisuride versus placebo identified no RCTs.[51] The third review (search date 1999, 1 RCT, 376 people with Parkinson's disease taking levodopa) found that pergolide significantly reduced daily "off" time (see glossary, p 1595) compared with placebo (mean difference 1.6 hours; $P < 0.001$), significantly reduced daily levodopa dose (mean reduction in dose: 235 mg/day with pergolide v 51 mg/day with placebo; $P < 0.001$), and improved activities of daily living scores (CIs not stated).[52] The fourth review (search date not stated, 4 RCTs, 669 people with Parkinson's disease taking levodopa) found that pramipexole versus placebo significantly reduced daily "off" time (WMD 1.8 hours, 95% CI 1.2 hours to 2.3 hours), reduced levodopa dose (WMD 115 mg, 95% CI 87 mg to 143 mg), and improved activities of daily living scores.[55] The fifth review (search date not stated, 1 RCT using sufficient dosage of ropinirole [8 mg three times daily], 149 people with Parkinson's disease taking levodopa) compared ropinirole versus placebo.[53] It found no significant difference with ropinirole versus placebo in "off" time (WMD 180 mg, 95% CI 106 mg to 253 mg) but found that ropinirole reduced the required dose of levodopa. Complete information on motor impairments and disability was not available. The sixth review (search date not stated, 3 RCTs, 268 people with Parkinson's disease taking levodopa) found no significant difference with cabergoline versus placebo in "off" time (WMD +1.1 hours, 95% CI –0.06 hours to +2.33 hours) but found that cabergoline significantly reduced the required dose of levodopa (WMD 150 mg, 95% CI 94 mg to 205 mg).[54] Small but significant benefits in Unified Parkinson's Disease Rating Score (UPDRS) (see glossary, p 1595), activities of daily living, and motor scores were seen with cabergoline in one study only. **Versus each other:** We found five systematic reviews.[56–60] The first systematic review (search date not stated, 1 RCT, 20 people) compared lisuride versus bromocriptine.[56] It found no significant difference in change in motor fluctuations (see glossary, p 1595) and the Columbia disability rating scale after 12 weeks (no quantitative data provided). Follow up may have been too short and the study too small to detect significant differences. The second systematic review (search date 1998, 3 RCTs, 293 people) compared pergolide versus bromocriptine.[57] It found that pergolide significantly increased the number of people with "marked or moderate improvement", as measured using a seven point clinician's global assessment scale, but found no significant difference in reduction in levodopa dose after 8–12 weeks (clinician's global assessment scale: 2 RCTs, "marked or moderate improvement", AR 43% with pergolide *v* 30% with bromocriptine; RR 1.45, 95% CI 1.08 to 1.95; difference in reduction in levodopa dose: 3 RCTs, WMD +3 mg/day, 95% CI –4 mg/day to +10 mg/day). Two of the RCTs found that pergolide significantly improved motor impairment compared with bromocriptine. The third systematic review (search date not stated, 1 RCT, 163 people) compared pramipexole versus bromocriptine.[58] It found that pramipexole reduced "off" time compared with bromocriptine (WMD 1.4 hours/day, 95% CI 0 hours/day to 2.8 hours/day). There were no differences in UPDRS or dyskinesias (see glossary, p 1595) (no quantitative data provided). The fourth systematic review (search date not stated, 3 RCTs, 482 people) compared ropinirole versus bromocriptine.[59] It found that ropinirole improved "off" time and levodopa dose reduction compared with bromocriptine after 8–25 weeks, but these differences were not significant ("off" time: WMD +0.8 hours/day, 95% CI –0.1 hours/day to +1.7 hours/day; difference in levodopa dose reduction: +50 mg/day, 95% CI –49 mg/day to +150 mg/day). The fifth systematic review (search date not stated, 5 RCTs, 1071 people) compared cabergoline versus bromocriptine.[60] Cabergoline improved "off" time compared with bromocriptine after 12–36 weeks, but the difference was not significant ("off" time: WMD +0.3 hours/day, 95% CI –0.1 hours/day to +0.7 hours/day). Four of the RCTs found no difference in motor scores or activities of daily living scores.

Harms: **Versus placebo:** The systematic reviews found that agonist treatment versus placebo significantly increased dopaminergic adverse effects (see glossary, p 1595).[50–55] In particular, dyskinesia was significantly increased with pergolide (OR 4.6, 95% CI 3.1 to 7.0), pramipexole (OR 2.1, 95% CI 1.5 to 2.9), and ropinirole (OR 2.9,

95% CI 1.4 to 6.2).[52,53,55] Withdrawal from treatment was significantly lower with pramipexole versus placebo (OR 0.64, 95% CI 0.44 to 0.93) but not with pergolide, ropinirole, or cabergoline.[52–54] **Versus each other:** Systematic reviews found no significant difference in adverse events with pergolide versus bromocriptine and pramipexole versus bromocriptine,[57,58] but nausea was significantly less frequent with ropinirole (OR 0.5, 95% CI 0.3 to 0.8).[59] Dyskinesias and confusion were reported as adverse events more commonly with cabergoline than bromocriptine, but there was no significant difference in the frequency of other dopaminergic adverse events (dyskinesia: OR 1.6, 95% CI 1.1 to 2.4; confusion: OR 2.0, 95% CI 1.1 to 3.8).[60]

Comment: We found no studies that directly compared the newer dopamine agonists.

QUESTION What are the effects of surgery in people with later Parkinson's disease?

OPTION PALLIDAL SURGERY

One systematic review found limited evidence that unilateral pallidotomy improved motor examination and activities of daily living compared with medical treatment. There is a high incidence of adverse effects with pallidotomy. One RCT found insufficient evidence to assess the effects of pallidotomy versus deep brain stimulation. We found no RCTs comparing pallidal deep brain stimulation versus medical treatment. One small RCT found insufficient evidence to assess the effects of pallidal deep brain stimulation versus subthalamic deep brain stimulation.

Benefits: **Pallidotomy versus medical treatment:** We found one systematic review (search date 1999, 2 RCTs) that evaluated mainly unilateral posteroventral pallidotomy (see glossary, p 1595) in people with advanced Parkinson's disease.[61] The first RCT in the systematic review, published only as an abstract, found that pallidotomy versus medical treatment improved tremor, bradykinesia, rigidity, gait, postural stability, and "off" time (see glossary, p 1595).[62] It found no difference in the need for medical treatment. The second RCT in the systematic review (37 people) compared unilateral pallidotomy versus medical treatment.[63] It found that pallidotomy improved "off" phase motor examination (Unified Parkinson's Disease Rating Score 3 [see glossary, p 1595]), activities of daily living (Barthel Index, UPDRS 2, and Schwab and England scale), but not pain on a visual analogue score at 6 months (UPDRS 3: decreased from 47 to 33 with pallidotomy *v* increased from 53 to 57 with medical treatment, $P < 0.001$; Barthel Index: increased by 2.5 with pallidotomy *v* decreased by 0.5 with medical treatment, $P = 0.004$; UPDRS 2: decreased from 30 to 21 with pallidotomy *v* increased from 32 to 35 with medical treatment, $P = 0.002$; Schwab and England scale: increased from 35 to 70 with pallidotomy *v* decreased from 35 to 30 with medical treatment, $P < 0.001$; pain score: decreased from 27 mm to 14 mm with pallidotomy *v* increased from 15 mm to 22 mm with medical treatment, $P = 0.13$; CIs not stated). **Pallidotomy versus pallidal**

deep brain stimulation: We found one systematic review (search date 2000, 1 RCT).[64] The RCT (13 people) in the systematic review found no significant difference between pallidotomy and deep brain stimulation (see glossary, p 1595) for symptoms, activities of daily living, and adverse effects over 3 months, but was too small to exclude clinically important differences.[65] **Pallidal deep brain stimulation versus medical treatment:** We found one systematic review (search date 2000) that identified no RCTs comparing pallidal deep brain stimulation versus medical treatment.[64] We found no subsequent RCTs. **Pallidal deep brain stimulation versus subthalamic deep brain stimulation:** We found one RCT (10 people) comparing bilateral pallidal deep brain stimulation versus bilateral subthalamic nucleus deep brain stimulation.[66] It found no difference in motor scores after 12 months (UPDRS 3 improvement: 39% with pallidal stimulation *v* 44% with subthalamic stimulation).

Harms: The first RCT in the review comparing pallidotomy versus medical treatment gave no information on adverse effects.[62] In the second RCT in the review, comparing pallidotomy versus medical treatment, 6/19 (31.5%) people who had unilateral pallidotomy had adverse effects persisting for 6 months after surgery, including dysarthria, dysphasia, facial paresis, and urinary incontinence.[63] We found three RCTs assessing neuropsychological, cognitive, or behavioural effects of pallidotomy versus medical treatment.[67–69] The first RCT (35 people) found that left sided, but not right sided, pallidotomy reduced verbal fluency.[67] The second RCT found subtle changes on measures of frontal lobe function after 6 months in people with unilateral pallidotomy.[68] The third RCT (33 people) found that surgery, particularly left sided surgery, reduced letter fluency compared with medical management at 3 months ($P = 0.011$).[69] One systematic review of case series (search date 1998) found that the incidence of permanent adverse effects of unilateral pallidotomy was 4–46%, with a risk of a serious complication (including death) of 3–10%.[70] Another systematic review of case series (search date 1998) estimated a 10–15% incidence of persistent adverse effects with unilateral pallidotomy.[71] One RCT (6 people) compared bilateral pallidotomy versus unilateral pallidotomy plus contralateral pallidal deep brain stimulation.[72] It found that all the three people with bilateral pallidotomy experienced severe adverse effects. This led to discontinuation of the study. Complication rates declined as surgeons developed experience in performing pallidotomy.[73] Adverse effects linked with deep brain stimulation include haemorrhage, lead displacement, visual deficit, speech, motor or sensory disturbances, psychosis, confusion, and disorientation. Follow up can be expensive and time consuming. Eventually, equipment or battery replacement may be needed, which will require further surgery.

Comment: One cohort study found that improvement after unilateral pallidotomy was maintained for 12 months.[74] One recent non-systematic review and consensus statement suggested that gait, balance disorders, and hypophonia were less responsive than other features of parkinsonism to surgery (no further data provided).[73] Transplants and implants of dopaminergic tissue remain experimental. Uncontrolled studies and limited RCT information suggest adverse effects may be more frequent after lesioning procedures than deep brain stimulation and are more likely to be permanent. Bilateral lesioning is likely to carry a high risk of adverse axial effects (see glossary, p 1595). Some surgeons propose that if bilateral procedures are required then deep brain stimulation rather than lesioning should be carried out on one side of the brain.

OPTION THALAMIC SURGERY

One systematic review identified no RCTs comparing thalamic surgery versus medical treatment. One RCT found that thalamic deep brain stimulation improved functional status and caused fewer adverse effects compared with thalamotomy.

Benefits: **Thalamotomy versus medical treatment:** We found two systematic reviews (search date 1999,[61] search date 1998[71]) that identified no RCTs of thalamotomy versus medical treatment for Parkinson's disease (see comment below). **Thalamic deep brain stimulation versus medical treatment:** We found one systematic review (search date 2000).[64] It found no RCTs of thalamic deep brain stimulation (see glossary, p 1595) versus medical treatment. We found no subsequent RCTs. **Thalamotomy versus thalamic deep brain stimulation:** We found one systematic review (search date 2000).[64] It identified one RCT (68 people with tremor, 45 of whom had Parkinson's disease), which compared thalamotomy versus thalamic deep brain stimulation.[75] Subgroup analysis in people with Parkinson's disease found that thalamic deep brain stimulation versus thalamotomy improved functional status after 6 months (change in Frenchay Activities Index: 0.8 with thalamotomy *v* 5.5 with deep brain stimulation, 95% CI for difference 1.2 to 8.0).

Harms: **Thalamotomy versus medical treatment:** Case series included in the second systematic review found that thalamotomy was associated with reversible complications (lasting < 3 months) in 36–61% of people and permanent complications, including speech disturbance, apraxia, and death, in 14–23%.[71] Bilateral thalamotomy carries a high risk of speech disturbance.[71] **Thalamotomy versus thalamic deep brain stimulation:** The RCT found that adverse effects were significantly less common with deep brain stimulation versus thalamotomy after 6 months (AR 47% with thalamotomy *v* 18% with deep brain stimulation; P = 0.02; CI not stated).[75]

Comment: The reviews found limited evidence from case series that thalamic surgery may not be as useful as pallidal or subthalamic surgery thalamotomy for parkinsonian features other than tremor.[61,71] The second systematic review did not describe fully the case series it identified, focusing on results from "key studies". See comment under pallidal surgery, p 1592.

OPTION SUBTHALAMIC SURGERY

One systematic review found no RCTs comparing subthalamic surgery with medical treatment. One small RCT comparing subthalamic deep brain stimulation with pallidal deep brain stimulation found no significant difference in motor scores.

Benefits: **Subthalamic deep brain stimulation versus medical treatment:** We found one systematic review (search date 2000) that identified no RCTs of subthalamic deep brain stimulation (see glossary, p 1595) versus medical treatment.[64] We found no subsequent RCTs. **Pallidal deep brain stimulation versus subthalamic deep brain stimulation:** See benefits of pallidal surgery, p 1591.

Harms: See comment under pallidal surgery, p 1592.

Comment: Larger and longer term RCTs are needed to compare the effects of pallidal versus subthalamic stimulation. A large RCT comparing quality of life and costs of subthalamic or pallidal lesioning and deep brain stimulation surgery versus best medical treatment is currently under way in the UK (Clarke C, personal communication, 2002).

QUESTION What are the effects of rehabilitation treatments in later Parkinson's disease?

OPTION PHYSIOTHERAPY

Two systematic reviews found insufficient evidence of the effects of physiotherapy in later Parkinson's disease.

Benefits: We found two systematic reviews.[76,77] The first review (search date 2000, 11 RCTs, 280 people with early or later Parkinson's disease) compared physiotherapy versus no treatment or versus inactive physiotherapy.[76] The review was unable to draw conclusions on the effects of physiotherapy in Parkinson's disease because of the small numbers of people, methodological flaws, different types of physiotherapy used, and the wide variety of outcome measures in the RCTs. The second systematic review (search date 1999, 8 RCTs included in the first review, 4 quasi-randomised studies) compared physiotherapy versus no treatment or versus other treatment (occupational therapy, regular exercises, non-specified psychological treatment).[77] It also found that methodological flaws of trials and trial heterogeneity made it difficult to draw conclusions on the effects of physiotherapy.[77]

Harms: The systematic reviews gave no information on adverse effects.[76,77]

Comment: Further, larger, well designed RCTs are required. A large UK RCT is in preparation (Clarke C, personal communication, 2003).

OPTION OCCUPATIONAL THERAPY

One systematic review found insufficient evidence of the effects of occupational therapy in later Parkinson's disease.

Benefits: We found one systematic review (search date 2000, 2 RCTs, 84 people with early or later Parkinson's disease).[78] One RCT in the review compared occupational therapy versus no treatment, and the other RCT compared occupational therapy plus physiotherapy versus physiotherapy alone. The review was unable to draw conclusions on the effects of occupational therapy because of the small number of people in the RCTs, methodological flaws, trial heterogeneity, and the variety of outcome measures used.[78]

Harms: The RCTs in the review gave no information on adverse effects.[78]

Comment: Further, larger, well designed RCTs are required. A UK RCT of occupational therapy in Parkinson's disease is in preparation (Clarke C, personal communication, 2003).

OPTION SPEECH AND LANGUAGE THERAPY FOR SPEECH DISTURBANCE

One systematic review found insufficient evidence of the effects of speech and language therapy for speech disturbance in later Parkinson's disease.

Benefits: We found one systematic review (search date 2000, 3 RCTs, 63 people) that compared speech and language therapy versus no treatment for speech disturbance.[79] It was unable to draw conclusions on the effects of speech and language therapy because of the small number of people, methodological flaws, and the variety of outcome measures used in the RCTs.

Harms: The RCTs in the review gave no information on adverse effects.[79]

Comment: Further, larger, well designed RCTs are required.

OPTION SWALLOWING THERAPY FOR DYSPHAGIA

One systematic review found no RCTs of swallowing therapy for dysphagia.

Benefits: We found one systematic review (search date 2000) of swallowing therapy for dysphagia, which did not identify any RCTs.[80]

Harms: We found no RCTs.

Comment: None.

GLOSSARY

Axial effects Changes affecting axial body sections, such as head and trunk, rather than the limbs.

Deep brain stimulation Prolonged focal electrical brain stimulation through a stereotactically implanted wire.

Dopaminergic adverse effects Include dyskinesia, hallucinations, and psychosis.

Dyskinesia Abnormal or involuntary writhing or jerky movements distinct from tremor.

Motor fluctuations Fluctuations in motor symptoms, such as bradykinesia, rigidity, and tremor, during a day. Response fluctuations are fluctuations in a person's overall response to treatment during a day.

"Off" time Periods when treatment is not working. "On" time is the period when treatment is working.

Pallidotomy Making a permanent surgical lesion, usually thermally or electrically, in the globus pallidum.

Unified Parkinson's Disease Rating Scale (UPDRS) A scale used to measure severity of Parkinson's Disease. It has six parts: mentation, behaviour, and mood (UPDRS 1); activities of daily living (UPDRS 2); motor examination (UPDRS 3); complications of treatment (UPDRS 4); a global disability staging score (UPDRS 5); and a global activities of daily living score (UPDRS 6).

Substantive changes

Selegiline Five RCTs added;[24–27,33] conclusions unchanged.

Pallidal surgery One RCT added;[69] conclusions unchanged.

REFERENCES

1. Hughes AJ, Daniel SE, Blankson S, et al. A clinico-pathologic study of 100 cases of Parkinson's disease. *Arch Neurol* 1993;50:140–148.
2. Zhang Z, Roman G. Worldwide occurrence of Parkinson's disease: an updated review. *Neuroepidemiology* 1993;12:195–208.
3. De Rijk MC, Tzourio C, Breteler MMB, et al. Prevalence of parkinsonism and Parkinson's disease in Europe: the EUROPARKINSON collaborative study. *J Neurol Neurosurg Psychiatry* 1997;62:10–15.
4. Ben-Shlomo Y. How far are we in understanding the cause of Parkinson's disease? *J Neurol Neurosurg Psychiatry* 1996;61:4–16.
5. De Rijk M, Breteler M, den Breeilnen J, et al. Dietary antioxidants and Parkinson's disease: the Rotterdam study. *Arch Neurol* 1997;54:762–765.
6. Hellenbrand W, Seidler A, Robra B, et al. Smoking and Parkinson's disease: a case-control study in Germany. *Int J Epidemiol* 1997;26:328–339.
7. Tzourio C, Rocca W, Breteler M, et al. Smoking and Parkinson's disease: an age-dependent risk effect? *Neurology* 1997;49:1267–1272.
8. Marder K, Tang M, Mejia H, et al. Risk of Parkinson's disease among first degree relatives: a community based study. *Neurology* 1996;47:155–160.
9. Jarman P, Wood N. Parkinson's disease genetics comes of age. *BMJ* 1999;318:1641–1642.
10. Lazzarini A, Myers R, Zimmerman T, et al. A clinical genetic study of Parkinson's disease: evidence for dominant transmission. *Neurology* 1994;44:499–506.
11. Gasser T, Müller-Myhsok B, Wszolek Z, et al. A susceptibility locus for Parkinson's disease maps to chromosome 2p13. *Nat Genet* 1998;18:262–265.
12. Tanner C, Ottman R, Goldman S, et al. Parkinson's disease in twins. An etiologic study. *JAMA* 1999;281:341–346.
13. Scott WK, Nance MA, Watts RL, et al. Complete genomic screen in Parkinson disease: evidence for multiple genes. *JAMA* 2001;286:2239–2244.
14. Martin ER, Scott WK, Nance MA, et al. Association of single-nucleotide polymorphisms of the tau gene with late-onset Parkinson disease. *JAMA* 2001;286:2245–2250.
15. Parkinson Study Group. Mortality in DATATOP: a multicenter trial in early Parkinson's disease. *Ann Neurol* 1998;43:318–325.
16. Rajput A, Uitti J, Offord K. Timely levodopa (LD) administration prolongs survival in Parkinson's disease. *Parkinson Relat Disord* 1997;3:159–165.
17. Clarke CE. Does levodopa therapy delay death in Parkinson's disease? A review of the evidence. *Mov Disord* 1995;10:250–256.
18. Hely MA, Morris JGL, Traficante R, et al. The Sydney multicentre study of Parkinson's disease: progression and mortality at 10 years. *J Neurol Neurosurg Psychiatry* 1999;67:300–307.
19. Morgante L, Salemi G, Meneghini F, et al. Parkinson disease survival. A population-based study. *Arch Neurol* 2000;57:507–512.
20. Fahn S, Elton L, for the UPDRS Development Committee. Unified Parkinson's disease rating scale. In: Fahn S, Marsden C, Calne D, et al, eds. *Recent developments in Parkinson's disease*, Vol. 2. Florham Park: Macmillan Healthcare Information, 1987:153–163.
21. Langston JW, Widner H, Goetz CG, et al. Core Assessment Program for Intracerebral Transplantations (CAPIT). *Mov Disord* 1992;7:2–13.
22. De Boer A, Wijker W, Speelman J, et al. Quality of life in people with Parkinson's disease: development of a questionnaire. *J Neurol Neurosurg Psychiatry* 1996;61:70–74.
23. Peto V, Jenkinson C, Fitzpatrick R, et al. The development and validation of a short measure of functioning and well being for individuals with Parkinson's disease. *Qual Life Res* 1995;4:241–248.
24. Tetrud JW, Langston JW. The effect of deprenyl (selegiline) on the natural history of Parkinson's disease. *Science* 1989;245:519–522.
25. Palhagen S, Heinonen E, Hagglund J, et al. Selegiline delays the onset of disability in *de novo* parkinsonian patients. *Neurology* 1998;51:520–525.
26. Allain H, Pollack P, Neukirch H, et al. Symptomatic effect of selegiline in *de novo* parkinsonian patients. *Mov Disord* 1993;8:S36–S40.
27. Myllala V, Sotaniemi K, Hakulinen P, et al. Selegiline as the primary treatment of Parkinson's disease-a long term double-blind study. *Acta Neurol Scand* 1997;95:211–218.
28. The Parkinson's Disease Study Group. Effects of tocopherol and deprenyl on the progression of disability in early Parkinson's disease. *N Engl J Med* 1993;328:176–183.
29. Olanow CW, Hauser RA, Gauger L, et al. The effect of deprenyl and levodopa on the progression of Parkinson's disease. *Ann Neurol* 1995;38:771–777.
30. Lees AJ, for the Parkinson's Disease Research Group of the United Kingdom. Comparison of therapeutic effects and mortality data of levodopa and levodopa combined with selegiline in people with early, mild Parkinson's disease. *BMJ* 1995;311:1602–1607.
31. Przuntek H, Conrad B, Dichgans J, et al. SELEDO: a 5-year long-term trial on the effect of selegiline in early Parkinsonian people treated with levodopa. *Eur J Neurol* 1999;6:141–150.
32. Larson JP, Boas J, Erdal JE, et al. Does selegiline modify the progression of early Parkinson's disease? Results from a five-year study. *Eur J Neurol* 1999;6:539–547.
33. The Italian Parkinson Study Group. A multicenter Italian randomised study on early treatment of Parkinson disease: comparison of L-dopa, L-deprenyl and dopaminoagonists. Study design and short term results. *Italian J Neurol Sci* 1992;13:735–739.
34. Olanow CW, Myllyla V, Sotaniemi K, et al. Effect of selegiline on mortality in people with Parkinson's disease. *Neurology* 1998;51:825–830.
35. Parkinson Study Group. Impact of deprenyl and tocopherol treatment for Parkinson's disease in DATATOP people requiring levodopa. *Ann Neurol* 1996;39:37–45.
36. Ben-Shlomo Y, Churchyard A, Head J, et al. Investigation by Parkinson's Disease Research Group of United Kingdom into excess mortality seen with combined levodopa and selegiline treatment in people with early, mild Parkinson's disease: further results of randomised trial and confidential inquiry. *BMJ* 1998;316:1191–1196.
37. Counsell C. Effect of adding selegiline to levodopa in early, mild Parkinson's disease. *BMJ* 1998;17:1586.
38. Thorogood M, Armstrong B, Nichols T, et al. Mortality in people taking selegiline: observational study. *BMJ* 1998;317:252–254.
39. Dupont E, Andersen A, Boas J, et al. Sustained-release Madopar HBS compared with standard Madopar in the long-term treatment of *de novo* Parkinsonian people. *Acta Neurol Scand* 1996;93:14–20.

40. Block G, Liss C, Reines S, et al. Comparison of immediate release and controlled release carbidopa/levodopa in Parkinson's disease. *Eur Neurol* 1997;37:23–27.
41. Ramaker C, van Hilten J. Bromocriptine versus levodopa in early Parkinson's disease. In: The Cochrane Library, Issue 4, 2002. Oxford: Update Software. Search date 1999; primary sources Cochrane Movement Disorders Group Specialised Register, Cochrane Controlled Trials Register, Medline, Embase, pharmaceutical companies, experts for unpublished studies, and hand searches of references and selected neurology journals.
42. Oertel WH. Pergolide versus levodopa monotherapy (PELMOPET). *Mov Disord* 2000;15(suppl 3):4.
43. Fahn S. Parkinson's disease, the effect of levodopa and the ELLDOPA trial. *Arch Neurol* 1999;56:529–535.
44. Ramaker C, Hilten JJ van. Bromocriptine/levodopa combined versus levodopa alone for early Parkinson's disease (Cochrane Review). In: The Cochrane Library, Issue 4, 2002. Oxford: Update Software. Search date 2001; primary sources Cochrane Movement Disorders Group Specialised Register, Cochrane Controlled Trials Register, Medline, Embase, pharmaceutical companies, experts for unpublished studies, and hand searches of references and selected neurology journals.
45. Rascol O, Brooks D, Korczyn A, et al. A five-year study of the incidence of dyskinesia in people with early Parkinson's disease who were treated with ropinirole or levodopa. *N Engl J Med* 2000;342:1484–1491.
46. Parkinson Study Group. Pramipexole versus levodopa as initial treatment for Parkinson's disease. *JAMA* 2000;284:1931–1938.
47. Rinne U. A 5-year double-blind study with cabergoline versus levodopa in the treatment of early Parkinson's disease. *Parkinsonism Relat Disord* 1999;5(suppl):84.
48. Rinne U. Lisuride, a dopamine agonist in the treatment of early Parkinson's disease. *Neurology* 1989;39:336–339.
49. Allain H, Destee A, Petit H, et al. Five-year follow-up of early lisuride and levodopa combination therapy versus levodopa monotherapy in de novo Parkinson's disease. *Eur Neurol* 2000;44:22–30.
50. Van Hilten J, Beek W, Finken M. Bromocriptine for levodopa-induced motor complications in Parkinson's disease. In: The Cochrane Library, Issue 4, 2002. Oxford: Update Software. Search date 1998; primary sources Cochrane Controlled Trials Register, Medline, Scisearch, pharmaceutical companies, experts for unpublished studies, and hand searches of references.
51. Clarke C, Speller J. Lisuride for levodopa-induced complications in Parkinson's disease. In: The Cochrane Library, Issue 4, 2002. Oxford: Update Software. Search date 1998; primary sources Medline, Embase, Cochrane Controlled Trials Register, pharmaceutical companies, and hand searches of references.
52. Clarke C, Speller J. Pergolide for levodopa-induced complications in Parkinson's disease. In: The Library, Issue 4, 2002. Oxford: Update Software. Search date 1999; primary sources Medline, Embase, Cochrane Controlled Trials Register, pharmaceutical companies, and hand searches of references.
53. Clarke C, Deane K. Ropinirole for levodopa-induced complications in Parkinson's disease. In: The Cochrane Library, Issue 4, 2002. Oxford: Update Software. Search date not stated; primary sources Cochrane Movement Disorders Group Specialised Register, Cochrane Controlled Trials Register, Medline, Embase, pharmaceutical companies, experts for unpublished studies, and hand searches of references and selected neurology journals.
54. Clarke C, Deane K. Cabergoline for levodopa-induced complications in Parkinson's disease. In: The Cochrane Library, Issue 4, 2002. Oxford: Update Software. Search date not stated; primary sources Medline, Embase, Cochrane Controlled Trials Register, hand searches of references and selected neurology journals, and contact with Pharmacia Upjohn.
55. Clarke C, Speller J, Clarke J. Pramipexole for levodopa-induced complications in Parkinson's disease. In: The Cochrane Library, Issue 4, 2002. Oxford: Update Software. Search date not stated; primary sources Cochrane Movement Disorders Group Specialised Register, Cochrane Controlled Trials Register, Medline, Embase, pharmaceutical companies, experts for unpublished studies, and hand searches of references and selected neurology journals.
56. Clarke CE, Speller JM. Lisuride versus bromocriptine for levodopa-induced complications in Parkinson's disease. In: The Cochrane Library, Issue 4, 2002. Oxford: Update Software. Search date not stated; primary sources Medline, Embase, Cochrane Controlled Trials Register, hand searches of the neurology literature, reference lists of identified studies, and contact with pharmaceutical companies.
57. Clarke C, Speller J. Pergolide versus bromocriptine for levodopa-induced motor complications in Parkinson's disease. In: The Cochrane Library, Issue 4, 2002. Oxford: Update Software. Search date 1998; primary sources Medline, Embase, Cochrane Controlled Trials Register, pharmaceuticals companies, and hand searches of references.
58. Clarke C, Speller J, Clarke J. Pramipexole versus bromocriptine for levodopa-induced complications in Parkinson's disease. In: The Cochrane Library, Issue 4, 2002. Oxford: Update Software. Search date not stated; primary sources Cochrane Movement Disorders Group Specialised Register, Cochrane Controlled Trials Register, Medline, Embase, pharmaceutical companies, experts for unpublished studies, and hand searches of references and selected neurology journals.
59. Clarke C, Deane K. Ropinirole versus bromocriptine for levodopa-induced complications in Parkinson's disease. In: The Cochrane Library, Issue 4, 2002. Oxford: Update Software. Search date not stated; primary sources Cochrane Movement Disorders Group Specialised Register, Cochrane Controlled Trials Register, Medline, Embase, pharmaceutical companies, experts for unpublished studies, and hand searches of references and selected neurology journals.
60. Clarke C, Deane K. Cabergoline versus bromocriptine for levodopa-induced complications in Parkinson's disease. In: The Cochrane Library, Issue 4, 2002. Oxford: Update Software. Search date not stated; primary sources Cochrane Movement Disorders Group Specialised Register, Cochrane Controlled Trials Register, Medline, Embase, pharmaceutical companies, experts for unpublished studies, and hand searches of references and selected neurology journals.
61. Development and Evaluation Committee. Report 105. *Pallidotomy, thalotomy and deep brain stimulation for severe Parkinson's disease.* Southampton: Wessex Institute for Health Research and Development, 1999. Search date 1999; primary sources Cochrane Library, Health

Technology Assessment database, Medline, Science Citation Index, Biosis, Embase, Index to Scientific and Technical Proceedings, Inspec, and Best Evidence.
62. Vitek J, Bakay R, Freeman A, et al. Randomised clinical trial of pallidotomy for Parkinson's disease. *Neurology* 1998;50(suppl 4):A80.
63. De Bie R, de Haan R, Nijssen P, et al. Unilateral pallidotomy in Parkinson's disease: a randomised, single-blind, multicentre trial. *Lancet* 1999;354:1665–1669.
64. Medical Services Advisory Committee. Deep brain stimulation for Parkinson's disease. Australian Department of Health and Ageing, Canberra, 2001. Search date 2000; primary sources Cochrane library, Medline, Psycinfo, Cinahl, Current Contents, PreMedline, Healthstar, Trip, and Australasian Medical Index.
65. Merello M, Nouzeilles MI, Kuzis G, et al. Unilateral radiofrequency lesion versus electrostimulation of posteroventral pallidum: a prospective randomized comparison. *Mov Disord* 1999;14:50–56.
66. Burchiel K, Anderson V, Favre J, et al. Comparison of pallidal and subthalamic nucleus deep brain stimulation for advanced Parkinson's disease: results of a randomized, blinded pilot study. *Neurosurgery* 1999;45:1375–1384.
67. Schmand B, de Bie R, Koning-Haanstra M, et al. Unilateral pallidotomy in PD. A controlled study of cognitive and behavioural effects. *Neurology* 2000;54:1058–1064.
68. Green J, McDonald W, Vitek J, et al. Neuropsychological and psychiatric sequelae of pallidotomy for PD. Clinical trial findings. *Neurology* 2002;58:858–865.
69. Green J, McDonald WM, Vitek JL, et al. Neuropsychological and psychiatric sequelae of pallidotomy for PD. *Neurology* 2002;58:858–865.
70. Gregory R. Posteroventral pallidotomy for advanced Parkinson's disease: a systematic review. *Neurol Rev Int* 1999;3:8–12. Search date 1998; primary sources not stated.
71. Hallett M, Litvan I. The Task Force on Surgery for Parkinson's Disease. Evaluation of surgery for Parkinson's disease. A report of the Therapeutics and Technology Assessment Subcommittee of the American Academy of Neurology. *Neurology* 1999;53:1910–1921. Search date 1998; primary sources Medline, Embase, Biosis.
72. Merello M, Starkstein S, Nouzeilles M, et al. Bilateral pallidotomy for treatment of Parkinson's disease induced corticobulbar syndrome and psychic akinesia avoidable by globus pallidus lesion combined with contralateral stimulation. *J Neurol Neurosurg Psychiatry* 2001;71:611–614.
73. Bronstein JM, DeSalles A, DeLong MR. Stereotactic pallidotomy in the treatment of Parkinson's disease. *Arch Neurol* 1999;56:1064–1069.
74. De Bie R, Schuurman P, Bosch D, et al. Outcome of unilateral pallidotomy in advanced Parkinson's disease: cohort study of 32 patients. *J Neurol Neurosurg Psychiatry* 2001;71:375–382.
75. Schuurman P, Bosch D, Bossuyt P, et al. A comparison of continuous thalamic stimulation and thalamotomy for suppression of severe tremor. *N Engl J Med* 2000;342:461–468.
76. Deane KHO, Jones D, Clarke CE, et al. Physiotherapy versus placebo or no intervention in Parkinson's disease. In: The Cochrane Library. Issue 4, 2002. Oxford: Update Software. Search date 2000; primary sources Medline, Embase, Cinahl, Isi-Sci, Amed, Mantis, Rehabdata, Rehadat, Gerolit, Pascal, Lilacs, MedCarib, Jicst-EPlus, Aim, IMEMR, Sigle, ISI-ISTP, Dissabs, Conference Papers Index, Aslib Index to Theses, Cochrane Library, the CentreWatch Clinical Trials listing service, the metaRegister of Controlled Trials, ClinicalTrials.gov, Crisp, Pedro, Niddr and NRR, and hand searches of references.
77. de Goede CJ, Keus SH, Kwakkel G, et al. The effects of physical therapy in Parkinson's disease: a research synthesis. *Arch Phys Med Rehab* 2001;2:509–515. Search date 1999; primary sources Medline, Cinahl, and hand searches of references.
78. Deane KHO, Ellis-Hill C, Clarke CE, et al. Occupational therapy for patients with Parkinson's disease. In: The Cochrane Library. Issue 4, 2002. Oxford: Update Software. Search date 2000; primary sources Medline, Embase, Cinahl, Isi-Sci, Amed, Mantis, Rehabdata, Rehadat, Gerolit, Pascal, Lilacs, MedCarib, Jicst-EPlus, Aim, IMEMR, Sigle, ISI-ISTP, Dissabs, Conference Papers Index, Aslib Index to Theses, Cochrane Library, the CentreWatch Clinical Trials listing service, the metaRegister of Controlled Trials, ClinicalTrials.gov, Crisp, Pedro, Niddr and NRR, and hand searches of reference.
79. Deane KHO, Whurr R, Playford ED, et al. Speech and language therapy for dysarthria in Parkinson's disease. In: The Cochrane Library Issue 4, 2002. Oxford: Update Software. Search date 2000; primary sources Medline, Embase, Cinahl, Isi-Sci, Amed, Mantis, Rehabdata, Rehadat, Gerolit, Pascal, Lilacs, MedCarib, Jicst-EPlus, Aim, IMEMR, Sigle, ISI-ISTP, Dissabs, Conference Papers Index, Aslib Index to Theses, Cochrane Library, the CentreWatch Clinical Trials listing service, the metaRegister of Controlled Trials, ClinicalTrials.gov, Crisp, Pedro, Niddr and NRR, and hand searches of references.
80. Deane KHO, Whurr R, Clarke CE, et al. Non-pharmacological therapies for dysphagia in Parkinson's disease. In: The Cochrane Library Issue 4, 2002. Oxford: Update Software. Search date 2000; Primary sources Medline, Embase, Cinahl, Isi-Sci, Amed, Mantis, Rehabdata, Rehadat, Gerolit, Pascal, Lilacs, MedCarib, Jicst-EPlus, Aim, IMEMR, Sigle, ISI-ISTP, Dissabs, Conference Papers Index, Aslib Index to Theses, Cochrane Library, the CentreWatch Clinical Trials listing service, the metaRegister of Controlled Trials, ClinicalTrials.gov, Crisp, Pedro, Niddr and NRR, and hand searches of reference.

Carl Clarke
Reader in Clinical Neurology
University of Birmingham, Birmingham, UK

A Peter Moore
Senior Lecturer in Neurology
University of Liverpool, Liverpool, UK

Competing interests: APM has been reimbursed by various manufacturers for attending and speaking at conferences, and for consulting. CC has been paid by various manufacturers of the drugs dealt with above for speaking at meetings and attending conferences.

Trigeminal neuralgia

Search date March 2003

Joanna M Zakrzewska and Benjamin C Lopez

QUESTIONS

INTERVENTIONS

See glossary, p 1608

Key Messages

- **Carbamazepine** One systematic review of three crossover RCTs found that carbamazepine increased pain relief compared with placebo. The review found that carbamazepine increased adverse effects (drowsiness, dizziness, constipation, and ataxia) compared with placebo. One small RCT provided insufficient evidence to compare tizanidine versus carbamazepine. One RCT found that pimozide reduced pain over 8 weeks compared with carbamazepine, but increased adverse effects (including hand tremors, memory impairment, and involuntary movements). One systematic review found one RCT of tocainide versus carbamazepine that was of insufficient quality.
- **Pimozide** One RCT found that pimozide reduced pain over 8 weeks compared with carbamazepine, but increased adverse effects (including hand tremors, memory impairment, and involuntary movements). Cardiac toxicity and sudden death have been reported with pimozide.
- **Baclofen** We found insufficient evidence on the effects of baclofen versus placebo or versus other active drugs.
- **Combined streptomycin and lidocaine nerve block** Small RCTs provided insufficient evidence about the effects of nerve block with streptomycin plus lidocaine compared with nerve block with lidocaine alone.

Trigeminal neuralgia

- **Lamotrigine** One systematic review provided insufficient evidence to compare lamotrigine versus placebo in people with trigeminal neuralgia.
- **Other drugs (phenytoin, clonazepam, sodium valproate, gabapentin, mexiletine, oxcarbazepine, topiramate)** We found insufficient evidence about the effects of these drugs in people with trigeminal neuralgia.
- **Peripheral laser treatment** We found insufficient evidence on the effects of peripheral laser treatment in people with trigeminal neuralgia.
- **Stereotactic radiosurgery** We found insufficient evidence about the effects of stereotactic radiosurgery in people with trigeminal neuralgia.
- **Tizanidine** One small RCT provided insufficient evidence to compare tizanidine versus carbamazepine.
- **Proparacaine eye drops** One RCT found no significant difference in pain at 30 days between placebo and a single application of proparacaine hydrochloride eye drops to the eye on the same side as the pain.
- **Tocainide** One systematic review found one RCT of tocainide versus carbamazepine which was of insufficient quality. The use of tocainide is limited by considerable harms (including serious haematological effects).
- **Cryotherapy of peripheral nerves; peripheral acupuncture; peripheral alcohol injection; peripheral injection of phenol; peripheral neurectomy; peripheral radiofrequency thermocoagulation** We found no RCTs about the effects of these interventions.

DEFINITION Trigeminal neuralgia is a characteristic pain in the distribution of one or more branches of the fifth cranial nerve. The diagnosis is made on the history alone, based on characteristic features of the pain. It occurs in paroxysms that last a few seconds to 2 minutes. The frequency of paroxysms is highly variable: from hundreds of attacks a day to long periods of remission that can last years. The pain is severe and described as intense, sharp, superficial, stabbing, burning, or like an electric shock. In any individual, the pain has the same character in different attacks. It is often triggered by touch in a specific area or by eating, talking, washing the face, or cleaning the teeth. Between paroxysms, the person is asymptomatic. Other causes of facial pain may need to be excluded.[1] In trigeminal neuralgia the neurological examination is usually normal.[2,3]

INCIDENCE/ PREVALENCE Most evidence about the incidence and prevalence of trigeminal neuralgia is from the USA.[4] The annual incidence (when age adjusted to 1980 age distribution of the USA) is 5.9/100 000 women and 3.4/100 000 men. The incidence tends to be slightly higher in women at all ages. The incidence increases with age. In men aged over 80 years the incidence is 45.2/100 000.[5] Other published surveys are small. One questionnaire survey of neurological disease in a single French village found one person with trigeminal neuralgia among 993 people.[6]

AETIOLOGY/ RISK FACTORS The cause of trigeminal neuralgia remains unclear.[7] It is more common in people with multiple sclerosis (RR 20.0, 95% CI 4.1 to 59.0).[5] Hypertension is a risk factor in women (RR 2.1, 95% CI 1.2 to 3.4) but the evidence is less clear for men (RR 1.53, 95% CI 0.30 to 4.50).[5] A study in the USA found that people with trigeminal neuralgia smoked less, consumed less alcohol, had fewer tonsillectomies, and were less likely than matched controls to be Jewish or an immigrant.[8]

PROGNOSIS One study found no reduction of 10 year survival with trigeminal neuralgia.[9] We found no evidence about the natural history of trigeminal neuralgia. The illness is characterised by recurrences and remissions. Many people have periods of remission with no pain for months or years.[3] Anecdotal reports suggest that in many people it becomes more severe and less responsive to treatment with time.[10] Most people with trigeminal neuralgia are initially managed medically, and a proportion eventually have a surgical procedure.[5] We found no good evidence about the proportion of people who require surgical treatment for pain control.

AIMS OF INTERVENTION To relieve pain with minimal adverse effects.

OUTCOMES Pain frequency and severity scores; measures of psychological distress; ability to perform normal activities; adverse effects.

METHODS *Clinical Evidence* search and appraisal March 2003. Author performed an additional hand search of her own bibliography.

QUESTION What are the effects of treatments on trigeminal neuralgia?

OPTION CARBAMAZEPINE

One systematic review of three crossover RCTs found that carbamazepine increased the proportion of people who had pain relief compared with placebo. The review found that carbamazepine increased adverse effects (drowsiness, dizziness, constipation, and ataxia) compared with placebo. One small RCT provided insufficient evidence to compare tizanidine versus carbamazepine. One RCT found that pimozide reduced pain over 8 weeks compared with carbamazepine, but increased adverse effects (including hand tremors, memory impairment, and involuntary movements). One systematic review found one RCT of tocainide versus carbamazepine that was of insufficient quality.

Benefits: **Versus placebo:** We found one systematic review (search date 1999, 3 crossover RCTs, 161 people with trigeminal neuralgia), which found that carbamazepine (for 5 days to 2 weeks) significantly increased the proportion of people having a "good" or "excellent" response compared with placebo (57% with carbamazepine *v* 18% with placebo; OR 4.8, 95% CI 3.4 to 6.9; NNT 3, 95% CI 2 to 4).[11] **Versus tizanidine:** See benefits of tizanidine, p 1602. **Versus pimozide:** See benefits of pimozide, p 1602. **Versus tocainide:** See benefits of tocainide, p 1603.

Harms: The review found that carbamazepine significantly increased adverse effects (drowsiness, dizziness, constipation, and ataxia) compared with placebo (NNH 3, 95% CI 2 to 7).[11] In the RCTs, significantly more people withdrew from the RCTs because of adverse effects with carbamazepine compared with placebo (NNH for withdrawal 24, 95% CI 14 to 112).[12] Adverse effects described in observational studies include rashes, leucopenia, and abnormal liver function tests.[13]

Comment: The RCTs used a crossover design, and one RCT[14] used multiple crossovers so that each individual was counted more than once when calculating the estimates of effectiveness in the systematic review.[11,12] The RCTs included in the systematic review were small and short term. All of the RCTs used simple measures for pain outcomes and no quality of life measures. Diagnostic criteria were not clearly stated. Previous treatment and duration of pain varied considerably. Long term effects of carbamazepine have been assessed only in open trials. We found one report (143 people with trigeminal neuralgia followed for up to 16 years) on the long term benefits of carbamazepine.[15] Initially carbamazepine was successful in 69% of participants, but by 5–16 years only 31 participants (22%) were still finding carbamazepine effective and 44% required additional or alternative treatment.

OPTION TIZANIDINE

One small RCT provided insufficient evidence to compare tizanidine versus carbamazepine.

Benefits: **Versus placebo:** We found no RCTs. **Versus carbamazepine:** We found one systematic review (search date 1999, 1 double blind RCT, 12 people).[11] It found that similar proportions of people rated tizanidine (≤ 18 mg/day) and carbamazepine (≤ 900 mg/day) as having "very good" efficacy (analysis not by intention to treat; 1/5 people with tizanidine *v* 4/6 with carbamazepine; P value not reported).

Harms: No adverse effects were reported but two people withdrew because of inadequate pain control.[11]

Comment: The RCT was too small to establish or exclude clinically important effects.

OPTION PIMOZIDE

One RCT found that pimozide reduced pain over 8 weeks compared with carbamazepine but increased adverse effects (including hand tremors, memory impairment, and involuntary movements). Cardiac toxicity and sudden death have been reported with pimozide.

Benefits: **Versus placebo:** We found no RCTs. **Versus carbamazepine:** We found one systematic review (search date 1999)[11] that identified one double blind crossover RCT[16] comparing pimozide versus carbamazepine in 48 people with trigeminal neuralgia who were refractory to other medical treatment. Precrossover results found that significantly more people achieved a large reduction in pain severity with 8 weeks of pimozide treatment compared with carbamazepine (total pain score reduction: results presented graphically, $P < 0.001$).[16]

Harms: The RCT found that pimozide significantly increased adverse effects compared with carbamazepine (40/48 [83%] with pimozide *v* 22/48 [46%] with carbamazepine; OR 7.8, 95% CI 3.7 to 20.0).[11] Adverse effects included hand tremors, memory impairment, and involuntary movements. The use of pimozide is restricted by its cardiac toxicity and by reports of sudden death.[13,17]

Comment: This was a well conducted multicentre trial using a variety of outcome measures. The crossover design limits interpretation of the results because untested assumptions are required to perform the statistical analyses.

OPTION TOCAINIDE

One systematic review found one RCT of tocainide versus carbamazepine that was of insufficient quality. The use of tocainide is limited by considerable harms (including serious haematological effects).

Benefits: **Versus placebo:** We found no RCTs. **Versus carbamazepine:** We found one systematic review (search date 1999, 1 RCT,[18] 12 people with trigeminal neuralgia).[11] The double blind, crossover RCT had weak methods and did not report precrossover results (see comment below).

Harms: The RCT reported that one person withdrew because of a skin rash and three people had other adverse effects.[18] The use of tocainide is limited by considerable harms (including severe haematological effects).[13,19]

Comment: In the RCT, combined analysis of precrossover and postcrossover results found that tocainide versus carbamazepine had no significant effect on the number of people who improved after treatment (figures not reported).[18] The available evidence is poor, but provides no support for the use of tocainide in trigeminal neuralgia.

OPTION LAMOTRIGINE

One systematic review provided insufficient evidence to compare lamotrigine versus placebo in people with trigeminal neuralgia.

Benefits: **Versus placebo:** We found one systematic review (search date 1999)[11] that identified one small crossover RCT (14 people)[20] comparing lamotrigine versus placebo. However, the RCT did not report precrossover results for global improvement (see comment below).

Harms: In the RCT, adverse effects with lamotrigine included dizziness, constipation, nausea, and drowsiness. It may also cause serious skin rash and allergic reactions. The total number of people reporting adverse effects was the same as with placebo (7/14 [50%] with lamotrigine *v* 7/14 [50%] with placebo).[20]

Comment: The RCT (double blind crossover, 14 people with refractory trigeminal neuralgia using either carbamazepine or phenytoin) found that lamotrigine versus placebo in addition to the current medication increased the proportion of people who improved after 2 weeks of treatment (postcrossover results: 10/13 [77%] with lamotrigine *v* 8/14 [57%] with placebo; ARI +20%, 95% CI –16% to +55%).[20] This RCT was a small study and lamotrigine was used in addition to existing treatment. The crossover design and short period of treatment limits interpretation.

OPTION BACLOFEN

We found insufficient evidence on the effects of baclofen versus placebo or versus other active drugs.

Benefits: **Versus placebo:** We found no RCTs of sufficient quality (see comment below). **Versus other active drugs:** We found no RCTs of sufficient quality (see comment below).

Harms: Baclofen is associated with transient sedation and loss of muscle tone. Abrupt discontinuation may cause seizures and hallucinations. One small, poor quality trial comparing racemic baclofen versus L-baclofen reported dizziness, confusion, or lethargy (6/15 [40%] v 1/15 [7%]; ARI 33%, 95% CI 3% to 64%; see comment below).[21]

Comment: **Versus placebo:** We found one controlled trial (double blind, crossover, 10 people, 4 using carbamazepine or phenytoin, not clearly randomised).[22] Postcrossover analysis found that baclofen compared with placebo in addition to pre-existing treatment increased the proportion of people with relief of pain after treatment for 2 weeks (7/10 [70%] with baclofen v 1/10 [10%] with placebo).[22] **Racemic versus L-baclofen:** We found one trial (double blind crossover, 15 people, not clearly randomised) that compared racemic (standard) baclofen versus L-baclofen over 2 weeks.[21] It found no significant difference in response (9/15 [60%] with L-baclofen v 6/15 [40%] with racemic baclofen; ARI +20%, 95% CI –16% to +56%). Some people included in the study were also taking other treatments, making interpretation difficult.

OPTION PROPARACAINE HYDROCHLORIDE EYE DROPS

One RCT found no significant difference in pain at 30 days between placebo and a single application of proparacaine hydrochloride eye drops to the eye on the same side as the pain.

Benefits: **Versus placebo:** We found no systematic review but found one double blind RCT (47 people with trigeminal neuralgia) of proparacaine hydrochloride versus placebo instilled for 20 minutes on the same side as the trigeminal neuralgia on one occasion only.[23] It found no significant reduction of pain after 3, 10, and 30 days (at 30 days: 6/25 [24%] improved with proparacaine v 5/22 [23%] with placebo; ARI +1.3%, 95% CI –23% to +26%).

Harms: None reported.

Comment: None.

OPTION OTHER DRUGS

We found insufficient evidence about effects of phenytoin, clonazepam, sodium valproate, gabapentin, mexiletine, oxcarbazepine, or topiramate in people with trigeminal neuralgia.

Benefits: We found no systematic review and no RCTs of sufficient quality examining the effects of phenytoin, clonazepam, sodium valproate, gabapentin, mexiletine, oxcarbazepine, or topiramate in people with trigeminal neuralgia (see comment below).

Harms: See harms of antiepileptic drugs under epilepsy, p 1508. Harms of mexiletine include dizziness, nausea, vomiting, confusion, and tremor.[24] The crossover RCT (see comment below) reported adverse effects with topiramate included irritability and diarrhoea (in 2 people) and fatigue/sedation, hyperactivity, nausea, abdominal cramps, lightheadedness, and cognitive impairment (in 1 person each).[25]

Comment: We found one double blind crossover RCT (3 people with trigeminal neuralgia) that compared 12 weeks of topiramate (25 mg/day titrated up to 600 mg/day) versus placebo.[25] Titration was by weekly telephone assessment of symptoms. Washout period between crossover was 2 weeks. The trial found that topiramate reduced pain (on a 10 point scale) compared with placebo in all three people ($P = 0.04$).[25] However, the trial was at high risk of detecting effects by chance. An extended confirmatory study in which two people continued to take medication for three 8 week segments (4 weeks of placebo and 4 weeks of topiramate assigned in random order) found no significant pain reduction with topiramate compared with placebo.[25] Concurrent medications continued during the study included carbamazepine and baclofen in one person, clonazepam and tricyclic antidepressants in one person, and carbamazepine and gabapentin in one person.[25]

OPTION CRYOTHERAPY OF PERIPHERAL NERVES

We found no RCTs on the effects of cryotherapy (see glossary, p 1608) in people with trigeminal neuralgia.

Benefits: We found no RCTs.

Harms: We found no RCTs.

Comment: We found many articles that reported studies of limited reliability, duplicated data, or included people with different types of pain.

OPTION NERVE BLOCK

We found no RCTs comparing nerve block versus placebo or no treatment. Small RCTs provided insufficient evidence about the effects of nerve block with streptomycin plus lidocaine compared with nerve block with lidocaine alone.

Benefits: **Nerve block versus placebo or no treatment:** We found no systematic review and no RCTs. **Local anaesthetic versus streptomycin plus local anaesthetic:** We found two RCTs comparing injections of streptomycin 1 g plus lidocaine (2 mL of 2% solution) versus lidocaine injections alone (1 injection weekly for 5 weeks).[26,27] The first RCT included 18 people with trigeminal neuralgia who had previously responded poorly to lidocaine injection alone (≤ 24 hours' pain relief from lidocaine alone). One person who did not gain pain relief from allocated treatment was excluded (see comment below). One week after the final injection, combined streptomycin plus lidocaine improved the chance of being pain free compared with lidocaine alone (AR for being pain free: 89% with combined injection *v* 38% with lidocaine alone; ARR 51%; CI not provided; P = 0.04). After 30 months the RCT found no significant difference between treatments (AR for being pain free: 33% with combined injection *v* 25% with lidocaine alone; ARR 8%; CI not provided; P = 0.38).[26] The second RCT compared weekly injections of streptomycin 1 g plus lidocaine (3 mL of 2% solution) versus lidocaine alone for 5 weeks in a randomised crossover design involving 20 people with idiopathic or traumatic trigeminal neuralgia. It found no significant short term differences between the groups in severity or frequency of pain as assessed clinically and from pain diaries.[27]

Harms: People found the injections painful and some refused to have further injections.[27] No sensory changes or other adverse effects were reported.

Comment: Neither trial reported the method of randomisation. One trial had short follow up and reliability of results may have been limited by selection bias (see benefits above).[27] Streptomycin was used on the assumption that it causes a long term peripheral nerve block.

OPTION PERIPHERAL ALCOHOL INJECTIONS

We found no RCTs on the effects of injecting peripheral nerves with alcohol in people with trigeminal neuralgia.

Benefits: We found no RCTs.

Harms: We found no RCTs.

Comment: None.

OPTION PERIPHERAL NEURECTOMY

We found no RCTs on the effects of peripheral neurectomy in people with trigeminal neuralgia.

Benefits: We found no RCTs.

Harms: We found no RCTs.

Comment: None.

OPTION PERIPHERAL RADIOFREQUENCY THERMOCOAGULATION

We found no RCTs on the effects of peripheral radiofrequency thermocoagulation in people with trigeminal neuralgia.

Benefits: We found no RCTs.

Harms: We found no RCTs.

Comment: None.

OPTION STEREOTACTIC RADIOSURGERY New

We found insufficient evidence about the effects of stereotactic radiosurgery in people with trigeminal neuralgia.

Benefits: We found no RCTs comparing stereotactic radiosurgery versus placebo or versus other treatments. We found one RCT comparing different radiosurgery regimens (see comment below).[28]

Harms: One RCT comparing two different radiosurgery regimens reported numbness (8/43 [19%] with two isocentres *v* 3/44 [7%] with one isocentre), mild paraesthesia (5/43 [12%] with two isocentres *v* 4/44 [9%] with one isocentre), and severe paraesthesia (1/43 [2%] with two isocentres *v* 0/44 [0%] with one isocentre; see comment below).[28]

Comment: One RCT (87 people with trigeminal neuralgia) compared radiosurgery using either one isocentre or two isocentres, the latter regimen to treat a longer length of the trigeminal nerve.[28] It found similar rates of maximal pain control (no pain with or without drugs: 29/44 [66%] with one isocentre *v* 28/43 [65%] with two isocentres) and pain control at final follow up (no pain with or without drugs: 20/44 [45%] with one isocentre *v* 23/43 [53%] with two isocentres).[28] The median follow up was 26 months (range 1–36 months).[28] People in the RCT took additional pain medication which was not specified. It reported more complications in the two isocentre group (see harms above), but pain outcomes were similar in both groups.[28] Typically, pain relief with radiosurgery is not immediate.

OPTION PERIPHERAL INJECTION OF PHENOL

We found no RCTs on the effects of peripheral nerve injection with phenol in people with trigeminal neuralgia.

Benefits: We found no RCTs.

Harms: We found no RCTs.

Comment: None.

OPTION PERIPHERAL ACUPUNCTURE

We found no RCTs on the effects of peripheral acupuncture in people with trigeminal neuralgia.

Benefits: We found no RCTs.

Harms: We found no RCTs.

Comment: None.

OPTION PERIPHERAL LASER TREATMENT

We found insufficient evidence on the effects of peripheral laser treatment (see glossary, p 1608) in people with trigeminal neuralgia.

Benefits: We found no RCTs of sufficient quality.

Harms: We found no RCTs of sufficient quality.

Comment: We found one RCT (35 people with trigeminal neuralgia) comparing helium neon laser (3 treatments/week for 10 weeks, 1 mW, 632.5 nm, 20 Hz applied for 20 seconds on skin overlying the trigger nerve and 30 seconds on painful areas of the face) versus sham treatment with apparatus that emitted no light.[29] The trial did not compare the two groups directly. However, it found that mean pain score significantly improved from baseline at weeks 6 and 7 with laser, but did not change significantly from baseline for any week with sham treatment. This reanalysis has limited reliability.

GLOSSARY

Cryotherapy After surgical exposure of the trigger nerve, three freeze–thaw cycles are applied under local anaesthesia and sedation as necessary.

Peripheral laser treatment Laser irradiation of skin overlying the trigger nerve.

REFERENCES

1. Anonymous. *Classification of chronic pain. Descriptors of chronic pain syndromes and definitions of pain terms.* Seattle: IASP Press, 1994.
2. Katusic S, Williams DB, Beard CM, et al. Epidemiology and clinical features of idiopathic trigeminal neuralgia and glossopharyngeal neuralgia: similarities and differences, Rochester, Minnesota, 1945–1984. *Neuroepidemiology* 1991;10:276–281.
3. Zakrzewska JM. *Trigeminal neuralgia.* London: WB Saunders, 1995.
4. Zakrzewska JM, Hamlyn PJ. Facial pain. In: Crombie IKCPR, Linton SJ, LeResche L, et al, eds. *Epidemiology of pain.* Seattle: IASP, 1999:171–202.
5. Katusic S, Beard CM, Bergstralh E, et al. Incidence and clinical features of trigeminal neuralgia, Rochester, Minnesota, 1945–1984. *Ann Neurol* 1990;27:89–95.
6. Munoz M, Dumas M, Boutros-Toni F, et al. A neuro-epidemiologic survey in a Limousin town. *Rev Neurol (Paris)* 1988;144:266–271.
7. Burchiel KJ. Pain in neurology and neurosurgery: tic douloureux (trigeminal neuralgia). In: Campbell JN, ed. *Pain 1996 – an updated review.* Seattle: IASP Press, 1996:41–60.
8. Rothman KJ, Monson RR. Epidemiology of trigeminal neuralgia. *J Chronic Dis* 1973;26:3–12.
9. Rothman KJ, Monson RR. Survival in trigeminal neuralgia. *J Chronic Dis* 1973;26:303–309.
10. Zakrzewska JM, Patsalos PN. Long term cohort study comparing medical (oxcarbazepine) and surgical management of infractable trigeminal neuralgia. *Pain* 2002; 95:259–266.
11. Wiffen P, Collins S, McQuay H, et al. Anticonvulsant drugs for acute and chronic pain. In: The Cochrane Library, Issue 1, 2003. Oxford: Update Software. Search date 1999; primary sources Medline, Embase, Sigle, Cochrane Controlled Trials Register, and hand searches of 40 medical journals and published reports.
12. McQuay H, Carroll D, Jadad AR, et al. Anticonvulsant drugs for management of pain: a systematic review. *BMJ* 1995;311:1047–1052. Search date 1994; primary sources Medline and hand searches of 40 medical journals, reference lists, and published reports.
13. Sweetman SC (Ed). *Martindale: the complete drug reference.* 33rd ed. London: Pharmaceutical Press, 2002.
14. Campbell FG, Graham JG, Zilkha KJ. Clinical trial of carbazepine (Tegretol) in trigeminal neuralgia. *J Neurol Neurosurg Psychiatry* 1966;29:265–267.
15. Taylor JC, Brauer S, Espir MLE. Long-term treatment of trigeminal neuralgia with carbamazepine. *Postgrad Med J* 1981;57:16–18.
16. Lechin F, van der Dijs B, Lechin ME, et al. Pimozide therapy for trigeminal neuralgia. *Arch Neurol* 1989;46:960–963.
17. Committee on Safety of Medicines/Medicines Control Agency. Cardiac arrhythmias with pimozide (Orap). *Current Problems* 1995;21:2.
18. Lindstrom P, Lindblom V. The analgesic effect of tocainide in trigeminal neuralgia. *Pain* 1987;28:45–50.
19. Denaro CP, Benowitz NL. Poisoning due to class 1B antiarrhythmic drugs. Lignocaine, mexiletine and tocainide. *Med Toxicol Adverse Drug Exp* 1989;4:412–428.
20. Zakrzewska JM, Chaudhry Z, Patton DW, et al. Lamotrigine in refractory trigeminal neuralgia: results from a double-blind placebo controlled crossover study. *Pain* 1997;73:223–230.
21. Fromm GH, Terrence CF. Comparison of L-baclofen and racemic baclofen in trigeminal neuralgia. *Neurology* 1987;37:1725–1728.
22. Fromm GH, Terrence CF, Chattha AS. Baclofen in the treatment of trigeminal neuralgia: double-blind study and long-term follow-up. *Ann Neurol* 1984;15:240–244.
23. Kondziolka D, Lemley T, Kestle JR, et al. The effect of single-application topical ophthalmic anesthesia in patients with trigeminal neuralgia. A randomized double-blind placebo-controlled trial. *J Neurosurg* 1994;80:993–997.
24. Wooten JM, Earnest J, Reyes J. Review of common adverse effects of selected antiarrhythmic drugs. *Crit Care Nurs Q* 2000;22:23–38.
25. Gilron I, Booher SL, Rowan JS, et al. Topiramate in trigeminal neuralgia: a randomized, placebo-controlled multiple crossover pilot study. *Clin Neuropharmacol* 2001;24:109–112
26. Stajcic Z, Juniper RP, Todorovic L. Peripheral streptomycin/lidocaine injections versus lidocaine alone in the treatment of idiopathic trigeminal neuralgia. A double blind controlled trial. *J Craniomaxillofac Surg* 1990;18:243–246.
27. Bittar GT, Graff-Radford SB. The effects of streptomycin/lidocaine block on trigeminal neuralgia: a double blind crossover placebo controlled study. *Headache* 1993;33:155–160.
28. Flickinger JC, Pollock BE, Kondziolka D, *et al.* Does increased nerve length within the treatment volume improve trigeminal neuralgia radiosurgery? A prospective double–blind, randomized study. *Int J Radiation Oncology Biol Phys* 2001;51:449–54.
29. Walker JB, Akhanjee LK, Cooney MM, et al. Laser therapy for pain of trigeminal neuralgia. *Clin J Pain* 1988;3:183–187.

Trigeminal neuralgia

Joanna M Zakrzewska
Barts and the London Queen Mary's
School of Medicine and Dentistry
London
UK

Benjamin C Lopez
Mr
Department of Neurosurgery
Barts and the London NHS Trust
London
UK

Competing interests: JMZ has been reimbursed by GlaxoWellcome (manufacturer of lamotrigine) for attending a conference and for conducting the lamotrigine RCT. BCL none declared.

Aphthous ulcers (recurrent)

Search date December 2002

Stephen Porter and Crispian Scully CBE

QUESTIONS

INTERVENTIONS

Key Messages

- **Chlorhexidine (but no effect on recurrence rates)** RCTs found that chlorhexidine gluconate mouth rinses increased the number of ulcer free days and reduced the severity of each episode of ulceration compared with control preparations, but did not affect the incidence of recurrent ulceration.
- **Topical corticosteroids** Nine small RCTs found no consistent difference in the incidence of new ulcers between topical corticosteroids and control preparations. They found weak evidence that topical corticosteroids may reduce the duration of ulcers and hasten pain relief.
- **Hexitidine** One RCT found no significant difference in the incidence or duration of ulceration between hexitidine mouthwash and a control mouthwash.

Clin Evid 2003;10:1610–1616.

DEFINITION Recurrent aphthous ulcers are superficial and rounded, with painful mouth ulcers usually occurring in recurrent bouts at intervals of a few days to a few months.[1]

INCIDENCE/ PREVALENCE The point prevalence of recurrent aphthous ulcers in Swedish adults has been reported as 2%.[1] Prevalence may be 5–10% in some groups of children. Up to 66% of young adults give a history consistent with recurrent aphthous ulceration.[1]

AETIOLOGY/ RISK FACTORS The causes of aphthous ulcers remain unknown. Associations with haematinic deficiency, infections, gluten sensitive enteropathy, food sensitivities, and psychological stress have rarely been confirmed. Similar ulcers are seen in Behçet's syndrome.

PROGNOSIS About 80% of people with recurrent aphthous ulcers develop a few ulcers smaller than 1 cm in diameter that heal within 5–14 days without scarring (the pattern known as minor aphthous ulceration). The episodes recur typically after an interval of 1–4 months. One in 10 sufferers has a more severe form (major aphthous ulceration), with lesions larger than 1 cm that may recur after a shorter interval and can cause scarring. Likewise, 1/10 people with such recurrent ulceration may have multiple minute ulcers (herpetiform ulceration).

AIMS OF INTERVENTION To reduce pain, frequency, and duration of ulceration with minimal adverse effects.

OUTCOMES Number of new ulcers appearing within a specified period, usually 4–8 weeks; ulcer day index (the sum of the number of ulcers each day over a period, usually 4–8 weeks, which indicates the severity of the episode and reflects the mean prevalence and duration of ulcers); symptom score based on subjective pain severity recorded in categories on a questionnaire (e.g. from 0–3, ranging from no pain to severe pain) or on a 10 cm visual analogue scale; mean duration of individual ulcers (difficult to determine because of uncertainty in detecting the point of complete resolution); number of ulcer free days during a specified period; preference of people for one treatment over another. The diameter of lesions is a proxy measure of these clinical outcomes.

METHODS *Clinical Evidence* search and appraisal December 2002.

QUESTION What are the effects of treatments for recurrent aphthous ulcers?

OPTION TOPICAL CORTICOSTEROIDS

Nine small RCTs found no consistent effect of topical corticosteroids on the incidence of new ulcers compared with control preparations. They found weak evidence that topical corticosteroids may reduce the duration of ulcers and hasten pain relief without causing notable local or systemic adverse effects.

Benefits: We found no systematic review, but found nine RCTs of corticosteroids versus placebo that reported relevant clinical outcomes in people with recurrent aphthous ulcers.[2–9] Overall, one RCT found larger effect sizes than the others.[2] **Incidence of new ulcers:** Five randomised crossover RCTs (102 people) found inconsistent effects on the incidence of new ulcers (see table 1, p 1615).[2,4,5] **Ulcer duration:** Six RCTs reported data on ulcer duration, but the data were not comparable.[3,4,6–9] Four RCTs reported the mean duration of ulcers and found no consistent effect (see table 1, p 1615).[3,4,7,9] One RCT found topical steroids versus control reduced ulcer duration (mean ulcer duration ≤ 6 days, AR 25/33 [76%] people receiving topical steroid *v* 14/30 [47%] with control preparations; ARI 29%, 95% CI 5% to 43%; RR 1.62, 95% CI 1.06 to 2.49; NNT 3, 95% CI 2 to 20).[6] One crossover RCT found that 13/15 people had shorter mean duration with topical steroid versus the control preparation.[8] **Ulcer days index:** Four RCTs found that topical steroids reduced the number of ulcer days compared with control;[2,4,5,7] the reduction was significant in two of the RCTs (see table 1, p 1615). **Symptom scores:** Four RCTs reported symptom scores with topical steroids versus control, but all presented their results in different ways.[6–9] The first RCT found that more people using steroids versus a control preparation had symptom relief (29/33 [88%] *v* 18/30 [60%]; ARI 27%, 95% CI 5% to 43%; RRI 46%, 95% CI 19% to 91%; NNT 4, 95% CI 2 to 20).[6] The second RCT (a crossover trial) found that topical steroids versus a control preparation reduced symptom scores but the results were not significant (2.77 *v* 3.54).[7] Another crossover trial found that 11/15 people using topical steroid versus the control preparation had lower pain scores.[8] A third crossover trial found that the pain score fell with time whether using topical steroids or control applications, but that the rate of fall was significantly faster when using topical steroids.[9] **User preference:** Two crossover trials found that more users preferred topical steroids than control preparations (20/26 [77%] in one study[4] and 10/17 [59%] in the other[6]).

Harms: All nine RCTs reported no serious adverse effects. Long term use of corticosteroid mouth rinses was occasionally associated with oral candidiasis (rate not specified). Limited studies of adrenal function found no evidence that 0.05% fluocinonide in adhesive paste and betamethasone-17-valerate mouth rinse caused adrenal suppression.[8,15] One RCT reported adrenal suppression in one man using betamethasone disodium phosphate.[5]

Comment: The trials differed in many ways: selection of people, type of topical corticosteroid and formulation used, control preparation used (although this was usually a base without topical steroid), duration of treatment, reported outcomes, and design (double or single blind, parallel group or crossover, use of washout period or not). Withdrawal rates were high. Most people in the trials had more severe ulceration than the average person with recurrent aphthous ulceration.

OPTION CHLORHEXIDINE AND SIMILAR AGENTS

RCTs found that chlorhexidine gluconate mouth rinses increased the number of ulcer free days and reduced the severity of each episode of ulceration, but did not effect the incidence of recurrent ulceration. Single RCTs found no significant benefit from hexitidine mouthwash or a proprietary antibacterial mouthwash compared with control mouthwashes.

Benefits: We found no systematic review but found five RCTs (203 people with recurrent aphthous ulceration) of chlorhexidine gluconate or similar preparations versus assumed inactive control preparations.[10–14] Four of the RCTs used a crossover design with a randomised sequence comparing a control preparation versus 1% chlorhexidine gel,[10] 0.2% chlorhexidine gel,[11] 0.2% chlorhexidine mouthwash,[12] or 0.1% hexetidine mouthwash.[13] One trial was a parallel group RCT of a proprietary antibacterial rinse versus a hydroalcoholic control.[14] **Incidence of ulceration:** All RCTs reported the number of ulcers as either the total number of ulcers or the number of new ulcers with each treatment (see table 1, p 1615). Only one of the five RCTs found that active treatment significantly reduced the number of ulcers.[11] Three RCTs found that the number of ulcers fell during the course of the study, irrespective of the treatment received.[12–14] The crossover trial that found a significant difference in numbers of ulcers did not overtly account for this effect.[11] However, data were available from only 12/26 people who were recruited, and it is not clear if there was a balanced sequencing of active and placebo treatments among these people. **Duration of ulceration:** The mean duration of individual ulcers was reported in four of the RCTs (see table 1, p 1615).[10,12–14] The mean duration of individual ulcers was reduced by active treatment in all four RCTs, but the difference was significant in only one RCT and the mean difference was less than 1 day in the others. **Ulcer days index:** Three RCTs reported the ulcer days index.[11–13] Both studies of chlorhexidine versus control found significant reduction in the ulcer day index (see table 1, p 1615).[11,12] One of these RCTs found that chlorhexidine versus an inert preparation significantly increased the number of ulcer free days from a mean of 17.5 to 22.9 over 6 weeks — an extra 5.4 ulcer free days per 6 weeks of treatment.[12] Another RCT found that hexitidine had no significant effect.[13] **Severity of pain:** All five RCTs reported severity scores.[10–14] Two RCTs found that chlorhexidine significantly reduced the mean severity of pain compared with an inert preparation.[10,11] One RCT of a proprietary antibacterial mouthwash versus the alcohol-containing control preparation found no significant difference between the treatment groups, but found a large improvement in clinical outcomes in both groups compared with baseline levels.[14] The evidence relating to other antibacterial agents such as triclosan will be reviewed in future *Clinical Evidence* updates.

Harms: The RCTs reported few adverse events. One RCT found that chlorhexidine had a bitter taste and was associated with brown staining of teeth and tongue and with nausea.[11]

Comment: Four of the RCTs used a crossover design. A consistent observation was that outcomes improved during the course of the trials irrespective of the treatment received. One of the studies did not make clear if the effect of sequencing had been allowed for.[11] The withdrawal rates in the crossover trials were high. The parallel group trial had fewer withdrawals: 106 people with recurrent aphthous ulceration were recruited and 96 completed the study. Analysis was not by intention to treat and the method of randomisation was not specified.[14] People recruited to the trials might not be typical of the average person with recurrent aphthous ulceration.

Aphthous ulcers (recurrent)

REFERENCES

1. Porter SR, Scully C, Pedersen A. Recurrent aphthous stomatitis. *Crit Rev Oral Biol Med* 1998;9:306–321.
2. Cooke BED, Armitage P. Recurrent Mikulicz's aphthae treatment with topical hydrocortisone hemisuccinate sodium. *BMJ* 1960;1:764–766.
3. Walter T, McFall JR. Effect of flurandrenolone on oral aphthae. *J Periodontol* 1968;39:364–365.
4. Browne RM, Fox EC, Anderson RJ. Topical triamcinolone acetonide in recurrent aphthous stomatitis. *Lancet* 1968;1:565–567.
5. MacPhee IT, Sircus W, Farmer ED, et al. Use of steroids in treatment of aphthous ulceration. *BMJ* 1968;2:147–149.
6. Merchant HW, Gangarosa LP, Glassman AB, et al. Betamethasone-17-benzoate in the treatment of recurrent aphthous ulcers. *Oral Surg Oral Med Oral Pathol* 1978;45:870–875.
7. Pimlott SJ, Walker DM. A controlled clinical trial of the efficacy of topically applied fluocinonide in the treatment of recurrent aphthous ulceration. *Br Dent J* 1983;154:174–177.
8. Thompson AC, Nolan A, Lamey P-J. Minor aphthous oral ulceration: a double-blind cross-over study of beclomethasone dipropionate aerosol spray. *Scot Med J* 1989;34:531–532.
9. Miles DA, Bricker SL, Razmus TF, et al. Triamcinolone acetonide versus chlorhexidine for treatment of recurrent stomatitis. *Oral Surg Oral Med Oral Pathol* 1993;75:397–402.
10. Addy M, Carpenter R, Roberts WR. Management of recurrent aphthous ulceration — a trial of chlorhexidine gluconate gel. *Br Dent J* 1976;141:118–120.
11. Addy M. Hibitane in the treatment of recurrent aphthous ulceration. *J Clin Periodontol* 1977;4:108–116.
12. Hunter L, Addy M. Chlorhexidine gluconate mouthwash in the management of minor aphthous stomatitis. *Br Dent J* 1987;162:106–110.
13. Chadwick B, Addy M, Walker DM. Hexetidine mouthrinse in the management of minor aphthous ulceration and as an adjunct to oral hygiene. *Br Dent J* 1991;171:83–87.
14. Meiller TF, Kutcher MJ, Overholser CD, et al. Effect of an antimicrobial mouthrinse on recurrent aphthous ulcerations. *Oral Surg Oral Med Oral Pathol* 1991;72:425–429.
15. Lehner T, Lyne C. Adrenal function during topical oral corticosteroid treatment. *BMJ* 1969;4:138–141.

Stephen Porter
Professor of Oral Medicine

Crispian Scully CBE
Dean and Professor of Special Needs Dentistry

Eastman Dental Institute for Oral Health Care Sciences
UCL, University of London
London
UK

Competing interests: None declared.

TABLE 1 Effects of treatments on different outcomes: results of RCTs (see text, p 1611).

Intervention	Ref	Participants	Treatment duration (weeks)	Outcomes		Effect (%)* (significance)
				Treatment	Control	
Incidence new ulcers (ulcers/week): topical corticosteroids versus inert preparations	2	17	8	0.51	1.15	–55% (P < 0.05)
	4	26	8	0.84	0.94	–11% (NS)
	5 pilot	8	4	2.07	1.85	+12% (NS)
	5 main	31†	4	0.73	0.82	–11% (NS)
	5	20	6	1.27	1.92	+6% (NS)
Mean ulcer duration (days): topical corticosteroids versus inert preparations	3	50	Until complete healing	6.00	6.00	0% (NS)
	4	26	8	8.07	8.94	–10% (NS)
	7	20	6	4.93	7.83	–37% (P < 0.001)
	9	19	12	5.93	5.92	0% (NS)
Ulcer days index: topical corticosteroids versus inert preparations	2	17	8	26.30	65.90	–60% (P < 0.01)
	4	26	8	58.30	71.30	–18% (NS)
	5 main	25	4	24.00	30.70	–22% (NS)
	7	20	6	48.30	70.60	–32% (P < 0.05)
Number of ulcers (ulcers/person/week): topical antibacterial versus presumed inert preparations	10	20	5	1.04	1.40	NS
	11	12	5	0.60	1.02	P < 0.05
	12	38	6	1.26	1.38	NS
	13	37	6	1.48	1.39	NS
	14	96	26	0.09	0.13	NS

TABLE 1 continued

Mean duration of ulcers (days): topical antibacterial versus inert preparation	10	20	5	4.80	7.80	P < 0.01
	12	38	6	5.02	5.78	NS
	13	37	6	6.64	6.80	NS
	14	96	26	Median fall in ulcer duration from start of trial 2.42 days	Median fall in ulcer duration from start of trial 1.58 days	NS
Ulcer days index: topical antibacterial versus inert preparations	11	12	5	9.50	17.00	P < 0.05
	12	38	6	42.80	52.30	P < 0.05
	13	37	6	79.70	65.70	NS

*Defined as difference between outcome measures for control and treatment, expressed as a fraction of the control.
†Each participant received one treatment for 4 weeks, a blank month, then another treatment with another drug. The trial compared an inert base, two local steroids and two other preparations. The figures given here are those during treatment with local steroids and with the inert base.
NS, not significant; ref, reference.

Burning mouth syndrome

Search date October 2002

John Buchanan and Joanna Zakrzewska

QUESTIONS

INTERVENTIONS

Key Messages

- **Cognitive behavioural therapy** One small RCT found that cognitive behavioural therapy in people with resistant burning mouth syndrome versus no cognitive behavioural therapy significantly reduced symptom intensity after 6 months.
- **Antidepressants; benzydamine hydrochloride; dietary supplementation; hormone replacement therapy in postmenopausal women** We found insufficient evidence on the effects of these interventions.

Burning mouth syndrome

DEFINITION Burning mouth syndrome is a psychogenic or idiopathic burning discomfort or pain affecting people with clinically normal oral mucosa in whom a medical or dental cause has been excluded.[1–3] Terms previously used to describe what is now called burning mouth syndrome include glossodynia, glossopyrosis, stomatodynia, stomatopyrosis, sore tongue, and oral dysaesthesia.[4] A survey of 669 men and 758 women randomly selected from 48 500 people aged between 20 and 69 years found that people with burning mouth also have subjective dryness (66%), take some form of medication (64%), report other systemic illnesses (57%), and have altered taste (11%).[5] Many studies of people with symptoms of burning mouth do not distinguish those with burning mouth syndrome (i.e. idiopathic disease) from those with other conditions (such as vitamin B deficiency), making results unreliable.

INCIDENCE/ PREVALENCE Burning mouth syndrome affects mainly women,[6–8] particularly after the menopause when its prevalence may be 18–33%.[9] One recent study in Sweden found a prevalence of 4% for the symptom of burning mouth without clinical abnormality of the oral mucosa (11/669 [2%] men, mean age 59 years; 42/758 [6%] women, mean age 57 years), with the highest prevalence (12%) in women aged 60–69 years.[5] Reported prevalence in general populations varies from 1%[10] to 15%.[6] Incidence and prevalence vary according to diagnostic criteria,[4] and many studies included people with the symptom of burning mouth rather than with burning mouth syndrome as defined above.

AETIOLOGY/ RISK FACTORS The cause is unknown, and we found no good aetiological studies. Hormonal disturbances associated with the menopause[7–9] and psychogenic factors (including anxiety, depression, stress, life events, personality disorders, and phobia of cancer) are possible causal factors.[11–13] Local and systemic factors (such as infections, allergies, ill fitting dentures,[12] hypersensitivity reactions,[14] and hormone and vitamin deficiencies[15–17]) may cause the symptom of burning mouth and should be excluded before diagnosing burning mouth syndrome.

PROGNOSIS We found no prospective cohort studies or other reliable evidence describing the natural history of burning mouth syndrome.[18] We found anecdotal reports of at least partial spontaneous remission in about half of people with burning mouth syndrome within 6–7 years.[12]

AIMS OF INTERVENTION To alleviate symptoms, with minimal adverse effects.

OUTCOMES Self reported relief of symptoms (burning mouth, altered taste, dry mouth); incidence and severity of anxiety and depression; quality of life using a validated ordinal scale.

METHODS *Clinical Evidence* search and appraisal October 2002. Keywords: burning mouth, burning mouth syndrome, dysaesthesia or dysaesthesia, stomatodynia or glossopyrosis, sore tongue, glossodynia, or glossalgia.

QUESTION What are the effects of treatments?

OPTION COGNITIVE BEHAVIOURAL THERAPY

One small RCT found that cognitive behavioural therapy relieved symptoms of burning mouth syndrome.

Benefits: We found one systematic review (search date 2000, 5 RCTs, 1 controlled trial, 384 people).[19] The review identified one small RCT (30 people with resistant burning mouth syndrome), which compared cognitive behavioural therapy (12–15 sessions of 1 h/wk) versus a control group who received similar attention but without the cognitive behavioural therapy sessions. It found that cognitive behavioural therapy significantly reduced the intensity of symptoms (measured on a visual analogue scale ranging from 1 = endurable to 7 = unendurable), and was still significant at 6 months' follow up (mean pretreatment score: 5.0 with cognitive behavioural therapy *v* 4.3 with placebo; mean score 6 months after treatment: 1.4 with cognitive behavioural therapy *v* 4.7 with placebo; $P < 0.001$; 4/15 [27%] with cognitive behavioural therapy *v* 0/15 [0%] with placebo people symptom free 6 months after treatment).[19]

Harms: The RCT provided no information on adverse effects.[19]

Comment: The trial was small and individual characteristics of the two groups were not described; therefore, the groups may not have been comparable. The visual analogue scale for assessing oral burning was not validated.[19]

OPTION HORMONE REPLACEMENT THERAPY IN POSTMENOPAUSAL WOMEN

We found insufficient evidence on the effects of hormone replacement therapy in postmenopausal women with burning mouth syndrome.

Benefits: We found one systematic review (search date 2000, 5 RCTs, 1 controlled trial, 384 people), which identified no RCTs of sufficient quality.[19]

Harms: Adverse effects of hormone replacement therapy are well documented (see oestrogens under menopausal symptoms, p 2138).

Comment: We found three non-randomised intervention studies with no clear diagnostic criteria or outcome measures.[20–22]

OPTION DIETARY SUPPLEMENTS

We found insufficient evidence from two small RCTs to draw reliable conclusions about the effects of alphalipoic acid in people with burning mouth syndrome. We found no RCTs evaluating other vitamin or coenzyme supplements.

Benefits: We found one systematic review (search date 2000)[19] and one subsequent RCT.[23] The review identified one RCT (42 people with burning mouth syndrome) comparing alphalipoic acid (600 mg/day for 20 days followed by 200 mg/day for 10 days) versus placebo (cellulose starch 100 mg/day for 30 days). It found that alphalipoic acid significantly increased the number of people reported to have "slight" or "decided" improvement in symptoms (AR 16/21 [76%] with alphalipoic acid *v* 3/14 [21%] with placebo; RR 0.28, 95% CI 0.13 to 0.61; NNT 2, 95% CI 1 to 3).[19] The subsequent RCT (60 people) compared alphalipoic acid (200 mg 3 times daily) versus placebo. After 2 months' treatment, it found that alphalipoic acid significantly increased the number of people reported to have "slight" or "decided" improvement, or complete resolution in symptoms (AR 29/30 [97%] with alphalipoic acid *v* 12/30 [40%] with placebo; $P < 0.0001$).[23] We found no RCTs in people with vitamin B deficiency and symptoms of burning mouth (see comment below).

Harms: The RCTs did not report adverse effects.[19,23]

Comment: The RCTs of alphalipoic acid were not clearly reported as blinded, and the subjective nature of the outcome used means that the results should be interpreted with caution.[19,23] People with vitamin B group deficiencies and symptoms of burning mouth should no longer be classified as having burning mouth syndrome (see definition, p 1618). One case control study in 70 people found that people with symptoms of burning mouth were more likely to have vitamin B deficiency (28/70 [40%] with vitamin B deficiency *v* 6/80 [8%] with no vitamin B deficiency).[16] One study of 16 people with vitamin deficiencies given vitamins or placebo found no improvement in symptoms.[17]

OPTION ANTIDEPRESSANTS

We found insufficient evidence on the effects of antidepressants in people with burning mouth syndrome.

Benefits: We found one systematic review (search date 2000).[19] **Clomipramine and mianserin:** The review identified one short term RCT (253 people with chronic idiopathic pain syndrome, including 77 people with burning mouth syndrome) comparing clomipramine versus mianserin versus placebo for 6 weeks.[19] After 6 weeks there was no significant improvement in any group. **Trazodone:** The review identified one double blind RCT (37 women with burning mouth syndrome) comparing trazodone (200 mg/day) versus placebo.[19] After 8 weeks there was no significant difference in pain or related symptoms between groups measured on a visual analogue scale (0 mm = best score and 100 mm = worst score). The mean pain on a visual analogue scale decreased in both groups at 8 weeks (from 59 to 45 with trazodone and from 47 to 34 with placebo). **Selective serotonin reuptake inhibitors versus amisulpride:** We found one small RCT (76 people), which found no significant difference among sertraline (50 mg/day), paroxetine (20 mg/day), and amisulpride (50 mg/day) for pain score at 8 weeks (pain assessed by 10 point visual analogue scale [higher score indicating more severe pain]; mean score at 8 weeks about 3 points in all groups; reduction in score from baseline about 4 points in all groups; P value not stated). However, the study may have lacked power to detect clinically important differences among treatments and lacked a placebo comparison.[24]

Harms: The first RCT did not report adverse effects.[19] In the second RCT, adverse effects caused 7/18 (39%) people taking trazodone to withdraw from the trial compared with 2/19 (10%) taking placebo. Adverse effects reported with trazodone were dizziness (11 people) and drowsiness (9 people).[19] Adverse effects of clomipramine, mianserin, and other antidepressants are documented elsewhere (see depressive disorders, p 1121). The RCT comparing selective serotonin reuptake inhibitors and amisulpride reported no serious adverse effects in any treatment group.[24]

Comment: The trial of clomipramine and mianserin versus placebo was too small to exclude an effect of treatment, did not use adequate diagnostic criteria, was of short duration, and had limited follow up.[19] Therefore, it does not provide sufficient evidence to determine the role of antidepressants in treating burning mouth syndrome. Although the trial of trazodone versus placebo was well conducted and used several pertinent outcome measures, including psychological ones, it was too small and brief to detect clinically important effects.[19] In the RCT comparing selective serotonin reuptake inhibitors versus amisulpride, 34 people had a concurrent psychiatric diagnosis.[24] The widespread use of antidepressants in burning mouth syndrome may be because of their effects on neuropathic pain,[25] and the association of burning mouth syndrome with generalised anxiety disorder, depression, and adverse life events.[26]

OPTION BENZYDAMINE HYDROCHLORIDE

We found insufficient evidence on the effects of benzydamine hydrochloride in burning mouth syndrome.

Benefits: We found one systematic review (search date 2000, 5 RCTs, 1 CCT, 384 people),[19] which identified one small RCT (30 people with burning mouth syndrome) comparing benzydamine hydrochloride (15 mL of 0.15% for 1 min 3 times daily for 4 wks) versus placebo versus no treatment. It found no significant difference among groups for symptoms (using a visual analogue scale), but the trial was too small to exclude a clinically important difference.[19]

Harms: No adverse effects were reported.

Comment: Inclusion criteria were well defined. The trial was incompletely blinded because the third group received no treatment.

REFERENCES

1. Fox H. Burning tongue glossodynia. *N Y State J Med* 1935;35:881–884.
2. Zakrzewska JM. The burning mouth syndrome remains an enigma. *Pain* 1995;62:253–257.
3. Van der Waal I. *The burning mouth syndrome.* 1st ed. Copenhagen: Munksgaard, 1990.
4. Merksey H, Bogduk N, eds. *Classification of chronic pain.* 2nd ed. Seattle: International Association for the Study of Pain Press, 1994.
5. Bergdahl M, Bergdahl J. Burning mouth syndrome: prevalence and associated factors. *J Oral Pathol Med* 1999;28:350–354.
6. Tammiala-Salonen T, Hiidenkarii T, Parvinen T. Burning mouth in a Finnish adult population. *Community Dent Oral Epidemiol* 1993;21:67–71.
7. Basker RM, Sturdee DW, Davenport JC. Patients with burning mouths. A clinical investigation of causative factors, including the climacteric and diabetes. *Br Dent J* 1978;145:9–16.
8. Grushka M. Clinical features of burning mouth syndrome. *Oral Surg Oral Med Oral Pathol Oral Radiol Endod* 1987;63:30–36.
9. Wardrop RW, Hailes J, Burger H, et al. Oral discomfort at the menopause. *Oral Surg Oral Med Oral Pathol Oral Radiol Endod* 1989;67:535–540.
10. Lipton JA, Ship JA, Larach-Robinson D. Estimated prevalence and distribution of reported orofacial pain in the United States. *J Am Dent Assoc* 1993;124:115–121.
11. Rojo L, Silvestre FJ, Bagan JV, et al. Psychiatric morbidity in burning mouth syndrome. Psychiatric

interview versus depression and anxiety scales. *Oral Surg Oral Med Oral Pathol Oral Radiol Endod* 1993;75:308–311.
12. Grushka M, Sessle BJ. Burning mouth syndrome. *Dent Clin North Am* 1991;35:171–184.
13. Lamey PJ, Lamb AB. The usefulness of the HAD scale in assessing anxiety in patients with burning mouth syndrome. *Oral Surg Oral Med Oral Pathol Oral Radiol Endod* 1989;67:390–392.
14. Bergdahl J, Anneroth G, Anneroth I. Clinical study of patients with burning mouth. *Scand J Dent Res* 1994;102:299–305.
15. Maragou P, Ivanyi L. Serum zinc levels in patients with burning mouth syndrome. *Oral Surg Oral Med Oral Pathol Oral Radiol Endod* 1991;71:447–450.
16. Lamey PJ, Allam BF. Vitamin status of patients with burning mouth syndrome and the response to replacement therapy. *Br Dent J* 1986;168:81–84.
17. Hugoson A, Thorstensson B. Vitamin B status and response to replacement therapy in patients with burning mouth syndrome. *Acta Odontol Scand* 1991;49:367–375.
18. Zakrzewska JM, Hamlyn PJ. Facial pain. In: Crombie IK, Croft PR, Linton SJ, et al, eds. *Epidemiology of pain.* Seattle: International Association for the Study of Pain Press, 1999:177–202.
19. Zakrewska JM, Glenny AM, Forsell H. Interventions for the treatment of burning mouth syndrome (Cochrane Review). In: The Cochrane Library, Issue 3, 2001. Oxford: Update Software. Search date 2000; primary sources Medline, Embase, The Cochrane Library, and The Cochrane Oral Health Group's Specialised Register.
20. Pisanty S, Rafaely B, Polshuk WZ. The effects of steroid hormones on buccal mucosa of menopausal women. *Oral Surg Oral Med Oral Pathol Oral Radiol Endod* 1975;40:346–353.
21. Ferguson MM, Carter J, Boyle P, et al. Oral complaints related to climacteric symptoms in oophorectomized women. *J R Soc Med* 1981;74:492–497.
22. Forabosco A, Crisculo M, Coukos G, et al. Efficacy of hormone replacement therapy in postmenopausal women with oral discomfort. *Oral Surg Oral Med Oral Pathol Oral Radiol Endod* 1992;73:570–574.
23. Femiano F, Scully C. Burning mouth syndrome (BMS): double blind controlled study of alpha-lipoic acid (thioctic acid) therapy. *J Oral Pathol Med* 2002:31:267–269.
24. Maina G, Vitalucci A, Gandolfo S, et al. Comparative efficacy of SSRIs and amisulpiride in burning mouth syndrome: A single–blind study. *J Clin Psychiatry* 2002;63:38–43
25. McQuay HJ, Tramer M, Nye BA, et al. A systematic review of antidepressants in neuropathic pain. *Pain* 1996;68:217–227.
26. Bogetto F, Maina G, Ferro G, et al. Psychiatric comorbidity in patients with burning mouth syndrome. *Psychosom Med* 1998;60:378–385.

John Buchanan
Specialist Registrar/Honorary Lecturer in Oral Medicine
The Eastman Dental Institute for Dental Health Care Sciences University College London
London
UK

Joanna Zakrzewska
Senior Lecturer/Honorary Consultant in Oral Medicine
St Bartholomew's and The Royal London School of Medicine and Dentistry
London
UK

Competing interests: None declared.

Candidiasis (oropharyngeal)

Search date February 2003

Caroline Pankhurst

QUESTIONS

INTERVENTIONS

PREVENTION

Beneficial

Antifungal prophylaxis in people undergoing cancer treatments 1626
Antifungal prophylaxis in people with advanced HIV disease .1633

Likely to be beneficial

Antifungal prophylaxis in immunocompromised infants and children 1629

Unknown effectiveness

Antifungal prophylaxis in people receiving tissue transplants.1627
Continuous prophylaxis versus intermittent treatment in people with HIV infection and acute episodes of oropharyngeal candidiasis (in preventing antifungal resistance). 1637
Preventive interventions in people with diabetes. 1631

TREATMENT

Beneficial

Antifungal treatment in immunocompetent and immunocompromised infants and children 1629
Oral suspension of systemically absorbed azoles in people with HIV infection 1636

Unknown effectiveness

Antifungal treatment for denture stomatitis 1631
Antifungal treatment in people undergoing chemotherapy, radiotherapy, or both treatments for cancer 1628
Denture hygiene 1632
Treatments in people with diabetes mellitus 1631

To be covered in future updates

Prevention and treatment in neonates
Treatment of systemic candidiasis

Key Messages

Prevention

- **Antifungal prophylaxis in people undergoing cancer treatments** One systematic review in people undergoing treatment for cancer found that antifungal drugs reduced the risk of oropharyngeal candidiasis compared with placebo or no treatment. One review found that drugs that were absorbed or partially absorbed via the gastrointestinal tract were more effective than non-absorbed drugs in preventing oral candidiasis.

Candidiasis (oropharyngeal)

- **Antifungal prophylaxis in people with advanced HIV disease** RCTs in people with HIV infection have found that daily or weekly antifungal prophylaxis with fluconazole, itraconazole, or nystatin reduces incidence and relapse of oropharyngeal candidiasis compared with placebo.
- **Antifungal prophylaxis in immunocompromised infants and children** One large RCT in immunocompromised infants and children found that fluconazole reduced the incidence of oropharyngeal candidiasis compared with oral nystatin or amphotericin B.
- **Antifungal prophylaxis in people receiving tissue transplants** Two small RCTs in people with liver transplant found no significant difference in the risk of oropharyngeal candidiasis between nystatin and fluconazole or clotrimazole. However, the trials may have lacked power to exclude clinically important differences. We found insufficient evidence from two RCTs about the effects of prophylactic chlorhexidine mouth rinse with or without nystatin compared with placebo in people receiving bone marrow transplant.
- **Continuous prophylaxis versus intermittent treatment in people with HIV infection and acute episodes of oropharyngeal candidiasis (in preventing antifungal resistance)** One RCT in people with HIV infection and acute episodes of oropharyngeal candidiasis found no significant difference in emergence of antifungal resistance between continuous antifungal prophylaxis with fluconazole and intermittent antifungal treatment with fluconazole.
- **Preventive interventions in people with diabetes** We found no systematic review or RCTs.

Treatments

- **Antifungal treatment in immunocompetent and immunocompromised infants and children** RCTs found that miconazole and fluconazole increased clinical cure of oropharyngeal candidiasis compared with nystatin in immunocompetent and immunocompromised infants and children.
- **Oral suspension of systemically absorbed azoles in people with HIV infection** RCTs have found that topical preparations of itraconazole, fluconazole, and clotrimazole effectively treat oropharyngeal candidiasis in people with HIV infection. One RCT found that fluconazole significantly reduced symptoms and signs of oropharyngeal candidiasis compared with topical nystatin.
- **Antifungal treatment for denture stomatitis** We found insufficient evidence from small RCTs to compare effects of antifungals versus placebo or versus each other for treating oropharyngeal candidiasis in people who wear dentures.
- **Antifungal treatment in people undergoing chemotherapy, radiotherapy, or both treatments for cancer** One systematic review found insufficient evidence from RCTs about the clinical effects of antifungals compared with placebo for treating oropharyngeal candidiasis in people undergoing chemotherapy or radiotherapy. It also found insufficient evidence about the effects of different antifungal agents or doses in people with oropharyngeal candidiasis who are receiving radiotherapy or chemotherapy.
- **Denture hygiene** We found insufficient evidence from RCTs to assess clinical effects on oropharyngeal candidiasis of mouth rinses, disinfectants, denture soaks, denture scrubbing, and microwave irradiation of dentures. Microwave treatment is not suitable for all dentures.
- **Treatments in people with diabetes mellitus** We found no RCTs assessing treatments for oral candidiasis in people with diabetes mellitus.

DEFINITION Oropharyngeal candidiasis is an opportunistic mucosal infection caused, in most cases, by *Candida albicans*. The four main types of oropharyngeal candidiasis are: (1) pseudomembranous (thrush), consisting of white discrete plaques on an erythematous background, located on the buccal mucosa, throat, tongue, or gingivae; (2) erythematous, consisting of smooth red patches on the hard or soft palate, dorsum of tongue, or buccal mucosa; (3) hyperplastic, consisting of white, firmly adherent patches or plaques, usually bilateral on the buccal mucosa; and (4) denture induced stomatitis, presenting as either a smooth or granular erythema confined to the denture bearing area of the hard palate and often associated with an angular cheilitis.[1] Symptoms vary, ranging from none to a sore and painful mouth with a burning tongue and altered taste. Oropharyngeal candidiasis can impair speech, nutritional intake, and quality of life.

INCIDENCE/ PREVALENCE Candida species are commensals in the gastrointestinal tract. Transmission occurs directly between infected people or on fomites (objects that can harbour pathogenic organisms). Candida is found in the mouth of 31–60% of healthy people.[2] Denture stomatitis associated with Candida is prevalent in 65% of denture wearers.[2] Oropharyngeal candidiasis affects 15–60% of people with haematological or oncological malignancies during periods of immunosuppression.[3] Oropharyngeal candidiasis occurs in 7–48% of people with HIV infection and in over 90% of those with advanced disease. In severely immunosuppressed people, relapse rates are high (30–50%) and usually occur within 14 days of stopping treatment.[4]

AETIOLOGY/ RISK FACTORS Risk factors associated with symptomatic oropharyngeal candidiasis include local or systemic immunosuppression, haematological disorders, broad spectrum antibiotic use, inhaled or systemic steroids, xerostomia, diabetes, and wearing dentures, obturators, or orthodontic appliances.[1,5] The same strain may persist for months or years in the absence of infection. In people with HIV infection, there is no direct correlation between the number of organisms and the presence of clinical disease. Symptomatic oropharyngeal candidiasis associated with *in vitro* resistance to fluconazole occurs in 5% of people with advanced HIV disease.[6] Resistance to azole antifungals is associated with severe immunosuppression ($\leq$ 50 CD4 cells/mm^3), more episodes treated with antifungal drugs, and longer median duration of systemic azole treatment.[7]

PROGNOSIS Untreated candidiasis persists for months or years unless associated risk factors are treated or eliminated. In neonates, spontaneous cure of oropharyngeal candidiasis usually occurs after 3–8 weeks.

AIMS OF INTERVENTION To resolve signs and symptoms of oropharyngeal candidiasis; to prevent or delay relapse in immunocompromised people; and to minimise drug induced resistance, with minimum adverse effects.

Candidiasis (oropharyngeal)

OUTCOMES Resolution of signs and symptoms; clinical cure; rate of recurrence on the basis of scoring of signs and symptoms. Many RCTs report the results of mycological culture but, whenever possible, this review has not used these intermediate outcomes because the relation between the clinical and mycological culture findings is uncertain.

METHODS *Clinical Evidence* search and appraisal February 2003 including a search for observational studies on dental hygiene. This was supplemented by a search of the author's library, selecting publications in English from 1975–2003. We included only systematic reviews and RCTs that specified oropharyngeal candidiasis in the protocol design and outcome measurements. RCTs dealing with oesophagitis and invasive, systemic candidal infections were excluded.

QUESTION **What are the effects of interventions to prevent and treat oropharyngeal candidiasis in adults receiving treatment causing immunosuppression?**

OPTION **ANTIFUNGAL PROPHYLAXIS IN PEOPLE RECEIVING CANCER TREATMENTS**

One systematic review found that absorbed antifungal drugs reduce the risk of oropharyngeal candidiasis compared with placebo or unabsorbed antifungals. It found that partially absorbed antifungal drugs reduce the risk of oropharyngeal candidiasis compared with placebo; however, there was significant heterogeneity among studies. The systematic review found no significant difference in adverse events between absorbed antifungal drugs and placebo or no treatment.

Benefits: We found one systematic review (search date 2001, 27 RCTS, 4137 people receiving chemotherapy or radiotherapy for cancer) that compared oral and topical antifungal prophylaxis versus placebo, no treatment, or another active intervention.[8] The drugs were categorised by absorption from the gastrointestinal tract. **Absorbed antifungals versus placebo:** The review found that absorbed antifungal drugs (ketoconazole, itraconazole, fluconazole) significantly reduced the risk of oral candidiasis compared with placebo or no drug treatment (7 RCTs; 1153 people; RR 0.45, 95% CI 0.32 to 0.64).[8] **Partially absorbed antifungals versus placebo:** The review found that partially absorbed antifungal drugs (miconazole, clotrimazole) significantly reduced the risk of oral candidiasis compared with placebo or no drug treatment (4 RCTs; 292 people; RR 0.13, 95% CI 0.06 to 0.27).[8] **Unabsorbed antifungals versus placebo:** The review found that there was no significant difference in the risk of oral candidiasis between unabsorbed drugs (nystatin alone, nystatin plus chlorhexidine, amphotericin B alone, or amphotericin B combined with nystatin, norfloxacin, natamycin, thymostimulin, or chlorhexidine) and placebo (8 RCTs; 382 people; RR 0.68, 95% CI 0.46 to 1.02).[8] However, the review found significant heterogeneity in the included studies ($P < 0.001$). **Absorbed versus unabsorbed antifungals:** The review found that absorbed antifungal drugs reduced the risk of oral candidiasis compared with unabsorbed antifungal drugs (7 RCTs; 2014 people; RR 0.40, 95% CI 0.21 to 0.76).[8]

Harms: The systematic review found no significant difference in adverse events between absorbed antifungal drugs and placebo (62/437 [14%] with absorbed antifungals *v* 52/434 [12%] with placebo; RR 1.18, 95% CI 0.84 to 1.66). The most common adverse events were abdominal pain, nausea, vomiting, and rash.[8]

Comment: None.

OPTION ANTIFUNGAL PROPHYLAXIS IN ADULTS WHO HAVE RECEIVED TISSUE TRANSPLANTS

Two small RCTs in people with liver transplant found no significant difference in the risk of oropharyngeal candidiasis between nystatin and fluconazole or clotrimazole. However, the trials may have lacked power to exclude clinically important differences. We found insufficient evidence from two RCTs about effects of prophylactic chlorhexidine mouth rinse with or without nystatin compared with placebo in people receiving bone marrow transplant.

Benefits: We found no systematic review. **In people receiving liver transplant:** We found two small RCTs in people with liver transplant comparing different antifungal agents for preventing oropharyngeal candidiasis.[9,10] The first RCT (143 people) found no significant difference in the risk of oropharyngeal candidiasis between fluconazole and nystatin at 28 days (rate of oropharyngeal candidiasis: 8/76 [11%] with fluconazole *v* 14/67 [21%] with nystatin; significance not stated).[9] The second RCT (34 people) found no significant difference in the risk of oropharyngeal candidiasis between clotrimazole and nystatin during hospital stay after transplantation (rate of oropharyngeal candidiasis: 1/17 [6%] with clotrimazole *v* 1/17 [6%] with nystatin; significance not stated).[10] However, the RCTs may have lacked power to exclude clinically important differences. **In people receiving bone marrow transplant:** We found two RCTs in people with neutropenia who had received bone marrow transplants.[11,12] The first RCT (51 people) found that chlorhexidine significantly reduced the risk of oropharyngeal candidiasis compared with placebo at 60 days (2/24 [8%] with chlorhexidine *v* 15/27 [56%] with placebo; ARR 47%, 95% CI 24% to 54%; RR 0.15, 95% CI 0.03 to 0.57; NNT 2, 95% CI 2 to 4).[11] The second RCT (86 adults with leukaemia and bone marrow transplant) found no significant difference in the development of oropharyngeal candidiasis between rinses containing saline alone, chlorhexidine alone, nystatin alone, or nystatin plus chlorhexidine (no statistical analysis available).[12]

Harms: There was no increased hepatotoxicity, cyclosporin interaction, or emergence of clinically relevant resistant strains reported in people receiving antifungal prophylaxis after liver transplantation.[9]

Comment: The RCTs of chlorhexidine found conflicting results about its effect on oropharyngeal candidiasis and mucositis,[11,12] but the second RCT had four parallel arms and was not powered to detect a clinically important difference.[12]

OPTION ANTIFUNGAL TREATMENT IN PEOPLE RECEIVING CHEMOTHERAPY AND RADIOTHERAPY

One systematic review found insufficient evidence from RCTs about clinical effects of antifungals compared with placebo for treating oropharyngeal candidiasis in people undergoing chemotherapy or radiotherapy, or about effects of different antifungal agents or doses in people with oropharyngeal candidiasis who are receiving radiotherapy or chemotherapy.

Benefits: We found one systematic review (search date 2001, 8 RCTs, 418 people with cancer receiving chemotherapy, radiotherapy, or both) that compared antifungal treatment of oral candidiasis versus placebo or another active intervention.[13] **Antifungals versus placebo:** The systematic review included two placebo controlled RCTs. The first small RCT (56 people) found that ketoconazole significantly decreased oral candidiasis compared with placebo at 14 days (persistence of oral candidiasis: 10/36 [28%] people with ketoconazole *v* 16/20 [80%] people with placebo; RR 0.35, 95% CI 0.20 to 0.61).[13] The second small RCT (13 people) included in the review found no significant difference in the proportion of people with oral candidiasis between clotrimazole and placebo.[13] The timing to outcome measurement was unclear.[13] This RCT may have lacked statistical power to detect a clinically important effect. **Versus different dosages:** One RCT (52 people) included in the review found no significant difference in clinically assessed cure of oral candidiasis between a 50 mg troche of clotrimazole and 10 mg of clotrimazole (persistence of oral candidiasis: 1/26 [4%] with clotrimazole 50 mg *v* 1/26 [4%] with clotrimazole 10 mg; RR 1.00, 95% CI 0.07 to 15.15).[13] The timing of outcome measurement was unclear.[13] **Absorbed drugs versus each other:** The systematic review found no significant difference in clinically assessed cure rates between different absorbed drugs (2 RCTs; persistence of oral candidiasis: 6/46 [13%] with fluconazole *v* 8/44 [18%] with ketoconazole/itraconazole; RR 0.72, 95% CI 0.27 to 1.88).[13] **Absorbed versus non-absorbed:** The review found three RCTs comparing absorbed and non-absorbed drugs. There was significant heterogeneity among the RCTs (P = 0.01).[13] One RCT found fluconazole significantly improved clinical cure rates compared with nystatin. One RCT found no significant difference between ketoconazole and nystatin in clinical or mycological cure rates. One RCT found fluconazole significantly improved cure rates when assessed clinically compared with amphotericin B.[13] Pooling the results of the three RCTs, the review found no significant difference between absorbed and non-absorbed drugs in clinical cure rates (3 RCTs; persistence of oral candidiasis: 16/105 [15%] with fluconazole/ketoconazole *v* 35/102 [34%] with amphotericin/nystatin; RR 0.50, 95% CI 0.11 to 2.27; random effects model). However, given the heterogeneity of the included studies, these results may not be robust. We found one subsequent RCT (268 people with head and neck cancer, 243 evaluated) which compared fluconazole oral suspension 50 mg once daily with amphotericin B oral suspension 0.5 mg three times daily for 7–14 days.[14] It found no significant difference in rates of clinical cure of oral candidiasis between fluconazole and amphotericin (clinical cure: 26/123 [21%] with fluconazole *v* 17/120 [14%] with amphotericin B).

Harms: The systematic review did not report on harms.[13]

Comment: In assessing outcomes, the review noted that few RCTs described the clinical criteria used.[13] The review concluded that there were insufficient trials to make strong recommendations for patient care, and that there was a need for further well designed, placebo controlled trials to assess the effectiveness of old and new interventions for treating oral candidiasis.[13]

QUESTION **What are the effects of interventions to prevent and treat oropharyngeal candidiasis in infants and children?**

OPTION **ANTIFUNGAL PREVENTION IN IMMUNOCOMPROMISED INFANTS AND CHILDREN**

One large RCT in immunocompromised infants and children has found that fluconazole significantly reduced the incidence of oropharyngeal candidiasis compared with oral nystatin, amphotericin B, or both. More people in the fluconazole group withdrew because of adverse events, though these numbers were small.

Benefits: We found no systematic review. We found one large, unblinded, multicentre RCT in 502 immunocompromised infants and children (aged 6 months to 17 years) about to undergo initial or repeat courses of chemotherapy or radiotherapy for haematological or oncological malignancies.[3] It found that fluconazole significantly reduced the incidence of oropharyngeal candidiasis compared with oral polyenes (nystatin, oral amphotericin B, or both) (3/236 [1%] with fluconazole *v* 15/249 [6%] with oral polyenes; RR 0.21, 95% CI 0.06 to 0.72; NNT 21, 95% CI 18 to 58).[3] Eighteen of the children from the multicentre RCT[3] were enrolled in a second, small RCT (50 children in total), which compared fluconazole versus oral nystatin for preventing oropharyngeal candidiasis.[15] The RCT found no significant difference in the incidence of oral candidiasis (2/25 [8%] with fluconazole *v* 3/25 [12%] with nystatin; P = 0.63). However, inclusion of pre-treated children may have biased results, and the study may have lacked power to exclude clinically important differences.

Harms: In the first RCT, adverse events caused 8/245 (3%) children on fluconazole to withdraw compared with 3/257 (1%) on oral polyenes.[3] In the second RCT, no children were withdrawn from the study, but three children treated with fluconazole reported nausea and abdominal discomfort and one reported pruritus.[15]

Comment: None.

OPTION **ANTIFUNGAL TREATMENT IN CHILDREN**

RCTs found that miconazole and fluconazole increased clinical cure of oropharyngeal candidiasis compared with nystatin in immunocompetent and immunocompromised infants and children.

Benefits: We found no systematic review. **Immunocompetent infants and children:** We found no placebo controlled RCTs. We found two RCTs in immunocompetent infants with oropharyngeal candidiasis, which compared miconazole gel and nystatin suspension and nystatin gel and one RCT which compared fluconazole and nystatin.[16–18] Both RCTs comparing miconazole and nystatin found that miconazole significantly increased the rate of clinical cure. The larger RCT (183 infants age < 1 year with signs of oropharyngeal candidiasis) found that miconazole gel had a significantly increased cure rate compared with nystatin (at day 5: cure rate 83/98 [85%] with miconazole gel 25 mg 4 times daily *v* 18/85 [21%] with nystatin suspension 100 000 U 4 times daily; $P < 0.0001$; at day 12: 97/98 [99%] with miconazole *v* 46/85 [54%] with nystatin; $P < 0.0001$).[16] The smaller RCT (95 infants, mean age 5 months, range 2–17 months with clinical oral thrush) found that miconazole gel significantly increased clinical cure at 14 days compared with two brands of nystatin gel preparation ($P = 0.0032$ and $P = 0.00068$).[17] One RCT (47 infants aged 1–12 months with clinical signs of oral candidiasis and culture positive for Candida species) compared nystatin oral suspension 100 000 IU/mL four times daily for 10 days versus fluconazole suspension 3 mg/kg once daily for 7 days.[18] It found that fluconazole significantly increased clinical cure compared with nystatin (36 infants evaluated; clinical cure: 15/15 [100%] with fluconazole *v* 6/19 [32%] with nystatin, $P < 0.0001$).[18] **Immunocompromised infants and children:** We found no placebo controlled RCTs. We found one multicentre RCT (32 centres, 182 immunocompromised infants and children aged 5 months to 14 years), which compared fluconazole suspension 3 mg/kg versus nystatin 400 000 U four times daily for 14 days.[19] It found that fluconazole significantly increased clinical cure rate compared with nystatin (78/86 [91%] with fluconazole *v* 37/73 [51%] with nystatin; RR 1.8, 95% CI 1.6 to 1.9; NNT 2, 95% CI 2 to 3).[19] In subgroup analyses of children with HIV infection, nystatin significantly increased clinical cure compared with fluconazole (clinical cure: 28/35 [80%] with fluconazole *v* 6/29 [21%] with nystatin), and for people with malignancy (clinical cure: 49/50 [98%] with fluconazole *v* 30/42 [71%] with nystatin). Clinical relapse rates after 2 weeks were similar (18% with fluconazole *v* 24% with nystatin).

Harms: **Immunocompetent infants and children:** The most common adverse events with both miconazole and nystatin were vomiting and, more rarely, diarrhoea, affecting less than 4.5% of infants.[16,17] **Immunocompromised infants and children:** Adverse events caused 2/94 (2%) children on fluconazole to withdraw versus 0/88 (0%) children on nystatin ($P = 0.04$).[19]

Comment: **Immunocompetent infants and children:** The RCTs were not blinded nor placebo controlled.[16–18] There is potential for observer bias, but the clinical results were corroborated by mycological findings, which were blinded.[16] The larger RCT was carried out in 26 general practices,[16] so it is representative of the context in which most otherwise healthy infants with oropharyngeal candidiasis would be treated, especially regarding adherence and cure rate. **Immunocompromised infants and children:** Participants included in the RCT were immunocompromised for different reasons: 64 had HIV infection, 92 had a malignancy, and 26 were receiving immunosuppressive treatment.[19]

QUESTION **What are the effects of interventions to prevent and treat oropharyngeal candidiasis in people with diabetes?**

OPTION **ANTIFUNGAL DRUGS**

We found insufficient evidence about prevention or treatment of oropharyngeal candidiasis in people with diabetes.

Benefits: We found no systematic review or RCTs.

Harms: We found no RCTs.

Comment: None.

QUESTION **What are the effects of interventions for oropharyngeal candidiasis in people with dentures?**

OPTION **ANTIFUNGAL DRUGS**

We found insufficient evidence from small RCTs to compare effects of antifungal agents versus placebo or versus each other for treating oropharyngeal candidiasis in people who wear dentures.

Benefits: We found no systematic review, but found several RCTs. **Versus placebo:** Five small RCTs compared topical oral antifungals versus placebo for the treatment of denture stomatitis.[20–24] The first small RCT (46 people) found that topical oral polyenes (nystatin, amphotericin B) significantly improved clinical cure of denture stomatitis after 4 weeks of treatment compared with placebo (nystatin *v* placebo, $P \leq 0.05$; amphotericin B *v* placebo, $P \leq 0.01$).[21] The second small RCT (22 people) found no significant difference between polyenes and placebo in the clinical appearance of denture stomatitis after 2 weeks of treatment, or 10 days after stopping treatment.[22] The third small RCT (49 people) found no significant difference between amphotericin B (with or without a hydrogen peroxide denture cleanser) and placebo in clinical cure.[20] The fourth small RCT (36 people) found no significant difference in the resolution of palatal symptoms between miconazole dental lacquer (applied to the fit surface of an upper denture as a single application) and a placebo lacquer at 14 days (symptom resolution: 54% with lacquer *v* 23% with placebo; RR 2.40, 95% CI 0.89 to 3.80).[23] The fifth small RCT (38 people) found that fluconazole significantly increased clinical improvement or cure rates compared with placebo at 2 and 4 weeks (at 2 weeks: 10/19 [53%] with fluconazole *v* 0/18 [0%] with placebo; $P < 0.001$; at 4 weeks: 5/19 [26%] with fluconazole *v* 0/19 [0%] with placebo; $P < 0.02$).[24] **Different antifungal treatments:** We found two RCTs.[25,26] The first small RCT (29 people) found no significant difference in clinical cure rate between fluconazole 50 mg daily for 14 days and amphotericin B lozenges plus denture cream for 28 days (84% with fluconazole *v* 90% with amphotericin B).[25] Clinical relapse was common in both groups at 12 weeks. The second RCT (multicentre; 305 elderly people, 176 with dentures) found no significant difference in clinical cure between fluconazole 50 mg and amphotericin B 0.5 g. Wearing dentures did not affect the response to antifungal treatment (clinical cure rate: 151/176 [86%] of denture wearers *v* 102/124 [82%] of non-denture wearers).[26] **Different modes of administration:** Two RCTs (41 people[27] and 33 people[28]) compared a single application of miconazole dental lacquer versus miconazole gel 2% applied to the denture four times daily. Neither RCT found a significant difference in palatal erythema (largest RCT, 14 days after treatment: 13/20 [65%] with lacquer *v* 16/21 [76%] with gel; RR of erythema with lacquer *v* gel: 0.85, 95% CI 0.42 to 1.20).[27,28]

Harms: None of the trials exclusively enrolling people with dentures were large enough to report reliably on adverse effects. In the large RCT of elderly people, 6/150 (4%) in the fluconazole arm and 0/155 (0%) in the amphotericin arm experienced adverse events, including diarrhoea, buccal bitterness, aggravation of pre-existing renal dysfunction (1 person, withdrawn from RCT), and increased liver transaminases (1 person, not withdrawn).[26]

Comment: Co-interventions included professional cleaning of the dentures at the start of the study, combined with advice on denture hygiene and advice not to wear the dentures while asleep at night. Because the fit surface of the denture may act as a reservoir of primary and recurrent infection, this cleaning and advice may explain the high clinical cure rate in the placebo groups. The RCTs comparing different antifungals were not sufficiently powered to detect clinically important differences.

OPTION DENTURE HYGIENE

We found insufficient evidence from RCTs to assess clinical effects on oropharyngeal candidiasis of mouth rinses, disinfectants, denture soaks, denture scrubbing, and microwave irradiation of dentures. Microwave treatment is not suitable for all dentures.

Benefits: We found no systematic review, but found four RCTs.[29–32] The first small crossover RCT (43 people aged 35–73 years) compared daily soaking of dentures in disinfectant (potassium persulphate 1%) versus placebo (water, peppermint, dye) for 4 weeks.[29] The results provided for the outcome of stomatitis were difficult to interpret and therefore no firm conclusions can be drawn. The second RCT (78 people with mild to moderate denture stomatitis) compared three treatments: mouth rinsing three times daily plus denture soaking once daily, using an antimicrobial mouth rinse; the same procedure, using a control mouth rinse, and weekly relining of the fit surface of the denture (to improve retention and reduce denture trauma) for 4 weeks.[30] It found that the antimicrobial mouth rinse significantly reduced symptoms of denture stomatitis compared with control mouth rinse ($P < 0.01$; absolute numbers not provided). The third, small RCT (34 people in long term care with acrylic dentures and a positive test for *C albicans*) compared microwave treatment (dentures scrubbed with antibacterial soap and water and then microwaved individually for 1 minute at 850 watts on days 1, 5, and 10) versus control treatment (dentures soaked in 0.2% chlorhexidine solution overnight for 14 days and scrubbed with antibacterial soap and water on days 1, 5, and 10).[31] Both groups also received the same course of topical antifungal medication (nystatin lozenges daily for 14 days). The RCT found no significant difference between treatments in the rates of dentures recolonised with *C albicans* after 3 months, although it may have lacked power to excluded a clinically important difference (RR 0.64, 95% CI 0.38 to 1.06). It found microwave treatment significantly decreased the proportion of people with infection of the oral mucosa on cytological smear after 3 months compared with control dental soak (RR 0.25, 95% CI 0.06 to 0.59).[31] The fourth small RCT (19 elderly, chronically ill, institutionalised people receiving nystatin pastilles 3 times daily) found no additional advantage from nystatin denture soaking solution (10 000 U/mL) compared with tap water as a soaking solution (all participants clinically cured at 7 days).[32]

Harms: The first two RCTs did not report on adverse effects.[29,30] In the microwave RCT, exposure time was decided arbitrarily.[31] In the RCT, exposure to microwave at 850 watts for 90 seconds seemed to damage the denture material.[31] The RCT noted microwave treatment may damage complete dentures that have been relined, repaired, or both by producing a bubble (pocketing) in the acrylic material, and porcelain teeth with metal retaining pins may cause the microwave to spark and scorch the denture material.[31] It noted microwave treatment was not suitable for all dentures and should be used with caution.[31] Microwave treatment cannot be used for chrome dentures or dentures with metal clasps.

Comment: We found no RCT evaluating the effect of removing dentures at night on preventing denture stomatitis. Two observational studies found a correlation between the prevalence of denture stomatitis and an unhealthy lifestyle (a global measure including dietary habits, physical activity, alcohol consumption, and smoking), wearing dentures at night, and poor oral hygiene.[33,34]

QUESTION What are the effects of interventions to prevent and treat oropharyngeal candidiasis in people with HIV infection?

OPTION CONTINUOUS ANTIFUNGAL PROPHYLAXIS

RCTs in people with HIV infection have found that daily or weekly antifungal prophylaxis with fluconazole, itraconazole, or nystatin significantly reduces incidence and relapse of oropharyngeal candidiasis compared with placebo.

Benefits: We found one systematic review (search date 2000).[35] The review was narrative in character and no data were pooled. We found 10 RCTs using different prophylaxis protocols with follow up of 3–29 months.[36–45] All RCTs enrolled people with AIDS, AIDS related complex, or CD4 cell counts less than or equal to 300 cells/mm^3. **Fluconazole versus placebo:** We found six RCTs that used daily or weekly regimens.[36,37,39–41,46] All six RCTs found that fluconazole significantly reduced oropharyngeal candidiasis compared with placebo. The first RCT (24 people) found that fluconazole 150 mg weekly reduced clinical relapse compared with placebo during 6 months of prophylaxis (relapse: 4/9 [44%] with fluconazole *v* 5/5 [100%] with placebo; P value not provided).[36] The second RCT (323 women with HIV infection) compared fluconazole 200 mg weekly and placebo and found similar results; fluconazole reduced the risk of recurrent oropharyngeal candidiasis over 29 months (RR 0.50, 95% CI 0.33 to 0.74).[37] The third RCT (84 people) found that fluconazole significantly reduced relapse compared with placebo (73 people; median time to relapse: 168 days with fluconazole *v* 37 days with placebo; P < 0.0001; relapse rate: 13/31 [42%] with fluconazole *v* 25/26 [96%] with placebo).[39] The fourth RCT (60 people) found that fluconazole 50 or 100 mg reduced relapse compared with no treatment at 137–215 days (58 people evaluated; rate of relapse: 11% with fluconazole 50 mg *v* 21% with fluconazole 100 mg *v* 95% with no treatment; significance not stated).[40] The fifth small RCT (25 people with 1–4 previous episodes of thrush, but none at baseline) found that fluconazole significantly reduced oral candidiasis compared with placebo at 12 weeks (0/12 [0%] with fluconazole *v* 8/13 [62%] with placebo; P = 0.002).[41] The sixth RCT (143 people) found that fluconazole reduced relapse compared with placebo (median time to relapse: 175 days with fluconazole *v* 35 days with placebo; P < 0.00001; freedom from relapse at 37 months: 26/67 [39%] with fluconazole *v* 7/71 [10%] with placebo).[46] **Itraconazole versus placebo:** We found three RCTs.[43–45] The first RCT (70 people) found that daily prophylaxis with itraconazole 200 mg for 24 weeks significantly reduced relapse rate (5/24 [21%] with itraconazole *v* 14/20 [70%] with placebo; ARR 49%, 95% CI 19% to 64%; NNT 2, 95% CI 2 to 5) and increased the time to relapse (median time to relapse: 10.4 weeks with itraconazole *v* 8.0 weeks with placebo; P = 0.001).[43] The second RCT (374 people) compared itraconazole 200 mg daily versus placebo.[44] The primary study end point was time to development of deep fungal infections. The study was terminated because of inadequate power (see comment below). The mean duration of study treatment was 448 days with itraconazole and 386 days with placebo. The RCT found that itraconazole significantly reduced the incidence of oral candidiasis and significantly prolonged the time to development of oral candidiasis compared with placebo (oral candidiasis: RR 0.33, CI not provided; P < 0.001, logistic regression; time to development of oral candidiasis: 508 days with itraconazole *v* 413 days with placebo; P < 0.001, log rank test; see comment below).[44] The third RCT (129 people) compared itraconazole 200 mg daily versus placebo.[45] The duration of follow up was 6–104 weeks in the itraconazole group and 5–104 weeks in the placebo group. The RCT found that itraconazole significantly reduced the proportion of people with two or more episodes of oral candidiasis compared with placebo (6/63 [10%] with itraconazole *v* 15/66 [23%] with placebo; P = 0.04).[45] **Nystatin versus placebo:** One RCT found that prophylaxis with one or two nystatin 200 000 U pastilles once daily over 20 weeks significantly delayed the onset of oropharyngeal candidiasis compared with placebo (HR 0.59, 95% CI 0.40 to 0.82; P < 0.001).[38] **Fluconazole versus clotrimazole:** One large RCT (428 people from 29 sites) that compared fluconazole 200 mg daily and clotrimazole 10 mg five times daily over 35 months found that fluconazole significantly reduced the recurrence of oropharyngeal candidiasis (5.7 episodes/100 person years with fluconazole *v* 38.1 episodes/100 person years with clotrimazole; P ≤ 0.001).[42]

Harms: In one RCT comparing two different daily doses of fluconazole versus no treatment, one person stopped fluconazole because of an allergic rash.[40] One RCT found no significant difference in adverse events between fluconazole and placebo (10/12 [83%] with fluconazole *v* 9/13 [69%] with placebo; P = 0.6).[41] One RCT comparing itraconazole and placebo found that 95% (177/187) of people with itraconazole and 95% (178/187) with placebo reported adverse events, the most frequent being gastrointestinal.[44] Most were classified as mild or moderate. Severe adverse events were reported by 38% of people with itraconazole and 36% of people with placebo. However, most adverse events were not considered to be related to study medication but, rather, related to HIV disease.[44] Study medication was withdrawn in 20% of people with itraconazole and 23% of people with placebo predominantly because of nausea and abdominal pain.[44] One RCT comparing itraconazole and placebo reported the most frequent adverse events were skin rashes (16/63 [25%] with itraconazole *v* 15/66 [23%] with placebo), mild anaemia (4/63 [6%] with itraconazole *v* 5/66 [8%] with placebo), and diarrhoea (3/63 [5%] with itraconazole *v* 5/66 [8%] with placebo).[45] One person discontinued treatment with itraconazole because of a skin rash, and concerns about hepatotoxicity resulted in treatment being discontinued in two people (1 with itraconazole and 1 with placebo). There was one case of Stevens–Johnson syndrome in a person also taking trimethoprim–sulfamethoxazole.[45] One RCT found no significant difference in rate of microbial resistance between fluconazole and placebo over 37 months (8/67 [12%] with fluconazole *v* 4/71 [6%] with placebo group, P = 0.20).[46] In the other RCTs, the most commonly reported adverse events were gastrointestinal symptoms, rash, and headache, but data on adverse effects were not presented in all the RCTs. Concomitant medication and severe underlying disease may have confounded attribution of adverse events.

Comment: Many of the RCTs were small and not blinded, and most did not adjust for confounding factors such as antiretroviral treatment and other established risk factors for oropharyngeal candidiasis. No RCTs used quality of life scores. The optimal dosage schedule and frequency of administration of preventive treatment have not been established. We found no RCTs comparing weekly and daily regimens of antifungal drugs. We found one RCT that compared two different doses of fluconazole.[40] It found no significant difference between 50 and 100 mg daily doses of fluconazole (oropharyngeal candidiasis: 2/18 [11%] with 50 mg *v* 4/19 [21%] with 100 mg; RR 0.53, 95% CI 0.09 to 2.09).[40] Subgroup analysis in the RCT comparing fluconazole to placebo, found that people with a history of oropharyngeal candidiasis had an absolute benefit of treatment with weekly fluconazole that was higher than in those with no history of infection (ARR 25.6/100 person years for those with previous infection *v* ARR 11.2/100 person years for those with no history of infection).[37] In the RCT comparing itraconazole versus placebo, too few deep fungal infections occurred to assess accurately the impact of itraconazole prophylaxis, and on the basis of statistical advice, the study was terminated.[44] Discontinuation rates were high and 145/187 (78%) of people with itraconazole versus 154/187 (82%) with placebo did not complete 2 years of medication.[44] Reasons for discontinuation were: withdrew consent (33 people with itraconazole *v* 46 with placebo); adverse event (31 with itraconazole *v* 29 with placebo); lost to follow up (17 with itraconazole *v* 11 with placebo); use of disallowed medication (15 with itraconazole *v* 3 with placebo); reached a study end point (5 with itraconazole *v* 11 with placebo); death (5 with itraconazole *v* 8 with placebo); elevated liver function test (2 with itraconazole *v* 3 with placebo); pregnancy (0 with itraconazole *v* 1 with placebo); and other (37 with itraconazole *v* 42 with placebo).[44] The extended time interval to relapse with itraconazole may reflect the introduction of highly active antiretroviral treatment.[44]

OPTION TOPICAL ANTIFUNGAL TREATMENT

RCTs have found that topical preparations of itraconazole, fluconazole, and clotrimazole effectively treat oropharyngeal candidiasis in people with HIV infection. One RCT found that fluconazole significantly reduced symptoms and signs of oropharyngeal candidiasis compared with topical nystatin.

Benefits: We found one systematic review (search date 2000).[35] The review was narrative in character and no data were pooled. We found five RCTs comparing topical (suspensions or pastilles) versus orally absorbed antifungals for treatment of oropharyngeal candidiasis in people with HIV infection, which included four RCTs identified by the review and one subsequent RCT.[47–51] Four RCTs found that itraconazole oral solution 100 or 200 mg used in a swish and swallow mode was as effective as topical fluconazole 100 mg once daily for 14 days or topical clotrimazole 10 mg five times daily.[47–49,51] Three of these RCTs achieved clinical response rates of over 90%.[47–49] The fifth RCT comparing fluconazole 100 mg daily and nystatin liquid for 14 days found that fluconazole significantly increased complete resolution of signs and symptoms of oropharyngeal candidiasis (60/69 [87%] with fluconazole *v* 36/69 [52%] with nystatin liquid; ARI 35%, 95% CI 22% to 42%; RR 1.67, 95% CI 1.42 to 1.80; NNT 3, 95% CI 2 to 5).[50]

Harms: The most frequently reported adverse effects were gastrointestinal symptoms (nausea, diarrhoea, and vomiting). Altered taste, dry mouth, headache, and rashes were also recorded.[47–50] In the other RCT, there were no withdrawals because of adverse effects.[51] On the basis of data from five RCTs (861 people), in which adverse events were considered to be drug induced and resulted in withdrawal from the study, adverse events were reported with fluconazole (4 people), itraconazole (14 people), clotrimazole (12 people), and nystatin (1 person).[42,47–50]

Comment: Once daily dosing is likely to increase adherence to treatment. Non-adherence was reported with clotrimazole because of the inconvenience of taking multiple doses.

QUESTION **Which treatments reduce the risk of acquiring resistance to antifungal drugs?**

OPTION **CONTINUOUS ANTIFUNGAL PROPHYLAXIS VERSUS INTERMITTENT ANTIFUNGAL TREATMENT**

One RCT in people with HIV infection and acute episodes of oropharyngeal candidiasis found no significant difference between continuous antifungal prophylaxis with fluconazole and intermittent antifungal treatment with fluconazole in terms of the emergence of antifungal resistance.

Benefits: We found no systematic review. We found one RCT comparing the effects of continuous prophylaxis with fluconazole versus intermittent treatment with fluconazole 200 mg daily on the development of acquired resistance in people with HIV infection and evidence of active oropharyngeal candidiasis over a mean follow up of 11 months.[52] Antifungal sensitivity testing followed the National Committee for Clinical Laboratory Standards guidelines.[53] The RCT found that continuous prophylaxis with fluconazole reduced median annual relapse rates compared with intermittent treatment (0 episodes/year with continuous prophylaxis *v* 4.1 episodes/year with intermittent treatment; $P \leq 0.001$). It also found that antifungal resistance developed in more people on continuous prophylaxis than on intermittent treatment, but the difference was not significant (9/16 [56%] with continuous *v* 13/28 [46%] with intermittent; $P = 0.75$).[52]

Harms: No adverse reactions were reported.

Comment: Optimal treatment regimens to reduce the risk of acquiring resistance have not been evaluated adequately. In a prospective observational study of protease inhibitor treatment, 93 people with HIV and with a history of recurrent oropharyngeal candidiasis were followed up for 1 year. Oropharyngeal candidiasis was diagnosed in 2/30 (7%) people given protease inhibitors and 23/63 (37%) given other treatment ($P \leq 0.001$; CI not provided).[54] Immunomodulating antiretroviral treatments (e.g. highly active antiretroviral treatment), by reducing the number of recurrences of oropharyngeal candidiasis, are acting indirectly as antifungal sparing agents, thereby reducing exposure to antifungals and the potential risk of resistance.

Substantive changes

Immunocompromised adults, antifungal prophylaxis One systematic review added;[8] conclusions unchanged.

Candidiasis (oropharyngeal)

Antifungal treatment in children One RCT added;[18] conclusions unchanged.
Prevention/treatment in HIV, continuous antifungal prophylaxis One RCT added;[46] conclusions unchanged.
Antifungal treatment One RCT added;[14] conclusions unchanged.

REFERENCES

1. Ellepola ANB, Samaranayake LP. Antimycotic agents in oral candidosis: an overview: 1. Clinical variants. *Dent Update* 2000;27:111–116.
2. Webb BC, Thomas CJ, Willcox MD, et al. Candida-associated denture stomatitis. Aetiology and management: a review. Part 3. Treatment of oral candidosis. *Aust Dent J* 1998;43:244–249.
3. Ninane JA. Multicentre study of fluconazole versus oral polyenes in the prevention of fungal infection in children with hematological or oncological malignancies. Multicentre study group. *Eur J Clin Microbiol Infect Dis* 1994;13:330–337.
4. Philips P, Zemcov J, Mahmood W, et al. Itraconazole cyclodextrin solution for fluconazole-refractory oropharyngeal candidiasis in AIDS: correlation of clinical response with *in vitro* susceptibility. *AIDS* 1996;10:1369–1376.
5. Wilson J. The aetiology, diagnosis and management of denture stomatitis. *B Dental J* 1998;185:380–384.
6. Rex JH, Rinald MG, Pfaler MA. Resistance of Candida species to fluconazole. *Antimicrob Agents Chemother* 1995;39:1–8.
7. Maenza JR, Keruly JC, Moore RD, et al. Risk factors for fluconazole-resistant candidiasis in human immuno-deficiency virus-infected patients. *J Infect Dis* 1996;173:219–225.
8. Worthington HV, Clarkson JE, Eden OB. Interventions for preventing oral candidiasis for patients with cancer receiving treatment. In: The Cochrane Library, Issue 1, 2003. Oxford: Update Software. Search date 2001; Primary sources Medline, Embase, Cinahl, Cancerlit, the Cochrane Controlled Trials Register, and the Cochrane Oral Health Group Specialist Register.
9. Lumbreras C, Cuervas-Mons V, Jara P, et al. Randomized trial of fluconazole versus nystatin for the prophylaxis of Candida infection following liver transplantation. *J Infect Dis* 1996;174:583–588.
10. Ruskin JD, Wood RP, Bailey MR, et al. Comparative trial of oral clotrimazole and nystatin for oropharyngeal candidiasis prophylaxis in orthotopic liver transplant patients. *Oral Surg Oral Med Oral Pathol Oral Radiol Endod* 1992;74:567–571.
11. Ferretti GA, Ash RC, Brown AT, et al. Control of oral mucositis and candidiasis in marrow transplantation: a prospective, double-blind trial of chlorhexidine digluconate oral rinse. *Bone Marrow Transplant* 1988;3:483–493.
12. Epstein JB, Vickars L, Spinelli J, et al. Efficacy of chlorhexidine and nystatin rinses in prevention of oral complications in leukemia and bone marrow transplantation. *Oral Surg Oral Med Oral Pathol Oral Radiol Endod* 1992;73:682–689.
13. Clarkson JE, Worthington HV, Eden OB. Interventions for treating oral candidiasis for patients with cancer receiving treatment. In: The Cochrane library, Issue 1, 2003. Oxford: Update Software. Search date 2001; primary sources Cochrane Oral Health Group Specialised Register, Cochrane Controlled Trials Register, Medline, and Embase. Reference lists from relevant articles were searched and the authors of eligible trials were contacted to identify trials.
14. Lefebvre JL, Domenge C. A comparative study of the efficacy and safety of fluconazole oral suspension and amphotericin B oral suspension in cancer patients with mucositis. *Oral Oncol* 2002;38:337–342.
15. Groll AH, Just-Nuebling G, Kurz M, et al. Fluconazole versus nystatin in the prevention of Candida infections in children and adolescents undergoing remission induction or consolidation chemotherapy for cancer. *J Antimicrob Chemother* 1997;40:855–862.
16. Hoppe J, Burr R, Ebeling H, et al. Treatment of oropharyngeal candidiasis in immunocompetent infants: a randomized multicenter study of miconazole gel vs. nystatin suspension. *Pediatr Infect Dis J* 1997;16:288–293.
17. Hoppe JE, Hahn H. Randomized comparison of two nystatin oral gels with miconazole oral gel for treatment of oral thrush in infants. Antimycotics study group. *Infection* 1996;24:136–139.
18. Goins RA, Ascher D, Waecker N, et al. Comparison of fluconazole and nystatin oral suspensions for treatment of oral candidiasis in infants. *Pediatr Infect Dis J* 2002;21:1165–1167.
19. Flynn PM, Cunningham CK, Kerkering T, et al. Oropharyngeal candidiasis in immunocompromised children: a randomized, multicenter study of orally administered fluconazole suspension versus nystatin. The multicenter fluconazole study group. *J Pediatr* 1995;127:322–328.
20. Walker DM, Stafford GD, Huggett R, et al. The treatment of denture stomatitis: evaluation of two agents. *Br Dent J* 1981;151:416–419.
21. Nairn RI. Nystatin and amphotericin B in the treatment of denture-related candidiasis. *Oral Surg Oral Med Oral Pathol Oral Radiol Endod* 1975;40:68–75.
22. Johnson GH, Taylor TD, Heid DW. Clinical evaluation of a nystatin pastille for treatment of denture-related oral candidiasis. *J Prosthet Dent* 1989;61:699–703.
23. Konsberg R, Axell T. Treatment of Candida-infected denture stomatitis with a miconazole lacquer. *Oral Surg Oral Med Oral Pathol Oral Radiol Endod* 1994;78:306–311.
24. Budtz-Jorgensen E, Holmstrup P, Krogh P. Fluconazole in the treatment of Candida-associated denture stomatitis. *Antimicrob Agents Chemother* 1988;32:1859–1863.
25. Bissell V, Felix DH, Wray D. Comparative trial of fluconazole and amphotericin B in the treatment of denture stomatitis. *Oral Surg Oral Med Oral Pathol Oral Radiol Endod* 1993;76:35–39.
26. Taillandier J, Esnault Y, Alemanni M, and the multicentre study group. A comparison of fluconazole oral suspension and amphotericin B oral suspension in older patients with oropharyngeal candidosis. *Age Ageing* 2000;29:117–123.
27. Budtz-Jorgensen E, Carlino P. A miconazole lacquer in the treatment of Candida-associated denture stomatitis. *Mycoses* 1994;37:131–135.
28. Parvinen T, Kokko J, Yli-Urpo A. Miconazole lacquer compared with gel in treatment of denture stomatitis. *Scand J Dental Res* 1994;102:361–366.
29. Mahonen K, Virtanen K, Larmas M. The effect of prosthesis disinfection on salivary microbial levels. *J Oral Rehabil* 1998;25:304–310.
30. DePaola LG, Minah GE, Elias SA, et al. Clinical and microbial evaluation of treatment regimens to reduce denture stomatitis. *Int J Prosthodont* 1990;3:369–374.

31. Banting DW, Hill SA. Microwave disinfection of dentures for the treatment of oral candidiasis. *Spec Care Dentist* 2001;21:4–8.
32. Banting DW, Greenhorn PA, McMinn JG. Effectiveness of a topical antifungal regimen for the treatment of oral candidiasis in older, chronically ill, institutionalized adults. *J Can Dent Assoc* 1995;61:199–195.
33. Sakki TK, Knuuttila ML, Laara E, et al. The association of yeasts and denture stomatitis with behavioral and biologic factors. *Oral Surg Oral Med Oral Pathol Oral Radiol Endod* 1997;84:624–629.
34. Fenlon MR, Sherriff M, Walter JD. Factors associated with the presence of denture related stomatitis in complete denture wearers: a preliminary investigation. *Eur J Prosthodont Restor Dent* 1998;6:145–147.
35. Patton LL, Bonito AJ, Shugars DA. A systematic review of the effectiveness of antifungal drugs for the prevention and treatment of oropharyngeal candidiasis in HIV positive patients. *Oral Surg Oral Med Oral Pathol Oral Radiol Endod* 2001;92:170–179. Search date 2000; primary sources Medline, Embase, and the Cochrane Library, and a manual check of reference lists of review articles.
36. Leen CLS, Dunbar EM, Ellis ME, et al. Once-weekly fluconazole to prevent recurrence of oropharyngeal candidiasis in patients with AIDS and AIDS-related complex: a double-blind placebo controlled study. *J Infect* 1990;21:55–60.
37. Schuman P, Capps L, Peng G, et al. Weekly fluconazole for the prevention of mucosal candidiasis in women with HIV infection. A randomized, double-blind, placebo-controlled trial. Terry Beirn community programs for clinical research on AIDS. *Ann Intern Med* 1997;126:689–696.
38. MacPhail LA, Hilton JF, Dodd CL, et al. Prophylaxis with nystatin pastilles for HIV-associated oral candidiasis. *J Acquir Immune Defic Syndr* 1996;12:470–476.
39. Marriott DJE, Jones PD, Hoy JF, et al. Fluconazole once a week as secondary prophylaxis against oropharyngeal candidiasis in HIV-infected patients. A double-blind placebo-controlled study. *Med J Aust* 1993;158:312–316.
40. Just-Nubling G, Gentschew G, Meissner K, et al. Fluconazole prophylaxis of recurrent oral candidiasis in HIV-positive patients. *Eur J Clin Microbiol Infect Dis* 1991;10:917–921.
41. Stevens DA, Greene SI, Lang OS. Thrush can be prevented in patients with acquired immunodeficiency syndrome and the acquired immunodeficiency syndrome-related complex. Randomized, double-blind, placebo-controlled study of 100 mg oral fluconazole daily. *Arch Intern Med* 1991;151:2458–2464.
42. Powderly WG, Finklestein DM, Feinberg J, et al. A randomised trial comparing fluconazole with clotrimazole troches for the prevention of fungal infection in patients with advanced human immunodeficiency virus infection. *N Engl J Med* 1995;332:700–705.
43. Smith D, Midgley J, Gazzard B. A randomised, double-blind study of itraconazole versus placebo in the treatment and prevention of oral or oesophageal candidosis in patients with HIV infection. *Int J Clin Pract* 1999;53:349–352.
44. Smith DE, Bell J, Johnson M, et al. A randomized, doubled-blind, placebo-controlled study of itraconazole capsules for the prevention of deep fungal infections in immunodeficient patients with HIV infection. *HIV Medicine* 2001;2:78–83.
45. Chariyalertsak S, Supparatpinyo K, Sirisanthana, T, et al. A controlled trial of itraconazole as primary prophylaxis for systemic fungal infections in patients with advanced human immunodeficiency virus infection in Thailand. *Clin Infect Dis* 2002;34:277–284.
46. Pagani JL, Chave JP, Casjka C, et al. Efficacy, tolerability and development of resistance in HIV-positive patients treated with fluconazole for secondary prevention of oropharyngeal candidiasis: a randomized, double-blind, placebo-controlled trial. *J Antimicrob Chemother* 2002;50:231–240.
47. Graybill JR, Vazquez J, Darouiche RO, et al. Randomized trial of itraconazole oral solution for oropharyngeal candidiasis in HIV/AIDS patients. *Am J Med* 1998;104:33–39.
48. Phillips P, De Beule K, Frechette G, et al. A double-blind comparison of itraconazole oral solution and fluconazole capsules for the treatment of oropharyngeal candidiasis in patients with AIDS. *Clin Infect Dis* 1998;26:1368–1373.
49. Murray PA, Koletar SL, Mallegol I, et al. Itraconazole oral solution versus clotrimazole troches for the treatment of oropharyngeal candidiasis in immunocompromised patients. *Clin Ther* 1997;19:471–480.
50. Pons V, Greenspan D, Lozada-Nur F, et al. Oropharyngeal candidiasis in patients with AIDS: randomized comparison of fluconazole versus nystatin oral suspensions. *Clin Infect Dis* 1997;24:1204–1207.
51. Linpiyawan R, Jittreprasert K, Sivayathorn A. Clinical trial: clotrimazole troche vs. itraconazole oral solution in the treatment of oral candidosis in AIDS patients. *Int J Dermatol* 2000;39:859–861.
52. Revankar SG, Kirkpatrick WR, McAtee RK, et al. A randomized trial of continuous or intermittent therapy with fluconazole for oropharyngeal candidiasis in HIV-infected patients: clinical outcomes and development of fluconazole resistance. *Am J Med* 1998;105:7–11.
53. National Committee for Clinical Laboratory Standards. Reference method for broth dilution antifungal susceptibility testing of yeasts: approved standard. Wayne, Penn: NCCLS, 1997 (document M27-A).
54. Cauda R, Tacconelli E, Tumbarello M, et al. Role of protease inhibitors in preventing recurrent oral candidiasis in patients with HIV infections: a prospective case control study. *J Acquir Immune Defic Syndr* 1999;21:20–25.

Caroline Pankhurst
Dr
Guy's, King's College, and St Thomas's Dental Institute, London, UK

Competing interests: None declared.

Halitosis

Search date April 2003

Bazian Ltd

QUESTIONS

INTERVENTIONS

See glossary, p 1643

Key Messages

- **Single-use mouthwash (short term benefit only)** Three small RCTs in people with confirmed halitosis found limited evidence that single-use mouthwash reduced odour unpleasantness and odour intensity between 1–8 hours after use compared with distilled water, saline rinse, or no treatment. One of these RCTs found no significant difference between single-use mouthwash and distilled water in odour unpleasantness or odour intensity after 24 hours.
- **Regular-use mouthwash** We found no RCTs on the effects of the regular use of mouthwash.
- **Artificial saliva; sugar free chewing gums; tongue cleaning, brushing, or scraping; zinc toothpastes** We found no RCTs on the effects of these interventions.

DEFINITION Halitosis is an unpleasant odour emitted from the mouth. It can be because of oral conditions including poor oral hygiene and periodontal disease or extraoral conditions including some respiratory and systemic diseases such as chronic sinusitis and bronchiectasis.[1,2] In this topic, we deal only with physiological halitosis, that is, confirmed persistent bad breath in the absence of systemic, periodontal, or gum disease. We have excluded halitosis due to underlying disease, which would require disease specific treatment, pseudo-halitosis (in people who believe they have bad breath but whose breath is not considered malodourous by others), and artificially induced halitosis (e.g. in studies requiring people to stop brushing their teeth). This topic is only applicable, therefore, to people in whom underlying causes have been ruled out, and in whom pseudo-halitosis has been excluded. There is no consensus regarding duration of bad breath for diagnosis of halitosis, although the standard organoleptic test (see glossary, p 1643) for bad breath involves smelling the breath on at least two or three different days.[1]

INCIDENCE/ PREVALENCE We found no reliable estimate of prevalence, although many authors report population prevalence of halitosis (physiological or because of underlying disease) to be about 50%.[1,3–5] One cross-sectional study of 491 people found that about 5% of people with halitosis have pseudo-halitosis and about 40% of people with halitosis have physiological bad breath not due to underlying disease.[6] We found no reliable data about age or sex distribution of physiological halitosis.

AETIOLOGY/ RISK FACTORS We found no reliable data about risk factors for physiological bad breath. Mass spectrometric and gas chromatographic analysis of expelled air from the mouth of people with any type of halitosis have shown that the main malodourants are volatile sulphur compounds including hydrogen sulphide, methyl mercaptan, and dimethyl suphide.[7,8]

PROGNOSIS We found no evidence on the prognosis of halitosis.

AIMS OF INTERVENTION To improve social functioning; to reduce embarrassment; to reduce odour with minimum adverse effects.

OUTCOMES Organoleptic test scores, other odour scales, quality of life scores, embarrassment scores, and social functioning scores. We excluded non-clinical outcomes such as gas chromatography and spectroscopy results and concentrations of compounds in exhaled air.

METHODS *Clinical Evidence* search and appraisal April 2003.

QUESTION **What are the effects of treatments in people with physiological halitosis?** New

OPTION **TONGUE CLEANING, BRUSHING, OR SCRAPING**

We found no RCTs on the effects of tongue cleaning, brushing, or scraping.

Benefits: We found no systematic review or RCTs.

Harms: We found no RCTs.

Comment: None.

OPTION MOUTHWASHES (CONTAINING ZINC, CHLORHEXIDINE, HYDROGEN PEROXIDE, OR OTHER ANTIMICROBIAL AGENTS)

We found no RCTs on the effects of the regular use of mouthwash. Three small RCTs in people with confirmed halitosis found limited evidence that single-use mouthwash reduced odour unpleasantness and odour intensity between 1–8 hours after use compared with distilled water, saline rinse, or no treatment. One of these RCTs found no significant difference between single-use mouthwash and distilled water in odour unpleasantness or odour intensity after 24 hours.

Benefits: **Regular-use mouthwash:** We found no systematic review and no RCTs on the regular use of mouthwash. **Single-use mouthwash:** We found three small RCTs that compared single-use mouthwash versus control or no treatment.[2,9,10] The first two RCTs compared single-use 0.1% chlorine dioxide mouthwash versus distilled water in healthy adults with confirmed oral malodour.[2,9] In both RCTs, three examiners scored unpleasant breath odour on a scale from +3 (very pleasant/fresh) to –3 (very unpleasant/stale) and odour intensity from 0 (no odour) to 4 (very strong odour). The first RCT (31 people) found that chlorine dioxide containing mouthwash significantly reduced odour unpleasantness score and odour intensity score at 2, 4, and 8 hours after treatment compared with distilled water (odour unpleasantness: –1.25 at baseline to –0.63 at 8 hours with chlorine dioxide mouthwash *v* –1.40 at baseline to –1.29 at 8 hours with distilled water, $P < 0.01$; odour intensity: 1.27 at baseline to 0.63 at 8 hours with chlorine dioxide containing mouthwash *v* 1.42 at baseline to 1.29 at 8 hours with distilled water, $P < 0.01$).[2] It found no significant difference in odour unpleasantness or intensity between groups at 24, 48, 72, and 96 hours. The second RCT (12 people, crossover design, 96 hour washout period) found that chlorine dioxide containing mouthwash significantly reduced odour unpleasantness score at 0.5, 1, 2, and 4 hours after treatment and odour intensity score at 2 and 4 hours after treatment compared with distilled water (odour unpleasantness: –1.25 at baseline to –0.61 at 4 hours with chlorine dioxide mouthwash *v* –1.06 at baseline to –1.08 at 4 hours with distilled water, $P < 0.01$; odour intensity: 1.14 at baseline to 0.81 at 4 hours with chlorine dioxide mouthwash *v* 1.11 at baseline to 1.19 at 4 hours with distilled water, $P = 0.03$).[9] The third RCT (62 people with confirmed halitosis) compared three treatments: test mouthwash (see comment below), saline rinse, and no treatment.[10] Three trained examiners rated breath odour from 0 (low odour) to 3 (high odour). It found that the test mouthwash significantly reduced odour compared with saline rinse and no treatment at 1, 2, and 3 hours (baseline to 3 hours: 1.63 to 1.03 with test mouthwash *v* 1.51 to 1.72 with saline rinse *v* 1.63 to 1.88 with no treatment, $P < 0.05$ for test mouthwash *v* saline rinse or no treatment).

Harms: The RCTs did not report harms.[2,9,10]

Comment: The third RCT did not report details of the composition of the mouthwash used.[10] Both RCTs of chlorine dioxide containing mouthwash were conducted by the same research group.[2,9]

OPTION SUGAR FREE CHEWING GUMS

We found no RCTs on the effects of sugar free chewing gum.

Benefits: We found no systematic review and no RCTs.

Harms: We found no RCTs.

Comment: None.

OPTION ZINC TOOTHPASTES

We found no RCTs on the effects of zinc toothpaste.

Benefits: We found no systematic review and no RCTs.

Harms: We found no RCTs.

Comment: None.

OPTION ARTIFICIAL SALIVA

We found no RCTs on the effects of artificial saliva.

Benefits: We found no systematic review and no RCTs.

Harms: We found no RCTs.

Comment: None.

GLOSSARY

Organoleptic test scores These are assigned by one or more examiners who sniff the person's exhaled breath on two or three different days. People having this examination should not have had antibiotics in the previous 3 weeks and should have refrained from eating garlic or onions and spicy foods for 48 hours and refrained from usual oral hygiene and smoking for the previous 12 hours.[1] Scoring systems vary among studies.

REFERENCES

1. Yaegaki K, Coil JM. Examination, classification, and treatment of halitosis; clinical perspectives. *J Can Dent Assoc* 2000;66:257–261.
2. Frascella J, Gilbert RD, Fernandez P, et al. Efficacy of a chlorine dioxide-containing mouthrinse in oral malodor. *Compend Contin Educ Dent* 2000;21:241–254.
3. Meningaud JP, Bado F, Favre E, et al. Halitosis in 1999 [in French]. *Rev Stomatol Chir Maxillofac* 1999;100:240–244.
4. Bollen CM, Rompen EH, Demanez JP. Halitosis: a multidisciplinary problem [in French]. *Rev Med Liege* 1999;54:32–36.
5. Tomas Carmona I, Limeres Posse J, Diz Dios P, et al. Extraoral etiology of halitosis. *Med Oral* 2001;6:40–47.
6. Delanghe G, Bollen C, van Steenberghe D, et al. Halitosis, foetor ex ore [in Dutch]. *Ned Tijdschr Tandheelkd* 1998;105:314–317.
7. Tonzetich J. Direct gas chromatographic analysis of sulphur compounds in mouth air in man. *Arch Oral Biol* 1971;16:587–597.
8. Kleinberg I, Westbay G. Oral malodor. *Crit Rev Oral Biol Med* 1990;1:247–259.
9. Frascella J, Gilbert R, Fernandez P. Odor reduction potential of a chlorine dioxide mouthrinse. *J Clin Dent* 1998;9:39–42.
10. Schmidt NF, Tarbet WJ. The effect of oral rinses on organoleptic mouth odor ratings and levels of volatile sulfur compounds. *Oral Surg Oral Med Oral Pathol* 1978;45:876–883.

Bazian Ltd
London, UK

Competing interests: None declared.

Postoperative pulmonary infections

Search date November 2002

Andrew Smith

QUESTIONS

INTERVENTIONS

See glossary, p 1650

Key Messages

- **Postoperative chest physiotherapy (deep breathing exercises)** One systematic review and one subsequent RCT have found that deep breathing exercises reduce postoperative pulmonary infections compared with control.
- **Epidural anaesthesia** Two systematic reviews have found that epidural anaesthesia with or without postoperative epidural analgesia reduces postoperative pulmonary infections compared with general anaesthesia with or without postoperative systemic analgesia. Neither review sought data on adverse effects. Subsequent and additional RCTs found inconsistent results.
- **Postoperative chest physiotherapy (incentive spirometry and intermittent positive pressure breathing)** Two RCTs found that incentive spirometry reduced pulmonary complications compared with control. One RCT found that intermittent positive pressure breathing reduced postoperative pulmonary complications compared with control.
- **Advice to stop smoking preoperatively** We found no RCTs about the effects of preoperative advice to stop cigarette smoking on postoperative pulmonary infections. Two observational studies found that people who smoked were more likely to develop postoperative pulmonary complications of all kinds than those who did not. One study suggested that people who had stopped smoking 6 months preoperatively reverted to the risk of those who had never smoked.

Clin Evid 2003;10:1644–1651.

DEFINITION A working diagnosis of postoperative pulmonary infection may be based on three or more new findings from: cough, phlegm, shortness of breath, chest pain, temperature above 38 °C, and pulse rate above 100/min.[1] In this topic, the diagnosis of pneumonia implies consolidation observed on a chest x ray.[2]

INCIDENCE/ PREVALENCE Reported morbidity for chest complications depends on how carefully they are investigated. One study found blood gas and chest radiograph abnormalities in about 50% of people after open cholecystectomy.[3] However, less than 20% of these had abnormal clinical signs and only 10% had a clinically significant chest infection. Another study estimated the incidence of pneumonia as 20%.[4] Another used a similarly strict definition and found the incidence was 23%.[5]

AETIOLOGY/ RISK FACTORS Risk factors include increasing age (> 50 years), cigarette smoking, obesity, thoracic or upper abdominal operations, and pre-existing lung disease.[6] One multivariate analysis did not confirm the association with cigarette smoking but suggested that longer preoperative hospital stay and higher grading on the American Society of Anesthesiologists' physical status scale (> 2) increased the risk of postoperative pulmonary complications.[5] Depression of the immune system may also contribute.[7]

PROGNOSIS In one large systematic review (search date 1997, 141 RCTs, 9559 people), 10% of people with postoperative pneumonia died.[8] If systemic sepsis ensues, mortality is likely to be substantial.[9] Pneumonia delays recovery from surgery and poor tissue oxygenation may contribute to delayed wound healing.

AIMS OF INTERVENTION To prevent the development of postoperative pulmonary infection; to minimise postoperative pain; to minimise adverse effects of treatment; to reduce mortality.

OUTCOMES Clinically diagnosed postoperative pulmonary infection (as in the definition above) and a variety of pain scales. Postoperative pulmonary complications are a commonly used outcome, but this combines pulmonary infections with other adverse outcomes.

METHODS *Clinical Evidence* search and appraisal November 2002 including a search for observational studies on preoperative advice to stop smoking.

QUESTION **What are the effects of preoperative advice to stop smoking?**

We found no RCTs about the effects of preoperative advice to stop cigarette smoking on postoperative pulmonary infections. Two observational studies found that people who smoked were more likely to develop pulmonary complications of all kinds than those who did not. One study suggested that people who had stopped smoking 6 months preoperatively reverted to the risk of those who had never smoked.

Benefits: We found one systematic review (search date 2001), which identified no RCTs.[10] We found no subsequent RCTs.

Harms: We found no RCTs.

Comment: One prospective observational study (200 people undergoing coronary artery bypass surgery) found that smokers were more likely than people who did not smoke to develop postoperative pulmonary complications of all types.[11] People who had stopped smoking 6 months preoperatively reverted to the risk of those who had never smoked. A benefit was seen only in people who had stopped smoking for 2 months or more. A later prospective cohort study (410 people undergoing a variety of elective procedures) found that current smokers were more likely to have postoperative pneumonia than those who had never smoked, but the differences were not tested statistically.[12] For all postoperative pulmonary complications, the odds ratio for developing complications for current smokers compared with those who had never smoked was 5.5 (95% CI 1.2 to 14.8). One multivariate analysis of postoperative pulmonary infections did not confirm the association with cigarette smoking.[5]

QUESTION What are the effects of different anaesthetic/analgesic techniques?

Two systematic reviews have found that epidural anaesthesia with or without postoperative epidural analgesia reduces postoperative pulmonary infections compared with general anaesthesia with or without postoperative systemic analgesia. Neither review sought data on adverse effects. Subsequent and additional RCTs found inconsistent results.

Benefits: We found two systematic reviews (search dates 1997[8] and 1996[13]), one additional RCT,[14] and three subsequent RCTs.[15–17] Both reviews found that regional analgesia/anaesthesia reduced the incidence of pulmonary infections compared with systemic anaesthesia/analgesia.[8,13] The first review (search date 1997) compared intraoperative neuraxial blockade (see glossary, p 1650) versus no neuraxial blockade (primarily general anaesthesia plus systemic analgesia).[8] The second systematic review (search date 1996) made three comparisons of postoperative epidural versus non-epidural anaesthesia/analgesia.[13] **Intraoperative regional versus general anaesthesia:** The first review found that neuraxial blockade significantly reduced postoperative pneumonia compared with general anaesthesia (28 RCTs; 149/4871 [3%] *v* 238/4688 [5%]; ARR 2%; RR 0.60, 95% CI 0.49 to 0.74; NNT 50, 95% CI 36 to 82).[8] The review found some evidence that the risk of developing pneumonia may be lower after thoracic epidural anaesthesia than after lumbar epidural or spinal anaesthesia. **Postoperative epidural local anaesthetic versus systemic opioid analgesia:** The second review (search date 1996) identified five RCTs (215 people; 3 RCTs in people undergoing cholecystectomy, 1 in people undergoing upper abdominal or hip surgery, and 1 in people undergoing upper abdominal surgery).[13] It found that postoperative epidural local anaesthesia significantly reduced the incidence of pulmonary infections compared with systemic opioids (RR 0.36, 95% CI 0.21 to 0.65; absolute figures not provided).[13] Sensitivity analysis found that exclusion of low quality trials did not alter these results. **Postoperative epidural opioid analgesia versus systemic opioid analgesia:** The second review (search date

1996, 5 RCTs, 547 people; 2 RCTs of thoracotomies, 2 of abdominal operations, 1 of upper abdominal surgery) found no significant difference in the rate of pulmonary infections between postoperative epidural and systemic opioids (RR 0.53, 95% CI 0.18 to 1.53; absolute figures not provided; see comment below).[13] **Postoperative epidural local anaesthetic plus analgesia versus systemic opioid analgesia:** The second review (search date 1996)[13] identified two RCTs[17,18] and we found one additional[14] and one subsequent RCT[15] comparing postoperative epidural local anaesthetic plus opioids versus postoperative systemic opioids. The first RCT identified by the review (163 people receiving general anaesthesia while undergoing abdominal surgery for cancer) compared postoperative epidural bupivacaine plus morphine versus postoperative intravenous fentanyl plus subcutaneous morphine. It found no significant difference in the rate of postoperative pulmonary infections between epidural local anasthesia plus analgesia and systemic analgesia (21/78 [31%] with epidural analgesia/anaesthesia *v* 23/75 [27%] systemic; RR 0.88, 95% CI 0.53 to 1.45; analysis not intention to treat; see comment below).[18] The second RCT identified by the review (53 people undergoing pulmonary resection) compared five different postoperative treatment strategies: epidural morphine plus epidural bupivacaine, epidural morphine alone, epidural bupivacaine alone, epidual saline, and systemic morphine.[19] It found no significant difference in rates of pneumonia between groups (2/11 [18%] with epidural morphine plus epidural bupivacaine *v* 3/12 [25%] with epidural morphine *v* 1/10 [10%] with epidural bupivacaine *v* 2/10 [20%] with epidural saline *v* 1/10 [10%] with systemic morphine; overall P = 0.86; see comment below). The additional RCT (46 elderly non-smokers undergoing major pancreatic and biliary surgery) found that postoperative epidural local anaesthetic plus opioid significantly reduced the incidence of pneumonia compared with systemic opioid (2/22 [9%] *v* 8/24 [33%]; P = 0.049).[14] The subsequent RCT (50 people undergoing thoracotomy) found no significant difference in postoperative pulmonary complications between epidural local anaesthetic plus opioids and intravenous patient controlled opioid (1/25 [4%] with epidural analgesia *v* 0/25 [0%] with patient controlled analgesia; see comment below).[15] Pneumonia was not separated out of pulmonary complications as a whole. **Other intraoperative/postoperative anaesthesia/analgesia combinations:** We found two subsequent RCTs.[16,17] The first RCT (24 people with chronic obstructive pulmonary disease undergoing upper abdominal or thoracic surgery) compared intraoperative general followed by postoperative systemic morphine versus intraoperative general plus epidural anaethesia followed by postoperative epidural bupivicaine plus morphine. It found no significant difference in the incidence of postoperative pulmonary infection between groups (reported as non-significant; no further data available; see comment below).[16] The second RCT (168 people undergoing elective abdominal aortic surgery) compared intropeperative general anaesthesia followed by either postoperative epidural or intravenous analgesia versus intraoperative thoracic epidural anaesthesia plus light general anaesthesia followed by either postoperative epidural or systemic analgesia (4 treatment groups).[17] It found no significant difference between groups in the incidence of postoperative pneumonia (see comment below).

Harms: The RCTs were not designed to look for information about harms of epidural anaesthesia.[8,13,16,17] However, one RCT found "mild reddening" of the epidural site in 16/25 people after an average of 5.6 days.[15] We found one large prospective French cohort study (30 413 epidural anaesthetics) of the incidence of harms from epidural analgesia.[20] This study estimated the frequency of cardiac arrest (usually owing to inadvertent intravascular injection of local anaesthetic) as 1/10 000; seizures (usually the same cause) as 1.3/10 000; neurological injury as 2/10 000; radiculopathy as 1.6/10 000; and paraplegia as 0.3/10 000.[20] There were no deaths attributable to epidural analgesia. In a large US prospective uncontrolled cohort study (1297 people receiving epidurals), 0.4% of people were judged to need naloxone to reverse the adverse effects of epidural opioids on breathing.[21] One case series reported three cases in which epidural analgesia was thought to contribute to the development of postoperative pressure sores.[22] Inadvertent dural puncture with the epidural needle can cause headache (frequency increases with gauge of needle).[23] Effective pain relief can delay recognition of surgical complications, such as anastomotic breakdown, peritonitis, or compartment compression syndrome of the legs.

Comment: Most of the individual RCTs were too small to detect a significant difference in postoperative pulmonary infections between treatments; only when RCTs were combined by meta-analysis was benefit apparent. The two systematic reviews differ in their approach. The first review sought aggregated benefit for all types of intraoperative neuraxial blockade compared with no neuraxial blockade and had more power.[8] The second review compared different kinds of postoperative epidural anaesthesia/analgesia; the smaller numbers of RCTs and people in each subgroup probably explain the lack of a significant effect for some of the regimens.[13] Although both reviews examined the effect of epidural anaesthesia on pulmonary infection after all types of surgery, sensitivity analyses were performed only in the later review.[8] One sensitivity analysis suggested that the overall benefits of regional anaesthesia in reducing all types of postoperative complications held for all types of surgery studied. The overall benefit of regional anaesthesia seemed independent of whether it was combined with general anaesthesia.

QUESTION **What are the effects of postoperative chest physiotherapy?**

One systematic review has found that postoperative chest physiotherapy reduces postoperative pulmonary complications compared with control. The review found most evidence for deep breathing exercises, but RCTs also found evidence of benefit with incentive spirometry and intermittent positive pressure breathing. One large subsequent RCT has also found that deep breathing exercises reduce postoperative pneumonia compared with control.

Benefits: We found two systematic reviews (search date 1992, 7 RCTs, 764 people;[24] and search date 2000, 2 RCTs, 212 people[25]) and two subsequent RCTs comparing physiotherapy versus control or no treatment.[26,27] The RCTs compared three methods of physiotherapy (incentive spirometry, deep breathing exercises, and intermittent positive pressure breathing [see glossary, p 1650]) on postoperative pulmonary complications. Only people undergoing any type of upper abdominal surgery were included. Not all of the included RCTs used pneumonia as an outcome. **Incentive spirometry:** Both reviews identified the same two RCTs of incentive spirometry versus control (details of control not stated in the reviews), but only the first review performed a meta-analysis.[24] It found that incentive spirometry significantly reduced the risk of postoperative pulmonary complications compared with control (212 people; OR 0.44, 95% CI 0.18 to 0.99; absolute numbers not provided). **Deep breathing/coughing exercises:** The first review[24] identified four RCTs (564 people) comparing deep breathing exercises versus control (details of control not stated in the review) and we found two subsequent RCTs comparing deep breathing exercises versus no treatment.[26,27] The review found that deep breathing exercises significantly reduced pulmonary complications compared with control (OR 0.43, 95% CI 0.27 to 0.63; absolute number not provided), but there was significant heterogeneity between trials. One of the four RCTs (60 people) used an outcome measure that could not in itself diagnose pulmonary infection. The first subsequent RCT (368 people undergoing major abdominal surgery) compared instruction to perform deep breathing exercises versus no physiotherapy instruction. Additional resistance training was given to people in the treatment group at high risk (defined as aged > 50 years or with one of the following: smoker or ex-smoker for < 12 months, body mass index > 30, pulmonary disease needing daily medication, or other coexisting medical condition). The RCT found that, in all people undergoing surgery, deep breathing exercises significantly reduced the risk of developing pneumonia compared with control (1/172 [0.6%] with deep breathing *v* 13/192 [6.8%] with control; RR 0.09, 95% CI 0.01 to 0.65; NNT 16, 95% CI 10 to 39). The relative risk of developing pneumonia in people at high risk was not given. The second subsequent RCT (120 people undergoing coronary artery surgery) compared two physiotherapy groups versus no treatment.[27] The RCT found low rates of chest infections in all groups (1/40 [2.5%] with no physiotherapy *v* 4/40 [10%] with instruction to perform deep breathing and coughing exercises *v* 1/40 [2.5%] with instruction to perform deep breathing and coughing exercises and more intensive attention from the physiotherapist). The RCT did not report formal statistical analysis because of the small number of complications. **Intermittent positive pressure breathing:** The first systematic review[24] identified one RCT[1] (172 people) comparing four interventions: intermittent positive pressure breathing; incentive spirometry; deep breathing exercises; and no treatment. It found that intermittent positive pressure breathing significantly reduced pulmonary complications compared with no treatment (10/45 [22%] with intermittent positive pressure breathing *v* 21/44 [48%] with no treatment; RR 0.5, 95% CI 0.2 to 0.9; NNT 4, 95% CI 3 to 18).[1]

Harms: The reviews gave no information on adverse effects.[24,25]

Comment: Some RCTs in the first review distinguished between people at low and high risk of pulmonary complications.[24] Individual RCTs in low risk people often did not find the benefits of physiotherapy that was seen when all RCTs were pooled. The two subsequent RCTs were conducted in people at lower risk of pulmonary infection.[26,27] The first review assessed study validity by two independent assessors using the following criteria: reproducibility of patient population and surgical procedure; comparability of groups; clear description of experimental manoeuvre; presence of control group; clear description of outcome measures; random allocation with blinding; withdrawals listed; prior estimate of study power; and some measure of test of compliance with treatment.[24]

GLOSSARY

The following three modalities of physiotherapy all count as methods to increase lung volume. Increasing lung volume is thought to cause a reduction in airways resistance and an improvement in ventilation:[28]

Deep breathing The person is instructed to breathe in deeply, comfortably, and slowly through the nose, and then sigh out through the mouth. Optimum conditions to ensure that deep breaths reach poorly ventilated dependent regions include accurate positioning, ensuring the person is comfortable and relaxed, avoiding distractions, and allowing the person to get their breath back after turning to avoid breathlessness.

Incentive spirometry The flow and volume achieved by a controlled and sustained deep breath can be encouraged by an incentive spirometer, which gives the person visual feedback on their performance. The same effect can theoretically be obtained without the device, but the incentive of using a tangible object may increase inhaled volume and produce more controlled flow.

Intermittent positive pressure breathing Assisted breathing with a pressure cycled ventilator triggered into inspiration by the user and allowing passive expiration. The user begins to inhale through the machine, which senses the breath and augments it by delivering gas to the user. When a preset pressure is reached, the machine stops delivering gas and allows the user to breathe out. In most devices, the inspiratory sensitivity, flow rate, and pressure can be varied to suit the user's needs, but some devices adjust the sensitivity and flow automatically.

Neuraxial blockade involves spinal or epidural anaesthesia.

REFERENCES

1. Celli BR, Rodriguez KS, Snider GL. A controlled trial of intermittent positive pressure breathing, incentive spirometry, and deep breathing exercises in preventing pulmonary complications after abdominal surgery. *Am Rev Respir Dis* 1984;130:12–15.
2. Hall JC, Tarala RA, Tapper J, et al. Prevention of respiratory complications after abdominal surgery: a randomised clinical trial. *BMJ* 1996;312:148–152.
3. Wirén FE, Janson L, Hellekant C. Respiratory complications after upper abdominal surgery. *Acta Chir Scand* 1981;147:623–627.
4. Garibaldi RA, Britt MR, Coleman ML, et al. Risk factors for postoperative pneumonia. *Am J Med* 1981;70:677–680.
5. Hall JC, Tarala RA, Hall JL, et al. A multivariate analysis of the risk of pulmonary complications after laparotomy. *Chest* 1991;99:923–927.
6. Christensen EF, Schultz P, Jensen OV, et al. Postoperative pulmonary complications and lung function in high-risk patients: a comparison of three physiotherapy regimens after upper abdominal surgery in general anaesthesia. *Acta Anaesthesiol Scand* 1991;35:97–104.
7. Sabiston DC Jr, ed. *Textbook of surgery: the biological basis of modern surgical practice*. Philadelphia: WB Saunders, 15th ed, 1997:345.
8. Rodgers A, Walker N, Schug S, et al. Reduction of postoperative mortality and morbidity with epidural or spinal anaesthesia: results from overview of randomised trials. *BMJ* 2000;321:1493–1497. Search date 1997; primary sources Medline, Embase, Current Contents, the Cochrane Library, and hand searches of reference lists from all identified papers and of selected conference proceedings and personal contact with authors.

9. Miller G, Ellis ME. Hospital-acquired pneumonia. In: Ellis M, ed. *Infectious diseases of the respiratory tract*. Cambridge: Cambridge University Press, 1998.
10. Møller A, Villebro N, Pedersen T. Interventions for preoperative smoking cessation. In: The Cochrane Library, Issue 1, 2002. Oxford: Update Software. Search date 2001: primary sources: Medline, Embase, and Cinhal.
11. Warner MA, Offord KP, Warner ME, et al. Role of preoperative cessation of smoking and other factors in postoperative pulmonary complications: a blinded prospective study of coronary artery bypass patients. *Mayo Clin Proc* 1989;64:609–616.
12. Bluman LG, Mosca L, Newman N, et al. Preoperative smoking habits and postoperative pulmonary complications. *Chest* 1998;113:148–152.
13. Ballantyne JC, Carr DB, deFerranti S, et al. The comparative effects of postoperative analgesic therapies on pulmonary outcome: cumulative meta-analyses of randomized controlled trials. *Anesth Analg* 1998;86:598–612. Search date 1996; primary sources Medline and hand searches of reference lists from relevant articles.
14. Barzoi G, Bianchi B, Mangiante G, et al. Hepato-biliary-pancreatic surgery in over 70-years-old patients: which is the best anaesthesiologic procedure? *Chir Ital* 1995;47:44–48.
15. Azad SC, Groh J, Beyer A, et al. Continuous epidural analgesia versus patient controlled intravenous analgesia for postthoracotomy pain. *Acute Pain* 2000;3:84–93.
16. Xue Z-G, Bai L, Jiang H. Combined epidural block with general anaesthesia in patients with chronic obstructive pulmonary disease. *J Shanghai Med Univ* 2000;27:302–305, 323.
17. Norris EJ, Beattie C, Perler BA, et al. Double-masked randomized trial comparing alternate combinations of intraoperative anesthesia and postoperative analgesia in abdominal aortic surgery. *Anaesthesiology* 2001;95:1054–1067.
18. Jayr C, Thomas H, Rey A, et al. Postoperative pulmonary complication: epidural analgesia using bupivacaine and opioids versus parenteral opioids. *Anesthesiology* 1993;78:666–676.
19. Logas W, El-Baz N, El-Ganzouri A, et al. Continuous thoracic epidural analgesia for postoperative pain relief following thoracotomy: a randomized prospective study. *Anesthesiology* 1987;67:787–791.
20. Auroy Y, Narchi P, Messiah A, et al. Serious complications related to regional anesthesia. *Anesthesiology* 1997;87:479–486.
21. Scott DA, Beilby DSN, McClymont C. Postoperative analgesia using epidural infusions of fentanyl with bupivacaine. *Anesthesiology* 1995;83:727–737.
22. Shah JL. Postoperative pressure sores after epidural anaesthesia. *BMJ* 2000;321:941–942.
23. Bromage PR. *Epidural analgesia*. Philadelphia: WB Saunders, 1978.
24. Thomas JA, McIntosh JM. Are incentive spirometry, intermittent positive pressure breathing and deep breathing exercises effective in the prevention of postoperative pulmonary complications after upper abdominal surgery? A systematic overview and meta-analysis. *Phys Ther* 1994;74:3–16. Search date 1992; primary sources Medline, Cinahl, and hand searches of reference lists from relevant articles and reference lists, and unpublished abstracts from a Consensus Exercise on Physical Therapy for the Surgical Patient 1989.
25. Overend TJ, Anderson C, Lucy, SD, et al The effect of incentive spirometry on postoperative pulmonary complications: a systematic review. *Chest* 2001;120:971–978. Search date 2000; primary sources Medline, Cinahl, HealthSTAR and Current Contents databases, and handsearches of reference lists from relevant articles.
26. Fagevik-Olsen M, Hahn I, Nordgren S, et al. Randomized controlled trial of prophylactic chest physiotherapy in major abdominal surgery. *Br J Surg* 1997;84:1535–1538.
27. Stiller K, Montarello J, Wallace M, et al. Efficacy of breathing and coughing exercises in the prevention of pulmonary complications after coronary artery surgery. *Chest* 1994;105:741–747.
28. Hough A. *Physiotherapy in respiratory care: a problem-solving approach.* London: Chapman and Hall, 1991.

Andrew Smith
Dept of Anaesthesia
Royal Lancaster Infirmary
Lancaster
UK

Competing interests: None declared.

Acute organophosphorus poisoning

Search date March 2003

Michael Eddleston, Surjit Singh, and Nick Buckley

QUESTIONS

INTERVENTIONS

*Based on consensus, RCTs would be considered unethical

See glossary, p 1661

Key Messages

- **Atropine** Consensus supports atropine treatment. Many case series have found that it reverses the early muscarinic effects of acute organophosphorus poisoning. We found no RCTs comparing atropine versus placebo, but such an RCT would now be considered unethical.
- **Benzodiazepines to control organophosphorus induced seizures** Consensus supports benzodiazepines for organophosphorus induced seizures. We found no RCTs comparing a benzodiazepine versus placebo or another anticonvulsant. It would now be unethical to conduct an RCT comparing benzodiazepines versus placebo.
- **Glycopyrronium bromide (glycopyrrolate)** One small RCT found no significant difference in death or ventilation rates between glycopyrronium bromide and atropine, but it may have lacked power to detect clinically important differences. Glycopyrronium bromide (glycopyrrolate) has been used instead of atropine because it is thought to have fewer adverse effects on the central nervous system.
- **Washing the poisoned person and removing contaminated clothes** Washing the poisoned person with warm water and soap and removing contaminated clothes after dermal and mucocutaneous exposure appears important and widely recommended, but this intervention has not been assessed in RCTs.

- **Gastric lavage** We found no RCTs assessing the role of gastric lavage in acute organophosphorus poisoning. If the procedure cannot be performed in sedated and intubated patients, the risk of harm due to aspiration is likely to surpass its potential benefits.
- **Milk or other home remedy immediately after ingestion** We found no RCTs on the effect of giving a "home remedy" soon after the ingestion.
- **Oximes** One systematic review found insufficient evidence about the effects of oximes in acute organophosphorus poisoning.
- **Ipecacuanha (ipecac)** We found no RCTs on the effects of ipecacuanha in acute organophosphorus poisoning. The significant risk of harm, although not quantified, probably outweighs any potential benefits.
- **Activated charcoal (single or multiple dose); α_2 adrenergic receptor agonists (clonidine); N-methyl-D-aspartate receptor antagonists; organophosphorus hydrolases; sodium bicarbonate** We found insufficient evidence about the effects of these interventions.

DEFINITION Acute organophosphorus poisoning occurs after dermal, respiratory, or oral exposure to either low volatility pesticides (e.g. chlorpyrifos, dimethoate) or high volatility nerve gases (e.g. sarin, tabun). Acetylcholinesterase (see glossary, p 1661) inhibition at synapses results in accumulation of acetylcholine and over-activation of acetylcholine receptors at the neuromuscular junction and in the autonomic and central nervous systems.[1] Early clinical features mainly involve the parasympathetic system: bradycardia, bronchorrhoea, miosis, salivation, lachrymation, defecation, urination, and hypotension. Features of neuromuscular junction (muscle weakness and fasciculations) and central nervous system (seizures, coma) involvement are also common at this stage. An intermediate syndrome has been described (cranial nerve palsies and proximal muscle weakness with preserved distal muscle power after resolution of early cholinergic symptoms), but its definition, pathophysiology, and incidence are still unclear. A late motor or motor/sensory peripheral neuropathy may also develop after recovery from acute poisoning with some organophosphorus compounds.[1]

INCIDENCE/ PREVALENCE Most cases occur in the developing world following occupational or deliberate exposure to organophosphorus pesticides.[2] Although data are sparse, organophosphates appear to be the most important cause of death from deliberate self poisoning worldwide.[3] In Sri Lanka, at least 17 000 cases of organophosphorus or carbamate poisoning occurred in 1999, resulting in 1700 deaths. More than 80% were intentional.[4] Case fatality rates across the developing world are commonly greater than 20%.[3] In Central America, occupational poisoning is more common than intentional poisoning and deaths are fewer.[5] Extrapolating from limited data, the World Health Organization has estimated that each year more than 200 000 people worldwide die from pesticide poisoning,[6] but these figures are old and widely contested.[2] Most deaths occur in Asia and organophosphorus pesticides probably cause at least 50% of cases.[3] Deaths from organophosphorus nerve gases occurred in Iran during the Iran–Iraq war.[7] Military or terrorist action with these chemical weapons remains possible. Twelve people died in a terrorist attack in Tokyo and thousands probably died in Iran after military or terrorist exposure.

AETIOLOGY/ RISK FACTORS	The widespread accessibility of pesticides in rural parts of the developing world makes them easy options for acts of self harm.[3] Occupational exposure is due to insufficient or inappropriate protective equipment in the use of toxic compounds.[2]
PROGNOSIS	There are no validated scoring systems for categorising severity or predicting outcome, although many have been proposed. The highly variable natural history and difficulty in determining ingested dose make predicting outcome for an individual inaccurate and potentially hazardous, because people admitted in good condition can deteriorate rapidly and require intubation and mechanical ventilation. Prognosis in acute self poisoning is likely to depend on dose and toxicity of the ingested organophosphorus (e.g. neurotoxicity potential, half life, rate of ageing [see glossary, p 1662], whether activation to the toxic compound is required [pro-poison — see glossary, p 1662], and whether dimethylated or diethylated [see comment under oximes, p 1659]).[8,9] Prognosis in occupational exposure is better because the dose is normally smaller and the route is dermal.
AIMS OF INTERVENTION	To prevent death; to reduce consciousness or respiratory arrest requiring intubation with or without ventilation, pneumonia, the intermediate syndrome (see definition above), and delayed polyneuropathy; and to reduce the period of ventilation and intensive care.
OUTCOMES	Rates of death, intubation, pneumonia; the intermediate syndrome; delayed polyneuropathy; and period of time requiring ventilation or intensive care.
METHODS	*Clinical Evidence* search and appraisal March 2003. The authors also searched Medline, Embase, and Cochrane databases; hand searched toxicological and Indian journals (search date November 2001); and contacted experts in the field to identify unpublished studies.

QUESTION What are the effects of treatments for acute organophosphorus poisoning?

OPTION DRINKING MILK OR OTHER HOME REMEDY SOON AFTER ORAL ORGANOPHOSPHORUS EXPOSURE

We found no RCTs on the effect of giving a "home remedy" soon after the ingestion.

Benefits: We found no systematic review, RCT, or cohort study for any form of home remedy.

Harms: We found no systematic review, RCT, or cohort study of complications.

Comment: The lay practice of giving a "home remedy" soon after the ingestion, before bringing the poisoned person to hospital, is common in many parts of the world. Problems may occur when large volumes of fluid are given "to dilute the poison". Gastric emptying of a fluid is proportional to volume. It is therefore believed that increasing the volume of fluid in the stomach increases the rate of emptying into the small bowel where the pesticide is absorbed. Giving fluids therefore risks speeding the onset of poisoning and causing respiratory arrest before the patient arrives at a healthcare facility. In contrast, a small volume highly lipid home remedy (such as unboiled eggs) may slow gastric emptying and may delay the onset of poisoning and respiratory failure until the patient has reached a healthcare facility.

OPTION WASHING THE POISONED PERSON AND REMOVING CONTAMINATED CLOTHES

We found no RCTs of washing the poisoned person and removing contaminated clothes. However, this appears to be an obvious way to reduce further dermal and mucocutaneous exposure and is widely recommended. Care should be taken to protect healthcare workers through gloves, aprons, and eye protection, with careful disposal of contaminated equipment and clothes.

Benefits: We found no systematic review and no RCTs.

Harms: We found no systematic review, RCT, or cohort study of complications in poisoned people or healthcare workers removing contaminated clothing from poisoned people. However, severe poisoning requiring intubation and mechanical ventilation has been reported in healthcare workers treating poisoned people.[10] No significant complications from the procedure for the initially poisoned person are envisaged, unless washing the poisoned person distracts caregivers from other priorities, such as resuscitation and careful observation for deterioration.

Comment: Absorbing organophosphorus compounds through the skin varies greatly, according to the volatility of the organophosphorus, its solvent, and the temperature and hydration of the skin.[11] Absorption of pesticides seems to be low, with studies of malathion, chlorpyrifos, and diazinon suggesting that less than 5% is absorbed and excreted in the urine.[12–14]

OPTION IPECACUANHA (IPECAC)

We found no RCTs on the effects of ipecacuanha (ipecac) in acute organophosphorus poisoning. The significant risk of harm, although not quantified, probably outweighs any potential benefits.

Benefits: We found no systematic review and no RCTs.

Harms: We found no systematic review, RCT, or cohort study of complications of ipecacuanha in people with acute organophosphorus poisoning, and no large, high quality RCT comparing ipecacuanha versus placebo in any form of poisoning that might have allowed calculation of complication rates. Complications of ipecacuanha may include aspiration, diarrhoea, ileus, dysrhythmias during vomiting, dystonia from treatment of vomiting, and haematemesis from vomiting.[15] Use of ipecacuanha in acute organophosphorus poisoning may be particularly hazardous because most organophosphorus compounds are dissolved in aromatic hydrocarbons, which cause serious harm if aspirated.[15]

Comment: One non-systematic review identified no human studies of ipecacuanha in people with organophosphorus poisoning.[15] One non-systematic review of ipecacuanha in all forms of poisoning found no evidence that it improved outcomes in poisoned people.[15] Administration of ipecacuanha may delay administration of activated charcoal and specific treatment for organophosphorus poisoning, in addition to increasing the risk of aspiration.

OPTION GASTRIC LAVAGE

We found no systematic review, RCT, or cohort study on the effects of gastric lavage in acute organophosphorus poisoning. If the procedure cannot be performed in sedated and intubated patients, the risk of harm due to aspiration is likely to surpass its potential benefits.

Benefits: We found no systematic review and no RCTs.

Harms: We found no systematic review, RCT, or cohort study assessing complications of gastric lavage in people with acute organophosphorus poisoning, and no large, high quality RCTs comparing gastric lavage versus placebo in any form of poisoning that allowed calculation of complication rates. Complications of gastric lavage may include aspiration, hypoxia, laryngeal spasm, and oesophageal perforation.[16] Complications are common when gastric lavage is performed in physically restrained, non-consenting patients as a routine procedure without careful control of the airway.

Comment: One non-systematic review identified no human studies of gastric lavage in people with organophosphorus poisoning.[16] One non-systematic review of gastric lavage in people with all forms of poisoning found no evidence that it improved outcome in poisoned people.[16] Gastric lavage may delay administering activated charcoal and specific treatment for organophosphorus poisoning. Anecdotal reports suggest that organophosphorus pesticides may remain in the gut for lengthy periods.[17] If studies indicate that a substantial proportion of organophosphorus remains in the stomach on admission to hospital, it may be appropriate to conduct an RCT to assess gastric lavage after protection of the airway.

OPTION ACTIVATED CHARCOAL (SINGLE OR MULTIPLE DOSE)

We found no systematic review, RCT, or cohort study on the effects of activated charcoal, in either single or multiple dose regimens, in acute organophosphorus poisoning.

Benefits: We found no systematic review, RCT, or cohort study.

Harms: We found no systematic review, RCT, or cohort study of complications in people with acute organophosphorus poisoning receiving activated charcoal and no large, high quality RCT comparing activated charcoal versus placebo in any form of poisoning that allowed calculation of complication rates. Complications of activated charcoal may include aspiration pneumonia, vomiting, diarrhoea, constipation, ileus, and reduced absorption of oral medication.[18–20] A large retrospective case series (878 people treated with multiple dose activated charcoal) suggests that rates of adverse events with multiple dose regimens (> 2 doses) are likely to be low (significant pulmonary aspiration in 6/878 [0.6%], 95% CI 0.1% to 1.1%).[21]

Comment: **Single dose regimens:** We found no human simulated overdose studies of single dose activated charcoal in organophosphorus poisoning.[18] Animal studies indicate that activated charcoal can bind to organophosphorus pesticides.[22] One non-systematic review of single dose activated charcoal in all forms of poisoning found no evidence that it improved outcomes in poisoned people.[18] **Multiple dose regimens:** We found no human studies of multiple dose activated charcoal in organophosphorus poisoning.[19] One non-systematic review of multiple dose activated charcoal in all forms of poisoning found no evidence that it improved outcomes in poisoned people.[19] Activated charcoal may reduce the efficacy of treatments given by mouth. A large RCT comparing single or multiple dose activated charcoal versus placebo in acute organophosphorus pesticide poisoning started in Sri Lanka in 2002, and the findings are expected to be reported in 2007.[23]

OPTION ATROPINE

Atropine is the mainstay of treatment, and many case series have found that it reverses the early muscarinic effects of acute organophosphorus poisoning. We found no RCTs comparing atropine versus placebo. It would now be considered unethical to perform such an RCT.

Benefits: We found no systematic review, RCT, or cohort study. Many case series have found that atropine reverses the early muscarinic effects of acute organophosphorus poisoning.[24]

Harms: We found no systematic review, RCT, or cohort study of complication rates in people with acute organophosphorus poisoning receiving atropine. Excessive treatment with atropine results in toxicity that is characterised by confusion and tachycardia.[24] In hypoxic people, supplemental oxygen may reduce toxicity caused by tachycardia with increased myocardial oxygen demand.

Comment: Atropine competes with excess acetylcholine at muscarinic acetylcholine receptors. We found no RCTs, but its effectiveness is now considered to be beyond question, so it would be unethical to perform an RCT comparing atropine versus placebo. The optimum dose of atropine has not been determined, but may vary among poisoned people because of variation in the dose taken and possibly because of co-administration of an oxime (oximes have been proposed to have anticholinergic action at high dose).[8] The first doses are given as boluses to reverse the muscarinic signs. Current recommendations are then to set up an atropine infusion.[8] Recent RCTs from India on the use of oximes have used an infusion of atropine sufficient to keep the pupils at mid-point, heart rate greater than 100 beats a minute, normal bowel sounds, clear lungs, and no bronchorrhoea.[25–28] The atropine dose regimen has not been compared with other regimens with different end points of atropinisation (see glossary, p 1662).

OPTION GLYCOPYRRONIUM BROMIDE (GLYCOPYRROLATE)

One small RCT found no significant difference in death or ventilation rates between glycopyrronium bromide and atropine, but it may have lacked power to detect clinically important differences. Glycopyrronium bromide (glycopyrrolate) has been used instead of atropine because it is thought to have fewer adverse effects on the central nervous system.

Benefits: We found no systematic review or RCT comparing glycopyrronium bromide versus placebo. It is unlikely that such a trial would be considered ethical unless glycopyrronium bromide and placebo were administered in addition to atropine. We found one small RCT (39 people) comparing glycopyrronium bromide versus atropine.[29] It found no significant difference between atropine and glycopyrronium bromide in death rates, need for ventilation, or respiratory infection (death rates: AR 1/22 [5%] with atropine *v* 2/17 [12%] with glycopyrronium; RR 0.39, 95% CI 0.04 to 3.91; need for ventilation: AR 8/22 [36%] with atropine *v* 6/17 [35%] with glycopyrronium; RR 1.03, 95% CI 0.44 to 2.41; respiratory infection: AR 12/22 [55%] with atropine *v* 5/17 [29%] with glycopyrronium; RR 1.86, 95% CI 0.81 to 4.25). The study may have lacked power to rule out clinically important differences in mortality rates, ventilation, or intermediate syndrome.

Harms: We found no systematic review, RCT, or cohort study of complication rates in people with acute organophosphorus poisoning receiving glycopyrronium bromide. Treatment with glycopyrronium bromide may result in peripheral anticholinergic effects such as tachycardia, dry mouth, and ileus.[30] When these symptoms arise, treatment is defined as excessive.

Comment: Glycopyrronium bromide has similar effects to atropine in humans, but is more selective for peripheral cholinergic synapses, resulting in less tachycardia and confusion than occur with atropine.[30] Animal studies have found that glycopyrronium bromide is less effective at controlling bradycardia and central nervous system complications of organophosphorus poisoning. It is not widely used. We found no large RCT comparing atropine versus glycopyrronium bromide. In some regions, glycopyrronium bromide is combined with atropine to limit the central stimulation produced by atropine.

OPTION OXIMES

One systematic review of two small RCTs found insufficient evidence on the effects of oximes in acute poisoning.

Benefits: We found one systematic review of oximes (search date 2002; 2 RCTs, 182 people; the inclusion criterion was any RCT of oximes in organophosphorus poisoned people).[9] Both RCTs focused on pralidoxime in pesticide poisoned people.[27,28] Neither of the two RCTs found any benefit of pralidoxime. The second RCT found that an infusion of 12 g pralidoxime over 3 days increased risks of death, intermediate syndrome, and requirement for ventilation compared with placebo (death: AR 16/55 [29%] with pralidoxime *v* 3/55 [5%]

with placebo; RR 5.3, 95% CI 1.7 to 17.3; intermediate syndrome: 36/55 [65%] with pralidoxime *v* 19/55 [35%] with placebo; RR 1.9, 95% CI 1.3 to 2.9; requirement for ventilation: 36/55 [67%] with pralidoxime *v* 22/55 [40%] with placebo; RR 1.7, 95% CI 1.1 to 2.4).

Harms: Neither RCT reported the incidence of complications in people with acute organophosphorus poisoning receiving oximes.[25–28] Complications of oximes include hypertension, cardiac dysrhythmias (including cardiac arrest with rapid administration), headache, blurred vision, dizziness, and epigastric discomfort.[31] Such adverse effects with pralidoxime have been reported only with either rapid administration or doses greater than 30 mg/kg bolus. It may be difficult to distinguish these adverse effects from the effects of organophosphorus. In one observational clinical study of a different oxime (obidoxime), a high dose regimen (8 mg/kg bolus, then 2 mg/kg/hour infusion) produced hepatitis in 3/12 people.[7] Two of six deaths were because of liver failure. The use of pralidoxime in eight people in the same study (dose 30 mg/kg bolus, and then 8 mg/kg/hour infusion) did not produce hepatitis. A more recently developed oxime (HI-6) has also been used in humans with no reported adverse effects.[32] We found no human studies that assessed the harms of giving oximes for carbamate poisoning (which presents with a similar cholinergic crisis but has a better prognosis).[1]

Comment: Oximes (such as pralidoxime, obidoxime, and HI-6) reactivate acetylcholinesterases (see glossary, p 1661) inhibited by organophosphorus poisoning.[8,9] Reactivation is limited by ageing (see glossary, p 1661) of the acetylcholinesterases and high concentrations of pesticides. Ageing of the acetylcholinesterases takes longer with diethyl organophosphorus compounds than with dimethyl organophosphorus compounds (120 hours *v* 12 hours). Oximes may therefore be effective for people presenting after about 12 hours if they have been exposed to a diethyl organophosphorus. Treatment may be beneficial if continued for as long as the person is symptomatic because it may take several days for the pesticide concentration to drop below the point at which the rate of reactivation surpasses reinhibition.[8,9] Both RCTs used doses of pralidoxime that are different from the regimen currently recommended by the World Health Organization (at least 30 mg/kg bolus, then 8 mg/kg/hour iv infusion).[27,28] The reporting of the methods was poor, and baseline differences in the second RCT suggested that more severely poisoned people might have been randomised to the intervention arm.[9] Post hoc analysis of the first RCT suggested that people receiving pralidoxime 1 g in the first 12 hours may be less likely to develop the intermediate syndrome than those receiving less than 1 g in the first 12 hours (29% *v* 51%; RR 0.58, 95% CI 0.27 to 1.26).[25] Studies in poisoned people indicate that oximes can reactivate acetylcholinesterase but have not been able to prove clinical benefit.[33] In vitro studies have also revealed mechanisms whereby oximes may be detrimental.[34] A large RCT will start in Sri Lanka in 2003–2004 and the findings are expected to be reported in 2007.[35]

OPTION ORGANOPHOSPHORUS HYDROLASES

We found no RCTs on the effects of organophosphorus hydrolases.

Benefits: We found no systematic reviews and no RCTs.

Harms: We found no systematic review, RCT, or cohort study.

Comment: Oxime efficacy is normally limited by the presence of high pesticide concentrations, which reinhibit acetylcholinesterases (see glossary, p 1661) that have been reactivated by the oximes.[9] A method of rapidly reducing pesticide concentrations could potentially allow oximes to be more effective. Animal studies have found that organophosphorus hydrolases (such as mammalian paraoxanase or the bacterial hydrolase isolated from *Pseudomonas* species) cleave organophosphorus compounds, lowering blood and tissue concentrations of organophosphorus.[36,37] These may prove beneficial for managing people with both pesticide and nerve gas organophosphorus poisoning.

OPTION SODIUM BICARBONATE

We found no RCTs on the effects of sodium bicarbonate in acute organophosphorus poisoning.

Benefits: We found no systematic review and no RCTs.

Harms: We found no systematic review, RCT, or cohort study of complications in people with acute organophosphorus poisoning receiving sodium bicarbonate. Dose dependent complications of sodium bicarbonate may include sodium and fluid overload and decreased oxygen delivery.[38]

Comment: Animal studies suggest that increasing the pH with sodium bicarbonate reduces mortality rates.[39,40] This effect is independent of correction of acidosis because it is seen in animals that are not acidotic. Studies conducted in Brazil[40] and Iran[7] have claimed good results in uncontrolled studies. The mechanism of action of sodium bicarbonate in organophosphorus poisoning is unknown. However, it is unclear whether the limited increase in pH that is possible in vivo is sufficient to make a significant difference in organophosphorus hydrolysis rates.

OPTION BENZODIAZEPINES

Diazepam is standard treatment for organophosphorus induced seizures. We found no RCTs comparing diazepam or other benzodiazepines versus placebo or another anticonvulsant. It would now be considered unethical to perform an RCT comparing benzodiazepines versus placebo in people with seizures.

Benefits: Many case series have reported that diazepam controls seizures in acute organophosphorus poisoning.[41]

Harms: We found no systematic review, RCT, or cohort study of complication rates in people with acute organophosphorus poisoning receiving diazepam. Excessive treatment with diazepam may result in respiratory depression requiring intubation and ventilation. However, this is also a direct complication of organophosphorus poisoning and it is difficult to distinguish between the two.[41]

Comment: Benzodiazepines such as diazepam, lorazepam, and midazolam are widely used for treating organophosphorus induced seizures. However, the seizures are believed to be started by excess acetylcholine in the brain following acetylcholinesterase (see glossary, p 1661) inhibition, with subsequent disruption of other neurotransmitter systems such as glutamate and catecholamine. Benziodiazepines work at γ-aminobutyric acid receptors. Other treatments may therefore be beneficial. Sufficient atropinisation (see glossary, p 1662) may help to manage organophosphorus induced seizures. Routine benzodiazepines before any seizure occurs has support from animal models, but we found no studies in humans.[42]

OPTION CLONIDINE

We found no RCTs on the effects of clonidine in acute organophosphorus poisoning.

Benefits: We found no systematic review and no RCTs.

Harms: We found no systematic review, RCT, or cohort study of complications in people with acute organophosphorus poisoning receiving clonidine. Complications of clonidine may include sedation, hypotension, bradycardia, and (with prolonged use) rebound hypertension.[43]

Comment: Clonidine inhibits the release of acetylcholine from cholinergic neurones and has α_2 adrenergic agonist effects. Animal studies have found that clonidine pretreatment improves survival after organophosphorus poisoning; combination with atropine was more than additive.[44] This treatment has not yet been studied in organophosphorus poisoning in humans.

OPTION N-METHYL-D-ASPARTATE RECEPTOR ANTAGONISTS

We found no RCTs on the effects of N-methyl-D-aspartate receptor antagonists in acute organophosphorus poisoning.

Benefits: We found no systematic review and no RCTs.

Harms: We found no systematic review, RCT, or cohort study of complications in people with acute organophosphorus poisoning receiving N-methyl-D-aspartate (NMDA) receptor antagonists. A dose ranging clinical study found that complications of NMDA receptor antagonists include dizziness, vomiting, nausea, stupor, agitation, and hallucinations.[45]

Comment: Primate studies have found that treating with NMDA receptor antagonists, such as gacyclidine, improves clinical recovery, reduces neural death, and improves electroencephalogram activity following organophosphorus poisoning.[46]

GLOSSARY

Acetylcholinesterase An enzyme that cleaves acetylcholine.

Ageing Esterases (such as acetylcholinesterase and neurotoxic target esterase) are inhibited by organophosphorus through phosphorylation. Inhibited acetylcholinesterase reactivates spontaneously at very slow rates; oximes speed up this reaction. However, phosphorylated acetylcholinesterase may lose an alkyl side chain non-enzymatically, leaving a hydroxyl group in its place ("ageing"). Regeneration is then no longer possible.

Atropinisation Administering atropine until it reaches sufficiently high blood levels to suppress cholinergic signs clinically.

Pro-poisons Some organophosphorus pesticides require activation in vivo to become toxic.

Rates of ageing The rate depends on the identity of the alkyl side chains on each organophosphorus. Those with two methyl groups will age faster than those with two ethyl groups and thus become unresponsive to oximes at an earlier time point.

Substantive changes

Activated charcoal One retrospective case series added;[21] conclusions unchanged.

REFERENCES

1. Ballantyne B, Marrs TC. Overview of the biological and clinical aspects of organophosphates and carbamates. In: Ballantyne B, Marrs TC, eds. *Clinical and experimental toxicology of organophosphates and carbamates*. Oxford: Butterworth Heinemann, 1992:3–14.
2. Karalliedde L, Eddleston M, Murray V. The global picture of organophosphate insecticide poisoning. In: Karalliedde L, Feldman F, Henry J, et al, eds. *Organophosphates and health*. London: Imperial Press, 2001:432–471.
3. Eddleston M. Patterns and problems of deliberate self-poisoning in the developing world. *Q J Med* 2000;93:715–731.
4. Sri Lankan Ministry of Health. *Annual Health Bulletin, Sri Lanka 1999*. Colombo: Ministry of Health, 2001.
5. Wesseling C, McConnell R, Partanen T, et al. Agricultural pesticide use in developing countries: health effects and research needs. *Int J Health Serv* 1997;27:273–308.
6. World Health Organization in collaboration with the United Nations Environment Programme. *Public health impact of pesticides used in agriculture*. Geneva: World Health Organization, 1990.
7. Balali-Mood M, Shariat M. Treatment of organophosphate poisoning. Experience of nerve agents and acute pesticide poisoning on the effects of oximes. *J Physiol Paris* 1998;92:375–378.
8. Johnson MK, Jacobsen D, Meredith TJ, et al. Evaluation of antidotes for poisoning by organophosphorus pesticides. *Emerg Med* 2000;12:22–37.
9. Eddleston M, Szinicz L, Eyer P, et al. Oximes in acute organophosphorus pesticide poisoning: a systematic review of clinical trials. *Q J Med* 2002;95:275–283. Search date 2002; primary sources Medline, Embase, The Cochrane Library, checking of reference lists, contact with experts, and a web search using Google.
10. Anonymous. Nosocomial poisoning associated with emergency department treatment of organophosphate toxicity: Georgia, 2000. *MMWR Morb Mortal Wkly Rep* 2001;49:1156–1158.
11. Riviere JE, Chang SK. Transdermal penetration and metabolism of organophosphate insecticides. In: Chambers JE, Levi PE, eds. *Organophosphates: chemistry, fate and effects*. San Diego: Academic Press, 1992:241–253.
12. Wester RC, Sedik L, Melendres J, et al. Percutaneous absorption of diazinon in humans. *Food Chem Toxicol* 1993;31:569–572.
13. Krieger RI, Dinoff TM. Malathion deposition, metabolite clearance, and cholinesterase status of date dusters and harvesters in California. *Arch Environ Contam Toxicol* 2000;38:546–553.
14. Griffin P, Mason H, Heywood K, et al. Oral and dermal absorption of chlorpyrifos: a human volunteer study. *Occup Environ Med* 1999;56:10–13.
15. American Academy of Clinical Toxicology, European Association of Poison Centres and Clinical Toxicologists. Position statement: ipecac syrup. *J Toxicol Clin Toxicol* 1997;35:699–709.
16. American Academy of Clinical Toxicology, European Association of Poison Centres and Clinical Toxicologists. Position statement: gastric lavage. *J Toxicol Clin Toxicol* 1997;35:711–719.
17. Futagami K, Otsubo K, Nakao Y, et al. Acute organophosphate poisoning after disulfoton ingestion. *J Toxicol Clin Toxicol* 1995;33:151–155.
18. American Academy of Clinical Toxicology, European Association of Poison Centres and Clinical Toxicologists. Position statement: single-dose activated charcoal. *J Toxicol Clin Toxicol* 1997;35:721–741.
19. American Academy of Clinical Toxicology, European Association of Poison Centres and Clinical Toxicologists. Position statement and practice guidelines on the use of multi-dose activated charcoal in the treatment of acute poisoning. *J Toxicol Clin Toxicol* 1999;37:731–751.
20. Mauro LS, Nawarskas JJ, Mauro VF. Misadventures with activated charcoal and recommendations for safe use. *Ann Pharmacother* 1994;28:915–924.
21. Dorrington CL, Johnson DW, Brant R, and the Multiple Dose Activated Charcoal Complication Study Group. The frequency of complications associated with the use of multiple-dose activated charcoal. *Ann Emerg Med* 2003;41:370–377.
22. Tuncok Y, Gelal A, Apaydin S, et al. Prevention of oral dichlorvos toxicity by different activated charcoal products in mice. *Ann Emerg Med* 1995;25:353–355.
23. University of Oxford. Acute organophosphate pesticide poisoning in Sri Lanka — management, complications and pharmacogenetics. ISRCTN02920054 allocated July 2002. http://www.controlled-trials.com/isrctn/trial/02920054/0/02920054.html (last accessed 19 August 2003).
24. Heath AJW, Meredith T. Atropine in the management of anticholinesterase poisoning. In: Ballantyne B, Marrs TC, eds. *Clinical and experimental toxicology of organophosphates and carbamates*. Oxford: Butterworth Heinemann, 1992:543–554.

25. Samuel J, Thomas K, Jeyaseelan L, et al. Incidence of intermediate syndrome in organophosphorus poisoning. *J Assoc Physic India* 1995;43:321–323.
26. Samuel J, Peter JV, Thomas K, et al. Evaluation of two treatment regimens of pralidoxime (1gm single bolus dose vs 12gm infusion) in the management of organophosphorus poisoning. *J Assoc Physic India* 1996;44:529–531.
27. Cherian AM, Jeyaseelan L, Peter JV, et al. *Effectiveness of pralidoxime in the treatment of organophosphorus poisoning — a randomised, double-blind, placebo-controlled clinical trial.* INCLEN Monograph series on Critical International Health Issues No. 7, 1997.
28. Cherian AM, Peter JV, Samuel J, et al. Effectiveness of P2AM (PAM — pralidoxime) in the treatment of organophosphorus poisoning. A randomised, double-blind, placebo-controlled trial. *J Assoc Physic India* 1997;45:22–24.
29. Bardin PG, van Eeden SF. Organophosphate poisoning: grading the severity and comparing treatment between atropine and glycopyrrolate. *Crit Care Med* 1990;18:956–960.
30. Ali-Melkkila T, Kanto J, Iisalo E. Pharmacokinetics and related pharmacodynamics of anticholinergic drugs. *Acta Anaesthesiol Scand* 1993;37:633–642.
31. Bismuth C, Inns RH, Marrs TC. Efficacy, toxicity and clinical uses of oximes in anticholinesterase poisoning. In: Ballantyne B, Marrs TC, eds. *Clinical and experimental toxicology of organophosphates and carbamates*. Oxford: Butterworth Heinemann, 1992:555–577.
32. Kusic R, Jovanovic D, Randjelovic S, et al. HI-6 in man: efficacy of the oxime in poisoning by organophosphorus insecticides. *Hum Exp Toxicol* 1991;10:113–118.
33. Worek F, Backer M, Thiermann H, et al. Reappraisal of indications and limitations of oxime therapy in organophosphate poisoning. *Hum Exp Toxicol* 1997;16:466–472.
34. Worek F, Eyer P, Kiderlen D, et al. Effect of human plasma on the reactivation of sarin-inhibited human erythrocyte acetylcholinesterase. *Arch Toxicol* 2000;74:21–26.
35. University of Oxford. Acute organophosphate pesticide poisoning in Sri Lanka – management, complications and pharmacogenetics. ISRCTN55264358 allocated July 2002. http://www.controlled-trials.com/isrctn/trial20/0/55264358.html (last accessed 19 August 2003).
36. Sogorb MA, Vilanova E. Enzymes involved in the detoxification of organophosphorus, carbamate and pyrethroid insecticides through hydrolysis. *Toxicol Lett* 2002;128:215–228.
37. Raushel FM. Bacterial detoxification of organophosphate nerve agents. *Curr Opin Microbiol* 2002;5:288–295.
38. Forsythe SM, Schmidt GA. Sodium bicarbonate for the treatment of lactic acidosis. *Chest* 2000;117:260–267.
39. Cordoba D, Cadavid S, Angulo D, et al. Organophosphate poisoning: modifications in acid base equilibrium and use of sodium bicarbonate as an aid in the treatment of toxicity in dogs. *Vet Hum Toxicol* 1983;25:1–3.
40. Wong A, Sandron CA, Magalhaes AS, et al. Comparative efficacy of pralidoxime vs sodium bicarbonate in rats and humans severely poisoned with O-P pesticide. *J Toxicol Clin Toxicol* 2000;38:554–555.
41. Sellstrom A. Anticonvulsants in anticholinesterase poisoning. In: Ballantyne B, Marrs TC, eds. *Clinical and experimental toxicology of organophosphates and carbamates*. Oxford: Butterworth Heinemann, 1992:578–586.
42. Murphy MR, Blick DW, Dunn MA, et al. Diazepam as a treatment for nerve agent poisoning in primates. *Aviat Space Environ Med* 1993;64:110–115.
43. van Zwieten PA. Centrally acting antihypertensive drugs. Present and future. *Clin Exp Hypertens* 1999;21:859–873.
44. Liu WF. A symptomatological assessment of organophosphate-induced lethality in mice: comparison of atropine and clonidine protection. *Toxicol Lett* 1991;56:19–32.
45. Lees KR, Dyker AG, Sharma A, et al. Tolerability of the low-affinity, use-dependent NMDA antagonist AR-R15896AR in stroke patients: a dose-ranging study. *Stroke* 2001;32:466–472.
46. Lallement G, Baubichon D, Clarencon D, et al. Review of the value of gacyclidine (GK-11) as adjuvant medication to conventional treatments of organophosphate poisoning: primate experiments mimicking various scenarios of military or terrorist attack by soman. *Neurotoxicology* 1999;20:675–684.

Michael Eddleston
Centre for Tropical Medicine
University of Oxford
Oxford
UK

Surjit Singh
Department of Internal Medicine
Postgraduate Institute of Medical
Education and Research
Chandigarh
India

Nick Buckley
Department of Clinical Pharmacology
and Toxicology
Canberra Hospital
Canberra
Australia

Competing interests: None declared.

Paracetamol (acetaminophen) poisoning

Search date November 2002

Nick Buckley and Michael Eddleston

QUESTIONS

INTERVENTIONS

Key Messages

- **Acetylcysteine** One systematic review in people with established paracetamol induced liver failure found that acetylcysteine versus placebo significantly reduced mortality at day 21. One observational study found that people given early treatment with acetylcysteine were less likely to develop liver damage than untreated historical controls.
- **Methionine** One systematic review found insufficient evidence on the effects of methionine on mortality. It found limited evidence that methionine reduced hepatotoxicity compared with supportive care.
- **Activated charcoal (single or multiple dose)** One systematic review found no evidence on the effects of activated charcoal, whether in single or multiple dose regimens, in paracetamol poisoning.
- **Gastric lavage** One systematic review found no evidence of the effects of gastric lavage in paracetamol poisoning.
- **Ipecacuanha** One systematic review found no evidence on the clinical effects of ipecacuanha in paracetamol poisoning.

DEFINITION Paracetamol poisoning occurs as a result of either accidental or intentional overdose with paracetamol (acetaminophen).

INCIDENCE/ PREVALENCE Paracetamol is the most common drug used for self poisoning in the UK.[1] It is also a common means of self poisoning in the rest of Europe, North America, and Australasia. An estimated 41 200 cases of poisoning with products containing paracetamol occurred in 1989–1990 in England and Wales, with a mortality of 0.40% (95% CI 0.38% to 0.46%). Overdoses owing to paracetamol alone result in an estimated 150–200 deaths and 15–20 liver transplants each year in England and Wales.

AETIOLOGY/ RISK FACTORS Most cases in the UK are impulsive acts of self harm in young people.[1,2] In one study of 80 people who had overdosed with paracetamol, 42 had obtained the tablets for the specific purpose of taking an overdose and 33 had obtained them less than 1 hour before the act.[2]

PROGNOSIS People with blood paracetamol concentrations above the standard treatment line (defined in the UK as a line joining 200 mg/L at 4 hours and 30 mg/L at 15 hours on a semilogarithmic plot) have a poor prognosis without treatment (see figure 1, p 1670).[3–5] In one study of 57 untreated people with blood concentrations above this line, 33 developed severe liver damage and three died.[4] People with a history of chronic alcohol misuse, use of enzyme inducing drugs, eating disorders, or multiple paracetamol overdoses may be at risk of liver damage with blood concentrations below this line.[6] In the USA, a lower line is used as an indication for treatment but we found no data relating this line to prognostic outcomes.[7] **Dose effect:** The dose ingested also indicates the risk of hepatotoxicity. People ingesting less than 125 mg/kg had no significant hepatotoxicity with a sharp dose dependent rise for higher doses.[8] The threshold for toxicity after acute ingestion may be higher in children, where a single dose of less than 200 mg/kg has not been reported to lead to death and rarely causes hepatotoxicity.[9] For people who present later than 24 hours or an unknown time after ingestion, several other prognostic indicators have been proposed, including half life, prothrombin time, and abnormal liver function tests.[10,11] These have not been validated prospectively.

AIMS OF INTERVENTION To prevent liver failure, liver transplantation, or death, with minimal adverse effects.

OUTCOMES Mortality, hepatotoxicity (most commonly defined by the objective criterion of blood aspartate aminotransferase > 1000 U/L), liver failure, or liver transplantation.

METHODS *Clinical Evidence* search and appraisal November 2002, including a search for observational studies. We also contacted experts in the field to identify unpublished studies.

QUESTION **What are the effects of treatments for acute paracetamol poisoning?**

OPTION **ACETYLCYSTEINE**

One systematic review found that in people with established paracetamol induced liver failure, acetylcysteine significantly reduced mortality and hypotension after 21 days compared with placebo. One observational study found that people given early treatment with acetylcysteine were less likely to develop liver damage than untreated historical controls.

Benefits: We found one systematic review (search date 2001, 1 RCT, 50 people with established paracetamol induced liver failure) that compared intravenous acetylcysteine (150 mg/kg over 15 minutes, 50 mg/kg over 4 hours, and then 100 mg/kg diluted in 5% dextrose over 16 hours, continued until death or recovery) versus a placebo infusion of 5% dextrose.[12] It found that after 21 days, acetylcysteine significantly reduced mortality compared with placebo (mortality: 13/25 [52%] with acetylcysteine *v* 20/25 [80%] with placebo; RR 0.65, 95% CI 0.43 to 0.99; NNT 4, 95% CI 2 to 16).

Harms: The systematic review found no evidence that quantified harms from acetylcysteine[12] and the RCT included did not specifically assess adverse outcomes and none were noted.[13] Four case series suggested that the incidence of adverse effects from intravenous acetylcysteine is 5–15%.[14–17] These were predominantly rash, urticaria, and occasionally more serious anaphylactoid reactions occurring with the initial "loading" dose. In most or all cases, adverse effects responded to temporary stopping of infusions and symptomatic treatment, and did not recur when treatment recommenced. Three deaths have been reported, two followed a 10-fold miscalculation of the dose of acetylcysteine and the other occurred in a person with severe asthma.[18,19] Adverse reactions seem to be more common in people with asthma and those who have non-toxic paracetamol concentrations.[16] Vomiting is common after oral acetylcysteine and occurred in 63% of people in one series despite previous administration of metoclopramide.[17] Oral acetylcysteine can also cause hypersensitivity and anaphylactoid reactions.[20]

Comment: In the RCT, allocation was concealed but treatment was not blinded.[13] There were differences between the groups in prognostic variables (prothrombin time, coma grade) and other treatments, but a possible confounding effect could not be assessed adequately because of the small size of the study. One observational study evaluated the effects of intravenous acetylcysteine in people presenting early to hospital.[4] It found that people treated within 10 hours of ingestion were less likely to develop liver damage than untreated historical controls (1/62 [2%] with treated people *v* 33/57 [58%] with untreated people). As a result, subsequent RCTs were considered unethical. A systematic review of numerous case series found evidence that acetylcysteine is beneficial in paracetamol poisoning.[14] For both oral and intravenous acetylcysteine, overall hepatotoxicity was worse if treatment was delayed beyond 8–10 hours (1% in those treated within 8 hours *v* 46% in those treated after 16 hours).[4,14] We found no RCTs of different regimens and no evidence of a difference between oral and intravenous routes of administration.[14] The optimal dose, route, and duration of treatment is unknown. Two recent observational studies comparing different protocols for intravenous[21] and oral[22] acetylcysteine did not find marked differences in outcomes.

OPTION ACTIVATED CHARCOAL (SINGLE OR MULTIPLE DOSE)

One systematic review found no evidence on the effects of activated charcoal, whether in single or multiple dose regimens, in paracetamol poisoning.

Benefits: One systematic review found no RCTs that examined clinical outcomes after paracetamol poisoning.[12]

Harms: The systematic review found no large study of complications in paracetamol poisoned people receiving single doses of activated charcoal.[12] Reported harms may include aspiration pneumonia, vomiting, diarrhoea, constipation, ileus, and interference with regular medications.[23]

Comment: **Single dose regimens:** One systematic review of simulated overdose studies in volunteers suggests that activated charcoal given within 2 hours of paracetamol ingestion decreases absorption by a variable amount and that this amount diminishes with time.[12] One cohort study in 450 consecutive people who had taken 10 g or more of paracetamol found that those who had been given activated charcoal were significantly less likely to have high risk blood paracetamol concentrations (OR 0.36, 95% CI 0.23 to 0.58).[3] The effect was seen only in those treated within 2 hours, and the study was not large enough to assess the effect of many potential confounders.[3] One non-systematic review of activated charcoal in all forms of poisoning found no evidence that activated charcoal improved outcome in poisoned people.[24] **Multiple dose regimens:** We found no studies of simulated overdose that evaluated multiple dose regimens in paracetamol poisoning. One non-systematic review of case series and reports of multiple dose regimens in all forms of poisoning found no evidence that multiple dose regimens improve outcomes in poisoned people.[25] The rapid absorption and short half life of paracetamol suggest a beneficial effect is unlikely.

OPTION GASTRIC LAVAGE

One systematic review found no evidence of the effects of gastric lavage in paracetamol poisoning.

Benefits: One systematic review found no RCTs or cohort studies that reported clinical outcomes.[12]

Harms: One systematic review found no large study of complications in paracetamol poisoned people receiving gastric lavage.[12] Harms may include aspiration of stomach contents, hypoxia, and oesophageal perforation.[26]

Comment: One systematic review of studies of simulated overdose in human volunteers suggests that gastric lavage carried out within 1 hour removes a variable number of paracetamol tablets and that the number diminishes with time.[12] One cohort study (450 consecutive people who took ≥10 g of paracetamol) found that those given activated charcoal were significantly less likely to have high risk blood paracetamol concentrations (OR 0.36, 95% CI 0.23 to 0.58).[3] The addition of gastric lavage did not decrease the risk further (OR 1.12, 95% CI 0.57 to 2.20). One non-systematic review of gastric lavage in all forms of poisoning found no evidence that gastric lavage improved outcome in poisoned people.[27]

OPTION IPECACUANHA

One systematic review found no evidence on the clinical effects of ipecacuanha in paracetamol poisoning.

Benefits: One systematic review found no evidence of clinical effects of ipecacuanha in paracetamol poisoning.[12]

Harms: A systematic review found no evidence that quantified harms from ipecacuanha in paracetamol poisoning.[12] Specific complications of ipecacuanha may include aspiration, diarrhoea, ileus, arrhythmia during vomiting, dystonia from treatment for vomiting, and haematemesis from vomiting.[26]

Comment: Human simulated overdose studies suggest that ipecacuanha given within 1 hour could reduce paracetamol absorption but no studies have shown a change in clinical outcome.[23] One non-systematic review of ipecacuanha in all forms of poisoning found no evidence that ipecacuanha improved outcome in poisoned people.[23] Administration of ipecacuanha may delay the administration of activated charcoal and oral antidotes.

OPTION METHIONINE

One systematic review found insufficient evidence on the effects of methionine on mortality. It found limited evidence that methionine reduced hepatotoxicity compared with supportive care.

Benefits: One systematic review (search date 2001, 1 RCT, 40 people with blood concentrations of paracetamol above the UK standard treatment line) compared 2.5 g of oral methionine (2.5 g 4 hourly for 4 doses), intravenous mercaptamine (formerly named cysteamine, prescribed at a dose of 3.6 g over 20 hours), and supportive care.[12] It found no significant effect on mortality (0 deaths with methionine *v* 0 deaths with mercaptamine *v* 1 with supportive care). Only 27 people had a liver biopsy. Fewer people suffered grade III hepatic necrosis (0/9 [0%] with methionine *v* 6/10 [60%] with supportive care) or had peak aspartate aminotransferase greater than 1000 U (1/13 [8%] with methionine *v* 8/13 [62%] with supportive care; RR 0.13, 95% CI 0.02 to 0.86; NNT 2, 95% CI 2 to 6).

Harms: The systematic review did not address harms from methionine.[12] No serious adverse effects associated with treatment were reported in the included RCT, but vomiting after administration of methionine occurred in 8/13 people (62%).[28] The incidence of adverse effects in the control group was not reported.

Comment: Interpretation of liver biopsy results from the RCT was difficult as not all people were tested and an intention to treat analysis was not possible. We found one case series in people treated with methionine in early and late paracetamol poisoning, but there was no untreated group for comparison.[29]

Substantive changes

Acetylcysteine One systematic review added[12] and one study describing harms added;[19] conclusions unchanged.
Methionine One systematic review added;[12] conclusions unchanged.
Ipecacuanha One systematic review added;[12] conclusions unchanged.
Activated charcoal One systematic review added;[12] conclusions unchanged.
Gastric lavage One systematic review added;[12] conclusions unchanged.

REFERENCES

1. Gunnell D, Hawton K, Murray V, et al. Use of paracetamol for suicide and non-fatal poisoning in the UK and France: are restrictions on availability justified? *J Epidemiol Community Health* 1997;51:175–179.
2. Hawton K, Ware C, Mistry H, et al. Paracetamol self-poisoning. Characteristics, prevention and harm reduction. *Br J Psychiatry* 1996;168:43–48.
3. Buckley NA, Whyte IM, O'Connell DL, et al. Activated charcoal reduces the need for *N*-acetylcysteine treatment after acetaminophen (paracetamol) overdose. *J Toxicol Clin Toxicol* 1999;37:753–757.
4. Prescott LF, Illingworth RN, Critchley JAJH, et al. Intravenous *N*-acetylcysteine: the treatment of choice for paracetamol poisoning. *BMJ* 1979;2:1097–1100.
5. Rumack BH, Matthew H. Acetaminophen poisoning and toxicity. *Pediatrics* 1975;55:871–876.
6. Vale JA, Proudfoot AT. Paracetamol (acetaminophen) poisoning. *Lancet* 1995;346:547–552.
7. Smilkstein MJ, Knapp GL, Kulig KW, et al. Efficacy of oral *N*-acetylcysteine in the treatment of acetaminophen overdose. Analysis of the National Multicentre Study (1976–1985). *N Engl J Med* 1988;319:1557–1562.
8. Prescott LF. Paracetamol overdosage. Pharmacological considerations and clinical management. *Drugs* 1983;25:290–314.
9. Caravati EM. Unintentional acetaminophen ingestion in children and the potential for hepatotoxicity. *J Toxicol Clin Toxicol* 2000;38:291–296.
10. Schiodt FV, Ott P, Christensen E, et al. The value of plasma acetaminophen half-life in antidote-treated acetaminophen overdosage. *Clin Pharmacol Ther* 2002;71:221–225.
11. James LP, Wells E, Beard RH, et al. Predictors of outcome after acetaminophen poisoning in children and adolescents. *J Pediatr* 2002;140:522–526.
12. Brok J, Buckley N, Gluud C. Interventions for paracetamol (acetaminophen) overdoses (Cochrane Review). In: The Cochrane Library, Issue 3, 2002. Oxford: Update Software. Search date 2001; primary sources Cochrane Hepato-Billiary Group Controlled Trials Register, Cochrane Controlled Trials Register, Medline, Embase, and hand searching of reference lists from RCTs, textbooks, review articles and meta-analyses, and personal contact with authors of relevant RCTs.
13. Keays R, Harrison PM, Wendon JA, et al. Intravenous acetylcysteine in paracetamol induced fulminant hepatic failure: a prospective controlled trial. *BMJ* 1991;303:1026–1029.
14. Buckley NA, Whyte IM, O'Connell DL, et al. Oral or intravenous *N*-acetylcysteine: which is the treatment of choice for acetaminophen (paracetamol) poisoning? *J Toxicol Clin Toxicol* 1999;37:759–767.
15. Chan TY, Critchley JA. Adverse reactions to intravenous *N*-acetylcysteine in Chinese patients with paracetamol (acetaminophen) poisoning. *Hum Exp Toxicol* 1994;13:542–544.
16. Schmidt LE, Dalhoff K. Risk factors in the development of adverse reactions to *N*-acetylcysteine in patients with paracetamol poisoning. *Br J Clin Pharmacol* 2001;51:87–91.
17. Wright RO, Anderson AC, Lesko SL, et al. Effect of metoclopramide dose on preventing emesis after oral administration of *N*-acetylcysteine for acetaminophen overdose. *J Toxicol Clin Toxicol* 1999;37:35–42.
18. Mant TG, Tempowski JH, Volans GN, et al. Adverse reactions to acetylcysteine and effects of overdose. *BMJ* 1984;289:217–219.
19. Appelboam AV, Dargan PI, Jones AL, et al. Fatal anaphylactoid reaction to *N*-acetylcysteine: caution in asthmatics. *J Toxicol Clin Toxicol* 2002;40:366–367.
20. Perry HE, Shannon MW. Efficacy of oral versus intravenous *N*-acetylcysteine in acetaminophen overdose: results of an open-label, clinical trial. *J Pediatr* 1998;132:149–152.
21. Dougherty T, Greene T, Roberts JR. Acetaminophen overdose: comparison between continuous and intermittent intravenous *N*-acetylcysteine 48-hour protocols. *Ann Emerg Med* 2000;36:S83.
22. Woo OF, Mueller PD, Olson KR, et al. Shorter duration of oral *N*-acetylcysteine therapy for acute acetaminophen overdose. *Ann Emerg Med* 2000;35:363–368.
23. Krenzelok EP, McGuigan M, Lheur P. Position statement: ipecac syrup. American Academy of Clinical Toxicology and European Association of Poisons Centres and Clinical Toxicologists. *J Toxicol Clin Toxicol* 1997;35:699–709.
24. Chyka PA, Seger D. Position statement: single-dose activated charcoal. American Academy of Clinical Toxicology; European Association of Poisons Centres and Clinical Toxicologists. *J Toxicol Clin Toxicol* 1997;35:721–741.
25. American Academy of Clinical Toxicology, European Association of Poison Centres, and Clinical Toxicologists. Position statement and practice

guidelines on the use of multi-dose activated charcoal in the treatment of acute poisoning. *J Toxicol Clin Toxicol* 1999;37:731–751.
26. Pond SM, Lewis-Driver DJ, Williams GM, et al. Gastric emptying in acute overdose: a prospective randomised controlled trial. *Med J Aust* 1995;163:345–349.
27. Vale JA. Position statement: gastric lavage. American Academy of Clinical Toxicology, European Association of Poisons Centres, and Clinical Toxicologists. *J Toxicol Clin Toxicol* 1997;35:711–719.
28. Hamlyn AN, Lesna M, Record CO, et al. Methionine and cysteamine in paracetamol (acetaminophen) overdose, prospective controlled trial of early therapy. *J Int Med Res* 1981;9:226–231.
29. Vale JA, Meredith TJ, Goulding R. Treatment of acetaminophen poisoning. The use of oral methionine. *Arch Intern Med* 1981;141:394–396.

Nick Buckley
Consultant Clinical Pharmacologist and Toxicologist
Canberra Hospital
Canberra
Australia

Michael Eddleston
Wellcome Trust Career Development Fellow
Centre for Tropical Medicine
University of Oxford
Oxford
UK

Competing interests: None declared.

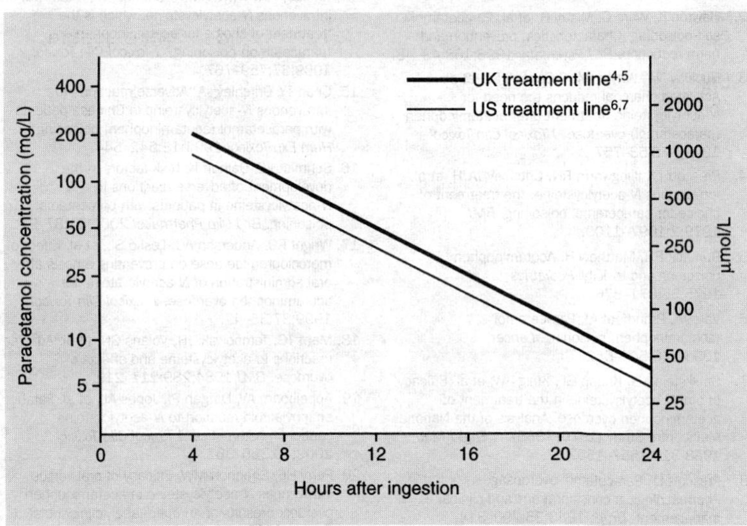

FIGURE 1 **Nomograms used to determine acetylcysteine or methionine treatment, based on the blood concentrations between 4 hours and 24 hours after ingestion of paracetamol. Published with permission (see text, p 1665).[3]**

Nausea and vomiting in early pregnancy

Search date November 2002

Richmal M Oates-Whitehead

QUESTIONS

INTERVENTIONS

See glossary, p 1681

Key Messages

Nausea and vomiting in pregnancy

- **Antihistamines (H1 antagonists)** Systematic reviews found limited evidence that antihistamines reduce nausea and vomiting, with no evidence of teratogenicity.
- **Cyanocobalamin (vitamin B_{12})** One systematic review has found that cyanocobalamin reduces vomiting episodes compared with placebo.
- **Ginger** Three RCTs found that ginger reduces nausea and vomiting in early pregnancy.
- **Pyridoxine (vitamin B_6)** Systematic reviews found limited evidence that pyridoxine reduces nausea but no evidence on the effect on vomiting.
- **Acupuncture** One RCT found that acupuncture improved nausea scores, retching, and wellbeing compared with no acupuncture, without increasing adverse effects. However, an improvement was found both with traditional acupuncture and sham acupuncture compared with no treatment after 3 weeks. A second RCT found that acupuncture had no more effect than sham acupuncture.
- **Dietary interventions (excluding ginger)** We found insufficient evidence to assess the effects of dietary interventions (excluding ginger).

- **P6 acupressure** One systematic review of small RCTs found limited evidence that P6 acupressure reduced morning sickness compared with sham acupressure or no intervention. Four additional RCTs found that P6 acupressure reduced duration, but not intensity, of nausea and vomiting. However, a further small RCT found acupressure bands to be less effective than placebo bands.
- **Phenothiazines** One systematic review found limited evidence that phenothiazines reduced the proportion of women with nausea and vomiting. However, results were not conclusive.

Hyperemesis gravidarum

- **Acupuncture** One randomised, crossover RCT in women with hyperemesis gravidarum found a faster reduction of nausea, as measured on a visual analogue scale, after active acupuncture compared with sham acupuncture. Episodes of vomiting were also reduced. However, we were unable to draw reliable conclusions from this small study.
- **Corticosteroids** One RCT found no significant improvement in persistent vomiting or readmission to hospital after 1 week of treatment with prednisolone compared with placebo in women with hyperemesis gravidarum. One RCT identified in two systematic reviews found no significant improvement in persistence of vomiting but found a reduction in admission to hospital compared with promethazine.
- **Corticotropins** One RCT found no significant improvement in nausea and vomiting with intramuscular corticotropin (adrenocorticotrophic hormone, ACTH).
- **Diazepam** One systematic review has found insufficient evidence on the effects of diazepam in women with hyperemesis gravidarum.
- **Dietary interventions (excluding ginger)** One crossover RCT in women with hyperemesis gravidarum found no significant difference in nausea and vomiting after 3 weeks between carob seed flour and placebo.
- **Ginger** One systematic review found insufficient evidence to assess the effects of ginger in hyperemesis gravidarum.
- **Ondansetron** We found insufficient evidence to assess the effects of ondansetron in hyperemesis gravidarum.

DEFINITION **Nausea and vomiting** are both common in early pregnancy. Most women do not require treatment. However, persistent vomiting and severe nausea can progress to hyperemesis if the woman is unable to maintain adequate hydration, and fluid and electrolytes as well as nutritional status are jeopardised. **Hyperemesis gravidarum** is a diagnosis of exclusion, characterised by prolonged and severe nausea and vomiting, dehydration, and body weight loss.[1] Laboratory investigation may show elevated plasma ketone levels in the absence of acidosis, low serum levels of sodium (hyponatraemia), potassium (hypokalaemia), a low serum urea level (hypouricaemia), metabolic hypochloraemic alkalosis (excess base alkali in the body fluids caused by chloride loss), and ketonuria (excessive ketones in the urine).

INCIDENCE/ PREVALENCE Nausea and vomiting are both common in pregnancy, with nausea affecting about 70% and vomiting affecting about 60% of women.[1] Symptoms commence between the fourth and the seventh week in 70% of the affected women.[2] Symptoms before the first missed period affect < 10% of pregnant women.[3] Vomiting ceases by the sixteenth week of pregnancy in about 90% of women.[1–3] Nausea and vomiting can occur at any time of the day and may be constant throughout the day, although it has been misleadingly termed "morning sickness".[1] The true incidence of hyperemesis gravidarum is not known. It has been documented to range from 0.3–2.0%; however, most authors report an incidence of 0.5%.[2]

AETIOLOGY/ RISK FACTORS The causes of nausea and vomiting in pregnancy are unknown. One theory, that they are caused by the rise in human chorionic gonadotrophin concentration, is compatible with the natural history of the condition, its severity in pregnancies affected by hydatidiform mole (see glossary, p 1681), and its good prognosis (see prognosis below).[4] The aetiology of hyperemesis gravidarum is also uncertain. Again, endocrine and psychological factors are suspected, but evidence is inconclusive.[4]

PROGNOSIS One systematic review (search date 1988, 11 studies) found that nausea and vomiting were associated with a reduced risk of miscarriage (6 studies, 14 564 women; OR 0.36, 95% CI 0.32 to 0.42), but found no association with perinatal mortality.[5] Nausea and vomiting and hyperemesis usually improve over the course of pregnancy, but one observational study (cross sectional) found that 13% of women reported that nausea and vomiting persisted beyond 20 weeks' gestation.[6]

AIMS OF INTERVENTION To reduce the symptoms of nausea and vomiting in early pregnancy; to reduce the incidence and duration of hyperemesis gravidarum; to reduce the adverse effects and possible teratogenic effects to the baby.

OUTCOMES Persistence, severity, or both of nausea and vomiting, morbidity and mortality to mother, incidence and duration of hospital stay of mother, readmission of mother, and evidence of teratogenic effects of treatments in the fetus/baby.

METHODS *Clinical Evidence* search and appraisal November 2002 plus an author updated search in the Cochrane Library Issue 2 2003, Medline, Embase, and Cinahl in April 2003.

QUESTION **What are the effects of treatment for nausea and vomiting in early pregnancy?**

OPTION **ACUPRESSURE**

One systematic review including small RCTs found limited evidence that P6 acupressure reduced morning sickness compared with sham acupressure or no intervention. Two further RCTs and two randomised crossover trials found that P6 acupressure reduced duration, but not intensity, of nausea and vomiting. However, a further small RCT found acupressure bands to be less effective than placebo bands.

Benefits: We found one systematic review (search date 2001, 4 RCTs, 661 women),[7] which identified the effects of P6 acupressure (see glossary, p 1681). The review found that acupressure (see glossary, p 1681) compared with placebo or sham acupressure reduced the proportion of women reporting morning sickness (2 RCTs, 404 women; OR 0.35, 95% CI 0.23 to 0.54).[7] However, the authors point out that the odds ratio may be an overestimate as the two trials that could not be included in the summary calculation[8,9] found no evidence of effect and one of these RCTs had the highest completion rate of all four trials (92%).[9] Three further RCTs and two randomised crossover trials were identified. One of the RCTs (97 women, 8–12 weeks' gestation) found that acupressure reduced duration of nausea and vomiting (WMD 1.89 hours/12 hour cycle, 95% CI 0.33 hours/12 hour cycle to 3.45 hours/12 hour cycle) but not intensity measured with a non-graded visual analogue scale ranging from zero to five (WMD +0.25 units, 95% CI −0.12 units to +0.62 units).[10] A further RCT (138 women randomised, 110 women analysed) found acupressure given by Seabands significantly reduced the frequency and severity of nausea (data were not given in a way to allow further statistical calculation).[11] One randomised crossover RCT (23 women randomised, 15 women analysed [65%]) showed a statistically significant improvement in the severity of nausea in favour of P6 acupressure measured with a 10 cm visual analogue scale (WMD 1.69 cm, 95% CI 0.32 cm to 3.06 cm).[12] A further randomised crossover trial (also 23 women randomised, 15 women analysed [65%]) found a statistically significant decrease in severity of nausea in favour of acupressure as reported on a visual analogue scale (data were not given in a way to allow further statistical calculation).[13] However, another RCT (30 women) using acupressure wristbands reported that placebo bands were more effective than treatment bands (incidence was not given so no further calculations can be made). The authors do admit that their study had several limitations including a small sample size, a sample not representative of the general population, and numerous other threats to both internal and external validity.[14]

Harms: None reported.

Comment: Conducting high quality trials in this area is difficult, because the condition tends to resolve spontaneously and interventions are difficult to mask and to control with credible placebos. The trial with the largest sample size[15] is subsequently described in a paper that questions the reliability of the randomisation.[16]

OPTION ACUPUNCTURE

One RCT found that acupuncture improved nausea scores, retching, and wellbeing compared with no acupuncture, without increasing adverse effects. However, an improvement was found with both traditional acupuncture and sham acupuncture compared with no treatment after 3 weeks. A second RCT found that acupuncture had no more effect than sham acupuncture.

Benefits: We found one RCT (593 women) comparing traditional acupuncture with P6 acupuncture, sham acupuncture, or no acupuncture on nausea and vomiting in early pregnancy.[17] At the end of the first week significantly more women were free of nausea with acupuncture (13/135 [10%] with acupuncture *v* 4/127 [3%] with no acupuncture; RR 0.93, 95% CI 0.88 to 0.99; NNT 15, CI not provided). Women who received P6 acupuncture reported less nausea from the second week of the trial ($P < 0.05$) and less dry retching ($P < 0.001$) from the third week compared with women in the no acupuncture control group. Women receiving sham acupuncture reported significantly less nausea ($P < 0.01$) and dry retching ($P < 0.001$) from the third week compared with women in the no acupuncture group. No differences in vomiting were found among the groups at any time.[17] A second RCT (55 women, 6–10 weeks' gestation) compared multi-site acupuncture with sham acupuncture.[18] There was strong evidence that nausea improved with time ($P < 0.001$) but no evidence of improvement associated with the intervention ($P = 0.9$) or an interaction between time and intervention ($P = 0.8$).[18]

Harms: A follow up study of the largest RCT found no differences between study groups in the incidence of perinatal outcome, congenital abnormalities, pregnancy complications, or other infant outcomes.[18]

Comment: The first RCT found a significant reduction in nausea with traditional acupuncture after the first week of treatment.[17] During the second week of treatment women receiving traditional acupuncture and PC6 acupuncture (see glossary, p 1681) had significant reduction of nausea scores compared with the no acupuncture group. During the third week, women receiving sham acupuncture also showed significant reduction of nausea scores compared with no acupuncture. The significant improvement in all groups receiving an intervention (traditional acupuncture, PC6 acupuncture, and sham acupuncture) makes it difficult to establish whether the results are influenced by placebo effect.[17]

OPTION ANTIHISTAMINES (H1 ANTAGONISTS)

Systematic reviews found limited evidence that antihistamines reduced nausea and vomiting, with no evidence of teratogenicity.

Benefits: We found two systematic reviews.[7,19] The most recent systematic review (search date 2001, 12 RCTs, 1505 women)[7] found that, compared with placebo, antihistamines as a group reduced nausea (timeframes not specified; OR 0.17, 95% CI 0.13 to 0.21). The earlier systematic review (search date 1998, 7 RCTs, 1190 women)[19] found that H1 antagonist antihistamines significantly reduced treatment failure (RR 0.34, 95% CI 0.27 to 0.43). However, the conclusions need to be interpreted with care because significant heterogeneity was found between studies.[19]

Harms: The first review (24 controlled studies, > 200 000 women between 1960 and 1991) found no increase in teratogenicity in women receiving antihistamines (RR 0.76, 95% CI 0.60 to 0.94).[19] The second review included three RCTs that gathered evidence on harms from 179 women.[7] It found that antihistamines significantly increased drowsiness (23/94 [24%] with antihistamines *v* 9/85 [11%] with placebo; RR 2.3, 95% CI 1.1 to 4.7; NNH 7, 95% CI 3 to 32).

Comment: The trials identified by the reviews were old and details on randomisation and concealment strategies were not provided.[7] The review combined results from trials in which different antihistamines (e.g.

buclizine, dimenhydrinate, doxylamine, hydroxyzine, meclozine) were compared with placebo. The earlier systematic review found important heterogeneity in the meta-analysis, which may be attributed to the variety of drugs included.[19] A preparation combining doxylamine plus dicycloverine plus pyridoxine assessed in the systematic reviews was found to reduce nausea and vomiting.[7] However, this preparation was withdrawn from the market in several countries after publication of papers suggesting teratogenicity, although such claims have subsequently been refuted.

OPTION CYANOCOBALAMIN (VITAMIN B_{12})

One systematic review has found that cyanocobalamin reduces vomiting episodes compared with placebo.

Benefits: We found one systematic review (search date 1998, 2 RCTs, 1018 women).[19] It found that cyanocobalamin (see glossary, p 1681) significantly reduced vomiting episodes compared with placebo (timeframes not specified; RR 0.49, 95% CI 0.28 to 0.86).[19]

Harms: The review found no adverse effects.[19]

Comment: It is believed that the combination of cyanocobalamin plus folic acid may prevent neural tube defects. The systematic review searched controlled trials addressing potential teratogenicity of cyanocobalamin and found none.[19] The conclusions of the systematic review are mostly based on one RCT that accounted for 1000 women and used a daily dose of a multivitamin compound that contained 4 μg of cyanocobalamin in each tablet.[20] The smaller RCT used a dose of cyanocobalamin of 25 μg orally, twice daily for 7 days (Jewell D, personal communication, 2001).

OPTION DIETARY INTERVENTIONS (EXCLUDING GINGER)

We found insufficient evidence to assess the effects of dietary interventions (excluding ginger).

Benefits: We found no systematic review or RCTs.

Harms: We found no systematic review or RCTs.

Comment: None.

OPTION GINGER

Three RCTs found that ginger reduces nausea and vomiting in early pregnancy.

Benefits: We found two RCTs and one randomised crossover trial examining the use of ginger as an antiemetic in early pregnancy. The first RCT (70 women) compared 250 mg of ginger in oral capsules taken four times daily, with placebo.[21] Ginger significantly reduced the proportion of women with vomiting after 4 days (12/32 [38%] with ginger *v* 23/35 [66%] with placebo; RR 0.57, 95% CI 0.34 to 0.95; NNT 4, 95% CI 2 to 12) and significantly reduced symptoms after 7 days (28/32 [88%] with ginger *v* 10/35 [29%] with placebo; RR 0.18, 95% CI 0.07 to 0.45; NNT 2, CI not provided).[21] The second RCT (26 women) compared 15 mL of ginger syrup containing 250 mg of ginger taken four times daily with placebo.[22] After 6 days, more women had stopped vomiting with ginger (8/12 [67%] with ginger *v* 2/10 [20%] with placebo; RR 0.42, 95% CI 0.18 to 0.98; NNT 2, CI not reported). The randomised crossover trial (30 women) compared 250 mg of ginger in oral capsules taken four times daily for 4 days, with placebo.[23] Ginger significantly reduced nausea and vomiting severity scores (P = 0.035, no raw data available).

Harms: We found no evidence about the harms of ginger. One RCT found no significant differences in spontaneous abortions with ginger compared with placebo (1/32 [3%] with ginger *v* 3/38 [8%] with placebo; P = 0.4), but the sample size may have been to small to rule out significant differences.[21]

Comment: Ginger used for the first RCT[21] and the randomised crossover trial[23] was derived from fresh ginger roots and given in capsules. The authors of the RCT warn that different presentations of ginger may have different magnitude of effects. The active ingredient that improves nausea and vomiting has not been isolated.[21]

OPTION PHENOTHIAZINES

One systematic review found limited evidence that phenothiazines reduced the proportion of women with nausea and vomiting. However, results were not conclusive.

Benefits: One systematic review (search date 1998, 3 RCTs, 398 women) found that phenothiazines compared with placebo reduced the proportion of women with nausea or vomiting (timeframes not specified; RR 0.31, 95% CI 0.24 to 0.42).[19] The results of this review should be interpreted with caution as the analysis combined results from different phenothiazines and one of the RCTs recruited women after the first trimester of pregnancy. After excluding this RCT, the review found reduced treatment failure (definition not provided) with phenothiazines (26/145 [18%] with phenothiazines *v* 89/139 [64%] with placebo; RR 0.28, 95% CI 0.19 to 0.41; NNT 3, 95% CI 2 to 3).[19]

Harms: The review assessed harms gathering evidence from seven controlled observational trials (78 440 women), which found no evidence of teratogenicity (RR 1.00, 95% CI 0.84 to 1.18).[19] However, harms of different phenothiazines vary, making it difficult to interpret a summary analysis.

Comment: The studies are old and lack sufficient information to appraise the quality of randomisation and allocation concealment. Only two RCTs provide support to the conclusions; therefore, conclusions should be drawn with caution.

OPTION PYRIDOXINE (VITAMIN B_6)

Systematic reviews of pyridoxine found limited evidence that pyridoxine reduced nausea score, but no evidence of an effect on vomiting.

Benefits: We found two systematic reviews.[7,19] The first review (search date 1998, 3 RCTs, 949 women) found that pyridoxine had similar "failure rates" compared with placebo (3 RCTs, 949 women; RR 0.97, 95% CI 0.78 to 1.20).[19] However, pyridoxine significantly improved nausea scores (2 RCTs, 395 women; WMD 0.92, 95% CI 0.44 to 1.40). The second systematic review (search date 2001, 2 RCTs, 392 women) compared pyridoxine versus placebo or no intervention.[7] It found that pyridoxine did not reduce vomiting (timeframes not specified; OR 0.91, 95% CI 0.60 to 1.38) but did reduce nausea (change in a 10 cm visual analogue scale; WMD 0.9 cm, 95% CI 0.4 cm to 1.4 cm).

Harms: The first systematic review searched for harms data (search date 1998, 1 cohort study, 1369 women). It found no significant increase in major fetal malformations attributable to pyridoxine (RR 1.05, 95% CI 0.60 to 1.84).[19]

Comment: The first review[19] included one RCT in which the nature of randomisation was unclear.[7] The remaining two RCTs were included in both reviews.[7,19] Treatment failure was defined in various subjective ways and included resolution or a clinically important improvement.[19]

QUESTION What are the effects of treatments for hyperemesis gravidarum?

OPTION ACUPUNCTURE New

One randomised crossover RCT found a faster reduction of nausea, as measured on a visual analogue scale, after active acupuncture compared with sham acupuncture. Episodes of vomiting were also reduced. However, we were unable to draw reliable conclusions from this study.

Benefits: We found one RCT (50 women) comparing P6 acupuncture with sham acupuncture.[24] All women were vomiting on the day of randomisation. The proportion of women vomiting on the third day (after the two acupuncture days) was less with acupuncture (7/17 [41%] with acupuncture *v* 12/16 [75%] with sham acupuncture; RR 0.55, 95% CI 0.29 to 1.04; NNT 3, 95% CI 2 to 45). No significant differences were found between groups with regard to food intake and the need for intravenous fluids.[24]

Harms: No adverse effects were reported.

Comment: The placebo treatment (sham acupuncture) used in the RCT was superficial acupuncture on an area away from a "real" acupuncture point. Needles were inserted only 1–2 mm in the skin. The authors of the RCT state that this kind of stimulation minimises the specific effects of acupuncture.[24] However, it may not be an entirely inert placebo, as some sensory stimulation does occur.

OPTION CORTICOTROPINS New

One RCT found no significant improvement in nausea and vomiting with intramuscular corticotropin (adrenocorticotrophic hormone, ACTH).

Benefits: We found two systematic reviews of corticotropins in hyperemesis, which identified the same RCT (search dates 1998[19] and 2001;[7] 1 RCT, 32 women). The RCT compared 0.5 mg of intramuscular corticotropin with placebo.[25] The was no significant difference between the treatment and placebo groups in nausea relief scores in a scale ranging from a score of 15 denoting a lack of nausea to 20 denoting the worst possible hyperemesis (WMD +0.6 mean relief score, 95% CI −1.65 to +2.85). No significant differences were found in the duration from commencement of treatment/placebo to stopping vomiting between the two groups and vomiting ceased in all women during the hospital stay. No significant differences between groups were found in the number of readmissions.

Harms: The systematic reviews reported no adverse effects.[7,19]

Comment: This RCT only provided data on intramuscularly administered corticotropin.[25]

OPTION CORTICOSTEROIDS

One RCT found no significant improvement in persistent vomiting or readmission to hospital after 1 week of treatment with prednisolone compared with placebo. One RCT identified in two systematic reviews found no significant improvement in persistence of vomiting but found a reduction in admission to hospital compared with promethazine.

Benefits: We found two systematic reviews of corticosteroids in hyperemesis, which identified the same RCTs (search dates 1998[19] and 2001[7]; 2 RCTs, 71 women) and one subsequent RCT.[26] **Versus placebo:** The one subsequent RCT (25 women with severe hyperemesis) compared oral prednisolone (20 mg twice daily) with placebo for 1 week.[26] Oral prednisolone had no significant effect on persistent vomiting (5/12 [42%] with prednisolone *v* 7/12 [58%] with placebo; RR 1.4 95% CI 0.6 to 3.2) or on subsequent readmission to hospital (5/12 [42%] with prednisolone *v* 8/12 [67%] with placebo; RR 1.6, 95% CI 0.7 to 3.5). **Versus promethazine:** One of the RCTs included in the systematic review compared oral methylprednisolone with promethazine (40 women admitted to hospital at < 16 weeks' gestation).[27] It found that methylprednisolone had no significant effect on persistence of vomiting when compared with promethazine (OR 1.56, 95% CI 0.25 to 9.94). However, there was a reduction in subsequent admission to hospital (0/17 [0%] with methylprednisolone *v* 5/18 [28%] with promethazine; OR 0.11, 95% CI 0.02 to 0.71).[7] The second RCT included in the systematic review assessed the effects of corticotropin versus placebo (see benefits of corticotropins, p 1679).[25]

Harms: The first review, which also included controlled observational studies (8 studies, 109 602 women), found no evidence of teratogenicity (RR 1.24, 95% CI 0.97 to 1.60).[19]

Comment: The rates of spontaneous resolution of symptoms in control groups were high. The possible benefit (based on a single small trial)[7] of methylprednisolone on preventing subsequent admission to hospital must be balanced against possible adverse effects of steroids given in the first trimester of pregnancy. The subsequent RCT was too small to rule out an important clinical effect.[26] A systematic search on the effects of promethazine will be included in future *Clinical Evidence* updates.

OPTION DIAZEPAM

One systematic review found insufficient evidence on the effects of diazepam in women with hyperemesis gravidarum.

Benefits: We found one systematic review (search date 2001, 1 RCT, 50 women admitted to hospital)[7] comparing intravenous fluids containing a multivitamin preparation with or without diazepam 20 mg daily. After symptoms settled, women were randomised to receive oral diazepam (5 mg twice daily) for 1 week or placebo. The trial found no difference in persistence of vomiting after 2 days of treatment (assessment not clearly specified; OR 0.64, 95% CI 0.10 to 4.19), but reported a difference in rates of readmission to hospital (4% with diazepam *v* 27% with placebo; detailed figures not provided)[7].

Harms: The trial did not report on adverse effects or acceptability of treatment.

Comment: The trials were too small to draw reliable conclusions. Rate of resolution in the control group was high and the effects of the vitamins used in the RCT are unknown.

OPTION DIETARY SUPPLEMENTS — CAROB SEED FLOUR

One crossover RCT found no significant difference in nausea and vomiting after 3 weeks between carob seed flour and placebo.

Benefits: We found one crossover RCT (43 women) which compared 1 g daily of a powder containing 96.5% carob seed flour plus 3.5% calcium lactate with placebo for 3 weeks.[28] It found no significant difference in relief of vomiting (subjective improvement: 20/34 [59%] with carob seed flour *v* 18/36 [50%] with placebo; RR 1.18, 95% CI 1.77 to 1.81).[28]

Harms: The RCT reported no adverse effects.[28]

Comment: The trial was conducted in 1966. It is unclear whether the composition of the soy flour commercially available products was the same when the RCT was conducted.[28]

OPTION GINGER

One systematic review found insufficient evidence to assess the effects of ginger in hyperemesis gravidarum.

Benefits: We found one systematic review (search date 2001, 1 crossover RCT, 27 women), which compared ginger 250 mg in oral capsules taken four times daily versus placebo.[7] After 4 days of treatment the RCT found no improvement in a hyperemesis score that evaluated the degree of nausea, vomiting, and weight loss (WMD +3.15, 95% CI –0.92 to +7.22).

Harms: The RCT reported no adverse effects.

Comment: The trial reported results before crossover but it was too small to make reliable conclusions.

OPTION ONDANSETRON

We found insufficient evidence to assess the effects of ondansetron in hyperemesis gravidarum.

Benefits: **Versus placebo:** We found no systematic review or RCTs. **Versus promethazine:** We found one systematic review (search date 2001, 1 RCT, 27 women admitted to hospital).[7] It compared ondansetron 10 mg versus promethazine 50 mg, both given by 50 mL solution over 30 minutes. Subsequent doses were given as needed every 8 hours until the woman was able to eat a bland diet. The review found no difference in persistence of vomiting between ondansetron and promethazine (2/15 [13%] with ondansetron *v* 3/12 [25%] with promethazine; OR 0.33, 95% CI 0.04 to 2.60).[7]

Harms: The RCT did not report on adverse effects.[7]

Comment: The study was too small to draw reliable conclusions.[7] A systematic search on the effects of promethazine will be included in future *Clinical Evidence* updates.

GLOSSARY

Acupressure Pressure applied to a specific point of the body. It does not require needles and can be administered by women themselves. Commercial products available include an elastic band to fit around the wrist with a plastic disc to apply pressure at the P6 point.
Cyanocobalamin Vitamin B_{12} produced for oral administration.
Hydatidiform mole A condition in which there is abnormal cystic development of the placenta. The uterus is often large for the duration of pregnancy and there may be vaginal bleeding, lack of fetal movement and fetal heart sounds, and severe nausea and vomiting. Rarer, but important, complications include haemorrhage, intrauterine infection, raised blood pressure, and persistent gestational trophoblastic disease, which may infiltrate local tissues or metastasise to distant sites.
P6 acupressure Pressure is applied at the P6 (Neiguan) point on the volar aspect of the wrist.
PC6 acupuncture The needle is applied at the PC6 point located near to the wrist crease.

Substantive changes

Ginger in nausea and vomiting Two RCTs added;[22,23] conclusions unchanged.
Acupressure in nausea and vomiting Four RCTs added;[11–14] conclusions unchanged.
Acupuncture in nausea and vomiting One RCT added;[24] conclusions relatively unchanged.
Dietary interventions other than ginger in hyperemesis gravidarum One RCT added;[28] conclusions unchanged.

REFERENCES

1. Nelson-Piercy C. Treatment of nausea and vomiting in pregnancy. When should it be treated and what can be safely taken? *Drug Saf* 1998;19:155–164.
2. Eliakim R, Abulafia O, Sherer DM. Hyperemesis gravidarum: a current review. *Am J Perinatol* 2000;17:207–218.
3. Gadsby R, Barnie-Adshead AM, Jagger C. A prospective study of nausea and vomiting during pregnancy. *Br J Gen Pract* 1993;43:245–248.
4. Baron TH, Ramirez B, Richter JE. Gastrointestinal motility disorders during pregnancy. *Ann Int Med* 1993;118:366–375.
5. Weigel MM, Weigel RM. Nausea and vomiting of early pregnancy and pregnancy outcome. A meta-analytical review. *Br J Obst Gynaecol* 1989;96:1312–1318. Search date 1988; primary sources Medline and hand searches of references cited in identified articles.
6. Whitehead SA, Andrews PLR, Chamberlain GVP. Characterisation of nausea and vomiting in early pregnancy: a survey of 1000 women. *J Obstet Gynaecol* 1992;12:364–369.
7. Jewell D, Young G. Interventions for nausea and vomiting in early pregnancy. In: The Cochrane Library, Issue 3, 2001. Oxford: Update Software. Search date 2001; primary sources Cochrane Pregnancy and Childbirth Group Trials Register and the Cochrane Controlled Trials Register.
8. Belluomini J, Litt RC, Lee KA, et al. Acupressure for nausea and vomiting of pregnancy: a randomized, blinded study. *Obstet Gynecol* 1994;84:245–248.
9. O'Brien B, Relyea MJ, Taerum T. Efficacy of P6 acupressure in the treatment of nausea and vomiting during pregnancy. *Am J Obstet Gynecol* 1996;174:708–715.
10. Norheim AJ, Pedersen EJ, Fønnebø V, et al. Acupressure treatment of morning sickness in pregnancy: a randomised, double-blind, placebo-controlled study. *Scand J Prim Health Care* 2001;19:43–47.
11. Steele NM, French J, Gatherer-Boyles J, et al. Effect of acupressure by Sea-Bands on nausea and vomiting of pregnancy. *J Obstet Gynecol Neonatal Nurs* 2001;30:61–70.
12. Bayreuther J, Lewith GT, Pickering R. A double-blind cross-over study to evaluate the effectiveness of acupressure at pericardium 6 (P6) in the treatment of early morning sickness (EMS). *Complement Therap Med* 1994;2:70–76.
13. Evans AT, Samuels SN, Marshall C, et al. Suppression of pregnancy-induced nausea and vomiting with sensory afferent stimulation. *J Reprod Med* 1993;38:603–606.
14. Stone CL. Acupressure wristbands for the nausea of pregnancy. *Nurse Pract* 1993;18:15.
15. Dundee JW, Sourial FBR, Ghaly RG, et al. P6 acupressure reduces morning sickness. *J R Soc Med* 1988;81:456–457.
16. Dundee J, McMillan C. Some problems encountered in the scientific evaluation of acupuncture emesis. *Acupunct Med* 1992;10:2–8.
17. Smith C, Crowther C, Beilby J. Pregnancy outcome following women's participation in a randomised controlled trial of acupuncture to treat nausea and vomiting in early pregnancy. *Complement Ther Med* 2002;10:78–83.
18. Knight B, Mudge C, Openshaw S, et al. Effect of acupuncture on nausea of pregnancy: a randomized, controlled trial. *Obstet Gynecol* 2001;97:184–188.
19. Mazzotta P, Magee LA. A risk–benefit assessment of pharmacological and nonpharmacological treatments for nausea and vomiting of pregnancy. *Drugs* 2000;59:781–800. Search date 1998; primary sources Medline, Pregnancy and Childbirth Module of the Cochrane Database of Systematic Reviews, hand searches of bibliographies of retrieved papers, standard toxicology text (Drugs in Pregnancy and Lactation), and personal contact with pharmaceutical companies, researchers, and clinicians in the fields of pharmacology, toxicology, obstetrics, and paediatrics.
20. Czeizel AE, Dudas I, Fritz G, et al. The effect of periconceptional multivitamin-mineral supplementation on vertigo, nausea and vomiting in the first trimester of pregnancy. *Arch Gynecol Obstet* 1992;251:181–185.
21. Vutyavanich T, Kraisarin T, Ruangsri R. Ginger for nausea and vomiting in pregnancy: randomized, double-masked, placebo-controlled trial. *Obstet Gynaecol* 97;2001:577–582.
22. Keating A, Chez RA. Ginger syrup as an antiemetic in early pregnancy. *Altern Ther Health Med* 2002;8:89–91.
23. Fischer-Rasmussen W, Kjaer SK, Dahl C, et al. Ginger treatment of hyperemesis gravidarum. *Eur J Obstet Gynecol Reprod Biol* 1990;38:19–24.
24. Carlsson CP, Axemo P, Bodin A, et al. Manual acupuncture reduces hyperemesis gravidarum: a placebo-controlled, randomized, single-blind, crossover study. *J Pain Symptom Manage* 2000;20:273–279.
25. Ylikorkala O, Kauppila A, Ollanketo ML. Intramuscular ACTH or placebo in the treatment of hyperemesis gravidarum. *Acta Obstet Gynecol Scand* 1979;58:453–455.
26. Nelson-Piercy C, Fayers P, de Swiet M. Randomised, double-blind, placebo-controlled trial of corticosteroids for the treatment of hyperemesis gravidarum. *Br J Obstet Gynaecol* 2001;108:9–15.
27. Safari HR, Fassett MJ, Souter IC, et al. The efficacy of methylprednisolone in the treatment of hypermesis gravidarum: a randomized, double-blind, controlled study. *Am J Obstet Gynecol* 1998;179:921–924.
28. General Practitioner's Research Group. Hyperemesis treated with a pharmacologically inert compound. *Practitioner* 1966;196:711–714.

Richmal Oates-Whitehead
Obstetrics & Gynaecology Epidemiologist
Royal College of Paediatrics
Editor Cochrane Acute Respiratory Infections Group, London, UK

Competing interests: None declared.

The following previous contributor of this topic would like to be acknowledged: David Jewell.

Pre-eclampsia and hypertension

Search date August 2002

Lelia Duley

QUESTIONS

INTERVENTIONS

See glossary, p 1696

Key Messages

Prevention

- **Antiplatelet drugs** One systematic review has found that, in women considered at risk of pre-eclampsia, antiplatelet drugs (mainly aspirin) versus placebo or no treatment significantly reduces the risk of pre-eclampsia, death of the baby, and delivery before 37 weeks, with no significant difference in other important outcomes. One small subsequent RCT found similar results. The systematic review found no evidence that aspirin versus placebo increased the risk of bleeding in mother or baby.
- **Calcium supplementation (in high risk women or those with low intake)** One systematic review has found that calcium supplementation (mainly 2 g daily) versus placebo significantly reduces the risk of pre-eclampsia, and significantly reduces the risk of having a baby with birth weight under 2500 g. There was no significant effect on the risk of stillbirth or perinatal death before discharge from hospital, caesarean section, or preterm delivery.
- **Magnesium supplementation** One systematic review found insufficient evidence about the effects of magnesium supplements on the risk of pre-eclampsia or its complications.
- **Other pharmacological interventions** Two RCTs comparing atenolol or glyceryl trinitrate patches versus placebo were too small to draw reliable conclusions.
- **Salt restriction** Limited evidence from one systematic review found no significant difference in the risk of pre-eclampsia with a low salt diet versus a normal diet.
- **Vitamin C and E** One RCT in high risk women found limited evidence that vitamins C and E versus placebo significantly reduced the risk of pre-eclampsia. However, we were unable to draw reliable conclusions about effects. We found insufficient evidence about effects on other clinical outcomes.
- **Evening primrose oil; fish oil** We found six RCTs of evening primrose and fish oil, which were too small to draw reliable conclusions.

Treatments

- **Aggressive versus expectant management for severe early onset pre-eclampsia** One systematic review based on two small RCTs found no evidence that aggressive management significantly reduced stillbirth or perinatal death rates compared with expectant management in babies born to mothers with severe early onset pre-eclampsia. However, it found that aggressive management increased rates of admission to neonatal intensive care and increased the risk of necrotising enterocolitis and respiratory distress in the baby compared with expectant management. We found insufficient evidence about effects of aggressive versus expectant management in the mother.
- **Antihypertensive drugs for mild to moderate hypertension** Two systematic reviews have found that antihypertensive agents versus placebo, no antihypertensive drug, or another antihypertensive drug significantly reduce the chance of developing severe hypertension, but found no clear effect on pre-eclampsia and perinatal death. Systematic reviews found that angiotensin converting enzyme inhibitors used in pregnancy were associated with fetal renal failure, and found that β blockers increased the risk of the baby being small for its gestational age.

- **Antihypertensive drugs for very high blood pressure (although insufficient evidence on best choice of agent)** One systematic review and one subsequent RCT in women with blood pressures high enough to merit immediate treatment found no evidence of a difference in the control of blood pressure by various antihypertensive drugs. The studies were too small to draw any further conclusions about the relative effects of different agents.
- **Antioxidants in severe pre-eclampsia** One RCT found insufficient evidence about the effects of a combination of vitamin E, vitamin C, and allopurinol versus placebo.
- **Bed rest for proteinuric hypertension** One systematic review found insufficient evidence about the effects of bed rest in hospital versus normal ambulation in hospital.
- **Bed rest/hospital admission** We found insufficient evidence about hospital admission, bed rest, or day care versus outpatient care or normal activities in hospital.
- **Choice of analgesia during labour with severe pre-eclampsia** One RCT found that epidural analgesia during labour versus intravenous patient controlled analgesia significantly reduced mean pain scores, but the clinical importance of the difference was unclear.
- **Hospital admission for non-proteinuric hypertension** One systematic review found no significant difference in any major outcome with hospital admission versus outpatient clinic assessment.
- **Magnesium sulphate for eclampsia (better than other anticonvulsants)** Systematic reviews have found that magnesium sulphate versus phenytoin, diazepam, or lytic cocktail significantly reduces further fits in women with eclampsia. All reviews found trends towards reduced maternal mortality with magnesium sulphate, although the benefit was not significant.
- **Plasma volume expansion in severe pre-eclampsia** One systematic review found insufficient evidence about the effects of plasma volume expansion versus no expansion.
- **Prophylactic magnesium sulphate in severe pre-eclampsia** One systematic review and one large RCT have found that prophylactic magnesium sulphate halves the risk of eclampsia compared with placebo in women with severe pre-eclampisa. The trials found no evidence of a difference between magnesium sulphate and placebo for rate of stillbirth or perinatal mortality in babies born to women with severe pre-eclampsia. A quarter of women reported mild adverse effects, mainly flushing.
- **Prophylactic diazepam in severe pre-eclampsia** One systematic review found insufficient evidence about effects of diazepam versus no anticonvulsants in women with severe pre-eclampsia.

DEFINITION Hypertension during pregnancy may be associated with one of several conditions. **Pregnancy induced hypertension** is a rise in blood pressure, without proteinuria, during the second half of pregnancy. **Pre-eclampsia** is a multisystem disorder, unique to pregnancy, which is usually associated with raised blood pressure and proteinuria. It rarely presents before 20 weeks' gestation. **Eclampsia** is one or more convulsions in association with the syndrome of pre-eclampsia. **Pre-existing hypertension** is known hypertension before pregnancy or raised blood pressure before 20 weeks' gestation. It may be essential hypertension or, less commonly, secondary to underlying disease.[1]

Pre-eclampsia and hypertension

INCIDENCE/ PREVALENCE Pregnancy induced hypertension affects 10% of pregnancies and pre-eclampsia complicates 2–8%.[2] Eclampsia occurs in about 1/2000 deliveries in developed countries.[3] In developing countries, estimates of the incidence of eclampsia vary from 1/100–1/1700.[4,5]

AETIOLOGY/ RISK FACTORS The cause of pre-eclampsia is unknown. It is likely to be multifactorial and may result from deficient placental implantation during the first half of pregnancy.[6] Pre-eclampsia is more common among women likely to have a large placenta, such as those with multiple pregnancy, and among women with medical conditions associated with microvascular disease, such as diabetes, hypertension, and collagen vascular disease.[7,8] Other risk factors include genetic susceptibility, increased parity, and older maternal age.[9] Cigarette smoking seems to be associated with a lower risk of pre-eclampsia, but this potential benefit is outweighed by an increase in adverse outcomes such as low birth weight, placental abruption, and perinatal death.[10]

PROGNOSIS The outcome of pregnancy in women with pregnancy induced hypertension alone is at least as good as that for normotensive pregnancies.[7,11] However, once pre-eclampsia develops, morbidity and mortality rise for both mother and child. For example, perinatal mortality for women with severe pre-eclampsia is double that for normotensive women.[7] Perinatal outcome is worse with early gestational hypertension.[7,9,11] Perinatal mortality also increases in women with severe essential hypertension.[12]

AIMS OF INTERVENTION To delay or prevent the development of pre-eclampsia and eclampsia, and to improve outcomes for women and their children. Once pre-eclampsia has occurred, to minimise morbidity and mortality for the woman and her child, and to ensure that health service resources are used appropriately.

OUTCOMES **For the woman:** Rates of pre-eclampsia (proteinuria and hypertension), eclampsia, death, severe morbidity (such as renal failure, coagulopathy, cardiac failure, liver failure, and stroke), placental abruption, and caesarean section; use of resources (such as dialysis, ventilation, admission to intensive care, or length of stay); adverse effects of treatment. **For the child:** Rates of death, intrauterine growth restriction, prematurity, and severe morbidity (such as intraventricular haemorrhage, respiratory distress syndrome, or asphyxia); measures of infant and child development (such as cerebral palsy or significant learning disability); use of resources (such as admission to special care nursery, ventilation, length of stay in hospital, and special needs in the community); adverse effects of treatment.

METHODS *Clinical Evidence* search and appraisal August 2002 and author search of the register of trials held by the Cochrane Pregnancy and Childbirth Group June 2002.

QUESTION **What are the effects of preventive interventions in women at high risk of pre-eclampsia?**

OPTION **ANTIPLATELET DRUGS**

One systematic review has found that, in women considered at risk of pre-eclampsia, antiplatelet drugs (mainly aspirin) versus placebo or no treatment significantly reduce the risk of pre-eclampsia, death of the baby, and delivery before 37 weeks, with no significant difference in other important outcomes. One small subsequent RCT found similar results. The systematic review found no evidence that aspirin versus placebo increased the risk of bleeding in mother or baby.

Benefits: We found one systematic review of antiplatelet agents (search date 1999, 39 RCTs, 30 563 women) and one subsequent small RCT.[13,14] **Versus placebo/no antiplatelet drug:** The systematic review found that, in women considered at risk of pre-eclampsia, antiplatelet agents reduced pre-eclampsia (32 RCTs: 975/14 743 women [6.6%] with antiplatelet *v* 1142/14 588 women [7.8%] with no antiplatelet; RR 0.85, 95% CI 0.78 to 0.92; NNT 59, 95% CI 59 to 167), premature delivery before 37 completed weeks (23 RCTs: 2447/14 169 women [17.3%] with antiplatelet *v* 2621/14 099 [18.6%] with no antiplatelet; RR 0.92, 95% CI 0.88 to 0.97; NNT 72, 95% CI 44 to 200), and baby deaths (30 RCTs: 383/15 091 women [2.5%] with antiplatelet *v* 439/15 002 [2.9%] with no antiplatelet; RR 0.86, 95% CI 0.75 to 0.98; NNT 250, 95% CI 95 to > 10 000).[13] There were no clear effects on other important outcomes. There was no effect of starting treatment before 20 weeks, and no significant difference in the relative risk reduction between women at high and low risk for pre-eclampsia and its complications. The benefit was greatest for women given more than 75 mg aspirin daily. The subsequent small RCT (placebo controlled, 90 women at high risk based on Doppler ultrasound of uterine arteries) found that low dose aspirin (0.5mg/kg daily) versus placebo significantly reduced the incidence of pre-eclampsia (4.7% *v* 23.3%; RR 0.2, 95% CI 0.05 to 0.86) and hypertension before 37 weeks (2.3% *v* 20.9%; RR 0.22, 95% CI 0.05 to 0.97).[14] **Versus each other:** Trials comparing one antiplatelet agent with another were too small for reliable conclusions.[13]

Harms: The systematic review found no evidence that aspirin increased the risk of bleeding for mother or baby.[13] Two studies followed up children of mothers enrolled in placebo controlled RCTs of aspirin versus placebo for 12–18 months.[15,16] It found no significant differences between aspirin versus placebo in hospital visits for congenital malformations, motor deficit, developmental delay, respiratory problems or bleeding problems; height or weight below the third centile; or bleeding rates in children of treated mothers.

Comment: Almost all studies used low dose aspirin (50–75 mg) and most were placebo controlled. The RCTs included women with a variety of risk factors, including a history of previous early onset disease, diabetes, or chronic hypertension, and were conducted in different countries in the developed and developing world. The number needed to treat values cannot be applied directly to different populations of women; the values stated represent estimates for women with a risk of pre-eclampsia that is an average over all the participants in the RCTs. The absolute benefit was higher (and the NNT lower) in women at higher risk of pre-eclampsia.

OPTION MATERNAL CALCIUM SUPPLEMENTATION

One systematic review has found that calcium supplementation (mainly 2 g daily) versus placebo significantly reduces the risk of pre-eclampsia, and significantly reduces the risk of having a baby with birth weight under 2500 g. There was no significant effect on the risk of stillbirth or perinatal death before discharge from hospital; caesarean section or preterm delivery.

Benefits: **Versus placebo:** We found one systematic review of calcium supplementation (search date 2001, 11 RCTs, 7203 women).[17] In the review, calcium (mainly 2 g daily) significantly reduced the risk of pre-eclampsia compared with placebo (11 RCTs: 197/3427 [6%] with calcium supplementation *v* 294/3452 [9%] with placebo; RR 0.68, 95% CI 0.57 to 0.81; NNT 38, 95% CI 26 to 67). Subgroup analysis found that the greatest effect was in women with low dietary calcium (27/907 [3%] with calcium supplementation *v* 90/935 [10%] with placebo for low dietary calcium compared with 169/2505 [7%] with calcium supplementation *v* 197/2517 [8%] with placebo for normal dietary calcium). Calcium supplementation significantly reduced the risk of having a baby with birth weight under 2500 g (234/3230 [7.2%] with calcium supplementation *v* 283/3261 [8.7%] with placebo; RR 0.83, 95% CI 0.71 to 0.98; NNT 67, 95% CI 36 to 1000). It found no significant effect of calcium supplements versus placebo on the risk of caesarean delivery, preterm delivery, or death of the baby. **Calcium and evening primrose oil versus placebo:** One small trial (48 women) did not provide sufficient evidence for reliable conclusions.[18]

Harms: After follow up of 518 children to 7 years of age, the review found no harms associated with maternal calcium supplements.[17]

Comment: Most trials in the systematic review were of good quality and included a wide range of women. They were conducted largely in the USA and South America. They included mainly women at low risk with adequate dietary calcium, so the number of women in the category who would benefit most from calcium supplementation was small. Several studies reported that adherence to treatment was between 60–90%.[17] The proportion of women taking 90–100% of all allocated treatment was low (20% in 1 study).[17]

OPTION OTHER DIETARY CHANGE

We found insufficient evidence from six small RCTs about effects on pre-eclampsia or preterm birth of fish oil; evening primrose oil or both versus placebo or each other. Systematic reviews have found insufficient evidence from small RCTs about effects on pre-eclampsia of reduced salt intake (to 20–50 mmol daily) or magnesium supplements. One RCT in high risk women has found that vitamins C and E supplements reduce the risk

of pre-eclampsia compared with placebo. One small RCT has found that supplementation with protein, fish oil, and calcium, plus rest in the left lateral position, reduces the risk of pre-eclampsia compared with iron supplementation.

Benefits: **Fish and evening primrose oil:** We found no systematic review. We found six RCTs of fish and evening primrose oil that were too small to draw reliable conclusions (3 RCTs compared fish oil *v* no supplement or placebo; 1 RCT compared evening primrose oil *v* fish oil *v* placebo; 1 RCT compared evening primrose oil plus fish oil *v* magnesium oxide *v* placebo; and 1 RCT compared evening primrose oil *v* placebo).[19–24] **Protein, fish oil, and calcium, plus rest in left lateral position:** We found one RCT (74 women with a positive roll over test (see glossary, p 1696) at 28–29 wks).[25] It compared protein (25 mg), fish oil (300 mg), and calcium (300 mg) three times a week plus 15 minutes rest in the left lateral position twice daily versus ferrous sulphate (105 mg) three times a week. It found a reduced risk of pre-eclampsia in the multiple supplements group (2/37 [5%] with multiple supplements *v* 16/37 [46%] with iron alone; RR 0.12, 95% CI 0.03 to 0.51; NNT 3, 95% CI 2 to 6). It was too small for reliable conclusions on other outcomes. **Reduced salt versus normal or high salt:** We found one systematic review (search date 1999, 2 RCTs, 600 women) comparing reduced salt with normal dietary salt.[26] It found no significant difference for rates of pre-eclampsia, although the trials may have lacked power to detect clinically important effects (RR 1.11, 95% CI 0.46 to 2.66). **Magnesium:** We found one systematic review (search date 2001, 2 RCTs, 474 women) reporting pre-eclampsia. The RCTs were too small for reliable conclusions.[27] **Vitamins C and E:** We found one RCT (283 high risk women) that found a significantly reduced risk of pre-eclampsia with vitamin C (1000 mg daily) and vitamin E (400 IU daily) versus placebo (11/141 [8%] with vitamins *v* 24/142 [17%] with placebo; RR 0.46, 95% CI 0.24 to 0.91; NNT 11, 95% CI 8 to 61).[28] The study was too small to provide reliable evidence about effects on other important outcomes.

Harms: **Fish oil:** One RCT (533 women) found no significant difference between fish oil versus olive oil or no supplement for rates of post-term delivery (RR 1.19, 95% CI 0.73 to 1.93) and postpartum haemorrhage (RR 1.21, 95% CI 0.76 to 1.92).[29] These outcomes were not reported in the other smaller studies. **Fish oil and evening primrose oil:** Vomiting was more commonly reported in the oil treated group, but numbers were not provided.[23] No other adverse events were reported. **Evening primrose oil:** These studies were too small for reliable conclusions. **Reduced salt:** We found no evidence of harmful effects in the trials.[26] **Magnesium:** There was no significant difference between the groups in the number of reported adverse effects (RR 0.84, 95% CI 0.65 to 1.08).[27] **Vitamins C and E:** We found little evidence about the safety of these vitamins at the high doses used in the RCT.[28]

Comment: The fish oil RCTs may have been difficult to blind because of the distinctive taste of fish oil. One study found that olive oil provided better masking than a no oil placebo.[29] The trials of salt restriction were conducted in the Netherlands, where advice to restrict salt intake during pregnancy has been routine for many years. Such advice is no longer widespread elsewhere. An updated systematic review of fish oil for prevention of pre-eclampsia will be available soon.[30]

OPTION OTHER PHARMACOLOGICAL AGENTS

We found two small RCTs. One compared atenolol versus placebo and the other compared glyceryl trinitrate patches versus placebo. Both were too small for any reliable conclusions.

Benefits: **Atenolol versus placebo:** We found one small RCT (68 women without hypertension selected because they had a cardiac output > 7.4 L/min), which found no significant reduction in the risk of pre-eclampsia with atenolol 100 mg daily (1/28 [4%] with atenolol *v* 5/28 [18%] with placebo; RR 0.20, 95% CI 0.02 to 1.60).[31] **Glyceryl trinitrate versus placebo:** One small RCT (40 women) found no significant difference between glyceryl trinitrate patches versus placebo (RR 1.13, 95% CI 0.35 to 3.60), but the confidence interval was wide.[32]

Harms: The RCT (68 women) of atenolol versus placebo found that mean birth weight was significantly lower with atenolol for a subgroup of primiparous women (mean difference 440 g; P = 0.02).[31]

Comment: Although the possible benefits of atenolol for prevention of pre-eclampsia remain unclear, the reduction in birth weight may be real. Concerns about the possible harmful effects of atenolol on fetal growth and development have been discussed for some time (see harms of antihypertensive agents, p 1692).[33,34]

QUESTION What are the effects of interventions in women who develop hypertension during pregnancy?

OPTION BED REST/HOSPITAL ADMISSION VERSUS DAY CARE

We found inadequate evidence about hospital admission, bed rest, or day care versus outpatient care or normal activities in hospital.

Benefits: **Bed rest/hospital admission versus no hospital admission:** We found two systematic reviews of hospital admission.[35,36] The first systematic review (search date 1993, 3 trials, 408 women) compared hospital admission versus outpatient clinic assessment for non-proteinuric hypertension and found no significant difference for any major outcome.[35] The second systematic review (search date 1993, 2 RCTs, 145 women with proteinuric hypertension) compared bed rest in hospital versus normal ambulation in hospital, but the trials were too small for any reliable conclusions.[36] **Antenatal day care units versus hospital admission:** We found one systematic review (search date 2001, 1 RCT, 54 women).[37] The RCT was too small for reliable conclusions.

Harms: It has been suggested that hospital admission increases the risk of venous stasis, thromboembolic disease, or infection, but we found no evidence in this context. In the trial of day care units, women preferred not to be admitted to hospital. We found no evidence from the other trials about the views of women and their families.

Comment: Trials of hospital admission and bed rest in hospital were conducted before widespread introduction of day care assessment units. Women with hypertension during pregnancy are now often seen in day care units, but only one small trial has compared day care assessment with assessment in an outpatient clinic. An updated systematic review of bed rest with or without hospitalisation is in preparation.[38]

OPTION ANTIHYPERTENSIVE AGENTS

Two systematic reviews have found evidence that antihypertensive agents may halve the risk of severe hypertension. The effects of antihypertensive agents on pre-eclampsia and on perinatal death are unclear. We were unable to draw reliable conclusions about any other important outcomes. It remains unclear whether treatment of mild to moderate hypertension during pregnancy is worthwhile with any antihypertensive agent compared with no treatment. Angiotensin converting enzyme inhibitors used in pregnancy are associated with fetal renal failure. β Blockers may increase the risk of the baby being small for its gestational age.

Benefits: We found two systematic reviews[39,40] and one subsequent RCT.[41] The first systematic review (search date 2000, 40 RCTs, > 3797 women with mild to moderate hypertension) included studies that compared any antihypertensive versus placebo or versus another antihypertensive.[39] The second systematic review (search date 2000, 27 RCTs, 2400 women) included only studies that compared β blockers versus no antihypertensive drug or versus another antihypertensive drug.[40] **Versus placebo or no antihypertensive:** The only significant effect was a reduced risk of developing severe hypertension (17 RCTs: RR 0.52, 95% CI 0.41 to 0.64; NNT 12, 95% CI 9 to 17), which was not reflected in other, more substantive, outcomes (pre-eclampsia: RR 0.99, 95% CI 0.84 to 1.18; perinatal death: RR 0.71, 95% CI 0.46 to 1.09).[39] **Versus other antihypertensive agents:** The systematic review[39] found no clear difference among any of these drugs for the risk of developing severe hypertension or pre-eclampsia. The review found that methyldopa versus other antihypertensive agents may increase the risk of the baby dying (14 RCTs: RR 0.49, 95% CI 0.24 to 0.99), but the RCTs were small and used weak methods, so that the difference may have arisen because of random error or bias. The small subsequent RCT (33 women) comparing alternative antihypertensive drugs found no significant differences in the risk of pre-eclampsia.[41]

Harms: The antihypertensive agents included in the systematic reviews[39,40] seem to be well tolerated during pregnancy, but adverse effects have not been reported in many RCTs. All antihypertensive drugs cross the placenta, but few trials reported possible adverse effects for the baby. The baby's risk of being small for its gestational age was increased if a β blocker was used to control the mother's hypertension (13 RCTs: RR 1.34, 95% CI 1.01 to 1.79).[40] Meta regression within a systematic review suggested that lowering blood pressure for women with mild or moderate hypertension may increase the risk of having a baby that is small for its gestational age.[42] One systematic review (search date 1999, 13 small RCTs in women with pre-existing chronic hypertension) found that angiotensin converting enzyme inhibitors used in the second or third trimester are associated with fetal renal failure.[43,44]

Comment: The RCTs were too small to exclude beneficial effects of antihypertensive agents. The trials had problems with their methods. Many were not placebo controlled, and few attempted to blind blood pressure measurement. Many important outcomes were reported by only a few studies. We found little evidence about adherence to treatment. One systematic review found that the effects of antihypertensive agents in women with pre-existing chronic hypertension were similar to those described above for women with pregnancy induced hypertension. The review did not establish or exclude benefit from treatment.[43,44]

QUESTION **What are the effects of interventions in women who develop severe pre-eclampsia or very high blood pressure during pregnancy?**

OPTION **ANTIHYPERTENSIVE DRUGS FOR VERY HIGH BLOOD PRESSURE**

One systematic review and one subsequent RCT found no evidence of a difference in the control of blood pressure by various antihypertensive drugs. Studies were too small for any further conclusions about relative effects of different agents. Ketanserin and diazoxide may be associated with more adverse effects than hydralazien and labetalol.

Benefits: We found one systematic review (search date 1998, 14 trials, 1200 women), which compared many agents (including hydralazine, labetalol, nifedipine, diazoxide, and ketanserin) mainly with hydralazine.[45] We also found one subsequent RCT.[46] The review found that all the active agents reduced blood pressure, but there was no significant evidence that one drug was better than another. The subsequent small RCT (126 women) compared nifedipine (8 mg sublingually) versus hydralazine (5 mg iv followed by further doses of 10 mg).[46] It found that nifedipine significantly delayed development of hypertensive crisis compared with hydralazine (median time to hypertensive crisis 3.1 h for nifedipine *v* 2.1 h for hydralazine; $P = 0.005$).

Harms: The use of ketanserin is associated with more persistent high blood pressure than hydralazine (RR 8.44, 95% CI 2.05 to 34.70), and labetalol is associated with less hypotension requiring treatment than diazoxide (RR 0.06, 95% CI 0.00 to 0.99).[45] Hypotension may compromise fetoplacental blood flow. Only four RCTs reported adverse effects, and frequency varied from 5–50%. Antihypertensives cross the placenta, but we found little evidence about effects on the baby.

Comment: Women in these studies had blood pressures high enough to merit immediate treatment, and many also had proteinuria or "severe pre-eclampsia". The trials were small and reported few outcomes other than control of blood pressure. In most trials there was no blinding after trial entry.

OPTION PLASMA VOLUME EXPANSION

One systematic review of plasma volume expansion versus no expansion found insufficient evidence to draw reliable conclusions.

Benefits: We found one systematic review (search date 2000, 3 RCTs, 61 women) evaluating colloid solutions compared with placebo or no infusion. The RCTs were too small for reliable conclusions but suggest that plasma volume expansion is not beneficial.[47]

Harms: RCTs found a non-significant increase in the risk of caesarean section (RR 1.5, 95% CI 0.8 to 2.9), and a non-significant increase in the need for additional treatment (RR 1.5, 95% CI 0.7 to 3.1) with plasma volume expansion versus placebo or no infusion.

Comment: These three RCTs all used a colloid rather than crystalloid solution. Two systematic reviews (search dates 1999) of plasma volume expansion in critically ill men and non-pregnant women have found an increased mortality with albumin (a colloid) when compared with either no expansion or crystalloid.[48,49]

OPTION ANTIOXIDANTS

We found insufficient evidence on the effects of antioxidants.

Benefits: We found no systematic review. We found one RCT (56 women) evaluating combined vitamin E, vitamin C, and allopurinol versus placebo.[50] It was too small for reliable conclusions to be drawn.

Harms: We found insufficient evidence for reliable conclusions.

Comment: Women in this study had severe pre-eclampsia at 24–32 weeks' gestation.

OPTION PROPHYLACTIC ANTICONVULSANTS FOR WOMEN WITH SEVERE PRE-ECLAMPSIA

One systematic review and one large RCT have found that prophylactic magnesium sulphate halves the risk of eclampsia compared with placebo in women with severe pre-eclampsia. The trials found no evidence of a difference between magnesium sulphate and placebo for rate of stillbirth or perinatal mortality in babies born to women with severe pre-eclampsia. A quarter of women reported mild adverse effects (mainly flushing). The review found insufficient evidence about effects of diazepam versus no anticonvulsants in women with severe pre-eclampsia.

Benefits: We found one systematic review (search date 1999, 10 RCTs, 3747 women)[51] and one subsequent RCT (10 141 women).[52] **Magnesium sulphate versus placebo or no anticonvulsant:** Meta-analysis of the five RCTs (11 390 women) that compared magnesium sulphate with placebo found that prophylactic magnesium sulphate halved the risk of eclampsia compared with placebo (43/5613 [0.8%] with magnesium sulphate *v* 107/5609 [1.9%] with placebo; RR 0.41, 95% CI 0.29 to 0.58; NNT 100 95%, CI 50 to 100). Prophylactic magnesium sulphate reduced maternal mortality compared with placebo, although results did not reach statistical significance (11/5393 [0.2%] with magnesium sulphate *v*

21/5379 [0.4%] with placebo; RR 0.53, 95% CI 0.26 to 1.09). For women randomised before delivery, there was no significant difference for rate of stillbirth or perinatal death (stillbirth: 424/5003 [8%] with magnesium sulphate v 426/4958 [8%] with placebo; RR 0.99, 95% CI 0.87 to 1.12; perinatal death: 538/4655 [12%] with magnesium sulphate v 541/4604 [12%] with placebo; RR 0.98, 95% CI 0.88 to 1.10).[51,52] **Diazepam versus no anticonvulsant:** One small RCT (59 women) compared diazepam versus no anticonvulsant; it was too small for any reliable conclusions.[51] **Magnesium sulphate versus phenytoin or diazepam:** Five RCTs (2439 women) have found that magnesium sulphate was better than phenytoin for preventing eclampsia (RR 0.05, 95% CI 0.00 to 0.84), but there was insufficient evidence for reliable conclusions about magnesium sulphate versus diazepam.[51]

Harms: In the subsequent RCT, a quarter of women experienced adverse effects (1201/4999 [24%] with magnesium sulphate v 228/4993 [5%] with placebo).[52] Specific effects included flushing (987/4999 [20%] v 98/4993 [2%]) and respiratory depression was rare (51/4999 [1%] with magnesium sulphate v 26/4993 [0.5%] with placebo). Meta-analysis of the five placebo controlled RCTs found that magnesium sulphate slightly increased caesarean section rates compared with placebo (2490/4969 [50%] with magnesium sulphate v 2329/4901 [48%] with placebo; RR 1.05, 95% CI 1.01 to 1.10; NNH 34, 95% CI 100 to 20). Compared with phenytoin, magnesium sulphate was also associated with an increased risk of caesarean section (RR 1.21, 95% CI 1.05 to 1.41; NNH 29, 95% CI 12 to 84).[51] One small RCT evaluated magnesium sulphate for preventing and treating preterm labour in women who did not have pre-eclampsia. It found an increase in infant mortality for babies born to these women. Many of the infants had very low birth weight (< 1500 g).[53]

Comment: Most of the data in these trials refers to women with relatively severe pre-eclampsia. One small study recruited only women with mild pre-eclampsia. Long term follow up of women and children in the large RCT is continuing.[52] Weak evidence from two case control studies suggests that magnesium sulphate may be associated with a decreased risk of cerebral palsy in babies weighing less than 1500 g.[54,55]

OPTION AGGRESSIVE MANAGEMENT FOR SEVERE EARLY ONSET PRE-ECLAMPSIA

One systematic review based on two small RCTs found no evidence that aggressive management significantly reduced stillbirth or perinatal death rates compared with expectant management in babies born to mothers with severe early onset pre-eclampsia. However, it found that aggressive management increased rates of admission to neonatal intensive care and increased the risk of necrotising enterocolitis and respiratory distress in the baby compared with expectant management. We found insufficient evidence about effects of aggressive versus expectant management in the mother.

Benefits: We found one systematic review (search date 2002, 2 RCTs, 133 women).[56] It found that, for the baby, there was no significant difference in rates of stillbirth or death after delivery for aggressive, interventional management versus expectant care (RR of death or stillbirth for interventional *v* expectant care 1.50, 95% CI 0.42 to 5.41). Babies of mothers in the aggressive management group were less likely to be small for gestational age than those in the expectant group (RR for aggressive *v* expectant management 0.36, 95% CI 0.14 to 0.90). The review found insufficient evidence about effects on maternal outcomes.

Harms: Aggressive management increased risks of respiratory distress syndrome, necrotising enterocolitis, and rate of admission to neonatal intensive care in babies born to mothers with severe pre-eclampsia (34/66 [52%] babies with respiratory distress syndrome with aggressive management *v* 15/67 [22%] with expectant care, RR 2.30, 95% CI 1.39 to 3.81; RR of necrotising colitis 5.5, 95% CI 1.04 to 29.56; RR admission to neonatal intensive care 1.32, 95% CI 1.13 to 1.55). We found insufficient evidence for reliable conclusions about effects of expectant management on maternal morbidity.

Comment: The women in these trials were at 28–34 weeks' gestation.

OPTION CHOICE OF ANALGESIA DURING LABOUR

One RCT in women with severe pre-eclampsia found that epidural analgesia during labour versus intravenous patient controlled analgesia significantly reduced mean pain scores, but the clinical importance of the difference was not clear.

Benefits: We found one RCT (105 women with severe pre-eclampsia) comparing intravenous patient controlled analgesia versus epidural analgesia.[57] Mean pain scores were significantly lower with an epidural but the clinical importance of the difference is unclear. The trial was too small for a reliable conclusion about other outcomes. We found no RCTs of other forms of intrapartum analgesia for this group of women.

Harms: Women allocated an epidural were more likely to have hypotension requiring intravenous ephedrine (5/56 [9%] with epidural *v* 0/60 [0%] with patient controlled analgesia).[57] Neonatal naloxone was more likely to be given following intravenous patient controlled analgesia (31/60 [54%] with intravenous patient controlled analgesia *v* 5/56 [9%] with epidural analgesia; RR 5.71, 95% CI 2.39 to 13.60; NNH 3, 95% CI 2 to 4). The trial was too small for reliable conclusions about other outcomes.

Comment: The name of the drug used for patient controlled analgesia was not stated.

QUESTION What is the best choice of anticonvulsant for women with eclampsia?

Systematic reviews have found that magnesium sulphate is better than phenytoin, diazepam, or lytic cocktail for preventing further fits in women with eclampsia. Although the effects on maternal mortality are not statistically significant, all reviews have found trends towards reduced risk with magnesium sulphate.

Benefits: **Versus diazepam:** We found one systematic review (search date 1999, 5 RCTs, 1236 women).[58] Magnesium sulphate versus diazepam reduced both maternal mortality (21/617 [3.4%] with magnesium sulphate *v* 36/619 [5.8%] with diazepam; RR 0.59, 95% CI 0.36 to 1.00) and further fits (71/618 [11%] *v* 160/618 [26%]; RR 0.45, 95% CI 0.35 to 0.58). There was no evidence of any differential effects on any other reported outcome. **Versus phenytoin:** We found one systematic review (search date 1999, 4 RCTs, 823 women)[59] and one subsequent small RCT.[60] Magnesium sulphate versus phenytoin reduced the risks of further fits (23/423 [5.4%] with magnesium sulphate *v* 73/422 [17%] with phenytoin; RR 0.32, 95% CI 0.21 to 0.50), pneumonia (RR 0.44, 95% CI 0.24 to 0.79), requirement for ventilation (RR 0.66, 95% CI 0.49 to 0.90), and admission to intensive care (RR 0.67, 95% CI 0.50 to 0.89).[59] Fewer babies died or stayed in a special baby care unit for more than 7 days with magnesium sulphate versus phenytoin (RR 0.77, 95% CI 0.63 to 0.95). The lower maternal death rate with magnesium sulphate compared with phenytoin was not significant, but the confidence interval was wide and a clinically important effect could not be excluded (RR 0.51, 95% CI 0.25 to 1.06). The small subsequent RCT (50 women) reported results consistent with those of the review.[60] **Versus lytic cocktail:** We found one systematic review (search date 2000, 2 RCTs, 199 women).[61] Magnesium sulphate versus lytic cocktail (see glossary, p 1696) significantly reduced further fits (4/96 [4%] with magnesium sulphate *v* 49/102 [48%] with lytic cocktail; RR 0.09, 95% CI 0.03 to 0.24), pneumonia (1/51 [2%] *v* 11/57 [19%]; RR 0.08, 95% CI 0.02 to 0.42), respiratory depression (0/96 [0%] *v* 8/102 [8%]; RR 0.12, 95% CI 0.02 to 0.91), and fetal or infant death (14/89 [16%] *v* 30/88 [34%]; RR 0.45, 95% CI 0.26 to 0.79). There was a non-significant reduction in maternal deaths (1/96 [1%] *v* 6/102 [6%]; RR 0.25, 95% CI 0.04 to 1.43).

Harms: **Versus diazepam:** We found no good evidence from RCTs about harms. **Versus phenytoin:** Clinical experience suggests that magnesium sulphate is safer than phenytoin. **Versus lytic cocktail:** Magnesium sulphate seems to be considerably safer than lytic cocktail.

Comment: Most information about the comparisons with diazepam and phenytoin comes from one large multicentre trial, in which adherence to treatment was 99%. The lytic cocktail trials included women with antepartum or postpartum eclampsia.

GLOSSARY

Lytic cocktail A mixture of pethidine, chlorpromazine, and promethazine.

Roll over test A test in which a woman lies on her left side for 15 minutes after which blood pressure is recorded. She then rolls into the supine position and, after 5 minutes, blood pressure is measured again. A rise in diastolic blood pressure in the supine position of more than 20 mm Hg is defined as abnormal. The value of this test has been questioned.

REFERENCES

1. Gifford RW, August P, Chesley LC, et al. National high blood pressure education program working group report on high blood pressure in pregnancy. *Am J Obstet Gynecol* 1990;163(5 Pt 1):1691–1712.
2. WHO international collaborative study of hypertensive disorders of pregnancy. Geographic variation in the incidence of hypertension in pregnancy. *Am J Obstet Gynecol* 1988;158:80–83.
3. Douglas K, Redman C. Eclampsia in the United Kingdom. *BMJ* 1994;309:1395–1400.
4. Crowther CA. Eclampsia at Harare maternity hospital. An epidemiological study. *S Afr Med J* 1985;68:927–929.
5. Bergström S, Povey G, Songane F, et al. Seasonal incidence of eclampsia and its relationship to meteorological data in Mozambique. *J Perinat Med* 1992;20:153–158.
6. Roberts JM, Redman CWG. Pre-eclampsia: more than pregnancy-induced hypertension. *Lancet* 1993;341:1447–1451.
7. Taylor DJ. The epidemiology of hypertension during pregnancy. In: Rubin PC, ed. *Hypertension in Pregnancy*. Amsterdam: Elsevier Science, 1988:223–240.
8. Sibai BM, Caritis S, Hauth J. Risks of preeclampsia and adverse neonatal outcomes among women with pregestational diabetes mellitus. National Institute of Child Health and Human Development Network of Maternal-Fetal Medicine Units. *Am J Obstet Gynecol* 2000;182:364–369.
9. MacGillivray I. *Pre-eclampsia. The hypertensive disease of pregnancy*. London: WB Saunders, 1983.
10. Conde-Agudelo A, Althabe F, Belizan JM, et al. Cigarette smoking during pregnancy and risk of preeclampsia: a systematic review. *Am J Obstet Gynecol* 1999;181:1026–1035. Search date 1998; primary sources Medline, Embase, Popline, Cinahl, Lilacs, and hand searches of proceedings of international meetings on pre-eclampsia and reference lists of retrieved articles.
11. Chamberlain GVP, Philip E, Howlett B, et al. *British Births*. London: Heinemann, 1970.
12. Sibai B, Lindheimer M, Hauth J, et al. Risk factors for preeclampsia, abruptio placentae, and adverse neonatal outcomes among women with chronic hypertension. *N Engl J Med* 1998;339:667–671.
13. Knight M, Duley L, Henderson-Smart DJ, et al. Antiplatelet agents for preventing and treating pre-eclampsia. In: The Cochrane Library, Issue 3, 2002. Oxford: Update Software. Search date 1999; primary sources Cochrane Pregnancy and Childbirth Group Trials Register and conference proceedings.
14. Vainio M, Kujansuu E, Iso-Mustajarvi M, et al. Low dose acetylsalicylic acid in prevention of pregnancy-induced hypertension and intrauterine growth retardation in women with bilateral uterine artery notches. *BJOG* 2002;109:161–167.
15. Grant A, Farrell B, Heineman J, et al. Low dose aspirin in pregnancy and early childhood development: follow up of the collaborative low dose aspirin study in pregnancy. *Br J Obstet Gynaecol* 1995;102:861–868.
16. Parazzini F, Bortolus R, Chatenoud L, et al. Follow-up of children in the Italian study of aspirin in pregnancy. *Lancet* 1994;343:1235.
17. Atallah AN, Hofmeyr GJ, Duley L. Calcium supplementation during pregnancy for preventing hypertensive disorders and related problems. In: The Cochrane Library, Issue 3, 2002. Oxford: Update Software. Search date 2001; primary source Cochrane Pregnancy and Childbirth Group Trials Register.
18. Herrera JA, Arevalo-Herrera M, Herrera S. Prevention of pre-eclampsia by linoleic acid and calcium supplementation: a randomized controlled trial. *Obstet Gynecol* 1998;91:585–590.
19. Salvig JD, Olsen SF, Secher NJ. Effects of fish oil supplementation in late pregnancy on blood pressure: a randomised controlled trial. *Br J Obstet Gynaecol* 1996;103:529–533.
20. Onwude JL, Lilford RJ, Hjartardottir H, et al. A randomised double blind placebo controlled trial of fish oil in high risk pregnancy. *Br J Obstet Gynaecol* 1995;102:95–100.
21. Bulstra-Ramakers MTE, Huisjes HJ, Visser GHA. The effects of 3 g eicosapentaenoic acid daily on recurrence of intrauterine growth retardation and pregnancy induced hypertension. *Br J Obstet Gynaecol* 1995;102:123–126.
22. Laivuori H, Hovatta O, Viinikka L, et al. Dietary supplementation with primrose oil or fish oil dose not change urinary excretion of prostacyclin and thromboxane metabolites in pre-eclamptic women. *Prostaglandins Leukot Essent Fatty Acids* 1993;49:691–694.
23. D'Almeida A, Carter JP, Anatol A, et al. Effects of a combination of evening primrose oil (gamma linolenic acid) and fish oil (eicosapentaenoic + docahexaenoic acid) versus magnesium, and versus placebo in preventing pre-eclampsia. *Women Health* 1992;19:117–131.
24. Moodley J, Norman RJ. Attempts at dietary alteration of prostaglandin pathways in the management of pre-eclampsia. *Prostaglandins Leukot Essent Fatty Acids* 1989;37:145–147.
25. Herrera JA. Nutritional factors and rest reduce pregnancy-induced hypertension and pre-eclampsia in positive roll-over test primigravidas. *Int J Gynaecol Obstet* 1993;41:31–35.
26. Duley L, Henderson-Smart D. Reduced salt intake compared to normal dietary salt, or high intake, in pregnancy. In: The Cochrane Library, Issue 3, 2002. Oxford: Update Software. Search date 1999; primary source Cochrane Pregnancy and Childbirth Group Trials Register.
27. Makrides M, Crowther CA. Magnesium supplementation in pregnancy. In: The Cochrane Library, Issue 3, 2002. Oxford: Update Software. Search date 2001; primary source Cochrane Pregnancy and Childbirth Group Trials Register.
28. Chappell LC, Seed PT, Briley AL, et al. Effect of antioxidants on the occurrence of pre-eclampsia in women at increased risk: a randomised trial. *Lancet* 1999;354:810–816.
29. Olsen SF, Sorensen JD, Secher NJ, et al. Randomised controlled trial of effect of fish oil supplementation on pregnancy duration. *Lancet* 1992;339:1003–1007.
30. Makrides M, Duley L, Olsen SF. Fish oil and other prostaglandin precursor supplementation during pregnancy for reducing pre-eclampsia, preterm birth, low birth weight and intrauterine growth restriction (Protocol for a Cochrane Review). In: The Cochrane Library, Issue 3, 2002. Oxford: Update Software.
31. Easterling TR, Brateng D, Schucker B, et al. Prevention of preeclampsia: a randomized trial of atenolol in hyperdynamic patients before onset of hypertension. *Obstet Gynecol* 1999;93:725–733.
32. Lees C, Valensise H, Black R, et al. The efficacy and fetal-maternal cardiovascular effects of transdermal glycerol trinitrate in the prophylaxis of

pre-eclampsia and its complications: a randomized double blind placebo controlled trial. *Ultrasound Obstet Gynaecol* 1998;12:334–338.

33. Butters L, Kennedy S, Rubin PC. Atenolol in essential hypertension during pregnancy. *BMJ* 1990;301:587–589.
34. Churchill D, Bayliss H, Beevers G. Fetal growth restriction. *Lancet* 1999;355:1366–1367.
35. Duley L. Hospitalisation for non-proteinuric pregnancy hypertension. In: Keirse MJNC, Renfrew MJ, Neilson JP, et al, eds. *Pregnancy and childbirth module*. In: The Cochrane Library, Issue 2, 1995. Oxford: Update Software. Search date 1993; primary source Cochrane Pregnancy and Childbirth Group Trials Register.
36. Duley L. Strict bed rest for proteinuric hypertension in pregnancy. In: Keirse MJNC, Renfrew MJ, Neilson JP, et al, eds. *Pregnancy and childbirth module*. In: The Cochrane Library, Issue 4, 1995. Oxford: Update Software. Search date 1993; primary source Cochrane Pregnancy and Childbirth Group Trials Register.
37. Kröner C, Turnbull D, Wilkinson C. Antenatal day care units versus hospital admission for women with complicated pregnancy. In: The Cochrane Library, Issue 3, 2002. Oxford: Update Software. Search date 2001; primary sources Cochrane Pregnancy and Childbirth Group Trials Register, Cochrane Controlled Trials Register, Cinahl, Current Contents, and conference proceedings.
38. Abalos E, Carroli G. Bed rest with or without hospitalisation for hypertension during pregnancy (Protocol for a Cochrane Review). In: The Cochrane Library, Issue 3, 2002. Oxford: Update Software.
39. Abalos E, Duley L, Steyn DW, et al. Antihypertensive drug therapy for mild to moderate hypertension during pregnancy. In: The Cochrane Library, Issue 3, 2002. Oxford: Update Software. Search date 2000; primary sources Cochrane Pregnancy and Childbirth Group Trials Register, Cochrane Controlled Trials Register, Medline, and Embase.
40. Magee LA, Duley L. Oral beta-blockers for mild to moderate hypertension during pregnancy. In: The Cochrane Library, Issue 3, 2002. Oxford: Update Software. Search date 2000; primary sources Cochrane Pregnancy and Childbirth Group Trial Register, Medline, and hand searches of reference lists.
41. Rudnicki M, Frolich A, Pilsgaard K, et al. Comparison of magnesium and methyldopa for the control of blood pressure in pregnancies complicated with hypertension. *Gynecol Obstet Invest* 2000;49:231–235.
42. Von Dadelszen P, Ornstein MP, Bull SB, et al. Fall in mean arterial pressure and fetal growth restriction in pregnancy hypertension: a meta-analysis. *Lancet* 2000;355:87–92. Search date 1997; primary sources Medline, Embase, hand searches of reference lists, *Hypertension and Pregnancy* 1992–1997, and a standard toxicology text.
43. Ferrer RL, Sibai BM, Mulrow CD, et al. Management of mild chronic hypertension during pregnancy: a review. *Obstet Gynecol* 2000;96:849–860. Search date 1999; primary sources 16 electronic databases, textbook references, and experts.
44. Mulrow CD, Chiquette E, Ferrer RL, et al. Management of chronic hypertension during pregnancy. Evidence Report/Technology Assessment No 14 (prepared by the San Antonio Evidence-based Practice Center based at the University of Texas Health Science Center at San Antonio under Contract No 290–97-0012). AHRQ Publication No 00-E011. Rockville, MD: Agency for Healthcare Research and Quality. August 2000. http://www.ahrq.gov/epcsums/pregsum.htm (last accessed 28 Jan 03). Search date 1999; primary sources 16 electronic databases, textbook references, and experts.
45. Duley L, Henderson-Smart DJ. Drugs for rapid treatment of very high blood pressure during pregnancy. In: The Cochrane Library, Issue 3, 2002. Oxford: Update Software. Search date 1998; primary source Cochrane Pregnancy and Childbirth Group Trials Register.
46. Aali BS, Nejad SS.Nifedipine or hydralazine as a first-line agent to control hypertension in severe preeclampsia. *Acta Obstet Gynecol Scand* 2002;81:25–30.
47. Duley L, Williams J, Henderson-Smart DJ. Plasma volume expansion for treatment of pre-eclampsia. In: The Cochrane Library, Issue 3, 2002. Oxford: Update Software. Search date 2000; primary source Cochrane Pregnancy and Childbirth Group Trials Register.
48. The Albumin Reviewers (Alderson P, Bunn F, Li Wan Po L, et al). Human albumin solution for resuscitation and volume expansion in critically ill patients. In: The Cochrane Library, Issue 3, 2002. Oxford: Update Software. Search date 1999; primary sources Cochrane Injuries Group Trials Register, Cochrane Controlled Trials Register, Medline, Embase, Bids Scientific and Technical Proceedings, hand searches of reference lists of trials and review articles, and personal contact with authors of identified trials.
49. Alderson P, Schierhout G, Roberts I, et al. Colloids versus crystalloids for fluid resuscitation in critically ill patients. In: The Cochrane Library, Issue 3, 2002. Oxford: Update Software. Search date 1999; primary sources Cochrane Clinical Trials Register, Medline, Embase, Bids Index to Scientific and Technical Proceedings, and reference lists of trials and review articles.
50. Gülmezoglu AM, Hofmeyr GJ, Oosthuizen MMJ. Antioxidants in the treatment of severe preeclampsia: a randomized explanatory study. *Br J Obstet Gynaecol* 1997;104:689–696.
51. Duley L, Gülmezoglu AM, Henderson-Smart D. Anticonvulsants for women with pre-eclampsia. In: The Cochrane Library, Issue 3, 2002. Oxford: Update Software. Search date 1999; primary source Cochrane Pregnancy and Childbirth Group Trials Register.
52. The Magpie Trial Collaboration Group. Do women with pre-eclampsia, and their babies, benefit from magnesium sulphate? The Magpie Trial: a randomised placebo-controlled trial. *Lancet* 2002;359:1877–1890.
53. Mittendorf R, Covert R, Boman J, et al. Is tocolytic magnesium sulphate associated with increased total paediatric mortality? *Lancet* 1997;350:1517–1518.
54. Nelson K, Grether JK. Can magnesium sulfate reduce the risk of cerebral palsy in very low birthweight infants? *Pediatrics* 1995;95:263–269.
55. Schendel DE, Berg CJ, Yeargin-Allsopp M, et al. Prenatal magnesium sulfate exposure and the risk of cerebral palsy or mental retardation among very low-birth-weight children aged 3 to 5 years. *JAMA* 1996;276:1805–1810.
56. Churchill D, Duley L. Interventionist versus expectant care for severe pre-eclampsia before term (Cochrane Review). In: The Cochrane Library, Issue 3, 2002. Oxford: Update Software. Search date 2002; primary sources Cochrane Pregnancy and Childbirth Group Trials Register, and Cochrane Controlled Trials Register.

57. Head BB, Owen J, Vincent Jr RD, et al. A randomized trial of intrapartum analgesia in women with severe preeclampsia. *Obstet Gynecol* 2002;99:452–457.
58. Duley L, Henderson-Smart D. Magnesium sulphate versus diazepam for eclampsia. In: The Cochrane Library, Issue 3, 2002. Oxford: Update Software. Search date 1999; primary source Cochrane Pregnancy and Childbirth Group Trials Register.
59. Duley L, Henderson-Smart D. Magnesium sulphate versus phenytoin for eclampsia. In: The Cochrane Library, Issue 3, 2002. Oxford: Update Software. Search date 1999; primary source Cochrane Pregnancy and Childbirth Group Trials Register.
60. Sawhney H, Sawhney IM, Mandal R, Subramanyam, Vasishta K. Efficacy of magnesium sulphate and phenytoin in the management of eclampsia. *J Obstet Gynaecol Res* 1999;25:333–338.
61. Duley L, Gulmezoglu AM. Magnesium sulphate versus lytic cocktail for eclampsia. In: The Cochrane Library, Issue 3, 2002. Oxford: Update Software. Search date 2000; primary sources Cochrane Pregnancy and Childbirth Group Trials Register and Cochrane Controlled Trials Register.

Lelia Duley
Obstetric Epidemiologist
Institute of Health Sciences
Oxford
UK

Competing interests: None declared.

Preterm birth

Search date January 2003

Bridgette Byrne and John J Morrison

QUESTIONS

INTERVENTIONS

To be covered in future updates

Effects of repeated doses of antenatal corticosteroid

Uterine activity monitoring for singleton and multiple pregnancies in prevention of preterm birth

Covered elsewhere in *Clinical Evidence*

Antibiotic treatment of bacterial vaginosis to prevent preterm birth: see bacterial vaginosis, p 1824.

See glossary, p 1713

Key Messages

- **Antenatal corticosteroids** One systematic review in women with anticipated preterm delivery has found that antenatal treatment with corticosteroids reduces the risk of respiratory distress syndrome, neonatal mortality, and intraventricular haemorrhage in preterm infants compared with placebo or no treatment.

Clin Evid 2003;10:1700–1715.

- **Antibiotic treatment for premature rupture of the membranes (prolongs gestation and may reduce infection, but unknown effect on perinatal mortality)** One systematic review in women with preterm premature rupture of membranes has found that antibiotics compared with placebo prolong pregnancy and reduce the risk of neonatal morbidity, such as neonatal infection, requirement for treatment with oxygen, and abnormal cerebral ultrasound. It found that co-amoxiclav (amoxicillin [amoxycillin] plus clavulanic acid) was associated with an increase in the incidence of neonatal necrotising enterocolitis.
- **Prophylactic cervical cerclage for women at risk of cervical incompetence** One large RCT has found that, in women presumed to have cervical incompetence, prophylactic cervical cerclage compared with no cerclage reduces preterm birth (< 33 weeks' gestation) but increases the risk of puerperal pyrexia. It found that 24 women would need to undergo cerclage to prevent one additional preterm delivery. A second RCT in women with cervix changes detected by ultrasound found that cerclage plus bed rest reduced deliveries before 34 weeks compared with bed rest alone. A third RCT found no significant difference in preterm birth between cerclage plus bed rest and bed rest alone when mid-trimester cervical change has been detected by transvaginal ultrasound.
- **Tocolytic treatment in threatened preterm labour** One systematic review and one subsequent RCT have found that atosiban, β_2 agonists, indometacin (indomethacin), and ethanol prolong pregnancy compared with placebo or no tocolytic, but they do not significantly reduce perinatal mortality or neonatal morbidity. Two systematic reviews found no significant difference in prolongation of pregnancy when comparing magnesium sulphate versus placebo or no tocolytics. Tocolytics increase maternal adverse effects, such as chest pain, nausea and vomiting, and dyspnoea. One systematic review has found that calcium channel blockers (mainly β_2 agonists) reduce deliveries within 48 hours, withdrawals caused by maternal adverse effects, and neonatal morbidity compared with other tocolytics.
- **Amnioinfusion for preterm rupture of the membranes** One systematic review found insufficient evidence about the effects of amnioinfusion.
- **Enhanced antenatal care programmes for socially deprived population groups/high risk groups** RCTs carried out in a range of countries found no significant difference between enhanced antenatal care and usual care in reducing the risk of preterm delivery.
- **Elective rather than selective caesarean delivery in preterm labour** One systematic review has found limited evidence that elective compared with selective caesarean delivery in women with preterm labour increases the risk of maternal morbidity, without clear evidence of benefit in neonatal morbidity or mortality.
- **Antibiotic treatment for preterm labour with intact membranes** One systematic review found that antibiotics do not prolong pregnancy and do not reduce perinatal mortality compared with placebo.
- **Thyrotropin releasing hormone before preterm delivery** One systematic review in women at risk of preterm birth has found no significant difference between thyrotropin releasing hormone plus corticosteroids and corticosteroids alone in improving neonatal outcomes. Thyrotropin releasing hormone plus corticosteroids increased maternal and fetal adverse events compared with corticosteroids alone.

Preterm birth

DEFINITION Preterm or premature birth is defined by the World Health Organization as delivery of an infant before 37 completed weeks of gestation.[1] There is no set lower limit to this definition, but 23–24 weeks' gestation is widely accepted,[1] which approximates to an average fetal weight of 500 g.

INCIDENCE/ PREVALENCE Preterm birth occurs in about 5–10% of all births in developed countries,[2–4] but in recent years the incidence seems to have increased in some countries, particularly the USA.[5] We found little reliable evidence for less developed countries that used the exact definition of premature birth. The rate in northwestern Ethiopia has been reported to vary between 11–22% depending on the age group studied, being highest in teenagers.[6]

AETIOLOGY/ RISK FACTORS About 30% of preterm births are unexplained and spontaneous.[4,7,8] The two strongest risk factors for idiopathic preterm labour (see glossary, p 1713) are low socioeconomic status and previous preterm delivery. Multiple pregnancy accounts for about another 30% of cases.[4,7] Other known risk factors include genital tract infection, preterm rupture of the membranes (see glossary, p 1713), antepartum haemorrhage, cervical incompetence, and congenital uterine abnormalities, which collectively account for about 20–25% of cases. The remaining cases (15–20%) are attributed to elective preterm delivery secondary to hypertensive disorders of pregnancy, intrauterine fetal growth restriction, congenital abnormalities, and medical disorders of pregnancy.[4,5,7,8]

PROGNOSIS Preterm labour usually results in preterm birth. One systematic review (search date not stated) of tocolysis compared with placebo found that about 27% of preterm labours spontaneously resolved and about 70% progressed to preterm delivery.[9] Observational studies have found that one preterm birth significantly raises the risk of another in a subsequent pregnancy.[10]

AIMS OF INTERVENTION To prevent preterm birth; to prolong the interval between threatened preterm labour and delivery; to optimise the condition of the fetus in preparation for delivery in order to improve neonatal outcome; to minimise maternal morbidity.

OUTCOMES The main clinical outcome is improved neonatal outcome, as indicated by perinatal (see glossary, p 1713) mortality, neonatal mortality, and morbidity (incidence of respiratory distress syndrome, intraventricular haemorrhage, necrotising enterocolitis, neonatal sepsis, and neonatal convulsions). An additional clinical outcome is incidence of maternal adverse effects. Proxy outcomes include duration of pregnancy, number of hours or days between onset of labour and delivery, and number of deliveries before 37 completed weeks of gestation.

METHODS *Clinical Evidence* search and appraisal January 2003.

QUESTION **What are the effects of preventive interventions in women at high risk of preterm delivery?**

OPTION **ENHANCED ANTENATAL CARE FOR SOCIALLY DEPRIVED WOMEN AND OTHER HIGH RISK GROUPS**

RCTs carried out in a range of countries found no significant difference between enhanced antenatal care and usual care in reducing the risk of preterm delivery.

Benefits: We found no systematic review. We found 11 RCTs.[11–21] All of the RCTs (carried out in Europe, USA, and Latin America; number of high risk women ranging from 150–2200) found no significant difference between enhanced antenatal care (see glossary, p 1713) and usual antenatal care in reducing preterm birth (see table 1, p 1715).

Harms: The RCTs gave no information on adverse effects.[11–21]

Comment: The definition of enhanced antenatal care varied.[11–21] Examples of enhanced antenatal care include increased number of antenatal visits, a bed rest programme including rest periods three times daily, home visits by midwives, fortnightly social worker counselling sessions, nutritional education, peer group education, and counselling by a psychologist.

OPTION **PROPHYLACTIC CERVICAL CERCLAGE IN WOMEN AT RISK OF CERVICAL INCOMPETENCE**

One large RCT has found that, in women presumed to have cervical incompetence, prophylactic cervical cerclage reduces preterm birth (< 33 weeks' gestation) compared with no cerclage, but significantly increases the risk of puerperal pyrexia. A second RCT in women with cervix changes detected by transvaginal ultrasound found that cerclage plus bed rest significantly reduced delivery before 34 weeks compared with bed rest alone. A third RCT found no significant difference in preterm birth between cerclage plus bed rest and bed rest alone when mid-trimester cervical change has been detected by transvaginal ultrasound.

Benefits: We found no systematic review. **When cervical changes have not been identified:** We found one multicentre RCT (1292 women with a history of early delivery or cervical surgery whose obstetricians were uncertain whether to advise cervical cerclage (see glossary, p 1713)) comparing cerclage versus no cerclage.[22] It found that cerclage significantly reduced the rate of delivery before 33 weeks' gestation (83/647 [13%] with cerclage *v* 110/645 [17%] with no cerclage; RR 0.75, 95% CI 0.57 to 0.98; NNT 24, 95% CI 14 to 275) but found no significant difference in the rate of deliveries occurring between weeks 33 and 36. **When cervical changes are present:** We found two RCTs of cervical cerclage when cervical change has been detected by transvaginal ultrasound.[23,24] The first RCT (35 women with cervical length < 25 mm and gestational age < 27 weeks) found that cerclage plus bed rest reduced delivery before 34 weeks compared with bed rest alone (0/19 [0%] with cerclage plus bed rest *v* 7/16 [44%] with bed rest alone; NNT 3, 95% CI 2 to 5; P = 0.002). It found no significant difference in neonatal survival between cerclage plus bed rest and bed rest alone (19/19 [100%] with cerclage plus bed rest v 13/16 [81%] with bed rest alone; ARR +0.19, 95% CI –0.02 to +0.43).[23] The second RCT (113 women between 16 and 24 weeks of gestation and distal cervix < 2.5 cm or membrane prolapse into endocervical canal at least 25% of cervical length) found that cerclage plus bed rest compared with bed rest alone did not significantly reduce delivery before 34 weeks (35% v 36%; P = 0.80), perinatal death (13% v 12%; P = 0.90), placental abruption (11% v 14%; P = 0.80), or chorioamnionitis (20% v 10%; P = 0.20).[24]

Harms: The RCT addressing prophylactic use of cerclage found that insertion of cervical sutures doubled the risk of puerperal pyrexia compared with no sutures (24/415 [6%] with cerclage v 11/405 [3%] with no cerclage; RR 2.13, 95% CI 1.06 to 4.15; NNH 33, 95% CI 12 to 607).[22] Information about puerperal pyrexia was collected only after 360 women had already been recruited to the trial. It was defined as a temperature of greater than 38 °C but uterine infection was mentioned as a possible cause of the pyrexia in only 13/24 (54%) in the cerclage group and 6/11 (55%) in the non-cerclage groups. The two RCTs looking at the use of cerclage when cervix changes have been detected by ultrasound gave no information on harms.[23,24]

Comment: The most common indication for entry to the RCT comparing cerclage versus no cerclage was a history of preterm delivery or second trimester miscarriage (74% of the cerclage group, 70% of the controls).[22] The two RCTs that examined cervical cerclage in the mid-trimester with documented cervical change differed in terms of patient selection and methodology.[23,24] Broad confidence intervals suggest that sample size may have been insufficient to rule out clinically important differences in neonatal mortality.

QUESTION What are the effects of interventions to improve outcome after preterm rupture of the membranes?

OPTION ANTIBIOTICS

One systematic review in women with preterm rupture of membranes has found that antibiotics prolong pregnancy and reduce the risk of neonatal morbidity, such as neonatal infection, requirement for treatment with oxygen, and abnormal cerebral ultrasound, compared with placebo. It found that co-amoxiclav (amoxicillin [amoxycillin] plus clavulanic acid) was associated with an increase in the incidence of neonatal necrotising enterocolitis.

Benefits: One systematic review (search date 2001, 13 RCTs, over 6000 women) found that antibiotics (including erythromycin, co-amoxiclav, benzylpenicillin, ampicillin, piperacillin, or clindamycin) compared with placebo significantly reduced the number of babies born within 48 hours (RR 0.7, 95% CI 0.72 to 0.83) and 7 days (RR 0.88, CI 0.84 to 0.92) following preterm premature rupture of the membranes (see glossary, p 1713).[25] It found that antibiotics compared with placebo significantly reduced the incidence of neonatal infection (RR 0.67, 95% CI 0.52 to 0.85), requirement for supplementary oxygen (RR 0.88, 95% CI 0.81 to 0.96), and abnormal cerebral ultrasound (RR 0.82, 95% CI 0.68 to 0.99), but found no significant difference in perinatal mortality with antibiotics compared with placebo (RR 0.92, 95% CI 0.75 to 1.12). Antibiotics significantly decreased maternal infection after delivery prior to discharge from hospital compared with placebo (RR 0.85, 95% CI 0.76 to 0.96).

Harms: The review found that co-amoxiclav was associated with a significantly increased risk of neonatal necrotising enterocolitis (2 RCTs: RR 4.6, 95% CI 1.98 to 10.72).[25]

Comment: Most of the RCTs in the review did not include antenatal administration of steroids but 77% of the women in one large RCT[26] received steroids. All but one of the RCTs in the review gave data on the percentage of withdrawals, which was always less than 20%.[25]

OPTION AMNIOINFUSION

One systematic review found insufficient evidence from one RCT about the effects of amnioinfusion compared with no amnioinfusion in improving neonatal outcomes after preterm rupture of the membranes.

Benefits: We found one systematic review (search date 2001, 1 RCT, 66 women) comparing amnioinfusion (see glossary, p 1713) versus no amnioinfusion.[27] It found no significant difference between amnioinfusion and no amnioinfusion in rates of caesarean section, low Apgar scores, p 1713, neonatal mortality, or endometritis.

Harms: No adverse effects were reported in the RCT identified by the review.[27]

Comment: The RCT was too small to detect clinically important changes in some of the outcomes (rates of caesarean section, neonatal mortality, and infectious morbidity) and had shortcomings in methods used (unspecified method of random assignment of women; blinding of treatment not possible).[27]

QUESTION What are the effects of treatments in threatened preterm labour?

OPTION TOCOLYTICS

One systematic review and one subsequent RCT have found that atosiban, β_2 agonists, indometacin, and ethanol prolong pregnancy compared with placebo or no tocolytic, but do not reduce perinatal mortality or neonatal morbidity. Two systematic reviews found no significant difference in prolongation of pregnancy when comparing magnesium sulphate with placebo or no tocolytics. Tocolytics increase maternal adverse effects, such as chest pain, nausea and vomiting, and dyspnoea. One systematic review has found that calcium channel blockers (mainly β_2 agonists) significantly reduce deliveries within 48 hours, withdrawals caused by maternal adverse effects, and neonatal morbidity compared with other tocolytics.

Benefits: We found a systematic review[28] and one subsequent RCT.[29] The systematic review (search date 1998, 18 RCTs, 2785 women in preterm labour [see glossary, p 1713]) compared different tocolytic drugs (β_2 agonists, magnesium sulphate, indometacin [indomethacin], atosiban, and ethanol) versus placebo or no tocolytic.[28] Three of the RCTs in the review included women with ruptured membranes. The most frequently evaluated tocolytic agent was the β agonist ritodrine (5 RCTs). The review found that β_2 agonists, indometacin, atosiban, and ethanol significantly delayed delivery following the onset of preterm labour for greater than 24 hours, 48 hours, and 7 days compared with placebo or no treatment. The subsequent RCT is described below.[29] **β_2 agonists versus placebo:** The systematic review (8 RCTs) found no significant difference between β_2 agonists and placebo or no treatment in perinatal (see glossary, p 1713) mortality (62/682 [9%] with β_2 agonists *v* 48/604 [8%] with placebo or no treatment; OR 1.08, 95% CI 0.72 to 1.62), incidence of respiratory distress syndrome (6 RCTs: 117/639 [18%] with β_2 agonists *v* 140/565 [25%] with placebo or no treatment; OR 0.76, 95% CI 0.57 to 1.01), birth weight less than 2500 g (5 RCTs: 332/601 [55%] with β_2 agonists *v* 332/525 [63%] with placebo or no treatment; OR 0.79, 95% CI 0.61 to 1.01), patent ductus arteriosus, necrotising enterocolitis, intraventricular haemorrhage, seizures, hypoglycaemia, or neonatal sepsis.[28] **Magnesium sulphate versus placebo:** The review (4 RCTs) found no significant difference between magnesium sulphate and placebo or no treatment in perinatal mortality (11/169 [6.5%] with magnesium sulphate *v* 7/182 [3.8%] with placebo or no treatment; OR 1.83, 95% CI 0.70 to 4.77) or in the incidence of respiratory distress syndrome (3 RCTs: 22/139 [16%] with magnesium sulphate *v* 22/153 [14%] with placebo or no treatment; OR 1.19, 95% CI 0.61 to 2.31).[28] It also found no significant difference between magnesium sulphate and placebo or no treatment in birth weight less than 2500 g, patent ductus arteriosus, necrotising enterocolitis, intraventricular haemorrhage, seizures, hypoglycaemia, or neonatal sepsis. The number of newborns assessed for these outcomes was small. A second systematic review (search date 2002) compared magnesium sulphate versus placebo, no treatment, and other tocolytics.[30] The studies included in the review comparing magnesium sulphate versus placebo, no treatment, or sedation are the same as those included in the initial review except for the addition of a study that compared magnesium sulphate versus barbiturate and bed rest.[31] The findings in the two reviews are comparable. **Indometacin versus placebo:** The first review (3 RCTs, 100 women) found no significant difference between indometacin and placebo or no treatment in perinatal mortality, respiratory distress syndrome, bronchopulmonary dysplasia, necrotising enterocolitis, neonatal sepsis, or low birth weight.[28] The number of newborns assessed for these outcomes may be too small to exclude a clinically important difference. **Atosiban:** The first systematic review (1 RCT, 114 newborns) found no significant difference between atosiban and placebo in the incidence of respiratory distress syndrome, patent ductus arteriosus, and hypoglycaemia.[28] The RCT may be too small to exclude a clinically important difference. One subsequent RCT (531 women) compared atosiban versus placebo.[29] In pregnancies of 28 weeks or over, it found that atosiban significantly prolonged pregnancy for up to 24 hours (150/203 [74%] with atosiban *v* 128/221 [58%] with placebo; RR 1.28, 95% CI 1.11 to 1.47; NNT 7, 95% CI 4 to 15), 48 hours (140/203 [69%] with atosiban *v* 122/221 [55%] with placebo; RR 1.25, 95% CI 1.08 to 1.45; NNT 8, 95% CI 5 to 23), and 7 days (131/203 [65%] with atosiban *v* 105/220 [48%] with placebo; RR 1.35, 95% CI 1.14 to 1.60; NNT 6, 95% CI 4 to 14) compared with placebo. **Calcium channel blockers versus other tocolytics:** We found no RCTs comparing calcium channel blockers versus placebo. We found one systematic review (search date 2002, 12 RCTs, 1029 women) comparing calcium channel blockers versus other tocolytics (mainly β agonists) for preterm labour.[32] The review found that calcium channel blockers significantly delayed delivery by 48 hours (9 RCTs, 761 women: 14/45 [31%] with calcium channel blocker *v* 10/44 [23%] with other tocolytics; RR 0.8, 95% CI 0.61 to 1.05) and by 7 days (4 RCTs, 453 women: 71/229 [31%] *v* 86/224 [38%]; RR 0.76, 95% CI 0.6 to 0.97), and reduced the incidence of delivery at less than 34 weeks' gestation (6 RCTs, 619 women: 107/311 [34%] *v* 122/308 [40%]; RR 0.83, 95% CI 0.69 to 0.99) compared with other tocolytics. Calcium channel blockers significantly reduced neonatal morbidity. Significant reductions were found for neonatal respiratory distress syndrome (9 RCTs, 763 newborns: 48/386 [12%] with calcium channel blocker *v* 72/377 [19%] with other tocolytics; RR 0.63, 0.46 to 0.88), necrotising enterocolitis (3 RCTs, 323 newborns: 1/166 [1%] *v* 8/157 [5%]; RR 0.21, 95% CI 0.05 to 0.96), and intraventricular haemorrhage (3 RCTs, 340 newborns: 19/173 [11%] *v* 31/167 [19%]; RR 0.59, 95% CI 0.36 to 0.98). No significant differences were found in perinatal mortality (10 RCTs, 810 newborns: 13/400 [3%] with calcium channel blocker *v* 7/410 [2%] with other tocolytics; RR 1.65, 95% CI 0.74 to 3.64).

Harms: **β_2 agonists:** The first systematic review compared β_2 agonists versus placebo or no treatment.[28] It found that β_2 agonists significantly increased maternal adverse effects, such as chest pain (2 RCTs: 39/406 [10%] with β_2 agonists *v* 3/408 [1%] with placebo or no treatment; OR 6.2, 95% CI 3.3 to 11.5), palpitations (3 RCTs: 200/420 [48%] with β_2 agonists *v* 19/423 [4%] with placebo or no treatment; OR 10.2, 95% CI 7.4 to 13.9), dyspnoea (2 RCTs: 55/406 [14%] with β_2 agonists *v* 4/408 [1%] with placebo or no treatment; OR 6.6, 95% CI 3.9 to 11.2), tremor (1 RCT: 138/352 [39%] with β_2 agonists *v* 13/356 [4%] with placebo or no treatment; OR 8.3, 95% CI 5.8 to 11.9), nausea (1 RCT: 72/352 [20%] with β_2 agonists *v* 42/356 [12%] with placebo or no treatment; OR 1.9, 95% CI 1.3 to 2.8), vomiting (2 RCTs: 48/366 [13%] with β_2 agonists *v* 29/371 [8%] with placebo or no treatment; OR 1.8, 95% CI 1.1 to 2.9), headache (2 RCTs: 84/366 [23%] with β_2 agonists *v* 22/371 [6%] with placebo or no treatment; OR 4.0, 95% CI 2.6 to 6.0), hyperglycaemia (1 RCT: 106/352 [30%] with β_2 agonists *v* 37/356 [10%] with placebo or no treatment; OR 3.4, 95% CI 2.4 to 4.9), and hypokalaemia (1 RCT: 138/352 [39%] with β_2 agonists *v* 23/356 [6%] with placebo or no treatment; OR 6.4, 95% CI 4.5 to 9.1), Frequently, these adverse effects necessitated discontinuation of treatment (3 RCTs: 25/88 [28%] with β_2 agonists *v* 0/86 with placebo or no treatment; OR 11.5, 95% CI 4.8 to 27.5). **Magnesium sulphate:** The first systematic review found that magnesium sulphate significantly increased the need to discontinue treatment compared with placebo or no treatment (3 RCTs: 10/137 [7%] with magnesium sulphate *v* 0/144 with placebo or no treatment; OR 8.36, 95% CI 2.36 to 29.61).[28] The second systematic review found that the grouped fetal, neonatal, and infant mortality was higher in the group of women allocated to magnesium sulphate (7 RCTs, 727 babies: 18/340 [5%] with magnesium sulphate *v* 6/387 [2%] with other tocolytics; RR 2.82, 95% CI 1.2 to 6.62).[30] **Indometacin:** The first systematic review found that indometacin significantly increased the incidence of postpartum haemorrhage compared with placebo or no treatment (1 RCT: 7/16 [44%] with indometacin *v* 2/18 [11%] with placebo or no treatment; OR 5.1, 95% CI 1.1 to 22.9), but there was no significant difference in nausea (1 RCT: 2/18 [11%] with indometacin *v* 0/18 with placebo or no treatment; OR 7.8, 95% CI 0.5 to 130.5) and chorioamnionitis (1 RCT: 2/15 [13%] with indometacin *v* 0/15 with placebo or no treatment; OR 7.9, 95% CI 0.5 to 133.3).[28] **Atosiban:** The first systematic review found increased nausea with atosiban compared with placebo or no treatment (2 RCTs: 33/306 [11%] with atosiban *v* 15/307 [5%] with placebo or no treatment; OR 2.3, 95% CI 1.3 to 4.1) but found no significant difference in vomiting (2 RCTs: 10/306 [3%] with atosiban *v* 13/307 [4%] with placebo or no treatment; OR 0.8, 95% CI 0.3 to 1.8).[28] Atosiban significantly reduced chest pain (2 RCTs: 3/306 [1%] with atosiban *v* 13/307 [4%] with placebo or no treatment; OR 0.3, 95% CI 0.1 to 0.8) and dyspnoea (1 RCT: 1/250 [0.4%] with atosiban *v* 7/251 [3%] with placebo or no treatment; OR 0.22, 95% CI 0.05 to 0.89) compared with placebo or no treatment. One subsequent RCT found that atosiban significantly increased injection site reactions after prolonged use (110/250 [44%] with atosiban *v* 58/251 [23%] with placebo; RR 1.90, 95% CI 1.46 to 2.48; NNH 4, 95% CI 3 to 7) and significantly increased withdrawal owing to adverse effects (16% with atosiban *v* 4% with placebo) compared with placebo.[29] There was a higher incidence of fetal mortality at less than 26 weeks' gestation with atosiban compared with placebo (10/27 [37%] with atosiban *v* 0/16 [0%] with placebo).[29] **Calcium channel blockers:** The systematic review on calcium channel blockers found that these are less likely to require discontinuation because of adverse effects compared with other tocolytics (10 RCTs, 833 women: 1/419 [0.2%] with calcium channel blocker *v* 29/414 [7.0%] with other tocolytics; RR 0.14, 95% CI 0.05 to 0.36).[32] The systematic review did not report specific adverse effects on calcium channel blockers.

Comment: False preterm labour presents a problem in analysis of the effects of tocolytic agents, but in 15/17 RCTs included in the first systematic review[28] the definition of preterm labour used for entry into the study included cervical dilatation, effacement, or change in the cervical condition in addition to uterine contractions.[33] This would minimise the potential confounding effect of spurious preterm labour. Combining results for all tocolytics was reasonable, based on the lack of evidence of the merits of one tocolytic over another.[28] Tocolytic rescue with ritodrine was used in the RCT comparing atosiban with placebo.[29] In this RCT, 24/246 (10%) women randomised to receive atosiban and 13/255 (5%) women randomised to receive placebo were recruited at less than 26 weeks' gestation. This may have contributed to a higher incidence of fetal mortality at less than 26 weeks' gestation in the atosiban group. Only 4/10 RCTs assessing perinatal mortality in the systematic review found any outcomes.[32] Broad confidence intervals in both the systematic review and the individual RCTs, suggest that these may have had insufficient power to detect important differences in mortality.

QUESTION What are the effects of elective compared with selective caesarean delivery for women in preterm labour?

One systematic review has found that elective compared with selective caesarean delivery increases the risk of maternal morbidity, and does not reduce neonatal morbidity or mortality. The RCTs may have been underpowered to detect a clinically important neonatal benefit.

Benefits: We found one systematic review (search date not stated, 6 RCTs, 122 women).[34] It found no significant difference in neonatal morbidity and mortality between elective caesarean delivery and selective caesarean (see glossary, p 1713) delivery (low Apgar score [see glossary, p 1713] at 5 minutes: OR 0.68, 95% CI 0.29 to 1.60; need for neonatal intubation: OR 0.58, 95% CI 0.26 to 1.31; intracranial haemorrhage: OR 0.86, 95% CI 0.2 to 3.67; perinatal death: OR 0.32, 95% CI 0.07 to 1.36).

Harms: The review found that major maternal complications were reported in 7/84 (8%) women, all after caesarean delivery, although one of these women was allocated to expectant management.[34] Maternal complications were therefore significantly higher in women allocated to elective caesarean compared with selective caesarean delivery (4 RCTs, 84 women: AR 6/44 [14%] with elective caesarean delivery *v* 1/40 [3%] with selective caesarean delivery; OR 6.18, 95% CI 1.27 to 30.1). Elective caesarean delivery may occasionally result in unnecessary preterm delivery; two women allocated to the selective delivery group did not deliver until some weeks after entry to one trial.

Comment: The neonatal confidence intervals in the systematic review suggest that RCTs were underpowered and no meaningful conclusions can be drawn on the neonatal effects of elective caesarean section.[34] The fetus presented by the breech in three of the studies. About a sixth of each group delivered by an alternative route, but the analysis was by intention to treat. Sample size of trials was small and most of the trials were terminated because of recruitment difficulties.

QUESTION What are the effects of interventions to improve outcome in preterm delivery?

OPTION CORTICOSTEROIDS BEFORE PRETERM DELIVERY

One systematic review in women with anticipated preterm delivery has found that antenatal treatment with corticosteroids reduces the risk of respiratory distress syndrome, neonatal mortality, and intraventricular haemorrhage in preterm infants compared with placebo or no treatment.

Benefits: We found one systematic review (search date 1996, 18 RCTs, > 3700 babies) in women experiencing anticipated preterm delivery (elective or after spontaneous onset of preterm labour [see glossary, p 1713]) comparing corticosteroids (β methasone, dexamethasone, or hydrocortisone) versus placebo or no treatment.[35] The review found that antenatal corticosteroids significantly reduced respiratory distress syndrome (18 RCTs, 3735 neonates: 292/1885 [15%] with corticosteroids *v* 439/1850 [24%] with placebo or no treatment; OR 0.52, 95% CI 0.44 to 0.62) compared with placebo or no treatment. Three RCTs (48 neonates) identified by the review found no significant difference between antenatal corticosteroids and placebo or no treatment in respiratory distress syndrome in neonates delivered before 28 weeks' gestation (7/17 [41%] with corticosteroids *v* 18/31 [58%] with placebo or no treatment; OR 0.64, 95% CI 0.16 to 2.50). Six RCTs identified by the review (349 neonates) found no significant difference between antenatal corticosteroids and placebo or no treatment in respiratory distress syndrome in babies delivered within less than 24 hours of initial treatment (45/176 [26%] with corticosteroids *v* 57/173 [33%] with placebo or no treatment; OR 0.70, 95% CI 0.43 to 1.16), and one RCT (42 neonates) identified by the review found no significant difference between antenatal corticosteroids and placebo or no treatment in respiratory distress syndrome in babies delivered within less than 48 hours of initial treatment (3/23 [13%] with corticosteroids *v* 6/19 [32%] with placebo or no treatment; OR 0.34, 95% CI 0.08 to 1.47). The review found that both β methasone and dexamethasone significantly reduced respiratory distress, but hydrocortisone did not. The small numbers of evaluable neonates from twin pregnancies did not allow a confident statement about the effects in multiple pregnancy. Antenatal corticosteroids significantly reduced neonatal mortality (14 RCTs: 129/1770 [7%] with corticosteroids *v* 204/1747 [12%] with placebo or no treatment; OR 0.60, 95% CI 0.48 to 0.75) and risk of intraventricular haemorrhage (diagnosed at autopsy: 7/446 [1.6%] with corticosteroids *v* 23/417 [5.5%] with placebo or no treatment; OR 0.29, 95% CI 0.14 to 0.61; diagnosed by ultrasound: 47/300 [16%] with corticosteroids *v* 77/296 [26%] with placebo or no treatment; OR 0.48, 95% CI 0.32 to 0.72) compared with placebo or no treatment. Antenatal corticosteroids did not significantly reduce the rates of necrotising enterocolitis (17/587 [3%] with corticosteroids *v* 27/567 [5%] with placebo or no treatment; OR 0.59, 95% CI 0.32 to 1.09) or chronic lung disease (38/204 [19%] with corticosteroids *v* 25/207 [12%] with placebo or no treatment; OR 1.57, 95% CI 0.87 to 2.84).[35]

Harms: The RCTs in the review found no strong evidence of any adverse effects of corticosteroids.[35] Subgroup analysis in one RCT in the review suggested that corticosteroids may be associated with death in hypertensive women, but no deaths in hypertensive women were observed in the other three RCTs in the review for which data were available.

Comment: The absence of a significant beneficial effect of corticosteroids on respiratory distress syndrome at less than 28 weeks' gestation may be because of the small numbers available for analysis at this gestation.[35] No RCTs in the review addressed the potentially harmful effects of repeated doses of antenatal corticosteroids, or whether one form of corticosteroid was more harmful than another, as a retrospective cohort study (883 babies delivered between 24 and 31 weeks' gestation) suggests.[36]

OPTION THYROTROPIN RELEASING HORMONE BEFORE PRETERM DELIVERY

One systematic review in women at risk of preterm birth found no difference in neonatal outcomes between thyrotropin releasing hormone plus corticosteroids and corticosteroids alone, and has found that thyrotropin releasing hormone plus corticosteroids increase maternal and fetal adverse events compared with corticosteroids alone.

Benefits: We found one systematic review (search date 1999, 11 RCTs, > 4500 women at risk of preterm birth taking antenatal corticosteroids) comparing thyrotropin releasing hormone (TRH) plus steroids versus steroids alone.[37] It found no significant difference between TRH plus steroids and steroids alone in gestational age at delivery (mean gestational age of 32 weeks in both groups), respiratory distress syndrome (676/1832 [37%] with TRH plus steroids *v* 640/1837 [35%] with steroids alone; RR 1.06, 95% CI 0.97 to 1.16), periventricular or intraventricular haemorrhage (282/1819 [16%] with TRH plus steroids *v* 262/1826 [14%] with steroids alone; RR 1.08, 95% CI 0.93 to 1.26), necrotising enterocolitis (56/1555 [4%] with TRH plus steroids *v* 61/1548 [4%] with steroids alone; RR 0.91, 95% CI 0.64 to 1.30), and death prior to hospital discharge (185/1842 [10%] with TRH plus steroids *v* 177/1852 [9%] with steroids alone; RR 1.05, 95% CI 0.86 to 1.27).

Harms: The review found that, in babies who received TRH plus steroids compared with steroids alone, TRH significantly increased the risk of low Apgar score (see glossary, p 1713) at 5 minutes (OR 1.8, 95% CI 1.14 to 1.92) and increased the requirement for assisted ventilation (OR 1.16, CI 1.02 to 1.29).[37] One RCT included in the review found a significant increase in motor delay (RR 1.31, 95% CI 1.09 to 1.56), motor impairment (RR 1.51, 95% CI 1.02 to 2.24), sensory impairment (RR 1.97, 95% CI 1.10 to 3.53), and social delay after 12 months (RR 1.25, 95% CI 1.03 to 1.51).[37] TRH plus steroids compared with steroids alone significantly increased maternal blood pressure (1 RCT: risk of an increase of 25 mm Hg in systolic blood pressure; 36/506 [7%] with TRH plus steroids *v* 20/505 [4%] with steroids alone; RR 1.80, 95% CI 1.05 to 3.06; risk of an increase of 15 mm Hg in diastolic blood pressure; 115/506 [23%] with TRH plus steroids *v* 71/505 [14%] with steroids alone; RR 1.62, 95% CI 1.24 to 2.12). Other maternal adverse effects included nausea (3 RCTs: 303/1175 [26%] with TRH plus steroids *v* 77/1195 [6%] with steroids alone; RR 3.92, 95% CI 3.13 to 4.92), vomiting (1 RCT: 40/506 [8%] with TRH plus steroids *v* 17/505 [3%] with steroids alone; RR 2.35, 95% CI 1.35 to 4.09), light-headedness (1 RCT: 139/506 [27%] with TRH plus steroids *v* 80/505 [16%] with steroids alone; RR 1.73, 95% CI 1.36 to 2.22), urgency of micturition (1 RCT: 115/506 [23%] with TRH plus steroids *v* 48/505 [10%] with steroids alone; RR 2.39, 95% CI 1.75 to 3.27), and facial flushing (3 RCTs: 397/1252 [32%] with TRH plus steroids *v* 149/1271 [12%] with steroids alone; RR 2.67, 95% CI 2.26 to 3.16).[37]

Comment: TRH regimens varied in the RCTs identified by the review.[37] Seven of the RCTs analysed by intention to treat.

OPTION ANTIBIOTICS IN PRETERM LABOUR WITH INTACT MEMBRANES

One systematic review found that antibiotics do not prolong pregnancy and do not reduce perinatal mortality compared with placebo, but they do reduce the incidence of maternal infection.

Benefits: We found one systematic review (search date 2002, 11 RCTs) comparing single or combined antibiotics versus placebo or no antibiotic in women in preterm labour (see glossary, p 1713) and with intact membranes.[38] Antibiotics did not delay delivery at 48 hours (4 RCTs, 6800 women: 509/4959 [10%] with antibiotics *v* 183/1841 [10%] without antibiotics; OR 1.04, 95% CI 0.89 to 1.23) or by 7 days (7 RCTs, 6957 women: 813/5044 [16%] *v* 337/1913 [18%]; OR 0.98, 95% CI 0.87 to 1.10). No significant differences were found in neonatal morbidity, respiratory distress syndrome (8 RCTs, 7104 newborns: 460/5112 [9%] with antibiotics *v* 194/1992 [10%] without antibiotics; RR 0.99, 95% CI 0.84 to 1.16), necrotising enterocolitis (6 RCTs, 6880 newborns: 62/5004 [1.2%] *v* 25/1876 [1.3%]; RR 1.06, 95% CI 0.64 to 1.73), and intraventricular haemorrhage (4 RCTs, 6717 newborns: 59/4921 [1.2%] *v* 30/1796 [1.7%]; RR 0.76, 95% CI 0.48 to 1.19), and there was no significant difference in perinatal mortality (9 RCTs, 7208 newborns: 140/5166 [2.7%] *v* 42/2042 [2.1%]; RR 1.22, 95% CI 0.88 to 1.70). A significant reduction was found in the incidence of maternal infection, namely chorioamnionitis and endometritis, with antibiotics compared with no antibiotics (9 RCTs, 7242 women: 456/5185 [9%] *v* 230/2057 [11%]; RR 0.74, 95% CI 0.64 to 0.87). Chorioamnionitis and endometritis were reduced with the use of β lactams alone (3 RCTs: 144/1635 [9%] with β lactams *v* 70/621 [11.3%] no antibiotics; RR 0.75, 95% CI 0.56 to 0.98) or in combination with a macrolide (4 RCTs: 165/1790 [9%] with β lactam plus macrolide *v* 97/773 [13%] with no antibiotics; RR 0.75, 95% CI 0.59 to 0.95), but they were not significantly reduced in women who received a macrolide alone (2 RCTs: 157/1653 [9%] with macrolide *v* 64/569 [11%] with no antibiotics; RR 0.81, 95% CI 0.62 to 1.07) or antibiotics used to treat anaerobic bacteria (3 RCTs: 5/155 [3%] with antianaerobic antibiotic *v* 6/139 [4%] with no antibiotic; RR 0.76, 95% CI 0.25 to 2.34).

Harms: There was a trend but not a statistically significant increase in neonatal deaths in the group receiving antibiotics (7 RCTs, 6877 newborns: 99/5005 [2.0%] with antibiotics *v* 24/1872 [1.3%]; RR 1.52, 95% CI 0.99 to 2.34).[38]

Comment: The ORACLE trial[39] dominated the review[38] because it was six times larger than all of the previous RCTs. It differed from the other RCTs because the diagnosis of preterm labour was made by each clinician (as distinct from the other studies, which used similar definitions of preterm labour including uterine contractions and cervical dilatation) and it was one of only two trials in the review in which antibiotics were administered orally and some women were recruited after 34 weeks. Tocolysis was used in 9/11 RCTs (56% in the ORACLE RCT) and 30–90% of women received corticosteroids.[38,39] Maternal choriomnionitis and endometritis is reduced by the prescription of prophylactic β lactam antibiotics but approximately 88% of women with threatened preterm birth and intact membranes would receive antibiotics unnecessarily for an infection that is easily diagnosed and treated.

GLOSSARY

Apgar score Clinical scoring method that assesses neonatal heart rate, respirations, tone, colour, and reflexes immediately after delivery.
Amnioinfusion Infusion of physiological saline or Ringer's lactate through a catheter transabdominally or transcervically into the amniotic cavity.
Cervical cerclage Insertion of a cervical suture, using non-absorbable suture material, circumferentially around the cervix. May be done transvaginally or transabdominally.
Elective caesarean section When the operation is done at a pre-selected time before the onset of labour, usually after 38 weeks' gestation.
Enhanced antenatal care Includes various programmes of increased medical, midwifery, psychological, social, and nutritional support during pregnancy.
Perinatal Refers to the period after 24 weeks' gestation and includes the first 7 days of postnatal life for the neonate.
Preterm labour Onset of labour (regular uterine contractions with cervical effacement and dilatation) in the preterm period.
Preterm rupture of membranes Leakage of amniotic fluid from the amniotic cavity during the preterm period owing to rupture of the fetal membranes.
Selective caesarean section When the operation is done after the onset of labour.

REFERENCES

1. Morrison JJ, Rennie JM. Clinical, scientific and ethical aspects of fetal and neonatal care at extremely preterm periods of gestation. *Br J Obstet Gynaecol* 1997;104:1341–1350.
2. Rush RW, Keirse MJNC, Howat P, et al. Contribution of preterm delivery to perinatal mortality. *BMJ* 1976;2:965–968.
3. Creasy RK. Preterm birth prevention: Where are we? *Am J Obstet Gynecol* 1993;168:1223–1230.
4. Burke C, Morrison JJ. Perinatal factors and preterm delivery in an Irish obstetric population. *J Perinat Med* 2000;28:49–53.
5. Goldenberg RL, Rouse DJ. Prevention of premature birth. *N Engl J Med* 1998;339:313–320.
6. Kumbi S, Isehak A. Obstetric outcome of teenage pregnancy in northwestern Ethiopia. *East Afr Med J* 1999;76:138–140.
7. Iannucci TA, Tomich PG, Gianopoulos JG. Etiology and outcome of extremely low-birth-weight infants. *Am J Obstet Gynecol* 1996;174:1896–1902.
8. Main DM, Gabbe SG, Richardson D, et al. Can preterm deliveries be prevented? *Am J Obstet Gynecol* 1985;151:892–898.
9. King JF, Grant A, Keisre MJNC, et al. β-mimetics in preterm labour: an overview of the randomised controlled trials. *Br J Obstet Gynaecol* 1988;95:211–222. Search date not stated; primary sources Oxford Database of Perinatal Trials, hand searched reference lists, and personal contacts.
10. Keirse MJNC, Rush RW, Anderson AB, et al. Risk of preterm delivery and/or abortion. *Br J Obstet Gynaecol* 1978;85:81–85.
11. Spencer B, Thomas H, Morris J. A randomized controlled trial of the provision of a social support service during pregnancy; the South Manchester Family Worker project. *Br J Obstet Gynaecol* 1989;96:281–288.

12. Mueller-Heubach E, Reddick D, Barrett B, et al. Preterm birth prevention: evaluation of a prospective controlled randomized trial. *Am J Obstet Gynecol* 1989;160:1172–1178.
13. Goldenberg R, Davis R, Copper R, et al. The Alabama birth prevention project. *Obstet Gynecol* 1990;75:933–939.
14. Blondel B, Breart G, Glado J, et al. Evaluation of the home-visiting system for women with threatened preterm labour. Results of a randomized controlled trial. *Eur J Obstet Gynaecol Reprod Biol* 1990;34:47–58.
15. Villar J, Farnot U, Barros F, et al. A randomized trial of psychosocial support during high-risk pregnancies. *N Engl J Med* 1992;327:1266–1271.
16. Collaborative Group on Preterm Birth Prevention. Multicenter randomized controlled trial of a preterm birth prevention program. *Am J Obstet Gynecol* 1993;169:352–366.
17. Moore ML, Meis PJ, Ernest JM, et al. A randomized trial of nurse intervention to reduce preterm and low birth weight births. *Obstet Gynecol* 1998;91:656–661.
18. Olds DL, Henderson CR Jr, Tatelbaum R, et al. Improving the delivery of prenatal care and outcomes of pregnancy: a randomized trial of nurse home visitation. *Pediatrics* 1986;77:16–28.
19. Koniak-Griffin D, Anderson NL, Verzemnieks I, et al. A public health nursing early intervention program for adolescent mothers: outcomes from pregnancy through 6 weeks postpartum. *Nursing Res* 2000;49:130–138.
20. Heins HC, Nance NW, McCarthy BJ, et al. A randomised trial of nurse–midwifery prenatal care to reduce low birth weight. *Obstet Gynecol* 1990;75:341–345.
21. Klerman LV, Ramey SL, Goldenberg RL, et al. A randomised controlled trial of augmented prenatal care for multiple-risk Medicaid eligible African American women. *Am J Public Health* 2001:91:105–111.
22. MRC/RCOG Working party on cervical cerclage. Final report of the Medical Research Council/Royal College of Obstetricians and Gynaecologists multicentre randomised trial of cervical cerclage. *Br J Obstet Gynaecol* 1993;100:516–523.
23. Althuisius SM, Dekker GA, Hummel P, et al. Final results of the Cervical Incompetence Prevention Randomised Cerclage Trial (CIPRACT): therapeutic cerclage with bed rest versus bed rest alone. *Am J Obstet Gynecol* 2001;185:1106 –1112.
24. Rust OA, Atlas RO, Reed J, et al. Revisiting the short cervix detected by transvaginal ultrasound in the second trimester: Why cerclage therapy may not help. *Am J Obstet Gynecol* 2001;185:1098–1105.
25. Kenyon S, Boulvain M. Antibiotics for preterm premature rupture of membranes. In: The Cochrane Library, Issue 2, 2002. Oxford: Update Software. Search date 2001; primary source Cochrane Pregnancy Childbirth Group Trials Register.
26. Kenyon SL, Taylor DJ, Tarnow-Mordi W. Broad-spectrum antibiotics for preterm, prelabour rupture of fetal membranes: the ORACLE I randomised trial. *Lancet* 2001;357:979–988.
27. Hofmeyr GJ. Amnioinfusion for preterm rupture of membranes. In: The Cochrane Library, Issue 1, 2003. Oxford: Update Software. Search date 2001; primary sources Cochrane Pregnancy and Childbirth Group Trials Register and Cochrane Register of Controlled Trials.
28. Gyetvai K, Hannah ME, Hodnett ED, et al. Tocolytics for preterm labor: A systematic review. *Obstet Gynecol* 1999;94:869–877. Search date 1998; primary sources Medline and Cochrane Register of Controlled Trials.
29. Romero R, Sibai BM, Sanchez-Ramos L, et al. An oxytocin receptor antagonist (atosiban) in the treatment of preterm labor: a randomized, double-blind, placebo-controlled trial with tocolytic rescue. *Am J Obstet Gynecol* 2000;182;1173–1183.
30. Crowther CA, Hiller JE, Doyle LW. Magnesium sulphate for preventing preterm birth in threatened preterm labour. In: The Cochrane Library, Issue 4, 2002. Oxford: Update Software. Search date 2002.
31. Ma L. Magnesium sulfate in prevention of preterm labour (translation). *Chung Hua I Hsueh Tsa Chih Taipei* 1992;72:158–161.
32. King JF, Flenady VJ, Papatsonis DNM, et al. Calcium channel blockers for inhibiting preterm labour. In: The Cochrane Library, Issue 1, 2003. Search date 2002; primary sources Cochrane Controlled Trials Register, Medline, Embase, Current Contents, hand searched relevant references, and contact with experts.
33. Hannah M, Amankwah K, Barret J, et al. The Canadian consensus on the use of tocolytics for preterm labour. J SOGC 1995;17:1089–1115.
34. Grant A, Penn ZJ, Steer PJ. Elective or selective caesarean delivery of the small baby? A systematic review of the controlled trials. *Br J Obstet Gynaecol* 1996;103:1197–1200. Search date not stated; primary sources not stated.
35. Crowley P. Prophylactic corticosteroids for preterm birth. In: The Cochrane Library, Issue 1, 2003. Oxford: Update Software. Search date 1996; primary sources Cochrane Pregnancy and Childbirth Group Trials Register.
36. Baud O, Foix-L'Helias L, Kaminski M, et al. Antenatal glucocorticoid treatment and cystic periventricular leukomalacia in very premature infants. *N Engl J Med* 1999;341:1190–1196.
37. Crowther CA, Alfirevic Z, Haslam RR. Prenatal thyrotropin-releasing hormone (TRH) for preterm birth. In: The Cochrane Library, Issue 1, 2003. Oxford: Update Software. Search date 1999; primary sources Cochrane Pregnancy and Childbirth Group Trials Register.
38. King J, Flenady V. Prophylactic antibiotic for inhibiting preterm labour with intact membranes. In: The Cochrane Library, Issue 1, 2003. Oxford: Update Software. Search date 2002; primary sources Cochrane Pregnancy and Childbirth Group Trials Register, personal contacts, and hand searched reference lists.
39. Kenyon SL, Taylor DJ, Tarnow-Mordi W. Broad-spectrum antibiotics for spontaneous preterm labour: the ORACLE II randomised trial. *Lancet* 2001;357:989–994.

Bridgette Byrne
Senior Lecturer in Obstetrics and Gynaecology
Royal College of Surgeons of Ireland
Coombe Women's Hospital
Dublin
Ireland

John J Morrison
Professor of Obstetrics and Gynaecology
Clinical Science Institute
University College Hospital
Galway
Ireland

Competing interests: None declared.

TABLE 1 **Summary of RCTs addressing enhanced care on preterm birth rates compared with usual care (see text, p 1703).**

Outcome	Absolute risks: Antibiotic	Absolute risks: Control	ARR (95% CI)	OR (95% CI)	NNT (95% CI)
Born within 48 hours of rupture	140/513 (27%)	207/545 (38%)	11% (6% to 16%)	0.6 (0.46 to 0.77)	9 (6 to 17)
Born within 7 days of rupture	283/483 (59%)	364/508 (72%)	14% (8% to 21%)	0.54 (0.41 to 0.70)	7 (5 to 13)
Chorio–amnionitis	122/736 (17%)	188/763 (25%)	8% (4% to 11%)	0.61 (0.47 to 0.79)	12 (9 to 24)
Neonatal infection	86/775 (11%)	127/799 (16%)	5% (2% to 8%)	0.62 (0.45 to 0.86)	18 (12 to 52)
Perinatal death	50/700 (7%)	53/732 (7%)	0.1% (–3% to +2%)	0.98 (0.66 to 1.47)	ND
Necrotising enterocolitis	43/611 (7%)	48/644 (7.5%)	0.4% (–2.9% to +2.7%)	0.93 (0.61 to 1.44)	ND

ND, no data.

Acute bronchitis

Search date February 2003

Peter Wark

QUESTIONS

INTERVENTIONS

Key Messages

- **Antibiotics versus placebo** One systematic review and one subsequent RCT have found that antibiotics modestly reduce cough at 1–2 weeks but found no significant difference in quality of life or impairment in normal activity compared with placebo. Antibiotics increased risk of adverse events such as nausea, vomiting, rash, headache, and vaginitis compared with placebo. Widespread antibiotic use may lead to bacterial resistance to antibiotics.
- **Antibiotics versus each other** RCTs found no significant difference in clinical improvement or cure between cefuroxime and amoxicillin (amoxycillin) or amoxicillin/clavulanic acid; among different cefalosporins; between azithromycin and clarithromycin; or between roxithromycin and amoxicillin. Two RCTs found that adverse effects were less common with cefuroxime than with amoxicillin/clavulanic acid.
- **Antihistamines** We found insufficient evidence about the effects of antihistamines compared with placebo in people with acute bronchitis.
- **β Agonists** One systematic review found no significant difference in cough or ability to return to work between β agonists and placebo in people with acute bronchitis. It found limited evidence from one small RCT that β agonists reduce cough compared with erythromycin. The review found that β agonists increase shaking and tremor compared with placebo or erythromycin.
- **Over the counter antitussives** RCTs found no significant difference in cough severity between codeine or dextromethorphan and placebo in children or adults with acute bronchitis. We found limited evidence from one RCT that moguisteine modestly reduced cough severity compared with placebo in adults, but was associated with more adverse gastrointestinal effects.
- **Over the counter expectorants** We found insufficient evidence about the effects of over the counter expectorants in people with acute bronchitis.

DEFINITION Acute bronchitis is transient inflammation of the trachea and major bronchi. Clinically, it is diagnosed on the basis of cough and occasionally sputum, dyspnoea, and wheeze. This review is limited to episodes of acute bronchitis in people with no pre-existing respiratory disease and excluding those with clinical or radiographic evidence of pneumonia.

INCIDENCE/ PREVALENCE Acute bronchitis affects 44/1000 adults (> 16 years old) per year, with 82% of episodes occurring in autumn or winter.[1] Acute bronchitis was the fifth most common reason to present to a general practitioner in Australia.[2]

AETIOLOGY/ RISK FACTORS Infection is believed to be the trigger for acute bronchitis. However, pathogens have been identified in fewer than 55% of people.[1] Community studies that attempted to isolate pathogens from the sputum of people with acute bronchitis found viruses in 8–23%, typical bacteria (*Streptococcus pneumoniae*, *Haemophilus influenzae*, *Moraxella catarrhalis*) in 45%, and atypical bacteria (*Mycobacterium pneumoniae*, *Chlamydia pneumoniae*, *Bordetella pertussis*) in 0–25%.[1,3,4]

PROGNOSIS Acute bronchitis is regarded as a mild self limiting illness but there are limited data on prognosis and complications such as chronic cough or progression to chronic bronchitis or pneumonia. One prospective longitudinal study reviewed 653 previously well adults who presented to suburban general practices over a 12 month period with symptoms of acute lower respiratory tract infection.[1] It found that within the first month of the illness 20% of people re-present to their general practitioner with persistent or recurrent symptoms. One prospective study of 138 previously well adults found that 34% had symptoms consistent with either chronic bronchitis or asthma 3 years after initial presentation with acute bronchitis.[5] It is also unclear whether acute bronchitis plays a causal role in the progression to chronic bronchitis or is simply a marker of predisposition to chronic lung disease.

AIMS OF INTERVENTION To improve symptoms associated with acute bronchitis; to reduce complications.

OUTCOMES Duration of symptoms, particularly cough, sputum production, and fever; quality of life scores; adverse effects of treatment; complications, especially chronic cough, pneumonia, and chronic bronchitis.

METHODS *Clinical Evidence* search and appraisal February 2003. We included people of any age or sex with acute bronchitis. We excluded trials conducted in people who had chronic respiratory disease or other acute respiratory diseases. We excluded non-systematic reviews, non-randomised trials, and RCTs of less than 4 days' treatment duration.

QUESTION **What are the effects of treatments for acute bronchitis in people without chronic respiratory disease?** New

OPTION **ANTIBIOTICS VERSUS PLACEBO**

One systematic review and one subsequent RCT have found that antibiotics modestly reduce cough at 1–2 weeks but found no significant difference in quality of life or impairment in normal activity compared with placebo. Antibiotics increased risk of adverse events such as nausea, vomiting, rash, headache, and vaginitis compared with placebo. Widespread antibiotic use may lead to bacterial resistance to antibiotics.

Benefits: We found one systematic review[6] and one subsequent RCT.[7] The systematic review (search date 2000, 9 RCTs; 750 people aged from 8 to over 65 years, including smokers, but excluding people with chronic bronchitis) compared antibiotics versus placebo.[6] Acute bronchitis was defined by cough, sputum production, or physician diagnosis. The antibiotics used were doxycycline in four RCTs, erythromycin in four RCTs, and sulphamethoxazole/trimethoprim in one RCT. The review found that antibiotics reduced the proportion of people with cough after 1–2 weeks and mean number of days with reported cough compared with placebo (people with cough, 4 RCTs: 47/143 [33%] with antibiotics *v* 67/132 [51%] with placebo; RR 0.64, 95% CI 0.49 to 0.85; WMD in number of days with cough, 5 RCTs: –0.58 days, 95% CI –1.16 days to –0.009 days). However, it found no significant difference between antibiotics and placebo in night time cough or productive cough after 1–2 weeks, or for days of impaired activity (night time cough, 3 RCTs: RR for antibiotics *v* placebo 0.76, 95% CI 0.45 to 1.3; productive cough, 7 RCTs: RR for antibiotics *v* placebo 0.97, 95% CI 0.82 to 1.16; WMD in days of impaired activity, 5 RCTs: –0.48 days, 95% CI –0.96 days to +0.01 days). The subsequent RCT (220 adults with a clinical diagnosis of acute bronchitis and no history of chronic lung disease) compared azithromycin versus vitamin C (as a placebo) for 5 days.[7] It found no significant difference between azithromycin and vitamin C in quality of life after 8 days (acute bronchitis specific health related quality of life score, ranging from 0 [not troubled at all] to 6 [extremely troubled]: 0.9 with azithromycin *v* 0.9 with vitamin C; difference adjusted for baseline score +0.03, 95% CI –0.2 to +0.26).

Harms: In the systematic review adverse events were significantly more common with antibiotics compared with placebo (7 RCTs, adverse events: 60/327 [18%] antibiotics *v* 38/316 [12%] with placebo; RR 1.48; 95% CI 1.02 to 2.14).[6] Adverse events included nausea, vomiting, headache, skin rash, and vaginitis.

Comment: Physicians may be more likely to prescribe antibiotics for smokers with acute bronchitis than for non-smokers (90% in smokers *v* 75% in non-smokers; $P < 0.05$).[8] Seven of the trials in the systematic review found that smoking status did not affect response to antibiotics.[6] Widespread antibiotic use in acute bronchitis may lead to bacterial resistance. The identified RCTs did not evaluate the effects of antibiotics on bacterial resistance.

OPTION ANTIBIOTICS VERSUS EACH OTHER

RCTs found no significant difference in clinical improvement or cure between cefuroxime and amoxicillin (amoxycillin) or amoxicillin/clavulanic acid; among different cefalosporins; between azithromycin and clarithromycin; or between roxithromycin and amoxicillin. Two RCTs found that adverse effects were less common with cefuroxime than with amoxicillin/clavulanic acid.

Benefits: We found no systematic review. **Cefuroxime versus amoxicillin:** We found one RCT (296 adults with clinically diagnosed acute bronchitis and no pre-existing lung disease) comparing cefuroxime 250 mg twice daily versus amoxicillin 250 mg three times daily for 7 days.[9] It found no significant difference in clinical cure rates between cefuroxime and amoxicillin at 72 hours post-treatment (109/143 [76%] with cefuroxime *v* 123/153 [80%] with amoxicillin; P = 0.8). **Cefuroxime versus amoxicillin/clavulanic acid:** We found 2 RCTs.[10,11] The first RCT (312 adults with clinically diagnosed acute bronchitis and no pre-existing lung disease) compared cefuroxime 250 mg twice daily versus amoxicillin/clavulanic acid 875/125 mg twice daily for 5 days.[10] It found no significant difference between cefuroxime and amoxicillin/clavulanic acid in self reported clinical improvement at 10–14 days (114/133 [86%] with cefuroxime *v* 128/142 90%] with amoxicillin/clavulanic acid; P = 0.27). The second RCT (537 people aged 12 years and older with clinically diagnosed acute bronchitis and no pre-existing lung disease) compared cefuroxime 250 mg twice daily for 5 days versus cefuroxime 250 mg twice daily for 10 days versus amoxicillin/clavulanic acid 500/125 mg three times daily for 10 days.[11] It found no significant difference between the groups in cure rates 1–3 days after completing treatment (84/177 [47%] with cefuroxime for 5 days *v* 100/177 [56%] with cefuroxime for 10 days *v* 116/183 [63%] with amoxicillin/clavulanic acid; cefuroxime for 5 days *v* cefuroxime for 10 days, P = 0.41; cefuroxime for 5 days *v* amoxicillin/clavulanic acid, P = 0.91; cefuroxime for 10 days *v* amoxicillin/clavulanic acid, P = 0.45). **Cefuroxime versus cefixime:** We found one RCT (465 children under 12 years old with clinically diagnosed acute bronchitis and no pre-existing lung disease) comparing cefuroxime 250 mg twice daily versus cefixime 400 mg once daily for 10 days.[12] It found no significant difference in clinical outcome between cefuroxime and cefixime after 14 days (proportion with satisfactory clinical outcome, as assessed by the treating general practioner: 130/148 [88%] with cefuroxime *v* 217/238 [91%] with cefixime; P = 0.8). It was not clear how "satisfactory clinical outcome" was defined. **Cefuroxime versus cefpodoxime:** We found one RCT (196 elderly people with clinically diagnosed acute purulent bronchitis and no pre-existing lung disease) comparing cefuroxime 250 mg twice daily versus cefpodoxime 200 mg twice daily.[13] It found no significant difference in physician rated satisfactory clinical response between cefuroxime and cefpodoxime after 10 days (86/95 [91%] with cefuroxime *v* 87/92 [95%] with cefpodoxime; P = 0.76). It was not clear how "satisfactory clinical outcome" was defined. **Azithromycin versus clarithromycin:** We found one RCT (214 adults with clinically diagnosed acute bronchitis and no pre-existing lung disease) comparing azithromycin 500 mg once daily for 2 days then 250 mg once daily for 3 days versus clarithromycin 250mg once daily for 5 days.[14] It found no significant difference between azithromycin and clarithromycin in clinical cure rates or relapse rates after 6–7 days (cure rate: 55/103 [53%] with azithromycin *v* 70/108 [65%] with clarithromycin, P = 0.4; relapse rate: 2/95 [2.1%] with azithromycin *v* 1/101 [1%] with clarithromycin, P = 0.5). **Roxithromycin versus amoxicillin:** We found one RCT (196 adults with clinically diagnosed acute bronchitis and no pre-existing lung disease) comparing roxithromycin 150 mg once daily versus amoxicillin 500 mg three times daily for 10 days.[15] It found no significant difference between roxithromycin and amoxicillin in the proportion with physician assessed improvement or cure (89/96 [93%] with roxithromycin *v* 88/96 [92%] with amoxicillin; P = 0.8).

Harms: **Cefuroxime versus amoxicillin:** The RCT did not report on adverse events.[9] **Cefuroxime versus amoxicillin/clavulanic acid:** The first RCT found that cefuroxime was associated with fewer adverse effects than was amoxicillin/clavulanic acid (16/133 [12%] with cefuroxime *v* 45/142 [32%] with amoxicillin/clavulanic acid; P = 0.001).[10] Most of the adverse effects were gastrointestinal. The second RCT found that a significantly lower proportion of people had gastrointestinal symptoms with cefuroxime than with amoxicillin/clavulanic acid (24/157 [15%] with cefuroxime for 5 days *v* 48/130 [37%] with amoxicillin/clavulanic acid; P < 0.01).[11] **Cefuroxime versus cefixime:** The RCT did not report on adverse events.[12] **Cefuroxime versus cefpodoxime:** The RCT found that the rate of adverse events was similar with cefuroxime and cefpodoxime (4/95 [4.2%] with cefuroxime *v* 6/92 [6.5%] with cefpodoxime; CI not reported).[13] Most of the adverse events were gastrointestinal. **Azithromycin versus clarithromycin:** The RCT found no significant difference between azithromycin and clarithromycin in adverse effects (17/105 [16%] with azithromycin *v* 13/109 [12%] with clarithromycin; P = 0.56).[14] **Roxithromycin versus amoxicillin:** The RCT gave no information on adverse effects.[15]

Comment: None.

OPTION β AGONISTS

One systematic review found no significant difference in cough or ability to return to work between β agonists and placebo in people with acute bronchitis. It found limited evidence from one small RCT that β agonists reduce cough compared with erythromycin. The review found that β agonists increase shaking and tremor compared with placebo or erythromycin.

Benefits: We found one systematic review (search date 2000; 2 RCTs in 109 children; 5 RCTs in 418 adults, both smokers and non-smokers).[16] People with pre-existing lung disease, with another acute respiratory disorder, or aged under 24 months were excluded. **Versus placebo:** Four of the RCTs included in the systematic review compared oral β agonists versus placebo; the other three RCTs compared inhaled β agonists versus placebo. Results from children and adults were analysed separately. The review found no significant difference in the proportion of children or adults with cough after 7 days (1 RCT, 59 children: 11/30 [37%] with β agonists *v* 12/29 [41%] with placebo; RR 0.89, 95% CI 0.47 to 1.65; 3 RCTs, 110 adults: RR 0.86, 95% CI 0.63 to 1.18). It also found no significant difference between β agonists and placebo in the proportion of adults unable to work after 4 days of treatment (2 RCTs, 149 adults: RR for β agonists *v* placebo 0.82, 95% CI 0.28 to 2.34). **Versus antibiotics:** The systematic review[16] identified one small RCT comparing inhaled β agonists versus oral erythromycin for 7 days. It found that β agonists significantly reduced the proportion of people with cough after 7 days compared with erythromycin (7/17 [41%] with inhaled β agonists *v* 15/17 [88%] with erythromycin; RR 0.47, 95% CI 0.26 to 0.85).

Harms: **Versus placebo:** The systematic review found no significant difference in shaking or tremor between β agonists and placebo in children, although shaking and tremor was increased (2 RCTs, 108 children: 6/55 [11%] with β agonists *v* 0/53 [0%] with placebo; RR undefined).[16] In adults, β agonists significantly increased shaking and tremor compared with placebo (3 RCTs, 211 adults: 58/105 [55%] with β agonists *v* 12/106 [11%] with placebo; OR 7.94, 95% CI 1.17 to 53.94; NNH 3, 95% CI 2 to 8). **Versus antibiotics:** The RCT identified by the review[16] found that β agonists increased tremor and shaking compared with erythromycin (6/17 [35%] with β agonists *v* 0/17 [0%] with erythromycin; RR 13.0, 95% CI 0.8 to 214.0). The RCT found no significant differences between β agonists and erythromycin in other adverse effects (2/23 [8.7%] with β agonists *v* 2/23 [8.7%] with erythromycin; RR 1.0, 95% CI 0.15 to 1.51).

Comment: None.

OPTION OVER THE COUNTER ANTITUSSIVES

RCTs found no difference in cough severity between codeine or dextromethorphan and placebo in children or adults with acute bronchitis. We found limited evidence from one RCT that moguisteine modestly reduced cough severity compared with placebo in adults, but was associated with more adverse gastrointestinal effects.

Benefits: We found one systematic review (search date 2000, 5 RCTs, 766 adults, 57 children) of over the counter medications in people with acute bronchitis.[17] The review did not perform a meta-analysis because of differences in preparations, outcomes, and duration of follow up. We excluded two of the 5 RCTs identified by the review because treatment duration was less than 4 days. **In children:** The review identified one RCT (57 children) that met our inclusion criteria.[18] It compared three treatments: dextromethorphan 15 mg once daily, codeine 10 mg once daily, and placebo. It found no significant difference between treatments in mean cough score after 3 days (reduction in mean cough score [range 0–4, higher score indicating more severe cough]: 2.2 with placebo *v* 2.1 with dextromethorphan *v* 2.2 with codeine; dextromethorphan *v* placebo, P = 0.4; codeine *v* placebo, P = 0.7). **In adults:** The review identified two RCTs that met our inclusion criteria.[19,20] The first (81 adults) compared codeine 30 mg four times daily versus placebo for 4 days.[19] It found no significant difference between codeine and placebo in mean cough severity score (higher score indicates worse cough, scale end points unclear) over a 5 day period (mean cough severity score: 17.2 with codeine *v* 18.0 with placebo; $P = 0.5$). The second RCT (108 adults) compared moguisteine 200 mg three times daily for 5 days versus placebo.[20] It found that moguisteine modestly reduced cough severity score compared with placebo (mean difference in cough score on a scale of 0–9 [higher score indicating more severe cough]: 0.5; $P < 0.05$).

Harms: **In children:** No additional adverse events were recorded with treatment compared with placebo (the event rates for each group were not reported). **In adults:** One of the RCTs found that moguisteine increased nausea, vomiting, and abdominal pain compared with placebo (13/58 [22%] with moguisteine *v* 5/58 [8.6%] with placebo; $P < 0.05$).[20]

Comment: The systematic review stated that it examined the effects of treatments in people with "upper respiratory tract infection" rather than "acute bronchitis".[17] However, the clinical criteria used to define this population were consistent with the definition of acute bronchitis used in this topic.

OPTION OVER THE COUNTER EXPECTORANTS

We found insufficient evidence about the effects of over the counter expectorants in people with acute bronchitis.

Benefits: We found one systematic review of over the counter medications for acute cough in people with acute bronchitis (search date 2000).[17] It found no RCTs that met our inclusion criteria. We found no subsequent RCTs.

Harms: We found no RCTs.

Comment: The systematic review stated that it examined the effects of treatments in people with "upper respiratory tract infection" rather than "acute bronchitis".[17] However, the clinical criteria used to define this population were consistent with the definition of acute bronchitis used in this topic.

OPTION ANTIHISTAMINES

We found insufficient evidence about the effects of antihistamines in people with acute bronchitis.

Benefits: We found one systematic review of over the counter medications in people with acute bronchitis (search date 2000).[17] The review identified one RCT (100 adult non-smokers) that met our inclusion criteria.[21] It compared terfenadine 100 mg twice daily versus placebo for 4 or 5 days. It found no significant difference in mean cough score between terfenadine and placebo at day 4 (mean cough score [range 0–3, higher scores indicating worse cough]: 0.8 with terfenadine *v* 0.65 with placebo; $P = 0.35$).

Harms: The RCT reported a low incidence of adverse events but failed to specify these.[21]

Comment: The systematic review stated that it examined the effects of treatments in people with "upper respiratory tract infection" rather than "acute bronchitis".[17] However, the clinical criteria used to define this population were consistent with the definition of acute bronchitis used in this topic.

REFERENCES

1. Macfarlane J, Holmes W, Gard P, et al. Prospective study of the incidence, aetiology and outcome of adult lower respiratory tract illness in the community. *Thorax* 2001;56:109–114.
2. Meza RA. The management of acute bronchitis in general practice results from the Australian morbidity and treatment survey. *Aust Fam Physician* 1994;23:1550–1553.
3. Boldy DAR, Skidmore SJ, Ayres JG. Acute bronchitis in the community: clinical features, infective factors, changes in pulmonary function and bronchial reactivity to histamine. *Respir Med* 1990;84:377–385.
4. Grayston JT, Aldous MB, Easton A, et al. Evidence that Chlamydia pneumoniae causes pneumonia and bronchitis. *J Infect Dis* 1993;168:1231–1235.
5. Jonsson JS, Gislason T, Gislason D, et al. Acute bronchitis and clinical outcome three years later: prospective cohort study. *Thorax* 1998;317:1433.
6. Smucny J, Fahey T, Becker L, et al. Antibiotics for acute bronchitis. In: The Cochrane Library, Issue 1, 2003. Oxford: Update Software. Search date 2000; primary sources Medline, Embase, Scisearch, Cochrane controlled trials register, hand searches of reference lists, and contact with study authors and drug manufacturers.
7. Evans AT, Husain S, Durairaj L, et al. Azithromycin for acute bronchitis: a randomised, double blind, controlled trial. *Lancet* 2002;359:1648–1654.
8. Oeffinger KC, Snell LM, Foster BM, et al. Treatment of acute bronchitis in adults. A national survey of family physicians. *J Fam Pract* 1998;46:469–475.
9. Shah SH, Shah IS, Turnbull G, et al. Cefuroxime axetil in the treatment of bronchitis: comparison with amoxicillin in a multicentre study in general practice patients. *Br J Clin Pract* 1994;48:185–189.
10. Henry DC, Ruoff GE, Noonan M, et al. Comparison of the efficacy and tolerabilityof short-course cefuroxime axetil and amoxicillin clavulanic acid in the treatment of secondary bacterial infections of acute bronchitis. *Clin Drug Invest* 1999;18:335–344.
11. Henry DC, Ruoff GE, Noonan M, et al. Effectiveness of short course therapy (5 days) with cefuroxime axetil in treatment of secondary bacterial infections of acute bronchitis. *Antimicrob Agents Chemother* 1995;39:2528–2534.
12. Arthur M, McAdoo M, Guerra J, et al. Clinical comparison of cefuroxime axetil with cefixime in the treatment of acute bronchitis. *Am J Ther* 1996;3:622–629.
13. Camus P, Beraud A, Phillip-Joet F, et al. Five days treatment of acute purulent bronchitis in the elderly with cefpodoxime proxetil. *Med Maladies Infect* 1994;24:681–685
14. Vincken W, Yernault JC. Efficacy and tolerability of clarithromycin versus azithromycin in the short course treatment of acute bronchitis. *Drug Invest* 1993:3;170–175.
15. Hopstaken RM, Nelemans P, Stobberingh EE, et al. Is roxithromycin better than amoxicillin in the treatment of acute lower respiratory tract infections in primary care? A double blind randomised controlled trial. *J Fam Pract* 2002;51:329–336.
16. Smucny J, Flynn C, Becker L, et al. Beta2 agonists for acute bronchitis. In: The Cochrane Library, Issue 1, 2003. Oxford: Update Software. Search date 2000; primary sources Cochrane library, Medline, Embase, Conference proceedings, and Science Citation Index.
17. Schroeder K, Fahey T. Over the counter medications for acute cough in children and adults in ambulatory settings. In: The Cochrane Library, Issue 1, 2003. Oxford: Update Software. Search date 2000; primary sources Cochrane library, Medline, Embase, UK Dept Health National Research Register and contact with study authors, and pharmaceutical companies.
18. Robinson RE, Cummings WB, Deffenbaugh ER. Effectiveness of guaifenesin as an expectorant: a co-operative double-blind study. *Curr Ther Res* 1977;22:284–296.
19. Eccles R, Morris S, Jawad M. Lack of effect of codeine in the treatment of cough associated with acute upper respiratory tract infection. *J Clin Pharmacol Ther* 1992;17:175–180.
20. Adams R, Hosie J, James I, et al. Antitussive activity and tolerability of moguisteine in patients with acute cough: a randomised double blind placebo controlled study. *Adv Ther* 1993;10:263–271.
21. Berkowitz RB, Tinkelman DG. Evaluation of oral terfenadine for treatment of the common cold. *Ann Allergy* 1991;67:593–597.

Peter Wark
Clinical Research Fellow
Brooke Laboratories
University of Southampton
Southampton
UK

Competing interests: None declared.

Community acquired pneumonia

Search date December 2002

Mark Loeb

QUESTIONS

INTERVENTIONS

TREATMENT

Beneficial

Antibiotics (amoxicillin, cephalosporins, macrolides, penicillin, quinolones) in hospital. 1728

Antibiotics (amoxicillin, cephalosporins, macrolides, penicillin, quinolones) in outpatient settings 1726

Likely to be beneficial

Prompt versus delayed administration of antibiotics in people admitted to intensive care with community acquired pneumonia 1732

Unknown effectiveness

Bottle blowing. 1731

Different antibiotic combinations in intensive care settings 1732

Guidelines for treating pneumonia (for clinical outcomes) 1732

Unlikely to be beneficial

Intravenous versus oral antibiotics in immunocompetent people in hospital without life threatening illness. 1730

PREVENTION

Beneficial

Pneumococcal vaccine in immunocompetent adults. . .1734

Likely to be beneficial

Influenza vaccine in elderly people 1733

Unknown effectiveness

Pneumococcal vaccine in chronically ill, immunosuppressed, or elderly people 1734

To be covered in future updates

Other antiviral treatments

Covered elsewhere in *Clinical Evidence*

Antivirals for influenza, p 867

Key Messages

Treatment

- **Antibiotics (amoxicillin, cephalosporins, macrolides, penicillin, quinolones) in hospital** RCTs that compared different oral or intravenous antibiotics in people admitted to hospital found clinical cure or improvement in 73–96% of people. Four RCTs found no significant difference in clinical cure or improvement among different antibiotics, and two RCTs found that quinolones may increase clinical cure compared with co-amoxiclav (amoxicillin plus clavulanic acid) or cephalosporins. However, most trials were small and were designed to show equivalence between treatments rather than superiority of one over another.

- **Antibiotics (amoxicillin, cephalosporins, macrolides, penicillin, quinolones) in outpatient settings** One systematic review that evaluated different oral antibiotics in outpatient settings has found clinical cure or improvement in over 90% of people regardless of antibiotic taken. Another systematic review found that azithromycin significantly reduced clinical failures over 6–21 days compared with other macrolides, cephalosporins, or penicillin. A third systematic review and a subsequent RCT found no significant difference in clinical cure or improvement between quinolones and amoxicillin, cephalosporins, or macrolides. Most trials were designed to show equivalence between treatments rather than superiority of one over another.
- **Prompt versus delayed administration of antibiotics in people admitted to intensive care with community acquired pneumonia** Two retrospective studies found that prompt administration of antibiotics improved survival. It probably would be unethical to perform an RCT of delayed antibiotic treatment.
- **Bottle blowing** One unblinded RCT in people receiving antibiotics and usual medical care found that bottle blowing physiotherapy plus early mobilisation plus encouragement to sit up regularly and take deep breaths reduced mean hospital stay compared with early mobilisation alone. It found no significant difference in duration of fever.
- **Different antibiotic combinations in intensive care settings** We found no RCTs that compared one combination of antibiotics versus another in intensive care units.
- **Guidelines for treating pneumonia (for clinical outcomes)** One systematic review that compared a guideline that incorporated early switch from intravenous to oral antibiotics and early discharge strategies (or both) versus usual care found no significant difference in clinical outcomes
- **Intravenous versus oral antibiotics in immunocompetent people in hospital without life threatening illness** Two RCTs in immunocompetent people admitted to hospital who did not have life threatening illness found no significant difference in clinical cure or mortality between intravenous and oral antibiotics (co-amoxiclav [amoxicillin plus clavulanic acid] or cefuroxime). The RCTs found that intravenous antibiotics may increase the length of hospital stay compared with oral antibiotics.

Prevention

- **Pneumococcal vaccine in immunocompetent adults** One systematic review found that pneumococcal vaccination reduced pneumococcal pneumonia in immunocompetent people compared with no vaccination.
- **Influenza vaccine in elderly people** We found no RCTs that assessed the effects of influenza vaccine in preventing community acquired pneumonia. Observational studies suggest that influenza vaccine may reduce the incidence of pneumonia and may reduce mortality.
- **Pneumococcal vaccine in chronically ill, immunosuppressed, or elderly people** One systematic review found no significant difference between pneumococcal vaccination and no vaccination in the incidence of pneumonia in elderly people or people likely to have an impaired immune system.

DEFINITION Community acquired pneumonia is pneumonia contracted in the community rather than in hospital. It is defined by clinical symptoms and signs, with radiological confirmation.

Community acquired pneumonia

INCIDENCE/ PREVALENCE In the northern hemisphere, community acquired pneumonia affects about 12/1000 people a year, particularly during winter and at the extremes of age (incidence: < 1 year old 30–50/1000 a year; 15–45 years 1–5/1000 a year; 60–70 years 10–20/1000 a year; 71–85 years 50/1000 a year).[1–6]

AETIOLOGY/ RISK FACTORS Over 100 microorganisms have been implicated in community acquired pneumonia, but most cases are caused by *Streptococcus pneumoniae* (see table 1, p 1737).[4–7] Smoking is probably an important risk factor.[8] One large cohort study in Finland (4175 people aged ≥ 60 years) suggested that risk factors for pneumonia in the elderly included alcoholism (RR 9.0, 95% CI 5.1 to 16.2), bronchial asthma (RR 4.2, 95% CI 3.3 to 5.4), immunosuppression (RR 3.1, 95% CI 1.9 to 5.1), lung disease (RR 3.0, 95% CI 2.3 to 3.9), heart disease (RR 1.9, 95% CI 1.7 to 2.3), institutionalisation (RR 1.8, 95% CI 1.4 to 2.4), and increasing age (≥ 70 years *v* 60–69 years; RR 1.5, 95% CI 1.3 to 1.7).[9]

PROGNOSIS Severity varies from mild to life threatening illness within days of the onset of symptoms. One systematic review of prognosis studies for community acquired pneumonia (search date 1995, 33 148 people) found overall mortality to be 13.7%, ranging from 5.1% for ambulant people to 36.5% for people who required intensive care.[10] The following prognostic factors were significantly associated with mortality: male sex (OR 1.3, 95% CI 1.2 to 1.4); pleuritic chest pain (OR 0.5, 95% CI 0.3 to 0.8, i.e. lower mortality); hypothermia (OR 5.0, 95% CI 2.4 to 10.4); systolic hypotension (OR 4.8, 95% CI 2.8 to 8.3); tachypnoea (OR 2.9, 95% CI 1.7 to 4.9); diabetes mellitus (OR 1.3, 95% CI 1.1 to 1.5); neoplastic disease (OR 2.8, 95% CI 2.4 to 3.1); neurological disease (OR 4.6, 95% CI 2.3 to 8.9); bacteraemia (OR 2.8, 95% CI 2.3 to 3.6); leucopenia (OR 2.5, 95% CI 1.6 to 3.7); and multilobar radiographic pulmonary infiltrates (OR 3.1, 95% CI 1.9 to 5.1).

AIMS OF INTERVENTION **Treatment:** To cure infection clinically, to reduce mortality, to alleviate symptoms, to enable return to normal activities, and to prevent recurrence, while minimising adverse effects of treatments. **Prevention:** To prevent onset of pneumonia.

OUTCOMES **Treatment:** Clinical cure, variably defined but usually defined as return to premorbid health status or complete absence of symptoms such as fever, chills, cough, dyspnoea or sputum production; improvement (relief of symptoms); admission to hospital; complications (empyema, endocarditis, lung abscess); death; adverse effects of antibiotics. **Prevention:** incidence of pneumonia, adverse effects of vaccination.

METHODS *Clinical Evidence* search and appraisal December 2002.

QUESTION **What are the effects of interventions in outpatient settings?**

OPTION **ANTIBIOTICS**

One systematic review that evaluated different oral antibiotics in outpatient settings has found clinical cure or improvement in over 90% of people regardless of antibiotic taken. Another systematic review found

that azithromycin significantly reduced clinical failures over 6–21 days compared with other macrolides, cephalosporins, or penicillin. A third systematic review and a subsequent RCT found no significant difference in clinical cure or improvement between quinolones and amoxicillin, cephalosporins, or macrolides. Most trials were designed to show equivalence between treatments rather than superiority of one over another.

Benefits: We found three systematic reviews[11–13] and one subsequent RCT.[14] The first systematic review (search date not stated, 9 RCTs, 1164 people) compared different oral antibiotics in outpatient settings.[11] Antibiotics evaluated were amoxicillin (amoxycillin) with and without clavulanate, macrolides, cephalosporins, and quinolones. The review did not perform a meta-analysis that directly compared antibiotics. Clinical cure or improvement was reported in over 90% of people regardless of antibiotic taken (no further data reported). **Azithromycin versus other macrolides, cephalosporins, or penicillins:** The second systematic review (search date 2000, 18 RCTs, 2 of which were included in the first review, 1664 people) found that, compared with other macrolides (clarithromycin, erythromycin, or roxithromycin, 13 RCTs), cephalosprorins (cefaclor, 2 RCTs), or penicillins (co-amoxiclav or penicillin, 3 RCTs), azithromycin significantly reduced clinical failures over 6–21 days (56/928 [6%] with azithromycin *v* 72/736 [10%] with other oral antibiotics; OR 0.63, 95% CI 0.42 to 0.95).[12] These results should be interpreted with caution as most of the RCTs were not blinded. **Quinolones versus amoxicillin, macrolides, or cephalosporins:** The third systematic review (search date 1999, 8 RCTs, none of which were included in the first or second review, 3131 people) found no significant difference in clinical success (cure or improvement) between quinolones (gatifloxacin, levofloxacin, moxifloxacin, sparfloxacin, and trovafloxacin) and high dose amoxicillin, cefaclor, cefpodoxime, ceftriaxone, ceftriaxone plus clarithromycin, cefuroxime axetil, clarithromycin, co-amoxiclav, erythromycin, or roxithromycin (ARR +1.7%, 95% CI −1.4% to +4.8%; no further data reported).[13] The subsequent RCT (299 people) compared oral clarithromycin (1000 mg daily) versus oral levofloxacin (500 mg daily).[14] It found no significant difference in clinical cure rates at 7 days between oral clarithromycin and levofloxacin (113/128 [88%] with clarithromycin *v* 107/124 [86%] with levofloxacin; RR 1.02, 95% CI 0.93 to 1.12).[14]

Harms: The first and third reviews gave no information on adverse effects.[11,13] The second review found that azithromycin significantly reduced withdrawals because of adverse effects compared with co-amoxiclav (no further data reported).[12] It also found limited evidence from indirect comparisons that withdrawals because of adverse effects were lower with azithromycin than with clarithromycin, erythromycin, or cefaclor. The subsequent RCT found no significant difference in the proportion of people who had adverse effects (primarily diarrhoea, nausea, and headache) with clarithromycin compared with levofloxacin (26% with clarithromycin *v* 20% with levofloxacin; reported as non-significant; CI not reported), although clarithromycin significantly increased taste disturbance (20/156 [13%] *v* 1/143 [0.7%]; $P < 0.001$).[14] Antibiotics can cause allergic reactions (including anaphylaxis), rash, gastrointestinal intolerance (nausea, vomiting, and diarrhoea), vaginal or oral candidiasis, and *Clostridium difficile* diarrhoea (including pseudomembranous colitis). Frequency of adverse effects varies with the antibiotic used.

Comment: Most trials were designed to show equivalence between treatments rather than superiority of one over another.

QUESTION **What are the effects of treatments in people admitted to hospital?**

OPTION **ANTIBIOTICS**

RCTs that compared different oral or intravenous antibiotics in people admitted to hospital found clinical cure or improvement in 73–96% of people. Four RCTs found no significant difference in clinical cure or improvement among different antibiotics, and two RCTs found that quinolones may increase clinical cure compared with co-amoxiclav (amoxicillin plus clavulanic acid) or cephalosporins. However, most trials were small, and were designed to show equivalence between treatments rather than superiority of one over another.

Benefits: We found no systematic review. RCTs found no clear evidence of a difference in clinical cure among different antibiotics. RCTs that compared different oral or intravenous antibiotics in people admitted to hospital found clinical cure or improvement in 73–96% of people. **Cephalosporins versus penicillin:** We found several RCTs that were too small, too old, or both, to be reliable given the changing sensitivity of organisms to antibiotics. One RCT (378 people) compared intravenous co-amoxiclav (amoxicillin plus clavulanic acid) followed by oral co-amoxiclav versus intravenous ceftriaxone followed by intramuscular ceftriaxone.[15] People in both groups also received intravenous erythromycin as decided by their physician (17/184 [9%] people taking co-amoxiclav and 25/194 [13%] people taking ceftriaxone). It found no significant difference in clinical cure at long term follow up, which was not specified (136/184 [73.9%] with co-amoxiclav *v* 144/194 [74.2%] with ceftriaxone; RR 0.99, 95% CI 0.88 to 1.12). **Quinolones versus high dose amoxicillin:** We found two multicentre double blind RCTs.[16,17] The first RCT (329 people in hospital in France, South Africa, and Switzerland) compared sparfloxacin 400 mg on day 1 followed by 200 mg once daily versus amoxicillin 1000 mg three times daily.[16] It found no significant difference in clinical cure at 14–21 days (133/159 [84%] with sparfloxacin *v* 144/170 [85%] with amoxicillin; RR 0.99, 95% CI 0.87 to 1.07).[16] It found that fewer people treated with sparfloxacin versus amoxicillin discontinued the drug at days 3, 4, or 5 because of a lack of response, but the difference did not reach significance (3/126 [2%] *v* 11/140 [8%]; RR 0.30, 95% CI 0.08 to 1.05). The second RCT (411 people with suspected pneumococcal pneumonia, 285 of whom were admitted to hospital) compared oral moxifloxacin 400 mg once daily versus oral amoxicillin 1000 mg three times daily.[17] It found no significant difference in clinical cure or improvement at 3–4 weeks after the end of 5–7 days' treatment (154/200 [77.0%] with moxifloxacin *v* 164/208 [78.8%] with amoxicillin; RR 0.97, 95%

CI 0.86 to 1.07). **Quinolones versus co-amoxiclav**: We found one multicentre RCT (628 people) that compared moxifloxacin 400 mg once daily (iv followed by oral) versus co-amoxiclav (amoxicillin plus clavulanic acid) 1.2 g intravenously followed by 625 mg orally three times daily with or without clarithromycin for 7–14 days.[18] It found that the moxifloxacin significantly increased the clinical cure rate at 5–7 days after treatment compared with co-amoxiclav (225/241 [93%] *v* 204/239 [85%]; P = 0.004).[18] **Quinolones versus cephalosporins:** We found one unblinded RCT (590 people, 280 of whom had been admitted to hospital) that compared oral or intravenous levofloxacin or both versus intravenous ceftriaxone or oral cefuroxime axetil, or both.[19] It found that levofloxacin significantly increased the proportion of people clinically cured or improved at 5–7 days compared with cephalosporins (96% with levofloxacin *v* 90% with cephalosporins; reported as significant; CI not reported). **Quinolones versus macrolides plus cephalosporins:** We found one multicentre open label RCT (236 people) that compared levofloxacin 500 mg daily (orally or intravenous) versus 500 mg intravenous azithromycin plus 1 g intravenous ceftriaxone for 2 days followed by an optional transition to 500 mg oral azithromycin.[20] It found no significant difference in clinical cure between groups (100/115 [87%] with levofloxacin *v* 97/121 [80%] with azithromycin plus ceftriaxone; RR 1.08, 95% CI 0.97 to 1.21).[20]

Harms: See also harms of antibiotics, p 1727. **Cephalosporins versus penicillin:** The RCT gave no information on adverse effects.[15] **Quinolones versus high dose amoxicillin:** The first RCT found that fewer people had gastrointestinal disturbances with sparfloxacin compared with amoxicillin (19 *v* 10; CI not reported).[16] Four people (2.5%) taking sparfloxacin withdrew because of adverse effects compared with two people (1.2%) taking amoxicillin (P value not reported). The second RCT found no significant difference in the proportion of people who had gastrointestinal adverse effects with moxifloxacin compared with amoxicillin (56/200 [28%] with moxifloxacin *v* 42/208 [20%] with amoxicillin; RR 1.39, 95% CI 0.98 to 1.97).[16] **Quinolones versus co-amoxiclav:** The RCT found similar rates of overall adverse effects (primarily nausea and diarrhoea) between moxifloxacin and co-amoxiclav (39% in both groups; CI not reported).[18] **Quinolones versus cephalosporins:** The RCT found that a similar proportion of people had gastrointestinal adverse effects (primarily nausea and diarrhoea) with levofloxacin compared with cephalosporins (5.8% levofloxacin *v* 8.5% with cephalosporins; absolute numbers and CI not reported).[19] **Quinolones versus macrolides plus cephalosporins:** The RCT found no significant difference in the rates of overall adverse effects (primarily gastrointestinal adverse effects) between levofloxacin and azithromycin plus ceftriaxone (6/113 [5%] *v* 11/118 [9%]; RR 0.57, 95% CI 0.22 to 1.49).[20]

Comment: Most trials were small and were designed to show equivalence between treatments rather than superiority of one over another. Although detection of penicillin resistant and multidrug resistant *S pneumoniae* is commonly reported, it is hard to enrol people with this infection in randomised studies. One study was carried out in areas with high prevalence of penicillin resistant *S pneumoniae*.[16] It found 8/135 (6.9%) isolates tested were resistant to penicillin,[16] but none showed high level resistance as measured by the minimum inhibitory concentration of penicillin (where pneumococcal strains with minimum inhibitory concentration ≥ 2 μg are termed highly resistant).[21] The trials in uncomplicated pneumonia may not apply to people with comorbidities such as meningitis.[21] There are also concerns about macrolide resistant *S pneumoniae,* but, so far, treatment failure in ambulatory people with community acquired pneumonia is uncommon.[22] In the RCT that compared levofloxacin versus cephalosporins, the route of administration was decided by the doctor, and it is unclear whether all participants who received intravenous antibiotics were admitted to hospital.[19] We found one retrospective review (12 945 people ≥ 65 years old in hospital with community acquired pneumonia).[23] It found that initial treatment with a second generation cephalosporin (cefuroxime) plus a macrolide (azithromycin, clarithromycin, or erythromycin), a non-pseudomonal third generation cephalosporin (ceftriaxone, cefotaxime, ceftizoxime) plus a macrolide, or a fluoroquinolone (ciprofloxacin, ofloxacin) reduced mortality at 30 days compared with initial treatment with a β-lactam/β-lactamase inhibitor (ampicillin plus sulbactam, ticarcillin plus clavulanic acid, piperacillin plus tazobactam) plus a macrolide, or an aminoglycoside plus another antimicrobial agent.[23] One retrospective cohort study found that people infected with penicillin resistant compared with non-penicillin resistant *S pneumoniae* were at greater risk of death in hospital (RR 2.1, 95% CI 1.0 to 4.3) and suppurative complications (RR 4.5, 95% CI 1.0 to 19.3).[24] From national surveillance data, penicillin resistant pneumonia was associated with significantly higher mortality after the first 4 days in hospital than non-penicillin resistant pneumonia.[25] These results should be interpreted with caution, however, as they may not account for confounding factors.

OPTION INTRAVENOUS VERSUS ORAL ANTIBIOTICS

Two RCTs in immunocompetent people admitted to hospital who did not have life threatening illness found no significant difference in clinical cure or mortality between intravenous and oral antibiotics (co-amoxiclav [amoxicillin plus clavulanic acid] or cefuroxime). The RCTs found that intravenous antibiotics may increase the length of hospital stay compared with oral antibiotics.

Benefits: We found no systematic review. We found two RCTs that compared oral versus intravenous antibiotics in people admitted to hospital with community acquired pneumonia.[26,27] The first RCT (541 people with lower respiratory tract infections, 40% of whom had chest radiographs that were compatible with pneumonia) compared three interventions: oral co-amoxiclav for 7 days, intravenous co-amoxiclav for 3 days followed by oral co-amoxiclav for 4 days, and intravenous cefotaxime for 3 days followed by oral cefuroxime for 4 days.[26] People were excluded if they had life threatening infection or were immunocompromised. At discharge from hospital, the RCT found no significant difference among groups in cure or improvement (142/181 [78%] with oral co-amoxiclav *v* 129/181 [71%] *v* 122/179 [68%]; P = 0.36 for all regimens *v* each other) or mortality (9/181 [5%] *v* 13/181 [7%] *v* 11/179 [6%]; P = 0.67 for all regimens *v* each other). However, it found that oral antibiotics significantly reduced hospital stay compared with intravenous antibiotics (proportion of people discharged within 3 days: 36/181 with oral antibiotics *v* 21/360 [6%] with intravenous antibiotics; P < 0.005).[26] The second RCT (73 people, no intention to treat analysis) assessed different duration of treatment with intravenous antibiotics.[27] It compared three interventions: 2 days of intravenous cefuroxime followed by 8 days of oral cefuroxime (group 1), 5 days of oral cefuroxime followed by 5 days of intravenous cefuroxime (group 2), or 10 days of intravenous cefuroxime (group three).[27] People were excluded if they had empyema, septic shock, or respiratory failure. It found no significant difference among groups in the proportion of people with clinical cure after 28 days (18/20 [90%] in group 1 *v* 17/20 [85%] in group 2 *v* 16/17 [94%] in group 3; reported as non-significant, no further data reported). However, it found that people in group 1 had a significantly shorter hospital stay compared with people in either of the other groups (6 days with group 1 *v* 8 days with group 2 *v* 11 days with group 3; reported as significant; CI not reported).[27]

Harms: The RCTs gave no information on adverse effects.[26,27]

Comment: Intravenous antibiotics are used in people who cannot take oral medication because of severe nausea or vomiting. A follow up study (96 people admitted to hospital with community acquired pneumonia) found clinical cure of pneumonia at 30 days in people who were switched from intravenous to oral antibiotics when they had been afebrile for 8 hours, symptoms of cough and shortness of breath were improving, white blood cell counts were returning to normal, and they could tolerate oral medication.[28]

OPTION BOTTLE BLOWING

One unblinded RCT in people who received antibiotics and usual medical care found that bottle blowing physiotherapy plus early mobilisation plus encouragement to sit up regularly and take deep breaths reduced mean hospital stay compared with early mobilisation alone. It found no significant difference in duration of fever.

Benefits: We found no systematic review. We found one RCT (145 people in hospital with community acquired pneumonia) that compared three interventions: early mobilisation alone, early mobilisation plus encouragement to sit up 10 times a day and take 20 deep breaths, and early mobilisation plus encouragement to sit up 10 times a day and blow bubbles through a plastic tube for 20 breaths into a bottle containing 10 cm of water (bottle blowing).[29] Participants concurrently received benzylpenicillin or phenoxymethylpenicillin and usual medical care independently of the study interventions. The RCT found that bottle blowing plus early mobilisation plus encouragement significantly reduced mean hospital stay compared with early mobilisation alone (5.3 *v* 3.9 days; P = 0.01). It found no significant difference among groups in duration of fever (2.3 with early mobilisation alone *v* 1.7 with encouragement to take deep breaths *v* 1.6 with bottle blowing; P = 0.28 for all groups *v* each other; see comment below).

Harms: The RCT gave no information on adverse effects.[29]

Comment: In the RCT, neither participants nor clinicians were blinded to the intervention.[29]

QUESTION What are the effects of treatments in people with community acquired pneumonia receiving intensive care?

OPTION DIFFERENT COMBINATIONS OF ANTIBIOTICS

We found no RCTs that compared one combination of antibiotics versus another in intensive care units (see comment below).

Benefits: We found no systematic review and no RCTs.

Harms: We found no RCTs.

Comment: Use of a combination of antibiotics is regarded as current best practice.

OPTION PROMPT VERSUS DELAYED ANTIBIOTIC TREATMENT

Two retrospective studies found that prompt administration of antibiotics improved survival. It probably would be unethical to perform an RCT of delayed antibiotic treatment.

Benefits: We found no systematic review and no RCTs (see comment below). One multicentre retrospective review (medical records of ≥ 14 000 people aged ≥ 65 years admitted to acute [emergency] care hospitals in the United States who were severely ill with community acquired pneumonia) found that antibiotics given within 8 hours of admission to hospital were associated with lower 30 day mortality (OR 0.85, 95% CI 0.75 to 0.96).[30] The review did not specify whether oral or intravenous antibiotics were given. Another retrospective study (39 people with serologically confirmed legionnaires' disease and clinically diagnosed community acquired pneumonia) examined outcome and time to start of treatment.[31] For the 10 people who died, the median delay between diagnosis of pneumonia and start of intravenous erythromycin was 5 days (range 1–10 days), and for those who survived it was 1 day (range 1–5 days; $P < 0.001$).

Harms: The retrospective studies gave no information on harms.[30,31]

Comment: It probably would be regarded as unethical to perform an RCT of delayed antibiotic treatment.

QUESTION What are the effects of guidelines on the treatment of community acquired pneumonia?

One systematic review that compared a guideline that incorporated early switch from intravenous to oral antibiotics and early discharge strategies (or both) versus usual care found no significant difference in clinical outcomes.

Benefits: We found one systematic review (search date 2000, 3 RCTs, 7 cohort studies) that compared a guideline incorporating early switch from intravenous to oral antibiotics and early discharge, or both, versus usual care.[32] It found no significant difference between groups in therapeutic success (not defined), readmission to hospital, admission to intensive care unit, complications, mortality, or any adverse outcome (no further data reported). It also found no significant difference between a guideline and usual care in mean length of hospital stay (mean 6.0 days with guideline *v* 7.6 days with usual care; $P = 0.05$).

Harms: The review found no significant difference in "any adverse outcome" (not specified) between a guideline and usual care (no further data reported).[32]

Comment: None.

QUESTION What are the effects of preventive interventions?

OPTION INFLUENZA VACCINE

We found no RCTs that assessed the effects of influenza vaccine in preventing community acquired pneumonia. Observational studies suggest that influenza vaccine may reduce the incidence of pneumonia and may reduce mortality.

Benefits: See comment below.

Harms: We found no RCTs (see comment below).

Comment: We found one systematic review of cohort studies (search date not stated, 20 studies) that compared influenza vaccine versus no vaccine.[33] It found that influenza vaccine significantly reduced the incidence of pneumonia (24 774 people; ARR 53%, 95% CI 35% to 66%) and significantly reduced mortality (29 928 people; ARR 68%, 95% CI 56% to 76%).[33] Timescales were not reported for any outcomes. Analysis of an administrative database (≥ 25 000 people aged ≥ 64 years) suggested that influenza vaccination reduced the rate of admission to hospital in people with pneumonia or influenza by 48–57% ($P < 0.01$).[34] We found one systematic review (search date 2000,[35] 1 RCT[36]) and one additional RCT that assessed the effects of influenza vaccine in preventing influenza and reducing mortality.[37–39] **Effects in vaccinated people:** The RCT (> 1800 people aged ≥ 60 years) identified by the review[35] compared split virion vaccine versus saline solution.[36] It found that vaccine versus placebo significantly reduced the incidence of clinical influenza at 5 months (AR 17/927 [1.8%] *v* AR 31/911 [3.4%]; RR 0.53, 95% CI 0.39 to 0.73).[36] The additional RCT (324 elderly residents of nursing homes) compared parenteral trivalent inactivated vaccine plus intranasal live attenuated cold adapted vaccine versus parenteral trivalent inactivated vaccine alone. It found that inactivated vaccine plus live attenuated vaccine versus inactivated vaccine alone significantly reduced the incidence of influenza A (9/162 [5.5%] for inactivated vaccine plus live attenuated vaccine *v* 24/169 [14.2%] for inactivated vaccine alone; RR 0.39, 95% CI 0.18 to 0.81; NNT 12, 95% CI 9 to 38).[37] **Effects of**

vaccinating healthcare workers: We found no systematic review but found two weak RCTs.[38,39] The first RCT (12 long term elderly care hospitals) compared the offer of vaccination of healthcare workers versus no offer of vaccination.[38] Of the healthcare workers offered vaccination, 653/1078 (60.6%) were vaccinated. In the hospitals where vaccination was offered to healthcare workers, more than 85% of residents had already been vaccinated compared with only one resident in the hospitals where vaccination was not offered to healthcare workers. This makes the results difficult to interpret. The RCT found that vaccination of healthcare workers versus no vaccination significantly reduced all cause mortality of elderly residents during one winter (50/490 [10.0%] residents in vaccine hospitals *v* 98/569 [17.2%] in non-vaccine hospitals; RR 0.59, 95% CI 0.42 to 0.82).[38] Another RCT (20 elderly care hospitals) compared influenza vaccination of healthcare workers versus no vaccination in a similar design to the previous RCT.[39] Of the healthcare workers offered vaccination, 620/1217 (50.9%) were vaccinated. In vaccine hospitals, 48% of residents versus 33% of residents in non-vaccine hospitals were already vaccinated. The RCT found that influenza vaccination of healthcare workers versus no vaccination significantly reduced all cause mortality of elderly people over 6 months (102/749 [13.6%] in vaccine hospitals *v* 154/688 [22.4%] in non-vaccine hospitals; RR 0.60, 95% CI 0.48 to 0.77; NNT 11, 95% CI 9 to 19).[39] A reduction in rates of influenza does not necessarily imply a reduction in rates of pneumonia. Two of the RCTs found that adverse effects included pain and tenderness at the site of injection.[38,39] Guillain-Barré syndrome was associated with 1/100 000 influenza vaccinations during the national vaccination programme against swine influenza in the USA in 1976, during which 45 million people were vaccinated.[40]

OPTION PNEUMOCOCCAL VACCINE

One systematic review found that pneumococcal vaccination reduced pneumococcal pneumonia in immunocompetent people compared with no vaccination. The review found no significant difference between pneumococcal vaccination and no vaccination in the incidence of pneumonia in elderly people or people likely to have an impaired immune system.

Benefits: We found one systematic review (search date 2000, 13 RCTs, > 45 000 people) that compared pneumococcal vaccination versus no vaccination.[41] It found that in immunocompetent people (3 RCTs, 21 152 African gold workers and Papua New Guinea highlanders), pneumococcal vaccination significantly reduced all cause pneumonia compared with no vaccination (3.1% *v* 6.5%; RR 0.56, 95% CI 0.47 to 0.66), pneumococcal pneumonia (0.5% v 3.1%; RR 0.16, 95% CI 0.11 to 0.23), pneumococcal bacteraemia (0.7% *v* 3.8%; RR 0.18, 95% CI 0.09 to 0.34), and pneumonia related mortality during one winter (1.1% *v* 1.6%; RR 0.70, 95% CI 0.50 to 0.96). In elderly people or people likely to have an impaired immune system (10 RCTs, 24 074 people), the review found no significant difference between pneumococcal vaccination and no vaccination in all cause pneumonia (7.0% *v* 6.8%; RR 1.08, 95% CI 0.92 to 1.27), pneumococcal pneumonia (1.7% *v* 1.9%; RR 0.88, 95% CI 0.72 to 1.07), pneumococcal bacteraemia (0.8% *v* 1.4%; RR 0.53, 95% CI 0.14 to 1.94), or pneumonia related mortality (1.0% *v* 1.1%; RR 0.93, 95% CI 0.72 to 1.20).

Harms: The systematic review found few RCTs that gave information on adverse effects.[41] One RCT in the review found that pneumococcal vaccination was associated with erythema and induration compared with no vaccination. Another RCT in the review found that pneumococcal vaccination increased sore arm, swollen arm, and fever compared with no vaccination.

Comment: A fifth of healthy elderly adults (mean age 71 years) do not have an antibody response to vaccination.[42] New conjugate pneumococcal vaccines are being evaluated. These have been shown to stimulate an antibody response in infants and have decreased the rate of carriage of resistant strains of *S pneumoniae*.[43,44] One retrospective cohort study (1898 elderly members of a staff healthcare organisation) found that pneumococcal vaccination was associated with lower risks of admission to hospital for pneumonia (adjusted RR 0.57, 95% CI 0.38 to 0.84) and lower mortality (adjusted RR 0.71, 95% CI 0.56 to 0.91).[45] The study found evidence of an additive effect for people who received both pneumococcal and influenza vaccinations during the influenza season (RR 0.28, 95% CI 0.14 to 0.58 for admission to hospital for pneumonia and influenza; RR 0.18, 95% CI 0.11 to 0.31 for death).

Substantive changes

Antibiotics (outpatients) One RCT added;[14] conclusions unchanged.

Antibiotics (hospital): quinolones versus co-amoxiclav One RCT found that moxifloxacin increased clinical cure compared with co-amoxiclav (amoxicillin plus clavulanic acid).[18]

Antibiotics (hospital): quinolones versus macrolides plus cephalosporins One RCT found no significant difference in clinical cure between levofloxacin and azithromycin plus ceftriaxone.[20]

REFERENCES

1. Foy HM, Cooney MK, Allan I, et al. Rates of pneumonia during influenza epidemics in Seattle, 1964–1975. *JAMA* 1979;241:253–258.
2. Murphy TF, Henderson FW, Clyde WA, et al. Pneumonia: an 11 year study in a pediatric practice. *Am J Epidemiol* 1981;113:12–21.
3. McConnochie KM, Hall CB, Barker WH. Lower respiratory tract illness in the first two years of life: epidemiologic patterns and costs in a suburban pediatric practice. *Am J Public Health* 1988;78:34–39.
4. Porath A, Schlaeffer F, Lieberman D. The epidemiology of community-acquired pneumonia among hospitalized adults. *J Infect* 1997;34:41–48.
5. Jokinen C, Heiskanen L, Juvonen H, et al. Incidence of community-acquired pneumonia in the population of four municipalities in eastern Finland. *Am J Epidemiol* 1993;137:977–988.
6. Houston MS, Silverstein MD, Suman VJ. Risk factors for 30-day mortality in elderly patients with lower respiratory tract infection. *Arch Intern Med* 1997;157:2190–2195.
7. Bartlett JG, Mundy LM. Community-acquired pneumonia. *N Engl J Med* 1995;333:1618–1624.
8. Almirall J, Gonzalez CA, Balanco X, et al. Proportion of community-acquired pneumonia attributable to tobacco smoking. *Chest* 1999;116:375–379.
9. Koivula I, Sten M, Makela PH. Risk factors for pneumonia in the elderly. *Am J Med* 1994;96:313–320.
10. Fine MJ, Smith MA, Carson CA, et al. Prognosis and outcomes of patients with community-acquired pneumonia: a meta-analysis. *JAMA* 1995;274:134–141. Search date 1995; primary sources Medline and handsearching of reference lists.
11. Pomilla PV, Brown RB. Outpatient treatment of community-acquired pneumonia in adults. *Arch Intern Med* 1994;154:1793–1802. Search date not stated; primary source Medline.
12. Contopoulos-Ioannidis DG, Ioannidis JPA, Chew P, et al. Meta-analysis of randomized controlled trials on the comparative efficacy and safety of azithromycin against other antibiotics for lower respiratory tract infections. *J Antimicrob*

Chemother 2001;48:691–703. Search date 2000; primary sources Embase, Medline, and Cochrane Controlled Trials Registry.

13. Metge CJ, Vercaigne L, Carrie A, et al. *The new fluoroquinolones in community-acquired pneumonia: clinical and economic perspectives. Technology overview no 5.* Ottawa: Canadian Coordinating Office for Health Technology Assessment, 2001. Search date 1999; primary sources Medline and Embase.
14. Gotfried MH, Dattani D, Riffer E, et al. A controlled, double-blind, multicenter study comparing clarithromycin extended-release tablets and levofloxacin tablets in the treatment of community-acquired pneumonia. *Clin Ther* 2002;24:736–751.
15. Roson B, Carratala J, Tubau F, et al. Usefulness of betalactam therapy for community-acquired pneumonia in the era of drug-resistant *Streptococcus pneumoniae*: a randomized study of amoxicillin-clavulanate and ceftriaxone. *Microb Drug Resist* 2001;7:85–96.
16. Aubier M, Verster R, Regamey C, et al and the Sparfloxacin European Study Group. Once-daily sparfloxacin versus high-dosage amoxicillin in the treatment of community-acquired, suspected pneumococcal pneumonia in adults. *Clin Infect Dis* 1998;26:1312–1320.
17. Petitpretz P, Arvis P, Marel M, et al. Oral moxifloxacin vs high-dosage amoxicillin in the treatment of mild-to-moderate, community-acquired, suspected pneumococcal pneumonia in adults. *Chest* 2001;119:185–195.
18. Finch R, Schurmann D, Collins O, et al. Randomized controlled trial of sequential intravenous and oral moxifloxacin compared with sequential i.v and oral co-amoxiclav with or without clarithromycin in patients with community-acquired pneumonia requiring initial parenteral treatment. *Antimicrob Agents Chemother* 2002;46:1746–1754.
19. File TM Jr, Segreti J, Dunbar L, et al. A multicenter, randomized study comparing the efficacy and safety of intravenous and/or oral levofloxacin versus ceftriaxone and/or cefuroxime axetil in treatment of adults with community-acquired pneumonia. *Antimicrob Agents Chemother* 1997;41:1965–1972.
20. Frank E, Liu J, Kinasewitz G, et al. A multicenter, open-label, randomized comparison of levofloxacin and azithromycin plus ceftriaxone in hospitalized adults with moderate to severe community-acquired pneumonia. *Clin Ther* 2002;24:1292–1308.
21. Friedland IR, McCracken GH Jr. Management of infections caused by antibiotic-resistant *Streptococcus pneumoniae*. *N Engl J Med* 1994;331:377–382.
22. Siegel RE. The significance of serum vs. tissue levels of antibiotics in the treatment of penicillin-resistant *Streptococcus pneumoniae* and community-acquired pneumonia. Are we looking in the wrong place? *Chest* 1999;116:535–538.
23. Gleason PP, Meehan TP, Fine JM, et al. Associations between initial antimicrobial therapy and medical outcomes for hospitalized elderly patients with pneumonia. *Arch Intern Med* 1999;159:2562–2572.
24. Metlay JP, Hofmann J, Cetron MS, et al. Impact of penicillin susceptibility on medical outcomes for adult patients with bacteremic pneumococcal pneumonia. *Clin Infect Dis* 2000;30:520–528.
25. Faikin DR, Schuchat A, Kolczak M, et al. Mortality from invasive pneumococcal pneumonia in the era of antibiotic resistance, 1995–1997. *Am J Public Health* 2000;90:223–229.
26. Chan R, Hemeryck L, O'Regan M, et al. Oral versus intravenous antibiotics for community-acquired lower respiratory tract infection in a general hospital: open randomised controlled trial. *BMJ* 1995;310:1360–1362.
27. Siegel RE, Halperin NA, Almenoff PL, et al. A prospective randomized study of inpatient IV antibiotics for community-acquired pneumonia: the optimal duration of therapy. *Chest* 1996;110:965–971.
28. Ramirez JA, Ahkee S. Early switch from intravenous antimicrobials to oral clarithromycin in patients with community acquired pneumonia. *Infect Med* 1997;14:319–323.
29. Bjorkqvist M, Wiberg B, Bodin L, et al. Bottle-blowing in hospital-treated patients with community-acquired pneumonia. *Scand J Infect Dis* 1997;29:77–82.
30. Meehan TP, Fine MJ, Krumholz HM, et al. Quality of care, process, and outcomes in elderly patients with pneumonia. *JAMA* 1997;278:2080–2084.
31. Heath CH, Grove DI, Looke DFM. Delay in appropriate therapy of *Legionella pneumonia* associated with increased mortality. *Eur J Clin Microbiol Infect Dis* 1966;15:286–290.
32. Rhew DC, Tu GS, Ofman J, et al. Early switch and early discharge strategies in patients with community-acquired pneumonia: a meta-analysis. *Arch Intern Med* 2001;161:722–727. Search date 2000; primary sources Medline, Healthstar, Embase, Cochrane Library, and Best Evidence.
33. Gross PA, Hermogenes AW, Sacks HS, et al. The efficacy of influenza vaccine in elderly persons: a meta-analysis and review of the literature. *Ann Intern Med* 1995;123:518–527. Search date not stated; primary source Medline.
34. Nichol KL, Margolis KL, Wuorenma J, et al. The efficacy and cost effectiveness of vaccination against influenza among elderly persons living in the community. *N Engl J Med* 1994;331:778–784.
35. Vu T, Farish S, Jenkins M, et al. A meta-analysis of influenza vaccine in persons aged 65 years and over living in the community. *Vaccine* 2002;20:1831–1836. Search date 2000; primary sources Medline, Biosis, Firstsearch, Bandolier, Cochrane Library, Current Contents, Effectiveness Matters, Derwent Drug File, American College of Physicians Journal Club, Database of Abstracts of Effectiveness, FluNet, CDC Influenza Home Page, Influenza Bibiography, several government Internet sites, hand searches of reference lists, and contact with prominent researchers in the field.
36. Govaert TM, Thijs CT, Masurel N, et al. The efficacy of influenza vaccination in elderly individuals: a randomized double-blind placebo-controlled trial. *JAMA* 1994;272:1661–1665.
37. Treanor JJ, Mattison HR, Dumyati G, et al. Protective efficacy of combined live intranasal and inactivated influenza A virus vaccines in the elderly. *Ann Intern Med* 1992;117:625–633.
38. Potter J, Stott DJ, Roberts MA, et al. Influenza vaccination of health care workers in long-term-care hospitals reduces the mortality of elderly patients. *J Infect Dis* 1997;175:1–6.
39. Carmen WF, Elder AG, Wallace LA, et al. Effects of influenza vaccination of health-care workers on mortality of elderly people in long-term care: a randomized controlled trial. *Lancet* 2000;355:93–97.
40. Betts RF. Influenza virus. In: Mandell GL, Bennett JE, Dolin R, eds. *Principles and practice of infectious diseases*. New York: Churchill Livingstone, 1995.
41. Moore RA, Wiffen PJ, Lipsky BA. Are the pneumococcal polysaccharide vaccines effective?

Meta-analysis of the prospective trials. *BMC Family Practice* 2000;1:1. http://www.biomedcentral.com/1471–2296/1/1 (last accessed 27 August 2003). Search date 2000; primary sources Cochrane Library, Medline, Embase, and handsearches of reference lists.

42. Rubins JB, Puri AKG, Loch J, et al. Magnitude, duration, quality and function of pneumococcal vaccine responses in elderly adults. *J Infect Dis* 1998;178:431–440.
43. Mbelle N, Wasas A, Huebner R, et al. Immunogenicity and impact on carriage of 9-valent pneumococcal conjugate vaccine given to infants in Soweto, South Africa. *Proceedings of the 37th Interscience Conference on Antimicrobial Agents and Chemotherapy; 1997 September*. Toronto: ASM Press, 1997.
44. Gesner M, Desidero D, Kim M, et al. *Streptococcus pneumoniae* in human immunodeficiency virus type 1 infected children. *Pediatr Infect Dis J* 1994;13:697–703.
45. Nichol KL, Baken L, Wuorenma J, Nelson A. The health and economic benefits associated with pneumococcal vaccination in elderly people with chronic lung disease. *Arch Intern Med* 1999;159:2437–2442.

Mark Loeb
Associate Professor
Departments of Pathology & Molecular Medicine and Clinical Epidemiology & Biostatistics
McMaster University
Hamilton
Canada

Competing interests: The author has received research grants from Bayer and Aventis and has attended conferences sponsored by Janssen Ortho and Aventis.

The following previous contributor of this topic would also like to be acknowledged: Thomas Marrie.

TABLE 1 **Causes of community acquired pneumonia (see text, p 1726).**

	USA (% of participants)*	UK (% of participants)†	Susceptibility (laboratory results)‡
Streptococcus pneumoniae	20–60	60–75	25% penicillin resistant, sensitive to quinolones
Haemophilus influenzae	3–10	4–5	30% ampicillin resistant, sensitive to cephalosporins or co-amoxiclav
Staphylococcus aureus	3–5	1–5	Methicillin resistant *S aureus* rare as cause of community acquired pneumonia
Chlamydia pneumoniae	4–6	ND	Sensitive to macrolides, tetracyclines, quinolones
Mycoplasma pneumoniae	1–6	5–18	Sensitive to macrolides, tetracyclines, quinolones
Legionella pneumophila	2–8	2–5	Sensitive to macrolides, tetracyclines, quinolones
Gram negative bacilli	3–10	Rare	
Aspiration	6–10	ND	
Viruses	2–15	8–16	

*Pooled data from 15 published reports from North America;[7] †data from British Thoracic Society;[7] ‡susceptibility data from recent studies.
ND, no data.

Spontaneous pneumothorax

Search date December 2002

John Cunnington

QUESTIONS

INTERVENTIONS

See glossary, p 1745

Key Messages

- We found insufficient evidence to determine whether any intervention is more effective than no intervention for spontaneous pneumothorax.

Treatment

- **Chest tube drainage** We found no RCTs comparing chest tube drainage versus observation. RCTs provided insufficient evidence to compare chest tube drainage versus needle aspiration.
- **Chest tube drainage plus suction** One small RCT found no significant difference in the rate of resolution whether chest tube drainage bottles were connected to suction or not, but the trial was too small to exclude a clinically important difference.
- **Needle aspiration** RCTs provided insufficient evidence to compare needle aspiration versus observation or chest tube drainage.
- **One way valves on chest tubes versus bottles with underwater seal** One RCT found no significant difference in rates of resolution between one way valves and drainage bottles with underwater seals, but it is likely to have been too small to detect a clinically important difference. It found that people treated with one way valves used less analgesia and spent less time in hospital than people treated with drainage bottles.
- **Small versus standard sized chest tubes** We found no RCTs comparing small versus standard sized chest tubes.

Preventing recurrence

- **Chemical pleurodesis** Two RCTs have found that adding chemical pleurodesis to chest tube drainage reduces the rate of recurrence of spontaneous pneumothorax compared with chest tube drainage alone, but one of the RCTs found that treatment can be painful. The RCTs found no significant difference in length of hospital stay. We found no RCTs comparing chemical versus surgical pleurodesis.
- **Surgical pleurodesis** One RCT found that thoracoscopic surgery with talc instillation reduced the rate of recurrence at 5 years compared with chest tube drainage. Another RCT found that video-assisted thoracoscopic surgery reduced hospital stay compared with thoracotomy. It found no significant difference in the rate of recurrence after 3 years, but the limited evidence cannot exclude a clinically important difference. We found no RCTs comparing surgical versus chemical pleurodesis.
- **Optimal timing of pleurodesis (after first, second, or third spontaneous pneumothorax)** We found no RCTs or good cohort studies assessing whether pleurodesis should take place after the first, second, or subsequent episodes of spontaneous pneumothorax.

DEFINITION A pneumothorax is air in the pleural space. A spontaneous pneumothorax occurs when there is no provoking factor, such as trauma, surgery, or diagnostic intervention. It implies a leak of air from the lung parenchyma through the visceral pleura into the pleural space.

INCIDENCE/ PREVALENCE In a survey in Minnesota, USA, the incidence of spontaneous pneumothorax was 7/100 000 for men and 1/100 000 for women.[1] Smoking increases the likelihood of spontaneous pneumothorax by 22 times for men and eight times for women. A dose–response relationship has been observed.[2]

AETIOLOGY/ RISK FACTORS Spontaneous pneumothorax can be primary (typically in young fit people and thought to be because of a congenital abnormality of the visceral pleura) or secondary (caused by underlying lung disease, typically occurring in older people with emphysema or pulmonary fibrosis).

PROGNOSIS Death from spontaneous pneumothorax is rare. Morbidity with pain and shortness of breath is common. Published recurrence rates vary. One cohort study in Denmark found that, after a first episode of primary spontaneous pneumothorax, 23% of people suffered a recurrence within 5 years, most within 1 year.[3] Recurrence rates had been thought to increase substantially after the first recurrence, but one retrospective case control study (147 military personnel) found that 28% of men with a first spontaneous pneumothorax had a recurrence; 23% of the 28% had a second recurrence; and 14% of that 23% had a third recurrence, giving a total recurrence rate of 35%.[4]

AIMS OF INTERVENTION To reduce morbidity; to restore normal function as quickly as possible; to prevent recurrence and mortality, with minimum adverse effects.

OUTCOMES Successful resolution of spontaneous pneumothorax after a stated period; time to full expansion of the lung; duration of hospital stay; time off work; harmful effects of treatments (pain, surgical emphysema, wound and pleural space infection); and rate of recurrence.

METHODS *Clinical Evidence* search and appraisal December 2002. Most of the literature consisted of uncontrolled case series.

QUESTION **What are the effects of treatments?**

OPTION **NEEDLE ASPIRATION**

RCTs provided insufficient evidence to compare needle aspiration versus observation or chest tube drainage.

Benefits: We found no systematic review. **Versus observation:** We found one RCT (21 people), which found faster resolution with needle aspiration compared with observation (time to full expansion was 3.2 weeks in 10 people with conservative treatment *v* 1.6 weeks in 8 people successfully treated with needle aspiration). However, two people randomised to needle aspiration required a chest tube.[5] The RCT did not assess the significance of the difference between groups. **Versus chest tube drainage:** We found three RCTs.[6–8] The first RCT (73 people) found that fewer people had immediate resolution of pneumothorax with needle aspiration compared with chest tube drainage (28/35 [80%] with needle aspiration *v* 38/38 [100%] with chest tube drainage; time not provided; 7 people initially treated with needle aspiration required subsequent chest tube drainage).[6] It found that, on average, people receiving needle aspiration spent significantly fewer days in hospital than people receiving chest tube drainage (3.2 days with needle aspiration *v* 5.3 days with chest tube drainage; $P = 0.005$).[6] It found no significant difference in the rate of recurrence at 1 year (5/30 [17%] with needle aspiration *v* 10/35 [29%] with chest tube drainage; ARR +12%, 95% CI –9% to +32%; RR 0.58, 95% CI 0.22 to 1.52). The second RCT (61 people) found that, at 24 hours, pneumothorax resolved in significantly fewer people with needle aspiration compared with chest tube drainage (22/33 [67%] with needle aspiration *v* 26/28 [93%] with chest tube drainage; ARR 26%, 95% CI 6% to 47%; RR of failure to resolve 0.72, 95% CI 0.55 to 0.93), but found no significant difference in the rate of recurrence at 3 months (6/33 [18%] with needle aspiration *v* 7/28 [25%] with chest tube drainage; ARR +7%, 95% CI –14% to +28%; RR 0.73, 95% CI 0.28 to 1.92).[7] The RCT was not designed to find a difference in duration of hospital stay because chest tube drainage was done on admission, whereas in most people needle aspiration was performed after 3 days of observation in hospital. The third RCT (60 people) found no significant difference between needle aspiration and chest tube drainage in immediate resolution rates (16/27 [59%] with needle aspiration *v* 21/33 [64%] with chest tube drainage; $P = 0.9$).[8] Resolution was defined for needle aspiration as complete or nearly complete lung expansion after manual aspiration, and for chest tube drainage as complete lung expansion and chest tube removal within 72 hours. It also found no significant difference between needle aspiration and chest tube drainage in mean hospital stay (mean 3.5 days with needle aspiration *v* 4.5 days with chest tube drainage; P = 0.20) or recurrence rate at 1 year (7/26 [26%] with needle aspiration *v* 9/33 [27%] with chest tube drainage; P = 0.9). The RCT is likely to have been too small to detect a clinically important difference in outcomes.

Harms: **Versus observation:** The RCT gave no information on adverse effects.[5] **Versus chest tube drainage:** The first RCT found that people treated with needle aspiration experienced significantly less pain on daily total pain scores during their hospital stay.[6] The second RCT found no significant difference in pain or dyspnoea between needle aspiration and chest tube drainage (reported as non-significant; results presented graphically).[7] The third RCT did not assess pain.[8]

Comment: The RCT of needle aspiration versus observation was published as a letter.[5] The results of this RCT are consistent with a large case series undertaken in the 1960s in which 88/119 (74%) people presenting to an outpatient chest clinic with spontaneous pneumothorax were managed successfully without intervention or hospital admission.[9]

OPTION CHEST TUBE DRAINAGE

We found no RCTs comparing chest tube drainage versus observation. RCTs provided insufficient evidence to compare chest tube drainage versus needle aspiration. We found no RCTs assessing small versus standard size tubes for chest drainage.

Benefits: We found no systematic review. **Versus observation:** We found no RCTs. **Versus needle aspiration:** See benefits of needle aspiration, p 1740. **Versus surgical pleurodesis:** See benefits of surgical pleurodesis, p 1744. **Small versus standard sized chest tubes:** We found no RCTs (see comment below).

Harms: **Versus needle aspiration:** See harms of needle aspiration, p 1741. **Small versus standard sized chest tubes:** We found no RCTs (see comment below).

Comment: **Small versus standard sized chest tubes:** Small gauge chest tubes are usually easier to insert. One non-randomised trial (44 people) compared small gauge (8 French gauge [see glossary, p 1745]) catheters versus standard chest tubes.[10] It found no significant difference in duration of drainage between groups (5 *v* 6 days; reported as non-significant, no further data provided). In people with large pneumothoraces (> 50% lung volume), successful resolution was significantly more likely with standard chest tubes than small gauge catheters (100% with standard tubes *v* 57% with small tubes; $P < 0.05$). No such difference was found in people with small (< 50%) pneumothoraces. The trial found that conventional chest tubes significantly increased the risk of subcutaneous emphysema (9/23 [39%] with conventional tubes *v* 0/21 [0%] with small tubes; $P < 0.05$) and pain compared with small gauge catheters.[10]

Spontaneous pneumothorax

OPTION ONE WAY VALVES ON CHEST TUBES

One RCT found no significant difference in rates of resolution between one way valves and drainage bottles with underwater seals, but it is likely to have been too small to detect a clinically important difference. It found that people treated with one way valves used less analgesia and spent less time in hospital than people treated with drainage bottles.

Benefits: We found no systematic review. We found one RCT (30 people with spontaneous pneumothorax and respiratory distress) comparing a chest tube (13 French gauge [see glossary, p 1745]) connected to a one way valve versus a chest tube (14 French gauge) connected to a drainage bottle with an underwater seal.[11] It found no significant difference in rate of resolution between groups (complete or nearly complete expansion 48 hours after treatment: 15/17 [88%] with one way valve *v* 11/13 [85%] with drainage bottle; ARI +4%, 95% CI –21% to +28%; RR 1.04, 95% CI 0.78 to 1.39), but fewer people treated with a one way valve required analgesia (5/17 [29%] with one way valve *v* 10/13 [77%] with drainage bottle; RR 0.38, 95% CI 0.17 to 0.85).[11] It found that one way valves significantly reduced hospital admissions compared with drainage bottles (5/17 [29%] with one way valve *v* 13/13 [100%] with drainage bottle; RR 0.29, 95% CI 0.14 to 0.61).[11]

Harms: The RCT found no significant difference in rates of complications between one way valves and drainage bottles with underwater seals (need for a second drain: 3/17 [18%] with one way valve *v* 1/13 [8%] with drainage bottle; skin emphysema 3/17 [18%] with one way valve *v* 3/13 [23%] with drainage bottle; reported as non-significant, no further data provided).[11]

Comment: None.

OPTION CHEST TUBE DRAINAGE PLUS SUCTION

One RCT found no significant difference in rate of resolution whether chest tube drainage bottles were connected to suction or not. However, the trial was too small to rule out a clinically important difference.

Benefits: **Versus chest tube drainage alone:** We found no systematic review, but found one RCT (53 people) comparing chest tube drainage using an underwater seal only versus drainage plus suction. Suction pressures ranged from 8–20 cm H_2O.[12] It found no significant difference in the proportion of people with full lung expansion by 10 days (13/23 [57%] with suction *v* 15/30 [50%] without suction; ARI +7%, 95% CI –21% to +34%; RR 1.13, 95% CI 0.68 to 1.88), but is likely to have been too small to exclude a clinically important difference.

Harms: We found no reports of adverse effects because of suction.

Comment: We found one RCT comparing suction versus no suction in 80 people with traumatic pneumothorax but because the mechanism of injury is different, the results could not be extrapolated to spontaneous pneumothorax.[13]

QUESTION **What are the effects of interventions to prevent recurrence?**

OPTION **CHEMICAL PLEURODESIS**

Two RCTs have found that adding chemical pleurodesis to chest tube drainage reduces the rate of recurrence of spontaneous pneumothorax compared with chest tube drainage alone, but one of the RCTs found that treatment can be painful. The RCTs found no significant difference in length of hospital stay. We found no RCTs comparing chemical versus surgical pleurodesis. We found no RCTs or high quality cohort studies assessing whether pleurodesis should be undertaken after the first, second, or subsequent episodes of pneumothorax.

Benefits: We found no systematic review. **Adding chemical pleurodesis to chest tube drainage versus chest tube drainage alone:** We found two RCTs[14,15] and one non-randomised trial (see comment below).[16] The first RCT (unblinded, 229 men with pneumothorax successfully treated by chest tube; mean age 54 years; 55% with chronic obstructive pulmonary disease) found that a chest tube plus intrapleural instillation of tetracycline significantly reduced the recurrence rate over 30 months compared with a chest tube alone (26/104 [25%] with tetracycline *v* 44/108 [41%] with the chest tube alone; ARR 16%, 95% CI 3% to 28%; RR 0.61, 95% CI 0.41 to 0.92). It found no significant difference between groups in length of hospital stay (5 days with tetracycline *v* 7 days with chest tube alone) or 5 year mortality (40/113 [35%] with tetracycline *v* 42/116 [36%] with chest tube alone; RR 0.98, 95% CI 0.62 to 1.38).[14] The second RCT (96 people treated with chest tube drainage) compared three groups: no further treatment, tetracycline pleurodesis, and talc pleurodesis.[15] Mean follow up was 4.6 years. It found that either type of chemical pleurodesis significantly reduced the pneumothorax recurrence rate over 4.6 years compared with no treatment (2/24 [8%] with talc pleurodesis *v* 3/23 [13%] with tetracycline pleurodesis *v* 9/25 [36%] with no treatment; ARR of recurrence with either form of pleurodesis 25%, 95% CI 6% to 45%; RR 0.64, 95% CI 0.12 to 3.48). It found no significant difference in mean hospital stay (mean 7 days with tetracycline *v* 6 days with talc or with chest tube alone; reported as non-significant, no further data provided). **Versus surgical pleurodesis:** We found no RCTs but found one non-randomised prospective study (see comment below).[16] **Optimal timing of pleurodesis:** We found no RCTs or high quality cohort studies comparing pleurodesis undertaken at different times (after the first, second, or subsequent episodes of spontaneous pneumothorax).

Harms: In the first RCT, 61/105 (58%) people reported intense chest pain on injection of tetracycline.[14] The second RCT found that similar proportions of people reported pain with chemical pleurodesis compared with chest tube alone (17/33 [52%] with tetracycline *v* 14/29 [48%] with talc *v* 18/34 [53%] with chest tube; no further data provided).[15] The non-randomised study (see comment below) gave no information on adverse effects.[16]

Comment: We found one non-randomised prospective study (213 people) comparing four interventions: chest tube drainage plus tetracycline pleurodesis (78 people), chest tube drainage alone (66 people), thoracotomy (28 people), and observation (38 people).[16] The mean follow up was 45 months. It found that chest tube drainage plus tetracycline pleurodesis significantly reduced the rate of recurrence compared with chest tube drainage alone or observation (6/66 [9%], excluding 8 treatment failures, 4 lost to follow up with tetracycline pleurodesis *v* 18/51 [36%], excluding 15 lost to follow up with chest tube alone *v* 10/28 [36%], excluding 10 lost to follow up with observation; $P < 0.05$ for both comparisons). It found no significant difference in recurrence rate between tetracycline pleurodesis and thoracotomy (6/66 [9%] with pleurodesis *v* 0/26 [0%], excluding 2 deaths with thoracotomy; $P = 0.13$). It found that tetracycline pleurodesis significantly increased the duration of hospital stay compared with chest tube drainage or observation alone (mean 10 days with tetracycline pleurodesis *v* 4 days with chest tube drainage or observation; $P < 0.01$). The trial provided no data on length of hospital stay with thoracotomy.[16] One observational study suggested that the 5 year recurrence rate after a first pneumothorax is about 28%, so there may be little reason to perform chemical pleurodesis after the first episode of pneumothorax.[4] There has been a consensus that pleurodesis is warranted after the second or third episode of pneumothorax. Even though the probability of success with pleurodesis is high, clinicians will have to weigh the likelihood of recurrence against the morbidity associated with the procedure.

OPTION SURGICAL PLEURODESIS

One RCT found that thoracoscopic surgery with talc instillation reduced the rate of recurrence at 5 years compared with chest tube drainage. Another RCT found that video-assisted thoracoscopic surgery reduced hospital stay compared with thoracotomy. It found no significant difference in the rate of recurrence after 3 years, but the limited evidence cannot exclude a clinically important difference. We found no RCTs comparing surgical versus chemical pleurodesis. We found no RCTs or high quality cohort studies assessing whether pleurodesis should be undertaken after the first, second, or subsequent episodes of pneumothorax.

Benefits: We found no systematic review. **Thoracoscopic surgery with talc instillation versus chest tube drainage:** We found one multicentre RCT (108 people with large primary spontaneous pneumothorax or primary spontaneous pneumothorax that had failed aspiration) that compared thoracoscopic surgery with talc instillation versus chest tube drainage.[17] It found that thoracoscopic surgery significantly reduced the recurrence rate at 5 years compared with chest tube drainage (3/59 [5%] with surgery *v* 16/47 [34%] with chest tube drainage; $P < 0.01$). It found similar length of hospital stay (mean 8.0 days with surgery *v* 7.4 days with drainage; no further data provided). **Video-assisted thoracoscopic surgery:** We found one RCT (60 people with primary spontaneous pneumothorax, either first recurrence or non-resolving first episode) that compared video-assisted thoracoscopic surgery versus thoracotomy.[18] It found that video-assisted surgery significantly reduced the use of analgesia and hospital stay compared with thoracotomy (hospital stay 6.5 days with video-assisted surgery *v* 10.7 days with thoracotomy; $P < 0.0001$). It found no significant difference in the rate of recurrence after 3 years (3/30 [10%] with video-assisted surgery *v* 0/30 [0%] with thoracotomy; ARR +10%, 95% CI −1% to +21%). **Versus chemical pleurodesis:** See benefits of chemical pleurodesis, p 1743. **Optimal timing of pleurodesis:** We found no RCTs or high quality cohort studies comparing surgical pleurodesis undertaken at different times (after the first, second, or subsequent episodes of spontaneous pneumothorax).

Harms: **Thoracoscopic surgery with talc instillation versus chest tube drainage:** The RCT did not establish a protocol for analgesia; four centres gave postoperative systemic opioids and three did not.[17] It found that thoracoscopic surgery modestly but significantly increased pain during the first 3 days compared with chest tube drainage (results presented graphically), but found no significant difference in pain between groups when people received systemic opioids.[17] **Versus chemical pleurodesis:** See harms of chemical pleurodesis, p 1743. **Video-assisted thoracoscopic surgery:** The RCT gave no information on adverse effects.[18]

Comment: The RCT comparing thoracoscopic surgery versus thoracotomy was too small to exclude a clinically important difference in recurrence rate.[18] One observational study suggested that the 5 year recurrence rate after a first pneumothorax is about 28%, so there may be little reason to perform pleurodesis after the first episode of pneumothorax.[4] There has been a consensus that surgical pleurodesis is warranted after the second or third episode of pneumothorax. Even though the probability of success with pleurodesis is high, clinicians will have to weigh the likelihood of recurrence against the morbidity associated with the procedure.

GLOSSARY

French gauge A measure of the size of a catheter or drainage tube defined (in France by JFB Charrière in 1842) to be the outside diameter of the tube in units of 1/3 mm. A 12 French gauge tube has an outer diameter of 4 mm. Sometimes the French gauge is called the Charrière (Ch) gauge.

Substantive changes

Needle aspiration One RCT added;[8] conclusions unchanged.

Surgical pleurodesis One RCT found that thoracoscopic surgery with talc instillation reduced the recurrence rate at 5 years compared with chest tube drainage.[17]

REFERENCES

1. Melton LJ, Hepper NG, Offord KP. Incidence of spontaneous pneumothorax in Olmsted County, Minnesota: 1950–1974. *Am Rev Respir Dis* 1979;120:1379–1382.
2. Bense L, Eklung G, Wiman LG. Smoking and the increased risk of contracting spontaneous pneumothorax. *Chest* 1987;92:1009–1012.
3. Lippert HL, Lund O, Blegvad S, et al. Independent risk factors for cumulative recurrence rate after first spontaneous pneumothorax. *Eur Respir J* 1991;4:324–331.
4. Voge VM, Anthracite R. Spontaneous pneumothorax in the USAF aircrew population: a retrospective study. *Aviat Space Environ Med* 1986;57:939–949.
5. Flint K, Al-Hillawi AH, Johnson NM. Conservative management of spontaneous pneumothorax. *Lancet* 1984;1:687–688.
6. Harvey J, Prescott RJ. Simple aspiration versus intercostal tube drainage for spontaneous pneumothorax in patients with normal lungs. British Thoracic Society Research Committee. *BMJ* 1994;309:1338–1339.

7. Andrivet P, Djedaini K, Teboul JL, et al. Spontaneous pneumothorax. Comparison of thoracic drainage vs immediate or delayed needle aspiration. *Chest* 1995;108:335–339.
8. Noppen M, Alexander P, Driesen P, et al. Manual aspiration versus chest tube drainage in first episodes of primary spontaneous pneumothorax: a multicenter, prospective, randomized pilot study. *Am J Respir Crit Care Med* 2002;165:1240–1244.
9. Stradling P, Poole G. Conservative management of spontaneous pneumothorax. *Thorax* 1966;21:145–149.
10. Kang YJ, Koh HG, Shin JW, et al. The effect of 8 French catheter and chest tube on the treatment of spontaneous pneumothorax. *Tuber Respir Dis* 1996;43:410–419.
11. Roggla M, Wagner A, Brunner C, et al. The management of pneumothorax with the thoracic vent versus conventional intercostal tube drainage. *Wien Klin Wochenschr* 1996;108:330–333.
12. So SY, Yu DYC. Catheter drainage of spontaneous pneumothorax: suction or no suction, early or late removal? *Thorax* 1982;37:46–48.
13. Davis JW, Mackersie RC, Hoyt DB, et al. Randomized study of algorithms for discontinuing tube thoracostomy drainage. *J Am Coll Surg* 1994;179:553–557.
14. Light RW, O'Hara VS, Moritz TE, et al. Intrapleural tetracycline for the prevention of recurrent spontaneous pneumothorax. Results of a Department of Veterans Affairs cooperative study. *JAMA* 1990;264:2224–2230.
15. Almind M, Lange P, Viskum K. Spontaneous pneumothorax: comparison of simple drainage, talc pleurodesis, and tetracycline pleurodesis. *Thorax* 1989;44:627–630.
16. Alfageme I, Moreno L, Huertas C, et al. Spontaneous pneumothorax. Long-term results with tetracycline pleurodesis. *Chest* 1994;106:347–350.
17. Tschopp J-M, Boutin C, Astoul P, et al. Talcage by medical thoracoscopy for primary spontaneous pneumothorax is more cost-effective than drainage: a randomised study. *Eur Respir J* 2002;20:1003–1009.
18. Ayed AK, Al-Din HJ. Video-assisted thoracoscopy versus thoracotomy for primary spontaneous pneumothorax: a randomized controlled trial. *Med Principles Pract* 2000;9:113–118.

John Cunnington
Associate Professor Medicine
McMaster University
Hamilton, Ontario
Canada

Competing interests: None declared.

Upper respiratory tract infection

Search date February 2003

Chris Del Mar and Paul Glasziou

QUESTIONS

INTERVENTIONS

Key Messages

- **Analgesia/anti-inflammatory drugs for symptom relief** One systematic review has found that analgesics or anti-inflammatory drugs reduce sore throat at 1–5 days compared with placebo.
- **Antibiotics for preventing (rare) complications of β haemolytic streptococcal pharyngitis** One systematic review has found that antibiotics prevent non-suppurative complications of β haemolytic streptococcal pharyngitis compared with no antibiotics, but in industrialised countries such complications are rare.
- **Antibiotics for reducing time to recovery in people with proven infection with *Haemophilus influenzae, Moraxella catarrhalis*, or *Streptococcus pneumoniae*** In a minority of people, upper respiratory tract infection is found to be caused by *H influenzae*, *M catarrhalis*, or *S pneumoniae*. One RCT found that, in these people, antibiotics increased recovery at 5 days compared with placebo. However, we have no methods currently of easily identifying this subgroup at first consultation.
- **Antihistamines for runny nose and sneezing** One systematic review has found that antihistamines reduce runny nose and sneezing after 2 days compared with placebo, but the clinical benefit is small.

- **Decongestants for short term relief of congestive symptoms** One systematic review found that a single dose of decongestant reduced nasal congestion over 3–10 hours compared with placebo.
- **Vitamin C** One systematic review found that vitamin C slightly reduced the duration of cold symptoms compared with placebo, but the benefit was small and may be explained by publication bias.
- **Antibiotics for reducing time to recovery in people with acute sore throat** One systematic review has found that antibiotics slightly improve symptoms at 6–8 days compared with placebo. Adverse effects (nausea, vomiting, headache, rash, vaginitis) were more common with antibiotics.
- **Echinacea for prevention** One systematic review found that, compared with no treatment, echinacea reduced the proportion of people who had one infection episode, but found insufficient evidence about the effects of echinacea compared with placebo.
- **Echinacea for treatment** Systematic reviews found limited evidence that some preparations of echinacea may improve symptoms compared with placebo, but we found insufficient evidence about the effects of any specific product.
- **Steam inhalation** One systematic review found insufficient evidence about the effects of steam inhalation.
- **Zinc (intranasal gel or lozenges)** Two RCTs found that zinc intranasal gel reduced the mean duration of cold symptoms compared with placebo, but the difference was significant in only one of the RCTs. Two systematic reviews found limited evidence that zinc gluconate or acetate lozenges may reduce duration of symptoms at 7 days, compared with placebo.
- **Antibiotics in people with colds** Systematic reviews found no significant difference between antibiotics and placebo in cure or general improvement at 6–14 days.
- **Decongestants for long term relief of congestive symptoms** One systematic review found insufficient evidence to assess the effects of longer use of decongestants. One case control study found weak evidence that phenylpropanolamine may increase the risk of haemorrhagic stroke.

DEFINITION Upper respiratory tract infection involves inflammation of the respiratory mucosa from the nose to the lower respiratory tree, but not including the alveoli. In addition to malaise, it causes localised symptoms that constitute several overlapping syndromes: sore throat (pharyngitis), rhinorrhoea (common cold), facial fullness and pain (sinusitis — see acute sinusitis, p 567), and cough (bronchitis — see acute broncitis, p 1716).

INCIDENCE/ PREVALENCE Upper respiratory tract infections, nasal congestion, throat complaints, and cough are responsible for 11% of general practice consultations in Australia.[1] Each year, children suffer about five such infections and adults two to three infections.[1–3]

AETIOLOGY/ RISK FACTORS Infective agents include over 200 viruses (with 100 rhinoviruses) and several bacteria. Transmission is mostly through hand to hand contact with subsequent passage to the nostrils or eyes rather than, as commonly perceived, through droplets in the air.[4] A systematic review of the risk factors for developing prolonged illness (especially tiredness) after infectious mononucleosis of five cohort studies of 531 adults showed that this occurred in 2–56% of people. The best predictor for tiredness was poor physical functioning immediately after the start of the illness; previous psychological factors were identified as unimportant in four studies and predictive in one.[5]

PROGNOSIS Upper respiratory tract infections are usually self limiting. Although they cause little mortality or serious morbidity, upper respiratory tract infections are responsible for considerable discomfort, lost work, and medical costs. Clinical patterns vary and overlap between infective agents. In addition to nasal symptoms, half of sufferers experience sore throat and 40% experience cough. Symptoms peak within 1–3 days and generally clear by 1 week, although cough often persists.[4]

AIMS OF INTERVENTION To relieve symptoms and to prevent suppurative and non-suppurative complications of bacterial infection, with minimal adverse effects from treatments.

OUTCOMES Cure rate; duration of symptoms; incidence of complications; incidence of adverse effects of treatment.

METHODS *Clinical Evidence* search and appraisal February 2003. We have excluded RCTs undertaken solely in people with experimentally induced upper respiratory tract infections.

QUESTION What are the effects of treatments?

OPTION ANTIBIOTICS

Systematic reviews found no significant difference between antibiotics and placebo in cure or general improvement at 6–14 days in people with colds. One additional RCT has found that, in people with proven infection with *H influenzae*, *M catarrhalis*, or *S pneumoniae* antibiotics versus placebo increases recovery at 5 days. However, we have no methods currently of easily identifying such people at first consultation. One systematic review has found that antibiotics slightly improve symptoms of sore throat at 6–8 days compared with placebo. One systematic review has found that antibiotics prevent non-suppurative complications of β haemolytic streptococcal pharyngitis compared with no antibiotics, but in industrialised countries such complications are rare. Adverse effects (nausea, vomiting, headache, rash, vaginitis) were more common with antibiotics.

Benefits: **Colds:** We found two systematic reviews.[6,7] The first review (search date 2001, 9 RCTs, 2249 people aged 2 months to 79 years with acute upper respiratory infections without complications [naturally acquired colds]) found no significant difference between antibiotics and placebo in general improvement or cure at 7 days (6 RCTs, 168/664 [25%] with antibiotics *v* 170/483 [35%] with placebo; RR 0.89, 95% CI 0.77 to 1.04).[6] The second review (search date not stated, 12 RCTs, 1699 children with naturally acquired upper respiratory tract symptoms in the previous 2 weeks) found no significant difference between antibiotics and placebo in the proportion of children with worse or unchanged clinical outcome at 6–14 days (6 RCTs with adequate data; 309/835 [37%] with antibiotics *v* 280/647 [43%] with placebo; RR 1.01, 95% CI 0.90 to

1.13; raw figures reported from table in paper), or with complications or progression (5 RCTs; 38/549 [6.9%] with antibiotics *v* 28/293 [9.5%] with placebo; RR 0.71, 95% CI 0.45 to 1.12).[7] One additional RCT (314 adults with naturally acquired colds for 1–30 days; < 7 days in 85% of people) comparing amoxicillin/clavulanic acid (co-amoxiclav) (375 mg 3 times daily) versus placebo found no overall difference in "cure" rates at 5 days (P value not reported).[8] However, it found that in the 61 people (20%) with positive sputum cultures for *H influenzae*, *M catarrhalis*, or *S pneumoniae* there was a significant difference in recovery at 5 days (27% with co-amoxiclav *v* 4% with placebo; P = 0.001). If such people could be identified at first consultation, then treating four of these people with antibiotic rather than placebo would result in an average of one more recovery at 5 days (NNT 4; CI not reported). However, we have no methods currently of easily identifying these people at first consultation. **Sore throat:** We found one systematic review (search date 1999, 25 randomised or quasi-randomised trials, 10 863 people with sore throat).[9] It found that, compared with placebo, antibiotics slightly but significantly reduced the proportion of people with symptoms of sore throat at 6–8 days (11 trials; 226/1739 [13%] with antibiotics *v* 199/1079 [18%] with placebo; RR 0.61, 95% CI 0.52 to 0.73), and shortened symptom duration by a mean of about 24 hours at day 3 and 16 hours at 1 week. It found that antibiotics significantly reduced the proportion of people who had developed rheumatic fever at 2 months compared with placebo (7 trials; 37/5287 [0.7%] with antibiotics *v* 74/4059 [1.8%] with placebo; RR 0.29, 95% CI 0.18 to 0.44). It also found that antibiotics significantly reduced otitis media at 14 days (5 trials; 11/2325 [0.5%] with antibiotics *v* 28/1435 [2.0%] with placebo; RR 0.26, 95% CI 0.14 to 0.49) and quincy at 2 months (6 trials; 2/1438 [0.1%] with antibiotics *v* 23/995 [2.3%] with placebo; RR 0.14, 95% CI 0.05 to 0.39). It found too few events to detect any possible protective effect of antibiotics against acute glomerulonephritis (0/2558 [0%] with antibiotics *v* 2/1834 [0.1%] with placebo).

Harms: Adverse effects such as nausea, vomiting, headache, rash, or vaginitis were more common in people taking antibiotics than placebo. For example, one review of antibiotics in people with bronchitis found one extra adverse effect for every 16 people treated.[10] We found no evidence of the size of the risk of antibiotic resistance or pseudomembranous colitis.

Comment: Because most upper respiratory tract infections are viral, the potential benefit from antibiotics is limited. Until rapid identification of those people likely to benefit is possible, the modest effects seen in trials must be weighed against the adverse effects of antibiotics, costs, and potential for inducing antibiotic resistance.

OPTION VITAMIN C

One systematic review found that vitamin C slightly reduced the duration of cold symptoms compared with placebo. However, the beneficial effect is small and may be explained by publication bias.

Benefits: We found one systematic review (search date not stated, 13 RCTs, 17 quasi-randomised or controlled trials identified by two previous systematic reviews[11,12]) that compared vitamin C 1 g or more daily versus placebo for naturally acquired colds.[13] It found that vitamin C reduced the duration of symptoms by about half a day compared with placebo (17 trials; 9365 people; WMD 0.44 days/cold episode, 95% CI 0.23 days/cold episode to 0.64 days/cold episode) representing about 15% fewer symptomatic days per episode.

Harms: The systematic review found no adverse effects associated with vitamin C.[13]

Comment: The beneficial effect reported in the review was small and might be explained by publication bias.

OPTION ZINC

Two systematic reviews found limited evidence that zinc gluconate or acetate lozenges may reduce duration of symptoms at 7 days compared with placebo. Two RCTs found that zinc intranasal gel reduced the mean duration of cold symptoms compared with placebo, but the difference was significant in only one of the RCTs.

Benefits: **Zinc lozenges:** We found two systematic reviews (search date 1997, 7 RCTs;[14] search date 1998, 8 RCTs[15]) comparing zinc lozenges (gluconate or acetate) versus placebo for the treatment of naturally acquired colds. The reviews had different inclusion criteria. Both reviews found that symptoms were unchanged at 3 and 5 days. At 7 days, the first review (7 RCTs, including 2 RCTs excluded from the second review because they were in people with experimentally induced colds, 754 people) found that zinc lozenges significantly reduced continuing symptoms at 7 days compared with placebo (random effects model; 14/93 [15%] with zinc *v* 46/94 [49%] with placebo; RR 0.31, 95% CI 0.18 to 0.52). However, the second review (8 RCTs, including 3 RCTs included in the first review and 1 RCT excluded from the first review on methodological grounds) found no significant difference between zinc lozenges and placebo in continuing symptoms at 7 days (OR 0.52, 95% CI 0.25 to 1.20; results presented graphically). The results at 7 days were statistically heterogeneous, which may be because the RCTs retrieved by the reviews used different zinc formulations; were undertaken in people with different types of virus; or because of other unknown factors. **Zinc intranasal gel:** We found two RCTs comparing intranasal zinc versus placebo.[16,17] The first RCT (213 people with naturally acquired colds of < 24 hours' duration) found that intranasal zinc significantly reduced overall symptom duration compared with placebo (mean duration 2.3 days with intranasal zinc *v* 9.0 days with placebo; $P < 0.05$).[16] The second RCT (160 people with naturally acquired colds of < 24 hours' duration) found no significant difference in overall symptom duration between intranasal zinc and placebo (mean duration 7 days for each group; $P = 0.45$).[17]

Harms: **Zinc lozenges:** The first review stated that, in some of the RCTs, a higher proportion of people had nausea, altered taste, dry mouth, abdominal pain, and headache with zinc lozenges than with placebo, but did not state whether the difference was significant.[14] The second review gave no information on adverse effects.[15] **Zinc intranasal gel:** The first RCT found that a similar proportion of people experienced a tingling or burning sensation with zinc intranasal gel compared with placebo (45/108 [42%] with zinc *v* 39/105 [37%] with placebo).[16] The second RCT found a similar proportion of people had adverse effects, including nausea, mouth or nasal irritation, abdominal pain, or headache with zinc intranasal gel compared with placebo (any adverse effect; 41/81 [51%] with zinc *v* 40/78 [52%] with placebo).[17]

Comment: None.

OPTION ECHINACEA

Systematic reviews found that some preparations of echinacea may be better than placebo or no treatment for cold treatment and prevention.

Benefits: **Treatment:** We found two systematic reviews (search date 1998, 8 RCTs;[18] search date 2000, 5 additional RCTs[19]) comparing echinacea versus placebo for naturally acquired upper respiratory tract infections. All RCTs included in the first review were double blind except one that was single blind.[18] Quantitative results could be extracted for only two RCTs on duration of illness, three RCTs for runny nose, and five RCTs for a summary symptom score. Results were not combined because of trial heterogeneity. All RCTs compared echinacea versus placebo, and one RCT also compared high versus low dose echinacea. Five RCTs found that echinacea significantly improved symptoms compared with placebo. One RCT found significant results for a subgroup only, and two RCTs found similar improvements in symptoms after treatment with echinacea compared with placebo.[18] The second review identified five further RCTs published after 1997. It also found that RCTs were heterogeneous and of poor quality and it reached the same conclusions as the first review.[19] **Prevention:** The first systematic review identified eight RCTs, with a total of almost 4000 people.[18] The placebo controlled RCTs varied considerably in quality of methods and preparation used, so results were not combined. Of the five placebo controlled RCTs, two found that echinacea significantly reduced the proportion of people who had at least one infection episode compared with placebo. One of these had large loss to follow up. The other placebo controlled RCTs found a non-significant reduction in the rate of infection. Meta-analysis of the three RCTs comparing echinacea versus no treatment found that significantly fewer people had one infection episode after taking echinacea (167/571 [29%] with echinacea *v* 292/566 [52%] with no treatment; RR 0.56, 95% CI 0.48 to 0.65). The three uncontrolled studies identified by the review all found a significant benefit.

Harms: Three of the eight treatment RCTs and four of the eight prevention RCTs reported adverse events. These were generally infrequent and not significantly different between echinacea and placebo. However, outside the trials, anaphylaxis has been reported with echinacea.[20]

Comment: Echinacea is not a single product. There are more than 200 different preparations based on different plants, different parts of the plant (roots, herbs, whole plant), and different methods of extraction. None of the trials were published in a Medline listed journal. The weakness of trial methods and differences in interventions make it difficult to draw conclusions about effectiveness. Large RCTs may be difficult because echinacea is not patentable and each producer controls a small share of the market. The authors of the systematic review received personal information about several unpublished studies that they were not able to include.

OPTION STEAM INHALATION

One systematic review found insufficient evidence about the effects of steam inhalation.

Benefits: We found one systematic review (search date 1999, 4 RCTs in people with naturally acquired colds, 2 RCTs in people with experimentally induced colds, 319 people) comparing steam inhalation at 40–47 °C versus sham inhalation (air at ≥30 °C).[21] The review could not perform a meta-analysis of all of the RCTs because of heterogeneity in populations, methods used to assess symptoms, and poor reporting in some of the RCTs. Pooling of data from two RCTs (146 people with naturally acquired colds) found limited evidence that steam inhalation significantly reduced the proportion of people with symptoms at the end of treatment compared with sham inhalation (29/77 [38%] with steam *v* 46/69 [68%] with control; RR 0.56, 95% CI 0.40 to 0.79). Another RCT that used a different method of assessing symptoms found no significant difference between steam inhalation and control in the proportion of people with improved symptoms at the end of treatment (no improvement in symptom score 23/45 [51%] with steam *v* 26/39 [67%] with control; RR 0.77, 95% CI 0.53 to 1.10), but may have been too small to exclude a clinically important difference.[21]

Harms: The RCTs identified by the review found no evidence of harms.[21] There may be a danger from spilling hot water and from nosocomial infections related to humidifier units.

Comment: None.

OPTION DECONGESTANTS

One systematic review found that, compared with placebo, decongestants reduced nasal congestion over 3–10 hours after a single dose, but found insufficient evidence to assess the effects of longer use of decongestants. One case control study found weak evidence that phenylpropanolamine may increase the risk of haemorrhagic stroke.

Benefits: We found one systematic review (search date 1999, 4 RCTs, 246 adults with naturally acquired colds).[22] It found that, compared with placebo, a single dose of nasal decongestant was moderately effective for the relief of nasal congestion over 3–10 hours (2 RCTs, 155 adults; WMD –0.12, 95% CI –0.19 to –0.16). It found no good evidence on the effects of repeated use over several days.

Harms: Information about harms was not sought actively or reported in the RCTs identified by the review.[22] One case control study compared the use of cold preparations containing phenylpropanolamine among 702 people with a history of haemorrhagic stroke versus 1376 control people with no history of stroke. The study found a non-significant trend towards increased haemorrhage stroke with phenylpropanolamine (RR 1.50, 95% CI 0.85 to 2.65).[23] However, the study was too small to make definitive conclusions.

Comment: The review found no RCTs in children.

OPTION ANTIHISTAMINES

One systematic review has found that antihistamines reduce runny nose and sneezing after 2 days compared with placebo, but the clinical benefit is small.

Benefits: One systematic review of previously unpublished individual patient data (search date not stated, 7 RCTs in adults with naturally acquired colds, 2 RCTs in adults with experimentally induced colds, 1757 adults) comparing antihistamines versus placebo found that antihistamines reduced the symptoms of runny nose and sneezing for the first 2 days of colds.[24] The effects were small. On a severity scale ranging from 0 (no symptoms) to 3 or 4 (severe symptoms), antihistamines reduced the score by about 0.25 (95% CI 0.10 to 0.40; results presented graphically) for runny nose on days 1 and 2, 0.15 (95% CI 0 to 0.30) for sneezing on day 1, and 0.30 (95% CI 0.15 to 0.45) for sneezing on day 2.

Harms: Harms were not actively looked for in RCTs,[24] but known harms of antihistamines include drowsiness and dry mouth.

Comment: None.

OPTION ANALGESICS OR ANTI-INFLAMMATORY DRUGS

One systematic review has found that analgesics or anti-inflammatory drugs reduce sore throat at 1–5 days compared with placebo.

Benefits: **Sore throat:** We found one systematic review (search date 1999, 12 RCTs of non-steroidal anti-inflammatory drugs [NSAIDs], 3 of paracetamol, 1 of steroids).[25] The RCTs found that all interventions were superior to placebo. Six RCTs (493 people) assessed the effects of NSAIDs only over 24 hours or less. The RCTs found consistently that NSAIDs reduced throat pain. Five RCTs (646 people) assessed the effects of NSAIDs over more than 24 hours. All of the RCTs found a significant reduction in symptoms over 2–5 days with NSAIDs versus placebo ($P < 0.05$ in all RCTs). Two RCTs (158 people) assessed the effects of paracetamol over 24 hours or less. One of these RCTs found a significant reduction in throat pain at 6 hours; the other found no significant difference. One RCT (154 people) assessed the effects of paracetamol over 2 days. It found a significant reduction in sore throat symptoms after 2 days ($P < 0.01$). One RCT comparing corticosteroid injection (dexamethasone 10 mg) versus placebo over 24 hours found a significant reduction in mean throat pain at 24 hours ($P < 0.05$). One RCT (243 adults in a 4 arm RCT) found short term benefits of NSAIDs in people with sore throat treated with flurbiprofen lozenges (3 different strengths: 0.5, 2.5, and 12.5 mg) compared with placebo.[26] Symptom relief scores improved with increasing strength of NSAID.

Harms: NSAIDs may increase the risk of gastrointestinal haemorrhage. One systematic review (search date not stated, 100 RCTs, 12 853 people) found a non-significant tendency towards a higher rate of haemorrhage (ARI for NSAIDs *v* placebo +0.7%, 95% CI –0.1% to +1.5%) and proved ulcer (ARI for NSAIDs *v* placebo +0.05%, 95% CI –0.01% to +0.11%) with NSAIDs compared with placebo (see non-steroidal anti-inflammatory drugs, p 1393).

Comment: None.

Substantive changes

Analgesics or anti-inflammatory drugs One new RCT;[26] conclusions unchanged.

REFERENCES

1. Fry J, Sandler G. *Common diseases. Their nature prevalence and care.* Dordrecht, The Netherlands: Kluwer Academic, 1993.
2. Tupasi TE, de Leon LE, Lupisan S, et al. Patterns of acute respiratory tract infection in children: a longitudinal study in a depressed community in Metro Manila. *Rev Infect Dis* 1990;12:S940–S949.
3. Cruz JR, Pareja G, de Fernandez A, et al. Epidemiology of acute respiratory tract infections among Guatemalan ambulatory preschool children. *Rev Infect Dis* 1990;12:1029S–1034S.
4. Lauber B. The common cold. *J Gen Intern Med* 1996;11:229–236.
5. Candy B, Chalder T, Cleare AJ, et al. Recovery from infectious mononucleosis: a case for more than symptomatic therapy? A systematic review. *Br J Gen Pract* 2002;52:844–851.
6. Arroll B, Kenealy T. Antibiotics for the common cold. In: The Cochrane Library, Issue 2, 2002. Oxford: Update Software. Search date 2001; primary sources Cochrane Controlled Trials Register, Medline, Embase, Family Medicine Database, reference lists in articles, and principal investigators.
7. Fahey T, Stocks N, Thomas T. Systematic review of the treatment of upper respiratory tract infection. *Arch Dis Child* 1998;79:225–230. Search date not stated; primary sources Medline, Embase, Science Citation Index, Cochrane Controlled Trials Register, authors of published RCTs, drug manufacturers, and hand searches of references.
8. Kaiser L, Lew D, Hirschel B, et al. Effects of antibiotic treatment in the subset of common-cold patients who have bacteria in nasopharyngeal secretions. *Lancet* 1996;347:1507–1510.
9. Del Mar CB, Glasziou PP, Spinks AB. Antibiotics for sore throat. In: The Cochrane Library, Issue 2, 2002. Oxford: Update Software. Search date 1999; primary sources Medline, Cochrane Library, and hand searches of reference lists of relevant articles.
10. Smucny J, Fahey T, Becker L, et al. Antibiotics for acute bronchitis. In: The Cochrane Library, Issue 2, 2002. Oxford: Update Software. Search date 2000; primary sources Medline, Embase, Science Citation Index, hand searches of reference lists of relevant trials, textbooks, and review articles.
11. Kleijnen J, Ter Riet G, Knipschild PG. Vitamin C and the common cold; review of a megadoses literature [in Dutch]. *Ned Tijdschr Geneeskd* 1989;133:1532–1535. Search date 1998; primary sources Medline and hand searches of references.
12. Hemila H. Vitamin C and the common cold. *Br J Nutr* 1992;67:3–16. Search date and primary sources not stated.
13. Douglas RM, Chalker EB, Treacy B. Vitamin C for preventing and treating the common cold. In: The Cochrane Library, Issue 2, 2002. Oxford: Update Software. Search date not stated; primary sources reviews by Kleinjen et al.[14] and Hemila.[15]
14. Marshall I. Zinc in the treatment of the common cold. In: The Cochrane Library, Issue 2, 2002. Oxford: Update Software. Search date 1997; primary sources Medline, Embase, the Cochrane Library, and hand searches of journals.
15. Jackson JL, Lesho E, Peterson C. Zinc and the common cold: a meta-analysis revisited. *J Nutrition* 2000;130(Suppl):1512S–1515S. Search date 1998; primary sources Medline, National Institute of Health database of funded studies, the Cochrane Randomised Clinical Trial database, and relevant papers.
16. Hirt M, Nobel S, Barron E. Zinc nasal gel for the treatment of common cold symptoms: a double-blind, placebo-controlled trial. *Ear Nose Throat J* 2000;79:778–782.
17. Belongia EA, Berg R, Liu K. A randomized trial of zinc nasal spray for the treatment of upper respiratory illness in adults. *Am J Med* 2001;111:103–108.
18. Melchart D, Linde K, Fischer P, et al. Echinacea for the prevention and treatment of the common cold. In: The Cochrane Library, Issue 2, 2002. Oxford: Update Software. Search date 1998; primary sources Medline, Embase, database of the Cochrane Acute Respiratory Infections Group, database of the Cochrane Field Complementary Medicine, Phytodok, bibliographies of existing reviews, and personal communications.
19. Giles JT, Palat CT III, Chien SH, et al. Evaluation of echinacea for treatment of the common cold. *Pharmacotherapy* 2000;20:690–697. Search date 2000; primary sources Medline, International Pharmaceutical Abstracts, Cambridge Scientific Abstracts Biological Sciences, Alt-Health Watch, Embase, and references from published articles.
20. Mullins RJ. Echinacea associated anaphylaxis. *Med J Aust* 1998;168:170–171.
21. Singh M. Heated, humidified air for the common cold. In: The Cochrane Library, Issue 2, 2002. Oxford: Update Software. Search date 1999; primary sources Medline, Embase, Current Contents, hand searches of review articles and reference lists, and contact with manufacturers.
22. Taverner D, Bickford L, Draper M. Nasal decongestants for the common cold. In: The Cochrane Library, Issue 2, 2002. Oxford: Update Software. Search date 1999; primary sources Medline, Embase, Current Contents, Cochrane Acute Respiratory Infectious Group's trials register, hand searches of reference lists, and personal contacts with known investigators and pharmaceutical companies.

23. Kernan WN, Viscoli CM, Brass LM, et al. Phenylpropanolamine and the risk of hemorrhagic stroke. *N Engl J Med* 2000;343:1826–1832.
24. D'Agostino RB Sr, Weintraub M, Russell HK, et al. The effectiveness of antihistamines in reducing the severity of runny nose and sneezing: a meta-analysis. *Clin Pharmacol Ther* 1998;64:579–596. Search date not stated; primary sources Medline and FDA unpublished clinical trials.
25. Thomas M, Del Mar C, Glaziou P. How effective are treatments other than antibiotics for acute sore throat? *Br J Gen Pract* 2000;50:817–820. Search date 1999; primary sources Medline and Cochrane Controlled Trials Registry.
26. Schachtel BP, Homan HD, Gibb IA, et al. Demonstration of dose response of flurbiprofen lozenges with the sore throat pain model. *Clin Pharmacol Ther* 2002;71:375–380.

Chris Del Mar
Professor of General Practice

Paul Glasziou
Director: Centre for Evidence-based Practice

Oxford University
Oxford
UK

Competing interests: None declared.

Asthma

Search date September 2002

J Mark FitzGerald and Bazian Ltd

QUESTIONS

INTERVENTIONS

To be covered in future updates

Allergen avoidance

Oral β_2 agonists

Theophyllines

Covered elsewhere in *Clinical Evidence*

Asthma and other wheezing disorders of childhood, p 314

*Categorisation based on consensus. RCTs are unlikely to be conducted.

See glossary, p 1776

Key Messages

In people with chronic asthma

- **Adding inhaled long acting β_2 agonists to inhaled corticosteroids in poorly controlled mild to moderate, persistent asthma (for symptom control)** RCTs have found that, in people with asthma that is poorly controlled with inhaled corticosteroids, adding regular long acting inhaled β_2 agonists significantly improves symptoms and lung function compared with adding placebo or a leukotriene antagonist. One systematic review and one additional RCT have found that adding regular doses of long acting inhaled β_2 agonists significantly improves lung function and symptoms and reduces rescue medication compared with increasing the dose of inhaled corticosteroids. However, one further RCT found that increasing inhaled corticosteroid dose reduced exacerbations compared with adding long acting inhaled β_2 agonists.
- **Adding leukotriene antagonists in people with mild to moderate, persistent asthma (*v* no added treatment)** RCTs in people taking β_2 agonists alone have found that leukotriene antagonists versus placebo significantly reduce asthma symptoms and β_2 agonist use. One systematic review and subsequent RCTs have found that adding leukotriene antagonists increased exacerbations, reduced lung function, and were less effective for symptom control compared with inhaled corticosteroids. Two RCTs have found that an inhaled corticosteroid plus a long acting β_2 agonist significantly improved symptoms, lung function, and exacerbations compared with a leukotriene antagonist at 12 weeks.
- **Adding leukotriene antagonists plus inhaled corticosteroids in people with mild to moderate, persistent asthma** One systematic review in people taking inhaled corticosteroids found no significant difference between leukotriene antagonists and placebo for exacerbation rates at 4–16 weeks. We found limited evidence from two RCTs that, in people with asthma that is poorly controlled with inhaled corticosteroids, adding a leukotriene antagonist was less effective for symptoms and lung function compared with adding a long acting β_2 agonist.
- **Inhaled short acting β_2 agonists as needed for symptom relief (as effective as regular use) in mild to moderate, persistent asthma** One systematic review and one subsequent RCT have found no significant difference between regular and as needed inhaled short acting β_2 agonists for clinically important outcomes.
- **Low dose, inhaled corticosteroids in mild, persistent asthma** Systematic reviews and RCTs have found that, in people with mild, persistent asthma, low doses of inhaled corticosteroids significantly improve symptoms and lung function compared with placebo or regular inhaled β_2 agonists.

In people with acute exacerbations of asthma

- **Continuous versus intermittent nebulised short acting β_2 agonists for acute asthma** One systematic review and one RCT have found no significant difference between continuous and intermittent nebulised short acting β_2 agonists for hospital admission rates in adults.
- **Education about acute asthma** One systematic review and one subsequent RCT found that education to facilitate self management of asthma in adults versus usual care significantly reduced hospital admission, unscheduled visits to the doctor, and days off work. However, a second subsequent RCT found no significant effect of asthma education for quality of life or social functioning at 6 months.

- **Helium–oxygen mixture for acute asthma** One systematic review found no significant difference for helium–oxygen mixture versus air or oxygen in pulmonary function tests at 60 minutes in adults and children with acute asthma.
- **Inhaled corticosteroids for acute asthma (better than placebo)** One systematic review has found that inhaled corticosteroids versus placebo given in the emergency department significantly reduces hospital admission rates in adults. One systematic review found no significant difference in relapse rates for oral versus inhaled steroids at 7–10 days.
- **Inhaled plus oral corticosteroids for acute asthma (as effective as oral corticosteroid alone)** One systematic review found no significant difference in relapse rates for inhaled plus oral corticosteroid versus oral corticosteroids up to 24 days.
- **Intravenous versus nebulised delivery of short acting β_2 agonists for acute asthma** One systematic review found that intravenous delivery of short acting β_2 agonists was no more effective than nebulised delivery in improving peak expiratory flow rate at 60 minutes.
- **Ipratropium bromide added to β_2 agonists for acute exacerbations** Two systematic reviews and one subsequent RCT have found that ipratropium bromide plus salbutamol versus salbutamol alone improves lung function and is likely to reduce hospital admission in people with severe acute asthma.
- **Magnesium sulphate for people with severe acute asthma** One systematic review and three subsequent RCTs found no significant difference between intravenous magnesium sulphate and placebo for hospital admission rates. However, we found limited evidence from one systematic review and two subsequent RCTs that intravenous magnesium versus placebo improved lung function compared with placebo in people with severe acute asthma.
- **Mechanical ventilation for people with severe acute asthma** We found no RCTs comparing mechanical ventilation with or without inhaled β_2 agonists versus no mechanical ventilation in people with severe acute asthma. Evidence from cohort studies support its use, although observational studies suggest that ventilation is associated with a high level of morbidity.
- **Oxygen supplementation for acute asthma** We found no systematic review or RCTs of oxygen in acute asthma. However, consensus opinion and pathophysiology suggest that its role is vital in acute asthma.
- **Short courses of systemic corticosteroids for acute exacerbations** Two systematic reviews and one subsequent RCT have found that early treatment with systemic corticosteroids reduces admission and relapse rates compared with placebo in people with acute asthma. One systematic review found no significant difference between oral and inhaled steroids for relapse rates at 7–10 days in adults with acute asthma.
- **Spacer devices for delivering inhaled medications from pressurised metered dose inhalers in acute asthma (as good as nebulisers)** One systematic review in people with acute, but not life threatening exacerbations of asthma found no significant difference with β_2 agonists delivered by spacer device/holding chamber versus nebulisers in rates of hospital admission, time spent in the emergency department, peak expiratory flow rate, or forced expiratory volume in 1 second.
- **Specialist versus generalist care for acute exacerbations** One systematic review found limited evidence that specialist versus generalist care improved outcomes in adults and children.

DEFINITION	Asthma is characterised by variable airflow obstruction and airway hyperresponsiveness. Symptoms include dyspnoea, cough, chest tightness, and wheezing. The normal diurnal variation of peak expiratory flow rate (see glossary, p 1776) is increased in people with asthma (see table 1, p 1781). **Chronic asthma** is defined here as asthma requiring maintenance treatment. Asthma is classified differently in the USA and UK (see table 1, p 1781). Where necessary, the text specifies the system of classification used.[1,2] **Acute asthma** is defined here as an exacerbation of underlying asthma requiring urgent treatment.
INCIDENCE/ PREVALENCE	Reported prevalence of asthma is increasing worldwide. About 10% of people have suffered an attack of asthma.[3–5] Epidemiological studies have also found marked variations in prevalence in different countries.[6,7]
AETIOLOGY/ RISK FACTORS	Most people with asthma are atopic. Exposure to certain stimuli initiates inflammation and structural changes in airways causing airway hyperresponsiveness and variable airflow obstruction, which in turn cause most asthma symptoms. There are a large number of such stimuli; the more important include environmental allergens, occupational sensitising agents, and respiratory viral infections.[8,9]
PROGNOSIS	**Chronic asthma:** In people with mild asthma, prognosis is good and progression to severe disease is rare. However, as a group, people with asthma lose lung function faster than those without asthma, although less quickly than people without asthma who smoke.[10] People with chronic asthma can improve with treatment. However, some people (possibly up to 5%) have severe disease that responds poorly to treatment. These people are most at risk of morbidity and death from asthma. **Acute asthma:** About 10–20% of people presenting to the emergency department with asthma are admitted to hospital. Of these, fewer than 10% receive mechanical ventilation.[11,12] Those who are ventilated are at 19-fold increased risk of ventilation for a subsequent episode.[13] It is unusual for people to die unless they have suffered respiratory arrest before reaching hospital.[14] One prospective study of 939 people discharged from emergency care found that 17% (95% CI 14% to 20%) relapsed by 2 weeks.[15]
AIMS OF INTERVENTION	To minimise or eliminate symptoms; to maximise lung function; to prevent exacerbations; to minimise the need for medication; to minimise adverse effects of treatment; and to provide enough information and support to facilitate self management of asthma.
OUTCOMES	Symptoms (daytime and nocturnal); lung function, in terms of peak expiratory flow rate and forced expiratory volume in 1 second (see glossary, p 1776); need for rescue medication such as inhaled β_2 agonists; variability of flow rates; activities of daily living; adverse effects of treatment.
METHODS	*Clinical Evidence* search and appraisal September 2002.

QUESTION **What are effects of treatments for chronic asthma?**

Bazian Ltd

OPTION **REGULAR VERSUS AS NEEDED INHALED SHORT ACTING β_2 AGONISTS IN ADULTS WITH MILD OR MODERATE ASTHMA**

One systematic review and one subsequent RCT have found no significant difference between regular and as needed inhaled short acting β_2 agonists for clinically important outcomes.

Benefits: We found one systematic review (search date not stated, 22 crossover RCTs, 8 parallel group RCTs)[16] and one subsequent RCT[17] comparing regular with as needed β_2 agonists. Results from crossover RCTs and parallel group RCTs were analysed separately. Only results from crossover RCTs were suitable for pooling. Most of the included studies did not allow the use of concurrent inhaled corticosteroids. The review found that morning peak expiratory flow rate (see glossary, p 1776) (PEFR) was not significantly different between regular versus as needed use (5 crossover RCTs, 437 adults: WMD 2.1 L/min, 95% CI –9.5 L/min to +13.6 L/min). Regular versus as needed β_2 agonists significantly increased evening PEFR (6 crossover RCTs, 874 adults: WMD 13.1 L/min, 95% CI 1.9 L/min to 24.3 L/min). As needed versus regular β_2 agonist significantly increased diurnal variation (see glossary, p 1776) of PEFR (2 crossover RCTs, 170 adults: 4.4%, 95% CI 4.3% to 4.5%) and pre-bronchodilator forced expiratory volume in 1 second (see glossary, p 1776) obtained at clinic visits (303 people: WMD 157 mL, 95% CI 123 mL to 192 mL). Use of rescue bronchodilator was measured in most of the RCTs that used a short acting β_2 agonist as a rescue agent. Results for an average 24 hour period showed that, when bronchodilators were given regularly, significantly less relief bronchodilator was used (2 crossover RCTs, 45 adults: WMD –0.68 puffs/day, 95% CI –1.30 puffs/day to –0.07 puffs/day). Two crossover RCTs (174 adults) identified by the review quantified exacerbation rates.[16] They found no significant difference between regular versus as needed use of β_2 agonists (SMD +0.10, 95% CI –0.11 to +0.31). One parallel group RCT (117 adults) identified by the review found that as needed versus regular use significantly improved symptom control over a 24 hour period (WMD 0.120 units, 95% CI 0.001 units to 0.239 units). No significant differences were found in quality of life.[16] The subsequent RCT (983 people with asthma in a general practice setting, 90% using regular inhaled corticosteroids) compared as needed versus regular salbutamol (see glossary, p 1776) (400 µg four times daily).[17] It found no significant difference with regular versus as needed salbutamol in the rate of exacerbations over 1 year (RR 0.96, 95% CI 0.80 to 1.15) or in morning PEFR (see comment below). Evening PEFR was significantly higher with regular salbutamol (WMD 10.7 L/min, 95% CI 6.7 L/min to 14.0 L/min) and diurnal variation of PEFR was also higher (WMD 3.3%, 95% CI 2.5% to 4.1%).[17]

Harms: The systematic review did not find any significant worsening of airways function after stopping regular treatment with β_2 agonists, and concluded that the small increase in lower airways reactivity with regular treatment was unlikely to be of any clinical importance.[16] Two case control studies found an association between increased asthma mortality and overuse of inhaled short acting β_2 agonists.[18,19] However, the evidence for this is not reliable because frequent use of β_2 agonists may simply indicate severe, uncontrolled asthma in high risk people. Other RCTs found that regular use of inhaled β_2 agonists was associated with transient rebound deterioration in airway hyperresponsiveness after stopping the medication[20] and increased allergen induced bronchoconstriction.[21] Tremor was commonly reported, but tolerance developed with more frequent use.[22]

Comment: In the subsequent RCT, 33% (323/983) of people randomised did not complete the RCT, reducing the power of the RCT to detect a significant difference between regular and as needed salbutamol.[17]

OPTION LOW DOSE INHALED CORTICOSTEROIDS IN PEOPLE WITH MILD, PERSISTENT ASTHMA

Systematic reviews and RCTs have found that, in people with mild, persistent asthma, low doses of inhaled corticosteroids significantly improve symptoms and lung function compared with placebo or regular inhaled β_2 agonists.

Benefits: **Versus placebo:** We found one systematic review (search date 1999, 6 RCTs, 393 people)[23] and five subsequent RCTs (1026 adults and adolescents)[24–28] of budesonide. We found one systematic review (search date 1999, 9 RCTs, 1800 people)[29] and one subsequent RCT (304 people aged ≥ 12 years)[30] of fluticasone. We found one systematic review (search date 1999, 6 RCTs, 492 people) of beclometasone (beclomethasone).[31] We found five additional RCTs (2187 adults and adolescents with mild, persistent asthma using the US classification; see table 1, p 1781) of low doses of triamcinolone,[32–35] flunisolide,[36] or mometasone.[37] The systematic reviews and RCTs all found that low dose inhaled corticosteroids versus placebo significantly improved lung function and symptoms, and reduced the need for short acting bronchodilators. The largest systematic review (search date 1999),[29] which compared fluticasone (≥ 100 μg/day) versus placebo, found that fluticasone significantly improved forced expiratory volume in 1 second (see glossary, p 1776) (WMD 0.41 L, 95% CI 0.35 L to 0.47 L); morning peak expiratory flow rate (see glossary, p 1776) (WMD 30 L/min, 95% CI 25 L/min to 35 L/min); use of inhaled β_2 agonists (WMD 1.36 puffs/day, 95% CI 1.0 puffs/day to 1.7 puffs/day); and the proportion of people who withdrew because of lack of efficiency compared with placebo over 4–12 weeks (RR 0.32, 95% CI 0.25 to 0.40).[29] **Versus β_2 agonists:** We found one systematic review (search date not stated; 5 RCTs; 3 comparing inhaled corticosteroids v placebo; 2 comparing inhaled corticosteroids v β_2

agonists; 141 adults with mild persistent asthma).[38] The review found that regular inhaled corticosteroids (≤ 2 drugs) versus regular β_2 agonists or placebo significantly improved lung function (overall weighted effect size for peak expiratory flow rate 0.59, 95% CI 0.32 to 0.84).

Harms: We found one systematic review (search date 2001, 2 RCTs) that examined effects of inhaled steroids on fracture rate.[39] It found no significant difference between conventional doses of inhaled steroids versus placebo for vertebral fracture rates (OR 1.87, 95% CI 0.50 to 7.03).[39] The second review (search date 1998) assessed the harms of inhaled corticosteroids and found that systemic adverse effects increased with dose.[40] It found that, although posterior subcapsular cataracts occur more frequently in people taking oral corticosteroids, most studies in adults provide no evidence that inhaled corticosteroids increase the risk once the confounding effect of oral corticosteroid use is removed.[40] The review found no significant effect of low dose inhaled corticosteroids on bruising or skin thickness.[40] The systematic review of fluticasone found that fluticasone significantly increased oral candidiasis compared with placebo (13/653 [2%] *v* 3/645 [0.5%]; RR 3.45, 95% CI 1.29 to 9.26).[29]

Comment: Two RCTs have found that inhaled corticosteroids delivered using chlorofluorocarbon-free propellants such as hydrofluoroalkane are effective at low dose for people with mild persistent asthma, but dose equivalence varies with each delivery system.[35,36] The dose of inhaled corticosteroid may need to be adjusted if a chlorofluorocarbon-free propellant is used.

OPTION — ADDITION OF LONG ACTING INHALED β_2 AGONISTS IN PEOPLE WITH MILD, PERSISTENT ASTHMA THAT IS POORLY CONTROLLED BY INHALED CORTICOSTEROIDS

RCTs have found that, in people with asthma that is poorly controlled with inhaled corticosteroids, adding regular long acting inhaled β_2 agonists significantly improves symptoms and lung function compared with adding placebo or a leukotriene antagonist. One systematic review and one additional RCT have found that adding regular doses of long acting, inhaled β_2 agonists significantly improves lung function and symptoms, and reduces rescue medication compared with increasing the dose of inhaled corticosteroids. However, one further RCT found that increasing inhaled corticosteroid dose reduced exacerbations compared with adding long acting inhaled β_2 agonists. We found insufficient evidence about effects of adding long acting inhaled β_2 agonists on mortality.

Benefits: **Versus placebo:** We found no systematic review. We found three RCTs (1400 people with moderate persistent asthma, uncontrolled by inhaled corticosteroids 250–2000 μg/day beclometasone diproprionate or equivalent) comparing regular long acting inhaled β_2 agonists versus placebo.[41–43] The RCTs found that twice daily salmeterol or formoterol (eformoterol) versus placebo improved quality of life scores, peak expiratory flow rate (PEFR), and forced expiratory volume in 1 second (see glossary, p 1776) (FEV_1) and reduced night awakening. In the largest RCT,[43] salmeterol versus placebo significantly improved the adjusted mean PEFR (398 L/min with salmeterol *v* 386 L/min with placebo; $P < 0.001$), and significantly increased the proportion of people who did not awaken at night (74% with salmeterol *v* 68% with placebo; $P < 0.05$). Exacerbation rates were not significantly different between the two groups in any of the RCTs (AR for severe exacerbations in the largest RCT:[43] 20.8% with salmeterol *v* 20.9% with placebo). **Versus increased use of inhaled corticosteroids:** We found one systematic review[44] and two additional RCTs.[45,46] The review (search date 1999, 9 double blind RCTs, 3685 people with symptomatic asthma on their current dose of inhaled steroids, duration 3–6 months) compared adding salmeterol versus increased use of inhaled corticosteroids (at least double the usual dose). It found that morning PEFR was significantly higher with salmeterol (3 months: WMD in PEFR 22 L/min, 95% CI 15 L/min to 30 L/min, $P < 0.001$; 6 months: WMD 28 L/min, 95% CI 19 L/min to 36 L/min). Salmeterol significantly increased days without symptoms (WMD at 6 months: 15 days, 95% CI 12 days to 18 days) and nights without symptoms (WMD at 6 months: 5 nights, 95% CI 3 nights to 7 nights). Salmeterol also significantly reduced the need for rescue medication. No increase in asthma exacerbations of any severity was found in the salmeterol group.[44] The first additional RCT (852 people taking low to moderate dose inhaled corticosteroids) compared adding formoterol, increasing the dose of inhaled corticosteroids, and increasing dose of corticosteroids plus adding formoterol.[45] It found that increased dose of corticosteroids significantly reduced severe exacerbations compared with adding formoterol at 1 year (AR 46% with increased corticosteroid *v* 67% with added formoterol; $P = 0.03$).[45] The second additional RCT (454 people with symptomatic asthma on their current dose of inhaled steroids) compared adding salmeterol (42 μg) plus fluticasone (88 μg twice daily) versus adding fluticasone (220 μg twice daily).[46] It found that salmeterol plus lower dose fluticasone versus higher dose fluticasone alone improved lung function, reduced the use of rescue β_2 agonists, and increased the proportion of symptom free days. **Versus addition of leukotriene antagonists:** We found three RCTs.[47–49] The first RCT (948 adults with symptomatic asthma on their current dose of inhaled steroids) that compared adding salmeterol (50 μg twice daily) versus adding montelukast (10 mg/day).[47] It found that salmeterol versus montelukast significantly increased the proportion of symptom free days (24% with salmeterol *v* 16% with montelukast; difference 8%, 95% CI 8% to 12%), improved lung function, and reduced the need for rescue medication and night time awakenings. It found no significant difference in the proportion of people with asthma exacerbations (26/476 [6%] *v* 23/472 [5%]; RR 1.12, 95% CI 0.65 to 1.93) over 12 weeks.[47] The second small RCT (65 people with moderate persistent asthma all using moderate or high dose inhaled steroid) compared three treatments: adding long acting β agonist formoterol (9 μg twice daily); adding leukotriene antagonist zafirlukast (20 mg twice daily); and adding a sustained release theophylline.[48] Additional short acting β agonists were allowed. It found no significant difference between adding formoterol and adding zafirlukast for lung function at 3 months (FEV_1 as % of predicted at 3 months 89.5% with added formoterol *v* 87.3% with added zafirlukast; $P > 0.05$).[48] However, the study may have lacked power to detect clinically important differences. The third RCT (429 people poorly controlled on inhaled corticosteroids) found that adding salmeterol (43 μg twice daily through a metered dose inhaler) versus adding zafirlukast (20 mg twice daily) found no significant difference in FEV_1 at 4 weeks (change from baseline in FEV_1 0.26 L with salmeterol v 0.23 L with zafirlukast, P = 0.004).[49] However, it found that salmeterol significantly improved symptom scores and reduced night time awakening compared with zafirlukast at 4 weeks (decrease in symptom scores 35% with salmeterol v 21% with zafirlukast; reduction in nocturnal awakenings 45% with salmeterol v 25% with zafirlukast).

Harms: Several studies have found that people taking regular doses of long acting, inhaled β_2 agonists develop tolerance to bronchodilatory effects[50–52] and may develop tremor. Regular use of long acting inhaled β_2 agonists has not been linked to deterioration in asthma control.[43–45]

Comment: We found no RCTs or other studies with sufficient power to assess the effect of regular use of long acting inhaled β_2 agonists on mortality.[53]

OPTION ADDING LEUKOTRIENE ANTAGONISTS ALONE IN PEOPLE WITH MILD TO MODERATE PERSISTENT ASTHMA

RCTs in people taking β_2 agonists alone have found that leukotriene antagonists versus placebo significantly reduce asthma symptoms and β_2 agonist use. One systematic review and subsequent RCTs have found that adding leukotriene antagonists increased exacerbations, reduced lung function, and were less effective for symptom control compared with inhaled corticosteroids. Two RCTs have found that an inhaled corticosteroid plus a long acting β_2 agonist significantly improved symptoms, lung function, and exacerbations compared with a leukotriene antagonist at 12 weeks.

Benefits: **Versus placebo:** We found no systematic review. We found three RCTs (1300 adults with asthma taking β_2 agonists alone), which compared adding leukotriene antagonists versus placebo for 13 weeks.[54–56] The RCTs all found that the inhaled leukotriene antagonist zafirlukast (20 mg twice daily) versus placebo significantly reduced daytime and night time asthma symptoms and β_2 agonist use. The largest RCT (762 people)[54] found that zafirlukast versus placebo significantly reduced daytime symptoms (symptom score 8.05 with zafirlukast v 9.45 with placebo; $P < 0.01$), night time awakenings (2.05/wk with zafirlukast v 2.52/wk with placebo; $P < 0.05$), and β_2 agonist use (3.1 puffs/day with zafirlukast v 3.0 puffs/day with placebo; $P < 0.01$). Morning forced expiratory volume in 1 second (see glossary, p 1776) (FEV_1) was significantly increased in people taking zafirlukast (morning FEV_1 improved by 7% with zafirlukast v 3% with placebo; $P < 0.01$).[54] **Versus inhaled corticosteroids:** We found one systematic review (search date 2002, 12 RCTs in adults, 2 RCTs in children, FEV_1 > 50% predicted)[57] and five subsequent RCTs.[58–62] The review compared various leukotriene antagonists (montelukast, pranlukast, zafirlukast) versus inhaled corticosteroids (beclomethasone, fluticasone) for 4–37 weeks.[57] It found that leukotriene antagonists versus corticosteroids increased risk of asthma exacerbations requiring systemic steroids (all leukotriene antagonists: 11 RCTs; significant heterogeneity among trials; RR 1.61, 95% CI 1.15 to 2.25). The review found no significant difference between leukotriene antagonists and inhaled corticosteroids for hospital admission rates for acute asthma (9 RCTs; RR 1.73, 0.64 to 4.73). It also found that leukotriene antagonists reduced symptom free days compared with inhaled corticosteroids at 6 weeks (3 RCTs; WMD 9%, 95% CI 5% to 13%).[57] The first subsequent RCT (533 adults with asthma who were symptomatic on β_2 agonists alone) compared fluticasone with montelukast for 24 weeks.[58] The second subsequent RCT (294 adults and children > 11 years of age previously treated with β_2 agonists alone) compared fluticasone (88 µg twice daily) versus zafirlukast (20 µg twice daily).[59] Both RCTs found no significant difference between leukotriene antagonists and inhaled corticosteroids groups for symptom scores.[58,59] The third subsequent RCT (522 non-smokers with persistent asthma) found that fluticasone propionate (88 µg twice daily) increased lung function and quality of life and decreased symptoms compared with oral montelukast (10 mg/day) at 24 weeks (mean improvement in FEV_1: 22% with fluticasone *v* 14% with montelukast, $P < 0.001$; mean improvement in asthma symptom score: 0.91 with fluticasone *v* 0.57 with montelukast, $P < 0.001$; mean increase in symptom free days: 34% with fluticasone *v* 20% with montelukast, $P < 0.001$; mean improvement in asthma quality of life questionnaire score 1.3 with fluticasone *v* 1.0 with montelukast, $P < 0.001$).[60] The fourth subsequent RCT (440 people aged ≥ 12 years, previously treated with inhaled steroids and short acting β agonists, FEV_1 60–80% of predicted) found that inhaled fluticasone (88 µg twice daily) versus zafirlukast (20 mg twice daily) increased lung function and symptom free days at 6 weeks (mean difference in morning FEV_1: 0.16 L, 95% CI 0.08 L to 0.24 L; increase in symptom free days 14%, 95% CI 7% to 21%).[61] The fifth subsequent RCT (45 non-smokers with mild asthma) compared three treatments: budesonide (400 µg twice daily), montelukast (10 mg/day), and budesonide plus montelukast (at the same doses).[62] It found no significant difference between budesonide versus montelukast for lung function at 16 weeks (increase in FEV_1: 2.1% with budesonide *v* 4.2 with montelukast; increase in forced vital capacity 3.1% with budesonide *v* 5.2% with montelukast; P values not reported).[62] **Versus inhaled corticosteroids plus long acting β_2 agonists:** We found no systematic review. We found two RCTs.[63,64] The first RCT (423 adults with symptomatic asthma taking short acting β_2 agonists) compared montelukast (20 mg once daily) versus fluticasone (100 µg) plus salmeterol (50 µg twice daily).[63] It found that adding fluticasone plus salmeterol significantly increased symptom free days and reduced exacerbations compared with adding montelukast alone at 12 weeks (increase in symptom free days from baseline 22% with montelukast *v* 49% with fluticasone plus salmeterol; WMD 27%, 95% CI 20% to 35%; 11 exacerbations with montelukast *v* 0 with fluticasone plus salmeterol; $P < 0.001$). The second RCT (432 people aged ≥ 15 years with persistent asthma, symptomatic on short acting β agonists) found that fluticasone (100 µg twice daily) plus salmeterol (50 µg twice daily) significantly increased lung function and reduced symptoms compared with oral montelukast (10 mg once daily) at 12 weeks (increase in FEV_1 27% with combination *v* 13% with montelukast, $P < 0.001$; increase in symptom free days 40% with combination *v* 27% with montelukast, $P < 0.017$).[64]

Harms: **Versus placebo in people not taking corticosteroids:** In the RCT comparing zafirlukast versus placebo, the incidence of adverse effects (predominantly pharyngitis and headache) was similar in both groups (350/514 [68%] with zafirlukast *v* 160/248 [65%] with placebo).[55] **Versus inhaled corticosteroids:** The systematic review found that leukotriene antagonists significantly increased the risk of "withdrawals for any cause" but there was no significant difference between treatments in withdrawal rates owing to adverse effects (12 RCTs; RR 1.2, 95% CI 0.9 to 1.7).[57] One RCT found no significant difference in between fluticasone and montelukast in adverse event rate.[60] One RCT found no significant difference between fluticasone and zafirlukast in adverse event rate (7% with fluticasone *v* 4% with zafirlukast, $P = 0.14$).[61] The most common adverse events were headache (2% for both fluticasone and zafirlukast), nausea (1% for fluticasone), and hoarseness (1% for fluticasone).

Comment: One systematic review (search date 2000) identified 22 cases of the Churg–Strauss Syndrome associated with anti-leukotriene treatment, but the total number of people exposed was not reported.[65]

OPTION ADDING LEUKOTRIENE ANTAGONISTS PLUS INHALED CORTICOSTEROIDS IN PEOPLE WITH MILD TO MODERATE PERSISTENT ASTHMA

One systematic review in people taking inhaled corticosteroids found no significant difference between leukotriene antagonists and placebo for exacerbation rates at 4–16 weeks. We found limited evidence from two RCTs that, in people with asthma that is poorly controlled with inhaled corticosteroids, adding a leukotriene antagonist was less effective for symptoms and lung function compared with adding a long acting β_2 agonist.

Benefits: **Versus placebo in people taking inhaled corticosteroids:** We found one systematic review (search date 2001, 12 RCTs in adults, 1 RCT in children with symptomatic asthma on their current dose of inhaled steroids).[66] It found no significant different for licensed doses of leukotriene antagonists (montelukast 5 or 10 mg/day, pranlukast 450 mg/day, zafirlukast 80 mg/day) versus placebo for exacerbations requiring systematic steroids at 4–16 weeks (2 RCTs: 20/466 [4%] with leukotriene antagonists *v* 33/468 [7%] with placebo; RR 0.61, 95% CI 0.36 to 1.05).[66] **Versus long acting β agonist in people taking inhaled corticosteroids:** See benefits of addition of long acting inhaled β_2 agonists in people with mild, persistent asthma that is poorly controlled by inhaled corticosteroids, p 1763.

Harms: **Versus placebo in people taking inhaled corticosteroids:** The systematic review found that higher than licensed dose leukotriene antagonists versus placebo significantly increased the risk of liver enzyme elevation (13/280 [5%] *v* 2/276 [0.7%]; RR 5.36, 95% CI 1.40 to 20.40).[66]

Comment: None.

QUESTION **What are the effects of treatments for acute asthma?**

Mark FitzGerald

OPTION **SPACER DEVICES/HOLDING CHAMBERS VERSUS NEBULISERS FOR DELIVERING β_2 AGONISTS IN ACUTE ASTHMA**

One systematic review found no significant difference in forced expiratory volume in 1 second, peak expiratory flow rate, hospital admissions, or time spent in the emergency department with nebulisers versus holding chambers plus metered dose inhalers for delivering β_2 agonists in people with acute but not life threatening asthma.

Benefits: We found one systematic review (search date 1999, 13 RCTs, non-hospitalised adults and children with acute asthma) comparing holding chambers plus metered dose inhalers versus nebulisers for delivering β_2 agonists.[67] Results in adults and children were analysed separately (see asthma and other wheezing disorders of childhood, p 314). In adults, there was no significant difference in rates of hospital admission (OR 1.12, 95% CI 0.45 to 2.76), length of time spent in the emergency department (WMD +0.02 h, 95% CI –0.40 h to +0.44 h), or in peak expiratory flow rate and forced expiratory volume in 1 second (see glossary, p 1776). There was still no significant difference when the three RCTs involving the most severely affected people (FEV_1 < 30% predicted) were included (WMD for FEV_1 holding chamber *v* nebuliser –1.5% predicted, 95% CI –8.3% to +5.3%). Symptoms were measured on different scales and findings could not be combined.

Harms: The review found no significant difference in heart rates with holding chambers versus nebulisers (WMD with holding chamber *v* nebuliser +1.6% of baseline, 95% CI –2.4% of baseline to +5.5% of baseline).[67]

Comment: The review found no evidence of publication bias.[67] To overcome possible dose confounding, the review was confined to studies that used multiple treatment doses titrated against the individuals' responses. As studies excluded people with life threatening asthma (see glossary, p 1776), results may not generalise to such people.

OPTION **SYSTEMIC CORTICOSTEROIDS FOR ACUTE ASTHMA**

Two systematic reviews and one subsequent RCT have found that early treatment with systemic corticosteroids reduce admission and relapse rates compared with placebo in people with acute asthma. One systematic review found no significant difference for oral versus inhaled steroids after emergency department discharge in relapse rates at 7–10 days in adults with acute asthma.

Benefits: **Versus placebo:** We found two systematic reviews[68,69] and one subsequent RCT.[70] The first review (search date 1991, 5 RCTs, 422 people) found that early use of systemic corticosteroids (oral, iv, or im) versus placebo in the emergency department significantly reduced hospital admissions (OR 0.47, 95% CI 0.27 to 0.79; no significant heterogeneity among RCTs, P = 0.72).[68] The second review (search date 2001, 7 RCTs, about 320 people) compared systematic steroids (im and oral) versus placebo after discharge from the emergency department.[69] It found that systemic corticosteroids significantly reduced relapse at 7–10 days and hospital readmissions within 7 days compared with placebo (relapse rates 5 RCTs, 345 people, RR 0.35, 95% CI 0.17 to 0.73, NNT 13, 95% CI 7 to 91; hospital readmissions 4 RCTs, 210 people, RR 0.32, 95% CI 0.11 to 0.94, NNT 16, 95% CI 7 to 125; no significant heterogeneity was found). Corticosteroids significantly reduced the use of β_2 agonists (WMD –3.3 puffs/day, 95% CI –5.5 puffs/day to –1.0 puffs/day). The review found no clear difference between intramuscular and oral corticosteroids.[69] The subsequent RCT (259 adults and children, all given nebulised salbutamol (see glossary, p 1776) for 5–20 minutes 1–3 times) compared single dose oral prednisolone (30 mg if aged < 5 years or 60 mg if > 5 years) versus placebo given in the emergency room or outpatient department.[70] It found that oral prednisone significantly reduced hospital admission rate compared with placebo (37/140 [26%] with prednisone *v* 50/119 [42%] with placebo, P < 0.01). **Versus inhaled steroids:** We found two systematic reviews.[71,72] The first review (search date 2000) found 4 RCTs in children but no RCTs in adults.[71] The second review (search date 2001, 4 RCTs, 772 adults and 22 children) compared oral corticosteroids (prednisone) versus high dose inhaled corticosteroids (≥ 2mg/day beclomethasone dipropionate or equivalent) in people with acute asthma after emergency department discharge.[72] It found no significant difference between oral and inhaled steroids for relapse rate at 7–10 days (OR relapse 1.00, 95% CI 0.66 to 1.52; no significant heterogeneity among trials; P = 0.88).

Harms: Systemic corticosteroids can cause the same adverse effects in asthma as in other diseases, even when administered for a short time (see asthma and other wheezing disorders of childhood, p 314).

Comment: One RCT (413 adults presenting to general practitioners with acute asthma) found no difference in rates of treatment failure with a short course of oral corticosteroids versus a high dose of inhaled fluticasone.[73] **Stopping treatment:** We found no systematic review but found 1 RCT (35 people admitted to hospital with acute asthma who received 40 mg prednisone for 10 days).[74] It found no significant difference in morning peak expiratory flow rate (see glossary, p 1776) with tapering of prednisone over 1 week versus abrupt stopping (mean increase in peak expiratory flow rate 45 L/min with tapering versus 43 L/min with abrupt stopping; P = 0.82).[74] **Optimal dose and duration of treatment:** We found no systematic review. One RCT (20 people) compared 1 week versus 2 weeks of oral prednisone after a 3 day course of intravenous methylprednisone and found no difference in peak expiratory flow rate and relapse rates.[75] The study was limited by its small sample size. The optimal duration of treatment is likely to depend on the individual, the severity of the exacerbation, and use of concomitant medications.

OPTION INHALED CORTICOSTEROIDS FOR ACUTE ASTHMA

One systematic review has found that inhaled corticosteroids versus placebo given in the emergency department significantly reduce hospital admission rates in adults. One systematic review found no significant difference in relapse rates for oral versus inhaled steroids at 7–10 days. One systematic review found no significant difference in relapse rates for inhaled plus oral corticosteroid versus oral corticosteroids up to 24 days.

Benefits: **Versus placebo:** We found one systematic review (search date 2001, 3 RCTs, 188 adults).[76] It found that inhaled corticosteroids given in the emergency department significantly reduced admission rates compared with placebo in people with acute asthma (OR 0.38, 95% 0.18 to 0.79). **Versus systemic steroids:** See benefits of systemic corticosteroids, p 1769. **Plus oral corticosteroids versus oral corticosteroids alone:** We found one systematic review (search date 1999, 3 RCTs, 909 adults).[77] It found no significant difference for inhaled plus oral corticosteroid versus oral corticosteroids alone in relapse rates at day 7–10 or day 20–24 (day 7–10: OR 0.72, 95% CI 0.48 to 1.10; day 20–24: OR 0.68, 95% CI, 0.46 to 1.02).[77]

Harms: The reviews found no significant differences in adverse effects between the groups, but one review commented that most of the RCTs identified gave little information on adverse effects apart from reporting that they were "rare".[77] See also harms of inhaled corticosteroids under asthma and other wheezing disorders of childhood, p 314.

Comment: None.

OPTION CONTINUOUS VERSUS INTERMITTENT SHORT ACTING β_2 AGONISTS FOR ACUTE ASTHMA

One systematic review and one RCT have found no significant difference between continuous and intermittent nebulised short acting β_2 agonists for hospital admission rates in adults.

Benefits: We found one systematic review (search date 2001, 6 RCTs, 393 adults)[78] and one additional RCT.[79] The review found no significant difference in admission rate between 1 hour of continuous versus 2 hours of intermittent nebulised albuterol (2.5–16 mg in first hour) after 1–3 hours (hospital admission rate: 2 RCTs; 80 adults; RR 0.68, 95% CI 0.33 to 1.38).[78] The included RCTs also used systemic steroids. The additional RCT similarly found no significant difference in lung function or rate of hospital admission for continuous versus intermittent salbutamol (see glossary, p 1776).[79]

Harms: Commonly reported mild adverse effects associated with frequent dosing include tachycardia, tremor, and headache. Metabolic abnormalities are less common and include hypokalaemia. One

RCT included in the review found the highest rate of adverse effects with high dose intermittent treatment. The most common adverse effect was tremor (24% with intermittent high dose, 20% with continuous high dose, 9% with hourly standard dose, and 3% with continuous standard dose).[80]

Comment: We found one RCT (46 adults in hospital), which addressed the slightly different, but related, question of regular nebulised salbutamol (5 mg every 4 h) versus on demand salbutamol (2.5–5 mg).[81] It found that on demand dosage significantly reduced hospital stay (3.7 days with on demand salbutamol *v* 4.7 days with regular salbutamol), the proportion of nebulisations (geometric mean 7.0 with on demand salbutamol *v* 14 with regular salbutamol; P = 0.003), and palpitations (P = 0.05).

OPTION INTRAVENOUS VERSUS NEBULISED DELIVERY OF SHORT ACTING β_2 AGONISTS FOR ACUTE ASTHMA

One systematic review comparing intravenous versus inhaled short acting β_2 agonists in the emergency department found no significant difference in peak expiratory flow rate at 60 minutes.

Benefits: We found one systematic review (search date not stated, 6 RCTs, 337 people) comparing intravenous versus inhaled short acting β_2 agonists.[82] Five of the RCTs used nebulised delivery of inhaled β_2 agonists, and one used intermittent positive pressure breathing. It found that intravenous versus inhaled β_2 agonists lowered peak expiratory flow rate (see glossary, p 1776) at 60 minutes, but the difference was not significant (WMD +24.7 L/min, 95% CI –2.9 L/min to +52 L/min). It found no significant difference in heart rate at 60 minutes with intravenous versus inhaled β_2 agonists (WMD +4.5 beats/min, 95% CI –4.9 beats/min to +14 beats/min).

Harms: The systematic review found no significant difference in the proportion of people with autonomic adverse effects (including palpitations, tachycardia, hypertension, tremor, headache, nausea, and vomiting) with intravenous versus inhaled β_2 agonists (53/153 [35%] with intravenous *v* 76/144 [53%] with inhaled; RR 1.46, 95% CI 0.46 to 4.68).[82]

Comment: None.

OPTION ADDITION OF IPRATROPIUM BROMIDE TO β_2 AGONISTS IN ACUTE ASTHMA

Two systematic reviews and one subsequent RCT have found that ipratropium bromide plus salbutamol versus salbutamol alone improves lung function and is likely to reduce hospital admission in people with severe acute asthma.

Benefits: We found two systematic reviews[83,84] and one subsequent RCT.[85] The first systematic review (search date 1999, 10 RCTs, 1483 people) found that inhaled ipratropium plus salbutamol (see glossary, p 1776) versus salbutamol alone significantly reduced hospital admissions (5 RCTs, 1186 people; OR 0.62, 95% CI 0.44 to 0.88; NNT 18, 95% CI 11 to 77).[83] Meta-analysis of the four RCTs that evaluated people with severe airflow obstruction

(FEV 1776)1> < 35%) found that additional treatment with ipratropium significantly improved FEV_1 over 90 minutes (effect size 0.38, 95% CI 0.05 to 0.67). The second systematic review (search date 1997, 10 RCTs, including 8 identified by the later reviews, 1377 people) found that adding ipratropium bromide versus salbutamol alone improved lung function, but also found no significant difference in hospital admissions, when assessing the same three RCTs.[84] The subsequent RCT (180 people with acute asthma, mean FEV_1 < 50%) compared salbutamol plus placebo versus salbutamol plus ipratropium.[85] It found that adding ipratropium significantly improved peak expiratory flow rate (see glossary, p 1776) (difference in improvement with ipratropium *v* placebo: 21%, 95% CI 3% to 38%) and FEV_1 (difference in improvement with ipratropium *v* placebo: 48%, 95% CI 20% to 76%). People taking ipratropium were significantly less likely to require hospital admission at the end of the 3 hour trial period (20% with ipratropium *v* 39% with placebo; P = 0.01).

Harms: The reviews and the subsequent RCT found no significant difference in adverse effects with the addition of ipratropium to salbutamol versus salbutamol alone.[83–85]

Comment: The authors of the second systematic review stated that only three RCTs reported data in sufficient detail to be included in the analysis of hospital admission rates.[84]

OPTION OXYGEN SUPPLEMENTATION FOR ACUTE ASTHMA

We found no systematic review or RCTs of oxygen in acute asthma. However, consensus opinion and pathophysiology suggest that its role is vital in acute asthma. One systematic review found no significant difference for helium–oxygen mixture versus air or oxygen in pulmonary function tests at 60 minutes for adults and children.

Benefits: **Oxygen alone:** We found no systematic review and no RCTs. **Plus helium versus air or oxygen:** We found one systematic review (search date 1999, 4 RCTs, 288 adults and children)[86] and one additional RCT.[87] The review found no significant difference for helium–oxygen mixture (80 : 20 or 70 : 30) versus air or oxygen in pulmonary function tests at 15–60 minutes (peak expiratory flow rate (see glossary, p 1776) as % of predicted: WMD –1.61 L/min, 95% CI –6.64 L/min to +3.41 L/min; P = 0.5). All included RCTs also used inhaled albuterol and corticosteroids. The additional RCT (27 people; peak expiratory flow rate < 250 L/min despite treatment, pulsus paradoxus (see glossary, p 1776) > 15 mm Hg) found that helium–oxygen mixture (80 : 20) versus air alone improved peak expiratory flow (results presented graphically).[87]

Harms: We found no evidence of adverse effects associated with oxygen alone. One RCT identified by the systematic review found one person became hypoxic with 70 : 30 helium–oxygen mixture.[86]

Comment: The most severe stages of acute asthma are respiratory failure, cardiopulmonary arrest, and death.[12,13] Studies of near fatal asthma suggest that hypoxia rather than arrhythmia account for asthma deaths. It seems reasonable that supplemental oxygen should continue to form a critical part of management even though we found no RCTs providing direct evidence for this. Peak flow readings vary depending on the viscosity of the gas being delivered (helium is less dense than oxygen so non-standardised measures of peak flow will increase relative to air, even if the mixture has no effect on airway narrowing). It was not clear in all RCTs whether peak flow readings were standardised for air and for helium–oxygen mixtures. Evidence for routine use of heliox as a therapeutic option in its own right is currently lacking.

OPTION MAGNESIUM SULPHATE FOR ACUTE ASTHMA

One systematic review and three subsequent RCTs found no significant difference between intravenous magnesium sulphate and placebo for hospital admission rates. We found limited evidence from one systematic review and two subsequent RCTs that intravenous magnesium versus placebo acutely improved lung function compared with placebo in people with severe acute asthma.

Benefits: **Intravenous magnesium sulphate:** We found one systematic review (search date 1998, 5 RCTs in adults, 2 RCTs in children, 665 people)[88] and three subsequent RCTs.[89–91] The review found no significant difference for intravenous magnesium sulphate versus placebo in hospital admissions (admission rates: OR 0.31, 95% CI 0.09 to 1.02; significant heterogeneity among trials). Prespecified subgroup analysis of adults with more severe airflow obstruction (5 RCTs, sample size not given; forced expiratory volume in 1 second [FEV_1] < 30% at presentation, failure to respond to initial treatment, or failure to improve beyond 60% in FEV_1 after 1 h) found magnesium sulphate significantly improved peak expiratory flow volume (see glossary, p 1776) and reduced rates of hospital admission compared with placebo (hospital admission rates: OR 0.10, 95% CI 0.04 to 0.27, no significant heterogeneity, P > 0.1).[88] The first subsequent RCT (33 evaluable people) found no significant difference in hospital admissions for intravenous magnesium sulphate versus placebo (18% with magnesium sulphate *v* 25% with placebo; RR 0.71, 95% CI 0.19 to 2.67).[89] The second subsequent RCT (42 people with acute asthma receiving inhaled bronchodilators and iv corticosteroids) found that intravenous magnesium sulphate versus placebo significantly improved peak expiratory flow rate (see glossary, p 1776) at 60 minutes (174 L/min with magnesium sulphate *v* 212 L/min with placebo; P = 0.04), but did not reduce the proportion of people admitted to hospital (5/18 [28%] with magnesium sulphate *v* 5/24 [21%] with placebo; RR 1.33, 95% CI 0.45 to 3.92).[90] The third subsequent RCT (248 adults, $FEV_1 \leq 30\%$ predicted, all previously treated with methylprednisone and nebulised albuterol) found that intravenous magnesium sulphate (2 g iv given in the emergency department) significantly improved lung function at 4 hours but found no significant difference in hospital admission rates compared with placebo (mean difference in FEV_1: 4.7% predicted, 95% CI 0.3% to 9.3%; P = 0.045; hospital admission rates 39/122[32%] with magnesium sulphate *v* 41/126 [32%] with placebo; P not reported).[91]
Nebulised magnesium sulphate: We found 1 RCT (35 people) that compared salbutamol (see glossary, p 1776) plus 0.9%

sodium chloride versus salbutamol plus magnesium sulphate through a nebuliser.[92] It found that magnesium sulphate versus 0.9% sodium chloride significantly increased peak expiratory flow rate (increase in peak expiratory flow rate after 10 min: 61% with magnesium sulphate *v* 31% with sodium chloride; difference 30%, 95% CI 3% to 56%; P = 0.03).

Harms: The RCTs did not specifically address harms.

Comment: Further studies are needed to clarify the role of intravenous magnesium sulphate in acute asthma. Two of the studies involved treatment with aminophylline and one with ipratropium, both of which have been found to affect hospital admission rates without affecting the degree of airflow obstruction.[93] The subgroup analysis in the systematic review and larger RCTs involved intergroup and intragroup analyses specified before the trial was conducted, and so provides reasonably strong evidence of an effect.

OPTION MECHANICAL VENTILATION FOR SEVERE ACUTE ASTHMA

We found no RCTs comparing mechanical ventilation with or without inhaled β_2 agonists versus no mechanical ventilation in people with severe acute asthma. Evidence from cohort studies support its use, although ventilation is associated with a high level of morbidity.

Benefits: **Versus no ventilation:** We found no systematic review or RCTs. **Plus inhaled β agonists versus mechanical ventilation:** We found one systematic review (search date 2001) that evaluated the role of inhaled β agonists for asthma in mechanically ventilated people.[94] It found no RCTs.

Harms: Mechanical ventilation is associated with hypotension, barotrauma, infection, and myopathy, especially when prolonged paralysis is required with muscle relaxants and systemic corticosteroids.[95] Adverse effects reported in one retrospective study of 88 episodes of mechanical ventilation were hypotension (20%), pulmonary barotrauma (14%), and arrhythmia (10%).[96]

Comment: Experience suggests that mechanical ventilation is a life saving intervention needed by a small minority of people with severe acute asthma. Cohort studies[97,98] and one case series[99] found fewer deaths with controlled hypoventilation versus ventilation in which carbon dioxide levels were normalised (for which historical cohorts and case series have reported mortality rates of 7.5–23.0%).[96,100–102] Non-invasive ventilation has been used in people with acute exacerbations of chronic obstructive lung disease,[103] but requires prospective validation in people with acute asthma. Future research should also focus on delivery of bronchodilators, optimal use of muscle relaxants, and dose of corticosteroids.

OPTION SPECIALIST VERSUS GENERALIST CARE FOR ACUTE ASTHMA

One systematic review found limited evidence that specialist versus generalist care may improve outcomes in people with acute asthma.

Benefits: We found one systematic review (search date 1995, 2 RCTs in adults and 2 RCTs in children, 10 observational studies).[104] It found limited evidence that specialist care versus generalist care may improve outcomes and that shared care (see glossary, p 1776) may be as effective as usual outpatient care.[104] The first RCT of adults in the review (801 people attending a UK outpatient clinic) excluded people with severe asthma.[104] It found no significant difference for integrated care versus regular outpatient care for most outcomes at 12 months (use of medication, primary care consultation, hospital admissions, restrictions on normal activity, psychological morbidity, patient satisfaction). The second RCT (245 adults admitted to emergency departments in the USA) found a significant reduction in emergency room visits at 2 weeks when educational information was provided by a nurses who themselves had asthma versus nurses who did not have asthma.[104]

Harms: The review did not report on harms of specialist versus generalist care.[104]

Comment: Many of the RCTs and observational studies in the systematic review were small.[104] One non-systematic review of RCTs and observational studies found that "expert based" care versus general care improved outcomes.[105] One quasi-randomised trial (based on day of attendance) identified by the non-systematic review referred people from the emergency department to specialist care versus routine general medical follow up.[106] It found that people receiving specialist care were significantly less likely to wake at night (OR 0.24, 95% CI 0.11 to 0.52), suffer relapse requiring emergency admission by 6 months (for 1 admission RR 0.56, 95% CI 0.34 to 0.95; for 2 admissions RR 0.30, 95% CI 0.16 to 0.60), or suffer multiple relapses. They were more likely to use inhaled corticosteroids (OR 3.6, 95% CI 1.9 to 6.6) and sodium cromoglycate (RR 2.2, 95% CI 1.9 to 2.5).

OPTION EDUCATION ABOUT ACUTE ASTHMA

One systematic review and one subsequent RCT found that education to facilitate self management of asthma in adults versus usual care significantly reduced hospital admission, unscheduled visits to the doctor, and days off work. However, a second subsequent RCT found no significant effect of asthma education for quality of life or social functioning at 6 months.

Benefits: We found one systematic review (search date 1999, 22 RCTs)[107] and two subsequent RCTs of adult self management of asthma.[108,109] The review found that education about asthma to facilitate self management, whether initiated from a specialist or generalist setting, significantly reduced hospital admission rates, unscheduled visits to the doctor, and days off work at the end of the study (hospital admission rates: RR 0.62, 95% CI 0.41 to 0.96; NNT 38, 95% CI 20 to 382; unscheduled visits to the doctor: RR 0.74, 95% CI 0.63 to 0.90; NNT 12, 95% CI 8 to 36; days off work: RR 0.75, 95% CI 0.63 to 0.90; NNT 7, 95% CI 5 to 13).[107] Best results were achieved in people who had written care plans.[107] The first subsequent RCT (105 people) compared three interventions: limited education (usual care plus teaching inhaler technique plus self care plan); structured education (structured asthma education programme in addition to limited education interventions); and usual care for 1 year.[108] It found no significant difference with limited education versus usual care in the proportion of unscheduled visits to the doctor, but found that structured education versus limited education or versus usual care significantly reduced unscheduled visits over the final 6 months of treatment (P = 0.03 with structured *v* limited education; P = 0.01 with structured education *v* usual care; results presented graphically). The second subsequent RCT (131 adults admitted to hospital with asthma).[109] It found no significant difference between an education programme (3 group sessions focused on improving self management skills) versus waiting list control on 12 out of 13 scales of health and social functioning at 6 months (115 people included in analysis; scales used were SF–36 and the Asthma Quality of Life Questionnaire).

Harms: The systematic review and subsequent RCTs gave no information on adverse effects.[107,108]

Comment: Despite the recent study, the weight of evidence from other published RCTs and systematic overviews supports the role of asthma education among asthma patients.

GLOSSARY

Diurnal variation A characteristic of people with asthma is increased variation in peak flow rates and forced expiratory volume in 1 second during the day. The diurnal variation is sometimes expressed as the difference between maximum and minimum values expressed as a fraction of the maximum value.

Forced expiratory volume in 1 second The volume breathed out in the first second of forceful blowing into a spirometer, measured in litres.

Life threatening asthma An attack of such severity that the person usually requires management in the emergency department. Some people require endotracheal intubation and, usually in the initial stages of resuscitation, cannot inhale bronchodilator treatment.

Peak expiratory flow rate The maximum rate that gas is expired from the lungs when blowing into a peak flow meter or a spirometer. It is measured at an instant, but the units are expressed as litres a minute.

Pulsus paradoxus A measure of the severity of asthma based on the difference in systolic pressure during inspiration and expiration. The blood pressure normally falls a little during inspiration (< 10 mm Hg), but in acute severe asthma (and in some other conditions) the fall of systolic pressure in inspiration is greater.

Salbutamol A short acting β_2 agonist known as albuterol in the USA.

Shared care Involves sharing care between outpatient specialist and general practitioner.

REFERENCES

1. National Heart, Blood and Lung Institute. National Asthma Education and Prevention Program. Expert Panel Report 2. Guidelines for the Diagnosis and Management of Asthma. NIH Publication No. 97–4051;July 1997:20.
2. British Thoracic Society Guidelines. *Thorax* 1997;52:S1–S2.
3. Kaur B, Anderson HR, Austin J, et al. Prevalence of asthma symptoms, diagnosis, and treatment in 12–14 year old children across Great Britain (international study of asthma and allergies in childhood, ISAAC UK). *BMJ* 1998;316:118–124.
4. Woolcock AJ, Peat JK. Evidence for an increase in asthma world-wide. *Ciba Found Symp* 1997;206:122–134.
5. Holgate ST. The epidemic of allergy and asthma. *Nature* 1999;402:B2–4.
6. The International Study of Asthma and Allergies in Childhood (ISAAC) Steering Committee. Worldwide variation in prevalence of symptoms of asthma, allergic rhinoconjunctivitis, and atopic eczema: ISAAC. *Lancet* 1998;351:1225–1232.
7. Burney P, Chinn DJ, Luczynska C, et al. Variations in the prevalence of respiratory symptoms, self-reported asthma attacks, and use of asthma

medication in the European Community Respiratory Health Survey. *Eur Respir J* 1996;9:687–695.
8. Duff AL, Platts-Mills TA. Allergens and asthma. *Pediatr Clin North Am* 1992;39:1277–1291.
9. Chan-Yeung M, Malo JL. Occupational asthma. *N Engl J Med* 1995;333:107–112.
10. Lange P, Parner J, Vestbo J, et al. A 15-year follow-up study of ventilatory function in adults with asthma. *N Engl J Med* 1998;339:1194–1200.
11. FitzGerald JM, Grunfeld A. Acute life-threatening asthma. In: FitzGerald JM, Ernst PP, Boulet LP, et al, eds. *Evidence based asthma management*. Decker: Hamilton, Ontario, 2000:233–244.
12. Nahum A, Tuxen DT. Management of asthma in the intensive care unit. In: FitzGerald JM, Ernst PP, Boulet LP, et al, eds. *Evidence based asthma management*. Decker: Hamilton, Ontario, 2000:245–261.
13. Turner MT, Noertjojo K, Vedal S, et al. Risk factors for near-fatal asthma: a case control study in patients hospitalised with acute asthma. *Am J Respir Crit Care Med* 1998;157:1804–1809.
14. Molfino NA, Nannimi A, Martelli AN, et al. Respiratory arrest in near fatal asthma. *N Engl J Med* 1991;324:285–288.
15. Emmerman CL, Woodruff PG, Cydulka RK, et al. Prospective multi-center study of relapse following treatment for acute asthma among adults presenting to the emergency department. *Chest* 1999;115:919–927.
16. Walters EH, Walters J. Inhaled short acting β_2 agonist use in asthma: regular versus as needed treatment. In: The Cochrane Library, Issue 4, 2001. Oxford: Update Software. Search date not stated; primary sources Cochrane Airways Group Asthma and Wheeze RCT register.
17. Dennis SM, Sharp SJ, Vickers MR, et al. Regular inhaled salbutamol and asthma control: the TRUST randomised trial. *Lancet* 2000;355:1675–1679.
18. Spitzer WO, Suissa S, Ernst P, et al. The use of β-agonists and the risk of death and near death from asthma. *N Engl J Med* 1992;326:501–506.
19. Crane J, Pearce N, Flatt A, et al. Prescribed fenoterol and death from asthma in New Zealand, 1981–1983: case-control study. *Lancet* 1989;1:917–922.
20. Kerrebijn KF, van Essen-Zandvliet EE, Neijens HJ. Effect of long-term treatment with inhaled corticosteroids and β-agonists on the bronchial responsiveness in children with asthma. *J Allergy Clin Immunol* 1987;79:653–659.
21. Cockcroft DW, McParland CP, Britto SA, et al. Regular inhaled salbutamol and airway responsiveness to allergen. *Lancet* 1993;342:833–837.
22. Ahrens RC. Skeletal muscle tremor and the influence of adrenergic drugs. *J Asthma* 1990;27:11–20.
23. Adams N, Bestall J, Jones PW. Budesonide for chronic asthma in children and adults (Cochrane Review). In: The Cochrane Library, Issue 4, 2001. Oxford: Update Software. Search date 1999; primary sources The Cochrane Airways Group Trial Register, reference lists of articles, contact with trialists and hand searches of abstracts of major respiratory society meetings (1997–1999).
24. Kemp J, Wanderer AA, Ramsdell J, et al. Rapid onset of control with budesonide Turbuhaler in patients with mild-to-moderate asthma. *Ann Allergy Asthma Immunol* 1999;82:463–471.
25. McFadden ER, Casale TB, Edwards TB, et al. Administration of budesonide once daily by means of Turbuhaler to subjects with stable asthma. *J Allergy Clin Immunol* 1999;104:46–52.
26. Miyamoto T, Takahashi T, Nakajima S, et al. A double-blind, placebo-controlled dose–response study with budesonide Turbuhaler in Japanese asthma patients. Japanese Pulmicort Turbuhaler study group. *Respirology* 2000;5:247–256.
27. Banov CH, Howland III WC, Lumry WR. Once-daily budesonide via Turbuhaler improves symptoms in adults with persistent asthma. *Ann Allergy Asthma Immunol* 2001;86:627–632.
28. O'Byrne PM, Barnes PJ, Rodriguez-Roisin R, et al. Low dose inhaled budesonide and formoterol in mild persistent asthma: the OPTIMA randomized trial. *Am J Respir Crit Care Med* 2001;164:1392–1397.
29. Adams N, Bestall J, Jones PW. Inhaled fluticasone proprionate for chronic asthma. In: The Cochrane Library, Issue 4, 2001. Oxford: Update Software. Search date 1999; primary sources The Cochrane Airways Group Trial Register, reference lists of articles, contact with trialists, and abstracts of major respiratory society meetings (1997–1999).
30. Wolfe JD, Selner JC, Mendelson LM, et al. Effectiveness of fluticasone propionate in patients with moderate asthma: a dose-ranging study. *Clin Ther* 1996;18:635–646.
31. Adams NP, Bestall JB, Jones PW. Inhaled beclomethasone versus placebo for chronic asthma (Cochrane Review). In: The Cochrane Library, Issue 4, 2001. Oxford: Update Software. Search date 1999; primary sources Cochrane Airways Group Trial Register, hand searches of journals, conference proceedings, and contact with pharmaceutical companies.
32. Bronsky E, Korenblat P, Harris AG, et al. Comparative clinical study of inhaled beclomethasone dipropionate and triamcinolone acetonide in persistent asthma. *Ann Allergy* 1998;80:295–302.
33. Bernstein DI, Cohen R, Ginchansky E, et al. A multicenter, placebo-controlled study of twice daily triamcinolone acetonide (800 μg per day) for the treatment of patients with mild-to-moderate asthma. *J Allergy Clin Immunol* 1998;101:433–438.
34. Ramsdell JW, Fish L, Graft D, et al. A controlled trial of twice daily triamcinolone oral inhaler in patients with mild-to-moderate asthma. *Ann Allergy* 1998;80:385–390.
35. Welch, M Bernstein D. A controlled trial of chlorofluorocarbon-free triamcinolone acetonide inhalation aerosol in the treatment of adult patients with persistent asthma. *Chest* 1999;116:1304–1312.
36. Corren J, Nelson H, Greos LS, et al. Effective control of asthma with hydrofluoroalkane flunisolide delivered as an extrafine aerosol in asthma patients. *Ann Allergy Asthma Immunol* 2001;87:405–411.
37. Nathan RA, Nayak AS, Grant DF, et al. Mometasone furoate; efficacy and safety in moderate asthma compared to beclomethasone dipropionate. *Ann Allergy Asthma Immunol* 2001;86:203–210.
38. Hatoum HT, Schumock GT, Kendzierski DL. Meta-analysis of controlled trials of drug therapy in mild chronic asthma: the role of inhaled corticosteroids. *Ann Pharmacother* 1994;28:1285–1289. Search date not stated; primary source Medline.
39. Jones A, Fay JK, Burr M, et al. Inhaled corticosteroid effects on bone metabolism in asthma and mild chronic obstructive pulmonary disease (Cochrane Review). In Cochrane Library, Issue 4, 2002. Oxford: Update Software. Search date 2001; primary sources Medline, Embase, Cinahl, Bids, Cochrane Controlled Trials Register,

Cochrane Airways Group trials register, electronic bibliographies of included studies, and contact with pharmaceutical companies.
40. Lipworth BJ. Systemic adverse effects of inhaled corticosteroid therapy; a systematic review and meta-analysis. *Arch Intern Med* 1999;159:941–955. Search date 1998; primary sources Medline, Embase, BIDS, and hand searches of bibliographies of retrieved articles and abstracts of respiratory and allergy based journals.
41. Kemp JP, Cook DA, Incaudo GA, et al. Salmeterol improves quality of life in patients with asthma requiring inhaled corticosteroids. *J Allergy Clin Immunol* 1998;101:188–195.
42. FitzGerald JM, Chapman KR, Della Cioppa G, et al. Sustained bronchoprotection, bronchodilatation, and symptom control during regular formoterol use in asthma of moderate or greater severity. *J Allergy Clin Immunol* 1999;103:427–435.
43. D'Urzo AD, Chapman KR, Cartier A, et al. Effectiveness and safety of salmeterol in nonspecialist practice settings. *Chest* 2001;119:714–719.
44. Shrewsbury S, Pyke S, Britton M. Meta-analysis of increased dose of inhaled steroid or addition of salmeterol in symptomatic asthma (MIASMA). *BMJ* 2000;320:1368–1373. Search date 1999; primary sources Medline, Embase, and GlaxoSmithKline databases.
45. Pauwels RA, Lofdahl C-G, Postma DS, et al. Effect of inhaled formoterol and budesonide on exacerbations of asthma. *N Engl J Med* 1997;337:1405–1411.
46. Baraniuk JM-J. Fluticasone alone or in combination with salmeterol vs triamcinolone in asthma. *Chest* 1999;116:625–632
47. Fish JE, Israel E, Murray JJ, et al. Salmeterol powder provides significantly better benefit than montelukast in asthmatic patients receiving concomitant inhaled corticosteroid therapy. *Chest* 2001;120:423–430.
48. Yurdakul AS, Calisir HC, Tunctan B, et al. Comparison of second controller medications in addition to inhaled corticosteroid in patients with moderate asthma. *Respir Med* 2002;96:322–329.
49. Chervinsky P, Nelson HS, Bernstein DI, et al. Comparison of mometasone furoate administered by metered dose inhaler with beclomethasone dipropionate. *Int J Clin Pract* 2002;56:419–425.
50. Cheung D, Timmers MC, Zwinderman AH, et al. Long-term effects of a long-acting β_2-adrenoceptor agonist, salmeterol, on airway hyperresponsiveness in patients with mild asthma. *N Engl J Med* 1992;327:1198–1203.
51. O'Connor BJ, Aikman SL, Barnes PJ. Tolerance to the nonbronchodilating effects of inhaled β_2-agonists in asthma. *N Engl J Med* 1992;327:1204–1208.
52. Nelson JA, Strauss L, Skowronski M, et al. Effect of long-term salmeterol treatment on exercise-induced asthma. *N Engl J Med* 1998;339:141–146.
53. Castle W, Fuller R, Hall J, et al. Serevent nationwide surveillance study: comparison of salmeterol with salbutamol in asthmatic patients who require regular bronchodilator treatment. *BMJ* 1993;306:1034–1037.
54. Fish JE, Kemp JP, Lockey RF, et al. Zafirlukast for symptomatic mild-to-moderate asthma: a 13-week multicenter study. *Clin Ther* 1997;19:675–690.
55. Suissa S, Dennis R, Ernst P, et al. Effectiveness of the leukotriene receptor antagonist zafirlukast for mild-to-moderate asthma. A randomized, double-blind, placebo-controlled trial. *Ann Intern Med* 1997;126:177–183.
56. Nathan RA, Bernstein JA, Bielory L, et al. Zafirlukast improves asthma symptoms and quality of life in patients with moderate reversible airflow obstruction. *Allergy Clin Immunol* 1998;102:935–942.
57. Ducharme FM, Hicks GC. Anti-leukotriene agents compared to inhaled corticosteroids in the management of recurrent and/or chronic asthma. In: The Cochrane Library, Issue 3, 2002. Oxford: Update Software. Search date 2002; primary sources Medline, Embase, and Cinahl.
58. Busse W, Raphael G, Galant S, et al. Low dose fluticasone propionate compared to montelukast for first-line treatment of persistent asthma: a randomized clinical trial. *J Allergy Clin Immunol* 2001;107:461–468.
59. Nathan RA, Bleecker ER, Kalberg C. A comparison of short-term treatment with inhaled fluticasone propionate and zafirlukast for patients with persistent asthma. *Am J Med* 2001;111:195–202.
60. Meltzer EO, Lockey RF, Friedman BF, et al. Efficacy and safety of low-dose fluticasone propionate compared with montelukast for maintenance treatment of persistent asthma. *Mayo Clin Proc* 2002;77:437–445.
61. Brabson JH, Clifford D, Kerwin E, et al. Efficacy and safety of low-dose fluticasone propionate compared with zafirlukast in patients with persistent asthma. *Am J Med* 2002;113:15–21.
62. Riccioni G, Ballone E, D'Orazio N, et al. Effectiveness of montelukast versus budesonide on quality of life and bronchial reactivity in subjects with mild-persistent asthma. *Int J Immunopathol Pharmacol* 2002;15:149–155.
63. Calhoun WJ, Nelson HS, Nathan RA, et al. Comparison of fluticasone propionate–salmeterol combination therapy and montelukast in patients who are symptomatic on short-acting β_2 agonists alone. *Am J Respir Crit Care Med* 2001;164:759–763.
64. Pearlman DS, White MV, Lieberman AK, et al. Fluticasone propionate/salmeterol combination compared with montelukast for the treatment of persistent asthma. *Ann Allergy Asthma Immunol* 2002;88:227–235.
65. Jamaleddine G, Diab K, Tabbarah Z, et al. Leukotriene antagonists and the Churg-Strauss syndrome. *Semin Arthritis Rheum* 2002;31:218–227. Search date 2000; primary source Medline.
66. Ducharme F. Addition of anti-leukotriene agents to inhaled corticosteroids for chronic asthma. In: The Cochrane Library. Issue 3, 2002. Oxford: Update Software. Search date 2001; primary sources Medline, Embase, Cinahl, reference lists of review articles and trials, contacted international headquarters of AL manufacturers, and ATS meeting abstracts (1998–2000).
67. Cates C. Holding chambers versus nebulisers for β agonist treatment of acute asthma. In: The Cochrane Library, Issue 3, 2002. Oxford: Update Software. Search date 1999; primary sources Cochrane Airways Review Group Register of Trials, Cochrane Controlled Trials Register, bibliographies of all included papers, and authors of included studies.
68. Rowe BH, Keller JL, Oxman AD. Effectiveness of steroid therapy in acute exacerbations of asthma: a meta-analysis. *Am J Emerg Med* 1992;10:301–310. Search date 1991; primary sources Medline, Science Citation Index, review articles, textbooks, experts, and primary authors.
69. Rowe BH, Spooner CH, Duchrame FM, et al. Corticosteroids for preventing relapse following acute exacerbations of asthma. In: The Cochrane Library, Issue 3, 2002. Oxford: Update Software.

Search date 2001; primary sources Cochrane Airways Review Group Register of Trials, Asthma, and Wheeze RCT Register.
70. Mahakalkar SM, Tibdewal S, Khobragade BP. Effect of a single dose of prednisolone on hospitalization in patients of acute bronchial asthma. *Ind J Med Sci* 2000;54:384–387.
71. Edmonds ML, Camargo CA Jr, Pollack CV, et al. Early use of inhaled corticosteroids in the emergency department treatment of acute asthma. In: The Cochrane Library, Issue 3, 2002. Search date 2000; primary sources The Cochrane Airways Review Group Register of Trials, hand searches of reference lists, conference abstracts, and contact with experts and pharmaceutical companies.
72. Edmonds ML, Camargo CA, Brenner BE, et al. Replacement of oral corticosteroids with inhaled corticosteroids in the treatment of acute asthma following emergency department discharge: a meta-analysis. *Chest* 2002;121:1798–1805. Search date 2001; primary sources Embase, Medline, Cinahl, hand searches of 20 respiratory journals and abstracts of meetings, Central, reference lists, and contact with authors and pharmaceutical companies.
73. Levy ML, Stevenson C, Maslen T. Comparison of a short course of oral prednisone and fluticasone propionate in the treatment of adults with acute exacerbations of asthma in primary care. *Thorax* 1996;51:1087–1092.
74. O'Driscoll BR, Kalra S, Wilson M, et al. Double-blind trial of steroid tapering in acute asthma. *Lancet* 1993;341:324–327.
75. Hasegaawa T, Ishihara K, Takakura S, et al. Duration of systemic corticosteroids in the treatment of asthma exacerbation: a randomized study. *Intern Med* 2000;39:794–797.
76. Edmonds ML, Camargo CA, Pollack CV, et al. The effectiveness of inhaled corticosteroids in the emergency department treatment of acute asthma: a meta-analysis. *Ann Emerg Med* 2002;40:145–154. Search date 2001; primary sources Embase, Medline, Cinahl, hand searches of 20 respiratory journals and abstracts of meetings, Central, reference lists, and contact with authors and pharmaceutical companies.
77. Edmonds ML, Camargo CA Jr, Saunders LD, et al. Inhaled steroids in acute asthma following emergency department discharge. The Cochrane Library, Issue 3, 2002. Oxford Software. Search date 1999; primary sources Cochrane Upper Airways Group register of controlled trials, hand searches of bibliographies, 20 respiratory journals, conference proceedings, and contact with authors of articles retrieved and pharmaceutical companies.
78. Rodrigo GJ, Rodrigo C. Continuous versus intermittent β agonists in the treatment of acute asthma. A systematic review with meta-analysis. *Chest* 2002;122:160–165. Search date 2001; primary sources Medline, Embase, Cinahl, Cochrane Controlled Trials Register, and bibliographies of trials and reviews.
79. Khine H, Fuchs SM, Saville AL. Continuous vs intermittent nebulized albuterol for emergency management of asthma. *Acad Emerg Med* 1969;3:1019–1024.
80. Shrestha M, Bidadi K, Gourlay S, et al. Continuous vs intermittent albuterol, at high and low doses, in the treatment of severe acute asthma in adults. *Chest* 1996;110:42–47.
81. Bradding P, Rushby I, Scullion J, et al. As required versus regular nebulized salbutamol for the treatment of acute severe asthma. *Eur Respir J* 1999;13:290–294.
82. Travers A, Jones AP, Kelly K, et al. Intravenous β_2-agonists for acute asthma in the emergency department. The Cochrane Library, Issue 3, 2002. Oxford Software. Search date not stated; primary sources Cochrane Airways Group Register, hand searches of 20 respiratory journals, bibliographies from included studies, and contact with authors and experts to identify eligible studies.
83. Rodrigo G, Rodrigo C, Burschtin O. Ipratropium bromide in acute adult severe asthma: a meta-analysis of randomized controlled trials. *Am J Med* 1999;107:363–370. Search date 1999; primary sources Medline, Current Contents, Science Citation Index, review articles, experts, pharmaceutical companies, Medical Editor's Trial Amnesty Register, and hand searches of references.
84. Stoodley RG, Aaron SD, Dales RE. The role of ipratropium bromide in the emergency management of acute asthma exacerbation: a metaanalysis of randomized clinical trials. *Ann Emerg Med* 1999;34:8–18. Search date 1997; primary sources Medline, Embase, Cinahl, Biological Abstracts, Cochrane Library, and Current Contents.
85. Rodrigo GJ, Rodrigo C. First-line therapy for adult patients with acute asthma receiving multiple dose protocol of ipratropium bromide plus albuterol in the emergency department. *Am J Respir Crit Care Med* 2000;161:1862–1868.
86. Rodrigo G, Rodrigo C, Pollack C, et al. Helium–oxygen mixture for non intubated acute asthma patients. *Cochrane Database Syst Rev* 2001;1. Search date 1999; primary sources Embase, Medline, Cinahl, hand searches of 20 relevant respiratory care journals, authors of all studies, references from included studies, reviews, and texts.
87. Manthous CA, Hall JB, Caputo MA, et al. Heliox improves pulsus paradoxus and peak expiratory flow in non-intubated patients with severe asthma. *Am J Respir Care Crit Care Med* 1995;151:310–314.
88. Rowe BH, Bretzlaff JA, Bourdon C, et al. Magnesium sulfate for treating exacerbations of acute asthma in the emergency department. In: The Cochrane Library, Issue 3, 2002. Oxford: Update Software. Search date 1998; primary sources Cochrane Airways Review Group Register of Trials, review articles, textbooks, experts, primary authors of included studies, and hand searches of references.
89. Boonyavoroakul C, Thakkinstian A, Charoenpan P. Intravenous magnesium sulfate in acute severe asthma. *Respirology* 2000;5:221–225.
90. Porter RS, Nester S, Braitman LE, et al. Intravenous magnesium is ineffective in adult asthma: a randomised trial. *Eur J Emerg Med* 2001;8:9–15.
91. Silverman RA, Osborn H, Runge J, et al. IV magnesium sulphate in the treatment of acute severe asthma: a multi centre randomized controlled trial. *Chest* 2002;122:489–497.
92. Nannini LJ, Pendino JC, Corna RA, et al. Magnesium sulfate as a vehicle for nebulized salbutamol in acute asthma. *Am J Med* 2000;108:193–197.
93. FitzGerald JM. Commentary: intravenous magnesium in acute asthma. *Evid Based Med* 1999;4:138.
94. Jones A, Rowe B, Peters J, et al. Inhaled beta-agonists for asthma in mechanically ventilated patients. *Cochrane Database Syst Rev* 2000;2:CD 001493. Search date 2001; primary sources Cochrane Airways Group Asthma and

Wheeze RCT register, reference lists from identified reports and reviews, and contact with colleagues, collaborators, and trialists.
95. Behbehani NA, Al-Mane FD, Yachkova Y, et al. Myopathy following mechanical ventilation for acute severe asthma: the role of muscle relaxants and corticosteroids. *Chest* 1999;115:1627–1631.
96. Williams TJ, Tuxen DV, Sceinkestel CD, et al. Risk factors for morbidity in mechanically ventilated patients with acute severe asthma. *Am Rev Respir Dis* 1992;146:607–615.
97. Darioli R, Perret C. Mechanical controlled hypoventilation in status asthmaticus. *Am Rev Respir Dis* 1984;129:385–387.
98. Menitove SM, Godring RM. Combined ventilator and bicarbonate strategy in the management of status asthmaticus. *Am J Med* 1983;74:898–901.
99. Higgins B, Greening AP, Crompton GK. Assisted ventilation in severe acute asthma. *Thorax* 1986;41:464–467.
100. Lam KN, Mow BM, Chew LS. The profile of ICU admissions for acute severe asthma in a general hospital. *Singapore Med J* 1992;33:460–462.
101. Mansel JK, Stogner SW, Petrini MF, et al. Mechanical ventilation in patients with acute severe asthma. *Am J Med* 1990;89:42–48.
102. Lim TK. Status asthmaticus in a medical intensive care unit. *Singapore Med J* 1989;30:334–338.
103. Keenan SP, Brake D. An evidence based approach to non invasive ventilation in acute respiratory failure. *Crit Care Clin* 1998;14:359–372.
104. Eastwood AJ, Sheldon TA. Organisation of asthma care: what difference does it make? A systematic review of the literature. *Quality Health Care* 1996;5:134–143. Search date 1995; primary sources Medline, CINAHL, HELMIS, Manchester Primary and Secondary Care Interface, Health Planning and Administration, DHSS databases, hand searches of references, and contact with experts.
105. Bartter T, Pratter MR. Asthma: better outcome at a lower cost? The role of the expert in the care system. *Chest* 1996;110:1589–1596.
106. Zeiger RS, Heller S, Mellon MH, et al. Facilitated referral to asthma specialist reduces relapses in asthma emergency room visits. *J Allergy Clin Immunol* 1991;87:1160–1168.
107. Gibson PG, Coughlan J, Wilson AJ, et al. Self-management education and regular practitioner review for adults with asthma. The Cochrane Library Issue 3, 2002. Search date 1999; primary sources Cochrane Airways Group Register of Trials, and hand searches of references.
108. Cote J, Bowie D, Robichaud P, et al Evaluation of two different educational interventions for adult patients consulting with an acute asthma exacerbation. *Am J Respir Crit Care Med* 2001;163:1415–1419.
109. Pereger TV, Sudre P, Muntner P, et al. Effect of patient education on self management skills and health status in patients with: a randomized controlled trial. *Am J Med* 2002;113:7–14.

J Mark FitzGerald
Respiratory Physician
and Director of Center
for Clinical Epidemiology and Evaluation
Vancouver General Hospital
Vancouver
Canada

Bazian Ltd
London
UK

Competing interests: MF has received honoraria for lectures and research funds from GlaxoSmithKline, Merck, AstraZeneca, Novartis, Boehringer Ingelheim, Byk Canada, Schering Canada, and 3M.

The following previous contributors of this topic would also like to be acknowledged: Chris Cates, Paul O'Byrne.

TABLE 1 **Classification of severity for chronic asthma (see text, p 1760).**

In the USA[1]

Asthma is classified by symptoms of severity. Using this system, even people with mild, intermittent asthma can develop severe exacerbations if exposed to appropriate stimuli.

Mild intermittent asthma	Symptoms less than weekly with normal or near normal lung function.
Mild persistent asthma	Symptoms more than weekly but less than daily with normal or near normal lung function.
Moderate persistent asthma	Daily symptoms with mild to moderate variable airflow obstruction.
Severe asthma	Daily symptoms and frequent night symptoms, and moderate to severe variable airflow obstruction.

In the UK[2]

Chronic asthma in ambulatory settings is graded according to the amount of medication required to keep symptoms controlled. People are classified according to whether, for symptom control, they need:

Step 1	Occasional β agonists for symptomatic relief.
Step 2	In addition, regular, inhaled anti-inflammatory agents (such as inhaled corticosteroids, cromoglycate, or nedocromil).
Step 3	In addition, high dose inhaled corticosteroids or low dose inhaled steroids plus long acting inhaled β_2 bronchodilator.
Step 4	In addition, high dose inhaled corticosteroids plus regular bronchodilators.
Step 5	In addition, regular oral corticosteroids.

Bronchiectasis

Search date October 2002

Bazian Ltd

QUESTIONS

INTERVENTIONS

Key Messages

- **Bromhexine** One systematic review found insufficient evidence to compare the effects of bromhexine versus placebo.
- **Inhaled steroids** One systematic review found insufficient evidence from two small RCTs about the effects of inhaled steroids versus placebo in people with bronchiectasis not due to a specific congenital disease.
- **Long acting β_2 agonists** One systematic review found no RCTs comparing long acting β_2 agonists versus placebo or other treatments in people with non-cystic fibrosis bronchiectasis.
- **Oral steroids** One systematic review found no RCTs comparing oral steroids versus placebo, no steroids, or other treatments in people with non-cystic fibrosis bronchiectasis.
- **Recombinant human deoxyribonuclease** One systematic review found insufficient evidence to compare the effects of recombinant human deoxyribonuclease versus those of placebo.

Clin Evid 2003;10:1782–1785.

DEFINITION Bronchiectasis is defined as irreversible widening of medium sized airways (bronchi) in the lung. It is characterised by inflammation, destruction of bronchial walls, and chronic bacterial infection. The condition may be limited to a single lobe or lung segment, or it may affect one or both lungs more diffusely. Clinically, the condition manifests as chronic cough and chronic overproduction of sputum (up to about 500 mL daily), which is often purulent.[1] People with severe bronchiectasis may have life threatening haemoptysis and may develop features of chronic obstructive airways disease, such as wheezing, chronic respiratory failure, pulmonary hypertension, and right sided heart failure.

INCIDENCE/ PREVALENCE We found few reliable data. Incidence has declined over the past 50 years and prevalence is low in higher income countries. Prevalence is much higher in poorer countries and is a major cause of morbidity and mortality.

AETIOLOGY/ RISK FACTORS Bronchiectasis is most commonly a long term complication of previous lower respiratory infections such as measles pneumonitis, pertussis, and tuberculosis. Foreign body inhalation and allergic, autoimmune, and chemical lung damage also predispose to the condition.[2] Underlying congenital disorders such as cystic fibrosis, cilial dysmotility syndromes, α_1 antitrypsin deficiency, and congenital immunodeficiencies may also predispose to bronchiectasis and may be of greater aetiological importance than respiratory infection in higher income countries. Cystic fibrosis is the most common congenital cause.

PROGNOSIS Bronchiectasis is a chronic condition with frequent relapses of varying severity. Long term prognosis is variable. Data on morbidity and mortality are sparse.[3] Bronchiectasis frequently coexists with other respiratory disease, making it difficult to distinguish prognosis for bronchiectasis alone.

AIMS OF INTERVENTION To alleviate symptoms; to reduce morbidity and mortality.

OUTCOMES **Primary outcomes:** Quality of life, admission to hospital, days off work, exacerbation and infection rates, haemoptysis, respiratory failure, mortality, and adverse effects of treatment. **Secondary outcomes:** Sputum volume and lung function indices. We reported secondary outcomes only if trials did not include primary outcomes.

METHODS *Clinical Evidence* search and appraisal October 2002.

QUESTION **What are the effects of pharmacological treatments in people with bronchiectasis but without cystic fibrosis?**

OPTION **MUCOLYTICS (BROMHEXINE AND DEOXYRIBONUCLEASE)**

One systematic review found insufficient evidence from three RCTs about the effects of mucolytics compared with those of placebo in people with non-cystic fibrosis bronchiectasis.

Benefits: We found one systematic review in people with non-cystic fibrosis bronchiectasis (search date 2001, 3 double blind RCTs, total number of participants not stated).[4] We found no subsequent RCTs.

Bromhexine: The review found one RCT comparing bromhexine (30 mg 3 times daily) versus placebo in 45 people with acute exacerbation of bronchiectasis (defined as morning cough and >20 mL sputum). It found that bromhexine reduced sputum volume versus placebo after about 2 weeks (weighted mean change in sputum volume with bromhexine *v* placebo: –21.5%, 95% CI –38.9% to –4.1%). The review found that bromhexine also improved some symptoms versus placebo (see comment below). **Recombinant human deoxyribonuclease (rhDNase):** The review found two RCTs comparing rhDNase aerosol versus placebo. The first (total number of participants not stated) found no significant difference between rhDNase (2.5 mg in 2.5 mL, once or twice daily) and placebo for lung function or infection rates (time to outcome not stated; infection rates reported for once daily dose: 4/21 with placebo *v* 0/21 with rhDNase; P > 0.1; no further numerical data reported). The second RCT similarly found no significant difference between rhDNase (twice daily for 24 wks) versus placebo for exacerbation rate (AR for exacerbation in 168 days: 0.66 with rhDNase *v* 0.56 with placebo; RR 1.17; CI not stated).

Harms: In one included trial, rhDNase (5 mg daily) increased the risk of influenza type symptoms compared with placebo (4 people with rhDNase *v* 0 with placebo).[4] Other adverse effects were not specifically reported.

Comment: One included RCT found that bromhexine significantly improved symptom scores versus placebo for "difficulty with expectoration", "cough", and "quality of sputum" after about 2 weeks.[4] The clinical importance of effects on these scores are uncertain.

OPTION INHALED STEROIDS

One systematic review found insufficient evidence from two small RCTs about the effects of inhaled steroids compared with those of placebo in people with bronchiectasis but without cystic fibrosis.

Benefits: We found one systematic review (search date 2001, 2 double blind RCTs, 54 people with bronchiectasis not due to congenital disease or focal airway obstruction).[5] The included RCTs compared inhaled steroids (beclomethasone 1500 µg daily or fluticasone 1000 µg daily) versus placebo. The systematic review pooled results and found no significant difference between inhaled steroids and placebo for symptom scores (75 mm visual analogue scale for steroids *v* placebo: mean improvement in cough score, 5 mm, 95% CI –28 to +38 mm; mean improvement in dyspnoea score, 4 mm, 95% CI –33 to +41 mm), lung function indices (improvement in forced expiratory volume in 1 s: 0.4 L/min, 95% CI –2.2 to +1.0 L/min; improvement in forced vital capacity: 0.6 L, 95% CI –0.1 to +1.3 L), or sputum volume (reduction in sputum volume: 0.2 mL daily, 95% CI –0.4 to +0.7 mL daily) after 4–6 weeks. The review reported that the RCTs lacked power to exclude clinically important effects. We found no subsequent RCTs.

Harms: Harms were not reported in the review.

Comment: None.

OPTION ORAL STEROIDS

One systematic review found no RCTs comparing oral steroids versus placebo, no steroids, or other treatments in people with non-cystic fibrosis bronchiectasis.

Benefits: We found one systematic review (search date 2002), which found no RCTs in people without cystic fibrosis.[6] We found no subsequent RCTs.

Harms: We found insufficient evidence to report on specific harms in people with bronchiectasis.

Comment: None.

OPTION LONG ACTING β_2 AGONISTS

One systematic review found no RCTs comparing long acting β_2 agonists versus placebo or other treatments in people with non-cystic fibrosis bronchiectasis.

Benefits: We found one systematic review (search date 2001), which found no RCTs in people without cystic fibrosis.[7] We found no subsequent RCTs.

Harms: We found insufficient evidence to report on specific harms in people with bronchiectasis.

Comment: None.

REFERENCES

1. Nicotra MB, Riveera M, Dale AM, et al. Clinical, pathophysiologic, and microbiologic characterization of bronchiectasis in an aging cohort. *Chest* 1995;108:955–961
2. Mysliwiec V, Pina JS. Bronchiectasis: the 'other' obstructive lung disease. *Postgrad Med* 1999;106:123–131.
3. Keistinen T, Saynajakangas O, Tuuponen T, et al. Bronchiectasis: an orphan disease with a poorly-understood prognosis. *Eur Respir J* 1997;10:2784–2787.
4. Crockett AJ, Cranston JM, Latimer KM, et al. Mucolytics for bronchiectasis (Cochrane Review). In: The Cochrane Library, Issue 4, 2002. Oxford: Update software. Search date 2001; primary sources Cochrane Airways Group register, contact with pharmaceutical manufacturers, contact with experts, handsearching of references.
5. Kolbe J, Wells A, Ram FSF. Inhaled steroids for bronchiectasis (Cochrane Review). In: The Cochrane Library, Issue 4, 2002. Oxford: Update Software. Search date 2001; primary sources Cochrane Airways Group register, contact with pharmaceutical manufacturers, contact with experts, handsearching of references.
6. Lasserson T, Holt K, Greenstone M. Oral steroids for bronchiectasis (stable and acute exacerbations) (Cochrane Review). In: The Cochrane Library, Issue 4, 2002. Oxford: Update Software. Search date 2002; primary sources Cochrane Controlled Trials Register, Medline, Embase, handsearching of references.
7. Sheikh A, Nolan D, Greenstone M. Long-acting beta-2-agonists for bronchiectasis (Cochrane Review). In: The Cochrane Library, Issue 4, 2002. Oxford: Update Software. Search date 2001; primary sources Cochrane Controlled Trials Register, Medline, Embase, handsearching of references.

Bazian Ltd
London
UK

Competing interests: None declared.

Chronic obstructive pulmonary disease

Search date October 2002

Huib Kerstjens and Dirkje Postma

QUESTIONS

INTERVENTIONS

See glossary, p 1801

*Extrapolated from studies of different types of pulmonary disease, including chronic obstructive pulmonary disease

Key Messages

- We found no evidence about effects of most interventions on progression of chronic obstructive pulmonary disease (measured by decline in lung function). However, we found good evidence from RCTs that inhaled corticosteroids do not prevent decline in lung function.
- **α_1 Antitrypsin infusion** One RCT in people with α_1 antitrypsin deficiency and moderate emphysema found no significant difference with α_1 antitrypsin infusion versus placebo in the decline in forced expiratory volume in 1 second (FEV_1) after 1 year.
- **Antibiotics** Two poor quality RCTs found no significant difference with antibiotics in frequency of exacerbations or decline in lung function over 5 years compared with placebo.

- **Deoxyribonuclease** We found no RCTs comparing long term effects of deoxyribonuclease versus placebo.
- **Inhaled anticholinergics** RCTs have found that inhaled anticholinergics versus placebo significantly improve FEV_1, exercise capacity, and symptoms. One large RCT found that adding ipratropium to a smoking cessation programme had no significant impact on decline in FEV_1 over 5 years. One RCT found that inhaled tiotropium (a long acting anticholinergic drug) reduced exacerbation and admission rates compared with placebo at 1 year.
- **Inhaled anticholinergics plus β_2 agonists** RCTs have found that combining a β_2 agonist with an anticholinergic drug for 2–12 weeks modestly but significantly improves FEV_1 compared with either drug alone. One RCT found that, when combined with an anticholinergic drug, a long acting β_2 agonist improved FEV_1 and peak expiratory flow rate significantly more than a short acting β_2 agonist.
- **Inhaled anticholinergics versus β_2 agonists** RCTs have found that 3 months of a short acting inhaled anticholinergic significantly improved forced expiratory volume in 1 second compared with short acting β_2 agonists. One RCT found that 6 months of a long acting inhaled anticholinergic significantly improved FEV_1 and quality of life compared with a long acting inhaled β_2 agonist. RCTs have found inconsistent evidence about effects of short acting inhaled anticholinergics versus long acting β_2 agonists over 3 months.
- **Inhaled β_2 agonists** RCTs found that inhaled β_2 agonists improve FEV_1 and symptoms compared with placebo after 1 week to 6 months' treatment.
- **Inhaled corticosteroids** RCTs have found no significant difference between inhaled corticosteroids and placebo in lung function (FEV_1) over 10 days to 10 weeks. However, large RCTs lasting at least 6 months suggested that inhaled steroids increased FEV_1 during the first 3–6 months of use, but we found evidence of no effect on subsequent decline in lung function. One systematic review found that long term inhaled steroids versus placebo reduced the frequency of exacerbations. Long term inhaled steroids may predispose to adverse effects, including osteoporosis, skin bruising, and oral candidiasis.
- **Long term domiciliary oxygen (in people with hypoxaemia)** RCTs found limited evidence that domiciliary oxygen versus no oxygen improved survival over 2 years in people with chronic obstructive pulmonary disease and hypoxaemia.
- **Oral corticosteroids** We found no evidence on long term benefits. One systematic review has found that oral corticosteroids for 2–4 weeks significantly improve lung function compared with placebo. Long term oral corticosteroids are associated with serious adverse effects, including osteoporosis and diabetes.
- **Oral versus inhaled corticosteroids** Three RCTs provided insufficient evidence about effects of oral versus inhaled corticosteroids over 2 weeks. Systemic corticosteroids are associated with serious adverse effects, including osteoporosis and diabetes.
- **Mucolytics** We found evidence from two systematic reviews that mucolytics versus placebo for 3–24 months may reduce the frequency and duration of exacerbations in people with chronic bronchitis. However, it is not clear whether these effects are generalisable to people with chronic obstructive pulmonary disease.

Chronic obstructive pulmonary disease

- **Theophyllines** One systematic review has found a slight but significant improvement in FEV_1 with theophyllines compared with placebo after 3 months. One large RCT has found that theophyllines significantly improve FEV_1 compared with placebo after 12 months of treatment. The usefulness of these drugs is limited by adverse effects and the need for monitoring of blood concentrations.

DEFINITION Chronic obstructive pulmonary disease (COPD) is characterised by chronic bronchitis or emphysema. Emphysema is abnormal permanent enlargement of the air spaces distal to the terminal bronchioles, accompanied by destruction of their walls and without obvious fibrosis. Chronic bronchitis is chronic cough or mucus production for at least 3 months in at least two successive years when other causes of chronic cough have been excluded.[1]

INCIDENCE/ PREVALENCE COPD mainly affects middle aged and elderly people. It is one of the leading causes of morbidity and mortality worldwide. In the USA, it affects about 14 million people and is the fourth leading cause of death. Both morbidity and mortality are rising. Estimated prevalence in the USA has risen by 41% since 1982, and age adjusted death rates rose by 71% between 1966 and 1985. All cause age adjusted mortality declined over the same period by 22% and mortality from cardiovascular diseases by 45%.[1] In the UK, physician diagnosed prevalence was 2% in men and 1% in women between 1990 and 1997.[2]

AETIOLOGY/ RISK FACTORS COPD is largely preventable. The main cause is exposure to cigarette smoke. The disease is rare in lifelong non-smokers (estimated incidence 5% in 3 large representative US surveys from 1971–1984), in whom "passive" exposure to environmental tobacco smoke has been proposed as a cause.[3,4] Other proposed causes include airway hyperresponsiveness, air pollution, and allergy.[5–7]

PROGNOSIS Airway obstruction is usually progressive in those who continue to smoke, resulting in early disability and shortened survival. Smoking cessation reverts the rate of decline in lung function to that of non-smokers.[8] Many people will need medication for the rest of their lives, with increased doses and additional drugs during exacerbations.

AIMS OF INTERVENTION To alleviate symptoms; to prevent exacerbations; to preserve optimal lung function; and to improve activities of daily living, quality of life, and survival.[9]

OUTCOMES Short and long term changes in lung function, including changes in forced expiratory volume in 1 second (see glossary, p 1801) (FEV_1); exercise tolerance; peak expiratory flow rate (see glossary, p 1801); frequency, severity, and duration of exacerbations; symptom scores for dyspnoea; quality of life; and survival.

METHODS *Clinical Evidence* search and appraisal October 2002. This review deals only with treatment of stable COPD and not with treatment of acute exacerbations. We were interested in the maintenance treatment of stable COPD; therefore, we did not include single dose or single day cumulative dose–response trials. In this review, short term treatment is defined as less than 6 months and long term as

6 months or over. There is consensus that 6 months is the absolute minimum duration of treatment required to assess effects on decline in lung function. Where RCTs were found, no systematic search for observational studies was performed.

QUESTION **What are the effects of maintenance treatment in stable chronic obstructive pulmonary disorder?**

OPTION **INHALED ANTICHOLINERGICS**

RCTs have found that inhaled anticholinergics versus placebo significantly improve forced expiratory volume in 1 second, exercise capacity, and symptoms. One large RCT found that adding ipratropium to a smoking cessation programme had no significant impact on decline in forced expiratory volume in 1 second over 5 years. One RCT found that inhaled tiotropium (a long acting anticholinergic drug) reduced exacerbation and admission rates compared with placebo at 1 year.

Benefits: **Short term short acting anticholinergics:** We found no systematic review that assessed effects on lung function. We found many small placebo controlled RCTs. Most found a significant effect in favour of ipratropium.[10–13] We found two large RCTs (276 people[14] and 405 people[15]) comparing ipratropium (36 μg 4 times daily) versus placebo or versus salmeterol for 12 weeks. In both RCTs, ipratropium versus placebo significantly improved baseline forced expiratory volume in 1 second (see glossary, p 1801) (FEV_1) but results were only presented graphically. We found one further RCT (780 people) comparing ipratropium (40 μg 4 times daily) versus placebo and versus formoterol (eformoterol) for 12 weeks.[16] It found that ipratropium versus placebo significantly improved FEV_1 (improvement in average FEV_1 over 12 h after medication 137 mL, 95% CI 88 mL to 186 mL). It found no significant difference in morning premedication peak expiratory flow rate (see glossary, p 1801), symptoms, quality of life scores, or need for rescue bronchodilators. We found one systematic review (search date 1999) assessing changes in exercise capacity with anticholinergic drugs versus placebo.[17] Meta-analysis was not performed because of heterogeneity in design and outcomes among studies. Sixteen of the 17 RCTs found that anticholinergic drugs improved exercise capacity compared with placebo. **Short term long acting anticholinergics:** We found three RCTs assessing effects on lung function of tiotropium (a long acting anticholinergic, 18 μg/day) versus placebo or versus ipratropium.[18–20] The first RCT (169 people) compared tiotropium versus placebo for 4 weeks. It found that tiotropium versus placebo significantly improved FEV_1 during the first 6 hours after treatment (mean improvement in FEV_1: +0.13 L with tiotropium *v* –0.02 L with placebo; $P < 0.05$), and significantly increased trough FEV_1 24 hours after the last dose (mean FEV_1: +0.07 L with tiotropium *v* –0.03 L with placebo; CI not provided; $P < 0.05$).[18] The second RCT (478 people) compared tiotropium versus placebo for 92 days. It found that tiotropium significantly improved FEV_1 during the first 3 hours after treatment ($P < 0.001$), increased the peak response (CI not provided;

$P < 0.001$; results presented graphically), and improved symptoms.[19] The third RCT (288 people, average age 65 years) compared tiotropium (18 μg/day) versus ipratropium (40 μg 4 times daily) for 13 weeks.[20] It found that tiotropium versus ipratropium significantly increased FEV_1 (mean FEV_1 6 h after treatment on first day: 0.24 L with tiotropium *v* 0.18 L with ipratropium; difference 0.06 L, 95% CI 0.02 L to 0.09 L), and significantly increased mean trough FEV_1 (0.15 L *v* 0.01 L with ipratropium; difference 0.13 L, 95% CI 0.09 L to 0.18 L). **Long term treatment with ipratropium or tiotropium:** We found three RCTs.[8,21,22] The first RCT (5887 smokers aged 35–60 years with spirometric signs of early chronic obstructive pulmonary disease [COPD]; FEV_1 75% predicted) compared three interventions over a 5 year period: an intensive 12 session smoking cessation programme combining behaviour modification and use of nicotine gum; the same smoking intervention programme plus ipratropium three times daily; or usual care. Although decline in FEV_1 was significantly slower in people in both smoking cessation groups compared with usual care, adding ipratropium had no significant effect (5 year mean cumulative decline in FEV_1 before bronchodilator: usual care 249 mL, 95% CI 236 mL to 262 mL; smoking programme plus ipratropium 188 mL, 95% CI 175 mL to 200 mL; smoking programme plus placebo 172 mL, 95% CI 159 mL to 185 mL). The second RCT (921 people) compared tiotropium (18 μg/day) versus placebo for 1 year.[21] It found that tiotropium significantly improved mean trough FEV_1 compared with placebo 3 and 24 hours after dosing (mean improvement compared with placebo at 3 h: 140–220 mL; P value not provided; at 24 h: 120–150 mL; $P < 0.01$). It also found that tiotropium significantly reduced exacerbations and hospital admissions compared with placebo (0.76 with tiotropium *v* 0.95 with placebo exacerbations per patient year, $P < 0.05$; admission to hospital for COPD exacerbation: 5.5% with tiotropium *v* 9.4% with placebo, $P < 0.05$).[21] The third RCT found that 1 year of tiotropium (18 μg/day) significantly improved trough FEV_1 and health related quality of life and reduced exacerbations compared with ipratropium (40 μg 4 times daily) at 1 year (improvement in FEV_1 with tiotropium *v* ipratropium: 150 mL, $P < 0.001$; quality of life: AR for 4 unit improvement in the St George's Respiratory Questionnaire 52% with tiotropium *v* 35% with ipratropium, $P = 0.001$; exacerbations in 1 year: 0.73 with ipratropium *v* 0.96 with ipratropium per patient year, $P = 0.006$).[22] It found no significant difference between tiotropium and ipratropium in admissions for COPD exacerbation at 1 year (7.3% with tiotropium *v* 11.7 % with ipratropium; $P = 0.11$).[22]

Harms: One RCT (233 people with asthma or COPD) found that continuous versus as needed treatment with bronchodilators (both ipratropium and fenoterol) caused a significantly faster decline in lung function (144 people, –0.07 L/year with continuous treatment *v* –0.02 L/year with as needed treatment; $P < 0.05$; CI not provided).[23] The first RCT of long term treatment found no significant difference between ipratropium and placebo in serious adverse events (cardiac symptoms, hypertension, skin rashes, and urinary retention; 1.2% with ipratropium *v* 0.8% with placebo), and dry mouth was the most common mild adverse effect.[8] The long term RCT comparing tiotropium versus placebo found similar rates of adverse effects, except for dry mouth (16.0 % with tiotropium *v* 2.7 % with placebo; $P < 0.05$).[21] Dry mouth was more common with tiotropium compared with ipratropium (6.1 with tiotropium *v* 12.1% with ipratropium; $P < 0.05$).[22]

Comment: RCTs of long term treatment found no evidence that people developed tachyphylaxis in response to the bronchodilating effect of ipratropium or tiotropium over a 1–5 year period.[8,21]

OPTION INHALED β_2 AGONISTS

RCTs have found that inhaled β_2 agonists for 1 week to 6 months significantly improve forced expiratory volume in 1 second and improve symptoms compared with placebo.

Benefits: **Short term treatment with short acting β_2 agonists:** We found one systematic review (search date 2002, 9 crossover RCTs, 264 people with stable chronic obstructive pulmonary disease) comparing short acting β_2 agonists versus placebo for at least 1 week.[24] It found that β_2 agonists delivered by metered dose inhaler slightly but significantly increased forced expiratory volume in 1 second (see glossary, p 1801) (FEV_1) compared with placebo (WMD 0.14 L, 95% CI 0.04 L to 0.25 L), and significantly improved daily breathlessness score (results reported as SMD; $P < 0.001$). There was no significant difference between treatments in exercise tolerance (4 RCTs), although the trials were small and results were heterogeneous. **Short term treatment with long acting β_2 agonists:** We found one systematic review (search date 2001, 8 RCTs of salmeterol, duration 4–16 wks, 979 people)[25] and four subsequent RCTs.[15,16,26,27] The review found no significant difference between salmeterol and placebo in FEV_1 (4 RCTs, 717 people; SMD +0.14 L, 95% CI –0.16 L to +0.44 L; see comment below).[25] Other outcomes could not be pooled. The first subsequent RCT (478 people) found that salmeterol (42 µg twice daily) versus placebo for 12 weeks significantly increased FEV_1 throughout the study period, but results were only presented graphically.[15] The second subsequent RCT (780 people) compared formoterol (12 µg *v* 24 µg twice daily) versus placebo and versus ipratropium for 12 weeks.[16] It found that both doses of formoterol versus placebo significantly improved FEV_1 (improvement in average FEV_1 over 12 h after medication, 12 µg formoterol *v* placebo 223 mL, 95% CI 174 L to 273 mL; 24 µg formoterol *v* placebo 194 mL, 95% CI 145 L to 243 mL). It also found that 12 or 24 mg formoterol versus placebo significantly improved quality of life scores (improvement in total score on St George's Respiratory Questionnaire, with 12 µg formoterol *v* placebo 5, $P < 0.001$; with 24 µg formoterol *v* placebo about 3–4, difference presented graphically, $P = 0.009$). The third subsequent RCT (692 people) compared formoterol (4.5, 9, or 18 µg twice daily) versus placebo for 12 weeks.[26] It found that all doses of formoterol significantly increased FEV_1 compared with placebo (results presented graphically). There was no dose–response effect for FEV_1. The RCT found that the two higher doses of formoterol significantly increased symptom free days compared with placebo (percentage increase in symptom free days compared with placebo +1.4%, 95% CI –2.7% to +5.4% with 4.5 μg formoterol, 4.7%, 95% CI 0.6% to 8.8% with 9 μg formoterol, and 5.7%, 95% CI 1.6% to 9.7% with 18 μg formoterol).[26] The fourth subsequent RCT (34 people, crossover design) compared effects of three interventions on exercise capacity: formoterol (4.5, 9, or 18 μg twice daily); ipratropium (80 μg 3 times daily); or placebo for 1 week.[27] It found that formoterol or ipratropium slightly but significantly increased time to exhaustion compared with placebo (10.94 min with 4.5 μg formoterol, $P < 0.0001$; 10.78 min with 9 μg formoterol, $P < 0.01$; 10.59 min with 18 μg formoterol, $P < 0.05$; 10.98 min with ipratropium, $P < 0.0001$; 10.20 min with placebo).[27] **Long term treatment with β_2 agonists:** We found no systematic review of long term treatment with short or long acting β_2 agonists versus placebo. We found one RCT (623 people) that compared salmeterol (50 μg twice daily) versus tiotropium and versus placebo for 6 months.[28] It found that salmeterol significantly improved mean pre-dose morning FEV_1 and average FEV_1 (0–12 h after dose) compared with placebo (mean improvement in mean pre-dose morning FEV_1 0.085 L, $P < 0.0001$; mean improvement in average FEV_1 0.138 L, $P < 0.0001$). However, the RCT found no significant improvement in symptom score (transition dyspnoea index) or health related quality of life score (St. George's respiratory questionnaire) compared with placebo.

Harms: In people with asthma, β_2 agonists have been linked to increased risk of death, worsened control of asthma, and deterioration in lung function.[29] One crossover RCT (53 people with chronic obstructive pulmonary disease, $FEV_1 < 70\%$ predicted) compared regular versus as needed treatment with the short acting inhaled β_2 agonist salbutamol for 3 months.[30] It found that regular versus as needed salbutamol doubled the total daily amount of salbutamol used (13 puffs/day [of which 8 puffs were the allocated regular dose] *v* 6 puffs/day with as needed treatment; significance not stated), with no significant difference in symptoms or lung function. The most common immediate adverse effect is tremor, which is usually worse in the first few days of treatment. High doses of β_2 agonists can reduce plasma potassium, cause dysrhythmia, and reduce arterial oxygen tension.[31] The risk of adverse events may be higher in people with pre-existing cardiac arrhythmias and hypoxaemia.[32] Two of the RCTs comparing salmeterol versus placebo over 12 weeks found no increase in any adverse events, but allowed rescue salbutamol.[14,15]

Comment: Many people report improvement in symptoms with bronchodilators that is not reflected by a change in FEV1>. Although the systematic review on long acting β_2 agonists showed no significant improvement in FEV_1,[25] two of the four included RCTs (412 people and 97 people) found significant effects, as did the three large subsequent RCTs. Additionally, the generalisability of the systematic review may be limited because RCTs were selected only if they excluded people with 15% or more airflow reversibility to a short acting β_2 agonist, whereas long term studies have found that up to two thirds of people with chronic obstructive pulmonary disease have at least 15% reversibility with β_2 agonists.[1,33]

OPTION INHALED ANTICHOLINERGICS PLUS β_2 AGONISTS

RCTs have found that combining a β_2 agonist with an anticholinergic drug for 2–12 weeks modestly but significantly improves bronchodilatation compared with either drug alone. One RCT found that, when combined with an anticholinergic drug, a long acting β_2 agonist improved forced expiratory volume in 1 second and peak expiratory flow rate significantly more than a short acting β_2 agonist. We found no RCTs of long term treatment with anticholinergics plus β_2 agonists versus placebo.

Benefits: **Short term treatment with anticholinergics plus short acting inhaled β_2 agonists:** We found six RCTs (705, 195, 652, 863, and 357 people with stable chronic obstructive pulmonary disease; 1 report combined the results from 2 RCTs) comparing the addition of ipratropium versus no additional ipratropium in people using standard dose short acting inhaled β_2 for 2 weeks to 3 months.[34–38] All found significant improvements in forced expiratory volume in 1 second (see glossary, p 1801) (FEV_1) of about 25% with the combination compared with either drug alone. **Short term treatment with anticholinergics plus long acting inhaled β_2 agonists:** One RCT (94 people) compared the long acting β_2 agonist salmeterol (50 µg twice daily) plus ipratropium (40 µg 4 times daily) versus salmeterol (50 µg twice daily) for 12 weeks.[39] It found that the combination versus the β_2 agonist alone significantly improved FEV_1 (mean improvement as a percentage of predicted FEV_1: 8% with combination *v* 5% with β_2 agonist; CI not provided; $P < 0.01$), and evening but not morning peak expiratory flow rate (see glossary, p 1801). It found no significant difference in daytime or night time symptoms.[40] **Short term treatment with anticholinergics plus long acting β_2 agonists versus anticholinergics plus short acting β_2 agonists:** One crossover RCT (172 people) compared ipratropium (40 µg 4 times daily) plus formoterol (12 µg twice daily) versus ipratropium (40µg 4 times daily) plus salbutamol (200 µg 4 times daily).[41] It found that formoterol plus ipratropium versus salbutamol plus ipratropium significantly improved FEV_1 and peak expiratory flow rate from baseline after 3 weeks of treatment (improvement in mean morning peak expiratory flow rate from baseline over the previous 7 days with formoterol 12 L/min, 95% CI 6 L/min to 19 L/min; improvement in premedication FEV_1 from baseline 116 mL, 95% CI 83 mL to 150 mL). **Long term treatment with anticholinergics plus inhaled β_2 agonists:** We found no systematic review or RCTs of long term treatment with anticholinergics plus β_2 agonists versus placebo.

Harms: The RCTs found no significant differences in adverse effects between treatments.[34–41]

Comment: None.

OPTION INHALED ANTICHOLINERGICS VERSUS β_2 AGONISTS

RCTs have found that 3 months of a short acting inhaled anticholinergic significantly improved forced expiratory volume in 1 second compared with short acting β_2 agonists. One RCT found that 6 months of a long

acting inhaled anticholinergic significantly improved forced expiratory volume in 1 second and quality of life compared with a long acting inhaled β_2 agonist. RCTs have found inconsistent evidence about effects of short acting inhaled anticholinergics versus long acting β_2 agonists over 3 months.

Benefits: We found no systematic review. **Short term treatment:** One non-systematic review (7 RCTs, 1445 people) compared ipratropium versus different short acting β_2 agonists for 90 days.[42] Lung function measurements were performed after withholding bronchodilators for at least 12 hours. It found that ipratropium versus β_2 agonists significantly improved mean forced expiratory volume in 1 second (see glossary, p 1801) (FEV_1) (28 mL increase with ipratropium *v* 1 mL decrease with β_2 agonist; CI not provided; $P < 0.05$). We found three subsequent RCTs comparing ipratropium versus β_2 agonists for 12 weeks.[14–16] The first two RCTs compared ipratropium (36 µg 4 times daily) versus salmeterol (42 µg twice daily).[14,15] The first RCT (411 people) found that salmeterol versus ipratropium significantly improved average FEV_1 at 4 and 8 weeks (CI not provided; $P < 0.005$), but not immediately after treatment or at 12 weeks.[14] The second RCT (405 people) found no significant difference in FEV_1 at any time.[15] The third RCT (780 people) compared three treatments: ipratropium; formoterol (12 µg *v* 24 µg twice daily); or placebo for 12 weeks.[16] It found that both doses of formoterol versus ipratropium significantly improved FEV_1 (improvement in average FEV_1 over 12 h after medication with 12 µg formoterol *v* with ipratropium 86 mL, 95% CI 37 mL to 136 mL; with 24 µg formoterol *v* ipratropium 57 mL, 95% CI 7 mL to 106 mL). Lower dose, but not higher dose, formoterol improved quality of life scores compared with ipratropium (improvement in total score on St George's Respiratory Questionnaire with 12 µg formoterol 3.79, $P < 0.001$; with 24 µg formoterol about 2, difference presented graphically, $P = 0.102$). **Long term treatment:** We found no systematic review comparing long term treatment with anticholinergics versus β_2 agonists. We found one RCT (623 people) comparing three treatments: tiotropium (18 µg/day); salmeterol (50 µg twice daily); or placebo for 6 months.[28] It found that tiotropium significantly improved mean pre-dose morning FEV_1; average FEV_1, and health related quality of life compared with salmeterol (improvement in mean pre-dose morning FEV_1 0.14 L with tiotropium *v* 0.09 L with salmeterol, $P < 0.01$; average FEV_1 [0–12 h after the dose] 0.08 L greater with tiotropium, $P < 0.001$; AR for 4 unit improvement in health related quality of life [St George's respiratory questionnaire] 51% with tiotropium *v* 40% with salmeterol, $P < 0.05$).

Harms: Adverse effects such as tremor and dysrhythmia associated with β_2 agonists seem to be more frequent than the adverse effects associated with anticholinergics, although the review provided no evidence for this.[42] The RCTs comparing salmeterol versus ipratropium found no significant difference in the frequency of adverse effects.[14,15] In the RCT of long term treatment, dry mouth was more frequent with tiotropium than with salmeterol or placebo (experienced by 10% with tiotropium, no further data provided).[28]

Comment: It has been suggested that older people experience greater bronchodilator response with anticholinergic drugs than with β_2 agonists, but we found no evidence for this.

OPTION THEOPHYLLINES

One systematic review has found a slight but significant improvement in forced expiratory volume in 1 second with theophyllines compared with placebo after 3 months. One large RCT found that theophyllines significantly improved forced expiratory volume in 1 second compared with placebo after 12 months treatment. The usefulness of these drugs is limited by adverse effects and the need for frequent monitoring of blood concentrations.

Benefits: **Short term treatment:** We found one systematic review (search date 2002, 20 small RCTs, 442 people) comparing theophyllines versus placebo for 1 week to 3 months.[43] It found that theophyllines slightly but significantly improved forced expiratory volume in 1 second (see glossary, p 1801) (FEV_1) compared with placebo (WMD 100 mL, 95% CI 40 mL to 160 mL). It found no significant difference in maximum walking distance (results presented as SMD).[43] **Long term treatment:** We found one RCT (854 people) comparing three treatments: open label theophylline, double blinded formoterol (12 or 24 µg twice daily), or placebo for 12 months.[44] It found that theophylline significantly improved FEV_1 compared with placebo (mean difference in FEV_1 with theophylline *v* placebo +120 mL, CI not provided; $P < 0.001$).

Harms: The RCTs identified by the review did not report adverse effects.[45] The therapeutic range for theophyllines is small, with blood concentrations of 10–15 mg/L required for optimal effects. Well documented adverse effects include nausea, diarrhoea, headache, irritability, seizures, and cardiac arrhythmias. These may occur within the therapeutic range.[46] One RCT found that people receiving theophylline were twice as likely to discontinue treatment compared with those taking placebo ($P < 0.002$).[44] Nausea was the most frequent adverse effect.

Comment: None.

OPTION ORAL CORTICOSTEROIDS

One systematic review of short term RCTs (usually 2–4 wks treatment) has found that oral corticosteroids versus placebo significantly improve lung function. We found no RCT of the effects of long term treatment with oral corticosteroids on lung function. Systemic corticosteroids are associated with serious adverse effects, including osteoporosis and induction of diabetes.

Benefits: **Short term treatment:** We found one systematic review (search date 1989, 10 RCTs, 445 people), which compared oral corticosteroids versus placebo in people with stable chronic obstructive pulmonary disease.[47] Treatment usually lasted 2–4 weeks. It found that significantly more people taking oral corticosteroids versus placebo had a 20% or greater improvement in baseline forced expiratory volume in 1 second (see glossary, p 1801) (WMD 10%, 95% CI 2% to 18%). When the other five RCTs were included, the difference in effect size was 11% (95% CI 4% to 18%). **Long term treatment:** We found no long term RCTs examining the effects of oral steroids on decline in lung function.

Harms: Many reviews have described the considerable harms of systemic corticosteroids, including osteoporosis and induction of diabetes.[48]

Comment: None.

OPTION INHALED CORTICOSTEROIDS

RCTs have found no significant difference between inhaled corticosteroids and placebo in lung function (forced expiratory volume in 1 second) over 10 days to 10 weeks. However, large RCTs lasting at least 6 months suggested that inhaled steroids increased forced expiratory volume in 1 second during the first 3–6 months of use, but we found evidence of no effect on subsequent decline in lung function. One systematic review found that long term inhaled steroids versus placebo reduced the frequency of exacerbations. Long term inhaled steroids may predispose to adverse effects, including osteoporosis, skin bruising, and oral candidiasis.

Benefits: **Short term treatment:** We found no systematic review. We found 10 RCTs of duration less than 6 months, summarised in one non-systematic review.[49] Nine short term trials (10 days to 10 wks, 10–127 people) found no significant improvement in lung function (forced expiratory volume in 1 s — FEV_1 — see glossary, p 1801) with inhaled steroids versus placebo. **Long term treatment:** We found two systematic reviews.[50,51] The first (search date 1996, 3 long term placebo controlled RCTs of inhaled steroids, 197 people treated for 2.0–2.5 years) examined lung function.[50] It found that inhaled steroids versus placebo significantly reduced the rate of deterioration in FEV_1 before bronchodilator (WMD 34 mL/year, 95% CI 5 mL/year to 63 mL/year). It found no significant difference in the rate of deterioration of FEV_1 after bronchodilator (WMD +39 mL/year, 95% CI –6 mL/year to +84 mL/year) or in the frequency of exacerbations. The second systematic review (search 2001, 9 RCTs of at least 6 months' duration, 3976 people) examined exacerbation rates.[51] It found that inhaled corticosteroids significantly reduced exacerbations compared with placebo (RR 0.70, 95% CI 0.58 to 0.84).[51] We found five RCTs examining lung function, which were published after the first review[50] (however, exacerbation rate results from these RCTs were included in the second review[51]).[52–56] The first subsequent RCT (281 people) found that fluticasone versus placebo significantly improved lung function (adjusted baseline daily peak expiratory flow rate 15 L/min with fluticasone *v* 2 L/min with placebo; $P < 0.001$).[52] The second RCT (290 people with mild airways obstruction, FEV_1 86% predicted) found no significant difference between budesonide (800 μg/day plus 400 μg/day for 6 months followed by 400 μg twice daily for 30 months) versus placebo for lung function.[53] The third RCT (1277 people, mean FEV_1 77% predicted; 912 people completed the trial) compared budesonide (800 μg/day) versus placebo for 3 years.[54] In the first 6 months of the study, FEV_1 improved in the budesonide group but decreased in the placebo group (rate of 17 mL/year with budesonide *v* 81 mL/year with placebo; CI not provided; P < 0.001). However, there was no effect on subsequent decline. The fourth RCT (751 people with more severe chronic obstructive pulmonary disease, FEV_1 50% predicted) compared fluticasone (500 μg twice daily for 3 years) versus placebo.[55] It found no effect on decline in lung function. The fifth RCT (1116 people with COPD, FEV_1 30–90% predicted) compared inhaled triamcinolone 600 μg twice daily versus placebo.[56] It found no significant difference between triamcinolone versus placebo in the rate of decline in FEV_1 after a mean duration of follow up of 40 months (mean 44.2 mL/year with triamcinolone *v* 47.0 mL/year with placebo; CI not provided; P = 0.50).

Harms: The systematic review of nine RCTs found that inhaled corticosteroids significantly increased risks of oropharyngeal candidiasis and skin bruising compared with placebo (candidiasis: RR 2.1, 95% CI 1.5 to 3.1; skin bruising RR 2.1, 95% CI 1.6 to 2.8).[51] The largest RCT identified by the review found that triamcinolone significantly reduced bone mineral density of the lumbar spine (P = 0.007) and femur (P = 0.001) compared with placebo.[56]

Comment: The RCTs in the systematic review[51] examined exacerbation frequency only as a secondary outcome.

OPTION ORAL VERSUS INHALED STEROIDS

Three RCTs provided insufficient evidence about effects of oral versus inhaled corticosteroids over 2 weeks. We found no RCTs of long term treatment with oral versus inhaled corticosteroids.

Benefits: We found no systematic review. **Short term treatment:** We found three RCTs comparing oral prednisolone versus inhaled beclometasone (beclomethasone) (12, 83, and 107 people).[57–59] All were double blind, placebo controlled crossover trials, with treatment periods of 2 weeks. One small RCT found no significant difference between the number of people responding to either or both treatments.[57] The other two RCTs found greater benefit with oral versus inhaled steroids. One found that forced expiratory volume in 1 second (see glossary, p 1801) rose from 0.65 L to 1.00 L with prednisolone versus 0.63 L to 0.80 L with beclometasone (CI not provided; P < 0.01). The other found that significantly more people responded to oral treatment (39/107 [36%] *v* 26/107 [24%]; CI not provided; P < 0.05).[58,59] **Long term treatment:** We found no RCTs.

Harms: None of the RCTs reported on adverse effects.[57–59]

Comment: One RCT included in the review recruited only people known to be responsive to oral steroids, and did not report severity of chronic obstructive pulmonary disease.[58] The other two RCTs included people with chronic obstructive pulmonary disease of duration more than 5 years and forced expiratory volume in 1 second less than 70% predicted.[57,59] All trials excluded people with evidence of reversible airflow obstruction.

OPTION MUCOLYTIC DRUGS

We found evidence from two systematic reviews that mucolytics versus placebo for 3–24 months may reduce the frequency and duration of exacerbations in people with chronic bronchitis. However, it is not clear whether these effects are generalisable to people with chronic obstructive pulmonary disease.

Benefits: **Long term treatment:** We found two systematic reviews.[60,61] However, not all included participants had chronic obstructive pulmonary disease. The first systematic review (search date 1999, 22 double blind RCTs, 2 RCTs in people with chronic obstructive pulmonary disease, 20 RCTs in people with chronic bronchitis not defined further; > 6000 people) found that mucolytics versus placebo for 3–6 months reduced significantly the average number of exacerbations (WMD –0.067 exacerbations/month, 95% CI –0.079 exacerbations/month to –0.055 exacerbations/month) and days of disability (WMD –0.56 days/month, 95% CI –0.77 to –0.35).[60] The second systematic review (search date 1995, 9 RCTs, 7 of which were included in the first review[60]) compared *N*-acetylcysteine versus placebo for 3–24 months.[61] It found an overall weighted effect size of 1.37 (95% CI 1.25 to 1.50), corresponding to a 23% reduction in exacerbations compared with placebo.

Harms: The first systematic review found no significant difference between mucolytics and placebo in the total number of adverse events.[60] Adverse effects of *N*-acetylcysteine were mainly mild gastrointestinal complaints.

Comment: Results of the reviews should be applied with caution.[60,61] It was unclear how many people included in the reviews had chronic obstructive pulmonary disease. In both reviews, there was significant heterogeneity among the RCTs, and symptom scores could not be pooled.[60,61] The effect of *N*-acetylcysteine in slowing the decline in lung function is being examined in a large European multicentre study (Dekhuijzen PNR, personal communication, 1999).

OPTION ANTIBIOTICS

We found no RCTs of antibiotics in short term treatment of stable chronic obstructive pulmonary disease. Two poor quality RCTs found no significant difference with antibiotics versus placebo in frequency of exacerbations or decline in lung function over 5 years.

Benefits: **Short term treatment:** We found no systematic review or RCTs. **Long term treatment:** We found no systematic review of antibiotics in people with stable chronic obstructive pulmonary disease, but found two RCTs.[62,63] The first RCT (497 people from 13 UK primary care clinics with chronic bronchitis, both with and without obstruction) compared four interventions: oxytetracycline plus chloramphenicol or sulphonamide; chloramphenicol or sulphonamide alone; oxytetracycline alone; or placebo over 5 years with oxytetracycline (0.5 mg/day for 3 years, increased to 0.5 mg twice daily in the fourth year, and 1 mg twice daily in the fifth year) versus chloramphenicol, sulphonamide, or placebo.[62] It found no significant difference in lung function or frequency of exacerbations with oxytetracycline versus chloramphenicol, sulphonamide, or placebo over 5 years (see comment below).[62] The second RCT (79 people) compared four interventions: tetracycline over the winter months for 5 years; placebo over winter for 5 years; tetracycline for two winters plus placebo for three winters; and placebo for two winters plus tetracycline for 3 years.[63] It found no significant difference between any of the treatment groups in mean frequency of exacerbations or decline in lung function, but may have been too small to exclude a clinically important difference.[63]

Harms: The RCTs did not report on harms.

Comment: The results of the first RCT should be interpreted with caution as it did not apply specific recruitment criteria and found evidence of heterogeneity in selection of people for the trial by each physician.[62] Doses of oxytetracycline were increased throughout the RCT because of lack of effect, which suggests that the benefits of double blinding may have been lost.[62]

OPTION DOMICILIARY OXYGEN TREATMENT

RCTs found limited evidence that domiciliary oxygen versus no oxygen improved survival over 2 years in people with chronic obstructive pulmonary disease and hypoxaemia. One RCT found that continuous treatment versus nocturnal treatment significantly reduced mortality over 24 months.

Benefits: **Long term treatment:** We found one systematic review (search date 2000, 5 RCTs).[64] The review could not perform a meta-analysis because of differences in trial design and participant selection. The first RCT (87 people), which compared daily oxygen for at least 15 hours versus no oxygen, found that domiciliary oxygen significantly reduced mortality over 5 years.[65] The second RCT (38 people with arterial desaturation at night) comparing nocturnal domiciliary oxygen versus room air found no significant difference in mortality at 3 years (figures not provided).[66] The third RCT (135 people with moderate hypoxaemia) identified by the review comparing oxygen versus no oxygen found no significant difference in survival at 3 years (HR 0.92, 95% CI 0.57 to 1.47; results presented graphically).[67] The fourth RCT (203 people) identified by the review compared continuous versus nocturnal domiciliary oxygen treatment. Continuous oxygen was associated with significant reduction in mortality over 24 months (22% with continuous *v* 41% with nocturnal oxygen; OR 0.45, 95% CI 0.25 to 0.81).[68] The fifth RCT (76 people with moderate daytime hypoxaemia [arterial pO_2 7.4–9.2 kPa] and significant nocturnal desaturation) comparing 2 years of nocturnal oxygen treatment versus placebo found no significant difference in survival.[69]

Harms: The systematic review did not report adverse effects.

Comment: Only one of the studies was double blinded. Domiciliary oxygen treatment seems to be more effective in people with severe hypoxaemia (arterial pO_2 < 8.0 kPa) than in people with moderate hypoxaemia or those who have arterial desaturation only at night.

OPTION α_1 **ANTITRYPSIN INFUSION**

We found no RCTs of short term treatment with α_1 antitrypsin. One RCT found no significant difference with α_1 antitrypsin versus placebo in the decline in forced expiratory volume in 1 second after 1 year in people with α_1 antitrypsin deficiency and moderate emphysema.

Benefits: We found no systematic review. **Short term treatment:** We found no RCTs. **Long term treatment:** We found one RCT (56 people with α_1 antitrypsin deficiency and moderate emphysema, forced expiratory volume in 1 second (see glossary, p 1801) [FEV_1] 30–80% predicted) comparing α_1 antitrypsin infusions (250 mg/kg) versus placebo infusion (albumin) given monthly for at least 3 years. It found no significant difference in the decline in FEV_1 after 1 year (decline in FEV_1 79 mL with α_1 antitrypsin v 59 mL with placebo; CI not provided; P = 0.25).[70]

Harms: The RCT reported no adverse effects in people taking α_1 antitrypsin or placebo.[70]

Comment: We found no clear evidence from observational studies on the effect of α_1 antitrypsin. For example, one cohort study (1048 people either homozygous for α_1 antitrypsin deficiency or with an α_1 antitrypsin concentration ≤ 11 µmol/L, with mean FEV_1 49 ± 30% predicted) compared weekly infusions of α_1 antitrypsin 60 mg/kg versus placebo for 3.5–7 years.[71] It found that α_1 antitrypsin significantly reduced mortality after an average of 5 years (RR of death 0.64, 95% CI 0.43 to 0.94). It found no significant difference between treatments in the decline in FEV_1, but in a subgroup of people with a mean FEV_1 of 35–49% predicted, α_1 antitrypsin significantly reduced the decline in FEV_1 (mean difference in FEV_1 0.08 L/year, 95% CI 0.003 L/year to 0.500 L/year; CI not provided; P = 0.03). A second cohort study (295 people homozygous for α_1 antitrypsin deficiency with FEV_1 < 65% predicted) compared 198 people who received weekly infusions of α_1 antitrypsin 60 mg/kg (duration not stated) versus 97 people who had never received α_1 antitrypsin. It found that α_1 antitrypsin significantly reduced the decline in FEV_1 (0.05 L/year with α_1 antitrypsin v 0.08 L/year with no α_1 antitrypsin; CI not provided; P = 0.02).[72]

OPTION **DEOXYRIBONUCLEASE**

We found no RCTs of deoxyribonuclease in people with chronic obstructive pulmonary disease.

Benefits: We found no systematic review or RCTs of deoxyribonuclease (DNase) specifically in people with chronic obstructive pulmonary disease (see comment below).

Harms: We found no RCTs.

Comment: **Short term treatment:** We found one RCT (349 people with bronchiectasis but not necessarily chronic airway obstruction) comparing DNase versus placebo given twice daily for 24 weeks.[73] It found that DNase significantly reduced forced expiratory volume in 1 second (see glossary, p 1801) (CI not provided; P ≤ 0.05), but found no significant difference in the frequency of exacerbations over 168 days (0.66/people with DNase *v* 0.56/people with placebo; RR 1.70, 95% CI 0.85 to 1.65). In people with cystic fibrosis, DNase treatment is used to degrade DNA that increases the viscosity of pulmonary secretions. However, we found no evidence that this mechanism is useful to people with chronic obstructive pulmonary disease and chronic sputum production.

GLOSSARY

Forced expiratory volume in 1 second (FEV_1) The volume breathed out in the first second of forceful blowing into a spirometer, measured in litres.

Peak expiratory flow rate The maximum rate that gas is expired from the lungs when blowing into a peak flow meter or a spirometer; the units are expressed as litres a minute.

REFERENCES

1. American Thoracic Society. Standards for the diagnosis and care of patients with chronic obstructive pulmonary disease: ATS statement. *Am J Respir Crit Care Med* 1995;152(5 pt 2)(suppl):77–120.
2. Soriano JB, Maier WC, Egger P, et al. Recent trends in physician diagnosed COPD in women and men in the UK. *Thorax* 2000;55:789–794.
3. Whittemore AS, Perlin SA, DiCiccio Y. Chronic obstructive pulmonary disease in lifelong nonsmokers: results from NHANES. *Am J Public Health* 1995;85:702–706.
4. Brunekreef B, Fischer P, Remijn B, et al. Indoor air pollution and its effects on pulmonary function of adult non-smoking women: III passive smoking and pulmonary function. *Int J Epidemiol* 1985;14:227–230.
5. Rijcken B, Weiss ST. Longitudinal analyses of airway responsiveness and pulmonary function decline. *Am J Respir Crit Care Med* 1996;154(suppl):246–249.
6. Dockery DW, Brunekreef B. Longitudinal studies of air pollution effects on lung function. *Am J Respir Crit Care Med* 1996;154(suppl):250–256.
7. O'Connor GT, Sparrow D, Weiss ST. The role of allergy and non-specific airway hyperresponsiveness in the pathogenesis of chronic obstructive pulmonary disease: state of the art. *Am Rev Respir Dis* 1989;140:225–252.
8. Anthonisen NR, Connett JE, Kiley JP, et al. Effects of smoking intervention and the use of an inhaled anticholinergic bronchodilator on the rate of decline of FEV_1: the lung health study. *JAMA* 1994;272:1497–1505.
9. Siafakas NM, Vermeire P, Pride NB, et al. Optimal assessment and management of chronic obstructive pulmonary disease (COPD): a consensus statement of the European Respiratory Society. *Eur Respir J* 1995;8:1398–1420.
10. Braun SR, McKenzie WN, Copeland W, et al. A comparison of the effect of ipratropium bromide and albuterol in the treatment of chronic obstructive airway disease. *Arch Intern Med* 1989;149:544–547.
11. Higgins BG, Powell RM, Cooper S, et al. Effect of salbutamol and ipratropium bromide on airway calibre and bronchial reactivity in asthma and chronic bronchitis. *Eur Respir J* 1991;4:415–420.
12. Ikeda A, Nishimura K, Koyama H, et al. Bronchodilating effects of combined therapy with clinical dosages of ipratropium bromide and salbutamol for stable COPD: comparison with ipratropium bromide alone. *Chest* 1995;107:401–405.
13. Ikeda A, Nishimura K, Koyama H, et al. Comparative dose–response study of three anticholinergic agents and fenoterol using a metered dose inhaler in patients with chronic obstructive pulmonary disease. *Thorax* 1995;50:62–66.
14. Mahler DA, Donohue JF, Barbee RA, et al. Efficacy of salmeterol xinafoate in the treatment of COPD. *Chest* 1999;115:957–965.
15. Rennard SI, Anderson W, ZuWallack R, et al. Use of a long-acting inhaled beta2-adrenergic agonist, salmeterol xinafoate, in patients with chronic obstructive pulmonary disease. *Am J Respir Crit Care Med* 2001;163:1087–1092.
16. Dahl R, Greefhorst LA, Nowak D, et al. Inhaled formoterol dry powder versus ipratropium bromide in chronic obstructive pulmonary disease. *Am J Respir Crit Care Med* 2001;164:778–784.
17. Liesker JJW, Wijkstra PJ, ten Hacken NHT, et al. A systematic review of the effects of bronchodilators on exercise capacity in patients with COPD. *Chest* 2002;121:597–608. Search date 1999; primary source Medline.
18. Littner MR, Ilowite JS, Tashkin DP, et al. Long-acting bronchodilation with once-daily dosing of tiotropium (Spiriva) in stable chronic obstructive pulmonary disease. *Am J Respir Crit Care Med* 2000;161:1136–1142.
19. Casaburi R, Briggs DD Jr, Donohue JF, et al. The spirometric efficacy of once-daily dosing with tiotropium in stable COPD: a 13-week multicenter trial. *Chest* 2000;118:1294–1302.
20. Van Noord JA, Bantje TA, Eland ME, et al. A randomised controlled comparison of tiotropium and ipratropium in the treatment of chronic obstructive pulmonary disease. The Dutch Tiotropium Study Group. *Thorax* 2000;55:289–294.
21. Casaburi R, Mahler DA, Jones PW, et al. A long-term evaluation of once-daily inhaled tiotropium in chronic obstructive pulmonary disease. *Eur Respir J* 2002;19:217–224.
22. Vincken W, van Noord JA, Greefhorst AP, et al. Improved health outcomes in patients with COPD during 1 yr's treatment with tiotropium. *Eur Respir J* 2002;19:209–216.
23. Van Schayck CP, Dompeling E, van Herwaarden CLA, et al. Bronchodilator treatment in moderate asthma or chronic bronchitis: continuous or on demand? A randomised controlled study. *BMJ* 1991;303:1426–1431.
24. Sestini P, Renzoni E, Robinson S, et al. Short-acting beta-2 agonists for stable chronic obstructive pulmonary disease. In: The Cochrane Library, Issue 4, 2002. Oxford: Update Software.

Search date 2002; primary sources Cochrane Airways Group database, and reference lists of review articles and retrieved studies.

25. Appleton S, Smith B, Veale A, et al. Long-acting beta-2 adrenoceptor agonists in stable chronic obstructive airways disease. In: The Cochrane Library, Issue 4, 2002. Oxford: Update Software. Search date 2001; primary sources Cochrane Airways Group Register to October 1998, hand searches of reference lists, and pharmaceutical companies contacted for unpublished studies.
26. Aalbers R, Ayres J, Backer V, et al. Formoterol in patients with chronic obstructive pulmonary disease: a randomized, controlled, 3-month trial. *Eur Respir J* 2002;19:936–943.
27. Liesker JJ, Van De Velde V, Meysman M, et al. Effects of formoterol (Oxis Turbohaler) and ipratropium on exercise capacity in patients with COPD. *Respir Med* 2002;96:559–566.
28. Donohue F, van Noord JA, Bateman ED, et al. A 6-month, placebo-controlled study comparing lung function and health status changes in COPD patients treated with tiotropium or salmeterol. *Chest* 2002;122:47–55.
29. O'Byrne PM, Kerstjens HAM. Inhaled β_2-agonists in the treatment of asthma. *N Engl J Med* 1996;335:886–888.
30. Cook D, Guyatt G, Wong E, et al. Regular versus as-needed short-acting inhaled beta-agonist therapy for chronic obstructive pulmonary disease. *Am J Respir Crit Care Med* 2001;163:85–90.
31. Hall IP, Tattersfield AE. Beta-agonists. In: Clark TJH, Godfrey S, Lee TH, eds. *Asthma*. 3rd ed. London: Chapman and Hall Medical, 1992:341–365.
32. Cazzola M, Imperatore F, Salzillo A, et al. Cardiac effects of formoterol and salmeterol in patients suffering from COPD with preexisting cardiac arrhythmias and hypoxemia. *Chest* 1998;114:411–415.
33. Anthonisen NR, Wright EC, and the IPPB Trial Group. Bronchodilator response in chronic obstructive pulmonary disease. *Am Rev Respir Dis* 1986;133:814–819.
34. Friedman M, Serby C, Menjoge S, et al. Pharmacoeconomic evaluation of a combination of ipratropium plus albuterol compared with ipratropium alone and albuterol alone in COPD. *Chest* 1999;115:635–641.
35. Levin DC, Little KS, Laughlin KR, et al. Addition of anticholinergic solution prolongs bronchodilator effect of beta 2 agonists in patients with chronic obstructive pulmonary disease. *Am J Med* 1996;100(1A;suppl):40–48.
36. Combivent Inhalation Solution Study Group. Routine nebulized ipratropium and albuterol together are better than either alone in COPD. *Chest* 1997;112:1514–1521.
37. Gross N, Tashkin D, Miller R, et al. Inhalation by nebulization of albuterol–ipratropium combination (Dey combination) is superior to either agent alone in the treatment of chronic obstructive pulmonary disease. Dey combination solution study group. *Respiration* 1998;65:354–362.
38. Campbell S. For COPD a combination of ipratropium bromide and albuterol sulfate is more effective than albuterol base. *Arch Intern Med* 1999;159:156–160.
39. Van Noord JM, de Munck DR, Bantje TA, et al. Long-term treatment of chronic obstructive pulmonary disease with salmeterol and the additive effect of ipratropium. *Eur Respir J* 2000;15:878–885.
40. Rutten van Molken M, Roos B, van Noord JA. An empirical comparison of the St George's Respiratory Questionnaire (SGRQ) and the Chronic Respiratory Disease Questionnaire (CRQ) in a clinical trial setting. *Thorax* 1999;54:995–1003.
41. D'Urzo AD, De Salvo MC, Ramirez-Rivera A, et al. In patients with COPD, treatment with a combination of formoterol and ipratropium is more effective than a combination of salbutamol and ipratropium: a 3-week, randomized, double-blind, within-patient, multicenter study. *Chest* 2001;119:1347–1356.
42. Rennard SI, Serby CW, Ghafouri M, et al. Extended therapy with ipratropium is associated with improved lung function in patients with COPD: a retrospective analysis of data from seven clinical trials. *Chest* 1996;110:62–70.
43. Ram FS, Jones PW, Castro AA, et al. Oral theophylline for chronic obstructive pulmonary disease. (Cochrane Review). In: The Cochrane Library, Issue 3, 2002. Oxford: Update Software. Search date 2002; primary sources: Cochrane Airways Group register and Cochrane Controlled Trials Register, Embase, LILACS, Medline, CINAHL, contact with experts, and handsearching of bibliographies.
44. Rossi A, Kristufek P, Levine BE, et al. Comparison of the efficacy, tolerability, and safety of formoterol dry powder and oral, slow-release theophylline in the treatment of COPD. *Chest* 2002;121:1058–1069.
45. Calverley PMA. Symptomatic bronchodilator treatment. In: Calverley PMA, Pride N, eds. *Chronic obstructive pulmonary disease*. London: Chapman and Hall, 1995:419–446.
46. Ramsdell J. Use of theophylline in the treatment of COPD. *Chest* 1995;107(suppl):206–209.
47. Callahan CM, Dittus RS, Katz BP. Oral corticosteroid therapy for patients with stable chronic obstructive pulmonary disease: a meta-analysis. *Ann Intern Med* 1991;114:216–223. Search date 1989; primary source Medline.
48. McEvoy CE, Niewoehner DE. Adverse effects of corticosteroid therapy for COPD: a critical review. *Chest* 1997;111:732–743.
49. Postma DS, Kerstjens HAM. Are inhaled glucocorticosteroids effective in chronic obstructive pulmonary disease? *Am J Respir Crit Care Med* 1999;160:66–71.
50. Van Grunsven PM, van Schayck CP, Derenne JP, et al. Long term effects of inhaled corticosteroids in chronic obstructive pulmonary disease: a meta-analysis. *Thorax* 1999;54:714–729. Search date 1996; primary sources Medline, Biosis, Online Contents, Glin, Cochrane Library, and Embase.
51. Alsaeedi A, Sin DD, McAlister FA. The effects of inhaled corticosteroids in chronic obstructive pulmonary disease: a systematic review of randomized placebo-controlled trials. *Am J Med* 2002;113:59–65. Search date 2001; primary sources Medline, Embase, Cinahl, Sigle, Cochrane Controlled Trial Register, and study bibliographies.
52. Paggiaro PL, Dahle R, Bakran I, et al. Multicentre randomised placebo-controlled trial of inhaled fluticasone propionate in patients with chronic obstructive pulmonary disease. *Lancet* 1998;351:773–780.
53. Vestbo J, Sorensen T, Lange P, et al. Long-term effect of inhaled budesonide in mild and moderate chronic obstructive pulmonary disease: a randomised controlled trial. *Lancet* 1999;353:1819–1823.
54. Pauwels RA, Lofdahl CG, Laitinen LA, et al. Long-term treatment with inhaled budesonide in persons with mild chronic obstructive pulmonary disease who continue smoking. European

Respiratory Society study on chronic obstructive pulmonary disease. *N Engl J Med* 1999;340:1948–1953.
55. Burge PS, Calverley PM, Jones PW, et al. Randomised, double blind, placebo controlled study of fluticasone propionate in patients with moderate to severe chronic obstructive pulmonary disease: the ISOLDE trial. *BMJ* 2000;320:1297–1303.
56. The Lung Health Study Research Group. Effect of inhaled triamcinolone on the decline in pulmonary function in chronic obstructive pulmonary disease. *N Engl J Med* 2000;343:1902–1909.
57. Robertson AS, Gove RI, Wieland GA, et al. A double-blind comparison of oral prednisolone 40 mg/day with inhaled beclomethasone dipropionate 1500 g/day in patients with adult onset chronic obstructive airways disease. *Eur J Respir Dis* 1986;69(suppl 146):565–569.
58. Shim CS, Williams MH. Aerosol beclomethasone in patients with steroid-responsive chronic obstructive pulmonary disease. *Am J Med* 1985;78:655–658.
59. Weir DC, Gove RI, Robertson AS, et al. Corticosteroid trials in non-asthmatic chronic airflow obstruction: a comparison of oral prednisolone and inhaled beclomethasone dipropionate. *Thorax* 1990;45:112–117.
60. Poole PJ, Black PN. Mucolytic agents for chronic bronchitis or chronic obstructive pulmonary disease. In: The Cochrane Library, Issue 1, 2002. Oxford: Update Software. Search date 1999; primary sources Cochrane Airways Group Register, and hand searches of reference lists.
61. Grandjean EM, Berthet P, Ruffmann R, et al. Efficacy of oral long-term *N*-acetylcysteine in chronic bronchopulmonary disease: a meta-analysis of published double-blind, placebo-controlled clinical trials. *Clin Ther* 2000;22:209–221. Search date 1995; primary sources Medline, hand searches of reference list, and personal contact with two experts.
62. Anonymous. Value of chemoprophylaxis and chemotherapy in early chronic bronchitis. A report to the Medical Research Council by their working party on trials of chemotherapy in early chronic bronchitis. *BMJ* 1966;5499:1317–1322.
63. Johnston RN, McNeill RS, Smith DH, et al. Five-year winter chemoprophylaxis for chronic bronchitis. *BMJ* 1969;4:265–269.
64. Crockett AJ, Moss JR, Cranston JM, et al. Domiciliary oxygen in chronic obstructive pulmonary disease. In: The Cochrane Library, Issue 1, 2002. Oxford: Update Software. Search date 2000; primary source Cochrane Airways Group Register.
65. Medical Research Council Working Party. Long term domiciliary oxygen therapy in chronic hypoxic cor pulmonale complicating chronic bronchitis and emphysema. *Lancet* 1981;1:681–686.
66. Fletcher EC, Luckett RA, Goodnight-White S, et al. A double-blind trial of nocturnal supplemental oxygen for sleep desaturation in patients with chronic obstructive pulmonary disease and a daytime PaO_2 above 60 mm Hg. *Am Rev Respir Dis* 1992;145:1070–1076.
67. Gorecka D, Gorzelak K, Sliwinski P, et al. Effect of long-term oxygen therapy on survival in patients with chronic obstructive pulmonary disease with moderate hypoxaemia. *Thorax* 1997;52:674–679.
68. Nocturnal Oxygen Therapy Trial Group. Continuous or nocturnal oxygen therapy in hypoxemic chronic obstructive lung disease: a clinical trial. *Ann Intern Med* 1980;93:391–398.
69. Chaouat A, Weitzenblum E, Kessler R, et al. A randomized trial of nocturnal oxygen therapy in chronic obstructive pulmonary disease patients. *Eur Respir J* 1999;14:1002–1008.
70. Dirksen A, Dijkman JH, Madsen F, et al. A randomized clinical trial of $alpha_1$-antitrypsin augmentation therapy. *Am J Respir Crit Care Med* 1999;160:1468–1472.
71. Anonymous. Survival and FEV_1 decline in individuals with severe deficiency of alpha1-antitrypsin. The Alpha-1-Antitrypsin Deficiency Registry Study Group. *Am J Respir Crit Care Med* 1998;158:49–59.
72. Seersholm N, Wencker M, Banik N, et al. Does alpha1-antitrypsin augmentation therapy slow the annual decline in FEV_1 in patients with severe hereditary alpha1-antitrypsin deficiency? Wissenschaftliche Arbeitsgemeinschaft zur Therapie von Lungenerkrankungen (WATL) alpha1-AT study group. *Eur Respir J* 1997;10:2260–2263.
73. O'Donnell AE, Barker AF, Ilowite JS, et al. Treatment of idiopathic bronchiectasis with aerosolized recombinant human DNase I. rhDNase Study Group. *Chest* 1998;113:1329–1334.

Huib Kerstjens
Pulmonary Physician

Dirkje Postma
Professor of Pulmonary Medicine

University Hospital Groningen
Groningen
The Netherlands

Competing interests: Both authors have received funding from the following manufacturers: AstraZeneca, the manufacturer of budesonide, terbutaline, formoterol; GlaxoSmithKline, the manufacturer of beclometasone, salbutamol, salmeterol, fluticasone; Boehringer Ingelheim, the manufacturer of fenoterol, ipratropium, tiotropium; and Novartis, the manufacturer of formoterol. DP has also received funding from Zambon, the manufacturer of *N*-acetylcysteine.

Lung cancer

Search date January 2003

Alan Neville

QUESTIONS

INTERVENTIONS

NON-SMALL CELL LUNG CANCER

Beneficial

Palliative chemotherapy with cisplatin or docetaxel containing regimens in stage 4 non-small cell lung cancer 1811

Thoracic irradiation plus chemotherapy versus irradiation alone in unresected stage 3 non-small cell lung cancer .1809

Unknown effectiveness

Hyperfractionated radiation treatment versus conventional radiotherapy in unresectable stage 3 non-small cell lung cancer 1810

Newer single drug or combined drug regimens in stage 4 non-small cell lung cancer (not clearly better than cisplatin or docetaxel based regimens) .1811

Preoperative chemotherapy in people with resectable stage 3 non-small cell lung cancer .1807

Unlikely to be beneficial

Postoperative chemotherapy in people with resected stage 1–3 non-small cell lung cancer .1807

SMALL CELL LUNG CANCER

Beneficial

Chemotherapy plus thoracic irradiation versus chemotherapy alone in limited stage small cell lung cancer 1816

Likely to be beneficial

Prophylactic cranial irradiation for people in complete remission with limited or extensive stage small cell lung cancer. 1818

Unknown effectiveness

Dose intensification of chemotherapy versus standard chemotherapy 1815

Likely to be ineffective or harmful

Oral etoposide versus combination chemotherapy in extensive stage small cell lung cancer. 1818

See glossary, p 1820

Key Messages

Non-small cell lung cancer

- **Palliative chemotherapy with cisplatin or docetaxel containing regimens in stage 4 non-small cell lung cancer** Systematic reviews in people with stage 4 non-small cell lung cancer have found that adding chemotherapy regimens containing cisplatin to best supportive care increases survival at 1 year compared with supportive care alone. Limited evidence from RCTs suggests that the adding chemotherapy to best supportive care may improve quality of life compared with best supportive care alone.

- **Thoracic irradiation plus chemotherapy versus irradiation alone in unresected stage 3 non-small cell lung cancer** Systematic reviews and one subsequent RCT in people with unresectable stage 3 non-small cell lung cancer have found that adding chemotherapy to irradiation improves survival at 2–5 years compared with irradiation alone. Another subsequent RCT has found no significant difference in median survival between radical radiotherapy plus chemotherapy and radiotherapy alone.
- **Hyperfractionated radiation treatment versus conventional radiotherapy in unresectable stage 3 non-small cell lung cancer** One systematic review in people with stage 3 non-small cell lung cancer found no significant difference between standard hyperfractionation and conventional radiotherapy in survival at 2 years. One RCT in people with stage 1–3B non-small cell lung cancer found that continuous, hyperfractionated, accelerated radiotherapy increased survival at 2 years compared with conventional radiotherapy.
- **Newer single drug or combined drug regimens in stage 4 non-small cell lung cancer (not clearly better than cisplatin or docetaxel based regimens)** One systematic review and subsequent RCTs in people with stage 3 and 4 non-small cell lung cancer found inconclusive evidence on the effects of single compared with combined chemotherapy. RCTs in people with stage 3 and 4 non-small cell lung cancer found no significant difference in survival at 1 year between first line platinum based and non-platinum based chemotherapy.
- **Preoperative chemotherapy in people with resectable stage 3 non-small cell lung cancer** One systematic review of small, weak RCTs and one subsequent RCT provided inconclusive evidence about the effects of preoperative chemotherapy in people with resectable stage 3 disease.
- **Postoperative chemotherapy in people with resected stage 1–3 non-small cell lung cancer** Systematic reviews and subsequent RCTs in people with completely resected stage 1–3 non-small cell lung cancer have found no significant difference in survival at 5 years between postoperative cisplatin based chemotherapy and surgery with or without concomitant radiotherapy, although subgroup analysis in one RCT suggests that postoperative chemotherapy may increase survival in people with stage 3 disease. One systematic review found that postoperative alkylating agents increased mortality compared with no postoperative chemotherapy.

Small cell lung cancer

- **Chemotherapy plus thoracic irradiation versus chemotherapy alone in limited stage small cell lung cancer** Two systematic reviews in people with limited stage small cell lung cancer have found that adding thoracic irradiation to chemotherapy improves survival at 3 years. However, one of these reviews has found that chemotherapy plus thoracic irradiation increases deaths related to treatment.
- **Prophylactic cranial irradiation for people in complete remission with limited or extensive stage small cell lung cancer** One systematic review in people in with small cell lung cancer in complete remission has found that, compared with no irradiation, prophylactic cranial irradiation improves survival at 3 years and reduces the risk of developing brain metastases. While long term cognitive dysfunction following cranial irradiation has been described in non-randomised studies, RCTs have not found a cumulative increase in neuropsychological dysfunction.

- **Dose intensification of chemotherapy versus standard chemotherapy** One systematic review found limited evidence that intensifying chemotherapy dose by either increasing the number of chemotherapy cycles, increasing chemotherapy dose, or increasing dose intensity per cycle may modestly improve survival compared with standard chemotherapy. However, additional RCTs have found inconclusive evidence about the effects of dose intensification on survival.
- **Oral etoposide versus combination chemotherapy in extensive stage small cell lung cancer** Two RCTs in people with extensive stage small cell lung cancer found that oral etoposide reduced survival compared with combination chemotherapy at 1 year. One RCT, in people with extensive stage small cell lung cancer who had not responded to induction combination chemotherapy, found no significant difference between oral etoposide and no further treatment in mortality at 3 years, although overall mortality was lower in people taking etoposide. RCTs found that etoposide may reduce nausea, alopecia and numbness in the short term compared with combination chemotherapy, but found no evidence that it offered better quality of life overall.

DEFINITION Lung cancer (bronchogenic carcinoma) is an epithelial cancer arising from the bronchial surface epithelium or bronchial mucous glands (see table 1, p 1823).

INCIDENCE/ PREVALENCE Lung cancer is the leading cause of cancer death in both men and women, affecting about 100 000 men and 80 000 women annually in the USA, and about 40 000 men and women in the UK. Small cell lung cancer constitutes about 20–25% of all lung cancers, the remainder being non-small cell lung cancers of which adenocarcinoma is now the most prevalent form.[1]

AETIOLOGY/ RISK FACTORS Smoking remains the major preventable risk factor, accounting for about 80–90% of all cases.[2] Other respiratory tract carcinogens have been identified that may enhance the carcinogenic effects of tobacco smoke, either in the workplace (e.g. asbestos and polycyclic aromatic hydrocarbons) or in the home (e.g. indoor radon).[3]

PROGNOSIS Lung cancer has an overall 5 year survival rate of 10–12%.[4] At the time of diagnosis, 10–15% of people with lung cancer have localised disease. Of these, half will have died at 5 years despite potentially curative surgery. Over half of people have metastatic disease at the time of diagnosis. People with non-small cell cancer who undergo surgery have a 5 year survival of 60–80% for stage 1 disease and 25–50% for stage 2 disease.[4] In people with small cell cancer, those with limited stage disease who undergo combined chemotherapy and mediastinal irradiation have a median survival of 18–24 months, whereas those with extensive stage disease who are given palliative chemotherapy have a median survival of 10–12 months.[4] About 5–10% of people with small cell lung cancer present with central nervous system involvement, and half develop symptomatic brain metastases by 2 years. Of these, only half respond to palliative radiation, and their median survival is less than 3 months.[4]

AIMS OF INTERVENTION To prolong life; to improve quality of life; and to provide palliation of symptoms, with minimum adverse effects of treatment.

OUTCOMES Survival; clinical response rates; disease related symptoms; adverse effects of treatment; quality of life. Despite recent progress in the development of valid instruments, measuring quality of life in people with lung cancer remains a serious challenge.[5,6]

METHODS *Clinical Evidence* search and appraisal January 2003. Unless stated otherwise, we have used the term stage 3 non-small cell lung cancer to refer to both stage 3A and stage 3B (see table 1, p 1823).

QUESTION **What are the effects of treatments for non-small cell lung cancer?**

OPTION **PRE- AND POSTOPERATIVE CHEMOTHERAPY IN PEOPLE WITH RESECTABLE NON-SMALL CELL LUNG CANCER**

One systematic review of small, weak RCTs and one subsequent RCT provided inconclusive evidence about the effects of preoperative chemotherapy in people with resectable stage 3 disease. Systematic reviews and subsequent RCTs in people with completely resected stage 1–3 non-small cell lung cancer have found no significant difference in survival at 5 years between postoperative cisplatin based chemotherapy and surgery with or without concomitant radiotherapy, although subgroup analysis in one RCT suggests that postoperative chemotherapy may increase survival in people with stage 3 disease. One systematic review found that postoperative alkylating agents increased mortality compared with no postoperative chemotherapy.

Benefits: **Preoperative chemotherapy:** We found one systematic review,[7] one non-systematic review,[8] and one subsequent RCT.[9] The systematic review (search date 1997, 4 RCTs, 204 people with technically resectable stage 3A non-small cell lung cancer) compared preoperative cisplatin based chemotherapy versus no chemotherapy.[7] It found that preoperative chemotherapy significantly reduced mortality at 2 years compared with no preoperative chemotherapy (two fully reported RCTs; AR 34/58 [59%] with preoperative chemotherapy *v* 54/62 [87%] with no chemotherapy; RR 0.67, 95% CI 0.42 to 0.89; NNT 4, 95% CI 2 to 11). One non-systematic review, which identified the same RCTs, suggested that this evidence is limited because the trials were small, staging was clinical rather than pathological, and treatment groups were not balanced for prognostic factors such as K-Ras mutations.[8] We found one subsequent RCT (355 people with resectable stages 1 [except T1N0] to 3A non-small cell lung cancer), which compared preoperative chemotherapy (two cycles of ifosfamide plus mitomycin plus cisplatin) versus primary surgery alone.[9] It found no significant difference in survival after 4 years follow up between preoperative chemotherapy and surgery alone in people with any disease stage or in people with stage 3 disease (median survival for any disease stage 37 months, 95% CI 26.7 months to 48.3 months with preoperative chemotherapy *v* 26.0 months, 95% CI 19.8months to 33.6 months, P = 0.15; RR for survival in people with stage 3 disease 1.04, 95% CI 0.68 to 1.60, P = 0.85). **Postoperative chemotherapy:** We found two systematic reviews[10,11] and one subsequent RCT.[12] The most recent review (search date 1998, 1 earlier systematic review)[10] did not fully describe the earlier identified review comparing postoperative cisplatin based chemotherapy versus no chemotherapy.[11] The earlier review (search date 1991, 14 RCTs, 1394 people with resected stage 1–3 non-small cell lung cancer) found no significant difference between postoperative cisplatin based chemotherapy and surgery alone in mortality at 5 years (8 RCTs; ARR +5%, 95% CI −1% to +10%; HR 0.87, 95% CI 0.74 to 1.02; P = 0.08).[11] However, it found that postoperative alkylating agents significantly increased mortality compared with surgery alone (5 RCTs; HR 1.15; CI not stated; P = 0.005; ARI of death at 5 years +5%, CI not stated). The subsequent RCT (70 people, stage 1–3B resected non-small cell lung cancer) compared postoperative chemotherapy (4 cycles of iv cyclophosphamide, vincristine, adriamycin and lomustine, followed by oral ftorafur) versus no chemotherapy for 1 year.[12] It found no significant difference in survival at 5 years between postoperative chemotherapy and no postoperative chemotherapy (49% with postoperative chemotherapy *v* 31% with no chemotherapy; P > 0.05, absolute numbers not provided).[12] A subgroup analysis in people with stage 3 non-small cell lung cancer (40 people with stage 3A, 9 with stage 3B) found that postoperative chemotherapy significantly increased survival at 5 years compared with no postoperative chemotherapy (44% with postoperative chemotherapy *v* 21% with no chemotherapy; P < 0.025, absolute numbers not provided). Results for people with stage 3A and 3B non-small cell lung cancer were not reported separately.[12] **Postoperative chemotherapy plus radiotherapy versus postoperative radiotherapy alone:** We found one systematic review (search date 1991, 7 RCTs, 807 people)[11] and one subsequent RCT.[12] The review found no significant difference in overall survival between adding postoperative chemotherapy to postoperative radiotherapy and postoperative radiotherapy alone (overall HR 0.98, CI not stated, P = 0.76; HR for 6 RCTs that used cisplatin based chemotherapy HR 0.94, CI not stated, P = 0.46; ARR for death at 5 years +2%, 95% CI −3% to +8%).[11] The subsequent RCT (488 people with completely resected stage 2 or 3A non-small cell lung cancer) compared postoperative radiotherapy with or without cisplatin plus etoposide.[13] It found no significant difference between postoperative chemotherapy plus radiotherapy and radiotherapy alone in median survival (37.9 months *v* 38.8 months; P = 0.56).

Harms: **Preoperative chemotherapy:** One RCT identified by the review, which compared preoperative chemotherapy versus no chemotherapy, found that chemotherapy was associated with grade III or IV neutropenia (80% of people), nausea and vomiting, diarrhoea, hypomagnesaemia, and alopecia (no further data provided).[7] **Postoperative chemotherapy:** The systematic review of postoperative cisplatin based chemotherapy gave no information on adverse effects.[11] One RCT (269 people) identified by the review, which compared four postoperative courses of cyclophosphamide plus adriamycin plus cisplatin versus no postoperative chemotherapy, found that only 53% of people allocated to postoperative chemotherapy completed all four courses.[14] Mild to severe gastrointestinal toxicity was reported in 88% of people receiving postoperative chemotherapy. A second RCT identified by the review reported similar toxicity.[15] Many adjuvant chemotherapy studies were published before serotonin receptor antagonist antiemetics were available.

Comment: The systematic review[7] examining effects of preoperative chemotherapy identified one interim report[16] of an RCT in 27 people, which was unsuitable for inclusion in the meta-analysis. The RCT found that preoperative chemotherapy significantly improved median survival after about 30 months follow up compared with no preoperative chemotherapy (median survival 28.7 months with preoperative chemotherapy *v* 15.6 months without; P = 0.095).[16] Larger trials of preoperative chemotherapy in people with stage 3A non-small cell lung cancer are needed. Most of the chemotherapy regimens in the postoperative RCTs identified by the reviews are no longer used, and more trials examining newer agents are needed.

OPTION ADDING CHEMOTHERAPY TO THORACIC IRRADIATION FOR UNRESECTABLE STAGE 3 NON-SMALL CELL LUNG CANCER

Systematic reviews and one subsequent RCT in people with unresectable stage 3 non-small cell lung cancer have found that adding chemotherapy to irradiation improves survival at 2–5 years compared with irradiation alone. Another subsequent RCT found no significant difference in median survival between radical radiotherapy plus chemotherapy and radiotherapy alone. Observational evidence suggests that, in people aged over 70 years with unresectable stage 3 non-small cell lung cancer, chemotherapy plus radiotherapy may reduce quality adjusted survival compared with radiotherapy alone. We found insufficient evidence about effects on quality of life.

Benefits: We found three systematic reviews[11,17,18] and two subsequent RCTs.[19,20] The first review (search date 1991, 22 RCTs, 3033 people with unresected stage 3 non-small cell lung cancer) found that chemotherapy plus thoracic irradiation significantly reduced mortality compared with radiotherapy alone (HR 0.90, 95% CI 0.83 to 0.97), with an absolute survival benefit of 3% with combined treatment compared with radiotherapy alone at 2 years.[11] The second review (search date 1995, 14 RCTs, including 9 RCTs identified by the first review and one RCT excluded from the first review because of poor methodology, 1887 people) found that a cisplatin based regimen plus radiotherapy significantly reduced mortality at 2 years compared with radiotherapy alone (OR 0.7, 95% CI 0.5 to 0.9).[17] The third review (search date 1995, 14 RCTs, including 11 RCTs identified by the first or second review, 2589 people) found that chemotherapy (primarily cisplatin based) plus radiotherapy significantly reduced mortality at 3 years compared with radiotherapy alone (RR 0.83, 95% CI 0.77 to 0.90).[18] The first subsequent RCT (458 people) compared 2 months of cisplatin plus vinblastine followed by standard radiotherapy versus either standard or hyperfractionated radiotherapy alone. It found that combined treatment significantly improved 5 year survival compared with radiotherapy alone (AR 8% with combined treatment v 5% with standard radiotherapy v 6% with hyperfractionated radiotherapy; P = 0.04 for combined v either comparison).[19] The second subsequent RCT (446 people) compared radical radiotherapy plus four cycles of mitomycin, ifosfamide, and cisplatin versus radical radiotherapy alone.[20] It found no significant difference in median survival between groups (11.7 months with combined treatment v 9.7 months with radiotherapy alone; P = 0.14). We found insufficient evidence about the effects of combining thoracic irradiation with chemotherapy on quality of life.

Harms: The reviews and RCTs gave no information on long term adverse effects of treatment.[11,17–20]

Comment: Radioprotector drugs and three-dimensional conformal radiotherapy are being investigated to reduce the toxicities of combined modality treatment.[21] One meta-analysis (6 prospective phase II or phase III studies) found that, in people aged over 70 years with unresectable stage 3 non-small cell lung cancer, chemotherapy plus radiotherapy significantly reduced quality adjusted survival compared with radiotherapy alone (10.8 months with chemotherapy plus radiotherapy v 13.1 months with standard radiotherapy; P < 0.01).[22]

OPTION HYPERFRACTIONATED RADIATION TREATMENT FOR UNRESECTABLE STAGE 3 NON-SMALL CELL LUNG CANCER

One systematic review in people with stage 3 non-small cell lung cancer found no significant difference between standard hyperfractionation and conventional radiotherapy in 2 year survival. One RCT in people with stage 1–3B non-small cell lung cancer found that continuous, hyperfractionated, accelerated radiotherapy increases 2 year survival compared with conventional radiotherapy.

Benefits: **Hyperfractionation:** We found one systematic review (search date 1999, 3 RCTs, 442 people with unresectable stage 3 non-small cell lung cancer) comparing standard hyperfractionation (not continuous, hyperfractionated, accelerated radiotherapy [CHART] — see glossary, p 1820) versus conventional radiotherapy.[23] It found no significant difference in 2 year survival between groups (OR 0.67, 95% CI 0.42 to 1.07; P = 0.09).[23] **CHART:** We found no systematic review or RCTs exclusively in people with stage 3 non-small cell lung cancer. One RCT (563 people with non-small cell lung cancer; 61% with stage 3A or 3B, 39% with stage 1 or stage 2) compared CHART versus conventional radiotherapy.[21] It found that, compared with conventional radiotherapy, CHART significantly reduced mortality at 2 years (AR 71% with CHART v 80% with conventional radiotherapy, HR 0.78, 95% CI 0.65 to 0.94; P = 0.008) and significantly improved local tumour control at 2 years (HR 0.79, 95% CI 0.63 to 0.98; P = 0.03).

Harms: Additional evidence on adverse effects was published subsequent to the RCT on CHART.[24] It found that, compared with conventional radiotherapy, significantly more people receiving CHART experienced pain on swallowing, heartburn (both of which were of brief duration), cough (P = 0.01), shortness of breath (P = 0.03), and dizziness (P = 0.03). It found no significant difference in long term morbidity.[21,24]

Comment: RCTs comparing CHART versus conventional radiotherapy or versus chemotherapy plus radiotherapy in people with stage 3 non-small cell lung cancer are under way.[23]

OPTION CHEMOTHERAPY IN STAGE 4 NON-SMALL CELL LUNG CANCER

Systematic reviews in people with stage 4 non-small cell lung cancer have found that adding chemotherapy regimens containing cisplatin to supportive care increases survival at 1 year compared with supportive care alone. Limited evidence from RCTs suggests that chemotherapy plus best supportive care may improve quality of life compared with best supportive care alone. One systematic review and five subsequent RCTs in people with advanced non-small cell lung cancer found inconclusive evidence on the effects of single compared with combined chemotherapy. RCTs provided insufficient evidence to compare first line platinum based versus non-platinum based chemotherapy.

Benefits: **First line chemotherapy versus supportive care:** We found three systematic reviews.[10,11,25] The most recent systematic review (search date 1998, 4 earlier systematic reviews)[10] did not fully describe the four earlier systematic reviews it identified, three of which included the same RCTs. The review did not perform a meta-analysis. The first review that performed a meta-analysis (search date 1991, 11 RCTs, 1190 people with advanced non-small cell lung cancer) compared supportive care plus chemotherapy versus supportive care alone.[11] It found that, in trials from the 1970s, long term alkylating agents plus supportive care did not significantly improve survival compared with supportive care alone (HR 1.26, 95% CI 0.96 to 1.66; P = 0.095). However, cisplatin containing regimens plus supportive care significantly increased survival at 1 year (HR 0.73; P < 0.0001) and increased median survival compared with supportive care alone (5.5 months with cisplatin containing regimens plus supportive care *v* 4 months with supportive care alone). It is not possible to deduce from these RCTs to what extent the observed effects are due to the cisplatin or to all the other drugs in the combinations studied. The second review[25] that performed a meta-analysis (search date not stated, 8 RCTs, 7 of which were included in the first review,[11] 712 people with advanced non-small cell lung cancer) comparing chemotherapy plus best supportive care versus best supportive care alone found that chemotherapy significantly reduced mortality at 6 months (OR 0.44, 95% CI 0.32 to 0.59).[25] The third review[10] identified four RCTs, which compared single agent chemotherapy plus best supportive care versus best supportive care alone, and assessed effects on quality of life.[26–29] Overall, the trials consistently found that chemotherapy plus best supportive care improved quality of life compared with best supportive care alone. The difference between groups was not significant in most trials, but they are likely to have been underpowered to detect a clinically important difference. The first RCT (207 people with stage 3B or 4 non-small cell lung cancer) found that adding docetaxel to supportive care significantly improved emotional functioning (assessed by European Organization for Research and Treatment of Cancer QLQ-C30 questionnaire $P = 0.01$, absolute numbers not provided), nausea and vomiting ($P = 0.04$), pain ($P < 0.01$) and dyspnea ($P = 0.02$) compared with supportive care alone.[26] It found no significant difference between groups in other measures of quality of life, although all scores, except those for diarrhoea, were improved in people taking docetaxel.[26] The second RCT (300 people with symptomatic locally advanced or metastatic non-small cell lung cancer, Karnofsky performance status 60–90) compared gemcitabine plus best supportive care versus best supportive care alone.[27] It found that people receiving gemcitabine had improved quality of life (assessed by European Organization for Research and Treatment of Cancer QLQ-C30 questionnaire) compared with people receiving best supportive care alone.[27] The RCT did not assess the significance of the difference between groups. The third RCT (157 people with stage 3B or stage 4 non-small cell lung cancer) found no significant difference in overall quality of life between paclitaxel plus supportive care and supportive care alone (assessed by the Rotterdam symptom checklist; lower scores indicate worse symptoms: –0.019 with paclitaxel *v* –0.017 with supportive care alone, $P = 0.242$), although scores improved in people taking paclitaxel.[29] The fourth RCT (191 people aged ≥ 70 years with stage 3B or stage 4 non-small cell lung cancer) found no significant difference in global health status between adding vinorelbine to supportive care and supportive care alone, although functional scale scores were higher in people taking vinorelbine (global health status assessed by European Organization for Research and Treatment of Cancer QLQ-C30 questionnaire, higher score indicates better function, mean difference in score +4.58, 95% CI –0.26 to +9.43).[26] Toxicity scores were also higher in people receiving vinorelbine compared with supportive care alone, but the difference was not significant. **First line single agent versus combined chemotherapy:** We found one systematic review (search date 1995–1996, 25 RCTs, 5156 people with stage 4 non-small cell lung cancer)[30] and five subsequent RCTs.[31–35] The review found no significant difference between platinum analogue or vinorelbine containing combination chemotherapy and platinum analogue or vinorelbine alone in 1 year survival (RR 1.10, 95% CI 0.94 to 1.43).[30] The first subsequent RCT (120 people with advanced non-small cell lung cancer aged > 70 years) found that gemcitabine plus vinorelbine significantly improved survival at median 14 months compared with vinorelbine alone (median survival 29 weeks with combined treatment *v* 18 weeks with single treatment; $P < 0.01$).[31] The second subsequent RCT (522 chemotherapy naive people with stage 3 or 4 non-small cell lung cancer) found that gemcitabine plus cisplatin significantly improved survival compared with cisplatin alone (median survival 9.1 months with combination treatment *v* 7.6 months; $P = 0.004$).[32] The third subsequent RCT (415 with histologically or cytologically confirmed stage 3–4 non-small cell lung cancer) found that cisplatin plus vinorelbine significantly improved survival compared with cisplatin alone (median survival 8 months with combination *v* 6 months; P = 0.002).[33] The fourth subsequent RCT (147 people with stage 3 or 4 non-small cell lung cancer) found no significant difference in median survival between cisplatin plus etoposide and gemcitabine (6.6 months with gemcitabine *v* 7.6 months with cisplatin plus etoposide; reported as non-significant, no further data provided).[34] The fifth RCT (169 people with unresectable stage 3B or stage 4 non-small cell lung cancer) compared single agent gemcitabine versus cisplatin plus vindesine.[35] It found that gemcitabine significantly increased the proportion of people with clinical benefit (based on visual analogue symptom scores, Karnofsky performance status and weight) compared with cisplatin plus vindesine (AR for clinical benefit 48.1% with gemcitabine *v* 28.9% with cisplatin plus vindesine; P = 0.003).[35] **First line platinum based versus non-platinum based chemotherapy:** We found no systematic review but found five RCTs.[36–40] The first RCT (441 people with stage 3 or 4 non-small cell lung cancer) compared docetaxel plus cisplatin versus docetaxel plus gemcitabine and found no significant difference in survival at 1 year (86/205 [42%] with docetaxel plus cisplatin *v* 78/201 [39%] with docetaxel plus gemcitabine; RR 1.08, 95% CI 0.84 to 1.33).[36] The second RCT (509 people with stage 3 or 4 non-small cell lung cancer) comparing paclitaxel plus carboplatin versus paclitaxel plus gemcitabine found no significant difference in median survival (10.4 months with paclitaxel plus carboplatin *v* 9.8 months with paclitaxel plus gemcitabine; P = 0.32).[37] The third RCT (90 people with stage 3 or 4 non-small cell lung cancer) found similar median survival time between paclitaxel plus carboplatin and paclitaxel plus gemcitabine (14.1 months with paclitaxel plus carboplatin *v* 12.6 months paclitaxel plus gemcitabine; CI not stated).[38] The fourth RCT (267 people with stage 3B or 4 non-small cell lung cancer) compared four regimens: paclitaxel plus carboplatin plus gemcitabine; paclitaxel plus carboplatin plus vinorelbine; paclitaxel plus gemcitabine; and gemcitabine plus vinorelbine.[39] It found no significant difference in survival at 1 year among groups (range 38–44%, reported as non-significant, no further data provided), but it is likely to have been too small to detect a clinically important difference among regimens.[39] The fifth RCT (284 people with stage 4 non-small cell lung cancer) compared three regimens: cisplatin plus carboplatin plus isfosfamide; cisplatin plus carboplatin plus gemcitabine; and isfosfamide plus gemcitabine.[40] It found no significant difference in median survival among groups, although people taking isfosfamide plus gemcitabine had longer median survival time compared with people taking a cisplatin containing regimen (P = 0.2). The RCT is likely to have been underpowered to detect a clinically important difference among regimens.[40] **Any second line chemotherapy:** We found one systematic review (search date not stated, 34 single agent studies and 24 combination regimen studies, 30 published only as an abstract).[41] The review found that results from studies were conflicting and was unable to draw conclusions because of the heterogeneity of participant selection in the studies, and the different definitions of people considered sensitive or refractory to treatment. **Second line single agent docetaxel:** We found one systematic review (search date 2000, 2 RCTs, 477 people resistant to platinum based combination chemotherapy).[42] Results of the RCTs were not combined because of trial heterogeneity. The first RCT identified by the review found that docetaxel 75 mg/m^2 significantly improved survival at 1 year compared with best supportive care (37% with docetaxel *v* 11% with supportive care; P = 0.003).[43] The second RCT identified by the review found that docetaxel significantly improved survival at 1 year compared with vinorelbine or ifosfamide (32% with docetaxel *v* 19% with vinorelbine or ifosfamide; P = 0.025).[44]

Harms: Over 50% of people with advanced lung cancer patients treated with chemotherapy reported alopecia, and gastrointestinal and haematological toxicity.[45] One non-systematic review found greater toxicity in people with Eastern Cooperative Oncology Group (ECOG) scale performance status 3 or 4 (see glossary, p 1820).[46] Subgroup analysis (64 people with ECOG scale performance status 2) from an RCT comparing four cisplatin based chemotherapy regimens found high rates of haematologic and gastrointestinal toxicity and low response rates after 1 year; as a result the enrolment of people with ECOG performance status 2 was discontinued (proportion of people who had any grade 3–4 toxicity: 30–60% of people taking paclitaxel plus cisplatin; 8–67% of people taking gemcitabine plus cisplatin; 12–59% of people taking docetaxel plus cisplatin; 27–33% of people taking paclitaxel plus carboplatin; response rate with any type of chemotherapy 14%, 95% CI 5.6% to 22.6%; median survival 4.1 months, 95% CI 0.2 months to 31.0 months).[47] **First line platinum based versus non-platinum based chemotherapy:** The first RCT, which compared docetaxel plus cisplatin versus docetaxel plus gemcitabine, found that docetaxel plus cisplatin significantly increased neutropenia (P = 0.01), nausea and vomiting (P = 0.001), and diarrhoea (P = 0.001).[36] The RCTs[37,38] comparing paclitaxel plus carboplatin versus paclitaxel plus gemcitabine found similar levels of haematogical toxicity between groups, although one RCT[38] found that paclitaxel plus carboplatin significantly increased grade 3 thrombocytopenia compared with paclitaxel plus gemcitabine. The fourth RCT found that gemcitabine plus vinorelbine significantly reduced non-haematologic toxicity (neuropathy, alopecia, nausea/emesis, diarrhoea, myalgia/arthralgia) compared with paclitaxel plus carboplatin plus gemcitabine; paclitaxel plus carboplatin plus vinorelbine; or paclitaxel plus gemcitabine (P < 0.05 for gemcitabine plus vinorelbine *v* any other regimen).[39]

Comment: For people with stage 4 non-small cell lung cancer, treatment options consist of either chemotherapy or symptomatic care, including palliative radiation. People with ECOG scale performance status 3 or 4 have usually been excluded from RCTs of lung cancer chemotherapy. One non-systematic review has found that carboplatin has comparable response rate to, but a better toxicity profile than, cisplatin in people with stage 4 non-small cell lung cancer.[48] One RCT (408 people with stage 3B or 4 non-small cell lung cancer) comparing carboplatin plus paclitaxel versus vinorelbine plus cisplatin found no significant difference in survival at 1 year (36% *v* 38%;

reported as non-significant), but found that vinorelbine plus cisplatin significantly increased withdrawal owing to toxicity (28% with vinorelbine plus cisplatin *v* 15% with carboplatin plus paclitaxel; P = 0.001).[49] Newer agents such as vinorelbine, gemcitabine, irinotecan, paclitaxel, and docetaxel produce objective responses in more than 20% of people with advanced lung cancer,[48] and combinations of some of these agents may be as effective and may cause less toxicity than platinum based regimens. Measuring quality of life in people with lung cancer remains a serious challenge. The systematic review comparing second line chemotherapy versus supportive care recommended that RCTs of second line chemotherapy report and analyse details of patient characteristics, response to first line treatment, and interval between last chemotherapy and recurrence.[41]

QUESTION **What are the effects of treatments for small cell lung cancer?**

OPTION **DOSE INTENSIFICATION OF CHEMOTHERAPY VERSUS STANDARD CHEMOTHERAPY**

One systematic review found limited evidence that intensifying chemotherapy dose by increasing the number of chemotherapy cycles, increasing chemotherapy dose, or increasing dose intensity per cycle may modestly improve survival compared with standard chemotherapy. However, additional RCTs have found inconclusive evidence about the effects of dose intensification on survival.

Benefits: We found one systematic review[50] (search date 2001, 20 RCTs, 5490 people most with extensive stage small cell lung cancer) and three additional RCTs[51–53] assessing dose or dose intensity of chemotherapy. Methods of dose intensification differed among RCTs. The review identified eight RCTs comparing an increased (12–14) versus a standard (5–6) number of cycles of chemotherapy; five RCTs comparing higher versus lower doses of chemotherapy; four RCTs comparing higher versus lower intensity chemotherapy, and three RCTs comparing changes in both dose per cycle and number of cycles of chemotherapy versus standard dose chemotherapy for standard number of cycles (see comment below). The review found that the median survival time was higher in people receiving dose intensification compared with standard chemotherapy (9.8 months *v* 11.5 months, significance not stated). The difference in median survival was increased if the two RCTs (of the three that altered both the dose per cycle and the total number of cycles of chemotherapy), which reduced the number of treatment cycles, were excluded (11.5 months with dose intensification *v* 8.7 months with standard chemotherapy, significance not stated). The first additional RCT (229 people with extensive stage small cell lung cancer) comparing dose intensive (cisplatin plus vincristine plus doxorubicin plus etoposide) versus standard chemotherapy (alternating cyclophosphamide, doxorubicin, vincristine plus cisplatin) found no significant difference in progression free survival (median 0.66 years in each group) or overall survival (0.98 *v* 0.91 years, reported as non-significant, no further data provided).[51] The second additional RCT (59 people with limited stage and 74 people with extensive stage small cell lung cancer) found no significant difference between paclitaxel plus cisplatin plus etoposide and cisplatin plus etoposide in survival at 1 year (AR 38.2% *v* 37%; P = 0.09).[52] The third additional RCT (233 people with extensive disease) found no significant difference in survival over 2 years with three different schedules of epirubicin, vindesine and ifosfamide (six 3 weekly cycles; six accelerated 2 weekly cycles with granulocyte macrophage colony stimulating factor [GM–CSF] support, and six accelerated 2 weekly cycles with oral co-trimoxazole) (2 year survival 5%–6%, P = 0.86).[53]

Harms: The review gave no information on adverse effects.[50] The additional RCTs found that, except in people with widespread extensive stage small cell lung cancer, adverse effects of chemotherapy were of short duration.[51–54] However, the first RCT found that dose intensive chemotherapy significantly increased deaths related to toxicity compared with standard chemotherapy (9/110 [8%] with dose intense treatment *v* 1/109 [1%] with standard chemotherapy; RR 8.9, 95% CI 1.1 to 69; NNH 14, 95% CI 7 to 60).[51] The second RCT also found that paclitaxel plus cisplatin plus etoposide significantly increased deaths related to toxicity compared with cisplatin plus etoposide (8/62 [13%] *v* 0/71 [0%]; P = 0.001).[52]

Comment: Dose escalation and intensification may modestly improve survival; however the only review of dose intensification available included four different variations of dose and cycle across 20 studies, making comparisons difficult. More research on alternative approaches to the treatment of small cell lung cancer is needed.

OPTION ADDING THORACIC IRRADIATION TO CHEMOTHERAPY IN LIMITED STAGE SMALL CELL LUNG CANCER

Two systematic reviews in people with limited stage small cell lung cancer have found that adding thoracic irradiation to chemotherapy versus chemotherapy alone improves survival at 3 years. However, one of these reviews has found that thoracic radiation plus chemotherapy increases death related to treatment compared with chemotherapy alone. One systematic review and six additional RCTs found insufficient evidence on the best timing, dose, and fractionation of radiation.

Benefits: We found two systematic reviews.[55,56] The first review (search date not stated, 13 RCTs, 2573 people with limited stage small cell lung cancer) found that radiation plus chemotherapy significantly increased 3 year survival compared with chemotherapy alone (AR 15% *v* 10%; P = 0.001).[55] The second review (search date not stated, 11 RCTs, 10 of which were included in the first review, 1911 people with limited stage small cell lung cancer) pooled data from nine of the RCTs (1521 people) and found that thoracic radiation plus chemotherapy significantly improved local control compared with chemotherapy alone (50% *v* 25%; ARI of improved local control 25%, 95% CI 17% to 34%).[56] **Timing of radiation:** We found one systematic review (search date 2000, 4 RCTs, 927 people with limited stage small cell lung cancer)[57] one additional[58] and two subsequent[59,60] RCTs, which compared early versus late addition of thoracic radiotherapy to chemotherapy. The review found no significant difference between early and late addition of radiotherapy in 5 year survival (AR 66/455 [14.5%] *v* 63/472 [13.2%]; RR 1.09, 95% CI 0.78 to 1.48).[57] The additional RCT, included in the review but not in the meta-analysis, found that early compared with late addition of radiotherapy significantly increased 5 year survival (30% *v* 15%; P = 0.03).[58] The first subsequent RCT (81 people with limited stage small cell lung cancer) compared early radiotherapy (given with the first cycle of chemotherapy) versus late radiotherapy (given with the fourth cycle of chemotherapy).[59] It found no significant difference between early and late chemotherapy in survival after median follow up of 35 months (median 17.5 months with early radiotherapy *v* 17 months with late radiotherapy; P = 0.6). The second subsequent RCT (231 people with limited stage small cell lung cancer receiving four cycles of cisplatin plus etoposide) compared early addition of thoracic radiotherapy (with the first cycle of chemotherapy [concurrent]) versus late (after the fourth cycle of chemotherapy [sequential]).[60] It found no significant difference in survival at 2, 3, or 5 years between concurrent and sequential radiotherapy (5 year survival 24% with concurrent *v* 18% with sequential; P = 0.097). Adjustments for prognostic factors, performance status, age and stage suggested that overall there was a significantly lower risk of death in people receiving concurrent rather than sequential radiotherapy (HR 0.70, 95% CI 0.52 to 0.94, P = 0.02).[60] **Dose:** One RCT (333 people with limited stage small cell lung cancer) found no significant difference between standard dose radiotherapy (25 Gy over 2 weeks) and high dose radiotherapy (37.5 Gy over 3 weeks) in overall survival over 3 years (P = 0.18; results presented graphically).[61] **Fractionation:** We found two RCTs.[62,63] One RCT found that hyperfractionation (twice daily treatment) compared with conventional fractionation (once daily treatment) significantly improved 5 year survival (26% with hyperfractionation *v* 16% with conventional fractionation; P = 0.04).[62] Another RCT comparing once daily irradiation versus twice daily irradiation found no significant difference in 3 year survival (34% with 50.4 Gy in 28 fractions daily *v* 29% with 48 Gy in 32 fractions twice daily; P = 0.46).[63]

Harms: The second systematic review found that thoracic radiation plus chemotherapy significantly increased death related to treatment compared with chemotherapy alone (29/884 [3.3%] *v* 12/841 [1.4%]; OR 2.54, 95% CI 1.90 to 3.18).[56] **Fractionation:** One RCT found that hyperfractionation increased the incidence of oesophagitis compared with conventional fractionation.[62]

Comment: Interest in adding thoracic irradiation to chemotherapy derives from the observation that local recurrence in the chest is a major cause of first treatment failure and carries an extremely poor prognosis. One non-systematic review suggested that chest irradiation reduced local failure rates and increased 3 year survival by 50%.[64] The reasons for this improvement have not been established but may include the early use of radiation plus chemotherapy rather than improvements in either modality alone.[65] The RCTs of early versus late addition of radiotherapy used different methods and do not provide strong evidence.[57–59] The different results may be explained by different rates of early toxicity from treatment and different rates of relapse in the central nervous system.

OPTION PROPHYLACTIC CRANIAL IRRADIATION IN LIMITED STAGE SMALL CELL LUNG CANCER

One systematic review in people with small cell lung cancer in complete remission has found that, compared with no irradiation, prophylactic cranial irradiation improves survival at 3 years and reduces the risk of developing brain metastases. Although long term cognitive dysfunction after cranial irradiation has been described in non-randomised studies, RCTs have not found a cumulative increase in neuropsychological dysfunction.

Benefits: We found one systematic review (search date 2000, 7 RCTs, 987 people with small cell lung cancer in complete remission) comparing cranial radiation versus no cranial radiation.[66] Of the people in the RCTs, 12% in the irradiation group and 17% in the no irradiation group had extensive stage small cell lung cancer at presentation. It found that, compared with no cranial irradiation, cranial irradiation significantly improved survival (RR of death at 3 years 0.84, 95% CI 0.73 to 0.97, corresponding to a 5.4% increase in survival) and increased disease free survival (RR of recurrence or death at 3 years 0.75, 95% CI 0.65 to 0.86). The review found that cranial irradiation versus no cranial irradiation significantly reduced the cumulative incidence of brain metastases (RR 0.46, 95% CI 0.38 to 0.57). Larger doses of radiation significantly reduced brain metastases ($P = 0.02$), but did not significantly improve survival ($P = 0.89$).

Harms: Non-randomised studies suggest that prophylactic cranial irradiation may lead to neuropsychological sequelae but the review was unable to assess this because adequate assessments were carried out in only two of the seven RCTs.[66] These two RCTs found no cumulative increase in neuropsychological dysfunction in individuals receiving prophylactic cranial irradiation. These RCTs and other non-randomised studies found that 24–60% of participants may have neuropsychological problems before treatment, and other studies have not accounted for potential confounding factors such as age, tobacco use, paraneoplastic syndromes, and neurotoxic chemotherapy effects.

Comment: The clinical importance of cognitive impairment after prophylactic cranial irradiation remains unclear. Differences in survival benefiting those patients receiving prophylactic cranial irradiation are small, reflecting the impact of other events not influenced by prophylactic cranial irradiation, for example other metastases or thoracic relapse.[67]

OPTION ORAL ETOPOSIDE IN EXTENSIVE STAGE SMALL CELL LUNG CANCER

Two RCTs in people with extensive stage small cell lung cancer found that oral etoposide reduced survival compared with combination chemotherapy at 1 year. One RCT, in people with extensive stage small

cell lung cancer who had not responded to induction combination chemotherapy, found no significant difference between oral etoposide and no further treatment in mortality at 3 years, although overall mortality was lower in people taking etoposide. RCTs found that etoposide may reduce nausea, alopecia and numbness in the short term compared with combination chemotherapy, but found no evidence that it offered better quality of life overall.

Benefits: **Versus combination chemotherapy:** We found no systematic review but found three RCTs.[68–70] The first RCT (155 people with extensive stage small cell lung cancer) compared oral etoposide 100 mg daily for 5 days versus combination chemotherapy.[68] It found that etoposide improved survival significantly less than combined chemotherapy at 1 year (9.8% with etoposide *v* 19.3% with combined chemotherapy; $P < 0.05$). It found similar median survival rates with etoposide compared with combination chemotherapy (4.8 months *v* 5.9 months, CI not stated) and found inconclusive results on quality of life. Acute nausea was significantly worse with combination chemotherapy ($P < 0.01$), but pain, appetite, general well-being, and mood were worse with oral etoposide ($P < 0.001$). Palliation of lung cancer symptoms was of significantly shorter duration with etoposide than with combination chemotherapy ($P < 0.01$).[68] The second RCT (339 people with extensive stage small cell lung cancer) comparing oral etoposide versus combination chemotherapy found that etoposide significantly reduced survival at mean 21 months (HR 1.35, 95% CI 1.03 to 1.70; $P = 0.03$; absolute numbers not provided).[69] The third RCT (233 people with extensive stage small cell lung cancer and Karnofsky performance status ≥ 50 who had not responded after four cycles of intravenous cisplatin, etoposide and ifosfamide) compared oral etoposide 50 mg/m^2 versus no further treatment for 3 months.[70] It found that oral etoposide significantly increased median progression free survival compared with no treatment (8.2 months with etoposide *v* 6.5 months with no treatment; $P = 0.0018$). It found no significant difference in overall survival at 3 years, although mortality was lower in people taking etoposide (9.1% with etoposide *v* 1.9% with no treatment; $P = 0.0704$).

Harms: The first RCT found that etoposide significantly reduced nausea in the short term (assessed by daily diary card; $P < 0.01$) compared with combination chemotherapy.[68] However, it found that combination chemotherapy significantly improved general well-being (assessed by daily diary card; $P < 0.01$) and overall quality of life (assessed by Rotterdam Symptom Checklist; $P < 0.01$) compared with etoposide.[68] The second RCT found that etoposide reduced alopecia and numbness compared with combination chemotherapy, but increased haematological adverse effects, particularly anaemia.[69] The third RCT found that oral etoposide was associated with alopecia and grade 3–4 toxicities, including myelosuppression (40% of people), anaemia (20%), and granulocytopenia (42%).[70] The RCT gave no comparative information about adverse effects in people receiving no treatment.

Comment: Treatment of extensive stage disease is palliative and because age has been identified as a prognostic factor in small cell lung cancer, studies have looked at outcomes in elderly people with limited and extensive stage disease and in people of all ages with a poor prognosis. Although small cell lung cancer is relatively sensitive to chemotherapy, extensive stage disease remains incurable. Median survival with treatment is 10–12 months, and as yet has been unaffected by high dose combination chemotherapy. Because of its lower acute toxicity, etoposide may be considered for elderly people with extensive stage disease or people with a poor prognosis.

GLOSSARY

Continuous, hyperfractionated, accelerated radiotherapy Radiotherapy given at a rate of two or more radiation fractions a day (each of smaller dose than conventionally fractionated doses). The number of fractions a week is gradually increased to shorten overall duration of treatment.

Performance status Expression used to describe functional status or wellness of participants in studies of cancer. There are two widely accepted scales: the Eastern Cooperative Oncology Group scale (0 = no symptoms; 1 = symptomatic but no extra time in bed; 2 = in bed less than 50% of the day, no work, can care for self; 3 = in bed more than 50% of day, not bedridden, minimal self care; 4 = completely bedridden), and the Karnofsky Scale of symptoms and disability (from 100% = no symptoms to 0% = dead).

Substantive changes

Pre- and postoperative chemotherapy in resectable non-small cell lung cancer One RCT added;[12] conclusions unchanged.

Chemotherapy in stage 4 non-small cell lung cancer Four RCTs comparing first line platinum versus non-platinum chemotherapy added;[37–40] conclusions unchanged.

Dose intensive chemotherapy versus standard chemotherapy One systematic review added.[50] Dose intensive chemotherapy versus standard chemotherapy recategorised from Unlikely to be beneficial to Unknown effectiveness.

Adding thoracic irradiation to chemotherapy in limited stage small cell lung cancer One RCT added;[59] conclusions unchanged.

Oral etoposide in extensive stage small cell lung cancer One RCT added;[70] conclusions unchanged.

REFERENCES

1. Travis WD, Travis LB, Devesa SS. Lung cancer. *Cancer* 1995;75(suppl 1):191–202.
2. American Thoracic Society/European Respiratory Society Pre-treatment evaluation of non-small cell lung cancer *Am J Respir Crit Care* 1997;156:320–332.
3. Schottenfeld D. Etiology and Epidemiology of Lung Cancer. In: Pass HI, Mitchell JB, Johnson DH et al, eds. *Lung Cancer, Principles and Practice* 2nd ed. Philadelphia: Lippincott Williams and Wilkins, 2000:376–388.
4. Ihde DC, Pass HI, Glatstein E. Lung cancer. In: DeVita VT Jr, Hellman S, Rosenberg SA, eds. *Cancer, principles and practice of oncology*, 5th ed. Philadelphia: Lippincott-Raven, 1997;849–959.
5. Montazeri A, Gillis CR, McEwen J. Quality of life in people with lung cancer: a review of literature from 1970 to 1995. *Chest* 1998;113:467–481.
6. Grilli R, Oxman AD, Julian JA. Chemotherapy for advanced non-small-cell lung cancer: how much benefit is enough? *J Clin Oncol* 1993;11:1866–1872. Search date 1991; primary source Medline.
7. Goss G, Paszat L, Newman T, et al. Use of preoperative chemotherapy with or without postoperative radiotherapy in technically resectable stage IIIA non-small cell lung cancer. *Cancer Prev Control* 1998;2:32–39. Search date 1997; primary sources Medline, hand searches of reference lists, and contact with experts.
8. Ramnath N, Hernandez FJ, Bepler G. Neoadjuvant chemotherapy for non-small-call lung cancer: Will the answer be in targeted chemotherapy. *Oncol Spect* 2002:1;27–34.
9. Depierre A, Milleron B, Moro-Sibilot D, et al. Pre-operative chemotherapy followed by surgery compared with primary surgery in resectable Stage I (except T1NO), II and IIIA non-small cell lung cancer. *J Clin Oncol* 2002;20:247–253.
10. Sorenson S, Glimelius B, Nygren P, et al. A systematic overview of chemotherapy effects in non-small cell lung cancer. *Acta Oncol* 2001;40:327–339. Search date 1998; primary sources Medline, Cancerlit, PDQ database, and handsearching of reference lists and the grey literature.
11. Non-Small Cell Lung Cancer Collaborative Group. Chemotherapy for non-small cell lung cancer. In: The Cochrane Library, Issue 4, 2002. Oxford: Update Software. Search date 1991; primary sources Medline, Cancerlit, hand search of meetings abstracts, bibliographies of books and specialist journals, consultation of trials registers

of National Cancer Institute, UK Coordinating Committee for Cancer Research, the Union Internationale Contre le Cancer, and discussion with trialists.

12. Guangchuan XU, Rong T, Lin P. Adjuvant chemotherapy following radical surgery for non-small-cell lung cancer: a randomized study on 70 patients. *Chin Med J* 2000;113:617–620.
13. Keller SM, Adak S, Wagner H, et al. A randomized trial of postoperative adjuvant therapy in patients with completely resected stage II or IIIA non-small-cell lung cancer. *N Engl J Med* 2000:343;1217–1222.
14. Feld R, Rubinstein L, Thomas PA, et al. Adjuvant chemotherapy with cyclophosphamide, doxorubicin, and cisplatin in patients with completely resected stage I non-small-cell lung cancer. *J Natl Cancer Inst* 1993;85:299–306.
15. Niiranen A, Niitamo-Korhonen S, Kouri M, et al. Adjuvant chemotherapy after radical surgery for non-small cell lung cancer: a randomized study. *J Clin Oncol* 1992;10:1927–1932.
16. Pass HI, Pogrebniak HW, Steinberg SM, et al. Randomized trial of neoadjuvant therapy for lung cancer: interim analysis. *Ann Thoracic Surg* 1992;53:992–998.
17. Marino P, Preatoni A. Randomized trials of radiotherapy alone versus combined chemotherapy and radiotherapy in stages IIIa and IIIb non small cell lung cancer. *Cancer* 1995;76:593–601. Search date 1995; primary sources Medline and manual search of references of review articles and abstracts.
18. Pritchard RS, Anthony SP. Chemotherapy plus radiotherapy compared with radiotherapy alone in the treatment of locally advanced, unresectable, non-small-cell lung cancer. *Ann Intern Med* 1996;125:723–729. Search date 1995; primary sources Medline and hand search of references of review articles and abstracts.
19. Sause W, Kolesar P, Taylor S, et al. Final results of phase III trial in regionally advanced unresectable non-small cell lung cancer: Radiation Therapy Oncology Group, Eastern Cooperative Oncology Group, and Southwest Oncology Group. *Chest* 2000;117:358–364.
20. Cullen MH, Billingham CM, Woodroffe AD, et al. Mitomycin, ifosfamide, and cisplatin in unresectable non-small-cell lung cancer: effects on survival and quality of life. *J Clin Oncol* 1999;17:3188–3194.
21. Saunders M, Dische S, Barrett A, et al. Continuous, hyperfractionated, accelerated radiotherapy (CHART) versus conventional radiotherapy in non-small cell lung cancer: mature data from the randomised multicentre trial. *Radiother Oncol* 1999;52:137–148.
22. Mousas B, Scott C, Sause W, et al. The benefit of treatment intensification is age and histology-dependent in patients with locally advanced non-small cell lung cancer (NSCLC): a quality-adjusted survival analysis of Radiation Therapy Oncology Group (RTOG) chemoradiation studies. *Int J Radiat Oncol Biol Phys* 1999;45:1143–1149.
23. Yu E, Lochrin C, Dixon P, et al. Altered fractionation of radical radiation therapy in the management of unresectable non-small-cell lung cancer. *Curr Oncol* 2000;7:98–109. Search date 1999; primary sources Medline, Cancerlit, PDQ database, and The Cochrane Library.
24. Bailey AJ, Parmar MKB, Stephens RJ. Patient-reported short-term and long-term physical and psychological symptoms: results of the continuous hyperfractionated accelerated radiotherapy (CHART) randomized trial in non-small cell lung cancer. *J Clin Oncol* 1998;16:3082–3093.
25. Marino P, Pampallona S, Preatoni A, et al. Chemotherapy versus supportive care in advanced non-small cell lung cancer: results of a meta-analysis of the literature. *Chest* 1994;106:861–865. Search date not stated; primary sources Medline and hand search of references from review articles and abstracts.
26. Elderly Lung Cancer Vinorelbine Study Group. Effects of vinorelbine on quality of life and survival of elderly patients with non-small cell lung cancer. *J Natl Cancer Inst* 1999;91:66–72.
27. Anderson H, Hopwood P, Stephens RJ, et al. Gemcitabine plus best supportive care (BSC) versus BSC in inoperable non-small cell lung cancer in a randomised trial with quality of life as the primary outcome. *Br J Cancer* 2000;83:447–453.
28. Roszkowski K, Pluzanska A, Krzakowski M, et al. A multicenter, randomised phase III study of docetaxel plus best supportive care versus best supportive care in chemo-naive patients with metastatic or non-resectable localised non-small cell lung cancer (NSCLC). *Lung Cancer* 2000;27:145–157.
29. Ranson M, Davidson N, Nicolson M, et al. Randomised trial of paclitaxel plus supportive care versus supportive care for patients with advanced non-small cell lung cancer. *J Natl Cancer Inst* 2000;92:1074–1080.
30. Lilenbaum RC, Langenberg P, Dickersin K. Single agent versus combination chemotherapy in patients with advanced non-small cell lung cancer: a meta-analysis of response, toxicity and survival. *Cancer* 1998;82:116–126. Search dates 1995–1996; primary sources Medline, Embase, handsearching of references, Physician Data Query from the National Cancer Institute, and expert consultation.
31. Frasci G, Lorusso V, Panza N, et al. Gemcitabine plus vinorelbine versus vinorelbine alone in elderly patients with advanced non-small cell lung cancer. *J Clin Oncol* 2000;18:2529–2536.
32. Sandler AB, Nemunaitis J, Denham C, et al. Phase III trial of gemcitabine plus cisplatin versus cisplatin alone in patients with locally advanced or metastatic non-small cell lung cancer. *J Clin Oncol* 2000;18:122–130.
33. Wozniak AG, Crowley JJ, Balcerzak SP, et al. Randomised trial comparing cisplatin with cisplatin plus vinorelbine in the treatment of advanced non-small cell lung cancer: a Southwest Oncology Group study. *J Clin Oncol* 1998;16:2459–2465.
34. ten Bokkel-Huinink WW, Bergman B, Chemaissani A, et al. Single-agent gemcitabine: an active and better tolerated alternative to standard cisplatin-based chemotherapy in locally advanced or metastatic non-small cell lung cancer. *Lung Cancer* 1999;26:85–94.
35. Vansteenkiste JF, Vanderbroek JE, Nackaerts KL, et al. Clinical-benefit response in advanced non-small cell lung cancer: A multicentre prospective randomized phase III study of single agent gemcitabine versus cisplatin-vindesine. *Ann Oncol* 2001;12:1221–1230.
36. Georgoulias V, Papadakis E, Alexopoulos A, et al. Platinum-based and non-platinum-based chemotherapy in advanced non-small cell lung cancer: a randomised multicentre trial. *Lancet* 2001;357:1478–1484.
37. Kosmidis P, Mylonakis N, Nicolaides C, et al. Paclitaxel plus carboplatin versus gemcitabine plus paclitaxel in advanced non-small-cell lung cancer: a phase III randomized trial. *J Clin Oncol* 2002;20:3578–3585.

38. Chen Y-M, Perng R-P, Lee Y-C, et al. Paclitaxel plus carboplatin, compared with paclitaxel plus gemcitabine, shows similar efficacy while more cost-effective: a randomised phase II study of combination chemotherapy against inoperable non-small-cell lung cancer previously untreated. *Ann Oncol* 2002;13:108–115.
39. Greco FA, Gray JR, Thompson DS, et al. Prospective randomized study of four novel chemotherapy regimens in patients with advanced non-small cell lung carcinoma. *Cancer* 2002;95:1279–1285.
40. Sculier JP, Lafitte JJ, Lecomte J, et al. A three-arm phase III randomised trial comparing combinations of platinum derivatives, ifosfamide and/or gemcitabine in stage IV non-small-cell lung cancer. *Ann Oncol* 2002;13:874–882.
41. Huisman C, Smit EF, Postmus PE. Second-line chemotherapy in relapsing or refractory non-small cell lung cancer: a review. *J Clin Oncol* 2000;18:3722–3730. Search date not stated; primary sources Medline and hand searches of the past five conference abstracts of the American Society of Clinical Oncology, European Cancer Conference, and the European Society of Medical Oncology.
42. Logan D, Laurie S, Markman BR, et al. The role of single-agent docetaxel as second-line treatment for advanced non-small cell lung cancer. *Curr Oncol* 2001;8:50–58. Search date 2000; primary sources Medline, Cancerlit, Cochrane Library, and hand search of reference lists of relevant articles.
43. Shepherd FA, Dancey J, Ramlau, et al. Prospective randomized trial of docetaxel versus best supportive care in patients with non-small-cell lung cancer previously treated with platinum-based chemotherapy. *J Clin Oncol* 2000;18:2095–2103.
44. Fossella FV, DeVore R, Kerr RN. Randomized phase III trial of docetaxel versus vinorelbine or ifosphamide in patients with advanced non-small cell lung cancer previously treated with platinum-containing regimens. *J Clin Oncol* 2000;18:2354–2362.
45. Le Chevalier T, Brisgand D, Douillard J-Y, et al. Randomized study of vinorelbine and cisplatin versus vindesine and cisplatin versus vinorelbine alone in advanced non-small cell lung cancer: results of a European multicenter trial including 612 people. *J Clin Oncol* 1994;12:360–367.
46. Bunn PA Jr, Kelly K. New chemotherapeutic agents prolong survival and improve quality of life in non-small cell lung cancer: a review of literature and future directions. *Clin Cancer Res* 1998;4:1087–1100.
47. Sweeney CJ, Zhu J, Sandler AB, et al. Outcome of patients with a performance status of 2 in Eastern Cooperative Oncology Group Study E1594. A Phase III trial in patients with metastatic non-small cell lung carcinoma. *Cancer* 2001;982:2639–2647.
48. Bunn PA Jr. Review of therapeutic trials of carboplatin in lung cancer. *Semin Oncol* 1989;16(S5):27–33.
49. Kelly K, Crowley J, Bunn PA, et al. Randomised phase III trial of paclitaxel plus carboplatin versus vinorelbine plus cisplatin in the treatment of patients with advanced non-small-cell lung cancer: a Southwest Oncology Group trial. *J Clin Oncol* 2001;19:3210–3218.
50. Tjan-Heijnen VCG, Wagener DJT, Postmus PE. An analysis of chemotherapy dose and dose-intensity in small-cell lung cancer: lessons to be drawn. *Ann Oncol* 2002;13:1519–1530. Search date 2001, primary sources Medline 1980–2001 and hand searches of reference lists of relevant articles.
51. Murray N, Livingston RB, Shepherd FA, et al. Randomised study of CODE versus alternating CAV/EP for extensive-stage small-cell lung cancer: an intergroup study of the National Cancer Institute of Canada clinical trials group and the Southwest Oncology Group. *J Clin Oncol* 1999;17:2300–2308.
52. Mavroudis D, Papadakis E, Veslemes M, et al. A multicenter randomized clinical trial comparing paclitaxel-cisplatin-etoposide versus cisplatin-etoposide as first-line treatment in patients with small-cell lung cancer. *Ann Oncol* 2001;12:463–470.
53. Sculier JP, Paessmans M, Reconte J, et al. A three-arm Phase III randomized trial assessing in patients with extensive disease small cell lung cancer, accelerated chemotherapy with support of hematological growth factor or oral antibiotics. *Br J Cancer* 2001;85:1444–1451.
54. Noda K, Nishikaa Y, Kawahara M, et al. Irinotecan plus cisplatin compared with etoposide plus cisplatin for extensive small cell lung cancer. *N Engl J Med* 2002;346:85–91.
55. Pignon JP, Arriagada R, Ihde DC, et al. A meta-analysis of thoracic radiotherapy for small-cell lung cancer. *N Engl J Med* 1992;327:1618–1624. Search date not stated; primary sources Medline and hand search of proceedings of key oncology meetings.
56. Warde P, Payne D. Does thoracic irradiation improve survival and local control in limited-stage small cell carcinoma of the lung? A meta-analysis. *J Clin Oncol* 1992;10:890–895. Search date not stated; primary sources Medline and Cancerline.
57. Okawara G, Gagliardi A, Evans WK, et al. The role of thoracic radiotherapy as an adjunct to standard chemotherapy in limited-stage small-cell lung cancer. *Curr Oncol* 2000;7:162–172. Search date 2000; primary sources Medline, Cochrane Library, Physician Data Query File, Cancerlit, and hand searches of conference proceedings.
58. Jeremic B, Shibamoto Y, Acimovic L, et al. Initial versus delayed accelerated hyperfracationated radiation therapy and concurrent chemotherapy in limited small-cell lung cancer. A randomised study. *J Clin Oncol* 1997;15:893–900.
59. Skarlos DV, Samantas E, Briassoulis E, et al. Randomized comparison of early versus late hyperfractionated thoracic irradiation concurrently with chemotherapy in limited disease small-cell lung cancer: A randomized phase II study of the Hellenic Cooperative Oncology Group (HeCOG). *Ann Oncol* 2001;12:1231–1238.
60. Takada M, Fukuoka M, Kawahara M, et al. Phase III study of concurrent versus sequential thoracic radiotherapy in combination with cisplatin and etoposide for limited-stage small-cell lung cancer: results of the Japan Clinical Oncology Group study 9104. *J Clin Oncol* 2002;20:3054–3060.
61. Coy P, Hodson I, Payne DG, et al. The effect of dose of thoracic irradiation on recurrence in patients with limited stage small cell lung cancer. Initial results of a Canadian multicentre randomized trial. *Int J Radiat Oncol Biol Phys* 1988;14:219–226.
62. Turrisi AT, Kim K, Blum R, et al. Twice-daily compared with once-daily thoracic radiotherapy in limited small-cell lung cancer treated concurrently with cisplatin and etoposide. *N Engl J Med* 1999;340:265–271.
63. Bonner JA, Sloan JA, Shanahan TG, et al. Phase III comparison of twice-daily split-course irradiation versus once-daily irradiation for patients with limited stage small-cell lung carcinoma. *J Clin Oncol* 1999;17:2681–2691.

64. Kumar P. The role of radiotherapy in the management of limited-stage small cell lung cancer: past, present, and future. *Chest* 1997;112(suppl):259–265.
65. Murray N, Coy P, Pater JL, et al. Importance of timing for thoracic irradiation in the combined modality treatment of limited-stage small-cell lung cancer. *J Clin Oncol* 1993;11:336–344.
66. Prophylactic Cranial Irradiation Overview Collaborative Group. Cranial irradiation for preventing brain metastasis of small cell lung cancer in patients in complete remission. In: The Cochrane Library, Issue 4, 2002. Oxford: Update Software. Search date 2000; primary sources Medline, Cancerlit, Excerpta Medica, Biosis, hand searches of meeting proceedings, the Physician Data Query clinical trial registry, and personal contact with investigators and experts.
67. Arriagada R, Le Chevalier T, Riviere A. Patterns of failure after prophylactic cranial irradiation in small-cell lung cancer: analysis of 505 randomized patients. *Ann Oncol* 2002;13:748–754.
68. Souhami RL, Spiro SG, Rudd RM, et al. Five day oral etoposide treatment for advanced small cell lung cancer: randomized comparison with intravenous chemotherapy. *J Natl Cancer Inst* 1997;89:577–580.
69. Medical Research Council Lung Cancer Working Party. Comparison of oral etoposide and standard intravenouis multidrug chemotherapy for small-cell lung cancer: a stopped multicentre randomised trial. *Lancet* 1996;348:563–566.
70. Hanna NH, Sandler AB, Loehrer PJ, et al. Maintenance daily oral etoposide versus no further therapy following induction chemotherapy with etoposide plus ifosfamide plus cisplatin in extensive small-cell lung cancer: a Hoosier Oncology Group randomized study. *Ann Oncol* 2002; 13:95–102.

Alan Neville
Professor
McMaster University
Hamilton
Canada

Competing interests: None declared.

TABLE 1 **Staging lung cancer (see text, p 1806).**

Non-small cell lung cancer

Stage	Definition*	5 year survival (%)
1	T1–T2, N0, M0	55–75
2	T1–T2, N1, M0	25–50
3A	T3, N0–N1, M0 or T1–T3, N2, M0	20–40
3B	T4, any N, M0 or any T, N3, M0	≤5
4	Any M1	≤5

Small cell lung cancer

Stage	Definition	Median survival
Limited stage disease	Tumour confined to one side of the chest, supraclavicular lymph nodes, or both	18–24 months†
Extensive stage disease	Defined as anything beyond limited stage	10–12 months‡

*M, metastases; N, nodes; T, tumour. †With combined chemotherapy and mediastinal irradiation. ‡With palliative chemotherapy.

Bacterial vaginosis

Search date November 2002

M Joesoef and George Schmid

QUESTIONS

INTERVENTIONS

TREATMENT

Beneficial

Antibacterial treatment in symptomatic non-pregnant women 1826

Likely to be beneficial

Antibacterial treatment (except intravaginal clindamycin) in pregnant women who have had a previous preterm birth 1828

Oral antibacterial treatment before surgical abortion . . . 1831

Unknown effectiveness

Antibacterial treatment before gynaecological procedures (other than abortion) 1831

Antibacterial treatment (except intravaginal clindamycin) in low risk pregnancy 1828

Likely to be ineffective or harmful

Treating pregnant women with intravaginal clindamycin cream. 1828

Treating pregnant women without bacterial vaginosis 1829

TREATING MALE SEXUAL PARTNER

Likely to be ineffective or harmful

Treating a woman's one steady male sexual partner with metronidazole or clindamycin. 1830

To be covered in future updates

Recurrent bacterial vaginosis

Key Messages

- Bacterial vaginosis may resolve spontaneously.

In non-pregnant women

- **Antibacterial treatment in symptomatic non-pregnant women** One systematic review found no significant difference between oral and intravaginal antibacterial drugs in cure rates after 5–10 days or at 4 weeks. Another systematic review has found that a 7 day course of twice daily oral metronidazole increases cure rates at 3–4 weeks compared with a single 2 g dose. Limited evidence from RCTs found no significant difference in cure rates with oral clindamycin versus oral metronidazole twice daily for 7 days, and no significant difference between once and twice daily dosing with intravaginal metronidazole gel. One RCT found no significant difference in cure rates at 35 days between intravaginal clindamycin ovules for 3 days and intravaginal clindamycin cream for 7 days.

In pregnant women

- **Antibacterial treatment (except intravaginal clindamycin) in pregnant women who have had a previous preterm birth** Limited evidence from a subgroup analysis in pregnant women with bacterial vaginosis who had a previous preterm birth found that oral antibacterial treatment reduced the risk of premature delivery compared with placebo. One small RCT in women with bacterial vaginosis who had a previous labour or midtrimester abortion found a higher rate of pre-term birth with oral metronidazole compared with placebo, but the group receiving metronidazole had higher previous antibacterial use and asymptomatic bacteriuria at baseline.
- **Antibacterial treatment (except intravaginal clindamycin) in low risk pregnancy** Two systematic reviews of antibacterial treatment versus placebo found no significant difference in the risk of preterm delivery.
- **Treating pregnant women with intravaginal clindamycin cream** Four RCTs found that intravaginal clindamycin cream versus placebo was associated with an increased risk of preterm delivery and low birth weight, but the increase was not significant.
- **Treating pregnant women without bacterial vaginosis** Subgroup analysis in two RCTs of pregnant women without bacterial vaginosis found that both intravaginal clindamycin cream and oral metronidazole plus erythromycin were associated with an increased risk of preterm delivery before 34 weeks of gestation compared with placebo, although the difference was significant in only one of the RCTs.

Preventing recurrence

- **Treating a woman's one steady male sexual partner with metronidazole or clindamycin** One systematic review has found that, in women receiving antibacterial agents, who have one steady male sexual partner, treating the partner with oral metronidazole or clindamycin does not reduce the woman's risk of recurrence.

Treatment before procedures

- **Oral antibacterial treatment before surgical abortion** RCTs consistently found that oral antibacterial treatment in women with bacterial vaginosis about to undergo surgical abortion was associated with a lower risk of pelvic inflammatory disease compared with placebo, but the difference was only significant in the largest RCT.
- **Antibacterial treatment before gynaecological procedures (other than abortion)** We found no RCTs on the effects of antibacterial treatment in women with bacterial vaginosis about to undergo gynaecological procedures other than abortion.

DEFINITION Bacterial vaginosis is a microbial disease characterised by an alteration in the bacterial flora of the vagina from a predominance of *Lactobacillus* species to high concentrations of anaerobic bacteria. Diagnosis requires three out of four features: the presence of clue cells; a homogenous discharge adherent to the vaginal walls; pH of vaginal fluid greater than 4.5; and a "fishy" amine odour of the vaginal discharge before or after addition of 10% potassium hydroxide. The condition is asymptomatic in 50% of infected women. Women with symptoms have an excessive white to grey, or malodorous vaginal discharge, or both; the odour may be particularly noticeable during sexual intercourse.

INCIDENCE/ PREVALENCE Bacterial vaginosis is the most common infectious cause of vaginitis, being about twice as common as candidiasis.[1] Prevalences of 10–61% have been reported among unselected women from a range of settings.[2] Data on incidence are limited but one study found that, over a 2 year period, 50% of women using an intrauterine contraceptive device had at least one episode, as did 20% of women using oral contraceptives.[3] Bacterial vaginosis is particularly prevalent among lesbians.[4]

AETIOLOGY/ RISK FACTORS The cause of bacterial vaginosis is not fully understood. Risk factors include new or multiple sexual partners[1,3,5] and early age of sexual intercourse,[6] but no causative microorganism has been shown to be transmitted between partners. Use of an intrauterine contraceptive device[3] and douching[5] have also been reported as risk factors. Infection seems to be most common around the time of menstruation.[7]

PROGNOSIS The course of bacterial vaginosis varies and is poorly understood. Without treatment, symptoms may persist or resolve in both pregnant and non-pregnant women. Recurrence after treatment occurs in about a third of women. The condition is associated with complications of pregnancy: low birth weight; preterm birth (pooled OR from 10 cohort studies: 1.8, 95% CI 1.5 to 2.6);[8] preterm labour; premature rupture of membranes; late miscarriage; chorioamnionitis (48% *v* 22%; OR 2.6, 95% CI 1.0 to 6.6);[9] endometritis after normal delivery (8.2% *v* 1.5%; OR 5.6, 95% CI 1.8 to 17.2);[10] endometritis after caesarean section (55% *v* 17%; OR 5.8, 95% CI 3.0 to 10.9);[11] and surgery to the genital tract. Women who have had a previous premature delivery are especially at risk of complications in pregnancy, with a sevenfold increased risk of preterm birth (24/428 [5.6%] in all women *v* 10/24 [41.7%] in women with a previous preterm birth).[12] Bacterial vaginosis can also enhance HIV acquisition and transmission.[13]

AIMS OF INTERVENTION To alleviate symptoms and to prevent complications relating to childbirth, termination of pregnancy, and gynaecological surgery, with minimal adverse effects; to reduce adverse neonatal outcomes.

OUTCOMES Preterm delivery; puerperal and neonatal morbidity and mortality; clinical or microbiological cure rates, usually at 1–2 weeks or 4 weeks after completing treatment.

METHODS *Clinical Evidence* search and appraisal November 2002. In addition, the authors used information from drug manufacturers.

QUESTION **What are the effects of different antibacterial regimens in non-pregnant women with symptomatic bacterial vaginosis?**

One systematic review found no significant difference in cure rates at 5–10 days or 4 weeks between oral and intravaginal antibacterial drugs. Another systematic review has found that a 7 day course of twice daily oral metronidazole versus a single 2 g dose increases cure rates. Limited evidence from RCTs found no significant difference in cure rates between oral clindamycin and oral metronidazole, and no significant difference

between once and twice daily dosing with intravaginal metronidazole gel. One RCT found no significant difference in cure rates at 35 days between 3 day treatment with intravaginal ovules versus 7 day treatment with intravaginal clindamycin cream.

Benefits: **Antibacterial versus placebo treatment:** We found one systematic review (search date 1996) that summarised the results of 4 RCTs comparing antibacterial versus placebo.[14] The systematic review found that the cumulative cure rate 25–39 days after completion of treatment was 82% with intravaginal clindamycin cream versus 35% with placebo. The cumulative cure rates for intravaginal metronidazole gel 4–16 days after completion of treatment was 81% compared with 17–27% with placebo. The relatively high cumulative cure rates with placebo treatment suggest that bacterial vaginosis could resolve spontaneously without treatment. **Oral versus intravaginal antibacterial treatment:** We found one systematic review (search date 1996, 5 RCTs) comparing oral and intravaginal formulations of metronidazole and clindamycin,[14] and one subsequent RCT.[15] Three RCTs were conducted in symptomatic non-pregnant women and two were conducted in symptomatic and asymptomatic non-pregnant women.[14] There was no significant difference in cumulative cure rates 5–10 days after completing treatment (86% for oral metronidazole 500 mg twice daily for 7 days *v* 85% for clindamycin vaginal cream 5 g at bedtime for 7 days *v* 81% for metronidazole vaginal gel 5 g twice daily for 5 days; P values and CI not provided). Four weeks after completing treatment, the cumulative cure rates were 78% for oral metronidazole versus 82% for clindamycin vaginal cream versus 71% for metronidazole vaginal gel. The subsequent RCT (399 women) of clindamycin vaginal cream versus oral metronidazole also found no significant difference in cure rates (68% for clindamycin cream *v* 67% for oral metronidazole; $P = 0.81$).[15] However, a large number of women were not included in the efficacy analysis, making interpretation of the results difficult (results reported on 233 women, many exclusions for different reasons). **Different oral antibacterial regimens:** We found one systematic review (search date 1996, 4 RCTs) comparing metronidazole 500 mg twice daily for 7 days versus a single 2 g dose of metronidazole,[14] and two additional RCTs comparing metronidazole 500 mg twice daily for 7 days versus clindamycin 300 mg twice daily for 7 days.[16,17] The systematic review found significantly higher cumulative cure rates at 3–4 weeks after completing treatment with 7 day metronidazole (82% with 7 days of metronidazole *v* 62% with single dose metronidazole; $P < 0.05$). The first additional RCT (143 symptomatic non-pregnant women) found no significant difference in cure rates within 7–10 days of starting treatment (women cured: 46/49 [94%] with clindamycin *v* 48/50 [96%] with metronidazole; RR 0.98, 95% CI 0.89 to 1.07).[16] A quarter of women were lost to follow up. The second RCT (96 non-pregnant women) found no significant difference in cure rates (39/41 [95%] with clindamycin *v* 41/44 [93%] with metronidazole; ARI 2%; RR 1.0, 95% CI 0.92 to 1.14).[17] **Different intravaginal antibacterial regimens:** We found two RCTs.[18,19] The first RCT (514 women) found no significant difference in effectiveness between once daily versus twice daily dosing of intravaginal metronidazole gel (118/207 [57%] with once daily gel v 129/209 [62%] with twice daily gel; RR 0.92, 95% CI 0.79 to 1.08).[18] The second RCT (662 women) compared 3 day treatment with intravaginal clindamycin ovules versus 7 day treatment with intravaginal clindamycin cream.[19] It found no significant difference in cure rates at 35 day assessment (134/238 [56%] with 3 day regimen v 113/224 [50%] with 7 day regimen; ARI 6%; RR 1.10, 95% CI 0.94 to 1.30).

Harms: The review of different oral antibacterial regimens found that adverse effects occurred in between a quarter and two thirds of women taking oral metronidazole, including mild to moderate nausea/dyspepsia, unpleasant metallic taste, headache, and dizziness.[14] Infrequent adverse effects from oral clindamycin included heartburn, nausea, vomiting, diarrhoea, constipation, headache, dizziness, and vertigo; the trials gave no data on frequency. Intravaginal clindamycin has been associated, rarely, with mild to severe colitis[20] and vaginal candidiasis. The RCT of once versus twice daily intravaginal metronidazole gel found no significant difference in frequency of adverse effects.[18] Comparison of results across RCTs found that yeast vulvovaginitis might be less common with intravaginal metronidazole than with oral metronidazole (4% for intravaginal[21] v 8–22% for oral[22]).

Comment: Intravaginal administration reduces systemic absorption and systemic adverse effects. Some women may prefer oral medication because it is more convenient. We found one RCT (61 women, 19 withdrew) that followed up women who had been treated for bacterial vaginosis with either clindamycin vaginal cream or oral metronidazole.[23] It found that more than 50% of women in both groups had recurrent bacterial vaginosis 2 months after treatment (exact figures and statistical analysis not provided).

QUESTION What are the effects of treatments in pregnant women with or without bacterial vaginosis?

Two systematic reviews of antibacterial treatment of bacterial vaginosis during pregnancy found no significant difference in the risk of preterm delivery. Subgroup analysis in women with bacterial vaginosis who had a previous preterm delivery found heterogeneous results, but most RCTs found that oral antibacterial treatment reduced the risk of preterm delivery. Four RCTs found an increase in preterm birth and low birth weight in women with bacterial vaginosis treated with clindamycin cream versus placebo. One small RCT, conducted in women with bacterial vaginosis who had a previous labour or midtrimester abortion, found a higher rate of preterm birth with oral metronidazole compared with placebo, but the group receiving metronidazole had higher previous antibacterial use and asymptomatic bacteriuria at baseline.

Benefits: We found two systematic reviews (search date 1999, 7 RCTs, 3613 women;[24] and search date not stated, 5 RCTs, 1508 women[25]). The first review included one RCT that was not included in the second review, and the second review contained three RCTs that were not included in the first review, two of which were published after the search date of the first review. **In low risk pregnancy:** Both reviews found no significant difference in the general population of women with bacterial vaginosis from antibacterial treatment versus placebo with respect to the rate of preterm delivery (< 37 weeks; ARR +0.1%, 95% CI –1.7% to +1.9%;[24] and RR 0.83, 95% CI 0.67 to 1.03[25]). **In women with previous preterm birth:** The first systematic review (5 RCTs, 440 women) included a subgroup analysis in women with a previous preterm birth from RCTs in general populations.[24] Four RCTs reported results for preterm delivery at less than 37 weeks. It found clustered results. Three RCTs found a reduction in the risk of preterm delivery (ARR 22%, 90% CI 13% to 31%) but one RCT found no reduction (ARI +8%, 90% CI –4% to +19%).

Harms: The second review found that adverse effects occurred in 4% of women receiving antibiotics for bacterial vaginosis.[25] **In women without bacterial vaginosis:** Two RCTs of antibiotic administration found an increase in preterm birth (before 34 weeks of gestation) in a subgroup of women without bacterial vaginosis who received intravaginal clindamycin cream versus placebo[26] or oral metronidazole and erythromycin versus placebo.[27] In the first RCT, differences between groups did not reach statistical significance (9/72 [12.5%] with clindamycin *v* 3/74 [4.1%] with placebo; recalculation by *Clinical Evidence*: ARI 8.4%; RR 3.1, 95% CI 0.9 to 10.9).[26] However, this RCT found a significantly increased risk of neonatal sepsis with clindamycin cream (5/83 [6%] with clindamycin *v* 0/85 [0%] with placebo; ARI 6.0%, 95% CI 0.5% to 13.3%). Subgroup analysis in the second RCT found no significant difference for preterm birth before 37 weeks of gestation (56/254 [22%] with metronidazole and erythromycin *v* 26/104 [25%] with placebo; RR 0.98, 95% CI 0.57 to 1.30) but found a significant difference for preterm birth before 34 weeks of gestation (34/254 [13%] with metronidazole and erythromycin *v* 5/104 [5%] with placebo; RR 2.8, 95% CI 1.2 to 6.0; NNH 12, 95% CI 4 to 136).[27] **In women with bacterial vaginosis:** Four RCTs[28–31] found an increase in preterm birth and low birth weight in women with bacterial vaginosis who received intravaginal clindamycin cream versus placebo. In all RCTs, the increase was not significant. In the second RCT, the rate of preterm birth (< 32 weeks of gestation) was higher with clindamycin cream than with placebo (16/340 [5%] with clindamycin *v* 9/341 [3%] with placebo; ARI +2.1%, 95% CI –0.8% to +5.1%; RR 1.78, 95% CI 0.80 to 3.98).[29] The rate of low birth weight was higher with clindamycin but the difference was not significant (30/334 [9%] with clindamycin cream *v* 23/338 [7%] with placebo; RR 1.32, 95% CI 0.78 to 2.22). In the third RCT the rate of preterm birth (< 37 weeks of gestation) was higher with clindamycin cream than with placebo (7/51 [14%] with clindamycin cream *v* 3/50 [6%] with placebo; RR 2.3, 95% CI 0.6 to 8.4).[30] In the fourth RCT the rate of preterm birth (< 37 weeks of gestation) was slightly higher with clindamycin cream than with placebo (9/187 [5%] with clindamycin cream *v* 7/188 [4%] with placebo; RR 1.29, 95% CI 0.49 to 3.40).[31] One small RCT (127 high risk women with bacterial vaginosis who had previous labour or midtrimester abortion) found a significantly higher rate of preterm birth (< 37 weeks of gestation) with oral metronidazole 400 mg twice daily for 2 days versus vitamin C 100 mg twice daily for 2 days given at less than 26 weeks of gestation (30/70 [43%] with metronidazole *v* 12/51 [24%] with vitamin C; ARI 19%, 95% CI 2% to 34%; RR 1.8, 95% CI 1.04 to

3.2, recalculated by *Clinical Evidence*; see comment below).[32] One large RCT (1953 women) found significantly more adverse effects with oral metronidazole versus placebo, particularly gastrointestinal symptoms (20.0% with metronidazole *v* 7.5% with placebo; CI not provided).[33]

Comment: The average quality of the trials in the systematic reviews was good. All trials reported loss to follow up between 1–17% for the various treatment groups.[25] In addition to an increased risk of preterm birth and neonatal sepsis with intravaginal clindamycin treatment,[26] one RCT reported an alteration of normal vaginal flora to flora consistent with bacterial vaginosis among women at high risk of preterm birth who were treated with clindamycin cream.[34] One small RCT that found a significantly higher rate of preterm birth with oral metronidazole versus vitamin C also reported significantly higher rates of antibiotic use and asymptomatic bacteriuria in the metronidazole versus the vitamin C group at baseline.[32] The finding of two different clusters of results for oral treatment of bacterial vaginosis among high risk women may be due to differences in treatment regimens. Of the three RCTs that found a reduction in preterm birth, two used the US Centers for Disease Control and Prevention recommended treatment of bacterial vaginosis in pregnancy (metronidazole 250 mg three times daily for 7 days). The other RCT used a lower dose of metronidazole (400 mg twice daily for 2 days) but found a reduction in preterm birth in a small subgroup analysis (17 women in each group). The two RCTs that found no reduction in preterm birth also used a lower dose of metronidazole (2 g single dose, repeated 48 hours later and 400 mg twice daily for 2 days). Thus, the difference in dose of treatment regimen may be responsible for differing results. To a lesser degree, differences in study population (symptomatic *v* asymptomatic), timing of treatment (early *v* late gestational age), and diagnosis of bacterial vaginosis (clinical *v* Gram stain diagnosis) may also have contributed to the differing results. Bacterial vaginosis is a condition of altered vaginal flora. There is a continuum of degrees of alteration of vaginal flora that women may have, and bacterial vaginosis may be defined differently according to the diagnostic criteria being used. Given this uncertainty, treatment policies may result in the treatment of some women who do not have, by all criteria, bacterial vaginosis. Thus, it is important to evaluate the harms of treatment among women who have unequivocal bacterial vaginosis.

QUESTION Does treating male partners prevent recurrence?

One systematic review has found that, in women receiving antibacterial agents, who have one steady male sexual partner, treating the partner with an oral antibacterial agent does not reduce the woman's risk of recurrence.

Benefits: We found one systematic review (search date not stated, 5 RCTs) evaluating the effect of treating male sexual partners of women with bacterial vaginosis on recurrence rates.[35] The review found that treatment of a sexual partner with metronidazole or clindamycin had no significant effect on recurrence rates in women with bacterial vaginosis also treated with metronidazole or clindamycin. The RCTs identified by the review assessed a variety of treatment regimens and populations but excluded women who were pregnant or who had coexistent vaginal infections. The systematic review did not attempt to test for heterogeneity between RCTs or to pool the results.

Harms: No harmful effects were reported.

Comment: The lack of evidence of effectiveness of both metronidazole and clindamycin suggests that anaerobes are unlikely to be the sole pathogenic agents linking bacterial vaginosis with sexual intercourse.

QUESTION What are the effects of treatment before gynaecological procedures?

In women with bacterial vaginosis who are about to undergo surgical abortion, three RCTs found a lower rate of pelvic inflammatory disease with oral or intravaginal antibacterial treatment versus placebo but the difference was significant only in the largest RCT. We found no RCTs on the effects of treatment before other gynaecological procedures, including abdominal hysterectomy, caesarean section, or insertion of an intrauterine contraceptive device.

Benefits: We found no systematic review. **Before surgical abortion:** We found three RCTs.[36–38] The first RCT (174 women with bacterial vaginosis) compared oral metronidazole 500 mg three times daily for 10 days versus placebo in women about to undergo surgical abortion.[36] Fewer women taking metronidazole developed pelvic inflammatory disease than those taking placebo, although the result did not reach significance (3/84 [4%] with metronidazole *v* 11/90 [12%] with placebo; RR 0.29, 95% CI 0.08 to 1.01). The second RCT (1655 women) compared intravaginal clindamycin cream versus placebo in women about to undergo surgical abortion.[37] It found that significantly fewer women treated with clindamycin had an infection after abortion (recalculation by *Clinical Evidence*: infection after abortion 3/181 [2%] with clindamycin cream *v* 12/181 [7%] with placebo; RR 0.25, 95% CI 0.07 to 0.87; NNT 20, 95% CI 11 to 409). The third RCT compared a single dose metronidazole suppository 2 mg versus placebo.[38] It found that metronidazole suppository was associated with a non-significantly lower rate of postoperative upper genital tract infection (12/142 [8%] with metronidazole *v* 21/131 [16%] with placebo; RR 0.52, 95% CI 0.27 to 1.02). **Before gynaecological surgery:** Bacterial vaginosis is associated with an increased risk of endometritis after caesarean section and vaginal cuff cellulitis after abdominal hysterectomy,[11,39] but we found no RCTs of antibacterial treatment in women before such surgery. **Before insertion of an intrauterine contraceptive device:** Bacterial vaginosis has been associated with pelvic inflammatory disease (see pelvic inflammatory disease, p 1871) in women using intrauterine contraceptive devices,[3] but we found no RCTs of antibacterial treatment in women with bacterial vaginosis before insertion of these devices.

Harms: The RCTs provided no information on adverse effects.[36]

Comment: None.

Bacterial vaginosis

Substantive changes

Treatment in pregnancy, harms One RCT added;[32] conclusions unchanged.

REFERENCES

1. Barbone F, Austin H, Louv WC, et al. A follow-up study of methods of contraception, sexual activity, and rates of trichomoniasis, candidiasis, and bacterial vaginosis. *Am J Obstet Gynecol* 1990;163:510–514.
2. Mead PB. Epidemiology of bacterial vaginosis. *Am J Obstet Gynecol* 1993;169:446–449.
3. Avonts D, Sercu M, Heyerick P, et al. Incidence of uncomplicated genital infections in women using oral contraception or an intrauterine device: a prospective study. *Sex Transm Dis* 1990;17:23–29.
4. Berger BJ, Kolton S, Zenilman JM, et al. Bacterial vaginosis in lesbians: a sexually transmitted disease. *Clin Infect Dis* 1995;21:1402–1405.
5. Hawes SE, Hillier SL, Benedetti J, et al. Hydrogen peroxide-producing lactobacilli and acquisition of vaginal infections. *J Infect Dis* 1996;174:1058–1063.
6. Hillier SL, Nugent RP, Eschenbach DA, et al. Association between bacterial vaginosis and preterm delivery of a low-birth-weight infant. *N Engl J Med* 1995;333:1737–1742.
7. Schwebke JR, Morgan SC, Weiss HL. The use of sequential self-obtained vaginal smears for detecting changes in the vaginal flora. *Sex Transm Dis* 1997;24:236–239.
8. Flynn CA, Helwig AL, Meurer LN. Bacterial vaginosis in pregnancy and the risk of prematurity: a meta-analysis. *J Fam Pract* 1999;48:885–892.
9. Hillier SL, Martius J, Krohn MA, et al. Case-control study of chorioamnionic infection and chorioamnionitis in prematurity. *N Engl J Med* 1988;319:972–975.
10. Newton ER, Prihoda TJ, Gibbs RS. A clinical and microbiologic analysis of risk factors for puerperal endometritis. *Obstet Gynecol* 1990;75:403–406.
11. Watts D, Krohn M, Hillier S, et al. Bacterial vaginosis as a risk factor for postcesarean endometritis. *Obstet Gynecol* 1990;75:52–58.
12. McDonald HM, O'Loughlin JA, Vigneswaran R, et al. Impact of metronidazole therapy on preterm birth in women with bacterial vaginosis flora (*Gardnerella vaginalis*): a randomised, placebo controlled trial. *Br J Obstet Gynaecol* 1997;104:1391–1397.
13. Schmid G, Markowitz L, Joesoef R, et al. Bacterial vaginosis and HIV infection [editorial]. *Sex Transm Infect* 2000;76:3–4.
14. Joesoef MR, Schmid GP. Bacterial vaginosis: review of treatment options and potential clinical indications for therapy. *Clin Infect Dis* 1999;28(suppl 1):S57–S65 Search date 1996; primary sources Medline, hand searches of text books about sexually transmitted diseases, meeting abstracts, and contact with drug manufacturers.
15. Paavonen J, Mangioni C, Martin MA, et al. Vaginal clindamycin and oral metronidazole for bacterial vaginosis: a randomized trial. *Obstet Gynecol* 2000;96:256–260.
16. Greaves WL, Chungafung J, Morris B, et al. Clindamycin versus metronidazole in the treatment of bacterial vaginosis. *Obstet Gynecol* 1988;72:799–802.
17. Aubert JM, Oliete S, Leira J. Treatment of bacterial vaginosis: clindamycin versus metronidazol. *Prog Obst Gin* 1994;37:287–292.
18. Livengood CH, Soper DE, Sheehan KL, et al. Comparison of once daily and twice daily dosing of 0.75% metronidazole gel in the treatment of bacterial vaginosis. *Sex Transm Dis* 1999;26:137–142.
19. Sobel J, Peipert JF, McGregor JA, et al. Efficacy of clindamycin vaginal ovule (3-day treatment) versus clindamycin vaginal cream (7-day treatment) in bacterial vaginosis. *Infect Dis Obstet Gynecol* 2001;9:9–15.
20. Trexler MF, Fraser TG, Jones MP. Fulminant pseudomembranous colitis caused by clindamycin phosphate vaginal cream. *Am J Gastroenterol* 1997;92:2112–2113.
21. Hillier SL, Lipinski C, Briselden AM, et al. Efficacy of intravaginal 0.75% metronidazole gel for the treatment of bacterial vaginosis. *Obstet Gynecol* 1993;81:963–967.
22. Schmitt C, Sobel JD, Meriwether C. Bacterial vaginosis: treatment with clindamycin cream versus oral metronidazole. *Obstet Gynecol* 1992;79:1020–1023.
23. Sobel JD, Schmitt C, Meriwether C. Long-term follow-up of patients with bacterial vaginosis treated with oral metronidazole and topical clindamycin. *J Infect Dis* 1993;167:783–784.
24. Guise J-M, Mahon SM, Aickin M, et al. Screening for bacterial vaginosis in pregnancy. *Am J Prevent Med* 2001;20:62–72. Search date 1999; primary sources Medline, Cochrane Controlled Trials Register, the Cochrane Library, hand searches of reference lists of selected publications, and personal contact with national experts.
25. Brocklehurst P, Hannah M, McDonald H. Interventions for treating bacterial vaginosis in pregnancy. In: The Cochrane Library, Issue 4, 2002. Oxford: Update Software. Search date not stated; primary sources Cochrane Pregnancy and Childbirth Group Specialised Register of Controlled Trials and Cochrane Controlled Trials Register.
26. Vermeulen GM, Bruinse HW. Prophylactic administration of clindamycin 2% vaginal cream to reduce the incidence of spontaneous preterm birth in women with an increased recurrence risk: a randomized placebo-controlled double-blind trial. *Br J Obstet Gynaecol* 1999;106:652–657.
27. Hauth JC, Goldenberg RL, Andrews WW, et al. Reduced incidence of preterm delivery with metronidazole and erythromycin in women with bacterial vaginosis. *N Engl J Med* 1995;333:1732–1736.
28. McGregor JA, French JI, Jones W, et al. Bacterial vaginosis is associated with prematurity and vaginal fluid mucinase and sialidase: results of a controlled trial of topical clindamycin cream. *Am J Obstet Gynecol* 1994;170:1048–1059.
29. Joesoef MR, Hillier SL, Wiknjosastro G, et al. Intravaginal clindamycin treatment for bacterial vaginosis: effect on preterm delivery and low birth weight. *Am J Obstet Gynecol* 1995;173:1527–1531.
30. Kurkinen-Raty M, Vuopala S, Koskela M, et al. A randomised controlled trial of vaginal clindamycin for early pregnancy bacterial vaginosis. *BJOG* 2000;107:1427–1432.
31. Kekki M, Kurki T, Pelkonen J, et al. Vaginal clindamycin in preventing preterm birth and peripartal infections in asymptomatic women with bacterial vaginosis: a randomized, controlled trial. *Obstet Gynecol* 2001;97:643–648.
32. Odendaal HJ, Popov I, Schoeman J, Smith M. Preterm labour: is bacterial vaginosis involved? *S Afr Med J* 2002;92:231–234.

33. Carey JC, Klebanoff MA, Hauth JC, et al. Metronidazole to prevent preterm delivery in pregnant women with asymptomatic bacterial vaginosis. *N Engl J Med* 2000;342:534–540.
34. Vermeulen GM, van Swet AA, Bruinse HW. Changes in the vaginal flora after two percent clindamycin vaginal cream in women at high risk of spontaneous preterm birth. *Br J Obstet Gynaecol* 2001;108:697–700.
35. Hamrick M, Chambliss ML. Bacterial vaginosis and treatment of sexual partners. *Arch Fam Med* 2000;9:647–648. Search date not stated; primary sources Medline and the Cochrane Library.
36. Larsson PG, Platz-Christensen JJ, Thejls H, et al. Incidence of pelvic inflammatory disease after first-trimester legal abortion in women with bacterial vaginosis after treatment with metronidazole: a double-blind, randomized study. *Am J Obstet Gynecol* 1992;166:100–103.
37. Larsson PG, Platz-Christensen JJ, Dalaker K, et al. Treatment with 2% clindamycin vaginal cream prior to first trimester surgical abortion to reduce signs of postoperative infection: a prospective, double-blinded, placebo-controlled, multicenter study. *Acta Obstet Gynecol Scand* 2000;79:390–396.
38. Crowley T, Low N, Turner A, et al. Antibiotic prophylaxis to prevent post-abortal upper genital tract infection in women with bacterial vaginosis: randomised controlled trial. *BJOG* 2001;108:396–402.
39. Soper DE, Bump RC, Hurt WG. Bacterial vaginosis and trichomoniasis vaginitis are risk factors for cuff cellulitis after abdominal hysterectomy. *Am J Obstet Gynecol* 1990;163:1016–1021.

M Joesoef
Medical Epidemiologist
National Center for HIV STD
and TB Prevention
Atlanta
USA

George Schmid
Medical Epidemiologist
Department of HIV/AIDS
World Health Organization
Geneva
Switzerland

Competing interests: None declared.

Genital chlamydial infection

Search date September 2002

Nicola Low and Frances Cowan

QUESTIONS

INTERVENTIONS

Key Messages

- Short term microbiological cure is the outcome used in most RCTs, but this may not mean eradication of *Chlamydia trachomatis*. Long term cure rates have not been studied extensively because of high default rates and difficulty in distinguishing persistent infection from reinfection due to re-exposure.

In men and non-pregnant women

- **Azithromycin (single dose)** One systematic review of short term RCTs has found no significant difference in microbiological cure of *C trachomatis* between a single dose of azithromycin versus a 7 day course of doxycycline, although the RCTs may have lacked power to detect a clinically important difference. Rates of adverse effects were similar.
- **Ciprofloxacin (multiple dose)** Two RCTs found that ciprofloxacin cured 63–92% of people. Meta-analysis found that ciprofloxacin versus doxycycline significantly increased microbiological failure.

- **Doxycycline, tetracycline, rosaramicin (multiple dose regimens)** Small RCTs with short term follow up and high withdrawal rates found that multiple dose regimens of tetracyclines (doxycycline, tetracycline) and macrolides (rosaramicin) achieve microbiological cure in at least 95% of people with genital chlamydia.
- **Erythromycin (multiple dose regimens)** Three small RCTs found that erythromycin achieved microbiological cure in 77–100% of people, with the highest cure rate with a 2 g versus a 1 g daily dose.
- **Ofloxacin, trovafloxacin, minocycline, lymecycline, clarithromycin, ampicillin, rifampicin (multiple dose regimens)** We found limited evidence on the effects of these regimens.

In pregnant women

- **Azithromycin (single *v* multiple dose antibiotics)** One systematic review has found that a single dose of azithromycin versus a 7 day course of erythromycin significantly increases microbiological cure. Two subsequent unblinded RCTs found no significant difference in cure rate between single dose azithromycin versus multiple dose amoxicillin.
- **Clindamycin (multiple dose)** One small RCT has found no significant difference in cure rates between clindamycin versus erythromycin.
- **Erythromycin, amoxicillin (multiple dose regimens)** One systematic review of one small RCT has found that erythromycin versus placebo significantly increased microbiological cure. The review found no significant difference between erythromycin and amoxicillin in microbiological cure, and high cure rates with both drugs.

DEFINITION Uncomplicated genital chlamydia is a sexually transmitted infection of the urethra in men, and of the endocervix, urethra (or both) in women that has not ascended to the upper genital tract. Infection is asymptomatic in up to 80% of women, but may cause non-specific symptoms, including vaginal discharge and intermenstrual bleeding. Infection in men causes urethral discharge and urethral irritation or dysuria, but may also be asymptomatic in up to half of cases.[1] Complicated chlamydia infection includes spread to the upper genital tract (causing pelvic inflammatory disease in women [see pelvic inflammatory disease, p 1871] and epididymo-orchitis in men) and extra genital sites, such as ocular infection.

INCIDENCE/ PREVALENCE Genital chlamydia is the most common bacterial sexually transmitted infection in developed countries. In the USA, over 642 000 cases of chlamydia were reported in the year 2000.[2] The prevalence of uncomplicated genital chlamydia in women attending general practice surgeries for a cervical smear in the UK is reported to be 3–5%.[3] Prevalence is highest in young adults. Reported rates in 16–19 year old women are about 940/100 000 in the UK,[4] 1000/100 000 in Sweden,[1] and 2500/100 000 in the USA.[5]

AETIOLOGY/ RISK FACTORS Infection is caused by the bacterium *C trachomatis* serotypes D–K. It is transmitted primarily through sexual intercourse.

PROGNOSIS In women, untreated chlamydial infection that ascends to the upper genital tract causes pelvic inflammatory disease in an estimated 30–40% of women.[6] Tubal infertility has been found to occur in about 11% of women after a single episode of pelvic inflammatory disease, and the risk of ectopic pregnancy is increased six- to sevenfold.[7] Ascending infection in men causes epididymitis, but evidence that this causes male infertility is limited.[8] Maternal to infant transmission can lead to neonatal conjunctivitis and pneumonitis in 30–40% of cases.[1] Chlamydia may coexist with other genital infections and may facilitate transmission and acquisition of HIV infection.[1] Untreated chlamydial infection persists symptomatically in most women for at least 60 days and for a shorter period in men.[9] Spontaneous remission also occurs but data are insufficient to determine the rate of clearance.[9]

AIMS OF INTERVENTION To eradicate *C trachomatis*; to prevent the development of upper genital tract infection; and to prevent further sexual transmission, with minimal adverse effects of treatment.

OUTCOMES The primary outcome is short term microbiological cure rate (calculated as the percentage of people attending a follow up visit at least 1 week after the end of antibiotic treatment who had a negative test for *C trachomatis*). Short term microbiological cure, which is the aim of treatment, may not mean eradication of *C trachomatis* because of the organism's prolonged life cycle. Some studies using DNA amplification techniques found that persistence of infection after successful antibiotic treatment does not appear to occur in people followed for up to 20 weeks.[9] However, long term cure rates have not been studied extensively because of high default rates and difficulty in distinguishing persistent infection from reinfection. Other outcomes include adverse effects of treatment, including effects on the fetus; pelvic inflammatory disease; and infertility.

METHODS *Clinical Evidence* search and appraisal September 2002. All relevant systematic reviews and masked clinical RCTs were included. Treatment RCTs for genital chlamydia usually compare a new antibiotic versus an existing regimen because placebo controlled RCTs would be considered unethical. Single trials usually have insufficient statistical power to establish equivalence but meta-analysis is often inappropriate because of differences in the antibiotics used. Therefore, we present the absolute cure rates for individual antibiotics, combining results across trials. We present the range of cure rates (with exact binomial CIs) or, if there was no evidence of statistical heterogeneity between RCTs, the summary cure rate (95% CIs) weighted by the standard error. Summary rates do not include cure rates of 100% because the standard error cannot be computed if there are no treatment failures. Where two or more RCTs compared the same regimens with no evidence of statistical heterogeneity, we used a fixed effects meta-analysis to calculate the summary odds ratio with 95% confidence intervals. Trial quality was assessed in terms of randomisation, blinding, and numbers of withdrawals from analysis.[10] RCTs with methodological limitations have been included but relevant problems are mentioned in the text. **Categorising interventions:** We considered a regimen beneficial if the summary cure rate from two or more RCTs was 95% or greater, as previously suggested,[11] and if the lower confidence limit was also above 90%. We found insufficient data to differentiate reinfections from persistent infections. We considered regimens to be likely (or unlikely) to be beneficial on the basis of positive (or negative) results from two or more RCTs, and of unknown effectiveness if there was only one RCT or if results were conflicting.

QUESTION **What are the effects of antibiotic treatment for men and non-pregnant women with uncomplicated genital chlamydial infection?**

OPTION **MULTIPLE DOSE ANTIBIOTICS VERSUS OTHER MULTIPLE DOSE ANTIBIOTICS**

Small RCTs in men and women with proven and presumed infection have found that tetracyclines (doxycycline and tetracycline) and macrolides (rosaramicin) achieve microbiological cure in 95% or more cases of genital chlamydia. Three small RCTs found that erythromycin achieved microbiological cure in 77–100% of people, with the highest cure rate with a 2 g versus a 1 g daily dose. Two RCTs found that ciprofloxacin cured 63–92% of people. Meta-analysis found that ciprofloxacin versus doxycycline significantly increased microbiological failure. We found limited evidence on the effectiveness of other macrolides, quinolones, and penicillins. The RCTs had short term follow up and high withdrawal rates.

Benefits: We found no systematic review. We found 22 RCTs reported to be double blind or with blinded outcome assessment comparing 19 different antibiotic regimens (see table A on web extra).[12–33] Results were similar in men and women and in populations with proven and presumed infection, so data were combined. **Doxycycline:** We found 11 RCTs (1434 men and women) comparing doxycycline with another antibiotic.[12–14,16–23] The cure rate was 100% in six RCTs and the weighted average 98% (95% CI 96% to 99%) in the other five. We found no RCTs comparing different regimens for doxycycline, but the most frequent schedule (in 6 RCTs) was 100 mg twice daily for 7 days. **Tetracycline:** The summary cure rate in four RCTs (201 men and women) comparing tetracycline hydrochloride (500 mg 4 times daily for 7 days) versus another antibiotic was 97% (95% CI 94% to 99%).[24–27] A *Clinical Evidence* meta-analysis of three RCTs[25–27] found that rates of treatment failure with rosaramicin compared with tetracycline were similar (OR 1.55, 95% CI 0.54 to 4.43; see figure A on web extra). **Erythromycin:** Cure rates with erythromycin stearate 1 g daily for 7 days (3 RCTs, 191 people) ranged from 77–95%,[30–32] and with erythromycin 2 g daily for 7 days (2 RCTs, 40 people) from 94–100%.[29,32] **Rosaramicin:** The summary cure rate from four RCTs (192 men and women) comparing rosaramicin versus another antibiotic was 97% (95% CI 94% to 99%).[25–28] **Ciprofloxacin:** In two RCTs (190 men and women) the cure rate for ciprofloxacin ranged from 63–92%.[20,21] Meta-analysis by *Clinical Evidence* found that failure of microbiological cure was significantly more frequent with ciprofloxacin than doxycycline (OR 5.0, 95% CI 1.2 to 10.0). A variety of other antibiotics (ofloxacin, trovafloxacin, minocycline, lymecycline, clarithromycin, ampicillin, rifampicin) were studied in single RCTs (see table A on web extra). No RCT measured the effect of antibiotics on pelvic inflammatory disease or infertility.

Harms: Reported adverse effects varied widely between RCTs but were mostly gastrointestinal (see table A on web extra). Adverse effects severe enough to stop treatment were infrequent. Photosensitivity, which is particularly associated with tetracyclines, was also reported to occur with sparfloxacin.[19]

Comment: Most RCTs were conducted in sexually transmitted diseases clinics, where follow up is difficult; in 7/14 RCTs with available data, more than 15% of randomised participants were not included in the analysis.[15,22,29–33] Most RCTs were small (3 had fewer than 40 people with chlamydia)[16,24,29] and many antibiotic regimens were compared so it is difficult to draw conclusions about relative efficacy. Only five RCTs reported that sexual partners of participants were offered treatment. Amoxicillin (amoxycillin) and ampicillin have not been adequately assessed in the treatment of genital chlamydia infection (see table A on web extra) because *in vitro* studies suggest that amoxicillin does not eradicate *C trachomatis*,[34] raising the concern that infection may persist and recrudesce *in vivo*.

OPTION SINGLE DOSE VERSUS DIFFERENT MULTIPLE DOSE ANTIBIOTICS

Short term RCTs have found no significant difference in microbiological cure of *C trachomatis* between a single dose of azithromycin versus a 7 day course of doxycycline, although the RCTs may have lacked power to detect a clinically important difference. Rates of adverse effects were similar.

Benefits: We found one systematic review (search date 1996, 9 blinded and unblinded RCTs, 1800 people) comparing azithromycin (1 g as a single dose) versus doxycycline (100 mg twice daily for 7 days) in people with proven or presumed genital chlamydia.[35] Data about laboratory diagnosed infection were available for five RCTs (554 men and women). Cure rates for single dose azithromycin ranged from 90–100% and for multiple dose doxycycline from 93–100%. Short term (2 wks) failure to achieve microbiological cure was more frequent with azithromycin than with doxycycline, but this was not statistically significant (4 RCTs, AR 22/301 [7.3%] azithromycin *v* 10/253 [4.0%] with doxycycline; OR recalculated by *Clinical Evidence* 1.83, 95% CI 0.87 to 3.87).

Harms: Short term adverse effects of both azithromycin and doxycycline were reported to be mild and similar between treatments.[35]

Comment: Azithromycin can be given in a single dose as directly observed treatment. More comparisons of azithromycin and doxycycline are needed to rule out a clinically important difference between them.

QUESTION What are the effects of treatment for pregnant women with uncomplicated genital chlamydial infection?

OPTION MULTIPLE DOSE ANTIBIOTICS VERSUS OTHER MULTIPLE DOSE ANTIBIOTICS

One systematic review of one small RCT has found erythromycin versus placebo significantly increases microbiological cure. The review found no significant difference between erythromycin and amoxicillin in microbiological cure, and high cure rates with both drugs.

Benefits: We found one systematic review (search date 1998, 11 blinded and unblinded RCTs, 1449 people).[36] **Erythromycin and amoxicillin:** The review found high rates of microbiological cure with both drugs but there was a non-significant higher cure rate with amoxicillin (amoxycillin) (3 RCTs; cure rates 182/199 [91%] with amoxicillin 500 mg 3 times daily for 7 days *v* 163/191 [85%] with erythromycin 500 mg 4 times daily for 7 days; RR for failure of cure with amoxicillin compared with erythromycin 0.59, 95% CI 0.34 to 1.03). One RCT found treatment with erythromycin was better than placebo (OR for failure of cure 0.15, 95% CI 0.08 to 0.28). **Clindamycin:** The review found one small RCT, which found no significant difference in cure rates between clindamycin and erythromycin (cure rate 38/41 [93%] *v* 31/37 [84%]; RR for failure of cure 0.45, 95% CI 0.12 to 1.7).[36]

Harms: Rates of adverse effects were similar for clindamycin and erythromycin, but adverse effects sufficient to stop treatment were less frequent with amoxicillin than erythromycin (OR 0.16, 95% CI 0.09 to 0.30). None of the RCTs gave information on adverse clinical outcomes in the offspring.

Comment: None.

OPTION SINGLE DOSE VERSUS DIFFERENT MULTIPLE DOSE ANTIBIOTICS

One systematic review has found that a single dose of azithromycin versus a 7 day course of erythromycin significantly increases microbiological cure. Two subsequent unblinded RCTs found no significant difference in cure rate between single dose azithromycin versus multiple dose amoxicillin.

Benefits: We found one systematic review (search date 1998, 4 non-blinded RCTs, 290 pregnant women),[36] and two subsequent RCTs.[37,38] The review compared a single dose of azithromycin (1 g) versus erythromycin (500 mg 4 times daily) for 7 days.[36] At first follow up visit, failure of microbiological cure was significantly less frequent with azithromycin than erythromycin (4 RCTs, 11/145 [8%] *v* 27/145 [19%]; RR 0.42, 95% CI 0.22 to 0.80).[36] There was no significant difference in the rate of premature delivery in one RCT (OR 0.75, 95% CI 0.28 to 2.04). The two subsequent unblinded RCTs both compared a single dose of azithromycin (1 g) versus 7 days of amoxicillin (500 mg).[37,38] The first RCT (39 pregnant women) found no significant difference in microbiological cure (failure to cure: 1/19 [5.2%] with azithromycin *v* 3/15 [20%] with amoxicillin [amoxyciilin]; OR 0.26, 95% CI 0.005 to 3.79).[37] The second RCT only reported the combined outcome of microbiological negative test and completion of all medication. It found no significant difference in outcome (32/55 [58%] with amoxicillin *v* 35/55 [63%] with azithromycin; RR 0.9, 95% CI 0.7 to 1.2).[38]

Harms: The systematic review found that azithromycin decreased the risk of an adverse effect sufficient to stop treatment compared with erythromycin (4/254 [1.6%] with azithromycin *v* 40/249 [16.6%] with erythromycin, RR 0.11, 95% CI 0.04 to 0.28).[36] Fetal anomaly was reported in one infant in each group. The first RCT of azithromycin versus amoxicillin found a greater proportion of people reported any adverse event with azithromycin but the difference was not significant (10/19 [52.6%] with azithromycin *v* 5/17 [29.4%] with amoxicillin, RR 1.8, 95% CI 0.8 to 4.2).[37] The second RCT also found more adverse effects with azithromycin but no significant difference (6/55 with azithromycin *v* 3/55 [5.5%] with amoxicillin, RR 0.5, 95% CI 0.1 to 1.9).[38] We found little good evidence on the effects of azithromycin on pregnancy outcomes.

Comment: Azithromycin can be given in a single dose as directly observed treatment.

REFERENCES

1. Holmes KK, Sparling PF, M rdh PA, et al, eds. *Sexually transmitted diseases*. 3rd ed. New York: McGraw Hill Inc, 1999.
2. Anonymous. Notifiable diseases/deaths in selected cities weekly information. *MMR Morb Mortal Wkly Rep* 2001;49:1168.
3. Stokes T. Screening for chlamydia in general practice: a literature review and summary of the evidence [review]. *J Public Health Med* 1997;19:222–232.
4. http://www.phls.co.uk/topics_az/hiv_and_sti/sti-chlamydia/epidemiology/epidemiology.htm(last accessed 17 February 2003).
5. US Department of Health and Human Services, Public Health Service. *Sexually Transmitted Disease Surveillance, 1999*. Atlanta: Centers for Disease Control and Prevention (CDC), September 2000.
6. Cates W Jr, Rolfs RT Jr, Aral SO. Sexually transmitted diseases, pelvic inflammatory disease, and infertility: an epidemiologic update. *Epidemiol Rev* 1990;12:199–220.
7. Weström L, Bengtsson LP, M rdh PA. Incidence, trends, and risks of ectopic pregnancy in a population of women. *BMJ* 1981;282:15–18.
8. Ness RB, Markovic N, Carlson CL, et al. Do men become infertile after having sexually transmitted urethritis? An epidemiologic examination [review]. *Fertil Steril* 1997;68:205–213.
9. Golden MR, Schillinger JA, Markowitz L, et al. Duration of untreated genital infections with *Chlamydia trachomatis*. A review of the literature. *Sex Transm Dis 2000;27:329–337.*
10. Chalmers I, Adams M, Dickersin K, et al. A cohort study of summary reports of controlled trials. *JAMA* 1990;263:1401–1405.
11. Clinical Effectiveness Group. National guideline for the management of *Chlamydia trachomatis* genital tract infection. *Sex Transm Infect* 1999;75(Suppl 1):4–8.
12. Nilsen A, Halsos A, Johansen A, et al. A double blind study of single dose azithromycin and doxycycline in the treatment of chlamydial urethritis in males. *Genitourin Med* 1992;68:325–327.
13. Steingrimsson O, Olafsson JH, Thórarinsson H, et al. Single dose azithromycin treatment of gonorrhea and infections caused by *C trachomatis* and *U urealyticum* in men. *Sex Transm Dis* 1994;21:43–46.
14. Stamm WE, Hicks CB, Martin DH, et al. Azithromycin for empirical treatment of the nongonococcal urethritis syndrome in men. A randomized double-blind study. *JAMA* 1995;274:545–549.
15. Brihmer C, M rdh PA, Kallings I, et al. Efficacy and safety of azithromycin versus lymecycline in the treatment of genital chlamydial infections in women. *Scand J Infect Dis* 1996;28:451–454.
16. Stein GE, Mummaw NL, Havlichek DH. A preliminary study of clarithromycin versus doxycycline in the treatment of nongonococcal urethritis and mucopurulent cervicitis. *Pharmacotherapy* 1995;15:727–731.
17. Romanowski B, Talbot H, Stadnyk M, et al. Minocycline compared with doxycycline in the treatment of nongonococcal urethritis and mucopurulent cervicitis. *Ann Intern Med* 1993;119:16–22.
18. Boslego JW, Hicks CB, Greenup R, et al. A prospective randomized trial of ofloxacin vs. doxycycline in the treatment of uncomplicated male urethritis. *Sex Transm Dis* 1988;15:186–191.
19. Phillips I, Dimian C, Barlow D, et al. A comparative study of two different regimens of sparfloxacin versus doxycycline in the treatment of non-gonococcal urethritis in men. *J Antimicrob Chemother* 1996;37(suppl A):123–134.
20. Hooton TM, Rogers ME, Medina TG, et al. Ciprofloxacin compared with doxycycline for nongonococcal urethritis. Ineffectiveness against *Chlamydia trachomatis* due to relapsing infection. *JAMA* 1990;264:1418–1421.
21. Jeskanen L, Karppinen L, Ingervo L, et al. Ciprofloxacin versus doxycycline in the treatment

of uncomplicated urogenital *Chlamydia trachomatis* infections. A double-blind comparative study. *Scand J Infect Dis Suppl* 1989;60:62–65.
22. McCormack WM, Dalu ZA, Martin DH, et al. Double-blind comparison of trovafloxacin and doxycycline in the treatment of uncomplicated Chlamydial urethritis and cervicitis. Trovafloxacin Chlamydial Urethritis/Cervicitis Study Group. *Sex Transm Dis* 1999;26:531–536.
23. Lassus AB, Virrankoski T, Reitamo SJ, et al. Pivampicillin versus doxycycline in the treatment of chlamydial urethritis in men. *Sex Transm Dis* 1990;17:20–22.
24. Lassus A, Juvakoski T, Kanerva L. Comparison between rifampicin and tetracycline in the treatment of nongonococcal urethritis in males with special reference to *Chlamydia trachomatis*. *Eur J Sex Transm Dis* 1984;2:15–17.
25. Lassus A, Allgulander C, Juvakoski T. Efficacy of rosaramicin and tetracycline in chlamydia-positive and -negative nongonococcal urethritis. *Eur J Sex Transm Dis* 1982;1:29–31.
26. Juvakoski T, Allgulander C, Lassus A. Rosaramicin and tetracycline treatment in *Chlamydia trachomatis*-positive and -negative nongonococcal urethritis. *Sex Transm Dis* 1981;8:12–15.
27. Brunham RC, Kuo CC, Stevens CE, et al. Therapy of cervical chlamydial infection. *Ann Intern Med* 1982;97:216–219.
28. Batteiger BE, Zwickl BE, French ML, et al. Women at risk for gonorrhea: comparison of rosaramicin and ampicillin plus probenecid in the eradication of *Neisseria gonorrhoeae*, *Chlamydia trachomatis* and genital mycoplasmas. *Sex Transm Dis* 1985;12:1–4.
29. Robson HG, Shah PP, Lalonde RG, et al. Comparison of rosaramicin and erythromycin stearate for treatment of cervical infection with *Chlamydia trachomatis*. *Sex Transm Dis* 1983;10:130–134.
30. Worm AM, Hoff G, Kroon S, et al. Roxithromycin compared with erythromycin against genitourinary chlamydial infections. *Genitourin Med* 1989;65:35–38.
31. Worm AM, Avnstorp C, Petersen CS. Erythromycin against *Chlamydia trachomatis* infections. A double blind study comparing 4- and 7-day treatment in men and women. *Dan Med Bull* 1985;32:269–271.
32. Linnemann CCJ, Heaton CL, Ritchey M. Treatment of *Chlamydia trachomatis* infections: comparison of 1- and 2-g doses of erythromycin daily for seven days. *Sex Transm Dis* 1987;14:102–106.
33. Paavonen J, Kousa M, Saikku P, et al. Treatment of nongonococcal urethritis with trimethoprim-sulphadiazine and with placebo. A double-blind partner-controlled study. *Br J Venereal Dis* 1980;56:101–104.
34. Kuo CC, Wang SP, Grayston JT. Antimicrobial activity of several antibiotics and a sulfonamide against *Chlamydia trachomatis* organisms in cell culture. *Antimicrob Agents Chemother* 1977;12:80–83.
35. Chlamydial STD treatment. *Bandolier* 1996;28:4–6. Search date 1996; primary source Medline. http://www.jr2.ox.ac.uk/bandolier/band28/b28-4.html (last accessed 17 February 2003).
36. Brocklehurst P, Rooney G. Interventions for treating genital *Chlamydia trachomatis* infection in pregnancy. In: The Cochrane Library, Issue 3, 2002. Oxford: Update Software. Search date 1998; primary sources Cochrane Pregnancy and Childbirth Review Group Specialised Register of Controlled Trials, and Cochrane Controlled Trials Register.
37. Jacobson GF, Autry AM, Kirby RS, et al. A randomized controlled trial comparing amoxicillin and azithromycin for the treatment of *Chlamydia trachomatis* in pregnancy. *Am J Obstet Gynecol* 2001;184:1352–1356.
38. Kacmar J, Cheh E, Montagno A, et al. A randomized trial of azithromycin versus amoxicillin for the treatment of *Chlamydia trachomatis* in pregnancy. *Infect Dis Obstet Gynecol* 2001;9:197–202.

Nicola Low
Department of Social Medicine
University of Bristol
Bristol
UK

Frances Cowan
Department of Sexually
Transmitted Diseases
Royal Free and
University College Medical School
London
UK

Competing interests: FC has received research and symposium funding from Glaxo Wellcome in relation to HSV research and from the NIMH for a community RCT of HSV prevention in Zimbabwe. NL none declared.

Genital herpes

Search date November 2002

Bazian Ltd

QUESTIONS

INTERVENTIONS

*Categorisation based on observational evidence

Key Messages

Treating first and recurrent episodes of genital herpes

- **Daily oral antiviral treatment in people with high rates of recurrence** RCTs have found that daily maintenance treatment with oral antiviral agents compared with placebo reduces the frequency of recurrences and improves psychosocial morbidity in people with frequent recurrence.
- **Oral antiviral treatment in first episodes** RCTs in people with a first episode of genital herpes have found that oral antiviral treatment versus placebo reduces the duration of symptoms, lesions, and viral shedding but found no significant difference in the time to recurrence or frequency of subsequent recurrences.

- **Oral antiviral treatment in people immunocompromised with HIV infection** We found no RCTs evaluating antiviral treatment for genital herpes in people immunocompromised with HIV infection.
- **Oral antiviral treatment taken at the start of a recurrence** One systematic review and one subsequent RCT have found that oral antiviral treatment taken at the start of a recurrence reduces the duration of lesions, symptoms, and viral shedding compared with placebo in people with recurrent genital herpes. RCTs found no significant differences among different antiviral agents.
- **Psychotherapy to reduce recurrence** One systematic review found insufficient evidence on the effects of psychotherapy on genital herpes recurrence.

Preventing transmission of herpes simplex virus

- **Abdominal delivery in women with genital lesions at term** We found insufficient evidence of the effects of abdominal delivery on mother to baby transmission of genital herpes. The procedure carries the risk of increased maternal morbidity and mortality.
- **Antiviral treatment to prevent sexual transmission** We found no good evidence on the effects of antiviral treatments to prevent sexual transmission.
- **Daily oral antiviral treatment in late pregnancy (36 or more wks of gestation) in women with a history of genital herpes** We found insufficient direct evidence about effects on neonatal infection. One systematic review and one subsequent RCT found that aciclovir reduced the rate of genital lesions at term in women with first or recurrent episodes of genital herpes simplex virus during pregnancy.
- **Female condoms** We found no good evidence on the effects of female condoms.
- **Male condom use to prevent sexual transmission to women** Limited evidence from a prospective cohort study suggested that male condom use reduced transmission of herpes simplex virus type 2 to women who had sexual partners with herpes simplex virus 2.
- **Male condom use to prevent transmission to men** One prospective cohort study found no significant difference between male condom use versus no condom use in preventing transmission of herpes simplex virus type 2 to men who had sexual partners with genital herpes.
- **Recombinant glycoprotein vaccine (gB2 and gD2)** One RCT found no significant difference between glycoprotein vaccine versus placebo for infection with herpes simplex virus 2. We found no good evidence on other forms of vaccination.
- **Serological screening and counselling in late pregnancy** The highest risk of mother to baby transmission is in women newly infected with genital herpes in late pregnancy. We found insufficient evidence of the effects of interventions to prevent infection in late pregnancy (such as serological screening and counselling).

DEFINITION Genital herpes is an infection with herpes simplex virus type 1 or type 2, causing ulceration in the genital area. Herpes simplex virus infections can be defined on the basis of virological and serological findings. Types of infection include **first episode primary infection**, which is herpes simplex virus in a person without prior herpes simplex virus type 1 or type 2 antibodies; **first episode non-primary infection**, which is herpes simplex virus type 2 in a person with prior herpes simplex virus type 1 antibodies or vice versa; **first**

recognised recurrence, which is herpes simplex virus type 2 (or type 1) in a person with prior herpes simplex virus type 2 (or type 1) antibodies; and **recurrent genital herpes**, which is caused by reactivation of latent herpes simplex virus.

INCIDENCE/ PREVALENCE Genital herpes infections are among the most common sexually transmitted diseases. Seroprevalence studies show that 22% of adults in the USA have herpes simplex virus type 2 antibodies.[1] A UK study found that 23% of adults attending sexual medicine clinics and 7.6% of blood donors in London had antibodies to herpes simplex virus type 2.[2] However, herpes simplex type 2 can cause other herpes infections such as ocular herpes.

AETIOLOGY/ RISK FACTORS Both herpes simplex virus type 1 and 2 can cause a first episode of genital infection, but herpes simplex virus type 2 is more likely to cause recurrent disease.[3] Most people with herpes simplex virus type 2 infection are not aware that they have genital herpes, as their symptoms are mild. However, these people can pass on the infection to sexual partners and newborns.[4,5]

PROGNOSIS Sequelae of herpes simplex virus infection include neonatal herpes simplex virus infection, opportunistic infections in immunocompromised people, recurrent genital ulceration, and psychosocial morbidity. Herpes simplex virus type 2 infection is associated with an increased risk of HIV transmission and acquisition.[6] The most common neurological complications are aseptic meningitis (reported in about 25% of women during primary infection) and urinary retention. The absolute risk of neonatal infection is high (41%, 95% CI 26% to 56%) in babies born to women who acquire infection near the time of labour[7,8] and low (< 3%) in women with established infection, even in those who have a recurrence at term. About 15% of neonatal infections result from postnatal transmission from oral lesions.

AIMS OF INTERVENTION To reduce the morbidity of the first episode; to reduce the risk of recurrent disease after a first episode; to prevent further transmission, with minimal adverse effects of treatment.

OUTCOMES Severity and duration of symptoms; healing time; duration of viral shedding; recurrence rates; psychosocial morbidity; rates of transmission; adverse effects of treatment.

METHODS *Clinical Evidence* search and appraisal November 2002. We also included preliminary results of clinical trials published in the abstracts of the *Interscience Conference on Antimicrobial Agents and Chemotherapy and International Society for STD Research*.

QUESTION **What are the effects of antiviral treatment in people with a first episode of genital herpes?**

RCTs have found that oral antiviral treatment versus placebo decreases the duration of lesions, symptoms, and viral shedding, and reduces neurological complications in people with first episode genital herpes. Limited data from two RCTs provide no evidence that oral antiviral treatment reduced the rate of recurrence compared with placebo. RCTs have found no evidence of a significant difference in clinical outcomes among aciclovir, valaciclovir, and famciclovir in people with a first episode of genital herpes.

Benefits: We found no systematic review. **Immediate effects:** We found five RCTs (350 men and women) of oral aciclovir for the treatment of first episode genital herpes.[9–13] The largest RCT (180 people) compared aciclovir (200 mg 5 times daily) versus placebo. It excluded 30 people from analysis (see comment below). Subgroup analysis (131 people with primary first episode genital herpes) found that aciclovir decreased the duration of viral shedding (median 2 days with aciclovir *v* 9 days with placebo), pain (5 days with aciclovir *v* 7 days with placebo), time to healing of lesions (12 days with aciclovir *v* 14 days with placebo), and reduced formation of new lesions (18% with aciclovir *v* 62% with placebo).[11] The other RCTs found similar results.[9,10,12,13] Neurological complications (aseptic meningitis and urinary retention) were also reduced. Numbers were small, so no precise estimates of effectiveness were available. **Different regimens:** We found two RCTs.[14,15] The first RCT (643 otherwise healthy adults with first episode genital herpes) compared oral valaciclovir (1000 mg twice daily) versus oral aciclovir (200 mg 5 times daily) for 10 days.[14] It found no significant differences between the two medications in any clinical or virological variables. The second RCT (951 adults with first episode genital herpes) compared three doses of oral famciclovir (125, 250, or 500 mg 3 times daily) versus oral aciclovir (200 mg 5 times daily).[15] It similarly found no significant differences among treatments. **Recurrence rates:** A meta-analysis of two small placebo controlled RCTs (61 people with first episode genital herpes) found no significant difference in time to recurrence or frequency of recurrence between people given oral aciclovir and those given placebo.[16] **Systemic versus topical treatment:** We found no direct randomised comparisons of oral, intravenous, or topical antiviral treatment.

Harms: Adverse effects (mostly headache and nausea) were rare and frequency was similar for aciclovir, valaciclovir, famciclovir, and placebo.

Comment: Oral aciclovir is more convenient than intravenous aciclovir.[17] A non-randomised comparison of results of different trials from one institution suggests that systemic treatment is more effective than topical.[17] The largest RCT of immediate treatment excluded 10 people for not completing the study protocol, 12 because of suspected past infection, and eight because herpes simplex virus was not isolated.[11]

QUESTION What interventions reduce the impact of recurrence?

OPTION ANTIVIRAL TREATMENT AT THE START OF RECURRENCE

One systematic review and one subsequent RCT have found that oral antiviral treatment taken at the start of a recurrence reduces the duration of lesions, symptoms, and viral shedding compared with placebo in people with recurrent genital herpes. RCTs found no significant differences among different antivirals.

Benefits: **Famciclovir versus placebo:** We found one systematic review (search date 1997, 1 RCT, 467 people with recurrent genital herpes) of famciclovir versus placebo.[18] The RCT found that oral famciclovir (125–500 mg twice daily) significantly reduced the duration of lesions (5 days with famciclovir *v* 4 days with placebo) and viral shedding (3 days with famciclovir *v* 2 days with placebo). **Valaciclovir versus placebo:** We found one systematic review (search date 1997, 1 RCT, 986 people) of valaciclovir versus placebo.[18] The RCT (987 people with recurrent genital herpes) found that self initiated oral valaciclovir (500 or 1000 mg twice daily) for 5 days versus placebo decreased the episode duration (4 days with valaciclovir *v* 6 days with placebo) and viral shedding (2 days with valaciclovir *v* 4 days with placebo), and increased the rate of aborted recurrences (31% with valaciclovir *v* 21% with placebo). **Aciclovir versus placebo:** We found one non-systematic review of several RCTs (more than 650 healthy adults with recurrent genital herpes) and one subsequent RCT.[19,20] The RCTs in the review evaluated 5 days of oral aciclovir (200 mg 5 times daily or 800 mg twice daily), started at the first sign of recurrence. Aciclovir versus placebo reduced the period of viral shedding (1 day with aciclovir *v* 2 days with placebo) and duration of lesions (5 days with aciclovir *v* 6 days with placebo).[19] The subsequent RCT (131 people with ≥3 recurrences in previous 12 months, observed for ≥1 recurrence).[20] It found that oral aciclovir (800 mg 3 times daily) versus placebo for 2 days significantly reduced the median duration of lesions, episodes, and viral shedding (median duration of lesions: 4 days with aciclovir *v* 6 days with placebo, $P = 0.001$; median duration of episodes: 4 days with aciclovir *v* 6 days with placebo, $P < 0.001$; median duration of viral shedding: 25 h with aciclovir *v* 58.5 h with placebo, $P = 0.04$).[20] **Valaciclovir versus aciclovir:** We found one systematic review (search date 1997, 2 RCTs, 1939 people) of oral valaciclovir versus aciclovir.[18] It found no significant difference in clinical outcomes between oral valaciclovir and aciclovir. **Famciclovir versus aciclovir:** We found one RCT (204 people with recurrent genital herpes), which found no significant difference in time to healing between oral famciclovir versus aciclovir (mean lesion healing time 5.1 days with famciclovir *v* 5.4 days with aciclovir, mean difference +0.3 days, 95% CI –0.3 to +0.8 days).[21]

Harms: Adverse effects (mostly headache and nausea) were rare, and frequency was similar for aciclovir, valaciclovir, famciclovir, and placebo.[18]

Comment: The benefit was found to be greater if the person with recurrent herpes initiated treatment at the first symptom or sign of a recurrence.[22] People can learn to recognise recurrences early on and should have an adequate supply of medication at home.

OPTION DAILY MAINTENANCE ANTIVIRAL TREATMENT

RCTs have found that daily maintenance treatment with oral antiviral agents compared with placebo reduces the frequency of recurrences and improves psychosocial morbidity in people with frequent recurrence.

Benefits: **Recurrence rates:** We found one systematic review of famciclovir and valaciclovir (search date 1997, 4 placebo controlled RCTs).[18] Two RCTs in the review evaluated treatment for 1 year. The first RCT

(1479 people with frequently recurring genital herpes) compared valaciclovir 250 mg (4 times daily); valaciclovir 250 mg (twice daily); valaciclovir 500 mg (4 times daily); valaciclovir 1000 mg (4 times daily); aciclovir 400 mg (twice daily); and placebo. It found that valaciclovir reduced recurrence compared with placebo (freedom from recurrence 48–50% with valaciclovir 1000 mg 4 times daily and aciclovir 400 mg twice daily; 40% with valaciclovir 500 mg 4 times daily; 22% with valaciclovir 250 mg 4 times daily *v* 5% with placebo).[23] The second RCT (455 people with frequently recurring genital herpes) compared famciclovir (250 mg twice daily), famciclovir (125 mg 3 times daily), famciclovir (250 mg 3 times daily) and placebo. It found that famciclovir increased median time to first recurrence compared with placebo (11 months with famciclovir 250 mg twice daily; 10 months with famciclovir 250 mg 3 times daily; 8 months with famciclovir 125 mg 3 times daily *v* 1.5 months with placebo).[24] One non-systematic review identified two small RCTs of aciclovir versus placebo for 1 year or more (107 people with a history of frequent recurrence ≥6/year).[19] The first RCT (32 people) of aciclovir (800 mg daily) versus placebo found that aciclovir reduced recurrence over 2 years (freedom from recurrence at 2 years: 5/18 [28%] with aciclovir *v* 0/14 [0%] with placebo; ARR 28%, 95% CI 1% to 51%). The second RCT similarly found that aciclovir (400 mg, twice daily) reduced recurrence compared with placebo over 1 year (freedom from recurrence at 1 year: 21/48 [44%] with aciclovir *v* 0/28 [0%] with placebo; ARR 44%, 95% CI 26% to 56%). We found one subsequent double blind, placebo controlled RCT (1146 adults), which also found that aciclovir reduced recurrence compared with placebo over 1 year (recurrence rate 1.7% with aciclovir *v* 12.5% with placebo; $P < 0.0001$).[25] Of 210 adults in the trial who completed 5 years of continuous treatment with aciclovir (400 mg twice daily), 53–70% were free of recurrence each year. **Viral shedding:** We found one RCT (34 women with recently acquired genital herpes simplex virus type 2 infection) of daily maintenance with aciclovir treatment versus placebo that assessed viral shedding in women.[26] Women obtained swabs for viral cultures daily for 70 days while receiving aciclovir (400 mg twice daily) or placebo. It found that aciclovir reduced viral shedding by 95% on days with reported lesions and by 94% on days without lesions. **Psychosocial morbidity:** We found one RCT (1479 people) that evaluated the effect of daily oral antiviral treatment on a genital herpes quality of life scale.[27] People receiving daily aciclovir or valaciclovir had significantly greater mean improvements from baseline than those receiving placebo.[28]

Harms: Daily treatment with aciclovir, famciclovir, and valaciclovir was well tolerated.[29] People taking aciclovir were followed for up to 7 years, and those taking famciclovir and valaciclovir for up to 1 year. Nausea and headache were infrequent, and participants rarely discontinued treatment because of adverse effects. We found no studies evaluating whether daily maintenance treatment increases high risk sexual behaviour. We found no evidence that daily treatment with aciclovir results in emergence of aciclovir resistant herpes simplex virus during or after stopping treatment in healthy adults.[29]

Comment: Viral shedding is an intermediate outcome, which reflects the risk of transmitting infection.

OPTION PSYCHOTHERAPY

One systematic review found that the effects of psychotherapy on the rate of genital herpes recurrence have not yet been adequately studied.

Benefits: We found one systematic review (search date 1991), which identified six poor quality studies of psychotherapeutic interventions in 69 people (4 studies had < 10 participants).[30] Interventions varied from hypnotherapy and progressive muscle relaxation to cognitive therapy and multifaceted intervention. The largest RCT (31 people with > 4 recurrences/year) compared psychosocial intervention, versus social support and versus waiting list. Participants receiving psychosocial intervention had significantly lower recurrence rates (6 recurrences/year) compared with the pretreatment frequency (11 recurrences/year) and with the other groups (11 recurrences/year).

Harms: No adverse effects were noted.[30]

Comment: Small numbers of people, inadequate controls, and subjective and retrospective assessment of recurrence frequency at baseline limit the usefulness of these studies.[30] Controlled studies that include prospective clinical evaluation of disease activity are needed.

QUESTION What are the effects of interventions to prevent transmission of herpes simplex virus?

OPTION CONDOMS

Limited evidence from one prospective cohort study suggested that male condom use may decrease the risk of sexual transmission of herpes simplex virus 2 among women who have a sexual partner disconcordant for herpes simplex virus 2. However, no benefit was found for preventing transmission among men.

Benefits: We found no RCTs. In a prospective cohort study (528 couples discordant for herpes simplex virus type 2 infection and followed for 18 months), use of condoms by men in more than 25% of sexual acts was associated with a lower risk of herpes simplex virus type 2 acquisition among women (adjusted HR 0.09, 95% CI 0.01 to 0.67) but not among men (adjusted HR 2.02, 95% CI 0.32 to 12.50).[31] Only 61% of couples ever used condoms during the study and only 8% used them consistently.

Harms: None reported.

Comment: Controlled trials of condoms for prevention of herpes simplex virus type 2 transmission are impractical. Even with routine counselling, many couples do not regularly use condoms. Trials of different methods of advising people to use condoms or providing condoms could be performed.

OPTION **ANTIVIRAL TREATMENT**

We found no good evidence on the effects of antiviral treatments on transmission.

Benefits: We found no RCTs examining effects on transmission. However, RCTs have shown that daily antiviral treatment decreases the frequency of clinical and subclinical viral shedding (see antiviral treatment at the start of recurrence, p 1845).

Harms: As for individual interventions (see harms of daily maintenance antiviral treatment, p 1847).

Comment: None.

OPTION **VACCINATION**

One RCT found no significant difference between a glycoprotein vaccine versus placebo in acquisition of genital herpes.

Benefits: We found one double blind RCT (2393 herpes simplex virus 2 and HIV seronegative people) of recombinant glycoprotein vaccine (gB2 and gD2) versus placebo.[32] It found no difference in vaccine efficacy (4.2 cases per 100 person years with glycoprotein vaccine *v* 4.6 cases per 100 person years with placebo; $P = 0.58$). It found no significant difference in the duration of initial genital herpes, or the frequency of subsequent recurrences in people who acquired genital herpes simplex virus infection.

Harms: We found no good evidence on harms.

Comment: None.

OPTION **ABDOMINAL DELIVERY TO PREVENT NEONATAL HERPES**

We found insufficient evidence for the effect of abdominal delivery on the risk of neonatal herpes. The procedure carries a risk of increased maternal morbidity and mortality.

Benefits: We found no systematic review and no RCTs that assessed the effects of abdominal delivery on the risk of mother to child transmission of herpes simplex virus. In the Netherlands, women with recurrent genital herpes at delivery have been allowed vaginal birth since 1987. This policy has not resulted in an increase in neonatal herpes (26 cases from 1981–1986 and 19 cases from 1987–1991).[8]

Harms: Abdominal delivery is associated with significant maternal morbidity and mortality. A study pooling data from different studies estimated that, for every two neonatal deaths from herpes simplex virus, a policy of abdominal delivery might cause one maternal death.[33]

Comment: Countries vary in their approach to obstetric management of women with recurrent genital herpes at term. In the USA and the UK, these women are advised to have an abdominal delivery, with its attendant risks to the mother. The absolute risk of neonatal infection is high (AR 41%, 95% CI 26% to 56%) in babies born to women who acquired infection near the time of labour[7,8] and low (AR < 3%) in women with established infection, even in those who have recurrence at term. Most women who acquire infection toward the end of pregnancy are undiagnosed, and most cases of neonatal herpes simplex virus infection are acquired from women without a history of genital herpes. The available evidence suggests that efforts to prevent neonatal herpes simplex virus infection should focus on preventing infection in late pregnancy.

OPTION ANTIVIRAL TREATMENT DURING PREGNANCY

We found insufficient direct evidence about effects of oral antivirals on neonatal infection. One systematic review and one subsequent RCT found that aciclovir reduced the rate of genital lesions at term in women with first or recurrent episodes of genital herpes simplex virus during pregnancy. We found insufficient evidence about adverse effects.

Benefits: We found one systematic review (search date 1996, 2 RCTs and 1 controlled study, 210 pregnant women near term with genital herpes)[8,34–36] of daily aciclovir versus placebo and one subsequent RCT.[37] The trials in the review differed in terms of the dose and duration of aciclovir and the populations enrolled. Abdominal delivery was performed in women with genital lesions at term. All three studies in the review found lower rates of abdominal delivery in women treated with aciclovir, although in two studies the effect was not significant (AR of abdominal delivery 4/21 [19%] with aciclovir *v* 10/25 [40%] with placebo, RR 0.48, 95% CI 0.17 to 1.30;[34] AR of abdominal delivery 6/46 [13%] with aciclovir *v* 15/46 [33%] with no treatment, RR 0.40, 95% CI 0.17 to 0.94, NNT 6, 95% CI 3 to 43;[36] and AR of abdominal delivery 7/31 [23%] with aciclovir *v* 10/32 [31%] with placebo, RR 0.72, 95% CI 0.32 to 1.66).[35] The subsequent RCT (231 women with genital herpes diagnosed either by positive culture of clinical diagnosis) found that aciclovir (400 mg 3 times daily) given from 36 weeks' gestation until delivery reduced clinically evident genital herpes at delivery compared with placebo (7/116 [6%] with aciclovir *v* 16/115 [14%] with placebo; $P = 0.046$; OR 0.40, 95% CI 0.13 to 1.08). It found no significant difference in rates of caesarean section for maternal herpes simplex infection between aciclovir and placebo (8/116 [7%] with aciclovir *v* 14/115 [12%] with placebo, OR 0.53, 95% CI 0.19 to 1.44). No neonate in either group had clinical herpes simplex infection.[37]

Harms: No adverse effects for women or newborns were reported, but the number of women was small. Rare adverse events, such as an increase in asymptomatic viral shedding or aciclovir related obstructive uropathy in the newborns, would be difficult to detect.

Comment: None.

OPTION SEROLOGICAL SCREENING AND COUNSELLING TO PREVENT ACQUISITION OF HERPES SIMPLEX VIRUS DURING PREGNANCY

We found insufficient evidence on the effects of serological screening and counselling during pregnancy on infection rates.

Benefits: We found no systematic review or RCTs that assessed either serological screening with type specific assays to identify women at risk for acquisition of herpes simplex virus infection in late pregnancy, or counselling to avoid genital–genital and oral–genital contact in late pregnancy.

Harms: We found insufficient evidence.

Comment: None.

QUESTION What are the effects of treatments in people with genital herpes and HIV infection?

OPTION ANTIVIRAL TREATMENTS

We found no RCTs evaluating antiviral treatment for genital herpes in people immunocompromised with HIV infection. However, evidence from other settings suggests that antivirals may be effective treatments of genital herpes in immunocompromised people.

Benefits: We found no systematic review and no RCTs on the treatment of first episode genital herpes in people with HIV infection. **Treatment of recurrence:** We found two RCTs.[38,39] One RCT (193 people on stable antiretroviral treatment) compared famciclovir (500 mg twice daily) versus aciclovir (400 mg 5 times daily) for 1 week.[38] It found no difference between the two drugs in mucocutaneous recurrence of herpes simplex virus. The other RCT (467 people) compared valaciclovir (1000 mg twice daily) versus aciclovir (200 mg 5 times daily) for 5 days.[39] It found no significant differences between the two drugs. **Prevention of recurrence:** We found two RCTs.[39,40] One crossover RCT (48 people with antibodies to HIV and herpes simplex virus; 38 with a history of genital herpes) compared famciclovir versus placebo over 8 weeks.[40] The results of the study are difficult to interpret (see comment below). The other RCT (1062 people with a median CD4 count of 320/mm^3) compared valaciclovir (500 mg twice daily) versus valaciclovir (1000 mg once daily) versus aciclovir (400 mg twice daily) over 1 year.[39] It found no significant difference between either dose of valaciclovir versus aciclovir, although recurrence was less likely with valaciclovir 500 mg twice daily than with the valaciclovir 1000 mg once daily (recurrence free at 48 wks 82% with 500 mg twice daily *v* 71% with 1000 mg once daily; $P < 0.05$).

Harms: Adverse effects (mostly headache and nausea) occurred with similar frequencies with aciclovir, valaciclovir, and famciclovir. Thrombotic microangiopathy, which has been reported in people receiving valaciclovir (8 g daily), has not been reported among 713 HIV infected people who received oral valaciclovir in daily doses of 250–1000 mg for up to 1 year (Wald A, personal communication, 2002).

Comment: Three of the four RCTs did not have a placebo control. Most studies compared new treatments with aciclovir rather than placebo. The crossover trial of famciclovir versus placebo was difficult to interpret because the withdrawal rate was high.[40] Although we found only limited evidence of an effect of antivirals for treatment of genital herpes in people with HIV infection, there was a consensus that antiviral treatment may be helpful, based on evidence from immunocompromised people who do not have HIV. Aciclovir has been found effective in immunocompromised populations. With the availability of effective treatments for HIV, trials of antiviral (antiherpes simplex virus) versus placebo may now be conducted. In HIV infected people, there is a markedly increased rate of herpes simplex virus shedding.[41] HIV has been recovered from genital herpes lesions.[42] We found no evidence on the effect of daily antiviral treatment on transmission of HIV to sexual partners.

REFERENCES

1. Fleming DT, McQuillan GM, Johnson RE, et al. Herpes simplex virus type 2 in the United States, 1976 to 1994. *N Engl J Med* 1997;337:1105–1111.
2. Cowan FM, Johnson AM, Ashley R, et al. Antibody to herpes simplex virus type 2 as serological marker of sexual lifestyle in populations. *BMJ* 1994;309:1325–1329.
3. Benedetti J, Corey L, Ashley R. Recurrence rates in genital herpes after symptomatic first-episode infection. *Ann Intern Med* 1994;121:847–854.
4. Mertz GJ, Schmidt O, Jourden JL, et al. Frequency of acquisition of first-episode genital infection with herpes simplex virus from symptomatic and asymptomatic source contacts. *Sex Transm Dis* 1985;12:33–39.
5. Whitley RJ, Kimberlin DW, Roizman B. Herpes simplex viruses. *Clin Infect Dis* 1998;26:541–553.
6. Wald A, Link K. Risk of HIV infection in HSV-2 seropositive persons: a meta-analysis. *J Infect Dis* 2002;185:45–52.
7. Brown ZA, Selke SA, Zeh J, et al. Acquisition of herpes simplex virus during pregnancy. *N Engl J Med* 1997;337:509–515.
8. Smith J, Cowan FM, Munday P. The management of herpes simplex virus infection in pregnancy. *Br J Obstet Gynaecol* 1998;105:255–268. Search date 1996; primary source Medline.
9. Nilsen AE, Aasen T, Halsos AM, et al. Efficacy of oral acyclovir in treatment of initial and recurrent genital herpes. *Lancet* 1982;2:571–573.
10. Corey L, Fife K, Benedetti JK, et al. Intravenous acyclovir for the treatment of primary genital herpes. *Ann Intern Med* 1983;98:914–921.
11. Mertz G, Critchlow C, Benedetti J, et al. Double-blind placebo-controlled trial of oral acyclovir in the first episode genital herpes simplex virus infection. *JAMA* 1984;252:1147–1151.
12. Mindel A, Adler MW, Sutherland S, et al. Intravenous acyclovir treatment for primary genital herpes. *Lancet* 1982;2:697–700.
13. Bryson YJ, Dillon M, Lovett M, et al. Treatment of first episodes of genital herpes simplex virus infections with oral acyclovir: a randomized double-blind controlled trial in normal subjects. *N Engl J Med* 1983;308:916–1920.
14. Fife KH, Barbarash RA, Rudolph T, et al. Valaciclovir versus acyclovir in the treatment of first-episode genital herpes infection: results of an international, multicenter, double-blind randomized clinical trial. *Sex Transm Dis* 1997;24:481–486.
15. Loveless M, Harris W, Sacks S. *Treatment of first episode genital herpes with famciclovir.* Programs and abstracts of the 35th Interscience Conference on Antimicrobial Agents and Chemotherapy. San Francisco, CA, 1995.
16. Corey L, Mindel A, Fife KH, et al. Risk of recurrence after treatment of first episode genital herpes with intravenous acyclovir. *Sex Transm Dis* 1985;12:215–218.
17. Corey L, Benedetti J, Critchlow C, et al. Treatment of primary first-episode genital herpes simplex virus infections with acyclovir: results of topical, intravenous and oral therapy. *J Antimicrob Chemother* 1983;12(Suppl B):79–88.
18. Wald A. New therapies and prevention strategies for genital herpes. *Clin Infect Dis* 1999;28:S4–S13. Search date 1997; primary source Medline.
19. Stone K, Whittington W. Treatment of genital herpes. *Rev Infect Dis* 1990;12(Suppl 6):610–619.
20. Wald A, Carrell D, Remington M, et al. Two-day regimen of acyclovir for treatment of recurrent genital herpes simplex virus type 2 infection. *Clin Infect Dis* 2002;34:944–948.
21. Chosidow O, Drouault Y, Leconte-Veyriac F, et al. Famciclovir versus aciclovir in immunocompetent patients with recurrent genital herpes infections: a parallel-groups, randomised, double-blind clinical trial. *Br J Dermatol* 2001;144:818–824.
22. Reichman RC, Badger GJ, Mertz GJ, et al. Treatment of recurrent genital herpes simplex infections with oral acyclovir: a controlled trial. *JAMA* 1984;251:2103–2107.
23. Reitano M, Tyring S, Lang W, et al. Valaciclovir for the suppression of recurrent genital herpes simplex virus infection: a large-scale dose range finding study. *J Infect Dis* 1998;178:603–610.
24. Diaz-Mitoma F, Sibbald RG, Shafran SD. Oral famciclovir for the suppression of recurrent genital herpes: a randomized controlled trial. *JAMA* 1998;280:887–892.
25. Goldberg L, Kaufman R, Kurtz T, et al. Continuous five-year treatment of patients with frequently recurring genital herpes simplex virus infection with acyclovir. *J Med Virol* 1993(Suppl 1);45–50.
26. Wald A, Zeh J, Barnum G, et al. Suppression of subclinical shedding of herpes simplex virus type 2 with acyclovir. *Ann Intern Med* 1996;124:8–15.
27. Doward LC, McKenna SP, Kohlmann T, et al. The international development of the RGHQoL: a quality of life measure for recurrent genital herpes. *Qual Life Res* 1998;7:143–153.
28. Patel R, Tyring S, Strand A, et al. Impact of suppressive antiviral therapy on the health related quality of life of patients with recurrent genital herpes infection. *Sex Transm Infect* 1999;75:398–402.
29. Fife KH, Crumpacker CS, Mertz GJ. Recurrence and resistance patterns of herpes simplex virus following stop of ≥ 6 years of chronic suppression with acyclovir. *J Infect Dis* 1994;169:1338–1341.
30. Longo D, Koehn K. Psychosocial factors and recurrent genital herpes: a review of prediction and psychiatric treatment studies. *Int J Psychiatry*

Med 1993;23:99–117. Search date 1991; primary sources Psychological Abstracts, Medline, and hand searches of reference lists.
31. Wald A, Langenberg A, Link K, et al. Effect of condoms on reducing the transmission of herpes simples virus type 2 from men to women. *JAMA* 2001;285:3100–6.
32. Corey L, Langenberg AG, Ashley R, et al. Recombinant glycoprotein vaccine for the prevention of genital HSV-2 infection: two randomised controlled trials. *JAMA* 1999;282:331–340.
33. Randolph A, Washington A, Prober C. Cesarean delivery for women presenting with genital herpes lesions. *JAMA* 1993;270:77–82.
34. Scott LL, Sanchez PJ, Jackson GL, et al. Acyclovir suppression to prevent Cesarean delivery after first-episode genital herpes. *Obstet Gynecol* 1996;87:69–73.
35. Brocklehurst P, Kinghorn G, Carney O, et al. A randomised placebo controlled trial of suppressive acyclovir in late pregnancy in women with recurrent genital herpes infection. *Br J Obstet Gynaecol* 1998;105:275–280.
36. Stray-Pedersen B. Acyclovir in late pregnancy to prevent neonatal herpes simplex [Letter] [see comments]. *Lancet* 1990;336:756.
37. Scott LL, Hollier LM, McIntire D, et al. Acyclovir suppression to prevent recurrent genital herpes at delivery. *Inf Dis Obstet Gynecol* 2002;10:71–77.
38. Romanowski B, Aoki FY, Martel AY, et al. Efficacy and safety of famciclovir for treating mucocutaneous herpes simplex infection in HIV-infected individuals. Collaborative Famciclovir HIV Study Group. *AIDS* 2000;14:1211–1217.
39. Conant MA, Schacker TW, Murphy RL, et al. International Valaciclovir HSV Study Group. Valaciclovir versus aciclovir for herpes simplex virus infection in HIV-infected individuals: two randomized trials. *Int J STD AIDS* 2002;13:12–21.
40. Schacker T, Hu HL, Koelle DM, et al. Famciclovir for the suppression of symptomatic and asymptomatic herpes simplex virus reactivation in HIV-infected persons. A double-blind, placebo-controlled trial. *Ann Intern Med* 1998;128:21–28.
41. Schacker T, Zeh J, Hu HL, et al. Frequency of symptomatic and asymptomatic HSV-2 reactivations among HIV-infected men. *J Infect Dis* 1998;178:1616–1622.
42. Schacker T, Ryncarz A, Goddard J, et al. Frequent recovery of HIV from genital herpes simplex virus lesions in HIV infected persons. *JAMA* 1998;280:61–66.

Bazian Ltd
London, UK

Competing interests: None declared.

The following previous contributor of this topic would also like to be acknowledged: Anna Wald.

Gonorrhoea

Search date January 2003

John Moran

QUESTIONS

INTERVENTIONS

Beneficial

Single dose regimens using selected cephalosporins or spectinomycin in uncomplicated infection in pregnant women 1857

Single dose regimens using selected fluoroquinolones, selected cephalosporins, or spectinomycin in uncomplicated infection* .1856

Likely to be beneficial

Selected injectable fluoroquinolones or selected injectable cephalosporins in disseminated infection** . .1858

Unknown effectiveness

Dual treatment for gonorrhoea and chlamydia infections in all people diagnosed with gonorrhoea .1859

*Based on comparisons of results across arms of different trials.

**Based only on non-RCT evidence and consensus.

Key Messages

- **Single dose regimens using selected cephalosporins or spectinomycin in uncomplicated infection in pregnant women** One systematic review has found that antibiotic treatment (amoxicillin [amoxycillin] plus probenecid, spectinomycin, ceftriaxone, and cefixime) is effective for curing gonorrhoea in pregnant women. We found no reports of serious adverse effects.
- **Single dose regimens using selected fluoroquinolones, selected cephalosporins, or spectinomycin in uncomplicated infection in men and non-pregnant women** One systematic review found limited evidence by combining cure rates across different arms of RCTs. It found that single dose regimens (ceftriaxone, ciprofloxacin, gatifloxacin, spectinomycin, azithromycin, ofloxacin, cefixime) achieve cure rates of 95% or higher in urogenital or rectal infection. Cure rates were lower (≤ 80%) for pharyngeal infection. Resistance to penicillins, tetracyclines, and sulphonamides is now widespread, and resistance to fluoroquinolones has become common in some geographic areas.

- **Selected injectable fluoroquinolones or selected injectable cephalosporins in disseminated infection** We found no RCTs assessing treatments for disseminated gonococcal infection published in the past 20 years, but there is strong consensus that multidose regimens using injectable cephalosporins or quinolones (except where quinolone-resistant *Neisseria gonorrhoeae* have been reported) are the most effective treatment. We found no reports of treatment failures with these regimens.
- **Dual treatment for gonorrhoea and chlamydia infections in all people diagnosed with gonorrhoea** Dual treatment for gonorrhoea and chlamydia infections is based on theory and expert opinion rather than on evidence from RCTs. The balance between benefits and harms will vary with the prevalence of coinfection in each population.

DEFINITION Gonorrhoea is caused by infection with *Neisseria gonorrhoeae*. In men, uncomplicated urethritis is the most common manifestation, with dysuria and urethral discharge. Less typically, signs and symptoms are mild and indistinguishable from chlamydial urethritis. In women, the most common manifestation is cervicitis, which produces symptoms (e.g. vaginal discharge, lower abdominal discomfort, and dyspareunia) in only half of the women. Coinfection with chlamydia is reported in 20–40% of people.[1,2]

INCIDENCE/ PREVALENCE Between 1975 and 1997 the incidence of reported gonorrhoea in the USA fell by 74%, reaching a nadir of 122/100 000 people. Since 1997 between 128 and 133 cases have been reported per 100 000 people each year.[3] Rates are highest in younger people. In 2001 the incidence was highest in women aged 15–19 years (703/100 000) and men aged 20–24 years (564/100 000). In England, Wales, and Northern Ireland, diagnoses of gonorrhoea have increased since 1994, reaching 256/100 000 for 20–24 year old males and 196/100 000 for 16–19 year old females in 2001.[4]

AETIOLOGY/ RISK FACTORS Most infections result from penile–vaginal, penile–rectal, or penile–pharyngeal contact. An important minority of infections are transmitted from mother to child during birth, which can cause ophthalmia neonatorum. Less common are ocular infections in older children and adults as a result of sexual exposure, poor hygiene, or the medicinal use of urine.

PROGNOSIS The natural history of untreated gonococcal infection is spontaneous resolution after weeks or months of unpleasant symptoms. During this time, there is a substantial likelihood of transmission to others and of complications developing in the infected individual.[5] In many women, the lack of readily discernible signs or symptoms of cervicitis means that infections go unrecognised and untreated. An unknown proportion of untreated infections causes local complications, including lymphangitis, periurethral abscess, bartholinitis, and urethral stricture; epididymitis in men; and in women involvement of the uterus, fallopian tubes, or ovaries causing pelvic inflammatory disease (see pelvic inflammatory disease, p 1871). Gonorrhoea is associated with pelvic inflammatory disease. One review found *N gonorrhoeae* was cultured from 8% to 32% of women with acute pelvic inflammatory disease in 11 European studies and from 27% to 80% of women in eight US studies.[6] The proportion of *N gonorrhoeae* infections in women that lead to pelvic inflammatory disease has not been well studied. However, one study of women exposed to men with gonorrhoea found that five out of 19 culture-positive women had pelvic inflammatory disease and another four of the 19 had uterine adnexal tenderness.[7] Pelvic inflammatory disease may lead to infertility (see pelvic inflammatory disease, p 1871). In some people, localised gonococcal infection may disseminate. A US study estimated the risk of dissemination to be 0.6% to 1.1% among women, whereas a European study estimated it to be 2.3–3%.[8,9] The same European study found a lower risk in men, estimated to be 0.4–0.7%.[9] When gonococci disseminate, they cause petechial or pustular skin lesions; asymmetrical arthropathies, tenosynovitis or septic arthritis; and, rarely, meningitis or endocarditis.

AIMS OF INTERVENTION To relieve symptoms; avoid complications; and prevent further transmission, with minimal adverse effects of treatment.

OUTCOMES Microbiological cure rates (number of infected people or infected sites culture-negative 1–14 days after treatment, divided by number of infected people or infected sites cultured 1–14 days after treatment).

METHODS *Clinical Evidence* search and appraisal January 2003. Additional PubMed search conducted by author March 2003. Key words: gonorrhoea and *N gonorrhoeae* infections, plus a search of references of key articles and books. Studies were excluded if they defined possible treatment failures as "reinfections", if they did not use end points based on microbiological cure, or if they were based on drug regimens unlikely to be of general use (e.g. those using antibiotic regimens that are toxic or to which resistance is now widespread).[10] The authors have not searched for, or included, papers published before 1981 as the susceptibility of *N gonorrhoea* changes over time. The results of particularly old clinical trials may be misleading because of intervening changes in susceptibility.

QUESTION What are the effects of treatments for uncomplicated infections in men and non-pregnant women?

One systematic review found limited evidence by combining cure rates across different arms of RCTs. It found that single dose regimens (ceftriaxone, ciprofloxacin, gatifloxacin, spectinomycin, azithromycin, ofloxacin, cefixime) achieve cure rates of 95% or higher in urogenital or rectal infection. Cure rates were lower (≤ 80%) for pharyngeal infection. Resistance to penicillins, tetracyclines, and sulphonamides is now widespread, and resistance to fluoroquinolones has become common in some geographic areas.

Benefits: **Uncomplicated urogenital, rectal, and pharyngeal infections:** We found one systematic review (search date 1993).[10] The results were updated to 2002 by the author of the review using the original methods (see table 1, p 1861) (Moran JS, personal communication, 2002). The original review identified studies (both RCTs and other clinical trials) published from 1981–1993 that used a single dose regimen based on an antimicrobial other than a β lactamase sensitive penicillin or a tetracycline.[10] The search retrieved studies with a total of 24 383 evaluable people. Combining results across arms of trials, 97% were cured on the basis of culture results. Sites of infection, when specified, included the cervix, urethra, rectum, and pharynx. Comparison of cure rates by site of infection found that cure rates were over 95% for all sites except the pharynx, for which they were about 80% (see table 1, p 1861).[13] **Eye infections:** We found no systematic review or RCTs (see comment below).

Harms: Single dose regimens using fluoroquinolones, third generation and extended spectrum cephalosporins, or spectinomycin are generally safe and well tolerated. The most important adverse effects are rare hypersensitivity reactions. Minor adverse effects are most troublesome for the 800 mg cefixime regimen[14,15] and the 2 g azithromycin regimen;[16] both cause frequent gastrointestinal upset. All the other doses found effective are associated with a low incidence of adverse outcomes. One large observational cohort study of azithromycin, cefixime, ciprofloxacin, and ofloxacin "in everyday use" found few serious adverse effects.[17] Quinolones may cause arthropathy in animals. One systematic review of harms (search date 2000) found no irreversible fluoroquinolone induced cartilage toxicity pathology after 0.3–10 months of follow up in 201 adolescents treated for between 7 and 270 days.[18]

Comment: There is good agreement between antigonococcal activity of antimicrobials *in vitro* and their efficacy in clinical trials. A large number of people were evaluated in a range of settings, suggesting that the results can be generalised. However, comparative results from different settings were not provided. Single dose regimens may make adherence more likely. The ceftriaxone and spectinomycin regimens require intramuscular injection. Resistance is now widespread for all penicillins, sulphonamides, and tetracyclines, and is becoming common for fluroquinolones in parts of Asia and the Pacific, including Hawaii and California.[4,19–21] Resistance to third generation and extended spectrum cephalosporins or spectinomycin is rarely reported (see table 2, p 1862). **Eye infections:** We found two small cohort studies of single dose ceftriaxone for gonococcal eye infections.[25,26] In the first study (12 adults with conjunctivitis), all people responded well to a single 1 g dose of ceftriaxone.[25] In the second study (21 neonates with gonococcal ophthalmia), eye swabs from all neonates were negative 24 hours after a single intramuscular 62.5 mg dose of ceftriaxone.[26]

QUESTION What are the effects of treatments for uncomplicated infections in pregnant women?

One systematic review has found that antibiotic treatment (amoxicillin [amoxycillin] plus probenecid, spectinomycin, ceftriaxone, and cefixime) is effective for curing gonorrhoea in pregnant women. We found no reports of serious adverse effects.

Benefits: We found one systematic review (search date 2001, 2 RCTs) of treatments of gonococcal infection during pregnancy.[27] One of the RCTs (267 pregnant women with positive cultures for gonorrhoea) compared amoxicillin (amoxycillin) plus probenecid versus spectinomycin versus ceftriaxone. Overall, it found no significant difference between regimens (failure to achieve cure 9/84 [10.7%] with amoxicillin *v* 4/84 [4.8%] with spectinomycin; RR 2.25, 95%

CI 0.72 to 7.02; 9/84 [10.7%] with amoxicillin *v* 4/84 [4.8%] with ceftriaxone; RR 2.25, 95% CI 0.72 to 7.02). However, the study may have lacked the power to detect clinically important effects. By site of infection, amoxicillin 3 g cured 91% of cervical infections, 85% of rectal infections, and 80% of pharyngeal infections; single dose ceftriaxone 250 mg cured 95% of rectal and cervical infections and 100% of pharyngeal infections; spectinomycin 2 g cured 97% of rectal and cervical infections and 83% of pharyngeal infections.[28] The second RCT (95 women with positive cultures for gonorrhoea) compared a single dose of ceftriaxone intramuscularly versus a single dose of cefixime orally.[27] It found that eradication rates were similar in the two groups: ceftriaxone 125 mg eradicated 96.8% (95% CI 89.0% to 99.6%) of cervical and rectal infections and 100% (95% CI 47.8% to 100%) of pharyngeal infections; and cefixime 400 mg eradicated 96% (95% CI 88.8% to 99.6%) of cervical and rectal infections and 100% (95% CI 54.1% to 100%) of pharyngeal infections.

Harms: The systematic review reported vomiting after treatment in 1/267 (0.4%) women included in one trial.[27] The second RCT reported soreness at the injection site among women receiving ceftriaxone and some "minor" malformations among their children, generally cosmetic (e.g. nevus, café au lait spots, skin tag; 10/60 [16.7%] with ceftriaxone *v* 7/62 [11.3%] with cefixime).[29] Because quinolones cause arthropathy in animals, their use is not recommended in pregnancy, although we found no reports of adverse effects of quinolones on pregnancy outcome in humans. One multicentre, prospective, controlled study (200 exposed women) found no evidence of adverse effects.[30] We found no evidence that the non-quinolone regimens listed above are less safe or less well tolerated by pregnant women than by men or non-pregnant women.

Comment: None.

QUESTION What are the effects of treatments for disseminated gonococcal infection?

We found no RCTs assessing treatments for disseminated gonococcal infection published in the past 20 years, but there is strong consensus that multidose regimens using injectable cephalosporins or quinolones (except where quinolone-resistant *N gonorrhoeae* have been reported) are the most effective treatment. We found no reports of treatment failures with these regimens.

Benefits: We found no systematic review and no RCTs of the treatment of disseminated gonococcal infection published in the past 20 years.

Harms: We found no reports of adverse effects of multidose regimens using injectable cephalosporins or quinolones in this context.

Comment: More than 100 clinical trials involving over 20 000 people have found that many single dose antimicrobial regimens cure uncomplicated infections more than 90% of the time.[10] Given the protracted natural history without treatment, this evidence suggests that treatment with these antimicrobial regimens is beneficial. Which regimens are most beneficial cannot be determined precisely because direct randomised comparisons of the best different regimens have not been performed. However, analysis of available trials supports the consensus that the most effective regimens are those using selected third generation or expanded spectrum cephalosporins and, except where resistance is common, those using selected fluoroquinolones or spectinomycin. We found no RCTs of antibiotic treatment in complicated gonorrhoea, but there is a strong consensus supporting the view that the most effective treatments for these conditions are multidose regimens using injectable cephalosporins or quinolones. Although we found no published data establishing the efficacy of this treatment, we found no reports of treatment failures.

QUESTION What are the effects of dual treatment for gonorrhoea and chlamydia infection?

Dual treatment with an antimicrobial effective against *Chlamydia trachomatis* is based on theory and expert opinion rather than evidence. The balance between benefits and harms from controlled trials will vary with the prevalence of coinfection in each population.

Benefits: We found no systematic review or RCTs.

Harms: We found no good evidence on the harms of dual treatment. Treatment for chlamydia can cause mild gastrointestinal distress, and there is the possibility that using a second drug could stimulate the emergence or spread of resistance in *N gonorrhoeae* or other bacteria.

Comment: Routine dual treatment has been advocated and implemented for the past 19 years, and is believed to have two potential benefits. Firstly, it is believed by some to have contributed to the decline in the prevalence of chlamydia infection observed in some populations. We found no evidence for any direct effect of dual treatment on chlamydia prevalence. Other factors may have contributed to reduced chlamydia prevalence (including widespread screening for asymptomatic chlamydia infection and changes in sexual behaviour), making it difficult to attribute decreases in the prevalence of chlamydia infection to any specific cause. Secondly, routine dual treatment may retard the spread of resistant gonococcal strains. Limited data from case reports support this belief. In the past, chlamydia testing was often unavailable, expensive, time consuming, and not highly sensitive, whereas dual treatment with a tetracycline, such as doxycycline, was safe and inexpensive. Chlamydia testing has now become more widely available, more affordable, quicker, and more sensitive, and the prevalence of chlamydia has fallen in some populations. Nevertheless, chlamydia is still found in 20–40% of people with gonorrhoea in many clinics.[1,2]

Substantive changes

Treatment of uncomplicated infection in men and non-pregnant women One systematic review added;[18] conclusions unchanged.

REFERENCES

1. Centers for Disease Control and Prevention. Sexually transmitted diseases treatment guidelines 2002. *MMWR Morb Mortal Wkly Rep* 2002;51:36–42.
2. Creighton S, Tenant-Flowers M, Taylor CB, et al. Co-infection with gonorrhoea and chlamydia: how much is there and what does it mean? *Int J STD AIDS* 2003;14:109–113.
3. Division of STD Prevention, Centers for Disease Control and Prevention. *Sexually transmitted disease surveillance, 2001*. Atlanta, Georgia: US Department of Health and Human Services, Centers for Disease Control and Prevention, September 2002. http://www.cdc.gov/std/stats (last accessed 27 June 2003).
4. PHLS, DHSS and PS, Scottish ISD(D)5 Collaborative Group. *Trends in sexually transmitted infections in the United Kingdom, 1996 to 2001*. London: Public Health Laboratory Service, 2002. http://www.phls.co.uk/topics_az/hiv_and_sti/sti-gonorrhoea/epidemiology/epidemiolgy.htm (last accessed 27 June 2003).
5. Hook EW, Handsfield HH. Gonococcal infections in the adult. In: Holmes KK, Mardh P-A, Sparling PF, et al, eds. *Sexually transmitted diseases* 3rd ed. New York: McGraw-Hill, 1999.
6. Cates WC Jr, Rolfs RT, Aral SG. Sexually transmitted diseases, pelvic inflammatory disease, and infertility: an epidemiologic update. *Epidemiol Rev* 1990;12:199–220.
7. Platt R, Rice PA, McCormack WM. Risk of acquiring gonorrhoea and prevalence of abnormal adnexal findings among women recently exposed to gonorrhoea. *JAMA* 1983;250:3205–3209.
8. Holmes KK, Wiesner PJ, Pedersen AHB. The gonococcal arthritis-dermatitis syndrome. *Ann Intern Med* 1971;75:470–471.
9. Barr J, Danielsson D. Septic gonococcal dermatitis. *BMJ* 1971;1:482–485.
10. Moran JS, Levine WC. Drugs of choice for the treatment of uncomplicated gonococcal infections. *Clin Infect Dis* 1995;20(suppl 1):47–65. Search date range 1981–1993; primary sources Medline, reference lists from retrieved articles, abstracts from the annual Interscience Conference on Antimicrobial Agents and Chemotherapy, and meetings of the International Society for Sexually Transmitted Disease Research.
11. Aplasca de los Reyes MR, Pato-Mesola V, et al. A randomized trial of ciprofloxacin versus cefixime for treatment of gonorrhea after rapid emergence of gonococcal ciprofloxacin resistance in the Philippines. *Clin Infect Dis* 2001;32:1313–1318.
12. Rahman M, Alam A, Nessa K, et al. Treatment failure with the use of ciprofloxacin for gonorrhea correlates with the prevalence of fluoroquinolone-resistant *Neisseria gonorrhoeae* strains in Bangladesh. *Clin Infect Dis* 2001;32:884–889.
13. Moran JS. Treating uncomplicated *Neisseria gonorrhoeae* infections: is the anatomic site of infection important? *Sex Transm Dis* 1995;22:39–47.
14. Handsfield HH, McCormack WM, Hook EW III, et al. The Gonorrhea Treatment Study Group. A comparison of single-dose cefixime with ceftriaxone as treatment for uncomplicated gonorrhea. *N Engl J Med* 1991;325:1337–1341.
15. Megran DW, LeFebvre K, Willets V, et al. Single-dose oral cefixime versus amoxicillin plus probenecid for the treatment of uncomplicated gonorrhea in men. *Antimicrob Agents Chemother* 1990;34:355–357.
16. Handsfield HH, Dalu ZA, Martin DH, et al. Azithromycin Gonorrhea Study Group. Multicenter trial of single-dose azithromycin vs. ceftriaxone in the treatment of uncomplicated gonorrhea. *Sex Transm Dis* 1994;21:107–111.
17. Wilton LV, Pearce GL, Mann RD. A comparison of ciprofloxacin, norfloxacin, ofloxacin, azithromycin and cefixime examined by observational cohort studies. *Br J Clin Pharmacol* 1996;41:277–284.
18. Burstein GR, Berman SM, Blumer JL, et al. Ciprofloxacin for the treatment of uncomplicated gonorrhea infection in adolescents: does the benefit outweigh the risk? *Clin Infect Dis* 2002;35(suppl 2):191–199. Search date 2000; primary sources Medline, and citation lists.
19. The WHO Western Pacific Region Gonococcal Antimicrobial Surveillance Programme. Surveillance of antibiotic resistance in *Neisseria gonorrhoeae* in the WHO Western Pacific Region, 2001. *Commun Dis Intell* 2002;26:541–545.
20. Ye S, Su X, Wang Q, et al. Surveillance of antibiotic resistance of *Neisseria gonorrhoeae* isolates in China, 1993–1998. *Sex Transm Dis* 2002;29:242–245.
21. Centers for disease Control and Prevention: Gonococcal isolate surveillance project annual report, 2001. In: *2001 Gonococcal isolate surveillance project (GISP) supplement*. Atlanta, Georgia: U.S. Department of Health and Human Services, 2002. http://www.cdc.gov/std/GISP2001/ (last accessed 27 June 2003).
22. Dan M, Poch F, Sheinberg B. High prevalence of high-level ciprofloxacin resistance in *Neisseria gonorrhoeae* in Tel Aviv, Israel: correlation with response to therapy. *Antimicrob Agents Chemother* 2002;46:1671–1673.
23. Public Health Laboratory Service. *The gonococcal resistance to antimicrobials surveillance programme annual report*, 2001. http://www.phls.co.uk/topics_az/hiv_and_sti/sti_gonorrhoea/epidemiology/grasp_report2001.pdf (last accessed 21 August 2003).
24. Fiorito S, Galarza P, Pagano I, et al. Emergence of high level ciprofloxacin resistant *Neisseria gonorrhoeae* strain in Buenos Aires, Argentina. Sex *Transm Infect* 2001;77:77.
25. Haimovici R, Roussel TJ. Treatment of gonococcal conjunctivitis with single-dose intramuscular ceftriaxone. *Am J Ophthalmol* 1989;107:511–514.
26. Hoosen AA, Kharsany AB, Ison CA. Single low-dose ceftriaxone for the treatment of gonococcal ophthalmia: implications for the national programme for the syndromic management of sexually transmitted diseases. *S Afr Med J* 2002;92:238–240.
27. Brocklehurst P. Antibiotics for gonorrhoea in pregnancy. In: The Cochrane Library, Issue 2, 2002. Oxford: Update Software. Search date 2001; primary sources Cochrane Pregnancy and Childbirth Group Register, and The Cochrane Controlled Trials Register.
28. Cavenee M, Farris J, Spalding T. Treatment of gonorrhea in pregnancy. *Obset Gynaecol* 1993;81:33–38.
29. Ramus RM, Sheffield JS, Mayfield JA, et al. A randomized trial that compared oral cefixime and intramuscular ceftriaxone for the treatment of gonorrhea in pregnancy. *Am J Obstet Gynecol* 2001;185:629–632.
30. Loebstein R, Addis A, Ho E, et al. Pregnancy outcome following gestational exposure to fluoroquinolones: a multicenter prospective controlled study. *Antimicrob Agents Chemother* 1998;42:1336–1339.

Gonorrhoea

John Moran
Medical Epidemiologist
Centers for Disease Control and Prevention
Atlanta
USA

Competing interests: None declared.

TABLE 1 **Effectiveness of selected single dose regimens in published clinical trials[10] and updated to 2002 (see text, p 1856).**

	Pharyngeal infections	Urogenital and rectal infections
Drug and dose	**% cured (95% CI)**	**% cured(95% CI)**
Ceftriaxone 250 mg	98.9 (94.0 to 100)	99.2 (98.8 to 99.5)
Ciprofloxacin 500 mg*	97.2 (85.5 to 99.9)	99.8 (98.7 to 100)
Ciprofloxacin 250 mg	88.5 (88.8 to 95.2)	98.7 (98.0 to 99.4)
Ceftriaxone† 125 mg	94.1 (85.6 to 98.4)	98.9 (97.9 to 99.8)
Gatifloxacin 600 mg	100 (82.3 to 100)	99.6 (97.7 to 100)
Spectinomycin 2 g	51.8 (38.7 to 64.9)	98.2 (97.6 to 99.9)
Azithromycin 2 g	100 (82.3 to 100)	99.2 (97.2 to 99.9)
Ofloxacin 400 mg	88.7 (68.8 to 97.8)	98.6 (97.8 to 99.4)
Gatifloxacin 400 mg	100 (63.1 to 100)	99.2 (97.1 to 99.9)
Cefixime 800 mg	80.0 (51.9 to 95.7)	98.4 (95.9 to 99.6)
Cefixime 400 mg	92.3 (74.9 to 99.1)	97.4 (95.9 to 98.6)

* Excludes two published clinical trials among people known to be at high risk of harbouring fluoroquinolone resistant strains; ciprofloxacin 500 mg cured only 48/72 (67%) of cervical infections in one trial [11] and 41/66 (62%) in the other.[12]
†Data have been updated to include those from eligible studies published between 1993 and 2001. Only those regimens that have been shown in published studies to cure more than 95% of uncomplicated urogenital and rectal infections (with a lower 95% confidence limit > 95%) have been selected.

TABLE 2 Reported resistance of *N gonorrhoeae* to antimicrobials (see text, p 1857).

Drug	Resistance
Sulphonamides	Widespread
Penicillins	Widespread
Tetracyclines	Widespread
Third generation cephalosporins (e.g. ceftriaxone, cefixime)	One report from China[20]
Spectinomycin	Rare
Quinolones	Asia: becoming very common, especially in the Far East (e.g. 80% in China, 64% in Japan, 54% in the Phillippines;[19] there are few data from the Middle East, but a high prevalence of resistance (61%) has been reported in Israel.[22]
	USA: in 2001, resistance to ciprofloxacin was reported in 0.4% of isolates from the mainland (0.2% in the mainland exclusive of California) and in 20% of isolates from Hawaii.[21]
	UK: among 2369 gonorrhoeae isolates from England and Wales tested in 2001, 3.1% were flouroquinolone resistant.[23]
	Australia and New Zealand; 13% and 10%, respectively.[19]
	South America: one fluoroquinolone resistant isolate reported[24]

Partner notification

Search date November 2002

Catherine Mathews, Nicol Coetzee, Merrick Zwarenstein, and Sally Guttmacher

QUESTIONS

INTERVENTIONS

See glossary, p 1869

Key Messages

- We found no good evidence on the effects of partner notification on relationships between patients and partners and, in particular, on the rate of violence, abuse, and abandonment of patient or partner.
- We found no studies comparing the effects of an intervention across different groups, such as people with different diseases or combinations of diseases, or people from different settings.
- **Contract referral (as effective as provider referral in people with syphilis)** One systematic review of one large RCT comparing different partner notification strategies in people with syphilis found no significant difference in the proportion of partners notified between provider referral and contract referral, when people receiving the contract referral option were given 2 days to notify their partners.
- **Offering a choice between provider and patient referral (v patient referral) in people with HIV** One systematic review of one RCT comparing different partner notification strategies found that, in people with HIV, offering a choice between provider referral (where the identity of the index patient was not revealed) and patient referral improved notification rates compared with offering patient referral alone.
- **Provider referral, or contract referral (v patient referral) in people with gonorrhoea or non-gonococcal urethritis (mainly chlamydia)** One systematic review has found that, for people with gonorrhoea, contract versus patient referral increased the rate of partners presenting for treatment. For people with non-gonococcal urethritis, one systematic review found that provider versus patient referral increased the proportion of partners notified and of positive partners detected per patient.

- **Adding telephone reminders and contract cards to patient referral; educational videos; information pamphlets; patient referral by different types of healthcare professionals; patient referral in HIV** We found insufficient evidence about the effects of these interventions in improving partner notification.

DEFINITION Partner notification is a process whereby the sexual partners of people with a diagnosis of sexually transmitted infection are informed of their exposure to infection. The main methods are patient referral, provider referral, contract referral, and outreach assistance (see glossary, p 1869).

INCIDENCE/ PREVALENCE A large proportion of people with sexually transmitted infections will have neither symptoms nor signs of infection. For example, 22–68% of men with gonorrhoea who were identified through partner notification were asymptomatic.[1] Partner notification is one of the two strategies to reach such individuals, the other strategy being screening. Managing infection in people with more than one current sexual partner is likely to have the greatest impact on the spread of sexually transmitted infections.[2]

PROGNOSIS We found no studies showing that partner notification results in a health benefit, either to the partner or to future partners of infected partners. Obtaining such evidence would be technically and ethically difficult. One RCT in asymptomatic women compared identifying, testing, and treating women at increased risk for cervical chlamydial infection versus usual care. It found these reduced incidence of pelvic inflammatory disease (RR 0.44, 95% CI 0.20 to 0.90).[3] This evidence suggests that partner notification, which also aims to identify and treat people who are largely unaware of infection, would provide a direct health benefit to partners who are infected.

AIMS OF INTERVENTION To prevent complications of infection in the partner; to prevent transmission to others; to prevent reinfection; and to identify social networks of people practising risky sexual behaviours.

OUTCOMES Partners identified; partners notified; partners presenting for care; partners testing positive; partners treated; rates of reinfection in the patient; incidence of sexually transmitted diseases in the population; harms to patient or partner, such as domestic violence and abuse; ethical outcomes (patient autonomy *v* beneficence). The main outcome presented in each option is the ratio of the number of partners notified to the number of index patients.

METHODS *Clinical Evidence* search and appraisal November 2002. We included RCTs comparing at least two alternative partner notification strategies. The outcome used in this summary was the absolute difference between the ratio of partners identified, notified, presenting for care, testing positive, or treated per index case. Assuming a Poisson distribution for the outcomes, the 95% confidence intervals were calculated using the normal approximation to the Poisson distribution. We excluded studies that did not allow us to extract data on people with specific sexually transmitted diseases, rather than on one of a range of sexually transmitted diseases.

QUESTION **What are the effects of different partner notification strategies in different groups of people?**

OPTION **IN PEOPLE WITH HIV INFECTION**

One systematic review of one RCT found that, for people with HIV infection, offering index patients a choice between provider referral (where the identity of the index patient is not revealed to the partner) and patient referral resulted in more partners being notified than offering patient referral alone. The systematic review found no good evidence on the effects of these strategies on relationships between patients and partners and, in particular, on the rate of violence, abuse, and abandonment of patient or partner.

Benefits: We found one systematic review (search date 2001, 1 RCT, 162 people who tested positive for HIV).[4] **Offering a choice between provider and patient referral versus patient referral:** The RCT (162 people who tested positive for HIV) compared provider referral with the choice between patient referral and provider referral (see glossary, p 1869). It was conducted at three public health departments in North Carolina, USA. Of those approached, the 46% who agreed to participate in the study were mostly men (69%), of whom most were homosexual or bisexual (76%). The choice between provider referral and patient referral significantly increased the likelihood that partners would be notified (rate of number of partners notified to number of index patients 78/39 [2.00] for the group with choice *v* 10/35 [0.29] for the patient referral group; rate increase 1.71, 95% CI 1.35 to 2.07). Thus, for every person offered provider referral compared with using patient referral there will be more than one additional partner notified (see figure A on web extra). **Contract referral:** We found no RCTs assessing contract referral (see glossary, p 1869) in people with HIV infection. **Outreach assistance:** The systematic review found one RCT, comparing patient referral versus outreach assistance (see glossary, p 1869) in people with HIV who were injecting drug users, the findings of which have yet to be reported fully.[4,5]

Harms: People's reluctance to disclose their HIV status to partners (see comment below) suggests expectation of harms from doing so. These and other potential harms are poorly understood. The systematic review found no good evidence on the effects of these strategies on relationships between patients and partners and, in particular, on the rate of violence, abuse, and abandonment of patient or partner.

Comment: The number of partners notified is an intermediate outcome. The number of infections in partners that are prevented or treated has not been assessed. Thus, the true benefits and harms of HIV partner notification are unknown. **Rates of disclosure:** One descriptive study (276 people attending for initial primary care for HIV infection in the USA) found that 40% of the respondents had not disclosed their HIV status to all partners over the preceding 6 months.[6] Individuals with more than one partner were significantly less likely to disclose to all partners. Only 42% of the non-disclosers reported that they used condoms all the time, which indicates that many partners were at risk of HIV infection. Another descriptive study conducted in the USA found that, even after repeated individual counselling of people with HIV infection and a 6 month opportunity to disclose HIV status, 30% had not informed any of their past partners and 29% had not informed any of their present partners.[7] **Patient preferences:** The RCT (162 people) comparing offering people a choice between provider and patient referral with patient referral alone found that, in the group with the choice, most partners (90%) were notified by the provider and only eight people by the index patient.[4] The RCT comparing patient referral versus outreach assistance[5] found, among people allocated to a choice, 82% chose to have the outreach team notify at least one partner, and the team was asked to notify 71% of all partners named by this group. One group in the USA attempted to compare contract referral with provider referral, but cross over between comparison groups made this impossible.[8] The results were therefore analysed as a series without comparison groups, where all patients were assigned to provider referral. The study included 1070 people, who reported having had 8633 partners in the past year. Of these partners, 1035 were successfully located, of whom 248 had previously tested positive for HIV, 560 were tested by the disease intervention specialist, 69 refused testing, and 158 were located by record search only. Of the 560 partners tested, 122 tested positive.

OPTION IN PEOPLE WITH GONORRHOEA OR CHLAMYDIA

One systematic review has found that, for people with gonorrhoea, contract versus patient referral increases the rate of partners presenting for treatment. One RCT also found that contract compared with patient referral increased the rate of positive partners detected. For people with non-gonococcal urethritis, one RCT found that provider versus patient referral increased the proportion of partners notified and of positive partners detected per patient. The systematic review found no good evidence on the effects of these strategies on relationships between patients and partners and, in particular, on the rate of violence, abuse, and abandonment of patient or partner.

Benefits: We found one systematic review (search date 2001, 2 RCTs of partner notification in people with gonorrhoea and 1 RCT in people with non-gonococcal urethritis).[4] **Gonorrhoea:** The two RCTs (2085 people with gonorrhoea) compared patient referral with contract referral (see glossary, p 1869). The first RCT (1898 people) found that contract referral significantly increased the number of partners assessed per index patient (392/632 [0.62 partners per index patient] with contract referral *v* 469/1266 [0.37] with patient referral; rate difference 0.25 partners per index patient, 95% CI 0.18 to 0.32). Positive gonorrhoea culture was significantly more likely in the contract referral group than in the patient referral group (233/632 [0.37 positive partners per index patient] with contract referral *v* 315/1266 [0.25] with patient referral; rate difference 0.12, 95% CI 0.06 to 0.18).[4] The second RCT (187 index patients) found contract referral was associated with a non-significantly higher proportion of partners assessed per index patient (119/94 [1.27] with contract referral *v* 107/93 [1.15] in the patient referral group; rate difference +0.12, 95% CI –0.2 to +0.44), and found no significant difference in the number of partners with positive gonorrhoea cultures per index patient.[4] (See figure B on web extra.) **Chlamydia:** One RCT (678 people with non-gonococcal urethritis) compared patient referral with provider referral (see glossary, p 1869). It found that provider referral significantly increased the proportion of partners assessed per patient (159/221 [0.72] with provider referral *v* 91/457 [0.20] with patient referral; rate difference 0.52, 95% CI 0.40 to 0.64). In this study, provider referral also significantly increased the proportion of partners with positive culture per index patient (20/221 [0.09] with provider referral *v* 14/457 [0.03] with patient referral; rate difference 0.06, 95% CI 0.02 to 0.10). Provider referral would have to be offered to two index patients with non-gonococcal urethritis for one additional partner to be assessed, and to 17 index patients to identify one additional partner with a positive culture. These findings are likely to over estimate the difference, as partners referred by index patients may have been assessed elsewhere.[4] (See figure C on web extra).

Harms: These are poorly understood. The systematic review found no good evidence on the effects of these strategies on relationships between patients and partners and, in particular, on the rate of violence, abuse, and abandonment of patient or partner.

Comment: One cohort study (265 urban, adolescent girls attending a clinic in Alabama, USA) found that, given the choice, people with gonorrhoea or chlamydia are about as likely to choose provider referral as patient referral.[9] Non-gonococcal urethritis is an old term used when gonorrhoea has been excluded but a positive diagnosis not made. The most common causative agent would be chlamydia.

OPTION IN PEOPLE WITH SYPHILIS

One systematic review of one large RCT found no significant difference between provider referral versus contract referral, when people receiving the contract referral option were given only 2 days in which to notify their partners. We found no RCTs assessing patient referral. The systematic review found no good evidence on the effects of these strategies on relationships between patients and partners and, in particular, on the rate of violence, abuse, and abandonment of patient or partner.

Benefits: We found one systematic review (search date 2001, 1 RCT, 1966 people diagnosed with syphilis in 3 US states).[4] It compared the proportion of partners per patient who were located, tested, tested positive, and treated, using three types of referral process: contract referral (see glossary, p 1869) (patients were given 2 days to notify partners themselves, before disease intervention specialists would notify them); provider referral (see glossary, p 1869) (immediate notification by an intervention specialist); and provider referral with the option of a blood test (immediate notification by an intervention specialist who had the option of performing a blood test if he or she thought that the partner would not seek medical attention despite being notified of exposure). There were no significant differences between the three groups: 1.2, 1.1, and 1.1 partners per patient were located; 0.92, 0.87, and 0.86 were tested; and 0.67, 0.61, and 0.62 were treated (CI not provided).[4]

Harms: These are poorly understood. The systematic review found no good evidence on the effects of these strategies on relationships between patients and partners and, in particular, on the rate of violence, abuse, and abandonment of patient or partner.

Comment: In the RCT, the investigators had no way of determining whether disease intervention specialists began actively seeking partners in the contract referral group before waiting 2 days, and they found some evidence of this.[4] Furthermore, the investigators speculated that people may have been allocated to groups not according to the randomisation schedule. These problems may compromise the validity of the study. The use of disease intervention specialists is an approach that may not be generalisable to other settings.

QUESTION **What can be done to improve the effectiveness of patient referral?**

OPTION **COUNSELLING PLUS CONTRACT REFERRAL CARDS AND TELEPHONE FOLLOW UP COMPARED WITH COUNSELLING ALONE**

One systematic review found one small RCT, which found no significant difference between counselling plus contract referral cards and telephone follow up versus counselling alone.

Benefits: We found one systematic review (search date 2001, 1 RCT).[4] One RCT (38 students from a university clinic in the USA) compared the use of counselling plus contract referral cards and telephone follow up of the index patient with counselling alone. It found no difference between the strategies in the rate of partners presenting for care. The trial also assessed adding a US$3 incentive to the referral card. Charges for clinic visits for patients and partners would be waived after successful recruitment of partners for treatment. This had no effect on the number of partners presenting for care.[4]

Harms: None reported.

Comment: None.

OPTION **DIFFERENT HEALTH PROFESSIONALS**

One systematic review found one RCT, which found no difference in the effects of patient referral by different healthcare professionals.

Benefits: We found one systematic review (search date 2001, 1 RCT).[4] One RCT (678 index patients) found that there was no difference between patient referral (see glossary, p 1869) using nurses who did not ask for partners' names and gave referral letters, and disease intervention specialists who took partners' names but no contact details, in terms of the number of partners with positive cultures who were identified (rate difference 0, 95% CI –0.03 to +0.03).[4]

Harms: None reported.

Comment: None.

OPTION INFORMATION PAMPHLETS

One RCT found insufficient evidence on information pamphlets compared with routine counselling.

Benefits: We found one systematic review (search date 2001, 1 unpublished RCT).[4] The unpublished RCT (1898 index patients), conducted in the USA, investigated the use of information pamphlets compared with a routine counselling interview alone. Providing patients with information pamphlets was as effective as the interview alone (rate difference 0, 95% CI −0.07 to +0.07). The two strategies were also equally effective in terms of the number of partners identified with a positive culture per index patient. However, the RCT combined two interventions: different health professionals and asking for partners' names, either of which may have affected the results.[4]

Harms: None reported.

Comment: None.

OPTION EDUCATIONAL VIDEOS

One RCT found no significant difference between educational videos versus standard care, but the outcome reported was potentially inappropriate.

Benefits: We found one systematic review (search date 2001, 1 RCT).[4] The RCT (902 people in the USA) compared a video taped story promoting partner notification versus standard care. No differences in the number of partners assessed were reported (figures not provided).[4] The RCT counted returned contract cards as the main outcome, which has not been shown to be a sensitive enough surrogate indicator for partners presenting for assessment.[10]

Harms: None reported.

Comment: None.

GLOSSARY

Contract referral (also known as conditional referral). Index patients are encouraged to inform their partners, with the understanding that health service personnel will notify those partners who do not visit the health service within a contracted time period.

Outreach assistance At the request of patients, partners are notified by members of an outreach team indigenous to the community, who do not disclose the name of the patient to the partners.

Patient referral Health service personnel encourage index patients to inform partners directly of their possible exposure to sexually transmitted infections.

Provider referral Third parties (usually health service personnel) notify partners identified by index patients, without disclosing the name of the patient to the partners.

REFERENCES

1. Holmes KK, Mardh PA, Sparling PF, et al, eds. *Sexually transmitted diseases*, 2nd ed. New York: McGraw-Hill, 1990:1083.
2. Fenton KA, Peterman TA. HIV partner notification: taking a new look. *AIDS* 1997;11:1535–1546.
3. Scholes D, Stergachis A, Heidrich FE, et al. Prevention of pelvic inflammatory disease by screening for cervical chlamydial infection. *N Engl J Med* 1996;21:1399–1401.
4. Mathews C, Coetzee N, Zwarenstein M, et al. Strategies for partner notification for sexually transmitted diseases. Cochrane Library, Issue 3, 002. Search date 2001; primary sources Medline, Embase, Psychological Abstracts, Sociological

Abstracts, Cochrane Controlled Trials Register, hand searches of the proceedings of International AIDS Conferences and the International Society for STD Research meetings, and personal contact with key experts.
5. Levy JA, Fox SE. The outreach-assisted model of partner notification with IDUs. *Public Health Rep* 1998;113(suppl 1):160–169.
6. Stein MD, Freedberg KA, Sullivan LM, et al. Sexual ethics: disclosure of HIV-positive status to partners. *Arch Intern Med* 1998;158:253–257.
7. Perry SW, Card CAL, Moffatt M, et al. Self-disclosure of HIV infection to sexual partners after repeated counseling. *AIDS Educ Prev* 1994;6:403–411.
8. Toomey KE, Peterman TA, Dicker LW, et al. Human immunodeficiency virus partner notification. *Sex Transm Dis* 1998;25:310–316.
9. Oh MK, Boker JR, Genuardi FJ, et al. Sexual contact tracing in adolescent chlamydial and gonococcal cervicitis cases. *J Adolesc Health* 1996;18:4–9.
10. Potterat JJ, Rothenberg R. The case-finding effectiveness of self-referral system for gonorrhea: a preliminary report. *Am J Public Health* 1977;67:174–176.

Nicol Coetzee
Senior Lecturer and Consultant
Department of Public Health
University of Cape Town
Cape Town
South Africa

Sally Guttmacher
Department of Health Studies
New York University
New York
USA

Catherine Mathews
Senior Scientist
Health Systems Unit
South African Medical Research Council
University of Cape Town
Cape Town
South Africa

Merrick Zwarenstein
Director, Health Systems Research Unit
Medical Research Council
Tygerberg
South Africa

Competing interests: None declared.

Pelvic inflammatory disease

Search date December 2002

Jonathan Ross

QUESTIONS

INTERVENTIONS

To be covered in future updates

Prevention

Key Messages

- **Antibiotics (symptoms improved and microbiological clearance in women with confirmed pelvic inflammatory disease)** One systematic review of observational studies and RCTs has found that several different antibiotic regimens (including parenteral clindamycin plus oral aminoglycoside; parenteral cefalosporin plus oral doxycycline with or without probenecid, ofloxacin, and co-amoxiclav) are similarly effective in relieving the symptoms of pelvic inflammatory disease, and achieve high rates of clinical and microbiological cure.
- **Different durations of antibiotic treatment** Systematic reviews found no good evidence on the optimal duration of treatment.
- **Empirical antibiotic treatment versus treatment guided by test results** We found no RCTs comparing empirical antibiotic treatment (before receiving results of microbiological tests) versus treatment that is guided by test results.
- **Oral versus parenteral antibiotics** Two RCTs found no significant difference between oral ofloxacin and parenteral cefoxitin plus doxycycline.
- **Outpatient versus inpatient antibiotic treatment** One RCT found no significant difference between outpatient treatment with intramuscular cefoxitin plus probenecid plus oral doxycycline versus inpatient treatment with parenteral antibiotics for recurrence, infertility, or ectopic pregnancy at 35 months.

Pelvic inflammatory disease

- **Routine antibiotic prophylaxis before intrauterine device insertion in women at high risk** We found no good evidence about antibiotic prophylaxis before intrauterine device insertion in women at high risk.
- **Routine antibiotic prophylaxis before intrauterine device insertion in women at low risk** One systematic review found no significant difference between routine prophylaxis with doxycycline versus placebo before intrauterine contraceptive device insertion in pelvic inflammatory disease in women at low risk of pelvic inflammatory disease.

DEFINITION Pelvic inflammatory disease (PID) is inflammation and infection of the upper genital tract in women, typically involving the fallopian tubes, ovaries, and surrounding structures.

INCIDENCE/ PREVALENCE The exact incidence of PID is unknown because the disease cannot be diagnosed reliably from clinical symptoms and signs.[1–3] Direct visualisation of the fallopian tubes by laparoscopy is the best single diagnostic test, but it is invasive and not used routinely in clinical practice. PID is the most common gynaecological reason for admission to hospital in the USA, accounting for 49/10 000 recorded hospital discharges. A diagnosis of PID is made in 1/62 (1.6%) women aged 16–45 years attending their primary care physician in England and Wales.[4] However, because most PID is asymptomatic, this figure underestimates the true prevalence.[1,5] A crude marker of PID in developing countries can be obtained from reported hospital admission rates, where it accounts for 17–40% of gynaecological admissions in sub-Saharan Africa, 15–37% in Southeast Asia, and 3–10% in India.[6]

AETIOLOGY/ RISK FACTORS Factors associated with PID mirror those for sexually transmitted infections: young age, reduced socioeconomic circumstances, African/Afro-Caribbean ethnicity, lower educational attainment, and recent new sexual partner.[2,7,8] Infection ascends from the cervix, and initial epithelial damage caused by bacteria (especially *Chlamydia trachomatis* and *Neisseria gonorrhoeae*) allows the opportunistic entry of other organisms. Many different microbes, including *Mycoplasma hominis* and anaerobes, may be isolated from the upper genital tract.[9] The spread of infection to the upper genital tract may be increased by vaginal douching and instrumentation of the cervix, but reduced by the barrier method and oral contraceptives compared with other forms of contraception.[10–13]

PROGNOSIS PID has a high morbidity; about 20% of affected women become infertile, 20% develop chronic pelvic pain, and 10% of those who conceive have an ectopic pregnancy.[2] We found no placebo controlled trials of antibiotic treatment. Uncontrolled observations suggest that clinical symptoms and signs resolve in a significant proportion of untreated women.[14] Repeated episodes of PID are associated with a four to six times increase in the risk of permanent tubal damage.[15] One case control study (76 cases and 367 controls) found that delaying treatment by even a few days is associated with impaired fertility (OR 2.6, 95% CI 1.2 to 5.9).[16]

AIMS OF INTERVENTION To alleviate the pain and systemic malaise associated with infection; to achieve microbiological cure; to prevent development of permanent tubal damage with associated sequelae, such as chronic pelvic pain, ectopic pregnancy, and infertility; and to prevent the spread of infection to others.

OUTCOMES Incidence and severity of acute symptoms and signs; microbiological cure of the upper genital tract; incidence of chronic pelvic pain, ectopic pregnancy, and infertility; rate of transmission to others.

METHODS *Clinical Evidence* search and appraisal December 2002.

QUESTION **What are the effects of empirical treatment versus treatment delayed until the results of microbiological investigations are known?**

OPTION **EMPIRICAL ANTIBIOTIC TREATMENT**

We found no good evidence on the effects of empirical treatment versus delayed antibiotic treatment for suspected pelvic inflammatory disease.

Benefits: We found no systematic review or RCTs comparing empirical versus delayed treatment.

Harms: We found no reliable evidence on harms.

Comment: Because there are no reliable clinical diagnostic criteria for pelvic inflammatory disease, early empirical treatment is common.[3] The positive predictive value of a clinical diagnosis is 65–90% compared with laparoscopy.[1–3] The absence of infection from the lower genital tract, where samples are usually taken, does not exclude pelvic inflammatory disease[2] and so may not influence the decision to treat. One case control study (76 cases and 367 controls) found that delaying treatment is associated with impaired fertility (OR 2.6, 95% CI 1.2 to 5.9).[16]

QUESTION **How do different antimicrobial regimens compare?**

One systematic review of observational studies and RCTs has found that several different antibiotic regimens (including parenteral clindamycin plus oral aminoglycoside; parenteral cefalosporin plus oral doxycycline with or without probenecid, ofloxacin, and co-amoxiclav) are similarly effective in resolving the acute symptoms and signs associated with pelvic inflammatory disease and for clinical and microbiological cure. We found no good evidence on the optimal duration of treatment. Two RCTs found no significant difference between oral ofloxacin versus parenteral cefoxitin and doxycycline. One RCT found no significant difference between outpatient treatment with intramuscular cefoxitin-probenecid and oral doxycycline versus parenteral antibiotics for recurrence, infertility, or ectopic pregnancy at 35 months.

Benefits: We found one systematic review (search date 1992, 21 studies),[17] aspects of which were subsequently updated (search date 1997, 26 studies, 1925 women).[18] The earlier review examined all antimicrobial regimens whereas the second review focused on antianaerobic treatment. The reviews evaluated 16 different antimicrobial regimens. The identified studies included case series and it is not possible to ascertain how many studies were RCTs from the aggregated data published in the reviews. Inclusion criteria were a diagnosis of pelvic inflammatory disease (clinical, microbiological, laparoscopic, or by endometrial biopsy) and microbiological testing for *C trachomatis* and *N gonorrhoeae*. The reviews found antibiotics were effective in relieving the symptoms associated with pelvic inflammatory disease, with clinical and microbiological cure rates of 88–100% (see table 1, p 1877). The only regimen that appeared to perform less well was oral metronidazole with doxycycline (see table 1, p 1877). However, the studies were of low power and apparent differences in efficacy may have been confounded by differences in disease severity among studies. **Duration of treatment:** The duration of treatment was not addressed, although the most common treatment period was 14 days. **Oral versus parenteral treatment:** The reviews did not analyse outcomes by oral or parenteral route of administration. Most regimens started with parenteral treatment and continued with oral treatment at different points. Two subsequent RCTs (249 and 72 women) compared oral ofloxacin versus parenteral cefoxitin and doxycycline. The RCTs found no significant difference in cure rates between groups (clinical cure rates about 95% for all treatments).[19,20] **Outpatient versus inpatient treatment:** We found one RCT (831 women with mild to moderate pelvic inflammatory disease) published after the review, which compared a single intramuscular dose of cefoxitin with oral probenecid followed by oral doxycycline given to outpatients versus inpatient admission for parenteral antibiotics.[21] It found no significant difference between treatments for tenderness, gonorrhoeal or chlamydial infection, or endometritis at 30 days (tenderness: 20.6% with outpatient treatment *v* 18.4% with inpatient treatment, P = 0.50; gonorrhoeal infection: 3.9% *v* 2.4%, P = 0.44; chlamydial infection: 2.7% *v* 3.6%, P = 0.52; endometritis 45.9% *v* 37.6%, P = 0.09). At 35 months, the study found no significant difference between treatments for pelvic inflammatory disease recurrence, chronic pelvic pain, infertility, or ectopic pregnancy (recurrence: 12.4% with outpatient treatment *v* 16.6% with inpatient treatment, P = 0.11; chronic pelvic pain: 33.7% *v* 29.8%, P = 0.27; infertility: 18.4% *v* 17.9%, P = 0.85; ectopic pregnancy: 1.0% *v* 0.3%, P = 0.37).[21]

Harms: The harms associated with treatment were not specifically addressed by the systematic reviews.[17,18] In two RCTs reporting adverse effects, withdrawal from treatment was uncommon (2/20 for doxycycline/metronidazole; 0/20 for pefloxacin/metronidazole; 0/16 for ciprofloxacin).[22,23] The RCT comparing outpatient treatment with inpatient parenteral treatment found no significant difference between treatments for adverse drug reactions (1.7% with outpatient treatment *v* 1.5% with inpatient treatment).[21]

Comment: We found little evidence about long term sequelae of pelvic inflammatory disease, adverse effects of treatment, treatment of pelvic inflammatory disease of differing severity, the effect of ethnicity, or the effects of tracing sexual contacts (see partner notification, p 1863). The risks of tubal occlusion and subsequent infertility relate to the severity of pelvic inflammatory disease before starting treatment,[24] and clinical improvement may not translate into preserved fertility.[25,26] The inclusion of observational studies in the systematic review without a sensitivity analysis may compromise the validity of the conclusions. In the review, reliable comparison of different drugs may be confounded by possible differences in disease severity among the included studies.

QUESTION **What are the effects of routine antibiotic prophylaxis to prevent pelvic inflammatory disease before intrauterine contraceptive device insertion?**

One systematic review found that routine prophylaxis with doxycycline versus placebo before intrauterine device insertion did not reduce the risk of pelvic inflammatory disease in women at low risk of pelvic inflammatory disease. We found no good evidence on the effects in women likely to be at high risk.

Benefits: We found one systematic review (search date 2002, 4 RCTs, 3598 women requesting intrauterine device insertion).[27] The RCTs compared a single dose of doxycycline (200 mg) versus placebo 1 hour before intrauterine device insertion. Meta-analysis in the review found no significant difference in the incidence of pelvic inflammatory disease (doxycycline *v* placebo OR 0.89, 95% CI 0.53 to 1.51). The rate of pelvic inflammatory disease in all women was low (0.5–1.6%). We found no RCTs on the effects in women at high risk of pelvic inflammatory disease.

Harms: The harms associated with treatment were not specifically addressed by the systematic review.[27] Nausea and vomiting has been reported with 17–28% of healthy volunteers on doxycycline, depending on the formulation administered.[28] See harms of antimicrobial regimens, p 1874.

Comment: In the populations included in the systematic review, the risk of pelvic inflammatory disease after intrauterine device insertion was low.[27] The occurrence of pelvic inflammatory disease in this group usually reflects the introduction of infection into the uterus during intrauterine device insertion and therefore will vary with the prevalence of sexually transmitted infections in the population. The confidence intervals are wide, suggesting that the study may have insufficient power to rule out a clinical important difference.

Substantive changes

Different antimicrobial regimens compared: One RCT added;[21] no evidence of clinically important differences between an outpatient and an inpatient antibiotic regimen.

REFERENCES

1. Morcos R, Frost N, Hnat M, et al. Laparoscopic versus clinical diagnosis of acute pelvic inflammatory disease. *J Reprod Med* 1993;38:53–56.
2. Metters JS, Catchpole M, Smith C, et al. *Chlamydia trachomatis: summary and conclusions of CMO's expert advisory group*. London: Department of Health, 1998.
3. Centers for Disease Control. 2002 guidelines for treatment of sexually transmitted diseases. Bethesda, Maryland: CDC, 1998, 2002. http://www.cdc.gov/std/treatment/TOC2002TG.htm (last accessed 26 March 2003).
4. Simms I, Rogers P, Charlett A. The rate of diagnosis and demography of pelvic inflammatory disease in general practice: England and Wales. *Int J STD AIDs* 1999;10:448–455.
5. Velebil P, Wingo PA, Xia Z, et al. Rate of hospitalization for gynecologic disorders among reproductive-age women in the United States. *Obstet Gynecol* 1995;86:764–769.
6. Kani J, Adler MW. Epidemiology of pelvic inflammatory disease. In: Berger GS, Weström L, eds. *Inflammatory disease*. New York: Raven Press, 1992.
7. Simms I, Catchpole M, Brugha R, et al. Epidemiology of genital chlamydia trachomatis in England and Wales. *Genitourin Med* 1997;73:122–126.
8. Grodstein F, Rothman KJ. Epidemiology of pelvic inflammatory disease. *Epidemiology* 1994;5:234–242.
9. Bevan CD, Johal BJ, Mumtaz G, et al. Clinical, laparoscopic and microbiological findings in acute salpingitis: report on a United Kingdom cohort. *Br J Obstet Gynaecol* 1995;102:407–414.
10. Wolner-Hanssen P, Eschenbach DA, Paavonen J, et al. Association between vaginal douching and acute pelvic inflammatory disease. *JAMA* 1990;263:1936–1941.
11. Jacobson L, Westrom L. Objectivized diagnosis of acute pelvic inflammatory disease. Diagnostic and prognostic value of routine laparoscopy. *Am J Obstet Gynecol* 1969;105:1088–1098.

12. Kelaghan J, Rubin GL, Ory HW, et al. Barrier-method contraceptives and pelvic inflammatory disease. *JAMA* 1982;248:184–187.
13. Wolner-Hanssen P, Eschenbach DA, Paavonen J, et al. Decreased risk of symptomatic chlamydial pelvic inflammatory disease associated with oral contraceptive use. *JAMA* 1990;263:54–59.
14. Curtis AH. Bacteriology and pathology of fallopian tubes removed at operation. *Surg Gynecol Obstet* 1921;33:621.
15. Hillis SD, Owens LM, Marchbanks PA, et al. Recurrent chlamydial infections increase the risks of hospitalization for ectopic pregnancy and pelvic inflammatory disease. *Am J Obstet Gynecol* 1997;176:103–107.
16. Hillis SD, Joesoef R, Marchbanks PA, et al. Delayed care of pelvic inflammatory disease as a risk factor for impaired fertility. *Am J Obstet Gynecol* 1993;168:1503–1509.
17. Walker CK, Kahn JG, Washington AE, et al. Pelvic inflammatory disease: metaanalysis of antimicrobial regimen efficacy. *J Infect Dis* 1993;168:969–978. Search date 1992; primary sources Medline, and bibliographies from reviews, textbooks, and references.
18. Walker CK, Workowski KA, Washington AE, et al. Anaerobes in pelvic inflammatory disease: implications for the Centers for Disease Control and Prevention's guidelines for treatment of sexually transmitted diseases. *Clin Infect Dis* 1999;28(suppl):29–36. Search date 1997; primary sources Medline, and bibliographies from reviews, textbooks, and references.
19. Martens MG, Gordon S, Yarborough DR, et al. Multicenter randomized trial of ofloxacin versus cefoxitin and doxycycline in outpatient treatment of pelvic inflammatory disease. Ambulatory PID Research Group. *South Med J* 1993;86:604–610.
20. Wendel GD, Cox SM, Bawdon RE, et al. A randomized trial of ofloxacin versus cefoxitin and doxycycline in the outpatient treatment of acute salpingitis. *Am J Obstet Gynecol* 1991;164:1390–1396.
21. Ness RB, Soper DE, Holley RL, et al. Effectiveness of inpatient and outpatient treatment strategies for women with pelvic inflammatory disease: results from the Pelvic Inflammatory Disease Evaluation and Clinical Health (PEACH) Randomized Trial. *Am J Obstet Gynecol* 2002;186:929–937.
22. Witte EH, Peters AA, Smit IB, et al. A comparison of pefloxacin/metronidazole and doxycycline/metronidazole in the treatment of laparoscopically confirmed acute pelvic inflammatory disease. *Eur J Obstet Gynecol Reprod Biol* 1993;50:153–158.
23. Heinonen PK, Teisala K, Miettinen A, et al. A comparison of ciprofloxacin with doxycycline plus metronidazole in the treatment of acute pelvic inflammatory disease. *Scand J Infect Dis* 1989;60(suppl):66–73.
24. Soper DE, Brockwell NJ, Dalton HP. Microbial etiology of urban emergency department acute salpingitis: treatment with ofloxacin. *Am J Obstet Gynecol* 1992;167:653–660.
25. Buchan H, Vessey M, Goldacre M, et al. Morbidity following pelvic inflammatory disease. *Br J Obstet Gynaecol* 1993;100:558–562.
26. Brunham RC, Binns B, Guijon F, et al. Etiology and outcome of acute pelvic inflammatory disease. *J Infect Dis* 1988;158:510–517.
27. Grimes DA, Schulz KF. Antibiotic prophylaxis for intrauterine contraceptive device insertion. In: The Cochrane Library, Issue 4, 2002. Oxford: Update Software. Search date 2000; primary sources Medline, Popline, Embase, lists of references, and contacted experts in the field.
28. Story MJ, McCloud PI, Boehm G. Doxycycline tolerance study. Incidence of nausea after doxycycline administration to healthy volunteers: a comparison of 2 formulations (Doryx' vs Vibramycin'). *Eur J Clin Pharmacol* 1991;40:419–421.

Jonathan Ross
Honorary Senior Lecturer
University of Birmingham
Birmingham
UK

Competing interests: None declared.

TABLE 1 **Cure rates for the antibiotic treatment of acute pelvic inflammatory disease: aggregated data from systematic reviews of RCTs and case series (see text, p 1873).[17,18]**

Drug regimen	Number of studies	Number of women	Cure rate (%) clinical/ microbiological*
Inpatient treatment (initially parenteral switching to oral)			
Clindamycin + aminoglycoside	11	470	91/97
Cefoxitin + doxycycline	8	427	91/98
Cefotetan + doxycycline	3	174	95/100
Ceftizoxime + tetracycline	1	18	88/100
Cefotaxime + tetracycline	1	19	94/100
Ciprofloxacin	4	90	94/96
Ofloxacin	1	36	100/97
Sulbactam/ ampicillin + doxycycline	1	37	95/100
Co-amoxiclav	1	32	93/–
Metronidazole + doxycycline	2	36	75/71
Outpatient treatment (oral unless indicated otherwise)			
Cefoxitin (im) + probenecid + doxycycline	3	219	89/93
Ofloxacin	2	165	95/100
Co-amoxiclav	1	35	100/100
Sulbactam/ampicillin	1	36	70/70
Ceftriaxone (im) + doxycycline	1	64	95/100
Ciprofloxacin + clindamycin	1	67	97/94

**N gonorrhoeae*, *C trachomatis*, or both, when detected in lower genital tract; im, intramuscular.

Cellulitis and erysipelas

Search date February 2003

Andrew Morris

QUESTIONS

INTERVENTIONS

Key Messages

- **Antibiotics** We found no RCTs comparing antibiotics versus placebo. RCTs comparing different antibiotic regimens found clinical cure in 50–100% of people at 4–30 days.
- **Different antibiotic regimens** RCTs comparing different antibiotic regimens were designed to test equivalence rather than to detect a clinically significant difference in cure rates between antibiotics.
- **Oral versus intravenous antibiotics; short versus long courses of antibiotics** We found no RCTs comparing oral antibiotics versus intravenous antibiotics, or different durations of antibiotics.
- **Treatment of predisposing factors to prevent recurrence** We found no RCTs or observational studies on the effects of treating predisposing factors for recurrence of cellulitis or erysipelas.

DEFINITION Cellulitis is a spreading bacterial infection of the dermis and subcutaneous tissues. It causes local signs of inflammation such as warmth, erythema, pain, lymphangitis, and frequently systemic upset with fever and raised white blood cell count. Erysipelas is a form of cellulitis and is characterised by pronounced superficial inflammation. The lower limbs are by far the most common sites, but any area can be affected. The term erysipelas is commonly used when the face is affected.

INCIDENCE/ PREVALENCE We found no specific data on the incidence of cellulitis, but cellulitis and abscess infections were responsible for 158 consultations per 10 000 person years at risk in the UK in 1991.[1] In 1985 in the UK, skin and subcutaneous tissue infections resulted in 29 820 hospital admissions and a mean occupancy of 664 hospital beds each day.[2]

AETIOLOGY/ RISK FACTORS The most common infective organisms for cellulitis and erysipelas in adults are streptococci (particularly *Streptococcus pyogenes*) and *Staphylococcus aureus*.[3] In children, *Haemophilus influenzae* is a frequent cause. Several risk factors for cellulitis and erysipelas have been identified in a case control study (167 cases and 294 controls): lymphoedema (OR 71.2, 95% CI 5.6 to 908.0), leg ulcer (OR 62.5, 95% CI 7.0 to 556.0), toe web intertrigo (OR 13.9, 95% CI 7.2 to 27.0), and traumatic wounds (OR 10.7, 95% CI 4.8 to 23.8).[4]

PROGNOSIS Cellulitis can spread through the bloodstream and lymphatic system. A retrospective case study of people admitted to hospital with cellulitis found that systemic symptoms such as fever and raised white blood cell count were present in up to 42% of cases at presentation.[5] Lymphatic involvement can lead to obstruction and damage of the lymphatic system that predisposes to recurrent cellulitis. Recurrence can occur rapidly or after months or years. One study found that 29% of people with erysipelas had a recurrent episode within 3 years.[6] Local necrosis and abscess formation can also occur. It is not known whether the prognosis of erysipelas differs from that of cellulitis. We found no evidence about factors that predict recurrence, or a better or worse outcome. We found no good evidence on the prognosis of untreated cellulitis.

AIMS OF INTERVENTION To reduce the severity and duration of infection; to relieve pain and systemic symptoms; to restore the skin to its premorbid state; to prevent recurrence; to minimise adverse effects of treatment.

OUTCOMES Duration and severity of symptoms (pain, swelling, erythema, and fever); clinical cure (defined as the absence of pain, swelling, and erythema); recurrence; adverse effects of treatment. We found no standard scales of severity in cellulitis or erysipelas.

METHODS *Clinical Evidence* search and appraisal February 2003. Where we found no RCTs, we included observational studies retrieved by the contributor's own search in June 1999.

QUESTION **What are the effects of antibiotics?**

We found no RCTs comparing antibiotics versus placebo, oral versus intravenous antibiotics, or different durations of treatment. RCTs comparing different antibiotic regimens found clinical cure in 50–100% of people at 4–30 days, but only one of the RCTs found a significant

difference in clinical cure between different antibiotics. However, most of the RCTs included only a small number of people with cellulitis or erysipelas, and were designed to test equivalence rather than to detect a clinically significant difference in cure rates between antibiotics.

Benefits: We found no systematic review. **Versus placebo:** We found no RCTs. **Oral versus intravenous antibiotics:** One small quasi-randomised trial (73 people with erysipelas in hospital with a body temperature > 38.5 °C and no suspected septicaemia; alternate allocation design) comparing oral with intravenous penicillin found no significant difference in clinical efficacy, which was assessed by indirect measures such as temperature fall, length of hospital stay, and absence from work.[7] No results were provided on relapse rates. **Different antibiotic regimens:** We found nine RCTs comparing different antibiotic regimens in people with various skin infections (see table 1, p 1882).[8–16] Two of the RCTs were conducted solely in people with cellulitis (192 people with moderate to severe cellulitis);[8,9] one RCT was conducted solely in people with erysipelas (69 people);[10] the other six RCTs were conducted in people with different skin infections and provided subgroup analysis of people with cellulitis or erysipelas.[11–16] One of the RCTs conducted solely in people with cellulitis (58 people with moderate to severe cellulitis) found that ceftriaxone significantly increased clinical cure after 4–6 days compared with flucloxacillin.[8] The other RCTs and the subgroup analyses found no significant difference between different antibiotics in clinical cure after 4–30 days.[8,10–16] However, most of the RCTs only included small numbers of people with cellulitis or erysipelas and were designed to test equivalence rather than to detect a clinically significant difference in cure rates between antibiotics. **Short versus long courses of antibiotics:** We found no RCTs comparing different durations of antibiotics.

Harms: In the quasi-randomised trial (73 people with erysipelas) comparing oral with intravenous penicillin, adverse events occurred in 15 people taking oral penicillin (rash 4, diarrhoea 7, abscess 4) and in 10 people taking intravenous penicillin (rash 2, diarrhoea 4, cannula phlebitis 4).[7] The RCT comparing flucloxacillin with ceftriaxone (58 people with moderate to severe cellulitis) found no significant difference in the proportion of people experiencing diarrhoea, nausea and vomiting, abdominal pain, or vaginal candidiasis (6/22 [27%] with flucloxacillin *v* 3/22 [14%] with ceftriaxone; RR 2.00, 95% CI 0.57 to 7.00).[8] The RCT comparing cefazolin plus probenecid versus ceftriaxone plus placebo (134 people with moderate to severe cellulitis) found no significant difference in the proportion of people who experienced adverse effects, including nausea and vomiting, diarrhoea, headache, and dizziness (14/67 [21%] with cefazolin plus probenecid *v* 7/67 [10%] with ceftriaxone plus placebo; RR 2.00, 95% CI 0.86 to 4.64).[9] The RCT comparing penicillin versus roxithromycin (69 people with erysipelas) found no significant difference in the proportion of people experiencing drug related rashes (2/38 [5%] with penicillin *v* 0/31 [0%] people with roxithromycin).[10] The RCTs comparing different antibiotics in a variety of skin infections gave no discrete information about adverse effects in people with cellulitis.[11–16]

Comment: None.

QUESTION Does the treatment of predisposing factors reduce recurrence?

We found no RCTs or observational studies on the effects of treatment of predisposing factors for recurrence of cellulitis or erysipelas.

Benefits: We found no systematic review, RCTs, or observational studies.

Harms: We found no RCTs.

Comment: Although there is a consensus that successful treatment of the predisposing factors reduces the risk of developing cellulitis/erysipelas (see aetiology, p 1879), we found no RCTs or observational studies to support or refute this.

REFERENCES

1. Office of Population Censuses and Surveys. *Morbidity statistics from general practice*. Fourth National Study. London: HMSO (series MB5), 1992, 272.
2. Department of Health, Department of Health and Social Security. *Hospital in-patient enquiry*. London: HMSO (series MB4), 1985, 16, 28.
3. Bernard P, Bedane C, Mounier M, et al. Streptococcal cause of erysipelas and cellulitis in adults. *Arch Dermatol* 1989;125:779–782.
4. Dupuy A, Benchikhi H, Roujeau J-C, et al. Risk factors for erysipelas of the leg (cellulitis): case-control study. *BMJ* 1999;318:1591–1594.
5. Aly AA, Roberts NM, Seipol K, et al. Case survey of management of cellulitis in a tertiary teaching hospital. *Med J Aust* 1996;165:553–556.
6. Jorup-Ronstrom C, Britton S. Recurrent erysipelas: predisposing factors and costs, of prophylaxis. *Infection* 1987;15:105–106.
7. Jorup-Ronstrom C, Britton A, Gavlevik K, et al. The course, costs and complications of oral versus intravenous penicillin therapy of erysipelas. *Infection* 1984;12:390–394.
8. Vinen J, Hudson B, Chan B, et al. A randomized comparative study of once-daily ceftriaxone and 6-hourly flucloxacillin in the treatment of moderate to severe cellulitis. Clinical efficacy, safety and pharmacoeconomic implications. *Clin Drug Invest* 1996;12:221–225.
9. Grayson ML, McDonald M, Gibson K, et al. Once-daily intravenous cefazolin plus oral probenecid is equivalent to once-daily ceftriaxone plus oral placebo for the treatment of moderate-to-severe cellulitis in adults. *Clin Infect Dis* 2002;34:1440–1448.
10. Bernard P, Plantin P, Roger H, et al. Roxithromycin versus penicillin in the treatment of erysipelas in adults: a comparative study. *Br J Dermatol* 1992;127:155–159.
11. Daniel R, Austad J, Debersaques J, et al. Azithromycin, erythromycin and cloxacillin in the treatment of infections of skin and associated soft tissues. *J Int Med Res* 1991;19:433–445.
12. Kiani R. Double-blind, double-dummy comparison of azithromycin and cephalexin in the treatment of skin and skin structure infections. *Eur J Clin Microbiol Infect Dis* 1991;10:880–884.
13. Tack KJ, Littlejohn TW, Mailloux G, et al. Cefdinir versus cephalexin for the treatment of skin and skin-structure infections. *Clin Ther* 1998;20:244–255.
14. Tassler H. Comparative efficacy and safety of oral fleroxacin and amoxicillin/clavulanate potassium in skin and soft tissue infections. *Am J Med* 1993;94:159S–165S.
15. Parish LC, Jungkind DL. Systemic anti-microbial therapy for skin and skin structure infections: comparison of fleroxacin and ceftazidime. *Am J Med* 1993;94:166S–173S.
16. Chan JC. Ampicillin-sulbactam versus cefazolin or cefoxitin in the treatment of skin and skin-structure infections of bacterial etiology. *Adv Ther* 1995;12:139–146.

Andrew Morris
Specialist Registrar in Dermatology
University Hospital of Wales
Cardiff
UK

Competing interests: None declared.

TABLE 1 **Different antibiotic regimens: results of comparative RCTs (see text, p 1880).**

Ref	Regimen	Participants	Clinical cure (significance)
8	iv ceftriaxone 1 g od for 7 days *v* iv flucloxacillin 1 g qds for a mean of 9 days	58 people with cellulitis	21/23 (92%) *v* 14/22 (64%) after 4–6 days (RR 1.43, 95% CI 1.02 to 2.02; NNT 4, 95% CI 2 to 17)
9	iv cefazolin 2 g od plus oral probenecid 1 g od *v* ceftriaxone 1 g od plus placebo for median 6–7 days	132 people with cellulitis	51/67 (76%) *v* 55/67 (82%) after 6–7 days (RR 0.93, 95% CI 0.78 to 1.10)
10	iv penicillin 2.5 MU 8 times daily followed by 6 MU orally od for mean 13 days *v* oral roxithromycin 150 mg bd for mean 13 days	69 people with erysipelas	29/38 (76%) *v* 26/31 (84%) after 30 days (RR 0.91, 95% CI 0.72 to 1.15)
11	Oral azithromycin total dose 1.5 g over 5 days *v* oral erythromycin 500 mg qds for 7 days	Subgroup analysis in 128 people with cellulitis	52/72 (72%) *v* 37/50 (74%) after 4–11 days (RR 0.97, 95% CI 0.78 to 1.21)
11	Oral azithromycin total dose 1.5 g over 5 days *v* oral cloxacillin 500 mg qds for 7 days	Subgroup analysis in 62 people with cellulitis	27/41 (66%) *v* 11/21 (52%) after 4–9 days (RR 1.26, 95% CI 0.79 to 2.00)
12	Oral azithromycin total dose 750 mg over 5 days *v* cefalexin 500 mg bd for 10 days	Subgroup analysis in 95 people with suspected cellulitis, 47 of whom had microbiologically proven cellulitis	12/24 (50%) *v* 14/23 (61%) after 11 days (RR 0.82, 95% CI 0.49 to 1.38)
13	Cefdinir 300 mg bd for 10 days *v* cefalexin 500 mg qds for 10 days	Subgroup analysis in 78 people with suspected cellulitis, 34 of whom had microbiologically proven cellulitis	In the 34 people with microbiologically proven cellulitis: 13/17 (76%) *v* 14/17 (82%) after 7–16 days (RR 0.93, 95% CI 0.66 to 1.31)

TABLE 1 continued

Ref	Regimen	Participants	Clinical cure (significance)
14	Oral amoxicillin/clavulanate potassium 125–500 mg tds *v* oral fleroxacin 400 mg od	Subgroup analysis in 11 people with cellulitis or erysipelas	7/7 (100%) *v* 4/4 (100%) after 3–9 days
15	iv fleroxacin 400 mg od *v* iv ceftazidime 0.52 g bd/tds	Subgroup analysis in 39 people with cellulitis	26/27 (96%) *v* 9/12 (75%) after 21 days (RR 1.28, 95% CI 0.92 to 1.78)
16	iv ampicillin/sulbactam 0.5–1 g qds *v* iv cefazolin 500 mg qds for 6–7 days	Subgroup analysis in 20 people with cellulitis	8/8 (100%) *v* 9/12 (75%) after 10 days

bd, twice daily; iv, intravenous; od, once daily; qds, four times daily; ref, reference; tds, three times daily.

Head lice

Search date February 2003

Ian Burgess

QUESTIONS

INTERVENTIONS

Key Messages

- **Insecticide based pharmaceutical products** One systematic review has found that permethrin and malathion both increase lice eradication rates compared with placebo. Limited evidence from another systematic review suggested that permethrin increased eradication rates compared with lindane.
- **Essential oils and other chemicals used as repellents** We found insufficient evidence on the effects of these interventions.
- **Herbal treatments** We found no RCTs that compared herbal treatment with placebo. One RCT found no significant difference in eradication rates between a herbal product (coconut, anise, and ylang ylang) and insecticide (permethrin, malathion, and piperonyl butoxide). However, results may not generalise to different concentrations of these components or to different herbal preparations.
- **Mechanical removal of lice or viable eggs by combing** We found inconclusive evidence from three RCTs about effects of combing instead of or in addition to insecticides.

DEFINITION Head lice are obligate ectoparasites of socially active humans. They infest the scalp and attach their eggs to the hair shafts. Itching, resulting from multiple bites, is not diagnostic but may increase the index of suspicion. Infestation can be diagnosed only by finding living lice. Eggs glued to hairs, whether hatched (nits) or unhatched, are not proof of active infection, because eggs may retain a viable appearance for weeks after death.

INCIDENCE/ PREVALENCE We found no studies on incidence and no recent published prevalence results from any developed country. Anecdotal reports suggest that prevalence has increased in the past few years in most communities in the UK and USA.

AETIOLOGY/ RISK FACTORS Observational studies indicate that infections occur most frequently in school children, although there is no proof of a link with school attendance.[1,2] We found no evidence that lice prefer clean hair to dirty hair.

PROGNOSIS The infection is almost harmless. Sensitisation reactions to louse saliva and faeces may result in localised irritation and erythema. Secondary infection of scratches may occur. Lice have been identified as primary mechanical vectors of scalp pyoderma caused by streptococci and staphylococci usually found on the skin.[3]

AIMS OF INTERVENTION To eliminate infestation by killing or removing all head lice and their eggs.

OUTCOMES Treatment success is given as the percentage of people completely cleared of head lice. There are no standard criteria for judging treatment success. Trials used different methods and, in many cases, the method was not stated. Few studies are pragmatic.

METHODS *Clinical Evidence* search and appraisal February 2003 The initial search was performed by the Cochrane Infectious Diseases Group at the Liverpool School of Tropical Medicine for a systematic review compiled in July 1998.[4]

QUESTION **What are the effects of treatment for head lice?**

OPTION **INSECTICIDE BASED PHARMACEUTICAL PRODUCTS**

One systematic review has found that permethrin and malathion both increase lice eradication rates compared with placebo. Limited evidence from another systematic review suggested that permethrin increased eradication rates compared with lindane.

Benefits: We found two systematic reviews.[4,5] The first systematic review (search date 1995, 7 RCTs, 1808 people) assessed 11 insecticide products, including lindane, carbaryl, malathion, permethrin, and other pyrethroids in various vehicles.[4] The subsequent systematic review (search date 2001, 4 RCTs, 345 children and adults) set stricter criteria for RCTs and rejected all but four RCTs,[5] and excluded studies on which the earlier review was based. **Versus placebo:** The second systematic review identified one RCT (63 people) comparing permethrin with placebo.[5] It found that permethrin (1% cream rinse) significantly increased eradication rates compared with placebo after 7 and 14 days (7 days: 29/29 [100%]

with permethrin v 3/34 [9%] with placebo; RR 11.3, 95% CI 3.9 to 33.4; 14 days: 28/29 [97%] with permethrin v 2/24 [8%] with placebo; RR 11.6, 95% CI 3.1 to 43.8; NNT 2, 95% CI 1 to 2). The second systematic review also identified one RCT (115 people) comparing malathion (0.5% alcoholic lotion) with placebo.[5] It found that malathion significantly increased eradication rates after 1 week compared with placebo (62/65 [95%] with malathion v 21/47 [45%] with placebo; RR 2.1, 95% CI 1.5 to 2.9; NNT 2, 95% CI 1 to 3). **Versus each other:** The first systematic review (7 RCTs, 726 people, search date 1995) found that permethrin (1% cream rinse) significantly increased eradication rates compared with lindane (1% shampoo) (lindane v permethrin; 2 RCTs; OR for not clearing head lice 15.2, 95% CI 8.0 to 28.8).[4] **Versus mechanical removal of lice:** See mechanical removal of lice or viable eggs by combing, p 1886.

Harms: Only minor adverse effects have been reported for most insecticides. The exception is lindane, where there are extensive reports of effects related to overdosing (treatment of scabies) and absorption (treatment of head lice). Transdermal passage of lindane occurs during treatment of head lice,[6] but we found no reports of adverse effects in this setting. We found no confirmed reports of adverse effects from the organophosphate malathion when used therapeutically.

Comment: Follow up for 6 days is inadequate, as the eggs take 7 days to hatch. Most investigators agree that a final examination after 14 days is appropriate for primary end point determination of cure. Three trials included in the most recent systematic review were conducted in developing countries where insecticide treatments were not regularly available.[5] This may have resulted in greater efficacy, because the insects may have had no previous exposure to the therapeutic agent. Studies *in vitro* suggest that other components of products (e.g. terpenoids and solvents) may be more effective pediculicides than the insecticide itself.[7] Resistance to one or more insecticides is now common.[8–10] One RCT (193 people) investigating resistance compared malathion (0.5% lotion with terpenoids) with phenothrin (0.3% lotion) in a community where lice were identified *in vitro* as being tolerant of phenothrin.[11] After 1 day, malathion increased lice eradication rates compared with phenothrin (louse free: 87/95 [92%] with malathion v 39/98 [40%] with phenothrin; RR 2.3, 95% CI 1.7 to 2.9) and this difference had increased by day 7 (90/95 [95%] with malathion v 38/98 [39%] with phenothrin; RR 2.4, 95% CI 1.8 to 3.2). However, some children not free from lice on day 1 had become louse free by day 7 in both groups, suggesting some parental intervention had influenced the results. This study suggests that resistance to pyrethroid insecticide may have influenced about 60% of the treatments.

OPTION MECHANICAL REMOVAL OF LICE OR VIABLE EGGS BY COMBING

We found inconclusive evidence from three RCTs about effects of combing instead of or in addition to insecticides.

Benefits: We found two RCTs that compared combing with an insecticide treatment and one RCT that compared an insecticide with and without combing.[12–14] The first RCT (72 people) compared "bug busting" (wet combing with conditioner) versus two applications of 0.5% malathion 7 days apart.[12] It found that malathion significantly improved lice eradication rates compared with "bug busting" 7 days after treatment (12/32 [38%] with "bug busting" *v* 31/40 [78%] with malathion; RR for "bug busting" *v* malathion 0.48, 95% CI 0.30 to 0.78; NNH 3, 95% CI 2 to 5).[12] The second RCT (30 people) compared "bug busting" versus two weekly applications of phenothrin lotion (concentration not specified) plus combing. It found that "bug busting" significantly increased eradication of head lice after 14 days compared with phenothrin (eradication rates: 8/15 [53%] with "bug busting" *v* 2/15 [13%] with phenothrin group; RR 4.0, 95% CI 1.0 to 15.8; NNT 3, 95% CI 2 to 17).[13] The third RCT (95 adults and children) compared combing with a metal louse/nit comb plus 1% permethrin cream rinse with permethrin cream rinse alone.[14] In both groups permethrin was applied by a community practitioner and if lice were found after 7 days a further application of permethrin was given. It found no significant difference in eradication rates with adjuvant combing compared with permethrin alone at 2, 8, and 15 days (louse free rates, at day 2: 49/59 [83%] with no combing *v* 24/33 [73%] with combing, RR 1.14, 95% CI 0.90 to 1.50; at day 8 before repeat treatment: 27/59 [46%] with no combing *v* 11/33 [33%] with combing, RR 0.92, 95% CI 0.60 to 1.40; at day 15: 47/60 [78%] with no combing *v* 24/33 [73%] with combing, RR 1.08, 95% CI 0.80 to 1.40). We found three RCTs comparing different pediculicides in combination with nit combing, but none included a non-combing control group.[15–17]

Harms: Apart from discomfort, we found no evidence of harms because of combing. Wet combing with conditioner may risk adverse reactions, which have been observed during normal cosmetic use, to hair conditioning agents.[18–22]

Comment: The first RCT looking at "bug busting" was designed be a pragmatic RCT with results that are applicable to normal practice.[12] In the second RCT interventions were applied by trained nurses. "Bug busting" involved the use of different graded combs and specific hair conditioner, while people in the phenothrin group used a single head lice comb and unspecified hair conditioners. The follow up strategy for the combing group differed from that offered to the lotion group.[13] This difference may introduce bias and confounding. One observational study compared two groups of children with louse eggs but no lice at initial assessment.[23] These children were followed to see if they developed active infestation over a period of 14 days. More children with five or more eggs within 6 mm of the scalp developed infestations compared with less than five eggs (infestation rates: 7/22 [32%] with ≥ 5 eggs *v* 2/28 [7%] with < 5 eggs; RR 4.45, 95% CI 1.02 to 19.30). The authors concluded that adequate follow up examinations are more likely to be productive than nit removal to prevent reinfestation.

OPTION HERBAL TREATMENTS

We found no RCTs that compared herbal products with placebo. One RCT found no significant difference in eradication rates between a herbal product (coconut, anise, and ylang ylang) and insecticide (permethrin, malathion, and piperonyl butoxide). However, results may not generalise to different concentrations of these components or to different herbal preparations.

Benefits: We found no RCTs that compared herbal products with placebo. We found one RCT (143 children) that compared a spray based on herbal oils (coconut, anise, and ylang ylang; concentrations unspecified) with an insecticide spray (0.5% permethrin, 0.25% malathion, and 2% piperonyl butoxide).[24] The herbal spray was used three times at 5 day intervals and the insecticide twice with 10 days between applications. It found no significant difference in eradication rates between the herbal product and insecticide (60/70 [86%] with herbal product *v* 59/73 [81%] with insecticide).

Harms: One RCT (143 children) found no clinically detectable adverse effects with either herbal oils (coconut, anise, and ylang ylang) or insecticide spray (permethrin, malathion, and piperonyl butoxide).[24]

Comment: Results may not generalise to different concentrations of these herbal ingredients or to other herbal products.

OPTION ESSENTIAL OILS AND OTHER CHEMICALS USED AS REPELLENTS

We found no systematic review, RCTs, or cohort studies on the effects of essential oils or other chemicals used as repellents (such as piperonal).

Benefits: We found no systematic review, RCTs, or cohort studies evaluating repellents.

Harms: We found no evidence of harms, although a potential for toxic effects has been recognised for several essential oils.[25]

Comment: None.

Substantive changes

Combing One RCT added;[14] conclusions unchanged.
Herbal treatments One RCT added;[24] conclusions unchanged.

REFERENCES

1. Burgess IF. Human lice and their management. *Adv Parasitol* 1995;36:721–342.
2. Gratz NG. *Human lice. Their prevalence, control and resistance to insecticides*. Geneva: World Health Organization, 1997.
3. Taplin D, Meinking TL. Infestations. In: Schachner LA, Hansen RC, eds. *Pediatric dermatology*, Vol 2. New York: Churchill Livingstone, 1988:1465–1493.
4. Vander Stichele RH, Dezeure EM, Bogaert MG. Systematic review of clinical efficacy of topical treatments for head lice. *BMJ* 1995;311:604–608. Search date 1995; primary sources Medline, International Pharmaceutical Abstracts, and Science Citation Index.
5. Dodd CS. Interventions for treating head lice (Cochrane Review). In: The Cochrane Library, Issue 1, 2003. Oxford: Update Software. Search date 2001; primary sources Cochrane Infectious Diseases Group Trials Register, Cochrane Controlled Trials Register, Medline, Embase, Science Citation Index, Biosis, Toxline and hand searches of reference lists from relevant articles and personal contact with pharmaceutical companies and UK and US Regulatory Authorities.
6. Ginsburg CM, Lowry W. Absorption of gamma benzene hexachloride following application of Kwell shampoo. *Pediatr Dermatol* 1983;1:74–76.
7. Burgess I. Malathion lotions for head lice: a less reliable treatment than commonly believed. *Pharm J* 1991;247:630–632.
8. Burgess IF, Brown CM, Peock S, et al. Head lice resistant to pyrethroid insecticides in Britain [letter]. *BMJ* 1995;311:752.

9. Pollack RJ, Kiszewski A, Armstrong P, et al. Differential permethrin susceptibility of head lice sampled in the United States and Borneo. *Arch Pediatr Adolesc Med* 1999;153:969–973.
10. Lee SH, Yoon KS, Williamson M, et al. Molecular analyses of *kdr*-like resistance in permethrin-resistant strains of head lice, *Pediculus capitis*. *Pestic Biochem Physiol* 2000;66:130–143.
11. Chosidow O, Chastang C, Brue C, et al. Controlled study of malathion and *d*-phenothrin lotions for *Pediculus humanus* var *capitis*-infested schoolchildren. *Lancet* 1994;334:1724–1727.
12. Roberts RJ, Casey D, Morgan DA, et al. Comparison of wet combing with malathion for treatment of head lice in the UK: a pragmatic randomised controlled trial. *Lancet* 2000;356:540–544.
13. Plastow L, Luthra M, Powell R, et al. Head lice infestation: bug busting vs. traditional treatment. *J Clin Nurs* 2001;10:775–783.
14. Meinking TL, Clineschmidt CM, Chen C, et al. An observer-blinded study of 1% permethrin creme rinse with and without adjunctive combing in patients with head lice. *J Pediatr* 2002;141:665–670.
15. Bainbridge CV, Klein GI, Neibart SI, et al. Comparative study of the clinical effectiveness of a pyrethrin-based pediculicide with combing versus a permethrin-based pediculicide with combing. *Clin Pediatr (Phila)* 1998;37:17–22.
16. Clore ER, Longyear LA. A comparative study of seven pediculicides and their packaged nit combs. *J Pediatr Health Care* 1993;7:55–60.
17. Hipolito RB, Mallorca FG, Zuniga-Macaraig ZO, et al. Head lice infestation: single drug versus combination therapy with one percent permethrin and trimethoprim/sulfamethoxazole. *Pediatrics* 2001;107:E30.
18. Korting JC, Pursch EM, Enders F, et al. Allergic contact dermatitis to cocamidopropyl betaine in shampoo. *J Am Acad Dermatol* 1992;27:1013–1015.
19. Niinimaki A, Niinimaki M, Makinen-Kiljunen S, et al. Contact urticaria from protein hydrolysates in hair conditioners. *Allergy* 1998;53:1070–1082.
20. Schalock PC, Storrs FJ, Morrison L. Contact urticaria from panthenol in hair conditioner. *Contact Dermatitis* 2000;43:223.
21. Pasche-Koo F, Claeys M, Hauser C. Contact urticaria with systemic symptoms caused by bovine collagen in hair conditioner. *Am J Contact Dermatol* 1996;7:56–57.
22. Stadtmauer G, Chandler M. Hair conditioner causes angioedema. *Ann Allergy Asthma Immunol* 1997;78:602.
23. Williams LK, Reichert A, MacKenzie WR, et al. Lice, nits, and school policy. *Pediatrics* 2001;107:1011–1015.
24. Mumcuoglu KY, Miller J, Zamir C, et al. The *in vivo* pediculicidal efficacy of a natural remedy. *Isr Med Ass J* 2002;4:790–793.
25. Veal L. The potential effectiveness of essential oils as a treatment for headlice, *Pediculus humanus capitis*. *Complement Ther Nurs Midwifery* 1996;2:97–101.

Ian Burgess
Director
Insect Research
& Development Limited
Cambridge
UK

Competing interests: IB has been a consultant to various makers of pharmaceutical products, alternative therapies, and combs for treating louse infestations.

Herpes labialis

Search date December 2002

Bazian Ltd

QUESTIONS

INTERVENTIONS

Key Messages

Prevention

- **Oral antiviral agents** Limited evidence from RCTs suggests that prophylactic oral antiviral agents may reduce the frequency and severity of attacks compared with placebo, but the optimal timing and duration of treatment is uncertain.
- **Sunscreen** We found limited evidence from two small crossover RCTs that ultraviolet sunscreen may reduce herpes recurrence compared with placebo.
- **Topical antiviral agents** We found no RCTs on the effects of topical antiviral agents used as prophylaxis.

Treatment

- **Oral aciclovir for first attack** One small RCT in children found that oral aciclovir reduced the mean duration of pain compared with placebo. Another small RCT in children found that oral aciclovir reduced the median time to healing compared with placebo.
- **Oral aciclovir for recurrent attack** Two RCTs found that oral aciclovir (if taken early in the attack) marginally reduced the duration of symptoms and pain compared with placebo.
- **Topical antiviral agents for recurrent attacks** We found limited evidence from RCTs that topical penciclovir or aciclovir reduced the duration of pain and symptoms compared with placebo.

Clin Evid 2003;10:1890–1896.

- **Topical anaesthetic agents** One small RCT found limited evidence that topical tetracaine reduced the mean time to scab loss compared with placebo. However, the clinical importance of this result is unclear.
- **Topical antiviral agents for first attack** We found no RCTs on the effects of topical antiviral agents.
- **Zinc oxide cream** One small RCT found limited evidence that zinc oxide cream reduced time to healing compared with placebo but found that it increased the risk of skin irritation.

DEFINITION Herpes labialis is a mild self limiting infection with herpes simplex virus type 1. It causes pain and blistering on the lips and perioral area (cold sores); fever and constitutional symptoms are rare. Most people have no warning of an attack, but some experience a recognisable prodrome.

INCIDENCE/ PREVALENCE Herpes labialis accounts for about 1% of primary care consultations in the UK each year; 20–40% of people have experienced cold sores at some time.[1]

AETIOLOGY/ RISK FACTORS Herpes labialis is caused by herpes simplex virus type 1. After the primary infection, which usually occurs in childhood, the virus is thought to remain latent in the trigeminal ganglion.[2] A variety of factors, including exposure to bright sunlight, fatigue, or psychological stress, can precipitate a recurrence.

PROGNOSIS In most people, herpes labialis is a mild, self limiting illness. Recurrences are usually shorter and less severe than the initial attack. Healing is usually complete in 7–10 days without scarring.[3] Rates of reactivation are unknown. Herpes labialis can cause serious illness in immunocompromised people.

AIMS OF INTERVENTION To reduce the frequency and severity of recurrent attacks; to speed healing of lesions; to reduce pain, with minimal adverse effects.

OUTCOMES Severity of symptoms, duration of symptoms, time to crusting of lesions, time to healing, rate of recurrence, and adverse effects of treatment.

METHODS *Clinical Evidence* search and appraisal December 2002. Keywords: herpes labialis, treatment, prevention, prophylaxis, controlled trial, and effectiveness.

QUESTION **What are the effects of interventions aimed at preventing attacks?**

OPTION **ORAL/TOPICAL ANTIVIRAL AGENTS**

Limited evidence from RCTs suggests that prophylactic oral antiviral agents may reduce the frequency and severity of attacks compared with placebo, but the optimal timing and duration of treatment is uncertain. We found no RCTs on the effects of topical antiviral agents used as prophylaxis.

Benefits: We found no systematic review. **Topical antiviral agents:** We found no good quality RCTs. **Oral antiviral agents:** We found four double blind, placebo controlled RCTs.[4–7] The first RCT (147 American skiers with a history of herpes labialis precipitated by ultraviolet light) found that prophylactic oral aciclovir (400 mg twice daily, beginning 12 hours before ultraviolet exposure) reduced frequency of attacks and duration of symptoms compared with placebo ($P < 0.05$).[4] The second RCT (239 Canadian skiers with a history of recurrent herpes labialis) found no significant difference in lesion occurrence between those who took aciclovir (800 mg twice daily, starting on the day before exposure to ultraviolet light for a minimum of 3 days to a maximum of 7 days) and those who took placebo (21/93 with aciclovir *v* 21/102 with placebo; $P = 0.92$).[5] The third RCT (20 people with recurrent herpes labialis) found that aciclovir (400 mg twice daily for 4 months) led to 53% fewer clinical recurrences than placebo ($P = 0.05$).[6] The fourth RCT (248 adults with a history of sun-induced recurrent herpes labialis) compared three different dosages of famciclovir (125 mg, 250 mg, and 500 mg) versus placebo.[7] Treatment was given three times daily for 5 days, beginning 48 hours after exposure to artificial ultraviolet light. The study found no significant difference in the number of lesions in the four groups, but increasing the dose of famciclovir significantly reduced the mean size ($P = 0.04$) and duration of lesions, in a dose–response relation. Compared with placebo, the 500 mg dose reduced the mean time to healing by 2 days ($P < 0.01$).

Harms: See harms under the effects of antiviral treatment for the first attack, p 1893.

Comment: All participants in the second RCT were allowed to use acetaminophen and encouraged to use sunscreen.[5]

OPTION SUNSCREEN

We found limited evidence from two small crossover RCTs that ultraviolet sunscreen may reduce herpes recurrence compared with placebo.

Benefits: We found no systematic review. We found two small, crossover RCTs.[8,9] The first RCT (38 people with a history of recurrent herpes) found that sunscreen significantly reduced recurrence compared with placebo at 6 days (recurrence 0/35 [0%] with sunscreen *v* 27/38 [71%] with placebo; $P < 0.001$).[8] The second RCT (19 people exposed to a pre-established dose of ultraviolet light in a laboratory) found that sunscreen significantly reduced recurrence compared with placebo at 6 days (11/19 [58%] with placebo *v* 1/19 [5%] with sunscreen; $P < 0.01$; see comment below).[9]

Harms: None reported.

Comment: The conclusions from the RCTs should be considered with care.[8,9] Crossover studies have important limitations, and the second RCT was conducted under artificial conditions.[9]

QUESTION What are the effects of antiviral treatment for the first attack of herpes labialis?

We found no RCTs on the effects of topical antiviral agents. One small RCT in children found that oral aciclovir reduced the mean duration of pain compared with placebo. Another small RCT in children found that oral aciclovir reduced the median time to healing compared with placebo.

Benefits: We found no systematic review. **Topical antiviral agents:** We found no RCTs. **Oral antiviral agents:** We found two small RCTs in children.[10,11] One double blind RCT (20 children having their first attack) found that oral aciclovir (200 mg five times daily) significantly reduced mean duration of pain and excess salivation (duration of pain: 4.3 days with aciclovir *v* 5.0 days with placebo; duration of excess salivation: 3.3 days with aciclovir *v* 5.0 days with placebo; $P < 0.05$).[10] The second RCT (72 children aged 1–6 years with herpes simplex gingivostomatitis of less than 3 days' duration) found that oral aciclovir (15 mg/kg five times daily for 7 days) significantly reduced the median time to healing compared with placebo (4 days with aciclovir *v* 10 days with placebo; median difference 6 days, 95% CI 4 days to 8 days).[11] We found no RCTs in adults.

Harms: Trials have found that topical aciclovir is associated with rash, pruritus, and irritation in some people, but no more frequently than placebo.[12–14] Oral aciclovir is excreted in breast milk. Aciclovir has been used to treat pregnant women with genital herpes, and one systematic review (search date 1996, three studies) found no evidence of adverse effects in women or newborn children (see antiviral treatment for genital herpes during pregnancy, p 1842).[14] Evidence is limited, however, and clinically important adverse effects cannot be ruled out.

Comment: Research in this area is difficult because people do not usually consult clinicians until they have had several attacks of herpes labialis.

QUESTION **Do treatments taken at the beginning of or during a recurrent attack reduce the duration or severity of symptoms?**

OPTION **ORAL/TOPICAL ANTIVIRAL AGENTS**

We found limited evidence from RCTs that topical penciclovir or aciclovir reduced the duration of pain and symptoms compared with placebo. Two RCTs found that oral aciclovir (if taken early in the attack) marginally reduced the duration of symptoms and pain compared with placebo.

Benefits: We found no systematic review. **Topical antiviral agents:** We found 12 RCTs (published in 11 papers) of antiviral creams or ointments.[12,13,15–23] The first RCT (double blind, 2209 people) found that penciclovir cream (twice hourly for 4 days) reduced healing time and duration of pain compared with placebo (median healing time: 4.8 days with penciclovir cream *v* 5.5 days with control cream; $P < 0.001$; median duration of pain: 3.5 days with penciclovir cream *v* 4.1 days control cream; $P < 0.001$).[18] The second small RCT (31 people aged > 17 years with recurrent herpes labialis) compared 5% aciclovir cream (10 people), 5% aciclovir in a liposomal vehicle (12 people), and drug free vehicle (nine people).[20] It found that aciclovir in liposomal vehicle versus drug free vehicle significantly reduced the mean time to crusting of the lesions (1.6 days for aciclovir in liposomes *v* 4.8 days for control; $P < 0.05$) but found no significant difference between aciclovir cream and the drug free vehicle (4.3 days for aciclovir cream *v* 4.8 days for control). The third double blind RCT (534 people) compared 1% penciclovir cream versus placebo.[21] It found that penciclovir significantly reduced the mean healing time of lesions compared with placebo (7.6 days with penciclovir *v* 8.8 days with placebo; $P < 0.01$). The fourth RCT (61 people) found no significant difference in the duration of pain and healing time between aciclovir and placebo (duration of pain: 1.2 days with aciclovir *v* 1.1 days with placebo; P value not reported).[12] The fifth crossover RCT (45 people) found no significant difference in duration of pain and healing time between aciclovir and placebo (healing time: 10 days with aciclovir *v* 13 days with placebo; P value not reported).[16] The sixth RCT (208 people) found no significant difference in duration of pain or healing time between aciclovir and placebo (duration of pain: 1.9 days with aciclovir *v* 2.1 days with placebo; $P = 0.30$; healing time: 7.2 days with aciclovir *v* 7.2 days with placebo; $P = 0.67$).[17] The seventh RCT found no significant difference in the duration of pain or healing time between aciclovir and placebo (duration of pain: 1.08 days with aciclovir *v* 1.04 with placebo; P value not reported; healing time: 8.9 days with aciclovir *v* 7.9 with placebo; P value not reported).[19] The eighth small crossover RCT (13 people with 31 lesions) found that aciclovir significantly reduced healing time compared with placebo (7 days with aciclovir *v* 8 days with placebo; $P < 0.05$).[13] The ninth small RCT (30 people) found that aciclovir significantly reduced healing time, but not duration of pain compared with placebo (healing time: 5.7 days with aciclovir *v* 8.3 days with placebo; $P = 0.022$; duration of pain: 1.7 days with aciclovir *v* 2.3 days with placebo; $P = 0.53$).[15] The 10th RCT (380 people) found that aciclovir cream significantly reduced healing time compared with placebo (9.0 days with aciclovir *v* 10.1 days with placebo; $P = 0.04$).[22] The 11th RCT (670 people) found that aciclovir significantly reduced healing time compared with placebo (4.3 days with aciclovir *v* 4.8 with placebo; $P = 0.010$).[23] The 12th RCT (673 people) found that aciclovir significantly reduced healing time compared with placebo (4.6 days with aciclovir *v* 5.2 days with placebo; $P = 0.007$).[23] **Oral antiviral agents:** We found two RCTs.[24,25] The first double blind RCT (174 adults with recurrent herpes labialis) found that oral aciclovir (400 mg five times daily for 5 days) taken early in the attack (when the person first experienced tingling) reduced the duration of symptoms compared with placebo (8.1 days with oral aciclovir *v* 12.5 days with placebo; $P = 0.02$).[24] The second double blind RCT (149 people) compared oral aciclovir taken within 12 hours of the onset of the first episode with placebo.[25] It found no significant difference in healing time or duration of pain between oral aciclovir and placebo (mean healing time: 7.23 days with acyclovir *v* 8.21 days with placebo; P value not reported; mean duration of pain: 1.12 days with acyclovir *v* 1.14 days with placebo; P value not reported).

Harms: See harms under the effects of antiviral treatment for the first attack, p 1893.

Comment: We found no RCTs that compared early versus delayed intervention, so no firm conclusions about timing of treatment can be drawn. Fifteen people in the second RCT later took part in a crossover study in which they received the two forms of aciclovir (in random order) separated by a washout period of at least 1 month.[20] The study found that aciclovir in liposomes significantly reduced the time to crusting of lesions compared with aciclovir cream (1.8 *v* 3.5 days; $P < 0.05$). Too few people in that study experienced pain to analyse statistically the impact of the preparations on discomfort. The 10th RCT was conducted under artificial conditions.[22] A number of the smaller trials that compared topical antiviral agents versus placebo found no significant effect of treatment; however, these studies may have lacked power to detect clinically important differences. No study found that topical antiviral agents were less effective than placebo, and two large RCTs found that topical antiviral agents were significantly more effective than placebo.

OPTION TOPICAL ANAESTHETIC AGENTS

One small RCT found limited evidence that topical tetracaine reduced the mean time to scab loss compared with placebo. However, the clinical importance of this result is unclear.

Benefits: We found no systematic review. One double blind RCT (72 people) found that 1.8% tetracaine (amethocaine) cream applied six times daily until scab loss occurred significantly reduced mean time to scab loss compared with placebo (5.1 days with tetracaine *v* 7.2 days with placebo; $P = 0.002$).[26] It also found that tetracaine cream significantly increased a subjective treatment benefit index (participants rated the benefits of their treatment daily; 1 = no benefit at all; 10 = very effective treatment) compared with placebo (7.3 with tetracaine *v* 5.9 with placebo; $P = 0.036$). However, the clinical importance of these results is unclear.

Harms: None reported.

Comment: See comment under antiviral agents for recurrent attacks, p 1894.

OPTION ZINC OXIDE CREAM

One small RCT found limited evidence that zinc oxide cream reduced time to healing compared with placebo but found that it increased the risk of skin irritation.

Benefits: One double blind RCT (46 people) found that zinc oxide/glycine (applied twice hourly during waking hours as soon as possible after the onset of an attack) significantly reduced time to healing compared with placebo (5.0 days with cream *v* 6.5 days with placebo; $P = 0.018$).[27]

Harms: The RCT reported adverse effects consisting of transient mild to moderate sensations of burning (7 [22%] people with zinc *v* 2 [7%] with placebo), itching (3 [9%] people with zinc *v* 1 [4%] with placebo), stinging (1 [3%] person with zinc *v* 1 [4%] with placebo), and tingling (1 [3%] person with zinc *v* 0 [0%] with placebo).[27] The RCT reported that all adverse effects resolved spontaneously. One person discontinued the active medication because of burning. One person discontinued the placebo because of lack of improvement.

Comment: See comment under antiviral agents for recurrent attacks, p 1894.

Herpes labialis

Substantive changes

Topical antiviral agents Three RCTs (two publications) added;[22,23] recategorised from Unknown effectiveness to Likely to be beneficial.

REFERENCES

1. Hodgkin K. *Towards earlier diagnosis: a guide to general practice*. Edinburgh: Churchill Livingstone, 1973.
2. Baringer SR, Swoveland P. Recovery of herpes simplex virus from human trigeminal ganglions. *N Engl J Med* 1973;288:648–650.
3. Bader C, Crumpacker CS, Schnipner LE, et al. The natural history of recurrent facial-oral infections with the herpes simplex virus. *J Infect Dis* 1978;138:897–905.
4. Spruance SL, Hammil ML, Hoge WS, et al. Acyclovir prevents reactivation of herpes labialis in skiers. *JAMA* 1988;260:1597–1599.
5. Raborn GW, Martel AY, Grace MG, et al. Oral acyclovir in prevention of herpes labialis: a randomized, double-blind, placebo controlled trial. *Oral Surg Oral Med Oral Pathol Oral Radiol Endod* 1998;85:55–59.
6. Rooney JF, Strauss SE, Mannix ML, et al. Oral acyclovir to suppress frequently recurrent herpes labialis: a double-blind, placebo controlled trial. *Ann Intern Med* 1993;118:268–272.
7. Spruance SL, Rowe NH, Raborn GW, et al. Peroral famciclovir in the treatment of experimental ultraviolet radiation-induced herpes simplex labialis: a double-blind, dose-ranging, placebo-controlled, multicenter trial. *J Infect Dis* 1999;179:303–310.
8. Rooney JF, Bryson Y, Mannix ML, et al. Prevention of ultraviolet-light-induced herpes labialis by sunscreen. *Lancet* 1991;338:1419–1421.
9. Duteil L, Queille-Roussel C, Loesche C, et al. Assessment of the effect of a sunblock stick in the prevention of solar-simulating ultraviolet light-induced herpes labialis. *J Dermatol Treat* 1998;9:11–14.
10. Ducoulombier H, Cousin J, DeWilde A, et al. La stomato-gingivite herpetique de l'enfant: essai a contolle aciclovir versus placebo [in French]. *Ann Pediatr* 1988;35:212–216.
11. Amir J, Harel L, Smetana Z, et al. Treatment of herpes simplex gingivostomatitis with aciclovir in children: a randomised double blind placebo controlled trial. *BMJ* 1997;314:1800–1803.
12. Raborn GW, Martel WT, Grace M, et al. Herpes labialis treatment with acyclovir modified aqueous cream: a double-blind randomized trial. *Oral Surg Oral Med Oral Pathol* 1989;67:676–679.
13. Fiddian AP, Ivanyi L. Topical acyclovir in the management of recurrent herpes labialis. *Br J Dermatol* 1983;109:321–326.
14. Smith J, Cowan FM, Munday P. The management of herpes simplex virus infection in pregnancy. *Br J Obstet Gynaecol* 1998;105:255–268. Search date 1996; primary sources Medline and hand searched references.
15. Van Vloten WA, Swart RNJ, Pot F. Topical acyclovir therapy in patients with recurrent orofacial herpes simplex infections. *J Antimicrob Chemother* 1983;12(suppl B):89–93.
16. Shaw M, King M, Best JM, et al. Failure of acyclovir ointment in treatment of recurrent herpes labiais. *BMJ* 1985;291:7–9.
17. Spruance SL, Schnipper LE, Overall JC, et al. Treatment of herpes simplex labialis with topical acyclovir in polyethylene glycol. *J Infect Dis* 1982;146:85–90.
18. Spruance SL, Rea TL, Thoming C, et al. Penciclovir cream for the treatment of herpes simplex labialis. *JAMA* 1997;277:1374–1379.
19. Raborn GW, McGraw WT, Grace MG, et al. Herpes labialis treatment with acyclovir 5 per cent ointment. *Sci J* 1989;55:135–137.
20. Horwitz E, Pisanty S, Czerninski R, et al. A clinical evaluation of a novel liposomal carrier for acyclovir in the topical treatment of recurrent herpes labialis. *Oral Surg Oral Med Oral Pathol Oral Radiol Endod* 1999;87:700–705.
21. Boon R, Goodman JJ, Martinez J, et al. Penciclovir cream for the treatment of sunlight-induced herpes simplex labialis: a randomized, double-blind, placebo-controlled trial. Penciclovir Cream Herpes Labialis Study Group. *Clin Ther* 2000;22:76–90.
22. Evans TG, Bernstein DI, Raborn GW, et al. Double-blind, randomized, placebo-controlled study of topical 5% acyclovir-1% hydrocortisone cream (ME-609) for treatment of UV radiation-induced herpes labialis. Antimicrob Agents Chemother 2002;46:1870–1874.
23. Spruance SL, Nett R, Marbury T, et al. Acyclovir cream for treatment of herpes simplex labialis: results of two randomized, double-blind, vehicle-controlled, multicenter clinical trials. Antimicrob Agents Chemother 2002;46:2238–2243.
24. Spruance SL, Stewart JC, Rowe NH, et al. Treatment of recurrent herpes simplex labialis with oral acyclovir. *J Infect Dis* 1990;161:185–190.
25. Raborn WG, McGraw WT, Grace M, et al. Oral acyclovir and herpes labialis: a randomized, double-blind, placebo-controlled study. *J Am Dental Assoc* 1987;115:38–42.
26. Kaminester LH, Pariser RJ, Pariser DM, et al. A double-blind, placebo-controlled study of topical tetracaine in the treatment of herpes labialis. *J Am Acad Dermatol* 1999;41:996–1001.
27. Godfrey H, Godfrey N, Godfrey J, et al. A randomized clinical trial on the treatment of oral herpes with topical zinc oxide/glycine. *Altern Ther Health Med* 2001;7:49–56.

Bazian Ltd
London
UK

Competing interests: None declared.

The following previous contributor of this topic would also like to be acknowledged: Graham Worrall.

Malignant melanoma (non-metastatic)

Search date February 2003

Philip Savage, Thomas Crosby, and Malcolm Mason

QUESTIONS

INTERVENTIONS

See glossary, p 1905

Key Messages

- **High dose adjuvant alfa interferon** One RCT has found that high dose alfa interferon extends the time to relapse at median follow up of 6.9 years compared with no adjuvant treatment, and may improve overall survival. However, another RCT found no significant difference in relapse rates or overall survival between high dose interferon and no adjuvant treatment. Toxicity (myelosuppression, hepatotoxicity, and neurotoxicity) and withdrawal rates were high.
- **Adjuvant vaccines in people with malignant melanoma** Four RCTs found no significant difference in survival between adjuvant vaccines and surgery alone or surgery plus placebo vaccine in people with malignant melanoma, but they may have been underpowered to detect a clinically important difference.
- **Low dose adjuvant alfa interferon** RCTs found inconsistent evidence on the effects of low dose alfa interferon compared with no adjuvant treatment on relapse free and overall survival. Toxicity occurred in 10% of people.
- **Sunscreens in prevention** We found no RCTs on the preventive effects of sunscreens. One systematic review of case control studies found inconclusive evidence about the effects of sunscreen for preventing malignant melanoma. However, consensus suggests that the appropriate use of sunscreen (to reduce excessive exposure to sunlight rather than to prolong the time spent in the sun) may reduce the risk of developing melanoma.
- **Surveillance to prevent recurrence** We found no RCTs of surveillance to prevent recurrence of malignant melanoma.

Malignant melanoma (non-metastatic)

- **Prophylactic lymph node dissection** One systematic review found no significant difference in survival at 5 years between elective lymph node dissection and delayed or no lymph node dissection in people with malignant melanoma without clinically detectable lymph node metastases.
- **Wide primary excision (no better than narrower excision)** RCTs found no significant difference in local recurrence rates or overall survival over 4–10 years between more radical local surgery (4–5 cm excision margins) and less radical surgery (1–2 cm excision margins). One RCT found that wide compared with narrow excision increased the need for skin grafting and the duration of hospital stay.

DEFINITION Cutaneous malignant melanoma is a tumour derived from melanocytes in the basal layer of the epidermis. After undergoing malignant transformation, the tumour becomes invasive by penetrating into and beyond the dermis.

INCIDENCE/ PREVALENCE Incidence in developed countries has increased by 50% in the past 20 years. Incidence varies in different populations (see table 1, p 1907) and is about 10-fold higher in white than in non-white populations. Despite the rise in incidence, death rates have flattened and even fallen in some populations (e.g. in women and young men in Australia).[1,2] During the same period there has been a sixfold increase in the incidence of melanoma *in situ*, suggesting earlier detection.

AETIOLOGY/ RISK FACTORS The number of common, atypical, and dysplastic naevi on a person's body correlates closely with the risk of developing malignant melanoma. A genetic predisposition probably accounts for 5–10% of all cases. Although the risk of developing malignant melanoma is higher in fair skinned populations living close to the equator, the relation between sun exposure, sunscreen use, and skin type and risk is not clear. Exposure to excessive sunlight and severe sunburn in childhood are associated with an increased risk of developing malignant melanoma in adult life. However, people do not necessarily develop tumours at sites of maximum exposure to the sun.

PROGNOSIS The prognosis of early malignant melanoma (stages I–III) (see table 2, p 1907) relates to the depth of invasion of the primary lesion, the presence of ulceration, and involvement of the regional lymph nodes, with the prognosis worsening with the number of nodes involved.[3] A person with a thin lesion (Breslow thickness [see glossary, p 1905] < 0.75 mm) and without lymph node involvement has a 3% risk of developing metastases and a 95% chance of surviving 5 years.[4] If regional lymph nodes are macroscopically involved then there is a 20–50% chance of surviving 5 years. Most studies have shown a better prognosis in women and in people with lesions on the extremities than in those with lesions on the trunk.

AIMS OF INTERVENTION To prevent melanoma; to detect melanoma earlier; to minimise extent of surgical treatment while still achieving cure of local disease; to optimise quality of life; and to eradicate occult micrometastatic disease, with minimum adverse effects.

OUTCOMES **Prevention:** Incidence of malignant melanoma; mortality from malignant melanoma; rates and severity of sunburn (proxy measure). **Primary excision:** Local recurrence; overall survival; requirement for skin grafting. **Lymph node dissection and adjuvant treatment:** Overall survival; disease free survival; quality of life; morbidity of disease treatment.

METHODS *Clinical Evidence* search and appraisal February 2003, and hand searches of reference lists of all review articles found and of the main oncological and dermatological textbooks performed by the authors in 1998.

QUESTION **What are the effects of interventions to prevent malignant melanoma?**

OPTION **SUNSCREENS**

We found no RCTs on the preventive effects of sunscreens. Systematic reviews of case control studies found inconclusive evidence about the effects of sunscreen use in preventing malignant melanoma. However, consensus suggests that the appropriate use of sunscreen (to reduce excessive exposure to sunlight rather than to prolong the time spent in the sun) may reduce the risk of developing melanoma.

Benefits: We found no RCTs assessing the effects of sunscreens in preventing malignant melanoma (see comment below). One RCT (588 people) found that a sunscreen significantly reduced the incidence or progression of solar keratosis compared with placebo.[5] Another RCT (87 people) found that people who used a sunscreen with a high sun protection factor (SPF 30) spent more hours in the sun than people who used sunscreen with a lower sun protection factor (SPF 10).[6]

Harms: We found no RCTs (see comment below).

Comment: We found two systematic reviews of retrospective cohort studies.[7,8] The first review (search date not stated, 8 case control studies) found conflicting results.[7] Two case control studies (522 people with malignant melanoma, 1039 controls) identified by the review found that people who "regularly" used sunscreen were less likely to develop melanoma than were people who "never" used sunscreen, but three case control studies (831 people with melanoma, 1550 controls) that adjusted for confounding factors (such as fair skin pigmentation, tendency to sunburn, and participation in water sports) found no association between sunscreen use and the development of melanoma. Three case control studies (1389 people with melanoma, 1991 controls) identified by the review found that regular use of sunscreen may be associated with an increased risk of developing melanoma compared with no use.[7] Another three case control studies found no significant difference between sunscreen use and no use in the risk of developing melanoma.[7] The second review (search date 1999, 11 case control studies, including 8 studies identified by the first review and 2 excluded from the first review because of methodological problems, 3681 cases, 5386 controls) found no significant difference in the risk of developing melanoma between people who "regularly", "often", or "always" used sunscreen and people who "never" used sunscreen (RR 1.11, 95% CI 0.37 to 3.32).[8] However, the review suggested that the results should be treated with caution because there was significant heterogeneity among the case control studies, and 8 of the 11 studies found that sunscreen use significantly increased the risk of melanoma compared with no sunscreen use.[8] Case control studies all have potential biases and confounding factors.[5] Although we found no prospective evidence, it would seem reasonable to take sensible precautions to avoid excessive exposure to sunlight, particularly in children and fair skinned individuals. A possible mechanism for the observed association between regular use of sunscreen and increased risk of developing melanoma may be that, because some sunscreens protect predominantly against ultraviolet B (which induces sunburn), people may spend more time exposed to higher doses of ultraviolet A.[6] Consensus suggests that sunscreens may have a role if used appropriately (SPF ≥ 15 and a star rating for ultraviolet A protection of 3–4), rather than being used to prolong the time spent in direct sunlight.

QUESTION Is there an optimal margin for primary excision of melanoma of different Breslow thicknesses?

One systematic review found no significant difference in overall survival over 4–10 years between more radical local surgery (4–5 cm excision margins) and less radical surgery (1–2 cm excision margins). Three RCTs found no significant difference in local recurrence rates between wider and narrower excision margins. One RCT found that wider versus narrower excision increased the need for skin grafting and the duration of hospital stay

Benefits: **Radical local surgery versus less radical surgery:** We found one systematic review (search date 2001, 4 RCTs, 2406 people with stage 1 and II melanoma [see comment below]).[9] It found no significant difference in overall survival at 5 years between narrower (1–2 cm) and wider (4–5 cm) excision margins (4 RCTs: 732/867 [84%] with narrower *v* 796/911 [87%] with wider; OR 0.79, 95% CI 0.61 to 1.04). The review[9] identified four RCTs[10–13] that assessed local recurrence, but it could not perform a meta-analysis for this outcome because of different durations of follow up among the trials (see table 3, p 1908).

Harms: One of the RCTs (612 people) found that narrow (1 cm) margin excision was associated with three local recurrences compared with wide margin excision, all in people with tumours 1–2 mm thick.[10] Local cure was achieved in two people with further surgery. Although not measured in the RCTs, there is potential for psychological and physical morbidity associated with further surgery after local recurrence.

Comment: Three of the RCTs identified by the review were in people with primary tumours of less than 2 mm Breslow thickness (see glossary, p 1905). We found one further RCT published only in abstract form that suggests that reducing the excision margin (from 3 cm to 1 cm) in people with >2 mm primary melanoma may be associated with increased risk of relapse and mortality (Savage P, personal communication, 2003). For current recommended excision margins see table 4, p 1909.[14,15]

QUESTION What are the effects of elective lymph node dissection in people with clinically uninvolved lymph nodes?

One systematic review found no significant difference in survival at 5 years between elective lymph node dissection and delayed or no lymph node dissection in people with malignant melanoma without clinically detectable lymph node metastases, although an effect within particular subgroups cannot be ruled out.

Benefits: We found one systematic review (4 RCTs, 1704 people with stage I and II melanoma with no clinical evidence of lymph node metastases [see comment below]) comparing elective lymph node dissection versus surgery deferred until the time of clinical recurrence.[16] It found no significant difference in mortality at 5 years between elective lymph node dissection and delayed or no lymph node dissection (3 RCTs: 197/768 [26%] with elective dissection *v* 219/765 [29%] with delayed or no dissection; OR 0.86, 95% CI 0.68 to 1.09; see comment below). Retrospective subgroup analyses in the RCTs found non-significant trends in favour of elective lymph node dissection in certain groups of people (those with intermediate thickness tumours, especially those < 60 years of age), but such analyses are subject to bias.[17–20]

Harms: The systematic review gave no information on harms.[16] One retrospective case series found that lymph node dissection was associated with temporary seroma (17%), wound infection (9%), wound necrosis (3%), and lymphoedema (20%).[21]

Comment: In about 20% of people who do not have clinically apparent lymph node involvement, the lymph nodes will contain occult micrometastases. None of the RCTs gave data on morbidity and quality of life in people undergoing lymph node dissection. Sentinel lymph node excision is an alternative to elective lymph node dissection. It involves using a dye or radioactive tracer to identify which nodes are draining the primary lesion. Excision biopsy is then used to determine whether the node is involved with metastatic disease, prior to considering a full lymph node dissection. Sentinel lymph node excision is currently being evaluated in clinical trials (Crosby T, personal communication, 2001).

QUESTION What are the effects of adjuvant treatment?

OPTION ALFA INTERFERON

One RCT has found that adjuvant treatment with high dose alfa interferon extends the time to relapse at median follow up of 6.9 years compared with no adjuvant treatment, and may improve overall survival. However, another RCT found no significant difference in relapse free or overall survival between high dose interferon and no adjuvant treatment. One

RCT found that high dose alfa interferon improved both relapse free and overall survival compared with ganglioside GM2 vaccine. RCTs found inconsistent evidence on the effects of low dose interferon compared with no adjuvant treatment on relapse free and overall survival. Toxicity (myelosuppression, hepatotoxicity, and neurotoxicity) and withdrawal rates were high.

Benefits: We found one systematic review[22] (search date 2001, 8 RCTs,[23–30] 3178 people) and one additional RCT[31] comparing high or low dose interferon alfa versus no adjuvant treatment, and one RCT comparing high dose interferon versus ganglioside GM2 vaccine.[32] The review could not perform a meta-analysis because of heterogeneity among the trials in dose and duration of interferon and stage of disease of participants.[22] **High dose versus no adjuvant treatment (observation):** The systematic review[22] identified two RCTs.[23,25] The first RCT (280 people with resectable stage IIB [primary lesions > 4 mm] or stage III melanoma) identified by the review compared high dose alfa interferon (20 MU/m^2/day iv for 1 month, followed by 10 MU/m^2 sc 3 times/week for 11 months) versus observation.[23] At a median follow up of 6.9 years, it found that alfa interferon significantly improved disease free survival (median 1.7 *v* 1.0 years; P = 0.023) and overall survival (median 3.8 *v* 2.8 years; P = 0.0237) compared with observation.[23] Retrospective subgroup analysis found prolonged quality of life adjusted survival in people receiving alfa interferon.[33] The clinical importance of this gain varied with the values assigned by people in the trial for the impact of treatment related toxicity and the impact of time with relapsed disease. The second RCT (262 people with completely resected stage I and II melanoma, primary tumours > 0.7 mm, lymph node negative) identified by the review compared high dose interferon (20 MU/m^2 im 3 times/week for 12 weeks) versus observation and found no significant difference in disease free survival (mean 2.4 years with alfa interferon *v* 2.2 years with observation; P = 0.19) or overall survival (median 6.6 years with alfa interferon *v* 5.0 years with observation; P = 0.40).[25] **High dose versus ganglioside GM2 vaccine:** We found one RCT (880 people with resected stage IIB and III melanoma) comparing high dose interferon (20 MU/m^2 iv 5 times/week for 4 weeks plus 10 MU/m^2 sc 3 times/week for 48 weeks) versus ganglioside GM2 vaccine.[32] It found that, compared with ganglioside vaccine, alfa interferon significantly improved both relapse free survival (98/385 [25%] with alfa interferon *v* 151/389 [39%] with ganglioside; HR 1.47, 95% CI 1.14 to 1.90) and overall survival (52/385 [14%] *v* 81/389 [21%]; HR 1.52, 95% CI 1.07 to 2.15) over a median follow up of 16 months. **Low dose versus no adjuvant treatment:** The review identified five RCTs,[26–30] and we found one additional RCT.[31] Three of the RCTs identified by the review were in people with stage II melanoma (primary tumours > 1.5 mm and lymph node negative).[26,27,29] The first RCT (489 people with stage II melanoma) identified by the review comparing low dose alfa interferon (3 MU sc 3 times/week for 18 months) versus no adjuvant treatment found that alfa interferon significantly increased relapse free survival over a median 5 years (HR 0.75, 95% CI 0.57 to 0.98; P = 0.035).[26] It found that overall survival rates after a median 5 years were higher with alfa interferon than with no adjuvant treatment, but the difference did not quite reach significance (HR 0.72, 95% CI 0.51 to 1.00; P = 0.059). The second RCT (311 people with stage II melanoma) identified by the review compared low dose alfa interferon (3 MU/day sc for 3 weeks and 3 times/week for 12 months) versus no adjuvant treatment after excision of the primary tumour.[27] At 41 months' follow up it found that alfa interferon significantly prolonged relapse free survival compared with no adjuvant treatment (P = 0.02). It found no significant difference in overall survival over 41 months between alfa interferon and no adjuvant treatment, but it may have been too small to exclude a clinically important difference (17/154 [11%] with alfa interferon *v* 21/157 [13%] with no adjuvant treatment; RR 0.82, 95% CI 0.45 to 1.50). The third RCT (654 people with stage II melanoma) identified by the review, published only in abstract form, found no significant difference in relapse free survival (P = 0.2) or overall survival (P = 1.0) at 4 years between low dose interferon (3 MU 3 times/week for 2 years or until recurrence) and observation.[29] The fourth RCT (96 people with stage II or III melanoma, primary tumours ≥ 3 mm Breslow thickness (see glossary, p 1905), or evidence of regional node involvement) identified by the review found no significant difference in relapse free survival or overall survival at a median follow up of 6 years between interferon (3 MU sc 3 times/week for 6 months) and observation, but it may have lacked power to exclude a clinically important difference.[30] The fifth RCT (424 people with stage III melanoma, lymph node metastases) compared low dose interferon (3 MU sc 3 times/week for 3 years) versus no adjuvant treatment.[28] It found no significant difference between low dose interferon and no adjuvant treatment in relapse free survival (28.4% with interferon *v* 27.5% with no adjuvant treatment; P = 0.50) or overall survival at 5 years (37% with interferon *v* 37% with no adjuvant treatment; P = 0.72). The additional RCT (830 people with stage II or III melanoma, primary tumours > 3 mm or lymph node involvement), published only as an abstract, compared low dose gamma or alfa interferon versus no adjuvant treatment for 12 months and found no significant difference in disease free survival (RR alfa interferon *v* no treatment 0.9, 95% CI 0.75 to 1.18; absolute numbers not provided) or overall survival at 6 years (reported as non-significant; no further data provided).[31] **High or low dose versus no adjuvant treatment:** One RCT (642 people with stage II or III primary or recurrent nodal involvement) identified by the review compared three interventions: high dose alfa interferon (20 MU/m^2/day iv 5 days/week for 1 month, followed by 10 MU/m^2 sc 3 times/week for 11 months); low dose alfa interferon (3 MU/m^2/day sc 3 times/week for 2 years); or observation.[24] It found that high dose interferon marginally but significantly improved relapse free survival over 5 years compared with observation (HR 1.28, 95% CI 1.00 to 1.65), but found no significant difference in overall survival (HR 1.0, 95% CI 0.75 to 1.33). It found no significant difference between low dose interferon and observation in relapse free survival (HR 1.19, 95% CI 0.93 to 1.53) or overall survival (HR 1.04, 95% CI 0.78 to 1.38) over 5 years.[24]

Malignant melanoma (non-metastatic)

Harms: Interferons commonly cause malaise, fevers, and flu-like symptoms. **High dose versus no adjuvant treatment (observation):** In the first RCT identified by the review, high dose alfa interferon also caused significant (> grade 3) myelosuppression in 24% of people, hepatotoxicity in 15% (including 2 deaths), and neurotoxicity in 28%. At 11 months, only 25% of participants were receiving more than 80% of the planned dose.[23] **Low dose versus no adjuvant treatment:** In the first RCT identified by the review, 10% of people taking low dose interferon suffered significant toxicity.[26] The fifth RCT identified by the review found that 162/225 (72%) taking low dose alfa interferon developed World Health Organization (WHO) grade 1 toxicity,[34] 54/225 (24%) WHO grade 2 toxicity, and 9/225 (4%) no toxicity.[28]

Comment: RCTs investigating the effects of sustained release pegylated alfa interferon are underway (Savage P, personal communication, 2003).

OPTION VACCINES

Four RCTs found no significant difference in survival between adjuvant vaccines and surgery alone or surgery plus placebo vaccine in people with malignant melanoma, but they may have been underpowered to detect a clinically important difference.

Benefits: Four RCTs found no significant difference in survival between adjuvant vaccines and surgery alone or surgery plus placebo vaccine, but may have been underpowered to detect a clinically important difference.[35–38] The first RCT (700 people with stage IIB or III primary or recurrent nodal involvement) compared adjuvant vaccine (prepared from vaccinia melanoma cell lysates) versus surgery alone.[35] It found no significant difference between adjuvant vaccine and surgery alone in relapse free survival (51% with adjuvant treatment *v* 47% with no treatment) or overall survival (60% with adjuvant treatment *v* 55% with no treatment; reported as non-significant, CI not stated) at 5 years or 10 years. The second RCT (689 people with completely resected stage II melanoma, primary tumour 1.5–4 mm Breslow thickness [see glossary, p 1905]) found no significant difference in relapse free survival at 5 years between adjuvant vaccine (allogeneic melanoma cell lysate) and surgery alone (66% with vaccine *v* 62% with no vaccine; P = 0.17).[36] The third RCT (217 people with resected stage III melanoma) compared adjuvant vaccinia melanoma oncosylate versus placebo vaccine (vaccinia virus).[37] Over 5 years, it found no significant difference between adjuvant melanoma vaccine and placebo vaccine in disease free survival (P = 0.61) or overall survival (P = 0.79, absolute results presented graphically). The fourth RCT (38 people with resected stage III melanoma) compared polyvalent melanoma vaccine versus placebo vaccine (human albumin).[38] It found that melanoma vaccine significantly increased time to recurrence compared with placebo vaccine (1.6 years with vaccine *v* 0.6 years with placebo vaccine; P = 0.03), but found no significant difference in overall survival at 3 years (53% with vaccine *v* 33% with placebo vaccine; reported as non-significant, CI not stated).

Harms: The first RCT found that melanoma vaccine was associated with erythema and ulceration at the injection site (47% of people), malaise (35%), and fever (20%).[35] The second RCT found that most people receiving melanoma vaccine had mild to moderate adverse effects and that 26 (9%) of people had severe adverse effects, including malaise, fatigue, visual complaints, fever, diarrhoea, thrombocytopenia, or skin rash.[36] The third RCT found that both melanoma vaccine and placebo vaccine were associated with erythema, swelling and tenderness at the injection site, headache, nausea, and fever.[37] The fourth RCT found that both vaccine and placebo vaccine were associated with skin reactions but found no other adverse effects.[38]

Comment: A different vaccine preparation was used in each RCT, making the results difficult to generalise.[35–38] More RCTs of vaccines and other active specific immunostimulants are needed.

OPTION SURVEILLANCE

We found no RCTs of surveillance to prevent recurrence of malignant melanoma.

Benefits: We found no systematic review or RCTs (see comment below).

Harms: We found no RCTs.

Comment: Retrospective studies found that people presented with symptomatic recurrent malignant melanoma regardless of whether they were taking part in an intensive follow up programme.[39] Thinner lesions (< 0.75 mm) may require longer surveillance because recurrence peaks at 5–10 years.[40]

GLOSSARY

Breslow thickness The vertical depth (in mm) to which the tumour has penetrated.

Substantive changes

Sunscreens One systematic review added;[8] conclusions unchanged.
Optimal excision margin One systematic review added;[9] conclusions unchanged.
Adjuvant vaccines One RCT added;[35] conclusions unchanged.

REFERENCES

1. International Agency for Research on Cancer. *Globocan 2000: cancer incidence, mortality and prevalence worldwide, version 1.0. IARC CancerBase No. 5*. Lyon: IARC Press, 2001.
2. Giles GG, Armstrong BK, Burton RC, et al. Has mortality from melanoma stopped rising in Australia? Analysis of trends between 1931 and 1994. *BMJ* 1996;312:1121–1125.
3. Balch CM, Buzaid AC, Soong SJ, et al. Final version of the American Joint Committee on Cancer staging system for cutaneous melanoma. *J Clin Oncol* 2001;19:3635–3648.
4. Balch CM, Smalley RV, Bartolucci AA, et al. A randomised prospective clinical trial of adjuvant *C. parvum* immunotherapy in 260 patients with clinically localized melanoma (stage I): prognostic factor analysis and preliminary results of immunotherapy. *Cancer* 1982;49:1079–1084.
5. Thompson SC, Jolley D, Marks R. Reduction of solar keratoses by regular sunscreen use. *N Engl J Med* 1993;329:1147–1151.
6. Autier P, Dore JF, Negrier S, et al. Sunscreen use and duration of sun exposure: a double-blind, randomized trial. *J Natl Cancer Inst* 1999;91:1304–1309.
7. Bastuji-Garin S, Diepgen TL. Cutaneous malignant melanoma, sun exposure, and sunscreen use: epidemiological evidence. *Br J Dermatol* 2002;146:24–30.Search date and primary sources not stated.
8. Huncharek M, Kupelnick B. Use of topical sunscreens and the risk of malignant melanoma: a meta-analysis of 9067 patients from 11 case-control studies. *Am J Public Health* 2002;92:1173–1177. Search date 1999, primary sources Medline, Cancerlit, Current Contents, and hand searches of bibliographies of published reports, review articles and textbooks.
9. Lens MB, Dawes M, Goodacre T, Bishop JA. Excision margins in the treatment of primary cutaneous melanoma: a systematic review of randomized controlled trials comparing narrow vs wide excision. *Arch Surg* 2002;137:1101–1105.
10. Veronesi U, Cascinelli N, Adamus J, et al. Thin stage I primary cutaneous malignant melanoma: comparison of excision with margins of 1 or 3 cm. *N Engl J Med* 1988;318:1159–1162.
11. Balch CM, Urist MM, Karakousis CP, et al. Efficacy of 2 cm surgical margins for

intermediate-thickness melanomas (1 to 4 mm): results of a multi-institutional randomized surgical trial. *Ann Surg* 1993;218:262–267.
12. Cohn-Cedermark G, Rutqvist LE, Andersson R, et al. Long term results of a randomized study by the Swedish melanoma study group on 2- versus 5 cm resection margins for patients with cutaneous melanoma with a tumour thickness of 0.8–2.0 mm. *Cancer* 2000;89:1495–1501.
13. Banzet P, Thomas A, Vuillemin E, et al. Wide versus narrow surgical excision in thin (*Proc Am Soc Clin Oncol* 1993;12:1320.
14. American Academy of Dermatology Association. Practice management: guidelines of care for primary cutaneous melanoma. American Academy of Dermatology Association, 2001. http://www.aadssociation.org/Guidelines/CutaneousMel.html (last accessed 25 June 2003).
15. European Society for Medical Oncology Guidelines Task Force. Minimal clinical recommendations for diagnosis, treatment and follow-up of cutaneous malignant melanoma. Lugano, Switzerland: European Society for Medical Oncology Guidelines Task Force, 2002. http://www.esmo.org/reference/referenceGuidelines/pdf/ESMO_17_cutaneous_malignant_melanoma.pdf (last accessed 25 June 2003).
16. Lens MB, Dawes M, Goodacre T, et al. Elective lymph node dissection in patients with melanoma: systematic review and meta-analysis of randomised controlled trials. *Arch Surg* 2002;137:458–461.
17. Balch CM, Soong SJ, Bartolucci AA, et al. Efficacy of an elective regional lymph node dissection of 1–4 mm thick melanomas for patients 60 years of age and younger. *Ann Surg* 1996;224:255–263.
18. Cascinelli N, Morabito A, Santinami M, et al. Immediate or delayed dissection of regional nodes in patients with melanoma of the trunk: a randomised trial. WHO Melanoma Programme. *Lancet* 1998;351:793–796.
19. Sim FH, Taylor WF, Ivins JC, et al. A prospective randomized study of the efficacy of routine elective lymphadenectomy in management of malignant melanoma: preliminary results. *Cancer* 1978;41:948–956.
20. Veronesi U, Adamus J, Bandiera DC, et al. Inefficacy of immediate node dissection in stage I melanoma of the limbs. *N Engl J Med* 1977;297:627–630.
21. Baas PC, Schraffordt KH, Koops H, et al. Groin dissection in the treatment of lower-extremity melanoma: short-term and long-term morbidity. *Arch Surg* 1992;127:281–286.
22. Lens MB, Dawes M. Interferon alfa therapy for malignant melanoma: a systematic review of randomised controlled trials. *J Clin Oncol* 2002;20:1818–1825.
23. Kirkwood JM, Strawderman MH, Erstoff MS, et al. Interferon alfa-2_b adjuvant therapy of high-risk resected cutaneous melanoma: the Eastern Cooperative Oncology Group trial EST 1684. *J Clin Oncol* 1996;14:7–17.
24. Kirkwood JM, Ibrahim JG, Sondak VK. High- and low-dose interferon Alfa-2_b in high risk melanoma: first analysis of intergroup trial E1690/S9111/C9190. *J Clin Oncol* 2000;18:2444–2458.
25. Creagan ET, Dalton RJ, Ahmann DL. Randomized, surgical adjuvant clinical trial of recombinant interferon alfa-2_b in selected patients with malignant melanoma. *J Clin Oncol* 1995;13:2776–2783.
26. Grob JJ, Dreno B, de la Salmoniere P, et al. Randomised trial of interferon alpha-2_a as adjuvant therapy in resected primary melanoma thicker than 1.5 mm without clinically detectable node metastases. French cooperative group on melanoma. *Lancet* 1998;351:1905–1910.
27. Pehamberger H, Peter Soyer H, Steiner A, et al. Adjuvant interferon alfa-2_a treatment in resected primary stage II cutaneous melanoma. *J Clin Oncol* 1998;16:1425–1429.
28. Cascinelli N, Belli F, Mackie RM, et al. Effect of long-term therapy with interferon alpha-2a in patients with regional node metastases from cutaneous melanoma: a randomised trial. *Lancet* 2001;358:866–869.
29. Hancock BW, Wheatley K, Harrison G, et al. Aim high adjuvant interferon in melanoma (high risk), a United Kingdom Co-ordinating Committee on Cancer Research (UKCCCR) randomised study of observation versus adjuvant low dose extended duration interferon alfa 2_a in high risk resected malignant melanoma. *Proc Am Soc Clin Oncol* 2001;20:1393.
30. Cameron DA, Cornbleet MC, Mackie RM, et al. Adjuvant interferon alpha 2b in high risk melanoma — the Scottish study. *Br J Cancer* 2001;84:1146–1149.
31. Kleeberg UR, Brocker EB, Lejeune F. Adjuvant trial in melanoma patients comparing rIFN-alfa to rIFN-gamma to Iscador to a control group after curative resection high risk primary (> 3 mm) or regional lymph node metastasis (EORTC 18871). *Eur J Cancer* 1999;35:S82.
32. Kirkwood JM, Ibrahim JG, Sosman JA, et al. High-dose interferon alfa2_b significantly prolongs relapse-free and overall survival compared with GM2-KLH/QS-21 vaccine in patients with resected stage IIB–III melanoma: results of the intergroup trial E1694/S9512/C509801. *J Clin Oncol* 2001;19:2370–2380.
33. Cole BF, Gelber RD, Kirkwood JM, et al. Quality-of-life-adjusted survival analysis of high-risk resected cutaneous melanoma: the Eastern Cooperative Oncology Group study. *J Clin Oncol* 1996;14:2666–2673.
34. Miller AB, Hoogstraten B, Staquet M, et al. Reporting results of cancer treatment. *Cancer* 1981;47:207–214.
35. Hersey P, Coates AS, McCarthy WH, et al. Adjuvant immunotherapy of patients with high-risk melanoma using vaccinia viral lysates of melanoma: results of a randomized trial. *J Clin Oncol* 2002;20:4181–4190.
36. Sondak VK, Liu PY, Tuthill RJ, et al. Adjuvant immunotherapy of resected, intermediate-thickness, node-negative melanoma with an allogeneic tumor vaccine: overall results of a randomized trial of the Southwest Oncology Group. *J Clin Oncol* 2002;20:2058–2066.
37. Wallack MK, Sivanandham M, Balch CM, et al. Surgical adjuvant active specific immunotherapy for patients with stage III melanoma: the final analysis of data from a phase III, randomized, double-blind, multicenter vaccinia melanoma oncolysate trial. *J Am Coll Surg* 1998;187:69–77.
38. Bystryn JC, Zeleniuch-Jacquotte A, Oratz R, et al. Double-blind trial of a polyvalent, shed-antigen, melanoma vaccine. *Clin Cancer Res* 2001;7:1882–1887.
39. Shumate CR, Urist MM, Maddox WA. Melanoma recurrence surveillance: patient or physician based? *Ann Surg* 1995;221:566–559.
40. Rogers GS, Kopf AW, Rigel DS, et al. Hazard-rate analysis in stage I malignant melanoma. *Arch Dermatol* 1986;122:999–1002.

Malignant melanoma (non-metastatic)

Thomas Crosby
Consultant Clinical Oncologist

Malcolm Mason
Professor of Clinical Oncology

Philip Savage
Consultant in Medical Oncology

Velindre Hospital
Cardiff
UK

Competing interests: None declared.

TABLE 1 **Melanoma incidence and mortality in different populations (see text, p 1898).[1]**

	New cases/year	ASR/100 000	Deaths/year	ASR/100 000
World	132 602	2.4	37 047	0.75
Australia	8706	40.51	950	4.8
China	2418	0.22	1390	0.13
India	2187	0.34	1274	0.17
UK	5773	6.14	1564	1.81
USA	40 646	13.27	7791	2.74

Reproduced with permission of IARCPress. GLOBOCAN 2000: Cancer Incidence, Mentality and Prevalence Worldwide, Version 1.0 IARC CancerBase No. 5. Lyon IARCPress, 2000 (http://www.iarc.fr)

TABLE 2 **Stage of malignant melanoma and 5 year survival (see text, p 1898).[3]**

Stage	Description	5 year survival (%)
IA	Primary tumour < 1 mm no ulceration	95
IB	Primary tumour < 1 mm with ulceration or 1–2 mm with no ulceration	90
IIA	Primary tumour 1–2 mm with ulceration or 2–4 mm with no ulceration	78
IIB	Primary tumour 2–4 mm with ulceration or >4 mm with no ulceration	63–67
IIC	Primary tumour >4 mm with ulceration	45
IIIA	Microscopic nodal involvement	63–70
IIIB	Microscopic nodal involvement	46–59
IV	Distant metastases	6.7–18.8

*In transit metastasis, a metastasis located between the primary tumour and the closest lymph node region. Reprinted with permission from the American Society of Clinical Oncology. Balch CM, Buzaid AC, Soong SJ et al. final version of the American Joint Committee of Cancer staging system for cutaneous melanoma. [Review][83 refs] Journal of Clinical Oncology. 19(16): 3635–48, 2001 Aug 15.

TABLE 3 RCTs for assessing radical versus less radical local surgery for malignant melanoma (see text, p 1900).[10–13]

Ref	Randomisation	Excision margin	Population	Relapse rates	Overall survival
10	Sealed envelopes, stratified blocks according to centre and previous treatment	(a) 1 cm margin (b) 3 cm margin	International multicentre RCT, 612 people with lesions < 2 mm thick	Local recurrence: 3/321 (1%) with 1 mm margin *v* 0/272 (0%) with 3 mm margin Regional node metastases as first relapse: 14/305 (5%) with 1 mm margin *v* 20/307 (7%) with 3 mm margin Distant metastases: 7/321 (2%) with 1 mm margin *v* 8/272 (3%) with 3 mm margin	4 year actuarial survival rate: 96.8% (305 people) with 1 cm margin *v* 96.0 (307 people) with 3 cm margin; P = 0.66
11	Strategy not described	(a) 2 cm margin (b) 2 cm margin plus elective node dissection (c) 4 cm margin (d) 4 cm margin plus elective node dissection	Multicentre RCT, 486 people in USA with 1–4 mm thickness lesion and no evidence of metastatic melanoma	Recurrence at median follow up of 72 months: 2/242 (0.8%) with 2 cm margin *v* 4/244 (1.7%) with 4 cm margin; P = NS A subgroup of all these people had elective node dissection as a co-intervention	Overall 5 year survival: 79.5% with 2 cm margin *v* 83.7% with 4 cm margin; P = NS
12	Telephone allocation using randomisation lists	(a) 2 cm margin (b) 5 cm margin	Multicentre RCT, 989 people in Sweden, with lesions 0.8–2.0 mm, followed for a median time of 11 years for survival, and 8 years for recurrence	First event local recurrence: 1/476 (0.2%) with 2 cm margin *v* 4/513 (1%) with 5 cm margin Distant metastases: 24/479 (5%) with 2 cm margin *v* 34/513 (7%) with 5 cm margin; HR 0.76, 95% CI 0.45 to 1.28; P = 0.29	Overall survival at a median of 8 year follow up: 117/476 (25%) with 2 cm margin: 134/513 (26%) with 5 cm margin; HR 0.96, 95% CI 0.75 to 1.24; P = 0.77
13	Not described	(a) 2 cm margin (b) 5 cm margin	Multicentre RCT, 319 people in Europe, with lesions < 2 mm, followed for a median 50 months	Recurrence: 14/153 (9%) with 2 cd margin *v* 21/166 (13%) with 5 cm margin; P = 0.31	Overall 5 year survival: 93% with 2 cm margin *v* 90% with 5 cm margin; P = 0.57

NS, not significant; Ref, reference.

TABLE 4 **Recommended clinical excision margins.**[14,15]

Tumour thickness *in situ*	Clinical excision margins
	0.5 cm
mm	1 cm
≥2 mm	2 cm

Reprinted from Sober AJ, Chuang TY, Duvic M. Guidelines of care for primary cutaneous melanoma. *J Am Acad Deratol* 2001;45:597–586. © 2001, with permission from the american acaemy of Dermatology, Inc.

Scabies

Search date January 2003

Godfrey Walker and Paul Johnstone

QUESTIONS

INTERVENTIONS

Key Messages

- **Permethrin** One systematic review has found that permethrin increases clinical and parasitic cure after 28 days compared with crotamiton. The systematic review found conflicting results with permethrin versus lindane. One subsequent RCT found limited evidence that permethrin increased clinical cure at 14 days compared with ivermectin.
- **Crotamiton** One systematic review found that crotamiton was less successfil in terms of clinical and parasite cure after 28 days compared with permethrin. One systematic review identified one RCT that found no significant difference between crotamiton and lindane in clinical cure rates at 28 days.
- **Oral ivermectin** One systematic review identified one RCT that found that ivermectin increased clinical cure rates after 7 days compared with placebo. Another small RCT identified by the review found no significant difference between ivermectin and benzyl benzoate in clinical cure rates at 30 days. One subsequent RCT found that, compared with benzyl benzoate, ivermectin increased clinical cure rates at 30 days. One systematic review identified one small RCT that found no significant difference between ivermectin and lindane in cure rates at 15 days. One subsequent RCT found no significant difference between ivermectin and lindane in failed clinical cure rates at 2 weeks, but it found that ivermectin decreased failed clinical cure rates at 4 weeks. One RCT found limited evidence that ivermectin reduced clinical cure rates at 14 days compared with permethrin. Experience suggests oral ivermectin is safe in younger adults being treated for onchocerciasis, but no such experience exists for children, and there have been reports of increased risk of death in elderly people.

Clin Evid 2003;10:1910–1918.

- **Lindane** One systematic review identified one RCT that found no significant difference between lindane and crotamiton in clinical cure rates at 28 days. The systematic review found conflicting results between lindane and permethrin after 28 days. Another small RCT identified by the review found no significant difference between lindane and ivermectin in cure rates at 15 days. One subsequent RCT found no significant difference between lindane and ivermectin in failed clinical cure rates at 2 weeks, but it found a higher proportion of people with failed clinical cure with lindane compared with ivermectin at 4 weeks. We found reports of rare, serious adverse effects such as convulsions.
- **Benzyl benzoate** One systematic review identified one small RCT that found no significant difference between benzyl benzoate and ivermectin in clinical cure rates at 30 days. One subsequent RCT found that benzyl benzoate reduced clinical cure at 30 days compared with ivermectin. One systematic review identified one RCT that found no significant difference between benzyl benzoate and sulphur ointment in clinical cure at 8 or 14 days.
- **Malathion** One systematic review found no RCTs on the effects of malathion. Case series have reported cure rates in scabies of over 80%.
- **Sulphur compounds** One systematic review identified one RCT that found no significant difference between sulphur ointment and benzyl benzoate in clinical cure at 8 or 14 days.

DEFINITION Scabies is an infestation of the skin by the mite *Sarcoptes scabiei*.[1] Typical sites of infestation are skin folds and flexor surfaces. In adults, the most common sites are between the fingers and on the wrists, although infection may manifest in elderly people as a diffuse truncal eruption. In infants and children, the face, scalp, palms, and soles are also often affected.

INCIDENCE/ PREVALENCE Scabies is a common public health problem with an estimated prevalence of 300 million cases worldwide, mostly affecting people in developing countries, where prevalence can exceed 50%.[2] In industrialised countries it is most common in institutionalised communities. Case studies suggest that epidemic cycles occur every 7–15 years and that these partly reflect the population's immune status.

AETIOLOGY/ RISK FACTORS Scabies is particularly common where there is social disruption, overcrowding with close body contact, and limited access to water.[3] Young children, immobilised elderly people, people with HIV/AIDS, and other medically and immunologically compromised people are predisposed to infestation and have particularly high mite counts.[4]

PROGNOSIS Scabies is not life threatening, but the severe, persistent itch and secondary infections may be debilitating. Occasionally, crusted scabies develops. This form of the disease is resistant to routine treatment and can be a source of continued reinfestation and spread to others. A search conducted by the author found no reports of spontaneous remission.

AIMS OF INTERVENTION To eliminate the scabies mites and ova from the skin; to cure pruritus (itching); to prevent reinfestation; to prevent spread to other people.

OUTCOMES **Clinical cure:** Number of visible burrows and papular and vesicular eruptions; pruritus. **Parasitic cure:** Presence of mites, ova, or faecal pellets in skin scrapings under a magnifying lens or microscope. Outcomes should be assessed 28–30 days after the start of treatment, which is the time it takes for lesions to heal and for any eggs and mites to reach maturity if treatment fails.

METHODS *Clinical Evidence* search and appraisal January 2003.

QUESTION **What are the effects of topical treatments?**

OPTION **PERMETHRIN**

One systematic review has found that permethrin increases clinical and parasitic cure after 28 days compared with crotamiton. The systematic review found conflicting results between permethrin and lindane. One subsequent RCT found limited evidence that permethrin increased clinical cure at 14 days compared with ivermectin.

Benefits: We found no RCTs that compared permethrin versus placebo. We found one systematic review (search date 1999, 6 RCTs)[5] and one subsequent RCT[6] comparing permethrin versus other topical and oral agents. **Versus crotamiton:** The review (2 RCTs, 194 people) found that permethrin compared with crotamiton significantly increased clinical cure rates after 28 days (2 RCTs; OR for failed clinical cure with permethrin *v* crotamiton 0.21, 95% CI 0.10 to 0.47) and significantly increased parasitic cure after 28 days (1 RCT; 94 people; OR for failed parasitic cure with permethrin *v* crotamiton 0.21, 95% CI 0.08 to 0.53).[5] It found no significant difference between permethrin and crotamiton in self reported pruritus (1 RCT: OR for itch persistence with permethrin *v* with crotamiton 0.38, 95% CI 0.12 to 1.19). **Versus lindane:** The systematic review identified four RCTs that compared permethrin with lindane.[5] Overall, the review found that permethrin appeared to be more effective than lindane in clinical cure after 28 days. However, it found significant trial heterogeneity ($P < 0.005$). Two RCTs (100 people; 52 people) included in the review found that permethrin compared with lindane significantly reduced clinical failure (OR for failed clinical cure of permethrin *v* lindane 0.14, 95% CI 0.05 to 0.43; and 0.19, 95% CI 0.05 to 0.70) whereas two RCTs (99 people; 467 people), including the largest RCT, found no significant difference between permethrin and lindane (OR for failed clinical cure of permethrin *v* lindane 0.8, 95% CI 0.21 to 3.14; and 0.93, 95% CI 0.60 to 1.42).[5] **Versus oral ivermectin:** We found one subsequent RCT that compared topical permethrin versus oral ivermectin.[6] The RCT (85 people attending an outpatient clinic in India) assessed clinical cure at 14 days, and if not assessed as completely cured at that time the same treatment was repeated. It found that permethrin significantly decreased failed clinical cure rate at 14 days compared with ivermectin (OR for failed clinical cure of permethrin *v* ivermectin 0.12, 95% CI 0.04 to 0.39).

Harms: One RCT identified by the review reported five people with adverse effects: two in the permethrin group (rash and possible diarrhoea) and three in the lindane group (pruritic rash, papules, and diarrhoea).[7] During 1990–1995, six adverse events were reported per 100 000 units distributed in the USA (1 central nervous system adverse effect reported per 500 000 units of permethrin distributed).[8] Resistance to permethrin seems to be rare[8] (see harms of lindane, p 1913).

Comment: None.

OPTION LINDANE

One systematic review identified one RCT that found no significant difference between lindane and crotamiton in clinical cure rates at 28 days. The systematic review found conflicting results with lindane compared with permethrin after 28 days. Another small RCT identified by the review found no significant difference between lindane and ivermectin in cure rates at 15 days. One subsequent RCT found no significant difference between lindane and ivermectin in failed clinical cure rates at 2 weeks, but found a higher proportion of people with failed clinical cure with lindane than with ivermectin at 4 weeks. We found reports of rare, serious adverse effects such as convulsions.

Benefits: We found no RCTs comparing lindane versus placebo. We found one systematic review (search date 1999, 6 RCTs)[5] comparing lindane versus other topical and oral agents, and one subsequent RCT comparing lindane versus ivermectin.[9] **Versus crotamiton:** One RCT (100 adults and children) identified by the review found no significant difference in clinical cure rates at 28 days (OR for failed clinical cure with crotamiton *v* lindane 0.41, 95% CI 0.15 to 1.10).[5] However, confidence intervals are broad and a clinically important difference cannot be ruled out. **Versus permethrin:** See benefits of permethrin, p 1912. **Versus oral ivermectin:** One RCT[10] (53 adults referred to hospital with scabies) identified by the review found no significant difference between lindane and ivermectin in clinical cure rates at 15 days (failed clinical cure 14/27 [52%] with lindane *v* 12/26 [46%] with oral ivermectin; RR 0.89, 95% CI 0.51 to 1.55).[5] One subsequent RCT compared topical lindane versus ivermectin.[9] It found no significant difference in failed clinical cure rates between lindane and ivermectin at 2 weeks (failed clinical cure rate 70/100 [70%] with ivermectin *v* 81/100 [81%] with lindane; RR 0.86, 95% CI 0.74 to 1.01) but it found that ivermectin significantly increased clinical cure rates at 4 weeks compared with lindane (failed clinical cure rate 43/100 [43%] with ivermectin *v* 64/100 [64%] with lindane; RR 0.67, 95% CI 0.51 to 0.88).

Harms: One RCT identified by the review reported five people with adverse effects: two in the permethrin group (rash and possible diarrhoea) and three in the lindane group (pruritic rash, papules, and diarrhoea).[7] One RCT identified by the review reported that six people taking lindane had headaches, and one person each had headache, hypotension, abdominal pain, and vomiting in the ivermectin group.[10] Case reports have reported rare severe adverse effects (e.g. convulsions, other long term neurological complications, and aplastic anaemia) particularly when lindane was applied to people with extensive skin diseases and to children.[11–13] Figures from the World Health Organization Collaborating Centre for International Drug Monitoring covering summary reports from 47 countries suggest that lindane is more toxic than other preparations (see comment below).[14] Five convulsions were reported in people on benzyl benzoate, two in people on crotamiton, 48 in people on lindane, two in people on malathion, and 19 in people on permethrin. Deaths reported on benzyl benzoate were none, crotamiton one, lindane four, malathion none, and permethrin five.[14] Resistance to lindane has been reported in many countries.[15]

Comment: Lindane was withdrawn from the market in the UK in 1995 because of concern about possible adverse effects. The evidence linking lindane with convulsions is suggestive but not conclusive.[11–14] It is difficult to draw firm conclusions on the relative occurrence of severe adverse effects of different preparations reported to the World Health Organization Collaborating Centre for International Drug Monitoring because of incomplete information on incidence in relation to use; however, lindane and permethrin appear possibly to be more likely to be related to rare severe adverse effects. Safety results from trials and observational studies need to be summarised, particularly regarding additional risks in infants and pregnant women.

OPTION CROTAMITON

One systematic review found that crotamiton was less successful in terms of clinical and parasitic cure after 28 days compared with permethrin. One systematic review identified one RCT that found no significant difference between crotamiton and lindane in clinical cure rates at 28 days.

Benefits: We found no RCTs comparing crotamiton versus placebo. We found one systematic review (search date 1999, 3 RCTs) comparing crotamiton versus other topical agents.[5] **Crotamiton versus permethrin:** See benefits of permethrin, p 1912. **Crotamiton versus lindane:** See benefits of lindane, p 1913.

Harms: The RCTs reported no serious adverse effects[5] (see harms of lindane, p 1913).

Comment: None.

OPTION MALATHION

One systematic review found no RCTs on the effects of malathion. Case series have reported cure rates in scabies of over 80%.

Benefits: We found one systematic review (search date 1999) that identified no RCTs.[5]

Harms: We found no RCTs (see harms of lindane, p 1913).

Comment: Case series suggest that malathion is effective in curing infestation with scabies, with a cure rate of over 80% of people at 4 weeks.[16–18] The safety results from trials and observational studies need to be systematically reviewed, particularly with regard to additional risks in infants and pregnant women.

OPTION BENZYL BENZOATE

One systematic review identified one small RCT that found no significant difference between benzyl benzoate and ivermectin in clinical cure rates at 30 days. One subsequent RCT found that benzyl benzoate reduced clinical cure at 30 days compared with ivermectin. One systematic review identified one RCT that found no significant difference between benzyl benzoate and sulphur ointment in clinical cure at 8 or 14 days.

Benefits: We found no RCTs comparing benzyl benzoate versus placebo. We found one systematic review (search date 1999, 2 RCTs, 202 people) comparing benzyl benzoate versus other agents[5] and one subsequent RCT comparing ivermectin and benzyl benzoate.[19] **Versus oral ivermectin:** The systematic review identified one RCT[20] and we found one subsequent RCT[19] (see benefits of oral ivermectin, p 1916). **Versus sulphur ointment:** One RCT identified by the review compared benzyl benzoate versus sulphur ointment (158 adults and children identified in a house to house survey of a semi-urban area of India).[21] It found no significant difference in the number of people with apparently cured lesions by 8 days (AR 68/89 [76%] with benzyl benzoate *v* 45/69 [65%] with sulphur ointment; RR 1.17, 95% CI 0.95 to 1.33) or by 14 days (AR 81/89 [91%] with benzyl benzoate *v* 67/69 [97%] with sulphur ointment; RR 0.94, 95% CI 0.86 to 1.01).

Harms: Both RCTs comparing benzyl benzoate versus oral ivermectin found that about a quarter of people treated with benzyl benzoate reported a transient increase in pruritus and dermatitis.[19,20] See harms of lindane, p 1913.

Comment: Non-randomised trials suggest benzyl benzoate has variable effectiveness (as low as 50%).[22,23] The low cure rate may be related to the concentration of the preparation and resistance of the mite to benzyl benzoate.

OPTION SULPHUR COMPOUNDS

One systematic review identified one RCT that found no significant difference between sulphur ointment and benzyl benzoate in clinical cure at 8 or 14 days.

Benefits: We found no RCTs comparing sulphur compounds versus placebo. **Versus benzyl benzoate:** We found one RCT (see benefits of benzyl benzoate, p 1915).[21]

Harms: Use of sulphur has been associated with increased local irritation in about a quarter of cases.[13]

Comment: None.

QUESTION What are the effects of systemic treatments?

OPTION ORAL IVERMECTIN

One systematic review identified one RCT that found that ivermectin increased clinical cure rates after 7 days compared with placebo. Another small RCT identified by the review found no significant difference between ivermectin and benzyl benzoate in clinical cure rates at 30 days. One subsequent RCT found that ivermectin increased clinical cure rates at 30 days compared with benzyl benzoate. One systematic review identified one small RCT that found no significant difference between ivermectin and lindane in cure rates at 15 days. One subsequent RCT found no significant difference between ivermectin and lindane in failed clinical cure rates at 2 weeks, but found that ivermectin increased clinical cure rates at 4 weeks. One RCT found limited evidence that ivermectin reduced clinical cure at 14 days compared with permethrin. Experience suggests that oral ivermectin is safe in younger adults being treated for onchocerciasis, but no such experience exists for children and there have been reports of increased risk of death in elderly people.

Benefits: We found one systematic review (search date 1999, 3 RCTs)[5] and three subsequent RCTs[6,9,19] comparing oral ivermectin versus placebo or other agents. **Versus placebo:** One RCT (55 young adults and children aged > 5 years) identified by the review found that oral ivermectin significantly increased clinical cure rates after 7 days compared with placebo (23/29 [79%] with oral ivermectin *v* 4/26 [15%] with placebo; RR 5.2, 95% CI 2.1 to 12.9; NNT 2, 95% CI 1 to 3).[5] **Versus benzyl benzoate:** One small RCT (44 adults and children) identified by the review found no significant difference in clinical cure rates at 30 days (16/23 [70%] with oral ivermectin *v* 10/21 [48%] with benzyl benzoate; RR 1.5, 95% CI 0.9 to 2.5).[20] One subsequent small RCT (58 adults and children) found that oral ivermectin significantly increased clinical cure rates at 30 days compared with benzyl benzoate (27/29 [93%] with oral ivermectin *v* 14/29 [48%] with benzyl benzoate; RR 1.9, 95% CI 1.3 to 2.8).[19] **Versus lindane:** See benefits of lindane, p 1913. **Versus permethrin:** See benefits of permethrin, p 1912.

Harms: One RCT identified by the review reported that six people had headaches in the lindane group (out of 27 people), and one person each had headache, hypotension, abdominal pain, and vomiting in the ivermectin group (out of 26 people).[10] One RCT reported no adverse effects for oral ivermectin, whereas 7/29 (24%) people taking benzyl benzoate had a mild to moderate increase in skin irritation by day 2 of treatment.[19] One RCT comparing ivermectin versus lindane reported one headache in the ivermectin group.[9] Oral ivermectin has been used widely in adults with onchocerciasis, and even with repeated doses serious adverse effects have been rare.[24,25] Summary reports to the World Health Organization Collaborating Centre for International Drug Monitoring from five countries indicate that it is associated with rare severe side effects, including three convulsions and eight deaths.[26] We found no good evidence about its safety in children. An increased risk of death has been reported among elderly people taking oral ivermectin for scabies in a long term care facility.[27] It is not clear whether this was caused by oral ivermectin, interactions with other scabicides (including lindane and permethrin), or other treatments such as psychoactive drugs. Other studies reported no such complications from its use in elderly people.[28]

Comment: Case series suggest that oral ivermectin may be effective when included in the treatment of hyperkeratotic crusted scabies (also known as Norwegian scabies)[29–31] and in people with concomitant HIV disease.[4] The RCT comparing oral ivermectin versus placebo assessed outcomes 7 days after the intervention was administered, which may be an insufficient time in which to achieve cure.[5]

REFERENCES

1. Meinking TL, Taplin D. Infestations. In: Schachner LA, Hansen RC, eds. *Pediatric dermatology*. New York: Churchill Livingston, 1995.
2. Stein DH. Scabies and pediculosis. *Curr Opin Pediatr* 1991;3:660–666.
3. Green M. Epidemiology of scabies. *Epidemiol Rev* 1989;11:126–150.
4. Meinking TL, Taplin D, Hermida JL, et al. The treatment of scabies with ivermectin. *N Engl J Med* 1995;333:26–30.
5. Walker GJA, Johnstone PW. Interventions for treating scabies. In: The Cochrane Library, Issue 4, 2002. Oxford: Update Software. Search date 1999; primary sources Medline, Embase, records of military trials from UK, USA, and Russia, and specialist register of the Cochrane Diseases Group.
6. Usha V, Gopalakrishnan Nair TV. A comparative study of oral ivermectin and topical permethrin cream in the treatment of scabies. *J Am Acad Dermatol* 2000;42:236–240.
7. Schultz MW, Gomez M, Hansen RC, et al. Comparative study of 5% permethrin cream and 1% lindane lotion for the treatment of scabies. *Arch Dermatol* 1990;126:167–170.
8. Meinking TL, Taplin D. Safety of permethrin vs lindane for the treatment of scabies. *Arch Dermatol* 1996;132:959–962.
9. Madan V, Jaskiran K, Gupta U, et al. Oral ivermectin in scabies patients: a comparison with 1% topical lindane lotion. *J Dermatol* 2001;28:481–484.
10. Chouela EN, Abeldano AM, Pellerano O, et al. Equivalent therapeutic efficacy and safety of ivermectin and lindane in the treatment of human scabies. *Arch Dermatol* 1999;135:651–655.
11. Hall RC, Hall RC. Long-term psychological and neurological complications of lindane poisoning. *Psychosomatics* 1999;40:513–517.
12. Nordt SP, Chew G. Acute lindane poisoning in three children. *J Emerg Med* 2000;18:51–53.
13. Elgart ML. A risk benefit assessment of agents used in the treatment of scabies. *Drug Saf* 1996;14386–393.
14. WHO Collaborating Centre for International Drug Monitoring. Reported adverse reactions to ectoparasiticodes, including scabicides, insecticides and repellents. Uppsala, Sweden, 2002. The WHO Collaborating Centre receives summary clinical reports from National Centres in countries participating in a collaborative programme. The information is not homogenous at least with respect to origin or likelihood that the pharmaceutical product caused the adverse reaction. The information does not represent the opinion of the World Health Organization.
15. Brown S, Belcher J, Brady W. Treatment of ectoparasitic infections: review of the English-language literature. *Clin Infect Dis* 1995;20(suppl 1):104–109.
16. Hanna NF, Clay JC, Harris JRW. *Sarcoptes scabiei* infestation treated with malathion liquid. *Br J Vener Dis* 1978;54:354.
17. Thianprasit M, Schuetzenberger R. Prioderm lotion in the treatment of scabies. *Southeast Asian J Trop Med Public Health* 1984;15:119–120.
18. Burgess I, Robinson RJF, Robinson J, et al. Aqueous malathion 0.5% as a scabicide: clinical trial. *BMJ* 1986;292:1172.
19. Nnoruka EN, Agu CE. Successful treatment of scabies with oral ivermectin in Nigeria. *Trop Doct* 2001;31:15–18.
20. Glaziou P, Cartel JL, Alzieu P, et al. Comparison of ivermectin and benzyl benzoate for treatment of scabies. *Trop Med Parasitol* 1993;44:331–332.
21. Gulati PV, Singh KP. A family based study on the treatment of scabies with benzyl benzoate and sulphur ointment. *Indian J Dermatol Venereol Lepr* 1978;44:269–273.
22. Kaur GA, Nadeswary K. Field trials on the management of scabies in Jengka Triangle, Pahang. *Med J Malaysia* 1980;35:14–21.
23. Haustein UF, Hlawa B. Treatment of scabies with permethrin versus lindane and benzyl benzoate. *Acta Derm Venereol* 1989;69:348–351.
24. Pacque M, Munoz B, Greene BM, et al. Safety of and compliance with community-based ivermectin therapy. *Lancet* 1990;335:1377–1380.
25. De Sole G, Remme J, Awadzi K, et al. Adverse reactions after large-scale treatment of onchocerciasis with ivermectin: combined results from eight community trials. *Bull World Health Organ* 1989;67:707–719.
26. WHO Collaborating Centre for International Drug Monitoring. Reported adverse reactions to ivermectin. Uppsala, Sweden, 2002. The WHO Collaborating Centre receives summary clinical reports from National Centres in countries participating in a collaborative programme. The information is not homogenous at least with respect to origin or likelihood that the pharmaceutical product caused the adverse reaction. The information does not represent the opinion of the World Health Organization.
27. Barkwell R, Shields S. Deaths associated with ivermectin treatment of scabies. *Lancet* 1997;349:1144–1145.

28. Diazgranados JA, Costa JL. Deaths after ivermectin treatment. *Lancet* 1997;349:1698.
29. Sullivan JR, Watt G, Barker B. Successful use of ivermectin in the treatment of endemic scabies in a nursing home. *Australas J Dermatol* 1997;38:137–140.
30. Aubin F, Humbert P. Ivermectin for crusted (Norwegian) scabies. *N Engl J Med* 1995;332:612.
31. Haas N, Henz BM, Ohlendorf D. Is single oral dose of ivermectin sufficient in crusted scabies? *Int J Dermatol* 2001;40:599.

Godfrey Walker
Specialist in Reproductive Health
UNFPA Country Technical Services Team
for Eastern Europe and Central Asia
Bratislava
Slovak Republic

Paul Johnstone
Director of Public Health, Visiting
Professor in Public Health
University of Teesside
Middlesbrough
UK

Competing interests: None declared.

Squamous cell carcinoma of the skin (non-metastatic)

Search date May 2003

Adèle Green and Robin Marks

QUESTIONS

INTERVENTIONS

PREVENTION

Likely to be beneficial

TREATMENT

Unknown effectiveness

See glossary, p 1923

Key Messages

Prevention

- **Sunscreens in prevention (daily *v* discretionary use)** One RCT in adults in a subtropical community in Queensland, Australia found that daily compared with discretionary use of sunscreen on the head, neck, arms, and hands reduced the incidence of squamous cell carcinoma after 4.5 years.
- **Sunscreens to prevent development of new solar keratoses (*v* placebo)** One RCT in people aged over 40 years living in Victoria, Australia who had previous solar keratoses (a risk factor for squamous cell carcinoma) found that daily sunscreen reduced the incidence of new solar keratoses after 7 months compared with placebo.

Treatment

- **Micrographically controlled surgery (compared with standard surgical excision)** We found no RCTs or observational studies of sufficient quality comparing the effects of micrographically controlled surgery versus standard primary surgical excision on local recurrence rates.
- **Optimal primary excision margin** We found no RCTs or observational studies of sufficient quality relating size of primary excision margin to local recurrence rate.
- **Radiotherapy after surgery (compared with surgery alone)** We found no RCTs or observational studies of sufficient quality comparing the effects of radiotherapy after surgery versus surgery alone on local recurrence rates.

Squamous cell carcinoma of the skin (non-metastatic)

DEFINITION Cutaneous squamous cell carcinoma is a malignant tumour of keratinocytes arising in the epidermis, showing histological evidence of dermal invasion.

INCIDENCE/ PREVALENCE Incidence rates are often derived from surveys because few cancer registries routinely collect notifications of squamous cell carcinoma of the skin. Incidence rates on exposed skin vary markedly around the world according to skin colour and latitude, and range from negligible rates in black populations and white populations living at high latitudes to rates of about 1000/100 000 in white residents of tropical Australia.[1]

AETIOLOGY/ RISK FACTORS People with fair skin colour who sunburn easily without tanning, people with xeroderma pigmentosum (see glossary, p 1923),[2–4] and those who are immunosuppressed[5] are susceptible to squamous cell carcinoma. The strongest environmental risk factor for squamous cell carcinoma is chronic sun exposure. Cohort and case control studies have found that the risk of squamous cell carcinoma is three times greater in people with fair skin colour, a propensity to burn on initial exposure to sunlight, or a history of multiple sunburns. Clinical signs of chronic skin damage, especially solar keratoses, are also risk factors for cutaneous squamous cell carcinoma.[3,4] In people with multiple solar keratoses (> 15), the risk of squamous cell carcinoma is 10–15 times greater than in people with no solar keratoses.[3,4]

PROGNOSIS Prognosis is related to the location and size of tumour, histological pattern, depth of invasion, perineural involvement, and immunosuppression.[6,7] A worldwide review of 95 case series, each comprising at least 20 people, found that the overall metastasis rate for squamous cell carcinoma on the ear was 11% and on the lip 14%, compared with an average for all sites of 5%.[7] A review of 71 case series found that lesions less than 2 cm in diameter compared with lesions greater than 2 cm have less than half the local recurrence rate (7% *v* 15%), and less than a third of the rate of metastasis (9% *v* 30%).[7]

AIMS OF INTERVENTION To prevent the occurrence of squamous cell carcinoma; to achieve cure by eradicating local disease including microinvasive disease; to reduce mortality.

OUTCOMES **Prevention:** Incidence of cutaneous squamous cell carcinoma; mortality from squamous cell carcinoma. **Primary excision:** Local recurrence; survival; cosmetic outcome. **Radiotherapy after surgery:** Local recurrence; regional recurrence; survival.

METHODS *Clinical Evidence* search and appraisal May 2003, including a search for observational studies. The authors performed a supplementary search in December 2002 of reference lists of all identified review articles and relevant sections of dermatology textbooks.

QUESTION **Does the use of sunscreen help to prevent cutaneous squamous cell carcinoma?**

Adèle Green

One RCT in people aged over 40 years living in Australia who had previous solar keratoses (a risk factor for squamous cell carcinoma) found that daily sunscreen for 7 months reduced the incidence of new solar keratoses compared with placebo. One RCT in adults in a subtropical community in Queensland, Australia found that daily compared with discretionary use of sunscreen on the head, neck, arms, and hands reduced the incidence of squamous cell carcinoma after 4.5 years.

Benefits: We found no systematic review. **Versus placebo:** One RCT (588 people with previous solar keratoses, aged > 40 years, living in Victoria, Australia) found that, compared with placebo, daily use of sunscreen significantly reduced the risk of new solar keratoses over 7 months (mean number of new lesions per person: 1.6 with sunscreen *v* 2.3 with placebo; RR 0.62, 95% CI 0.54 to 0.71), and significantly increased lesion remission (OR 1.5, 95% CI 1.3 to 1.8).[8] **Daily versus discretionary use:** One RCT (1621 adults in a subtropical community in Queensland, Australia) compared daily sunscreen (sun protection factor 15+) versus sunscreen at their usual discretionary rate.[9] People allocated to daily sunscreen were told to apply it to the head, neck, arms, and hands every morning and to reapply it after heavy sweating, bathing, or long sun exposure. They were reminded of this advice every 3 months by research staff when sunscreen supplies were replenished. The RCT found that daily sunscreen significantly reduced the incidence of squamous cell carcinoma tumours after 4.5 years compared with discretionary sunscreen (22 people with 28 new squamous cell carcinomas with daily sunscreen *v* 25 people with 46 new squamous cell carcinomas with discretionary sunscreen use; RR 0.61, 95% CI 0.46 to 0.81). Subgroup analysis found no significant difference between people with a history of skin cancer and those without.[9] However, confidence intervals were wide, suggesting that the subgroup analysis may have lacked sufficient power to rule out a clinically important difference.

Harms: Daily sunscreen caused contact allergy in a small proportion of users (< 10%)[8,10] and skin irritation in a variable proportion of users (2–15%).[8,9,10] In the placebo controlled RCT, no people tested were allergic to the active ingredients of sunscreen, but irritant reactions both to active sunscreen and the control base cream were observed.[8,10] The RCT of regular versus discretionary use found that daily sunscreen use was not associated with greater sun exposure, including recreational exposure.[9] However, another RCT assessing sun exposure times among young adults who used sunscreen while intentionally exposing themselves to the sun ("sunbathing") found that a sun protection factor 30 sunscreen compared with a sun protection factor 10 sunscreen was associated with significantly longer exposure times.[11]

Comment: In a long term prevention trial with skin cancer as the outcome, placebo sunscreen may be regarded as unethical. It would also be difficult to mask treatment allocation.

Squamous cell carcinoma of the skin (non-metastatic)

QUESTION What is the optimal margin for primary excision of cutaneous squamous cell carcinoma?

Robin Marks

We found no RCTs or observational studies of sufficient quality relating size of primary excision margin to local recurrence rate.

Benefits: We found no systematic review or RCTs assessing different excision margins at any sites measuring local recurrence (see comment below).

Harms: We found no RCTs. As with all kinds of surgery, there is a potential for tissue destruction and scarring — particularly of vital structures such as eyelids, lip margins, and motor and sensory nerves.

Comment: One prospective case series using micrographically controlled surgery (see glossary, p 1923) assessed excision margins in relation to histological extension of the tumour and found a 95% clearance rate of squamous cell carcinomas less than 2 cm in diameter with a margin of 4 mm of normal skin, and a 96% clearance rate of tumours greater than 2 cm with a margin of 6 mm.[12] The sites of scalp, ears, eyelid, nose, and lip were found to have more deeply invasive tumours. Numerous case series suggest that primary excision of cutaneous squamous cell carcinoma has a likelihood of local recurrence varying from 5–20% depending on tumour size, site, histopathological differentiation, perineural involvement, and depth of invasion.[7,13–18]

QUESTION Does micrographically controlled surgery result in lower rates of local recurrence than standard primary excision?

We found no RCTs or observational studies of sufficient quality comparing the effects of micrographically controlled (Mohs') surgery versus standard primary surgical excision on local recurrence rates.

Benefits: We found no systematic review or RCTs (see comment below).

Harms: Although we found no RCTs, it is thought that with all kinds of surgery there is potential for tissue destruction and scarring particularly of vital structures such as eyelids, lip margins, and motor and sensory nerves. However, Mohs' microscopic surgery (see glossary, p 1923) is considered more tissue sparing because of its specificity in determining the amount of normal surrounding tissue removed.

Comment: A review of case series since 1940 suggested a local recurrence rate of 3% after Mohs' surgery compared with 8% after primary excision of cutaneous squamous cell carcinoma. However, the evidence must be treated with caution because of differing study quality, the long time period covered, and potential differences between people treated with Mohs' surgery and those treated with non-Mohs' surgery.[7] A site specific comparison found lower 5 year local recurrence rates after Mohs' surgery than after primary excision for squamous cell carcinoma of the lip (2% with Mohs' *v* 16% with primary excision) and of the ear (5% with Mohs' *v* 19% with primary excision).[7]

QUESTION **Does radiotherapy after surgery effect local recurrence of cutaneous squamous cell carcinoma?**

Adèle Green

We found no RCTs or observational studies of sufficient quality comparing the effects of radiotherapy after surgery versus surgery alone on local recurrence rates.

Benefits: We found no systematic review or RCTs (see comment below).

Harms: Although not measured, there is the potential for long term scar deterioration with postradiation depigmentation and gradual development of chronic radiodermatitis, including telangiectasiae, thinning of the skin, and hyperkeratosis (see glossary, p 1923).

Comment: In rare instances, squamous cell carcinomas cannot be excised completely and these have recurrence rates of over 50%.[19,20] Case series of inadequately excised squamous cell carcinomas, especially those with microscopic perineural invasion (see glossary, p 1923) found at the time of curative surgery, have reported recurrence rates of 20–25% after 5 years when surgery was followed by radiotherapy.[21,22] Ability to detect advanced perineural invasion can be enhanced by computerised tomography or magnetic resonance imaging.[23]

GLOSSARY

Hyperkeratosis Increased scaling on the surface of the skin.

Micrographically controlled surgery Does not use standard excision margins as the basis for achieving tumour clearance. The visible tumour and a thin margin of apparently normal skin are removed, mapped, and examined microscopically using a specialised sectioning technique at the time of surgery, and the surgery continues until there is microscopic confirmation of complete tumour clearance, at which stage the wound is closed.[24]

Perineural invasion Tumour invasion along (not in) a nerve.

Radiodermatitis Chronic non-malignant changes in the skin due to excessive radiation.

Telangiectasiae Permanently dilated small blood vessels in the skin.

Xeroderma pigmentosum An inherited disorder with defective repair of DNA damage caused by ultraviolet radiation, resulting in sun related skin cancers of all types at an early age.

REFERENCES

1. Buettner PG, Raasch BA. Incidence rates of skin cancer in Townsville, Australia. *Int J Cancer* 1998;78:587–593.
2. Bouwes Bavinck JN, Claas FH, Hardie DR, et al. The risk of skin cancer in renal transplant recipients in Queensland, Australia: a follow-up study. *Transplantation* 1996;15:715–721.
3. English DR, Armstrong BK, Kricker A, et al. Demographic characteristics, pigmentary and cutaneous risk factors for squamous cell carcinoma: a case-control study. *Int J Cancer* 1998;76:628–634.
4. Green A, Battistutta D, Hart V, et al, the Nambour Study Group. Skin cancer in a subtropical Australian population: incidence and lack of association with occupation. *Am J Epidemiol* 1996;144:1034–1040.
5. Kraemer KH, Lee MM, Andrews AD, et al. The role of sunlight and DNA repair in melanoma and nonmelanoma skin cancer. The xeroderma pigmentosum paradigm. *Arch Dermatol* 1994;130:1018–1021.
6. Johnson TM, Rowe DE, Nelson BR, et al. Squamous cell carcinoma of the skin (excluding lip and oral mucosa). *J Am Acad Dermatol* 1992;26:467–484.
7. Rowe DE, Carroll RJ, Day CL. Prognostic factors for local recurrence, metastasis, and survival rates in squamous cell carcinoma of the skin, ear, and lip. *J Am Acad Dermatol* 1992;26:976–990.
8. Thompson SC, Jolley D, Marks R. Reduction of solar keratoses by regular sunscreen use. *N Engl J Med* 1993;329:1147–1151.
9. Green A, Williams G, Neale R, et al. Daily sunscreen application and betacarotene

supplementation in prevention of basal cell and squamous-cell carcinomas of the skin: a randomised controlled trial. *Lancet* 1999;354:723–729.
10. Foley P, Nixon R, Marks R, et al. The frequency of reactions to sunscreens: results of a longitudinal population-based study on the regular use of sunscreens in Australia. *Br J Dermatol* 1993;128:512–518.
11. Autier P, Dore JF, Negrier S, et al. Sunscreen use and duration of sun exposure: a double blind randomised trial. *J Natl Cancer Inst* 1999;15:1304–1309.
12. Brodland DG, Zitelli JA. Surgical margins for excision of primary cutaneous squamous cell carcinoma. *J Am Acad Dermatol* 1992;27:241–248.
13. de Visscher JGAM, Botke G, Schakenradd JACM, et al. A comparison of results after radiotherapy and surgery for stage 1 squamous cell carcinoma of the lower lip. *Head Neck* 1999:526–530.
14. Ashby MA, Smith J, Ainslie J, et al. Treatment of nonmelanoma skin cancer at a large Australian Center. *Cancer* 1989;6:1863–1871.
15. Eroglu A, Berberoglu U, Berreroglu S. Risk factors related to locoregional recurrence in squamous cell carcinoma of the skin. *J Surg Oncol* 1996;61:124–130.
16. McCombe D, MacGill, Ainslie J, et al. Squamous cell carcinoma of the lip: a retrospective review of the Peter MacCallum Cancer Institute experience 1979–88. *Aust NZ J Surg* 2000;70:358–361.
17. Yoon M, Chougule P, Dufresne R, et al. Localised carcinoma of the external ear is an unrecognised aggressive disease with a high propensity for local regional recurrence. *Am J Surg* 1992;164:574–577.
18. Zitsch RP, Park CW, Renner GJ, et al. Outcome analysis for lip carcinoma. *Otolaryngol Head Neck Surg* 1995;113:589–596.
19. Glass RL, Perez-Mesa C. Management of inadequately excised epidermoid carcinoma. *Arch Surg* 1974;108:50–51.
20. Glass RL, Spratt JS, Perez-Mesa C. The fate of inadequately excised epidermoid carcinoma of the skin. *Surg Gynaecol Obstet* 1966;122:245–248.
21. Shimm DS, Wilder RB. Radiation therapy for squamous cell carcinoma of the skin. *Am J Clin Oncol* 1991;14:381–386.
22. McCord MW, Mendenhall WM, Parsons JT, et al. Skin cancer of the head and neck with clinical perineural invasion. *Int J Radiat Oncol Biol Phys* 2000;47:89–93.
23. Williams LS, Mancuso AA, Mendenhall WM. Perineural spread of cutaneous squamous and basal cell carcinoma: CT and MR detection and its impact on patient management and prognosis. *Int J Radiat Oncol Biol Phys* 2001;49:1061–1069.
24. Holmkvist KA, Roenigk RK. Squamous cell carcinoma of the lip treated with Mohs' micrographic surgery: outcome at 5 years. *J Am Acad Dermatol* 1998;38:960–966.

Adèle Green
Professor
Queensland Institute of Medical Research
Brisbane
Australia

Robin Marks
Professor
University of Melbourne
Melbourne
Australia

Competing interests: AG none declared. RM has undertaken studies in association with 3M Pharmaceuticals on the value of topically applied imiquimod in the management of actinic (solar) keratoses and basal cell carcinoma.

Warts

Search date January 2003

Michael Bigby, Sam Gibbs, Ian Harvey, and Jane Sterling

QUESTIONS

INTERVENTIONS

See glossary, p 1937

Key Messages

Treatments

- **Topical treatments containing salicylic acid** One systematic review has found that simple topical treatments containing salicylic acid increase complete wart clearance, successful treatment, or loss of one or more warts after 6–12 weeks compared with placebo. The review identified two RCTs, which found no significant difference between cryotherapy and salicylic acid in wart clearance at 3–6 months.
- **Cryotherapy** One systematic review of two small RCTs found no significant difference between cryotherapy and placebo in the proportion of people with wart clearance after 2–4 months. However, the RCTs may have been too small to detect a clinically important difference. Meta-analysis of two larger RCTs found limited evidence of equivalence between cryotherapy and salicylic acid in wart clearance at 3–6 months. One RCT found that aggressive cryotherapy compared with gentle cryotherapy increased the proportion of people with wart clearance after 1–3 months.
- **Contact immunotherapy (dinitrochlorobenzene)** One systematic review has found that contact immunotherapy with dinitrochlorobenzene increases wart clearance compared with placebo.
- **Carbon dioxide laser** One systematic review identified no RCTs about the effects of carbon dioxide laser.

- **Cimetidine** Three small RCTs found insufficient evidence about the effects of cimetidine compared with placebo for wart clearance after 12 weeks, and one RCT found insufficient evidence about the effects of cimetidine compared with local treatments. One RCT found that levamisole plus cimetidine increased wart clearance compared with cimetidine alone.
- **Distant healing** One RCT found insufficient evidence about the effects of distant healing on wart clearance.
- **Hypnotic suggestion** We found no RCTs on the effects of hypnotic suggestion in clearance of warts.
- **Inosine pranobex** One RCT found insufficient evidence about the effects of inosine pranobex on wart clearance.
- **Intralesional bleomycin** RCTs found conflicting evidence on the effects of intralesional bleomycin.
- **Levamisole** Two RCTs and one CCT found insufficient evidence about the effects of levamisole compared with placebo on the clearance of warts. One RCT found that levamisole plus cimetidine wart clearance at 12 weeks compared with cimetidine alone.
- **Photodynamic treatment** RCTs found insufficient evidence about the effects of photodynamic treatment on wart clearance.
- **Pulsed dye laser** One RCT found insufficient evidence about the effects of pulsed dye laser in number of warts cured.
- **Surgical procedures** One systematic review identified no RCTs about the effects of surgical procedures on wart clearance.
- **Systemic interferon α** We found no RCTs of sufficient quality about systemic interferon α.
- **Homeopathy** Two RCTs found no significant difference between homeopathy and placebo in wart clearance after 8–18 weeks.

DEFINITION Non-genital warts are an extremely common, benign, and usually self limiting skin disease. Infection of epidermal cells with the human papillomavirus results in cell proliferation and a thickened, warty papule on the skin. Any area of skin can be infected, but the most common sites involved are the hands and feet. Genital warts are not covered in this review.

INCIDENCE/ PREVALENCE There are few reliable, population based data on the incidence and prevalence of common warts. Prevalence probably varies widely between different age groups, populations, and periods of time. Two large population based studies found prevalence rates of 0.84% in the USA[1] and 12.9% in Russia.[2] Prevalence rates are highest in children and young adults, and two studies in school populations have shown prevalence rates of 12% in 4–6 year olds in the UK[3] and 24% in 16–18 year olds in Australia.[4]

AETIOLOGY/ RISK FACTORS Warts are caused by human papillomavirus, of which there are over 70 different types. They are most common at sites of trauma, such as the hands and feet, and probably result from inoculation of virus into minimally damaged areas of epithelium. Warts on the feet can be acquired from common bare foot areas. One observational study (146 adolescents) found that the prevalence of warts on the feet was 27% in those that used a communal shower room compared with 1.3% in those that used the locker room.[5] Hand warts are also an occupational risk for butchers and meat handlers. One cross-sectional survey (1086 people) found that the prevalence of hand warts was 33% in abattoir workers, 34% in retail butchers, 20% in engineering fitters, and 15% in office workers.[6] Immunosuppression is another important risk factor. One observational study in immunosuppressed renal transplant recipients found that at 5 years or longer after transplantation 90% had warts.[7]

PROGNOSIS Non-genital warts in immunocompetent people are harmless and usually resolve spontaneously as a result of natural immunity within months or years. The rate of resolution is highly variable and probably depends on several factors, including host immunity, age, human papillomavirus type, and site of infection. One cohort study (1000 children in long stay accommodation) found that two thirds of warts resolved without treatment within a 2 year period.[8] One systematic review (search date 2000, 17 RCTs) comparing local treatments with placebo found that about 30% of people using placebo (range 0–73%) had no warts after about 10 weeks (range 4–24 weeks).[9]

AIMS OF INTERVENTION To eliminate warts, with minimal adverse effects.

OUTCOMES Wart clearance (generally accepted as complete eradication of warts from the treated area); adverse effects of treatment; recurrence.

METHODS *Clinical Evidence* search and appraisal January 2003 and hand searches by the contributors.

QUESTION What are the effects of treatments?

OPTION INTRALESIONAL BLEOMYCIN

Sam Gibbs, Ian Harvey, and Jane Sterling

RCTs found conflicting evidence on the effects of intralesional bleomycin. Two RCTs found that intralesional bleomycin compared with placebo increased the number of warts cured after 6 weeks. One RCT found no significant difference between bleomycin and placebo in the proportion of people with wart clearance after 30 days, and another RCT found weak evidence that bleomycin cured fewer warts than placebo after 3 months. A fifth RCT found no significant difference between different concentrations of bleomycin in the number of warts cured after 3 months.

Benefits: We found one systematic review (search date 2000, 5 RCTs, 159 people).[9] The review did not perform a meta-analysis because of trial heterogeneity. **Versus placebo:** Four RCTs (133 people) identified by the review compared intralesional bleomycin with placebo.[10–13] The first RCT (24 adults with warts unsuccessfully treated for >3 months) compared bleomycin 0.1% with saline placebo.[10] Matched pairs of warts on the left and right hand side of the body were injected with bleomycin or saline. It found that bleomycin compared with placebo significantly increased the proportion of people with a more favourable response (not defined) after 6 weeks (21/24 [88%] with bleomycin *v* 3/24 [13%] with placebo; $P < 0.001$) and increased the number of warts cured after

6 weeks (34/59 [58%] with bleomycin v 6/59 [10%] with placebo; P < 0.001).[10] The second RCT (16 people) found that bleomycin 0.1% compared with placebo significantly increased the number of warts cured at 6 weeks (31/38 [82%] with bleomycin v 16/46 [34%] with placebo; P < 0.001).[11] The third RCT (62 adults) compared four groups: bleomycin 0.1% in saline; bleomycin 0.1% in oil; saline placebo; and sesame oil placebo.[12] It found no significant difference between individual groups (P value not provided) but combined results for bleomycin compared with combined results for placebo found significantly fewer warts cured with bleomycin after 3 months (4/22 [18%] with bleomycin in saline + 5/22 [23%] with bleomycin in oil v 8/19 [42%] with saline placebo + 5/11 [46%] with sesame oil placebo, P = 0.018).[12] The fourth RCT (31 people), which compared 0.1% bleomycin versus placebo, found no significant difference in the proportion of people with wart clearance after 30 days (15/16 [94%] with bleomycin v 11/15 [73%] with placebo; RR 1.28, 95% CI 0.92 to 1.78).[13] **Different concentrations of bleomycin:** One RCT (26 adults) found no significant difference between bleomycin 0.25%, bleomycin 0.5%, and bleomycin 1.0% in the proportion of warts cured after 3 months (11/15 [73%] with 0.25% v 26/30 [86%] with 0.5% v 25/34 [74%] with 1.0%; P > 0.05).[14]

Harms: **Versus placebo:** In the first RCT, one person withdrew because of pain during injection and one withdrew because of pain after injection.[10] The third RCT reported dullness, pain, swelling, or bleeding in 19/62 (31%) of all participants but did not specify which treatment they received.[12] The other RCTs found that pain was experienced by most participants (no further data provided).[11,14] In two of the RCTs, local anaesthetic was used routinely before the injection of bleomycin.[11,13] **Different concentrations of bleomycin:** The RCT comparing different concentrations of bleomycin reported pain at the injection site in most participants, irrespective of dose (no further data provided).[14]

Comment: The results of two of the RCTs should be interpreted with caution as they randomised people but analysed number of warts cured rather than proportion of people cured.[11,12] In the RCT comparing different concentrations of bleomycin, the disparity in the number of warts assessed in each group could be explained by the exclusion of warts that spontaneously regressed from the analysis, and by a high withdrawal rate in participants receiving bleomycin 0.25%.[14]

OPTION CARBON DIOXIDE LASER

Sam Gibbs, Ian Harvey, and Jane Sterling

One systematic review identified no RCTs on the effects of carbon dioxide laser.

Benefits: One systematic review (search date 2000) identified no RCTs.[9]

Harms: We found no RCTs.

Comment: None.

OPTION CIMETIDINE

Michael Bigby

Three small RCTs found insufficient evidence on the effects of cimetidine compared with placebo for wart clearance after 12 weeks, and one RCT found insufficient evidence on the effects of cimetidine compared with local treatments. One RCT found that levamisole plus cimetidine increased wart clearance compared with cimetidine alone.

Benefits: We found no systematic review. **Versus placebo:** We found three small RCTs.[15–17] The first RCT (39 people aged > 15 years), which compared cimetidine 2400 mg daily versus placebo, found no significant difference in the proportion of people with wart clearance after 12 weeks (5/19 [26%] with cimetidine *v* 1/20 [5%] with placebo; RR 3.14, 95% CI 0.75 to 5.66).[15] The second RCT (54 people), which compared cimetidine (400 mg three times daily) versus placebo, found no significant difference in the proportion of people with wart clearance after 12 weeks (10/36 [27%] with cimetidine *v* 4/18 [22%] with placebo; RR 1.3, 95% CI 0.5 to 3.4).[16] The third RCT (70 women and children), which compared cimetidine 25–40 mg/kg versus placebo, found no significant difference in the proportion of people with wart clearance after 3 months (9/35 [26%] with cimetidine *v* 8/35 [23%] with placebo; RR 1.1, 95% CI 0.5 to 2.6).[17] **Versus local treatments:** One RCT (13 people) compared cimetidine 30–40 mg/kg versus topical treatment (cryotherapy (see glossary, p 1937), salicylic acid, and other [not specified]).[18] It found no significant difference between cimetidine and topical treatments in the proportion of people with wart clearance after 8 weeks (2/6 [33%] with cimetidine *v* 3/7 [42%] with topical treatments; RR 0.78, 95% CI 0.19 to 3.21). **Cimetidine plus levamisole:** See levamisole, p 1934.

Harms: Two of the RCTs, which compared cimetidine versus placebo, found no adverse effects associated with cimetidine.[16,17] The third RCT found no significant difference between cimetidine and placebo in the proportion of people with gastrointestinal symptoms, fatigue, dyspnoea, or hair thinning (5/19 [26%] with cimetidine *v* 5/21 [24%] with placebo).[15] In the RCT comparing cimetidine with local treatments, 1/6 [17%] people taking cimetidine developed watery, green diarrhoea, and 1/6 [17%] had a rash and abdominal pain.[18]

Comment: The RCTs may have been too small to exclude a clinically important difference between treatments.[15–18]

OPTION CRYOTHERAPY

Sam Gibbs, Ian Harvey, and Jane Sterling

One systematic review of two small RCTs found no significant difference between cryotherapy and placebo in wart clearance after 2–4 months. However, the RCTs may have been too small to detect a clinically important difference. Meta-analysis of two larger RCTs found limited evidence of equivalence between cryotherapy and salicylic acid in wart clearance at 3–6 months. One RCT found that aggressive cryotherapy compared with gentle cryotherapy increased the proportion of people with wart clearance after 1–3 months.

Benefits: We found one systematic review (search date 2000, 13 RCTs, 1389 people).[9] **Versus placebo or versus no treatment:** The review found no significant difference between cryotherapy (see glossary, p 1937) and topical placebo cream or no treatment in the proportion of people with wart clearance at 2–4 months (2 RCTs, 69 people: 11/31 [35%] with cryotherapy v 13/38 [34%] with placebo or no treatment; RR 0.95, 95% CI 0.49 to 1.84).[9] **Versus photodynamic treatment:** One RCT (28 adults receiving topical salicylic acid) identified by the review compared cryotherapy with four different types of photodynamic treatment (see glossary, p 1937) (white light photodynamic treatment 3 times; white light photodynamic treatment once; red light photodynamic treatment 3 times; and blue light photodynamic treatment 3 times).[19] It found that cryotherapy reduced the number of warts significantly less than white light or red light photodynamic treatment after 4–6 weeks (20% with cryotherapy v 73% with white photodynamic treatment 3 times, $P < 0.01$ v 71% with white photodynamic treatment once, P value not provided v 42% with red light photodynamic treatment 3 times, $P = 0.03$). **Versus salicylic acid:** The review found no significant difference between cryotherapy and salicylic acid in the proportion of people with wart clearance at 3–6 months (2 RCTs, 320 people: 107/165 [65%] with cryotherapy v 96/155 [62%] with salicylic acid; RR 1.04, 95% CI 0.88 to 1.22).[9] **Aggressive versus gentle cryotherapy (defined by length of freeze):** Four RCTs (592 adults) identified by the review found that aggressive compared with gentle cryotherapy significantly increased the proportion of people with wart clearance after 1–3 months (159/304 [52%] with aggressive cryotherapy v 89/288 [31%] with gentle cryotherapy; RR 1.68, 95% CI 1.37 to 2.06; NNT 5, 95% CI 4 to 7).[9] Definitions of aggressive and gentle differed and some RCTs included warts that were resistant to treatment and others did not. **Interval between freezes:** Three RCTs (313 people) identified by the review found no significant difference between cryotherapy at 2, 3, or 4 weekly intervals in wart clearance at the end of the trial (not specified).[9] **Number of freezes:** One RCT (115 people not cured after 3 months of 3 weekly cryotherapy) identified by the review found no significant difference between no further treatment and prolonging cryotherapy for a further 3 months in the proportion of people with wart clearance (after a total of 6 months: 43% with no further treatment v 38% with prolonged cryotherapy; no further data available to calculate RR).[9]

Harms: **Versus photodynamic treatment:** In the RCT comparing cryotherapy versus photodynamic treatment, one person receiving cryotherapy withdrew because of pain.[19] Photodynamic treatment was associated with burning and itching during the first few minutes of treatment and mild discomfort throughout treatment in all participants. **Interval between freezes:** One RCT identified by the review found that cryotherapy at 1 weekly intervals was associated with pain, blistering, or both in 29% of people; at 2 weekly intervals in 7%; and at 3 weekly intervals in 0% (no further data provided).[20] **Aggressive versus gentle cryotherapy:** One RCT identified by the review found that aggressive compared with gentle cryotherapy significantly increased pain or blistering (64/100 [64%] with aggressive cryotherapy *v* 44/100 [44%] with gentle cryotherapy; RR 1.44, 95% CI 1.14 to 1.75; NNH 5, 95% CI 3 to 16).[21] Five participants withdrew from the aggressive group and one from the gentle group because of pain and blistering.

Comment: The evidence from available RCTs about cryotherapy is both limited and contradictory. Heterogeneity of study design, methodology, and the populations included make it extremely difficult to draw firm conclusions.[9] For instance, some RCTs identified by the review included all types of warts on the hands and feet in all age groups, whereas others were more selective and simply looked at hand warts, or excluded certain groups such as mosaic plantar warts or warts that were resistant to treatment. Of particular note is the likelihood that wart clinic populations used for these studies might have had very different characteristics in different periods of time. For instance, hospital based studies carried out in the 1970s in the UK would have included a higher proportion of participants with warts that had never been treated before, which have a greater chance of cure, spontaneous resolution, or both. In the 1980s and 1990s more people with warts were being treated in primary care; consequently the people included in hospital based RCTs were more likely to have warts that were resistant to treatment, with correspondingly lower cure rates.

OPTION DISTANT HEALING

Michael Bigby

One RCT found insufficient evidence on the effects of distant healing on wart clearance.

Benefits: We found no systematic review. One double blind RCT (84 people) compared distant healing versus no treatment (see comment below).[22] Wart clearance was not reported. It found no significant difference between distant healing and no treatment in proportion of warts at 6 weeks (increase of 0.2 warts with healing *v* decrease of 1.1 warts with no treatment; P = 0.25) or in mean change in size of three representative warts.

Harms: The RCT gave no information on adverse effects.[22]

Comment: In the RCT, ten experienced healers located within 150 miles of the area in which participants lived performed distant healing for 6 weeks, which was defined as a flow/channelling/projection of energy between healer and participant at a distance.[22]

OPTION HOMEOPATHY

Michael Bigby

Two RCTs found no significant difference between homeopathy and placebo in the proportion of people with wart clearance after 8–18 weeks.

Benefits: We found no systematic review but found two RCTs comparing homeopathy and placebo.[23,24] The first RCT (174 people), which compared homeopathy (Thuya 30CH, antimony crudum 7CH, nitricium acidum 7CH for 6 weeks) and placebo found no significant difference in the proportion of people with wart clearance after 18 weeks (16/80 [20%] with homeopathy *v* 20/82 [24%] with placebo; ARR +4%, 95% CI –8% to +17%).[23] The second RCT (67 people) found no significant difference between homeopathy (individually selected regimen) and placebo in the proportion of people with wart clearance after 8 weeks (5/34 [15%] with homeopathy *v* 1/33 [3%] with placebo; RR 4.85, 95% CI 0.60 to 39.35).[24]

Harms: The first RCT found no significant difference between homeopathy and placebo in the proportion of people with stomach ache, loose stools, fatigue, and acne (2/86 [2%] with homeopathy *v* 4/88 [5%] with placebo; RR 0.51, 95% CI 0.10 to 2.72).[23] The second RCT gave no information on adverse effects.[24]

Comment: Performing RCTs of homeopathic treatment is difficult because a major principle of homeopathy is to individualise treatment to the overall condition of the person. One RCT overcame this difficulty by allowing practitioners to evaluate all participants prior to randomisation and select homeopathic regimens appropriate to each of their overall conditions.[24] Participants were then randomised to their individually selected regimen (10 different regimens were used) or to placebo.

OPTION HYPNOTIC SUGGESTION

Michael Bigby

We found no RCTs on the effects of hypnotic suggestion in the clearance of warts.

Benefits: We found no systematic review or RCTs that assessed the effects of hypnotic suggestion on complete wart clearance.

Harms: The RCTs of loss of one wart gave no information on adverse effects.[25,26]

Comment: **Loss of one wart:** Three RCTs, two of which are reported in the same article, assessed the effects of hypnotic suggestion on the loss of one wart.[25,26] The first RCT (40 people) compared four treatments: hypnotic suggestion; topical salicylic acid; topical placebo; and no treatment (see comment below).[25] Participants were given a 10 minute hypnotic induction procedure involving interrelated suggestions for sleep, drowsiness, and entering hypnosis, followed by a 2 minute suggestion of wart regression imagery repeated again after 30 seconds. Participants were then awakened and instructed to practice their wart regression imagery twice daily for 6 weeks.[25] It found that hypnotic suggestion compared with salicylic acid, topical placebo, or no treatment, significantly increased the proportion of people with loss of one wart at 6 weeks (6/10 [60%] with hypnosis *v* 0/10 [0%] with salicylic acid *v* 1/10 [10%] with topical placebo *v* 3/10 [30%] with no treatment; $P < 0.05$). The second RCT (64 people) compared three treatments: hypnotic suggestion, sham laser, and no treatment (see comment below).[26] It used the same procedure for hypnotic suggestion as the first RCT, except people were given a 5 minute hypnotic induction.[26] The cold laser placebo group in the RCT received two 4 minute treatments with a simulated laser and were told to count their warts daily and assess whether they experienced any sensations in their warts. It found that hypnosis compared with no treatment significantly increased the proportion of people with loss of one wart after 6 weeks (11/22 [50%] with hypnosis v 2/17 [12%] with no treatment; $P < 0.01$). It found that a higher proportion of people treated with hypnosis compared with sham treatment lost at least one wart but the difference was not significant (11/22 [50%] with hypnosis v 6/24 [25%] with sham treatment; $P = 0.06$). Participants who lost warts had significantly more warts at baseline than those who did not lose warts ($P < 0.01$).[26] The third RCT (76 people) compared four groups: hypnotic suggestion, hypnotic suggestion plus relaxation, suggestion alone, and no treatment (see comment below).[26] It used the same hypnotic suggestion as the second RCT. The hypnotic suggestion plus relaxation group received a 5 minute relaxation procedure involving interrelated suggestions for relaxation and comfort instead of the induction procedure, and the suggestion alone group received suggestions for wart regression without the hypnotic induction procedure.[26] It found that hypnotic suggestion versus no treatment significantly increased the proportion of people who lost warts after 6 weeks (4/19 [21%] with hypnotic suggestion v 0/19 [0%] with no treatment; $P < 0.05$), but found no significant difference between hypnotic suggestion plus relaxation and no treatment (2/19 [11%] with hypnotic suggestion plus relaxation v 0/19 [0%] with no treatment; no further data provided).

OPTION CONTACT IMMUNOTHERAPY

Sam Gibbs, Ian Harvey, and Jane Sterling

One systematic review has found that contact immunotherapy (see glossary, p 1937) with dinitrochlorobenzene increases wart clearance compared with placebo.

Benefits: We found one systematic review (search date 2000, 2 RCTs, 80 people).[9] It found that dinitrochlorobenzene 2% solution followed by 1% solution significantly increased the proportion of people with wart clearance at the end of the trial compared with placebo (32/40 [80%] with dinitrochlorobenzene v 15/40 [38%] with placebo; RR 1.88, 95% CI 1.27 to 2.79). The end of trial was 4 months in one RCT and unspecified in the other.[9]

Harms: The systematic review gave no information on adverse effects.[9] One of the RCTs identified by the review found that 6/20 (30%) of participants developed an inflammatory reaction to dinitrochlorobenzene 2% solution only after the second application, but that all of these people subsequently experienced significant local irritation with or without blistering when they were treated with dinitrochlorobenzene 1% solution.[27] No-one withdrew from the study.

Comment: None.

OPTION INOSINE PRANOBEX

Michael Bigby

One RCT found insufficient evidence about the effects of inosine pranobex on wart clearance.

Benefits: We found no systematic review. We found one RCT (50 people aged > 12 years receiving topical salicylic acid and cryotherapy [see glossary, p 1937]), which compared inosine pranobex (1 g 3 times daily for 1 month) versus placebo.[28] It found no significant difference in the proportion of people with wart clearance at 6 months (9/24 [38%] with inosine pranobex *v* 9/26 [35%] with placebo; RR 1.08, 95% 0.52 to 2.27).[28]

Harms: One person taking inosine pranobex developed a sore throat.[28]

Comment: The RCT could have been too small to exclude a clinically important difference between treatments.

OPTION SYSTEMIC INTERFERON α

Michael Bigby

We found no RCTs of sufficient quality on systemic interferon α.

Benefits: We found no systematic review and no RCTs of sufficient quality.

Harms: We found no RCTs.

Comment: None.

OPTION LEVAMISOLE

Michael Bigby

Two RCTs and one CCT found insufficient evidence on the effects of levamisole compared with placebo on clearance of warts. One RCT found that levamisole plus cimetidine increased wart clearance at 12 weeks compared with cimetidine alone.

Benefits: We found no systematic review. **Versus placebo:** We found two RCTs and one CCT.[29–31] The first RCT (60 people), which compared levamisole (150 mg 3 times weekly for 10 weeks) versus placebo, found no significant difference in the proportion of people with wart clearance after 3 months (5/29 [17%] with levamisole *v* 6/31 [19%] with placebo; RR 0.89, 95% CI 0.30 to 2.61).[29] The second RCT (32 people), which compared levamisole (2.5 mg/kg 2 days/week) versus placebo, found no significant difference in wart clearance after 8 weeks (7/14 [50%] with levamisole *v* 10/18 [55%] with placebo; RR 0.90, 95% CI 0.46 to 1.75).[30] **Levamisole plus cimetidine:** One RCT (48 people) found that levamisole (150 mg twice weekly) plus cimetidine (30 mg/kg daily divided into 3 doses) versus cimetidine alone 30 mg/kg daily significantly increased the proportion of people with wart clearance at 12 weeks (15/24 [62%] with cimetidine plus levamisole *v* 8/24 [33%] with cimetidine alone; RR 1.78, 95% CI 1.01 to 2.49).[32]

Harms: The RCTs and CCT of levamisole versus placebo gave no information on adverse effects.[29–31] In the RCT that compared cimetidine plus levamisole versus cimetidine alone, two people taking cimetidine plus levamisole withdrew because of severe nausea.[32] One person taking cimetidine plus levamisole and one person taking cimetidine alone experienced change in taste and constitutional symptoms (fatigue, weakness, and myalgia).[32]

Comment: One CCT (40 people), which compared levamisole (5 mg/kg for 3 days every 2 weeks) versus placebo, found that levamisole significantly increased the proportion of people with wart clearance after 5 months (12/20 [60%] with levamisole *v* 1/20 [5%] with placebo; RR 12.0, 95% CI 1.7 to 83.8).[31] The RCTs may have been too small to detect a clinically important difference between treatments.[29,30] The lack of randomisation in the CCT means that the results should be interpreted with caution.[31]

OPTION PHOTODYNAMIC TREATMENT

Sam Gibbs, Ian Harvey, and Jane Sterling

RCTs found insufficient evidence on the effects of photodynamic treatment on wart clearance.

Benefits: We found one systematic review (search date 2000, 4 RCTs, 240 people)[9] and one subsequent RCT.[33] **Versus placebo:** The review could not perform a meta-analysis because of trial heterogeneity; one of the RCTs identified assessed complete wart clearance, the others assessed proportion of warts cured.[9] The first RCT (52 people) in the review compared proflavine photodynamic treatment (see glossary, p 1937) or neutral red photodynamic treatment versus placebo in a left/right hand design.[34] Matched pairs of warts on the left and right hands were treated with photodynamic treatment or placebo. It found no significant difference between proflavine photodynamic treatment and neutral red photodynamic treatment in the proportion of people with wart clearance after 8 weeks (10/27 [37%] with proflavine photodynamic treatment *v* 10/23 [43%] with neutral red photodynamic treatment; RR 0.85, 95% CI 0.43 to 1.68). In all those who responded to treatment, the warts on the placebo treated side also resolved.[34] The second RCT in the review (45 adults with warts unsuccessfully treated for > 3 months), which compared aminolaevulinic acid photodynamic treatment versus placebo photodynamic treatment, found that aminolaevulinic acid photodynamic treatment significantly increased the proportion of warts cured after 18 weeks (64/114 [56%] with aminolaevulinic acid photodynamic treatment *v* 47/113 [42%] with placebo photodynamic treatment; $P < 0.05$).[35] One subsequent RCT (67 people with warts unsuccessfully treated for > 12 months who had received keratolytic ointment under an occlusive dressing for 7 days) compared aminolaevulinic acid photodynamic treatment three times versus placebo photodynamic treatment.[33] It found that aminolaevulinic acid photodynamic treatment compared with placebo significantly increased the number of warts cured after 4 months (48/64 [75%] with aminolaevulinic acid photodynamic treatment *v* 13/57 [23%] with placebo; $P < 0.01$). **Versus cryotherapy:** See glossary, p 1937. The review identified one RCT (see cryotherapy *v* photodynamic treatment, p 1930). **Versus salicylic acid plus creosote:** One RCT (120 people) identified by the review found no significant difference between methylthioninium chloride (methylene blue)/dimethyl sulfoxide (dimethyl sulphoxide) photodynamic treatment versus salicylic acid plus creosote in the proportion of people with wart clearance after 8 weeks (5/65 [8%] with methylthioninium chloride/dimethyl sulfoxide *v* 8/55 [15%] with salicylic acid; RR 0.54, 95% CI 0.19 to 1.55).[36]

Harms: **Versus placebo:** One of the RCTs identified by the review found that aminolaevulinic acid photodynamic treatment versus placebo significantly increased the risk of painful warts (light–unbearable pain) immediately after treatment.[35] Burning and itching continued for up to 48 hours in some participants and 3/30 (10%) withdrew because of pain during treatment. The subsequent RCT found that participants receiving aminolaevulinic acid photodynamic treatment experienced a burning sensation or slight pain during treatment, and moderate swelling and mild erythema of the treated area 24 hours after treatment.[33] **Versus cryotherapy:** See cryotherapy v photodynamic treatment, p 1930.

Comment: Differences in trial methodology makes it difficult to draw conclusions.[9]

OPTION PULSED DYE LASER

Sam Gibbs, Ian Harvey, and Jane Sterling

One RCT found insufficient evidence on the effects of pulsed dye laser.

Benefits: We found one systematic review (search date 2000, 1 RCT).[9] The RCT (40 people using daily topical salicylic acid, 194 warts) in the review compared pulsed dye laser versus cryotherapy (see glossary, p 1937) or cantharidin.[37] All treatments were used at monthly intervals up to a maximum of four times. It found no difference between pulsed dye laser versus cryotherapy or cantharidin in complete wart clearance at the end of the study (66% with pulsed dye laser *v* 70% with either cryotherapy or cantharidin). Fifteen of the 35 participants were contacted by telephone at an average of 11 months after treatment. It found no significant difference between pulsed dye laser versus cryotherapy or cantharidin in the proportion of these people who had recurrence of at least one wart (3/10 [30%] with pulsed dye laser *v* 2/5 [40%] with either cryotherapy or cantharidin; RR 0.75, 95% CI 0.18 to 3.14).[37]

Harms: The RCT found that no significant adverse events occurred in either treatment group.[37]

Comment: None.

OPTION TOPICAL TREATMENTS CONTAINING SALICYLIC ACID

Sam Gibbs, Ian Harvey, and Jane Sterling

One systematic review has found that simple topical treatments containing salicylic acid increase complete wart clearance, successful treatment, or loss of one or more warts after 6–12 weeks compared with placebo. The review identified two RCTs, which found no significant difference between cryotherapy and salicylic acid in wart clearance at 3–6 months.

Benefits: We found one systematic review (search date 2000, 9 RCTs, 816 people) of topical salicylic acid.[9] **Versus placebo or no treatment:** The review (6 RCTs, 376 people) found that salicylic acid compared with placebo significantly increased the proportion of people with either complete wart clearance, successful treatment (not defined), or loss of one or more warts after 6–12 weeks (144/191 [75%] with salicylic acid *v* 89/185 [48%] with placebo; RR 1.55, 95% CI 1.32 to 1.82; NNT 4, 95% CI 3 to 6) (see comment below). **Versus cryotherapy:** See glossary, p 1937. We found two RCTs (see cryotherapy v salicylic acid, p 1930). **Versus photodynamic treatment:** See glossary, p 1937. We found one RCT (see photodynamic treatment *v* salicylic acid, p 1935).

Harms: Some of the RCTs identified by the review found that salicylic acid was associated with minor skin irritation.[9]

Comment: Trial heterogeneity and poor quality of the RCTs included in the review mean that the pooled results should be treated with caution.[9] However, sensitivity analysis found that removal of the two RCTs that did not use complete warts clearance did not significantly alter the results.

OPTION SURGICAL PROCEDURES

Sam Gibbs, Ian Harvey, and Jane Sterling

One systematic review identified no RCTs on the effects of surgical procedures on wart clearance.

Benefits: One systematic review (search date 2000) identified no RCTs.[9]

Harms: We found no evidence.

Comment: None.

GLOSSARY

Contact immunotherapy Contact sensitisers such as dinitrochlorobenzene, diphencyprone, and squaric acid dibutyl ester result in allergic dermatitis, which stimulates an immune reaction in close proximity to the wart.

Cryotherapy A destructive treatment based on the targeted freezing of tissue using liquid nitrogen, dimethyl ether propane, or carbon dioxide snow. Liquid nitrogen achieves the lowest temperatures and is now the most commonly used agent.

Photodynamic treatment Combines the application of a photosensitising substance (usually aminolaevulinic acid) to the wart and subsequent irradiation with wavelengths of light that are absorbed by the photosensitising substance and lead to destruction of the target tissue.

Substantive changes

Topical treatments containing salicylic acid Reinterpretation of the evidence, categorisation changed to Beneficial.

REFERENCES

1. Johnson ML, Roberts J. Skin conditions and related need for medical care among persons 1–74 years. *US Department of Health Education and Welfare Publication* 1978;1660:1–26.
2. Beliaeva TL. The population incidence of warts. *Vestn Dermatol Venerol* 1990;2:55–58.
3. Williams HC, Pottier A, Strachan D. The descriptive epidemiology of warts in British schoolchildren. *Br J Dermatol* 1993;128:504–511.
4. Kilkenny M, Merlin K, Young R, et al. The prevalence of common skin conditions in Australian school students: 1. Common, plane and plantar viral warts. *Br J Dermatol* 1998;138:840–845.
5. Johnson LW. Communal showers and the risk of plantar warts. *J Fam Pract* 1995;40:136–138.
6. Keefe M, al-Ghamdi A, Coggon D, et al. Cutaneous warts in butchers. *Br J Dermatol* 1995;132:166–167.
7. Leigh IM, Glover MT. Skin cancer and warts in immunosuppressed renal transplant recipients. *Recent Results Cancer Res* 1995;139:69–86.
8. Massing AM, Epstein WL. Natural history of warts. *Arch Dermatol* 1963;87:303–310.
9. Gibbs S, Harvey I, Sterling J, et al. Local treatments for cutaneous warts: systematic review. *BMJ* 2002;325:461–464 [see comments]. Search date 2000; primary sources Medline, Embase, Cochrane Controlled Trials Register, hand searched references, and contact with pharmaceutical companies and experts.

10. Bunney MH, Nolan MW, Buxton PK, et al. The treatment of resistant warts with intralesional bleomycin: a controlled clinical trial. *Br J Dermatol* 1984;111:197–207.
11. Rossi E, Soto JH, Battan J, et al. Intralesional bleomycin in verruca vulgaris. Double-blind study. *Dermatol Rev Mex* 1981;25:158–165.
12. Munkvad M, Genner J, Staberg B, et al. Locally injected bleomycin in the treatment of warts. *Dermatologica* 1983;167:86–89.
13. Perez Alfonzo R, Weiss E, Piquero Martin J. Hypertonic saline solution vs intralesional bleomycin in the treatment of common warts. *Dermatol Venez* 1992;30:176–178.
14. Hayes ME, O'Keefe EJ. Reduced dose of bleomycin in the treatment of recalcitrant warts. *J Am Acad Dermatol* 1986;15:1002–1006.
15. Rogers CJ, Gibney MD, Siegfried EC, et al. Cimetidine therapy for recalcitrant warts in adults: is it any better than placebo? *J Am Acad Dermatol* 1999;41:123–127.
16. Karabulut AA, Sahin S, Eksioglu M. Is cimetidine effective for nongenital warts: a double-blind, placebo-controlled study [letter]. *Arch Dermatol* 1997;133:533–534.
17. Yilmaz E, Alpsoy E, Basaran E. Cimetidine therapy for warts: a placebo-controlled, double-blind study. *J Am Acad Dermatol* 1996;34:1005–1007.
18. Bauman C, Francis JS, Vanderhooft S, et al. Cimetidine therapy for multiple viral warts in children [see comments]. *J Am Acad Dermatol* 1996;35:271–272.
19. Stender IM, Lock-Anderson J, Wulf HC. Recalcitrant hand and foot warts successfully treated with photodynamic therapy with topical 5-aminolaevulinic acid: a pilot study. *Clin Exp Dermatol* 1999;24:154–159.
20. Bourke JF, Berth-Jones J, Hutchinson PE. Cryotherapy of common viral warts at intervals of 1, 2 and 3 weeks. *Br J Dermatol* 1995;132:433–436.
21. Connolly M, Basmi K, O'Connell M, et al. Cryotherapy of viral warts: a sustained 10-s freeze is more effective than the traditional method. *Br J Dermatol* 2001;145:554–557.
22. Harkness EF, Abbot NC, Ernst E. A randomized trial of distant healing for skin warts [see comments]. *Am J Med* 2000;108:448–452.
23. Labrecque M, Audet D, Latulippe LG, et al. Homeopathic treatment of plantar warts [see comments]. *CMAJ* 1992;146:1749–1753.
24. Kainz JT, Kozel G, Haidvogl M, et al. Homoeopathic versus placebo therapy of children with warts on the hands: a randomized, double-blind clinical trial [see comments]. *Dermatology* 1996;193:318–320.
25. Spanos NP, Williams V, Gwynn MI. Effects of hypnotic, placebo, and salicylic acid treatments on wart regression. *Psychosom Med* 1990;52:109–114.
26. Spanos NP, Stenstrom RJ, Johnston JC. Hypnosis, placebo, and suggestion in the treatment of warts. *Psychosom Med* 1988;50:245–260.
27. Rosado-Cancino MA, Ruiz-Maldonado R, Tamayo L, et al. Treatment of multiple and stubborn warts in children with 1-chloro-2,4-dinitrobenzene (DNCB) and placebo. *Dermatol Rev Mex* 1989;33:245–252.
28. Benton EC, Nolan MW, Kemmett D, et al. Trial of inosine pranobex in the management of cutaneous viral warts. *J Dermatol Treat* 1991;1:295–297.
29. Morales-Caballero HG, Ruiz MR, Tamayo L. Levamisole in the treatment of warts (double blind study). *Dermatologia* 1978;22:20–25.
30. Saul A, Sanz R, Gomez M. Treatment of multiple viral warts with levamisole. *Int J Dermatol* 1980;19:342–343.
31. Amer M, Tosson Z, Soliman A, et al. Verrucae treated by levamisole. *Int J Dermatol* 1991;30:738–740.
32. Parsad D, Saini R, Negi KS. Comparison of combination of cimetidine and levamisole with cimetidine alone in the treatment of recalcitrant warts. *Australas J Dermatol* 1999;40:93–95.
33. Fabbrocini G, Di Constanzo MP, Riccardo AM, et al. Photodynamic therapy with topical delta-aminolaevulinic acid for the treatment of plantar warts. *J Photochem Photobiol* 2001;61:30–34.
34. Veien NK, Genner J, Brodthagen H, et al. Photodynamic inactivation of *Verrucae vulgares*. II. *Acta Derm Venereol* 1977;57:445–447.
35. Stender IM, Na R, Fogh H, et al. Photodynamic therapy with 5-aminolaevulinic acid or placebo for recalcitrant foot and hand warts: randomised double-blind trial. *Lancet* 2000;355:963–966.
36. Stahl D, Veien NK, Wulf HC. Photodynamic inactivation of virus warts: a controlled clinical trial. *Clin Exp Dermatol* 1979;4:81–85.
37. Robson KJ, Cunningham NM, Kruzan KL. Pulsed dye laser versus conventional therapy for the treatment of warts: a prospective randomized trial. *J Am Acad Dermatol* 2000;43:275–280.

Michael Bigby
Assistant Professor of Dermatology
Harvard Medical School
Boston, Massachusetts
USA

Sam Gibbs
Consultant Dermatologist
Ipswich Hospital NHS Trust
Ipswich
UK

Ian Harvey
Professor of Epidemiology
and Public Health
University of East Anglia
Norwich
UK

Jane Sterling
Honorary Consultant Dermatologist
Addenbrooke's NHS Trust
Cambridge
UK

Competing interests: None declared.

Wrinkles

Search date April 2003

Miny Samuel, Rebecca Brooke, and Christopher Griffiths

QUESTIONS

INTERVENTIONS

See glossary, p 1951

Key Messages

Prevention

- **Sunscreens; vitamins (vitamin C and vitamin E)** We found no RCTs on the effects of these interventions in preventing wrinkles.

Treatment

- **Tazarotene (0.1% strength more beneficial than lower strength or placebo)** Two RCTs in people with moderately photodamaged skin found that tazarotene cream improved fine wrinkling compared with placebo at 24 weeks. One RCT found no significant difference between tazarotene cream and tretinoin in fine wrinkling at 24 weeks.
- **Tretinoin (for fine wrinkles after 6 months)** RCTs in people with mild to moderate photodamage found that topical tretinoin applied for up to 48 weeks improved fine wrinkles compared with vehicle cream, but the effect on coarse wrinkles differed among studies. Three RCTs in people with moderate to severe photodamage found that topical tretinoin (0.01–0.02%) applied for 6 months improved fine and coarse wrinkles on the face compared with vehicle cream. Common short term adverse effects with tretinoin included itching, burning, and erythema. Skin peeling was the most common persistent adverse effect, which was most frequent and severe at 12–16 weeks.

- **Isotretinoin** In people with mild to severe photodamage, two RCTs found that isotretinoin cream improved fine and coarse wrinkles after 36 weeks compared with vehicle cream. Severe facial irritation occurred in 5–10% of people using isotretinoin.
- **Carbon dioxide laser** We found no RCTs comparing carbon dioxide laser versus placebo or no treatment. We found insufficient evidence from small RCTs about the effects of carbon dioxide laser compared with dermabrasion, chemical peel, or other laser treatments.
- **Dermabrasion** We found no RCTs comparing dermabrasion versus placebo or no treatment. Three small RCTs in women with perioral wrinkles found no significant difference between dermabrasion and carbon dioxide laser in improvement in wrinkles at 4–6 months. Adverse effects were commonly reported. Erythema was reported in all three RCTs, two of which found that erythema was more common with laser than with dermabrasion.
- **Facelift** We found no RCTs on the effects of facelifts.
- **Oral natural cartilage polysaccharides** One RCT found no significant difference between an oral preparation of cartilage polysaccharide and placebo in wrinkle appearance at 3 months. Smaller RCTs found that oral cartilage polysaccharide reduced fine, moderate, or severe wrinkles compared with placebo. However, these studies were small and of limited reliability. We found limited evidence that some preparations may be more effective than others.
- **Retinyl esters** We found no systematic review or RCTs of retinyl esters that evaluated clinical outcomes.
- **Topical antioxidants (ascorbic acid)** One poor quality RCT found limited evidence that an ascorbic acid formulation compared with a vehicle cream applied daily to the face for 3 months improved fine and coarse wrinkles. Stinging and erythema were common but were not analysed by treatment group. We were unable to draw reliable conclusions from this study.
- **Topical natural cartilage polysaccharides** One small RCT found that a topical commercial preparation of natural cartilage polysaccharide reduced the number of fine and coarse wrinkles at 120 days compared with placebo. However, we were unable to draw reliable conclusions from this study.

DEFINITION Wrinkles, also known as rhytides, are visible creases or folds in the skin. Wrinkles less than 1 mm in width and depth are defined as fine wrinkles and those greater than 1 mm are coarse wrinkles. Most RCTs have studied wrinkles on the face, forearms, and hands.

INCIDENCE/ PREVALENCE We found no information on the incidence of wrinkles alone, only on the incidence of skin photodamage (see glossary, p 1951), which includes a spectrum of features such as wrinkles, hyperpigmentation, tactile roughness, and telangiectasia. The incidence of ultraviolet light associated skin disorders increases with age and develops over several decades. One Australian study (1539 people aged 20–55 years living in Queensland) found moderate to severe photoageing in 72% of men and 47% of women under 30 years of age.[1] The severity of photoageing was significantly greater with increasing age, and was independently associated with solar keratoses ($P < 0.01$) and skin cancer ($P < 0.05$). Wrinkling was more common in people with white skin, especially skin phototypes I and II. One study reported that the incidence of photodamage in European and North American populations with Fitzpatrick skin types I, II, and III (see glossary, p 1951) is about 80–90%.[2] We found few reports of photodamage in black skin (phototypes V and VI).

AETIOLOGY/ RISK FACTORS Wrinkles may be caused by intrinsic factors (e.g. ageing, hormonal status, and intercurrent diseases) and by extrinsic factors (e.g. exposure to ultraviolet radiation and cigarette smoke). These factors contribute to epidermal thinning, loss of elasticity, skin fragility, and creases and lines in the skin. The severity of photodamage varies with skin type, which includes skin colour and the capacity to tan.[3] One review of five observational studies found that facial wrinkles in men and women were more common in smokers than in non-smokers.[4] It also found that the risk of moderate to severe wrinkles in lifelong smokers was more than twice that in current smokers (RR 2.57, 95% CI 1.83 to 3.06). Oestrogen deficiency may contribute to wrinkles in postmenopausal women.[5]

PROGNOSIS Although wrinkles cannot be considered a medical illness requiring intervention, concerns about ageing may commonly affect quality of life. Such concerns are likely to be influenced by geographical differences, culture, and personal values. In some cases concerns about physical appearance can lead to difficulties with interpersonal interactions, occupational functioning, and self esteem.[6] In societies in which the ageing population is growing and a high value is placed on the maintenance of a youthful appearance, there is a growing preference for interventions that ameliorate the visible signs of ageing.

AIMS OF INTERVENTION To prevent skin wrinkling; to improve fine and coarse wrinkling in adults; to minimise adverse effects of treatment; to improve quality of life.

OUTCOMES Physician and patient evaluation of wrinkles, and adverse effects of treatment. We excluded RCTs based solely on non-clinical outcomes, such as histological assessment, photography, or optical profilometry. Quality of life was not reported in any trial.

METHODS *Clinical Evidence* search and appraisal April 2003. Most RCTs recruited people with moderate to severe photodamage and wrinkles, rather than people with wrinkles alone.

QUESTION **What are the effects of interventions to prevent skin wrinkles?**

OPTION **SUNSCREENS**

We found no RCTs on the effects of sunscreens in preventing wrinkles.

Benefits: We found no systematic review or RCTs.

Harms: We found no RCTs.

Comment: We found two non-systematic reviews that reported the effects of sunscreens on the incidence of photodamage and skin cancer but they did not assess the effect of sunscreens in preventing wrinkles.[7,8]

OPTION VITAMINS

We found no RCTs on the effects of vitamins C or E on wrinkles.

Benefits: We found no systematic review or RCTs.

Harms: We found no RCTs.

Comment: None.

QUESTION What are the effects of treatments for skin wrinkles?

OPTION TOPICAL ANTIOXIDANTS

One poor quality RCT found limited evidence that an ascorbic acid formulation compared with a vehicle cream applied daily to the face for 3 months improved fine and coarse wrinkling. Stinging and erythema were common but were not quantified according to treatment. We were unable to draw reliable conclusions from this study.

Benefits: We found no systematic review. We found one small and brief crossover RCT (28 people, age 36–72 years, with mild to moderate photodamage [see glossary, p 1951]) comparing topical ascorbic acid (0.5 mL) in a vehicle cream versus the vehicle cream alone applied once daily for 12 weeks.[9] Only 19 people completed the trial. Participants were randomly assigned to treatments to the left and right sides of the face. Improvement was assessed by investigators with reference to pretreatment photographs, and graded as "much improved", "improved", "no change", or "worse". Analysis, not by intention to treat, found that significantly more people had improvement in fine and course wrinkles with ascorbic acid at 12 weeks (fine wrinkles 16/19 [84%] *v* 3/19 [15.8%]; P = 0.02; coarse wrinkles 13/19 [68%] *v* 6/19 [32%]; P = 0.01). The RCT also found that significantly more participants reported improvement in wrinkles with ascorbic acid than with vehicle cream (number of people reporting wrinkles as being "slightly improved", "improved", or "much improved": 16/19 [84%] *v* 3/19 [16%]; RR 5.33, 95% CI 1.85 to 15.34).

Harms: Adverse effects in the RCT, which were not quantified by treatment given, included stinging in 11 people (55%), erythema in five people (24%), and dry skin in one person (0.05%).[9] Symptoms responded to moisturisation and usually resolved within the first 2 months of treatment.

Comment: The RCT is limited by its small sample size and short duration, and by the high withdrawal rate (9/28 [32%]), which compromises the validity of the results.[9]

OPTION TRETINOIN

RCTs in people with mild to moderate photodamage found that topical tretinoin applied for up to 48 weeks improved fine wrinkles compared with vehicle cream but the effect on coarse wrinkles differed among studies. Three RCTs in people with moderate to severe photodamage found that topical tretinoin (0.01%–0.02%) applied for 6 months improved fine and

coarse wrinkles on the face compared with vehicle cream. Common short term adverse effects with tretinoin included itching, burning, and erythema. Skin peeling was the most common persistent adverse effect, which was most frequent and severe at 12–16 weeks.

Benefits: We found no systematic review. **Versus vehicle cream:** We found 12 double blind, vehicle controlled RCTs (see table A on web extra).[10–20] Seven of the RCTs included people with mild to moderate photodamage with Fitzpatrick skin types I–III (see glossary, p 1951). Three of the RCTs (in 2 published articles) included people with moderate to severe photodamage (see glossary, p 1951).[19,20] All three found that tretinoin cream improved fine and coarse facial wrinkles at 24 weeks. The remaining two RCTs did not clearly define the extent of photodamage. The RCTs compared tretinoin (0.1%, 0.05%, 0.02%, 0.01%, 0.025%, and 0.001%) once daily, three times weekly, or once weekly versus a vehicle cream for 12–48 weeks. All of the RCTs that examined higher strength creams (tretinoin 0.1%, 0.05%, and 0.02%) found that tretinoin significantly improved fine wrinkles compared with vehicle cream. Two of three RCTs examining lower strength creams (tretinoin 0.01% and 0.001%) found a significant reduction in fine wrinkles compared with vehicle cream.[15,18] One RCT found no significant difference between lower strength tretinoin cream and vehicle cream.[17] Assessment of improvement by the participants and investigators was consistent although the degree of improvement varied. The effect on coarse wrinkles was inconsistent.

Harms: Overall, the most common adverse effects reported after the application of tretinoin were dry skin/peeling, which were most frequent and severe after 12–16 weeks and tended to be persistent; and itching, burning/stinging, and erythema, which peaked during the first 2 weeks and decreased with time. One RCT found that erythema and scaling occurred in a significantly greater proportion people using tretinoin 0.1% than in those using tretinoin 0.025% (16/36 [44%] *v* 5/39 [13%]; RR 3.47, 95% CI 1.41 to 8.49).[19] Two RCTs, described in one report, found that more people reported skin irritation for tretinoin cream versus placebo, but that irritation was generally mild and well tolerated (skin irritation 20% with tretinoin *v* 7% with vehicle in 1 RCT, and 38% with tretinoin *v* 11% with vehicle in the other RCT).[20] Signs and symptoms of skin irritation (erythema, peeling, dryness, burning, or stinging) tended to peak during the first 4 weeks of the trial period. We found individual case reports of congenital defects associated with topical tretinoin used during the first trimester of pregnancy.[21,22] We found one observational study that identified 215 case histories of women who used tretinoin cream for acne during the first trimester of pregnancy and compared them with 430 age matched, non-exposed women who delivered infants at the same hospital.[23] It found no significant difference in the incidence of major congenital disorders (1.9% *v* 2.6%; RR 0.7, 95% CI 0.2 to 2.3).

Comment: The RCTs were limited by small sample sizes, short duration, and inconsistencies among investigator and participant assessments.[10–19]

OPTION RETINYL ESTERS

We found no RCTs of retinyl esters that evaluated clinical outcomes.

Benefits: We found no systematic review or RCTs that evaluated clinical outcomes.

Harms: We found no RCTs.

Comment: None.

OPTION ISOTRETINOIN

In people with mild to severe photodamage, two RCTs found that isotretinoin cream improved fine and coarse wrinkles after 36 weeks compared with vehicle cream. Severe facial irritation occurred in 5–10% of people using isotretinoin.

Benefits: We found no systematic review. We found two RCTs (see table B on web extra).[24,25] The first RCT (776 people in 17 US centres, aged 20–76 years, with mild to moderate facial photodamage [see glossary, p 1951]) compared isotretinoin 0.05% applied once daily for 12 weeks followed by 0.1% for another 24 weeks versus vehicle cream for 36 weeks.[24] Assessment of photodamage performed by a physician was graded on a 100 mm visual analogue scale (0 = no change from baseline; +50 mm = improvement; and –50 mm = worse). Photographs taken at baseline were compared with photographs taken after 12, 24, and 36 weeks. Only 613 people (79%) remained in the study at 36 weeks and analysis was not by intention to treat. Physician assessment at 36 weeks found that isotretinoin compared with vehicle cream significantly improved overall skin appearance and fine wrinkles (see table B on web extra). Participant assessment found no significant difference between treatments in overall skin appearance, but isotretinoin significantly improved fine wrinkles. Pretreatment and post-treatment photographs were also assessed by five dermatologists; all found that isotretinoin significantly improved fine wrinkles (see table B on web extra). The second RCT (800 people in 20 European centres, mean age 53.5 years, Fitzpatrick skin types I–IV [see glossary, p 1951] with moderate/severe facial photodamage, mild to severe photodamage of the forearms and hands) compared isotretinoin 0.1% versus vehicle cream for 36 weeks.[25] The methods employed in the trial were the same as those in the first RCT. Physician assessment at 36 weeks found that isotretinoin significantly improved overall appearance, fine and coarse wrinkles of the face, and fine wrinkles of the forearms and hands compared with vehicle cream (see table B on web extra). Participant and panel assessment found consistent results.

Harms: The first RCT reported that severe tolerability reactions, which were unspecified, occurred in "less than 5% of people" taking isotretinoin.[24] More people using isotretinoin withdrew from the study because of local irritation (5 *v* 1). The second RCT found that facial symptoms were more common in people using isotretinoin than in those using vehicle cream (erythema 65% *v* 26%, peeling 54% *v*

8%, burning 64% v 16%, and pruritus 45% v 13%).[25] Severe facial irritation occurred in 5–10% of people, causing 3.6% of people to discontinue treatment. Irritation usually occurred during the first few weeks of treatment and was alleviated by emollients or brief interruption of treatment.

Comment: None.

OPTION TAZAROTENE

One RCT in people with moderately photodamaged skin found that tazarotene cream (0.1%, 0.05%, 0.025%, and 0.01%) improved fine wrinkling compared with placebo at 24 weeks but found no significant difference between tazarotene cream and tretinoin. A second RCT found that tazarotene 0.1% improved both fine and coarse wrinkling at 24 weeks compared with placebo cream.

Benefits: We found no systematic review. We found two RCTs.[26,27] The first RCT (349 men and women aged ≥ 18 years with Fitzpatrick skin types I–IV [see glossary, p 1951]) compared tazarotene (0.1%, 0.05%, 0.025%, and 0.01%), placebo cream, and tretinoin (0.05%) applied once daily for 24 weeks.[26] **Versus tretinoin:** The RCT found no significant difference in fine wrinkling assessed monthly for 24 weeks between tretinoin and any concentration of tazarotene (percentage of people improved at least 1 grade on a 6 point scale for fine wrinkling at 24 weeks, results presented graphically: about 58% for tretinoin v about 40–55% for tazarotene; P value not reported).[26] **Versus vehicle cream:** The RCT found a significant improvement for all concentrations of tazarotene (0.1%, 0.05%, 0.025%, and 0.01%) in fine wrinkling at 24 weeks compared with placebo (percentage of people improved at least 1 grade on a 6 point scale for fine wrinkling, results presented graphically: about 40% for 0.025% tazarotene, about 45% for 0.01% tazarotene, and about 55% for 0.05% and 0.1% tazarotene v 18% for placebo; $P < 0.05$).[26] The second RCT (563 men and women aged 18 years or older with Fitzpatrick skin types I–IV) compared tazarotene 0.1% versus placebo cream applied once daily for 24 weeks.[27] Tazarotene was significantly more effective than placebo in improving both fine and coarse wrinkling after 24 weeks (percentage of people improved at least 1 grade on a 5 point scale for both fine and coarse wrinkling at 24 weeks, results presented graphically: fine wrinkling about 42% with tazarotene v about 18% with placebo, $P < 0.001$; coarse wrinkling about 15% with tazarotene 0.1% v about 8% with placebo, $P < 0.001$).

Harms: Adverse events were reported by most people in the first RCT (249/349 [71.3%]).[26] Most were considered to be treatment related. The most frequent adverse events were signs and symptoms of local skin irritation, such as mild to moderate desquamation, burning sensation, erythema, pruritus, and dry skin. "Severe" treatment related adverse events were reported by fewer than 3% of people in the 0.1%, 0.05%, and 0.01% tazarotene groups and by 5% in the tretinoin 0.05% group. In the second RCT adverse events were reported mainly during the first 2 weeks of therapy.[27] The main adverse events were desquamation (105/283 [37.1%] with tazarotene *v* 8/280 [2.9%] with placebo), erythema (84/283 [29.7%] with tazarotene *v* 6/280 [2.1%] with placebo), and burning (82/283 [29%] with tazarotene *v* 1/280 [0.4%] with placebo).

Comment: None.

OPTION TOPICAL NATURAL CARTILAGE POLYSACCHARIDES

One small RCT found that a topical preparation of cartilage polysaccharide reduced fine and coarse wrinkles at 120 days compared with placebo. However, we were unable to draw reliable conclusions from this study.

Benefits: We found no systematic review. **Versus placebo:** We found one double blind RCT (30 women, aged 40–60 years, with moderate to severe facial wrinkles) comparing a topical 1% cartilage polysaccharide twice daily for 120 days on one side of the face versus placebo on the other.[28] It found that active treatment significantly increased the number of women with no shallow (< 1 mm), moderate (1 mm), or deep (> 1 mm) wrinkles after 120 days (treatment *v* placebo: no shallow wrinkles 30/30 *v* 0/30; no moderate wrinkles 27/30 *v* 0/30; no deep wrinkles 5/30 *v* 2/30; overall $P < 0.001$). The clinical importance of these results is unclear (see comment below).

Harms: No adverse effects were reported by any of the participants in the RCT.[28]

Comment: The RCT is limited by its small sample size and by potential difficulties with concealment of allocation.[28] Application of creams to each side of the face may result in contamination (one side receiving treatment intended for the other side).

OPTION ORAL NATURAL CARTILAGE POLYSACCHARIDES

One RCT found no significant difference between an oral preparation of cartilage polysaccharide and placebo in wrinkle appearance at 3 months. Smaller RCTs reported that oral cartilage polysaccharide reduced fine, moderate, or severe wrinkles compared with placebo. However, these studies were small and of limited reliability. We found limited evidence that some preparations may be more effective than others.

Benefits: We found no systematic review. **Versus placebo:** We found three RCTs.[29–31] The first, a double blind RCT (144 people, aged 35–50 years, with Fitzpatrick skin type II or III and mild to moderate photoageing [see glossary, p 1951]), compared a commercial preparation of a cartilage polysaccharide (Imedeen® 400 or 200 mg/day) versus placebo for 3 months.[29] It found no significant difference between either dose of active treatment and placebo in face or eye wrinkles, as assessed by investigator or subject analyses on a 10 cm visual analogue scale and by assessment of photographs by a dermatologist. The second RCT (30 women, aged 40–60 years, with moderate to severe wrinkles) compared a different commercial oral cartilage polysaccharide preparation (Vivida® 500 mg/day) versus placebo for 90 days.[30] Assessment of wrinkles was measured by the investigator on a three point scale (0 = absent; 1 = moderate; 2 = severe). The RCT found that treatment significantly reduced the number of women with moderate or severe wrinkles at 45 days (overall $P < 0.01$) and at 90 days ($P < 0.001$) compared with placebo. The third RCT (30 women, aged 35–60 years, with Fitzpatrick skin types II or III and mild to moderate wrinkles) compared a preparation of 750 mg marine fish cartilage with antioxidant mix (*Ginkgo biloba*, flavonoids, *Centella asiatica*) daily versus placebo (soybean oil) for 8 weeks.[31] A trained investigator assessed clinical outcome on a 0–9 scale (0 = no signs; 9 = severe signs; based on assessment of dryness, pigmentation, skin tone, and fine superficial wrinkles). It was not clear whether results were directly compared between groups. However, the RCT reported that, at 8 weeks, treatment significantly improved superficial fine wrinkles from baseline whereas placebo did not (results presented graphically: wrinkle score 5.5 at baseline and 4.5 at 8 weeks with treatment; 5.4 at baseline and 5.1 at 8 weeks with placebo). **Versus each other:** One double blind RCT (30 women, aged 40–60 years, with moderate to severe wrinkles) compared two commercial preparations.[32] Participants were given Vivida® 500 mg daily or Imedeen® 380 mg daily for 90 days. At 90 days, the RCT found that Vivida® significantly increased the number of women with no wrinkles (10/15 [66%] *v* 3/15 [20%]) and reduced the number of women with severe wrinkles (0/15 [0%] *v* 7/15 [47%]; overall $P < 0.01$) compared with Imedeen®. It found no significant difference in the number of women with moderate wrinkles (5/15 [33%] *v* 5/15 [33%]; RR 1.0, 95% CI 0.4 to 2.7).

Harms: The first RCT found no significant difference between Imedeen® and placebo in adverse effects (23/96 [24%] *v* 10/48 [21%]; $P > 0.05$).[29] Acne and seborrhoea were the most common skin related events (24/38 [63%]) and oedema and weight increase were the most frequently reported non-skin related events (18/47 [38%]), but the proportions attributable to active treatment or placebo were not specified. The second RCT reported that "some" people taking Vivida® developed mild pimples during the first 3–4 weeks.[30] The third RCT reported that some people experienced epigastric discomfort (numbers or treatment arm not reported), but no other adverse effects were reported.[31] In the final RCT, 33% of people using Vivida® had mild facial pimples during the first 3–4 weeks compared with no adverse effects in the Imedeen® group.[32]

Comment: In the RCT of Vivida® versus placebo, the grading of wrinkling is unusual in that wrinkles were graded as severe, moderate, or absent, without a grading of "mild".[30] One might have expected that wrinkles would have reduced from moderate/severe to mild rather than to absent. The RCTs are small, and the possibility of publication bias cannot be excluded. It is not clear whether the RCT of marine fish cartilage with antioxidant was blinded.[31] The available evidence is inadequate to assess accurately the effects of oral cartilage preparations.

OPTION DERMABRASION

We found no RCTs comparing dermabrasion versus placebo or no treatment. Three small RCTs in women with perioral wrinkles found no significant difference between dermabrasion and carbon dioxide laser in improvement in wrinkles at 4–6 months. Adverse effects were commonly reported. Erythema was reported in all three RCTs, two of which found that erythema was more common with laser than with dermabrasion.

Benefits: **Versus placebo/control:** We found no RCTs. **Versus carbon dioxide (CO_2) laser:** We found three RCTs comparing dermabrasion versus a CO_2 laser.[33–35] The first RCT (20 women, 48–76 years old with moderate/severe wrinkles of the upper lip, Fitzpatrick skin types I–III [see glossary, p 1951]) compared dermabrasion with a coarse diamond fraize versus CO_2 laser to the left or right upper lip.[33] Upper lip wrinkles were graded as 0 (none) to 5 (severe) by an independent investigator before treatment and 6 months later. The average pretreatment wrinkle score was 4.3 for the laser side and 4.4 for the dermabrasion side. The RCT found no significant difference in wrinkle score between treatments at 6 months (areas retaining wrinkle score of 4/5: 1/19 [5%] with dermabrasion *v* 2/19 [11%] with laser; P = 0.22). The second RCT (15 women, 46–73 years old with perioral wrinkles, Fitzpatrick skin types I–III) compared dermabrasion versus a CO_2 laser to the left and right sides of the perioral area.[34] The mean pretreatment wrinkle score on both sides of the perioral area was 3.73 (1 = mild; 5 = severe). The RCT found no significant difference in mean post-treatment wrinkle score at 4 months, as assessed by the investigator (2.64 with laser *v* 2.79 with dermabrasion; P = 0.35). The third RCT (20 women, 44–74 years old with perioral wrinkles, moderate to severe photodamage [see glossary, p 1951], Fitzpatrick skin type not specified) compared dermabrasion versus a CO_2 laser to the left or right sides of the perioral area.[35] Photographs of participants assessed by plastic surgeons were graded in terms of improvement in wrinkles (0 = no improvement to 5 = best improvement) at 1 and 6 months after treatment. The RCT found that laser significantly improved the wrinkle score at 1 month (2.33 *v* 2.01; P = 0.002) but not at 6 months (2.55 *v* 2.22; P = 0.02) compared with dermabrasion. The RCT also found that significantly more women rated a greater improvement in wrinkles with laser than with dermabrasion at 6 months (13/20 [65%] *v* 3/20 [15%]; P = 0.001; 4 women reported no difference).

Harms: In the first RCT, 85% of women had erythema on the upper lip, which was similar on sides of the face treated with CO_2 laser and dermabrasion 1 month after treatment.[33] In 10% of people the erythema was worse on the laser treated side, and in 5% it was worse on the dermabraded side. The average duration of erythema was 2.5 months for both treatments. One woman developed a hypertrophic scar on the dermabraded side. Three people developed herpetic lesions several days after treatment, despite valaciclovir prophylaxis. Other complications such as pain, oedema, eczema, and whiteheads resolved either spontaneously or with minimal treatment. The second RCT found that erythema was significantly increased on the laser side compared with the dermabrasion side at 1 month ($P = 0.003$) but not at 4 months ($P = 0.15$).[34] The third RCT found that laser significantly increased erythema at 1 month compared with dermabrasion ($P < 0.001$).[35] Also, significantly more people reported that "post-treatment drainage" was worse with laser than with dermabrasion (10/20 [50%] *v* 2/20 [10%]; $P = 0.002$).

Comment: The RCTs found inconsistent results, were small, and may not have been powered to detect a significant difference between treatments.[33–35] The RCTs varied in their grading of wrinkles, and in participant and investigator assessments. The available evidence is insufficient to define the effects of dermabrasion for wrinkles.

OPTION CARBON DIOXIDE LASER

We found no RCTs comparing carbon dioxide laser versus placebo or no treatment. We found insufficient evidence from small RCTs about the effects of carbon dioxide laser compared with dermabrasion, chemical peel, or other laser treatments.

Benefits: We found no systematic review. **Versus placebo/no treatment:** We found no RCTs. **Versus dermabrasion:** See benefits of dermabrasion, p 1948. **Versus chemical peel:** We found one double blind RCT (20 women, aged 51–71 years, with upper lip wrinkles, Fitzpatrick skin types I–III [see glossary, p 1951]) comparing a carbon dioxide (CO_2) laser versus a phenol chemical peel.[36] At the start of the RCT, photographs of each participant were graded by an independent investigator in terms of the severity of upper lip wrinkles (0 = none; 5 = severe). Participants were then randomly assigned to receive laser treatment on one side of the upper lip and chemical peel on the other. The RCT found that CO_2 laser was less effective than chemical peel at 6 months (wrinkle score reduced from 4.30 to 1.11 with laser *v* 4.20 to 0.47 with chemical peel; mean difference in post-treatment score 0.54; $P < 0.03$; see comment below). A second RCT (24 men and women, aged 43–73 years, with Fitzpatrick skin types I–III) compared CO_2 laser versus trichloroacetic acid chemical peel applied to opposite sides of the face.[37] It found that CO_2 laser was more effective than chemical peel for reducing severity of periorbital wrinkles after 6 months (severity assessed by independent blinded investigator on a 5 point scale [0 = none; 5 = severe]: score improved from 4.00 to 1.75 with laser treatment *v* from 4.13 to 3.29 with chemical peel; $P < 0.001$). **Versus erbium:YAG laser:** We found three RCTs.[38–40] The first RCT (21 women, aged 39–74 years, with upper lip wrinkles, Fitzpatrick skin types I–IV) compared variable pulse erbium:YAG laser (see glossary, p 1951) versus CO_2 laser to the left or right sides of the upper lip.[38] Photographs and digital images of participants were recorded preoperatively and at intervals up to 2 months after treatment. The RCT found that there was a greater overall improvement (which was not defined) in wrinkles with CO_2 laser than with erbium:YAG laser (improvement: 63% *v* 54%; P value not reported). The second RCT (13 people [12 were women] aged 30–80 years, with perioral or periorbital wrinkles, Fitzpatrick skin types I–III) compared treatment with one pass pulsed CO_2 laser versus four passes erbium:YAG laser to periorbital or perioral sites or both.[39] Each participant received CO_2 laser on one side of the face and erbium:YAG laser on the other by random allocation. Wrinkles were graded from 0 (absent) to 8 (severe) based on photographs. The RCT found no significant difference between treatments for wrinkle improvement (time to outcome not stated; average improvement in wrinkle scores from baseline about 1–2 points in both groups; P value for difference not reported). However, the RCT might have been too small to exclude a clinically important difference. The third RCT (21 people [19 were women] aged 18–90 years, with perioral or periorbital wrinkles, Fitzpatrick skin types I–III) compared variable pulse erbium:YAG laser versus CO_2 laser to the left or right sides of the face by alternate allocation.[40] Photographs of participants were taken preoperatively and at 1 week, 2 weeks, 2 months, and 6 months. Investigators and participants were not blinded to treatment allocation, but a blinded panel of dermatologists also assessed outcomes. The RCT found that CO_2 laser improved wrinkles significantly more than erbium:YAG laser at 6 months (measured by aggregate of investigators', participants', and panel's assessments; $P < 0.03$; further data not reported; see comment below). **Versus CO_2 laser plus variable pulse erbium:YAG laser:** We found one double blind RCT.[41] The RCT (20 people, aged 42–72 years with upper lip wrinkles, Fitzpatrick skin types I–III) compared CO_2 laser versus CO_2 laser plus variable pulse erbium:YAG laser to right or left sides of the upper lip. Photographs recorded before treatment and at intervals after treatment for up to 4 months were graded by investigators, but no details of grading were provided. The RCT found no significant difference in improvement in perioral wrinkles at 4 months (67.5% with laser alone *v* 68.5% with combination; P value not reported).

Harms: **Versus chemical peel:** The first RCT found that 55% of people had erythema and/or coagulum on the upper lip; in 35% of people this was more severe on the chemical peel side, and in 10% it was more severe on the laser treated side.[36] One person developed an 8 mm hypertrophic scar on the phenol treated side. Herpes simplex infection was reported in three people, which responded to valaciclovir (treatment side not reported). The second RCT found that the erythema lasted for a mean of 4.5 months after laser treatment and 2.5 months after chemical peel.[37] Scarring developed in 13/24 (52%) people with laser treatment and 3/24 (12.5%) with chemical peel. All scars improved or resolved after treatment with topical silicone paste or intralesional steroids. Contact dermatitis to bacitracin–polymyxin B ointment occurred in four participants. This resolved after switching topical therapy to petrolatum and a low potency topical steroid. Hypopigmentation developed in 6/24 (25%) participants in the CO_2 laser treated arm but resolved or improved by the end of the study (no other data given). Milia formation was also relatively common during the prolonged healing phase but resolved or improved with tretinoin or manual extraction (no data reported). **Versus erbium:YAG laser:** In the first RCT postoperative erythema occurred with both treatments, but there was no significant difference (P value not reported).[38] Only one person was reported to have mild hyperpigmentation at around

4 weeks after treatment with erbium:YAG laser, which had cleared by 3 months. The second RCT found that postoperative erythema was significantly less frequent with CO_2 laser than with erbium:YAG laser at 2 weeks ($P < 0.04$) but rates were similar at 2 and 6 months.[39] The RCT found no significant difference between treatments for rates of hyperpigmentation. The third RCT found that both treatments were associated with erythema (at 2 weeks AR 67% with erbium:YAG laser *v* 95% with CO_2 laser; at 2 months AR 24% with erbium:YAG laser *v* 62% with CO_2 laser; at 6 months AR for mild erythema 0% with erbium:YAG laser *v* 10% with CO_2 laser).[40] Hypopigmentation (5% with erbium:YAG laser *v* 43% with CO_2 laser; $P < 0.05$) and hyperpigmentation (24% with erbium:YAG laser *v* 29% with CO_2 laser) were seen. Hyperpigmentation resolved spontaneously in all cases within 6 months. **Versus CO_2 laser plus variable pulse erbium:YAG laser:** One RCT reported no significant difference between treatments for erythema or pain.[41]

Comment: The effects of chemical peels and CO_2 lasers are likely to be dependent on the expertise of the dermatological surgeon, and therefore results may not generalise to different populations.[36] The difference in outcomes was not expressed dichotomously, and the clinical importance of the mean “0.54 units” difference in wrinkle score with CO_2 laser compared with chemical peel is difficult to interpret. The available evidence is too weak to define the effects of CO_2 laser on wrinkles.[36] The results of the third RCT comparing CO_2 versus erbium:YAG laser should be interpreted with caution because the participants and investigators were not blinded to treatment allocation.[40]

OPTION FACELIFT

We found no systematic review or RCTs on the effects of facelifts.

Benefits: We found no systematic review and no RCTs.

Harms: We found no RCTs.

Comment: The effectiveness and safety of facelift surgery is likely to depend on the expertise of the surgeon.

GLOSSARY

Erbium:YAG laser An yttrium aluminium garnet laser.

Fitzpatrick skin phototype classification I = always burns easily, never tans; II = always burns easily, tans minimally; III = burns moderately, tans gradually (light brown); IV = burns minimally, always tans well (brown); V = rarely burns, tans profusely (dark brown); VI = never burns, deeply pigmented (black).

Mild/moderate/severe photodamage A spectrum of features including wrinkles, hyperpigmentation, tactile roughness, and telangiectasia. Usually measured on a scale from 0–9 (0 = none; 1–3 = mild; 4–6 = moderate; and 7–9 = severe).

Substantive changes

Tazarotene One RCT added;[27] intervention recategorised from Likely to be beneficial to Beneficial.

Oral polysaccharides One RCT added;[31] conclusions unchanged.

Carbon dioxide laser One RCT added;[37] conclusions unchanged.

REFERENCES

1. Green AC. Premature aging of the skin in a Queensland population. *Clin Exp Dermatol* 1991;155:473–478.
2. Maddin S, Lauharanta J, Agache P, et al. Isotretinoin improves the appearance of photodamaged skin: results of a 36-week, multicenter, double-blind, placebo-controlled trial. *J Am Acad Dermatol* 2000;42:56–63.
3. Nagashima H, Hanada K, Hashimoto I. Correlation of skin phototype with facial wrinkle formation. *Photodermatol Photoimmunol Photomed* 1999;15:2–6.
4. Grady D, Ernster V. Does cigarette smoking make you ugly and old? *Am J Epidemiol* 1992;135:839–842.
5. Affinito P, Palomba S, Sorrentino C, et al. Effects of postmenopausal hypoestrogenism on skin collagen. *Maturitas* 1999;15:239–247.
6. Gupta MA, Gupta AK. Photodamaged skin and quality of life: reasons for therapy. *J Dermatol Treat* 1996;7:261–264.
7. Alsarraaf R. Outcomes research in facial plastic surgery: a review and new directions. *Aesthetic Plast Surg* 2000;24:192–197.
8. Boyd AS, Naylor M, Cameron GS, et al. The effects of chronic sunscreen use on the histologic changes of dermatoheliosis. *J Am Acad Dermatol* 1995;33:941–946.
9. Traikovich SS. Use of topical ascorbic acid and its effects on photodamaged skin topography. *Arch Otolaryngol Head Neck Surg* 1999;125:1091–1098.
10. Weiss JS, Ellis CN, Headington JT, et al. Topical tretinoin improves photoaged skin. *JAMA* 1988;259:527–532.
11. Leyden JJ, Grove GL, Grove MJ, et al. Treatment of photodamaged facial skin with topical tretinoin. *J Am Acad Dermatol* 1989;21:638–644.
12. Lever L, Kumar P, Marks R. Topical retinoic acid for treatment of solar damage. *Br J Dermatol* 1990; 122:91–98.
13. Barel AO, Delune M, Clarys P, et al. Treatment of photodamaged facial skin with topical tretinoin: a blinded, vehicle-controlled half-side study. *Nouv Dermatol* 1995;14:585–591.
14. Lowe PM, Woods J, Lewis A, et al. Topical tretinoin improves the appearance of photo damaged skin. *Australas J Dermatol* 1994;35:1–9.
15. Weinstein GD, Nigra TP, Pochi PE, et al. Topical tretinoin for treatment of photodamaged skin. *Arch Dermatol* 1991;127:659–665.
16. Salagnac V, Leonard F, Lacharriere Y, et al. Topical treatment of actinic aging with vitamin A acid at various concentrations. *Rev Fr Gynecol Obstet* 1991;86:458–460.
17. Olsen EA, Katz HI, Levine N, et al. Tretinoin emollient cream: a new therapy for photodamaged skin. *J Am Acad Dermatol* 1992;26:215–224.
18. Andreano J, Bergfeld WF, Medendorp SV. Tretinoin emollient cream 0.01% for the treatment of photoaged skin. *Cleve Clin J Med* 1993;60:49–55.
19. Griffiths CEM, Kang S, Ellis CN, et al. Two concentrations of topical tretinoin (retinoic acid) cause similar improvement of photoaging but different degrees of irritation. *Arch Dermatol* 1995;131:1037–1044.
20. Nyirady J, Bergfeld W, Ellis C, et al. Tretinoin cream 0.02% for the treatment of photodamaged facial skin: A review of 2 double-blind clinical studies. *Cutis* 2001;68:135–143.
21. Lipson AH, Collins F, Webster WS. Multiple congenital defects associated with maternal use of topical tretinoin. *Lancet* 1993;341:1352–1353.
22. Camera G, Pregliasco P. Ear malformation in baby born to mother using tretinoin cream. *Lancet* 1992;339:687.
23. Jick SS, Terris BZ, Jick H. First trimester topical tretinoin and congenital disorders. *Lancet* 1993;341:1181–1182.
24. Sendagorta E, Lesiewicz J, Armstrong RB. Topical isotretinoin for photodamaged skin. *J Am Acad Dermatol* 1992;27:S15–S18.
25. Maddin S, Lauharanta J, Agache P, et al. Isotretinoin improves the appearance of photodamaged skin: results of a 36-week, multicenter, double blind, placebo-controlled trial. *J Am Acad Dermatol* 2000;42:56–63.
26. Kang S, Leyden JJ, Lowe NJ, et al. Tazarotene cream for the treatment of facial photodamage. *Arch Dermatol*.2001;137:1597–1604.
27. Phillips TJ, Gottlieb AB, Leyden JJ, et al. Efficacy of 0.1% tazarotene cream for the treatment of photodamage. *Arch Dermatol* 2002;138:1486–1493.
28. Lassus A, Eskelinen A, Santalahti J. The effect of Vivida® cream as compared with placebo cream in the treatment of sun-damaged or age-damaged facial skin. *J Int Med Res* 1992;20:381–391.
29. Kieffer ME, Efsen J. Imedeen® in the treatment of photoaged skin: an efficacy and safety trial over 12 months. *J Eur Acad Dermatol Venereol* 1998;11:129–136.
30. Eskelinen A, Santalahti J. Special natural cartilage polysaccharides for the treatment of sun-damaged skin in females. *J Int Med Res* 1992;20:99–105.
31. Distante F, Scalise F, Rona C, et al. Oral fish cartilage polysaccharides in the treatment of photoageing: biophysical findings. *Int J Cosmet Sci* 2002;24:81–87.
32. Eskelinen A, Santalahti J. Natural cartilage polysaccharides for the treatment of sun-damaged skin in females: a double-blind comparison of Vivida® and Imedeen®. *J Int Med Res* 1992; 20:227–233.
33. Gin I, Chew J, Rau KA, et al. Treatment of upper lip wrinkles: a comparison of the 950 μsec dwell time carbon dioxide laser to manual tumescent dermabrasion. *Dermatol Surg* 1999;25:468–474.
34. Holmkvist KA, Rogers GS. Treatment of perioral rhytides. *Arch Dermatol* 2000;136:725–731.
35. Kitzmiller WJ, Visscher M, Page DA, et al. A controlled evaluation of dermabrasion versus CO_2 laser resurfacing for the treatment of perioral wrinkles. *Plast Reconstr Surg* 2000;106:1366–1372.
36. Chew J, Gin I, Rau KA, et al. Treatment of upper lip wrinkles: a comparison of 950 μsec dwell time carbon dioxide laser with unoccluded baker's phenol chemical peel. *Dermatol Surg* 1999; 25:262–266.
37. Reed JT, Joseph AK, Bridenstine JB. Treatment of periorbital wrinkles. *Dermatol Surg* 1997;23:643–648.
38. Newman JB, Lord JL, Ash K, et al. Variable pulse erbium:YAG laser skin resurfacing of perioral rhytides and side-by-side comparison with carbon dioxide laser. *Lasers Surg Med* 2000;26:208–214.
39. Ross EV, Miller C, Meehan K, et al. One-pass CO_2 versus multiple-pass Er:YAG laser resurfacing in the treatment of rhytides: a comparison side-by-side study of pulsed CO_2 and Er:YAG lasers. *Dermatol Surg 2001;27:709–715.*
40. Khatri KA, Ross V, Grevelink LM, et al. Comparison of Erbium:YAG and carbon dioxide lasers in resurfacing of facial rhytides. *Arch Dermatol* 1999;135:391–397.
41. McDaniel DH, Lord J, Ash K, et al. Combined CO_2/Erbium:YAG laser resurfacing of peri-oral rhytides and side-by-side comparison with carbon dioxide laser alone. *Dermatol Surg* 1999;25:285–293.

Wrinkles

Miny Samuel
EBM Analyst
NMRC Clinical Trials & Epidemiology Research Unit, Singapore

Rebecca Brooke
Research Fellow
Dermatology Centre
University of Manchester School of Medicine, Manchester, UK

Christopher Griffiths
Professor of Dermatology
University of Manchester, Manchester, UK

Competing interests: MS and RB none declared. CG has been a paid consultant to Johnson & Johnson, the manufacturers of tretinoin; he has also received fees for speaking from Johnson & Johnson.

Insomnia

Search date November 2002

Bazian Ltd

QUESTIONS

INTERVENTIONS

See glossary, p 1957

Key Messages

Treatments in older people

- **Cognitive behavioural therapy** One systematic review identified one small RCT, which found that individual or group cognitive behavioural therapy improved sleep quality more than no treatment at 3 months, although mean sleep quality scores were consistent with continuing insomnia both with and without treatment.
- **Exercise programmes** One systematic review identified one small RCT. It found that sleep quality improved following a 16 week programme of regular, moderate intensity exercise four times weekly versus no treatment.
- **Timed exposure to bright light** One systematic review found no RCTs about the effects of timed bright light exposure versus other treatments or no treatment.

DEFINITION Insomnia is defined by the US National Institutes of Health as experience of poor quality sleep, with difficulty in initiating or maintaining sleep, waking too early in the morning, or failing to feel refreshed. Chronic insomnia is defined as insomnia occurring for at least three nights per week for 1 month or more.[1] Primary insomnia is defined as chronic insomnia without specific underlying medical or psychiatric disorders such as sleep apnoea, depression, or dementia.

INCIDENCE/ PREVALENCE Across all adult age groups, up to 40% of people have insomnia.[2] However, prevalence increases with age, with estimates ranging from 31–38% in people aged 18–64 years to 45% in people aged 65–79 years.[3]

AETIOLOGY/ RISK FACTORS The aetiology of insomnia is uncertain. The risk of primary insomnia increases with age and may be related to age associated changes in circadian rhythms. Psychological factors and lifestyle changes may exacerbate perceived effects of age associated changes in sleep patterns, leading to reduced satisfaction with sleep.[4] Other risk factors in all age groups include hyperarousal, chronic stress, and daytime napping.[1,5]

PROGNOSIS We found few reliable data on long term morbidity and mortality in people with primary insomnia. Primary insomnia is a chronic and relapsing condition.[6] Likely consequences include reduced quality of life and increased risk of accidents due to daytime sleepiness. People with primary insomnia may be at greater risk of dependence on hypnotic medication, depression, dementia, and falls, and may be more likely to require residential care.[6,7]

AIMS OF INTERVENTION To improve satisfaction with sleep; to prevent sleepiness and improve functional ability during the daytime.

OUTCOMES Quality of life; self report of sleep satisfaction; sleep quality scales such as the Pittsburgh Sleep Quality Index (PSQI) (see glossary, p 1957); performance on attentional task tests; daytime functioning scales such as the Stanford Sleepiness Scale and the Epworth Sleepiness Scale. We excluded measures that record only time or duration of sleep, or wakefulness in the comments, because each of these measures may not directly correlate with symptoms

METHODS *Clinical Evidence* search and appraisal November 2002. Only studies examining the effects of treatments in people with chronic primary insomnia were included.

QUESTION **What are the effects of non-drug treatments in older people?**

OPTION **COGNITIVE BEHAVIOURAL THERAPY**

One systematic review identified one small RCT, which found that individual or group cognitive behavioural therapy versus no treatment improved sleep quality more than no treatment at 3 months, although mean sleep quality scores were consistent with continuing insomnia at 3 months both with and without treatment.

Benefits: We found one systematic review (search date 2002, 6 RCTs, 282 people with primary insomnia, at least 80% of whom were ≥ 60 years old).[8] Only one of the included RCTs (36 people) reported on outcomes relevant to the present review. It found that group or individual cognitive behavioural therapy (see glossary, p 1957) significantly improved Pittsburgh Sleep Quality Index scores (see glossary, p 1957) versus no treatment both immediately after treatment and at 3 months (mean improvement in score for cognitive behavioural therapy consisting of sleep hygiene, stimulus control, sleep restriction, muscle relaxation, and sleep education *v* no treatment: immediately after treatment 2.8, 95% CI 0.2 to 5.4; at 3 months 4, 95% CI 1.4 to 6.7). However, final mean scores in both groups were consistent with continuing insomnia (insomnia defined as score > 5; score 6.2 with cognitive behavioural treatment *v* 10.2 with no treatment after 3 months).

Harms: The systematic review did not report on harms.[8]

Comment: In the RCT, Pittsburgh Sleep Quality Index was assessed by investigators who were blind to treatment allocation.[8] We found one subsequent RCT (75 adults), in which 45% of participants were older than 55 years.[9] It compared three treatments: cognitive behavioural therapy (sleep education, stimulus control, and restrictions on time spent in bed); relaxation therapy; and a placebo treatment that involved listening to descriptions of neutral activities before going to bed. The trial did not separate results for different age groups. Overall, it found no significant differences among treatments for symptoms (100 point insomnia symptom questionnaire).

OPTION EXERCISE PROGRAMMES

One systematic review identified one small RCT, which found that sleep quality improved after a 16 week programme of regular, moderate intensity exercise four times weekly versus no treatment.

Benefits: We found one systematic review (search date 2002, 1 RCT, 43 people with primary insomnia, at least 80% of whom were ≥ 60 years old).[10] The included RCT compared 16 weeks of regular moderate intensity exercise (30–40 min walking or low impact aerobics 4 times weekly) versus no treatment. It found that, after completion, the exercise programme significantly improved Pittsburgh Sleep Quality Index more than did no treatment (mean improvement in score for exercise programme *v* control: 3.4, 95% CI 1.9 to 5.4). We found no subsequent RCTs.

Harms: The systematic review did not report on harms.[10]

Comment: None.

OPTION TIMED EXPOSURE TO BRIGHT LIGHT

One systematic review found no RCTs about the effects of timed bright light exposure versus other or no treatment.

Benefits: We found one systematic review that compared the effects of timed bright light exposure versus other or no treatment in people aged 60 years and over (search date 2001).[11] It identified no RCTs. We found no RCTs published after the review.

Harms: The review did not report on harms.[11]

Comment: None.

GLOSSARY

Cognitive behavioural therapy The following cognitive behavioural therapies were considered in this review: stimulus control, sleep hygiene education, muscle relaxation, sleep restriction, and cognitive therapy. Stimulus control consists of measures to control the stimuli that affect sleep, such as establishing a standard wake up time, getting out of bed during long periods of wakefulness, and eliminating non-nocturnal sleep. Sleep hygiene education informs people about lifestyle modifications that may impair or enhance sleep, such as avoiding alcohol, heavy meals, and exercise before bed, and aims to alter expectations about normal sleep durations. Muscle relaxation involves sequential muscle tensing and relaxing. Sleep restriction reduces the time spent in bed to increase the proportion of time spent asleep while in bed. Cognitive therapy aims to identify and alter beliefs and expectations about sleep and sleep onset (for example, beliefs about "necessary" sleep duration). Cognitive behavioural therapy may be undertaken on a one-to-one basis (individual therapy) or with a group of people (group therapy).

Pittsburgh Sleep Quality Index (PSQI) A validated 21 point scale (0 = best, 21 = worst) to measure subjective sleep quality. A score above 5 indicates insomnia.

REFERENCES

1. National Heart, Lung and Blood Institute Working Group on Insomnia. Insomnia: assessment and management in primary care. *Am Fam Physician* 1999;59:3029–3038.
2. Liljenberg B, Almqvist M, Hetta J, et al. Age and the prevalence of insomnia in adulthood. *Eur J Psychiatry* 1989;3:5–12.
3. Mellinger GD, Balter MB, Uhlenhuth EH. Insomnia and its treatment. *Arch Gen Psychiatry* 1985;42:225–232.
4. Bliwise DL. Sleep in normal aging and dementia. *Sleep* 1993;16:40–81.
5. National Center on Sleep Disorders Research Working Group. Recognizing problem sleepiness in your patients. *Am Fam Physician* 1999;59:937–944.
6. Reynolds CF, Buysse DJ, Kupfer DJ. Treating insomnia in older adults: taking a long term view *JAMA* 1999;281:1034–1035
7. Cricco M, Simonsick EM, Foley DJ. The impact of insomnia on cognitive functioning in older adults. *J Am Geriatr Soc* 2001;49:1185–1189.
8. Montgomery P, Dennis J. Cognitive behavioural interventions for sleep problems in adults aged 60+ (Cochrane Review). In: The Cochrane Library, Issue 4, 2002. Oxford: Update Software. Search date 2002; primary sources Medline, Embase, Cinahl, PsychINFO, The Cochrane Library, National Research Register, handsearching of references and trial reports and contacts with experts.
9. Edinger JD, Wohlgemuth WK, Radtke RA, et al. Cognitive behavioural therapy for treatment of chronic primary insomnia: a randomized controlled trial. *JAMA* 2002;285:1856–1864.
10. Montgomery P, Dennis J. Physical exercise for sleep problems in adults aged 60+ (Cochrane Review). In: The Cochrane Library, Issue 4, 2002. Oxford: Update Software. Search date 2002; primary sources Medline, Embase, Cinahl, PsychINFO, The Cochrane Library, National Research Register, handsearching of references and trial reports and contacts with experts.
11. Montgomery P, Dennis J. Bright light therapy for sleep problems in adults aged 60+ (Cochrane Review). In: The Cochrane Library, Issue 4, 2002. Oxford: Update Software. Search date 2001; primary sources Medline, Embase, Cinahl, PsychINFO, The Cochrane Library, National Research Register, handsearching of references and trial reports and contacts with experts.

Bazian Ltd
London
UK

Competing interests: None declared.

Sleep apnoea

Search date December 2002

Michael Hensley and Cheryl Ray

QUESTIONS

INTERVENTIONS

See glossary, p 1968

Key Messages

- **Nasal continuous positive airway pressure in moderate to severe obstructive sleep apnoea-hypopnoea syndrome (OSAHS)** Systematic reviews and subsequent RCTs have found that nasal continuous positive airway pressure reduces daytime sleepiness, improves vigilance and cognitive functioning, and reduces depression in people with moderate to severe OSAHS after 3–9 months compared with placebo, oral appliances, or no treatment.
- **Nasal continuous positive airway pressure in mild OSAHS** One systematic review of four RCTs in people with mild OSAHS found no significant difference between nasal continuous positive airway pressure and conservative treatment or placebo tablets in daytime sleepiness, but found significant improvement in some measures of cognitive performance at about 4 weeks. One subsequent RCT found no significant difference between nasal continuous positive pressure plus conservative treatment and conservative treatment alone for daytime sleepiness or functional or cognitive outcomes, but found significant improvement in sleep apnoea-hypopnoea related symptoms at 3 and 6 months.
- **Oral appliance in mild OSAHS** One RCT found that oral appliances that produce mandibular advancement reduced apnoea and hypopnoea, but had no significant effect on daytime sleepiness or quality of life compared with uvulopalatopharyngoplasty in people with mild OSAHS.
- **Oral appliance in moderate to severe OSAHS** RCTs have found that oral appliances that produce anterior advancement of the mandible reduce daytime sleepiness and sleep disordered breathing at 1–4 weeks in people with moderate to severe OSAHS compared with no treatment or control oral appliances.
- **Weight loss in mild OSAHS** One systematic review found no RCTs on the effects of weight loss in people with mild OSAHS.

- **Weight loss in moderate to severe OSAHS** One systematic review found no RCTs on the effects of weight loss in people with moderate to severe OSAHS.

DEFINITION Obstructive sleep apnoea-hypopnoea syndrome (OSAHS) is abnormal breathing during sleep that causes recurrent arousals, sleep fragmentation, and nocturnal hypoxaemia. It is associated with daytime sleepiness, impaired vigilance and cognitive functioning, and reduced quality of life.[1,2] Criteria for the diagnosis of significant sleep disordered breathing (see glossary, p 1969) have not been rigorously assessed, but have been set by consensus and convention.[3,4] Diagnostic criteria have variable sensitivity and specificity. For example, an apnoea/hypopnoea index (see glossary, p 1968) of 5–20 episodes an hour is often used to define borderline to mild OSAHS, 20–35 to define moderate OSAHS, and more than 35 to define severe OSAHS.[5] However, people with upper airway resistance syndrome (see glossary, p 1969) have an index below five episodes an hour,[6] and many healthy elderly people have an index greater than five episodes an hour.[7] In an effort to obtain an international consensus, new criteria have been proposed but have not been widely used.[8] The most pragmatic test for clinically significant OSAHS is to show clinical improvement in daytime symptoms after treatment for sleep disordered breathing. In this topic, the criteria for OSAHS include apnoeas and hypopnoeas (see glossary, p 1968) caused by upper airway obstruction. Central sleep apnoea and sleep associated hypoventilation syndromes are not covered here.

INCIDENCE/ PREVALENCE The Wisconsin Sleep Cohort Study of over 1000 people (mean age 47 years) in North America found a prevalence of apnoea/hypopnoea index greater than five episodes an hour in 24% of men and 9% of women, and of OSAHS with an index greater than five plus excessive sleepiness in 4% of men and 2% of women.[9] There are international differences in the occurrence of OSAHS, for which obesity is considered to be an important determinant.[10] Ethnic differences in prevalence have also been found after adjustment for other risk factors.[7,10] Little is known about the burden of illness in developing countries.

AETIOLOGY/ RISK FACTORS The site of the upper airway obstruction in the OSAHS is around the level of the tongue, soft palate, or epiglottis. Disorders that predispose to either narrowing of the upper airway or reduction in its stability (e.g. obesity, certain craniofacial abnormalities, vocal cord abnormalities, and enlarged tonsils) have been associated with an increased risk of OSAHS. It has been estimated that a 1 kg/m^2 increase in body mass index (3.2 kg for a person 1.8 m tall) leads to a 30% increase (95% CI 13% to 50%) in the relative risk of developing abnormal sleep disordered breathing (apnoea/hypopnoea index ≥ 5/hour) over a period of 4 years.[10] Other strong associations include increasing age and sex (male to female ratio is 2 : 1). Weaker associations include menopause, family history, smoking, and night time nasal congestion.[10]

PROGNOSIS The long term prognosis of people with untreated severe OSAHS is poor with respect to quality of life, likelihood of motor vehicle accidents, hypertension, and possibly cardiovascular disease and premature mortality.[11] Unfortunately, the prognosis of both treated and untreated OSAHS is unclear.[7] The limitations in the evidence include bias in the selection of participants, short duration of follow up, and variation in the measurement of confounders (e.g. smoking, alcohol use, and other cardiovascular risk factors). Treatment is widespread, making it difficult to find evidence on prognosis for untreated OSAHS. Observational studies support a causal association between OSAHS and systemic hypertension, which increases with the severity of OSAHS (OR 1.21 for mild OSAHS to 3.07 for severe OSAHS).[11] OSAHS increases the risk of motor vehicle accidents three- to sevenfold.[11,12] It is associated with increased risk of premature mortality, cardiovascular disease, and impaired neurocognitive functioning.[11]

AIMS OF INTERVENTION To minimise or eliminate symptoms of daytime sleepiness; to improve vigilance and quality of life; to reduce or abolish the increased risk of motor vehicle accidents and cardiovascular events; to enhance compliance with treatment; to minimise adverse effects of treatment.

OUTCOMES **Daytime sleepiness:** Subjective and objective measures such as Epworth Sleepiness Scale, Multiple Sleep Latency Test, and Maintenance of Wakefulness Test. **Quality of life:** General measures such as the Medical Outcomes Study 36-item Short Form Health Survey and the General Health Questionnaire; measures of mood such as the Hospital Anxiety and Depression Scale, the Beck Depression Inventory, and the Profile of Mood States; measures of energy and vitality such as the 36-item Short Form SF-36 energy scale, the UWIST Mood Adjective Checklist, and the energy and vitality scale of the Nottingham Health Profile. Disease specific quality of life measures include the Functional Outcomes of Sleep Questionnaire. **Cognitive performance measures:** Steer Clear, Trailmaking Test B, Digit Symbol Substitution, and Paced Auditory Serial Addition-2 Second Timing. **Mortality and morbidity:** For example, road traffic accidents, hypertension, stroke, cardiac failure, and ischaemic heart disease. **Intermediate outcomes:** Measures of the degree of disturbed breathing during sleep, such as the number of apnoeas and hypopnoeas an hour (apnoea/hypopnoea index), the frequency of arousals, and the degree of sleep fragmentation. Details of validated outcome measures for daytime sleepiness, quality of life and cognitive performance are listed in table 1, p 1972.[13–25]

METHODS *Clinical Evidence* search and appraisal December 2002 and ongoing additional hand searches by the author. Different RCTs have used slightly different definitions of OSAHS. An attempt has been made to provide some details of the definitions used. Further clarification will be attempted in future *Clinical Evidence* updates.

QUESTION What are the effects of treatment of moderate to severe obstructive sleep apnoea-hypopnoea syndrome?

OPTION NASAL CONTINUOUS POSITIVE AIRWAY PRESSURE IN MODERATE TO SEVERE OBSTRUCTIVE SLEEP APNOEA-HYPOPNOEA SYNDROME

Systematic reviews and subsequent RCTs have found that nasal continuous positive airway pressure reduces daytime sleepiness, improves vigilance and cognitive functioning, and reduces depression compared with placebo, oral appliances, or no treatment in people with moderate to severe obstructive sleep apnoea-hypopnoea syndrome.

Benefits: **Versus no treatment:** We found one systematic review (search date 1999, 1 RCT) comparing nasal continuous positive airway pressure (CPAP — see glossary, p 1968) versus control for 3 months.[5] The included RCT (105 people with severe obstructive sleep apnoea-hypopnoea syndrome [OSAHS], mean apnoea/hypopnoea index [see glossary, p 1968] 56/hour, and mean Epworth Sleepiness Scale 12) did not compare effects of nasal CPAP versus control directly. However, it found that nasal CPAP significantly reduced daytime sleepiness from baseline, whereas the control treatment did not (mean Epworth Sleepiness Scale was reduced from 12.1 to 5.6 with nasal CPAP, $P < 0.01$, CI not reported; and was reduced from 11.4 to 10.6 with control, NS).[26]

Versus sham/subtherapeutic nasal CPAP: We found one systematic review (search date 1999, 1 RCT),[5] one report of 6 month follow up from the RCT identified by the review,[27] and three subsequent RCTs,[28–30] which compared nasal CPAP versus sham/subtherapeutic nasal CPAP (see glossary, p 1969). The RCT identified by the systematic review (107 people with moderate to severe OSAHS) found that nasal CPAP significantly reduced daytime sleepiness at 1 month compared with sham/subtherapeutic nasal CPAP (mean improvement in Epworth Sleepiness Scale with CPAP *v* control 7.0, $P < 0.0001$, CI not reported; mean improvement in Maintenance of Wakefulness Test with CPAP *v* control 6.75 min, $P = 0.005$).[31] The first subsequent RCT (55 people with moderate to severe sleep disordered breathing [see glossary, p 1969], all with an apnoea/hypopnoea index > 30/hour [average > 50/hour], but with no or very little complaint of excessive daytime sleepiness [average Epworth Sleepiness Scale was 7/24, normal is < 10/24]) found no significant difference in daytime sleepiness after 6 weeks between nasal CPAP and sham nasal CPAP (change in Epworth Sleepiness Scale: 1, 95% CI 0 to 2 with nasal CPAP *v* 1, 95% CI 0 to 2 with sham nasal CPAP).[28] It also found no significant difference in a range of measures of cognitive functioning or in 24 hour blood pressure readings. The second subsequent RCT (59 men with an Epworth Sleepiness Scale > 10 and moderate to severe OSAHS; 48 people included in this RCT were also included in the RCT[31] described above) compared the effects of nasal CPAP versus sham nasal CPAP on simulated driving performance for 1 month.[29] It found that nasal CPAP significantly reduced daytime sleepiness compared with sham nasal CPAP (subjective measures: $P = 0.0006$; objective measures: $P = 0.003$; CI not reported). The third subsequent RCT (45 people with moderate to severe OSAHS) found that nasal CPAP significantly reduced daytime sleepiness and functional outcomes compared with sham nasal CPAP after 6 weeks (mean change in Epworth Sleepiness Scale –9.48 with nasal CPAP *v* –2.27 with sham nasal CPAP, $P < 0.001$; mean change in sleep apnoea-hypopnoea syndrome related symptoms score –18.48 with nasal CPAP *v* –4.45 with sham nasal CPAP, $P < 0.001$; mean change in Functional Outcomes of Sleep Questionnaire [general productivity domain] 3.99 with nasal CPAP *v* 0.50 with sham nasal CPAP, $P < 0.05$; and mean change in Functional Outcomes of Sleep Questionnaire [vigilance domain] 8.52 with nasal CPAP *v* 3.44 with sham nasal CPAP, $P < 0.01$).[30] **Versus oral placebo tablets:** We found one systematic review[32] and one subsequent RCT[33] comparing nasal CPAP versus oral placebo tablets. The systematic review (search date 2001, 3 crossover RCTs, 82 people) compared nasal CPAP versus oral placebo tablets in people with moderate OSAHS.[32] The RCTs in the systematic review were found to have some methodological shortcomings. The review found no significant difference in sleep latency between nasal CPAP and oral placebo tablets (Multiple Sleep Latency Test: WMD +0.90 minutes, 95% CI –0.84 minutes to +2.62 minutes) or cognitive functioning (Steer Clear: WMD –5.04, 95% CI –20.1 to +10.0).[32] The subsequent RCT (68 people with moderate to severe OSAHS, apnoea/hypopnoea index range 15–129/hour, Epworth Sleepiness Scale range 6–24) compared nasal CPAP versus oral placebo tablets over 4 weeks.[33] It found that nasal CPAP significantly reduced daytime sleepiness over 4 weeks compared with oral placebo tablets (Epworth Sleepiness Scale 10.1 with nasal CPAP *v* 12.5 with placebo tablets; $P = 0.001$) and quality of life (Functional Outcomes of Sleep Questionnaire total score 12.4 with nasal CPAP *v* 11.6 with placebo tablets; $P = 0.01$).[33] **Versus oral appliances:** We found one systematic review (search date 2001,[32] 60 people, 3 RCTs[34–36]) and one subsequent RCT, which compared nasal CPAP with oral appliances (see glossary, p 1968) (removable mandibular advancement devices).[37] The systematic review found that nasal CPAP significantly improved apnoea/hypopnoea index compared with oral appliance (WMD –7.3/hour, 95% CI –10.0/hour to –4.7/hour).[32] One RCT included in the review found no significant difference in sleepiness between nasal CPAP and oral appliances.[36] Overall, the review found that people preferred an oral appliance over nasal CPAP (OR 9.5, 95% CI 4.3 to 21.1). However, the trial results were significantly heterogeneous.[32] The subsequent RCT (48 people with a mean apnoea/hypopnoea index of 31 ± 26/hour and Epworth Sleepiness Scale of 14 ± 4; crossover design) found that CPAP significantly improved apnoea/hypopnoea index, symptoms, functional outcomes and aspects of quality of life after 8 weeks compared with mandibular repositioning splint (apnoea/hypopnoea index: 8 with CPAP *v* 15 with splint; Epworth Sleepiness Scale: 8 *v* 12; symptoms: 17 *v* 11; effectiveness rating: 5 *v* 7; Functional Outcomes of Sleep Questionnaire: 13 *v* 14; SF–36 mental component: 48 *v* 52; health transition scores: 2.9 *v* 2.4; P for all these outcomes < 0.01). However, objective sleepiness, cognitive performance, and preference for treatments were not significantly different between treatments.[37]

Harms: Neither of the systematic reviews summarised any harmful effects found in the RCTs that were reviewed.[5,32] One systematic review (search date 1999) reported a high prevalence of minor adverse effects from nasal CPAP treatment, the most common being dry mouth, nose, and throat (40%).[5] We found one case series (52 consecutive people with severe OSAHS, mean oxygen desaturation index 43/hour), in which the occurrence of nasopharyngeal symptoms was studied systematically before and after nasal CPAP.[38] It found that nasopharyngeal symptoms were common before nasal CPAP in OSAHS (nasal dryness 74%, sneezing 51%, blocked nose 43%, and rhinorrhoea 37%) and increased during nasal CPAP (sneezing 75% and rhinorrhoea 57%), with greater discomfort in winter. Other adverse effects of nasal CPAP include local effects of the mask on the nasal bridge, mask discomfort, nasal congestion, rhinitis, sore eyes, headache, chest discomfort, and noise disturbance.

Comment: The RCTs have problems with their methods and with applicability of results. First, severity of sleep disordered breathing (using apnoea/hypopnoea index, etc.) is not a good guide to severity of daytime sleepiness, which is a major symptom.[28] Second, it is not clear whether the sham or subtherapeutic CPAP used in some "placebo" groups are truly inactive treatments. Third, RCT evidence reports short term symptomatic outcomes only, rather than longer term complications, such as mortality, motor vehicle accident rate, hypertension, stroke, and ischaemic heart disease.

OPTION WEIGHT LOSS IN MODERATE TO SEVERE OBSTRUCTIVE SLEEP APNOEA-HYPOPNOEA SYNDROME

We found no RCTs on the effect of weight loss in people with moderate to severe obstructive sleep apnoea-hypopnoea syndrome.

Benefits: We found one systematic review (search date 2000), which identified no RCTs on the effect of weight loss in people with obstructive sleep apnoea-hypopnoea syndrome (OSAHS); see comment below.[39]

Harms: We found no RCTs on the effects of weight loss in people with OSAHS.

Comment: One review of the effect of body weight in OSAHS found no RCTs but included case series in which weight loss, especially that achieved by surgery, was associated with improvement, mainly in people with severe OSAHS.[40] Large relative improvements in apnoea/hypopnoea index (see glossary, p 1968) (−72% to −98%) were found after a weight loss of 30–70% of initial weight.[40] It seems that weight loss has the potential to benefit obese persons with OSAHS. There is consensus that advice about weight reduction is an important component of management. However, weight loss is difficult and advice may need to be combined with nasal continuous positive airway pressure (see glossary, p 1968) in people with moderate and severe OSAHS.

OPTION ORAL APPLIANCES IN MODERATE TO SEVERE OBSTRUCTIVE SLEEP APNOEA-HYPOPNOEA SYNDROME

RCTs have found that oral appliances that produce anterior advancement of the mandible reduce daytime sleepiness and sleep disordered breathing at 1–4 weeks in people with moderate to severe obstructive sleep apnoea-hypopnoea syndrome compared with no treatment or control oral appliances.

Benefits: **Versus no treatment:** We found no systematic review but found one RCT.[41] The RCT (crossover, 24 people with moderate obstructive sleep apnoea-hypopnoea syndrome [OSAHS]; mean apnoea/hypopnoea index [see glossary, p 1968] 26.7 and significant daytime sleepiness [Epworth Sleepiness Scale 11.9]) compared two different oral appliances (see glossary, p 1968) that produced mandibular advancement versus no treatment for 1 week each. It found that, after 1 week, both oral appliances significantly reduced daytime sleepiness and sleep disordered breathing (see glossary, p 1969) compared with no treatment (daytime sleepiness: Epworth Sleepiness Scale 9.0, 95% CI 6.5 to 11.0 with first oral appliance; 9.0, 95% CI 6.5 to 10.0 with second oral appliance; and 13.5, 95% CI 9.5 to 16.0 with no oral appliance; $P < 0.01$ for each oral appliance *v* no oral appliance; apnoea/hypopnoea index: 8.7, 95% CI 5.8 to 11.6 with first oral appliance; 7.9, 95% CI 4.8 to 11.0 with second oral appliance; 22.6, 95% CI 16.5 to 28.7 with no oral appliance; $P < 0.05$ for each oral appliance *v* no oral appliance). It also found that oral appliance versus no treatment significantly reduced interference with daily tasks, snoring frequency and loudness, and improved performance ability and energy level compared with no treatment. **Versus control oral appliances:** We found three RCTs comparing an oral appliance that produced anterior advancement of the mandible (removable mandibular advancement device) versus an oral appliance that did not (control intervention).[42–44] The first RCT (24 adults with loud snoring and severe OSAHS) found that mandibular advancement device significantly reduced daytime sleepiness compared with control after 2 weeks (Epworth Sleepiness Scale –3.8 with mandibular advancement device *v* –0.5 with control oral appliance; $P < 0.005$).[42] There was a significant withdrawal rate, with only 10 people in the mandibular advancement group and eight people in the control group providing outcome data after 2 weeks of treatment. The second RCT (crossover study, 28 people with moderate to severe OSAHS [average apnoea/hypopnoea index 27/hour]) compared a mandibular advancement splint versus control (oral appliance that did not advance the mandible) for 1 week each.[43] It found that mandibular advancement splint significantly reduced daytime sleepiness and apnoea/hypopnoea index compared with control oral appliance (Epworth Sleepiness Scale 3.9 with mandibular advancement splint *v* 10.1 with control oral appliance, $P < 0.01$, CI not reported; apnoea/hypopnoea index: 14/hour with mandibular advancement splint *v* 30/hour with control oral appliance, $P < 0.0001$, CI not reported). The third RCT[44] (85 patients, 14 women with mean Epworth Sleepiness Scale of 11, crossover design) found that an active mandibular advancement splint significantly increased sleep latency and improved sleepiness compared with an inactive mandibular advancement splint at 4 weeks (decrease in sleep latency for active v inactive treatment: 1.2 minutes, 95% CI 0.3 minutes to 2.1 minutes; improvement in Epworth Sleepiness Scale for active v inactive treatment: 2 points, 95% CI 1 point to 3 points; proportion of people with normal Epworth Sleepiness score: 82% with active v 62% with inactive, $P < 0.01$). **Versus nasal continuous positive airway pressure:** See glossary, p 1968. See benefits of nasal continuous positive airway pressure in moderate to severe OSAHS, p 1961.

Harms: **Versus no treatment:** The RCT did not report on adverse effects.[41] One small series (22 people involved in the RCT) investigated adverse effects over 12–30 months.[45] It found that adverse effects were common (mucosal dryness [86%], tooth discomfort [59%], and hypersalivation [55%]) but did not require discontinuation of treatment. **Versus control oral appliances:** The first RCT did not report on adverse effects.[42] The second RCT reported the following adverse effects: excessive salivation (50%), gum irritation (20%), mouth dryness (46%), jaw discomfort (12.5%), and tooth grinding (12.5%).[43] Those adverse effects were described as mild to moderate, lasting less than 3 weeks, and not preventing the use of the mandibular advancement splint.

Comment: Oral appliances are commonly used for snoring. We found one systematic review (search date 1994, 304 people with mean apnoea/hypopnoea index in the severe range, 21 publications, 19 case series), which found that about 70% of people had a 50% or greater reduction in apnoea/hypopnoea index.[46] There is insufficient evidence about long term effectiveness and adverse effects. One RCT (24 people, crossover design), which compared an oral appliance with a small bite opening (4 mm) versus one with a larger opening (14 mm) found no significant difference in sleep disordered breathing or Epworth Sleepiness Scale.[47]

QUESTION What are the effects of treatment for mild obstructive sleep apnoea-hypopnoea syndrome?

OPTION NASAL CONTINUOUS POSITIVE AIRWAY PRESSURE IN MILD OBSTRUCTIVE SLEEP APNOEA-HYPOPNOEA SYNDROME

One systematic review of four RCTs in people with mild obstructive sleep apnoea-hypopnoea syndrome found no significant difference between nasal continuous positive airway pressure and conservative treatment or placebo tablets in daytime sleepiness, but found significant improvement in some measures of cognitive performance at about 4 weeks. One subsequent RCT found no significant difference between nasal continuous positive pressure plus conservative treatment and conservative treatment alone for daytime sleepiness or functional or cognitive outcomes, but found significant improvement in sleep apnoea-hypopnoea related symptoms at 3 and 6 months.

Benefits: **Versus no treatment:** We found no RCTs. **Versus conservative treatment or oral placebo tablets:** We found one systematic review[5] and one subsequent RCT.[48] The systematic review (search date 1999, 4 RCTs, 208 people with mild obstructive sleep apnoea-hypopnoea syndrome [OSAHS]) compared nasal continuous positive airway pressure (CPAP — see glossary, p 1968) versus conservative treatment (sleep hygiene and advice about weight reduction) or oral placebo tablets for at least 4 weeks.[5] It found no significant difference between nasal CPAP and conservative treatment or oral placebo tablets in daytime sleepiness (1 RCT:[49] mean reduction in Epworth Sleepiness Scale –0.57, 95% CI –1.39 to +0.25; 3 RCTs:[50–52] Multiple Sleep Latency Test, graphical representation; mean effect about 0 with 95% CI of about ±0.7). It found no significant difference between nasal CPAP and conservative treatment or oral placebo tablets in two measures of cognitive performance, but found significant improvement in two other measures of cognitive performance (no significant difference in Steer Clear, 2 RCTs;[49,50] or Digit Symbol Substitution, 2 RCTs;[49,51] significant improvement in Trailmaking Test B, 3 RCTs:[49–51] $P = 0.003$; 2 RCTs, Paced Auditory Serial Addition-2 Second Timing:[49,50] $P < 0.0001$; CI not reported). The review found no significant difference between nasal CPAP and oral placebo tablets for quality of life and anxiety measures, but found significant improvement for depression and for energy and vitality (quality of life: 2 RCTs, 36-item Short Form general perception);[49,51] anxiety measures (2 RCTs, Hospital Anxiety and Depression Scale);[49,50] depression (2 RCTs, Hospital Anxiety and Depression Scale;[49,50] 1 RCT, Beck Depression Inventory;[51] combined $P = 0.0004$); energy and vitality (2 RCTs, 36-item Short Form vitality;[49,51] 1 RCT, UWIST Mood Adjective Checklist Energetic Arousal Score;[50] combined $P = 0.013$; 1 RCT, energy/fatigue subscore of MOD;[52] $P < 0.05$). The three RCTs that reported a symptom score (in-house questionnaires using an analogue scale) showed a significant benefit of appliance over placebo (combined $P = 0.006$).[49–51] We found one subsequent RCT (142 people with mild OSAHS) comparing nasal CPAP plus conservative treatment (sleep hygiene and weight loss) versus conservative treatment alone.[48] It found that nasal CPAP plus conservative treatment significantly reduced symptoms at 3 and 6 months compared with conservative treatment alone (sleep apnoea-hypopnoea syndrome related symptom score 14 with nasal CPAP plus conservative treatment *v* 19 with conservative treatment alone; $P < 0.001$). However, it found no significant difference between nasal CPAP plus conservative treatment in daytime sleepiness or functional outcomes at 3 and 6 months compared with conservative treatment alone (results not by intention to treat, 17 people excluded; Epworth Sleepiness Scale 10.5 with nasal CPAP plus conservative treatment *v* 12.0 with conservative treatment alone; $P = 0.67$ at 3 months; 9.6 with nasal CPAP plus conservative treatment *v* 11.8 with conservative treatment alone; $P = 0.11$ at 6 months; Multiple Sleep Latency Test not reported at 3 months; 10 minutes with nasal CPAP plus conservative treatment *v* 11 minutes with conservative treatment alone, $P = 0.87$; Functional Outcomes of Sleep Questionnaire score 106 with nasal CPAP plus conservative treatment *v* 102 with conservative treatment alone at 3 and at 6 months, $P = 0.29$ at 3 months and $P = 0.06$ at 6 months). The RCT also found no significant difference between treatments in several measures of cognitive function at 3 or 6 months (e.g. Steer Clear score 10% in both groups at 3 months, P = 0.65; 8% in both groups at 6 months, P = 0.88). **Versus oral appliances:** We found no reliable RCTs.

Harms: The systematic review grouped mild and moderate to severe OSAHS for reporting of adverse effects (see harms of nasal continuous positive airway pressure in moderate to severe OSAHS, p 1963).[5] The subsequent RCT did not report on harms.[48]

Comment: People with mild OSAHS find nasal CPAP less acceptable. People with an apnoea/hypopnoea index (see glossary, p 1968) below 15/hour have been found to have half the long term use of nasal CPAP compared with people with an apnoea/hypopnoea index greater than 15/hour.[53] In the RCT published after the review, adherence by people with mild OSAHS was moderately high (4.8 hours/day).[48] Treatment acceptance was also good (62% of people who finished the trial chose to continue CPAP).

OPTION — WEIGHT LOSS IN MILD OBSTRUCTIVE SLEEP APNOEA-HYPOPNOEA SYNDROME

One systematic review found no RCTs on the effect of weight loss in people with mild obstructive sleep apnoea-hypopnoea syndrome.

Benefits: We found one systematic review (search date 2000), which found no RCTs on the effect of weight loss in people with obstructive sleep apnoea-hypopnoea syndrome (see comment below).[39]

Harms: We found no RCTs on the effect of weight loss in people with mild obstructive sleep apnoea-hypopnoea syndrome.

Comment: We found one large population based cohort study (690 people with sleep disordered breathing [see glossary, p 1969], including those who did not qualify for diagnosis of obstructive sleep apnoea-hypopnoea syndrome) that evaluated sleep disordered breathing at 4 year intervals over 10 years.[54] It found an association between changes in weight and apnoea/hypopnoea index (see glossary, p 1968) (weight gain of 10% was associated with an increase in apnoea/hypopnoea index of 32% [95% CI 20% to 45%]; weight loss of 10% was associated with a decrease in apnoea/hypopnoea index of 26% [95% CI 18% to 34%]).

OPTION — ORAL APPLIANCES IN MILD OBSTRUCTIVE SLEEP APNOEA-HYPOPNOEA SYNDROME

One RCT found that oral appliances that produce mandibular advancement reduced apnoea and hypopnoea, but had no significant effect on daytime sleepiness or quality of life compared with uvulopalatopharyngoplasty in people with mild obstructive sleep apnoea-hypopnoea syndrome.

Benefits: **Versus surgical treatment (uvulopalatopharyngoplasty):** We found three reports comparing an oral appliance (see glossary, p 1968) (producing anterior advancement of the mandible) versus uvulopalatopharyngoplasty.[55–57] However, they were all related to the same RCT of 95 people with mild obstructive sleep apnoea-hypopnoea syndrome (mean apnoea/hypopnoea index (see glossary, p 1968) 18.2/hour, 95% CI 15.7/hour to 20.8/hour in oral appliance group; 20.4/hour, 95% CI 17.4/hour to 23.3/hour in the uvulopalatopharyngoplasty group). Successful treatment was defined as a reduction in apnoea/hypopnoea index to less than 10/hour. The RCT found that the oral appliance significantly improved the apnoea/hypopnoea index compared with uvulopalatopharyngoplasty at 12 months (78% improved with oral appliance *v* 51% with uvulopalatopharyngoplasty; $P < 0.05$; CI not reported). It found no significant difference between oral appliance and uvulopalatopharyngoplasty in daytime sleepiness (as measured using 5 questions, with a 5 point scale for each),[55] quality of life (Minor Symptoms Evaluation Profile), or vitality, contentment, and sleep.[57] The uvulopalatopharyngoplasty group had a better contentment score.

Harms: The RCTs on oral appliances have generally been too brief to evaluate clinically important adverse effects. See harms of oral appliances in moderate to severe obstructive sleep apnoea-hypopnoea syndrome, p 1965.

Comment: Oral appliances are used commonly for people with snoring with or without mild sleep apnoea (see glossary, p 1968). Although the number and duration of trials are not ideal, there is consensus that oral appliances are effective.[58]

GLOSSARY

Apnoea Absence of airflow at the nose and mouth for at least 10 seconds. Sometimes defined indirectly in terms of oxygen desaturation index (impact on pulse oximetry saturation is measured as the number of occasions an hour when oxygen saturation falls by ≥4%). Apnoeas may be "central", in which there is cessation of inspiratory effort, or "obstructive", in which inspiratory efforts continue but are ineffective because of upper airway obstruction.

Apnoea/hypopnoea index The sum of apnoeas and hypopnoeas per hour of sleep. Although the generally accepted cut off point for "normal" is an index of five per hour, there are several definitions of normal, of which at least four are applicable to the situation of sleep disordered breathing: levels that are inside the range found in a "normal" (i.e. healthy) population; levels that are well removed from those found in a target disorder such as obstructive sleep apnoea-hypopnoea syndrome; levels that are not associated with a significant risk of disease and disability; and levels for which there is evidence of a significant benefit of treatment.[4]

Continuous positive airway pressure (CPAP) Involves applying positive pressure from a blower motor to the upper airway through tubing and a soft nasal mask or a facemask. It provides a "pneumatic splint" to the upper airway. Because nasal delivery is the most common in the published literature, we refer to "nasal CPAP".

Hypopnoea A major reduction (> 50%) in airflow at the nose and mouth for at least 10 seconds. A smaller reduction in airflow may be accepted as hypopnoea if it is associated with either an arousal or a reduction in oxygen saturation of 4% or more.

Oral appliance The term "oral appliance" is generic for devices that are placed in the mouth in order to change the position of the mandible, tongue, and other structures in the upper airway to reduce snoring or the upper airway obstruction of obstructive sleep apnoea-hypopnoea syndrome. Specific types are referred to as mandibular advancement devices or splints.

Sham/subtherapeutic nasal continuous positive airway pressure This involves the use of the nasal mask and continuous positive airway pressure machine, but with inadequate pressure generated to overcome upper airway obstruction during sleep.

Sleep disordered breathing Can be described as apnoeas (no airflow for 10 s or more) or hypopnoeas (markedly reduced airflow for 10 s or more). The choice of 10 seconds is by convention. The usual measure of the degree of sleep disordered breathing is the apnoea/hypopnoea index. Features of sleep disordered breathing include snoring, witnessed episodes of absent breathing (apnoeas), abnormal breathing during sleep, nocturnal hypoxaemia, and abnormal sleep architecture.

Upper airway resistance syndrome Measurement of inspiratory effort by oesophageal pressure shows recurrent episodes of increased inspiratory effort that maintain stable ventilation but are associated with arousals and sleep fragmentation. These episodes are also referred to as respiratory effort related arousal events.[8] More recent techniques of measuring nasal air flow can show changes consistent with upper airway resistance syndrome without the need for an oesophageal pressure catheter.[59]

Substantive changes

Nasal CPAP in moderate to severe OSAHS: One RCT added;[37] conclusions unchanged.

Oral appliances in moderate to severe OSAHS: One RCT added;[44] conclusions unchanged.

Nasal CPAP in mild OSAHS: One RCT added;[53] conclusions unchanged.

REFERENCES

1. Gastaut H, Tassarini CA, Duron B. Polygraphic study of the episodic diurnal and nocturnal (hypnic and respiratory) manifestations of the Pickwick syndrome. *Brain Res* 1965;2:167–186.
2. Bassari AG, Guilleminault C. Clinical features and evaluation of obstructive sleep apnea hypopnea syndrome. In: Kryger MH, Roth T, Dement WC, eds. *Principles and practice of sleep medicine*. Philadelphia, PA: WB Saunders, 2000:869–878.
3. Ross SD, Sheinhait IA, Harrison KJ, et al. Systematic review and meta-analysis of the literature regarding the diagnosis of sleep apnea. *Sleep* 2000;23:519–532.
4. Sackett DL, Straus SE, Richardson WS, et al. *Evidence-based medicine. How to practice and teach EBM*. Edinburgh: Churchill Livingstone, 2000:69–70.
5. National Health and Medical Research Council of Australia. *Effectiveness of nasal continuous airway pressure (nCPAP) in obstructive sleep apnoea in adults*. National Health and Medical Research Council of Australia, 2000. http://www.health.gov.au/nhmrc/publications/pdf/hpr21.pdf(last accessed 4 July 2003). Search date 1999; primary sources Medline, Cochrane Library, some Health Technology Assessment websites, Centre for Reviews and Dissemination website, Veteran Affairs Research website, hand searches of reference lists of review articles, and personal contact with experts.
6. Guilleminault C, Stoohs R, Clerk A, et al. A cause of excessive daytime sleepiness. The upper airway resistance syndrome. *Chest* 1993;104:781–787.
7. Lindberg E, Gislason T. Epidemiology of sleep-related obstructive breathing. *Sleep Med Rev* 2000;4:411–433.
8. American Academy of Sleep Medicine Task Force (Flemons W, Chair). Sleep-related breathing disorders in adults: recommendations for syndrome definition and measurement techniques in clinical research. *Sleep* 1999;22:667–689.
9. Young T, Palta M, Dempsey J, et al. The occurrence of sleep-disordered breathing among middle-aged adults. *N Engl J Med* 1993;328:1230–1235.
10. Young TB, Peppard P. Epidemiology of obstructive sleep apnea. In: McNicholas WT, Phillipson EA, eds. *Breathing disorders in sleep*. London, UK: WB Saunders, 2002:31–43.
11. Redline S. Morbidity, mortality and public health burden of sleep apnea. In: McNicholas WT, Phillipson EA, eds. *Breathing disorders in sleep*. London, UK: WB Saunders, 2002:222–235.
12. George CFP. Reduction in motor vehicle collisions following treatment of sleep apnoea with nasal CPAP. *Thorax* 2001;56:508–512.
13. Johns MW. A new method for measuring daytime sleepiness: the Epworth Sleepiness Scale. *Sleep* 1991;14:540–545.
14. Carskadon MA, Dement WC, Mitler MM, et al. Guidelines for the Multiple Sleep Latency Test (MSLT): a standard measure of sleepiness. *Sleep* 1986;9:519–524.
15. Poceta JS, Timms RM, Jeong DU, et al. Maintenance of Wakefulness Test in obstructive sleep apnea syndrome. *Chest* 1992;101:893–897.
16. Ware JE and Sherbourne CD. The MOS 36–item short form health survey (SF–36). 1. Conceptual framework and item selection. *Med Care* 1992;30:473–483.
17. NFER website: http://www.nfer-nelson.co.uk/ghq/ghq28.htm
18. Zigmond AS, Snaith RP. The Hospital Anxiety and Depression Scale. *Acta Psychiatr Scand* 1983;67:361–370.

19. Beck AT, Ward CH, Mendelson M, et al. An inventory for measuring depression. *Arch Gen Psychiatry* 1961;4:561–571.
20. McNair D, Lorr M, Droppleman L. *EITS manual for the profile of mood states*. San Diego: Educational and Industrial Test Services, 1971.
21. Matthews G, Jones DM, Chamberlin AG. Refining the measurement of mood: The UWIST Mood Adjective Checklist. *Br J Psychol* 1990;81:17–42.
22. Hunt SM, McEwen J, McKenna SP. Measuring health stats: a new tool for clinicians and epidemiologists. *J R Coll Gen Pract* 1985;35:185–88.
23. Weaver TE, Laizner AM, Evans LK, et al. Instrument to measure functional status outcomes for disorders of excessive sleepiness. *Sleep* 1997;20:835–43.
24. Findley LJ, Fabrizio MJ, Knight H, et al. Driving simulator performance in patients with sleep apnea. *Am Rev Respir Dis* 1989;140:529–530.
25. Weaver TE. Outcome measurement in sleep medicine practice and research. Part 2: assessment of neurobehavioral performance and mood. *Sleep Med Rev* 2001;5:223–236.
26. Ballester E, Badia JR, Hernandez L, et al. Evidence of the effectiveness of continuous positive airway pressure in the treatment of sleep apnea/hypopnea syndrome. *Am J Respir Crit Care Med* 1999;159:495–501.
27. Jenkinson C, Davies RJ, Mullins R, et al. Long-term benefits in self-reported health status of nasal continuous positive airway pressure therapy for obstructive sleep apnoea. *QJ Med* 2001;94:95–99.
28. Barbe F, Mayoralas LR, Duran J, et al. Treatment with continuous airway pressure is not effective in patients with sleep apnea but no daytime sleepiness. A randomised, controlled trial. *Ann Intern Med* 2001;134:1015–1023.
29. Hack M, Davies RJ, Mullins R, et al. Randomised prospective parallel trial of therapeutic versus subtherapeutic nasal continuous positive airway pressure on simulated steering performance in patients with obstructive sleep apnoea. *Thorax* 2000;55:224–231.
30. Montserrat JM, Ferrer M, Hernandez L, et al. Effectiveness of CPAP treatment in daytime function in sleep apnea syndrome: a randomized controlled study with an optimized placebo. *Am J Respir Crit Care Med* 2001;164:608–613.
31. Jenkinson C, Davies RJO, Mullins R, et al. Comparison of therapeutic and subtherapeutic nasal continuous positive airway pressure for obstructive sleep apnoea: a randomised prospective parallel trial. *Lancet* 1999;353:2100–2105.
32. Wright J, Cates C, White J. Continuous positive airways pressure for obstructive sleep apnoea. In: The Cochrane Library, Issue 4, 2002. Oxford: Update Software. Search date 2001; primary sources Medline, Embase, Cinahl, hand searches of reference lists of identified papers, and personal contact with researchers and clinical experts.
33. Faccenda JF, Mackay TW, Boon NA, et al. Randomised placebo-controlled trial of continuous positive airway pressure on blood pressure in the sleep apnea-hypopnea syndrome. *Am J Respir Crit Care Med* 2001;163:344–348.
34. Clark GT, Blumenfeld I, Yoffe N, et al. A crossover study comparing the efficacy of continuous airway pressure with anterior mandibular positioning devices on patients with obstructive sleep apnea. *Chest* 1996;109:1477–1483.
35. Ferguson KA, Ono T, Lowe AA, et al. A randomized crossover study of an oral appliance vs nasal-continuous positive airway pressure in the treatment of mild-moderate obstructive sleep apnea. *Chest* 1996;109:1269–1275.
36. Ferguson KA, Ono T, Lowe AA, et al. A short term controlled trial of an adjustable oral appliance for the treatment of mild to moderate obstructive sleep apnoea. *Thorax* 1997;52:362–368.
37. Engleman HM, McDonald JP, Graham D, et al. Randomized crossover trial of two treatments for sleep apnea/hypopnea syndrome: continuous positive airway pressure and mandibular repositioning splint. *Am J Respir Crit Care Med* 2002;166:855–859.
38. Brander PE, Soirinsuo M, Lohela P. Nasopharyngeal symptoms in patients with obstructive sleep apnea syndrome. *Respiration* 1999;66:128–135.
39. Shneerson J, Wright J. Lifestyle modification of obstructive sleep apnoea. In: The Cochrane Library, Issue 4, 2002. Oxford: Update Software. Search date 2000; primary sources Cochrane Airways Group Trials Register, Medline, Embase, Cinahl, and hand searches of reference lists of review articles.
40. Barvaux VA, Aubert G, Rodenstein DO. Weight loss as a treatment for obstructive sleep apnoea. *Sleep Med Rev* 2000;4:435–452.
41. Bloch KE, Iseli A, Zhang JN, et al. A randomized, controlled crossover trial of two oral appliances for sleep apnea treatment. *Am J Respir Crit Care Med* 2000;162:246–251.
42. Hans MG, Nelson S, Luks VG, et al. Comparison of two dental devices for treatment of obstructive sleep apnea syndrome (OSAS). *Am J Orthod Dentofac Orthop* 1997;111:562–570.
43. Mehta A, Qian J, Petocz P, et al. A randomized controlled study of a mandibular advancement splint for obstructive sleep apnea. *Am J Respir Crit Care Med* 2001;163:1457–1461.
44. Gotsopoulos H, Chen C, Qian J, et al. Oral appliance therapy improves symptoms in obstructive sleep apnea: a randomized, controlled trial. *Am J Respir Crit Care Med* 2002;166:743–748.
45. Fritsch KM, Iselli A, Russi EW, et al. Side effects of mandibular advancement devices for sleep apnea treatment. *Am J Respir Crit Care Med* 2001;164:813–818.
46. Schmidt-Nowra W, Lowe A, Wiegand L, et al. Oral appliance for the treatment of snoring and obstructive sleep apnea: a review. *Sleep* 1995;18:501–510. Search date 1994; primary sources Medline and consultation with experts.
47. Pitsis AJ, Darendeliler MA, Gotsopoulos H, et al. Effect of vertical dimension on efficacy of oral appliance therapy in obstructive sleep apnea. *Am J Respir Crit Care Med* 2002;166:860–864.
48. Monasterio C, Vidal S, Duran J, et al. Effectiveness of continuous positive airway pressure in mild sleep apnea-hypopnea syndrome. *Am J Respir Crit Care Med* 2001;164:939–943.
49. Engleman HM, Kingshott RN, Wraith PK, et al. Randomised placebo-controlled crossover trial of continuous positive airway pressure for mild sleep apnea/hypopnea syndrome. *Am J Respir Crit Care Med* 1999;159:461–467.
50. Engleman HM, Martin SE, Deary IJ, et al. Effect of CPAP therapy on daytime function in patients with mild sleep apnoea/hypopnoea syndrome. *Thorax* 1997;52:114–119.
51. Barnes M, Houston D, Worsnop CJ, et al. A randomised controlled trial of CPAP in mild obstructive sleep apnea. *Am J Respir Crit Care Med* 2002;165:773–780.
52. Redline S, Adams N, Strauss ME, et al. Improvement of mild sleep-disordered breathing

with CPAP compared with conservative therapy. *Am J Respir Crit Care Med* 1998;157:858–865.
53. McArdle N, Dvereux G, Heidarnejad H, et al. Long-term use of CPAP therapy for sleep apnea/hypopnea syndrome. *Am J Respir Crit Care Med* 1999;159:1108–1114.
54. Peppard PE, Young T, Dempsey J, et al. Longitudinal study of moderate weight change and sleep-disordered breathing. *JAMA* 2000;284:3015–3021.
55. Wilhelmsson B, Tegelberg A, Walker-Engstrom ML, et al. A prospective randomized study of a dental appliance compared with uvulopalatopharyngoplasty in the treatment of obstructive sleep apnoea. *Acta Otolaryngol* 1999;119:503–509.
56. Tegelberg A, Wilhelmsson B, Walker-Engstrom ML, et al. Effects and adverse events of a dental appliance for treatment of obstructive sleep apnoea. *Swed Dent J* 1999;23:117–126.
57. Walker-Engstrom ML, Wilhelmsson B, Tegelberg A, et al. Quality of life assessment of treatment with dental appliance or UPPP in patients with mild to moderate obstructive sleep apnoea. A prospective randomized 1-year follow-up study. *J Sleep Res* 2000;9:303–308.
58. Ferguson K. Oral appliance therapy for obstructive sleep apnea. Finally evidence you can sink your teeth into (editorial). *Am J Resp Crit Care Med* 2001;163:1294–1295.
59. Ayappa I, Norman RG, Krieger AC, et al. Non-invasive detection of respiratory effort-related arousals (RERAs) by a nasal cannula/pressure transducer system. *Sleep* 2000;23:763–761.

Michael Hensley
Professor of Medicine
University of Newcastle
Newcastle, NSW
Australia

Cheryl Ray
Data Manager
Newcastle Sleep Disorders Centre
Royal Newcastle Hospital
Newcastle, NSW
Australia

Competing interests: None declared.

TABLE 1 **Validated outcome measures (see text, p 1960).**

Outcome measure (abbreviation)	Description	Scoring
Epworth sleepiness scale (ESS)[13]	Questionnaire developed to measure the general level of sleepiness by the likelihood of falling asleep in eight common situations	The score for each question ranges from 0 (no likelihood of falling asleep) to 3 highly likely to fall asleep). A lower score indicates less daytime sleepiness in the last week. Maximum score 24 Normal < 10 Severe > 16–24
Multiple Sleep Latency test (MSLT)[14]	A daytime sleep laboratory based test in which the patient is asked to try and fall asleep when placed in a quiet dark room for 20 minutes at 2-hourly intervals. Monitoring is by electroencephalography. The time between lights out and sleep onset (sleep latency) is measured in minutes. The mean value of 4–5 test sleeps in the day is calculated. The mean sleep latency is considered an "objective" sleep measure of daytime sleepiness. A reduced score indicates an increase in daytime sleepiness.	Mean adult sleep latency of < 5 minutes is indicative of pathological sleepiness Mild 5–7 minutes Borderline 8–9 minutes Normal ≥ 10 minutes
Maintence of Wakefulness Test (MWT)[15]	Similar to the MSLT, but the patient is asked to stay awake during the 20 minutes in a dark room	Sleep latencies of < 20 minutes are indicative of pathological sleepiness
Quality of life		
Medical Outcomes Survey Short form 36 (SF–36)[16]	A short form health survey that measures generic health related quality of life. The instrument is used widely to evaluate Health Related Quality of Life across various populations It is a 36 item questionnaire comprising eight health concepts : physical functioning; role limitations due to physical health problems; bodily pain; social functioning; general mental health; role limitations due to emotional problems; vitality, energy or fatigue; general health perceptions	Most of the 36 items are scored on a 3–6 point Likert scale. Scaling for different questions includes ranges from excellent to poor; limited a lot to not limited at all; not at all to extremely; and otheres. A higher score reflects a better health related quality of life

TABLE 1 continued

Outcome measure (abbreviation)	Description	Scoring
General Health Questionnaire – 28 (GHQ–28)[17]	A self administered screening test, designed to identify short term changes in mental health. The most popular of the GHQ, it has 28 questions, seven in each sub–scale of depression, anxiety, social dysfunction and somatic symptoms	Four subscores as well as a total score are obtained. The higher the score the more severe the condition. A 4 point scoring system ranges from a "better/healthier than normal" option, through a "same as usual" and a "worse/more than usual" to a "much worse/more than usual" option
Hospital Anxiety and Depression scale (HADS)[18]	A 14 item questionnaire designed to identify clinical depression and anxiety. Seven items conceptually assess depression and seven items were derived from psychic manifestations of anxiety neurosis	Overall level of severity of each mood on a 4 point scale (0–3). A score of 8 is clinically significant, a score of 11 or more is highly clinically significant
Beck Depression Inventory (BDI)[19]	A measurement of clinical depression with 21 statements regarding a symptom associated with depression (e.g. appetite, mood, sense of failure)	Scores range from 0, indicating the absence of the particular symptom, to 3 for most severe
Profile of Mood States (POMS)[20]	A self report designed to measure six dimensions of mood, which include: tension–anxiety; depression–dejection; anger–hostility; vigour–activity; fatigue–inertia; and confusion– bewilderment. It consists of 65 short phrases describing feeling and mood, with respondents asked to indicate mood readtions for the "past week including today" or for shorter periods such as "right now"	A five point Likert type scale ranging from 0 for no mood reaction to 5, indicating extreme mood reaction
University of Wales Institute of Science and Technology (UWIST) Mood adaptive checklist (UMACL)[21]	A measurement of mood with four subscales: hedonic tone, anger, tense arousal, and energetic arousal. Except for anger, which only has positively loaded items, each one is made up of a combination of positively loaded and negatively loaded items	The final score is the result of adding the positively loaded answers and subtracting the negatively loaded answers

TABLE 1 continued

Outcome measure (abbreviation)	Description	Scoring
Nottingham Health Profile (NHP) [22]	Generic health related quality of life measure made up of 38 items that can be used to produce scores for six domains of health, including: physical mobility (8 items), pain (8 items), social isolation (5 items), emotional reactions (9 items), energy (3 items) and sleep (5 items)	Yes/No answers and domain scores ranging from 0 to 100. Mean score is calculated across all items within each domain. Overall score is the mean across all items. The higher the score the greater the health problem
Functional Outcomes of Sleep Questionnaire (FOSQ) [23]	A sleep specific functional measure designed to evaluate the impact of sleep disorders and excessive sleepiness. Thirty five items represent five subscales: activity level, vigilance, intimacy and sexual relationships, general productivity, and social outcome	Individual scores of each subscale are obtained and summated to produce a global score. The lower the score the greater the dysfunction as a result of sleepiness. Four levels of response: no difficulty, a little, moderate, or extreme plus non–participation. Scored on a 5 point Likert scale
Cognitive performance measures		
SteerClear (SC)[24]	A computer program designed to simulate a long, mundane highway drive and to characterise the decrements in driving ability. The patient is required to avoid obstacles that randomly appear on a two lane highway by pressing a single computer key. Performance on this 30 minute task is reflected by the number of obstacles passed and the number hit	Reducing the number of obstacles hit reflects improved vigilance
Trailmaking B tests (TTB)[25]	A test for broad cognitive performance that uses the connect a dot concept requiring the patient to draw lines from circle to circle to consecutively link numbers and letters in the quickest time possible	Better cognitive performance is indicated by a reduction in score, which reflects the time taken to complete the task
Digit Symbol Substitution (DSS)[25]	Cognitive speed is tested by matching individually presented symbols to their numbers using a reference key	Improved speed of performance is reflected by an increased score
Paced Auditory Serial Addition Task – 2 second timing (PASAT–2)[25]	A test of auditory attention and concentration by evaluating the time taken to add up numbers presented every 2 seconds	An increase in the score indicates improved ability to maintain

Breast cancer (metastatic)

Search date January 2003

Stephen Johnston and Justin Stebbing

QUESTIONS

INTERVENTIONS

Likely to be ineffective or harmful

High dose chemotherapy (*v* standard chemotherapy) as first line treatment 1988

Progestins (*v* aromatase inhibitors) as second line treatment . .1983

*Not based on RCT evidence

See glossary, p 1997

Key Messages

- **Anthracycline based regimens (CAF) containing doxorubicin as first line treatment** RCTs have found that combination chemotherapy regimens containing an anthracycline, such as doxorubicin (CAF), versus other regimens as first line treatment increase response rates, time to progression, and survival.
- **Classical combination first line chemotherapy (CMF)** One systematic review has found that classical combination chemotherapy as first line treatment increases response rate and survival compared with modified CMF regimens.
- **First line chemotherapy plus monoclonal antibody (in women with overexpressed HER2 neu oncogene)** One RCT found that, in women whose tumours overexpress HER2, standard chemotherapy plus the monoclonal antibody trastuzumab as first line treatment increased the time to disease progression, objective response, and overall survival compared with standard chemotherapy alone.
- **Selective aromatase inhibitors as first line hormonal treatment in postmenopausal women** RCTs have found that the aromatase inhibitor anastrozole as first line treatment in metastatic postmenopausal breast cancer is at least as effective as tamoxifen in reducing time to disease progression, and found that the aromatase inhibitor letrozole was superior to tamoxifen in reducing time to disease progression.
- **Selective aromatase inhibitors as second line hormonal treatment in postmenopausal women** RCTs in postmenopausal women who have relapsed during or after treatment with tamoxifen have found that the selective aromatase inhibitors anastrozole, letrozole, and exemestane increase overall survival at 2–3 years, and are associated with fewer adverse effects compared with progestins or the non-selective aromatase inhibitor aminoglutethamide. Two RCTs found that anastrozole was as effective as fulvestrant for delaying progression.
- **Tamoxifen as first line treatment in oestrogen receptor positive disease** RCTs have found that antioestrogens such as tamoxifen prolong remission in women with oestrogen receptor positive metastatic breast cancer.
- **Radiotherapy for spinal cord compression** We found no RCTs. Retrospective analyses found that early radiotherapy improved outcomes, but fewer than 10% of people walked again if severe deterioration of motor function occurred before radiotherapy.
- **Radiotherapy plus appropriate analgesia for bone metastases** We found no RCTs comparing radiotherapy versus no treatment or versus bisphosphonates. We found limited evidence from non-randomised studies that persistent and localised bone pain can be treated successfully in over 80% of women with radiotherapy plus concomitant appropriate analgesia (from non-steroidal anti-inflammatory drugs to morphine and its derivatives). RCTs found no evidence that short courses are less effective for pain relief than long courses of radiotherapy. One RCT found that different fractionation schedules can be used to treat neuropathic bone pain effectively.

- **Radiotherapy plus high dose steroids in spinal cord compression** One small RCT found that adding high dose steroids to radiotherapy improved the chance of walking after 6 months.
- **Bisphosphonates for bone metastases** RCTs in women receiving standard chemotherapy for bone metastases secondary to metastatic breast cancer found that adding bisphosphonates reduced and delayed skeletal complications compared with adding placebo. None of the RCTs found an impact on overall survival.
- **Combined gonadorelin analogues and tamoxifen as first line treatment in premenopausal women** RCTs (in premenopausal women with oestrogen receptor positive metastatic breast cancer) have found that first line treatment with gonadorelin analogues plus tamoxifen improves response rates, overall survival, and progression free survival compared with gonadorelin analogues alone.
- **Radiotherapy to control cerebral and choroidal metastases** We found no RCTs. Retrospective studies suggest that whole brain radiation improves general neurological function in some women with brain metastases secondary to breast cancer, and that radiotherapy benefits some women with choroidal metastases.
- **Taxane based chemotherapy as first line treatment (compared with single agent)** One RCT found that doxorubicin-paclitaxel (AT) improved response rate compared with either doxorubicin or paclitaxel alone, but found no significant difference in overall survival. One RCT found no significant difference between doxorubicin-paclitaxel and doxorubicin-cyclophosphamide in survival or response rate.
- **Taxanes for anthracycline resistant disease** We found limited evidence that taxanes may improve response rates compared with CMF or continued doxorubicin, especially in anthracycline resistant disease. One RCT found no significant difference in progression or overall survival between docetaxel and 5-fluorouracil plus vinorelbine given as second line chemotherapy.
- **Capecitabine for anthracycline resistant disease** One RCT found no significant difference in progression or response rate between capecitabine and paclitaxel following anthracycline failure.
- **Semisynthetic vinca alkaloids for anthracycline resistant disease** One RCT found no significant difference in survival or quality of life between vinorelbine plus docetaxel versus vinorelbine alone. One RCT found no significant difference in progression or overall survival between docetaxel and 5-fluorouracil plus vinorelbine given as second line chemotherapy. One RCT found that second line vinorelbine improved survival and reduced progression compared with melphalan.
- **Ovarian ablation as first line treatment in premenopausal women (*v* tamoxifen)** One systematic review and one subsequent RCT in premenopausal women found no significant difference in response rate, duration of response, or survival with ovarian ablation (surgery or irradiation) versus tamoxifen as first line treatment. Ovarian ablation is associated with substantial adverse effects such as hot flushes and "tumour flare".
- **Progestins (*v* tamoxifen, beneficial as first line treatment in women with bone pain or anorexia)** RCTs found no significant difference in response rates, remission rates, or survival between progestins and tamoxifen as first line treatment, but found that progestins increased adverse effects, including nausea, weight gain, and exacerbations of hypertension. One RCT found that

medroxyprogesterone versus tamoxifen improved bone pain. Observational evidence suggests that progestins may increase appetite, weight gain, and well being.

- **High dose chemotherapy (v standard chemotherapy) as first line treatment** One systematic review found no significant difference in overall survival or progression free survival between high dose chemotherapy (requiring haematopoeitic cell transplant) and standard dose chemotherapy. It found that high dose chemotherapy increased treatment related morbidity and mortality compared with standard chemotherapy.
- **Progestins (v aromatase inhibitors) as second line treatment** RCTs have found that, in postmenopausal women with metastatic breast cancer who have relapsed on adjuvant tamoxifen or progressed during first line treatment with tamoxifen, the selective aromatase inhibitors anastrozole, letrozole, and exemestane prolong survival compared with progestins or aminoglutethimide, with minimal adverse effects.

DEFINITION Metastatic or advanced breast cancer is the presence of disease at distant sites such as the bone, liver, or lung. It is not treatable by primary surgery and is currently considered incurable. However, young people with good performance status may survive for 15 to 20 years.[1] Symptoms may include pain from bone metastases, breathlessness from spread to the lung, and nausea or abdominal discomfort from liver involvement.

INCIDENCE/ PREVALENCE Breast cancer is the second most frequent cancer in the world (1.05 million people) and is by far the most common malignant disease in women (22% of all new cancer cases). Worldwide, the ratio of mortality to incidence is about 36%. It ranks fifth as a cause of death from cancer overall (although it is the leading cause of cancer mortality in women — the 370 000 annual deaths represent 13.9% of cancer deaths in women). In the USA, metastatic breast cancer causes 46 000 deaths, and in the UK causes 15 000 deaths.[2] It is the most prevalent cancer in the world today and there are an estimated 3.9 million women alive who have had breast cancer diagnosed in the past 5 years (compared, for example, with lung cancer, where there are 1.4 million alive). The true prevalence of metastatic disease is high because some women live with the disease for many years. Since 1990, there has been an overall increase in incidence rates of about 1.5% annually.[3]

AETIOLOGY/ RISK FACTORS The risk of metastatic disease relates to known prognostic factors in the original primary tumour. These factors include oestrogen receptor negative disease, primary tumours 3 cm or more in diameter, and axillary node involvement — recurrence occurred within 10 years of adjuvant chemotherapy for early breast cancer (see glossary, p 1997) in 60–70% of node positive women and 25–30% of node negative women in one large systematic review.[4]

PROGNOSIS Prognosis depends on age, extent of disease, and oestrogen receptor status. There is also evidence that overexpression of the product of the HER2/neu oncogene, which occurs in about a third of women with metastatic breast cancer, is associated with a worse prognosis.[5] A short disease free interval (see glossary, p 1997) (e.g. < 1 year) between surgery for early breast cancer and developing metastases suggests that the recurrent disease is likely to be resistant to adjuvant treatment (see glossary, p 1997).[6] In women who receive no treatment for metastatic disease, the median survival from diagnosis of metastases is 12 months.[7] The choice of first line treatment (see glossary, p 1997) (hormonal or chemotherapy) is based on a variety of clinical factors (see table 1, p 2002).[8–11] In many countries, such as USA, Canada and some countries in Europe, there is evidence of a decrease in death rates in recent years. This probably reflects improvements in treatment (and therefore improved survival) as well as earlier diagnosis.[2,12]

AIMS OF INTERVENTION To relieve symptoms, prolong life, and improve quality of life, with minimal adverse effects.

OUTCOMES Symptoms; progression free survival; overall objective response rate; complete response; partial response (see glossary, p 1998); duration of response; disease stabilisation; time to progression of disease (progression defined as > 25% increase in lesion size or the appearance of new lesions); quality of life;[13] improvement in performance status (according to validated scales of daily functioning/activity);[14] adverse effects and toxicity of treatment;[15] and overall survival. Response to treatment is a surrogate outcome measure for assessing the effects of treatment on survival or quality of life. The link between clinical and proxy outcomes has not been clearly validated. Women who respond to treatment are more likely to experience improved symptomatic relief, performance status, and survival.[16–18] One recent prospective study (300 women with metastatic breast cancer) found a significant relationship between improvement and objective response for three symptoms, in particular cancer pain, shortness of breath, and abnormal mood. Symptom improvement was greatest in those women who had a complete or partial response.[19]

METHODS *Clinical Evidence* search and appraisal January 2003. We looked for good quality systematic reviews that used the outcome measures listed above. Where we found no good systematic reviews, we included relevant randomised phase III trials using these outcomes. Studies presented only in abstract form were discarded. Response to treatment is often assessed in an unblinded fashion, introducing the possibility of bias. We found few trials of good quality that reported on symptoms or quality of life.

QUESTION What are the effects of first line treatments?

OPTION ANTIOESTROGENS (TAMOXIFEN)

RCTs have found that antioestrogens such as tamoxifen prolong remission in women with oestrogen receptor positive metastatic breast cancer.

Benefits: We found no systematic review. Non-systematic reviews published in 1986 and 1991 identified 86 RCTs in 5353 women with metastatic breast cancer unselected for oestrogen receptor status. The overall objective response rate to tamoxifen (see glossary, p 1998) was 34%. Disease stabilisation was achieved in a further 20%, and overall the median duration of response was 12–18 months.[8,9] The likelihood of responding to tamoxifen was highest (60–70%) in postmenopausal women with oestrogen receptor positive disease (see comment below).[10,11] **Versus ovarian ablation in premenopausal women:** See ovarian ablation in premenopausal women, p 1981.

Harms: **Minor adverse effects:** Tamoxifen is well tolerated in women with metastatic breast cancer; fewer than 3% of women discontinued tamoxifen as a result of toxicity.[20] Reported adverse effects included minor gastrointestinal upset (8%), hot flushes (27%), and menstrual disturbance in premenopausal women (13%).[21] **Tumour flare:** During the first few weeks of treatment, tumour flare occurred in fewer than 5% of women. For those with bone metastases, this may have resulted in increased pain or symptomatic hypercalcaemia. **Relapse:** Most women who initially respond to tamoxifen eventually progress and develop acquired resistance to tamoxifen, although they may still respond to further hormonal interventions.[22]

Comment: The choice of first line treatment (hormonal or chemotherapy [see glossary, p 1998]) is based on a variety of clinical factors (see table 1, p 2002).[8–11] **Antioestrogens:** An emerging problem is that many women have already received adjuvant tamoxifen for early breast cancer or have developed metastatic disease while still taking tamoxifen, and are thus considered resistant to it. Effective second line treatment (see glossary, p 1998) hormonal drugs, such as selective aromatase inhibitors (see glossary, p 1997), are now used after tamoxifen failure (see selective aromatase inhibitors in postmenopausal women, p 1983), and RCTs have compared these drugs with tamoxifen as first line treatment (see selective aromatase inhibitors as first line treatment in postmenopausal women, p 1982). New non-steroidal antioestrogens (toremifene, idoxifene, raloxifene) and steroidal antioestrogens (fulvestrant) are more selective than tamoxifen and may have fewer long term adverse effects. RCTs comparing some of these drugs with tamoxifen as first line hormonal treatment in metastatic breast cancer are in progress. So far, one RCT in 658 women has found no evidence of clear clinical superiority of toremifene over tamoxifen.[23]

OPTION PROGESTINS (MEDROXYPROGESTERONE; MEGESTROL)

RCTs found no significant difference in response rates, remission rates, or survival between progestins and tamoxifen as first line treatment, but found that progestins increased adverse effects, including nausea, weight gain, and exacerbations of hypertension. One RCT found that medroxyprogesterone versus tamoxifen improved bone pain. Observational evidence suggests that progestins may increase appetite, weight gain, and well being.

Benefits: We found one systematic review (search date 1991, 7 RCTs, 801 women with metastatic breast cancer) comparing medroxyprogesterone versus tamoxifen (see glossary, p 1998),[24] and one subsequent RCT.[25] The review found no significant difference in response rates (35–54%), remission rates, or survival between the two groups. Benefits of progestins (see glossary, p 1998) included an analgesic effect (assessed using questionnaires), especially on painful bone metastases,[26] increased appetite, weight gain, and a feeling of wellbeing. The subsequent RCT (166 women) found that medroxyprogesterone increased the rate of response of bone metastases compared with tamoxifen (33% v 13%; P = 0.01), although it found no significant difference in survival.[25]

Harms: Women taking medroxyprogesterone experienced more adverse effects than women taking tamoxifen.[27] These were common at higher doses and included nausea (14%), weight gain (56%), vaginal bleeding (10%), and exacerbation of hypertension. In women with lymphangitis carcinomatosis, progestins may exacerbate symptoms of breathlessness.[28]

Comment: In view of the lack of evidence of greater benefit, and the evidence of greater harm, progestins are reserved for second or third line hormonal treatment (see glossary, p 1998) in women with advanced breast cancer who have not responded to tamoxifen.

OPTION OVARIAN ABLATION IN PREMENOPAUSAL WOMEN

One systematic review and one subsequent RCT in premenopausal women found no significant difference in response rate, duration of response, or survival between ovarian ablation (surgery or irradiation) and tamoxifen as first line treatment. Ovarian ablation is associated with substantial adverse effects such as hot flushes and "tumour flare".

Benefits: **Versus tamoxifen:** We found one systematic review (search date not stated, 4 RCTs, 220 premenopausal women) comparing tamoxifen (see glossary, p 1998) versus ovarian ablation (carried out by either surgery or irradiation),[29] and one subsequent RCT.[30] There was no significant difference between treatments in response rate, response duration, or survival. The subsequent RCT (39 premenopausal women) comparing initial treatment with tamoxifen or ovarian ablation found similar results (OR for progressive disease (see glossary, p 1998) 0.71, 95% CI 0.37 to 1.38; median survival 2.35 years with tamoxifen, 2.46 years with ovarian ablation; P = 0.98; OR for death 1.07, 95% CI 0.55 to 2.06).[30] **Different methods of ovarian ablation:** We found two RCTs comparing gonadorelin analogues (see glossary, p 1998) versus surgical ovariectomy or irradiation. They found no significant difference in survival between treatments.[31,32]

Harms: Adverse effects include hot flushes (75% with gonadorelin analogues, 46% with surgical ovariectomy) and "tumour flare" (16% with gonadorelin analogues).[31] In addition, surgical ovariectomy requires an operation and anaesthetic.

Comment: None.

OPTION COMBINED GONADORELIN ANALOGUES PLUS TAMOXIFEN IN PREMENOPAUSAL WOMEN

Stephen Johnston

One non-systematic review has found that, in premenopausal women, combined treatment with a gonadorelin analogue and tamoxifen improves response rates, overall survival, and progression free survival compared with a gonadorelin analogue alone.

Benefits: We found one non-systematic review (4 RCTs, 506 women) that found combined endocrine treatment with gonadorelin analogues plus tamoxifen significantly improved both progression free survival (see glossary, p 1998) (HR 0.70, 95% CI 0.58 to 0.85; P = 0.0003) and overall survival (HR 0.78, 95% CI 0.63 to 0.96; P = 0.02) compared with a gonadorelin analogue alone.[33] The overall response rate was also significantly higher for combined treatment (OR 0.67; P = 0.03).

Harms: Although the meta-analysis did not analyse differences in tolerability, the largest of the individual trials found there was no significant difference in expected hormonal adverse effects (hot flushes, vaginal discharge) between the combined treatment and gonadorelin analogues alone.

Comment: We found that combined endocrine treatment in metastatic breast cancer has been shown to be beneficial over single agent treatment. Attention is now turning to see if there is any additional benefit from complete oestrogen deprivation in premenopausal women using ovarian ablation with gonadorelin analogues combined with aromatase inhibitors (see glossary, p 1997).

OPTION SELECTIVE AROMATASE INHIBITORS AS FIRST LINE HORMONAL TREATMENT IN POSTMENOPAUSAL WOMEN

Stephen Johnston and Justin Stebbing

RCTs have found that the aromatase inhibitor anastrozole as first line treatment in metastatic postmenopausal breast cancer is at least as effective as tamoxifen in reducing time to disease progression, and found that the aromatase inhibitor letrozole was superior to tamoxifen in reducing time to disease progression.

Benefits: **Anastrozole:** We found two RCTs comparing anastrozole versus tamoxifen (see glossary, p 1998).[34,35] The larger RCT (668 women) found no significant difference in time to disease progression (HR 0.99, 95% CI 0.86 to 1.12) or response rate (32.9% anastrozole *v* 32.6% tamoxifen).[34] The smaller RCT (353 women) found that anastrozole significantly prolonged time to progression (HR for progression, tamoxifen *v* anastrozole 1.44, 95% CI 1.16 to 1.82).[35] Neither trial reported on the effect on survival. **Letrozole:** One RCT (907 women) found that letrozole significantly improved the time to disease progression (HR 0.70, 95% CI 0.60 to 0.82; P = 0.0001) and tumour response rate (P = 0.0006) compared with tamoxifen.[36] In women who had received prior adjuvant tamoxifen but stopped at least 12 months before study entry, letrozole significantly improved response rate compared with tamoxifen rechallenge (HR for response, tamoxifen *v* letrozole 0.64, 95% CI 0.41 to 0.98). Women with visceral disease as the dominant site of metastases had a significantly greater chance of response to letrozole than tamoxifen (HR for response, tamoxifen *v* letrozole 0.37, 95% CI 0.26 to 0.53).[36]

Harms: In both anastrozole trials, anastrozole was associated with reduced thromboembolism and vaginal bleeding compared with tamoxifen (thromboembolic events: 4.8% with anastrozole *v* 7.3% with tamoxifen;[34] vaginal bleeding: 4.1% *v* 8.2%[35]). In the letrozole trial, the frequency of adverse events was similar with letrozole and tamoxifen.[36]

Comment: These RCTs[34–36] have confirmed that the selective third generation aromatase inhibitors (see glossary, p 1997) are more efficacious than tamoxifen, with a similar if not better safety profile. These treatments may, therefore, replace tamoxifen as the first line endocrine treatment of choice for postmenopausal women with oestrogen receptor positive metastatic breast cancer. Results from the letrozole trials suggest an early survival advantage for women treated with letrozole rather than tamoxifen, which was not seen on further follow up owing to the prospective crossover of a large number of patients at progression (Mouridsen H et al, San Antonio Breast Cancer Symposium, 2001).[37]

QUESTION What are the effects of second line hormonal treatment in women who have not responded to tamoxifen?

OPTION PROGESTINS

RCTs have found that progestins are less effective in second line treatment than selective aromatase inhibitors and have more adverse effects.

Benefits: **Versus selective aromatase inhibitors:** See selective aromatase inhibitors in postmenopausal women, p 1983.

Harms: **Versus selective aromatase inhibitors:** See selective aromatase inhibitors in postmenopausal women, p 1984.

Comment: In women who are not responding to tamoxifen, progestins (see glossary, p 1998) may have a role in increasing feelings of wellbeing and relieving anorexia.

OPTION SELECTIVE AROMATASE INHIBITORS IN POSTMENOPAUSAL WOMEN

RCTs have found that, in postmenopausal women with metastatic breast cancer who have relapsed on adjuvant tamoxifen or progressed during first line treatment with tamoxifen, the selective aromatase inhibitors anastrozole, letrozole, and exemestane prolong survival compared with progestins aminoglutethimide, with fewer adverse effects. Two RCTs found that anastrozole was as effective as fulvestrant for delaying progression. The evidence suggests that selective aromatase inhibitors are more effective and better tolerated than previous standard second line treatment with a progestin or the non-selective aromatase inhibitor aminoglutethimide, and are most effective in oestrogen receptor positive women.

Benefits: **Anastrozole:** A meta-analysis of the two randomised phase III trials comparing anastrozole versus megestrol (764 postmenopausal women with metastatic breast cancer unresponsive to tamoxifen (see glossary, p 1998), median age 65 years, 70% oestrogen receptor positive, 30% oestrogen receptor status unknown) found no significant difference in objective response rates (10.3% *v* 7.9%), or in the proportion of women whose disease was stabilised for 6 months (25.1% *v* 26.1%).[38] A subsequent analysis after a median of 31 months' follow up found a significant improvement in overall survival with anastrozole (HR for death 0.78; P = 0.02), with an absolute improvement in 2 year survival from 46–56% (P = 0.02) and an improvement in median survival of 4 months (from 22.5–26.7 months).[39] We found two RCTs comparing anastrozole versus fulvestrant.[40,41] The first RCT (400 postmenopausal women with locally advanced or metastatic breast cancer who had progressed on endocrine treatment) found that fulvestrant increased median time to progression compared with anastrozole, although the difference was not significant (median time to progression 5.4 months with fulvestrant *v* 3.4 months with anastrozole; HR 0.92; 95% CI 0.74 to 1.14).[40] Among 70 women who responded to treatment, fulvestrant increased duration of response compared with anastrozole (19 months *v* 10.8 months; P = 0.01). The second RCT (451 postmenopausal women with locally advanced or metastatic breast cancer who had progressed on endocrine treatment) found no significant difference between fulvestrant and anastrozole in time to progression (median time 5.5 months with fulvestrant *v* 5.1 months with anastrozole; HR 0.98, 95% CI 0.80 to 1.21).[41] **Exemestane:** Exemestane is currently being evaluated in phase III trials.[42] One RCT (769 women) found that exemestane significantly improved median survival time, median duration of treatment success, and time to progression compared with megestrol (median survival time: not reached with exemestane *v* 123 weeks with megestrol; P = 0.039; median duration of overall success [complete response/partial response or stable disease ≥ 24 weeks]: 60.1 *v* 49.1 weeks; P = 0.025; time to tumour progression: 20.3 *v* 16.6 weeks; P = 0.037).[43] Compared with megestrol, there were similar or greater improvements in pain control, tumour related signs and symptoms, and quality of life with exemestane.[43] **Letrozole:** Two large RCTs compared letrozole (0.5 mg or 2.5 mg) versus megestrol (551 women)[44] and aminoglutethimide (555 women).[45] Both trials were in postmenopausal women with metastatic breast cancer unresponsive to tamoxifen (median age 64–65 years, 55% oestrogen receptor positive, 45% oestrogen receptor status unknown). Letrozole 2.5 mg significantly increased the response rate, duration of response, and time to treatment failure compared with megestrol (response: HR 1.82, 95% CI 1.02 to 3.25; treatment failure: HR 0.77, 95% CI 0.61 to 0.99).[44] Compared with aminoglutethimide, letrozole improved overall survival and progression (overall survival: HR 0.64, 95% CI 0.49 to 0.85; progression: HR 0.72, 95% CI 0.57 to 0.92).[45]

Harms: The selective aromatase inhibitors (see glossary, p 1997) were generally well tolerated and associated with fewer adverse events than aminoglutethimide or progestins. **Anastrozole:** In the RCTs, anastrozole 1 mg increased minor gastrointestinal disturbance (nausea or change in bowel habit) compared with megestrol (29% *v* 21%; P = 0.005), but reduced weight gain (AR for ≥ 5% weight gain: 13% v 34%; $P < 0.0001$).[38] Both RCTs comparing anastrozole versus fulvestrant found that both treatments were well tolerated.[40,41] The second of these reported that 1.3% of people stopped anastrozole because of adverse effects, compared with 3.2% taking fulvestrant (significance not stated).[41] **Exemestane:** In the RCTs, progestin increased adverse events compared with exemestane (45.8% v 39.1%). The most frequently reported adverse events with exemestane were low grade hot flushes (12.6%), nausea (9.2%), and fatigue (7.5%). In the RCT comparing exemestane versus megestrol, both drugs were well tolerated, although grade 3 or 4 weight changes (> 10% weight gain) were more common with megestrol (17.1% v 7.6%; $P = 0.001$).[43] **Letrozole:** Compared with megestrol, letrozole (2.5 mg) reduced serious cardiovascular adverse events and reduced weight gain (AR for cardiovascular adverse events: 2% v 11%; AR for ≥ 5% weight gain: 19% v 30%).[44] Compared with aminoglutethimide, letrozole (2.5 mg) reduced skin rash and serious drug related adverse events (skin rash: 3% v 11%; serious drug related adverse events: 0% v 3%).[45]

Comment: The evidence indicates greater efficacy and tolerability of anastrozole and letrozole over megestrol acetate or aminoglutethimide. There is a consensus that they are agents of choice as second line hormonal treatment in postmenopausal women no longer responding to tamoxifen. An ongoing RCT is comparing anastrozole versus letrozole in this context (Rose C et al, personal communication, 1999). A trial conducted in 2000 has evaluated the activity of exemestane in metastatic breast cancer after failure of non-steroidal aromatase inhibitors.[46] A total of 241 people were enrolled; 56% had received aminoglutethimide, 19% anastrozole, and 17% letrozole. Exemestane produced objective responses in 7% of treated women, including 8% of women after failure of treatment with aminoglutethimide and 5% after failure of other non-steroidal aromatase inhibitors (anastrozole, letrozole, and vorozole), and an overall success rate (complete response plus partial response plus no change for 24 weeks or longer) of 24%. Women who do not respond to anastrozole or letrozole may respond to exemestane.

QUESTION What are the effects of first line chemotherapy?

OPTION NON-TAXANE COMBINATION CHEMOTHERAPY

We found no RCTs comparing combination chemotherapy versus no chemotherapy in women with metastatic breast cancer. Trials comparing one type of chemotherapy versus another found that first line chemotherapy was associated with an objective tumour response in 40–60% of women, with a median response duration of 6–12 months irrespective of menopausal or oestrogen receptor status. A small proportion of women achieve complete remission, which may persist for an extended length of time (see high dose chemotherapy, p 1989). One systematic review has found that classical combination chemotherapy as first line treatment increases response rate and survival compared with

modified CMF regimens. RCTs have found that combination chemotherapy regimens containing an anthracycline, such as doxorubicin (CAF), versus other regimens as first line treatment increase response rates, time to progression, and survival.

Benefits: **Versus best supportive care:** We found no systematic review and no RCTs comparing first line chemotherapy versus palliative (best supportive) care in women with metastatic breast cancer. **Different chemotherapy regimens:** We found one systematic review (search date 1997, 189 RCTs, 31 510 women) evaluating different chemotherapy (see glossary, p 1997) and endocrine regimens.[20] **"Classical" versus modified CMF:** In the largest RCT (254 postmenopausal women with metastatic breast cancer who had received no prior chemotherapy) the classical CMF (see glossary, p 1997) regimen significantly improved survival and response rate compared with a modified version, in which all three drugs were given intravenously every 3 weeks (response rate 48% *v* 29%; P = 0.03: median survival 17 *v* 12 months; P = 0.016).[47] One RCT (133 women who had received no prior chemotherapy) found that standard dose CMF significantly improved both response rate (30% *v* 11%; P = 0.03) and symptom control compared with low dose CMF.[48] **CAF versus CMF:** One systematic review (search date not stated) found that regimens containing doxorubicin increased response rate, time to progression, and survival compared with other regimens.[49] However, two RCTs comparing CAF (see glossary, p 1997) versus non-anthracycline based regimens (CMF) found no evidence of improved survival.[50,51] **Standard versus modified CAF regimens:** Two large multicentre trials of CAF (containing doxorubicin) versus FEC (see glossary, p 1997), a modified anthracycline based regimen containing epirubicin, found no significant difference in response rates (263 women, response rate 52% *v* 50%;[52] 497 women, response rate 56% *v* 54%[53]). One RCT (249 women) comparing standard CAF (containing doxorubicin) versus a modified, better tolerated anthracycline based regimen containing mitoxantrone (mitozantrone) found that the regimen containing doxorubicin significantly prolonged the time to progression (3.2 *v* 5.3 months; P = 0.03) and increased median survival (10.9 *v* 15.2 months; P = 0.003).[54] **CAF or modified CAF versus mitoxantrone and vinorelbine (MV):** One RCT (281 women) compared MV versus either CAF or FEC. It found no significant difference in response rates among treatments (35% for MV *v* 33% for CAF or FEC). Subgroup analysis in women who had received prior adjuvant treatment found that MV significantly improved response rate and progression free survival compared with other treatments (response rate: 33% *v* 13%; P = 0.025; progression free survival: 9 months *v* 6 months; P = 0.014).[55]

Harms: The toxicity profiles of different combination chemotherapy regimens vary. In RCTs, anthracycline based regimens (CAF) and non-anthracycline based regimens (CMF) are equally associated with haematological toxicity,[51] but CAF is more likely to be associated with alopecia (34% *v* 22%) and severe nausea and vomiting (17% *v* 7%; P = 0.05). Other studies reported the incidence of greater than grade 3 alopecia (complete hair loss) to be 55–61% with CAF, which was significantly higher than with either mitoxantrone or epirubicin (FEC).[53,54] In one of the trials comparing CAF versus FEC, FEC was associated with fewer episodes of greater than or equal to grade 2 neutropenia (10% *v* 13.1%), and significantly lower rates of nausea and vomiting (7.8% *v* 13.3%; $P < 0.01$), and no cardiotoxicity (8 women taking CAF discontinued treatment because of cardiac dysfunction compared with none taking FEC).[52] MV was associated with less nausea and vomiting and alopecia than CAF or FEC, although myelosuppression was greater ($P = 0.001$).

Comment: The optimal duration of chemotherapy for metastatic breast cancer is unknown, although a more recent systematic review (search date not stated; 65 publications reporting 97 treatment comparisons) has found that more, rather than fewer, cycles of chemotherapy given at appropriate doses improved survival (ratio of median survivals 1.23, 95% CI 1.01 to 1.49; $P = 0.01$).[56] The choice of first line treatment (see glossary, p 1997) (hormonal or chemotherapy) is based on a variety of clinical factors (see table 1, p 2002).[8–11] In one RCT (231 women undergoing first line treatment, 60% oestrogen receptor positive, remainder unknown) women were randomised to receive either chemotherapy (CAF) or chemotherapy plus hormonal treatment (see glossary, p 1998) (CAF plus tamoxifen and fluoxymesterone). Response rates and time to treatment failure were similar for women who received chemo–hormonal therapy compared with chemotherapy alone (time to treatment failure 13.4 months *v* 10.3 months; $P = 0.087$).[57] The effect on time to treatment failure was just significant for women who were oestrogen receptor positive compared with those who were negative (17.4 months *v* 10.3 months; $P = 0.048$). Oestrogen receptor status had no effect on overall survival. The choice of a specific drug or regimen is based on which drugs have already been given as adjuvant treatment (see glossary, p 1997), together with the likelihood of benefit balanced against a given drug's adverse effects and tolerability profile. Retrospective series in sequential decades (from 1950–1980) have compared the survival of women from the time of diagnosis with metastatic breast cancer. They suggest that the introduction of chemotherapy has improved median survival by about 9 months (from 12 months without treatment to 21 months with treatment).[7,58] This median survival conceals a bimodal distribution of benefit, with the 40–60% of women who respond to treatment achieving survival of 1 year or greater, and the non-responders experiencing little or no survival benefit. With the increasing use of adjuvant chemotherapy,[59] more women who develop metastatic disease will have received combination chemotherapy. In the treatment of metastatic breast cancer, better quality of life scores predict better outcome (this is not the case in adjuvant treatment).[60] In one RCT (283 women with metastatic breast cancer) evaluating quality of life as a primary end point, no significant differences were found between women randomised to receive either docetaxel or sequential methotrexate and fluorouracil. This suggests that choice of treatment should be based on expected clinical effect.[61] This may influence the likelihood of response to further treatment.[6,62] The prevention of nausea and vomiting caused by chemotherapy has been studied in one RCT

(619 women). It compared placebo versus dexamethasone versus dexamethasone plus ondansetron following chemotherapy. In people who did not have acute nausea and vomiting with chemotherapy, dexamethasone alone was found to provide adequate protection against delayed nausea and vomiting.[63]

OPTION TAXANE BASED COMBINATION CHEMOTHERAPY New

One RCT found that doxorubicin-paclitaxel improved response rate compared with either doxorubicin or paclitaxel alone, but found no significant difference in overall survival. One RCT found no significant difference between doxorubicin-paclitaxel and doxorubicin-cyclophosphamide in survival or response rate.

Benefits: **Doxorubicin-paclitaxel versus either drug alone:** One RCT (739 women) compared three treatments: doxorubicin alone, paclitaxel alone, and doxorubicin-paclitaxel (AT) plus G-CSF support.[64] It found that AT improved overall response rate and time to treatment failure compared with doxorubicin or paclitaxel alone (overall response rate 47% with AT *v* 34% with paclitaxel *v* 36% with doxorubicin; $P = 0.017$ for doxorubicin *v* AT; $P = 0.006$ for paclitaxel *v* AT; median time to treatment failure 8.2 months with AT *v* 6.3 months with paclitaxel *v* 6.0 months with doxorubicin; $P = 0.0022$ for doxorubicin *v* AT; $P = 0.0567$ for paclitaxel *v* AT). It found no significant difference in overall survival between combination chemotherapy and single agent therapy (median survival 19.1 months with doxorubicin, 22.5 months with paclitaxel, 22.4 months with AT; $P = 0.60$ for doxorubicin *v* paclitaxel, $P = 0.82$ for doxorubicin *v* AT; $P = 0.49$ for paclitaxel *v* AT). **Doxorubicin-paclitaxel versus doxorubicin-cyclophosphamide:** One RCT (275 women, who had not previously been treated with anthracycline) compared AT and doxorubicin-cyclophosphamide (AC).[65] It found no significant difference between AT and AC in progression free survival, response rate or median overall survival (progression free survival: 20.6 months with AT *v* 20.5 months with AC; $P = 0.49$; response rate: 58% for AT *v* 54% for AC, $P = 0.51$; overall survival: median 6 months in both groups, $P = 0.65$).

Harms: The RCT comparing AT versus single agent chemotherapy found that grade 4 or 5 infection or neutropenic fever were less common with single agent therapy than with AT (no further data provided).[64] In the RCT comparing AC versus AT, febrile neutropenia was more common with AT than with AC (32% with AT *v* 9% with AC; $P < 0.001$).[65]

Comment: None.

OPTION HIGH DOSE VERSUS STANDARD DOSE CHEMOTHERAPY

One systematic review found no significant difference in overall survival or progression free survival between high dose chemotherapy (requiring haematopoeitic transplant) and standard dose chemotherapy. It found that high dose chemotherapy increased treatment related morbidity and mortality compared with standard chemotherapy.

Benefits: We found one systematic review (search date 2002; 5 RCTs of first line high dose chemotherapy plus bone marrow or stem cell transplant; 740 women).[66] It found no significant difference in overall survival or progression free survival between high dose and standard dose chemotherapy (overall survival at 5 years: RR 1.28, 95% CI 0.72 to 2.27; progression free survival at 5 years: RR 1.21, 95% CI 0.40 to 3.69).

Harms: The review found that high dose chemotherapy increased treatment related death compared with standard dose chemotherapy (10 treatment related deaths with high dose *v* none with standard dose; RR 5.70, 95% CI 1.30 to 25).[66] It found that high dose chemotherapy significantly increased leucopenia; diarrhoea; cardiotoxicity; thrombocytopenia, and anaemia (leucopenia: RR 1.97, 95% CI 1.58 to 2.45; diarrhoea: RR 22.0, 95% CI 3.05 to 159; cardiotoxicity RR 3.15, 95% CI 1.15 to 8.59; thrombocytopenia: RR 19.5, 95% CI 7.49 to 50.8; anaemia: RR 11.3, 95% CI 4.80 to 26.8).[66]

Comment: Fifteen years' follow up of women with metastatic breast cancer treated with standard dose FAC (see glossary, p 1997) found that 263/1581 (16.6%) women achieved a complete response and that median time to progression was 2 years; 19% of these women remained free of disease at 5 years.[18] Any long term remissions associated with high dose chemotherapy in metastatic disease must be interpreted in the context of these figures. It remains to be seen if certain women, for example those with a complete response after standard dose chemotherapy, may benefit from subsequent high dose.[67,68] Although haematological support with colony stimulating growth factors (see glossary, p 1997) has reduced complications from high dose chemotherapy, non-haematological toxicity to the gastrointestinal tract and nervous system remain dose limiting. There is a recognised mortality with high dose chemotherapy (3%), although this is lower than in the early days of this approach.

QUESTION **What are the effects of first line chemotherapy in combination with a monoclonal antibody?**

OPTION **TRASTUZUMAB**

One RCT found that trastuzumab increased the clinical benefit of first line chemotherapy in metastatic breast cancer in those women whose tumours overexpress HER2. The main adverse effect observed was cardiac dysfunction in women who received an anthracycline plus trastuzumab.

Benefits: We found no systematic review and no RCT comparing trastuzumab versus no treatment. **Versus chemotherapy alone:** One RCT (469 women with HER2 overexpression) compared standard chemotherapy alone versus standard chemotherapy (see glossary, p 1997) plus trastuzumab. Women who had not previously received postoperative chemotherapy with an anthracycline were treated with doxorubicin (or epirubicin) and cyclophosphamide with or without trastuzumab. Women who had previously received postoperative anthracycline were treated with paclitaxel with or without trastuzumab. Adding trastuzumab to chemotherapy significantly prolonged the time to disease progression (7.4 months *v* 4.6 months; P < 0.001), increased objective response (50% *v* 32%; P < 0.001), and improved overall survival (25.1 months *v* 20.3 months; P = 0.046).[69] We found one subsequent report examining quality of life in some of the women included in this RCT (see comment below).[70]

Harms: Cardiac dysfunction occurred in 27% of women given anthracycline, cyclophosphamide, and trastuzumab versus 8% given anthracycline and cyclophosphamide alone; 13% with paclitaxel and trastuzumab; and 1% of those given paclitaxel alone. Symptoms usually improved with standard medical management, although two women died from cardiac dysfunction. About 25% of women had chills, fever, or both during the initial infusion; no episodes of anaphylaxis occurred.

Comment: Trastuzumab based combination treatment was effective at reducing the relative risk of death by 20% at a median follow up of 30 months. Few studies have shown that adding a single agent improves survival to this degree. Cardiac toxicity appears only significant in people concurrently receiving an anthracycline. The most appropriate treatment duration in responders is unclear. We found one subsequent report of the RCT comparing trastuzumab plus chemotherapy versus chemotherapy alone.[70] It reported on quality of life among 400 of the enrolled 469 women and found that trastuzumab plus chemotherapy significantly improved reported global quality of life scores compared with chemotherapy alone (rate of improvement of quality of life assessed with European Organisation for Research and Treatment Care Quality of Life Questionnaire: 51% improved with trastuzumab and chemotherapy *v* 36% with chemotherapy alone; P < 0.05). We found one RCT comparing two different dosing regimens of trastuzumab as first line treatment in 114 women with HER2 overexpressing metastatic breast cancer. It found no significant difference between the high dose regimen (8 mg/kg loading dose followed by 4 mg/kg weekly) and low dose regimen (4 mg/kg loading dose followed by 2 mg/kg weekly) for time to progression or time to death (median time to progression 3.5 months with high dose, 95% CI 3.3 to 5.5 months *v* 3.8 months, 95% CI 2.4 to 5.5 months; median survival 22.9 months, 95% CI 16.0 months to 37.1 months *v* 25.8 months, 95% CI 13.3 to 34.7 months).[71] Adverse effects included asthenia (23%), fever (22%), nausea (14%), and cardiac dysfunction (2%).

QUESTION What are the effects of second line chemotherapy?

OPTION TAXANES

We found limited evidence that taxanes may improve response rates compared with CMF or continued doxorubicin, especially in anthracycline resistant disease. One RCT found no significant difference in progression or overall survival between docetaxel and 5-fluorouracil plus vinorelbine given as second line chemotherapy.

Benefits: We found no systematic review and no RCTs comparing taxanes with no treatment. One non-systematic review of RCTs and other studies concluded that, in women with anthracycline resistant disease, second line treatment (see glossary, p 1998) with paclitaxel was associated with response rates ranging from 6–48%.[72] The taxane paclitaxel has been compared in two RCTs with both doxorubicin (331 women)[73] and CMF based chemotherapy (see glossary, p 1997) (209 women).[74] The response rates were higher with doxorubicin than paclitaxel (41% *v* 25%; P = 0.003), yet compared with CMF based chemotherapy, there was a modest survival advantage with paclitaxel in a multivariate analysis (median survival 17.3 *v* 13.9 months; P = 0.025). One RCT (392 women with anthracycline resistant metastatic disease) compared the taxane docetaxel (100 mg/m^2 iv every 3 weeks) versus a standard relapse treatment of mitomycin (12 mg/m^2) plus vinblastine (6 mg/m^2).[75] Docetaxel was associated with a significantly higher response rate (30% *v* 11.6%; P < 0.001), longer time to progression (median 19 weeks *v* 11 weeks; P = 0.001), and longer overall survival (11.4 months *v* 8.7 months; P = 0.0097). Another RCT (283 women with anthracycline resistant metastatic disease) comparing docetaxel versus methotrexate and fluorouracil found a similar improvement for docetaxel both in response rate (42% *v* 19%; P < 0.001) and time to progression (median 6 months *v* 3 months; P = 0.006).[76] In a separate RCT (326 women who had not responded to an alkylating regimen [CMF] either in the adjuvant setting or as first line treatment), docetaxel was associated with a significantly higher response rate than single drug doxorubicin (43% *v* 21%; P = 0.003).[77] **Versus semi synthetic vinca alkaloids:** We found one RCT (176 women after anthracycline therapy failure) comparing docetaxel versus 5-fluorouracil plus vinorelbine.[78] It found no significant difference between treatments in time to progression or overall survival (median time to progression 5.1 months with docetaxel *v* 6.5 months with 5-fluorouracil plus vinorelbine; P = 0.34; median overall survival 16.0 months with docetaxel *v* 15.0 months with 5-fluorouracil plus vinorelbine; P value not stated).[78] **Versus capecitabine:** See capecitabine, p 1993.

Harms: Paclitaxel was better tolerated than doxorubicin with a lower incidence of febrile neutropenia (7% *v* 20%; P < 0.001) and grade 3/4 vomiting (2% *v* 13%; P < 0.001), although there was a higher incidence of sensory neurotoxicity (5% *v* 0%; P < 0.001).[73] Likewise, compared with CMF based chemotherapy, paclitaxel was associated with significantly less febrile neutropenia and infection (10% *v* 27%; P = 0.001), and nausea and vomiting, but significantly more alopecia, sensory neuropathy, and myalgia and arthralgia (P < 0.0001).[74] Docetaxel is associated with moderate to severe haematological toxicity; 89% of women experienced grade 3/4 neutropenia in the phase III study compared with 69% given mitomycin plus vinblastine,[75] although the incidence of febrile neutropenia with docetaxel was only 9%. Other specific toxicities associated with docetaxel include alopecia, neurotoxicity, arthralgia, and occasionally fluid retention. Hypersensitivity reactions can be avoided by premedication with corticosteroids and histamine H_2 receptor antagonists. The RCT comparing docetaxel versus

5-fluorouracil plus vinorelbine found that 5-fluorouracil and vinorelbine significantly increased severe thrombocytopenia and severe stomatitis compared with docetaxel (severe thrombocytopenia 10% *v* 1%, P = 0.02; severe stomatitis: 40% *v* 5%, P < 0.0001). Docetaxel significantly increased grade 3/4 neutropenia compared with 5-fluorouracil and vinorelbine (82% *v* 67%, P = 0.02).[78]

Comment: The taxanes (see glossary, p 1997), paclitaxel and docetaxel, have an established role as second line treatment in advanced breast cancer, especially in people with disease progression despite a previous anthracycline based regimen, with evidence in some RCTs for a survival advantage over other available options. Trials are in progress to determine the efficacy and tolerability of taxanes in combination with anthracyclines as first line treatment (see glossary, p 1997), although there are concerns about cardiac toxicity. At present, the indication for docetaxel remains as a single drug for second line treatment, especially in anthracycline resistant disease, although definitive results on improvement in quality of life are awaited.

OPTION SEMISYNTHETIC VINCA ALKALOIDS

One RCT found no significant difference in survival or quality of life between vinorelbine plus docetaxel and vinorelbine alone. One RCT found no significant difference in progression or overall survival between docetaxel and 5-fluorouracil plus vinorelbine given as second line chemotherapy. One RCT found that second line vinorelbine improved survival and reduced progression compared with melphalan.

Benefits: We found no systematic review and no RCTs comparing treatment with no treatment. One RCT compared vinorelbine plus 5-fluorouracil versus docetaxel (see benefits of taxanes, p 1991).[78] One RCT (303 women, first or second line treatment, no previous vinca alkaloid or anthracycline treatment) compared doxorubicin combined with vinorelbine versus doxorubicin alone. The response rates, quality of life scores, and overall survival were not significantly improved with combined chemotherapy in this setting.[79] Vinorelbine has single agent activity with response rates of 20–33%, including in women with anthacycline resistant metastatic disease.[72] One RCT (183 women with anthracycline resistant disease) found increased time to progression and survival with vinorelbine 30 mg/m^2 weekly compared with intravenous melphalan (median survival 35 *v* 31 weeks; P < 0.001).[80]

Harms: Vinorelbine is associated with minimal toxicity compared with anthracycline based chemotherapy (FAC/FEC (see glossary, p 1997)), with considerably lower rates of nausea (8% *v* 16%; P = 0.03) and grade 3 alopecia (7% *v* 30%; P = 0.0001), although haematological toxicity that delayed treatment was more frequent (27% *v* 17%).[81]

Comment: Vinorelbine seems to have a favourable toxicity profile, but results from phase III trials are awaited. Vinorelbine associated with protracted infusional fluorouracil is an active and well tolerated regimen (overall response rate 61.4%, 95% CI 50.9% to 70.9%), and further trials are under way.[82] One uncontrolled study of vinorelbine plus gemcitabine twice weekly found an objective response rate of 54%.[83]

OPTION CAPECITABINE

One RCT found no significant difference in progression or response rate between capecitabine and paclitaxel following anthracycline failure.

Benefits: We found one systematic review (search date 2000) assessing the oral fluoropyrimidine capecitabine in metastatic breast cancer,[84] which identified one RCT (42 women) comparing capecitabine versus paclitaxel as second or third line treatment following anthracycline failure. It found no significant difference between treatments in response rate or time to disease progression.

Harms: The most commonly reported grade 3/4 toxicities were hand–foot syndrome (13%), diarrhoea (12%), and stomatitis (4%).[84]

Comment: Promising activity has been seen with capecitabine in paclitaxel–refractory, heavily pretreated women,[85] and the low toxicity profile, together with evidence of efficacy, all warrant further investigation of this drug as an alternative to more toxic second or third line chemotherapy schedules. It has been suggested that the effectiveness of docetaxel may be increased by the addition of capecitabine,[86] and RCTs are under way.

QUESTION What are the effects of treatments for bone metastases?

OPTION BISPHOSPHONATES

Three placebo controlled RCTs in women with metastatic breast cancer and bone involvement have found that adding bisphosphonates to standard treatment reduces and delays skeletal complications, but have no effect on survival.

Benefits: We found no systematic review. **Versus placebo:** Three double blind RCTs in women with metastatic breast cancer who had bone involvement compared the addition of bisphosphonates (see glossary, p 1997) versus placebo to standard treatment (either chemotherapy or hormonal treatment [see glossary, p 1997]).[87–89] The first RCT (380 women with at least 1 lytic bone lesion who also received chemotherapy) found that intravenous pamidronate (90 mg as a 2 hourly infusion every month for 12 cycles) significantly prolonged the median time to the first skeletal complication (13.1 months *v* 7.0 months; P = 0.005).[87] Significantly fewer women taking pamidronate developed skeletal complications (43% *v* 56%; P = 0.008), and there was a significantly reduced requirement for radiotherapy to treat painful sites of bone disease (19% *v* 33%; P = 0.01). In an updated analysis in women who completed 2 years of treatment, those taking placebo were more than twice as likely to suffer a fracture than those taking pamidronate (OR 2.3, 95% CI 1.5 to 3.5).[90] The second RCT (173 women with bone metastases who may also have received either chemotherapy or hormonal treatment) found that the addition of oral clodronate (1600 mg daily) significantly reduced hypercalcaemic episodes (23% *v* 35%; $P < 0.01$) and vertebral fractures (84 *v* 124 per 100 women years; $P < 0.025$).[88] The third RCT (372 women with at least 1 lytic bone lesion who also received hormonal treatment) found that pamidronate significantly prolonged the median time to the first skeletal complication (10.4 months *v* 6.9 months; $P = 0.049$).[89] Significantly fewer women taking pamidronate developed skeletal complications (2.4 *v* 3.8 events a year; $P = 0.008$), and there was a significantly reduced need for radiotherapy to treat painful sites of bone disease (25% *v* 34%; $P = 0.042$). None of the three trials found an effect on overall survival. **Versus radiotherapy:** We found no RCTs.

Harms: In the first RCT, intravenous pamidronate was well tolerated with no serious adverse events in women treated for up to 2 years.[87] One of the 185 women taking pamidronate developed symptomatic hypocalcaemia. Myalgia and arthralgia were more common in women taking pamidronate. Oral clodronate can be associated with minor gastrointestinal disturbance, but the RCT reported this in fewer than 5% of women.[87]

Comment: Large RCTs are in progress in the adjuvant setting to see whether these agents may delay or prevent the development of bone metastases. The American Society of Clinical Oncology released recent guidelines on the use of bisphosphonates, stating that this treatment reduces the rate of bone complications (although not mortality) in women with lytic bone disease who may or may not also be receiving systemic treatment (chemotherapy or endocrine treatment).[91] It remains unclear exactly when to start or stop treatment, which may affect the costs involved.[92] Although these effects are likely to improve quality of life, this outcome has not been formally evaluated. We found no evidence that bisphosphonates improve survival.

OPTION RADIOTHERAPY

We found limited evidence from non-randomised studies that persistent and localised bone pain can be successfully treated with radiotherapy plus analgesics in over 80% of cases. Longer courses and wide fields are rarely required, and adverse effects are minimal. The RCTs found no evidence that single fraction regimens (usually 8 Gy) were less effective than fractionated regimens.

Benefits: We found no systematic review and no RCTs comparing radiotherapy versus no treatment or versus bisphosphonates (see glossary, p 1997) (see comment below). **Pain control:** Questionnaire studies found that control of pain was successful in over 80% of women who received radiotherapy for bone metastases, with concomitant use of appropriate analgesia according to the World Health Organization ladder (this moves upwards from non-steroidal anti-inflammatory drugs and paracetamol to mild opiates through to morphine and its derivatives).[93] **Cranial nerve compression:** In people with skull base metastases causing cranial nerve involvement, retrospective studies suggest that radiotherapy leads to improvement in 50–80% of women, which is usually maintained.[94] **Different radiotherapy regimens:** We found two RCTs comparing different radiotherapy regimens. These found no significant differences between short courses (8 Gy as a single fraction) and longer courses (e.g. 20 Gy/5 fractions or 30 Gy/10 fractions).[95,96] Studies of accelerated fractionation schedules (e.g. twice daily treatments for 5 days) have failed to show any benefit over conventional regimens in the control of disease secondary to metastatic breast cancer.[97] Published interim results from one RCT (270 women) have found that different fractionation regimens can be used to treat neuropathic bone pain effectively.[98]

Harms: Adverse effects of radiotherapy for bone metastases include nausea and vomiting.[97] Higher dose fractions a day produce more toxic effects.

Comment: Randomised comparisons against no treatment or placebo would be considered unethical in palliative care, and even RCTs comparing one treatment versus another are difficult to undertake because it is reasonable to try many different options in order to make a woman comfortable. Rating of success of end of life care is difficult. Usual outcomes, such as response rates and survival duration, do not apply.[99]

QUESTION **What are the effects of treatments for spinal cord, cerebral, and choroidal metastases?**

OPTION **SPINAL CORD COMPRESSION**

Spinal cord compression is an emergency. Retrospective studies suggest that early radiotherapy preserves function. One small RCT suggested that adding high dose steroids improved the chance of walking 6 months after radiotherapy for spinal cord compression.

Benefits: We found no systematic review. **Radiotherapy:** Retrospective analyses found an improvement with early radiotherapy, but fewer than 10% of people walked again if severe deterioration of motor function occurred before radiotherapy.[100] **Addition of high dose steroids:** One blinded RCT (57 women) evaluated addition of high dose steroids to radiotherapy. It found that more women were walking 6 months after receiving intravenous dexamethasone 96 mg bolus followed by 96 mg orally for 3 days compared with those who received no steroids (59% *v* 33%).[101]

Harms: In the RCT of high dose steroids, significant adverse effects caused withdrawal from treatment in 11% of people.[101] Use of lower doses of glucocorticoids in the control of symptoms from cerebral metastases may result in short term agitation and the longer term development of Cushingoid facies.

Comment: See comment under radiotherapy, p 1995.

OPTION CEREBRAL METASTASES

Evidence from retrospective studies suggests that symptoms from cerebral metastases can be successfully controlled with radiotherapy.

Benefits: We found no systematic review and no RCTs comparing one form of treatment with another. **Radiotherapy:** Retrospective studies suggest that whole brain radiation produces general improvement in neurological function in 40–70% of women with brain metastases secondary to breast cancer.[102] **Different radiotherapy regimens:** One RCT (544 symptomatic people) that compared two whole brain radiotherapy schedules (30 Gy/10 fractions *v* 12 Gy/2 fractions) found no evidence that the response rate or duration of response in people with multiple brain metastases were improved with higher doses of radiation compared with the shorter regimen.[97] **Surgical resection:** A retrospective cohort study nested in one RCT (859 women) found that there may be some beneficial effect in a small subgroup of people.[103] **Intrathecal chemotherapy:** We found no evidence that meningeal infiltration responds to intrathecal chemotherapy.

Harms: Adverse effects of radiotherapy in the treatment of cerebral metastases include hair loss and somnolence.[97] Higher dose fractions a day produce more toxic effects.

Comment: See comment under radiotherapy, p 1995. There is a consensus that raised intracranial pressure associated with cerebral metastases is best managed by dexamethasone given immediately with anticonvulsants to control seizures if necessary.

OPTION CHOROIDAL METASTASES

Evidence from retrospective studies suggests that symptoms from choroidal metastases can be successfully controlled with radiotherapy.

Benefits: We found no systematic review and no RCTs. External beam radiotherapy prevents functional loss and doses of about 40 Gy in total are used.[104] Retrospective studies suggest that radiotherapy benefits 70% of people.[105]

Harms: People with choroidal metastases who are treated with radiotherapy may lose the sight in that eye. Optic atrophy and proliferative radiation retinopathy are possible late complications.

Comment: See comment under radiotherapy, p 1995. Generally, choroidal metastases occur later than metastases to other organs. Choroidal metastasis is considered a poor prognostic sign; most people die within 6 months of diagnosis. Systemic chemotherapy can induce partial or complete remission of metastatic choroidal breast carcinoma.[106] Recent retrospective studies have shown that krypton red or argon green laser photocoagulation is feasible, easy, rapid, and effective for small choroidal breast carcinoma.[107] Women with deteriorating vision are likely to benefit from emergency assessment and treatment for choroidal metastases.

GLOSSARY

Adjuvant treatment This usually refers to systemic chemotherapy or hormonal treatment, or both, taken after removal of a primary tumour (in this case, surgery for early breast cancer), with the aim of killing any remaining micrometastatic tumour cells and thus preventing recurrence.

Anthracycline resistance This applies to people who have received at least one chemotherapeutic regimen with anthracyclines (doxorubicin or epirubicin) in either an adjuvant setting or for metastatic disease. Primary resistance to an anthracycline is defined as progressive disease during or within 6 months after completion of adjuvant anthracycline. People without any documented tumour response to first line chemotherapy that included anthracyclines for metastatic disease are also classified as having primary resistance. Secondary resistance is defined as disease progression after a documented clinical response to first line chemotherapy with anthracyclines for metastatic disease. Secondary resistance can be further divided into three categories, as follows: (1) absolute resistance, or disease progression during treatment with regimens that contained anthracyclines after a period of response; (2) relative resistance, or disease progression within 6 months after completion of the chemotherapy; and (3) sensitive regrowth, or disease progression more than 6 months after completion of the chemotherapy.[108]

Aromatase inhibitors Drugs that block the conversion of androgens into oestrogens. Aminoglutethimide, anastrozole, and letrozole are non-steroidal aromatase inhibitors. Formestane and exemestane are steroidal aromatase inhibitors. Anastrozole, formestane, exemestane, and letrozole are selective inhibitors of oestrogen synthetase, which is a part of the aromatase enzyme system. Aminoglutethimide also inhibits adrenal steroid production. These drugs cause oestrogen suppression in postmenopausal women.

Bisphosphonates (pamidronate, clodronate) Bone specific palliative drugs that inhibit osteoclast induced bone resorption associated with breast cancer metastases.

Chemotherapy Treatment with cytotoxic drugs.

Colony stimulating growth factors Naturally occurring cytokines that stimulate development of different cell lines.

Combination chemotherapy regimens Use of different combinations of cytotoxic drugs:

CAF Cyclophosphamide (500 mg/m^2 iv), doxorubicin (50 mg/m^2 iv), and fluorouracil (500 mg/m^2 iv) every 3 weeks for up to six cycles of treatment are given, depending on response.

Classical CMF Cyclophosphamide (100 mg/m^2 orally days 1–14), methotrexate (40 mg/m^2 iv days 1 and 8), and fluorouracil (600 mg/m^2 iv days 1 and 8) every 4 weeks for up to six cycles of treatment are given, depending on response.

FAC Fluorouracil, doxorubicin, and cyclophosphamide every 3 weeks for up to six cycles of treatment are given, depending on response.

FEC Fluorouracil, epirubicin, and cyclophosphamide every 3 weeks for up to six cycles of treatment are given, depending on response.

Complete response Disappearance of all known lesions on two separate measurements at least 4 weeks apart.

Disease free interval Time between surgery for early breast cancer (see below) and metastatic breast cancer developing.

Early breast cancer Operable disease, restricted to the breast and sometimes to local lymph nodes.

First line treatment Initial treatment for a particular condition that has previously not been treated. For example, first line treatment for metastatic breast cancer may include chemotherapy or hormonal treatment, or both.

Gonadorelin analogues (Also called LHRH agonists.) These are synthetic peptides that occupy the receptors for gonadorelin in the pituitary gland. Continuous administration of gonadorelin agonists may initially increase the release of luteinising hormone, but continuous administration blocks the physiological pulsatile luteinising hormone release and this causes a fall in oestrogen levels.
Hormonal treatment Includes treatment with antioestrogens such as tamoxifen, aromatase inhibitors, and progestins.
Overall objective response rate The proportion of treated people in whom a complete (see above) or partial response (see below) is observed.
Partial response More than a 50% reduction in the size of lesions.
Progestins (medroxyprogesterone, megestrol) The antitumour effects of progestins may be mediated by a direct action on tumour cells, or an indirect effect on the pituitary–ovarian/adrenal axes.
Progression free survival (or time to progression) Interval between diagnosis of metastatic disease and diagnosis of progression (see below).
Progressive disease More than a 25% increase in the size of lesions, or the appearance of new lesions.
Second line treatment Treatment given after relapse following first line treatment (see above).
Tamoxifen An oral, non-steroidal, competitive oestrogen receptor antagonist.
Taxanes Drugs derived from the Pacific yew tree *Taxus brevifolia*, such as paclitaxel and docetaxel.

Substantive changes

High dose versus standard dose chemotherapy One systematic review added;[66] conclusions unchanged.
Second line chemotherapy One RCT added;[78] conclusions unchanged.
Second line hormonal therapy Two RCTs added;[40,41] conclusions unchanged.

REFERENCES

1. Hortobagyi GN. Can we cure limited metastatic breast cancer? *J Clin Oncol* 2002;20:620–623.
2. Pisani P, Parkin DM, Ferlay J. Estimates of the worldwide mortality from eighteen major cancers in 1985. Implications for prevention and projections of future burden. *Int J Cancer* 1993;55:891–903.
3. Parkin MD. Global cancer statistics in the year 2000. *Lancet Oncol* 2001;2:533–543.
4. Early Breast Cancer Trialists' Collaborative Group. Polychemotherapy for early breast cancer: an overview of the randomised trials. *Lancet* 1998;352:930–942. Search date 1995; studies were identified using lists prepared by three international cancer research groups, by searching the international Cancer Research Data Bank, meeting abstracts and references of published trials, and by consulting experts.
5. Slamon DJ, Clark GM, Wong SG, et al. Human breast cancer: correlation of relapse and survival with amplification of the HER-2/neu oncogene. *Science* 1987;235:177–182.
6. Rubens RD, Bajetta E, Bonneterre J, et al. Treatment of relapse of breast cancer after adjuvant systemic therapy. *Eur J Cancer* 1994;30A:106–111.
7. Cold S, Jensen NV, Brincker H, et al. The influence of chemotherapy on survival after recurrence in breast cancer: a population based study of patients treated in the 1950s, 1960s, and 1970s. *Eur J Cancer* 1993;29A:1146–1152.
8. Jackson IM, Litherland S, Wakeling AE. Tamoxifen and other antioestrogens. In: Powels TJ, Smith IE, eds. *Medical management of breast cancer*. London: Martin Dunitz, 1997:51–59.
9. Arafah BM, Pearson OH. Endocrine treatment of advanced breast cancer. In: Jordan VC, ed. *Estrogen/antiestrogen action and breast cancer therapy*. Madison: University of Wisconsin Press, 1986:417–429.
10. McGuire WL. Hormone receptors: their role in predicting prognosis and response to endocrine therapy. *Semin Oncol* 1978;5:428–443.
11. Kuss JT, Muss HB, Hoen H, Case LD. Tamoxifen as initial endocrine therapy for metastatic breast cancer: long term follow-up of two Piedmont Oncology Association (POA) trials. *Breast Cancer Res Treat* 1997;42:265–274.
12. Olsen O, Gotzsche PC. Cochrane review on screening for breast cancer with mammography. *Lancet* 2001;358:1340–1342.
13. Coates A, Gebski V, Signori D. Prognostic value of quality-of-life scores during chemotherapy for advanced breast cancer. *J Clin Oncol* 1992;10:1833–1838.
14. European Organisation for Research and Treatment of Cancer (EORTC). *A practical guide to EORTC studies*. Brussels: EORTC Data Center, 1996:126.
15. Miller AB, Hoogstraten B, Staquet M, et al. Reporting results of cancer treatment. *Cancer* 1981;47:207–214.
16. Baum M, Priestman T, West RR, et al. A comparison of subjective responses in a trial comparing endocrine with cytotoxic treatment in advanced carcinoma of the breast. In: Mouridsen HT, Palshof T, eds. *Breast cancer — experimental and clinical methods*. London: Pergamon Press, 1980:223–228.

17. Bernhard J, Thurlimann B, Schmitz SF, et al. Defining clinical benefit in postmenopausal patients with breast cancer under second-line endocrine treatment: Does quality of life matter? *J Clin Oncol* 1999;17:1672–1679.
18. Greenberg PA, Hortobagyi GN, Smith TL, et al. Long-term follow-up of patients with complete remission following combination chemotherapy for metastatic breast cancer. *J Clin Oncol* 1996;14:2197–2205.
19. Geels P, Eisenhauer E, Bezjak A, et al. Palliative effect of chemotherapy: objective tumor response is associated with symptom improvement in patients with metastatic breast cancer. *J Clin Oncol* 2000;18:2395–2405.
20. Fossati R, Confalonieri C, Torri V, et al. Cytotoxic and hormonal treatment for metastatic breast cancer: a systematic review of published randomised trials involving 31 510 women. *J Clin Oncol* 1998;16:3439–3460. Search date 1997; primary sources Medline, Embase, and hand search of reference lists from retrieved articles and lists from relevant meetings.
21. Litherland S, Jackson IM. Antioestrogens in the management of hormone-dependent cancer. *Cancer Treat Rev* 1988;15:183–194.
22. Johnston SRD. Acquired tamoxifen resistance in human breast cancer — potential mechanisms and clinical implications. *Anti Cancer Drugs* 1997;8:911–930.
23. Hayes DF, Van Zyl JA, Goedhals L, et al. Randomised comparison of tamoxifen and two separate doses of toremifene in postmenopausal patients with metastatic breast cancer. *J Clin Oncol* 1995;13:2556–2566.
24. Parazzini F, Colli E, Scatigna M, Tozzi L. Treatment with tamoxifen and progestins for metastatic breast cancer in postmenopausal women: a quantitative review of published randomised clinical trials. *Oncology* 1993;50:483–489. Search date 1991; primary sources Medline and hand searching reference lists of articles identified.
25. Muss HB, Case DL, Atkins JN, et al. Tamoxifen versus high-dose oral medroxyprogesterone acetate as initial endocrine therapy for patients with metastatic breast cancer: a Piedmont Oncology Association study. *J Clin Oncol* 1994;12:1630–1638.
26. Pannuti F, Martoni A, Murari G, et al. Analgesic activity of medroxyprogesterone acetate in cancer patients: an anti-inflammatory mediated activity? *Int J Tissue React* 1985;7:505–508.
27. Ingle JN, Ahmann DL, Green SJ. Randomised clinical trial of megesterol acetate versus tamoxifen in paramenopausal or castrated women with advanced breast cancer. *Am J Clin Oncol* 1982;5:155–160.
28. Panutti F, Martoni A, Zamagni C, et al. Progestins. In: Powles TJ, Smith IE, eds. *Medical management of breast cancer*. London: Martin Dunitz, 1997:95–107.
29. Crump M, Sawka CA, DeBoer G, et al. An individual patient-based meta-analysis of tamoxifen versus ovarian ablation as first-line endocrine therapy for premenopausal women with metastatic breast cancer. *Breast Cancer Res Treat* 1997;44:201–210. Search date not stated; primary sources Medline, CancerLit, hand searches of bibliographies of related publications, and personal contact with principal investigators of unpublished trials.
30. Sawka CA, Pritchard KI, Shelley W, et al. A randomised crossover trial of tamoxifen versus ovarian ablation for metastatic breast cancer in premenopausal women: a report of the National Cancer Institute of Canada clinical trials group trial MA1. *Breast Cancer Res Treat* 1997;44:211–215.
31. Taylor CW, Green S, Dalton WS, et al. Multicenter randomised clinical trial of goserelin versus surgical ovariectomy in premenopausal patients with receptor-positive metastatic breast cancer: an intergroup study. *J Clin Oncol* 1998;16:994–999.
32. Boccardo F, Rubagotti A, Perotta A, et al. Ovarian ablation versus goserelin with or without tamoxifen in pre-perimenopausal patients with advanced breast cancer: results of a multicentric Italian study. *Ann Oncol* 1994;5:337–342.
33. Klijn JGN, Blamey RW, Boccardo F, et al. Combined tamoxifen and luteinising hormone-releasing hormone (LHRH) agonist versus LHRH agonist alone in premenopausal advanced breast cancer; a meta-analysis of four randomised trials. *J Clin Oncol* 2001;19:343–353.
34. Bonneterre J, Thurlimann B, Robertson JFR, et al. Anastrozole versus tamoxifen as first-line therapy for advanced breast cancer in 668 postmenopausal women: results of the tamoxifen or arimidex randomised group efficacy and tolerability study. *J Clin Oncol* 2000;18:3748–3757.
35. Nabholtz JM, Buzdar A, Pollak M, et al. Anastrozole is superior to tamoxifen as first-line therapy for advanced breast cancer in postmenopausal women: results of a North American multicentre randomised trial. *J Clin Oncol* 2000;18:3758–3767.
36. Mouridsen H, Gershanovich M, Sun Y, et al. Superior efficacy of letrozole (Femara) versus tamoxifen as first-line therapy for post-menopausal women with advanced breast cancer; results of a phase III study of the International Letrozole Breast Cancer Group. *J Clin Oncol* 2001:19;2596–2606.
37. Mouridsen H, Sun Y, Gershanovich M, et al. Final survival analysis of the double-blind, randomized, multinational phase III trial of letrozole (Femara®) compared to tamoxifen as first-line hormonal therapy for advanced breast cancer. Program of the 24th Annual San Antonio Breast Cancer Symposium, San Antonio, December 10–13, 2001. http://www.sabcs.org (last accessed 1 May 2003).
38. Buzdar A, Jonat W, Howell A, et al. Anastrozole, a potent and selective aromatase inhibitor, versus megesterol acetate in post-menopausal women with advanced breast cancer; results of overview analysis of two phase III trials. *J Clin Oncol* 1996;14:2000–2011.
39. Buzdar A, Jonat W, Howell A, et al. Significant improved survival with arimidex (anastrozole) versus megesterol acetate in postmenopausal advanced breast cancer; updated results of two randomised trials. *Proc Am Soc Clin Oncol* 1997;16:A545.
40. Osborne CK, Pippen J, Jones SE, et al. Double-blind randomised trial comparing the efficacy and tolerability of fulvestrant versus anastrozole in postmenopausal women with advanced breast cancer progressing on prior endocrine therapy. *J Clin Oncol* 2002;20:3386–3395.
41. Howell A, Robertson JF, Quaresma Albano J, et al. Fulvestrant, formerly ICI 182,780, is as effective as anastrozole in postmenopausal women with advanced breast cancer progressing after prior endocrine treatment. *J Clin Oncol* 2002;20:3396–3403.
42. Jones S, Vogel C, Arkhipov A, et al. Multicenter phase II trial of exemestane as third-line hormonal

therapy of postmenopausal women with metastatic breast cancer. *J Clin Oncol* 1999;17:3418–3425.
43. Kaufman M, Bajetta E, Dirix LY, et al. Exemestane is superior to megestrol acetate after tamoxifen failure in postmenopausal women with advanced breast cancer: results of a phase III randomised double-blind trial. *J Clin Oncol* 2000;18:1399–1411.
44. Dombernowsky P, Smith IE, Falkson G, et al. Letrozole, a new oral aromatase inhibitor for advanced breast cancer: double-blind randomised trial showing a dose effect and improved efficacy and tolerability compared with megesterol acetate. *J Clin Oncol* 1998;16:453–461.
45. Gershanovich M, Chaudri HA, Campos D, et al. Letrozole, a new oral aromatase inhibitor: randomised trial comparing 2.5 mg daily, 0.5 mg daily and aminoglutethimide in postmenopausal women with advanced breast cancer. *Ann Oncol* 1998;9:639–645.
46. Lønning PE, Bajetta E, Murray R, et al. Activity of exemestane in metastatic breast cancer after failure of nonsteroidal aromatase inhibitors: a phase II trial. *J Clin Oncol* 2000;18:2234–2244.
47. Engelsman E, Klijn JCM, Rubens RD, et al. "Classical" CMF versus a 3-weekly intravenous CMF schedule in postmenopausal patients with advanced breast cancer. *Eur J Cancer* 1991;27:966–970.
48. Tannock IF, Boyd NF, DeBoer G, et al. A randomised trial of two dose levels of cyclophosphamide, methotrexate and fluorouracil chemotherapy for patients with metastatic breast cancer. *J Clin Oncol* 1988;6:1377–1387.
49. A'Hern RP, Smith IE, Ebbs SR. Chemotherapy and survival in advanced breast cancer: the inclusion of doxorubicin in Cooper type regimens. *Br J Cancer* 1993;67:801–805. Search date not stated; primary sources CancerLit and communication with colleagues.
50. Cummings FJ, Gelman R, Horton J. Comparison of CAF versus CMFP in metastatic breast cancer: analysis of prognostic factors. *J Clin Oncol* 1985;3:932–940.
51. Smalley RV, Lefante J, Bartolucci A, et al. A comparison of cyclophosphamide, adriamycin, and 5-fluorouracil (CAF) and cyclophosphamide, methotrexate, 5-fluorouracil, vincristine, and prednisolone (CMFVP) in patients with advanced breast cancer. *Breast Cancer Res Treat* 1983;3:209–220.
52. French Epirubicin Study Group. A prospective randomised phase III trial comparing combination chemotherapy with cyclophosphamide, fluorouracil, and either doxorubicin or epirubicin. *J Clin Oncol* 1988;6:679–688.
53. Italian Multicentre Breast Study with Epirubicin. Randomised phase III study of fluorouracil, doxorubicin, and cyclophosphamide in advanced breast cancer: an Italian multicentre trial. *J Clin Oncol* 1988;6:976–982.
54. Stewart DJ, Evans WK, Shepherd FA, et al. Cyclophosphamide and fluorouracil combined with mitozantrone versus doxorubicin for breast cancer: superiority of doxorubicin. *J Clin Oncol* 1997;15:1897–1905.
55. Namer M, Soler-Michel P, Turpin F. Results of a phase III prospective randomised trial comparing mitoxantrone and vinorelbine in combination with standard FAC/FEC in front-line therapy of metastatic breast cancer. *Eur J Cancer* 2001;37:1132–1140.
56. Stockler M, Wilcken NR, Ghersi D, et al. Systematic reviews of chemotherapy and chemotherapy and endocrine therapy in metastatic breast cancer. *Cancer Treat Rev* 2000;26:151–168. Search date not stated; primary source Medline.
57. Sledge GW, Hu P, Torney D, et al. Comparison of chemotherapy with chemohormonal therapy as first-line therapy for metastatic, hormone sensitive breast cancer. An Eastern Cooperative Oncology Group Study. *J Clin Oncol* 2000;18:262–266.
58. Ross MB, Buzdar AU, Smith TL, et al. Improved survival of patients with metastatic breast cancer receiving combination chemotherapy. *Cancer* 1985;55:341–346.
59. Goldhirsch A, Glick JH, Gelber RD, et al. International consensus panel on the treatment of primary breast cancer. *J Natl Cancer Inst* 1998;90:1601–1608.
60. Coates AS, Hurny C, Peterson HF, et al. Quality of life scores predict outcome in metastatic but not early breast cancer. *J Clin Oncol* 2000;18:3768–3774.
61. Hakamies-Blomquist L, Luoma M, Sjostrom J, et al. Quality of life in patients with metastatic breast cancer receiving either docetaxel or sequential methotrexate and 5-fluorouracil. A multicenter randomised phase III trial by the Scandinavian breast group. *J Clin Oncol* 2000;36:1411–1417.
62. Houston SJ, Richards MA, Bentley AE, et al. The influence of adjuvant chemotherapy on outcome after relapse for patients with breast cancer. *Eur J Cancer* 1993;29A:1513–1518.
63. The Italian Group for Antiemetic Research. Dexamethasone alone or in combination with ondansetron for the prevention of delayed nausea and vomiting induced by chemotherapy. *N Engl J Med* 2000;342:1554–1559.
64. Sledge GW, Neuberg D, Bernado P, et al. A phase III trial of doxorubicin, paclitaxel and the combination of doxorubicin and paclitaxel as front-line chemotherapy for metastatic breast cancer: an intergroup trial (E1193). *J Clin Oncol* 2003;21:588–592.
65. Bignazoli L, Cufer T, Bruning P, et al. Doxorubicin and paclitaxel versus doxorubicin and cyclophosphamide as first line chemotherapy in metastatic breast cancer. *J Clin Oncol* 2002;20:3114–3121.
66. Farquhar C, Basser R, Hetrick S, et al. High dose chemotherapy and autologous bone marrow or stem cell transplantation versus conventional chemotherapy for women with metastatic breast cancer. In: The Cochrane Library, Issue 1, 2003. Oxford: Update Software. Search date 2002; primary sources Cochrane Breast Cancer Group database and cooperative research groups' websites, Medline, Embase, American Society of Clinical Oncology, and Cochrane Library.
67. Hortobagyi GN, Bodey GP, Buzdar AU, et al. Evaluation of high-dose versus standard FAC chemotherapy for advanced breast cancer in protected environment units; a prospective randomised trial. *J Clin Oncol* 1987;5:354–364.
68. Bastholt L, Dalmark M, Gjedde S, et al. Dose-response relationship of epirubicin in the treatment of post-menopausal patients with metastatic breast cancer: a randomised study of epirubicin at four different dose-levels performed by the Danish Breast Cancer Co-operative Group. *J Clin Oncol* 1996;14:1146–1155.
69. Slamon DJ, Leyland-Jones B, Shak S, et al. Use of chemotherapy plus a monoclonal antibody against HER2 for metastatic breast cancer that overexpresses HER2. *New Engl J Med* 2001;344:783–792.
70. Osoba D, Slamon DJ, Burchmore M, et al. Effects on quality of life of combined trastuzumab and

chemotherapy in women with metastatic breast cancer. *J Clin Oncol* 2002;20:3106–3113.

71. Vogel CL, Cobleigh MA, Tripathy D, et al. Efficacy and safety of trastuzumab as a single agent in first-line treatment of HER2-overexpressing metastatic breast cancer. *J Clin Oncol* 2002;20:719–726.
72. Vermoken JB, Ten Bokkel Huinick WW. Chemotherapy for advanced breast cancer: the place of active new drugs. *Breast* 1996;5:304–311.
73. Paridaens R, Bignazoli L, Bruning P, et al. Paclitaxel versus doxorubicin as first-line single agent chemotherapy for metastatic breast cancer; an EORTC randomised study with cross-over. *J Clin Oncol* 2000;18:724–733.
74. Bishop JF, Dewar J, Toner GC, et al. Initial paclitaxel improves outcome compared with CMFP combination chemotherapy as front-line therapy in untreated metastatic breast cancer. *J Clin Oncol* 1999;17:2355–2364.
75. Nabholtz JM, Senn HJ, Bezwoda WR, et al. Prospective randomised trial of docetaxel vs mitomycin plus vinblastine in patients with metastatic breast cancer progressing despite previous anthracycline-containing chemotherapy. *J Clin Oncol* 1999;17:1413–1424.
76. Sjosrom J, Blomqvist C, Mouridsen H, et al. Docetaxel compared with sequential methotrexate and 5-fluorouracil in patients with advanced breast cancer after anthracycline failure; a randomised phase III study with cross-over on progression by the Scandinavian Breast Group. *Eur J Cancer* 1999;35:1194–1201.
77. Chan S, Friedrichs K, Noel D, et al. Prospective randomised trial of docetaxel versus doxorubicin in patients with metastatic breast cancer. *J Clin Oncol* 1999;35:2341–2354.
78. Bonneterre J, Roche H, Monnier A, et al. Docetaxel vs 5-fluorouracil plus vinorelbine in metastatic breast cancer after anthracycline therapy failure. *Br J Cancer* 2002;87:1210–1215.
79. Norris B, Pritchard KI, James K, et al. Phase III comparative study of vinorelbine combined with doxorubicin versus doxorubicin alone in disseminated metastatic/recurrent breast cancer: National Cancer Institute of Canada Clinical Trials Group Study MA8. *J Clin Oncol* 2000;18:2385–2394.
80. Jones S, Winer E, Vogel C, et al. Randomised comparison of vinorelbine and melphalan in anthracycline-refractory advanced breast cancer. *J Clin Oncol* 1995;13:2567–2574.
81. Namer M, Soler-Michel P, Mefti F, et al. Is the combination FAC/FEC always the best regimen in advanced breast cancer? Utility of mitoxantrone and vinorelbine association as an alternative: results from a randomised trial [abstract]. *Breast Cancer Res Treat* 1997;46:94(A406).
82. Berruti A, Sperone P, Bottini A. Phase II study of vinorelbine with protracted fluorouracil infusion as a second or third line approach for advanced breast cancer patients previously treated with anthracyclines. *J Clin Oncol* 2000;18 (19):3370–3377.
83. Stathopoulus GP, Rigatos SK, Pergantas N, et al. Phase II trial of biweekly administration of vinorelbine and gemcitabine in pretreated advanced breast cancer. *J Clin Oncol* 2002;20:37–41.
84. Tomiak E, Verma S, Levine M, et al. Use of capecitabine in stage IV breast cancer: an evidence summary. *Curr Oncol* 2000;7:84–90. Search date 2000; primary sources Medline, Cancerlit, Cochrane, PubMed, United States Food and Drug Administration website, Physician Query Database, Clinical Trials Listing service, hand searches of proceedings of the American Society of Clinical Oncology, and contact with Hoffmann-La Roche.
85. Blum JL, Jones SE, Buzdar AU, et al. Multicenter phase II study of capecitabine in paclitaxel-refractory metastatic breast cancer. *J Clin Oncol* 1999;17:485–493.
86. Diasio RB. An evolving role for oral fluoropyrimidine drugs. *J Clin Oncol* 2002;20:894–896.
87. Hortobagyi GN, Theriault RL, Porter L, et al. Efficacy of pamidronate in reducing skeletal complications in patients with breast cancer and lytic bone metastases. *N Engl J Med* 1996;335:1785–1791.
88. Paterson AHG, Powles TJ, Kanis JA, et al. Double-blind controlled trial of oral clodronate in patients with bone metastases from breast cancer. *J Clin Oncol* 1993;11:59–65.
89. Theriault RL, Lipton A, Hortobagyi GN. Pamidronate reduces skeletal morbidity in women with advanced breast cancer and lytic bone lesions; a randomised placebo controlled trial. *J Clin Oncol* 1999;17:846–854.
90. Hortobagyi GN, Theriault RL, Lipton A, et al. Long-term prevention of skeletal complications of metastatic breast cancer with pamidronate. *J Clin Oncol* 1998;16:2038–2044.
91. Hillner BE, Ingle JN, Berenson JR, et al. American Society of Clinical Oncology guideline on the role of bisphosphonates in breast cancer: American Society of Oncology Bisphosphonates Expert Panel. *J Clin Oncol* 2000;18:1378–1391.
92. Hillner BE, Weeks JC, Desch CE, et al. Pamidronate in prevention of bone complications in metastatic breast cancer; a cost-effectiveness analysis. *J Clin Oncol* 2000;18:72–79.
93. World Health Organization. *Cancer pain relief*. Geneva: WHO, 1996.
94. Hall SM, Budzar AV, Blumenschein GR. Cranial nerve palsies in metastatic breast cancer due to osseous metastasis without intracranial involvement. *Cancer* 1983;52:180–184.
95. Bone Trial Working Party. 8 Gy single fraction radiotherapy for the treatment of metastatic skeletal pain: randomised comparison with a multifraction schedule over 12 months of patient follow-up. *Radiother Oncol* 1999;52:111–121.
96. Price P, Hoskin PJ, Easton D, et al. Prospective randomised trial of single and multifraction radiotherapy schedules in treatment of painful bony metastases. *Radiother Oncol* 1986;6:247–255.
97. Priestman TJ, Dunn J, Brada M, et al. Final results of the Royal College of Radiologists' trial comparing two different radiotherapy schedules in the treatment of brain metastases. *Clin Oncol* 1996;8:308–315.
98. Roos DE, O'Brien PC, Smith JG, et al. A role for radiotherapy in neuropathic bone pain: preliminary response rates from a prospective trial. *Int J Radiat Oncol Biol Phys* 2000;46:975–981.
99. Bretscher N. Care for dying patients: what is right? *J Clin Oncol* 2000;18:233–234.
100. Rades D, Blach M, Nerreter V, et al. Metastatic spinal cord compression. Influence of time between onset of motor deficits and start of irradiation on therapeutic effect. *Strahlenther Onkol* 1999;175:378–381.
101. Sorensen S, Helweg-Larsen S, Mouridsen H, et al. Effect of high-dose dexamethasone in carcinomatous metastatic spinal cord compression treated with radiotherapy: a randomised trial. *Eur J Cancer* 1994;30A:22–27.

102. Cancer Guidance Subgroup of the Clinical Outcomes Group. *Improving outcomes in breast cancer. The research evidence*. London: NHS Executive, 1996.
103. Diener-West M, Dobbins TW, Phillips TL, et al. Identification of an optimal subgroup for treatment evaluation of patients with brain metastases using RTOG study 7916. *Int J Radiat Oncol Biol Phys* 1989;16:669–673.
104. Ratanatharathorn V, Powers WE, Grimm J, et al. Eye metastasis from carcinoma of the breast: radiation treatment and results. *Cancer Treat Rev* 1991;18:261–276.
105. Piccone MR, Maguire AM, Fox KC, et al. Choroidal metastases. Case 1: breast cancer. *J Clin Oncol* 1999;17:3356–3358.
106. Hortobagyi GN. Treatment of breast cancer. *N Engl J Med* 1998;339:974–984.
107. Levinger S, Merin S, Seigal R, et al. Laser therapy in the management of choroidal breast tumor metastases. *Ophthalmic Surg Lasers* 2001;32:294–299.
108. Ando M, Watanabe T, Nagata K, et al. Efficacy of docetaxel 60 mg/m^2 in patients with metastatic breast cancer according to the status of anthracycline resistance. *J Clin Oncol* 2001;19:336–342.

Stephen Johnston
Senior Lecturer in Medical Oncology

Justin Stebbing
MRC Clinical Training Fellow

The Royal Marsden NHS Trust, London, UK

Competing interests: None declared.

TABLE 1 **Clinical factors that predict response to hormonal treatment in metastatic breast cancer, based on results of RCTs (see text, p 1978).[8–11]**

Factors predictive of good response to hormonal treatment

Postmenopausal status
Disease limited to soft tissue sites (skin, nodes)
Oestrogen receptor positive tumour
Long disease free interval since primary treatment for early breast cancer (> 18–24 months)

Factors making initial hormonal treatment less appropriate

Symptomatic visceral metastases (e.g. lymphangitis carcinomatosis or progressive liver metastases)
Oestrogen receptor negative tumour
Short disease free interval (12–18 months)
Relapse on adjuvant tamoxifen (unless oestrogen receptor positive tumour and other features predictive of good response)

Breast cancer (non-metastatic)

Search date October 2002

J Michael Dixon, Kate Gregory, Stephen Johnston, and Alan Rodger

QUESTIONS

INTERVENTIONS

DUCTAL CARCINOMA *IN SITU*

Likely to be beneficial

OPERABLE BREAST CANCER

Beneficial

Likely to be beneficial

Trade off between benefits and harms

Unknown effectiveness

See glossary, p 2028

Key Messages

Ductal carcinoma in situ

- **Radiotherapy after breast conserving surgery (reduces recurrence)** RCTs found that radiotherapy reduced the risk of local recurrence and invasive carcinoma, with no evidence of an effect on survival.
- **Tamoxifen plus radiotherapy after breast conserving surgery (reduces recurrence)** One RCT has found that adjuvant tamoxifen significantly reduces breast cancer events in women who have undergone wide excision and radiotherapy, but found no significant difference in overall survival at about 6 years.

Primary operable breast cancer

- **Adjuvant chemotherapy** One systematic review has found that adjuvant chemotherapy versus no chemotherapy significantly reduces rates of recurrence and improves survival at 10 years. The benefit seems to be independent of nodal or menopausal status, although the absolute improvements are greater in women with node positive disease, and probably greater in younger women.
- **Adjuvant tamoxifen** One systematic review has found that adjuvant tamoxifen taken for up to 5 years reduces the risk of recurrence and death in women with oestrogen receptor positive tumours irrespective of age, menopausal status, nodal involvement, or the addition of chemotherapy. Tamoxifen slightly increases the risk of endometrial cancer, but we found no evidence of an overall adverse effect on non-breast cancer mortality.
- **Anthracycline regimens as adjuvant chemotherapy** One systematic review has found that adjuvant regimens containing an anthracycline significantly reduce recurrence, and significantly improve survival compared with a standard multidrug chemotherapy (CMF) regimen at 5 years.

- **Axillary clearance (no evidence of survival benefit and increased morbidity compared with axillary sampling)** RCTs found no significant difference in survival at 5–10 years between axillary clearance versus axillary sampling, axillary radiotherapy, or sampling plus radiotherapy combined. One systematic review of mainly poor quality evidence found that the risk of arm lymphoedema was highest with axillary clearance plus radiotherapy, lower with axillary sampling plus radiotherapy, and lowest with sampling alone.
- **Axillary radiotherapy** One systematic review has found that axillary radiotherapy versus axillary clearance significantly reduces isolated local recurrence, and has found no significant difference in mortality or overall recurrence at 10 years. One systematic review of mainly poor quality evidence found that radiotherapy plus axillary surgery was associated with arm lymphoedema.
- **Breast conserving surgery (similar survival to more extensive surgery)** Systematic reviews and long term results of included RCTs have found that, providing all local disease is excised, more extensive surgery does not increase survival up to 20 years. More extensive local resection in breast conserving surgery gives worse cosmetic results.
- **Chemotherapy plus tamoxifen** One RCT found that adding chemotherapy (CMF) to tamoxifen significantly improves survival at 5 years.
- **Enhanced dose regimens of adjuvant chemotherapy** RCTs found no significant improvement from enhanced dose regimens.
- **Neoadjuvant chemotherapy (reduces mastectomy rates v adjuvant chemotherapy; no evidence of effect on survival)** RCTs have found that neoadjuvant versus adjuvant chemotherapy reduces mastectomy rates, but found no significant difference in survival at 4–10 years.
- **Ovarian ablation in premenopausal women** One systematic review has found that in women less than 50 years of age, ovarian ablation versus no ablation significantly improves survival for at least 15 years.
- **Prolonged chemotherapy (8–12 months v 4–6 months)** One systematic review found no additional benefit from prolonging adjuvant chemotherapy from 4–6 to 8–12 months.
- **Radical mastectomy (no greater survival than less extensive surgery)** Systematic reviews and long term follow up of one RCT have found no significant difference between radical, total, supraradical, or simple mastectomy in survival up to 25 years. More extensive surgery results in greater mutilation.
- **Radiotherapy after breast conserving surgery (reduces local recurrence; no evidence of effect on survival)** One systematic review has found that adding radiotherapy to breast conserving surgery significantly reduces the risk of isolated local recurrence and loss of a breast, but does not increase survival at 10 years. Rates of survival and local recurrence are similar with radiotherapy plus either breast conserving surgery or mastectomy.
- **Radiotherapy after mastectomy in node positive disease, large tumours, or where lymphovascular invasion is present** One systematic review has found that radiotherapy to the chest wall after mastectomy reduces the risk of local recurrence by about two thirds and the risk of death from breast cancer at 10 years, but found no evidence of effect on overall 10 year survival. One review of retrospective data found that greater axillary node involvement, larger tumour size, higher histological grade, presence of lymphovascular invasion, and involvement of tumour margins reduced the chance of successful

treatment. Radiotherapy may be associated with late adverse effects, which are rare, including pneumonitis, pericarditis, arm oedema, brachial plexopathy, and radionecrotic rib fracture.

- **Radiotherapy after mastectomy in women at high risk of local recurrence** RCTs in high risk women receiving adjuvant chemotherapy after mastectomy have found that radiotherapy versus no radiotherapy significantly reduces local recurrence and increases survival at 10–15 years. Radiotherapy may be associated with late adverse effects, which are rare, including pneumonitis, pericarditis, arm oedema, brachial plexopathy, and radionecrotic rib fracture.
- **Radiotherapy after mastectomy in women not at high risk of local recurrence** One systematic review has found that radiotherapy to the chest wall after mastectomy reduces the risk of local recurrence by about two thirds and the risk of death from breast cancer at 10 years, but found no evidence of effect on overall 10 year survival. Radiotherapy may be associated with late adverse effects, which are rare, including pneumonitis, pericarditis, arm oedema, brachial plexopathy, and radionecrotic rib fracture.
- **Radiotherapy to the internal mammary chain** One RCT found no significant difference in overall survival or breast cancer specific survival at 2–3 years between radiotherapy versus no radiotherapy to the internal mammary chain. Treatment may increase radiation induced cardiac morbidity.
- **Radiotherapy to the ipsilateral supraclavicular fossa** We found insufficient evidence about the effects of irradiation of the ipsilateral supraclavicular fossa on survival. RCTs have found that radiotherapy reduces the risk of supraclavicular fossa nodal recurrence.
- **Total nodal radiotherapy in high risk disease** RCTs have found that, in women with high risk disease, total nodal irradiation versus no irradiation improves survival. An earlier systematic review found reduced locoregional recurrence, but no evidence of improved survival.

Locally advanced breast cancer

- **Chemotherapy (cyclophosphamide/methotrexate/fluorouracil or anthracycline based regimens)** We found no evidence that the cytotoxic, multidrug chemotherapy regimen (CMF) improves survival, disease free survival, or long term locoregional control.
- **Radiotherapy** For locally advanced breast cancer that is rendered operable, small RCTs found that radiotherapy or surgery as sole local treatments have similar effects on response rates, duration of response, and overall survival.
- **Radiotherapy after attempted curative surgery** One RCT found weak evidence that radiotherapy after attempted curative surgery versus no further local treatment may reduce local and regional recurrence.
- **Surgery** For locally advanced breast cancer that is rendered operable, small RCTs found that surgery or radiotherapy as sole local treatments have similar effects on response rates, duration of response, and overall survival.
- **Tamoxifen plus radiotherapy (*v* radiotherapy)** One RCT found that hormone treatment plus radiotherapy versus radiotherapy alone significantly improved locoregional recurrence at 6 years and improved median survival at 8 years.

DEFINITION **Ductal carcinoma *in situ*** is a non-invasive (see glossary, p 2029) tumour characterised by the presence of malignant cells in the breast ducts but with no evidence that they breach the basement membrane and invade into periductal connective tissues. **Invasive breast cancer** can be separated into three main groups: early (see glossary, p 2028) or operable breast cancer, locally advanced disease, and metastatic breast cancer (see, p 1975). **Operable breast cancer** is apparently restricted to the breast and sometimes to local lymph nodes and can be removed surgically. Although these women do not have overt metastases at the time of staging (see glossary, p 2029), they remain at risk of local recurrence and of metastatic spread. They can be divided into those with tumours greater than 4 cm with multifocal cancers that can be treated by mastectomy, and those with tumours less than 4 cm with unifocal cancers that can be treated by breast conserving surgery (see glossary, p 2028). **Locally advanced breast cancer** is defined according to the TNM staging system of the UICC TNM system (see glossary, p 2029)[1] as stage III B (includes T4 a–d; N2 disease, but absence of metastases). It is a disease presentation with evidence (clinical or histopathological) of skin, or chest wall involvement, or axillary nodes matted together by tumour extension, or a combination of these features. **Metastatic breast cancer** is presented in a separate topic (see, p 1975).

INCIDENCE/ PREVALENCE Breast cancer affects 1/10–1/11 women in the UK and causes about 21 000 deaths a year. Prevalence is about five times higher, with over 100 000 women living with breast cancer at any one time. Of the 15 000 new cases of breast cancer a year in the UK, most will present with primary operable disease.[2]

AETIOLOGY/ RISK FACTORS The risk of breast cancer increases with age, doubling every 10 years up to the menopause. Risk factors include an early age at menarche, older age at menopause, older age at birth of first child, family history, atypical hyperplasia, excess alcohol intake, radiation exposure to developing breast tissue, oral contraceptive use, postmenopausal hormone replacement therapy, and obesity. Risk in different countries varies fivefold. The cause of breast cancer in most women is unknown. About 5% of breast cancers can be attributed to mutations in the genes *BRCA1* and *BRCA2*.[3]

PROGNOSIS **Primary carcinoma** of the breast is potentially curable. The risk of relapse depends on various clinicopathological features, including axillary node involvement, oestrogen receptor status, and tumour size. Tumour size, axillary node status, histological grade, and oestrogen receptor status provide the most significant prognostic information. Seventy per cent of women with operable disease are alive 5 years after diagnosis and treatment (adjuvant drug treatment is given to most women after surgery). Risk of recurrence is highest during the first 5 years, but the risk remains even 15–20 years after surgery. Those with node positive disease have a 50–60% chance of recurrence within 5 years, compared with 30–35% for node negative disease. Recurrence at 10 years, according to one large systematic review,[4] is 60–70% compared with 25–30% of node negative women. The prognosis for a disease free survival (see glossary, p 2028) at 5 years is worse for stage III B (33%) than that for stage III A (71%). Five year overall survival is 44% for stage III B and 84% for stage III A.[5] Poor survival and high rates of local recurrence characterise locally advanced breast cancer (see glossary, p 2028).

AIMS OF INTERVENTION To improve survival; to prevent local or regional node recurrence; to obtain prognostic information on the type and extent of tumour and the status of the axillary lymph nodes; to optimise cosmetic results and minimise psychosocial impact; to minimise adverse effects of treatment; and to maximise quality of life.

OUTCOMES Survival; rates of local and regional recurrence; rates of mastectomy after breast conserving treatment; rates of development of metastases; cosmetic outcomes; quality of life; incidence of adverse effects of treatment, including upper limb lymphoedema.

METHODS *Clinical Evidence* search and appraisal October 2002.

QUESTION **What are the effects of interventions after breast conserving surgery for ductal carcinoma *in situ*?**

OPTION **RADIOTHERAPY**

Alan Rodger and Mike Dixon

Two RCTs found that radiotherapy is associated with a reduced risk of local recurrence and invasive carcinoma, but with no evidence of an effect on survival.

Benefits: We found no systematic review but found two RCTs comparing radiotherapy (see glossary, p 2029) with no radiotherapy after surgery for ductal carcinoma *in situ* (DCIS). The first RCT (814 women) found no significant difference in survival at 8 years with radiotherapy, but a significant reduction in risk of local recurrence (survival 95% with radiotherapy *v* 94% with no radiotherapy; local recurrence 12.1% with radiotherapy *v* 26.8% with no radiotherapy; $P < 0.0005$; risk of recurrent DCIS 8.2% with radiotherapy *v* 13.4% with no radiotherapy; $P = 0.007$; risk of invasive carcinoma 3.9% with radiotherapy *v* 13.4% with no radiotherapy; $P < 0.0001$).[6] The second RCT (1002 women) found, at median follow up of 4.25 years, significantly lower recurrence of DCIS in women given radiotherapy.[7] At 4 years, local relapse free survival was more likely with surgery plus radiotherapy than with surgery alone (91% with surgery plus radiotherapy *v* 84% with surgery alone; $P = 0.005$; HR 0.62, 95% CI 0.44 to 0.87). More women were free of DCIS recurrence after 4 years with radiotherapy but the difference was not significant (95% with surgery plus radiotherapy *v* 92% with surgery alone; HR 0.65, 95% CI 0.43 to 1.03). There was a significant reduction in invasive recurrence (96% with surgery plus radiotherapy *v* 92% with surgery alone; HR 0.60, 95% CI 0.37 to 0.97).[7]

Harms: One RCT found an increase in contralateral breast cancer associated with radiotherapy at 4 years (3% with surgery plus radiotherapy *v* 1% with surgery alone; HR 2.57, 95% CI 1.24 to 5.33).[7]

Comment: Ongoing RCTs are evaluating radiotherapy in all grades of DCIS. Subset analyses may be required to identify subgroups of women who benefit most from radiotherapy after breast conserving surgery (see glossary, p 2028).

OPTION TAMOXIFEN PLUS RADIOTHERAPY

Mike Dixon and Alan Rodger

One RCT found that adjuvant tamoxifen reduced breast cancer events in women who have undergone wide excision and radiotherapy, but found no evidence of an effect on survival.

Benefits: We found no systematic review. We found one RCT in women with ductal carcinoma *in situ* treated with wide excision and radiotherapy, which compared adjuvant tamoxifen (see glossary, p 2029) (20 mg/day) with placebo for 5 years in 1804 women.[8] At median follow up of 74 months, there were fewer breast cancer events with tamoxifen than placebo (OR 0.63, 95% CI 0.47 to 0.83), and fewer invasive ipsilateral or contralateral breast cancers (OR 0.57, 95% CI 0.38 to 0.85). However, there was no significant difference in overall survival (RR 0.88, 95% CI 0.33 to 2.28).

Harms: One RCT found a higher, but non-significant rate of endometrial cancers associated with tamoxifen (RR 3.4, 95% CI 0.6 to 33.4).[8]

Comment: RCTs of tamoxifen in ductal carcinoma *in situ* are under way. Results of one of these RCTs are expected to be published shortly (Dixon M, personal communication, 2002).

QUESTION What are the effects of neoadjuvant chemotherapy in the management of primary breast cancer?

Kate Gregory and Stephen Johnston

Five RCTs found no difference in survival with neoadjuvant chemotherapy versus adjuvant chemotherapy.

Benefits: We found no systematic review. We found five RCTs of neoadjuvant chemotherapy versus adjuvant chemotherapy (see glossary, p 2028).[9–13] The first RCT (272 women with tumours > 3 cm in whom mastectomy was indicated) compared preoperative (neoadjuvant) EVMTV (epirubicin, vincristine, mitomycin-C, thiotepa, vindesine) chemotherapy versus mastectomy followed by EVMTV regimen. At an initial median follow up of 34 months, a significant survival difference was reported in favour of neoadjuvant chemotherapy (85% with preoperative EVMTV *v* 95% with mastectomy + EVMTV; P = 0.04).[9] However, the final analysis at 124 months showed that the survival improvement was no longer significant, with survival of about 55% in both groups.[14] The second RCT (414 women) compared four cycles of FAC (see glossary, p 2028) chemotherapy given either preoperatively or postoperatively. At 54 months' follow up, the primary (neoadjuvant) chemotherapy group had a better overall survival (86% with preoperative *v* 68% with postoperative; P = 0.039);[10] however, a subsequent analysis at 105 months did not show a long term survival benefit.[15] The third RCT (309 women) compared four cycles of MM (mitoxantrone [mitozantrone], methotrexate) chemotherapy, then surgery, then four cycles of MM versus surgery, then eight cycles of MM. At 48 months' follow up, there was no difference in survival between the neoadjuvant and adjuvant groups (84% with neoadjuvant *v* 82% with adjuvant, not significant).[11] The third, and largest

RCT (NSABP-18), in which 1523 women were randomised to four cycles of adriamycin (doxorubicin) plus cyclophosphamide (AC) either preoperatively or postoperatively, found identical survival rates (67%) in the two groups at 60 months.[12] The fifth RCT (698 women) compared four cycles of fluorouracil, epirubicin, and cyclophosphamide given either preoperatively or postoperatively. It found no significant difference between preoperative versus postoperative chemotherapy in overall survival (82% with preoperative *v* 84% with postoperative, HR 1.16, 95% CI 0.83 to 1.63), progression free survival (65% with preoperative *v* 70% with postoperative; HR 1.15, 95% CI 0.89 to 1.48), or locoregional recurrence at 4 years (21.5% with preoperative *v* 17.8% with postoperative; HR 1.13, 95% CI 0.70 to 1.81).[13]

Harms: We found no evidence that neoadjuvant chemotherapy has a negative impact on survival.

Comment: We found no evidence to support the use of neoadjuvant chemotherapy to improve the chances of survival for operable breast cancers outside the context of an RCT.

QUESTION What is the effect of neoadjuvant chemotherapy on mastectomy rates?

Several RCTs have found that neoadjuvant chemotherapy leads to a marked reduction in the mastectomy rate.

Benefits: **Neoadjuvant versus adjuvant chemotherapy:** We found no systematic review but found three RCTs, which found a lower rate of mastectomy in women who had received neoadjuvant chemotherapy compared with women receiving adjuvant chemotherapy (see glossary, p 2028). **MM regimen:** One RCT in the UK (309 women receiving MM [mitoxantrone, methotrexate] chemotherapy) found that neoadjuvant versus adjuvant chemotherapy significantly reduced the mastectomy rate (13% with neoadjuvant *v* 28% with adjuvant; $P < 0.005$).[16] **AC (adriamycin [doxorubicin], cyclophosphamide) regimen:** In the second RCT (1523 women), breast conservation rates were lower in the adjuvant arm (60% with adjuvant *v* 67% with neoadjuvant), although this was not significant.[12] **FAC regimen:** See glossary, p 2028. One RCT assessed 272 women at diagnosis in terms of the recommended surgical procedure, and two of three women who were initially advised to have mastectomy were able to have breast conserving surgery (see glossary, p 2028) after neoadjuvant chemotherapy.[17]

Harms: None of the RCTs reported a significantly higher local recurrence rate with neoadjuvant chemotherapy compared with adjuvant chemotherapy.[9,11,12]

Comment: With an increased number of conservative operations being performed after downstaging by neoadjuvant chemotherapy for large primary tumours, there are theoretical concerns that this may result in an increased rate of local recurrence. Neoadjuvant chemotherapy can lead to a reduction in the requirement for mastectomy and as such an increase in breast conservation surgery. In the three RCTs of women with operable breast cancer receiving breast conserving surgery, this has not been associated with a significant increase in the rate of local recurrence.[12,16,17]

QUESTION **What are the effects of different regimens used in the neoadjuvant setting?**

We found no evidence that any one of the common neoadjuvant chemotherapy regimens improves survival, recurrence, or quality of life.

Benefits: We found no systematic review. We found one non-systematic review and five additional RCTs comparing adjuvant to neoadjuvant chemotherapy (see glossary, p 2029) using a variety of regimens.[11,12,18–21] Most studies used anthracycline (see glossary, p 2028) based regimens, which are of proven benefit in the adjuvant setting.[18] **AC regimen:** One RCT treated women with AC (adriamycin [doxorubicin], cyclophosphamide) and found an objective response rate (complete or partial clinical response) of 79%.[12] **MM regimen:** MM (mitoxantrone, methotrexate) in the UK RCT gave an overall objective response rate (see glossary, p 2029) of 85%.[11] Three RCTs compared different neoadjuvant regimens. **FAC regimen versus paclitaxel:** An RCT (174 women in the US) compared conventional FAC (see glossary, p 2028) versus single agent paclitaxel, and found similar response rates in both groups (79% with FAC *v* 80% with paclitaxel), with no significant difference in survival rates.[19] **Comparison between MPEMi, MPEpiE, and MPEpiV regimens:** A European RCT (101 women treated with three different combinations: MPEMi [methotrexate, cisplatin, etoposide, mitomycin-C], MPEpiE [methotrexate, cisplatin, epirubicin, etoposide], and MPEpiV [methotrexate, cisplatin, epirubicin, vincristine]) found the response to be 89%, with no significant differences between the groups.[20] **Sequencing of anthracycline based chemotherapy and docetaxel:** We found two RCTs.[22,23] The first RCT (104 women who had achieved complete or partial clinical response to four cycles of cyclophosphamide, adriamycin [doxorubicin], vincristine, and prednisolone [CVAP]) compared a further four cycles of CVAP versus four cycles of docetaxel.[22] It found that further treatment with docetaxel significantly improved clinical complete response rate compared with further CVAP (clinical complete response rate 85% with docetaxel *v* 64% with CVAP; $P = 0.03$).[22] In the second RCT (2411 people), all participants received four cycles of AC and were then randomly allocated to three regimens: surgery alone, four cycles of docetaxel followed by surgery, or surgery followed by four cycles of docetaxel. Preliminary results of this RCT found that, at the time of surgery, preoperative docetaxel improved clinical complete response rate compared no preoperative docetaxel (65% with docetaxel *v* 40% with no docetaxel; $P < 0.001$).[23] Final results, which will also examine effects of postoperative docetaxel, are awaited. **Navelbine based regimens:** We found no fully published RCTs (see comment below). **Comparison between routes of administration:** We found one Japanese study comparing routes of administration.[21] It compared no neoadjuvant treatment, neoadjuvant intravenous epirubicin, or intra-arterial epirubicin. Response rates were higher in women receiving intra-arterial epirubicin versus intravenous epirubicin (68% with intra-arterial epirubicin *v* 36% with iv epirubicin; $P < 0.05$); however, this was not associated with a survival benefit.

Harms: **FAC versus paclitaxel:** In the RCT in the USA comparing FAC with paclitaxel, rates of septic neutropenia (53% with paclitaxel *v* 21% with FAC) and granulocyte colony stimulating factor usage (56% with paclitaxel *v* 25% with FAC) were higher in women taking paclitaxel.[19]

Comment: More work is needed to determine the optimal regimen for neoadjuvant treatment. We found little evidence in the literature comparing different combinations, but anthracycline based combinations probably remain the treatment of choice. Ongoing RCTs are investigating the role of taxane sequencing after anthracycline based treatment (NSABP-27), and anthracycline in combination with fluorouracil infusion. **Navelbine based regimens:** We found one RCT (published as an abstract, 147 women), which compared AC, navelbine plus mitoxantrone (NM), and navelbine plus epirubicin (NE). Response rates were 65% with AC, 73% with NM, and 86% with NE. The time to outcome was not stated. The trial is ongoing although NM has been stopped because of haematological toxicity.[24]

QUESTION Is the extent of surgery related to outcome in early invasive breast cancer?

Mike Dixon and Alan Rodger

We found good evidence from two systematic reviews and long term follow up of included RCTs that more extensive surgery does not improve outcomes in women with early invasive breast cancer, providing that all local disease is excised. Cosmetic appearance is worse with more extensive surgery.

Benefits: **Comparisons between supraradical, radical, and total mastectomy:** We found one systematic review (search date not stated, 5 RCTs, 2090 women with operable breast cancer) comparing supraradical mastectomy with radical mastectomy, radical with total mastectomy (see glossary, p 2029), and supraradical with total mastectomy.[25] It found no significant difference in risk of death over 10 years (ARR of more extensive *v* less extensive surgery +0.02, 95% CI –0.04 to +0.08). **Comparisons between radical, total, and simple mastectomy:** The same review included four RCTs comparing either radical with simple mastectomy (3 RCTs) or total with simple mastectomy (1 RCT) in 1296 women with operable breast cancer.[25] Meta-analysis found no significant difference in risk of death over 10 years (ARR for more extensive *v* less extensive surgery +2%, 95% CI –5% to +9%). One included RCT (1079 women) comparing radical mastectomy and total mastectomy with or without axillary radiotherapy (see glossary, p 2028) has now reported 25 year follow up results.[26] It found no significant difference in survival between total and radical mastectomy (in women with negative nodes: HR for total mastectomy + radiotherapy (see glossary, p 2029) v radical mastectomy 1.08, 95% CI 0.91 to 1.28; HR for total mastectomy without radiotherapy v radical mastectomy 1.03, 95% CI 0.87 to 1.23; in women with positive nodes: HR for total mastectomy + radiotherapy v radical mastectomy 1.06, 95% CI 0.89 to 1.27).[26] **Mastectomy versus breast conservation:** We found two systematic reviews.[25,27] One review (search date 1995)[27] analysed data on 10 year survival from six RCTs comparing breast conservation with mastectomy. Meta-analysis of data from five of the RCTs (3006 women) found no significant difference in the risk of death at 10 years (OR v mastectomy 0.91, 95% CI 0.78 to 1.05). The sixth RCT used different protocols. Where more than half of node positive women in both mastectomy and breast conservation groups received adjuvant nodal radiotherapy (see glossary, p 2028), both groups had similar survival rates. Where fewer than half of node positive women in both groups received adjuvant nodal radiotherapy, survival was better with breast conservation (OR v with mastectomy 0.69, 95% CI 0.49 to 0.97). In the second review (search date not stated, 9 RCTs, 4981 women potentially suitable for breast conserving surgery (see glossary, p 2028)) all participants received postoperative radiotherapy.[25] Meta-analysis found no significant difference in risk of death over 10 years (RRR for breast conservation compared with mastectomy +2%, 95% CI –5% to +9%). It also found no significant difference in rates of local recurrence (6 RCTs in 3107 women; RRR mastectomy v breast conservation +4%, 95% CI –4% to +12%). Two RCTs included in the reviews have now reported 20 year follow up results.[28,29] The first RCT (701 women with breast cancer < 2 cm diameter) found no significant difference between radical mastectomy and quadrantectomy (see glossary, p 2029) for all cause mortality at 20 years (death rate about 42% in both groups; P = 1.0).[28] The second RCT (1851 women) compared lumpectomy (see glossary, p 2028) alone, lumpectomy plus breast irradiation, and total mastectomy.[29] It found no significant difference between lumpectomy and total mastectomy for mortality at 20 years (HR lumpectomy alone v mastectomy 1.05, 95% CI 0.90 to 1.23; HR lumpectomy + irradiation v mastectomy 0.97, 95% CI 0.77 to 1.06).[29] **Different extents of local excision in breast conservation:** We found no systematic review. We found one RCT (705 women) comparing lumpectomy with quadrantectomy.[30] There were significantly more local recurrences with lumpectomy than with quadrantectomy (7% with lumpectomy v 2% with quadrantectomy), but a major factor associated with local recurrence in the lumpectomy group was incomplete excision (see comment below).[31] We found no RCTs comparing wide local excision (complete excision microscopically) with quadrantectomy.

Harms: More extensive surgery results in greater mutilation. Between 60–90% of women having breast conservation have an excellent or good cosmetic result (median 83%, 95% CI 67% to 87%).[30,32–40] The single most important factor influencing cosmetic outcome is the volume of tissue excised; the larger the amount of tissue excised the worse the cosmetic result.[30] The RCT of different extents of local excision in breast conservation found that, in a subset of 148 women, there was a significantly higher rate of poor cosmetic outcome with quadrantectomy (RR *v* lumpectomy 3.1, 95% CI 1.2 to 8.1).[30] Only isolated small studies have shown no correlation between extent of surgical excision and cosmesis.[38]

Comment: The link between completeness of excision and local recurrence after breast conservation has been evaluated in 16 centres. In 13 of these, incomplete excision was associated with an increased relative risk of local recurrence compared with complete excision (estimated median RRI 3.4%, 95% CI 2.6% to 4.6%).[31] The three centres not reporting increased rates of local recurrence after incomplete excision gave much higher doses of local radiotherapy (65–72 Gy) to people with involved margins. Two centres also used re-excision, and women with involved margins had only focal margin involvement.

QUESTION What are the effects of different radiotherapy regimens in operable breast cancer?

Alan Rodger and Mike Dixon

OPTION RADIOTHERAPY AFTER BREAST CONSERVING SURGERY

One systematic review has found that radiotherapy reduces the risk of isolated local recurrence and loss of a breast, but does not increase 10 year survival compared with breast conserving surgery alone. Similar rates of survival and local recurrence are achieved with breast conserving surgery plus radiotherapy as with mastectomy.

Benefits: **Versus breast conserving surgery alone:** See glossary, p 2028. We found one systematic review (search date not stated, 4 RCTs, 382–1450 women),[25] comparing surgery plus radiotherapy (see glossary, p 2029) with surgery alone. All four RCTs began before 1985 and used megavoltage x rays. Pooled data from RCTs reporting sites of local recurrence (781 women) found that women with isolated local recurrence were less likely to have received radiotherapy (OR 0.25, 95% CI 0.16 to 0.34). Even an RCT limited to "good prognosis disease" (tumour ≤2 cm, node negative, 381 people) found a significantly lower local relapse rate with radiotherapy at 5 and 10 years (5 years: relapse rate with radiotherapy 2.3%, 95% CI 1% to 4.3%; no radiotherapy 18.4%, 95% CI 12.5% to 24.2%).[41] Ten year data found that radiotherapy was associated with significantly lower local recurrence rates (8.5%, 95% CI 3.9% to 13.1% with radiotherapy *v* 24%, 95% CI 17.6% to 30.4% with no radiotherapy), but no significant difference in overall survival (77.5% with radiotherapy *v* 78% with no radiotherapy).[42] One subsequent RCT (585 people) also found that after 6 years the proportion of women free of locoregional disease and with breast conservation was higher with radiotherapy (93.8% with radiotherapy *v* 81.3% with no radiotherapy).[43] Pooled data from all four RCTs found no significant difference in 10 year survival (80.1% with radiotherapy *v* 78.9% with no radiotherapy). **Versus mastectomy:** The systematic review identified nine RCTs (4891 women) comparing breast radiotherapy after breast conserving surgery with simple or modified radical mastectomy (see glossary, p 2029) in women with invasive breast cancer.[25] It found no difference in survival rates at 10 years (22.9% with radiotherapy after breast conserving surgery *v* 22.9% with radical mastectomy; CI values not provided) or in local recurrence (6.2% radiotherapy after breast conserving surgery *v* 5.9% radical mastectomy from pooled data from 6 RCTs, 3107 women).[25]

Harms: The RCTs and systematic review included in a consensus document published in 1998 (mainly of women undergoing breast conserving surgery or mastectomy with variation in radiotherapy techniques, doses, and fractionation) reported two severe adverse effects of radiotherapy: acute pneumonitis (0.7–7.0%) and pericarditis (0–0.3%); and the following long term adverse effects: significant arm oedema (1% without axillary dissection), radionecrotic rib fracture (1.1–1.5%), and brachial plexopathy (0–1.8%).[44] The risk and severity of adverse effects increased with volume irradiated, total dose received, dose per fraction, previous surgery (e.g. axillary dissection), and radiotherapy techniques that caused overlap in irradiated tissues. The review found an increased risk of non-breast cancer death (OR 1.24, 95% CI 1.09 to 1.43).[25] One systematic review (search date not stated)[45] of 10 RCTs found that the excess of non-breast cancer deaths after chest wall radiotherapy was caused by cardiac deaths resulting from the radiotherapy, but recent RCTs with data beyond 10 years did not find an excess of cardiac deaths.[46–48] A more recent systematic review (search date not stated, 40 RCTs in early breast cancer with meta-analysis of 10 and 20 year results) confirms a reduction in local recurrence of two thirds, a reduction in breast cancer mortality, but an increase in other, particularly vascular, mortality.[49] Overall, 20 year survival was 37.1% with radiotherapy versus 35.9% for controls (two sided P value = 0.06). Studies assessing cosmetic results have mainly been retrospective using poorly validated outcomes. The effects of social, psychological, and financial disruptions from attending 5–6 weeks of radiotherapy have not been addressed clearly. There is an extremely low reported incidence of radiation induced malignancy, usually soft tissue sarcomas, in the irradiated breast.

Comment: The four RCTs comparing breast conserving surgery with and without radiotherapy, as well as retrospective case series, found that prognostic factors for local recurrence after breast conserving surgery include positive tumour margins, an extensive intraduct component, younger age, lymphovascular invasion, histological grade, and systemic treatment. The only consistent independent risk factor is avoiding radiotherapy. Although there is no published evidence of a difference in survival at 10 years, recent results from the Fifth Early Breast Cancer Trialists' Group meeting suggest a reduction in breast cancer death in women having breast surgery with radiotherapy versus no radiotherapy (6100 women; 3.9% [SE 1.2%] increase in survival) (Dixon M, personal communication 2001).

OPTION **RADIOTHERAPY AFTER MASTECTOMY**

RCTs have found that radiotherapy to the chest wall after mastectomy reduces the risk of local recurrence by about two thirds, and reduces the risk of death from breast cancer at 10 years compared with mastectomy alone.

Benefits: We found one systematic review (search date not stated, 32 RCTs) comparing mastectomy with mastectomy followed by radiotherapy (see glossary, p 2029) to the chest wall.[25] Five RCTs were of mastectomy alone (4541 women), four of mastectomy and axillary clearance (3286 women), and 23 of mastectomy and axillary clearance (6699 women) (see glossary, p 2028). The review found that radiotherapy reduced local recurrence by two thirds and slightly reduced breast cancer mortality (OR 0.94, 95% CI 0.88 to 1.00), but found no significant difference in overall survival (OR 0.98, 95% CI 0.93 to 1.03).[25] **Versus mastectomy plus adjuvant chemotherapy or tamoxifen alone:** Two subsequent RCTs in high risk women receiving adjuvant (see glossary, p 2028) chemotherapy (CMF; see glossary, p 2029) after mastectomy compared irradiation to the chest wall and peripheral lymphatics with no radiotherapy.[46,47] One found radiotherapy reduced relative locoregional relapse rates by 56% (RR 0.44, 95% CI 0.26 to 0.77), and the other by 76% (AR 58% with radiotherapy *v* 14% no radiotherapy).[46,47] One RCT found that survival at 10 years was higher with radiotherapy (54%, 95% CI 51% to 58% with radiotherapy *v* 45%, 95% CI 42% to 48% with no radiotherapy).[47] The other, smaller RCT found a 29% relative reduction in mortality at 15 years with radiotherapy (RR 0.71, CI 0.51 to 0.99), although when these results were pooled with the results of the review no significant difference in overall mortality was detected (OR 0.96, 95% CI 0.91 to 1.01).[25,46,50,51] Another RCT in high risk postmenopausal women who had a mastectomy and received tamoxifen (see glossary, p 2029) 30 mg daily for 1 year, compared irradiation of the chest wall and peripheral lymphatics versus no radiotherapy. It found that radiotherapy reduced local or regional recurrence (as first site of recurrence) from 35% to 8%. Overall survival at 10 years was higher with radiotherapy (45%, 95% CI 41% to 49% with radiotherapy *v* 36%, 95% CI 33% to 40% with no radiotherapy).[50] We found no evidence that reduction in relative risk of local recurrence was affected by age, nodal status, receptor status, tumour grade, or tumour size, nor that the effect of radiotherapy on mortality varied significantly with extent of surgery, type of radiotherapy (megavoltage or orthovoltage), years the RCTs commenced or completed recruitment, or whether systemic treatment was given.[51]

Harms: See harms of radiotherapy after breast conserving surgery, p 2015. Three RCTs of postmastectomy total nodal irradiation (see glossary, p 2029) in high risk disease found no significant increase in cardiac mortality.[46–48,50]

Comment: The RCTs in the large systematic review were heterogeneous, in part because they began when RCT methods were less developed.[25] They varied in randomisation processes, areas irradiated, use of systemic treatment, radiotherapy doses, fractionation, and treatment schedules. We found little good evidence to identify which women should have postmastectomy radiotherapy to prevent local recurrence. One review of retrospective data found that extent of axillary node involvement, larger tumour size, higher histological grade, presence of lymphovascular invasion, and involvement of tumour margins reduced the chance of successful treatment.[51–54]

OPTION RADIOTHERAPY TO THE INTERNAL MAMMARY CHAIN

We found no direct evidence that radiotherapy to the internal mammary chain improved overall survival or breast cancer specific survival. Treatment may increase radiation induced cardiac morbidity.

Benefits: We found no systematic review. We found one RCT (270 women treated with breast conserving surgery and radiotherapy (see glossary, p 2029)), which compared internal mammary chain irradiation with no internal mammary chain irradiation.[55] At median follow up of 2.7 years there was no significant difference in relapse or survival (numbers not provided).

Harms: See harms of radiotherapy after breast conserving surgery, p 2014. Radiotherapy to the internal mammary chain is more likely to affect the heart compared with other types of radiotherapy.

Comment: The risk of internal mammary chain node involvement is related to the location and size of the primary tumour and, most importantly, histopathological axillary nodal status. Up to 30% of women with axillary involvement will also exhibit internal mammary chain nodal metastases. Central or medial breast cancers are more likely to metastasise to the internal mammary chain, as are larger tumours.[56,57] The risk of internal mammary chain recurrence is low, and after modified radical mastectomy (see glossary, p 2029) alone is 2%.[58] Modern radiotherapy planning and delivery should involve an assessment of the position and depth of the internal mammary chain nodes to be treated (using computerised tomography or ultrasound), and computer assisted placement, arrangement, and determination of dose distribution, technologies unavailable at the time of most RCTs included in the reviews.[25,45] Recent indirect evidence from RCTs suggests improved survival from nodal irradiation (including radiation to the internal mammary chain) after modified radical mastectomy combined with systemic treatment.[46,47,50] Another RCT of internal mammary chain irradiation has started recently (sponsored by the European Organisation for Research and Treatment of Cancer [EORTC]).

OPTION RADIOTHERAPY TO THE IPSILATERAL SUPRACLAVICULAR FOSSA

We found insufficient evidence to assess the impact on survival of irradiation of the ipsilateral supraclavicular fossa. RCTs have found that radiotherapy is associated with reduced risk of supraclavicular fossa nodal recurrence. Morbidity associated with irradiation of the supraclavicular fossa is rare and, where it occurs, is mild and temporary.

Benefits: We found no systematic review or RCTs on radiotherapy (see glossary, p 2029) to the ipsilateral supraclavicular fossa. One systematic review (search date not stated) found that postoperative radiotherapy was associated with reduced locoregional recurrence: see radiotherapy after breast conserving surgery, p 2014; radiotherapy after mastectomy, p 2016; and radiotherapy to internal mammary chain irradiation, p 2017.[25] RCTs indicate reduced recurrence in the supraclavicular fossa. One RCT in postmenopausal women at high risk of local recurrence who received tamoxifen (see glossary, p 2029) after mastectomy found that radiotherapy was associated with lower recurrence in the supraclavicular fossa at median follow up of 123 months (9/689 [1.3%] with radiotherapy *v* 37/686 [5.4%] with no radiotherapy).[50]

Harms: The acute morbidity of irradiation to the supraclavicular fossa is mild and includes temporary upper oesophagitis in nearly all women. The risk of radiation pneumonitis increases with the volume of lung irradiated. Treatment irradiates the lung apex in addition to any lung included in the breast or chest wall fields. Possible late morbidity includes brachial plexopathy but this should not exceed 1.8% if attention is paid to limiting total dose to 50 Gy, the limiting of the dose per fraction to 2 Gy or less, and avoiding field junction overlaps.[44,59] Late apical lung fibrosis is common and usually of no clinical importance. Demyelination of the cervical cord is an extremely rare complication of supraclavicular fossa radiotherapy.

Comment: None.

OPTION TOTAL NODAL RADIOTHERAPY

Three RCTs found that total nodal irradiation improved survival in high risk disease. An earlier systematic review found reduced locoregional recurrence, but no evidence of improved survival.

Benefits: One systematic review (search date not stated) included RCTs of total nodal irradiation (see glossary, p 2029) to the internal mammary chain, supraclavicular fossa, and axilla.[25] It found that postoperative radiotherapy (see glossary, p 2029) was associated with reduced locoregional recurrence, but no evidence of improved 10 year survival.[25] However, three RCTs found improved overall survival in women with high risk disease who had a mastectomy, axillary dissection, and systemic adjuvant (see glossary, p 2028) treatment, if total nodal postoperative radiotherapy was given.[46,47,50]

Harms: See harms of radiotherapy to the internal mammary chain, p 2017, supraclavicular fossa, p 2018, and axilla, p 2023. The three RCTs found no increase in cardiac mortality because of radiotherapy.[46–48,50]

Comment: None.

QUESTION What are the effects of adjuvant systemic treatment?

Stephen Johnston

OPTION ADJUVANT COMBINATION CHEMOTHERAPY

One systematic review has found that adjuvant chemotherapy reduces rates of recurrence and improves survival for women with early breast cancer. The benefit seems to be independent of nodal or menopausal status, although the absolute improvements are greater in those with node positive disease, and probably greater in younger women. The review found no evidence of a survival advantage from additional months of combination chemotherapy using two or more drugs, nor did RCTs find survival advantage from increased or reduced dosages of combination chemotherapy. Regimens containing anthracycline may modestly improve outcomes compared with the standard CMF regimen.

Benefits: **Versus no chemotherapy:** We found one systematic review (search date not stated, 47 RCTs, 18 000 women) comparing prolonged combination chemotherapy (see glossary, p 2028) with no chemotherapy.[60] Chemotherapy was associated with significantly lower rates of any kind of recurrence (women aged < 50 years, OR 0.65, 95% CI 0.61 to 0.69; women aged 50–69 years, OR 0.80, 95% 0.72 to 0.88) and death from all causes (women aged < 50 years, OR 0.73, 95% CI 0.68 to 0.78; women aged 50–69 years, OR 0.89, 95% CI 0.86 to 0.92). Proportional benefits were similar for women with node negative and node positive disease. Ten year survival according to nodal and age group is summarised (see table 1, p 2033). **Duration of treatment:** The same review identified 11 RCTs (6104 women), which compared longer regimens (doubling duration of chemotherapy from between 4 and 6 months to 8 and 12 months) with shorter regimens.[60] It found no additional benefit from longer treatment duration. **Different doses:** Several RCTs found no significant improvement from enhanced dose regimens, whereas others found little difference from untreated controls when suboptimal doses were used.[61,62] **Anthracycline regimens versus standard CMF regimen:** The systematic review identified 11 RCTs (5942 women) comparing regimens containing anthracycline (including the drugs adriamycin [doxorubicin] or 4-epidoxorubicin) with standard CMF (see glossary, p 2029) regimens.[60] It found a significant reduction in recurrence rates in those on anthracycline regimens (P = 0.006), and a modest but significant improvement in 5 year survival (72% with anthracycline *v* 69% with CMF regimen; P = 0.02).

Harms: **Acute adverse effects:** Adverse effects include nausea and vomiting, hair loss, bone marrow suppression, fatigue, and gastrointestinal disturbance. Prolonged chemotherapy is more likely to be associated with lethargy and haematological toxicity (anaemia and neutropenia), and anthracycline regimens cause complete hair loss. **Long term adverse effects:** Fertility and ovarian function may be permanently affected by chemotherapy, especially in women aged over 40 years, although for some women with hormone dependent cancer, reduced ovarian function may contribute to the benefit of adjuvant (see glossary, p 2028) treatment. Other potential long term risks include induction of second cancers (especially haematological malignancies, although the risk is very low), and cardiac impairment with cumulative anthracycline dosages. Provided the cumulative dose of adriamycin (doxorubicin) does not exceed 300–350 mg/m^2, the risk of congestive heart failure is less than 1%.

Comment: The absolute benefits of these regimens need to be balanced against their toxicity for different women. RCTs of high dose chemotherapy with haematological support (bone marrow transplantation or peripheral stem cell support) are under way in women with high risk disease (at least 10 positive lymph nodes), although one RCT did not find survival advantage for high dose treatment.[63,64] New and highly active cytotoxic agents such as the taxanes are being examined with anthracyclines either in combination or sequence. Alternating sequences of cytotoxic agents may prove an effective way of circumventing acquired drug resistance and thus enhancing the efficacy of a regimen, such as the Milan regimen (see glossary, p 2029) of single agent anthracycline followed by standard CMF chemotherapy.[65]

OPTION ADJUVANT TAMOXIFEN

One systematic review has found that adjuvant tamoxifen taken for up to 5 years reduces the chance of recurrence and death in postmenopausal women, and in women with oestrogen receptor positive tumours irrespective of age, menopausal status, nodal involvement, or the addition of chemotherapy. Five years of treatment seems better than shorter durations, but available evidence does not find benefit associated with prolongation beyond 5 years. Tamoxifen carries a slightly increased risk of endometrial cancer, but we found no evidence of an overall adverse effect on non-breast cancer mortality.

Benefits: **Versus placebo:** We found one systematic review (search date not stated, 55 RCTs, 37 000 women), which compared adjuvant tamoxifen (see glossary, p 2029) with placebo.[66] It found that 5 years of adjuvant tamoxifen had a similar effect on recurrence and long term survival in all age groups, irrespective of menopausal status or age. Overall tamoxifen for 5 years reduced the annual risk of recurrence by 47%, and of death by 26%. **Oestrogen receptor status:** Five years of tamoxifen treatment was associated with a greater reduction in the recurrence rate for women with oestrogen receptor positive rather than negative tumours (RRR 50% with oestrogen receptor positive *v* 6% with oestrogen receptor negative), and with a slightly greater reduction in the risk of 10 year recurrence in women with node positive compared with node negative disease (ARR 14.9% with oestrogen receptor positive *v* 15.2% with oestrogen receptor negative). **Duration of treatment:** The review found significantly greater reductions in recurrence with increasing duration of adjuvant tamoxifen (RRR 26% for 5 years of tamoxifen use *v* 12% for 1 year; $P < 0.0001$).[66] The absolute improvement in 10 year survival from 5 years of tamoxifen is tabulated (see table 2, p 2033). One RCT (3887 women) comparing 2 and 5 years of treatment found similar results.[67] The effects of prolonged treatment beyond 5 years are unclear. In the largest RCT in the systematic review, 1153 women who had completed 5 years of tamoxifen were randomised to either placebo or 5 more years of tamoxifen.[66,68] Disease free survival (see glossary, p 2028) after 4 years of further follow up was greater for those who switched to placebo rather than continued tamoxifen (92% with placebo *v* 86% with continued tamoxifen; P = 0.003), although there was no significant difference in overall survival. Other studies found no detrimental effect or improvement in continuing tamoxifen beyond 5 years.[69]

Harms: One systematic review found an increased hazard ratio for endometrial cancer with tamoxifen (average HR 2.58, 95% CI 2.23 to 2.93).[66] For 5 years of tamoxifen treatment, this resulted in a cumulative risk over 10 years of two deaths (95% CI 0 to 4) per 1000 women. There was no evidence of an increased incidence of other cancers, nor of non-breast cancer related deaths (i.e. cardiac or vascular), although one extra death per 5000 women years of tamoxifen was attributed to pulmonary embolus. Bone loss was found in premenopausal women (1.4% bone loss a year) but not in postmenopausal women, because of the partial agonist effects of tamoxifen.[70] There were mixed effects on cardiovascular risk, with significant reductions in low density lipoprotein cholesterol associated with a reduced incidence of myocardial infarction in some studies, but an increased risk of thrombosis. Overall, no effect has been found on non-breast cancer mortality (HR 0.99 95% CI 0.88 to 1.16).[66]

Comment: The risk to benefit ratio may vary between women, with oestrogen receptor negative women deriving little benefit. Even in oestrogen receptor positive women, any benefit on breast cancer could be offset with prolonged treatment (beyond 5 years), by drug resistance, and by adverse effects on the endometrium. Two multicentre RCTs of tamoxifen duration are in progress (Cancer Research Campaign, personal communication, 2000); however, because of concerns about long term toxicity with tamoxifen (see harms above) and in the absence of further definitive data, current clinical practice has been to recommend tamoxifen for 5 years.[71] For women with completely oestrogen receptor negative disease, the overall benefit of adjuvant tamoxifen needs further research.

OPTION COMBINED CHEMOTHERAPY PLUS TAMOXIFEN

One RCT has found that adding chemotherapy to tamoxifen improved survival.

Benefits: We found no systematic review. We found one RCT (2306 women with lymph node negative, oestrogen receptor positive early breast cancer), which compared tamoxifen alone versus tamoxifen plus CMF chemotherapy (see glossary, p 2029).[72] It found that adding chemotherapy to tamoxifen caused a further absolute improvement in disease free survival (see glossary, p 2028) (at 5 years' follow up 90% with tamoxifen + chemotherapy *v* 85% with tamoxifen alone; P = 0.006), and in overall survival (97% with tamoxifen + chemotherapy *v* 94% with tamoxifen alone; P = 0.03).

Harms: Adding CMF chemotherapy to tamoxifen was associated with a greater incidence of grade 3/4 neutropenia (9% with tamoxifen + chemotherapy *v* 0% with tamoxifen alone), greater than or equal to grade 2 nausea (35% with tamoxifen + chemotherapy *v* 4% with tamoxifen alone), moderate/severe alopecia (35.6% with tamoxifen + chemotherapy *v* 0.4% with tamoxifen alone), and thromboembolism/phlebitis (7.5% with tamoxifen + chemotherapy *v* 2.1% with tamoxifen alone).[72]

Comment: None.

OPTION OVARIAN ABLATION

One systematic review has found that ovarian ablation significantly improves long term survival in women aged under 50 years with early breast cancer.

Benefits: We found one systematic review (search date not stated, 12 RCTs with at least 15 years' follow up, 2102 premenopausal women) comparing ovarian ablation (see glossary, p 2029) by irradiation or surgery with no ablation.[73] Significantly more women with ovarian ablation survived (52% with ablation *v* 46% with no ablation; P = 0.001), and survived recurrence free (45% with ablation *v* 39% with no ablation; P = 0.0007). Benefit was independent of nodal status.

Harms: We found no good evidence on long term adverse effects. Concerns exist about late sequelae of ovarian ablation, especially effects on bone mineral density and cardiovascular risk. Acute adverse effects are likely to be menopausal symptoms.

Comment: Five of the RCTs compared ovarian ablation plus chemotherapy with chemotherapy alone.[73] In these, the absolute benefit of ablation was smaller than in RCTs of ovarian ablation alone. It may be that cytotoxic chemotherapy itself suppresses ovarian function, making the effect of ablation difficult to detect in combined RCTs. When only premenopausal women were considered in the absence of chemotherapy, there was a 27% improvement in the odds of recurrence free survival. RCTs are under way of reversible oophorectomy using gonadotrophin releasing hormone analogues, which would allow preservation of fertility in younger women with oestrogen receptor positive tumours.

QUESTION What are the effects of axillary clearance, sampling, or radiotherapy in women with operable primary breast cancer?

Mike Dixon and Alan Rodger

RCTs found no evidence that axillary clearance is associated with improved survival compared with axillary node sampling, axillary radiotherapy, or sampling plus radiotherapy combined. One systematic review of mainly poor quality evidence found that the risk of arm lymphoedema was highest with axillary clearance plus radiotherapy, lower with axillary sampling plus radiotherapy, and lowest with sampling alone.

Benefits: **Versus axillary sampling:** We found no systematic review but found one RCT (466 women) in women undergoing breast conserving surgery (see glossary, p 2028). It found that axillary sampling was associated with improved survival compared with axillary clearance (see glossary, p 2028), but the difference was not significant (estimated 5 year survival 88.6% with axillary sampling *v* 82.1% with axillary clearance).[74] Rates of node positivity were similar in both groups. **Versus axillary radiotherapy:** We found one systematic review (search date not stated, 8 RCTs, 4370 women) comparing axillary clearance (level I, II, and III dissection) versus axillary radiotherapy (see glossary, p 2028). It found no significant difference in mortality at 10 years (54.7% with axillary clearance *v* 54.9% with axillary radiotherapy) or in rates of recurrence (OR 1.01). Radiotherapy (see glossary, p 2029) was associated with fewer isolated local recurrences (OR 15%, 95% CI 7% to 22%).[25] **Versus sampling plus radiotherapy:** We found no systematic review. Two RCTs compared axillary clearance (level I, II, and III dissection) with sampling followed by radiotherapy in women with involved axillary nodes. They found no significant difference in local, axillary, or distant recurrence.[74,75] **Axillary clearance plus radiotherapy:** We found no studies assessing the effect of radiotherapy in addition to axillary clearance (level I and II, or level I, II, and III dissection) in regional control of disease.

Harms: **Axillary clearance:** Adverse effects of axillary surgery include seroma formation, arm swelling, damage to the intercostobrachial nerve, and shoulder stiffness. We found one RCT comparing the morbidity of different axillary procedures.[74] It compared complete axillary clearance (level I, II, and III dissection) with four node axillary sampling followed by radiotherapy if the nodes were involved. The rate of arm swelling was higher after clearance than after sampling whether or not women received postoperative radiotherapy (at 3 years, forearm girth was significantly greater; $P = 0.005$). After removal of axillary drains, between a quarter and half of women who had undergone a level I and II, or level I, II, and III axillary dissection developed seromas requiring aspiration. **Axillary radiotherapy:** One RCT comparing clearance with sampling plus radiotherapy for node positive disease found significantly reduced shoulder movement with radiotherapy, even though the shoulder joint was not irradiated.[74] At 6 months, both groups had significantly reduced shoulder movement compared with women receiving axillary sampling alone ($P < 0.004$). However, by 3 years, the axillary clearance group had improved and was not significantly different from the sampling group. **Arm lymphoedema:** One Australian systematic review (search date 1996) of lymphoedema prevalence, risks, and management found that, although current information is of poor quality, the combination of axillary dissection (to or beyond level II) and axillary radiotherapy (see glossary, p 2028) was associated with a risk of lymphoedema of 12–60%, with most studies suggesting that at least a third of women are affected.[76] Studies of axillary sampling followed by irradiation found lower rates (between 6–32%), and for axillary sampling alone, lower still (between

0–21%). Studies of dissection beyond level I found rates between 0–42%, with most studies reporting a rate of 20–30% 1 year after operation.[76] In women who receive axillary radiotherapy without axillary surgery, the overall lymphoedema rate is about 8%.

Comment: **Axillary staging:** Both clearance and sampling provide important prognostic information on which decisions on local and systemic treatment can be based. Further RCTs of less invasive and potentially less morbid staging procedures such as sentinel node biopsy are underway. A decision on axillary management should be based on the risk of involvement of axillary nodes (which varies according to tumour size, grade, and the presence of vascular/lymphatic invasion), and potential treatment related morbidity. Two retrospective cohort studies found that level I dissection accurately assessed axillary lymph node status, providing that at least 10 nodes were removed.[77,78] One RCT found that a sample of four nodes provided sufficient information to categorise an axilla as histologically positive or negative.[79] Removal of nodes at level I and level II, or removal of all nodes below the axillary vein (level I, II, and III), accurately stages the axilla.[77,78] RCTs comparing sentinel node biopsy with axillary node clearance and sampling are currently under way, and results of these will be incorporated in future *Clinical Evidence* updates (Dixon M, personal communication, 2000).

QUESTION What are the effects of interventions in locally advanced breast cancer (stage III B)?

Alan Rodger

OPTION LOCAL TREATMENT FOR LOCALLY ADVANCED BREAST CANCER

Two small RCTs including women with locally advanced disease (stage III B) found that, for locally advanced breast cancer that is rendered operable, radiotherapy or surgery as sole local treatments have similar effects on response rates, duration of response, and overall survival. One RCT found weak evidence that, if surgery is possible and is carried out, postoperative radiotherapy will reduce locoregional recurrence. Local skin toxicity (acute and late) after radiotherapy is greater in locally advanced breast cancer than after treatment for less advanced disease, because of the need for a higher radiation dose to skin.

Benefits: We found no systematic review of the role of radiotherapy (see glossary, p 2029) in locally advanced (stage III B) breast cancer. We found seven RCTs, including women with stage III B, which compared radiotherapy versus no radiotherapy.[47,50,80–84] Other management options varied across these RCTs. Most RCTs were small, but included more than stage III B women. **Postoperative radiotherapy versus no further local treatment after surgery:** We found two RCTs.[80,83] In one of these RCTs[80] preoperative and postoperative chemo-endocrine treatment was given to all women who also had a mastectomy and half the women were randomised to postmastectomy radiotherapy to the chest wall and regional lymphatics (45–50 Gy in 5 wks). However, 43% of the 184 women were excluded with more exclusions in the radiotherapy group, and it is impossible to ascertain what percentage of women were stage III B. There were numerous chemotherapy complications, including one death. The RCT found no significant difference in local or distant failures, but found that overall crude survival was significantly higher with no radiotherapy versus radiotherapy (28.7 months with no radiotherapy *v* 21.7 months with radiotherapy; $P < 0.05$). Conclusions cannot be drawn from this RCT. The second RCT of operable locally advanced breast cancer (see glossary, p 2028) (332 women who were recurrence free after modified radical mastectomy (see glossary, p 2029) and 6 cycles of chemo-hormone treatment; 38% stage T4 and 14% N2)[82] compared postoperative radiotherapy versus no further treatment. It found no significant difference in time to relapse (4.7 years with radiotherapy *v* 5.2 years with no further treatment), and median overall survival (8.3 years with radiotherapy *v* 8.1 years with no further radiotherapy). Radiotherapy reduced locoregional sites as first recurrence by 9%. **Postmastectomy radiotherapy in women having systemic treatment after surgery:** Two RCTs of "high risk breast cancer" (including women with stage III B disease) studied postmastectomy radiotherapy in women having systemic treatment after surgery.[47,50] The postmenopausal RCT separated some T4 tumours by skin invasion (14%).[50] For those receiving postmastectomy radiotherapy with tamoxifen (see glossary, p 2029), 8% developed local recurrence versus 34% receiving tamoxifen alone (5 year disease free survival (see glossary, p 2028): 41% with radiotherapy *v* 37% with tamoxifen; 10 year disease free survival: 23% with radiotherapy *v* 22% with tamoxifen; 5 year survivals: 51% with radiotherapy *v* 61% with tamoxifen; 10 year survivals: 31% with radiotherapy *v* 27% with tamoxifen). However, the studies used small and retrospective subgroups, making conclusions uncertain. **Surgery alone versus radiotherapy alone:** Two RCTs compared surgery alone versus radiotherapy alone as local treatment.[81,82] In one RCT (113 women with stage III breast cancer, 67% stage III B) women were given chemotherapy and 81% became operable; then 87 women were randomised to surgery or to radiotherapy.[81] After local treatment, a further 2 years of chemotherapy was given. Both groups had similar duration of disease control (29.2 months with surgery *v* 24.4 months with radiation; $P = 0.5$), similar overall median survival (39.3 months with surgery *v* 39 months with radiation), and similar sites of first relapse. In the other RCT (132 women, 91% stage III B, 9% stage III A) all women received chemotherapy before randomisation to either surgery or radiotherapy.[81] Total response rate was 75% in each group. Duration of remission was not significantly different (15 months with surgery *v* 22 months with radiotherapy; $P = 0.58$). Survival was similar at 4 years (52 months with radiotherapy *v* 49.1 months with surgery). **Low dose radiotherapy versus tamoxifen:** A small RCT (143 women)[84] compared low dose radiotherapy (40 Gy in 15 fractions) versus tamoxifen (20 mg twice daily). Women were given the alternative treatment on relapse. The RCT found no significant difference in response rates ($P = 0.34$), duration of response ($P = 0.76$), or survival ($P = 0.38$).

Harms: The type of harms from radiotherapy for locally advanced breast cancer were similar to those from radiotherapy after mastectomy or breast conserving surgery (see glossary, p 2028). However, in stage III B disease with skin involvement (T4 b, c, d), the skin is usually given a higher dose of radiotherapy. In addition, a higher dose (60 Gy) is often given to more of the breast volume. Acute skin toxicity (including moist desquamation) and late skin toxicity (pigmentation and telangiectasia) are also more likely than in women without skin involvement.

Comment: The lack of good quality, large RCTs addressing directly stage III B breast cancer and the role of radiotherapy render it difficult to draw firm conclusions on its value. Such RCTs are small and have varying approaches to management. From the results of two RCTs,[81,82] it can be concluded that in terms of overall response (which includes the response from local treatments such as surgery, radiotherapy, or both, and the effects of any initial systemic treatment), duration of that response, and overall survival, there is no advantage of either surgery alone or radiotherapy alone as sole local treatment over the other. It is more difficult to detail the possible benefits of postoperative radiotherapy in women whose locally advanced breast cancers have been rendered operable by systemic treatment and who have undergone surgery, usually modified radical mastectomy. It is likely that such postoperative radiotherapy will reduce the risk of local (and regional if nodal areas are irradiated) recurrence. It is not possible to conclude that it will affect survival.

OPTION SYSTEMIC TREATMENT FOR LOCALLY ADVANCED BREAST CANCER

We found no evidence that cytotoxic chemotherapy of cyclophosphamide, methotrexate, and fluorouracil, or an anthracycline based multidrug regimen improved survival, disease free survival, or long term locoregional control in locally advanced breast cancer. One RCT found evidence that hormone treatment plus radiotherapy versus radiotherapy alone improves survival in locally advanced breast cancer. One RCT found that chemotherapy, hormone treatment, or both, delayed locoregional recurrence.

Benefits: We found no systematic review. **Radiotherapy versus radiotherapy plus systemic chemotherapy:** We found three RCTs,[85–87] which compared radiotherapy (see glossary, p 2029) versus radiotherapy plus systemic treatment (hormone treatment, chemotherapy, or both). One RCT (410 women, most stage III B)[85] compared radiotherapy versus radiotherapy plus chemotherapy (CMF (see glossary, p 2029)) (for 12 cycles) versus radiotherapy plus hormone treatment (ovarian irradiation for premenopausal women, tamoxifen (see glossary, p 2029) for postmenopausal women) versus radiotherapy plus both chemotherapy and hormone treatment. Both chemotherapy (P = 0.0002) and hormone treatment (P = 0.0007) significantly delayed locoregional recurrence. Combined chemotherapy and hormone treatment had the largest effect (P = 0.0001). Locoregional recurrence at 6 years was reduced (about 60% with radiotherapy *v* about 50% with added chemotherapy or hormonal therapy). The effect on distant metastases was similar but less marked. Significantly increased median survival was found only with hormone treatment (4.3 years with hormone treatment v 3.3 years without hormone treatment, after 8 years HR death 0.75, 95% CI 0.59 to 0.96; median survival 3.8 years with chemotherapy v 3.6 years without chemotherapy, HR 0.84, 95% CI 0.66 to 1.08). Another RCT (118 women with stage III B breast cancer)[86] compared radiotherapy versus radiotherapy plus chemotherapy (CMF for 12 cycles) plus tamoxifen versus chemotherapy (CMF alternating with adriamycin [doxorubicin] and vincristine — AV) followed by radiotherapy and then further similar chemotherapy and tamoxifen. The radiotherapy in the third arm delivered a lower dose to the skin and a lower total dose. After a minimum follow up of 14 years, the RCT found no significant difference in survival, disease free survival (see glossary, p 2028), or locoregional control. The 10 year survival rates were 13% with radiotherapy alone; 21% with radiotherapy, CMF, and tamoxifen; and 28% for radiotherapy plus CMF, AV, and tamoxifen. Differences in 10 year survival were +8% (95% CI –9% to +25%) for radiotherapy versus radiotherapy, CMF, and tamoxifen; and 15% (95% CI 3% to 33%) for radiotherapy versus radiotherapy plus CMF, AV, and tamoxifen. There was no significant difference between the two arms with chemotherapy. Adding CMF and tamoxifen and adding CMF, AV, and tamoxifen significantly increased disease free survival compared with radiotherapy alone at 10 years (4% with radiotherapy alone v 15% in each of the other groups; ARI for each of the other groups v radiotherapy alone 12%, 95% CI 1% to 25%). Local recurrence was similar in the three arms (42% with radiotherapy alone v 45% with radiotherapy plus CMF and tamoxifen v 49% with radiotherapy plus CMF, AV, and tamoxifen). The third RCT (52 women with T4 breast cancer)[87] compared an anthracycline (see glossary, p 2028) chemotherapy regimen before radiotherapy versus similar radiotherapy alone. The combined treatment arm achieved a higher initial locoregional control rate (complete response 78.6% with chemotherapy regimen before radiotherapy v 45.8% with radiotherapy alone; P = 0.03). However, the number of women free of locoregional spread at death or last follow up was similar (57% with chemotherapy regimen before radiotherapy v 50% with radiotherapy alone). Overall survival and time to distant recurrence were not significantly different. **Multimodal treatment versus hormone treatment:** One RCT (108 women)[88,89] compared multimodal treatment (preoperative chemotherapy, surgery, radiotherapy, and tamoxifen) versus initial hormone treatment plus subsequent salvage treatments upon tumour progression. The objective remission after 6 months was higher with multimodal treatment than with tamoxifen alone (31/54 [57%] with multimodal treatment v 19/53 [36%] with tamoxifen alone; OR 2.4, 95% CI 1.1 to 5.0).[88] However, at a median follow up of 52 months, there was no significant difference in survival, the development of metastases, the time to metastases, or uncontrolled local disease. Women with oestrogen receptor positive tumours had a higher objective response rate (49% with oestrogen receptor positive v 7% with oestrogen receptor negative tumours; P value not provided), and increased survival (numbers not provided).[89]

Breast cancer (non-metastatic)

Harms: In many RCTs harms of treatment were not reported (see harms of adjuvant combination chemotherapy, p 2019).

Comment: The lack of large RCTs and the frequent inclusion of less locally advanced disease (T3) with locally advanced breast cancer (see glossary, p 2028) defined here as stage III B make it difficult to draw conclusions. There is, however, no evidence from the studies using CMF chemotherapy or various regimens incorporating anthracyclines that cytotoxic chemotherapy improves survival, disease free survival, or long term locoregional control in stage III B breast cancer.

GLOSSARY

Adjuvant treatment This usually refers to systemic chemotherapy, hormonal treatment, or both, taken by people after removal of a primary tumour (in this case, surgery for early breast cancer), with the aim of killing any remaining micrometastatic tumour cells and thus preventing recurrence.

Advanced breast cancer Operable locally advanced breast cancer (stage III A) is T3 (tumours > 5 cm) and N1 (non-matted involved axillary nodes). Locally advanced breast cancer (stage III B) is M0 with T4 (skin or chest wall infiltration by tumour), N2 (matted axillary nodes)/N3 (internal mammary node involvement) disease, or both, not classified as non-invasive or early invasive breast cancer. Metastatic breast cancer (stage IV) is M1 (any supraclavicular fossa node involvement or distant metastases to bone, lung, liver, etc.) with any combination of tumour and node parameters.

Anthracyclines Are also known as cytotoxic antibiotics, and are used as adjuvant treatment with radiotherapy. Examples of anthracyclines are aclarubicin, daunorubicin, adriamycin (doxorubicin), epirubicin, and idarubicin.

Axillary clearance Clearance of level I, II, and usually level III axillary lymph nodes. Level I nodes are lateral to the pectoralis minor muscle, level II nodes are under it, and level III nodes are medial to it at the apex of the axilla.

Axillary radiotherapy This usually includes irradiation of the supraclavicular fossa. Irradiation of this area incorporates some underlying lung that increases the risk of radiation pneumonitis. By increasing the volume of the lung irradiated, compared with chest wall or breast radiotherapy alone, the risk of acute pneumonitis is increased.

Axillary sampling Aims to remove the four largest, most easily palpable axillary lymph nodes, for histological examination.

Breast conserving surgery Surgery that consists of lumpectomy (minimal free margins), wide local excision (wider free margins), or segmental or quadrant resection (usually with very wide free margins).

CMF (classical) Chemotherapy regimen containing cyclophosphamide, methotrexate, and fluorouracil (5-FU).

Combination chemotherapy Two or more cytotoxic drugs given intravenously every 3–4 weeks for 4–6 months.

Disease free survival Means being alive with no local or distant recurrence or contralateral disease.

Early invasive breast cancer (stage I or II) is M0 with T1 or T2 (tumour diameter ≤ 5 cm, no involvement of skin or chest wall) and N0 or N1 (mobile axillary nodes); or M0 with T3 (tumour diameter > 5 cm, no skin or chest wall involvement), but only N0.

FAC Chemotherapy regimen containing fluorouracil (5-FU), adriamycin (doxorubicin), and cyclophosphamide.

Lumpectomy Gross tumour excision.

Milan regimen A sequential regimen of single agent anthracycline followed by CMF.

Neoadjuvant chemotherapy (also known as primary medical treatment.) Involves the use of chemotherapy to treat breast cancer before locoregional treatment (surgery and or radiotherapy) to the breast to downstage large primary cancers that would require mastectomy to improve chances of survival.

Non-invasive breast cancer (stage 0) is Tis (carcinoma *in situ*, intraductal carcinoma, lobular carcinoma *in situ*, or Paget's disease of the nipple with no associated tumour); N0 (no axillary nodal involvement); and M0 (no metastases).

Ovarian ablation Surgical, medical, or radiation induced suppression of ovarian function in premenopausal women.

Overall objective response rate The proportion of treated people in whom a complete response (disappearance of all known lesions on 2 separate measurements at least 4 wks apart), or partial response (> 50% reduction in the size of lesions) is observed.

Quadrantectomy Tumour excised with at least 2 cm of normal surrounding breast tissue and with a segment of breast tissue from the periphery of the breast to the nipple.

Radical mastectomy Removal of breast and pectoralis major and minor muscles and axillary contents.

Radiotherapy Part of initial local and regional treatment. In early stage disease it may be an adjunct to surgery; in locally advanced disease (T4, N2) it may be the sole locoregional treatment. Radiotherapy may be delivered to the breast or postmastectomy chest wall, as well as to the lymphatic areas of the axilla, supraclavicular fossa, or internal mammary node chain.

Staging of breast cancer A detailed description by tumour, nodal, and metastatic parameters at a particular time (TNM).[1] These are amalgamated into broader categories called stages (0–IV). Stages can be aggregated into even broader categories (non-invasive, early invasive, and advanced breast cancer) (see table 3, p 2033).

Supraradical mastectomy Removal of breast, pectoralis major and minor muscles, axillary contents, and internal mammary chain of nodes.

Tamoxifen A non-steroidal anti-oestrogen taken as daily oral tablets, usually for between 2–5 years.

TNM staging system See "staging of breast cancer" above.

Total mastectomy Removal of breast.

Total nodal irradiation Radiotherapy to the regional lymph nodes, including supraclavicular, infraclavicular, axillary nodes, and internal mammary nodes in the upper intercostal spaces.

UICC system International Union against Cancer.

REFERENCES

1. UICC International Union Against Cancer. *TNM classification of malignant tumours* 5th ed. Sobin LH, Wittekind CH, eds. New York: Wiley–Liss, 1997.
2. CRC. Breast Cancer Factsheet. 1996.
3. Easton D, Ford D. Breast and ovarian cancer incidence in BRCA-1 mutation carriers. *Am J Hum Genet* 1995;56:265–271.
4. Carter CL, Allen C, Henson DE. Relation of tumour size, lymph node status and survival in 24 740 breast cancer cases. *Cancer* 1989;63:181–187.
5. Hortobagyi GN, Ames FC, Buzdar AU, et al. Management of stage III primary breast cancer with primary chemotherapy, surgery and radiation therapy. *Cancer* 1988;62:2507–2516.
6. Fisher B, Dignam J, Wolmark N, et al. Lumpectomy and radiation therapy for the treatment of intraductal breast cancer: findings of the National Surgical Adjuvant Breast and Bowel Project B-17. *J Clin Oncol* 1998;16:441–452.
7. Julien JP, Bijker N, Fentiman IS, et al. Radiotherapy in breast-conserving treatment for ductal carcinoma *in situ*; first results of EORTC randomised Phase III trial 10853. *Lancet* 2000;355:528–533.
8. Fisher B, Dignam J, Wolmark N, et al. Tamoxifen in treatment of intraductal breast cancer: National Surgical Adjuvant Breast and Bowel Project B-24 randomised controlled trial. *Lancet* 1999;353:1993–2000.
9. Mauriac L, Durand M, Avril A, et al. Effects of primary chemotherapy in conservative treatment of breast cancer patients with operable tumours larger than 3 cm: results of a randomised trial in a single centre. *Ann Oncol* 1991;2:347–354.
10. Scholl SM, Fourquet A, Asselain B, et al. Neoadjuvant versus adjuvant chemotherapy in

premenopausal patients with tumours considered too large for breast conserving surgery: preliminary results of a randomised trial. *Eur J Cancer* 1994;30A:645–652.
11. Powles TJ, Hickish TF, Makris A, et al. Randomized trial of chemoendocrine therapy started before or after surgery for treatment of primary breast cancer. *J Clin Oncol* 1995;13:547–552.
12. Fisher B, Bryant J, Wolmark N, et al. Effect of preoperative chemotherapy on the outcome of women with operable breast cancer. *J Clin Oncol* 1998;16:2672–2685.
13. Van der Hage JA, van de Velde CJ, Julien JP, et al. Pre-operative chemotherapy in primary operable breast cancer: results from the European Organisation for Research and Treatment of Cancer Trial 10902. *J Clin Oncol* 2001;19:4224–4237.
14. Mauriac L, MacGrogan G, Avril A, et al. Neoadjuvant chemotherapy for operable breast carcinoma larger than 3 cm: a unicentre randomized trial with a 124-month median follow-up. Institut Bergonie Bordeaux Groupe Sein (IBBGS). *Ann Oncol* 1999;10:47–52.
15. Broet P, Scholl S, De la Rochrfordiere A, et al. Short and long term effects on survival in breast cancer patients treated by primary chemotherapy: an updated analysis of a randomised trial. *Breast Cancer Res Treat* 1999;58:151–156.
16. Makris A, Powles TJ, Ashley SE, et al. A reduction in the requirements for mastectomy in a randomized trial of neoadjuvant chemoendocrine therapy in primary breast cancer. *Ann Oncol* 1998;9:1179–1184.
17. Avril A, Faucher A, Bussieres E, et al. Resultats a 10 ans d'un essai randomise de chimiotherapie neo-adjuvante dans les cancers du sein de plus de 3 cm. *Chirurgie* 1998;123:247–256.
18. Early Breast Cancer Trialists Collaborative Group. Polychemotherapy for early breast cancer: an overview of the randomised trials. *Lancet* 1998;352:930–942.
19. Buzdar AU, Singletary SE, Theriault RL, et al. Prospective evaluation of paclitaxel versus combination chemotherapy with fluorouracil, doxorubicin, and cyclophosphamide as neoadjuvant therapy in patients with operable breast cancer. *J Clin Oncol* 1999;17:3412–3417.
20. Cocconi G, Bisagni G, Ceci G, et al. Three new active cisplatin-containing combinations in the neoadjuvant treatment of locally advanced and locally recurrent breast carcinoma: a randomized phase II trial. *Breast Canc Res Treat* 1999;56:125–132.
21. Takatsuka Y, Yayoi E, Kobayashi T, et al. Neoadjuvant intra-arterial chemotherapy in locally advanced breast cancer: a prospective randomised study. *Jpn J Clin Oncol* 1994;24:20–25.
22. Smith IC, Heys SD, Hutcheon A, et al. Neoadjuvant chemotherapy in breast cancer: significantly enhanced response with docetaxel. *J Clin Oncol* 2002;20:1456–1466.
23. D'Orazio AI, O'Shaughnessy J, Seidman AD. Neoadjuvant docetaxel augments the efficacy of preoperative docetaxel/cyclophosphamide in operable breast cancer: first results of NSABP-27. *Clin Breast Cancer* 2002;2;266–268.
24. Webb A, Smith IE, Ahern R. A randomised phase II trial of pre-operative navelbine/epirubicin (NE) versus navelbine/mitozantrone (NM) versus adriamycin/cyclophosphamide (AC) for early breast cancer. *Eur J Cancer* 2001;37:174.
25. Early Breast Cancer Trialists' Collaborative Group. Effects of radiotherapy and surgery in early breast cancer: an overview of the randomised trials. *N Engl J Med* 1995;333:1444–1455. Search date not stated; primary sources individual patient data from trials that began before 1985, trials identified from lists from national cancer bodies, the International Cancer Research Data Bank, hand searches of conference proceedings and reference lists, and personal contact with investigators.
26. Fisher B, Jeong J-H, Anderson S, et al. Twenty-five year follow-up of a randomized trial comparing radical mastectomy, total mastectomy, and total mastectomy followed by irradiation. *New Engl J Med* 2002;347:567–575.
27. Morris AD, Morris RD, Wilson JF, et al. Breast conserving therapy versus mastectomy in early stage breast cancer: a meta-analysis of 10 year survival. *Cancer J Sci Am* 1997;3:6–12. Search date 1995, primary source Medline.
28. Veronesi U, Cascinelli N, Mariani L, et al. Twenty-year follow-up of a randomised study comparing breast-conserving surgery with radical mastectomy for early breast cancer. *N Engl J Med* 2002;347:1227–1232.
29. Fisher B, Andeson S, Bryant J, et al. Twenty-year follow-up of a randomised trial comparing total mastectomy, lumpectomy and lumpectomy plus irradiation for the treatment of invasive breast cancer. *N Engl J Med* 2002;347:1233– 1241.
30. Sacchini V, Luini A, Tana S, et al. Quantitative and qualitative cosmetic evaluation after conservative treatment for breast cancer. *Eur J Cancer* 1991;27:1395–1400.
31. Smitt NC, Nowels KW, Zdeblick MJ, et al. The importance of the lumpectomy surgical margin status in long-term results of breast conservation. *Cancer* 1995;76:259–267.
32. Wazer DE, DiPetrillo T, Schmidt-Ullrich R, et al. Factors influencing cosmetic outcome and complication risk after conservative surgery and radiotherapy for early-stage breast carcinoma. *J Clin Oncol* 1992;10:356–363.
33. Abner AL, Recht A, Vicini FA, et al. Cosmetic results after surgery, chemotherapy and radiation therapy for early breast cancer. *Int J Radiat Oncol Biol Phys* 1991;21:331–338.
34. Dewar JA, Benhamou S, Benhamou E, et al. Cosmetic results following lumpectomy axillary dissection and radiotherapy for small breast cancers. *Radiother Oncol* 1988;12:273–280.
35. Rochefordiere A, Abner A, Silver B, et al. Are cosmetic results following conservative surgery and radiation therapy for early breast cancer dependent on technique? *Int J Radiat Oncol Biol Phys* 1992;23:925–931.
36. Sneeuw KA, Aaronson N, Yarnold J, et al. Cosmetic and functional outcomes of breast conserving treatment for early stage breast cancer 1: comparison of patients' ratings, observers' ratings and objective assessments. *Radiother Oncol* 1992;25:153–159.
37. Ash DV, Benson EA, Sainsbury JR, et al. Seven year follow-up on 334 patients treated by breast conserving surgery and short course radical postoperative radiotherapy: a report of the Yorkshire Breast Cancer Group. *Clin Oncol* 1995;7:93–96.
38. Lindsey I, Serpell JW, Johnson WR, et al. Cosmesis following complete local excision of breast cancer. *Aust N Z J Surg* 1997;67:428–432.
39. Touboul E, Belkacemi Y, Lefranc JP, et al. Early breast cancer: influence of type of boost (electrons vs iridium-192 implant) on local control and cosmesis after conservative surgery and radiation therapy. *Radiother Oncol* 1995;34:105–113.

40. Halyard MY, Grado GL, Schomber PJ, et al. Conservative therapy of breast cancer: the Mayo Clinic experience. *Am J Clin Oncol* 1996;19:445–450.
41. Liljegren G, Holmberg L, Adami HO, et al, for the Uppsala– rebro Breast Cancer Study Group. Sector resection with or without postoperative radiotherapy for stage I breast cancer: five year results of a randomised trial. *J Natl Cancer Inst* 1994;86:717–722.
42. Liljegren G, Holmberg J, Bergh, J, et al, and the Uppsala– rebro Breast Cancer Study Group. 10-year results after sector resection with or without postoperative radiotherapy for stage I breast cancer: a randomized trial. *J Clin Oncol* 1999;17:2326–2333.
43. Forrest AP, Stewart HJ, Everington D, et al, on behalf of the Scottish Cancer Trials Breast Group. Randomised controlled trial of conservation therapy in breast cancer: 6 year analysis of the Scottish trial. *Lancet* 1996;348:708–713.
44. Steering Committee on Clinical Practice Guidelines for the Care and Treatment of Breast Cancer. A Canadian consensus document. *Can Med Assoc J* 1998;158(suppl 3):1–84.
45. Cuzick J, Stewart H, Rutqvist L, et al. Cause-specific mortality in long term survivors of breast cancer who participated in trials of radiotherapy. *J Clin Oncol* 1994;12:447–453. Search date not stated; primary source cause specific mortality data from unconfounded randomised trials began before 1975 (trial identification methods not stated.).
46. Ragaz J, Jackson SM, Le N, et al. Adjuvant radiotherapy and chemotherapy in node-positive premenopausal women with breast cancer. *N Engl J Med* 1997;337:956–962.
47. Overgaard M, Hansen PS, Overgaard J, et al. Postoperative radiotherapy in high-risk premenopausal women with breast cancer who receive adjuvant chemotherapy. *N Engl J Med* 1997;337:949–955.
48. Hojris I, Overgaard M, Christensen JJ, et al. Morbidity and mortality of ischaemic heart disease in high-risk breast-cancer patients after adjuvant postmastectomy systemic treatment with or without radiotherapy: analysis of DBCG 82b and 82c randomised trials. Radiotherapy Committee of the Danish Breast Cancer Cooperative Group. *Lancet* 1999;354:1425–1430.
49. Early Breast Cancer Trialists Collaborative Group. Favourable and unfavourable effects on long-term survival of radiotherapy for early breast cancer: an overview of the randomised trials. Early Breast Cancer Trialists' Collaborative Group. *Lancet* 2000;355:1757–1770. Search date not stated; primary sources individual patient data from trials that began before 1990, trials identified from lists from national cancer bodies, the International Cancer Research Data Bank, hand searches of conference proceedings and reference lists, and personal contact with investigators.
50. Overgaard M, Jensen MB, Overgaard J, et al. Postoperative radiotherapy in high risk postmenopausal breast cancer patients given adjuvant tamoxifen: Danish Breast Cancer Cooperative Group DBCG 82c randomised trial. *Lancet* 1999;353:1641–1648.
51. Ghersi D, Simes J. Draft report of effectiveness of postmastectomy radiotherapy and risk factors for local recurrence in early breast cancer. Report to NHMRC National Breast Cancer Centre, Sydney, 1998.
52. O'Rourke S, Gaba MH, Morgan D, et al. Local recurrence after simple mastectomy. *Br J Surg* 1994;81:386–389.
53. Fowble B, Gray R, Gilchrist K, et al. Identification of a subset of patients with breast cancer and histologically positive nodes who may benefit from postoperative radiotherapy. *J Clin Oncol* 1988;6:1107–1117.
54. Houghton J, Baum M, Haybittle JL. Role of radiotherapy following total mastectomy in patients with early breast cancer: the closed trials working party of the CRC breast cancer trials group. *World J Surg* 1994;18:117–122.
55. Kaija H, Maunu P. Tangential breast irradiation with or without internal mammary chain irradiation: results of a randomised trial. *Radiother Oncol* 1995;36:172–176.
56. Handley R. Carcinoma of the breast. *Ann R Coll Surg Engl* 1975;57:59–66.
57. Veronesi U, Cascinelli NM, Bufalino R, et al. Risk of internal mammary lymph node metastases and its relevance on prognosis in breast cancer patients. *Ann Surg* 1983;198:681–684.
58. Veronesi U, Valagussa P. Inefficacy of internal mammary node dissection in breast cancer surgery. *Cancer* 1981;47:170–175.
59. Bates T, Evans RGB. Report of the Independent Review commissioned by The Royal College of Radiologists into brachial plexus neuropathy following radiotherapy for breast cancer. London: Royal College of Radiologists, 1995.
60. Early Breast Cancer Trialists' Collaborative Group. Polychemotherapy for early breast cancer: an overview of the randomised trials. *Lancet* 1998;352:930–942. Search date not stated; primary sources individual patient data from trials that began before 1990, trials identified from lists from national cancer bodies, the International Cancer Research Data Bank, hand searches of conference proceedings and reference lists, and personal contact with investigators.
61. Fisher B, Anderson S, Wickerham DL, et al. Increased intensification and total dose of cyclophosphamide in a doxorubicin-cyclophosphamide regimen for the treatment of primary breast cancer: findings from national surgical adjuvant breast and bowel project B-22. *J Clin Oncol* 1997;15:1858–1869.
62. Wood WC, Budman DR, Korzun AH. Dose and dose intensity of adjuvant chemotherapy for stage II, node-positive breast carcinoma. *N Engl J Med* 1994;330:1253–1259.
63. Peters WP, Ross M, Vredenburgh JJ, et al. High-dose chemotherapy and autologous bone marrow support as consolidation after standard-dose adjuvant chemotherapy for high-risk primary breast cancer. *J Clin Oncol* 1993;11:1132–1143.
64. Rodenhuis S, Richel DJ, Van der Wall E, et al. Randomised trial of high-dose chemotherapy and haemopoietic progenitor-cell support in operable breast cancer with extensive axillary lymph-node involvement. *Lancet* 1998;352:515–521.
65. Bonadonna G, Zambeti M, Valagussa P. Sequential or alternating doxorubicin and CMF regimens in breast cancer with more than three positive nodes. *JAMA* 1995;273:542–547.
66. Early Breast Cancer Trialists' Collaborative Group. Tamoxifen for early breast cancer: an overview of the randomised trials. *Lancet* 1998;351:1451–1467. Search date not stated; primary sources individual patient data from trials that began before 1990, trials identified from lists from national cancer bodies, the International Cancer Research Data Bank, hand searches of conference proceedings and reference lists, and personal contact with investigators.
67. Swedish Breast Cancer Cooperative Group. Randomised trial of two versus five years of

adjuvant tamoxifen for post-menopausal early stage breast cancer. *J Natl Cancer Inst* 1996;88:1543–1549.
68. Fisher B, Dignam J, Bryant J, et al. Five versus more than five years of tamoxifen therapy for breast cancer patients with negative lymph nodes and estrogen receptor-positive tumours. *J Natl Cancer Inst* 1996;88:1529–1542.
69. Stewart HJ, Forrest AP, Everington D, et al. Randomised comparison of 5 years of adjuvant tamoxifen with continuous therapy for operable breast cancer. *Br J Cancer* 1996;74:297–299.
70. Powles TJ, Hickish T, Kanis JA, et al. Effect of tamoxifen on bone mineral density measured by dual-energy x-ray absorptiometry in healthy premenopausal and postmenopausal women. *J Clin Oncol* 1996;14:78–84.
71. Swain SM. Tamoxifen: the long and short of it. *J Natl Cancer Inst* 1996;88:1510–1512.
72. Fisher B, Dignam J, Wolmark N, et al. Tamoxifen and chemotherapy for lymph node-negative, estrogen receptor-positive breast cancer. *J Natl Cancer Inst* 1997;89:1673–1682.
73. Early Breast Cancer Trialists' Group. Ovarian ablation in early breast cancer: overview of the randomised trials. *Lancet* 1996;348:1189–1196. Search date not stated; primary sources individual patient data from trials that began before 1990, trials identified from lists from national cancer bodies, the International Cancer Research Data Bank, hand searches of conference proceedings and reference lists, and personal contact with investigators.
74. Chetty U, Jack W, Prescott RJ, et al. A. Management of the axilla in operable breast cancer treated by breast conservation: a randomised controlled trial. *Br J Surg* 2000;87:163–169.
75. Stelle RJC, Forrest APM, Gibson R, et al. The efficacy of lower axillary sampling in obtaining lymph node status in breast cancer: a controlled randomised trial. *Br J Surg* 1985;72:368–369.
76. Browning C, Redman S, Pillar C, et al. NHMRC National Breast Cancer Centre, Sydney 1998. Lymphoedema: prevalence risk factors and management: a review of research. Search date 1996; primary sources Medline, hand searches of article references, personal contact with key resources of article references, and personal contact with key resources.
77. Axelsson CK, Mouridzsen HT, Zedeler K. Axillary dissection at level I and II lymph nodes is important in breast cancer classification. *Eur J Cancer* 1992;28A:1415–1418.
78. Kiricuta CI, Tausch J. A mathematical model of axillary lymph node involvement based on 1446 complete axillary dissections in patients with breast carcinoma. *Cancer* 1992;69:2496–2501.
79. Steele RJC, Forrest APM, Givson T, et al. The efficacy of lower axillary sampling in obtaining lymph node status in breast cancer: a controlled randomised trial. *Br J Surg* 1985;72:368–369.
80. Papaioannou A, Lissaios B, Vasilaros S, et al. Pre- and post-operative chemoendocrine treatment with or without post-operative radiotherapy for locally advanced breast cancer. *Cancer* 1983;51:1284–1290.
81. Perloff M, Lesnick G J, Korzun A, et al. Combination chemotherapy with mastectomy or radiotherapy for stage III breast carcinoma: a Cancer and Leukaemia Group B Study. *J Clin Oncol* 1988;6:261–269.
82. De Lena M, Varini M, Zucali R, et al. Multimodal treatment for locally advanced breast cancer. Results of chemotherapy–radiotherapy versus chemotherapy–surgery. *Cancer Clin Trials* 1981;4:229–236.
83. Olson JE, Neuberg D, Pandya KJ, et al. The role of radiotherapy in the management of operable locally advanced breast carcinoma: results of a randomised trial by the Eastern Co-operative Oncology Group. *Cancer* 1997;79:1138–1149.
84. Willsher PC, Robertson JF, Armitage NC, et al. Locally advanced breast cancer: long term results of a randomised trial comparing primary treatment with tamoxifen or radiotherapy in post-menopausal women. *Eur J Surg Oncol* 1996;22:34–37.
85. Bartelink H, Rubens RD, Van der Schueren E, et al. Hormonal therapy prolongs survival in irradiated locally advanced breast cancer: a European Organisation for Research and Treatment of Cancer randomised Phase III trial. *J Clin Oncol* 1997;15:207–215.
86. Koning C, Hart G. Long term follow up of a randomised trial on adjuvant chemotherapy and hormonal therapy in locally advanced breast cancer. *Int J Rad Oncol Biol Phys* 1998;41:397–400.
87. Rodger A, Jack WJL, Hardman PDJ, et al. Locally advanced breast cancer: report of a phase II study and subsequent Phase III trial. *Br J Cancer* 1992;65:761–765.
88. Willsher PC, Robertson JF, Chan SY, et al. Locally advanced breast cancer: early results of a randomised trial of multimodal therapy versus initial hormone therapy. *Eur J Cancer* 1997;33:45–49.
89. Tan SM, Cheung KL, Willsher PC, et al. Locally advanced primary breast cancer: medium term results of a randomised trial of multimodal therapy versus initial hormone therapy. *Eur J Cancer* 2001;37:2331–2338.

J Michael Dixon
Senior Lecturer in Surgery
Western General Hospital
Edinburgh
UK

Kate Gregory
Consultant Medical Oncologist
Royal Southampton Hospital
Southampton
UK

Stephen Johnston
Senior Lecturer in Medical Oncology
The Royal Marsden NHS Trust
London
UK

Alan Rodger
Professor of Radiation Oncology
William Buckland Radiotherapy Centre
The Alfred Hospital Monash University
Melbourne
Australia

Competing interests: None declared.

TABLE 1 Ten year survival with combination chemotherapy versus placebo, according to nodal and age/menopausal status: results of a systematic review of RCTs (see text, p 2019).[60]

	Control (%)	Chemotherapy (%)	Absolute benefit (%)	SD (%)	Significance (two sided)
Age < 50 years					
Node +ve	41.4	53.8	+12.4	2.4	P < 0.0001
Node –ve	71.9	77.6	+5.7	2.1	P = 0.01
Age 50–69 years					
Node +ve	46.3	48.6	+2.3	1.3	P = 0.001
Node –ve	64.8	71.2	+6.4	2.3	P = 0.0025

SD, standard deviation.

TABLE 2 Ten year survival in women treated with tamoxifen for 5 years compared with control treatment (no tamoxifen): results of a systematic review (see text, p 2020).[66]

	Control (%)	Tamoxifen (%)	Absolute benefit (%)	SD (%)	Significance (two sided)
Node +ve	50.5	61.4	+10.9	2.5	P < 0.00001
Node –ve	73.3	78.9	+5.6	1.3	P < 0.00001

SD, standard deviation.

TABLE 3 Staging of breast cancer (the individual terms are explained in the glossary).[1]

	TNM			Stage
Non-invasive	Tis	N0	M0	0
Early invasive	T1–2	N0–1	M0	I, II A or B
	T3	N0	M0	II B
Advanced				
Locally advanced	Tany	N2	M0	III A
	T3	N1–2	M0	III A
	T4	N0–3	M0	III B
	Tany	N3	M0	III B
Metastatic	Tany	Nany	M1	IV

Breast pain

Search date November 2002

Nigel Bundred

Key Messages

- **Low fat, high carbohydrate diet** One small RCT found that advice to follow a low fat, high carbohydrate diet compared with general dietary advice reduced self reported breast swelling and breast tenderness at 6 months.
- **Danazol** One RCT found that danazol compared with placebo reduced cyclical breast pain after 12 months, but increased adverse effects (weight gain, deepening of the voice, menorrhagia, and muscle cramps). It found no significant difference in pain relief between 6 months treatment with danazol and tamoxifen.
- **Gestrinone** One RCT found that gestrinone compared with placebo reduced breast pain after 3 months, but increased adverse effects (greasy skin, hirsutism, acne, reduction in breast size, headache, and depression).
- **Tamoxifen** Three RCTs found limited evidence that tamoxifen is more effective than placebo at reducing breast pain. Two of the RCTs found more hot flushes and vaginal discharge with tamoxifen compared with placebo. The third RCT did not report on adverse events. One RCT found no significant difference in pain relief between tamoxifen and danazol. One RCT found fewer adverse effects with a lower dose of 10 mg compared with a higher dose of 20 mg.
- **Lisuride maleate** One RCT with weak methods found that lisuride maleate (a dopamine agonist) compared with placebo reduced breast pain over 2 months.
- **Tibolone** One small RCT found limited evidence that tibolone reduced breast pain after 1 year compared with hormone replacement therapy.

- **Bromocriptine** Two RCTs found limited evidence that bromocriptine (a dopamine agonist) compared with placebo reduced breast pain. Both RCTs found a higher incidence of adverse effects with bromocriptine compared with placebo. Adverse events included nausea, dizziness, postural hypotension, and constipation.
- **Hormone replacement therapy** One small RCT found limited evidence that women taking hormone replacement therapy had more breast pain after 1 year than women taking tibolone.
- **Progesterones** Two small crossover RCTs found no significant difference between progesterones and placebo in breast pain.
- **Antibiotics; diuretics; evening primrose oil; gonadorelin analogues (luteinising hormone releasing hormone analogues); progestogens; pyridoxine; vitamin E** We found no RCTs on the effects of these interventions.

DEFINITION Breast pain can be differentiated into cyclical mastalgia (worse before a menstrual period) or non-cyclical mastalgia (unrelated to the menstrual cycle).[1,2] Cyclical pain is often bilateral, usually most severe in the upper outer quadrants of the breast, and may be referred to the medial aspect of the upper arm.[1–3] Non-cyclical pain may be caused by true breast pain or chest wall pain located over the costal cartilages.[1,2,4] Specific breast pathology and referred pain unrelated to the breasts are not included in this definition.

INCIDENCE/ PREVALENCE Up to 70% of women develop breast pain in their lifetime.[1,2] Of 1171 US women attending a gynaecology clinic, 69% suffered regular discomfort, which was judged as severe in 11% of women, and 36% had consulted a doctor about breast pain.[2]

AETIOLOGY/ RISK FACTORS Breast pain is most common in women aged 30–50 years.[1,2]

PROGNOSIS Cyclical breast pain resolves spontaneously within 3 months of onset in 20–30% of women.[5] The pain tends to relapse and remit, and up to 60% of women develop recurrent symptoms 2 years after treatment.[1] Non-cyclical pain responds poorly to treatment but may resolve spontaneously in about 50% of women.[1]

AIMS OF INTERVENTION To reduce breast pain and improve quality of life.

OUTCOMES Breast pain score based on the number of days of severe (score 2) or moderate (score 1) pain experienced in each menstrual cycle; visual analogue score of breast pain, heaviness, or breast tenderness; questionnaires.

METHODS *Clinical Evidence* search and appraisal November 2002 using the following keywords: breast tenderness, discomfort, pain, mastalgia, and mastodynia. Overall, the evidence was poor and some studies with weaker methods were included when higher quality evidence was not found, as indicated in the text. Studies were included whatever the definition of breast pain, as indicated in the text.

QUESTION **What are the effects of treatments for breast pain?**

OPTION LOW FAT, HIGH CARBOHYDRATE DIET

One small RCT found that advice to follow a low fat, high carbohydrate diet compared with general dietary advise reduced self reported breast swelling and tenderness at 6 months more than general dietary advice.

Benefits: We found no systematic review. We found one RCT (21 women attending a clinic in Canada with severe cyclical mastalgia for at least 5 years), which compared instruction to reduce fat content of the diet (to 15% of total calorie intake, while increasing complex carbohydrates to maintain calorie intake) versus general dietary advice (the principles for a healthy diet based on Canada's Food Guide, but not counselled to modify the fat content of their diet) for 6 months.[6] One woman in each group withdrew and was excluded from the analysis. Over 6 months, self reported breast swelling was significantly reduced in women with low fat, high carbohydrate diet versus general dietary advice (breast swelling at 6 months: 5/10 [50%] with low fat diet *v* 9/9 [100%] with general diet; NNT 2, 95% CI 2 to 5). Reported tenderness was significantly reduced in women receiving low fat dietary advice compared with those receiving general dietary advice at 6 months (6/10 [60%] with low fat diet *v* 9/9 [100%] with general diet; NNT 3, 95% CI 2 to 9). However, it found no significant difference in breast swelling, tenderness, and nodularity on physical examination at 6 months (6/10 [60%] with low fat diet *v* 2/9 [22%] with general diet; RR 2.7, 95% CI 0.8 to 4.1).[6]

Harms: The small RCT reported no adverse effects.[6]

Comment: Diets can be difficult to sustain in the long term.

OPTION EVENING PRIMROSE OIL

We found insufficient evidence on the effects of evening primrose oil.

Benefits: We found no systematic review and no good quality RCTs.

Harms: Poor quality RCTs found that adverse effects causing treatment discontinuation were similar with evening primrose oil and placebo (3%), and were largely caused by abdominal bloating.[5,7]

Comment: In one RCT, 72 women received evening primrose oil or placebo for 3 months followed by 3 months of evening primrose oil.[7] It reported that pain, tenderness, and lumpiness improved in cyclical but not non-cyclical breast pain. However, the methods of the trial were poor and included post hoc revision of the inclusion criteria, subgroup analysis, exclusion of withdrawals, and the use of baseline comparisons (with the best response seen in women who were symptomatically worse at baseline). We found one survey of randomised and open studies; however, data were reported as overall summary figures, which makes specific data extraction impossible.[5] In the UK, the Committee for Safety of Medicines has withdrawn the prescription licence from evening primrose oil because of lack of efficacy but it is still available over the counter.[8]

OPTION DANAZOL

One RCT found that danazol reduced cyclical breast pain after 12 months compared with placebo, but increased adverse effects (weight gain, deepening of the voice, menorrhagia, and muscle cramps). It found no significant difference in pain relief between 6 months of treatment with danazol and tamoxifen.

Benefits: We found no systematic review. We found one good quality three arm outpatient based RCT in 93 women with severe cyclical mastalgia.[9] **Versus placebo:** The RCT compared three treatments over 6 months: danazol (200 mg/day), tamoxifen (10 mg/day), and placebo. It found that significantly more women achieved greater than 50% pain relief at the end of treatment with danazol versus placebo (pain relief: 21/32 [66%] with danazol *v* 11/29 [38%] with placebo; RR 1.7, 95% CI 1.0 to 2.9; NNT 4, 95% CI 2 to 29). After 12 months of treatment, the difference remained significant (pain relief after 1 year: 12/32 [38%] with danazol *v* 0/29 [0%] with placebo; NNT 3, 95% CI 2 to 5). **Versus tamoxifen:** See tamoxifen, p 2039. The same RCT found no significant difference in pain relief after 6 months of treatment with danazol compared with tamoxifen (21/32 [66%] with danazol *v* 23/32 [72%] with tamoxifen; RR 0.9, 95% CI 0.7 to 1.3).[9]

Harms: Adverse effects were reported in more women taking danazol than placebo.[9] These included a significant increase in weight gain (10/32 [31%] with danazol *v* 1/29 [3%] with placebo; P = 0.006), and non-significant increases for deepening of the voice (4/32 [13%] with danazol *v* 0/29 [0%] with placebo; P = 0.11), menorrhagia (4/32 [13%] with danazol *v* 0/29 [0%] with placebo; P = 0.11), and muscle cramps (3/32 [9%] with danazol *v* 0/29 [0%] with placebo; P = 0.24).[9]

Comment: Although we found no direct evidence, there is consensus that once a response is achieved, adverse effects can be avoided by reducing the dose of danazol to 100 mg daily and confining treatment to the 2 weeks preceding menstruation.[9,10] Non-hormonal contraception is essential with danazol when given in 200 mg doses, as danazol has deleterious androgenic effects in the fetus.[11]

OPTION BROMOCRIPTINE

Two RCTs found limited evidence that bromocriptine (a dopamine agonist) reduced breast pain compared with placebo. Both RCTs found a higher incidence of adverse effects with bromocriptine compared with placebo. Adverse events included nausea, dizziness, postural hypotension, and constipation.

Benefits: We found no systematic review but found two RCTs.[12,13] The first outpatient based, European RCT (272 premenopausal women with diffuse fibrocystic disease of the breast) compared bromocriptine (2.5 mg twice daily) with placebo.[12] After 3 and 6 months it found that bromocriptine significantly improved symptoms compared with placebo on self assessed visual analogue scoring of breast pain, tenderness, and heaviness (results presented graphically).[12] Results have to be approached with care as overall withdrawal rates were high (see comment below). The second RCT (10 women) used a crossover design, and also found that bromocriptine significantly reduced pain compared with placebo ($P < 0.02$).[13]

Harms: The larger RCT found that adverse effects were significantly more frequent with bromocriptine than with placebo (61/135 [45%] with bromocriptine *v* 41/137 [30%] with placebo; RR 1.5, 95% CI 1.1 to 1.9; NNH 7, 95% CI 4 to 29).[13] Withdrawals related to adverse effects were more frequent in women taking bromocriptine (15/135 [11%] with bromocriptine *v* 8/137 [6%] with placebo; RR 1.9, 95% CI 0.8 to 4.3). Adverse reactions included nausea (32% with bromocriptine *v* 13% with placebo), dizziness (12% with bromocriptine *v* 7% with placebo), postural hypertension, and constipation.[12] Overall, withdrawal rates were high (see comment below). The second RCT found that nausea and dizziness occurred in 8/10 (80%) women on bromocriptine compared with 0/10 (0%) on placebo.[13] Strokes and death have been reported after use of bromocriptine to inhibit lactation, and the US Food and Drug Administration has withdrawn its license for this indication.[14]

Comment: Bromocriptine is now used rarely because frequent and intolerable adverse effects at the therapeutic dose outweigh the benefits for this indication. In the larger RCT, analysis was not intention to treat and overall withdrawal rates were high (withdrawals: 49/135 [36%] with bromocriptine *v* 36/137 [26%] with placebo; RR 1.4, 95% CI 1.0 to 2.0).[12]

OPTION LISURIDE MALEATE

One RCT with weak methods found that lisuride maleate (a dopamine agonist) reduced breast pain over 2 months compared with placebo.

Benefits: One double blind RCT (60 women with premenstrual breast pain) comparing lisuride maleate (200 µg/day) versus placebo over 2 months found significant improvement in visual analogue scores for pain (improved scores in 27/30 [90%] with lisuride maleate *v* 10/30 [33%] with placebo; RR 2.7, 95% CI 1.6 to 4.5; NNT 2, 95% CI 2 to 3) (see comment below).[15]

Harms: During the first month of treatment, nausea was more frequently reported by women taking lisuride maleate; however, the difference was not significant (women reporting nausea: 5/30 [17%] with lisuride maleate *v* 3/30 [10%] with placebo; RR 1.7, 95% CI 0.4 to 6.4).[15]

Comment: Allocation was carried out in blocks of 10 consecutive women. Tablet coding for active treatments and placebo differed, potentially confounding any treatment effect. Response to treatment was defined as a reduction greater than 25% from the baseline score during the first month, or greater than 50% during the second month.[15]

OPTION HORMONE REPLACEMENT THERAPY IN BREAST PAIN

One small RCT found limited evidence that people taking hormone replacement therapy had more breast pain after 1 year than women taking tibolone.

Benefits: We found no systematic review. **Versus placebo:** We found no RCTs. **Versus tibolone:** One RCT (44 postmenopausal women) compared hormone replacement therapy (transdermal oestrogen patches 50 µg twice weekly for 3 weeks/month, plus progestogen 5 mg/day for 12 days/month/cycle) versus tibolone (2.5 mg/day) versus no treatment.[16] The RCT found significantly more breast pain in women on hormone replacement therapy versus tibolone after 1 year (increase of breast pain as assessed by questionnaire: 53% with hormone replacement therapy *v* 5% with tibolone; P < 0.02).[16]

Harms: The RCT did not report on adverse effects.[16] See harms of hormone replacement therapy under secondary prevention of ischaemic cardiac events, p 188.

Comment: Tibolone is a synthetic steroid reported to have oestrogenic, progestogenic, and weak androgenic properties, which can be used as a form of hormone replacement therapy.[17]

OPTION TAMOXIFEN

Three RCTs found limited evidence that tamoxifen is more effective than placebo at reducing breast pain. Two of the RCTs found more hot flushes and vaginal discharge with tamoxifen compared with placebo. The third RCT did not report on adverse events. One RCT found no significant difference in pain relief between tamoxifen and danazol. One RCT found fewer adverse effects with a lower dose of 10 mg compared with a higher dose of 20 mg.

Benefits: We found no systematic review. **Versus placebo:** We found three RCTs.[9,18,19] One double blind RCT (60 premenopausal women with cyclical breast pain) compared tamoxifen (20 mg/day) with placebo.[19] It found that significantly more women experienced pain relief (measured by visual analogue scale over 3 months) with tamoxifen compared with placebo (22/31 [71%] with tamoxifen *v* 11/29 [38%] with placebo; RR 1.9, 95% CI 1.1 to 3.1; NNT 3, 95% CI 2 to 13). The second RCT (93 women) compared tamoxifen, danazol, and placebo.[9] It found that significantly more women with tamoxifen achieved a good outcome (> 50% reduction in mean pain score) at the end of treatment, 6 months later, and 12 months later compared with placebo (pain relief after 6 months of treatment: 23/32 [72%] with tamoxifen *v* 11/29 [38%] with placebo; RR 1.9, 95% CI 1.1 to 3.2; NNT 3, 95% CI 1 to 10). The third RCT (88 women, aged 22–44 years) found that 8 months of tamoxifen increased the number of women who achieved complete recovery compared with placebo (outcome not clearly defined) (complete recovery, 40/44 [90%] with tamoxifen *v* 0/44 [0%] with placebo).[18] **Dose response:** One RCT (301 women with cyclical breast pain for > 6 months) compared 10 mg versus 20 mg daily doses of tamoxifen from days 15–25 in the menstrual cycle for 3 months. It found no significant difference in pain relief (127/155 [82%] with 10 mg *v* 107/142 [75%] with 20 mg; RR 1.09, 95% CI 0.96 to

1.18).[20] Another RCT (60 women) compared 10 mg versus 20 mg daily doses of tamoxifen for 3 and 6 months in cyclical and non-cyclical mastalgia.[21] Three month response rates were similar (pain relief: 12/14 [86%] with 10 mg *v* 14/15 [93%] with 20 mg; RR 0.9, 95% CI 0.4 to 1.1). **Versus other treatments:** One RCT found no significant difference in pain relief between tamoxifen and danazol (see versus other drugs under benefits of danazol, p 2037).[9]

Harms: The first two RCTs found that hot flushes and vaginal discharge were more common with 20 mg tamoxifen daily than with placebo. However, differences were not significant.[18,19] The first RCT found more hot flushes (8/31 [26%] with tamoxifen *v* 3/29 [10%] with placebo; ARI 16%; RR 2.5, 95% CI 0.7 to 8.5) and vaginal discharge (5/31 [16%] with tamoxifen *v* 2/29 [7%] with placebo; ARI 9.2%; RR 2.3, 95% CI 0.5 to 11.0).[19] The second RCT found more hot flushes and vaginal discharge with tamoxifen 20 mg daily compared with placebo (hot flushes 8/32 [25%] with tamoxifen *v* 3/29 [10%] with placebo; RR 2.4, 95% CI 0.7 to 8.3; vaginal discharge 5/32 [16%] with tamoxifen *v* 2/29 [7%] with placebo; RR 2.3, 95% CI 0.5 to 10.8).[9] See adverse effects of tamoxifen under treatment of breast cancer, p 2003. The third RCT did not report any significant adverse events but these were not defined.[18] One meta-analysis of the four largest breast cancer prevention trials found that tamoxifen used long term at 20 mg daily was associated with venothromboembolism.[22] **Dose response:** Adverse effects occurred more frequently with the 20 mg dose than with the 10 mg dose between days 15–25 of the menstrual cycle.[20,21] The largest RCT found that adverse effects were reported more frequently with the 20 mg dose than with the 10 mg dose (adverse effects: 94/142 [66%] with 20 mg/day *v* 80/155 [52%] with 10 mg/day; RR 1.28, 95% CI 1.06 to 1.56; NNT 6, 95% CI 3 to 28).[20] Adverse effects were primarily hot flushes (AR 54/142 [38%] with 20 mg/day *v* 33/155 [21%] with the 10 mg/day; RR 1.79, 95% CI 1.24 to 2.58; NNH 6, 95% CI 3 to 16) and gastrointestinal disturbances (AR 54/142 [38%] with 20 mg/day *v* 30/155 [19%] with 10 mg/day; RR 1.97, 95% CI 1.34 to 2.88; NNH 6, 95% CI 4 to 12).

Comment: Tamoxifen is not licensed for mastalgia in the UK or the USA. There is consensus to limit its use to no more than 6 months at a time under expert supervision and with appropriate non-hormonal contraception because of the high incidence of adverse effects. Tamoxifen is contraindicated in pregnancy because of potential teratogenicity.[23]

OPTION GONADORELIN ANALOGUES (LUTEINISING HORMONE RELEASING HORMONE ANALOGUES)

We found no systematic review or RCTs on the effects of gonadorelin analogues (e.g. goserelin) in women with breast pain.

Benefits: We found no systematic review or RCTs.

Harms: Adverse effects of goserelin can include hot flushes (90%), headaches (57%), nausea and vomiting (29%), depression and irritability (24%), loss of libido (37%), and amenorrhoea (100%).[24]

Comment: None.

OPTION **SYNTHETIC STEROIDS (GESTRINONE, TIBOLONE)**

One RCT found that gestrinone relieved breast pain more than placebo, but increased adverse effects (greasy skin, hirsutism, acne, reduction in breast size, headache, and depression). One small RCT found that tibolone reduced breast pain more than hormone replacement therapy after 1 year.

Benefits: We found no systematic review. **Versus placebo:** We found one double blind, outpatient based RCT (145 premenopausal women with cyclical breast pain) comparing gestrinone (2.4 mg twice weekly) with placebo.[25] It found that gestrinone reduced breast pain more than placebo after 3 months (using visual analogue score where 0 = no pain, 100 = worst pain; pain score reduced from 59.5 to 11.0 with gestrinone *v* 58.2 to 36.7 with placebo; $P < 0.0001$). **Versus hormone replacement therapy:** See hormone replacement therapy versus tibolone, p 2039.[16]

Harms: **Versus placebo:** The RCT found that adverse effects were significantly more common with gestrinone than placebo (at least 1 adverse effect, 41% with gestrinone *v* 14% with placebo; ARI 27%; RR 2.96, 95% CI 1.70 to 4.40). Adverse effects included greasy skin (13 with gestrinone *v* 2 with placebo); hirsutism (10 with gestrinone *v* 3 with placebo); acne (9 with gestrinone *v* 2 with placebo); intermenstrual bleeding (7 with gestrinone *v* 0 with placebo); voice change (5 with gestrinone *v* 1 with placebo); reduced libido (5 with gestrinone *v* 3 with placebo); reduction in breast size (3 with gestrinone *v* 0 with placebo); headache (4 with gestrinone *v* 0 with placebo); depression (2 with gestrinone *v* 0 with placebo); and tiredness (2 with gestrinone *v* 0 with placebo).[25] **Versus hormone replacement therapy:** The RCT comparing tibolone versus hormone replacement therapy did not report adverse effects.[16]

Comment: Gestrinone is a synthetic steroid, reported to have androgenic, antioestrogenic, and antiprogestogenic properties.[17]

OPTION **PROGESTERONES**

Two small crossover RCTs found no significant difference in breast pain between progesterones and placebo.

Benefits: We found two RCTs.[26,27] The first RCT (crossover, 26 women with cyclical breast pain of at least 6 months' duration) treated all included women with daily 20 mg tablets of medroxyprogesterone acetate for 6 months, followed by a 2 month observation period. Women with persistent symptoms were then randomly allocated to oral medroxyprogesterone acetate (20 mg tablets) or placebo given from day 10–26 of the menstrual cycle, for 3 months and then switched group (crossover) for the remaining 3 months.[26] The RCT found no significant differences in the visual analogue scale for pain at the end of each phase before and after the crossover (data presented graphically). The overall withdrawal rate was 15%.[26] The second RCT (crossover, 80 women with breast pain of at least 2 months' duration) identified women who were able to keep an updated diary with visual analogue scales of pain for 2 months and then randomised them to daily applications of cream with progesterone 1% versus placebo, from the 10th day of the cycle to the beginning of the next cycle, for 3 months. The pre-crossover analysis found no significant difference in pain scores between progesterone and placebo cream (numerical results not available).[27]

Harms: The first RCT found that five women reported adverse effects while on medroxyprogesterone acetate, five while on placebo, and one with both. Symptoms were mostly vague premenstrual symptoms.[26] No further details were provided. The second RCT did not report harms.[27]

Comment: The second RCT provided insufficient details about the analysis. Withdrawals involved 7/32 (22%) women.[27] Both RCTs have small sample size, significant withdrawals, and a selection phase, which may restrict the generalisibility of the evidence.[26,27]

OPTION PROGESTOGENS

We found no RCTs on the effects of progestogens in women with breast pain.

Benefits: We found no systematic review or good quality RCTs.

Harms: We found no RCTs.

Comment: None.

OPTION OTHER AGENTS

We found no RCTs of the effects of pyridoxine, diuretics, antibiotics, or vitamin E compared with placebo for the treatment of breast pain.

Benefits: We found no systematic review or good quality RCTs on the effects of other agents.

Harms: We found no RCTs.

Comment: None.

Substantive changes

Tamoxifen One RCT added;[18] conclusions unchanged.

REFERENCES

1. Gateley CA, Mansel RE. Management of the painful and nodular breast. *Br Med Bull* 1991;47:284–294.
2. Ader DN, Shriver CD. Cyclical mastalgia: prevalence and impact in an outpatient breast clinic sample. *J Am Coll Surg* 1997;185:466–470.
3. Harding C, Osundeko O, Tetlow L, et al. Hormonally-regulated proteins in breast secretions are markers of target organ sensitivity. *Br J Cancer* 2000;2:354–360.
4. Maddox PR, Harrison BJ, Mansel RE, et al. Non-cyclical mastalgia: improved classification and treatment. *Br J Surg* 1989;76:901–904.
5. Pye JK, Mansel RE, Hughes LE. Clinical experience of drug treatments for mastalgia. *Lancet* 1985;1:373–377.
6. Boyd NF, McGuire V, Shannon P, et al. Effect of a low-fat high-carbohydrate diet on symptoms of cyclical mastopathy. *Lancet* 1988;2: 128–132.
7. Preece PE, Hanslip JI, Gilbert L, et al. Evening primrose oil (Efamol) for mastalgia. In: Horrobin D, ed. *Clinical uses of essential fatty acids*. Montreal: Eden Press, 1982:147–154.
8. What's new: Epogam and Efamast (gamolenic acid) — withdrawal of marketing authorisations. www.mca.gov.uk/whatsnew/epogam.htm (last accessed 8 May 2003).
9. Kontostolis E, Stefanidis K, Navrozoglou I, et al. Comparison of tamoxifen with danazol for treatment of cyclical mastalgia. *Gynecol Endocrinol* 1997;11:393–397.

10. Maddox PR, Harrison BJ, Mansel RE. Low-dose danazol for mastalgia. *Br J Clin Pract* 1989;68:43–47.
11. Anonymous. Danazol. In: *The ABPI compendium of data sheets and summaries of product characteristics*. London: Datapharm Publications, 1999–2000:1395.
12. Mansel RE, Dogliotti L. European multicentre trial of bromocriptine in cyclical mastalgia. *Lancet* 1990;335:190–193.
13. Blichert-Toft M, Anderson AN, Henrikson OB, et al. Treatment of mastalgia with bromocriptine: a double blind crossover study. *BMJ* 1979;1:237.
14. Arrowsmith-Lowe T. Bromocriptine indications withdrawn. *FDA Med Bull* 1994;24:2.
15. Kaleli S, Aydin Y, Erel CT, et al. Symptomatic treatment of premenstrual mastalgia in premenopausal women with lisuride maleate: a double-blind placebo-controlled randomized study. *Fertil Steril* 2001;75:718–723.
16. Colacurci N, Mele D, De Franciscis P, et al. Effects of tibolone on the breast. *Eur J Obs Gyn Rep Bio* 1998;80:235–238.
17. Parfitt K, ed. *Martindale. The complete drug reference*, 32nd ed. London: Pharmaceutical Press, 1999:1447–1448.
18. Grio R, Cellura A, Geranio R, et al. Clinical efficacy of tamoxifen in the treatment of premenstrual mastodynia. *Minerva Ginecol* 1998;50:101–103.
19. Fentiman IS, Caleffi M, Brame K, et al. Double-blind controlled trial of tamoxifen therapy for mastalgia. *Lancet* 1986;1:287–288.
20. GEMB Group. Tamoxifen therapy for cyclical mastalgia: dose randomised trial. *Breast* 1997;5:212–213.
21. Fentiman IS, Hamed H, Caleffi M, et al. Dosage and duration of tamoxifen treatment for mastalgia: a controlled trial. *Br J Surg* 1988;75:845–846.
22. Cuzick J, Powles T, Veronesi U, et al. Overview of the main outcomes in breast cancer prevention trials *Lancet* 2003;361:296–300.
23. Anonymous. Nolvadex. In: *The ABPI compendium of data sheets and summaries of product characteristics*. London: Datapharm Publications Ltd, 1999–2000:1799.
24. Hamed H, Caleffi M, Chaudary MA, et al. LHRH analogue for treatment of recurrent and refractory mastalgia. *Ann R Coll Surg Engl* 1990;72:221–224.
25. Peters F. Multicentre study of gestinone in cyclical breast pain. *Lancet* 1992;339:205–208.
26. Maddox PR, Harrison BJ, Horobin JM, et al. A randomised controlled trial of medroxyprogesterone acetate in mastalgia. *Ann R Coll Surg Engl* 1990;72:71–76.
27. McFadyen IJ, Raab GM, Macintyre CC, et al. Progesterone cream for cyclic breast pain. *BMJ* 1989;298:931.

Nigel Bundred
Professor in Surgical Oncology
University of Manchester Department of Surgery
South Manchester University Hospital
Manchester
UK

Competing interests: The author has received reimbursement by AstraZeneca, the maker of tamoxifen, for attending several conferences and running education programmes. The author has also received support by Searle Pharmacia for attending and speaking at symposia.

Candidiasis (vulvovaginal)

Search date March 2003

Des Spence

QUESTIONS

INTERVENTIONS

To be covered in future updates

Complementary and alternative treatments (lactobacilli, tea tree oil, *Solanum nigrescens*, stockings *v* tights)

Treatments in post-menopausal women

Treatments in pregnant women

Treatments in women with diabetes mellitus

Treatments in women with HIV infection

See glossary, p 2055

Key Messages

Acute vulvovaginal candidiasis

- **Intravaginal imidazoles** RCTs found that intravaginal imidazoles (butoconazole, clotrimazole, miconazole, or terconazole) reduced persistent symptoms of vulvovaginal candidiasis after 9–38 days compared with placebo, and found no clear evidence that effects differ among the various intravaginal imidazoles. RCTs found no clear evidence of any difference in persistent symptoms between shorter and longer durations of treatment (1–14 days). RCTs found no significant difference in symptoms between intravaginal imidazoles and oral fluconazole, itraconazole, or ketoconazole. RCTs found that intravaginal imidazoles were associated with less nausea, headache, and abdominal pain but more vulvar irritation and vaginal discharge than oral fluconazole or oral ketoconazole. Two RCTs provided insufficient evidence to compare intravaginal imidazoles versus intravaginal nystatin.

- **Oral fluconazole** We found no RCTs comparing oral fluconazole versus placebo or no treatment. One systematic review found no significant difference in persistent symptoms of vulvovaginal candidiasis over 1–12 weeks between oral fluconazole or oral itraconazole and intravaginal imidazoles, and found that oral fluconazole was associated with more nausea, headache, and abdominal pain but less vulvar irritation and vaginal discharge than intravaginal imidazoles. One weak RCT provided insufficient evidence to compare oral fluconazole versus oral itraconazole. One systematic review found no significant difference in persistent symptoms of vulvovaginal candidiasis or in adverse effects between oral fluconazole and oral ketoconazole.
- **Oral itraconazole** One RCT found that oral itraconazole reduced persistent symptoms of vulvovaginal candidiasis at 1 week after treatment compared with placebo. One systematic review found no significant difference in persistent symptoms over 1–12 weeks between oral itraconazole or oral fluconazole and intravaginal imidazoles. One weak RCT provided insufficient evidence to compare oral itraconazole versus oral fluconazole.
- **Intravaginal nystatin** One RCT found that intravaginal nystatin reduced the proportion of women with a poor symptomatic response after 14 days' treatment compared with placebo. Two RCTs provided insufficient evidence to compare intravaginal nystatin versus intravaginal imidazoles. We found no RCTs comparing intravaginal nystatin versus oral fluconazole, itraconazole, or ketoconazole.
- **Oral ketoconazole** We found no RCTs comparing oral ketoconazole versus placebo or no treatment. RCTs found no significant difference between oral ketoconazole and intravaginal imidazoles in persistent symptoms of vulvovaginal candidiasis and found that oral ketoconazole may cause more nausea, fatigue, and headaches but less vulvar irritation. One systematic review found no significant difference in persistent symptoms or adverse effects between oral ketoconazole and oral fluconazole. Case reports have associated ketoconazole with a low risk of fulminant hepatitis (1/12 000 courses of treatment with oral ketoconazole).

Recurrent vulvovaginal candidiasis

- **Regular prophylaxis with oral itraconazole** One RCT found that regular prophylaxis with oral itraconazole reduced the rate of symptomatic recurrence of vulvovaginal candidiasis over 6 months compared with placebo.
- **Intermittent or continuous prophylaxis with oral ketoconazole** One RCT found that oral ketoconazole, reduced symptomatic recurrence of vulvovaginal candidiasis over 6 months compared with placebo. This benefit is associated with an increased risk of harms, including rare cases of fulminant hepatitis (1/12 000 courses of treatment with oral ketoconazole).
- **Regular prophylaxis with intravaginal imidazoles** Two RCTs provided insufficient evidence about the effects of regular prophylaxis with intravaginal clotrimazole versus placebo in preventing recurrence of vulvovaginal candidiasis. One RCT found no significant difference in the number of episodes of symptomatic vaginitis over 6 months between regular prophylaxis with intravaginal clotrimazole and treatment as required, although women who took regular prophylaxis had fewer episodes. The RCT was too small to exclude a clinically important difference. More women preferred treatment as required. One RCT found insufficient evidence about the effects of regular prophylaxis with intravaginal clotrimazole versus oral itraconazole.

- **Regular prophylaxis with oral fluconazole** We found no RCTs about the effects of regular prophylaxis with oral fluconazole in preventing symptomatic recurrence of vulvovaginal candidiasis.
- **Treating a male sexual partner** Two RCTs found no significant difference between treating and not treating a woman's male sexual partner in the resolution of the woman's symptoms of vulvovaginal candidiasis over 1–4 weeks or in the rate of symptomatic recurrence. The women in the RCTs were not selected because of a history of recurrent vulvovaginal candidiasis.

DEFINITION **Vulvovaginal candidiasis** is symptomatic vaginitis (inflammation of the vagina), which often involves the vulva, caused by infection with a *Candida* yeast. Predominant symptoms are vulvar itching and abnormal vaginal discharge (which may be minimal, a "cheese like" material, or a watery secretion). Differentiation from other forms of vaginitis requires the presence of yeast on microscopy of vaginal fluid. **Recurrent vulvovaginal candidiasis** is commonly defined as four or more symptomatic episodes a year.[1]

INCIDENCE/ PREVALENCE Vulvovaginal candidiasis is the second most common cause of vaginitis (after bacterial vaginosis). Estimates of its incidence are limited and often derived from women who attend hospital clinics. At least one episode of vulvovaginal candidiasis occurs during the lifetime of 50–75% of all women. Vulvovaginal candidiasis is diagnosed in 5–15% of women who attend sexually transmitted disease and family planning clinics.[1] About half of the women who have an episode develop recurrent vulvovaginal candidiasis.[2]

AETIOLOGY/ RISK FACTORS *Candida albicans* accounts for 85–90% of cases of vulvovaginal candidiasis. Development of symptomatic vulvovaginal candidiasis probably represents increased growth of yeast that previously colonised the vagina without causing symptoms. Risk factors for vulvovaginal candidiasis include pregnancy (RR 2–10), diabetes mellitus, and systemic antibiotics. The evidence that different types of contraceptives are risk factors is contradictory. The incidence of vulvovaginal candidiasis rises with initiation of sexual activity, but we found no direct evidence that vulvovaginal candidiasis is sexually transmitted.[3–5]

PROGNOSIS We found few descriptions of the natural history of untreated vulvovaginal candidiasis. Discomfort is the main complication and can include pain while passing urine or during sexual intercourse. Balanitis (see glossary, p 2055) in male partners of women with vulvovaginal candidiasis can occur, but it is rare.

AIMS OF INTERVENTION To alleviate symptoms with minimal adverse effects from treatment.

OUTCOMES **Acute vulvovaginal candidiasis:** clinical cure rates, either measured in the short term (5–15 days) or medium term (3–6 weeks) after treatment. The definition of clinical cure varies among RCTs but often includes both complete resolution of symptoms and negative culture of *Candida*. **Recurrent vulvovaginal candidiasis:** symptomatic recurrence.

METHODS *Clinical Evidence* search and appraisal March 2003, and personal contact with the medical information department of Bristol Myers Squibb to retrieve an RCT on nystatin.[6] We included only those RCTs in which most participants were from the target population (for example, to answer the questions for non-pregnant women, we sought RCTs that excluded pregnant women or RCTs in which pregnant women represented < 20% of the participants). We excluded studies of women with HIV infection. Many RCTs excluded women with diabetes mellitus. We included RCTs only if recruitment was restricted to women with both symptoms of vaginal candidiasis and laboratory confirmation of candidal infection. Studies of asymptomatic women with vaginal colonisation by *Candida* species were excluded.

QUESTION **What are the effects of treatments for acute vulvovaginal candidiasis in non-pregnant women?**

OPTION **INTRAVAGINAL IMIDAZOLES**

RCTs found that intravaginal imidazoles (butoconazole, clotrimazole, miconazole, or terconazole) reduced persistent symptoms of vulvovaginal candidiasis after 9–38 days compared with placebo and found no clear evidence that effects differ among the various intravaginal imidazoles. RCTs found no clear evidence of any difference in persistent symptoms between shorter and longer durations of treatment (1–14 days). RCTs found no significant difference in symptoms between intravaginal imidazoles and oral fluconazole, itraconazole, or ketoconazole. RCTs found that intravaginal imidazoles were associated with less nausea, headache, and abdominal pain but more vulvar irritation and vaginal discharge than oral fluconazole or oral ketoconazole. Two RCTs provided insufficient evidence to compare intravaginal imidazoles versus intravaginal nystatin.

Benefits: **Versus placebo:** We found one systematic review (search date 1993,[7] 3 RCTs[8–10]) and three additional RCTs (see table A on web extra).[11–13] The systematic review did not perform a meta-analysis.[7] Five RCTs found that, compared with placebo, intravaginal imidazoles (butoconazole, clotrimazole, miconazole, or terconazole) significantly reduced persistent symptoms of vaginal candidiasis at 9–38 days after treatment.[8–10,12,13] However, only two of these RCTs[12,13] provided intention to treat results. The sixth RCT (95 women) found no significant difference in symptoms after 5 weeks between clotrimazole and placebo, but results were not intention to treat findings and the follow up rate was very low (62/95 [65%]).[11] **Versus each other:** We found one systematic review (search date 1993,[7] 12 RCTs[8,9,14–23]) and 22 additional RCTs (see table B on web extra).[24–45] Many of the RCTs were too small to exclude clinically important differences in outcomes. The populations selected by each RCT varied considerably in the prevalence of prognostic risk factors (such as diabetes mellitus or a history of recurrent attacks in the previous year), and a variety of outcomes were assessed. The RCTs provided no clear evidence of any consistent difference in effectiveness among the different imidazoles. **Duration of treatment:** We found one systematic review (search date 1993, 13 RCTs)[7] and nine additional RCTs comparing regimens that used the same intravaginal imidazole for different durations.[9,14,16,20,46–61] The RCTs found no consistent difference in the proportion of women with persistent symptoms, but they were too small to exclude a clinically important difference. **Versus oral fluconazole or oral itraconazole:** See benefits of oral fluconazole, p 2049. **Versus oral ketoconazole:** See benefits of oral ketoconazole, p 2050. **Versus intravaginal nystatin:** We found two RCTs.[24,62] The first RCT (70 women) found no significant difference between clotrimazole (100 mg for 14 days) and high strength nystatin vaginal cream (1 million IU, once daily for 7 days) in the proportion of women with persistent symptoms after 4 weeks (2/33 [6%] with nystatin *v* 1/37 [3%] with clotrimazole; OR 2.24, 95% CI 0.23 to 22.40).[24] The second RCT (292 women) compared six interventions: intravaginal clotrimazole, intravaginal econazole, intravaginal miconazole, oral miconazole plus intravaginal nystatin, oral nystatin plus intravaginal nystatin, and intravaginal nystatin alone.[62] It found no significant difference among interventions in symptomatic relapse over 6 months (18/53 [34%] with intravaginal clotrimazole *v* 16/34 [47%] with intravaginal econazole *v* 18/80 [22%] with intravaginal miconazole *v* 6/31 [19%] with oral miconazole plus intravaginal nystatin *v* 14/49 [28%] with oral nystatin plus intravaginal nystatin *v* 26/45 [58%] with intravaginal nystatin alone; reported as non-significant; CI not reported). The RCT is likely to have been underpowered to detect a clinically important difference among treatments.[62]

Harms: **Versus placebo:** In the RCTs of intravaginal imidazoles versus placebo, most women did not report any adverse effects.[8–13] The most common adverse effect was vulvar irritation. Most RCTs did not report frequencies of specific adverse effects in women who took placebo. In one RCT, adverse effects were more common in women who took oral placebo than in women who used intravaginal imidazole (nine adverse events, mainly nausea and headache, in 22 women who received oral placebo *v* one episode of irritation in 23 women who used intravaginal imidazole).[10] **Versus oral fluconazole or oral itraconazole:** See harms of oral fluconazole, p 2049. **Versus intravaginal nystatin:** The first RCT found no adverse effects in women who took intravaginal clotrimazole or intravaginal nystatin.[24] The second RCT gave no information on adverse effects.[62]

Comment: Most RCTs were small and many had weak methods (poorly described randomisation, inadequate concealment and blinding, and definitions of cure based on mycology results rather than symptoms). We excluded all RCTs that defined cure only on the basis of mycology results. Trials in women who obtain intravaginal imidazoles over the counter are needed.

OPTION ORAL FLUCONAZOLE

We found no RCTs comparing oral fluconazole versus placebo or no treatment. One systematic review found no significant difference in persistent symptoms of vulvovaginal candidiasis over 1–12 weeks between oral fluconazole or oral itraconazole and intravaginal imidazoles and found that oral fluconazole was associated with more nausea, headache, and abdominal pain but less vulvar irritation and vaginal discharge than intravaginal imidazoles. One weak RCT provided

insufficient evidence to compare oral fluconazole versus oral itraconazole. One systematic review found no significant difference in persistent symptoms of vulvovaginal candidiasis or in adverse effects between oral fluconazole and oral ketoconazole.

Benefits: **Versus placebo:** We found no systematic review or RCTs. **Versus intravaginal imidazoles:** We found one systematic review (search date 2000, 7 RCTs, 1247 women) that found no significant difference between oral fluconazole or oral itraconazole and intravaginal imidazoles (clotrimazole, miconazole, econazole) in persistent symptoms at 5–15 days (124/627 [20%] with oral fluconazole or itraconazole *v* 121/620 [20%] with intravaginal imidazoles; RR 1.00, 95% CI 0.95 to 1.06) or at 2–12 weeks (74/432 [17%] with oral fluconazole or itraconazole *v* 71/404 [18%] with intravaginal imidazoles; RR 1.04, 95% CI 0.95 to 1.07).[63] **Versus oral itraconazole:** We found no systematic review but found one RCT (86 women) that found no significant difference between oral fluconazole 150 mg in a single dose and oral itraconazole 200 mg daily for 3 days in the proportion of women cured at 7 days (13/38 [34%] with fluconazole *v* 16/32 [50%] with itraconazole; P = 0.18) or at 21 days (18/38 [47%] *v* 17/32 [53%]; P = 0.63; see comment below).[64] **Versus oral ketoconazole:** See benefits of oral ketoconazole, p 2050. **Versus intravaginal nystatin:** We found no RCTs.

Harms: **Versus intravaginal imidazoles:** Two large RCTs identified by the review[63] found that oral fluconazole may be associated with increased nausea, headache, and abdominal pain compared with intravaginal imidazoles.[65,66] The first RCT (429 women) found that single dose 150 mg oral fluconazole significantly increased adverse effects over 14 days compared with intravaginal clotrimazole 100 mg daily for 7 days (59/217 [27%] with oral fluconazole *v* 37/212 [17%] with intravaginal clotrimazole; OR 1.75, 95% CI 1.11 to 2.75; NNH 11, 95% CI 6 to 54).[65] The individual events that were more common with oral fluconazole were headache (12% *v* 9%), abdominal pain (7% *v* 3%), and nausea (4% *v* 0%). The second RCT (235 women) found that oral fluconazole significantly increased nausea and other gastrointestinal symptoms compared with intravaginal econazole (9/121 [7%] *v* 2/114 [2%]; OR 3.55, 95% CI 1.06 to 11.90), but intravaginal econazole significantly increased local vulvar burning and vaginal discharge (3/121 [2%] with oral fluconazole *v* 25/114 [22%] with intravaginal econazole; OR 0.16, 95% CI 0.07 to 0.35).[66] A third RCT (369 women) identified by the review found very few adverse effects with either oral fluconazole or clotrimazole (8/188 [4%] *v* 9/181 [5%]).[67] A fourth RCT (double blind, 81 women) identified by the review found no significant difference between oral itraconazole and intravaginal econazole in the proportion of women who had adverse effects (4/40 [10%] with itraconazole *v* 8/41 [20%] with econazole; OR 0.48, 95% CI 0.14 to 1.61).[68] **Versus oral itraconazole:** The RCT found that oral fluconazole and oral itraconazole were associated with similar rates of adverse effects, including gastrointestinal disturbances, pelvic pain, insomnia, anxiety, and rash.[64] **Versus oral ketoconazole:** See harms of oral ketoconazole, p 2051.

Comment: **Versus oral itraconazole:** In the first RCT, women who received oral fluconazole had significantly higher baseline symptom scores than women who received oral itraconazole (9.03 *v* 7.03; P = 0.003); this makes the results difficult to interpret.[64]

OPTION ORAL ITRACONAZOLE

One RCT found that oral itraconazole reduced persistent symptoms at 1 week after treatment compared with placebo. One systematic review found no significant difference in persistent symptoms over 1–12 weeks between oral itraconazole or oral fluconazole and intravaginal imidazoles. One weak RCT provided insufficient evidence to compare oral itraconazole versus oral fluconazole.

Benefits: **Versus placebo:** We found one systematic review (search date 2000),[63] which identified one RCT (90 women) that compared three interventions: oral itraconazole, oral clotrimazole, and placebo.[10] The RCT found that oral itraconazole (200 mg daily for 3 days) significantly reduced the proportion of women with persistent symptoms at 1 week after treatment compared with placebo (13/48 [27%] with itraconazole *v* 12/22 [55%] with placebo; $P < 0.05$).[10] **Versus intravaginal imidazoles:** See benefits of oral fluconazole, p 2049. **Versus oral fluconazole:** See benefits of oral fluconazole, p 2049. **Versus oral ketoconazole:** We found no RCTs. **Versus intravaginal nystatin:** We found no RCTs.

Harms: **Versus placebo:** The RCT identified by the review[63] found that itraconazole significantly increased the proportion of women who had adverse effects compared with intravaginal clotrimazole (17/50 [34%] with itraconazole *v* 1/23 [4%] with clotrimazole; OR 4.83, 95% CI 1.55 to 15.1); the adverse effects with increased frequency were nausea (14%), headache (12%), dizziness (6%), and bloating (6%).[10] **Versus intravaginal imidazoles:** See harms of oral fluconazole, p 2049.

Comment: None.

OPTION ORAL KETOCONAZOLE

We found no RCTs comparing oral ketoconazole versus placebo or no treatment. RCTs found no significant difference between oral ketoconazole and intravaginal imidazoles in persistent symptoms and found that oral ketoconazole may cause more nausea, fatigue, and headaches but less vulvar irritation. One systematic review found no significant difference in persistent symptoms or adverse effects between oral ketoconazole and oral fluconazole. Case reports have associated ketoconazole with a low risk of fulminant hepatitis (1/12 000 courses of treatment with oral ketoconazole).

Benefits: **Versus oral placebo:** We found no systematic review or RCTs. **Versus intravaginal imidazoles:** We found one systematic review (search date 1993,[7] 4 RCTs,[69–72] 280 women) and three additional RCTs[73–75] (see table C on web extra). The systematic review concluded that oral treatment is as effective as topical treatment at eliminating *Candida* but did not compare clinical outcomes.[7] Six RCTs found no significant difference in persistent symptoms at

1–4 weeks between oral ketoconazole and intravaginal clotrimazole, miconazole, or tioconazole,[69–74] and one RCT found that significantly more women had persistent symptoms at 4 weeks with oral ketoconazole than with intravaginal isoconazole.[75] **Versus oral itraconazole:** We found no RCTs. **Versus oral fluconazole:** We found one systematic review (search date 1993,[7] 1 RCT,[76] 183 women). The RCT found no significant difference between ketoconazole (400 mg daily for 5 days) and oral fluconazole (1 dose of 150 mg) in the proportion of women with persistent symptoms after 5–16 days (17/72 [24%] with ketoconazole v 17/80 [21%] with fluconazole; OR 1.15, 95% CI 0.53 to 2.45) or after 27–62 days (14/72 [19%] with ketoconazole v 14/76 [18%] with fluconazole; OR 1.07, 95% CI 0.47 to 2.43).[76] **Versus intravaginal nystatin:** We found no RCTs.

Harms: Observational studies have found that asymptomatic elevation of liver enzymes is common in people who take oral ketoconazole, and fulminant hepatitis was observed in about 1/12 000 courses of treatment.[77] **Versus intravaginal imidazoles:** Most of the RCTs gave little information on adverse effects.[69–73,75] In these RCTs, thirteen women who took oral ketoconazole had nausea, fatigue, headaches, or abdominal pain, and two women who used intravaginal clotrimazole had vulvar irritation or vaginal bleeding. One RCT (151 women) found that oral ketoconazole increased rates of headache (23% v 4%), nausea (22% v 1%), abdominal discomfort (14% v 7%), and fatigue (7% v 2%; CIs not reported) compared with intravaginal clotrimazole.[74] **Versus oral fluconazole:** The RCT (183 women) found that nausea was reported by similar proportions of women who took oral fluconazole as those who took oral ketoconazole (9/92 [10%] with fluconazole v 13/91 [14%] with ketoconazole; CI not reported).[76]

Comment: The possibility of rare but serious hepatitis has led to a consensus that the risks associated with oral ketoconazole may outweigh its benefits in women with vulvovaginal candidiasis.

OPTION INTRAVAGINAL NYSTATIN

One RCT found that intravaginal nystatin reduced the proportion of women with a poor symptomatic response after 14 days' treatment compared with placebo. Two RCTs provided insufficient evidence to compare intravaginal nystatin versus intravaginal imidazoles. We found no RCTs that compared intravaginal nystatin versus oral fluconazole, itraconazole, or ketoconazole.

Benefits: **Versus placebo:** We found no systematic review but found one RCT that compared intravaginal nystatin versus placebo.[6] The RCT (double blind, 50 women) found that, compared with placebo, intravaginal nystatin (500 000 IU twice daily for 14 days) significantly reduced the proportion of women with a symptomatic response categorised as "poor" (2/25 [8%] with nystatin v 10/25 [40%] with placebo; ARR 32%, 95% CI 8% to 56%; OR 0.18, 95% CI 0.05 to 0.65; NNT 3, 95% CI 2 to 12). **Versus intravaginal imidazoles:** See benefits of intravaginal imidazoles, p 2047. **Versus oral fluconazole, itraconazole, or ketoconazole:** We found no RCTs.

Harms: **Versus placebo:** The RCT found no reports of adverse effects among 52 women who used intravaginal nystatin.[6]

Comment: None.

QUESTION **What are the effects of treatments for recurrent vulvovaginal candidiasis in non-pregnant women?**

OPTION **REGULAR PROPHYLAXIS WITH INTRAVAGINAL IMIDAZOLES**

Two RCTs provided insufficient evidence about the effects of regular prophylaxis with intravaginal clotrimazole compared with placebo in preventing recurrence of vulvovaginal candidiasis. One RCT found no significant difference in the number of episodes of symptomatic vaginitis over 6 months between regular prophylaxis with intravaginal clotrimazole and treatment as required, although women who took regular prophylaxis had fewer episodes. The RCT was too small to exclude a clinically important difference. More women preferred treatment as required. One RCT found insufficient evidence about the effects of regular prophylaxis with intravaginal clotrimazole versus oral itraconazole.

Benefits: **Versus placebo:** We found one systematic review (search date 1993,[7] 2 RCTs,[78,79] 89 women with recurrent vulvovaginal candidiasis) that compared intravaginal clotrimazole 500 mg monthly versus intravaginal placebo monthly for 6 months. Both RCTs found that intravaginal clotrimazole reduced the proportion of women with symptomatic recurrence over 6 months compared with placebo, although in one RCT the difference was significant and in the other RCT it was not.[78,79] **Versus as required treatment:** We found one crossover RCT (unblinded, 23 women with recurrent vaginal candidiasis) that compared regular prophylactic intravaginal clotrimazole 500 mg each month versus intravaginal clotrimazole 500 mg at the onset of symptoms for 12 months.[80] It found that women who took regular clotrimazole had fewer symptomatic episodes of vaginitis over 6 months than women who took clotrimazole as required, but the difference was not significant (2.2 episodes per woman with regular treatment *v* 3.7 with as needed treatment; P = 0.05). It found that significantly more women preferred treatment as required compared with prophylactic treatment (17/23 [74%] *v* 4/23 [17%]; P = 0.001). The RCT is likely to have been too small to exclude a clinically important difference. **Versus oral itraconazole:** See benefits of oral itraconazole, p 2053.

Harms: See harms of intravaginal imidazoles, p 2048.

Comment: None.

OPTION **REGULAR PROPHYLAXIS WITH ORAL FLUCONAZOLE**

We found no RCTs about the effects of regular prophylaxis with oral fluconazole in prevention of recurrent vulvovaginal candidiasis.

Benefits: We found no systematic review or RCTs.

Harms: We found no RCTs.

Comment: None.

OPTION REGULAR PROPHYLAXIS WITH ORAL ITRACONAZOLE

One RCT found that regular prophylaxis with oral itraconazole reduced the rate of symptomatic recurrence of vulvovaginal candidiasis over 6 months compared with placebo. One RCT found insufficient evidence about the effects of regular prophylaxis with oral itraconazole versus intravaginal clotrimazole.

Benefits: We found no systematic review. **Versus placebo:** One RCT (single blind, 114 women with recurrent vulvovaginal candidiasis) found that regular prophylaxis with oral itraconazole (400 mg monthly) significantly reduced recurrence of symptoms of vulvovaginal candidiasis compared with placebo (recurrence during 6 months' follow up: 20/55 [36%] with itraconazole *v* 34/53 [64%] with placebo; ARR 28%, 95% CI 9% to 47%; OR 0.33, 95% CI 0.16 to 0.71; NNT 4, 95% CI 3 to 11).[83] After discontinuation of oral itraconazole, recurrence rates were similar.[83] **Versus intravaginal imidazoles:** We found one RCT (unblinded, 44 women) that compared oral itraconazole (200 mg twice weekly) versus intravaginal clotrimazole (200 mg twice weekly) for 6 months.[84] One woman withdrew from itraconazole treatment and five withdrew from clotrimazole treatment. The RCT found that oral itraconazole versus intravaginal clotrimazole increased the proportion of women with symptomatic recurrences over 6 months (7/21 [33%] with itraconazole *v* 0/17 [0%] with clotrimazole; see comment below). **Versus as required treatment:** We found no RCTs.

Harms: The first RCT gave no information on adverse effects (see oral itraconazole, p 2050).[83]

Comment: **Versus intravaginal imidazoles:** The results of the RCT are difficult to interpret because it was unblinded, and the unbalanced withdrawal from the RCT could explain the observed difference between groups.[84]

OPTION ORAL KETOCONAZOLE

One RCT found that oral ketoconazole, reduced symptomatic recurrence of vulvovaginal candidiasis over 6 months compared with placebo. This benefit is associated with an increased risk of harms, including rare cases of fulminant hepatitis (1/12 000 courses of treatment with oral ketoconazole).

Benefits: **Versus placebo:** We found one systematic review (search date 1993,[7] 1 RCT,[85] 63 women). The RCT (74 women) compared three interventions: intermittent oral ketoconazole (400 mg daily for 5 days of each menstrual cycle), continuous low dose ketoconazole (100 mg daily for 6 months), and placebo over 6 months.[85] It found that intermittent oral ketoconazole significantly reduced symptomatic recurrence over 6 months compared with placebo (6/21 [29%] with intermittent ketoconazole *v* 15/21 [71%] with placebo; OR 0.19, 95% CI 0.06 to 0.62). It also found that continuous low dose oral ketoconazole reduced symptomatic recurrence over 6 months compared with placebo (1/21 [5%] with continuous ketoconazole v 15/21 [71%] with placebo; OR 0.06, 95% CI 0.02 to 0.22). **Versus intravaginal imidazoles:** We found no RCTs. **Regular prophylaxis versus as required treatment:** We found no RCTs.

Harms: Ketoconazole is associated with an increased frequency of gastrointestinal adverse effects and case reports of rare fulminant hepatitis (see ketoconazole, p 2050).

Comment: The possibility of rare but serious hepatitis has led to a consensus that the risks associated with oral ketoconazole may outweigh its benefits in women with vulvovaginal candidiasis.

OPTION — EFFECTS OF TREATING A MALE SEXUAL PARTNER IN WOMEN WITH RECURRENT VULVOVAGINITIS

Two RCTs found no significant difference between treating and not treating a woman's male sexual partner in the resolution of the woman's symptoms of vulvovaginal candidiasis over 1–4 weeks or in the rate of symptomatic recurrence. The women in the RCTs were not selected because of a history of recurrent vulvovaginal candidiasis.

Benefits: We found no systematic review but found two RCTs.[81,82] In the first RCT (40 women with acute vulvovaginal candidiasis and their male partners), all the women received oral itraconazole 100 mg daily for 5 days.[81] Their male partners were randomised to receive oral itraconazole 100 mg daily for 5 days or placebo. The RCT found no significant difference between treating the male partner with oral itraconazole and placebo in the proportion of women with persistent symptoms after 30 days (2/19 [11%] with partners who received itraconazole *v* 4/18 [22%] with partners who received placebo; OR 0.43, 95% CI 0.08 to 2.43). The second RCT (117 women with acute or recurrent vaginal candidiasis and their male partners) treated all of the women with oral ketoconazole 200–600 mg daily for 3 days. Their male partners were randomised to oral ketoconazole 400 mg daily versus placebo for 3 days. The RCT found no significant difference in the proportion of women cured 1 week after treatment (48/57 [84%] with partners receiving ketoconazole *v* 53/60 [88%] with partners receiving placebo; OR 0.71, 95% CI 0.25 to 2.02) or the proportion of initially cured women who relapsed by 4 weeks after treatment (13/48 [27%] with ketoconazole *v* 19/53 [36%] with placebo; OR 0.67, 95% CI 0.29 to 1.54; see comment below).

Harms: The RCTs gave no information on harms.[81,82]

Comment: The women in the RCTs were not selected because of a history of recurrent vulvovaginal candidiasis.[81,82] The definition of "cured" and "relapsed" in the second RCT is not clear, but it seems to be a combination of improved symptoms and negative cultures.[82] Only a small number of men in the RCT had any penile symptoms, and these were distributed equally between the ketoconazole and placebo groups.

GLOSSARY

Balanitis is inflammation of the glans of the penis. The foreskin is often involved (balanoposthitis).

REFERENCES

1. Sobel JD. Vulvovaginal candidiasis. In: Holmes KK MP-A, Sparling PF, Lemon SM, et al, eds. *Sexually transmitted diseases*. New York: McGraw-Hill, 1999:629–639.
2. Sobel JD, Faro S, Force RW, et al. Vulvovaginal candidiasis: epidemiologic, diagnostic, and therapeutic considerations. *Am J Obstet Gynecol* 1998;178:203–211.
3. Foxman B. The epidemiology of vulvovaginal candidiasis: risk factors. *Am J Public Health* 1990;80:329–331.
4. Geiger AM, Foxman B, Sobel JD. Chronic vulvovaginal candidiasis: characteristics of women with *Candida albicans*, *C glabrata* and no *Candida*. *Genitourin Med* 1995;71:304–307.
5. Geiger AM, Foxman B, Gillespie BW. The epidemiology of vulvovaginal candidiasis among university students. *Am J Public Health* 1995;85:1146–1148.
6. Isaacs JH. Nystatin vaginal cream in monilial vaginitis. *Illinois Med J* 1973;3:240–241.
7. Reef SE, Levine WC, McNeil MM, et al. Treatment options for vulvovaginal candidiasis, 1993. *Clin Infect Dis* 1995;20:S80–S90. Search date 1993; primary sources Medline and hand search of two textbooks.
8. Thomason JL, Gelbart SM, Kellett AV, et al. Terconazole for the treatment of vulvovaginal candidiasis. *J Reprod Med* 1990;35:992–994.
9. Brown D Jr, Henzl MR, LePage ME, et al. Butoconazole vaginal cream in the treatment of vulvovaginal candidiasis: comparison with miconazole nitrate and placebo. *J Reprod Med* 1986;31:1045–1048.
10. Stein GE, Mummaw N. Placebo-controlled trial of itraconazole for treatment of acute vaginal candidiasis. *Antimicrob Agents Chemother* 1993;37:89–92.
11. Bro F. Single-dose 500-mg clotrimazole vaginal tablets compared with placebo in the treatment of *Candida vaginitis*. *J Fam Pract* 1990;31:148–152.
12. Fleury F, Hodgson C. Single-dose treatment of vulvovaginal candidiasis with a new 500mg clotrimazole vaginal tablet. *Adv Ther* 1984;1:349–356.
13. Guess EA, Hodgson C. Single-dose topical treatment of vulvovaginal candidiasis with a new 500mg clotrimazole vaginal tablet. *Adv Ther* 1984;1:137–145.
14. Franklin R. Seven-day clotrimazole therapy for vulvovaginal candidiasis. *South Med J* 1978;71:141–143.
15. Corson SL, Kapikian RR, Nehring R. Terconazole and miconazole cream for treating vulvovaginal candidiasis. *J Reprod Med* 1991;36:561–567.
16. Kjaeldgaard A. Comparison of terconazole and clotrimazole vaginal tablets in the treatment of vulvovaginal candidosis. *Pharmatherapeutica* 1986;4:525–531.
17. Stein GE, Gurwith D, Mummaw N, et al. Single-dose tioconazole compared with 3-day clotrimazole treatment in vulvovaginal candidiasis. *Antimicrob Agents Chemother* 1986;29:969–971.
18. Kaufman RH, Henzl MR, Brown D Jr, et al. Comparison of three-day butoconazole treatment with seven-day miconazole treatment for vulvovaginal candidiasis. *J Reprod Med* 1989;34:479–483.
19. Droegemueller W, Adamson DG, Brown D. Three-day treatment with butoconazole nitrate for vulvovaginal candidiasis. *Obstet Gynecol* 1984;64:530–534.
20. Jacobson JB, Hajman AJ, Wiese J. A new vaginal antifungal agent — butoconazole nitrate. *Acta Obstet Gynecol Scand* 1985;64:241–244.
21. Hajman AJ. Vulvovaginal candidosis: comparison of 3-day treatment with 2% butoconazole nitrate cream and 6-day treatment of 1% clotrimazole cream. *J Int Med Res* 1988;16:367–375.
22. Adamson GD, Brown D Jr, Standard JV, et al. Three-day treatment with butoconazole vaginal suppositories for vulvovaginal candidiasis. *J Reprod Med Obstet Gynecol* 1986;31:131–132.
23. Bradbeer CS, Mayhew SR, Barlow D. Butaconazole and miconazole in treating vaginal candidiasis. *Genitourin Med* 1985;61:270–272.
24. Cassar NL. High-potency nystatin cream in the treatment of vulvovaginal candidiasis. *Curr Ther Res* 1983;34:305–310.
25. Glasser A. Single-dose treatment of vaginal mycoses. Effectiveness of clotrimazole and econazole. *Fortschr Med* 1986;104:259–262.
26. Gastaldi A. Treatment of vaginal candidiasis with fenticonazole and miconazole. *Curr Ther Res Clin Exp* 1985;38:489–493.
27. Gabriel G, Thin RN. Clotrimazole and econazole in the treatment of vaginal candidosis. A single-blind comparison. *Br J Ven Dis* 1983;59:56–58.
28. Amrouni B, Pereiro M, Florez A, et al. A phase III comparative study of the efficacies of flutrimazole versus clotrimazole for the treatment of vulvovaginal candidiasis. *J Mycol Med* 2000;10:62–65.
29. Arendt J. Terconazole versus clotrimazole cream in vulvovaginal candidiasis. *Adv Ther* 1989;6:287–294.
30. Gouveia DC, Jones Da Silva C. Oxiconazole in the treatment of vaginal candidiasis: single dose versus 3-day treatment with econazole. *Pharmatherapeutica* 1984;3:682–685.
31. Brewster E, Preti PM, Ruffmann R, et al. Effect of fenticonazole in vaginal candidiasis: a double-blind clinical trial versus clotrimazole. *J Int Med Res* 1986;14:306–310.
32. Balsdon M-J. Comparison of miconazole-coated tampons with clotrimazole vaginal tablets in the treatment of vaginal candidosis. *Br J Ven Dis* 1981;57:275–278.
33. Bradbeer CS, Thin RN. Comparison of econazole and isoconazole as single dose treatment for vaginal candidosis. *Genitourin Med* 1985;61:396–398.
34. Brown D Jr, Binder CL, Gardner HL, et al. Comparison of econazole and clotrimazole in the treatment of vulvovaginal candidiasis. *Obstet Gynecol* 1980;56:121–123.
35. Brown D, Henzl MR, Kaufman RH, et al. Butoconazole nitrate 2% for vulvovaginal candidiasis. *J Reprod Med* 1999;44:933–938.
36. Cohen L. Single dose treatment of vaginal candidosis: comparison of clotrimazole and isoconazole. *Br J Ven Dis* 1984;60:42–44.
37. Dellenbach P, Thomas J-L, Guerin V, et al. Topical treatment of vaginal candidosis with sertaconazole and econazole sustained-release suppositories. *Int J Gynecol Obstet* 2000;71:S47–S52.
38. Wiest W, Azzollini E, Ruffmann R. Comparison of single administration with an ovule of 600 mg

fenticonazole versus a 500 mg clotrimazole vaginal pessary in the treatment of vaginal candidiasis. *J Int Med Res* 1989;17:369–372.
39. Palacio-Hernanz A, Sanz-Sanz F, Rodriquez-Noriega A. Double-blind investigation of R-42470 (terconazole cream 0.4%) and clotrimazole (cream 1%) for the topical treatment of mycotic vaginitis. *Chemioterapia* 1984;3:192–195.
40. Lolis D, Kanellopoulos N, Liappas I, et al. Double-blind evaluation of miconazole tampons, compared with clotrimazole vaginal tablets, in vaginal candidiasis. *Clin Ther* 1981;4:212–216.
41. Studd JW, Dooley MM, Welch CC, et al. Comparative clinical trial of fenticonazole ovule (600 mg) versus clotrimazole vaginal tablet (500 mg) in the treatment of symptomatic vaginal candidiasis. *Curr Med Res Opin* 1989;11:477–484.
42. Herbold H. Comparative studies to the clinical efficacy of two 1-dose-therapies of vaginal candidosis. *Med Welt* 1985;36:255–257.
43. Lappin MA, Brooker DC, Francisco CA, et al. Effect of butoconazole nitrate 2% vaginal cream and miconazole nitrate 2% vaginal cream treatments in patients with vulvovaginal candidiasis. *Infect Dis Obstet Gynecol* 1996;4:323–328
44. Lebherz TB, Goldman L, Wiesmeier E, et al. A comparison of the efficacy of two vaginal creams for vulvovaginal candidiasis, and correlations with the presence of *Candida* species in the perianal area and oral contraceptive use. *Clin Ther* 1983;5:409–416.
45. Stettendorf S, Benijts G, Vignali M, et al. Three-day therapy of vaginal candidiasis with clotrimazole vaginal tablets and econazole ovules: a multicenter comparative study. *Chemotherapy* 1982;28:87–91.
46. Wolfson N, Samuels B, Hodgson C, et al. One-day management of vulvovaginal candidiasis. *J La State Med Soc* 1987;139:27–29.
47. Lebherz T, Guess E, Wolfson N. Efficacy of single- versus multiple-dose clotrimazole therapy in the management of vulvovaginal candidiasis. *Am J Obstet Gynecol* 1985;152:965–968.
48. Fleury F, Hughes D, Floyd R. Therapeutic results obtained in vaginal mycoses after single-dose treatment with 500 mg clotrimazole vaginal tablets. *Am J Obstet Gynecol* 1985;152:968–970.
49. Loendersloot EW, Goormans E, Wiesenhaan PE, et al. Efficacy and tolerability of single-dose versus six-day treatment of candidal vulvovaginitis with vaginal tablets of clotrimazole. *Am J Obstet Gynecol* 1985;152:953–955.
50. Wolfson N, Samuels B, Riley J. A three-day treatment regimen for vulvovaginal candidiasis. *J La State Med Soc* 1982;134:28–31.
51. Oates JK, Davidson F. Treatment of vaginal candidiasis with clotrimazole. *Postgrad Med J* 1974;50:99–102.
52. Lebherz TB, Ford LC, Kleinkopf V. A comparison of a three-day and seven-day clotrimazole regimen for vulvovaginal candidiasis. *Clin Ther* 1981;3:344–348.
53. Robertson WH. Vulvovaginal candidiasis treated with clotrimazole cream in seven days compared with fourteen day treatment with miconazole cream. *Am J Obstet Gynecol* 1978;132:321–323.
54. Pasquale SA, Lawson J, Sargent EC Jr, et al. A dose–response study with Monistat cream. *Obstet Gynecol* 1979;53:250–253.
55. Floyd R, Hodgson C. One-day treatment of vulvovaginal candidiasis with a 500-mg clotrimazole vaginal tablet compared with a three-day regimen of two 100-mg vaginal tablets daily. *Clin Ther* 1986;8:181–186.
56. Hughes D, Kriedman T, Hodgson C. Treatment of vulvovaginal candidiasis with a single 500-mg clotrimazole vaginal tablet compared with two 100-mg tablets daily for three days. *Curr Ther Res Clin Exp* 1986;39:773–777.
57. Mizuno S, Cho N. Clinical evaluation of three-day treatment of vaginal mycosis with clotrimazole vaginal tablets. *J Int Med Res* 1983;11:179–185.
58. Milsom I, Forssman L. Treatment of vaginal candidosis with a single 500-mg clotrimazole pessary. *Br J Ven Dis* 1982;58:124–126.
59. Westphal J. Treatment of *Candida mycoses* of the vulva and vagina with clotrimazole. Comparison of single-dose and six-day therapy. *Fortschr Med* 1988;106:445–448.
60. Upmalis DH, Cone FL, Lamia CA, et al. Single-dose miconazole nitrate vaginal ovule in the treatment of vulvovaginal candidiasis: two single-blind, controlled studies versus miconazole nitrate 100mg cream for 7 days. *J Women's Health Gender-based Medicine* 2000;9:421–429.
61. Wiest W, Ruffmann R. Short-term treatment of vaginal candidiasis with fenticonazole ovules: a three dose schedule comparative trial. *J Int Med Res* 1987;15:319–325.
62. Dennerstein GJ, Langley R. Vulvovaginal candidiasis: treatment and recurrence. *Aust N Z J Obstet Gynaecol* 1982;22:231–233.
63. Watson MC, Grimshaw JM, Bond CM, et al. Oral versus intra-vaginal imidazole and triazole anti-fungal treatment of uncomplicated vulvovaginal candidiasis (thrush). In: The Cochrane Library, Issue 4. Oxford: Update Software, 2001. Search date 2000; primary sources Cochrane Library, Medline, Embase, Cochrane Collaboration Sexually Transmitted Disease Group Specialised Register of Controlled Trials, hand search of reference lists, and UK manufacturers of antifungal drugs.
64. De Punzio C, Garutti P, Mollica M, et al. Fluconazole 150 mg single dose versus itraconazole 200 mg per day for 3 days in the treatment of acute vaginal candidiasis: a double-blind randomized study. *Eur J Obs Gynecol Reprod Biol* 2003;106:193–197.
65. Sobel JD, Brooker D, Stein GE, et al. Single oral dose fluconazole compared with conventional clotrimazole topical therapy of *Candida vaginitis*. *Am J Obstet Gynecol* 1995;172:1263–1268.
66. Osser S, Haglund A, Weström L. Treatment of vaginal candidiasis: a prospective randomized investigator-blind multicenter study comparing topically applied econazole with oral fluconazole. *Acta Obstet Gynecol Scand* 1991;70:73–78.
67. Anon. A comparison of single-dose oral fluconazole with 3-day intravaginal clotrimazole in the treatment of vaginal candidiasis. *Br J Obstet Gynaecol* 1989;96:226–232.
68. Timonen H, Hartikainen-Vahtera P, Kivijarvi A, et al. A double-blind comparison of the effectiveness of itraconazole oral capsules with econazole vaginal capsules in the treatment of vaginal candidosis. *Drug Invest* 1992;4:515–520.
69. Puolakka J, Tuimala R. Comparison between oral ketoconazole and topical miconazole in the treatment of vaginal candidiasis. *Acta Obstet Gynecol Scand* 1983;62:575–577.
70. Rohde-Werner H. Topical tioconazole versus systemic ketoconazole treatment of vaginal candidiasis. *J Int Med Res* 1984;12:298–302.
71. Bingham JS. Single blind comparison of ketoconazole 200 mg oral tablets and clotrimazole 100 mg vaginal tablets and 1% cream in treating acute vaginal candidosis. *Br J Ven Dis* 1984;60:175–177.
72. Miller PI, Humphries M, Grassick K. A single-blind comparison of oral and intravaginal treatments in

acute and recurrent vaginal candidosis in general practice. *Pharmatherapeutica* 1984;3:582–587.
73. Comninos A, Kapellakis I, Pikouli-Giannopoulou P, et al. Double-blind evaluation of ketoconazole comparatively with clotrimazole in vaginal candidiasis. *Curr Ther Res* 1984;36:100–104.
74. Sobel JD, Schmitt C, Stein G, et al. Initial management of recurrent vulvovaginal candidiasis with oral ketoconazole and topical clotrimazole. *J Reprod Med* 1994;39:517–520.
75. Farkas B, Simon N. Ergebnisse einer Vergleichsstudie mit einem oral und einem lokal zu applizierenden Antimykotikum bei Vaginalmykosen. *Mykosen* 1984;27:554–561.
76. Kutzer E, Oittner R, Leodolter S, et al. A comparison of fluconazole and ketoconazole in the oral treatment of vaginal candidiasis: report of a double-blind multicentre trial. *Eur J Obstet Gynecol Reprod Biol* 1988;29:305–313.
77. Lake-Bakaar G, Scheuer PJ, Sherlock S. Hepatic reactions associated with ketoconazole in the United Kingdom. *BMJ* 1987;294:419–422.
78. Roth AC, Milsom I, Forssman L, et al. Intermittent prophylactic treatment of recurrent vaginal candidiasis by postmenstrual application of a 500 mg clotrimazole vaginal tablet. *Genitourin Med* 1990;66:357–360.
79. Sobel JD. Clotrimazole treatment of recurrent and chronic and chronic candida vulvovaginitis. *Obstet Gynecol* 1989;73:330–334.
80. Fong IW. The value of prophylactic (monthly) clotrimazole versus empiric self-treatment in recurrent vaginal candidiasis. *Genitourin Med* 1994;70:124–126.
81. Calderon-Marquez JJ. Itraconazole in the treatment of vaginal candidosis and the effect of treatment of the sexual partner. *Rev Inf Dis* 1987;9:S143–S145.
82. Bisschop MP, Merkus JM, Scheygrond H, et al. Co-treatment of the male partner in vaginal candidosis: a double-blind randomized control study. *Br J Obstet Gynaecol* 1986;93:79–81.
83. Spinillo A, Colonna L, Piazzi G, et al. Managing recurrent vulvovaginal candidiasis. Intermittent prevention with itraconazole. *J Reprod Med* 1997;42:83–87.
84. Fong IW. The value of chronic suppressive therapy with itraconazole versus clotrimazole in women with recurrent vaginal candidiasis. *Genitourin Med* 1992;68:374–377.
85. Sobel JD. Recurrent vulvovaginal candidiasis. A prospective study of the efficacy of maintenance ketoconazole therapy. *N Engl J Med* 1986;315:1455–1458.

Des Spence
Dr
General Practice
Glasgow University
Glasgow
Scotland

Competing interests: None declared.

The following previous contributor of this topic would also like to be acknowledged: Jeanne Marrazo.

Dysmenorrhoea

Search date February 2003

Michelle Proctor and Cynthia Farquhar

QUESTIONS

INTERVENTIONS

See glossary, p 2074

Key Messages

- **Non-steroidal anti-inflammatory drugs (other than aspirin)** Two systematic reviews have found that naproxen, ibuprofen, mefenamic acid, valdecoxib, and rofecoxib reduce pain compared with placebo. It remains unclear from direct comparisons which non-steroidal anti-inflammatory drugs have better efficacy or safety. One systematic review found that naproxen reduced pain more and was associated with fewer adverse effects than co-proxamol. It also found that mefenamic acid reduced symptoms more than co-proxamol.
- **Aspirin, paracetamol, and compound analgesics** One systematic review found that aspirin was more effective for pain relief than placebo, but less effective than naproxen or ibuprofen. The review found no significant difference between paracetamol compared with placebo, aspirin, or ibuprofen in pain relief, although some of the RCTs may have been too small to rule out clinically important differences. It found limited evidence that co-proxamol reduced pain compared with placebo.
- **Magnesium** One systematic review found limited evidence from two out of three small RCTs that magnesium reduced pain after 5–6 months compared with placebo. A third RCT found no significant difference.
- **Thiamine** One large RCT identified by a systematic review found that thiamine reduced pain after 60 days compared with placebo.
- **Toki-shakuyaku-san (herbal remedy)** One systematic review found limited evidence that toki-shakuyaku-san reduced pain after 6 months compared with placebo and that it reduced the need for additional medication with diclofenac.
- **Topical heat** One RCT found topical heat (about 39 °C) treatment to be as effective as ibuprofen and more effective than placebo in reducing pain.

- **Transcutaneous electrical nerve stimulation** One systematic review found limited evidence from small RCTs that high frequency transcutaneous electrical nerve stimulation reduced pain compared with placebo transcutaneous electrical nerve stimulation. We found insufficient evidence from small RCTs to assess effects of low frequency transcutaneous electrical nerve stimulation compared with other or no treatment.
- **Vitamin E** One RCT found limited evidence that vitamin E reduced pain compared with placebo.
- **Acupuncture** One systematic review of one small RCT found insufficient evidence to compare acupuncture with placebo or no treatment.
- **Behavioural interventions** We found insufficient evidence from two poor quality RCTs about the effects of behavioural interventions.
- **Combined oral contraceptives** One systematic review found insufficient evidence about the effects of combined oral contraceptives versus placebo for pain relief.
- **Fish oil** One small RCT identified by a systematic review and one additional RCT found limited evidence that fish oil reduced pain and symptoms after 1–3 months compared with placebo.
- **Herbal remedies (other than toki-shakuyaku-san)** We found no RCTs of other herbal remedies.
- **Surgical interruption of pelvic nerve pathways** One small RCT found limited evidence suggesting that laparoscopic uterine nerve ablation increased pain relief compared with diagnostic laparoscopy. Another RCT found that laparoscopic uterine nerve ablation reduced pain at 12 months compared with laparoscopic presacral neurectomy. It found no significant difference in pain relief between treatments at 3 months. It also found increased constipation with laparoscopic uterine nerve ablation.
- **Vitamin B_{12}** We found no RCTs that compared vitamin B_{12} with placebo. One small RCT found insufficient evidence for vitamin B_{12} compared with advice to follow a low fat vegetarian diet.
- **Spinal manipulation** One systematic review has found inconclusive evidence on the effects of spinal manipulation compared with placebo or no treatment in pain relief.

DEFINITION Dysmenorrhoea is painful menstrual cramps of uterine origin. It is commonly divided into primary dysmenorrhoea (pain without organic pathology) and secondary dysmenorrhoea (pelvic pain associated with an identifiable pathological condition, such as endometriosis [see endometriosis, p 2079] or ovarian cysts). The initial onset of primary dysmenorrhoea is usually shortly after menarche (6–12 months) when ovulatory cycles are established. Pain duration is commonly 8–72 hours and is usually associated with the onset of menstrual flow. Secondary dysmenorrhoea can also occur at any time after menarche, but may arise as a new symptom during a woman's fourth and fifth decade, after the onset of an underlying causative condition.[1]

INCIDENCE/ PREVALENCE Variations in the definition of dysmenorrhoea make it difficult to determine prevalence precisely. However, various types of study have found a consistently high prevalence in women of different ages and nationalities. One systematic review (search date 1996) of the prevalence of chronic pelvic pain, summarising both community and hospital surveys, estimated prevalence to be 45–95%.[2] Reports focus on adolescent girls and generally include only primary dysmenorrhoea, although this is not always specified. Studies of prevalence are summarised in table 1, p 2077.

AETIOLOGY/ RISK FACTORS A longitudinal study of a representative sample of women born in 1962 found that severity of dysmenorrhoea was significantly associated with duration of menstrual flow (average duration of menstrual flow was 5.0 days for women with no dysmenorrhoea and 5.8 days for women with severe dysmenorrhoea: where severe dysmenorrhoea was defined as pain that did not respond well to analgesics and clearly inhibited daily activity; $P < 0.001$; WMD –0.80, 95% CI –1.36 to –0.24); younger average menarcheal age (13.1 years in women without dysmenorrhoea *v* 12.6 years in women with severe dysmenorrhoea; $P < 0.01$; WMD 0.50, 95% CI 0.09 to 0.91); and cigarette smoking (41% of smokers and 26% of non-smokers experienced moderate or severe dysmenorrhoea).[9] There is also some evidence of a dose–response relationship between exposure to environmental tobacco smoke and increased incidence of dysmenorrhoea.[10]

PROGNOSIS Primary dysmenorrhoea is a chronic recurring condition that affects most young women. Studies of the natural history of this condition are sparse. One longitudinal study in Scandinavia found that primary dysmenorrhoea often improves in the third decade of a woman's reproductive life, and is also reduced after childbirth.[9] We found no studies that reliably examined the relationship between the prognosis of secondary dysmenorrhoea and the severity of underlying pathology such as endometriosis.

AIMS OF INTERVENTION To relieve pain from dysmenorrhoea, with minimal adverse effects.

OUTCOMES Pain relief, measured either by a visual analogue scale (see glossary, p 2075), other pain scales, or as a dichotomous outcome (pain relief achieved yes/no); overall improvement in dysmenorrhoea measured by change in dysmenorrhoeic symptoms either self reported or observed, quality of life scales, or other similar measures such as the Menstrual Distress or Menstrual Symptom Questionnaires; adverse effects of treatment (incidence and type of adverse effects); proportion of women requiring analgesics in addition to their assigned treatment; proportion of women reporting activity restriction or absences from work or school and hours or days of absence as a more selective measure.

METHODS *Clinical Evidence* search and appraisal February 2003.

QUESTION What are the effects of treatments for dysmenorrhoea?

OPTION ACUPUNCTURE

One systematic review of one small RCT found insufficient evidence to compare acupuncture with placebo or no treatment.

Benefits: We found one systematic review of acupuncture for primary dysmenorrhoea (search date 2001, 1 RCT, 43 women).[11] The RCT included in the systematic review compared weekly acupuncture during three menstrual cycles a month for 3 months versus three other treatments: placebo acupuncture (see glossary, p 2075); monthly medical visits; or no medical visits. Outcomes were assessed after 3 months using non-validated pain scales and symptom questionnaires, and improvement was defined as a reduction in pain by more than half the admission score. It found that acupuncture significantly increased the proportion of women with reduced pain compared with other treatment (10/11 [91%] with acupuncture *v* 4/11 [36%] with placebo acupuncture *v* 1/10 [10%] with monthly medical visits *v* 2/11 [18%] with no medical treatment; $P < 0.05$ for acupuncture *v* all other treatments).

Harms: The RCT identified by the review did not address harms of acupuncture.[12]

Comment: The scale used to assess outcomes in the RCT identified by the review does not seem to be validated.[11] We found no evidence of statistical adjustment for multiple comparisons (such as Bonferroni's correction) in the published paper.[12] The review identified a second RCT comparing different modalities of acupuncture.[11]

OPTION ASPIRIN, PARACETAMOL, AND COMPOUND ANALGESICS

One systematic review found that aspirin was more effective for pain relief than placebo, but less effective than naproxen or ibuprofen. The review found no significant difference between paracetamol compared with placebo, aspirin, or ibuprofen in pain relief, although some of the RCTs may have been too small to rule out clinically important differences. It found limited evidence that co-proxamol reduced pain compared with placebo.

Benefits: We found one systematic review (search date 1997, 13 RCTs) of the effects of analgesics in primary dysmenorrhoea (see table 2, p 2078), which compared analgesics versus placebo, versus each other, or versus non-steroidal anti-inflammatory drugs.[13] **Aspirin versus placebo:** The review identified eight RCTs comparing aspirin versus placebo (486 women, 650 mg 4 times daily). The review found that aspirin was significantly more effective than placebo for pain relief (proportion of women with at least moderate pain relief, 5 RCTs: RR 1.60, 95% CI 1.12 to 2.29; NNT 10, 95% CI 5 to 50). It also found no significant difference between aspirin and placebo in the need for additional medication or restriction of daily activity and absence from work (additional medications, 3 RCTs: RR 0.79, 95% CI 0.58 to 1.08; restriction of activity, 3 RCTs: RR 0.82, 95% CI 0.64 to 1.04; absence from work, 1 RCT: RR 1.28, 95% CI 0.24 to 6.76).[13] **Paracetamol versus placebo:** One RCT identified by the review found no significant difference between paracetamol (500 mg 4 times daily) and placebo in pain relief (proportion of women with at least moderate pain relief; 35 women; RR 1.00, 95% CI 0.28 to 3.63).[13] **Co-proxamol versus placebo:** One RCT identified by the review found that co-proxamol (see glossary, p 2074) significantly increased the proportion of women with at least moderate pain relief compared with placebo (72 women; 650 mg/65 mg 4 times daily; RR 3.72, 95% CI 2.13 to 6.52).[13] **Paracetamol versus aspirin:** One RCT (35 women) identified by the review compared aspirin (500 mg 4 times daily) versus paracetamol (500 mg 4 times daily). It found no significant difference in pain relief (10 cm visual analogue scale (see glossary, p 2075): median change from baseline 1.6 cm, 95% CI 0.4 cm to 3.3 cm with paracetamol *v* 1.2 cm, 95% CI 0 cm to 2.7 cm with aspirin). **Aspirin or paracetamol or co-proxamol versus non-steroidal anti-inflammatory drugs:** See benefits of non-steroidal anti-inflammatory drugs, p 2062.

Harms: The most common adverse effects described by the review were nausea or abdominal discomfort, headaches, and dizziness.[13] Adverse effects occurred in 7–17% of women taking aspirin versus 3–17% of women taking placebo. The review found no difference between aspirin or paracetamol compared with placebo in the frequency of adverse effects (any adverse effect for aspirin *v* placebo: RR 1.31, 95% CI 0.79 to 2.17; any adverse effect for paracetamol *v* placebo: RR 1.00, 95% CI 0.36 to 2.75).

Comment: Most RCTs included in the systematic review were short (usually only 1 menstrual cycle on each treatment), small, and used a crossover design without a washout period. All of the RCTs (except 1 of co-proxamol versus naproxen) used double blinding. All the RCTs used oral administration of treatment in the form of tablets or capsules. Negative RCTs may have been too small to rule out clinically important differences.

OPTION NON-STEROIDAL ANTI-INFLAMMATORY DRUGS (OTHER THAN ASPIRIN)

Two systematic reviews and subsequent RCTs have found that naproxen, ibuprofen, mefenamic acid, valdecoxib, and rofecoxib reduced pain compared with placebo. It remains unclear from direct comparisons which non-steroidal anti-inflammatory drugs have better efficacy or safety. One systematic review found that naproxen reduced pain more and was associated with fewer adverse effects than co-proxamol. It also found that mefenamic acid reduced symptoms more than co-proxamol.

Benefits: We found two systematic reviews[13,14] and six subsequent RCTs of the effects of non-steroidal anti-inflammatory drugs (NSAIDs) in primary dysmenorrhoea.[15–20] The first systematic review (search date 1997, 46 RCTs, 2733 women) evaluated the effects of naproxen (23 RCTs, 1728 women), ibuprofen (18 RCTs, 748 women), and mefenamic acid (5 RCTs, 257 women).[13] The second systematic review (search date not stated, 1 RCT) assessed rofecoxib, a cyclo-oxygenase-2 selective NSAID, versus placebo or versus naproxen in people with primary dysmenorrhoea.[14] **Versus placebo:** The first systematic review found that all three NSAIDs significantly increased proportion of women with at least moderate pain relief compared with placebo (naproxen, 13 RCTs: RR 3.17, 95% CI 2.72 to 3.67; NNT 3, 95% CI 2 to 4; ibuprofen, 9 RCTs: RR 2.41, 95% CI 1.58 to 3.68; NNT 3, 95% CI 2 to 4; mefenamic acid, 3 RCTs: RR 2.03, 95% CI 1.65 to 2.48; NNT 3, 95% CI 2 to 5). The use of additional analgesics was significantly reduced for all NSAIDs versus placebo. Women taking naproxen were 60% less likely to use additional analgesics (10 RCTs; RR 0.4, 95% CI 0.3 to 0.4); those taking ibuprofen were 70% less likely (2 RCTs; RR 0.23,

95% CI 0.13 to 0.41); and those on mefenamic acid were 35% less likely (1 RCT; RR 0.65, 95% CI 0.52 to 0.80). Restriction of daily life was significantly less for naproxen and ibuprofen (naproxen, 1 RCT: RR 0.65, 95% CI 0.52 to 0.80; ibuprofen, 3 RCTs: RR 0.26, 95% CI 0.16 to 0.42). Absence from work or school was significantly reduced with naproxen but not with ibuprofen (naproxen, 7 RCTs: RR 0.29, 95% CI 0.13 to 0.66; ibuprofen, 1 RCT: RR 0.14, 95% CI 0.02 to 1.10).[13] The RCT identified by the second review (127 women) compared four treatments: rofecoxib 25 mg/day; rofecoxib (50 mg loading dose then 25 mg/day); naproxen sodium (550 mg every 12 hours); and placebo over four consecutive cycles.[14] It found that both doses of rofecoxib and naproxen provided more pain relief compared with placebo (pain relief measured by combining the TOPAR8 scales over 4 menstrual cycles [total pain relief scores to 8 hours]; $P < 0.006$ for all treatments *v* placebo). The first subsequent RCT (69 women) found that niflumic acid (750 mg/day for 3 days) significantly increased the proportion of women who had complete remission or more than 50% remission of pain on day 3 of treatment compared with placebo (26/30 [87%] with niflumic acid *v* 15/31 [48%] with placebo; RR 1.73, 95% CI 1.17 to 2.57; NNT 3, 95% CI 2 to 5).[15] The second subsequent RCT (crossover design; 57 women) compared four treatments: bromfenac (10 or 50 mg/day), naproxen (550 mg loading dose, then 275 mg repeat doses 4 hourly as needed), and placebo.[16] It found that women taking bromfenac (10 or 50 mg/day) or naproxen had significantly less pain than women taking placebo after three days of treatment in one cycle ($P < 0.05$ for all comparisons *v* placebo). The third subsequent RCT (crossover design; 52 women) compared six hourly doses of dexketoprofen 12.5 or 25 mg, racemic ketoprofen 25 mg, and placebo.[17] It found that after 1 day of treatment pain relief was better in the three treatment groups compared to placebo ($P < 0.05$ for all treatment groups *v* placebo). The fourth subsequent RCT (crossover design; 24 women) found that lysine clonixinate or ibuprofen increased the proportion of women with total pain relief compared with placebo (10/24 [42%] with lysine clonixinate *v* 9/24 [38%] with ibuprofen *v* 2/24 [8%] with placebo; active treatment versus placebo; $P < 0.001$).[18] However, results were difficult to interpret because no pre-crossover results were reported. The sixth subsequent RCT (crossover design; 96 women) compared valdecoxib (20 mg or 40 mg every 12 hours) versus naproxen sodium (550 mg every 12 hours) versus placebo.[20] It found that valdecoxib significantly reduced pain 8 and 12 hours after the first dose compared with placebo ($P < 0.01$ for 20 mg dose and $P < 0.001$ for 40 mg dose). It also found that naproxen sodium significantly reduced pain compared with placebo ($P < 0.001$). However, results were difficult to interpret because no pre-crossover results were reported. **Comparison of NSAIDs:** The first systematic review identified 5 RCTs comparing different NSAIDs.[13] Three RCTs identified by the review found no significant difference in pain relief between naproxen (550 mg loading dose followed by 275 mg) and ibuprofen (400 mg) (proportion of women with at least moderate pain relief: pooled RR 1.1, 95% CI 0.8 to 1.5). One RCT identified by the review found that naproxen (550 mg loading dose followed by 275 mg) significantly increased pain relief compared with mefenamic acid (500 mg followed by 250 mg) (proportion of women with at least moderate pain relief: RR 2.4, 95% CI 1.4 to 4.1). Another RCT identified by the review found no significant difference in pain relief between ibuprofen 400 mg and mefenamic acid 250 mg (no RR or P values provided). The second subsequent RCT (crossover design; 57 women) compared bromfenac 50 mg/day, bromfenac 10 mg/day, naproxen sodium (550 mg loading dose, then 275 mg repeat doses 4 hourly as needed), and placebo measuring outcomes with a categorical scale (described in the study, no information of validation).[16] No significant differences were found in pain scores between the three treatment groups after day one of treatment ($P > 0.05$). The third subsequent RCT (crossover design; 52 women) compared six hourly doses of dexketoprofen 12.5 mg, dexketoprofen 25 mg, racemic ketoprofen 25 mg, and placebo using a visual analogue scale (see glossary, p 2075).[17] It found no difference in pain scores between the three treatment groups after 3 days of treatment in one cycle ($P > 0.05$), and all treatments reduced pain significantly more than placebo ($P < 0.05$). The fourth subsequent RCT (crossover design; 24 women) found no significant difference in the proportion of women with total pain relief between lysine clonixinate and ibuprofen (10/24 [42%] with lysine clonixinate *v* 9/24 [38%] with ibuprofen; $P > 0.05$). However, results were difficult to interpret because no pre-crossover results were reported. The fifth subsequent RCT (308 women) compared nimesulide 100 mg and diclofenac 50 mg taken up to three times daily as needed over two menstrual cycles. It found no significant difference in the proportion of women who rated the treatment as "good" or "very good" at the end of each menstrual cycle (85.5% with nimesulide *v* 81.0% with diclofenac; RR 1.05, 95% CI 0.95 to 1.16).[19] The sixth subsequent RCT (crossover design; 96 women) found no significant difference in pain relief between valdecoxib 40 mg and naproxen sodium 550 mg ($P > 0.05$). However, results were difficult to interpret because no pre-crossover results were reported.[20] **Versus aspirin or paracetamol:** The first systematic review identified three RCTs comparing NSAIDs versus aspirin or paracetamol.[13] It found that both naproxen (275 mg 4 times daily) and ibuprofen (400 mg 4 times daily) reduced pain more than aspirin (650 mg 4 times daily) (excellent or moderate pain relief: naproxen *v* aspirin, 1 RCT: RR 2.29, 95% CI 1.09 to 4.79; ibuprofen *v* aspirin, 1 RCT: RR 1.90, 95% CI 1.13 to 2.78). It found no significant difference in pain relief between ibuprofen and paracetamol (1 RCT, results presented graphically).[13] **Versus co-proxamol:** The first systematic review identified three RCTs comparing NSAIDs versus co-proxamol (see glossary, p 2074).[13] One RCT identified by the review compared mefenamic acid (500 mg 3 times daily) versus co-proxamol (650 mg/65 mg 3 times daily). It found that mefenamic acid was significantly more effective in reducing dysmenorrhoea related symptoms than co-proxamol ($P < 0.01$). Mefenamic acid also reduced the need for additional medication compared with co-proxamol (mean number of tablets of additional medication 2.6 with mefenamic acid *v* 6.8 with co-proxamol; P value not provided).

The RCT found no difference between treatments in absence from work or school. Two RCTs (98 women) identified by the review compared naproxen (275 mg 3 times daily) versus co-proxamol (650 mg/65 mg 3 times daily). Neither RCT found a significant difference in pain severity.[13]

Harms: The most commonly reported adverse effects in the RCTs identified by the review were nausea, dizziness, and headaches.[13] Naproxen significantly increased the number of adverse effects compared with placebo (number of RCTs not specified; RR 1.45, 95% CI 1.03 to 2.04). The review found no difference between ibuprofen and placebo in the number of adverse effects (RR 1.12, 95% CI 0.85 to 1.47) or between mefenamic acid and placebo (RR 0.59, 95% CI 0.28 to 1.23). The review also found that co-proxamol significantly increased adverse effects compared with naproxen (23–58% with co-proxamol *v* 15–25% with naproxen; RR 1.94, 95% CI 1.11 to 3.41). It also found that naproxen significantly increased adverse effects compared with placebo (RR 1.45, 95% CI 1.03 to 2.04) and marginally increased nausea (RR 2.71, 95% CI 1.00 to 7.36). The second RCT (57 women) found adverse effects in 13/57 (23%) women taking bromfenac 50 mg, 15/57 (26%) women taking bromfenac 10 mg, 20/57 (35%) women taking naproxen (550 mg loading dose, then 275 mg repeat doses 4 hourly as needed), and 19/57 (33%) women taking placebo.[16] The fifth RCT (308 women) found gastrointestinal adverse effects in 7/149 (4.8%) women taking nimesulide and 16/155 (10.3%) women taking diclofenac.[19] The systematic review of rofecoxib[14] did not describe fully the adverse effects found in the RCT it identified.[21] The RCT found that minor adverse effects including nausea and dry mouth were reported by: 4/127 (3%) with placebo; 7/127 (6%) with rofecoxib (25 mg followed by 25 mg/day); 13/127 (11%) with rofecoxib (50 mg followed by 25 mg/day); and 11/127 (9%) with naproxen sodium (550 mg twice daily for 3 days) ($P < 0.05$ for rofecoxib [50 mg followed by 25 mg/day] *v* placebo).[21] The RCT (crossover design; 96 women) that compared valdecoxib (20 or 40 mg every 12 hours) versus naproxen sodium (550 mg every 12 hours) versus placebo reported minor adverse events in all groups.[20] Adverse events included abdominal pain, diarrhoea, dizziness, fever, headache, nausea, and pain. People taking valdecoxib 20 mg reported 27 adverse events (16 were headache). Those taking valdecoxib 40 mg reported 19 adverse events (9 were headaches). People taking naproxen sodium reported 12 adverse events (8 were headaches) and people taking placebo reported 23 adverse events (20 were headaches). However, results were difficult to interpret because no pre-crossover results were reported.

Comment: All the RCTs identified by the review used oral treatment.[13] NSAIDs can be given as suppositories, which seem to have a similar effect on overall pain relief but less effect than oral treatment for spasmodic pain.[22] Most RCTs in the first systematic review used a crossover design without a washout period and were brief (usually only 1 menstrual cycle/treatment). Nine of the included RCTs did not blind the researchers to treatment allocation. Many of the trials on NSAIDs were sponsored by the pharmaceutical industry. The pain relief figures used above (see benefits above) refer to RCTs that include women with primary dysmenorrhoea only. However, some of the figures regarding the use of additional medication included data from women with undefined dysmenorrhoea. A systematic review with stricter inclusion criteria and methodological quality assessment is underway.[23] Some RCTs used a scale with categories (categorical scale) to measure outcomes.[16,18] There is no evidence that those scales were validated. Variations in pain measured in the categorical scales were summarised using parametric statistics, making those results difficult to interpret.[16,18] The second systematic review also identified one crossover clinical trial (63 women) that compared rofecoxib (50 mg loading dose then 25 mg/day), naproxen (550 mg every 12 hours), and placebo as needed.[14] It found no difference in outcomes between rofecoxib and naproxen, but found that rofecoxib significantly reduced pain as measured by TOPAR8 scores ($P < 0.002$) and time to remedication ($P < 0.009$) compared with placebo.

OPTION BEHAVIOURAL INTERVENTIONS

We found insufficient evidence from two poor quality RCTs about the effects of behavioural interventions.

Benefits: We found no systematic review. We found two small RCTs on behavioural interventions (see glossary, p 2074). One involved relaxation and imagery for women with congestive or spasmodic (see glossary, p 2075) dysmenorrhoea,[24] and the other involved aerobic exercise for women with primary dysmenorrhoea.[25] **Relaxation treatment:** The first RCT (69 women) compared relaxation treatment plus positive imagery regarding menstruation versus self directed group discussion about menstruation versus waiting list control. The groups were divided into women with congestive or spasmodic dysmenorrhoea using the Menstrual Symptom Questionnaire. It found that in women with spasmodic or congestive dysmenorrhoea, relaxation treatment significantly improved symptoms compared with waiting list control ($P < 0.01$). However, it found that only the women with spasmodic dysmenorrhoea experienced significantly less pain with relaxation compared with group discussion or waiting list control ($P < 0.001$).[24] **Aerobic exercise:** The second RCT (36 women) comparing a training group that participated in 30 minutes of exercise 3 days a week with a sedentary control group found that aerobic exercise significantly lowered Menstrual Distress Questionnaire scores ($P < 0.05$; results presented graphically).[25]

Harms: The RCTs gave no information on adverse effects.

Comment: Both RCTs were small and of poor methodological quality.[24,25] In one RCT, spasmodic dysmenorrhoea was defined as spasms of pain mainly in the abdomen, and congestive dysmenorrhoea was defined as a dull aching pain in the lower abdomen and other areas of the body.[24] However, the classification of dysmenorrhoea into spasmodic and congestive categories is no longer commonly used and has little meaning.[25] The RCT (36 women) comparing aerobic exercise with a sedentary control analysed results for the 26 women (72%) who completed the trial (11 in the exercise group and 15 in the control group).[25] A systematic review is underway.[26]

OPTION COMBINED ORAL CONTRACEPTIVES

One systematic review found insufficient evidence of the effects of oral contraceptives for pain relief.

Benefits: We found one systematic review of combined oral contraceptives for primary dysmenorrhoea (search date 1999, 5 RCTs, 379 women).[27] It found no significant difference between medium dose oestrogen (> 35 μg) plus first or second generation progestogens compared with placebo in pain relief at 1–3 months (4 RCTs, 320 women; RR 1.40, 95% CI 0.58 to 3.42). It found that oral contraceptives reduced the proportion of women absent from work or school compared with placebo but the difference was of borderline statistical significance (1 RCT; 19/49 [39%] with contraceptives *v* 24/40 [60%] with placebo; RR 0.65, 95% CI 0.42 to 1.00).[27]

Harms: The review found no significant difference between combined oral contraceptives and placebo in adverse effects, such as nausea, vomiting, depression, and abdominal pain (1 RCT, 89 women: 15/49 [31%] with contraceptives *v* 8/40 [20%] with placebo; RR 1.53, 95% CI 0.72 to 3.24).[27] The results of two RCTs are difficult to interpret and could not be included in the meta-analysis of adverse effects performed by the review because the RCTs randomised menstrual cycles and not women.[28,29] One small RCT (18 women) identified by the review comparing combined oral contraceptives with placebo found that more women receiving oral contraceptives experienced breakthrough bleeding (2/12 [17%] with contraceptives *v* 0/6 [0%] with placebo).[28] Another RCT (59 women) identified by the review found that combined oral contraceptives increased weight gain, nausea, and vomiting compared with placebo (no further data provided).[29]

Comment: Most of the RCTs identified by the review had weak methods.[27] Because of the small number of included trials and participants, the results of the systematic review are sensitive to the statistical methods of calculation used. One of the RCTs identified by the review could not be included in the meta-analysis because of poor reporting of data.[29] All of the RCTs identified by the review used oral contraceptives that are no longer commonly prescribed, so the results may not be applicable to women today who take different preparations.[27]

OPTION FISH OIL

One small RCT identified by a systematic review and one additional RCT found limited evidence that fish oil reduced pain and symptoms after 1–3 months compared with placebo.

Benefits: **Versus placebo:** We found one systematic review (search date 2000, 1 RCT, 42 women)[30] and one additional RCT[31] that compared fish oil versus placebo. The RCT (crossover design; 42 women) identified by the review compared fish oil capsules with placebo twice daily for 1 month. It found that menstrual symptom scores were significantly lower with fish oil compared with placebo but this refers to the average of the two groups after the allocated treatments were crossed over.[30] Less additional medication (ibuprofen 200 mg) was used in the fish oil group (mean 4.7 tablets with fish oil v 10.1 with placebo; P = 0.015). One additional RCT (78 women) compared four interventions: fish oil (0.5–1.0 g 5 times daily); fish oil plus vitamin B_{12}; seal oil (higher in saturated fat than fish oil); and placebo for a minimum of 3 months.[31] It found that pain measured on a visual analogue scale (see glossary, p 2075) significantly decreased only in the fish oil with vitamin B_{12} group (reduction in mean scores: fish oil –0.15, fish oil plus vitamin B_{12} –0.73, seal oil –0.2, placebo –0.19; P = 0.015 for fish oil plus vitamin B_{12} v placebo). However, all three active treatment groups experienced significant change in the number of other menstrual symptoms and the amount of interference with daily activities (P < 0.05).

Harms: **Versus placebo:** One RCT (42 women) identified by the review found that two women taking fish oils reported nausea and one woman reported acne.[30] No adverse effects were reported in women receiving placebo.

Comment: Both RCTs included women with dysmenorrhoea and no additional health problems.[30,31] This could include women with either primary or secondary dysmenorrhoea.

OPTION MAGNESIUM

One systematic review found limited evidence from two out of three small RCTs that magnesium reduced pain after 5–6 months compared with placebo. The third RCT found no significant difference between treatments.

Benefits: **Versus placebo:** We found one systematic review (search date 2000, 3 RCTs).[30] The first RCT (50 women) identified by the review compared magnesium aspartate three times daily with placebo. It found that magnesium aspartate significantly increased the proportion of women without pain after 6 months compared with placebo (21/25 [84%] with magnesium v 7/25 [28%] with placebo; RR 3.0, 95% CI 1.6 to 5.8; NNT 2, 95% CI 2 to 3). The second RCT (27 women) identified by the review found no significant difference between magnesium (5 mmol 3 times daily) and placebo in reducing pain as measured by visual analogue scale (see glossary, p 2075) pain scores, or in the number of ibuprofen tablets taken after 6 months (P = 0.07; no further data provided). The third RCT (21 women) identified by the review found that magnesium (500 mg/day during menses) significantly reduced pain after 5 months compared with placebo (P < 0.01).[30]

Harms: One RCT identified by the review found that magnesium significantly increased the proportion of women who experienced intestinal discomfort and other minor adverse effects compared with placebo (5/25 [20%] with magnesium v 0/25 [0%] with placebo; NNH 5, 95% CI 2 to 38), although relief of these symptoms occurred when the dose was reduced from three to two tablets daily.[30]

Comment: None.

OPTION THIAMINE

One large RCT identified by a systematic review has found that thiamine reduces pain after 60 days compared with placebo.

Benefits: We found one systematic review (search date 2000, 1 RCT).[30] The RCT identified by the review (crossover, 556 Indian adolescents attending school) compared thiamine 100 mg/day with placebo for 3 months. It found that thiamine significantly increased the proportion of women with no pain before crossover after 60 days compared with placebo (142/277 [51%] with thiamine *v* 0/279 [0%] with placebo; NNT 2, 95% CI 2 to 3).[18] After completion of the RCT, 87% of all women experienced no pain.

Harms: The review did not report any harms of thiamine.[30]

Comment: None.

OPTION VITAMIN B_{12}

One small RCT found insufficient evidence for vitamin B_{12} compared with a low fat vegetarian diet.

Benefits: **Versus dietary change:** We found no systematic review. We found one RCT (crossover design; 33 women) that compared a supplement tablet containing vitamin B_{12} (0.02 mg/day) with advice to follow a low fat vegetarian diet.[32] However, results were difficult to interpret because no pre-crossover results were reported.

Harms: The RCT comparing a vitamin B_{12} tablet with advice to follow a low fat vegetarian diet found that stomach upset, slight nausea, burping, and a bad taste in the mouth were reported by eight women across the different treatment groups.[32] No additional information was reported in the trial.

Comment: The RCT comparing vitamin B_{12} with dietary advice may have been too small to rule out clinically important differences.[32]

OPTION VITAMIN E

One RCT found limited evidence that vitamin E reduced pain compared with placebo.

Benefits: We found one systematic review (search date 2000, 1 RCT)[30] and one subsequent RCT.[33] **Versus placebo:** The subsequent RCT (100 women, aged 16–18 years) compared vitamin E (500 units/day for 5 days/cycle, which is about 333 mg) with placebo.[33] It found that vitamin E reduced pain significantly more than placebo (median visual analogue scale (see glossary, p 2075) pain scores, 3.5 with vitamin E *v* 4.3 with placebo; $P = 0.02$). **Vitamin E plus ibuprofen versus ibuprofen alone:** One RCT identified by the review (crossover design; 50 women) compared vitamin E (100 mg/day for 20 days before menses) plus ibuprofen (400 mg 3 times daily at the outset of painful menstruation) versus ibuprofen alone (400 mg 3 times daily at the onset of pain).[30] It found no significant difference between vitamin E plus ibuprofen and ibuprofen alone in pain relief (23/26 [88%] with vitamin E plus ibuprofen *v* 17/24 [71%] with ibuprofen; RR 1.25, 95% CI 0.93 to 1.67).

Harms: The RCTs did not report harms.[30,33]

Comment: None.

OPTION HERBAL REMEDIES

One systematic review found limited evidence that toki-shakuyaku-san reduced pain after 6 months compared with placebo and that it reduced the need for additional medication with diclofenac.

Benefits: We found one systematic review (1 RCT, search date 2000, 50 women) comparing a herbal remedy versus placebo.[30] It found that the Japanese herbal remedy toki-shakuyaku-san (2.5 g 3 times daily) significantly reduced pain as measured by a visual analogue scale (see glossary, p 2075) after 6 months compared with placebo ($P < 0.005$), and reduced the need for additional medication (diclofenac sodium) ($P < 0.01$; results presented graphically).

Harms: The RCT gave no information on adverse effects.[30]

Comment: Toki-shakuyaku-san is a mixture of six herbs, including angelica and peony root. Allocation method is not clearly described in the RCT.[30]

OPTION SPINAL MANIPULATION

One systematic review has found inconclusive evidence on the effects of spinal manipulation compared with placebo or no treatment for pain relief.

Benefits: We found one systematic review (search date 2000, 5 RCTs) comparing spinal manipulation versus placebo or no treatment.[34] The review did not perform a meta-analysis because of heterogeneity. The first RCT (11 women) identified by the review compared high velocity, low amplitude manipulation (see glossary, p 2074) versus no treatment versus placebo manipulation (see glossary, p 2075). It found no significant difference between HVLA in pain relief after 1 month compared with either no treatment or placebo (7/8 [87%] with HVLA *v* 0/2 [0%] with no treatment; RR 5.00, 95% CI 0.39 to 63.85; 7/8 [87%] with HVLA *v* 0/1 [0%] with placebo treatment; RR 3.33, 95% CI 0.30 to 37.42). The second RCT identified by the review (44 women) comparing HVLA with placebo manipulation found that HVLA significantly reduced pain intensity as measured by a 10 cm visual analogue scale (see glossary, p 2075) pain score after one treatment and one menstrual cycle (WMD −1.41, 95% CI −2.55 to −0.27). The third RCT (138 women) identified by the review found no difference between HVLA and placebo manipulation in pain as measured by mean change in visual analogue scale pain score after one menstrual cycle (WMD +2.08, 95% CI −3.20 to +7.36). The fourth RCT (12 women) identified by the review found that HVLA improved pain after one treatment during one menstrual cycle compared with placebo manipulation (no further data provided). The fifth RCT (26 women) identified by the review compared 3 months of Toftness manipulation (see glossary, p 2075) with placebo manipulation.[34] It found that manipulation significantly reduced pain intensity after 6 months compared with placebo, but not at 3 months (WMD at 6 months −1.40, 95% CI −2.21 to −0.59; WMD at 3 months 2.20, 95% CI 1.38 to 3.02).[34]

Harms: One RCT identified by the review (138 women) found no significant difference between HVLA and placebo manipulation in the proportion of women experiencing soreness in the lower back region within 48 hours of the intervention (3/69 [4%] with HVLA *v* 2/69 [3%] with placebo; RR 1.50, 95% CI 0.26 to 8.70).[34] Soreness resolved within 24 hours. No other adverse effects were reported. The other RCTs identified by the review gave no information on adverse effects.

Comment: The overall methodological quality of the RCTs identified by the review was good: low withdrawal rate (2%), adequate randomisation method, blinding of the outcome assessor, and potential blinding of the participants as the control procedure was similar to the treatment.

OPTION TRANSCUTANEOUS ELECTRICAL NERVE STIMULATION

One systematic review found limited evidence from small RCTs that high frequency transcutaneous electrical nerve stimulation reduced pain compared with placebo transcutaneous electrical nerve stimulation. We found insufficient evidence from small RCTs to assess effects of low frequency, transcutaneous electrical nerve stimulation compared with other or no treatment.

Benefits: We found one systematic review including women with primary dysmenorrhoea (search date 2001, 8 RCTs, 172 women).[11] **High frequency transcutaneous electrical nerve stimulation (TENS) versus placebo TENS:** It found that high frequency TENS (see glossary, p 2075) significantly increased pain relief compared with placebo TENS as measured by subjective assessment or by a visual analogue scale (see glossary, p 2075) (pain relief by subjective assessment, 2 RCTs, 53 women: OR 7.2, 95% CI 3.1 to 16.5; pain relief by visual analogue scale range 0–100 [0 meaning no pain relief and 100 total pain relief] 1 RCT, 18 women: WMD 45.0 scale units, 95% CI 22.5 scale units to 67.5 scale units). The review found no significant difference in the proportion of women needing additional analgesics between high frequency TENS and placebo TENS (1 RCT, 64 women: OR 0.3, 95% CI 0.1 to 1.1). It also found no significant difference in the number of analgesic tablets taken between high frequency TENS and placebo TENS (1 RCT, 24 women, mean number of tablets taken each day 6.92 with high frequency TENS *v* 6.78 with placebo, WMD +0.1 tablets, 95% CI −2.1 tablets to +2.4 tablets). It found no difference between high frequency and placebo TENS in absence from work or school as measured by the number of lost hours each menstrual cycle (1 RCT, 24 women: WMD +0.04 hours, 95% CI −0.4 hours to +0.5 hours). **Low frequency TENS versus placebo TENS:** The review found no significant difference in pain relief between low frequency TENS and placebo TENS (pain relief by subjective assessment, 2 RCTs, 29 women: OR 1.3, 95% CI 0.4 to 4.1; pain relief by visual analogue scale 0–100, 1 RCT, 18 women: WMD +24.1 scale units, 95% CI −2.9 scale units to +51.1 scale units). One additional RCT (24 women) that could not be included in the meta-analysis because of the way in which results were reported found that pain relief was significantly increased by low frequency TENS compared to placebo TENS ($P < 0.05$). Low frequency TENS reduced the number of additional tablets of analgesic used compared with placebo TENS

(1 RCT, 24 women; WMD −3.1 tablets, 95% CI −5.5 tablets to −0.7 tablets). However, there was no difference between the two groups for hours of absence from work or school (1 RCT, 24 women; WMD −0.2 hours, 95% CI −0.6 hours to +0.2 hours). **Low frequency TENS versus placebo tablets:** The review found no difference in pain relief between low frequency TENS and placebo tablets (1 RCT, 21 women; OR 2.9, 95% CI 0.4 to 24.4). One additional RCT (20 women) that could not be included in the meta-analysis found low frequency TENS increased pain relief compared to placebo tablets ($P < 0.05$). **High frequency TENS versus low frequency TENS:** The review found that high frequency TENS was more effective than low frequency TENS for pain relief measured by subjective assessment (1 RCT, 21 women; OR 3.9, 95% CI 1.1 to 13.0), but not for pain relief measured with a visual analogue scale (1 RCT, 18 women; WMD +21, 95% CI −4.4 to +46). One additional RCT that could not be included in the meta-analysis found that low frequency TENS versus high frequency TENS significantly reduced pain ($P < 0.05$). The review found that low frequency TENS versus high frequency TENS significantly reduced the number of additional analgesic tablets taken (WMD 3.2 tablets, 95% CI 0.5 tablets to 5.9 tablets). There was no difference between the two groups for the outcome of absence from work or school (WMD +0.2 hours, 95% CI −0.2 hours to +0.6 hours). **TENS versus non-steroidal anti-inflammatory drugs:** One RCT (32 women) comparing high frequency TENS, ibuprofen, and placebo found that high frequency TENS was significantly less effective than ibuprofen in achieving pain relief (14/32 [44%] with TENS *v* 24/32 [75%] using ibuprofen; OR 0.26, 95% CI 0.09 to 0.75).[35] Another unblinded RCT (12 women, crossover) found no significant difference between naproxen and high frequency/high intensity TENS in pain relief (data presented in graphic form but no OR or P values provided) but both significantly reduced pain from baseline ($P < 0.001$).[36]

Harms: Adverse effects of muscle vibrations, tightness, headaches, and slight burning or redness after use were experienced by four women on treatment and none on placebo (OR 10.0, 95% CI 0.5 to 199.0; $P = 0.12$).[35] In the unblinded crossover RCT, 10/12 (83%) women considered TENS to be temporarily painful but were prepared to accept this effect for the pain relief achieved.[36] None of the 12 women reported any adverse effects during treatment with naproxen. One RCT found that 4/32 (13%) women using high frequency TENS experienced muscle vibrations, tightness, headaches after use, and slight redness or burning of the skin (OR 8.2, 95% CI 1.1 to 60.9). There were no reported adverse effects from low frequency TENS or placebo TENS. The systematic review identified one RCT comparing high frequency TENS and naproxen reported an increase in the number of adverse effects experienced by participants (OR 26.7, 95% CI 5.5 to 130.9). In the TENS group, 10/12 (83%) experienced pain from the treatment whereas those taking naproxen reported no adverse effects. The women who reported pain from TENS stated that they were prepared to accept the short term pain from the treatment in return for relief of dysmenorrhoea.[11]

Comment: None.

OPTION TOPICAL HEAT

One RCT found topical heat (about 39 °C) treatment to be as effective as ibuprofen and significantly more effective than placebo for pain relief.

Benefits: We found no systematic review. We found one efficacy RCT (see glossary, p 2074) (84 volunteer women with moderate or greater pain in at least four of their last six cycles who experienced pain relief with non-prescription analgesics and a history consistent with a diagnosis of primary dysmenorrhoea) of topically applied heat that used a double dummy (see glossary, p 2074) design with a heated or unheated patch and oral ibuprofen or placebo.[37] An abdominal patch (heated to 38.9 °C or unheated) was applied for about 12 hours daily for 2 days from the start of menses. In addition, oral medication (placebo or ibuprofen 400 mg) was given three times daily for 2 days. There were four treatment groups: heated patch plus placebo, heated patch plus ibuprofen, unheated patch plus placebo, and unheated patch plus ibuprofen. Pain relief was measured on a scale from 0 to 5; 0 was no relief and 5 complete relief of pain. After 2 days of treatment, significant pain relief was obtained with the heated patch plus placebo (mean pain score 3.27; $P < 0.001$), the heated patch plus ibuprofen (mean pain score 3.55; $P < 0.001$), and the unheated patch plus ibuprofen (mean pain score 3.07; $P = 0.001$) compared with the unheated patch plus placebo group (mean pain score 1.95). There was no difference in pain relief between the heated patch plus ibuprofen and the unheated patch plus ibuprofen groups ($P = 0.09$). However, the "time to noticeable pain relief" was significantly shorter for the heated patch plus placebo compared to the unheated patch plus placebo group (median 1.5 hours with heated patch plus placebo *v* 2.79 hours with unheated patch plus placebo; $P = 0.01$; no further data were provided).

Harms: The RCT found that women with a heated patch were more likely to report pinkness or redness of the skin than those with an unheated patch at the end of day 2 after women had used the patch for 12 continuous hours (23/40 [58%] with a heated patch *v* 5/41 [12%] with an unheated patch; OR 9.74, 95% CI 3.16 to 30.04). All women reported normal skin 3–7 days after starting treatment.

Comment: Participants in the RCT included volunteer women. Disease in these women may have a different pattern and response to treatment than disease in women seeking health care.

OPTION SURGICAL TREATMENTS

One small RCT found limited evidence suggesting that laparoscopic uterine nerve ablation increased pain relief compared with diagnostic laparoscopy. Another RCT found that laparoscopic uterine nerve ablation reduced pain at 12 months compared with laparoscopic presacral neurectomy but found no significant difference in pain relief between treatments at 3 months. It also found increased constipation with laparoscopic uterine nerve ablation.

Benefits: We found one systematic review (search date 1998, 6 RCTs) of surgical pelvic nerve interruption for primary and secondary dysmenorrhoea.[38] Only two of the six RCTs included women with primary dysmenorrhoea. Meta-analysis was not performed because of RCT heterogeneity. One RCT identified by the review (21 women) compared laparoscopic uterine nerve ablation (see glossary, p 2074) with diagnostic laparoscopy and found that LUNA significantly increased pain relief at 3 months (OR 15.5, 95% CI 2.9 to 83.0) and at 12 months (OR 10.9, 95% CI 1.5 to 77.0). The other RCT (68 women) found no significant difference between LUNA and laparoscopic presacral neurectomy (see glossary, p 2074) in pain relief at 3 months' follow up (OR 0.7, 95% CI 0.2 to 2.7). However, at 12 months' follow up, the LPSN group had significantly better pain relief scores (OR 0.26, 95% CI 0.10 to 0.71).[38]

Harms: One RCT identified by the review found that LPSN versus LUNA increased constipation (31/33 [94%] with LPSN *v* 0/35 [0%] with LUNA; RR 0.01, 95% CI 0 to 0.24).[38]

Comment: Two larger RCTs of LUNA are underway, and data will be included in an update of the systematic review (Proctor M, personal communication, 2002).[39] We found a second relevant systematic review but we have not included it because it includes lower levels of evidence, such as case studies.[40]

GLOSSARY

Behavioural interventions Treatments that attempt modification of thought and beliefs (cognition) about symptoms and pain, modification of behavioural or physiological responses to symptoms, pain, or both.

Co-proxamol Non-proprietary label for a dextropropoxyphene hydrochloride and paracetamol combination. The most common presentation is tablets containing dextropropoxyphene hydrochloride 32.5 mg and paracetamol 325 mg.

Double dummy Design pertaining to an RCT in which multiple treatments are compared (usually against a placebo) and the treatments have dissimilar presentation. Each participant will receive either active treatment or placebo for each treatment. Because multiple treatments are being compared (at least two), it allows identification of treatment effects against placebo as well as the additive effects of treatments.

Efficacy trial A trial designed to study if an intervention works in ideal conditions (e.g. when people receive treatments exactly as prescribed). In contrast, effectiveness trials evaluate the effects of treatments in "real life" conditions. Analysis in efficacy trials usually involves only the participants who had full compliance with the therapeutic scheme. The applicability of the results from efficacy trials may be limited because conditions were artificial and hence response may be different in real life situations.

High velocity, low amplitude manipulation (HVLA) A technique of spinal manipulation that uses high velocity, low amplitude thrusts to manipulate vertebral joints. The technique is designed to restore motion to a restricted joint and improve function. The physician positions the person at the barrier of restricted motion and then gives a rapid, accurate thrust in the direction of the restricted barrier to resolve the restriction and improve motion.

Laparoscopic presacral neurectomy (LPSN) Involves the total removal of the presacral nerves lying within the boundaries of the interiliac triangle. This procedure interrupts most of the cervical sensory nerve fibres and is used to diminish uterine pain.

Laparoscopic uterine nerve ablation (LUNA) Involves laparoscopic surgery to transect (usually they are cut and then electrocauterised) the uterosacral ligaments at their insertion into the cervix. This procedure interrupts most of the cervical sensory nerve fibres and is used to diminish uterine pain.

Placebo acupuncture Also known as sham acupuncture, a commonly used control intervention involving the use of acupuncture needles to stimulate non-acupuncture points in areas outside of Chinese meridians. These points can be identified by a point detector as areas of the skin that do not have skin electrical activity similar to acupuncture points. There is some disagreement over correct needle placement, as placement of a needle in any position may elicit some biological response that can complicate interpretation of results.

Placebo manipulation Also known as sham manipulation, it is a control intervention. The main principle is to use a non-therapeutic level of torque. There are two common techniques for placebo manipulation. In one, thrust is administered but the posture of the participant is such that the mechanical torque of the manipulation is substantially reduced. In the other, an activator adjusting tool is used, which can make spinal adjustments using spring recoil, where the spring is set so no force is exerted in the spine.

Toftness manipulation A low force technique of chiropractic adjusting that uses a sensometer to detect sites of abnormal electromagnetic radiation, and to determine which sites to adjust. Adjustment is then delivered using a metered, handheld pressure applicator.

Transcutaneous electrical nerve stimulation (TENS) Electrodes are placed on the skin and different electrical pulse rates and intensities are used to stimulate the area. Low frequency TENS (also referred to as acupuncture-like TENS) usually consists of pulses delivered at 1–4 Hz at high intensity so they evoke visible muscle fibre contractions. High frequency TENS (conventional TENS) usually consists of pulses delivered at 50–120 Hz at a low intensity, so there are no muscle contractions.

Visual analogue scale A commonly used scale in pain assessment. It is a 10 cm horizontal or vertical line with word anchors at each end, such as "no pain" and "pain as bad as it could be". The person is asked to make a mark on the line to represent pain intensity. This mark is converted to distance in millimetres from the "no pain" anchor to give a pain score that can range from 0–100.

Spasmodic dysmenorrhoea Spasms of acute pain that typically begin on the first day of menstruation.[41]

Congestive dysmenorrhoea A dull aching pain in the lower abdomen as well as other areas of the body that may begin several days before menstruation and can include other premenstrual symptoms such as irritability.[41]

Substantive changes

Non-steroidal anti-inflammatory drugs (other than aspirin) One RCT added;[20] conclusions unchanged.

REFERENCES

1. Fraser I. Prostaglandins, prostaglandin inhibitors and their roles in gynaecological disorders. *Bailliere's Clinical Obstet Gynaecol* 1992;6:829–857.
2. Zondervan KT, Yudkin PL, Vessey MP, et al. The prevalence of chronic pelvic pain in the United Kingdom: a systematic review. *Br J Obstet Gynaecol* 1998;105:93–99. Search date 1996; primary sources Medline, Embase, and Psychlit.
3. Harlow SD, Park M. A longitudinal study of risk factors for the occurrence, duration and severity of menstrual cramps in a cohort of college women. *Br J Obstet Gynaecol* 1996;103:1134–1142.
4. Campbell MA, McGrath PJ. Use of medication by adolescents for the management of menstrual discomfort. *Arch Pediatr Adolesc Med* 1997;151:905–913.
5. Robinson JC, Plichta S, Weisman CS, et al. Dysmenorrhoea and the use of oral contraceptives in adolescent women attending a family planning clinic. *Am J Obstet Gynecol* 1992;166:578–583.
6. Andersch B, Milsom I. An epidemiologic study of young women with dysmenorrhea. *Am J Obstet Gynecol* 1982;144:655–660.
7. Pedron Neuvo N, Gonzalez-Unzaga LN, De Celis-Carrillo R, et al. Incidence of dysmenorrhoea and associated symptoms in women aged 12–24 years. *Ginecol Obstet Mex* 1998;66:492–494.

8. Klein JR, Litt IF. Epidemiology of adolescent dysmenorrhea. *Pediatrics* 1981;68:661–664.
9. Sundell G, Milsom I, Andersch B. Factors influencing the prevalence and severity of dysmenorrhoea in young women. *Br J Obstet Gynaecol* 1990;97:588–594.
10. Chen C, Cho SI, Damokosh AI, et al. Prospective study of exposure to environmental tobacco smoke and dysmenorrhea. *Environ Health Perspect* 2000;108:1019–1022.
11. Proctor ML, Smith CA, Farquhar CM, et al. Transcutaneous electrical nerve stimulation and acupuncture for primary dysmenorrhoea. In: The Cochrane Library, Issue 2, 2002. Oxford: Update Software. Search date 2001; primary sources Cochrane Controlled Trials Register, Medline, Embase, Cinahl, Bio extracts, Psychlit, SportDiscus, Cochrane Complementary Medicine Field's Register of Controlled Trials (CISCOM), and hand searches of citation lists.
12. Helms JM. Acupuncture for the management of primary dysmenorrhea. *Obstet Gynecol* 1987;69:51–56.
13. Zhang WY, Li Wan Po A. Efficacy of minor analgesics in primary dysmenorrhoea: a systematic review. *Br J Obstet Gynaecol* 1998;105:780–789. Search date 1997; primary sources Medline, Embase, and Science Citation Index.
14. Weaver AL. Rofecoxib: clinical pharmacology and clinical experience. *Clin Ther* 2001;23:1323–1338. Search date not stated; primary sources Medline, Embase, relevant web sites, and hand searches of proceedings of relevant scientific meetings.
15. Legris M, Duhon R, Larue F, et al. Double-blind placebo-controlled study of the efficacy of niflumic acid (750 mg/day in three divided doses) in dysmenorrhea. *Rev Fr Gynecol Obstet* 1997;92:288–296.
16. Mehlisch DR, Fulmer RI. A crossover comparison of bromfenac sodium, naproxen sodium, and placebo for relief of pain from primary dysmenorrhea. *J Womens Health* 1997;6:83–92.
17. Ezcurdia M, Cortejoso FJ, Lanzon R, et al. Comparison of the efficacy and tolerability of dexketoprofen and ketoprofen in the treatment of primary dysmenorrhea. *J Clin Pharmacol* 1998;38:65S–73S.
18. Di Girolamo G, Gimeno MA, Faletti A, et al. Menstrual prostaglandin and dysmenorrhea: modulation by non-steroidal antiinflammatory drugs. *Medicina* 1999;59:259–264. [In Spanish]
19. Facchinetti F, Piccinini F, Sgarbi L, et al. Nimesulide in the treatment of primary dysmenorrhea: a double-blind study versus diclofenac. *Drugs Today* 2001;37:39–45.
20. Daniels SE, Talwalker S, Torri S, et al. Valdecoxib, a cyclooxygenase-2-specific inhibitor, is effective in treating primary dysmenorrhea. *Obstet Gynecol* 2002;100:350–358.
21. Morrison BW, Daniels SE, Kotey P, et al. Rofecoxib, a specific cyclooxygenase-2 inhibitor, in primary dysmenorrhea: a randomized controlled trial. *Obstet Gynecol* 1999;94:504–508.
22. Ylikorkala O, Puolakka J, Kauppila A. Comparison between naproxen tablets and suppositories in primary dysmenorrhea. *Prostaglandins* 1980;20:463–468.
23. Proctor ML, Sinclair OJ, Farquhar CM, et al. Non-steroidal anti-inflammatory drugs for primary dysmenorrhoea (Protocol for a Cochrane Review). In: The Cochrane Library, Issue 2, 2002. Oxford: Update Software.

24. Chesney MA, Tasto DL. The effectiveness of behavior modification with spasmodic and congestive dysmenorrhea. *Behav Res Ther* 1975;13:245–253.
25. Israel RG, Sutton M, O'Brien KF. Effects of aerobic training on primary dysmenorrhea symptomatology in college females. *J Am Coll Health* 1985;33:241–244.
26. Proctor ML, Murphy PA, Pattison HM, et al. Behavioural interventions for primary and secondary dysmenorrhoea (Protocol for a Cochrane Review). In: The Cochrane Library, Issue 2, 2002. Oxford: Update Software.
27. Proctor ML, Roberts H, Farquhar C. Combined oral contraceptives for primary dysmenorrhoea. In: The Cochrane Library, Issue 2, 2002. Oxford, Update Software. Search date 1999; primary sources Medline, Embase, Cinahl, Cochrane Controlled Trials Register, and hand searches of citation lists.
28. Nakano R, Takemura H. Treatment of function dysmenorrhoea: a double-blind study. *Acta Obstet Gynaecol Jpn* 1971;18:41–44.
29. Matthews AE, Clarke JE. Double-blind trial of a sequential oral contraceptive (Sequens) in the treatment of dysmenorrhoea. *J Obstet Gynaecol Br Commonw* 1968;75:1117–1122.
30. Proctor ML, Murphy PA. Herbal and dietary therapies for primary and secondary dysmenorrhoea. In: The Cochrane Library, Issue 2, 2002. Oxford: Update Software. Search date 2000; primary sources Medline, Embase, Cinahl, Psychlit, Bioabstracts, Cochrane Controlled Trials Register, and hand searches of citation lists.
31. Deutch B, Jorgensen EB, Hansen JC. Menstrual discomfort in Danish women reduced by dietary supplements of omega-3 PUFA and B12 (fish oil or seal oil capsules). *Nutr Res* 2000;20:621–631.
32. Barnard ND, Scialli AR, Hurlock D, et al. Diet and sex-hormone binding globulin, dysmenorrhea, and premenstrual symptoms. *Obstet Gynecol* 2000;95:245–250.
33. Ziaei S, Faghihzadeh S, Sohrabvand F, et al. A randomised placebo-controlled trial to determine the effect of vitamin E in treatment of primary dysmenorrhoea. *BJOG* 2001;108:1181–1183.
34. Proctor ML, Hing W, Johnson TC, et al. Spinal manipulation for primary and secondary dysmenorrhoea. In: The Cochrane Library, Issue 2, 2002. Oxford: Update Software. Search date 2000; primary sources Medline, Embase, Cinahl, Psychlit, Bioabstracts, SportDiscus, Cochrane Controlled Trials Register, and hand searches of citation lists.
35. Dawood MY, Ramos J. Transcutaneous electrical nerve stimulation (TENS) for the treatment of primary dysmenorrhea: a randomized crossover comparison with placebo TENS and ibuprofen. *Obstet Gynecol* 1990;75:656–660.
36. Hedner N, Milsom I, Eliasson T, et al. Tens bra vid smatsam mens. [TENS is effective in painful menstruation.] *Lakartidningen* 1996;93:1219–1222. [in Swedish]
37. Akin MD, Weingand KW, Hengehold DA, et al. Continuous low-level topical heat in the treatment of dysmenorrhea. *Obstet Gynecol* 2001;97:343–349.
38. Proctor ML, Farquhar CM, Sinclair OJ, et al. Surgical interruption of pelvic nerve pathways for primary and secondary dysmenorrhoea. In: The Cochrane Library, Issue 2, 2002. Oxford: Update Software. Search date 1998; primary sources Medline, Embase, Cochrane Controlled Trials Register, and hand searches of citation lists and conference proceedings.
39. Birmingham Women's Health Care NHS Trust. An RCT to assess the efficacy of laparoscopic

uterosacral nerve ablation (LUNA) in the treatment of chronic pelvic pain. *The National Research Register*. 2002;4:N0047063419. http://www.update-software.com/national/provUpdate.htm (last accessed 8 July 2003).

40. Khan KS, Khan SF, Nwosu CR, et al. Laparoscopic uterosacral nerve ablation in chronic pelvic pain: an overview. *Gynaecol Endosc* 1999;8:257–265. Search date 1997; primary sources Medline, Embase, and Science Citation Index.

41. Rosenwaks Z, Jones GS, Henzl MR, et al. Naproxen sodium, aspirin, and placebo in primary dysmenorrhoea. Reduction of pain and blood levels of prostaglandin-F2-alpha metabolite. *Am J Obstet Gynecol* 1981:140;592–598.

Michelle Proctor
Cochrane Review Group Co-ordinator

Cynthia Farquhar
Professor

School of Medicine
University of Auckland
Auckland
New Zealand

Competing interests: None declared.

TABLE 1 **Prevalence of dysmenorrhoea: results of community and hospital surveys (see text, p 2059).[3–8]**

Study population	Population size	Location	Year	Prevalence
College students aged 17–19 years[3]	165	USA	1996	72% (13% severe)
High school students aged 14–21 years[4]	291	Canada	1997	93% (5% severe)
Adolescents attending an inner city family planning clinic[5]	308	USA	1992	80% (18% severe)
Women from an urban population aged 19 years[6]	596	Sweden	1982	73% (15% severe)
Students aged 12–24 years[7]	1066	Mexico	1998	52–64%
Adolescents aged 12–17 years[8]	2699	USA	1981	60% (14% severe)

TABLE 2 Effects of aspirin, paracetamol, and compound analgesics for dysmenorrhoea: results of a systematic review (see text, p 2061).[13]

Comparison	Usual dosage	Number of RCTs	Number of women	Pain relief	Adverse effects	Conclusion
Aspirin *v* placebo	650 mg four times daily	8	486	RR 1.60 (95% CI 1.12 to 2.29)	More frequent on aspirin (7–17% *v* 3–17% on placebo; RR 1.3, 95% CI 0.79 to 2.17)	Aspirin more effective than placebo (NNT 10, 95% CI 5 to 50)
Aspirin *v* paracetamol	650 mg *v* 500 mg four times daily	1	35	Median pain relief: paracetamol 1.6 (95% CI 0.4 to 3.3); aspirin 1.2 (95% CI 0 to 2.7)	NA	No significant difference
Aspirin *v* naproxen	650 mg *v* 275 mg four times daily	1	32	RR 2.29 (95% CI 1.09 to 4.79)	NA	Naproxen more effective than aspirin
Aspirin *v* ibuprofen	650 mg *v* 400 mg four times daily	1	56	RR 1.9 (95% CI 1.13 to 2.78)	NA	Ibuprofen more effective than placebo
Paracetamol *v* placebo	500 mg four times daily	1	35	RR 1.00 (95% CI 0.28 to 3.63)	No significant difference (RR 1.00, 95% CI 0.36 to 2.75)	No significant difference
Paracetamol *v* ibuprofen	1000 mg *v* 400 mg three times daily	1	67	RR 0.86 (95% CI 0.68 to 1.10)	NA	No significant difference
Co-proxamol *v* placebo	650 mg/65 mg four times daily	1	72	RR 3.72 (95% CI 2.13 to 6.52)	NA	Co-proxamol more effective than placebo
Co-proxamol *v* naproxen	650 mg/65 mg *v* 275 mg three times daily	2	98	P > 0.05 (no other data could be obtained from the report)	More frequent on co-proxamol (23–58% *v* 15–25% on naproxen; RR 1.94, 95% CI 1.11 to 3.41)	No significant difference
Co-proxamol *v* mefenamic acid	650 mg/65 mg *v* 500 mg three times daily	1	30	P < 0.01 (no other evidence can be obtained from the trial)	NA	Mefenamic acid more effective than co-proxamol

NA, not available.

Endometriosis

Search date October 2002

Cynthia Farquhar

QUESTIONS

INTERVENTIONS

See glossary, p 2089

Key Messages

In women with pain attributed to endometriosis

- We found no RCTs comparing medical and surgical treatments.

- **Hormonal treatment at diagnosis (danazol, medroxyprogesterone, gestrinone, gonadorelin [gonadotrophin releasing hormone — GnRH] analogues)** Small systematic reviews and small RCTs have found that hormonal treatments (except for dydrogesterone) reduce pain attributed to endometriosis compared with placebo, and are all similarly effective.
- **Combined oral contraceptive pill** One systematic review found that combined low dose oral contraceptive significantly reduced dysmenorrhoea compared with goserelin during 6 months of treatment, but all women improved 6 months after stopping treatment. Two RCTs found no significant difference with combined oral contraceptives in overall pain relief compared with gonadorelin analogues.
- **Combined ablation of endometrial deposits and uterine nerve** One RCT found that laparoscopic ablation of deposits plus laparoscopic uterine nerve ablation reduced pain more than diagnostic laparoscopy at 6 months.
- **Cystectomy for ovarian endometrioma (better than drainage)** One RCT found that cystectomy reduced pain caused by ovarian endometrioma at 2 years compared with drainage. Complication rates were similar.
- **Postoperative hormonal treatment after conservative surgery** RCTs have found that postoperative hormonal treatment with danazol or medroxyprogesterone for 6 months reduces pain and delays the recurrence of pain at 12 and 24 months compared with placebo. One RCT found no significant difference in recurrence of pain between combined oral contraceptives and placebo at 6 months. Adverse effects of hormonal treatment are common and include hot flushes and bone loss with gonadorelin analogues and androgenic adverse effects with danazol.
- **Dydrogesterone** Systematic reviews have found no significant difference in pain at 6 months with dydrogesterone given at two different doses in the luteal phase compared with placebo.
- **Laparoscopic ablation of endometrial deposits without ablation of the uterine nerve** We found no systematic reviews or RCTs assessing the effects of laparoscopic ablation of endometrial deposits without ablation of the uterine nerve.
- **Laparoscopic uterine nerve ablation** One systematic review found insufficient evidence on the effects of laparoscopic uterine nerve ablation in women with pain attributed to endometriosis.
- **Postoperative hormonal treatment after oophorectomy** One RCT in women who previously had an oophorectomy found insufficient evidence on the effects of hormone replacement therapy in recurrence of endometriosis compared with no treatment.
- **Preoperative hormonal treatment** Two RCTs found insufficient evidence on the effects of preoperative hormonal treatments in pain attributed to endometriosis.

In women with subfertility

- **Cystectomy for ovarian endometrioma (better than drainage)** One RCT found that cystectomy increased pregnancy rates compared with drainage in women with subfertility caused by ovarian endometrioma. Complication rates were similar.
- **Laparoscopic ablation/excision of endometrial deposits** One systematic review found that laparoscopic surgery increased cumulative pregnancy rates compared with diagnostic laparoscopy after 9–12 months. We found no RCTs comparing medical and surgical treatments.

- **Hormonal treatment at diagnosis (danazol, medroxyprogesterone acetate, gonadorelin [GnRH] analogues)** One systematic review and one subsequent RCT found no significant difference between hormonal treatments and placebo in rates of pregnancy at 4–6 months.
- **Postoperative hormonal treatment (gonadorelin analogues and decapeptyl) after conservative surgery** RCTs found no significant difference between gonadorelin analogues and placebo after conservative surgery in rates of pregnancy or time to conception. Adverse effects of hormonal treatment are common and include hot flushes and bone loss with gonadorelin analogues and androgenic adverse effects with danazol.

DEFINITION Endometriosis is characterised by ectopic endometrial tissue, which can cause dysmenorrhoea, dyspareunia, non-cyclical pelvic pain, and subfertility. Diagnosis is made by laparoscopy. Most endometrial deposits are found in the pelvis (ovaries, peritoneum, uterosacral ligaments, pouch of Douglas, and rectovaginal septum). Extrapelvic deposits, including those in the umbilicus and diaphragm, are rare. Severity of endometriosis (see glossary, p 2089) is defined by the American Fertility Society: this review uses the terms mild (stage I and II), moderate (stage III), and severe (stage IV).[1] Endometriomas are cysts of endometriosis within the ovary.

INCIDENCE/ PREVALENCE In asymptomatic women, the prevalence of endometriosis ranges from 2–22%, depending on the diagnostic criteria used and the populations studied.[2–5] In women with dysmenorrhoea, the incidence of endometriosis ranges from 40–60%, and in women with subfertility from 20–30%.[3,6,7] The severity of symptoms and the probability of diagnosis increase with age.[8] Incidence peaks at about 40 years of age.[9] Symptoms and laparoscopic appearance do not always correlate.[10]

AETIOLOGY/ RISK FACTORS The cause of endometriosis is unknown. Risk factors include early menarche and late menopause. Embryonic cells may give rise to deposits in the umbilicus, whereas retrograde menstruation may deposit endometrial cells in the diaphragm.[11,12] Use of oral contraceptives reduces the risk of endometriosis, and this protective effect persists for up to 1 year after their discontinuation.[9]

PROGNOSIS We found two RCTs in which laparoscopy was repeated in women treated with placebo.[13,14] Over 6–12 months, endometrial deposits resolved spontaneously in up to a third of women, deteriorated in nearly half, and were unchanged in the remainder.

AIMS OF INTERVENTION To relieve pain (dysmenorrhoea, dyspareunia, and other pelvic pain) and to improve fertility, with minimal adverse effects.

OUTCOMES American Fertility Society scores for size and number of deposits;[1] recurrence rates; time between stopping treatment and recurrence; rate of adverse effects of treatment. **In women with pain:** Relief of pain, assessed by the Visual Analogue Scale ranging from 0 to 10, and subjective improvement. **In women with subfertility:** Cumulative pregnancy rate, live birth rate. **In women undergoing surgery:** Ease of surgical intervention (rated as easy, average, difficult, or very difficult).[15]

METHODS *Clinical Evidence* search and appraisal October 2002. The authors also sought RCTs by electronic searching of databases, hand searching of 30 key journals, searching the reference lists of other RCTs, and identifying unpublished studies from abstracts, proceedings, and pharmaceutical companies. They used the search strategy and database of the Cochrane Menstrual Disorders and Subfertility Group, updated on a monthly basis, to identify RCTs on Medline and Embase. They included RCTs that used adequate diagnostic criteria for inclusion of participants (endometriosis diagnosed either by laparoscopy or laparotomy in association with dysmenorrhoea, dyspareunia, other pelvic pain, or infertility) and clinical outcomes (see outcomes above). Studies of assisted reproductive technologies were not included. Trials comparing different hormonal treatments of the same class were not included.

QUESTION What are the effects of hormonal treatments given following diagnosis?

Four small systematic reviews and two additional RCTs have found that all different hormonal treatments, except for dydrogesterone, reduce pain attributed to endometriosis compared with placebo while the person remains on treatment, but relapses are common after treatment stops. One systematic review and one subsequent RCT found no evidence that hormonal treatments improve fertility. Adverse effects of hormonal treatments are common. One systematic review found that combined low dose oral contraceptive reduced dysmenorrhoea compared with goserelin during 6 months' treatment, but all women improved 6 months after stopping treatment.

Benefits: **In women with pain attributed to endometriosis:** We found four systematic reviews (search dates 1998,[16] 2000,[17] and 2001[18,19]) and two subsequent RCTs[20,21] comparing 6 months of continuous ovulation suppression (using danazol, gestrinone, depot medroxyprogesterone acetate, dydrogesterone, oral contraceptives, gonadorelin analogues, or cyproterone acetate) versus placebo or no treatment. The reviews found that when compared with placebo, all treatments were effective at reducing severe and moderate pain at 6 months, except dydrogesterone, which, given at two different dosages in the luteal phase, showed no evidence of effect. The first systematic review identified seven RCTs (nearly 400 women) comparing danazol versus gonadorelin analogues.[16] It found no significant difference in pain or in resolution of endometrial deposits after 6 months of treatment compared with placebo. One included RCT (49 women) compared low dose combined oral contraceptives (30 μg ethinyl oestradiol) versus gonadorelin analogues.[22] It found no significant difference in rate of relief for all types of pain, except menstrual pain, for which oral contraceptives were better. In women who received 12 months of the gonadorelin agonist, leuprolide, and who received norethisterone with or without oestrogen, pain relief was maintained for the duration of treatment and up to 8 months after treatment was stopped.[23,24] The second systematic review identified one RCT (269 women) comparing danazol 200 mg daily versus gestrinone 2.5 mg twice weekly.[25] It found no significant difference in pain reduction with danazol compared with gestrinone.

The review also included two RCTs assessing depot medroxyprogesterone acetate (140 women).[17] The larger RCT (80 women) compared depot medroxyprogesterone acetate (150 mg every 3 months) versus combined oral contraceptive plus danazol 50 mg daily. It found that depot medroxyprogesterone acetate was more effective at reducing dysmenorrhoea, but not any other outcomes. The third systematic review (1 RCT, 35 women) compared danazol versus placebo.[18] It found that danazol significantly reduced pain compared with placebo (WMD –5.7, 95% CI –7.5 to –3.9). The fourth systematic review (1 RCT, 57 women with laparoscopically diagnosed endometriosis and moderate or severe pain) found that cyclic low dose monophasic combined oral contraceptive used in a conventional manner was less effective for relief of dysmenorrhoea than goserelin 3.6 mg subcutaneous depot formulation monthly for 6 months. After 6 months of follow up without treatment, all women improved (at the end of treatment: 21/24 [88%] with combined oral contraceptive *v* 0/25 [0%] with goserelin; OR 33.1, 95% CI 10.8 to 101.0; at the end of follow up: 24/24 [100%] with combined oral contraceptive *v* 25/25 [100%] with goserelin). No significant difference was found between the oral contraceptive pill and a goserelin in the relief of dyspareunia or non-menstrual pain at the end of treatment (OR 0.93, 95% CI 0.25 to 3.53).[19] The first subsequent RCT (102 women) compared 12 months of combined oral contraceptive versus 4 months of combined oral contraceptive versus 8 months of gonadorelin analogues. It found no difference in pain (either menstrual or non-menstrual) at 12 months.[21] The second subsequent RCT (double blind, 48 women with endometriosis treated for 6 months and followed for 1 year after allocation) assessed quality of life in addition to relief of pain. It found an improvement in symptoms attributable to endometriosis and sleep disturbances and anxiety–depression scores in women treated with either gonadorelin analogues or medroxyprogesterone acetate compared with baseline measurements.[22] **In women with subfertility attributed to endometriosis:** We found one systematic review (search date 1996, 4 RCTs, 244 women with "visually diagnosed" endometriosis attempting conception for more than 12 months)[26] and one subsequent RCT.[14] The trials assessed 6 months' treatment with danazol, medroxyprogesterone, or gonadorelin analogues compared with placebo. The review found no significant effect on pregnancy rates with danazol (likelihood of pregnancy, danazol *v* placebo, RR 0.90, 95% CI 0.66 to 1.21). The subsequent RCT (100 infertile women) found no significant difference in pregnancy rates between medroxyprogesterone 50 mg daily and placebo (after 16 weeks: 0 pregnancies with medroxyprogesterone *v* 3 with placebo).[14]

Harms: **Gonadorelin (gonadotrophin releasing hormone) analogues:** The first systematic review found that gonadorelin analogues were associated with more hot flushes than placebo (about 80% with gonadorelin analogues *v* 30% with placebo, RR 2.7, 95% CI 1.5 to 4.8) and more headaches (33% gonadorelin analogues *v* 10% with placebo, RR 3.6, 95% CI 1.1 to 11.5).[16] Gonadorelin analogues are associated with hypo-oestrogenic symptoms, such as hot flushes and vaginal dryness. RCTs have found that adding oestrogen, progestogens, or tibolone significantly relieves hot flushes caused by gonadorelin analogues (reducing symptom scores by 50% or more).[15,23,24,27,28] The fourth systematic review found that compared to combined oral contraceptives, women receiving goserelin (a gonadorelin analogue) reported higher incidence of insomnia (0/28 [0%] with combined oral contraceptives *v* 7/29 [24%] with goserelin; OR 0.11, 95% CI 0.02 to 0.53) and vaginal dryness (0/28 [0%] with combined oral contraceptives *v* 5/29 [17%] with goserelin; OR 0.12, 95% CI 0.02 to 0.74).[19] **Danazol:** In one RCT of 6 months' postoperative danazol 100 mg daily compared with no treatment, danazol was associated with more adverse effects: spotting (12% with danazol *v* 7% with no treatment), bloating (16% with danazol *v* 9% with no treatment), headache (21% with danazol *v* 13% with no treatment), and weight gain (22% with danazol *v* 14% with no treatment) (see postoperative hormonal treatment, p 2086).[29] **Gestrinone:** One RCT identified by the second systematic review[17] found a significantly higher frequency of hot flushes with gestrinone compared with gonadorelin analogues; other trials found greater frequency of greasy skin and hirsutism compared with danazol, but less reduction in breast size, muscle cramps, and hunger. **Medroxyprogesterone:** The RCTs assessing hormonal treatment at diagnosis of endometriosis gave no information on adverse effects of medroxyprogesterone. One RCT (28 women with previous laparoscopic surgery) found more adverse events with depot medroxyprogesterone acetate compared with danazol plus combined oral contraceptives: amenorrhoea (20% with medroxyprogesterone acetate *v* 0% with danazol plus combined oral contraceptives), breakthrough bleeding (15% with medroxyprogesterone acetate *v* 0% with danazol plus combined oral contraceptives), spotting (65% with medroxyprogesterone acetate *v* 10% with danazol plus combined oral contraceptives); bloating (63% with medroxyprogesterone acetate *v* 28% with danazol plus combined oral contraceptives), and weight gain (53% with medroxyprogesterone acetate *v* 30% with danazol plus combined oral contraceptives).[30]

Comment: The RCTs were mainly small with no long term follow up. Trials comparing different hormonal treatments of the same class were not included. The RCT addressing quality of life had high withdrawal rates (18/48 [38%]).[22] It has been suggested that bone loss associated with prolonged use of gonadorelin analogue (12 months) may be prevented by using norethisterone with and without oestrogen.[25]

QUESTION What are the effects of surgical treatments?

OPTION LAPAROSCOPIC UTERINE NERVE ABLATION

One systematic review found insufficient evidence on the effects of laparoscopic uterine nerve ablation in women with pain attributed to endometriosis.

Benefits: We found one systematic review (search date 1998, 2 RCTs, 132 women with endometriosis, stages I–III [see glossary, p 2089], age range 18–40 years).[29] It found no significant difference in pain relief between laparoscopic uterine nerve ablation and laparoscopic treatment without laparoscopic uterine nerve ablation. The largest trial (81 women) identified by the review found that satisfaction with treatment was high in both groups (73% with control *v* 68% with laparoscopic uterine nerve ablation).

Harms: The RCTs gave no information on adverse effects.[29] Potential harms include denervation of pelvic structures and uterine prolapse.

Comment: The RCTs included in the review may have been too small to exclude a significant effect.[29]

OPTION LAPAROSCOPIC ABLATION OF ENDOMETRIAL DEPOSITS

One systematic review in women with pain attributed to endometriosis found limited evidence that ablation of deposits plus laparoscopic uterine nerve ablation reduced pain at 6 months compared with diagnostic laparoscopy, and that reduction persisted for several years in more than half the women. Another systematic review found that laparoscopic surgery increased fertility after 9–12 months compared with diagnostic laparoscopy in women with subfertility attributed to mild or moderate endometriosis.

Benefits: We found two systematic reviews (search dates 1999[31] and 2001[32]). The first systematic review was of women with pain associated with endometriosis[31] and the second one of women with subfertility associated with endometriosis.[32] **In women with pain attributed to endometriosis:** The systematic review included one RCT (63 women with mild to moderate (see glossary, p 2089) endometriosis) comparing ablation of deposits plus laparoscopic uterine nerve ablation and diagnostic laparoscopy.[31,33,34] It found that ablation plus laparoscopic uterine nerve ablation reduced pain at 6 months (median decrease in pain score 2.85 with ablation *v* 0.05 with diagnostic laparoscopy; $P = 0.01$), and that 55% continued to have pain improvement 5 years later.[31,33,34] **In women with subfertility attributed to endometriosis:** We found one systematic review (search date 2001, 2 RCTs, 437 women with subfertility attributed to mild or moderate endometriosis).[32] It found that laparoscopic ablation/excision of mild to moderate endometriotic deposits significantly increased pregnancy rates compared with diagnostic laparoscopy alone in women with subfertility attributed to mild or moderate endometriosis (ongoing pregnancy at 20 weeks or live birth: 2 RCTs, 437 women; OR 1.64, 95% CI 1.05 to 2.57).[32] **Laser compared with diathermy ablation:** We found no RCTs.

Harms: The systematic review of women with subfertility found that operative complications were significantly higher with laparoscopic surgery compared with diagnostic laparoscopy alone. Only one RCT reported on adverse events and four women (3 in the surgery group) had minor intraoperative complications but none required laparotomy or transfusion as a result (OR 2.69, 95% CI 0.38 to 19.30). Sixteen women (6% with laparoscopic surgery *v* 4% with diagnostic laparoscopy; raw data not provided) reported minor postoperative complications.[32] Other potential harms include adhesions, reduced fertility, and damage to other pelvic structures.

Comment: The number of trials and the total number of women randomised is small and further trials would be welcome. A further RCT of laparoscopic uterine nerve ablation is underway in Auckland, New Zealand. One hundred and ten women were randomised and 12 months' follow up data were due by the end of 2002 (Farquhar C, personal communication, 2003). The systematic review assessing pregnancy rates in women with subfertility attributed to endometriosis found that women were followed for 36 weeks after laparoscopy, but does not state the follow up time for the other included RCT.[32]

QUESTION What are the effects of hormonal treatment after conservative surgery?

RCTs have found that 6 months of postoperative hormonal treatment with danazol or gonadorelin analogues reduces pain and delays the recurrence of pain compared with placebo. Treatment for 3 months or treatment with combined oral contraceptives does not seem to be effective. RCTs found no evidence of an effect of postoperative hormonal treatment on fertility after conservative surgery. Adverse effects of hormonal treatment are common and include hot flushes and bone loss with gonadorelin analogues and androgenic adverse effects with danazol.

Benefits: We found no systematic review. We found seven placebo controlled RCTs, and one RCT comparing expectant management of medical treatment in women who had undergone surgery for endometriosis (4 RCTs of gonadorelin analogues, 2 RCTs of danazol, 1 RCT of combined oral contraceptive, and 1 RCT comparing danazol to depot medroxyprogesterone acetate and to expectant management).[29,35–41] We found one RCT comparing low dose continuous cyproterone acetate and continuous monophasic oral contraceptive pill.[42] **In women with pain attributed to endometriosis:** One RCT (77 women with moderate to severe endometriosis) compared postoperative danazol 600 mg daily to placebo for 3 months after surgery. It found no significant difference in pain relief 6 months after finishing treatment (moderate to severe pain: 7/31 [23%] with danazol *v* 9/29 [31%] with no treatment; RR 0.73, 95% CI 0.31 to 1.70).[36] A second RCT (28 women with moderate endometriosis who had undergone conservative surgery followed by monthly injections of decapeptyl for 6 months) compared danazol 100 mg daily for 6 months to expectant management.[29] It found that danazol significantly reduced pain at both 12 months ($P < 0.01$) and 24 months ($P < 0.05$). Overall recurrence at 24 months was 44% with danazol compared with 67% with expectant management ($P < 0.05$). A third RCT (60 women with mild to severe (see glossary, p 2089) endometriosis) found that postoperative danazol 600 mg daily or medroxyprogesterone 100 mg daily for 180 days reduced pain more than placebo at 6 months.[37] Four RCTs assessed gonadorelin analogues.[35,36,39,41] The first RCT (75 women with endometriosis stages I and II) compared 3 months' treatment with nafarelin versus placebo in women who had laparotomy as part of their endometriosis treatment, and were followed for 12 months. It found no difference in pain relief at 12 months.[35] The second RCT (89 women with endometriosis stages III and IV) compared monthly intramuscular leuprolide acetate depot injections for 3 months versus expectant management with 36 months of follow up in women after laparoscopic conservative surgery.[41] It found no significant difference in pain (moderate to severe pain recurrence during follow up, 10/44 [23%] with gonadorelin analogue v 11/45 [24%] with no treatment; cumulative pain recurrence rates at 18 months, 23% with gonadorelin analogue v 29% with no treatment; log rank test not significant) or fertility (pregnancies: 5/15 [33%] with gonadorelin analogue v 6/15 [40%] with no treatment; P > 0.05; cumulative pregnancy rates at 30 months presented in survival analysis graph; log rank test not significant). The two larger RCTs (109 women[38] and 269 women[39] with mild to moderate symptomatic endometriosis after conservative surgery) assessed 6 months of treatment (nafarelin 200 μg twice daily for 6 months and followed for 24 months;[38] and open label allocation of 3.6 mg of subcutaneous goserelin versus expectant management with 2 years of follow up[39]) found that gonadorelin analogues significantly reduced pain scores (P = 0.008)[38] and delayed the recurrence of pain by more than 12 months.[38,39] One small RCT (70 women) comparing combined oral contraceptives to placebo postoperatively for 6 months found no reduction in the recurrence of pain associated with endometriosis[39] (mean follow up 22 months; recurrences 2/33 [6%] with oral contraceptives v 1/35 [3%] with no treatment; RR 2.1, 95% CI 0.2 to 22.3).[40] One RCT (open label, 90 women with recurrent pelvic pain of more than 6 months' duration after complete surgical eradication of endometriosis) compared low dose continuous cyproterone acetate versus continuous monophasic oral contraceptive pill.[42] It found that both treatments were similarly effective and safe in women with modest and severe pain.[42] It found no significant difference between treatments in the proportion of women who were satisfied with treatment (33/45 [73%] with cyproterone acetate v 30/45 [67%] with oral contraceptive; RR 1.1, 95% CI 0.8 to 1.4). **In women with subfertility attributed to endometriosis:** Three of the RCTs (28, 75, and 269 women, all stages of endometriosis) assessed the effects of postoperative hormonal treatment (decapeptyl and gonadorelin analogues) versus placebo on fertility and found no difference in pregnancy rates or time to conception.[29,35,39]

Harms: See harms of hormonal treatments, p 2083.

Comment: The RCTs were mainly small with no long term follow up.

QUESTION **What are the effects of hormonal treatment on women with endometriosis who have had oophorectomy (with or without hysterectomy)**

One RCT in women who previously had an oophorectomy found insufficient evidence on the effects of hormone replacement therapy compared with no treatment.

Benefits: We found no systematic review. We found one RCT (172 women who previously had bilateral salpingo-oophorectomy for any reason with or without hysterectomy) comparing HRT (115 women) versus no treatment (57 women).[43] HRT consisted of two weekly 1.5 mg oestradiol patches and 200 mg daily of micronised progesterone given orally during 14 days followed by a 16 day interval free of treatment. HRT was started 4 weeks after the salpingo-oophorectomy. It found no significant difference in recurrence rates at a mean of 45 months (0/57 [0%] without HRT *v* 4/115 [4%] with HRT; ARI +3.5%, 95% CI –3.2% to +8.6%).

Harms: The RCT found that surgical reinterventions were more frequent with HRT but this difference was not significant (2.6% with HRT *v* 0% with no HRT; OR 4.5, 95% CI 0.4 to 60.0).[43] The risk factors for recurrence were women who had endometriotic peritoneal involvement > 3 cm (2.4% recurrence a year with HRT *v* 0.3% with no HRT) and incomplete surgery (22.2% with HRT *v* 1.9% with no HRT).

Comment: The RCT had insufficient power to rule out clinically important differences.[43]

QUESTION What are the effects of preoperative hormonal treatment?

One RCT found no significant difference in ease of surgery with preoperative treatment with gonadorelin (gonadotrophin releasing hormone) analogues compared with no treatment. One RCT found no significant difference in the difficulty of surgery with preoperative treatment with gonadorelin analogues. Both treatments measured subjective assessment by the surgeon.

Benefits: We found no systematic review but found two RCTs.[42,44] Both compared 3 months' preoperative treatment with a gonadorelin analogue with no treatment. The first RCT (75 women with moderate or severe [see glossary, p 2089] endometriosis)[42] assessed ease of surgery as judged subjectively by the surgeon. It found no significant difference in ease of surgery between women receiving 200 μg of intranasal nafarelin compared with no preoperative nafarelin (Easy to treat: 14/25 [56%] with nafarelin *v* 10/28 [36%] without nafarelin; RR 1.60, 95% CI 0.86 to 2.90).[42] The second RCT assessed whether surgeons would describe a surgery to be moderately or very difficult. It found no significant differences in surgeons' ratings for women receiving gonadorelin analogues compared with women with no treatment (14/20 [70%] with gonadorelin analogues *v* 20/27 [74%] with no treatment; RR 0.94, 95% CI 0.60 to 1.50).[44]

Harms: Adverse events were frequently experienced both in women receiving preoperative gonadorelin analogues and those receiving no treatment (at least one adverse event: 18/21 [86%] with gonadorelin analogue *v* 21/27 [78%] with no treatment; *Clinical Evidence* recalculation: RR 1.1, 95% CI 0.8 to 1.4). The most frequently reported adverse effects were hot flushes and headaches, and these happened only in women receiving gonadorelin analogue (hot flushes 13/21 [62%], headaches 6/21 [29%]).[44] See harms of hormonal treatments, p 2083.

Comment: The trial may have been too small to exclude a clinically significant effect.

QUESTION What are the effects of treatments for ovarian endometrioma?

OPTION LAPAROSCOPIC DRAINAGE VERSUS LAPAROSCOPIC CYSTECTOMY

One RCT found that pain and fertility improved more with cystectomy compared with drainage, with no evidence of a difference in complication rates.

Benefits: We found no systematic review. We found one RCT (64 women) comparing laparoscopic cystectomy to laparoscopic drainage and coagulation.[45] **In women with pain attributed to endometrioma:** The RCT found that cystectomy versus drainage significantly reduced recurrence of pain at 2 years (OR 0.2, 95% CI 0.1 to 0.8) and increased the pain free interval after operation (median interval; 19 months with cystectomy *v* 9.5 months with drainage; $P < 0.05$).[45] **In women with subfertility attributed to endometrioma:** The RCT found that compared with drainage, cystectomy significantly increased the pregnancy rate (67% with cystectomy *v* 24% with drainage; OR 8.3, 95% CI 1.2 to 59.0).[45]

Harms: The RCT reported no intraoperative or postoperative complications in either group.[45]

Comment: None.

GLOSSARY

Severity of endometriosis Determination of the stage or degree of endometrial involvement is based on a weighted point scale of arbitrary estimations, evaluating the degree of involvement of the peritoneum, ovaries, and tubes.[1] According to the allocated score, endometriosis is categorised as:

Mild (stage I and II) 1–15 points
Moderate (stage III) 16–40 points
Severe (stage IV) > 40 points

Substantive changes

Hormonal treatments following diagnosis Two systematic reviews updated[18,19] and a report of long term follow up of an RCT added;[24] conclusions unchanged.
Laparoscopic deposit ablation Two systematic reviews added; one in women with pain[31] and the other one in women with subfertility attributed to endometriosis;[32] conclusions unchanged.
Preoperative hormonal treatments One RCT added;[44] conclusions unchanged.

REFERENCES

1. American Fertility Society. Revised American Fertility Society (RAFS) classification of endometriosis. *Fertil Steril* 1985;43:351–352.
2. Mahmood TA, Templeton A. Prevalence and genesis of endometriosis. *Hum Reprod* 1991;6:544–549.
3. Gruppo Italiano per lo studio dell'endometriosi. Prevalence and anatomical distribution of endometriosis in women with selected gynaecological conditions: results from a multicentric Italian study. *Hum Reprod* 1994;9:1158–1162.
4. Moen MH, Schei B. Epidemiology of endometriosis in a Norwegian County. *Acta Obstet Gynecol Scand* 1997;76:559–562.
5. Eskenazi B, Warner ML. Epidemiology of endometriosis. *Obstet Gynecol Clin North Am* 1997;24:235–258.
6. Ajossa S, Mais V, Guerriero S, et al. The prevalence of endometriosis in premenopausal women undergoing gynecological surgery. *Clin Exp Obstet Gynecol* 1994;21:195–197.
7. Waller KG, Lindsay P, Curtis P, et al. The prevalence of endometriosis in women with infertile partners. *Eur J Obstet Gynecol Reprod Biol* 1993;48:135–139.
8. Berube S, Marcoux S, Maheux R. Characteristics related to the prevalence of minimal or mild endometriosis in infertile women. Canadian Collaborative Group on Endometriosis. *Epidemiology* 1998;9:504–510.

9. Vessey MP, Villard-Mackintosh L, Painter R. Epidemiology of endometriosis in women attending family planning clinics. *BMJ* 1993;306:182–184.
10. Vercellini P, Trespidi L, DeGiorgi O, et al. Endometriosis and pelvic pain: relation to disease stage and localization. *Fertil Steril* 1996;65:299–304.
11. Rock JA, Markham SM. Pathogenesis of endometriosis. *Lancet* 1992;340:1264–1267.
12. McLaren J, Prentice A. New aspects of pathogenesis of endometriosis. *Curr Obstet Gynaecol* 1996;6:85–91.
13. Cooke ID, Thomas EJ. The medical treatment of mild endometriosis. *Acta Obstet Gynecol Scand Suppl* 1989;150:27–30.
14. Harrison RF, Barry-Kinsella C. Efficacy of medroxyprogesterone treatment in infertile women with endometriosis: a prospective, randomized, placebo-controlled study. *Fertil Steril* 2000;74:24–30.
15. Compston JE, Yamaguchi K, Croucher PI, et al. The effects of gonadotrophin-releasing hormone agonists on iliac crest cancellous bone structure in women with endometriosis. *Bone* 1995;16:261–267.
16. Prentice A, Deary AJ, Goldbeck-Wood S, et al. Gonadotrophin releasing hormone analogues for pain associated with endometriosis. In: The Cochrane Library, Issue 2, 2001. Oxford: Update Software. Search date 1998; primary sources Medline, Embase, Cochrane Controlled Trials Register, and unpublished trials by UK distributors of gonadotrophin releasing hormone analogues.
17. Prentice A, Deary AJ, Bland E. Progestogens and antiprogestogens for pain associated with endometriosis. In: The Cochrane Library, Issue 2, 2001. Oxford: Update Software. Search date 2000; primary sources Medline, Embase, and Cochrane Controlled Trials Register.
18. Selak V, Farquhar C, Prentice A, et al. Danazol versus placebo for the treatment of endometriosis. In: The Cochrane Library, Issue 4, 2001. Oxford: Update Software. Search date 2001; primary sources Medline, Embase, Cochrane Controlled Trials Register, and hand searches of journals and conference proceedings.
19. Moore J, Kennedy S, Prentice A. Modern combined oral contraceptives for the treatment of painful symptoms associated with endometriosis. In: The Cochrane Library, Issue 4, 2002. Oxford: Update Software. Search date 2001; primary sources Medline, Embase, and Cochrane Controlled Trials Register.
20. Parazzini F, Di Cintio E, Chatenoud L, et al. Estroprogestin vs. gonadotrophin agonists plus estroprogestin in the treatment of endometriosis-related pelvic pain: a randomized trial. Gruppo Italiano per lo Studio dell'Endometriosis. *Eur J Obstet Gynecol Reprod Biol* 2000;88:11–14.
21. Bergqvist A, Theorell T. Changes in quality of life after hormonal treatment of endometriosis. *Acta Obstet Gynecol Scand* 2001;80:628–637.
22. Vercellini P, Trespidi L, Colombo A, et al. A gonadotropin-releasing hormone agonist versus a low-dose oral contraceptive for pelvic pain associated with endometriosis. *Fertil Steril* 1993;60:75–79.
23. Hornstein MD, Surrey ES, Weisberg GW, et al. Leuprolide acetate depot and hormonal add-back in endometriosis: a 12-month study. Lupron Add-Back Study Group. *Obstet Gynecol* 1998; 91:16–24.
24. Surrey ES, Hornstein MD. Prolonged GnRH agonist and add-back therapy for symptomatic endometriosis: long-term follow-up. *Obstet Gynecol* 2002;99:709–719
25. Bromham DR, Bookere MW, Rose R, et al. Updating the clinical experience in endometriosis: the European perspective. *B J Obstet Gynaecol* 1995(suppl);102:12–16.
26. Hughes E, Fedorkow D, Collins J, et al. Ovulation suppression versus placebo in the treatment of endometriosis. In: The Cochrane Library, Issue 2, 2001. Oxford: Update Software. Search date 1996; primary sources Medline, Embase, Cochrane Controlled Trials Register, and hand searches of journals and conference proceedings.
27. Gregoriou O, Konidaris S, Vitoratos N, et al. Gonadotropin-releasing hormone analogue plus hormone replacement therapy for the treatment of endometriosis: a randomized controlled trial. *Int J Fertil Womens Med* 1997;42:406–411.
28. Taskin O, Yalcinoglu AI, Kucuk S. Effectiveness of tibolone on hypoestrogenic symptoms induced by goserelin treatment in patients with endometriosis. *Fertil Steril* 1997;67:40–45.
29. Proctor M, Farquhar CM, Sinclair O, et al. Surgical interruption of pelvic nerve pathways for primary and secondary dysmenorrhoea. In: The Cochrane Library, Issue 2, 2001. Oxford: Update Software. Search date 1998; primary sources Medline, Embase, Cochrane Controlled Trials Register, and hand searches of journals, conference proceedings, and references.
30. Morgante G. Low-dose danazol after combined surgical and medical therapy reduces the incidence of pelvic pain in women with moderate and severe endometriosis. *Hum Reprod* 1999;14:2371–2374.
31. Jacobson TZ, Barlow DH, Garry R, et al. Laparoscopic surgery for pelvic pain associated with endometriosis (Cochrane Review). In: The Cochrane Library, Issue 4, 2002. Oxford: Update Software. Search date 1999; primary sources Medline, Embase, The Cochrane Menstrual Disorders and Subfertility Group's Specialised Register of controlled trials, and the National Research Register.
32. Jacobson TZ, Barlow DH, Koninckx PR, et al. Laparoscopic surgery for subfertility associated with endometriosis (Cochrane Review). In: The Cochrane Library, Issue 4, 2002. Oxford: Update Software. Search date 2001; primary sources The Cochrane Menstrual Disorders and Subfertility Group's specialised register of trials, Cochrane Controlled Trials Register, the National Research Register, Medline, Embase, and reference lists of articles.
33. Sutton CJG, Ewen SP, Whitelaw N, et al. A prospective, randomised, double-blind, controlled trial of laser laparoscopy in the treatment of pelvic pain associated with minimal, mild and moderate endometriosis. *Fertil Steril* 1994;62:696–700.
34. Sutton CJG, Pooley AS, Ewen SP. Follow-up report on a randomised, controlled trial of laser laparoscopy in the treatment of pelvic pain associated with minimal to moderate endometriosis. *Fertil Steril* 1997;68:170–174.
35. Parazzini F, Fedele L, Busacca M, et al. Postsurgical medical treatment of advanced endometriosis: results of a randomized clinical trial. *Am J Obstet Gynecol* 1994;171:1205–1207.
36. Bianchi S, Busacca M, Agnoli B, et al. Effects of 3 month therapy with danazol after laparoscopic surgery for stage III/IV endometriosis: a randomized study. *Hum Reprod* 1999;14:1335–1337.
37. Telimaa S, Ronnberg L, Kauppila A. Placebo-controlled comparison of danazol and

high-dose medroxyprogesterone acetate in the treatment of endometriosis after conservative surgery. *Gynecol Endocrinol* 1987;1:363–371.
38. Hornstein MD, Hemmings R, Yuzpe AA, et al. Use of nafarelin versus placebo after reductive laparoscopic surgery for endometriosis. *Fertil Steril* 1997;68:860–864.
39. Vercellini P, Crosignani PG, Fadini R, et al. A gonadotrophin-releasing hormone agonist compared with expectant management after conservative surgery for symptomatic endometriosis. *Br J Obstet Gynaecol* 1999;106:672–677.
40. Muzii L, Marana R, Caruana P, et al. Postoperative administration of monophasic combined oral contraceptives after laparoscopic treatment of ovarian endometriosis: a prospective, randomized trial. *Am J Obstet Gynecol* 2000;183:588–592.
41. Busacca M, Somigliana E, Bianchi S, et al. Post-operative GnRH analogue treatment after conservative surgery for symptomatic endometriosis stage III–IV: a randomized controlled trial. *Hum Reprod* 2001;16:2399–2402.
42. Audebert A, Descampes P, Marret H, et al. Pre or post operative medical treatment with nafarelin in Stage III–IV endometriosis: a French multicentered study. *Eur J Obstet Gynecol Reprod Biol* 1998;79:145–148.
43. Vercellini P, De Giorgi O, Mosconi P, et al. Cyproterone acetate versus a continuous monophasic oral contraceptive in the treatment of recurrent pelvic pain after conservative surgery for symptomatic endometriosis. *Fertil Steril* 2002;77:52–61.
44. Shaw R, Garry R, McMillan L, et al. A prospective randomized open study comparing goserelin (Zoladex) plus surgery and surgery alone in the management of ovarian endometriomas. *Gynaecol Endosc* 2001;10:151–157.
45. Beretta P, Franchi M, Ghezzi F, et al. Randomised clinical trial of two laparoscopic treatments of endometriomas: cystectomy versus drainage and coagulation. *Fertil Steril* 1998;709:1176–1180.

Cynthia Farquhar
Professor
School of Medicine
University of Auckland
Auckland
New Zealand

Competing interests: None declared.

Fibroids (uterine myomatosis, leiomyomas)

Search date August 2002

Anne Lethaby and Beverley Vollenhoven

QUESTIONS

INTERVENTIONS

To be covered in future updates

Acupuncture/integrative medicines

Covered elsewhere in *Clinical Evidence*

Menorrhagia: many women with fibroids experience symptoms of heavy menstrual bleeding (see menorrhagia, p 2151)

*Based on consensus.

See glossary, p 2104

Key Messages

Medical treatment alone

- **Gonadorelin analogues alone** RCTs have found that gonadorelin analogues reduce fibroid related symptoms compared with placebo, but are associated with important adverse effects. One RCT found that nafarelin versus placebo significantly increased amenorrhoea at 12 weeks. One systematic review found insufficient evidence to compare nafarelin versus buserelin. One RCT found that higher versus lower doses of nafarelin significantly increased amenorrhoea at 16 weeks. Two RCTs found that nafarelin versus placebo significantly reduced bone density from baseline after 16 weeks' treatment, but that bone density returned to pretreatment levels 6 months after treatment was stopped. Two RCTs found that hot flushes were significantly more common with nafarelin versus placebo or buserelin.

- **Gonadorelin analogue plus combined oestrogen and progestogen** We found insufficient evidence from one small RCT to compare effects on fibroid related symptoms of gonadorelin analogue plus combined oestrogen and progestogen versus gonadorelin analogues plus progesterone alone.
- **Gonadorelin analogues plus progestogen** One small RCT found that leuprorelin (leuprolide) acetate plus progesterone significantly reduced heavy bleeding compared with leuprorelin acetate alone. Two small RCTs found that gonadorelin analogue plus progesterone significantly reduced the proportion of women with hot flushes compared with gonadorelin analogue alone.
- **Gonadorelin analogue plus tibolone** One small RCT found no significant difference with gonadorelin analogue alone versus gonadorelin analogue plus tibolone on uterine and fibroid size and fibroid related symptoms.
- **Non-steroidal anti-inflammatory drugs** We found insufficient evidence from two small RCTs about the effects of non-steroidal anti-inflammatory drugs on heavy menstrual bleeding in women with uterine fibroids.
- **Gestrinone; levonorgestrel intrauterine system; mifepristone** We found no RCTs on the effects of these interventions.

Preoperative medical treatment

- **Gonadorelin analogues** One systematic review and one additional RCT have found that gonadorelin analogues versus placebo or no treatment given at least 3 months before fibroid surgery increase haemoglobin and haematocrit, and reduce uterine and pelvic symptoms and blood loss during surgery. Women having hysterectomy are more likely to have a vaginal rather than an abdominal procedure after gonadorelin treatment. However, women are more likely to experience adverse hypo-oestrogenic effects from preoperative treatment.

Effects of surgical treatments

- **Abdominal hysterectomy** We found no RCTs. There is consensus that abdominal hysterectomy is superior to no treatment in reducing fibroid related symptoms.
- **Laparoscopic assisted vaginal hysterectomy** We found no RCTs comparing long term effects of laparoscopic assisted vaginal hysterectomy versus other treatments. One small RCT found limited evidence that women having laparoscopically assisted vaginal hysterectomy had shorter recovery and less postoperative pain compared with women having total abdominal hysterectomy.
- **Laparoscopic myomectomy (compared with abdominal myomectomy)** One RCT found that laparoscopic myomectomy versus abdominal myomectomy resulted in lower postoperative pain, and a shorter recovery time.
- **Thermal balloon endometrial ablation** We found no RCTs comparing thermal balloon ablation versus non-surgical treatment or versus hysterectomy. One RCT compared thermal balloon ablation versus rollerball endometrial ablation in women with fibroids smaller than the average size of a 12 week pregnancy, all of whom had been pretreated with gonadorelin analogues. It found no significant difference between thermal balloon and rollerball ablation in hysterectomy rates, amenorrhoea rates, pictorial bleeding assessment chart score,

or haemoglobin at 12 months. It found that thermal balloon ablation reduced operation time and intraoperative complication rate compared with rollerball ablation. About one third of women reported being "not very satisfied" with either operation.

DEFINITION Fibroids (uterine leiomyomas) are benign tumours of the smooth muscle cells of the uterus. Women with fibroids can be asymptomatic or can present with menorrhagia (30%), dysmenorrhoea, pelvic pain, pressure symptoms, infertility, and recurrent pregnancy loss.[1] However, much of the data describing the relationship between the presence of fibroids and symptoms are based on uncontrolled studies that have assessed the effect of myomectomy (see glossary, p 2104) on the presenting symptom.[2]

INCIDENCE/ PREVALENCE The reported incidence of fibroids varies from 5.4–77% depending on the method of diagnosis (the gold standard is histological evidence). A random sample of 335 Swedish women aged 25–40 years was reported to have an incidence of fibroids of 5.4% (95% CI 3.0% to 7.8%) based on transvaginal ultrasound examination. The prevalence of these tumours increased with age (age 25–32 years: 3.3%, 95% CI 0.7% to 6.0%; 33–40 years: 7.8%, 95% CI 3.6% to 12%).[3] Based on postmortem examination of women, 50% were found to have these tumours.[4] Gross serial sectioning at 2 mm intervals of 100 consecutive hysterectomy specimens revealed the presence of fibroids in 77%. These women were having hysterectomies for reasons other than fibroids.[5] The incidence of fibroids in black women is three times greater than that in white women, based on ultrasound or hysterectomy diagnosis.[6] Submucosal fibroids have been diagnosed in 6–34% of women having a hysteroscopy for abnormal bleeding, and in 2–7% of women having infertility investigations.[7]

AETIOLOGY/ RISK FACTORS The cause of uterine fibroids is unknown. It is known that each fibroid is of monoclonal origin and arises independently.[8,9] Factors thought to be involved include the sex steroid hormones oestrogen and progesterone as well as the insulin-like growth factors, epidermal growth factor and transforming growth factor. Risk factors for fibroid growth include nulliparity and obesity. There is a risk reduction to a fifth with five term pregnancies, compared with nulliparous women ($P < 0.001$).[10] Obesity increases the risk of fibroid development by 21% with each 10 kg weight gain ($P = 0.008$).[10] Factors associated with reduced incidence of fibroids include cigarette smoking and hormonal contraception. Women who smoke 10 cigarettes a day have an 18% lowered risk of fibroid development compared with non-smokers ($P = 0.036$).[10] The combined oral contraceptive pill reduces the risk of fibroids with increasing duration of use compared with never users (users for 4–6 years: OR 0.8, 95% CI 0.5 to 1.2; users for ≥ 7 years: OR 0.5, 95% CI 0.3 to 0.9).[11] Women who have used injections containing 150 mg depot medroxyprogesterone acetate also have a reduced incidence compared with women who have never used (OR 0.44, 95% CI 0.36 to 0.55).[12]

PROGNOSIS There are few data on the long term untreated prognosis of these tumours, particularly in women who are asymptomatic at diagnosis. One small case control study reported that in a group of 106 women treated with observation alone over 1 year there was no significant change in symptoms and quality of life over that time.[13]

AIMS OF INTERVENTION To reduce menstrual bleeding; prevent or correct iron deficiency anaemia; reduce pressure symptoms; reduce pelvic pain; and induce a change in fertility status with minimal adverse effects.

OUTCOMES Menstrual blood flow (assessed objectively [mL/cycle] or subjectively); haemoglobin and haematocrit concentration; pregnancy rate; relief of pelvic pain, pressure, or both (measured by a validated scale or subjective report); reduction in fibroid and uterine volume. Some of the outcomes relate to surgery: ease of surgery; complication rates during and after surgery; blood loss during surgery; duration of surgery; length of hospital stay; rate of blood transfusions; probability of transverse versus vertical incisions during surgery; probability of vaginal versus abdominal hysterectomy; change in quality of life; recurrence rate; satisfaction rate.

METHODS *Clinical Evidence* search and appraisal August 2002.

QUESTION What are the effects of medical treatments?

OPTION GONADORELIN ANALOGUES (GNRHA) WITHOUT HORMONE REPLACEMENT THERAPY

RCTs have found that gonadorelin analogues reduce fibroid related symptoms compared with placebo, but are associated with important adverse effects. One RCT found that nafarelin versus placebo significantly increased amenorrhoea at 12 weeks. One systematic review found insufficient evidence to compare nafarelin versus buserelin. One RCT found that higher versus lower doses of nafarelin significantly increased amenorrhoea at 16 weeks. Two RCTs found that nafarelin versus placebo significantly reduced bone density from baseline after 16 weeks' treatment, but that bone density returned to pretreatment levels 6 months after treatment was stopped. Two RCTs found that hot flushes were significantly more common with nafarelin versus placebo or buserelin.

Benefits: **Versus placebo:** We found one systematic review of nafarelin (search date 1997, 1 RCT, 101 women).[14] The RCT identified by the systematic review found that intranasal nafarelin (200 μg twice daily) versus placebo significantly increased the proportion of women with amenorrhoea at 3 months (33/64 [51%] women amenorrhoeic with nafarelin *v* 3/37 [8%] with placebo, $P \leq 0.05$).[14] **Versus other gonadorelin analogues:** We found one systematic review (search date 1997) that identified one RCT (211 women enrolled) comparing intranasal nafarelin versus intranasal buserelin.[14] The RCT found that nafarelin (200 μg twice daily) versus buserelin (300 μg 3 times daily) significantly increased haemoglobin at 16 weeks (haemoglobin 12.8 g/dL with nafarelin *v* 12.3 g/dL with buserelin; $P = 0.03$). However, the RCT did not describe the clinical importance of this difference. **Versus**

different doses: We found one systematic review (search date 1997) that identified one RCT (257 women) comparing different doses of nafarelin (50 µg, 100 µg, 200 µg, and 400 µg twice daily).[14] The RCT found that higher versus lower doses of nafarelin significantly increased the proportion of women who were amenorrhoeic at 16 weeks (women amenorrhoeic 41/59 [69.5%] with 50 µg *v* 46/54 [85.2%] with 100 µg *v* 40/48 [83.3%] with 200 µg *v* 52/57 [91.2%] with 400 µg; P = 0.0053 for dose response effect). **Different modes of administration:** We found no systematic review and no RCTs that measured effects on clinical outcomes (see comment below). **Versus GnRHa plus hormonal treatment:** See benefits of GnRHa plus hormone replacement therapy, p 2097.

Harms: **Versus placebo:** The systematic review identified two RCTs, which found that nafarelin (200 µg) versus placebo reduced bone density by 2.5% from baseline after 16 weeks' treatment.[14] Six months after treatment was withdrawn, bone density had increased to values that were not significantly different from baseline. Many women reported hot flushes during nafarelin treatment (rates ranged from 39% to 100% across 5 RCTs in the review). One RCT found that hot flushes were more common with nafarelin versus placebo (61% women with nafarelin *v* 36% with placebo; P = 0.02).[14] **Versus other gonadorelin analogues:** The RCT identified by the review found that a significantly higher proportion of women had hot flushes with nafarelin versus buserelin (38.5% with nafarelin *v* 23.4% with buserelin; P = 0.025), but this caused few to discontinue treatment (data not provided).[14]

Comment: **Versus placebo:** We found four additional RCTs (154 women) comparing gonadorelin analogues versus placebo.[15–18] All had important methodological weaknesses. The first RCT (13 participating centres, 128 women, 24 wks' treatment) had high withdrawal rates, precluding reliable comparison of treatments.[15] It found that leuprorelin versus placebo was associated with vasomotor flushes, vaginitis, arthralgia/myalgia, asthenia, peripheral oedema, nausea, and insomnia (see table 1, p 2107).[15] The RCT found no significant difference with nafarelin versus placebo in the risk of developing emotional lability/nervousness, depression, headaches, or decreased libido, although sample size may have been insufficient to rule out clinically significant differences for all these outcomes (see table 1, p 2107).[15] The second RCT (38 premenopausal women) did not assess clinical outcomes.[16] The other two RCTs were too small to yield reliable results (12 women[17] and 15 women[18]). Two of these RCTs found that fibroids returned to their previous size after stopping treatment.[15,16] **Versus other gonadorelin analogues:** We found four additional small RCTs (171 women in total).[19–22] Two RCTs compared two different doses of leuprorelin (leuprolide) acetate (1.88 mg *v* 3.75 mg every 4 wks for 24 wks).[19,20] The third RCT compared buserelin (1.8 mg every 4 wks) versus leuprorelin (1.88 mg every 4 wks) by subcutaneous injection.[21] The fourth RCT compared triptorelin standard dose treatment plus three different types of dosage regimen.[22] None of these RCTs compared clinical outcomes among treatment groups, but one RCT reported that all participants experienced partial or complete relief from symptoms throughout their treatment.[19]

Different modes of administration: We found three RCTs (96 women) comparing intranasal versus subcutaneous gonadorelin analogues, none of which reported quantitative results for clinical outcomes. One RCT reported that all women had a subjective improvement in their subsequent menstrual symptoms after 6 months' treatment, especially menorrhagia and dysmenorrhoea, but no figures were provided.[23] The RCTs found no differences in uterine and fibroid shrinkage according to how gonadorelin analogue treatment was given.[23–25]

OPTION GONADORELIN ANALOGUES (GNRHA) PLUS HORMONE REPLACEMENT THERAPY

One small RCT found that leuprorelin (leuprolide) acetate plus progesterone hormone replacement therapy versus leuprorelin acetate alone significantly reduced heavy bleeding and two small RCTs found that gonadorelin analogue plus progesterone versus gonadorelin analogue alone reduced the proportion of women with hot flushes. One small RCT found no significant difference with gonadorelin analogue alone versus gonadorelin analogue plus tibolone on uterine and fibroid size and fibroid related symptoms. We found insufficient evidence from one small RCT to compare effects on fibroid related symptoms of gonadorelin analogue plus oestrogen–progestogen hormone replacement therapy versus gonadorelin analogues plus progesterone only hormone replacement therapy.

Benefits: **Gonadorelin analogue plus progestogen versus gonadorelin analogue alone:** We found no systematic review but we found one RCT (41 women).[26] It found that that leuprorelin (leuprolide) acetate plus progesterone significantly reduced heavy bleeding compared with leuprorelin acetate plus placebo (18/21 [86%] women with heavy bleeding with added progesterone *v* 11/20 [55%] with added placebo; RR 1.6, 95% CI 1.0 to 2.4). **Gonadorelin analogue plus tibolone versus gonadorelin alone:** We found one RCT (50 women) that found no significant difference with gonadorelin analogue plus tibolone versus gonadorelin analogue plus placebo on uterine and fibroid size and fibroid related symptoms at 6 months (mean uterine volume 415 cm^3 with added tibolone *v* 386 cm^3 with added placebo; mean fibroid volume 139 cm^3 *v* 133 cm^3; symptom intensity on a visual analogue scale from 0–10: 3.3 *v* 3.5 for pelvic pressure; 2.0 *v* 2.5 for pelvic pain; 3.0 in both groups for urinary frequency; P for all comparisons reported as non-significant).[27] **Gonadorelin analogue plus progestogen versus gonadorelin plus combined oestrogen and progestogen:** We found one RCT (51 women) that compared gonadorelin analogues plus progestogen hormone replacement therapy (HRT) versus gonadorelin analogues plus combined oestrogen–progestogen HRT over a 2 year period.[28] After 3 months of leuprorelin treatment, there was a significant decrease in the mean uterine volume in both groups compared with baseline estimates (416 cm^3 with oestrogen–progestogen HRT *v* 440 cm^3 with progestogen alone HRT; CI of the difference not available). After 21 months of treatment with oestrogen–progestogen HRT, the mean uterine volume was reduced (414 cm^3 with oestrogen–progestogen HRT *v* 647 cm^3 with progestogen alone

HRT; CI not provided). Most women experienced a reduction in fibroid related symptoms (statistical comparison between groups not reported). Menorrhagia improved or resolved in 85%, pelvic pressure in 63%, and pelvic pain in 100% of participants.

Harms: **Gonadorelin analogue plus progestogen versus gonadorelin analogue alone:** One RCT (24 women) found that gonadorelin analogue plus medroxyprogesterone acetate versus gonadorelin analogue alone significantly reduced vasomotor symptoms ($P < 0.05$; raw data not provided).[29] One RCT (16 women) found that leuprorelin acetate plus progestogen HRT versus leuprorelin acetate alone significantly reduced the proportion of women with hot flushes (1/9 [11%] with progestogen HRT *v* 6/7 [86%] with placebo HRT; RR 0.13, 95% CI 0.02 to 0.84).[30] **Gonadorelin analogue plus tibolone versus gonadorelin analogue alone:** After 6 months' treatment, gonadorelin analogue plus tibolone versus gonadorelin analogue alone significantly reduced the mean number of hot flushes each day (1.5 with tibolone *v* 4.6 with placebo; $P < 0.01$; data presented graphically).[27] The RCT also found that that the significant reduction in bone mineral density after 6 months' treatment with gonadorelin alone was prevented with the concurrent administration of tibolone (mean difference $P < 0.01$).[27] The risk of fractures was not assessed. See also gonadorelin analogues without hormonal replacement therapy, p 2095.

Comment: Most of the RCTs were small. There is insufficient evidence to determine the optimum HRT regimen that minimises the adverse effects of gonadorelin analogues.

OPTION NON-STEROIDAL ANTI-INFLAMMATORY DRUGS

Two small RCTs found insufficient evidence about the effects of non-steroidal anti-inflammatory drugs in women with uterine fibroids.

Benefits: We found two small RCTs, which assessed the effects of non-steroidal anti-inflammatory drugs (ibuprofen and naproxen) on heavy menstrual bleeding in women with fibroids.[31,32] The first RCT (25 women with menorrhagia; 11 with fibroids) found no significant difference in menstrual blood loss between naproxen and placebo in women with fibroids (total menstrual blood loss over 4 cycles 221 mL with placebo *v* 196 mL with naproxen; CI and P value not stated).[31] The second RCT (24 women; 10 with fibroids) similarly found no significant difference between ibuprofen (600–1200 mg/day) versus placebo in women with fibroids (total menstrual blood loss over 2 cycles about 130 mL in all groups; P value not stated).[32]

Harms: See harms under the non-steroidal anti-inflammatory drugs topic, p 1393.

Comment: Both RCTs may have been underpowered to assess an effect on clinical outcomes.[31,32]

OPTION GESTRINONE

We found no RCTs on the effects of gestrinone on fibroid related symptoms. Androgenic adverse effects limit its use.

Benefits: We found no systematic review and no RCTs of the effect of gestrinone on clinical outcomes (see comment below).

Harms: Two uncontrolled trials found that gestrinone was associated with seborrhoea and acne, which increased with duration of treatment.[33,34] One RCT found that after 1 year of treatment, seborrhoea affected 71–93% of women, and acne was reported by 31–63% of women after 2 years of treatment. Myalgia and arthralgia, mild hirsutism, hoarseness, and increased libido were also reported. Body weight also increased after 2 years of treatment, from a mean of 57.4 kg to 60.9 kg, with no differences between groups. These changes reversed when treatment was discontinued.

Comment: We found two uncontrolled trials (197 women) that compared the mode of administration in reducing uterine volume.[33,34] The effects of gestrinone were assessed as comparisons with baseline values. After 3 months of treatment in one trial, 76–86% of participants reported amenorrhoea. Pelvic pain was resolved in 76–98% of women. Haemoglobin increased from a mean of 12.38 g/dL to 13.26 g/dL and haematocrit increased from 36.9% to 38.4%. Gestrinone needs to be adequately evaluated against other drugs or placebo.

OPTION MIFEPRISTONE

We found no RCTs about the effects of mifepristone.

Benefits: We found no systematic review or RCTs.

Harms: Mild atypical hot flushes were reported in 28–40% of women in one observational study.[35]

Comment: None.

OPTION LEVONORGESTREL INTRAUTERINE SYSTEM

One systematic review identified no RCTs. We found no additional RCTs.

Benefits: **Versus no treatment:** One systematic review (search date 2000) identified no RCTs.[36] We found no additional RCTs.

Harms: The review identified no RCTs.

Comment: None.

QUESTION In women scheduled for fibroid surgery, what are the effects of preoperative medical treatments?

OPTION GONADORELIN ANALOGUES (GNRHA)

One systematic review has found that gonadorelin analogues versus placebo or no treatment for at least 3 months before fibroid surgery increase haemoglobin concentration and haematocrit, and reduce uterine and pelvic symptoms. One RCT found that gonadorelin versus lynestrenol pretreatment significantly increased postoperative haematocrit. However, women are more likely to experience adverse hypo-oestrogenic effects from preoperative treatment such as hot flushes, vaginal symptoms,

sweating, and withdrawal from treatment. Preoperative gonadorelin also reduces blood loss and the rate of vertical incisions during laparotomy. Women having hysterectomy are more likely to have a vaginal rather than an abdominal procedure after gonadorelin analogue pretreatment.

Benefits: **Versus placebo or no treatment:** We found one systematic review(search date 2000, 21 RCTs, 1886 women)[37] and one additional RCT.[38] The systematic review assessed gonadorelin analogue pretreatment (given at least 3 months before surgery) compared with placebo or no treatment, in separate categories: before surgery; during and after myomectomy (see glossary, p 2104); and during and after hysterectomy. Where possible, meta-analysis was performed. The systematic review found that pretreatment with gonadorelin analogues versus placebo or no treatment improved haemoglobin concentration (9 RCTs, 541 women: WMD 0.98 g/dL, 95% CI 0.74 g/dL to 1.22 g/dL) and haematocrit (4 RCTs, 138 women: 3.14%, 95% CI 1.78% to 4.51%). Pelvic symptoms significantly improved when measured on a symptom scale (pelvic symptom score [see glossary, p 2104]: 3 RCTs, 372 women: WMD −2.12, 95% CI −2.38 to −1.87). Women receiving gonadorelin analogue pretreatment versus no pretreatment had a significantly lower risk of no improvement (1 RCT: OR 0.38, 95% CI 0.22 to 0.60). Pretreatment with gonadorelin analogue versus placebo or no treatment significantly reduced intraoperative blood loss estimated by measuring the weight of swabs and the volume of blood collected in receptacles (8 RCTs, 263 women: WMD 67 mL, 95% CI 44 mL to 91 mL during myomectomy; 6 RCTs, 419 women: WMD 58 mL, 95% CI 40 mL to 76 mL during hysterectomy). The duration of operation in women pretreated with gonadorelin analogue undergoing hysterectomy was significantly shorter (7 RCTs: WMD 6.6 min, 95% CI 2.3 min to 10.9 min) and hospital stay was shorter (4 RCTs: WMD 1 day, 95% CI 0.9 days to 1.2 days). Gonadorelin analogue pretreatment versus placebo or no treatment significantly reduced vertical incision rate in women having laparotomy (myomectomy 1 RCT, 28 women: OR 0.11, 95% CI 0.02 to 0.75; hysterectomy 4 RCTs, 529 women: OR 0.36, 95% CI 0.23 to 0.55). There was also an indication that hysterectomy was subjectively graded by the surgeons as "not as difficult" in the pretreated women (2 RCTs: OR 0.73, 95% CI 0.25 to 0.97). A significantly higher proportion of these women also converted to a vaginal procedure (3 RCTs: OR 4.7, 95% CI 3.0 to 7.5). The review found that pretreated versus non-pretreated women maintained marginally but significantly higher postoperative blood counts (postoperative haemoglobin: 3 RCTs, 240 women: WMD 0.8 g/dL, 95% CI 0.5 g/dL to 1.1 g/dL) for both types of surgery and higher haematocrit levels after hysterectomy (2 RCTs, 173 women: WMD 1.8%, 95% CI 1.1% to 2.4%), although the clinical significance of these results is unclear. One small additional RCT (24 women) assessed pregnancy rate in infertile women who had undergone myomectomy for fibroids at a mean follow up of 13 months.[39] Pregnancy rate was higher for pretreated versus non-pretreated women, although the difference was not significant (AR 7/11 [64%] for pretreated *v* 6/13 [46%] for non-pretreated; RR 1.4, 95% CI 0.7 to 2.9). The RCT may have been too small to detect a clinically important difference. **Versus other pretreatments:** One RCT (56 women enrolled, 42 women analysed) compared leuprorelin (leuprolide) with lynestrenol pretreatment.[40] It found that the decrease in postoperative haematocrit was significantly lower with leuprorelin versus lynestrenol (WMD −7.8%, 95% CI −14.0% to −1.3%). The RCT had a 25% withdrawal rate.

Harms: The review found that women pretreated with gonadorelin analogues versus placebo or no treatment were significantly more likely to experience hypo-oestrogenic symptoms, such as hot flushes (534 women: OR 6.5, 95% CI 4.6 to 9.2), change in breast size (261 women: OR 7.7, 95% CI 2.4 to 24.9), and vaginal symptoms (534 women: OR 4.0, 95% CI 2.1 to 7.6).[37] Women were also more likely to withdraw from treatment because of adverse events (4 RCTs, 628 women: OR 2.5, 95% CI 1.0 to 5.9). The systematic review identified two small RCTs that evaluated long term follow up in women having myomectomy. In one of these, 24 women were checked for fibroid recurrence at 6 months and 63% of the pretreated group had a recurrence of their fibroids compared with 13% of the control group. Fibroid recurrence 2–3 years after surgery was over 50% in the 18 women from the second RCT, but no significant differences were found. No other harms were assessed.

Comment: The RCTs were not evaluated individually as pooled measures of effect were calculated in the systematic review. **Versus other pretreatments:** One RCT was not included in the systematic review because the outcome of avoiding scheduled hysterectomy was assessed in the gonadorelin analogues group only.[38]

QUESTION What are the effects of surgical treatments?

OPTION LAPAROSCOPICALLY ASSISTED VAGINAL HYSTERECTOMY

We found no RCTs comparing long term effects of laparoscopically assisted vaginal hysterectomy versus other treatments. One small RCT found limited evidence that women having laparoscopically assisted vaginal hysterectomy had shorter recovery and less postoperative pain compared with women having total abdominal hysterectomy.

Benefits: We found no systematic review. We found no RCTs comparing laparoscopically assisted vaginal hysterectomy (LAVH) versus no intervention or sham surgery. We found one RCT (62 women with symptomatic fibroids scheduled for hysterectomy) comparing the effects of LAVH versus total abdominal hysterectomy (TAH) (see glossary, p 2105) on operating time, blood loss, complications (not clearly specified), febrile morbidity, postoperative analgesic requirement, and hospital stay.[41] Overall, it found that LAVH significantly reduced operating time, hospital stay, and analgesic use compared with TAH (mean operating time 135 min with LAVH *v* 120 min with TAH; $P = 0.001$; mean hospital stay 3.8 days *v* 5.8 days; $P < 0.001$; analgesic use for > 24 h postoperatively 23% *v* 77%; CI not reported). Post hoc subgroup analyses found limited evidence that relative effects of LAVH and TAH depended on uterine weight (see comment below).

Harms: No major complications were reported, although there was insufficient information to determine which complications were addressed.

Comment: **In women with uterus estimated to weigh 500 g or less:** Subgroup analysis of the RCT in 41 women with uteri estimated to weigh 500 g or less in the preoperative assessment had comparable operating times (130 min on average with LAVH *v* 120 min with TAH) but less postoperative pain and shorter recovery compared with the TAH group.[41] Sonograms were used to estimate uterine weight. Analgesia requirement was reduced with LAVH (1/20 [5%] for LAVH *v* 6/11 [55%] for TAH; RR 0.09, 95% CI 0.01 to 0.67; NNT 2: 95% CI 1 to 6). Hospital stay was also reduced with LAVH (3.8 days, 95% CI 3.2 days to 4.0 days with LAVH *v* 5.8 days, 95% CI 5.0 days to 6.4 days with TAH; P < 0.0001). **In women with uterus estimated to weigh more than 500 g:** Subgroup analysis of the RCT in 21 women with uteri weighing more than 500 g found that LAVH was associated with a shorter recovery but a longer operating time compared with TAH, and a 27% rate of conversion to laparotomy. Mean operating time was increased with LAVH (150 min, 95% CI 125 min to 173 min with LAVH *v* 108 min, 95% CI 83 min to 120 min with TAH; P = 0.002). Mean hospital stay was reduced with LAVH (4.0 days, 95% CI 3.9 days to 5.8 days with LAVH *v* 6 days, 95% CI 5.8 days to 6.0 days with TAH). Conversion to laparotomy was not significantly different between LAVH and TAH (3/11 [27%] with LAVH *v* 0/20 [0%] with TAH), although the sample size was insufficient to rule out a clinically important difference.[41] **Extrapolating results of hysterectomy for other disorders:** Other RCTs have compared different types of hysterectomy in heterogeneous groups of participants but results from these RCTs are not generalisable to women with fibroids.

OPTION LAPAROSCOPIC MYOMECTOMY

Limited evidence from RCTs suggests that laparoscopic myomectomy versus abdominal myomectomy is associated with less postoperative pain and fever, and shorter recovery time.

Benefits: We found no systematic review. We found no RCTs against no intervention or sham surgery. We found two RCTs comparing laparoscopic myomectomy (see glossary, p 2104) versus myomectomy by laparotomy.[42,43] The first RCT (40 women with < 5 myomas and the size of the largest myoma < 7 cm) found no differences in surgical time, blood loss, or postoperative complications (fever). Women undergoing laparoscopic myomectomy reported a lower intensity of postoperative pain (unlabelled scale), required less analgesia, and had a shorter recovery time than women undergoing myomectomy by laparotomy. Two days after surgery, a significantly smaller proportion of women required analgesia with laparoscopic myomectomy versus abdominal myomectomy (analgesia free women: 17/20 [85%] with laparoscopy *v* 3/20 [15%] with laparotomy; RR 5.7, 95% CI 2.0 to 16.4; NNT 2, 95% CI 1 to 3), and by day 15 more women were fully recovered after laparoscopic myomectomy (18/20 [90%] with laparoscopy *v* 1/20 [5%] with laparotomy; RR 18.0, 95% CI 2.7 to 122.0; NNT 2, 95% CI 1 to 2). The second

RCT (131 women with at least 1 myoma ≥5 cm)[43] found no differences in surgical time. However, it found a greater drop in haemoglobin with abdominal versus laparoscopic myomectomy (1.33 g/dL with laparoscopy *v* 2.17 g/dL with laparotomy; CI not provided; $P < 0.001$). Women who had laparoscopic versus abdominal myomectomy were marginally but significantly less likely to experience postoperative fever (8/66 [12%] with laparoscopy *v* 17/65 [26%] with laparotomy; RR 0.46, 95% CI 0.22 to 1.00; NNT 9, 95% CI 4 to 116) and were more likely to have a shorter hospital stay (75.6 h with laparoscopy *v* 142.8 h with laparotomy; CI not provided; $P < 0.001$). Pregnancy rate after surgery did not differ between groups.

Harms: No major complications were reported in the two RCTs.[42,43] Transfusions were more frequent in the laparotomy group but the difference did not reach statistical significance (transfusion risk: 0/66 [0%] with laparoscopic myomectomy *v* 3/65 [5%] with laparotomy; ARR –0.05, 95% CI –0.13 to +0.02).

Comment: Other RCTs have compared different types of hysterectomy in heterogeneous groups of participants but results from these RCTs are not generalisable to women with fibroids.

OPTION ABDOMINAL HYSTERECTOMY

We found no RCTs comparing abdominal hysterectomy versus no treatment or sham surgery, but there is consensus that it is superior to no treatment in improving fibroid related symptoms. One RCT found limited evidence that women having total abdominal hysterectomy versus laparoscopically assisted vaginal hysterectomy had longer recovery times and more postoperative pain.

Benefits: We found no systematic review. We found no RCTs against no intervention or sham surgery (see comment below). We found one RCT comparing abdominal hysterectomy versus laparoscopically assisted vaginal hysterectomy (see benefits of laparoscopically assisted vaginal hysterectomy, p 2101 and benefits of laparoscopic myomectomy, p 2102).[41]

Harms: See harms under laparoscopically assisted vaginal hysterectomy, p 2102 and laparoscopic myomectomy, p 2103.

Comment: There is consensus that abdominal hysterectomy is superior to no treatment in improving fibroid related symptoms.

OPTION THERMAL BALLOON ABLATION

We found no RCTs comparing thermal balloon ablation versus non-surgical treatment or hysterectomy. One RCT compared thermal balloon ablation versus rollerball endometrial ablation in women with fibroids smaller than the average size of a 12 week pregnancy, all of whom had been pretreated with gonadorelin analogues. It found no significant difference with thermal balloon versus rollerball ablation in hysterectomy rates, amenorrhoea rates, pictorial bleeding assessment

chart score, or haemoglobin at 12 months. It found that thermal balloon ablation reduced operation time and intraoperative complication rate compared with rollerball ablation. About one third of women reported being "not very satisfied" with either operation.

Benefits: **Versus non-surgical treatment:** We found no RCTs. **Versus other surgical treatment:** We found no RCTs comparing thermal balloon ablation (see glossary, p 2105) versus hysterectomy. We found one RCT (96 women with fibroids smaller than the average size of a 12 wk pregnancy who had received 2 month of preoperative treatment with gonadorelin analogues) that compared thermal balloon ablation versus rollerball endometrial ablation (see glossary, p 2105).[44] Thermal balloon ablation was performed by staff surgeons or supervised residents under local intracervical and paracervical anaesthesia with intravenous sedation. Rollerball ablation was performed under general anaesthesia by experienced surgeons. The RCT found no significant difference with thermal balloon ablation versus rollerball endometrial ablation in hysterectomy rates, amenorrhoea rates, pictorial bleeding assessment chart score (see glossary, p 2104), or haemoglobin at 12 months (women undergoing hysterectomy: 4/45 [9%] with thermal balloon *v* 4/48 [8%] with rollerball; amenorrhoea: 5 women with thermal balloon *v* 8 women with rollerball; mean decrease in pictorial bleeding assessment chart score: 343 with thermal balloon *v* 345 with rollerball; mean increase in haemoglobin: 2.7 g/dL with thermal balloon *v* 3.0 g/dL with rollerball; P values reported as non-significant for all comparisons; no further data provided). Operating time was significantly shorter in the thermal balloon group compared to the rollerball group (11.5 min with thermal balloon *v* 37.3 min with rollerball, $P < 0.0001$). About a third of women in both groups reported that they were "not very satisfied" with their operation (33% with thermal balloon *v* 39% with rollerball).[44]

Harms: The RCT found that a significantly higher proportion of women had intraoperative complications with rollerball ablation versus thermal balloon ablation (5/45 [11%] with rollerball *v* 0/48 [0%] with thermal balloon, $P < 0.05$; 2 women had fluid overload, 2 had major bleeding and 1 had injury to the cervix).[44] It found no significant difference with rollerball ablation versus thermal balloon ablation in postoperative complications (3 women in each group) or postoperative pain score at 12 hours.

Comment: None.

GLOSSARY

Myomectomy Removal of fibroids from the uterus. The mode of removal may be abdominal, laparoscopic, or hysteroscopic.

Pelvic score scale An ordinal scale that adds the results of pelvic pain and pelvic pressure. Each symptom is evaluated in a scale ranging of 0–3, where 0 means absence of pain, and increasing numbers represent mild, moderate, and severe pain. Because both results are added, absence of symptoms is represented by a 0 and severe pain and pelvic pressure by 6. We found no data on validation of the scale. However, it is commonly used in studies evaluating pelvic pain.

Pictorial bleeding assessment chart (PBAC) Used to measure menstrual bleeding. Validation studies indicate that a PBAC score of 100–185 is suggestive of menorrhagia (heavy menstrual bleeding) which is objectively defined by the alkaline haematin test as a menstrual blood loss greater than 80 mL.

Rollerball endometrial ablation Destruction of the endometrium using electrical coagulation with a rollerball electrode applied through the cervical os.

Thermal balloon ablation Destruction of the endometrium using pressure from a balloon catheter inserted through the cervical os and then filled with fluid to a pressure of 160–180 mm Hg and heated to about 87°C.

Total abdominal hysterectomy Open operation through the abdominal wall to remove the uterus. In some situations, this is performed in conjunction with a bilateral salpingo-oophorectomy, the removal of both ovaries and fallopian tubes.

REFERENCES

1. Buttram VC, Reiter RC. Uterine leiomyomata: etiology, symptomatology and management. *Fertil Steril* 1981;6:433–445.
2. Lumsden MA, Wallace EM. Clinical presentation of uterine fibroids. *Baillieres Clin Obstet Gynaecol* 1998;12:177–195.
3. Borgfeldt C, Andolf E. Transvaginal ultrasonographic findings in the uterus and the endometrium: low prevalence of leiomyoma in a random sample of women age 25–40 years. *Acta Obstet Gynecol Scand* 2000;79:202–207.
4. Thompson JD, Rock JA, eds. *Te Linde's Operative Gynecology*, 7th edition. 1992, JB Lippincott Company: London, Hagerstrom.
5. Cramer SF, Patel A. The frequency of uterine leiomyomas. *Am J Clin Pathol* 1990;90:435–438.
6. Schwartz SM, Marshall LM, Baird DD. Epidemiologic contributions to understanding the etiology of uterine leiomyomata. *Environ Health Perspect* 2000;108:821–827.
7. Farquhar C, Arroll B, Ekeroma A, et al. An evidence-based guideline for the management of uterine fibroids. *Aust N Z J Obstet Gynaecol* 2001;41:125–140.
8. Townsend DE, Sparkes RS, Baluda MC, et al. Unicellular histogenesis of uterine leiomyomas as determined by electrophoresis of glucose-6-phosphate dehydrogenase. *Am J Obstet Gynecol* 1970;107:1168–1174.
9. Hashimoto K, Azuma C, Kamiura S, et al. Clonal determination of uterine leiomyomas by analyzing differential inactivation of the X-chromosome-linked phosphoglycerokinase gene. *Gynecol Obstet Invest* 1995;40:204–208.
10. Ross RK, Pike MC, Vessey MP, et al. Risk factors for uterine fibroids: reduced risk associated with oral contraceptives. *BMJ* 1986;293:359–363.
11. Chiaffarino F, Parazzini F, La Vecchia C, et al. Use of oral contraceptives and uterine fibroids: results from a case-control study. *Br J Obstet Gynaecol* 1999;106:857–860.
12. Lumbiganon P, Rugpao S, Phandhu-Fung S, et al. Protective effect of depot-medroxyprogesterone acetate on surgically treated uterine leiomyomas: a multicentre-case control study. *Br J Obstet Gynaecol* 1995;103:909–914.
13. Carlson KJ, Miller BA, Fowler FJ Jr. The Maine Women's Health Study: II. Outcomes of nonsurgical management of leiomyomas, abnormal bleeding, and chronic pelvic pain. *Obstet Gynecol* 1994;83:566–572.
14. Minaguchi H, Wong JM, Snabes MC. Clinical use of nafarelin in the treatment of leiomyomas. A review of the literature. *J Reprod Med* 2000;45:481–489. Search date 1997; primary sources Medline, Refline, bibliographies, relevant journals, and abstracts from conferences and other meetings.
15. Friedman AJ, Hoffman DI, Comite F, et al. Treatment of leiomyomata uteri with leuprolide acetate depot: a double-blind, placebo-controlled, multicenter study. *Obstet Gynecol* 1991;77:720–725.
16. Friedman AJ, Harrison-Atlas D, Barbieri RL, et al. A randomized placebo-controlled double-blind study evaluating the efficacy of leuprolide acetate depot in the treatment of uterine leiomyomata. *Fertil Steril* 1989;51:251–254.
17. Schlaff WD, Zerhouni EA, Huth JA, et al. A placebo-controlled trial of a depot gonadotropin-releasing hormone analogue (leuprolide) in the treatment of uterine leiomyomata. *Obstet Gynecol* 1989;74:856–862.
18. Espinos JJ, Marti A, Asins E, et al. Efectos de dos dosis de un analogo de la GnRH (leuprorelina depot) sobre la miomatosis uterina. *Clin Invest Gin Obst* 1993;20:382–387.
19. Watanabe Y, Nakamura G, Matsuguchi H, et al. Efficacy of a low-dose leuprolide acetate depot in the treatment of uterine leiomyomata in Japanese women. *Fertil Steril* 1992;58:66–71.
20. Watanabe Y, Nakamura G. Effects of two different doses of leuprolide acetate depot on uterine cavity area in patients with uterine leiomyomata. *Fertil Steril* 1995;63:487–490.
21. Takeuchi H, Kobori H, Kikuchi I, et al. A prospective randomised study comparing endocrinological and clinical effects of two types of GnRH agonists in cases of uterine leiomyomas or endometriosis. *J Obstet Gynecol Res* 2000;26:325–331.
22. Broekmans FJ, Hompes PG, Heitbrink MA, et al. Two-step gonadotropin-releasing hormone agonist treatment of uterine leiomyomas: standard-dose therapy followed by reduced-dose therapy. *Am J Obstet Gynecol* 1996;175:1208–1216.
23. Vollenhoven BJ, Shekleton P, McDonald J, et al. Clinical predictors for buserelin acetate treatment of uterine fibroids: a prospective study of 40 women. *Fertil Steril* 1990;54:1032–1038.
24. Friedman AJ, Barbieri RL, Benacerraf BR, et al. Treatment of leiomyomata with intranasal or subcutaneous leuprolide, a gonadotropin-releasing hormone agonist. *Fertil Steril* 1987;48:560–564.
25. Costantini S, Anserini P, Valenzano M, et al. Luteinizing hormone-releasing hormone analog therapy of uterine fibroid: analysis of results obtained with buserelin administered intranasally and goserelin administered subcutaneously as a monthly depot. *Eur J Obstet Gynaecol Reprod Biol* 1990;37:63–69.
26. Scialli AR, Jestila KJ. Sustained benefits of leuprolide acetate with or without subsequent medroxyprogesterone acetate in the nonsurgical management of leiomyomata uteri. *Fertil Steril* 1995;64:313–320.
27. Palomba S, Affinito P, Giovanni MD, et al. A clinical trial of the effects of tibolone administered with gonadotropin-releasing hormone analogues for the treatment of uterine leiomyomata. *Fertil Steril* 1998;70:111–118.
28. Friedman AJ, Daly M, Juneau-Norcross M, et al. Long-term medical therapy for leiomyomata uteri: a prospective, randomized study of leuprolide

acetate depot plus oestrogen-progestin or progestin 'add-back' for 2 years. *Hum Reprod* 1994;9:1618–1625.

29. Caird LE, West CP, Lumsden MA, et al. Medroxyprogesterone acetate with Zoladex for long-term treatment of fibroids: effects on bone density and patient acceptability. *Hum Reprod* 1997;2:436–440.
30. Friedman AJ, Barbieri RL, Doubilet PM, et al. A randomized double-blind trial of a gonadotropin releasing-hormone agonist (leuprolide) with or without medroxyprogesterone acetate in the treatment of leiomyomata uteri. *Fertil Steril* 1988;49:404–409.
31. Ylikorkala O, Pekonen F. Naproxen reduces idiopathic but not fibromyoma-induced menorrhagia. *Obstet Gynecol* 1986;68:10–12.
32. Makarainen L, Ylikorkala O. Primary and myoma-associated menorrhagia: role of prostaglandins and effects of ibuprofen. *Br J Obstet Gynaecol* 1986;93:974–978.
33. Coutinho EM, Goncalves MT. Long-term treatment of leiomyomas with gestrinone. *Fertil Steril* 1989;51:939–946.
34. Coutinho EM, Boulanger GA, Goncalves MT. Regression of uterine leiomyomas after treatment with gestrinone, an antiestrogen, antiprogesterone. *Am J Obstet Gynecol* 1986;155:761–767.
35. Mahajan DK, London SN. Mifepristone (RU486): a review. *Fertil Steril* 1997;68:967–976.
36. Ikomi A, Pepra EF. Efficacy of the levonorgestrel intrauterine system in treating menorrhagia: actualities and ambiguities. *J Fam Plann Reprod Health Care* 2002;28:99–100.
37. Lethaby A, Vollenhoven B, Sowter M, et al. Preoperative GnRH analogue therapy before hysterectomy or myomectomy for uterine fibroids. In: The Cochrane Library, Issue 4, 2000. Oxford: Update Software. Search date 2000; primary sources the Cochrane Menstrual Disorders and Subfertility Group Register of Trials, Medline, Embase, the National Research Register, the National Library of Medicine's Clinical Trials Register, and Current Contents. Published trials were also identified from citation lists of review articles and direct contact with drug companies for unpublished trials. In most cases, the first author of each included trial was contacted for additional information.
38. Parazzini F, Bortolotti A, Chiantera V, et al. Goserelin acetate to avoid hysterectomy in pre-menopausal women with fibroids requiring surgery. *Eur J Obstet Gynecol Reprod Biol* 1999;87:31–33.
39. Campo S, Garcea N. Laparoscopic myomectomy in premenstrual women with and without preoperative treatment using gonadotrophin-releasing hormone analogues. *Hum Reprod* 1999;14:44–48.
40. Verspyck E, Marpeau L, Lucas C. Leuprorelin depot 3.75 mg versus lynestrenol in the preoperative treatment of symptomatic uterine myomas: a multicentre randomised trial. *Eur J Obstet Gynecol Reprod Biol* 2000;89:7–13.
41. Ferrari MM, Berlanda N, Mezzopane R, et al. Identifying the indications for laparoscopically assisted vaginal hysterectomy: a prospective, randomised comparison with abdominal hysterectomy in patients with symptomatic uterine fibroids. *Br J Obstet Gynaecol* 2000;107:620–625.
42. Mais V, Ajossa S, Guerriero S, et al. Laparoscopic versus abdominal myomectomy: a prospective, randomized trial to evaluate benefits in early outcome. *Am J Obstet Gynecol* 1996;174:654–658.
43. Seracchioli R, Rossi S, Govoni F, et al. Fertility and obstetric outcome after laparoscopic myomectomy of large myomata: a randomised comparison with abdominal myomectomy. *Hum Reprod* 2000;15:2663–2668.
44. Soysal ME, Soysal SK, Vicdan K. Thermal balloon ablation in myoma-induced menorrhagia under local anesthesia. *Gynecol Obstet Invest* 2001;51:128–133.

Anne Lethaby
Cochrane Menstrual Disorders and Subfertility Group
Auckland
New Zealand

Beverley Vollenhoven
Department of Obstetrics and Gynaecology
Monash University
Clayton, Victoria
Australia

Competing interests: None declared.

TABLE 1 Harms of gonadorelin versus placebo (see text, p 2096).[15]

Harms	Gonadorelin			Placebo				
	Outcome	Population	%	Outcome	Population	%	RR*	95% CI*
Vasomotor flushes	52	63	83%	5	65	8%	10.7	4.6 to 25.1
Vaginitis	11	63	17%	0	65	0%		
Arthralgia/mialgia	9	63	14%	0	65	0%		
Asthenia	10	63	16%	3	65	5%	3.4	0.97 to 996
Peripheral oedema	7	63	11%	1	65	2%	7.2	0.9 to 57
Insomnia	6	63	10%	0	65	0%		
Nausea	6	63	10%	1	65	2%	6.2	0.8 to 50
Emotional ability /nervousness	5	63	8%	1	65	2%	5.2	0.6 to 42.9
Depression	7	63	11%	2	65	3%	3.6	0.8 to 16.7
Headaches	18	63	29%	13	65	20%	1.4	0.8 to 2.7
Decreased libido	2	63	3%	0	65	0%		

*Clinical Evidence recalculation.

Infertility and subfertility

Search date October 2002

Kirsten Duckitt

QUESTIONS

INTERVENTIONS

To be covered in future updates

Counselling

Covered elsewhere in *Clinical Evidence*

See endometriosis, p 2079
See erectile dysfunction, p 1003
See fibroids, p 2092
See pelvic inflammatory disease, p 1871

See glossary, p 2130

Clin Evid 2003;10:2108–2137.

Key Messages

In women with infertility caused by ovulation disorders

- **Clomifene** One systematic review has found that clomifene significantly increases pregnancy rate compared with placebo in women who ovulate infrequently. Four other studies comparing clomifene versus tamoxifen have found no significant difference in ovulation or pregnancy rates. One RCT found that clomifene plus metformin significantly increased pregnancy rate compared with clomifene alone after 6 months' treatment.
- **Cyclofenil** One RCT found no significant difference in pregnancy rates with cyclofenil versus placebo.
- **Gonadotrophins** One systematic review found no significant difference between human menopausal gonadotrophins and urofollitropin (urofollitrophin, urinary follicle stimulating hormone) in pregnancy rates. Two RCTs found no significant difference in cumulative pregnancy or live birth rates with follitropin (recombinant follicle stimulating hormone) versus urofollitropin. The review found that urofollitropin versus human menopausal gonadotrophins significantly reduced the risk of ovarian hyperstimulation syndrome, although this was confined to women who were not treated with concomitant gonadotrophin releasing hormone analogues. Observational evidence suggests that gonadotrophins may be associated with an increased risk of non-invasive ovarian tumours and multiple pregnancies.
- **Laparoscopic ovarian drilling** One systematic review and one subsequent small RCT found no significant difference in pregnancy rate with laparoscopic ovarian drilling versus gonadotrophins, but found that laparoscopic ovarian drilling significantly reduced rates of multiple pregnancies.
- **Pulsatile gonadotrophin releasing hormone** One systematic review found insufficient evidence on the effects of pulsatile gonadotrophin releasing hormone treatment.

In women with tubal infertility

- **In vitro fertilisation** We found no RCTs of in vitro fertilisation versus no treatment. One RCT found that immediate versus delayed in vitro fertilisation significantly increased numbers of pregnancies and live births. Three RCTs found no significant difference in numbers of live births with in vitro fertilisation versus intracytoplasmic sperm injection. Observational evidence suggests that adverse effects associated with in vitro fertilisation include multiple pregnancies and ovarian hyperstimulation syndrome.
- **Selective salpingography plus tubal catheterisation** We found no RCTs on the effects of selective salpingography plus tubal catheterisation.
- **Tubal flushing with oil soluble media** One systematic review found that tubal flushing with oil soluble media versus no intervention increased pregnancy rate. The review found that tubal flushing with oil soluble media increased the live birth rate compared with flushing with water soluble media.
- **Tubal flushing with water soluble media** One systematic review found no RCTs of tubal flushing with water soluble media versus no intervention. It found that tubal flushing with water soluble media decreased live birth rate compared with flushing with oil soluble media.

- **Tubal surgery (before in vitro fertilisation)** One systematic review in women undergoing in vitro fertilisation has found that tubal surgery significantly increases pregnancy and live birth rates compared with no treatment or medical treatment. Another review found no significant difference in pregnancy rates between different types of tubal surgery. One systematic review found no significant difference in pregnancy rates with tubal surgery plus additional treatments versus tubal surgery alone to prevent adhesion formation (steroids, dextran, noxytioline).

In women with infertility caused by endometriosis

- **Drug-induced ovarian suppression** One systematic review found no significant difference in pregnancy rates between drugs that induce ovarian suppression versus placebo. The review found that ovulation suppression agents cause adverse effects, including weight gain, hot flushes, and osteoporosis, and that danazol may cause dose related weight gain and androgenic effects.
- **Intrauterine insemination plus gonadotrophins** One RCT found that intrauterine insemination plus gonadotrophins significantly increased live birth rates compared with no treatment. A second RCT found no significant difference in birth rates between expectant management versus intrauterine insemination plus pituitary down regulation plus gonadotrophins. A third RCT found that intrauterine insemination plus gonadotrophins significantly increased pregnancy rates compared with intrauterine insemination alone after the first treatment cycle.
- **In vitro fertilisation** We found no RCTs in women with endometriosis related infertility.
- **Laparoscopic surgical treatment** Two RCTs found inconsistent evidence about effects on pregnancy and live birth rates of laparoscopic surgery compared with diagnostic laparoscopy.

In couples with male factor infertility

- **Donor insemination** We found no good evidence on the effects of donor insemination.
- **Intracytoplasmic sperm injection plus in vitro fertilisation** One systematic review found insufficient evidence on the effects of intracytoplasmic sperm injection plus in vitro fertilisation versus in vitro fertilisation alone.
- **Intrauterine insemination** Two systematic reviews have found that intrauterine insemination significantly increases pregnancy rate compared with intracervical insemination or natural intercourse.
- **In vitro fertilisation versus gamete intrafallopian transfer** One RCT found insufficient evidence on the effects of in vitro fertilisation versus gamete intrafallopian transfer.

In couples with unexplained infertility

- **Clomifene** One systematic review found limited evidence that clomifene versus placebo significantly increased rates of pregnancy per cycle.
- **Fallopian tube sperm perfusion (*v* intrauterine insemination)** One systematic review and one subsequent RCT have found that fallopian tube sperm perfusion significantly increases pregnancy rates compared with intrauterine insemination.
- **Gamete intrafallopian transfer** We found no RCTs of gamete intrafallopian transfer versus no treatment. RCTs found conflicting effects on pregnancy rates of gamete intrafallopian transfer versus other treatments (intrauterine insemination, timed intercourse, and in vitro fertilisation).

- **Intrauterine insemination (plus ovarian stimulation treatment)** Two systematic reviews and one subsequent RCT in couples undergoing ovarian stimulation treatment have found that intrauterine insemination significantly increases pregnancy rates compared with timed intercourse or intracervical insemination. One systematic review found no significant difference with intrauterine insemination versus timed intercourse or intracervical insemination in pregnancy rates, but found that adding ovarian stimulation to any of the three interventions significantly increased pregnancy rate per cycle. One systematic review and one subsequent RCT have found that fallopian tube sperm perfusion significantly increased pregnancy rates compared with intrauterine insemination. One systematic review found no significant difference between intrauterine insemination with or without ovarian stimulation versus in vitro fertilisation for live birth rate.
- **In vitro fertilisation** One systematic review found no significant difference between in vitro fertilisation and expectant management for pregnancy rate. It found no significant difference between in vitro fertilisation versus gamete intrafallopian transfer or versus intraterine insemination with or without ovarian stimulation for live birth rate.

DEFINITION Normal fertility has been defined as achieving a pregnancy within 2 years by regular sexual intercourse.[1] However, many define infertility as the failure to conceive after 1 year of unprotected intercourse. Infertility can be primary, in couples who have never conceived, or secondary, in couples who have previously conceived. Infertile couples include those who are sterile (who will never achieve a natural pregnancy) and those who are subfertile (who could eventually achieve a pregnancy).

INCIDENCE/ PREVALENCE Although there is no evidence of a major change in the prevalence of infertility, many more couples are seeking help than previously. Currently, about 1/7 couples in industrialised countries will seek medical advice for infertility.[2] Rates of primary infertility vary widely between countries, ranging from 10% in Africa to about 6% in North America and Europe.[1] Reported rates of secondary infertility are less reliable.

AETIOLOGY/ RISK FACTORS In the UK, nearly a third of infertility cases are unexplained. The rest are caused by ovulatory failure (27%), low sperm count or quality (19%), tubal damage (14%), endometriosis (5%), and other causes (5%).[3]

PROGNOSIS In developed countries, 80–90% of couples attempting to conceive are successful after 1 year and 95% after 2 years.[3] The chances of becoming pregnant vary with the cause and duration of infertility, the woman's age, the couple's previous pregnancy history, and the availability of different treatment options.[4,5] For the first 2–3 years of unexplained infertility, cumulative conception rates remain high (27–46%) but decrease with increasing age of the woman and duration of infertility. The background rates of spontaneous pregnancy in infertile couples can be calculated from longitudinal studies of infertile couples who have been observed without treatment.[4]

AIMS OF INTERVENTION To achieve the delivery of one healthy baby; to reduce the distress associated with infertility.

OUTCOMES Live births, miscarriages, multiple pregnancies, incidence of ovarian hyperstimulation syndrome (see glossary, p 2131), satisfaction with services and treatments, acceptance of childlessness if treatment is unsuccessful, and pregnancy rate. Pregnancy rate is an intermediate outcome, but one that is important in itself to many people. Ovulation is an intermediate outcome. A large number of pregnancies in infertile couples will occur spontaneously without treatment.[4] Effectiveness of treatments for infertility should be assessed on the basis of pregnancy rates over and above the spontaneous pregnancy rates, otherwise the impacts of treatments may be overestimated.

METHODS *Clinical Evidence* search and appraisal February 2002. **Crossover design:** For infertility, RCTs with a crossover design may overestimate the treatment effect because pregnancies occurring in the first half of the trial will remove couples from the second half.[6] Crossover trials were included in some systematic reviews where no or few RCTs using a parallel group design were available. Ideally, only data from the first half of the trial, before crossover, should be used. However, a study that used a computer model to compare the results of crossover and parallel designed trials suggests that any overestimation may be clinically irrelevant.[7]

QUESTION **What are the effects of treatments for infertility caused by ovulation disorders?**

OPTION **CLOMIFENE**

One systematic review has found that clomifene versus placebo significantly increases the likelihood of pregnancy in women who ovulate infrequently. Four other studies comparing clomifene versus tamoxifen have found no significant difference in ovulation rates or number of pregnancies. One RCT found that clomifene plus metformin versus clomifene alone significantly increased the pregnancy rate per woman after 6 months' treatment.

Benefits: **Versus placebo:** We found one systematic review (search date not stated, 3 crossover RCTs), which compared clomifene (clomiphene) (50–200 mg) versus placebo in 217 cycles in women who ovulate infrequently (see table 1, p 2136).[8] It found that clomifene versus placebo significantly increased the chance of pregnancy (OR 3.4, 95% CI 1.2 to 9.5). **Versus tamoxifen:** We found no systematic review, but found four studies (2 RCTs, 1 quasi-randomised study, and 1 observational study; 197 anovulatory or infrequently ovulating women; see comment below).[29,35–37] The first RCT (86 anovulatory women aged < 40 years) compared tamoxifen (maximum 60 mg daily) versus clomifene (maximum 150 mg daily).[35] It found no significant difference in the overall rate of ovulation (50/113 [44%] ovulatory cycles with tamoxifen *v* 41/91 [45%] ovulatory cycles with clomifene; $P > 0.05$; see comment below) or the number of pregnancies (10/46 [22%] with tamoxifen *v* 6/40 [15%] with clomifene; RR 1.7, 95% CI 0.7 to 4.2). Three other studies found similar results.[29,36,37] **Versus other drug combinations:** We found no systematic review but found one RCT (90 infertile women with polycystic ovary syndrome, infrequent menstruation, high insulin levels, and body mass indexes > 28), which compared clomifene (at its lowest effective dose; see comment below) plus metformin (500 mg orally 3 times daily) versus clomifene alone (at its lowest effective dose; see comment below).[38] The RCT found that clomifene plus metformin significantly increased pregnancy rates per person after 6 months' treatment (13/45 [29%] with clomifene plus metformin v 4/45 [9%] with clomifene alone; RR 3.3, 95% CI 1.2 to 9.2; NNT 5, 95% CI 3 to 22).

Harms: **Ovarian cancer:** In a cohort study of 3837 infertile women, 11 women were found to have ovarian cancer.[39] In 135 women that were randomly selected as a subcohort from these 3837 women, there was an 11-fold increase in risk of ovarian cancer in women using clomifene for 12 or more cycles (RR 11.1, 95% CI 1.5 to 82.3). The association was present for both gravid and nulligravid women, and for infertile women both with ovulatory disorders and with infertility from other causes. Subsequent studies have found no association between clomifene and ovarian cancer.[40–43] **Multiple pregnancy:** Multiple pregnancy occurs in 2–13% of women with all causes of infertility taking clomifene compared with a spontaneous multiple pregnancy rate of about 1–2% of women in North American and European populations.[44,45] In a 1 year survey in the UK, 25/44 (57%) triplet pregnancies reported were attributable to clomifene.[46] Clomifene was also implicated in two of the eight sets of quadruplets and quintuplets reported. **Ovarian hyperstimulation syndrome:** See glossary, p 2131. Clomifene tends to cause only mild ovarian hyperstimulation that does not require treatment.

Comment: Clomifene was first introduced in the 1960s and most of the trials testing its efficacy took place in the 1970s before more recent quality standards for RCTs were established. Three of the studies comparing clomifene versus tamoxifen based estimates of pregnancy rates on fewer than 30 pregnancies.[29,35,37] In the first RCT comparing tamoxifen versus clomifene, the different number of treatment cycles between groups could potentially bias the results.[35] In the RCT comparing clomifene plus metformin versus clomifene alone, the dose of clomifene was initially 50 mg daily for 5 days and only increased to 100 mg or 150 mg daily for 5 days if the lower dose was insufficient to enable ovulation to be triggered with human chorionic gonadotrophin.[38] With regard to the cohort study, 5/11 (45%) people with ovarian cancer were diagnosed with borderline epithelial tumours that had low malignant potential, and two with granulosa cell tumours that had different embryological, pathological, and epidemiological features from epithelial tumours.[39] Borderline and malignant tumours pose different risks that are not easy to combine and excluding the two granulosa cell tumours from the number of ovarian cancers found diminishes the increased risk attributed to clomifene treatment.

OPTION CYCLOFENIL

One RCT found no significant difference in pregnancy rates with cyclofenil versus placebo.

Benefits: **Versus placebo:** We found one RCT (213 women with either ovulatory disorders or unexplained infertility) comparing three cycles of cyclofenil (800 mg daily) versus placebo from days 4–8 of the ovulatory cycle.[47] It found no significant difference in cumulative pregnancy rates (26/114 [23%] with cyclofenil *v* 21/99 [21%] with placebo; RR 1.1, 95% CI 0.7 to 1.8).

Harms: The RCT did not report on adverse effects.[47]

Comment: Only 123/213 (58%) women in the RCT had ovulatory disorders and the results for these women were not presented separately.[47] The RCT does not, therefore, exclude a possible benefit of cyclofenil.

OPTION GONADOTROPHINS

One systematic review found no significant difference between human menopausal gonadotrophins and urofollitropin (urofollitrophin, urinary follicle stimulating hormone) in pregnancy rates. Two RCTs found no significant difference in cumulative pregnancy rates or numbers of live births with follitropin (recombinant follicle stimulating hormone) versus urofollitropin. The review found that urofollitropin versus human menopausal gonadotrophins significantly reduced the risk of ovarian hyperstimulation syndrome, although this was confined to women who were not treated with concomitant gonadotrophin releasing hormone analogues. Observational evidence suggests that gonadotrophins may be associated with an increased risk of non-invasive ovarian tumours and multiple pregnancies.

Benefits: **Versus placebo:** We found no RCTs. **Versus clomifene (clomiphene):** We found no RCTs. **Human menopausal gonadotrophins versus urofollitropin:** We found one systematic review (search date not stated, 14 RCTs, 388 women with subfertility associated with polycystic ovarian syndrome), which compared human menopausal gonadotrophins versus urofollitropin.[18] It found no significant difference in pregnancy rates (OR 0.8, 95 % CI 0.4 to 1.5). **Follitropin versus urofollitropin:** We found no systematic review but found two RCTs comparing urofollitropin versus follitropin.[48,49] The first RCT (172 women with clomifene resistant, normogonadotrophic anovulation) found no significant difference with follitropin versus urofollitropin in cumulative ovulation rates (95% with follitropin *v* 96% with urofollitropin), cumulative pregnancy rates (27% with follitropin *v* 24% with urofollitropin), or miscarriage rates (31% with follitropin *v* 32% with urofollitropin).[48] A second smaller RCT (51 women with clomifene resistant, normogonadotrophic anovulation) found similar results, although a significantly lower total dose and shorter duration of follitropin was used to achieve ovulation.[49] **Versus laparoscopic ovarian drilling:** See glossary, p 2130. See benefits of laparoscopic ovarian drilling, p 2115.

Harms: **Ovarian cancer:** One case control study (200 women with ovarian cancer and 408 area matched controls) found that women with non-invasive ovarian tumours were more than three times more likely to have been exposed to an ovulation induction agent (adjusted OR 3.5, 95% CI 1.2 to 10.1), particularly to human menopausal gonadotrophins (adjusted OR 9.4, 95% CI 1.7 to

52.1).[43] Women with invasive ovarian tumours were no more likely to have been exposed to any ovulation induction agents. **Multiple pregnancy:** Multiple pregnancy occurs in 29% of women with polycystic ovaries when conventional regimens of gonadotrophins are used to induce ovulation.[28] **Ovarian hyperstimulation:** The systematic review (search date not stated, 7 RCTs) found that urofollitropin versus human menopausal gonadotrophins significantly reduced the risk of ovarian hyperstimulation (OR 0.3, 95% CI 0.2 to 0.7).[18] However, this effect was only present where no concomitant gonadotrophin releasing hormone (GnRH) analogue was used (5 RCTs; OR 0.2, 95% CI 0.1 to 0.5). The review found that concomitant use of a GnRH analogue increased the risk of ovarian hyperstimulation (2 RCTs; OR 3.2, 95% CI 1.5 to 6.7). The RCT (172 women) comparing urofollitropin versus follitropin found no significant difference in the risk of multiple pregnancy or ovarian hyperstimulation syndrome, although the low event rates found with either treatment limit the usefulness of the result.[48]

Comment: Despite not being placebo controlled, trials of gonadotrophins often included women who were not ovulating and, therefore, provide some evidence that treatment is effective.[18] Avoiding gonadotrophins may reduce the risk of multiple pregnancy and ovarian hyperstimulation syndrome. Follitropin is not derived from human tissues.

OPTION LAPAROSCOPIC OVARIAN DRILLING

One systematic review and one subsequent small RCT found no significant difference with laparoscopic ovarian drilling versus gonadotrophins in pregnancy rates, but found that laparoscopic ovarian drilling significantly reduced rates of multiple pregnancies.

Benefits: We found one systematic review (search date 2001, 4 RCTs, 303 women with anovulatory clomifene [clomiphene] resistant polycystic ovary syndrome)[19] (see table 1, p 2136) and one subsequent RCT (see comment below).[50] The review found no significant difference with laparoscopic ovarian drilling (see glossary, p 2130) versus gonadotrophins in pregnancy rates after 12 months' follow up (OR 1.42, 95% CI 0.84 to 2.42).[19] The subsequent RCT (18 women with polycystic ovarian syndrome who had failed to ovulate after treatment with clomifene or purified follicle stimulating hormone) compared laparoscopic ovarian drilling versus a gonadotrophin releasing hormone analogue plus a combined oral contraceptive.[50] All the women also received three cycles of follitropin plus intrauterine insemination. The RCT found no significant difference in the number of pregnancies (5/10 [50%] with ovarian laser drilling *v* 5/8 [63%] with GnRH plus combined oral contraceptive; RR 0.8, 95% CI 0.4 to 1.8).

Harms: The systematic review found that laparoscopic ovarian drilling versus gonadotrophins significantly reduced rates of multiple pregnancies (OR 0.16, 95% CI 0.03 to 0.98).[19] Adverse effects associated with laparoscopic ovarian drilling include the risks of general anaesthesia, postoperative adhesion formation,[51] and pelvic infection.[52] We found no evidence to support the suggestion that laparoscopic drilling increases the long term risk of premature ovarian failure. Laparoscopic drilling is thought not to increase the risk of multiple pregnancy as it usually induces spontaneous ovulation, in contrast to the multifollicular ovulation that may be induced by the use of gonadotrophins.

Comment: The trials of laparoscopic ovarian drilling included women who were not ovulating and, therefore, provide some evidence that treatment is effective despite the lack of placebo controls.[19,50]

OPTION PULSATILE GONADOTROPHIN RELEASING HORMONE

One systematic review found insufficient evidence on the effects of pulsatile gonadotrophin releasing hormone treatment.

Benefits: We found one systematic review (search date not stated, 3 RCTs, 29 women with subfertility and clomifene resistant polycystic ovary syndrome) that compared pulsatile gonadotrophin releasing hormone (GnRH) versus another treatment to induce ovulation.[53] The RCTs included in the review described four different comparisons, were small (each reporting 1–4 pregnancies), and of short duration (1–3 cycles), and so provided insufficient evidence to assess the value of pulsatile GnRH in polycystic ovary syndrome.

Harms: One retrospective analysis (229 cycles in 71 women) compared pulsatile GnRH versus gonadotrophins alone, and found no significant difference in multiple pregnancy rates after six cycles.[54] However, 75% of the multiple pregnancies in the gonadotrophin group were triplets or higher order multiple pregnancies, whereas all multiple pregnancies in the GnRH group were twins.

Comment: Pulsatile GnRH is used in women with anovulation caused by low serum gonadotrophins and oestrogen concentrations (hypogonadotropic hypogonadism). Hypogonadotropic hypogonadism is a well defined condition and so evidence from case series should be generalisable to most affected women. Case series (256 anovulatory women with hypogonadotropic hypogonadism undergoing 1043 treatment cycles) found cumulative pregnancy rates of 59–73% at 6 months and 81–92% at 12 months.[55–57] Only one series reported the live birth rate; this was 65% after 12 treatment cycles.[55]

QUESTION What are the effects of treatments for tubal infertility?

OPTION SELECTIVE SALPINGOGRAPHY PLUS TUBAL CATHETERISATION

We found no RCTs on the effects of selective salpingography plus tubal catheterisation.

Benefits: We found no systematic review and no RCTs.

Harms: Observational studies have found that tubal perforation, which does not seem to be clinically important, occurred in 2%, and ectopic pregnancy in 3–9% of women undergoing selective salpingography and tubal catheterisation.[58,59]

Comment: One systematic review (search date not stated) combined data from 10 cohort and other observational studies of selective salpingography and tubal cannulation (482 women), and four observational studies of hysteroscopic cannulation for proximal tubal blockage (133 women).[58] It found that hysteroscopy versus selective salpingography and tubal catheterisation was associated with a higher pregnancy rate (pregnancies exceeding 20 wks' gestation: 65/133 [49%] with hysteroscopy *v* 103/482 [21%] with salpingography). None of the observational studies included an untreated group, so it is not possible to estimate the treatment related pregnancy rate over and above the spontaneous pregnancy rate. Tubal patency and pregnancy without treatment have been reported in women diagnosed with bilateral proximal tube obstruction.[60]

OPTION TUBAL FLUSHING

One systematic review found no RCTs of tubal flushing with water soluble media versus no intervention. It found that tubal flushing with oil soluble media versus no intervention increased the chance of pregnancy. The review found that tubal flushing with oil soluble versus water soluble media increased the live birth rate.

Benefits: We found no RCTs reporting solely on women with tubal infertility. We found one systematic review (search date 2001, 8 RCTs, 1706 women) that evaluated flushing of the woman's fallopian tubes with oil or water soluble media in couples with infertility.[61] **Versus no intervention:** The review found no RCTs comparing tubal flushing with water soluble media versus no intervention.[61] It found that tubal flushing with oil soluble media versus no intervention significantly increased the chance of pregnancy (2 RCTs; 224 women; OR 3.57, 95% CI 1.76 to 7.23). **Oil soluble versus water soluble media:** The review found no significant difference between tubal flushing with oil soluble versus water soluble media for chance of pregnancy, although oil soluble media versus water soluble media sigificantly increased the chance of live birth (live birth: 2 RCTs; 951 women; OR 1.49, 95% CI 1.05 to 2.11; pregnancy: 5 RCTs; 1241 women; OR 1.23, 95% CI 0.95 to 1.60).

Harms: **Versus no intervention:** The RCTs included in the review did not report on miscarriage, ectopic pregnancy, procedural pain, or short or long term procedural complications.[61] **Oil versus water soluble media:** The systematic review found that oil versus water soluble media reduced procedural pain and procedural complications (pain: 2 RCTs; 834 women; OR 0.40, 95% CI 0.28 to 0.57; procedural complications: 4 RCTs; 1357 women; OR 0.22, 95% CI 0.14 to 0.34).[61] It found no significant difference for miscarriage or ectopic pregnancy (miscarriage per pregnancy: 1 RCT; 158 women; OR 0.82, 95% CI 0.41 to 1.64; ectopic pregnancy: 2 RCTs; 562 women; OR 0.49, 95% CI 0.10 to 2.42).

Comment: RCTs comparing oil soluble versus water soluble media were statistically heterogeneous.[61] The RCTs were not solely in women with tubal infertility and so may also be relevant to couples with unexplained infertility. One RCT included in the review only included women with unexplained infertility or mild endometriosis.[62]

OPTION **TUBAL SURGERY**

One systematic review in women undergoing in vitro fertilisation has found that tubal surgery versus no treatment or medical treatment significantly increases the chance of becoming pregnant and significantly increases the live birth rate. Another review found no significant difference in pregnancy rates between different types of tubal surgery. One systematic review found no significant difference with tubal surgery plus additional treatments versus tubal surgery alone to prevent adhesion formation (steroids, dextran, and noxytioline) in pregnancy rates.

Benefits: **Versus no treatment or medical treatment:** We found one systematic review (search date 2000, 3 RCTs, 295 women with hydrosalpinges undergoing in vitro fertilisation [IVF]; see comment below), which found that tubal surgery versus no treatment or medical treatment (see comment below) significantly increased the chances of becoming pregnant (OR 1.75, 95% CI 1.07 to 2.86) and significantly increased the live birth rate (OR 2.13, 95% CI 1.24 to 3.65).[63] **Different types of tubal surgery versus each other:** We found three systematic reviews (search date not stated, 8 RCTs [see comment below];[64] search date not stated, 5 RCTs, 588 women;[65] search date not stated, 10 RCTs, 1086 women[66]). Two RCTs (130 women) identified by the first review found no significant difference with CO_2 laser adhesiolysis (see glossary, p 2130) versus diathermy adhesiolysis in numbers of pregnancies (16/30 [53%] with laser *v* 17/33 [52%] with diathermy; RR 1.04, 95% CI 0.65 to 1.67) or with CO_2 laser salpingostomy versus diathermy salpingostomy in numbers of pregnancies (26/75 [35%] with laser *v* 16/60 [27%] with diathermy; RR 1.30, 95% CI 0.77 to 2.19).[64] One RCT (72 women) identified by the first review found no significant difference with the use of an operating microscope versus magnifying lenses (loupes) during microsurgical reversal of sterilisations in pregnancies after 2 years (26/36 [72%] with microscope *v* 28/36 [78%] with loupes; OR 0.75, 95% CI 0.26 to 2.15).[64] The second systematic review compared postoperative hydrotubation or second look laparoscopy (see glossary, p 2131) plus adhesiolysis after tubal surgery versus control.[65] It found that all the studies were either poor quality or underpowered. It found insufficient evidence to support the routine practice of hydrotubation (1 RCT; OR 1.12, 95% CI 0.57 to 2.21) or second look laparoscopy (2 RCTs; OR 0.96 95% CI 0.44 to 2.07) after tubal surgery. The third systematic review compared tubal surgery plus additional treatments to prevent adhesion formation (steroids, dextran, and noxytioline) versus tubal surgery alone.[66] It found no significant difference in pregnancy rates with tubal surgery plus steroids (systemic or intraperitoneal) versus no steroids (4 RCTs; OR 1.10, 95% CI 0.74 to 1.64), tubal surgery plus dextran (intraperitoneal) versus no dextran (3 RCTs; OR 0.65, 95% CI 0.37 to 1.14), or tubal surgery plus noxytioline (intraperitoneal) versus no noxytioline (1 RCT; OR 0.67, 95% CI 0.30 to 1.47). **Versus IVF:** We found no RCTs (see comment below). **Proximal tubal blockage:** We found no RCTs (see comment below).

Harms: The systematic review comparing tubal surgery versus no treatment or medical treatment found no significant difference in the rate of ectopic pregnancy (OR 0.42, 95% CI 0.08 to 2.14), miscarriage per pregnancy (OR 0.49, 95% CI 0.16 to 1.52), or treatment related complications (OR 5.80, 95% CI 0.35 to 96.79).[63] Tubal surgery involves general anaesthesia and admission to hospital. There is a risk of ectopic pregnancy caused by pre-existing tubal damage; rates of 7–9% have been reported, compared with 1–3% with IVF.[9,10] IVF carries the risk of multiple pregnancy and ovarian hyperstimulation syndrome (see harms of IVF under treatments for infertility caused by ovulation disorders, p 2120).

Comment: Success rates with tubal surgery depend on the severity and site of disease. The best figures from surgery in women with distal tubal occlusion are live birth rates of 20–30%, with rates of up to 60% reported for the less common proximal occlusion.[11–16] **Versus no treatment or medical treatment:** In the systematic review comparing tubal surgery versus non-surgical treatment, although a variety of different surgical techniques were used, laparoscopic unilateral or bilateral salpingectomy were the most common (numerical data not provided).[63] **Different types of tubal surgery versus each other:** One systematic review (search date not stated, 7 observational studies, 279 women with proximal tubal blockage) compared microsurgery (275 women) versus macrosurgery (see glossary, p 2131) (104 women).[58] It found that microsurgery significantly increased pregnancy rates (RR 2.2, 95% CI 1.5 to 3.2). One of the systematic reviews comparing different techniques for pelvic surgery versus each other included non-randomised studies if there was an appropriate control group and no RCT evidence available.[64] Of the eight RCTs included in the review, five used outdated surgical techniques, were small, and had problems relating to methods of randomisation. These data precede recent improvements in case selection and laparoscopic training. **Versus IVF:** Case series of tubal surgery have been compared with large databases of couples undergoing IVF.[11,67–71] These found that tubal surgery was as effective as IVF in women with filmy adhesions, mild distal tubal occlusion, or proximal obstruction. If successful, tubal surgery allows women to have more pregnancies without further medical intervention and without the risks associated with IVF.[72]

OPTION IN VITRO FERTILISATION

We found no RCTs of in vitro fertilisation versus no treatment. One RCT found that immediate versus delayed in vitro fertilisation significantly increased numbers of pregnancies and live births. Three RCTs found no significant difference in numbers of live births with in vitro fertilisation versus intracytoplasmic sperm injection. Observational evidence suggests that adverse effects associated with in vitro fertilisation include multiple pregnancies and ovarian hyperstimulation syndrome.

Benefits: We found no systematic review. **In vitro fertilisation (IVF) versus no treatment:** We found no RCTs. **Immediate versus delayed IVF:** We found one RCT (399 couples with any cause of infertility; the couples who received delayed IVF acted as untreated controls for at least 6 months), which found that immediate IVF versus delayed IVF (see glossary, p 2130) significantly increased the numbers of pregnancies (33/190 [17%] with immediate IVF *v* 13/163 [8%] with delayed IVF; RR 2.18, 95% CI 1.19 to 4.0), and significantly increased the numbers of live births (22/190 [12%] with immediate IVF *v* 8/163 [5%] with delayed IVF; RR 2.36, 95% CI 1.08 to 5.16).[73] **Versus tubal surgery:** See benefits of tubal surgery, p 2118. **Versus intracytoplasmic sperm injection:** One RCT (415 couples with non-male factor infertility) found no significant difference with IVF versus intracytoplasmic sperm injection in pregnancy rates (72/224 [32%] with IVF *v* 53/211 [25%] with intracytoplasmic sperm injection; RR 1.30, 95% CI 0.95 to 1.73).[74] Two other small RCTs (167 couples in total) found similar results.[75,76]

Harms: **Multiple pregnancy:** Two RCTs did not report on multiple pregnancy rates,[73,75] and two RCTs lacked the statistical power required to detect significant differences in multiple pregnancy rates between treatments. However, of the 6450 live births following IVF in the UK in 1998–1999, 31% were multiple, including 235 (3.6%) sets of triplets and two sets of quadruplets.[30] In the UK, the number of embryos that can be replaced is restricted to three. In the USA, where there are no such restrictions, 15 367 live births included 38% multiple births, 6% of which were triplets and above.[77] **Ovarian hyperstimulation syndrome:** Severe ovarian hyperstimulation syndrome (see glossary, p 2131) occurs in 0.5–2.0% of all IVF cycles.[78] Ovarian hyperstimulation syndrome rates were not reported in the RCTs above.[73,75] **Obstetric outcome:** We found one systematic review (search date 1998, 42 high quality observational studies) that compared obstetric outcome in mothers receiving IVF versus either a population-based control group or a selected control group matched for different variables.[79] It found that children born after IVF had a considerably higher risk of being born preterm and with a lower birth weight than children conceived naturally, although this was likely to be because of the high incidence of multiple births and maternal characteristics such as nulliparity, increased age, previous infertility, and obstetric history (absolute numbers not provided). There was no evidence of an increased overall incidence of congenital malformations in children born after conventional IVF or after embryo cryopreservation.

Comment: The success of IVF is influenced by a woman's age, duration of infertility, and previous pregnancy history. Pregnancy rates are highest between the ages of 25 and 35 years and decline steeply after 35 years.[5] Similar clinics, which describe the same methods, report different success rates for IVF. In the UK, the live birth rate per IVF cycle varies from 0–28% with an average of 19.5% if intracytoplasmic sperm injection cycles are also taken into account.[30] The equivalent average figure in the USA is 25%, but again results vary between centres.[77,80] In the UK, larger centres (≥ 200 cycles a year) report slightly higher live birth rates than smaller centres (20% per cycle started compared with 16%).[81] Such a difference has not been consistently reported in the USA.

QUESTION **What are the effects of treatment for infertility associated with endometriosis?**

OPTION **DRUG-INDUCED OVARIAN SUPPRESSION**

One systematic review has found no significant difference in pregnancy rates between drugs that induce ovarian suppression versus either placebo or danazol. The review found that ovulation suppression agents cause adverse effects that include weight gain, hot flushes, and osteoporosis, and that danazol may cause dose related weight gain and androgenic effects.

Benefits: We found one systematic review (search date not stated, 13 RCTs).[82] **Versus placebo:** The review identified five RCTs (244 women with visually diagnosed endometriosis who had been attempting conception for < 12 months) comparing ovulation suppression agents (medroxyprogesterone, gestrinone, combined oral contraceptive pills, and gonadotrophin releasing hormone analogues) versus placebo and found no significant difference in pregnancy rates (OR 0.8, 95% CI 0.5 to 1.4).[82] **Versus danazol:** The review identified eight RCTs (658 similar women with visually diagnosed endometriosis who had been attempting conception for < 12 months), which compared ovulation suppression versus danazol and found no significant difference in pregnancy rates (OR compared with danazol 1.2, 95% CI 0.9 to 1.7).[82] **Versus surgery:** See benefits of surgical treatment, p 2122.

Harms: The review found that ovulation suppression agents caused adverse effects that included weight gain, hot flushes, and osteoporosis.[82] Adverse effects of danazol were dose related and included an average weight gain of 2–4 kg with 3 months' treatment, androgenic effects such as acne, seborrhoea, hirsutism, voice changes, and general complaints, including irritability, musculoskeletal pains, and tiredness. Hot flushes and breast atrophy were sometimes observed. Most of these adverse effects were reversible on stopping treatment.[83]

Comment: In the review, three of the trials used a combination of clomifene with other infertility drugs.[82] Treatment using ovulation suppression could waste valuable time for women who are trying to get pregnant, as the opportunity for spontaneous conceptions is lost during treatment.

OPTION **INTRAUTERINE INSEMINATION PLUS GONADOTROPHINS**

One RCT found that intrauterine insemination plus gonadotrophins versus no treatment significantly increased live birth rates. A second RCT found no significant difference in birth rates with intrauterine insemination plus pituitary down regulation plus gonadotrophins versus expectant management. A third RCT found that intrauterine insemination plus gonadotrophins versus intrauterine insemination alone significantly increased pregnancy rates after the first treatment cycle.

Benefits: We found no systematic review but found three RCTs.[84–86] The first RCT (104 couples) compared intrauterine insemination plus gonadotrophins (53 couples, 127 cycles) versus no treatment (50 couples, 184 cycles).[84] It found that intrauterine insemination plus gonadotrophins significantly increased live birth rates (14/53 [26%] with intrauterine insemination plus gonadotrophins *v* 4/50 [8%] with no treatment; RR 3.3, 95% CI 1.2 to 9.4; NNT 6, 95% CI 3 to 28). The second RCT (49 women with minimal or mild endometriosis) comparing three cycles of pituitary down regulation plus gonadotrophins plus intrauterine insemination versus 6 months of expectant management found no significant difference in birth rates (7/24 [29%] with intrauterine insemination *v* 5/25 [20%] with expectant management; RR 1.5, 95% CI 0.5 to 4.0).[85] When combined, these two RCTs show an overall twofold increase in live birth rates with intrauterine insemination plus gonadotrophins versus expectant management over a similar time period (RR *v* no treatment 2.3, 95% CI 1.1 to 4.6). The third RCT (119 couples with primary pelvic or cervical factor infertility for a mean of 3.7 years) compared alternate cycles of gonadotrophins plus intrauterine insemination versus intrauterine insemination alone.[86] It found that gonadotrophins plus intrauterine insemination versus intrauterine insemination alone significantly increased the pregnancy rate after the first treatment cycle (11/58 [19%] with gonadotrophins plus intrauterine insemination *v* 0/61 [0%] with intrauterine insemination alone; NNT 5, 95% CI 4 to 14). The 119 couples were subsequently followed up longitudinally and it was found that, in the 57 couples with a diagnosis of endometriosis, gonadotrophins plus intrauterine insemination versus intrauterine insemination alone significantly increased the probability of pregnancy over a total of 127 cycles (RR 5.1, 95% CI 1.1 to 22.5).

Harms: No cases of severe ovarian hyperstimulation or hospital admission were reported in the first or third RCTs.[84,86] In the second RCT, one severe case (1/24 [4%]), one moderate case (1/24 [4%]), and three mild cases (3/24 [13%]) of ovarian hyperstimulation syndrome were reported.[85]

Comment: None.

OPTION SURGICAL TREATMENT

Two RCTs that compared laparoscopic surgery versus diagnostic laparoscopy found inconsistent results for differences in numbers of pregnancies and live births.

Benefits: **Versus placebo or ovarian suppression:** We found no RCTs (see comment below). **Laparoscopic surgery versus diagnostic laparoscopy:** We found two RCTs (in a total of 442 infertile women with minimal or mild endometriosis) comparing laparoscopic surgery (ablation or resection of endometriosis) versus diagnostic laparoscopy.[21,22] In the larger RCT (341 women), laparoscopic surgery versus diagnostic laparoscopy significantly increased the probability of pregnancy occurring within 36 weeks and lasting longer than 20 weeks (50/172 [29%] with laparoscopic surgery *v* 29/169 [17%]; RR 1.7, 95% CI 1.2 to 2.6; NNT 8, 95% CI 4 to 41; see comment below).[21] The smaller RCT (101 women) found no significant difference between laparoscopic surgery versus diagnostic laparoscopy in live birth rates after 1 year (10/51 [20%] with laparoscopic surgery *v* 10/45 [22%] with diagnostic laparoscopy; RR 0.90, 95 % CI 0.41 to 1.92).[22] See laparoscopic ablation of endometrial deposits under endometriosis, p 2079.

Harms: The risks and morbidity of surgery under general anaesthesia, and of postoperative adhesion formation, should be balanced against the adverse effects of treatments involving ovarian suppression or stimulation. One multicentre series of 29 966 diagnostic and operative gynaecological laparoscopies found a mortality of 3.3/100 000 laparoscopies and a complication rate of 3.2/1000 laparoscopies.[23]

Comment: We found one systematic review (search date not stated)[24] and one non-systemic review,[25] which together identified 21 cohort studies and one quasi-randomised trial in a total of 3879 women with all stages of endometriosis. Interventions were laparoscopic or open surgery versus medical treatment or no treatment. Surgical treatment versus medical or no treatment significantly increased pregnancy rates (RR 1.4, 95% CI 1.3 to 1.5), although there was no significant difference between laparoscopic and open surgery (RR 0.9, 95% CI 0.8 to 1.0).[25] In women with mild or minimal endometriosis, analysis of pooled data found that laparoscopic surgery versus danazol or no treatment significantly increased pregnancy rates (OR 2.7, 95% CI 2.1 to 3.5).[25] In the larger RCT, comparing laparoscopic surgery versus diagnostic laparoscopy, 48/341 (14%) women who received laparoscopic surgery for their endometriosis also had peri-adnexal adhesions treated, which may have affected their fertility.[21]

OPTION IN VITRO FERTILISATION

We found no RCTs in women with endometriosis related infertility undergoing in vitro fertilisation treatment.

Benefits: We found no systematic review or RCTs.

Harms: See harms of in vitro fertilisation under treatments for tubal infertility, p 2120.

Comment: We found two retrospective cohort studies in women undergoing in vitro fertilisation comparing women with endometriosis versus women with different stages of endometriosis or other causes of infertility, which found no significant differences in pregnancy rates.[26,87] We found one systematic review (search date 1999, 22 non-randomised studies) that examined effects of endometriosis versus other cause of infertility on in vitro fertilisation outcome.[88] It found that women with endometriosis were less likely to become pregnant than women with infertility due to blocked or damaged tubes (pregnancy assessed by human chorionic gonadotrophin levels; adjusted OR 0.56, 95% CI 0.44 to 0.70). There is a need for properly controlled prospective randomised studies that present their results for different stages of endometriosis using a validated classification system. Comparisons with assisted reproductive techniques are also required.

QUESTION **What are the effects of treatments for male infertility?**

OPTION **INTRAUTERINE INSEMINATION**

Two systematic reviews have found that intrauterine insemination versus intracervical insemination or natural intercourse significantly increases pregnancy rates per cycle.

Benefits: We found two systematic reviews (search date not stated[33] and search date 1996–1997[89]). The first review (10 RCTs, 2082 treatment cycles in couples with male infertility) found that intrauterine insemination versus intracervical insemination or natural intercourse significantly increased the pregnancy rate per cycle (6.5% with intrauterine insemination *v* 3.1% with intracervical insemination or timed natural intercourse; OR 2.2, 95% CI 1.4 to 3.4).[33] The second review (17 RCTs; 3662 completed treatment cycles in couples with male subfertility) found that intrauterine insemination versus timed intercourse significantly increased pregnancy rates both in natural cycles (OR 2.4, 95% CI 1.5 to 3.8) and in controlled ovarian hyperstimulation (see glossary, p 2131) cycles (OR 2.1, 95% CI 1.3 to 3.5).[89] The review found that intrauterine insemination in controlled cycles versus timed intercourse in natural cycles also significantly increased the probability of conception (OR 6.2, 95% CI 2.4 to 16.5), but found no significant difference with intrauterine insemination in controlled cycles versus intrauterine insemination in natural cycles (OR 1.8, 95% CI 1.0 to 3.3).[80]

Harms: Apart from the risks of ovarian hyperstimulation syndrome and multiple pregnancy associated with ovarian stimulation, intrauterine insemination may increase the likelihood of infection and may cause discomfort.[90] However, data from RCTs are scarce.

Comment: We found three RCTs that addressed the optimum number of inseminations in controlled ovarian stimulation cycles. Two RCTs found that two inseminations performed in the pre-ovulatory and peri-ovulatory periods produced significantly higher pregnancy rates than one peri-ovulatory insemination.[91,92] The other RCT found a non-significant increase in pregnancy rates with two similarly timed inseminations.[93] One small crossover RCT addressed the timing of insemination in clomifene stimulated cycles. It found similar pregnancy rates per cycle whether insemination was timed with a urinary luteinising hormone kit or whether ultrasound monitoring with human chorionic gonadotrophin induction of ovulation was used.[94]

OPTION **INTRACYTOPLASMIC SPERM INJECTION PLUS IN VITRO FERTILISATION**

One systematic review found insufficient evidence on the effects of intracytoplasmic sperm injections plus in vitro fertilisation versus in vitro fertilisation alone.

Benefits: **Versus in vitro fertilisation (IVF) alone:** We found one systematic review (search date not stated, 10 RCTs, 437 couples; see comment below), which compared intracytoplasmic sperm injection

(ICSI) plus IVF versus IVF alone (8 RCTs compared ICSI plus IVF *v* conventional IVF; 1 RCT compared ICSI plus IVF *v* subzonal sperm injection; and 1 RCT compared ICSI plus IVF *v* additional IVF).[95] For couples with normal semen, the review found no significant difference with ICSI plus IVF versus IVF alone in fertilisation rates per retrieved oocyte or pregnancy rates, but found that ICSI plus IVF versus IVF alone significantly increased fertilisation rates per inseminated oocyte (combined OR 1.4, 95% CI 1.2 to 1.7). For couples with borderline semen (concentration 10–20 million/mL, motility 30–50%, morphology 4–14% normal forms) the review found that ICSI plus IVF versus IVF alone significantly increased fertilisation rates per oocyte retrieved (OR 3.79, 95% CI 2.97 to 4.85) and fertilisation rates per oocyte inseminated (OR 3.9, 95% CI 3.0 to 5.2). For couples with poor semen (concentration < 10 million/mL, motility < 30%, morphology < 4% normal forms), two RCTs identified by the review found that ICSI plus IVF versus subzonal sperm injection or additional IVF improved fertilisation outcomes.

Harms: Observational studies have found conflicting reports of congenital abnormalities[27,96] and sex chromosomal abnormalities in children born after ICSI (see comment below).[97,98]

Comment: The review used the proxy outcome of fertilisation rates, and eight RCTs included in the review used randomisation strategies based on oocytes or metaphase II oocytes.[95] Many couples have a strong preference for a child genetically related to both partners.[99] The data on congenital and chromosome abnormalities with ICSI are constantly being revised as experience increases.

OPTION IN VITRO FERTILISATION VERSUS GAMETE INTRAFALLOPIAN TRANSFER

One RCT found insufficient evidence on the effects of in vitro fertilisation versus gamete intrafallopian transfer.

Benefits: We found no systematic review. We found one RCT (13 couples with male infertility), which found no significant difference with in vitro fertilisation versus gamete intrafallopian transfer in numbers of pregnancies (2/7 [29%] with in vitro fertilisation *v* 2/6 [33%] with gamete intrafallopian transfer; RR 1.20, 95% CI 0.23 to 5.95).[100]

Harms: See harms of in vitro fertilisation under treatments for tubal infertility, p 2120.

Comment: None.

OPTION DONOR INSEMINATION

We found no good evidence on the effects of donor insemination.

Benefits: **Versus no treatment:** We found no systematic review or RCTs in couples with male infertility that compared donor insemination versus no treatment or other interventions.

Harms: We found no good evidence.

Comment: One systematic review (search date 1996, 12 RCTs, 2215 treatment cycles) found limited evidence that intrauterine insemination of frozen donor sperm versus intracervical insemination of donor sperm increased pregnancy rates.[90] The review included RCTs that were poor in their methodology, contained several different treatment variations making direct comparisons difficult, and included a mixture of women with and without fertility problems. Data are available from large databases, but it is sometimes unclear whether ovarian stimulation was used in addition to donor insemination. The live birth rate per cycle in the UK Human Fertilisation and Embryology Authority database (based on 7136 women) was 9%.[30] Similar rates are reported from the French donor insemination database (23 700 women over 4 years), with a mean pregnancy rate of 10.3% per cycle, and the Sheffield database (UK, 343 women, 980 treatment cycles), with an 11.3% overall live birth rate.[31,32] Comparisons of donor insemination versus no treatment or other interventions may be inappropriate as, for many couples, donor insemination is not an acceptable option. RCTs have tended to concentrate on comparisons between different techniques of donor insemination.

QUESTION What are the effects of treatment for unexplained infertility?

OPTION CLOMIFENE

One systematic review found limited evidence that clomifene versus placebo significantly increased rates of pregnancy per cycle.

Benefits: We found one systematic review (search date 2000, 5 RCTs, 4 using crossover designs; 458 cycles in women with unexplained infertility), which found that clomifene (clomiphene) versus placebo significantly increased pregnancy rates per cycle (OR 2.5, 95% CI 1.4 to 4.6; see comment below).[101] When only cycles before crossover were analysed (which was only possible with the data from 3 of these trials), the positive effect increased (OR 5.0, 95% CI 1.8 to 14.3).

Harms: See harms of clomifene under treatments for infertility caused by ovulation disorders, p 2113.

Comment: The systematic review[101] excluded one RCT because of the risk of selection bias with a pseudo-random allocation method based on odd or even chart numbers.[102] The other RCTs identified by the review were generally of poor quality and it is possible that, if one further medium sized RCT was performed, the direction of the overall effect found with meta-analysis could change again.[101] The review highlighted important differences between the trials: two RCTs included women with surgically treated endometriosis, one included only couples with primary infertility, and one included couples with a short duration of infertility (median of 28 months). Three of the RCTs included co-intervention with intrauterine insemination or cervicovaginal insemination. The RCTs also differed in their design (4 were crossover trials) and in the quality of randomisation (only 1 used properly concealed randomisation). The authors of the review commented that as the baseline cycle fecundity of the women included in these trials would only be about 1–2%, even with clomifene their cycle fecundity would be unlikely to exceed 5%.[101]

OPTION INTRAUTERINE INSEMINATION

Two systematic reviews and one subsequent RCT in couples undergoing ovarian stimulation treatment have found that intrauterine insemination versus timed intercourse or intracervical insemination significantly increases the rate of pregnancy. One systematic review has found no significant difference with intrauterine insemination versus timed intercourse or intracervical insemination in pregnancy rates, but has found that the addition of ovarian stimulation to any of the three interventions significantly increases pregnancy rate per cycle. One systematic review and one subsequent RCT have found that fallopian tube sperm perfusion versus intrauterine insemination significantly increases pregnancy rates. One systematic review found no significant difference between intrauterine insemination with or without ovarian stimulation versus in vitro fertilisation for live birth rate.

Benefits: **Versus timed intercourse or intracervical insemination:** We found three systematic reviews,[33,34,103] and one subsequent RCT,[104] in couples with unexplained infertility. The first review (search date not stated, 8 RCTs, number of treatment cycles not stated) compared intrauterine insemination plus ovarian stimulation with gonadotrophins versus timed intercourse plus ovarian stimulation with gonadotrophins.[103] It found that intrauterine insemination plus ovarian stimulation significantly increased the likelihood of pregnancy (OR 2.4, 95% CI 1.4 to 3.9). The second review (search date 1997, 7 RCTs, 980 treatment cycles) compared intrauterine insemination plus ovarian stimulation with gonadotrophins versus timed intercourse plus ovarian stimulation with gonadotrophins.[34] It found that intrauterine insemination plus ovarian stimulation significantly increased the pregnancy rate per cycle (110/549 [20%] with intrauterine insemination *v* 49/431 [11%] with timed intercourse; RR 0.20, 95% CI 0.08 to 0.31). The third systematic review (search date not stated, 7 RCTs, 934 treatment cycles) compared intrauterine insemination versus timed intercourse or intracervical insemination.[33] Four RCTs used gonadotrophins, two used clomifene (clomiphene), and three used no ovarian stimulation. The review found no significant difference with intrauterine insemination versus intracervical insemination or timed intercourse in pregnancy rates (OR 1.5, 95% CI 1.0 to 2.2). The review also found that the addition of ovarian stimulation with gonadotrophins to any of the three interventions significantly increased the overall pregnancy rates (45/249 [18%] with intrauterine insemination or favourable timed intracervical insemination or natural intercourse plus gonadotrophin stimulation *v* 9/108 [8%] with intrauterine insemination or favourable timed intracervical insemination or natural intercourse alone; RR 2.17, 95% CI 1.10 to 4.28; NNT 11, 95% CI 7 to 58). The subsequent RCT (932 couples) compared intracervical insemination alone, intrauterine insemination alone, intracervical insemination plus ovarian stimulation, and intrauterine insemination plus ovarian stimulation for four cycles or until pregnancy was achieved.[104] It found that intrauterine insemination plus ovarian stimulation versus intracervical insemination significantly increased the chance of becoming pregnant (OR 3.2, 95% CI 2.0 to 5.3). The RCT also found pregnancy rates of 14/233 (6%) with intracervical insemination, 35/234 (15%) with intrauterine insemination, 26/234 (11%) with ovarian stimulation plus intracervical insemination, and 54/231 (23%) with ovarian stimulation plus intrauterine insemination.[104] **Versus intrauterine insemination plus ovarian stimulation:** We found one RCT (932 couples), which found that intrauterine insemination plus ovarian stimulation versus intrauterine insemination alone significantly increased the chance of becoming pregnant (OR 1.7, 95% CI 1.2 to 2.6).[104] **Versus fallopian tube sperm perfusion:** See glossary, p 2130. See benefits of fallopian tube sperm perfusion, p 2129. **Versus gamete intrafallopian transfer:** See benefits of gamete intrafallopian transfer, p 2129. **Versus in vitro fertilisation (IVF):** See IVF for unexplained infertility, p 2130.

Harms: In the RCT (258 couples) comparing intrauterine insemination versus IVF, multiple pregnancy rates were 4% with intrauterine insemination in natural cycles, 29% with intrauterine insemination in stimulated cycles, and 21% with IVF (see harms of gonadotrophins, p 2114).[102] Mild ovarian hyperstimulation syndrome (see glossary, p 2131) occurred in two women in the stimulated intrauterine insemination group, and severe ovarian hyperstimulation syndrome occurred in three women in the IVF group. Apart from the risks of ovarian hyperstimulation syndrome and multiple pregnancy, intrauterine insemination may increase the likelihood of infection and may be associated with some discomfort. However, data from RCTs are scarce. One RCT (97 couples with unexplained infertility) compared low dose, step up follicle stimulating hormone (FSH) versus a conventional FSH regimen combined with intrauterine insemination.[105] There was no significant difference in pregnancy rates (7/49 [14%] with low dose FSH and intrauterine insemination v 7/48 [15%] with conventional FSH and intrauterine insemination; RR 0.98, 95% CI 0.37 to 2.58), but low dose FSH versus conventional FSH significantly reduced the number of women with ovarian hyperstimulation syndrome (4/49 [8%] with low dose FSH v 13/48 [27%] with conventional FSH; RR 0.30, 95% CI 0.11 to 0.86; NNT 6, 95% 3 to 28), and ovarian hyperstimulation syndrome requiring hospitalisation (0% v 16.7%). However, the low dose regimen did not completely prevent multiple pregnancies.

Comment: Only three of the RCTs were common to all three systematic reviews. One of the reviews scored the included studies for validity.[34] They scored from 49–70% when 100% was taken as the ideal study. The evidence from RCTs for timing and the optimum number of inseminations per cycle is conflicting (see benefits of intrauterine insemination under treatments for infertility associated with endometriosis, p 2123).

OPTION FALLOPIAN TUBE SPERM PERFUSION

One systematic review and one subsequent RCT have found that fallopian tube sperm perfusion versus intrauterine insemination significantly increases pregnancy rates.

Benefits: **Versus intrauterine insemination:** We found one systematic review (search date not stated, 5 RCTs in couples with unexplained infertility)[106] and one subsequent RCT, which compared fallopian tube sperm perfusion (see glossary, p 2130) versus intrauterine insemination.[107] All five RCTs in the review used gonadotrophins or gonadotrophins plus clomifene, and in total 293 cycles of intrauterine insemination and 317 cycles of fallopian tube sperm perfusion were assessed. The review found that fallopian tube sperm perfusion versus intrauterine insemination significantly increased pregnancy rate per cycle (70/317 [22%] with fallopian tube sperm perfusion *v* 38/293 [13%] with intrauterine insemination; RR 1.70, 95% CI 1.19 to 2.44; NNT 11, 95% CI 7 to 33). The subsequent RCT (132 cycles in 65 couples) found that fallopian tube sperm perfusion versus intrauterine insemination significantly increased pregnancy rates per cycle (16/66 [24%] with fallopian tube sperm perfusion *v* 6/66 [9%] with intrauterine insemination; RR 2.67, 95% CI 1.11 to 6.40; NNT 7, 95% CI 4 to 38) and significantly increased pregnancy rates per person (16/33 [48%] with fallopian tube sperm perfusion *v* 6/32 [19%] with intrauterine insemination; RR 2.59, 95% CI 1.16 to 5.77; NNT 4, 95% CI 2 to 9) after a maximum of three treatment cycles.[107]

Harms: See harms of intrauterine insemination, p 2128. The systematic review did not report on harms.[106] The subsequent RCT reported that complications, including cervical bleeding, vasovagal episodes, uterine cramping, or pelvic infections, were not reported with either treatment.[107]

Comment: None.

OPTION GAMETE INTRAFALLOPIAN TRANSFER

We found no RCTs of gamete intrafallopian transfer versus no treatment. RCTs found conflicting results with gamete intrafallopian transfer versus other treatments (intrauterine insemination, timed intercourse, and in vitro fertilisation in pregnancy rates).

Benefits: **Versus no treatment:** We found no systematic review or RCTs. **Versus intrauterine insemination or timed intercourse:** We found no systematic review. We found three RCTs (283 couples with unexplained infertility).[108–110] The first RCT compared gamete intrafallopian transfer (GIFT) versus ovarian stimulation plus either timed intercourse or timed cervical donor insemination and found no significant difference in pregnancy rates (2/24 [8%] with GIFT cycles *v* 2/15 [13%] with ovarian stimulation; RR 0.63, 95% CI 0.10 to 3.98).[108] Of the other two RCTs, one found that GIFT versus ovarian stimulation plus intrauterine insemination increased pregnancy rates, and the other found no significant difference in pregnancy rates.[109,110] **Versus in vitro fertilisation:** See benefits of in vitro fertilisation for the treatment of unexplained infertility, p 2130.

Harms: Potential harms include the risks attributable to general anaesthesia and laparoscopy. Multiple pregnancy rates vary with the number of oocytes transferred.[110]

Comment: One prospective cohort study (99 treatment cycles, 53 couples) found that GIFT versus no treatment increased numbers of pregnancies.[111] GIFT, unlike in vitro fertilisation, gives no diagnostic information regarding fertilisation, and involves a laparoscopy and general anaesthetic, both of which are usually avoided with in vitro fertilisation. Success rates decrease with increasing age.[112,113]

OPTION IN VITRO FERTILISATION

One systematic review found no significant difference between in vitro fertilisation and expectant management for pregnancy rate in people with unexplained infertility. It found no significant difference between in vitro fertilisation versus gamete intrafallopian transfer or versus intraterine insemination with or without ovarian stimulation for live birth rate.

Benefits: We found one systematic review (search date 2001, 5 RCTs, 353 women).[114] **Versus expectant management:** The review found no significant difference between in vitro fertilisation and expectant management for clinical pregnancy rate (1 RCT; 35 women; OR 0.3, 95% CI 0.02 to 3.67).[114] **Versus intrauterine insemination:** Three included RCTs found no significant difference in live birth rate between IVF versus intrauterine insemination with or without ovarian stimulation (without ovarian stimulation; 1 RCT; 113 women; OR for live birth 1.96, 95% CI 0.88 to 4.36; with ovarian stimulation; 1 RCT; 118 women; OR 1.15, 95% CI 0.55 to 2.42).[114] **Versus gamete intrafallopian transfer:** The review found no significant difference between in vitro fertilisation and gamete intrafallopian transfer for live birth rate (1 RCTs; 69 women; OR 2.57, 95% CI 0.93 to 7.08).[114]

Harms: See harms of in vitro fertilisation under treatments for tubal infertility, p 2120.

Comment: The RCTs included in the systematic review may lack power to detect clinically important differences between treatments.

GLOSSARY

Adhesiolysis Division of adhesions, which are bands of scar tissue that form after infection or surgery.

Delayed in vitro fertilisation In vitro fertilisation treatment after 6 months of being assessed in an infertility clinic after at least 12 months of infertility.

Fallopian tube sperm perfusion Fallopian tube sperm perfusion is based on a pressure injection of 4 mL sperm suspension with an attempt to seal the cervix to prevent semen reflux. It attempts to ensure a sperm flushing of the fallopian tubes and an overflowing of the inseminate into the pouch of Douglas.

Hydrotubation Flushing of the fallopian tubes through the cervix and uterine cavity to remove surgical debris and reduce the incidence of tubal reocclusion.

Immediate in vitro fertilisation In vitro fertilisation treatment within 6 months of being assessed in an infertility clinic after at least 12 months of infertility.

Laparoscopic ovarian drilling Ovarian drilling can be performed laparoscopically by either cautery or laser vapourisation (using CO_2, argon, or Nd:YAG lasers), which are used to create multiple perforations (about 10 holes/ovary) of the ovarian surface and stroma (inner area of the ovary). This is thought to cause ovulation by restoring the intra-ovarian hormonal environment to normal, which in turn beneficially affects the hypothalamic–pituitary–ovarian axis.

Macrosurgery Surgery without dedicated optical magnification.

Microsurgery Surgery involving optical magnification to allow the use of much finer instruments and suture material in addition to a non-touch technique, with the aim of minimising tissue handling and damage.

Ovarian hyperstimulation syndrome Can occur in mild, moderate, and severe forms. Mild ovarian hyperstimulation syndrome is characterised by fluid accumulation, as shown by weight gain, abdominal distension, and discomfort. Moderate ovarian hyperstimulation syndrome is associated with nausea and vomiting, ovarian enlargement, abdominal distension, discomfort, and dyspnoea. Severe ovarian hyperstimulation syndrome is a life threatening condition, in which there is contraction of the intravascular volume, tense ascites, pleural and pericardial effusions, severe haemoconcentration, and the development of hepatorenal failure. Deaths have occurred, caused usually by cerebrovascular thrombosis, renal failure, or cardiac tamponade.

Second look laparoscopy Laparoscopy performed some time after tubal surgery (either open or laparoscopic) with the aim of dividing adhesions relating to the initial procedure.

REFERENCES

1. European Society for Human Reproduction and Embryology. Guidelines to the prevalence, diagnosis, treatment and management of infertility, 1996. *Hum Reprod* 1996;11:1775–1807.
2. Schmidt L, Munster K. Infertility, involuntary infecundity, and the seeking of medical advice in industrialized countries 1970–1992: a review of concepts, measurements and results. *Hum Reprod* 1995;10:1407–1418.
3. Effective Health Care. The management of subfertility. *Effective Health Care Bulletin* 1992;3:13. Search date and primary sources not stated.
4. Collins JA, Burrows EA, Willan AR. The prognosis for live birth among untreated infertile couples. *Fertil Steril* 1995;64:22–28.
5. Templeton A, Morris JK. IVF — factors affecting outcome. In: Templeton A, Cooke ID, O'Brien PMS, eds. *35th RCOG study group evidence-based fertility treatment*. London: RCOG Press, 1998.
6. Khan KS, Daya S, Collins JA, et al. Empirical evidence of bias in infertility research: overestimation of treatment effect in crossover trials using pregnancy as the outcome measure. *Fertil Steril* 1996;65:939–945.
7. Cohlen BJ, Te Velde ER, Looman CW, et al. Crossover or parallel design in infertility trials? The discussion continues. *Fertil Steril* 1998;70:40–45.
8. Hughes E, Collins J, Vandekerckhove P. Clomiphene citrate for ovulation induction in women with oligo-amenorrhoea (Cochrane Review) In: The Cochrane Library, Issue 3, 2002. Oxford: Update Software. Search date not stated; primary source Cochrane Subfertility Group Register of Controlled Trials.
9. Holst N, Maltau JM, Forsdahl F. Handling of tubal infertility after introduction of in vitro fertilization: changes and consequences. *Fertil Steril* 1991;55:140–143.
10. Vilos GA, Verhoest CR, Martin JS, Economic evaluation of in vitro fertilization-embryo transfer and neosalpingostomy for bilateral tubal obstruction. *J Soc Obstet Gynecol Can* 1998;20:139–147.
11. Winston RM, Margara RA. Microsurgical salpingostomy is not an obsolete procedure. *Br J Obstet Gynaecol* 1991;98:637–642.
12. Singhal V, Li TC, Cooke ID. An analysis of factors influencing the outcome of 232 consecutive tubal microsurgery cases. *Br J Obstet Gynaecol* 1991;98:628–636.
13. Marana R, Quagliarello J. Distal tubal occlusion: microsurgery versus in vitro fertilization: a review. *Int J Fertil* 1988;33:107–115.
14. Meirow D, Schenker JG. Appraisal of Gift. *Eur J Obstet Gynecol Reprod* 1995;58:59–65.
15. Marana R, Quagliarello J. Proximal tubal occlusion: microsurgery versus IVF: a review. *Int J Fertil* 1988;33:338–340.
16. Patton PE, Williams TJ, Coulam CB. Results of microsurgical reconstruction in patients with combined proximal and distal occlusion: double obstruction. *Fertil Steril* 1987;47:670–674.
17. Wahab M, Li TC, Cooke ID. Reversal of sterilization versus IVF. *J Obstet Gynaecol* 1997;17:180–185.
18. Nugent D, Vandekerckhove P, Hughes E, et al. Gonadotrophin therapy for ovulation induction in subfertility associated with polycystic ovarian syndrome. In: The Cochrane Library, Issue 3, 2002. Oxford: Update Software. Search date not stated; primary sources Subfertility Register of Controlled Trials, Medline, and bibliographies of identified studies.
19. Farquhar C, Vandekerckhove P, Arnot M, et al. Laparoscopic "drilling" by diathermy or laser for ovulation induction in anovulatory polycystic ovary syndrome (Cochrane Review). In: The Cochrane Library, Issue 3, 2002. Oxford: Update Software. Search date 2001; primary source Cochrane Menstrual Disorders and Subfertility Group Register of Controlled Trials.
20. RCOG Infertility Guideline Group. *The Management of Infertility in Secondary Care*. London: RCOG, 1998.

21. Marcoux S, Maheux R, Berube S. Laparoscopic surgery in infertile women with minimal or mild endometriosis. *N Engl J Med* 1997;337:217–222.
22. Parazzini F. Ablation of lesions or no treatment in minimal-mild endometriosis in infertile women: a randomized trial. Gruppo Italiano per lo Studio dell'Endometriosi. *Hum Reprod* 1999;14:1332–1334.
23. Chapron C, Querleu D, Bruhat M, et al. Surgical complications of diagnostic and operative gynaecological laparoscopy: a series of 29 966 cases. *Hum Reprod* 1998;13:867–872.
24. Hughes EG, Fedorkow DM, Collins J. A quantitative overview of controlled trials in endometriosis-associated infertility. *Fertil Steril* 1993;59:963–970. Search date not stated; primary sources Medline, Science Citation Index, abstracts from scientific meetings, and hand searches of relevant trials and personal contacts.
25. Adamson GD, Pasta DJ. Surgical treatment of endometriosis-associated infertility: meta-analysis compared with survival analysis. *Am J Obstet Gynecol* 1994;171:1488–1504.
26. Geber S, Paraschos T, Atkinson G, et al. Results of IVF in patients with endometriosis: the severity of the disease does not affect outcome or the incidence of miscarriage. *Hum Reprod* 1995;10:1507–1511.
27. Kurinczuk J, Bower C. Birth defects in infants conceived by intracytoplasmic sperm injection: an alternative interpretation. *BMJ* 1997;315:1260–1265.
28. Wang CF, Gemzell C. The use of human gonadotrophins for the induction of ovulation in women with polycystic ovarian disease. *Fertil Steril* 1980;33:479–486.
29. Buvat J, Buvat-Herbaut M, Marcolin G, et al. Antiestrogens as treatment of female and male infertilities. *Horm Res* 1987;28:219–229.
30. Human Fertilisation and Embryology Authority. Annual Report 2000. London: HFEA, 2000.
31. Le Lannou D, Lansac J. Artificial procreation with frozen donor sperm: the French experience of CECOS. In: Barratt CLR, Cooke ID, eds. *Donor insemination*. Cambridge: Cambridge University Press, 1993;152–169.
32. Cooke ID. Donor insemination — timing and insemination method. In: Templeton A, Cooke ID, O'Brien PMS, eds. *35th RCOG Study Group evidence-based fertility treatment*. London: RCOG Press, 1998.
33. Ford WCL, Mathur RS, Hull MGR. Intrauterine insemination: is it an effective treatment for male factor infertility? *Balliere Clin Obstet Gynecol* 1997;11:691–710. Search date not stated; primary sources Medline, BIDS, and manual scanning of leading reproductive journals.
34. Zeyneloglu HB, Arici A, Olive DL, et al. Comparison of intrauterine insemination with timed intercourse in superovulated cycles with gonadotrophins: a meta-analysis. *Fertil Steril* 1998;69:486–491. Search date 1997; primary sources Medline, and hand searches of bibliographies of relevant publications and review articles.
35. Boostanfar R, Jain JK, Mishell DR Jr, et al. A prospective randomized trial comparing clomiphene citrate with tamoxifen citrate for ovulation induction. *Fertil Steril* 2001;75:1024–1026.
36. Messinis IE, Nillius SJ. Comparison between tamoxifen and clomiphene for induction of ovulation. *Acta Obstet Gynecol Scand* 1982;61:377–379.
37. Gerhard I, Runnebaum B. Comparison between tamoxifen and clomiphene therapy in women with anovulation. *Arch Gynecol* 1979;227:279–288.
38. El Biely MM, Habba M. The use of metformin to augment the induction of ovulation in obese infertile patients with polycystic ovary syndrome. *Middle East Fertil Soc J* 2001;6:43–49.
39. Rossing MA, Daling JR, Weiss NS, et al. Ovarian tumours in a cohort of infertile women. *N Engl J Med* 1994;331:771–776.
40. Venn A, Watson L, Lumley J, et al. Breast and ovarian cancer incidence after infertility and IVF. *Lancet* 1995;346:995–1000.
41. Parazzini F, Negri E, La Vecchia C, et al. Treatment for infertility and risk of invasive epithelial ovarian cancer. *Hum Reprod* 1997;12:2159–2161.
42. Mosgaard BJ, Lidegaard O, Kjaer SK, et al. Infertility, fertility drugs, and invasive ovarian cancer: a case-control study. *Fertil Steril* 1997;67:1005–1012.
43. Shushan A, Paltiel O, Iscovich J, et al. Human menopausal gonadotrophin and the risk of epithelial ovarian cancer. *Fertil Steril* 1996;65:13–18.
44. Dunn A, Macfarlane A. Recent trends in the incidence of multiple births and associated mortality in England and Wales. *Arch Dis Child Fetal Neonatal Ed* 1996;75:F10–F19.
45. State-specific variation in rates of twin births — United States, 1992–1994. *MMWR Morb Mortal Wkly Rep* 1997;46:121–125.
46. Levene MI, Wild J, Steer P. Higher multiple births and the modern management of infertility in Britain. British Association of Perinatal Medicine. *Br J Obstet Gynecol* 1992;99:607–613.
47. Cabau A, Krulik DR. Stérilités de cause hormonale et stérilitées inexpliquées. Traitement par le cyclofenil. Etude controlée à double insu. *J Gynécol Obstet Biol Reprod* 1990;19:96–101.
48. Coelingh-Bennink HJ, Fauser BC, Out HJ. Recombinant follicle-stimulating hormone (FSH; Puregon) is more efficient than urinary follicle stimulating hormone (Metrodin) in women with clomiphene-resistant, normogonadotrophic, chronic anovulation: a prospective, multicenter, assessor-blind, randomized, clinical trial. European Puregon collaborative anovulation study group. *Fertil Steril* 1998;69:19–25.
49. Yarali H, Bukulmez O, Gurgan T. Urinary follicle stimulating hormone (FSH) versus recombinant FSH in clomiphene citrate resistant normogonadotropic, chronic anovulation: a prospective randomised study. *Fertil Steril* 1999;72:276–281.
50. Muenstermann U, Kleinstein J. Long-term GnRH analogue treatment is equivalent to laparoscopic laser diathermy in polycystic ovarian syndrome patients with severe ovarian dysfunction. *Hum Reprod* 2000;15:2526–2530.
51. Greenblatt E, Casper R. Adhesion formation after laparoscopic ovarian cautery for polycystic ovarian syndrome: lack of correlation with pregnancy rates. *Fertil Steril* 1993;60:766–770.
52. Deans A, Wayne C, Toplis P. Pelvic infection: a complication of laparoscopic ovarian drilling. *Gynaecol Endoscopy* 1997;6:301,en303.
53. Bayram N, Van Wely M, Vandekerckhove P, et al. Pulsatile luteinising hormone releasing hormone for ovulation induction in subfertility associated with polycystic ovary syndrome. In: The Cochrane Library, Issue 3, 2002. Oxford: Update Software. Search date not stated; primary sources Cochrane Menstrual Disorders and Subfertility Group Register of Controlled Trials and hand searches of reference lists of included trials.
54. Martin KA, Hall JE, Adams JM, et al. Comparison of exogenous gonadotropins and pulsatile gonadotropin-releasing hormone for induction of ovulation in hypogonadotropic amenorrhea. *J Clin Endocrinol Metab* 1993;77:125–129.

55. Balen AH, Braat DD, West C, et al. Cumulative conception and live birth rates after the treatment of anovulatory infertility: safety and efficacy of ovulation induction in 200 patients. *Hum Reprod* 1994;9:1563–1570.
56. Braat DD, Schoemaker R, Schoemaker J. Life table analysis of fecundity in intravenously gonadotropin-releasing hormone-treated patients with normogonadotropic and hypogonadotropic amenorrhea. *Fertil Steril* 1991;55:266–271.
57. Filicori M, Flamigni C, Dellai P, et al. Treatment of anovulation with pulsatile gonadotropin-releasing hormone: prognostic factors and clinical results in 600 cycles. *J Clin Endocrinol Metab* 1994;79:1215–1220.
58. Honore GM, Holden AE, Schenken RS. Pathophysiology and management of proximal tubal blockage. *Fertil Steril* 1999;71:785–795. Search date not stated; primary sources Medline and Science Citation Index.
59. Thurmond AS. Pregnancies after selective salpingography and tubal recanalization. *Radiology* 1994;190:11–13.
60. Marana R. Proximal tubal obstruction: are we overdiagnosing and overtreating? *Gynaecol Endoscopy* 1992;1:99–101.
61. Johnson N, Vandekerckhove P, Watson A, et al. Tubal flushing for subfertility. In: *The Cochrane Library,* Issue 3, 2002. Oxford:Update Software. Search date 2001; primary sources The Menstrual Disorders & Subfertility Group's Specialised Register of clinical trials, Medline, Embase, Biological Abstracts, , the National Research Register (NRR), the Clinical Trials Register, search of citation lists of included trials, eligible studies and relevant review articles, contact with authors of trials eligible for inclusion, and search of abstract booklets from scientific meetings.
62. Nugent D, Watson AJ, Killick SR, et al. A randomized controlled trial of tubal flushing with lipiodol for unexplained infertility. *Fertil Steril* 2002;77:173–175.
63. Johnson NP, Mak W, Sowter MC. Surgical treatment for tubal disease in women due to undergo in vitro fertilisation. In: The Cochrane Library, Issue 3, 2002. Oxford: Update Software. Search date 2000; primary sources Cochrane Menstrual Disorders and Subfertility Group Register of Controlled Trials, Medline, Embase, Psychlit, Current Contents, Biological Abstracts, Social Sciences Index, and the National Research Register.
64. Watson A, Vandekerckhove P, Lilford R. Techniques for pelvic surgery in subfertility (Cochrane Review). In: The Cochrane Library, Issue 3, 2002. Oxford: Update Software. Search date not stated; primary source Cochrane Menstrual Disorders and Subfertility Group Register of Controlled Trials.
65. Johnson NP, Watson A. Postoperative procedures for improving fertility following pelvic reproductive surgery. In: The Cochrane Library, Issue 3, 2002. Oxford: Update Software. Search date not stated; primary source Cochrane Menstrual Disorders and Subfertility Group Register of Controlled Trials.
66. Watson A, Vandekerckhove P, Lilford R. Liquid and fluid agents for preventing adhesions after surgery for subfertility (Cochrane Review). In: *The Cochrane Library*, Issue 3, 2002. Oxford: Update Software. Search date not stated; primary source Cochrane Menstrual Disorders and Subfertility Group Register of Controlled Trials.
67. Filippini F, Darai E, Benifla JL, et al. Distal tubal surgery: a critical review of 104 laparoscopic distal tuboplasties [in French]. *J Gynecol Obstet Biol Reprod* 1996;25:471–478 (review in French).
68. Donnez J, Casanas-Roux F. Prognostic factors of fimbrial microsurgery. *Fertil Steril* 1986;46:200–204.
69. Tomazevic T, Ribic-Pucelj M, Omahen A, et al. Microsurgery and in vitro fertilization and embryo transfer for infertility resulting from pathological proximal tubal blockage. *Hum Reprod* 1996;11:2613–2617.
70. Wu CH, Gocial B. A pelvic scoring system for infertility surgery. *Int J Fertil* 1988;33:341–346.
71. Oelsner G, Sivan E, Goldenberg M, et al. Should lysis of adhesions be performed when in vitro fertilization and embryo transfer are available? *Hum Reprod* 1994;9:2339–2341.
72. Gillett WR, Clarke RH, Herbison GP. First and subsequent pregnancies after tubal surgery: evaluation of the fertility index. *Fertil Steril* 1998;68:1033–1042.
73. Jarrell J, Labelle R, Goeree R, et al. In vitro fertilization and embryo transfer: a randomized controlled trial. *Online J Curr Clin Trials* 1993;2:Doc 73.
74. Bhattacharya S, Hamilton MP, Shaaban M, et al. Conventional in-vitro fertilisation versus intracytoplasmic sperm injection for the treatment of non-male-factor infertility: a randomised controlled trial. *Lancet* 2001;357:2075–2079.
75. Bukulmez O, Yarali H, Yucel A, et al. Intracytoplasmic sperm injection versus in vitro fertilization for patients with a tubal factor as their sole cause of infertility: a prospective, randomized trial. *Fertil Steril* 2000;73:38–42.
76. Poehl M, Holagschwandtner M, Bichler K, et al. IVF-patients with nonmale factor "to ICSI" or "not to ICSI" that is the question? *J Assist Reprod Genet* 2001;18:205–208.
77. Centers for Disease Control and Prevention. US Department of Health and Human Services. 1998 Assisted Reproductive Technology Success Rates. National Summary and Clinic Reports. December 2000.
78. Brinsden PR, Wada I, Tan SL, et al. Diagnosis, prevention and management of ovarian hyperstimulation syndrome. *Br J Obstet Gynaecol* 1995;102:767–772.
79. Wennerholm U, Bergh C. Obstetric outcome and follow-up of children born after in vitro fertilization (IVF). *Hum Fertil* 2000;3:52–64. Search date 1998; primary source Medline.
80. Chapko KM, Weaver MR, Chapko MK, et al. Stability of in vitro fertilization-embryo transfer success rates from the 1989,1990, and 1991 clinic-specific outcome assessments. *Fertil Steril* 1995;64:757–763. Search date not stated; primary source Medline.
81. Human Fertilisation and Embryology Authority. The Patients' Guide to IVF Clinics. London: HFEA, 2000.
82. Hughes E, Fedorkow D, Collins J, et al. Ovulation suppression for endometriosis. In: The Cochrane Library, Issue 3, 2002. Oxford: Update Software. Search date not stated; primary source Cochrane Subfertility Group Register of Controlled Trials.
83. Dockeray CJ, Sheppard BL, Bonnar J. Comparison between mefenamic acid and danazol in the treatment of established menorrhagia. *Br J Obstet Gynaecol* 1989;96:840–844.
84. Tummon IS, Asher LJ, Martin JSB, et al. Randomized controlled trial of superovulation and insemination for infertility associated with minimal or mild endometriosis. *Fertil Steril* 1997;68:8–12.
85. Fedele L, Bianchi S, Marchini M, et al. Superovulation with human menopausal gonadotrophins in the treatment of infertility associated with endometriosis: a controlled randomised study. *Fertil Steril* 1992;58:28–31.

86. Nulsen JC, Walsh S, Dumez S. A randomised and longitudinal study of human menopausal gonadotrophin with intrauterine insemination in the treatment of infertility. *Obstet Gynaecol* 1993;82:780–786.
87. Olivennes F, Feldberg D, Liu H-C, et al. Endometriosis: a stage by stage analysis — the role of in vitro fertilization. *Fertil Steril* 1995;64:392–398.
88. Barnhart K, Dunsmoor-Su R, Coutifaris, C. Effect of endometriosis on in vitro fertilization. *Fertil Steril* 2002;77:1148–1155. Search date 1999; primary sources Medline and manual search of references.
89. Cohlen BJ, Vandekerckhove P, Te Velde ER, et al. Timed intercourse versus intra-uterine insemination with or without ovarian hyperstimulation for subfertility in men. In: The Cochrane Library, Issue 3, 2002. Oxford: Update Software. Search date 1996/1997; primary sources Medline, Embase, DDFU, Biosis, SciSearch, hand searching, and conference abstracts.
90. O'Brien P, Vandekerckhove P. Intra-uterine versus cervical insemination of donor sperm for subfertility. In: The Cochrane Library, Issue 3, 2002. Oxford: Update Software. Search date 1996; primary source Cochrane Subfertility Group Specialist Register of Controlled Trials.
91. Ragni G, Maggioni P, Guermandi E, et al. Efficacy of double intrauterine insemination in controlled ovarian hyperstimulation cycles. *Fertil Steril* 1999;72:619–622.
92. Silverberg KM, Johnson JV, Olive DL, et al. A prospective, randomized trial comparing two different intrauterine insemination regimens in controlled ovarian hyperstimulation cycles. *Fertil Steril* 1992;576:357–361.
93. Ransom MX, Blotner MB, Bohrer M, et al. Does increasing frequency of intrauterine insemination improve pregnancy rates significantly during superovulation cycles? *Fertil Steril* 1994;61:303–307.
94. Zreik TG, Garcia-Velasco JA, Habboosh MS, et al. Prospective, randomized, crossover study to evaluate the benefit of human chorionic gonadotrophin-timed versus urinary luteinising hormone-timed intrauterine inseminations in clomiphene citrate-stimulated treatment cycles. *Fertil Steril* 1998;71:1070–1074.
95. Van Rumste MME, Evers JLH, Farquhar CM, et al. Intra-cytoplasmic sperm injection versus partial zona dissection, subzonal insemination and conventional techniques for oocyte insemination during IVF. In: The Cochrane Library, Issue 3, 2002. Oxford: Update Software. Search date not stated; primary source Cochrane Menstrual Disorders and Subfertility Group Specialist Register of Controlled Trials.
96. Bonduelle M, Legein J, Buyesse A, et al. Prospective follow up study of 423 children born after intracytoplasmic sperm injection. *Hum Reprod* 1996;11:1558–1564.
97. Bonduelle M, Legein J, Derde M, et al. Comparative follow-up study of 130 children born after ICSI and 130 children born after IVF. *Hum Reprod* 1995;10:3327–3331.
98. Velde E, Van Baar A, Van Kooije R. Concerns about assisted reproduction. *Lancet* 1998;351: 1524–1525.
99. De Wert G. Ethics of intracytoplasmic sperm injection: proceed with care. *Hum Reprod* 1998;13(suppl 1):219–227.
100. Leeton J, Healy D, Rogers P. A controlled study between the use gamete intrafallopian transfer (GIFT) and in vitro fertilization and embryo transfer in the management of idiopathic and male infertility. *Fertil Steril* 1987;48:605–607.
101. Hughes E, Collins J, Vandekerckhove P. Clomiphene citrate for unexplained subfertility in women. In: The Cochrane Library, Issue 3, 2002. Oxford: Update Software. Search date 2000; primary sources Cochrane Menstrual Disorders and Subfertility Review Group Specialist Register of Controlled Trials, Medline, Embase, and Cinahl.
102. Fujii S, Fukui A, Fukushi Y, et al. The effects of clomiphene citrate on normally ovulatory women. *Fertil Steril* 1997;68:997–999.
103. Hughes EG. The effectiveness of ovulation induction and intrauterine insemination in the treatment of persistent infertility: a meta-analysis. *Hum Reprod* 1997;12:1865–1872. Search date not stated; primary source Cochrane Menstrual Disorders and Subfertility Group Specialist Register of Controlled Trials.
104. Guzick DS, Carson SA, Coutifaris C, et al. Efficacy of superovulation and intrauterine insemination in the treatment of infertility. National Cooperative Reproductive Medicine Network. *N Engl J Med* 1999;340:177–183.
105. Sengoku K, Tamate K, Takaoka Y, et al. The clinical efficacy of low-dose step-up follicle stimulating hormone administration for treatment of unexplained infertility. *Hum Reprod* 1999;14:349–353.
106. Trout SW, Kemmann E. Fallopian sperm perfusion versus intrauterine insemination: a randomized controlled trial and meta-analysis of the literature. *Fertil Steril* 1999;71:881–885. Search date not stated; primary source Medline.
107. Ricci G, Nucera G, Pozzobon C, et al. A simple method for fallopian tube sperm perfusion using a blocking device in the treatment of unexplained infertility. *Fertil Steril* 2001;76:1242–1248.
108. Hogerzeil HV, Spiekerman JCM, De Vries JWA, et al. A randomized trial between GIFT and ovarian stimulation for the treatment of unexplained infertility and failed artificial insemination by donor. *Hum Reprod* 1992;7:1235–1239.
109. Murdoch AP, Harris M, Mahroo M, et al. Gamete intrafallopian transfer (GIFT) compared with intrauterine insemination in the treatment of unexplained infertility. *Br J Obstet Gynaecol* 1991;98:1107–1111.
110. Wessels PHX, Cronje HS, Oosthuizen AP, et al. Cost-effectiveness of gamete intrafallopian transfer in comparison with induction of ovulation with gonadotrophins in the treatment of female infertility: a clinical trial. *Fertil Steril* 1992;57:163–167.
111. Murdoch AP, Harris M, Mahroo M, et al. Is GIFT (gamete intrafallopian transfer) the best treatment for unexplained infertility? *Br J Obstet Gynaecol* 1991;98:643–647.
112. Rombauts L, Dear M, Breheny S, et al. Cumulative pregnancy rates and live birth rates after gamete intra-fallopian transfer. *Hum Reprod* 1997;12:1338–1342.
113. Society for Assisted Reproductive Technology and the American Society for Reproductive Medicine. Assisted reproductive technology in the United States and Canada: 1995 results generated from the American Society for Reproductive Medicine/Society for Assisted Reproductive Technology Registry. *Fertil Steril* 1998;69:389–398.
114. Pandian Z, Bhattacharya S, Nikolaou D, et al. In vitro fertilisation for unexplained subfertility. In: *The Cochrane Library,* Issue 3, 2002. Oxford:Update Software. Search date 2001;

primary sources Cochrane Menstrual Disorders and Subfertility Group's trials register, the Cochrane Controlled Trials Register, Medline, Embase, reference lists of articles, handsearch of relevant conference proceedings, and contact with researchers in the field.

Kirsten Duckitt
Consultant Obstetrician and Gynaecologist
John Radcliffe Hospital
Oxford
UK

Competing interests: None declared.

TABLE 1 **Comparative success rates of treatments for infertility: evidence from RCTs and observational studies (see text, p 2112).**

Treatment	Live birth rates	Pregnancy rates	Adverse effects
All causes of infertility			
IVF (per treated cycle)	UK 15%; US 20%[5]	59–77% (with 3–5 treatment cycles)[8]	Ectopic pregnancy: 1–3%[9,10]
GIFT (per cycle) (not including tubal infertility)	23% [14]	ND	
Infertility caused by ovulation disorders			
Clomifene to induce ovulation in amenorrhoeic women (after 2–4 cycles of treatment)		Ovulation rate 61%, pregnancy rate 14%[8]	Risk of ovarian cancer, unproved. MP: 2–13%, mostly twins.[28] OHSS: infrequent and mild
Gonadotrophins to induce ovulation in clomifene resistant PCOS (per cycle)		27–40%[3,18] FSH 27%[18]	Risk of ovarian cancer, unproved. MP: 29%[29] OHSS: 4%
Laparoscopic drilling (cumulative rate 1–2 years after treatment)		48%[19,20]	Risks of laparoscopy, general anaesthesia, and adhesions. Risk of premature ovarian failure unproved
Tubal infertility			
Tubal surgery for distal occlusion (cumulative rate 2 years after surgery)[11–13]	20–30%		Risks of general anaesthesia. Ectopic pregnancy: 7–9%[9,10]
Tubal surgery for proximal occlusion (cumulative rate)	40–60%[15,16]		
Reversal of female sterilisation (cumulative live birth rate 1–2 years after surgery)	50–90%[17] depending on method used for sterilisation		

TABLE 1 continued

Treatment	Live birth rates	Pregnancy rates	Adverse effects
Infertility associated with endometriosis			
Surgery (per cycle)		13–38%†[21–26]	Risks of surgery and general anaesthesia (for laparoscopic surgery). Mortality 3.33/100 000; complication rate 3.2/1000[23]
Male infertility			
IUI ± ovarian stimulation (per cycle)		6.5%[33]	
ICSI plus IVF (per cycle)	20%[5]		
Donor insemination* (per cycle)	9–12%[30–32]		No adverse effects if no ovarian stimulation is given, but child is not male partner's genetic offspring
Unexplained infertility			
IUI ± ovarian stimulation (per cycle)		9–12% without stimulation; 19–20% with[33,34]	

*Using frozen donor sperm in women without female factor or with corrected female factor infertility; †Over spontaneous rate.
FSH, follicle stimulating hormone; GIFT, gamete intrafallopian transfer; ICSI, intracytoplasmic sperm injection; IUI, intrauterine insemination; IVF, in vitro fertilisation; MP, multiple pregnancy; ND, no data; OHSS, ovarian hyperstimulation syndrome; PCOS, polycystic ovary syndrome.

Menopausal symptoms

Search date November 2002

Edward Morris and Janice Rymer

QUESTIONS

INTERVENTIONS

Key Messages

- **Progestogens (at high doses, in reducing vasomotor symptoms)** One systematic review and six additional RCTs have found that progestogens with or without oestrogens reduce vasomotor symptoms compared with placebo. We found no good quality evidence on other outcomes, including quality of life.
- **Tibolone** RCTs have found that tibolone improves vasomotor symptoms and sexual function compared with placebo. Two RCTs found that tibolone improved sexual function compared with hormone replacement therapy, However, we found insufficient evidence from RCTs about effects on vasomotor symptoms and vaginal dryness compared with hormone replacement therapy.
- **Phyto-oestrogens** We found limited evidence from RCTs that phyto-oestrogens reduced vasomotor symptoms compared with placebo.
- **Antidepressants** We found no RCTs on the effects of antidepressants on menopausal symptoms.
- **Clonidine** One small RCT found that transdermal clonidine reduced the number and intensity of hot flushes after 8 weeks compared with placebo. However, we were unable to draw reliable conclusions from that study.
- **Testosterone** We found no reliable RCTs evaluating testosterone alone. We found limited evidence from RCTs that testosterone plus oestrogens may improve vasomotor symptoms compared with oestrogen alone. However, we were unable to draw reliable conclusions from these studies.
- **Oestrogens** One systematic review and three subsequent RCTs have found that oestrogen with or without progestogens improves vasomotor symptoms. Two systematic reviews and four subsequent RCTs have found that oestrogen reduces the incidence of urinary tract infection and improves urogenital symptoms. One systematic review found that oestrogens reduced depressed mood. Four RCTs have found that oestrogen improves quality of life in the short term. Important adverse effects include breast cancer, endometrial cancer, stroke and thromboembolic disease.

DEFINITION Menopause is defined as the end of the last menstrual period. A woman is deemed to be postmenopausal 1 year after her last period. For practical purposes most women are diagnosed as menopausal after 1 year of amenorrhoea. Menopausal symptoms often begin in the perimenopausal years.

INCIDENCE/ PREVALENCE In the UK, the mean age for the start of the menopause is 50 years and 9 months. The median onset of the perimenopause is 45.5–47.5 years. One Scottish survey (6096 women aged 45–54 years) found that 84% of women had experienced at least one of the classic menopausal symptoms, with 45% finding one or more symptoms a problem.[1]

AETIOLOGY/ RISK FACTORS Urogenital symptoms of menopause are caused by decreased oestrogen concentrations, but the cause of vasomotor symptoms and psychological effects is complex and remains unclear.

PROGNOSIS Menopause is a physiological event. Its timing may be determined genetically. Although endocrine changes are permanent, menopausal symptoms such as hot flushes, which are experienced by about 70% of women, usually resolve with time.[2] Some symptoms, however, such as genital atrophy, may remain the same or worsen.

AIMS OF INTERVENTION To reduce or prevent menopausal symptoms; and to improve quality of life, with minimum adverse effects.

OUTCOMES Frequency and severity of vasomotor, urogenital, and psychological symptoms; quality of life.

METHODS *Clinical Evidence* search and appraisal November 2002. We included only systematic reviews and RCTs that met *Clinical Evidence* quality criteria. Many of the RCTs included were crossover trials, which may have important limitations (see *Clinical Evidence* glossary). Where results are reported only for comparisons with pretreatment values, they have been omitted because these comparisons may be influenced in many (often unquantifiable) ways by other factors apart from treatment effect.

QUESTION What are the effects of medical treatments?

OPTION OESTROGENS

One systematic review and three subsequent RCTs have found that oestrogen with or without progestogens improves vasomotor symptoms. Two systematic reviews and four subsequent RCTs have found that oestrogen reduces the incidence of urinary tract infection and improves urogenital symptoms. One systematic review found that oestrogen improved depressed mood. Four RCTs have found that oestrogen improves quality of life in the short term. However, important adverse effects include increased risk of breast cancer, endometrial cancer, stroke and thromboembolic disease.

Benefits: **Vasomotor symptoms:** We found one systematic review[3] and three subsequent RCTs.[4–6] The systematic review (search date 2000, 21 RCTs, 2511 women) compared oral oestrogens at varying doses with or without progestogens versus placebo.[3] The review found that oestrogen significantly reduced hot flushes compared with placebo (6 RCTs, 371 women: RR of a hot flush in one week 0.23, 95% CI 0.12 to 0.42; WMD −15.7, 95% CI −20.0 to −11.5 flushes/week). It also found that oestrogen significantly reduced the number of women with hot flushes at the end of the study compared with placebo (8 RCTs, 1240 women: 139/906 [15%] with oestrogen *v* 158/334 [47%] with placebo; RR 0.37, 95% CI 0.30 to 0.45; NNT 4, 95% CI 3 to 4). There was a wide variation in the frequency of hot flushes in both control and treatment groups among the RCTs (range of means for each RCT 0.9–13.8 flushes/week with oestrogen *v* 12.6–33.5 with placebo). The first subsequent RCT (361 women) compared nasal and transdermal oestrogen.[4] It found that both 300 μg nasal oestrogen daily and 500 μg transdermal oestrogen daily significantly reduced the total number of daily hot flushes and menopausal symptoms as assessed by the Kupperman index (see glossary, p 2147) after 12 weeks. We found no comparisons between treatments. The second subsequent RCT (2673 women entered, 2152 analysed) compared eight combinations of different doses of oral conjugated equine oestrogen (0.625 mg, 0.45 mg, and 0.3 mg) either alone or plus different doses of medroxyprogesterone acetate (2.5 mg or 1.5 mg) with placebo.[5] It found that daily doses of 0.3 mg, 0.45 mg, or 0.625 mg conjugated equine oestrogens (with or without medroxyprogesterone acetate 2.5 mg/day) significantly reduced vasomotor symptoms from weeks 3–12, as assessed using diary cards to record number and severity of hot flushes, compared with placebo ($P < 0.05$). There was no significant difference in the number or severity of hot flushes between different doses of medroxyprogesterone acetate. There were significant reductions in the number of hot flushes with oestrogen alone by week 3, and for 0.625 mg conjugated oestrogen alone compared with the 0.45 mg and 0.3 mg oestrogen dosages (data presented graphically). The third subsequent RCT (165 women) compared two doses of intranasal estradiol (oestradiol; 150 or 300 μg/day) versus placebo over 12 weeks.[6] Symptoms were assessed with diaries and the Kupperman index. It found that both doses of oestrogen reduced moderate to severe symptoms at 12 weeks compared with placebo (mean reduction from baseline in number of moderate to severe vasomotor symptoms per day: 9.39 with 300 μg estradiol *v* 7.86 with 150 μg estradiol *v* 5.22 with placebo; $P = 0.002$ for high dose *v* placebo and $P < 0.001$ for low dose *v* placebo). **Urogenital system:** We found two systematic reviews (search date 1995, 6 RCTs[7] and search date 1998, 6 RCTs, 334 people[8]) and four subsequent RCTs.[6,9–11] The first systematic review found that oestrogen improved urogenital symptoms regardless of route (no figures available).[7] The second systematic review found a significant reduction in the incidence of urinary tract infection with oral or vaginal oestrogen hormone replacement therapy (HRT) compared with placebo or no treatment (OR for infection when not using HRT 2.51, 95% CI 1.48 to 4.25).[8] Vaginal oestrogens were superior to oral oestrogens in reducing urinary tract infections ($P < 0.008$). The first subsequent RCT (136 women) found that low dose transdermal oestrogen (25 μg/day) plus norethisterone acetate significantly reduced vaginal dryness and dyspareunia compared with placebo over 6 months ($P < 0.001$).[9] The second subsequent RCT (145 women) found that low dose estradiol (oestradiol) was associated with a higher number of days without vaginal dryness at weeks 9–12 compared with placebo (86% with 1 mg estradiol v 76% with 0.5 mg estradiol v 74% with placebo), but significance was not tested.[10] The third RCT (multicentre, 84 women treated for 24 weeks, 20% withdrawals) found that an estradiol ring significantly increased relief from dyspareunia compared with placebo (90% with estradiol ring v 45% with placebo; P = 0.028).[11] The fourth RCT (165 women) compared the effects of two doses of intranasal estradiol (150 or 300 μg/day) versus placebo on dyspareunia and "urinary troubles" (measured on a visual analogue scales).[6] It found that the 150 μg dose significantly reduced symptoms compared with placebo at 12 weeks (P < 0.001), and that the 300 μg dose significantly reduced urogenital symptoms compared with placebo at 4 weeks (P = 0.014). **Psychological symptoms:** We found one systematic review (search date 1995, 14 RCTs including several crossover RCTs, 12 cohort studies), which found that oestrogen reduced depressed mood (measured using different scales) among menopausal women compared with placebo or no treatment (P < 0.0001).[12] Duration of treatment ranged from 1 month to 2 years. We found no RCTs of oestrogen treatment in women with clinically proven depression. We found one systematic review (search date 1996, 10 controlled trials, and 9 observational studies) of the effects of oestrogen on cognitive function in postmenopausal women and in women with Alzheimer's disease.[13] The review found that studies were too weak to allow reliable conclusions to be drawn. An additional crossover RCT (62 women) found a significant reduction in subjective sleep problems compared with placebo over 7 months (P < 0.01).[14] **Quality of life:** We found no systematic review. We found four RCTs (639 women, 3 placebo controlled,[15–17] 2 with added progestogen[17,18]), all of which found significant improvement in quality of life among women treated with oestrogen compared with baseline or placebo. The largest RCT (223 postmenopausal women in Sweden) found a significant improvement in quality of life (P = 0.0003) and wellbeing (P = 0.003) with estradiol transdermal patches (50 μg/24 hours) versus placebo patches after 12 weeks.[16]

Harms: Women often report an increase in weight when starting oestrogen, but we found no evidence from RCTs that oestrogen causes significant weight gain in the long term. One systematic review (search date 1998) of 22 studies has found no effect of either unopposed or combined hormone replacement therapy (HRT) on body weight.[19] The most important long term adverse effects are increased risk of venous thromboembolic disease (see hormone replacement therapy under secondary prevention of ischaemic cardiac events, p 188), endometrial cancer, and breast cancer.[19–22] One systematic review (search date not stated) reanalysed 51 studies (> 160 000 women) of the relation between oestrogen (as HRT) and breast cancer.[23] It found that the relative risk of breast cancer increased by 2.3% (95% CI 1.1% to 3.6%) each year in women using HRT. Five or more years after HRT was stopped, there was no significant excess of breast cancer. One systematic review (search date not stated) of the effects of HRT (18 RCTs, 5247 women) found significant risks of endometrial hyperplasia in women taking unopposed oestrogen (RR 8.14, 95% CI 1.05 to 63.1 for 6 months of treatment; RR 37.0, 95% CI 9.3 to 147 for 36 months of treatment).[22] The review also found significant reductions in the incidence of hyperplasia when women are given progestogens, either cyclically or continuously, with continuous combined HRT having the greatest effect at 36 months (RR 0.17, 95% CI 0.02 to 1.26). Several large RCTs including a total of more than 20 000 women have recently reported the effects of long term HRT on major diseases such as breast cancer, endometrial cancer, colorectal cancer, coronary heart disease, stroke, pulmonary embolus and fractured neck of femur. Four of these studies were recently meta-analysed.[24] For women receiving HRT, the relative risk of developing breast cancer was 1.27 (95% CI 1.03 to 1.56), pulmonary embolism 2.16 (95% CI 1.47 to 3.18), colorectal cancer 0.64 (95% CI 0.45 to 0.92), fractured neck of femur 0.72 (95% CI 0.52 to 0.98), endometrial cancer 0.76 (95% CI 0.45 to 1.31), and coronary heart disease 1.11 (95% CI 0.96 to 1.30).

Comment: Based on the evidence of important adverse effects, there has been a change in prescribing attitude toward HRT. Before starting HRT, it is now considered important for prescribers to discuss with women the excess risks associated with HRT.

OPTION PROGESTOGENS

We found good evidence from one systematic review and six additional RCTs that progestogens with or without oestrogen reduce vasomotor symptoms compared with placebo. We found no good quality evidence on other outcomes, including quality of life.

Benefits: **Vasomotor symptoms:** We found no systematic review of progestogens alone versus placebo. We found one systematic review (search date 2000, 21 RCTs, 2511 women, follow up for 3–36 months) of oestrogen alone versus oestrogens at varying doses and routes of administration with or without progestogens, including lower dose preparations,[3] four additional RCTs of progestogens versus placebo,[25–28] and two additional RCTs of progestogens versus other interventions.[29,30] The systematic review found a significant reduction in the severity of hot flushes in users of oestrogen alone and users of both oestrogen and progesterone, but the reduction in hot flush severity was greater in those taking progesterone and oestrogen (OR 0.1, 95% CI 0.06 to 0.19) than in those taking oestrogen alone (OR 0.35, 95% CI 0.22 to 0.56).[3] The four RCTs versus placebo (three of them < 1 year in duration) found that progestogens significantly reduced vasomotor symptoms (see table 1, p 2150).[25–28] The fifth RCT (43 menopausal women) compared oestrogen alone with progesterone (150 mg depot medroxyprogesterone for 25 days/month).[29] It found no significant difference between treatments in vasomotor symptoms at 3 months (no decrease in vasomotor symptoms in 18% of women in each group, P value not reported). The sixth additional RCT (351 women) compared oestrogen alone versus oestrogen plus progestogen.[30] It found a reduction in hot flushes with both preparations with small differences between them (figures not provided). **Urogenital system:** We found no RCTs evaluating the effects of progestogens alone on urinary incontinence, the lower genital tract, or libido. **Psychological symptoms:** We found no RCTs. **Quality of life:** We found no studies of progestogen alone on quality of life. One RCT (351 women) compared cyclical progestogen plus oestrogen versus oestrogen alone and found no significant difference in quality of life between treatments at 6 months ($P < 0.001$).[30]

Harms: We found three RCTs that evaluated harms of progestogens.[31–33] The first RCT (321 women who had undergone hysterectomy and were already taking conjugated oestrogen) compared continuous progestogen (norgestrel) versus placebo.[31] It found no difference in symptoms (including weight gain and bloating). The second RCT (875 women) compared various oestrogen/progestogen combinations over 3 years.[32] It found that additional progestogen increased breast discomfort (OR 1.92, 95% CI 1.16 to 3.09). Neither RCT found evidence of an effect on cardiovascular events. The third crossover RCT (51 women receiving 2 mg estradiol) compared adverse effects of medroxyprogesterone acetate 10 mg versus norethisterone 1 mg.[33] It found that medroxyprogesterone acetate induced significantly fewer negative mood symptoms and more positive mood symptoms in women without a history of premenstrual syndrome than did norethisterone, but that medroxyprogesterone acetate induced more physical symptoms, such as breast tenderness and bloating, than did norethisterone.

Comment: Progestogens are seldom given alone, which makes it hard to isolate their effects. When given without oestrogen, doses of progestogens were high, the lowest dose being 20 mg medroxyprogesterone acetate daily. We found one further RCT that compared depomedroxyprogesterone acetate versus placebo, but the disparity in size between the experimental and control groups (57 *v* 12 women) and lack of detail on randomisation strategies make the results difficult to interpret.[34] Three of the placebo controlled RCTs had crossover comparisons, which make conclusions difficult to interpret.[25–27]

OPTION TIBOLONE

RCTs have found that tibolone improves vasomotor symptoms and sexual function compared with placebo. Two RCTs found that tibolone improved sexual function compared with hormone replacement therapy. However, we found insufficient evidence from RCTs about effects of tibolone on vasomotor symptoms and vaginal dryness compared with oestrogen.

Benefits: We found no systematic review. **Vasomotor symptoms:** We found three RCTs. One RCT compared tibolone with placebo[35] and two RCTs compared tibolone with oestrogen/progestogen combinations.[36,37] The first RCT (82 women with menopausal symptoms) found that tibolone significantly reduced vasomotor symptoms at 16 weeks compared with placebo (39% reduction in mean score; $P = 0.001$).[35] The second RCT (437 women with menopausal symptoms) compared combined oestrogen/progestogen versus tibolone.[36] It found that the combined oestrogen/progestogen regimen significantly reduced hot flushes over 48 weeks compared with tibolone ($P = 0.01$). The third RCT (235 postmenopausal women) found no significant difference in vasomotor symptoms between combined oestrogen/progestogen and tibolone at 52 weeks (figures not available).[37] **Urogenital system:** We found three RCTs.[36,38–40] The first RCT (437 women) found that tibolone significantly improved vaginal dryness compared with continuous hormone replacement therapy after 48 weeks of treatment assessed using a five point scoring system (vaginal dryness: for tibolone 2.16 at baseline to 1.33 post-treatment *v* for hormone replacement therapy 2.12 at baseline to 1.27 at post-treatment; for change from baseline $P < 0.001$).[36] The RCT also found that tibolone improved sexual satisfaction as measured with McCoy's Sex Scale Questionnaire compared with estradiol (oestradiol) plus norethisterone ($P < 0.05$).[38] The second RCT (50 women attending a university gynaecology clinic) found that tibolone significantly improved sexual desire and coital frequency as measured by a questionnaire compared with conjugated oestrogen ($P < 0.05$ for both).[39] The third RCT (crossover, 38 women) found that tibolone significantly increased sexual fantasies ($P < 0.03$) and arousability over 3 months compared with placebo ($P < 0.01$).[40] We found no RCTs examining the effects on urinary incontinence. **Psychological symptoms:** We found no RCTs. **Quality of life:** We found no RCTs.

Harms: We found no evidence on adverse effects from RCTs. One non-randomised controlled trial found that the main adverse effect of tibolone was breakthrough bleeding, which occurred in about 10% of users.[41] We found no good evidence of androgenic adverse effects, such as hair growth and greasiness of the skin. Two RCTs of short term use found a 33% reduction in plasma high density lipoproteins with tibolone,[42,43] although the long term effects on cardiovascular disease are unknown.

Comment: None.

OPTION PHYTO-OESTROGENS

We found limited evidence from RCTs that phyto-oestrogens reduced vasomotor symptoms compared with placebo.

Benefits: We found no systematic review. **Vasomotor symptoms:** We found seven placebo controlled RCTs.[44–50] The first RCT (58 postmenopausal women) compared soy flour (which contains phyto-oestrogens) with wheat flour for 12 weeks.[44] It found no significant difference between soy flour and wheat flour in hot flushes at 12 weeks (reduction in hot flushes: 40% with soy flour *v* 25% with wheat flour; $P = 0.82$). The second RCT (crossover, 51 women) compared a daily dietary supplement containing no phyto-oestrogens versus a supplement containing 34 mg soy protein.[45] It found that soy protein reduced the severity ($P < 0.001$) but not the frequency of vasomotor symptoms at 6 weeks. The third RCT (unblinded crossover, 51 women) compared isoflavone 40 mg daily versus placebo.[46] It found no significant difference between isoflavone and placebo in vasomotor symptoms assessed after 12 weeks by flush count (mean hot flush count: 3.72 in 46 women receiving placebo *v* 4.22 in 42 women receiving isoflavone; SMD –0.5, 95% CI –8.9 to +7.9) and Greene climacteric scale (mean: 7.23 in 42 women with isoflavone *v* 6.93 in 46 women with placebo; SMD −0.3, 95% CI −19.2 to +18.6; data recalculated by *Clinical Evidence*). The fourth RCT (39 women) found that soy flour significantly reduced mean flushes per week compared with placebo (45% reduction with soy flour *v* 25% with placebo tablets after 12 weeks; P < 0.01), although it should be noted that the women taking soy extract had a greater number of vasomotor symptoms at baseline than the placebo group.[47] The fifth RCT (94 women) found no significant difference between soy protein and placebo at 3 months for vasomotor symptoms as assessed using a four point subjective rating scale.[48] The sixth RCT (177 women) found that a 50 mg daily dose of an isoflavone extract significantly reduced hot flush severity over 12 weeks compared with placebo (P = 0.01).[49] There was no significant difference between groups in hot flush frequency. The seventh RCT (80 women) found that 100 mg soy isoflavone daily significantly reduced menopausal symptoms compared with placebo (change in Kupperman index [see glossary, p 2147] from baseline to 16 weeks: for isoflavone 44.6 at baseline to 24.9 at 16 weeks *v* for placebo 40.3 at baseline to 41.6 at 16 weeks; difference between treatments P < 0.01).[50] **Other symptoms:** One RCT (94 women) found no significant difference between soy protein and placebo at 3 months for psychological, musculoskeletal, and genitourinary symptoms as assessed using a four point subjective rating scale.[48] **Quality of life:** We found no RCTs.

Harms: We found no evidence of significant adverse effects.

Comment: Few studies have specifically investigated adverse effects of phyto-oestrogens. Results of studies are difficult to interpret because phyto-oestrogen preparations are not standardised. One recent RCT (80 women) compared effects of 100 mg soy isoflavone daily versus placebo on blood pressure, plasma glucose, serum lipid and lipoprotein concentrations, and endometrial thickness.[50] It found that phyto-oestrogens reduced serum total cholesterol and low density lipoprotein compared with placebo (P < 0.01).

OPTION CLONIDINE

One small RCT found that transdermal clonidine reduced the number and intensity of hot flushes after 8 weeks compared with placebo. However, we were unable to draw reliable conclusions from this study.

Benefits: We found no systematic review. **Vasomotor symptoms:** One RCT (30 women) found that transdermal clonidine (3.5 cm^2 patch delivering 0.1 mg clonidine/day for 7 days) significantly reduced the number of women with hot flushes at 8 weeks and increased the number of women perceiving a reduction in severity of the hot flushes compared with placebo (women reporting reduction in number of hot flushes: 12/15 [80%] with clonidine *v* 5/14 [35%] with placebo; RR 2.4, 95% CI 1.1 to 4.7; NNT 3, 95% CI 2 to 12; women reporting reduction in severity of hot flushes: 11/15 [73%] with transdermal clonidine *v* 4/14 [29%] with placebo; RR 2.7, 95% CI 1.09 to 6.6; NNT 3, 95% CI 2 to 5).[51] **Psychological symptoms:** We found no RCTs. **Quality of life:** We found no RCTs.

Harms: The RCT found no significant difference in the incidence of adverse effects between placebo and clonidine.[51] The analysed adverse effects included transient local skin reactions (4/15 [27%] with clonidine patch *v* 3/14 [21%] with placebo; RR 1.2, 95% CI 0.34 to 4.6). No women complained of mouth dryness or drowsiness.

Comment: One RCT included in previous versions of *Clinical Evidence* has now been excluded because it failed to produce a pre-crossover analysis.[52] Transdermal patches of clonidine are not widely available. Results may not be generalisable; extrapolating results to oral clonidine is potentially misleading.

OPTION TESTOSTERONE

We found no reliable RCTs evaluating testosterone alone. We found limited evidence from RCTs that testosterone plus oestrogens may improve vasomotor symptoms compared with oestrogen alone. However, we were unable to draw reliable conclusions from these studies.

Benefits: We found no systematic review. **Vasomotor symptoms:** We found no RCTs against placebo or evaluating testosterone alone in women with menopausal symptoms. We found two RCTs of testosterone/oestrogen combinations.[53,54] The first RCT (93 postmenopausal women) compared oestrogen alone (0.625 mg/day or 1.25 mg/day) versus oestrogen plus methyltestosterone (1.25 mg/day or 2.5 mg/day).[53] It found that the addition of a small dose of methyltestosterone significantly reduced hot flushes ($P = 0.008$) and the dose of oestrogen needed to control menopausal symptoms. The second RCT (40 women) found no significant difference in vasomotor symptoms with estradiol (oestradiol) alone compared with estradiol plus testosterone after 2 and 6 months of treatment (numbers not provided).[54] **Urogenital system:** We found one RCT of a testosterone/oestrogen combination[54] and one of testosterone alone.[55] The first RCT (40 women) found no significant difference between estradiol alone and estradiol plus testosterone in level of self reported sexual enjoyment and desire.[54] The second RCT (crossover, 53 surgically menopausal women) compared oestrogen alone, testosterone/oestrogen, testosterone and placebo.[55] It found that, while receiving both testosterone/oestrogen and testosterone alone, women reported significantly improved levels of sexual desire ($P < 0.01$), sexual arousal ($P < 0.01$), and number of sexual fantasies ($P < 0.01$) during the treatment months. **Psychological symptoms:** We found no RCTs. **Quality of life:** We found no RCTs.

Harms: We found no evidence from RCTs or other controlled studies on the incidence of androgenic adverse effects with testosterone in women with menopausal symptoms.

Comment: The crossover RCT addressing urogenital symptoms did not provide an analysis prior to crossover.[55] Results are therefore likely to be confounded by carry-over effects of treatments.

OPTION ANTIDEPRESSANTS

We found no RCTs on the effects of antidepressants on menopausal symptoms.

Benefits: We found no systematic review or RCTs that specifically addressed the effects of antidepressants on menopausal symptoms or quality of life in menopausal women.

Harms: We found no evidence on adverse effects in postmenopausal women. Antidepressants as a group can cause many central nervous system adverse effects, including sedation and agitation, as well as urinary and vision problems, liver dysfunction, and cardiac dysrhythmias (see antidepressants under depressive disorders, p 1121).

Comment: None.

GLOSSARY

Kupperman index A numerical index that scores 11 menopausal symptoms: hot flushes, paraesthesia, insomnia, nervousness, melancholia, vertigo, weakness, arthralgia or myalgias, headache, palpitations, and formication. Each symptom is rated from 0 to 3 according to severity and symptoms are then weighted and the total sum calculated. The maximum score is 51 points.

Substantive changes

Oestrogens One RCT[6] and one meta-analysis added; [24] intervention recategorised from Beneficial to Trade off between benefits and harms.

Phyto-oestrogens One RCT added;[50] conclusions unchanged.

REFERENCES

1. Porter M, Penney G, Russell D, et al. A population based survey of women's experience of the menopause. *Br J Obstet Gynaecol* 1996;103:1025–1028.
2. Hagsta TA, Janson PO. The epidemiology of climacteric symptoms. *Acta Obstet Gynecol Scand* 1986;134(suppl):59.
3. MacLennan A, Lester S, Moore V. Oral oestrogen replacement therapy versus placebo for hot flushes. In: The Cochrane Library, Issue 2, 2001. Oxford: Update Software. Search date 2000; primary sources Medline, Embase, Cinahl, and hand searched relevant journals and conference abstracts.
4. Lopes P, Merkus HMWM, Nauman J, et al. Randomized comparison of intranasal and transdermal estradiol. *Obstet Gynecol* 2000;96:906–912.
5. Utian WH, Shoupe D, Bachmann G, et al. Relief of vasomotor symptoms and vaginal atrophy with lower doses of conjugated equine estrogens and medroxyprogesterone acetate. *Fertil Steril* 2001;75:1065–1079.
6. Rozenbaum H, Chevallier O, Moyal M, et al. Efficacy and tolerability of pulsed estrogen therapy: a 12-week double-blind placebo-controlled study in highly symptomatic postmenopausal women. *Climacteric* 2002;5:249–258.
7. Cardozo L, Bachmann G, McClish D, et al. Meta-analysis of estrogen therapy in the management of urogenital atrophy in postmenopausal women: second report of the hormones and urogenital therapy committee. *Obstet Gynecol* 1998;2:722–727. Search date 1995; primary sources Medline, Excerpta Medica, Biosis, and hand searched journals.
8. Cardozo L, Lose G, McClish D, et al. A systematic review of estrogens for recurrent urinary tract infections: third report of the hormones and urogenital therapy (HUT) committee. *Int Urogynecol J Pelvic Floor Dysfunct* 2001;12:15–20. Search date 1998; primary sources Excerpta Medica, Medline, Science Citation Index, and hand-searching relevant journals.
9. Mattsson LA. Clinical experience with continuous combined transdermal hormone replacement therapy. *J Menopause* 1999;6:25–29.
10. Notelovitz M, Mattox JH. Suppression of vasomotor and vulvovaginal symptoms with continuous oral 17β-estradiol. *Menopause* 2000;7:310–317.
11. Casper F, Petri E. Local treatment of urogenital atrophy with an estradiol-releasing vaginal ring: a comparative and a placebo-controlled multicenter study. Vaginal Ring Study Group. *Int Urogynecol J Pelvic Floor Dysfunct* 1999;10:171–176.
12. Zweifel JE, O'Brien WH. A meta-analysis of the effect of HRT upon depressed mood. *Psychoneuroendocrinology* 1997;22:189–212. Search date 1995; primary sources Psychological Abstracts, Medline, and hand searches of Dissertation Abstracts International.
13. Haskell SG, Richardson ED, Horwitz RI. The effect of ORT on cognitive function in women: a critical review of the literature. *J Clin Epidemiol* 1997;50:1249–1264. Search date 1996; primary sources Medline and hand searched reference lists.
14. Polo-Kantola P, Erkkola R, Irjala K, et al. Effect of short-term transdermal estrogen replacement therapy on sleep: a randomized, double-blind crossover trial in postmenopausal women. *Fertil Steril* 1999;71:873–880.
15. Wiklund I, Karlberg J, Mattsson L. Quality of life of postmenopausal women on a regimen of transdermal estradiol therapy: a double-blind placebo-controlled study. *Am J Obstet Gynecol* 1993;168:824–830.
16. Karlberg J, Mattsson L, Wiklund I. A quality of life perspective on who benefits from estradiol replacement therapy. *Acta Obstet Gynecol Scand* 1995;74:367–372.

17. Derman RJ, Dawood MY, Stone S. Quality of life during sequential hormone replacement therapy — a placebo-controlled study. *Int J Fertil Menopausal Stud* 1995;40:73–78.
18. Hilditch JR, Lewis J, Ross AH, et al. A comparison of the effects of oral conjugated equine estrogen and transdermal estradiol-17 β combined with an oral progestin on quality of life in postmenopausal women. *Maturitas* 1996;24:177–184.
19. Norman RJ, Flight IHK, Rees MCP. Oestrogen and progestogen hormone replacement therapy for peri-menopausal and post-menopausal women: weight and body fat distribution. In: The Cochrane Library, Issue 2, 2001. Search date 1998; primary sources Medline, Embase, Current Contents, Biological Abstracts, Cinahl, citation lists, and contact with authors of eligible trials retrieved.
20. Grady D, Sawaya G. Postmenopausal hormone therapy increases risk of deep vein thrombosis and pulmonary embolism. *Am J Med* 1998;105:41–43.
21. Barrett-Connor E. Fortnightly review: hormone replacement therapy. *BMJ* 1998;317:457–461.
22. Lethaby A, Farquhar C, Sarkis A, et al. Hormone replacement therapy in postmenopausal women: endometrial hyperplasia and irregular bleeding. In: The Cochrane Library, Issue 2, 2001. Oxford: Update Software. Search date not stated; primary sources Cochrane Menstrual Disorders and Subfertility Group Trials Register, Medline, Embase, Current Contents, Biological Abstracts, Social Sciences Index, Psychlit, Cinahl, hand searched citation lists, and contact with drug companies and trials authors.
23. Collaborative Group on Hormonal Factors in Breast Cancer. Breast cancer and hormone replacement therapy: collaborative reanalysis of data from 51 epidemiological studies of 52 705 women with breast cancer and 108 411 women without breast cancer. *Lancet* 1997;350:1047–1059. Search date and primary sources not stated; the authors collected epidemiological data on 52 705 women with breast cancer and 108 411 women without breast cancer from 51 studies identified from literature searches, review articles, and discussions with colleagues.
24. Beral V, Banks E, Reeves G. Evidence from randomized trials on the long-term effects of hormone replacement therapy. *Lancet* 2002;360:942–944.
25. Loprinzi CL, Michalak JC, Quella SK, et al. Megestrol acetate for the prevention of hot flashes. *N Engl J Med* 1994;331:347–352.
26. Aslaksen K, Frankendal B. Effect of oral MPA on menopausal symptoms on patients with endometrial carcinoma. *Acta Obstet Gynecol Scand* 1982;61:423–428.
27. Schiff I, Tulchinsky D, Cramer D, et al. Oral medroxyprogesterone in the treatment of postmenopausal symptoms. *JAMA* 1980;244:1443–1445.
28. Leonetti HB, Longo S, Anasti JN. Transdermal progesterone cream for vasomotor symptoms and postmenopausal bone loss. *Obstet Gynecol* 1999;94:225–228.
29. Lobo RA, McCormick W, Singer F, et al. DMPA compared with conjugated oestrogens for the treatment of postmenopausal women. *Obstet Gynecol* 1984;63:1–5.
30. Reginster JY, Zartarian M, Colau JC. Influence of nomogestrel acetate on the improvement of the quality of life induced by estrogen therapy in menopausal women. *Contracept Fertil Sex* 1996;24:847–851.
31. Medical Research Council's General Practice Research Framework. Randomised comparison of oestrogen versus oestrogen plus progesterone hormone replacement therapy in women with hysterectomy. *BMJ* 1996;312:473–478.
32. Greendale GA, Reboussin BA, Hogan P, et al. Symptom relief and side effects of postmenopausal hormones: results from the postmenopausal estrogen/progestin interventions trial. *Obstet Gynecol* 1998;92:982–988.
33. Reginster JY, Zartarian M, Colau JC. Influence of nomogestrel acetate on the improvement of the quality of life induced by estrogen therapy in menopausal women. *Contracept Fertil Sex* 1996;24:847–851.
34. Bjorn I, Bixo M, Noid KS, et al. Negative mood changes during hormone replacement therapy: a comparison between two progestogens. *Am J Obstet Gynecol* 2000;183:1419–1426.
35. Kicovic PM, Cortes-Prieto J, Luisi M, et al. Placebo-controlled cross-over study of effects of Org OD14 in menopausal women. *Reproduction* 1982;6:81–91.
36. Hammar M, Christau S, Nathorst-Boos J, et al. A double-blind, randomised trial comparing the effects of tibolone and continuous combined hormone replacement therapy in postmenopausal women with menopausal symptoms. *Br J Obstet Gynaecol* 1998;105:904–911.
37. Al Azzawi F, Wahab M, Habiba M, et al. Continuous combined hormone replacement therapy compared with tibolone. *Obstet Gynecol* 1999;93:258–264.
38. Nathorst-Boos J, Hammar M. Effect on sexual life — a comparison between tibolone and a continuous estradiol-norethisterone acetate regimen. *Maturitas* 1997;26:15–20.
39. Kokcu A, Cetinkaya MB, Yanik F, et al. The comparison of effects of tibolone and conjugated estrogen- medroxyprogesterone acetate therapy on sexual performance in postmenopausal women. *Maturitas* 2000;36:75–80.
40. Laan E, Van Lunsen RHW, Everaerd W. The effects of tibolone on vaginal blood flow, sexual desire and arousability in postmenopausal women. *Climacteric* 2001;4:28–41.
41. Morris EP, Wilson POG, Robinson J, et al. Long term effects of tibolone on the genital tract in postmenopausal women. *Br J Obstet Gynaecol* 1999;106:954–959.
42. Benedek-Jaszmann LJ. Long-term placebo-controlled efficacy and safety study of Org OD14 in climacteric women. *Maturitas* 1987;1:25–33.
43. Walker ID, Davidson JF, Richards A, et al. The effect of the synthetic steroid Org OD14 on fibrinolysis and blood lipids in postmenopausal women. *Thromb Haemost* 1985;53:303–305.
44. Murkies AL, Lombard C, Stauss BJ, et al. Dietary flour supplementation decreases postmenopausal hot flushes: effect of soy and wheat. *Maturitas* 1995;21:189–195.
45. Washburn S, Burke GL, Morgan T, et al. Effect of soy protein supplementation on serum lipoproteins, blood pressure, and menopausal symptoms in perimenopausal women. *Menopause* 1999;6:7–13.
46. Baber RJ, Templeman C, Morton T, et al. Randomized placebo-controlled trial of an isoflavone supplement and menopausal symptoms in women. *Climacteric* 1999;2:85–92.
47. Scambia G, Mango D, Signorile PG, et al. Clinical effects of a standardized soy extract in postmenopausal women: a pilot study. *Menopause* 2000;7:105–111.
48. Kotsopoulos D, Dalais FS, Liang Y-L, et al. The effects of soy protein containing phytoestrogens on menopausal symptoms in postmenopausal women. *Climacteric* 2000;3:161–167.

49. Upmalis DH, Lobo R, Bradley L, et al. Vasomotor symptom relief by soy isoflavone extract tablets in postmenopausal women: a multicenter, double-blind, randomized, placebo-controlled study. *Menopause* 2000;7:236–242.
50. Han KK, Soares JM Jr, Haidar MA, et al. Benefits of soy isoflavone therapeutic regimen on menopausal symptoms. *Obstet Gynecol* 2002;99:389–394.
51. Nagamani M, Kelver ME, Smith ER. Treatment of menopausal hot flashes with transdermal administration of clonidine. *Am J Obstet Gynecol* 1987;156:561–565.
52. Edington RF, Chagnon JP. Clonidine (Dixarit) for menopausal flushing. *Can Med Assoc J* 1980;123:23–26.
53. Simon J, Klaiber E, Wiita B, et al. Differential effects of estrogen-androgen and estrogen-only therapy on vasomotor symptoms, gonadotropin secretion, and endogenous androgen bioavailability in postmenopausal women. *Menopause* 1999;6:138–146.
54. Dow MG, Hart DM, Forrest CA. Hormonal treatments of sexual unresponsiveness in postmenopausal women: a comparative study. *Br J Obstet Gynaecol* 1983;90:361–366.
55. Sherwin BB, Gelfand MM, Brender W. Androgen enhances sexual motivation in females: a prospective crossover study of sex steroid administration in the surgical menopause. *Psychosom Med* 1985;47:339–351.

Edward Morris
Consultant in Obstetrics and Gynaecology
Norfolk and Norwich University Hospital
Norwich
UK

Janice Rymer
Senior Lecturer/Consultant in Obstetrics and Gynaecology
Guy's, King's and St Thomas' Medical School
London
UK

Competing interests: JR has been sponsered to attend conferences by Organan, Solvay healthcare Ltd, Wyeth, Novo Nordish, Janssen-Cilag and Servier. JR has also received research funding from Organon and Novo Nordish, and consultancy fees from Organon, Wyeth, Janssen-Cilag and Pifzer. EM has been sponsored to attend conferences and has received speakers' fees from Eli Lilly, Organon, Novo Nordisk, Astra Zeneca and Pharmacia.

TABLE 1 Placebo controlled RCTs evaluating the effect of progestogens on vasomotor symptoms (see text, p 2142).

Trial	Total participants	Comparison	Duration	Outcome	Difference	Effect
Loprinzi [25]	163	Oral medroxyprogesterone acetate 200 mg twice daily versus placebo (crossover)	9 weeks	50% reduction in daily hot flush frequency at 4 weeks (pre-crossover)	34/48 (71%) with medroxyprogesterone acetate *v* 12/49 (24%) with placebo	RR 2.9, 95% CI 1.71 to 4.89; NNT 3, 95% CI 2 to 4
Aslaksen [26]	21	Oral medroxyprogesterone acetate 100 mg twice daily versus placebo (crossover)	24 weeks	Free from hot flushes at end of study	18/21 (86%) with medroxyprogesterone acetate *v* 7/21 (33%) with placebo	RR for no flush 2.6, 95% CI 1.37 to 4.83; NNT 2, 95 % CI 2 to 3
				Free from sweating	18/21 (86%) with medroxyprogesterone acetate *v* 3/21 (14%) with placebo	RR for no sweating 6.0, 95% CI 2.1 to 17.4; NNT 2, 95% CI 1 to 2
Schiff [27]	27	Oral medroxyprogesterone acetate 20 mg daily versus placebo (crossover)	24 weeks	% reduction in hot flushes at 12 week crossover to alternative treatment	74% with medroxyprogesterone acetate *v* 26% with placebo	$P < 0.05$
Leonetti [28]	102	Transdermal progesterone cream 20 mg versus placebo	1 year	Improvement or resolution of vasomotor symptoms as determined by review of weekly symptom diaries	25/30 (83%) with transdermal progesterone *v* 26/47 (55%) with placebo	RR 1.5, 95% CI 1.1 to 2.0; NNT 4, 95% CI 2 to 9

Menorrhagia

Search date February 2003

Kirsten Duckitt and Keri McCully

QUESTIONS

INTERVENTIONS

See glossary, p 2167

Key Messages

Treatments

- **Endometrial thinning before hysteroscopic surgery** One systematic review has found that preoperative gonadorelin (gonadotrophin releasing hormone) analogues reduce moderate or heavy periods and increase amenorrhoea compared with placebo, no preoperative treatment, or preoperative danazol. We found insufficient evidence about effects of preoperative danazol or progestogens compared with placebo or no preoperative treatment.
- **Hysterectomy (*v* endometrial destruction) after medical failure** Systematic reviews have found that hysterectomy reduces menstrual blood loss and the number of women requiring further operations, and increases satisfaction compared with endometrial destruction. RCTs found no differences in effectiveness between different types of hysterectomy. One large cohort study reported major or minor complications in about a third of women undergoing hysterectomy.

- **Non-steroidal anti-inflammatory drugs** One systematic review has found that non-steroidal anti-inflammatory drugs reduce mean menstrual blood loss compared with placebo. One systematic review found no significant difference in menstrual blood loss between mefenamic acid and naproxen, or between non-steroidal anti-inflammatory drugs and oral progestogens, oral contraceptives, or progesterone releasing intrauterine devices.
- **Tranexamic acid** Systematic reviews have found that tranexamic acid reduces menstrual blood loss compared with placebo or other drugs (oral progestogens, mefenamic acid, etamsylate, flurbiprofen, and diclofenac). Adverse effects of tranexamic acid include leg cramps and nausea, which occur in about a third of women using this drug. One long term population based observational study found no evidence that tranexamic acid increases the risk of thromboembolism.
- **Hysteroscopic versus non-hysteroscopic endometrial destruction after medical failure** One systematic review found that hysteroscopic methods of endometrial destruction increased amenorrhoea at 12 months compared with non-hysteroscopic methods. We found no consistent evidence of a difference in amenorrhoea or satisfaction rates among different types of hysteroscopic procedure. RCTs found that complications, such as infection, haemorrhage, or uterine perforation occurred in up to 15% of women undergoing endometrial destruction.
- **Danazol** Systematic reviews found limited evidence that danazol reduced blood loss compared with placebo, luteal phase oral progestogens, mefenamic acid, naproxen, or oral contraceptives, but found that danazol increased adverse effects compared with either non-steroidal anti-inflammatory drugs or oral progestogens.
- **Combined oral contraceptives** One systematic review found insufficient evidence about effects of oral contraceptives in women with menorrhagia.
- **Endometrial resection versus medical treatment** One systematic review and one additional RCT found no consistent evidence of a difference in blood loss or satisfaction between transcervical endometrial resection and medical treatment. RCTs found that complications, such as infection, haemorrhage, or uterine perforation occurred in up to 15% of women undergoing endometrial destruction.
- **Etamsylate** We found insufficient evidence from one systematic review about effects of etamsylate compared with placebo, mefenamic acid, aminocaproic acid, or tranexamic acid.
- **Intrauterine progestogens** We found no systematic review or RCTs comparing intrauterine progestogens versus placebo. Two systematic reviews and three subsequent RCTs found conflicting evidence about menstrual blood loss, satisfaction rates, and quality of life scores with levonorgestrel releasing intrauterine devices compared with other treatments (endometrial resection, thermal balloon ablation, norethisterone, medical treatment, non-steroidal anti-inflammatory drugs, and hysterectomy).
- **Oral progestogens (longer cycle)** We found no RCTs comparing oral progestogens versus placebo. One RCT identified by a systematic review found no significant difference in menstrual blood loss between a longer treatment cycle of oral progestogen and a levonorgestrel releasing intrauterine device.
- **Oral progestogens in luteal phase only** We found no RCTs comparing oral progestogens versus placebo. One systematic review has found that luteal phase oral progestogens increase mean menstrual blood loss compared with danazol, tranexamic acid, or a progesterone releasing intrauterine device.

- **Dilatation and curettage after medical failure; gonadorelin (gonadotrophin releasing hormone) analogues; myomectomy after medical failure** We found no RCTs on the effects of these interventions.

DEFINITION Menorrhagia is defined as heavy but regular menstrual bleeding. Idiopathic ovulatory menorrhagia is regular heavy bleeding in the absence of recognisable pelvic pathology or a general bleeding disorder. Objective menorrhagia is taken to be a total menstrual blood loss of 80 mL or more in each menstruation.[1] Subjectively, menorrhagia may be defined as a complaint of regular excessive menstrual blood loss occurring over several consecutive cycles in a woman of reproductive years.

INCIDENCE/ PREVALENCE In the UK, 5% of women (aged 30–49 years) consult their general practitioner each year with menorrhagia.[2] In New Zealand, 2–4% of primary care consultations by premenopausal women are for menstrual problems.[3]

AETIOLOGY/ RISK FACTORS Idiopathic ovulatory menorrhagia is thought to be caused by disordered prostaglandin production within the endometrium.[4] Prostaglandins may also be implicated in menorrhagia associated with uterine fibroids, adenomyosis, or the presence of an intrauterine device. Fibroids have been reported in 10% of women with menorrhagia (80–100 mL/cycle) and 40% of those with severe menorrhagia (≥ 200 mL/cycle).[5]

PROGNOSIS Menorrhagia limits normal activities and causes iron deficiency anaemia in two thirds of women proved to have objective menorrhagia.[1,6,7] One in five of all women in the UK and one in three women in the USA have a hysterectomy before the age of 60 years; menorrhagia is the main presenting problem in at least 50% of these women.[8–10] About 50% of the women who have a hysterectomy for menorrhagia are found to have a normal uterus.[11]

AIMS OF INTERVENTION To reduce menstrual bleeding; improve quality of life; and prevent or correct iron deficiency anaemia, with minimum adverse effects. Women may regard amenorrhea as a benefit or a harm of treatment depending on their perspective.

OUTCOMES Menstrual blood flow (assessed objectively [mL/cycle] or subjectively); haemoglobin concentration; quality of life; patient satisfaction; incidence of adverse drug effects; and incidence of postoperative complications. Whether a particular percentage reduction in menstrual blood loss is considered clinically important will depend on pretreatment menstrual loss and the individual woman's perception of acceptable menstrual loss.

METHODS *Clinical Evidence* search and appraisal February 2003. The author also hand searched reference lists of non-systematic reviews and studies obtained from the initial search, and recent issues of key journals.

QUESTION What are the effects of medical treatments?

OPTION NON-STEROIDAL ANTI-INFLAMMATORY DRUGS

One systematic review has found that non-steroidal anti-inflammatory drugs reduce mean menstrual blood loss compared with placebo. One systematic review found no significant difference in menstrual blood loss between mefenamic acid and naproxen, or between non-steroidal anti-inflammatory drugs and oral progestogens, oral contraceptives, or progesterone releasing intrauterine devices.

Benefits: **Versus placebo:** We found one systematic review (search date 1996, 12 RCTs, 313 women) comparing non-steroidal anti-inflammatory drugs (NSAIDs: mefenamic acid, naproxen, meclofenamic acid, ibuprofen, and diclofenac) versus placebo.[3] Treatment was taken only during menstruation, but doses varied depending on the drug used. The review found that NSAIDs significantly reduced mean menstrual blood loss compared with placebo (WMD for blood loss for all NSAIDs *v* placebo –35 mL, 95% CI –43 mL to –27 mL). **Versus other NSAIDs and other drugs:** We found one systematic review (search date 2001, 16 RCTs) comparing different NSAIDs versus each other, and NSAIDs versus other drugs.[12] It found no significant difference in menstrual blood loss between mefenamic acid and naproxen (WMD for blood loss +21.0 mL, 95% CI –5.9 mL to +47.9 mL); between NSAIDs and oral progestogens given in the luteal phase (WMD for blood loss –23.0 mL, 95% CI –46.6 mL to +0.625 mL); between NSAIDs and the combined oral contraceptive (WMD for blood loss +25.3 mL, 95% CI –22.3 mL to +72.8 mL), or between NSAIDs and a progesterone releasing intrauterine device (WMD for blood loss –4.0 mL, 95% CI –31.2 mL to +23.2 mL). However, many of these comparisons may have lacked power to exclude clinically important differences between treatments.

Harms: The reviews found that commonly reported adverse effects included headaches and gastrointestinal disturbances, including indigestion, nausea, vomiting, and diarrhoea.[3,12] These occurred in at least 50% of women taking NSAIDs in the RCTs that reported data on adverse effects, but similar levels of adverse effects were found in placebo cycles (see non-steroidal anti-inflammatory drugs, p 1393).

Comment: NSAIDs have the additional benefit of relieving dysmenorrhoea (see dysmenorrhoea, p 2058).

OPTION TRANEXAMIC ACID

Systematic reviews have found that tranexamic acid reduces menstrual blood loss compared with placebo or other drugs (oral progestogens, mefenamic acid, etamsylate, flurbiprofen, and diclofenac). Adverse effects of tranexamic acid include leg cramps and nausea, which occur in about a third of women using this drug. One long term population based observational study found no evidence that tranexamic acid increases the risk of thromboembolism.

Benefits: **Versus placebo:** We found two systematic reviews.[3,13] The first review (search date 1996, 5 RCTs, 153 women) found that tranexamic acid (250–500 mg 4 times daily during menstruation) significantly reduced mean menstrual blood loss compared with placebo (WMD −52 mL; other results and significance presented graphically).[3] Few studies in the review measured patient satisfaction. The second systematic review (search date 1997, 7 RCTs) identified two RCTs that compared tranexamic acid (1 g 4 times daily) or a prodrug of tranexamic acid (Kabi 2161, 1.2 g twice daily) versus placebo.[13] It found that either active drug significantly reduced mean menstrual blood loss compared with placebo (WMD −94 mL, 95% CI −151 mL to −37 mL). **Versus other drugs:** We found two systematic reviews.[3,13] One review (search date 1997) found that tranexamic acid significantly reduced mean menstrual blood loss compared with luteal phase oral progestogens or mefenamic acid (WMD for tranexamic acid *v* oral progestogens −111 mL, 95% CI −179 mL to −44 mL; WMD for tranexamic acid *v* mefenamic acid −73 mL, 95% CI −123 mL to −23 mL).[13] The second review (search date 1996) did not pool data from several RCTs comparing tranexamic acid versus other drugs.[3] The RCTs consistently found that tranexamic acid significantly improved outcomes compared with mefenamic acid, etamsylate (ethamsylate), flurbiprofen, diclofenac, and norethisterone. One of the RCTs (46 women) identified by the review found that tranexamic acid significantly reduced limitations on social activities (proportion of people who reported reduced limitation of social activities compared with placebo cycles: 67% with tranexamic acid *v* 45% with norethisterone) and increased the proportion of people with improved sex life (proportion of people reporting improved sex life compared with placebo cycles: 46% with tranexamic acid *v* 15% with norethisterone) compared with norethisterone.[14]

Harms: Nausea and leg cramps occur in a third of women taking tranexamic acid. One systematic review (search date 1997) found no increase in gastrointestinal adverse effects compared with either placebo or other drugs.[13] Isolated case reports have suggested a risk of thromboembolism associated with tranexamic acid, but a large population based study over 19 years found no evidence that this was higher than expected in the normal population.[15]

Comment: Unlike non-steroidal anti-inflammatory drugs, tranexamic acid has no effect on dysmenorrhoea.

OPTION ETAMSYLATE

We found insufficient evidence from one systematic review about effects of etamsylate compared with placebo, mefenamic acid, aminocaproic acid, or tranexamic acid.

Benefits: We found one systematic review (search date not stated, 4 RCTs) comparing etamsylate (ethamsylate) versus placebo, mefenamic acid, aminocaproic acid, or tranexamic acid.[16] Most results were presented as comparison with baseline. However, one RCT (double blind, 81 women; see comment below) identified by the review compared three treatments directly: etamsylate, tranexamic acid, and mefenamic acid. The RCT found that both tranexamic acid and mefenamic acid significantly reduced mean menstrual blood loss compared with etamsylate (WMD tranexamic acid *v* etamsylate −97 mL, 95% CI −140 mL to −54 mL; WMD mefenamic acid *v* etamsylate −51 mL, 95% CI −96 mL to −6 mL). The review found that etamsylate achieved an overall reduction in menstrual blood loss compared with baseline of 13% (95% CI 11% to 15%), which may not be clinically significant.[16]

Harms: The review found no significant difference in the rate of adverse effects (nausea, headaches, and dizziness) between different drug regimens, and these adverse effects seldom caused women to withdraw from studies.[16]

Comment: The RCT reported that 27% of women had withdrawn from the study before its completion, and made no adjustment for the multiple treatment comparisons involved.[17]

OPTION DANAZOL

Systematic reviews found limited evidence that danazol reduced blood loss compared with placebo, luteal phase oral progestogens, mefenamic acid, naproxen, or oral contraceptives, but found that danazol increased adverse effects compared with either non-steroidal anti-inflammatory drugs or oral progestogens.

Benefits: We found two systematic reviews (search date 2001, 9 RCTs, 353 women;[18] search date 1996, 3 RCTs, 127 women;[3] see comment below) comparing danazol versus placebo, other medical treatments, or different doses of danazol. **Versus placebo:** The first review identified one RCT (66 women), which compared danazol versus placebo. It found that danazol significantly improved blood loss scores from baseline whereas placebo had no significant effect at 3 months.[18] However, it was unclear how this result was calculated. The second review found that danazol (200 mg daily continuously for 2–3 months) significantly reduced mean menstrual blood loss compared with placebo (WMD danazol *v* placebo −108 mL; CI presented graphically).[3] **Versus other drugs:** The first review found that danazol reduced blood loss more than progestogens (OR for mean blood loss < 80 mL at the end of the intervention 7.20; 95% CI 1.28 to 40.40), non-steroidal anti-inflammatory drugs (WMD for mean menstrual blood loss −96.7 mL, 95% CI −138.0 mL to −54.6 mL), and the combined oral contraceptive pill, although confidence intervals were wide. Results were based on a small number of trials, all of which were small and may have lacked power to detect clinically important effects.[18] We found no randomised trials comparing danazol with tranexamic acid or the levonorgestrel releasing intrauterine system. **Different danazol regimens:** The first review included two small RCTs that compared different danazol regimens: standard dose danazol 200 mg daily; lower dose danazol 100 mg daily; and a reducing dose regimen.[18] It found no significant differences in blood loss (WMD for mean menstrual blood loss +33.5 mL, 95% CI −32.4 mL to +99.4 mL), frequency of adverse events (OR for number of women reporting adverse events 1.13, 95% CI 0.14 to 9.07), or duration of menstruation (WMD for duration of menstruation +1.3 days, 95% CI –0.76 days to +3.36 days) when a dose of 200 mg daily was compared with a reducing dose regimen.

Harms: The first review found that adverse events were more frequent with danazol than non-steroidal anti-inflammatory drugs (OR 7.0, 95% CI 1.7 to 28.2) or progestogens (OR 4.05, 95% CI 1.6 to 10.2). However, the review reported no significant differences in adherence to treatment.[18] RCTs included in the review reported that danazol may be associated with weight gain; androgenic effects such as acne, seborrhoea, hirsutism, and voice changes; and general complaints including irritability, musculoskeletal pains, and tiredness. Hot flushes and breast atrophy can sometimes occur. Most of these adverse effects are reversible on cessation of treatment (see harms of hormonal treatments under endometriosis, p 2079, and harms of danazol under breast pain, p 2034).

Comment: The second systematic review comparing danazol with placebo had less rigorous inclusion criteria and included two RCTs that were excluded by the first review.[3] Women using danazol may be advised to use barrier methods of contraception because of potential virilisation of the fetus if pregnancy occurs during treatment with this drug.

OPTION COMBINED ORAL CONTRACEPTIVES

One systematic review found insufficient evidence about effects of oral contraceptives in women with menorrhagia.

Benefits: We found one systematic review (search date 1997), which identified one small RCT (38 women) comparing a combined oral contraceptive versus danazol, mefenamic acid, or naproxen.[19] It found no significant difference between any of the treatments (doses not provided) but was too small to rule out a clinically important difference.

Harms: Minor adverse effects are common and include nausea, headache, breast tenderness, changes in body weight, hypertension, changes in libido, and depression.

Comment: One non-randomised controlled trial (164 women) found that a 50 mg oral contraceptive pill led to a 53% reduction in menstrual blood loss compared with baseline.[20] The trial also found that aminocaproic acid (85 women) led to a 54% reduction and tranexamic acid (172 women) led to a 47% reduction in menstrual blood loss.[20] Two longitudinal case control studies found that women taking the contraceptive pill were less likely than those not taking the pill to experience heavy menstrual bleeding or anaemia.[21,22]

OPTION ORAL PROGESTOGENS

We found no RCTs comparing oral progestogens with placebo. One systematic review has found that luteal phase oral progestogens increase mean menstrual blood loss compared with danazol, tranexamic acid, or a

progesterone releasing intrauterine device. One RCT identified by the review found no significant difference in menstrual blood loss between a longer treatment cycle of oral progestogen and a levonorgestrel releasing intrauterine device.

Benefits: **Versus placebo:** We found no RCTs. **Versus other drugs:** We found one systematic review (search date not stated; 7 RCTs), which compared four treatments: luteal phase oral progestogens, danazol, tranexamic acid, and progesterone releasing intrauterine devices (IUDs).[23] It found that oral progestogens significantly increased mean menstrual blood loss compared with any of the other treatments (progestogen *v* danazol WMD −56 mL, 95% CI −96 mL to −15 mL; progestogen *v* tranexamic acid WMD −111 mL, 95% CI −179 mL to −44 mL; and progestogen *v* progesterone releasing IUD WMD −51 mL, 95% CI −84 mL to −18 mL). The review also found that luteal phase oral progestogens significantly increased the proportion of women who reported a greater self assessed menstrual blood loss after treatment compared with danazol (2 RCTs: 19/28 [68%] with luteal phase progestogens *v* 8/26 [31%] with danazol; RR 2.2, 95% CI 1.2 to 4.1; NNH 2, 95% CI 1 to 9).[23] **Longer treatment cycle:** We found one systematic review (search date not stated).[23] One RCT (48 women) identified by the review found no significant difference with a longer regimen of oral progestogen (norethisterone, 21 days/cycle) versus a levonorgestrel releasing IUD in menstrual blood loss (94 mL with oral norethisterone *v* 104 mL with levonorgestrel IUD).

Harms: Two systematic reviews (search dates not stated) found that adverse effects (including headache, breast tenderness, premenstrual symptoms, and gastrointestinal disturbances) were reported in a third to a half of the women who received oral progestogens.[16,23] In the RCT that compared longer treatment cycle with oral progestogens with a levonorgestrel releasing IUD, 56% of women did not feel "well" or "very well" on the treatment and 22% elected to continue with treatment after the 3 months of the study.[23]

Comment: None.

OPTION INTRAUTERINE PROGESTOGENS

We found no systematic review or RCTs comparing intrauterine progestogens with placebo. Two systematic reviews and three subsequent RCTs found conflicting evidence about menstrual blood loss, satisfaction rates, and quality of life scores with levonorgestrel releasing intrauterine devices compared with other treatments (endometrial resection, thermal balloon ablation, norethisterone, medical treatment, non-steroidal anti-inflammatory drugs, and hysterectomy).

Benefits: We found no systematic review or RCTs comparing intrauterine progestogens with placebo. Two systematic reviews (search date 1999, 5 RCTs;[24] search date 1999, 5 RCTs[25]) and three subsequent RCTs compared intrauterine progestogens with other treatments.[26–28] The second review identified four of the RCTs in the first review and one additional RCT.[25] **Progesterone releasing intrauterine device (IUD):** The first systematic review found one

RCT that compared four different treatments: a progesterone releasing IUD 65 μg daily, danazol, mefenamic acid, or norethisterone.[24] The review did not compare treatments with each other, but found that all treatments reduced menstrual blood loss compared with baseline values. **Levonorgestrel releasing IUD:** Both reviews found four RCTs that examined the effects of levonorgestrel releasing IUDs 20 μg daily.[24] Two RCTs (60 and 70 women) identified by the reviews compared levonorgestrel releasing IUDs versus transcervical endometrial resection, using the pictorial blood loss assessment chart (see glossary, p 2167).[24,25] The reviews found no significant difference between treatments in mean blood loss (endometrial resection *v* levonorgestrel IUD WMD +12.2 mL, 95% CI −1.9 mL to +26.3 mL) or satisfaction rates (satisfaction rate 94% with endometrial resection *v* 85% with levonorgestrel IUD; P = NS) after 12 months.[24] The third RCT (44 women) identified by the reviews found no significant difference between norethisterone (15 mg daily, day 5 to day 26 of cycle) and levonorgestrel releasing IUDs in reduction of blood loss or rates of satisfaction (median reduction from baseline 6 mL/cycle with norethisterone *v* 20 mL/cycle with levonorgestrel; satisfaction data not stated).[24,25] The fourth RCT (56 women) identified by the reviews found that levonorgestrel releasing IUDs significantly increased the number of women who cancelled their hysterectomy after 6 months of treatment compared with medical treatment and improved all the quality of life scores that were assessed (cancelled hysterectomy: 18/28 [64%] with levonorgestrel releasing IUD *v* 4/28 [14%] with medical treatment; RR 4.5, 95% CI 1.7 to 11.6).[24,25] Details of medical treatment and results of quality of life assessment were not provided. The additional RCT (35 women) identified by the second review compared three groups: a levonorgestrel releasing IUD, flurbiprofen, and tranexamic acid (see comment below).[25] It found that a levonorgestrel releasing IUD significantly reduced mean menstrual flow after 12 months compared with both other treatments (mean menstrual blood flow reduction: 96% with levonorgestrel *v* 21% with flurbiprofen, $P < 0.001$; 96% with levonorgestrel *v* 44% with tranexamic acid, $P < 0.01$). The first subsequent RCT (236 women) compared a levonorgestrel releasing IUD with hysterectomy (see comment below).[26] It found no significant difference in health related quality of life, general health state, anxiety, depression (results presented graphically; significance data not provided), or in haemoglobin concentration (135 g/L with levonorgestrel *v* 132 g/L with hysterectomy; significance data not provided), although both treatments significantly improved these outcomes compared with baseline levels after 12 months. The second subsequent RCT (59 women) found that a levonorgestrel releasing IUD significantly decreased the number of women judged to have been successfully treated after 12 months compared with endometrial resection (treatment success defined as a pictorial blood loss assessment chart score of ≤ 75; 20/30 [67%] with a levonorgestrel releasing IUD *v* 26/29 [90%] with endometrial resection; RR 1.35, 95% CI 1.02 to 1.78; NNT 5, 95% CI 3 to 26).[27] The third subsequent RCT (72 women) compared a levonorgestrel releasing IUD versus thermal balloon ablation (see glossary, p 2167).[28] It found that thermal balloon ablation increased success rate (defined as a pictorial blood loss assessment chart score of ≤ 75) compared with levonorgestrel releasing IUD, but found no significant difference between treatments in haemoglobin at 1 year (success rate: 97% with thermal balloon ablation *v* 77% with levonorgestrel releasing IUD, neither CI nor P values for comparison were reported; increase in haemoglobin: 3.9 g/dL with thermal balloon ablation *v* 3.7 g/dL with levonorgestrel releasing IUD, neither CI nor P values for comparison were reported).

Harms: There are concerns that progesterone releasing IUDs increase rates of ectopic pregnancy, although the RCTs identified by the reviews did not report this adverse effect.[24,25] The first review found that most adverse effects in women using a levonorgestrel releasing IUD were typical of progestogens (bloating, weight gain, breast tenderness).[24] One RCT included in the review found that levonorgestrel releasing IUD significantly increased the number of women reporting at least one adverse effect compared with transcervical endometrial resection (56% with levonorgestrel releasing IUD *v* 26% with transcervical endometrial resection; RR 2.2, 95% CI 1.2 to 3.0).[29] One further trial found that levonorgestrel releasing IUDs significantly increased the proportion of women who were amenorrhoeic after 3 months of treatment compared with norethisterone (32% with levonorgestrel releasing IUDs *v* 0% with norethisterone).[30] The other main adverse effect reported with levonorgestrel releasing IUDs was irregular, although not usually heavy, menstrual bleeding.[24] RCTs looking at the contraceptive effect of levonorgestrel releasing IUDs in younger women found that during the first few months of use the total number of bleeding days (including menstrual bleeding, intermenstrual bleeding, and spotting) increased in most women.[31] However, most women bled lightly for only 1 day a month and about 15% were amenorrhoeic after 12 months.[32] One RCT (72 women) found that levonorgestrel releasing IUD significantly increased adverse effects compared with thermal balloon ablation (adverse effects: 58.3% with levonorgestrel releasing IUD *v* 22.2% with thermal balloon ablation, $P < 0.05$).[28] Adverse effects with levonorgestrel releasing IUD included spotting (6 women), mastalgia (5 women), weight gain (10 women), mood swings (2 women), bloating (8 women), acne–greasy skin (7 women), nausea (4 women), headache and leg pain (1 woman), and lost IUD (1 woman). Adverse effects with thermal balloon included mastalgia (1 woman), weight gain (4 women), mood swings (1 woman), bloating (1 woman), dysmenorrhoea (2 women), and lower abdominal pain (1 woman). The RCT also found a higher pain score 12 hours after surgery with thermal balloon ablation compared with IUD (no results provided).[28]

Comment: In the additional RCT (35 women) identified by the second review, the first 20 women were given a levonorgestrel releasing IUD and the following 15 women were randomised in a crossover design to receive either flurbiprofen or tranexamic acid.[25] The first subsequent RCT (236 women) found that 24/119 (20%) women who received a levonorgestrel releasing IUD had a hysterectomy, 10/119 (8%) women had the IUD removed, and 3/119 (3%) women were lost to follow up after 12 months.[26] The RCT also found that women had the levonorgestrel releasing IUD removed because of intermenstrual bleeding (94%), heavy bleeding (40%), hormonal symptoms

(17%), or a combination of symptoms. Long term follow up on women with menorrhagia is required to assess continuation rates, satisfaction, and whether surgical treatment is avoided or just postponed. The trials that considered long term bleeding patterns were mainly in women under 40 years of age. It is not yet known whether these results can be extrapolated to older women with menorrhagia.

OPTION **GONADORELIN (GONADOTROPHIN RELEASING HORMONE) ANALOGUES**

We found no good evidence on the effects of gonadorelin analogues.

Benefits: We found no systematic review or RCTs.

Harms: We found no RCTs (see comment below).

Comment: A few small non-randomised studies have looked at gonadorelin analogues in menorrhagia. Others have looked at their effects in women with fibroids or on thinning the endometrium before ablation or resection. Adverse effects of gonadorelin analogues are mainly caused by reduced oestrogens. Hormone replacement to counteract hypo-oestrogenism has been tried with limited success to reduce hot flushes.[33] Bone demineralisation occurs in most women after 6 months of treatment but is reversible after treatment is stopped.[34] Contraception whilst using these drugs is not guaranteed.[35]

QUESTION **What are the effects of surgical treatments if medical treatments fail?**

OPTION **DILATATION AND CURETTAGE**

We found no good evidence on the effects of dilatation and curettage.

Benefits: We found no systematic review or RCTs.

Harms: Observational evidence suggest that dilatation and curettage may cause adverse effects including uterine perforation and cervical laceration as well as the usual risks of general anaesthesia.[36]

Comment: Dilatation and curettage still plays a part in the investigation of menorrhagia. We found one uncontrolled cohort study (50 women) that measured blood loss before and after dilatation and curettage.[37] It found a reduction in menstrual blood loss immediately after the procedure, but losses returned to previous levels or higher by the second menstrual period.

OPTION **HYSTERECTOMY**

Systematic reviews have found that hysterectomy reduces menstrual blood loss and the number of women requiring further operations, and increases participant satisfaction compared with endometrial destruction. RCTs found no difference in effectiveness between different types of hysterectomy. One large cohort study reported major or minor complications in about a third of women undergoing hysterectomy.

Benefits: **Versus endometrial destruction:** We found two systematic reviews (search dates 1996[3] and not stated[38]). Both identified the same five RCTs (708 premenopausal women) comparing hysterectomy versus endometrial destruction (transcervical endometrial resection or laser ablation — see glossary, p 2167). The reviews found that hysterectomy significantly reduced menstrual blood loss, and significantly increased the proportion of women with a reduction in menstrual blood loss after 12 months (3 RCTs; 220/220 [100%] with hysterectomy *v* 191/220 [87%] with endometrial destruction; NNT 8, 95% CI 6 to 13). However, the reviews reported that the differences in reduction in blood loss between treatments seemed to narrow with longer follow up, possibly because of re-treatment in the endometrial ablation group or because of menopause. The reviews also found that women were more satisfied with hysterectomy than endometrial ablation after 12 months compared with hysterectomy (RR 0.93, 95% CI 0.89 to 0.99) and after 2 years (RR for being "moderately" or "very" satisfied with endometrial ablation *v* hysterectomy: 0.87, 95% CI 0.81 to 0.94).[3,38] Two RCTs included in the reviews found no significant difference between treatments in satisfaction rates after 3 and 4 years. The reviews found that endometrial destruction significantly increased the number of women requiring repeat surgery compared with hysterectomy (after 12 months, 5 RCTs: 1/320 [0.3%] with hysterectomy *v* 54/386 [14%] with endometrial destruction; RR 44.8, 95% CI 6.2 to 321.8; after 4 years, 1 RCT: 1/95 [1%] with hysterectomy *v* 39/102 [38%] with endometrial destruction; RR 36.3, 95% CI 5.1 to 259.2), but found that endometrial destruction significantly reduced the duration of surgery (–23 minutes), duration of hospital stay (–5 days), and time to return to work (–4.5 weeks). **Different techniques:** We found no systematic review. Five small RCTs (total of 334 women) compared abdominal, vaginal, or laparoscopic hysterectomy.[39–43] They found no evidence of a difference in effectiveness or complication rates. However, operating and recovery times varied.

Harms: Large population based analyses stratified by age have found that mortality after hysterectomy for non-malignant conditions is about 1/2000 in women aged under 50 years.[44] When compared with endometrial destruction, hysterectomy increased the risk of sepsis, blood transfusion, urinary retention, anaemia, pyrexia, vault and wound haematoma, and cautery of hypergranulation before hospital discharge. One large, prospective cohort study of hysterectomy for non-malignant conditions found combined major and minor complication rates (mainly infectious morbidity) of 25% for vaginal hysterectomy and 43% for abdominal hysterectomy.[45] It is possible that the difference seen was attributable to the prevalence and efficacy of prophylactic antibiotic use among the vaginal hysterectomy group. Prophylactic antibiotics are used more routinely in both groups nowadays.

Comment: None.

OPTION ENDOMETRIAL DESTRUCTION (RESECTION OR ABLATION)

Systematic reviews have found that endometrial destruction increases menstrual blood loss and the need for further operations and reduces participant satisfaction compared with hysterectomy. One systematic review found that hysteroscopic methods of endometrial destruction increased amenorrhoea at 12 months compared with non-hysteroscopic methods. We found no consistent evidence of a difference in amenorrhoea or satisfaction rates among different types of hysteroscopic procedure. We found no consistent evidence of a difference in blood loss or satisfaction between transcervical endometrial resection and medical treatment. RCTs found that complications, such as infection, haemorrhage, or uterine perforation occurred in up to 15% of women undergoing endometrial destruction.

Benefits: **Versus hysterectomy:** See benefits of hysterectomy, p 2162. **Hysteroscopic resection or ablation versus non-hysteroscopic techniques:** We found one systematic review (search date 2001, 8 RCTs, 1595 premenopausal women)[46] and two subsequent RCTs.[47,48] Hysteroscopic methods included in the review were laser ablation, rollerball ablation, transcervical endometrial resection (see glossary, p 2167), and vaporising electrode ablation. Non-hysteroscopic methods included thermal uterine balloon therapy, multielectrode balloon ablation, microwave ablation (see glossary, p 2167), and heated saline. All methods reduced menstrual blood loss compared with baseline assessment. The review found that hysteroscopic ablation significantly increased amenorrhoea at 12 months compared with non-hysteroscopic ablation (amenorrhoea: OR 0.76, 95% CI 0.60 to 0.90). The review found no significant difference between hysteroscopic and non-hysteroscopic methods in satisfaction rate, inability to work, and subsequent requirement for additional surgery or pictorial blood loss assessment chart (see glossary, p 2167) results after 12 months. Among hysteroscopic techniques the review found no significant difference in rates of amenorrhoea between laser ablation and transcervical resection.[49] The review also found no significant difference with vaporising electrode ablation in amenorrhoea rate, satisfaction rate, or pictorial blood loss assessment chart results after 12 months. The first subsequent RCT (120 women, 113 followed up at 5 years) found no significant difference between transcervical endometrial resection and rollerball ablation in reduction in bleeding, hysterectomy rates, or satisfaction at 5 years (median number of days bleeding in 3 months 18 days with resection *v* 16 days with rollerball ablation; hysterectomy 8/59 [14%] with resection *v* 10/61 [16%] with rollerball ablation, $P > 0.05$; would recommend procedure to a friend 46 women with resection *v* 49 women with rollerball ablation, the number of women responding to this question was not reported by treatment group, $P > 0.05$).[47] The second subsequent RCT (82 women) found that transcervical endometrial resection significantly increased recurrent bleeding and reoperation rate at 2 years compared with thermal ablation (68 women included in analysis; recurrent bleeding 24.2% with endometrial resection *v* 8.5% with thermal ablation; reoperation 15.1% with endometrial resection *v* 5.7% with thermal ablation).[48] It also found higher satisfaction rates with thermal ablation at 1 and 2 years (2 years: health excellent or good 79.9% with thermal ablation *v* 60.5% with endometrial resection). **Resection versus medical treatment:** We found one systematic review (search date 1999, 2 RCTs, 60 and 70 women) comparing transcervical endometrial resection versus levonorgestrel releasing intrauterine devices,[24] and one additional RCT (187 women) comparing transcervical endometrial resection versus medical treatment (not including a levonorgestrel releasing intrauterine device).[50] The systematic review found that resection reduced the blood loss from baseline significantly more than levonorgestrel releasing intrauterine devices, but had no significant effect on mean blood loss or satisfaction rates after 12 months (for numerical results see intrauterine progestogens, p 2158). The additional RCT (187 women) found that transcervical endometrial resection versus a variety of medical treatments (oral progestogens, combined oral contraceptive, tranexamic acid, danazol, or hormone replacement therapy plus non-steroidal anti-inflammatory drug) significantly increased total satisfaction at 5 years (not intention to treat analysis, 144 women followed up to 5 years; AR for total satisfaction 61% with resection *v* 39% with medical management; ARR 21%, 95% CI 4% to 37%; see comment below).[50]

Harms: Intraoperative complications include uterine perforation, haemorrhage, and fluid overload from the distension medium. Immediate postoperative complications include infection, haemorrhage, and, rarely, bowel injury. Complication rates in the RCTs included in the systematic review above ranged from 0% to 15%.[46] One large prospective survey of 10 686 women undergoing endometrial destructive procedures in the UK found an immediate complication rate of 4%.[49] Intraoperative emergency procedures were performed in 1%, and two procedure related deaths occurred. Newer non-hysteroscopic methods of endometrial destruction have been evaluated only in small numbers of women and, although complications in the RCTs seem minimal, safety data for routine use are awaited. The first subsequent RCT (120 women) found no significant difference in complication rates at 5 years between transcervical endometrial resection and rollerball ablation (only data for infections were reported 6/59 [10%] infections with resection *v* 9/61 [15%] with coagulation, P not reported).[47] Prophylactic antibiotics were given to 48/74 [65%] having resection compared with 35/61 [57%] having coagulation. The second subsequent RCT (82 women) found that transcervical endometrial resection increased short and long term complications compared with thermal ablation (intraoperative complications 5/42 [12%] with endometrial resection *v* 0/40 [0%] with thermal ablation).[48] Intraoperative complications of endometrial resection included open hysterectomy for uterine perforation (2 women).

Comment: The additional RCT comparing resection with medical treatment (187 women) comparing transcervical endometrial resection with a variety of medical treatments reported that at 5 years, 90% of women had stopped medical treatment or had other treatments in addition. At 5 years, 77% of women in the medical group received either transcervical endometrial resection or hysterectomy and 27% of women in the transcervical resection group subsequently had repeat surgery.[50] The review found that hysteroscopic ablation significantly increased the duration of procedure compared with non-hysteroscopic ablation and significantly increased the number of times general anaesthesia was required although equipment failure was more likely with non-hysteroscopic methods (duration of procedure: WMD 8.4 minutes, 95% CI 6.8 minutes to 10.1 minutes; general anaesthesia required: OR 6.8, 95% CI 4.5 to 10.4; equipment failure: OR 4.1, 95% CI 1.1 to 15.0).[46] The review found no significant difference in complication rates between hysteroscopic and non-hysteroscopic methods. Among hysteroscopic techniques the review found that laser ablation significantly increased procedural length compared with transcervical resection (WMD 9.15 minutes, 95% CI 7.20 minutes to 11.10 minutes), and significantly increased rates of equipment failure (OR 6.0, 95% CI 1.7 to 20.9) and fluid overload (fluid overload: OR 5.2, 95% CI 1.5 to 18.4).[49] The review found that vaporising electrode ablation reduced duration of surgery compared with transcervical resection (WMD 1.50 minutes, 95% CI 0.35 minutes to 2.65 minutes).

OPTION MYOMECTOMY

We found no good evidence on the effects of myomectomy.

Benefits: We found no systematic review. **Open versus laparoscopic myomectomy:** We found no RCTs or other studies in women with menorrhagia that measured menstrual blood loss. **Hysteroscopic myomectomy:** We found no RCTs.

Harms: Intraoperative complications for hysteroscopic myomectomy are similar to those with endometrial destructive procedures that use a hysteroscope (see harms of endometrial destruction, p 2164). The main complication of open myomectomy is haemorrhage, making a hysterectomy necessary.

Comment: One uncontrolled study (15 women, 10 with additional symptoms) reported objective measures of menstrual blood loss.[51] Mean menstrual blood loss, assessed preoperatively and at 3 and 6 months postoperatively, was significantly reduced (261 mL at baseline, 76 mL at 3 months, and 57 mL at 6 months). The study found a significant reduction in pain scores and menstrual duration, despite the fibroids removed measuring only 1–4 cm. RCTs are needed that use objective assessment of menstrual blood loss. This is especially important in the evaluation of surgical procedures because of the greater difficulty in blinding.

QUESTION What are the effects of endometrial thinning before endometrial destruction?

One systematic review has found that preoperative gonadorelin (gonadotrophin releasing hormone) analogues reduce moderate or heavy periods and increase amenorrhoea compared with placebo, no preoperative treatment, or preoperative danazol. We found insufficient evidence about effects of preoperative danazol or progestogens compared with placebo or no preoperative treatment.

Benefits: We found one systematic review (search date 2001, 12 RCTs, 1179 women)[52] and one subsequent RCT evaluating medical treatment to thin the endometrium before endometrial destruction for menorrhagia.[53] **Gonadorelin (gonadotrophin releasing hormone) analogues versus placebo/no treatment:** Eight RCTs (618 women) identified by the review compared gonadorelin analogues with placebo or no treatment. The review found that gonadorelin analogues significantly increased the rate of postoperative amenorrhoea at 24 months or longer and significantly reduced the risk of continued moderate or heavy periods after 6–12 months (amenorrhoea, 2 RCTs: RR 1.62, 95% CI 1.04 to 2.52; moderate or heavy periods, 4 RCTs: RR 0.74, 95% CI 0.59 to 0.92). The review found no significant difference in patient satisfaction or the likelihood of undergoing further surgery. **Gonadorelin analogues versus danazol:** Three RCTs (340 women) identified by the review compared gonadorelin analogues (goserelin or decapeptyl) with danazol. The review found that gonadorelin analogues significantly increased postoperative amenorrhoea (RR 1.57, 95% CI 1.06 to 2.33; NNT 5.9).[52] **Danazol versus no treatment:** The review identified two small RCTs and we found one subsequent RCT.[52,53] Both RCTs identified by the review found no significant difference in amenorrhoea between danazol and placebo at 12 and 24 months (1 RCT, 50 women: RR 1.31, 95% CI 0.82 to 2.08; 1 RCT, 20 women: RR 3.00, 95% CI 0.79 to 11.44). The subsequent RCT (132 women) found no significant difference in amenorrhoea between danazol and placebo at 1 year (129 women analysed; amenorrhoea rate: 49% with danazol *v* 52% with placebo, CI and P values not reported).[53] **Progestogens versus no treatment:** Two RCTs included in the review (70 women) compared progestogens with no hormonal medication. They found no significant difference in amenorrhoea at 2 years after endometrial destruction (RR 0.75, 95% CI 0.36 to 1.54).[52] **Progestogens versus other medical treatments:** One RCT included in the review (40 women) compared four groups: progestogens, gonadorelin analogues, danazol, and no treatment. The trial was too small to allow firm conclusions to be drawn.[52]

Harms: The review found no significant difference between goserelin and either placebo or no treatment in intraoperative uterine perforations (2/266 [0.8%] with goserelin *v* 1/275 [0.4%] with no treatment/placebo; RR 2.01, 95% CI 0.19 to 22.67).[52] The review found that goserelin significantly increased hot flushes, depression, and vaginal dryness and reduced libido compared with danazol. Oily skin, hirsutism, and weight gain were significantly more common with danazol. The review also found that danazol significantly increased withdrawal due to adverse effects compared with goserelin (11/139 [8%] with danazol *v* 1/566 [0.2%] with goserelin; RR 44.80, 95% CI 5.83 to 344.00).

Comment: None of the RCTs included in the review used objective measures of postoperative menstrual blood loss.[52] Rates of withdrawal or loss to follow up were low in all studies. One systematic review found that gonadorelin analogues significantly reduced both the duration of surgery and operative difficulty (duration of surgery, 3 RCTs: WMD –4.8 minutes, 95% CI –6.5 minutes to –3.0 minutes; difficulty during procedure, 2 RCTs: RR 0.32, 95% CI 0.22 to 0.46).[52] The review also found that gonadorelin analogues significantly reduced the duration of surgery compared with danazol. It found no significant difference in operative difficulty (amenorrhoea RR 1.57, 95% CI 1.06 to 2.33; NNT 5.9; duration of surgery, 3 RCTs: WMD –3.9 minutes, 95% CI –6.1 minutes to –1.7 minutes; operative difficulty RR 0.68, 95% CI 0.31 to 1.51).[52] The subsequent RCT (132 women) found that danazol reduced operating time compared with placebo (25.7 minutes with danazol *v* 33.6 minutes with placebo, $P < 0.001$).[53]

GLOSSARY

Laser ablation A hysteroscopic procedure in which endometrium is destroyed under direct vision by a laser beam.

Microwave endometrial ablation A procedure in which a microwave probe is passed through the cervix into the uterine cavity. When activated it is moved slowly from side to side over the whole surface of the uterine cavity in order to destroy the endometrium.

Multielectrode balloon ablation A procedure in which an inflatable device with electrodes on the outside is inserted into the uterine cavity through the cervix. The electrodes make contact with the endometrium and cause necrosis.

Pictorial blood loss assessment chart (PBAC) A semi-quantitative assessment of menstrual blood loss based on women filling in the number and appearances of their sanitary protection and size of blood clots on a pictorial chart. Scores of 100 or more equate to a menstrual blood loss of 80 mL or more.[54]

Rollerball ablation A hysteroscopic procedure in which endometrium is destroyed under direct vision by diathermy applied by a rollerball.

Thermal uterine balloon therapy/thermal ablation A procedure in which a balloon catheter is passed through the cervix into the uterine cavity. The balloon is then filled with fluid, which is heated to about 87 °C, and left for 8 minutes. This causes necrosis of the endometrium.

Transcervical endometrial resection A hysteroscopic procedure in which endometrium is removed under direct vision by using an electrosurgical loop.

Substantive changes

Intrauterine progestogens One RCT added;[28] conclusions unchanged.

Endometrial destruction (resection or ablation) Two RCTs added;[47,48] conclusions unchanged.

Preoperative endometrial thinning One RCT added;[53] conclusions unchanged.

REFERENCES

1. Hallberg L, Hogdahl A, Nilsson L, et al. Menstrual blood loss – a population study: variation at different ages and attempts to define normality. *Acta Obstet Gynecol Scand* 1966;45:320–351.
2. Vessey MP, Villard-Mackintosh L, McPherson K, et al. The epidemiology of hysterectomy: findings in a large cohort study. *Br J Obstet Gynaecol* 1992;99:402–407.
3. Working Party of the National Health Committee New Zealand. *Guidelines for the management of heavy menstrual bleeding*. Wellington: Ministry of Health, 1998. (Available from The Ministry of Health, 133 Molesworth Street, PO Box 5013, Wellington, New Zealand.) Search date 1996; primary sources Medline, Embase, Current Contents, Biological Abstracts, Social Sciences Index, Psychlit, and Cinahl.
4. Smith SK, Abel MH, Kelly RW, et al. A role for prostacyclin (PGI_2) in excessive menstrual bleeding. *Lancet* 1981;1:522–524.
5. Rybo G, Leman J, Tibblin R. Epidemiology of menstrual blood loss. In: Baird DT, Michie EA, eds. *Mechanisms of menstrual bleeding*. New York: Raven Press, 1985:181–193.
6. Alexander DA, Naji AA, Pinion SB, et al. Randomised trial comparing hysterectomy with endometrial ablation for dysfunctional uterine bleeding: psychiatric and psychosocial aspects. *BMJ* 1996;312:280–284.
7. Coulter A, Peto V, Jenkinson C. Quality of life and patient satisfaction following treatment for menorrhagia. *Fam Pract* 1994;11:394–401.
8. Coulter A, McPherson K, Vessey M. Do British women undergo too many or too few hysterectomies? *Soc Sci Med* 1988;27:987–994.
9. Pokras R, Hufnagel VG, NCHS. Hysterectomies in the United States, 1965–84. Hyattsville, Maryland: US Department of Health and Human

Services, Public Health Service, CDC, 1987; DHHS publication no. (PHS)87–1753. (Vital and health statistics; series 13, no. 92).
10. Coulter A, Kelland J, Long A. The management of menorrhagia. *Effective Health Care Bull* 1995;9:1–14.
11. Clarke A, Black N, Rowe P, et al. Indications for and outcome of total abdominal hysterectomy for benign disease: a prospective cohort study. *Br J Obstet Gynaecol* 1995;102:611–620.
12. Lethaby A, Augood C, Duckitt K. Nonsteroidal anti-inflammatory drugs for heavy menstrual bleeding In: The Cochrane Library, Issue 1, 2003. Oxford: Update Software. Search date 2001; primary sources Cochrane Menstrual Disorders and Subfertility Group trials register, Medline, Embase, Psychlit, Current Contents, Biological Abstracts, Social Sciences Index, Cinahl, reference lists, and drug companies.
13. Lethaby A, Farquhar C, Cooke I. Antifibrinolytics for heavy menstrual bleeding (Cochrane review). In: The Cochrane Library, Issue 1, 2003. Oxford: Update Software. Search date 1997; primary sources Cochrane Menstrual Disorders and Subfertility Group trials register, Medline, Embase, and hand searches of reference lists from experts and drug companies.
14. Preston JT, Cameron IT, Adams EJ, et al. Comparative study of tranexamic acid and norethisterone in the treatment of ovulatory menorrhagia. *Br J Obstet Gynaecol* 1995;102:401–406.
15. Rybo G. Tranexamic acid therapy is effective treatment in heavy menstrual bleeding: clinical update on safety. *Ther Adv* 1991;4:1–8.
16. Coulter A, Kelland J, Peto V, et al. Treating menorrhagia in primary care. An overview of drug trials and a survey of prescribing practice. *Int J Technol Assess Health Care* 1995;11:456–471. Search date not stated; primary sources Medline and Embase.
17. Bonnar J, Sheppard BL. Treatment of menorrhagia during menstruation: randomised controlled trial of etamsylate, mefenamic acid, and tranexamic acid. *BMJ* 1996;313:579–582.
18. Beaumont H, Augood C, Duckitt K, et al. Danazol for heavy menstrual bleeding (Cochrane Review). In: The Cochrane Library, Issue 1, 2003. Oxford: Update Software. Search date 2001; primary sources Medline, Embase, Current Contents, Cinahl, National Research Register, Menstrual Disorders and Subfertility Group's Specialised Register, reference lists and authors contacted.
19. Iyer V, Farquhar C, Jepson R. Oral contraceptive pills for heavy menstrual bleeding. In: The Cochrane Library, Issue 1, 2003. Oxford: Update Software. Search date 1997; primary source Cochrane Register of Controlled Trials.
20. Nilsson L, Rybo G. Treatment of menorrhagia. *Am J Obstet Gynecol* 1971;5:713–720.
21. Ramcharan S, Pellegrin FA, Ray MR, et al. The Walnut Creek contraceptive drug study — a prospective study of the side effects of oral contraceptives. Vol III. An interim report: a comparison of disease occurrence leading to hospitalization or death in users and nonusers of oral contraceptives. *J Reprod Med* 1980;25:345–372.
22. Royal College of General Practitioners. *Oral contraceptives and health*. London: Pitman Medical, 1974.
23. Lethaby A, Irvine G, Cameron I. Cyclical progestogens for heavy menstrual bleeding (Cochrane review). In: The Cochrane Library, Issue 1, 2003. Oxford: Update Software. Search date not stated; primary sources Cochrane Menstrual Disorders and Subfertility Group trials register, Medline, Embase, Psychlit, Current Contents, Biological Abstracts, Social Sciences Index, Cinahl, and reference lists.
24. Lethaby AE, Cooke I, Rees M. Progesterone/progestogen intrauterine releasing systems for heavy menstrual bleeding. In: The Cochrane Library, Issue 1, 2003. Oxford: Update Software. Search date 1999; primary sources Cochrane Menstrual Disorders and Subfertility Group trials register, Medline, Embase, and experts contacted.
25. Stewart A, Cummins C, Gold L, et al. The effectiveness of the levonorgestrel-releasing intrauterine system in menorrhagia: a systematic review. *Br J Obstet Gynaecol* 2001;108:74–86. Search date 1999; primary sources Medline, Cinahl, Embase, Cochrane Library, Best Evidence, BMJ website archive facility, various internet search engines, hand searches of the *J Family Plan* and *The Diplomate*, and personal contact with Schering Health Care Ltd and the Royal College of Obstetricians and Gynaecologists Audit Unit.
26. Hurskainen R, Teperi J, Rissanen P, et al. Quality of life and cost-effectiveness of levonorgestrel-releasing intrauterine system versus hysterectomy for treatment of menorrhagia: a randomised trial. *Lancet* 2001;357:273–277.
27. Istre O, Trolle B. Treatment of menorrhagia with the levonorgestrel intrauterine system versus endometrial resection. *Fertil Steril* 2001;76:304–309.
28. Soysal M, Soysal S, Ozer S. A randomized controlled trial of levonorgestrel releasing IUD and thermal balloon ablation in the treatment of menorrhagia. *Zentralbl Gynakol* 2002;124:213–219.
29. Crosignani PG, Vercellini P, Mosconi P, et al. Levonorgestrel-releasing intrauterine device versus hysteroscopic endometrial resection in the treatment of dysfunctional uterine bleeding. *Obstet Gynecol* 1997;90:257–263.
30. Irvine GA, Campbell-Brown MB, Lumsden MA, et al. Randomised comparative study of the levonorgestrel intrauterine system and norethisterone for the treatment of idiopathic menorrhagia. *Br J Obstet Gynaecol* 1998;105:592–598.
31. Long-acting progestogen-only contraception. *Drug Ther Bull* 1996;34:93–96.
32. Luukkainen T. The levonorgestrel-releasing IUD. *Br J Fam Plann* 1993;19:221–224.
33. Thomas EJ, Okuda KJ, Thomas NM. The combination of a depot gonadotrophin releasing hormone agonist and cyclical hormone replacement therapy for dysfunctional uterine bleeding. *Br J Obstet Gynaecol* 1991;98:1155–1159.
34. Eldred JM, Haynes PJ, Thomas EJ. A randomized double blind placebo controlled trial of the effects on bone metabolism of the combination of nafarelin acetate and norethisterone. *Clin Endocrinol* 1992;37:354–359.
35. Pickersgill A, Kingsland CR, Garden AS, et al. Multiple gestation following gonadotrophin releasing hormone therapy for the treatment of minimal endometriosis. *Br J Obstet Gynaecol* 1994;101:260–262.
36. Smith JJ, Schulman H. Current dilatation and curettage practice: a need for revision. *Obstet Gynecol* 1985;65:516–518.
37. Haynes PJ, Hodgson H, Anderson AB, et al. Measurement of menstrual blood loss in patients complaining of menorrhagia. *Br J Obstet Gynaecol* 1977;84:763–768.
38. Lethaby A, Sheppers S, Cooke I, et al. Endometrial resection and ablation versus

hysterectomy for heavy menstrual bleeding. In: The Cochrane Library, Issue 1, 2003. Oxford: Update Software. Search date not stated; primary sources Cochrane Menstrual Disorders and Subfertility Group trials register, Medline, Embase, Psychlit, Current Contents, Biological Abstracts, Social Sciences Index, and Cinahl.
39. Phipps JH, John M, Nayak S. Comparison of laparoscopically assisted vaginal hysterectomy and bilateral salpingo-oophorectomy with conventional abdominal hysterectomy and bilateral salpingo-oophorectomy. *Br J Obstet Gynaecol* 1993;100:698–700.
40. Raju KS, Auld BJ. A randomised prospective study of laparoscopic vaginal hysterectomy versus abdominal hysterectomy each with bilateral salpingo-oophorectomy. *Br J Obstet Gynaecol* 1994;101:1068–1071.
41. Richardson RE, Bournas N, Magos AL. Is laparoscopic hysterectomy a waste of time? *Lancet* 1995;345:36–41.
42. Summitt RL Jr, Stovall TG, Lipscomb GH, et al. Randomized comparison of laparoscopy-assisted vaginal hysterectomy with standard vaginal hysterectomy in an outpatient setting. *Obstet Gynecol* 1992;80:895–901.
43. Langebrekke A, Eraker R, Nesheim B, et al. Abdominal hysterectomy should not be considered as primary method for uterine removal. *Acta Obstet Gynecol Scand* 1996;75:404–407.
44. Carlson KJ. Outcomes of hysterectomy. *Clin Obstet Gynecol* 1997;40:939–946.
45. Dicker RC, Greenspan JR, Strauss LT, et al. Complications of abdominal and vaginal hysterectomy among women of reproductive age in the United States. The Collaborative Review of Sterilization. *Am J Obstet Gynecol* 1982;144:841–848.
46. Lethaby A, Hickey M. Endometrial destruction techniques for heavy menstrual bleeding (Cochrane Review). In: The Cochrane Library, Issue1, 2003. Oxford: Update Software. Search date 2001; primary sources Conchrane Controlled Trials Register, Medline, Embase, Current Contents, Biological Abstracts, Psychlit, Cinahl, Register of Cochrane Menstrual Disorders and Subfertility Group, reference lists of articles, contacted pharmaceutical companies, and experts in the field.
47. Boujida VH, Philipsen T, Pelle J, et al. Five-year follow-up of endometrial ablation: endometrial coagulation versus endometrial resection. *Obstet Gynecol* 2002;99:988–992.
48. Pellicano M, Guida M, Acunzo G, et al. Hysteroscopic transcervical endometrial resection versus thermal destruction for menorrhagia: a prospective randomized trial on satisfaction rate. *Am J Obstet Gynecol* 2002;187:545–550.
49. Overton C, Hargreaves J, Maresh M. A national survey of the complications of endometrial destruction for menstrual disorders: the MISTLETOE study. Minimally invasive surgical techniques — laser, endothermal or endoresection. *Br J Obstet Gynaecol* 1997;104:1351–1359.
50. Cooper KG, Jack SA, Parkin DE, et al. Five-year follow up of women randomised to medical management or transcervical resection of the endometrium for heavy menstrual loss: clinical and quality of life outcomes. *Br J Obstet Gynaecol* 2001;108:1222–1228.
51. Broadbent JAM, Magos AL. Menstrual blood loss after hysteroscopic myomectomy. *Gynaecol Endoscop* 1995;4:41–44.
52. Sowter MC, Singla AA, Lethaby A. Pre-operative endometrial thinning agents before endometrial destruction for heavy menstrual bleeding (Cochrane review). In: The Cochrane Library, Issue 1, 2003. Oxford: Update Software. Search date 2001; primary sources Cochrane Menstrual Disorders and Subfertility Group trials register, Medline, Embase, Psychlit, Biological Abstracts, Cinahl, reference lists, authors of conference abstracts, Zeneca Pharmaceuticals, and Sanofi Winthrop.
53. Kriplani A, Manchanda R, Nath J, et al. A randomized trial of danazol pretreatment prior to endometrial resection. *Eur J Obstet Gynecol Reprod Biol* 2002;103:68–71.
54. Higham JM, O'Brien PMS, Shaw RW. Assessment of menstrual blood loss using a pictorial chart. *Br J Obstet Gynaecol* 1990;97:734–739.

Kirsten Duckitt
Consultant Obstetrician and Gynaecologist

Keri McCully
Specialist Registrar Obstetrics and Gynaecology

John Radcliffe Hospital
Oxford
UK

Competing interests: None declared.

Ovarian cancer

Search date October 2002

Hani Gabra, Charles Redman, and Jennifer Byrom

QUESTIONS

INTERVENTIONS

See glossary, p 2180

Key Messages

- We found insufficient evidence on the effects of any treatments on quality of life.
- **Adding platinum to chemotherapy regimens** One systematic review has found that adding platinum to any non-platinum regimen significantly improves survival, particularly if platinum is added to a combination regimen.
- **Adding paclitaxel to platinum regimens** One systematic review and one additional RCT have found that adding paclitaxel to platinum based chemotherapy improves progression free survival and overall survival after primary surgery for advanced ovarian cancer.

Clin Evid 2003;10:2170–2183.

- **Combination platinum regimens versus combination non-platinum regimens** Seven RCTs have compared combination platinum regimens versus many different non-platinum combination regimens. Most RCTs have found that platinum regimens improve outcomes, although benefits and harms depend on the regimens being compared. None have found that platinum significantly decreased progression free survival or overall survival.
- **Combination platinum regimens versus single agent platinum regimens** One systematic review and three additional RCTs found no evidence that combination platinum based regimens improved progression free or overall survival compared with single agent platinum regimens.
- **Carboplatin plus paclitaxel versus carboplatin plus docetaxel** We found no reliable RCTs comparing the effects of carboplatin plus paclitaxel versus carboplatin plus docetaxel.
- **Paclitaxel plus cisplatin versus paclitaxel plus carboplatin** One RCT found no significant difference in progression free or overall survival between paclitaxel plus cisplatin versus paclitaxel plus carboplatin, although it may have lacked power to exclude clinically important effects.
- **Routine interval debulking after primary surgery plus chemotherapy** One RCT found that interval debulking after primary surgery plus chemotherapy improved overall survival over about 3.5 years compared with chemotherapy alone. A second RCT found that interval debulking had no significant effect on survival, but it was probably underpowered to detect a clinically important effect.
- **Routine second look surgery** Two RCTs found no evidence that routine second look surgery improves overall survival compared with watchful waiting in women undergoing chemotherapy after primary surgery for advanced ovarian cancer.
- **Primary surgery versus no surgery; primary surgery plus chemotherapy versus chemotherapy alone** We found no RCTs.

DEFINITION Ovarian tumours are classified according to the assumed cell type of origin (surface epithelium, stroma, or germ cells). Most malignant ovarian tumours (85–95%) are derived from the epithelium of the ovarian surface, and are thus termed epithelial.[1] These can be further grouped into histological types (serous, mucinous, endometroid, and clear cell). Epithelial ovarian cancer is staged using the FIGO classification (see table A on web extra). This review concerns only advanced epithelial ovarian cancer, which is regarded as FIGO stages II–IV.

INCIDENCE/ PREVALENCE The worldwide annual incidence of ovarian cancer exceeds 140 000.[2] Rates vary between countries. Differences in reproductive patterns, including age of menarche and menopause, gravidity, breast feeding, and use of the oral contraceptive pill may contribute to this variation. Rates are highest in Scandinavia, northern America, and the UK; and lowest for Africa, India, China, and Japan.[3] In the UK, ovarian cancer is the fourth most common malignancy in women and is the leading cause of death from gynaecological cancers, with a lifetime risk of about 2%.[4] In the UK, the incidence was 5174 in 1988[5] and 6880 in 1998.[6] The incidence of ovarian cancer seems to be stabilising in some other countries, and in some affluent countries (Finland, Denmark, New Zealand, and the USA) rates are declining.

AETIOLOGY/ RISK FACTORS	Risk factors include increasing age, family history of ovarian cancer, low fertility, use of fertility drugs, and low parity.[7–11] Case control studies found that using the combined oral contraceptive pill for more than 5 years was associated with a 40% reduction in the risk of ovarian cancer.[3,7,12,13]
PROGNOSIS	Over 80% of women present with advanced disease, and the overall 5 year survival rates are poor (< 30%).[6] For advanced disease the major independent prognostic factors seem to be stage, and residual tumour mass after surgery.
AIMS OF INTERVENTION	To prolong survival and reduce disability, and to minimise adverse effects.
OUTCOMES	Mortality; disease free survival; disease related symptoms; quality of life; adverse effects of treatment.
METHODS	*Clinical Evidence* search and appraisal October 2002. RCTs with greater than 20% withdrawal or with less than 18 months' follow up were excluded.

QUESTION **What are the effects of surgery for ovarian cancer that is advanced at first presentation**

OPTION **PRIMARY SURGERY**

We found no RCTs in women with advanced ovarian cancer comparing the effects of primary surgery versus no surgery, or primary surgery plus chemotherapy versus chemotherapy alone.

Benefits: **Primary surgery alone versus no surgery:** We found one systematic review (search date not stated), which found no RCTs comparing primary debulking (see glossary, p 2180) surgery versus no surgery.[1] We found no subsequent RCT. **Primary surgery plus chemotherapy versus chemotherapy alone:** We found no systematic review and no RCT.

Harms: We found no RCT.

Comment: None.

OPTION **ROUTINE SECOND LOOK SURGERY**

Two RCTs found no significant difference in survival between routine second look surgery and watchful waiting in women undergoing chemotherapy after primary surgery for advanced ovarian cancer.

Benefits: **Primary surgery plus chemotherapy with or without second look surgery:** We found two RCTs in women with advanced ovarian cancer.[14,15] The first RCT (102 women in complete remission after primary debulking surgery [see glossary, p 2180] and first line chemotherapy of cisplatin plus cyclophosphamide or doxorubicin plus cyclophosphamide every 3 weeks for 5 cycles) compared second look surgery (see glossary, p 2180), which included visual inspection and biopsy, versus watchful waiting.[14] Complete remission before trial entry was confirmed by clinical and biochemical assessment, computed tomography, and laparoscopy. The RCT found no significant difference between interventions for overall survival after 60 months (AR for survival 65% with second look laparotomy *v* 78% with watchful waiting; CI not provided; P = 0.14). The second RCT (166 women, after primary debulking surgery plus cisplatin every 3 weeks for 5 cycles) compared three groups.[15] One group had a second look laparotomy (which included visual inspection, cytology of any free fluid, total hysterectomy, bilateral salpingo-oophorectomy, omentectomy, and multiple biopsies, followed by oral chlorambucil [12 courses of 0.2 mg/kg daily for 14 days]). The second group received second look laparotomy and pelvic irradiation. The third group received chlorambucil without second look surgery. The RCT found no significant difference among groups for overall survival after 46 months (median survival time 21 months, 95% CI 11 months to 31 months with second look laparotomy plus chlorambucil; 15 months, 95% CI 11 months to 19 months with second look laparotomy and pelvic irradiation; 17 months, 95% CI 8 months to 26 months with chlorambucil without second look surgery).

Harms: The first RCT did not report harms.[14] The second RCT reported that one woman died of a cerebrovascular accident 10 days after second look laparotomy.[15] Other reported surgical complications were ileus, wound infection, urinary and respiratory tract infection, and anaemia (rates not reported).

Comment: None.

OPTION ROUTINE INTERVAL DEBULKING

One RCT found that interval debulking after primary surgery plus chemotherapy improved overall survival over about 3.5 years compared with chemotherapy without debulking. A second RCT found that interval debulking had no significant effect on survival, but it was probably underpowered to detect a clinically important effect

Benefits: **Primary surgery plus chemotherapy with or without interval debulking:** We found two RCTs.[16,17] The first RCT (319 women with non-progressive disease after 3 cycles of cisplatin and cyclophosphamide chemotherapy after primary surgery) compared interval debulking (see glossary, p 2180) versus continued chemotherapy.[16] All women had residual tumour diameter of greater than 1 cm after primary surgery. It found that interval debulking significantly improved progression free and overall survival after a median of 3.5 years (278 women; median progression free survival 18 months with interval debulking *v* 13 months without, P = 0.01; median overall survival 26 months *v* 20 months, P = 0.01; adjusted HR for death for interval debulking *v* no interval debulking 0.77, 95% CI 0.50 to 0.90).[16] The second RCT (79 women with advanced ovarian cancer with residual tumour of at least 2 cm maximal diameter after primary surgery) compared interval debulking after primary surgery and response to chemotherapy versus continued chemotherapy without interval debulking.[17] Chemotherapy consisted of either ciaplatin plus cyclophosphamide or ciaplatin plus bleomycin plus doxorubicin followed by escalating cyclophosphamide. Of the women allocated to interval debulking, 11 had non-responsive or progressive disease after three cycles of chemotherapy and were excluded from surgery. Interval debulking (which could include hysterectomy, oophorectomy, and omentectomy) was undertaken at a median of 13 weeks after primary surgery. The RCT found no significant difference between interval debulking versus no interval debulking for overall survival after 48 months' median follow up, but may have lacked power to exclude a clinically important effect (intention to treat analysis: median survival 15 months with interval debulking v 12 months without; HR 0.71, 95% CI 0.44 to 1.33).

Harms: The second RCT found that among 26 women who received interval debulking, 11 received a blood transfusion, two developed intestinal fistulae, and one developed a deep vein thrombosis.[17]

Comment: None.

QUESTION **What are the effects of cytotoxic chemotherapy for ovarian cancer that is advanced at first presentation?**

OPTION **PLATINUM BASED REGIMENS**

One systematic review has found that adding platinum to a range of non-platinum regimens improves survival after surgery in women with advanced ovarian cancer. However, it found no significant benefit in the subgroup of RCTs that added platinum to single-agent non-platinum regimens. Seven additional RCTs have compared combination platinum regimens with many different non-platinum combination regimens. Most of these have found that platinum regimens improve outcomes, although benefits and harms depend on the regimens being compared. None found that platinum decreased progression free or overall survival. One systematic review and three additional RCTs found no evidence that combination platinum based regimens improved progression free or overall survival compared with single agent platinum regimens.

Benefits: **Platinum versus non-platinum chemotherapy:** We found one systematic review (search date 1998, 37 RCTs)[18] and six additional RCTs[19–24] in women with advanced ovarian cancer. The review identified 11 RCTs (1329 women with advanced ovarian cancer) comparing single agent non-platinum chemotherapy versus platinum based combination chemotherapy. It found no significant difference between these types of regimen for overall survival (9 RCTs; HR 0.93, 95% CI 0.83 to 1.05; P = 0.23; estimated ARR for 2 and 5 year survival with single agent non-platinum versus combination platinum +3%, 95% CI –2% to +7%). The review also identified nine RCTs (1704 women) assessing the effects of adding platinum to a chemotherapy regimen. Meta-analysis found that adding platinum to any regimen significantly reduced the risk of death (death with platinum added to any regimen, HR 0.88, 95% CI 0.79 to 0.98; estimated ARR of death 5%, 95% CI 1% to 8% at 2 and 5 years). Within this group, adding platinum to combination regimens also reduced risk of death (HR 0.85, 95% CI 0.74 to 0.97). However, meta-analysis of RCTs that added platinum to a single agent found no significant effect on risk of death, although results of trials were statistically heterogeneous (death with platinum added to single agent, HR 0.93, 95% CI 0.78 to 1.10).[18] The first additional RCT (171 women) compared a single platinum agent (cisplatin, 75 mg/m^2 every 28 days for 6 cycles) versus a single non-platinum agent (thiotepa, 60 mg loading dose im followed by 10 cycles of 30 mg im every 14 days).[19] It found that cisplatin versus thiotepa significantly improved progression free survival after 110 months' median follow up (median progression free survival 10.5 months with cisplatin *v* 6.3 months with thiotepa, $P = 0.025$; HR for thiotepa *v* cisplatin 1.64, 95% CI 1.17 to 2.30). Cisplatin versus thiotepa did not significantly improve overall survival (median overall survival 20 months with cisplatin *v* 14 months with thiotepa, $P = 0.155$; AR for survival at 8 years 10.6% *v* 7.4%, CI and P value not stated). The second additional RCT (228 women) found that adding cisplatin (50 mg/m^2 every 3–4 weeks) to 12 cycles of doxorubicin plus cyclophosphamide with or without Bacillus Calmette-Guérin significantly improved overall survival (median survival 17.8 months with cisplatin *v* 9.9 months without cisplatin; $P < 0.005$).[20] The third RCT (169 women) compared 12 cycles at four weekly intervals of ciaplatin (60 mg/m^2/cycle) plus melphalan (1 mg/kg/cycle) versus hexamethylmelamine, doxorubicin, and cyclophosphamide.[21] It found no significant difference between treatments for overall survival (153 women; median survival 29.6 months with platinum *v* 26.4 months without; P value not stated) but the trial may have lacked power to exclude a clinically important difference.[21] The fourth RCT (120 women) similarly found no significant difference between hexamethylmelamine, doxorubicin, and cyclophosphamide versus cisplatin, doxorubicin, and cyclophosphamide for overall survival after 10 years (median survival 126 months without platinum *v* 138 months with platinum; $P = 0.54$).[22] The fifth RCT (83 women) compared 12 cycles at four weekly intervals of doxorubicin (60 mg/m^2) plus cyclophosphamide (750 mg/m^2) combined with either cisplatin (80 mg/m^2) or with vincristine (1.4 mg/m^2). It found that the platinum based regimen increased progression free and overall survival compared with the non-platinum regimen after 5 years (median progression free survival 14 months with platinum *v* 10 months without platinum, $P < 0.05$; median overall survival 24 months with platinum *v* 15 months without platinum, $P < 0.01$).[23] The sixth RCT (186 women) compared hexamethylmelamine, cyclophosphamide, methotrexate, and 5-fluorouracil versus a regimen that alternated between cyclophosphamide plus hexamethylmelamine and doxorubicin plus cisplatin.[24] It found that the platinum versus the non-platinum regimen improved progression free and overall survival after about 50 months (median progression free survival 19.5 months with platinum *v* 6.8 months without platinum, $P < 0.0001$; median overall survival 30.7 months with platinum *v* 19.6 months without platinum, $P < 0.002$). **Single agent platinum versus combined platinum chemotherapy:** We found one systematic review (search date 1998, 9 RCTs in 1095 women with advanced ovarian cancer)[18] and three additional RCTs in women with advanced ovarian cancer.[25–27] The review found no significant difference between treatments for risk of death (HR 0.91, 95% CI 0.80 to 1.05).

Separate analyses of cisplatin and carboplatin containing regimens found similar results (HR of death for single agent *v* combination cisplatin regimens 0.86, 95% CI 0.73 to 1.02; HR of death for single agent *v* combination carboplatin regimens 1.05, 95% CI 0.82 to 1.35). The first additional RCT (multicentre; 1526 women; 36% of women < 55 years old) compared six cycles of cyclophosphamide (500 mg/m^2), doxorubicin (50 mg/m^2), and cisplatin (50 mg/m^2) versus three weekly carboplatin alone ([{glomerular filtration rate multiplied by 5} + 25] mg).[26] After a median follow up of 35 months, it found no significant difference between treatments for progression free survival or overall survival (for progression free survival HR for combined treatment *v* carboplatin alone 0.92, 95% CI 0.81 to 1.04; for overall survival 1.00, 95% CI 0.86 to 1.16). The second additional RCT (611 women aged < 75 years) compared cisplatin alone (50 mg/m^2) weekly for nine cycles versus cisplatin (75 mg/m^2) plus cyclophosphamide (750 mg/m^2) three weekly for six cycles.[26] It found similar rates between groups for 3 year progression free and overall survival (3 year progression free survival 33.8% with cisplatin alone *v* 35.1% with combined treatment, CI and P values not stated; 3 year overall survival 44.1% with cisplatin alone *v* 44.6% with combined treatment, CI not provided, P = 0.96). The third RCT (176 women) compared six four weekly courses of cisplatin alone (75 mg/m^2) versus cisplatin (50 mg/m^2) plus cyclophosphamide (500 mg/m^2). It found no significant difference between treatments for progression free survival or overall survival after a median of 10 years (median progression free survival 11.9 months with single *v* 10.0 months with combination, P = 0.092; median overall survival 21.5 months with single *v* 19.4 months with combination, P = 0.1299).[27] We found one further RCT that was reported as a conference abstract (see comment below).

Harms: **Platinum versus non-platinum chemotherapy:** The first systematic review did not report adverse effects.[18] One additional RCT found that 1/85 (1%) women taking cisplatin versus thiotepa stopped cisplatin because of weakness and dizziness.[19] The RCT comparing ciaplatin and melphalan versus hexamethylmelamine, doxorubicin, and cyclophosphamide found that haematological toxicity was more common with the platinum regimen (white cells < 3000/m^3, P < 0.0001; platelets < 75 000/m^3, P < 0.0001; anaemia, P = 0.001).[9] The RCT comparing doxorubicin plus cyclophosphamide combined with either vincristine or cisplatin reported that platinum increased haematological toxicity (rates not stated).[23] One cohort analysis of two RCTs comparing platinum and non-platinum regimens found that grade 3 nausea and vomiting (see table 1, p 2183), mild renal toxicity, and neurotoxicity were significantly more common with platinum containing regimens compared with non-platinum regimens (AR grade 3 nausea and vomiting about 6–10% with platinum regimens *v* 4% with non-platinum, P = 0.004; AR any renal toxicity 17–20% with platinum *v* 4% with non-platinum, P value not stated; AR neurotoxicity 1–4% with platinum *v* 0% with non-platinum, P value not stated).[29] We found one analysis of data from two RCTs (387 women with advanced ovarian cancer) comparing hexamethylmelamine plus cyclophosphamide plus methotrexate plus 5-fluorouracil with or without cisplatin, or with cyclophosphamide plus cisplatin.[30] After median follow up of 45 months, it found that neurotoxicity was more common and more severe with regimens that included platinum versus those without platinum (AR for any neurotoxicity 47% with platinum *v* 25% without platinum; AR for grade 2–3 neurotoxicity 25% with platinum *v* 3% without platinum; CI and P values not stated). **Single agent platinum versus combined platinum chemotherapy:** The systematic review did not report adverse effects.[18] In the RCT comparing carboplatin alone versus cyclophosphamide plus doxorubicin plus cisplatin, 875 women (57%) were assessed for adverse effects.[25] Leucopenia, hair loss, and nausea and vomiting were more common with combination treatment versus carboplatin alone (AR for leucopenia 36% with combination *v* 10% with carboplatin alone; AR for hair loss 70% with combination *v* 4% with carboplatin alone; AR for nausea and vomiting 20% with combination *v* 9% with carboplatin alone). Thrombocytopenia was more common with carboplatin (AR 6% with combination *v* 16% with carboplatin alone). Renal, cardiac, and neurotoxicity were rare in both groups (1–2% in both groups for each category).

Comment: **Single agent platinum versus combined platinum chemotherapy:** We found one RCT (120 women with advanced ovarian cancer) reported as a conference abstract, which compared six cycles of cisplatin plus cyclophosphamide versus three cycles of epirubicin plus ifosfamide followed by four cycles of cisplatin.[31] It found no significant differences between treatments for relapse free or overall survival (relapse free survival at 3 years 24% with cisplatin plus cyclophosphamide *v* 41% with epirubicin plus ifosfamide plus cisplatin, CI and P values not stated; median overall survival 141 weeks with cisplatin plus cyclophosphamide *v* 172 weeks with epirubicin plus ifosfamide plus cisplatin, CI and P values not stated).[31]

OPTION TAXANES

One systematic review and one additional RCT have found that adding paclitaxel to platinum based chemotherapy improves progression free and overall survival compared with platinum based chemotherapy alone after primary surgery in women with advanced ovarian cancer. One RCT found no significant difference in progression free or overall survival between paclitaxel plus carboplatin versus paclitaxel plus cisplatin, although it may have lacked power to exclude clinically important effects. We found no reliable RCTs comparing docetaxel plus carboplatin versus paclitaxel plus carboplatin.

Benefits: **Adding paclitaxel to platinum:** We found one systematic review[32] and one additional RCT[33] in women with advanced ovarian cancer. The systematic review (search date not stated, 3746 women) included one published RCT[34] and three unpublished RCTs, two of which have since been published.[35,36] The first included RCT (386 women) compared cisplatin (75 mg/m^2) combined with either cyclophosphamide or paclitaxel (135 mg/m^2).[34] It found that cisplatin plus paclitaxel versus cisplatin plus cyclophosphamide improved progression free survival and overall survival (median progression free survival: 18 months with cisplatin plus paclitaxel *v*

13 months with cisplatin plus cyclophosphamide, $P < 0.001$; median overall survival: 38 months with cisplatin plus paclitaxel *v* 24 months with cisplatin plus cyclophosphamide, $P < 0.001$).[34] The second included RCT (680 women), which has since been published,[35] compared cisplatin (75 mg/m^2) combined with either cyclophosphamide or paclitaxel (175 mg/m^2). It found that cisplatin plus paclitaxel versus cisplatin plus cyclophosphamide significantly improved progression free survival and overall survival (median progression free survival 17 months with cisplatin plus paclitaxel *v* 12 months with cisplatin plus cyclophosphamide, $P = 0.001$; median survival 35 months with cisplatin plus paclitaxel *v* 25 months with cisplatin plus cyclophosphamide, $P = 0.001$). The third included RCT (614 women), which has also since been published,[36] compared three treatments: cisplatin alone (100 mg/m^2), paclitaxel alone (200 mg/m^2), and paclitaxel (135 mg/m^2) followed by cisplatin (75 mg/m^2). It found no significant difference between cisplatin alone versus cisplatin plus paclitaxel for progression free survival or overall survival after median follow up of 61 months (progression free survival: median 16 months with cisplatin alone *v* 14 months with cisplatin plus paclitaxel, HR 1.06, 95% CI 0.90 to 1.30; overall survival: median 30 months with cisplatin alone *v* 27 months with cisplatin plus paclitaxel, HR 0.99, 95% CI 0.80 to 1.23). The fourth RCT in the review, which is still unpublished (2974 women), compared three treatments: paclitaxel (175 mg/m^2) plus carboplatin, carboplatin alone, and cyclophosphamide plus doxorubicin plus cisplatin. It found no difference in progression free survival or overall survival between paclitaxel plus carboplatin versus carboplatin alone after 24 months (progression free survival: estimated RR 1.02, CI not provided; overall survival: estimated RR 1.1, CI not provided). A full report of the trial is in press (Gabra H, personal communication, 2002). We found one additional RCT[33] (45 women) comparing cisplatin (75 mg/m^2) plus either paclitaxel (175 mg/m^2) or cyclophosphamide (750 mg/m^2). It found that cisplatin plus paclitaxel versus cisplatin plus cyclophosphamide significantly increased time to relapse and increased relapse free survival after 25 months (38 women; median time to relapse 17.5 months with cisplatin plus paclitaxel *v* 9.9 months with cisplatin plus cyclophosphamide, CI and P value not stated; P value for difference in relapse free survival = 0.001, mean values and CI not provided). **Paclitaxel plus carboplatin versus paclitaxel plus cisplatin:** One RCT (208 women) compared at least six cycles of paclitaxel (175 mg/m^2 over 3 hours) combined with either cisplatin (75 mg/m^2) or carboplatin ([{glomerular filtration rate multiplied by 5} + 25] mg).[37] It found that treatments had different adverse effects (see harms below), but found no significant differences between treatments for progression free survival or overall survival after a median of 37 months (median progression free survival 16 months in both groups, HR 1.07, 95% CI 0.78 to 1.48; median overall survival 30 months with paclitaxel plus cisplatin *v* 32 months with paclitaxel plus carboplatin, HR 0.85, 95% CI 0.59 to 1.24). We found several further RCTs reported as conference abstracts (see comment below). **Carboplatin plus paclitaxel or docetaxel:** We found no RCTs with sufficient follow up for inclusion (see comment below).

Harms: **Adding paclitaxel to platinum:** The systematic review found that reporting of adverse effects was not consistent among trials.[32] It presented results from two RCTs, which found that adding paclitaxel to platinum based regimens did not significantly increase haematological toxicity, fever, or anaemia (any haematological toxicity [1 RCT] RR about 1, 95% CI about 0.8 to 1.3; anaemia [1 RCT] RR 1.10, 95% CI 0.57 to 2.13; fever [1 RCT] RR 16.38 in favour of non-paclitaxel regimen, 95% CI 0.83 to 284). Compared with platinum alone, infection was more common with paclitaxel plus platinum, but less common with cyclophosphamide plus doxorubicin plus platinum (1 RCT; compared with platinum alone, RR 3.38, 95% CI 2.15 to 5.32; compared with cyclophosphamide plus doxorubicin plus platinum RR 0.59, 95% CI 0.40 to 0.86). Nausea and vomiting was reported in 7–18% of women receiving paclitaxel and hair loss was reported in 68–77% of women receiving paclitaxel. Cardiac toxicity was not reported in the included RCTs. One of the RCTs included in the review (614 women)[36] found that neutropenia, hair loss, and fever were more common with paclitaxel or paclitaxel plus cisplatin versus cisplatin alone ($P < 0.001$). Another included RCT found that grades 3 and 4 muscle pain (see table 1, p 2183), neurosensory and neuromotor symptoms, and hair loss were more common with cisplatin plus paclitaxel than cisplatin plus cyclophosphamide (AR muscle pain 6% with cisplatin plus paclitaxel *v* 0% with cisplatin plus cyclophosphamide; neurosensory symptoms 19.6% with cisplatin plus paclitaxel *v* 1% with cisplatin plus cyclophosphamide; neuromotor symptoms 5% with cisplatin plus paclitaxel *v* 0.6% with cisplatin plus cyclophosphamide; hair loss 51% with cisplatin plus paclitaxel *v* 21% with cisplatin plus cyclophosphamide; CI and P values not stated).[35] Grade 3 and 4 leucopenia (see table 1, p 2183), anaemia, and thrombocytopenia were less common with cisplatin plus paclitaxel than cisplatin plus cyclophosphamide (AR, CI, and P values not stated). Febrile neutropenia rates were similar between groups (AR 3% for both groups). **Paclitaxel plus carboplatin versus paclitaxel plus cisplatin:** The RCT comparing paclitaxel plus cisplatin versus paclitaxel plus carboplatin found no significant differences between treatments for rates of hair loss, fever, mucositis, diarrhoea, allergic reaction, cardiorespiratory complications, skin reactions, muscle or joint pain, constipation, fever, or renal toxicity. However, after six cycles of treatment, grade 4 nausea and vomiting (see table 1, p 2183) was more common with paclitaxel plus cisplatin (AR 17% with paclitaxel plus cisplatin *v* 14% with paclitaxel plus carboplatin; $P < 0.01$). Grade 3–4 thrombocytopenia and grade 4 granulocytopenia (see table 1, p 2183), were more common with paclitaxel plus carboplatin (AR for grade 3–4 thrombocytopenia 6% with paclitaxel plus carboplatin *v* 1% with paclitaxel plus cisplatin, $P < 0.01$; AR for grade 4 granulocytopenia 40% with paclitaxel plus carboplatin *v* 23% with paclitaxel plus cisplatin, $P < 0.01$).[37] We found several other RCTs reported as conference abstracts (see comment below).

Comment: **Paclitaxel plus carboplatin or paclitaxel plus cisplatin:** The first abstract reported preliminary safety data among 488 women from a trial comparing cisplatin plus paclitaxel versus carboplatin plus paclitaxel in 797 women.[38] Grade 3–4 haematological toxicity (see table 1, p 2183), was more common with the carboplatin regimen and non-haematological toxicity other than hair loss was more common with the cisplatin regimen. A second abstract from the same trial found no significant difference between treatments for progression free or overall survival after 2 years' median follow up ($P > 0.05$).[39] The third abstract reported a trial comparing paclitaxel plus carboplatin versus paclitaxel plus alternating cisplatin and carboplatin in 164 women. It found no significant differences for disease free or overall survival ($P = 0.4$ for both outcomes).[40] **Carboplatin plus paclitaxel or docetaxel:** We found one ongoing RCT (1077 women from 83 centres),[41] which will compare effects of six cycles of carboplatin ([{glomerular filtration rate multiplied by 5} + 25] mg) combined with either paclitaxel (175 mg/m^2) or docetaxel (75 mg/m^2). **Paclitaxel plus carboplatin versus carboplatin or cyclophosphamide plus doxorubicin plus cisplatin:** We found one ongoing RCT (2075 women).[42]

GLOSSARY

Debulking is removal of a major proportion of the tumour. Initial and primary debulking both refer to front line surgery (up front surgery).

Interval debulking is a second operation to remove residual tumour after a specified number of cytotoxic chemotherapy cycles, which is then followed by further chemotherapy.

Routine second look surgery is a "second look" operation to assess the response to cytotoxic chemotherapy.

REFERENCES

1. Allen DG, Heintz AP, Touw FW. A meta-analysis of residual disease and survival in stage III and IV carcinoma of the ovary. *Eur J Gynaecol Oncol* 1995;16:349–356. Search date not stated; primary sources literature search of Silver-Platter 3.1, hand searches, and personal communications.
2. Beral V. The epidemiology of ovarian cancer. In: Sharp F, Soutter WP, eds. *Proceedings of the Seventeenth Study Group of the Royal College of Obstetricians and Gynaecologists in Conjunction with the Helene Harris Memorial Trust*. London: RCOG, 1987:21–31.
3. Banks E, Beral V, Reeves G. The epidemiology of ovarian cancer: a review. *Int J Gynecol Cancer* 1997;7:425–438.
4. Parkin DM, Laara E, Muir CS. Estimates of the worldwide frequency of sixteen major cancers in 1980. *Int J Cancer* 1988;41:184–197.
5. Blake P, Lambert H, Crawford R. Cancer of the ovary and fallopian tube. In: Blake P, Lambert H, Crawford R, eds. Gynaecological oncology. A guide to clinical management. Oxford: Oxford University Press, 1998:12–44.
6. Cancer Statistics: Cancer Research Campaign, 2002. http://www.cancerresearchuk.org/aboutcancer/statistics/incidence. Last accessed 13 May 2003.
7. Whittemore AS, Harris R, Itnyre J. Characteristics relating to ovarian cancer risk: collaborative analysis of 12 US case-control studies. II. Invasive epithelial ovarian cancers in white women. Collaborative Ovarian Cancer Group. *Am J Epidemiol* 1992;136:1184–1203.
8. Yancik R. Ovarian cancer. Age contrasts in incidence, histology, disease stage at diagnosis and mortality. *Cancer* 1993;71:517–523.
9. Adami H-O, Hseih C-C, Lambe M, et al. Parity, age at first childbirth, and risk of ovarian cancer. *Lancet* 1994;344:1250–1254.
10. Rossing MA, Daling JR, Weiss NS, et al. Ovarian tumours in a cohort of infertile women. *New Engl J Med* 1994;331:771–776.
11. Venn A, Watson L, Bruinsma F, et al. Risk of cancer after use of fertility drugs with in-vitro fertilisation. *Lancet* 1999;354:1586–1590.
12. Mant JWF, Vessey MP. Ovarian and endometrial cancers. In: Doll R, Fraumeni JF Jr, Muir CS, eds. *Trends in cancer incidence and mortality*. Plainview, NY: Cold Spring Harbor Laboratory Press, 1994:287–307.
13. Booth M, Beral V, Smith P. Risk factors for ovarian cancer: a case-control study. *Br J Cancer* 1989;60:592–598.
14. Nicoletto MO, Tumolo S, Talamini R, et al. Surgical second look in ovarian cancer: a randomized study in patients with laparoscopic complete remission — a Northeastern Oncology Cooperative Group-Ovarian Cancer Cooperative Group Study. *J Clin Oncol* 1997;15:994–999.
15. Luesley D, Lawton F, Blackledge G, et al. Failure of second-look laparotomy to influence survival in epithelial ovarian cancer. *Lancet* 1988;2:599–603.

16. Van der Burg ME, van Lent M, Buyse M, et al. The effect of debulking surgery after induction chemotherapy on the prognosis in advanced epithelial ovarian cancer. Gynecological Cancer Cooperative Group of the European Organization for Research and Treatment of Cancer. *New Engl J Med* 1995;332:629–634.
17. Redman CW, Warwick J, Luesley DM, et al. Intervention debulking surgery in advanced epithelial ovarian cancer. *Br J Obstet Gynaecol* 1994;101:142–146.
18. Advanced Ovarian Cancer Trialists Group. Chemotherapy for advanced ovarian cancer. In: The Cochrane Library, Issue 1, 2002. Oxford: Update Software. Search date 1998; primary sources Medline, Cancerlit, the trial registers produced by the National Cancer Institute (Physicians Data Query) and the United Kingdom Co-ordinating Committee on Cancer Research, hand searches of relevant meeting proceedings, and contact with experts in the field and pharmaceutical companies.
19. Dorum A, Kristensen GB, Trope C. A randomised study of cisplatin versus thiotepa as induction chemotherapy in advanced ovarian carcinoma. *Eur J Cancer* 1994;30A:1470–1474.
20. Alberts DS, Mason-Liddil N, O'Toole RV, et al. Randomized Phase III trial of chemoimmunotherapy in patients with previously untreated stages III and IV suboptimal disease ovarian cancer: a Southwest Oncology Group Study. *Gynecol Oncol* 1989;32:8–15.
21. Edwards CL, Herson J, Gershenson DM, et al. A prospective randomized clinical trial of melphalan and cis-platinum versus hexamethylmelamine, adriamycin, and cyclophosphamide in advanced ovarian cancer. *Gynecol Oncol* 1983;15:261–277.
22. Sessa C, Colombo N, Bolis G, et al. Randomized comparison of hexamethylmelamine, adriamycin, cyclophosphamide (HAC) vs. cisplatin, adriamycin, cyclophosphamide (PAC) in advanced ovarian cancer: long-term results. *Cancer Treat Rev* 1991;18(suppl A):37–46.
23. Krommer CF, Szalai JP. Cyclophosphamide, adriamycin and cisplatin (CAP) versus cyclophosphamide, adriamycin and vincristin (CAV) in the treatment of advanced ovarian cancer: a randomized study. *Ann Oncol* 1992;3:37–39.
24. Neijt JP, Bokkel Huinink WW, van der Burg ME, et al. Randomised trial comparing two combination chemotherapy regimens (Hexa-CAF vs CHAP-5) in advanced ovarian carcinoma. *Lancet* 1984;2:594–600.
25. The ICON Collaborators. ICON2: randomised trial of single-agent carboplatin against three-drug combination of CAP (cyclophosphamide, doxorubicin, and cisplatin) in women with ovarian cancer. ICON Collaborators. International Collaborative Ovarian Neoplasm Study. *Lancet* 1998;352:1571–1576.
26. Bolis G, Favalli G, Danese S, et al. Weekly cisplatin given for 2 months versus cisplatin plus cyclophosphamide given for 5 months after cytoreductive surgery for advanced ovarian cancer. *J Clin Oncol* 1997;15:1938–1944.
27. Marth C, Trope C, Vergote IB, et al. Ten-year results of a randomised trial comparing cisplatin with cisplatin and cyclophosphamide in advanced, suboptimally debulked ovarian cancer. *Eur J Cancer* 1998;34:1175–1180.
28. US Food and Drug Administration. Center for Drug Evaluation and Research. http://www.fda.gov/cder/cancer/toxicityframe.htm. Last accessed 13 May 2003.
29. Sevelda P, Dittrich CH, Kurz CH, et al. Prospective randomized trial of sequential alternating chemotherapy in advanced ovarian carcinoma. *Onkologie* 1992;15:288–292.
30. van der Hoop RG, van der Burg ME, Bokkel Huinink WW, et al. Incidence of neuropathy in 395 patients with ovarian cancer treated with or without cisplatin. *Cancer* 1990;66:1697–1702.
31. Bella M, Cocconi A, Mambrini A, et al. The concept of a medical debulking in advanced ovarian carcinoma before cisplatin treatment. Final results of a prospective randomized trial. *Tumori* 1998;84(supp 54): A146.
32. Lister-Sharp D, McDonagh MS, Khan KS, et al. A rapid and systematic review of the effectiveness and cost-effectiveness of the taxanes used in the treatment of advanced breast and ovarian cancer. *Health Technol Assess* 2000;4:17–115. Search date not stated; primary sources Medline, Embase, Cancerlit, Cochrane Controlled Trials Register, National Research Register, and contact with researchers and review groups.
33. Smith-Sorensen B, Kaern J, Holm R, et al. Therapy effect of either paclitaxel or cyclophosphamide combination treatment in patients with epithelial ovarian cancer and relation to TP53 gene status. *Br J Cancer* 1998;78:375–381.
34. McGuire WP, Hoskins WJ, Brady MF, et al. Cyclophosphamide and cisplatin compared with paclitaxel and cisplatin in patients with stage III and stage IV ovarian cancer. *New Engl J Med* 1996;334:1–6.
35. Piccart MJ, Bertelsen K, James K, et al. Randomized intergroup trial of cisplatin–paclitaxel versus cisplatin–cyclophosphamide in women with advanced epithelial ovarian cancer: three-year results. *J Natl Cancer Inst* 2000;92:699–708.
36. Muggia FM, Braly PS, Brady MF, et al. Phase III randomized study of cisplatin versus paclitaxel versus cisplatin and paclitaxel in patients with suboptimal stage III or IV ovarian cancer: a gynecologic oncology group study. *J Clin Oncol* 2000;18:106–115.
37. Neijt JP, Engelholm SA, Tuxen MK, et al. Exploratory Phase III study of paclitaxel and cisplatin versus paclitaxel and carboplatin in advanced ovarian cancer. *J Clin Oncol* 2000;18:3084–3092.
38. Mobus V, Schoder W, Luck HJ, et al. Cisplatin/paclitaxel vs carboplatin/paclitaxel as first-line chemotherapy in ovarian cancer: an AGO study group Phase III trial. *Ann Oncol* 1998;9:173.
39. Shröeder W, DuBois A, Kuhn W, et al. Treatment of patients with advanced ovarian cancer (FIGO IIB-IV) with cisplatin/paclitaxel or carboplatin/paclitaxel — an interim analysis of the AGO study protocol ovar-3. *Eur J Cancer* 1999; 35 supp 4: S231, abstr 908.
40. Skarlos DV, Aravantinos G, Kosmidis P, et al. Paclitaxel with carboplatin versus paclitaxel with carboplatin alternating with cisplatin as first-line chemotherapy in advanced epithelial ovarian cancer: preliminary results of a Hellenic Cooperative Oncology Group study. *Semin Oncol* 1997;24:S15.
41. Vasey PA. First results of the SCOTROC trial: a Phase III comparison of paclitaxel–carboplatin and docetaxel–carboplatin as first line chemotherapy for epithelial ovarian cancer. *Proc ASCO* 2001;84:170–178.
42. Harper P. A randomised comparison of paclitaxel (T) and carboplatin (J) versus a control arm of single agent carboplatin (J) or CAP (cyclophosphamide, doxorubicin, cisplatin): 2075 patients randomised into the 3rd International Collaborative Ovarian Neoplasm Study [abstract]. *Proc ASCO* 1999;18:A1375.

Hani Gabra
Clinical Scientist and Consultant Medical Oncologist
Cancer Research UK
Edinburgh Oncology Unit
Western General Hospital
Edinburgh
UK

Charles Redman
Consultant Gynaecological Oncologist
Department of Obstetrics and Gynaecology
City General Hospital
Stoke-on-Trent
UK

Jennifer Byrom
Lecturer in Gynaecological Oncology
Academic Department of Obstetrics and Gynaecology
Birmingham Women's Hospital
Birmingham
UK

Competing interests: HG has been reimbursed by Schering-Plough, the manufacturers of Caelyx, for attending the ASCO conference on two occasions. He has received fees for consulting from Schering-Plough and he has received funds to cover costs of the South East Scotland Gynae-Cancer network Annual Meeting from Aventis (manufacturers of Taxotere), Bristol Myers (manufacturers of Taxol and Carboplatin), Merck (distributors of Hycamtin), Schering-Plough (manufacturers of Caelyx), and Merck. He has received research support from Aventis for Scottish Gynae Cancer Trials Group clinical trials. CR and JB none declared.

TABLE 1 Adverse effects of chemotherapy — Common Toxicity Criteria (see text, p 2176).[28] Published with permission.

Toxicity grade	0	1	2	3	4
Blood and bone marrow					
WBC (10^9/L)	≥ 4.0	3.0–3.9	2.0–2.9	1.0–1.9	< 1.0
Platelets (10^9/L)	WNL	75.0 normal	50.0–74.9	25.0–49.9	< 25.0
Haemoglobin (g/L)	WNL	10.0 normal	8.0–10.0	6.5–7.9	< 6.5
Granulocytes and bands (10^9/L)	≥ 2.0	1.5–1.9	1.0–1.4	0.5–0.9	< 0.5
Lymphocytes (10^9/L)	≥ 2.0	1.5–1.9	1.0–1.4	0.5–0.9	< 0.5
Nausea					
	None	Able to eat	Oral intake significantly decreased	No significant intake, requiring iv fluids	
Vomiting					
	None	1 episode in 24 hours over pretreatment	≥ 6 episodes in 24 hours over pretreatment; or need for iv fluids	Requiring parenteral nutrition; or physiological consequences requiring intensive care; haemodynamic collapse	
Muscle pain					
	None	Mild pain not interfering with function	Moderate pain: pain or analgesics interfering with function, but not interfering with activities of daily living	Severe pain: pain or analgesics severely interfering with activities of daily living	Disabling

iv, intravenous; WBC, white blood cells; WNL, within normal limits.

Premenstrual syndrome

Search date October 2002

Katrina Wyatt

QUESTIONS

INTERVENTIONS

See glossary, p 2200

Key Messages

- **Bromocriptine (breast symptoms only)** RCTs have found limited evidence that bromocriptine relieves breast tenderness compared to placebo, although adverse effects are common.
- **Cognitive behavioural therapy** RCTs found that cognitive behavioural therapy significantly reduced premenstrual symptoms compared to control treatments, but the evidence is insufficient to define the size of an effect.
- **Danazol** RCTs have found that danazol significantly reduces premenstrual symptoms compared to placebo, but has important adverse effects associated with masculinisation when used continuously in the long term.
- **Diuretics** RCTs have found that spironolactone improves symptoms of premenstrual syndrome including breast tenderness and bloating, compared to placebo. Two RCTs have found that metolazone or ammonium chloride versus placebo reduce premenstrual swelling and weight gain.

- **Exercise** One RCT has found that aerobic exercise significantly improves premenstrual symptoms compared to placebo. Another RCT has found that high intensity aerobic exercise improves symptoms significantly more than low intensity.
- **Gonadorelin analogues** RCTs have found that gonadorelin analogues (GnRH in previous nomenclatrues) significantly reduce premenstrual symptoms compared to placebo. RCTs have found that gonadorelin plus oestrogen plus progestogen (addback treatment) improves symptom scores less than that gonadorelin analogue alone but more than placebo. One small RCT found a similar reduction in symptom scores with gonadorelin analogue plus tibolone compared to gonadorelin analogue alone. Treatment with gonadorelin analogues for more than 6 months carries a significant risk of osteoporosis, limiting their usefulness for long term treatment.
- **Hysterectomy with or without bilateral oophorectomy** We found no RCTs. Observational studies have found that hysterectomy plus bilateral oophorectomy is curative. Hysterectomy alone may reduce symptoms, but evidence is limited because of the difficulty in providing controls. The risks are those of major surgery. Infertility is an irreversible consequence of bilateral oophorectomy.
- **Non-selective serotonin reuptake inhibitor antidepressants/anxiolytics** RCTs have found that non-selective serotonin reuptake inhibitor antidepressants and anxiolytic drugs significantly improve at least one symptom of premenstrual syndrome compared to placebo, but a proportion of women stop treatment because of adverse effects. We found insufficient evidence from small RCTs about effects of β blockers and lithium.
- **Non-steroidal anti-inflammatory drugs** RCTs found that prostaglandin inhibitors significantly improved a range of premenstrual symptoms but did not reduce premenstrual breast pain, compared to placebo.
- **Oestrogens** Limited evidence from small RCTs suggests that oestradiol improves symptoms compared to placebo, but the magnitude of any effect remains unclear.
- **Oral contraceptives** RCTs found limited evidence that oral contraceptives improved premenstrual symptoms compared to placebo.
- **Progesterone** One systematic review of progesterone has found a small but significant improvement in overall premenstrual symptoms and no increase in the frequency of withdrawals caused by adverse effects, compared to placebo. However, the improvement is unlikely to be clinically important. It remains unclear whether the route or timing of administration of progesterone is important.
- **Progestogens** We found insufficient evidence from one small RCT about the effects of progestogens compared to placebo.
- **Pyridoxine** One systematic review of poor quality RCTs found insufficient evidence about the effects of pyridoxine (vitamin B_6). In the review, an analysis of weak RCTs suggested that pyridoxine significantly reduced symptoms compared to placebo. Additional RCTs with weak methods found conflicting evidence on the effects of pyridoxine.
- **Selective serotonin reuptake inhibitors** One systematic review and subsequent RCTs have found that selective serotonin reuptake inhibitors significantly improve premenstrual symptoms, but cause frequent adverse events compared to placebo.
- **Tibolone** One small RCT found limited evidence that tibolone improved premenstrual symptom score compared to placebo (multivitamins).

- **Chiropractic treatment; dietary supplements; endometrial ablation; evening primrose oil; laparoscopic bilateral oophorectomy; reflexology; relaxation treatment** We found insufficient evidence about the effects of these interventions.

DEFINITION A woman has premenstrual syndrome if she complains of recurrent psychological or somatic symptoms (or both) occurring specifically during the luteal phase of the menstrual cycle, and resolving by the end of menstruation (see table 1, p 2203).[1]

INCIDENCE/ PREVALENCE Premenstrual symptoms occur in 95% of all women of reproductive age; severe, debilitating symptoms (premenstrual syndrome) occur in about 5% of those women.[1]

AETIOLOGY/ RISK FACTORS The aetiology is unknown, but hormonal and other (possibly neuroendocrine) factors probably contribute.[2,3] There may be enhanced sensitivity to progesterone, possibly caused by a deficiency of serotonin.[2]

PROGNOSIS Except after oophorectomy, symptoms usually recur when treatment is stopped.

AIMS OF INTERVENTION To improve or eliminate physical and psychological symptoms; to minimise the impact on normal functioning, interpersonal relationships, and quality of life; to minimise adverse effects of treatment.

OUTCOMES **Symptom severity:** There is no consensus on how this should be assessed. One review of premenstrual syndrome outcomes found 65 different questionnaires or scales, measuring 199 different symptoms or signs.[4]

METHODS The initial search strategy was adapted from the Cochrane Collaboration's Menstrual Disorders and Subfertility Group.[5] *Clinical Evidence* search and appraisal October 2002. We included systematic reviews and subsequent RCTs that (1) diagnosed premenstrual syndrome by validated scales prior to randomisation; (2) used a pre-randomisation placebo cycle to exclude women with a non-specific response; (3) contained sufficient cycles to allow for symptom variability between cycles. Few trials fulfilled these criteria. The wide range of diagnostic scales, outcome criteria, and dosing regimens made comparison between trials difficult. We excluded reviews that systematically searched electronic databases but did not use overt criteria to appraise the results.[6]

QUESTION **What are the effects of treatments for women with premenstrual syndrome?**

OPTION **ANXIOLYTICS/NON-SELECTIVE SEROTONIN REUPTAKE INHIBITOR ANTIDEPRESSANTS**

RCTs have found that non-selective serotonin reuptake inhibitor antidepressants and anxiolytic drugs versus placebo significantly improve at least one symptom of premenstrual syndrome, but a proportion of women stop treatment because of adverse effects. We found insufficient evidence from small RCTs about effects of β blockers and lithium.

Benefits: We found no systematic review. We found 14 RCTs of antidepressant and anxiolytic drugs for premenstrual syndrome. Most (9/14 [64%]) reported significant improvement of one or more symptoms. **Alprazolam:** Five RCTs (150 women) compared alprazolam (0.25–2.25 mg daily) versus placebo.[7–11] The RCT using the lowest dose (0.25–0.75 mg daily) found no significant reduction in premenstrual symptoms, but four RCTs using a higher dose (≥ 0.75 mg daily) found significant reduction of symptoms. **Buspirone:** Two small RCTs (17 women,[12] 41 women[13]) found significant symptom reduction with buspirone (25 mg daily,[12] 10–20 mg daily[13]) versus placebo. **Non-selective serotonin reuptake inhibitors antidepressants:** Four small RCTs of antidepressants versus placebo (81 women) found variable results: two RCTs of clomipramine (25–75 mg daily) versus placebo found significant reduction of premenstrual symptoms, but RCTs of buproprion[14] and desipramine[15] found no significant reduction. We found no meta-analysis; inconsistent results among RCTs may have arisen by chance. **β blockers:** Three RCTs found variable results. Two small RCTs (27 women) found significant symptom improvement with atenolol versus placebo at lower doses (25 mg daily) but no significant difference with higher doses (100 mg daily).[16,17] The third RCT (30 women) found significant reduction of severe premenstrual headaches with propranolol (20–40 mg daily during luteal phase) versus placebo.[18] **Lithium:** One RCT (19 women) found no significant difference in premenstrual symptoms with lithium carbonate (750–1000 mg daily) versus placebo.[19]

Harms: Adverse effects such as drowsiness, nausea, anxiety, and headache led to problems with adherence to treatment in most of the trials.[7,11,20,21] **Alprazolam:** Drowsiness and sedation were found in about 50% of women, as well as lower rates of headache and nausea. **Antidepressants:** Adverse effects were frequent and more women withdrew when taking antidepressants than when taking placebo (11/81 [14%] with antidepressants *v* 6/81 [7%] with placebo).[14,15,20,22] Common adverse effects reported were dry mouth, fatigue, nausea, and dizziness. **Lithium:** Tremor, weakness, and gastrointestinal disturbances resulted in 4/19 (21%) withdrawals from the RCT. **Other interventions:** The other trials did not report specific adverse effects.

Comment: The evidence is limited, but is consistent with at most a small benefit from antidepressants/anxiolytics in premenstrual syndrome, which is countered by frequent adverse effects.

OPTION BROMOCRIPTINE

RCTs have found limited evidence that bromocriptine versus placebo relieves premenstrual breast tenderness, although adverse effects are common.

Benefits: We found no systematic review. One survey of 14 trials found no evidence that bromocriptine versus placebo improved overall symptom scores in premenstrual syndrome, although it found limited evidence of improvement in premenstrual mastalgia.[23]

Harms: Bromocriptine has a high incidence of adverse effects, including nausea, dizziness, headache, weight increase, and swelling.[24–26] The survey did not include any mention of adverse effects, which on analysis of individual trials are well documented.[23] There have been very rare case reports of stroke and death following bromocriptine treatment to prevent lactation.[27]

Comment: None.

OPTION CHIROPRACTIC MANIPULATION

One systematic review found insufficient evidence about the effects of chiropractic treatment in women with premenstrual syndrome.

Benefits: We found one systematic review (search date 2000, 1 RCT, 45 women).[28] The placebo controlled crossover RCT found a significant decrease in premenstrual syndrome scores with chiropractic treatment (3 sessions premenstrually over 3 cycles) versus placebo. Women who received placebo first did not experience significant additional improvement when they were switched to chiropractic treatment.

Harms: None reported.

Comment: The RCT had a high withdrawal rate (25/45 [56%] completed). Women improved most with whatever treatment they had first (real or sham treatment). The evidence is insufficient to define the effects of chiropractic treatment in women with premenstrual syndrome.

OPTION COGNITIVE BEHAVIOURAL THERAPY

RCTs have found significant reduction of premenstrual symptoms with cognitive behavioural therapy versus control treatments, but the evidence is insufficient to define the size of any effect.

Benefits: **Versus control treatments:** We found no systematic review. Seven RCTs compared a treatment with cognitive behavioural content versus some type of control treatment.[29–35] Four of the RCTs (112 women) found significant reduction of symptoms with cognitive behavioural therapy versus a dummy treatment (relaxation, activity through movement, or information focused treatment) or versus a waiting list group. The abstract of the seventh RCT (41 women 19–40 years old) compared cognitive restructuring intervention (self monitoring, educational, and coping skills training phases), support (general discussion on menstrual symptoms), and assessment only (no treatment). Women were followed for 3 months and treatments were offered during the second month during four weekly sessions that lasted 1 hour. It found that after 3 months all women had improved, experiencing fewer and less severe symptoms and taking less medication (figures not provided in the abstract).[35]

Harms: None reported.

Comment: It is difficult to design appropriate control treatments and to maintain blinding of allocation for cognitive behavioural therapies, but studies using both dummy and waiting list controls have found significant benefits. Several trials noted benefits of cognitive behavioural therapy over the medium to long term. Cognitive behavioural therapy may be appropriate only for a motivated subgroup of women.

OPTION DANAZOL

RCTs have found that danazol versus placebo significantly reduces premenstrual symptoms, but has important adverse effects associated with masculinisation when used continuously in the long term.

Benefits: We found no systematic review but found six RCTs.[36–41] **Continuous danazol:** Four RCTs (3 crossover, 144 women with premenstrual syndrome) found significant symptom reduction with danazol given continuously (over 3 cycles) versus placebo.[36–38,40] Many women withdrew before the trial finished (see harms of danazol below). **Luteal phase danazol:** Two RCTs gave danazol in the luteal phase only.[39,41] One RCT found that danazol versus placebo significantly reduced overall symptoms. The other, larger trial found danazol versus placebo significantly reduced premenstrual breast pain only.[39,41]

Harms: **Continuous danazol:** More people withdrew from the studies when given danazol than when given placebo (e.g. in 1 parallel RCT, withdrawals: 12/30 [40%] with danazol *v* 1/10 [10%] with placebo; RR 4.0, 95% CI 0.6 to 27; NNH 3, 95% CI 1 to 9).[37] The initial severity of the premenstrual symptoms was higher among women who withdrew than among women who remained in the RCTs (see comment below). Observational studies have described masculinisation (deepening of the voice, hirsutism) and weight gain with long term use of danazol (see harms of danazol under breast pain, p 2034). Plasma lipid levels can change, leading to concern that the cardiovascular risk may be increased. Osteoporosis seems not to be a risk. **Luteal phase danazol:** The two RCTs did not find a significantly higher rate of short term adverse effects with danazol than with placebo. Long term adverse effects were not assessed.[39,41]

Comment: It seems clear that danazol is capable of reducing premenstrual symptoms (many women who remained in the RCTs had some types of symptom eradicated by danazol, but fewer did with placebo). However, the magnitude of the danazol effect is less certain because some of the mean improvement in symptom scores can be attributed to the withdrawal of women with worse symptoms. The RCTs did not report intention to treat analyses.

OPTION DIETARY SUPPLEMENTS

One systematic review found insufficient evidence on the effects of calcium and magnesium supplements versus placebo in women with premenstrual syndrome.

Benefits: We found one systematic review (search date 2000).[28] **Magnesium supplements:** The systematic review (3 RCTs, 144 women) found unclear results with magnesium supplements versus placebo for premenstrual syndrome symptoms. One RCT found an improvement in overall premenstrual syndrome symptoms, one found no effect, and the third found significant improvement of bloating. The review did not perform a meta-analysis. **Calcium supplements:** The systematic review (2 RCTs, 557 women) found that calcium supplements (1–1.2 g daily for 3 cycles) versus placebo significantly reduced overall symptoms (including breast tenderness and swelling, headaches, and abdominal cramps).[28]

Harms: None reported.

Comment: **Calcium supplements:** Both RCTs were performed by the same research unit. The smaller RCT had a high withdrawal rate and compliance with treatment was poor. The second, larger RCT did not exclude other treatments of premenstrual symptoms during the trial.[28]

OPTION DIURETICS

RCTs have found that spironolactone versus placebo improves symptoms of premenstrual syndrome including breast tenderness and bloating. Two RCTs have found limited evidence that metolazone or ammonium chloride versus placebo reduce premenstrual swelling and weight gain. One RCT found insufficient evidence about the effects of chlorthalidone versus placebo or lithium on premenstrual symptoms.

Benefits: **Spironolactone:** We found no systematic review but found four RCTs (210 women) that compared spironolactone versus placebo.[42–45] Three RCTs found significant reduction of symptoms with spironolactone (100 mg daily) versus placebo, and one RCT[44] found no significant difference. Two RCTs found that significantly more women had improved irritability[45] and overall symptoms, including breast tenderness and bloating[43] with spironolactone than with placebo (14/17 [82%] with spironolactone *v* 9/16 [56%] with placebo; RR 1.46, 95% CI 0.90 to 2.38; NNT 4, 95% CI 2 to 292;[43] and 20/26 [77%] with spironolactone *v* 11/21 [52%] with placebo; RR 1.47, 95% CI 0.93 to 2.32; NNT 4, 95% CI 2 to 85[45]). **Metolazone:** One RCT (crossover design, 46 women with premenstrual swelling or weight gain, 33 completed) found significant reduction of premenstrual symptoms with luteal phase metolazone (1, 2.5, and 5 mg daily) versus placebo.[46] There was no significant difference in effect among doses. **Chlorthalidone:** One RCT (crossover design, 25 women) found that similar numbers of women felt "much better" over eight menstrual cycles on a global rating scale of premenstrual symptoms with chlorthalidone versus placebo or lithium.[47] However, the RCT did not diagnose premenstrual syndrome prior to randomisation, and it may have been too small to detect a clinically important difference in symptoms. **Ammonium**

chloride: One RCT (22 women with premenstrual weight gain) found significantly more weight loss on days 20–23 with a diuretic on sale to the general public in the USA (ammonium chloride 325 mg plus caffeine 100 mg 6 times daily for days 18–24) versus placebo.[48]

Harms: **Spironolactone:** Adverse effects were reported in only one RCT: two people reported palpitations while on spironolactone. **Metolazone:** Women on metolazone (5 mg) complained of severe adverse effects (excessive diuresis and weakness).[46] Other adverse effects include nausea, dizziness, palpitations, excess diuresis, and weakness.[48]

Comment: Diuretics are widely used in the belief that many symptoms of premenstrual syndrome are the direct consequence of fluid retention; we found little evidence of water retention in most women with premenstrual syndrome.

OPTION ENDOMETRIAL ABLATION

We found no RCTs about the effects of endometrial ablation in premenstrual syndrome.

Benefits: We found no systematic review or RCTs.

Harms: We found insufficient evidence.

Comment: Studies of women with menorrhagia have claimed that endometrial ablation may relieve symptoms of premenstrual syndrome. However, effects in women with premenstrual syndrome alone remain unclear.

OPTION EVENING PRIMROSE OIL

One systematic review of poor quality RCTs found insufficient evidence about the effects of evening primrose oil.

Benefits: We found one systematic review (search date 1993, 7 RCTs, 329 women).[49] Although some trials found a small beneficial effect, the number of women included in the RCTs was low. Weak methods and different outcome measures prevented meta-analysis. The authors concluded that there was insufficient evidence to define the effects of evening primrose oil in women with premenstrual syndrome.

Harms: Few adverse effects have been reported. There are rare reports of evening primrose oil causing seizures in people with epilepsy.[50]

Comment: Only five of the trials in the review clearly indicated that they were randomised. Evening primrose oil is one of the most popular "self help" remedies for premenstrual syndrome.

OPTION EXERCISE

One RCT has found that aerobic exercise versus placebo significantly improves premenstrual symptoms. Another RCT has found that high intensity aerobic exercise improves symptoms significantly more than low intensity exercise.

Benefits: We found no systematic review, but found two abstracts of RCTs.[51,52] The first RCT (32 women with premenstrual syndrome diagnosed prior to randomisation) found significantly improved symptoms with high intensity aerobic exercise versus low intensity exercise.[51] The second RCT (30 women with premenstrual syndrome) found significant reduction of premenstrual symptoms with both low intensity aerobic exercise (40% maximum effort for 45 mins, 3 times weekly, for 3 cycles) versus placebo weekly and with moderate intensity aerobic exercise (70% maximum effort for 45 mins, 3 times weekly, for 3 cycles) versus placebo.[52]

Harms: Harms were not mentioned in the abstracts of the RCTs.[51,52]

Comment: Both reports[51,52] were available to us only as abstracts. Further details may be available in future *Clinical Evidence* updates.

OPTION GONADORELIN (GNRH) ANALOGUES (BUSERELIN, GOSERELIN, LEUPRORELIN)

RCTs have found that gonadorelin analogues (GnRH) significantly reduce premenstrual symptoms compared to placebo. RCTs have found that gonadorelin plus oestrogen plus progestogen (addback treatment) improves symptom scores less than that gonadorelin analogue alone but more than placebo. One small RCT found similar reduction in symptom scores with gonadorelin analogue plus tibolone compared to gonadorelin analogue plus placebo. Treatment with gonadorelin analogues for more than 6 months carries a significant risk of osteoporosis, limiting their usefulness for long term treatment.

Benefits: We found no systematic review. **Gonadorelin analogues versus placebo:** We found 10 RCTs[53–62] of gonadorelin (GnRH) analogues versus placebo. All 10 trials diagnosed premenstrual syndrome before randomisation. Seven of the RCTs used a crossover design. Nine of the RCTs found a significant reduction in premenstrual symptoms with gonadorelin analogues versus placebo (typically, by 3 months symptom scores fell to about 50% of their initial value with a gonadorelin analogue *v* 10% decline with placebo[61]). **Gonadorelin analogues plus oestrogen and progestogen:** Three of the RCTs (78 women) compared gonadorelin analogues plus oestrogen and progestogen (addback treatment) versus placebo or gonadorelin analogue alone.[57,58,61] Two of the RCTs were small (8 women[57] and 10 women[58]). The largest RCT (60 women, 41 completed the 6 month study) found that gonadorelin plus addback treatment produced a fall in symptom scores that was intermediate between that produced by gonadorelin analogue alone and placebo (irritability symptom score at baseline 2 in all groups; change in score after 6 months: –0.37 with placebo *v* –0.64 with gonadorelin analogue plus addback *v* –1.03 with gonadorelin analogue alone; $P < 0.05$).[61] **Gonadorelin analogue plus tibolone versus gonadorelin analogue alone:** We found one RCT (30 women with severe premenstrual syndrome (see glossary, p 2200)), which found no difference in symptom scores after 8 weeks with gonadorelin analogue plus tibolone versus gonadorelin analogue plus placebo (irritability scores: changed from 7.3 to 3.3 with gonadorelin analogue plus tibolone *v* from 8.4 to 4.0 with gonadorelin analogue alone).[63]

Harms: A large proportion of the women in the RCTs experienced adverse effects. Commonly reported adverse effects include hot flushes, night sweats, nausea, decreased libido, pruritus, bronchospasm, and headache.[53,54,56,60,62] In one typical RCT, over 6 months' withdrawals from the RCT were common (7/20 [35%] with placebo *v* 9/21 [43%] with gonadorelin plus addback treatment *v* 3/19 [16%] with gonadorelin analogue alone).[61]

Comment: A truly double blind RCT of gonadorelin analogues would be hard to conduct because women receiving these agents experience amenorrhoea. Treatment with gonadorelin analogues for more than 6 months carries significant risk of osteoporosis, limiting their usefulness for long term treatment.[64]

OPTION HYSTERECTOMY WITH OR WITHOUT OOPHORECTOMY

We found no RCTs. Observational studies have found that hysterectomy plus bilateral oophorectomy is curative. Hysterectomy alone may reduce symptoms, but evidence is limited because of the difficulty in providing controls. The risks are those of major surgery. Infertility is an irreversible consequence of bilateral oophorectomy.

Benefits: We found no systematic review and no RCTs.

Harms: We found no systematic review or RCT, but potential risks include those associated with major surgery.[65]

Comment: Cohort studies have described a reduction in the symptoms of premenstrual syndrome after hysterectomy.[66,67] However, without a control group, it is impossible to know how much of the observed response is attributable to the hysterectomy itself or to a non-specific placebo response that is seen in most RCTs of premenstrual syndrome. Other cohort studies have found almost complete eradication of the symptoms of premenstrual syndrome after hysterectomy plus bilateral oophorectomy.[68,69] Surgery is rarely used but may be indicated if there are coexisting gynaecological problems.

OPTION LAPAROSCOPIC BILATERAL OOPHORECTOMY

We found no RCTs on the effects of laparoscopic bilateral oophorectomy in women with premenstrual syndrome.

Benefits: We found no systematic review or RCTs.

Harms: We found insufficient evidence.

Comment: After oophorectomy, oestrogen replacement treatment and cyclical progesterone (to prevent endometrial hyperplasia and carcinoma) are often used. Progesterone may restimulate premenstrual syndrome.

OPTION LOW DOSE OESTROGENS

Limited evidence from three small RCTs suggests benefit from oestradiol (oestrogen) compared to placebo, but the magnitude of any effect remains unclear.

Benefits: We found no systematic review but found three RCTs (71 women) of oestrogen versus placebo.[70–72] All trials diagnosed premenstrual syndrome before randomisation. The first RCT (11 women) found no significant difference in symptoms with oral conjugated equine oestrogens (0.6 mg from day 15 until menses) versus placebo over three cycles (9 women had worse symptoms with oestrogen *v* 2 women with placebo).[70] The second RCT (crossover, 40 women, 35 completed) compared oestradiol (200 μg transdermal patches changed every 3 days throughout the cycle) versus placebo for three cycles.[71] Oral norethisterone (5 mg daily) was added from day 19–26 for all women. Women were randomly allocated to a sequence of treatment (active for 3 cycles then placebo for 3 cycles, or the reverse). Both groups improved during the first three cycles. After the crossover, significant further improvement was seen with women switching from placebo to active treatment, but the symptoms of women switching from active treatment to placebo deteriorated to the level they were at the start of the RCT. The third RCT (crossover design, 20 women with migraine just before or during menses, 18 completed) found that oestradiol (oestradiol gel 1.5 mg daily to the skin for 7 days over 3 cycles) versus placebo reduced the number of cycles with menstrual migraine (8/26 [31%] of the oestradiol cycles *v* 26/27 [96%] of placebo cycles; RR 0.32, 95% CI 0.18 to 0.57; NNT 1.5, 95% CI 1.1 to 2.0).[72]

Harms: Adverse effects included mastalgia, nausea, weight gain, headache, and change in cycle length. The patch trial also reported skin irritation and skin pigmentation. Similar numbers of women withdrew on active treatment compared with placebo (3/71 [4%] with active treatment *v* 2/71 [3%] with placebo).[71]

Comment: Oestrogens may improve premenstrual symptoms. To avoid endometrial hyperplasia and adenocarcinoma, a 12 day progestogen course is needed every 28 days. Progestogen may induce premenstrual syndrome symptoms in some women. To avoid this systemic effect, progestogen may be given locally (using a levonorgestrel intrauterine device or progesterone gel). We found no RCTs evaluating this approach. We found one report of an ongoing RCT (80 women) comparing cyclical oestradiol and medroxyprogesterone versus placebo in women with premenstrual syndrome and depressive symptoms.[73]

OPTION NON-STEROIDAL ANTI-INFLAMMATORY DRUGS

RCTs have found benefit from non-steroidal anti-inflammatory drugs compared to placebo for a range of premenstrual symptoms.

Benefits: We found no systematic review. **Mefenamic acid:** We found five RCTs,[74–78] but only three diagnosed premenstrual syndrome prior to randomisation.[74,75,78] One RCT (37 women) found significantly more women preferred mefenamic acid (1.5 g daily in the luteal phase for 1 cycle) than placebo (23/37 [62%] with mefenamic acid *v* 6/37 [16%] with placebo; RR 3.8, 95% CI 1.8 to 8.3; NNT 3, 95% CI 2 to 4).[74] The frequency of irritability was significantly lower with mefenamic acid than with placebo (11/36 [31%] *v* 24/33 [73%]; RR 0.42, 95% CI 0.25 to 0.72; NNT 3, 95% CI 2 to 4).[74] The other

RCT (crossover design, 19 women) found significantly improved physical and mood symptoms with three cycles of mefenamic acid versus placebo.[75] **Naproxen sodium:** Two RCTs diagnosed premenstrual syndrome before randomisation. One RCT (34 women) found significant reduction of pain symptoms with naproxen sodium (550 mg twice daily for days 21–4 in 3 cycles) versus placebo.[79] The other RCT (crossover design, 42 women randomised, 21 completed) found significant reduction of physical symptoms of premenstrual syndrome with naproxen sodium (500 mg twice daily for 6 cycles) versus placebo.[80]

Harms: Adverse effects included nausea, gastrointestinal disturbances, and rashes.[74–76]

Comment: None.

OPTION ORAL CONTRACEPTIVES

Two RCTs found limited evidence that oral contraceptives versus placebo improved premenstrual symptoms.

Benefits: We found no systematic review but found two RCTs,[81,82] which diagnosed premenstrual syndrome prior to randomisation. The first RCT (82 women) found significant reduction with triphasic oral contraceptive for three cycles versus placebo in premenstrual breast pain and bloating. Oral contraceptives were no better than placebo for mood symptoms. The second RCT (82 women with severe premenstrual syndrome (see glossary, p 2200)) found significant reduction in some premenstrual symptoms (appetite, acne, and food cravings) with an experimental oral contraception (ethinyloestradiol 30 μg plus drospirenone 3 mg over 3 cycles) versus placebo.[82] Other symptom scores were improved with oral contraception, but the differences were not significant.[82]

Harms: Spotting, nausea, cramps, breast pain, and decreased libido were more commonly reported on active treatment compared with placebo. More women withdrew because of adverse effects with active treatment than with placebo (13 *v* 1).[81]

Comment: Some women develop premenstrual syndrome-like symptoms for the first time when taking the oral contraceptive pill. Anecdotal evidence suggests that oral contraceptives may be beneficial in premenstrual syndrome.[83–85] Continuous combined regimens (those without a 1 wk break) should, in theory, suppress ovulation and provide symptom relief, but we found no published trials.

OPTION PROGESTERONE

One systematic review of progesterone versus placebo has found a small but significant improvement in overall premenstrual symptoms and no increase in the frequency of withdrawals caused by adverse effects. However, the improvement is unlikely to be clinically important. It remains unclear whether the route or timing of administration of progesterone is important.

Benefits: We found one systematic review (search date 2000, 10 RCTs, 531 women with previously diagnosed premenstrual syndrome).[86] Six of the RCTs were crossover studies. The review found a small improvement in overall premenstrual symptoms for women taking progesterone versus control treatments over 2–6 months (standardised mean differences –0.028, 95% CI –0.017 to –0.040; no heterogeneity of pooled results). Two RCTs (116 completed) used oral progesterone and seven RCTs (296 completed) used progesterone suppositories. One crossover RCT (25 women) compared oral progesterone versus progesterone pessaries versus placebo, and was analysed as if it was two studies. Six of the 10 RCTs administered the progesterone in the luteal phase of the menstrual cycle.

Harms: Some RCTs reported adverse effects such as abdominal pain, nausea, headache, vaginal pruritus, dizziness, drowsiness, excessive bleeding, and dysmenorrhoea.[86] Withdrawal because of adverse effects was not increased significantly by progesterone (OR 1.66, 95% CI 0.43 to 6.79).

Comment: The systematic review[86] did not specify whether results after the crossovers had been included in the analyses. The authors of the systematic review argued that the very small improvement in overall symptoms was statistically significant, but clinically unimportant. The observed change in symptoms was small compared with that produced by selective serotonin reuptake inhibitors (see selective serotonin reuptake inhibitors, p 2198). Subgroup analysis found a small but significant improvement of symptoms with oral progesterone (3 RCTs), and a small but significant deterioration of symptom suppositories or pessaries (8 RCTs). Oral micronised progesterone is not available in many countries.[86] The systematic review tabulated the adverse effects reported with progesterone and placebo, but did not specify how many women were in the five RCTs that reported harms.

OPTION PROGESTOGENS (SYNTHETIC PROGESTERONE-LIKE DRUGS)

We found insufficient evidence about the effects of progestogens versus placebo.

Benefits: We found one systematic review (search date 2000, 3 RCTs, 319 women) of progestogens versus placebo.[86] Two RCTs were crossover studies. One RCT compared medroxyprogesterone versus norethisterone versus placebo and was analysed as if it were two RCTs. The systematic review found a small but significant reduction of premenstrual symptoms with progestogens versus placebo (standardised mean differences –0.036, 95% CI –0.059 to –0.014). However, results may not be reliable (see comments below).

Harms: None of the RCTs reported a detailed analysis of adverse effects.[86] The systematic review found no significant difference with progestogens versus placebo in withdrawals from the RCTs because of adverse events (OR 1.65, 95% CI 0.86 to 3.21).[7] The most common adverse effects associated with progestogens are nausea, breast discomfort, headache, and menstrual irregularity.

Comment: The systematic review[86] did not specify how the results of the crossover studies were analysed (in particular, whether results after the crossover were included). The review stated that it found no heterogeneity of the results from the four RCTs, but published a figure that appears to show disagreement among the studies (3 significantly favouring progestogen and 1 significantly favouring placebo).

OPTION PYRIDOXINE (VITAMIN B_6)

A systematic review of poor quality RCTs found that the evidence was insufficient to define the effects of pyridoxine versus placebo in women with premenstrual syndrome. In the review, an analysis of nine weak RCTs suggested a significant reduction of symptoms with pyridoxine versus placebo. Three additional RCTs with weak methods found conflicting evidence of the benefits of pyridoxine.

Benefits: We found one systematic review[87] and three additional RCTs.[18,88,89] The systematic review (search date 1998, 9 RCTs, 940 women with premenstrual syndrome) found no high quality RCTs comparing pyridoxine (either as a single supplement or as part of a multivitamin supplement) with placebo.[88] The pooled odds ratio for relief of overall premenstrual syndrome symptoms was 2.32 (95% CI 1.95 to 2.54) with pyridoxine (over 2–4 months) versus placebo. There was no dose related response. One additional RCT compared pyridoxine with *Vitex agnus castus*. It found that both treatments improved symptoms.[89] Another RCT with weak methods found no improvement over placebo,[18] whereas the third additional RCT found a significant improvement.[90]

Harms: High doses of pyridoxine (> 200 mg daily) have been associated with a reversible peripheral neuropathy.[88] The review found few reports of adverse events in the RCTs.

Comment: One of the RCTs is being translated.[90] Further details will be added in future *Clinical Evidence* updates.

OPTION REFLEXOLOGY

One systematic review of one RCT found insufficient evidence about the effects of reflexology versus sham reflexology in premenstrual syndrome.

Benefits: We found one systematic review (search date 2000, 1 RCT, 50 women).[28] The RCT found significant reduction of premenopausal symptoms with reflexology (1 weekly session over 2 cycles) versus sham reflexology.

Harms: None mentioned.

Comment: Only 35 women completed the RCT. Reflexology involved manual pressure to specific reflex areas of the body, but the sham treatment comprised uneven tactile stimulation of alternative areas (shoulder, elbow, or nose). The allocated intervention was not concealed to those assessing the outcomes or to participants. The evidence is insufficient to define the effects of reflexology in women with premenstrual syndrome.

OPTION RELAXATION TREATMENT

RCTs found insufficient evidence on the effects of relaxation treatment in premenstrual syndrome.

Benefits: We found one systematic review (search date 2000, 2 RCTs, 101 women).[28] The first RCT found significant reduction of physical symptoms with muscular relaxation treatment versus reading leisure material or charting symptoms. The second RCT compared muscle relaxation versus massage, but did not compare the reduction in symptoms produced by each treatment. Both groups improved compared with baseline symptoms.

Harms: None mentioned.

Comment: Most studies of relaxation techniques have used them as an adjunct to other treatment. The evidence is insufficient to define the effects of relaxation in women with premenstrual syndrome.

OPTION SELECTIVE SEROTONIN REUPTAKE INHIBITORS

One systematic review and subsequent RCTs have found that selective serotonin reuptake inhibitors significantly improve premenstrual symptoms, but cause frequent adverse events compared to placebo.

Benefits: We found one systematic review,[91] one additional report of an RCT in the review,[92] and two subsequent RCTs.[93,94] The systematic review (search date not stated, 15 RCTs, 904 women with premenstrual syndrome) found significant improvement in overall symptoms with selective serotonin reuptake inhibitors (SSRIs) versus placebo (WMD –1.07, 95% CI –1.38 to –0.75).[91] There was no significant difference in symptom improvement between continuous and intermittent dosing. The review did not report absolute proportions of women who had improved symptoms with SSRIs. A large RCT that was included in the review subsequently reported the proportion of women who had improved physical symptoms (observer rated scale of physical symptoms, including breast tenderness, bloating, headache, joint and muscle pain).[92] The first RCT (320 women with severe premenstrual syndrome (see glossary, p 2200) diagnosed before randomisation) found significant reduction of physical premenstrual symptoms with fluoxetine for six cycles versus placebo (substantial reduction of physical premenstrual symptoms: 11/95 [12%] with fluoxetine 20 mg *v* 13/85 [15%] with fluoxetine 60 mg *v* 4/94 [4%] with placebo; ARR fluoxetine *v* placebo 9.1%, 95% CI 1.5% to 16.7%; NNT 11 women treated for 6 cycles for 1 woman to have a substantial reduction in symptoms). No difference in physical premenstrual symptoms was found between the two doses of fluoxetine (20 mg *v* 60 mg daily; OR 0.73, 95% CI 0.31 to 1.71). The subsequent RCT (164 women with severe premenstrual syndrome diagnosed before randomisation) found significant improvement of overall premenstrual symptoms with venlafaxine (50–200 mg daily for 4 cycles) versus placebo (≥ 50% reduction in daily total symptom score: 41/68 [60%] with venlafaxine *v* 26/75 [35%] with placebo; ARR 25%, 95% CI 9% to 42%; NNT 4).[93] The second RCT (multicentre, 260 women with severe premenstrual syndrome and regular menstrual cycles who were not using hormonal contraception, in 20 different cities of the US, diagnosed prior to randomisation) compared fluoxetine (10 mg daily) and fluoxetine (20 mg) versus placebo. Treatments were started 14 days before the expected date of menses and stopped the first day of bleeding. It found that 20 mg of fluoxetine versus placebo produced significant improvement of overall premenstrual symptoms (breast tenderness, bloating, headache and joint/muscle pain as assessed with the Daily Record of Severity Problems total luteal scores). No detailed figures were provided for comparisons between groups. The RCT found an improvement in symptoms with a dose of 10 mg of fluoxetine.[94]

Harms: Common adverse effects were nausea, drowsiness/fatigue, nervousness, insomnia, headache, and sexual dysfunction (see table 2, p 2203).[91] The frequency of adverse events is similar to that seen with SSRIs in other populations.[92] The systematic review found that withdrawal because of adverse effects was more likely with SSRIs than with placebo (OR 2.4, 95% CI 1.6 to 3.7).[91] Adverse effects were more likely with the higher dose of fluoxetine.[92] The second RCT found no significant differences between groups in adverse effects such as dyspepsia, dysphagia, metrorrhagia, agitation, headache, insomnia, and nausea. However, decreased libido was more frequent reported with fluoxetine (placebo: 0%; 10 mg: 5.8%; 20 mg: 9.3%; $P = 0.007$). In contrast, accidental injury (definiton not specified) happened more frequently with placebo (6.8% with placebo; 0% with fluoxetine 10 mg; 1.2% with fluoxetine 20 mg; $P = 0.019$).[94]

Comment: SSRIs used in the RCTs were fluoxetine (7 RCTs), sertraline (5 RCTs), citalopram (1 RCT), fluvoxamine (1 RCT), and paroxetine (1 RCT).[91] Venlafaxine is described as an inhibitor of serotonin and norepinephrine (noradrenaline) uptake. The systematic review found significant heterogeneity of the results ($P < 0.0001$), but the results were robust and did not depend on the type of meta-analysis (fixed effects or random effects). Many of the harms attributed to treatment were frequent, and some (nervousness, headache, insomnia) were similar to the typical symptoms of premenstrual syndrome. However, the net effect of SSRI antidepressants versus placebo was a significant reduction of total symptom scores.[91,93] The second RCT[94] screened 1276 women and randomised 260. Reasons for exclusion included placebo response, physician decision, consent withdrawal, non-compliance to collect data in a digital diary. Of the randomised women, 218/260 (84%) finished the study.[94]

OPTION TIBOLONE

One small RCT found limited evidence of benefit from tibolone versus multivitamins.

Benefits: We found no systematic review but found one small RCT (18 women).[88] It found that tibolone for 3 months versus multivitamins (placebo) significantly improved premenstrual symptom scores (mean improvement in symptom score: –55% with tibolone *v* –10% with placebo; $P < 0.05$).

Harms: No adverse effects were reported.

Comment: The RCT was too small to offer reliable conclusions.

GLOSSARY

Severe premenstrual syndrome The definition of severe premenstrual syndrome varies among RCTs, but in recent studies[92,93] standardised criteria have been used to diagnose one variant of severe premenstrual syndrome (termed the Premenstrual Dysphoric Disorder), based on at least five symptoms, including one of four core psychological symptoms (from a list of 17 physical and psychological symptoms), being severe premenstrually and mild or absent postmenstrually. The 17 symptoms are depression, feeling hopeless or guilty, anxiety/tension, mood swings, irritability/persistent anger, decreased interest, poor concentration, fatigue, food craving or increased appetite, sleep disturbance, feeling out of control or overwhelmed, poor coordination, headache, aches, swelling/bloating/weight gain, cramps, and breast tenderness.

REFERENCES

1. O'Brien PMS. Premenstrual syndrome. London: Blackwell Science, 1987.
2. Rapkin AJ, Morgan M, Goldman L, et al. Progesterone metabolite allopregnanolone in women with premenstrual syndrome. *Obstet Gynecol* 1997;90:709–714.
3. O'Brien PMS. Helping women with premenstrual syndrome. *BMJ* 1993;307:1471–1475.
4. Budeiri DJ, Li WP, Dornan JC. Clinical trials of treatments of premenstrual syndrome: entry criteria and scales for measuring treatment outcomes. *Br J Obstet Gynaecol* 1994;101:689–695
5. Cochrane Menstrual Disorders and Subfertility Group. Search strategy for specialist registrar (Collaborative Review Groups). In: The Cochrane Library, Issue 4. Oxford: Update software, 1999.
6. Frackiewicz EJ, Shiovitz TM. Evaluation and management of premenstrual syndrome and premenstrual dysphoric disorder. *J Am Pharm Assoc* 2001;41:437–447. Search date 2001; primary sources Medline and hand searches of bibliographies of retrieved articles.
7. Freeman EW, Rickels K, Sondheimer SJ, et al. A double-blind trial of oral progesterone, alprazolam, and placebo in treatment of severe premenstrual syndrome. *JAMA* 1995;274:51–57.
8. Schmidt PJ, Grover GN, Rubinow DR. Alprazolam in the treatment of premenstrual syndrome: a double-blind, placebo-controlled trial. *Arch Gen Psychiatry* 1993;50:467–473.
9. Harrison WM, Endicott J, Rabkin JG, et al. Treatment of premenstrual dysphoria with alprazolam and placebo. *Psychopharmacol Bull* 1987;23:150–153.
10. Smith S, Rinehart JS, Ruddock VE, et al. Treatment of premenstrual syndrome with alprazolam: results of a double-blind, placebo-controlled, randomized crossover clinical trial. *Obstet Gynecol* 1987;70:37–43.
11. Harrison WM, Endicott J, Nee J. Treatment of premenstrual dysphoria with alprazolam: a controlled study. *Arch Gen Psychiatry* 1990;47:270–275.
12. Rickels K, Freeman E, Sondheimer S. Buspirone in treatment of premenstrual syndrome. *Lancet* 1989;1:777.
13. Landen M, Eriksson O, Sundblad C, et al. Compounds with affinity for serotonergic receptors in the treatment of premenstrual dysphoria: a comparison of buspirone, nefazodone and placebo. *Psychopharmacologia* 2001;155:292–298.
14. Pearlstein TB, Stone AB, Lund SA, et al. Comparison of fluoxetine, buproprion, and placebo in the treatment of premenstrual dysphoric disorder. *J Clin Psychopharmacol* 1997;17:261–266.
15. Sundblad C, Hedberg MA, Eriksson E. Clomipramine administered during the luteal phase reduces the symptoms of premenstrual syndrome: a placebo-controlled trial. *Neuropsychopharmacology* 1993;9:133–145.
16. Rausch JL, Janowsky DS, Golshan S, et al. Atenolol treatment of late luteal phase dysphoric disorder. *J Affect Disord* 1988;15:141–147.
17. Parry BL, Rosebthal NE, James SP, et al. Atenolol in premenstrual syndrome: A test of the melatonin hypothesis. *Psychiatry Res* 1991;37:131–138.
18. Diegoli MSC, DaFonseca AM, Diegoli CA, et al. A double-blind trial of four medications to treat severe premenstrual syndrome. *Int J Gynecol Obstet* 1998;62:63–67.
19. Singer K, Cheng R, Schou M. A controlled evaluation of lithium in the premenstrual tension syndrome. *Br J Psychiatry* 1974;124:50–51.
20. Sundblad C, Modigh K, Andersch B, et al. Clomipramine effectively reduces premenstrual irritability and dysphoria: a placebo-controlled trial. *Acta Psychiatr Scand* 1992;85:39–47.
21. Harrison WM, Endicott J, Nee J. Treatment of premenstrual depression with nortriptyline: a pilot study. *J Clin Psychiatry* 1989;50:136–139.
22. Freeman EW, Rickels K, Sandheimer SJ, et al. Differential response to antidepressants in women with premenstrual syndrome/premenstrual dysphoric disorder. *Arch Gen Psychiatry* 1999;56;932–939.
23. Andersch B. Bromocriptine and premenstrual symptoms: a survey of double blind trials. *Obstet Gynecol Surv* 1983;38:643–646.
24. Ylostalo P, Kauppila A, Puolakka J, et al. Bromocriptine and norethisterone in the treatment of premenstrual syndrome. *Obstet Gynecol* 1982;59:292–298.
25. Graham JJ, Harding PE, Wise PH, et al. Prolactin suppression in the treatment of premenstrual syndrome. *Med J Aust* 1978;2:18–20.
26. Kullander S, Svanberg L. Bromocriptine treatment of the premenstrual syndrome. *Acta Obstet Gynecol Scand* 1979;58:375–378.
27. Arrowsmith-Lowe T. Bromocriptine indications withdrawn. *FDA Med Bull* 1994;24:2.
28. Stevinson C, Ernst E. Complementary/alternative therapies for premenstrual syndrome: a systematic review of randomized controlled trials. *Am J Obstet*

Gynecol 2001;185:227–235. Search date 2000, primary sources Medline, Embase, Biosis, Cinahl, PsychoINFO, and the Cochrane Library Ciscom.
29. Morse C, Dennerstein L, Farrell E. A comparison of hormone therapy, coping skills training and relaxation for the relief of premenstrual syndrome. *J Behav Med* 1991;14:469–489.
30. Kirkby RJ. Changes in premenstrual symptoms and irrational thinking following cognitive-behavioural coping skills training. *J Consult Clin Psychol* 1994;62:1026–1032.
31. Blake F, Salkovskis P, Gath D, et al. Cognitive therapy for premenstrual syndrome: a controlled trial. *J Psychosom Res* 1998;45:307–318.
32. Corney RH, Stanton R, Newell R. Comparison of progesterone, placebo and behavioural psychotherapy in the treatment of premenstrual syndrome. *J Psychosom Obstet Gynaecol* 1990;11:211–220.
33. Christensen AP, Oei TPS. The efficacy of cognitive behaviour therapy in treating premenstrual dysphoric changes. *J Affect Disord* 1995;33:57–63.
34. Taylor D. Effectiveness of professional-peer group treatment: symptom management for women with PMS. *Res Nursing Health* 1999:22;496–511.
35. Arlane M. The use of a cognitive restructuring intervention in the treatment of premenstrual syndrome: A controlled study. *Dissert Abstracts Int* 1986;47:381.
36. Gilmore DH, Hawthorn RJ, Hart DM. Danol for premenstrual syndrome: a preliminary report of a placebo-controlled double-blind study. *J Int Med Res* 1985;13:129–130.
37. Watts JF, Butt WR, Logan ER. A clinical trial using danazol for the treatment of premenstrual tension. *Br J Obstet Gynaecol* 1987;94:30–34.
38. Deeny M, Hawthorn R, McKay HD. Low dose danazol in the treatment of the premenstrual syndrome. *Postgrad Med J* 1991;67:450–454.
39. Sarno APJ, Miller EJJ, Lundblad EG. Premenstrual syndrome: beneficial effects of periodic, low-dose danazol. *Obstet Gynecol* 1987;70:33–36.
40. Hahn PM, Van Vugt DA, Reid RL. A randomized, placebo-controlled, crossover trial of danazol for the treatment of premenstrual syndrome. *Psychoneuroendocrinology* 1995;20:193–209.
41. O'Brien PMS, Abukhalil IEH. Randomised controlled trial of the management of premenstrual syndrome and premenstrual mastalgia using luteal phase only danazol. *Am J Obstet Gynecol* 1999;180:18–23.
42. Hellberg D, Claesson B, Nilsson S. Premenstrual tension: a placebo-controlled efficacy study with spironolactone and medroxyprogesterone acetate. *Int J Gynaecol Obstet* 1991;34:243–248.
43. Wang M, Hammarback S, Lindhe BA, et al. Treatment of premenstrual syndrome by spironolactone: a double-blind, placebo-controlled study. *Acta Obstet Gynecol Scand* 1995;74:803–808.
44. Burnet RB, Radden HS, Easterbrook EG, et al. Premenstrual syndrome and spironolactone. *Aust N Z J Obstet Gynaecol* 1991;31:366–368.
45. Vellacott ID, Shroff NE, Pearce MY, et al. A double-blind, placebo-controlled evaluation of spironolactone in the premenstrual syndrome. *Curr Med Res Opin* 1987;10:450–456.
46. Werch A, Kane RE. Treatment of premenstrual tension with metolazone: a double-blind evaluation of a new diuretic. *Curr Ther Res Clin Exp* 1976;19:565–572.
47. Mattsson B, von Schoultz B. A comparison between lithium, placebo and a diuretic in premenstrual tension. *Acta Psychiatr Scand Suppl* 1974;255:75–84.
48. Hoffman JJ. A double blind crossover clinical trial of an OTC diuretic in the treatment of premenstrual tension and weight gain. *Curr Ther Res* 1979;26:575–580.
49. Budeiri D, Li WP, Dornan JC. Is evening primrose oil of value in the treatment of premenstrual syndrome? *Control Clin Trials* 1996;17:60–68. Search date 1993; primary sources Science Citation Index, Medline, Dissertation Abstracts, and companies who marketed evening primrose oil were approached for any published or unpublished trials.
50. Vaddadi KS. The use of gamma-linolenic acid and linoleic acid to differentiate between temporal lobe epilepsy and schizophrenia. *Prostaglandins Med* 1981;6:375–379.
51. Lemos D. The effects of aerobic training on women who suffer from premenstrual syndrome. *Dissert Abstracts Int* 1991;52:563.
52. Bibi KW. The effects of aerobic exercise on premenstrual syndrome symptoms. *Dissert Abstracts Int* 1995;56:6678.
53. Freeman EW, Sondheimer SJ, Rickels K. Gonadotrophin-releasing hormone agonist in the treatment of premenstrual symptoms with and without ongoing dysphoria: a controlled study. *Psychopharmacol Bull* 1997;33:303–309.
54. Brown CS, Ling FW, Andersen RN, et al. Efficacy of depot leuprolide in premenstrual syndrome: effect of symptom severity and type in a controlled trial. *Obstet Gynecol* 1994;84:779–786.
55. Helvacioglu A, Yeoman RR, Hazelton JM, et al. Premenstrual syndrome and related hormonal changes. Long-acting gonadotrophin releasing hormone agonist treatment. *J Reprod Med* 1993;38:864–870.
56. Muse KN, Cetel NS, Futterman LA, et al. The premenstrual syndrome. Effects of "medical ovariectomy". *N Engl J Med* 1984;311:1345–1349.
57. Mortola JF, Girton L, Fischer U. Successful treatment of severe premenstrual syndrome by combined use of gonadotrophin-releasing hormone agonist and estrogen/progestin. *J Clin Endocrinol Metab* 1991;72:252A–252F.
58. Mezrow G, Shoupe D, Spicer D, et al. Depot leuprolide acetate with estrogen and progestin add-back for long-term treatment of premenstrual syndrome. *Fertil Steril* 1994;62:932–937.
59. Hammarback S, Backstrom T. Induced anovulation as treatment of premenstrual tension syndrome: a double-blind cross-over study with GnRH-agonist versus placebo. *Acta Obstet Gynecol Scand* 1988;67:159–166.
60. West CP, Hillier H. Ovarian suppression with the gonadotrophin-releasing hormone agonist goserelin (Zoladex) in management of the premenstrual tension syndrome. *Hum Reprod* 1994;9:1058–1063.
61. Leather AT, Studd JWW, Watson NR, et al. The treatment of severe premenstrual syndrome with goserelin with and without 'add-back' estrogen therapy: a placebo-controlled study. *Gynecol Endocrinol* 1999;13:48–55.
62. Sundstrom I, Nyberg S, Bixo M, et al. Treatment of premenstrual syndrome with gonadotrophin-releasing hormone agonist in a low dose regimen. *Acta Obstet Gynecol Scand* 1999;78:891–899.
63. Di Carlo C, Palomba S, Tommaselli GA, et al. Use of leuprolide acetate plus tibolone in the treatment of severe premenstrual syndrome. *Fertil Steril* 2001;75:380–384.
64. Studd J, Leather AT. The need for add-back with gonadotrophin-releasing hormone agonist therapy. *Br J Obstet Gynaecol* 1996;103 Suppl 14:1–4.

65. Shaw RW, Soutter WP, Stanton SL. Gynaecology. New York: Churchill Livingstone, 1997.
66. Metcalf MG, Braiden V, Livesey JH, et al. The premenstrual syndrome: amelioration of symptoms after hysterectomy. *J Psychosom Res* 1992;36:569–584.
67. Osborn M, Gath D. Psychological and physical determinants of premenstrual symptoms before and after hysterectomy. *Psychol Med* 1990;20:565–572.
68. Casper RF, Hearn MT. The effect of hysterectomy and bilateral oophorectomy in women with severe premenstrual syndrome. *Am J Obstet Gynecol* 1990;162:105–109.
69. Casson P, Hahn PM, Van Vugt DA, et al. Lasting response to ovariectomy in severe intractable premenstrual syndrome. *Am J Obstet Gynecol* 1990;162:99–105.
70. Dhar V, Murphy BE. Double-blind randomized crossover trial of luteal phase estrogens (Premarin) in the premenstrual syndrome (PMS). *Psychoneuroendocrinology* 1990;15:489–493.
71. Watson NR, Studd JW, Savvas M, et al. Treatment of severe premenstrual syndrome with oestradiol patches and cyclical oral norethisterone. *Lancet* 1989;2:730–732.
72. de Lignieres B, Vincens M, Mauvais-Jarvis P, et al. Prevention of menstrual migraine by percutaneous oestradiol. *BMJ* 1986;293:1540.
73. Panay N. Treatment of depressive symptoms in women diagnosed as having premenstrual syndrome (PMS) with long cycle hormone replacement therapy (TridestraR). National Research Register, 1999.
74. Mira M, McNeil D, Fraser IS, et al. Mefenamic acid in the treatment of premenstrual syndrome. *Obstet Gynecol* 1986;68:395–398.
75. Jakubowicz DL, Godard E, Dewhurst J. The treatment of premenstrual tension with mefenamic acid: analysis of prostaglandin concentrations. *Br J Obstet Gynaecol* 1984;91:78–84.
76. Wood C, Jakubowicz D. The treatment of premenstrual symptoms with mefenamic acid. *Br J Obstet Gynaecol* 1980;87:627–630.
77. Gunston KD. Premenstrual syndrome in Cape Town. Part II: a double-blind placebo-controlled study of the efficacy of mefenamic acid. *S Afr Med J* 1986;70:159–160.
78. Budoff PW. No more menstrual cramps and other good news. New York: GP Putman and Sons, 1980.
79. Facchinetti F, Fioroni L, Sances G, et al. Naproxen sodium in the treatment of premenstrual symptoms: a placebo-controlled study. *Gynecol Obstet Invest* 1989;28:205–208.
80. Budoff PW. Use of prostaglandin inhibitors in the treatment of PMS. *Clin Obstet Gynecol* 1987;30(2):453–464.
81. Graham CA, Sherwin BB. A prospective treatment study of premenstrual symptoms using a triphasic oral contraceptive. *J Psychosom Res* 1992;36:257–266.
82. Freeman EW, Kroll R, Rapkin A, et al. Evaluation of a unique oral contraceptive in the treatment of premenstrual dysphoric disorder. *J Womens Health Gend Based Med* 2001;10:561–569.
83. Cullberg J. Mood changes and menstrual symptoms with different gestagen/estrogen combinations: a double blind comparison with a placebo. *Acta Psychiatr Scand* Suppl 1972; 236:1–86.
84. Morris NM, Udry JR. Contraceptive pills and day-by-day feelings of well-being. *Am J Obstet Gynecol* 1972;113:763–765.
85. Silbergeld S, Brast N, Noble EP. The menstrual cycle: a double blind study of symptoms, mood and behaviour and biochemical variables using Enovid and placebo. *Psychosom Med* 1971;33:411–428.
86. Wyatt K, Dimmock P, Jones P, et al. Efficacy of progesterone and progestogens in management of premenstrual syndrome: systematic review. *BMJ* 2001;323:776–780. Search date 2000; primary sources Embase, Medline, PsychINFO, the Cochrane controlled trial register, hand searches, and pharmaceutical companies who manufacture progesterone preparations.
87. Wyatt KM, Dimmock PW, O'Brien PMS. Vitamin B6 therapy: a systematic review of its efficacy in premenstrual syndrome. *BMJ* 1999;318:1375–1381. Search date 1998; primary sources Medline, Psychlit, and Cinahl.
88. Taskin O, Gokdeniz R, Yalcinoglu A, et al. Placebo-controlled cross-over study of effects of tibolone on premenstrual symptoms and peripheral beta-endorphin concentrations in premenstrual syndrome. *Hum Reprod* 1998;13:2402–2405.
89. Lauritzen CH, Reuter HD, Repges R, et al. Treatment of premenstrual tension syndrome with vitex agnus castus, controlled double blind study vs pyridoxine. *Phytomedicine* 1994;4:183–189.
90. Lauritzen C. Die behandling des premenstreullen syndoms. Doppelblind studie mi hochdosertem vitamin B6 gegen placebo. *Z Allg Med* 1988;64:275–278.
91. Dimmock PW, Wyatt KM, Jones PW, et al. Efficacy of selective serotonin–reuptake inhibitors in premenstrual syndrome: A systematic. *Lancet* 2000;356:1131–1136. Search date not stated; primary sources Medline, Embase, PsychLit, Cinahl, Cochrane Controlled Trials Register, and reference lists of retrieved articles.
92. Steiner M, Romano SJ, Babcock S, et al. The efficacy of fluoxetine in improving physical symptoms associated with premenstrual dysphoric disorder. *Br J Obstet Gynaecol* 2001;108:462–468.
93. Freeman EW, Rickels K, Yonkers KA, et al. Venlafaxine in the treatment of premenstrual dysphoric disorder. *Obstet Gynecol* 2001;98:737–744.
94. Cohen LS, Miner C, Brown E, et al. Premenstrual Daily Fluoxetine for Premenstrual Dysphoric Disorder: A placebo-controlled clinical trial using computerized diaries. *Obstet Gynecol* 2002;100:435–44.

Katrina Wyatt
Lecturer in Health Services Research
Exeter and North Devon Research and Development Support Unit, Exeter, UK

Competing interests: None declared.

The following previous contributors of this topic would also like to be acknowledged: P Dimmock, and PMS O'Brien.

TABLE 1 **Commonly reported symptoms in women with premenstrual syndrome (see text, p 2186).[2]**

Psychological symptoms	Irritability, depression, crying/tearfulness, anxiety, tension, mood swings, lack of concentration, confusion, forgetfulness, unsociableness, restlessness, temper outbursts/anger, sadness/blues, loneliness
Behavioural symptoms	Fatigue, dizziness, sleep/insomnia, decreased efficiency, accident prone, sexual interest changes, increased energy, tiredness
Physical symptoms: pain	Headache/migraine, breast tenderness/soreness/pain/swelling (collectively known as premenstrual mastalgia), back pain, abdominal cramps, general pain
Physical symptoms: bloatedness and swelling	Weight gain, abdominal bloating or swelling, oedema of arms and legs, water retention
Appetite symptoms	Increased appetite, food cravings, nausea

TABLE 2 **Frequency of adverse events with selective serotonin reuptake inhibitors versus placebo in women with premenstrual syndrome (see text, p 2199).[91–93]**

Symptom	Systematic review[91]	RCT[93]
Nausea	66/323 (20%) *v* 13/222 (6%) NNH = 7	34/77 (45%) *v* 10/80 (13%) NNH = 3
Insomnia	56/323 (17%) *v* 17/222 (8%) NNH = 11	26/77 (34%) *v* 13/80 (16%) NNH = 6
Dizziness	32/323 (10%) *v* 46/222 (21%) NNT = 9	25/77 (32%) *v* 4/80 (4%) NNH = 4
Fatigue	46/323 (14%) *v* 24/222 (11%) NS	18/77 (23%) *v* 13/80 (16%) NS
Headache	24/323 (7%) *v* 16/222 (7%) NS	16/77 (21%) *v* 23/80 (29%) NS
Dry mouth	41/323 (13%) *v* 13/222 (6%) NNH = 15	13/77 (17%) *v* 6/80 (8%) NS
Sexual dysfunction	23/323 (7%) *v* 6/222 (3%) NNH = 23	12/77 (16%) *v* 0/80 (0%) NNH = 7

NS, not significant.

Pyelonephritis in non-pregnant women

Search date November 2002

Bazian Ltd

QUESTIONS

INTERVENTIONS

*Not based on placebo controlled RCTs. Such studies are likely to be considered unethical.

Key Messages

- **Intravenous antibiotics (ampicillin, co-trimoxazole) in women admitted to hospital with uncomplicated infection** We found no RCTs comparing intravenous antibiotics versus no antibiotics. However, consensus holds that these drugs are effective, and it is unlikely that such an RCT would now be performed. We found insufficient evidence to compare clinical effects of different intravenous regimens.
- **Oral antibiotics (co-trimoxazole, co-amoxiclav, or a fluoroquinolone) for women with uncomplicated infection** We found no RCTs comparing oral antibiotics versus no antibiotics. However, consensus holds that these drugs are effective, and it is unlikely that such an RCT would now be performed. One systematic review and one subsequent RCT in women with uncomplicated pyelonephritis have found no consistent differences among oral co-trimoxazole, co-amoxiclav, or fluoroquinolones (ciprofloxacin, norfloxacin, levofloxacin, or lomefloxacin) in bacteriological or clinical cure rates.
- **Inpatient versus outpatient management** We found no RCTs comparing inpatient versus outpatient management of women with acute uncomplicated pyelonephritis.

Pyelonephritis in non-pregnant women

DEFINITION Acute pyelonephritis, or upper urinary tract infection, is an infection of the kidney characterised by pain when passing urine, fever, flank pain, nausea, and vomiting. White blood cells are almost always present in the urine and occasionally white blood cell casts are also seen on urine microscopy. Uncomplicated infection occurs in an otherwise healthy person without any other underlying disease. Complicated pyelonephritis occurs in people with structural or functional urinary tract abnormalities or additional diseases. People with acute pyelonephritis may also be divided into those able to take oral antibiotics and without signs of sepsis who may be managed at home, and those requiring treatment delivered by injection whilst in hospital.

INCIDENCE/ PREVALENCE In the USA, there are 250 000 cases of acute pyelonephritis a year.[1] Worldwide prevalence and incidence are unknown.

AETIOLOGY/ RISK FACTORS Pyelonephritis is most commonly caused when bacteria in the bladder ascend the ureters and invade the kidneys. In some cases, this may result in bacteria entering and multiplying in the bloodstream.

PROGNOSIS Complications include sepsis, infection that spreads to other organs, renal impairment, and renal abscess. Conditions such as underlying renal disease, diabetes mellitus, and immunosuppression may worsen prognosis, but we found no good long term evidence about rates of sepsis or death among such people.

AIMS OF INTERVENTION To reduce the duration and severity of symptoms; to prevent or minimise potential complications, with minimum adverse effects.

OUTCOMES Urine culture after treatment; signs and symptoms of infection; rates of complications of infection; and adverse effects of treatment.

METHODS *Clinical Evidence* search and appraisal November 2002. We excluded studies that were primarily in men, pregnant women, and people with complicated pyelonephritis.

QUESTION What are the effects of treatments for acute pyelonephritis?

OPTION ORAL ANTIBIOTICS (CO-TRIMOXAZOLE, CO-AMOXICLAV, OR A FLUOROQUINOLONE) FOR WOMEN WITH UNCOMPLICATED INFECTION

We found no RCTs comparing oral antibiotics versus no antibiotics. However, consensus holds that these drugs are effective, and it is unlikely that such an RCT would now be performed. One systematic review and one subsequent RCT in women with uncomplicated pyelonephritis have found no consistent differences among oral co-trimoxazole, co-amoxiclav, or a fluoroquinolone (ciprofloxacin, norfloxacin, levofloxacin, or lomefloxacin) in bacteriological or clinical cure rates.

Benefits: **Versus placebo:** We found no systematic review or RCTs. **Versus other oral antibiotics:** We found one systematic review (search date 1991, 9 RCTs, 470 men and non-pregnant women) (see table 1, p 2209),[2] and one subsequent RCT[3] comparing different oral antibiotics in acute pyelonephritis. Five RCTs identified by the review were conducted in people outside hospital and four in people admitted to hospital. The studies were conducted in the USA, Europe, and Peru. All RCTs included in the review included more women than men. Most excluded people with complicating factors such as structural abnormalities of the urinary tract, additional diseases, pregnancy, or signs of possible sepsis. All but one of the RCTs in the review found no significant difference between different antibiotics in rates of early cure (negative urine culture within 7–10 days), and six of the RCTs found no significant difference in rates of late cure (negative urine culture 2–4 weeks or more after stopping treatment). However, several of the individual RCTs included were too small to rule out a significant difference between antibiotic regimens. The subsequent RCT (186 people with acute uncomplicated pyelonephritis treated at home) compared oral levofloxacin (250 mg/day for 10 days) versus either oral ciprofloxacin (500 mg twice daily for 10 days) or oral lomefloxacin (400 mg/day for 14 days) and found similar clinical cure rates for all three antibiotics (92% with levofloxacin *v* 88% with ciprofloxacin *v* 80% with lomefloxacin; extraction of absolute numbers and significance testing not possible).[3] **Versus intravenous antibiotics:** We found no RCTs in women with uncomplicated pyelonephritis.

Harms: The subsequent RCT reported adverse effects in 3/124 (2%) people taking levofloxacin, 6/80 (8%) people taking ciprofloxacin, and 3/55 (5%) people taking lomefloxacin.[3] Gastrointestinal symptoms were common with both ciprofloxacin and levofloxacin, whereas rash was the most common adverse effect with lomefloxacin. One of the 186 people discontinued treatment (lomefloxacin) because of adverse effects.[3]

Comment: The lack of evidence in women with pyelonephritis comparing oral antibiotics versus placebo reflects the fact that RCTs in this area would be considered unethical. Calculated cure rates from the systematic review comparing the oral antibiotic regimens are likely to overestimate rates that would be achieved in clinical practice because many people were excluded, including those who experienced adverse effects, had growth of resistant bacteria on initial culture, or did not adhere to treatment.[2] The high rate of ampicillin resistance found in laboratory tests has led to consensus that ampicillin and amoxicillin (amoxycillin) are not recommended in pyelonephritis. We found no direct evidence to confirm or refute this view. Ampicillin and amoxicillin were found in the trials to have cure rates comparable with other antibiotics, but the studies were too small to exclude clinically important differences. We found one RCT (376 adults with complicated urinary tract infection or uncomplicated pyelonephritis; 57% women) comparing oral gatifloxacin versus oral ciprofloxacin.[4] It was unclear what proportion of study participants were women with uncomplicated pyelonephritis. About half of all participants were included in the analysis, making results difficult to interpret.

OPTION **INTRAVENOUS ANTIBIOTICS (AMPICILLIN, CO-TRIMOXAZOLE) IN WOMEN ADMITTED TO HOSPITAL WITH UNCOMPLICATED INFECTION**

We found no RCTs comparing intravenous antibiotics versus no antibiotics. However, consensus holds that these drugs are effective, and it is unlikely that such an RCT would now be performed. We found insufficient evidence to compare clinical effects of different intravenous regimens.

Benefits: **Versus placebo:** We found no systematic review and no RCTs. **Versus other intravenous antibiotics:** We found no systematic review. We found one RCT (85 women admitted to hospital for acute uncomplicated pyelonephritis; see comment below), which compared intravenous ampicillin (1 g every 6 hours) versus intravenous co-trimoxazole (160 mg/800 mg twice daily), initiated before culture results were known.[5] Both regimens were combined with intravenous gentamicin and followed by oral treatment with either ampicillin or co-trimoxazole. The RCT found that all the women who completed the trial displayed a satisfactory clinical response (defined as all symptoms related to the infection having resolved during treatment), and found no significant difference in the number of women with a recurrence of bacteria in the urine after 28 days between ampicillin and co-trimoxazole (1/20 [5%] with ampicillin *v* 2/27 [7%] with co-trimoxazole; RR 0.70, 95% CI 0.07 to 6.94). We found no other adequately designed RCTs comparing treatments that included intravenous quinolones, cephalosporins, broad spectrum β lactams, or co-trimoxazole. **Plus oral antibiotics:** We found one RCT (118 women admitted with acute uncomplicated pyelonephritis), which compared a single dose of intravenous tobramycin (2 mg/kg) plus oral ciprofloxacin (500 mg twice daily for 10 days) versus oral ciprofloxacin plus intravenous placebo (0.9% saline solution).[6] Clinical success or failure was categorised, with failure defined as the persistence of fever or pain after 48 hours of treatment. The RCT found no significant difference in rates of clinical success between intravenous tobramycin plus oral ciprofloxacin and oral ciprofloxacin plus placebo (58/60 [97%] with intravenous tobramycin plus oral ciprofloxacin *v* 54/58 [93%] with oral ciprofloxacin plus placebo; RR 1.04, 95% CI 0.95 to 1.13). **Versus oral antibiotics:** We found no RCTs in women with uncomplicated pyelonephritis.

Harms: The RCT comparing intravenous regimens found no significant difference in the total number of possible medication related adverse effects between treatments (10/32 [32%] with ampicillin *v* 13/39 [33%] with co-trimoxazole; RR 0.90, 95% CI 0.48 to 1.85).[6] Common adverse effects with ampicillin include rash, diarrhoea, and vaginitis, and with co-trimoxazole include nausea, vomiting, and vaginitis. The RCT comparing intravenous tobramycin plus ciprofloxacin versus ciprofloxacin plus placebo reported "no undesirable side effects were observed".[6] No further details were provided.

Comment: RCTs comparing antibiotics versus placebo would be considered unethical in women with uncomplicated pyelonephritis. The RCT comparing intravenous regimens reported that 47/85 (55%)

women completed the trial to the 28 days' follow up assessment; 14/42 (33%) women receiving ampicillin were infected with ampicillin resistant isolates and were withdrawn from the study.[5] There is a consensus view that the choice of empirical antibiotics should take into account the setting, medical history of the patient, Gram stain of the urine, previous infecting organism, and local antibiotic sensitivities. We found one RCT (258 adults with complicated urinary tract infection or either uncomplicated or complicated pyelonephritis; 58% women) comparing intravenous ertapenem versus intravenous ceftriaxone.[7] It was unclear what proportion of study participants were women with uncomplicated pyelonephritis, and less than three quarters of all participants were included in the analysis, making results difficult to interpret.

OPTION INPATIENT VERSUS OUTPATIENT MANAGEMENT

We found no RCTs comparing inpatient versus outpatient management of women with acute uncomplicated pyelonephritis.

Benefits: We found no systematic review and no RCTs.

Harms: We found no RCTs.

Comment: Hospitals might be able to provide closer monitoring and supervision of people with pyelonephritis than can be provided outside hospital. However, we found no RCTs to clarify whether treatment in hospital delivers any benefit in terms of outcomes or whether there is an increased risk of harm from hospital treatment.

REFERENCES

1. Stamm WE, Hooton TM, Johnson JR. Urinary tract infection: from pathogenesis to treatment. *J Infect Dis* 1989;15:400–406.
2. Pinson AG, Philbrick JT, Lindbeck GH, et al. Oral antibiotic therapy for acute pyelonephritis: a methodologic review of the literature. *J Gen Intern Med* 1992;7:544–553. Search date 1991; primary sources Medline and Current Contents.
3. Richard GA, Klimberg IN, Fowler CL, et al. Levofloxacin versus ciprofloxacin versus lomefloxacin in acute pyelonephritis. *Urology* 1998;52:51–55.
4. Cox CE, Marbury TC, Pittman WG, et al. A randomized, double-blind, multicenter comparison of gatifloxacin versus ciprofloxacin in the treatment of complicated urinary tract infection and pyelonephritis. *Clin Ther* 2002;24:223–236.
5. Johnson JR, Lyons MF, Pearce W, et al. Therapy for women hospitalized with acute pyelonephritis: a randomized trial of ampicillin versus trimethoprim–sulfamethoxazole for 14 days. *J Infect Dis* 1991;163:325–330.
6. Le Conte P, Simon N, Bourrier P, et al. Acute pyelonephritis. Randomized multicentre double-blind study comparing ciprofloxacin with combined ciprofloxacin and tobramycin [French]. *Presse Med* 2001;30:11–15.
7. Jimenez-Cruz F, Jasovich A, Cajigas J, et al. A prospective, multicenter, randomized, double-blind study comparing ertapenem and ceftriaxone followed by appropriate oral therapy for complicated urinary tract infections in adults. *Urology* 2002;60:16–22.

Bazian Ltd
London
UK

Competing interests: None declared.

The following previous contributors of this topic would also like to be acknowledged: Lisa Chew, Stephan Finn, Ruth Jepson, and Bruce Cooper.

TABLE 1 Oral antibiotic treatment for acute pyelonephritis: results of RCTs (see text, p 2205).[2]

Oral antibiotic regimens	Total number of people	Early cure* rates %	Late cure* rates %	P value
Amoxicillin 500 mg three times daily for 14 days	16	NA	94	NS
Co-trimoxazole 160 mg/800 mg twice daily for 14 days	12	NA	92	
Norfloxacin 400 mg twice daily for 10 days	14	100	86	NS
Co-trimoxazole 160 mg/800 mg twice daily for 10 days	10	100	90	
Ampicillin 500 mg four times daily for 10 days	8	88	NA	NS
Cefaclor 250 mg twice daily for 10 days	6	67	NA	
Norfloxacin 400 mg twice daily for 7 days or longer	3	67	NA	NS
Co-trimoxazole 160 mg/800 mg twice daily for 7 days or longer	12	92	NA	
Co-amoxiclav 250 mg/125 mg three times daily for 10 days	54	94	85	P = 0.02 for late cure; NS for early cure
Co-trimoxazole 160 mg/800 mg twice daily for 10 days	50	82	64	
Ampicillin 500 mg four times daily for 2 or 6 weeks	17	100	47	P = 0.004 for late cure; NS for early cure
Co-trimoxazole 160 mg/800 mg twice daily for 2 or 6 weeks	22	100	91	
Amoxicillin 2000 mg one time dose then 1000 mg twice daily for 9 days	22	100	100	NS
Amoxicillin 750 mg three times daily for 12 days	23	96	87	
Cefetamet 2000 mg once daily or 1000 mg twice daily for 10–15 days	28	93	79	NS
Cefadroxil 1000 mg twice daily for 10–15 days	22	73	52	
Norfloxacin 400 mg twice daily for 14 days	76	91	82	P < 0.0001 for both early and late cures
Cefadroxil 1000 mg twice daily for 14 days	75	59	44	

*Early cure: negative urine culture within 7–10 days of starting treatment; late cure: negative urine culture 2–4 weeks or more after stopping treatment. NA, not available; NS, not significant. Pinson AG, Philbrick JT, Lindbeck GH, et al. Oral antibiotic therapy for acute pyelonephritis; a methodologic review of the literature. *J Gen Intern Med* 1992;7:544–553. Reprinted by permission of Blackwell Science, Inc.

Recurrent cystitis in non-pregnant women

Search date April 2003

Adriana Wechsler

QUESTIONS

INTERVENTIONS

Key Messages

- **Continuous antibiotic prophylaxis (trimethoprim, co-trimoxazole, nitrofurantoin, cefaclor, or a quinolone)** RCTs have found that continuous antibiotic prophylaxis for 6–12 months with trimethoprim, co-trimoxazole, nitrofurantoin, cefaclor, or a quinolone reduces rates of recurrent cystitis compared with placebo, and have found no consistent difference in recurrence rates among different continuous regimens. One RCT comparing continuous daily antibiotic prophylaxis versus postcoital antibiotic prophylaxis found no significant difference in rates of positive urine culture after 1 year.
- **Postcoital antibiotic prophylaxis (co-trimoxazole, nitrofurantoin, or a quinolone)** RCTs have found that co-trimoxazole, nitrofurantoin, or a quinolone up to 2 hours after sexual intercourse reduces the rates of cystitis compared with placebo. One RCT comparing continuous daily antibiotic prophylaxis versus postcoital antibiotic prophylaxis found no significant difference in rates of positive urine culture after 1 year.
- **Cranberry juice and cranberry products** One systematic review of two weak RCTs provided insufficient evidence to assess cranberry juice and other cranberry products in women with recurrent cystitis.
- **Prophylaxis with methenamine hippurate** One systematic review of weak RCTs provided insufficient evidence to assess methenamine hippurate (hexamine hippurate) in women with recurrent cystitis.
- **Single dose self administered co-trimoxazole** One small RCT that single dose, self administered co-trimoxazole started at the onset of cystitis symptoms was less effective in reducing recurrence rates over 1 year than continuous co-trimoxazole prophylaxis. However, evidence was too limited to draw firm conclusions.

DEFINITION Cystitis is an infection of the lower urinary tract, which causes pain when passing urine, and causes frequency, urgency, haematuria, or suprapubic pain not associated with passing urine. White blood cells and bacteria are almost always present in the urine. The presence of fever, flank pain, nausea, or vomiting suggests pyelonephritis (upper urinary tract infection) (see pyelonephritis in non-pregnant women, p 2204). Recurrent cystitis may be either a reinfection (after successful eradication of infection) or a relapse after inadequate treatment.

INCIDENCE/ PREVALENCE The incidence of cystitis among premenopausal sexually active women is 0.5–0.7 infections per person year,[1] and 20–40% of women will experience cystitis during their lifetime. Of those, 20% will develop recurrence, almost always (90% of cases) because of reinfection rather than relapse. Rates of infection fall during the winter months.[2]

AETIOLOGY/ RISK FACTORS Cystitis is caused by uropathogenic bacteria in the faecal flora that colonise the vaginal and periurethral openings, and ascend the urethra into the bladder. Prior infection, sexual intercourse, and exposure to vaginal spermicide are risk factors for developing cystitis.[3,4]

PROGNOSIS We found little evidence on the long term effects of untreated cystitis. One study found that progression to pyelonephritis was infrequent, and that most cases of cystitis regressed spontaneously, although symptoms sometimes persisted for several months.[5] Women with a baseline rate of more than two infections a year, over many years, are likely to have ongoing recurrent infections.[6]

AIMS OF INTERVENTION To prevent recurrent cystitis in women predisposed to frequent infections, with minimal adverse effects of treatment.

OUTCOMES Rate of infection based on symptoms and urine culture.

METHODS *Clinical Evidence* search and appraisal January 1998 to April 2003. We reviewed all systematic reviews and RCTs comparing different forms of prophylaxis, or comparing prophylaxis versus placebo in non-pregnant women with a history of recurrent cystitis. We excluded studies in populations consisting mainly of men or pregnant women.

QUESTION **Which interventions prevent further recurrence of cystitis in women experiencing at least two infections per year?**

OPTION **CONTINUOUS ANTIBIOTIC PROPHYLAXIS (TRIMETHOPRIM, CO-TRIMOXAZOLE, NITROFURANTOIN, CEFACLOR, OR A QUINOLONE)**

RCTs have found that continuous antibiotic prophylaxis for 6–12 months with trimethoprim, co-trimoxazole, nitrofurantoin, cefaclor, or a quinolone reduces rates of recurrent cystitis compared with placebo, and have

found no consistent difference in recurrence rates among different continuous regimens. One RCT comparing postcoital versus continuous daily antibiotic prophylaxis found no significant difference in rates of positive urine culture after 1 year.

Benefits: We found no systematic review. We found eight RCTs (in women with at least 2 episodes of cystitis per year) comparing different regimens for continuous antibiotic prophylaxis lasting 6–12 months (see table 1, p 2217).[7–14] **Versus placebo or no treatment:** Four of the RCTs (225 women) found that active treatment (co-trimoxazole, nitrofurantoin, or a quinolone) significantly reduced rates of cystitis compared with placebo or no treatment.[7–9] **Versus each other:** One RCT (72 women) found that women taking oral nitrofurantoin (100 mg at night) compared with oral trimethoprim (100 mg at night) had significantly fewer episodes of cystitis after 12 months ($P < 0.05$; absolute numbers not reported).[10] Four other RCTs compared different antibiotic regimens versus each other and found no significant difference in numbers of infections among treatments over 6–12 months.[7,11–13] **Versus postcoital prophylaxis:** One RCT (135 women) compared daily oral ciprofloxacin (125 mg) versus postcoital (within 2 hours of sexual intercourse) oral ciprofloxacin (125 mg) (see benefits of postcoital prophylaxis, p 2213). It found no significant difference in the number of positive urine cultures after 1 year (27/239 [11%] positive urine cultures with daily prophylaxis *v* 32/254 [13%] with postcoital prophylaxis; RR 0.9, 95% CI 0.55 to 1.45).[8]

Harms: Rates of adverse effects in the RCTs ranged from 7–40% for trimethoprim, 0–40% for nitrofurantoin, 5% for cefaclor, 7–21% for norfloxacin, and 13% for ciprofloxacin.[7–9,11–13] The most common adverse effects for all agents were gastrointestinal symptoms, rash, and yeast vaginitis. One cohort study (see comment below) reported no significant adverse effects in women taking trimethoprim, co-trimoxazole, or nitrofurantoin, even when treatment continued for as long as 5 years. The development of bacterial resistance from continuous antibiotic prophylaxis was rare. However, the number of co-trimoxazole resistant infections increased during the latter part of the study.[2]

Comment: Many of the RCTs were not placebo controlled or blinded, and had small study populations. However, most of the reported rates of infection in the RCTs comparing different antibiotic regimens versus each other were much less than 0.6 per person year, suggesting that they were all effective in reducing the rate of infection in people with a history of recurrent cystitis.[7,10–13] These studies were not powered to exclude a clinically important difference between treatments, and adjustments were not made for confounding factors such as frequency of sexual intercourse. We found one cohort study (51 non-pregnant women with a baseline rate of more than 2 urinary tract infections a year over many years), which compared continuous treatment with three different antibiotics (trimethoprim, co-trimoxazole, or nitrofurantoin) for more than 12 months.[2] It found that all were effective in preventing both cystitis and pyelonephritis for over 112 person years.

OPTION POSTCOITAL ANTIBIOTIC PROPHYLAXIS

RCTs have found that co-trimoxazole, nitrofurantoin, or a quinolone up to 2 hours after sexual intercourse reduces the rates of cystitis compared with placebo. One RCT comparing postcoital versus continuous daily antibiotic prophylaxis found no significant difference in rates of cystitis after 1 year.

Benefits: We found no systematic review. **Versus placebo or no treatment:** We found four RCTs (in women with at least 2 episodes of cystitis per year) comparing postcoital (within 2 hours of sexual intercourse) antibiotic regimens versus placebo or no treatment evaluated over 6–14 months.[8,15–17] All four RCTs found that active treatment (co-trimoxazole, nitrofurantoin, or a quinolone) significantly reduced rates of cystitis (see table 2, p 2218). **Versus continuous daily prophylaxis:** See benefits of continuous antibiotic prophylaxis, p 2212.

Harms: Rates of adverse effects were as follows: co-trimoxazole 18%, ciprofloxacin 6%, and nitrofurantoin less than 1%.[8,15–17] The most common adverse effects for all agents were gastrointestinal symptoms, rash, and yeast vaginitis.

Comment: Only one of the studies was placebo controlled and blinded.[15] Adjustments were not made for confounding factors such as frequency of sexual intercourse.

OPTION SINGLE DOSE SELF ADMINISTERED CO-TRIMOXAZOLE

One small RCT found that single dose, self administered co-trimoxazole started at the onset of cystitis symptoms was less effective in reducing recurrence rates over 1 year than continuous co-trimoxazole prophylaxis. However, evidence was too limited to draw firm conclusions.

Benefits: We found no systematic review but found one RCT (38 non-pregnant women with 2 or more culture documented urinary tract infections in the previous 12 months; see comment below).[18] The RCT compared continuous oral co-trimoxazole prophylaxis (40 mg/200 mg) versus single dose, self administered co-trimoxazole (40 mg/200 mg) to be taken at the onset of cystitis symptoms. It found that single dose co-trimoxazole was significantly less effective in reducing the number of episodes of cystitis compared with continuous co-trimaxazole (2.2 infections per person year with treatment at onset of symptoms *v* 0.22 infections per person year with continuous prophylaxis; $P < 0.001$; see comment below).

Harms: The RCT reported a total of eight adverse reactions; five in women taking continuous antibiotic prophylaxis compared with three in women taking single dose treatment (CI not reported).[18] Adverse reactions included mild nausea, abdominal pain, rash, mouth ulcers, and yeast vulvovaginitis.

Comment: The RCT reported that 10/38 (26%) women did not complete the full study protocol, and it is not clear whether analysis of results was by intention to treat.[18] It found that the women were almost always able to diagnose their own episodes of cystitis from symptoms (positive predictive value 92%). The higher rate of cystitis in women using single dose prophylaxis is to be expected because treatment was only administered after the onset of symptoms.

OPTION CRANBERRY JUICE AND CRANBERRY PRODUCTS

One systematic review of two weak RCTs provided insufficient evidence to assess cranberry juice and other cranberry products in women with recurrent cystitis.

Benefits: We found one systematic review (search date 2001, 2 RCTs, 211 women) comparing cranberry juice or other cranberry products versus placebo in the prevention of urinary tract infections (see comment below).[19] The first RCT (19 women with recurrent cystitis) included in the review compared cranberry capsules versus placebo (see comment below). The review reported 21 infections among 10 women who completed the study; six of these infections occurred in women taking cranberry capsules (the number of infections/women in the different groups was not reported; significance testing not possible). The second RCT (192 elderly women) compared cranberry juice versus placebo and found that cranberry juice significantly reduced the rate of infection (defined as ≥100 000 organisms/mL of urine plus white blood cells in the urine; OR 0.42, $P = 0.004$; see comment below).

Harms: The review gave no information on adverse effects.[19]

Comment: The RCTs identified by the review were small, with high withdrawal rates (47% in the first RCT and 20% in the second RCT), and the lack of intention to treat analyses in either trial may mean that they overestimated the effectiveness of cranberry juice and products.[19] High withdrawal rates suggest that long term adherence may be difficult to achieve.

OPTION PROPHYLAXIS WITH METHENAMINE HIPPURATE

One systematic review of weak RCTs provided insufficient evidence to assess methenamine hippurate (hexamine hippurate) in women with recurrent cystitis.

Benefits: We found one systematic review (search date 2000, 3 RCTs, 372 women) comparing methenamine hippurate versus placebo or antibiotics.[20] The review concluded that there was insufficient evidence about effects of methenamine hippurate (see comment below).

Harms: We found no reliable RCTs.

Comment: The review found three RCTs comparing methenamine hippurate versus placebo or versus antibiotics in women with recurrent urinary tract infection.[20] All had important problems with their methods, principally that each participant could contribute more than once to assessment of recurrence rate.[21–23] Two of the included RCTs were small (30 and 52 women with recurrent lower urinary tract infection).[21,22] Both found that methenamine hippurate reduced recurrence compared with placebo (monthly recurrence rate 0.03–0.08 episodes per month with methenamine hippurate *v* 0.25–0.34 episodes per month with placebo; CI not reported).[21,22] The largest of the RCTs (290 people [92% women] with recurrent urinary tract infection) also included women with chronic pyelonephritis. It found that methenamine hippurate reduced recurrence of cystitis compared with placebo after 1 year (recurrence was observed on 34% of tests in women receiving methenamine hippurate *v* 63.2% with placebo; CI not reported).[23]

Substantive changes

Continuous antibiotic prophylaxis (trimethoprim, co-trimoxazole, nitrofurantoin, cefaclor, or a quinolone) One RCT added;[14] conclusions unchanged.

REFERENCES

1. Hooton TM, Scholes D, Hughes JP, et al. A prospective study of risk factors for symptomatic urinary tract infection in young women. *N Engl J Med* 1996;335:468–474.
2. Stamm WE, McKevitt M, Roberts PL, et al. Natural history of recurrent urinary tract infections in women. *Rev Infect Dis* 1991;13:77–84.
3. Fihn SD, Latham RH, Roberts P, et al. Association between diaphragm use and urinary tract infection. *JAMA* 1985;254:240–245.
4. Fihn SD, Boyko EJ, Normand EH, et al. Association between use of spermicide-coated condoms and *Escherichia coli* urinary tract infection in young women. *Am J Epidemiol* 1996;144:512–520.
5. Mabeck CE. Treatment of uncomplicated urinary tract infection in non-pregnant women. *Postgrad Med J* 1972;48:69–75.
6. Stamm WE, Counts GW, McKevitt M, et al. Urinary prophylaxis with trimethoprim and trimethoprim-sulfamethoxazole: efficacy, influence on the natural history of recurrent bacteriuria and cost control. *Rev Infect Dis* 1982;4:450–455.
7. Stamm WE, Counts GW, Wagner KF, et al. Antimicrobial prophylaxis of recurrent urinary tract infections: a double-blind placebo-controlled trial. *Ann Intern Med* 1980;92:770–775.
8. Melekos MD, Asbach HW, Gerharz E, et al. Post-intercourse versus daily ciprofloxacin prophylaxis for recurrent urinary tract infections in premenopausal women. *J Urol* 1997;157:935–939.
9. Nicolle LE, Harding GKM, Thompson M, et al. Prospective, randomized, placebo-controlled trial of norfloxacin for the prophylaxis of recurrent urinary tract infection in women. *Antimicrob Agents Chemother* 1989;33:1032–1035.
10. Brumfitt W, Smith GW, Hamilton-Miller JMT, et al. A clinical comparison between macrodantin and trimethoprim for prophylaxis in women with recurrent urinary infection. *J Antimicrob Chemother* 1985;16:111–120.
11. Raz R, Boger S. Long-term prophylaxis with norfloxacin versus nitrofurantoin in women with recurrent urinary tract infection. *Antimicrob Agents Chemother* 1991;35:1241–1242.
12. Brumfitt W, Hamilton-Miller JMT, Smith GW, et al. Comparative trial of norfloxacin and macrocrystalline nitrofurantoin (Macrodantin) in the prophylaxis of recurrent urinary tract infection in women. *Q J Med* 1991;81:811–820.
13. Brumfitt W, Hamilton-Miller JMT. A comparative trial of low-dose cefaclor and macrocrystalline nitrofurantoin in the prevention of recurrent urinary tract infection. *Infection* 1995;23:98–102.
14. Martorana C, Giberti C, Damonte P: Preventive treatment of recurring cystitis in women. Double-blind randomised study using cinoxacin and placebo. *Minerva Urol Nefrol* 1984;36:43–49.
15. Stapleton A, Latham RH, Johnson C, et al. Postcoital antimicrobial prophylaxis for recurrent urinary tract infection: a randomized, double-blind placebo-controlled trial. *JAMA* 1990;264:703–706.
16. Pfau A, Sacks TG. Effective postcoital quinolone prophylaxis of recurrent urinary tract infection in women. *J Urol* 1994;152:136–138.
17. Pfau A, Sacks T, Englestein D. Recurrent urinary tract infections in premenopausal women: prophylaxis based on an understanding of the pathogenesis. *J Urol* 1983;129:1153–1156.
18. Wong ES, McKevitt M, Running K, et al. Management of recurrent urinary tract infections with patient-administered single-dose therapy. *Ann Intern Med* 1985;102:302–307.
19. Jepson RG, Mihaljevic L, Craig J. Cranberries for preventing urinary tract infections. In: The Cochrane Library, Issue 3, 2002. Oxford: Update Software. Search date 2001; primary sources Cochrane Collaboration Field in Complementary Medicine Registry of randomised trials, Cochrane Controlled Trials Register (CCTR) and CENTRAL, Psychlit, LILACS, Cinahl, Medline, Embase, Biological Abstracts, Current Contents, the Internet, hand searches of reference lists of review articles and relevant trials, conference abstracts from relevant meetings, and personal contact with companies involved with the manufacture of cranberry preparations.
20. Lee B, Bhuta T, Craig J, et al. Methenamine hippurate for preventing urinary tract infections. In: The Cochrane Library, Issue 3, 2002. Oxford: Update Software. Search date 2000; primary sources Cochrane Controlled Trials Register, Medline, Embase, Cinahl, Current Contents, reference lists of review articles, and retrieved trials. The manufacturers of methenamine salts were contacted for unpublished studies, and contact was made with known investigators in the area.
21. Hoivik HO, Gundersen R, Osmundsen K, et al. Prevention of recurrent cystitis in fertile women. A double-blind comparison of hiprex and placebo in general practice. [Norwegian]. *Tidsskr Nor Laegeforen* 1984;104:1150–1152.

Recurrent cystitis in non-pregnant women

22. Gundersen R, Hoivik HO, Osmundsen K. Frequent cystitis in elderly women. A double-blind comparison of hiprex and placebo in general practice. [Norwegian]. *Tidsskr Nor Laegeforen* 1986;106:2048–2049.

23. Kasanen A, Junnila SY, Kaarsalo E, et al. Secondary prevention of recurrent urinary tract infections. Comparison of the effect of placebo, methenamine hippurate, nitrofurantoin and trimethoprim alone. *Scand J Infect Dis* 1982;14:293–296.

Adriana Wechsler
Assistant Professor of Medicine
Baylor College of Medicine
Houston, Texas
USA

Competing interests: None declared

The following previous contributors of this topic would also like to be acknowledged: Lisa Chew, Bruce Cooper, Stephan Finn, Ruth Jepson, and Bazian Ltd

TABLE 1 Continuous antimicrobial prophylactic regimens for recurrent urinary tract infections: results of RCTs (see text, p 2212).

Study design	Total number of people	Regimen	Duration of prophylaxis (months)	Infections per patient year	P value
Placebo controlled RCT[7]	60	Placebo Co-trimoxazole (40 mg/200 mg) at bedtime Nitrofurantoin 100 mg at bedtime Nitrofurantoin 100 mg at bedtime	6	2.80 0.15 0.14 0	< 0.001 (drug treatment *v* placebo)
No treatment controlled and comparative RCT[8]	135	Without prophylaxis Ciprofloxacin 125 mg postcoital Ciprofloxacin 125 mg daily	12	3.62–3.66 0.043 0.031	< 0.001
Placebo controlled RCT[9]	30	Placebo Norfloxacin 200 mg at bedtime	12	1.6 0	< 0.001
Comparative RCT[10]	72	Trimethoprim 100 mg at bedtime Nitrofurantoin 100 mg bedtime	12	1.00 0.17	< 0.05
Comparative RCT[11]	94	Norfloxacin 200 mg at bedtime Nitrofurantoin 50 mg at bedtime	6	0.04 0.60	= 0.05
Comparative RCT[12]	88	Norfloxacin 200 mg at bedtime Nitrofurantoin 100 mg at bedtime	12	0.002 0.003	Not reported
Comparative RCT[13]	97	Cefaclor 250 mg at bedtime Nitrofurantoin 50 mg at bedtime	12	0.006 0.006	Not reported
Placebo controlled RCT[14]	40	Cinoxacin 500 mg at bedtime	6		< 0.001 Cimoxacin *v* placebo

TABLE 2 **Postcoital regimens for recurrent urinary tract infections: results of RCTs (see text, p 2213).**

Study design	Total number of people	Regimen	Duration of prophylaxis (months)	Infections per patient year	P value
Placebo controlled RCT[15]	27	Placebo	6	3.6	= 0.0001
		Postcoital co-trimoxazole 40 mg/20 mg		0.3	
Comparative RCT[16]	33	Without prophylaxis	14	6.13	= 0.0000
		Postcoital prophylaxis with either ofloxacin 100 mg, norfloxacin 200 mg, or ciprofloxacin 125 mg		0.02	
Comparative RCT[8]	135	Without prophylaxis	12	3.62–3.66	< 0.0001
		Ciprofloxacin 125 mg daily		0.031	
		Ciprofloxacin 125 mg postcoital		0.043	
Comparative RCT[17]	56	Without prophylaxis	12	4.6	< 0.001
		Postcoital prophylaxis with either			
		Co-trimoxazole 80 mg/400 mg		0	
		Nitrofurantoin 50–100 mg		0.1	

Bites (mammalian)

Search date July 2002

Iara Marques de Medeiros and Humberto Saconato

QUESTIONS

INTERVENTIONS

*No RCT evidence, but there is consensus that treatment is likely to be beneficial.

See glossary, p 2224

Key Messages

- **Antibiotics for treatment of infected mammalian bites** We found no RCTs of antibiotics versus placebo for infected mammalian bites. However, there is consensus that antibiotics are likely to be beneficial.
- **Antibiotic prophylaxis** Limited evidence from one systematic review found no significant difference with antibiotics versus control in the infection rate in people bitten by a dog, cat, or human in the preceding 24 hours. Meta-analysis according to the site of the wound found that antibiotics significantly reduced infections of the hand. One small RCT in the review found that in people with human bites, antibiotics versus control significantly reduced the rate of infection.
- **Comparative effectiveness of different antibiotics for treatment of infected mammalian bites** One RCT in people with infected and uninfected animal and human bites comparing penicillin with or without dicloxacillin versus amoxicillin/clavulanic acid found no significant difference in failure rate (which was undefined).
- **Debridement, irrigation, and decontamination** We found no reliable studies assessing debridement, irrigation, decontamination measures, or serum infiltration in the wound. However, there is consensus that such measures are likely to be beneficial.
- **Education to prevent bites** We found no RCTs of the effect of education programmes on the incidence of mammalian bites. One RCT found that an educational programme versus no education in school children significantly increased precautionary behaviour around dogs.

- **Education to prevent bites in specific occupational groups** We found no RCTs of education to prevent bites in specific occupational groups.
- **Primary wound closure** One poor quality RCT comparing primary wound closure versus no closure in people with dog bites found no significant difference in the incidence of infection, but the RCT was too small to exclude clinically important effects.
- **Tetanus toxoid after mammalian bites** We found no evidence on the effects of tetanus toxoid in preventing tetanus after human or animal bites.

DEFINITION Bite wounds are mainly caused by humans, dogs, or cats. They include superficial abrasions (30–43%), lacerations (31–45%), and puncture wounds (see glossary, p 2224) (13–34%).[1]

INCIDENCE/ PREVALENCE In areas where rabies is poorly controlled among domestic animals, dogs account for 90% of reported mammalian bites compared with less than 5% in areas where rabies is well controlled. In the USA, an estimated 3.5–4.7 million dog bites occur each year.[2] About one in five people bitten by a dog seek medical attention, and 1% of those require admission to hospital.[3,4] Between a third and half of all mammalian bites occur in children.[5]

AETIOLOGY/ RISK FACTORS In over 70% of cases, people are bitten by their own pets or by an animal known to them. Males are more likely to be bitten than females, and are more likely to be bitten by dogs, whereas females are more likely to be bitten by cats.[2] One study found that children under 5 years old were significantly more likely than older children to provoke animals before being bitten.[6] One study of infected dog and cat bites found that the most commonly isolated bacteria was *Pasteurella*, followed by *Streptococcus*, *Staphylococcus*, *Moraxella*, *Corynebacterium*, and *Neisseria*.[7] Mixed aerobic and anaerobic infection was more common than anaerobic infection alone.

PROGNOSIS In the USA, dog bites cause about 20 deaths a year.[8] In children, dog bites frequently involve the face, potentially resulting in severe lacerations, and scarring.[9] Rabies, a life threatening viral encephalitis, may be contracted as a consequence of being bitten or scratched by a rabid animal. More than 99% of human rabies is in developing countries where canine rabies is endemic.[10]

AIMS OF INTERVENTION To prevent mammalian bites; to prevent or achieve rapid resolution of complications after mammalian bites, with minimal adverse effects.

OUTCOMES **Prevention:** Incidence of mammalian bites. **Prophylaxis:** Rate of infection after mammalian bites, incidence of tetanus. **Treatment:** Cure rate of infection due to mammalian bites.

METHODS *Clinical Evidence* search and appraisal July 2002. In addition, we searched Web of Science (Science Citation Index to October 2001). Observational studies were used when systematic reviews or RCTs were not found.

QUESTION What are the effects of interventions to prevent mammalian bites?

OPTION EDUCATION

We found no RCTs of the effect of education programmes on the incidence of mammalian bites. One RCT found that an educational programme compared with no education in school children increased precautionary behaviour around dogs. We found no RCTs of education to prevent bites in specific occupational groups.

Benefits: We found no systematic review. **In the general population:** We found no RCTs on the effect of education programmes on the incidence of mammalian bites. One RCT (346 school children aged 7–8 years in 8 primary schools in Sydney, Australia) cluster randomised schools to either an educational programme or no education.[11] The educational programme consisted of one 30 minute lesson demonstrating behavioural techniques around dogs, such as how to recognise friendly, angry, or frightened dogs; how to approach dogs and owners when wanting to pat a dog; and how to use a precautionary and protective body posture when approached or knocked over by a dog. After 10 days, children were videotaped for 10 minutes while playing in school grounds where a dog was leashed. The trial found that children in schools receiving education were significantly less likely to pat the dog without hesitation and try to excite it (118/149 [79%] *v* 18/197 [9%]; RR 0.16, 95% CI 0.064 to 0.20). **In specific occupational groups:** We found no RCTs.

Harms: The RCT did not report on adverse effects.[11]

Comment: The RCT was brief and reported only the proxy outcome of behaviour modification. The effect of such a programme on the incidence of dog bites in the long term is unclear.

QUESTION What are the effects of measures to prevent complications from mammalian bites?

OPTION IMMUNISATION AGAINST TETANUS

We found insufficient evidence on the effects of tetanus toxoid or tetanus immunoglobulin in preventing tetanus after human or animal bites.

Benefits: **Tetanus toxoid:** We found no RCTs or cohort studies. **Tetanus immunoglobulin:** We found no RCTs or cohort studies.

Harms: We found no evidence.

Comment: General measures to prevent tetanus, such as cleaning the wound, removing debris, excision (except on the face), irrigation, and excision and removal of skin flaps around puncture wounds, may be beneficial. However, we found no evidence to confirm or refute this. We found no RCTs on the effects of passive immunisation using tetanus immunoglobulin.

OPTION ANTIBIOTIC PROPHYLAXIS

The effects of antibiotic prophylaxis in preventing complications of mammalian bites remain unclear. Limited evidence from one systematic review found that, when all causes and sites of mammalian bite were combined, there was no evidence of a difference in infection rate between antibiotics compared with placebo. Meta-analysis according to the site of the wound found that antibiotics significantly reduced infections of the hand. One small RCT in the review found that in people with human bites, antibiotics significantly reduced the rate of infection compared with placebo.

Benefits: We found one systematic review (search date 2001, 7 RCTs and 1 quasi-randomised controlled trial, 522 people bitten by dogs, cats, or humans in the preceding 24 h) comparing prophylactic antibiotics versus placebo or no treatment.[12] There was significant heterogeneity between trials. The review found no significant difference in infection rate with antibiotics compared with placebo after dog, cat, or human bites (OR 0.49, 95% CI 0.15 to 1.58; timescale not specified). When the results were analysed for each wound site (hands, trunk, arms, or head/neck), antibiotics significantly reduced infections of the hand only (3 RCTs: 2% with antibiotics *v* 28% with control; OR 0.10, 95% CI 0.01 to 0.86; NNT 4, 95% CI 2 to 50). **Animal bites:** The review identified six RCTs (463 people) of dog bites and found no significant difference in infection rate with antibiotics compared with control (10/225 [4%] with antibiotics *v* 13/238 [5%] with control; OR 0.74, 95% CI 0.30 to 1.85). The review identified one small RCT of cat bites (12 people), which found no significant difference in infection rate with antibiotics compared with control (4/6 [67%] with antibiotics *v* 0/5 [0%] with control; $P < 0.06$).[12] **Human bites:** The review included one RCT of human bites (48 people with uncomplicated bites on the hand in the preceding 24 h) comparing oral cephalosporin versus intravenous cephalosporin plus penicillin versus placebo. All participants received debridement, irrigation, and sterile dressing and remained in hospital for 5 days. It found that antibiotics by either route significantly reduced the number of people with wound infection compared with placebo (0/33 [0%] with oral or iv antibiotics *v* 7/15 [47%]; $P < 0.05$; timescale not specified).[12]

Harms: The review did not report on adverse effects.[12]

Comment: Most of the RCTs were small and gave insufficient information about allocation concealment and randomisation. Some studies were not double blind, and four studies had withdrawal rates greater than 10%.[12] The effects of antibiotic prophylaxis in preventing complications of mammalian bites remain unclear. Only a few studies analysed the effect of antibiotics on specific wound types (lacerations, puncture (see glossary, p 2224), or avulsions).[12]

OPTION PRIMARY WOUND CLOSURE

One poor quality RCT comparing primary wound closure versus no closure in people with dog bites found no significant difference in the incidence of infection, but the RCT was too small to exclude clinically important effects.

Benefits: We found no systematic review. We found one RCT comparing primary wound closure versus no closure (96 people bitten by dogs in the preceding 24 h).[13] All wounds were debrided and irrigated, and tetanus immunisation was updated, but no antibiotics were given. In uncomplicated lacerations (see glossary, p 2224), closure was performed by an experienced nurse; in complicated lacerations closure was performed by a specialist. The RCT found no difference in the incidence of infection with closed compared with open wounds (7/92 [8%] with closed *v* 6/77 [8%] with open; RR 0.98, 95% CI 0.33 to 2.62; timescale not specified). There were significantly more infections of the hand compared with the rest of the body (69% with hand *v* 31% with rest of body), but there was no difference between closure and non-closure groups in the rate of hand infection (5/9 [56%] with closure *v* 4/9 [44%] with non-closure).

Harms: The RCT did not report on adverse effects.[13]

Comment: Although the RCT found no increased risk of infection with primary wound closure, further RCTs are required to confirm this conclusion, and also to evaluate if wound closure may increase the risk of rabies.

OPTION DEBRIDEMENT, IRRIGATION, AND DECONTAMINATION

We found no reliable studies assessing debridement, irrigation, decontamination measures, and serum infiltration in the wound. However, there is consensus that such measures are likely to be beneficial.

Benefits: We found no RCTs or good cohort studies.

Harms: We found no evidence.

Comment: It would be regarded as unethical to conduct an RCT comparing debridement, irrigation, and decontamination versus no treatment.

QUESTION What are the effects of treatments for infected mammalian bites?

OPTION ANTIBIOTICS

We found no RCTs comparing antibiotics versus placebo for infected mammalian bites. One RCT in people with infected and uninfected animal and human bites found no significant difference in failure rate (which was undefined) with penicillin, with or without dicloxacillin, compared with amoxicillin/clavulanic acid.

Benefits: We found no systematic review. **Versus placebo:** We found no RCTs. **Versus other antibiotics:** We found one RCT (61 people bitten in the preceding 10 days; 48 by animals, 13 by humans) comparing penicillin with or without dicloxacillin versus amoxicillin (amoxycillin)/clavulanic acid.[10] Treatment was given for 5 days in people bitten less than 8 hours previously or in those without clinical infection (34 people), and for 10 days in people bitten more than 8 hours previously or with clinical infection (27 people). All wounds received usual care and were left closed or open at the discretion of the attending physician. Before inclusion, 27 people already had clinical signs of infection (see comment below). The RCT found no significant difference in failure rate (which was undefined) with penicillin/dicloxacillin compared with amoxicillin/clavulanic acid (1/31 [3%] *v* 3/30 [10%]; RR 0.32, 95% CI 0.03 to 2.54; timescale not specified).

Harms: Adverse effects were significantly more common in people using amoxicillin/clavulanic acid compared with penicillin/dicloxacillin (13/31 [42%] *v* 3/30 [10%]; RR 4.2, 95% CI 1.5 to 7.4; NNH 3, 95% CI 2 to 19). Diarrhoea was the most common adverse event (9/31 [29%] with amoxicillin/clavulanic acid *v* 1/30 [3%] with penicillin/dicloxacillin; RR 8.71, 95% CI 1.34 to 23.3; NNH 4, 95% CI 1 to 79).[10]

Comment: Interpretation of the results is difficult as the main outcome measure of "failure rate" was not defined. Also, failure rates were not separated according to whether people had infected or uninfected wounds at inclusion.

GLOSSARY

Abrasion The scraping or rubbing away of a small area of skin or mucous membrane.

Laceration Occurs when the skin, soft tissues, or both are torn by the crushing and shearing forces produced on impact; characterised by ragged, irregular margins, surrounding contusion, marginal abrasion, and tissue bridging in the wound depths.

Puncture A wound caused by perforation of the skin with a sharp point.

REFERENCES

1. Dire DJ. Emergency management of dog and cat bite wounds. *Emerg Med Clin North Am* 1992;10:719–736.
2. Overall KL, Love M. Dog bites to humans — demography, epidemiology, injury and risk. *JAMA* 2001;218:1923–1934.
3. Sacks JJ, Kresnow M, Houston B. Dog bites: how big a problem? *Injury Prev* 1996;2:52–54.
4. Quinlan KP, Sacks JJ. Hospitalizations for dog bite injuries. *JAMA* 1999;281:232–233.
5. Fishbein DB, Bernard KW. Rabies virus. In: *Mandell, Douglas and Bennett's principles and practice of infectious diseases*. 4th ed. Vol 2:1527–1543. New York: Churchill Livingstone.
6. Avner JR, Baker MD. Dog bites in urban children. *Pedriatrics* 1991;88:55–57.
7. Talan DA, Citron DM, Abrahamian FM, et al. Bacteriologic analysis of infected dog and cat bites. Emergency Medicine Animal Bite Infection Study Group. *N Engl J Med* 1999;340:85–92.
8. Sacks JJ, Sattin RW, Bonzo SE. Dog bite-related fatalities from 1979 through 1988. *JAMA* 1989;262:1489–1492.
9. Karlson TA. The incidence of facial injuries from dog bites. *JAMA* 1984;251:3265–3267.
10. Goldstein EJC, Reinhardt JF, Murray PM, et al. Outpatient therapy of bite wounds. Demographic data, bacteriology, and prospective, randomized trial of amoxicillin/clavulanic acid versus penicillin +/– dicloxacillin. *Int J Dermatol* 1987;26:123–127.
11. Chapman S, Cornwall J, Righetti J, et al. Preventing dog bites in children: randomised controlled trial of an educational intervention. *BMJ* 2000;320:1512–1513.
12. Medeiros I, Saconato H. Antibiotic prophylaxis for mammalian bites (Cochrane Review). In: The Cochrane Library, Issue 4, 2002. Oxford: Update Software. Search date 2001; primary sources Medline, Embase, Lilacs, and the Cochrane Controlled Trials Register.
13. De Melker HE, De Melker RA. Dog bites: publications on risk factors, infections, antibiotics and primary wound closure. *Ned Tijdschr Geneesd* 1996;140:709–713.
14. Maimaris C, Quinton DN. Dog-bite lacerations: a controlled trial of primary wound closure. *Arch Emerg Med* 1988;5:156–161.

Iara Marques de Medeiros

Humberto Saconato

Universidade Federal do Rio Grande do NorteNatal, Brazil

Competing interests: None declared.

Venous leg ulcers

Search date March 2003

E Andrea Nelson, Nicky Cullum, and June Jones

QUESTIONS

INTERVENTIONS

See glossary, p 2237

Key Messages

Treatment

- **Compression** One systematic review has found that compression heals more venous leg ulcers than no compression. We found insufficient evidence from RCTs to compare the effects of different types of multilayer compression, or multilayer high compression versus short stretch bandages. One systematic review found that multilayer compression increased ulcer healing compared with single layer bandages.
- **Pentoxifylline** One systematic review and two subsequent RCTs have found that oral pentoxifylline increases the proportion of ulcers healed over 6–12 months compared with placebo.

- **Cultured allogenic bilayer skin replacement** One RCT found that cultured allogenic bilayer skin replacement increased the proportion of ulcers healed after 6 months compared with a non-adherent dressing.
- **Flavonoids** Two RCTs found that flavonoids increased ulcer healing compared with placebo or standard care.
- **Peri-ulcer injection of granulocyte–macrophage colony stimulating factor (GM-CSF)** One RCT found that peri-ulcer injection of GM-CSF increased the proportion of ulcers healed after 13 weeks' treatment compared with placebo.
- **Sulodexide** Two RCTs found that sulodexide plus compression increased the proportion of ulcers healed after 60–90 days' treatment compared with compression alone.
- **Systemic mesoglycan** One RCT found that systemic mesoglycan plus compression increased the proportion of ulcers healed after 24 weeks' treatment compared with compression alone.
- **Antimicrobial agents; aspirin; debriding agents; foam, film, or alginate (semi-occlusive) dressings versus simple dressings in the presence of compression; intermittent pneumatic compression; low level laser treatment; oral rutosides; oral zinc; skin grafting; thromboxane α_2 antagonists; topical calcitonin gene related peptide plus vasoactive intestinal polypeptide; topical keratinocyte growth factor 2; topical mesoglycan; topical negative pressure; ultrasound; vein surgery** We found insufficient evidence about the effects of these interventions on ulcer healing.
- **Hydrocolloid dressings versus simple low adherent dressings in the presence of compression** One systematic review found that, in the presence of compression, hydrocolloid dressings did not heal more venous leg ulcers than simple, low adherent dressings.
- **Topically applied autologous platelet lysate** One RCT found no significant difference in time to healing of ulcers after 9 months between topically applied autologous platelet lysate and placebo.

Preventing recurrence

- **Compression** We found limited evidence that compression reduced recurrence, and that non-compliance with compression is a risk factor for recurrence.
- **Rutoside; stanozolol; vein surgery** We found insufficient evidence about the effects of these interventions on ulcer recurrence.

DEFINITION Definitions of leg ulcers vary, but the following is widely used: loss of skin on the leg or foot that takes more than 6 weeks to heal. Some definitions exclude ulcers confined to the foot, whereas others include ulcers on the whole of the lower limb. This review deals with ulcers of venous origin in people without concurrent diabetes mellitus, arterial insufficiency, or rheumatoid arthritis.

INCIDENCE/ PREVALENCE Between 1.5 and 3/1000 people have active leg ulcers. Prevalence increases with age to about 20/1000 in people aged over 80 years.[1]

AETIOLOGY/ RISK FACTORS Leg ulceration is strongly associated with venous disease. However, about a fifth of people with leg ulceration have arterial disease, either alone or in combination with venous problems, which may require specialist referral.[1] Venous ulcers (also known as varicose or stasis ulcers) are caused by venous reflux or obstruction, both of which lead to poor venous return and venous hypertension.

PROGNOSIS People with leg ulcers have a poorer quality of life than age matched controls because of pain, odour, and reduced mobility.[2] In the UK, audits have found wide variation in the types of care (hospital inpatient care, hospital clinics, outpatient clinics, home visits), in the treatments used (topical agents, dressings, bandages, stockings), in healing rates, and in recurrence rates (26–69% in 1 year).[3,4]

AIMS OF INTERVENTION To promote healing; to reduce recurrence; to improve quality of life, with minimal adverse effects.

OUTCOMES Ulcer area; number of ulcers healed; number of ulcer free limbs; recurrence rates; number of new ulcer episodes; number of ulcer free weeks or months; number of people who are ulcer free; frequency of dressing/bandage changes; quality of life; adverse effects of treatment.

METHODS *Clinical Evidence* search and appraisal March 2003.

QUESTION What are the effects of treatments?

OPTION COMPRESSION

One systematic review has found that compression heals more venous leg ulcers than no compression. We found insufficient evidence from RCTs to compare the effects of different types of multilayer compression, or multilayer high compression versus short stretch bandages. One systematic review found that multilayer compression increased ulcer healing compared with single layer bandages.

Benefits: **Compression versus no compression:** We found one systematic review (search date 2000, 6 RCTs, 260 people) comparing compression versus no compression.[5] It found that compression (e.g. elastomeric multilayer high compression bandages, short stretch bandages, double layer bandages, compression hosiery, or Unna's boot — see glossary, p 2238) healed more venous leg ulcers than no compression (e.g. dressing alone). The RCTs were heterogeneous, using different forms of compression in different settings and populations. The results were not pooled. The results of individual RCTs consistently favoured compression. **Elastomeric versus non-elastomeric multilayer compression:** The systematic review[5] identified three RCTs (273 people), and we found one subsequent RCT (112 people)[6] comparing elastomeric multilayer high compression bandages versus non-elastomeric multilayer compression. Meta-analysis of all four RCTs (Nelson EA, Cullum N, Jones J, personal communication, 2002) found no significant difference in the proportion of people whose ulcers healed with 12–26 weeks of high compression compared with non-high compression bandages (RR 1.30, 95% CI 0.94 to 1.82). **Multilayer high compression versus short stretch bandages:** The systematic review[5] identified four small RCTs (search date 2000, 167 people), and we identified one subsequent RCT (112 people).[7] The systematic review found no significant difference in healing rates between multiplayer high compression and short stretch bandages (RR 1.10, 95% CI 0.78 to 1.55).[5] Meta-analysis of all five RCTs (Nelson EA, Cullum N, Jones J, personal communication, 2003; 279 people) found no significant difference in healing rates between multilayer high compression and short stretch bandages (RR 1.0, 95% CI 0.81 to 1.24). The lack of power in these small studies means that a clinically important difference cannot be excluded. **Multilayer high compression versus single layer bandage:** The systematic review identified four RCTs (280 people) comparing multilayer high compression versus a single layer of bandage.[5] It found a significant increase in the proportion of people whose reference ulcer had healed with multilayer compression compared with single layer bandages (82/139 [59%] *v* 59/141 [42%]; RR 1.41, 95% CI 1.12 to 1.77; NNT for variable periods of treatment 6, 95% CI 4 to 18) (see table 1, p 2240). **Multilayer high compression versus each other:** The systematic review identified three RCTs (285 people) comparing different elastic layered bandage regimens versus four layer bandage regimens, and we found two subsequent RCTs (294 people).[5,8,9] Meta-analysis of all five RCTs (Nelson et al, personal communication, 2003) found no significant difference in healing rates between the systems (RR for healing 0.98, 95% CI 0.89 to 1.09).

Harms: High levels of compression applied to limbs with insufficient arterial supply, or inexpert application of bandages, can lead to tissue damage and, at worst, amputation.[10] Complication rates were rarely reported in RCTs. One observational study (194 people) found that four layer compression bandaging for several months was associated with toe ulceration in 12 (6%) people.[11]

Comment: People thought to be suitable for high compression bandages are those with clinical signs of venous disease (ulcer in the gaiter region, from the upper margin of the malleolus to the bulge of the gastrocnemius; staining of the skin around an ulcer; or eczema), no concurrent diabetes mellitus or rheumatoid arthritis, and adequate arterial supply to the foot as determined by ankle/brachial pressure index. The precise ankle/brachial pressure index below which compression is contraindicated is often quoted as 0.8; however, many RCTs used the higher cut off of 0.9.[5] Effectiveness is likely to be influenced by the ability of those applying the bandage to generate safe levels of compression. Bandages may be applied by the person with the leg ulcer, their carer, nurse, or doctor. We found no comparisons of healing rates between specialist and non-specialist application of compression. Training improves bandaging technique among nurses.[12] Bandages containing elastomeric fibres can be applied weekly as they maintain their tension over time. Bandages made of wool or cotton, or both, such as short stretch bandages, may need to be reapplied more frequently as they do not maintain their tension.

OPTION INTERMITTENT PNEUMATIC COMPRESSION

We found insufficient evidence from one small RCT about the effects of intermittent pneumatic compression compared with compression bandages. One RCT found that intermittent pneumatic compression plus compression bandaging improved ulcer healing at 3 months compared with compression bandaging alone, but two other RCTs found no significant difference in healing at 6 months.

Benefits: **Intermittent pneumatic compression versus compression bandaging:** We found two systematic reviews (search dates 2001, 1 RCT, 16 people).[13,14] The RCT found no significant difference in the proportion of people with healed ulcers over 2–3 months between intermittent pneumatic compression (see glossary, p 2237) and compression (0/10 *v* 0/6), but the RCT was probably too small to exclude a clinically important difference. **Intermittent pneumatic compression plus compression bandaging versus compression bandaging alone:** We found two systematic reviews (search dates 2001).[13,14] The more comprehensive review identified three small RCTs (115 people).[13] It did not perform a meta-analysis because of clinical and methodological heterogeneity among the trials. The first RCT (45 people) found that intermittent pneumatic compression plus graduated compression stockings significantly increased the proportion of people with healed ulcers at 3 months compared with graduated compression stockings alone (10/21 [48%] *v* 1/24 [4%]; RR 11.4, 95% CI 1.6 to 82). The second RCT (53 people) found no significant difference between intermittent pneumatic compression plus elastic stockings and Unna's boot (see glossary, p 2238) in the proportion of people healed at 6 months (20/28 [71%] *v* 15/20 [75%]; RR 0.95, 95% CI 0.67 to 1.34). The third RCT (22 people) found no significant difference in healing at 6 months between intermittent pneumatic compression plus Unna's boot and Unna's boot alone (12/12 [100%] *v* 8/10 [80%]; RR 1.25, 95% CI 0.92 to 1.70).[13]

Harms: The RCTs identified by the review gave no information on adverse effects.[13]

Comment: Availability may vary widely in different healthcare settings. Treatment can be delivered in the home, in outpatient clinics, or in the hospital ward. RCTs have evaluated the use of intermittent pneumatic pressure for 1 hour twice weekly and 3–4 hours daily. Treatment requires resting for 1–4 hours daily, which may reduce quality of life. One RCT (45 people) identified by a systematic review found that a few people were not able to use the pump for 4 hours every day.[14]

OPTION DRESSINGS AND TOPICAL AGENTS

One systematic review found insufficient evidence on the effects of semi-occlusive dressings (foam, film, or alginate) compared with simple dressings, in the presence of compression. The review found that, in the presence of compression, hydrocolloid dressings did not heal more venous leg ulcers than simple, low adherent dressings. The review found insufficient evidence from small, heterogeneous RCTs about the effects

of topical agents, such as growth factors, compared with inert comparators. One RCT found that cultured allogenic bilayer skin replacement increased complete ulcer healing at 6 months compared with simple dressings. One small RCT found no significant difference in the proportion of people with healed ulcers after 12 weeks iontophoretic treatment with calcitonin gene related peptide plus vasoactive intestinal polypeptide versus placebo. One RCT found no significant difference after 9 months in time to healing between topical autologous platelet lysate and placebo. We found insufficient evidence from one small RCT to compare topical mesoglycan versus placebo. One RCT found no significant difference in ulcer healing between topical keratinocyte growth factor 2 and placebo after 12 weeks. One systematic review found insufficient evidence on the effects of topical negative pressure. One systematic review found insufficient evidence on the effects of antimicrobial agents compared with placebo or standard care. One systematic review found insufficient evidence on the effects of debriding agents compared with traditional dressings.

Benefits: **Foam, film, or alginate (semi-occlusive) dressings compared with simple dressings, in the presence of compression:** We found one systematic review (search date 1997, 5 RCTs) comparing semi-occlusive dressings (foam, film, alginates) versus simple dressings (such as paraffin-tulle or knitted viscose dressings).[15] Two comparisons of foam dressings versus simple dressings; two of film dressings versus simple dressings; and one comparing an alginate versus a simple dressing found no evidence of benefit. However, the RCTs were too small (10–132 people, median 60) to detect anything but a very large difference in effectiveness. **Hydrocolloid (occlusive) dressings compared with simple low adherent dressings, in the presence of compression:** We found one systematic review (search date 1997), which identified nine RCTs comparing hydrocolloid dressings versus simple dressings in the presence of compression.[15] A pooled analysis of seven RCTs (714 people) found no evidence of benefit. **Comparisons between occlusive or semi-occlusive dressings:** The same systematic review identified 12 small RCTs comparing different occlusive or semi-occlusive dressings.[15] It found no significant difference in healing rates between dressings, or insufficient data were provided to calculate their significance. We found one subsequent RCT comparing hydrocolloid versus hydrocellular dressings, which found no significant difference in healing rates.[16] **Topical agents (e.g. growth factors) versus inert comparators:** The same systematic review identified 16 RCTs comparing topical agents (such as growth factors, cell suspensions, oxygen free-radical scavengers) versus either placebo or standard care in the treatment of venous leg ulcers.[15] It found insufficient evidence to recommend any topical agent. The studies were small (9–233 people, median 45) and heterogeneous; therefore, results could not be pooled. We found five subsequent RCTs, which are described below.[17–21] **Cultured allogenic bilayer skin replacement versus non-adherent dressing:** The first subsequent RCT (293 people) found that a cultured allogenic bilayer skin replacement (see glossary, p 2237), containing both epidermal and dermal components, significantly increased the proportion of ulcers healed completely in 6 months compared with a non-adherent dressing (92/146 [63%] *v* 63/129

[49%]; RR 1.29, 95% CI 1.04 to 1.60; NNT for 6 months' treatment 7, 95% CI 4 to 41) (see table 1, p 2240).[17] **Topical calcitonin gene related peptide plus vasoactive intestinal polypeptide versus placebo:** The second subsequent RCT (66 people) compared calcitonin (salcatonin) gene related peptide plus vasoactive intestinal polypeptide administered by iontophoresis (see glossary, p 2237) with placebo iontophoresis.[18] It found no significant difference in the proportion of people with healed ulcers after 12 weeks' treatment (11/33 [37%] *v* 6/33 [28%]; RR 1.83, 95% CI 0.77 to 4.38), but may have been too small to exclude a clinically important difference.[18] **Topical mesoglycan:** The third subsequent RCT (40 people) of topically applied mesoglycan, a profibrinolytic agent, found no evidence of benefit.[19] **Topically applied autologous platelet lysate:** The fourth subsequent RCT (86 people) found no difference after 9 months in time to healing between topical autologous platelet lysate and placebo.[20] **Topical recombinant human keratinocyte growth factor 2:** The fifth subsequent RCT (94 people) compared topically applied recombinant human keratinocyte growth factor 2 (repifermin 20 or 60 $\mu g/cm^2$) versus placebo (beneath compression).[21] The RCT found no significant difference in rates of complete ulcer healing ulcers between human keratinocyte growth factor 2 and placebo after 12 weeks (32% with 20 μg dose *v* 38% with 60 μg dose *v* 29% with placebo, for all doses of human keratinocyte growth factor 2 *v* placebo P = 0.57). **Topical negative pressure:** We found one systematic review (search date 2000, 2 small RCTs, 34 people).[22] One of the RCTs included some people with venous leg ulcers. It found no clear evidence of benefit of topical negative pressure (see glossary, p 2238), but the RCTs may have been too small to exclude a clinically important difference in outcomes. **Antimicrobial agents versus placebo or standard care:** We found one systematic review (search date 1997, 14 RCTs) comparing antimicrobial agents versus either placebo agents or standard care.[23] The RCTs were small (25–153 people, median 56), of poor quality, and no firm conclusions could be drawn. **Debriding agents:** We found one systematic review (search date 1997) comparing debriding agents versus traditional agents.[24] The review did not perform a meta-analysis specifically in people with venous leg ulcers.[24] Six RCTs (277 people) identified by the review compared dextranomer polysaccharide bead dressings with traditional dressings, but only two RCTs reported complete ulcer healing. Data pooling of these RCTs (137 ulcers) found no significant difference in the proportion of ulcers completely healed over 3 weeks (RR 2.15, 95% CI 0.34 to 13.3), but the size of the trials meant that a clinically important difference cannot be excluded (Nelson EA, Cullum N, Jones J, personal communication, 2002). Seven RCTs (451 people) identified by the review compared cadexomer iodine with traditional dressings, but only three RCTs reported complete ulcer healing. Data pooling of these RCTs (181 ulcers) found that cadexomer iodine healed significantly more ulcers than traditional dressings (31/60 *v* 15/75; RR 2.03, 95% CI 1.21 to 3.43), but the ulcers were smaller in people treated with cadexomer iodine, and results must be treated with caution as four RCTs could not be included in the data pooling. Two RCTs identified by the review compared enzymatic preparations with traditional dressings (52 ulcers) and found no evidence of a difference in ulcer healing rates.[24] Four RCTs identified by the review compared debriding agents versus each other, two compared cadexomer iodine versus dextranomer (69 people), one compared cadexomer iodine versus hydrogel (95 people), and one compared dextranomer versus hyaluronic acid (50 people). The RCTs found no significant difference in ulcer healing with different debriding agents, but may have been too small to detect a clinically important difference.[24]

Harms: It is unlikely that low adherent primary wound dressings cause harm, although dressings containing iodine may affect thyroid function if used over large surface areas for extended periods.[25] Many people (50–85%) with venous leg ulcers have contact sensitivity to preservatives, perfumes, or dyes.[26] **Topical recombinant human keratinocyte growth factor 2:** One RCT (94 people) found no significant difference in adverse effects (leg pain, pruritus, skin ulcer, rash abrasion, reopening of venous ulcer) between repifermin and placebo.[21] However, this study may have lacked power to detect a clinically important difference between groups.

Comment: Simple primary dressings maintain a moist environment beneath compression bandages by preventing loss of moisture from the wound.[27]

OPTION ULTRASOUND

One systematic review found insufficient evidence about the effects of therapeutic ultrasound in the treatment of venous leg ulcers.

Benefits: We found one systematic review (search date 1999, 7 RCTs, 470 people) comparing therapeutic ultrasound (see glossary, p 2238) with no ultrasound or sham ultrasound for venous leg ulcers.[28] Ultrasound improved ulcer healing in all studies, but a significant difference was found in only four of the seven RCTs, and heterogeneity precluded pooling the seven RCTs.

Harms: Mild and severe erythema, local pain, and small areas of bleeding were reported in trials included in the review.[29,30]

Comment: None.

OPTION SYSTEMIC DRUG TREATMENTS

One systematic review and two subsequent RCTs have found that oral pentoxifylline increases ulcer healing over 6–12 months in people receiving compression compared with placebo. Two RCTs found that flavonoids increased the proportion of ulcers healing compared with placebo or standard care. One RCT found that injections of granulocyte macrophage-colony stimulating factor increased complete healing compared with placebo. Two RCTs found that sulodexide plus compression increased the proportion of ulcers healed after 60–90 days' treatment compared with compression alone. One RCT found that systemic mesoglycan plus compression increased the proportion of

ulcers healed after 24 weeks treatment compared with compression alone. RCTs found insufficient evidence on the effects of oral thromboxane α_2 antagonists, aspirin, oral rutosides, or oral zinc supplements.

Benefits: **Pentoxifylline:** We found one systematic review (search date 2001, 9 RCTs, 572 people)[31] and two subsequent RCTs.[32,33] The systematic review compared pentoxifylline (oxpentifylline) (1200 mg or 2400 mg daily) versus placebo or versus other treatments, with or without compression.[31] It found that, in the presence of compression, pentoxifylline significantly increased the proportion of people with healed ulcers over 8–24 weeks compared with placebo (5 RCTs: 155/243 [64%] *v* 96/204 [47%]; RR 1.30, 95% CI 1.10 to 1.54; NNT for 6 months' treatment 6, 95% CI 4 to 14) (see table 1, p 2240). One RCT identified by the review found no evidence of benefit for pentoxifylline compared with defibrotide in people receiving compression.[31] The two subsequent RCTs compared pentoxifylline (400 mg three times daily) and placebo in people receiving compression.[32,33] The first RCT (172 people, 160 analysed) found that pentoxifylline for 6 months significantly increased rates of complete healing compared with placebo (55/82 [67%] with pentoxifylline *v* 24/78 [30.7%] with placebo; $P < 0.02$).[31] The second subsequent RCT (85 people, 80 analysed) found that pentoxifylline for 12 months significantly increased rates of complete healing compared with placebo (complete healing: 36/41 [88%] with pentoxifylline *v* 17/39 [44%] with placebo; $P < 0.02$).[33] **Flavonoids:** We found two RCTS, which compared micronised purified flavonoid fraction 1 g/day plus standard care with standard management alone.[34,35] When pooled in a random effects model (Nelson EA, Cullum N, Jones J, personal communication, 2001), flavonoids healed significantly more ulcers than placebo (100/206 [48%] with flavonoids *v* 53/189 [28%] with placebo; RR 1.80, 95% CI 1.20 to 2.70).[34,35] **Peri-ulcer injection of granulocyte macrophage–colony stimulating factor versus placebo:** One RCT (60 people) found that a 4 week course of injections around the ulcer of granulocyte–macrophage colony stimulating factor (400 μg) significantly increased the proportion of people whose ulcers had completely healed after 13 weeks' treatment compared with placebo (23/39 [59%] *v* 4/21 [19%]; RR 3.21, 95% CI 1.23 to 8.34; NNT for 13 weeks' treatment 2, 95% CI 1 to 7) (see table 1, p 2240).[36] **Sulodexide:** We found two RCTs (330 people).[37,38] They found that sulodexide (daily im injection for 20 or 30 days and then orally for 70 or 30 days) plus compression treatment significantly increased the proportion of ulcers healed after 60–90 days' treatment compared with compression alone (33% with compression alone *v* 54% with sulodexide plus compression; RR for healing 1.65, 95% CI 1.27 to 2.15; NNT 4, 95% CI 3 to 9) (Nelson EA, Cullum N, Jones J, personal communication 2003) (see table 1, p 2240).[37,38] **Systemic mesoglycan:** We found one RCT (183 people) comparing systemic mesoglycan (daily im injection for 21 days and then orally for 21 weeks) plus compression versus placebo plus compression.[39] It found that systemic mesoglycan significantly increased the proportion of people with healed ulcers after 24 weeks' treatment compared with placebo (82/92 [89%] *v* 69/91 [76%]; RR 1.17, 95% CI 1.03 to 1.35).

Thromboxane α_2 antagonists: We found one RCT (165 people) of an oral thromboxane α_2 antagonist versus placebo. It found no significant difference in the proportion of ulcers healed (54% v 55%).[40] **Oral zinc:** We found one systematic review (search date 1997, 5 RCTs, 151 people) comparing daily doses of 440–660 mg oral zinc sulphate versus placebo. The review found no evidence of benefit for oral zinc.[41] **Aspirin:** We found one small RCT of aspirin (300 mg daily, enteric coated) versus placebo. It found aspirin increased ulcer healing rates compared with placebo (38% v 0%), but the RCT had several methodological weaknesses so the result should be treated with caution.[42] **Rutosides:** We found one report of two RCTs.[43] The RCTs (total of 119 people) compared two different doses of oral hydroxyethyl rutosides (500 mg and 1000 mg twice daily) with placebo.[43] The RCTs found no significant difference between either dose of rutosides and placebo in rates of complete ulcer healing at 12 weeks (1 RCT, 55 people, 48 analysed: 12/23 [52%] with 1 g/day rutoside v 7/25 [28%] with placebo, P = 0.087; results for the other RCT were not reported). The RCTs may have been too small to detect a clinically important difference.

Harms: **Pentoxifylline:** The systematic review of pentoxifylline found that pentoxifylline increased adverse effects compared with placebo, although the difference was not significant (RR 1.25, 95% CI 0.87 to 1.80).[30] Nearly half of the adverse effects were gastrointestinal (dyspepsia, vomiting, or diarrhoea). Adverse effects of flavonoids, such as gastrointestinal disturbance, were reported in 10% of people. **Rutosides:** One report of two RCTs (119 people) found no significant difference in adverse effects between rutosides and placebo (no details were presented).[43] However, they may have lacked power to detect a clinically important difference between the groups.

Comment: Sulodexide is not widely available, and daily injections may be unacceptable to some people.

OPTION VEIN SURGERY

One RCT found insufficient evidence of the effects of vein surgery on ulcer healing.

Benefits: We found no systematic review. We found one RCT (47 people) comparing vein surgery (perforator ligation) versus no surgery or surgery plus skin grafting.[44] It found no difference in the proportion of ulcers healed after 1 year, or in the rate of ulcer healing. The RCT may have been too small to rule out a beneficial effect.

Harms: Vein surgery carries the usual risks of surgery and anaesthesia.

Comment: Several operative approaches are commonly used, including perforator ligation, saphenous vein stripping, and a combination of both procedures.

OPTION SKIN GRAFTING

One systematic review found insufficient evidence of the effects of skin grafting on ulcer healing.

Benefits: We found one systematic review (search date 1999, 6 RCTs, 197 people) of skin grafts (autografts or allografts) for venous leg ulcers.[45] In five RCTs, people also received compression bandaging; two RCTs (98 people) evaluated split thickness autografts; three RCTs (92 people) evaluated cultured keratinocyte allografts; and one RCT (7 people, 13 ulcers) compared tissue engineered skin (artificial skin) with split thickness skin grafts. We found insufficient evidence to determine whether skin grafting increased the healing of venous ulcers.[45]

Harms: Taking a skin graft leaves a wound that itself requires management and may cause pain. We found no evidence of harm from tissue engineered skin.

Comment: None.

OPTION LOW LEVEL LASER TREATMENT

Systematic reviews and two subsequent small RCTs found insufficient evidence of the effects of low level laser treatment on ulcer healing.

Benefits: We found two systematic reviews and two subsequent RCTs.[46–49] The first review (search date 1998) identified four RCTs (139 people).[46] Two RCTs compared low level laser treatment (see glossary, p 2238) versus sham treatment and found no significant difference in healing rates over 12 weeks (17/44 [39%] *v* 14/44 [32%]; RR 1.21, 95% CI 0.73 to 2.03). One three-arm RCT (30 people) identified by the review compared laser treatment versus laser treatment plus infrared light or versus non-coherent, unpolarised red light. It found that significantly more ulcers healed completely after 9 months' treatment in the group receiving a combination of laser and infrared light compared with non-coherent, unpolarised red light (12/15 [80%] *v* 5/15 [33%]; RR 2.4, 95% CI 1.12 to 5.13). The fourth RCT identified by the review compared laser and ultraviolet light and found no significant difference in healing over 4 weeks.[46] The second review (search date 1999, 5 RCTs)[47] identified but did not fully describe the four RCTs identified by the first review. The review did not perform a meta-analysis. The additional RCT identified by the review (9 people, 12 venous leg ulcers) compared low level laser treatment with sham treatment and found limited evidence that ulcer area reduction was greater with laser over 10 weeks (25% of ulcer area remained unhealed in people receiving laser *v* 85% in people receiving sham treatment).[47] The RCT did not assess complete ulcer healing. The first subsequent small RCT (15 people) compared laser therapy plus phototherapy once weekly for 4 weeks versus sham therapy.[48] It found no significant difference between laser and sham in ulcer area at 12 weeks. The second small subsequent RCT (65 people) compared laser, sham laser, and no treatment (although it is unclear if the "no additional treatment" was established by randomisation).[49] It found no significant difference between treatments in the change in area of ulceration (reduction in area: 4.25 cm^2 (27%) with laser *v* 5.21 cm^2 (39%) with sham laser *v* 2.98 cm^2 (18%) with no treatment; P value not reported).

Harms: Eye protection is required when using some types of laser as the high energy beam may lead to damage of the retina.

Venous leg ulcers

Comment: The laser power, wavelength, frequency, duration, and follow up of treatment were different for all of the studies. The subsequent RCTs may have lacked power to detect clinically important differences between laser and sham treatment.

QUESTION **What are the effects of interventions to prevent recurrence?**

OPTION **COMPRESSION**

We found limited evidence that compression reduced recurrence, but non-compliance with compression is a risk factor for recurrence.

Benefits: **Versus no compression:** We found one systematic review of compression hosiery versus no compression (search date 2000, no identified RCTs),[50] and one subsequent RCT.[51] The RCT (153 people) found that wearing compression stockings significantly reduced recurrence at 6 months compared with not wearing compression stockings (21% *v* 46%; RR 0.46, 95% CI 0.28 to 0.76; NNT for 6 months' treatment 2, 95% CI 2 to 5).[51] **Versus other forms of compression:** We found one systematic review (search date 2000, 2 RCTs).[50] One RCT (166 people) compared two brands of UK Class 2 stockings (see comment below) and found no significant difference in recurrence. The larger RCT (300 people) compared Class 2 and Class 3 stockings (see comment below). With intention to treat analysis, the RCT found no significant reduction in recurrence after 5 years with high compression hosiery (UK Class 3) compared with moderate compression hosiery (UK Class 2). This analysis may underestimate the effectiveness of the Class 3 hosiery because a significant proportion of people changed from Class 3 to Class 2. Both RCTs found that non-compliance with compression hosiery was associated with recurrence.

Harms: The application of high compression to limbs with reduced arterial supply may result in ischaemic tissue damage and, at worst, amputation.[31]

Comment: Compression hosiery is classified according to the magnitude of pressure exerted at the ankle; the UK classification states that Class 2 hosiery is capable of applying 18–24 mm Hg pressure and Class 3 is capable of applying 25–35 mm Hg pressure at the ankle. Other countries use different classification systems. Hosiery reduces venous reflux by locally increasing venous pressure in the legs relative to the rest of the body. This effect only takes place while hosiery is worn. The association between non-compliance with compression and recurrence of venous ulceration provides some indirect evidence of the benefit of compression in prevention. People are advised to wear compression hosiery for life and may be at risk of pressure necrosis from their compression hosiery if they subsequently develop arterial disease. Regular reassessment of the arterial supply is considered good practice, but we found no evidence about the optimal frequency of assessment. Other measures designed to reduce leg oedema, such as resting with the leg elevated, may be useful.

OPTION **SYSTEMIC DRUG TREATMENT**

One systematic review found insufficient evidence on the effects of rutoside or stanozolol on ulcer recurrence.

Benefits: We found one systematic review (search date 1997, 2 RCTs, 198 people) comparing stanozolol or rutoside with placebo in the prevention of leg ulcer recurrence.[52] **Rutoside:** The first RCT (139 people) identified by the review found no significant difference between rutoside and placebo in recurrence at 18 months (32% *v* 34%; P = 0.93; no raw data available to calculate CI). **Stanozolol:** The second RCT (60 people) identified by the review found no significant difference between stanozolol and placebo for 6 months in recurrence at the end of the study (length of follow up not specified; recurrence in 7/25 [28%] legs with stanozolol *v* 4/23 [17%]; RR 1.61, 95% CI 0.54 to 4.79).[52]

Harms: Stanozolol is an anabolic steroid; adverse effects include acne, hirsutism, amenorrhoea, oedema, headache, dyspepsia, rash, hair loss, depression, jaundice, and changes in liver enzymes. Tolerance of rutoside was reported to be good; adverse effects include headache, flushing, rashes, and mild gastrointestinal disturbances.[53]

Comment: None.

OPTION **VEIN SURGERY**

One RCT identified by a systematic review found insufficient evidence on the effects of vein surgery on ulcer recurrence.

Benefits: We found one systematic review (search date 1997, 1 RCT, 30 people).[52] The identified RCT, which was poorly controlled, compared surgery plus compression hosiery versus compression hosiery alone for prevention of recurrence. It found a reduced rate of recurrence when surgery was carried out in addition to the use of compression hosiery (5% *v* 24%; RR 0.21, 95% CI 0.03 to 0.80).

Harms: Vein surgery has the usual risks of surgery and anaesthesia.

Comment: The results of the RCT should be interpreted with caution because it was small and poorly controlled.[52] The RCT randomised legs rather than people.

GLOSSARY

Cultured allogenic bilayer skin replacement Also called human skin equivalent. This is made of a lower (dermal) layer of bovine collagen containing living human dermal fibroblasts and an upper (epidermal) layer of living human keratinocytes.

Elastomeric multilayer high compression bandages Usually a layer of padding material followed by one to three additional layers of elastomeric bandages.

Intermittent pneumatic compression External compression applied by inflatable leggings or boots either over, or instead of, compression hosiery or bandages. A pump successively inflates and deflates the boots to promote the return of blood from the tissues. Newer systems have separate compartments in the boots so that the foot is inflated before the ankle, which is inflated before the calf.

Iontophoresis The delivery of an ionic substance by application of an electrical current.

Low level laser treatment Application of treatment energy (< 10 J/cm^2) using lasers of 50 mW or less.
Short stretch bandages Minimally extensible bandages usually made of cotton with few or no elastomeric fibres. They are applied at near full extension to form a semi-rigid bandage.
Therapeutic ultrasound Application of ultrasound to a wound, using a transducer and a water based gel. Prolonged application can lead to heating of the tissues but, when used in wound healing, the power used is low and the transducer is constantly moved by the therapist so that the tissue is not significantly heated.
Topical negative pressure Negative pressure (suction) applied to a wound through an open cell dressing (e.g. foam, felt).
Unna's boot An inner layer of zinc oxide impregnated bandage, which hardens as it dries to form a semi-rigid layer against which the calf muscle can contract. It is usually covered in an elastomeric bandage.

Substantive changes

Compression Two RCTs added;[8,9] conclusions unchanged.
Intermittent pneumatic compression One systematic review added;[14] conclusions unchanged.
Dressings and topical agents One RCT added;[21] conclusions unchanged.
Systemic drug treatments Two RCTs added;[32,33] conclusions unchanged.
Systemic drug treatments One report of two RCTs added;[43] conclusions unchanged.
Low level laser treatment Two RCTs added;[48,49] conclusions unchanged.
Systemic drug treatments, sulodexide One RCT added;[38] conclusions changed from Unknown effectiveness to Likely to be beneficial.

REFERENCES

1. Callam MJ, Ruckley CV, Harper DR, et al. Chronic ulceration of the leg: extent of the problem and provision of care. *BMJ* 1985;290:1855–1856.
2. Roe B, Cullum N, Hamer C. Patients' perceptions of chronic leg ulceration. In: Cullum N, Roe B, eds. *Leg ulcers: nursing management.* Harrow: Scutari, 1995:125–134.
3. Roe B, Cullum N. The management of leg ulcers: current nursing practice. In: Cullum N, Roe B, eds. *Leg ulcers: nursing management.* Harrow: Scutari, 1995:113–124.
4. Vowden KR, Barker A, Vowden P. Leg ulcer management in a nurse-led, hospital-based clinic. *J Wound Care* 1997;6:233–236.
5. Cullum N, Nelson EA, Fletcher AW, et al. Compression bandages and stockings in the treatment of venous leg ulcers. In: The Cochrane Library, Issue 1, 2002. Oxford: Update Software. Search date 2000; primary sources 19 electronic databases, hand searches, and personal contacts.
6. Meyer F, Burnand KG, McGuiness C, et al. Randomized clinical RCT comparing the efficacy of two bandaging regimens in the treatment of venous leg ulcer. *Br J Surg* 2002;89:40–44.
7. Partsch H, Damstra RJ, Tazelaar DJ, et al. Multicentre, randomised controlled RCT of four-layer bandaging versus short-stretch bandaging in the treatment of venous leg ulcers. *VASA* 2001;30:108–113.
8. Vowden KR, Mason A, Wilkinson D, et al. Comaprison of the healing rates and complications of three four-layer bandage regimens. *J Wound Care* 2000;9:269–272.
9. Meyer FJ, Burnand KG, Lagattolla NRF, et al. More venous leg ulcers are healed by three-layer paste than by four-layer bandages: a randomised, controlled, prospective study. Proceedings of the First World Wound Healing Congress, 74–75, 2000. Australian Wound Management Association.
10. Callam MJ, Ruckley CV, Dale JJ, et al. Hazards of compression treatment of the leg: an estimate from Scottish surgeons. *BMJ* 1987;295:1382.
11. Chan CLH, Meyer FJ, Hay RJ, et al. Toe ulceration associated with compression bandaging: observational study. *BMJ* 2001;323;1099.
12. Nelson EA, Ruckley CV, Barbenel J. Improvements in bandaging technique following training. *J Wound Care* 1995;4:181–184.
13. Mani R, Vowden K, Nelson EA. Intermittent pneumatic compression for treating venous leg ulcers. In: The Cochrane Library, Issue 1, 2002. Oxford: Update Software. Search date 2001; primary sources The Cochrane Wound Group Trials Register and hand searches of journals, relevant conference proceedings and citations within obtained reviews and papers and personal contact with relevant companies.
14. Berliner E, Ozbilgin B, Zarin DA. A systematic review of pneumatic compression for treatment of chronic venous insufficiency and venous ulcers. *J Vasc Surg* 2003;37:539–44. Search date 2001; primary source Medline, Embase, Amed, hand searches from reference lists and suggestions from experts.
15. Bradley M, Cullum N, Nelson EA, et al. Dressings and topical agents for healing of chronic wounds: a systematic review. *Health Technol Assess* 1999;3 No17(Pt2). Search date 1997; primary sources Cochrane Library, Medline, Embase, and Cinahl.
16. Seeley J, Jensen JL, Hutcherson J. A randomised clinical study comparing a hydrocellular dressing

to a hydrocolloid dressing in the management of pressure ulcers. *Ostomy Wound Manage* 1999;45:39–47.

17. Falanga V, Margolis D, Alvarez O, et al. Rapid healing of venous ulcers and lack of clinical rejection with an allogeneic cultured human skin equivalent. Human Skin Equivalent Investigators Group. *Arch Dermatol* 1998;134:293–300.
18. Gherardini G, Gurlek A, Evans GRD, et al. Venous ulcers: improved healing by iontophoretic administration of calcitonin gene-related peptide and vasoactive intestinal polypeptide. *Plast Reconstr Surg* 1998;101:90–93.
19. La Marc G, Pumilia G, Martino A. Effectiveness of mesoglycan topical treatment of leg ulcers in subjects with chronic venous insufficiency. *Minerva Cardioangiol* 1999;47:315–319.
20. Stacey MC, Mata SD, Trengove NJ, et al. Randomised double-blind placebo controlled RCT of autologous platelet lysate in venous ulcer healing. *Eur J Vasc Endovasc Surg* 2000;20:296–301.
21. Robson MC, Phillips TJ, Falanga V, Odenheimer DJ, Parish LC, Jensen JL, and Steed DL. Randomized trial of topically applied repifermin (recombinant human keratinocyte growth factor–2) to accelerate wound healing in venous ulcers. *Wound Repair Regen* 2001;9:347–352.
22. Evans D, Land L. Topical negative pressure for treating chronic wounds. In: The Cochrane Library, Issue 1, 2002. Oxford: Update Software. Search date 2000; primary sources Cochrane Wounds Group specialised register, experts, relevant companies, and a hand search.
23. O'Meara S, Cullum N, Majid M, et al. Systematic reviews of wound care management: (3) antimicrobial agents for chronic wounds. *Health Technol Assess* 2000;4(No 21):1–237. Search date 1997; primary sources Cochrane Library, Medline, Embase, and Cinahl.
24. Bradley M, Cullum N, Sheldon T. The debridement of chronic wounds: a systematic review. *Health Technol Assess*, 1999; 3 (17 Pt 1). Search date 1997; primary sources 19 electronic databases (including the Cochrane Wounds Group Specialised Register) and hand searches of specialist wound care journals, conference proceedings and bibliographies of retrieved relevant publications and personal contact with appropriate companies and an advisory panel of experts.
25. Thomas S. *Wound management and dressings.* London: Pharmaceutical Press, 1990.
26. Cameron J, Wilson C, Powell S, et al. Contact dermatitis in leg ulcer patients. *Ostomy Wound Manage* 1992;38:10–11.
27. Wu P, Nelson EA, Reid WH, et al. Water vapour transmission rates in burns and chronic leg ulcers: influence of wound dressings and comparison with in vitro evaluation. *Biomaterials* 1996;17:1373–1377.
28. Flemming K, Cullum N. Therapeutic ultrasound for venous leg ulcers. In: The Cochrane Library, Issue 1, 2002. Oxford: Update Software. Search date 1999; primary sources Cochrane Wounds Group specialised register, and hand searches of citation lists.
29. Peschen M, Vanscheidt W. Low frequency ultrasound of chronic venous leg ulcers as part of an out-patient treatment [abstract]. In: Cherry GW, Gottrup F, Lawrence JC, et al. *Fifth European Conference on Advances in Wound Management.* 271. 96. Macmillan.
30. Weichenthal M, Mohr P, Stegmann W, et al. Low-frequency ultrasound treatment of chronic venous ulcers. *Wound Repair Regen* 1997;5:18–22.
31. Jull AB, Waters J, Arroll B. Oral pentoxifylline for treatment of venous leg ulcers. In: The Cochrane Library, Issue 1, 2002. Oxford: Update Software. Search date 2001; primary sources Cochrane Peripheral Vascular Diseases and Wounds Group, specialised registers, hand searches of reference lists, relevant journals and conference proceedings, personal contact with manufacturer of pentoxifylline, and experts in the field.
32. Belcaro G, Cesarone MR, Nicolaides AN, et al. Treatment of venous ulcers with pentoxifylline: a 6-month randomized double-blind placebo controlled trial. *Angiology* 2002;53:S45–S47.
33. De Sanctis MT , Belcaro G, Cesarone MR, et al. Treatment of venous ulcers with pentoxfylline: a 12-month double-blind placebo controlled trial. Microcirculation and healing. *Angiology* 2002;53:S49–S51.
34. Guilhou JJ, Dereure O, Marzin L, et al. Efficacy of Daflon 500 mg in venous leg ulcer healing: a double-blind, randomized, controlled versus placebo RCT in 107 patients. *Angiology* 1997;48:77–85.
35. Glinski W, Chodynicka B, Roszkiewicz J, et al. The beneficial augmentative effect of micronised purified flavonoid fraction (MPFF) on the healing of leg ulcers: an open, multicentre, controlled randomised study. *Phlebology* 1999;14:151–157.
36. Da Costa RM, Ribeiro Jesus FM, Aniceto C, et al. Randomized, double-blind, placebo-controlled, dose-ranging study of granulocyte–macrophage colony stimulating factor in patients with chronic venous leg ulcers. *Wound Repair Regen* 1999;7:17–25.
37. Scondotto G, Aloisi D, Ferrari P, et al. Treatment of venous leg ulcers with sulodexide. *Angiology* 99;50:883–889.
38. Coccheri S, Scondotto G, Agnelli G, et al. Randomised, double blind, Multicentre, placebo controlled study of sulodexide in the treatment of venous leg ulcers. *Thromb Haemost* 2002;87:947–952.
39. Arosio E, Ferrari G, Santoro F, et al. A placebo-controlled, double blind study of mesoglycan in the treatment of chronic venous ulcers. *Eur J Vasc Endovas Surg* 2001;22:365–372.
40. Lyon RT, Veith FJ, Bolton L, et al. Clinical benchmark for healing of chronic venous ulcers. Venous Ulcer Study Collaborators. *Am J Surgery* 1998;176:172–175.
41. Wilkinson EAJ, Hawke CI. Does oral zinc aid the healing of chronic leg ulcers? A systematic literature review. *Arch Dermatol* 1998;134:1556–1560. Search date 1997; primary sources Medline, Embase, Cinahl, Science Citation Index, Biosis, British Diabetic Association Database, Ciscom, Cochrane Controlled Register of Clinical RCTs, Dissertation Abstracts, Royal College of Nursing Database, electronic databases of ongoing research, hand searches of wound care journals and conference proceedings, and contact with manufacturer of zinc sulphate tablets.
42. Layton AM, Ibbotson SH, Davies JA, et al. Randomised RCT of oral aspirin for chronic venous leg ulcers. *Lancet* 1994;344:164–165.
43. Schultz–Ehrenburg U and Müller B . Two multicentre clinical trials of two different dosages of O–β–Hydroxyethyl)–Rutosides in the treatment of leg ulcers. *Phlebology* 1993; 8(suppl 1):29–30.
44. Warburg FE, Danielsen L, Madsen SM, et al. Vein surgery with or without skin grafting versus conservative treatment for leg ulcers. *Acta Dermatol Vereol* 1994;74:307–309.
45. Jones JE, Nelson EA. Skin grafting for venous leg ulcers. In: The Cochrane Library, Issue 1, 2002. Oxford: Update Software. Search date 1999;

primary sources Cochrane Wounds Group specialised register, hand searches of reference lists, relevant journals, conference proceedings, and personal contact with experts in the field.
46. Flemming K, Cullum N. Laser therapy for venous leg ulcers. In: The Cochrane Library, Issue 1, 2002. Oxford: Update Software. Search date 1998; primary sources 19 electronic databases, hand searches of journals, conference proceedings, and bibliographies.
47. Schneider WL, Hailey D. Low level laser therapy for wound healing. Alberta Heritage Foundation Report 1999. Search date 1999; primary sources Medline, HealthStar, Embase, Dissertation Abstracts, Current Contents, Cinahl, Cochrane Library, the Internet.
48. Lagan KM, McKenna T, Witherow A, et al. Low-intensity laser therapy/combined phototherapy in the management of chronic venous ulceration: a placebo-controlled study. *J Clin Laser Med Surg* 2002;20:109–116.
49. Franek A, Krol P, Kucharzewski M. Does low output laser stimulation enhance the healing of crural ulceration? Some critical remarks. *Med Eng Phys* 2002;24:607–615.
50. Cullum N, Nelson EA, Flemming K, et al. Systematic reviews of wound care management: (5) beds; (6) compression; (7) laser therapy, therapeutic ultrasound, electrotherapy and electromagnetic therapy. *Health Technol Assess* 2001;5(9). Search date 2000; primary sources Cochrane Wounds Group specialised register, 19 electronic databases (up to December 1999), and hand searches of relevant journals, conferences and bibliographies of retrieved publications, and personal contact with manufacturers and an advisory panel of experts.
51. Vandongen YK, Stacey MC. Graduated compression elastic stockings reduce lipodermatosclerosis and ulcer recurrence. *Phlebology* 2000;15:33–37.
52. Cullum N, Fletcher A, Semlyen A, et al. Compression therapy for venous leg ulcers. *Qual Health Care* 1997;6:226–231. Search date 1997; primary sources 18 databases, including Medline, Embase, Cinahl with no restriction on date, hand searches of relevant journals, conference proceedings, and correspondence with experts to obtain unpublished papers.
53. Taylor HM, Rose KE, Twycross RG. A double-blind clinical RCT of hydroxyethylrutosides in obstructive arm lymphoedema. *Phlebology* 1993;8(suppl 1):22–28.

E Andrea Nelson
Senior Research Fellow
Centre for Evidence Based Nursing
Department of Health Sciences
University of York
York
UK

Nicky Cullum
Professor
Centre for Evidence Based Nursing
Department of Health Sciences
University of York
York
UK

June Jones
Clinical Nurse Specialist
Southport and Formby PCT
Southport
UK

Competing interests: EAN has been reimbursed for attending symposia by Smith and Nephew, Huntleigh Healthcare Ltd, Convatec, and Johnson & Johnson. EAN and NC are applicants on a RCT of compression bandages for which Beiersdorf UK Ltd provided RCT related education. JJ has been reimbursed for attending symposia by 3M.

TABLE 1 NNTs for healing of leg ulcers (see text, p 2227).

Intervention	NNT (95% CI)
Elastomeric multilayer compression *v* non-elastomeric multilayer compression bandages	5 (3 to 12)[5]
Multilayer high compression *v* single layer compression bandages	6 (4 to 18)[5]
Pentoxifylline 400 mg three times a day *v* placebo (concurrent use of compression)	6 (4 to 14)[31]
Peri-ulcer injection of GM–CSF (400 μg) *v* placebo	2 (1 to 17)[36]
Cultured allogenic bilayer skin equivalent *v* non-adherent dressing	7 (4 to 41)[17]
Sulodexide plus compression *v* compression alone	4 (3 to 9)[37,38]

GM–CSF, granulocyte–macrophage colony stimulating factor.

Note

When looking up a class of drug, the reader is advised to also look up specific examples of that class of drug where additional entries may be found. The reverse situation also applies. Abbreviations used: CVD, cardiovascular disease; HRT, hormone replacement therapy; IVF, in vitro fertilisation; MI, myocardial infarction; NSAIDs, non-steroidal anti-inflammatory drugs; STD, sexually transmitted disease.

INDEX

Subject index

Subject index

Subject index

Subject index

Subject index

Clinical evidence comments

Clinical Evidence is an evolving resource and we welcome any feedback on the content of this issue and suggestions for future issues.

Please photocopy and complete this form, then return it to us.

For UK and rest of world - Fax: + 44 (0) 20 7383 6242, mail: BMJ Clinical Evidence, BMJ Publishing Group, BMA House, Tavistock Square, London WC1H 9JR, UK

For North and South America - Fax: 1-240-646-7005, mail: BMJ Clinical Evidence, PO Box 512, Annapolis Jct, MD20701-0512, USA

Alternatively, email us at CEfeedback@bmjgroup.com

Name: ....

Address: ....

....

....Email: ....

Position

- ☐ GP/Primary Care Physician
- ☐ Hospital Doctor/Specialist Physician
- ☐ Pharmacist
- ☐ Resident/Registrar
- ☐ Nurse
- ☐ PAM
- ☐ Manager
- ☐ Press
- ☐ Researcher
- ☐ Administrator
- ☐ Librarian
- ☐ Medical Student
- ☐ Member of Public/Patient Support Group
- ☐ Other.........................

1. Comments concerning the selection of studies

Section...

Topic ....

Reference ....

Comment...

....

....

2. Suggestions for future issues

....

....

....

3. Other comments/questions

....

....

....

inical
idence
ıbscribe
today

UK
& rest
f world

Tel:
4 (0)20 7383 6270

Fax:
4 (0)20 7383 6402

Email:
Esubscriptions@
bmjgroup.com

lorth &
South
merica
only

Tel:
-373-2897 toll free/
-240-646-7000

Fax:
-240-646-7005

Email:
evid@pmds.com

inicalevidence.com

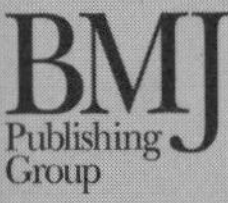

Clinical evidence
Subscription Card

Clinical Evidence **Publication: Six monthly** **ISSN: 1462-3846 (Full)**
ISSN: 1475-9225 (Concise)

Annual Subscription rates to full print and concise editions (Issues 10 & 11):

PLEASE TICK/CHECK ONE

For 2 full print copies per year, plus online access at no additional cost:

Personal:	£100 ☐	€160 ☐	US$160 ☐	Can$220 ☐
Student/Nurse:	£45 ☐	€70 ☐	US$70 ☐	Can$100 ☐

(Students: please supply proof of student status.
Nurses: please provide your registration no. ....)

For 2 full print copies:

Institutional:	£210 ☐	€335 ☐	US$335 ☐	Can$460 ☐

For 2 concise copies (including mini CD-ROM) per year, plus online access at no additional cost:

Personal:	£90 ☐	€145 ☐	US$145 ☐	Can$200 ☐
Student/Nurse:	£40 ☐	€65 ☐	US$65 ☐	Can$90 ☐

(Students: please supply proof of student status.
Nurses: please provide your registration no. ....)

For 2 concise copies (including mini CD-ROM) per year:

Institutional:	£190 ☐	€305 ☐	US$305 ☐	Can$420 ☐

Special discount rates available online for combined purchase of full print and concise editions.

Institutions may purchase online site licences separately.
Visit our website for further details.
Euro rate applicable to Eurozone only.
US dollar rate applicable to USA only.
Canadian dollar rate applicable to Canada only.

Important: If you are from one of the countries listed below you must add tax to the quoted price, unless you can provide a registration number now **(not Canada):**

Registration number ....

Use the following information to identify what tax percentage applies to your order and insert the full rate including tax in the cheque or credit card payment space overleaf:

Tax Information: Italy & Spain-4%IVA, Ireland-12.5%VAT, Germany-7%MWS, Belgium-6%TVA/BTW, France-19.6%TVA and Canada-7%GST/HST

PLEASE TURN OVER TO COMPLETE YOUR PAYMENT DETAILS

10BIC2

Clinical evidence
Payment Details

PLEASE TICK/CHECK

For UK and Eurozone:

☐ I enclose a cheque for £/€__________ made payable to British Medical Journal

For North America:

☐ I enclose a check for $__________ made payable to BMJ Publishing Inc.

(Sterling cheques to be drawn on a UK bank account, Euro cheques on a Eurozone bank account, US dollar cheques on a USA bank account and Canadian dollar cheques on a Canadian bank account)

☐ Charge my credit card £/$/€...

American Express/Visa/Mastercard/Delta/Switch ***(Circle as appropriate)***

Start issue from December 2003 (Issue 10)

Cardholders No

☐☐☐☐ ☐☐☐☐ ☐☐☐☐ ☐☐☐☐ ☐☐☐

Expiry/Expiration Date:........................ Issue No. ....
(Switch card holders only)

Signature: ....

Name: ....

Title/Profession: ....

Specialty: ....

Address: ....

....

....

Country: .... Post/Zip code: ....

E-Mail Address: ....

If the credit card account holders address differs, please advise:

....

....

....

☐ Please tick/check if you do not wish your data to be used for direct marketing purposes

RETURN TO:

(for UK and rest of world)

BMJ Publishing Group, Journals Marketing Department, PO Box 299, London WC1H 9TD, UK
Tel: +44 (0)20 7383 6270 Fax: +44 (0)20 7383 6402

OR **(for North & South America)**

BMJ-Clinical Evidence, PO Box 512, Annapolis Jct., MD 20701-0512, USA
Tel: 1-800-373-2897(toll free)/1-240-646-7000 Fax: 1-240-646-7005

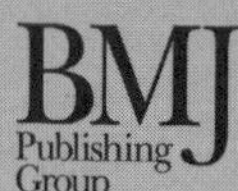

Estimating cardiovascular risk and treatment benefit

Adapted from the New Zealand guidelines on management of dyslipidaemia[1] and raised blood pressure[2] by Rod Jackson

Appendix 1

How to use these colour charts

The charts help the estimation of a person's absolute risk of a cardiovascular event and the likely benefit of drug treatment to lower cholesterol or blood pressure. For these charts, cardiovascular events include: new angina, myocardial infarction, coronary death, stroke or transient ischaemic attack (TIA), onset of congestive cardiac failure, or peripheral vascular syndrome.

There is a group of patients in whom risk can be assumed to be high (>20% in 5 years) without using the charts. They include those with symptomatic cardiovascular disease (angina, myocardial infarction, congestive heart failure, stroke, TIA, and peripheral vascular disease), or left ventricular hypertrophy on ECG.

To estimate a person's absolute 5 year risk:

- Find the table relating to their sex, diabetic status (on insulin, oral hypoglycaemics, or fasting blood glucose over 8 mmol/L), smoking status, and age. The age shown in the charts is the mean for that category, i.e. age 60 = 55 to 65 years.
- Within the table find the cell nearest to the person's blood pressure and total cholesterol : HDL ratio. For risk assessment it is enough to use a mean blood pressure based on two readings on each of two occasions, and cholesterol measurements based on one laboratory or two non-fasting Reflotron measurements. More readings are needed to establish the pre-treatment baseline.
- The colour of the box indicates the person's 5 year cardiovascular disease risk (see below).

Notes: (1) People with a strong history of CVD (first degree male relatives with CVD before 55 years, female relatives before 65 years) or obesity (body mass index above 30 kg/m^2) are likely to be at greater risk than the tables indicate. The magnitude of the independent predictive value of these risk factors remains unclear — their presence should influence treatment decisions for patients at borderline treatment levels. (2) If total cholesterol or total cholesterol : HDL ratio is greater than 8 then the risk is at least 15%. (3) Nearly all people aged 75 years or over also have an absolute cardiovascular risk over 15%.

Charts reproduced with permission from The National Heart Foundation of New Zealand. Also available on http://www.nzgg.org.nz/library/gl_complete/bloodpressure/table1.cfm.

REFERENCES

1. Dyslipidaemia Advisory Group. 1996 National Heart Foundation clinical guidelines for the assessment and management of dyslipidaemia. *NZ Med J* 1996;109:224–232.
2. National Health Committee. Guidelines for the management of mildly raised blood pressure in New Zealand: Ministry of Health National Health Committee Report, Wellington, 1995.

RISK LEVEL	5 year CVD risk (non-fatal and fatal)	**BENEFIT (1)** CVD events prevented per 100 treated for 5 years*	**BENEFIT (2)** Number needed to treat for 5 years to prevent one event*
Very High	>30%	>10 per 100	<10
	25–30%	9 per 100	11
	20–25%	7.5 per 100	13
High	15–20%	6 per 100	16
Moderate	10–15%	4 per 100	25
Mild	5–10%	2.5 per 100	40
	2.5–5%	1.25 per 100	80
	<2.5%	<0.8 per 100	>120

*Based on a 20% reduction in total cholesterol or a reduction in blood pressure of 10–15 mm Hg systolic or 5–10 mm Hg diastolic, which is estimated to reduce CVD risk by about a third over 5 years.

Estimating cardiovascular risk and treatment benefit

RISK LEVEL: MEN

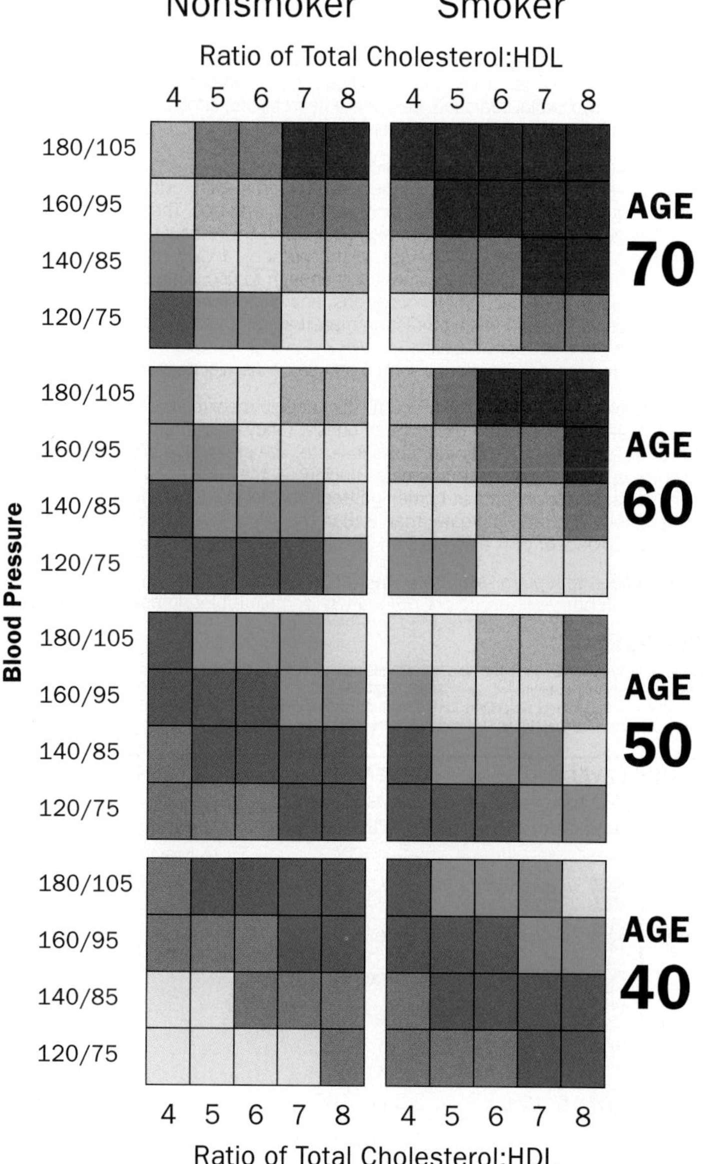

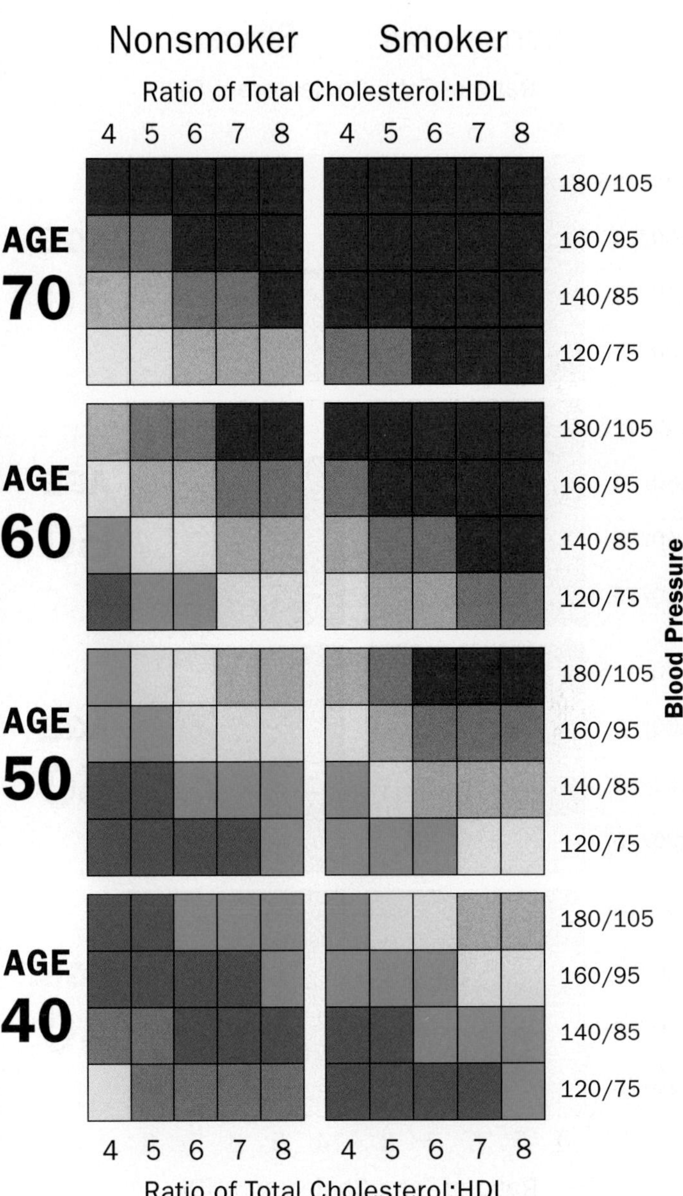
DIABETES
Nonsmoker
Smoker
Ratio of Total Cholesterol:HDL
4 5 6 7 8 4 5 6 7 8
AGE 70
AGE 60
AGE 50
AGE 40
180/105
160/95
140/85
120/75
Blood Pressure
4 5 6 7 8 4 5 6 7 8
Ratio of Total Cholesterol:HDL

Estimating cardiovascular risk and treatment benefit

RISK LEVEL: WOMEN

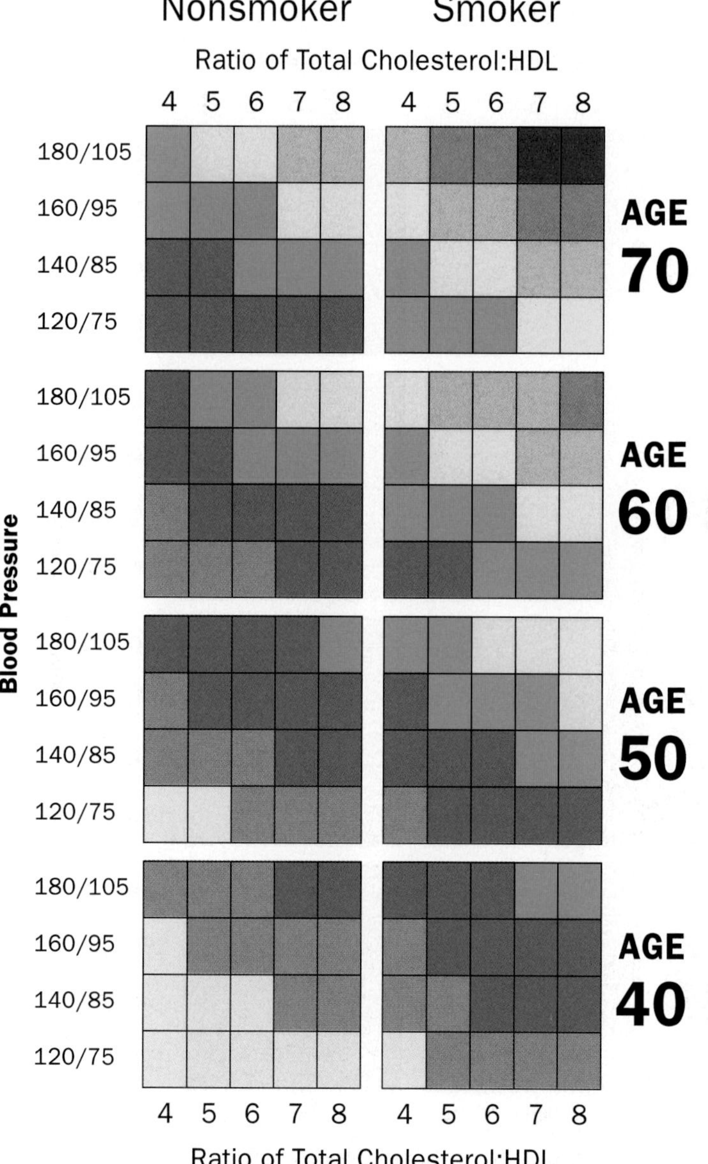

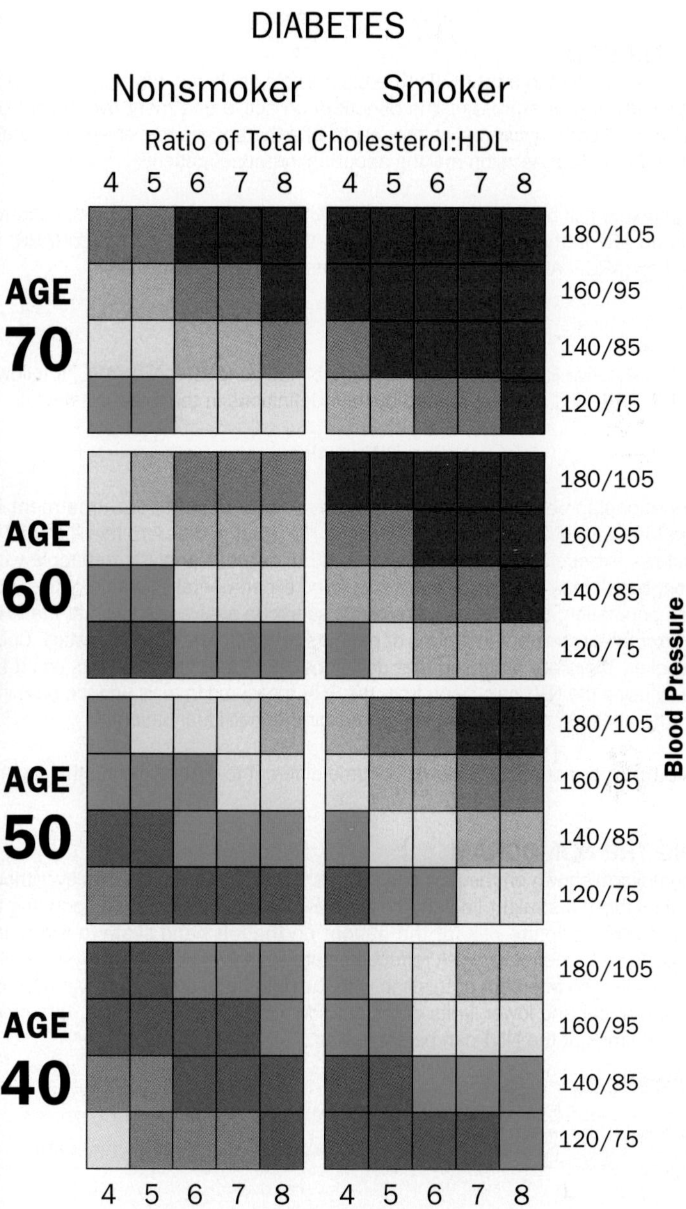
DIABETES
Nonsmoker
Smoker
Ratio of Total Cholesterol:HDL
4 5 6 7 8 4 5 6 7 8
AGE 70
AGE 60
AGE 50
AGE 40
180/105
160/95
140/85
120/75
Blood Pressure
4 5 6 7 8 4 5 6 7 8
Ratio of Total Cholesterol:HDL

The number needed to treat: adjusting for baseline risk

Appendix 2

Adapted with permission from Chatellier et al, 1996[1]

BACKGROUND

The number needed to treat (NNT) to avoid a single additional adverse outcome is a meaningful way of expressing the benefit of an active treatment over a control. It can be used both to summarise the results of a therapeutic trial or series of trials and to help medical decision making about an individual patient.

If the absolute risk of adverse outcomes in a therapeutic trial is ARC in the control group and ART in the treatment group, then the absolute risk reduction (ARR) is defined as (ARC – ART). The NNT is defined as the inverse of the ARR:

$$\text{NNT} = 1/(\text{ARC} - \text{ART})$$

Since the Relative Risk Reduction (RRR) is defined as (ARC – ART)/ARC, it follows that NNT, RRR, and ARC are related by their definitions in the following way:

$$\text{NNT} \times \text{RRR} \times \text{ARC} = 1$$

This relationship can be used to estimate the likely benefits of a treatment in populations with different levels of baseline risk (that is different levels of ARC). This allows extrapolation of the results of a trial or meta-analysis to people with different baseline risks. Ideally, there should be experimental evidence of the RRR in each population. However, in many trials, subgroup analyses show that the RRR is approximately constant in groups of patients with different characteristics. Cook and Sackett therefore proposed that decisions about individual patients could be made by using the NNT calculated from the RRR measured in trials and the baseline risk in the absence of treatment estimated for the individual patient.[2]

The method may not apply to periods of time different to that studied in the original trials.

USING THE NOMOGRAM

The nomogram shown on the next page allows the NNT to be found directly without any calculation: a straight line should be drawn from the point corresponding to the estimated absolute risk for the patient on the left hand scale to the point corresponding to the relative risk reduction stated in a trial or meta-analysis on the central scale. The intercept of this line with the right hand scale gives the NNT. By taking the upper and lower limits of the confidence interval of the RRR, the upper and lower limits of the NNT can be estimated.

REFERENCES

1. Chatellier G, Zapletal E, Lemaitre D, *et al*. The number needed to treat: a clinically useful nomogram in its proper context. *BMJ* 1996;321:426–429.
2. Cook RJ, Sackett DL. The number needed to treat: a clinically useful measure of treatment effect. *BMJ* 1995;310:452–454.

The number needed to treat

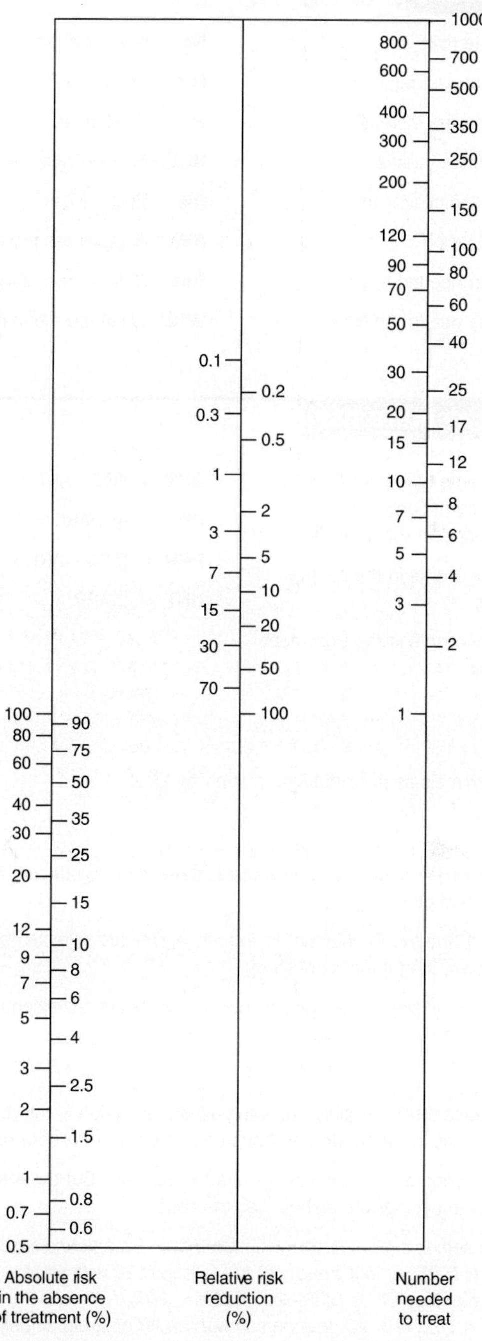

FIGURE **Nomogram for calculating the number needed to treat. Published with permission.[1]**

Abbreviations

AR Absolute risk
ARR Absolute risk reduction
ARI Absolute risk increase
CI Confidence interval
CCT Controlled clinical trial
HR Hazard ratio
NNH Number needed to harm
NNT Number needed to treat
NS Not significant
OR Odds ratio
P P value
RCT Randomised controlled trial
RR Relative risk
RRI Relative risk increase
RRR Relative risk reduction
WMD Weighted mean difference

How to calculate risk

AR = # events (good or bad) in treated or control groups/ # people in that group

ARC = AR of events in the control group

ART = AR of events in the treatment group

ARR = ARC – ART

RR = ART/ARC = 1 – RRR

RRR = (ARC – ART)/ARC = 1 – RR

NNT = 1/ARR

To express decimals as percentages, multiply by 100.

If:

the RR (or OR) = 1, or the CI includes 1, there is no significant difference between treatment and control groups

the RR > 1 and the CI does not include 1, events are significantly more likely in the treatment than the control group

the RR < 1 and the CI does not include 1, events are significantly less likely in the treatment than the control group

RR of 0.8 means a RRR of 20% (meaning a 20% reduction in the relative risk of the specified outcome in the treatment group compared with the control group).

RRR is usually constant across a range of absolute risks. But the ARR is higher and the NNT lower in people with higher absolute risks.

Example: If a person's AR of stroke, estimated from his age and other risk factors (see appendix 1), is 0.25 without treatment but falls to 0.20 with treatment, the ARR is 25%–20% = 5%; the RRR is (25%–20%)/25% = 20%;
and the NNT is 1/0.05 = 20. In a person with an AR of stroke of only 0.025 without treatment, the same treatment will still produce a 20% RRR, but treatment will reduce her AR of stroke to 0.020, giving a much smaller ARR of 2.5%–2% = 0.5%, and a NNT of 200.